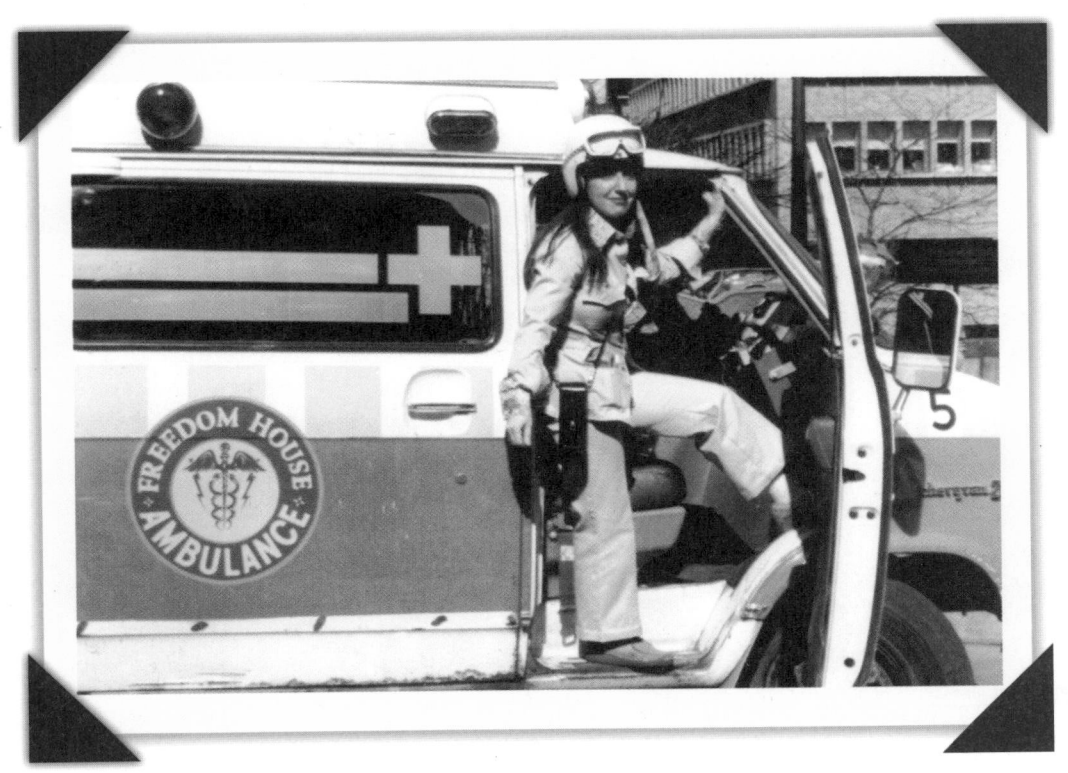

Dedicated to:

Nancy L. Caroline, MD

"The Mother of Paramedics"

1944–2002

AAOS

Sixth Edition

Nancy Caroline's
Emergency
Care in the Streets

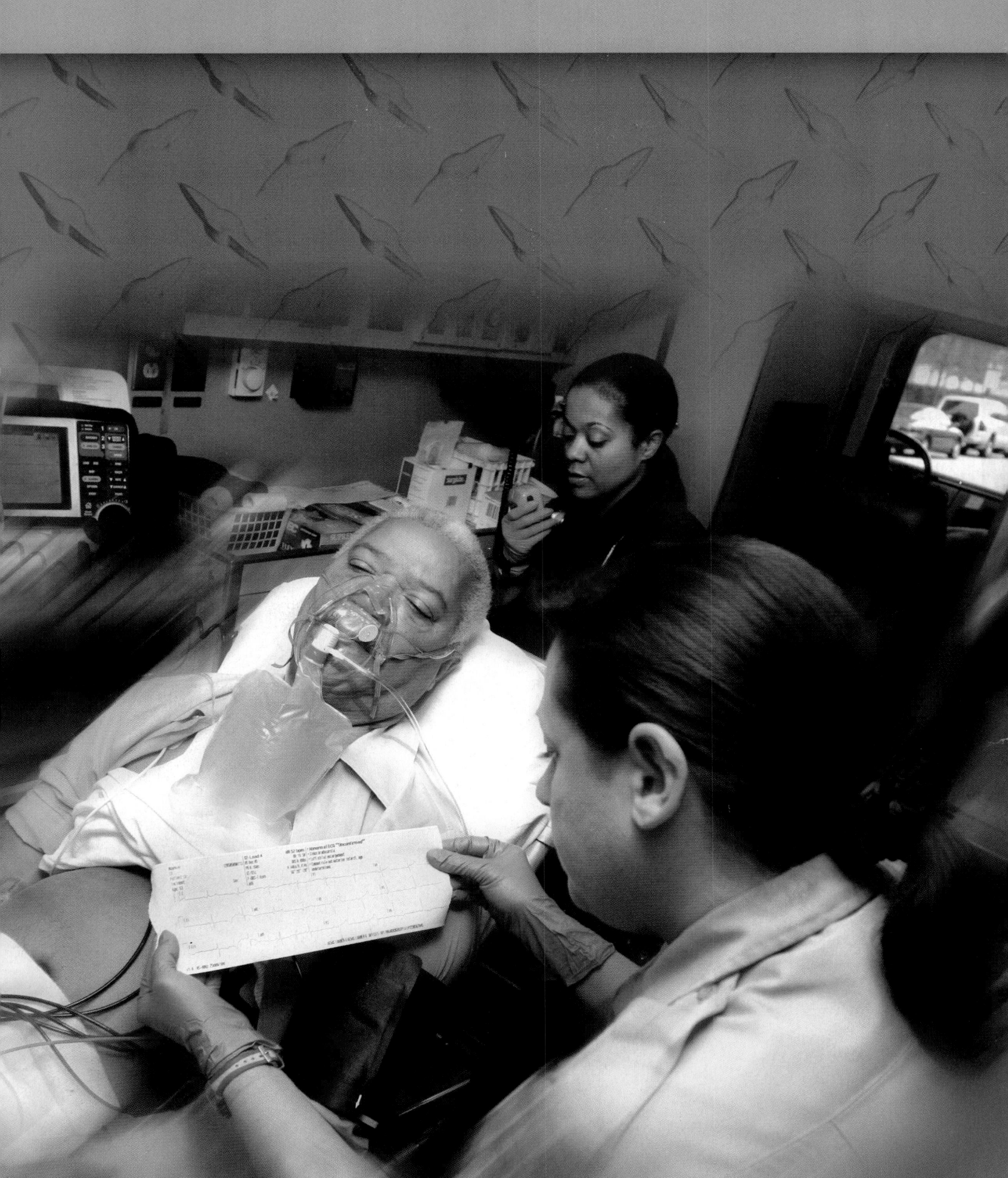

AAOS

Sixth Edition

Nancy Caroline's
Emergency
Care in the Streets

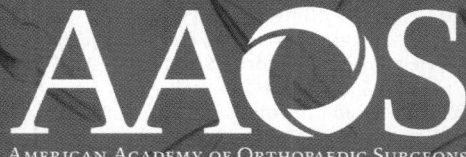

AMERICAN ACADEMY OF ORTHOPAEDIC SURGEONS

Author:

Nancy L. Caroline, MD

Series Editor:

Andrew N. Pollak, MD, FAAOS

Editors:

Bob Elling, MPA, NREMT-P   Mike Smith, BS, MICP

JONES AND BARTLETT PUBLISHERS

Sudbury, Massachusetts

BOSTON   TORONTO   LONDON   SINGAPORE

Jones and Bartlett Publishers

World Headquarters
Jones and Bartlett Publishers
40 Tall Pine Drive
Sudbury, MA 01776
978-443-5000
info@jbpub.com
www.EMSzone.com

Jones and Bartlett Publishers Canada
6339 Ormindale Way
Mississauga, ON L5V 1J2
Canada

Jones and Bartlett Publishers International
Barb House, Barb Mews
London W6 7PA
United Kingdom

Jones and Bartlett's books and products are available through most bookstores and online booksellers. To contact Jones and Bartlett Publishers directly, call 800-832-0034, fax 978-443-8000, or visit our website, www.jbpub.com.

Substantial discounts on bulk quantities of Jones and Bartlett's publications are available to corporations, professional associations, and other qualified organizations. For details and specific discount information, contact the special sales department at Jones and Bartlett via the above contact information or send an email to specialsales@jbpub.com.

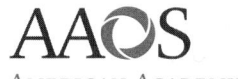

AMERICAN ACADEMY OF
ORTHOPAEDIC SURGEONS

Production Credits

Chief Executive Officer: Clayton Jones
Chief Operating Officer: Donald W. Jones, Jr
President, Higher Education and Professional Publishing: Robert Holland
V.P., Sales and Marketing: William J. Kane
V.P., Production and Design: Anne Spencer
V.P., Manufacturing and Inventory Control: Therese Connell
Publisher, Public Safety: Kimberly Brophy
Acquisitions Editor, EMS: Christine Emerton
Managing Editor: Carol Guerrero

Editor: Jennifer S. Kling
Associate Managing Editor: Amanda Green
Associate Managing Editor: Janet Morris
Editorial Assistant: Amanda Brandt
Editorial Assistant: Justin Keogh
Senior Production Editor: Susan Schultz
Production Editor: Karen Ferreira
Photo Research Manager/Photographer: Kimberly Potvin
Director of Marketing: Alisha Weisman
Interior Design: Anne Spencer and Kristin Ohlin

Cover Design: Kristin Ohlin
Cartoons: Nick Bertozzi
Composition: Shepherd, Inc.
Text Printing and Binding: Courier Kendallville
Cover Printing: Courier Kendallville
Cover Photograph: Jones and Bartlett Publishers, Courtesy of MIEMSS
Back cover photograph: Photo by Bachrach, all rights reserved
Photos of Nancy L. Caroline provided in loving memory by her mother, Zelda Caroline.

ISBN-13: 978-0-7637-8172-9

The procedures and protocols in this book are based on the most current recommendations of responsible medical sources. The American Academy of Orthopaedic Surgeons and the publisher, however, make no guarantee as to, and assume no responsibility for, the correctness, sufficiency, or completeness of such information or recommendations. Other or additional safety measures may be required under particular circumstances.

This textbook is intended solely as a guide to the appropriate procedures to be employed when rendering emergency care to the sick and injured. It is not intended as a statement of the standards of care required in any particular situation, because circumstances and the patient's physical condition can vary widely from one emergency to another. Nor is it intended that this textbook shall in any way advise emergency personnel concerning legal authority to perform the activities or procedures discussed. Such local determinations should be made only with the aid of legal counsel.

Notice: The patients described in "You are the Provider," "Assessment in Action," and "Points to Ponder" throughout this text are fictitious.

Library of Congress Cataloging-in-Publication Data
Elling, Bob.
  Nancy Caroline's emergency care in the streets. -- 6th ed. / Bob Elling, Michael G. Smith, Andrew N. Pollak.
      p. ; cm.
  Rev. ed. of: Emergency care in the streets / Nancy L. Caroline. 5th ed. c1995.
  Includes bibliographical references and index.
  Single Volume: ISBN-13: 978-0-7637-2907-3 (hardcover); ISBN-10: 0-7637-2907-8 (hardcover)
  Volume 1: ISBN-13: 978-0-7637-4238-6; ISBN-10: 0-7637-4238-4; Volume 2: ISBN-13: 978-0-7637-4239-3;
  ISBN-10: 0-7637-4239-2; Volume 3: ISBN-13: 978-0-7637-4240-9; ISBN-10: 0-7637-4240-6
  1. Medical emergencies. 2. Emergency medical technicians. I. Smith, Mike
(Michael Gordon), 1952- II. Pollak, Andrew N. III. Caroline, Nancy L.
Emergency care in the streets. IV. Title. V. Title: Emergency care in the
streets.
  [DNLM: 1. Emergency Treatment. 2. Emergency Medical Services. 3.
Emergency Medical Technicians. WB 105 E46n 2007]
  RC86.7.C38 2007
  616.02'5--dc22
6048   2006103366
Printed in the United States of America
13 12 11 10   10 9 8 7 6 5 4

Additional illustration and photo credits appear on page C.1, which constitutes a continuation of the copyright page.

Brief Contents

Contents

Section 5 Medical 26.3

Appendices A.2

Paramedic Skill Drills

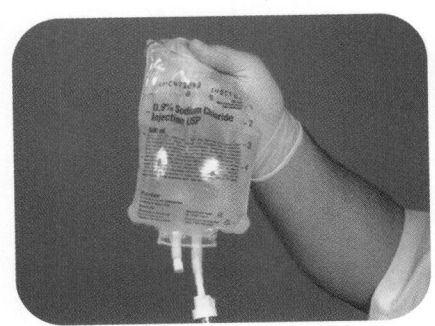
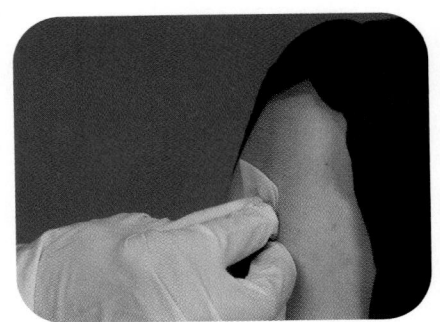
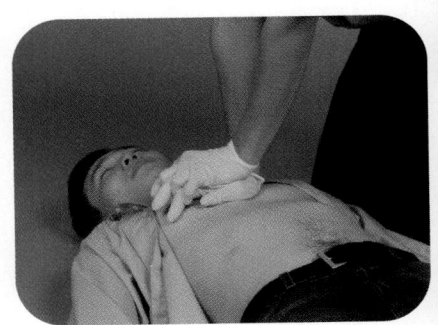

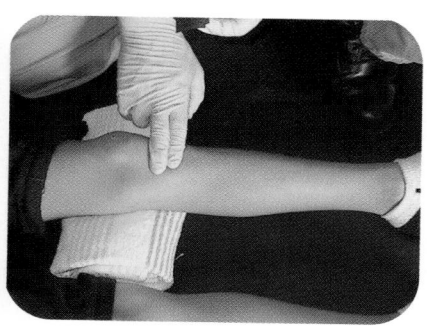
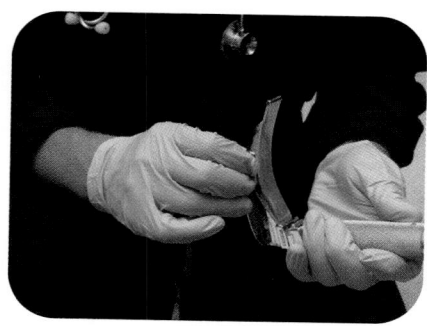
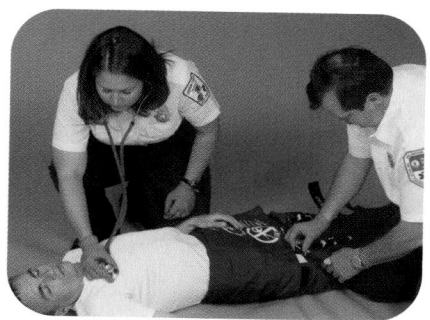

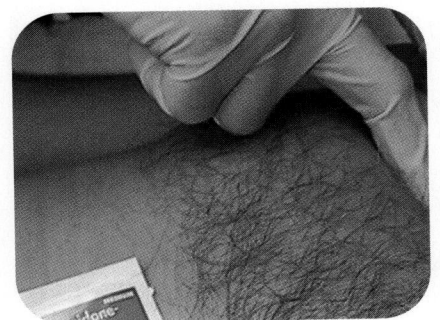
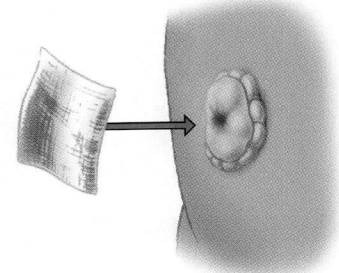
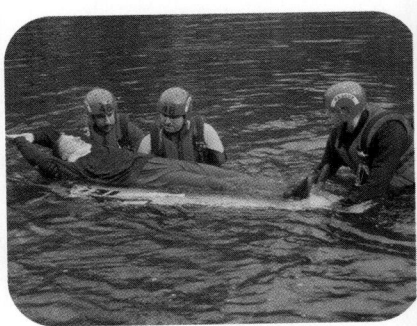

Resource Preview

CAROLINE'S BACK!

THINK BACK TO THE TIME when paramedics did not exist; when "drivers" simply brought patients to the hospital; when the EMS industry was in its infancy. This was the time before Dr. Nancy Caroline.

Then Nancy Caroline wrote the first national standard curriculum for paramedic training, which she translated into the first paramedic textbook. You are holding the sixth edition of that groundbreaking textbook.

Join us in welcoming back Dr. Caroline's legacy, *Emergency Care in the Streets!* This *Sixth Edition* honors Dr. Caroline's work with the clear, fun, understandable writing style for which she was known.

Chapter Resources

A multitude of fun, dynamic features have been incorporated to make learning more engaging, in the spirit of Dr. Caroline's approach. The following pages show you the features to help you learn—from case studies to skill drills to an interactive website. On Dr. Caroline's behalf, the American Academy of Orthopaedic Surgeons wishes you a successful and rewarding paramedic career!

Chapter Objectives

National Standard Curriculum objectives are provided for each chapter with corresponding page references.

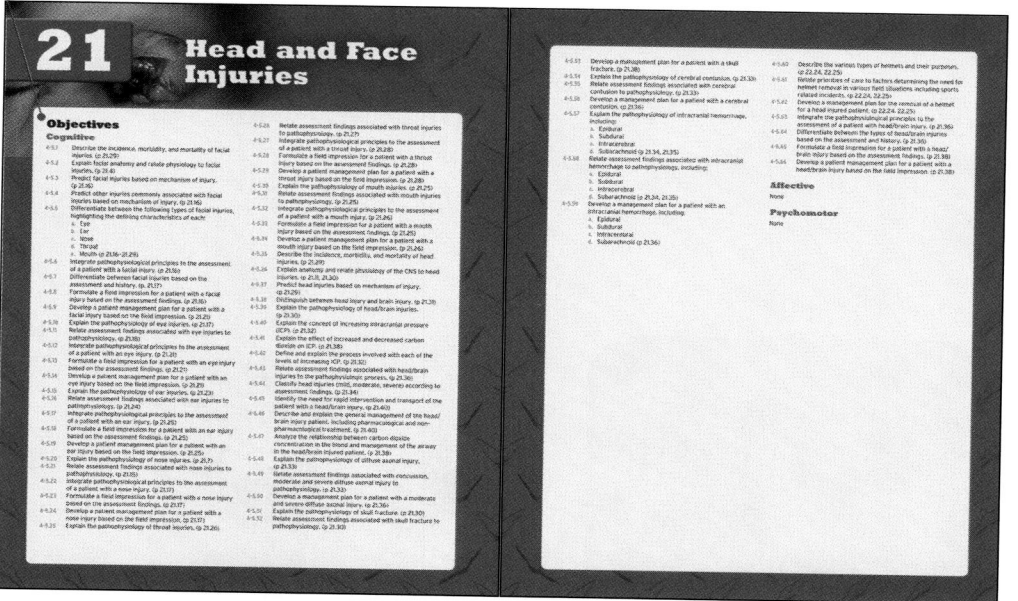

You are the Provider

Each chapter contains a progressive case study to make students start thinking about what they would do if they encounter a similar case in the field. This feature is a valuable learning tool that encourages critical thinking skills.

The case study introduces patients and follows their progress from dispatch to delivery at the emergency department. The case becomes progressively more detailed as new medical information is presented.

A summary of the case study concludes the chapter.

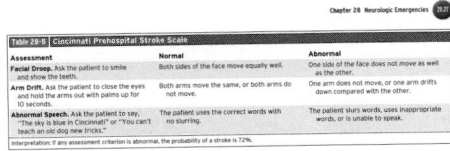

Notes from Nancy

Provide words of wisdom from Dr. Nancy Caroline.

Special Considerations

Discuss the specific needs and emergency care of special populations, including pediatric patients, geriatric patients, and special needs patients.

Skill Drills

Provide written step-by-step explanations and visual summaries of important skills and procedures.

Documentation and Communication

Provide advice on how to document patient care and tips on how to communicate with other health care professionals.

In the Field

Discuss practical applications of material for use in the field.

Controversies

Highlight issues that may be under debate in the EMS community.

Vital Vocabulary

Terms are easily identified and defined within the text. A comprehensive vocabulary list follows each chapter.

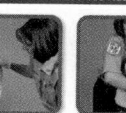

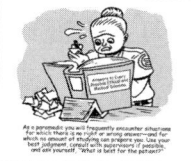

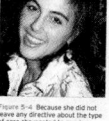

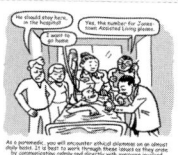

Prep Kit

End-of-chapter activities reinforce important concepts and improve students' comprehension.

Ready for Review

Summarize chapter content in a comprehensive bulleted list.

Assessment in Action

Promote critical thinking with case studies and provide discussion points for classroom presentation.

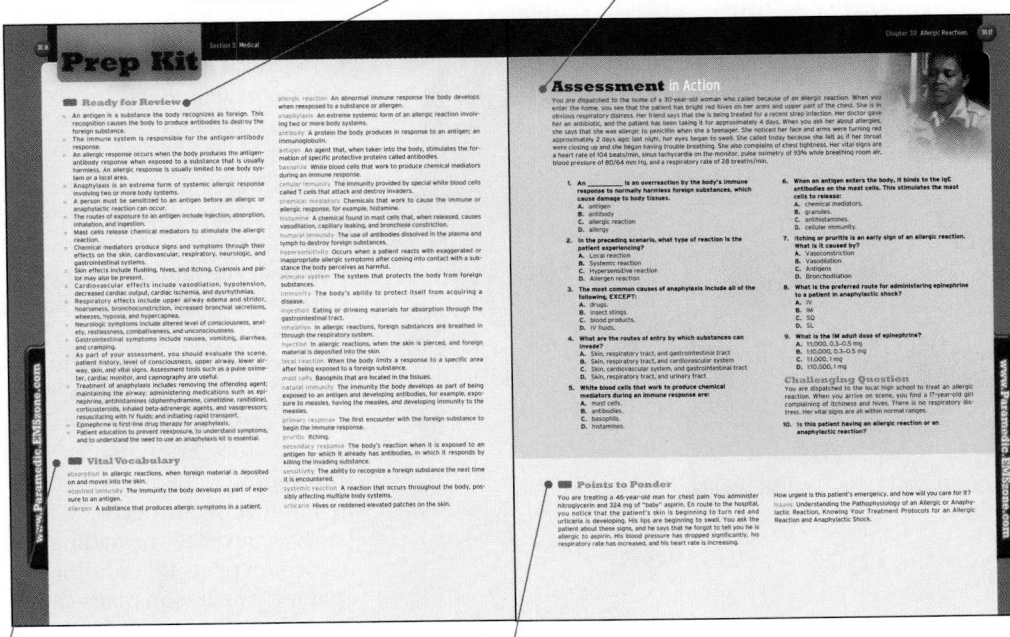

Vital Vocabulary

Provide key terms and definitions from the chapter.

Points to Ponder

Tackle cultural, ethical, and legal issues through case studies.

Paramedic Practical Skills Review DVD

Your Resource to Passing the Paramedic Practical Examination

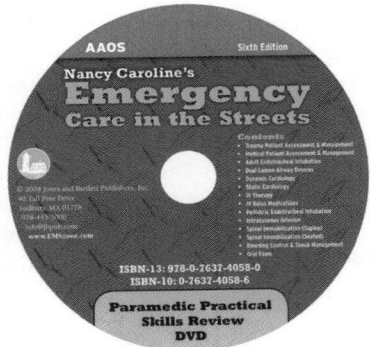

ISBN-13: 978-0-7637-4058-0
ISBN-10: 0-7637-4058-6

This DVD walks you through the skills that you must successfully complete as part of the national paramedic practical examination process. These skills include:

- Trauma Patient Assessment & Management
- Medical Patient Assessment & Management
- Adult Endotracheal Intubation
- Dual Lumen Airway Devices
- Dynamic Cardiology
- Static Cardiology
- IV Therapy
- IV Bolus Medications
- Pediatric Endotracheal Intubation
- Intraosseous Infusion
- Spinal Immobilization (Supine)
- Spinal Immobilization (Seated)
- Bleeding Control & Shock Management
- Oral Exam

With this DVD, you will learn how to perform each skill successfully and will find helpful information, tips, and pointers designed to facilitate your progression through the practical examination. For each skill, you will find:

- Objectives
- Equipment
- Key steps to perform to successfully complete the skill
- Critical errors that will result in failure

Instructor Resources

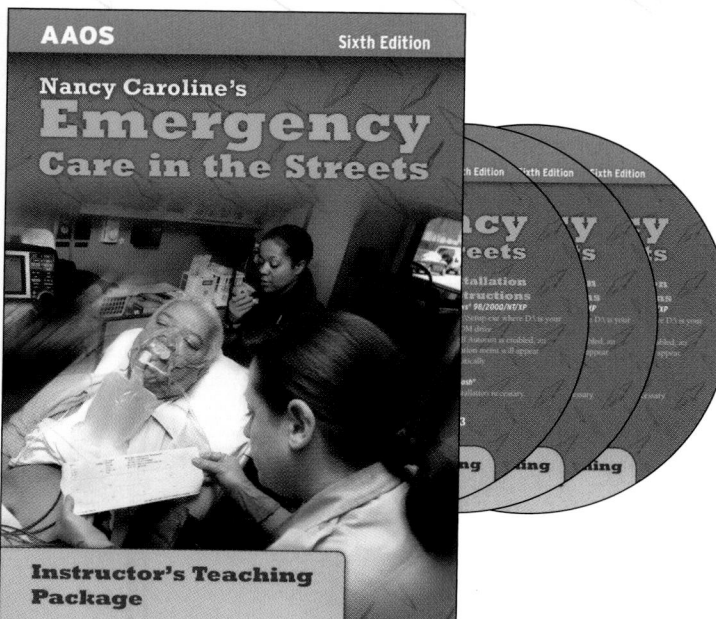

ISBN-13: 978-0-7637-5175-3
ISBN-10: 0-7637-5175-8

This robust package contains everything needed to instruct a dynamic paramedic course. The CD-ROMs in the package contain:

- **Instructor's manual**, providing you with creative ideas and tools to enhance your presentation. For each chapter, this indispensable manual contains:
  - Objectives with page references
  - Support materials
  - Enhancements
  - Teaching tips
  - Readings and preparation
  - Presentation overview with suggested teaching times
  - Lesson plans and corresponding PowerPoint slide text
  - Skill drill evaluation sheets
  - Answers to all end-of-chapter student questions found in the text
  - Activities and assignments
- **PowerPoint presentations**, providing you with educational and engaging presentations. Following the content of the chapter, the slides also contain case studies and images throughout. The presentations can be modified and edited to meet your needs.
- **Lecture outlines**, providing you with complete, ready-to-use lesson plans that outline all of the topics covered in the chapter. The lesson plans can be modified and edited to fit your course.
- **Image and table bank**, providing you with many of the images and tables found in the text. You can use them to incorporate more images into the PowerPoint presentations, make handouts, or enlarge a specific image for further discussion.
- **Test bank**, providing you with multiple-choice general knowledge and critical thinking questions, similar to those found on national certification exams. With the test bank, you can originate tailor-made classroom exams and quizzes quickly and easily by selecting, editing, organizing, and printing an exam along with an answer key, that includes page references to the text.
- **Skill sheets**, allowing you to track students' skills and conduct skill proficiency exams.
- **National Registry Skill Sheets**

The resources found in the Instructor's Package have been formatted so that you can seamlessly integrate them into the most popular course administration tools. Please contact Jones and Bartlett Publishers technical support at 1-800-832-0034 at any time with questions.

Student Resources

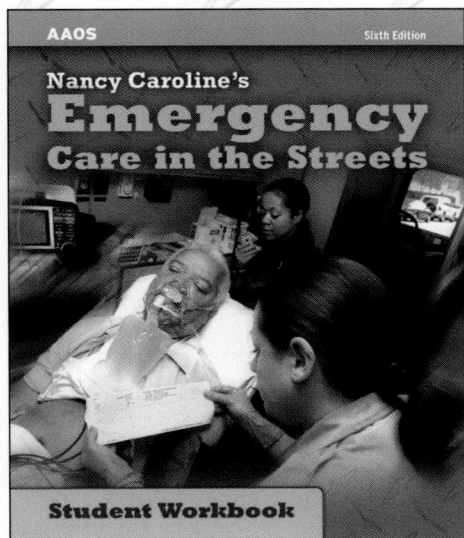

ISBN-13: 978-0-7637-4412-0
ISBN-10: 0-7637-4412-3

Dr. Caroline trained her paramedics to be well-rounded, compassionate, quick-thinking problem solvers. This workbook will help students become great paramedics!

Critical thinking skills are further developed through:
- Fun and engaging case studies
- ECG Interpretation exercises
- "What Would You Do?" scenarios

Comprehension of the course material is aided through:
- Skill drill activities
- Anatomy labeling exercises
- Medical vocabulary building exercises

Fun is ensured with these activities:
- Crossword puzzles
- Secret messages
- Word finds

The Workbook comes complete with an answer key, page references, and a student resources CD-ROM for further study.

Technology Resources

www.Paramedic.EMSzone.com

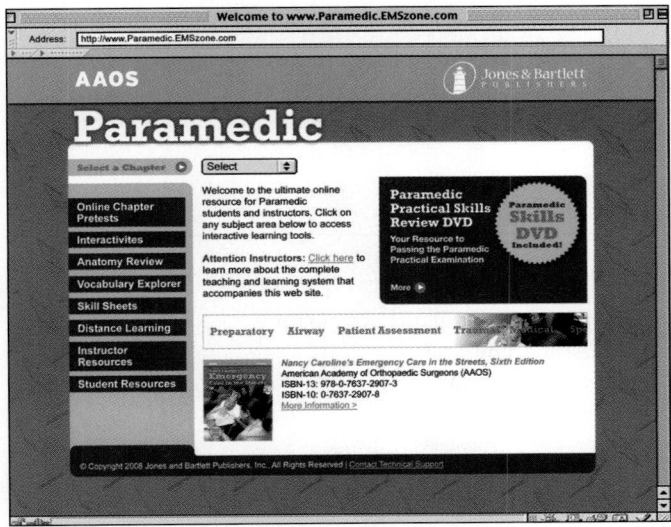

This site has been specifically designed to complement *Nancy Caroline's Emergency Care in the Streets, Sixth Edition* with interactivities and simulations to help students become great paramedics. Some of the resources available include:

- **Chapter pretests** prepare students for training. Each chapter has a pretest and provides instant results, feedback on incorrect answers, and page references for further study.
- **Interactivities** allow your students to experiment with the most important skills and procedures in the safety of a virtual environment.
- **Anatomy review** provides interactive anatomical figure labeling exercises to reinforce students' knowledge of human anatomy.
- **Vocabulary explorer** is a virtual dictionary. Here, students can review key terms, test their knowledge of key terms through flashcards, and complete exercises.
- **Skill sheets** provide both National Registry Skill Sheets and skill evaluation sheets from the textbook.

Acknowledgments

AAOS
AMERICAN ACADEMY OF
ORTHOPAEDIC SURGEONS

The American Academy of Orthopaedic Surgeons and Jones and Bartlett Publishers would like to thank past editors, contributors, and reviewers of *Emergency Care in the Streets*.

Editorial Board

Bob Elling, MPA, NREMT-P
Hudson Valley Community
    College
Andrew Jackson University
Colonie EMS Department
Times Union Center EMS
Colonie, New York

Andrew N. Pollak, MD, FAAOS
Medical Director, Baltimore
    County Fire Departments
Associate Professor, University of
    Maryland School of Medicine
Baltimore, Maryland

Stephen J. Rahm, NREMT-P
EMS Professions Educator
Bulverde-Spring Branch EMS
Spring Branch, Texas

Mike Smith, BS, MICP
Program Chair, Emergency
    Medical and Health Services
Tacoma Community College
Tacoma, Washington

Editors and Authors

SECTION 1

Section Editor: David Gurchiek, MS, NREMT-P
Paramedic Program Director
Montana State University-Billings
Billings, Montana

Authors

Chapter 1: Don Kimlicka, NREMT-P, CCEMT-P
EMS Coordinator, Saint Clare's Hospital
Weston, Wisconsin
Field Paramedic, Great Divide EMS
Cable, Wisconsin

Chapter 2: Anne Austin, EMT-P, AAS
Flint River Technical College
Thomaston, Georgia

Chapter 2: Thom Dick, NREMT-B
Platte Valley EMS
Brighton, Colorado

Chapter 3: Keith Griffiths
President, The RedFlash Group
Encinitas, California

Chapter 4: W. Ann Maggiore, JD, NREMT-P
Butt Thornton & Baehr PC
Albuquerque, New Mexico

Chapter 5: W. Ann Maggiore, JD, NREMT-P
Butt Thornton & Baehr PC
Albuquerque, New Mexico

Chapter 6: Jeffrey Morse, MD
Medical Director, Paramedic Education Program
Tacoma Community College
Tacoma, Washington

Chapter 7: Geoffrey T. Miller, EMT-P
University of Miami Miller School of Medicine
Miami, Florida

Chapter 7: Shaun Froshour, NREMT-P
Public Safety Management Solutions
Telford, Pennsylvania

Chapter 8: David Gurchiek, MS, NREMT-P
Paramedic Program Director
Montana State University-Billings
Billings, Montana

Chapter 8: Stephen J. Rahm, NREMT-P
EMS Professions Educator
Bulverde-Spring Branch EMS
Spring Branch, Texas

Chapter 9: Howard E. Huth, III, BA, EMT-P
Chief of Operations
Western Turnpike Rescue Squad
Guilderland, New York

Chapter 10: Thom Dick, NREMT-B
Platte Valley EMS
Brighton, Colorado

Chapter 10: Charles R. Jones, BA, CC-EMTP/TA, CAS, CHS-III
Prairie Township Fire Protection District
Lee's Summit, Missouri

SECTION 2

Section Editor: Stephen J. Rahm, NREMT-P
EMS Professions Educator
Bulverde-Spring Branch EMS
Spring Branch, Texas

Authors

Chapter 11: Stephen J. Rahm, NREMT-P
EMS Professions Educator
Bulverde-Spring Branch EMS
Spring Branch, Texas

SECTION 3

Section Editor: Mike Smith, BS, MICP
Program Chair, Emergency Medical and Health Services
Tacoma Community College
Tacoma, Washington

Authors

Chapter 12: Mike Smith, BS, MICP
Program Chair, Emergency Medical and Health Services
Tacoma Community College
Tacoma, Washington

SECTION 3, continued

Chapter 13: John F. Elder, EMT-P, CCEMT-P
Director of Clinical Services
Emergicon, L.L.C.
Emergency Medical Consultants
Fort Worth, Texas

Chapter 13: Jonathan S. Halpert, MD, FACEP, REMT-P
Director of EMS Affairs
St. Peter's Hospital
Albany, New York

Chapter 14: Mike Smith, BS, MICP
Program Chair, Emergency Medical and Health Services
Tacoma Community College
Tacoma, Washington

Chapter 15: Mike Smith, BS, MICP
Program Chair, Emergency Medical and Health Services
Tacoma Community College
Tacoma, Washington

Chapter 16: Melissa M. Doak, NREMT-P
York County Department of Fire and Life Safety
Yorktown, Virginia

SECTION 4

Section Editor: Bob Elling, MPA, NREMT-P
Hudson Valley Community College
Andrew Jackson University
Colonie EMS Department
Times Union Center EMS
Colonie, New York

Section Editor: Connie J. Mattera, RN, MS, TNS, EMT-P
Northwest Community Hospital, EMS Department
Arlington Heights, Illinois

Authors

Chapter 17: Samuel A. Getz Jr, BS, NREMT-P
President and CEO
EMS/QA Systems Consulting Service
Austintown, Ohio

Chapter 17: Edward K. Rodriguez, MD-PhD
Chief, Orthopaedic Trauma Service
Beth Israel Deaconess Medical Center
Boston, Massachusetts

Chapter 18: Bob Elling, MPA, NREMT-P
Hudson Valley Community College
Andrew Jackson University
Colonie EMS Department
Times Union Center EMS
Colonie, New York

Chapter 19: Chad E. Brocato, DHSc, REMT-P
Deerfield Beach Fire-Rescue
Deerfield Beach, Florida

Chapter 20: Charles Bortle, MEd, NREMT-P, RRT
Director EMS Education
Albert Einstein Medical Center
Philadelphia, Pennsylvania

Chapter 20: Jennifer McCarthy, MAs, MICP
Assistant Professor–Union County College
Paramedic Program Director
Cranford, New Jersey

Chapter 20: Mark A. Merlin, DO, EMT-P, FACEP
EMS Medical Director
Assistant Professor of Emergency Medicine
Robert Wood Johnson Medical School
Robert Wood Johnson University Hospital
New Brunswick, New Jersey
Chair, MICU Advisory Board, New Jersey Department of Health and
    Senior Service
Medical Director, New Jersey EMS/Disaster Medicine Fellowship
Medical Director, New Jersey EMS Physician Response Program
"MD-1" New Jersey
EMS Task Force
Medical Director, Union County College Paramedic Program

Chapter 21: Stephen J. Rahm, NREMT-P
EMS Professions Educator
Bulverde-Spring Branch EMS
Spring Branch, Texas

Chapter 22: Debra Lee, MD
Medical Director, Prehospital Care and Emergency Preparedness
St. Vincent's Hospital–Manhattan
New York, New York

Chapter 23: John Freese, MD
EMS Medical Director–Manhattan
OLMC Medical Director
EMS Fellowship Co-Director
New York City Fire Department
New York, New York

Chapter 24: Samuel A. Getz Jr, BS, NREMT-P
President and CEO
EMS/QA Systems Consulting Service
Austintown, Ohio

Chapter 24: Robert S. Levy, MD
Instructor of Emergency Medicine
Robert Wood Johnson Medical School
New Jersey EMS/Disaster Medicine Fellow
New Brunswick, New Jersey

Chapter 24: Mark A. Merlin, DO, EMT-P, FACEP
EMS Medical Director
Assistant Professor of Emergency Medicine
Robert Wood Johnson Medical School
Robert Wood Johnson University Hospital
New Brunswick, New Jersey
Chair, MICU Advisory Board, New Jersey Department of Health and
    Senior Service
Medical Director, New Jersey EMS/Disaster Medicine Fellowship
Medical Director, New Jersey EMS Physician Response Program
"MD-1" New Jersey
EMS Task Force
Medical Director, Union County College Paramedic Program

Chapter 25: Matthew J. Belan, MD, MBA
Department of Anesthesiology and Critical Care Medicine
The Johns Hopkins Hospital
Baltimore, Maryland
First Lieutenant, Fire Suppression
White Marsh Volunteer Fire Company
Baltimore County, Maryland

Chapter 25: Michael D. Panté, NREMT-P
Somerset Medical Center
Somerville, New Jersey

SECTION 5

Section Editor: Bob Elling, MPA, NREMT-P
Hudson Valley Community College
Andrew Jackson University
Colonie EMS Department
Times Union Center EMS
Colonie, New York

Authors

Chapter 26: Charles Bortle, MEd, NREMT-P, RRT
Director EMS Education
Albert Einstein Medical Center
Philadelphia, Pennsylvania

Chapter 27: Bruce Butterfras, MS-Ed, LP
The University of Texas Health Science Center at San Antonio
San Antonio, Texas

Chapter 27: Deborah J. McCoy-Freeman, BS, RN, NREMT-P
EMS Education Specialist, Prehospital Care
University of Pittsburgh Medical Center
Pittsburgh, Pennsylvania

Chapter 28: Charles W. Sowerbrower, MEd, NREMT-P, NCEMSE
Sinclair Community College
Dayton, Ohio

Chapter 29: Don Kimlicka, NREMT-P, CCEMT-P
EMS Coordinator, Saint Clare's Hospital
Weston, Wisconsin
Field Paramedic, Great Divide EMS
Cable, Wisconsin

Chapter 29: J. Michael Morrow, MICP, CICP
Aeromed International
Bethel, Alaska
Airborne Critical Care
Smithfield, North Carolina

Chapter 30: Ann Bellows, RN, NREMT-P, EdD
Director of Clinical Services Southwest MedEvac
Las Cruces, New Mexico

Chapter 31: Charles W. Sowerbrower, MEd, NREMT-P, NCEMSE
Sinclair Community College
Dayton, Ohio

Chapter 32: George E. Perry, EdD, NREMT-P
Blue Ridge Community and Technical College
Martinsburg, West Virginia

Chapter 33: Mike Smith, BS, MICP
Program Chair, Emergency Medical and Health Services
Tacoma Community College
Tacoma, Washington

Chapter 34: Don Kimlicka, NREMT-P, CCEMT-P
EMS Coordinator, Saint Clare's Hospital
Weston, Wisconsin
Field Paramedic, Great Divide EMS
Cable, Wisconsin

Chapter 35: Frederick "Fritz" Fuller, REMT-P, PA-C, BS
Thurston County Fire District #1
Rochester, Washington
Department of Emergency Medicine
Providence Centralia Hospital
Cantralia, Washington

Chapter 36: Katherine H. West, BSN, MSEd, CIC
Infection Control Consultant
Infection Control/Emerging Concepts, Inc.
Manassas, Virginia

Chapter 37: Chris Stratford, RN, BS, EMT-I
University of Utah Health Sciences
Health Promotion and Education Department
EMS Programs
Salt Lake City, Utah

Chapter 38: Charles R. Jones, BA, CC-EMT-P/TA, CAS, CHS-III
Prairie Township Fire Protection District
Lee's Summit, Missouri

Chapter 39: Charles R. Jones, BA, CC-EMT-P/TA, CAS, CHS-III
Prairie Township Fire Protection District
Lee's Summit, Missouri

SECTION 6

Authors

Chapter 40: Patricia Chess, MD
Golisano Children's Hospital at Strong
University of Rochester Medical Center
Rochester, New York

Chapter 40: Nirupama Laroia, MD
Director, Special Care Nursery, Rochester General Hospital
Associate Professor, Department of Pediatrics/Neonatology
Golisano Children's Hospital at Strong
University of Rochester Medical Center
Rochester, New York

Chapter 40: Yogangi Malhotra, MD
Golisano Children's Hospital at Strong
University of Rochester Medical Center
Rochester, New York

Chapter 41: Dena Brownstein, MD, FAAP
Division of Emergency Medicine
Children's Hospital and Regional Medical Center
Associate Professor, Pediatrics
University of Washington
Seattle, Washington

Chapter 41: Kimberly P. Stone, MD, MS, MA
Division of Emergency Medicine
Children's Hospital and Regional Medical Center
Seattle, Washington

Chapter 42: Samuel A. Getz Jr, BS, NREMT-P
President and CEO
EMS/QA Systems Consulting Service
Austintown, Ohio

Chapter 42: Michael D. Panté, NREMT-P
Somerset Medical Center
Somerville, New Jersey

Chapter 42: Jim Upchurch, MD, MA, NREMT-P
Indian Health Service
Big Horn County EMS
Crow Agency, Montana

Chapter 43: Daniel Doherty, NREMT-P
Disaster Preparedness Unit
NYS DOH Bureau of Emergency Services
Albany, New York

SECTION 6, continued

Chapter 44: Lori L. Bisping, NREMT-P
Emergency Medical Specialist
City of DuPont Fire Department
DuPont, Washington

Chapter 44: Annmary E. Thomas, MEd, NREMT-P
Community College of Philadelphia
Philadelphia, Pennsylvania

Chapter 45: Deborah Kufs, MS, RN, NREMT-P
Institute for Prehospital Emergency Medicine
Hudson Valley Community College
Troy, New York

SECTION 7

Section Editor: David L. Seabrook, MPA, EMT-P
Captain, Vancouver Fire Department
Vancouver, Washington

Authors

Chapter 46: Anne Austin, EMT-P, AAS
Flint River Technical College
Thomaston, Georgia

Chapter 47: Doyle Dennis, NREMT-P
Education Coordinator
Acadian Ambulance & Air Med Services, Inc.
Houma, Louisiana

Chapter 48: Donell Harvin, MPA, NREMT-P
NYC EMS
New York, New York

Chapter 49: Norm Rooker, EMT-P
Ouray County EMS
Ouray Mountain Rescue Team
Ouray, Colorado

Chapter 49: Hank R. Christen, Jr, MPA
Consultant
Mary Esther, Florida

Chapter 50: David L. Seabrook, MPA, EMT-P
Captain, Vancouver Fire Department
Vancouver, Washington

Chapter 51: Dennis R. Krebs, NREMT-P
Senior Operations Specialist
Division of Special Operations
Johns Hopkins Medical Institutions
Department of Emergency Medicine
Baltimore, Maryland

APPENDICES

Appendix A: Bob Elling, MPA, NREMT-P
Hudson Valley Community College
Andrew Jackson University
Colonie EMS Department
Times Union Center EMS
Colonie, New York

Appendix B: Bob Elling, MPA, NREMT-P
Hudson Valley Community College
Andrew Jackson University
Colonie EMS Department
Times Union Center EMS
Colonie, New York

Medication Formulary

Geoffrey T. Miller, EMT-P
University of Miami Miller School of Medicine
Miami, Florida

Shaun Froshour, NREMT-P
Public Safety Management Solutions
Telford, Pennsylvania

Peter A. Dillman, EdD, EMT-P
Director, EMS
St. Vincent Health
Indianapolis, Indiana

Contributors

Trisha Appelhans
Recruitment & Enrollment Coordinator
Division of EMS Education
Medical University of Ohio at Toledo
Toledo, Ohio

Vicki Bacidore, RN, MSN, ACNP-BC
Loyola Emergency Medical Services
Loyola University Medical Center
Maywood, Illinois

Darrin M. Batty, AEMT-P
Public Safety Training Facility
Monroe Community College
Rochester, New York

Jeffery L. Beinke, MBA-HCM, BS, REMT-P
EMS Program Coordinator
Forsyth Technical Community College
Winston-Salem, North Carolina

Garry Briese
Executive Director
International Association of Fire Chiefs
Fairfax, Virginia

Tom Carpenter, NREMT-P, CCEMT-P
EMS Educator
Gundersen Lutheran Emergency Medical
  Services Educator
Caledonia, Minnesota

Julie Chase, BS, NREMT-P
EMS Training Officer
Loudoun County Department of Fire, Rescue
  and Emergency Management
Leesburg, Virginia

Kathleen E. Curran, MICP
Robert Wood Johnson University Hospital at
  Rahway
Rahway, New Jersey

Mike Dymes, NREMT-P
Durham Technical Community College
Durham, North Carolina

Mickey Eisenberg, MD, PhD
King County EMS
Seattle, Washington

Jill E. Hobbs
Editor
Waltham, Massachusetts

Susan M. Hohenhaus, MA, RN, FAEN
Duke University Health Systems
Durham, North Carolina

Jay Keefauver, Founder
National Academy for Prehospital Care
Freemont, Nebraska

Rick Kimball, NREMT-P
Operations Supervisor
Erway Ambulance Service
Elmira, New York

Contributors, continued

Gregg C. Lord, BA, NREMT-P
Associate Director and Co-investigator
National EMS Preparedness Initiative
The Homeland Security Policy Institute
The George Washington University
Washington, DC

Patricia Maher, MPA, EMT-P
Daytona Beach Community College
EVAC Ambulance
Dayton Beach, Florida

Brittany Ann Martinelli, MHSc, BSRT, NREMT-P
Santa Fe Community College Institute for
    Public Safety
Gainesville, Florida

Lynette S. McCullough, MPH, EMT-P
Griffin Technical College
Griffin, Georgia

Scott F. McConnell, FP-C, NREMT-P, MICP, CCEMT-P
JeffSTAT EMS Education
Thomas Jefferson University
Philadelphia, Pennsylvania

David McEvoy, MS, NREMT-P
Missoula Emergency Services
Aerie Backcountry Medicine
Missoula, Montana

Eugene Nagel
Winter Haven, Florida

Cynthia Osborne
New Mexico State University–Alamogordo
EMS Department
Alamogordo, New Mexico

Deborah L. Petty, BS, EMT-P, I/C
St. Charles County Ambulance District
Saint Peter's, Missouri

Randy Price, A/As, NREMT-P
Instructor/Continuing Education Program
    Coordinator
EMS Science Department
Catawba Valley Community College
Hickory, North Carolina

Sabra Raulston, NREMT-P
Abingdon Volunteer Rescue Squad
Gloucester Point, Virginia

Bernadette A. Royce, BA, FF/EMT-P
Osceola County Fire Rescue
Valencia Community College
Orlando, Florida

Joan Scheffer, EMT-B/WEMT, CRNFA
Aerie School for Backcountry Medicine
Missoula, Montana

Jeffrey J. Spencer, BS, EMT-P
Higher Education Officer
Director or Paramedic Education
LaGuardia Community College/CUNY
Long Island City, New York

Ron Stewart
Medical Humanities Program
Faculty of Medicine
Dalhousie University
Halifax, Nova Scotia
Canada

Barbara O. Ward, BA, MA
Editor
Norfolk, Massachusetts

Reviewers

Anne Austin, EMT-P, AAS
Flint River Technical College
Thomaston, Georgia

Vicki Bacidore, RN, MS
Loyola University Medical Center
Program for Prehospital Medicine
Maywood, Illinois

Tod Baker, EMT-P, EMSI
EMS Academy, Cleveland Clinic
Cleveland, Ohio

Leaugeay C. Barnes, BS, CC/NREMT-P
Oklahoma City Community College
Oklahoma City, OK

Tim Barnett, BA, NREMT-P
Kanawha County Emergency Ambulance
    Authority
Charleston, West Virginia

Jeff C. Bates, BSHS, NREMT-P
Idaho State University
Boise, Idaho

Edward Bays, BS, NREMT-P
Marshall Community and Technical College
Huntington, West Virginia

Jeffery L. Beinke, MBA-HCM, BS, REMT-P
EMS Program Coordinator
Forsyth Technical Community College
Winston-Salem, North Carolina

Michael D. Berg, AAS, NREMT-P
Captain
Charlottesville-Albemarle Rescue Squad
Charlottesville, Virginia

Robert Bernini, REMT-P
Harrisburg Area Community College
Harrisburg, Pennsylvania

Paul A. Bishop
Monroe Community College
Rochester, New York

Christopher Black
Eastern Arizona College
Thatcher, Arizona

Michael Blakeney, RN, MSN, EMS Educator I, II, III
Eastern Kentucky University
Richmond, Kentucky

Cynthia Branscum BS, EMT-P, MICT Instructor/Coordinator
Cowley County Community College
Winfield, Kansas

Sheri K. Brenner, NREMT-P
College of Emergency Services
Beaverton, Oregon

Michael Brooks
Manatee Technical Institute, Richard T.
    Conrad M.D. Medical and Dental Building
Bradenton, Florida

David Bryant, BS, EMT-P, I/C
Northeast State Community College
Blountville Tennessee

Katrina Bryant, NREMT-P, BS HS
East Central Community College
Decatur, Mississippi

Brian K. Bugbee, CCT, NREMT-P
Perrysburg Township Fire/EMS
Perrysburg, Ohio

Michael A. Buldra, MEd, NREMT-P
Eastern New Mexico University-Roswell
Roswell, New Mexico

Ken Bullwinkle, RN, BSN, PHRN, CEN, CCRN
Nursing Education Department
Crozer-Chester Medical Center
Upland, Pennsylvania

Brandon Burgess, BAS, NREMT-P
EMT/Fire Service Department
Phoenix College
Phoenix, Arizona

Robert Butcher, EMSI, EMT-P
Cincinnati State Technical and Community
    College
Cincinnati, Ohio

Bruce Butterfras, MS-Ed, LP
The University of Texas Health Science
    Center at San Antonio
San Antonio, Texas

Daniel Carlascio, NREMT-P, CCEMT-P
Loyola University Medical Center
Maywood, Illinois

Wesley Carter, NREMT-P
Lenoir County EMS
Lenoir Community College
Kinston, North Carolina

Chris G. Caulkins, MPH, FF/EMT-P
Century College
White Bear Lake, Minnesota

Joseph Chappell, AAS
Paramedics and Fire Science Paramedic
    Instructor BRTC
Black River Technical College
Pocahontas, Arkansas

Tony C. Cipolla, NREMT-P
Louisville Fire Rescue
Louisville, Kentucky

Reviewers, continued

Julie Coffman
Alabama Fire College
Tuscaloosa, Alabama

DeMoss Collins, FF/NREMT-P
Faculty, Brookhaven College Emergency
    Medical Services Program
Farmers Branch, Texas

Harvey Conner, AS, NREMT-P
Oklahoma City Community College EMS
    Program
Oklahoma City, Oklahoma

Roy E. Cox Jr, DEd, EMT-P
Educator and Patient Care Coordinator
City of Pittsburgh Dept. of Public Safety,
    Bureau of EMS
Faculty at Point Park University & Drexel
    University
Pittsburgh, Pennsylvania

Keith Cox, BS, NREMT-P
Joint Special Operations Medical Training
    Center
Fort Bragg, North Carolina

Anthony Cuda
Community College of Allegheny County
Pittsburgh, Pennsylvania

Peter E. Cunnius, Sr, MS, RNc, NREMT-P
Drexel University Goodwin College of
    Professional Studies
Philadelphia, Pennsylvania

Lyndal M. Curry, MA, NREMT-P
University of South Alabama
Mobile, Alabama

Joseph A. DeAngelis, NREMT-P, CCEMT-P
EMS Educator
Community College of Rhode Island – Liston
    Campus
Providence, Rhode Island

Christopher DeMorse, AAS, CC/NREMT-P
Northwest-Shoals Community College
Muscle Shoals, Alabama

Doyle Dennis, NREMT-P
Education Coordinator
National EMS Academy
Houma, Louisiana

Katherine Deskins, BS, EMT-P
EMS Coordinator
Southern West Virginia Community College
Mount Gay, West Virginia

Terry DeVito, RN, EMT-P, MEd, EMSI
Capital Community College
Hartford, Connecticut

Melissa M. Doak, NREMT-P
York County Department of Fire and Life
    Safety
Yorktown, Virginia

Brian R. Dose, FF/EMT-P
Ottawa Fire Department
Ottawa, Illinois
EMS Instructor
Illinois Valley Community College
Oglesby, Illinois

Lt. Doug Driscoll, EMT-P, AS
EMS Training Officer
Orlando Fire Department
Daytona Beach Community College
Orlando, Florida

John Dudte, MPA, MICT
The George Washington University
Washington, DC

Tim Duncan, RN, CCRN, CEN, CFRN, EMT-P
Flight Nurse
St. Vincent Mercy Medical Center Life Flight
Toledo, Ohio

Mike Dymes, NREMT-P
Durham Technical Community College
Durham, North Carolina

Patricia A. Edwards, BA, NREMT-P CCEMT-P, I/C
White River Valley Ambulance
Bethel, Vermont

Peter D. Eikenberry, NREMT-P
University of Maryland
Maryland Fire and Rescue Institute, ALS
    Division
College Park, Maryland

Richard Ellis, BSOE, NREMT-P
United States Air Force (Air Force Reserve
    Command)
Robins AFB, Georgia

Phil Ester, BA, CCEMT-P, NREMT-P
Red Carpet Emergency Medical Training
    Consortium
Woodward, Oklahoma

Bruce Evans
Community College of Southern Nevada
Henderson, Nevada

Michael Fisher, AHS, NREMT-P
Program Director
Greenville Technical College
Greenville, South Carolina

Jim Floyd, MEd, WEMT, PI, CTC
EMS Program Manager–St. Vincent Hospital
Indianapolis, Indiana

Steven K. Frye, BS, NREMT-P
University of Maryland
Maryland Fire and Rescue Institute
College Park, Maryland

Tony Garcia
Texas Engineering Extension Service
College Station, Texas

John Garrett, Jr, BS, MSN, MPH, CHI
Community Health Associates, LLC
Atlanta, Georgia

Scott Garrett, NREMT-P
Upstate EMS Council
Greenville, South Carolina

Daniel R. Gerard, MS, RN, EMT-P
Professor/Adjunct Faculty
The George Washington University
Washington D.C.

Daniel E. Glick, BPS, AEMT-CC
Queensbury, New York

Steven D. Glow, MSN, FNP, RN, CEN, EMT-P
Montana State University College of Nursing
Missoula, Montana

Robin Goede, FF/NREMT-P, BA, AAS
St. Louis Community College
St. Louis, Missouri

Matthew Goodman, NREMT-P
California Institute of Emergency Medical
    Training
Long Beach California

Jeffrey R. Grunow, MSN, NREMT-P
Weber State University
Assistant Professor and Chair, Emergency
    Care and Rescue Department
Ogden, Utah

Janie Gunnell, BA Ed, EMT-P
Florida State Fire College
Nassau County Fire/Rescue
Ocala, Florida

Adam L. Harrell, NREMT-P
Halifax County Rescue Squad, Inc.
Halifax, Virginia

Cathy E. Harris, RN, BS, CFRN, CMTE, NREMT-P, PI
Parkview Hospital
Fort Wayne, Indiana

Eryq Hastings, NREMT-P
Tri-City Meds
Pinal County, Arizona

Thomas Herron, EMT-P
Cape Fear Community College
Wilmington, North Carolina

Attila Hertelendy, MS, MHSM, NREMT-P, CCEMT-P, ACP
University of Mississippi Medical Center
Jackson, Mississippi

Jonathan R. Hockman, EMSIC, NREMT-P
Goldrush Consulting
Livonia, Michigan

Lindi Holt, PhD, NREMT-P
Clarian Health/Methodist Hospital
Indianapolis, Indiana

Mark A. Huckaby, NREMT-P
Grant Medical Center LifeLink
Columbus, Ohio

Sandy Hunter, MA, NREMT-P
Associate Professor, Paramedic Program,
    Eastern Kentucky University
Richmond, Kentucky

Rebecca Jackson, AAS, EMT-P/IC
Schoolcraft College
Garden City, Michigan

C.H. Johnson, DVM, EMT-P
Medical Coordinator, Mountain Rescue
    Aspen
EMS, ACLS Instructor, Aspen Ambulance
    District
Aspen, Colorado

Reviewers, continued

Mark D. Johnson, BS, Paramedic
EMS Program Director
Front Range Community College
Boulder County Campus
Longmont, Colorado

Jason Joling, FF/NREMT-P, CCEMT-P
Wisconsin Rapids Fire Department
EMS Instructor, Mid State Technical College
Wisconsin Rapids, Wisconsin

Don Jones, BS, NREMT-P
Avera McKennan School of EMS
Sioux Falls, South Dakota

Scott C. Jones, MBA, EMT-P
Victor Valley College
Victorville, California

Edward J. Kalinowski, MEd, DrPH
Department of Emergency Medical Services
University of Hawaii
Honolulu, Hawaii

Sue A. Kartman
Madison Area Technical College
Madison, Wisconsin

Walter Kelch, NREMT-P
Harrisburg Area Community College
Harrisburg, Pennsylvania

William R. Kerney, MA, EMT-P-A
Community College of Southern Nevada
Las Vegas, Nevada

Timothy M. Kimble, NREMT-P
Culpeper Co. Emergency Services
Rappahannock EMS Council
EMS Training Staff
Fredericksburg, Virginia

Shawn Koser, ATS, NREMT-P
Captain
Columbus Division of Fire
Columbus, Ohio

John A. Kubincanek, EMT-P, AA, EMSI
Cuyahoga Community College
Cleveland, Ohio

Al M. Landry, AS, NREMT-P
National EMS Academy
Lafayette, Louisiana

John Lewis, MEd, NREMT-P
Paramedic Program Director
Brigham Young University—Idaho
Rexburg, Idaho

Larry Macy, NREMT-P
Western Wyoming Community College
Rock Springs, Wyoming

Patty Maher, MPA, EMT-P
Daytona Beach Community College
Daytona Beach, Florida

Ric Maloney
Sacramento Metropolitan Fire District
Sacramento, California

Paul M. Maniscalco, MPA, EMT-P
Deputy Chief/Paramedic (retired), FDNY
Sr. Research Scientist and Principal
  Investigator
The George Washington University
  Homeland Security Policy Institute
Washington, District of Columbia

Mark L. Marchetta, BS, RN, NREMT-P
Director EMS Education
Aultman Health Foundation
Canton, Ohio

Andrew Margolies, EMT-P/CIC
Paramedic Program
State University of New York at Stony Brook
Stony Brook, New York

Brittany Martinelli, MHSc, RRT-NPS, NREMT-P
Santa Fe Community College
Gainesville, Florida

Bill Maser, BEd
Independent Educational Contractor
British Columbia, Canada

Vicki May, MEd, LP
Houston Community College
Houston, Texas

Lynette S. McCullough, MPH, EMT-P
Griffin Technical College
Griffin, Georgia

Gene McDaniel, BS, NREMT-P
Phoenix College
Phoenix, Arizona

Craig McElhaney, NREMT-P
Lead Paramedic Instructor
Broward Community College
Fort Lauderdale, Florida

Matthew McQuisten
Avera McKennan Hospital and University
Sioux Falls, South Dakota

William M. Mehbod, BS, EMT-P
Bethesda Hospital Paramedic Training
  Program
Cincinnati, Ohio

Jeffrey J. Messerole, Paramedic
Director of Clinical Services
Lakes Regional Healthcare
Spirit Lake, Iowa

Steve Monsam, NREMT-P, BS
Community Ambulance Service of Minot
Minot, North Dakota

Pete Moreno Jr, NREMT-LP, AAS
Texas State Technical College
Harlingen, Texas

John L. Morrissey, NREMT-P
New York State EMS Program
Syracuse, New York

Diana Neubecker, RN, BSN, EMT-P
Northwest Community EMS System
Arlington Heights, Illinois

Julie Marie Nordyke, MICP, WEMT-P
Adjunct Faculty
University of Alaska Fairbanks – Chukchi
  Campus
Lotzebue, Alaska

Bruce Nepon, MA, NREMT-P
Delaware Technical and Community College
Dover, Delaware

Jeanne O'Brien, RN, MN
Paramedic Instructor
Harborview Paramedic Training Program
Seattle, Washington

Dr. Laurie Oelslager, EdD, AHA Regional Faculty, NREMT-P
South Central College
Mankato, Minnesota

Cynthia Osborne
New Mexico State University – Alamogordo
EMS Department
Alamogordo, New Mexico

Michael D. Panté, NREMT-P
Somerset Medical Center
Somerville, New Jersey

David M. Patton, Paramedic
Emergency Medical Sciences Training
  Institute
Stockton, California

Randall Perkins, EMT-P
Paramedic Program Director, AHA Regional
  Faculty
Scottsdale Community College
Scottsdale, Arizona

Jerry L. Peters, BS, EMT-P
Good Fellowship Amblance and Training
  Institute
West Chester, Pennsylvania

Deborah Petty
St. Charles County Ambulance District
Saint Peter's, Missouri

Christian Phelps, RN, BS, CEN, NREMT-P
Southwestern Vermont Medical Center
Bennington, Vermont

Kyle Pierce, BA, LP
Austin Community College
Austin, Texas

Carol Pillsbury, EMT-P, I/C
Tri-County EMS
Lewiston, Maine

Andrew H. Popick, BPA, NREMT-P
Battalion Chief, Town of Davie Fire Rescue
Core Emergency Medical Skills Instructor,
  University of Miami Miller School of
  Medicine
Gordon Center for Research in Medical
  Education
Adjunct EMS Instructor and ACLS Program
  Coordinator, Broward Community College
Davie, Florida

Merle D. Potter, NREMT-P
Casper College
Casper, Wyoming

Reviewers, continued

Randy Price, NREMT-P, A/As
Gaston County EMS
Gastonia, North Carolina

Mark J. Reed, BA Ed, BA FSA, NREMT-P, C-FP
Lieutenant/Paramedic, Columbia River Fire and Rescue
St. Helens, Oregon
Flight Paramedic, Life Flight Network
EMS Instructor, Portland Community College
Portland, Oregon

Brian Reiselbara, BA, MICP
Chief Flight Paramedic, Maniilaq MedFlight
Kotzebue, Alaska

Lt. Timothy Robinson, BS, EMT-P
Concord Fire Department
New England EMS Institute
Concord, New Hampshire

James R. Ross, Jr, FF/EMT-P
Training Manager
Washington Township Fire Department
Dublin, Ohio
Clinical Coordinator
Franklin County Firefighters
EMS Education
Grant Medical Center
Columbus, Ohio

Bernadette A. Royce, BA, FF/EMT-P
Osceola County Fire Rescue
Valencia Community College
Orlando, Florida

Jose V. Salazar, MPH, NREMT-P
Loudoun County Department Fire, Rescue and Emergency Management
Leesburg, Virginia

Jeff Scheulen, REMT-P
Washington Hospital Center
Washington, DC

Patrick Sennett, EMT-P
Advocate Health Care
Good Samaritan EMS System
Downers Grove, Illinois

Valerie Simonds, MS, RN, NREMT-P
Anne Arundel Community College
Arnold, Maryland

Gursarn Singh, BS, NREMT-P
AHA Regional Faculty
University of Arkansas at Monticello College of Technology
McGehee, Arkansas

Lillian Urban Slater, RN, NREMT-P
Barton County Community College
Ellis County EMS
Hays, Kansas

David H. Sloane AS, NREMT-P
Georgetown Scott County EMS
Georgetown Kentucky

Michael L. Smith, MPA, BA, EMS Senior Instructor
Washington State DOH/EMS
Tumwater, Washington

Scott A. Smith, RN, BSN, BA, CFRN, CEN, NREMT-P, I/C
Maine Department of Public Safety, Bureau of EMS
Augusta, Maine

Todd Soard, IEMR-P, NREMT-P, PhD
Emergency Educational Institute
Coral Springs, Florida

Jeffrey J. Spencer, BS, EMT-P
Higher Education Officer
Director of Paramedic Education
LaGuardia Community College/CUNY
Long Island City, New York

Lisa Starr, NREMT-P, EMS-I
Southeast Community College
Lincoln, Nebraska

Nerina J. Stepanovsky, MSN, RN, EMT-P, Program Director
St. Petersburg College EMS Program
St. Petersburg, Florida

Charles G. Stutzman, NREMT-P, BS
Susquehanna Health
Williamsport, Pennsylvania

Gilbert N. Taylor, FF/NREMT-P, I/C
Institute for Emergency Medical Education (a division of IEME International, Inc.)
Bourne, Massachusetts

Pamela N. Taylor, EMT-P, PI
St. Vincent Hospital
Indianapolis, Indiana

Edward G. Teevan, BA, RI EMS- I/C
Dayville, Connecticut

Susan I. Valdez, RN, EMT-P
Northeastern University
Burlington, Massachusetts

Mary Alice Vanhoy, RN, MSN, CEN, NREMT-P
Shore Health System, Chesapeake College
Easton, Maryland

George F. Vannatta, BS, EMT-P
Mercy School of Emergency Medical Services
Des Moines, Iowa

Eileen Van Orden, MICP, NREMT-P
Hudson Community College
Jersey City, New Jersey

Robert Vroman, BS, NREMT-P
HealthONE EMS
Englewood, Colorado

Mitchell R. Waite, PhD, CFO, EFO, NREMT-P, CCEMT-P
Paramedic Director, Wisconsin Rapids Fire Department
EMS Instructor, Mid State Technical College
Wisconsin Rapids, Wisconsin

Laura L. Walker, DM, NREMT-P
Tidewater EMS Council, Inc.
Norfolk, Virginia

Brad D. Weilbrenner, AS, NREMT-P
Rockingham Regional Ambulance
Nashua, New Hampshire

Stanley E. Whiteway, EMT-P, I/C
Dyersburg State Community College
Dyersburg, Tennessee

David A. Yarmesch, AAS, EMT-P
Cleveland Clinic EMS Academy
Cleveland, Ohio

Alan W. L. Young, MICT, BA, MPH
Kapiolani Community College—University of Hawaii
Honolulu, Hawaii

Joseph R. Yow, MA, EMT-P
Guilford Technical Community College
Jamestown, North Carolina

Suzan A. Zehner, NREMT-I/LPN
University of Alaska
Fairbanks, Alaska
Medical Training Institute
Anchorage, Alaska

Lawrence S. Zicherman, MPA, NREMT-P, I/C
Emergency Training and Consulting
Greenville, North Carolina

Jason J. Zigmont, BS, NREMT-P
Center for Public Safety Education
Middletown, Connecticut

Biography

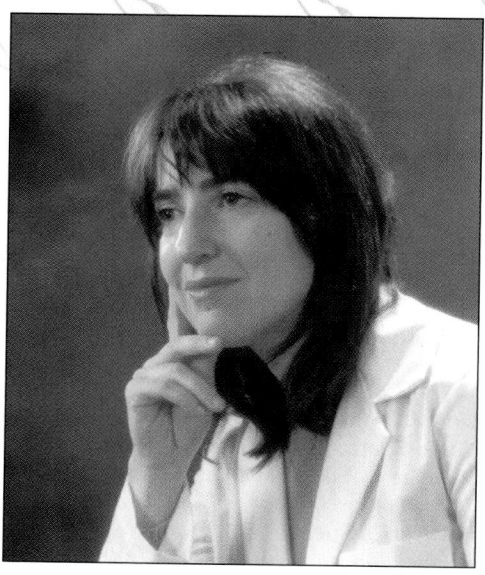

Nancy L. Caroline, MD

Nancy L. Caroline, MD, was only 58 when she died of multiple myeloma in 2002, but her spirit will never leave Emergency Medical Services. She has often been rightly called the Mother of Paramedics because of her dedication to paramedic education.

No physician can be more revered, yet Nancy never used the academic titles to which she was most entitled—everyone from a first year EMT to a distinguished leader called Dr. Caroline, simply, "Nancy."

Nancy Lee Caroline was born in a Boston suburb to Leo and Zelda Caroline in 1944. Nancy had a strong social conscience, and devoted her life to medicine, teaching, and her patients.

Nancy's medical career began at the age of 15 in the pathology laboratory of the famous Benjamin Castleman, MD, at Massachusetts General Hospital. However, Dr. Castleman was unable to pay her for her services, because she was not of legal age to be working for money. Nancy went on to do actual medical research in Dr. Castleman's laboratory, long before she entered college.

Nancy chose to major in linguistics at Radcliffe College. Not surprisingly, it continued to be a point of pride for her to develop a knowledge of the languages in whatever country she was working. She went on to receive her MD from Case Western Reserve University in 1977.

After finishing her residency in Cleveland, Nancy took a fellowship in Critical Care Medicine at the University of Pittsburgh. Beginning in 1974, the late Peter Safar, MD, was overseeing a US Department of Transportation grant to create a curriculum for paramedics. Much of Safar's work began to be delegated to (or, perhaps, seized upon by) the young Dr. Caroline. Because of this work, Nancy served as an advisor to President Gerald Ford on EMS.

Dr. Safar offered Nancy an opportunity, as medical director of Freedom House Enterprises Ambulance Service, to train paramedics chosen from a group of African-American men who did not have a chance to complete their high school educations. Nancy was extremely successful—so successful that she was asked to write a curriculum for paramedic training, a curriculum that was published as *Emergency Care in the Streets*.

Nancy, proud of her Jewish heritage, took an opportunity to emmigrate to Israel as the first medical director of Magen David Adom, Israel's Red Cross society. During her first months in the country, Nancy rose early to attend the extensive Hebrew lessons required of new immigrants, then spent her late afternoons and evenings training the first Israeli paramedics. She would then take a bus home, where she would spend a few precious hours working on the first edition of *Emergency Care in the Streets*.

After her tenure at Magen David Adom came to an end in 1981, Nancy relocated to Nairobi, Kenya, to become Senior Medical Officer of the African Medical and Research Foundation (AMREF), the foundation that oversees the famous Flying Doctor service.

One of Nancy's many duties at AMREF was writing a health advice column for the local newspaper, called "Ask Dr. AMREF." Nancy's famous sense of humor made the column "must" read in Nairobi. Nancy reported that one reader had all the males on the AMREF staff quite concerned when he began: "Everyone knows that a normal male can go six times in an evening."

No one who ever met her will ever forget her sense of humor, nowhere more evident than in her publications:

Nancy made the editors of a proper Bostonian publishing firm gasp when she wore a hardhat with a revolving red light when she came to call.

Nancy won permission to publish the first cartoon on the cover of the *Journal of the American Medical Association* for her article on the curative power of chicken soup. The cartoonist, her brother Peter, said he was sure it would be the last.

Nancy lost an argument with her editors to have a series of case studies for paramedics called *The Pulseless Man in the Topless Bar*. The case book became *Ambulance Calls* instead—to her undisguised loathing.

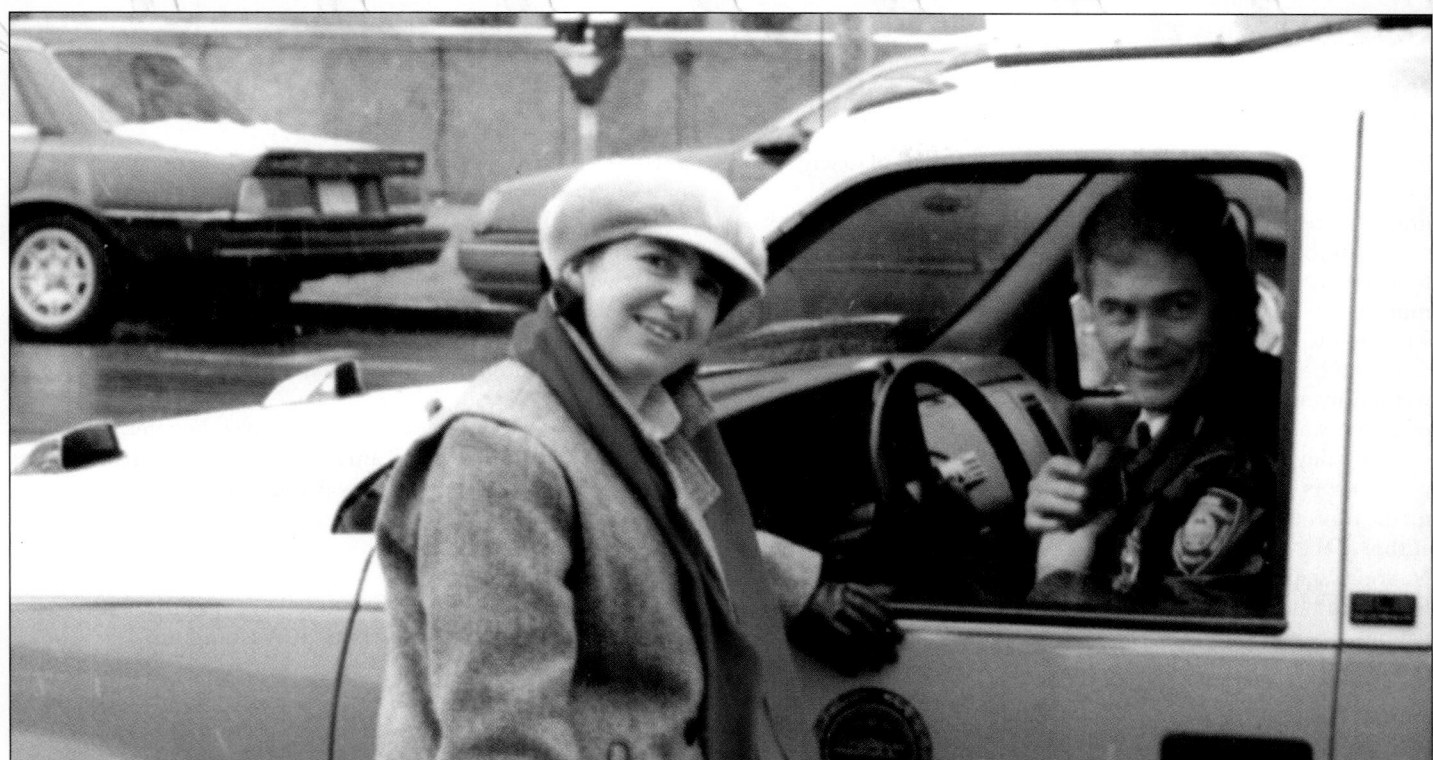

During much of her life, Nancy would return to the United States to visit her mother Zelda and her brother Peter. But, on her trips home, Nancy always found time to ride with working paramedics in several cities, to listen to their ups and downs, and to determine what real paramedics needed in the updates of *Emergency Care in the Streets*.

When she became aware of the awful famine that overtook Ethiopia in the early 1980s, Nancy became a consultant for the League of Red Cross Societies, writing a handbook on basic life support and running classes on first aid for African nations.

Nancy worked with the Ethiopian Orthodox Church to provide better nourishment and health care to children in over 600 orphanages, setting up small-scale agricultural projects to feed Africans. In addition, Nancy served as director of medical programs for the American Joint Distribution Committee in Addis Ababa.

During Nancy's time in Ethiopia, she had to return to the United States for a family emergency. Nancy discovered the only way she could get a plane to the United States was with a substantial cash payment for a ticket. The Christian Bishop of the Ethiopian Orthodox Church, to whom Nancy reported on the orphanages, personally got Nancy on a plane to Boston in short order.

Returning to Israel in 1987, she served as medical consultant for the Center for Educational Technology and for AMREF, developing training materials in emergency medicine and writing correspondence courses for rural health workers in Africa. She also served as an adjunct professor at the University of Pittsburgh's medical school, and, while volunteering in the Department of Oncology in Tel Hashomer, Nancy collaborated

with Alexander Waller, MD, on a *Handbook of Palliative Care in Cancer.*

Nancy settled in Metulla, Israel. She realized there was a need for special care in north Israel for people with advanced cancer. In 1995, she founded the Hospice of the Upper Galilee (HUG). In 2002, she married geneticist and molecular biologist Lazarus Astrachan.

Nancy left the world too soon, but few people have done more to leave the world a better place. Despite all her accomplishments, however, the compliment that meant the most to her was to be called the "Mother of Paramedics." Nancy was, no doubt, the best mother paramedics could have.

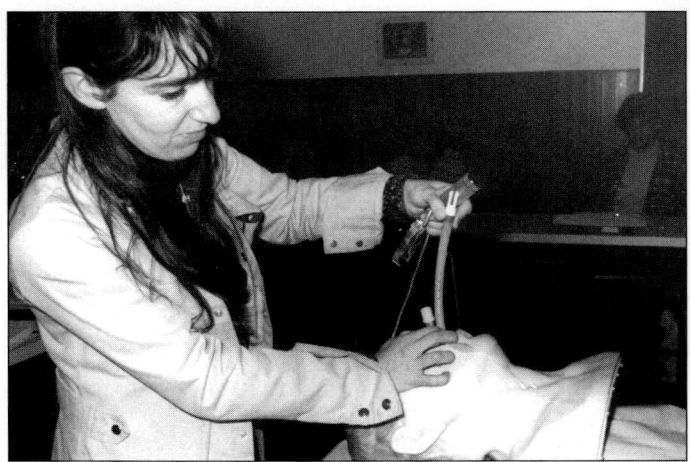

Foreword

for the Sixth Edition of *Emergency Care in the Streets*

Nancy Caroline, the author of the first five editions of *Emergency Care in the Streets,* and I went to medical school together. After graduation, our careers took different paths, but we always stayed in touch until her untimely death a few years ago. Her letters to me were masterpieces of wit, erudition, and plain common sense. For those reasons, I have kept every letter that she wrote to me. I mention this because the first edition of *Emergency Care in the Streets* was a masterpiece and could only have been written by someone with her combination of street savvy, experience, and creative writing ability.

In today's era of information overload, it can be easy to forget that everything has a beginning. And the beginning of paramedic training was *Emergency Care in the Streets.* Nancy was the author of the original United States Department of Transportation National Standard Curriculum for Paramedics which she translated into her *Emergency Care in the Streets.* For the first time, paramedics had a complete body of knowledge, encapsulated in a textbook filled with medical wisdom and peppered with humor. Publication of this book was a groundbreaking event.

Above all, Nancy was a compassionate, sensitive person. She always tried to instill these qualities into her students and in her writing. Remember that whatever your patient's underlying condition, be it a cut finger or a cardiac episode, your patient will be frightened, anxious, and in distress. Your patient needs your wisdom, knowledge, skills, care, comfort, and compassion.

I have seen *Emergency Care in the Streets* become better and better with each edition and am proud to see the enhancements in this the sixth edition. I know Nancy would have been even prouder.

Mickey Eisenberg, MD, PhD
Medical Director, King County Emergency Medical Services
Professor of Medicine, University of Washington

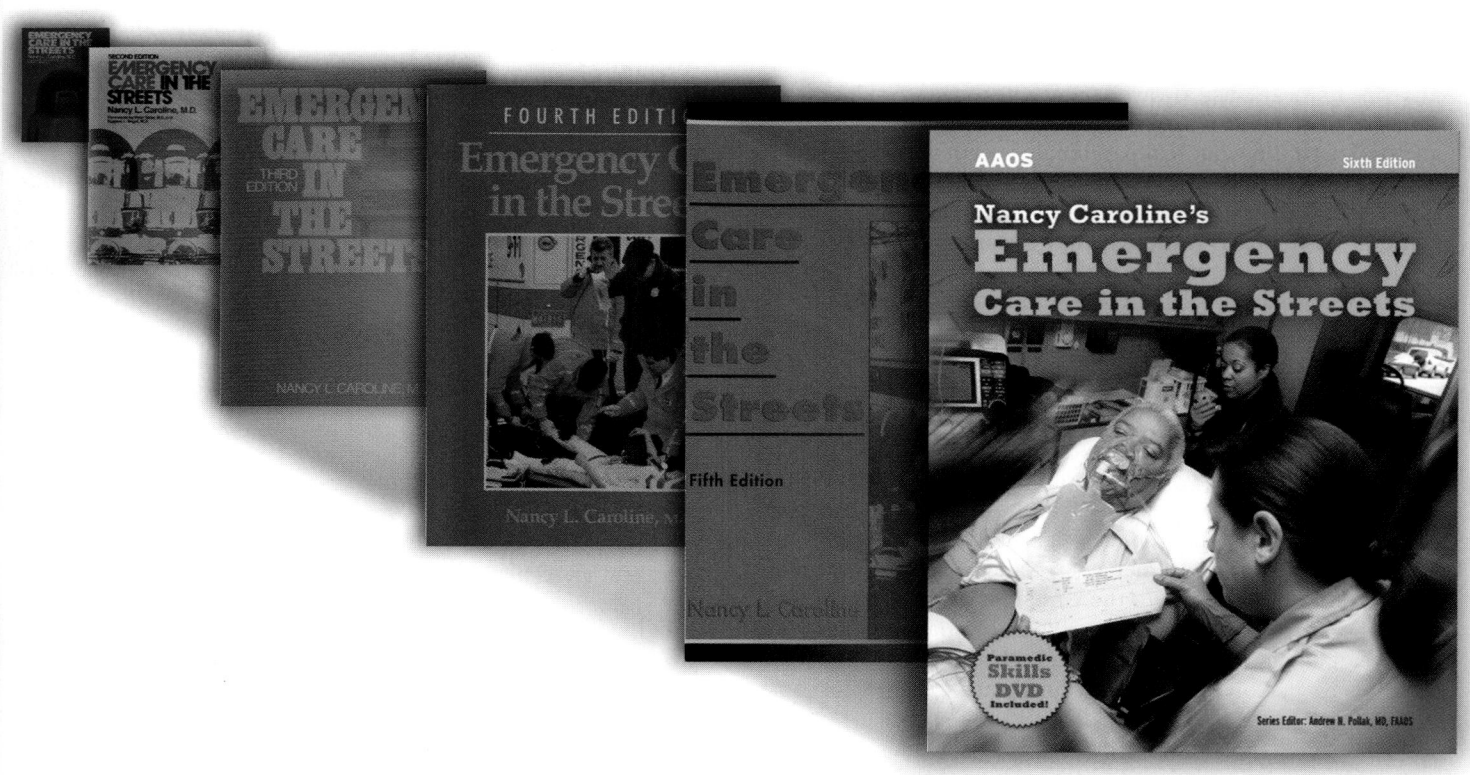

Preface

Publisher's Note:
The American Academy of Orthopaedic Surgeons and Jones and Bartlett Publishers are pleased to present Dr. Nancy L. Caroline's teaching philosophy in this abridged version of her preface from the Fifth Edition of *Emergency Care in the Streets*. This is the philosophy that has guided the development of the Sixth Edition.

In the late autumn of 1974, when Dr. Peter Safar talked me into leaving my relatively calm and secure enclave in the intensive care unit for the world of emergency care outside the hospital, I didn't know I was getting myself mixed up in a revolution. The revolution was in the immediate care of the critically ill and injured, and unwittingly I was being shipped off to the front lines, to marshal a new type of medical shock troops that went by the name of paramedics. My job presumably was to teach those troops the sophisticated techniques of advanced life support, but I had a great deal to learn from them as well. The first time I climbed into a sewer to do a resuscitation, I realized there were lots of things they never told me in medical school.

Nonetheless, I was in good hands. My teachers were veteran emergency medical technicians of the Freedom House Ambulance Service and were also very special human beings. They had been recruited by Dr. Safar in 1967 from among the "unemployables" of Pittsburgh's mean streets and had been among the first ambulance personnel in the country to receive training in advanced life support. They were tough, skilled, compassionate, and professional.

For many months, I rode the ambulances with them. While they learned more emergency medicine, I learned the special stresses and constraints of rendering care outside the controlled conditions of a hospital: CPR in a crowded restaurant, childbirth in the lingerie section of a department store, splinting at the bottom of an elevator shaft, intravenous infusions inside a wrecked automobile. It was an education for all concerned— for the EMTs, for me, and also for the public, who were in those days unaccustomed to the idea that the emergency room had sprouted wheels and definitive care could now begin at the scene.

Out of that experience, the first edition of *Emergency Care in the Streets* was born, together with the first United States Department of Transportation (USDOT) curriculum for paramedics. Since then, the USDOT curriculum has been completely revised, and the revolution in immediate care of the ill and injured has become commonplace on the streets and byways of the United States and many other countries. The paramedic is no longer a strange new creature on the public scene, but rather has become an accepted and respected member of the medical community.

Nonetheless, the revolution isn't over yet. Many things are still changing out on the streets. Paramedics are better trained today and are deploying a variety of skills that were not part of the original curriculum.

There is only one certainty in the field of medicine, and that is that things change. At any time, new research and new data may overthrow some of our most cherished and firmly held concepts. That is another reason why this book—like other

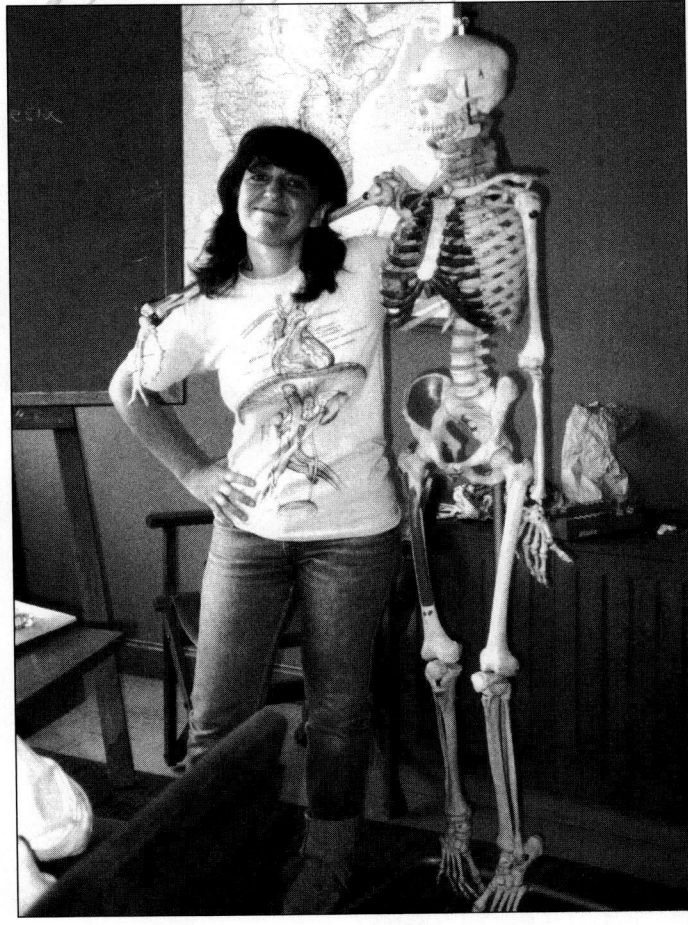

books in the medical field—must undergo periodic revision. It is likely, therefore, that also during the lifetime of this edition, there will be changes in the theory and practice relating to emergency medical care. For that reason, this text (or any other text, for that matter) should not be regarded as the "last word" on every subject. It is, rather, an attempt to give the paramedic a firm grounding in the fundamental concepts—a basis on which to build through a professional lifetime of learning. The treatment recommendations presented here reflect, as much as possible, the current medical consensus. But that consensus may change, and local practice may differ. The paramedic, therefore, should keep abreast of new developments in prehospital emergency care through the professional journals in the field and should be guided in his or her practice by the policies of the local EMS system.

Looking back now on the days I spent riding ambulances full time, I realize they were the best days I have known in medicine. They were days of adventure and challenge and the shared pride in having done a tough job well. I learned a lot from the paramedics, and this book belongs to them.

Dr. Nancy Caroline
Pittsburgh, Pennsylvania
1995

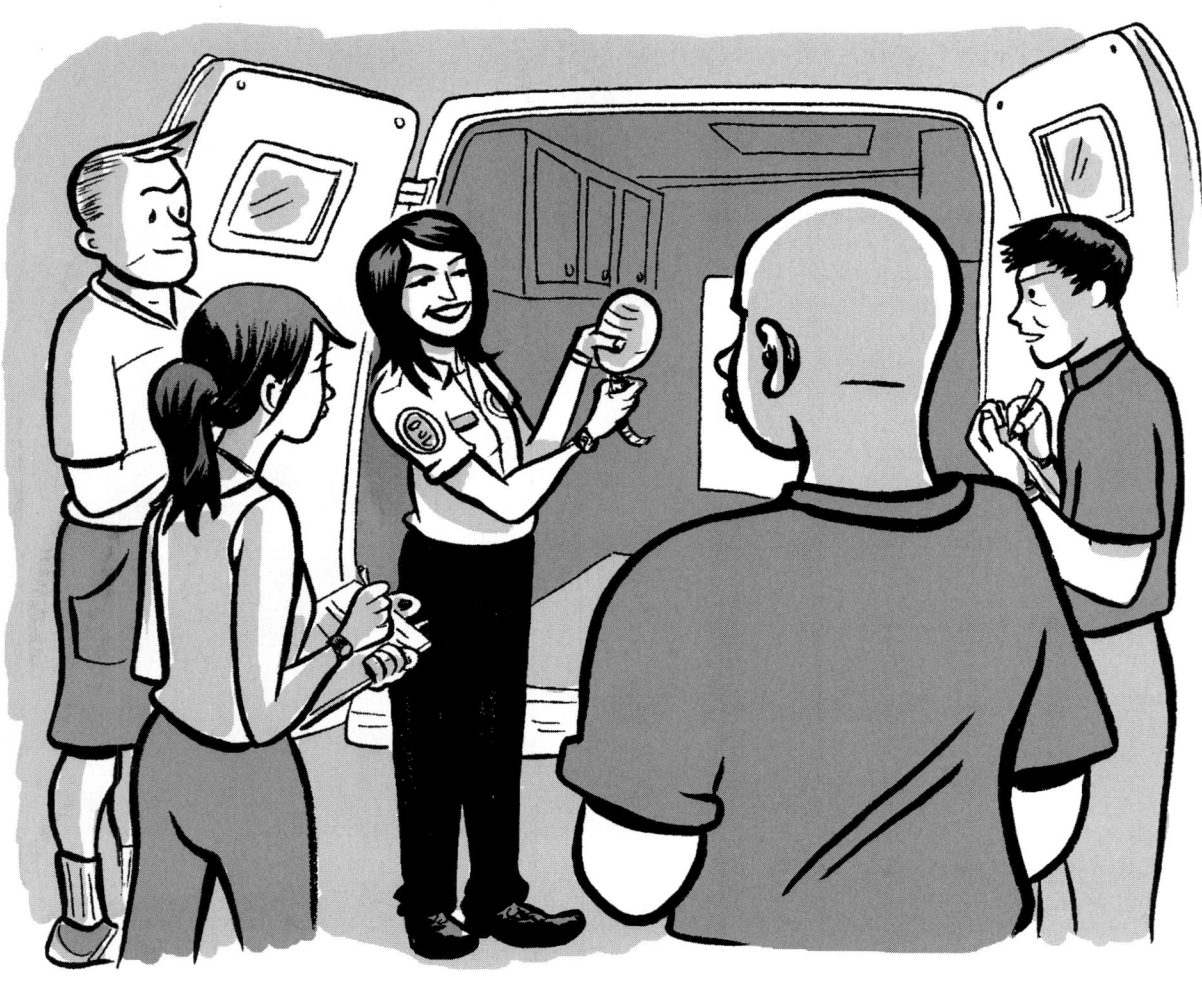

"If they really want to be paramedics, then we can teach them."

—Eugene Nagel, MD

Preparatory

Section 1

Section Editor: David Gurchiek, MS, NREMT-P

Objectives

Cognitive

1-1.1 Define the following terms:
a. EMS Systems
b. Licensure
c. Certification
d. Registration
e. Profession
f. Professionalism
g. Health care professional
h. Ethics
i. Peer review
j. Medical direction
k. Protocols (p 1.5)

1-1.2 Describe key historical events that influenced the development of national Emergency Medical Services (EMS) systems. (p 1.5)

1-1.3 Identify national groups important to the development, education, and implementation of EMS. (p 1.6)

1-1.4 Differentiate among the four nationally recognized levels of EMS training/education, leading to licensure/certification/registration. (p 1.9)

1-1.5 Describe the attributes of a paramedic as a health care professional. (p 1.9)

1-1.6 Describe the recognized levels of EMS training/education, leading to licensure/certification in his or her state. (p 1.11)

1-1.7 Explain paramedic licensure/certification, recertification, and reciprocity requirements in his or her state. (p 1.11)

1-1.8 Evaluate the importance of maintaining one's paramedic license/certification. (p 1.11)

1-1.9 Describe the benefits of paramedic continuing education. (p 1.10)

1-1.10 List current state requirements for paramedic education in his/her state. (p 1.10)

1-1.11 Discuss the role of national associations and of a national registry agency. (p 1.11)

1-1.12 Discuss current issues in his/her state impacting EMS. (p 1.11)

1-1.13 Discuss the roles of various EMS standard setting agencies. (p 1.6)

1-1.14 Identify the standards (components) of an EMS System as defined by the National Highway Traffic Safety Administration. (p 1.7)

1-1.15 Describe how professionalism applies to the paramedic while on and off duty. (p 1.11)

1-1.16 Describe examples of professional behaviors in the following areas: integrity, empathy, self-motivation, appearance and personal hygiene, self-confidence, communications, time management, teamwork and diplomacy, respect, patient advocacy, and careful delivery of service. (p 1.12)

1-1.17 Provide examples of activities that constitute appropriate professional behavior for a paramedic. (p 1.12)

1-1.18 Describe the importance of quality EMS research to the future of EMS. (p 1.17)

1-1.19 Identify the benefits of paramedics teaching in their community. (p 1.14)

1-1.20 Describe what is meant by "citizen involvement in the EMS system." (p 1.14)

1-1.21 Analyze how the paramedic can benefit the health care system by supporting primary care to patients in the out-of-hospital setting. (p 1.15)

1-1.22 List the primary and additional responsibilities of paramedics. (p 1.13)

1-1.23 Describe the role of the EMS physician in providing medical direction. (p 1.15)

1-1.24 Describe the benefits of medical direction, both online and off-line. (p 1.15)

1-1.25 Describe the process for the development of local policies and protocols. (p 1.15)

1-1.26 Provide examples of local protocols. (p 1.15)

1-1.27 Discuss prehospital and out-of-hospital care as an extension of the physician. (p 1.9)

1-1.28 Describe the relationship between a physician on the scene, the paramedic on the scene, and the EMS physician providing on-line medical direction. (p 1.7)

1-1.29 Describe the components of continuous quality improvement. (p 1.16)

1-1.30 Analyze the role of continuous quality improvement with respect to continuing medical education and research. (p 1.16)

1-1.31 Define the role of the paramedic relative to the safety of the crew, the patient, and bystanders. (p 1.13)

1-1.32 Identify local health care agencies and transportation resources for patients with special needs. (p 1.13)

1-1.33 Describe the role of the paramedic in health education activities related to illness and injury prevention. (p 1.14)

1-1.34 Describe the importance and benefits of research. (p 1.17)

1-1.35 Explain the EMS provider's role in data collection. (p 1.17)

1-1.36 Explain the basic principles of research. (p 1.17)

1-1.37 Describe a process of evaluating and interpreting research. (p 1.18)

Affective

1-1.38 Assess personal practices relative to the responsibility for personal safety, the safety of the crew, the patient, and bystanders. (p 1.13)

1-1.39 Serve as a role model for others relative to professionalism in EMS. (p 1.12)

1-1.40 Value the need to serve as the patient advocate inclusive of those with special needs, alternate life styles, and cultural diversity. (p 1.12)

1-1.41 Defend the importance of continuing medical education and skills retention. (p 1.10)

1-1.42 Advocate the need for supporting and participating in research efforts aimed at improving EMS systems. (p 1.15)

1-1.43 Assess personal attitudes and demeanor that may distract from professionalism. (p 1.12)

1-1.44 Value the role that family dynamics plays in the total care of patients. (p 1.12)

1-1.45 Advocate the need for injury prevention, including abusive situations. (p 1.13)

1-1.46 Exhibit professional behaviors in the following areas: integrity, empathy, self-motivation, appearance and personal hygiene, self-confidence, communications, time management, teamwork and diplomacy, respect, patient advocacy, and careful delivery of service. (p 1.12)

Psychomotor

None

Introduction

Early in the emergency medical services (EMS) system development, the role of a responder was to identify an individual who was ill or injured and rapidly transport the person to a facility, often called "scoop and swoop." Today that has changed dramatically because of the expectations of communities and findings in research. As a paramedic you will encounter many different situations, from life threatening to simply lending an ear to a person just needing a listener. People you meet in the field may evaluate you on what they see on television, read in published articles, or your treatment of a loved one. Remember this: "Upon becoming a licensed paramedic, one must not lose recognition of the fact that it is a privilege, and not a right, to treat someone who is perhaps experiencing one of the worst moments in their lives. Along with that privilege comes a responsibility to continually educate and train oneself. You would expect no less from someone responding to your family."
—Dr. Rob Puls, DC, CCEMT-P

EMS System Development

Pre-20th Century

The modern-day EMS system is a relatively new profession when compared with many other professions   Figure 1-1 ▶ . Way back in the Babylon of 1700 BC, the medical care professional went to the patient's home, and the Code of Hammurabi (the king who invented rule by law) spelled out protocols and reimbursements for medical care—including punishment for malpractice   Figure 1-2 ▶ .

Sending the care provider to the patient was the way it was done until Napoleon's time. In the 1790s Jean Larrey, a physician, developed *ambulances volantes,* or flying ambulances. Care was brought to patients in the field as quickly as possible.

The first documented ambulance service was started in 1869 by the New York City Health Department.

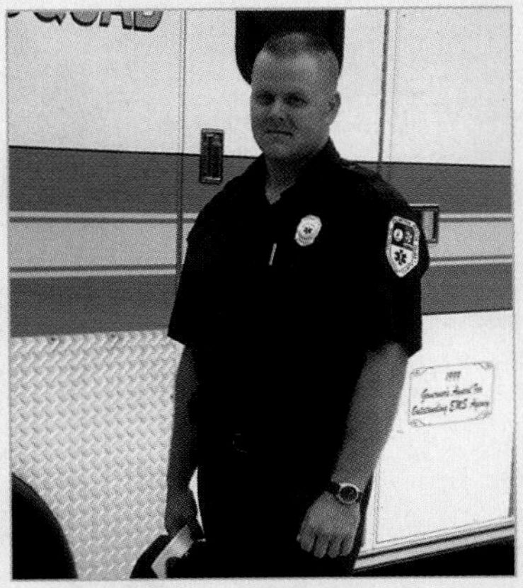

Figure 1-1 Today's prehospital care professionals are highly trained to provide a wide variety of medical services to the public.

The 20th Century and Modern Technology

World Wars I and II saw the development of ambulance corps to rapidly care for and remove injured persons from the battlefields to take them to hospitals far from the front. But, during the 1950s and the Korean War, military medical researchers recognized that bringing the hospital closer to the field would give patients a better chance of surviving   Figure 1-3 ▶ . Helicopters, another new technology, brought patients to Mobile Army Surgical Hospitals (M*A*S*H units) that helped thousands survive.

In the late 1950s and early 1960s, however, the focus moved back to bringing the hospital to the patient in Northern Ireland, Germany, and Eastern European countries. Mobile

You are the Provider Part 1

You are dispatched to an episode of syncope at a local church. En route to the scene, the dispatcher informs you that your patient is an older woman who was reported by family members to have fainted during a church ceremony. She is now conscious and complaining of shortness of breath and light-headedness. Because the location of this call is 15 minutes from your station, additional responders who are closer to the scene have also been dispatched.

EMT-Bs quickly arrive on the scene to find a 70-year-old woman surrounded by members of her family, including her grandchildren, the eldest of whom was getting married. Her family members believe she is "just worn out," and think that she should go home and rest. In a brief radio report, the EMT-Bs provide you with this updated information. Shortly after arriving at the scene, you introduce yourself to the patient and perform an intial assessment.

Initial Assessment	Recording Time: 0 Minutes
Appearance	Noticeably diaphoretic and pale
Level of consciousness	Conscious but confused
Airway	Patent
Breathing	Increased respirations; adequate depth
Circulation	Very weak radial pulse

1. How is patient care initiated for this or any call?
2. What role do dispatchers play in patient care?

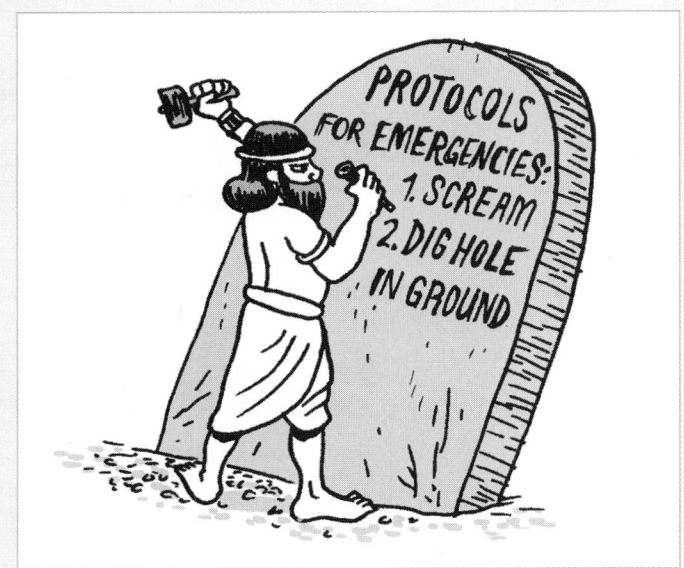

Figure 1-2

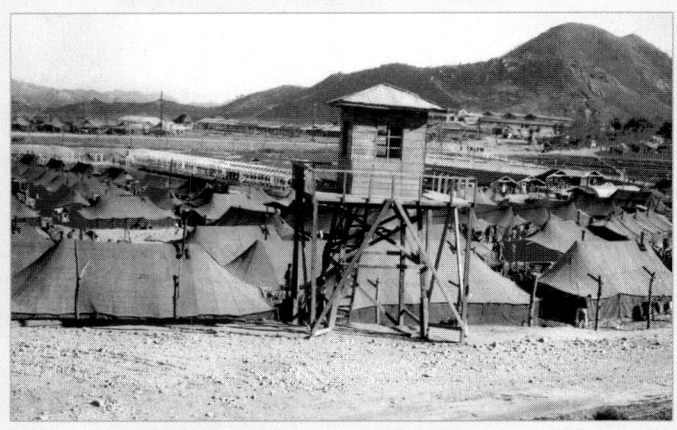

Figure 1-3 Temporary hospitals, such as this one in use during the Korean War, were set up to provide more rapid care for the injured.

Table 1-1	Critical Points

- Develop collaborative strategies to identify and address community health and safety issues.
- Align the financial incentives of EMS and other health care providers and payers.
- Participate in community-based prevention efforts.
- Develop and pursue a national EMS research agenda.
- Pass EMS legislation in each state to support innovation and integration.
- Allocate adequate resources for medical direction.
- Develop information systems that link EMS across its continuum.
- Determine the costs and benefits of EMS to the community.
- Ensure nationwide availability of 9-1-1 as the emergency telephone number.
- Ensure that all calls for emergency help are automatically accompanied by location-identifying information.

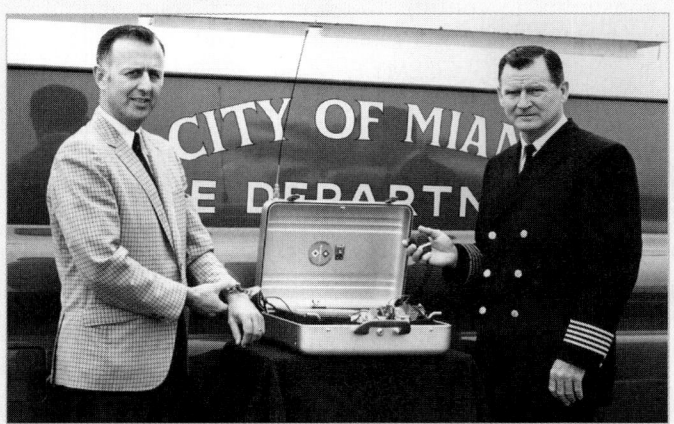

Figure 1-4 Dr Eugene Nagel, widely considered the father of paramedicine, provided much-needed leadership to the developing field of EMT training. Here he is shown (at left) in 1967 with Chief Larry Kenney of the Miami Fire Department, with the first telemetry package to be used by paramedics.

intensive care units (MICUs) were staffed by specially trained physicians riding these units. The idea quickly spread to the United States, but US physicians were in short supply, and those physicians who were interested had minimal expertise to venture into the prehospital area. So a question was asked "Can a nonphysician be trained to perform advanced medical skills?" The answer was "Yes."

In 1966 the National Academy of Science and the National Research Council released a "White Paper" entitled "Accidental Death and Disability: The Neglected Disease of Modern Society," in which they outlined 10 critical points Table 1-1 ▶ . From these points the National Highway Safety Act was instituted in 1966. In this act the US Department of Transportation (US DOT) was created, providing authority and financial support for the development of basic and advanced life support programs. The first EMT textbook, *Emergency Care and Transportation of the Sick and Injured,* was published by the American Academy of Orthopaedic Surgeons (AAOS) in 1971.

In 1969, the same year the basic training course for EMTs was released, Dr Eugene Nagel, then of Miami, Fla, began training fire fighters from the Miami Fire Department with advanced emergency skills Figure 1-4 ▲ . Dr Nagel took the use of advanced emergency treatment one step further. He developed a telemetry system that enabled fire fighters to transmit a patient's electrocardiogram to physicians at Jackson Memorial Hospital and to receive radio instructions from the physicians regarding what measures to take. Dr Nagel is often called the "Father of Paramedicine."

In 1973 the Emergency Medical Services System Act defined 15 required components Table 1-2 ▶ of an EMS system, with emphasis on regional development and trauma care. The act provided a structure and uniformity to the EMS system that came out of pioneering programs in Miami, Seattle, and Pittsburgh, and the Illinois Trauma System (Dr. David Boyd).

Table 1-2	Required Components

- Integration of health services
- EMS research
- Legislation and regulation
- System finance
- Human resources
- Medical direction
- Education systems
- Public education
- Prevention
- Public access
- Communication systems
- Clinical care
- Information systems
- Evaluation

Table 1-3	System Elements

1. Regulation and policy
2. Resource management
3. Human resources and training
4. Transportation
5. Facilities
6. Communication
7. Public information and education
8. Medical direction
9. Trauma systems
10. Evaluation

Many cities set up individual advanced EMS training, and regions added their own spin to what they thought was the essential standard of care, but it wasn't until 1977 that the first National Standard Curriculum for paramedics was developed by the US DOT. This first paramedic curriculum was based on the work of Dr Nancy Caroline.

Through the 1980s and 1990s, changes continued in EMS while the number of trained personnel grew. Federal funding and staff were reduced, and the responsibility for funding EMS was transferred to the states. The National Highway Traffic Safety Administration (NHTSA) developed "10 System Elements" Table 1-3 ▶ in an effort to sustain EMS systems. The rapid advancement slowed greatly after this change in responsibility, primarily because of funding issues. Although it was made clear that the federal funding being provided was just "seed money" and that long-term local funding strategies needed to be developed, many states apparently believed that the federal dollars wouldn't go away. Unfortunately, they did. Several other major legislative initiatives also came about in

this time frame such as the EMS for Children (EMS-C) program grant funding in 1984. In 1986 an amendment was made to the Public Safety Officers Benefit Act in which families of Fire and EMS providers were compensated if the provider was killed in the line of duty. As progress continued into the 1990s, trauma systems started making headway.

Controversies

Many communities initially fought against ambulance drivers "playing doctor," or in other words, becoming paramedics. Now, even the smallest communities expect access to advanced life support (ALS)-trained personnel.

The EMS System

The modern-day EMS system is a complex network of coordinated services providing various levels of care to a community. These services work in unison to meet both the growing and standing needs of the citizens in the community in which they reside. You as a paramedic are part of this network; therefore,

You are the Provider Part 2

As you perform a focused history and physical exam, your partner takes the patient's vital signs. Her pulse rate and blood pressure concern you, and you apply the cardiac monitor. As you question the patient and her family about her medical history and events that have occurred during today's festivities, you immediately note an arrhythmia.

Vital Signs	Recording Time: 5 Minutes
Level of consciousness	Conscious but confused
Skin	Diaphoretic, pale, and cool
Pulse	180 beats/min, regular and weak
Blood pressure	80/42 mm Hg
Respirations	24 breaths/min; adequate depth
Sao$_2$	95% on 15 L/min using a nonrebreathing mask
ECG	Ventricular tachycardia

3. What care can EMT-Bs provide for this patient?

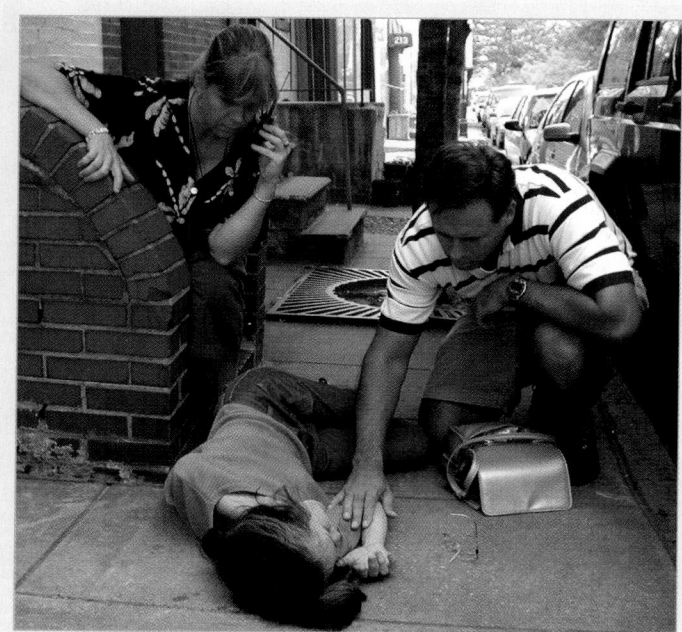

Figure 1-5 One of your roles as a paramedic is educating the public about how to first respond to an emergency, before medical help has arrived.

you must stay active in your community to be able to meet the ever-changing needs.

The EMS network begins with citizen involvement in the complex EMS system. The public needs to be taught how to recognize that an emergency exists, how to activate the EMS system, and how basic care can be provided before EMS arrives ` Figure 1-5 ▲ `. Remember that the public's idea of an emergency may be drastically different from yours.

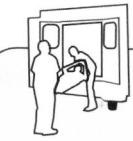

In the Field

A patient may only experience once what a paramedic may experience hundreds of times. Understand the patient's anxiety.

When you are called to a "sick person" at 2 AM who only has a common cold and can't sleep, there is no reason to become angry at the patient, your career, or your EMS system. Instead, use this time to educate the public by offering sympathy and insight on cold treatment, and, perhaps tactfully discuss why a cold is not an emergency. Remember, a paramedic is a public servant. You will often respond to non-emergent calls.

When the public activates the EMS system, their first contact is usually a dispatcher. Requirements for dispatcher training vary greatly from state to state. Dispatchers are limited in interpreting an emergency and in extracting appropriate information from a stressed caller. Once on scene, you have to

determine what is really going on, which in many cases is a far cry from what dispatch told you. Despite this or limited information, you, as a paramedic, will develop your care plan for the patient and decide on the appropriate transport method and receiving facility for your patient.

Being active in your community will keep you on top of the best local resources. When you are drawing up a potential care plan, you will ask yourself, "Does the receiving facility have the resources needed for this patient?" When you are active in your community, you will know the answer. If the answer is no, the next question, "Is there an appropriate facility within a reasonable distance?" will also be a part of your community knowledge. And of course, you will remember that your patients have the ultimate decision regarding where they go.

There are currently several levels of providers in the EMS system. Each level has a scope of practice, as outlined by the US DOT. The scope of practice is reevaluated from time to time and may change as a result. Let's take a look at these various levels.

Special Considerations

EMS systems must be capable of handling many different situations including obstetric, pediatric, and geriatric emergencies. Proper procedures, drug dosages, and even assessment techniques are often different in children, adults, and older people.

The Dispatcher

The dispatcher plays a key role in an EMS call. He or she must receive and enter all information on the call, interpret the information, and in turn, relay it to the appropriate resources ` Figure 1-6 ▼ `. In some locations the dispatcher may be

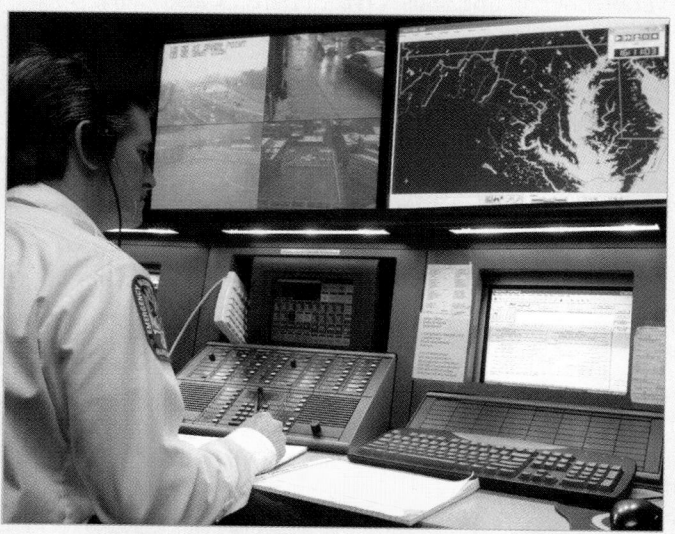

Figure 1-6 The dispatcher coordinates the entire rescue effort. He or she interprets a caller's information and then sends appropriate personnel and resources to the scene.

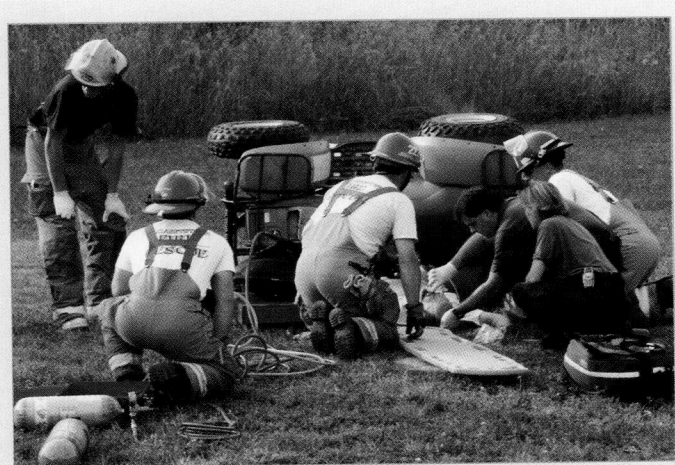

Figure 1-7 The first responder is critical for providing the initial emergency patient care, particularly when medical personnel must travel long distances to a scene.

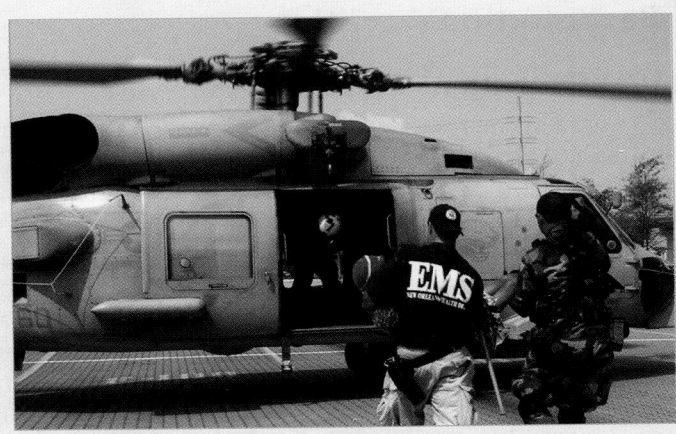

Figure 1-8 EMTs were a critical part of the massive evacuation efforts following Hurricane Katrina in 2005.

trained as an emergency medical dispatcher (EMD), which charges these individuals with the added task of giving simple medical direction (ie, CPR, bleeding control, etc) to a caller in hopes that this care may benefit the patient until EMS personnel are on scene.

First Responder

Not all states have this as a certification and/or licensing level, and for those states that do, there can be considerable variability in requirements. In the generic use of the term, a first responder is usually a person trained in CPR and/or first aid. As a paramedic, one of your jobs will be to familiarize yourself with the level of training of first responders in your EMS system.

From an EMS point of view, a first responder has completed a National Standard Curriculum course. This training should make the first responder capable of recognizing the seriousness of a patient's condition, administering appropriate basic care, and relaying information to the paramedic. First responders are an essential level of provider to the EMS system, especially in rural areas **Figure 1-7 ▲**.

The EMT-Basic

In most states the EMT-Basic (EMT-B) is the backbone and primary provider level in many EMS systems. This is also the level of certification required for you prior to entering your paramedic training program.

In some states EMT-Bs may be trained in advanced airway intervention, limited medication administration, and intravenous fluid (IV) therapy; however, EMT-Bs with this expanded scope of practice are still considered EMT-Bs. In EMS, the highest number of trained and certified individuals are EMT-Bs **Figure 1-8 ▶**.

The EMT-Intermediate

The skill level for the EMT-Intermediate (EMT-I) saw a significant change in 1999, when a major revision of the 1985 curriculum took place. The US DOT placed a number of common emergency skills previously only performed by a paramedic under the umbrella of the EMT-I. These skills include IV therapy, cardiac monitoring, and advanced airway procedures. The number of individuals trained and certified at the EMT-I level remains low.

Controversies

Some argue that in an urban setting all that is needed are EMT-Is rather than paramedics, while others argue that EMT-Is perform ALS skills without having adequate academic preparation and should be phased out. The jury is still out on whether this particular level of training will become an attractive option for jurisdictions and EMS providers.

The EMT-Paramedic

Currently the EMT-Paramedic (EMT-P) is the highest skill level at which you can be either certified or licensed at the state or national level. In 1998, the US DOT paramedic curriculum underwent major revisions and the level of training and skills increased greatly. Although you may hold a license or certification independently, states still require paramedics to function directly under the guidance of a licensed physician and to be affiliated with a paramedic-level service.

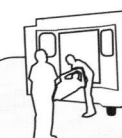

In the Field

The best paramedics will keep up-to-date on basic life support skills as well as advanced life support skills.

Paramedic Education

Initial Education

Education may vary state to state, but for the most part all states base their paramedic education programs on the US DOT EMT-Paramedic National Standard Curriculum. The National EMS Education and Practice Blueprint (from NHTSA) and its recommended competencies also have an impact on paramedic programs. One of the major recommendations is the inclusion of a college-level anatomy and physiology course as part of many training programs today. The National EMS Education and Practice Blueprint outlines the bare-bones minimum of what a paramedic must know to practice, including cognitive (knowledge) objectives, psychomotor (skills) objectives, and affective (attitude) objectives. States require varying hours of training, but the national average falls between 1,000 and 1,200 hours of combined classroom, clinical, and field education. Some leaders want to structure education so that the paramedic designation is achieved through an associate degree program. A distinct benefit of this is that it can give paramedics credits that could be used in achieving higher level college degrees.

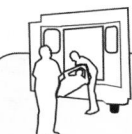

In the Field

The number of calls you go on isn't the deciding factor on how much more training you need.

Continuing Education

Most states require that paramedics show proof of hours spent in continuing education programs. Such programs keep you up-to-date on new research findings and new techniques and

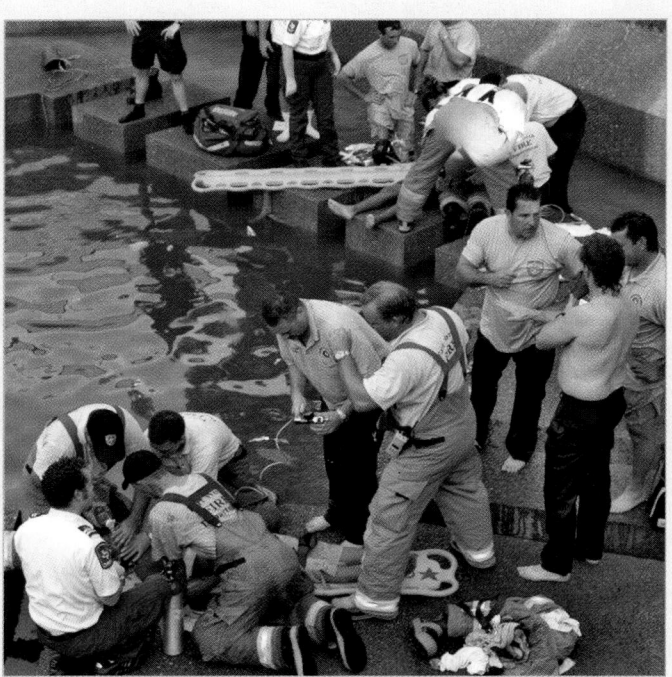

Figure 1-9 Continuing education can keep you up-to-date on technological improvements that are continually made available to EMT-Ps.

skills, and they knock the rust off of skills you seldom use **Figure 1-9 ▲** . Continuing education can also showcase current issues in your state that impact you and your system's ability to provide quality emergency medical care. Continuing education can be enjoyable and it should be. Whenever possible, you should attend conferences and seminars, ideally with some of them being out of your region and/or state, which helps

You are the Provider Part 3

Your paramedic partner asks the patient whether she has any allergies to medication and then administers an appropriate dose of Versed for sedation. You simultaneously prepare your equipment for synchronized cardioversion and explain to the patient what you must do and what she should expect. You advise the other responders to be prepared for deterioration of the patient's condition and to notify the receiving facility of her condition and the treatment she has received. Having successfully converted your patient's heart rhythm, you take another set of vital signs.

Reassessment	Recording Time: 10 Minutes
Level of consciousness	A (Alert to person, place, and day)
Skin	Pink, warm, and dry
Pulse	88 beats/min, regular and strong
Blood pressure	130/60 mm Hg
Respirations	16 breaths/min and unlabored
Sao_2	99% on 15 L/min using a nonrebreathing mask
ECG	Sinus rhythm

4. What are the advantages of having a paramedic partner?

5. Is there one team member who is more important than another?

Table 1-4	National EMS Organizations

- National Highway Traffic Safety Administration (NHTSA)
- National Association of Emergency Medical Service Physicians (NAEMSP)
- National Association of State EMS Directors (NASEMSD)
- National Association of EMS Educators (NAEMSE)
- National Registry of EMTs (NREMT)
- National Association of EMTs (NAEMT)
- Emergency Medical Services for Children (EMS-C)
- American College of Emergency Physicians (ACEP)
- American Ambulance Association (AAA)
- National Association of State EMS Training Coordinators
- International Flight Paramedics Association

broaden your knowledge base. It is certainly worth attending conferences that may not be designed for paramedics, such as those targeted at physicians. Keep up with reading EMS journals. Another great resource for paramedics is the surprising number of Internet-based continuing education providers; however, be sure that these programs meet your state or national requirements. Get everyone on your service involved in postrun critiques—they can be very beneficial in identifying problem areas in your practice.

No matter what requirements are mandated by the state licensing agency, responsibility for continuing medical education ultimately rests with each individual paramedic. You are the only person who knows which subjects have become alarmingly foggy in your memory and which procedures leave you feeling as if you have ten thumbs. And you are the person who will have to live with the questions and doubts that inevitably arise after something goes wrong in the field. Continuing medical education is a way to help make sure that things *don't* go wrong.

National EMS Group Involvement

Many national and state organizations exist, and many invite EMT-P membership. These organizations do have an impact on the future direction of EMS, so it is very important for you to become involved in them. You will also be able to access many valuable resources to help you develop yourself and your service area and to improve your problem-solving skills. One of the common goals of many national organizations is to promote uniformity of EMS standards and practice throughout the nation. Some of these organizations are listed in Table 1-4 ▲.

Licensure, Certification, and Registration

Upon completing a paramedic training program, you will be required to be licensed and/or certified to practice your profes-

sion. Performing functions as a paramedic prior to this is unlawful, or to be more specific, considered practicing medicine without a license. State and local guidelines determine whether you are going to be licensed or certified when you complete your paramedic training. There are subtle differences between licensure and certification, which are discussed in Chapter 4. For all intents and purposes, these are essentially the same. Throughout this chapter, to avoid repetition, when we talk about being certified it means the same as holding a license.

Although holding a license shows that you have successfully completed a training program and met the requirements to achieve such license, it does not mean that you can perform as a paramedic without the supervision of your service's physician medical director. Agencies (state, local, and national) still require that paramedics receive medical direction. The concept and principles of medical control will be discussed later in the chapter.

Finally, you may be required to be registered as well as licensed. Registration means that records of your training, state or local licensure, and recertification will be held by a recognized board of registration.

Additionally, some states require that paramedic graduates come from an accredited paramedic program. The Committee on Accreditation of Educational Programs for the EMS Professions (CoAEMSP) is the only accrediting agency for paramedic programs. The mission of the CoAEMSP is to continuously improve the quality of EMS education through accreditation and recognition services for the full range of EMS professions.

Reciprocity

Be aware that each state has different licensing or certification requirements and procedures. Granting certification to a provider from another state or agency is known as reciprocity. More than 40 states recognize National Registry certification as part of their reciprocity process. For reciprocity to be granted to an individual EMT or paramedic, most states will require you to hold current state certification and to be in good standing as well as having National Registry certification. Several states will require you to challenge their requirements; in other words, you may be required to go through that state's written and/or practical evaluations prior to reciprocity being granted. Others may request your training program transcript and continuing education hours.

Professionalism

During your paramedic education and training process, you learn a vast amount of information designed to make you a health care professional, practicing at the paramedic level. A profession is a field of endeavor that requires a specialized set of knowledge, skills, and expertise, often gained after lengthy training.

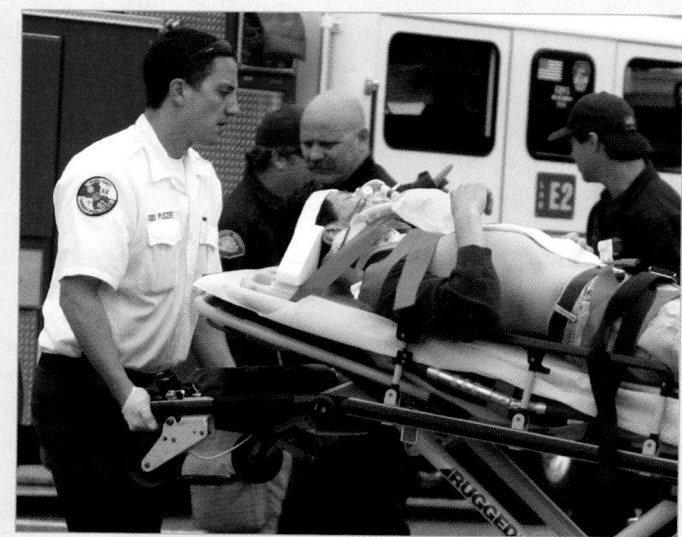

Figure 1-10 Adopting a professional attitude and appearance is a critical part of working with the public and earning their trust.

As a paramedic, you will be trained at length for certification with standards, competencies, and continuing education requirements.

A paramedic is considered a health care professional. The attributes of a health care professional are that he or she:

- Conforms to the same standards of other health care professions.
- Provides quality patient care.
- Instills pride in the profession.
- Strives continuously for high standards.
- Earns respect from others in the profession.
- Meets societal expectations of the profession whether on or off duty.

As a paramedic, you will be trained for certification using standards, competencies, and continuing education requirements. The paramedic profession has expected standards and performance parameters as well as a code of ethics. Collectively, these are the standards by which you will be measured as a paramedic.

As a paramedic you must remind yourself that you are in a highly visible role in your community   Figure 1-10 ▲ . Professional image and behavior must be a top priority. You are a representative of the agency, city, county, district, or state you work in. Sometimes, people will make a negative judgment within the first 10 seconds of meeting you. As a paramedic you will be meeting new people as an everyday part of your career. To provide the best possible care, you must establish and maintain credibility and instill confidence. As you walk into a situation, never forget that a big part of your job is to continually show that you are truly concerned for the well-being of your patients and their families. Your appearance is also of utmost importance—it has more impact than you may think. It is not appropriate to arrive at a call in dirty clothes, with dirty hands, and smelling offensively. You must look and act like a professional at all times.

Notes from Nancy

The role of paramedic entails new prestige, but it also imposes new responsibilities. Paramedics are entrusted with the lives of other human beings, and there is no more awesome or sacred responsibility than that. Your education as a paramedic must not stop with this text. You must continue to read and study and ask questions, to refine your knowledge and skills, so that you may give to each patient the best of which you are capable. You must learn to conduct yourself with humility, to accept criticism, to learn from mistakes as well as from triumphs, and to demand of yourself and your colleagues nothing less than the best. For only then will the title of paramedic signify what it is meant to signify: a commitment to other human beings.

Other attributes of professionalism as a paramedic include:

- **Integrity.** The single most important attribute. Be open, honest, and truthful with your patients.
- **Empathy.** Show your patients, their families, and other health care professionals that you identified and understand their feelings.
- **Self-motivation.** You should have an internal drive for excellence, which is often a driving force to ensure that you always behave in a professional manner. You will need to continuously educate yourself, accept constructive feedback, and perform with minimal supervision.
- **Communications.** You must be able to express and exchange your ideas, thoughts, and findings with other professional colleagues. Make conscious reminders to yourself when interacting with patients and their families to listen well and speak directly, without using confusing medical terms   Figure 1-11 ▶ .
- **Teamwork and respect.** Teamwork is required in EMS. On every call, everyone involved must work together to achieve a common goal—to provide the best possible prehospital care to ensure the overall well-being of your patient. Most often in the field, the paramedic is the team leader. A team leader will not undermine his or her team, but instead will help guide and support the team, remaining flexible and open for change at any moment and communicating at an appropriate place and time with other members of the team to resolve problems. You must always be as respectful of others as you would expect them to be with you.
- **Patient advocate.** You must always act in the best interest of the patient while respecting his or her wishes and beliefs, regardless of your own. This includes patients with special needs or those with different lifestyles, values, and cultures from your own. Never allow your personal feelings about a patient to have an impact on the care you provide. Respect those you serve. While you need to communicate to do your job, be sure that you maintain a high level of confidentiality.

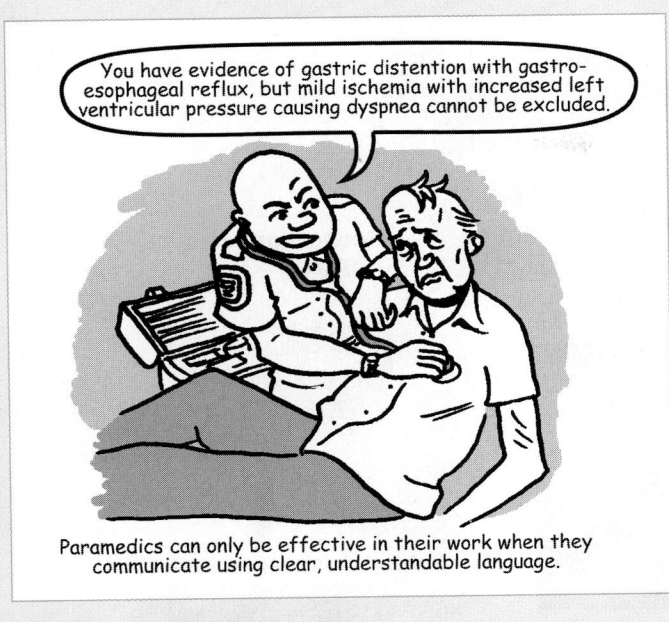

Figure 1-11

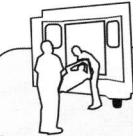

In the Field

For safety, avoid wearing long necklaces, dangling earrings, or other jewelry that could interfere with your work.

Roles and Responsibilities

So what does it actually mean to be a paramedic? What are my roles? What am I responsible for? These are questions that you should ask yourself throughout your career. The EMS system continues to grow and mature, and with those changes will come new roles and additional responsibilities. Some of the primary responsibilities are shown in Figure 1-12 ▶ and include:

- **Preparation.** Be prepared physically, mentally, and emotionally. Keep up your knowledge and skill abilities. Be sure you have the appropriate equipment for your call and that it is in good working order.
- **Response.** Responding to the event in a timely, safe manner is very important. High speed—running "hot" without due regard to the safety of you, your partner, your patient, and persons on the highway (even if they should get out of your way but don't)—is not acceptable.
- **Scene management.** Ensuring your own safety and the safety of your team is the first priority. You must also ensure the patient's safety and the safety of any bystanders. Part of your preparation before you reach the scene should include assessing the situation; the nature of the call will give valuable information. Preparing for scene safety starts with the use of personnel protective equipment such as gloves and goggles. The paramedic often sets the example for safety to the members of the EMS team who might believe that running hot is running safe.
- **Patient assessment and care.** An appropriate organized assessment based on the principles you will learn in this book should be performed on all patients. You will need to recognize and prioritize the patient's needs on the basis of the injuries he or she has sustained or the illness that most urgently needs treatment.
- **Management and disposition.** A paramedic must follow protocols signed off by the medical director. Sometimes,

Whatever details you have about your patient, do your best not to talk in front of anyone who is not on your team. When you talk to members of your team, do so quietly and with appropriate respect. Your role in patient advocacy means you should always be on the lookout for spousal or child abuse and elder neglect. Make sure you communicate your findings to the appropriate authorities.

- **Injury prevention.** A paramedic is in the unique position of seeing the patient's surroundings prior to transport. If you can spot a potential hazard (such as a loose rug at the top of the stairs), use your diplomatic skills and talk about your findings to the patient or a family member. You may prevent a potential injury. Discuss the importance of using bike helmets, safety belts, and child car seats whenever you can. It is another way of preventing injuries.
- **Careful delivery of service.** A paramedic must deliver the highest quality patient care. Pay careful attention to detail and continuously evaluate and reevaluate your performance. Use other medical professionals as resources, not adversaries. Follow policies, protocols, and procedures as well as the orders of your superiors.

You are the Provider Part 4

Your patient's pulse has decreased, blood pressure has increased, and she no longer feels short of breath or light-headed. Her skin signs are much improved, with color returning to her cheeks. Your paramedic partner administers lidocaine, 1 mg/kg of body weight, as well as a maintenance infusion of 2 mg/min. Your patient and her entire family thank you and your partner in the emergency department for your help. You feel gratified to know that all of your hard work has paid off.

6. Why is it important to keep skills and knowledge current?

7. Why is it important to practice these skills as a team?

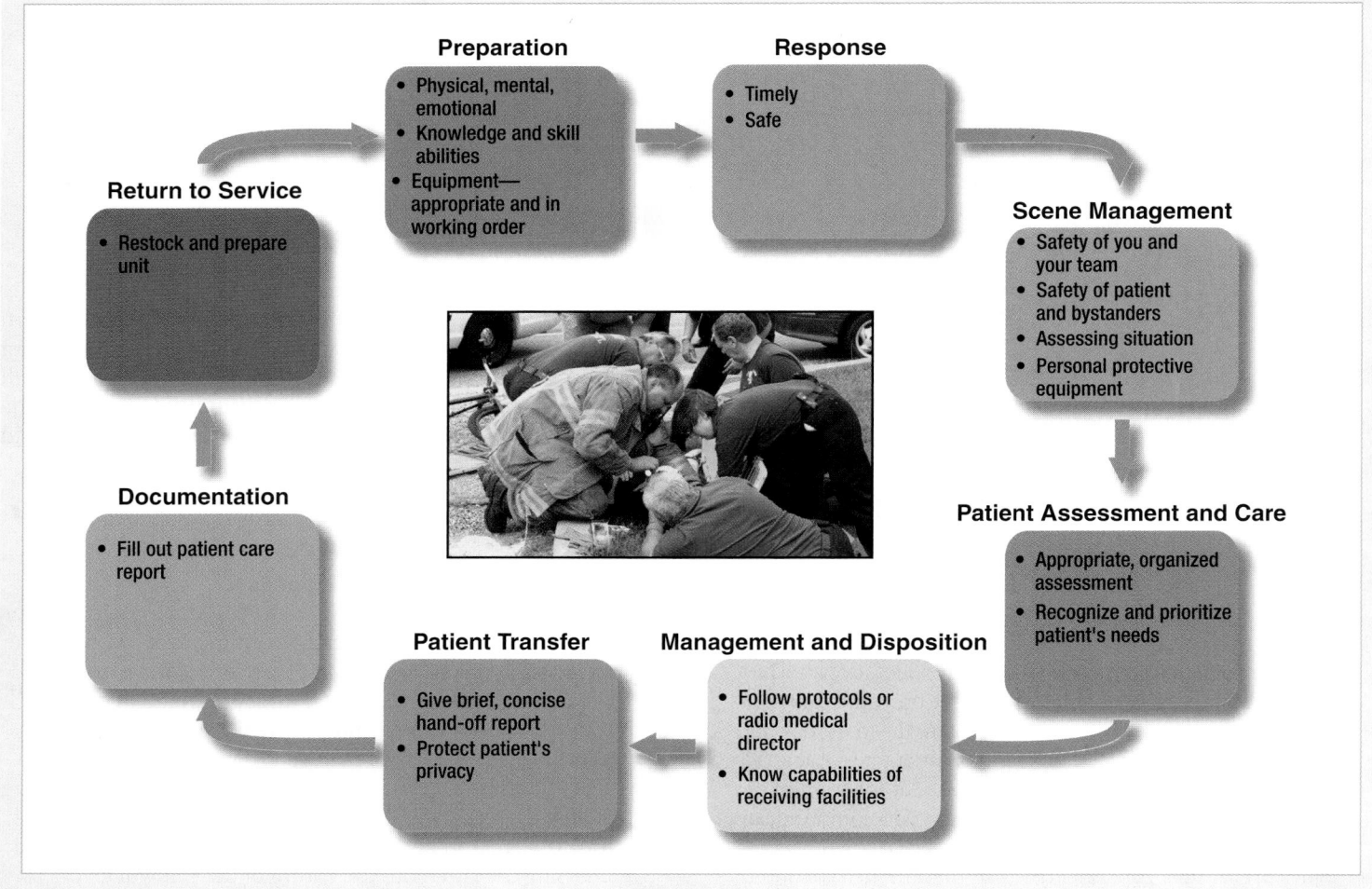

Figure 1-12 Paramedics follow an important sequence of procedures for each emergency call.

however, when you are in the field, you will discover that the protocols might not cover the situation you are in. This is the time that you must radio your medical director for orders. Having a good working relationship with your medical director is critical. You are the eyes, ears, and touch of the medical director. Situations that require a variance of protocol or a decision outside of your scope of practice need to be communicated with your medical director. You must also make the appropriate transport and destination decisions, often with the cooperation of other medical professionals. For example, a patient with carbon monoxide poisoning may need to be transported to a hospital with a hyperbaric chamber. Know the capabilities of all receiving facilities with which you may interact; this will assist you in making the right decisions for your patient. You might not know where the nearest *unoccupied* hyperbaric chamber is, so use your radio and ask.

■ **Patient transfer.** Once you arrive at the receiving facility, continue to act as a patient advocate and give the appropriate facility staff a brief, concise hand-off report.

Once again, use discretion so that you protect your patient's privacy.

■ **Documentation.** After you transfer the patient, it is extremely important that a patient care report be filled out immediately. The report serves as a legal record of what you did in the field. Physicians must document their care of patients—so must you. Guidelines for documentation will be covered later in this text.

■ **Return to service.** Every person on the EMS team is responsible for restocking and preparing the unit as quickly as possible for the next call. Failure to do so can bring about nasty legal consequences if another call comes in and the unit is not fully restocked and ready to respond.

You are looked upon as a health care professional, so take advantage. Educate the public about what you do and its importance. Get involved with prevention, community, and leadership activities whenever possible **Figure 1-13 ▶** . Never miss an opportunity to teach the community about prevention of injury and illness. Explain to people how to appropriately use your services. For those areas where trained EMS staff are few and far between, use your abilities to promote programs that get the

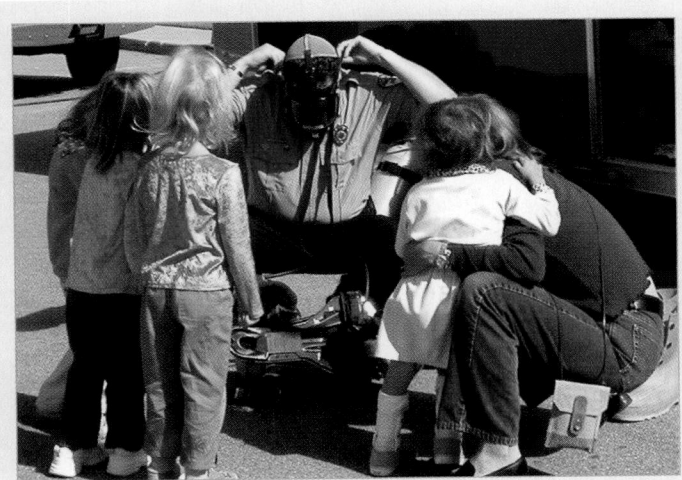

Figure 1-13 Part of your role as a public servant is to interact with and educate the public.

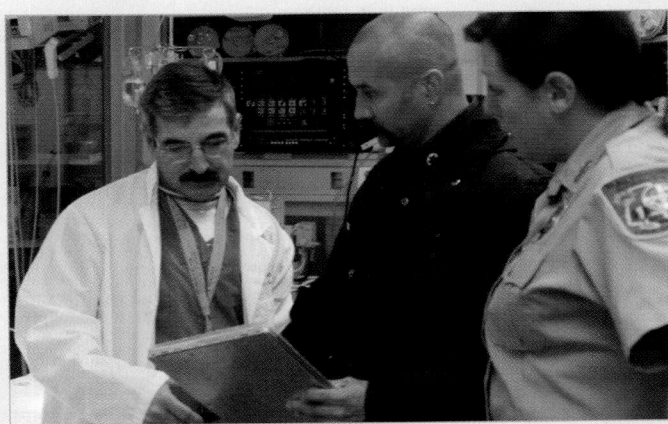

Figure 1-14 Physicians work closely with paramedics through all stages of a patient run. Here, EMS personnel hand off the patient report to the attending emergency department physician.

Documentation and Communication

Documentation of equipment repairs and checks is nearly as important as documenting patient care.

public involved in CPR, one of the major determinants of whether or not a person in cardiac arrest will live or die.

In some regions, paramedics have other health care responsibilities such as working in clinics, free-standing emergency facilities, and hospitals. Home visits by paramedics under direct medical control are being considered.

Providers of all EMS levels need to be advocates for prehospital health care, which often means setting out a well thought-out campaign for EMS. Research your community, look at the strengths and weaknesses of the system, and develop plans for initiatives to improve the system. Many people lack the understanding of what EMS does and recognition of how vital your job can be when a loved one is unexpectedly taken ill. Many programs on television today give the public only a very small insight into the true world of EMS. Some of these programs use unrealistic events or show unrealistic outcomes or inappropriate behavior on the part of EMS providers. By involving yourself in your communities, you can both educate and advocate. It is up to all of us to educate the media and public of the truths in "our world." We must all strive to stay at the top of our profession. Continue your education, become a mentor for new EMS professionals, and conduct research activities.

Medical Direction

The quickest distinction in the differences among levels of EMS training is that the paramedic carries out invasive procedures—procedures that otherwise are performed only by

physicians or other advanced practitioners. The law, however does not give the paramedic independent authority to act. Physicians who are educated about the levels and the extent of the training of EMS personnel play a vital role in running a service Figure 1-14 ▲ . The role of an EMS medical director includes:

- Educating and training personnel.
- Participating in the selection of new personnel.
- Participating in equipment selection.
- Developing clinical protocols in cooperation with other EMS personnel who are considered experts in the field.
- Developing and assisting in a quality improvement program.
- Providing input into patient care.
- Interfacing between EMS systems and other health care agencies.
- Serving as an EMS advocate to the community.
- Serving as the "medical conscience" of the EMS system.

The medical director also provides online (either by radio or by electronic communication) and off-line medical control. The benefit to online medical control is that it provides immediate and specific patient care resources, allows telemetry transmission, allows for continuous quality improvement, and can render on-scene assistance. Off-line medical control allows for the development of protocols, standing orders, procedures, and training. A protocol is a treatment plan for a specific illness or injury. A standing order is a type of protocol that is a written document signed by the EMS system's medical director that outlines specific directions, permissions, and sometimes prohibitions regarding patient care that is rendered prior to contacting medical control (for example, defibrillation). Protocols are usually developed in conjunction with national standards. For example, EMS personnel use the American Heart Association advanced cardiac life support algorithms as a protocol for cardiac patients (discussed in detail in Chapter 27). Protocols also

In the Field

In some cases you may encounter a physician on scene. If the physician is familiar with EMS protocols or happens to be your medical director, it can be a great help. But you may be caught between what the physician on the scene wants and the protocols that your medical director has given your service. Remember that you work with your physician medical director and you must adhere to the local protocols and standing orders.

You must not lose your cool should the physician on the scene demand medical control of the situation.

Politely explain that all your actions must be in accordance with your EMS medical director's protocols. Point out that you can only transfer care of the patient to an onsite physician if that physician is now taking full responsibility for the patient and he or she will be present during transport, riding with the patient in your ambulance to the emergency department, as well as signing for any orders given.

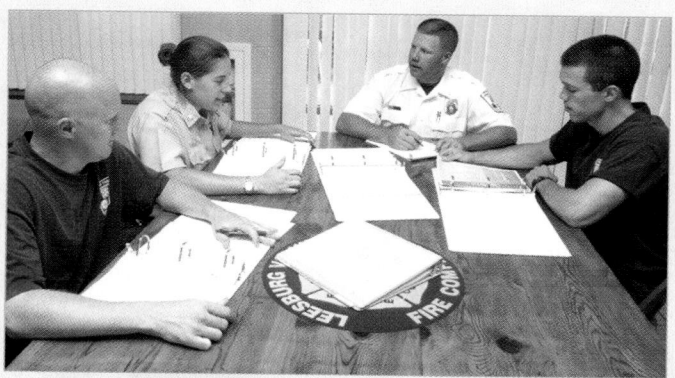

Figure 1-15 Peer reviews should be seen as a constructive part of paramedic practice.

dictate what type of equipment and supplies are approved and needed as well as minimum expectations of personnel. The medical director also plays a role after the ambulance run. Medical directors help with patient care report review or even personally perform such reviews to assure continuous quality improvement.

Improving System Quality

Making a good thing better should always be part of your paramedic career. A tool often used to continually evaluate your care is called continuous quality improvement (CQI). Quality assurance is another process that evaluates problems and finds solutions. CQI is a process of assessing for ongoing improvement without waiting for a problem to arise first. When properly developed and followed, a CQI program can help you and your service.

The process of CQI is dynamic, and your EMS system should develop a structure before a CQI assessment program is started. A good CQI process should include the following:

- Identify any system-wide problem(s).
- Conduct an in-depth review of the problem(s).
- Aid the problem(s) and develop a remedy(ies).
- Develop an action plan for correction of problems.
- Enforce the plan of action.
- Reexamine the problem.
- Identify excellence in patient care.
- Look for modifications that need to be made to protocols and standing orders.
- Identify situations that are currently not addressed by protocols and standing orders.

Although it may not be feasible, all ambulance runs should be reviewed. First and foremost the focus of CQI needs to be on improving patient care.

Some services will choose to do quality assurance as *peer review* **Figure 1-15 ▲** . Peer review can be a good learning experience if the people doing the reviewing have good guidelines to follow and you keep an open mind. No matter how good your education and training, you will still make mistakes and miss things from time to time. When a peer reviewer finds things you can improve, you should look at it as an educational tool. In an ideal system, the members of the peer review team rotate on and off, meaning that you at some point in time will also serve as a reviewer yourself. Caution: never use this process as a tool to demean or belittle a fellow paramedic. Nor should you discuss your findings with anyone who is not identified as part of the review process. Be professional.

A comprehensive CQI program can help to prevent problems from arising by evaluating day-to-day operations and identifying possible stress points in these operations. These may include:

- Medical direction issues.
- Training.
- Communications.
- Prehospital treatment.
- Transportation issues.
- Financial issues.
- Receiving facility review.
- Dispatch.
- Public information and education.
- Disaster planning.
- Mutual aid.

EMS Research

In the early years of EMS, many standards relating to professionalism, protocols, training, and equipment were developed from "great ideas" or direct experience. The standards for EMS research are now similar to those in any other medical profession. The public of today expects that you, as a paramedic, will do what is medically proven to work in research findings.

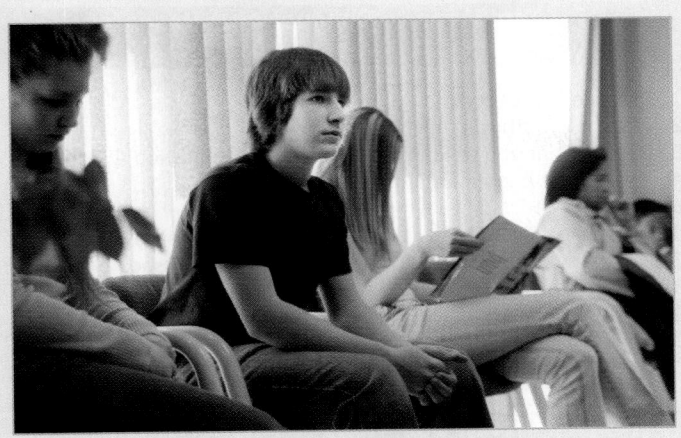

Figure 1-16 Often, medical subjects are paid to participate in research projects. The greater the number of participants, the more reliable the findings.

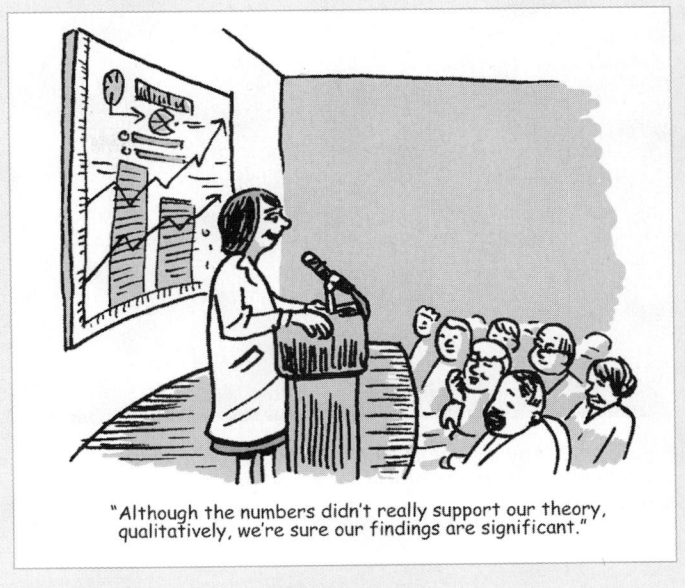

"Although the numbers didn't really support our theory, qualitatively, we're sure our findings are significant."

Figure 1-17

Quality EMS research has many benefits for the future. In all health care fields, research determines the effectiveness of treatment—what works and what doesn't. Because funding for EMS continues to be a problem, it is important that paramedics initiate research and prove that emergency services are necessary.

When you begin your research project, use some form of institutional review board (IRB). In 1966, the US Public Health Service outlined the requirements of reviews that would make them eligible for federal funding. The first part of research is to identify a specific problem or question. Even if the topic of your project has been researched before, this does not mean you can't revisit it. Sometimes research findings can be flawed and your process may identify flaws or enhance previous research findings. The next step is to decide on what style of research you wish to perform, which may include:

- **Descriptive research.** Research that is basically observation only, where no attempt to change or alter an event occurs.
- **Experimental research.** When a skill, new product, or general idea is used in a trial phase, and the effects are evaluated.
- **Prospective research.** Research that defines a clear problem or question prior to gathering data.
- **Retrospective research.** Research that is based on currently available data.
- **Cross-sectional research.** Research that is based on a group of individuals over an outlined time frame.

Your next step is to outline the group or groups of individuals necessary for the research **Figure 1-16 ▲** . Once the group(s) is identified you may wish to refine the group further, such as giving a specific age bracket, medical condition, or gender. As an example, you may wish to study men between the ages of 20 and 30 who have asthma. Once the list of eligible subjects is identified you should randomly choose who will be part of the research. There are many different ways you can achieve this. You may wish to have the computer generate a list

of subjects or groups (systematic sampling) or you can set time frame parameters (alternative time sampling). Finally, the least preferred or accurate would be to assign subjects to a specific person or crew (convenience sampling). Even in the best cases, sampling errors can occur. Not everyone will be included in the study, or there may be individuals in the study who meet criteria but still aren't the best representation.

Parameters should be identified in research. They outline the type of individuals who are appropriate for the study. One other tool to use is "blinding," in which subjects are not told the specifics of the project. There are single-, double-, and triple-blinded studies where one, two, or all parties are blinded, respectively. When participants of the research project are advised of all aspects of the project, it is known as an unblinded study.

As your research continues, data will be acquired. You can achieve statistics either in a descriptive or inferential format. Descriptive statistics can also be performed in either a qualitative or quantitative style. The qualitative method does not use numerical information and is the least accurate **Figure 1-17 ▲** . The quantitative approach adds several other possible variables to the research: mean, median, and mode. For example, the mean age of study participants in a study on asthma in men who are between 20 and 30 years old is the average age of the subjects, the median is the midpoint age of the subjects, and the mode is the most frequent age of the subjects. Finally, standard deviation outlines how much those scores in each set will differ from the mean.

As in many aspects of a profession, there are ethical items to consider. When you decide on a research project you must ensure that the risks will not outweigh the benefits. You must acquire consent from the subject(s) and be certain their rights and welfare are adequately protected **Figure 1-18 ▶** . More information on consent will be covered later in this text.

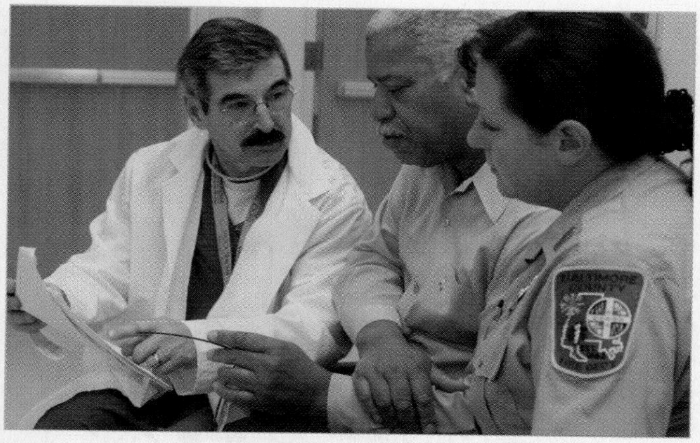

Figure 1-18 Any individual who participates in a research study should be well informed of the goals and parameters of the project.

Table 1-5	Ten Steps to Conducting a Research Project

1. Prepare a question.
2. Write a hypothesis.
3. Decide what you will measure and the best method to use.
4. Outline the population you will use.
5. Identify expected study limitations.
6. Acquire approval of the study by an institutional review board.
7. Obtain needed consent from the population(s) used.
8. Gather data.
9. Analyze your data.
10. Decide what you will do with your final research product.

Table 1-6	Fifteen Questions to Answer When Evaluating and Interpreting Research

1. Was the research peer reviewed?
2. What was the research hypothesis?
3. Was the study approved by an institutional review board and conducted ethically?
4. What was the population being studied?
5. What were the inclusion and exclusion criteria?
6. What method was used to acquire a sample of patients?
7. How many groups were the patients divided into?
8. How were the patients assigned to the groups?
9. What type of data was gathered?
10. Did the study have enough patients involved?
11. Are there any confounding variables unaccounted for?
12. Were the data analyzed correctly?
13. Is your conclusion logically based from the data?
14. Will it apply in local EMS systems?
15. Were the patients similar to those in your local EMS system?

All research projects have the following format:

- **Introduction.** Outlines a brief background of the research, including previous studies, reasons for the study, and a hypothesis of the project.
- **Methods.** Includes a specific description of the project so it can be replicated. This part will outline inclusion and exclusion criteria.
- **Results.** Describes the findings of the project.
- **Discussion.** Details the results of your findings along with the limitations placed on the project and gives ideas you may have that could improve the project next time.
- **Conclusion.** Provides a final summary of information you have outlined in the introduction, methods, results, and discussion sections.

Table 1-5 ▶ lists the steps for conducting a research project. **Table 1-6 ▶** provides 15 questions to answer when evaluating and interpreting research.

You are the Provider Summary

1. How is patient care initiated for this or any call?

Patient care most often comes with a phone call to 9-1-1, or if the 9-1-1 system does not exist in your service area, with a call to the police or fire department. Educational programs provided by local fire and EMS agencies are vital in guiding the public in how to recognize an emergency, how to access emergency services, and how to provide basic first aid, including cardiopulmonary resuscitation (CPR) and automated external defibrillator (AED) use. If your community has not yet asked for outreach programs, you should initiate them.

2. What role do dispatchers play in patient care?

Without dispatchers, appropriate medical, fire, and police resources would not be allocated properly. Dispatchers are highly skilled individuals who are able to calm callers, gather pertinent information regarding the location and nature of the incident, and in some cases provide instruction in basic first aid over the phone. All of these actions are essential in providing care to the sick and injured.

3. What care can EMT-Bs provide for this patient?

EMT-Bs can provide essential life-saving care by administering oxygen, splinting, controlling bleeding, providing CPR, and using AEDs. Some EMT-Bs have expanded scopes of practice that allow a broader range of skills, depending on local protocols or regulations.

4. What are the advantages of having a paramedic partner?

Some systems provide two paramedics on ALS units, while others do not. Having a paramedic partner is especially helpful when you first begin your career. Some days you will notice that finding a vein for an IV line and opening an airway for an endotracheal tube are more difficult, even for the most seasoned provider. Having a partner there to help you is especially advantageous, and your partner can also serve as a sounding board for your ideas and concerns. It is important to note that not all systems run an ambulance with two paramedics; instead, your team may include one paramedic and one other-level provider such as an EMT-B, so you must be prepared to function as the only paramedic.

5. Is there one team member who is more important than another?

No team member is any more important than another. It is very important to treat all team members with respect—they are all essential in providing quality patient care. You, as a paramedic, might be the most highly trained person on the scene, but you must remember your professional demeanor, which includes good manners. Providing quality care is a team effort, and it serves us well to remember that our purpose is to provide the best patient care possible. In the end, if we don't get our act together, only one person pays the true price—the patient we are committed to serve.

6. Why is it important to keep skills and knowledge current?

One of the challenging aspects of being a paramedic is that it is an ever-changing field. Medical research projects track positive and negative impacts of prehospital care. As technology changes and as more information is assessed about using medications and applying patient care techniques, your treatment in the field will continue to change and improve.

7. Why is it important to practice these skills as a team?

Because teamwork is an essential element of emergency medicine, it is extremely important to practice working as a team. As each member knows what is expected to meet patient needs, the more effective and efficient care becomes. An efficient team working together will boost the image of the service in the opinion of the patient, the patient's family members, and the public.

■ Ready for Review

- World Wars I and II saw the development of ambulance corps to rapidly care for and remove those injured from the battlefields.
- During the Korean and Vietnam Wars, wounded soldiers could be saved by using helicopters to rapidly remove them from the battlefields to a medical unit.
- In 1966 the National Academy of Science and the National Research Council released a "White Paper" outlining 10 critical points.
  - From these points the National Highway Safety Act was instituted in 1966.
  - The US Department of Transportation was also created.
- The public needs to be taught how to recognize that an emergency exists, how to activate the EMS system, and how to perform basic care until EMS arrives.
- The highest level of EMS training is the paramedic level. At this level, personnel may perform invasive procedures under the direction of medical control.
- Continuing education programs expose paramedics to new research findings and refresh their skills and knowledge.
- Paramedics are required to be licensed and/or certified.
- The paramedic profession contains expected standards and performance parameters as well as a code of ethics.
- Some of the primary paramedic responsibilities include:
  - Preparation
  - Response
  - Scene management
  - Patient assessment and care
  - Management and disposition
  - Patient transfer
  - Documentation
  - Return to service
- The medical director provides online and off-line medical control.
- Research helps bring together the findings of many professionals involved in EMS and brings forth a consensus of what EMS personnel should or should not do.
- Quality assurance and continuous quality improvement are tools paramedics use to evaluate the care they provide to patients.

■ Vital Vocabulary

alternative time sampling Time parameters that are set during a research project.

blinding The method of not giving the specifics of a project to the individuals participating in a research or study.

certified A title given when a person has shown that he or she has met requirements based on knowledge of certain facts.

convenience sampling A type of research in which subjects are manually assigned to a specific person or crew, rather than being randomly assigned; the least-preferred component of research.

cross-sectional research A type of research in which information is gathered from a group of individuals over a specific time frame.

descriptive research A type of research in which an observation of an event is made, but without attempts to alter or change it.

emergency medical services (EMS) A health care system designed to bring immediate on-scene care to those in need along with transport to a definitive medical care facility.

ethical A behavior expected by an individual or group following a set of rules.

experimental research Describes a new product, skill, or idea that is undergoing research and will be trialed, with the effects evaluated.

health care professional A person who follows specific professional attributes that are outlined in this profession.

inferential A research format that uses a hypothesis to prove one finding from another.

institutional review board (IRB) A group or institution that follows a set of requirements for review that were devised by the US Public Health Service.

licensed Similar to certified, a person who has shown a degree of competency in a specific occupation and is granted ability to function through a governmental body.

mean The average number in a given research project.

median The midpoint number in a given research project.

medical direction Direction given to an EMS service or provider by a physician.

mobile intensive care units (MICUs) An early title given to an ambulance-style unit.

mode The most common number in any given research project.

off-line medical control Medical direction given through a set of protocols, policies, and/or standards.

online medical control Medical direction given in real time to an EMS service or provider.

parameters Outlined measures that may be difficult to obtain in a research project.

profession A specialized set of knowledge, skills, and/or expertise.

professional A person who follows expected standards and performance parameters in a specific profession.

prospective research Specific reason a task or research will be performed before it is started.

protocol A treatment plan developed for a specific illness or injury.

qualitative A type of descriptive statistic in research that does not use numerical information.

quantitative A type of measurement in research that uses a mean, median, and mode.

randomly A way of choosing subjects for a research project without specific reasons.

reciprocity The process of granting licensing or certification to a provider from another state or agency.

registration Giving information that will be stored in some form of record book.

retrospective research Research performed from current available information.

sampling errors Expected errors that occur in the sampling phase of research.

standard deviation In research this outlines how much change from the mean is expected.

standing order A type of protocol that is a written document signed by the EMS system's medical director that outlines specific directions, permissions, and sometimes prohibitions regarding patient care that is rendered prior to contacting medical control.

systematic sampling A computer-generated list of subjects or groups for research.

trauma systems The collaboration of prehospital and in-hospital medicine that focuses on optimizing the use of resources and assets of each with a primary goal of reducing the mortality and morbidity of trauma patients.

unblinded study A type of study in which the subjects are advised of all aspects of the study.

Assessment in Action

You are in training to become a paramedic. You are not yet certified, but you do run rescue with a local rescue squad as an EMT-B.

You come upon a car crash near your home. No rescue personnel or police are on scene yet. You have your own personal "jump bag" with rescue supplies in your vehicle, including advanced life support supplies you would use as a paramedic. There are two patients, both with significant injuries. They were both unrestrained in the vehicle. One patient is having noticeable trouble breathing.

1. **Even though you are not "on duty," what should you do first in this situation, assuming a bystander has already called for help?**
   A. Call 9-1-1.
   B. Put on gloves and any other personal protective equipment you may need.
   C. Call medical control and get permission to treat the patient.
   D. Assess the ABCs.

2. **Which of the following are you *allowed* to do based on the training you already have?**
   A. C-spine stabilization, pressure to stop bleeding, talk to victims to calm them and let them know what to expect.
   B. Put a c-collar in place, bandage bleeding wounds, use a Combitube if necessary to help the patient who is having trouble breathing.
   C. Help stop bleeding, and intubate if necessary.
   D. Call medical control and ask for permission to treat patients as necessary, including intubation.

3. **If a physician arrives and offers to help, is it appropriate to turn over care to that physician?**
   A. Yes, a physician is a higher authority than you are.
   B. Yes, but only if the physician is willing to take responsibility for the patients, including riding with them to the hospital and signing paperwork.
   C. No, you are not authorized to turn over care until an ALS unit arrives.
   D. It is the option of the EMS crew that arrives on scene.

4. **When EMS arrives on scene, it is your responsibility to:**
   A. explain quickly and accurately your assessments and any treatment or intervention you have administered.
   B. help prepare the patient(s) for transport in any way you can under the direction of the paramedic on scene.
   C. maintain patient care unless the person on scene has the same authority as you or higher.
   D. all of the above

5. **Are you legally allowed to perform ANY paramedic treatments in this situation?**
   A. Yes
   B. No

6. **Because you are not on duty, is it appropriate to tell the patient "everything will be fine," or do anything else you would not be allowed to do in uniform while working with your agency?**
   A. Yes, you're not on duty, so those sets of rules do not apply. You are acting as a Good Samaritan.
   B. No, you are a health professional whether on duty or off duty, which means being professional at all times.

Challenging Questions

7. **Being a paramedic is not just a job you work during a shift. You are always a paramedic, being a role model for the public at all times. With the increase in television shows that do not always accurately depict the roles of health care providers, do you feel it is your responsibility to educate the public in every situation possible as to what the EMS field is truly like, correct misconceptions, and give an accurate portrayal of what you are responsible for and capable of as a paramedic?**

8. **You are called to the scene of a two-car crash with serious injuries to the drivers and passengers of both vehicles. You call for additional assistance, but know it will be several minutes until more help arrives. Someone stops, and offers his assistance. He does seem to be knowledgeable in what needs to be done for the victims of the accident. Should you enlist his help in stabilizing your patients? Why or why not?**

▮ Points to Ponder

You and your crew are called to a scene in which a car has hit a power pole. Active power lines are down around the vehicle, and the driver seems to be unconscious.

Is your first priority the injured patient, or the safety of yourself and your crew?

Issues: Scene Safety, Patient Care, Patient Access.

www.Paramedic.EMSzone.com

2 The Well-Being of the Paramedic

Objectives

Cognitive

1-2.1   Discuss the concept of wellness and its benefits. (p 2.3)

1-2.2   Define the components of wellness. (p 2.3)

1-2.3   Describe the role of the paramedic in promoting wellness. (p 2.4)

1-2.4   Discuss the components of wellness associated with proper nutrition. (p 2.4)

1-2.5   List principles of weight control. (p 2.4)

1-2.6   Discuss how cardiovascular endurance, muscle strength, and flexibility contribute to physical fitness. (p 2.5)

1-2.7   Describe the impact of shift work on circadian rhythms. (p 2.5)

1-2.8   Discuss how periodic risk assessments and knowledge of warning signs contribute to cancer and cardiovascular disease prevention. (p 2.6)

1-2.9   Differentiate proper from improper body mechanics for lifting and moving patients in emergency and nonemergency situations. (p 2.6)

1-2.10   Describe the problems that a paramedic might encounter in a hostile situation and the techniques used to manage the situation. (p 2.22)

1-2.11   Given a scenario involving arrival at the scene of a motor vehicle collision, assess the safety of the scene and propose ways to make the scene safer. (p 2.23)

1-2.12   List factors that contribute to safe vehicle operations. (p 2.19)

1-2.13   Describe the considerations that should be given to:
a. Using escorts
b. Adverse environmental conditions
c. Using lights and siren
d. Proceeding through intersections
e. Parking at an emergency scene (p 2.19)

1-2.14   Discuss the concept of "due regard for the safety of all others" while operating an emergency vehicle. (p 2.20)

1-2.15   Describe the equipment available for self-protection when confronted with a variety of adverse situations. (p 2.20)

1-2.16   Describe the benefits and methods of smoking cessation. (p 2.5)

1-2.17   Describe the three phases of the stress response. (p 2.10)

1-2.18   List factors that trigger the stress response. (p 2.9)

1-2.19   Differentiate between normal/healthy and detrimental reactions to anxiety and stress. (p 2.11)

1-2.20   Describe the common physiological and psychological effects of stress. (p 2.10)

1-2.21   Identify causes of stress in EMS. (p 2.13)

1-2.22   Describe behavior that is a manifestation of stress in patients and those close to them and how these relate to paramedic stress. (p 2.11)

1-2.23   Identify and describe the defense mechanisms and management techniques commonly used to deal with stress. (p 2.10)

1-2.24   Describe the components of critical incident stress management (CISM). (p 2.18)

1-2.25   Provide examples of situations in which CISM would likely be beneficial to paramedics. (p 2.18)

1-2.26   Given a scenario involving a stressful situation, formulate a strategy to help cope with the stress. (p 2.18)

1-2.27   Describe the stages of the grieving process (Kubler-Ross). (p 2.15)

1-2.28   Describe the needs of the paramedic when dealing with death and dying. (p 2.16)

1-2.29   Describe the unique challenges for paramedics in dealing with the needs of children and other special populations related to their understanding or experience of death and dying. (p 2.17)

1-2.30   Discuss the importance of universal precautions and body substance isolation practices. (p 2.20)

1-2.31   Describe the steps to take for personal protection from airborne and bloodborne pathogens. (p 2.20)

1-2.32   Given a scenario in which equipment and supplies have been exposed to body substances, plan for the proper cleaning, disinfection, and disposal of the items. (p 2.21)

1-2.33   Explain what is meant by an exposure and describe principles for management. (p 2.22)

Affective

1-2.34   Advocate the benefits of working toward the goal of total personal wellness. (p 2.4)

1-2.35   Serve as a role model for other EMS providers in regard to a total-wellness lifestyle. (p 2.3)

1-2.36   Value the need to assess his/her own lifestyle. (p 2.8)

1-2.37   Challenge him/herself to each wellness concept in his/her role as a paramedic. (p 2.4)

1-2.38   Defend the need to treat each patient as an individual, with respect and dignity. (p 2.9)

1-2.39   Assess his/her own prejudices related to the various aspects of cultural diversity. (p 2.12)

1-2.40   Improve personal physical well-being through achieving and maintaining proper body weight, regular exercise, and proper nutrition. (p 2.14)

1-2.41   Promote and practice stress management techniques. (p 2.10)

1-2.42   Defend the need to respect the emotional needs of dying patients and their families. (p 2.15)

1-2.43   Advocate and practice the use of personal safety precautions in all scene situations. (p 2.20)

1-2.44   Advocate and serve as a role model for other EMS providers relative to body substance isolation practices. (p 2.20)

Psychomotor

1-2.45   Demonstrate safe methods for lifting and moving patients in emergency and non-emergency situations. (p 2.7)

1-2.46   Demonstrate the proper procedures to take for personal protection from disease. (p 2.20)

Introduction

Jake Owens is a veteran paramedic who has been in EMS for more than 25 years. Jake has arthritis in his knees and hips, and his back is chronically stiff and sore. He avoids most kinds of exercise because everything he has tried hurts.

When Jake ran his first EMS call, few people thought about provider wellness. The slogan of the times was "the patient always comes first." Every third day, Jake was assigned to 24-hour shifts that were so busy, few staffers bothered to cook. Jake and most of his colleagues resorted to fast food while they were on duty, often putting off eating until their last late-night run when they were ravenous. They ate large portions and gulped down large soft drinks and great volumes of coffee to get them through their nights.

Ambulance cots typically had to be lifted into and out of ambulances, with or without patients. Two people managed that job by themselves, because there were no first responders. The only way a provider could load or unload one of those cots was by lifting from the side. To avoid straining his or her back, a provider would try to stand very close to the cot, spreading his or her thighs widely and lifting with the hands between the knees, about 18″ apart. The whole procedure put a lot of stress on the lifter's knees and hips.

Between calls, most crews sat and waited—or slept, bracing themselves for repeated wake-up calls. Many smoked more than a pack of cigarettes a day. Providers were generally young (usually in their early 20s) with no plans to stay in medical caregiving. Like most people their age, they gave little thought to the long-term consequences of their on-duty lifestyle. But many of them developed life-altering injuries.

Even an expert in human occupational health care could not have devised a more torturous test of human mind or body. Thirty years ago no research project tracked the injuries or the impact of sleep loss and bad eating and exercise habits on ambulance crews. The research about the impact of stress on all health care providers has blossomed in 30 years, culminating in a better understanding of (and hopefully the prevention of) the damage to the physical and mental health of the dedicated professionals on either side of the emergency department door.

Paramedics need to know how to ensure their own well-being and to share what they have learned with other professionals and the public.

Components of Well-Being

Wellness is a baseline state of adjustment to the rigors of life that makes us happy and pain-free most of the time, often brings us

You are the Provider Part 1

You are the "newbie" of your crew. Your supervisor has paired you with a veteran paramedic, who is knowledgeable but somewhat cranky. You and your partner have had a long day. Just as you sit down to eat dinner, you are dispatched to a nonemergency transport from a local nursing care facility. As you get up from the table, your partner lets out a big sigh and mumbles something under his breath.

When you arrive, you are greeted by one of the care center's registered nurses. She tells you this patient is being transported for evaluation by his physician and, as she begins to tell you about the patient's recent history of illness, your partner says, "That's OK. We've got it. Do you have the guy's chart?" She quickly hands you the patient's medical file, and you enter the room to find a morbidly obese 55-year-old man. You estimate his weight to be about 400 pounds. You take an initial set of vital signs.

As your partner is readying the gurney, you ask him if it would be a good idea to call for additional help. He tells you, "No, let's just get this over with."

Initial Assessment	Recording Time: 0 Minutes
Appearance	Eyes open, no apparent distress
Level of consciousness	A (Alert to person, place, and day)
Airway	Open
Breathing	Adequate rate and tidal volume
Circulation	Radial pulse present
Vital Signs	
Skin	Warm, pink, and dry
Pulse	90 beats/min, regular and strong
Blood pressure	160/94 mm Hg
Respirations	22 breaths/min
Sao_2	94% on 2 L/min nasal cannula

1. What is your main concern at the moment?
2. What concerns do you have, if any, regarding your partner's behavior?
3. Does your partner's attitude have any effect on patient care?

joy, and generally produces interactions with others that are mutually supportive and fulfilling (Figure 2-1 ▾). Wellness has at least three dimensions: the physical, the mental, and the emotional. Many people believe that a fourth dimension, the spiritual, is also essential.

Physical Well-Being

Health care providers have known for years that they are less likely to get hurt if they show up in shape for the work. Your muscle strength, the flexibility of your joints, your cardiac endurance, your emotional equilibrium, your posture (both sitting and standing), your state of hydration, the quality of the foods you eat, and even the amount of sleep you get affect your quality of life. And each of these factors directly impacts the likelihood that you will get through a shift without injury and be able to deal with the mental stress inherent in the job. Let's take a closer look at these factors.

Nutrition

Supervisors and schedule planners understand a lot more about scheduling for good nutrition and hydration today than they did 30 years ago. Even food and drink containers have improved (along with the interiors of vehicles, which now provide space for them). Researchers learned a lot about the consequences of poor nutrition—cardiac illness, type 2 diabetes, obesity, and possibly even Alzheimer's disease. But many EMS providers still work 24-hour shifts,

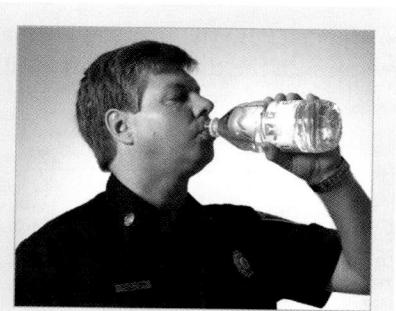

Figure 2-1 Because of the special demands of their job, paramedics must be continually focused on staying both physically and emotionally healthy.

sometimes without scheduled meal breaks. The EMS system is clearly challenged.

Many years ago, nutritional education in schools suggested eating foods from the four main food groups (fruits and vegetables, meats, grains, and dairy products) in carefully prescribed amounts. Research has shown that one size does not fit all, and people must adjust their diets to meet their individual energy needs.

According to the 2005 Dietary Guidelines for Americans, it is important to balance calorie intake with the energy needs of the individual. A sedentary individual will not need the same quantities of food as the person who is physically active. For instance, the new standards say that a man between the ages of 19 and 30 years with a sedentary lifestyle should consume 2,400 calories a day. If he is active, the intake rises to 3,000 calories a day. The US Department of Agriculture (USDA) Food Pyramid also recommends the following minimum servings from each of the following food groups (Figure 2-2 ▾):

- **Fruits.** Four servings a day
- **Vegetables.** Five servings a day
- **Grains.** 6-oz equivalents a day (1-oz equivalents can be one slice of bread, 1 cup of dry cereal, or ½ cup of cooked rice or pasta)
- **Meat and beans.** 5.5-oz equivalents a day (1-oz equivalents can be 1 oz of cooked lean meats, poultry, or fish; ¼ cup of cooked dry beans; 1 tbsp of peanut butter; or ½ oz of nuts or seeds)
- **Dairy.** 3 cups of milk a day
- **Oils.** 6 tsp a day

So, what is the best way for a paramedic to sustain energy? Perhaps the best answer to nutrition is to plan your meals before you report for duty. You can keep yourself better hydrated by carrying bottled water instead of buying soft drinks, and minimizing your intake of caffeine. You can stay better nourished and more alert by carrying numerous small snacks (like raisins, nuts, and fruits) you can eat slowly. Taking these steps will also save you lots of money. This is better than speed-eating big, expensive, high-fat meals.

Weight Control

EMS fieldwork demands active people who can quickly and accurately observe, assess, access, cope with, and control chaotic situations. Staying fit is a necessity in public service. Patterns of living you develop in your youth are hard to modify in later life—and impose lasting effects on your overall health.

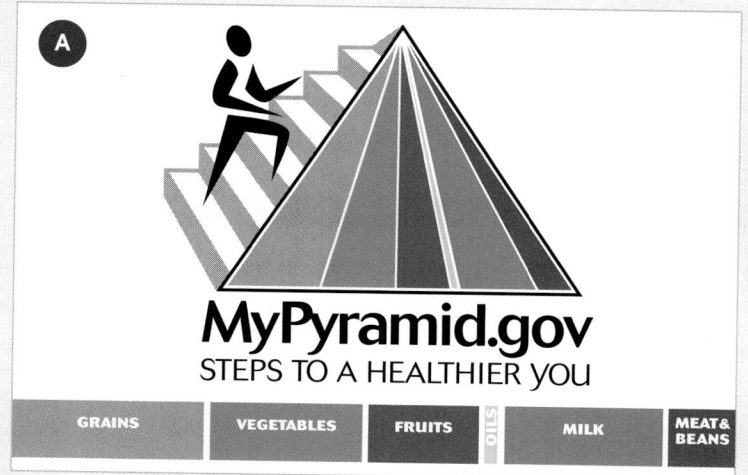

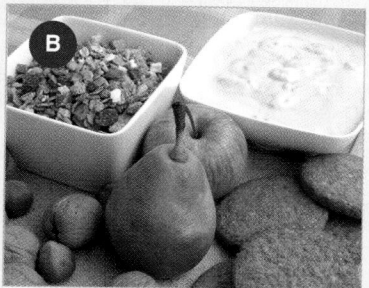

Figure 2-2 The USDA's Food Pyramid (**A**) emphasizes a healthy balance of grains, fruits, vegetables, and dairy products (**B**). Health bars, smoothies, and energy drinks provide a quick, healthy alternative to fast foods.

MyPyramid.gov
STEPS TO A HEALTHIER YOU

| GRAINS | VEGETABLES | FRUITS | OILS | MILK | MEAT & BEANS |

The 2005 Dietary Guidelines encourage lowering calorie intake, increasing physical activity, and making wiser food choices. The Guidelines discourage crash-dieting and instead recommend "eating fewer calories while increasing physical activity [as] the keys to controlling body weight."

However, gradual weight reduction, like an exercise program, requires you to plan your meals and your breaks. Rather than taking coffee breaks, some paramedics take breaks by walking or doing other forms of aerobic activity. These EMS providers often split a meal between two people when they eat in a restaurant, and they are hearty eaters of salad, vegetables, and fresh-caught broiled fish. You too can do this, with some planning. If you have to eat out, you could order oatmeal or cold cereal for breakfast, a salad (with dressing on the side) and soup for lunch, and roast turkey for dinner.

Exercise

Regular vigorous exercise is closely linked to your body weight, nutritional status, and hydration, and has been shown to improve your sleep, sex life, mental capacity, ability to cope with stress, and overall long-term health. The best exercise program for you depends on your personal preferences. It should be something you enjoy and should be targeted at maintaining, or improving, three areas: your cardiovascular endurance, your flexibility, and your physical strength. More specifically, it should involve enough moderate to vigorous daily physical activity to keep you from gaining weight.

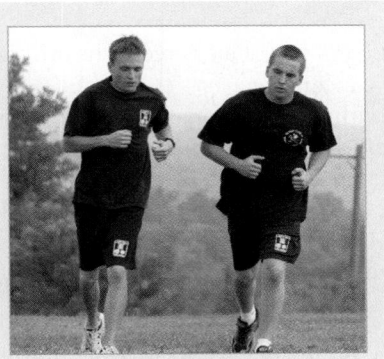

Figure 2-3 Regular exercise—apart from the work you do on calls—should be part of your daily or weekly routine.

It is recommended that adults engage in at least 30 minutes of moderate to vigorous physical activity most days of the week to help build optimal cardiovascular endurance. Working in a busy unit, you probably feel that you get that workout on every run. Back at the station, it is very tempting to prop your feet up and vegetate until the next call. But to stay in good physical condition, you need to find a healthy balance between full-out physical activity (when you are "running hot") and no activity at all Figure 2-3 ▲ . Most employers realize this and provide their employees with workout equipment to use on each shift.

You should know your target heart rate and attempt to reach this goal every time you exercise. To find your target heart rate, calculate the following:

1. Measure your resting heart rate.
2. Subtract your age from 220. This total is your estimated maximum heart rate.

3. Subtract your resting heart rate from your maximum heart rate. Multiply that figure by 0.7.
4. Add this figure to your resting heart rate.

For example, a 40-year-old man has a resting heart rate of 70 beats/min. Calculations would be as follows:

1. **Resting heart rate.**
   70 beats/min
2. **Maximum heart rate.**
   $220 - 40 = 180$ beats/min
3. **Maximum heart rate minus resting heart rate multiplied by 0.7.**
   $180 - 70 = 110 \times 0.7 = 77$
4. **Target heart rate.**
   $77 + 70 = 147$ beats/min

In the Field

Being a paramedic in the field is physically and mentally demanding. Following simple guidelines for nutrition, exercise, and mental health will greatly enhance and prolong your career. Recruiting others you work with to join a health maintenance plan that includes these elements will foster teamwork as well as help maintain a balance between your career and your health.

Smoking

If you don't already, *please* don't start! If you do, *please* stop! Not only does this habit fly in the face of everything EMS is about, it also produces many of the most terrible cardiovascular and pulmonary disasters that caregivers in our field confront during the span of our careers. In addition, it sets an awful example for the public—especially to people who have breathing disorders such as asthma. And it makes us look and smell (*Yes, smell!*) like anything but professional caregivers.

Are you a smoker who is trying to quit? Several strategies can help you. First, try to cultivate a relationship with a mentor who was once truly addicted to smoking but who has successfully quit. Use that person as a support,

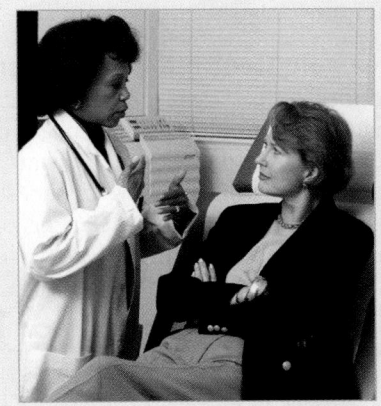

Figure 2-4 Both traditional and alternative health care providers offer a variety of ways to help smokers deal with nicotine addiction.

and draw on his or her advice and encouragement. There are also programs that attack a smoker's psychological dependency. These programs may include instructions and audiotapes, and provide ongoing support. Other options include psychotherapy, hypnotism, and acupuncture.

Talk to your primary care physician. Your doctor should be familiar with more techniques (Figure 2-4 ◄). All of these solutions are cheaper than cigarettes and their attendant health risks.

Circadian Rhythms and Shift Work

EMS imposes schedules on paramedics that conflict with the body's circadian rhythms, or natural timing system. These rhythms are controlled by special areas of the brain, called the suprachiasmatic nuclei, which govern our "internal clocks." Ignoring our circadian rhythms can cause some of us to experience consistent difficulty with sleep, higher thought functions, physical coordination, and even with social functions. You can have trouble focusing during some times of the day or night (so that you simply cannot function as a paramedic) if you don't know what your natural rhythms are, try hard to understand them, and determine a schedule that is best for you. Research on circadian rhythms is only beginning to appear in medical journals, suggesting that some day we might be able to alter our internal clock.

Some tips for dealing with shift work:
- Avoid caffeine.
- Eat healthy meals and try to eat at the same times every day.
- Keep a regular sleep schedule.

The most important point for all paramedics is: don't overlook the need for rest, whatever your rhythms (Figure 2-5 ►). Many EMS providers depend on overtime as part of their normal income. But a paramedic who has been awake and working for 18 to 20 hours straight is only human, and needs rest. In some states, even interns and residents on 13-hour shifts have had mandated changes in their schedules. You cannot continue to operate an emergency vehicle or administer medications without necessary sleep.

Periodic Health Risk Assessments

Besides sleep, diet, exercise, hydration, and all the other things that make up a healthy lifestyle, you need to be aware of your hereditary factors. Consider what you might know about your immediate family's and your ancestors' health. Alzheimer's disease, chemical addiction, cancer, cardiac illness, hypertension, migraine, mental illness, and stroke all feature prominent

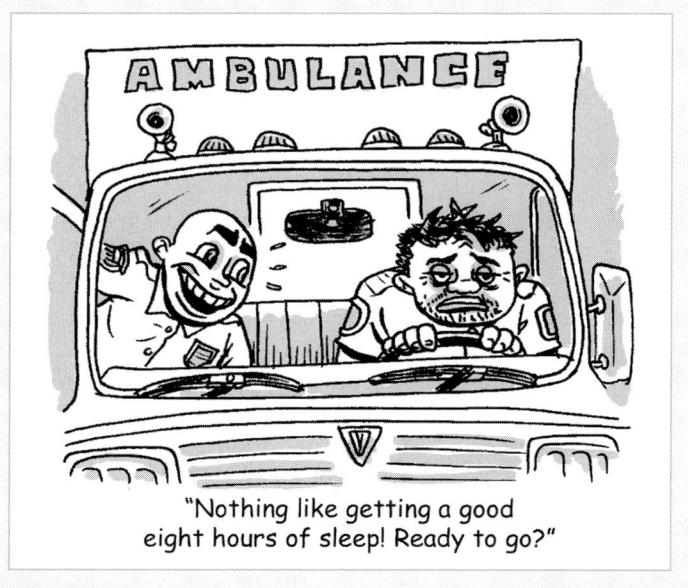

"Nothing like getting a good eight hours of sleep! Ready to go?"

Figure 2-5

hereditary factors. The most common of all heredity health risk factors are heart disease and cancer.

Share this information with your personal physician. Your physician is bound by the same oath of confidentiality that you are. Work with him or her to set up a schedule for health assessments, building them into your routine physical check-ups. Your physician should be your ally in screening for these diseases and in assessing your lifestyle as well as your heredity.

Body Mechanics

A professional weight lifter typically performs a 30-minute warm-up routine before he or she lifts his or her personal maximum weight. Obviously, that's not an option in any emergency service. But there are a number of habits you can develop that are sure to reduce your exposure to damage from lifting your maximum weight. They include the following:
- *Minimize the number of total body-lifts you have to perform.* When patients need to be lifted, they need to be lifted. But remember that you risk an injury every time you do it. A patient with an arm laceration can stand for a moment while someone rolls the cot behind him or her and then helps the patient sit down. Another thing: you can cut your total number of lifts from ground level by

You are the Provider Part 2

As you pull the patient across to the cot, you feel a slight twinge in your lower back. You hope it's nothing, and prepare to lift your end of the gurney. As you lift, although you are using proper lifting techniques, you feel a sharp pain in the area of your lumbar spine. You are fairly certain you've just hurt yourself. You tell your partner, who replies, "OK. Well, let's just get this guy to his appointment, and then we'll call the shift captain." Reservedly, you agree, but you must still load the patient in the ambulance.

4. Is this the best course of action?
5. What is the best way to handle this situation?
6. What factors could affect your decisions?

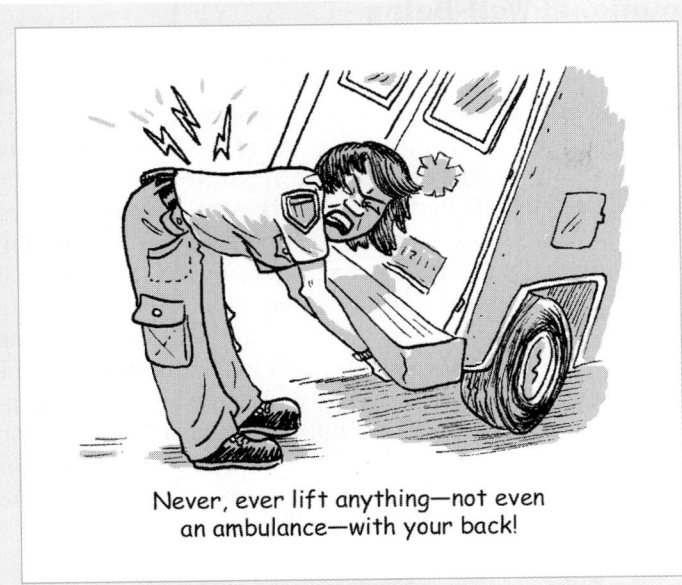

Never, ever lift anything—not even an ambulance—with your back!

Figure 2-6

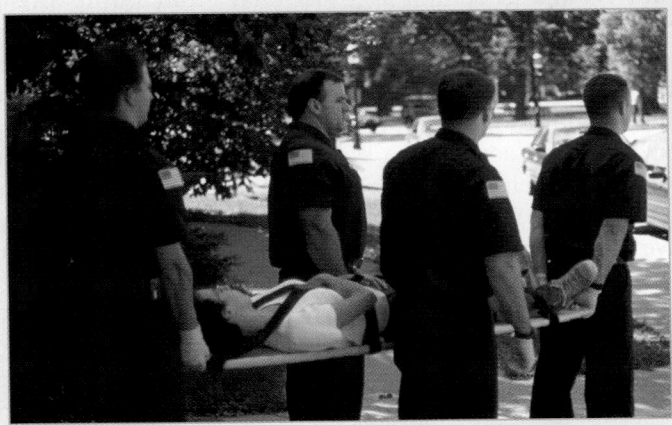

Figure 2-7 Never hesitate to ask for help from your coworkers, or to provide it when you are asked.

having the ambulance cot ready in a hands-height position—never fully lowered. That way, you bend down only once—to lift the patient on a backboard or accessory stretcher (scoop/basket). Then, stand where you are and ask a bystander to roll the cot underneath the backboard or accessory stretcher. (Don't forget, anytime you walk, you are balancing on only one foot at a time.)

- *Coordinate every lift in advance.* Make sure that every member of the team knows what you expect him or her to do. Just as important, make sure the patient knows it as well. The last thing you want is for him or her to panic in midlift and grab someone around the neck, throwing everyone off balance.
- *Minimize the total amount of weight you have to lift.* If you have access to a second person who can help lift and load at the foot end of the cot, why not ask for his or her help? Additionally, consider taking unnecessary equipment off the cot prior to loading or unloading it.
- *Never lift with your back,* not ever. Anyone who has spent a few years in EMS has made this mistake at least a few times, citing the pressure of the moment. That pressure can be a career-ender, unless you're lucky. You cannot trust luck. The human back is a great weight bearer, but it's a terrible lifter. To protect your back, follow these precautions Figure 2-6 ▲ :
  - Always keep your back in a straight, upright position and lift without twisting.
  - When lifting, spread your legs about shoulder-width apart and place your feet so that your center of gravity is properly balanced.
  - Hold your back upright as you bring your upper body down by bending your legs.

- Lift by raising your upper body and arms and by straightening your legs until you are standing.
  - Always lift with your legs, not with your back!
- *Don't carry what you can put on wheels.* Get the ambulance, and the cot, as close to the patient as you can. Use a stair chair if you have to. (Tip: If you have access to a wheelchair, and the stairs are not too narrow, remember that a wheelchair makes a better stair chair than a stair chair!)
- *Ask for help any time,* without embarrassment or hesitation—and offer it liberally to others. Anytime you need to move a patient who cannot or should not walk, consider the possibility of asking an extra person to help you Figure 2-7 ▲ . That's not laziness. It's good sense, and it almost always enhances your body mechanics.

Mental Well-Being

EMS can be a challenging and demanding profession because paramedics are no less vulnerable to diseases and injuries than their patients. Paramedics, like the loved ones of their patients, can be frazzled by the stress of addressing the immediate and inflexible needs of others.

Mild stress can be a good thing, because it can enhance your mental acuity. But overwhelming stress can push us into fight-or-flight syndrome, a physiologic response to a profound stressor, featuring increased sympathetic tone and resulting in dilation of the pupils, increased heart rate, dilation of the bronchi, mobilization of glucose, shunting of blood away from the gastrointestinal tract, and increasing blood flow to the cerebrum and skeletal muscles. It helps you deal with the situation right now, but can lead to crushing physical and mental strain if you do not learn appropriate coping skills.

Let's say you need to get away from a marauding grizzly bear. Your body quickly modifies its performance to enable you to run from the bear. It borrows blood from your gastrointestinal tract and cerebrum, and shunts the blood to your skeletal muscles, your adrenal glands, your lungs, and your reptilian brain (your cerebellum and medulla). Your pupils dilate, enhancing your night vision. You become a running machine—at least for a short time. But you do that at the expense of your higher mental faculties. Your speech becomes clumsy. With those big pupils, you forfeit your depth perception and visual acuity. Your skeletal muscles perform well but, for the time being, you don't feel most kinds of pain such as muscle strain. You lose your fine motor control, so you might have trouble performing motions that require manual dexterity, for example loading a gun or threading a bow and arrow as defense against the bear! You might experience a case of the jitters. And all of that would occur in less than 20 seconds. Your body is preparing you for trouble. You need coping strategies for behavior that would be most effective in dealing with the situation.

A paramedic needs to be a great observer and a sharp thinker with a two-fisted grip on his or her emotions. Is there a way to control your reactions? It can be difficult, because some events are simply overwhelming. But there are some immediate and long-term techniques that you can use. Remember, the most important thing you can do in modeling your behavior is to plan for it. Try any or all of these techniques long before you feel yourself melting down in the field.

You can look and act the part of a professional; take pride in what you do. Caring for people is an ancient pursuit, perhaps the oldest in history. Remind yourself that the world is full of caregivers who do what they do without support, rewards, or recognition from anyone—much less payment. Accept that you are a caregiver with a trust from the public you serve. Because the public elects the officials who certify you, you are responsible to that public in the same way as any other health care professional.

And remember, EMS is a lot bigger than your job, but your life is much bigger than EMS. Keep your lifelong perspective as broad as possible by cultivating relationships with people who are not part of EMS.

Emotional Well-Being

Any professional caregiver needs to have a natural interest in and liking for people. The key to remaining happy in the lifelong practice of critical care medicine is making a deliberate effort to create a healthy balance between life at work and life away. Although many practitioners become very involved in EMS and very dedicated to it, EMS should never be a caregiver's whole life.

EMS does satisfy some of its practitioners' deeply felt needs—especially the need for self-esteem. But, as a popular saying goes, "Don't love something that can't love you back." In fact, many EMS practitioners will say that the more energy you pour into EMS, the more energy it will require to deal with the stress of its importance to you. Why? Because, as another popular saying goes, "Nobody gets out of here alive." Patients can die, regardless of how good their paramedics, nurses, or trauma surgeons are. And you need to recognize that patient death is not your fault, unless you allow your skills, education, or professionalism to decay.

One practical way caregivers manage their balance is by allowing the misfortunes of patients and their families to remind them, year after year, how fortunate they are. Another technique is to faithfully keep a scrapbook. Every thank-you note from a patient or family member goes into that scrapbook and later serves as a reminder that most people appreciate what their field providers do for them.

Develop and nourish your realization that the same situational awareness that you develop in yourself shift after shift as an EMS provider can help you to see and appreciate many kinds of beauty in the world around you.

Good health care providers are sensitive people **Figure 2-8 ▶**. They have to be. But part of the price of that trait is that they tend to get their feelings hurt, maybe a little more easily than the average person. They can also be needy, fussy, emotional, and demanding of their leaders. Those are all traits to watch for in colleagues who need to be reminded from time to

You are the Provider Part 3

Because you are on probation, you are afraid to contradict your partner. You assist him in loading the patient into the ambulance, and you are now in great pain. It is all you can do to focus on caring for your patient. He is stable and in a position of comfort. You wish the same statement held true for you. After reading his medical chart, you notify the receiving facility of the incoming patient, pertinent information, and estimated time of your arrival.

Vital Signs	Recording Time: 15 Minutes
Skin	Warm, pink, and dry
Pulse	90 beats/min, regular and strong
Blood pressure	162/94 mm Hg
Respirations	22 breaths/min
Sao$_2$	95% on 2 L/min nasal cannula

7. What decisions could you have made to prevent this situation?
8. Has patient care been affected?

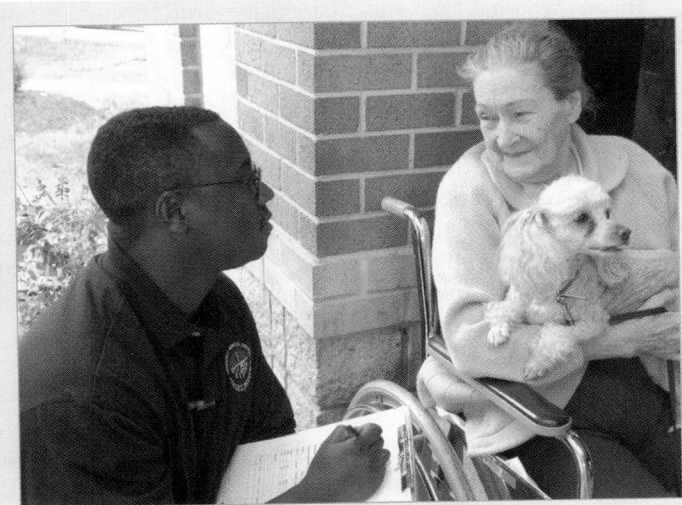

Figure 2-8 One thing that draws people to work as a paramedic is the pleasure of interacting closely with people.

time that they're valuable and that what they do matters. You need to remember that too. You should also speak up when you notice that colleagues are not taking care of themselves. You may feel uncomfortable about broaching the subject, but letting them know that you are worried about them can make a difference.

Spiritual Well-Being

Human spirituality is an unseen dimension of human experience. Some people address it with formal religion, but those who do not may still recognize the existence of supernatural power and even of one or more divine entities. Few experienced emergency medical workers deny the possibility of a plane of life beyond our understanding. This possibility may have been reinforced from witnessing the effectiveness of the portable defibrillator, which seems to interrupt the death process, giving EMS providers credible and consistent stories from patients.

Medical care supports the dignity and value of life, and the sacredness of individuals. It is essential for you to respect the beliefs of others—those you work with, and patients and their families—to whom those beliefs can be all-important. Your respect for patients' beliefs will also help you in managing effective patient care. Many EMS providers describe a rich sense of their own spirituality that keeps their lives in good perspective.

▌Stress

All of us have experienced the effects of stress at one time or another. In fact, virtually every human activity involves some degree of stress—sometimes pleasant, sometimes unpleasant, sometimes mild, sometimes intense. And virtually all living creatures are equipped with some sort of inborn stress reaction that enables them to deal effectively with their environment. Hans Selye, MD, PhD, considered the "father of stress theory,"

has defined biologic stress as the "nonspecific response of the body to any demand made upon it."

So, stress is a reaction of the body to any agent or situation (stressor) that requires the individual to adapt. Adaptation of one sort or another is necessary all the time, for growth, for development, or just for meeting the demands of everyday life. By itself, then, stress is neither a good thing nor a bad thing, nor should all stress be avoided. After all, self-preservation, one of the most basic requirements of life,

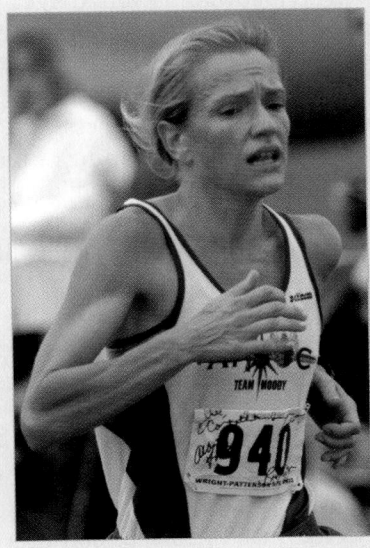

Figure 2-9 Some types of stress, called eustress, are positive and help push us to greater achievements.

would be impossible without a stress-alarm mechanism. Think about that grizzly we talked about earlier. That mechanism also serves you in other ways, for example, motivating you to study for examinations!

It is important to distinguish between injurious and noninjurious stress responses. Selye, for that reason, has classified stress into two categories: eustress (positive stress), the kind of stress that motivates an individual to achieve; and distress (negative or injurious stress), the stress that a person finds overwhelming and debilitating (**Figure 2-9 ▲**). In the rest of this chapter, when we speak about stress, we shall in fact be talking about distress, the negative kind of stress.

Documentation and Communication

People from certain cultures and some older patients may believe that showing emotion is a sign of weakness. They may not show the emotions you may readily see in other people in the same situations. Do not assume because they don't indicate stress in the usual ways that they are not distressed. Try to read their body language and hear what they are saying. Also make sure they understand you.

What Triggers Stress

The stress response often begins with events that are perceived as threatening or demanding, but the specific events that trigger the reaction vary enormously from individual to individual. One person may go into a cold sweat even at the *thought* of air travel, while another de-stresses among the clouds piloting an airplane. Learned attitudes strongly affect the situations people find stressful.

The following factors trigger stress in the vast majority of people:

- Loss of a loved one (death of a spouse or family member or going through a divorce) or of a valued possession
- Personal injury or illness
- Major life event (starting or finishing school, marriage, pregnancy, or having children leave home)
- Job-related stress (conflicts with others, excessive responsibility, the possibility of losing your job, or changing a job)

To deal effectively with stress, each of us needs to make a personal appraisal of the stress triggers in his or her life and take action to minimize their effects.

The Physiology of Acute Stress

One of the fundamental models for stress evolved from studies of how humans and other animals responded to threats. It was observed that when a person or a laboratory animal was confronted with a situation that he or she perceived as threatening, a standard series of physiologic reactions was triggered, whatever the threat (this is why Selye referred to stress as a nonspecific response).

Typically, these physiologic reactions prepare the animal for fight-or-flight syndrome by activating the sympathetic nervous system. We will discuss the sympathetic nervous system in Chapter 22. The sympathetic nervous system is the part of the autonomic, or involuntary, nervous system that prepares the body to deal with an emergency.

Generally, the first stage of the stress response is an alarm reaction, which occurs within a fraction of a second after being confronted with a strong stimulus—for instance, a sudden loud noise. The alarm reaction begins with a quick alert response, in which you immediately stop whatever you are doing and focus on the source of the stimulus **Figure 2-10**.

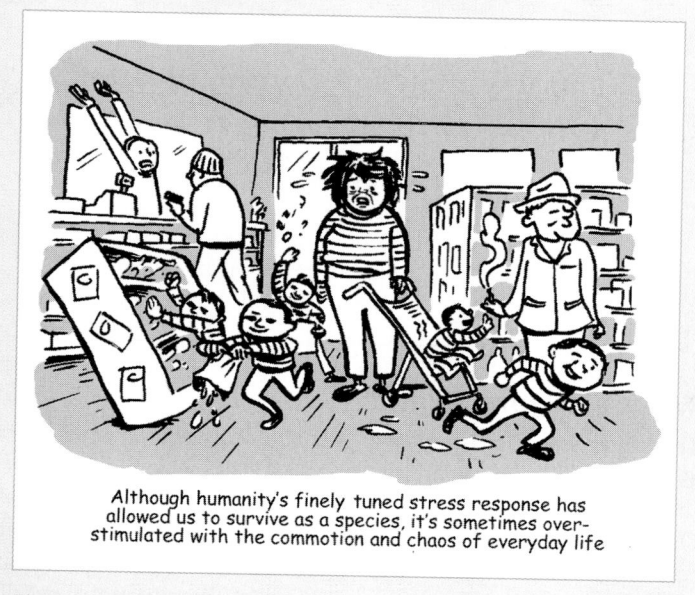

Although humanity's finely tuned stress response has allowed us to survive as a species, it's sometimes over-stimulated with the commotion and chaos of everyday life

Figure 2-10

Anyone who has ever startled a grazing deer remembers how the deer exhibited an alert response: it stopped grazing, looked toward the sound that had startled it, and stood absolutely still. Along with the alert response, there is sudden stimulation of the sympathetic nervous system, producing constricted blood vessels, increased heart rate, dilated pupils, erect hair follicles, increased perspiration, and a variety of other physiologic effects. Indeed, we often describe our reactions to a stressful experience in terms of the sympathetic nervous system: "My heart was pounding in my chest." "I broke out in a cold sweat." These are all part of the body's fight-or-flight response to a perceived threat.

For most animals, the fight-or-flight response is a very useful and adaptive mechanism, mobilizing them either to defend themselves (fight) or to run away (flight) in the face of possible danger. Taking either of these steps dissipates the stress, and the animal then goes through a stage of relaxation ("I breathed a sigh of relief when it was over.") and finally returns to its original internal balance. In the modern world, however, the automatic fight-or-flight response to stressful circumstances is probably not as useful as it was in an earlier stage of evolution. Most of the stressors that humans face today are not best solved by fighting or running away.

When a loved one dies or when you lose a job, there is no fight-or-flight outlet for the stress. Under such circumstances, stress becomes chronic, placing our bodies in a continuous, unrelieved state of alert, possibly leading eventually to exhaustion and ill health.

It's important to point out that the stress response is normal. Many people misunderstand the normal physiologic reactions to stressors and interpret the body's preparations for fight or flight as signs of disease, which only serves to increase the level of anxiety. It's essential for paramedics to learn to recognize the symptoms of the stress response, because chronic stress can exact a high toll when it goes unrecognized and unrelieved.

Coping With Your Own Stress

Some early warning signs of your own stress include heart palpitations, rapid breathing, chest tightness, and sweating. Learn to feel yourself entering your fight-or-flight mode. You may notice rapid breathing and breathlessness, unnecessary shouting, and use of curse words that you would not normally use. You may also feel yourself perspiring despite the weather. It is important to the care of your patients that you try keeping calm to help control the fight-or-flight mechanism in emergencies. Take appropriate action. Initial management techniques include the following steps:

1. **Controlled breathing.** On emergency calls, controlled breathing or taking deep breaths in through the nose and out through the mouth may be the least obvious way to control your anxiety.
2. **Reframing.** Reframing is using your head to look at the situation from a different viewpoint. Instead of thinking "I can't do this," reframe your thoughts to "I trust my training, I can do this."

3. **Progressive relaxation.** After the call, you may find yourself still stressed. Progressive relaxation is a strategy in which you tighten and then relax specific muscle groups to initiate muscle relaxation throughout the body.

Other coping strategies include focusing on the immediate situation while on duty. Off duty, remind yourself (even aloud, although not within the hearing of a patient or his or her loved ones), "I will do my very best, but what I can do to help may not be enough" Figure 2-11 ▼ .

Coffee is not your friend in avoiding stress reactions. Avoid excessive amounts of stimulants such as caffeine. Faithfully get enough rest, and avoid alcohol during the 24 hours before a duty day. Exercise vigorously and regularly, especially during the 12 hours preceding a shift. Find plenty of things to laugh and joke about, and find compatible partners at work.

A sense of skepticism is valuable to a paramedic, but don't let yourself become cynical and judgmental. Don't spend too long in environments where people don't care about EMS, and avoid prolonged or frequent assignments with cynical people. Study routinely, and keep your certifications and Continuing Education Units up-to-date. The social element of continuing education is invaluable in managing stress.

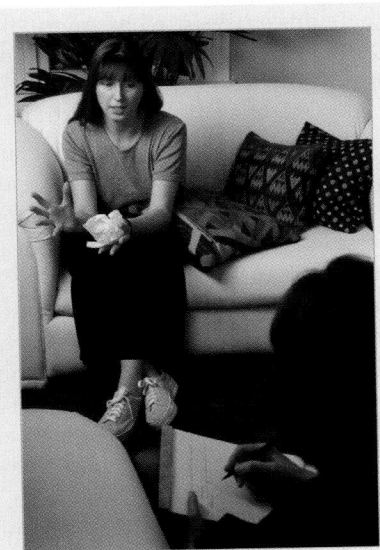

Figure 2-11 Consulting with a professional counselor or therapist can be an important part of dealing with stress and maintaining your emotional well-being.

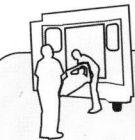

In the Field

Learn to look for signs of stress in your coworkers and patients. Early discovery can often prevent the situation from worsening.

How People React to Stressful Situations

Anyone—the patient, the family, bystanders, or health care professionals—who confronts critical illness or injury responds in some way to the stresses of each emergency.

Responses of Patients to Illness and Injury

Patients' responses to emergencies are determined by their personal methods of adapting to stress. It will help you as a paramedic to recognize certain common patterns of coping. If the emergency is a medical illness, most people first become aware

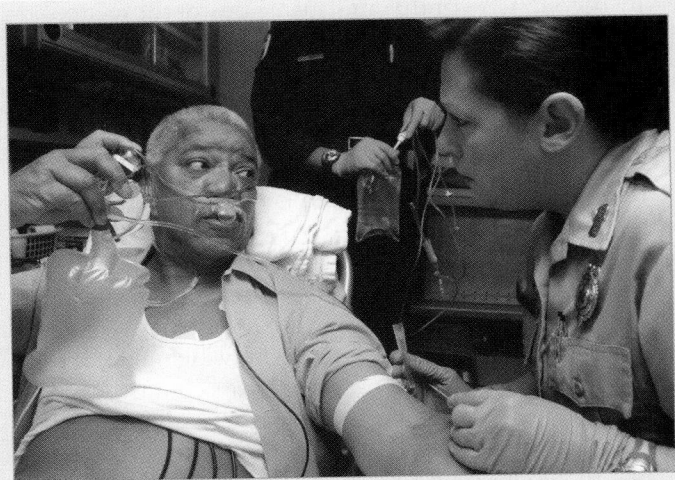

Figure 2-12 The sudden loss of control a patient feels when being treated during an emergency can lead to surprising and sometimes extreme reactions.

of some painful or unpleasant sensations and perhaps a decrease in energy and strength as well. The common response to that awareness is anxiety. Some people exhibit their anxiety by denying it; others become irritable or angry. Once the patient accepts that he or she is ill or injured, any of several common reactions may occur:

- **Fear.** Patients in these situations have realistic fears, such as fear of pain, disability, or death (or fear of their economic effects).
- **Anxiety.** Patients can also experience diffuse anxiety, often stemming from a feeling of helplessness. People who find themselves transformed into patients experience a loss of control. They must place themselves in the hands of a stranger who they must depend on completely and whose competence they cannot really evaluate. People whose self-esteem depends on being active, independent, and aggressive are particularly vulnerable to anxiety when they become ill or injured.
- **Depression.** Depression is a natural response to loss. The patient with a critical illness or injury has lost some bodily function as well as some control. The patient who has had a stroke, for example, may have lost the ability to move an arm or leg on one side of the body and even the ability to speak. It is only natural to feel depressed under such circumstances.
- **Anger.** Anger is one of the most difficult problems for many caregivers to deal with. Suppose a paramedic arrives at the scene of a collision and starts tending immediately to the patient, but the patient becomes hostile and abusive Figure 2-12 ▲ . The paramedic's natural tendency, under the circumstances, is to think, "Here I am trying to save this guy's life, and he's dumping all over me. Well, he can just go straight to blazes." It is crucial, therefore, to understand that often people respond to discomfort or limitation of function

by becoming resentful and suspicious of those around them. A patient who feels angry may vent anger on the rescuer by becoming impatient and irritable or excessively demanding, simply because the rescuer is the most convenient target. A *professional* caregiver realizes in these circumstances that the patient's anger stems from fear and discomfort, and is not really directed at the rescue team.

- **Confusion.** Confusion is especially common among older patients, in whom illness or injury may precipitate disorientation. Such confusion is furthered by the presence of unfamiliar people and equipment, which may seem overwhelming. When a patient appears confused, therefore, it is very important to explain carefully at the outset who you are and what your mission is; thereafter, you should keep up a running commentary on what you are doing to help orient the patient to your role.

In addition to experiencing the reactions just described, most people who have a sudden illness or injury will mobilize one or more psychologic <u>defense mechanisms</u>. Patients and EMS providers usually employ these defense mechanisms automatically and subconsciously as a way of relieving personal stress. Here are some examples:

- **Denial.** Many patients tend to ignore or diminish the seriousness of their medical emergencies, because of the anxiety they cause. Denial is often evident in a tendency to dismiss all symptoms with words such as *only* or *a little* (for example, the middle-aged man with chest pain who says, "I'm fine, I'm fine. It's only a little indigestion."). When a patient tries to minimize his or her symptoms in that way, it may be necessary to find a reliable informant among the patient's family or friends so you can obtain more details.
- **Regression.** Regression is a return to an earlier age level of behavior or emotional adjustment. Regression is often evident in children under stress; for instance, a 10-year-old who sailed through his toilet-training years earlier may suddenly start wetting the bed at night after a stressful experience. Adults too can revert to more childish behaviors under stress. Indeed, when people are injured or become ill, their roles as patients *force* them into a state of dependency, very much like children.
- **Projection.** Projection is attributing your own (sometimes unacceptable) feelings, motives, desires, or behavior to others. Patients who express vehement indignation or anger at the behavior of others can unconsciously be denying their own "bad" behavior by attributing it to other people.
- **Displacement.** Displacement occurs when someone redirects an emotion from the original cause of the emotion (like a cardiac problem) to a more immediate substitute (like a paramedic). Displacement is often the operative mechanism when patients express anger at the paramedic. In reality, patients are angry at someone else— themselves, a family member, fate, God—but they unconsciously redirect their anger toward the stranger who comes to provide medical care. A professional caregiver recognizes that, and accepts it without complaint.

As noted, most of the psychological stress responses are not under your patients' conscious control. Injured patients who respond with anger toward the paramedic often have no perspective on their unpleasant behavior. The reaction is automatic for the stressed patient.

Just as patients have their own ways of reacting to stress, you have subconscious expectations of how the patient *should* behave when stressed. You might expect a child to cry or to reach out to someone for comfort. But do you allow or tolerate that same reaction in adults?

Often, reactions to illness or injury are rooted in the patient's culture. We live in a multicultural society. Some cultures may openly exhibit their anxieties in what might be termed inappropriate behavior in another culture. You will not be able to manage patient care well if you do not respect the culture of your patient.

For example, many patients may react to a situation in what you may think of as quite an emotional way. They may take comfort in having many family members around them for support. This can be quite overwhelming if you come from a cultural background where people are often rather stoic.

Many Americans place great emphasis on making eye contact, having a firm handshake, and respecting personal space. Some patients may not make eye contact with you because, in their culture, lowered eyes show deference to your authority and uniform. Many people are not comfortable with physical contact (even with their own health care provider) until they have developed a rapport. Obtain permission, if possible, before any hands-on encounters. It is difficult to learn about another culture in an emergency situation, but we need to recognize cultural differences. Learn the cultural differences of the populations you serve, realizing that the reactions you see are only different, not wrong or abnormal **Figure 2-13 ▾** .

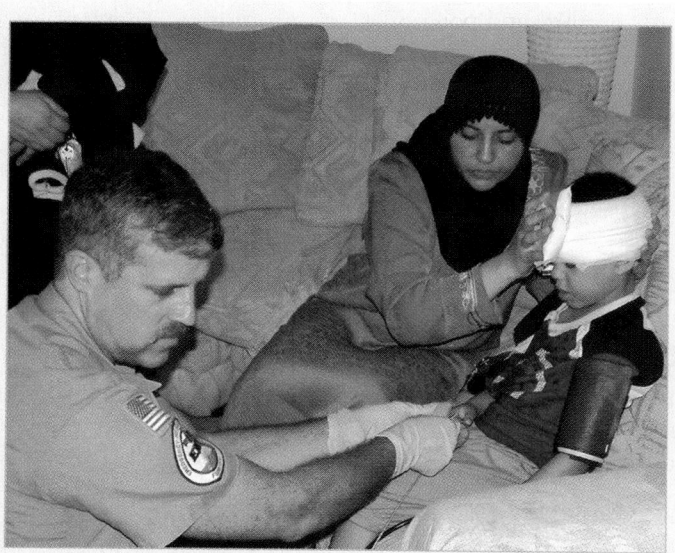

Figure 2-13 Particularly when serving people whose backgrounds are different from your own, you must always maintain an open, nonjudgmental attitude.

Responses of Family, Friends, and Bystanders

Bystanders and family members can exhibit many of the responses that patients exhibit. Family members can be anxious, panicky, or—especially if they are struggling with guilt—angry. Suppose you are called to care for a 4-year-old child who has been struck by a car. The parents of the child are at the scene. Consciously or unconsciously, they feel guilty for what has happened; they may believe, deep down, that if they had kept a closer eye on the child, he or she would not have run out into the street. But, using the mechanisms of projection and displacement, the parents express their guilty feelings as aggression and/or anger toward the rescuers.

They may demand instant action or put pressure on you to move immediately to the hospital. Especially galling may be their implications that you are not competent to handle the situation ("Hurry up and get her to the hospital so that she can be seen by a *doctor!*"). The paramedic needs to recognize that the patient's family and friends

Notes from Nancy

Remember, in emergency situations, everyone is under stress.

have concerns too and that their behavior, however irritating, arises from distress. Step back emotionally from the situation for a moment. Keep your cool. Reassure the patient's family or friends that there is radio contact with the physician at all times and that you are working under the physician's guidance in the best interests of the patient. Whether dealing with the behavior of the patient or of those around him or her, the paramedic must constantly remain aware of the distress that lies behind the behavior. When you are summoned to an emergency, it will never be a festive party. You are entering a situation in which *everyone is under stress,* and you cannot guarantee that people are going to behave appropriately. People who are ordinarily calm and polite in everyday life may not be calm and polite in an emergency. But if *you* can stay calm and polite, no matter what is going on around you, you can improve the behavior of everyone else at the scene, including your own.

Special Considerations

When children are seriously ill or injured, family members and other people at the scene may become frantic. You need to remain calm and confident in your skills, as this may be all that is needed to provide reassurance to everyone at the scene. Remind yourself (and, if you can, the anxious people around you) that scientific studies indicate that paramedic care and stabilization will improve the patient's chances of a positive outcome.

Responses in Multiple-Casualty Incidents

In a situation involving multiple casualties, such as a train derailment, building collapse, or natural disaster (such as a tornado, flood, or earthquake), both victims and bystanders may react by becoming dazed, disorganized, or overwhelmed. The American Psychiatric Association has identified five categories of reactions in such circumstances. In general, people with these reactions should be removed from the scene.

- **Anxiety.** The normal reactions to such incidents are signs of extreme anxiety, including sweating, trembling, weakness, nausea, and sometimes vomiting. People experiencing this response can recover fully within a few minutes and provide useful assistance if properly directed. EMS personnel are not immune to this type of reaction. If you see one of your crew looking a little shaky, the best remedy is to give him or her a specific task ("Get this IV started.").

- **Blind panic.** A more worrisome reaction is blind panic, in which the individual's judgment seems to disappear entirely. Blind panic is particularly dangerous because it is "catchy," and it may precipitate mass panic among others present. For this reason, a panicky bystander needs to be separated quickly from others and, if at all possible, placed under the supervision of a calmer person.

- **Depression.** Depression is seen in the individual who sits or stands in a numbed, dazed state. The depressed bystander needs to be brought back to reality and removed from the scene.

- **Overreaction.** People who overreact tend to talk compulsively, joke inappropriately, become overly active, and race from one task to another without accomplishing anything useful. The person who is overreacting needs to be removed from the area where casualties are being treated.

- **Conversion hysteria.** In conversion hysteria, the patient subconsciously converts anxiety into a bodily dysfunction; he or she may be unable to see or hear or may become paralyzed in an extremity.

We shall go into more detail on how to cope with bystanders in Chapter 48 where we discuss mass-casualty incidents.

Responses of the Paramedic

Health care professionals are not immune to the stresses of emergency situations, and it is to be expected that those dealing with the critically ill and injured will experience a multitude of feelings, not all of them pleasant. The paramedic may feel angry at the demands of the family or the patient, anxious in the face of life-threatening injuries, defensive at inferences he or she is not competent to handle the situation, sad in response to the death of a patient, or any number of these sensations at the same time. These feelings are all perfectly natural, but it is preferable to keep them to yourself during an emergency. An attitude of outward calm and confidence on your part will do much to relieve the anxieties of others at the scene—and that too is part of the paramedic's therapeutic role.

One reaction that is common among health care professionals is a feeling of irritation at the patient who does not appear to be particularly ill. That reaction is especially prevalent among emergency personnel, who are psychologically geared to deal with life-threatening and catastrophic cases and who therefore tend to regard an apparently minor complaint as a burdensome annoyance. Try hard to remember that people define their own emergencies. Also, consider the possibility that people who call 9-1-1 with seemingly minor complaints are not calling for something minor at all—like the woman who called 9-1-1 because she couldn't get to sleep. Her problem was that it was her first night back home after the funeral of her husband—at Arlington National Cemetery, by the way. She was scared to death of her first night alone in that bed, thousands of miles away from the body of her husband, and she had no one else to call. Anyone who has ever been truly alone knows what an emergency that can be. These victims are not abusing us. They're precisely the ones we're here for.

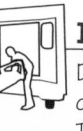

In the Field

Do not assume that seemingly nonemergency complaints are not a sign of something wrong. Tunnel vision can cause many mistakes in patient assessments and ultimately in their outcomes.

Burnout

What's this? We've scarcely started the paramedic course, and already we're talking about burnout! Why should we start worrying now about something that may (or may not) happen 10 years down the line?

We need to consider burnout now—at the earliest stage of paramedic training—because now is the time to start developing attitudes and habits that will help prevent burnout, whether 1 year or 20 years down the line.

The dictionary defines <u>burnout</u> as the exhaustion of physical or emotional strength. Burnout is, in fact, a consequence of chronic, unrelieved stress. The paramedic's job, by its very nature, is full of potential stresses. There are the obvious stresses imposed by having to deal, day after day, with mutilating trauma or catastrophic illness. There are, as well, more subtle stresses associated with interpersonal relations, pay, prestige, fringe benefits, and other issues. These complaints and stresses are, no doubt, legitimate. But burnout does not occur solely because of stress. Burnout develops because of the way a person *reacts* to stress.

One person's eustress may be another's distress **Figure 2-14 ▶**. The reason is that distress is a *learned* reaction, based on the way an individual perceives and interprets the world around him or her. In other words, distress is nearly always the result of what a person *believes*. Some beliefs are more likely than others to produce stress. Here are some beliefs that are common among EMS personnel:

- I have to be perfect all the time.
- My safety depends on being able to anticipate every possible danger.
- I am totally responsible for what happens to patients; if they die, it is wholly my fault.
- If there's something I don't know, people will think less of me.
- A good paramedic never makes mistakes.

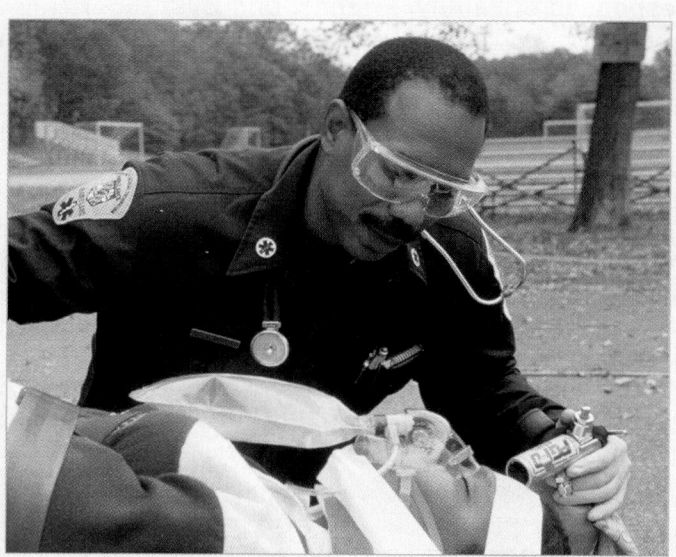

Figure 2-14 Dealing with stress as a paramedic requires the ability to emotionally distance yourself from the situation, and accepting the limits of what you can personally do.

These perfectionist beliefs are very likely to produce stress. They are also false beliefs. Prevention and relief of stress among EMS personnel begin with the recognition that such beliefs are unrealistic and invalid.

Like many of the conditions we will study in this textbook, burnout is also a sort of illness. And like any other illness, it has signs and symptoms. Learn to look for the symptoms of burnout in yourself and in your coworkers. These symptoms are warning signals, telling you to stop and reexamine your beliefs and your ways of responding to stress. Symptoms of impending burnout include:

- Chronic fatigue and irritability
- Cynical, negative attitudes
- Lack of desire to report to work
- Emotional instability (crying easily, flying off the handle without provocation, laughing inappropriately)
- Changes in sleep patterns (insomnia or sleeping more than usual), and waking without feeling refreshed
- Feelings of being overwhelmed or being helpless or hopeless
- Loss of interest in hobbies
- Decreased ability to concentrate
- Declining health—having lots of colds, stomach upsets, and muscle aches and pains (especially headaches or backaches)
- Constant tightness in your muscles
- Overeating, smoking, or abusing drugs or alcohol

It is preferable, of course, not to wait until symptoms of burnout develop. There are paramedics who have been in the field for 20 years and show no signs whatsoever of burnout, who still report to work every day with the same enthusiasm they did as rookies. What is their secret? In general, the paramedics who do not suffer burnout are those who have learned to respect and value *themselves.* That is not as easy as it sounds. The type of person who chooses to become a paramedic is usually altruistic—someone who puts the needs of others ahead of his or her own needs. In theory, that is very laudable. But in fact, no one can give their best to others for very long if they ignore their own personal needs.

Practically speaking, what does it mean to respect and value yourself? How can you translate that attitude into concrete action? Some of the steps you can take to protect yourself from burnout are summarized in **Table 2-1 ▶**.

Coping With Death and Dying

We all deal with death (remember the quote, "Nobody gets out of here alive"?). What do you say to people who know they're dying? What do you say to a bereaved parent or spouse? How do you deal with your own feelings when a patient has died while under your care? These are all questions we need to be able to answer for ourselves eventually, and it can take a lifetime to sort them out.

Death in the Western hemisphere is generally regarded as a very traumatic experience, something to be feared and postponed as long as possible. It's not that way everywhere in the world. It may help you to know that many seasoned paramedics reveal in candid discussion that they are not afraid to die. Think about it. The average person's only experience with death has been the death of a loved one. It was a rare event. Chances are it was surprising, it was frightening, and it was painful for the survivor.

As a paramedic, you will be there when a lot of people are born and you will be there when a lot of them die. Every one of these encounters is an honor—a most private moment in someone's life, to which you and a small number of your coworkers are invited. Why an honor? Because, in many cultures, these moments are a holy time. And because you are meeting someone for the very first time in his or her life—or seeing him or her alive for the very last time. Many of the latter group will exhibit great dignity with their passing, and perhaps show you how to die well someday.

You don't need to experience great frustration because you tried to resuscitate someone and he or she died anyway. For you to resuscitate someone, everything has to go just right. As a paramedic, you will have the opportunity to help a great many people, but you will not be involved in many successful resuscitations, even in the course of a long career. Accept your profession as a calling, and be fulfilled by it. Keep a good grip on your ego, and you will find that "losing" someone will rarely be an issue for you.

What follows here are some general guidelines and techniques for dealing with the dying, their families, and your own stress.

Stages of the Grieving Process

In her classic study, *On Death and Dying,* Elisabeth Kubler-Ross, MD, defined five stages through which grieving people—usually the dying, but sometimes their survivors—often proceed

TABLE 2-1	Nancy's Guidelines for Preventing Burnout

1. Paramedic heal thyself! Take care of your own health.
   - Get enough rest.
   - Eat a balanced diet.
   - Get regular physical exercise—at least 30 minutes of aerobic activity (walking, running, or swimming) three to four times a week.
   - Don't abuse your body. Smoking, overindulgence in alcohol, taking recreational drugs, or self-prescribing any other drugs are all forms of self-abuse.
2. Give yourself some "me" time every day. Some of the most stress-resistant paramedics are those who have learned the techniques of meditation and can thereby escape now and then to a quiet place within themselves. Try different methods of meditation or relaxation and see which one works best for you.
3. Learn how to relax **Figure 2-15 ▼**.
   - Take time for hobbies.
   - Engage in social activities with people not involved in EMS.
   - Leave your job behind when your shift is over.
4. Do not make unreasonable demands on yourself.
   - Forget the idea that you have to be perfect. No one is perfect. If you do the best job you can, that is good enough.
   - You don't have to be right all the time. Accept the fact that now and then you will make a mistake—and that the world will not come to an end on account of it.
5. Do not make unreasonable demands on others.
6. Stay in touch with your feelings.
   - Find someone you can talk to. Share the stress.
   - Cry when you need to. There's no shame in being sad sometimes.
7. Learn techniques for shedding stress while on duty. Don't let stress accumulate.
8. Debrief after tough calls.

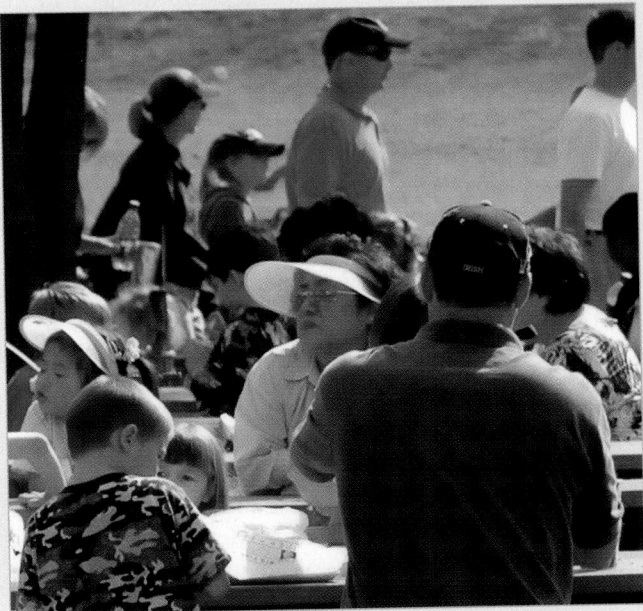

Figure 2-15 One of the best ways of dealing with the stress of working as a paramedic is to invest in relationships and activities outside of work that are meaningful to you.

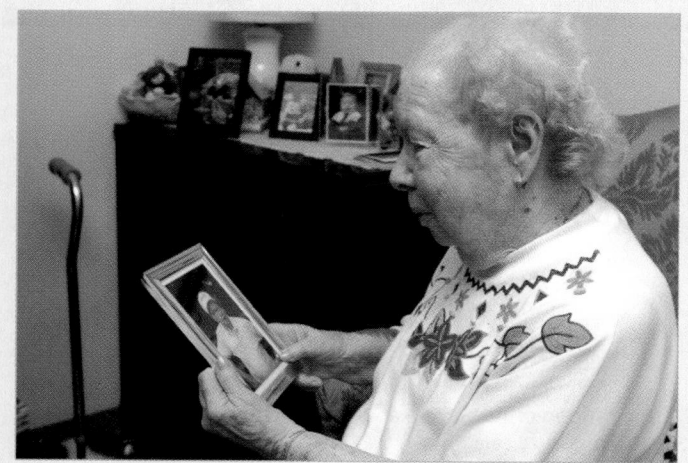

Figure 2-16 People usually go through a lengthy process of grieving before fully accepting the death of a loved one.

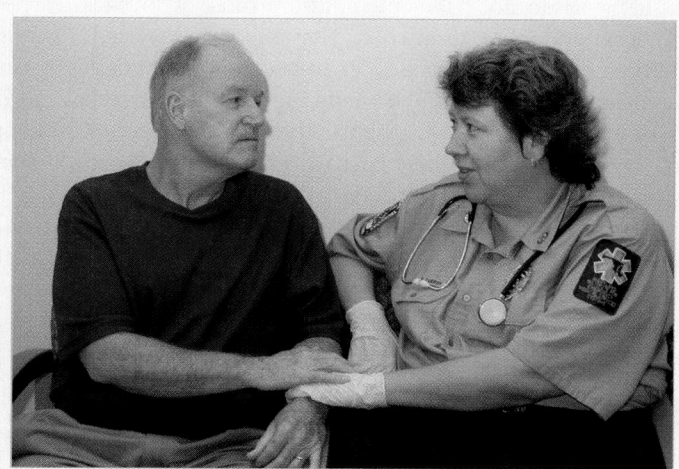

Figure 2-17 Be aware that each patient will have different ways of dealing with his or her immediate situation. Some may be relieved to talk openly about how they feel, while others may have a greater sense of privacy or stoicism.

Figure 2-16 ▲ . Each of these stages in some way helps the dying or their family members adapt to their own reality. It helps to be aware of these stages, and to consider the behavior of dying patients or their families in the context of the grieving process.

- **Stage 1: Denial.** We have already mentioned denial as a mechanism by which people attempt to ignore a problem or pretend it does not exist. Denial is a way of buffering bad news until we can mobilize the resources to deal with that news more effectively.
- **Stage 2: Anger.** When people can no longer deny the reality of a situation, anger over the loss replaces denial. They may ask, "Why me?" and displace their anger randomly to those around them. As we mentioned earlier, such anger may be very difficult for health care personnel to deal with, and it is necessary again and again to remind yourself, "This patient (or this family member) is not really angry at me. She is angry at the hand life has just dealt her."
- **Stage 3: Bargaining.** When anger does not change the painful reality of a situation, people may resort to bargaining, that is, trying to make some sort of deal in hopes of postponing the inevitable ("If I can just live long enough to see my daughter's wedding, then I'll die in peace.").
- **Stage 4: Depression.** When bargaining fails to change the reality of a loss and people must come to terms with dying, there is suddenly an enormous sense of loss. They may become very quiet. Other people may make the mistake of trying to "cheer them up" at this point. But the people who have experienced the loss typically do not *want* to be cheered up. They want permission to express their sorrow—in words, in tears, or in what Kubler-Ross calls "the silence that goes beyond words." Acknowledge their loss and sadness, and if they act like they want to cry, offer some tissues or a towel and encourage them to "let it out." If they seem to want a hug, offer it. If they seem to just

want to be quiet by themselves, do what you can to accommodate that as well. But try hard not to steer their behaviors in any way unless their behavior is harmful.
- **Stage 5: Acceptance.** In the final stage of grief, people who are dying prepare to disengage from the world around them. They shed their fears and most of their other feelings as well and begin to loosen the ties that bind them to the living. When the dying enter this acceptance stage, it is often the family that is in need of the most help.

Dealing With the Dying Patient

People who are dying generally know, at the very least, that their situation is serious; they may, in fact, be well aware that they are dying and may want to talk about it. Many health care professionals are reluctant to discuss death with patients, mostly because of their own anxiety about the subject. So they try to maintain an attitude of cheery reassurance ("Everything is going to be all right."), when they both know that everything will *not* be all right. The message patients get is that the subject of dying is taboo and that they'd better keep their feelings about dying to themselves. In fact, perhaps the most important thing you can do for dying patients is to let them know that it's OK to talk about it. There are many ways of doing so. You don't need to come right out and ask, "Do you want to talk about dying?" It's enough to say, "If there's anything worrying you, I'd be glad to listen."

Having made the offer to listen, be prepared to do so. Let patients talk as much as they wish **Figure 2-17 ▲** . Make some physical contact. Hold their hand, put a hand on their shoulder, or make some other unmistakable gesture of empathy.

What if patients come straight out and ask you, "Am I going to die?" There is no simple answer as to how to reply to that question, but the answer should acknowledge the seriousness of their condition without taking away all hope. For example, you might say, "You seem to have had a severe heart attack. We're going to give you the best care available, but the situation *is* serious." For patients who know they are dying, it may be a great relief to have someone else acknowledge the fact and thereby give them permission to talk about it.

Dying patients also need to feel that they still have some control over their life. When people lose all control over their life, they may lose a large measure of their dignity and self-respect. As much as possible, explain to them what you are doing and allow them to participate in the treatment. Ask them if there is anyone they would like you to contact or if they have any special instructions they want conveyed to someone. If they *do* ask you to convey a message, *write it down* word-for-word as they state it to you.

Experience tells us that people who know they're going to die usually don't *ask* you if they are going to die. They look you in the eye and *tell* you, "I think I'm going to die." People who ask tend to be fairly stable, but that doesn't mean they're not scared to death. If they appear to be doing OK, let them know that, and tell them not to be afraid, that you've "got them."

Dealing With a Grieving Family

Suppose you are called to the scene where a child has been run over by a truck. You can see at a glance that the child is dead and beyond hope of resuscitation—his skull has been smashed open and his brains are all over the street. Two police officers are restraining the child's mother, who is crying hysterically.

The fact that there is nothing you can do for the child does *not* mean that the call is over. There is another "patient" at the scene—the child's mother—and the call is not over until you have done all you can for her **Figure 2-18 ▾** .

What kinds of things *can* you do for a grieving family? How can you help them begin the process of dealing with their loss? Here are a few guidelines:

- Do *not* try to hide the body of the deceased from the family, even if the body has been badly mutilated. (*Do* hide

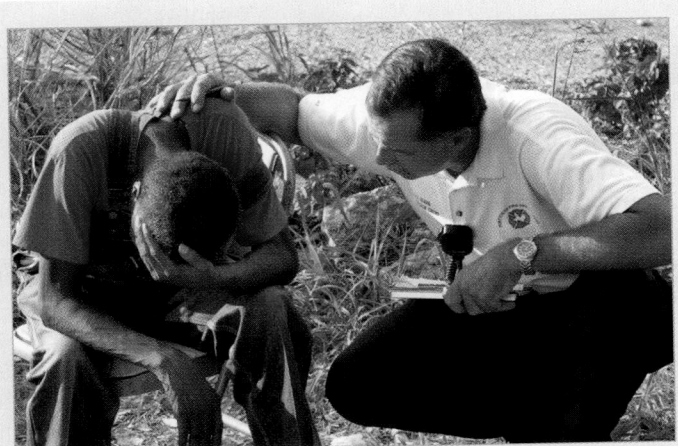

Figure 2-18 While on the scene, one of your responsibilities is to help family members through the initial period after the death of a loved one.

it from the general public, however.) People who are prevented from seeing the body of a loved one may later have enormous difficulty working through their grief, for they may not be able to get beyond their denial.

- For similar reasons, do not use euphemisms for death, such as "expired" or "passed away." The family needs to hear the word "dead."

- Do not be in a hurry to clear away all your resuscitation equipment. Let the family see the equipment before you start tidying up and packing away your gear, so that they will know that everything possible was done to try to save the patient.

- Give the family some time with the remains, especially when the victim is a child. If the death occurred in a public place—as in the hypothetical motor vehicle crash described—move the remains into the ambulance and let the family be alone with the body there. Give them a chance to say goodbye in their own way.

- Try to arrange for further support. Recruit a neighbor to come over, or offer to call the family's clergy.

- Accept the family's right to experience a variety of feelings—guilt, shock, denial, or anger. And when family members do respond with anger, remind yourself yet again, "They aren't really angry at *me*."

Dealing With a Grieving Child

You need to be particularly sensitive to the emotional needs of children and how they differ depending on their age group. Children up to 3 years of age will be aware that something has happened and people are sad. Family members should be advised to try to maintain the child's routine. They should also watch for irritability and monitor the child's eating and sleeping patterns. Children 3 to 6 years of age believe that death is temporary and may continually ask when the person will return. Family members should be informed that the child may feel responsible for the death and may worry that everyone else they love may also die. The family should emphasize to the child that he or she was not responsible for the death and also that it's OK to cry when you are sad.

Children 6 to 9 years of age may mask their feelings in an effort to not look babyish. Family members should discuss the normal feelings of grieving with the child. Also, they should not hesitate to cry in front of the child. This will convey to the child that crying is acceptable behavior after the loss of a loved one.

Children 9 to 12 years of age may want to know details surrounding the incident. Family members should encourage the sharing of feelings and memories to facilitate the grieving process.

After the Call Is Over

Some kinds of calls can be real shockers, like the Oklahoma City bombing or the World Trade Center attack. In those cases, everyone involved in the call is likely to experience some heavy-duty feelings. If these feelings stay bottled up, there may be all sorts of problems later. Every ambulance service, therefore, needs to develop routine procedures for debriefing after any call that involved the death of a patient. All those who participated in the call need a chance to sit down together, in an atmosphere of confidentiality, and air their feelings about what happened.

By definition, a critical incident is one that overwhelms the ability of an EMS worker or an EMS system to cope with the experience, either at the scene or later. It has become standard practice for EMS systems in the United States and abroad to deploy specially trained teams to conduct critical incident stress debriefings (CISDs) with emergency personnel who have been involved in particularly traumatic calls or other painful incidents. A CISD is usually held within 24 to 72 hours of the incident. Although public safety organizations have used CISDs for more than 20 years, there is no evidence that they are effective, or that their effects are not actually harmful. The sorts of incidents that are apt to require debriefing include:

- Serious injury or death of a fellow worker in the line of duty
- Suicide of a fellow worker
- Multiple-casualty incidents, such as an airliner crash or train wreck
- Serious injury or death of a child
- Intense media attention to an incident

It is impossible to predict how any given person will react to a particular incident. A call that may be very disturbing to one paramedic may not bother his or her partner at all. People should be offered opportunities to debrief but debriefings should never be forced upon them.

Controversies

There are definitely two sides of the fence on the effectiveness of CISD. Psychology professionals and EMS professionals alike have debated this issue for some time now. Take part in a debriefing whenever you can. Be open-minded about the experience and then draw your own conclusion as to which side of the fence you are on.

Posttraumatic Stress Disorder

Most calls should not disrupt your normal life functions. But, depending on a number of variables, some especially traumatic calls can preoccupy even well-adjusted providers for weeks or even months afterward. This is called posttraumatic stress disorder (PTSD). Most paramedics never experience it, but it's what CISDs were developed to prevent. Let your superiors know if you experience one or more of the following signs of PTSD:

- You have trouble getting an incident out of your thoughts.
- You keep having flashbacks of an incident.
- You have nightmares or other sleep disturbances after an incident.
- Your appetite is not the same after an incident.
- After an incident, you laugh or cry for no good reason.
- You find yourself withdrawing from coworkers and family members after an incident.

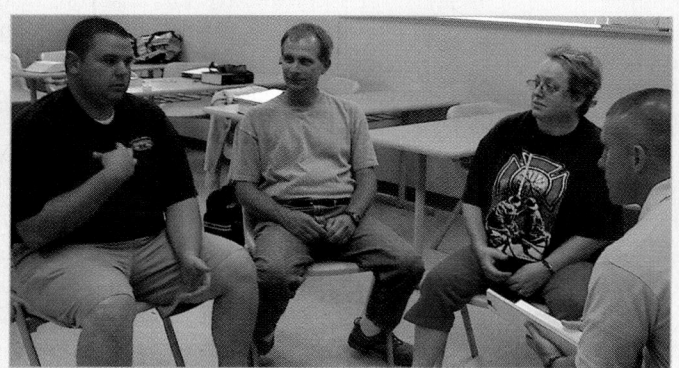

Figure 2-19 A debriefing with colleagues after an especially traumatic or difficult call can help everyone voice their feelings.

The purpose of a CISD is to accelerate the normal recovery process and to help EMS personnel realize that they are normal people having normal reactions to *ab*normal events **Figure 2-19 ▲**. As mentioned, many EMS systems have CISD management teams to provide support after a traumatic call—and sometimes even during the incident itself. The intervention may take the form of a brief (usually about 30 minutes) defusing session right after the call, in which all who were involved in the incident are offered an opportunity to express their feelings about what happened. As the name implies, a defusing session is intended to remove the explosive potential from a situation and thereby prevent more serious psychological consequences later on.

A formal debriefing is usually coordinated by one or more professional counselors 24 to 72 hours after an incident, when it becomes clear that the incident has had a serious impact and is causing persistent symptoms among the crew. A debriefing usually takes about 3 hours, and is conducted away from the workplace and in a confidential atmosphere so participants can feel free to say what's on their minds.

▌Emergency Vehicle Operations

An emergency vehicle is a four-sided billboard that communicates to the public all the time, whether we realize it or not. It communicates our respect for—or lack of respect for—the safety of others. It communicates our courtesy—or complete lack of it. And it communicates our concern for the comfort and safety of that patient and caregiver in the compartment—or our complete lack of it.

A paramedic's first job is to come home safe to loved ones. There are plenty of paramedics (some whose careers span 20 or 30 years) who have never been involved in an ambulance collision, and not by dumb luck. They understand that safety is deliberate. They understand that operating an ambulance is a public trust. And they never forget that driving an ambulance is dangerous.

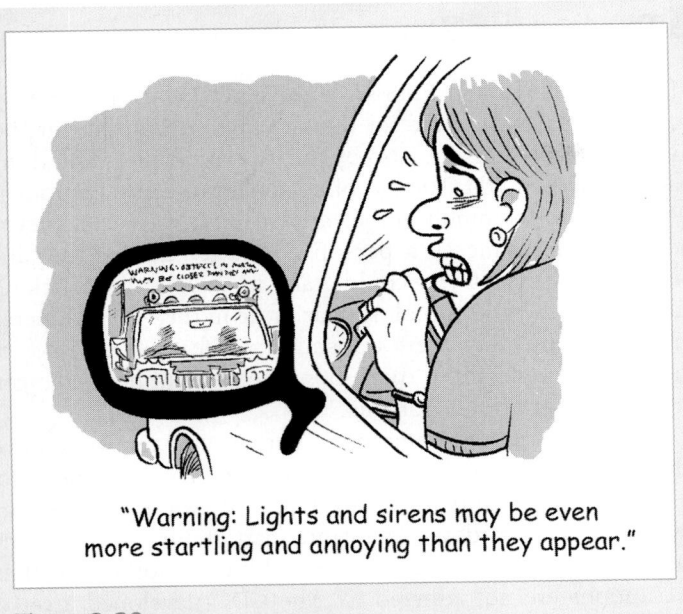

"Warning: Lights and sirens may be even more startling and annoying than they appear."

Figure 2-20

Here are some proven safety tips you can use in your daily driving:

1. Think of your warning equipment as tools you can use to *ask for* (never demand) the right of way.

2. Always allow for the incompetence of other drivers.

3. Come to a full and complete stop when you encounter an opposing signal. Proceed only after you have given other drivers time and cause to anticipate your intentions.

4. Expect some drivers to panic **Figure 2-20 ▲**. If that happens, turn off your siren, switch on the personal address system, and politely say, "Please pull to the right and stop. Thank you." Repeat it in case they don't understand you the first time.

5. Remember, other drivers may not immediately hear your siren when you are traveling at freeway speed. Stay far enough behind other drivers so they can see your lights in their rear-view mirrors. Anticipate that, when they notice you, their first instinct will be to slam on their brakes.

6. As frustrating as it may be, control your emotions when it appears that a driver is refusing to yield. Avoid reacting to the situation, which will cause you to lose your cool and potentially worsen it.

Documentation and Communication

When considering transporting a patient with lights and siren on, ask yourself, "Can I justify the potential risk to my safety, my patient's safety, and the safety of others to save a few minutes?" Make sure you can legitimately justify why you transported emergently and document the need to do so.

Besides the general use of lights and the siren, some additional aspects of operating an emergency vehicle deserve special mention.

Using Escorts

When you find yourself responding in tandem with an escort vehicle, remember that the average driver is not likely to understand that one vehicle is escorting another. Most drivers have not had a course in emergency driving. Typically, drivers on a street or highway hear one siren and, especially in their rear-view mirrors, will see only the first vehicle in a convoy. Deliberately using an escort is not only a bit pompous, but also dangerous. Do yourself a favor. Minimize the number of times you use any warning equipment and the number of vehicles on a given response. You'll live longer, and so will the public.

Adverse Environmental Conditions

Most of us have enough trouble keeping ourselves visible and trying to predict other drivers' behavior on clear, sunny days. Add a little bad weather, fog, blowing dust, or slippery asphalt and the average driver can be overwhelmed. Try to be as careful, alert, and predictable for other drivers as you can under the circumstances. When you lose even the slightest visibility, be super observant and expect the worst decision-making from your fellow travelers. In fact, don't even trust yourself under these conditions. Drive slowly, carefully, and remember to sign up for emergency driving classes long before winter, the hurricane season, the wildfire season, or whatever weather torments the EMS providers in your region.

Parking at Emergency Scenes

Many of us were taught years ago that when we park in traffic, we should shield ourselves with our equipment and aim the front wheels into traffic. That works fine if you're in law

You are the Provider Part 4

Your partner drives to the ambulance entrance of the hospital. It takes every ounce of your concentration to aid your partner in unloading the patient. You tell yourself that you can finish the call but, as you and your partner lower the gurney to the height of the hospital bed, you are unable to hold up your end. It drops to the floor, and the patient drops with it. Although he appears to be uninjured, the patient screams loudly and immediately threatens to sue you. Your partner now seems to be injured, and the hospital staff members appear to be horrified at what has just transpired.

9. What parts of this situation were preventable?

10. Beyond the physical injuries, what other damage has occurred?

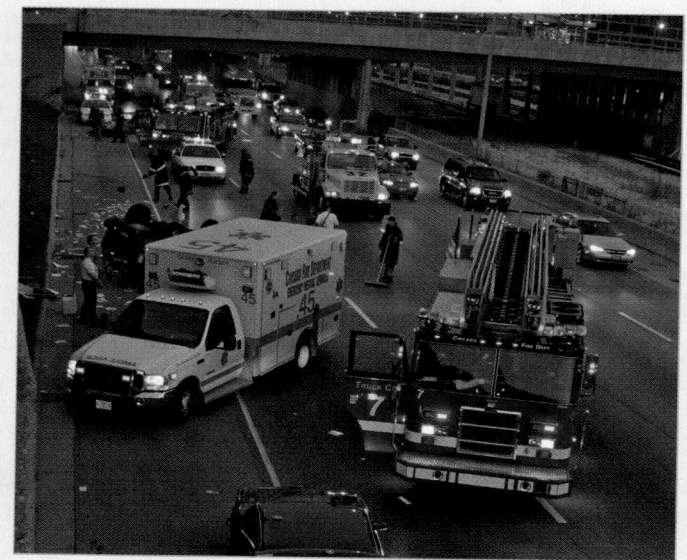

Figure 2-21 Place your vehicle where it can be seen, out of traffic, and where the patient can be easily transported into and out of the vehicle.

enforcement and you need the illumination from your head-lamps anyway, or if you're doing fire suppression and you have access to a front-facing water outlet. But it does you no good at all if you're going to end up loading an ambulance, because ambulances load from the rear. Protect your back; park in the best position for loading Figure 2-21 ▲.

There is an exception, and that's if the ambulance happens to be the first equipment on the scene. Just remember: it will need to be moved later on. (Chapter 46 provides a more detailed discussion of this situation.)

Due Regard for the Safety of Others

Everything that makes us EMS providers belongs to the public. Our certificates do. Our equipment does. So do the radio frequencies we use everyday, and the roads we travel. And so does our occasional prerogative to override certain traffic laws in order to do our jobs. Anyone who operates an emergency vehicle needs to have profound respect for the pain EMS drivers can inflict on the public by driving too fast, or by insisting on the right-of-way.

People who have abused this privilege tell us that no teacher can possibly describe the horror they felt on the morning after causing a fatality (especially the death of a coworker). These events are always horrible, and they can usually be traced to something that took no more than a couple of seconds to occur. There is no "undo" button in EMS driving, and no amount of shock or grief can ever give us those seconds back.

While speed is sometimes perceived as the essence of EMS, rest secure in this advice: knowledge is the essence of professional EMS. As you become a paramedic, you will have the most training and the most experience of any EMS provider. Be professional.

Protecting Yourself

Much has changed in EMS since the early 1990s. For one, we have become more aware of the fact that we can be hurt not just by flying bullets but also by the invisible bullets found in a patient's body fluids. The use of personal protective equipment (PPE) was not common in the early years. It was a status symbol to see how messy a person could get during the shift because that meant you could "take it" and keep on ticking. Surgeons in the 1800s took similar pride in their messy operating aprons, but they were transmitting infectious diseases by the score. Paramedics in the 2000s take pride in not endangering themselves or their patients.

Face it, there are some nasty germs out there nowadays. Thanks to the research and reporting done by the Centers for Disease Control and Prevention (CDC), we are now more aware that biohazards are an integral part of our profession and can have long-term effects on the health care worker if certain precautions are not adhered to. The CDC developed a set of universal precautions for health care workers to use in treating patients. EMS follows body substance isolation (BSI) precautions rather than relying on universal precautions. BSI differs from universal precautions in that it is designed to approach all body fluids as being potentially infectious. In observing universal precautions, you assume that only blood and certain body fluids pose a risk for transmission of hepatitis B and human immunodeficiency virus (HIV).

Use the personal tools that are at your disposal that are designed not only to protect you from your sick patients but to protect them from you! In addition to these tools, consider adopting a practice that doesn't necessarily involve tools, but has proven its worth over the years. Wash your hands!

Personal Protective Equipment and Practices

At a minimum, each ambulance should be equipped with certain PPE, not just because it is the law under the Occupational Safety and Health Administration (OSHA), but because it is an important part of safety for yourself. At a minimum, you should have access to gloves, facial protection (masks and eyewear), gowns, and N95 respirators. The following paragraphs explain the importance of using infection control practices.

Wear Gloves

Gloves are absolutely essential on any EMS call, and some patient encounters warrant more than one set of gloves for a caregiver, depending on the procedure, the patient's history, and the environment Figure 2-22 ▶. Anytime you intubate or start an IV, consider following that with a new set of gloves before loading the patient and jumping aboard that ambulance. Gloves are a good idea anytime you sanitize the ambulance too or even handle the cleaning rags. Sterile gloves should be reserved for clean or sterile patient care procedures; they're substantially more expensive than examination gloves. And whatever you've been doing with them, take off your gloves before you drive.

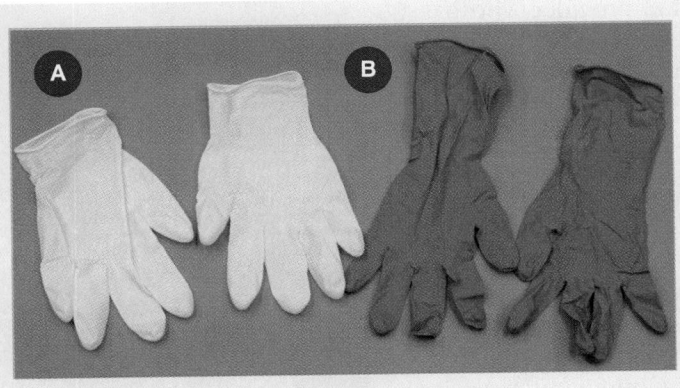

Figure 2-22 Two commonly used types of gloves are (A) latex and (B) nitrile.

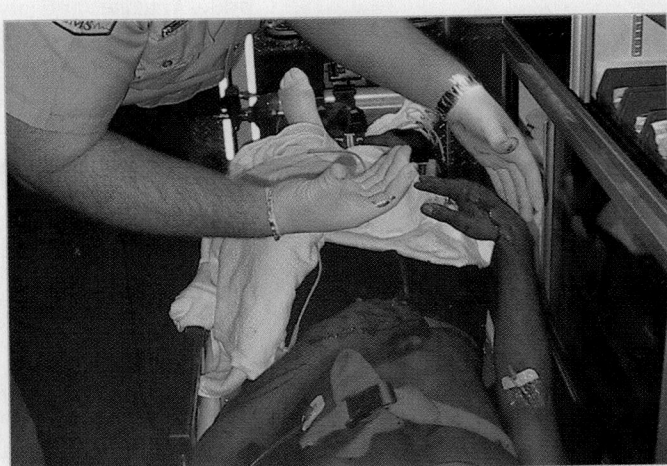

Figure 2-23 Paramedics always need to protect themselves from contact with any type of body fluids.

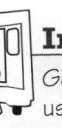
In the Field

Get used to washing your hands before and after using the bathroom, before ingesting anything by mouth, before getting into your personal car, and before and after any physical contact between you and a patient or an instrument.

Any advanced medical text on infection control starts with "wash your hands" and ends with it, too.

When you do wash your hands, wash them vigorously with antibacterial soap for at least 30 seconds before rinsing with clean water. If you don't have access to soap and water, carry waterless hand cleaner wipes in your ambulance and use them instead. Isopropyl alcohol, the active ingredient they contain, is a very effective bactericide.

Whatever else you do, wash your hands.

Wash Your Hands
Wash your hands, routinely and often. Long before it was common practice for field caregivers (or any clinical workers) to wear gloves during nonsterile procedures, we learned to wash our hands—sometimes more than 30 times a day, depending on our caseloads. Turn that into a habit. Habits are reliable, even when we're stressed.

Use Lotion
To replenish the natural oils you wash off your skin, and to keep the skin on your hands from cracking, use hand lotion several times a day both on and off duty. For you guys, it's not sissy stuff; it's good sense. Your skin is a very effective barrier to pathogens, as long as it hasn't been breached by the drying effects of frequent washing. And the job of a professional caregiver warrants frequent washing.

Use Eye Protection
Many seasoned paramedics make it their standard practice to wear antisplash eyewear throughout any patient contact. That's a good idea. It's an absolute necessity during suctioning or

intubation procedures. In fact, during intubation, it may be a good idea to use a face shield instead.

Consider Wearing a Mask
Have a cold? Wear a mask—not only to protect your patients and your coworkers from you, but to protect you from additional infections while you are in a weakened state. Have a bad cold? Stay home.

Protect Your Body
Masks and gowns are appropriate whenever you deal with a patient who is extremely messy or bloody Figure 2-23 ▲. A 30-gallon trash bag can be used as a two-armed glove to slide a patient from a couch or bed onto an ambulance cot if the patient is covered with feces, urine, or blood. Once the patient has been moved, the crew can simply turn the bag inside-out, squeeze the air out of it, tie a knot in its open end, and place it in a hazardous materials bag.

Incontinence bar-riers should be laid out on a surface when the patient is leaking any type of fluid or has skin lesions.

N95 Respirators
Read some of the recent statistics by the CDC regarding tuberculosis (TB) and you will realize that this is one of the most common diseases contracted by breathing in germs. The CDC and world public health associations estimate that 1.7 *billion* people are affected with TB worldwide, with 3 million deaths a year. The chance of getting the TB bacillus makes it that much more important to wear the N95 respirator Figure 2-24 ▶ and not just a simple surgical mask.

Clean Your Ambulance and Equipment
Sanitize your patient compartment surfaces frequently, but especially the ambulance cot, the bench seat, the grab rails, the deck and deck hardware, and the interior and exterior areas around the door handles. These surfaces should be cleaned daily and after every call. The same is true for the door hardware inside (and outside) the cab, the steering wheel and gear-shift lever, the emergency

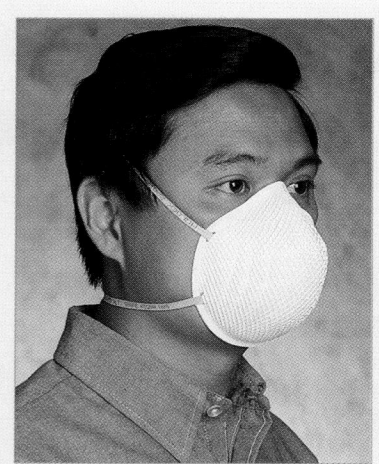

Figure 2-24 Specially designed respirator masks, such as the N95 respirator, protect against infection from tuberculosis bacteria.

brake release, and anything else that you or your coworkers may have handled while wearing contaminated gloves. Remove the cot mounts at least once a week to get rid of the dried blood and vomit that tends to accumulate there. It produces an odor that can make some people sick, and it attracts insects such as flies. Clean this area more often if you have had messy calls. Sanitize the phones and microphones as a matter of routine—especially the ones in the patient compartment, which you surely handle while wearing contaminated gloves.

Sanitize or replace your pen often. You typically handle it several times during every call, with your gloves on. Then, you handle it after the call, after you've washed your hands. Likewise, sanitize your stethoscope with alcohol after every call.

Decontamination of equipment and supplies that have been exposed to body substances requires a different cleansing routine than just soap and water. First, any piece of equipment that is intended for single use should be discarded in an appropriate hazardous materials bag. Second, use a commercial disinfecting agent on any piece of equipment that has had direct contact with the patient's skin. Bleach diluted in water (1:10) can also be used as a disinfecting agent. Disinfecting kills many of the microorganisms on the surface of your equipment.

To kill all microorganisms, sterilization by using a commercial sterilizing chemical or pressurized steam is needed. Tools, such as a laryngoscope blade, that come in direct contact with the interior of a patient's body must be sterilized after use.

Properly Dispose of Sharps

Disposal containers (large for the ambulance and small for carry-in gear) for sharps, such as needles and blades, are essential to protect crews against needle sticks or cuts **Figure 2-25 ▶**.

Consider Wearing Body Armor

Body armor can be bulky, expensive, and uncomfortable. It's not nearly as protective against bullets or knives as are self-protective avoidance strategies. But it can protect the wearer from many kinds of chest and abdominal trauma such as those that occur during extrications and in emergency vehicle collisions.

Management of an Exposure

In the event that you have been exposed to a patient's blood or body fluids, follow your local EMS guidelines. Generally, any EMS provider who has been exposed should do the following:

- Wash the affected area immediately with soap and water.
- Comply with all reporting requirements.
- Get a medical evaluation.
- Obtain proper immunization boosters.
- Document the incident, including the actions taken to reduce chances of infection.

Hostile Situations

Until very recently, EMS providers were routinely thrust without assistance into situations involving hostile patients who needed to be restrained, treated, and transported against their will. There is no more dangerous prospect than confronting someone like that without special equipment and plenty of help. A position statement by the National Association of EMS Physicians in December 2003 outlined for the first time an official endorsement of the rights to safety not only of patients but also of their field caregivers. In addition, most modern jurisdictions ask their EMS providers to stand back until police have defused these situations (using electric stun devices if necessary).

But EMS providers are also exposed to other kinds of hostile situations. If the element of hostility is known or can be anticipated in advance, EMS crews and their first responders should never be allowed to arrive on scene first. Discipline yourself to scrutinize all information that comes to you from others, and keep yourself on "yellow alert" any time you are on duty. Specifically, beware any call dispatched as a fight, stabbing, shooting, domestic disturbance, "person down," or "unknown medical aid." Every one of these calls is suspicious and warrants an initial response by police **Figure 2-26 ▶**. In addition, you should have the prerogative to ask for a police response to any call that your intuition says is violent. Whether or not you ask for police backup may depend on your knowledge of the response area and your analysis of the information you receive from your communications center.

Do not be afraid of being less than a good caregiver if you ask for police to go in first. You will not be able to treat your patient if you are hurt.

You will surely find that your intuition is a reliable tool that warrants your trust; and it will become more and more sensitive as you gain experience and additional training. Every EMS provider should read a book called *The Gift of Fear:*

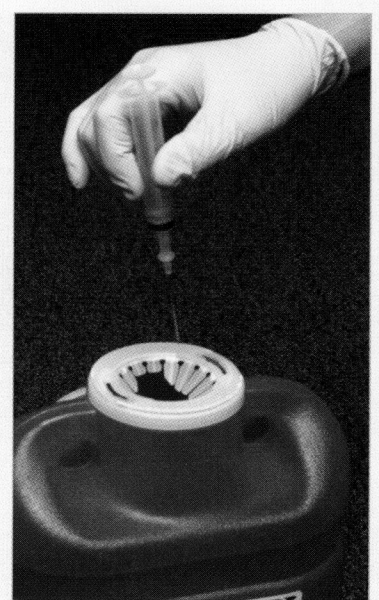

Figure 2-25 Any needles or blades must be disposed of in special containers.

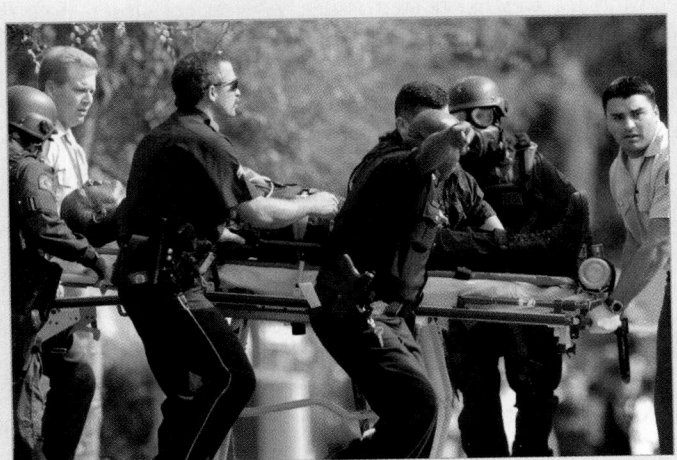

Figure 2-26 Do not hesitate to call for law enforcement if anyone's safety is in question.

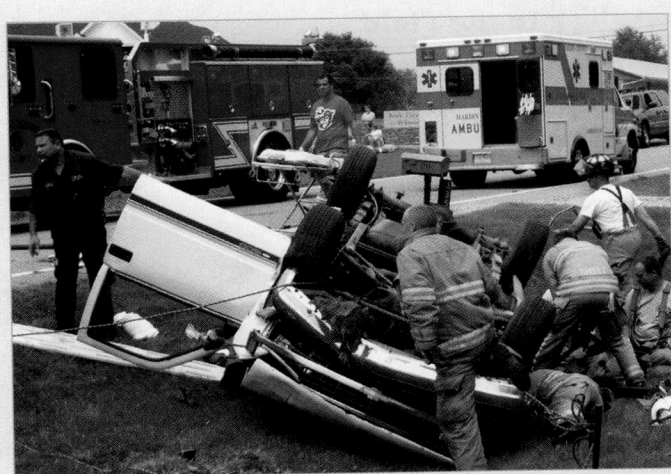

Figure 2-27 At a busy accident scene, it is important to place your vehicle in a safe, visible location, and to minimize the risk of any additional accidents.

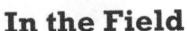

In the Field

Some of the most dangerous calls are those that are not obviously dangerous. The most worrisome calls are those with limited or vague information from the caller. If someone refuses to give information to a dispatcher, it may be because of something they are trying to hide.

Survival Signals That Protect Us From Violence, by Gavin De Becker. It explains how your intuition picks up on small details that your rational side discounts. Intuition is often not the product of your imagination, but of your ability to process small details almost outside of your awareness.

Once you are in contact with a hostile patient, try hard to listen a lot more than you talk. Avoid arguing. Concentrate on de-escalating his or her emotions, because people who are upset don't listen well and they don't reason well either. (Remember fight-or-flight?) Many hostile patients who started out willing to go to the hospital became unwilling because a crew member couldn't resist a "witty" comment.

Learn and use verbal judo. You can learn more about verbal judo by reading *Verbal Judo: Redirecting Behavior With Words,* by George J. Thompson. Verbal judo is a discipline for communication and negotiation that parallels the characteristics of judo, the martial art. As you may know, there are hard forms and soft forms of the martial arts. Judo is a soft form. It's designed to deflect energy or simply move out of its way, rather than inflict it yourself.

Remember that anytime you're on someone else's turf, they have a clear advantage. You can expect them to know everything about their environment while you know nothing (including locations of weapons). Volatile patients in their home environment are much more dangerous there than anywhere else—especially in poor lighting.

Finally, some situations get out of hand due to the paramedic's inability to communicate effectively and build a rapport. Show empathy and understanding on the scene, and you will develop the trust of your patients. Knowledge of diverse cultures plays a major role in effective communication. "Know your audience" is not just a catch phrase for entertainers. The more you know about the people you serve, the more likely you will know their customs and expectations. You must also be diligent in your pursuit of treating all patients with respect and dignity. Put your personal prejudices aside every time you step on the scene.

Traffic Scenes

The most dangerous kinds of calls you will run are the everyday ones, because you naturally get comfortable with them. But regardless of where you are, autos move at high speeds, may carry hazardous substances, and may crash into one another in locations that are both dangerous for you and sure to attract spectators. It is important to stay aware of your surroundings, even the familiar ones that you see day in and day out.

Like any scene, your approach to traffic scenes always begins with your familiarity with the response area and your awareness of what the system's other public servants have been doing for the past few hours (because we know you've been paying attention to their frequencies!). This is critical information, because it lets you know your best routing and who might be available to help you with traffic control, air support, hazardous materials, terrain issues, and potential destinations.

Traffic may be only one of the many hazards at the scene of a motor vehicle collision Figure 2-27 ▲ . The undercarriage of our units are quite hot, especially after traveling 5 to 10 minutes to get to a scene. Parking a hot, running unit on the side of the road in dry grass is just inviting a grass fire. Watch where you park, and the type of material you park over, very carefully. If you arrive at a scene in the early morning hours, before the sun starts heating up, and park over a liquid spill long enough, it may trigger combustion of the liquid. Sometimes we create our own hazards by carelessly throwing equipment and its packaging all around us at the scene. Not only can people trip over them but we often lose pieces because they get kicked under the vehicles.

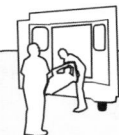

In the Field

If you are the first unit arriving on the scene, do a scene assessment and notify other responding units of any actual or potential hazards that may be present. Your first job is to ensure the safety of the EMS crew—including yourself.

Remember that your primary concern at any scene is safety; safety for yourself as well as for those around you. Identify as many hazards as you can before even leaving your unit. Reviewing the scene before leaving your vehicle goes a long way toward identifying hazards such as fire, unstable vehicles or buildings, unruly crowds, or hazardous materials.

Begin making physical observations a mile or so before you approach the scene. Watch the traffic, pay attention to the wind direction, look for smoke, and begin planning for evolving dark-ness and for weather-related issues. As you get closer, note the kinds of vehicles and obstacles involved. Make an educated guess about what may have happened. If someone is not yet handling traffic, decide how to control the flow of traffic initially (sometimes it can be a lot more important than medicine at first).

How big an incident do you have, both in size and scope? Are you dealing with commercial carriers of industrial products? What resources will you need immediately? What is the topography? Where will fluids drain naturally? Remember that if you do not have fire on the scene now, it could start quickly as some kinds of fuel begin leaking on hot metal exhaust systems or as a result of electrical arcing.

Where do you eventually want to park? What will your working space be? These are all important considerations, and they will be covered in more detail in Section 7. For now, concentrate more on seeing and protecting the whole scene and not so much on what's wrong with individual patients.

You are the Provider Summary

1. What is your main concern at the moment?

Your main concern should be the safety of yourself, your partner, and, finally, your patient. Lifting patients of this size should be performed by an adequate number of responders (no less than four). Your patient is stable, so there is no need for immediate action.

2. What concerns do you have, if any, regarding your partner's behavior?

It's possible that your partner is having a bad day, is generally disagreeable, or is suffering from burnout. Because you do not know him well yet, it is hard to determine definitively. Employee assistance programs are in existence to aid responders when they are overwhelmed and in need of help.

3. Does your partner's attitude have any effect on patient care?

He dropped the ball on obtaining essential information regarding this patient's medical history and, most likely, his attitude has affected his patient care on other calls. People suffering from burnout can be more likely to cut corners, make mistakes, and experience problems with coworkers, other medical professionals, and patients. Depending on their condition, these responders may also have difficulty in their personal lives as well.

4. Is this the best course of action?

The best course of action was your first reaction, to call for additional resources. This is appropriate whenever you feel that the number of ambulances, supplies, equipment, or personnel that you have on the scene is inadequate.

5. What is the best way to handle this situation?

Although you might experience grumbling and resistance from your partner, you should tell him that you feel it is unsafe for you and your partner to lift this patient without additional personnel. If you stress the issue of safety, he will likely cooperate with your suggestion.

6. What factors could affect your decisions?

When you are newly hired, no matter how supportive the agency is that you work for, you will be under pressure to perform well. Most agencies have a probationary period for new members during which you can be fired for any reason, or for no reason at all. Obviously, this is a source of stress. No matter how much you are concerned about your employee evaluation, you must put safety first.

7. What decisions could you have made to prevent this situation?

You could have called for additional resources despite the complaints of your partner. You could have requested aid from other employees within the nursing facility. Certified nursing assistants are familiar with appropriate lifting techniques, and with some communication, could aid you in safely moving and lifting the patient. Some departments forbid any nondepartmental personnel from engaging in activities such as this, so always follow local standard operating guidelines.

8. Has patient care been affected?

Obviously, you must obtain information regarding this patient's medical history and reason for transport. To do otherwise could place the patient at risk. Because the patient's condition was stable, patient care was not jeopardized a great deal. However, if the patient's condition changed rapidly and you were not able to care for the patient because of your own pain, patient care could very well have been compromised.

9. What parts of this situation were preventable?

This situation was entirely avoidable. Don't hesitate to protect yourself. In the end, it was your responsibility to speak up regardless of whether or not it would create an uncomfortable situation with your partner.

10. Beyond the physical injuries, what other damage has occurred?

Because you chose to be agreeable rather than use your common sense and instincts, you not only hurt yourself but also your partner and possibly the patient. Beyond the physical injuries and their associated costs (treatment, rehabilitation, and lost work hours and the resultant overtime), you have damaged the image of your department. This last type of injury is very difficult to fix. The patient will remember what happened, and may choose to sue you, your partner, the department, the city, and the hospital. Depending on what transpires, word of this story could travel to outside parties, including local or national newspapers and/or Web sites.

Prep Kit

■ Ready for Review

- Paramedics need to know how to ensure their own well-being.
- Wellness has at least three dimensions: physical, mental, and emotional. It is important to keep all three dimensions healthy and balanced.
- Nutrition plays a key role in maintaining day-to-day energy and maintaining a healthy body for life.
- Practice proper lifting techniques to protect your body and lengthen your career.
  - Minimize the number of total body-lifts you have to perform.
  - Coordinate every lift in advance.
  - Minimize the total amount of weight you have to lift.
  - Never lift with your back.
  - Don't carry what you can put on wheels.
  - Ask for help anytime, without embarrassment or hesitation, and offer it liberally to others.
- Learn how to effectively control stress so that it does not affect your wellness. Take appropriate action. Initial management techniques include:
  - Controlled breathing
  - Reframing
  - Progressive relaxation
- A patient's reaction to stress may include fear, anxiety, depression, anger, confusion, denial, regression, projection, and displacement. Most of these reactions are not under the patient's conscious control. Remember, under emergency situations, everyone is under stress.
- Health care professionals are not immune to the stresses of emergency situations and experience a multitude of feelings, not all of them pleasant. These feelings are normal, but it is better to keep them to yourself during an emergency.
- Burnout is a consequence of chronic, unrelieved stress. Perfectionist beliefs are likely to produce stress.
- As a paramedic, you will be present when a lot of people are born and you will be there when a lot of people die. Every one of these encounters is an honor.
- The patient who is dying may be aware of that fact, and may want to talk about it. One of the most important things you can do for a dying patient is to let him or her know that it is OK to talk about it. Be prepared to listen and provide empathy.
- Critical incident stress debriefings (CISDs) are provided to emergency personnel who have been involved in traumatic calls or other painful incidents.
- An emergency vehicle is an instrument that can either earn its crew a living or kill them. It deserves respect and it warrants understanding.
- Protect yourself by washing your hands; using hand lotion; wearing gloves, eye protection, and a mask and gown (when necessary); cleaning your ambulance and equipment; and properly disposing of sharps.
- Decontamination of equipment and supplies that have been potentially exposed to body substances require a different cleansing routine than just soap and water; sterilization may be required.
- Keep yourself on "yellow alert" while you are on duty. Do not be afraid to ask for the police to enter a scene first. You will not be able to treat a patient if you or your partner is hurt.
- The most dangerous calls are your everyday ones because you become comfortable with them and let down your guard.
- Your primary concern at any scene is safety—safety for yourself as well as those around you.

■ Vital Vocabulary

alarm reaction The body's first, "startle" response to a stressor.

alert response The first reaction in the alarm reaction, in which you immediately stop whatever you are doing and focus on the source of the stimulus.

blind panic A fear reaction in which a person's judgment seems to disappear entirely; it is particularly dangerous because it may precipitate mass panic among others.

body substance isolation (BSI) An infection control concept and practice that assumes that all body fluids are potentially infectious.

burnout The exhaustion of physical or emotional strength.

conversion hysteria A reaction in which a person subconsciously transforms his or her anxiety into a bodily dysfunction; the person may be unable to see or hear or may become partially paralyzed.

critical incident An event that overwhelms the ability to cope with the experience, either at the scene or later.

critical incident stress debriefings (CISDs) A confidential peer group discussion in which specially trained teams work with emergency personnel who have been involved in traumatic calls or other painful incidents; CISDs usually occur within 24 to 72 hours of the incident.

defense mechanisms Psychological ways to relieve stress; they are usually automatic or subconscious. Defense mechanisms include denial, regression, projection, and displacement.

denial An early response to a serious medical emergency, in which the severity of the emergency is diminished or minimized. Denial is the first coping mechanism for people who believe they are going to die.

displacement Redirection of an emotion from yourself to another person.

distress A type of stress that a person finds overwhelming and debilitating.

eustress A type of stress that motivates an individual to achieve.

fight-or-flight syndrome A physiologic response to a profound stressor that helps one deal with the situation at hand; features increased sympathetic tone and resulting in dilation of the pupils, increased heart rate, dilation of the bronchi, mobilization of glucose, shunting of blood away from the gastrointestinal tract and cerebrum, and increased blood flow to the skeletal muscles.

posttraumatic stress disorder (PTSD) A delayed stress reaction before an incident, often the result of one or more unresolved issues concerning the incident.

projection Blaming unacceptable feelings, motives, or desires on others.

regression A return to more childish behavior while under stress.

stress A nonspecific response of the body to any demand made upon it.

stressor Any agent or situation that causes stress.

universal precautions Protective measures that have traditionally been developed by the Centers for Disease Control and Prevention (CDC) for use in dealing with objects, blood, body fluids, or other potential exposure risks of communicable disease.

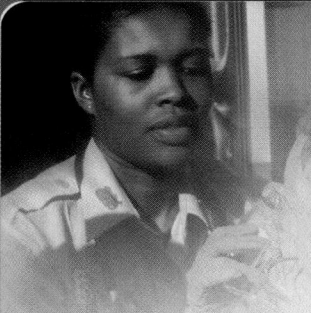

Assessment in Action

On duty, paramedics are expected to be able to perform all the functions of their job. This includes lifting, handling stress, prioritizing patient care, assessing the situation quickly and accurately, keeping themselves and their crew safe, controlling chaotic situations, and dealing with grieving family members. In order to do all of these things, paramedics must take care of themselves outside of the job. They need to keep physically fit, know safe lifting techniques, maintain flexibility, eat right, and much more, as suggested in this book. The following questions pertain to taking care of yourself in order to perform your job at the highest level you can.

1. **Wellness has how many defined dimensions?**
   - A. Two—physical and mental
   - B. Three—physical, mental, emotional
   - C. Three—physical, mental, and spiritual
   - D. Four—physical, mental, emotional, and spiritual

2. **Which of these is NOT recommended for EMS providers to help themselves stay fit and prepared for their job duties?**
   - A. Carrying bottled water instead of buying soft drinks during shifts
   - B. Making sure to take vitamins daily
   - C. Eating several small, nutritious snacks
   - D. Minimizing intake of caffeine

3. **During any given shift you go on approximately seven calls that involve moving quickly, lifting patients, and other related movement. Does this meet the criteria for "regular vigorous exercise"?**
   - A. Yes. It gets your heart rate up and exercises various muscles several times during shifts.
   - B. No. Regular vigorous exercise means approximately 30 minutes of cardiovascular exercise involving various muscle groups four to five times a week.

4. **What is the suggested exercise program for EMS providers?**
   - A. Muscle size improvement, cardiovascular endurance, and lifting capabilities
   - B. Cardiovascular endurance, flexibility, and physical strength
   - C. Flexibility, increasing amounts of weight able to be lifted, and cardiovascular endurance
   - D. Physical strength, cardiovascular strength, and concentration on developing muscles most frequently injured in EMS

5. **True or false? Fight-or-flight syndrome can always help in EMS by giving you the energy boost you need to handle a crisis situation.**
   - A. True
   - B. False

6. **True or false? There is good stress (eustress) and bad stress (distress).**
   - A. True
   - B. False

7. **Which one of the following is NOT a reaction identified as occurring in multiple-casualty incidents?**
   - A. Overreaction—talking or joking inappropriately or racing from one task to another without accomplishing anything
   - B. Blind panic—person's judgment seems to disappear entirely
   - C. Coping—finding small ways to cope with a situation
   - D. Conversion hysteria—patient or bystander subconsciously converts own anxiety into a bodily dysfunction

8. **A patient with serious internal injuries asks you point blank, "Am I going to die?" What would be the best response to this question?**
   - A. Be honest, and say that the outlook is not good.
   - B. Reassure her that things will be fine.
   - C. Be honest but reserved. Assure her that you and all other medical personnel will do your very best to take care of her, but that the situation is serious.
   - D. Avoid the question by explaining each procedure you perform on the way to the hospital.

9. **Which of the following is NOT a suggested guideline for helping a grieving family cope with their loved one's death?**
   - A. Do not try to hide the body of their loved one from them; give them time alone with the body if requested.
   - B. Do not be in a hurry to clear away all resuscitation equipment that was used. Let them see everything possible was done to save their loved one.
   - C. Use softer words to present the information, such as "he passed away" or "he's expired."
   - D. Accept any feelings the family may go through in your presence, including anger directed toward you.

Challenging Questions

10. **If you cannot easily stay up late at night, be alert during the night, or get up early, can you still successfully work in EMS?**

11. **List some activities and approaches that will help you keep a positive perspective while working in a stressful field.**

12. **A common reaction among EMS providers is irritation at being called to help a patient who does not seem particularly ill. When you receive this kind of call, what should you consider?**

Points to Ponder

You are called to the home of a frequent caller for the general complaint of "not feeling well." This person usually calls when she is depressed and lonely, and does not usually have any medical conditions that you can treat. Sometimes, after talking, she says she feels better and refuses transport. Your partner is familiar with her as well. Because of past situations, your partner says you should take your time getting to the scene, neither of you should waste a pair of gloves going in because she is never ill or injured, and the two of you should get through the call as quickly as possible so that you can respond to those who actually need help.

Should you listen to your partner? Should you wear gloves?

Issues: Treating Each Patient, Serving as a Role Model for Scene Safety, Empathy, Working With Other Providers.

3 Illness and Injury Prevention

Objectives

Cognitive

1-3.1 Describe the incidence, morbidity, and mortality of unintentional and alleged unintentional events. (p 3.5)

1-3.2 Identify the human, environmental, and socioeconomic impact of unintentional and alleged unintentional events. (p 3.4)

1-3.3 Identify health hazards and potential crime areas within the community. (p 3.9)

1-3.4 Identify local municipal and community resources available for physical, socioeconomic crises. (p 3.12)

1-3.5 List the general and specific environmental parameters that should be inspected to assess a patient's need for preventative information and direction. (p 3.7)

1-3.6 Identify the role of EMS in local municipal and community prevention programs. (p 3.9)

1-3.7 Identify the local prevention programs that promote safety for all age populations. (p 3.12)

1-3.8 Identify patient situations where the paramedic can intervene in a preventative manner. (p 3.14)

1-3.9 Document primary and secondary injury prevention data. (p 3.3)

Affective

1-3.10 Value and defend tenets of prevention in terms of personal safety and wellness. (p 3.13)

1-3.11 Value and defend tenets of prevention for patients and communities being served. (p 3.3)

1-3.12 Value the contribution of effective documentation as one justification for funding of prevention programs. (p 3.15)

1-3.13 Value personal commitment to success of prevention programs. (p 3.14)

Psychomotor

1-3.14 Demonstrate the use of protective equipment appropriate to the environment and scene. (p 3.13)

Injury Prevention and EMS

Several years ago, San Diego paramedic Paul Maxwell went on a drowning call. A 2-year-old boy had wandered away from a day care facility and fallen into a neighbor's backyard pool. Despite everyone's best efforts, he could not be resuscitated. The mother was inconsolable and her cries haunted the paramedic. Maxwell wondered how such tragedies could be prevented—if he could help it, he never wanted to go on another call like that again. Doing a little investigation, and looking up incidents on his EMS system's database, he discovered a pattern of increased drownings in his region. Maxwell made the decision to get involved. In cooperation with his EMS agency, he contacted other groups in his community with an interest in child safety. Using his system's data and motivated by his firsthand knowledge of the suffering that such a death inflicts, Maxwell began a coordinated and successful effort to reduce backyard pool drownings in his community, through both legislation and education. Although the reduction in drownings was incentive enough for Maxwell, he was recognized with a special award by the state of California.

More than a few paramedics have been motivated by their field experiences to work actively on prevention. Throughout the country, EMS providers are taking the lead or providing support in a wide variety of interventions—specific prevention measures or activities designed to increase positive health and safety outcomes ▶ Figure 3-1 ▶ . From beginnings such as these, EMS has emerged as a strong advocate—and practitioner—of injury prevention. Few practitioners see the scene of an injury as a whole: the physical situation, the design flaws in home or highway, and the tragic stress of trauma.

EMS providers, of course, participate in illness prevention such as flu inoculation programs or blood pressure monitoring. However, illness prevention programs are often well-focused by physicians and public health officials. This chapter focuses on injury because of your unique field perspective on injuries. Few providers in a hospital or a physician's office are conscious of the physical situation of an accident site for example, or the number of times an incident has occurred at that site. You are uniquely aware. The principles and techniques for illness prevention are not substantially different from those for injury prevention. If you discover a need for a prevention program—perhaps some of your elderly patients might not be getting their influenza or pneumococcal vaccines—by all means, apply the principles.

Common Roots

Injury prevention shares the common root of EMS: the historic National Academy of Sciences/National Research Council 1966 study, "Accidental Death and Disability: The Neglected Disease of Modern Society." The commission noted that just as EMS could help with trauma after an event, injury prevention initiatives could help before an accident happened.

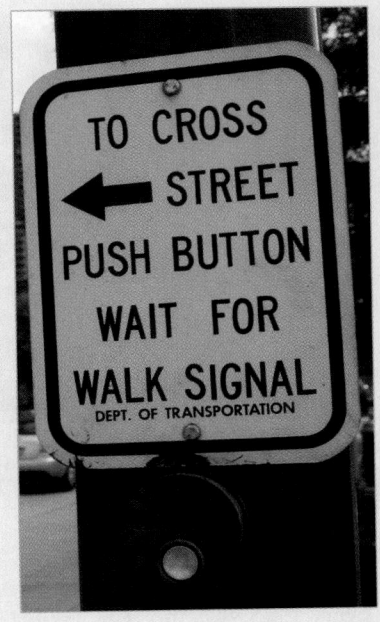

Figure 3-1 Many rules of public safety exist because of the persistent efforts of medical professionals and other involved citizens.

Strengthening this link, the broader definition of injury prevention has always included EMS. Primary injury prevention is defined as keeping an injury from ever occurring. EMS traditionally has focused on secondary injury prevention, reducing the effects of an injury that has already happened. (For the inquiring mind, a third area, tertiary prevention, is defined as the effort to rehabilitate a person who has survived an injury.)

In 1996 the *Consensus Statement on the EMS Role in Primary Injury Prevention* was published. Representing every imaginable EMS constituency, the authors of the statement made clear that primary injury prevention is an "essential" activity "that must

You are the Provider Part 1

For the third time in as many months you respond to a call in the same stretch of highway—a winding road along the top of a river gorge. Too many times, the patient is a drunk driver who couldn't negotiate the curve and plunged over the side, unimpeded by guardrails. More often than not, the driver is not wearing a seat belt. The tragic scenario plays itself out: the driver is thrown from the vehicle, and he or she is severely injured. Your EMS team has a long and treacherous extrication, working on a steep hillside. Everyone on the team knows it will be dangerous. No one has to say it, but you know that the whole team is tempted to think: "Stupid drunks."

This time the driver is a man in his mid-twenties. He will live, but appears to have suffered severe head and neck injuries and may never walk again. Later you find out he has a wife and two children, and was coming home after having a few beers at a local tavern after work. By all accounts he is a loving father and husband. He made a mistake, you think, but did he deserve this? After paramedic training, you now wonder, what can I do to prevent another tragedy like this?

1. Why should you consider getting involved in preventing these injuries?
2. What are the risk factors associated with the injuries described here?

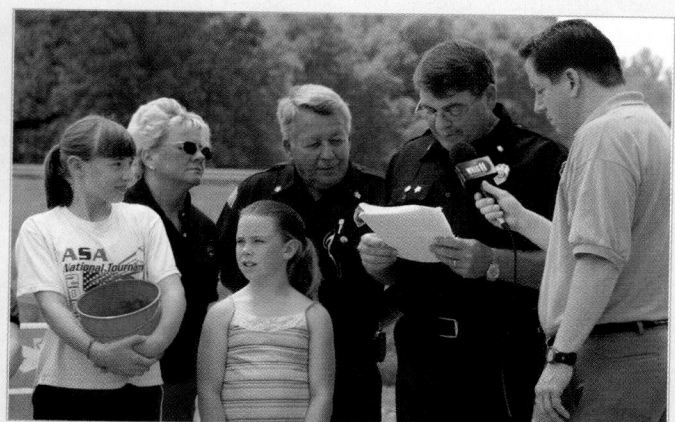

Figure 3-2 Embracing the full role of a paramedic means being involved in the concerns of your community.

be undertaken by the leaders, decision-makers, and providers of every EMS system." The 1998 US DOT Paramedic National Standard Curriculum, created by consensus with EMS educators, researchers, and practitioners, calls for specific training in primary injury prevention.

Notes from Nancy

In addition to being a health care provider, the paramedic—like any other health professional—must also be a health *educator*. Teaching helps the paramedic keep his or her own skills sharp; at the same time, teaching *identifies* the paramedic as a resource person in the community.

Of course, the number one priority for paramedics is to be prepared to respond and treat the injuries that will inevitably occur in their communities. And all providers in particularly busy systems will find that time for prevention initiatives will be limited. However, there is a role for every EMS provider, at some level, in primary injury prevention **Figure 3-2 ▲**. This includes, first and foremost, teaching others in the health care system and the public *why* you see an injury reoccurring at the same place.

Documentation and Communication

Do not forget special population groups in your safety and prevention programs. For instance, you may find different illness and injury patterns related to ethnicity and can present these topics through your programs. Have printed materials available in all languages throughout your community. Do not neglect people with physical and developmental challenges. Do your best to get the word out in every way possible.

Why EMS Should Be Involved

Leaders in both EMS and the prevention field offer the following rationale:

- EMS providers are widely distributed in the population.
- EMS providers reflect the composition of the community they serve.
- In many rural communities, the EMT might be the most medically sophisticated person.
- If properly coordinated, EMS would provide a formidable resource in the effort to reduce the overall injury burden.
- EMS providers are high-profile role models.
- EMS providers are perceived as champions of their patients.
- EMS providers are welcome in schools and other environments conducive to delivering the prevention message.
- Since they face the results of injuries everyday, EMS providers are perceived as authorities on injury and prevention. (A paramedic talking to a city council about drowning prevention legislation, relating a true story about the suffering he or she witnessed, can be an extremely effective teacher.)

Injuries as Public Health Threat

Injuries, according to the National Center for Injury Prevention and Control, part of the Centers for Disease Control and Prevention (CDC), are "the intentional or unintentional damage to the person resulting from acute exposure to thermal, mechanical, electrical, or chemical energy or from the absence of such essentials as heat or oxygen." Historically, injuries were not grouped together. Instead, they were reported under distinct umbrellas, which made it difficult to let the lay population see just how widespread injuries truly are **Figure 3-3 ▶**. Grouping injuries as a common health problem makes it possible to consider the breadth and depth of the problem. It has enabled public health officials and other care providers to call attention to important problems and target more effective interventions.

Intentional injuries, such as assaults or suicide, are included in the definition. EMS can often play a supporting role here too, but can usually have a greater impact in preventing unintentional injuries.

How big a problem are injuries in the United States? To many health experts, it is the largest public health problem facing the country today. According to data collected by the

Special Considerations

With a growing geriatric population, a good fall prevention program may be one of the keys to preventing an overload of the health care system. Evaluate all community options available to the older population in your area and bridge any gaps with programs to meet their needs and prevent injuries related to falls.

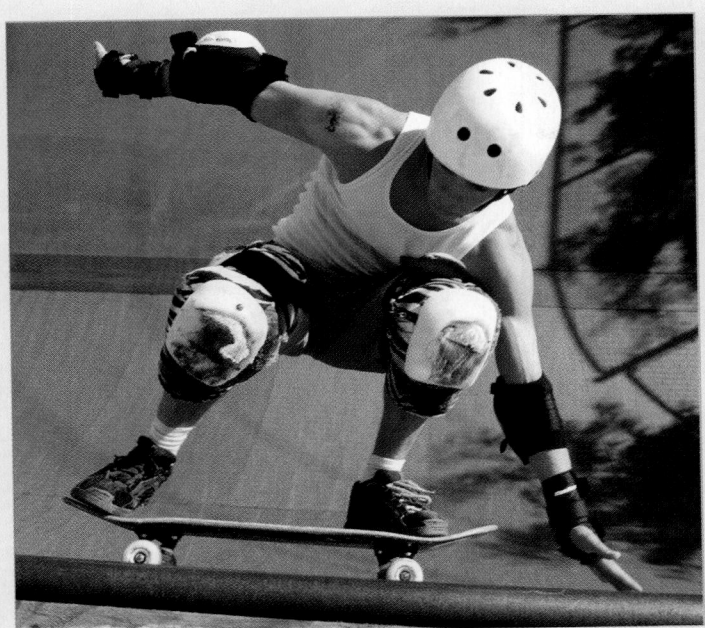
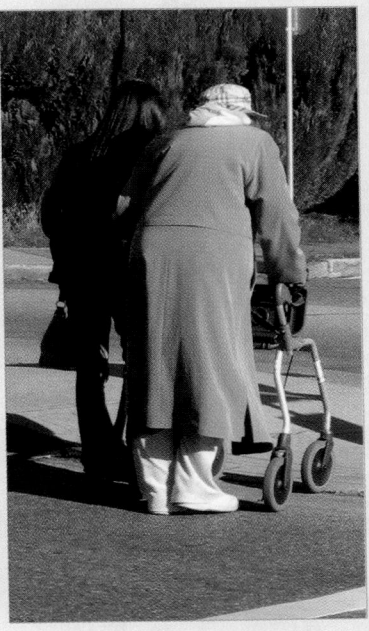

Figure 3-3 Injuries affect people of all age groups and physical abilities. For each potential injury, there are appropriate preventative measures that can and should be taken.

- About 4,292,000 visits to the emergency department were related to motor vehicle crashes.
- Approximately 44,065 deaths were caused by motor vehicle crashes.

Table 3-1 ▶ shows the top 10 causes of death in the United States in 2002. This information is extremely important in understanding how injury impacts different age groups. From ages 1 to 44 years, unintentional injuries are the leading killer. For all ages combined, unintentional injuries are the fifth leading killer behind heart disease, cancer, cerebrovascular events (stroke), and the effects of bronchitis, emphysema, and asthma.

How much do these injuries cost society, above and beyond the tremendous personal suffering? It is estimated unintentional injuries account for more than $200 billion. There is another concept that researchers are using to measure the cost to society: <u>years of potential life lost</u>. It works like this: assume a productive work life until age 65, and deduct the year of death from that age. Thus, an 18-year-old who dies in a car crash has lost 47 years of potential productive work life, while someone who dies of a stroke at age 63 years has lost 2 years. Because injuries are a leading cause of death in the young, it quickly adds up **Figure 3-5 ▶**. This method allows a comparison of the years of productive work life lost, disease by disease. This method can measure how many years of usefulness to society a child killed in an accident could have had, comparing those years to those of an older person who, for example, had a myocardial infarction. The value of the comparison is to teach members of your community that the prevention of a childhood accident is of great importance to the community. **Figure 3-6 ▶** compares years of potential productive work life lost by injury to other causes of death.

It's easier to measure death rates than to measure nonfatal (<u>morbidity</u>) injury rates because visits to clinics, emergency departments, doctors' offices, and other places for treatment

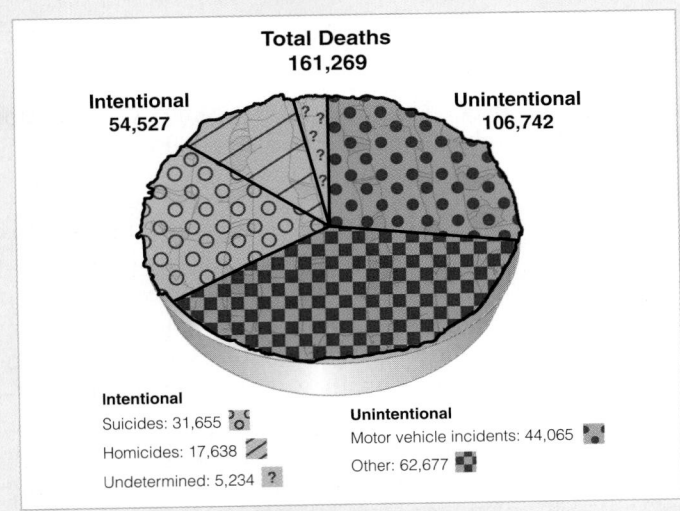

Total Deaths
161,269

Intentional
54,527

Unintentional
106,742

Intentional
Suicides: 31,655
Homicides: 17,638
Undetermined: 5,234

Unintentional
Motor vehicle incidents: 44,065
Other: 62,677

Figure 3-4 The vast majority of injuries that occur are unintentional—particularly accidents related to driving.

National Center for Health Statistics, in 2002 (the latest available year for figures) **Figure 3-4 ▲**:

- There were a total of 178.2 million injury-related visits to physician offices, emergency departments, and outpatient clinics.
- In total, 161,269 people died as a result of injury.
- Of those, 106,742 died of unintentional injuries and 54,527 died of intentional injuries (31,655 suicides and 17,638 homicides; 5,234 deaths were undetermined).

In the Field

Unintentional falls are the third leading cause of unintentional death behind motor vehicle crashes and suicide by firearm. The nonfatal injury rate for falls is higher than any other single type of injury.

Table 3-1	Top 10 Causes of Death in 2002

1. Heart disease
2. Cancer
3. Stroke
4. Chronic, lower respiratory disease
5. Unintentional injuries
6. Diabetes
7. Influenza and pneumonia
8. Alzheimer's disease
9. Kidney disease
10. Septicemia

Source: Adapted from National Center for Health Statistics/National Vital Statistics System, 2002.

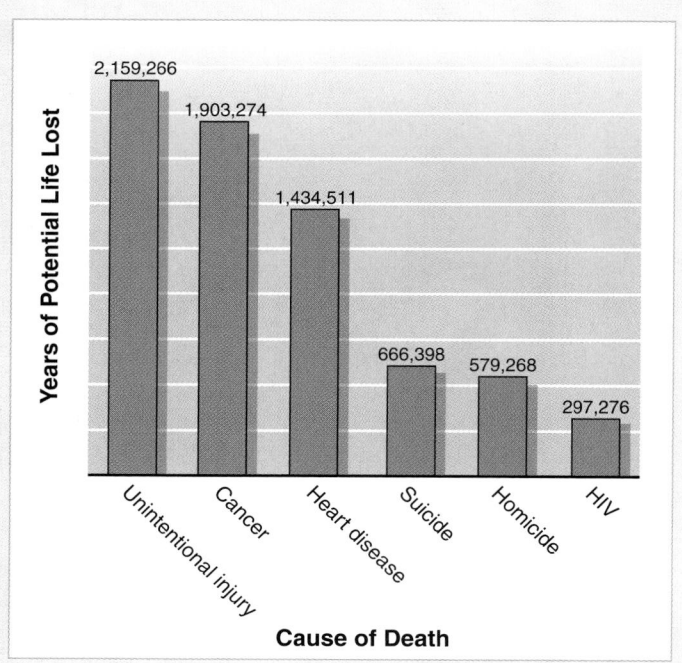

Figure 3-6 Years of potential life lost categorized by cause of death.

Source: Adapted from National Center for Health Statistics/National Vital Statistics System, 2002, United States.

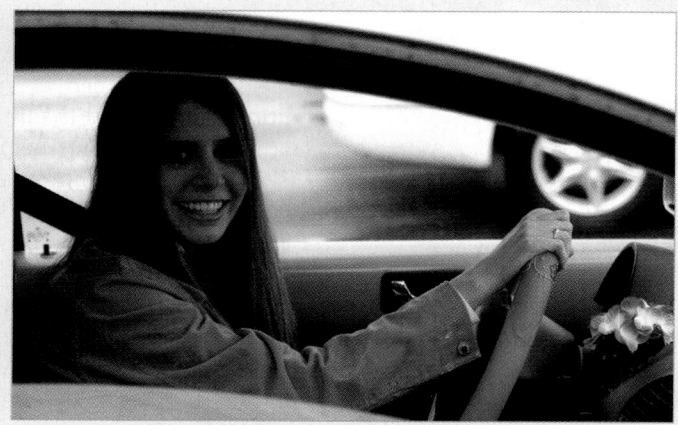

Figure 3-5 The regular use of a seat belt can have a dramatic effect on the number of years of potential life lost—particularly in younger age groups.

are scattered in a number of agencies and professional groups. On an average day, more than 110 million people will judge their injuries to be severe enough to seek treatment in an emergency department.

Principles of Injury Prevention

The 4 Es of Prevention

An injury risk is a potentially hazardous situation in which the well-being of people can be harmed. Interventions need to combine *education* with three other types of interventions: *enforcement, engineering/environment,* and *economic incentives.* These are commonly referred to as the 4 Es of injury preven-

tion (Figure 3-7 ▶). The most effective injury prevention efforts reflect a combination of these interventions.

Education

Most paramedics know that people can behave in ways that cause them to become injured or put others at risk. Many people do not know and therefore cannot assess the risk of doing something—"I didn't know it was unsafe to put my baby's seat in the front passenger seat." Or people know the risk—"I won't wear seat belts, they are too uncomfortable"—and disregard it anyway. Through education we can often inform people about potential dangers and then act to persuade them to change risky behavior. Show moms and dads how to use an infant car seat. Tell people about the horrors of being thrown from a vehicle.

To be effective, messages need to be tailored to very specific groups and reinforced with meaningful rewards. Educational techniques that seem to be particularly promising include the use of contracts or participant commitment, incentives, behavioral feedback, and modeling.

You are the Provider Part 2

You decide your best course of action is to enlist the help of law enforcement officers. They know vehicle crash prevention and detect patterns in highway death and injury. You decide to call your local law enforcement agencies to begin your quest to minimize death and disability resulting from motor vehicle crashes at this particular stretch of road.

3. Which law enforcement agencies could you contact?
4. Who else might be able to help you in assessing road conditions?

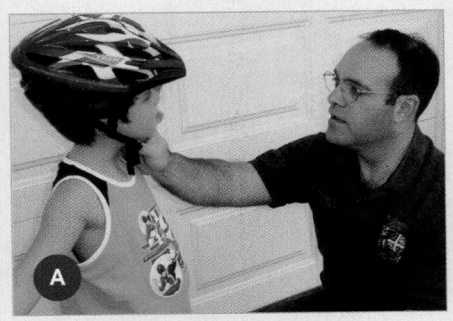
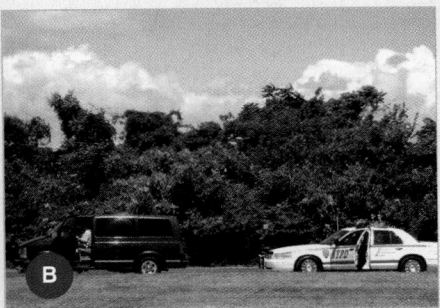
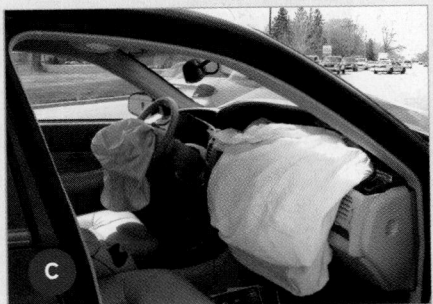
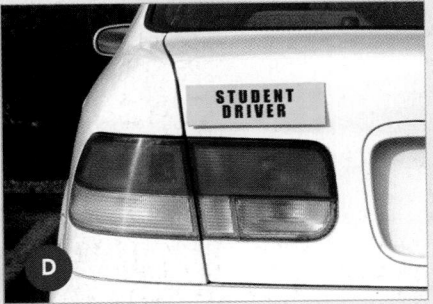

Figure 3-7 **A.** The four Es of injury prevention start with education. **B.** and **C.** Enforcement and engineering/environment contribute as well. **D.** Economic incentives, such as lower insurance rates for young drivers who have taken approved driver education programs, complete the picture.

Engineering/Environment

Most EMS providers know spots where adding guardrails or smoothing out dangerous curves in a road could prevent collisions. Changing the design of products or spaces such as roads can offer automatic protection from injury, often without any conscious change of behavior by the individual. These are called passive interventions.

For example, making child-resistant bottles is a passive intervention that reduces poisonings, and can be more effective than trying to keep the bottle out of children's reach. Strategies to change the environment can include social, legal, political, and cultural approaches. Environmental modifications, which are often expensive, usually happen when the community's awareness of the problem is raised, causing that community to accept responsibility for change.

Economic Incentives

Economic self-interest—saving money on health care costs or insurance rate reduction for careful drivers—provides monetary incentives to reinforce safe behavior. The threat of lawsuits (and significant monetary damages) often causes manufacturers to improve the safety of consumer products—an economic loss that serves as an incentive to change behavior. Organizations also recognize the value of offering free or subsidized safety products (bike helmets, fire extinguishers, safety locks) to encourage use.

However, despite your best efforts, some members of your community may know about a risk but their behavior will not necessarily change. There are even some paramedics who refuse to wear seat belts on their rigs! A crucial advantage of any educational effort is that it can pave the way to legislative and environmental/technological changes.

Enforcement

Behavior can be forced to change by law (that is why it is called law enforcement). Legislation/regulation formulates rules that require individuals, manufacturers, and governments to comply with certain safety practices. Legislation is made by elected government bodies enacting laws that require safe practices. Regulations are made by bureaucracies or agencies that set policies and establish procedures that control the manufacture, sale, and/or use of products. Litigation sets policy when lawsuits are brought against manufacturers or distributors of dangerous products. For example, product liability litigation can encourage manufacturers to remove dangerous products from the market or make them safer. All these measures have been shown to be helpful in enforcement of safety regulations.

The Value of Automatic Protections

Passive interventions—those that do not require a conscious decision to act—are often the most successful of all interventions. This approach is also referred to as automatic protection. Examples include the use of sprinkler systems in commercial buildings, air bags in automobiles, or the use of softer, yielding materials for playground surfaces. These measures provide 24-hour protection without requiring a conscious action or decision on the part of the user.

Consider the following injury prevention strategies, comparing education to automatic protection, in the case of head and chest injuries of drivers in motor vehicle crashes:

- **Option 1.** Educate people to buckle up every time they drive.
- **Option 2.** Require that car manufacturers install automatic seat belts and air bags.

The automatic protection offered by option 2 is more likely to reduce injuries because people do not have to do anything to protect themselves each time they are at risk. Again, however, a combination of approaches—education, enforcement, engineering/environmental modifications, and economic incentives—will result in the most effective strategy.

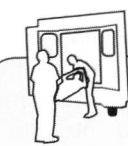

In the Field

The less the personal effort required, the greater the chance that the interventions will be successful.

Note that education is still an important aspect of the above examples. Motor vehicle passengers need to know that air bags do not replace the need for seat belts.

Models for Injury Prevention

A variety of visual models have been created to describe a health problem and how to approach it. The public health model identifies and seeks to control three factors: the host, the agent, and the environment. The public health model triumphed in the prevention and control of diseases such as malaria and polio, sometimes by attacking only two parts of the model. For example, to prevent malaria, you might develop a vaccine, spray pesticides to kill mosquitoes, and/or drain swamps to keep mosquitoes from breeding. These approaches target the host (people), the agent (mosquitoes), and the environment (swamps).

The public health model has been applied to a variety of injury problems. If you add the 4 Es of injury prevention, you can think through appropriate strategies for each part of the model (the host, the agent, and the environment). **Figure 3-8 ▶** sets out the three parts of the public health model using the example of bicycle-auto collisions.

The Haddon Matrix

William Haddon, Jr, MD, the National Highway Traffic Safety Administration's first director, had a mandate to find ways to prevent people from being killed and injured on the nation's highways. Haddon created a matrix that identified several principles of injury prevention. The matrix proved so successful in helping researchers think about injuries, that it was named after Haddon: the Haddon matrix.

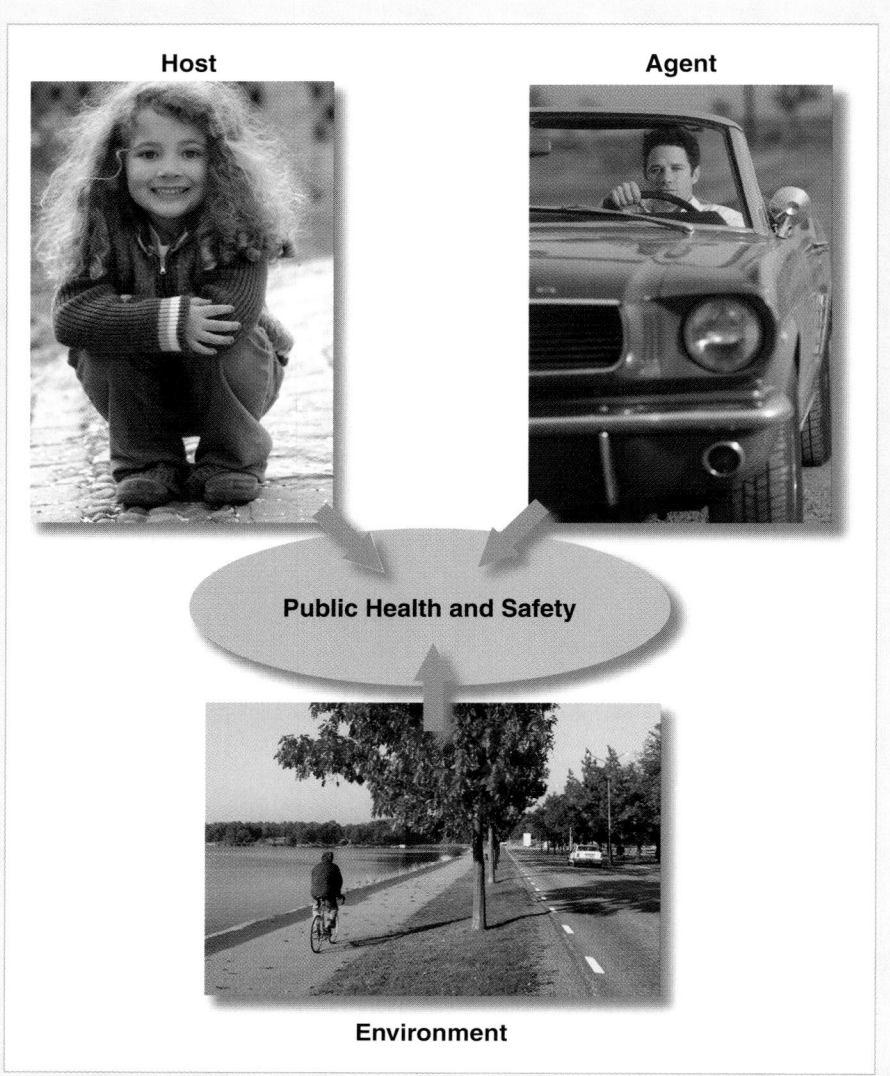

Figure 3-8 For bicycle-auto collisions, the public health model suggests the need to educate the child (*host*) and driver (*agent*) about safety, minimize the danger of serious injury through the required use of helmets, and perhaps create independent bike paths to separate children from traffic (*environment*).

Haddon added the factor of *time* to the previous models used to address the causes of injury. The host, agent, and environment are seen as factors that interact over time to cause injury. These factors correspond to three phases of the event: pre-event, event, and post-event. The matrix uses nine separate components to analyze the injury. The Haddon matrix encourages creative thinking in understanding the causes of and potential interventions for injury. **Table 3-2 ▶** shows a Haddon matrix for the example of bicycle-auto collisions.

Most EMS providers are trained to respond to the post-event—the period of time after an injury has already occurred. The 9-1-1 call is received by the emergency medical dispatcher who sends a service unit to the scene. There, the team members administer emergency care, a form of secondary intervention that can change the outcome, severity, or result of the event.

You can use the Haddon matrix to trigger your fellow EMS providers and others in the community to think about and plan for strategies before the 9-1-1 call comes through. The pre-event phase can get everyone brainstorming about everything that can be done to prevent an injury from occurring. The event phase can get all people involved thinking about interventions to minimize an injury at the time of the event. The post-event phase can address ways to lessen the severity of the injury once it has occurred.

Injury prevention requires broad and innovative thinking to be most successful. The Haddon matrix helps you to think through which interventions can be effective at certain points in time. Addressing injury prevention within the context of a timeline—pre-event, event, and post-event—can expand our problem-solving capabilities beyond the answer of more education.

Table 3-2	Childhood Motor Vehicle Occupant Injuries Using the Haddon Matrix		
	Host (Human)	**Agent (Car Seat/Vehicle)**	**Environment**
Pre-event	• Wear seat belt and use car seat at all times. • Make sure babysitter, day care, and extended family members use car seat. • Drive defensively. • Reduce driving during high-risk times, such as rush hour, holiday weekends, or high-speed long distance travel.	• Maintain up-to-date recall information on car seats. • Manufacture easy-to-use car seats. • Provide 3-point seat belts in rear seating positions. • Regulate good maintenance and safety features of vehicle.	• Enforce seat belt and car seat laws. • Encourage safer roads with lower speeds, breakaway poles, and medians. • Encourage low-cost car seat programs. • Conduct media and education campaigns about seat belts, car seats, drunk driving, and enforcement.
Event	• Driver maintains control of vehicle. • Driver is belted. • Child is restrained.	• Seat belts and correctly used car seats restrain and protect. • Vehicle design provides crash protection.	• Breakaway signs and light poles are in place. • Guardrails and medians are in place.
Post-event	• Bystanders are trained in first response. • EMS personnel are expertly trained in treating pediatric injuries as well as car seat and seat belt extrications.	• Ambulances are outfitted with up-to-date supplies and equipment designed for children.	• Roadside call boxes are in place. • 9-1-1 and emergency medical dispatch systems are in place. • Adequate road shoulders for emergency use are in place. • There is quality EMS response and transport. • A trauma center is nearby.

Blaming the parent for lack of supervision or the driver for going too fast does not generate solutions to the problem of childhood injury. You can generate solutions with physical and measurable attributes using the Haddon matrix as a guide.

Injury Surveillance

Surveillance in injury prevention does *not* mean watching over a criminal suspect! In injury prevention, it means watching over society by collecting and analyzing injury data. Injury surveillance is the ongoing, systematic collection, analysis, and interpretation of injury data essential to the planning, implementation, and evaluation of public health practice Figure 3-9 ▶ . These data are collected and then carefully disseminated to individuals or organizations who can use the data to affect change. The final link in the surveillance chain is the application of these data to interventions aimed at preventing injuries.

A strong surveillance system is fundamental to creating an effective injury prevention program. To do the most good, you

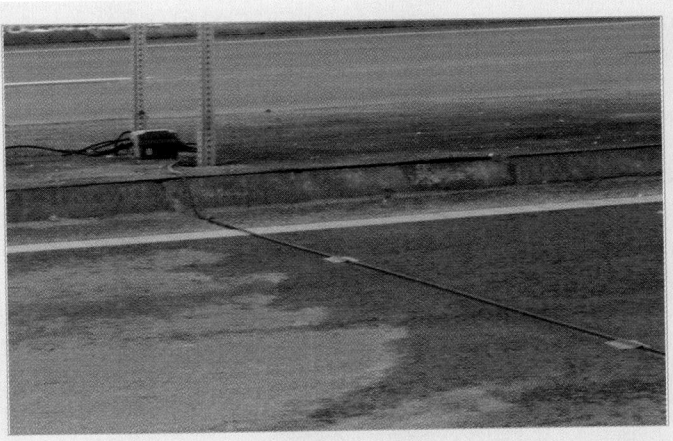

Figure 3-9 One type of surveillance that is familiar to anyone who drives is the use of technology that can tally the number of cars using a particular roadway.

need to know who is being injured, where, and by what mechanism. The news media may focus on a dramatic incident where a dozen people are severely injured, but surveillance data might show that a commonplace, but less newsworthy injury (such as falls among older people) is a greater threat to the community and more easily remedied. As part of the health system, paramedics need to triage their focus on injury prevention. Do not let the headlines be your guide.

Controversies

There is a theory that says if people keep falling off a mountain you should put a fence around the mountain to keep people from climbing it. Another theory says that you should tear down the mountain so that people can't fall off it. Yet another theory says that if you educate people on safe climbing you can prevent them from falling. Finally, there are some who believe an ambulance should be parked at the base of the mountain to save the people who keep falling. So goes the controversy of injury and potential interventions.

Getting Started in Your Community

An abundance of problems faces every community. Each community requires the assessment of the problems that are

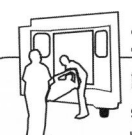

impairing the health of the largest number of people. Otherwise, you may be overwhelmed with the enormity of the task.

There is a good chance that, eventually, you can roll up your sleeves and dig in to remedy even the problems that arise from the social conditions causing some injuries. But it will give you and your community a good feeling to address a problem that will have the maximum impact on the community's well-being.

Recognizing Injury Patterns in Your Community

To be effective in prevention, you need to understand the patterns of injuries that occur in your community and learn the characteristics of its population and environment and the types of risks that are present. Your regional or state EMS department or public health office will have the most data about injury statistics and is a good starting place to gather information. Many states have this information on the Internet. There are a wide variety of other resources readily available online, including detailed information about specific problems, case studies, and expert assistance.

Intentional Injuries

Intentional injuries include suicides and suicide attempts, homicides, nonfatal batterings, violent assaults on women (including rapes and spousal abuse), and child and elder abuse.

Assaults are more likely to be fatal in the United States than in any other developed country `Figure 3-10 ▾`. In 1997

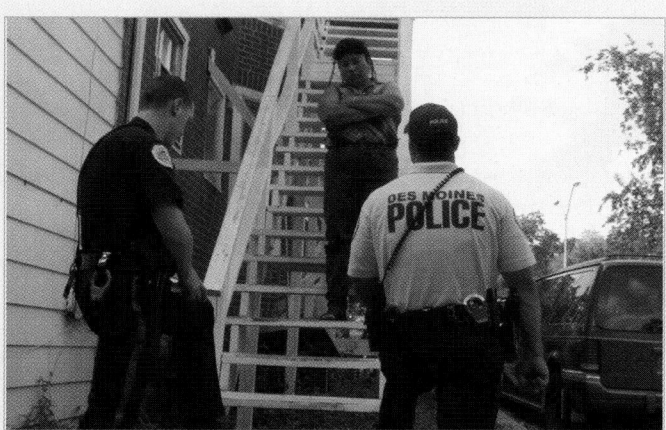

Figure 3-10 Intentional injuries include all cases of domestic and child abuse. As citizens and medical professionals, we are obligated to report all incidents of abuse or potentially abusive situations.

there were 19,491 homicides and 30,535 suicides. It is estimated there are nearly 7 million intentional injuries inflicted each year. Researchers are studying the causes of intentional violence in the United States. Certain factors emerge as numerically connected with intentional violence: being male, access to firearms, alcohol abuse, history of childhood abuse, mental illness, and poverty. These are all risk factors—characteristics that increase the chances of disease or injury.

It is often overwhelming to consider solutions when the challenges are linked to deeply rooted social ills. How can EMS personnel prevent intentional violence when it is clear that the scope of the problem is a wide one?

One way EMS providers have played important supporting roles in programs that seek to reduce suicide, domestic violence, and child abuse is by carefully reporting data and noting risk factors while on the scene. Also, EMS providers can be taught to identify injuries and risk factors associated with domestic violence or child abuse, and report them to the proper channels.

Remember, you are about to become a paramedic. What you do, your expectations of yourself, and your role will filter down to the other members of your crew. Being a conscientious observer will set an example.

Unintentional Injuries

Unintentional injuries have no premeditation; we often call them accidents. `Table 3-3 ▾` shows the top 10 causes of deaths from injury in 2001. Motor vehicle traffic incidents account for the most unintentional deaths (40%), followed by suicides by firearm, falls, poisonings, homicides by firearm, suffocations, and fires and burns. Almost all motor vehicle deaths are classified as unintentional.

Table 3-3	Top 10 Causes of Death From Injury in 2001
1. Unintentional motor vehicle traffic incidents	
2. Suicides by firearm	
3. Unintentional falls	
4. Unintentional poisonings	
5. Homicides by firearm	
6. Unintentional injuries, unspecified	
7. Suicides by suffocation	
8. Unintentional suffocations	
9. Suicides by poisoning	
10. Unintentional fires and burns	

Source: Adapted from National Center for Health Statistics/National Vital Statistics Systems, 2001.

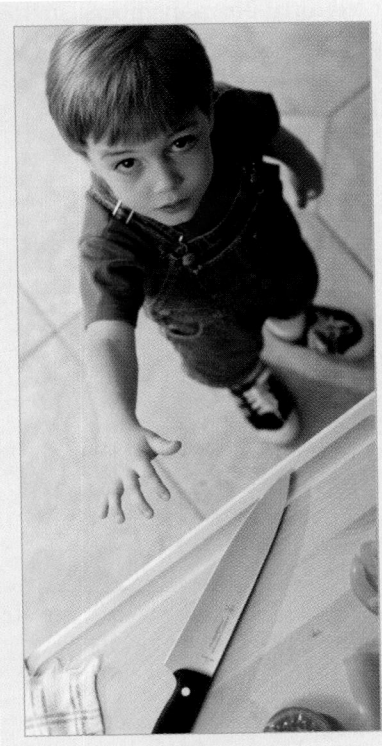

Figure 3-11 Children are at higher risk of sustaining serious injuries from an accident. Parents should always be aware of the potential dangers in reach of a child.

Unintentional Injuries in Children

Many prevention programs have been strongly linked to children, for good reason. Each year 20% to 25% of *all* children sustain an injury sufficiently severe to require medical attention, miss school, and/or require bed rest. Their developing bodies, including a larger head in proportion to the body, thinner skin, and a smaller airway, put them at higher risk of injury and of being more seriously affected by the injury than adults. Each year more than 14 million injured children require medical treatment **Figure 3-11** ◂ .

Grants, partners, and commercial sponsors support car seat inspections or donations of bike helmets for children because communities recognize that children are at risk. An additional reason to focus on children's issues is the "pass-along effect." Other family members benefit from the message too, such as when a third-grader insists that Daddy buckle up too.

EMS for Children (EMSC) is a federal initiative that provides millions of dollars in funding to a wide variety of prevention and research programs. The National Safe Kids Campaign has more than 260 coalitions in all 50 states dedicated to reducing childhood injuries. Both have excellent web sites, easily found by looking up their names in a search engine.

Risk Factors for Children

Children at greatest risk of injury are of lower socioeconomic status. The patterns of injury will differ from community to community, but just as the poorest children statistically are at risk of contracting a physiologic disease, they are also at risk of injury.

The CDC reports that home injuries of children occur most frequently where there is/are:

- Water, such as in the kitchen or bathroom, or a backyard swimming pool.
- Intense heat, such as in the kitchen or a backyard barbecue.
- Toxic agents, such as in the kitchen, bathroom, garage, or in a purse.
- High potential "energy," such as in stairwells or loaded firearms.

Many community members have a common belief that schools have become more violent and that intentional injuries are an increasing threat to students. However, *unintentional* injuries—accidents—still represent a much greater threat to health.

School injuries occur most frequently during sports activities, industrial arts classes, and on playgrounds. Each year about 200,000 preschool and elementary children have injuries while playing on playgrounds.

With the wide variety of injuries affecting children, how do we prioritize prevention efforts? Experts in public health suggest focusing on injuries that have high mortality (death) rates or hospitalization rates, that have a high long-term disability rate, or that have effective countermeasures. The highest priorities are assigned to those types of injuries that are common, severe, and readily preventable.

Community Organizing

Those in EMS who have created successful prevention programs give the following advice as you build your team and create an implementation plan:

- Identify a lead person to coordinate the effort.
- Build as broad a base of support as possible.
- Create a realistic time line for any project, keeping in mind that most must be ongoing to be effective.
- Gather data and facts that pinpoint who is being injured where, with what, and how frequently.
- Choose goals and objectives that are SMART—Simple, Measurable, Accurate, Reportable, and Trackable; build consensus in the community on the need for action.
- Make sure you understand the religious, ethnic, cultural, and language challenges that you may face in implementing an intervention.
- Don't reinvent the wheel—seek out others who have had success with similar interventions or who have expertise in public health.
- Anticipate opposition and expect some losses; turf battles are common but not inevitable.

You are the Provider Part 3

You have enlisted the help of many different organizations who are now as determined as you are to minimize the recurrence of crashes in this stretch of road. They aid you in performing assessments of the area and making plans to prevent crashes.

5. What groups are potential partners to enlist in a prevention program in this situation?

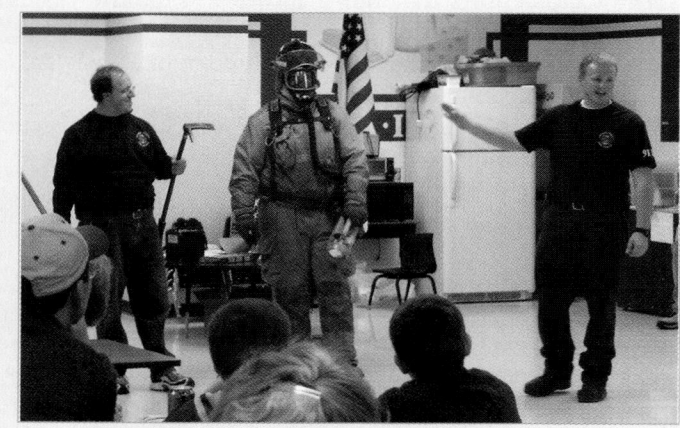

Figure 3-12 An example of an injury prevention program is training to avoid injury in the event of a fire in the home.

- As you lobby to legislators, be brief in phone calls, visits, and testimony.
- Set up your program so that you can measure results and make changes as needed.
- Establish self-sustaining funding sources.
- Keep a sense of humor and persist—change doesn't happen overnight.

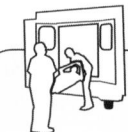

In the Field

For your first project, start small with realistic goals.

The Five Steps to Developing a Prevention Program

This step-by-step approach to establishing an injury prevention program, as advocated by the EMSC program, emphasizes the need to carefully establish goals and objectives, with measurable outcomes. (Although the following discusses childhood prevention programs, the methods can be applied to other age groups and their problems.)

1. Conduct a Community Assessment

Bring individuals and groups together to assess what is already being accomplished in your region and to establish what resources (expertise, time, money) are potentially available. Make sure to invite people who represent the community at large, in all its diversity, including survivors of injuries and their families **Figure 3-12 ▲** . Potential partners include:

- EMS groups (private and public ground and air ambulance services, fire departments and fire fighter unions, volunteer services, rescue squads, lifeguards)
- Law enforcement (police departments and police officers, unions, sheriff's office, highway patrol, training academies)
- School groups (parent-teacher associations, student clubs, school boards, faculty)

- The media (management, editorial board members, staff reporters)
- Public health officials and health care providers (groups representing emergency physicians and nurses, pediatricians, managed care organizations, hospitals, clinics)
- Members of the business community (including those related to insurance, cars, sports, home improvements, safety equipment, local chambers of commerce)
- Religious organizations, civic groups, and service clubs (such as the Kiwanis and the Boy Scouts and Girl Scouts)
- Sports-related organizations (such as Little Leagues or YMCAs)
- Local chapters of nonprofit groups (such as SAFE KIDS Coalitions, Mothers Against Drunk Driving [MADD], the American Red Cross, the American Alzheimer's Association)
- Local and national celebrities, community leaders, and elected officials
- Research groups (such as those at state universities, private colleges, community colleges)

2. Define the Injury Problem

On the basis of the community assessment and the data you've been able to gather, define the problem in specific quantifiable terms. For example, you should be able to answer the following questions for your community:

- What are the most frequent causes of fatal and nonfatal childhood injuries?
- What populations (by age, location, and other characteristics) are at highest risk of these injuries? When and where are they occurring?
- Using the Haddon matrix, what other factors are associated with these causes?
- What, if anything, is already being done to prevent these injuries?
- Is there an effective intervention available? What resources do you have in order to develop, implement, and evaluate different interventions?

3. Set Goals and Objectives

Goals Make this a broad, general statement about the long-term changes the prevention initiatives are designed to make. (For example, a goal can be to decrease preventable injuries to children on the community's roadways.)

Objectives Make these specific, time-limited, and quantifiable. There are two types: process objectives (1,000 child safety seats will be distributed to low income families within the next 18 months) and outcome (impact) objectives (the bicycle safety program will increase the rate of helmet use by children younger than 18 years from 30% to 50% within the next 18 months).

4. Plan and Test Interventions

Interventions are the actions you take to accomplish your goals and objectives. Using the 4 Es of prevention and the Haddon matrix, brainstorm options. Consider the resources you have available to commit, and make sure you have thoroughly reviewed what others have already done. You may find communities have had success with similar interventions in similar populations. In that case, you can reliably duplicate their efforts as a process objective. (For example, other groups have shown that bike helmets reduce head injuries; you then need only to demonstrate increased usage of helmets in your targeted population.) Experienced prevention specialists also suggest that you be keenly aware of timing and cultural considerations as you plan your intervention. Getting a sample group together and testing the intervention before actually rolling out the entire program usually helps to improve your chances of success.

5. Implement and Evaluate Interventions

To be credible, your intervention needs to be established so that the results can be measured quantitatively; that is, a formal evaluation will definitely tell you whether you met your goals and objectives. One EMS group knew from previous surveys that the seat belt usage rate in their community was well below the national average. They established an objective of improving seat belt usage in their community by 50%. Working with the department of public health in their state, they enacted a series of prevention programs. To measure the effectiveness of different interventions, they put volunteers at selected intersections around the city. They physically counted with a clicker every belted and nonbelted motorist who stopped in front of them. This is extremely important so that your experience can be shared with others. You want to spend your time and resources on efforts you can *show* make a difference. There is a science to planning, implementing, and evaluating an intervention. Seek out others who have knowledge and experience in this facet of injury prevention; it will make for a better program.

Finally, be aware that many if not most interventions demand ongoing attention to be effective. Those EMS providers who had initial success in reducing backyard drownings saw the numbers go back up a few years after the initial burst of publicity and after enthusiasm for the interventions began to wane. Legislation to fence pools worked well but did not eliminate the problem. They had to gear back up to reestablish the educational interventions that had worked so well originally. Consider building long-term maintenance into any plan to continue the momentum of your program.

Funding a Prevention Program

Ideally, emergency services should have the resources and motivation to include primary prevention activities in their normal operating budget. As a relatively new expansion of the EMS mission, this likely will take time. But motivated services and individuals have found a variety of innovative ways to secure resources including:

- Partnering with the local media to create prevention messages, especially related to seasonal injuries or hazards.
- Seeking grants from regional, state, or national organizations, such as the EMSC program. (A good place to start is to contact your state EMS office about grant programs.)

- Seeking sponsorships from local nonprofit service organizations or commercial firms, including fire, EMS, and Kiwanis organizations, and car dealerships **Figure 3-13 ▶**.

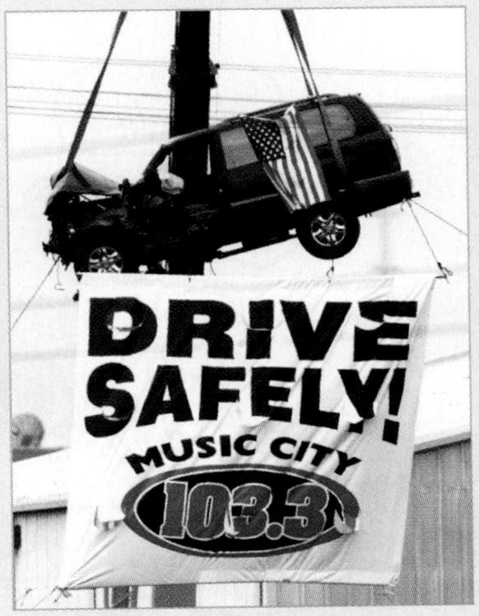

Networking with other organizations interested in prevention often provides greater leverage in seeking grants or sponsorships. Perhaps the EMS provider donates the time of volunteers and is a credible voice in the community, whereas the partner provides organizational resources and knowledge about establishing a scientifically credible injury intervention.

Figure 3-13 Like any successful ad campaign, a public safety program needs to continually remind the public of its message.

How Every Provider Can Be Involved

Taking care of patients is the number one job of paramedics. Some won't have the time or inclination to get involved in every aspect of the primary injury prevention measures discussed here. However, there are certain things paramedics can and should do, starting with preventing their own injuries.

Primary injury prevention begins at home, so to speak, by taking care of yourself and at the same time presenting a role model for others in your service and for the community in general. Do you always wear seatbelts, on and off duty? Do you drive safely? Have you prepared yourself physically for the rigors of the job? Do you practice safe lifting techniques? Do you always wear appropriate protective equipment? Do you always maintain scene safety? Your employer will have policies regarding many of these safety issues, but it's up to you to implement them and to take seriously the risks you face everyday on and off the job. Refer back to Chapter 2 to review the appropriate use of personal protective equipment and practices.

Responding to the Call

Perhaps the most ironic, if not most tragic, of all injuries are those caused when an ambulance collides with another vehicle while speeding to a scene, only to find out later the original call was not serious or even one requiring transport. Studies have shown that very few calls demand the use of siren and lights, and many departments now require all ambulances to stop at every stop sign or red light *on every call,* and to maintain strict speed control **Figure 3-14 ▶**. Prioritized dispatch systems using certified EMS dispatchers can provide sophisticated

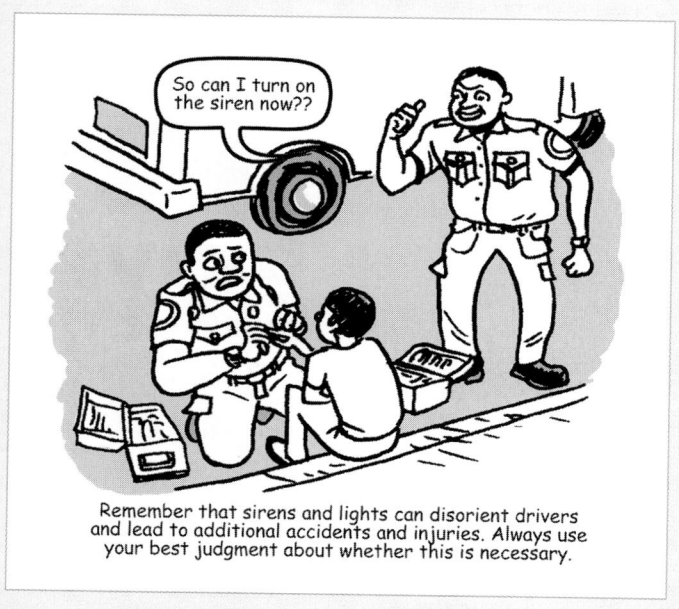

"So can I turn on the siren now??"

Remember that sirens and lights can disorient drivers and lead to additional accidents and injuries. Always use your best judgment about whether this is necessary.

Figure 3-14

assessments of the need for different levels of response and can improve scene safety while reducing the need for unnecessary responses.

You can provide leadership within your own department for primary injury prevention by advocating policies or equipment that provide a safer environment or initiatives such as an EMS wellness program. At the same time, you can be a role model by how you personally approach the multitude of decisions you face each day regarding the risks of injury. It is impossible to be a credible advocate for injury prevention if you don't practice what you preach.

Education for EMS Providers

Every EMS provider should understand the fundamentals of injury prevention. This can easily be the focus of a continuing education program. Some states sponsor injury prevention workshops geared specifically to EMS providers. Contact your state EMS office to see if a workshop can be scheduled for your area, or contact your local public health office to see what training resources it might have available. There are also

excellent self-paced courses and additional information available online.

The "Teachable Moment"

You're on the scene at the site of a collision between two vehicles. The injuries aren't serious, and you notice one of the passengers wasn't wearing a seatbelt. As you prepare him for transport, you look him in the eye and say, "You were very lucky this time . . . the other vehicle didn't hit you square. I've seen plenty of very bad injuries from collisions less serious than this. You really need to wear your seatbelt *every* time you get in the car. It'll save your life."

This was a teachable moment. Educators tell us that there are times when we are more receptive to accepting advice than others. A near-miss like this makes people realize their vulnerability and the true risk of their behavior—and the lesson is more likely to stick. The EMS provider is in the perfect position to articulate and reinforce this message. However, you must use good judgment and be sensitive to the situation. Lecturing a parent immediately after a child has been seriously injured is not going to be effective. What makes a teachable moment?

- The injuries are such that the parents, companions, or the patients themselves will be receptive to the message; you're aware of how ethnic and religious differences must temper the message.
- The scene is conducive to delivering such a message in a nonthreatening, nonjudgmental way. You're not intruding inappropriately or causing embarrassment that could lead to the opposite reaction.
- There is a definitive prevention measure that could have helped, such as using a seatbelt, correct installation of a car seat, wearing a helmet, or keeping firearms locked and safe. Vague advice is less likely to have a lasting effect.

Collection and Analysis of Data

In the opening paragraph of this chapter, we referred to data about backyard drownings. The importance of collecting data in measuring trends, validating interventions, assessing resources, and ultimately persuading others to act cannot be overestimated. For the EMS provider, this process starts with the prehospital care report, often approached as a necessary evil by many in the field. Standardized coding of incidents is

You are the Provider Part 4

Much to your disappointment, you are dispatched to the same familiar stretch of road for another motor vehicle crash. Because of your hard work and successful changes to local protocol, members of the flight crew are simultaneously dispatched, and will land in the designated landing zone unless you cancel their response. You arrive to find one male patient who has suffered head injuries and has an altered level of consciousness. You successfully extricate the patient, take spinal precautions, and successfully initiate IVs as well as endotracheal intubation. Just as you finish securing the endotracheal tube, the flight team arrives and now assumes patient care efforts. The patient is flown to a nearby trauma center where his head injuries are successfully treated. He makes a full recovery.

6. What other common types of injuries can be easily avoided?

7. Some might question your obligation to this issue. What is your response?

In the Field

The best teachable moments are those that convey positive reinforcement. If people are wearing seat belts properly and survive a collision with little or no injuries, tell them, "It's a good thing you had your seatbelts on." You will notice smiles on their faces and they will remember your statement forever.

required to collect useful data from far-flung sources. By accurately (and legibly) describing the details of the scene, the external mechanism of injury, the nature of the injury, and the use or absence of protective devices, EMS providers can supply important evidence of the scope of a problem and help in monitoring trends.

As a prevention advocate, assess your current prehospital care report to see if it can be modified to be a better tool. Are there ways for the information to be gathered more quickly? Can the information put into a computerized database be promptly updated, easily accessed, and searched? Get involved in local, state, or national database systems. Often, much information is being gathered, but agencies aren't consistent or timely in the process, aren't sharing data, or don't have it on a common database. For the injury prevention field, the accurate and timely col-

lection of data is critically important. In EMS, our goal is to put resources into those prevention interventions that can do the most good. This requires documenting injuries and monitoring trends that can be tied to the effects of interventions.

Conclusion

Injury prevention is a complex but rewarding field. Many veteran EMS providers have embraced a leadership role in primary prevention after witnessing too many episodes of needless suffering. These leaders recognize their unique role and use their positions to support interventions that make a difference. In their own lives and in their workplace, every EMS provider should be proactive in primary injury prevention, whether reducing the odds of a back injury by keeping fit, using proper lifting techniques and protective gear, or taking advantage of a teachable moment with a patient.

Many extend this interest further, reaching out in their communities to become involved as leaders or supporters of a wide variety of prevention programs. They find personal satisfaction and professional fulfillment in the challenge of learning a new field, interacting with a new set of colleagues, and reducing the suffering of those they serve.

You are the Provider Summary

1. Why should you consider getting involved in preventing these injuries?

EMS providers should be patient advocates. If you can aid the general public in the prevention of foreseeable injuries, it is your duty to intervene.

2. What are the risk factors associated with the injuries described here?

Risk factors include driving under the influence, failure to use seat belts, and the age and sex of the driver (as young men typically drive faster and more aggressively than their female and older male counterparts).

3. Which law enforcement agencies could you contact?

The state patrol, county sheriff's office, and other local law enforcement agencies are all appropriate to contact. They will likely have prevention programs and vehicle accident experts on staff who may assist you in minimizing motor vehicle crashes on this stretch of road.

4. Who else might be able to help you in assessing road conditions?

The Department of Transportation and the National Highway Traffic Safety Administration are also appropriate agencies to contact.

5. What groups are potential partners to enlist in a prevention program in this situation?

You might also consider contacting other service groups in your community who have a desire to combat drunk driving such as MADD and other organizations.

6. What other common types of injuries can be easily avoided?

Injuries involving children, including vehicle crashes and bicycle-related trauma, are also common. There are many programs already designed to target these audiences (for example, dispensing free car seats to new parents and donating bike helmets to children, for those who cannot afford to buy them).

7. Some might question your obligation to this issue. What is your response?

Most people become involved in emergency services because they have a strong desire to help others. As a paramedic, you are responsible to your patients and your community. You should serve as an advocate for those people who cannot care for themselves. This is just another way to perform this service and to have a positive impact on the citizens you serve.

Prep Kit

Ready for Review

- Many paramedics have been motivated by their field experience to work actively on injury prevention.
- The 1966 National Academy of Sciences/National Research Council study, "Accidental Death and Disability: The Neglected Disease of Modern Society," noted that EMS could help with trauma after an event, and injury prevention could help prevent an accident before it happens.
- The 1996 *Consensus Statement on the EMS Role in Primary Injury Prevention* emphasized that primary injury prevention is an essential activity of EMS.
- EMS can play a supporting role in preventing intentional injuries and can have an even larger impact in preventing unintentional injuries.
- The years of potential life lost concept is another way to measure the cost of unintentional injury to society. It assumes that an average productive work life continues for 65 years. The age of death is deducted from 65, leaving the years of potential life lost.
- The 4 Es of injury prevention are:
  - Education
  - Enforcement
  - Engineering/environment
  - Economic incentives
- Automatic protections do not include a conscious decision to act and include air bags in automobiles.
- The Haddon matrix uses nine separate components to analyze injury. It encourages creative thinking in understanding the causes and potential interventions for injury.
- Injury surveillance is the ongoing systematic collection, analysis, and interpretation of injury data essential to the planning, implementation, and evaluation of public health practice.
- Paramedics need to triage their focus on injury prevention—do not let the headlines be your guide.
- The five steps to developing a prevention program are:
  - Conduct a community assessment.
  - Define the injury problem.
  - Set goals and objectives.
  - Plan and test interventions.
  - Implement and evaluate interventions.
- Primary injury prevention begins at home by taking care of yourself and presenting a role model for others in your service and in the community.
- The best teachable moments are those that convey positive reinforcement.
- The importance of collecting data in measuring trends, validating interventions, assessing resources, and ultimately persuading others to act cannot be overestimated.

Vital Vocabulary

evaluation Collection of the methods, skills, and activities necessary to determine whether a service or program is needed, likely to be used, conducted as planned, and actually helps people.

goals The end points toward which intervention efforts are directed. A statement of changes sought in an injury problem, stated in broad terms.

Haddon matrix A framework developed by William Haddon, Jr, MD as a method to generate ideas about injury prevention that address the host, agent, and environment and their impact in the pre-event, event, and post-event phases of the injury process.

implementation plan A strategy for carrying out an intervention. Includes goals, objectives, activities, evaluation measures, resource assessment, and time line.

injuries Any unintentional or intentional damage to the body resulting from acute exposure to thermal, mechanical, electrical, or chemical energy or from the absence of such essentials as heat or oxygen.

injury risk A potentially hazardous situation that puts people in a position in which they could be harmed.

injury surveillance The ongoing systematic collection, analysis, and interpretation of injury data essential to the planning, implementation, and evaluation of public health practice.

intentional injuries Injuries that are purposefully inflicted by a person on himself or herself or on another person. Examples include suicide or attempted suicide, homicide, rape, assault, domestic abuse, elder abuse, and child abuse.

interventions Specific prevention measures or activities designed to meet a program objective. Categories include education/behavior change, enforcement/legislation, engineering/technology, and economic incentives.

morbidity Number of nonfatally injured or disabled people. Usually expressed as a rate, meaning the number of nonfatal injuries in a certain population in a given time period divided by the size of the population.

mortality Deaths caused by injury and disease. Usually expressed as a rate, meaning the number of deaths in a certain population in a given time period divided by the size of the population.

objectives Specific, time-limited, and quantifiable statements that summarize an expected result of an intervention.

outcome (impact) objectives State the intended effect of the program on participants or on the community in such terms as the participants' increased knowledge, changed behaviors or attitudes, or decreased injury rates.

passive interventions Something that offers automatic protection from injury, often without requiring any conscious change of behavior by the individual; child-resistant bottles and air bags are some examples.

primary injury prevention Keeping an injury from occurring.

process objectives State how a program will be implemented, describing the service to be provided, the nature of the service, and to whom it will be directed.

risk factors Characteristics of people, behaviors, or environments that increase the chances of disease or injury. Some examples are alcohol use, poverty, or gender.

secondary injury prevention Reducing the effects of an injury that has already happened.

unintentional injuries Injuries that occur without intent to harm (commonly called accidents). Some examples are motor vehicle crashes, poisonings, drownings, falls, and most burns.

years of potential life lost A way of measuring and comparing the overall impact of deaths resulting from different causes. It is calculated based on a fixed age minus the age at death. Usually the fixed age is 65 or 70 or the life expectancy of the group in question.

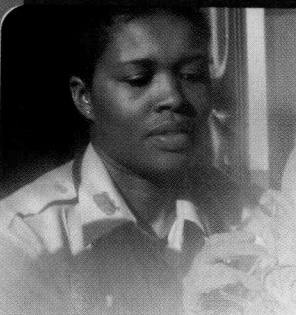

Assessment in Action

Each year, more than 110 million injuries will be serious enough for the injured person to seek medical care through EMS or an emergency department. There are several things, besides treating injuries, that the paramedic can do to cut down on the number of injuries sustained each year. There is also information about injuries that is important for all paramedics to know. The following questions concern the information that is important to know, and what things paramedics and other health care professionals can do to cut down on the number of injuries sustained each year.

1. **Paramedics are responsible for many duties. However, what is the number one priority of paramedics in their community?**
   A. To be ready to stop and help, whether off duty or on duty.
   B. To be prepared to respond and treat injuries that will inevitably occur in their community.
   C. To make sure their skills are always up-to-date.
   D. To make sure they are good role models in their community.

2. **Injuries are defined by the National Center for Injury Prevention and Control as:**
   A. intentional or unintentional.
   B. resulting from exposure to thermal, mechanical, electrical, or chemical energy.
   C. resulting from the absence of essentials such as heat or oxygen.
   D. all of the above.

3. **One way to measure the cost of injuries to society and the full impact of injury and disease is by using the concept of years of potential life lost. This means:**
   A. assume a productive life until age 65 years for all people, then deduct the year of age at death.
   B. estimate how long that person would have lived given his or her socioeconomic background and genetic makeup, then subtract that number from his or her age at death.
   C. factor in all the patient's health issues at the time of death and estimate how long he or she may have lived based on that information.
   D. compare the cost to society of injuries versus other diseases.

4. **The most successful interventions need to combine education with three other factors. What are they?**
   A. Enforcement, persuasion, modeling of safe behavior
   B. Legislation, litigation, regulation
   C. Regulatory change, behavioral feedback, economic incentives
   D. Enforcement, engineering/environment, economic incentives

5. **The public health model identifies three influences that cause a health problem. What are they?**
   A. Disease, heredity, lifestyle
   B. Host, agent, environment
   C. Accidents, homicides, suicides
   D. Noneducation, bad lifestyle choices, not using safety measures such as seat belts

6. **A doctor developed a method to help find ways to prevent people from being killed on highways. He identified several principles of injury prevention and summarized them in a matrix. The host, agent, and environment are seen as factors that interact over time to cause injury. The factors correspond to three phases of the event: pre-event, event, post-event. The matrix discusses nine separate components that contribute to injury. This matrix encourages creative thinking in understanding injury causes and potential interventions. Who was this person, and what is the matrix called?**
   A. William Haddon, Jr, MD; the Haddon matrix
   B. Paul Maxwell; the Maxwell matrix
   C. Ricardo Martinez, MD; the Martinez matrix
   D. Frank Holden; the Holden matrix

7. **Passive interventions in preventing injuries are things such as:**
   A. making seat belt use a law and adding guardrails to certain roads.
   B. putting safety caps on medicine bottles and putting air bags in cars.
   C. offering monetary discounts for safe driving records.
   D. offering educational classes such as CPR and safe babysitting classes often.

Challenging Questions

8. **You are given the statistics for accidental falls in your town, and asked to develop a plan that may reduce the number of falls, given your experience as a paramedic. What are some ideas you can come up with to help reduce the number of falls in your area in the upcoming year?**

9. **What could you and other health care professionals do to decrease the number of people in your area who contract diseases such as chickenpox, tuberculosis (TB), hepatitis, and influenza?**

Points to Ponder

For the fourth time in 3 weeks, you are called to a specific place on a winding highway for a one-car accident. There are no streetlights on this highway, no reflectors to help drivers see how winding it is, and the speed limit is 45 mph.

What can you do to try to prevent further accidents on this particular stretch of highway?

Issues: Personal Commitment to Prevention, Valuing Personal Safety and Wellness, Teaching Prevention in Your Community.

4

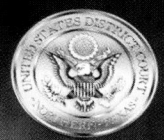

Medical and Legal Issues

Objectives

Cognitive

1-4.1   Differentiate between legal and ethical responsibilities. (p 4.3)

1-4.2   Describe the basic structure of the legal system in the United States. (p 4.4)

1-4.3   Differentiate between civil and criminal law as it pertains to the paramedic. (p 4.4)

1-4.4   Identify and explain the importance of laws pertinent to the paramedic. (p 4.6)

1-4.5   Differentiate between licensure and certification as they apply to the paramedic. (p 4.12)

1-4.6   List the specific problems or conditions encountered while providing care that a paramedic is required to report, and identify in each instance to whom the report is to be made. (p 4.18)

1-4.7   Define the following terms:
- a. Abandonment
- b. Advance directives
- c. Assault
- d. Battery
- e. Breach of duty
- f. Confidentiality
- g. Consent (expressed, implied, informed, involuntary)
- h. Do not resuscitate (DNR) orders
- i. Duty to act
- j. Emancipated minor
- k. False imprisonment
- l. Immunity
- m. Liability
- n. Libel
- o. Minor
- p. Negligence
- q. Proximate cause
- r. Scope of practice
- s. Slander
- t. Standard of care
- u. Tort (p 4.4–4.15)

1-4.8   Differentiate between the scope of practice and the standard of care for paramedic practice. (p 4.7)

1-4.9   Discuss the concept of medical direction, including off-line medical direction and online medical direction, and its relationship to the standard of care of a paramedic. (p 4.7)

1-4.10   Describe the four elements that must be present in order to prove negligence. (p 4.10)

1-4.11   Given a scenario in which a patient is injured while a paramedic is providing care, determine whether the four components of negligence are present. (p 4.10)

1-4.12   Given a scenario, demonstrate patient care behaviors that would protect the paramedic from claims of negligence. (p 4.10)

1-4.13   Explain the concept of liability as it might apply to paramedic practice, including physicians providing medical direction and paramedic supervision of other care providers. (p 4.6)

1-4.14   Discuss the legal concept of immunity, including Good Samaritan statutes and governmental immunity, as it applies to the paramedic. (p 4.9)

1-4.15   Explain the importance and necessity of patient confidentiality and the standards for maintaining patient confidentiality that apply to the paramedic. (p 4.13)

1-4.16   Differentiate among expressed, informed, implied, and involuntary consent. (p 4.14)

1-4.17   Given a scenario in which a paramedic is presented with a conscious patient in need of care, describe the process used to obtain consent. (p 4.14)

1-4.18   Identify the steps to take if a patient refuses care. (p 4.15)

1-4.19   Given a scenario, demonstrate appropriate patient management and care techniques in a refusal of care situation. (p 4.15)

1-4.20   Describe what constitutes abandonment. (p 4.12)

1-4.21   Identify the legal issues involved in the decision not to transport a patient, or to reduce the level of care being provided during transportation. (p 4.12)

1-4.22   Describe how hospitals are selected to receive patients based on patient need and hospital capability and the role of the paramedic in such selection. (p 4.8)

1-4.23   Differentiate between assault and battery and describe how to avoid each. (p 4.5)

1-4.24   Describe the conditions under which the use of force, including restraint, is acceptable. (p 4.16)

1-4.25   Explain the purpose of advance directives relative to patient care and how the paramedic should care for a patient who is covered by an advance directive. (p 4.12)

1-4.26   Discuss the responsibilities of the paramedic relative to resuscitation efforts for patients who are potential organ donors. (p 4.12)

1-4.27   Describe the actions that the paramedic should take to preserve evidence at a crime or accident scene. (p 4.18)

1-4.28   Describe the importance of providing accurate documentation (oral and written) in substantiating an incident. (p 4.18)

1-4.29   Describe the characteristics of a patient care report required to make it an effective legal document. (p 4.18)

1-4.30   Given a scenario, prepare a patient care report, including an appropriately detailed narrative. (p 4.18)

Affective

1-4.31   Advocate the need to show respect for the rights and feelings of patients. (p 4.13)

1-4.32   Assess his/her personal commitment to protecting patient confidentiality. (p 4.13)

1-4.33   Given a scenario involving a new employee, explain the importance of obtaining consent for adults and minors. (p 4.14)

1-4.34   Defend personal beliefs about withholding or stopping patient care. (p 4.11)

1-4.35   Defend the value of advance medical directives. (p 4.12)

Psychomotor

None

Introduction

All medical providers provide care under laws—like many human activities in a democracy. When you become a paramedic, you, too, will be governed by a set of laws affecting how you must treat patients. Your ethical responsibilities, which will be discussed in Chapter 5, differ from legal obligations. Ethics are principles, personal or societal, that determine what is right and wrong. One of the major differences between law and ethics is that laws have sanctions for violation that are enforceable **Figure 4-1 ▼**. Laws define our obligations and protect our rights and the rights of others. A paramedic responding to an emergency works within a framework of several types of laws that are set down by either (or both) the federal government or the state government:

- Motor vehicle laws for the operation of an emergency vehicle
- EMS legislation
- Medical licensing statutes and regulations
- Civil and criminal statutes about touching, treating, transporting, and possibly injuring another person

It is essential, therefore, that the paramedic have a basic understanding of laws applicable to prehospital emergency care. Failing to perform the job within the law can result in civil liability (malpractice suits against EMS providers are increasing) or even criminal liability. It may also result in regulatory action within your state—a disciplinary hearing, for example—or action by your agency and medical director.

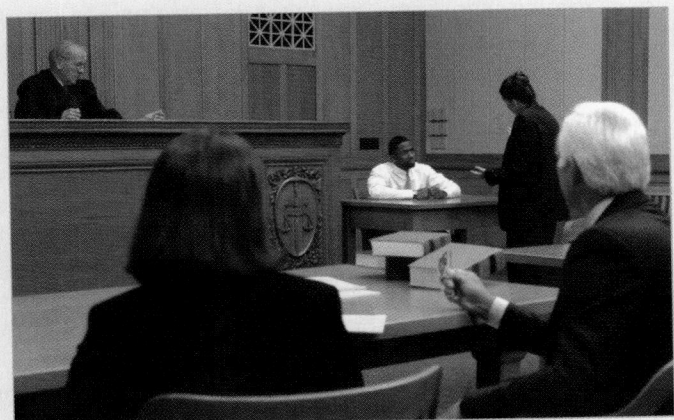

Figure 4-1 Unlike ethics, laws are enforceable rules that all citizens are obliged to follow. Paramedics are sometimes called into court to testify and provide evidence regarding cases under investigation or that are being litigated.

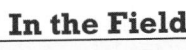
In the Field

Without question, the best legal protection is to provide a careful, detailed patient assessment and appropriate medical care, followed by complete and accurate documentation.

In this chapter, we shall review the more important legal concepts affecting the paramedic. However, this text is only a framework to help your understanding. It cannot substitute for competent legal advice because many laws and legal obligations will differ from state to state. Contact an attorney who specializes in the representation of medical professionals if you need legal advice related to your practice.

You are the Provider Part 1

You are dispatched to an unknown medical problem at a nearby private residence. As you arrive, the patient's wife greets you at the door. She tells you that her husband is a diabetic and that "his sugar must be low." She tells you that he is in the basement and refuses to come upstairs to have something to eat.

As you walk down the basement stairs, you see a 45-year-old man with his back toward you. You call out his name and tell him you are here because his wife is worried that his blood sugar is low. He doesn't acknowledge you. As you attempt to walk in front of him to get eye contact, he takes a swing at you. Unfortunately, you are forced to defend yourself by attempting to restrain the patient. Your partner tries to assist you while simultaneously calling for law enforcement.

Initial Assessment	Recording Time: 0 Minutes
Appearance	Back to you, shoulders raised, fists clenched
Level of consciousness	Conscious
Airway	Open
Breathing	Rapid and deep
Circulation	Unable to assess; patient is combative

1. List the clues that were available to tip you off as to the potential for this patient to become violent.
2. What would be the best course of action at this point?

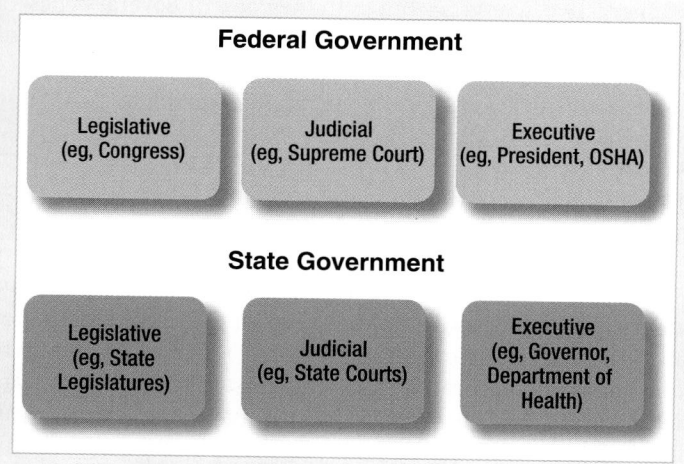

Federal Government

| Legislative (eg, Congress) | Judicial (eg, Supreme Court) | Executive (eg, President, OSHA) |

State Government

| Legislative (eg, State Legislatures) | Judicial (eg, State Courts) | Executive (eg, Governor, Department of Health) |

Figure 4-2 Both federal and state governments enact and review legislation that is specific to paramedics and their practice.

In the Field

Many state EMS offices have web sites with information on laws that affect first responders, EMTs, and paramedics. It is a good idea to review the laws of the state in which you are working.

The Legal System in the United States

Although many of our laws are derived from English common law, we have both federal (the big people in Washington, DC) and state governments (the folks in your state capital) who make, administer, and interpret laws that affect paramedics.

There are three branches of government at each level **Figure 4-2 ▲** . The legislative branch, made up of elected officials (Congress at the federal level; state legislatures at the state level), actually make the laws. The judicial branch (consisting of the court system) enforces and interprets laws, and resolves disputes based on interpretation of laws. Courts have a number of levels as well, including trial courts and appellate courts.

The third branch—the executive or administrative branch—reports to the president (in Washington, DC) or the governor (in your state capital) and is made up of various cabinets and agencies (the bureaucrats) that carry out and administer the laws. The agencies often use regulations to establish how things should be done. Agencies such as the Occupational Safety and Health Administration (OSHA) at the federal level, and the Department of Health at the state level, are examples of parts of the administrative branch.

All states now have some type of enabling EMS legislation that sets out the framework for the EMS system. In addition, there may be administrative regulations that are set forth by state agencies or county governments that regulate the practice of paramedics. It is vital for paramedics to know and understand the laws and administrative regulations that affect their practice in their home state.

Types of Law

Two kinds of law govern paramedics in court: civil law, under which a patient can sue you for a perceived injury, and criminal law, in which the state will prosecute for breaking a legal statute. Malpractice suits are tried under civil law; many misuses of drugs will be tried under criminal law.

A substantial part of civil law is concerned with establishing liability, or responsibility. When a person experiences an injury and seeks redress for that injury, the judicial process must determine who was responsible. For example, a patient or (if the patient died) the survivor of a patient may be dissatisfied with the medical care the patient received. The patient or survivor may feel that inadequate care led to a bad outcome. People have a constitutional right to take legal action against the doctor, nurse, paramedic, or other involved parties. However, the person who is suing must prove that the medical providers he or she is suing caused harm by failing to provide medical care that met the accepted standards. A bad outcome alone does not necessarily mean the medical provider was negligent; however, the patient or survivor has to prove all of the elements of negligence before a lawsuit will be successful.

A legal action of that sort is called a civil suit—that is, an action instituted by a private individual or corporation (the plaintiff) against another private individual or corporation (the defendant)—and the wrongful act that gives rise to a civil suit is called a tort. The objective of a civil suit is usually some sort of compensation (damages) for the injury the plaintiff sustained.

In medical liability cases, the plaintiff usually seeks monetary compensation for physical suffering, mental anguish, hospital and medical bills, and sometimes loss of earnings or earning capacity. To succeed in a civil suit, the plaintiff need only show that a preponderance of the believable evidence favors his or her position, and only 9 of the 12 jurors must agree.

Most often, lawsuits against EMS providers result from emergency vehicle collisions. In Chapter 3, you learned about the importance of safe driving to your personal health and well-being. You should also be aware that safe driving is a key to preventing lawsuits. Vehicle crashes are all too common and, each year, cause serious harm to patients, bystanders, and EMS providers, as well as expensive property damage **Figure 4-3 ▶** .

However, other kinds of lawsuits against EMS providers are on the rise each year. Many of these suits involve dispatch and transport issues in cases where a response is delayed, or a patient is not transported and his or her condition subsequently deteriorates. Others involve the quality of the medical care provided by the EMS providers, especially paramedics.

Sometimes the same allegedly wrongful or harmful act that gave rise to a civil suit may also elicit criminal prosecution. A criminal prosecution is an action taken by the government

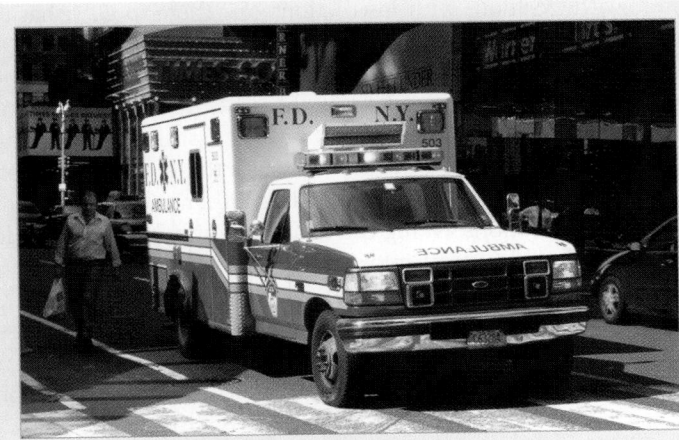

Figure 4-3 The majority of civil suits against paramedics arise from emergency vehicle collisions.

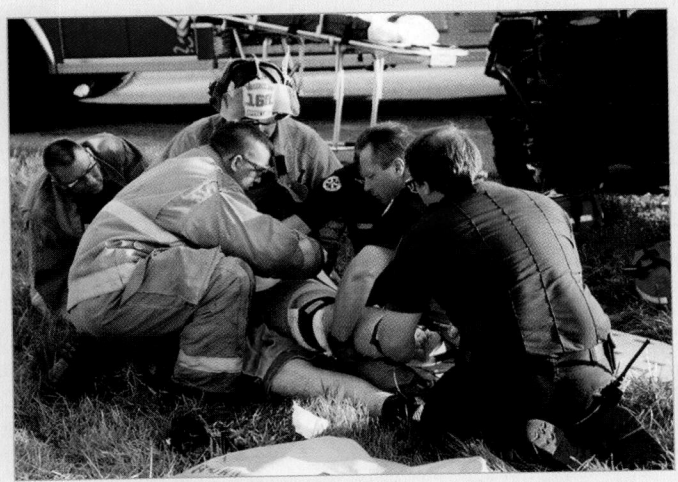

Figure 4-4 Your best prevention against any legal action is to keep the needs of your patient as your top priority.

against a person the prosecutors feel has violated criminal laws. In a criminal case, the government must prove guilt beyond all reasonable doubt to 12 jurors: If it does so, the defendant can be fined or imprisoned or both.

The criminal laws most likely to apply to prehospital care include assault, battery, and false imprisonment. All of these are criminal actions resulting from complaints about a paramedic's behavior such as using improper restraining methods, not asking a patient if you may touch him or her before making physical contact, or transporting a patient without his or her consent **Figure 4-4 ▲**.

Assault, battery, and false imprisonment may also be grounds for a civil suit, although suits of this nature against EMS providers are rare. But you should know that assault is said to occur when a person (the EMS provider) instills the fear

of immediate bodily harm or breach of bodily security to another (the patient)—whether or not the threat of harm is actually carried out. Battery occurs when the defendant (the EMS provider) touches another person (the patient) without his or her consent. Here are rough working definitions of the difference: saying "I'm going to kick your teeth in" is assault; actually kicking the person's teeth in is battery. Clearly just about any act of medical treatment performed without consent may be considered assault or battery or both, for such acts constitute a threat to the patient's bodily security ("Now I'm going to stick you with this needle. . . .") and an unsanctioned contact with the patient's body.

False imprisonment occurs when a person is intentionally and unjustifiably detained against his or her will. In prehospital care, charges of false imprisonment may arise if a paramedic transports a patient without the patient's consent or uses restraints in a wrongful manner. As we shall see later in this chapter, a paramedic's best protection against these charges is to obtain informed consent for almost everything you do. All medical care providers need to get informed consent, but you will need some guidelines and tips (which come later in this chapter) that most hospital-based personnel don't need to think about.

Paramedics may also be sued for defamation, which is intentionally making a false statement through written or verbal communication that injures a person's good name or reputation. Libel is making a false statement in the written form that injures a person's good name. When you write your patient care report, avoid using terms that may be considered insulting or offensive, such as "the patient appears to be drunk." Whatever your personal views, think about the way in which your run report would read in court. Don't let any thoughtless comments become evidence against you.

Slander is verbally making a false statement that injures a person's good name. Once again, avoid using terms that could be considered offensive to the patient when passing along prehospital care information to emergency department personnel. Keep in mind always that your patient is very likely a son or daughter, a husband or wife, a brother or sister, or even a father or mother. How would you like information about members of your own family to be treated when information is relayed to the hospital?

How Laws Affect the Paramedic

EMS, as we know it, has been in existence for about 30 years. However, over the last 10 years, the media and public education have made the public very aware of what to expect from the local EMS system. If citizens perceive your response as delayed or your efforts as incompetent, they will often file lawsuits seeking compensation for injuries they believe were caused by inadequate EMS care. If you do not explain to your patients why you were delayed, or why a procedure is difficult, you leave yourself open to unasked questions. In the case of health care providers, that silent criticism can lead to the courtroom.

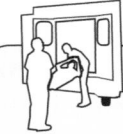

In the Field

Being courteous, honest, and professional will prevent most patients from complaining or filing lawsuits.

The Legal Process: Anatomy of a Lawsuit

A civil suit begins when a dissatisfied patient contacts an attorney, who then files a document for a lawsuit (called a complaint) on behalf of the patient with a local court. The complaint will contain the general allegations against the paramedic (let's say it's you) and the EMS system, but may not contain very much specific information about what the patient thinks went wrong. The patient's attorney (or his or her staff) must hand deliver a copy of the complaint, and a notice called a summons, to all persons or agencies named in the lawsuit, notifying them of the complaint and the need to respond. From start to finish, a lawsuit may take several years. Because the lawsuit may not begin until several years after the paramedic sees the patient, good documentation is essential to defending a lawsuit.

In EMS, your attorney will usually be assigned to you by the insurance company that handles claims for your employer, whether it is a government or private agency. The response, or answer to the complaint, will be filed by your lawyer. Once the complaint is filed and you (through your lawyer) have answered, a period known as the discovery period begins. The discovery period can last anywhere from a few months to more than 2 years **Figure 4-5**. During the discovery period, the attorneys on both sides seek to find out as much about the case as possible. They will exchange written questions that must be answered by the parties under oath, and they will also exchange documents, such as the patient's medical record, and take depositions, or statements taken under oath. You should stay in touch with your lawyer during this time and ask for a full explanation of everything that is happening. Your lawyer will also prepare

you for a deposition, with instructions on where to go, what to wear, and how to respond to certain types of questions.

Attorneys may also file motions, which are requests for the court to take an action, and argue them before the judge. Your attorney will seek to have the lawsuit dismissed by filing motions. The plaintiff's attorney may ask the court to rule on certain portions of the claim by filing other motions. Either side may file motions asking the court to compel the other side to produce documents or information that is being withheld.

Most civil cases are resolved during a settlement process because it is very expensive and time-consuming to take a case through trial. Settlement processes involve the parties and their lawyers in mediation, which is a conference set up to see if the parties can agree on a dollar amount that will resolve the case, or an arbitration, which is a minitrial in which a single arbitrator or a panel of arbitrators will make a decision based on the evidence presented by both sides.

If the case does not resolve itself during a settlement process, it will proceed to trial. During a trial, the judge rules on what the law is and the jury decides what the facts are. Trial juries can be very unpredictable; if they perceive that EMS has failed to meet community standards, large monetary damage awards can result.

Notes from Nancy

Probably the most important law affecting paramedics is one that doesn't appear in any of the statute books; it is the *law of doing what is best for the patient.*

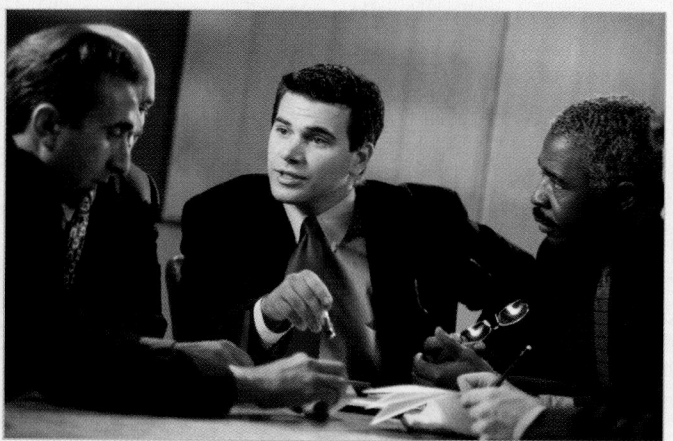

Figure 4-5 The process of a lawsuit can take years, and because of expenses associated with a trial, can result in out-of-court settlements.

Legal Accountability of the Paramedic

A variety of laws and ordinances, many of which differ considerably from state to state, regulate the actions of the paramedic. However, the most important premise affecting paramedics is one that doesn't appear in any of the statute books; it is the *rule of doing what is best for the patient.* Paramedics are trained in emergency medical care, not law. Every decision regarding patient care that a paramedic makes, therefore, should be based on the standards of good medical care—*not* on the possible legal consequences. When you do what is best for the patient, it is unlikely you will run afoul of the law—and even if you do get sued, your defense will be greatly enhanced if you have always kept the patient's best interest in mind.

Paramedics always have the responsibility to act in a reasonable and prudent manner and to provide appropriate care and transportation consistent with their education and training, their medical director's protocols, and the transport protocols in their EMS system.

The Paramedic and the Medical Director

The relationship between the paramedic and the medical director is complex and often not well understood. Ultimately, the

Documentation and Communication

If you must deviate from your protocols because of unusual circumstances, consult with online medical control and make sure you document it well on your patient care report.

paramedic has three lines of authority to answer to: the medical director, the licensing agency, and the employer. Although there is some overlap, it is important to keep these distinctions in mind. State EMS legislation usually requires that the paramedic perform advanced life-support procedures and skills only under the supervision of a physician. Legislation may also require the EMS system to have a medical director. Although the medical director is in a supervisory relationship with the paramedic, legally speaking, the paramedic is not the agent of the physician.

The acts of the paramedic, therefore, are not the actions of the physician, and the paramedic will be held accountable for his or her own actions. However, the medical director can be held legally accountable for failing to supervise the paramedic closely enough, or failing to take action when the paramedic's performance is not up to standard. The medical director may restrict the paramedic's practice, or even withdraw supervision entirely from a paramedic if he or she does not believe the paramedic is performing as he or she should. The medical director may also require certain remedial training if the paramedic is weak in some areas of practice. Although the medical director's remedial requirements may ultimately result in employment actions, medical directors are generally not held legally responsible for disciplinary actions taken by employers.

Many of the paramedic's activities require an order from a licensed physician. Orders may be given by radio (online medical control) or instead may be defined by protocols, or standing orders (off line medical control), but, in any case, the paramedic is not at liberty to disregard or reverse a physician's order unless, for some reason, the paramedic truly believes that carrying out the order will harm the patient. That fact may give rise to difficult situations, such as instances where paramedics find themselves at the scene of an emergency together with a physician who may not be knowledgeable in prehospital emergency care. Under those circumstances, the paramedics may feel that the orders of the on-scene physician are inappropriate. However, paramedics are on shaky legal ground if they choose to disregard a physician's orders, assuming the physician is licensed in that state and the order is appropriate. To avoid conflicts in such situations, it is best to ask the service medical director to develop protocols ahead of time defining the paramedic's relationship with the medical director of the service and with other physicians in the community, including bystander physicians. A physician is not required to ride in with EMS unless he or she has performed procedures above the level of the EMS providers, or has otherwise assumed responsibility for

patient care. Always be sure that the physician is licensed in your state, and document the physician's name and contact information, before allowing him or her to provide patient care. When conflicts do arise between paramedics and physician bystanders in the field, online medical control, not the paramedic, should resolve them.

EMS-Enabling Legislation

Most states now have what is called EMS-enabling legislation, defining how EMS is structured and designating responsibilities to government agencies. These laws also provide the state's framework for the paramedic's actual practice—what you are permitted to do in the field. For example, EMS legislation may define the need for a medical director, and may also define the scope of practice for the different levels of EMS personnel. The paramedic must be familiar with the EMS legislation in his or her state and any regulations that flow from those statutes.

Administrative Regulations

Administrative regulations—set forth by bureaucracies at the state and federal levels—also affect and define the specific rules under which paramedics practice. For example, regulations may set out the precise skills and medications to be used by each level of EMS provider. Regulations—usually developed by either the state's Department of Health or the county agency responsible for regulating EMS practice—may further define the paramedic's role in emergency medical care of patients. Regulations may also define the requirements for licensure or certification, renewal requirements, continuing education requirements, and a list of behaviors that may subject paramedics to suspension or revocation of their license or certification.

If a paramedic provides less than adequate care, or fails to meet the requirements for recertification, the administrative agency may also take action against that paramedic's license. A license is not a right, but rather a privilege, granted by a government agency, allowing the paramedic to provide care to its citizens. Failure to abide by the regulations can have serious consequences.

Scope of Practice

The scope of practice for paramedics may be spelled out in that state's EMS legislation or regulations. The scope of practice is care that a paramedic is permitted to perform according to the state under its license or certification; however, a local medical director may not permit a paramedic to perform all of the skills or give all of the medications for which he or she is licensed or certified.

A paramedic carrying out procedures for which he or she is not authorized under the enabling legislation is practicing outside his or her scope of practice, which may be considered negligence or, in some states, even a criminal offense. The scope of practice should not be confused with the standard of care, which is what a reasonable paramedic in a similar situation would do. This is discussed later in this chapter.

Medical Practice Act

In most states physicians and other health care practitioners are enabled to function through the provisions of a Medical Practice Act. This act usually defines the minimum qualifications of those who may perform various health services, defines the skills that each type of practitioner is legally permitted to use, and establishes a means of certification for different categories of health care professionals. The paramedic should become familiar with the terms of the Medical Practice Act in his or her region.

Health Insurance Portability and Accountability Act

Few health care providers have not been inundated with information about the Health Insurance Portability and Accountability Act (HIPAA), which provides stringent privacy requirements for patient information. The act was enacted in 1996 and provides for criminal sanctions as well as civil penalties for releasing a patient's private medical information in an unauthorized manner. Medical information can be disclosed only if it is necessary for a patient's treatment or for payment or medical/billing operations. HIPAA requires each EMS agency to have a privacy officer responsible for ensuring that all protected health information (PHI) that the service deals with, in either written or electronic form, not be released in an unauthorized manner. This means you must be aware of where written information is at all times, and you cannot casually discuss a patient where just anyone might overhear—like in an elevator Figure 4-6 ▶ .

It is no longer acceptable for EMS patient care reports to sit in the public area of the fire station, or to be easily accessible to anyone who does not need to know the information for the reasons stated above. It is also unacceptable to discuss a patient's PHI in a public forum without that patient's consent. "War stories" told by paramedics may subject paramedics to liability. Similarly, you must use caution when the media or the public is riding with your service to ensure that PHI is not disclosed without the patient's consent. If your service receives a subpoena for a patient's PHI, be sure to notify legal counsel before releasing a patient's medical record to anyone.

Emergency Medical Treatment and Active Labor Act

The Emergency Medical Treatment and Active Labor Act (EMTALA) was enacted in 1986 to combat the practice of

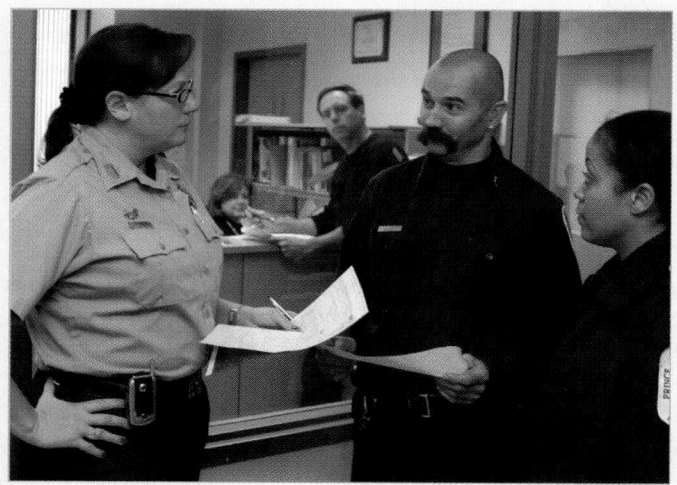

Figure 4-6 Remember that the HIPAA law guarantees a patient's confidentiality at all times. Be careful never to discuss a patient's condition in public.

"patient dumping" and pays particular attention to the practice of sending women in labor to distant hospitals. (Patient dumping occurs when a hospital emergency department denies medical screening or stabilizing treatment, or if it inappropriately transfers an individual whose condition is not stable). EMTALA can be enforced because it regulates hospitals that receive Medicare funding. EMTALA also doles out stiff fines for hospitals and doctors who violate its provisions. If that is not enough, EMTALA further allows private individuals to sue for violations of the act.

EMTALA guarantees a medical screening exam, and treatment to stabilize any emergency medical conditions found, to any patient presenting to a hospital that has an emergency department Figure 4-7 ▶ . It prohibits discrimination for any reason, although most often EMTALA violations occur because a patient has no medical insurance and may be unable to pay his or her bill. Some urgent care centers may also be covered by EMTALA. Although EMTALA does not directly regulate paramedics, EMS is often the vehicle—both figuratively and literally—by which patient dumping takes place.

EMTALA also regulates patient transfers and applies to both the sending and receiving facilities, so paramedics will get a close view of EMTALA during patient transfers. Paramedics should be certain never to transfer a patient who needs care that falls outside their scope of practice, and to be sure the

You are the Provider Part 2

You feel that for the safety of yourself and your partner you must leave the home. With only two of you, you are not able to safely restrain this patient, who continues to attempt to punch, bite, and kick. Because the patient is combative, you are unable to obtain vital signs.

3. Could your actions be considered abandonment?
4. What other courses of action, if any, could be taken?

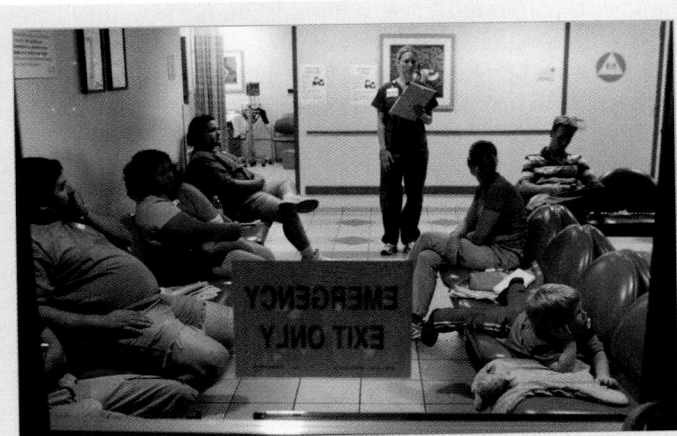

Figure 4-7 EMTALA legislation guarantees that every patient must receive basic medical treatment—regardless of his or her ability to pay for medical treatment when it is received.

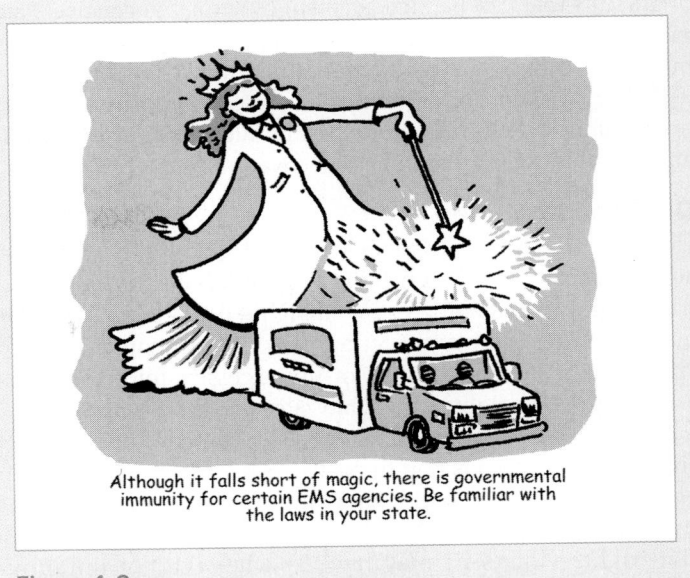

Although it falls short of magic, there is governmental immunity for certain EMS agencies. Be familiar with the laws in your state.

Figure 4-8

patient really is stable enough to transfer. Should a patient need a higher level of care, it is the responsibility of the transferring hospital to provide someone to ride along (a nurse, respiratory therapist, or even a physician). Paramedics should also be certain to receive all appropriate paperwork before setting out on a patient transfer, including all pertinent medical records, lab results, x-rays, and other documents. When arriving at the receiving hospital, that hospital should have a bed ready for the patient, after agreeing to accept the patient.

EMTALA issues are regulated by the Centers for Medicare and Medicaid Services (CMS) and carry severe monetary penalties, up to and including loss of Medicare funding, for hospitals that fail to comply. EMTALA has complex language that appears to be medical language but is actually legal language. For example, an emergency medical condition under EMTALA means what most paramedics would call an acute situation. CMS has recently frowned on the practice of stacking ambulances at emergency departments with patients waiting to be seen.

Emergency Vehicle Laws

Most states have specific statutes that define an emergency vehicle and what traffic should do when one approaches. Although these laws vary somewhat from state to state, it is important to remember that these statutes still require emergency vehicles to be operated in a safe and prudent manner. Laws governing emergency vehicle operation do not authorize speeding or running red lights, or driving the vehicle in an unsafe manner which can put the public at risk. Most state laws establish a higher standard for the emergency vehicle operator by making him or her responsible for operating the vehicle with due regard for the safety of all others. If a crash occurs, EMS providers will often be found at fault in civil cases brought against the drivers. Worse, if you are the driver, you might also be charged criminally for such situations. Although it is important for paramedics to know the laws of their state about emergency vehicle operation, it is also important to

remember that the blue star of life on the side of your vehicle and flashing red lights on top do not exempt you from defensive driving and common courtesy.

Immunity: Good Samaritan Legislation

All but 13 states have some form of Good Samaritan law designed to provide immunity from liability to any member of the community who stops and helps at the scene of an emergency. Although the laws were initially passed to encourage the public to help at emergency scenes, many of these statutes also operate to provide some protection for EMS personnel who are off duty and assist at an emergency. The laws of most states limit the legal protection provided: the emergency care must be given *free of charge* (gratuitously). An EMT or paramedic providing emergency care while on duty is not, therefore, protected under Good Samaritan laws. As a general rule, if a paramedic has a legal duty to a patient, the Good Samaritan law will not protect him or her.

Most Good Samaritan laws also require that persons responding to an emergency do all that they can, *within their knowledge*, to support and sustain life and to prevent further injury. The paramedic is not expected to function as a physician; but the paramedic is expected to deploy those skills that any other paramedic with similar training would use under the same or similar circumstances.

Courts have not been generous in applying the Good Samaritan law during routine EMS work. Courts have been applying the concept of immunity only during emergencies.

Other Kinds of Immunity
Governmental Immunity

An abiding principal of English law is that you cannot sue the queen (or king) because "the queen can do no wrong." In the United States, this concept, called sovereign immunity, has taken the form of legislation that identifies only limited types of lawsuits that can be filed against government agencies. Paramedics working for government agencies, such as a fire department, also have some governmental immunity for their actions Figure 4-8 ◄ . The immunity statutes may also set limited time frames in which lawsuits can be filed, and may limit the amount of money a plaintiff can recover.

Qualified Immunity

However, this immunity does not cover civil rights violations, and attorneys have begun filing lawsuits against public sector paramedics for violating the civil rights of their patients. The most common complaint occurs when EMS personnel improperly restrain a violent patient, or use excessive force to restrain a patient. Civil rights suits may also be filed when a paramedic's conduct deviates so far from the standard of care that a civil rights violation is said to occur.

Paramedics who work or volunteer for public agencies, such as fire departments, who are sued by patients alleging civil rights violations may have another type of immunity called qualified immunity. Under this doctrine, the paramedic is only held liable when the plaintiff can show that the paramedic violated a clearly established law of which the paramedic should have known. This kind of immunity, of course, does not apply to tort cases.

▉ Negligence and Protection Against Negligence Claims

Unless there is some type of immunity, nothing can protect the paramedic from liability for gross negligence, a serious charge. Negligence occurs when a series of events happen:

- The paramedic—or, in some cases, the EMS system—had a legal duty to the patient. For example, a paramedic hired to serve a community has a legal duty to the citizens of that community.
- There was a breach of duty; that is, the person accused of negligence failed to act as another person with similar training would have acted under the same or similar circumstances. Breach of duty may involve doing *less* than one was trained to do (an error of omission—for example, a paramedic who fails to splint an injured extremity) or doing *more* than one was trained to do (an error of commission—for example, a paramedic who stitches up a laceration).
- The failure to act appropriately was the proximate cause (the first event in a chain of events) that caused the plaintiff's injury.
- Harm resulted.

Paramedics and the EMS systems in which they work are protected from liability as long as they perform according to the standards expected of paramedics and EMS systems. The paramedic's best protection is to behave in all circumstances according to established procedures and standards set by national agencies (such as the National Highway Traffic Safety Administration, with its guidelines for ambulance design and equipment). Although those standards are not law, they can be introduced as evidence in litigation and may affect the outcome of a suit. It is therefore in your best interest to make sure that your vehicle is maintained in optimal condition and equipped according to prevailing standards.

A big part of negligence is whether or not there is "foreseeability." This concept implies that the injury, or harm, could have been predicted, or known in advance, and therefore could have been avoided if the proper precautions had been taken. It is foreseeable that giving an incorrect dosage of a drug will result in harm to a patient just as it is foreseeable that running a red light while en route to a call may result in a crash.

Elements of Negligence
Duty

Duty is prescribed by the law: it is what we must do (as EMS providers) and how we must do it. Without question, our first duty as EMS providers is to do no further harm to a patient. As the Latin phrase (which is thought to have originated with Hippocrates) states: *Primum non nocere* (First, do no harm).

The first element of negligence a patient must prove for a lawsuit to be successful is that of duty. The definitive *Black's Law Dictionary* defines duty, as it is understood in medical negligence, as "an obligation, to which law will give recognition and effect, to conform to a particular standard of conduct towards another." *Black's Law Dictionary* goes on to say that if one fails to perform according to that standard "he becomes subject to liability to the person to whom the duty is owed for any injury sustained by that person of which the conduct is the legal cause."

A great deal of confusion surrounds the concept of legal duty in EMS. For example, many paramedics think that they have a legal obligation to stop at roadside crashes simply because they are paramedics. However, in all but a few states, this is not the case. Although a paramedic may feel an ethical obligation to stop and assist, the law in most states does not require it. When the paramedic is working a shift, however, or signed up for a particular shift on a volunteer squad, he or she is obligated to respond to calls during that period.

Popular EMS folklore also says that if you put a sticker that says "paramedic" on your vehicle, this somehow invokes a legal responsibility to stop at all emergencies. But once again, this is not the case Figure 4-9 ▶ . However, if the paramedic does stop to assist, he or she has a legal duty to perform within the standard of care. If you do stop, there is a further legal duty not to abandon the patient once treatment has begun. It is important to know what your legal obligations are when you are off duty. If you live in a state where you must stop for a collision, you need to know that, too.

The concept of duty extends to the paramedic's duties to himself or herself as well. Each of you has an obligation to keep up your licensure or certification, to attend continuing education courses, and to maintain your skills. In addition, you have a duty to maintain your health and psychological well-being so that you will be both mentally and physically prepared for the rigors of your job in prehospital patient care.

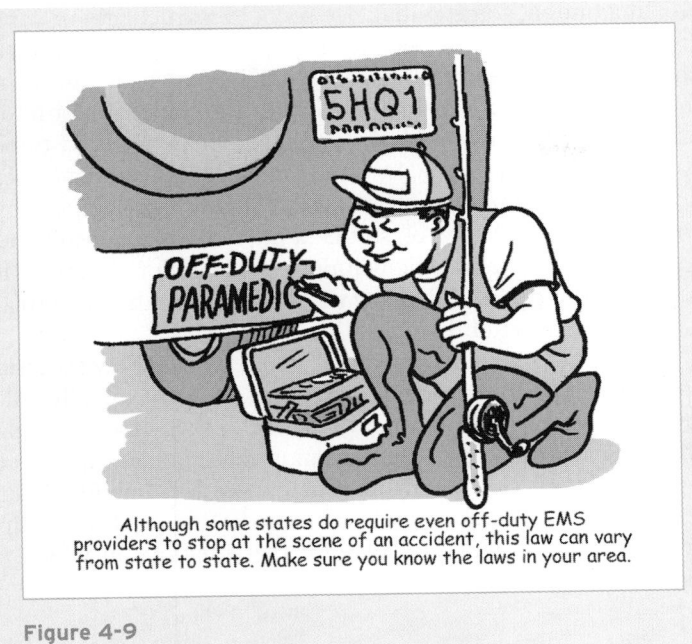

Although some states do require even off-duty EMS providers to stop at the scene of an accident, this law can vary from state to state. Make sure you know the laws in your area.

Figure 4-9

Further, you have a duty to check your equipment at the beginning of each shift and to take action to ensure that all equipment is functioning properly. Finally, you have a duty to honor your patient's rights to privacy, and their rights to refuse or limit the care you provide.

In addition, not just individual paramedics but EMS agencies—and even entire EMS systems—can be held to a legal duty. EMS agencies have a duty to respond to calls for aid and to use mutual aid resources appropriately if their own call volume is too heavy to allow response within an appropriate time frame. Some EMS agencies may operate with contracts that specify legal duties, such as minimum response times.

Legal duty is a concept in the law that tells us what our standards of practice are. It is an unpredictable legal concept, often defined in the context of a case tried in a court of law. But the concept of legal duty is used by attorneys defending EMS providers. For example, in a lawsuit against an off-duty paramedic who stopped at an accident to render aid, the paramedic's attorney may attempt to show that the paramedic had no duty to the patient, but instead provided assistance he or she was not required by law to provide.

Remember, lawyers are often trained to work from the most general defense to the most specific elements of the case. Lack of legal duty is a general defense, that, however general, may still be true.

Breach of Duty

The second element a patient must prove for a lawsuit to be successful is that the paramedic failed to perform within the standard of care. The standard of care is what a reasonable paramedic, in the same or similar situation, would have done. In a lawsuit, a jury will listen to the testimony of expert witnesses on both sides and ultimately decide whether the paramedic's care was reasonable or not. These expert witnesses will provide a number of sources on which to base their testimony about whether the paramedic's care was reasonable. Those sources will include their own training and experience; the paramedic's training, experience, and continuing education; textbooks; protocols; national standards; standard operating procedures; and the patient care report. (Good documentation will go a long way to prove your high standards of care.)

Some states differentiate between ordinary negligence and gross negligence. How high a standard of care a paramedic will be held to varies from one state to another. Some states provide immunity for all but the poorest care given by the paramedic. This immunity usually comes in the form of a Good Samaritan law.

In states that follow a gross negligence standard, a lawsuit against a paramedic will not be successful unless that paramedic has seriously departed from the accepted standards. Actions are grossly negligent if they are found to be willful or wanton under the law. This is a very difficult standard for a plaintiff to meet. Usually, either intentional conduct or recklessness is essential to a finding of willful or wanton conduct. For example, Ohio has defined willful and wanton misconduct as "the intent, purpose or design to injure another" or "an intentional disregard of a clear duty or definite rule of conduct; a purpose not to discharge that duty; or the performance of wrongful acts with the knowledge of the likelihood of resulting injury." Other states have defined it as "reckless disregard," "utter indifference," or "conscious disregard" for the safety of others. Usually, if the paramedic can convince the jury that he or she acted in good faith, this will be a defense to a claim of gross negligence.

In other states, a plaintiff will only have to show ordinary negligence. This can be a failure to act or a simple mistake that causes harm to a patient. It is much easier for a plaintiff to prove negligence under the ordinary negligence standard.

Proximate Cause

Even in cases where the paramedic had a legal duty to the patient, and the paramedic breached the standard of care, a plaintiff must still link the act that fell below the standard of care directly to his or her injury by showing that the act (or failure to act) proximately caused the harm. *Black's Law Dictionary* defines proximate cause as "that which, in a natural and continuous sequence, unbroken by any intervening cause, produces injury, and without which the result would not have occurred." Simply stated, a plaintiff will have to prove that the paramedic's improper action, or failure to act, was the cause of his or her injury.

Failure to secure a patient on a backboard can be the proximate cause of severing the spinal cord. Proving that an act, or a failure to act, proximately caused an injury is the most difficult part of a lawsuit to prove. It is also the part that defense attorneys spend a great deal of their time on. For example, if paramedics are treating a patient from a car crash who has a spinal cord injury and, during patient care, they drop the stretcher, the patient may try to show that his or her injury resulted from the dropped stretcher and not from the crash itself. Careful documentation of the patient's neurologic status at the time you first encounter him or her will be essential to your defense.

Harm

The final element plaintiffs must prove in a negligence lawsuit is that they were harmed. Although physical injury is usually part of any lawsuit for medical negligence, patients also may claim damages for emotional distress, loss of income, loss of enjoyment of life, loss of spousal consortium, loss of household services, and loss of future earning capacity. They will have to show that the paramedic's actions proximately caused each of these kinds of damage.

Abandonment

Abandonment is a form of negligence that involves the termination of care without the patient's consent. The term also implies that the patient had a continuing need for medical treatment and that the abrupt termination of treatment was the cause of subsequent injury or death. Therefore, once you have responded to an emergency, you may not leave a patient in need of medical treatment until another competent health care professional with an equal or higher level of training has taken responsibility for that patient's care. Shocking as it may seem, on more than one occasion, a critically ill or injured patient was left in a busy emergency department by EMS providers, and the patient died before emergency department personnel took note of the patient. It is the responsibility of the paramedic to stay with the patient until proper transfer of care has taken place.

Proper transfer of care means transfer of care to another health care professional, not to a gurney or a clerk! Thus, if you arrive at a busy emergency department with a seriously ill patient, you may have to remain with the patient until emergency department personnel are free to attend to him or her.

Busy emergency departments may direct you to leave your patient in a triage station or waiting area. The hospital personnel may not know that, under law, this practice would be considered abandonment. Be firm with the hospital personnel about staying with your patient, unless they will start a proper transfer of care. Paramedics should not leave patients in any area of the hospital where they will not be attended to and assessed by medical personnel. You must never leave a patient without giving a full report to a physician, physician assistant, or nurse.

It is also very important that you leave a copy of your report with the emergency department physician or nurse who is taking over care of your patient. Although many busy services complain that this is impossible, you must leave a written report so that the emergency department physician and staff will know what your findings were in the field, what medications you may have given the patient, and what procedures you may have performed.

It is important to remember, however, that there are some situations in which transport may not be needed, but that do not constitute abandonment. EMS systems are subjected to calls for service for patients who may not really need treatment or transportation. Your local medical director should provide protocols for these situations.

In addition, some ambulance services, particularly in rural areas, may have mixed personnel (providers of various levels) and may not have a full staff of paramedics at all times. In those areas, even if a paramedic makes the initial response, if only basic care is required, the paramedic may not need to be part of the transport crew for situations where the patient does not need advanced care. If in doubt, this is best decided by contacting medical control, so that a physician can consult and confirm that the paramedic will not be needed for transport. It is the kind of decision that always benefits from the proverbial "two heads are better than one."

Many EMS systems provide a tiered response, with basic life support (BLS) providers reaching the patient quickly, followed by advanced life support (ALS). If a BLS crew responds and makes an improper determination that a patient does not need ALS care, the system may be exposed to liability. Your service needs to work with every provider involved to set up protocols that provide guidance for the situations in which a BLS crew may cancel an incoming ALS crew.

Advance Directives

An advance directive is a written document that expresses the wants, needs, and desires of a patient in reference to his or her future medical care. Advance directives state what medical care the patient wants or doesn't want when the patient is unable to express his or her wishes. Living wills, do not resuscitate (DNR) orders, and organ donation orders are all advance directives.

Whether or not EMS personnel are bound by advance directives is totally a function of state law—and such laws, like those that cover DNR orders, for example, are very strict, often limited to terminal patients in nursing homes or hospice care. More often than not, you will be required to treat. But you must learn what the laws are in your state, and follow them.

A do not resuscitate (DNR) order is an advance directive that describes which life-sustaining procedures should be performed in the event of a sudden deterioration in a patient's medical condition. For patients who have been identified as organ donors and are critically ill or injured, you may be required to perform some procedures before potential organ procurement, after the patient is deceased. If your EMS system does not already have a protocol for organ donation, assist it in developing protocols to keep organs viable. It is your responsibility to contact your online medical control for consultation and direction on local prehospital organ procurement procedures.

The ethics of advance directives and organ procurement will be discussed in detail in Chapter 5.

▮ Licensure and Certification

The terms licensure and certification are often confused because, in some states, paramedics are considered licensed but in others certified. Certification generally means only evidence of a certain level of training, such as a certificate of completion from a course or school. It is really simply evidence that an individual has a certain level of credentials based on hours of training and examination. It does not address anything more than minimum competency. Licensure, on the other hand, is the privilege to practice at a carefully defined level, usually granted by a government agency or local authority, such as a state health department or county EMS authority. Often, these agencies themselves give licensing examinations.

It is important to remember that, although certain rights do come with a license, a license itself is a privilege granted by a government authority only on certain conditions, and the paramedic must comply with the government's requirements for professional behavior, continuing education, and licensure renewal, or risk losing that privilege. Those rights may not be conferred in states that certify, rather than license, paramedics.

Discipline and Due Process

The rights that come with a license (and with some certificates as well) include what is known as a property interest in your license, because paramedics earn their living by working under their license. However, if a paramedic commits an infraction that jeopardizes that license, he or she may be subjected to a licensure action. The agency that granted the license may seek to restrict, suspend, or even revoke the privilege to practice.

When an administrative agency proposes a licensing action in a state that licenses paramedics, the paramedic has a right to due process. Due process is a right to a fair procedure for the action the agency proposes to take. Due process has two components: *Notice* and the *Opportunity to be Heard*. Notice means that the agency must notify the paramedic of the actions that allegedly constitute the infraction. This usually happens by way of a certified letter containing a *Notice of Contemplated Action*. The letter will inform the paramedic of the proposed action to be taken and the sections of the regulations the agency is alleging he or she has violated. The letter will also inform the paramedic of a right to a hearing and the procedure for requesting a hearing. The hearing provides an opportunity for the paramedic to tell his or her side of the story. If the licensing agency still believes that it has grounds for the licensure action after the hearing, it will send a *Notice of Final Action*. The paramedic may also have appeal rights if a final action is taken against his or her license.

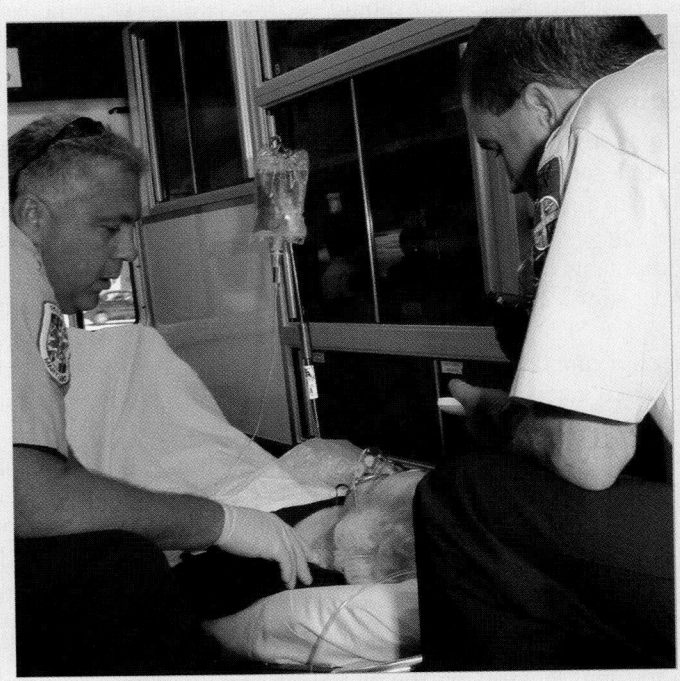

Figure 4-10 When communicating with a patient, be sensitive to his or her point of view, and the environment in which you choose to communicate.

Paramedic–Patient Relationships

Confidentiality

The paramedic has an ongoing duty to maintain the confidentiality of the private information shared by the patient Figure 4-10 ▲. It is important not to disclose any of the patient's medical information to anyone who does not have a need to know it. As mentioned previously, HIPAA is a strict federal law governing the disclosure of patient information. Some states also have laws pertaining to patient confidentiality; a breach of that confidentiality may provide a means for patients to sue for unauthorized release of their medical information.

Be careful *where* you talk about patients too. You must do your best, even at the scene of a crash or in the halls or elevators of hospitals, not to confer in front of bystanders.

You are the Provider Part 3

You exit the house, and wait in the locked ambulance for arrival of law enforcement personnel. The patient's wife runs from the home and pleads with you to return inside as her husband is punching through a glass cabinet in the basement. You explain to her that she should wait with you outside until police officers arrive.

5. Was any part of this situation avoidable?
6. What would be helpful in handling this situation?

As a paramedic, you should become familiar with the laws in your state that are applicable to your EMS operations.

Consent and Refusal

The concepts of consent and refusal can be traced back to the Magna Carta and are clearly embodied in the US Constitution. Prior to providing emergency medical care, you must obtain the consent of the patient. Any touching of a patient's body without his or her consent may give rise to charges of assault and battery. The concept of consent is predicated on patients who are of legal age and who possess the capacity to make medical care decisions that are appropriate for themselves. This is called decision-making capacity. Patients with decision-making capacity have the right to refuse all or part of the emergency medical care offered to them. There are two types of consent that the paramedic must be familiar with: informed consent and implied consent.

Informed consent must be obtained from every adult patient who has decision-making capacity. Informed consent has two elements.

First, you must tell patients what it is you are proposing to do to them. Before you touch patients, and particularly before you perform any invasive procedure, you must ensure that the patients understand what it is you propose to do to them, and what potential risks the procedure carries. There are a number of things that can get in the way of giving patients the information they need to make their decision, such as language barriers, their emotional state, and their mental abilities. It is usually best to get patients somewhere quiet (such as the back of your EMS unit), where you can calm them down and explain, in a manner they can understand, the nature and extent of the procedure to be performed and the possible risks involved.

Second, patients must give you permission to touch them in the manner you have proposed. This may be done verbally, or by actions such as rolling up a sleeve so that you can take their blood pressure. It is very important that you document how you obtained informed consent in case legal issues arise later. Expressed consent is a type of informed consent that occurs when the patient does something, either by telling you or by taking some sort of action, that demonstrates giving you permission to provide care.

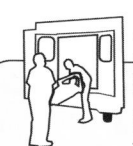

In the Field

Never tell patients that you are going to do a procedure. Instead, ask them if you can perform the procedure and explain to them why they need it.

The other kind of consent is implied consent. In unconscious adults, or in adults who are too ill or injured to consent to emergency lifesaving treatment, their consent is implied. In those cases, the paramedic assumes that the patients would want care because of the severity of their condition. Generally,

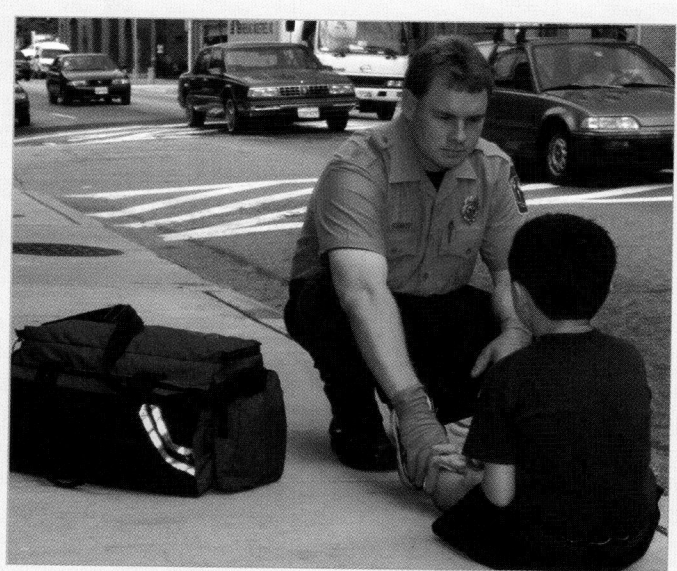

Figure 4-11 Whenever you are dealing with a young child, explain to him or her the need for treatment, and consult his or her parent or guardian.

when you encounter patients who are seriously injured or extremely ill, they will not have decision-making capacity and their consent to treatment may be implied.

There is nothing in law called *involuntary consent*. Some EMS personnel have been taught the concept of involuntary consent, a term that has been incorrectly applied to describe the permission granted by law enforcement or a legal guardian to treat someone who is under arrest (or otherwise in custody), incapacitated, a minor, or for other reasons. This term is an oxymoron, because consent can *never* be involuntary.

Minors present special issues for the paramedic. Because minors have no legal status, they cannot either consent to or refuse medical care. In the case of children and adults who have legal guardians, consent must be obtained, if possible, from a parent or legal guardian of the patient. If the parent or guardian is not available, emergency treatment to sustain life may be undertaken without consent under the doctrine of implied consent. A great deal of confusion surrounds the issue of emancipated minors. Emancipated minors are under the legal age in a given state but because of other circumstances can be legally treated as adults. Although the question of who is an emancipated minor can only be answered by state law, most states recognize any minor who has been emancipated by court order as an adult. Other states add criteria such as marriage, pregnancy, or active military service. Emancipated minors may be treated as adults for purposes of consent or refusal.

Overall, obtaining consent for adults and children may be somewhat difficult for the new paramedic **Figure 4-11 ▲**. A patient or a guardian of a child may not want you to assess and treat for a variety of reasons. However, as a patient advocate you will need to be aware of potential problems for obtaining permission and be prepared to discuss the need for care.

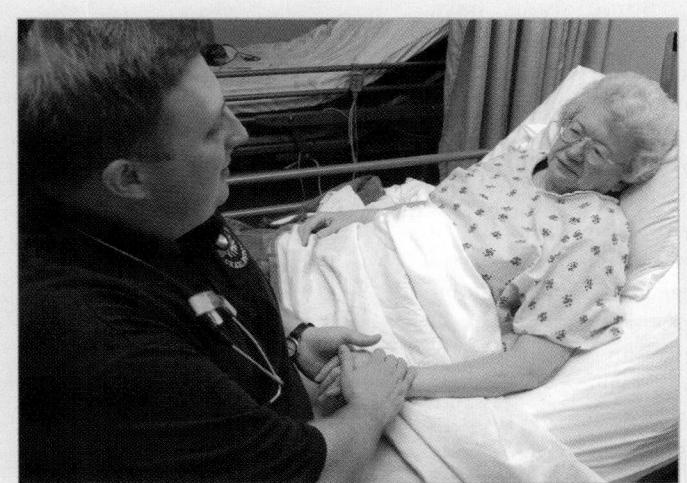

Figure 4-12 When a conscious patient with decision-making capability makes a decision, you must respect that decision.

Decision-Making Capacity: The Prerequisite for Consent and Refusal

Refusals, like consent, must be informed refusals, and all the same prerequisites apply. Patients must have decision-making capacity in order to be able to refuse care. Decision-making capacity is the ability of patients to understand the information you are providing to them, coupled with the ability to process that information and make a choice regarding medical care that is appropriate for them. Paramedics have a number of tools to use in evaluating patients' decision-making capacity, but the best one is their ability to talk to patients to find out whether patients understand what is happening to them. In addition, if pulse oximetry and blood glucose measurements are outside normal ranges, they can provide measurable information regarding patients' ability to understand and communicate. Detailed documentation of decision-making capacity is important to show that patients were able to understand your proposed plan of care.

If a conscious patient with decision-making capacity refuses to consent to treatment, that person may not be treated without a court order Figure 4-12 ▲ . In such instances, the paramedic should consult with medical control for instructions. The most prudent approach is for the paramedic to inform the person in a calm and sympathetic manner of the possible consequences of refusing treatment. Bear in mind that many people who refuse medical treatment do so out of fear and emotional distress, and the patient's distress needs to be recognized and dealt with in an understanding way.

It is *not* appropriate nor is it in your interest as an advocate to consider the person who refuses treatment a "bad patient" and to behave in a hostile or aggressive manner toward him or her. Remember, you are at the scene to help the patient, so try to find out what is bothering the patient and why he or she is rejecting help, and always respect their rights.

Bear in mind that some patients refuse treatment as a way of denying that they have a problem—such as the middle-aged macho man with chest pain who refuses treatment in order to deny the possibility that he may be experiencing a heart attack. A sympathetic ear and a little reassurance will often convert the problem patient into someone you can help. Remember the phrase: "It never hurts to have these things checked out."

Sometimes having patients talk by radio or telephone with medical control may be helpful. If, however, after your best efforts to talk with patients about their situation and to explain the possible consequences of refusing treatment, they still decline care, there is little more that you can do. Even at that point, though, do not close any doors. Let patients know that, should they change their mind, you will be willing and ready to help them because that is your job.

Maintain a courteous, sympathetic attitude. Let patients know that your chief concern is their well-being. Let patients know that it is all right to change their mind. Urge patients to seek further medical evaluation by the doctor of their choice. Help them make concrete plans for follow-up. Sometimes patients will consent to transport but not consent to treatment; others may consent to treatment but refuse transport. If patients refuse transport, try to make sure that someone will be with them after you leave and always advise them to call back for help if needed.

Once again, documentation of patient refusals is critically important should litigation arise in which the patient claims the paramedic abandoned him or her. Document carefully, including the patient's history, all findings of your physical examination and mental status examination, the patient's stated reasons for refusing care, and all advice given to the patient, including explanations of the risks of refusing care. It is also important to note how much time you spent attempting to provide care. The report should be signed by the patient and, preferably, by an impartial observer (for example, a police officer, if present). The purpose of a witness/observer is to *hear* the exchange of the information, not just to sign a piece of paper with his or her name. Soliciting for signatures from others on the scene who may not have been paying attention to your conversation or the information exchanged with the patient may pose legal issues. Soliciting for a signature just to fill in your report is not useful and could be harmful.

Prehospital refusal forms look like the answer to documentation of a particularly difficult problem for paramedics. However, the forms must be backed up with action. Legally, a paramedic must have undertaken the process of attempting to obtain informed consent to treat the patient. Just because a patient has signed a refusal form does not mean that the patient has given you an informed refusal. You must have informed the

Notes from Nancy

If you place the welfare of the patient ahead of all other considerations, you will rarely if ever commit an unethical act in medical care.

patient of what you propose to do to care for him or her, and the potential risks of refusing that care, in a manner he or she is capable of understanding.

It is often frustrating and difficult for the paramedic, like any other health care provider, to accept the fact that a patient may refuse all or part of care. However, it is important to respect a patient's rights, regardless of whether it is contrary to your beliefs or what you think you should be doing. Courts have upheld patient refusals when paramedics carefully documented a patient's decision-making capacity, and their explanation of the possible consequences of refusing care.

A problem sometimes arises in determining whether a person who refuses care or transport to a hospital has decision-making capacity. Suppose, for example, you are called to help a patient who has had a seizure in a downtown store. By the time you arrive, the seizure is over, and the patient is conscious. She says she is all right, and she refuses to go to the hospital. You smell alcohol on her breath. Does that patient possess the decision-making capacity to refuse treatment? To make that determination, you need to spend a little time evaluating the patient. You should explain to her, "I can't let you go until I've checked you over and until you talk to me enough to convince me that you're OK and that you understand your situation."

In general, any patient with altered mental status or unstable vital signs probably cannot be considered able to refuse transport to the hospital. The paramedic must become proficient in establishing whether a patient has decision-making capacity in a very short time frame, and with minimal information. The criteria for determining mental competence should be spelled out in detail in the protocols of every ambulance service. As a rule, such criteria will include the following:

- The patient is oriented to person, place, and day.
- The patient responds to questions appropriately.
- There is no significant mental impairment from alcohol, drugs, head injury, or other organic illness. (Ask family members, if present, whether the patient is behaving the way he or she normally does.) What constitutes significant mental impairment is a judgment call that is very subjective.
- The patient demonstrates to you that he or she understands the nature of his or her condition and the risks of not going to the hospital for immediate care. This can only be done after a thorough explanation of the patient's condition, and the risks of refusal.
- The patient can describe a reasonable plan for follow-up care.
- Oxygen saturation levels are within normal limits.
- Blood glucose levels are within normal limits `Figure 4-13 ▶`.

When patients have a potentially life-threatening illness or injury and there is any doubt as to their decision-making capacity, it is always preferable to transport them to the hospital even if it is against their will. The decision to allow a potentially impaired patient to refuse treatment is a *medical* decision, requiring judgment and experience. That decision is best made by a doctor in the hospital, not by a paramedic on the street.

Some states have enacted emergency transportation statutes that permit EMS personnel to transport patients against their will under very narrow circumstances. These statutes are designed to protect paramedics who make a good faith judgment that patients cannot make an informed decision because they do not have decision-making capacity. In 1993, New Mexico passed a law that permits transport without consent if:

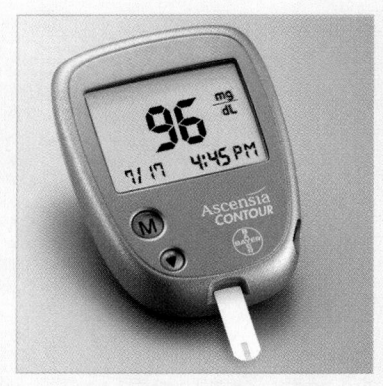

Figure 4-13 Remember that a patient's decision-making ability can be affected by the intake of alcohol or drugs, and by abnormal blood glucose or oxygen saturation levels.

- There is online medical control.
- The provider is at least an EMT-Basic.
- The provider has made a good faith judgment.
- The patient is incapable of making an informed decision.
- The patient is reasonably likely to suffer death or disability without medical intervention.

In the Field

The potential legal consequences of using reasonable force to bring a patient to the hospital (false imprisonment) are far less serious than the consequences—legal and medical—of a bad outcome (wrongful death or malpractice) if a patient in need of care is released at the scene. It is always preferable to err on the side of transporting a patient but, in all cases, confer first with online medical control.

Psychiatric emergencies present particularly vexing problems of consent. When a person's life is not in danger, a police officer is generally the only individual given the authority to restrain and transport that person against his or her will. An EMS system should not do so except at the express request of the police. Notably, neither a physician nor the patient's family may, in most regions, authorize such transport; they may authorize involuntary *commitment*, but their authority does not extend to the forcible transport of a patient against his or her will. Therefore, it is essential for every EMS service to establish protocols, based on local laws, for dealing with the mentally disturbed patient who refuses transport. In many instances, the participation of the police will be required, and the role of each agency involved should be clearly defined beforehand.

Use of Force: Violent Patients and Using Restraints

The use of force by paramedics against patients has been the cause of numerous lawsuits in recent years. However, in the reality of today's EMS practice, the paramedic will encounter violent patients who must be restrained in order to protect the patients themselves and to protect those who are trying to care for them.

Under the law, paramedics can use force only in response to a patient's use of force against them. If the paramedic is attacked, he or she may defend himself or herself against the attack. However, the use of temporary disabling sprays, knives, or firearms are generally outside the scope of the paramedic's practice and are usually prohibited by the EMS agency. The amount of force that is allowed under the law is either equal to or slightly greater than the force offered by the patient, and must be in response to the patient's actions. Violence against EMS providers is on the rise. It is always acceptable—nay, almost obligatory—for paramedics to refuse to enter a dangerous and unsecured situation, or for paramedics to leave a situation that becomes violent, until law enforcement can secure the scene and make it safe for paramedics to enter.

In situations requiring patient restraint for medical reasons, it is important to understand that a paramedic may only restrain patients when they are a danger to themselves or to others **Figure 4-14 ▶**. Violence can be the result of hypoxia, hypoglycemia, mental illness, brain injury, drug abuse or overdose, alcohol, or a variety of other underlying medical and psychiatric causes. Specific medical protocols should cover what is considered appropriate in your EMS system for restraining patients, and should spell out what medications or devices are allowed for use in restraining patients. Many EMS systems now use medications, such as benzodiazepines or antipsychotics, to calm patients who are violent and need transportation to a hospital to discover the underlying medical or psychiatric cause of their outbursts.

Transportation

Patients should be transported to the hospital of their choice when possible and reasonable; however, most EMS systems have

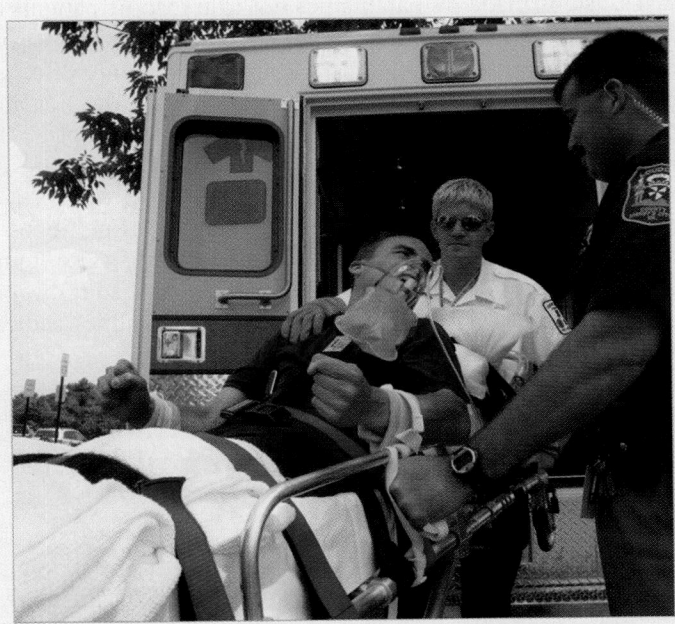

Figure 4-14 Use restraint only when absolutely necessary to ensure your own safety and that of the patient. Remember that it takes several strong people to fully restrain a patient, ideally.

protocols that direct paramedics to transport certain types of patients to particular hospitals. The capability of each hospital to care for particular kinds of patients should guide the EMS system in developing transport protocols. Transportation of patients to a facility that does not have the ability to care for their particular illness or injury can result in liability for the paramedic.

You are the Provider Part 4

Law enforcement arrives at the scene and successfully restrains your patient, who now has multiple lacerations on his face, arms, and torso. You are able to control major bleeding, initiate an IV, and provide dextrose to raise his blood glucose level. You transport him to the nearest appropriate hospital for further treatment of his injuries. Just as you transfer his care to emergency department staff, the patient's wife bursts through the emergency department doors, screaming at you and your partner and threatening to file a lawsuit. She says, "You abandoned my husband! Now look at him! This is all your fault!"

Reassessment	Recording Time: 20 Minutes
Level of consciousness	A (Alert to person, place, and day)
Skin	Warm, pink, and moist
Pulse	100 beats/min; strong and regular
Blood pressure	112/64 mm Hg
Respirations	24 breaths/min; adequate depth
Sao$_2$	98% on oxygen at 6 L/min via nasal cannula
Blood glucose	120 mg/dL

7. Can she prove negligence?
8. Can she file a lawsuit?

Decisions made by paramedics not to transport patients at all have been the subject of litigation. A number of studies have demonstrated that paramedics should not be compelled to decide which patients need to be transported to the hospital for any health problems. Paramedics, indeed the whole EMS system, do not have access to sophisticated diagnostic tools or radiography in the prehospital setting. Failure to transport a patient whose condition later deteriorates can bring about a lawsuit that is difficult to defend. Again, most EMS systems have protocols outlining when it is acceptable not to transport a patient, and many require consultation with online medical control.

Crime Scene and Emergency Scene Responsibilities

When handling a situation involving a death, or any potential crime scene, remember that it may take law enforcement officials some time to figure out whether the scene involved a suicide, homicide, or some other form of criminal activity. It is important for paramedics to use extreme caution and not disturb or destroy potential evidence.

If the scene is a vehicle crash, don't move anything unless you have to—including broken glass, pieces of metal, or even a beer can. Leave dead bodies where they are until a coroner or medical examiner arrives to investigate.

If the incident scene is indoors, don't touch anything you don't have to touch, such as telephones or doorknobs, because of the risk of eliminating fingerprints. Carefully document any statements made by witnesses and get their contact information. Limit the number of EMS personnel who enter the scene, as each person who enters further contaminates what may later turn out to be a crime scene.

Remember that in rape cases the victim may carry vital pieces of evidence, such as fiber or hair, on his or her body—take care to protect this evidence.

If the scene involves a death, stay with the body until the police arrive, and protect the scene from contamination by bystanders, family members, media, or additional EMS personnel.

In most jurisdictions, a paramedic is not legally authorized to pronounce a patient dead. If you have any doubt about the possibility of saving the patient, initiate resuscitation and transport him or her to the hospital.

Documentation

Importance of Documentation

Even the most skilled and conscientious health care professional may eventually have to go to court as a witness or defendant in a civil or criminal action. The paramedic's best protection in court is a *thorough and accurate medical record*. This cannot be overstressed. The information recorded should con-

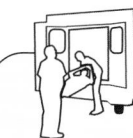

In the Field

Be aware that at crime scenes the perpetrator may still be at or near the scene and could be a factor in when and how you care for your patient.

tain only a record of the facts of what your findings and patient treatment entailed. Remember, you are at the scene and the emergency department physician is not; therefore, you can assist greatly by painting a picture of what you experienced at the scene. Whenever a paramedic cares for a patient in the field, a careful, detailed record should be made of at least the following information, which are the characteristics of an effective patient care report:

- **Date and times.** The time the call was received, the time of your arrival at the scene, the time of your departure from the scene, and the time of your arrival at the hospital.
- **History.** Information elicited from the patient and bystanders. If you are quoting patients or bystanders directly, identify them and put their statements in quotation marks.
- **Observations.** Observations of the scene, particularly if they suggest how the injury took place.
- **Physical examination.** Give a detailed description of your assessments. Include all pertinent negatives, for example, any part of the body you examine and find to be normal.
- **Treatment.** Be precise! Do not write, for example, "IV therapy was given." Write "An IV was initiated under orders from Dr Smith with an 18-gauge Angiocath and D_5W to a keep-open rate."
- **Changes.** Note any changes in the patient's status while under your care.

Documentation and Communication

For syncope, pertinent negatives include (but are not limited to) the patient denying that he or she has had recent diarrhea, vomiting, or tarry or bloody stools.

Patient Care Report

The following is an example of a thorough patient care report:

EXAMPLE   PATIENT CARE REPORT

BLS 7 responded to a 911 dispatch for a possible heart attack @ a private residence. Arrived @ 3235 1st avenue @ 12:55 to find a 73 y/o female complaining that her grandson "is causing her to have a heart attack." Next-door neighbor, crew from engine 6, & grandson are on scene. Neighbor called 911-dispatch center.

Subjective
Chief Complaint: Chest Pain
Pt states sudden onset while arguing c̄ grandson. She feels this may have triggered the pain because she was quite upset.

EXAMPLE PATIENT CARE REPORT

She has taken 2 of her own NTG in the last 15 minutes s̄ relief. Describes chest pain as crushing to the left side of her chest radiating to her jaw & left arm. Rates it a 9 on 1-10 scale & states it began 1 hour ago. She also complains of some sweating & SOB. States she has ∅ allergies to meds, has medical history of chest pain & takes NTG for relief. States while having lunch, she got into an argument c̄ grandson & started having chest pain. Denies any nausea, vomiting, or dizziness. Grandson stated, "She fell in the kitchen." Pt repeatedly denies falling. ∅ evidence of trauma noted on assessment.

Objective
Arrived to find pt sitting on front steps of home, c̄ O2 by NRB 15 lpm being administered by fire fighters. Pt appears to be in moderate distress, anxious, holding her hand to her chest & unable to sit still. Airway–clear. Breathing–lungs clear equal bilaterally, c̄ good tidal volume, equal rise/fall of chest & ∅ noted accessory muscle use. Circulation–strong/regular radial pulse, skin pale/cool/clammy. Disability–alert, able to speak full/clear sentences.
Head–3″ laceration below left eye c̄ swelling & redness left side of face, ∅ other trauma noted. Pupils–equal and reactive, Chest–intact, ∅ noted change to chest pain c̄ palpation or inspiration. Abd–soft non-tender, Extremities– +PMS in all extremities c̄ equal hand grips. Posterior Body– spinal assessment reveals spinal area non-tender, ∅ numbness/tingling/weakness or loss of sensation in any extremity. Baseline Vitals: BP-128/80, P-88, R-20. Refer to vital signs data boxes for times and reassessment.

Analysis
Possible: Cardiac Chest Pain

Rule out: Head / C-Spine Injury

Plan
12:55– Arrive, initial assessment, spinal immobilization equipment applied with no change to PMS post immobilization, vitals assessed, continue O2 at 15 lpm/NRM. Pt states oxygen is not helping her chest pain. Pt agrees to treatment & transport.

13:04– Confirm that NTG is pts, was prescribed by her physician, & she has taken 2 c̄ last one being > 5 minutes ago. Dressed wound with 4x4.

13:06– Paramedic Jones assisted pt in administration of 1 sublingual 0.4 mg NTG tab.

13:10– Moved pt to ambulance, en route to hospital.

13:15– Reassess, pt states the pain is now a "3" on 1-10 scale, she states "SOB is now gone." Skin color is improved, pt appears more relaxed.

13:17– Vitals reassessed with no change. Pt removed O2 mask stated "I don't need or want this anymore." Explained to pt significant importance of O2 with chest pain and potential for condition to worsen if oxygen is discontinued. Pt still refused NRM or nasal cannula.

13:20– Arrive ED, pt care transferred & report given to RN Turner.

Complete your records as soon as possible after the call. Even a few hours later, the details may become vague in your memory. Write legibly in ink. Be as precise and detailed as possible. Document everything you did, and everything about your examination and reassessment of the patient. Remember, *if you don't document it, you can't prove you did it.* Your patient care report becomes a permanent part of the patient's record. It is also a legal document and reflects on its author.

Neatness counts! A sloppy, incomplete record suggests to the reader (and to the court!) that the care of the patient may also have been sloppy and incomplete Figure 4-15 . Such records are red flags to plaintiff's attorneys who consider them an invitation to file suit. Take the time to make your records accurate and thorough. Document any unusual events, including equipment failures, interference by bystanders, getting lost, or other problems you encounter either on the way to or at the scene. These problems should be documented factually and objectively. All crew members—not just the one writing the report—should sign the report legibly, and denote their crew numbers.

There are some things a paramedic should never do in a medical record. It is not the place for creative writing. The medical record is not the place for flippant or derogatory remarks about a patient. At the very least, you could live to regret your error when your remarks are read out loud in a court of law. Do not use the medical record to blame another medical provider for an adverse event. Find another outlet for your opinions, medical or otherwise. The medical record is the worst possible place to voice frustrations with the administration of the EMS system. You will only hurt, not help, any systems issues that may arise in the course of a lawsuit.

Your Report Becomes Part of the Medical Record
Always leave a copy of your written report at the emergency department. It is critical for you to leave a written record of your field treatment of the patient to ensure continuity of care in the emergency department Figure 4-16 . The emergency department staff needs to know how you encountered the patient, what treatment you rendered, and any changes in the patient's condition resulting from your care. Failure to leave a copy of the report can result in duplication of treatment, or a lack of understanding of what precipitated the emergency call. That copy of your report will become a part of the patient's permanent medical record. Paramedics in busy services who race out the door without leaving a record of their care leave themselves open for problems with the legal system, if not the hospital. Remember, many hospitals caution all health care providers against verbal orders. Verbal records are unprofessional.

Retention of Medical Records
Your run reports should be maintained for a period generally described by state law. Providers should never keep personal copies of patient care reports because of the confidential nature of the information contained.

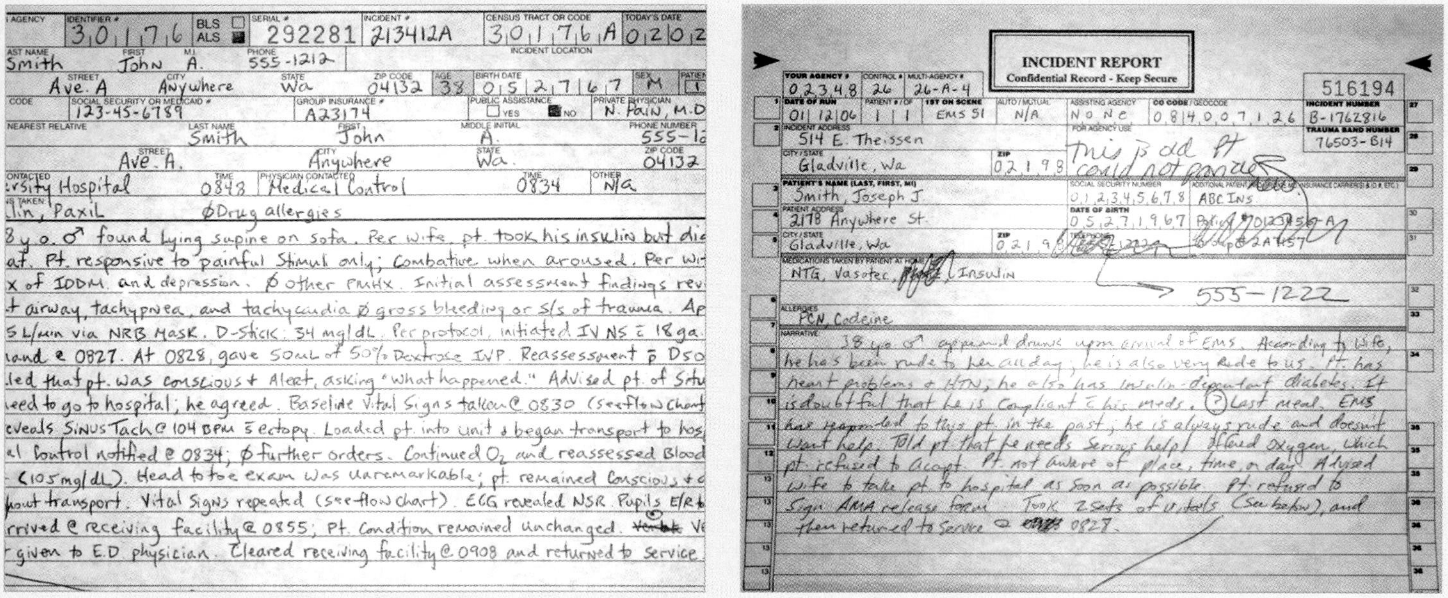

Figure 4-15 Filing a patient care report is a critical part of your responsibilities as a paramedic. **A.** Proper documentation **B.** Improper documentation. Particularly if you sense that there might be legal complications with a patient, take extra time and care to submit a thorough report.

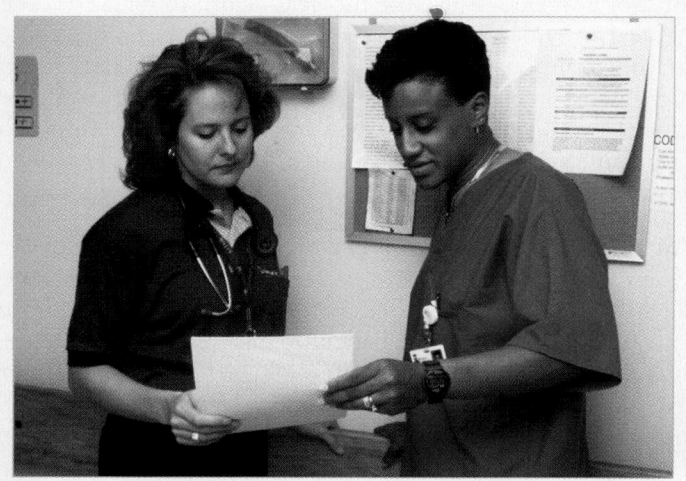

Figure 4-16 Part of ensuring competent and continuous care for each patient is making sure that the patient's report is handed over to appropriate medical personnel at the hospital.

Reportable Cases

Each state has its own requirements regarding categories of cases that must be reported to the appropriate authorities. These cases include some of the most difficult a paramedic will see.

Virtually every state has laws requiring EMS providers to report suspected child abuse. It is essential for you to be familiar with the reporting requirements of your own state.

The obligation to report is most frequently applied to the following categories of cases:

- Neglect or abuse of children
- Neglect or abuse of older people
- Domestic violence
- Injury sustained during the commission of a felony, or specific injuries considered to be of suspicious origin (such as gunshot wounds or stab wounds)
- Drug-related injuries
- Childbirth occurring outside a licensed medical facility
- Rape
- Animal bites
- Certain communicable diseases

As noted, reporting requirements vary widely from state to state. Learn the laws of your state and observe the reporting obligations that apply to you.

Special Considerations

Elder abuse is as prevalent as child abuse in our society. Do not forget to be observant and report any suspicious signs or symptoms to the proper authorities.

Coroner and Medical Examiner Cases

Every EMS system should have a list of procedures for coroner and medical examiner cases Figure 4-17 ▸. Although the coroner's law varies somewhat from state to state, generally you should notify the police of all coroner cases, including:

1. Obvious or suspected homicide
2. Obvious or suspected suicide
3. Any other violent or sudden, unexpected death
4. Death of a prison inmate

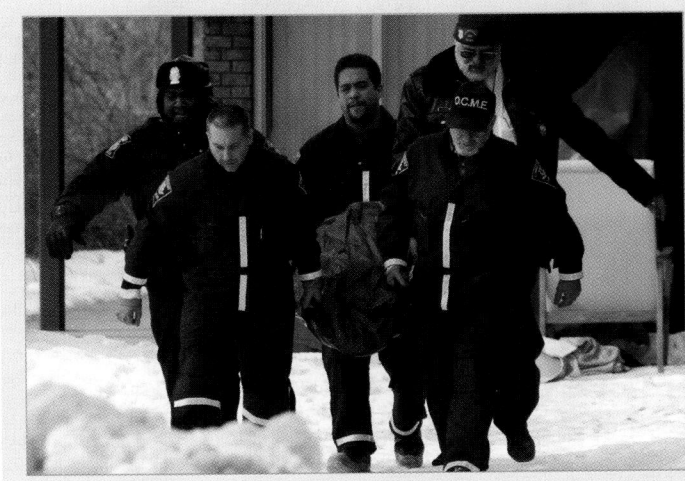

Figure 4-17 In any situation involving the death of an individual, paramedics should contact the police or coroner with pertinent details depending on local protocols.

You are the Provider Summary

1. What clues, if any, were available to tip you off as to the potential for this patient to become violent?

Most often, body language is a bigger indicator of potential violence than words that patients use. This patient had his back to you with his shoulders raised and fists clenched. These are all indications of impending violence. If you have no indication that the scene is unsafe, and you find yourself in a situation such as this one, maintain a safe distance, never allow the patient to come between you and your exit, call for law enforcement, and immediately leave the scene if you feel you or your partner are in danger.

2. What would be the best course of action at this point?

Your best course of action is to leave the immediate area. It takes, at minimum, four trained personnel to safely restrain a patient (one for each limb). Because you do not have these resources immediately available, you are not able to safely restrain this patient. Unfortunately, violence can erupt very quickly, and it is imperative not to enter a scene you believe is unsafe or to put yourself or your partner in harm's way.

3. Could your actions be considered abandonment?

Technically, you left the patient after you had initiated contact. However, you were unable to render required medical care because of the patient's combative behavior. You remained ready to provide necessary treatment as soon as the patient had been properly restrained. It could be argued that you should have responded with an adequate number of staff and/or law enforcement because the details of the call were unknown. This could be construed as a grey area, depending on the interpreter.

4. What other courses of action, if any, could be taken?

When you are unsure as to the intent of the patient, or suspect that the patient could become violent, you should avoid any physical movement or verbal statements that may induce anger. It would have been more prudent to slowly initiate contact rather than immediately attempting to gain eye contact.

5. Was any part of this situation avoidable?

As part of your training, you will learn that the brain is very sensitive to lowered levels of blood glucose and blood oxygen. Hypoglycemic and hypoxic states can cause significant deterioration in mental status, sometimes accompanied by bizarre or combative behavior. Be on the lookout for these things when dealing with known diabetics who have apparent low blood glucose levels.

6. What would be helpful in handling this situation?

The more information that can be obtained regarding the details of the incident prior to your arrival, the greater chance you have of avoiding a situation such as this one. However, for reasons stated earlier, this may not be possible. Be prepared for the unexpected.

7. Can she prove negligence?

If it could be proved that you should have known that the patient was likely to become violent, then negligence could be proven. For instance, if this patient had a history of becoming violent and you did not immediately request appropriate additional resources, then there could be a legitimate claim of negligence.

8. Can she file a lawsuit?

Yes. People can and do file lawsuits for many reasons. The best method of protection is to always follow local protocols, document each call thoroughly, and act in the patient's best interest. Doing these things will minimize chances of a successful lawsuit against you. This does not, however, prevent a lawsuit from occurring.

Prep Kit

Ready for Review

- Paramedics operate in a community that exposes them to professional liability. Failing to perform their job as expected within the medical community, the legal community, and the regulations of the jurisdiction in which they function will expose them to civil and/or criminal liability.
- The foundation of our legal system is our federal government. There are three branches of government: executive, judicial, and legislative.
- There are two types of law: civil and criminal.
  - Civil cases result in monetary damages.
  - Criminal cases result in incarceration of an individual.
- Paramedics are particularly susceptible to charges of assault and battery. Assault is when you instill the fear of bodily harm. Battery is when you (as a paramedic) unlawfully touch another without his or her consent.
- False imprisonment can occur when a paramedic restrains a patient against his or her will. Protection against this charge can exist only if appropriate documentation and policy exist regarding the specific call.
- Defamation, slander, and libel present risks to paramedics when they make statements, either verbal or written, that injure a person's good name. Saying a patient looks drunk is inappropriate. Paramedics should describe the behavior that reflects their concerns.
- Lawsuits follow a general process that starts with a complaint or notice of complaint, a response or answer by the defendant, discovery, settlement discussions, and trial process.
- Paramedics are subject to multiple legal jurisdictions, including state law, state regulations, local medical protocol, and departmental policy.
- Medical directors have a supervisory relationship over paramedics.
- Your activities function as an extension of a series of medical directions from the medical director that are either online or offline. These directives are binding on paramedics unless they believe that they will cause harm to the patient.
- State legislation enables paramedics to practice in every state. It is the responsibility of paramedics to understand the statutes of the state in which they practice.
- State laws define scope of practice for the paramedic, which specifies the limits of practice allowed under the Medical Practice Act.
- HIPAA was enacted to protect patient information from unlawful and unnecessary dissemination.
- EMTALA is another federal law designed to prevent hospital emergency departments from turning patients away for any reason. Paramedics must be sure that the patients they are transporting from one facility to another have been managed in accordance with EMTALA.
- Emergency vehicle operations must be done in a manner that protects the public from further injury. No call can justify driving in a manner that endangers the public.
- You may provide care when off duty and in most jurisdictions be protected under the Good Samaritan laws. Paramedics must remember that they are only protected if they perform within their training and education and if they do not receive any compensation.
- You can be protected under certain governmental immunity clauses. These protections may not be valid if the paramedics have committed negligence or if the paramedics are deemed to be liable personally.

- Negligence occurs only when four processes have occurred:
  - Duty to act. The paramedic must have had a duty to act.
  - Breach of duty. The paramedic did not fulfill that duty.
  - Proximate cause. The paramedic's breach of duty caused the plaintiff's injury.
  - Injury resulted. An injury occurred as a result of the above.
- As the highest level of prehospital care providers, paramedics must ensure that they do not abandon their patients. Abandonment can occur anytime paramedics turn over their patients inappropriately or to a level of care lesser than themselves.
  - Documentation is the only methodology to prevent the appearance of abandonment.
- Patients have the right to determine their own care. Paramedics must understand their legal limitations based on any advance directives issued by the patient.
- Do not resuscitate (DNR) orders are a specific form of advance directive that generally define the care a patient wants when lifesaving procedures are required. A DNR order is *not* a "do-not-care-for-the-patient" order.
- State jurisdictions issue paramedics either licenses or certificates. Paramedics must understand that the licensure or certification is a privilege extended by the governing authority that allows paramedics to practice within the enacting legislation.
- All patients of sound mind have the legal right under the US Constitution to privacy, consent, and refusal. Paramedics cannot infringe on these inalienable rights unless they believe that patients are not of sound mind and pose a detriment to themselves or others.
- You must obtain informed consent from patients prior to any medical process including examination.
- You must get expressed consent from patients before initiating treatment.
- Implied consent is said to exist when patients are unable to answer for themselves and paramedics deem that treatment is required.
- Minors pose challenges that local jurisdictions must address before a call occurs. In general, if the patient is a minor, the minor has neither the right to consent to care nor the right to refuse it. Paramedics must always take responsibility for minors.
- Documentation is the lifeblood of a paramedic. All calls should have documentation that reflects what occurred. The documentation must include any and all demographics, times, history of events, physical examinations, treatment processes, and changes.
- Documentation is a legal form that will be used against you if you are part of a legal action.
- Patient refusals pose a large potential legal liability to paramedics. The only protection against a civil suit over a refusal will be the documentation that the paramedic produces at the time of the incident.
  - A refusal signature without narrative and evidence of a physical examination is worthless.
- Paramedics must plan to protect themselves and their partners from violence. Understanding local law enforcement protocols and having local medical protocols for the restraint of patients by both physical and chemical methods are necessary.
- Crime scenes present the intersection between EMS and law enforcement. Paramedics have an obligation to assist the law enforcement community in preservation of evidence and documentation of scenes or actions that may later be introduced on behalf of a criminal prosecution.

■ Vital Vocabulary

abandonment Abrupt termination of contact with the patient without giving the patient sufficient opportunity to find another suitable health care professional to take over his or her medical treatment.

advance directive A written document that expresses the wants, needs, and desires of a patient in reference to future medical care; examples include living wills, do not resuscitate (DNR) orders, and organ donation.

assault To create in another person a fear of immediate bodily harm or invasion of bodily security.

battery Any act of touching another person without that person's consent.

civil suit An action instituted by a private individual or corporation against another private individual or corporation.

consent Agreement by the patient to accept a medical intervention.

criminal prosecution An action instituted by the government against a private individual for violation of criminal law.

damages Compensation for injury awarded by a court.

decision-making capacity The patient's ability to understand and process the information you give him or her about your proposed plan of care.

defamation Intentionally making a false statement, through written or verbal communication, which injures a person's good name or reputation.

defendant In a civil suit, the individual against whom a legal action is brought.

do not resuscitate (DNR) order A type of advance directive that describes which life-sustaining procedures should be performed in the event of a sudden deterioration in a patient's medical condition.

due process A right to a fair procedure for a legal action against a person or agency; has two components: *Notice* and *Opportunity to be Heard*.

duty Legal obligation of public and certain other ambulance services to respond to a call for help in their jurisdiction.

emancipated minor A person who is under the legal age in a given state but, because of other circumstances, is legally considered an adult.

EMTALA The Emergency Medical Treatment and Active Labor Act enacted in 1986 to combat the practice of patient dumping (hospitals refusing to admit seriously ill patients or women in labor who could not pay, forcing EMS providers to dump the patients at another hospital). EMTALA regulates hospitals that receive Medicare funding and severely fines hospitals or doctors who violate its provisions.

ethics A set of values in society that differentiates right from wrong.

expressed consent A type of informed consent that occurs when the patient does something, either through words or by taking some sort of action, that demonstrates permission to provide care.

false imprisonment The intentional and unjustified detention of a person against his or her will.

Good Samaritan law A statute providing limited immunity from liability to persons responding voluntarily and in good faith to the aid of an injured person outside the hospital.

gross negligence Negligence that is willful, wanton, intentional, or reckless; a serious departure from the accepted standards.

HIPAA The Health Insurance Portability and Accountability Act that was enacted in 1996, providing for criminal sanctions as well as for civil penalties for releasing a patient's protected health information (PHI) in a way not authorized by the patient.

immunity Legal protection from penalties that could normally be incurred under the law.

implied consent Assumption on behalf of a person unable to give consent that he or she would have done so.

informed consent A patient's voluntary agreement to be treated after being told about the nature of the disease, the risks and benefits of the proposed treatment, alternative treatments, or the choice of no treatment at all.

liability A finding in civil cases that the preponderance of the evidence shows the defendant was responsible for the plaintiff's injuries.

libel Making a false statement in written form that injures a person's good name.

Medical Practice Act An act that usually defines the minimum qualifications of those who may perform various health services, defines the skills that each type of practitioner is legally permitted to use, and establishes a means of certification for different categories of health care professional.

negligence Professional action or inaction on the part of the health care worker that does not meet the standard of ordinary care expected of similarly trained and prudent health care practitioners and that results in injury to the patient.

ordinary negligence Negligence that is a failure to act, or a simple mistake that causes harm to a patient.

plaintiff In a civil suit, the individual who brings a legal action against another individual.

proximate cause The specific reason that an injury occurred; one of the items that must be proven in order for a paramedic to be held liable for negligence.

qualified immunity Protection in which the paramedic is only held liable when the plaintiff can show that the paramedic violated clearly established law of which he or she should have known.

scope of practice What a state permits a paramedic practicing under its license or certification to do.

slander Verbally making a false statement that injures a person's good name.

standard of care What a reasonable paramedic with training would do in the same or a similar situation.

tort A wrongful act that gives rise to a civil suit.

Assessment in Action

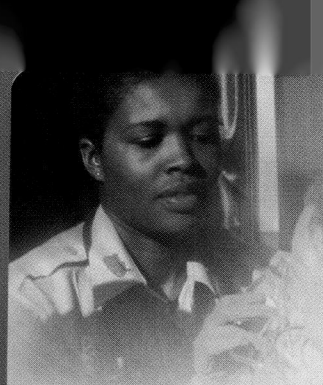

You are called to a scene in which a man with altered mental status is bleeding heavily from an open cut on his forehead. The neighbors called 9-1-1 after seeing him in his yard where he was having trouble walking and attempting to mow the lawn in the pouring rain. When you arrive, the man is angry that someone called 9-1-1. He insists that he's fine. He has no memory of how he may have cut his head, isn't making sense, and seems confused. He refuses to let you examine him, refuses to answer any questions, and refuses transport. What would be the appropriate response to the following questions?

1. **Can treating this patient without his consent be considered assault and/or battery?**
   A. Yes
   B. No

2. **What is the difference between *assault* and *battery*?**
   A. Assault is physical contact in a harmful way; battery is severe injury.
   B. Assault is verbal or other threats that instill fear in someone; battery is actually touching someone without their consent.
   C. Assault is verbal threats actually carried out; battery is physically harming someone without any kind of warning to that person.
   D. Assault is physical only; battery is verbal only.

3. **True or false? The scope of practice for a paramedic may vary significantly from state to state.**
   A. True
   B. False

4. **True or false? The medical director has the authority to prevent a paramedic from performing certain skills that he or she is licensed or certified to perform if he or she feels like doing so for some reason.**
   A. True
   B. False

5. **You cannot discuss anything regarding the man in the scenario because of the HIPAA law, which:**
   A. protects the privacy of medical information, insurance information, and any other privacy issues affecting the patient within the health care system.
   B. requires criminal sanctions against anyone who releases private health care information regarding a patient.
   C. requires civil penalties for anyone who uses protected health information in an unauthorized manner.
   D. requires that no personal patient information be released over the radio.

6. **The man tells you that one of the reasons he is refusing transport is lack of medical insurance. How does the EMTALA act relate to this?**
   A. It regulates hospitals that receive Medicare funding, and makes sure patients are stable enough to be transferred to another facility.
   B. It makes sure women in labor are taken to the farthest possible hospital.
   C. It allows private individuals to sue when they are taken to a hospital they didn't want to go to.
   D. It combats the practice of patient dumping, preventing discrimination for any reason, and regulates patient transfers, applying to both sending and receiving facilities.

7. **True or false? If your agency is part of a government agency, you cannot be sued for wrongdoing as a paramedic working for that agency.**
   A. True
   B. False

8. **The elements that must be proven for a negligence lawsuit to be successful are:**
   A. duty; breach of duty; proximate cause; and harm.
   B. duty; breach of duty; harm; and abandonment.
   C. breach of duty; harm; abandonment; and proximate cause.
   D. abandonment and breach of duty.

9. **You must obtain consent—either implied or informed (except in some cases)—to do which of the following?**
   A. Touch a patient, treat a patient, transport a patient
   B. Transport a patient
   C. Treat and transport a patient
   D. None of the above

10. **True or false? A patient with some, or all, of the following, is not able to refuse care.**
    - Patient is not oriented to person, place, and time.
    - Patient demonstrates that he or she does not understand his or her condition or the need for medical attention.
    - It is obvious that the patient is impaired as a result of alcohol or drugs.
    - The patient has an obvious head injury and is not answering questions appropriately.
    A. True
    B. False

11. **What is the paramedic's BEST protection in court, no matter what the charge or case against him or her?**
    A. A good attitude and proper maintenance of skills
    B. His or her reputation, professionally and personally
    C. A thorough and accurate medical record on all patients treated
    D. An exceptional memory of all calls and patients treated

Challenging Questions

12. **You and your crew have transported a patient with minor injuries from a car crash. The emergency department is very busy. Your rescue squad is understaffed. It is a rainy night. You pull aside a nurse and give your report. The nurse says he'll get to her as soon as possible. You leave a copy of the run report at the nurses station and leave the patient on the stretcher. What are you doing wrong that you could be sued for later?**

13. **You are called to a scene of domestic violence. The man who attacked his wife has been taken into custody by local police, who are still on the scene. However, the man has injuries that you know require stitches. He is refusing care. The officers tell you that you can treat and transport him (in their presence) based on the concept of involuntary consent. Why is this not acceptable reasoning? (There is more than one reason.)**

■ Points to Ponder

You and your partner are dispatched to a dying patient who has a valid advance directive per your EMS system. In this advance directive the patient requests that no resuscitative measures be taken. The only care requested is comfort care.

A hospice volunteer is on scene and has requested transport to the hospital. The patient's daughter, who is the medical power of attorney, is also on scene. She was unaware that the volunteer phoned EMS and is refusing to let you and your partner transport the patient to the hospital. The family members are very upset and becoming angry, repeating over and over "she just wanted to die in the bed her husband died in 40 years ago." They state, "This is difficult enough without you here," and they want you to leave.

Did the volunteer have the right to call EMS without speaking to the family first, in particular the medical power of attorney? Does the medical power of attorney have the right to refuse transporting the patient to the hospital? How do you and your partner resolve these issues?

Issues: Defending the Patient's Right to Die With Dignity, Defending the Value of Advance Directives.

5 Ethical Issues

Objectives

Cognitive

1-5.1   Define ethics. (p 5.3)
1-5.2   Distinguish between ethical and moral decisions. (p 5.3)
1-5.3   Identify the premise that should underlie the paramedic's ethical decisions in out-of-hospital care. (p 5.4)
1-5.4   Analyze the relationship between the law and ethics in EMS. (p 5.5)
1-5.5   Compare and contrast the criteria that may be used in allocating scarce EMS resources. (p 5.8)
1-5.6   Identify the issues surrounding the use of advance directives in making a prehospital resuscitation decision. (p 5.5)
1-5.7   Describe the criteria necessary to honor an advance directive in your state. (p 5.6)

Affective

1-5.8   Value the patient's autonomy in the decision-making process. (p 5.5)
1-5.9   Defend the following ethical positions:
   a. The paramedic is accountable to the patient.
   b. The paramedic is accountable to the medical director.
   c. The paramedic is accountable to the EMS system.
   d. The paramedic is accountable for fulfilling the standard of care. (p 5.6)

1-5.10   Given a scenario, defend or challenge a paramedic's actions concerning a patient who is treated against his/her wishes. (p 5.6)
1-5.11   Given a scenario, defend a paramedic's actions in a situation where a physician orders therapy the paramedic feels to be detrimental to the patient's best interests. (p 5.6)

Psychomotor

None

Medical Ethics

Ethics is the philosophy of right and wrong, of moral duties, and of ideal professional behavior. Morality is a code of conduct that can be defined by society, religion, or a person, affecting character, conduct, and conscience.

Paramedics need to be ethical in their practice and be aware of their own moral standards in their daily work. Do not assume that your patients share your moral standards. Your moral standards may conflict with your patients' wishes or your patients' best interests, and it is important that you put your patients' interests before your own Figure 5-1 ▾.

Many times, however, the word *ethics* becomes blurred with the word *morals*. Morality is what *you* think about an issue and ethics are the foundations for the actions you take.

Medical ethics (sometimes called bioethics) is a discipline within ethics that discusses and debates the health care of human beings, your patients. Your understanding of medical ethics must be formed as a part of, and consistent with, the general codes of the health care professional Figure 5-2 ▾. Throughout the ages, there have been many published codes of ethics for health professionals. The Oath of Geneva, drafted by the World Medical Association in 1948, provides a good example; it is the oath taken by many medical students on completion of their studies, at the time of being admitted to the medical profession:

> "I solemnly pledge myself to consecrate my life to the service of humanity; I will give to my teachers the respect and gratitude which is their due; I will practice my profession with conscience and dignity; the health of my patient will be my first consideration; I will respect the secrets which are confided in me; I will maintain by all the means in my power the honor and noble traditions of the medical profession; my colleagues will be my brothers; I will not permit considerations of religion, nationality, race, party politics, or social standing to intervene between my duty and my patient; I will maintain the utmost respect for human life from the time of conception; even under threat, I will not make use of my medical knowledge contrary to the laws of humanity. I make these promises solemnly, freely and upon my honor."

Very similar principles underlie the more detailed *Code of Ethics for Emergency Medical Technicians,* which was issued by

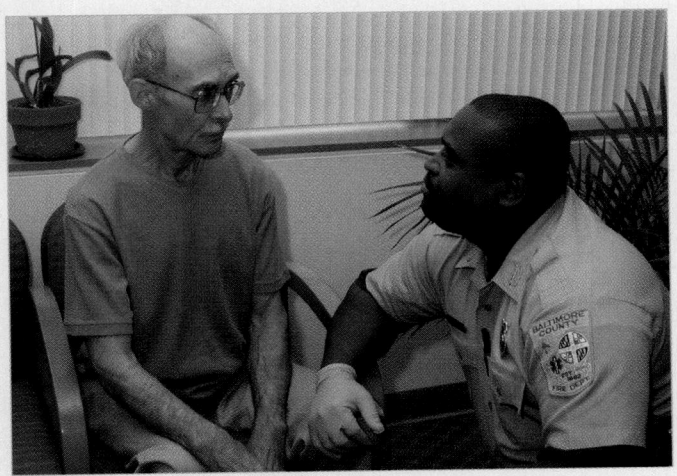

Figure 5-1 As a paramedic serving a diverse public, you will frequently work with people who have cultural backgrounds that are different from your own. Work to set aside your own personal beliefs when making decisions on the patient's behalf.

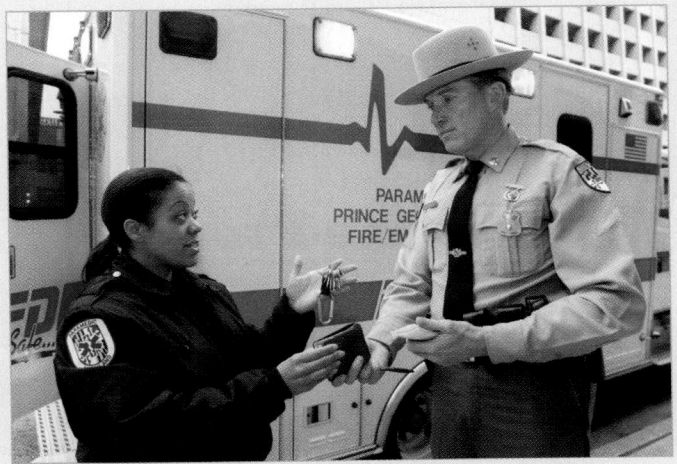

Figure 5-2 When people call 9-1-1, they trust you not only with providing proper medical care, but also with using sound ethical judgment—including the safeguarding of their personal possessions.

You are the Provider Part 1

You are dispatched to 1625 Lance Lane for a 50 year-old-man with an unknown medical problem. En route to the scene, the dispatcher informs you that "CPR is in progress." Your estimated time of arrival to the scene is approximately 15 minutes, but you feel confident this patient has a good chance for survival because your primary service area has a tiered-response system.

In a brief radio report, EMTs advise you that this was a witnessed cardiac arrest. The patient complained of chest pain just prior to collapse, and CPR was started immediately by a family member. No other information is provided. When you ask whether electrical therapy with the AED has been administered, no one replies. You find this odd, and wonder if something is wrong.

1. Are career and volunteer staffing held to the same standards of patient care?
2. If sensitive information needs to be relayed regarding patient care, what other communication options should the EMTs have available?

the National Association of Emergency Medical Technicians in 1978 and is still in effect today:

"Professional status as an Emergency Medical Technician is maintained and enriched by the willingness of the individual practitioner to accept and fulfill obligations to society, other medical professionals, and the profession of Emergency Medical Technician. As an Emergency Medical Technician, I solemnly pledge myself to the following code of ethics:

- The fundamental responsibility of the Emergency Medical Technician is to conserve life, to alleviate suffering, and to promote health.
- The Emergency Medical Technician provides services based on human need, with respect for human dignity, unrestricted by considerations of nationality, race, creed, or status.
- The Emergency Medical Technician does not use professional knowledge and skill in any enterprise detrimental to the public good.
- The Emergency Medical Technician respects and holds in confidence all information of a confidential nature obtained in the course of professional work unless required by law to divulge such information.
- The Emergency Medical Technician as a citizen understands and upholds the laws and performs the duties of citizenship; as a professional person, the Emergency Medical Technician has a particular responsibility to work with other citizens and health professionals in promoting efforts to meet the health needs of the public.
- The Emergency Medical Technician maintains professional competence and demonstrates concern for the competence of other members of the medical profession.

- The Emergency Medical Technician assumes responsibility in defining and upholding standards of professional practice and education. The Emergency Medical Technician assumes responsibility for individual professional actions and judgment, both in dependent and independent emergency functions and knows and upholds the laws that affect the practice of the Emergency Medical Technician.
- The Emergency Medical Technician has the responsibility to participate in the study of and action on matters of legislation affecting Emergency Medical Technicians and emergency service to the public.
- The Emergency Medical Technician adheres to standards of personal ethics that reflect credit upon the profession.
- The Emergency Medical Technician may contribute to research in relation to a commercial product or service, but does not lend professional status to advertising, promotion, or sales.
- The Emergency Medical Technician, or groups of Emergency Medical Technicians, who advertise professional services, do so in conformity with the dignity of the profession.
- The Emergency Medical Technician has an obligation to protect the public by not delegating to a person less qualified any service which requires the professional competence of an Emergency Medical Technician.
- The Emergency Medical Technician works harmoniously with, and sustains confidence in, Emergency Medical Technician associates, the nurse, the physician, and other members of the health team.
- The Emergency Medical Technician refuses to participate in unethical procedures and assumes the responsibility to expose incompetence or unethical conduct in others to the appropriate authority."

You are the Provider Part 2

When you arrive, you learn that the AED could not be used because the battery failed. The EMTs were from a volunteer agency, and no one had been assigned that weekend to check the equipment because it was a holiday and everyone was gone. They ask you not to tell anyone, and promise it will never happen again.

You don't have time to become involved in a detailed discussion, but gather information pertinent to caring for your patient. As you proceed to the hospital, the patient's wife identifies herself, tells you that she is an RN and asks if she can ride with you to the hospital. En route to the receiving facility, she asks you why the AED failed to operate.

Initial Assessment	Recording Time: 15 Minutes
Level of consciousness	U (Unresponsive)
Airway	Patent
Breathing	Bag-mask ventilations
Circulation	Carotid pulse detected with compressions
Vital Signs	
Skin	Cool, mottled with blue mucosa
Blood pressure	None
Sao₂	Unable to obtain
ECG	Asystole in three leads
Pupils	Fixed and dilated

3. Is it ever appropriate to conceal information regarding patient care?
4. How should you answer the wife's question?
5. How and when should you address her concerns?

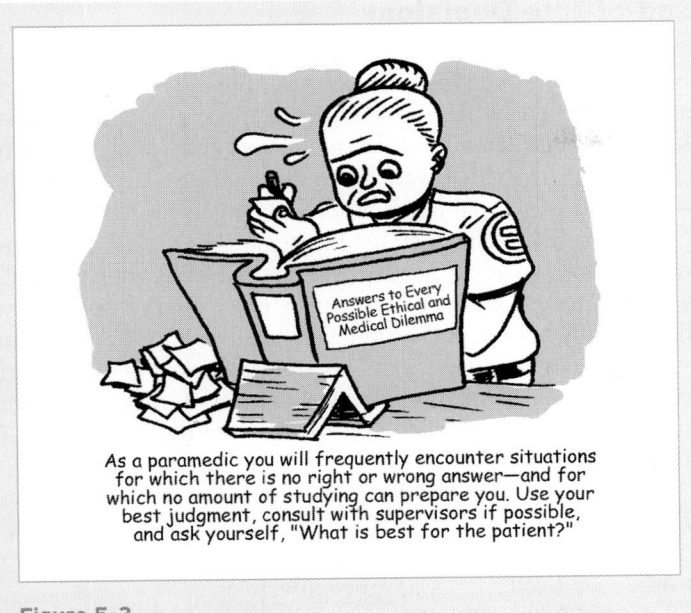

As a paramedic you will frequently encounter situations for which there is no right or wrong answer—and for which no amount of studying can prepare you. Use your best judgment, consult with supervisors if possible, and ask yourself, "What is best for the patient?"

Figure 5-3

These oaths, and others like them, are simply an amplification of a very basic concept: concern for the welfare of others. All of the various codes of right and wrong must ultimately arise from that concern, and it is a safe generalization that *if you place the welfare of the patient ahead of all other considerations, you will rarely if ever commit an unethical act in medical care* `Figure 5-3 ▲` . It would be impossible to enumerate here all the ethical dilemmas with which you may at one time or another be faced in your work as a paramedic. However, if each time you are confronted with a dilemma of right and wrong you ask yourself, "What is in the best interest of the *patient?*" you will be on firm footing.

Controversies

Some religious beliefs influence a patient's decision about being treated and may be different from what you think is best for a patient. Patients sometimes refuse standard life-saving therapies and treatments based on their religious convictions.

Patient's Rights: Autonomy

As you learned in the previous chapter, patients have the right to direct their own care and to decide how they want their end of life medical care provided to them. This right, known as patient autonomy, has come to the forefront of medical ethics.

As medical technology has made the line between life and death more imprecise, a number of high-profile cases have brought the issue of patient autonomy to the forefront of the medical ethics debate in the past 20 years. Most recently, the Terry Schiavo case demonstrated that courts will ultimately support the right of a patient, or their closest relative, to make end-of-life decisions `Figure 5-4 ▼` . Unfortunately Terry Schiavo did not leave written advance directives, which ultimately put the case in the hands of the courts (state and federal). Patients' decisions may not be accepted by other members of the public or other members of the patient's family, but it is important for the paramedic to remember that our Constitution gives each of us the right to make decisions about our own medical care. Patients may well make decisions, such as refusals of treatment, that the paramedic does not agree with, but the paramedic must respect that patient's wishes, assuming the patient has decision-making capacity. Ethics has become the subject of many paramedic discussions because paramedics find themselves in the unique position of being accountable to more systems than the average health care provider in trying to respect the wishes of the patient `Figure 5-5 ▼` . The EMS system, your medical director, the EMS or ambulance service you work for, and your community's standard of care can compete with the wishes of the patient. These competing interests can create an ethical

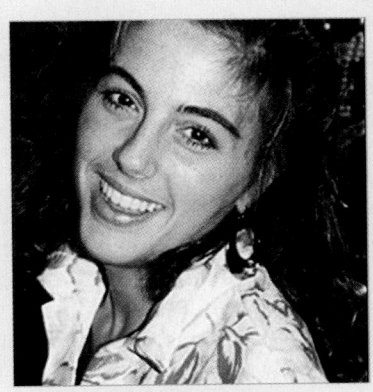

Figure 5-4 Because she did not leave any directive about the type of care she wanted to receive, Terry Schiavo's case became a battleground between family members who held different viewpoints about care of the terminally ill.

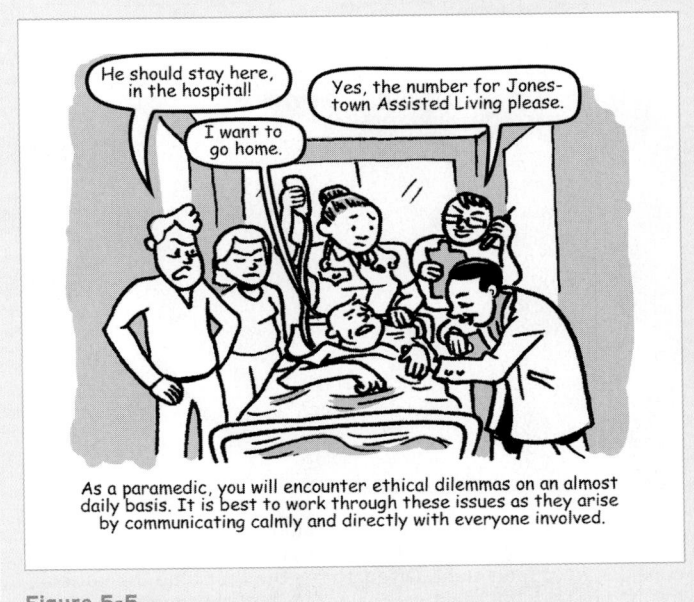

As a paramedic, you will encounter ethical dilemmas on an almost daily basis. It is best to work through these issues as they arise by communicating calmly and directly with everyone involved.

Figure 5-5

conflict that you will want to resolve. How? Communicate, communicate, communicate. Occasionally, a physician will give an order that the paramedic feels is detrimental to the patient's best interests. It is important for the paramedic to discuss why he or she feels that way with the physician immediately. Remember, you are often in a better position to see what is going on with the patient, and a big part of your job is to communicate fully with the physician. A paramedic should never perform a procedure or administer a medication that he or she believes will be detrimental to the patient. If a physician, for example, mistakenly asks you to perform a procedure in which you are not trained, it is important for you to ask the physician to repeat that order. However, if the dispute is not resolved, you need to be a patient advocate and act in the patient's best interest. If the doctor is insistent, there are several ways to handle the problem: (1) Tell the doctor that your standing orders are never to perform this procedure; can he or she suggest another alternative? (2) If you are not working with your medical director, tell the doctor that you can only perform the procedure if your medical director approves. None of these are even half as good as having a good, trusting relationship between you as a paramedic and the staff of the emergency department. Communicate!

A situation that is much more common is the necessity of treating patients against their wishes. Usually, these patients do not have decision-making capacity and therefore consent is implied. If your patient is the proverbial "guy who doesn't want to admit he's having an MI," you must use your best diplomatic negotiating skills to persuade him to come with you to the hospital [Figure 5-6 ▾]. These situations should be covered in protocols and discussed regularly and in detail with your physician medical director. Involve the patient's family, your supervisor, and medical control in persuasion of what is best for the patient.

End-of-Life Decisions

Paramedics will often deal with patients at the very end of their lives. It is a unique trust in EMS, and these patients, and their families, should be treated with the utmost respect and empathy. Paramedics should never think: "Why did they bother to call 9-1-1 if they don't want us to do anything?" (An example, by the way, of the paramedic moral code getting in the way of the paramedic's medical ethics.) Instead, you must understand that the family of a dying patient, even one under hospice care, may not know how to check a pulse, and may not understand that difficult, agonal respirations may continue for hours before a patient actually dies. Many people have never been with someone at the moment of death. You have. If information and support is what they called you for, be sure they receive it—it is part of your job.

There are two major concepts that direct prehospital care about end-of-life decisions: the do not resuscitate (DNR) order and the advance directive. The living will and durable power of attorney are two types of advance directives.

Paramedics need to be aware that advance directives differ from state to state. Not only do the 50 states disagree on *how* to let health care providers know what a patient's wishes are, but there is no common agreement on *what* can be done for a patient and on *who* can execute the DNR order. In some states, a DNR order may restrict any advanced life support care, while others provide for comfort care, including pain medications and oxygen therapy. In Colorado, a person designated as the medical durable power of attorney can revoke a resuscitation directive. However, in Montana the patient or physician are the only ones who can revoke a resuscitation directive. Because of these differences, paramedics must be versed in their own local and state protocols and regulations.

DNR Orders

During the last decade, DNR orders were finally recognized in the prehospital setting [Figure 5-7 ▾]. EMS has now joined

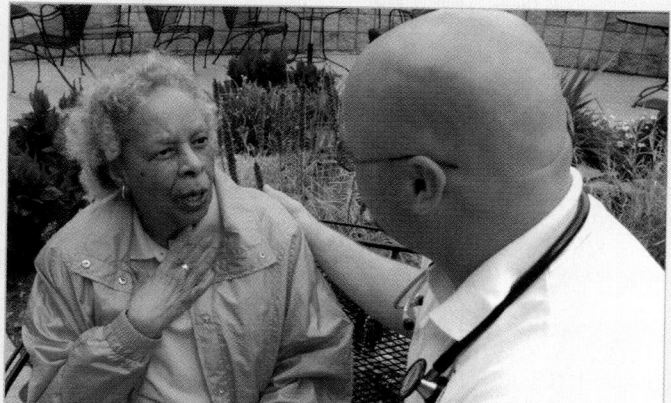

Figure 5-6 Remember that the decision to accept medical treatment is a difficult one. Give the patient time to think and to consider what feels right. Often, this is the first time the patient has had to face the reality of his or her medical condition.

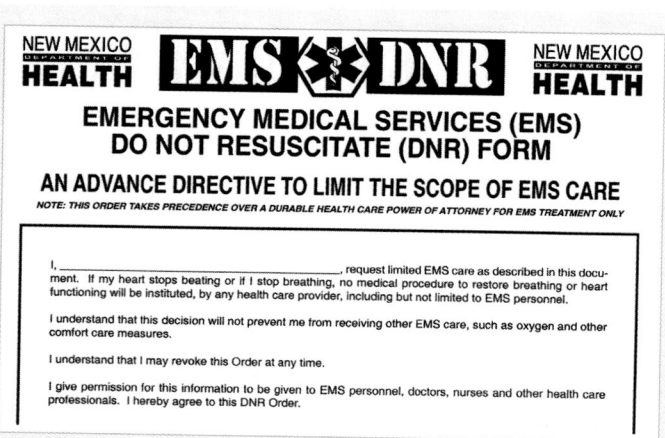

NEW MEXICO DEPARTMENT OF HEALTH   EMS✦DNR   NEW MEXICO DEPARTMENT OF HEALTH

EMERGENCY MEDICAL SERVICES (EMS) DO NOT RESUSCITATE (DNR) FORM

AN ADVANCE DIRECTIVE TO LIMIT THE SCOPE OF EMS CARE

NOTE: THIS ORDER TAKES PRECEDENCE OVER A DURABLE HEALTH CARE POWER OF ATTORNEY FOR EMS TREATMENT ONLY

I, _____, request limited EMS care as described in this document. If my heart stops beating or if I stop breathing, no medical procedure to restore breathing or heart functioning will be instituted, by any health care provider, including but not limited to EMS personnel.

I understand that this decision will not prevent me from receiving other EMS care, such as oxygen and other comfort care measures.

I understand that I may revoke this Order at any time.

I give permission for this information to be given to EMS personnel, doctors, nurses and other health care professionals. I hereby agree to this DNR Order.

Figure 5-7 Do not resuscitate (DNR) orders can apply for a patient before he or she is taken to a hospital. Make sure you are familiar with the specific legalities of DNR orders in your area.

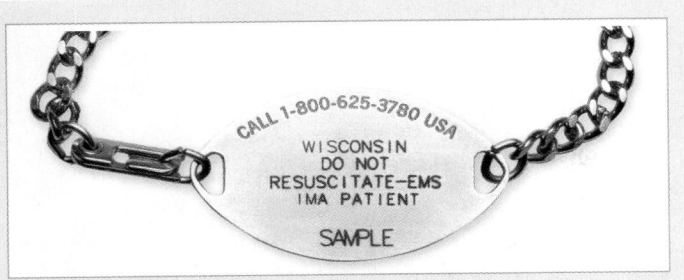

Figure 5-8 Medical ID bracelets can provide access to vital information about a patient, including important medical conditions and possible DNR orders. In the case of MedicAlert®, the EMS provider can obtain stored patient information from the MedicAlert Foundation.

the medical community in recognizing that patients have the same rights to direct their care, and to refuse care, outside the hospital that they do inside the hospital. Many states now have DNR forms specific to EMS, and most states have laws that govern the process of dying and what rights patients have to direct that process.

Although the technicalities may vary from state to state, EMS DNR orders are written orders designed to tell EMS providers when resuscitation is or is not appropriate. States have their own procedure for how to recognize a valid DNR order. Some states rely on a written physician order (which might not be available to the EMS provider), while others may require the patient to wear a bracelet or necklace. In some cases, such jewelry indicates that the patient has consented to the release of stored information, such as the patient's DNR status, to medical personnel (Figure 5-8 ▲). In some states, DNR orders expire within a specified time frame, and must be renewed in order to remain valid, while others may have no expiration date. You should be familiar with the documents used in your state, and what you are expected to do if the documents are not available.

You, the paramedic, should avoid imposing your own moral code on a patient whose value system may be very different from your own. Paramedics will be called to assist with dying patients with varied cultural beliefs and should be prepared to respect a patient's wishes even if the patient's lifestyle or religious beliefs differ greatly from the paramedic's.

Paramedics are likely to encounter confusing scenarios when the DNR paperwork may not be immediately available. It is permissible to begin resuscitation efforts, and then to discontinue them if and when the paperwork is confirmed. In other situations, the paperwork may be present, but family members may disagree with the DNR order and insist that you begin resuscitation. In these situations, avoid any hostile encounters while carrying out the patient's wishes to the best of your ability. Contact medical control in confusing situations involving resuscitation questions.

Advance Directives: Living Wills and Health Care Power of Attorney

Advance directives are generally executed while the patient has decision-making capacity. Advance directives may be given orally, as well as in writing; however, the written form is preferred as there may be disputes among family members about the patient's stated wishes. The extent to which an oral directive will be honored will vary from situation to situation.

The living will and the health care power of attorney (also called a durable power of attorney) are types of advance directives in which a patient can express his or her wishes regarding end of life medical care. These directives are sometimes called health care "durable" powers of attorney because they remain in effect once a patient loses decision-making capacity. Living wills generally require some kind of precondition to activate, such as a terminal illness or an irreversible coma, for them to become active. The living will should spell out exactly what kind of treatment a patient wishes to be given, should he or she be incapacitated. Such a living will often contains a health care power of attorney, which designates another person to make health care decisions for the patient at any time the patient is unable to make those decisions (eg, a spouse, partner, adult sibling, or parent). The person designated to make

In the Field

Do not be confused: A living will is not the same as a DNR order. The living will allows for decisions to be made regarding DNR orders if a patient becomes incapacitated or unable to make his or her own decisions.

You are the Provider Part 3

After you arrive at the hospital your patient is pronounced dead. At this point, there is no way for you to know whether the patient could have been saved with the prompt use of the AED. You contact your shift supervisor, notify him of this issue and contact your medical program director to report the incident to her. You then carefully document all of the pertinent patient care information in the medical incident report.

6. Beyond the documentation required to complete the medical incident report, what else should you document and how?

7. Why is it important to completely and concisely document a call, especially a call such as this one?

8. What is the purpose of continuous quality improvement?

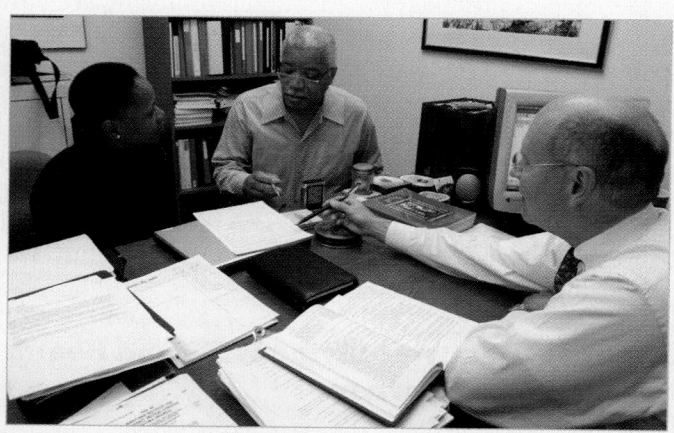

Figure 5-9 A surrogate decision maker (often a child or other close relative) is frequently designated when a person draws up a living will.

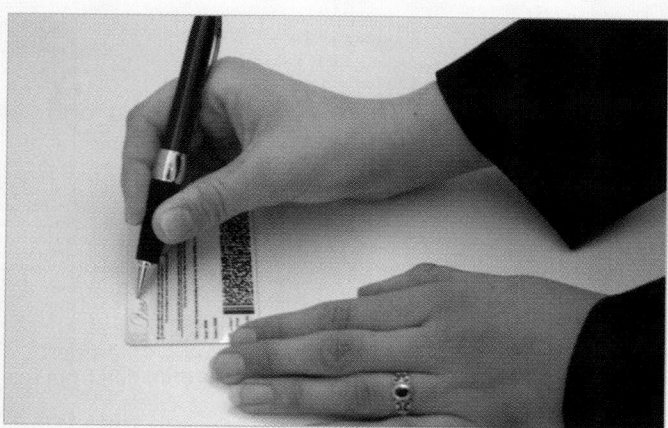

Figure 5-10 Most states have an organ donation form on the reverse side of the driver's license.

decisions does not have to be a relative, but may be someone close to the patient who understands his or her wishes.

The person who makes the health care decisions for another, who carries the power of attorney, is often called the surrogate decision maker 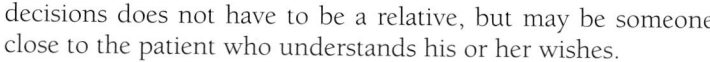 **Figure 5-9 ▲** . The surrogate decision maker is legally obligated to make decisions as the patient would want, and has presumably discussed these decisions with the patient.

If you are unsure of the time of a cardiac arrest, begin care and immediately contact medical control to discuss termination of the resuscitative effort.

Organ Donation

A major issue in medical ethics involves the potential for patients with mortal injuries to donate organs. Donor organs are badly needed within the medical system, with patients waiting years for a match.

Whether or not a patient should be kept alive for the sole purpose of organ donation is an issue that paramedics should discuss with their medical director and local hospital system. The parameters for viable organs should be clearly spelled out within the individual EMS system. You should also understand the state law concerning organ donation: a patient must have witnessed informed consent, usually in writing.

In general, major organs such as kidneys and livers are not appropriate for organ donation after prolonged hypotension or CPR. However, other tissue such as corneas and skin may be valuable. Many states have programs that allow patients to agree to organ donation by making a notation on their driver's license **Figure 5-10 ▲** . If the patient's wishes regarding organ donation are not known, consent should be obtained from a family member before any arrangements are made to keep a patient alive solely for purposes of organ donation.

Another resource that might be available to your system are workshops offered by organ transplant teams and EMS leaders as continuing education for paramedics in order to make you aware of the vital role of EMS in securing transplants.

Withholding or Withdrawing Resuscitation

Modern bioethical guidelines rely on the use of common sense and reasonable judgment in deciding when to stop CPR and resuscitation efforts, as well as when it is appropriate for paramedics to decline to initiate them at all. Numerous medical studies have shown that resuscitation of medical as well as trauma patients is sometimes futile at the onset or may become futile at some point. Futile resuscitation efforts—interventions

You are the Provider Part 4

An internal investigation was initiated by your EMS director to determine the appropriate course of action regarding this call. You learn that evidence normally gathered by this agency's AED, including an audio recording of the event, as well as a cardiac strip, are now missing. Without these pieces to the puzzle, the investigation comes to a halt.

You receive a call from one of the EMTs who responded, and he tells you that he witnessed one of the other EMTs destroying the evidence. Even more unnerving, he tells you this has happened before. He is a fairly new provider and is afraid that he will be kicked out of the agency if anyone learns that he called you.

9. What should you do?

10. Can EMS departments be sued? Can EMS providers be sued?

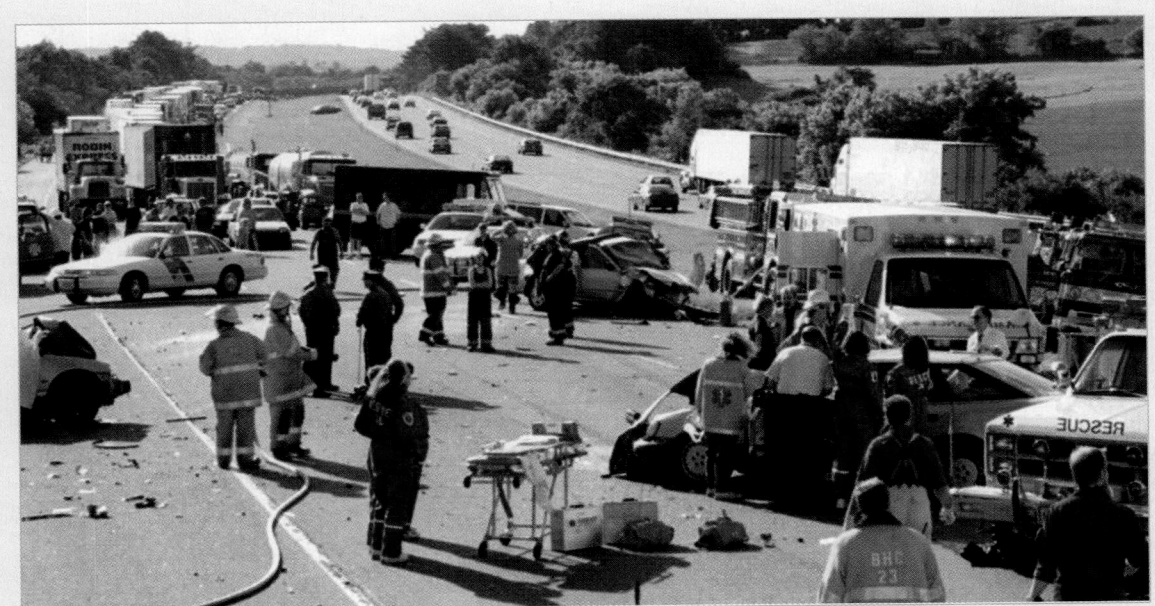

Figure 5-11 Although our instincts are always to try to sustain life at whatever cost, sometimes it is clear that resuscitation efforts will be futile, and should be withheld per local protocols.

resuscitation efforts may be indications for cessation of resuscitative efforts in the field.

These decisions are particularly difficult and emotional when dealing with pediatric patients, although again modern medical guidelines weigh against prolonged resuscitation efforts. Studies have shown that paramedics feel particularly uncomfortable about terminating resuscitation in children. "Working a code" simply because the patient is a child who has experienced sudden infant death syndrome (SIDS) may not be legally or ethically appropriate and may actually cause a family additional suffering when they are led to believe that the child may have a chance of survival. Paramedics tend to be action-oriented people who feel that they must "do something" (remember, this is *your* moral code). However, there are some situations in which a paramedic can do more for the grieving family than for the patient who has died, and ethically, you should be prepared to support the family. It can be the hardest part of the job.

Training, a review of the available literature, and open discussions about what is medically appropriate in a given EMS system should provide guidance and ease concerns about this difficult situation. Once again, continuing education on the topic of futility in resuscitation could help you look at this particularly difficult issue from many sides.

Do not try to judge whether or not interventions are futile totally by yourself. Communicate, communicate. Ultimately, medical interventions and lifesaving attempts may also prolong suffering or fail to return a patient to a meaningful life. You need guidance from medical control. In order to judge whether a cardiac arrest is the natural end of a life or a reversible response to a treatable medical event requires a thorough understanding of all the consequences of a particular intervention. You are not playing God. You are considering

that studies have shown do not benefit patients—are not medically or ethically indicated Figure 5-11.

Paramedics, especially those working in rural and wilderness situations, will need to carefully consider the time it will take for a patient to reach definitive care at the hospital.

Generally the focus is on providing approximately 15 minutes of your best efforts at resuscitation. If after this time there has not been a return of spontaneous circulation or there are no extenuating medical circumstances (eg, overdose, submersion, hypothermia), termination of the resuscitation should be seriously considered and efforts turned toward helping other survivors. Of course, local protocols must also be followed.

Each state has different laws that may define the role of the paramedic in resuscitation issues. In some states, a paramedic may be able to "pronounce" death, while in other states, only a medical investigator or physician may do so. What your state requires of you as a paramedic will affect how you practice your profession when you encounter a patient for whom resuscitation will be futile.

Some of these common sense guidelines include frank discussions of when it is appropriate for paramedics not to begin even the most basic life support. Although local protocols will ultimately guide the paramedic's practice, situations where a DNR order is present, where the patient is obviously dead (livor/rigor mortis, or has sustained injuries incompatible with life), are situations where it may be appropriate to withhold initial resuscitation interventions. Blunt trauma arrest, prolonged response times, and lengthy medical

Notes from Nancy
The paramedic's best protection in court is a thorough and accurate medical record.

Documentation and Communication
Imagine what it would be like to have a family emergency while visiting another country. How difficult would it be for you to trust their medical system knowing it is different than what you are use to?

the treatment benefit to your patient, who might be beyond your help. Communicate.

Ethics and EMS Research

EMS practices have largely grown up as the rest of EMS—with "grass roots" effort and precious little research to confirm the effectiveness of the procedures used in the prehospital setting. Properly randomized, controlled studies in EMS are not common, but they are emerging. Paramedics must remember that the first principle of medical practice is to do no harm, and continue to seek further education about the effectiveness of EMS practice. Some of EMS care still relies on anecdotal experience that is unsupported by research. Some EMS procedures, however well-intentioned, prove *not* to be helpful to patients, and you must as a health care provider act on those recommendations as well. EMS studies on the critically ill or injured patients without their informed consent is a true ethical dilemma—many of the patients a paramedic sees in practice are critically ill or injured. These patients are usually unable to give consent, and their physical state is so compromised that even if they are conscious, they may not be able to absorb information to give *informed* consent. Continue to make yourself aware of how researchers are handling this issue, and other ethical debates concerning patients in research.

Ethics in the EMS Workplace: Accountability

Paramedics must be accountable for their actions at all times—accountable to the patient, to the EMS medical director, and to the EMS system as a whole. At all times, the paramedic is obligated to meet the expectations of the community, including highly ethical behavior. How a paramedic handles teamwork, his or her attitude on the job, justice and respect for patient autonomy as well as a patient's cultural and lifestyle diversity will ultimately shape that paramedic's career. Each paramedic must consider what type of a paramedic he or she wants to become **Figure 5-12 ▶**. New paramedics may want to choose a mentor whose style and professionalism they strive to emulate.

Professional ethics are extremely important as EMS continues to struggle to be recognized and funded in the same manner as the other medical professions. Immature, unprofessional behavior and criminal acts, such as sexual misconduct,

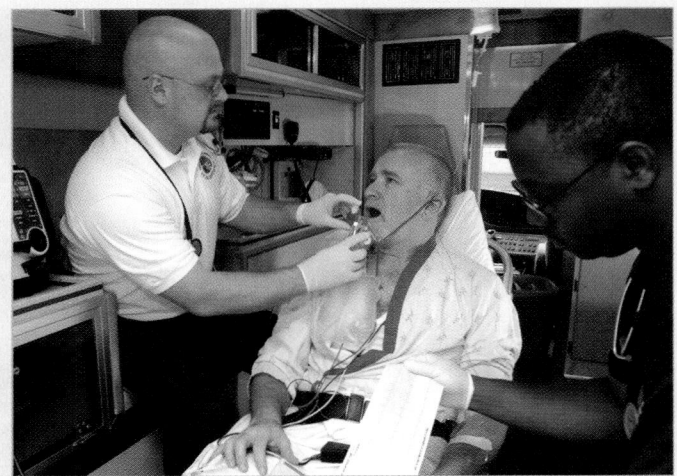

Figure 5-12 One of the best ways to hone your skills as a paramedic is to find a good mentor whose work ethic and attitude you admire.

substance abuse, patient abuse, and harassment of coworkers, have no place in an emerging profession. Off-duty misconduct can, and does, affect a paramedic's reputation and may affect his or her employment as well. News stories that depict EMS personnel engaged in any immature or illegal activities serve to lessen the public's confidence in the services we provide. Illegal drug use or selling drugs, inappropriate use of emergency vehicles, inappropriate visitors entertained at the station, and use of alcohol on duty are strictly forbidden.

Paramedics also may not stand by silently and watch as other EMS providers engage in misbehavior if they care about their patients, their coworkers, and the EMS system as a whole. Misconduct should be promptly reported to the appropriate chain of command. Similarly, paramedics are obligated to report medical errors they make or witness to the medical director as soon as possible.

Paramedics who choose to become patient advocates, who participate in and actively seek out the very best in training and professional development, and who put the good of the team above their own personal aspirations will ultimately succeed and be rewarded with a fulfilling career in EMS. Human beings seem to perform best when they share themselves and work towards an end much greater than themselves. You probably would not be reading this text if you were not that kind of person. But you must remember, EMS is an evolving specialty, and the future of it lies in your hands.

You are the Provider Summary

1. Are career and volunteer staffing held to the same standards of patient care?

Ideally, they should be held to the same patient care standards, but occasionally they are not. This is unfortunate because the patient and the patient's family are often unaware of who gets paid and who doesn't. They want a professional—someone who looks and acts the part of a lifesaving team member. Professionalism includes all facets of response and preparation for response. Both volunteer and career paramedics can and should function as professionals at all times.

2. If sensitive information needs to be relayed regarding patient care, what other communication options should the EMS providers have available?

It is never appropriate to ignore an incoming EMS provider's radio questions regarding patient care or other pertinent information. We've all been in situations where we feel that information needs to be communicated in a discreet manner. Use a landline or cellular phone even if it is only to let the provider know you need to relay information face-to-face. Failure to communicate to an incoming responder will lead the crew to wonder whether the radio system is malfunctioning, you are ignoring them, or something else is wrong.

3. Is it ever appropriate to conceal information regarding patient care?

No. It is never acceptable to cover up mistakes or omissions in patient care. To do so could jeopardize the patient's life and your professional future. Ideally, no mistakes should be made in the field, but they can and do happen. If you should find yourself in this situation, immediately report any mistakes or other concerns to the appropriate medical authority.

4. How should you answer the wife's question?

Don't lie. Give her factual information, and stick to what you know. If you are unsure, tell her you don't know but that you will look into the matter to ensure she receives accurate information.

5. How and when should you address her concerns?

Because you are actively caring for her husband, now is not the time to discuss what has occurred during the call. Ideally, a physician should explain any patient care procedures or complications regarding her husband's care in an environment that is quiet, private, and much less stressful. Adhere to your local standard operating procedures and other protocols for interacting with patient's family members. If none are in place regarding a specific issue, use common sense and sensitivity.

6. Beyond the documentation required to complete the medical incident report, what else should you document and how?

You should also fill out an addendum or memo that will not be directly attached to the medical incident report. This type of formal note should include all related information not appropriate to include in a medical document, such as comments from providers, conditions, items you noticed at the scene, or other important information that you believe is pertinent. Ensure that this is a typed document that includes names, dates, times, witnesses, and references to other appropriate documents. Stick to factual information, and write this as though it could also be subpoenaed at a later time.

7. Why is it important to accurately, concisely, and completely document a call, especially a call such as this one?

All your documentations should reflect a professional image. Misspellings, illegible handwriting, and major omissions all point to one thing—you are not a professional. It can be argued that if your documentation is poor, so is your patient care. Always document with the anticipation that one day a lawyer might have your medical incident report enlarged for a jury to inspect. More important than this, however, should be your strong desire to provide complete verbal and written reports to ensure your patient has exceptional continuity of care.

8. What is the purpose of continuous quality improvement?

Continuous quality improvement exists to keep EMS providers on the right track and should involve an informal and formal method for evaluating all calls and flagging those that need review. As providers, we all benefit from reviewing calls, learning what we did right and what can improve. It is our responsibility to ensure that we work within the guidelines of national accepted standards and the local protocols as set forth by the oversight physician.

9. What should you do?

Obviously, you must keep this individual's name private. His concern regarding a backlash is a valid one. However, you must report this information immediately to your supervisor and medical program director so that corrective action can be taken. Explain to the EMT what course of action you must take, but that you will protect his identity.

10. Can EMS departments be sued? Can EMS providers be sued?

Yes! Absolutely! Both can be tried in civil and criminal courts. Don't assume that your department has an insurance policy that will cover your legal fees and other court judgments should you be sued as an individual provider. They may or may not. Depending on your work situation, it may be a wise idea to keep an insurance policy separate from your employer, and your best method for avoiding litigation is to provide the best patient care possible. With that being said, individuals can and do sue individuals and departments—big and small.

Prep Kit

■ Ready for Review

■ Paramedics who maintain a good, well-rounded general ethical code in their daily lives will be able to carry that through to their profession.

■ Paramedics who are concerned for the welfare of others will rarely commit an unethical act in their professional career.

■ Paramedics need to keep in mind that all patients have the right to make their own decisions regarding their medical care, regardless of the paramedic's personal or professional views.

■ Empathy and compassion are part of a paramedic's job.

■ Patients often decide on medical care and treatment issues prior to an emergency. Paramedics need to be familiar with DNR orders, living wills, health care powers of attorney, surrogate decisions, and organ donations.

■ Futile resuscitation efforts, which a paramedic may encounter, need to be addressed and considered prior to an emergency event. Weighing various ethical issues prior to their occurrence can help prevent and reduce suffering in our patient population.

■ Paramedics who strive to become an advocate for their communities and carry a high sense of accountability will not only have a rewarding career, but will also be able to make the right ethical decisions regardless of whether they are encountered in the field, with coworkers, or in their daily lives.

■ Vital Vocabulary

advance directive A directive from the patient, either orally or in writing, describing his or her wishes for medical treatment.

ethics The philosophy of right and wrong.

health care power of attorney A legal document that allows another person to make health care decisions for the patient, including withdrawal or withholding of care, when the patient is incapacitated.

living will A type of advance directive, generally requiring a precondition for withholding resuscitation when the patient is incapacitated.

morality Pertaining to conscience, conduct, and character.

patient autonomy The right to direct one's own care, and to decide how you want your end-of-life medical care provided.

surrogate decision maker A person designated by a patient to make health care decisions for them when they are unable to make decisions for themselves.

■ Points to Ponder

The more time you spend with your new partner, the more you think he may have a substance abuse problem that is getting worse. He is having trouble remembering things and making quick decisions on the job, which is a "have to" in EMS. You see him taking pills often, but nothing you recognize. When you question him even subtly, he gets defensive and angry. His actions may cause a mistake in the field, or put someone in danger. You like him, and he's a good partner when he isn't affected by whatever he is taking, and you don't want to get him in trouble.

What do you do?

Issues: Working With Other Providers, Accountability to the EMS System and the Patient, Maintaining and Encouraging the Standard of Care.

Assessment in Action

You are dispatched to a messy scene—a two-vehicle, one motorcycle crash in the pouring rain. When you arrive, you see that the motorcycle driver was not wearing a helmet. The passengers in one of the vehicles were not wearing seatbelts, and the inside of the vehicle smells strongly of alcohol.

When you check on the motorcycle driver, he is not breathing and has a partially crushed skull. You are not sure how long he has not been breathing. The head injury may mean that if you revive him, he will be brain damaged.

1. **Do you initiate resuscitation?**
   A. Yes
   B. No

2. **In the car are teenagers who you recognize from a lecture you recently gave on the importance of seatbelts and not drinking and driving. They are conscious and alert, but most of them have some kind of injury. How do you handle this situation?**
   A. As you would any other trauma call, but less gently. Comment on how careless they were and tell them they could have prevented this if they had used common sense.
   B. Take care of them last. They were obviously the reason the crash happened in the first place.
   C. Make them feel as guilty as you can. Tell them the motorcycle driver is most likely dead, and the people in the other car have been hurt by their carelessness.
   D. Assume nothing, and treat all the patients as you would in any trauma call—gently, compassionately, and quickly.

3. **You and a fellow coworker disagree on how to treat one victim of the crash. Your coworker is talking loudly in front of the patient and bystanders. One patient is beginning to wonder if he is in competent hands. What do you do?**
   A. Remind the coworker that you are the paramedic, and therefore what you say goes, period.
   B. Take the coworker aside and professionally (and quietly) explain that the scene is not a place to have disagreements, you are in charge, you are accepting responsibility, and you can discuss your differences after the call.
   C. Explain to the patient that you are the more experienced EMS worker and your coworker has an inferiority complex. Give the coworker a mundane task to do with a different patient to get him out of your way.
   D. Tell the coworker to shut up, and ignore him as you take care of the patient in the way you feel is appropriate.

4. **The medical director gives you an order to give one of the patients 2 mg of morphine for pain. The patient says he is not in that much pain, and although he is not allergic to narcotics, he doesn't like the effect they have on him. Should you follow the medical director's order?**
   A. Give the medical director the information the patient has shared with you, and ask that he reconsider his order.
   B. Tell the patient that the medical director is your boss, and what he says has to be done.
   C. Tell the medical director you will administer the morphine, but don't actually administer it to the patient.
   D. Tell the patient that he may not be in much pain yet, but he will, and the medical director knows best.

5. **On an off-duty Friday night, some friends call and ask you to a party. You don't have a designated driver, and you can't stay out too late because you have a shift in the morning. What do you do?**
   A. Go out and have a good time; life is short. You can drive slowly on the way home and be very careful because it's not too far from your house.
   B. If you go, don't drink. You have a reputation to uphold.
   C. Go, but drink very little, so you're only driving under the influence a little, not a lot.
   D. Just make sure you're completely sober before hitting the road home.

6. **The older woman in the second vehicle tells you she has a terminal illness. When she begins having chest pains, she requests that you do nothing to save her if she should go into cardiac arrest. She does not have her DNR orders with her, however. She is relatively calm, and seems to be of sound mind in making her decision. She does not even want the ECG put on her. What do you do?**
   A. Comply with her wishes if she is competent to make the decision.
   B. You cannot comply with her request unless she has her DNR order with her.
   C. Tell her that you must hook up the ECG machine and treat her until she is at the hospital, where she and a doctor can decide what is best.
   D. Call medical control, explain the situation, and ask for advice.

7. **You find out that the motorcycle driver is an organ donor. Medical control told you a few seconds ago *not* to initiate CPR based on his severe head injury and lack of breathing. What do you do?**
   A. Call medical control and ask about keeping his body alive until his organs can be donated.
   B. Go with what medical control said earlier.
   C. Find out from a close family member what his wishes were, if possible, and follow his wishes if they were known.
   D. Keep his body alive so they can be given to someone who needs them. The fact that his driver's license says that he is an organ donor is enough to cover any liability.

Challenging Questions

You are called to the scene of a two-car crash involving several teenage girls. They all claim to be injured only slightly. One of the members of your team jokingly says that in any trauma, the rule is to "strip them" and check them thoroughly. You know they should have a complete physical exam—many patients don't feel other injuries until the adrenaline of the situation has worn off. However, you also know that at least one person on your team is hinting at taking advantage of the situation.

8. **Do you give the patients a thorough exam, while also giving your coworker(s) a cheap thrill?**

9. **Do you point out to your coworker(s) that what they are doing is unethical and unprofessional, and has no place in the field of EMS?**

10. **Do you report what you saw and heard to the chain of command after the incident is taken care of?**

6

Pathophysiology

This chapter on pathophysiology has been adapted from *Paramedic: Pathophysiology* (Bob Elling, Mikel A. Rothenberg, MD, and Kirsten M. Elling, 2006, Jones and Bartlett Publishers). It is dedicated to the late Dr. Rothenberg, who, like Dr. Caroline, spent his life helping health care providers understand the complexity of the human body in crisis and injury.

Objectives

Cognitive

1-6.1   Discuss cellular adaptation. (p 6.7)

1-6.2   Describe cellular injury and cellular death. (p 6.15)

1-6.3   Describe the factors that precipitate disease in the human body. (p 6.19)

1-6.4   Describe the cellular environment. (p 6.7)

1-6.5   Discuss analyzing disease risk. (p 6.19)

1-6.6   Describe environmental risk factors. (p 6.19)

1-6.7   Discuss combined effects and interaction among risk factors. (p 6.19)

1-6.8   Describe aging as a risk factor for disease. (p 6.19)

1-6.9   Discuss familial diseases and associated risk factors. (p 6.19)

1-6.10   Discuss hypoperfusion. (p 6.26)

1-6.11   Define cardiogenic, hypovolemic, neurogenic, anaphylactic and septic shock. (p 6.27)

1-6.12   Describe multiple organ dysfunction syndrome. (p 6.30)

1-6.13   Define the characteristics of the immune response. (p 6.33)

1-6.14   Discuss induction of the immune system. (p 6.34)

1-6.15   Discuss fetal and neonatal immune function. (p 6.42)

1-6.16   Discuss aging and the immune function in the elderly. (p 6.42)

1-6.17   Describe the inflammation response. (p 6.38)

1-6.18   Discuss the role of mast cells as part of the inflammation response. (p 6.38)

1-6.19   Describe the plasma protein system. (p 6.39)

1-6.20   Discuss the cellular components of inflammation. (p 6.39)

1-6.21   Describe the systemic manifestations of the inflammation response. (p 6.38)

1-6.22   Describe the resolution and repair from inflammation. (p 6.40)

1-6.23   Discuss the effect of aging on the mechanisms of self-defense. (p 6.42)

1-6.24   Discuss hypersensitivity. (p 6.42)

1-6.25   Describe deficiencies in immunity and inflammation. (p 6.45)

1-6.26   Describe homeostasis as a dynamic steady state. (p 6.5)

1-6.27   List types of tissue. (p 6.4)

1-6.28   Describe the systemic manifestations that result from cellular injury. (p 6.15)

1-6.29   Describe neuroendocrine regulation. (p 6.10)

1-6.30   Discuss the inter-relationships between stress, coping, and illness. (p 6.46)

5-9.9   Identify the characteristics of the inflammatory process. (p 6.38)

5-9.10   Identify the difference between cellular and humoral immunity. (p 6.33)

5-9.11   Identify alterations in immunologic response. (p 6.42)

5-9.16   Describe the function of coagulation factors, platelets and blood vessels necessary for normal coagulation. (p 6.39)

5-9.18   Identify blood groups. (p 6.44)

5-9.19   Describe how acquired factor deficiencies may occur. (p 6.45)

5-9.20   Define fibrinolysis. (p 6.39)

Affective

1-6.31   Advocate the need to understand and apply the knowledge of pathophysiology to patient assessment and treatment. (p 6.3)

Psychomotor

None

Introduction

The human body is made up of cells, tissues, and organs, which function in a constantly changing microenvironment. The study of living organisms with regard to their origin, growth, structure, behavior, and reproduction is known as biology. Pathophysiology refers to the study (*logos*) of the functioning of the organism (*physiology*) in the presence of suffering/disease (*pathos*). When the normal condition or functioning of the cellular systems breaks down in response to stressors, and the systems can no longer maintain homeostasis, disease may result. Determining the etiology (cause) of this disease process often helps the paramedic identify a reasonable approach to both evaluation and initial treatment of the patient.

To understand how disease may alter cellular function, it is first necessary to understand normal cellular structure and function. This chapter begins by reviewing the structure and function of the cellular system and environment. Following that review is a discussion of how alterations of the environment and its normal homeostasis may result in the state of disease. Next, the impact of genetics on the development of disease states, the role of immunity and self-defense mechanisms in protecting the organism from disease, the states of inflammation and shock, and the role of stress on the development of disease are described and discussed in detail.

Review of the Basic Cellular Systems

Cells

The cell is the basic self-sustaining unit of the human body. As cells grow and mature, they become specialized (eg, kidney cells) through the process of differentiation. Groups of cells form tissues, various types of tissues make up organs, and groups of organs constitute organ systems.

Nearly all cells of higher organisms, except mature red blood cells and platelets, have three main components: the cell membrane, the cytoplasm containing the internal components or organelles, and a nucleus.

The cell membrane consists of fat and protein. It surrounds the cell and protects the internal components within the cytoplasm.

In the Field

Chemically, fatty compounds—like those in the cell membrane—are neutral (uncharged), whereas electrolytes (sodium and potassium) are water-based (charged). Fats are soluble in oil but not in water. Thus, for a charged molecule to enter through a cell membrane, it has to travel through a special pathway. These transport channels—the so-called ion channels—consist of protein-lined pores that are specifically sized for each substance (calcium and potassium). Local anesthetics (eg, lidocaine) and antiarrhythmic drugs (eg, amiodarone) exert their effects by blocking ion channels.

The organelles, which are found within the cell's cytoplasm (fluid), operate in a cooperative and organized fashion to maintain the life of the cell. They include the following components Figure 6-1 ▶ :

Ribosomes contain RNA and protein. They interact with RNA from other parts of the cell, joining amino acid chains together to form proteins. When ribosomes attach to endoplasmic reticulum, they create rough endoplasmic reticulum.

You are the Provider Part 1

You are complaining to your partner about how taking a pathophysiology review class has nothing at all to do with being a paramedic when you are called to a local dialysis center for an unknown medical emergency. You are met by a patient care technician who takes you to a 67-year-old woman who appears to be in moderate distress. The nurse caring for the patient states that 30 minutes into dialysis, the patient's blood pressure dropped to 86/44 and she became short of breath. They immediately stopped therapy and called 9-1-1. This occurred approximately 15 minutes prior to your arrival. The nurse further mentions that the patient has a fever of 102.4°F. When questioned, the patient tells you that she missed her last two dialysis sessions because she was not feeling well. She admits to having malaise and a fever for 3 days. She further complains of pain in her right forearm at the site of the dialysis shunt and slight shortness of breath. The patient denies experiencing chest pain, nausea, vomiting, abdominal pain, or dizziness.

Initial Assessment	Recording Time: 0 Minutes
Appearance	Awake and anxious
Level of consciousness	A (Alert to person, place, and day)
Airway	Open
Breathing	Slightly elevated rate with accessory muscle use noted
Circulation	Weak radial pulses with pale, warm, moist skin

1. What are some of the potential complications that can occur from missing dialysis?
2. Does renal disease affect other organ systems?

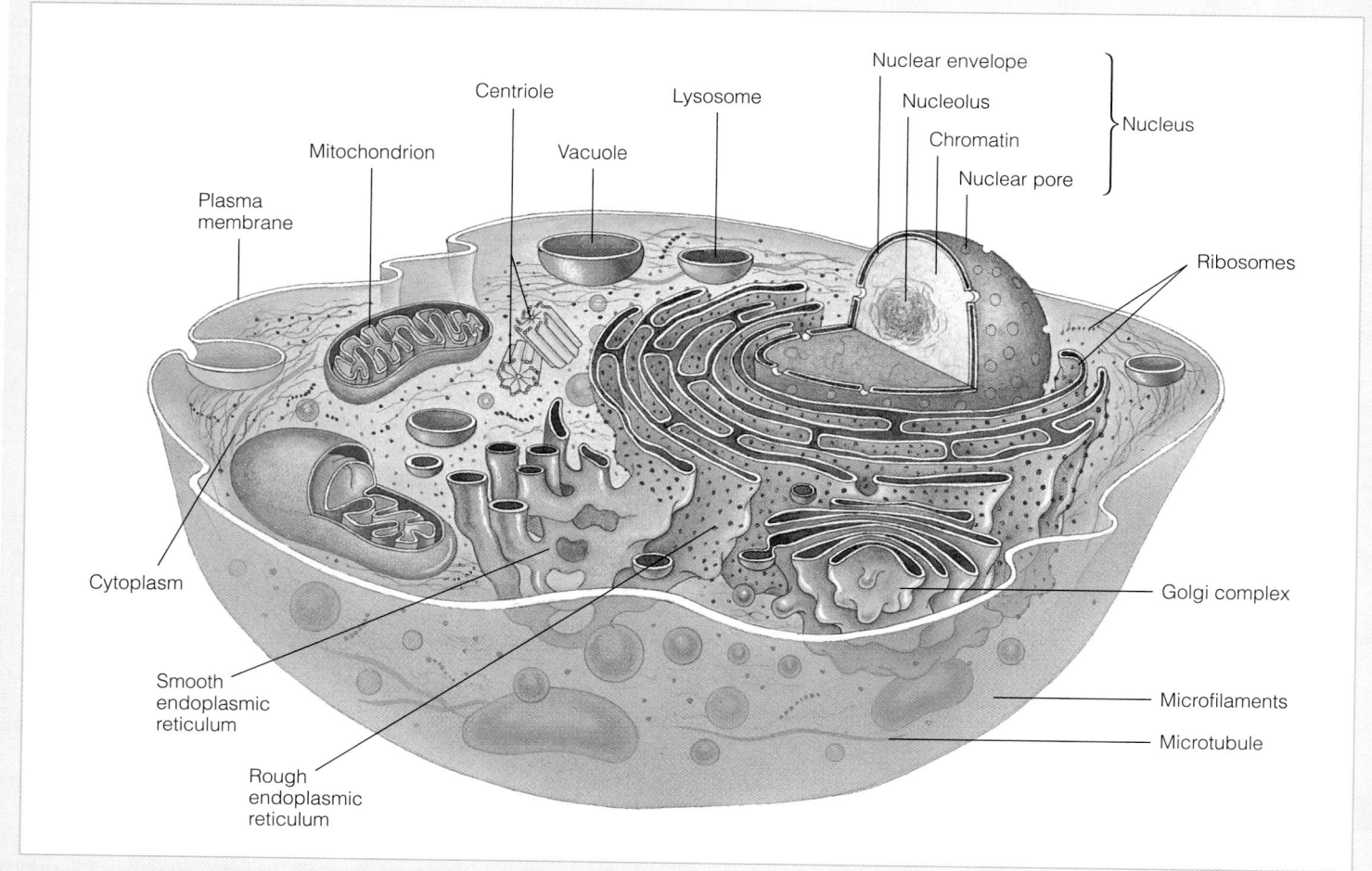

Figure 6-1 The structure of a cell. The cell is divided into nuclear and cytoplasmic compartments. The cytoplasm is packed with organelles, the structures in which the cell carries out many functions.

The *endoplasmic reticulum* is a network of tubules, vesicles, and sacs. Rough endoplasmic reticulum is involved in building proteins. Smooth endoplasmic reticulum is involved in building lipids (fats), such as those found in the cell membranes and those found in carbohydrates.

The *Golgi complex* is located near the nucleus of the cell. It is involved in the synthesis and packaging of various carbohydrates (sugar) and complex protein molecules such as enzymes.

Lysosomes are membrane-bound vesicles that contain digestive enzymes. These enzymes function as an intracellular digestive system, breaking down bacteria and organic debris that have been taken into the cell.

Similar to lysosomes, *peroxisomes* are found in high concentrations in the liver and neutralize toxins such as alcohol.

Mitochondria are small, rod-like organelles that function as the metabolic center of the cell. They produce adenosine triphosphate (ATP), which is the major energy source for the body.

The nucleus contains the genetic material, called chromatin, and the nucleoli, which are rounded, dense structures that contain ribonucleic acid (RNA). The RNA is responsible for controlling the cellular activities. The nucleus is surrounded by a membrane called the nuclear envelope; the nucleus itself is embedded in the cytoplasm.

Tissues

Tissues are composed of groups of similar cells that work together for a common function. There are four types of tissues: epithelial, connective, muscle, and nerve tissue.

Epithelium covers the external surfaces of the body. Epithelial tissue also lines hollow organs within the body, such as the intestines, blood vessels, and bronchial tubes. In addition to providing a protective barrier, epithelial tissues play roles in the absorption of nutrients in the intestines and the secretion of various body substances. For example, the sweat glands in the dermis layer of the skin—specifically, the stratified squamous epithelial cells—produce a solution containing urea and salt. In contrast, the simple columnar epithelium lines the small intestine and absorbs nutrients from the foods we eat. The epithelial cells that line the inside of blood vessels are called endothelial cells; they regulate the flow of blood through the vessel as well as clotting of the blood (coagulation).

Connective tissue binds the other types of tissue together. Extracellular matrix is a nonliving substance consisting of protein fibers, nonfibrous protein, and fluid that separates connective tissue cells from one another. Collagen is the major protein within the extracellular matrix. At least 12 types of collagen exist, with types I, II, and III being the most abundant. Alterations in collagen structure resulting from abnormal genes or abnormal processing of collagen proteins result in numerous diseases (eg, scurvy). Bone and cartilage are subtypes of connective tissue. Adipose tissue is a special type of connective tissue that contains large amounts of lipids (fat).

Muscle tissue is characterized by its ability to contract. It is enclosed by fascia, which is the layer of fibrous connective tissue that separates individual muscles. Muscles overlie the framework of the skeleton and are classified in terms of both their structure and their function. Structurally, muscle tissue is either striated (ie, microscopic bands or striations can be seen) or nonstriated (also called smooth). Functionally, muscle is either voluntary (consciously controlled) or involuntary (not normally under conscious control).

The three types of muscle are skeletal muscle (striated voluntary), cardiac muscle (striated involuntary), and smooth muscle (nonstriated involuntary). Most of the muscles used voluntarily in day-to-day activities are skeletal muscles. The heart consists of cardiac muscle and has the ability to both contract and generate impulses. Smooth muscle lines most glands, digestive organs, lower airways, and vessels. When a patient's brain senses the need to respond to an environmental stimulus by vasoconstriction, the vessels in the periphery react. For example, the smooth muscle in the bronchioles may vasoconstrict during an asthma attack, leading to wheezing and difficulty moving air out of the lungs. Smooth muscle is also responsible for constriction and dilation of the pupil of the eye when it is exposed to changes in light levels.

Nerve tissue is characterized by its ability to transmit nerve impulses. The central nervous system (CNS) consists of the brain and the spinal cord. Peripheral nerves extend from the brain and spinal cord, exiting from between the vertebrae to various parts of the body.

Neurons are the main conducting cells of nerve tissue, and the cell body of the neuron is the site of most cellular functions. Dendrites receive electrical impulses from the axons of other nerve cells and conduct them toward the cell body, whereas axons typically conduct electrical impulses away from the cell body. Each neuron has only one axon, but it may have several dendrites. Nerve cells are separated by a gap called the synapse. Electrical impulses travel down the nerve and trigger the release of neurotransmitters, which carry the impulse from axon to dendrite.

Homeostasis

Adaptive responses to various stimuli allow the cells and tissues to respond and function in stressful environments, in a constant effort to preserve a degree of stability or equilibrium.

This adaptation process is known as homeostasis (from the Greek words for "same" and "steady"); it is also called the *dynamic steady state.*

Homeostasis is maintained in the body because normal regulatory systems are counterbalanced by counter-regulatory systems. Thus, for every cell, tissue, or organ that performs one function, there is always at least one component that performs the opposing function. For example, the autonomic nervous system consists of the sympathetic and parasympathetic components, which act to speed up or slow down the activity of target organs. Other homeostatic mechanisms include the body's control of its internal temperature despite fluctuations in the external temperature, the regulation of pH and acid–base balance in the body, and the balance of water or hydration in the cells and body of the organism.

Regulatory systems communicate within the body mainly at the cellular level. Cells communicate electrochemically through a process called cell signaling, in which they release molecules (such as hormones) that bind to proteins called receptors, located on the surface of the receiving cells. This signaling triggers chemical reactions in the receiving cells that lead to a biological action. When the action is completed, the opposing system "turns off" the action through a process called feedback inhibition or negative feedback Figure 6-2 ▶.

The thermostat mechanism in a home is a good example of a feedback mechanism. In the middle of the winter, heat is constantly being lost through the house's windows, doors, and any poorly insulated areas. The thermostat detects this decrease in temperature and signals the furnace to produce heat to rewarm the house. Once the temperature rises to a certain point, the thermostat gives negative feedback to the furnace, causing it to shut down to prevent overheating. This feedback process keeps the house temperature within a selected range Figure 6-3 ▶. Similarly, the body is constantly generating heat through its cellular processes. Five primary mechanisms help the body eliminate excess temperature or heat: convection, conduction, radiation, evaporation, and respiration. In short, the body's thermostat works to balance the generation of heat with the processes of heat elimination.

The human body maintains homeostasis by balancing what it takes in with what it puts out. For example, the body takes in chemicals and electrolytes, food, and water. It utilizes the nutrients, proteins, sugars, and oxygen and then eliminates the unnecessary chemicals and byproducts through respiration (carbon dioxide), urine and sweat (excess liquids), and feces (solid waste). Figure 6-4 ▶ illustrates this normal balance.

When normal cell signaling is interrupted, disease occurs. The normal counterbalances within the body are rendered ineffective, such that normal regulatory systems begin to operate autonomously. The system stops providing critical negative feedback; instead, it gives unopposed positive feedback.

Excessive output can rapidly upset homeostasis (eg, severe diarrhea kills millions of children each year in some nations, and severe perspiration can cause excessive water loss and dehydration). Likewise, changes in input can alter homeostasis

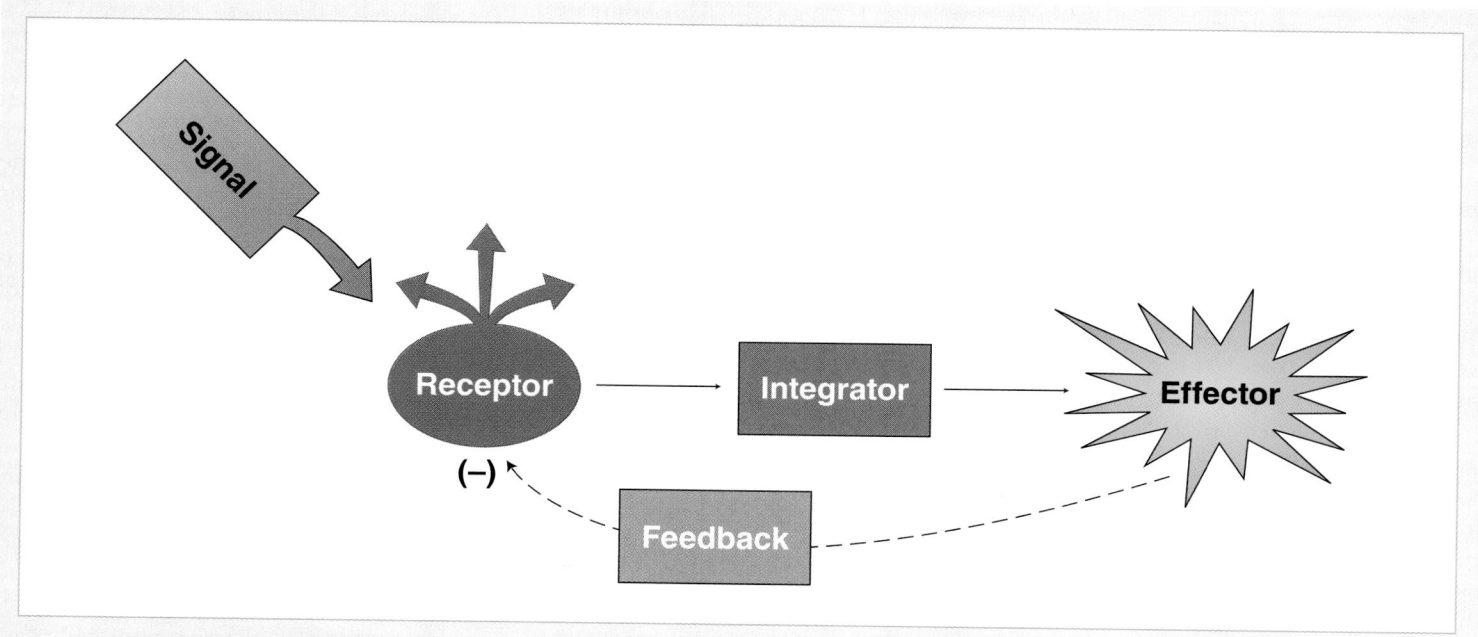

Figure 6-2 Most cellular communication includes a component of negative feedback in which the product of a reaction feeds back information about its own "assembly line," thereby stopping its own production.

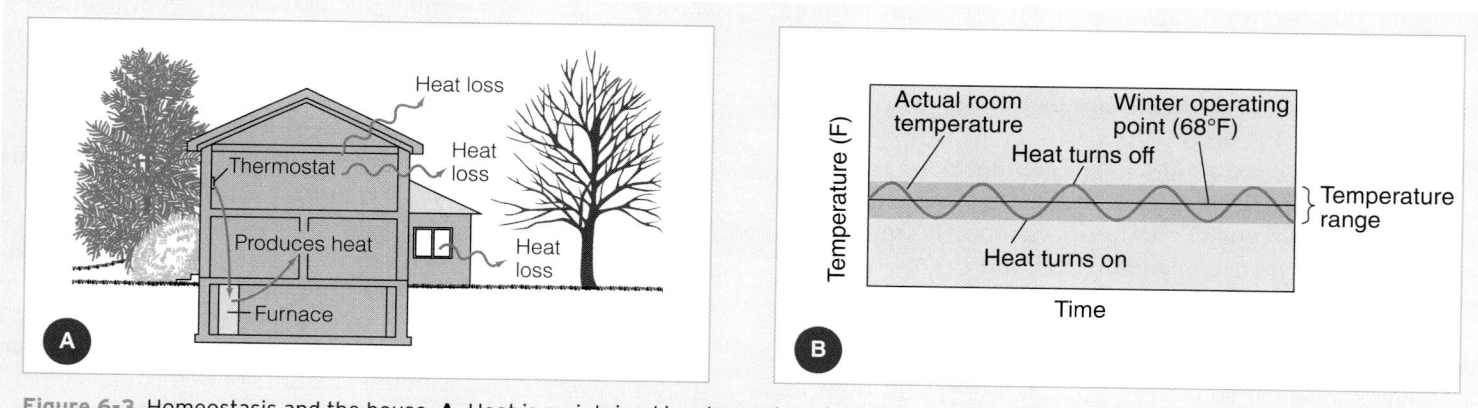

Figure 6-3 Homeostasis and the house. **A.** Heat is maintained in a house by a furnace, which compensates for heat loss. The thermostat monitors the internal temperature and switches the furnace on and off in response to temperature changes. **B.** A hypothetical temperature graph showing temperature fluctuation around the set point.

(eg, going without water for 3 or more days can be life-threatening, and excess salt intake can cause hypertension) **Figure 6-5** ►.

The degree of fluid imbalance required to alter homeostasis and result in illness depends on the patient's size, age, and underlying medical conditions. In healthy adults, loss of more than 30% of total body fluid is required, but a loss of only 10% to 15% of total body fluid in a small child could easily result in symptoms. For this reason, fluid therapy is part of the basics of resuscitation.

Ligands

Ligands are molecules that are either produced by the body (endogenous) or given as a drug (exogenous), and that bind any receptor, anywhere, leading to any reaction. In addition to medications, common ligands include hormones, neurotransmitters, and electrolytes.

Hormones are substances that are formed in very small amounts in one specialized organ or group of cells and then carried to another organ or group of cells in the same organism to perform regulatory functions. Endocrine hormones (eg,

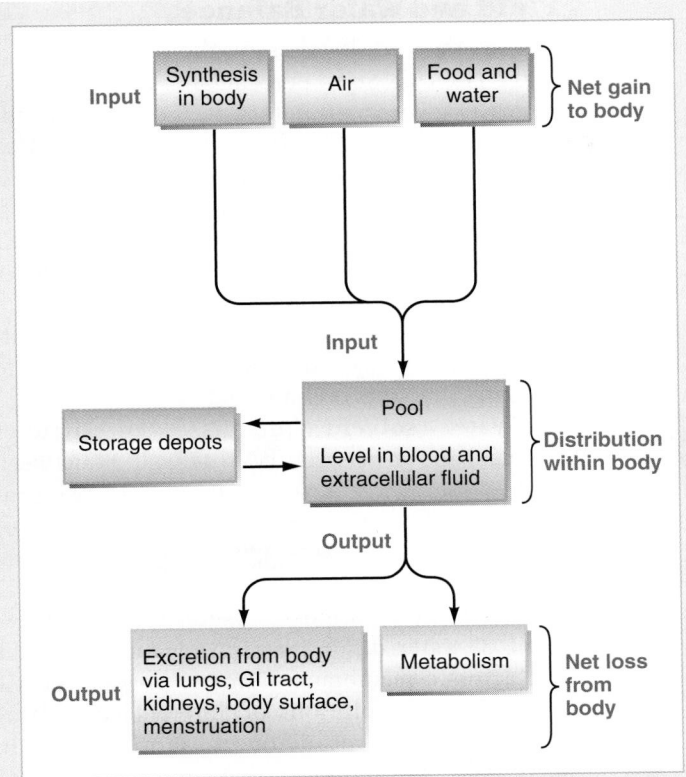

Figure 6-4 Generalized view of the homeostatic system. Inputs and outputs are balanced to maintain more or less constant levels of chemical and physical parameters.

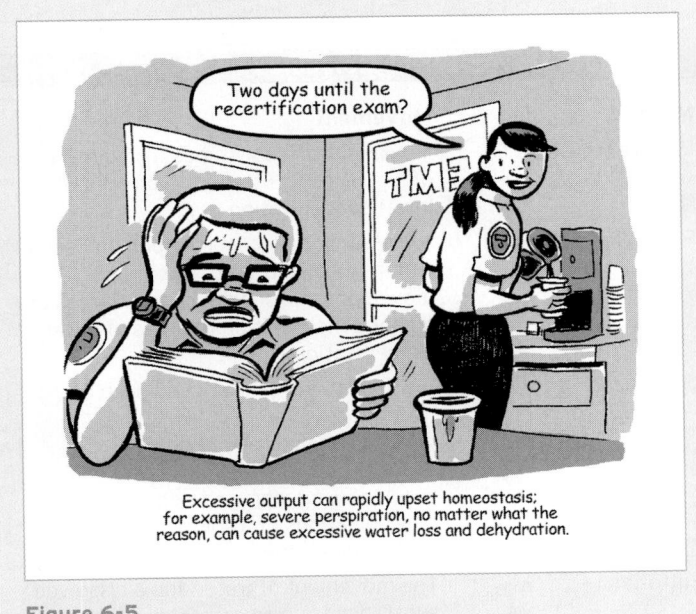

Excessive output can rapidly upset homeostasis; for example, severe perspiration, no matter what the reason, can cause excessive water loss and dehydration.

Figure 6-5

thyroid hormones, adrenal steroids) are carried to their target organ or cell group in the blood. Exocrine hormones reach their target via a specific duct that opens into an organ; examples of exocrine secretions include stomach acids and perspiration. Paracrine hormones (eg, histamine, the hormone released

during allergic and inflammatory reactions) diffuse through intracellular spaces to reach their target. If the hormone acts on the cell that secreted it, it is called an autocrine hormone.

Neurotransmitters are proteins that affect signals between cells of the nervous system. For example, acetylcholine, which aids in the movement of nerve impulses from neuron to neuron, is a neurotransmitter.

Electrolytes play an important role in cell signaling as well as generating the nervous system's action potential. Examples of electrolytes commonly found in the body include sodium, potassium, calcium, and chloride.

Adaptations in Cells and Tissues

When cells are exposed to adverse conditions, they go through a process of adaptation in an attempt to protect themselves from injury. In some situations, the cells change permanently; in others, they change their structure and function only temporarily.

Atrophy is a decrease in cell size due to a loss of subcellular components, which in turn leads to a decrease in the size of the tissue and organ. The actual number of cells remains unchanged. The decreased size represents an attempt to cope with a new steady state with less-than-favorable conditions or a lack of use. For example, a casted, immobilized limb will shrink in size due to disuse atrophy.

Hypertrophy is an increase in the size of the cells due to synthesis of more subcellular components, which in turn leads to an increase in tissue and organ size. For example, the left ventricle in the heart may hypertrophy owing to chronic high resistance pressures from hypertension (elevated blood pressure).

Hyperplasia is an increase in the actual number of cells in an organ or tissue, usually resulting in an increase in the size of the organ or tissue. For example, a callous represents hyperplasia of the keratinized layer of the epidermis of the foot in response to increased friction or trauma.

Dysplasia is an alteration in the size, shape, and organization of cells. It is most often found in epithelial cells that have undergone irregular, atypical changes in response to chronic irritation or inflammation. For example, dysplasia is strongly associated with the development of cancer in the cervix of women who are exposed to human papillomavirus and in the respiratory tracts of smokers.

Metaplasia refers to the reversible, cellular adaptation in which one adult cell type is replaced by another adult cell type. For example, the ciliated and secretory epithelium in the airways of smokers may be replaced by squamous metaplasia.

The Cellular Environment

Distribution of Body Fluids

The cellular environment refers to the distribution of cells, molecules, and fluids throughout the body. This environment changes with aging, exercise, pregnancy, medications, disease,

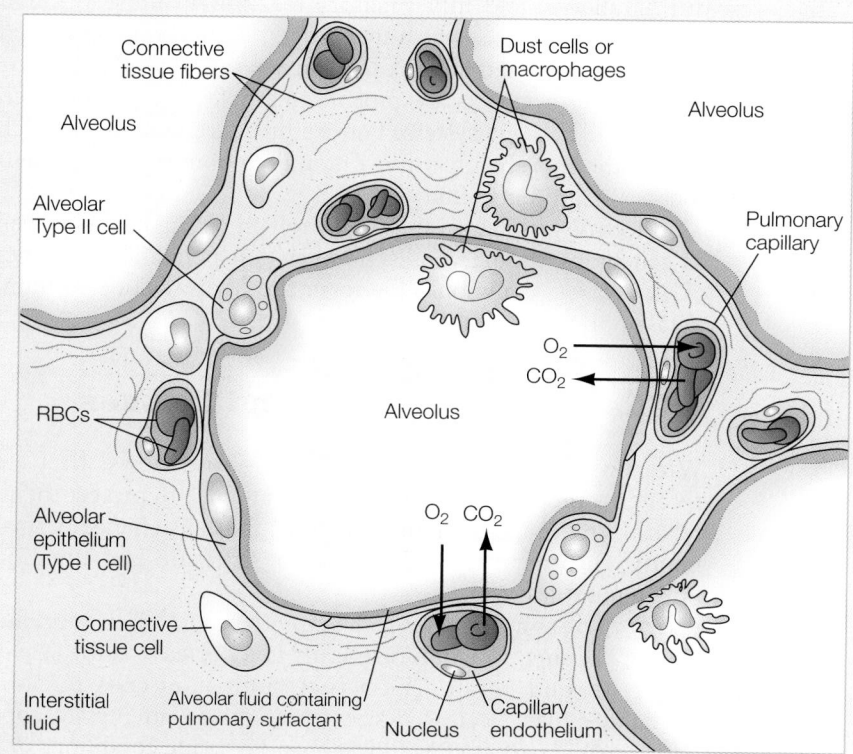

Figure 6-6 Close-up of the alveolus. Oxygen diffuses out of the alveolus and into the capillary. Carbon dioxide diffuses in the opposite direction, entering the alveolar air that is expelled during exhalation. Note the location of the interstitial fluid.

Fluid and Water Balance

The average adult takes in about 2,500 mL of water per day. Sixty percent of this fluid intake occurs by drinking. Another 30% comes from the water in foods, such as fruits. The remaining 10% is a byproduct of cellular metabolism. Most water (60%) is lost in the form of urine; 28% is lost through the skin and lungs; 6% is lost in the feces; and 6% is lost through sweat. The amount of water lost through sweating is highly variable—for example, in hot environmental conditions or during periods of rigorous exercise, it is possible to lose large amounts of fluid.

Water (solvent) and dissolved particles (solutes) move between cells as well as between blood vessels and connective tissues. The two general methods of movement are passive transport and active transport Table 6-1 ▼ .

Water moves between intracellular and extracellular fluid by osmosis. Osmosis is the movement of water down its concentration gradient and across a membrane. Osmotic pressure develops when two solutions of different concentrations are separated by a semipermeable membrane. Water moves from the region of low osmotic pressure to the region of higher osmotic pressure Figure 6-7 ▶ . When you compare the two solutions, the solution with a higher solute

and injury. Body fluids contain water, sodium, chloride, potassium, calcium, phosphorus, and magnesium.

Approximately 50% to 70% of the total body weight is fluid (a component also known as the total body water). The average male is 60% fluid; the average female is 50% fluid. Body fluid is classified into two main types: intracellular fluid (45% of body weight) and extracellular fluid (15% of body weight). (In terms of the total body water volume—as compared to body weight—approximately 75% of the body's fluid is intracellular, and the remaining 25% is extracellular.) The extracellular fluid can be further classified into interstitial fluid (10.5% of body weight; see Figure 6-6 ▲), which surrounds tissue cells and includes cerebrospinal fluid and synovial fluid, and intravascular fluid (4.5% of body weight), which is found within the blood vessels but outside the cells themselves.

Special Considerations

Total body water changes throughout a person's lifetime. At birth, a healthy, full-term infant will have approximately 80% total body water; in older people, total body water may constitute only 45% of body weight. For this reason, dehydration can be a serious concern in geriatric patients.

Table 6-1	Movement of Molecules
Method	**Movement**
Passive transport diffusion	Movement of a substance from an area of higher concentration to an area of lower concentration.
Facilitated diffusion	A transport molecule ("helper" molecule) within the membrane helps the movement of a substance from areas of higher concentration to areas of lower concentration.
Osmosis	The movement of a solvent, such as water, from an area of low solute concentration to one of high concentration through a selectively permeable membrane to equalize concentrations of a solute on both sides of the membrane.
Filtration	The movement of water and a dissolved substance from an area of high pressure to an area of low pressure.
Active transport	Movement via "pumps" or transport molecules that require energy and move substances from an area of low concentration to an area of high concentration.

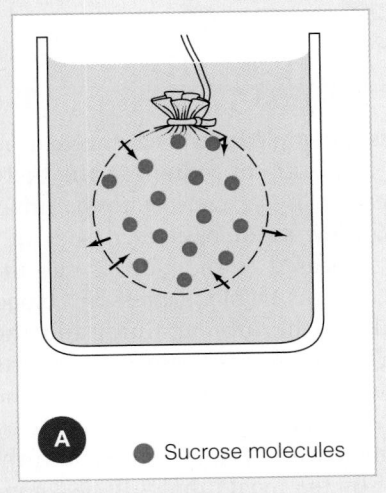

● Sucrose molecules

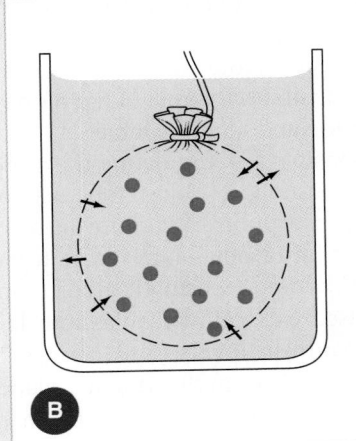

Figure 6-7 Osmosis is the diffusion of water molecules from a region of higher water concentration (or low solute concentration) to one of lower water concentration (or high solute concentration) across a selectively permeable membrane. **A.** To demonstrate the process, immerse a bag of sugar water in a solution of pure water. **B.** Water diffuses into the bag (toward the lower water concentration).

concentration has a higher osmotic pressure and is referred to as a hypertonic solution. The solution with a lower solute concentration has a lower osmotic pressure and is referred to as a hypotonic solution. Solutions with equal solute concentrations are called isotonic solutions (ie, 0.9% NaCl or lactated Ringer's solution).

Intracellular fluid volume is controlled in two ways: by the proteins and organic compounds that cannot escape through the cell membrane and by the sodium–potassium (Na^+/K^+) membrane pump. Most intracellular substances are negatively charged and so attract positively charged ions, including potassium. Because all of these substances are osmotically active, they can pull water into the cell—even until the cell ruptures. The Na^+/K^+ pump is responsible for keeping this situation in check and maintaining the cell's electrical potential by continuously removing three Na^+ ions from the cell for every two K^+ ions that are moved back into the cell. If this pump is impaired due to insufficient potassium in the body, sodium accumulates and causes the cells to swell.

Plasma

Plasma, which makes up about 55% of the blood, is composed of 91% water and 9% plasma proteins. Plasma proteins include albumin, which maintains osmotic pressure; globulin; fibrinogen; and prothrombin, which assists with clotting. Water moves between plasma and interstitial fluid based on conditions known as Starling's forces. Under normal conditions, the amount of fluid filtering outward through the arterial ends of the capillaries equals the amount of fluid that is returned to the circulation by reabsorption at the venous ends of the capillaries.

The equilibrium between the capillary and the interstitial space is controlled by four forces: capillary hydrostatic pressure, capillary colloidal osmotic pressure, tissue hydrostatic pressure, and tissue colloidal osmotic pressure. Capillary hydrostatic pressure pushes water out of the capillary into the interstitial space. Because the pressure is higher on the arterial end than the venous end, more water is pushed out of the capillary on the arterial end and more water is reabsorbed on the venous end. Capillary colloidal osmotic pressure is generated by dissolved proteins in the plasma that are too large to penetrate the capillary membrane. Tissue hydrostatic pressure opposes the pushing of fluids from the capillary into the interstitial space. Tissue colloidal osmotic pressure pulls fluid into the interstitial space.

Capillary and membrane permeability plays an important role in the movement of fluid and the emergence of edema in the surrounding tissues. If permeability increases, capillaries and membranes are more likely to leak. If permeability decreases, capillaries and membranes are less likely to leak.

Alterations in Water Movement: Edema

Edema occurs when excess fluid builds up in the interstitial space. Peripheral edema (eg, in the ankles and feet) is the most common form. Severe edema may be caused by long-standing lymphatic obstruction. If the patient is bedridden, edema may occur in the sacral area (sacral edema). Ascites is the abnormal accumulation of fluid in the peritoneal cavity.

Edema may have any of several causes:

- Increased capillary pressure—arteriolar dilation (eg, allergic reactions, inflammation), venous obstruction (eg, hepatic obstruction, heart failure, thrombophlebitis), increased vascular volume (eg, heart failure), increased levels of adrenocortical hormones, premenstrual sodium retention, pregnancy, environmental heat stress, or the effects of gravity from prolonged standing.
- Decreased colloidal osmotic pressure in the capillaries—decreased production of plasma proteins (eg, liver disease, starvation, severe protein deficiency) or increased loss of plasma proteins (eg, protein-losing kidney diseases, extensive burns).

Notes from Nancy

The cardinal sign of overhydration is edema.

In the Field

The clinical manifestations of edema may be either local or generalized. Patients may have pulmonary edema for cardiac reasons, or edema may present following near-drowning (submersion) or a narcotic overdose. Excess fluid in the lungs (eg, acute pulmonary edema) impairs the diffusion of oxygen into pulmonary capillaries, making the patient hypoxic. Patients can literally drown in their own fluids if they do not receive proper care.

- Lymphatic vessel obstruction due to infection; disease of the lymphatic structures or their removal (eg, mastectomy and removal of lymph nodes may lead to edema in the upper extremity). In this case, the amount of fluid leaving the arterial end of capillaries does not equal the amount of fluid that returns in the venous side of the capillaries. Hence, more fluid leaves the arterial sides, where the mean forces favoring outward movement are slightly higher, and the additional fluid is picked up by the lymphatic system.

Fluid and Electrolyte Balance

Water balance in the body is maintained through a variety of factors, of which the thirst mechanism and release of anti-diuretic hormone (ADH) are the most important. The renin-angiotensin-aldosterone system also plays a role in water homeostasis. The body's state of hydration is monitored continuously by three types of receptors:

- *Osmoreceptors* monitor extracellular fluid osmolarity. Sensors for these receptors are located primarily in the hypothalamus. When the extracellular fluid osmolarity is too high, they stimulate the production of ADH.
- *Volume-sensitive receptors* are located in the atria. When the intravascular fluid volume increases, the atria are stretched, leading to the release of natriuretic proteins.
- *Baroreceptors* are found primarily in the carotid artery, aorta, and kidneys. They are sensitive to changes in blood pressure.

The most potent stimulation for the release of ADH is an increase in blood osmolarity. When osmolarity increases, the pituitary gland releases ADH, also known as vasopressin. ADH stimulates the kidneys to resorb water, decreasing the blood's osmolarity.

Sodium and Chloride Balance

Sodium is the most common cation (ie, positively charged ion) in the body. The average adult has 60 mEq of sodium for each kilogram of body weight (2.2 lb = 1 kg). Most of the body's sodium is found in the extracellular fluid, but a small amount is found in the intracellular fluid. Intracellular sodium is transported out of the cell by the sodium–potassium pump because a resting cell membrane is relatively impermeable to sodium. Sodium also plays an important role in the regulation of the body's acid–base balance (sodium bicarbonate buffer system).

Sodium is taken in with foods. As little as 500 mg per day meets the body's needs. In the United States, the average adult ingests between 6 and 15 g of sodium per day.

Sodium is regulated primarily by the renin-angiotensin-aldosterone system (RAAS) and by natriuretic proteins. The RAAS is a complex feedback mechanism responsible for the kidney's regulation of sodium in the body. When sodium is present in excess, it is excreted into the urine; when the body sodium levels are low, the kidneys resorb sodium.

Renin is a protein that is released by the kidneys into the bloodstream in response to changes in blood pressure, blood flow, the amount of sodium in the tubular fluid, and the glomerular filtration rate. When renin is released, it converts the plasma protein angiotensinogen to angiotensin I. In the lungs, angiotensin I is converted rapidly to angiotensin II by angiotensin-converting enzyme (ACE). Angiotensin II, in turn, stimulates sodium resorption by the renal tubules. It also constricts the renal blood vessels, slowing kidney blood flow and decreasing the glomerular filtration rate. As a result, less sodium is filtered into the urine and more sodium is resorbed in the blood. **Figure 6-8 ▶** illustrates the role of the kidneys in the regulation of blood pressure and blood volume.

Angiotensin II is also responsible for stimulating the secretion of the adrenal hormone aldosterone. Aldosterone acts on the kidneys to increase the reabsorption of sodium into the blood and enhance the elimination of potassium in the urine. In addition to the stimulation by angiotensin II, aldosterone release is stimulated by increased extracellular potassium levels, decreased extracellular sodium levels, and release of adrenocorticotropic hormone (ACTH) from the pituitary gland.

Whereas activation of the RAAS leads to retention of sodium and water, production of natriuretic proteins increases when there is too much sodium and water in the body. Natriuretic proteins inhibit ADH and promote excretion of sodium and water by the kidneys.

Chloride is an important anion, or negatively charged ion, that when combined with sodium makes ordinary table salt. When placed in water, the compound will separate into its original ionic form. It assists in regulating the acid–base balance, especially the pH of the stomach, and is involved in the osmotic pressure of the extracellular fluid. Table salt, milk, eggs, and meats all contain chloride. It is often the case that where sodium goes, chloride follows.

Alterations in Sodium, Chloride, and Water Balance

Changes in water content can cause a cell to either shrink or swell. Tonicity refers to the tension exerted on a cell due to

Notes from Nancy

When you eat a bag of potato chips, you ingest a very large quantity of salt. Acutely, the body responds by holding on to water (hence urine output temporarily declines). In normal individuals, the kidneys and other regulatory mechanisms soon straighten things out.

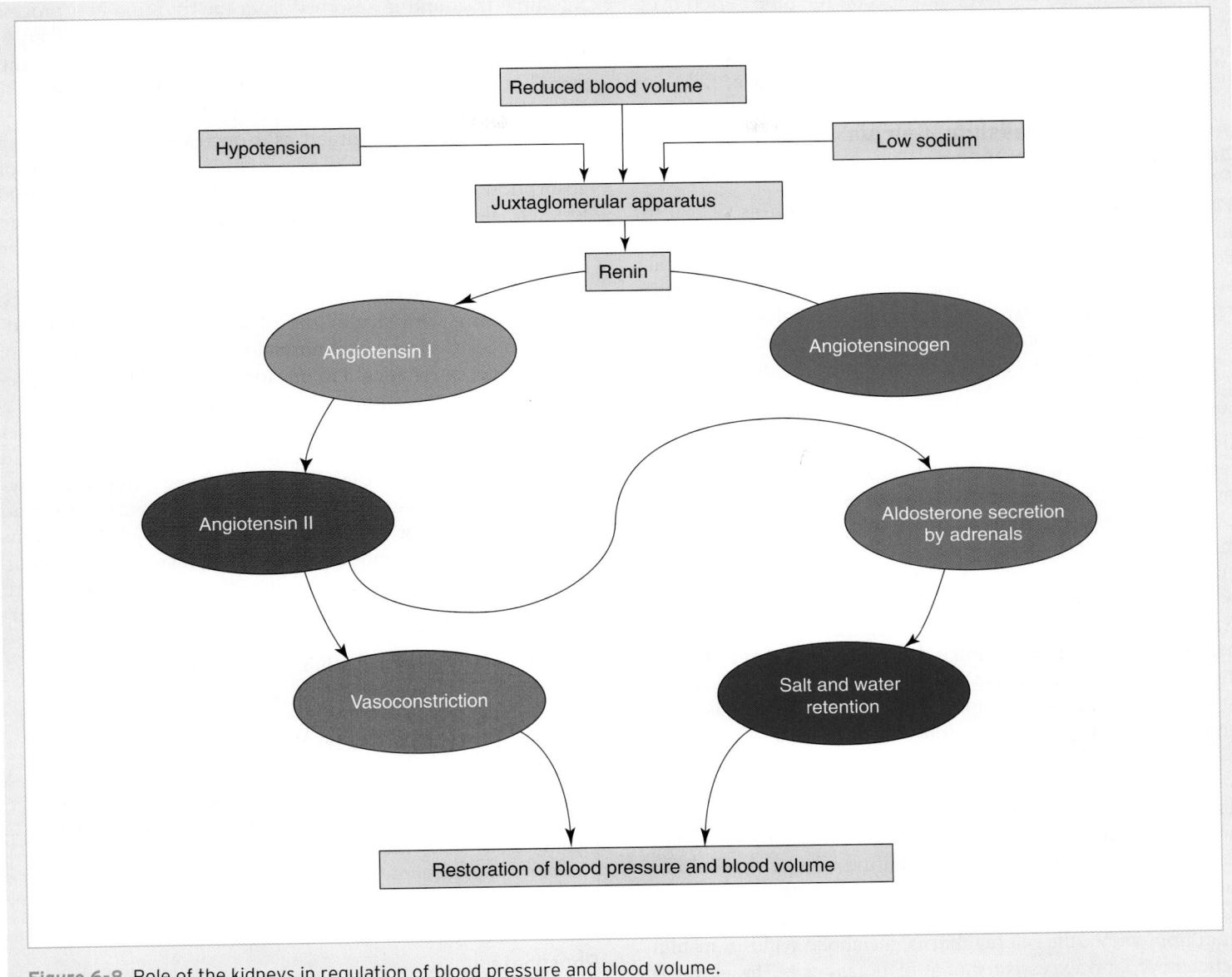

Figure 6-8 Role of the kidneys in regulation of blood pressure and blood volume.

water movement across the cell membrane. When cells are placed in an isotonic solution (ie, one with the same osmolarity as intracellular fluid—280 mOsm/L), they neither shrink nor swell. When cells are placed in a hypertonic solution, water is pulled out of the cells and they shrink. When cells are placed in a hypotonic solution, they swell.

An isotonic fluid deficit is a decrease in extracellular fluid with proportionate losses of sodium and water. An isotonic fluid excess is a proportionate increase in both sodium and water in the extracellular fluid compartment; common causes include kidney, heart, and liver failure. Manifestations of these problems depend on the serum sodium level. When dehydration exists, orthostatic hypotension and decreased urine output (oliguria) are common. Hyperthermia, delirium, and coma may be seen with very high sodium levels (> 160 mEq/L).

A hypertonic fluid deficit is caused by excess body water loss without a proportionate sodium loss (a relative water loss exists). The result is hypernatremia, which is clinically defined as a serum sodium level greater than 148 mEq/L and a serum osmolarity greater than 295 mOsm/kg. A hypotonic fluid deficit is caused by excessive sodium loss with less water loss (a relative water excess exists). This results in hyponatremia, which is characterized by a serum sodium level less than 135 mEq/L and a serum osmolarity less than 280 mOsm/kg.

Causes of hypernatremia and hyponatremia may include excess sweating from hot environmental conditions or exercise as well as gastrointestinal losses through vomiting, diarrhea, inappropriate intravenous fluids, or diuretics. Some patients have nausea and headaches, and others go on to develop seizures and coma. Clinical findings typically depend not only on the absolute sodium level, but also on the time period over which the abnormality developed. Patients who become hyponatremic over a period of days tend to have fewer symptoms than individuals who develop the abnormality acutely.

Alterations in Potassium, Calcium, Phosphate, and Magnesium Balance
Potassium
Potassium (K⁺), as the major intracellular cation, is critical to many functions of the cell. Potassium is necessary for neuromuscular control, regulation of the three types of muscles (skeletal, smooth, and cardiac), acid–base balance, intracellular enzyme reactions, and maintenance of intracellular osmolarity. The normal serum level of potassium is in the range of 3.5 to 5.0 mEq/L.

Hypokalemia is defined as a decreased serum potassium level. Common causes include decreased potassium intake, potassium shifts into the cells (eg, insulin, alkalosis, beta-adrenergic stimulation such as with epinephrine), renal potassium losses (eg, increased aldosterone activity, diuretics), and extrarenal potassium losses (eg, vomiting, diarrhea, laxatives). Muscular weakness, fatigue, and muscle cramps are the most frequent complaints in mild to moderate hypokalemia. Flaccid paralysis, hyporeflexia, and tetany may occur with very low levels of potassium (< 2.5 mEq/L). The ECG shows decreased amplitude and broadening of T waves, prominent U waves, premature ventricular contractions and other arrhythmias (eg, torsade de pointes), and depressed ST segments. Although acute hypokalemia can be treated with IV potassium supplementation, this therapy is rarely undertaken in the prehospital setting.

Hyperkalemia is an elevated serum potassium level. Common causes include spurious causes (repeated fist-clenching during phlebotomy, with release of potassium from forearm muscles; specimen drawn from an arm with a potassium infusion), decreased excretion (renal failure, drugs that inhibit potassium excretion [spironolactone, ACE inhibitors, nonsteroidal anti-inflammatory drugs (NSAIDs)]), shifts of potassium from within the cell (eg, burns, metabolic acidosis, insulin deficiency), and excessive intake of potassium. The elevated potassium level interferes with normal neuromuscular function, leading to muscle weakness and, rarely, flaccid paralysis. ECG changes occur in fewer than half of patients with a serum potassium level greater than 6.5 mEq/L and include peaked T waves, widening of the QRS complex, and arrhythmias (eg, ventricular tachycardia).

Hyperkalemia can be life-threatening due to its cardiac manifestations; therefore, it should be treated in the prehospital setting. Calcium administered intravenously immediately antagonizes cardiac conduction abnormalities. Bicarbonate, insulin, and albuterol shift potassium into the cells during a 15- to 30-minute period.

Calcium
The majority (98%) of the body's calcium is found in the bone and teeth. This element provides strength and stability for the collagen and ground substance that forms the matrix of the skeletal system. Calcium enters the body through the gastro-intestinal tract and is absorbed from the intestine in a process that depends on the presence of vitamin D **Figure 6-9**. Vitamin D is largely obtained through exposure to sunlight, stored in the bone, and ultimately excreted by the kidney. The normal serum calcium level is 8.5 to 10.5 mg/100 mL.

Hypocalcemia is defined as a decreased serum calcium level. Causes of hypocalcemia include decreased intake or absorption (eg, malabsorption, vitamin D deficit), increased loss (eg, alcoholism, diuretic therapy), and endocrine disease (eg, hypoparathyroidism, sepsis). Symptoms reflect the increased excitation of the neuromuscular and cardiovascular systems. Spasm of skeletal muscle causes cramps and tetany. Laryngospasm with stridor can obstruct the airway. Convulsions can occur as well as abnormal sensations (paresthesias) of the lips and extremities. Prolongation of the QT interval predisposes to the development of ventricular arrhythmias.

Hypercalcemia is an increased serum calcium level. Causes include increased intake or absorption (eg, excess antacid ingestion), endocrine disorders (eg, primary hyperparathyroidism, adrenal insufficiency), neoplasms (eg, cancers), and miscellaneous causes (eg, diuretics, sarcoidosis). Symptoms include constipation and frequent urination (polyuria). Stupor, coma, and renal failure may develop in severe cases. Treatment of the underlying cause is the mainstay of dealing with hypercalcemia. On an acute basis, volume replacement with boluses of 0.45% or 0.9% normal saline may be helpful.

In the Field
In the presence of tetany, arrhythmias, or seizures, 10% IV calcium gluconate (10 to 20 mL) administered over 10 to 15 minutes is indicated. Oral calcium and vitamin D preparations are appropriate in moderate or asymptomatic cases.

Phosphate
Phosphate is primarily an intracellular anion and is essential to many body functions.

Hypophosphatemia is characterized by a decrease in serum phosphate levels. Causes include decreased supply or absorption (eg, starvation, malabsorption, blocked absorption [aluminum-containing antacids]), excessive loss of phosphate ion (eg, diuretics, hyperparathyroidism, hyperthyroidism, alcoholism), intracellular shift of phosphorus (eg, administration of glucose, anabolic steroids, oral contraceptives, respiratory alkalosis, salicylate poisoning), electrolyte abnormalities (eg, hypercalcemia, hypomagnesemia, metabolic acidosis), and abnormal losses followed by inadequate repletion (eg, diabetic ketoacidosis, chronic alcoholism). Symptoms include muscle weakness, decreased deep tendon reflexes, mental obtundation, and confusion. Weakness is common. Acute, severe hypophosphatemia can lead to acute hemolytic anemia and increased susceptibility to infection. Muscle death (rhabdomyolysis) may also occur. Treatment involves oral replenishment

LOW BLOOD CALCIUM		HIGH BLOOD CALCIUM	
Increase PTH secretion and calcitriol formation		**Secrete calcitonin**	**Decrease PTH secretion and calcitriol formation**
Parathyroid gland secretes PTH. Increased PTH levels stimulate calcitriol (vitamin D₃) production in the kidney	**Thyroid/Parathyroid** 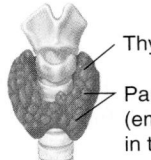 Thyroid — Parathyroid (embedded in the thyroid)	Thyroid gland secretes calcitonin	PTH formation slows and PTH levels drop. Decreased PTH levels slow calcitriol formation
Absorb more dietary calcium	**Small intestine**	**Absorb less dietary calcium**	
Calcitriol increases intestinal absorption of calcium and phosphorus	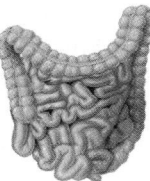	No major effect – calcitonin slightly inhibits calcium absorption	Decreased calcitriol slows intestinal absorption of calcium and phosphorus
Retain calcium	**Kidney**	**Excrete calcium**	
PTH and calcitriol increase calcium reabsorption in the kidney, thus decreasing calcium excretion	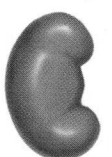	No major effect – calcitonin slightly increases calcium excretion	Decreased PTH and calcitriol levels increase calcium excretion
Move calcium from bone to bloodstream	**Bone**	**Move calcium from bloodstream to bone**	
PTH and calcitriol work together to stimulate osteoclast activity. The osteoclasts resorb bone, releasing calcium into the bloodstream	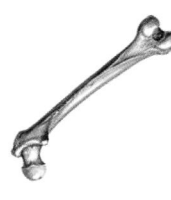	Calcitonin inhibits the activity of osteoclasts, shifting the balance toward the deposition of calcium in bone	Decreased PTH and calcitriol levels slow osteoclast activity and breakdown of bone
RAISE BLOOD CALCIUM		**LOWER BLOOD CALCIUM**	

Figure 6-9 Regulation of blood calcium levels. Calcitonin has only a weak effect on calcium ion concentration. It is fast-acting, but any decrease in calcium ion concentration triggers the release of parathyroid hormone (PTH), which almost completely overrides the calcitonin effect. In prolonged calcium excess or deficiency, the parathyroid mechanism is the most powerful hormonal mechanism for maintaining normal blood calcium levels.

in mild to moderate cases. Severe cases and symptomatic patients require IV phosphate replacement.

Hyperphosphatemia is defined as an increased serum phosphate level. Causes include massive loading of phosphate into the extracellular fluid (eg, excess vitamin D, laxatives or enemas containing phosphate, IV phosphate supplements, chemotherapy, metabolic acidosis) and decreased excretion into the urine (eg, renal failure, hypoparathyroidism, excessive growth hormone [acromegaly]). Symptoms vary widely, but may include tremor, paresthesia, hyporeflexia, confusion, seizures, muscle weakness, stupor, coma, hypotension, heart failure, and prolonged QT interval. Treatment of the underly-

ing cause and of any accompanying hypocalcemia is the most common therapeutic approach. Saline boluses (forced diuresis) are often helpful.

Magnesium

Magnesium is the second most abundant intracellular cation, after potassium. About 50% of the body's magnesium is stored in the bones, 49% in the body cells, and the remaining 1% in the extracellular fluid. Normal serum levels are 1.5 to 2.0 mEq/L.

Hypomagnesemia is defined as a decreased serum magnesium level. Causes include diminished absorption or intake (eg, malabsorption, chronic diarrhea, laxative abuse, malnutrition), increased renal loss (eg, diuretics, hyperaldosteronism, hyper-calcemia, volume expansion), and miscellaneous causes (eg, diabetes, respiratory alkalosis, pregnancy). Common symptoms are weakness, muscle cramps, and tremor. Patients develop marked neuromuscular and central nervous system hyperirritability with tremors and jerking. There may be hypertension, tachycardia, and ventricular arrhythmias. In some patients, confusion and disorientation are prominent features. Treatment consists of IV fluids containing magnesium.

Hypermagnesemia is an increased serum magnesium level. It is almost always the result of kidney insufficiency and the inability to excrete the amount of magnesium taken in from food or drugs, especially antacids and laxatives. Symptoms include muscle weakness, decreased deep tendon reflexes, mental obtundation, and confusion. Weakness is common, and respiratory muscle paralysis or cardiac arrest is possible.

Acid–Base Balance

The measurement of hydrogen ion concentration of a solution is called pH. Normal body functions depend on an acid–base balance that remains within the normal physiologic pH range of 7.35 to 7.45. The mathematical formula for calculating pH is $pH = -log [H^+]$, where "log" refers to the base-10 logarithm and $[H^+]$ refers to the hydrogen ion concentration. Changes in the pH are exponential, not linear. For example, a change in the pH from 7.40 to 7.20 results in a 10^2 (ie, 100-fold) change in the acid concentration.

To maintain the delicate acid–base balance, the body relies on its buffer systems. Buffers are molecules that modulate changes in pH. In the absence of buffers, the addition of acid to a solution will cause a sharp change in pH. In the presence of a buffer, the pH change will be moderated or may even be unnoticeable in the same situation. Because acid production is the major challenge to pH homeostasis, most physiologic buffers combine with H^+.

Buffer systems include proteins, phosphate ions, and bicarbonate (HCO_3^-). The large amounts of bicarbonate produced from the carbon dioxide (CO_2) made during metabolism create the body's most important extracellular buffer system. Hydrogen and bicarbonate ions combine to form carbonic acid, which readily dissociates into water and carbon dioxide:

$$H^+ + HCO_3^- \Leftrightarrow H_2CO_3 \Leftrightarrow H_2O + CO_2$$

In the bicarbonate buffer system, excess acid (H^+) combines with bicarbonate (HCO_3^-), forming H_2CO_3. This compound rapidly dissociates into water and CO_2, which is then exhaled. Because the acid is eliminated as water and CO_2, the total pH does not change significantly. A similar process occurs with the production of metabolic base (bicarbonate).

Acidosis Versus Alkalosis

When the buffering capacity of the body is exceeded, acid–base imbalances occur. A blood pH greater than 7.45 is called alkalosis; a blood pH less than 7.35 is called acidosis.

If the pH is too low (acidosis), neurons become less excitable and CNS depression results. Patients become confused and disoriented. If CNS depression progresses, the respiratory centers cease to function, leading to the person's death.

If pH is too high (alkalosis), neurons become hyperexcitable, firing action potentials at the slightest signal. This condition first manifests as sensory changes, such as numbness or tingling, then as muscle twitches. If alkalosis is severe, muscle twitches turn into sustained contractions (tetanus) that paralyze respiratory muscles.

Disturbances of acid–base balance are associated with disturbances in potassium balance, in part because of the kidney transport system that moves H^+ and K^+ in opposite directions. In acidosis, the kidneys excrete H^+ and resorb K^+. Conversely, when the body goes into a state of alkalosis, the kidneys resorb H^+ and excrete K^+. A potassium imbalance usually shows up as disturbances in excitable tissues, especially the heart.

Metabolic Versus Respiratory Acid–Base Imbalances

Acid–base disturbances are classified into two general categories: metabolic and respiratory. Each is then broken down into acidosis and alkalosis.

Metabolic acidosis is an accumulation of abnormal acids in the blood for any of several reasons (eg, sepsis, diabetic ketoacidosis, salicylate poisoning). Initially, the $Paco_2$ (partial pressure of carbon dioxide) is not affected, but the pH is decreased. Later, the body compensates for the metabolic abnormality by hyperventilating, leading to excretion of CO_2 and compensatory respiratory alkalosis. For example, patients with diabetic ketoacidosis often experience *Kussmaul respirations* (deep, rapid, sighing ventilations), in which they hyperventilate to "blow off" CO_2 and decrease the acidosis.

Metabolic alkalosis is rarely seen in an acute condition, but is very common in chronically ill patients, especially those undergoing nasogastric suction. It involves either a buildup of excess metabolic base (eg, chronic antacid ingestion) or a loss of normal acid (eg, through vomiting or nasogastric

In the Field

Respiratory compensation for metabolic problems (acidosis or alkalosis) occurs *rapidly* and is relatively predictable. Metabolic compensation for respiratory problems (acidosis or alkalosis), if it occurs at all, takes hours to days. Compensation returns the pH toward normal. Acutely, compensation is never complete. Chronic compensation, as in chronic obstructive pulmonary disease (COPD), often does result in a completely normal pH.

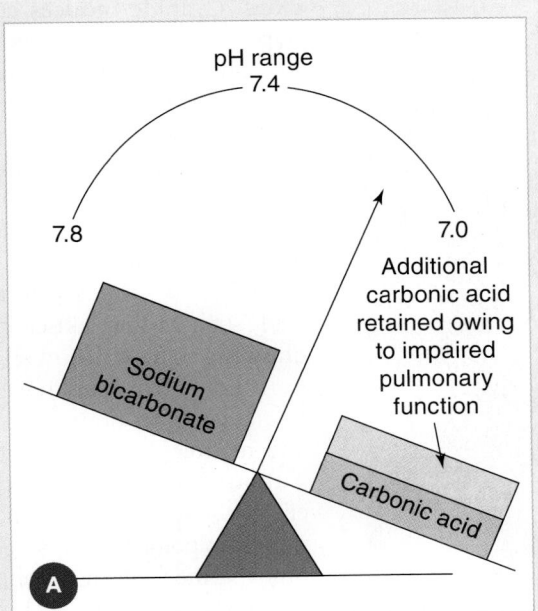

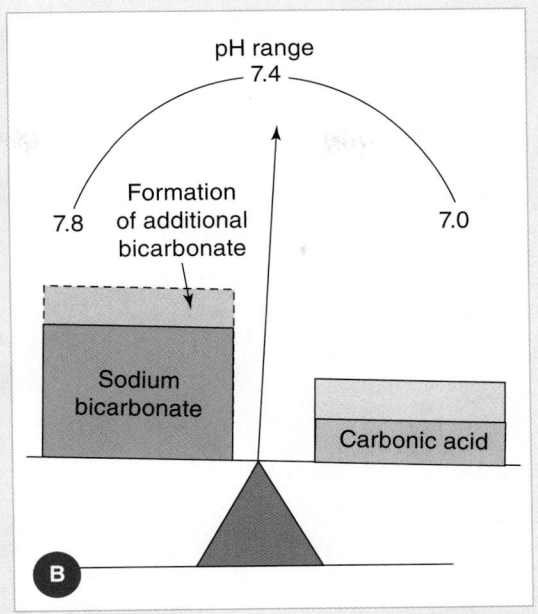

Figure 6-10 **A.** Derangement of acid-base balance in respiratory acidosis. **B.** Compensation by formation of additional bicarbonate.

Figure 6-11 ▶ . This damage often results in a change in cell shape and function. Functional changes may include an inability to use oxygen appropriately, development of intracellular acidosis, accumulation of toxic waste products, and an inability to metabolize nutrients.

Damage and functional changes in individual cells often have an impact on the entire organism. In some cases, only minor systemic abnormalities are noted, such as fever. At other times, entire organ systems fail and the patient's situation becomes critical (eg, kidney failure). Because all body systems are connected in some manner, dysfunction in one system inevitably affects other systems. When the homeostatic balance in the body is upset, the "scales" can shift in an unfavorable direction.

Cell injury may, up to a point, be repaired with proper treatment. Irreversible injury occurs once cells have passed the "point of no return," after which no treatment will help. Cell death is followed by necrosis, a process in which the cell breaks down. The cell membrane becomes abnormally permeable, leading to an influx of electrolytes and fluids. The cell and its organelles swell. Lysosomes also release enzymes that destroy intracellular components. These processes occur both during and after actual cell death.

suctioning). The pH is high and the Pa_{CO_2} unchanged initially. On a chronic basis, the body compensates by slowing ventilation and increasing the Pa_{CO_2}, thereby creating a compensatory respiratory acidosis.

Respiratory acidosis occurs when CO_2 retention leads to increased Pa_{CO_2} levels. It also occurs in situations of hypoventilation (eg, heroin overdose) or intrinsic lung diseases (eg, asthma or COPD) Figure 6-10 ▲ .

Excessive "blowing off" of CO_2 with a resulting decrease in the Pa_{CO_2} causes respiratory alkalosis. Although often called hyperventilation, many potentially serious diseases (eg, pulmonary embolism, acute myocardial infarction, severe infection, diabetic ketoacidosis) may be responsible for increased ventilatory levels.

Cell Injury

Cellular injury may result from various causes, such as hypoxia (lack of oxygen), ischemia (hypoxia due to lack of blood supply), chemical injury, infectious injury, immunologic (hypersensitivity) injury, physical damage (mechanical injury), and inflammatory injury. The manifestations of cell injury and death depend on how many and which types of cells are damaged.

Manifestations of cellular injury occur at both the microscopic (structural) and the functional levels. Common microscopic abnormalities (eg, those observed in the cardiac cell undergoing necrosis from hypoxemia for an extended period of time) include cell swelling, rupture of cell membranes or nuclear membranes, and breakdown of nuclear material (chromosomes)

Hypoxic Injury

Hypoxic injury is a common—and often deadly—cause of cellular injury. It may result from decreased amounts of oxygen in the air or loss of hemoglobin function (eg, carbon monoxide poisoning), a decreased number of red blood cells (eg, bleeding), disease of the respiratory or cardiovascular system (eg, COPD), or loss of cytochromes (mitochondrial proteins that convert oxygen to ATP, like that seen in cyanide poisoning).

Although hypoxia by itself has deleterious effects on cells, the damage does not stop there. Cells that are hypoxic for more than a few seconds produce mediators (substances) that may damage other local or distant body locations. The result is a positive feedback cycle in which mediators lead to more cell damage, which leads to more hypoxia, which leads to further mediator production, and so forth.

The earliest and most dangerous mediators produced by cells in response to hypoxia are free radicals. These molecules are missing one electron in their outer shell. The presence of an odd, unpaired electron results in chemical instability

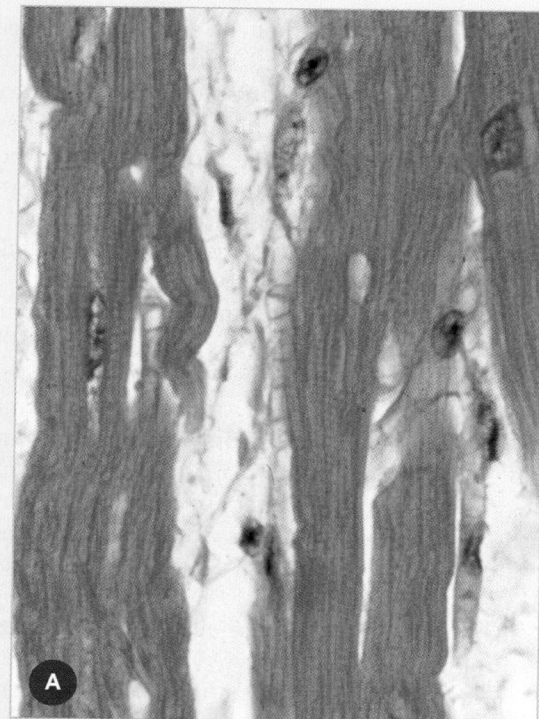
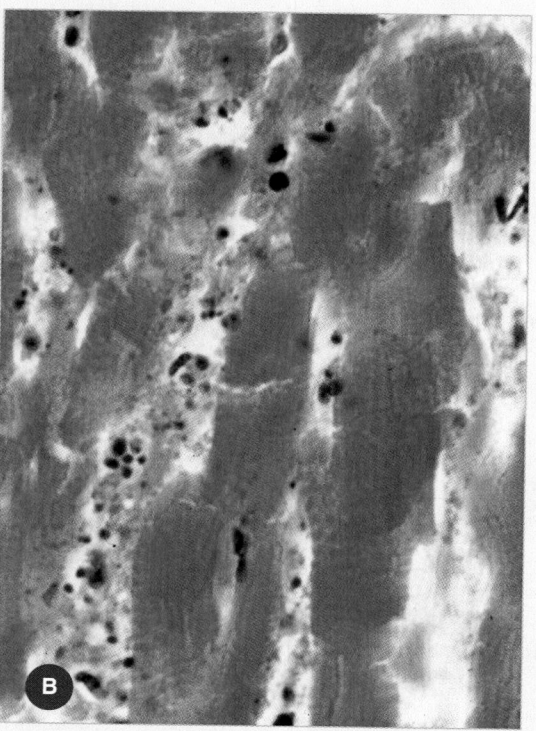

Figure 6-11 Comparison of cardiac muscle fibers. **A.** With necrotic fibers. **B.** Note fragmentation of fibers, loss of nuclear staining, and fragmented bits of nuclear debris. When the cell is injured it swells, resulting in nuclear membrane rupture and breakdown of the nuclear material (original magnification, ×400).

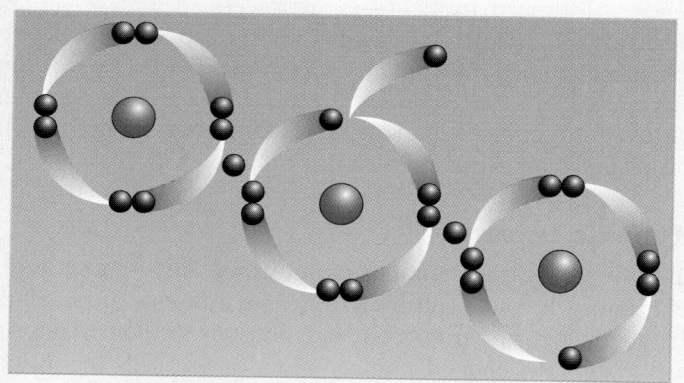

Figure 6-12 Free radicals are missing one electron in their outside orbit. This molecular structure results in chemical instability. Each black dot represents an electron in the outer shell.

Figure 6-12 ▲ . Free radicals randomly attack cells and membranes in an attempt to "steal back" the missing electron. The result is widespread and potentially deadly tissue damage.

Chemical Injury

A variety of chemicals may injure and ultimately destroy cells, including poisons, lead, carbon monoxide, ethanol, and pharmacologic agents. Common poisons include cyanide and pesti-

cides. Cyanide induces cell hypoxia by blocking oxidative phosphorylation in the mitochondria and preventing the metabolism of oxygen. Pesticides block an enzyme, acetylcholinesterase, thereby preventing proper transmission of nerve impulses.

Chronic ingestion of lead, such as that caused by chewing on windowsills painted with lead-based paint, leads to brain injury and neurologic dysfunction. Although all of lead's toxic effects cannot be tied together neatly by pointing to a single unifying mechanism, its ability to substitute for calcium (molecules of lead and calcium are a similar size) is a common factor in many of its toxic actions. Mostly likely lead is "mistaken" for calcium in vital biochemical reactions, leading to abnormal results and dysfunction.

Carbon monoxide binds to hemoglobin, preventing adequate oxygenation of the tissues. Low levels cause nausea, vomiting, and headache. Higher levels result in death.

In lower doses, ethanol causes the well-known effects of inebriation. Higher doses result in severe CNS depression, hypoventilation, and cardiovascular collapse.

Some pharmacologic agents produce toxic products when they are metabolized in the body, especially in "overdose conditions." Acetaminophen (Tylenol), in doses of more than 140 mg/kg in an adult, results in acute overdose, causing the accumulation of toxic intermediates that poison the liver and may lead to death.

Infectious Injury

Infectious injury to cells occurs as a result of an invasion of either bacteria or viruses. Bacteria may cause injury either by direct action on cells or by the production of toxins. Viruses often initiate an inflammatory response that leads to cell damage and patient symptoms.

Virulence measures the disease-causing ability of a microorganism. The pathogenicity of any particular microorganism is a function of its ability to reproduce and cause disease within the human body. In particular, the growth and survival of bacteria in the body depend on the effectiveness of the body's own defense mechanisms and the bacteria's ability to resist those mechanisms. A depressed immune system is less able to fight off microorganisms that the body perceives as harmful; populations with weaker immune systems may include newborn infants, elderly patients, diabetics, and people with cancer or other chronic diseases.

Bacteria

Many bacteria possess a capsule that protects them from ingestion and destruction by <u>phagocytes</u>—cells (eg, white blood cells) that engulf and consume foreign material such as microorganisms and cellular debris **Figure 6-13 ▾** . Not all bacteria are encapsulated, however. *Mycobacterium tuberculosis,* for example, lacks a capsule, yet stubbornly resists destruction; it can be transported by phagocytes throughout the body. Gram-positive bacteria are distinguished by very thick cell walls composed of many layers of peptidoglycan (amino acids and sugar); conversely, the cell walls of gram-negative bacteria consist largely of lipids. The pathogenic qualities of gram-negative bacteria, which include the microorganism that causes bubonic plague, make them especially problematic for humans.

Bacteria also produce exotoxins or endotoxins—substances such as enzymes or toxins—that can injure or destroy cells. Staphylococci, streptococci, and *Clostridium tetani,* for example, secrete exotoxins into the medium surrounding the cell. Endotoxins are lipopolysaccharides that are part of the cell walls of gram-negative bacteria. When large amounts of endotoxins are present in the body, a person may develop septic shock.

When cells are injured, circulating white blood cells are attracted to the site of injury. White blood cells release endogenous <u>pyrogens</u>, which then cause a fever to develop. Indeed, the body's most common reaction to the presence of bacteria is inflammation. Some bacteria have the ability to produce hypersensitivity reactions. The proliferation of microorganisms in the blood is called bacteremia or sepsis.

Viruses

Viruses are intracellular parasites that take over the metabolic processes of the host cell and then use the cell to help them replicate. A virus consists of a nucleic acid core of either RNA or DNA. Surrounding the viral core is a layer of protein known as the capsid, which protects the virus from phagocytosis. Some viruses have an additional protective coat known as the envelope.

The replication of a virus occurs inside the host cell because viruses do not contain any of their own organelles. Viral infection of a host cell leads to a decreased synthesis of macromolecules that are vital to the host cell. Unlike bacteria, however, viruses do not produce exotoxins or endotoxins.

There may be a symbiotic relationship between a virus and normal cells that results in a persistent unapparent infection. Viruses have been known to evoke a strong immune response and can rapidly produce an irreversible, lethal injury in highly susceptible cells, as is the case with acquired immunodeficiency syndrome (AIDS).

Immunologic and Inflammatory Injury

Inflammation is a protective response that can occur even without bacterial invasion. Infection is characterized by an invasion of microorganisms that causes cell or tissue injury, which leads to the inflammatory response. The immune system protects the body by providing defenses to attack and remove foreign organisms such as bacteria or viruses.

Cellular membranes may be injured when they come in direct contact with the cellular and chemical components of the immune or inflammatory process, such as phagocytes (neutrophils and macrophages), histamine, antibodies, and lymphokines. In such a case, potassium leaks out of the damaged cell and water flows inward, causing the cell to swell. The nuclear envelope, organelle membranes, and cell membrane may all rupture, leading to cell death. The degree of swelling and chance of membrane rupture depend on the severity of the immune and inflammatory responses.

Other Injurious Factors

Genetic factors that may damage cells include chromosomal disorders, premature development of atherosclerosis, and obesity (in some cases). There are two ways an abnormal gene may develop in an individual: by mutation of the gene during meiosis, which affects the newly formed fetus, or by heredity. In trisomy 21 (Down syndrome), the child is born with an extra chromosome, usually number 21.

Good nutrition is required to maintain good health and assist the cells in fighting off disease. Nutritional disorders that can injure cells and the organism as a whole include obesity, malnutrition, vitamin excess or deficiency, and mineral excess or deficiency. These conditions can lead to alterations in physical growth, mental and intellectual retardation, and even death in some circumstances.

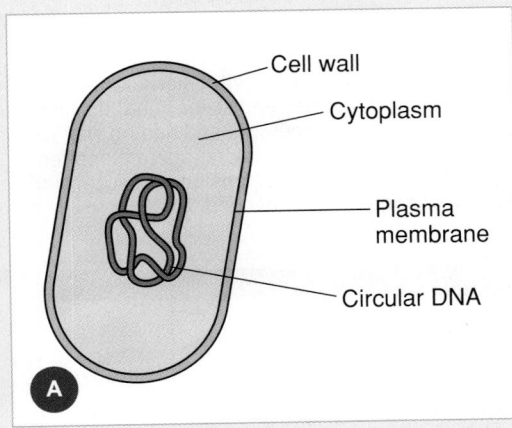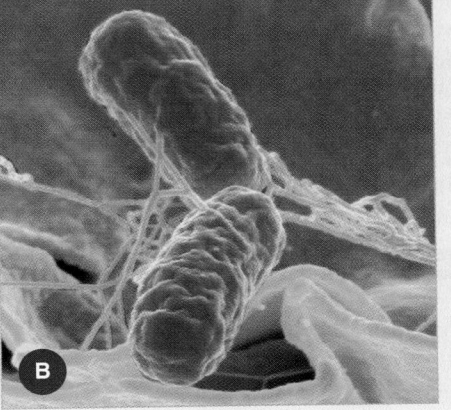

Figure 6-13 General structure of a bacterium. **A.** Bacteria come in many shapes and sizes, but all have a circular strand of DNA, cytoplasm, and a plasma membrane. A cell wall surrounds the membrane in many bacteria. **B.** An electron micrograph of salmonella bacteria. Many bacteria have a capsule that protects them from ingestion and destruction by phagocytes.

Physical agents, such as heat, cold, and radiation, may also cause cell injury—for example, burns, frostbite, radiation sickness, and tumors. The degree of cell injury that results is determined by both the strength of the agent and the length of exposure.

Apoptosis

Apoptosis is normal cell death. It is unique in that it is genetically programmed into the cell as a part of normal development, organogenesis, immune function, and tissue growth. It plays a normal role in aging, early development, menses, lactating breast tissue, thymus involution, and red blood cell turnover.

During apoptosis, cells exhibit characteristic nuclear changes, and they typically die in well-defined clusters rather than in a random fashion. The molecular mechanism underlying apoptosis involves the activation of genes that code for proteins known as caspases. These proteins are essentially cellular "cyanide"—in essence, their production leads to cell suicide. Unlike in the case of cell death from disease processes, proteins and DNA undergo controlled degradation that allows their remnants to be taken up and reused by neighboring cells. In this way, apoptosis allows the body to eliminate a cell but still "recycle" many of its components. Pathologically, areas that have undergone apoptotic death do not show any evidence of inflammation. In contrast, an inflammatory response is typically observed when cells undergo necrosis from hypoxia or cellular toxins.

Apoptosis can be activated prematurely by pathologic factors such as cell injury. This sort of premature stimulation results in early cell death, which occurs in some forms of heart failure. Another example of pathologic apoptosis is the death of hepatocytes (liver cells) in patients with viral hepatitis. The dying cells form lumps of chromatin known as Councilman's bodies. Factors that inhibit the normal course of apoptosis result in unwanted cellular proliferation, as in cancer and rheumatoid arthritis (uncontrolled synovial tissue proliferation). **Figure 6-14 ▾** illustrates the process by which cancerous cells develop from normal cells.

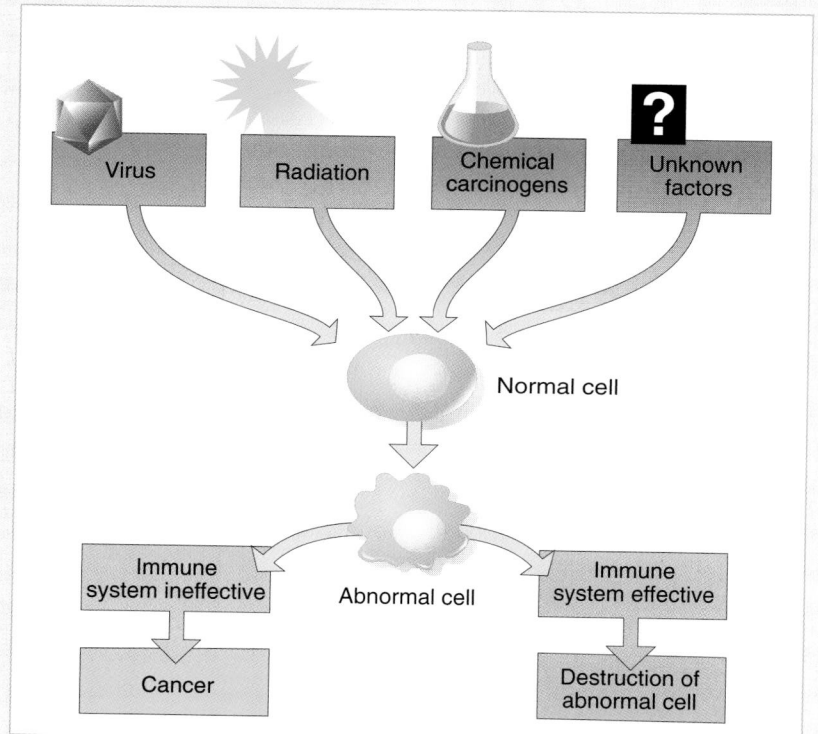

Figure 6-14 The onset of cancer. Viruses and other factors induce a normal cell to become abnormal. When the immune system is working effectively, it destroys the abnormal cells, so no cancer develops. When abnormal cells evade the immune system, they form a tumor and then may become a spreading cancer.

You are the Provider Part 2

You ask your partner to place the patient on 100% oxygen via a nonrebreathing mask and get a set of baseline vital signs while you begin to question her regarding her current illness and past medical history. The patient tells you that she has end-stage renal disease and requires dialysis every other day. She was unable to make it to her last appointment because she did not feel well and had no way to get there. She did not call her physician, stating that she thought she could "shake off this bug." She had been taking acetaminophen (Tylenol) every 4 hours for the fever and the pain in her forearm. Her past medical history is significant for hypertension, a myocardial infarction in 2003, and congestive heart failure. Daily medications include Captopril, aspirin, and nitroglycerin as needed.

Vital Signs	Recording Time: 5 Minutes
Skin	Pale, warm, and moist
Pulse	140 beats/min, regular; weak radial
Blood pressure	86/50 mm Hg
Respirations	28 breaths/min, accessory muscle use, rales auscultated half way up the back bilaterally
Sao$_2$	93% on nonrebreathing mask at 15 L/min of supplemental oxygen

3. What should you monitor your patient for?

4. Which interventions should you consider at this point, if any?

Abnormal Cell Death

If the injury leading to cell degeneration is of sufficient intensity and duration, irreversible cell injury will lead to cell death. Necrosis is the result of the morphologic changes that occur following cell death in living tissues. It may be either simple necrosis (coagulation) or derived necrosis.

Simple necrosis refers to areas of necrosis where the gross and microscopic tissue and some of the cells are recognizable. It may be caused by acute ischemia, acute toxicity (eg, from heavy metals), or direct physical injury (eg, from caustic chemicals and burns).

Derived necrosis includes caseation necrosis, dry gangrene, fat necrosis, and liquefaction necrosis. Caseation necrosis is manifested by the loss of all features of the tissue and cells, so that they come to resemble cheese when viewed through a microscope. Dry gangrene results from invasion and putrefaction of necrotic tissue, after the blood supply is compromised to the tissue and the tissue undergoes coagulation necrosis. Fat necrosis results from the destruction of fat cells, usually by enzymes (ie, pancreatic proteases and lipases). Liquefaction necrosis results from coagulation necrosis followed by liquefaction necrosis of tissues and invasion by putrefying bacteria that grow rapidly in a warm moist environment; the bacteria then produce lytic enzymes and gas.

Genetics and Familial Disease

Factors Causing Disease

Genetic, environmental, age-related, and sex-associated factors can all cause disease. Genetic factors are present at birth and are passed on through a person's genes to future generations. Environmental factors include microorganisms, immunologic and toxic exposures, personal habits and lifestyle, exposures to chemicals, the physical environment, and the psychosocial environment.

Age and sex-associated factors interact with a combination of genetic and environmental factors, lifestyle, and anatomic or hormonal differences. The risk of a particular disease often depends on the patient's age. For example, newborns are at greater risk of certain diseases because their immune systems are not fully developed (see Chapter 41). Teenagers are at high risk of other diseases due to trauma, drugs, and alcohol. The older we become, the greater the risk of cancer, heart disease, stroke, and Alzheimer's disease (see Chapter 42). Some diseases are more prevalent in men, such as lung cancer, gout, and Parkinson's disease. Women are more likely to have osteoporosis, rheumatoid arthritis, and breast cancer.

Some uncontrollable factors (eg, genetics) influence a disease process, but many other factors can be controlled. For example, behaviors such as smoking, drinking alcohol, poor nutrition (eg, excessive fat, salt, and sugar intake; insufficient intake of protein, fruits, vegetables, and fiber), lack of exercise, and stress can all be modified.

Analyzing Disease Risk

Analyzing disease risk involves consideration of disease rates and disease risk factors (both causal and noncausal). All studies of a disease should consider the incidence, prevalence, and mortality of the disease. The incidence is the frequency of disease occurrence (eg, one in four patients has this disease). The prevalence is the number of cases in a particular population over time (eg, last year, more than 100,000 patients had this disease). The mortality is the number of deaths from a disease in a given population (eg, 1 in 50 affected individuals in the United States with this disease will die).

Risk factors, age, and sex differences often interact. For example, suppose a person has a genetic tendency toward coronary artery disease; the risk of myocardial infarction or sudden death is higher in this individual even if he or she exercises regularly and has no other risk factors. A person who smokes heavily but has no other risk factors may have a similarly elevated risk.

Common Familial Diseases and Associated Risk Factors

The terms *genetic risk* and *familial tendency* are often used interchangeably. A true genetic risk is one that is passed through generations by inheritance of a gene. In contrast, with a familial tendency, diseases may "cluster" in family groups despite lack of evidence for heritable gene-associated abnormalities.

Table 6-2 ▶ lists some of the traits and diseases carried on human chromosomes. Autosomal recessive is a pattern of inheritance that involves genes located on autosomes (any chromosome other than sex chromosomes). A person needs to inherit two copies of a particular form of such a gene to show that trait. A parent who carries the gene for an autosomal recessive trait but does not display the trait has a 25% chance of passing the inherited condition to his or her child if the other parent is also a carrier for the trait. If both parents actually have the inherited condition, then all of their children will have the condition. Hemochromatosis, which causes people to accumulate too much iron in their bodies, shows an autosomal recessive pattern of inheritance—a person must inherit a copy of the hemochromatosis gene from each parent to develop the disease.

In autosomal dominant inheritance, a person needs to inherit only one copy of a particular form of a gene to show that trait; it does not matter which form of the gene is inherited from the other parent. A parent has at least a 50% chance of passing on an autosomal dominant inherited condition to his or her child. Familial adenomatous polyposis, which places people at extremely high risk of developing colon cancer, shows an autosomal dominant pattern of inheritance.

Immunologic Disorders

Immunologic diseases are caused by either hyperactivity or hypoactivity of the immune system. Most immunologic diseases that exhibit familial tendencies involve an overactive immune system—for example, allergies, asthma, and rheumatic fever. Often there is significant overlap between causative factors, including the patient's environment. **Table 6-3 ▾** lists common respiratory diseases that may be caused by environmental pollutants, viruses, or bacteria.

Allergies are acquired following initial exposure to a stimulant, known as an allergen. Repeated exposures cause the immune system to react to the allergen **Figure 6-15 ▸**. Although the clinical presentation varies, it usually includes swelling and itching, runny nose, coughing, sneezing, wheezing, and nasal congestion. A person who has an allergic tendency is said to be atopic. Environmental conditions may also increase a person's susceptibility toward an allergic reaction.

Asthma is a chronic inflammatory condition resulting in intermittent wheezing and excess mucus production. Nearly 60% of attacks are precipitated by viral infections. Allergies account for another 20% of asthma attacks, with stress and emotions causing the remainder. In addition to the familial component, chromosomal differences in certain individuals may enhance their susceptibility to asthma.

Rheumatic fever is an inflammatory disease that occurs primarily in children. This disease results from a delayed reaction to an untreated streptococcal infection of the upper respiratory tract (eg, strep throat). Symptoms, which appear several weeks after the acute infection, may include fever, abdominal pain, vomiting, arthritis, palpitations, and chest pain. Recurrent episodes of rheumatic fever may cause permanent myocardial damage, especially to the cardiac valves. A family history of acute rheumatic fever may predispose an individual to the disease.

Cancer

Cancer includes a large number of malignant growths (neoplasms). The prognosis often depends on the extent of its spread (metastasis) and the effectiveness of treatment.

Table 6-2 | Traits and Diseases Carried on Human Chromosomes

Autosomal recessive

Albinism	Lack of pigment in eyes, skin, and hair
Cystic fibrosis	Pancreatic failure, mucus buildup in lungs
Sickle cell anemia	Abnormal hemoglobin leading to sickle-shaped red blood cells that obstruct vital capillaries
Tay-Sachs disease	Improper metabolism of gangliosides in nerve cells, resulting in early death
Phenylketonuria	Accumulation of phenylalanine in blood; results in mental retardation
Attached earlobe	Earlobe attached to skin of the neck
Hyperextendable thumb	Thumb bends past 45° angle

Autosomal dominant

Achondroplasia	Dwarfism resulting from a defect in epiphyseal plates of forming long bones
Marfan's syndrome	Defect manifest in connective tissue, resulting in excessive growth and aortic rupture
Widow's peak	Hairline coming to a point on forehead
Huntington's disease	Progressive deterioration of the nervous system beginning in late 20s or early 30s; results in mental deterioration and early death
Brachydactyly	Disfiguration of hands, shortened fingers
Freckles	Permanent aggregations of melanin in the skin

Table 6-3 | Common Respiratory Diseases

Disease	Pathology/Symptoms	Cause	Treatment
Emphysema	Breakdown of alveoli; shortness of breath	Smoking and air pollution	Administer oxygen to relieve symptoms; quit smoking; avoid polluted air. No known cure.
Chronic bronchitis	Coughing, shortness of breath	Smoking and air pollution	Quit smoking; move out of polluted area; if possible, move to warmer, drier climate.
Acute bronchitis	Inflammation of the bronchi; yellow mucus coughed up; shortness of breath	Many viruses and bacteria	If bacterial, take antibiotics, cough medicine; use vaporizer.
Sinusitis	Inflammation of the sinuses; mucus discharge; blockage of nasal passageways; headache	Many viruses and bacteria	If bacterial, take antibiotics and decongestant tablets; use vaporizer.
Laryngitis	Inflammation of larynx and vocal cords; sore throat; hoarseness; mucus buildup and cough	Many viruses and bacteria	If bacterial, take antibiotics, cough medicine; avoid irritants, such as smoke; avoid talking.
Pneumonia	Inflammation of the lungs ranging from mild to severe; cough and fever; shortness of breath at rest; chills; sweating; chest pains; blood in mucus	Bacteria, viruses, or inhalation of irritating gases	Consult physician immediately; go to bed; take antibiotics, cough medicine; stay warm.
Asthma	Constriction of bronchioles; mucus buildup in bronchioles; periodic wheezing; difficulty breathing	Allergy to pollen, some foods, food additives; dandruff from dogs and cats; exercise	Use inhalants to open passageways; avoid irritants.

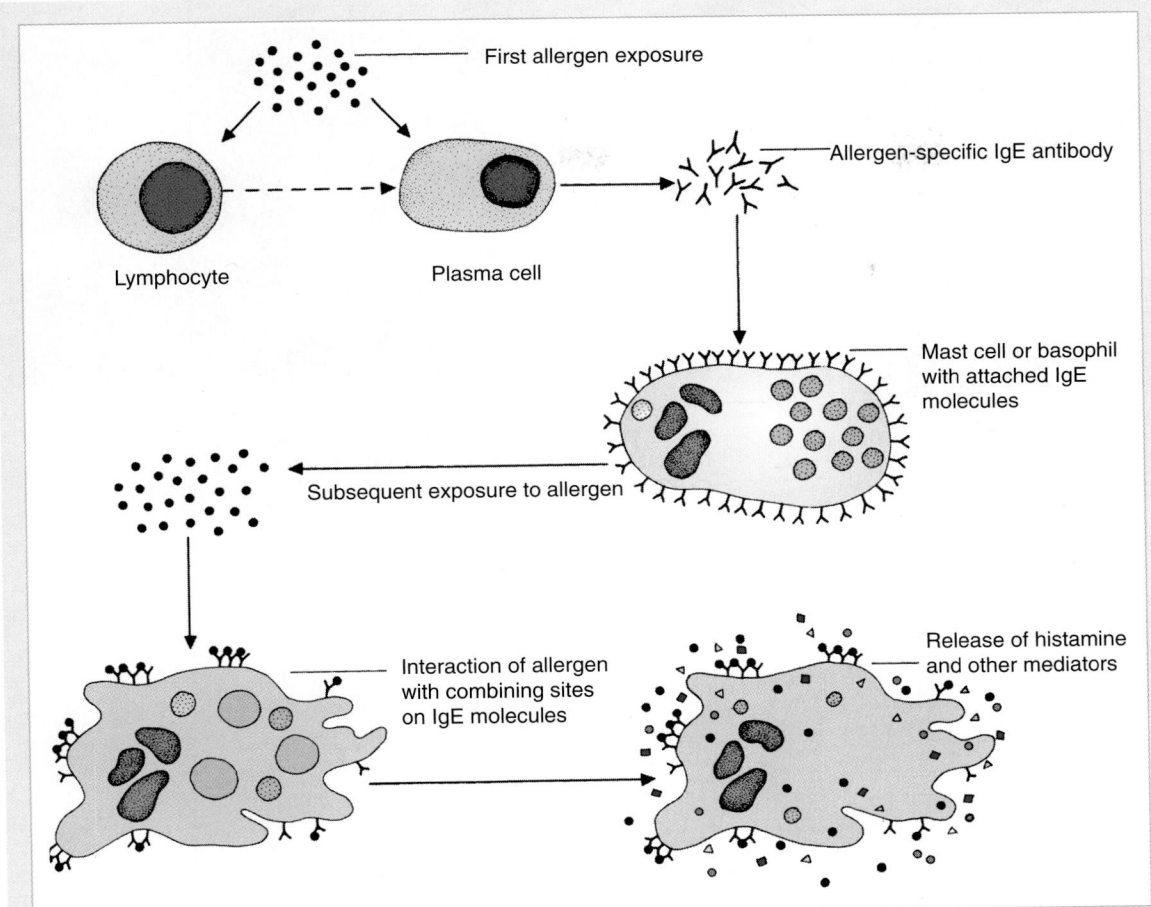

Figure 6-15 Pathogenesis of allergy. First, exposure to an allergen induces formation of specific IgE antibodies in susceptible individuals, which then bind to mast cells and basophils by the nonantigen receptor end of the molecule. Subsequent exposure to the same allergen leads to antigen-antibody interaction, liberating histamine and other mediators from mast cells and basophils. These mediators induce allergic manifestations.

(figure labels:) First allergen exposure · Allergen-specific IgE antibody · Lymphocyte · Plasma cell · Mast cell or basophil with attached IgE molecules · Subsequent exposure to allergen · Interaction of allergen with combining sites on IgE molecules · Release of histamine and other mediators

Lung cancer is the leading cause of death due to cancer in the United States. The major risk factor is cigarette smoking. Research has identified eight alterations in the genetic material of lung cancers that suggest a genetic tendency to develop the disease. Other predisposing factors include exposure to asbestos, coal products, and other industrial and chemical products. Symptoms include cough, difficulty breathing, blood-tinged sputum, and repeated infections. Treatment depends on the type, site, and extent of the cancer and may include surgery, chemotherapy, and/or radiotherapy.

Breast cancer is the most common type of cancer occurring among women and accounts for as many as 178,700 newly diagnosed cases and 48,000 deaths each year in the United States. Women whose first-degree relatives (ie, parent, sister, or daughter) have breast cancer are 2.1 times more likely to develop the disease. Risk varies with the age at which the affected relative was diagnosed; the younger the age at occurrence, the greater the risk posed to relatives. Approximately 5% to 10% of patients with breast cancer demonstrate a pattern of autosomal dominant inheritance, in which cancer predisposi-

tion is transmitted from generation to generation. The susceptibility may be inherited through either the mother's or the father's side of the family.

Early symptoms of breast cancer are usually detected by the woman during breast self-examination and include a small, painless lump, thick or dimpled skin, or a change in the nipple Figure 6-16 ▸. Later symptoms include nipple discharge, pain, and swollen lymph glands in the axilla. Treatment depends on the location, size, and metastasis of the tumor.

Colorectal cancer is the third most common type of cancer in both males and females, accounting for a combined 131,600 newly diagnosed cases and 55,000 deaths in the United States each year. Relatives of people who have had colorectal cancer are more likely to develop the disease themselves, and parents can pass on to their children changes in certain genes that can lead to colorectal cancer. Symptoms may be minimal, consisting only of small amounts of blood in the stool. Treatment involves surgery and sometimes chemotherapy. Periodic rectal examinations and colonoscopy are recommended for adults older than 40 years to detect the disease at an early stage.

Endocrine Disorders

Diabetes mellitus is one of the most significant endocrine diseases. This chronic disorder of metabolism is associated with either partial insulin secretion or total lack of insulin secretion by the pancreas, which in turn affects the patient's ability to utilize glucose. Symptoms include excessive thirst and urination, weight abnormalities, and presence of excessive sugar in the urine and the blood.

Ketoacidosis-prone (type 1) diabetes is also known as insulin-dependent diabetes mellitus because patients need exogenous insulin to survive. Nonketoacidosis-prone (type 2) diabetes is called non–insulin-dependent diabetes, even though many type 2 diabetics require exogenous insulin injections. Both forms have a hereditary predisposition. There is no cure

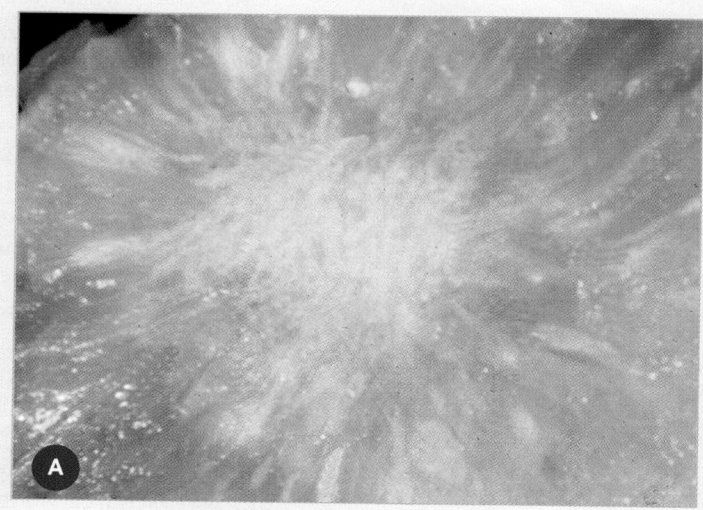

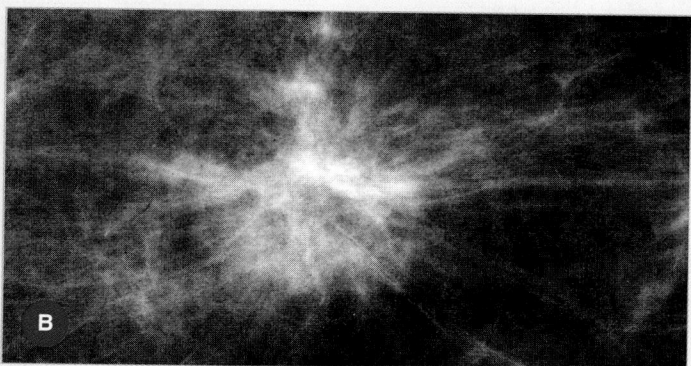

Figure 6-16 Breast carcinoma. **A.** Cross-section of breast biopsy specimen. The tumor appears as a firm, poorly circumscribed mass that infiltrates the surrounding fatty breast tissue. **B.** Appearance of breast carcinoma in a mammogram. The tumor appears as a white area with infiltrating margins.

for type 1 diabetes (other than pancreas transplantation) at the present time; type 2 diabetes can occasionally be brought under control with weight loss.

Hematologic Disorders

Hemolytic anemia is characterized by increased destruction of red blood cells. This disorder has a number of causes, such as an Rh factor blood transfusion reaction, a disorder of the immune system, or exposure to chemicals (eg, benzene and bacterial toxins). Figure 6-17 ▸ depicts how the body handles iron. Hemolytic anemia following aspirin overdose or penicillin treatment is rare; it is much more common, albeit still rare, with sulfa drugs used to treat urinary tract infection (eg, Septra or Bactrim [trimethoprim-sulfamethoxazole]). An inherited enzyme deficiency (glucose-6-phosphatase dehydrogenase deficiency) markedly increases a person's susceptibility to sulfa drug-induced hemolytic anemia.

Hemophilia is an inherited disorder characterized by excessive bleeding. It is a sex-linked condition, occurring only in males, and is passed from asymptomatic mothers to sons. In this disorder, one of the blood-clotting proteins (usually factor VIII) necessary for normal blood coagulation is missing or is present in abnormally low amounts. Patients experience greater than usual blood loss in dental extractions and following simple injuries. They may also bleed into joints and, rarely, into

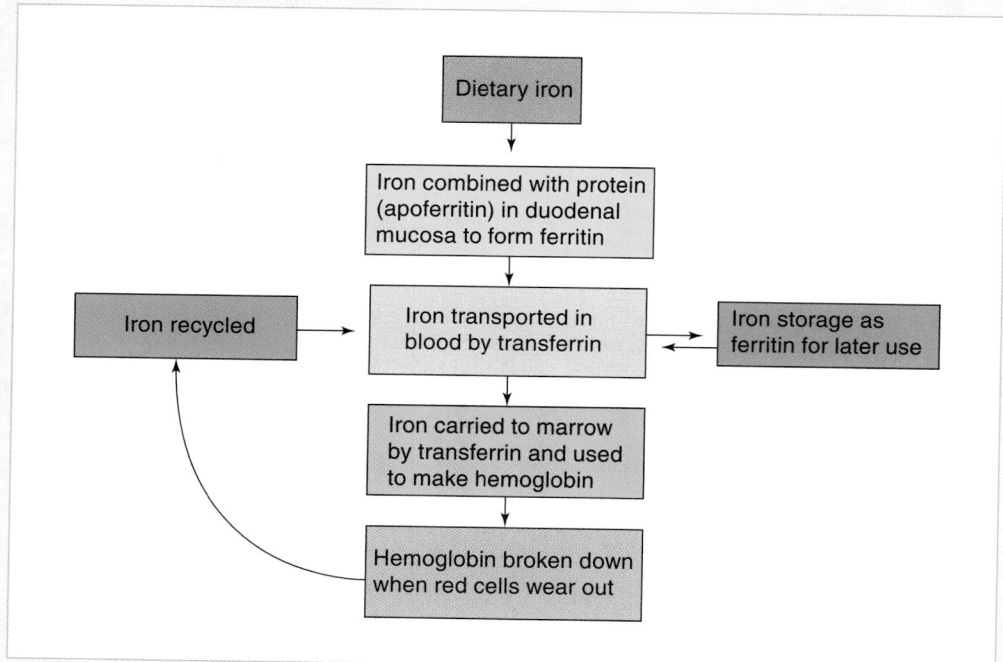

Figure 6-17 Iron uptake, transport, storage, and utilization for hemoglobin synthesis. Most of the iron used for hemoglobin synthesis is recycled from worn-out red cells. Chronic blood loss removes iron-containing cells from the circulation, and the iron contained in the red cells can no longer be recycled to make hemoglobin; this leads to iron deficiency anemia.

the brain. Treatment consists of administration of missing blood-clotting factors.

Hemochromatosis is an inherited (autosomal recessive) disease in which the body absorbs more iron than it needs. The excess iron is stored in various organs, including the liver, kidney, and pancreas. Hemochromatosis can lead to diabetes, heart disease, liver disease, arthritis, impotence, and a bronzed skin color.

These symptoms can be avoided by regularly drawing blood (phlebotomy).

Cardiovascular Disorders

Several cardiovascular disorders are known to follow specific patterns of inheritance. Still others have strong familial tendencies (eg, coronary heart disease).

Long QT syndrome is a cardiac conduction system abnormality that results in a prolongation of the QT interval on the ECG. Because most long QT syndromes are inherited in an autosomal dominant manner, all first-degree relatives must also be screened. Sometimes these syndromes are associated with congenital hearing loss, hypertrophic cardiomyopa-

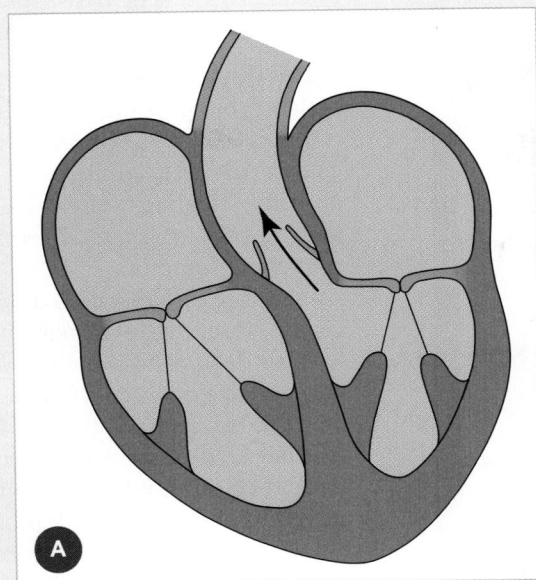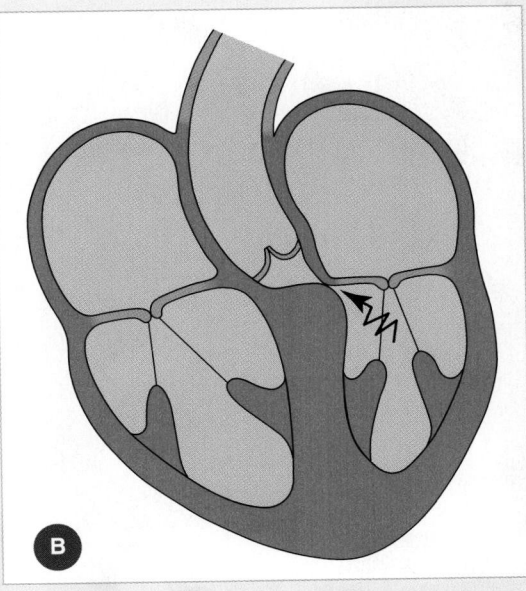

Figure 6-18 Comparison of normal cardiac function with malfunction characteristic of hypertrophic cardiomyopathy. **A.** Normal heart, illustrating unobstructed flow of blood from left ventricle into aorta during ventricular systole. **B.** Hypertrophic cardiomyopathy, illustrating obstruction to outflow of blood from left ventricle by hypertrophied septum, which impinges on the anterior leaflet of mitral valve.

thy, or mitral valve prolapse. Patients are at risk for palpitations and ventricular arrhythmias, especially torsade de pointes. Many patients are asymptomatic until they have an arrhythmia, causing either syncope or sudden death. Always consider syncope under the following conditions to be due to a life-threatening arrhythmia until proven otherwise:

- Exercise-induced syncope
- Syncope associated with chest pain
- A history of syncope in a close family member (ie, parent, sibling, or child)
- Syncope associated with startle (eg, loud noises such as phones or alarm clocks)

Cardiomyopathy is a general term for diseases of the myocardium (heart muscle) that ultimately progress to heart failure, acute myocardial infarction, or death. These diseases cause the heart muscle to become thin, flabby, dilated, or enlarged. One variant, hypertrophic cardiomyopathy, is autosomal-dominant hereditary. The main feature of hypertrophic cardiomyopathy is an excessive thickening of the heart muscle (hypertrophy means to thicken or grow excessively); see **Figure 6-18 ▲**. In addition, microscopic examination of the heart muscle shows that it is abnormal. Patients may have shortness of breath, chest pains, palpitations, or syncope; sudden cardiac death is also possible. Beta blockers are effective treatment in some patients. Others require surgery or an automatic implantable cardiac defibrillator designed to deliver a shock to the heart.

Mitral valve prolapse (MVP; also referred to as a floppy mitral valve) is relatively common, affecting 2.5% of males and 7.6% of females. There is a familial tendency toward MVP, albeit usually in association with other cardiovascular condi-

tions. The mitral valve leaflets balloon into the left atrium during systole. MVP is often a benign, symptomless condition but may be symptomatic (eg, chest pain, fatigue, dizziness, dyspnea, or palpitations). Generally, the only physical finding is a "clicking" sound heard during cardiac auscultation. Cardiac arrhythmias develop in a small number of patients.

Sometimes MVP leads to mitral regurgitation (also called mitral insufficiency), in which a large amount of blood leaks backward through the defective valve. Mitral regurgitation can lead to thickening or enlargement of the heart wall, caused by the extra pumping the heart must do to make up for the backflow of blood. It sometimes causes people to feel tired or short of breath. Mitral regurgitation usually can be treated with medication, but some people need surgery to repair or replace the defective valve.

Coronary heart disease, often called coronary artery disease, is caused by impaired circulation to the heart. Typically, patients have occluded coronary arteries from atherosclerotic plaque buildup. The effects can range from ischemia to infarction and necrosis (death) of the myocardium. Almost half of all cardiovascular deaths result from coronary heart disease. This condition has a familial tendency; significant risk factors for coronary artery disease development include having a father who had an acute myocardial infarction or died suddenly before 55 years of age and having a mother who died before 65 years of age. Other risk factors include hypercholesterolemia, cigarette smoking, hypertension (high blood pressure), age, and diabetes.

Hypercholesterolemia is an elevation of the blood cholesterol level. The blood cholesterol level is further divided into

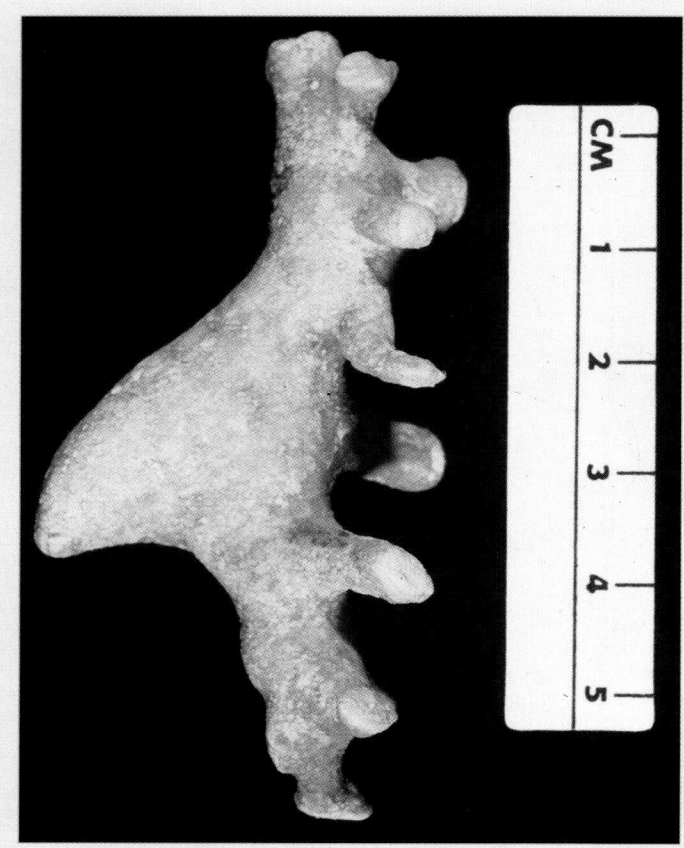

Figure 6-19 Large staghorn-shaped kidney stone.

high-density lipoproteins (HDL; "good cholesterol") and low-density lipoproteins (LDL; "bad cholesterol"). Despite having a normal total cholesterol level, persons with abnormally low levels of HDL and/or elevations of LDL are at an increased risk of coronary heart disease.

Renal Disorders

Gout is an abnormal accumulation of uric acid due to a defect in metabolism. As a result of this defect, uric acid accumulates in the blood and joints, causing pain and swelling of the joints, especially the big toe. Often, the patient has fever and chills. Gout is more common among men than women and usually has a genetic basis. If left untreated, it causes destructive tissue changes in the joints and kidneys. Treatment includes diet and drugs to reduce inflammation and to increase the excretion of uric acid or decrease its formation.

Kidney stones are small masses of uric acid or calcium salts that form in any part of the urinary system (eg, kidney, ureter, or bladder). Often—although not always—stones cause severe pain, nausea, and vomiting when the body attempts to pass them. Although most stones are small, occasionally they become large enough to adopt the internal contours of the kidney Figure 6-19 ▲ . Researchers have found a gene that causes the intestines to absorb too much calcium, which can lead to the formation of kidney stones. Uric acid stones also often have a genetic basis. Some are small enough to pass in the urine, with or without pain; others must be removed surgically.

Gastrointestinal Disorders

Malabsorption disorders result from defects in the function of the bowel wall that prevent normal absorption of nutrients. The result is a complex of symptoms, including loss of appetite, bloating, weight loss, muscle pain, and stools with high fat content. Diarrhea, which may be bloody, may also be a prominent symptom.

Lactose intolerance is a defect or deficiency of the enzyme lactase, resulting in an inability to digest lactose (milk sugar). Lactase deficiency, which appears to be due to an abnormal gene, affects between 30 and 50 million people in the United States alone, and nearly three fourths of the world's population is believed to be lactose intolerant. Symptoms include bloating, flatulence, abdominal discomfort, nausea, and diarrhea on ingestion of milk and milk products.

Ulcerative colitis is a serious chronic inflammatory disease of the large intestine and rectum. This disease, which shows a familial tendency, is characterized by recurrent episodes of abdominal pain, fever, chills, and profuse diarrhea, with stools containing pus, blood, and mucus. Treatment consists of anti-inflammatory agents, including corticosteroids. Severe cases may require surgery with removal of parts of the intestinal tract. Patients are at increased risk for developing cancer of the colon.

Crohn's disease is a chronic inflammatory condition affecting the colon and/or terminal part of the small intestine. It is believed to be associated with as-yet-undetermined gene abnormalities. Symptoms include frequent episodes of non-bloody diarrhea, abdominal pain, nausea, fever, weakness, and weight loss. Treatment is by anti-inflammatory agents, antibiotics, and proper nutrition.

Peptic ulcer disease is characterized by circumscribed erosions (ulcerations) in the mucous membrane lining of the gastrointestinal tract—specifically, in the esophagus, stomach, duodenum, or jejunum. Peptic ulcers may result from excess acid production or from a breakdown in the normal mechanisms protecting the mucous membranes. Although this disease appears to have a genetic component, a major contributor to its development is infection with the bacterium *Helicobacter pylori*—the observed familial patterns appear to be due to shared infections with *H pylori*. Symptoms include gnawing pain, which is often worse when the stomach is empty, after the person eats certain foods, or when the patient is under stress. Treatment includes avoidance of irritants (eg, tobacco, alcohol, irritating foods), antibiotics, and drugs to decrease acidity. In refractory cases, surgery may be necessary.

Gallstones (cholethiasis) are stone-like masses in the gallbladder or its ducts caused by precipitation of substances contained in bile (eg, cholesterol, bilirubin). Factors that contribute to their formation include abnormalities in the composition of bile, stasis of bile, and inflammation of the gallbladder with many gallstones. Gallstones may be asymptomatic, but cause symptoms when they obstruct the flow of bile. Small stones that are able to pass into the common duct produce indigestion and biliary colic. Biliary colic pain is sudden in onset and increases steadily to its maximum in approximately 1 hour. The pain is located in the upper right quadrant or the epigastric area and may be referred to the back. Larger stones may cause jaundice (yellow skin and sclerae). Although genetic factors are responsible for at least 30% of symptomatic gallstone disease, heredity probably plays an even larger role in gallstone pathogenesis, because data based on symptomatic gallbladder disease underestimate the true prevalence in the population.

Obesity is an unhealthy accumulation of body fat that has many deleterious side effects, both medical and social. Health risks associated with obesity include hypertension, hyperlipidemia, cardiovascular disease, glucose intolerance, insulin resistance, diabetes, gallbladder disease, infertility, and cancer of the endometrium, breast, prostate, and colon. Although some people likely have a genetic predisposition to obesity, the roles of specific genes in its development have yet to be determined.

Neuromuscular Disorders

Although environmental contributions are highly likely, certain neuromuscular disorders have a familial and genetic basis. Huntington's disease (also called Huntington's chorea), for example, is a hereditary condition (autosomal dominant) characterized by progressive chorea (involuntary rapid, jerky motions) and mental deterioration, leading to dementia. Symptoms usually first appear in the third or fourth decade of life and progress to death, often within 15 years.

Muscular dystrophy is a generic term for a group of hereditary diseases of the muscular system characterized by weakness and wasting of groups of skeletal muscles, leading to increasing disability. The various forms differ in age of onset, rate of progression, and mode of genetic transmission. Duchenne's muscular dystrophy is a sex-linked recessive disease (affecting only males); symptoms first appear around the age of 4 years. Progressive wasting of leg and pelvic muscles produces a waddling gait and abnormal curvature of the spine, progressing to inability to walk and confinement to a wheelchair, usually by age 12 years. There is no specific treatment, and death, usually from heart disorders, often results by age 20 years.

Multiple sclerosis is a progressive disease in which nerve fibers of the brain and spinal cord lose their myelin cover. Although it is not directly inherited, there is a familial predisposition in some cases, suggesting a genetic influence on susceptibility. The disease usually begins in early adulthood and progresses slowly, with periods of remission and exacerbation. Early symptoms include abnormal sensations in the face or extremities, weakness, and visual disturbances (such as double vision), which progress to ataxia (lack of coordination), abnormal reflexes, tremors, difficulty in urination, and difficulty in walking. Depression is also common. There is no specific treatment or cure, but corticosteroids and other drugs are used to treat symptoms.

Alzheimer's disease affects nearly 4 million Americans. Although its cause is unknown, the disease results in cortical atrophy and loss of neurons in the frontal and temporal lobes of the brain; in addition, ventricular enlargement occurs due to the loss of brain tissue. Histologic changes in the brain of an Alzheimer's patient include neurofibrillary tangles and senile plaques Figure 6-20 ▶ . Studies of the genetics of inherited early-onset Alzheimer's have been linked to mutations on three genes.

Clinical manifestations of Alzheimer's disease occur in three distinct stages. Stage 1 is characterized by memory loss, lack of spontaneity, subtle personality changes, and disorientation to time and date. Stage 2 features impaired cognition and

You are the Provider Part 3

You perform a physical exam on the patient while your partner prepares an IV set-up. Your physical exam is significant for the following findings: positive jugular vein distention; use of accessory muscles in the neck and shoulders to assist respirations; pitting edema of both lower extremities; and an area surrounding the shunt site on the right arm approximately 4″ in diameter that is red, swollen, and hot to the touch. As you are completing your assessment, the patient begins to complain of feeling lightheaded. You lower the head of the dialysis chair to a 60° angle, initiate an IV using a 18-gauge catheter in the left antecubital, and begin a fluid bolus of 200 mL.

Reassessment	Recording Time: 10 Minutes
Skin	Pale, warm, and moist
Pulse	140 beats/min, regular; weak radial
ECG	Narrow complex tachycardia with tall T waves
Blood pressure	78/44 mm Hg
Respirations	28 breaths/min labored
SaO_2	93% on nonrebreathing mask at 15 L/min of supplemental oxygen
Pupils	Equal and reactive to light

5. Is the patient going into shock? If so, what type?
6. Why is a fluid bolus appropriate in this setting?

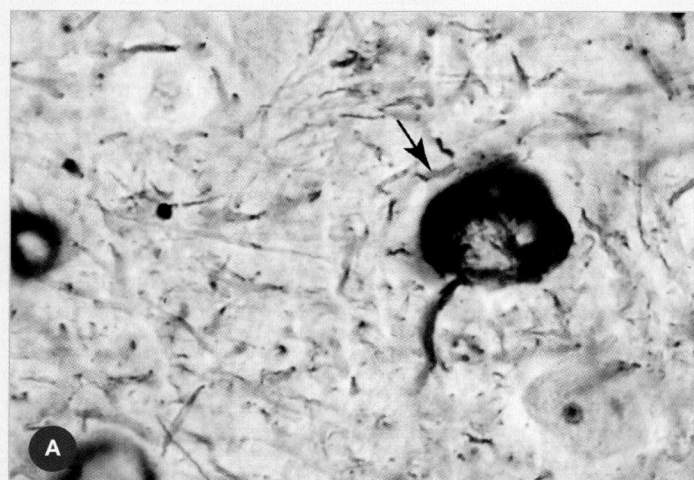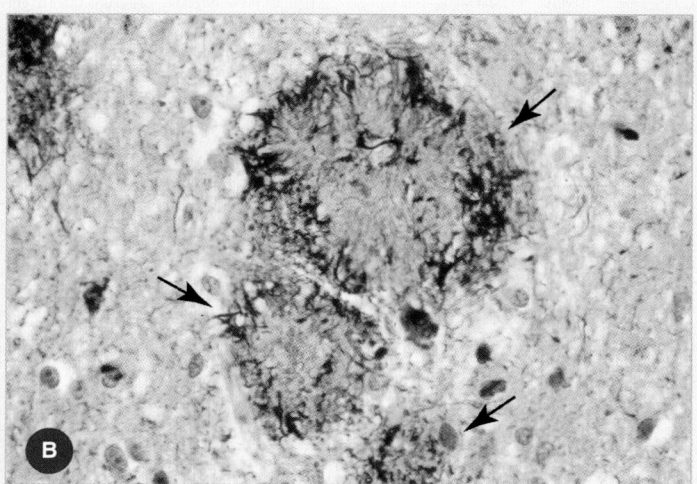

Figure 6-20 Alzheimer's disease. **A.** Thickened neurofilaments encircle and obscure the nuclei of nerve cells (arrow), forming a neurofibrillary tangle (original magnification, ×400). **B.** Three senile plaques (arrows) composed of broken masses of thickened neurofilaments (original magnification, ×100).

Special Considerations

Never assume that new or worsening confusion in a geriatric patient is due purely to Alzheimer's disease, without first considering potentially correctable causes such as new medications, infections, or myocardial infarction. An "apparent" emotional, psychological, or behavioral problem may have an organic cause, especially in the geriatric population.

abstract thinking, restlessness and agitation, wandering, inability to carry out activities of daily living, impaired judgment, and inappropriate social behavior. Stage 3 involves indifference to food, inability to communicate, urinary and fecal incontinence, and seizures.

Psychiatric Disorders

Some common psychiatric disorders appear to have a familial, and perhaps even genetic, component. For example, schizophrenia comprises a group of mental disorders characterized by gross distortions of reality (psychoses), withdrawal from social contacts, and disturbances of thought, language, perception, and emotional response. Its symptoms are highly varied but may include apathy, catatonia or excessive activity, bizarre actions, hallucinations, delusions, and rambling speech. Although the cause of schizophrenia has not been identified, a combination of hereditary or genetic predisposing factors is likely in most cases.

Manic-depressive disorder (also known as bipolar disorder or manic-depressive psychosis) is a mental disorder characterized by episodes of mania and depression. One or the other phase may be dominant at a given time, and the phases may alternate or aspects of both phases may be present at the same time. The higher rates of bipolar disorder among relatives, identical twins, and biologic parents versus adoptive parents have been cited as evidence of the role of genetics in this disorder; the risk within the general population as a whole is approximately 1%. Treatment consists of psychotherapy plus antidepressants and tranquilizers.

Hypoperfusion

Perfusion is defined as delivery of oxygen and nutrients and removal of wastes from the cells, organs, and tissues by the circulatory system. Evaluation of a patient's level of organ perfusion is important in emergency care, especially in diagnosing shock. Hypoperfusion occurs when the level of tissue perfusion decreases below normal.

When the body senses tissue hypoperfusion, it sets compensatory mechanisms into motion. In some cases, this action is sufficient to stabilize the patient. In other cases, the hypoperfusion overwhelms the normal compensatory mechanisms and the patient's condition progressively deteriorates ⟨ Table 6-4 ▸ ⟩.

In response to hypoperfusion, the body releases catecholamines (ie, epinephrine and norepinephrine), which

Documentation and Communication

The terms *shock* and *hypoperfusion* are usually synonymous, at least when they are applied to multiple body systems. Localized hypoperfusion, such as from arterial occlusion, is *not* shock.

Table 6-4	Signs and Symptoms in the Phases of Hypoperfusion	
Compensated	**Decompensated**	
■ Agitation, anxiety, restlessness	■ Altered mental status (verbal to unresponsive)	
■ Sense of impending doom	■ Hypotension	
■ Weak, rapid (thready) pulse	■ Labored or irregular breathing	
■ Clammy (cool, moist) skin	■ Thready or absent peripheral pulses	
■ Pallor with cyanotic lips	■ Ashen, mottled, or cyanotic skin	
■ Shortness of breath	■ Dilated pupils	
■ Nausea, vomiting	■ Diminished urine output (oliguria)	
■ Delayed capillary refill in infants and children	■ Impending cardiac arrest	
■ Thirst		
■ Normal blood pressure		

produce vasoconstriction (increased systemic vascular resistance). In addition, the RAAS is activated and antidiuretic hormone is released from the pituitary gland. Together these actions trigger salt and water retention as well as peripheral vasoconstriction, thereby increasing blood pressure and cardiac output. Depending on the severity of the insult, variable amounts of fluid will shift from the interstitial tissues into the vascular compartment. The spleen also releases some red blood cells that are normally sequestered there, to augment the oxygen-carrying capacity of the blood. The overall response of the initial compensatory mechanisms is to increase the preload (venous return), stroke volume, and heart rate. The result is usually an increase in cardiac output and myocardial oxygen demand.

As hypoperfusion persists, the myocardial oxygen demand continues to increase. Eventually, the above-normal compensatory mechanisms can no longer keep up with the demand. Myocardial function worsens, with decreased cardiac output and ejection fraction. Tissue perfusion decreases, leading to impaired cell metabolism. Often, the blood pressure decreases, especially in progressive hypoperfusion. Fluid may leak from the blood vessels, causing systemic and pulmonary edema. At this point, other signs of hypoperfusion may be present, such as dusky skin, oliguria, and impaired mentation.

Types of Shock

Shock is an abnormal state associated with inadequate oxygen and nutrient delivery to the metabolic apparatus of the cell, resulting in impairment of cell metabolism and inadequate perfusion of vital organs (see Chapter 18). Once a certain level of tissue hypoperfusion is reached, cell damage proceeds in a similar manner regardless of the type of initial insult. Impairment of cellular metabolism prevents the body from properly using oxygen and glucose at the cellular level. Cells revert to anaerobic metabolism, which causes increased lactic acid production and metabolic acidosis, decreased oxygen affinity for hemoglo-

bin, decreased ATP production, changes in cellular electrolytes, cellular edema, and release of lysosomal enzymes. Glucose impairment leads to elevated blood glucose levels due to release of catecholamines and cortisol. In addition, fat breakdown (lipolysis) with ketone formation may occur.

Shock can occur due to inadequacy of the central circulation (eg, the heart and the great vessels) or of the peripheral circulation (the remaining vessels, including the microscopic circulation [eg, arterioles, venules, and capillaries, as illustrated in Figure 6-21]). From a mechanistic approach, two types of shock are distinguished: central and peripheral. Central shock consists of cardiogenic shock and obstructive shock. Peripheral shock includes hypovolemic shock and distributive shock.

Cardiogenic shock occurs when the heart cannot circulate enough blood to maintain adequate peripheral oxygen delivery. In the case of ischemic heart disease, this requires loss of 40% or more of functioning myocardium. The most common cause of cardiogenic shock is myocardial infarction, either as a single event or by cumulative damage. Other forms of cardiac dysfunction may also result in cardiogenic shock (ie, large ventricular septal defect or hemodynamic significant arrhythmias) (see Chapter 27).

Obstructive shock occurs when blood flow becomes blocked in the heart or great vessels. In pericardial tamponade Figure 6-22 , diastolic filling of the right ventricle is impaired due to significant amounts of fluid in the pericardial sac surrounding the heart, leading to a decrease in the cardiac output. Aortic dissection leads to a false lumen (aortic opening), with loss of normal blood flow Figure 6-23 . A left atrial tumor may obstruct flow between the atrium and ventricle and decrease cardiac output. Obstruction of either the superior or inferior vena cava (vena cava syndrome) decreases cardiac output by decreasing venous return. A large pulmonary embolus (blood clot in the lung) or a tension pneumothorax (lung collapse) may prevent adequate blood flow to the lungs, resulting in inadequate venous return to the left side of the heart.

In hypovolemic shock, the circulating blood volume is unable to deliver adequate oxygen and nutrients to the body. Two types of hypovolemic shock—exogenous and endogenous—are possible, depending on where the fluid loss occurs. The most common type of exogenous hypovolemic shock is external bleeding (eg, from an open wound); it may also result from loss of plasma volume caused by diarrhea or vomiting. Endogenous hypovolemic shock occurs when the fluid loss is contained within the body.

Distributive shock occurs when there is widespread dilation of the resistance vessels (small arterioles), the capacitance vessels (small venules), or both. The circulating blood

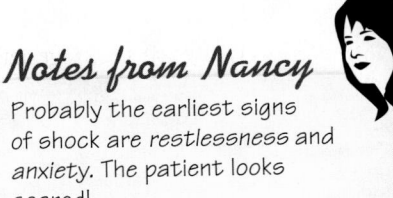

Notes from Nancy
Probably the earliest signs of shock are restlessness and anxiety. The patient looks scared!

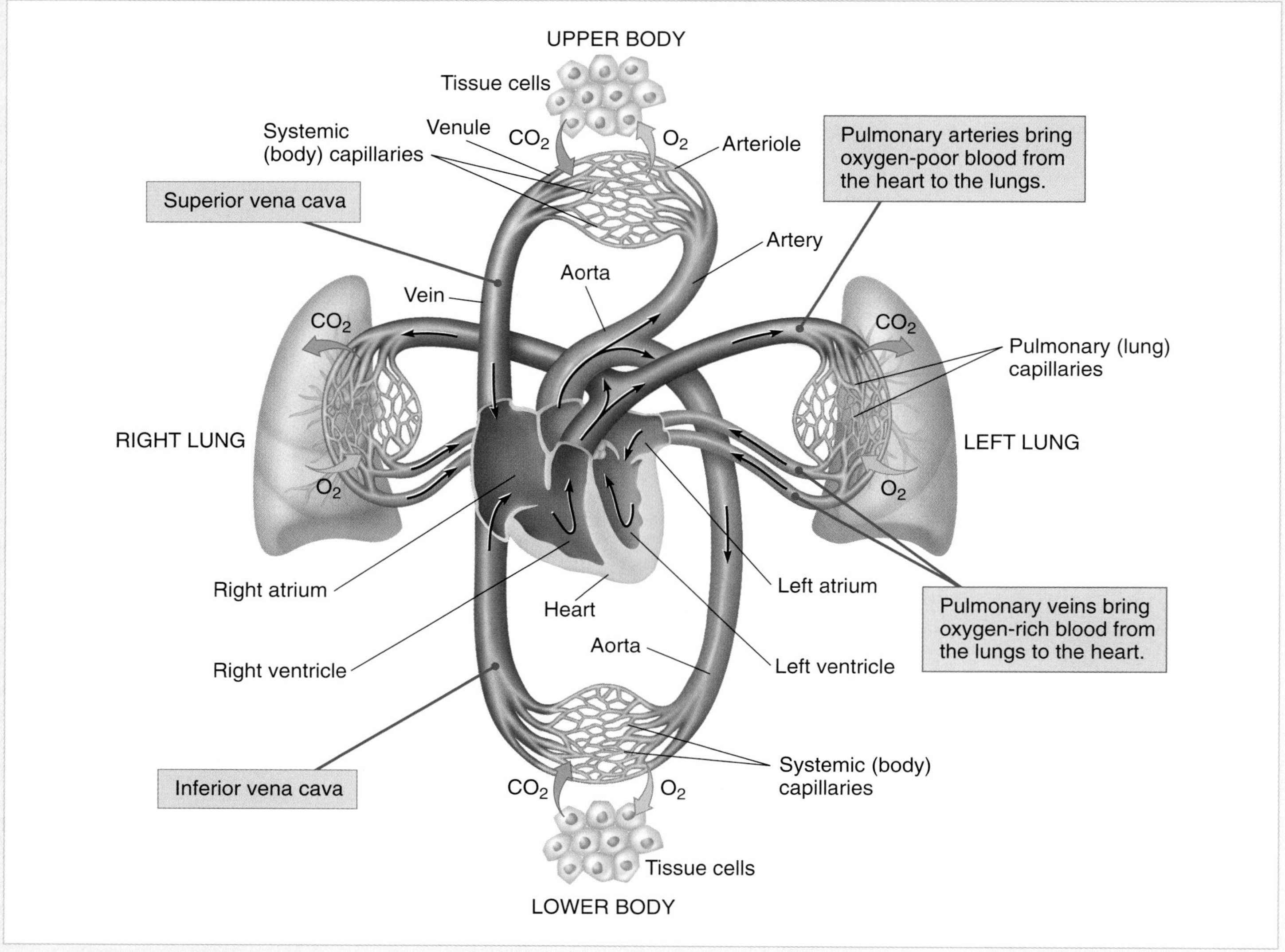

UPPER BODY

Tissue cells

Systemic (body) capillaries

Venule

CO_2

O_2

Arteriole

Superior vena cava

Pulmonary arteries bring oxygen-poor blood from the heart to the lungs.

Vein

Aorta

Artery

CO_2

O_2

RIGHT LUNG

LEFT LUNG

CO_2

Pulmonary (lung) capillaries

O_2

Right atrium

Left atrium

Heart

Pulmonary veins bring oxygen-rich blood from the lungs to the heart.

Right ventricle

Aorta

Left ventricle

Inferior vena cava

CO_2

O_2

Systemic (body) capillaries

Tissue cells

LOWER BODY

Figure 6-21 The circulatory system includes the heart, arteries, veins, and interconnecting capillaries. The capillaries—the smallest vessels—connect with venules and arterioles. At the center of the system, and providing its driving force, is the heart.

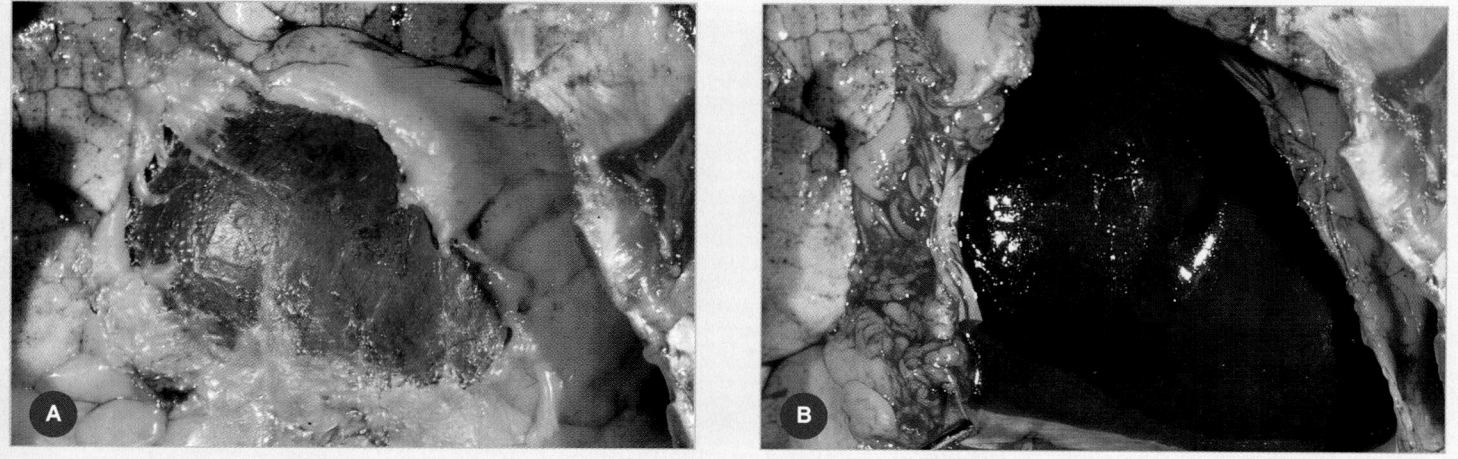

Figure 6-22 Cardiac tamponade secondary to myocardial rupture. **A.** Distended pericardial sac. **B.** Pericardial sac opened, showing clotted blood surrounding the heart, which compressed the heart and prevented filling of the right ventricle in diastole.

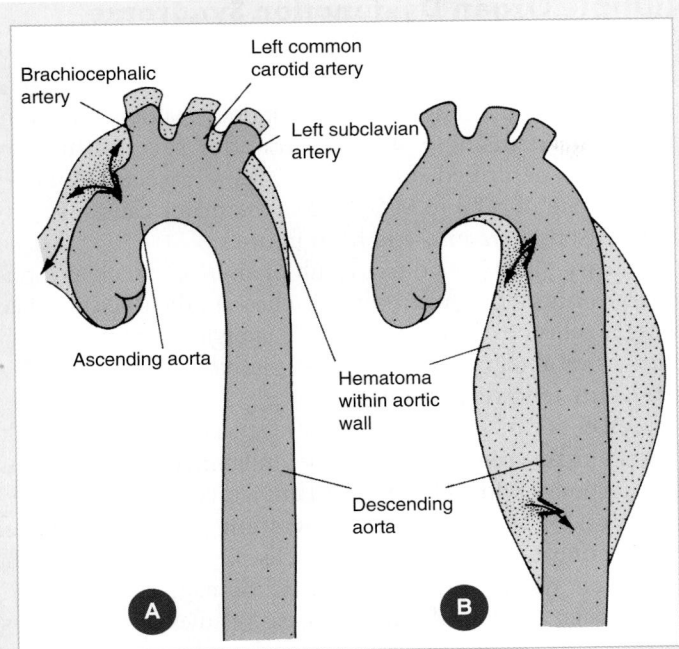

Figure 6-23 Sites of thoracic aortic dissection. **A.** A tear in the ascending aorta causes both proximal and distal dissection. **B.** A tear in the descending aorta may cause extensive distal dissection.

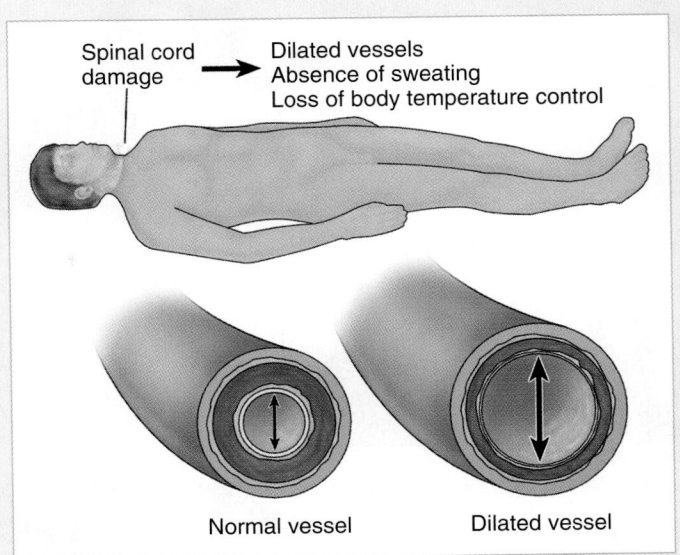

Figure 6-24 Damage to the spinal cord can cause significant injury to the part of the nervous system that controls the size and muscle tone of blood vessels. If the muscles in the blood vessels are cut off from their impulses to contract, then the vessels dilate widely, increasing the size and capacity of the vascular system. The blood in the body can no longer fill the enlarged vessels, resulting in inadequate perfusion and neurogenic shock.

volume then "pools" in the expanded vascular beds, and tissue perfusion decreases. The three most common types of distributive shock are anaphylactic shock, septic shock, and neurogenic shock **Figure 6-24 ▶**.

In anaphylactic shock, histamine and other vasodilator proteins are released upon exposure to an allergen. Anaphylaxis is also accompanied by wheezing and urticaria (hives). The result is widespread vasodilation that causes distributive shock and blood vessels that continue to leak. Fluid leaks out of the blood vessels into the interstitial spaces, resulting in intravascular hypovolemia.

Septic shock occurs as a result of widespread infection, usually bacterial. Complex interactions occur between the bacterial invader and the body's defense systems. Initially, the body's own defense mechanisms may keep the infection at bay. If the normal immune mechanisms become overwhelmed, the body produces a multitude of substances that cause vasodila-

tion and decreased cardiac output. If left untreated, the result is multiple organ dysfunction syndrome and often death.

Neurogenic shock usually results from spinal cord injury. The effect is loss of normal sympathetic nervous system tone and vasodilation. Often patients have fluid-refractory hypotension due to the degree of vasodilation.

Management of Shock

All types of shock are characterized by reduced cardiac output, circulatory insufficiency, and rapid heartbeat. Although low blood pressure is classically associated with shock, it is a late sign, especially in children. In compensated shock, the systolic blood pressure is within the normal range; in decompensated shock, the systolic blood pressure is less than the fifth percentile for the age.

Clinically, determining the presence or absence of shock requires the evaluation of the presence and volume of the peripheral pulses, and assessment of end-organ perfusion and function. Strength of the peripheral pulses is related to both stroke volume of the heart and pulse pressures. Peripheral pulses should be readily palpable if the person is not in shock, although cold environments or obesity may compromise the presence or strength of these pulses. Skin perfusion in the normal individual results in warm, dry, and pink extremities, fingers, and toes, whereas shock may result in slow, delayed, or prolonged capillary refill time. To test the capillary refill time, briefly squeeze the toe or finger, then look for return of pink color. A normal capillary refill time is less than 2 seconds

In the Field

In anaphylaxis, interstitial fluid may cause significant swelling. In some cases, this swelling may occlude the upper airway, resulting in a life-threatening condition. Recurrent large areas of subcutaneous edema of sudden onset, usually disappearing within 24 hours, are called angioedema. This condition is seen mainly in young women, frequently as a result of allergy to food or drugs.

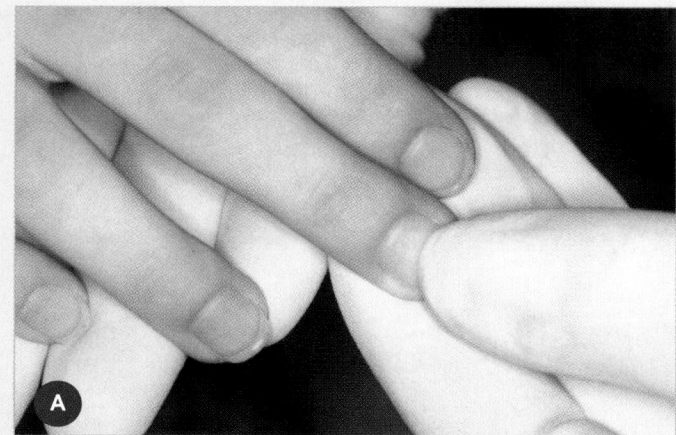

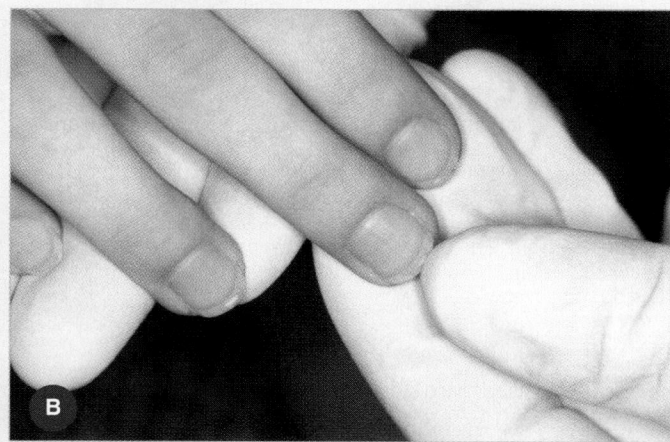

Figure 6-25 Testing capillary refill time. **A.** To test capillary refill, gently compress the fingertip until it blanches. **B.** Release the fingertip and count until it returns to its normal pink color.

In the Field

A possible exception to the rule of IV fluid therapy is hypovolemic shock caused by ongoing bleeding. Some studies suggest that fluid therapy to maintain the systolic blood pressure at approximately 80 mm Hg may be safer for the patient than attempting restoration of normotension, which may aggravate ongoing bleeding. As always, follow your local protocols.

after blanching of the toe or finger, whereas a person in shock may have a capillary refill time of more than 2 seconds Figure 6-25 ▲ . Mottling, pallor, peripheral or central cyanosis, and delayed capillary refill may signal the presence of shock, whereas altered mental status is an indication of inadequate brain tissue perfusion.

Treatment primarily addresses the underlying condition (see Chapter 18).

Multiple Organ Dysfunction Syndrome

Multiple organ dysfunction syndrome (MODS) is a progressive condition usually characterized by concurrent failure of several organs, such as the lungs, liver, and kidneys, along with some clotting mechanisms, which occurs after severe illness or injury. First described in 1975, MODS is associated with a mortality rate of 60% to 90%, and is the major cause of death following sepsis, trauma, and burn injuries.

Primary MODS is a direct result of an insult, such as a pulmonary contusion from striking the chest on the steering wheel during a collision. Secondary MODS is organ dysfunction that occurs as an integral component to the patient's response (eg, renal failure following trauma).

MODS occurs when injury or infection (eg, septic shock) triggers a massive systemic immune, inflammatory, and coagulation response with release of inflammatory mediators. Overactivation of the complement system further increases inflammation and damage to the cells. Overactivation of the coagulation system due to endothelial damage causes uncontrolled coagulation in the microscopic venules and arterioles, which in turn results in microvascular thrombus formation and tissue ischemia. MODS also activates the kallikrein/kinin system, resulting in the release of bradykinin, a potent vasodilator. Vasodilation leads to tissue hypoperfusion and may also contribute to hypotension.

The net outcome of the activation of these systems is maldistribution of systemic and organ blood flow. Often tissues attempt to compensate for this problem by accelerating their metabolism. The result is an oxygen supply and demand imbalance with tissue hypoxia, including tissue hypoperfusion, exhaustion of the cells' fuel supply (ATP), metabolic failure, lysosome breakdown, anaerobic metabolism, and acidosis and impaired cellular function.

MODS typically develops hours to days following resuscitation. Its signs and symptoms include hypotension, insufficient tissue perfusion, uncontrollable bleeding (coagulopathy), and multisystem organ failure. Patients may develop a low-grade fever from the inflammatory response, tachycardia, and dyspnea. They may also be difficult to oxygenate due to the presence of acute lung injury and adult respiratory distress syndrome. During a 14- to 21-day period, renal and liver failure can develop in these patients, along with collapse of the gastrointestinal and immune systems. Cardiovascular collapse and death typically occur within days to weeks of the initial insult.

The Body's Self-defense Mechanisms

The immune system includes all structures and processes associated with the body's defense against foreign substances and disease-causing agents. The body has three lines of defense: anatomic barriers, the inflammatory response, and the immune response.

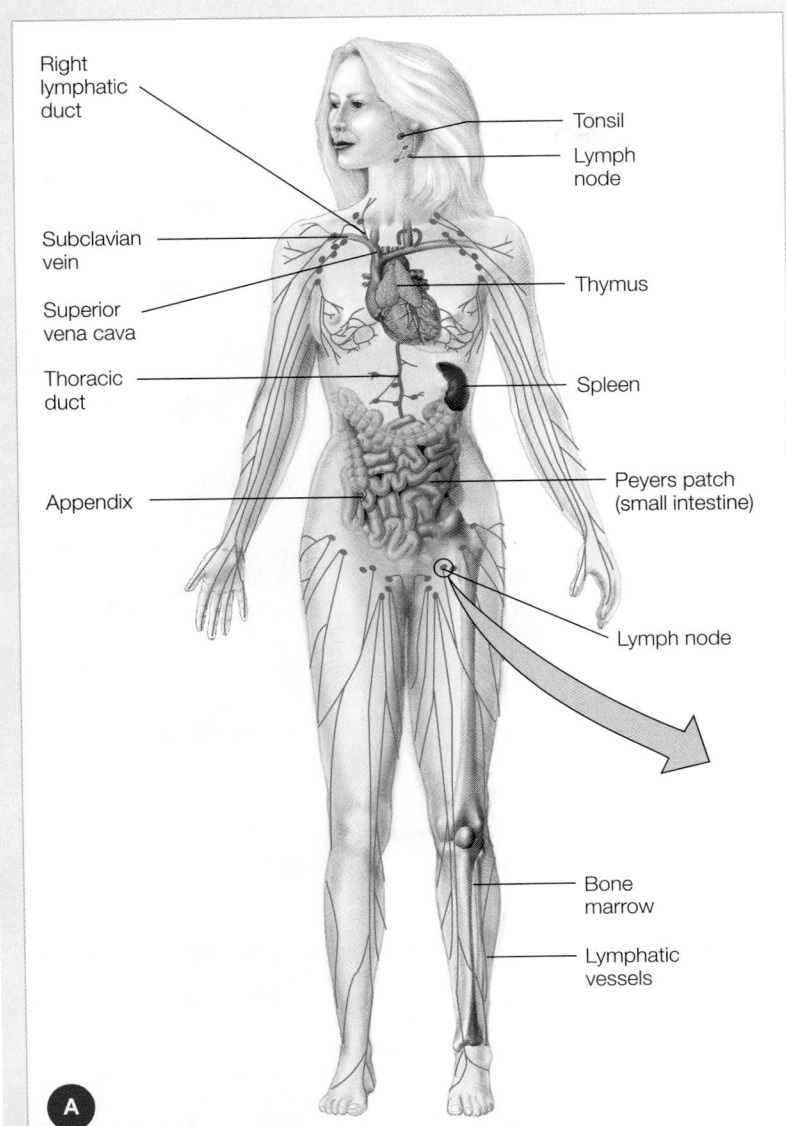

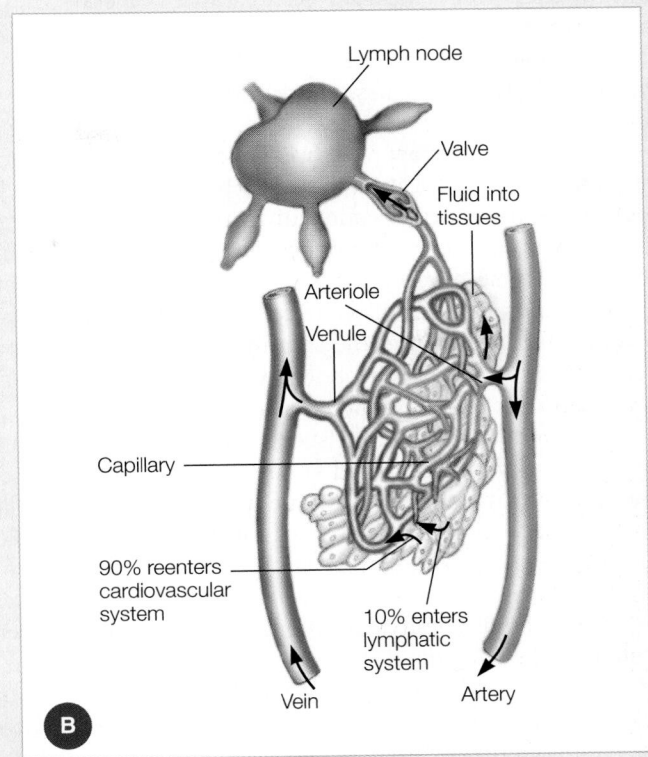

Figure 6-26 The lymphatic system. **A.** The lymphatic system consists of vessels that transport lymph and excess tissue fluid back to the circulatory system. **B.** Lymph is picked up by lymphatic capillaries that drain into larger vessels. Like the veins, the lymphatic vessels contain valves that prohibit backflow. Lymph nodes are interspersed along the vessels and filter the lymph.

Several anatomic barriers decrease the chances of bodily invasion by foreign substances. The skin serves as a major deterrent. Hairs in the upper respiratory tract (the nose) and the lining of the lower respiratory tract (cilia-covered epithelial cells) help repel foreign matter, especially small particles and some bacteria. Acid in the stomach prevents many infectious agents from entering the body via the gastrointestinal tract.

The inflammatory response is a response of the tissues of the body to irritation or injury characterized by pain, swelling, redness, and heat. White blood cells of various types are a major component of this response.

The immune response is the body's defense reaction to any substance that is recognized as foreign. Often, this response is directed toward invading microbes, such as bacteria or viruses. It is also triggered by foreign bodies (eg, a splinter) and even abnormal growths in the cells (eg, a tumor). The immune response involves only one type of white blood cells, namely lymphocytes.

The inflammatory reaction and the immune response are independent processes, although they often occur simultaneously. Inflammation can be present without activation of the immune response, and vice versa.

Not all invaders can be destroyed by the body's immune system. In some cases, the best compromise the body can reach is to control the damage and keep the invader from spreading. Often, the immune system succeeds in preventing severe disease following infection. When the normal systems become overwhelmed or fail, serious disease occurs.

Anatomy of the Immune System

The lymphatic system is a network of capillaries, vessels, ducts, nodes, and organs that helps maintain the fluid environment of the body by producing lymph and conveying it through the body Figure 6-26 ▲. The immune system has two anatomic components: the lymphoid tissues and the cells that are responsible for the immune response.

Lymphoid tissues are distributed throughout the body. The two primary lymphoid tissues are bone marrow and the thymus gland. Bone marrow is specialized soft tissue found within bone. Red bone marrow, which is widespread in the bones of children and is found in some adult bones (eg, sternum and ribs), is essential for formation of mature blood cells; it produces B lymphocytes. T lymphocytes originate from precursor cells in the bone marrow, leave the bone marrow, and mature in the thymus gland. This bilobed gland—located below the thyroid gland and behind the sternum—is prominent at birth, increases in size until the body reaches puberty, and then shrinks and decreases in functional activity during adulthood.

In secondary lymphoid tissues (ie, encapsulated and unencapsulated diffuse lymphoid tissues), mature immune cells interact with invaders and initiate a response. Encapsulated lymphoid tissues consist of the lymph nodes and the spleen. Lymph nodes (lymph glands) are small structures that filter lymph and store lymphocytes; they are concentrated in areas of the body such as the axillae, groin, and neck. The spleen is located on the left side of the body, posterior and lateral to the stomach (left upper quadrant); it monitors the blood, destroys worn-out red blood cells, and traps foreign invaders. The diffuse lymphoid tissues are scattered throughout the body.

Lymph is a thin, watery fluid that bathes the tissues of the body; it circulates through lymph vessels and is filtered in lymph nodes. Lymphatic capillaries unite to form the lymph vessels, which eventually coalesce and empty their contents into the central venous circulation (Figure 6-27 ▶). Most lymph empties into the superior vena cava via the thoracic duct, located on the left side of the thorax. The remaining lymph enters the right subclavian vein via three or four lymphatic ducts.

Clusters of lymphoid tissue are associated with the skin and the respiratory, urinary, gastrointestinal, and reproductive tracts. These tissues, which are collectively termed mucosal-associated lymphoid tissue (MALT), contain immune cells that are in a position to intercept pathogens before they reach the general circulation. The tonsils are perhaps the best-known type of MALT. Unencapsulated lymphoid tissue is particularly prominent in the gastrointestinal tract. Called the gut-associated lymphoid tissue (GALT), this tissue lies just under the inner lining of the esophagus and intestines.

The primary cells of the immune system are the white blood cells, or leukocytes. There are five general types (Table 6-5 ▶):

- Basophils contain histamine granules and other substances that are released during inflammatory and allergic responses. They account for less than 1% of the leukocytes but are essential to the nonspecific immune response to inflammation because they release histamine and other chemicals that dilate blood vessels.
- Eosinophils release substances that damage or kill parasitic invaders. They also play a major role in mediating the

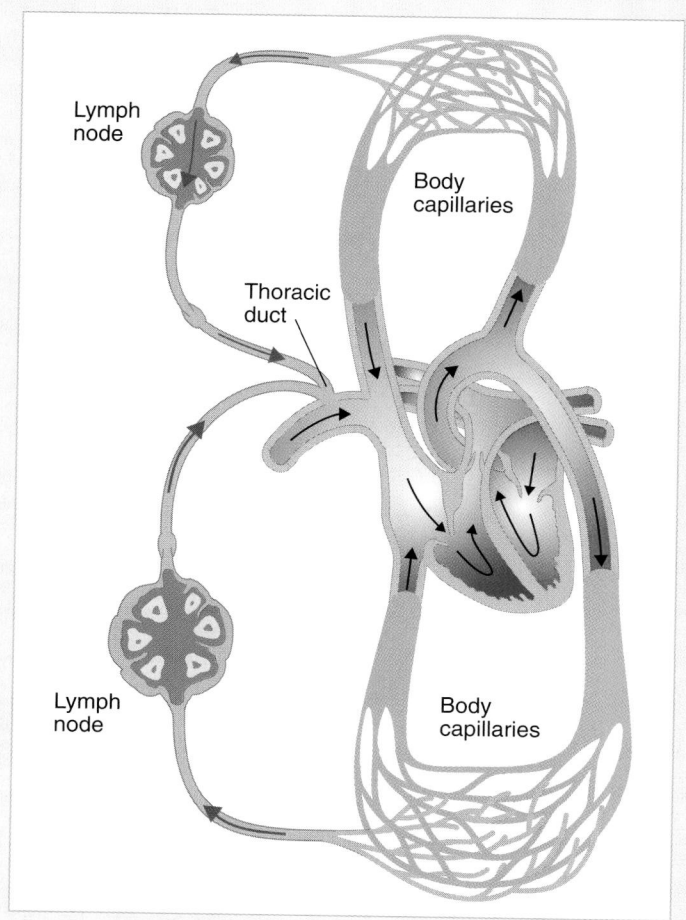

Figure 6-27 The interrelationship of the lymphatic system and the circulatory system. Blood fluid passes out of the arteries in the upper and lower parts of the body, and then enters a system of lymphatic ducts that arise in the tissues. The fluid, called lymph, passes through lymph nodes and on the right side makes its way back to the general circulation via the thoracic duct. Lymph vessels from the left upper quadrant join the thoracic duct and empty into the left subclavian vein. Lymph vessels from the right upper quadrant join together to form the right lymphatic duct, which empties into the right subclavian vein.

allergic response. These white blood cells, which account for 1% to 3% of the leukocytes, release chemoactive substances that can result in severe bronchospasm.
- Neutrophils are the most abundant white blood cells, accounting for 55% to 70% of the leukocytes. They have a segmented nucleus and are often called polymorphonuclear leukocytes ("polys"). Neutrophils are largely responsible for protecting the body against infection and are key components of the first response to foreign body invasion. They are readily attracted by foreign antigens, which they destroy by engulfing and digesting the antigens (phagocytosis).
- Monocytes mature in the blood during their first 24 hours and then travel to the tissues, where they differentiate into macrophages. Macrophages function primarily as

Table 6-5	Types of White Blood Cells			
Name	**Description**	**Concentration (number of cells/mm³)**	**Life Span**	**Function**
Neutrophil	Approximately twice the size of red blood cells; multilobed nucleus; clear-staining cytoplasm	3,000–7,000	6 hours to a few days	Phagocytizes bacteria
Eosinophil	Approximately same size as neutrophil; large pink-stained granules; bilobed nucleus	100–400	8-12 days	Phagocytizes antigen-antibody complex; attacks parasites
Basophil	Slightly smaller than neutrophil; contains large, purple cytoplasmic granules; bilobed nucleus	20–50	A few hours to a few days	Releases histamine during inflammation
Monocyte	Larger than neutrophil; cytoplasm grayish-blue; no cytoplasmic granules; U- or kidney-shaped nucleus	100–700	Lasts many months	Phagocytizes bacteria, dead cells, and cellular debris
Lymphocyte	Slightly smaller than neutrophil; large, relatively round nucleus that fills the cell	1,500–3,000	Can persist many years	Involved in immune protection, either attacking cells directly or producing antibodies

scavengers for the tissues. Monocytes and macrophages represent one of the first lines of defense in the inflammatory process.

■ Lymphocytes and their derivatives mediate the acquired immune response. Although most lymphocytes are found in the lymphoid tissues, many are found in circulating lymph and blood as well. There are two basic types: B lymphocytes and T lymphocytes.

Mast cells resemble basophils but do not circulate in the blood. They are found in the connective tissues, beneath the skin, in the gastrointestinal mucosa, and in the mucosal membranes of the respiratory system. Mast cells play a role in allergic reactions, immunity, and wound healing.

Characteristics of the Immune Response

The native and acquired immune responses protect the body from potentially infectious agents (eg, viruses, bacteria) and foreign substances that have gained access to the body through the skin or the lining of internal organs.

Native immunity (also called natural or innate immunity) is a nonspecific cellular and humoral (antibody) response that operates as the first line of defense against pathogens. Most native immunity is associated with the initial inflammatory response.

Acquired immunity (also called adaptive immunity) is a highly specific, inducible, discriminatory, and unforgetting method by which armies of cells respond to an immune stimulant. It arises when the body is exposed to a foreign substance or disease and produces antibodies to that invader. Passive acquired immunity is the receipt of preformed antibodies to fight or prevent an infection. Typically passive acquired immunity lasts for a much shorter period of time than active acquired immunity. Examples include transplacental and colostrum (the mother's initial milk to her infant, which is

loaded with antibodies); transmission of maternal antibodies, which protect newborn infants until their own immune system matures sufficiently to take over; and injection of immunoglobulin (a concentrated form of antibodies obtained from donors).

The primary (initial) immune response takes place during the first exposure to an antigen (a foreign substance). It may or may not result in clinical symptoms. Sometimes, the initial response of the body is to produce an antibody that causes symptoms on subsequent exposures. The secondary (amnestic) immune response occurs upon repeat exposure to a foreign substance. The body has already developed a "memory" for that substance, so a reaction occurs upon reexposure to it.

The beginning (induction) phase of the immune response occurs when a part of the immune system recognizes an antigen. Antigens may be either immunogenic (ie, elicit an immune response) or nonimmunogenic (do not elicit an immune response). An antibody binds a specific antigen so that the complex can attach itself to specialized immune cells that either ingest the complex to destroy it or release biologic mediators such as histamine to induce an allergic/inflammatory response. The specific features of the antigen–antibody interaction depend on the foreign substance involved **Figure 6-28 ▶**.

An immunogen is an antigen that activates immune cells to generate an immune response against itself. Thus, an immunogen is an antigen, but an antigen is not necessarily an immunogen. A hapten is a substance that normally does not stimulate an immune response but that can be combined with an antigen and, at a later time, initiate a specific antibody response on its own.

Humoral Immune Response

In humoral immunity, B-cell lymphocytes produce antibodies, which then react with a specific antigen, as shown in **Figure 6-29 ▶**.

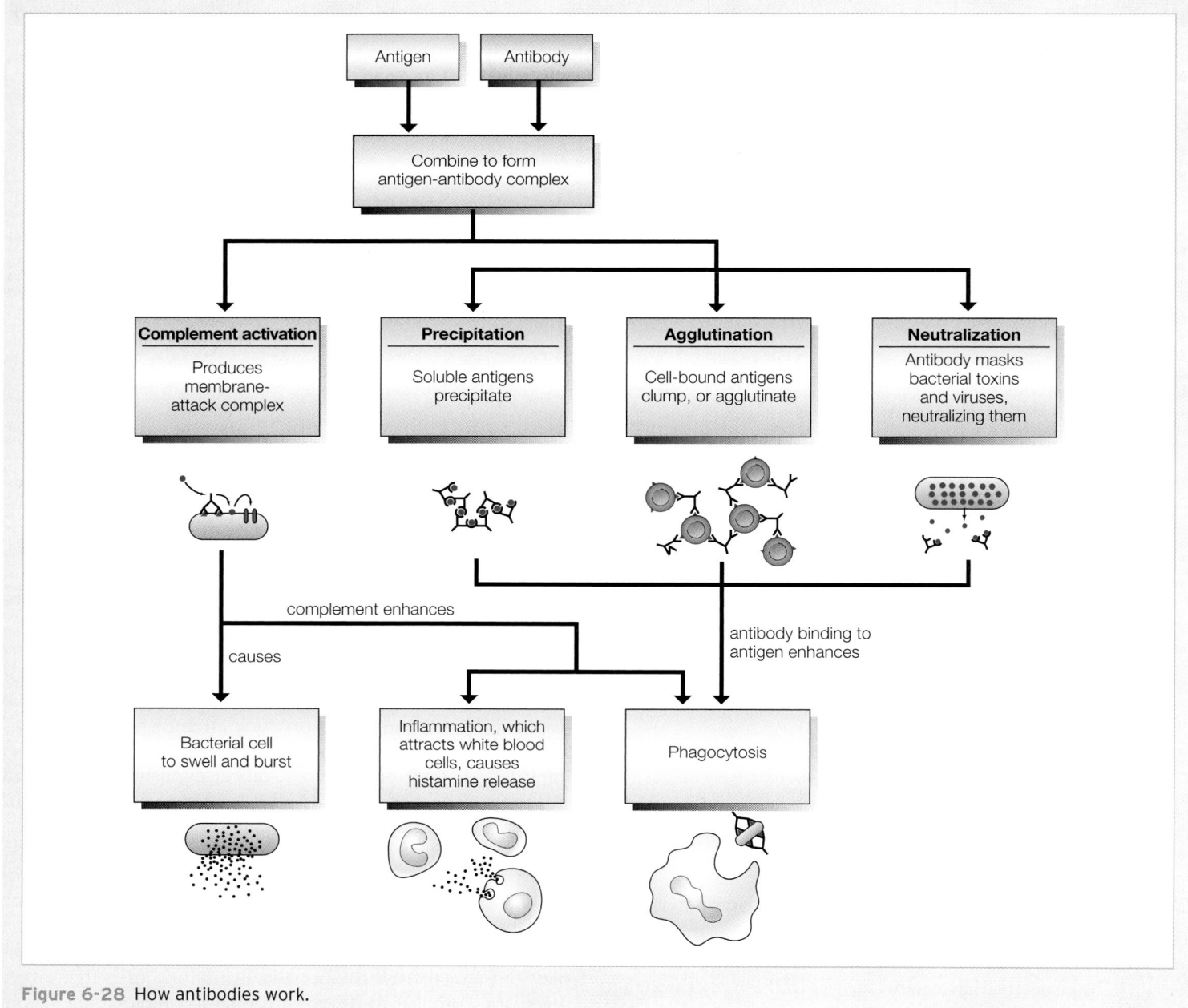

Figure 6-28 How antibodies work.

B Lymphocytes

Like all blood cells, B cells are born in the bone marrow, where they are descended from stem cells. The clonal selection theory holds that each B cell makes antibodies that have only one type of antigen-binding region and, therefore, are specific for a particular antigen, known as the cognate antigen. Antibodies are found on the surface of B cells, where they are able to recognize the presence of their cognate antigens. When a B cell recognizes the cognate antigen, it proliferates to make more identical B cells in an exponential fashion, each of which can make antibodies that recognize the same antigen.

For B cells to produce antibodies, they must first be activated. The most common way this occurs is via helper T cells:

1. A macrophage engulfs the antigen via phagocytosis. It digests the antigen, pushing the discarded particles to the cell surface. These remnants interact with the B cell and a helper T cell.

2. The antigen binds to both the B cell and the helper T cell, activating both.

3. The activated helper T cell secretes a lymphokine, a substance that stimulates the B cells to produce a clone. A clone is a group of identical cells formed from the same parent cell. The clone comprises two types of identical cells that have different functions: plasma cells, which make the antibodies, and memory cells, which "remember" the initial encounter with the antigen.

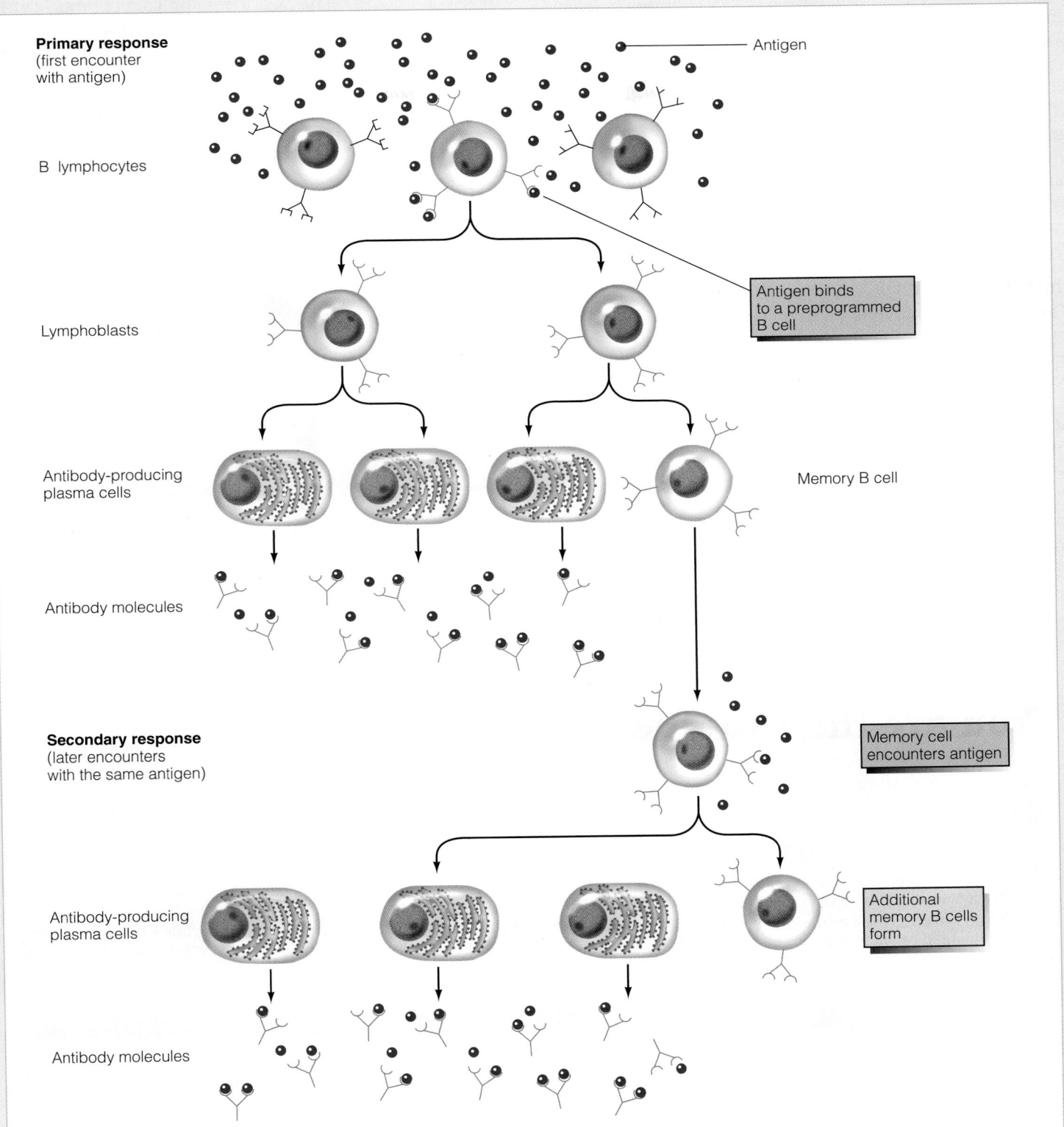

Figure 6-29 B-cell activation. Immunocompetent B cells are stimulated by the presence of an antigen, producing an intermediate cell, the lymphoblast. The lymphoblasts divide, producing plasma cells and some memory B cells. Memory B cells respond to subsequent antigen encroachment, yielding a rapid secondary response.

The human body distinguishes between foreign substances and its own cells and tissues by means of the major histocompatibility complex (MHC). A group of genes located on a single chromosome, the MHC permits an individual who is capable of generating an immune response to distinguish *self* from *nonself* (ie, what is foreign). The human leukocyte antigen (HLA) gene complex is the human MHC and is present in all nucleated human cells. It codes for numerous antigens that are unique to an individual. When the immune system "sees" these particular antigens, it recognizes them as "self" and no immune response occurs.

Immunoglobulins

The antibodies secreted by B cells are called immunoglobulins (this text uses use the terms *immunoglobulins* and *antibodies* interchangeably, unless otherwise stated). These Y-shaped proteins consist of a crystallizable fragment (Fc) portion and two antigen-binding fragment (Fab) regions that bind only a specific antigen. The basic antibody molecule has four chains linked into a Y-shape. Each side of the Y is identical, with one light chain attached to one heavy chain

Figure 6-30 ▾ . The two arms, or Fab regions, contain antigen-binding sites. The stem, or Fc region, determines to which of the five immunoglobin classes an antibody belongs Figure 6-31 ▶ .

Most antibodies are found in the plasma, where they make up about 20% of the plasma proteins in a healthy individual.

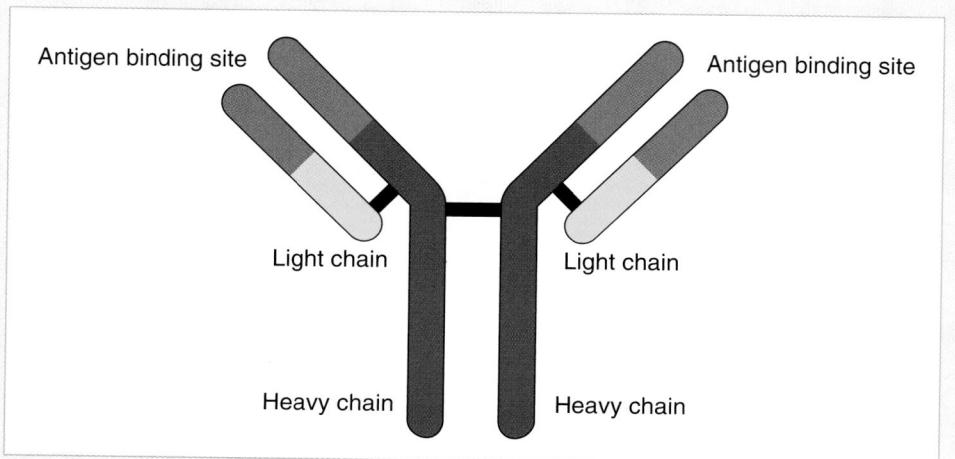

Figure 6-30 Structure of an immunoglobulin molecule.

You are the Provider Part 4

You prepare the patient for transport, noting that her breathing is still labored. She tells you that she is less lightheaded after the first 100 mL of saline has been administered; however, she still complains of being "short-winded." You contact the hospital for further orders, advising an estimated time of arrival of 8 minutes. The emergency department physician has no further orders at this time.

Upon your arrival at the emergency department, you notice that the dialysis nurse is already preparing for Mrs. Jensen. The emergency room physician explains to you that the physical findings are compatible with the beginning of septic shock due to an infection at the shunt site in addition to being volume-overloaded secondary to missed dialysis. He also suspects that Mrs. Jensen's potassium level will be high because of the tall T waves present on the ECG.

When you return to the emergency department that evening with another patient, you check up on Mrs. Jensen. She's resting comfortably in the medical intensive care unit, where she is being treated for sepsis, congestive heart failure, and hyperkalemia (her level was 6.7 mEq/L!). After the day's experience, you decide that studying pathophysiology is beneficial after all!

Reassessment	Recording Time: 15 Minutes
Skin	Pale, warm, and moist
Pulse	150 beats/min, regular; weak radial
ECG	Narrow complex tachycardia with tall T waves
Blood pressure	84/56 mm Hg
Respirations	26 breaths/min labored
Sao_2	93% on nonrebreathing mask at 15 L/min of supplemental oxygen
Pupils	Equal and reactive to light

7. How did the inflammatory process manifest itself in this patient?

8. What are other signs and symptoms of hyperkalemia?

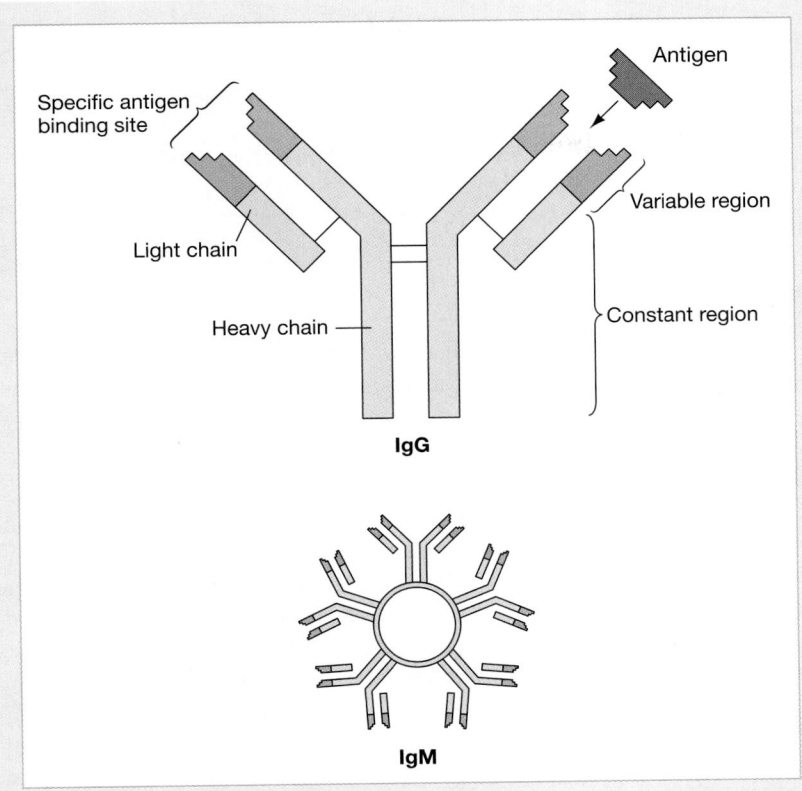

Figure 6-31 General structure of an antibody.

Antibodies make antigens more visible to the immune system in three ways:

- Antibodies act as opsonins. In opsoninization, an antibody coats an antigen to facilitate its recognition by immune cells. Antibodies are not toxic by themselves, but they label antigens so that other immune cells will attack them.
- Antibodies cause antigens to clump for easier phagocytosis (precipitation, also known as agglutination).
- Antibodies bind to and inactivate some toxins produced by bacteria. Macrophages can then ingest and destroy the inactivated toxins.

Antibodies are divided into five general classes of immunoglobulins Table 6-6 ▶ . Fetal immunity is a passive acquired immunity that is derived primarily from maternal IgG and IgM antibodies. Following delivery, these antibodies persist until the neonate's own B cells take over. A substantial number of antibodies are also transferred through breast milk, which is one of many reasons why experts favor breastfeeding.

Cell-Mediated Immune Response

In cell-mediated immunity, T-cell lymphocytes recognize antigens and contribute to the immune response in two major ways: (1) by secreting cytokines that attract other cells or (2) by becoming cytotoxic and killing infected or abnormal cells. There are four subgroups of T cells:

- *Killer T cells* (also called cytotoxic T cells) destroy the antigen. Cytotoxic T cells help rid the body of cells that

have been infected by viruses as well as cells that have been transformed by cancer. They are also responsible for the rejection of tissue and organ grafts.

- *Helper T cells* activate many immune cells, including B cells and other T cells (also called T4 or CD4+ cells).
- *Suppressor T cells* (also called T8 or CD8+ cells) suppress the activity of other lymphocytes so they do not destroy normal tissue.
- *Memory T cells* remember the reaction for the next time it is needed.

During the cell-mediated response, macrophages ingest pathogens. When a macrophage digests a pathogen, it releases small particles of antigen. This antigen pushes its way to the macrophage surface, where it is recognized by specific T cells. Other T cells, such as helper T cells and killer T cells, bind to the antigen and macrophage, destroying the invader.

Cellular Interactions in the Immune Response

There are remarkable similarities in how the body responds to different kinds of immune challenges. Although the details depend on the particular challenge, the basic pattern is the same—the innate response starts first and is then reinforced by the more specific acquired response. These two pathways are interconnected.

Consider what happens when bacteria enter the body. If the bacteria are not encapsulated, macrophages begin to ingest them immediately. If the bacteria are encapsulated, antibodies

Table 6-6	General Classes of Immunoglobulins
IgG	The most common immunoglobulin. Accounts for 75% of the antibodies in the blood. Found in lymph, synovial fluid, peritoneal fluid, cerebrospinal fluid, and breast milk. IgG is the only immunoglobulin that crosses the placenta, giving infants immunity in the first few months of life.
IgA	Accounts for 15% of the antibodies in the blood. Also found in tears, saliva, respiratory tract secretions, and the stomach. IgA combines with a protein in the mucosa and defends body surfaces against invading microorganisms.
IgM	Accounts for 5% to 10% of the antibodies in the blood and is the dominant antibody in ABO (blood type) incompatibilities. IgM is the initial antibody formed in most infections.
IgE	Accounts for less than 1% of the antibodies in the blood and is associated with allergic reactions. When mast cell receptors combine with IgE and antigen, the mast cells degranulate and release chemical mediators such as histamine.
IgD	Accounts for less than 1% of the antibodies in the blood. The physiologic role of IgD is unclear.

(opsonins) must coat the capsule before they can be ingested by phagocytes.

Components of the cell wall then activate the complement system. Some components of the activated complement system, termed chemotaxins, attract leukocytes from the circulation to help fight the infection. The complement cascade ends with the formation of a set of proteins called the membrane attack complex (MAC). These molecules insert themselves into the bacterial membrane, weakening those areas in the membrane. Ions and water enter the cell through the weakened areas, leading to lysis of the bacterium (a chemical process that does not involve immune cells).

If antibodies to the bacteria are already in the body, they will help the innate response by acting as opsonins and neutralizing bacterial toxins. Although it often takes several days, memory B cells attracted to the infection site will be activated if they encounter an antigen they recognize. If the infection is new to the body (preexisting antibodies are not present), B cells will be activated. Combined with helper T cells and cytokine release, antibodies are produced and memory B and T cells are formed.

T-cell and B-cell function is deficient in older patients. Depressed lymphocyte function is accompanied by a decrease in macrophage activity. Therefore, older people are more prone to experience infections and recover slowly. In addition, older people have increased levels of autoantibodies (antibodies directed against the patient), which partly explains why older people are prone to autoimmune disease.

Acute and Chronic Inflammation

Inflammation is a dynamic process that, once initiated, triggers a complex cascade of events involving both local and systemic events. The two most common causes of inflammation are infection (eg, bacterial or viral) and injury.

The acute inflammatory response involves both vascular and cellular components. After transient arteriolar constriction, the arterioles dilate, allowing an influx of blood under increased pressure. This active hyperemia (increased intravascular pressure) causes the blood vessel to expand; as in a balloon that is being inflated, the vessel walls become thinner. The higher pressure combined with increased vessel wall permeability causes fluid to leak into the interstitial spaces (edema). When enough fluid has escaped into the surrounding area and the intravascular pressure has been released, the vessel wall contracts and the outflow slows, leading to stasis of blood in the capillaries.

A variety of blood cells participate in tissue inflammatory reactions: white blood cells (leukocytes), platelets, mast cells, and plasma cells (B lymphocytes that create antibodies). Specific cell types include neutrophils, monocytes, lymphocytes, eosinophils, basophils, and activated platelets. Chemical mediators, primarily produced by the mast cells, account for the vascular and cellular events that occur during the acute inflam-

In the Field

Corticosteroids can decrease the initial inflammatory response, which is a necessary part of wound healing. They also increase the risk of wound infection owing to their immunosuppressive activity. This consideration is important in diabetic patients because of their propensity to develop wound infections.

matory response. Cell-derived mediators include histamine, arachidonic acid derivatives, and cytokines (eg, interleukins, tumor necrosis factor).

Mast Cells

Mast cells play a major role in inflammation. During inflammation, they degranulate and release a variety of substances. The major stimuli for the degranulation of mast cells during the inflammatory response are physical injury (eg, trauma), chemical agents (eg, bacterial toxins), and immunologic substances (eg, interaction of an antigen and an IgE antibody).

Following their degranulation, mast cells release vasoactive amines. The most important of these substances, histamine and serotonin, increase vascular permeability, cause vasodilation, and can cause bronchoconstriction, nausea, and vomiting. Because histamine is a preformed vasodepressor amine that is stored in mast cells, it can be released quickly, so its actions are seen early in the inflammatory response. Mast cells also synthesize chemotactic factors that attract neutrophils (neutrophil chemotactic factor) and eosinophils (eosinophilic chemotactic factor).

Mast cells also synthesize leukotrienes. Leukotrienes—also known as slow-reacting substances of anaphylaxis (SRS-A)—are a family of biologically active compounds derived from arachidonic acid. The clinically important leukotrienes participate in host defense reactions and pathophysiologic conditions that paramedics commonly see in the field, such as immediate hypersensitivity and inflammation. Leukotrienes have potent actions on many parts of the body, including the cardiovascular, pulmonary, immune, and central nervous systems, and the gastrointestinal tract.

Leukotrienes are primarily endogenous mediators of inflammation. They contribute to the signs and symptoms seen in acute inflammatory responses, including responses resulting from the interaction of allergens with IgE antibodies on mast cells. Certain leukotrienes are bronchoconstrictors, stimulate airway mucus secretion, and are very potent at increasing the permeability of postcapillary venules (including those in the bronchial circulation), thereby causing plasma protein exudation (oozing out of the tissue) and edema. Certain leukotrienes may also promote eosinophil migration into the airways of animals and asthmatic patients, and they may also increase bronchial hyperresponsiveness through an action on sensory nerves.

Finally, mast cells synthesize prostaglandins. These substances, which are derived from arachidonic acid, comprise a group of about 20 lipids that are modified fatty acids attached to a five-member ring. Prostaglandins are found in many vertebrate tissues, where they act as messengers involved in reproduction, the inflammatory response to infection, and pain. Aspirin and NSAIDs inhibit prostaglandin synthesis, leading to reduced inflammation and pain.

Plasma Protein Systems

The plasma-derived mediators that modulate the inflammatory process are called plasma protein systems. They include the complement system, the coagulation (clotting) system, and the kinin system. The interaction of these systems is vital to a normal inflammatory response. Each system consists of a cascade of biochemical reactions such that as one compound is produced, it catalyzes the formation of the next compound—much like knocking over a line of dominos.

Complement System

The complement system is a group of plasma proteins that attract white blood cells to sites of inflammation, activate white blood cells, and directly destroy cells. The central compound in this complement cascade is called C3. C3 is produced by one of the two "complement pathways": the classic pathway or the alternate pathway. The classic pathway starts when an antigen–antibody complex binds to a complement component (C1); activation of this pathway is dependent on the presence of antibodies. The alternate pathway can be triggered by bacterial toxins and does not need antibodies to be activated.

Regardless of which pathway is taken, the main products are the same: C3b, anaphylatoxins, and the MAC. C3b coats bacteria, making it easier for macrophages to engulf them. Anaphylatoxins (C3a, C4a, and C5a) stimulate smooth-muscle contraction and increase vascular permeability by stimulating the release of histamine from mast cells and platelets. The MAC is a set of complement proteins (C5b, C6, C7, C8, and C9) that bind to form a hollow tube, much like a short straw, that can puncture into the plasma membrane of a cell. In this way, transmembrane channels are formed that allow ions, water, and other small molecules to pass through, resulting in loss of cellular osmolarity and death of the cell.

Coagulation System

The coagulation system plays a vital role in the formation of blood clots in the body and facilitates repairs to the vascular tree. Inflammation triggers the coagulation cascade, initiating a complex series of reactions that result in the formation of fibrin. Fibrin is the protein that polymerizes (bonds) to form the fibrous component of a blood clot. The various coagulation factors are counterbalanced by a variety of inhibitors, so that the coagulation is restricted to one area. Simultaneously, the fibrinolysis cascade is activated to dissolve the fibrin and create fibrin split products (ie, fragments of the dissolving clot).

Kinin System

The kinin system leads to the formation of the vasoactive protein bradykinin from kallikrein. Kallikrein is an enzyme that is normally found in blood plasma, urine, and body tissue in an inactive state. When it becomes activated, it can dilate blood vessels, influence blood pressure, modulate salt and water excretion by the kidneys, and influence cardiac remodeling after acute myocardial infarction. Bradykinin increases vascular permeability, dilates blood vessels, contracts smooth muscle, and causes pain when injected into the skin.

The kinin system is spurred into action by the activation of Hageman factor (coagulation factor XII). (**Table 6-7 ▶** lists the various coagulation factors.) In addition to its role in the kinin system, Hageman factor participates in the clotting, fibrinolytic, and complement cascades. Its activators include bacterial lipopolysaccharides and endotoxin. Activated factor XII triggers the intrinsic clotting cascade, which occurs when blood is exposed to collagen or other substances. For example, when a blood vessel is cut, the skin cells are damaged and the blood comes in contact with collagen. The extrinsic clotting cascade is activated by substances released from injured cells when tissue damage occurs.

Cellular Components of Inflammation

The goal of the cellular component of acute inflammatory response is for inflammatory cells—namely, polymorphonuclear neutrophils (PMNs)—to arrive at the sites within tissue where they are needed. This process involves two major stages: an intravascular phase and an extravascular phase. During the intravascular phase, leukocytes move to the sides of blood vessels and attach to the endothelial cells. During the extravascular phase, leukocytes travel to the site of inflammation and kill organisms. The cellular event sequence is as follows:

1. **Margination.** Loss of fluid from the blood vessels into the inflamed or infected tissue causes the blood left in the vessels to have increased viscosity, which slows the flow of blood and produces stasis. PMNs, which usually travel toward the center of the vessel, settle toward the sides of the vessel as the blood flow slows down. As stasis develops, leukocytes also move (marginate) toward the sides of blood vessels, where they bump into the endothelial cells and bind to them. Stress can lead to demargination of some white blood cells, which stimulates the bone marrow to produce more white blood cells, which in turn increases the white blood cell count.
2. **Activation.** Mediators of inflammation trigger the appearance of selectins and integrins on the surfaces of endothelial cells and PMNs, respectively.
3. **Adhesion.** PMNs attach to endothelial cells, as mediated by selectins and integrins.
4. **Transmigration (diapedesis).** The PMNs permeate through the vessel wall, moving into the interstitial space.
5. **Chemotaxis.** PMNs move toward the site of inflammation in response to chemotactic factors that are released by

Table 6-7	Coagulation Factors	
Factor Number	**Name**	**Functions**
I	Fibrinogen	Protein synthesized in liver; converted into fibrin in stage 3
II	Prothrombin	Protein synthesized in liver (requires vitamin K); converted into thrombin in stage 2
III	Tissue thromboplastin	Released from damaged tissue; required in extrinsic stage 1
IV	Calcium ions	Required throughout entire clotting sequence
V	Proaccelerin (labile factor)	Protein synthesized in liver; required to form prothrombin activator in both intrinsic and extrinsic stage 1
VII	Serum prothrombin conversion accelerator (stable factor, proconvertin)	Protein synthesized in liver (requires vitamin K); functions in extrinsic stage 1
VIII	Antihemophilic factor (antihemophilic globulin)	Protein synthesized in liver; required for intrinsic stage 1
IX	Plasma thromboplastin component	Protein synthesized in liver (requires vitamin K); required for intrinsic stage 1
X	Stuart factor (Stuart-Prower factor)	Protein synthesized in liver (requires vitamin K); required to form prothrombin activator in both intrinsic and extrinsic stage 1
XI	Plasma thromboplastin antecedent	Protein synthesized in liver; required for intrinsic stage 1
XII	Hageman factor	Protein required for intrinsic stage 1
XIII	Fibrin-stabilizing factor	Protein required to stabilize the fibrin strands in stage 3

bacteria or formed from activated complement, chemokines, or arachidonic acid derivatives (eg, leukotrienes) in response to cell injury. **Figure 6-32** ▸ illustrates the inflammatory response.

Cellular Products of Inflammation

Cytokines are products of cells that affect the function of other cells. Monocytes release monokines, and lymphocytes release lymphokines.

Interleukins include IL-1 (interleukin-1) and IL-2 (interleukin-2), which attract white blood cells to the sites of injury and bacterial invasion. Interferon is a protein produced by cells when they are invaded by viruses. This cytokine is released into the bloodstream or intercellular fluid to induce healthy cells to manufacture an enzyme that counters the infection.

Lymphokines stimulate leukocytes. Macrophage-activating factor stimulates macrophages to help engulf and destroy foreign substances. Migration inhibitory factor keeps white blood cells at the site of infection or injury until they can perform their designated task.

Injury Resolution and Repair

Normal wound healing involves four steps—repair of damaged tissue, removal of inflammatory debris, restoration of tissues to a normal state, and regeneration of cells. Healing after tissue injury or loss caused by inflammation depends on the type of cells that make up the affected organ. Labile cells divide continuously, so organs derived from these cells (eg, skin or intestinal mucosa) heal completely. Stable cells are replaced by regeneration from remaining cells, which are stimulated to enter mitosis. These cells are found in the liver and kidney. Permanent cells, such as nerve cells and cardiac myocytes, cannot be replaced; scar tissue is laid down instead.

Wounds may heal by either primary or secondary intention. Healing by primary intention occurs in clean wounds with opposed margins (eg, a clean surgical wound). First, blood fills the defect and coagulates, forming a scab, which is a mesh-like structure composed of fibrin and fibronectin. If the inflammatory process was severe, tissue may be destroyed and require repair. Next, macrophages remove cellular debris and secrete growth factors. These growth factors stimulate angiogenesis and growth of fibroblasts, leading to the formation of granulation tissue. The epithelium then regenerates, covering the surface defect. Deposition of collagen results in fibrous union. By the end of the first week, 10% of the preoperative strength is regained. Scar maturation occurs as collagen cross-linking takes place. By the end of 3 months, 80% of the normal tensile strength of the tissue has been restored.

Healing by secondary intention occurs in large gaping or infected wounds. Wounds that heal by secondary intention have a more pronounced and prolonged inflammatory phase, causing the neutrophils to persist for days. They also have more abundant granulation tissue. Wound contraction is mediated by myofibroblasts, which help to draw the margins of the wound closer to each other as time passes.

Factors that can lead to dysfunctional wound healing may be either local or systemic. Local factors include infection (when the body's healing efforts are diverted to fight off the cause of the infection); an inadequate blood supply (as in diabetes) that produces tissue hypoxia, which slows wound

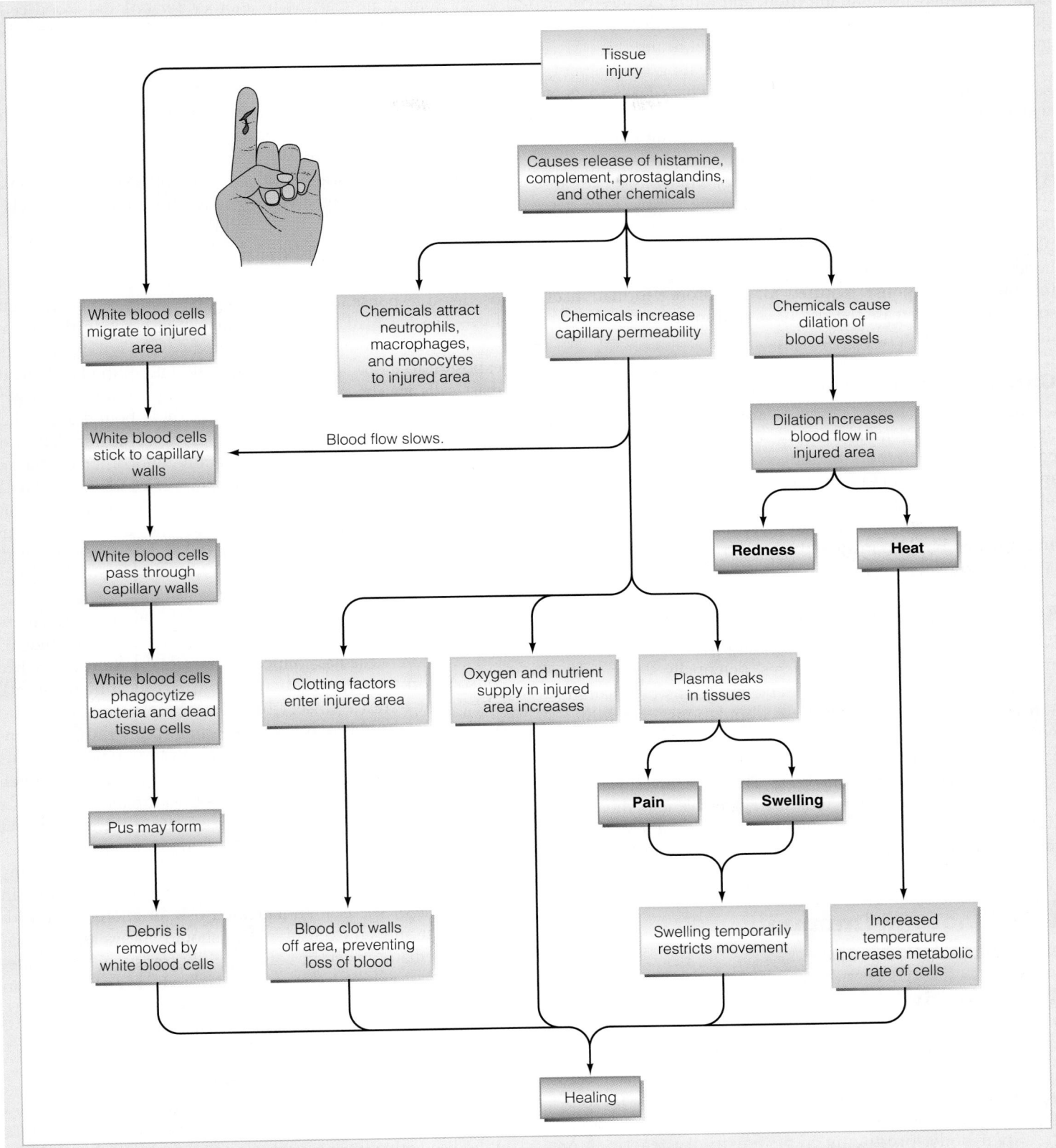

Figure 6-32 The inflammatory response.

healing and may promote infection; and foreign bodies (when present in a wound, they stimulate acute and chronic inflammation, both of which interfere with wound healing).

Systemic factors that influence the healing of a patient's wounds include poor nutritional intake, which leads to poor scar formation and suppression of the immune system, and hematologic abnormalities (proper wound healing requires the presence of adequate numbers of white blood cells). Patients who have impaired bone marrow stores of white blood cells are susceptible to infection and often heal more slowly. Both diabetes and AIDS affect the cells of the immune system, which plays a direct role in wound healing, and increase the likelihood of wound infection. Corticosteroids suppress the initial inflammatory response required for the proper formation of scar tissue and increase the risk of wound infection by slowing the immune system response.

Chronic Inflammation Responses

Chronic inflammation responses are usually caused by an unsuccessful acute inflammatory response due to a foreign body, persistent infection, or antigen. They are associated with an infiltrate containing monocytes and lymphocytes, and usually involve tissue destruction and repair (or scar formation). The vascular events are similar to those that take place in acute inflammation but also include the growth of new blood vessels (a process known as angiogenesis).

Age and the Inflammatory Response

Both newborns and geriatric patients often exhibit relative impairment of their immune systems, potentially slowing their inflammatory response. As a consequence, signs of inflammation may be more subtle in these populations. In addition, wound healing often takes longer, especially in the geriatric patient. The immune system is not fully developed until the child is between 2 and 3 years of age. Therefore, investigation of a fever in younger children must be aggressive and thorough. Many experts recommend hospital admission for a temperature greater than 100.4°F in a child younger than 3 months.

▌Variances in Immunity and Inflammation

Hypersensitivity

Hypersensitivity is any bodily response to any substance to which a patient has increased sensitivity. It is a generic term for a variety of reactions. Allergy is a hypersensitivity reaction to the presence of an agent (allergen). Autoimmunity is the production of antibodies or T cells that work against the tissues of one's own body, producing hypersensitivity reactions or autoimmune disease (as in systemic lupus). Isoimmunity is the formation of T cells or antibodies directed against the antigens on another person's cells (typically after the transplantation of an organ or tissues). A blood transfusion reaction is an example of an isoimmune reaction to another person's red blood cells. The destruction of cells by antibodies or T cells may be either an autoimmune or an isoimmune reaction.

Mechanisms of Hypersensitivity

A hypersensitivity reaction may be immediate, occurring within seconds to minutes, or delayed, occurring hours to days after exposure to an antigen. The speed of symptom evolution depends on the antigen and the type of response the body mounts against it. Hypersensitivity reactions are typically classified into four types: I, II, III, and IV.

Type I Hypersensitivity Reactions

A type I hypersensitivity reaction is an acute reaction that occurs in response to a stimulus (eg, bee sting, penicillin, shellfish). The mechanism involves interaction between the stimulus (antigen) and a preformed antibody of the IgE type. At first exposure to a specific antigen, specific IgE antibodies bind to mast cells via the nonspecific region (Fc) portion. Upon secondary exposure to the same antigen, these bound antibodies are cross-linked by the antigen, resulting in degranulation of the mast cell, and release of histamine and other mediators Figure 6-33 ▸. The released histamine feeds back on both mast cells and eosinophils, leading to the release of additional histamine and other mediators. The severity of the symptoms that a particular patient develops depends on the extent of mediator release.

The degree of severity of hypersensitivity reactions varies from very severe and life-threatening reactions, such as anaphylaxis, to less severe reactions, such as allergic rhinitis (edema and irritation of the nasal mucosa), bronchial asthma (bronchial constriction, mucus production, and airway inflammation), wheal and flare (ie, insect bite leading to vasodilation and swelling), and mild food allergy (leading to diarrhea, gastrointestinal distress, and vomiting). A propensity to type I reactions may be diagnosed through skin tests (eg, patch test, scratch test) and other laboratory procedures (measurement of specific IgE antibody levels). Treatment is avoidance of the antigen, but desensitizing injections may be helpful in severe cases.

Nevertheless, it is impossible to predict how severe any given reaction will be. If a person has had a severe reaction in the past, he or she is at an increased risk for another one with subsequent antigen exposures. You should always assume that an IgE-mediated reaction could rapidly transition into a life-threatening event. These reactions need to be treated quickly in the field, and most prehospital providers are trained to administer epinephrine by using an EpiPen auto-injector or by giving a subcutaneous injection.

Type II Hypersensitivity Reactions

Type II hypersensitivity reactions are cytotoxic (cell destructive) and classically involve the combination of IgG or IgM antibodies with antigens on the cell membrane. Cells are lysed (destroyed), either by complement fixation or by other antibodies. This process also destroys many of the body's healthy cells. Histamine release from mast cells is not involved, and IgG-mediated allergic responses occur within a few hours of

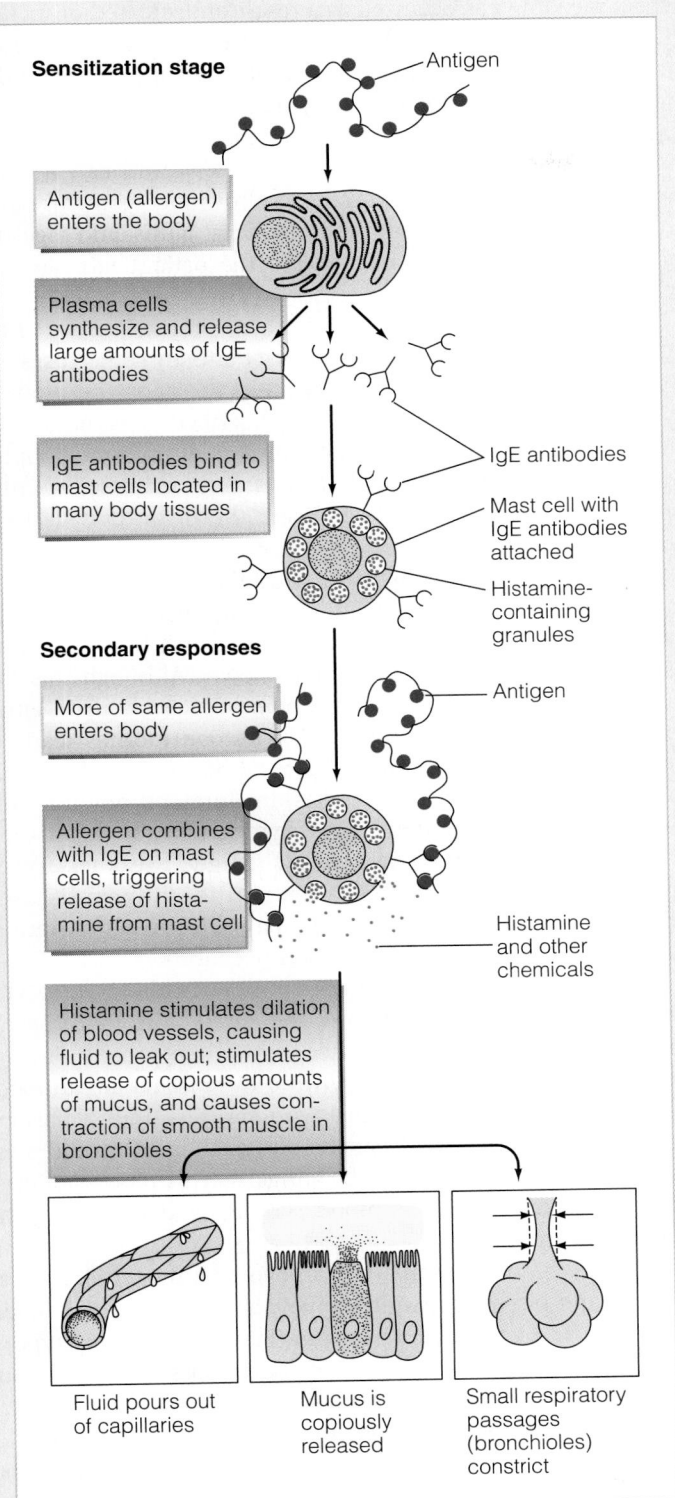

Sensitization stage

Antigen

Antigen (allergen) enters the body

Plasma cells synthesize and release large amounts of IgE antibodies

IgE antibodies bind to mast cells located in many body tissues

IgE antibodies

Mast cell with IgE antibodies attached

Histamine-containing granules

Secondary responses

More of same allergen enters body

Antigen

Allergen combines with IgE on mast cells, triggering release of histamine from mast cell

Histamine and other chemicals

Histamine stimulates dilation of blood vessels, causing fluid to leak out; stimulates release of copious amounts of mucus, and causes contraction of smooth muscle in bronchioles

Fluid pours out of capillaries

Mucus is copiously released

Small respiratory passages (bronchioles) constrict

Figure 6-33 Type I allergic reaction. The antigen stimulates the production of massive amounts of IgE, a type of antibody produced by plasma cells; the IgE, in turn, attaches to mast cells. This is a sensitization stage. When the antigen enters again, it binds to the IgE antibodies on the mast cells, triggering a massive release of histamine and other chemicals. Histamine causes blood vessels to dilate and become leaky, and it promotes increased production of mucus in the respiratory tract. Mast cell degranulation may also cause bronchospasm in some people.

antigen exposure. Examples of IgG-mediated responses include transfusion reactions and newborn hemolytic disease.

Type III Hypersensitivity Reactions

Type III hypersensitivity responses involve primarily IgG antibodies that form immune complexes with antigen to recruit phagocytic cells, such as neutrophils, to a site where they can release inflammatory cytokines. Since histamine release from mast cells is not involved, IgG-mediated allergic responses occur within a few hours of antigen exposure. Reactions may be systemic or localized.

The systemic form is called serum sickness and results from a large, single exposure to an antigen, such as horse antibody serum. Antigen–antibody complexes formed in the bloodstream are then deposited in sites around the body, most notably in the kidney, with resultant inflammatory reactions (eg, serum sickness from penicillin). Signs and symptoms of serum sickness may include fever, malaise, rashes, joint aches, lymphademopathy, and splenomegaly.

The localized form of type III response is called an Arthus reaction. Arthus reactions consist of a circumscribed area of vascular inflammation (vasculitis). An example of an Arthus reaction is farmer's lung (a hypersensitivity pneumonitis), which is a local hypersensitivity reaction in the lung to molds that grow on hay.

Type IV Hypersensitivity Reactions

Type IV allergic responses, also known as cell-mediated hypersensitivity, are primarily mediated by soluble molecules that are released by specifically activated T cells. These reactions are classified into two subtypes: delayed hypersensitivity and cell-mediated cytotoxicity.

Delayed hypersensitivity involves lymphocytes and macrophages. T cells respond to an antigen and activate CD4 (a helper T cell) lymphocytes. These lymphocytes release mediators that are designed to destroy the foreign substance. Examples include contact hypersensitivity to poison ivy, or the local induration due to mononuclear cell infiltrates from a PPD (tuberculin) skin test.

Cell-mediated cytotoxicity involves only sensitized T cells (CD8 lymphocytes or T killer cells). These cells kill the antigen-bearing target cells rather than activating the CD4 lymphocyte to do so. Examples include the body's response to viral infections, tumor immune surveillance, and the mechanism by which transplant rejection occurs.

Targets of Hypersensitivity

The immune system targets different molecules, depending on the type of hypersensitivity reaction. In allergic reactions, the target is an antigen or allergen. Allergens are substances that cause a hypersensitivity reaction, such as those listed in **Table 6-8 ▶**.

In autoimmune reactions, the target is a person's own tissues. For reasons that are unclear, normal tolerance of "self" tissues breaks down and the immune system treats the body's own tissues as foreign.

Graves' disease is an autoimmune disease caused by thyroid-stimulating or thyroid-growth immunoglobulins.

Table 6-8	Allergens That Can Cause Hypersensitivity Reactions	
Type	**Examples**	
Inhalants	Pollen, dust, smoke, fungi, plastic, odors	
Foods	Eggs, milk, wheat, chocolate, strawberries	
Drugs	Aspirin, antibiotics, serums, codeine	
Infectious agents	Bacteria, viruses, fungi, animal parasites	
Contactants	Animals, plants, metals, chemicals	
Physical agents	Light, pressure, radiation, heat and cold	

These antibodies activate receptors for thyroid-stimulating hormone, causing increased activity by the thyroid gland. In addition to hyperthyroidism, Graves' disease is associated with characteristic eye changes—lid retraction, stare, and exophthalmus (protrusion of the eyes)—and skin changes (pretibial myxedema—localized edematous skin in the pretibial area).

Type 1 diabetes mellitus is also considered an autoimmune disease. Although the exact insult is unknown (but is suspected to be a viral infection), some agent stimulates the body to produce autoantibodies against beta cells in the pancreas that produce insulin. The result is a deficiency of insulin, and diabetes.

Rheumatoid arthritis is a chronic systemic disease that affects the entire body. One of the most common forms of arthritis, it is characterized by inflammation of the synovium (the connective tissue membrane lining the joint) with resulting pain, stiffness, warmth, redness, and swelling. Inflammatory cells release enzymes that cause damage to bone and cartilage. The involved joint can lose its shape and alignment, resulting in pain and loss of movement. Rheumatoid arthritis is associated with the formation of rheumatoid factor—that is, IgM antibodies to tissue IgG. In the joints, the synovial membrane is thickened due to infiltration of inflammatory cells (lymphocytes).

Myasthenia gravis is an acquired autoimmune disease that is characterized by autoimmune attack on the nerve–muscle junction. The circulating autoantibodies cause abnormal muscle fatigability and typically involve the smallest motor units first, such as the extraocular muscles. This produces ptosis (droopy eyelid) and diplopia (double vision). Other muscles may be involved, causing problems with swallowing (dysphagia). Characteristically, repeated contraction of the affected muscles makes the symptoms worse. Two thirds of patients with myasthenia gravis have thymic abnormalities, with the most common being thymic hyperplasia. A minority of patients have a tumor of the thymus, called a thymoma.

Immune thrombocytopenia purpura (ITP) is a blood disorder in which the patient forms antibodies to blood platelets that cause their destruction. Thrombocytopenia describes a decrease in blood platelets; purpura are purplish areas of the skin and mucous membranes (such as the lining of the mouth)

where bleeding has occurred as a result of decreased or ineffective platelets. Some cases of ITP are caused by drugs, whereas others are associated with infection, pregnancy, or immune disorders such as systemic lupus erythematosus. About half of all cases are classified as "idiopathic" (ie, the cause is unknown).

Bleeding is the main symptom of ITP and can include bruising and tiny red dots on the skin or mucous membranes. In some instances, bleeding from the nose, gums, and digestive or urinary tracts may occur. Rarely, the patient has bleeding within the brain.

Treatment of idiopathic ITP is based on the severity of the symptoms and the patient's platelet count. In some cases, no therapy is needed. In most cases, drugs that alter the immune system's attack on the platelets are prescribed, such as corticosteroids (eg, prednisone) and IV infusions of immunoglobulin. Another treatment that usually results in an increased number of platelets is removal of the spleen, the organ that destroys antibody-coated platelets.

Systemic lupus erythematosus (SLE) is a chronic autoimmune disease with many manifestations. In this disease, the body's own immune system is directed against the body's own tissues. The etiology of SLE is not known. Although this disease is more common in young women, it can occur in either sex at any age. The production of autoantibodies leads to immune complex formation. These immune complexes can then be deposited in glomeruli, skin, lungs, synovium, and mesothelium, among other places. Symptoms include arthritis, a red rash over the nose and cheeks, fatigue, weakness, fever, and photosensitivity. Glomerulonephritis (kidney disease), pericarditis, anemia, and neuritis may develop. In addition, many SLE patients develop renal complications.

Rh factor is an antigen that is present in the erythrocytes (red blood cells) of about 85% of the population. Erythrocytes contain antigens on their surface, which are proteins recognized by the immune system. Within the plasma are antibodies, which are proteins that react with antigens. Individuals are classified as having one of four blood types based on the presence or absence of these specific antigens. This process of classification is referred to as blood typing, or determining the ABO blood group.

Type A blood contains erythrocytes with type A surface antigens and plasma containing type B antibodies; type B blood contains type B surface antigens and plasma containing type A antibodies. Type AB blood contains both types of antigens but the plasma contains no ABO antibodies. Type O contains neither A nor B antigens but contains both A and B plasma antibodies. A person's blood type determines which type of blood he or she may receive in a blood transfusion.

Rh blood groups involve a complex of antigens first discovered in rhesus monkeys. The presence of any of the 18 separate Rh antigens makes an individual's blood Rh positive. If an individual with Rh negative blood were to be exposed to Rh positive blood, antibodies to the antigens could be produced.

Persons who have the factor are designated Rh-positive; those who lack the factor are termed Rh-negative. Blood for transfusions must be classified in terms of its Rh factor, as well as the ABO blood group, to prevent possible incompatibility reactions. If an Rh-negative person receives Rh-positive blood, for example, hemolysis and anemia can result. A similar reaction can occur if an Rh-negative mother exposes her Rh-positive fetus to antibodies to the factor.

Immune and Inflammation Deficiencies

Immunodeficiency is an abnormal condition in which some part of the body's immune system is inadequate, and consequently resistance to infectious disease is decreased. It may be congenital or acquired.

Congenital Immunodeficiencies

Patients with severe combined immunodeficiency disease have defects that involve lymphoid stem cells. As a consequence, both T cells (cellular immunity) and B cells (humoral immunity) are affected. Patients are at risk for infection with all types of organisms (eg, bacteria, mycobacteria, fungi, viruses, parasites). There are two forms of this disease, both of which are inherited.

X-linked agammaglobulinemia is one of the most common forms of primary immunodeficiency. This disease, which affects male infants, is caused by a defect in the differentiation of pre-B cells into B cells. The result is markedly decreased levels of all immunoglobulins and of mature B lymphocytes. T lymphocytes, however, function normally. Patients develop recurrent pyrogenic infections, but have no problems with fungal and viral infections because their cell-mediated immunity is unaffected. These infections first emerge in affected infants at about 6 months of age when maternal immunoglobulin levels have decreased.

Isolated deficiency of IgA is probably the most common form of immunodeficiency. This disease results from a block in the terminal differentiation of B lymphocytes. Most patients are asymptomatic, but some may develop chronic sinus infections. Patients also have an increased incidence of autoimmune disease.

Acquired Immunodeficiencies

Any nutritional deficiency can hamper normal immune function and the inflammatory response. Nutritional deficiencies may depress bone marrow function and diminish white blood cell development Figure 6-34 ▶ . A lack of protein in the diet, for example, decreases the liver's ability to manufacture inflammatory mediators and plasma proteins.

The stress of trauma can also cause immunodeficiency. Other contributors to this condition may include hypoperfusion or shock, mediator production, damage to vital organs, and the decreased nutrition occurring during trauma states.

Iatrogenic (treatment-induced) immunodeficiency is most frequently caused by drugs. Corticosteroids, whether taken orally or inhaled, suppress the immune system. Often, this results in therapeutic benefit to the patient. In a small number of patients, however, the resulting immunosuppression leads to other diseases (eg, tuberculosis). Usually physicians are very careful about the prescribed duration of this therapy because of

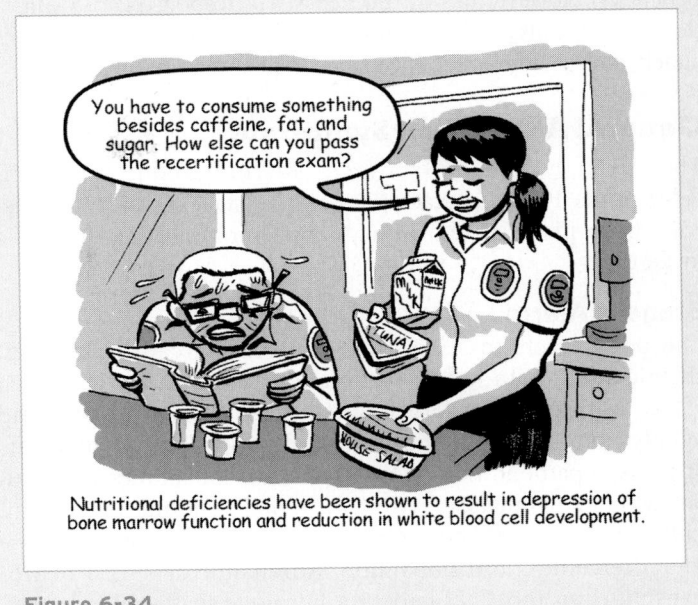

Nutritional deficiencies have been shown to result in depression of bone marrow function and reduction in white blood cell development.

Figure 6-34

its potential for adverse effects. In addition, idiosyncratic reactions to antibiotics may result in bone marrow suppression, as is the case with chemotherapeutic drugs for cancer. Many cases of bone marrow suppression in cancer are direct and predictable side effects of chemotherapy, and not true idiosyncratic, "out of the blue" reactions.

Physical or mental stress has been shown to decrease white blood cell and lymphocyte function. It may also lead to decreased production of various antibodies.

AIDS is an immunodeficiency disease that is caused by the RNA retrovirus HIV (human immunodeficiency virus). HIV binds to the CD4 surface protein of helper T cells, infects these cells, and kills them. Their destruction causes decreased humoral and cell-mediated reactions.

Treatment of Immunodeficiencies

Replacement therapy is available for some types of immunodeficiencies (eg, common variable immunodeficiency). Intravenous gamma globulin has been used in the therapy of a number of immunologic disorders of the nervous system, especially myasthenia gravis and inflammatory neuropathies, with considerable success. Bone marrow transplantation may restore immune competence in persons with acquired causes of immunodeficiency, such as following chemotherapy for cancer. In the future, gene therapy may be useful for treatment of both congenital and acquired causes of immunodeficiency.

Stress and Disease

Stress is the medical term for a wide range of strong external stimuli, both physiologic and psychological, that can cause a physiologic response. Usually, the response to stress is appropriate and beneficial. However, an unchecked stress response can result in deleterious outcomes, including chemical dependency, heart attack, stroke, depression, headache, and abdominal pain.

General Adaptation Syndrome

The general adaptation syndrome, a term introduced by Hans Selye in the 1920s, characterizes a three-stage reaction to stressors, both physical (eg, injury) and emotional (eg, loss of a loved one).

Stage 1: Alarm

The body reacts to stress first by releasing catecholamines, chemical compounds derived from the amino acid tyrosine that act as hormones or neurotransmitters. They are produced mainly from the adrenal medulla and the postganglionic fibers of the sympathetic nervous system. Catecholamines are soluble, so they circulate dissolved in blood. The most abundant catecholamines are epinephrine (adrenaline), norepinephrine (noradrenaline), and dopamine. Adrenaline acts as a neurotransmitter in the CNS and as a hormone in the blood. Noradrenaline is primarily a neurotransmitter of the peripheral sympathetic nervous system but is also present in the blood (mostly through "spillover" from the synapses of the sympathetic system).

Normally, the "fight-or-flight" response that occurs in the alarm reaction prepares the body to deal with stress, but it can also weaken the immune system, leading to infection.

Stage 2: Resistance

Stage 2, the resistance stage, is the body's way of adapting to stressors. It does so primarily by stimulating the adrenal gland to secrete two types of corticosteroid hormones that increase the blood glucose level and maintain blood pressure: glucocorticoids and mineralocorticoids. The most significant glucocorticoid in the body is cortisol, which controls carbohydrate, fat, and protein metabolism. Cortisol also has potent anti-inflammatory actions. Mineralocorticoids (predominantly aldosterone) control electrolyte and water levels in the body, mainly by promoting sodium retention by the kidney.

Continuation of stress and accompanying corticosteroid release eventually leads to fatigue, lapses in concentration, irritability, and lethargy.

Stage 3: Exhaustion

After a long period of stress, the person enters the exhaustion stage. The adrenal glands become depleted, leading to decreased blood glucose levels. The result is decreased stress tolerance, progressive mental and physical exhaustion, illness, and collapse. At this point, the body's immune system is compromised, significantly reducing a person's ability to resist disease. Heart attack, high blood pressure, or severe infection may result.

Effects of Chronic Stress

The hypothalamic-pituitary-adrenal axis (HPA axis) is a major part of the neuroendocrine system that controls reactions to stress. The HPA axis triggers a set of interactions among the glands, hormones, and parts of the midbrain that mediate the general adaptation syndrome. Continued stress, however, leads to loss of these normal control mechanisms. As a result, the adrenals continue to produce cortisol, which exhausts the stress mechanism and leads to fatigue and depression. Cortisol also interferes with serotonin activity, furthering the depressive effect.

Consistently high cortisol levels lead to suppression of the immune system through increased production of interleukin-6, an immune system messenger. Not surprisingly, then, research indicates that stress and depression have a negative effect on the immune system. Reduced immunity renders the body more susceptible to everything from colds and flu to cancer. For example, the incidence of serious illness, including cancer, is significantly higher among people who have suffered the death of a spouse in the previous year. Although severe, prolonged stress does not cause death directly, it does cause the body to lose its ability to fight disease in its effort to manage the stress. Stress also causes the body to release fat and cholesterol into the bloodstream, which in turn leads to clogging of the arteries and may eventually result in heart attack or stroke.

Many people start drinking alcohol to excess to combat their stress. Other manifestations of chronic stress include depression, headaches, insomnia, ulcers, and asthma. Fortunately, this immune suppression process can be corrected with psychotherapy, medication, or any number of other positive influences that restore hope and a feeling of self-esteem. The ability of human beings to recover from adversity is remarkable.

You are the Provider Summary

1. What are some of the potential complications that can occur from missing dialysis?

Patients who have end-stage renal disease depend on dialysis to take on the workload of the kidneys, such as being a filter for toxins and maintaining proper fluid balance and electrolyte balance. An interruption in these vital functions can lead to the development of problems such as congestive heart failure, myocardial infarction, pulmonary edema, arrhythmias, electrolyte imbalances, and medication toxicity.

2. Does renal disease affect other organ systems?

Yes; all organ systems are affected by renal failure. Patients can develop problems similar to those experienced by diabetics and patients with hypertension. For example, patients with renal disease often develop problems with peripheral neuropathy, gastrointestinal disturbances, and anemia.

3. What should you monitor your patient for?

The patient is presenting with a number of issues, any of which could potentially lead to problems. First and foremost, she is hypotensive and in respiratory distress. You need to keep a watchful eye on her blood pressure and respiratory status, being prepared to intubate if necessary. The tall T waves on the ECG are characteristic of hyperkalemia. The heart does not play nice in an environment in which the potassium is out of line. Frequently check the monitor for the development of ventricular arrhythmias such as premature ventricular contractions, ventricular tachycardia, and ventricular fibrillation.

4. Which interventions should you consider at this point, if any?

At this point, Mrs. Jensen is receiving high-flow supplemental oxygen. The patient definitely requires cardiac monitoring and intravenous access for possible fluid and medication administration.

5. Is the patient going into shock? If so, what type?

Yes; the patient is going into shock, but which type can be a little tricky. We know from her clinical presentation that septic shock is a possibility due to the signs of infection at the shunt site. With a history of a past myocardial infarction and congestive heart failure, cardiogenic shock cannot be ruled out as a possible cause.

6. Why is a fluid bolus appropriate in this setting?

Hypotension is a common side effect of dialysis that can result from the change in fluid and/or electrolyte distribution. Most patients will respond favorably to a small fluid bolus (200 to 250 mL) returning fluid back to the blood vessels. This small amount of fluid should not have a negative effect in the respiratory status of your patient.

7. How did the inflammatory process manifest itself in this patient?

The inflammatory process manifested itself in both local and systemic effects. Local effects include the development of redness, swelling, tenderness, and heat at the shunt site. Systemic involvement of the inflammatory process is seen in the presence of fever.

8. What are other signs and symptoms of hyperkalemia?

Patient's who have hyperkalemia may also present with irritability, abdominal distention, nausea, diarrhea, oliguria, weakness, or paralysis. Good history taking will help you clue into this serious electrolyte imbalance and initiate therapy!

Prep Kit

▬ Ready for Review

- All cells except red blood cells and platelets have three main components: a nucleus, cytoplasm, and a cell membrane.
- There are four major tissue types: epithelial tissue; connective tissue, muscle tissue, and nervous tissue.
- When cells are exposed to adverse conditions, they go through a process of adaptation (which can be temporary or permanent) to protect themselves from injury. Examples of adaptations include atrophy, hypertrophy, hyperplasia, dysplasia, and metaplasia.
- The cellular environment refers to the distribution of cells, molecules, and fluids throughout the body. It changes with aging, exercise, pregnancy, medications, disease, and injury. Body fluids contain water, sodium, chloride, potassium, calcium, phosphorus, and magnesium.
- pH is a measurement of hydrogen ion concentration. Normal body functions depend on an acid–base balance that remains within the normal physiologic pH range of 7.35 to 7.45.
- Cellular injury results from causes such as chemical exposure, infectious agents, immunologic responses, inflammatory responses, prolonged periods of hypoxia, genetic factors, nutritional imbalances, and physical agents.
- Age- and sex-associated factors interact with a combination of genetic and environmental factors, lifestyle, and anatomic or hormonal differences to cause disease.
- Analyzing disease risk involves consideration of disease rates (incidence, prevalence, mortality) and disease risk factors (causal and noncausal). These risk factors, age, and sex differences interact to influence an individual's level of risk.
- A true genetic risk is passed through generations on a gene. In contrast, a familial tendency may "cluster" in family groups despite lack of evidence for heritable gene-associated abnormalities. In autosomal dominant inheritance, a person needs to inherit only one copy of a particular form of a gene to show that trait. In autosomal recessive inheritance, the person must inherit two copies of a particular form of a gene to show the trait.
- Immunologic diseases occur because of hyperactivity or hypoactivity of the immune system. Allergies are acquired following initial exposure to a stimulant, known as an allergen. Repeated exposures cause a reaction by the immune system to the allergen.
- Perfusion is the delivery of oxygen and nutrients to cells, organs, and tissues through the circulatory system. Hypoperfusion occurs when the level of tissue perfusion falls below normal.
- Shock is an abnormal state associated with inadequate oxygen and nutrient delivery to the metabolic apparatus of the cell, resulting in an impairment of cell metabolism.
- Multiple organ dysfunction syndrome (MODS) is a progressive condition usually characterized by combined failure of several organs, such as the lungs, liver, and kidney, along with some clotting mechanisms. It occurs after severe illness or injury.
- The immune system includes all of the structures and processes that mount a defense against foreign substances and disease-causing agents. The body has three lines of defense: anatomic barriers, the inflammatory response, and the immune response.
- The immune system has two anatomic components: the lymphoid tissues of the body and the cells that are responsible for the immune response.
- The primary cells of the immune system are the white blood cells, or leukocytes.
- There are two general types of immune response: native and acquired.
- Immunity may be either humoral or cell-mediated.
- The antibodies secreted by B cells are called immunoglobulins. Antibodies make antigens more visible to the immune system in three ways: by acting as opsonins, by making antigens clump, and by inactivating bacterial toxins.

- The inflammatory response is a reaction of the tissues of the body, triggered by cellular injury, to irritation or injury that is characterized by pain, swelling, redness, and heat.
- The two most common causes of inflammation are infection and physical agents.
- Cytokines are products of cells that affect the functioning of other cells; they include interleukins, lymphokines, and interferon.
- Chronic inflammatory responses are usually caused by an unsuccessful acute inflammatory response after the invasion of a foreign body, persistent infection, or antigen.
- Normal wound healing involves four steps: repair of damaged tissue, removal of inflammatory debris, restoration of tissues to a normal state, and regeneration of cells.
- Wounds may heal by either primary or secondary intention.
- Hypersensitivity is an increased bodily response to any substance to which the person is abnormally sensitive. A hypersensitivity reaction may be immediate, occurring within seconds to minutes, or delayed, occurring hours to days after exposure to the antigen.
- Immunodeficiency may be congenital or acquired.
- Stress does not cause death directly, but it can permit diseases that ultimately lead to the patient's death to flourish.
- The general adaptation syndrome describes the body's short-term and long-term reactions to stress.

▬ Vital Vocabulary

acidosis A blood pH of less than 7.35.

acquired immunity A highly specific, inducible, discriminatory, and permanent method by which literally armies of cells respond to an immune stimulant.

activation Mediators of inflammation trigger the appearance of molecules known as selectins and integrins on the surfaces of endothelial cells and PMNs, respectively.

active hyperemia The dilation of arterioles after transient arteriolar constriction, which allows influx of blood under increased pressure.

adhesion The attachment of PMNs to endothelial cells, mediated by selectins and integrins.

adipose tissue A connective tissue containing large amounts of lipids.

alkalosis A blood pH greater than 7.45.

allergen Any substance that causes a hypersensitivity reaction.

allergy Hypersensitivity reaction to the presence of an agent (allergen) that is intrinsically harmless.

anaphylactic shock A severe hypersensitivity reaction that involves bronchoconstriction and cardiovascular collapse.

angiogenesis The growth of new blood vessels.

antibodies Proteins secreted by certain immune cells that bind antigens to make them more visible to the immune system.

antigen A foreign substance recognized by the immune system.

apoptosis Normal, genetically programmed cell death.

Arthus reaction A localized reaction involving vascular inflammation in response to an IgG-mediated allergic response.

asthma A chronic inflammatory lower airway condition resulting in intermittent wheezing and excess mucus production.

atopic The medical term for having an allergic tendency.

atrophy A decrease in cell size due to a loss of subcellular components.

autoantibodies Antibodies directed against the patient.

autocrine hormone A hormone that acts on the cell that has secreted it.

autoimmunity The production of antibodies or T cells that work against the tissues of a person's own body, producing autoimmune disease or a hypersensitivity reaction.

autosomal dominant A pattern of inheritance that involves genes that are located on autosomes or the nonsex chromosomes. You only need to inherit a single copy of a particular form of a gene to show the trait.

autosomal recessive A pattern of inheritance that involves genes located on autosomes or the nonsex chromosomes. You must inherit two copies of a particular form of a gene to show the trait.

axon Part of the neuron that conducts the impulses away from the cell body.

basophils Approximately 1% of the leukocytes, they are essential to nonspecific immune response to inflammation due to their role in releasing histamine and other chemicals that dilate blood vessels.

bone marrow Specialized tissue found within bone.

buffers Molecules that modulate changes in pH to keep it in the physiologic range.

capillary refill time A test done on the fingers or toes by briefly squeezing the toe or finger, then evaluating the time it takes for the pink color to return.

cardiogenic shock A condition caused by loss of 40% or more of the functioning myocardium; the heart is no longer able to circulate sufficient blood to maintain adequate oxygen delivery.

cell-mediated immunity Immune process by which T-cell lymphocytes recognize antigens and then secrete cytokines (specifically lymphokines) that attract other cells or stimulate the production of cytotoxic cells that kill the infected cells.

cell signaling The process by which cells communicate with one another.

central shock A term that describes shock secondary to central pump failure, it includes both cardiogenic shock and obstructive shock.

chemotaxins Components of the activated complement system that attract leukocytes from the circulation to help fight infections.

chemotaxis The movement of additional white blood cells to an area of inflammation in response to the release of chemical mediators, such as neutrophils, injured tissue, and monocytes.

coagulation system The system that forms blood clots in the body and facilitates repairs to the vascular tree.

complement system A group of plasma proteins whose function is to do one of three things: attract leukocytes to sites of inflammation, activate leukocytes, and directly destroy cells.

connective tissue Tissue that serves to bind various tissue types together.

cytokines Products of cells that affect the function of other cells.

dendrites Part of the neuron that receives impulses from the axon and contains vesicles for release of neurotransmitters.

distributive shock Occurs when there is widespread dilation of the resistance vessels (small arterioles), the capacitance vessels (small venules), or both.

dysplasia An alteration in the size, shape, and organization of cells.

endocrine hormones Hormones that are carried to their target or cell group in the bloodstream.

endothelial cells Specific types of epithelial cells that serve the function of lining the blood vessels.

eosinophils Cells that make up approximately 1% to 3% of the leukocytes, which play a major role in allergic reactions and bronchoconstriction in an asthma attack.

epithelium Type of tissue that covers all external surfaces of the body.

etiology The cause of a disease process.

exocrine hormones Hormones that are secreted through ducts into an organ or onto epithelial surfaces.

feedback inhibition Negative feedback resulting in the decrease of an action in the body.

fibrin A whitish, filamentous protein formed by the action of thrombin on fibrinogen. Fibrin is the protein that polymerizes (bonds) to form the fibrous component of a blood clot.

fibrinolysis cascade The breakdown of fibrin in blood clots, and the prevention of the polymerization of fibrin into new clots.

free radicals Molecules that are missing one electron in their outer shell.

general adaptation syndrome A three-stage description of the body's short-term and long-term reactions to stress.

gut-associated lymphoid tissue (GALT) The lymphoid tissue that lies under the inner lining of the esophagus and intestines.

hapten A substance that normally does not stimulate an immune response but can be combined with an antigen and at a later point initiate an antibody response.

helper T cells A type of T lymphocyte that is involved in both cell-mediated and antibody-mediated immune responses. It secretes cytokines that stimulate the B cells and other T cells.

hemochromatosis An inherited disease in which the body absorbs more iron than it needs and stores it in the liver, kidneys, and pancreas.

hemolytic anemia A disease characterized by increased destruction of the red blood cells. It can occur from an Rh factor reaction, exposure to chemicals, or a disorder of the immune system.

hemophilia An inherited sex-linked disorder characterized by excessive bleeding.

histamine A vasoactive amine that increases vascular permeability and causes vasodilation.

homeostasis is a term derived from the Greek words for "same" and "steady." All organisms constantly adjust their physiologic processes in an effort to maintain an internal balance.

hormones Proteins formed in specialized organs or glands and carried to another organ or group of cells in the same organism. Hormones regulate many body functions, including metabolism, growth, and temperature.

humoral immunity The immunity that utilizes antibodies made by B-cell lymphocytes.

hypercalcemia A condition in which calcium levels are elevated.

hypercholesterolemia An elevated blood cholesterol level.

hyperkalemia An elevated blood serum potassium level.

hypermagnesemia An increased serum magnesium level.

hypernatremia A blood serum sodium level greater than 148 mEq/L and a serum osmolarity greater than 295 mOsm/kg.

hyperphosphatemia An elevated blood serum phosphate level.

hyperplasia An increase in the actual number of cells in an organ or tissue, usually resulting in an increase in size of the organ or tissue.

hypersensitivity A generic term for bodily responses to a substance to which a patient is abnormally sensitive.

hypertonic solution A solution with an osmolarity greater than intracellular fluid.

hypertrophy An increase in the size of the cells due to synthesis of more subcellular components, leading to an increase in tissue and organ size.

hypocalcemia A decreased serum calcium level.

hypokalemia A decreased blood serum potassium.

hypomagnesemia A decreased serum magnesium level.

hyponatremia A blood serum sodium level that is below 135 mEq/L and a serum osmolarity that is less than 280 mOsm/kg.

hypoperfusion A condition that occurs when the level of tissue perfusion decreases below that needed to maintain normal cellular functions.

hypophosphatemia A decreased blood serum phosphate level.

hypothalamic-pituitary-adrenal (HPA) axis A major part of the neuroendocrine system that controls reactions to stress. It is the mechanism for a set of interactions among glands, hormones, and parts of the midbrain that mediate the general adaptation syndrome.

hypotonic solution A solution with an osmolarity lower than intracellular fluid.

hypovolemic shock A condition that occurs when the circulating blood volume is inadequate to deliver adequate oxygen and nutrients to the body.

immune response The body's defense reaction to any substance that is recognized as foreign.

immune system The body system that includes all of the structures and processes designed to mount a defense against foreign substances and disease-causing agents.

immunodeficiency An abnormal condition in which some part of the body's immune system is inadequate, and consequently resistance to infectious disease is decreased.

immunogen An antigen that activates immune cells to generate an immune response against itself.

immunoglobulins Antibodies secreted by the B cells.

incidence The frequency with which a disease occurs.

inflammatory response A reaction by tissues of the body to irritation or injury, characterized by pain, swelling, redness, and heat.

interferon Protein produced by cells in response to viral invasion. Interferon is released into the bloodstream or intercellular fluid to induce healthy cells to manufacture an enzyme that counters the infection.

interleukins Chemical substances that attract white blood cells to the sites of injury and bacterial invasion.

isoimmunity Formation of antibodies or T cells that are directed against antigens or another person's cells.

isotonic solution A solution with the same osmolarity as intracellular fluid (280 mOsm/L).

kinin system A general term for a group of polypeptides that mediate inflammatory responses by stimulating visceral smooth muscle and relaxing vascular smooth muscle to produce vasodilation.

leukocytes The white blood cells responsible for fighting off infection.

leukocytosis Elevation of the white blood cell count often due to inflammation.

leukotrienes Arachidonic acid metabolites that function as chemical mediators of inflammation. Also known as slow-reacting substances of anaphylaxis (SRS-A).

ligand Any molecule that binds a receptor leading to a reaction.

lymph A thin, watery fluid that bathes the tissues of the body.

lymphatic system A network of capillaries, vessels, ducts, nodes, and organs that helps to maintain the fluid environment of the body by producing lymph and transporting it through the body.

lymphocytes The white blood cells responsible for a large part of the body's immune protection.

lymphokines Cytokines released by lymphocytes, including many of the interleukins, gamma interferon, tumor necrosis factor beta, and chemokines.

macrophages Cells that developed from the monocytes that provide the body's first line of defense in the inflammatory process.

margination Loss of fluid from the blood vessels into the tissue, causing the blood left in the vessels to have an increased viscosity, which in turn slows the flow of blood and produces stasis.

mast cells The cells that resemble basophils but do not circulate in the blood. Mast cells play a role in allergic reactions, immunity, and wound healing.

membrane attack complex (MAC) Molecules that insert themselves into the bacterial membrane, leading to weakened areas in the membrane.

metaplasia A reversible, cellular adaptation in which one adult cell type is replaced by another adult cell type.

mitochondria The metabolic center or powerhouse of the cell. They are small and rod-shaped organelles.

monocytes Mononuclear phagocytic white blood cells derived from myeloid stem cells. They circulate in the bloodstream for about 24 hours and then move into tissues to mature into macrophages.

mortality The number of deaths from a disease in a given population.

mucosal-associated lymphoid tissue (MALT) The lymphoid tissue associated with the skin and the respiratory, urinary, and reproductive traits as well as the tonsils.

multiple organ dysfunction syndrome (MODS) A progressive condition usually characterized by combined failure of several organs, such as the lungs, liver, and kidney, along with some clotting mechanisms, which occurs after severe illness or injury.

native immunity A nonspecific cellular and humoral response that operates as the body's first line of defense against pathogens.

negative feedback The concept that once the desired effect of a process has been achieved, further action is inhibited until it is needed again; also called feedback inhibition.

neurogenic shock This condition usually results from spinal cord injury. The effect is loss of normal sympathetic nervous system tone and vasodilation.

neurotransmitters Proteins that transmit signals between cells of the nervous system.

neutrophils Cells that make up approximately 55% to 70% of the leukocytes responsible in large part for the body's protection against infection. They are readily attracted by foreign antigens and destroy them by phagocytosis.

nucleus A cellular organelle that contains the genetic information. The nucleus controls the function and structure of a cell.

obstructive shock This occurs when there is a block to blood flow in the heart or great vessels.

oliguria Decreased urine output.

opsoninization Occurs when an antibody coats an antigen to facilitate its recognition by immune cells.

organelles Internal cellular structures that carry out specific functions for the cell.

osmosis The movement of water down its concentration gradient across a membrane.

paracrine hormones Hormones that diffuse through intracellular spaces to their target.

pathophysiology The study of how normal physiologic processes are affected by disease.

perfusion The delivery of oxygen and nutrients to the cells, organs, and tissues of the body. Also involves the removal of wastes.

pericardial tamponade Impairment of diastolic filling of the right ventricle due to significant amounts of fluid in the pericardial sac surrounding the heart, leading to a decrease in the cardiac output.

peripheral nerves All of the nerves of the body extending from the brain and spinal cord.

peripheral shock A term that describes shock secondary to peripheral circulatory abnormalities—includes both hypovolemic shock and distributive shock.

pH The measure of acidity or alkalinity of a solution.

phagocyte A kind of cell that engulfs and consumes foreign material such as microorganisms and debris.

phagocytosis Process in which one cell eats or engulfs a foreign substance to destroy it.

polymorphonuclear neutrophils (PMNs) A type of white blood cell formed by bone marrow tissue that possesses a nucleus consisting of several parts or lobes connected by fine strands; a variety of leukocyte.

polyuria Frequent and plentiful urination.

prevalence The number of cases of a disease in a specific population over time.

prostaglandins A group of lipids that act as chemical messengers.

pyrogens Chemicals or proteins that travel to the brain and affect the hypothalamus, and stimulate a rise in the body's core temperature.

renin-angiotensin-aldosterone system (RAAS) A complex feedback mechanism responsible for the kidney's regulation of sodium in the body.

Rh factor An antigen present in the erythrocytes (red blood cells) of about 85% of people.

ribonucleic acid (RNA) Nucleic acid associated with controlling cellular activities.

septic shock This occurs as a result of widespread infection, usually bacterial. Untreated, the result is multiple organ dysfunction syndrome (MODS) and often death.

serotonin A vasoactive amine that increases vascular permeability to cause vasodilation.

serum sickness A condition in which antigen antibody complexes formed in the bloodstream deposit in sites around the body, most notably in the kidney, with resultant inflammatory reactions.

slow-reacting substances of anaphylaxis (SRS-A) Biologically active compounds derived from arachidonic acid called leukotrienes.

T killer cells Cells released during a type IV allergic reaction that kill antigen-bearing target cells.

tonicity Tension exerted on a cell due to water movement across the cell membrane.

transmigration (diapedesis) The PMNs permeate through the vessel wall, moving into the interstitial space.

urticaria Multiple small, raised areas on the skin that may be one of the warning signs of impending anaphylaxis. Also known as hives.

vasculitis An inflammation of the blood vessels.

vasoactive amines Substances such as histamine and serotonin that increase vascular permeability.

virulence A measure of the disease-causing ability of a microorganism.

Points to Ponder

You have a new partner for the day and you respond to a "difficulty breathing" call. Once there, your patient advises that he has an "autoimmune disease." Your partner leans over to you and says quietly, "Oh no, this guy has AIDS and we're going to get it."

How are you going to explain this patient's medical condition to your partner without doing so in front of your patient?

Issues: Bloodborne Pathogens, Autoimmune Diseases, Universal Precautions.

Assessment in Action

You have responded to a 40-year-old male patient who crashed on his motorcycle. The patient is wearing a helmet and is conscious but agitated and restless. You notice a large amount of blood on the ground around the patient's lower body. As you complete your assessment, you find the patient has an unstable pelvis and an open femur fracture. Your initial vital signs are blood pressure, 136/70 mm Hg; pulse, 100 beats/min; and respiration, 16 breaths/min. You know your patient has lost a considerable amount of blood and are concerned the patient may start exhibiting signs of shock.

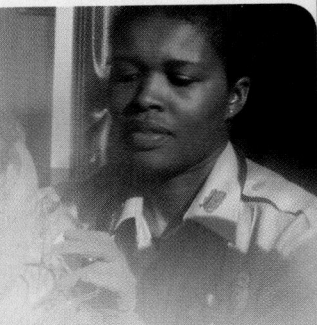

1. **What are the two types of shock?**
   A. Arterial and venous
   B. Central and peripheral
   C. Hypovolemic and systemic
   D. Peripheral and distributive

2. **What type of shock involves fluid loss?**
   A. Anaphylactic
   B. Cardiogenic
   C. Hypovolemic
   D. Septic

3. **What are the two types of hypovolemic shock and which one is exhibited by this patient?**
   A. Exogenous and endogenious
   B. Aerobic and anerobic
   C. Kallikrein and kinin
   D. Angiotensin and aldosterone

4. **Based on your assessment of this patient, his agitation, anxiety, and restlessness may be a sign of:**
   A. decompensated shock.
   B. compensated shock.
   C. neurogenic shock.
   D. distributive shock.

5. **Which adult blood pressure reading would represent decompensated shock?**
   A. The systolic blood pressure is greater than 5% for the age range
   B. The systolic blood pressure is less than 5% for the age range
   C. The diastolic blood pressure is greater than 5% for the age range
   D. The diastolic blood pressure is less than 5% for the age range

6. **A normal capillary refill time should be:**
   A. more than 4 seconds.
   B. 3 to 4 seconds.
   C. greater than 2 seconds.
   D. less than 2 seconds.

Challenging Question

7. **Your unit has a pair of MAST (military antishock trousers) in the inventory. Since your patient has an obvious pelvic injury and a decompensated blood pressure, should you use them?**

7 Pharmacology

Objectives

Cognitive

1-7.1 Describe historical trends in pharmacology. (p 7.3)
1-7.2 Differentiate among the chemical, generic (nonproprietary), and trade (proprietary) names of a drug. (p 7.5)
1-7.3 List the four main sources of drug products. (p 7.5)
1-7.4 Describe how drugs are classified. (p 7.8)
1-7.5 List the authoritative sources for drug information. (p 7.5)
1-7.6 List legislative acts controlling drug use and abuse in the United States. (p 7.6)
1-7.7 Differentiate among Schedule I, II, III, IV, and V substances. (p 7.7)
1-7.8 List examples of substances in each schedule. (p 7.7)
1-7.9 Discuss standardization of drugs. (p 7.8)
1-7.10 Discuss investigational drugs, including the Food and Drug Administration (FDA) approval process and the FDA classifications for newly approved drugs. (p 7.8)
1-7.11 Discuss special consideration in drug treatment with regard to pregnant, pediatric and geriatric patients. (p 7.9)
1-7.12 Discuss the paramedic's responsibilities and scope of management pertinent to the administration of medications. (p 7.10)
1-7.13 Review the specific anatomy and physiology pertinent to pharmacology with additional attention to autonomic pharmacology. (p 7.11)
1-7.14 List and describe general properties of drugs. (p 7.14)
1-7.15 List and describe liquid and solid drug forms. (p 7.15)
1-7.16 List and differentiate routes of drug administration. (p 7.16)
1-7.17 Differentiate between enteral and parenteral routes of drug administration. (p 7.17)
1-7.18 Describe mechanisms of drug action. (p 7.19)
1-7.19 List and differentiate the phases of drug activity, including the pharmaceutical, pharmacokinetic, and pharmacodynamic phases. (p 7.21)
1-7.20 Describe the process called pharmacokinetics, pharmacodynamics, including theories of drug action, drug-response relationship, factors altering drug responses, predictable drug responses, iatrogenic drug responses, and unpredictable adverse drug responses. (p 7.18, 7.21)
1-7.21 Differentiate among drug interactions. (p 7.22)
1-7.22 Discuss considerations for storing and securing medications. (p 7.23)
1-7.23 List the component of a drug profile by classification. (p 7.24)
1-7.24 List and describe drugs that the paramedic may administer according to local protocol. (p 7.24)
1-7.25 Integrate pathophysiological principles of pharmacology with patient assessment. (p 7.33)
1-7.26 Synthesize patient history information and assessment findings to form a field impression. (p 7.33)
1-7.27 Synthesize a field impression to implement a pharmacologic management plan. (p 7.34)
1-7.28 Assess the pathophysiology of a patient's condition by identifying classifications of drugs. (p 7.24)

Affective

1-7.29 Serve as a model for obtaining a history by identifying classifications of drugs. (p 7.33)
1-7.30 Defend the administration of drugs by a paramedic to effect positive therapeutic effects. (p 7.10)
1-7.31 Advocate drug education through identification of drug classifications. (p 7.24)

Psychomotor

None

Introduction

The goal of emergency pharmacology in the prehospital setting is to use medications to reverse, prevent, or control various diseases and illnesses, chronic and acute. To achieve this goal, prehospital providers must be able to interpret a patient's history and physical findings, formulate a management plan, and incorporate appropriate treatment modalities, including pharmacology and medication administration. Medication errors are the leading cause of patient safety errors in health care. For this reason, medications must always be delivered according to the *six rights:* the Right patient, the Right dose, the Right route, the Right time, the Right medication, and the Right patient care report (PCR) documentation ⬛ Table 7-1 ▸ . This chapter will aid you in understanding the medications used to treat specific medical problems, how they are administered to achieve therapeutic and nontoxic levels, and their actions, absorption, and elimination, while keeping in mind the six rights of medication administration.

All medications are poisons if they are given to the wrong patient or in toxic quantities. For this reason, paramedics and health care personnel must have a strong understanding of pharmacology and use great caution when administering medications to patients. In this chapter, the drugs and doses mentioned comply with nationally accepted guidelines. Paramedics must become familiar with the specific medications, uses, and doses that are used in their systems as approved by the medical director. The medications discussed in this chapter may not be administered without authorization of medical direction through approved standing orders or by direct verbal communication with an authorized medical control physician.

Historical Trends in Pharmacology

The use of chemical compounds to treat illnesses is an ancient practice. Records of medication use date back thousands of years from the use of plants and minerals to today's modern and ever-changing methods of synthetic and laboratory-engineered medications. The study of medications and their effect or actions on the body is called pharmacology.

Ancient Health Care

Ancient Egyptian health care was heavily influenced by spiritual beliefs. It did, however, incorporate basic first-aid techniques to treat obvious external injuries. Ancient doctors also used chemical compounds to treat certain ailments. In fact, documents have been found containing formularies for more than 700 medications.

The Pre-Renaissance and Post-Renaissance Periods

During the medieval period, doctors had no concept of viruses or bacteria or their infectious properties. People relied on the idea that sickness represented punishment for one's sins. Attempts to treat ailments centered on approaches intended to counteract the presenting symptoms. Presenting symptoms were categorized based on their moisture and temperature: Blood was hot and wet, phlegm was cold and wet, black bile was cold and dry, and yellow bile was hot and dry. According to the prevailing theory of the time, when a person became sick, one of these four items was out of balance. Phlegm, for example, needed to be counteracted by its opposite, yellow

You are the Provider Part 1

You and your partner are on your way back to the station when you are called to an assisted-living facility for an unknown medical. Upon arrival, you are met in the lobby by the patient's son, who brings you back to the apartment. The door to the apartment is open when you get there, and you see an older man sitting on a recliner in the living room. As you approach him and introduce yourself, you note that he is pale and slightly diaphoretic. He tells you that he has been feeling "skips in his chest" for the past couple of hours and that he becomes extremely lightheaded when he stands. He also says he feels "a little winded" and states that his vision "is off." He denies having any chest pain, headaches, or any other symptoms. He states that he takes heart medications but cannot recall what they are. His son recalls that his father keeps a list of his medications and medical history on an index card in his wallet.

Initial Assessment	Recording Time: 0 Minutes
Appearance	Awake and ill-appearing
Level of consciousness	A (Alert to person, place and day)
Airway	Open and clear
Breathing	Slightly elevated rate with adequate chest rise and volume
Circulation	Weak, irregular radial pulses with pale, cool, moist skin

1. What are some potential differential diagnoses?
2. What types of medications might your patient be taking?

Table 7-1 | The Six Rights of Medication Administration

1. Right patient

Although you will typically treat one patient at a time, sometimes you may have to manage multiple patients. It is critical to confirm the identity of a patient before administering any medication—especially when patients are unconscious or are unable to communicate (because of extremes of age, altered consciousness, or other factors). Always make an attempt to have the patient confirm his or her identity verbally, or confirm the identity of the patient yourself through identification devices (bracelets, ID cards). A critical issue, as identified in your SAMPLE history, is to ensure that the patient does not have allergies to the medication(s) you intend to give **Figure 7-1 ▶** .

2. Right medication

Administration of the wrong medication is the most common pharmacology-related error. Several factors may lead to "wrong medication" errors, including similar labeling and packaging, similar names and storage practices, and poor communication. Always repeat back (echo) the medication order, and confirm that the packaging matches the intended order. Avoid using abbreviations, verify the route of administration, and always recheck the order before administration.

3. Right dose

Dosages of nearly every medication depend on patient-specific factors (such as condition, weight, age); the actual dosage called for is often not equal to the amount supplied in an ampule or prefilled syringe in the prehospital setting. Therefore, you will have to calculate the patient's specific dose. When calculating the correct dose, always recheck your math and, if possible, have your partner recheck and verify the final dose.

4. Right route

Many medications can be administered by a variety of routes; the optimal route depends on the patient's condition and the speed with which the medication needs to take effect. Errors can occur when medication doses and routes are confused. For example, intravenous (IV) drip doses can be different concentrations than the same medication injected into an IV as a bolus. Another important route-related issue is the patient's condition. If a patient is in profound shock, you must consider how well the medication will be absorbed and distributed to target tissues. Choosing the right route makes a big difference in allowing the medication to have the correct effect.

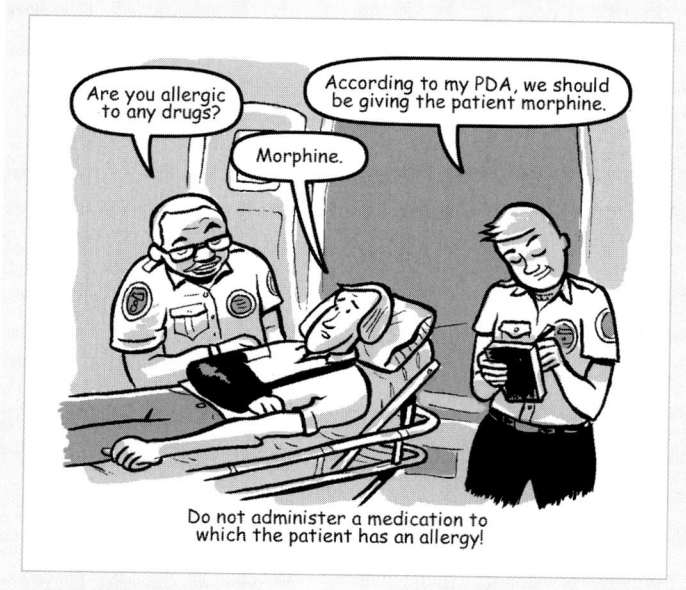

Do not administer a medication to which the patient has an allergy!

Figure 7-1

5. Right time

Because all medications take a certain amount of time to take effect and may have the potential to interfere with other medications, you must always follow the recommended guidelines for the proper frequency of medication administration. Evaluate the patient's condition before and after you administer any medication, and document any noted response or change in the patient's condition. Also remember that some medications require a specific administration frequency to maintain a therapeutic level.

6. Right documentation and reporting

Because paramedics frequently transfer care of a patient to other health care providers, it is critical to document in writing the medications administered, the dose, when they were administered, and what kinds of changes the patient has experienced. Whenever possible, communicate this information in writing, on the PCR, and in a verbal report to the next level of care.

---

bile. Therefore, the patient would need to take a prescription made from plants and animals that were hot and dry and likely contained a fair amount of bile. After the Renaissance, medication use took on a slightly more scientific approach. Through the process of observation, early health care providers began to recognize—albeit to a limited extent—that certain compounds (such as plants and minerals) were effective for treating some ailments and ineffective for others.

Modern Health Care

The modern pharmaceutical industry began in the 19th century with the discovery of highly active medicinal compounds

that could be manufactured most efficiently on a large scale. Today, pharmaceuticals form the basis of a $243 billion industry. Thanks to the thousands of <u>drugs</u> currently in use and the new drugs approved on a daily basis, health care has made tremendous strides in our ability to care for sick and injured people. Although not every condition has a cure, virtually all diseases can be treated to some degree with medications.

Pharmaceuticals can be expected to continue to make great strides in all aspects of disease treatment. As cancer rates continue to rise, treatments and cures for this set of diseases are the focus of much research. Remarkable progress continues to be made in the prevention and treatment of heart disease and stroke. The pharmaceutical industry is likely to continue expanding into biotechnology, including the use of compounds to target specific proteins or DNA. Ideally, work on the molecular level will lead to the eradication of some of the leading killers of today.

Medication Names

A medication is a drug that has been approved by the government agency that regulates pharmaceuticals (in the United States, the Food and Drug Administration, or FDA) for the purpose of curing or reducing the symptoms of an illness or medical condition or to assist in the diagnosis, treatment, or prevention of a disease. A drug may also be given in an attempt to alter the disease process itself.

Medications may be available either with or without a prescription. Prescription-only medicines (POM) are available at a pharmacy and may be purchased only with a physician's prescription. In contrast, over-the-counter (OTC) medications do not require a prescription and are available in many places—pharmacies, convenience stores, and grocery stores, for example—without special restrictions. Prescription-only medicines can be given OTC status only if they are considered safe enough that most people will not hurt themselves accidentally by taking the medication as instructed.

Pharmaceutical companies invest more than $34 billion each year in research and development. Not surprisingly, they are eager to protect their investments by obtaining patents on their new drugs. A patent gives its holder exclusive rights to produce and sell the drug until the patent expires. After it loses its patent, the medication may then be available as a generic drug (nonpatented) from multiple sources.

Because thousands of medications are already on the market and more emerge every year (hundreds are approved each year in the United States alone), a systematic way of naming them is essential. All medications are assigned four names: chemical, generic, trade, and official.

- The chemical name describes the drug's chemical makeup—that is, its composition and molecular structure.
- The generic name (or nonproprietary name) is a general name for a drug. Although it is not manufacturer-specific, the generic name is usually created by the company that first manufactures the chemical. The generic name is generally derived from the chemical name but is shorter and simpler.
- The trade name (or brand name) is the unique name under which the original manufacturer registers the new drug with the FDA. Use of the "registered" symbol (®) in the upper-right corner of the trade name indicates that it has been registered as a trademark; a trade name may also be signified by capitalizing the name. If a given drug is

marketed by a number of manufacturers, it may have several trade names. Some familiar trade names include Lipitor (a cholesterol-lowering medication), Zyrtec (used to treat common allergies), and Xanax (used to treat anxiety disorders).

- Once the generic name has been approved by the US Adopted Names Council and the drug has been approved by the FDA, the name is listed in the *United States Pharmacopeia* (USP) and becomes the drug's official name. It is designated by the addition of the initials "USP" following the name.

To see how this naming system works, consider the names given to amiodarone, an important antidysrrhythmic carried by paramedics:

- Chemical name: 2-butyl-3-benzofuranyl 4-[2-(diethylamino)-ethoxy]-3,5-diiodophenyl ketone hydrochloride
- Generic name: amiodarone
- Trade names: Cordarone, Pacerone
- Official name: amiodarone USP

In this text, we will refer to drugs by their generic names. When a drug is widely known by its trade name, the trade name will be capitalized and placed in parentheses in this text after the generic name—for example, diazepam (Valium), norepinephrine (Levophed), furosemide (Lasix), naloxone (Narcan), and oxytocin (Pitocin).

Sources of Drugs

The drugs we use are derived from four principal sources: animal, vegetable, mineral, and synthetic compounds Figure 7-2 . Plant sources of drugs include a variety of roots, leaves, flowers, and seeds. For example, digitalis, which is used in the treatment of heart failure, is prepared from the dried leaves of a wildflower called purple foxglove. In contrast, insulin, a medication taken by diabetics, is usually prepared from the pancreas of animals (primarily pigs). Armour, a thyroid medication, is derived from desiccated pig thyroid. Minerals used in the treatment of medical problems include calcium, iron, and magnesium. Drugs that are manufactured synthetically include synthetic forms of vitamins, steroids, narcotics, and many others.

Sources of Drug Information

In addition to standard continuing education, you should stay abreast of newly approved medications and current research. Drug information may be obtained from many sources, many of which are available in print and electronic formats. Table 7-2 discusses some of the most up-to-date and reliable resources.

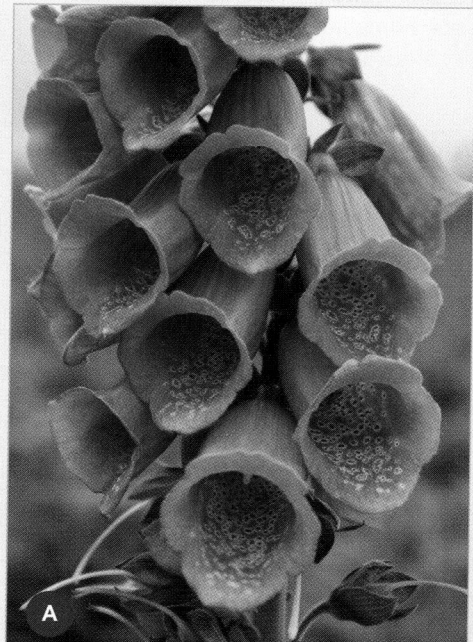

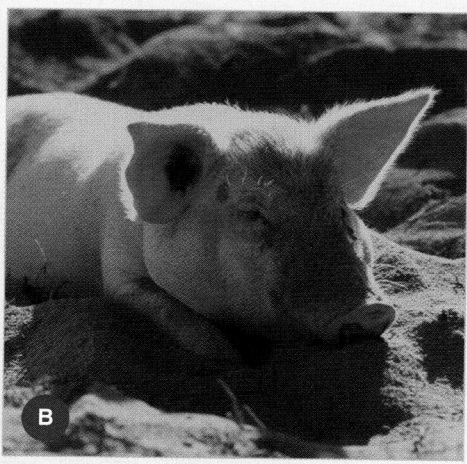

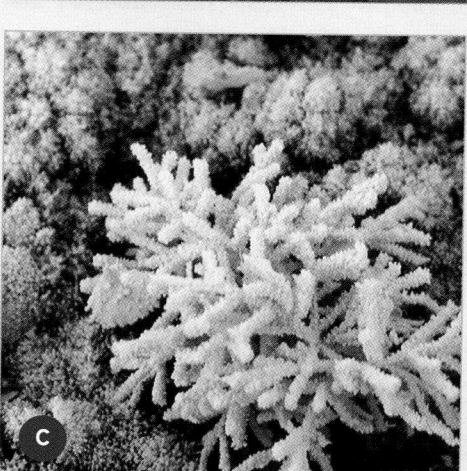

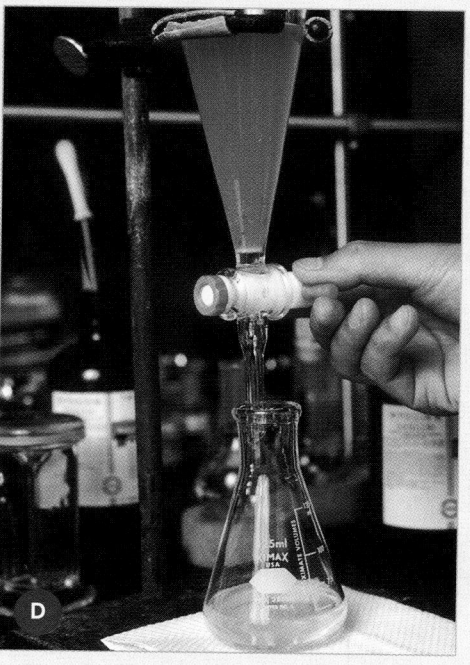

Figure 7-2 Drug sources and examples. **A.** Plant source. **B.** Animal source. **C.** Mineral source. **D.** Laboratory source.

US Regulation of Pharmaceuticals

The manufacture of pharmaceuticals in the United States and most other countries is subject to a variety of laws and regulations. The goal of these laws and regulations is to protect consumers. In particular, they prohibit manufacturers from making false claims about their drugs' benefits or advising patients to administer the drugs incorrectly. They also seek to protect patients from drugs that might cause harm and require drug manufacturers to publish information about side effects and known potential harmful effects of their products.

Laws and regulations also outline standards for drug manufacture to ensure that drugs produced by different manufacturers are of uniform strength and purity. In the United States, these drug standards are published in the *United States Pharmacopeia* and the *National Formulary*. In addition, several federal laws have been enacted to protect consumers (patients) from unsafe substances and unscrupulous manufacturers and distributors.

Drug-Related Legislation

The *Pure Food Act* (1906) was the first federal legislation in the United States aimed at protecting the public from mislabeled, poisonous, or otherwise harmful foods, medications, and alcoholic beverages. It required little more than the labeling of drugs, and it was replaced by more comprehensive legislation in 1938.

The *Food, Drug and Cosmetic Act* (1938, amended in 1952 and 1962) added several new provisions:

- Required drug makers to label their products, indicating whether they contain potentially habit-forming substances and to include warnings about possible side effects
- Authorized the creation of the FDA, discussed later in this chapter
- Mandated that dangerous drugs could be dispensed only with a prescription from a physician, dentist, or veterinarian

The *Harrison Narcotic Act* (1914) regulated the import, manufacture, prescription, and sale of several nonnarcotic

In recent years, the Internet has emerged as an invaluable resource for drug information. Familiarize yourself with reputable and reliable Internet resources. Software versions of some of these resources, such as Epocrates, are available for notebook computers, personal digital assistants (PDAs), and pocket personal computers. No matter which format you use, be sure to research the resource's accuracy before relying on the information. The most accurate sites are updated and then revised in your download site (for example, your PDA) on a regular basis.

Table 7-2	Sources of Drug Information
Source	**Description**
US FDA Center for Drug Evaluation and Research (CDER)	Mission is to ensure that safe and effective drugs are available in the United States
Physician's Desk Reference	Compiles data on most medications available in the United States; uses the information on file with the FDA; includes all of the necessary information on indications, dosages, contraindications, and adverse reactions. The book's size makes it difficult for use on an ambulance, but CD-ROM versions make it more accessible in the field.
Hospital formulary	A list of drugs, dosage forms, package sizes, and drug strengths stocked by hospitals and pharmacies; published as a quick reference to assist the physician and nursing staffs; divided into four general sections: introduction, therapeutic index, drug monographs, and general reference
Drug inserts	Printed document included in the packaging provided by the drug's manufacturer; generally the same information submitted and approved by the FDA; when available, serves as a valuable reference; should not be confused with the information provided by a pharmacy when a patient receives a prescription, which is useful in obtaining information pertaining to a drug but is not necessarily all inclusive
AMA Drug Evaluation	A nonofficial compendium that provides another source of useful and miscellaneous drug information for pharmacists and medical practitioners; includes generic and trade names; information may not be limited to drugs approved for use by the FDA

drugs and cocaine, opium, and their derivatives. Precise record keeping about the dispensing of controlled drugs and registration of distributors, such as pharmacists, are required. Penalties—namely, fines and imprisonment—are specified for illegal possession or distribution of controlled drugs.

The *Narcotic Control Act* (1956) increased the penalties for violation of the Harrison Act, made the possession of heroin illegal, and outlawed the acquisition and transportation of marijuana.

In 1970, Congress enacted the *Controlled Substances Act,* comprehensive legislation dealing with narcotic and non-

narcotic drugs that have a potential for abuse. This act specifies requirements for registration, procurement, storage, distribution, and record keeping for these drugs and penalties for failure to comply with these requirements. The drugs covered by the Controlled Substances Act are classified into five categories, or *schedules,* according to their abuse potential:

- **Schedule I.** These drugs have the highest abuse potential and a propensity for severe dependence; none of them has any accepted medical application. In general, Schedule I drugs are completely outlawed. On very rare occasions, and under the strictest control by the FDA and Drug Enforcement Agency (DEA), these drugs may be used for research, analysis, and instruction only. Examples are heroin, lysergic acid diethylamide (LSD), marijuana, methylenedioxymethamphetamine (MDMA), psilocybin, and mescaline.
- **Schedule II.** These drugs have a very high abuse potential and may lead to severe addiction, but they have a lower propensity for addiction than Schedule I drugs. Examples are amphetamines, opiates, cocaine, meperidine hydrochloride (Demerol), and short-acting barbiturates.
- **Schedule III.** The narcotics listed in Schedule III (limited opioids combined with noncontrolled substances such as hydrocodone-acetaminophen combination [Vicodin] and acetaminophen [Tylenol] with codeine) have a lower potential for abuse than Schedule I and II drugs. These drugs may lead to low or moderate physical dependence or high psychologic dependence.
- **Schedule IV.** These drugs have a low abuse potential compared with Schedule III drugs and have limited dependence potential. Examples are phenobarbital, chloral hydrate, diazepam (Valium), and lorazepam (Ativan).
- **Schedule V.** Schedule V drugs (which include some opioids) have the lowest potential for abuse of all controlled substances, although they may lead to limited dependence. Examples include cough syrups containing codeine.

In the Field

It is important for you to become familiar with "street" names of these commonly used and abused drugs. Most users will not tell you they took methylenedioxymethamphetamine; most likely you will hear terms like ecstasy or XTC. Research or look up these common street terms.

Some states have enacted their own laws or regulations related to the use, storage, and handling of controlled substances. If the state law is more stringent than the federal law, the state law takes precedence.

Manufacturing-Related Regulations

Federal legislation also focuses on guaranteeing standardization of doses. Standardization assures patients that when they take a medication with a stated amount of the active ingredient, they will, in fact, receive that amount of the drug. Clearly, no one would want to be prescribed a certain dose of a drug and find that the actual medication contained twice (or half) the amount of active ingredient stated on the drug's label. For a drug to carry the USP label, the amount of active ingredients must be within 95% to 105% of that stated on the label. For example, if the label says "300 mg of amiodarone," the medication must contain between 285 mg and 315 mg of the drug.

The pharmaceutical manufacturers and the FDA use two techniques to analyze the content of a drug: assays and bioassays. An assay is an analysis of the drug itself to evaluate its potency. A bioassay is a procedure for determining the concentration, purity, and/or biological activity of a substance by measuring its effect on an organism, tissue, cell, or enzyme.

Government Agencies That Regulate Drugs

Today, regulation of drugs in the United States falls under the jurisdiction of several agencies:

- The FDA enforces the Food, Drug and Cosmetic Act. As part of its responsibilities, the FDA is charged with determining the safety and efficacy of drugs before they are allowed to enter the US market.
- The DEA, formerly the Bureau of Narcotics and Dangerous Drugs, was created by the Federal Controlled Substances Act of 1970. The DEA, which is a division of the Justice Department, is responsible for executing the provisions of the Controlled Substances Act, including the registration of physicians who are permitted to dispense controlled substances.
- The Public Health Service regulates biologic products—that is, medications made from living organisms such as antitoxins and vaccines.
- The Federal Trade Commission (FTC) monitors drug advertising and ensures that it is not misleading or inappropriate. More recently, the FTC has become involved in making recommendations to the FDA regarding direct-to-consumer (DTC) advertisements. The FTC found that DTC advertisements "generally benefit consumers" but stated that DTC ads should contain a "major statement of drug risks along with adequate provision for more complete risk information."

■ The Drug-Approval Process

New drugs are constantly being developed. The commercialization process, however, takes years—the average time for a drug to be developed, tested, and approved is about 9 years. In some cases, manufacturers spend most of those 9 years developing a drug only to find out that the drug does not work as envisioned or is too dangerous for human consumption.

All new drugs must go through animal studies and clinical trials in humans before they are approved for distribution.

Animal Studies

Animal studies are designed to identify tissues and organs sensitive to the drug's actions and to elucidate the drug's pharmacodynamic and pharmacokinetic properties. Testing in at least two animal species is required by law. After successful completion of animal studies, an investigational new drug may enter clinical trials in humans.

Clinical Trials

Clinical trials proceed in four phases:

- **Phase I.** The new drug is tested in healthy volunteers to compare human data with those in animals, to determine safe doses of the drug, and to assess its safety.
- **Phase II.** These trials are performed in homogenous populations of patients (50 to 300 patients). In double-blind studies, one group receives the drug and the other group receives a placebo. These studies are designed to evaluate the drug's efficacy and safety and to establish which form is the most effective dose.
- **Phase III.** In these clinical trials, the drug is made available to a larger group of patients (several thousand). These studies, which usually last several years, evaluate the drug's efficacy and monitor the nature and incidence of side effects.
- **Phase IV.** After successful completion of Phase III clinical trials, the drug company can apply to the FDA for approval to market the drug. Phase IV trials compare the new drug with others on the market and examine the drug's long-term efficacy and cost-effectiveness.

FDA Classification of Newly Approved Drugs

In an effort to effectively and accurately categorize medications, the Center for Drug Evaluation and Research (CDER) at the FDA uses a streamlined process to assign a numeric and letter classification to aid in the approval process. The classifications used by CDER reflect the type of drug being submitted and its intended uses.

Numeric classifications:

1. A new molecular drug: A completely new medication that is not derived from an existing drug
2. A new salt of a previously approved drug (not a new molecular drug): A new medication that is derived from an existing drug
3. A new formulation of a previously approved drug (not a new salt *or* a new molecular drug): A drug that has already been created and approved, but the manufacturer has made some changes to the medication
4. A new combination of two or more drugs: The combining of two or more medications can make administration easier by reducing the number of pills needed.
5. An already marketed drug product (for example, a duplication, a new manufacturer): Often seen when a

manufacturer's patent is expired and generic versions are produced

6. A new indication or claim for a drug that is already being marketed (including drugs that switch from prescription to OTC): It is not unusual for additional benefits to be found beyond those originally stated.

7. A drug that is already marketed with no new drug application: For medications that are already in use but that are not classified according to this system

Letter classifications describe the review priority of the drug:

S Standard review for drugs that are similar to currently available drugs

P Priority review for drugs that represent significant advances over treatments that currently exist

Other designations include the following:

O Orphan drugs

AA Drugs indicated for acquired immunodeficiency syndrome, or AIDS, and human immunodeficiency virus (HIV)-related disease

E Drugs developed or evaluated under special procedures to treat life-threatening or severely debilitating illnesses

Special Considerations in Drug Therapy

Pregnant Patients

Administration of any medication to a pregnant woman poses two pharmacologic challenges: It can alter the mother's anatomy and physiologic functions, and it has the potential to directly harm the fetus. For this reason, you must be familiar with how a particular medication might affect the fetus before

you consider giving it to a pregnant patient. The FDA has developed a rating scale regarding the risk to the mother and fetus for medications; categories include A, B, C, D, and X. (An explanation of these ratings can be found in the medication reference materials mentioned earlier.) In the field, you must be able to quickly evaluate the risks versus the benefits of the drug's administration. Does the potential benefit to the mother outweigh the risk to the fetus? If the drug is the only option for saving the mother's life, then that consideration would be paramount. When in doubt, contact medical control to discuss the situation.

To see how the twin concerns of mother and fetus play into your decision to administer a particular medication, let's examine the profile for amiodarone:

- **Drug:** Amiodarone (Cordarone). An antiarrhythmic
- **Category:** D, crosses placenta. There are no adequate human studies of effects on the mother or fetus. Congenital hypothyroidism has been described in the second trimester (the drug is 38% iodine by weight). Fetal bradycardia.
- **Breastfeeding:** Excretion into breast milk is significant. Elimination half-life is 58 days. The American Academy of Pediatrics has classified amiodarone as a drug "for which the effect on nursing infants is unknown but may be of concern."
- **Neonatal side effects:** May accumulate in infant with breastfeeding. Possible hypothyroidism.

Pediatric Patients

Medications have much different effects in adults than they do in children—whether the pediatric patient is a newborn, a neonate, an infant, or a toddler. In particular, infants do not achieve the same level of hepatic function as adults until they reach about 6 months of age; as a consequence, babies have a

You are the Provider Part 2

You ask your partner to place the patient on 100% oxygen via nonrebreathing mask and obtain a set of vital signs while you begin to question the patient further about his current illness and past medical history. The patient's son explains that his father was discharged from the hospital last week for problems associated with his heart. He hands you an index card that contains his father's medical history and list of medications. You note that the patient has a history of atrial fibrillation, congestive heart failure, and stable angina. Daily medications include digoxin, 0.125 mg every morning; Coumadin, 3 mg every morning; Lasix, 60 mg with breakfast and 60 mg at bedtime; Cardizem CD, 240 mg every morning; and nitroglycerin as required for chest pain. As you are looking over the list, the son pulls you over to side of the room and quietly expresses his concern about his father's medication compliance, as he has noticed that his father can be forgetful and may be taking his medication more often than it is prescribed.

Vital Signs	Recording Time: 5 Minutes
Skin	Pale, cool, and moist
Pulse	45 beats/min, irregular; weak radial
Blood pressure	72/50 mm Hg
Respirations	24 breaths/min, rales auscultated at bases
Sao$_2$	96% on nonrebreathing mask at 15 L/min of supplemental oxygen

3. What type of drug is Cardizem and how does it work?

> **Special Considerations**
>
> Pediatric and geriatric patients often have slower absorption and elimination times, necessitating modification of the doses administered. Pregnant patients are limited in the medications they can take because of risk to the fetus.

sharply reduced metabolic capacity. Similarly, the products of metabolism in children can vary from those seen in adults, which may sometimes result in unexpected responses. At the same time, children can metabolize some medications much more quickly than adults do, so they may require relatively higher doses or more frequent administration of some medications. The incomplete development of the gastrointestinal tract in young infants slows absorption of oral medications and delays elimination, so the same medication would be more potent in an infant than in an adult.

Geriatric Patients

The changes in pharmacokinetics in geriatric patients are comparable to those observed in young children. In elderly people, hepatic functions and gastrointestinal activity slow, which in turn delays absorption and elimination. In addition, geriatric patients are often taking several medications; these concomitant therapies may interact and modify one another's effects. Furthermore, because they may have a large number of medications to be taken and alterations in their normal mental status, geriatric patients may unintentionally overdose on a particular drug or forget to take it.

■ The Scope of Management

Safe and Effective Drug Administration

One of the principal areas in which your activities differ from those of EMT-Bs is in the administration of a long list of pharmacologic agents. Such agents have lifesaving and life-endangering potential, depending on how they are used. The wrong drug or the wrong dose of the right drug can kill a patient as effectively as a lethal weapon. For this reason, you must be intimately familiar with the pharmacologic agents used in the field—their indications and contraindications, their side effects, and their dangers. Nowhere in emergency care can ignorance or careless-

> **In the Field**
>
> The ever-growing variety of medications available makes it impossible for you to know everything about each drug. Do not hesitate to contact medical direction or consult a reference guide when faced with a medication you are not intimately familiar with.

ness on the part of paramedics do so much harm as in the administration of drugs. As a paramedic, you will be responsible for ensuring that administration of medications in the field is safe, therapeutic, and effective.

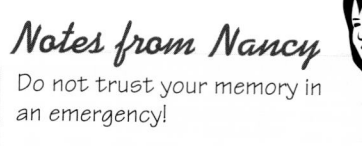

Legal, Moral, and Ethical Responsibilities

When administering medications to a patient, you are legally responsible for the appropriate use and documentation of that therapy. Even if another paramedic prepares the medication and hands a syringe to you to administer, you are still the person responsible. Always have a clear understanding of which medication you are administering and why you are administering it.

Put yourself in the shoes of your patient. How much confidence would you have in the person providing your care if he or she did not have a complete understanding of each drug, when to use it, and how it works? In addition to the obvious legal responsibility, we have a moral and ethical responsibility to ensure that we administer drugs safely.

The following guidelines will help you fulfill your responsibilities.

- Make certain you understand the precautions and contraindications associated with each medication. In addition, consider the precautions and contraindications as they relate to this case.
- Practice proper administration techniques. The manner in which you administer the medication will directly affect how the drug works and may prevent complications such as infection.
- Know the side effects associated with the particular medication, and understand how to observe for, and document, side effects experienced by your patient. Being familiar with the medication's classification will assist you in understanding its side effects.
- Understand the pharmacokinetics and pharmacodynamics of the medications.

As health care has evolved in the prehospital setting, the list of medications administered by paramedics has expanded in tandem. Keeping abreast of all the information is a challenge that you will face throughout your entire career. Do not hesitate

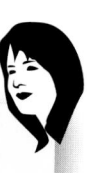

to use references to refresh your memory. Having appropriate material readily available will prove beneficial, especially when you need to make important decisions.

Try to obtain concise yet thorough information about the patient's medication use. It is essential to get an accurate list of the patient's current prescribed medications because this list may reveal clues about the patient's medical history. It is also necessary for deciding appropriate drug therapy so that you may avoid potentially dangerous drug interactions. Determine what, if any, OTC medications the patient may have taken. Find out if the patient is taking any recreational drugs, vitamins, herbal remedies, or folk medicines. All of these substances can have significant interactions with the medications used in emergency settings—and they may even be the culprit causing the patient's current condition.

Finally, remember that the patient has the right to refuse treatment. Be sure to fully inform your patient about the care that you are giving, including any medications that may be administered and the potential effects and side effects that the patient may experience.

Pharmacology and the Nervous System

Medications administered as part of the care provided in the prehospital setting exert their effects largely by acting on the nervous system. For this reason, it is critical that you understand the functioning of the nervous system as it relates to pharmacology.

Anatomically, the nervous system is made up of the central nervous system (CNS; the brain and spinal cord) and various types of peripheral nerves. The two major types of peripheral nerves are the afferent nerves (Latin: ad, "to" + ferre, "to bear"), which carry sensory impulses from all parts of the body to the brain, and the efferent nerves (Latin: efferns, "to bring out"), which carry messages from the brain to the muscles and all other organs of the body.

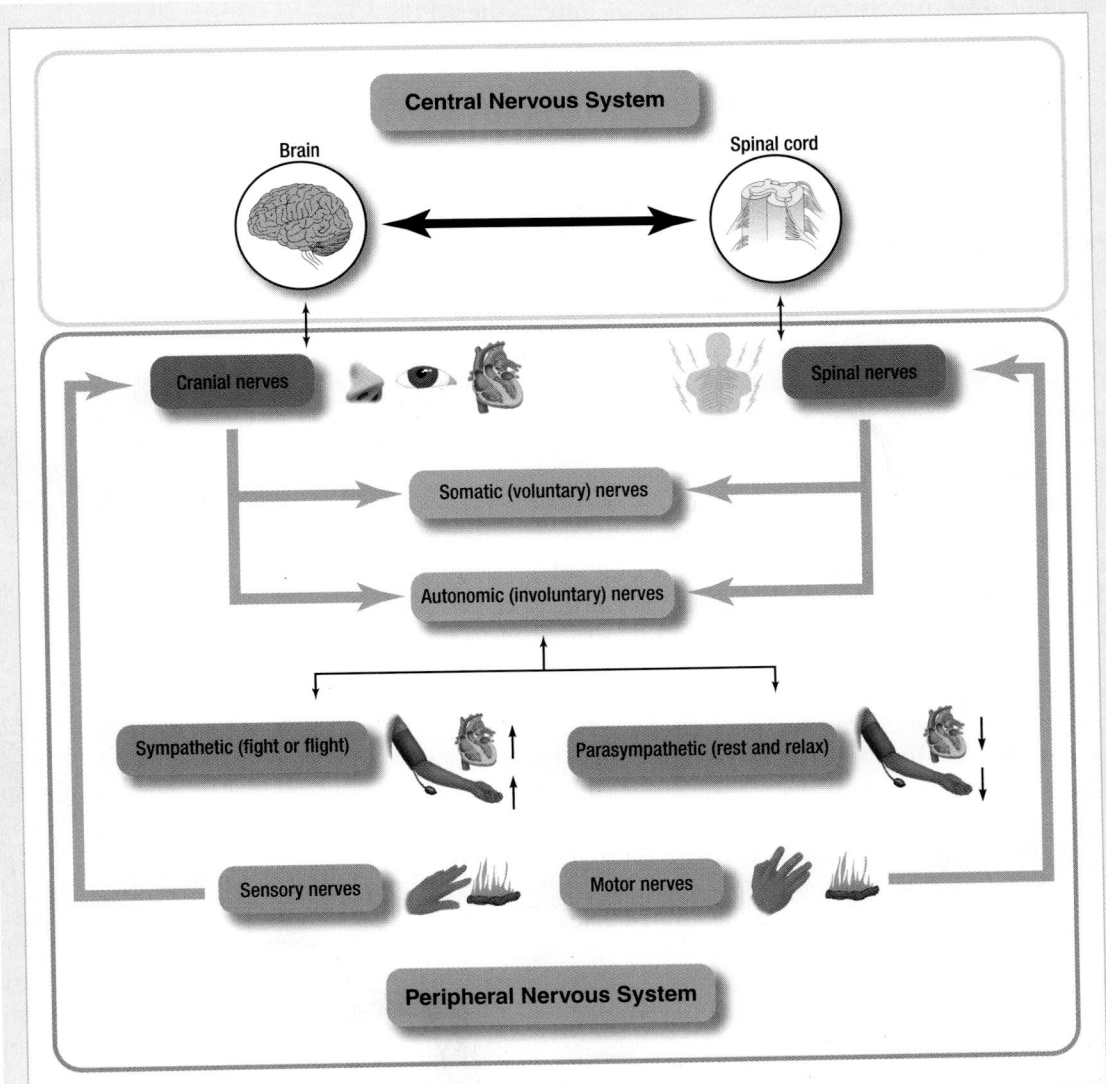

Figure 7-3 Organization of the nervous system.

Functionally, the nervous system is divided into two primary components **Figure 7-3**: the CNS and the peripheral nervous system (PNS).

Central Nervous System

The CNS functions as the control center for all other nervous system functions. One can easily think of the CNS like the CPU (central processing unit) in a home computer. The CPU in a computer carries out all calculations, coordinating a wide array of incoming and outgoing information from the many cables and connections of the computer. The CNS receives input from many receptors throughout the body, interprets the stimulus received via these sensory neurons, and makes decisions and directs actions to be carried out at target sites and organs throughout the body. These messages are then sent back out to the body via motor neurons or effectors, which carry out the desired action in various muscles and glands throughout the body. Computers work in a similar manner—the CPU interprets data from the keyboard, mouse, disk drives, and so forth and makes decisions and produces output actions such as printing. The whole system is connected by cables that function like the efferent and afferent nerves, sending and receiving information back and forth between the various components.

Peripheral Nervous System

The peripheral nervous system (PNS) consists of all nervous tissue outside of the brain and spinal cord and is separated into two divisions: the somatic nervous system and the autonomic nervous system (ANS). The ANS is particularly vulnerable to the administration of prehospital medications. It is considered to be "automatic" or involuntary because we cannot control its functioning or force functions under its control to happen or not happen.

The autonomic nervous system (ANS) sends sensory impulses from internal structures (such as blood vessels, the heart, and organs of the chest, abdomen, and pelvis) through afferent autonomic nerves to the brain. Afferent neurons are an essential element in reflex regulation of the ANS. The responses to these stimuli sent by afferent neurons are carried back to the organ systems by efferent autonomic nerves, which cause appropriate responses from the organs of the body to change the way they are functioning or behaving. The ANS transmits nerve impulses from the CNS to effector organs through two types of neurons: preganglionic and postganglionic. The preganglionic neurons originate in the CNS, emerge through the brain stem or spinal cord, and make connections at ganglia (groupings of nerve cell bodies located in the PNS). Ganglia act as relay stations through which a ganglionic transmitter relays the impulse to the postganglionic neurons. The postganglionic neurons terminate and stimulate the effector organs (such as smooth muscle, glands, and cardiac muscle) **Figure 7-4 ▶**.

To see how this system works, consider what happens when specialized sensory organs in the carotid sinus and aortic arch detect the pressure within each of these areas. This stimulus is signaled to the CNS via afferent neurons, causing the efferent branch of the system to respond and effecting pressure changes within the system.

The ANS is divided into two further subsystems: the sympathetic nervous system and the parasympathetic nervous system. These two systems have opposing effects on the body.

Sympathetic Nervous System

The sympathetic nervous system, responsible for the fight-or-flight response, is the dominant system during periods of stress

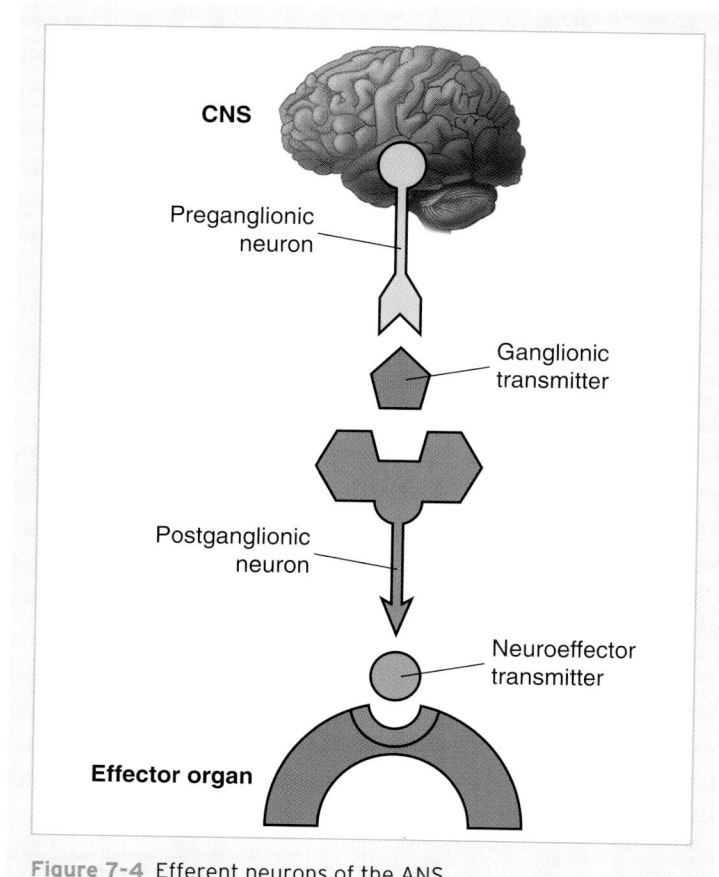

Figure 7-4 Efferent neurons of the ANS.

and activity. It is also a key player in the regulation of hypoglycemia, hypothermia, and trauma.

The sympathetic nerves have their origins in the thoracic and lumbar sections of the spinal cord. They exit the spinal cord through the spinal nerves, which then extend to two types of ganglia: sympathetic chain ganglia and collateral ganglia. Working through these ganglia, the sympathetic nervous system increases heart rate and blood pressure, the release of energy stores throughout the body, and blood flow to the skeletal muscles and heart by diverting flow from the skin and other internal organs. Sympathetic stimulation also results in dilation of the pupils and bronchioles of the respiratory system. The net goal of sympathetic stimulation is to provide the body with energy, oxygen, and the ability to react to stressful situations. The primary chemical messengers of the sympathetic nervous system are norepinephrine and epinephrine. The nerve fibers that release norepinephrine are referred to as adrenergic nerve fibers.

To better understand how sympathetic influences are working, let's look at the heart. The heart rate and force of contraction in response to stress are primarily under the control of the sympathetic nervous system. Sympathetic nerve fibers stimulate all parts of the atria and ventricles. Stimulation of the sympathetic nervous system releases epinephrine, a primary chemical messenger that activates a specific type of receptor in

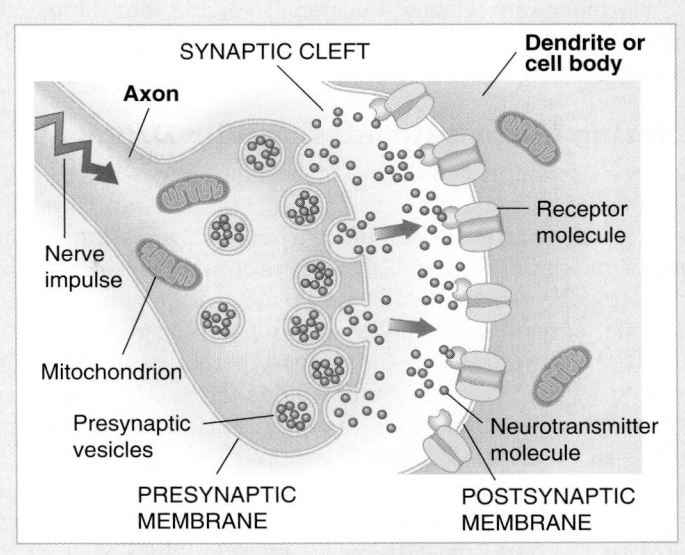

Figure 7-5 A synaptic cleft.

the heart known as the beta-1 adrenergic receptor. Epinephrine affects the heart by increasing the rate of contraction, the conduction velocity, and the force of contraction in the ventricular muscle. The result: increased systemic heart rate and blood pressure. The same actions occur when you administer an injection of epinephrine; this effect is referred to as a *sympathomimetic* response.

Parasympathetic Nervous System

The parasympathetic nervous system is the dominant system during periods of rest and relaxation. It sometimes is referred to as the rest-and-digest system. The nerves associated with the parasympathetic system have their origins in the brain stem and sacral segments of the spinal cord. The nerves from the brain stem pass through four of the cranial nerves: oculomotor (III), facial (VII), pharyngeal (IX), and vagus (X). These nerves innervate most of the body, including the eyes, salivary glands, ears, lungs, and abdominal organs. The sacral segments innervate the kidneys, urinary bladder, sexual organs, and the terminal large intestine.

To see how the sympathetic and parasympathetic nervous systems work in conjunction, consider the effect of these two systems on the heart. The heart, like most major organs and glands, receives sympathetic and parasympathetic stimuli. The sympathetic stimulus increases the heart rate and contractility of the muscle; the parasympathetic impulses decrease the rate and contractility. The constant tug-of-war between these two sets of stimuli determines the final heart rate and contractility status.

Neurochemical Transmission

Neurotransmission is the process of chemical signaling between cells. This process involves several steps. Let's look at a cholinergic neuron to describe the process. A cholinergic neuron is one that releases the chemical acetylcholine (ACh).

The first step involves the synthesis of ACh. Here choline is taken from extracellular fluid, along with sodium, into the neuron where it is turned into ACh. Second, the ACh is stored in vesicles in the nerve terminal. Third involves the release of ACh from the nerve ending. This occurs when an action potential

arrives at the nerve ending, stimulating the voltage-sensitive channels to open and release ACh into the synaptic gap (the space between the cell membrane of an axon terminal and of the target cell with which it synapses, also called the *synaptic cleft*) Figure 7-5 ▲. The fourth step involves binding of released ACh to a receptor. Once ACh is released from the synaptic vesicles, it diffuses across the synaptic space and binds to receptors on the next, or target, cell. The binding of ACh to the receptor causes a response within the cell, and a new nerve impulse is initiated.

Receptors are unique molecular structures or sites on the surface or interior of a cell that bind with substances such as hormones, drugs, and neurotransmitters. Receptors are highly specialized and, in most cases, respond only to a particular substance. It is easy to think of the receptor-neurotransmitter relationship like a lock and key. If every neurotransmitter stimulated every receptor, there would be tremendous competition and confusion within the body's cells.

The fifth step involves the degradation of ACh. Once the new nerve impulse is initiated, an enzyme called acetylcholinesterase (AChE) is released, which breaks ACh into choline and acetate. The sixth and final step is the recycling of choline by the neurons so that it can be made into ACh for a subsequent action or transmission.

Other Receptors

In addition to neurotransmission, other methods of chemical signaling occur through local mediators and the secretion of hormones. Most cells in the body secrete chemicals that may act at the local area and stimulate changes in their immediate environment. Nearly all of these locally released chemicals are destroyed or removed by the cells and do not enter blood circulation and create changes throughout the entire body. A good example of a local mediator is histamine.

Hormones are secreted by specialized cells into the bloodstream. Hormones are transported throughout the entire body and have a broad range of effects at various target tissues.

Altering Neurotransmission With Drugs

In some cases and conditions, it becomes necessary to alter normal neurotransmission. This can be accomplished by using drugs that mimic or inhibit neurotransmission. Some medications inhibit the release of neurotransmitters, and others block the receptor sites along the neural pathway. For example, contamination involving organophosphates (pesticides) alters neural transmissions. In this case, the ACh released by the organophosphate binds to the AChE, making it ineffective. The final result is overstimulation of the nerves due to an excess of ACh in the synaptic cleft. In this case, a medication is needed to break the bond between the organophosphate and AChE so that AChE can break down the ACh and terminate the nerve stimulation. The drug of choice is 2 PAM chloride, which is effective at cleaving the organophosphate from AChE and allowing it to break down the excess ACh, terminating nerve stimulation and returning it to a normal state. There are many medications that can alter normal neurotransmission.

Selective Drug Action: Nicotinic and Muscarinic Receptors

Nicotinic receptors are present in many tissues in the body, including the CNS and the PNS. These receptors function at the neuromuscular junctions of somatic muscles, and stimulation causes muscular contraction. Nicotinic receptors are triggered by the neurotransmitter ACh, but they are also opened by nicotine. Nicotinic effects are those of sympathetic overactivity and neuromuscular dysfunction and include tachycardia, hypertension, dilated pupils, muscle fasciculation (involuntary contractions or twitching of groups of muscle fibers), and muscle weakness.

Muscarinic receptors are found throughout the body as subcomponents of the CNS and ANS **Figure 7-6 ▶**. The primary neurotransmitters for muscarinic receptors are ACh and muscarine. Muscarinic effects result in parasympathetic overactivity and include bradycardia, miosis (pinpoint pupils), sweating, blurred vision, excessive lacrimation (tearing), excessive bronchial secretions, wheezing, shortness of breath, coughing, vomiting, abdominal cramping, diarrhea, and urinary and fecal incontinence. Atropine is a

common medication that is given in the prehospital setting to reverse the effects of muscarinic overstimulation.

■ General Properties of Medications

Drugs adjust or influence the body's existing functions; they usually do not provide the body with functions it does not already have. To exert their effects, they must interact with various cells and tissues in the body, and they typically work through several mechanisms of action rather than relying on a single action. In most cases, medications may bind to a receptor site and trigger a stimulus; in some cases, they change the chemical properties of cells and tissues. They may also combine with other chemicals within cells or organ systems to aid in elimination or bind to receptors to alter the normal metabolic functions of cells and tissues.

Receptors are specialized target molecules that are present on the surface of cells or within the cell. They bind a medication and mediate its pharmacologic effect. Medications may interact with a variety of receptor sites—for example, enzymes, nucleic acids, and membranous receptors. Once the medication and the receptor site bind, a biologic response follows. The magnitude of this response is directly proportional to the number of these drug-receptor sites.

The attraction between a medication and its receptors is referred to as affinity. The stronger the affinity between the two, the stronger the resulting bond. In some cases, different medications have affinity for the same receptor site; however, it is unlikely that both will bind with the same strength, which means that one medication inevitably takes priority.

A medication that stimulates a response in a receptor site is called an agonist. The strength of its effect depends on the

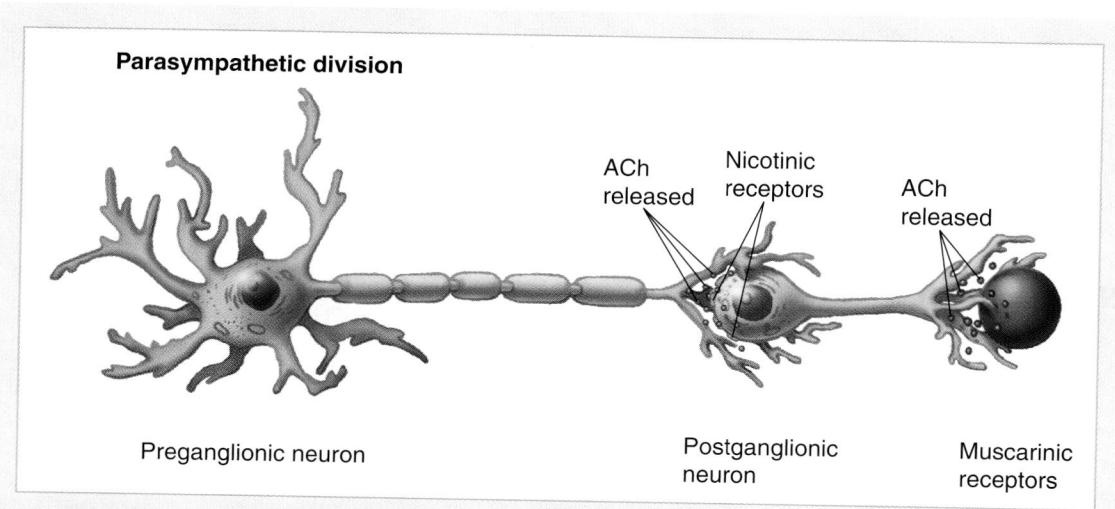

Parasympathetic division

ACh released   Nicotinic receptors   ACh released

Preganglionic neuron   Postganglionic neuron   Muscarinic receptors

Figure 7-6 Muscarinic receptors are present on some sympathetic and all parasympathetic target tissues.

concentration of the agonist at the receptor site, which is in turn determined by the dose administered and the drug's rate of absorption, distribution, and metabolism.

Drug Forms

Drugs come in many forms, solid and liquid, each of which has special properties. In the field, you will use only a limited subset of the drug forms described herein.

Liquid Drug Forms

- **Solution.** A liquid containing one or more chemical substances entirely dissolved, usually in water, for example, normal saline solution (The majority of medications used by paramedics are solutions.)
- **Suspension.** Preparation of a finely divided drug intended to be (or already) incorporated in a suitable liquid, for example, methylprednisolone, supplied as a powder requiring the addition of sterile water (Note: All bottles containing suspensions must be shaken thoroughly before use because their ingredients tend to separate on standing.)
- **Fluid extract.** Concentrated form of a drug prepared by dissolving the crude drug in the fluid in which it is most readily soluble; standardized such that 1 milliliter (mL) contains 1 gram (g) of the drug, for example, many herbal supplements and remedies, such as saw palmetto
- **Tincture.** Dilute alcoholic extract of a drug such as tincture of iodine, used as a skin antiseptic
- **Spirits.** Preparation of a volatile substance dissolved in alcohol, such as spirits of ammonia, formerly used to rouse people from fainting through its noxious odor
- **Syrup.** Drug suspended in sugar and water to improve its taste, such as cough syrup and syrup of ipecac
- **Elixir.** Syrup with alcohol and flavoring added, such as cough medicines, particularly those formulated for children
- **Milk.** Aqueous suspension of an insoluble drug, such as milk of magnesia
- **Emulsion.** Preparation of one liquid (usually an oil) distributed in small globules in another liquid (usually water), for example, some preparations of diazepam (Valium); often used as lubricants
- **Liniments and lotions.** Preparations of drugs for external use, usually to relieve discomfort such as pain or itching or to protect the skin, for example, calamine lotion

Solid Drug Forms

- **Extract.** A concentrated preparation of a drug made by putting the drug into solution (in alcohol or water) and evaporating the excess solvent until the concentration reaches a prescribed standard, for example, liver extract, which has been used in the treatment of anemia, prepared

by dissolving ground mammalian liver and allowing the solvent to evaporate; extract is then incorporated into a tablet or capsule
- **Powder.** A drug that has been ground into pulverized form, for example, mixtures of powdered sodium bicarbonate and calcium carbonate, used as an antacid in the treatment of ulcers; example in prehospital care: activated charcoal powder
- **Pill.** A drug shaped into a ball or oval to be swallowed; often coated to disguise an unpleasant taste, for example, ferrous sulfate (iron), often given in the form of coated pills to patients with anemia
- **Capsule.** A cylindrical gelatin container enclosing a dose of medication, for example, many over-the-counter pain medications, such as acetaminophen (Tylenol)
- **Pulvule.** Resembles a capsule, but it is not made of gelatin and does not separate; usually are proprietary forms of a drug, such as propoxyphene hydrochloride (Darvon)
- **Tablet.** A powdered drug that has been molded or compressed into a small disk, such as aspirin tablets; example in prehospital care: nitroglycerin tablets
- **Suppository.** A drug mixed in a firm base that melts at body temperature and is shaped to fit the rectum, urethra, or vagina; may be used for local action (for example, glycerin suppositories to promote evacuation of the rectum) or for systemic effect (for example, diazepam [Valium] suppositories to treat seizure disorders and status epilepticus in children)
- **Ointment.** A semisolid preparation for external application to the body, usually containing a medicinal substance, for example, neomycin ointment, a topical antibiotic
- **Patch.** A medication impregnated into a membrane or adhesive that is applied onto the surface of the skin, for example, nitroglycerin patch **Figure 7-7 ▼**

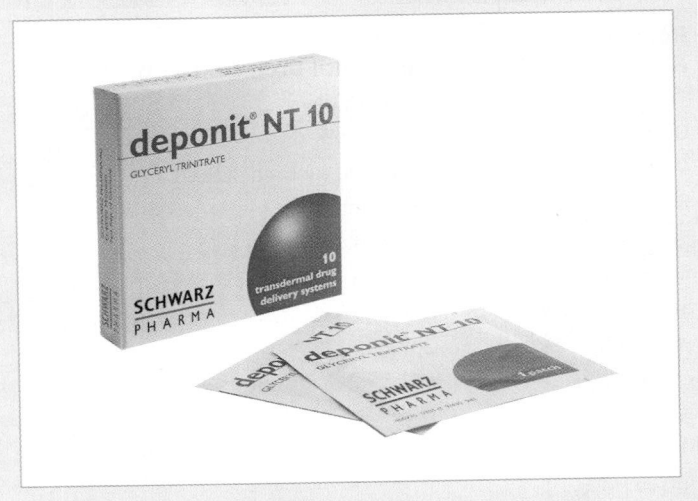

Figure 7-7 Nitroglycerin patch.

Gaseous Drug Forms

Medications may also come in the form of a vapor. Gaseous medications are primarily used in operating suite anesthesia. To create the gas, a medication in liquid form is placed into a machine that promotes vaporization. The vapors are inhaled by the patient to induce anesthesia. An example of a medication administered as a vapor is sevoflurane (Ultane).

■ Overview of the Routes of Drug Administration

Rates of Drug Absorption

How you choose to administer a drug—that is, the mode of administration—affects the rate at which the body absorbs the drug and, ultimately, the onset of its therapeutic effects. The action of a drug, especially the speed with which it works, is also influenced by the way it enters the body—that is, the route of administration. Obviously, drugs injected directly into the circulation, such as IV or intraosseous (IO) injections, enter the bloodstream the most rapidly. Nearly as fast is the absorption across the respiratory mucosa when drugs are sprayed down an endotracheal tube or breathed in from an inhaler. Other mucosal surfaces, such as those found in the rectum, provide for rapid absorption as well, albeit at an unpredictable rate. Intramuscular (IM) injection is slower because the drug must be picked up from the muscles by the circulating blood; the same is true of subcutaneous (SC) injections, which are absorbed more slowly than IM injections. Near the slowest end of the scale are drugs administered orally (PO). The slowest absorption of all is across intact skin.

Table 7-3 ▾ summarizes the rates of absorption. Note that the route of administration that is appropriate for one drug

Table 7-3	Rates of Absorption by Different Routes
Route of Administration	**Time Until Drug Takes Effect***
Topical	Hours to days
Oral	30–90 min
Rectal	5–30 min (unpredictable)
SC injection	15–30 min
IM injection	10–20 min
Sublingual tablet	3–5 min
Sublingual injection	3 min
Inhalation	3 min
Endotracheal	Unknown; unpredictable
IO	60 s
IV	30–60 s
Intracardiac	15 s
*In a healthy person with normal perfusion.	

may be unsuitable for another drug, so for any given drug it is essential to know the routes by which it may be given.

Local or Systemic Effects

Drugs may produce their effects locally, systemically, or both. Local effects result from the direct application of a drug to a tissue—for example, when you apply a lotion to the skin to relieve itching. Systemic effects occur after the drug is absorbed by any route and distributed by the bloodstream; they almost invariably involve more than one organ, although the response of one or another organ may predominate.

The action of a drug is rarely a completely fixed property of the medication. Instead, the effect of any given drug typically varies depending on the patient, the dose, the route by which the drug is given, and the drug's metabolic rate.

■ Routes of Drug Administration

The routes of administration are classified into three categories based on how the medication is absorbed and distributed: percutaneous, enteral, and parenteral. Medications given via the percutaneous routes are applied to and absorbed through the skin or mucous membranes. Enteral medications are administered and absorbed somewhere along the gastrointestinal tract, most commonly orally. Any route of administration that does not cause the drug to be absorbed through the skin, mucous membranes, or gastrointestinal tract is considered parenteral. The actual route of administration you select in the field is dependent on the medication and the intended effect.

Percutaneous Routes

Percutaneous routes of medication administration are those for any medication that is absorbed through the skin or through a mucous membrane. Drugs may be applied topically—that is, on the surface of the body. Ordinarily, the intact skin is an effective barrier to absorption of drugs, but some drugs have been specially prepared to cross the barrier at a very slow rate, so the route is useful for sustained release of drugs for a long period. Thus, some patients take nitroglycerin in the form of a cream rubbed into the skin or a patch pasted onto the skin. Estrogens (female hormones) are also sometimes given in the form of a patch.

Administration via the transdermal route is generally performed by placing medication directly onto the patient's skin. It is also easily controlled by simply removing and wiping the medication from the skin, which causes the effect to quickly subside. Although the rate of absorption is consistent, steady, and predictable, it can be affected by the thickness of the skin and the presence of scar tissue at the site of administration. It can also be affected by the amount of peripheral circulation. Conditions that decrease peripheral circulation, such as hypothermia and hypotension, will lead to a slower rate of absorption. In a febrile patient, the rate of absorption would be much quicker than anticipated.

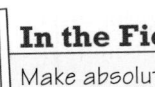

In the Field

Make absolutely certain you use body substance isolation when administering any medication, particularly topical drugs. If the medication can be absorbed into the patient's skin, it can be absorbed into yours as well.

Administering medications through mucous membranes is becoming increasingly popular in the prehospital setting. This route allows for the medication to be absorbed at a moderate to rapid rate. Sublingual (SL) administration refers to giving a medication—nitroglycerin, for example—under the tongue. Drugs given sublingually are usually rapidly absorbed, with effects becoming apparent within a few minutes. The buccal route (between the cheeks and gums) may be used to give glucose gel to a hypoglycemic diabetic patient. The nasal route is an increasingly popular way to aerosolize and administer medications. Naloxone given intranasally, for example, is quickly absorbed into the blood vasculature in the nasopharynx. Although this route of administration is less commonly used in the prehospital setting, drops may be placed in the eye to be absorbed in the conjunctival sac or in the ear (aurally) to fight infection or minimize pain.

The pulmonary route of drug administration is used to deliver medications directly to the pulmonary system through inhalation or injection. In the inhalation route, the drug is placed in a nebulizer that reduces it to a mist, which the patient then breathes in. In the lungs, the drug is absorbed into the bronchioles and alveolar sacs. Paramedics can also administer medications through an endotracheal tube, placing it in liquid form into the bronchioles and alveolar sacs to be absorbed. Only certain medications are suitable to be given via the endotracheal tube. NAVEL is a handy mnemonic that will help you recall which drugs can be delivered in this way: Naloxone, Atropine, Vasopressin, Epinephrine, and Lidocaine. If medications are given via the endotracheal route, the dose must be doubled to achieve the same effects as if given intravenously. Currently, the endotracheal tube route is not recommended in cardiac arrest because the effectiveness of medication absorption is questionable at best. The IV and IO routes are preferred in these cases. Specific routes and the steps of administration are discussed further in Chapter 8.

Enteral Routes

Medications that are given via one of the enteral routes are absorbed somewhere along the gastrointestinal tract. Most patients take their daily medications at home by the oral route (per os, or PO) because that route is painless, convenient, and economical. Drugs taken by mouth are absorbed at an unpredictable but generally slow rate from the stomach and intestines—usually somewhere between 30 and 90 minutes. Because absorption is slow and unpredictable, drugs are rarely given by the oral route in emergency situations. The

one exception is aspirin for patients suspected of having acute coronary syndrome (ACS); its administration requires an adequate level of consciousness to prevent aspiration, however. In some cases, you may need to administer medications via a gastric tube, which allows for access directly to the gastrointestinal system.

Drugs may be administered rectally for their local effect; they may also be given rectally because they are irritating if given orally or because the patient cannot take an oral medication (for example, if vomiting). In the prehospital setting, the rectal route can be considered if quick IV access is impractical. The extreme vascularity of the rectum promotes rapid but sometimes unpredictable absorption. Medications administered rectally (per rectum, or PR) generally do not pass through the liver and, therefore, are not subjected to hepatic alterations.

Parenteral Routes

Parenteral routes include those in which medications are administered via any route other than the alimentary canal (digestive tract), skin, and mucous membranes. They are generally administered via syringes and needles. In most cases, parenteral routes allow for the fastest absorption rate.

The IV route is the most rapidly effective—but also the most dangerous route of administration. Drugs given intravenously go directly into the bloodstream and to the target organs, without any appreciable delay in absorption. Thus, IV injection enables you to deliver a known quantity of drug over a known period; that is, it allows the most accurate control of dosage. It is a dangerous route, however, precisely because the entire dose of the drug is delivered in one blast, so a toxic reaction is much more likely. Absorption of an IV drug usually takes about 30 to 60 seconds. The absorption rate will be slowed in heart failure (because of the longer circulation time). In cardiac arrest with CPR in progress, an IV drug will take 3 to 4 times longer than usual to reach its target organ because the cardiac output is only one third of the normal rate. As a consequence, it will take at least 1 or 2 minutes after giving an emergency drug during CPR to ensure that the drug has circulated adequately. Always prepare to administer a medication in cardiac arrest by drawing it up ahead of time. Administer drugs during compression cycles to enhance distribution whenever possible, and never interrupt compressions to administer a medication during cardiac arrest. In general, IV drugs should be given *slowly*, unless you receive contrary orders. In the field, it is unacceptable to administer a medication by direct venipuncture because this technique may result in infiltration of the drug. Infiltration is the escape of fluid into the surrounding tissue, which causes a localized area of edema, and is discussed in more detail in Chapter 8.

The intraosseous (IO) route is becoming increasingly popular in the prehospital setting. This route has long been used for pediatric patients, but with the advent of convenient devices for adult use, it is quickly becoming a standard when quick IV access is not practical. Any medication that can be given intravenously can be given intraosseously. The rate of absorption and time of onset have been shown to be identical if not better because the medicine enters a noncollapsible channel with rapid flow into the central circulation.

Drugs given by the intramuscular (IM) route take longer to act than those given intravenously because they must first be absorbed from the muscle into the bloodstream. By the same token, IM medications have a longer duration of action than IV drugs because they are absorbed gradually during a period of minutes to hours. Obviously, absorption of medications given by the IM or SC route depends on adequate blood flow to muscles and peripheral tissues, which is not the case in shock or cardiac arrest. Therefore, IM injections should be given only to patients with adequate perfusion.

An IM injection usually involves volumes of about 1 to 5 mL and is given into the deltoid muscle of the upper arm (the preferred site for prehospital applications) or into the upper outer quadrant of the gluteus muscle of the buttocks. (The technique for IM injection is described later in this chapter.) The use of the deltoid muscle of the arm has the advantage that the rate of drug absorption can be slowed in case of an adverse reaction. Should dyspnea, dizziness, itching, edema,

urticaria, wheezing, or any other sign of an allergic reaction develop following an IM (or SC) injection in the arm, you should immediately fasten a constricting band proximal to the injection site and then manage the patient as described in Chapter 30.

With the subcutaneous (SC or SQ) route, a small amount (usually less than 2 mL) of drug is injected into the fat or connective tissue beneath the skin. Medications administered by this route are absorbed more slowly and over a more prolonged period than when they are given intravenously; the peak drug effect usually occurs within about 30 minutes. The SC route is used to administer epinephrine in asthmatic attacks of mild to moderate severity. These injections are usually given under the skin of the upper outer arm, anterior thigh, or abdomen.

Pharmacokinetics

Every medication has varying effects on the body. Pharmacokinetics is the study of the metabolism and action of medications within the body, with particular emphasis on the time required for absorption, duration of action, distribution in the body, and method of excretion.

Absorption

Absorption of medications refers to the transfer of a medication from its site of administration into the body to specific target organs

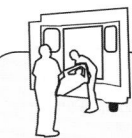

In the Field

Do not give IM or SC injections to patients with impaired peripheral perfusion.

You are the Provider Part 3

You perform a physical exam on the patient while your partner prepares an IV set up. You document the following findings: positive JVD; rales auscultated at the bases; slight swelling around the ankles; and a slow, irregular, weak pulse. You ask the patient to describe his vision problems. He explains that for the past 2 days his sight has been blurry and objects have had a yellow-green circle around them. He jokingly tells you that this blurriness interferes with him being able to complete the morning crossword puzzle and watch his game shows at night.

You establish an 18-gauge IV in the right AC and begin to administer a 200-mL fluid bolus. Before leaving for the hospital you perform a 12-lead ECG, which shows atrial fibrillation at a rate in the 40s with frequent PVCs. Recalling the information on cardiac medication from a recent in-service you know that both digoxin and Cardizem CD can lower the heart rate. You also know that the patient is symptomatic from the low heart rate and PVCs. Unsure of how to proceed with treatment, you decide to contact medical control for guidance.

Reassessment	Recording Time: 10 Minutes
Skin	Pale, cool, and moist
Pulse	42 beats/min, irregular; weak radial
ECG	Atrial fibrillation with a slow ventricular response and frequent PVCs
Blood pressure	78/44 mm Hg
Respirations	24 breaths/min, slight increase work of breathing
Sao_2	96% on nonrebreathing mask at 15 L/min of supplemental oxygen
Pupils	Equal and reactive to light

4. Does the patient present with signs and symptoms of possible drug toxicity? If so, which medications are in question?

5. What treatment will increase the patient's blood pressure?

and tissues. The ultimate goal is for the medication to reach a therapeutic concentration in the bloodstream. Achieving this therapeutic concentration depends partially on the rate and extent to which the drug is absorbed. The rate and extent are, in turn, dependent on the ability of the medication to cross the cell membrane.

Mechanisms of Medication Absorption

A medication may cross the cell's membrane by one of two mechanisms: active transport or passive diffusion (discussed in Chapter 8). In active transport, specialized proteins that span the membrane of a cell facilitate the movement of the medication inside target tissues and cells. This energy-dependent process uses a carrier-mediated mechanism to assist the medication into the cell and can move the drug across the concentration gradient (from an area of lower concentration to an area of higher concentration). In contrast, passive diffusion (also known as absorption) of a medication does not use energy or carrier-mediated mechanisms. Instead, medications move from an area of high concentration to an area of low concentration. Lipid-soluble medications move easily across most cell membranes, as do water-soluble drugs via aqueous channels.

Blood Flow and Medication Absorption

A properly functioning circulatory system greatly enhances the rate of medication absorption. If the body area to which a medication is applied (for example, transdermal route) or injected (for example, IM route) has a good vascular system and a rich blood supply, the rate of absorption is enhanced. In contrast, areas of the body with poor blood supply or particular routes of administration (for example, SC route) may be associated with a delay in the rate of absorption. As mentioned earlier, medications administered via the IV route are immediately passed throughout the circulatory system, absorbed, and delivered to target tissues and organs. In patients in profound states of shock or circulatory compromise, absorption may be delayed with any of the administration methods.

Surface Areas and Medication Absorption

All medications must pass through nontarget cells to reach their intended receptor target; these nontarget cells may include the skin, mucosa, and intestinal tissue. The larger the surface area that is available to the medication as a "launching pad," the greater the amount of absorption and the more quickly the medication can reach its target and take effect.

Another factor affecting the absorption rate is the nature of the cells that the medication is trying to pass through. Single layers of cells, like the tissue of the intestines, readily transport medications. In contrast, multilayer tissues like the skin require more time for absorption.

Medication Concentration and Absorption

The concentration of the medication administered affects its absorption as well. Pharmaceutical manufacturers use this fact to their advantage—for example, by altering a medication's coating to tweak the ultimate rate of absorption. Medications that are administered in high doses are generally absorbed more quickly than medications that are administered at lower doses.

When medications are administered to a patient, they eventually become distributed throughout the entire body. Thus, the higher the concentration in the body, the greater the absorption. For this reason, giving very high concentrations or doses to speed absorption is not a good idea. Once a medication is administered, it will continue to circulate in the body and affect its target receptors until the drug is eliminated. Typically, when continued doses are required, two approaches to administration are used. First a loading dose—a large dose of the same concentration that temporarily exceeds the body's ability to eliminate the medication—is given to quickly reach a therapeutic level. It is followed by a maintenance dose—a smaller dose administered over time and intended to maintain a therapeutic level of the medication at the receptor site. Loading doses are typically based on the volume of distribution, which takes into account the patient's weight; maintenance doses are selected based on the body's ability to eliminate the medication.

Environmental pH and Medication Absorption

Most medications are weak acids or weak bases. Once in solution, they become ionized (electrically charged). Most medications reach a state of equilibrium between their ionized and nonionized forms, facilitating their absorption. The pH of a medication affects its ability to ionize. Medications that are weak acids are able to ionize much better in an alkaline environment, whereas medications that are weak bases are able to ionize more completely in an acidic environment.

Medications administered by any route inevitably undergo side reactions—that is, reactions with nontarget cells and tissues—before they reach their intended destination. A critical consideration for the effectiveness of any drug is how much of it is still active by the time it reaches its target organ. This property, called the drug's bioavailability, must be taken into account when selecting the dose to ensure that enough medication is being absorbed at the target organ to achieve the desired effect.

Distribution

Medication distribution is the process by which a medication moves throughout the body. Blood is the primary distribution vehicle. Factors that change the way blood flows through the body will change the way medications are transported to the target tissue. If the patient's overall cardiac output is diminished, the medication will not move as quickly. Along the same lines, if blood is not moving efficiently to a particular part of the body, the distribution may be slowed. For example, if the patient is cold, the blood is shunted away from the skin and peripheral extremities. In such a case, an antibiotic intended to fight an infection in the foot will not arrive at that area as quickly as intended.

The only way a medication molecule can actually be used by the body is if it is not bound with anything else—that is, it must be "free drug." Because of this, the extent to which the medication binds with nontarget cells affects its intensity and duration of action. Not all of the medication molecules are floating around the blood at the same time. Medications have a tendency to collect in certain areas of the body that act as storage sites. Typically, drugs will become bound to fat, muscle tissue, and bone, thereby limiting the amount of medication that is free in the bloodstream. In particular, lipid-soluble medications have a high affinity for adipose (fat) tissue. As a consequence, low blood flow may allow for their extended retention in the adipose tissue. Still other medications have an unusual affinity for bone tissue. Molecules of these drugs will accumulate after the drug is absorbed onto the bone crystal surface.

In contrast, while roaming around the body in the bloodstream, the medication may become bound to plasma proteins. Such a drug-protein complex cannot be used by the body, so its formation lowers the therapeutic concentration of the drug. The amount of free drug is always proportional to the amount of bound drug. Thus, as the free drug is used and eliminated, the drug-protein complexes break down and release more free drug to replace what has been used.

In particular, molecules of a medication may become bound to the plasma protein known as albumin. Albumin, which is too large to diffuse out of the bloodstream, essentially kidnaps drug molecules, making them ineffective. Albumin is not in endless supply, however. Furthermore, other medications may be competing to bind to the same albumin. As such, the amount of free drug is influenced by the amount of available albumin. Some conditions may cause a decrease in the albumin levels, particularly those that involve decreased liver functions. Even if the albumin levels are normal, the amount of affinity for albumin that one medication has compared with another can affect free-drug levels (think of it like magnets and a metal screw for the albumin, with one magnet being stronger than the other).

Other aspects of the body may also prevent medication molecules from being distributed to certain tissue. The blood-brain barrier is a single layer of capillary endothelial cells. It allows only lipid-soluble medications to enter the brain and cerebrospinal fluid. In a pregnant patient, the placental barrier consists of membrane layers separating blood vessels of the mother and the fetus. Much like the blood-brain barrier, the placental barrier does not permit most non–lipid-soluble medications to pass to the fetus. This is not an impregnable barrier, however; some non–lipid-soluble medications can cross the placental barrier, so you must understand which medications can be given to a pregnant patient and in which situations.

Biotransformation

The manner in which the body metabolizes medications is referred to as biotransformation. It occurs in one of two ways: by transforming the medication into a metabolite or by making the medication more water soluble. Only medication molecules that are in a free-drug form are able to be biotransformed.

Drug manufacturers use this fact to their advantage when creating medications, known as prodrugs, that become active only *after* they undergo biotransformation. Most of the biotransformation takes place in the liver. The endoplasmic reticulum of hepatocytes contains the enzymes primarily responsible for biotransformation.

The biotransformation of a medication directly affects the route chosen to deliver a medication. All blood that comes from the gastrointestinal tract must pass through the liver before moving on to the rest of the body. This gives the liver the opportunity to partially or completely inactivate drugs long before they reach the intended target tissue, a scenario known as the first-pass effect. Because of the first-pass effect, some medications can be given only parenterally. For example, insulin must always be given subcutaneously—never orally. The liver would completely inactivate insulin if it were to undergo the first-pass effect, making it useless. Even medications that are not completely inactivated by the first-pass effect sometimes require a higher dose when given orally to ensure that enough of the drug survives to have a therapeutic effect.

Liver enzymes can act on a drug in two ways, or phases. In phase 1, the enzymes may oxidize the drug or bind it with oxygen molecules. The enzymes may also hydrolyze the medication, decomposing it by a reaction with water. In either case, the medication becomes more soluble with water. In phase 2, the medication molecules combine with a chemical found in the body; this interaction is known as a conjugation reaction. Phase 1 and phase 2 allow the drug to move to the next stage, excretion.

Excretion

In excretion, the body eliminates the remnants of the drug, which could be toxic or inactive metabolites. (Recall that the liver may have inactivated at least some of the drug through biotransformation.) Excretion occurs primarily through the kidneys via three mechanisms:

- **Glomerular filtration.** A passive process in which blood flows through the glomeruli of the kidneys. These structures are bundles of capillaries within a capsule. A differential in pressure forces wastes away from the blood into the capsule where it is transported for excretion via the urine.
- **Tubular secretion.** An active transport process in which medications are bound to specific transporters aiding in their elimination.
- **Partial reabsorption.** This occurs when some amount of the drug is reabsorbed after being filtered.

The same factors that affect absorption can also affect excretion, particularly the environmental pH—in this case, the pH of the urine. In this case, if the medication is acidic in an alkaline urine, the medication will more readily move into the urine for excretion. Conversely, an alkaline medication in an acidic urine environment will also readily move to the urine. The closer the pH, the slower the medication will be excreted.

Once a blood clot has formed, a <u>fibrinolytic agent</u> may be administered to dissolve the thrombus and prevent it from breaking off and entering the bloodstream, where it might do further damage. Fibrinolytic agents actually promote the digestion of fibrin. The use of fibrinolytic medications in the prehospital setting remains controversial and, in some circumstances, other forms of reperfusion therapy may be indicated.

Antihyperlipidemic Medications

Although the significance of high cholesterol as an indicator for heart disease remains a topic of discussion, many doctors prefer to treat hyperlipidemia (high cholesterol) in an effort to stave off future problems for their patients. Several types of medications are available to control cholesterol levels. HMG (3-hydroxy-3-methylglutaryl) coenzyme A reductase inhibitors—commonly referred to as statins—are especially popular choices. These medications disrupt the cholesterol production pathway in the body.

Mucokinetic and Bronchodilator Drugs

Serious respiratory emergencies often arise from severe narrowing of any portion of the respiratory tract. The respiratory tract is lined by smooth muscle fibers that influence the diameter of the airway. Control of the smooth muscles is maintained by the ANS. Namely, the parasympathetic nervous system stimulates the airway to constrict, whereas the sympathetic nervous system causes the airway diameter to dilate. Sympathetic stimulation is a result of epinephrine stimulation of the beta-2 receptors.

Many respiratory emergency treatments attempt to expand the respiratory tract by using sympathomimetic medications. These medications are classified according to their effects on the receptors. Some medications are nonselective: They affect alpha, beta-1, and beta-2 receptors alike. Stimulation of alpha receptors reduces vasoconstriction, which in turn reduces mucosal edema. Stimulation of beta-1 receptors increases the patient's heart rate and the force of myocardial contraction. Most beneficial to patients with respiratory issues, stimulation of the beta-2 receptors produces bronchodilation and vasodilation.

Complications arise when patients with respiratory emergencies eventually experience decreased amounts of oxygen to the vital organs, including the heart. As nonselective sympathomimetics begin exerting their effects, the increased heart rate and greater force of contraction lead to a higher demand for oxygen—but, of course, oxygen is already in short supply in a respiratory emergency. For this reason, it is preferable to treat respiratory emergencies with medications specific to beta-2 receptors. Such drugs produce smaller increases in heart rate and force of contraction and, thereby, dramatically decreases the body's rate of oxygen consumption.

A second-line treatment in a respiratory emergency is the class of drugs known as <u>xanthines</u>. These drugs relieve airway constriction by relaxing the smooth muscles of the bronchioles and stimulating cardiac muscles to work harder, thereby increasing blood flow. They also stimulate the CNS—in fact, one notable xanthine is the well-known CNS stimulant, caffeine.

Other respiratory medications suppress the inflammatory response that typically causes acute distress for patients with restrictive airway diseases. In the acute care setting, steroids—including methylprednisolone (Solu-Medrol) and dexamethasone (Decadron)—can be administered for this purpose.

Oxygen and Miscellaneous Respiratory Drugs

Oxygen is the most commonly used medication in the prehospital setting. And it is, in fact, a medication—which means it has appropriate and inappropriate uses and some side effects. Supplementary oxygen therapy is covered in depth in Chapter 11.

Patients may be taking a gamut of medications to treat respiratory problems, depending on their symptoms. Especially during the cold and influenza seasons, use of OTC decongestant medications is common. Try to find out what medications your patient is taking, and know the effects that these drugs may have on other medications and the signs and symptoms they can produce. Although each decongestant varies slightly in terms of its mechanism of action, all such medications seek to reduce tissue edema, facilitate drainage, and maintain the patency of the sinuses. For example, pseudoephedrine, a sympathomimetic, can cause the expected responses associated with medications in this class.

Unfortunately, the fact that these and other medications are readily available sometimes leads to their illicit use. People looking for a high have been known to overdose on decongestants—particularly dextromethorphan, pseudoephedrine, and diphenhydramine.

Drugs Affecting the Gastrointestinal System

Several classes of medications that target the gastrointestinal system are available; the exact choice of drug depends on the specific complaint. Patients experiencing nausea and vomiting may be treated in the prehospital setting with antiemetic medications. Promethazine, which is technically classified as an antihistamine and a sedative, has significant antiemetic effects and may sometimes be administered to relieve a patient's nausea. Like other antihistamines, this drug works as a competitive antagonist, blocking histamines from binding to H-1 receptors. **Table 7-4 ▶** lists other gastrointestinal agents.

Eye Medications

Ophthalmic (eye) medications are virtually always administered in the form of drops directly to the eye. The exact treatment depends on the patient's particular condition but often includes anti-infective agents and drugs intended to reduce swelling (such as NSAIDs and steroids). Ophthalmic administration of medications in the prehospital setting is generally limited to anesthetic purposes to relieve isolated irritation or to ease flushing of the eye. Tetracaine (Pontocaine) is a topical anesthetic used with a Morgan lens to flush debris or contamination from the eye. Tetracaine reduces the pain and discomfort that may be associated with these injuries.

Table 7-4	Gastrointestinal Agents
Agent(s)	**Action**
Antacids	Neutralize stomach acid, used to relieve acid indigestion, upset stomach, "sour stomach," and heartburn; typically are OTC preparations, for example, Mylanta, Tums, Maalox, and milk of magnesia
Antiflatulents	Prevent or are used to treat excessive gas in the intestinal tract, for example, Gas-X and simethicone
Digestants	Used to aid in or stimulate the digestive process; for example, lactase, used by people who are intolerant to dairy products
Antiemetics	Prevent or arrest vomiting, for example, include promethazine (Phenergan), prochlorperazine (Compazine), metoclopramide (Reglan), trimethobenzamide (Tigan), and ondansetron (Zofran)
Cannabinoids	Provide relief to people whose chemotherapy drug causes *minimal* nausea and vomiting; believed to work in an area of the brain thought to be partly responsible for causing nausea and vomiting; mild drowsiness, dizziness, and euphoria are common side effects
Emetics	Used to promote or cause vomiting, for example, syrup of ipecac
Cytoprotective agents	Predominantly used to treat peptic ulcer disease; provide protection to the lining of the stomach and the duodenum to allow ulcers to heal
H_2-receptor antagonists	Reduce acid production in the stomach; act by blocking acid-producing cells in the stomach, for example, include cimetidine (Tagamet) and esomeprazole (Nexium)
Laxatives	Stimulate loosening, relaxation, or evacuation of the bowels; sometimes abused by patients with eating disorders and can lead to profound dehydration if taken improperly; often used for in-hospital management of ACS patients to avoid vagal stimulation during bowel movements
Antidiarrheals	Used to prevent or treat diarrhea and frequently found as OTC preparations

Patients may be prescribed antiglaucoma drugs that are used to treat glaucoma, an eye disease characterized by abnormally high intraocular fluid pressure, damaged optic disc, hardening of the eyeball, and partial to complete loss of vision. Common examples include demecarium (Humorsol), echothiophate iodide (Phospholine iodide), and isoflurophate (Floropryl). All of these agents are prepared as eye solutions or ointments. Other agents include mydriatic and cycloplegic agents. Mydriatic agents are used to dilate the pupils, and cycloplegics are used in the treatment and evaluation of eye problems and include tropicamide (Mydriacyl), cyclopentolate (Cyclogyl), and topical atropine. Several other medications used in the prehospital setting are contraindicated in the presence of glaucoma, so having an idea of which medications the patient may be taking for this condition will assist you in making appropriate decisions about your patient's care.

Ear Medications

Much like ophthalmic medications, medications affecting the ear (otic) are generally administered in the form of drops directly to the ear. The exception occurs in the rare case of a significant infection of the ear, which may require systemic antimicrobial medications. Most otic medications have anti-infective and anti-inflammatory effects. Prehospital administration of otic medications is not indicated.

Drugs Affecting the Pituitary Gland

Although not used in the prehospital setting, medications are available to treat pituitary disorders. These drugs may be administered to shrink or eradicate pituitary tumors. They can also block the pituitary gland from making too much hormone.

Drugs Affecting the Parathyroid and Thyroid Glands

Thyroid disorders are not an uncommon finding in patients treated by paramedics. There are two medical options for treating thyroid disorders: Medications suppress the activity of the thyroid (used in hyperthyroidism) or replace missing thyroid hormones (used in hypothyroidism). Levothyroxine (Synthroid) is a popular medication used to replace the hormones missing in hypothyroidism.

Drugs Affecting the Adrenal Cortex

Most of the treatment for disorders of the adrenal cortex involves the use of corticosteroids. Corticosteroids have anti-inflammatory properties and can have profound metabolic effects.

Drugs Affecting the Pancreas

A variety of medications are available to affect the pancreas. Still others may not act on the pancreas directly, but rather alter the way insulin (produced by the pancreas) is utilized by the body.

To directly affect the pancreas, sulfonylureas increase insulin secretion from the pancreatic beta cells. This medication is effective only if patients have residual beta cell function. Insulin sensitivity is increased by thiazolidinediones and biguanides, which are oral hypoglycemic agents.

Drugs for Labor and Delivery

The use of medications for women in labor is generally limited to situations in which the delivery is abnormal or complicated, which is relatively rare. Of course, if the labor were normal, you probably would not be there. The medications administered in this situation have one of two effects: precipitating labor or inhibiting labor. Currently, only one FDA-approved medication to facilitate labor is available, oxytocin (Pitocin). Oxytocin is a naturally occurring hormone that has multiple reproductive functions. Boosting the levels of oxytocin increases the force and frequency of contractions. This drug is also used to reduce postpartum hemorrhage.

If labor begins before the baby is fully developed or if the labor is causing danger to the mother or baby, medications with tocolytic properties can be used. Tocolytic medications suppress the force and frequency of uterine contractions. Magnesium sulfate is the medication most commonly used for this purpose. It relaxes the smooth muscles, including those located in the uterus. Terbutaline is a beta agonist that has also been used as a tocolytic agent.

Drugs Affecting the Reproductive System

Medications and the Male Reproductive System

With the exception of antibiotics and antivirals for specific infections, a majority of the medications prescribed to affect the male reproductive system are intended to treat erectile dysfunction. Although you will not need to be involved in the treatment of erectile dysfunction, you need to be aware of whether the patient is being treated because of the complications that can arise in prehospital care. Phosphodiesterase inhibitors—for example, sildenafil (Viagra), vardenafil (Levitra), and tadalafil (Cialis)—are commonly prescribed to relax the smooth muscles of the corpora cavernosa and induce vasodilation. Using other vasodilatory medications, particularly nitroglycerin, within 24 to 48 hours of having taken a phosphodiesterase inhibitor can have serious implications for the patient's blood pressure. Always ask patients if they have used erectile dysfunction medications before administering nitroglycerin to avoid profound hypotension Figure 7-8 ▸ .

Medications and the Female Reproductive System

Female reproductive medications perform a variety of functions, from contraception to promoting conception. Most of the medications carry out their functions by altering the reproductive hormones. Contraceptive medications contain synthetic hormones that trick the body into believing the ovary has already released an ovum, which in turn prevents an ovum from being released for fertilization. Antibiotics and antifungal medications may be used for specific conditions. Involvement of paramedics in administering medications affecting the female reproductive system is not indicated.

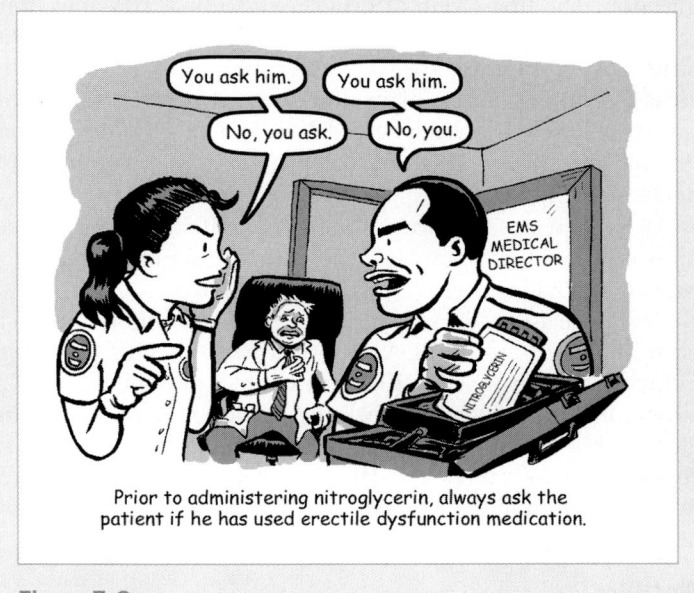

Prior to administering nitroglycerin, always ask the patient if he has used erectile dysfunction medication.

Figure 7-8

You are the Provider Part 4

You make contact with medical control, where the physician advises you to administer 500 mg of calcium chloride IV and closely monitor the patient's vital signs. Upon safe transfer of the patient at the hospital the physician explains that the patient is likely experiencing the effects of digitalis and calcium channel blocker toxicity.

Reassessment	Recording Time: 15 Minutes
Skin	Pink, warm, and dry
Pulse	74 beats/min, irregular; strong radial
ECG	Atrial fibrillation
Blood pressure	118/84 mm Hg
Respirations	22 breaths/min
Sao₂	98% on nonrebreathing mask at 15 L/min of supplemental oxygen
Pupils	Equal and reactive to light

6. What does it mean when a medication has a low therapeutic index?

7. What occurs when one drug potentiates a second drug?

Antineoplastic Drugs

Antineoplastic medications are designed to combat cancer. Most chemotherapy medications are antineoplastic drugs that work by targeting the DNA within the cancerous cells. As yet, these medications do not have the ability to single out cancerous cells, so their systemic side effects are typically significant. As paramedics, we are called to care for cancer patients from time to time; an understanding of their condition and treatments will assist you in treating them effectively.

Drugs Used in Infectious Diseases and Inflammation

Drugs Used to Treat HIV Infection

The FDA has approved a number of drugs for treating HIV infection. The first group of drugs used to treat HIV infection, called nucleoside reverse transcriptase inhibitors, interrupts the virus during an early stage of replication (that is, when the virus is making copies of itself). These drugs may slow the spread of HIV in the body and delay the acquisition of opportunistic infections. This class of drugs is also referred to as nucleoside analogs.

A second class of drugs for treating HIV infection, called protease inhibitors, interrupts the virus during replication at a later step in its life cycle.

A new class of drugs, known as fusion inhibitors, has also been approved by the FDA as a treatment for HIV infection. Enfuvirtide (Fuzeon, or T-20), for example, prevents the HIV-1 virus from entering immune cells by blocking the merger of the virus with the cell membranes. This drug is designed for use in combination with other anti-HIV treatment. It reduces the level of HIV infection in the blood and may be active against HIV that has become resistant to current antiviral treatment schedules.

Antibiotics

Antibiotic medications are actually a subclassification of antimicrobial medications. Antibiotics are themselves classified into several categories based on their composition and the types of bacteria they target. Not all antibiotics affect all types of infections. Antibiotics generally work by killing the bacteria (bactericidal) or by preventing multiplication of the bacteria and thereby allowing the body's immune system to overcome the infectious invaders. Many patients are allergic to certain antibiotics. Thus, although we do not administer antibiotics in the prehospital setting, we should ascertain specific medication allergies of our patients.

Antifungal, Antiviral, and Antiparasitic Medications

Treating fungal infections in humans, particularly systemic infections, can be much more difficult than treating bacterial or viral infections. The basic cellular structure is nearly identical between humans and fungi. Because antimicrobial medications target a specific structure within the infective organism, it is a challenge to identify a medication that will not harm human cells as well. One difference between human and fungal cells is

that fungal cells use ergosterol instead of cholesterol as part of the cellular wall. Polyene medications cause the fungal cells' contents to leak out, causing them to die. Two other classes of antifungal medications, the imidazoles and the triazoles, work by inhibiting certain enzymes, thereby blocking fungal cell wall synthesis.

Antiviral medications work by a variety of mechanisms. Some antiviral medications inhibit the replication of RNA and DNA in the virus. Others inhibit the penetration and uncoating of the virus in the host cell. Still others can act as prodrugs, boosting the effectiveness of other antiviral medications given concurrently.

Antiparasitic medications target parasites (organisms that live in or on the living tissue of a host organism at the expense of that host). For example, nitazoxanide (Alinia) is an antiparasitic medication used to treat diarrhea caused by infection with *Giardia lamblia;* this intestinal parasite causes giardiasis. Approximately 2.5 million cases of giardiasis occur each year in the United States. **Table 7-5 ▾** lists types of antifungal, antiviral, and antiparasitic agents.

Nonsteroidal Anti-inflammatory Drugs

The NSAIDs are designed to reduce pain, inflammation, and fever. They work by inhibiting the cyclooxygenase (COX) enzymes, which produce the chemical prostaglandin; prostaglandin, in turn, promotes pain, inflammation, and fever. There are two COX enzymes, known as COX-1 and COX-2. Some NSAIDs can be nonselective or semiselective in targeting only the COX-2 enzymes. It has been shown that COX-2 medications are associated with a lower incidence of bleeding and ulcers.

Aspirin differs slightly from other NSAIDs in that it targets the COX-1 enzymes to reduce platelet aggregation, which

Table 7-5	Antifungal, Antiviral, and Antiparasitic Agents
Agent(s)	**Action**
Antimalarial	Any drug used to prevent or treat malaria: chloroquine, an antimalarial drug used to treat malaria and amebic dysentery; mefloquine hydrochloride (Larium and Mephaquin), an antimalarial drug effective in cases that do not respond to chloroquine and said to produce harmful neuropsychiatric effects in some people; primaquine and quinine, bitter alkaloids extracted from cinchona bark
Antituberculous	A group of medications used in the treatment of tuberculosis, including isoniazid, rifampicin, pyrazinamide, and ethambutol
Antiamebiasis	Medications used to treat amebas in the body
Anthelmintics	Medications used to treat parasitic intestinal worms
Leprostatic	A group of medications used in the treatment and management of leprosy

provides great benefit in patients who are suspected of having a myocardial infarction. This selectivity also explains why you cannot substitute another NSAID such as ibuprofen, which targets COX-2 to a much greater extent, for aspirin in this situation.

Uricosuric Drugs

Uric acid is found in the blood and is excreted by the kidneys. If uric acid levels are too high, this chemical can be deposited in the form of solid crystals in the joints—a condition known as gout. Uricosuric medications are designed to lower the uric acid levels in the blood by increasing its excretion by the kidneys into the urine.

Serums, Vaccines, and Other Immunizing Agents

Serums, vaccines, and other immunizing agents all fall into the immunobiologic medications category. Immunizations can consist of antigens (vaccines, toxoids) or antibodies (immune globulins, antitoxins). A toxoid is a modified bacterial toxin that has been made nontoxic but retains the ability to stimulate the formation of antibodies. A vaccine, a suspension of whole (live or inactivated) or fractionated bacteria or viruses that have been made nonpathogenic, is given to induce an immune response and prevent disease.

Drugs Affecting the Immunologic System

Patients who undergo organ transplantation or have an autoimmune disease are often prescribed immunosuppressant medications. Immunosuppressants are intended to inhibit the body's ability to attack the "foreign" organ or, in the case of autoimmune diseases, the medications inhibit the body's attack on itself. These drugs are generally derived from fungi or bacteria and tend to have a complicated mechanism of action. Put succinctly, they inhibit lymphocytes and T cells from carrying out their immune functions.

Dermatologic Drugs

A wide variety of afflictions can affect a patient's skin, from infections to cancer. The specific medication used will be determined by the condition itself. Although several systemic medications can be used to treat dermatologic disorders, a majority of the drugs used will be applied topically. In addition, medications used to affect other areas of the body can be given through the skin (that is, transdermally). Nitroglycerin for patients with chest pain and fentanyl for pain management, for example, are commonly encountered medications that are administered transdermally.

Vitamins and Minerals

Vitamins and minerals are necessary substances that allow for normal metabolism, growth and development, and cellular function. Patients may be taking vitamin and mineral supplements to replace deficient items or as a preventive measure.

Vitamins affect a wide variety of functions, but one particular we focus on in the prehospital setting is thiamine (vitamin B_1). Thiamine aids in converting carbohydrates into energy. People with alcoholism, among others, have a propensity to be deficient in this vitamin. It is sometimes appropriate to give thiamine intravenously to patients with risk factors for thiamine deficiency before administering dextrose in an attempt to facilitate effective metabolism.

Fluids and Electrolytes

Several types of IV fluids may be administered to patients. Crystalloid solutions are typically used in the prehospital setting and can be isotonic, hypotonic, or hypertonic. Isotonic solutions provide a stable medium for the administration of medication and provide effective fluid and electrolyte replacement. Hypertonic solutions help provide nutrition. Hypotonic solutions are beneficial in dehydration situations but not in hypovolemic cases. In addition to crystalloids, you may administer colloid solutions to your patients. IV fluids are discussed in detail in Chapter 8.

Antidotes and Overdoses

The management of overdose reflects the agent that the patient has consumed. Antidotes can function antagonistically by blocking receptor sites that would otherwise be stimulated by the agent. They can transform the agent into an inert, non-hazardous form to facilitate excretion. Alternatively, they may bind to the agent to prohibit its absorption into the bloodstream. Overdoses and their antidotes are discussed in depth in Chapter 33.

■ Tying It All Together

As you review the various classifications of medications on the preceding pages, you will probably ask yourself why you need to know all of these because you don't administer them in the prehospital setting. And that is a very good question.

The answer is that there is a tremendous amount of information that can be obtained about your patient's current condition and medical history based on the medications taken. Having an understanding of which types of medications have specific functions allows you to more effectively assess your patient's condition(s). If your patient is unresponsive and you find a spilled bottle of nitroglycerin tablets, what will you suspect? Knowing what nitroglycerin is used for and the effects it has on the body allows you to significantly narrow down the possible conditions your patient might have.

In addition to the assessment of the current condition, you can also gather significant information about the patient's medical history. Again, a general understanding of the uses and effects of different medications provides the clues you need to obtain a large portion of the patient's medical history even when the patient is unable to answer. Furthermore, it is common for patients to forget about a medical condition or not consider it a medical *problem*. For example, a patient may tell you that you he does not have high blood pressure, but when you review his prescription medications, you find labetalol. Because you know that labetalol is often used to treat hypertension, you question him again. He may respond this way: "I don't have high blood pressure because that medication lowers it." This proves to be very useful information that you might have missed had you not understood the classifications of medications.

In addition, a patient's medications may alter the clinical presentation of some conditions. As you probably already know, a patient who is in hypovolemic shock will have an increased pulse rate followed by a decrease in blood pressure. What do you think you will see in a patient with hypovolemic shock but who is taking a prescription medication intended to block beta adrenergic receptors?

Once you have an idea of the condition the patient has and know the medical history, you can begin to develop your pharmacologic treatment plan. Understanding the classifications of medications has a role in this situation as well. You need to develop a treatment plan that will treat the patient's condition while considering the negative effects and interactions with the patient's other medications.

You are the Provider Summary

1. What are some potential differential diagnoses?

Your patient presents with a combination of symptoms: palpitations, mild shortness of breath and visual disturbances. Looking at this trio of symptoms, cardiac problems such as a silent MI, high blood pressure, and abnormal heart rate or rhythm are good possibilities. The mention that he has a history of "heart problems" also helps to tip the scale in this direction.

2. What types of medications might your patient be taking?

There are a variety of different types of medications that he could be taking for heart problems—including a diuretic, a beta blocker, a calcium channel blocker, or an ACE inhibitor.

3. What type of drug is Cardizem and how does it work?

Cardizem is a calcium channel blocker. This drug lowers blood pressure by decreasing peripheral vascular resistance. It helps decrease the work load of the heart by diminishing myocardial and smooth muscle contraction. Calcium channel blockers are also effective in the management of fast cardiac rhythm disturbances because of their ability to decrease the conduction of electrical impulses through the heart.

4. Does the patient present with signs and symptoms of possible drug toxicity? If so, which medications are in question?

Yes, drug toxicity, specifically digoxin and Cardizem, is a possibility. When taken in excess, either medication can cause a significant drop in a patient's hemodynamic status, which explains the problems with the heart rate and blood pressure, but what about the vision disturbances? One of the other side effects of digoxin toxicity is visual disturbances, including the presence of a yellow-green halo around objects and blurred vision.

5. What treatment will increase the patient's blood pressure?

In this case the best treatment is to reverse the effects of the calcium channel blocker, Cardizem, by administering calcium chloride.

6. What does it mean when a medication has a low therapeutic index?

The therapeutic index measures the safety of the drug. It is calculated by dividing the lethal dose 50 (LD_{50}) by the effective dose 50 (ED_{50}). The closer the answer is to 1, the more harmful the drug is. Since the therapeutic index for digoxin is close to one, the amount of medication between a normal dose and a toxic dose is very small, making it easy for toxic levels to develop. Because of this, patients who take digoxin frequently have their blood levels checked to make sure that they are within the therapeutic range.

7. What occurs when one drug potentiates a second drug?

When potentiation occurs, the effect of one drug increases the effect of another. In your patient, the administration of Cardizem increased the amount of digoxin in the blood, leading to the increased effects of digoxin and an increased chance of toxicity.

Ready for Review

- In the prehospital setting, the goal of emergency pharmacology is to use medications to reverse, prevent, or control various diseases and illnesses, chronic and acute.
- Medications must always be delivered according to the *six rights*: the Right patient, the Right dose, the Right route, the Right time, the Right medication, and Right documentation on your PCR.
- A medication is a drug that has been approved by the government agency that regulates pharmaceuticals for the purpose of curing or reducing the symptoms of an illness or medical condition or to assist in the diagnosis, treatment, or prevention of a disease. A drug may also be given in an attempt to alter the disease process.
- The manufacture of pharmaceuticals in the United States and most other countries is subject to a variety of laws and regulations that aim to prohibit manufacturers from making false claims about their drugs' benefits and advising patients to administer the drugs incorrectly.
- Drugs are derived from four principal sources: animal, vegetable, mineral, and synthetic compounds.
- Special considerations exist when administering medications to pregnant women, children, and older people.
- Paramedics are legally responsible for the appropriate use of medications and documentation of medication therapy. Always have a clear understanding of which medication you are administering and why you are administering it.
- Medications administered as part of the care provided in the prehospital setting exert their effects largely by acting on the nervous system.
- The peripheral nervous system is separated into two divisions: the somatic nervous system and the ANS. The ANS is particularly vulnerable to the administration of prehospital medications. It is considered to be "automatic" or involuntary because we cannot control its functioning or force functions under its control to happen or not happen. The sympathetic nervous system, which gives the fight-or-flight response, is the dominant system during periods of stress and activity. The parasympathetic nervous system is the dominant system during periods of rest and relaxation.
- Neurotransmission is the process of chemical signaling between cells.
- Receptors are unique molecular structures or sites on the surface or interior of a cell that bind with substances such as hormones, drugs, and neurotransmitters. Receptors are highly specialized and, in most cases, respond only to a particular substance, much like a lock and key.
- Normal neurotransmission can be altered by using drugs that mimic or inhibit neurotransmission. Some medications inhibit the release of neurotransmitters, and others work by blocking the receptor sites along the neural pathway.
- Drugs adjust or influence the body's existing functions by interacting with various cells and tissues in the body, and they typically work through several mechanisms of action rather than relying on a single action. In most cases, medications may bind to a receptor site and trigger a stimulus; in some cases, they change the chemical properties of cells and tissues. They may also combine with other chemicals within cells or organ systems to aid in elimination or bind to receptors to alter the normal metabolic functions of cells and tissues.
- Drugs are available in a wide array of forms, including liquids, solids, and vapors. In the field, you use only a limited subset of drug forms.
- The mode of administration affects the rate at which the body absorbs the drug, and the route of administration affects the speed with which a drug works.
- Local effects result from the direct application of a drug to a tissue. Systemic effects occur after the drug is absorbed by any route and distributed by the bloodstream.
- The routes of administration are classified into three categories based on how the medication is absorbed and distributed: percutaneous (applied to and absorbed through the skin), enteral (absorbed somewhere along the gastrointestinal tract), and parenteral (any route of administration that does not cause the drug to be absorbed through the skin, mucous membranes, or gastrointestinal tract).
- Every medication has varying effects on the body. The study of the metabolism and action of medications within the body is called pharmacokinetics, which focuses particularly on the time required for absorption, duration of action, distribution in the body, and method of excretion.
- A medication's ability to reach a therapeutic concentration in the bloodstream depends partially on the rate and extent to which the drug is absorbed. Rate and extent are dependent on the ability of the medication to cross the cell membrane, which occurs by active transport or passive diffusion.
- Blood is the primary distribution vehicle for medications. Factors that change the way blood flows through the body will change the way medications are transported to the target tissue.
- Biotransformation, or the way in which the body metabolizes medications, occurs by transforming the medication into a metabolite or by making the medication more water-soluble.
- Excretion occurs primarily through the kidneys via glomerular filtration, tubular secretion, and partial reabsorption.
- Medications cause their action on the body by binding to a receptor site, changing the physical properties of cells, chemically combining with other chemicals, or altering a normal metabolic pathway.
- The drug-response relationship correlates the amount of medication given and the response it causes.
- Factors affecting how patients react to medications include age, weight, sex, environment, time of administration, condition of the patient (overall state of health), genetic factors, and psychologic factors.
- Every medication has some side effects that are known and anticipated, although occasionally unanticipated adverse reactions (iatrogenic responses) are seen.
- Extremes of temperature, exposure to direct sunlight, or excessive humidity may decrease the potency of some medications or degrade the actual molecular components and make the medication inactive.
- Understanding drug profiles will help you select the most appropriate medication for your patients.
- Classifications of drugs are based on the effect the drugs will have on a particular part of the body or on a specific condition.

Vital Vocabulary

absorption The process by which a medication's molecules are moved from the site of entry or administration into the body and into systemic circulation.

adrenal medulla The inner portion of the adrenal glands that synthesizes, stores, and eventually releases epinephrine and norepinephrine.

adrenergic Pertaining to nerves that release the neurotransmitter norepinephrine or noradrenaline (such as adrenergic nerves, adrenergic response). The term also pertains to the receptors acted on by norepinephrine, that is, the adrenergic receptors.

afferent nerves The nerves that carry sensory impulses from all parts of the body to the brain.

affinity The force attraction between medications and receptors causing them to bind together.

agonist A substance that mimics the actions of a specific neurotransmitter or hormone by binding to the specific receptor of the naturally occurring substance.

analgesia The absence of the sensation of pain.

analgesics A classification for medications that relieve pain, or induce analgesia.

anesthetic A type of medication intended to induce a loss of sensation to touch or pain.

angiotensin converting enzyme (ACE) inhibitors Medications that suppress the conversion of angiotensin I to angiotensin II.

angiotensin II receptor antagonists Medications that are similar to ACE inhibitors but work by selectively blocking angiotensin II at their receptor sites.

antagonist A molecule that blocks the ability of a given chemical to bind to its receptor, preventing a biologic response.

antiarrhythmic medications The medications used to treat and prevent cardiac rhythm disorders.

antibiotic medications The medications that fight bacterial infection by killing the bacteria or by preventing multiplication of the bacteria to allow the body's immune system to overcome them.

anticholinergic Of or pertaining to the blocking of acetylcholine receptors, resulting in inhibition of transmission of parasympathetic nerve impulses.

anticoagulant drugs The medications used to prevent intravascular thrombosis by preventing blood coagulation in the vascular system.

anticonvulsant medications The medications used to treat seizures, which are believed to work by inhibiting the influx of sodium into cells.

antihypertensives The medications used to control blood pressure.

antineoplastic medications The medications designed to combat cancer.

antiplatelet agents The medications that interfere with the collection of platelets.

autonomic nervous system (ANS) The component of the peripheral nervous system that sends sensory impulses from internal structures (such as blood vessels, the heart, and organs of the chest, abdomen, and pelvis) through afferent autonomic nerves to the brain.

barbiturates Any medications of a group of barbituric acid derivatives that act as central nervous system depressants and are used as sedatives or hypnotics.

benzodiazepines Any medications of a group of psychotropic agents used as antianxiety, muscle relaxants, sedatives, or hypnotics.

bioavailability The amount of a medication that is still active once it reaches its target tissue.

biologic half-life The time it takes the body to eliminate half of the drug.

biotransformation A process by which a medication is chemically converted to a different compound or metabolite.

buccal route A medication route in which medication is administered between the cheeks and gums.

calcium channel blockers The medications that suppress arrhythmias, provide more oxygen to the heart via coronary artery dilation, and reduce peripheral vascular resistance.

capsule A cylindrical gelatin container enclosing a dose of medication.

cardiac glycosides A classification of medications that naturally occur in plant substances and that block certain ionic pumps in the heart cells' membranes, which indirectly increases calcium concentrations; an example is digoxin.

chemical name A description of the drug's chemical composition and molecular structure.

cholinergic Fibers in the parasympathetic nervous system that release a chemical called acetylcholine.

chronotropic Affecting the rate of rhythmic movements, such as the heartbeat. A positive chronotropic effect would result in increasing the heart rate.

CNS stimulants Any medications or agents that increase brain activity.

contraindications In health care, conditions or factors that increase the risk involved in using a particular drug, carrying out a medical procedure, or engaging in a particular activity.

cross-tolerance A form of drug tolerance in which patients who take a particular medication for an extended period can build up a tolerance to other medications in the same class.

cumulative effect An effect that occurs when several successive doses of a medication are administered or when absorption of a medication occurs faster than excretion or metabolism.

depolarizing neuromuscular blocking agents Medications designed to keep muscles in a contracted state.

distribution The movement and transportation of a medication throughout the bloodstream to tissues and cells of the body and, ultimately, to its target receptor.

diuretic medications The medications designed to promote elimination of excess salt and water by the kidneys.

dopaminergic receptors The receptors believed to cause dilation of the renal, coronary, and cerebral arteries.

dromotropic Relating to or influencing the conductivity of nerve fibers or cardiac muscle fibers.

drugs Any chemical compounds that may be used on humans to help in diagnosis, treatment, cure, mitigation, or prevention of disease or other abnormal conditions.

duration of action How long the medication concentration can be expected to remain above the minimum level needed to provide the intended action.

efferent nerves The nerves that carry messages from the brain to the muscles and all other organs of the body.

elixir A syrup with alcohol and flavoring added.

emulsion A preparation of one liquid (usually an oil) distributed in small globules in another liquid (usually water).

enteral routes The medication administration routes in which medications are absorbed somewhere along the gastrointestinal tract.

excretion The elimination of toxic or inactive metabolites from the body. This is primarily done by the kidneys, intestines, lungs, and assorted glands.

extract A concentrated preparation of a drug made by putting the drug into solution (in alcohol or water) and evaporating off the excess solvent to a prescribed standard.

fibrinolytic agents The only medications available to dissolve blood clots after they have already formed; the drugs promote the digestion of fibrin.

fluid extract A concentrated form of a drug prepared by dissolving the crude drug in the fluid in which it is most readily soluble.

ganglia Groupings of nerve cell bodies located in the peripheral nervous system.

generic drug A medication that is not patented.

generic name A general name for a drug that is not manufacturer-specific; usually the name given to the drug by the company that first manufactures it.

hypnosis Altered consciousness often caused by hypnotic drugs, which are used to induce sleep.

iatrogenic response An adverse condition inadvertently induced in a patient by the treatment given.

idiosyncrasy An abnormal (and usually unexplained) reaction by a person to a medication, to which most other people do not react.

immunobiologic medications The medications that include serums, vaccines, and other immunizing agents.

immunosuppressant medications The medications intended to inhibit the body's ability to attack the "foreign" organ or, in the case of autoimmune diseases, the medications that inhibit the body's attack on itself.

indications The reasons or conditions for which the medication is given.

inotropic affecting the contractility of muscle tissue, especially cardiac muscle.

interference A direct biochemical interaction between two drugs.

intramuscular (IM) route A method of delivering a medication into the muscle of the body. This is accomplished by placing a needle into a muscle space and injecting the medication into the tissue.

intraosseous (IO) route A method of delivering a medication into the marrow cavity of a bone. This is accomplished by placing a rigid needle into the marrow cavity and flushing a medication into the space.

liniments Liquid preparations of drugs for external use, usually to relieve some discomfort (such as pain, itching) or to protect the skin.

local anesthesia A type of anesthesia that causes a loss of sensation to touch or pain at a specific isolated spot on the body where a procedure is to take place.

local effects The effects that result from the direct application of a drug to a tissue, for example when lotions are applied to the skin to relieve itching.

loop diuretics Medications that inhibit the reabsorption of sodium and calcium ions and that can cause an excessive loss of potassium.

mechanism of action The way in which a medication produces the intended response.

medication A licensed drug taken to cure or reduce symptoms of an illness or medical condition or as an aid in the diagnosis, treatment, or prevention of a disease or other abnormal condition.

milk In the context of pharmacology, an aqueous suspension of an insoluble drug.

muscarinic cholinergic antagonists Medications that block acetylcholine exclusively at the muscarinic receptors; an example is atropine.

neuromuscular blocking agents Medications that affect the parasympathetic nervous system by inducing paralysis.

neurotransmission The process of chemical signaling between cells.

nicotinic cholinergic antagonists Medications that block the acetylcholine only at nicotinic receptors.

nonbarbiturate hypnotics Medications designed to sedate without the side effects of a barbiturate.

nondepolarizing neuromuscular blocking agents Medications designed to cause temporary paralysis by binding in a competitive but nonstimulatory manner to part of the ACh receptor. Do not cause fasciculations.

nonopioid analgesics Medications designed to relieve pain without the side effects of opioids.

nonspecific agents Medications that produce effects on different cells through a variety of mechanisms. Generally classified by the focus of action or specific therapeutic use.

nonsteroidal anti-inflammatory drugs (NSAIDs) Medications with analgesic and fever reducing properties.

official name The name listed in the United States Pharmacopeia (USP) once the generic name has been approved by the United States Adopted Name Council and the drug has been approved by the US Food and Drug Administration.

ointment A semisolid preparation for external application to the body, usually containing a medicinal substance.

onset of action The time needed for the concentration of the medication at the target tissue to reach the minimum effective level.

opioid agonist-antagonists Medications designed to relieve pain without the side effects of opioids.

opioid agonists Chemicals that are similar to or derived from the opium plant.

opioid antagonists A classification of medications that reverses the effects of opioid drugs.

para-aminophenol derivatives Medications designed to reduce fevers and relieve pain.

parenteral routes Medication routes in which medications are administered via any route other than the alimentary canal (digestive tract), skin, or mucous membranes.

patch A solid medication impregnated into a membrane or adhesive that is applied to the surface of the skin.

percutaneous routes The medication routes of any medication absorbed through the skin or a mucous membrane.

peripheral nervous system (PNS) Consists of all nervous tissue outside of the brain and spinal cord and is subdivided into two divisions, the *somatic* and *autonomic* nervous systems.

pharmacodynamics The branch of pharmacology that studies reactions between medications and living structures, including the processes of body responses to pharmacologic, biochemical, physiologic, and therapeutic effects.

pharmacokinetics The study of the metabolism and action of medications with particular emphasis on the time required for absorption, duration of action, distribution in the body, and method of excretion.

pharmacology The branch of medicine dealing with the actions of drugs in the body—therapeutic and toxic effects—and development and testing of new drugs and new uses of existing ones.

pill A drug shaped into a ball or oval to be swallowed; often coated to disguise an unpleasant taste.

potentiation In health care, the effect of increasing the potency or effectiveness of a drug or other treatment; may occur by administering two medications concurrently, and one increases the effect of the other.

powder A drug that has been ground into pulverized form.

pulmonary route A medication route in which medication is administered directly to the pulmonary system through inhalation or injection.

pulvule A solid medication form that resembles a capsule but it is not made of gelatin and does not separate.

regional anesthesia A type of anesthesia that focuses on a particular portion of the body, such as the legs or the arms.

sedation An effect in which the patient experiences decreased anxiety and inhibition.

side effects Reactions that can manifest as signs or symptoms that are not desired but are expected based on how the medication works.

skeletal muscle relaxants Medications that provide relief of skeletal muscle spasms.

sodium channel blockers Antiarrhythmic medications that slow conduction through the heart.

solution A liquid containing one or more chemical substances entirely dissolved, usually in water.

specific agents Medications that bring about an identifiable mechanism with unique receptors for the agent.

spirits A preparation of a volatile substance dissolved in alcohol.

stimulants An agent that increases the level of body activity.

subcutaneous (SC or SQ) route A medication route in which injections are given beneath the skin into the fat or connective tissue immediately underlying it.

sublingual (SL) A medication route in which medication is administered under the tongue.

summation effect The process whereby multiple medications can produce a response that the individual medications alone do not produce.

suppository A drug mixed in a firm base that melts at body temperature and is shaped to fit the rectum, urethra, or vagina.

suspension A preparation of a finely divided drug intended to be (or already) incorporated in a suitable liquid.

sympathetic blocking agent An antihypertensive medication that decreases cardiac output and rennin secretions.

sympathomimetics The medications administered to stimulate the sympathetic nervous system.

synergism An interaction of two or more medications that results in an effect that is greater than the sum of their effects if taken independently.

syrup A drug suspended in sugar and water to improve its taste.

systemic anesthesia A type of anesthesia often done through the inhalation of volatile vaporized liquids and predominantly reserved for operating room use; also called general anesthesia.

systemic effects The effects that occur after the drug is absorbed by any route and distributed by the bloodstream; almost invariably involve more than one organ.

tablet A powdered drug that has been molded or compressed into a small disk.

tachyphylaxis A condition in which the patient rapidly becomes tolerant to a medication.

termination of action The amount of time after the medication's concentration falls below the minimum effective level until it is eliminated from the body.

therapeutic The desired or intended action of a medication.

therapeutic index The ratio of a drug's lethal dose for 50% (LD_{50}) of the population to its effective dose for 50% (ED_{50}) of the population; a medication's margin of safety.

thiazides A type of diuretic medication that specifically controls the sodium and water quantities excreted by the kidneys.

tincture A dilute alcoholic extract of a drug.

tolerance A physiologic response that requires a patient to take an increased medication dose to produce the same effect that formerly was produced by the lower dose.

toxoid A modified bacterial toxin that has been made nontoxic but retains the ability to stimulate the formation of antibodies.

trade name The brand name registered to a specific manufacturer or owner; also called proprietary name.

transdermal route A medication route generally performed by placing medication directly onto the patient's skin.

uricosuric medications The medications designed to lower the uric acid level in the blood by increasing the excretion by the kidneys into the urine.

vaccine A suspension of whole (live or inactivated) or fractionated bacteria or viruses that have been made nonpathogenic; given to induce an immune response and prevent disease.

vapor A gaseous medication form primarily used in operating room anesthesia.

vasodilator medications The medications that work on the smooth muscles of the arterioles and/or the veins.

xanthines A classification of medications that affect the respiratory smooth muscle and that relax bronchiole smooth muscles, stimulate cardiac muscle, and stimulate the central nervous system.

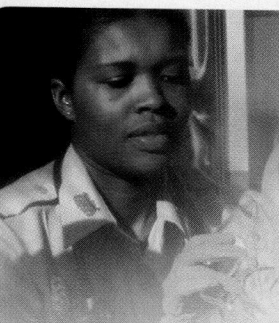

Assessment in Action

You and your partner have responded to a call for chest pain. The patient is a 68-year-old man who describes the pain as being a 20 on a 1-to-10 scale with 10 being the worst pain ever. As your partner connects the patient to the monitor, you start gathering your patient's history. The patient has had a previous cardiac event and has been prescribed a "beta blocker."

1. **What is the primary action of a beta blocker?**
   A. It reduces the adrenergic stimulation of the beta receptors in the heart.
   B. It increases the adrenergic stimulation of the beta receptors in the heart.
   C. It reduces the cholinergic stimulation of the beta receptors in the heart.
   D. It increases the cholinergic stimulation of the beta receptors in the heart.

2. **You decided to give your patient salicylic acid once you determine that he is not allergic to it. Salicylic acid is a(n):**
   A. calcium channel blocker.
   B. sympathomimetic.
   C. antiplatelet agent.
   D. antihypertensive.

3. Your patient has not taken any of his own nitroglycerin, so you decide to give him a dose of yours. How are you going to deliver the medication?
   A. IV push
   B. Sublingual
   C. Intramuscular
   D. Subcutaneous

4. How long should it take for the nitroglycerin to take effect through this route of administration?
   A. 15 to 20 minutes
   B. 10 to 15 minutes
   C. 5 to 10 minutes
   D. Less than 5 minutes

5. Your patient is still having substantial chest pain after the nitroglycerin, and you decide that he will benefit greatly from analgesia. Which medication is an analgesic?
   A. Morphine
   B. Narcan
   C. Oxygen
   D. Albuterol

6. What is a specific cardiac action of the analgesic mentioned in question 5 that should benefit this patient?
   A. It has a chronotropic action that slows the heart rate.
   B. It decreases the workload on the heart.
   C. It increases the workload on the heart.
   D. It decreases ectopic beats.

Challenging Question

7. If this patient had taken three doses of his own nitroglycerin, would you still give him three doses of yours?

▆ Points to Ponder

You respond outside of your response area to a mutual aid request from a neighboring jurisdiction for a cardiac arrest. When you arrive on the scene, you find that a local engine company arrived ahead of you. The local engine company crew has a paramedic on board and has secured the airway and inserted an IV line. You introduce yourself and your EMT partner to the crew and assume responsibility for administering the medications. You ask your partner to hand you some epinephrine. Your partner pulls the unfamiliar drug box over and starts rummaging through looking for a particular color of label, which he cannot find. All of the medications are unboxed and stored in elastic loops in a soft-sided pack. You look back at your partner to see what the hold-up is and you see the medication pack.

Are all medication boxes standardized by the color of the box? Who has the responsibility to select the correct medication?

Issues: Working With Other Responders, Properly Administering Medication.

8

Vascular Access and Medication Administration

Objectives

Cognitive

1-8.1   Review the specific anatomy and physiology pertinent to medication administration. (p 8.3)

1-8.2   Review mathematical principles. (p 8.28)

1-8.3   Review mathematical equivalents. (p 8.29)

1-8.4   Differentiate temperature readings between the Centigrade and Fahrenheit scales. (p 8.30)

1-8.5   Discuss formulas as a basis for performing drug calculations. (p 8.30)

1-8.6   Discuss applying basic principles of mathematics to the calculation of problems associated with medication dosages. (p 8.28)

1-8.7   Describe how to perform mathematical conversions from the household system to the metric system. (p 8.28)

1-8.8   Describe the indications, equipment needed, technique used, precautions, and general principles of peripheral venous or external jugular cannulation. (p 8.18)

1-8.9   Describe the indications, equipment needed, technique used, precautions, and general principles of intraosseous needle placement and infusion. (p 8.23)

1-8.10   Discuss legal aspects affecting medication administration. (p 8.33)

1-8.11   Discuss the "six rights" of drug administration and correlate these with the principles of medication administration. (p 8.33)

1-8.12   Discuss medical asepsis and the differences between clean and sterile techniques. (p 8.35)

1-8.13   Describe use of antiseptics and disinfectants. (p 8.35)

1-8.14   Describe the use of universal precautions and body substance isolation (BSI) procedures when administering a medication. (p 8.35)

1-8.15   Differentiate among the different dosage forms of oral medications. (p 8.36)

1-8.16   Describe the equipment needed and general principles of administering oral medications. (p 8.36)

1-8.17   Describe the indications, equipment needed, techniques used, precautions, and general principles of administering medications by the inhalation route. (p 8.36)

1-8.18   Describe the indications, equipment needed, techniques used, precautions, and general principles of administering medications by the gastric tube. (p 8.36)

1-8.19   Describe the indications, equipment needed, techniques used, precautions, and general principles of rectal medication administration. (p 8.38)

1-8.20   Differentiate among the different parenteral routes of medication administration. (p 8.38)

1-8.21   Describe the equipment needed, techniques used, complications, and general principles for the preparation and administration of parenteral medications. (p 8.39)

1-8.22   Differentiate among the different percutaneous routes of medication administration. (p 8.50)

1-8.23   Describe the purpose, equipment needed, techniques used, complications, and general principles for obtaining a blood sample. (p 8.23)

1-8.24   Describe disposal of contaminated items and sharps. (p 8.35)

1-8.25   Synthesize a pharmacologic management plan including medication administration. (p 8.9)

1-8.26   Integrate pathophysiological principles of medication administration with patient management. (p 8.3)

Affective

1-8.27   Comply with paramedic standards of medication administration. (p 8.33)

1-8.28   Comply with universal precautions and body substance isolation (BSI). (p 8.35)

1-8.29   Defend a pharmacologic management plan for medication administration. (p 8.33)

1-8.30   Serve as a model for medical asepsis. (p 8.35)

1-8.31   Serve as a model for advocacy while performing medication administration. (p 8.28)

1-8.32   Serve as a model for disposing contaminated items and sharps. (p 8.36)

Psychomotor

1-8.33   Use universal precautions and body substance isolation (BSI) procedures during medication administration. (p 8.35)

1-8.34   Demonstrate cannulation of peripheral or external jugular veins. (p 8.14, 8.18)

1-8.35   Demonstrate intraosseous needle placement and infusion. (p 8.25)

1-8.36   Demonstrate clean technique during medication administration. (p 8.35)

1-8.37   Demonstrate administration of oral medications. (p 8.36)

1-8.38   Demonstrate administration of medications by the inhalation route. (p 8.53)

1-8.39   Demonstrate administration of medications by the gastric tube. (p 8.37)

1-8.40   Demonstrate rectal administration of medications. (p 8.38)

1-8.41   Demonstrate preparation and administration of parenteral medications. (p 8.40)

1-8.42   Demonstrate preparation and techniques for obtaining a blood sample. (p 8.23)

1-8.43   Perfect disposal of contaminated items and sharps. (p 8.53)

Introduction

Vascular access is often needed in emergency medicine for patients in hemodynamically unstable condition and in need of intravenous (IV) fluids, various medications, or both. A number of techniques are used to gain vascular access in the pre-hospital setting, including cannulation of a peripheral extremity vein, external jugular vein cannulation, and intraosseous infusion. In critically ill or injured patients, survival often depends on your ability to obtain vascular access quickly and effectively. Because these procedures are invasive, you must be proficient, yet cautious. Significant harm to the patient can result from improper technique and/or insufficient knowledge of the medication(s) being administered.

This chapter begins with an overview of fluids and electrolytes—balanced and imbalanced—and the processes of osmosis and diffusion. Next, it discusses the various types of IV solutions used in the prehospital setting and the techniques of IV therapy and intraosseous infusion. Finally, it describes the mathematical principles used in pharmacology, calculating medication doses (bolus and maintenance infusion), and the various routes for administering medications.

Fluids and Electrolytes

The human body is composed mostly of water, which provides the environment in which the chemical reactions necessary to life take place. Water also serves as a transport medium for nutrients, hormones, and waste materials. The total body water (TBW) con-

stitutes 60% of the weight of an adult man and is distributed among the following compartments Figure 8-1 ▶ :

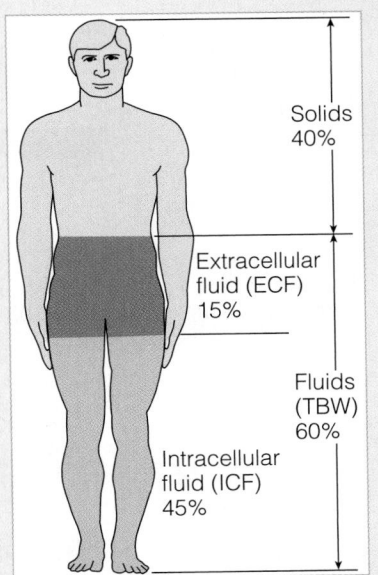

- Intracellular fluid (ICF) is the water contained inside the cells; it normally accounts for 45% of body weight.
- Extracellular fluid (ECF), the water outside the cells, accounts for 15% of body weight and is further divided into two types of fluids:
  - Interstitial fluid, the water bathing the cells, accounts for about 10.5% of body weight. The interstitial fluid also includes special fluid collections, such as cerebrospinal fluid and intraocular fluid.
  - Intravascular fluid (plasma), the water within the blood vessels, carries red blood cells, white blood cells, and vital nutrients. Intravascular fluid normally accounts for about 4.5% of body weight.

Figure 8-1 Distribution of water throughout the body.

You are the Provider Part 1

You are dispatched to the home of a 70-year-old woman who has diabetes. A neighbor found her lying on a couch in her living room. The neighbor tells you she tried to wake up the patient, but was unable to do so. The patient appears to be unconscious; she is pale and noticeably diaphoretic. She is breathing, but her respirations are rapid and shallow.

Your general impression of the patient and her environment reveals no signs of injury. After carefully moving the patient to the floor, you perform an initial assessment. Your partner opens the jump kit in preparation for treatment.

Initial Assessment	Recording Time: 0 Minutes
Level of consciousness	U (Unresponsive)
Airway	Patent; airway is clear of secretions
Breathing	Respirations, rapid and shallow
Circulation	Radial pulses, rapid and weak; skin, pale and diaphoretic; no gross bleeding

1. Is this a medical patient or a trauma patient?
2. What are your initial priorities of care?
3. What is the most appropriate initial airway management for this patient?
4. Does this patient require immediate medication therapy?

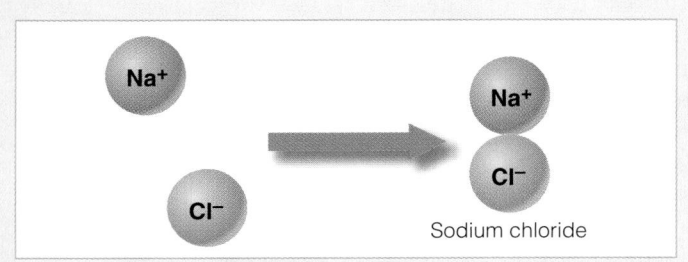

Figure 8-2 When sodium (Na⁺) and chloride (Cl⁻) unite, they form salt (sodium chloride [NaCl]).

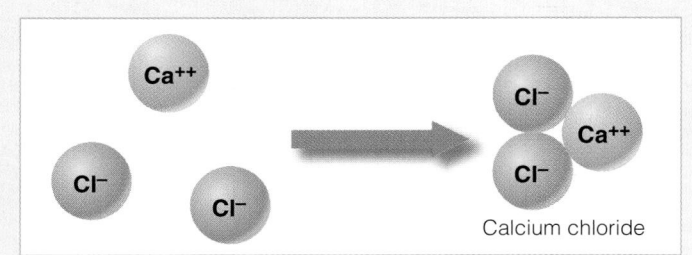

Figure 8-3 A doubly charged (bivalent) cation such as calcium (Ca⁺⁺) needs two anions.

The fluids in the body are composed of dissolved elements and water, a combination known as a solution. A solution is a mixture of two things:

- Solvent. The fluid that does the dissolving, or the solution that contains the dissolved components
- Solute. The dissolved particles contained in the solvent

Water in the body serves as the universal solvent, dissolving a variety of solutes. These solutes can be classified as electrolytes or nonelectrolytes.

Electrolytes

Atoms carry charges—some positive, some negative. Two or more atoms that bond together form a molecule. When atoms bond together, they share and disperse their charges throughout the molecule. Organic molecules contain carbon atoms—for example, table sugar ($C_6H_{12}O_6$). By contrast, inorganic molecules do not contain carbon—for example, table salt (NaCl). Inorganic molecules give rise to electrolytes (so called because of their ability to conduct electricity) when they dissociate in water into their charged components.

Electrolytes, also called ions, are reactive and dangerous if left to circulate in the body. The body, however, uses the energy stored in these charged particles. Electrolytes help to regulate everything from water levels to cardiac function and muscle contractions. Water in the body stabilizes the electrolyte charges so that the electrolytes can aid in the metabolic functions that are necessary for life.

Each electrolyte has a unique property or value to the body. If the electrolyte has an overall *positive* charge, it is called

a cation; if it has an overall *negative* charge, it is called an anion. The major cations of the body include sodium, potassium, calcium, and magnesium; bicarbonate, chloride, and phosphorus are the major anions.

The unit of measurement for electrolytes is the milliequivalent (mEq); it represents the chemical combining power of the ion and is based on the number of available ionic charges in an electrolyte solution. One milliequivalent of any cation is able to react completely with 1 mEq of any anion. For example, sodium (Na⁺) is a singly charged (monovalent) cation, and chloride (Cl⁻) is a singly charged anion. Thus 1 mEq of Na⁺ will react with 1 mEq of Cl⁻ to form NaCl—ordinary table salt **Figure 8-2 ◄**. Calcium (Ca⁺⁺) has two positive charges (bivalent); thus the Ca⁺⁺ ion represents 2 mEq and reacts completely with 2 mEq of a singly charged anion **Figure 8-3 ◄**.

Sodium

Sodium (Na⁺) is the principal extracellular cation needed to regulate the distribution of water throughout the body in the intravascular and interstitial fluid compartments. Its role in maintaining adequate cellular perfusion gives rise to the saying, "Where sodium goes, water follows."

Potassium

About 98% of all the body's potassium (K⁺) is found inside the cells of the body, making it the principal intracellular cation. Potassium plays a major role in neuromuscular function and in the conversion of glucose into glycogen. Cellular potassium levels are regulated by insulin. The sodium-potassium (Na⁺-K⁺) pump is helped by the presence of insulin and epinephrine. Low potassium levels—hypokalemia—in the serum (blood plasma) can lead to decreased skeletal muscle function, gastrointestinal disturbances, and alterations in cardiac function. High potassium levels in the serum—hyperkalemia—can lead to hyperstimulation of neural cell transmission, resulting in cardiac arrest.

Calcium

Calcium (Ca⁺⁺) is the principal cation needed for bone growth. It also plays an important part in the functioning of heart muscle, nerves, and cell membranes and is necessary for proper blood clotting.

Low serum calcium levels—hypocalcemia—can lead to overstimulation of nerve cells. Signs and symptoms of hypocalcemia include skeletal muscle cramps, abdominal cramps, carpopedal spasms, hypotension, and vasoconstriction.

High serum calcium levels—hypercalcemia—can lead to decreased stimulation of nerve cells. Signs and symptoms of hypercalcemia include skeletal muscle weakness, lethargy, ataxia, vasodilation, and hot, flushed skin.

Magnesium

Magnesium (Mg⁺⁺) has an important role as a coenzyme in the metabolism of proteins and carbohydrates. In addition, it acts in a manner similar to calcium in controlling neuromuscular irritability.

Bicarbonate

Bicarbonate (HCO_3^-) levels are the determining factor between acidosis and alkalosis in the body. Bicarbonate is the primary buffer used in all circulating body fluids.

Chloride

Chloride concentration is a primary determinant of stomach pH. It also regulates extracellular fluid levels.

Phosphorus

Phosphorus (P) is an important component in adenosine triphosphate (ATP), the body's powerful energy source.

Nonelectrolytes

The body also contains solutes that have no electrical charge. These nonelectrolytes include glucose and urea. The normal concentration of glucose in the blood, for example, is 70 to 110 milligrams (mg) per 100 milliliters (mL).

Fluid and Electrolyte Movement

Water and electrolytes move among the body's fluid compartments according to some basic chemical and biologic tenets. One governing principle is that unequal concentrations on different sides of a cell membrane will move to balance themselves equally on both sides of the membrane. Balance across a cell membrane has two components:

- Balance of compounds (for example, water and electrolytes) on either side of the cell membrane
- Balance of charges [the positive (+) or negative (−) charges carried on the atoms] on either side of the cell membrane

When concentrations of charges or compounds are greater on one side of the cell membrane than on the other side, a gradient is created. The natural tendency for materials is to flow from an area of higher concentration to one of lower concentration, establishing a concentration gradient. Gradients are categorized according to the type of material that flows down them: Chemical compounds flow down chemical gradients; electrical currents flow down electrical gradients. The process of flowing down a gradient depends on whether the cell membrane will allow the material to pass through it. Certain compounds can travel freely across the cell membrane (a kinetically favorable situation that requires little energy), whereas others require active transport across the membrane because of the size of the compound or because of an incompatible charge.

Diffusion

When compounds or charges concentrated on one side of a cell membrane move across it to an area of lower concentration, the process is called diffusion. To visualize this situation, imagine that too many people show up for a theater performance. The management decides to open another seating area to accommo-date the crowd. Patrons (charges or compounds) are concentrated in a small area (the cell) outside the door (the cell membrane) leading to the new seating area. When the theater manager opens the door, patrons can move through it (selective cell membrane permeability) from the congested area (down a concentration gradient). The patrons spread themselves out evenly (diffuse) throughout the total area, with some choosing to stay behind in the original seating area as others move into the new area, until all have an equal amount of room.

Filtration

Filtration, another type of diffusion, is commonly used by the kidneys to clean blood. Water carries dissolved compounds across the cell membranes of the tubules of the kidney. The tubule membrane traps these dissolved compounds but lets the water pass through in much the same way that a coffee filter traps the grounds as water passes through it. This cleans the blood of wastes and removes the trapped compounds from circulation so they can be flushed out of the body. The antidiuretic hormone (ADH) prevents the loss of water from the kidneys by causing its reabsorption into the tubules.

Active Transport

Often, the cell must maintain an imbalance of compounds across its membrane to achieve some metabolic purpose. For example, in the sodium-potassium pump, the cell uses sodium outside the cell and potassium inside the cell for depolarization. To maintain this imbalance, the cell must use energy in the form of ATP and actively transport compounds across its membrane. Even though active transport demands a high-energy expenditure, its benefits outweigh the initial use of ATP. Pumping sodium out of the cell and potassium into the cell has the added benefit of moving glucose into the cell at the same time.

Osmosis

As noted earlier, fluid compartments in the body are separated from one another by membranes, such as the cell membranes and the membranes lining blood vessels. The concentration of fluid in those compartments—that is, the number of solute particles—is chiefly influenced by the process called osmosis. If two solutions are separated by a semipermeable membrane (eg, a cell membrane), water will flow across the membrane *from* the solution of *lower* solute concentration *to* the solution of *higher* solute concentration. The net effect is to equalize the solute concentrations on both sides of the membrane.

The effects of osmotic pressure on a cell constitute the tonicity of the solution Figure 8-4 ▸ . Tonicity reflects the concentration of sodium in a solution and the movement of water in relation to the sodium levels inside and outside the cell.

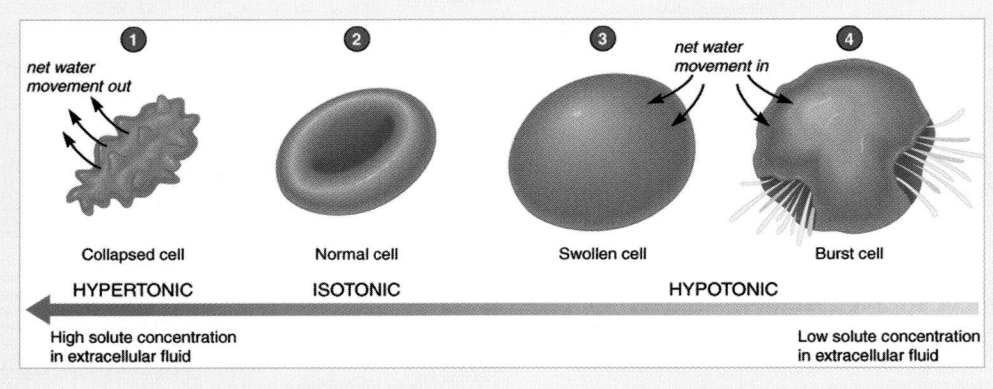

net water movement out

Collapsed cell   Normal cell   Swollen cell   Burst cell

HYPERTONIC   **ISOTONIC**   **HYPOTONIC**

net water movement in

High solute concentration in extracellular fluid   Low solute concentration in extracellular fluid

Figure 8-4 Tonicity.

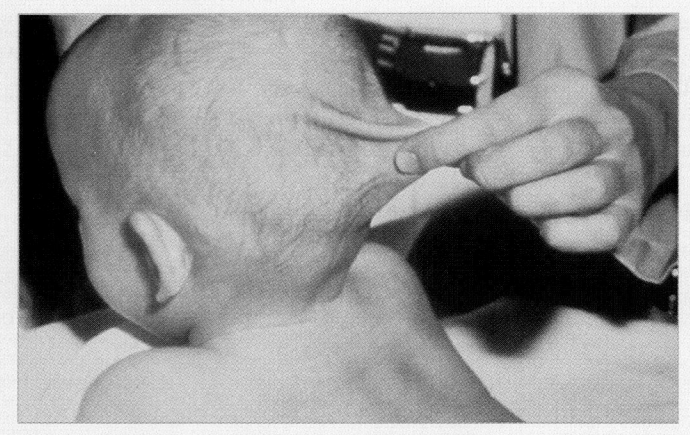

Figure 8-5 Skin tenting is a sign of dehydration.

Abnormal States of Fluid and Electrolyte Balance

The healthy body maintains a delicate balance between intake and output of fluids and electrolytes, ensuring that the internal environment remains fairly constant. The internal environment's resistance to change is called homeostasis. The ill or injured body, however, may be unable to maintain homeostasis, and excesses or deficits of fluids and electrolytes may occur. You need to know when IV fluids are indicated, what kinds of fluids are required in different situations, and when IV fluids can be dangerous. Although verbal orders or protocols will largely govern the use of IV fluids in the field, you must still use your judgment when administering IV fluids. At a minimum, you must know enough to question orders that seem inappropriate and to function independently should radio communications fail during an emergency situation.

A healthy person loses approximately 2 to 2.5 L of fluid daily through urine output and through the lungs (exhalation) and skin. These losses are replaced by intake of fluids and by nutrients that are partially converted to water in their metabolism. In illness, abnormal states of hydration may occur in which intake and output are no longer in balance.

Dehydration

Dehydration is defined as inadequate total systemic fluid volume **Figure 8-5**. It is usually a chronic condition of elderly or very young people and may take days to manifest. As fluid is lost from the vascular compartment, the body reacts by shifting interstitial fluid into the vascular area; fluid also shifts from the intracellular to the extracellular compartments. As a consequence, a total systemic fluid deficit occurs.

Signs and symptoms of dehydration include decreased level of consciousness, postural hypotension, tachypnea, dry mucous membranes, tachycardia, poor skin turgor, and flushed, dry skin. Causes of dehydration include diarrhea, vomiting, gastrointestinal drainage, hemorrhage, and insufficient fluid or food intake.

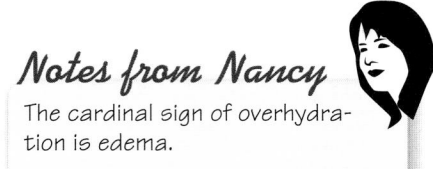

Notes from Nancy

The cardinal sign of overhydration is edema.

Overhydration

When the body's total systemic fluid volume increases, overhydration occurs. Fluid fills the vascular compartment, filters into the interstitial compartment, and is forced from the engorged interstitial compartment into the intracellular compartment. This fluid backup can lead to death **Figure 8-6**.

Signs and symptoms of overhydration include shortness of breath, puffy eyelids, edema, polyuria, moist crackles (rales), and acute weight gain. Causes of overhydration include unmonitored IVs, kidney failure, and prolonged hypoventilation.

■ IV Fluid Composition

The use of IV fluids can significantly alter the patient's condition and facilitate patient treatment. Each bag of IV solution must be sterile and safe; therefore, each bag of IV solution is individually sterilized **Figure 8-7**. The compounds and ions dissolved in the solutions are identical to the ones found in the body.

Sodium is used as the benchmark to calculate a solution's tonicity. The concentration of sodium in the cells of the body is approximately 0.9%. Altering the concentration of sodium in the IV solution, therefore, can move the water into or out of any fluid compartment in the body.

Types of IV Solutions

There are five basic types of IV solutions: isotonic, hypotonic, hypertonic, crystalloid, and colloid. IV fluids use combinations of these solutions to create the desired effects inside the body.

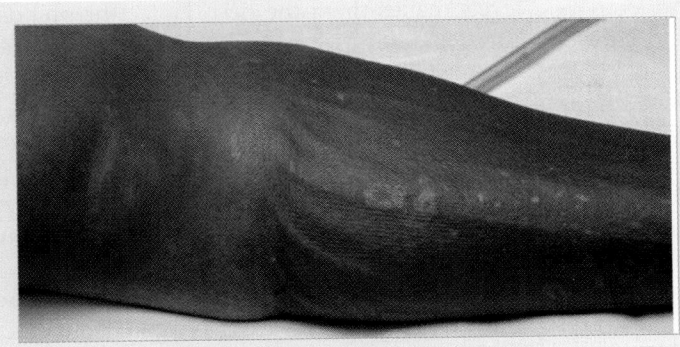

Figure 8-6 In an overhydrated patient, fluid backup occurs.

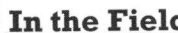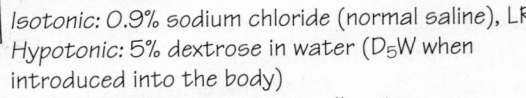

In the Field

Isotonic: 0.9% sodium chloride (normal saline), LR
Hypotonic: 5% dextrose in water (D₅W when introduced into the body)
Hypertonic: 2.0% saline, blood products, albumin

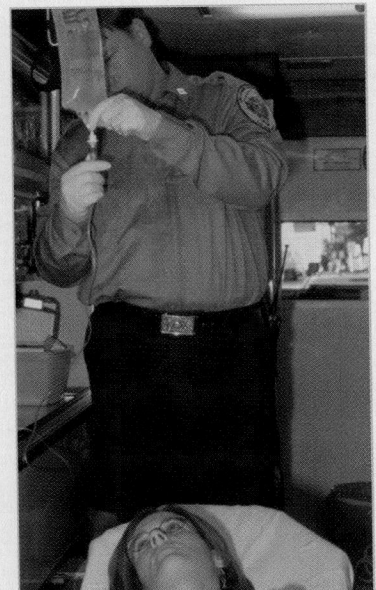

Figure 8-7 Each bag of IV solution must be sterile and safe.

Fluid movement across a cell membrane resulting from hypertonic, isotonic, and hypotonic solutions is illustrated in **Figure 8-8** . IV fluids introduced into the circulatory system can affect the tonicity of the extracellular fluid, resulting in dire consequences unless care is used.

Isotonic Solutions

Isotonic solutions such as normal saline (0.9% sodium chloride) have almost the same osmolarity (concentration of solute) as serum and other body fluids. As a consequence, isotonic solutions expand the contents of the intravascular compartment without shifting fluid to or from other compartments, or changing cell shape—an important consideration when dealing with hypotensive or hypovolemic patients. When administering isotonic solutions, you must be careful to avoid fluid overloading. Patients with hypertension and congestive heart failure are at greatest risk of this problem. The extra fluid increases preload, which in turn increases the workload of the heart, creating fluid backup in the lungs.

Lactated Ringer's (LR) solution is generally used in the field for patients who have lost large amounts of blood. It contains lactate, which is metabolized in the liver to form bicarbonate—the key buffer that combats the intracellular acidosis associated with severe blood loss. LR solution should not be given to patients with liver problems because they cannot metabolize the lactate.

D₅W, 5% dextrose in water, is a unique type of isotonic solution. As long as it remains in the bag, it is considered an isotonic solution. Once it is administered, however, the dextrose is quickly metabolized, and the solution becomes hypotonic.

Hypotonic Solutions

A hypotonic solution has an osmolarity less than that of serum. When this fluid is placed in the vascular compartment, it begins diluting the serum. Soon the serum osmolarity is less than that of the interstitial fluid; water is pulled from the vascular compartment into the interstitial fluid compartment, causing cells to swell and possibly burst from the increased intracellular osmotic pressure.

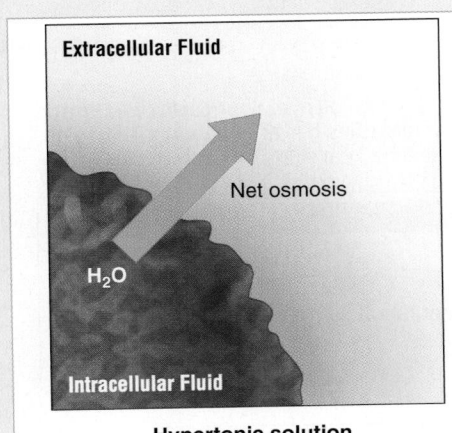
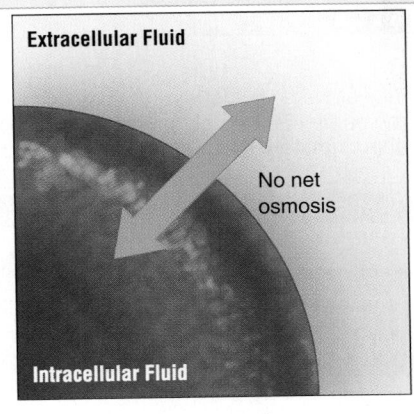
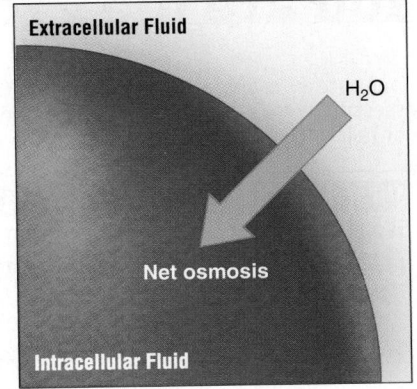

Figure 8-8 Fluid movement with hypertonic, isotonic, and hypotonic solutions.

Hypotonic solutions hydrate the cells while depleting the vascular compartment. They may be needed for a patient who is receiving dialysis because dialysis therapy dehydrates the cells.

Hypotonic solutions can cause a sudden fluid shift from the intravascular space to the cells, leading to cardiovascular collapse and increased intracranial pressure from shifting fluid into the brain cells. For example, giving D5W for an extended period can increase intracranial pressure. This makes hypotonic solutions dangerous for patients with stroke or any head trauma. Administering these solutions to patients with burns, trauma, malnutrition, or liver disease is also hazardous because these patients are at risk for developing third spacing, an abnormal fluid shift into the interstitial compartment.

Hypertonic Solutions

A hypertonic solution has an osmolarity higher than that of serum, meaning that the solution has more ionic concentration than serum and pulls fluid and electrolytes from the intracellular and interstitial compartments into the intravascular compartment. The danger is that the cells may collapse from the increased extracellular osmotic pressure. Hypertonic solutions shift body fluids into the vascular spaces and help stabilize blood pressure, increase urine output, and reduce edema. These fluids are rarely, if ever, used in the prehospital setting.

Often the term "hypertonic" is used to refer to solutions that contain high concentrations of proteins. These proteins have the same effect on fluid as sodium. Careful monitoring is needed to guard against fluid overloading when using hypertonic fluids, especially with patients with impaired heart or kidney function. Also, hypertonic solutions should not be given to patients with diabetic ketoacidosis or others at risk of cellular dehydration.

Crystalloid Solutions

Crystalloid solutions are dissolved crystals (eg, salts or sugars) in water. The ability of these fluids to cross membranes and alter fluid levels makes them the best choice for prehospital care of injured patients who need body fluid replacement. When you use an isotonic crystalloid for fluid replacement to support blood pressure after blood loss, remember the 3-to-1 replacement rule: *3 mL of isotonic crystalloid solution is needed to replace 1 mL of patient blood.* This amount is needed because approximately two thirds of the infused isotonic crystalloid solution will leave the vascular spaces in about 1 hour.

When you replace lost volume, it is imperative to remember that crystalloid solutions cannot carry oxygen. Boluses of 20 mL/kg should be given to maintain perfusion (ie, radial pulses, adequate mental status) but not to raise blood pressure to the patient's normal level. Increasing blood pressure too much with IV solutions not only dilutes remaining blood volume, thereby decreasing the proportion of hemoglobin, but also may increase internal bleeding by interfering with hemostasis—the body's internal blood-clotting mechanism.

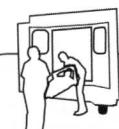

In the Field

Isotonic crystalloid solutions—normal saline and LR—replace lost volume but do not carry oxygen. Replace lost volume to maintain perfusion, but recognize the need for rapid transport.

Colloid Solutions

Colloid solutions contain molecules (usually proteins) that are too large to pass out of the capillary membranes and, therefore, remain in the vascular compartment. These very large protein molecules give colloid solutions a very high osmolarity. As a result, they draw fluid from the interstitial and intracellular compartments into the vascular compartments. Colloid solutions work very well in reducing edema (eg, in pulmonary or cerebral edema)

You are the Provider Part 2

Your partner is appropriately managing the patient's airway. The patient remains unconscious and unresponsive. Your rapid head-to-toe assessment reveals no gross injury or bleeding. The patient is wearing a medic-alert bracelet that identifies her as a diabetic. The neighbor tells you that she just spoke with the patient approximately 1 hour earlier and she was fine. Baseline vital signs reveal the following:

Vital Signs	Recording Time: 5 Minutes
Blood pressure	100/60 mm Hg
Pulse	120 beats/min, weak and regular
Respirations	30 breaths/min and shallow (baseline); your partner is assisting ventilation with a bag-mask device and 100% oxygen
Sao₂	99% (with assisted ventilation and 15 L/min of oxygen)
Skin	Cool, pale, and moist

5. Given the patient's history, what additional assessment should you perform?
6. When starting an IV for this patient, what solution should you use?

while expanding the vascular compartment. They could cause dramatic fluid shifts and place the patient in considerable danger if they are not administered in a controlled setting. For this reason, colloids are rarely used in the prehospital setting. Examples of colloids are albumin, dextran, Plasmanate, and hetastarch (Hespan).

Oxygen-Carrying Solutions

Obviously, the best fluid to replace lost blood is whole blood. Unlike the crystalloid and colloid solutions, whole blood contains hemoglobin, which carries oxygen to the body's cells. On occasion (eg, aeromedical transports, mass-casualty incidents), O-negative blood—a universally compatible blood type—may be used outside a hospital setting. However, because of the refrigeration requirements and other storage issues, general use of whole blood is impractical in the prehospital setting.

Synthetic blood substitutes, which do have the ability to carry oxygen, are being researched and, in some places, field-tested. They show great potential for improving the way you treat patients who have lost large amounts of blood. Not only would these synthetic blood substitutes expand circulating volume, but they also would carry and deliver oxygen to the part of the body that needs it the most—the cell.

■ IV Techniques and Administration

Intravenous means "within a vein." Intravenous (IV) therapy involves cannulation of a vein with a catheter to access the patient's vascular system. It is one of the most invasive techniques you will perform as a paramedic. Peripheral vein cannulation involves cannulating veins of the periphery—that is, veins that can be seen and/or palpated (eg, veins of the hand, arm, or lower extremity and the external jugular vein).

The most important point to remember about IV therapy is to keep the IV equipment sterile. Forethought and attention to detail will help prevent mental and procedural errors while starting the IV. One way to ensure proper technique is to develop a routine to follow as you assemble the appropriate equipment.

Assembling Your Equipment

To avoid delays and IV site contamination, gather and prepare all your equipment before you attempt to start an IV. In some cases, the patient's condition may make full preparation difficult, so working as a team becomes critical. The members of your own crew, by anticipating your needs, often make the assembly of IV equipment possible.

Choosing an IV Solution

When choosing the most appropriate IV solution, you must identify the needs of your patient. Ask yourself these questions:

- Is the patient's condition critical?
- Is the patient's condition stable?
- Does the patient need fluid replacement?
- Will the patient need medications?

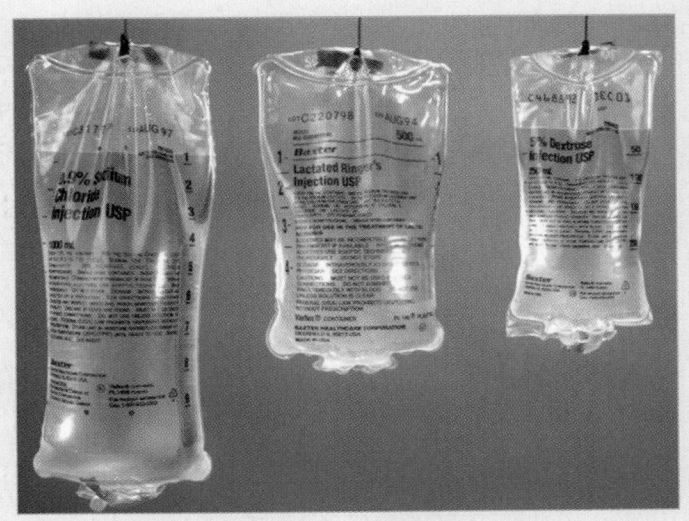

Figure 8-9 IV solution bags come in different fluid volumes.

In the prehospital setting, the choice of IV solution is usually limited to two isotonic crystalloids, normal saline and LR solution. D_5W is often reserved for administering medication because the presence of dextrose has the potential to alter fluid and electrolyte levels in the body.

Each IV solution bag is wrapped in a protective sterile plastic bag and is guaranteed to remain sterile until the posted expiration date. Once the protective wrap is torn and removed, however, the IV solution must be used within 24 hours. The bottom of each IV bag has two ports: an injection port for medication and an access port for connecting the administration set. A removable pigtail protects the sterile access port. Once this pigtail is removed, the bag must be used immediately or discarded.

IV solution bags come in different fluid volumes Figure 8-9 ▲ . Volumes commonly used in hospitals are 1,000 mL, 500 mL, 250 mL, 100 mL, and 50 mL; the more common prehospital volumes are 1,000 mL and 500 mL. The smaller volumes (250 mL and 100 mL) typically contain D_5W or saline and are used for mixing and administering maintenance medication infusions.

Choosing an Administration Set

An administration set moves fluid from the IV bag into the patient's vascular system. IV administration sets are sterile as long as they remain in their protective packaging. Each set has a piercing spike protected by a plastic cover. Once this spike is exposed and the seal surrounding the cap is broken, the set must be used immediately or discarded.

On most drip sets, a number on the package indicates the number of drops it takes for a milliliter of fluid to pass through the orifice and into the drip chamber Figure 8-10 ▶ . Administration sets come in two primary sizes: microdrip and macrodrip. Microdrip sets allow 60 gtt (drops) per milliliter (mL)

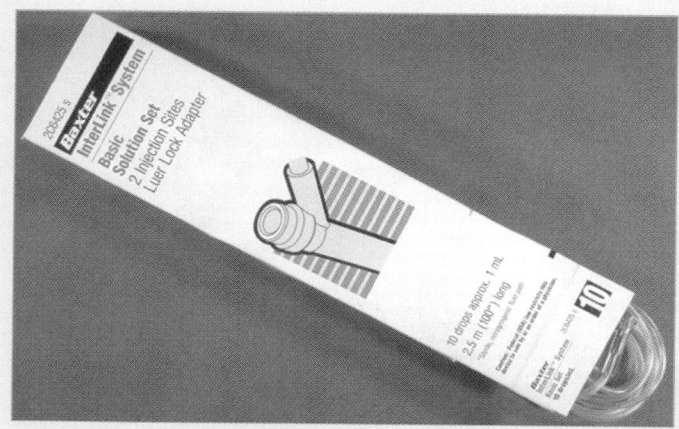

Figure 8-10 The number visible on the drip set refers to the number of drops it takes for a milliliter of fluid to pass through the orifice and into the drip chamber.

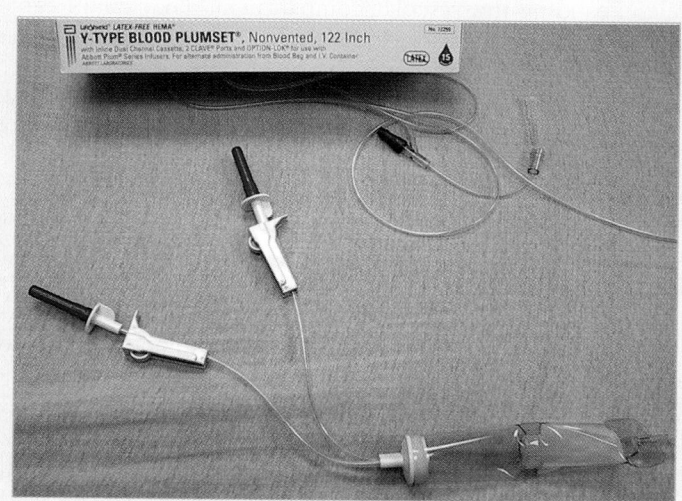

Figure 8-11 Most blood sets have dual piercing spikes that allow two bags of fluid to be used at once for the same patient.

through the needlelike orifice inside the drip chamber. They are ideal for medication administration or pediatric fluid delivery because it is easy to control their fluid flow. Macrodrip sets allow 10 or 15 gtt/mL through a large opening between the piercing spike and the drip chamber. They are best used for rapid fluid replacement.

Preparing an Administration Set

After choosing the IV administration set and the IV solution bag, verify the expiration date of the solution and check for solution clarity. Prepare to spike the bag with the administration set. The steps for this procedure are shown here and illustrated in (**Skill Drill 8-1 ▶**):

1. Remove the rubber pigtail found on the end of the IV bag by pulling on it. The bag is still sealed and will not leak until the piercing spike punctures this port. Remove the protective cover from the piercing spike. (Remember, this spike is sterile!) (**Step 1**).

2. Slide the spike into the IV bag port until you see fluid enter the drip chamber (**Step 2**).

3. Allow the solution to run freely through the drip chamber and into the tubing to prime the line and flush the air out of the tubing (**Step 3**).

4. Twist the protective cover on the opposite end of the IV tubing to allow air to escape. Do not remove this cover yet, because the cover keeps the tubing end sterile until it is needed. Let the fluid flow until air bubbles are removed from the line before turning the roller clamp wheel to stop the flow (**Step 4**).

5. Go back and check the drip chamber; it should be only half-filled. The fluid level must be visible to calculate drip rates. If the fluid level is too low, squeeze the chamber until it fills; if the chamber is too full, invert the bag and the chamber and squeeze the chamber to empty the fluid back into the bag (**Step 5**). Hang the bag in an appropriate location with the end of the IV tubing easily accessible.

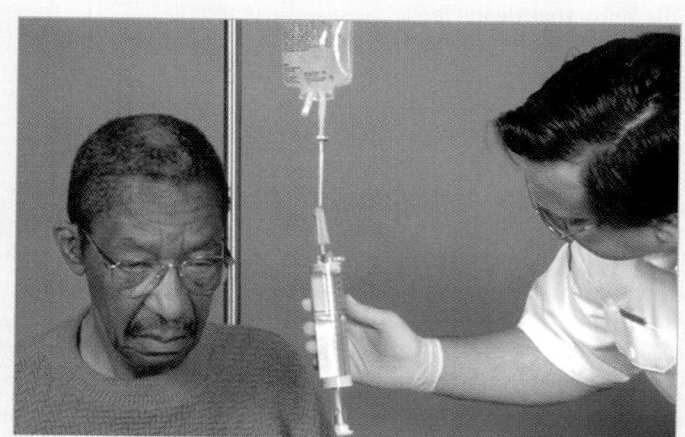

Figure 8-12 Volutrol administration set.

Other Administration Sets

Blood tubing is a macrodrip administration set that is designed to facilitate rapid fluid replacement by manual infusion of multiple IV bags or IV and blood replacement combinations. Most blood tubing administration sets have dual piercing spikes that allow two bags of fluid to be used simultaneously for the same patient (**Figure 8-11 ▲**). The central drip chamber has a special filter designed to filter the blood during transfusions.

Fluid control for pediatric patients and certain geriatric patients is very important. A microdrip set called a Volutrol (or Buretrol) allows you to fill a 100- or 200-mL calibrated drip chamber with a specific amount of fluid and administer only that amount to avoid inadvertent fluid overload (**Figure 8-12 ▲**). These are commonly used in pediatric patients. A proximal roller clamp enables you to shut off the Volutrol drip chamber from the IV bag. If the patient needs additional fluids, simply open the proximal roller clamp and fill the Volutrol with more fluid.

Skill Drill 8-1: Spiking the Bag

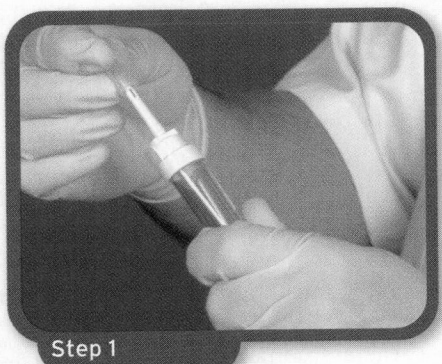

Step 1

Pull on the rubber pigtail on the end of the IV bag to remove it. Remove the protective cover from the piercing spike.

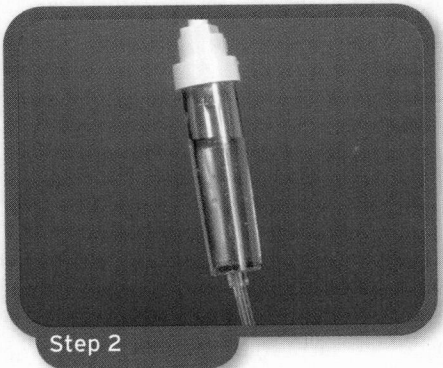

Step 2

Slide the spike into the IV bag until you see fluid enter the drip chamber.

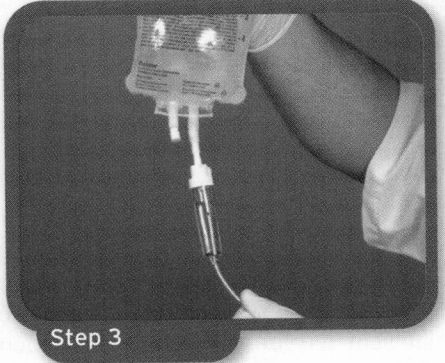

Step 3

Allow the solution to run freely through the drip chamber and into the tubing to prime the line and flush the air out of the tubing.

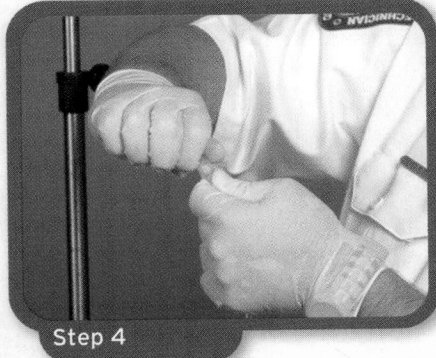

Step 4

Twist the protective cover of the opposite end of the IV tubing to allow air to escape. Do not remove this cover yet. Let the fluid flow until air bubbles are removed from the line before turning the roller clamp wheel to stop the flow.

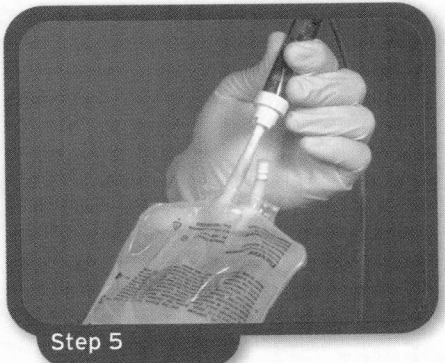

Step 5

Check the drip chamber; it should be only half-filled. If the fluid level is too low, squeeze the chamber until it fills; if the chamber is too full, invert the bag and the chamber and squeeze the chamber to empty the fluid back into the bag. Hang the bag in an appropriate location.

Choosing an IV Site

It is important to select the most appropriate vein for IV catheter insertion. Avoid areas of the vein that contain valves because a catheter will not pass through these areas easily and the needle may cause damage. Valves can be recognized as small bumps located in the vein. Use the following criteria to select a vein:

- Locate the vein section with the straightest appearance **Figure 8-13 ▶**.
- Choose a vein that has a firm, round appearance or is springy when palpated.
- Avoid areas where the vein crosses over joints.
- Avoid edematous extremities and any extremity with a dialysis fistula or on the side a mastectomy was done.

If IV therapy is being given for a life-threatening illness or injury, this choice is often limited to the areas that remain open during hypoperfusion. Otherwise, limit IV access to the more distal areas of the extremities: *Start distally, work proximally.* If the most distal site ruptures or infiltrates, you can move up the extremity to the next appropriate site. Because failed cannulation brings the possibility of leakage into the surrounding tissues, any fluid introduced immediately below an

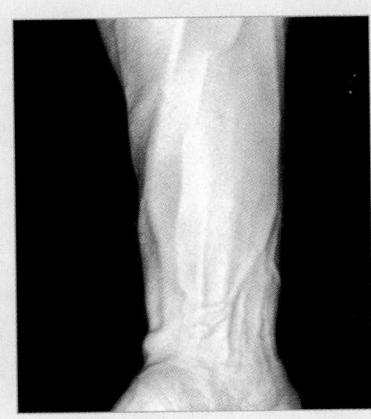

Figure 8-13 Look for veins that are relatively straight and spring back when palpated.

open wound has the potential to enter the tissue and cause damage.

Large protruding arm veins can be deceiving in terms of their ease of cannulation. Often these bulging veins can roll from side to side during a cannulation attempt, causing you to miss the vein. A remedy is to apply manual traction to the vein to lock it into position. Traction techniques differ depending on the location chosen for cannulation. Hold hand veins in place by pulling the skin over the vein taut with the thumb of your free hand as you flex the patient's hand **Figure 8-14 ▼**. Stabilize wrist veins by flexing the wrist and pulling the skin taut over the vein. Applying lateral traction to the vein with your free hand can stabilize veins in the forearm and antecubital areas. Stabilizing and cannulating the external jugular vein requires a different approach (discussed later in this chapter).

The patient's opinion should also be considered when selecting an IV site because he or she may know an IV location that has worked in the past. Avoid attempts to insert an IV in an extremity if it shows signs of trauma, injury, or infection; if it has an arteriovenous shunt for renal dialysis; or if it is on the same side a mastectomy was done. Also, pay careful attention to areas of the vein that have track marks; they are usually a sign of sclerosis caused by frequent cannulation or puncture of the vein, for example from IV drug abuse.

Some protocols allow IV cannulation of leg veins. Use caution when cannulating veins in these areas because they can place the patient at greater risk of venous thrombosis and subsequent pulmonary embolism.

Choosing an IV Catheter

Catheter selection should reflect the purpose of the IV, the age of the patient, and the location for the IV. The most common types used in the prehospital setting are over-the-needle catheters and butterfly catheters. An over-the-needle catheter **Figure 8-15 ▼** is a Teflon catheter inserted *over* a hollow needle (eg, Angiocath, Terumo, Jelco). A butterfly catheter is a hollow, stainless steel needle with two plastic wings to facilitate its handling **Figure 8-16 ▼**. Through-the-needle catheters (Intracaths) are plastic catheters inserted *through* a hollow needle; these catheters are rarely used in the prehospital setting.

Table 8-1 ▶ lists the advantages and disadvantages of over-the-needle catheters. These catheters are preferred for use in the prehospital setting for infusing IV fluids or medications in adults and children. They are more readily secured, are less cumbersome than the butterfly catheter, and allow for greater patient movement without the need to immobilize the entire limb.

Table 8-2 ▶ lists the advantages and disadvantages of butterfly catheters.

Over-the-needle catheters come in different gauges and lengths **Figure 8-17 ▶**. The smaller the gauge of the catheter, the larger the diameter. Thus a 14-gauge catheter is of larger diameter than a 22-gauge catheter; 14 gauge is the largest, 27 gauge is the smallest. The larger the diameter, the more fluid that can be delivered through it. The most common lengths are 1¼″ and 2¼″.

Select the largest-diameter catheter that will fit the vein you have chosen or that will be the most appropriate and comfortable for the patient. An 18- or 20-gauge catheter is usually a good size for adults who do not need fluid replacement. Metacarpal veins of the hand can usually accommodate 18- or

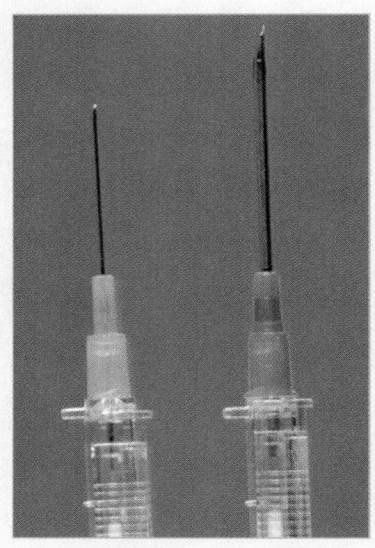

Figure 8-15 Over-the-needle catheters.

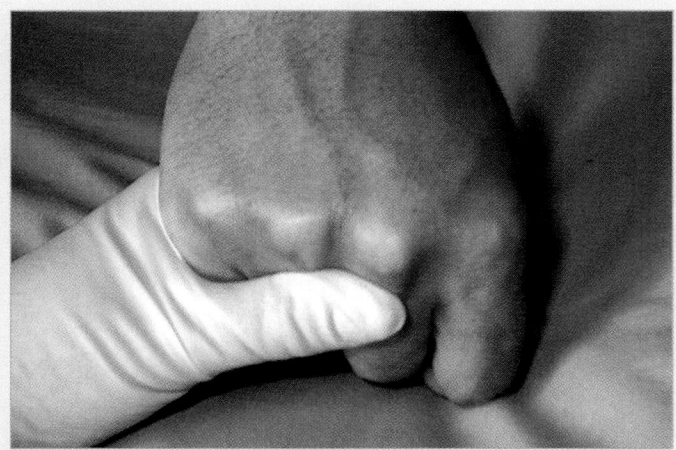

Figure 8-14 Hold hand veins in place by pulling the skin over the vein taut with the thumb of your free hand as you flex the patient's hand.

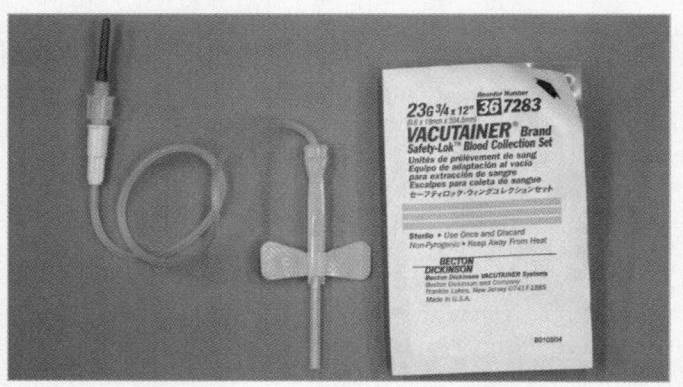

Figure 8-16 Butterfly catheter.

In the Field

As a general rule, you should start distally and work your way up the patient's extremity when starting an IV. For patients who need rapid fluid replacement, are in cardiac arrest, or are otherwise hemodynamically unstable, however, you should use the antecubital vein. Unlike other extremity veins (eg, hand, forearm), this vein is usually visible and easier to palpate. A neck vein or an adult IO are other options.

Special Considerations

If you are using an over-the-needle catheter to start an IV in a pediatric patient, choose among the 20-, 22-, 24-, or 26-gauge catheters, depending on the child's age. Butterfly catheters can be placed in the same locations as over-the-needle catheters and in visible scalp veins in pediatric patients. Scalp veins are best used in young infants.

Table 8-1	Advantages and Disadvantages of Over-the-Needle Catheters	
Advantages	**Disadvantages**	
■ Less likely to puncture the vein than a butterfly catheter ■ More comfortable once in position ■ Radiopaque for easy identification during x-ray	■ Risk of sticking the paramedic with contaminated needle as it is withdrawn ■ More difficult to insert than other devices ■ Possibility of catheter shear	

Table 8-2	Advantages and Disadvantages of Butterfly Catheters	
Advantages	**Disadvantages**	
■ Easiest venipuncture device to insert ■ Useful for scalp veins in infants and in small, difficult veins in geriatric patients for obtaining blood samples ■ Small, short needles	■ May easily cause infiltration ■ Possible blood cell damage when drawing blood through the butterfly catheter ■ Small-gauge needles limit fluid flow	

20-gauge catheters. A 14- or 16-gauge catheter should be used when the patient requires fluid replacement (eg, for hypovolemic shock). You should be able to insert a 14- or 16-gauge catheter into an antecubital vein or external jugular vein in the average adult.

In recent years, an attempt has been made to create over-the-needle catheters that minimize the risk of a <u>contaminated stick</u>—when a paramedic punctures his or her skin with the same catheter that was used to cannulate the vein of a patient. For example, some of these newer catheters offer automatic needle retraction after insertion, usually accomplished with a locking slide mechanism or a spring-loaded slide mechanism.

Inserting the IV Catheter

Each paramedic has a unique technique to insert an IV, and you should observe many different techniques to determine what works best for you. Two considerations, however, apply to *any* technique: (1) Keep the beveled side of the catheter up when inserting the needle in a vein Figure 8-18 ▾ , and (2) maintain adequate traction on the vein during cannulation.

Apply a constricting band above the site you have chosen for the insertion to allow blood to fill the veins. This creates additional vascular pressure to engorge the veins with blood below the band. It should be snug enough to significantly diminish venous flow but should not hamper arterial flow. The constricting band should be left in place only long enough to complete the IV insertion, obtain blood samples (if needed),

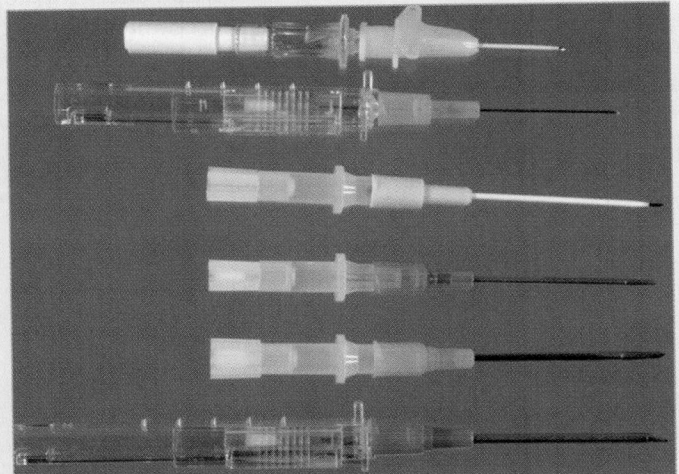
Figure 8-17 Note the difference in the lengths and diameters of over-the-needle catheters.

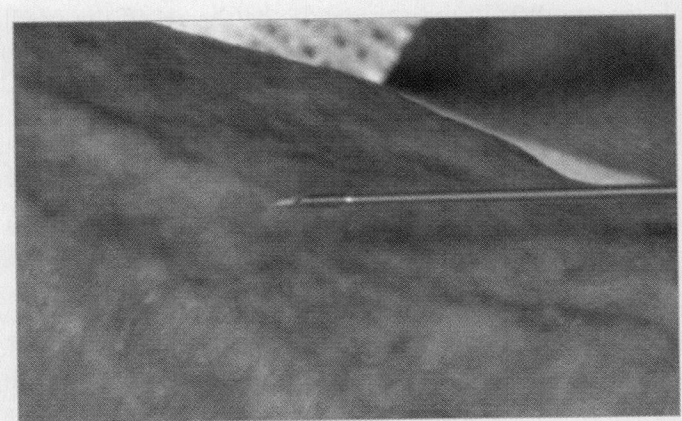
Figure 8-18 Keep the beveled side of the catheter up when inserting the needle into a vein.

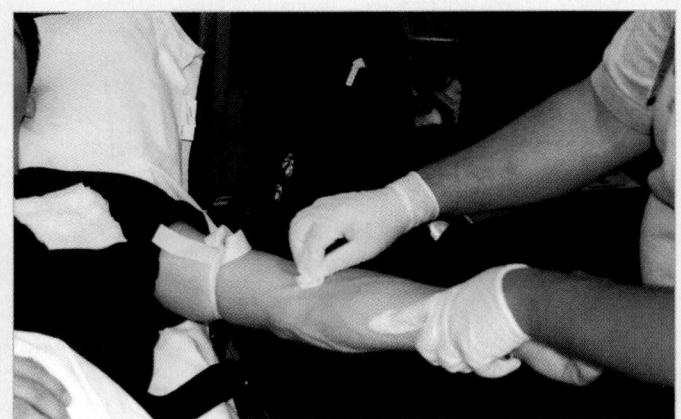

Figure 8-19 When cleansing the site for IV cannulation, use the first alcohol pad or iodine swab to clean in a circular motion from the inside out, then use the second to wipe straight down the center of the vein.

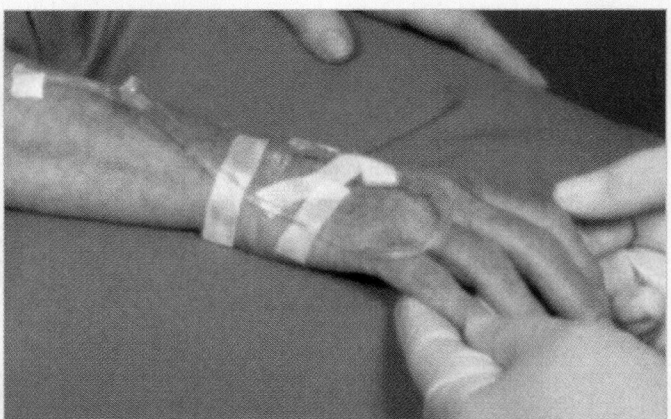

Figure 8-20 Tape the area so that the catheter and tubing are securely anchored.

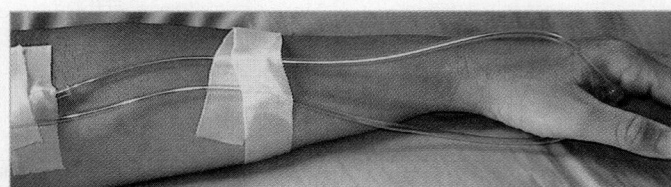

Figure 8-21 Loosely wrap the IV line around the patient's thumb and secure it to the forearm.

and attach the line. *Do not leave the constricting band in place while you assemble IV equipment.*

Constricting bands can be difficult to manage, especially if you are wearing gloves. You should develop a technique that will allow you to release the constricting band with a small tug on one end. Items that can be used as constricting bands include a Penrose drain, a blood pressure cuff, or in a pinch, surgical hose.

Once you have selected an insertion site, prep it with an alcohol or iodine swab Figure 8-19 ▲ . Apply gentle downward or lateral traction on the vein with your free hand while holding the catheter, bevel side up, in your dominant hand. Take care as you apply traction to avoid collapsing the vein. Begin by establishing an insertion angle of about 45°. Advance the catheter through the skin until the vein is pierced (you should see a flash of blood in the catheter flash chamber); then immediately drop the angle down to about 15° and advance the catheter a few more centimeters to ensure the catheter sheath is in the vein. Slide the sheath off the needle and into the vein; do not advance the needle too far because it can lacerate the vein. After the catheter is fully advanced, apply pressure to the vein just proximal to the end of the indwelling catheter, remove the needle, and dispose of it in a sharps container, or in the case of other style catheters, trigger the shielding device.

Securing the Line

Once the catheter is in position and the contents of the IV bag are flowing properly, you must secure the IV. Tape the area so that the catheter and tubing are securely anchored in case of a sudden pull on the line Figure 8-20 ▶ . Tear the tape before you start the IV, because you will need one hand to stabilize the site while you tape the IV. Double back the tubing to create a loop that will act as a shock absorber if the

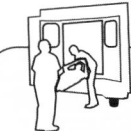

In the Field

Iodine helps to make veins more visible in dark-skinned people. As with any patient, make sure the patient is not allergic to iodine.

line is pulled accidentally. Cover the insertion site with sterile gauze, and secure it with tape or use a commercially manufactured device (eg, Veniguard, Opsite). Avoid circumferential taping around any extremity, as it may impair circulation.

The steps for establishing vascular access are as follows Skill Drill 8-2 ▶ :

1. Choose the appropriate fluid, and examine the bag for clarity and expiration date.

   Make sure that no particles are floating in the fluid and that the fluid is appropriate for the patient's condition.

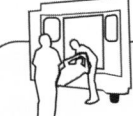

In the Field

To further stabilize the IV line, loosely wrap it around the patient's thumb and secure it to the forearm Figure 8-21 ▲ . This will prevent disruption of the IV if the line is pulled.

2. Choose the appropriate drip set, and attach it to the fluid. A macrodrip set (eg, 10 gtt/mL) should be used for a patient who needs volume replacement; a microdrip set (eg, 60 gtt/mL) should be used for a patient who needs a medication route.

3. Fill the drip chamber by squeezing it (Step 1).

4. Flush or "bleed" the tubing to remove any air bubbles by opening the roller clamp (Step 2). Make sure no errant bubbles are floating in the tubing.

5. Tear the tape before venipuncture, or have a commercial device available (Step 3).

6. Apply gloves before making contact with the patient. Palpate a suitable vein (Step 4). Veins should be "springy" when palpated. Stay away from areas that are hard when palpated.

7. Apply the constricting band above the intended IV site (Step 5). It should be placed approximately 6″ to 10″ above the intended site.

8. Clean the area using aseptic technique. Use an alcohol pad to cleanse in a circular motion from the inside out. Use a second alcohol pad to wipe straight down the center (Step 6).

9. Choose the appropriately sized catheter, twist the catheter to break the seal. Do not advance the catheter upward, as this may cause the needle to shear the catheter. Examine the catheter and discard it if you discover any imperfections (Step 7). Occasionally you will find "burrs" on the edge of the catheter.

10. Insert the catheter at an angle of approximately 45° with the bevel up while applying distal traction with the other hand (Step 8). This traction will stabilize the vein and help to keep it from "rolling" as you stick.

11. Observe for "flashback" as blood enters the catheter (Step 9). The clear chamber at the top of the catheter should fill with blood when the catheter enters the vein. If you note only a drop or two, you should gently advance the catheter farther into the vein.

12. Occlude the catheter to prevent blood leaking while removing the stylet (Step 10). Place the thumb of the hand not holding the catheter over the end of the catheter that is currently situated inside the vein to prevent blood running out when you remove the needle. With practice, you will be able to feel the catheter.

13. Immediately dispose of all sharps in the proper container (Step 11).

14. Attach the prepared IV line (Step 12).

15. Remove the constricting band (Step 13).

16. Open the IV line to ensure fluid is flowing and the IV is patent. Observe for any swelling or infiltration around the IV site (Step 14). If the fluid does not flow, check whether the constriction band has been released. If infiltration is noted, immediately stop the infusion and remove the catheter while holding pressure over the site to prevent bleeding.

17. Secure the catheter with tape or a commercial device (Step 15).

18. Secure IV tubing and adjust the flow rate while monitoring the patient (Step 16).

Documentation and Communication

To document an IV, you need to include four things:
- The gauge of the needle
- The site (for example, left forearm, left external jugular)
- The type of fluid you are administering
- The rate at which the fluid is running

For example, if you initiated an IV in the left antecubital fossa with an 18-gauge catheter and are infusing normal saline at a rate of 120 mL per hour, the documentation should appear as follows:

18g IV L ac c̄ NS @ 120 mL/h

In the Field
Helpful IV Hints
- Allow the arm to hang off the stretcher.
- Pat or rub the area.
- Apply chemical heat packs for about 60 seconds.
- If you meet resistance from a valve, elevate the extremity.
- After two misses, let your partner try (Figure 8-22 ▶).
- Try sticking without a constricting band if the IV keeps infiltrating.
- Never pull the catheter back over the needle.
- The more IVs you perform, the more proficient you will become.

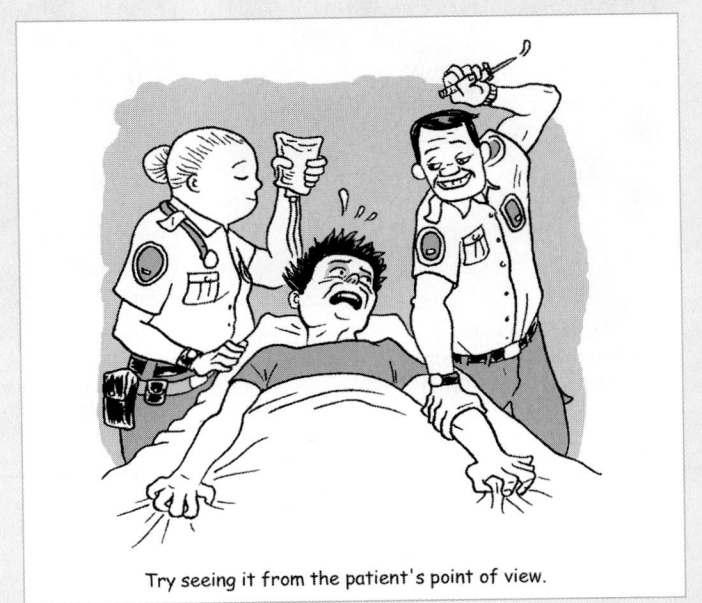

Try seeing it from the patient's point of view.

Figure 8-22

Skill Drill 8-2: Obtaining Vascular Access

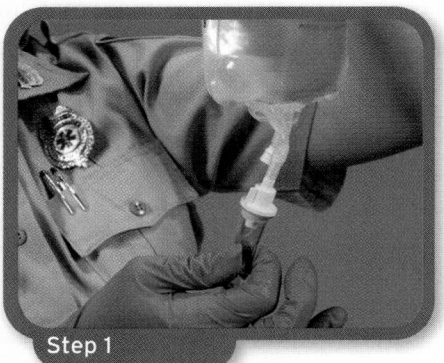

Step 1

Fill the drip chamber by squeezing it.

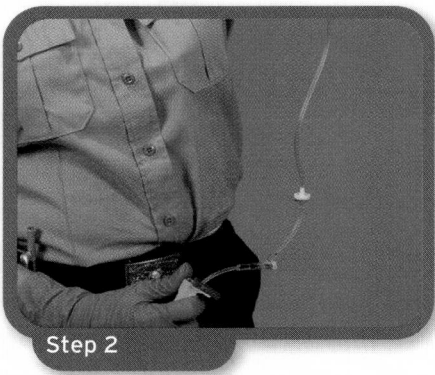

Step 2

Flush or "bleed" the tubing to remove any air bubbles by opening the roller clamp.

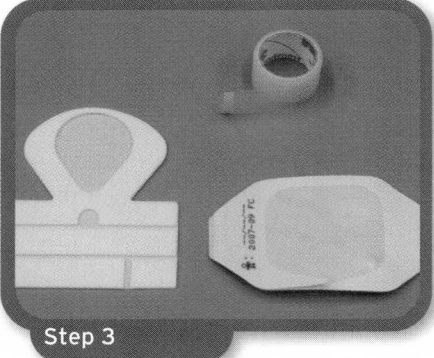

Step 3

Tear the tape before venipuncture, or have a commercial device available.

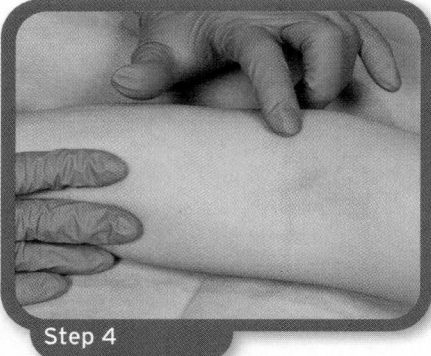

Step 4

Apply gloves before making contact with the patient. Palpate a suitable vein.

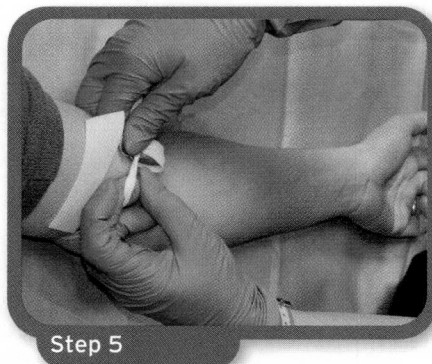

Step 5

Apply the constricting band above the intended IV site.

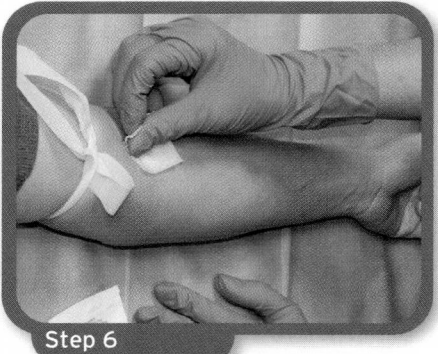

Step 6

Clean the area using aseptic technique. Use an alcohol pad to cleanse in a circular motion from the inside out. Use a second alcohol pad to wipe straight down the center.

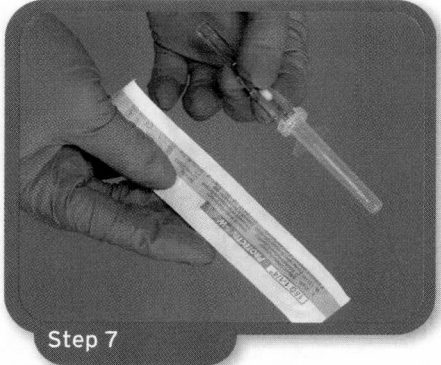

Step 7

Choose the appropriately sized catheter, and examine it for any imperfections.

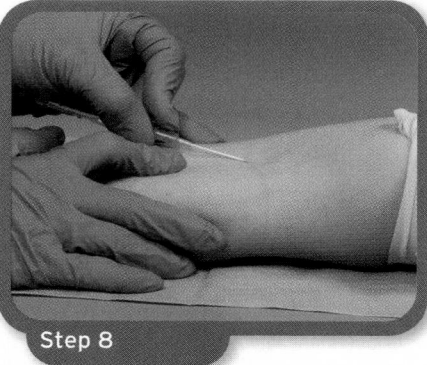

Step 8

Insert the catheter at an angle of approximately 45° with the bevel up while applying distal traction with the other hand.

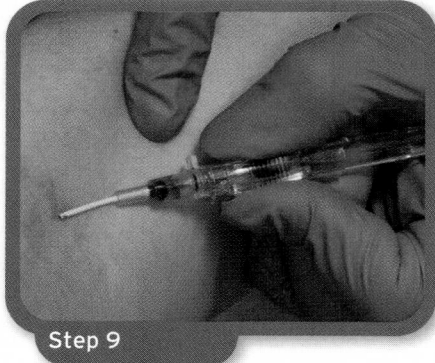

Step 9

Observe for "flashback" as blood enters the catheter.

Skill Drill 8-2: Obtaining Vascular Access (*continued*)

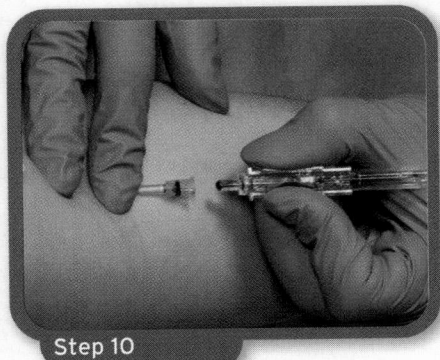

Step 10

Occlude the catheter to prevent blood leaking while removing the stylet.

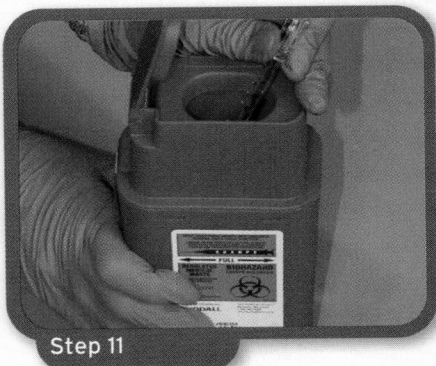

Step 11

Immediately dispose of all sharps in the proper container.

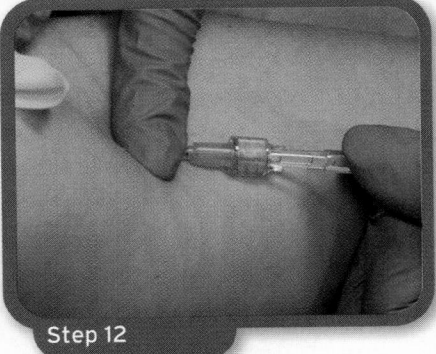

Step 12

Attach the prepared IV line.

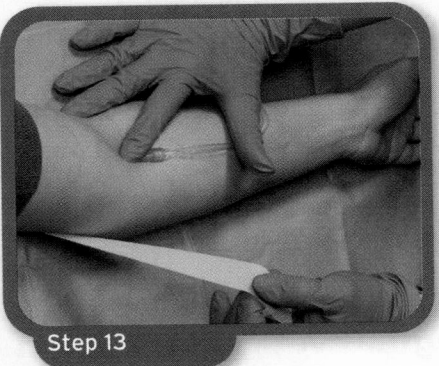

Step 13

Remove the constricting band.

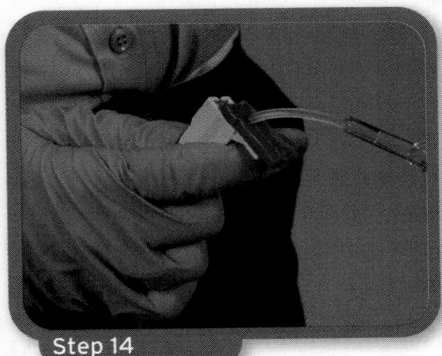

Step 14

Open the IV line to ensure fluid is flowing and the IV is patent. Observe for swelling or infiltration around the IV site.

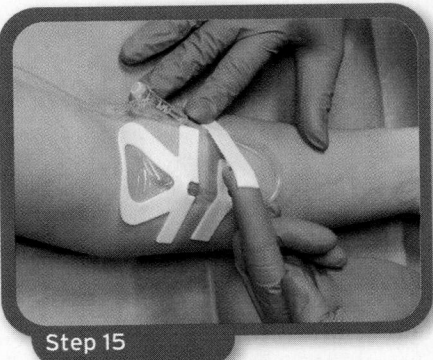

Step 15

Secure the catheter with tape or a commercial device.

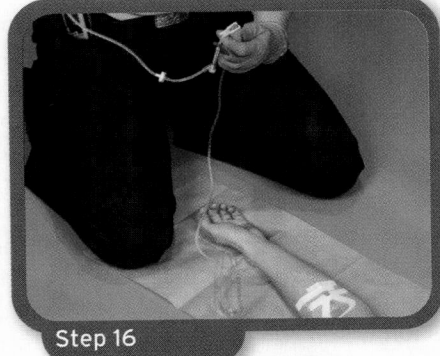

Step 16

Secure the IV tubing and adjust the flow rate while monitoring the patient.

In the Field

Saline locks (buff caps) are a way to maintain an active IV site without running fluids through the vein. These access ports are used primarily for patients who do not need additional fluids but who may need rapid medication delivery (eg, in case of congestive heart failure or pulmonary edema). A saline lock is attached to the end of an IV catheter and filled with approximately 2 mL of normal saline to keep blood from clotting at the end of the catheter **Figure 8-23 ▼**. Because this is a sealed-access site, the saline remains in the port without entering the vein, preventing clotting. These devices are also known as intermittent (INT) sites because they eliminate the need to reestablish an IV each time the patient needs medication or fluid.

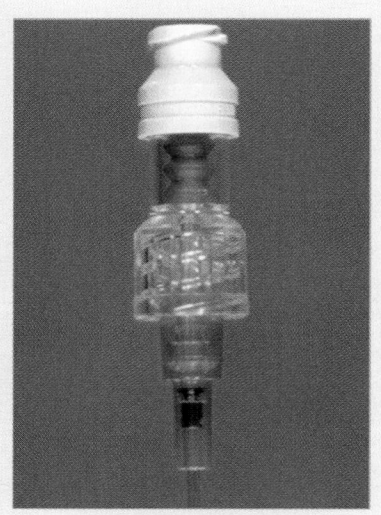

Figure 8-23 A saline lock is attached to the end of an IV catheter and filled with approximately 2 mL of normal saline to keep blood from clotting at the end of the catheter.

Changing an IV Bag

You may have to change the IV bag for some patients, particularly those who require larger volumes of IV fluid (ie, for hypovolemic shock). Do not allow an IV fluid bag to become *completely* depleted of fluid. Change the bag when about 25 mL of fluid is left.

There are two important points to remember when changing an IV bag. First, like the initial setup of the IV bag and administration set (see Skill Drill 8-1), replacing the IV bag is a sterile process. If the equipment becomes contaminated, replace it and use new equipment. Second, never allow the administration set to become depleted of fluid; always ensure that some fluid remains in the drip chamber and tubing of the set. This simple action will prevent air from entering the patient's vein.

The steps for changing an IV fluid bag are as follows:

1. Stop the flow of fluid from the depleted bag by closing the roller clamp.
2. Prepare the new IV bag by removing the pigtail from the piercing spike port. Inspect the new bag of IV fluid for clarity and discoloration and to ensure that the expiration date has not passed.
3. Remove the piercing spike from the depleted bag and insert it into the port on the new bag. *Do not touch the piercing spike of the administration set.*
4. Ensure that the drip chamber is appropriately filled, and then open the roller clamp and adjust the fluid rate accordingly.

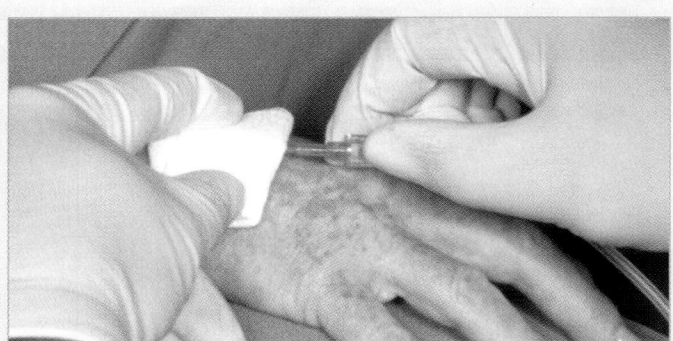

Figure 8-24 When removing a catheter and IV line, pull gently and apply pressure to control bleeding.

Discontinuing the IV Line

To discontinue the IV line, shut off the flow from the IV with the roller clamp. Gently peel the tape back toward the IV site. As you get closer to the site and the catheter, stabilize the catheter while you loosen the remaining tape holding the catheter in place. Do not remove the IV tubing from the hub of the catheter. Fold a 4″ × 4″ piece of gauze and place it over the site, holding it down while you pull back on the hub of the catheter. Gently pull the catheter and the IV line from the patient's vein while applying pressure to control bleeding **Figure 8-24 ▲**.

External Jugular Vein Cannulation

The external jugular (EJ) vein **Figure 8-25 ▶** runs downward and obliquely backward behind the angle of the jaw until it pierces the deep fascia of the neck just above the middle of the clavicle. It ends in the subclavian vein, where valves retard backflow of blood. The EJ vein is fairly large and usually easy to cannulate; however, because the vein lies so near the surface of the skin, it rolls if the vein is not appropriately anchored during cannulation. It is also very near other vessels (such as the carotid artery) that may be damaged during cannulation.

You should exhaust all other means of cannulating a peripheral vein (ie, in the arm or hand) before attempting cannulation of the EJ vein. Although it is a "peripheral" vein, more risks are associated with cannulation of this vein—namely, inadvertent puncture of the carotid artery, a *rapidly* expanding hematoma if infiltration occurs, and air embolism.

Follow these steps to cannulate the external jugular vein:

1. Place the patient in a supine, head-down position to fill the jugular vein. Turn the patient's head to the side opposite the intended venipuncture site. ***Always** feel carefully for a pulse before cannulating an external jugular vein. It is imperative not to pierce the carotid artery.*
2. Appropriately cleanse the venipuncture site.
3. Occlude the jugular vein with your finger, distal to the catheter insertion site, to facilitate backflow of blood; this will allow the vein to become more visible.

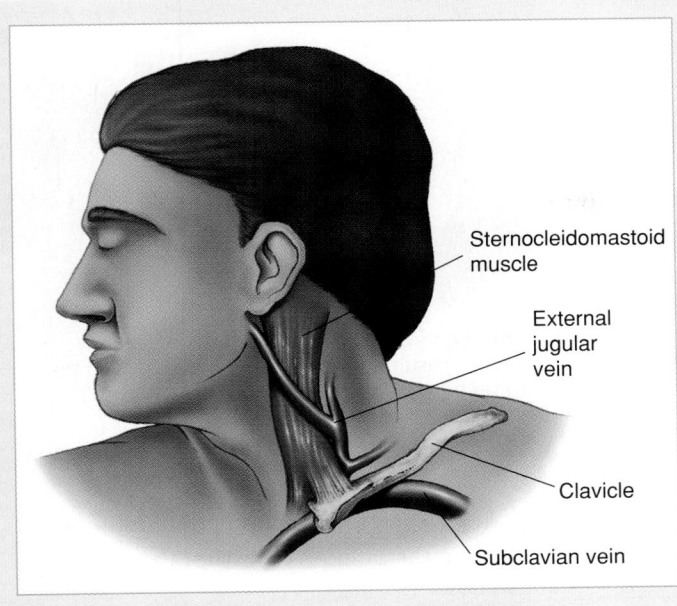

Figure 8-25 Anatomy of the external jugular vein.

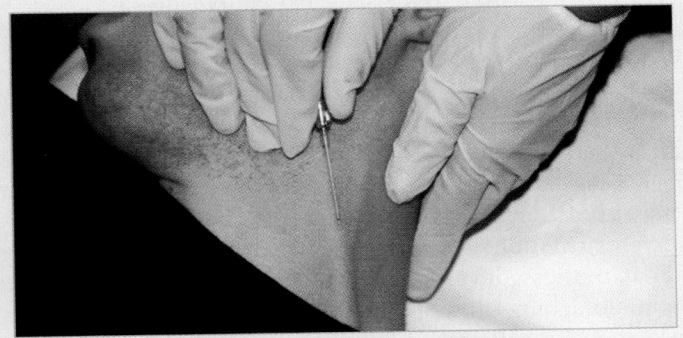

Figure 8-26 The external jugular vein requires a specific insertion site midway between the angle of the jaw and the midclavicular line with the catheter pointed toward the shoulder on the same side as the venipuncture.

4. Align the catheter in the direction of the vein, with the point aimed toward the shoulder on the side of the venipuncture Figure 8-26 ▲.
5. Make the puncture midway between the angle of the jaw and the midclavicular line. Stabilize the vein by placing a finger lightly on top of it just above the clavicle.
6. Proceed as described for cannulation of a peripheral vein. *Do not let air enter the catheter once it is in the vein.*
7. Tape the line securely but do *not* put circumferential dressings around the neck.

Factors Affecting IV Flow Rates

Several factors can influence the flow rate of an IV. For example, if the IV bag is not hung high enough, the flow rate will not be sufficient. Perform the following checks after completing IV administration and whenever a flow problem occurs:

- *Check the IV fluid.* Thick, viscous fluids such as blood products and colloid solutions infuse slowly and may be diluted to help speed delivery. Cold fluids run more slowly than warm fluids. If possible, warm IV fluids before administering them in a cold environment.
- *Check the administration set.* Macrodrips are used for rapid fluid delivery; microdrips deliver a more controlled flow.
- *Check the height of the IV bag.* The IV bag must be hung high enough to overcome gravity. Hang it as high as possible.
- *Check the type of catheter used.* The larger the diameter of the catheter (the smaller the number—for example a 14-gauge is of larger diameter than a 20-gauge), the more fluid can be delivered.
- *Check the constricting band.* Do not leave the constricting band on the patient's arm after completing the IV.

Potential Complications of IV Therapy

Problems associated with IVs can be categorized as local or systemic reactions. Local reactions include problems such as infiltration and thrombophlebitis. Systemic complications include allergic reactions and circulatory overload.

Local IV Site Reactions

Most local reactions require that you discontinue the IV and reestablish the IV in the opposite extremity. Examples of local reactions include infiltration; thrombophlebitis; occlusion; vein irritation; hematoma; nerve, tendon, or ligament damage; and arterial puncture.

Infiltration

Infiltration is the escape of fluid into the surrounding tissue, which causes a localized area of edema. Causes of infiltration include the following problems:

- The IV passes completely through the vein and out the other side.
- The patient moves excessively.
- The tape used to secure the IV becomes loose or dislodged.
- The catheter is inserted at too shallow an angle and enters only the fascia surrounding the vein (this problem is more common with IVs in larger veins, such as those in the upper arm and neck).

Signs and symptoms of infiltration include edema at the catheter site, continued IV flow after occlusion of the vein above the insertion site, and patient complaints of tightness and pain around the IV site.

If infiltration occurs, discontinue the IV and reestablish it in the opposite extremity or in a more proximal location on the same extremity. Apply direct pressure over the swollen area to reduce further swelling or bleeding into the tissue. Avoid wrapping tape around the extremity, as it could create a constricting band.

Thrombophlebitis

Infection and thrombophlebitis (inflammation of the vein and the presence of a clot) may occur in association with venous cannulation; both conditions are most frequently caused by lapses in aseptic technique. Thrombophlebitis is commonly encountered in patients who abuse drugs as well as in patients who are receiving long-term IV therapy in a hospital or hospice setting or with vein-irritating solutions (eg, dextrose solutions, which have a very low pH, or hypertonic solutions of any sort). It can also be produced by mechanical factors, such as excessive motion of the IV needle or catheter after it has been placed.

Thrombophlebitis is usually manifested by pain and tenderness along the vein and redness and edema at the venipuncture site. These signs generally do not appear until after several hours of IV therapy, so you are unlikely to see a case of thrombophlebitis in the field setting unless you are doing an interhospital transport of a patient with an established IV. In such a case, stop the infusion and discontinue the IV at that site. Warm compresses applied to the site may provide some relief.

It is far better to prevent thrombophlebitis or infection than to treat it afterward. To prevent thrombophlebitis, take the following measures:

- Use a povidone-iodine preparation to scrub and disinfect the skin over the venipuncture site; then do a final wipe with an alcohol swab. Make certain the site is dry before initiating the venipuncture.
- Always wear gloves when doing a venipuncture.
- After inserting the catheter, cover the puncture site with a sterile dressing.
- Anchor the catheter and tubing securely to prevent motion of the catheter within the vein.

Occlusion

Occlusion is the physical blockage of a vein or catheter. If the flow rate is not sufficient to keep fluid moving out of the catheter tip such that blood enters the catheter, a clot may form and occlude the flow. The first sign of an occlusion is a decreasing drip rate or the presence of blood in the IV tubing. With a positional IV site, fluid flows at different rates depending on the position of the catheter within the vein; these differences can produce occlusions. Positional IVs may be necessary because of proximity to a valve or because of patient movement that allows the line to become physically blocked, such as resting on the line or crossing arms. Occlusion may also develop if the IV bag nears empty and the patient's blood pressure overcomes the flow, causing fluid backup in the line.

If occlusion occurs, follow the steps shown in **Skill Drill 8-3 ▸** to determine whether the IV should be reestablished:

1. Select and assemble a sterile 10-mL syringe and large-gauge needle **Step 1** .
2. Select an injection port closest to the IV site, and swab it with an alcohol wipe.
3. Insert the needle into the injection port **Step 2** .

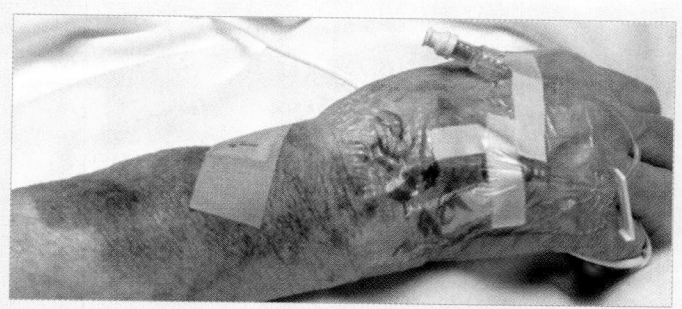

Figure 8-27 Hematomas can be caused by the improper removal of a catheter, resulting in pooling of blood around the IV site, leading to tenderness and pain.

4. Pinch the line in between the injection port and IV bag.
5. Gently pull back on the plunger to disrupt the occlusion and reestablish flow.
6. If flow is reestablished, ensure that the rate is sufficient.
7. If you are unable to reestablish flow, discontinue the IV and reestablish it in the opposite extremity or at a proximal location in the same extremity **Step 3** .

Vein Irritation

Occasionally, a patient will experience vein irritation from the IV fluid. Patients who have this problem often complain immediately that the solution is bothering them (ie, tingling, stinging, itching, and burning). In such cases, observe the patient closely in case an allergic reaction to the fluid develops.

Vein irritation is usually caused by a too-rapid infusion rate. If redness develops at the IV site—a sign suggesting thrombophlebitis—discontinue the IV and save the equipment for later analysis. Reestablish the IV in the other extremity with new equipment in case the old equipment contained unseen contaminants.

Hematoma

A hematoma is an accumulation of blood in the tissues surrounding an IV site, often resulting from vein perforation or improper catheter removal. Blood can be seen rapidly pooling around the IV site, leading to tenderness and pain **Figure 8-27 ▲** . Patients with a history of vascular diseases (including diabetes) and patients taking certain medications (eg, corticosteroids or a blood thinner like Coumadin) can have a predisposition to vein rupture or to hematoma development with IV insertion.

If a hematoma develops while you are attempting to insert a catheter, stop and apply direct pressure to help minimize bleeding. If a hematoma develops after a successful catheter insertion, evaluate the IV flow and the hematoma. If the hematoma appears to be controlled and the flow is not affected, monitor the IV site and leave the line in place. If the hematoma develops as a result of discontinuing the IV, apply direct pressure with a 4″ × 4″ gauze pad to the site.

Skill Drill 8-3: Determining Whether an IV Is Viable

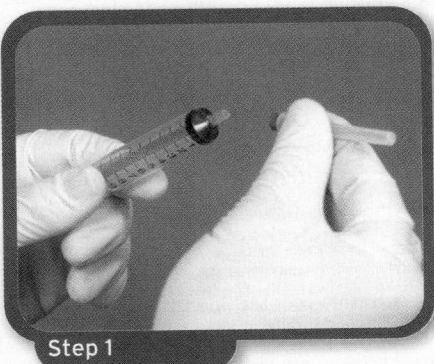

Step 1

Select and assemble a sterile 10-mL syringe and large-gauge needle.

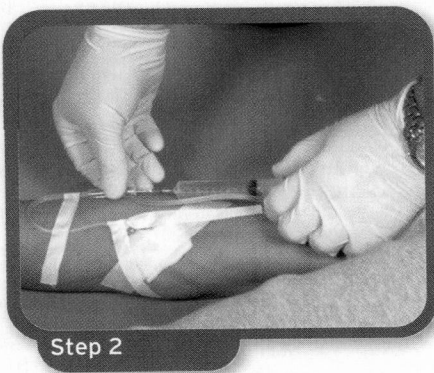

Step 2

Select an injection port near the IV site, and swab it with an alcohol wipe.
Insert the syringe into the port.

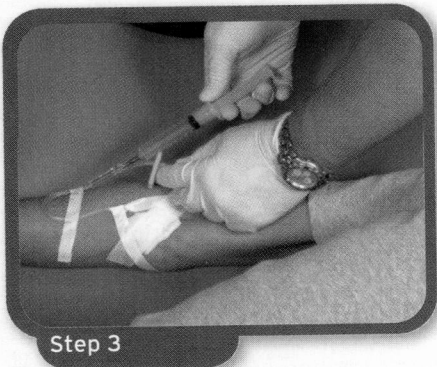

Step 3

Pinch the line in between the injection port and IV bag.
Gently pull back on the plunger to disrupt the occlusion and reestablish flow. If flow is reestablished, ensure that the rate is sufficient.
If the occlusion does not dislodge, discontinue the IV and reestablish it in the opposite extremity or at a proximal location on the same extremity.

Nerve, Tendon, or Ligament Damage

Improper identification of anatomic structures around the IV site can lead to perforation of tendons, ligaments, and nerves. Selecting an IV site located near joints increases the risk for perforation of these structures. When this type of injury occurs, patients will experience sudden and severe shooting pain. Numbness or tingling in the extremity after the incident is common. Immediately remove the catheter and select another IV site.

Arterial Puncture

You may accidentally puncture the wrong blood vessel if the vein selected for cannulation lies near an artery. *The risk of arterial puncture is especially high when cannulating an external jugular vein—be careful!* If you insert a catheter into an artery by mistake, bright red blood will spurt back through the catheter. The blood's color and its flow characteristics will alert you to your error. *Immediately withdraw the catheter, and apply direct pressure over the puncture site for at least 5 minutes or until bleeding stops.*

To avoid cannulating an artery, always check for a pulse in any vessel you intend to cannulate. Under normal circumstances, veins are near the skin surface and arteries lie much deeper. On occasion, an anatomic anomaly occurs and the vessels become transpositioned, resulting in an artery being very superficial.

Systemic Complications

Systemic complications can evolve from reactions or complications associated with IV insertion. They usually involve other body systems and can be life-threatening. If the IV line is established and patent in such a patient, do not remove it because it may be needed for treatment. Potential systemic complications include allergic reactions, pyrogenic reactions, circulatory overload, air embolus, vasovagal reactions, and catheter shear.

Allergic Reactions

Often, allergic reactions associated with IV therapy are minor. However, anaphylaxis—a potentially life-threatening condition—is possible and must be treated aggressively. Allergic reactions can result from a person's unexpected sensitivity to an IV fluid or medication. Such sensitivity could be unknown to the patient, so you must maintain vigilance with any IV for a possible allergic reaction.

The patient presentation depends on the extent of the reaction. Common signs and symptoms of an allergic reaction include itching (pruritus), shortness of breath, edema of face and hands, urticaria (hives), bronchospasm, and wheezing.

If an allergic reaction occurs, discontinue the IV and remove the solution. Leave the catheter in place as an emergency medication route. Attach a saline lock, if available.

Notify medical control immediately, and maintain an open airway. Monitor the patient's ABCs and vital signs. Keep the solution or medication for evaluation by the hospital (Chapter 30 covers allergic reactions and anaphylaxis in more detail).

Pyrogenic Reactions

Pyrogens are foreign proteins capable of producing fever. Their presence in the infusion solution or administration set may induce a pyrogenic reaction, which is characterized by an abrupt temperature elevation (as high as 106°F [41.1°C]) with severe chills, backache, headache, weakness, nausea, and vomiting. Occasionally vascular collapse occurs, with all the signs and symptoms of shock. The reaction usually begins within 30 minutes after the IV infusion has been started.

If you observe *any* signs of such a reaction—for example, if the patient complains of a headache or backache after you have started running fluids—*stop the infusion immediately!* Start a new IV in the other arm with a *fresh infusion solution,* and remove the first IV. If the patient is showing signs of shock, treat as any other case of shock.

Pyrogenic reactions can be largely avoided by inspecting the IV bag carefully before use. If the bag has any leaks or if the fluid looks cloudy or discolored, select another bag.

Circulatory Overload

Healthy adults can handle as much as 2 to 3 extra liters of fluid without compromise. Problems occur, however, when the patient has cardiac, pulmonary, or renal dysfunction; these types of dysfunction do not tolerate any additional demands from increased circulatory volume. The most common cause of circulatory overload in the prehospital setting is failure to readjust the drip rate after flushing an IV line immediately after insertion. Always monitor the IV to ensure the proper drip rate. If available, consider using a Volutrol (Buretrol) administration set for patients who are at risk for circulatory overload.

Signs and symptoms of circulatory overload include dyspnea, jugular vein distention, and hypertension. Crackles (rales) are often heard when evaluating breath sounds. Acute peripheral edema can also be an indication of circulatory overload.

To treat a patient with circulatory overload, slow the IV rate to keep the vein open and raise the patient's head to ease respiratory distress. Administer high-flow oxygen, and monitor vital signs and breathing adequacy. Contact medical control immediately, because certain drugs can be given to reduce the circulatory volume.

Air Embolus

Healthy adults can tolerate as much as 200 mL of air introduced into the circulatory system. For patients who are already ill or injured, however, *any* air introduced into the IV line can present a problem. Properly flushing an IV line will help eliminate the likelihood of air embolus. Although IV bags are designed to collapse as they empty to help prevent this problem, this collapse does not always occur. Be sure to replace empty IV bags with full ones.

> **Special Considerations**
>
> It is easy to overload older patients who need large amounts of IV fluids. Administer small boluses of fluid (200 to 300 mL), and check breath sounds before and after each bolus to ensure that the lungs remain "dry."

If your patient begins developing respiratory distress with unequal breath sounds, consider the possibility of an air embolus. Other associated signs and symptoms include cyanosis (even in the presence of high-flow oxygen), signs and symptoms of shock, loss of consciousness, and respiratory arrest.

Treat a patient with a suspected air embolus by placing the patient on his or her left side with the head down to trap any air inside the right atrium or right ventricle, administering 100% oxygen, and rapidly transporting to the closest appropriate facility. Be prepared to assist ventilation if the patient experiences inadequate breathing.

Vasovagal Reactions

Some patients have anxiety concerning needles or the sight of blood. Such anxiety may cause vasculature dilation, leading to a drop in blood pressure and patient collapse. Patients can present with anxiety, diaphoresis, nausea, and syncopal episodes.

Treatment for patients with vasovagal reactions (also known as "vagaling down") centers on treating them for shock:

1. Place patient in shock position.
2. Apply high-flow oxygen.
3. Monitor vital signs.
4. Establish an IV in case fluid resuscitation is needed.

Catheter Shear

Catheter shear occurs when part of the catheter is pinched against the needle, and the needle slices through the catheter, creating a free-floating segment. The catheter segment can then travel through the circulatory system and possibly end up in the pulmonary circulation, causing a pulmonary embolus. Treatment involves surgical removal of the sheared tip. If you suspect a catheter shear, place the patient in a left lateral recumbent position with his legs down and his head up to try to keep the catheter remnant out of the pulmonary circulation.

Catheter hubs are radiopaque (ie, they appear white in an x-ray) to aid in diagnosing this type of problem. Never rethread a catheter. Dispose of the used one and select a new catheter.

Patients who have experienced catheter shear with pulmonary artery occlusion present with sudden dyspnea, shortness of breath, and possibly

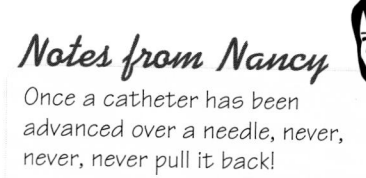

Notes from Nancy

Once a catheter has been advanced over a needle, never, never, never pull it back!

diminished breath sounds. Their symptoms mimic the presentation of an air embolus and can be treated the same way. Such patients need continued IV access, and you must try to obtain an IV site in the other extremity.

Obtaining Blood Samples

If blood samples are needed—usually at the request of the hospital for laboratory analysis—you should obtain them at the same time you start the IV. If you have difficulty drawing blood, however, stop and finish the IV.

To obtain blood samples when starting an IV, you will need the following equipment:

- 15- or 20-mL syringe
- 18- or 20-gauge needle
- Self-sealing blood tubes

The blood-tube tops usually come in red, blue, green, and lavender, and should be filled in that order. Use the following mnemonic to help remember the order for filling the tubes: Red Blood Gives Life. The *red*-topped tube contains no additives and is intended to clot if blood typing is needed. The *blue*-topped tube contains the preservative EDTA and is used to help determine a patient's prothrombin time and partial thromboplastin time (values that are used to calculate the patient's blood clotting time). The *green*-topped tube is filled with heparin to prevent clotting and is used to evaluate the patient's electrolyte and glucose levels. *Lavender*-topped tubes are filled with sodium citrate and are often used for a complete blood count, including hematocrit and hemoglobin values.

After the IV catheter is in place, occlude the catheter and remove the constricting band. Attach a 15- or 20-mL syringe to the hub of the IV catheter and draw the necessary amount of blood. *Do not leave the constricting band on while drawing blood with the syringe; doing so may cause waste products to build up in the blood and could skew laboratory test results.* Detach the syringe after the required amount of blood has been obtained, attach the IV tubing, and begin the infusion. Attach an 18- or 20-gauge needle to the syringe, fill the blood tubes with the necessary amount of blood, and immediately dispose of the syringe and needle in a puncture-proof sharps container. *Exercise extreme caution when filling blood tubes with this technique; you are handling a "live" needle!*

If IV therapy is not indicated but blood samples are required, you can obtain them by using a cylindrical device that attaches to an 18- or 20-gauge sampling needle (a Vacutainer). The blood tubes are inserted into the Vacutainer after the needle it is attached to has entered the vein. To obtain blood using a Vacutainer, follow these steps:

1. Apply a constricting band, and locate a suitable vein—typically, the antecubital vein. Follow body substance isolation (BSI) precautions.
2. Prep the vein as you would when starting an IV—use an alcohol prep or iodine swab, and cleanse the area in a

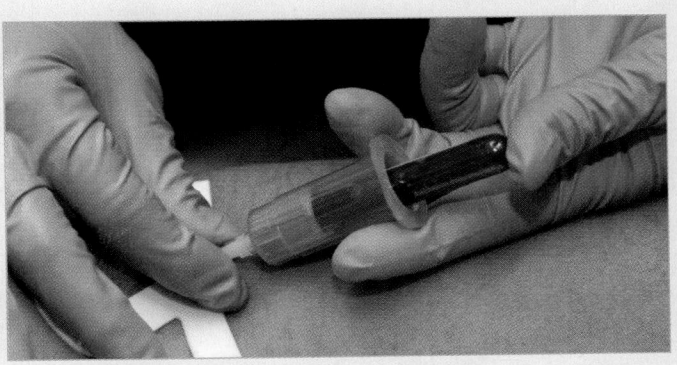

Figure 8-28 Obtaining blood samples with a Vacutainer.

circular motion, starting from the inside and working your way out.

3. Insert the needle (already attached to the Vacutainer) into the vein.
4. Remove the constricting band, and insert blood tubes into the Vacutainer to obtain the necessary amount of blood **Figure 8-28 ▲** .
5. Remove the needle from the vein, and apply direct pressure.
6. Dispose of the needle in a puncture-proof sharps container.
7. Label all the tubes with patient's name, the date, the time, and your name as soon as possible to avoid mixing tubes with those of another patient.

Once the blood tubes are filled, gently turn them back and forth several times to mix the anticoagulant and blood evenly. The exception is the red-topped tube, which is intended to separate the serum from the other blood components. Avoid shaking this tube after the blood has clotted, because the motion may destroy the sample.

For blood tubes to be viable for testing, they must be at least three fourths full. Follow local protocols for the types of blood tubes to fill.

Intraosseous Infusion

Intraosseous means "within the bone." Intraosseous (IO) infusion is a technique of administering fluids, blood and blood products, and medications into the intraosseous space of a long bone, usually the proximal tibia.

Long bones consist of a shaft (diaphysis), the ends (epiphyses), and the growth plate (epiphyseal plate) **Figure 8-29 ▶** .

The intraosseous (IO) space collectively comprises the spongy cancellous bone of the epiphyses and the medullary cavity of the diaphysis. Its vasculature drains into the central circulation by a network of venous sinuses and canals.

When a patient is in shock, cardiac arrest, or an otherwise hemodynamically compromised condition, peripheral veins

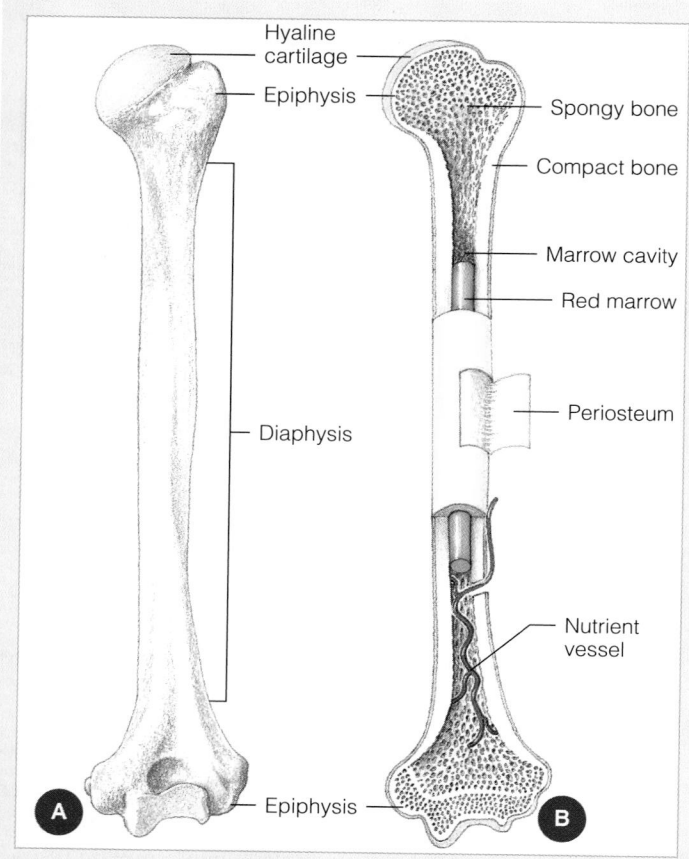

Figure 8-29 The components of a long bone. **A.** The humerus. Note the long shaft and dilated ends. **B.** Longitudinal section of the humerus showing compact bone, cancellous (spongy) bone, and marrow.

often collapse, making IV access extremely difficult, if not impossible. However, the IO space remains patent, unless the patient has suffered trauma to its bony structure (eg, a fracture). For this reason, the IO space is commonly referred to as a "noncollapsible vein." It quickly absorbs IV fluids and medications and rapidly gets them to the central circulation—as rapidly as is possible with the IV route. Anything that can be given via the IV route—crystalloids, medications, and blood and blood products—can be given via the IO route.

IO infusion is indicated when you are unable to obtain IV access in a critically ill or injured patient (eg, in profound shock, cardiac arrest, or status epilepticus). Historically, IO infusion was reserved for children younger than 6 years when IV access could not be obtained within 3 attempts or 90 seconds. Although this still holds true, IO infusion has also been approved by the US Food and Drug Administration as an alternative means of establishing vascular access in critically ill or injured adults.

Equipment for IO Infusion

Several products are used for placing an IO needle into the IO space: manually inserted IO needles, the F.A.S.T.1, the EZ-IO,

and the Bone Injection Gun (BIG). Use of these devices requires specialized training and thorough familiarity with each device's features, functionality, and clinical application. If your EMS system uses any of these devices, follow local protocols regarding their application.

Manually inserted IO needles (ie, Jamshedi needle, Cook catheter) were the original devices used for establishing IO access in children and are still widely used in the prehospital setting. They consist of a solid boring needle (trocar) inserted through a sharpened hollow needle   Figure 8-30 ▾ . The IO needle is pushed into the bone with a screwing, twisting action. Once the needle pops through the bone, the solid needle is removed, leaving the hollow steel needle in place. The IV tubing is attached to this catheter.

Because manually inserted IO needles are long, rest at a 90° angle to the bone, and are easily dislodged, they require full and careful immobilization. Stabilization is critical for these lines to maintain adequate flow. Stabilize the IO needle in the same manner that you would any impaled object.

The F.A.S.T.1 (First Access for Shock and Trauma) was the first IO device approved for use in adults; *it is not used in children.* Four design elements allow for this device's IO placement in the sternum: an infusion tube and subcutaneous portal, an introducer, a target/strain relief patch, and a protective dome   Figure 8-31 ▾ . The company that developed the F.A.S.T.1 chose sternum placement based on the ease of locating the manubrium and the easier penetration than other bones.

The EZ-IO features a hand-held battery-powered driver, to which a special IO needle is attached   Figure 8-32 ▸ . This device is used to insert an IO needle into the

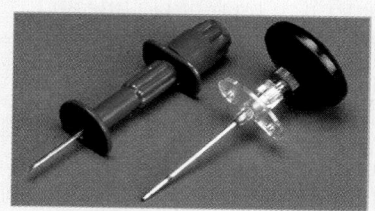

Figure 8-30 Manually inserted IO needles.

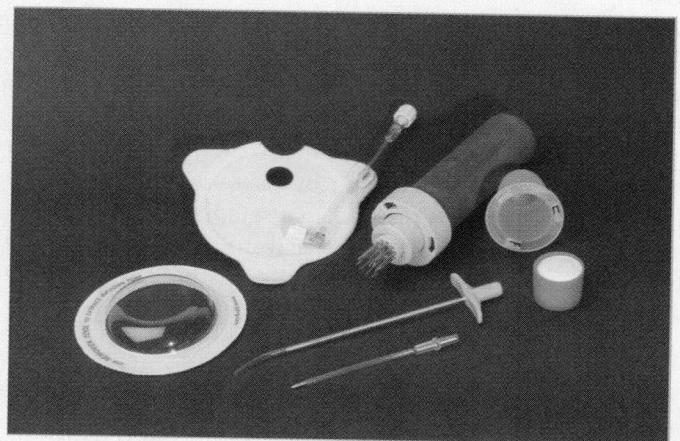

Figure 8-31 F.A.S.T.1 sternal IO device.

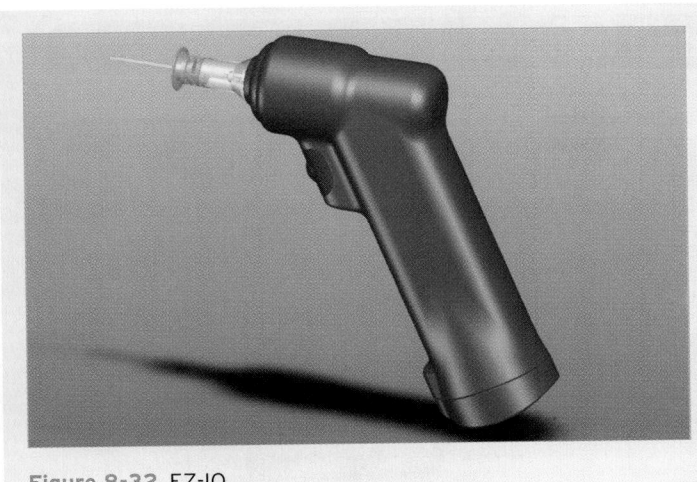

Figure 8-32 EZ-IO.

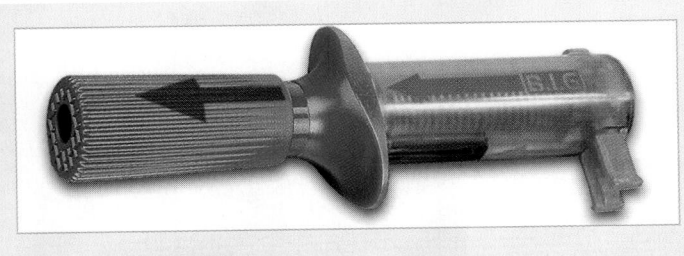

Figure 8-33 Adult BIG.

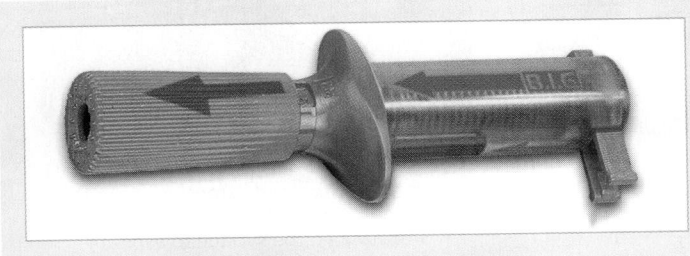

Figure 8-34 Pediatric BIG.

proximal tibia of adults and children when IV access is difficult or impossible to obtain. The battery-powered driver of the EZ-IO is universal, but different sizes of needles are available for adults and children.

The <u>Bone Injection Gun (BIG)</u> is a spring-loaded device that is used to insert an IO needle into the proximal tibia of adult and pediatric patients. It comes in an adult size **Figure 8-33 ▲** and a pediatric size **Figure 8-34 ▲**, though both versions offer the same operational features.

Performing IO Infusion

The technique for performing IO infusion requires proper anatomic landmark identification. The flat bone of the proximal tibia—the most commonly used site—is located medial to the tibial tuberosity, the bony protuberance just below the knee.

Follow these steps to perform IO infusion using a manually inserted IO needle **Skill Drill 8-4 ▶**.

1. Check the selected IV fluid for proper fluid, clarity, and expiration date. Look for discoloration and for particles floating in the fluid. If found, discard the bag and choose another bag of fluid.

2. Select the appropriate equipment, including an IO needle, syringe, saline, and extension set **Step 1**. A three-way stopcock may also be used to facilitate easier fluid administration.

3. Select the proper administration set. Connect the administration set to the bag.
   Prepare the administration set. Fill the drip chamber and flush the tubing. Make sure all air bubbles are removed from the tubing.

4. Prepare the syringe and extension tubing.

5. Cut or tear the tape. This can be done at any time before IO puncture.

6. Take BSI precautions **Step 2**. *This must be done before IO puncture.*

7. Identify the proper anatomic site for IO puncture **Step 3**. When using the BIG in an adult, go 2 cm from the tibial tuberosity toward the inner leg, and then 1 cm up toward the knee. When using the EZ-IO, go down 2 cm from the patella to the tibial tuberosity, then 1 cm toward the inner leg. It is important to avoid penetrating the epiphyseal (growth) plate in children. When using the BIG in a child, go 1 to 2 cm from the tibial tuberosity toward the inner leg, and then 1 cm down toward the foot.

8. Cleanse the site appropriately. Follow aseptic technique by cleansing in a circular manner from the inside out.

9. Perform the IO puncture, by first stabilizing the tibia, then placing a folded towel under the knee, and finally holding in a manner to keep your fingers away from the site of puncture.

10. Insert the needle at a 90° angle to the leg. Advance the needle with a twisting motion until a "pop" is felt **Step 4**. Unscrew the cap, and remove the stylet from the needle **Step 5**.

11. Attach the syringe and extension set to the IO needle. Pull back on the syringe to aspirate blood and particles of bone marrow to ensure proper placement.

12. Slowly inject saline to ensure proper placement of the needle. Watch for extravasation, and stop the infusion immediately if it is noted. It is possible to fracture the bone during insertion of the IO. If this happens, you should remove the IO and switch to the other leg.

13. Connect the administration set and adjust the flow rate as appropriate **Step 6**. Fluid does not flow as rapidly through an IO catheter as through an IV line; therefore, crystalloid boluses should be given with a syringe in children and a pressure infuser device in adults.

14. Secure the needle with tape, and support it with a bulky dressing. Stabilize in place in the same manner that an

Skill Drill 8-4: IO Infusion

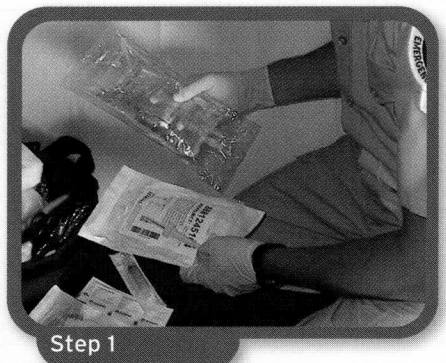
Step 1

Check selected IV fluid for proper fluid, clarity, and expiration date.
Select the appropriate equipment, including an IO needle, syringe, saline, and extension tubing.
Select the proper administration set. Connect the administration set to the bag. Prepare the administration set, syringe, and extension tubing.

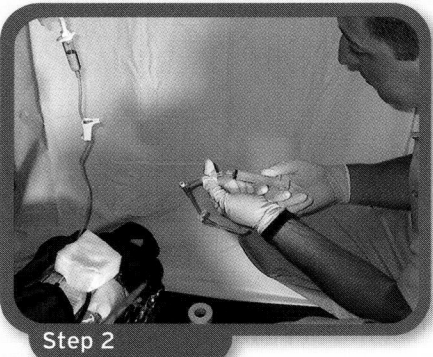
Step 2

Take BSI precautions.

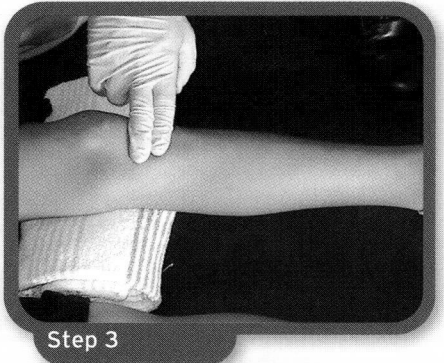
Step 3

Identify the proper anatomic site for IO puncture.

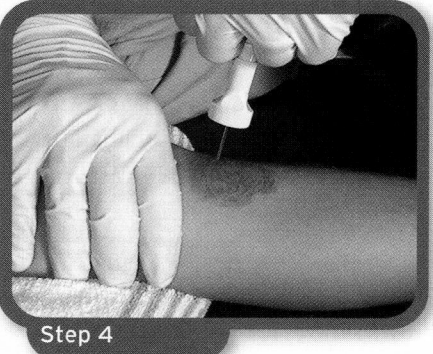
Step 4

Cleanse the site appropriately.
Stabilize the tibia, and insert the needle at a 90° angle, advancing it with a twisting motion until a "pop" is felt.

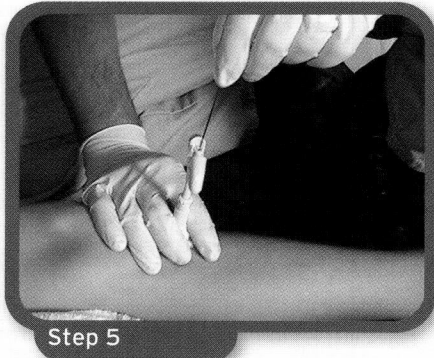
Step 5

Unscrew the cap, and remove the stylet from the needle.

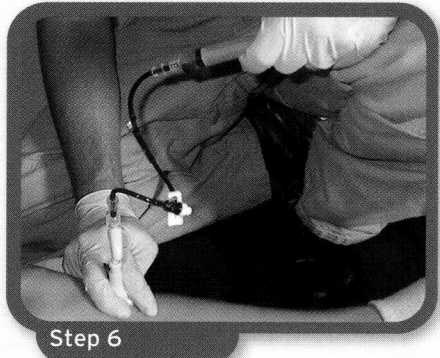
Step 6

Attach the syringe and extension set to the IO needle.
Pull back on the syringe to aspirate blood and particles of bone marrow to ensure proper placement.
Slowly inject saline to ensure proper placement of the needle.
Watch for extravasation, and stop the infusion immediately if it is noted.
Connect the administration set, and adjust the flow rate as appropriate.

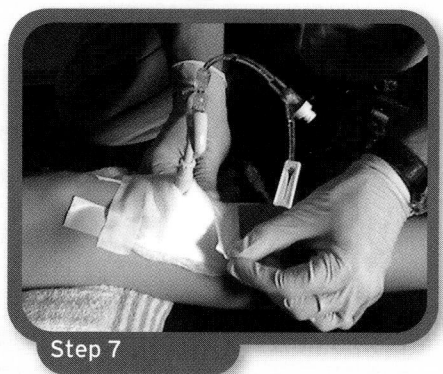
Step 7

Secure the needle with tape, and support it with bulky dressing.

impaled object is stabilized. Use bulky dressings around the catheter, and tape securely in place. Be careful not to tape around the entire circumference of the leg, as this could impair circulation and potentially result in compartment syndrome (Step 7).

15. Dispose of the needle in the proper container.

Potential Complications of IO Infusion

If proper technique is used (ie, proper anatomic landmark identification, aseptic technique), IO infusion is associated with a relatively low complication rate. The same potential complications associated with IV therapy—thrombophlebitis, local irritation, allergic reaction, circulatory overload, and air embolism—can occur with IO infusion, as well as several others unique to this method of infusion.

Extravasation occurs when the IO needle does not rest in the IO space, but rather rests outside the bone (because the bone was missed completely or is fractured). In such a case, IV fluid will collect in the soft tissues. The risk of extravasation can be reduced significantly by using the proper insertion technique: *Insert the IO needle at a 90° angle to the bone.* Extravasation should be suspected if the infusion does not run freely or if the site—especially the posterior aspect of the leg—rapidly becomes edematous. If this occurs, discontinue the infusion immediately and reattempt insertion in the opposite leg. Undetected extravasation could result in compartment syndrome.

Osteomyelitis is inflammation of the bone and muscle caused by an infection. According to several studies, osteomyelitis occurs in fewer than 0.6% of IO insertions.

Failure to identify the proper anatomic landmark can damage the growth plate, potentially resulting in long-term bone growth abnormalities in children.

If your insertion technique is too forceful, or if you use an IO needle that is too large for the patient's age or size, fractures can occur.

Through-and-through insertion occurs when the IO needle passes through *both* sides of the bone. To avoid this, stop inserting the needle when you feel a pop. If you feel a "pop, pop," you have likely passed the needle through both sides of the bone. Remove the needle and attempt insertion on the opposite extremity.

A pulmonary embolism (PE) can occur if particles of bone, fat, or marrow find their way into the systemic circulation and lodge in a pulmonary artery. Suspect a PE if the patient experiences acute shortness of breath, pleuritic chest pain, and cyanosis.

Contraindications to IO Infusion

Cannulation of a peripheral vein remains the preferred route for administering IV fluids and medications. If a functional IV line is available—in a pediatric patient or an adult—IO cannulation is *not* indicated. Other contraindications to IO cannulation and infusion include fracture of the bone intended for IO cannulation, osteoporosis, osteogenesis imperfecta (a

In the Field

With the exception of the F.A.S.T.1 sternal IO device, all IO devices—manual, spring-loaded, and battery-powered—are primarily used to insert an IO needle into the IO space of the proximal tibia. However, other anatomic locations, such as the distal tibia and distal femur, may also be acceptable locations for IO needle insertion.

congenital disease resulting in fragile bones), and bilateral knee replacements (obviously more relevant in adults).

Calculating Fluid Infusion Rates

Once the IV or IO catheter is in place, you need to adjust the flow rate according to the patient's clinical condition or as dictated by medical control. To do so, you must know the following information:

- The volume to be infused
- The period over which it is to be infused
- The properties of the administration set you are using—that is, how many drops per milliliter (gtt/mL) it delivers

Documentation and Communication

When you start an IV for the purpose of administering a medication, you should set the flow rate just slow enough to keep the vein patent. This slow flow rate can be documented using the acronym KVO, which stands for Keep Vein Open, or TKO, which stands for To Keep Open.

By knowing in advance the volume to be infused, the period over which it will be infused, and the properties of the administration set, you can easily calculate the flow rate:

$$\text{gtt/min} = \frac{\text{volume to be infused} \times \text{gtt/mL of administration set}}{\text{total time of infusion } \textit{in minutes}}$$

For example, suppose the physician orders an infusion of 1 L (1,000 mL) of normal saline to be infused in 4 hours, and the macrodrip administration set provides 10 gtt/mL:

Total volume to be infused = 1,000 mL
gtt/mL of the administration set = 10
Time of infusion (in minutes) = 240

$$gtt/min = \frac{1,000\ mL \times 10\ gtt/mL}{240\ minutes} = \text{approximately } 42\ gtt/min$$

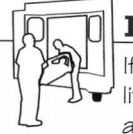

In the Field

If the physician orders a specific number of milliliters to be administered per hour (mL/h), a quick and easy way to calculate the number of drops per minute (gtt/min) is to divide the number of milliliters per hour:

- By 6, if using a macrodrip that provides 10 gtt/mL
- By 4, if using a macrodrip that provides 15 gtt/mL
- By 1, if using a microdrip set that provides 60 gtt/mL

▋Medication Administration

Before administering any medication to a patient, you must have a thorough understanding of how the medication will affect the human body—negatively and positively. This includes familiarity with the medication's mechanism of action, indications, contraindications, side effects, routes of administration, pediatric and adult doses, and antidotes (if available) for adverse reactions (see Chapter 7).

The first rule of medicine is *primum non nocere,* "The first thing (is) to do no harm." For example, administering the drug atropine to a patient with asymptomatic bradycardia could result in undesirable tachycardia and potential hemodynamic compromise. As a result, you have caused harm to the patient who otherwise did not need the drug. It is, therefore, paramount to ensure that a particular drug is clearly indicated to treat the patient's condition.

You must also have an understanding of basic math for pharmacology to calculate the appropriate medication dose. This section begins with a review of basic mathematical principles as they apply to pharmacology and concludes with the various methods of medication administration.

Drug doses and flow rate calculations are often sources of confusion for many prehospital personnel, yet they are skills you will need to utilize frequently in the field and during your initial training while practicing at skill stations. As a paramedic, you must learn to quickly and accurately calculate medication doses to maximize the chance for a positive patient outcome. Disastrous results, including death, may be the outcome if you administer an inappropriate drug or dose, give it by the wrong route, or give the medication too rapidly or too slowly.

Mathematical Principles Used in Pharmacology

The Metric System

The metric system is a decimal system based on multiples of ten Figure 8-35 ▼ . In this system, the basic unit of length is the meter (m), the basic unit of volume is the liter (L), and the basic unit of weight is the gram (g). Prefixes indicate the fraction of the base being used. Commonly used prefixes, from smallest to largest, include *micro-* (0.000001), *milli-* (0.001), *centi-* (0.01), and *kilo-* (1,000).

Drugs are supplied in a variety of weights and volumes, and you will be required to convert those weights to volume to administer the appropriate dose of a medication to your patient. Table 8-3 ▶ lists the symbols of weight and volume, with their respective abbreviations, that are used in the metric system. Table 8-4 ▶ lists the metric units of weight and volume and their equivalents.

Weight and Volume Conversion

To administer the appropriate dose of a medication to a patient, you must be able to convert larger units of weight to smaller ones (for example, g to mg) and larger units of volume to smaller ones (for example, L to mL). Conversely, you must be able to convert smaller units of weight to larger ones (for example, mg to g) and smaller units of volume to larger ones (for example, mL to L).

Drugs are packaged in different units of weight and volume. However, the weight (for example, µg, mg, g) and volume (for example, mL) of the drug to be administered usually comprise only a fraction of the total amount of its packaged form. For example, a physician may order 50 mg of a drug for a patient, but the drug is packaged in grams. Therefore, you must be able to convert grams to milligrams and then determine how much volume is required to achieve the desired dose.

Weight Conversion

Converting weight is simply a matter of multiplying or dividing by 1,000 *or* moving the decimal point three places to the right or left.

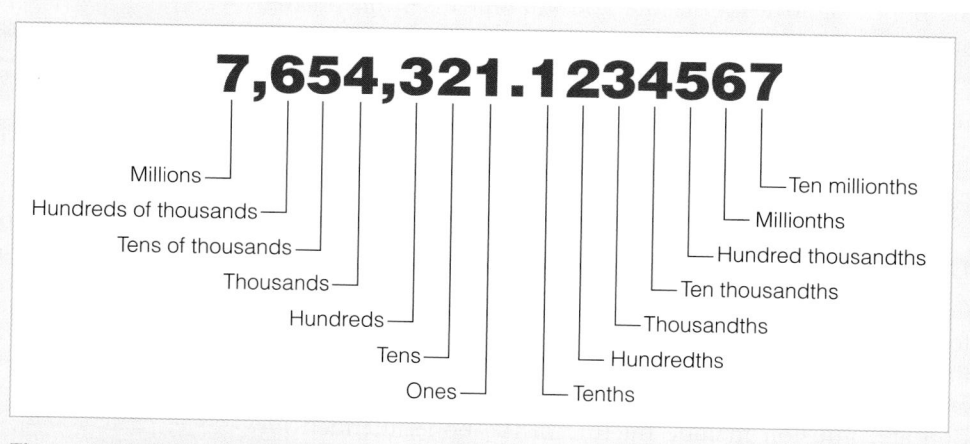

Figure 8-35 Decimal scale.

Table 8-3	Symbols Used in the Metric System

Symbols of weight (smallest to largest)

- microgram = µg (or mcg)
- milligram = mg
- gram = g (or gm)
- kilogram = kg

Symbols of volume (smallest to largest)

- milliliter = mL
- deciliter = dL
- liter = L

Table 8-4	Metric Units and Their Equivalents

Units of weight (smallest to largest)

- 1 µg = 0.001 mg
- 1 mg = 1,000 µg
- 1 g = 1,000 mg
- 1 kg = 1,000 g

Units of volume (smallest to largest)

- 1 mL = 1 cc*
- 100 mL = 1 dL
- 1,000 mL = 1 L

*One milliliter (mL) of water weighs 1 g and occupies 1 cubic centimeter (cc) of volume. Thus a mL and a cc both express one one-thousandth of a liter and are, therefore, equivalent expressions.

To convert a larger unit of weight to a smaller one, *multiply* the larger unit of weight by 1,000 *or* move the decimal point three places to the *right*:

> **EXAMPLE**
>
> Converting 2 g to mg (2 g = X mg)
>
> 2 g × 1,000 = 2,000 mg *or* 2.000 g = 2,000 mg
> →

To convert a smaller unit of weight to a larger one, *divide* the smaller unit of weight by 1,000 *or* move the decimal point three places to the *left*:

> **EXAMPLE**
>
> Converting 200 µg to mg (200 µg = X mg)
>
> 200 µg ÷ 1,000 = 0.2 mg *or* 200.0 µg = 0.2 mg
> ←

Volume Conversion

In the prehospital setting, you will usually deal with only two measurements of volume: milliliters and liters. The formula is the same as for converting units of weight: Divide or multiply by 1,000 *or* move the decimal point three places to the left or right.

When converting a smaller unit of volume to a larger one, *divide* the smaller unit of volume by 1,000 *or* move the decimal point three places to the *left*:

> **EXAMPLE**
>
> Converting 100 mL to L (100 mL = X L)
>
> 100 mL ÷ 1,000 = 0.1 L *or* 100.0 mL = 0.1 L
> ←

To convert a larger unit of volume to a smaller one, *multiply* the larger unit of volume by 1,000 *or* move the decimal point three places to the *right*:

> **EXAMPLE**
>
> Converting 1.5 L to mL (1.5 L = X mL)
>
> 1.5 L × 1,000 = 1,500 mL *or* 1.500 L = 1,500 mL
> →

Converting Pounds to Kilograms

The only apothecary-to-metric conversion that you will likely make in the field is from pounds (apothecary) to kilograms (metric). It would be a luxury—and an unusual event—if your patients were able to tell you how much they weighed in kilograms (kg). If the patient is able to tell you his or her weight in pounds, great! For patients who do not know their weight in pounds or who are unconscious and unable to provide you with this information, you must do the following:

1. Estimate the patient's weight in pounds (lb).
2. Convert pounds to kilograms (kg).

Although many of the drugs given in emergency medicine are administered in a standard dose (eg, 1 mg of epinephrine), others are administered based on the patient's weight in kilograms (eg, 1 to 1.5 mg/kg of lidocaine). In addition, most drugs administered to pediatric patients are based on their weight in kilograms.

Two formulas can be used to convert pounds to kilograms. Use whichever one is easiest for you to remember.

> *Formula 1: Divide the patient's weight in pounds by 2.2*
> *(1 kg = 2.2 lb)*

For example, when converting a 170-lb man's weight to kilograms, the formula would be as follows:

> 170 lb ÷ 2.2 = 77.27 kg

Because the value following the decimal point in this example is less than 0.5, you may round the patient's weight in kilograms to 77. If the value after the decimal point had been greater than 0.5, you would round the weight in kilograms to 78. Although this may seem negligible, it is good practice to administer the *most* appropriate amount of the drug to the patient.

> Formula 2: Divide the patient's weight in pounds by 2 and subtract 10% of that number

For example, when converting a 120-lb woman's weight to kilograms, the formula would be as follows:

> Step 1: 120 lb ÷ 2 = 60
> Step 2: 60 × 10% = 6
> Step 3: 60 − 6 = 54 kg
> NOTE: This formula provides an approximate weight and is not exact.

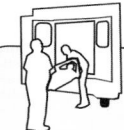
In the Field

Carry a calculator or EMS field guide to assist you in converting pounds to kilograms or when calculating a drug dosage.

Other Systems of Measurement

The apothecary system was formerly used by physicians and pharmacists but has been largely replaced by the metric system. It is based on 480 grains (gr) to 1 oz and 16 oz to 1 lb. The grain (gr) is the basic unit of weight and is approximately the weight of a drop of water. The minim is the unit of volume and is approximately the volume of a drop of water. Additional units of volume are the pint (pt), quart (qt), and gallon (gal). Fractions are used in the apothecary system.

You may also encounter the household system, which consists of measurements such as drops, teaspoons, tablespoons, and cups. This system is rarely, if ever, used for drug dosage calculation or administration in the prehospital setting.

The Fahrenheit and Celsius (or centigrade) temperature scales are commonly used to measure temperature. On the Celsius scale, water freezes at 0° and boils at 100°. On the Fahrenheit scale, water freezes at 32° and boils at 212°. Normal body temperature is 98.6° Fahrenheit (37° Celsius). Values on each of these scales can easily be interconverted by using the following equations:

- To convert Fahrenheit to Celsius: Subtract 32, then multiply by 0.555 (5/9)

> 98.6°F − 32 × 0.555 = 36.9 (37°C)

- To convert Celsius to Fahrenheit: Multiply by 1.8 (9/5), then add 32

> 37°C × 1.8 + 32 = 98.6°F

Calculating Medication Doses

There are multiple formulas for calculating medication doses. This chapter focuses on those formulas that most students find easy to understand. For other calculation formulas, you are encouraged to consult with your instructor. The method of drug dose calculation demonstrated in this chapter is based on the following three factors:

- Desired dose
- Concentration of the drug available (dose on hand)
- Volume to be administered

Desired Dose

The desired dose (ie, the drug order) is the amount of a drug that the physician orders you to give to a patient. It may be expressed as a standard dose (eg, 5 mg of diazepam [Valium], 25 g of 50% dextrose) or as a specific number of micrograms, milligrams, or grams per kilogram of body weight (eg, 1 to 1.5 mg/kg of lidocaine [Xylocaine]).

Drug Concentrations

After receiving a drug order (desired dose), you must determine how much of the drug that you have available. In other words, you must know its concentration—the total weight (μg, mg, or g) of the drug contained in a specific amount of volume (mL or L). Sometimes this information is printed on the label of the drug container (eg, Drug X at a concentration of 5 mg/mL); other containers may list the total weight and total volume of the drug separately (eg, 50 mg of drug Y in 10 mL). The following are examples of common prepackaged drug concentrations:

- Lidocaine, 100 mg/10 mL
- Epinephrine, 1 mg/10 mL
- Furosemide, 40 mg/4 mL
- Adenosine, 6 mg/2 mL
- 50% dextrose, 25 g/50 mL

In the preceding examples, notice that the drugs are contained in different volumes of solution. *To administer a drug, you must know the weight of the drug that is present in **1 mL**.* This information will tell you the concentration of the drug that you have on hand. The formula for calculating this is as follows:

> Total weight of the drug ÷ total volume in milliliters
> = weight per milliliter

By using this formula, you can easily calculate how much of the drug is contained in each milliliter.

EXAMPLE

Lidocaine, 100 mg/10 mL

> 100 mg (total weight) ÷ 10 mL (total volume) = 10 mg/mL

Things become a bit trickier when the label of the drug lists the drug concentration as a percentage—for example, "1% Xylocaine." What *percentage* means in terms of drug concentration is the number of *grams present in 100 mL*. Thus 1% Xylocaine contains 1 g of drug in every 100 mL (1 dL). By dividing the numerator and denominator by 100, we arrive at a concentration of 10 mg/mL:

$$\frac{1\,g}{100\,mL} = \frac{1{,}000\,mg}{100\,mL} = 10\,mg/mL$$

Documentation and Communication

To prevent errors when documenting decimals, write 0.2 mg or 2 mg instead of .2 mg or 2.0 mg, which could easily be mistaken for 2 mg or 20 mg, respectively.

Volume To Be Administered

After determining the concentration of the drug present in each milliliter, you must calculate how much volume is needed to give the amount of the drug ordered (desired dose). Use the following formula to calculate the volume to be administered:

Desired dose (mg) ÷ concentration of drug on hand (mg/mL)
= volume to be administered

EXAMPLE 1

Medical control orders you to administer 5 mg of diazepam (Valium) to your patient for sedation. You have a vial of diazepam, which contains 20 mg in 5 mL. How many milliliters of diazepam must you give to achieve the ordered dose of 5 mg?

Step 1: Determine the concentration (in mg/mL).

20 mg ÷ 5 mL = 4 mg/mL (concentration)

Step 2: Determine how much volume to administer.

5 mg (desired dose) ÷ 4 mg/mL (concentration) = **1.25 mL**

EXAMPLE 2

You are ordered to administer 12.5 g of dextrose to a hypoglycemic patient. You have a prefilled syringe of 50% dextrose containing 25 g in 50 mL. How many milliliters of dextrose will you give?

Step 1: Determine the concentration (in g/mL).

25 g ÷ 50 mL = 0.5 g/mL (concentration)

Step 2: Determine how much volume to administer.

12.5 g (desired dose) ÷ 0.5 g (500 mg)/mL (concentration) = **25 mL**

Weight-Based Drug Doses

As mentioned earlier, some medication doses are based on the patient's weight in kilograms. Determining the appropriate dose for the patient requires simply adding one step to the formula we just discussed—conversion of the patient's weight in pounds to kilograms. Remember, 1 kg = 2.2 lb.

EXAMPLE

A 7-year-old girl requires 0.02 mg/kg of atropine to treat symptomatic bradycardia. You have a prefilled syringe of atropine containing 1 mg in 10 mL. The child's mother tells you that she weighs 60 lb. How many milligrams will you give to this child (that is, what is the desired dose)? How much volume will you give to achieve the required dose?

Step 1: Convert the child's weight in pounds to kilograms.

Formula 1: 35 lb ÷ 2.2 = 15.9 kg (round to 16 kg)
Formula 2: 35 lb ÷ 2 − 10% = 15.75 kg (round to 16 kg)

Step 2: Determine the desired dose.

0.02 mg × 16 kg = 0.32 mg (round to 0.3 mg [desired dose])

Step 3: Determine the concentration.

1 mg ÷ 10 mL = 0.1 mg/mL (concentration)

Step 4: Determine how much volume to administer.

0.3 mg (desired dose) ÷ 0.1 mg/mL (concentration) = **3 mL**

Calculating the Dose and Rate for a Medication Infusion

Non–Weight-Based Medication Infusions

Following the administration of certain drugs, you may need to begin a continuous infusion to maintain a therapeutic blood level of the drug to prevent a recurrence of the condition. Medication infusions are usually ordered to be administered over a specified period, usually per minute.

To calculate a continuous medication infusion that is not weight-based, you must know the following information in advance:

- The desired dose (μg/min or mg/min)
- The properties of the administration set you are using (eg, microdrip [60 gtt/mL])

You will use the same formula to calculate a drug dose as previously discussed. Then, however, you will calculate the desired dose to be administered continuously—usually a certain number of micrograms (μg) or milligrams (mg) per minute.

For example, suppose you have just administered 75 mg of lidocaine to your patient in cardiac arrest, after which time the cardiac rhythm converts to a perfusing rhythm. Medical control then orders you to begin a continuous lidocaine infusion at 2 mg/min. You must determine at how many drops per minute (gtt/min) to set the IV drip rate to deliver the 2 mg/min desired dose. To do so, you will add a certain amount of lidocaine into a bag of IV fluid. For demonstrative purposes, we will add 2 g (2,000 mg) of lidocaine to a 500-mL bag of normal saline, a common combination. The formula to calculate the continuous infusion rate is as follows:

Step 1: Determine the concentration.

2 g (2,000 mg) of lidocaine ÷ 500 mL of normal saline
= 4 mg/mL (concentration)

Step 2: Determine the amount of volume to infuse per minute (mL/min).

For this calculation, you must recall the desired dose—in this case, 2 mg/min. To determine the number of mL/min, you perform the following calculation:

2 mg *(desired dose)* ÷ 4 mg/mL *(concentration)* = 0.5 mL/min

Step 3: Determine how many drops per minute (gtt/min) at which to set the IV flow rate.

For this calculation, you must know the number of drops per milliliter (gtt/mL) that your IV administration set delivers—a microdrip (60 gtt/mL) or a macrodrip (10 or 15 gtt/mL). For a microdrip administration set (typically used when administering a continuous medication infusion), the number of drops per minute for the IV flow rate would be calculated as follows:

0.5 mL/min × 60 gtt/mL ÷ total time in minutes (1) = 30 gtt/min

Weight-Based Medication Infusions

Some continuous medication infusions are based on the patient's weight in kilograms. Dopamine, for example, is typically administered in a range of 5 to 20 µg/kg/min. By using the previously discussed formula and factoring in the patient's weight in kilograms to determine the desired dose, we will calculate the IV drip rate for a 70-kg patient who requires a continuous dopamine infusion at 5 µg/kg/min. For demonstrative purposes, we will add 800 mg of dopamine to a 500-mL bag of normal saline, a common combination.

Step 1: Determine the desired dose.

5 µg/kg/min × 70 kg = 350 µg/min *(desired dose)*

Step 2: Determine the concentration.

800 mg (800,000 µg) of dopamine ÷ 500 mL of normal saline = 1.6 mg/mL *(concentration)*

The caveat here is that dopamine is administered in *micrograms,* not milligrams. Therefore, we must convert the 1.6 mg/mL concentration to µg/mL. Recall that to convert a larger unit of weight to a smaller one, you must multiply by 1,000 *or* move the decimal point three places to the *right;* in other words, 1.6 mg is equal to *1,600 µg.*

Step 3: Determine the amount of volume to infuse per minute (mL/min).

Again, you must recall the desired dose—in this case, 350 µg/min. To determine the number of mL/min, the calculation continues as follows:

350 µg *(desired dose)* ÷ 1,600 µg/mL *(concentration)* = 0.22 mL/min

Step 4: Determine how many drops per minute (gtt/min) at which to set the IV flow rate.

Again, you must know the properties of the administration set you are using. In this example, we will use the microdrip (60 gtt/mL). The number of drops per minute for the IV flow rate would be calculated as follows:

0.22 mL/min × 60 gtt/mL ÷ total time in minutes (1) = 13.2 gtt/min (round to 13 gtt/min)

▮ Pediatric Drug Doses

There are numerous methods for determining the appropriate dose of medication for a pediatric patient. Many paramedics use length-based resuscitation tape measures **Figure 8-36 ▾**; others carry an EMS field guide with tables or charts specific to pediatric patients. Most drugs used in pediatric emergency medicine are based on the child's weight in kilograms. With the exception of the obviously smaller doses and volumes, the calculations for pediatric drug dosing and medication infusions are the same as they are for adults.

▮ Medical Direction

Medication administration is governed by your local protocols and/or online medical direction. The medical director for your service may allow the administration of certain medications as long as the patient meets certain criteria.

For example, for an unconscious diabetic patient with a confirmed blood glucose reading of 40 mg/dL, the paramedic may be allowed by written protocols (standing orders) to administer 50% dextrose (D_{50}). Standing orders are a form of

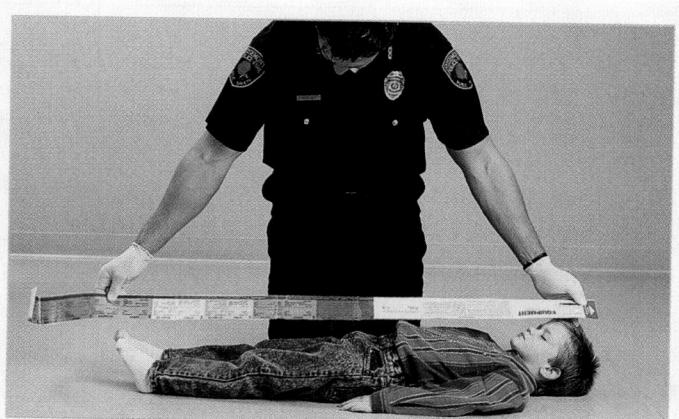

Figure 8-36 Use of a length-based resuscitation tape measure is one method of calculating pediatric drug doses. The tape measure estimates the child's weight (up to 34 kg) based on his or her length.

off-line or indirect medical control, in which the paramedic performs certain predefined procedures before contacting the physician.

Some EMS system medical directors may not allow paramedics to perform certain procedures (for example, administering medications) before making contact with him or her. This is referred to as online (direct) medical control.

Local policies and procedures are designed to guide you in specific situations. When questions or unusual situations arise—even if you function primarily by standing orders—contact medical control for direction. *Never make a hasty critical decision without consulting with medical control first!*

Paramedic's Responsibility Associated With Drug Orders

The danger of something going wrong when administering a drug—for example, administering the wrong drug or the wrong dose of a drug—can be minimized by following a set procedure that incorporates a number of safety precautions:

1. Make sure the base physician understands the situation. The decision to order the administration of any given drug is complex, involving such considerations as the patient's age, weight, clinical status, allergy history, concomitant medical problems, and other drugs he or she may be taking. Thus, it is critical that you obtain and communicate complete and accurate information about the patient to enable the physician to make prudent and correct decisions about drug administration.

2. Make sure you understand the physician's orders clearly. If the orders are unclear or seem—on the basis of your knowledge—to be in error (for example, dosage more than the usual range, an unusual route of administration), *ask the physician to repeat the order.* Do not assume that the doctor is infallible, especially at 3:00 AM.

3. Always repeat any orders, word for word, back to the physician before administering a medication, to confirm that you received and understood the order accurately. In the repetition, state the *name of the drug,* the *dose,* and the *route* by which it is to be given. As a paramedic, you are just as responsible for the administration of the drug and its possible consequences as the physician giving the order, so be absolutely certain which drug is to be administered, in what dose, and by which route. If your partner does not hear the exchange of information, you should repeat the order to him or her as an additional safety measure.

4. If the patient is conscious, or if there is another reliable source of information, confirm that the patient is not allergic to the drug that has been ordered.

5. Read the label carefully as you take the vial or syringe from its box and again before you give the drug. Note the *drug concentration* printed on the label and the drug's *date of expiration.*

6. Check for defects in the vial, preloaded syringe, or ampule, and make sure that the fluid inside is not cloudy,

discolored, or precipitated. Check whether the container itself appears to be cracked or damaged. If the medication looks suspicious in any way, do *not* use it.

7. If you have orders to administer more than one drug, make sure that the drugs are compatible. Some drugs will not mix with others. For example, if sodium bicarbonate ($NaHCO_3$) is mixed with calcium chloride (CaCl), an insoluble precipitate, calcium carbonate ($CaCO_3$), will form in the solution. Should any cloudiness occur after a drug has been injected into IV tubing, *clamp the tubing immediately* and replace it with a new administration set.

8. Notify the physician when the medication has been administered.

9. Monitor the patient for possible adverse side effects.

10. Dispose of the syringe and needle safely. Do *not* try to recap the needle, for the likelihood is quite high of sticking yourself in the process; rather, dispose of the needle and syringe in a sharps container.

Notes from Nancy
Never guess what the physician has ordered. When in doubt, ask.

The "Six Rights" of Drug Administration

If given inappropriately, some medications can have lethal effects. Paramedics are dedicated to helping others, not harming them. Before giving *any* drug, review the "six rights" of medication administration:

- Right patient
- Right drug
- Right dose
- Right route
- Right time
- Right documentation

Verify that this is indeed the *right patient.* In multipatient situations, reconfirm the patient's name and compare it with the wrist band or triage tag.

Read the drug label at least three times before administration to ensure that you have the *right drug:*

1. When it is still in the drug box it came in
2. When you prepare the drug for administration
3. Before actually administering the drug to the patient

You are responsible for knowing the appropriate doses for the medications you carry on your ambulance. You are also responsible for accurately calculating the appropriate dose of the drug. Always recheck your drug calculations before administration to ensure that you are administering the *right dose.*

It is imperative that you know the *right route* for the drug or drugs that you are about to administer. A drug given by an inappropriate route—even if it is the right drug—could have disastrous and possibly fatal consequences.

Knowledge of the indications, contraindications, therapeutic effects, side effects, and appropriate doses for each of the drugs that you carry on your ambulance is critical to safe patient care.

Based on the patient's clinical presentation, you must know the *right time* to administer a medication (that is, when the medication is indicated). Of equal if not greater importance is knowing when *not* to administer a medication (that is, when the medication is contraindicated). Furthermore, some of the medications you carry on the ambulance have specific intervals for repeated doses; you must be aware of these drugs and the appropriate intervals at which they are administered.

Recall the adage, "If you did not document it, you did not do it." Always document the following information on the patient care report after administering a medication:

- Name of the drug
- Dose of the drug
- Time you administered the drug
- Route of administration
- Your name or the paramedic who administered the drug
- Patient's response to the medication, whether positive or negative

Documentation and Communication

If you administer a controlled substance to your patient (eg, morphine, midazolam [Versed], fentanyl), document the amount of medication that you gave to the patient and the amount of medication that you wasted (did not give to the patient). Have your partner or supervisor witness (actually see) you wasting the medication. Both of you should sign the form—you as the paramedic who administered and wasted the medication—and your partner or supervisor who witnessed your actions.

Local Drug Distribution System

Before responding to an EMS call, you must ensure that all equipment on the ambulance is fully functional; this verification is made during your check of the ambulance at the beginning of your shift. All medications must be checked to ensure that they are not expired or damaged and that they are readily available in the right quantity. You must be thoroughly familiar with the system used to exchange and replace outdated or damaged drugs in your EMS system.

You are also responsible for the documentation and security of all controlled substances carried on your ambulance, including accounting for all controlled substances that were wasted (ie, residual medication that was not administered to the patient). Follow the specific policies and procedures of your local drug distribution, security, and accountability system.

Medical Asepsis

Medical asepsis is the practice of preventing contamination of the patient by using aseptic technique. This method of

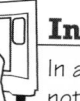

In the Field

In addition to ensuring that medications have not expired or become contaminated, you must ensure that the medications are kept at the recommended temperatures while stored in your ambulance. Refer to the package insert for the medication for this information.

You are the Provider Part 3

Your partner obtains a blood glucose reading of 38 mg/dL. You initiate an IV line of normal saline with an 18-gauge catheter and set the rate to keep the vein open (KVO). A police officer arrives at the scene and obtains additional information from the neighbor. You quickly reassess the patient.

Reassessment	Recording Time: 9 Minutes
Level of consciousness	Unresponsive
Airway and breathing	Airway remains patent; ventilation is assisted by bag-mask device and 100% oxygen
Blood pressure	104/64 mm Hg
Pulse	118 beats/min, weak and regular
Sao_2	99% (with assisted ventilation)
Blood glucose	38 mg/dL

The patient requires 50% dextrose (D_{50}) to treat her hypoglycemia. You open the box, remove the drug, and prepare to administer it.

7. What does the "%" in 50% dextrose mean?

8. What is the concentration of D_{50} that you have on hand?

9. What are the "six rights" of medication administration?

cleansing is intended to prevent contamination of a site when performing an invasive procedure such as starting an IV or administering a medication. Medical asepsis may be accomplished through the use of sterilization of equipment, antiseptics, or disinfectants.

Clean Technique Versus Sterile Technique

Some of the equipment you will use in the field has been sterilized for patient safety. For example, some medications have been packaged using <u>sterile</u> technique. Sterile technique refers to the destruction of all living organisms and is achieved by using heat, gas, or chemicals.

Because it is almost impossible to maintain a sterile environment in the field, you must practice medical asepsis to reduce the risk of contamination and infection. Examples of medical asepsis include handwashing, wearing gloves, and keeping equipment as clean as possible. For example, the site on a patient's hand that has been cleaned with iodine and alcohol before starting an IV is said to be "medically clean."

If you open an IV catheter package and the IV catheter inadvertently falls to the ground or otherwise comes in contact with a contaminated surface, discard it and use a new IV catheter. If you have already cleaned the injection port on the IV tubing where you intend to inject a medication and you inadvertently touch the cleaned injection port, recleanse the port before injecting the medication. You must always make a *conscious* effort to prevent contamination—whether handling equipment, supplies, or the patient. This is the cornerstone of maintaining a medically clean environment.

Antiseptics and Disinfectants

<u>Antiseptics</u> are used to cleanse an area before performing an invasive procedure such as IV therapy or medication administration. Even though antiseptics are capable of destroying pathogens, they are not toxic to living tissues. Isopropyl alcohol (rubbing alcohol) and iodine are the two most common antiseptics you will use in the field.

<u>Disinfectants</u>, by contrast, are toxic to living tissues; therefore, you should never use them on a patient. Use disinfectants only on nonliving objects such as the inside of the ambulance, laryngoscope blades, and other nondisposable equipment. Examples of common disinfectants include Virex, Cidex, and Microcide.

▮ BSI Precautions and Contaminated Equipment Disposal

Body Substance Isolation

The first rule of BSI is to treat any body fluid as being potentially infectious. Many patients who harbor infectious diseases may be asymptomatic and/or unaware that they are infected. As a paramedic, you owe it to yourself to protect yourself by

taking the proper BSI precautions when starting an IV or administering a medication. Minimum BSI precautions for these procedures include wearing gloves and protective eyewear (ie, goggles, face shield). If blood splattering is possible, full facial protection is indicated.

According to the Centers for Disease Control and Prevention, handwashing is the *most* effective way to prevent the spread of disease. It should be a routine practice for you, between all patients. Note, however, that handwashing alone will not prevent you from being infected; use the appropriate BSI precautions as dictated by the situation.

Disposal of Contaminated Equipment

After an IV catheter or needle has penetrated a patient's skin, it is contaminated. Considering the fact that accidental needlesticks are the most common route for disease transmission in the health care setting, you must always handle contaminated equipment carefully and dispose of it immediately and properly. <u>Sharps</u> are any contaminated item that can cause injury. Sharps include IV needles and catheters, broken ampules or vials, and anything else that can penetrate or lacerate the skin.

Immediately dispose of all sharps in a puncture-proof sharps container that bears a biohazard logo

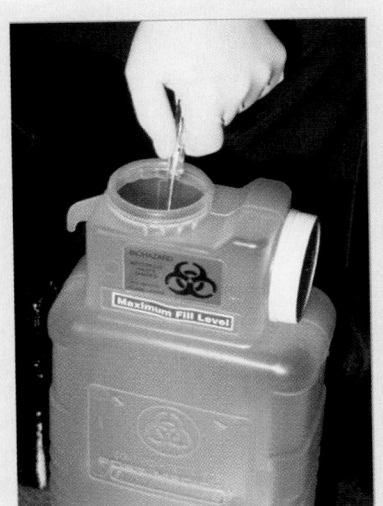

Figure 8-37 ▶. Sharps containers should be readily accessible; place at least two in the back of the ambulance so that your handling of needles, catheters, and other sharps is kept to a minimum amount of time. In addition, you should have a smaller sharps container in your jump kit for immediate disposal of sharps while not in the ambulance.

Figure 8-37 Always dispose of sharp objects or blood-filled items in a puncture-proof sharps container.

Table 8-5 ▶ lists some safe practices that will minimize your risk of an inadvertent needlestick. As always, follow your agency's exposure control plan.

▮ Enteral Medication Administration

The <u>enteral route</u> refers to any route in which medication is absorbed through some portion of the gastrointestinal tract. Enteral medication routes include the oral, gastric tube, and rectal administration routes.

Table 8-5	Minimizing Your Risk of a Needlestick

- *Immediately* dispose of all sharps in a puncture-proof sharps container. *Do not* drop the sharps on the floor for later disposal, and *do not* attempt to recap a needle and syringe before placing it in the sharps container.
- When possible, perform all invasive procedures at the scene. If your patient's condition warrants starting an IV or administering a medication en route to the hospital, *use extreme caution.* Although most paramedics become proficient at starting IVs in the back of a moving ambulance, it may be necessary to have your partner briefly stop the ambulance, especially if you are traveling over rough terrain.
- Recap needles *only* as an absolute last resort. If you must recap a needle, use the one-handed technique. Place the needle cover on a stationary surface, then slide the needle—with one hand—into the needle cap.

Oral Medication Administration

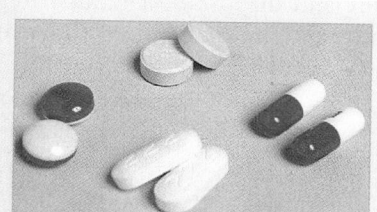

Figure 8-38 Tablets and capsules, oral medications typically taken by mouth, enter the bloodstream through the digestive system.

Most patients take their daily medications at home by the oral route (PO [per os]). Forms of solid and liquid oral medications include capsules, timed-release capsules, lozenges, pills, tablets, elixirs, emulsions, suspensions, and syrups **Figure 8-38 ▲** (see Chapter 7).

Drugs taken by mouth are absorbed at a slow rate from the stomach and intestines—usually somewhere between 30 and 90 minutes. Because absorption is slow, drugs are rarely given by the oral route in the prehospital setting.

To give oral medications, you may use a small medicine cup, a medicine dropper, a teaspoon, an oral syringe, or a nipple. Gather the appropriate equipment for the form of medication you are administering. Check for indications, contraindications, precautions, and review the six rights before administering any medication.

Follow these steps when administering an oral medication **Figure 8-39 ▶**.

1. Take BSI precautions.
2. Determine the need for the medication based on patient presentation.
3. Obtain a focused history and physical exam, including any drug allergies.
4. Follow standing orders, or contact medical control for permission.
5. Check the medication to be sure it is the right medication, it is not cloudy or discolored, and its expiration date has not passed.
6. Determine the appropriate dose. If using a liquid medication, pour the desired amount into a calibrated cup.

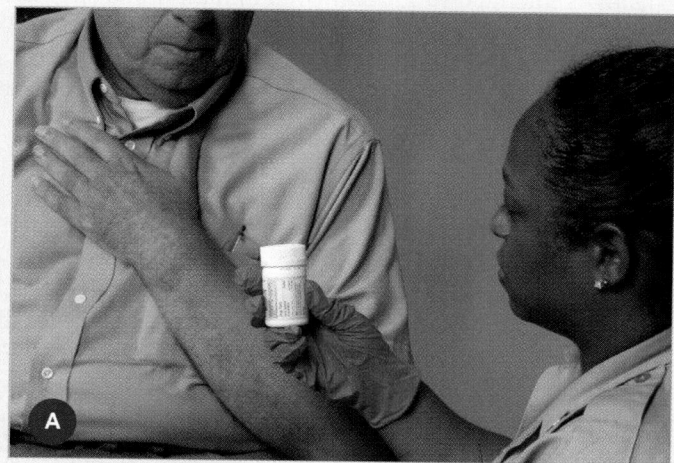

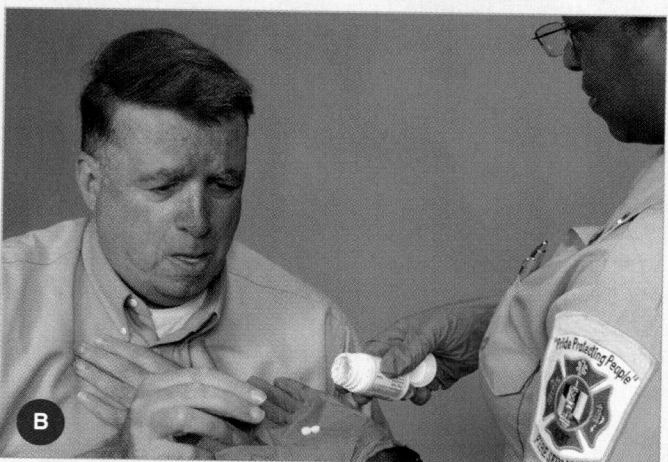

Figure 8-39 Administering an oral medication. **A.** Check the medication and its expiration date. **B.** Have the patient take the medication. Provide a glass or cup of water if necessary.

7. Instruct the patient to swallow the medication with water, if administering a pill or tablet.
8. Monitor the patient's condition, and document the medication given, route, time of administration, and response of the patient.

Gastric Tube Medication Administration

Gastric tubes (orogastric or nasogastric) are occasionally inserted in the prehospital setting to decompress the stomach. However, gastric tube placement also provides a route for enteral medication administration. Although most medications given via the gastric tube are administered in a hospital setting, activated charcoal for certain toxic ingestions—particularly in patients with a depressed swallowing mechanism or decreased level of consciousness—is the most likely scenario in which a gastric tube would be used as a medication route in the prehospital setting. Chapter 11 describes insertion of orogastric and nasogastric tubes. Follow these steps to administer

Skill Drill 8-5: Administering Medication via the Gastric Tube

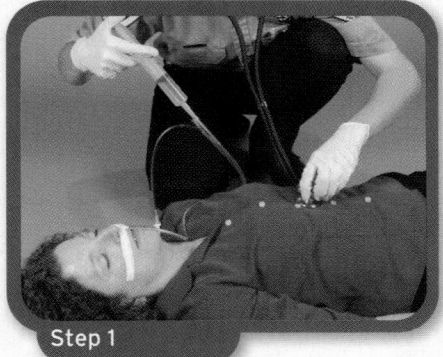

Step 1

Attach a 60-mL syringe to the proximal end of the gastric tube, and slowly inject air into the tube while auscultating over the epigastrium to confirm proper placement.

For further confirmation of correct tube placement, aspirate with the syringe and observe for gastric contents.

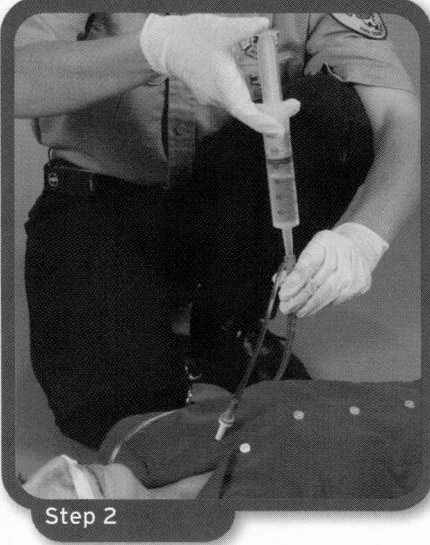

Step 2

Inject 30 to 60 mL of normal saline into the gastric tube to irrigate the tube.

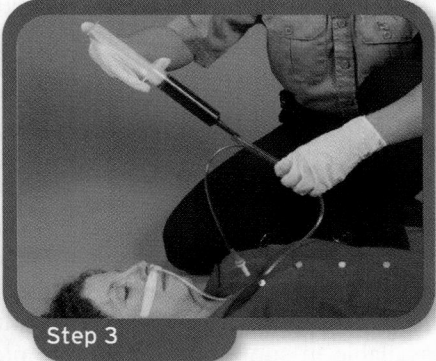

Step 3

Inject the appropriate amount of medication into the gastric tube.

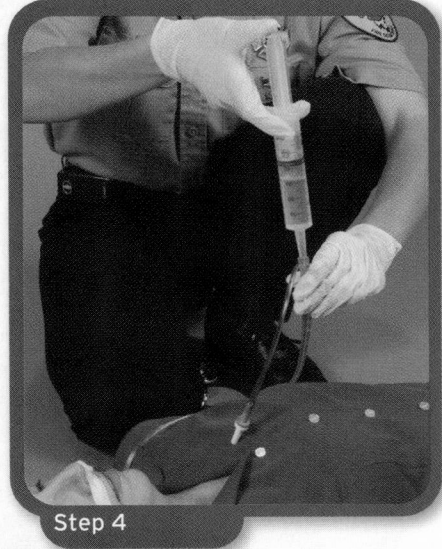

Step 4

Flush the gastric tube with 30 to 60 mL of normal saline to ensure dispersal of the drug into the stomach.

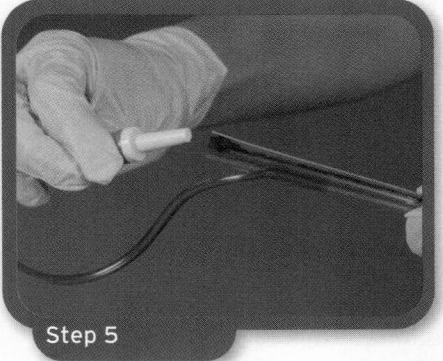

Step 5

Clamp off the proximal end of the gastric tube; do not reattach the tube to suction.

Monitor the patient for adverse reactions, and repeat the medication dose if indicated.

medications via the gastric tube after the tube has been inserted **Skill Drill 8-5 ▲**.

1. Take BSI precautions.
2. Confirm proper gastric tube placement. Attach a 60-mL cone-tipped syringe to the gastric tube and slowly inject air as you or your partner auscultates over the epigastrium **Step 1**.

   To further confirm proper placement, withdraw on the plunger of the syringe and observe for the return of gastric contents in the tube. Leave the gastric tube open to air.

3. Draw up 30 to 60 mL of normal saline into the syringe, and irrigate the gastric tube **Step 2**. If you meet resistance, ensure that the tube is not kinked.
4. Draw up the appropriate amount of medication, and slowly inject it into the gastric tube **Step 3**.
5. Inject 30 to 60 mL of normal saline into the gastric tube following administration of the medication **Step 4**. This will ensure that the tube is flushed and that the patient has received the entire dose of the medication.

6. Clamp off the proximal end of the gastric tube (Step 5). Do not attach the gastric tube to suction because this will result in removal of the medication from the stomach. Monitor the patient for adverse reactions. Repeat the medication dose if indicated.

Rectal Medication Administration

Certain drugs may be administered rectally if you are unable to establish IV or IO access. In the field, diazepam (Valium) can be administered rectally in pediatric patients because IV access can be challenging enough under normal circumstances, and even more so when the child is having a seizure. Because the rectal mucosa is highly vascular, medication absorption is rapid and predictable (Figure 8-40 ▾). Certain antiemetic medications are available in suppository form (eg, promethazine [Phenergan]), and under certain circumstances, you might be asked to administer them. A suppository is a drug mixed in a firm base that melts at body temperature and is shaped to fit the rectum.

Follow these steps to administer a drug via the rectal route:

1. Take BSI precautions.

2. Determine the need for the medication based on patient presentation.

3. Obtain a focused history and physical exam, including any drug allergies.

4. Follow standing orders, or contact medical control for permission.

5. Determine the appropriate dose, and check that the medication is the right medication, there is no cloudiness or discoloration, and the expiration date has not passed.

6. When inserting a suppository, use a water-soluble gel for lubrication. Insert the suppository into the rectum approximately 1″ to 1½″ while instructing the patient to relax and not to bear down.

7. For medications in liquid form, some modifications are needed. You may use a nasopharyngeal airway or a small endotracheal tube as your delivery device.

- Lubricate the end of the nasal airway or endotracheal tube with a water-soluble gel, and gently insert it approximately 1″ to 1½″ into the rectum (Figure 8-41 ▾).
- Instruct the patient to relax and not to bear down.
- With a *needleless* syringe, gently push the medication through the tube.
- Once the medication has been delivered, remove and dispose of the tube or syringe in an appropriate container.

8. Monitor the patient's condition, and document the medication given, route, time of administration, and response of the patient.

▌Parenteral Medication Administration

The parenteral route refers to any route other than the gastrointestinal tract. Parenteral routes for medication administration

In the Field

Diazepam (Valium) is available in a specially designed container, which is marketed under the name Diastat. The distal end of the container is tapered, which facilitates insertion into the rectum. This feature eliminates the need for syringes or other methods of injecting the medication into the rectum.

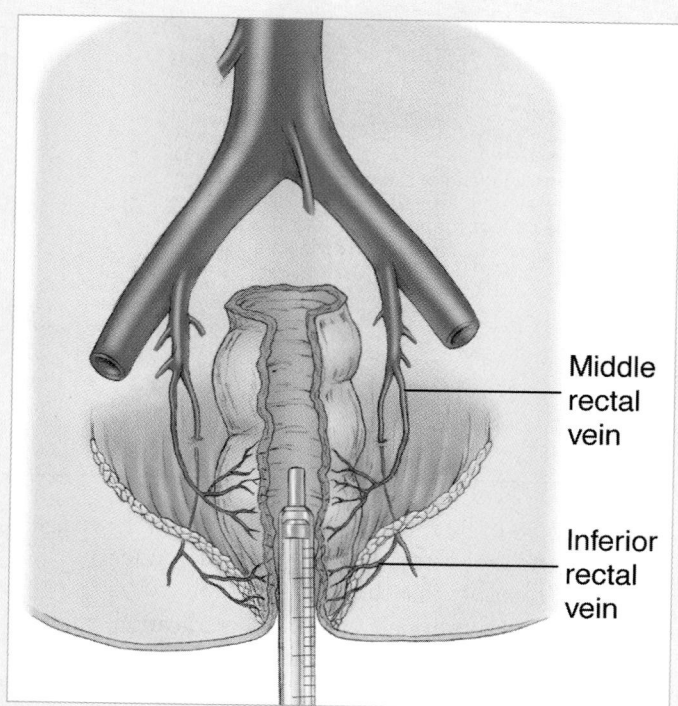

Figure 8-40 The rectal mucosa is highly vascular. It rapidly and predictably absorbs medications.

- Middle rectal vein
- Inferior rectal vein

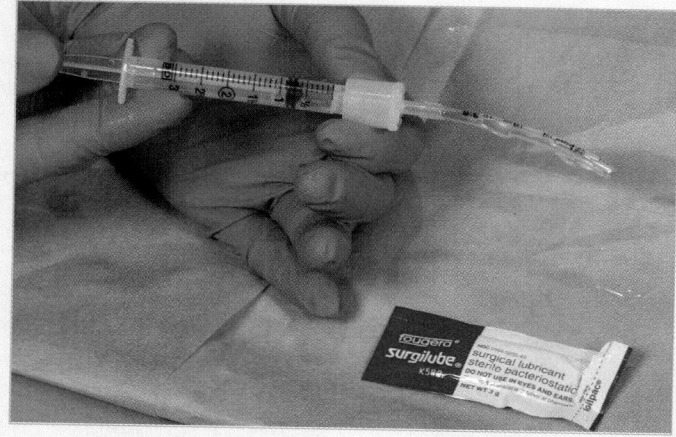

Figure 8-41 Syringe attached to an endotracheal tube.

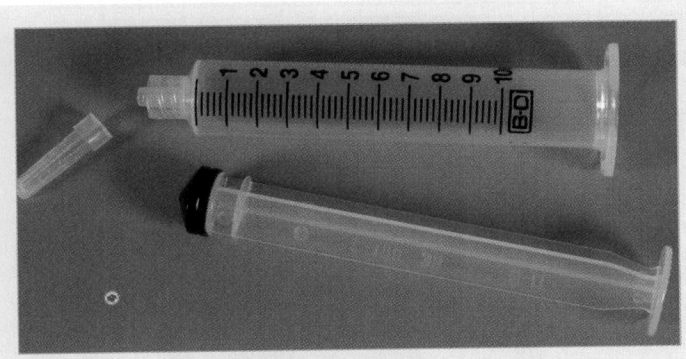

Figure 8-42 A syringe consists of a plunger, body or barrel, flange, and tip.

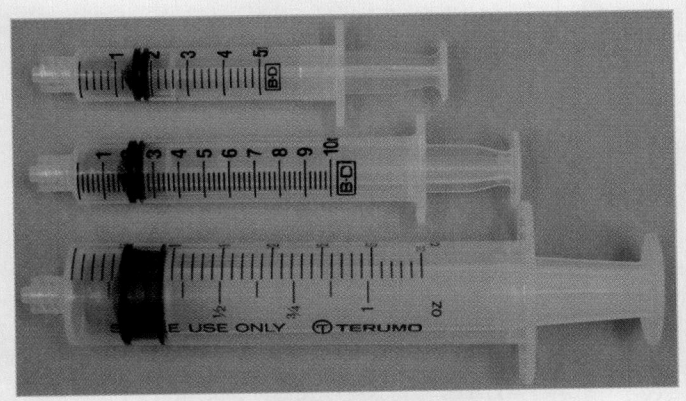

Figure 8-43 Syringes come in a variety of sizes. Some come with needles already attached, others without needles attached.

include the intradermal, subcutaneous, intramuscular, intravenous, intraosseous, and percutaneous routes. Compared with enterally administered medications (eg, oral, gastric tube), parenterally administered medications are absorbed into the central circulation more quickly and at a more predictable rate, thus achieving their therapeutic effects faster. Of the parenteral drug routes, IV administration is the route most commonly used in the prehospital setting and generally is the quickest route for getting medication into the central circulation.

Syringes and Needles

A variety of needles and syringes are used for administering parenteral medications. Most syringes come prepackaged in color-coded packs with a needle already attached. The needles and syringes may also be packaged separately. Syringes consist of a plunger, body or barrel, flange, and tip ▸ Figure 8-42 ▴ . Most syringes are marked with 10 calibrations per milliliter on one side of the barrel, where each small line represents 0.1 mL; the other side of the barrel is marked in minims. Syringes vary from 1 mL to 60 mL; the 3-mL syringe is the one most commonly used for injections. Syringe selection is based on the volume of medication that you will administer ▸ Figure 8-43 ▴ .

Hypodermic needle lengths vary from ⅜" to 2" for standard injections. As with IV catheters, the <u>gauge</u> of the nee-

dle refers to the diameter: The smaller the number, the larger the diameter. Common needle gauges range from 18 to 26. The needle gauge used depends on the route of parenteral medication administration. Smaller-gauge needles, for example, are used for subcutaneous injections, whereas larger-gauge needles are used for intramuscular and IV injections.

The proximal end of the needle, or hub, attaches to the standard fitting on the syringe. The distal end of the needle is beveled.

Packaging of Parenteral Medications

Ampules

<u>Ampules</u> are breakable sterile glass containers that are designed to carry a single dose of medication ▸ Figure 8-44 ▸ . They may contain as little as 1 mL or as much as 10 mL, depending on the medication.

When drawing a medication from an ampule, follow the steps in ▸ Skill Drill 8-6 ▸ .

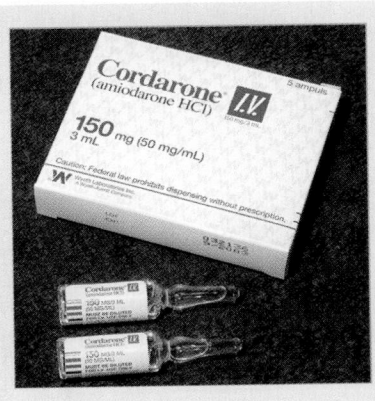

Figure 8-44 Ampules.

1. Check the medication to be sure that the expiration date has not passed and that it is the correct drug and concentration.
2. Shake the medication into the base of the ampule. If some of the drug is stuck in the neck, gently thump or tap the stem ▸ Step 1 ▸ .
3. Using a 4" × 4" gauze pad or an alcohol prep, grip the neck of the ampule and snap it off. Drop the stem in the sharps container ▸ Step 2 ▸ .
4. Insert the needle into the ampule without touching the outer sides of the ampule. Draw the solution into the syringe, and dispose of the ampule in the sharps container ▸ Step 3 ▸ .
5. Hold the syringe with the needle pointing up, and gently tap the barrel to loosen air trapped inside and cause it to rise ▸ Step 4 ▸ . Press gently on the plunger to dispel any air bubbles ▸ Step 5 ▸ .
6. Recap the needle using the one-handed method.

Vials

<u>Vials</u> are small glass or plastic bottles with a rubber-stopper top; they may contain single or multiple doses of a medication ▸ Figure 8-45 ▸ . When using a vial of medication, you must first determine how much of the drug you will need and how many doses are in the vial.

For a single-dose vial, you will draw up the entire amount in the vial. For multiple-dose vials, you should draw up only the amount needed. Remember that once you remove

Skill Drill 8-6: Drawing Medication From an Ampule

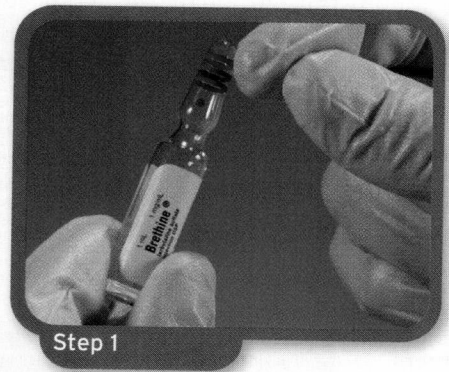

Step 1

Gently tap the stem of the ampule to shake medication into the base.

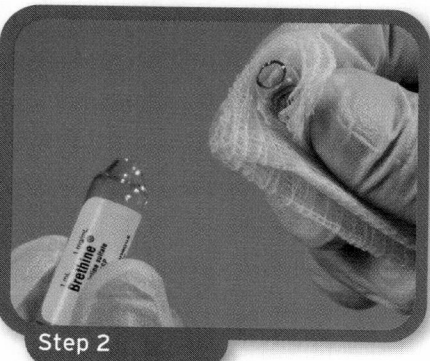

Step 2

Grip the neck of the ampule using a 4″ × 4″ gauze pad, and snap the neck off.

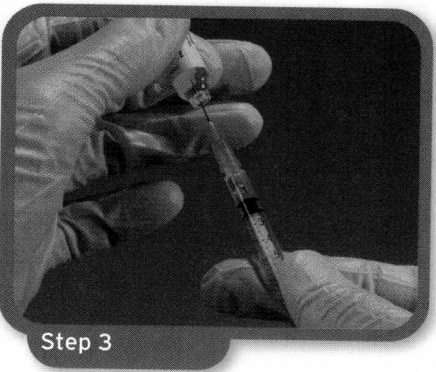

Step 3

Without touching the outer sides of the ampule, insert the needle into the medication in the ampule, and draw the solution into the syringe.

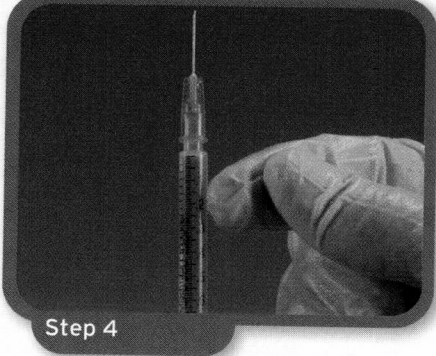

Step 4

Holding the syringe with the needle pointing up, gently tap the barrel to loosen air trapped inside.

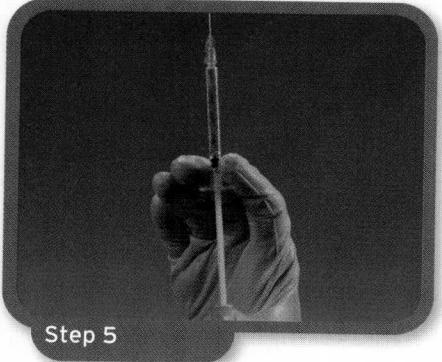

Step 5

Gently press on the plunger to dispel any air bubbles, and recap the needle using the one-handed method.

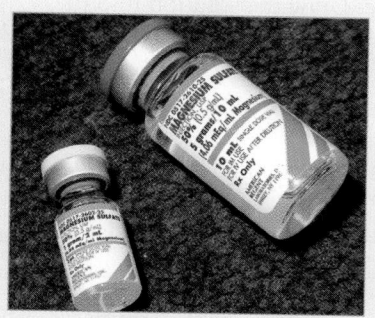

Figure 8-45 Vials (single-dose and multidose).

the cover from a vial, it is no longer sterile. If you need a second dose, clean the top of the vial with alcohol before withdrawing the medication.

Some medications that are stored in vials may need to be reconstituted, such as methylprednisolone sodium succinate (Solu-Medrol) and glucagon. Glucagon is stored in two vials, one with the powdered form of the drug and the other with sterile water. Drug reconstitution involves injecting the sterile water (or provided diluent) from one vial into the vial that contains the powder, thereby making a solution for injection. To reconstitute the contents of two vials, draw the fluid out of the first vial and inject it into the vial that contains the powder. Shake the vial vigorously to mix the medication before drawing out the contents for administration.

Solu-Medrol is stored in a Mix-o-Vial, a single vial divided into two compartments by a rubber stopper **Figure 8-46 ▶**. To reconstitute a drug that is

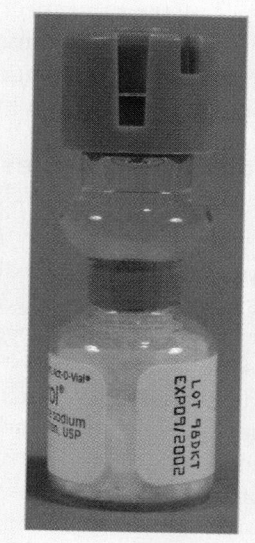

Figure 8-46 A Mix-o-Vial.

Skill Drill 8-7: Drawing Medication From a Vial

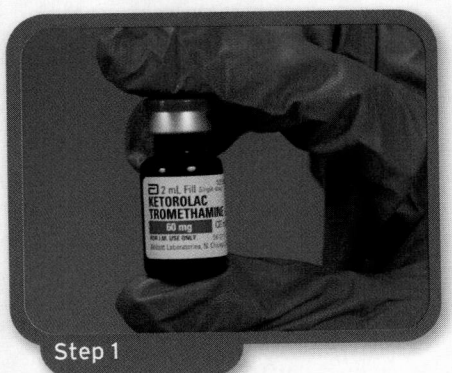

Step 1

Check the medication and its expiration date.

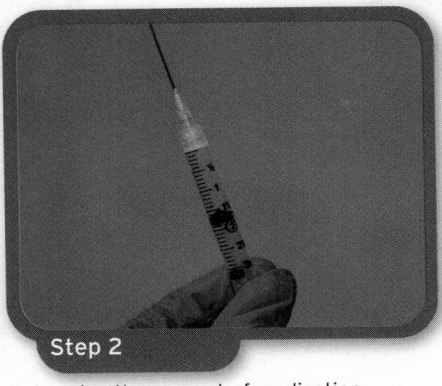

Step 2

Determine the amount of medication needed, and draw that amount of air into the syringe.

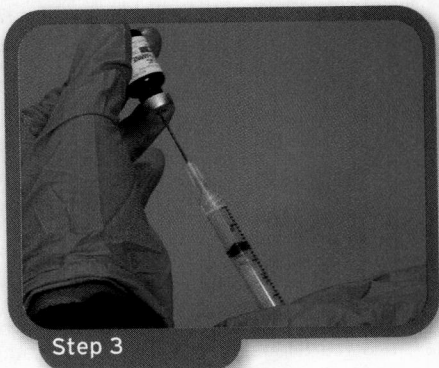

Step 3

Invert the vial, and insert the needle through the rubber stopper. Expel the air in the syringe into the vial, and then withdraw the amount of medication needed.

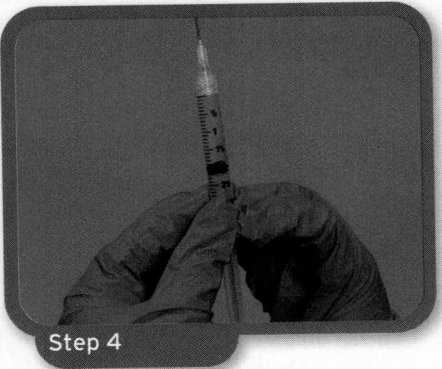

Step 4

Withdraw the needle, and expel any air in the syringe.

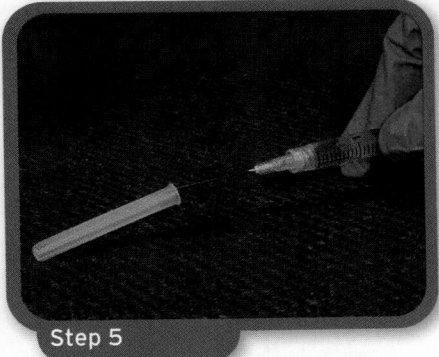

Step 5

Recap the needle using the one-handed method.

---

contained in a Mix-o-Vial, squeeze the two vials together, which releases the center stopper and allows the contents to mix. Shake vigorously to mix the contents before drawing out the medication.

When drawing medication from a vial, follow the steps in **Skill Drill 8-7 ▲**.

1. Check the medication to be sure that the expiration date has not passed and that it is the correct drug and concentration **Step 1**.

2. Remove the sterile cover, or clean the top with alcohol if the vial was previously opened.

3. Determine the amount of medication that you will need, and draw that amount of air into the syringe **Step 2**. Allow a little extra room to expel some air while removing air bubbles.

4. Invert the vial, and insert the needle through the rubber stopper into the medication. Expel the air in the syringe into the vial and then withdraw the amount of medication needed **Step 3**.

5. Once you have the correct amount of medication in the syringe, withdraw the needle from the vial and expel any air in the syringe **Step 4**.

6. Recap the needle using the one-handed method **Step 5**.

Prefilled Syringes

Prefilled syringes are packaged in tamper-proof boxes. Two types of prefilled syringes exist: those that are separated into a glass drug cartridge and a syringe, **Figure 8-47 ▶**, and pre-assembled prefilled syringes **Figure 8-48 ▶**. These syringes are designed for ease of use. After all, it is much easier and quicker to use a prefilled syringe when you are treating a patient in cardiac arrest than it is to draw up each individual dose.

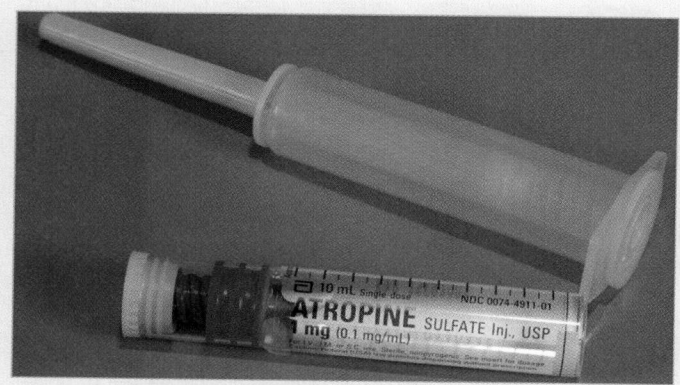

Figure 8-47 Two-part prefilled syringes are separated into a glass drug cartridge and a syringe (for example, Bristojet).

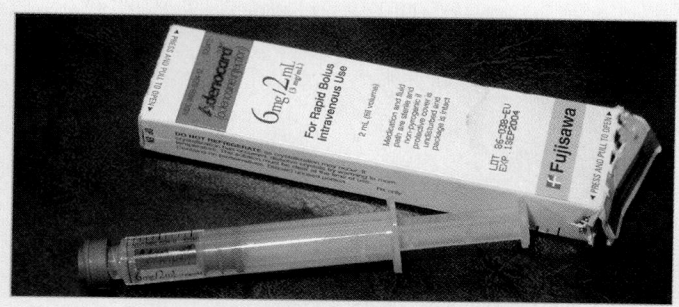

Figure 8-48 Preassembled prefilled syringe.

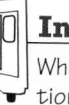

In the Field

Whenever you use a needle to draw up medication from an ampule or vial, hold the syringe against your palm with the needle pointing up and draw the ampule or vial down onto the needle using the thumb and forefinger of the palm the syringe is braced against to avoid sticking yourself. This especially applies if you are in a moving ambulance.

To assemble the two-part prefilled syringe, pop the yellow caps off of the syringe and the drug cartridge, insert the drug cartridge into the barrel of the syringe, and screw them together. Remove the needle cover, and expel air in the manner previously described. Follow the steps for the route the medication is to be given.

Single-dose disposable medication cartridges that are inserted into a reusable syringe are also available. These syringes are commonly referred to as Tubex, Abojext, and Carpuject syringes **Figure 8-49 ▶**.

Intradermal Medication Administration

Intradermal injections involve administering a small amount of medication—typically less than 1 mL—into the dermal layer,

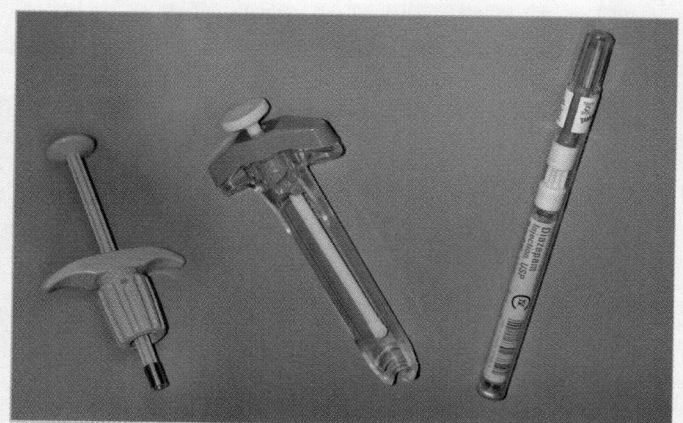

Figure 8-49 Reusable syringes (left). Disposable medication cartridge (right).

just beneath the epidermis. The technique involves the use of a 1-mL syringe (for example, a tuberculin syringe) and a 25- to 27-gauge, ⅜″ to 1″ needle.

When selecting a site for an intradermal injection, you should avoid areas that contain superficial blood vessels to minimize the risk of systemic medication absorption. Because of their high visibility and relative lack of hair, the most common anatomic locations for intradermal injections are the anterior forearm and upper back.

Medications administered intradermally have a very slow rate of absorption; there is minimal to no systemic distribution. The medication remains locally collected at the site of the injection. Unless you are anesthetizing the skin before establishing an IV, you will rarely use the intradermal route to administer medications in the prehospital setting. Instead, these injections are typically given in a physician's office or in the hospital to test a patient for allergies or to perform a PPD (purified protein derivative)—a skin test for tuberculosis.

Follow these steps to administer a medication via the intradermal route:

1. Take BSI precautions.
2. Determine the need for the medication based on patient presentation.
3. Obtain a focused history and physical exam, including any drug allergies and vital signs.
4. Follow standing orders, or contact medical control for permission.
5. Check the medication to ensure that it is the correct one, that it is not cloudy or discolored, and that the expiration date has not passed, and determine the appropriate amount to give for the correct dose.
6. Advise the patient of potential discomfort while explaining the procedure.
7. Assemble and check equipment needed: alcohol preps and a 1-mL syringe with a 25- to 27-gauge, ⅜″ or 1″ needle. Draw up the correct dose of medication.

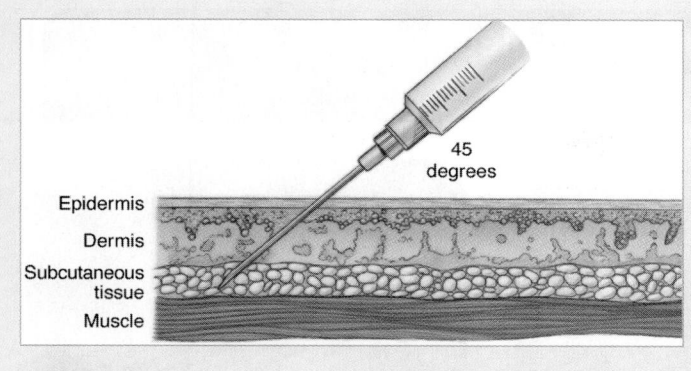

Figure 8-50 A subcutaneous injection is below the dermis and above the muscle.

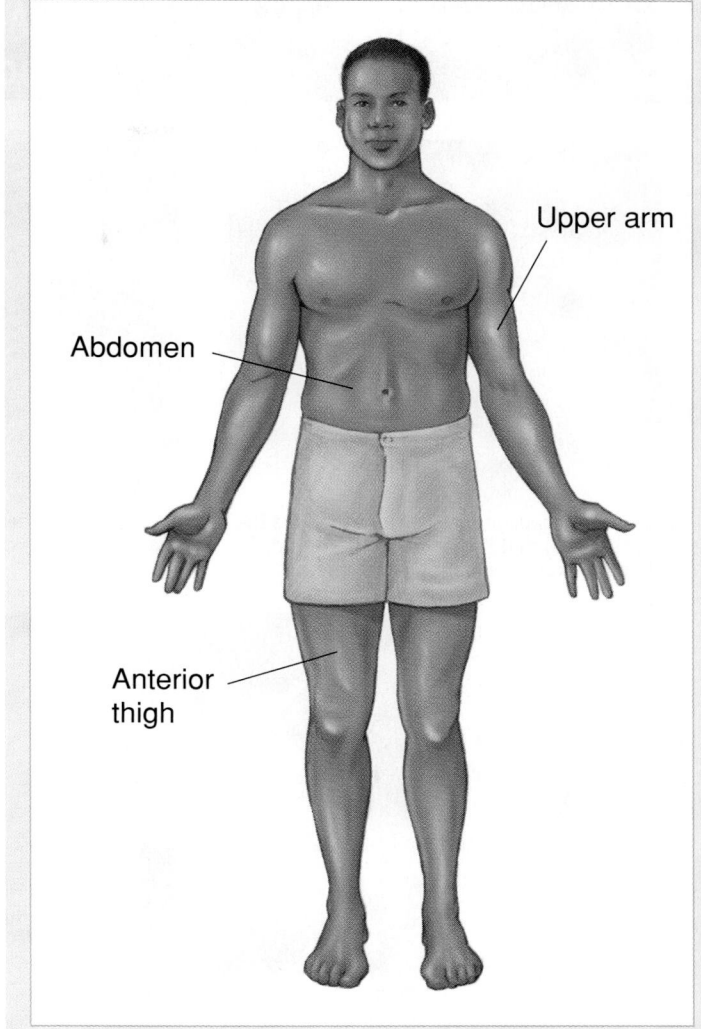

Figure 8-51 Common sites for subcutaneous injections.

8. Cleanse the area for administration using aseptic technique.
9. Pull the skin taut with your nondominant hand.
10. Insert the needle at a 10° to 15° angle with the bevel up.
11. Slowly inject the medication while observing for the formation of a wheal, or small bump, which indicates that the medication is collecting in the intradermal tissue.
12. Remove the needle. Immediately dispose of the needle and syringe in the sharps container.
13. Monitor the patient's condition, and document the medication given, route, administration time, and response of the patient.

Subcutaneous Medication Administration

Subcutaneous (SC) injections are given into the loose connective tissue between the dermis and the muscle layer (Figure 8-50 ▲). Volumes of a drug administered subcutaneously are usually 1 mL or less. The injection is performed using a 24- to 26-gauge ½″ to 1″ needle. Common sites for SC injections—in both adults and children—include the upper arms, anterior thighs, and the abdomen (Figure 8-51 ▶). Patients who take insulin injections usually vary the sites owing to the multiple (usually daily) injections they require.

Follow the steps in (Skill Drill 8-8 ▶) to administer a medication via the subcutaneous route:

1. Take BSI precautions.
2. Determine the need for the medication based on patient presentation.
3. Obtain a focused history and physical exam, including any drug allergies and vital signs.
4. Follow standing orders, or contact medical control for permission.
5. Check the medication to ensure that it is the correct one, that it is not cloudy or discolored, and that the expiration date has not passed, and determine the appropriate amount and concentration for the correct dose (Step 1).
6. Advise the patient of potential discomfort while explaining the procedure.

7. Assemble and check equipment needed: alcohol preps and a 3-mL syringe with a 24- to 26-gauge needle. Draw up the correct dose of medication (Step 2).
8. Cleanse the area for the administration (usually the upper arm or thigh) using aseptic technique (Step 3).
9. *Pinch the skin* surrounding the area, advise the patient of a stick, and insert the needle at a *45° angle*.
10. Pull back on the plunger to aspirate for blood. The presence of blood in the syringe indicates you may have entered a blood vessel. In such a case, remove the needle, and hold pressure over the site. Discard the syringe and needle in the sharps container. Prepare a new syringe and needle, and select another site.
11. If there is no blood in the syringe, inject the medication and remove the needle. Immediately dispose of the needle and syringe in the sharps container (Step 4).

Skill Drill 8-8: Administering Medication via the Subcutaneous Route

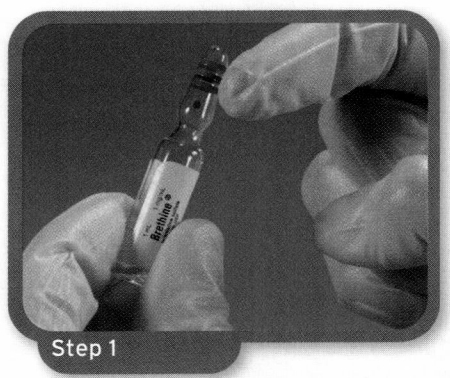

Step 1

Check the medication to ensure that it is the correct one, that it is not discolored, and that the expiration date has not passed.

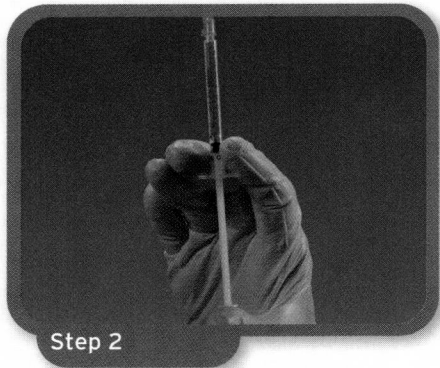

Step 2

Assemble and check the equipment. Draw up the correct dose of medication.

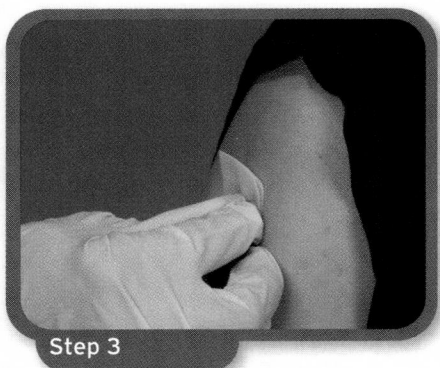

Step 3

Using aseptic technique, cleanse the injection area.

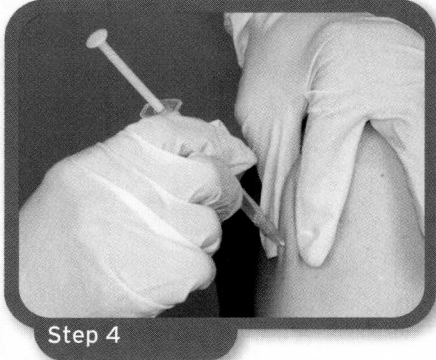

Step 4

Pinch the skin surrounding the area, and insert the needle at a 45° angle. Pull back on the plunger to aspirate for blood. If there is no blood, inject the medication, remove the needle, and hold pressure over the area. Immediately dispose of the needle and syringe in the sharps container.

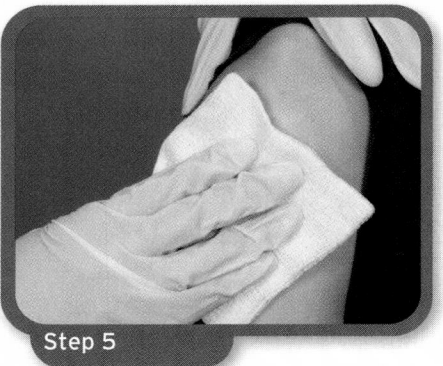

Step 5

To disperse the medication, rub the area in a circular motion. Monitor the patient's condition.

---

12. To disperse the medication through the tissue, rub the area in a circular motion with your gloved hand.
13. Properly store any unused medication.
14. Monitor the patient's condition, and document the medication given, route, administration time, and response of the patient (Step 5).

Intramuscular Medication Administration

Intramuscular (IM) injections are given by penetrating a needle through the dermis and subcutaneous tissue and into the muscle layer (Figure 8-52 ▸). This technique allows administration of a larger volume of medication (up to 5 mL) than the subcutaneous route. Because there is also

the potential for damage to nerves due to the depth of the injection, it is important to choose the appropriate site. Common anatomic sites for IM injections for adults and children include the following:

- **Vastus lateralis muscle**—the large muscle on the lateral side of the thigh.
- **Rectus femoris muscle**—the large muscle on the anterior side of the thigh.
- **Gluteal area**—the buttocks, specifically the upper lateral aspect of either side.
- **Deltoid muscle**—the muscle of the upper arm that covers the prominence of the shoulder. The site for injection is approximately 1½″ to 2″ below the acromion process on the lateral side (Figure 8-53 ▸).

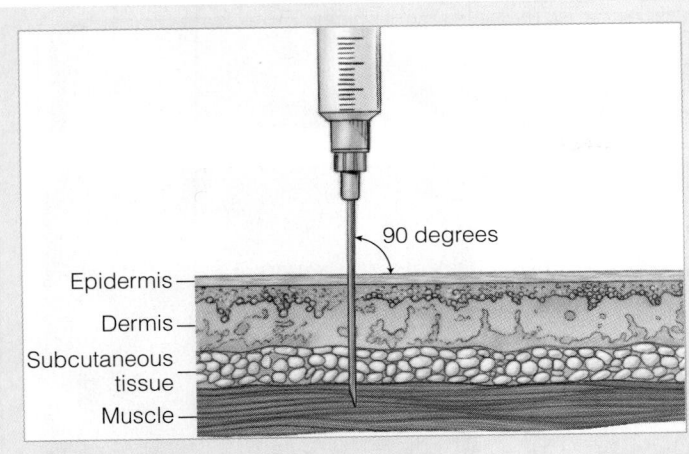

Figure 8-52 An intramuscular injection is below the dermis and subcutaneous layer and into the muscle.

4. Follow standing orders, or contact medical control for permission.
5. Check the medication to ensure that it is the correct one, that it is not cloudy or discolored, and that the expiration date has not passed, and determine the appropriate amount and concentration for the correct dose (**Step 1**).
6. Advise the patient of potential discomfort while explaining the procedure.
7. Assemble and check equipment needed: alcohol preps and a 3- to 5-mL syringe with a 21-gauge, 1″ or 2″ needle. Draw up the correct dose of medication (**Step 2**).
8. Cleanse the area for administration (usually the upper arm or the hip) using aseptic technique (**Step 3**).
9. *Stretch the skin* over the cleansed area, advise the patient of a stick, and insert the needle at a *90° angle*.
10. Pull back on the plunger to aspirate for blood. The presence of blood in the syringe indicates you may have entered a blood vessel. In such a case, remove the needle, and hold pressure over the site. Discard the syringe and needle in the sharps container. Prepare a new syringe and needle, and select another site.
11. If there is no blood in the syringe, inject the medication and remove the needle. Immediately dispose of the needle and syringe in the sharps container (**Step 4**).
12. To disperse the medication through the tissue, rub the area in a circular motion with your gloved hand (**Step 5**).
13. Store any unused medication properly.
14. Monitor the patient's condition, and document the medication given, route, administration time, and response of the patient.

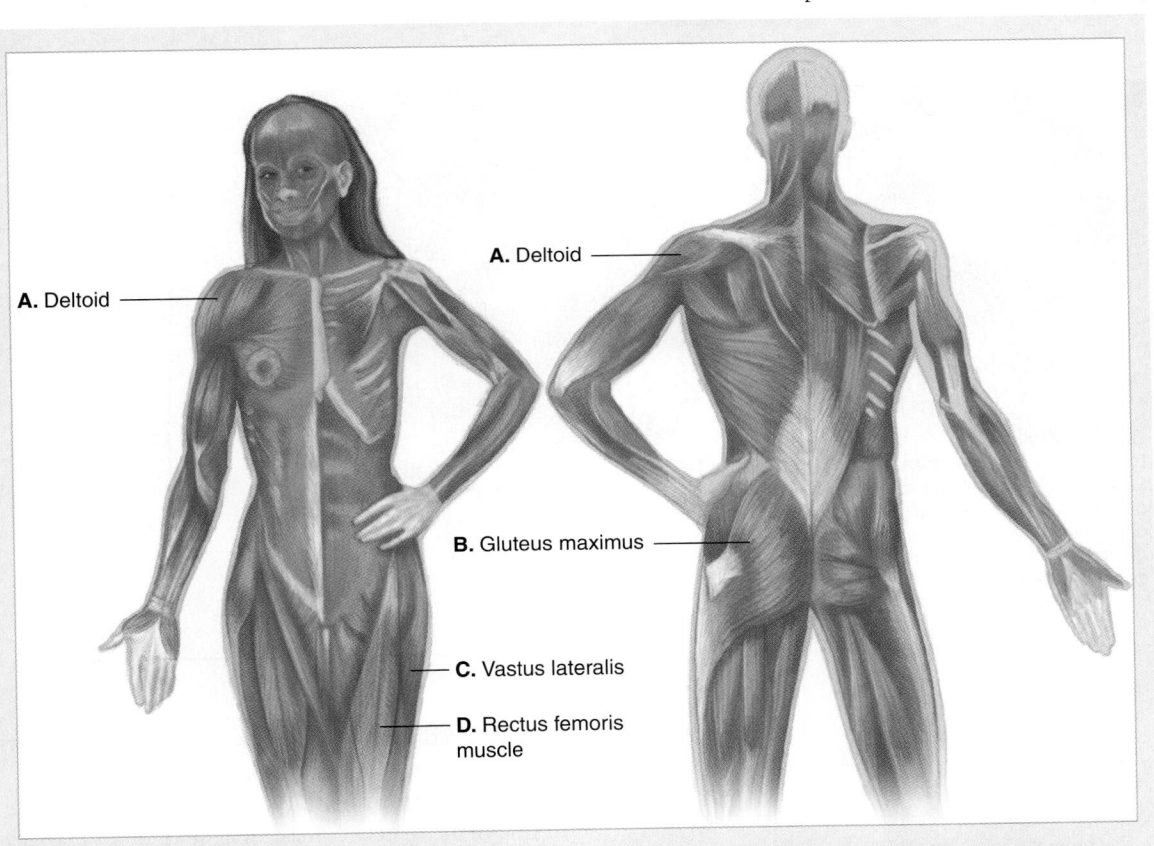

Figure 8-53 Common sites for intramuscular injections. **A.** Deltoid muscle. **B.** Gluteal area. **C.** Vastus lateralis muscle. **D.** Rectus femoris muscle.

Follow the steps in (**Skill Drill 8-9** ▸) to administer a medication via the intramuscular route:
1. Take BSI precautions.
2. Determine the need for the medication based on patient presentation.
3. Obtain a focused history and physical exam, including any drug allergies and vital signs.

IV Bolus Medication Administration

The IV route places the drug directly into the circulatory system. It is the fastest route of medication administration because it bypasses most barriers to drug absorption. As a result, *there is no room for error with IV administration.* (See "Potential Complications

Skill Drill 8-9: Administering Medication via the Intramuscular Route

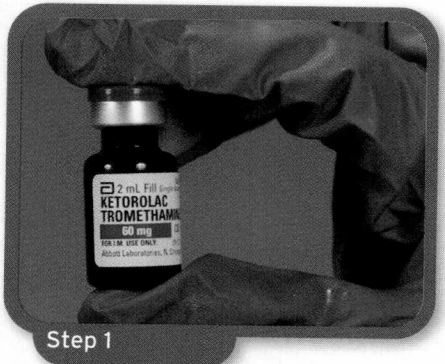

Step 1

Check the medication to ensure that it is the correct one, that it is not discolored, and that its expiration date has not passed.

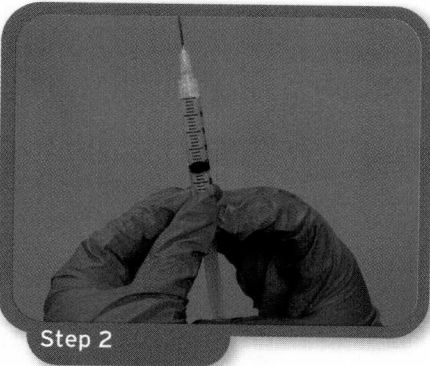

Step 2

Assemble and check the equipment. Draw up the correct dose of medication.

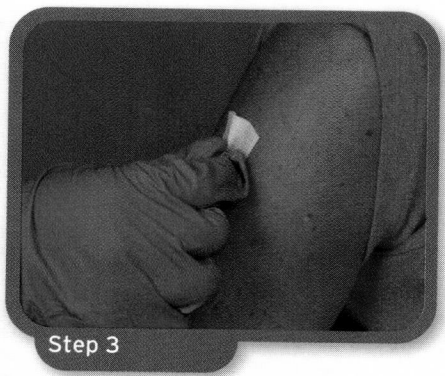

Step 3

Using aseptic technique, cleanse the injection area.

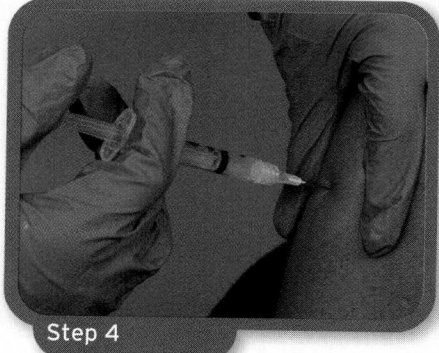

Step 4

Stretch the skin over the area, and insert the needle at a 90° angle. Pull back on the plunger to aspirate for blood. If there is no blood, inject the medication and remove the needle. Immediately dispose of the needle and syringe in the sharps container.

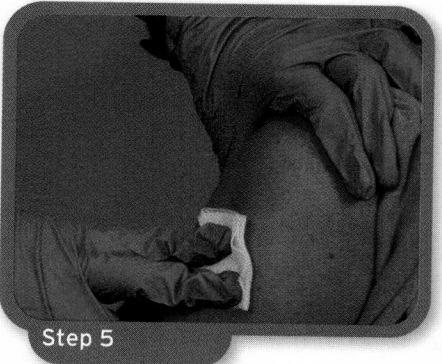

Step 5

To disperse the medication, rub the area in a circular motion. Monitor the patient's condition.

In the Field

Effective absorption of medications administered by the subcutaneous and intramuscular routes requires adequate peripheral perfusion. This is clearly not the case in patients in profound shock or cardiac arrest. Therefore, subcutaneous and intramuscular injections should not be given to patients with inadequate perfusion.

of IV Therapy" earlier in this chapter for details on what can go wrong.) Drugs are administered by direct injection with a needle and syringe into an established peripheral IV line. Many services now use needleless systems to provide protection against needle-

sticks. When using a needleless system, the syringe simply screws into the injection port of the administration set (IV tubing).

A <u>bolus</u> is a single dose, usually given by the IV route. When given in one mass, it may consist of a small or large quantity of a drug and can be given rapidly or slowly, depending on the drug. Some medications, such as lidocaine and amiodarone, require an initial bolus and then may require a continuous IV infusion to maintain a therapeutic level of the drug.

Follow the steps in **Skill Drill 8-10 ▶** when administering a medication via the IV bolus route:

1. Take BSI precautions.
2. Determine the need for the medication based on patient presentation.
3. Obtain a focused history and physical exam, including any drug allergies and vital signs.

4. Follow standing orders, or contact medical control for permission.

5. Check the medication to ensure that it is the correct one, that it is not cloudy or discolored, and that the expiration date has not passed, and determine the appropriate amount and concentration for the correct dose.

6. Explain the procedure to the patient and the need for the medication.

7. Assemble needed equipment, and draw up medication. Expel any air in the syringe. Draw up 20 mL of normal saline to use as a flush for the medication.

8. Cleanse the injection port with alcohol, or remove the protective cap if using the needleless system (Step 1).

9. Insert the needle into the port, and pinch off the IV tubing proximal to the administration port. Failure to shut off the line will result in the medication taking the pathway of least resistance and flowing into the bag instead of into the patient.

10. Administer the correct dose of the medication at the appropriate rate. Some medications must be administered very quickly, while others must be pushed slowly to prevent adverse effects (Step 2).

11. Place the needle and syringe into the sharps container.

Skill Drill 8-10: Administering Medication via the Intravenous Bolus Route

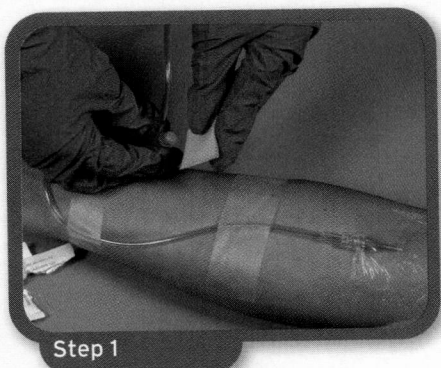

Step 1

Assemble and check the equipment. Cleanse the injection port, or remove the protective cap if using the needleless system.

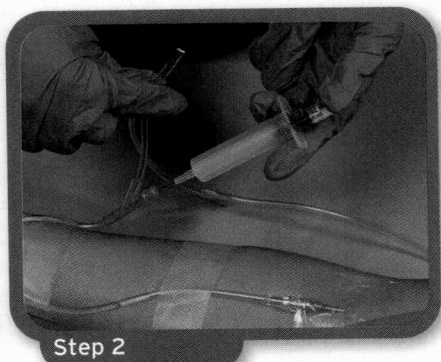

Step 2

Insert the needle into the port, and pinch off the IV tubing proximal to the administration port. Administer the correct dose at the appropriate rate.

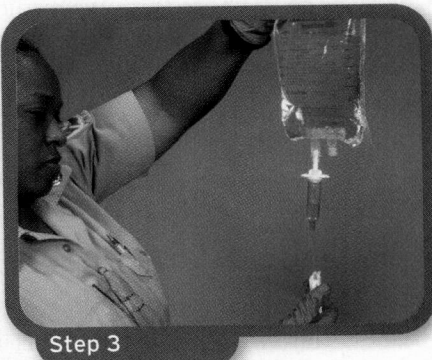

Step 3

Unclamp the IV line to flush the medication into the vein, allowing it to run briefly wide open, or flush with a 20-mL bolus of normal saline. Readjust the IV flow rate to the original setting, and monitor the patient's condition.

You are the Provider Part 4

After administering 50 mL of 50% dextrose, the patient's level of consciousness rapidly improves. She pushes the bag and mask away from her face but will tolerate a nonrebreathing mask. She is obviously confused about what happened, but consents to EMS transport to the hospital. You apprise her of the events that transpired and reassess her. Your partner retrieves the stretcher from the ambulance.

Reassessment	Recording Time: 12 Minutes
Level of consciousness	A (Alert to person, place, and day)
Airway and breathing	Airway remains patent; respirations, 18 breaths/min with adequate depth
Blood pressure	112/70 mm Hg
Pulse	88 beats/min, strong and regular
Sa_{O_2}	99% (with 100% oxygen)
Blood glucose	80 mg/dL

10. Does this patient require an additional dose of 50% dextrose?

11. Does this patient require an IV bolus of normal saline?

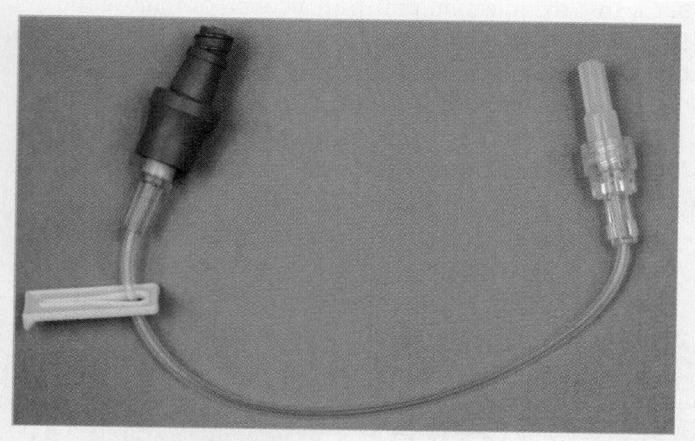

Figure 8-54 Saline lock.

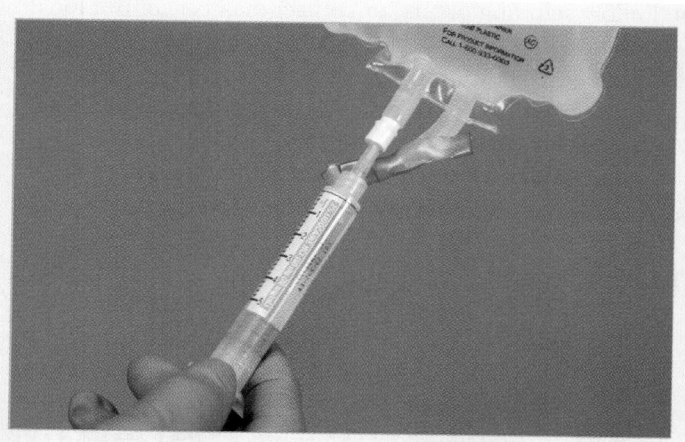

Figure 8-55 Adding medication to an IV bag.

12. Unclamp the IV line to flush the medication into the vein. Allow it to run briefly wide open, or flush with a 20-mL bolus of normal saline.

13. Readjust the IV flow rate to the original setting (Step 3).

14. Properly store and label any unused medication.

15. Monitor the patient's condition, and document the medication given, route, time of administration, and response of the patient.

As discussed earlier in this chapter, saline locks are used for patients who are not in need of IV fluid boluses but may need medication therapy. Follow these steps to administer a medication through a saline lock (Figure 8-54 ▲):

1. Take BSI precautions.

2. Determine the need for the medication based on patient presentation.

3. Obtain a focused history and physical exam, including any drug allergies and vital signs.

4. Follow standing orders, or contact medical control for permission.

5. Check the medication to ensure that it is the correct one, that it is not cloudy or discolored, and that the expiration date has not passed, and determine the appropriate amount and concentration for the correct dose.

6. Explain the procedure to the patient and the need for the medication.

7. Assemble needed equipment, and draw up the medication. Draw up 20 mL of normal saline to use as a flush for the medication.

8. Cleanse the injection port with alcohol, or remove the protective cap if using the needleless system.

9. Insert the needle into the port while holding it carefully, or screw the syringe onto the port.

10. Pull back slightly on the syringe plunger, and observe for blood return. If blood appears, slowly inject the medication, watching for infiltration. If resistance is felt, or if the patient complains of any discomfort, discontinue

administration immediately. A new site will need to be established.

11. Place the needle and syringe into the sharps container.

12. Clean the port, and insert the needle with the syringe containing the flush.

13. Flush the saline lock, and place the needle in the sharps container.

14. Store any unused medication properly.

15. Monitor the patient's condition, and document the medication given, route, time of administration, and response of the patient.

Adding Medication to an IV Bag

Certain medications are added to the IV solution itself to be administered as a maintenance infusion—for example, dopamine, lidocaine, and epinephrine. All of these medications require careful titration to achieve the desired effect.

The steps for adding medication to an IV bag are as follows:

1. Check the fluid in the IV bag for clarity or discoloration, and ensure that the expiration date has not passed.

2. Check the *drug name* on the ampule, vial, or prefilled syringe. Check the *concentration of the drug* it contains (for example, µg/mL or mg/mL).

3. *Compute the volume* of the drug to be added to the IV bag. Draw up that amount in a syringe (if a prefilled syringe is used, note the proportion of the volume of the syringe required).

4. Cleanse the medication injection port on the IV bag with an alcohol swab.

5. Inject the desired volume of medication into the IV bag by puncturing the rubber stopper on the medication injection port (Figure 8-55 ▲).

6. Withdraw the needle, and dispose of the needle and syringe in the sharps container. Agitate the IV bag gently to ensure that the added drug is well mixed in the solution.

7. *Label the IV bag* with the name of the medication added, the amount added, the concentration of medication in the

In the Field

Medications that are used for maintenance infusions (for example, lidocaine and dopamine) are commonly premixed and prepackaged, which eliminates the need to calculate and draw up the appropriate amount of medication to add to the bag. However, you must still be aware of the concentration (for example, μg/mL or mg/mL) of drug in the premixed solution and the appropriate maintenance infusion rate.

IV bag (for example, μg/mL or mg/mL), the date and time, and your name.

8. Attach the IV administration set, and prepare the IV bag as discussed earlier in this chapter.

Electromechanical Infusion Pumps

When administering a medication maintenance infusion, you should use an electromechanical infusion pump, if available. The infusion pump can also be used to deliver IV fluid maintenance infusions in children and elderly patients to minimize the risk of a "runaway IV" and subsequent circulatory overload.

Most infusion pumps allow you to set the parameters of medication administration—drug concentration and volume to be infused—and will then calculate the appropriate infusion rate. This feature allows for precise medication dosing, minimizing the risk of delivering too little or too much medication.

Electromechanical infusion pumps deliver fluids or medications via positive pressure. Although medications delivered in this manner can result in infiltration of a vein, most infusion pumps are equipped with an alarm that indicates a change in the flow pressure. Other common safety features include alarms that alert you to the presence of occlusion (eg, air in the tubing) or depletion of the medication. Some infusion pumps are designed to accommodate the IV tubing to regulate the flow of IV fluids or medications (Figure 8-56 ▾), whereas others are designed to accommodate a needleless syringe (Figure 8-57 ▸).

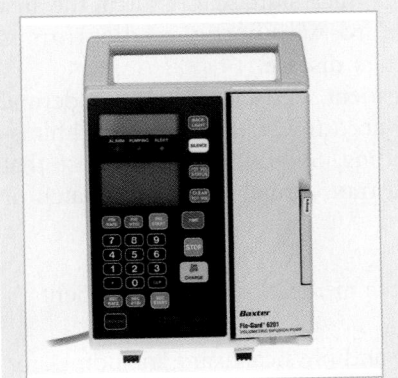

Figure 8-56 Infusion pump that accommodates IV tubing.

IO Medication Administration

The IO route is used for critically ill or injured children and adults when IV access is difficult or impossible to obtain. Any fluid or medication that may be given through an IV line—bolus or maintenance infusion—can be given by the IO route. Shock, status epilepticus, and cardiac arrest are but a few of the reasons for establishing IO access. Unlike with an IV line, fluid does not flow well into the bone because of resistance; therefore, it is necessary to use a large syringe to infuse the fluid. A pressure infuser device—a sleeve placed around the IV bag and inflated to force fluid from the IV bag—should be used when infusing fluids in adults.

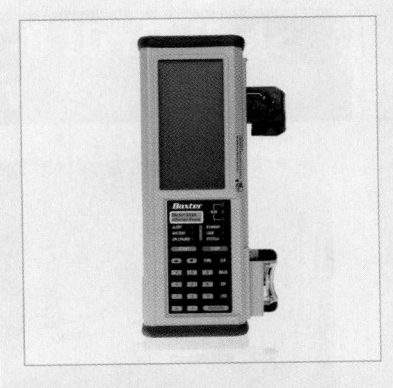

Figure 8-57 Syringe-type infusion pump.

Complications of using the IO route are similar to those of the IV route. Along with the complications discussed earlier in this chapter, there is also the potential for compartment syndrome if fluid leaks outside the bone and into the osteofascial compartment.

Follow the steps in Skill Drill 8-11 ▸ to administer a medication via the IO route:

1. Take BSI precautions.
2. Determine the need for the medication based on patient presentation.
3. Obtain a focused history and physical exam, including any drug allergies and vital signs.
4. Follow standing orders, or contact medical control for permission.
5. Check the medication to ensure that it is the correct one, that it is not cloudy or discolored, and that the expiration date has not passed, and determine the appropriate amount and concentration for the correct dose.
6. Explain the procedure to the patient and/or parent and the need for the medication.
7. Assemble needed equipment, and draw up the medication. Also draw up 20-mL of normal saline for a flush (Step 1).
8. Cleanse the injection port of the extension tubing with alcohol, or remove the protective cap if using the needleless system (Step 2).
9. Insert the needle into the port, and clamp off the IV tubing proximal to the administration port. This is usually managed with a three-way stopcock. Failure to shut off the line will result in the medication taking the pathway of least resistance and flowing into the bag instead of into the patient.
10. Administer the correct dose of the medication at the proper push rate. Some medications must be administered very quickly, while others must be pushed slowly to prevent adverse effects (Step 3).
11. Place the needle and syringe into the sharps container.

Skill Drill 8-11: Administering Medication via the IO Route

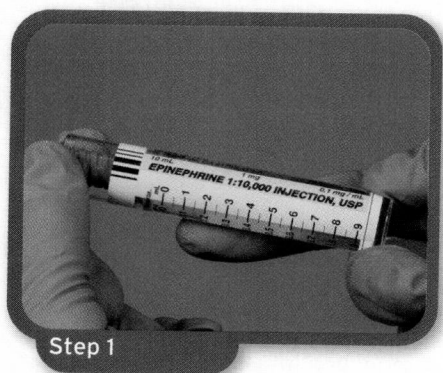

Step 1

Check the medication to ensure that it is the correct one, that it is not discolored, and that the expiration date has not passed.
Assemble the equipment, and draw up the medication. Draw up 20-mL of normal saline for a flush.

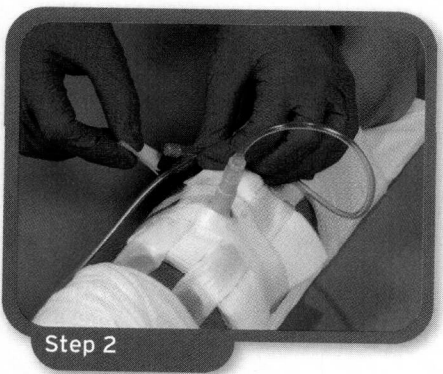

Step 2

Cleanse the injection port, or remove the protective cap if using the needleless system.

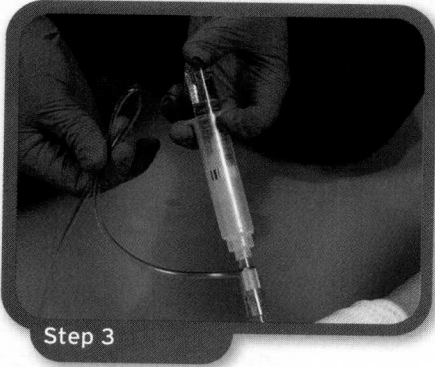

Step 3

Insert the needle into the port, and pinch off the IV tubing proximal to the administration port. Administer the correct dose at the proper push rate.

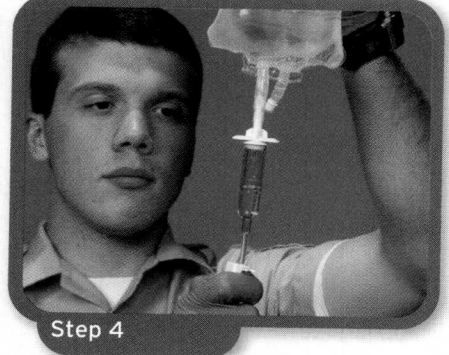

Step 4

Unclamp the IV line to flush the medication into the vein, allowing it to run briefly wide open, or flush with a 20-mL bolus of normal saline.
Readjust the IV flow rate to the original setting, and monitor the patient's condition.

12. Unclamp the IV line to flush the medication into the vein. Flush with at least a 20-mL bolus of normal saline.

13. Readjust the IV flow rate to the original setting.

14. Store any unused medication properly.

15. Monitor the patient's condition, and document the medication given, route, time of administration, and response of the patient (Step 4).

Percutaneous Medication Administration

With percutaneous routes of administration, medications are applied to and absorbed through the skin and mucous membranes. Because percutaneously administered medications bypass the gastrointestinal tract, their absorption is more predictable. Percutaneous routes of medication administration include the transdermal, sublingual, buccal, ocular, aural, and nasal routes.

Transdermal Medication Administration

Transdermal medications are applied topically—that is, on the surface of the body. Ordinarily, intact skin is an effective barrier to absorption of drugs. However, some drugs have been specially prepared to cross that barrier at a very slow steady rate, so the transdermal route is useful for the sustained release of certain medications.

Nitroglycerin, estrogen, nicotine, and analgesic patches, for example, are applied to the skin and release medications over a specified period. Creams, lotions, and pastes (eg, nitroglycerin paste, corticosteroid cream) are also transdermally administered medications.

Factors that can increase the speed of transdermal absorption include administration of too much of the medication (ie, inadvertent or intentional overdose) and thin or nonintact skin. Decreased speed of transdermal absorption can be caused by factors such as thick skin, scar tissue in the area to which the medication is applied, and peripheral vascular disease.

Other than assisting a patient with his or her transdermal medication, there is rarely a need to use this route of administration in the prehospital setting. Should a situation arise that requires you to administer a transdermal medication patch or paste, follow these steps:

1. Take BSI precautions.

2. Determine the need for the medication based on patient presentation.

3. Obtain a focused history and physical exam, including any drug allergies and vital signs.

4. Follow standing orders, or contact medical control for permission.

5. Check the medication patch or cream to ensure that it is the correct one and that the expiration date has not passed, and determine the appropriate amount for the correct dose.

6. Explain the procedure to the patient and the need for the medication.

7. Clean and dry the area of the skin where the medication will be applied.

8. Apply the medication to the area in accordance with the manufacturer's specifications.

9. Monitor the patient's condition, and document the medication given, route, time of administration, and response of the patient.

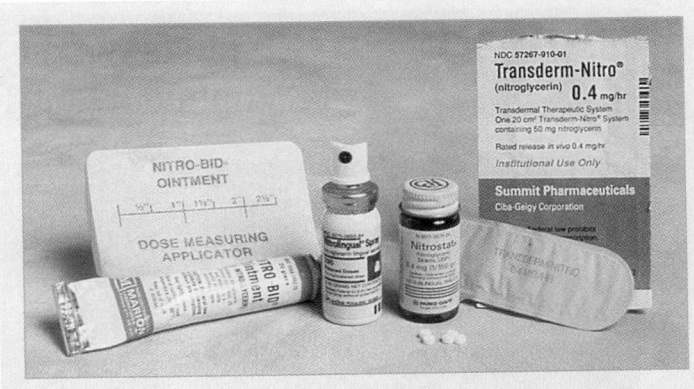

Figure 8-58 Nitroglycerin is often given sublingually as a spray or a tablet. It is also available as a transdermal patch or paste and can be administered as an IV drip as well.

In the Field

During assessment of your patient, look for transdermal medication patches, especially narcotic and nitroglycerin patches, which can result in hypotension. If the patient is already in a hemodynamically unstable condition, narcotics and nitroglycerin may complicate the clinical picture.

Sublingual Medication Administration

The sublingual (under the tongue) region is highly vascular, so medications given via the sublingual route are rapidly absorbed. Sublingually administered medications, relative to enterally administered medications, get into the circulation much faster. Nitroglycerin—spray or tablet—is a drug that is most commonly administered via the sublingual route 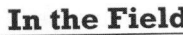 **Figure 8-58 ▶**.

Drugs may also be *injected* into the network of veins (venous plexus) under the tongue (strictly speaking, that is another form of intravenous injection). This technique is especially useful for giving narcotic antagonists to patients who have overdosed on heroin because finding a suitable vein in such patients may be nearly impossible.

To administer a sublingual medication, follow these steps **Skill Drill 8-12 ▶**.

1. Take BSI precautions.
2. Determine the need for the medication based on patient presentation.
3. Obtain a focused history and physical exam, including any drug allergies and vital signs.
4. Follow standing orders, or contact medical control for permission.
5. Check the medication to ensure that it is the correct one and that its expiration date has not passed, and determine the appropriate amount for the correct dose.
6. Ask the patient to rinse his or her mouth with a little water if the mucous membranes are dry (Step 1).

7. Explain the procedure, and ask the patient to lift his or her tongue. Place the tablet or spray the dose under the tongue, or ask the patient to do so.
8. Advise the patient not to chew or swallow the tablet, but to let it dissolve slowly.
9. Monitor the patient's condition, and document the medication given, route, administration time, and response of the patient (Step 2).

Buccal Medication Administration

The buccal region, which is also highly vascular, lies in between the cheek and gums. Most medications administered via the buccal route are in the form of tablets. Unlike the sublingual route, you will rarely administer medications via the buccal route in the prehospital setting.

To administer a medication via the buccal route, follow these steps:

1. Take BSI precautions.
2. Determine the need for the medication based on patient presentation.
3. Obtain a focused history and physical exam, including any drug allergies and vital signs.
4. Follow standing orders, or contact medical control for permission.
5. Check the medication to ensure that it is the correct one and that its expiration date has not passed, and determine the appropriate amount for the correct dose.
6. Explain the procedure to the patient and the need for the medication.
7. Place the medication in between the patient's cheek and gum, or ask the patient to do so.
8. Advise the patient not to chew or swallow the tablet, but to let it dissolve slowly.
9. Monitor the patient's condition, and document the medication given, route, administration time, and response of the patient.

Skill Drill 8-12: Administering Medication via the Sublingual Route

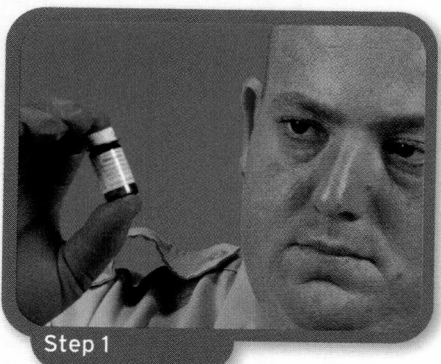

Step 1

Check the medication for drug type and its expiration date, and determine the appropriate amount for the correct dose.

Have the patient rinse his or her mouth with a little water if the mucous membranes are dry.

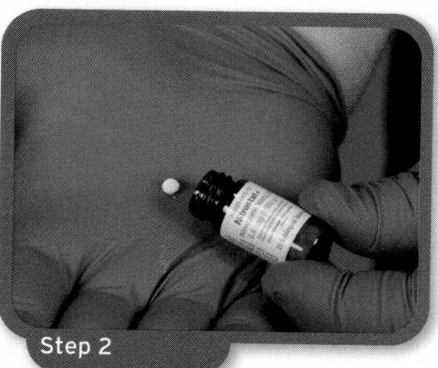

Step 2

Explain the procedure to the patient, and ask the patient to lift his or her tongue. Place the tablet or spray the dose underneath the tongue, or have the patient do so.

Advise the patient not to chew or swallow the tablet, but to let it dissolve slowly.

Monitor the patient, and document the medication given, the route, administration time, and the response of the patient.

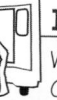

In the Field

Wear gloves when administering nitroglycerin. Otherwise, the medication can be absorbed through your skin.

Ocular Medication Administration

Drops or ointments are commonly administered via the ocular route. Ocular medications are typically administered for pain relief, allergies, drying of the eyes, or infections. Other than assisting a patient with his or her ocular medication or irrigating a patient's eyes following a toxic exposure, none of the medications used in the prehospital setting are administered via the ocular route.

If a patient asks you to assist him or her with ocular medication administration, follow these steps:

1. Take BSI precautions.
2. Confirm that the medication is prescribed to the patient.
3. Place the patient in a supine position, or have the patient place his or her head back and look up.
4. *Without touching the eyeball,* expose the conjunctiva by gently pulling down on the lower eyelid.
5. Administer the required amount of medication on the conjunctival sac by using an eye dropper. Do not apply the medication directly on the eyeball.
6. Advise the patient to close his or her eyes for 1 to 2 minutes.
7. Document the medication name, dose, and administration time.

Aural Medication Administration

Certain medications—mainly antibiotics, analgesics, and ear-wax removal preparations—are administered via the mucous membranes of the aural (ear) canal. As with ocular medications, the aural route is rarely, if ever, used in the prehospital setting.

If you are asked by the patient to assist in administering his or her aural medication, follow these steps:

1. Take BSI precautions.
2. Confirm that the medication is prescribed to the patient.
3. Place the patient on his or her side with the affected ear facing up.
4. Expose the ear canal by pulling the ear up and back (adults) or down and back (infants and children).
5. Administer the medication in the appropriate dose with a medicine dropper.
6. Document the medication name, dose, and administration time.

Intranasal Medication Administration

Intranasal (within the nose) medications include nasal spray for congestion or solutions to moisten the nasal mucosa. In recent years, this route of medication administration has become increasingly more popular in the prehospital setting. Intranasally administered medications are rapidly absorbed, providing a more rapid onset of action than IM injections. Administration of emergency medications via the intranasal route is performed with a mucosal atomizer device (MAD) **Figure 8-59 ▶**. The MAD attaches to a syringe and allows you to spray (atomize) select medications into the nasal mucosa.

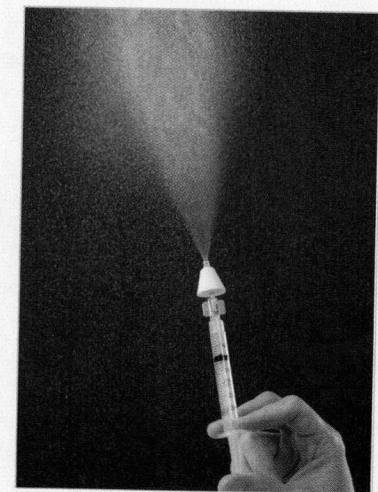

Figure 8-59 Mucosal atomizer device (MAD).

Owing to the molecular structure of drugs, only a few emergency medications can be given intranasally, including naloxone (Narcan) and midazolam (Versed). Follow local protocol, or consult with medical control about the appropriate doses of these medications and any other medications that may be administered intranasally.

To administer a drug via the intranasal route, follow these steps:

1. Take BSI precautions.
2. Determine the need for the medication based on patient presentation.
3. Obtain a focused history and physical exam, including any drug allergies and vital signs.
4. Follow standing orders, or contact medical control for permission.
5. Check the medication to ensure that it is the correct one, that it is not cloudy or discolored, and that the expiration date has not passed.
6. Draw up the appropriate dose of medication in the syringe.
7. Attach the mucosal atomizer device to the syringe.
8. Explain the procedure to the patient (or to a relative if the patient is unconscious) and the need for the medication.
9. Spray *half* of the medication dose into each nostril.
10. Dispose of the atomizer device and syringe in the appropriate container.
11. Monitor the patient's condition, and document the medication given, route, time of administration, and response of the patient.

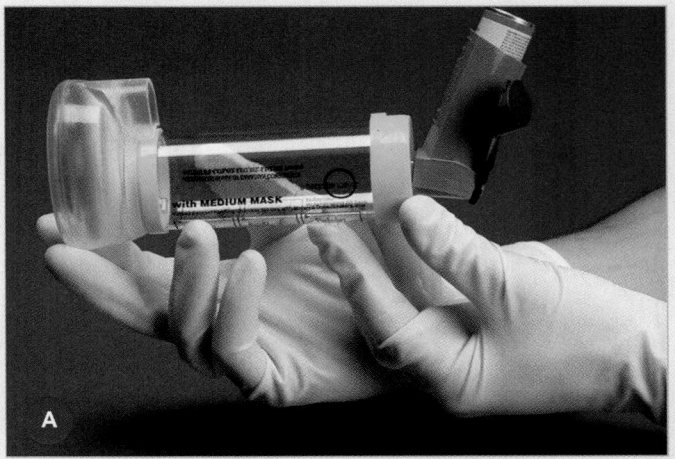

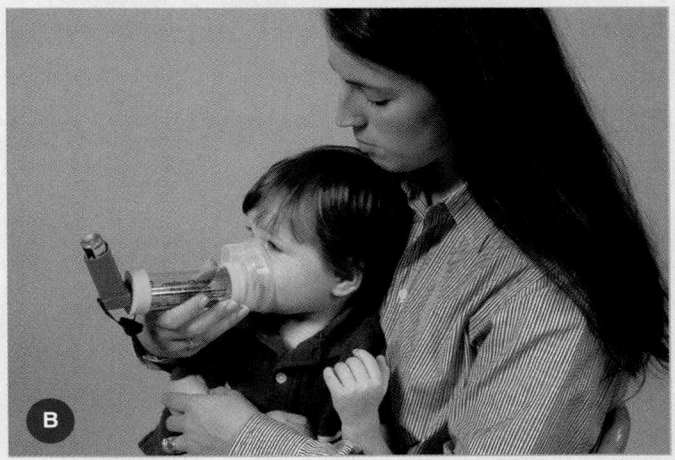

Figure 8-61 **A.** In children, an MDI and spacer can be used with or without a mask. **B.** Children as young as 6 months can use a mask and spacer device.

Medications Administered by the Inhalation Route

Nebulizer and Metered-Dose Inhaler

Many medications used in the treatment of respiratory emergencies are administered via the inhalation route. The most common inhaled medication is oxygen. Beta₂ agonist bronchodilators (eg, albuterol [Ventolin, Proventil], isoetharine [Bronkosol], metaproterenol [Alupent]) are often administered in the prehospital setting for patients experiencing respiratory distress caused by certain obstructive airway diseases, such as asthma, bronchitis, and emphysema. Other medications, such as ipratropium bromide (Atrovent)—an anticholinergic bronchodilator—are also administered via the inhalation route. Check your drug reference guide or the package insert for the indications, contraindications, and precautions before giving any of these medications.

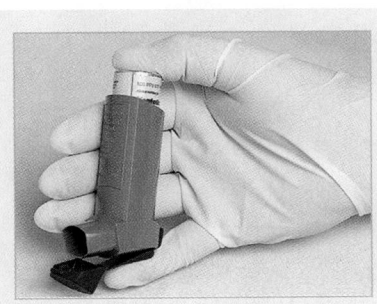

Figure 8-60 Some medications are inhaled into the lungs with an MDI so that they can be absorbed quickly into the bloodstream.

A patient with a history of respiratory problems will usually have a metered-dose inhaler (MDI) to use on a regular basis or as needed Figure 8-60 ◄ . Medications administered by the MDI can be delivered through a mouthpiece held by the patient or by a mask—with or without a spacer device—for young children and patients who are unable to hold the mouthpiece Figure 8-61 ▲ .

For more severe problems, liquid bronchodilators may be aerosolized in a nebulizer for inhalation. Small-volume nebulizers (also called updraft or hand-held nebulizers) are the most commonly used method of administration of inhaled medications in the prehospital setting Figure 8-62 ► . Oxygen or a compressed air source is connected to the nebulizer to produce the aerosolized mist.

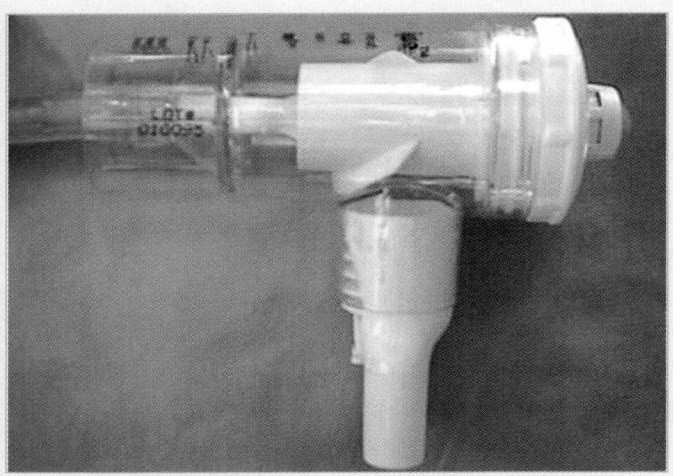

Figure 8-62 A small-volume nebulizer is used to deliver medications via aerosolized mist.

9. With the MDI or hand-held nebulizer in position, instruct the patient on the proper way to breathe. Have the patient breathe as deeply as possible and hold his or her breath for 3 to 5 seconds before exhaling. Continue to coach the patient as needed.

10. Monitor the patient's condition, and document the medication given, route, time of administration, and response of the patient to the medication (Step 4).

11. Cardiac monitoring is essential when administering a beta agonist. If cardiac dysrhythmias are noted, stop the administration of the medication, administer high-flow oxygen, and contact medical control.

Some patients with respiratory emergencies may be breathing inadequately (ie, inadequate tidal volume, fast or slow respiratory rate) and will not be able to effectively inhale beta-agonist medications into the lungs via a nebulizer or an MDI. In this case, assist with bag-mask ventilation and attach a small-volume nebulizer to the ventilation device. Place a short

Follow the steps in Skill Drill 8-13 ▶ to administer a medication via small-volume nebulizer:

1. Take BSI precautions.
2. Determine the need for an inhaled bronchodilator based on patient presentation.
3. Obtain a focused history and physical exam, including any drug allergies and vital signs.
4. Follow standing orders, or contact medical control for permission.
5. Check the medication and its expiration date. Make sure that you have the right medication and that it is not cloudy or discolored (Step 1).
6. If the medication is in a premixed package, add it to the bowl of the nebulizer. If it is not premixed, add the medication to the bowl and mix it with the specified amount of normal saline, usually 3 mL (Step 2).
7. Connect the T piece with the mouthpiece to the top of the bowl, or the mask to the bowl, and connect it to the oxygen tubing.
8. Set the flowmeter at 6 L/min to produce a steady mist (Step 3).

Skill Drill 8-13: Administering a Medication via Small-Volume Nebulizer

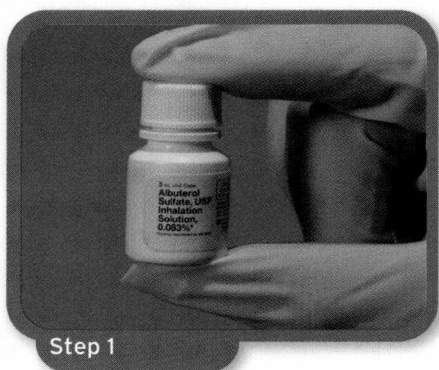

Step 1

Check the medication and the expiration date.

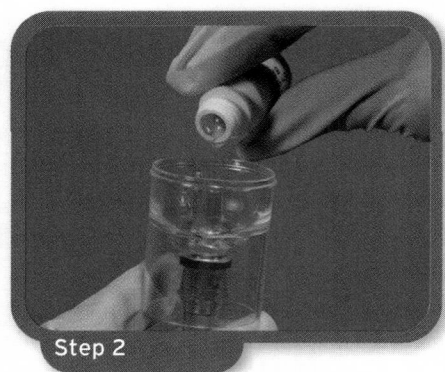

Step 2

Add premixed medication to the bowl of the nebulizer.

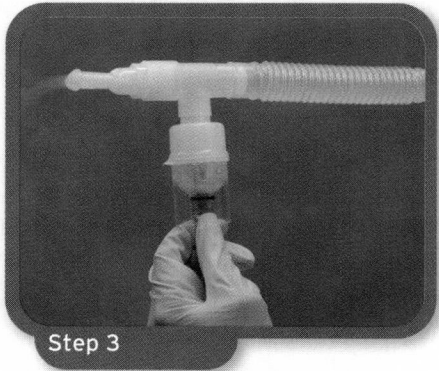

Step 3

Connect the T piece with the mouthpiece to the top of the bowl, connect it to the oxygen tubing, and set the flowmeter at 6 L/min.

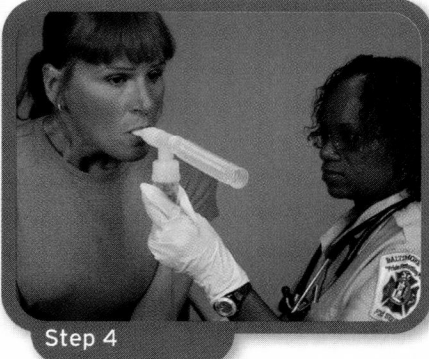

Step 4

Instruct the patient to breathe as deeply as possible and hold his or her breath for 3 to 5 seconds before exhaling. Monitor the patient for effects.

Controversies

In the past, nebulizers were considered the preferred method of delivering beta-agonist medications for the treatment of asthma attacks. Recent studies, however, have shown that MDIs—especially when used with spacing devices—are at least as effective as nebulizers and have several distinct advantages:

- MDIs are *more convenient* than nebulizers. They do not require any setup time or a source of compressed gas.
- MDIs are *more reliable* than nebulizers. With a nebulizer, one cannot be certain that the patient is getting the full dose of the drug. MDIs deliver a more consistent amount of drug aerosol.
- Because most people with asthma use MDIs at home, using the MDI in an emergency provides an excellent opportunity to *educate the patient* in proper use of the device. Studies have shown that more than half of patients using MDIs at home employ an incorrect and ineffective technique. Showing a patient the correct technique and demonstrating its effectiveness can improve the outcome of subsequent asthma attacks.

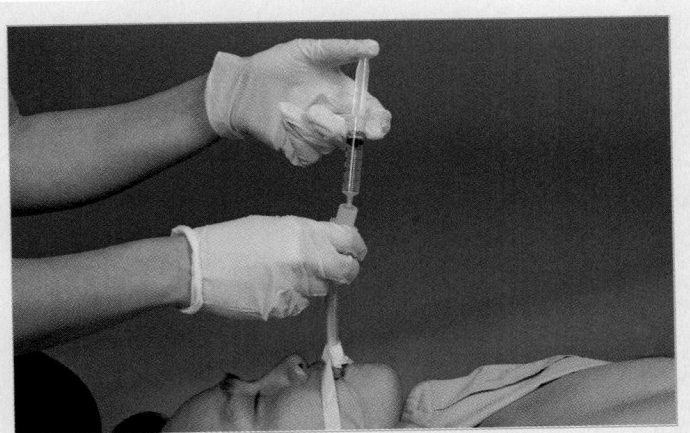

Figure 8-63 Administering medication via the ET tube.

piece of corrugated tubing—separated by a T piece to connect the nebulizer to—between the bag and mask or endotracheal tube if the patient is intubated.

Endotracheal Medication Administration

If IV or IO access is unavailable, certain resuscitative medications can be administered down the endotracheal (ET) tube. For the medication to be adequately dispersed throughout the tracheobronchial tree, you must administer 2 to 2.5 times the standard IV dose. *Only* four medications should be given down the ET tube; they can easily be remembered by the mnemonic LEAN: Lidocaine, Epinephrine, Atropine, Narcan.

To administer medications via the ET tube, follow these steps:

1. Draw up the appropriate dose of the medication to be administered as your partner ventilates the patient. Dilute the appropriate dose of the medication in 10 mL of normal saline.
2. Disconnect the bag-mask device from the ET tube, and rapidly instill the medication down the ET tube **Figure 8-63 ◂** .
3. Immediately reconnect the bag-mask device to the ET tube, and ventilate the patient briskly to facilitate passage of the drug down the trachea and into the lungs.

Controversies

Although current practice calls for administering certain resuscitative medications via the ET tube, recent studies have suggested that this route of medication administration may not be particularly effective. Follow local protocols, or contact medical control as needed regarding endotracheal drug administration.

Rates of Medication Absorption

The speed at which a drug is absorbed is directly related to the route by which it is given. Obviously, drugs injected directly into the bloodstream (ie, as IV or IO injections) gain access to the central circulation the fastest. Oral medications take longer to achieve their therapeutic effects, because they must be absorbed through the gastrointestinal tract first. **Table 8-6 ▾** summarizes the various medication routes and their rates of absorption.

Table 8-6	Medication Routes and Rates of Absorption
Route of Administration	**Onset of Action***
Intraosseous	30–60 s
Intravenous	30–60 s
Endotracheal	2–3 min[†]
Inhalation	2–3 min
Sublingual	3–5 min
Intramuscular injection	10–20 min
Subcutaneous injection	15–30 min
Rectal	5–30 min
Oral	30–90 min
Topical	Minutes to hours

*In a healthy person with adequate perfusion.

[†]Recent data suggest that ET drug administration may be less effective than previously thought, especially in poor perfusion states.

You are the Provider Summary

1. Is this a medical patient or a trauma patient?

You have not obtained enough information to be able to establish whether this is a medical patient or a trauma patient. Your index of suspicion should increase for the potential for trauma in this case, especially because no one witnessed the events preceding the patient's condition. Further assessment of the patient and her surroundings is required. If there is *any* potential for trauma, then treat her accordingly (ie, spinal motion restriction precautions). Paramedics should not be too hasty to "label" a patient as being a medical or trauma patient; this requires a careful assessment. Some patients have *both* medical and traumatic elements to their condition.

2. What are your initial priorities of care?

Immediate care for this patient involves carefully moving her to the floor (with spinal precautions if trauma is suspected) and performing an initial assessment. This is the most important aspect of initial patient care. You *must* be able to *rapidly identify and correct* immediate threats to life. This patient is unresponsive; clearly, her condition requires immediate treatment.

3. What is the most appropriate initial airway management for this patient?

The patient is unconscious and unresponsive, so you must immediately ensure that her airway is open and clear of secretions. Furthermore, her respirations are rapid and shallow (reduced tidal volume). Initial airway management should include inserting an oral or nasal airway adjunct and assisting ventilation with bag-mask ventilation and 100% oxygen. Rapid, shallow respirations will result in decreased minute volume. If this is not *immediately* treated, significant hypoxia and acidosis will develop.

4. Does this patient require immediate medication therapy?

Other than 100% oxygen, which you have already administered, further assessment is required before determining whether medication therapy is indicated. Although the patient's history of diabetes and clinical presentation are highly suggestive of hypoglycemia, they are not conclusive. In some diabetic patients, it may be difficult to differentiate between hypoglycemia and hyperglycemia, especially if the patient is unconscious.

5. Given the patient's history, what additional assessment should you perform?

Obviously, you should test the blood glucose level of any unconscious patient—with or without a history of diabetes. This is especially true if you observe signs suggesting hypoglycemia. Adequate glucose to the brain is just as critical as oxygen; without it, permanent brain damage or death can occur. Because hypoglycemia is an easily correctable condition, rapid blood glucose testing should be performed and, if needed, treated immediately.

6. When starting an IV for this patient, what solution should you use?

An isotonic crystalloid (most often normal saline) is the fluid of choice for the vast majority of patients that you will treat in the prehospital setting. A D_5W solution (or any glucose-containing solution) should not be used in patients with diabetes. D_5W is a more appropriate choice when mixing a medication to deliver in a maintenance infusion. Patients with diabetic ketoacidosis, for example, are typically dehydrated from the osmotic diuresis caused by excess blood glucose levels. Isotonic crystalloids, because they remain in the vascular space for longer periods, are needed for rehydration and maintenance of adequate perfusion.

7. What does the "%" in 50% dextrose mean?

In terms of medication concentration, *percent* refers to the number of grams present in 100 mL (1 dL) of volume. Therefore, 50% dextrose contains a concentration of 50 g (50,000 mg) of dextrose in 100 mL of volume. Since 50% dextrose is dispensed in a 50 mL volume, there are 25 g of medication in the container.

8. What is the concentration of D_{50} that you have on hand?

The concentration on hand represents the total amount of weight (μg, mg, or g) present in 1 mL. D_{50} represents 50 g of dextrose in 100 mL of volume. However, because D_{50} is contained in only 50 mL, you have only 25 g of dextrose in one pre-filled syringe. To determine the concentration on hand, divide the total number of milligrams (25 g = 25,000 mg) by the total volume (50 mL): 25,000 mg ÷ 50 mL = 500 mg/mL.

9. What are the "six rights" of medication administration?

Before administering any medication, you must review the six rights to ensure that safe and effective patient care is given: (1) right patient, (2) right drug, (3) right dose, (4) right route, (5) right time, and (6) right documentation. You can cause further harm to the patient if a drug—even if it's the right drug—is given at the wrong time, by an inappropriate route, or in the wrong dose.

10. Does this patient require an additional dose of 50% dextrose?

Based on a post-D_{50} glucose reading of 80 mg/dL and the patient's obvious clinical improvement, additional doses of D_{50} are not indicated. However, the question remains as to why her blood glucose level dropped initially. Ask further questions to explore this issue, such as when she last ate, what she ate (if she ate), if she took her insulin and how much, and if she has any other medical problems. During transport, continue to monitor the patient's level of consciousness and reassess her blood glucose level as needed.

11. Does this patient require an IV bolus of normal saline?

The IV line can remain at a KVO rate; there is no need for fluid boluses. At present, the patient's vital signs indicate hemodynamic stability. Her heart rate, which was 120 beats/min initially, was likely due to a sympathetic nervous system discharge in response to hypoglycemia, not hypovolemia. Following administration of the D_{50}, the patient's heart rate promptly recovered. No mechanism for volume loss has been identified (eg, vomiting, diarrhea).

Prep Kit

Ready for Review

- The cellular environment contains charged ions, called electrolytes, that are used by the cell for different purposes. These electrolytes include sodium, potassium, calcium, bicarbonate, chloride, and phosphorus. Their electrical charges must remain in balance on either side of the cell membrane.

- There must be a balance of compounds on either side of the cell membrane. If an imbalance occurs, the cell can move chemicals or charges across its membrane by various methods, including osmosis, diffusion, active transport, and filtration.

- Understanding the workings of the intracellular and extracellular chemicals and charges will provide you with a better foundation for understanding why different types of IV solutions are administered for different conditions.

- Techniques for gaining vascular access include cannulation of a peripheral extremity vein, cannulation of the external jugular vein, and cannulation of the IO space. Although the ultimate goal of vascular access is to be able to administer fluids and medications, each of these techniques requires a different approach and must be practiced frequently for initial and ongoing proficiency.

- Several different IV administration sets exist, and you must know which one is most appropriate for a given patient condition. Microdrip sets (60 gtt/mL) are commonly used for medication infusions. Macrodrip sets (10 or 15 gtt/mL) are used when the patient requires IV fluid boluses to treat dehydration, hypovolemic shock, and other states of hemodynamic instability.

- You must consider two factors when choosing an IV catheter: gauge and length. The larger the gauge (the smaller the number), and the shorter the length, the more fluid that can be infused through it. Over-the-needle catheters are the most commonly used IV catheters in the prehospital setting.

- Cannulation of a peripheral extremity vein is the preferred initial means of establishing vascular access. If it is unsuccessful and the patient is critically ill or injured, proceed with IO cannulation without delay. External jugular vein cannulation is usually attempted only after all other techniques of gaining vascular access have failed.

- IO cannulation and infusion are no longer reserved for children only; they can also be used to establish emergency vascular access in adults. The IO space, which acts like a sponge, quickly absorbs fluids and medications and rapidly transports them to the central circulation.

- Although peripheral veins often collapse when a patient is in shock or cardiac arrest, the IO space tends to remain patent. Thus IO cannulation and infusion—in children and adults—may be life-saving measures if peripheral venous access is not possible. Any fluid or medication that can be administered via the IV route can be administered via the IO route and can travel to the central circulation just as rapidly.

- You must be thoroughly familiar with the equipment you are using when performing IO cannulation. Follow local protocols and attend in-service training regarding the specific equipment used for IO cannulation in your EMS system.

- Use aseptic technique when performing any invasive procedure to minimize the risk of patient contamination. Always use BSI precautions when performing an invasive procedure to maximize your own safety.

- Along with the dispensing of medications comes the responsibility to be thoroughly familiar with each medication carried on your ambulance. Carry an EMS field guide or other reference to look up unfamiliar drugs or to confirm the doses and routes of drugs that you are familiar with. Remember: *First do no harm.*

- Good math skills and a thorough understanding of the metric system are imperative to providing the right dose of a drug to your patient. The six rights of medication are right patient, right drug, right dose, right route, right time, and right documentation. Administering the wrong drug, using the wrong route, or giving the wrong dose can have disastrous effects.

- All equipment used in the administration of medications must be kept sterile to prevent contamination of the patient. Use proper BSI precautions to protect yourself. Needleless systems have made older needle systems increasingly obsolete, as the former systems decrease the incidence of needlesticks.

- As a paramedic, you must be familiar with the various routes of medication administration, including the proper use of equipment and proper anatomic locations for administration via each route.

- Enteral medication administration includes the administration of all drugs that may be given through any portion of the gastrointestinal tract. The parenteral route includes any method of drug administration that does not pass through the gastrointestinal tract.

- The IV and IO routes are the fastest routes of medication administration; the oral and transdermal (topical) routes are the slowest.

- When in doubt, always follow local protocols or contact medical control as needed for direction when administering a medication. *Never make a hasty critical decision before consulting with a physician!*

Vital Vocabulary

access port A sealed hub on an administration set designed for sterile access to the IV fluid.

acidosis A pathologic condition resulting from the accumulation of acids in the body.

administration set Tubing that connects to the IV bag access port and the catheter to deliver IV fluid.

alkalosis A pathologic condition resulting from the accumulation of bases in the body.

ampules Small glass containers that are sealed and the contents sterilized.

anion An ion that contains an overall negative charge.

antecubital The anterior aspect of the elbow.

anticoagulant A substance that prevents blood from clotting.

antidiuretic hormone (ADH) A hormone produced by the pituitary gland that signals the kidneys to prevent excretion of water.

antiseptics Chemicals used to cleanse an area before performing an invasive procedure, such as starting an IV; not toxic to living tissues; examples include isopropyl alcohol and iodine.

aseptic technique A method of cleansing used to prevent contamination of a site when performing an invasive procedure, such as starting an IV.

ataxia A staggered walk or gait.

aural Pertaining to the ear.

bivalent An ion that contains two charges.

blood tubing A special type of macrodrip administration set designed to facilitate rapid fluid replacement by manual infusion of multiple IV bags or IV-blood replacement combinations.

bolus A term used to describe "in one mass"; in medication administration, a single dose given by the IV or IO route; may be a small or large quantity of the drug.

Bone Injection Gun (B.I.G.) A spring-loaded device that is used for inserting an IO needle into the proximal tibia in adult and pediatric patients.

buccal Between the cheek and gums.

www.Paramedic.EMSzone.com

butterfly catheter A rigid, hollow, venous cannulation device identified by its plastic "wings" that act as anchoring points for securing the catheter.

cannulation The insertion of a catheter, such as into a vein to allow for fluid flow.

carpopedal spasms Hand or foot spasms; usually the result of hyperventilation or hypocalcemia.

catheter shear Occurs when a needle is reinserted into the catheter, and it slices through the catheter, creating a free-floating segment.

cation An ion that contains an overall positive charge.

Celsius scale A scale for measuring temperature in which water freezes at 0° and boils at 100°.

colloid solutions Solutions that contain molecules (usually proteins) that are too large to pass out of the capillary membranes and, therefore, remain in the vascular compartment.

concentration The total weight of a drug contained in a specific volume of liquid.

concentration gradient The natural tendency for substances to flow from an area of higher concentration to an area of lower concentration, within or outside the cell.

contaminated stick The puncturing of an emergency care provider's skin with a needle or catheter that was used on a patient.

crystalloid solutions Solutions of dissolved crystals (for example, salts or sugars) in water; contain compounds that quickly dissociate in solution.

D_5W An intravenous solution made up of 5% dextrose in water.

dehydration Depletion of the body's systemic fluid volume.

depolarization The rapid movement of electrolytes across a cell membrane that changes the cell's overall charge. This rapid shifting of electrolytes and cellular charges is the main catalyst for muscle contractions and neural transmissions.

desired dose The amount of a drug that the physician orders for a patient; the drug order.

diaphysis The shaft of a long bone.

diffusion A process in which molecules move from an area of higher concentration to an area of lower concentration.

diluent A solution (usually water or normal saline) used for diluting a medication.

disinfectants Chemicals used on nonliving objects to kill organisms; toxic to living tissues; examples include Virex, Cidex, and Microcide.

drip chamber The area of the administration set where fluid accumulates so that the tubing remains filled with fluid.

drug reconstitution Injecting sterile water or saline from one vial into another vial containing a powdered form of the drug.

electrolytes Charged atoms or compounds that result from the loss or gain of an electron. These are ions that the body uses to perform certain critical metabolic functions.

enteral route A route of medication administration that involves the medication passing through a portion of the gastrointestinal tract.

epiphyseal plate The growth plate of a bone; a major site of bone development during childhood.

epiphyses The ends of a long bone.

external jugular (EJ) vein Large neck vein that is lateral to the carotid artery.

extracellular fluid (ECF) The water outside the cells; accounts for 15% of body weight.

EZ-IO A hand-held, battery-powered driver to which a special IO needle is attached; used for insertion of the IO needle into the proximal tibia of children and adults.

Fahrenheit scale A scale for measuring temperature in which water freezes at 32° and boils at 212°.

fascia The fiberlike connective tissue that covers arteries, veins, tendons, and ligaments.

F.A.S.T.1 A sternal IO device used in adults; stands for First Access for Shock and Trauma.

flash chamber The area of an IV catheter that fills with blood to help indicate when a vein is cannulated.

gastric tubes Tubes that are commonly inserted in patients in the prehospital setting to decompress the stomach; can also be used to administer certain enteral medications.

gauge The internal diameter of an IV catheter or needle.

gtt A unit of measure that indicates drops.

hematoma An accumulation of blood in the tissues beneath the skin; a potential complication of IV therapy.

hemostasis The body's natural blood-clotting mechanism.

homeostasis The balance of all body systems of the body; also known as homeostatic balance.

hypercalcemia A high serum calcium level.

hyperkalemia A high serum potassium level.

hypertonic solution A solution that has a greater concentration of sodium than does the cell; the increased osmotic pressure can draw water out of the cell and cause it to collapse.

hypocalcemia A low serum calcium level.

hypokalemia A low serum potassium level.

hypotonic solution A solution that has a lower concentration of sodium than does the cell; the increased osmotic pressure lets water flow into the cell, causing it to swell and possibly burst.

infiltration The escape of fluid into the surrounding tissue; the result of vein perforation during IV cannulation.

inhalation Breathing into the lungs; a medication delivery route.

interstitial fluid The water bathing the cells; accounts for about 10.5% of body weight; includes special fluid collections, such as cerebrospinal fluid and intraocular fluid.

intracellular fluid (ICF) The water contained inside the cells; normally accounts for 45% of body weight.

intradermal the layer of the dermis, just beneath the epidermis; a medication delivery route.

intramuscular (IM) Into a muscle; a medication delivery route.

intranasal Within the nose.

intraosseous Within the bone.

intraosseous (IO) infusion A technique of administering fluids, blood and blood products, and medications into the intraosseous space of a long bone, usually the proximal tibia.

intraosseous (IO) space The spongy cancellous bone of the epiphyses and the medullary cavity of the diaphysis, collectively.

intravascular fluid Plasma; the water within the blood vessels, which carries red blood cells, white blood cells, and vital nutrients; normally accounts for about 4.5% of body weight.

intravenous Within a vein.

intravenous (IV) therapy Cannulation of a vein with an IV catheter to access the patient's vascular system.

ionic concentration The amount of charged particles found in a particular area.

ions Charged atoms or compounds that results from the loss or gain of an electron.

isotonic crystalloids Intravenous solutions that do not cause a fluid shift into or out of the cell; examples include normal saline and lactated Ringer's solutions.

isotonic solution A solution that has the same concentration of sodium as does the cell. In this case, water does not shift, and no change in cell shape occurs.

lactated Ringer's (LR) solution A sterile isotonic crystalloid IV solution of specified amounts of calcium chloride, potassium chloride, sodium chloride, and sodium lactate in water.

local reactions Reactions that occur in a localized area; a potential complication of IV therapy.

macrodrip sets Administration sets named for the large orifice between the piercing spike and the drip chamber; allow for rapid fluid flow into the vascular system; allow 10 or 15 gtt/mL, depending on the manufacturer.

medical asepsis A term applied to the practice of preventing contamination of the patient by using aseptic technique.

metabolic Pertaining to the breakdown of ingested foodstuffs into smaller and smaller molecules and atoms that are used as energy sources for cellular function.

metered-dose inhaler (MDI) A pressurized canister that delivers a specific dose of a medication; commonly used for beta-agonist bronchodilators.

metric system A decimal system based on tens for the measurement of length, weight, and volume.

microdrip sets Administration sets named for the small needlelike orifice between the piercing spike and the drip chamber; allow for carefully controlled fluid flow and are ideally suited for medication administration; allow for 60 gtt/mL.

milliequivalent (mEq) Unit of measure for electrolytes.

Mix-o-Vial A single vial divided into two compartments by a rubber stopper; Solu-Medrol is stored this way.

monovalent An ion that contains one charge.

mucosal atomizer device (MAD) A device that attaches to the end of a syringe that is used to spray (atomize) certain medications via the intranasal route.

nebulizer A device for producing a fine spray or mist that is used to deliver inhaled medications.

nonelectrolytes Solutes that have no electrical charge; include glucose and urea; measured in milligrams (mg).

normal saline A solution of 0.9% sodium chloride; an isotonic crystalloid.

occlusion Blockage, usually of a tubular structure such as a blood vessel or IV catheter.

ocular Pertaining to the eye.

online (direct) medical control Type of medical control in which the paramedic is in direct contact with a physician, usually via two-way radio or telephone.

osmolarity The ability to influence the movement of water across a semipermeable membrane.

osmosis The movement of water across a semipermeable membrane (for example, the cell wall) from an area of lower to higher concentration of solute molecules.

osteogenesis imperfecta A congenital bone disease that results in fragile bones.

osteomyelitis Inflammation of the bone and muscle caused by infection.

overhydration An increase in the body's systemic fluid volume.

over-the-needle catheter A Teflon (plastic) catheter inserted over a hollow needle.

parenteral route A route of medication administration that involves any route other than the gastrointestinal tract.

Penrose drain A type of surgical drain often used as a constricting band.

percutaneous Through the skin or mucous membrane.

peripheral vein cannulation Cannulating veins of the periphery, that is, those that can be seen and/or palpated. Examples of peripheral veins include those of the hand, arm, and lower extremity and the external jugular vein.

piercing spike The hard, sharpened plastic spike on the end of the administration set designed to pierce the sterile membrane of the IV bag.

postural hypotension Symptomatic drop in blood pressure related to the patient's body position; detected by measuring pulse and blood pressure while the patient is lying supine, sitting up, and standing. An increase in pulse rate and a decrease in blood pressure in any one of these positions is considered a positive sign for this condition.

prefilled syringes Medication syringes that are prepackaged and prepared with a specific concentration.

pressure infuser device A sleeve that is placed around the IV bag and inflated to force fluid to flow from the IV bag and into the tubing.

pulmonary embolism A blood clot or foreign matter trapped within the pulmonary circulation.

pyrogenic reaction A reaction characterized by an abrupt temperature elevation (as high as 106° F [41° C]) with severe chills, backache, headache, weakness, nausea, and vomiting; a potential complication of IV or IO therapy.

radiopaque Feature of an IV catheter (or any other object) that allows it to appear on an x-ray.

saline locks Special types of IV devices that eliminate the need to hang a bag of IV fluid; also called a buff cap or INT (intermittent); commonly used for patients who do not require fluid boluses but may require medication therapy.

self-sealing blood tubes Glass tubes with self-sealing rubber caps; used to obtain blood samples for laboratory analysis.

sharps Any contaminated item that can cause injury; includes IV needles and catheters, broken ampules or vials, or anything else that can penetrate or lacerate the skin.

sodium-potassium (Na$^+$-K$^+$) pump The mechanism by which the cell brings in two potassium (K$^+$) ions and releases three sodium (Na$^+$) ions.

solute The dissolved particles contained in the solvent.

solution Combination of dissolved elements (solutes) and water (solvent).

solvent The fluid that does the dissolving, or the solution that contains the dissolved components.

standing orders A form of off-line or indirect medical control, in which the paramedic performs certain predefined procedures before contacting the physician.

sterile The destruction of all living organisms; achieved by using heat, gas, or chemicals.

subcutaneous (SC) Into the tissue between the skin and muscle; a medication delivery route.

sublingual Under the tongue; a medication delivery route.

syncopal episodes Fainting; brief losses of consciousness caused by transiently inadequate blood flow to the brain.

systemic complications Reactions that affect systems of the body.

third spacing The shifting of fluid into the tissues, creating edema.

thrombophlebitis Inflammation of a vein.

through-the-needle catheters Plastic catheters inserted through a hollow needle; referred to as Intracaths.

tonicity The osmotic pressure of a solution, based on the relationship between sodium and water inside and outside the cell, that takes advantage of their chemical and osmotic properties to move water to areas of higher sodium concentration.

total body water (TBW) Total amount of water in the human body; accounts for approximately 60% of the weight of an average man; divided into various compartments.

track marks The visible scars from repeated cannulation of a vein; commonly associated with illicit drug use.

transdermal Across the skin; a medication delivery route.

tubules Sections of the kidney where the filtration of wastes, electrolytes, and water is controlled.

Vacutainer A cylindrical device that attaches to an 18- or 20-gauge sampling needle; accommodates self-sealing blood tubes when obtaining blood samples.

venous thrombosis The development of a stationary blood clot in the venous circulation.

vials Small glass or plastic bottles that contain medication; may contain single or multiple doses.

Volutrol A special type of microdrip set that features a 100- or 200-mL calibrated drip chamber; used for fluid regulation in patients prone to circulatory overload, such as pediatric and elderly patients; also called a Buretrol.

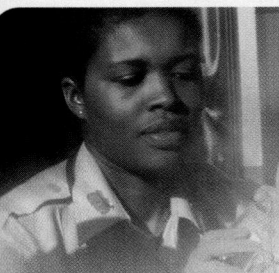

Assessment in Action

You and your partner are dispatched to an apartment complex because of a possible overdose. Law enforcement personnel are already present and radio you that the scene is secure. When you enter the apartment, you find the patient, a 30-year-old man, unconscious on the couch. With the assistance of law enforcement personnel, you and your partner quickly move the patient to the floor and perform an initial assessment. The patient has sonorous respirations and a slow, weak radial pulse. There is no gross bleeding or evidence of trauma.

1. How will you treat this patient initially?
   A. Apply oxygen via nonrebreathing mask.
   B. Suction his oropharynx for 15 seconds.
   C. Provide bag-mask ventilation and 100% oxygen.
   D. Manually open his airway and insert an airway adjunct.

2. Your EMT-B partner assesses the patient's respirations and notes that they are slow and shallow. What should you direct him to do?
   A. Apply a nonrebreathing mask set at 15 L/min.
   B. Provide bag-mask ventilation and 100% oxygen.
   C. Assess the patient's oxygen saturation with a pulse oximeter.
   D. Help you prepare to perform immediate endotracheal intubation.

3. Following additional assessment of the patient, you suspect a narcotic overdose. While your partner continues to manage the patient's airway, you prepare to establish vascular access. Which of the following statements regarding vascular access is MOST correct?
   A. You should immediately insert an IO catheter into the patient's proximal tibia.
   B. External jugular vein cannulation is preferred when patients are deeply unconscious.
   C. 5% dextrose in water (D_5W) is the fluid of choice for patients who may require volume expansion.
   D. The antecubital vein is the preferred vein to use when starting an IV on a critically ill or injured patient.

4. Which of the following IV catheters will allow you to deliver the greatest amount of volume in the *shortest* period?
   A. 14-gauge, 1¼″ catheter
   B. 14-gauge, 2¼″ catheter
   C. 16-gauge, 1½″ catheter
   D. 18-gauge, 2¼″ catheter

5. Vascular access has been obtained. Your protocols call for the administration of naloxone (Narcan) in a dose of 2 mg. You have a prefilled syringe of naloxone that contains 10 mg in 5 mL. How many milliliters of naloxone will you administer to achieve the desired dose of 2 mg?
   A. 1 mL
   B. 2 mL
   C. 3 mL
   D. 4 mL

6. Compared with medications administered via the enteral route, parenteral medications:
   A. must be instilled through a gastric tube.
   B. can be delivered only by the IV route.
   C. do not pass through the gastrointestinal tract.
   D. reach the central circulation at a much slower rate.

7. Which of the following medication routes has the *slowest* rate of absorption?
   A. Intravenous
   B. Transdermal
   C. Subcutaneous
   D. Intramuscular

8. **Shortly after administering naloxone to your patient, the IV line infiltrates. You obtain a blood glucose reading of 40 mg/dL and must administer glucagon via the IM route. However, glucagon must be reconstituted before being administered. What does drug reconstitution involve?**
   A. Administration of the drug during a period of at least 5 seconds
   B. Delivering the medication in the form of a maintenance infusion
   C. Diluting the drug with at least 5 mL of normal saline or sterile water
   D. Adding diluent to the powdered form of the drug to make a solution

Challenging Questions

A 54-year-old male is found unconscious in his home by a close friend. The patient is unresponsive, breathing slowly and shallowly, and is bradycardic. As your partner begins ventilation assistance with a bag-mask device and 100% oxygen, you find a bottle of hydrocodone—a potent narcotic analgesic—on an adjacent table. The prescription was filled 2 days prior and is now empty. According to the friend, the patient recently had bilateral knee replacements, and was prescribed the medication for pain relief. He further states that the patient has "emotional problems." Recognizing that the patient will require naloxone (Narcan), you attempt to establish a peripheral IV line, but are unsuccessful after several attempts. Your partner reports that she is not having difficulty with bag-mask ventilation.

9. **Should you intubate this patient?**

10. **What alternate medication routes are available to administer the Narcan?**

Points to Ponder

You and your partner are treating a 35-year-old man with a headache. The patient is conscious and alert and denies chest pain or shortness of breath. His blood pressure is 130/84 mm Hg, heart rate is 44 beats/min and regular, and respirations are 16 breaths/min and unlabored. Further assessment reveals that the patient's skin is pink, warm, and dry, and his lungs are clear to auscultation bilaterally. The cardiac monitor reveals sinus bradycardia at 40 beats/min.

An IV line is established and set at a keep vein open (KVO) rate. As you are obtaining the patient's medical history, your paramedic partner administers 1 mg of atropine sulfate to the patient. Following administration of the atropine, the patient experiences tachycardia at a rate of 130 beats/min and becomes anxious and nauseous. However, his symptoms have resolved by the time you arrive at the hospital.

Analyze this situation and explain what happened.

Issues: Recognizing a Patient in Stable Versus Unstable Condition, Understanding the Need to Verify the "Six Rights" of Medication Administration, Documenting and Reporting a Medication Error.

9 Human Development

Objectives

Cognitive

1-10.1   Compare the physiological and psychosocial characteristics of an infant with those of an early adult. (p 9.3)

1-10.2   Compare the physiological and psychosocial characteristics of a toddler with those of an early adult. (p 9.7)

1-10.3   Compare the physiological and psychosocial characteristics of a pre-school child with those of an early adult. (p 9.7)

1-10.4   Compare the physiological and psychosocial characteristics of a school-aged child with those of an early adult. (p 9.8)

1-10.5   Compare the physiological and psychosocial characteristics of an adolescent with those of an early adult. (p 9.9)

1-10.6   Summarize the physiological and psychosocial characteristics of an early adult. (p 9.10)

1-10.7   Compare the physiological and psychosocial characteristics of a middle aged adult with those of an early adult. (p 9.10)

1-10.8   Compare the physiological and psychosocial characteristics of a person in late adulthood with those of an early adult. (p 9.11)

Affective

1-10.9   Value the uniqueness of infants, toddlers, pre-school, school aged, adolescent, early adulthood, middle aged, and late adulthood physiological and psychosocial characteristics. (p 9.3–9.13)

Psychomotor

None

Introduction

One of the most interesting things about humans is that we evolve—not just as a species, but also as people over our life span. Paramedics must be aware of both the obvious and subtle changes that a person undergoes physically and mentally at various stages of life and understand how these changes might alter the approach to patient care.

Infants

As any parent can attest, infants (1 month to 1 year) develop at a startling rate [Figure 9-1 ▶]. Neonates (birth to 1 month) are covered in detail in Chapter 40: *Neonatology*.

Physical Changes

Vital Signs

[Table 9-1 ▶] lists the normal ranges of vital signs for various age groups. The younger the person, the faster the pulse rate and respirations. At birth, a pulse rate of 90 to 180 beats/min and a respiratory rate of 30 to 60 breaths/min are considered normal. After about a half hour, an infant's heart rate often drops to around 120 beats/min and the respiratory rate adjusts to between 30 to 40 breaths/min. Tidal volume in infants starts at 6 to 8 mL/kg. By age 1 year, the volume increases to 10 to 15 mL/kg.

Blood pressure directly corresponds to the patient's weight, so it typically increases with age. At birth, the average systolic blood pressure of an infant is 50 to 70 mm Hg. By 1 year of age, it is in the range of 70 to 95 mm Hg.

Weight

An infant usually weighs 6½ to 8 lb (3 to 3.5 kg) at birth. After birth, infants usually lose 5% to 10% of their birth weight due to the loss of fluid in the first week. Then they normally gain weight in their second week of life. From here on, infants grow at a rate of about 30 g per day, doubling their weight by 4 to 6 months and tripling it by age 1 year.

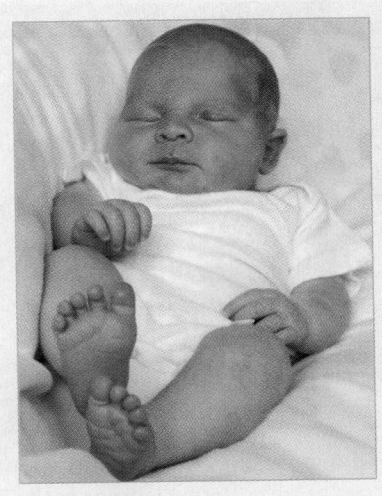
Figure 9-1 An infant.

Cardiovascular System

Prior to birth, fetal circulation occurs through the placenta, which is connected to the ductus venosus and ductus arteriosus. Just after birth, the ductus venosus constricts and closes.

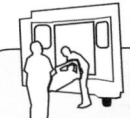
In the Field

Infants often land head first when they fall because their heads account for 25% of their total body weight. Also, most infants cannot stretch out their arms in time to cushion or slow their fall. Keep this point in mind when considering spinal immobilization on an infant.

You are the Provider Part 1

You and your partner have just finished checking your rig when you hear the dispatcher: "Ambulance 5281, respond to 1425 Washington Avenue for a 16-year-old female complaining of abdominal pain."

When you arrive at the residence, you are greeted by an anxious man who introduces himself as the patient's father. While holding his terrified and screaming 2-year-old son, he cries, "My daughter's upstairs in her bedroom with her mom. I think her appendix burst!" Upon entering the patient's bedroom, you introduce yourself and see the patient curled in a fetal position on the floor, writhing in pain and complaining of nausea. She moans, "My stomach hurts, please help me!" You begin your initial assessment of the patient as her parents watch intently over your shoulder.

Initial Assessment	Recording Time: 0 Minutes
Appearance	Fetal position, obvious distress
Level of consciousness	A (Alert to person, place, and day)
Airway	Open
Breathing	24 breaths/min and adequate
Circulation	Strong radial pulses at 118 beats/min, no external bleeding

1. What are your differential diagnoses given the information provided?
2. How would you approach your patient interview?
3. What could explain the slightly elevated patient respirations and pulse?

Table 9-1	Vital Signs at Various Ages			
Age	Pulse Rate (beats/min)	Respirations (breaths/min)	Blood Pressure (mm Hg)	Temperature (°F)
Newborn (0 to 1 month)	90 to 180	30 to 60	50 to 70	98 to 100
Infant (1 month to 1 year)	100 to 160	25 to 50	70 to 95	96.8 to 99.6
Toddler (1 to 3 years)	90 to 150	20 to 30	80 to 100	96.8 to 99.6
Preschool age (3 to 6 years)	80 to 140	20 to 25	80 to 100	98.6
School age (6 to 12 years)	70 to 120	15 to 20	80 to 110	98.6
Adolescent (12 to 18 years)	60 to 100	12 to 16	90 to 110	98.6
Early adult (19 to 40 years)	70	12 to 20	90 to 140	98.6
Middle adult (41 to 60 years)	70	12 to 20	90 to 140	98.6
Late adult (61 and older)	Depends on health	Depends on health	Depends on health	98.6

As a consequence, the infant's blood pressure changes, and the foramen ovale, an opening in the septum of the heart, closes. The ductus arteriosus also constricts and closes, resulting in circulation through the pulmonary system and the veins and arteries (rather than through the placenta) as well as increased vascular resistance and decreased pulmonary resistance **Figure 9-2 ▶**.

Pulmonary System

Prior to an infant's first breath, the lungs have never been inflated. An infant's first breath is therefore forceful—it has to be!

Infants are primarily "nose breathers" for the first month of their lives. Infants younger than 6 months are particularly prone to nasal congestion, which can cause viral upper respiratory infections. If you receive a call for a baby choking, always make sure the infant's nasal passages are clear and unobstructed by mucus.

The rib cages of infants are less rigid than those of older humans, and the ribs sit horizontally. This explains the diaphragmatic breathing ("belly breathing") in infants.

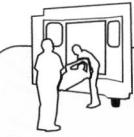

In the Field

When you are counting respirations in an infant, count the number of times the abdomen rises instead of concentrating solely on the chest rise.

Two other important anatomic points related to an infant's airway, when compared with an adult's, are the proportionally large size of the tongue and the proportionally shorter and narrower airway. As a result of these factors, infants can much more easily occlude their airway than older children or adults can.

In the Field

Keep the infant's unique airway anatomy in mind when you are selecting an appropriate upper airway adjunct, the proper advanced airway, and the most appropriate sized endotracheal tube.

When providing bag-mask ventilations to an infant, you need to be aware that an infant's lungs are fragile. Ventilations that are too forceful can result in trauma from pressure, or barotrauma.

Renal System

Infants can become easily dehydrated because their kidneys usually cannot produce concentrated urine. An infant's urine consists mainly of water, which can cause the child to develop electrolyte imbalances.

Immune System

While in the womb, infants collect antibodies from the maternal blood. For the first year of life, the infant maintains some of the mother's immunities, so he or she has naturally acquired passive immunities. Infants can also receive antibodies via breastfeeding, further bolstering their immune system.

Nervous System

Although the infant's nervous system is developed at birth, its evolution continues after birth. For example, the newborn lacks the ability to localize and isolate a particular response to sensation. Motor and sensory development are most developed in the cranial nerves, which control blinking, sucking, and gag reflexes.

An infant is born with certain reflexes. The moro reflex (startle reflex) happens when an infant is caught off guard by something or someone; the infant opens his or her arms wide, spreads the fingers, and seems to grab at things. A palmar grasp occurs when an object is placed into the infant's palm. The rooting reflex takes place when something touches an infant's cheek; the infant will instinctively turn his or her head toward the touch. In conjunction with the sucking reflex, which occurs when an infant's lips are stroked, these reflexes are often tested when feeding.

An infant's fontanelles allow the head to be molded **Figure 9-3 ▶** —for example, when the newborn passes through the birth canal. These three or four bones of the skull eventually bind together and form suture joints within 18 months of birth. If the anterior fontanelle is sunken, the infant is most likely dehydrated.

Perhaps the neurologic development that is of most interest to parents is the development of a sleep pattern. Some

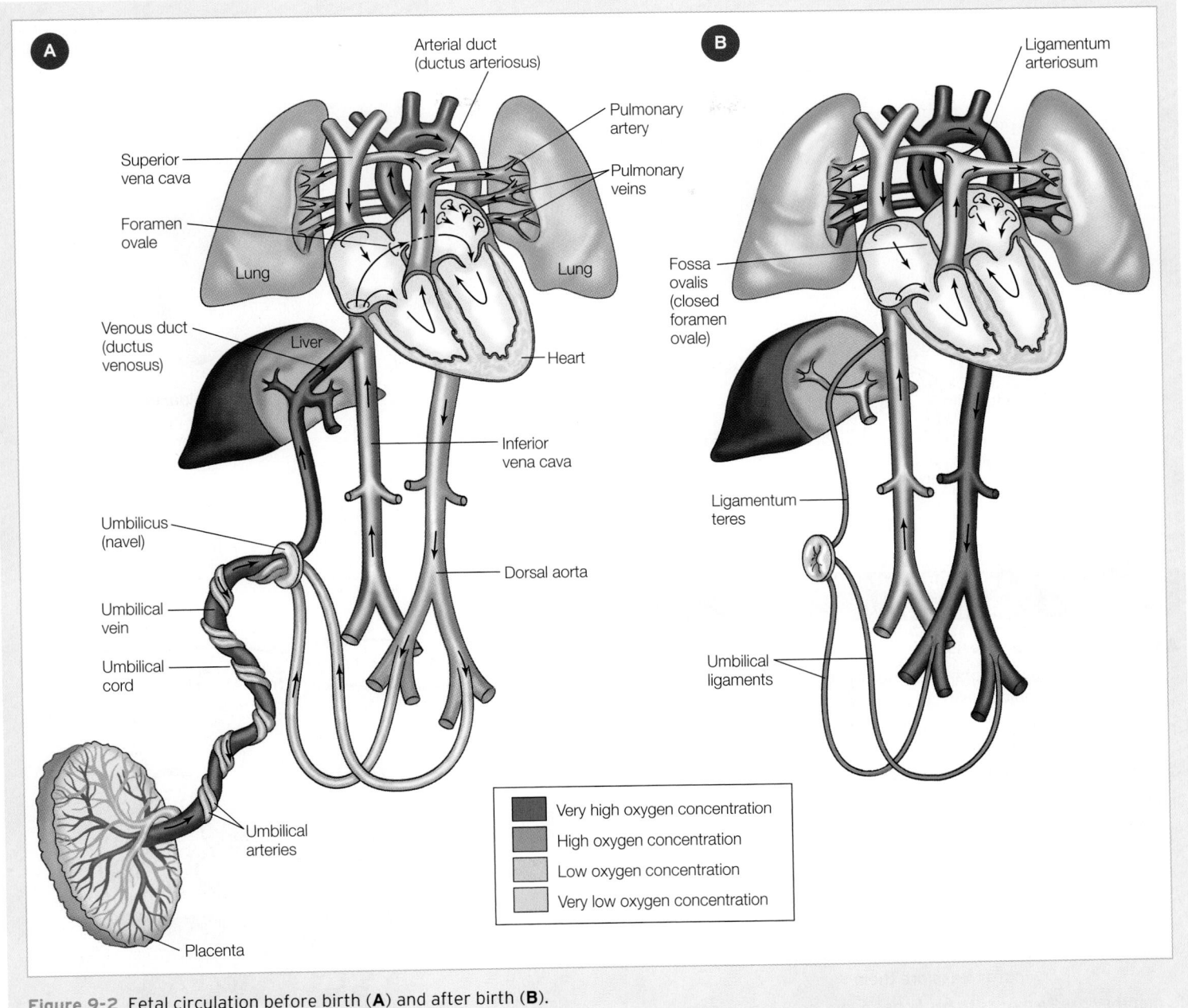

Figure 9-2 Fetal circulation before birth (**A**) and after birth (**B**).

physicians suggest that parents wake infants every few hours for both feeding and safety (eg, to guard against sudden infant death syndrome [SIDS]). Others suggest that infants should be left to sleep so that they can adjust to family life and develop a circadian rhythm, ideally within 4 months after birth. (For more information on SIDS, see Chapter 41.)

Musculoskeletal System

Growth plates, located on either end of an infant's bone, aid in lengthening a child's bones. Epiphyseal plates, or secondary bone-growing plates, are also present. Bones grow in thickness by building on themselves. In contrast, an infant's muscles account for approximately 25% of his or her total weight.

Psychosocial Changes

An infant's psychosocial development begins at birth and continues to evolve as the infant interacts with and reacts to the environment. Parents often obsess about whether their child is developing within the socially accepted norms. **Table 9-2** ▶ outlines typical ages at which major psychosocial changes are noticed.

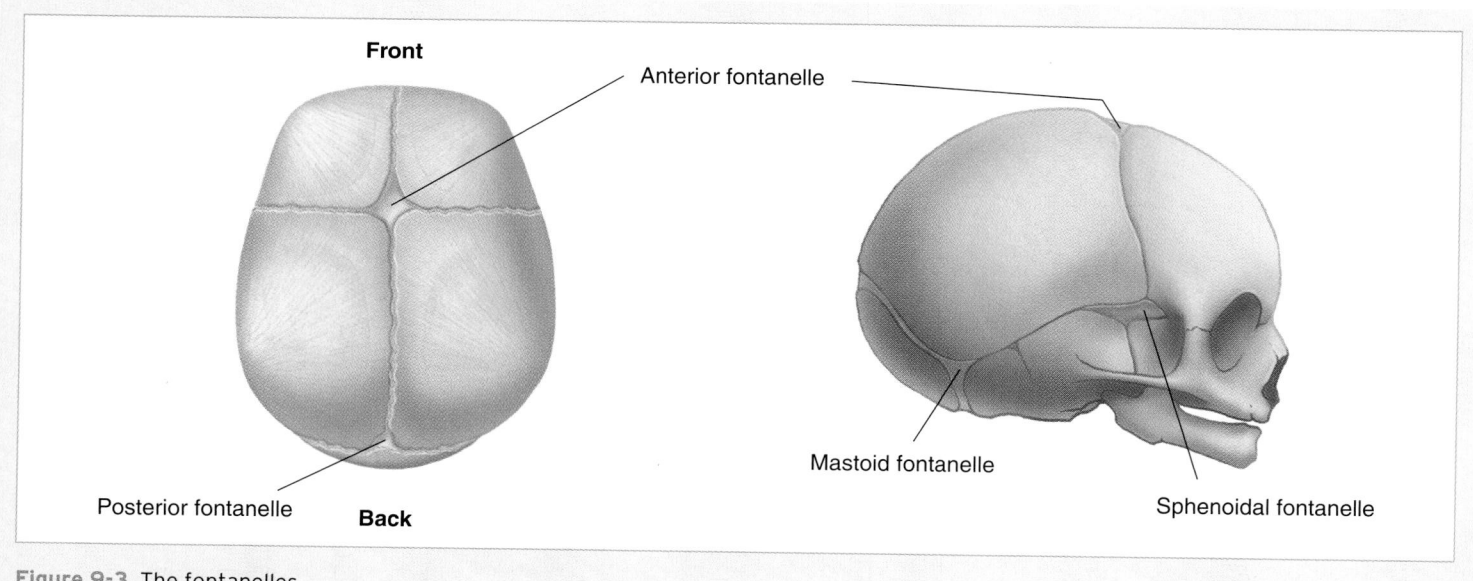

Figure 9-3 The fontanelles.

Table 9-2	Noticeable Characteristics at Various Ages	
Age	**Characteristic**	
2 months	Can recognize familiar faces; able to track objects with the eyes	
3 months	Can bring objects to the mouth; can smile and frown	
4 months	Reaches out to people; drools	
5 months	Sleeps through the night; can tell family from strangers	
6 months	Teething begins, sits upright in a chair, one-syllable words spoken	
7 months	Afraid of strangers, mood swings	
8 months	Responds to "no"; can sit alone; plays peek-a-boo	
9 months	Pulls himself or herself up; places objects in mouth to explore them	
10 months	Responds to his or her name; crawls efficiently	
11 months	Starts to walk without help; frustrated with restrictions	
12 months	Knows his or her name; can walk	

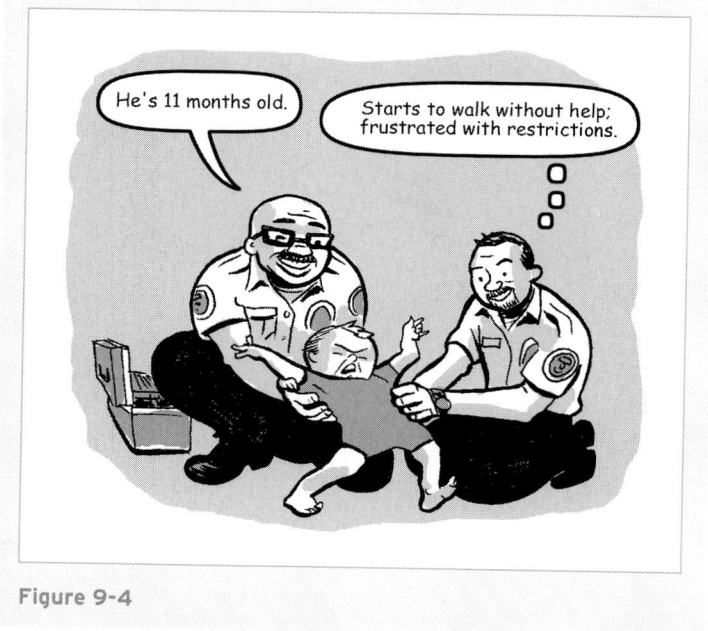

Figure 9-4

In most infants, the primary method of communicating distress is through crying **Figure 9-4 ▶** . Parents can often tell what is upsetting their child simply by listening to the tone of the child's crying—that is, they know the difference between tears for anger, frustration, pain, fear, hunger, discomfort, and sleepiness. Infants occasionally make another distinct cry—an alarming distressed cry. This cry may be heard when an unexpected event occurs, causing a situational crisis for the infant.

The key to having a happy, healthy infant is spending time with the child. Nevertheless, infants often have their own timetable as to when they will become attached to their parents and other family members. Bonding, or the formation of a close, personal relationship, is usually based on a secure attachment. A secure attachment occurs when an infant understands that parents or caregivers will be responsive to his or her needs. This realization encourages a child to reach out and explore, knowing that his or her parents will provide a "safety net."

Another type of attachment, referred to as <u>anxious avoidant attachment</u>, is observed in infants who are repeatedly rejected. These children develop an isolated lifestyle where they do not have to depend on the support and care of others.

<u>Trust and mistrust</u> refers to a stage of development from birth to about 18 months of age. Most infants desire that their world be planned, organized, and routine. When their caregivers and parents provide this environment for them, the infant gains trust in those individuals. The opposite also holds true Figure 9-5 .

Toddlers and Preschoolers

Physical Changes

In <u>toddlers</u> (ages 1 to 3 years Figure 9-6) and <u>preschoolers</u> (ages 3 to 6 years Figure 9-7), the heart rate and respiratory rate are slower than the corresponding vital signs in infants, whereas the systolic blood pressure is higher (approximately 100 mm Hg). At the same time, weight gain should level off.

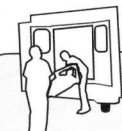

In the Field

When dealing with patients who are very young, try to keep their routine the same by keeping family and familiar items nearby.

A toddler's cardiovascular system isn't dramatically different from that of an adult. A toddler's lungs continue to develop more bronchioles and alveoli. Although toddlers and preschoolers have more lung tissue, they do not have well-developed lung musculature. This anomaly prevents them from sustaining deep or rapid respirations for an extended period of time.

The loss of passive immunity in the immune system is possibly the most obvious development at this stage of human life. "Colds" often develop that may manifest as gastrointestinal distress or upper respiratory tract infections. As toddlers spend

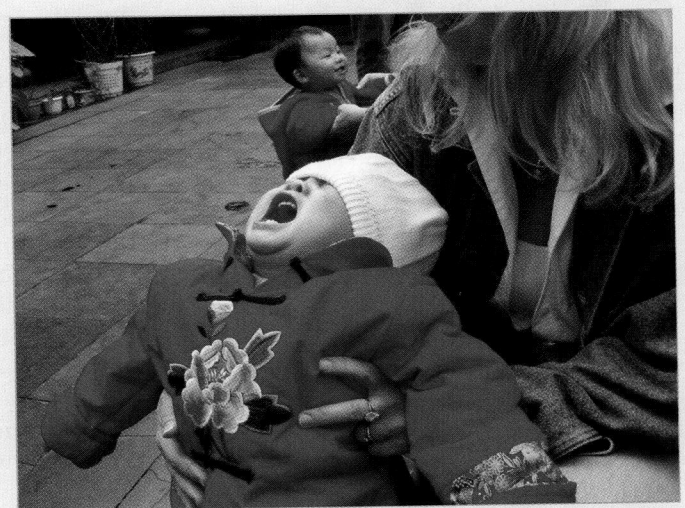

Figure 9-5 If an infant perceives that his or her parents or caregivers will not provide an organized, routine environment, the infant can develop behavioral problems.

You are the Provider Part 2

You apply supplemental high-flow oxygen to your patient, place her in a position of comfort, and begin your focused assessment and history. Your assessment reveals right-sided lower abdominal pain rated as 9 on a 10-point scale, with radiation to the back and groin. You continue to ask your patient questions about her history. Her father provides answers about her prior knee surgery a few years ago, and the fact that she takes fexofenadine and albuterol for her allergies and asthma.

When you ask the patient about her last menstrual period, you discover that she is taking extended-cycle birth control pills for regulation of her menstrual cycle and that her last period was a little less than 2 months ago. Per her medication schedule, her next menstrual period is due in about a month and a half. When you ask the patient whether there is any chance she may be pregnant, she adamantly denies the possibility, and her father is insulted that you would ask such a question.

Assessment	Recording Time: 10 Minutes
Skin	Pale, warm, and moist
Pulse	118 beats/min
Blood pressure	130/88 mm Hg
Respirations	24 breaths/min
Sao$_2$	100% on 15 L/min nonrebreathing mask on supplemental oxygen

4. What are your differential diagnoses now?
5. What is your next step in treatment of this patient?
6. Do you allow the parent to ride in the compartment of the ambulance along with the patient?

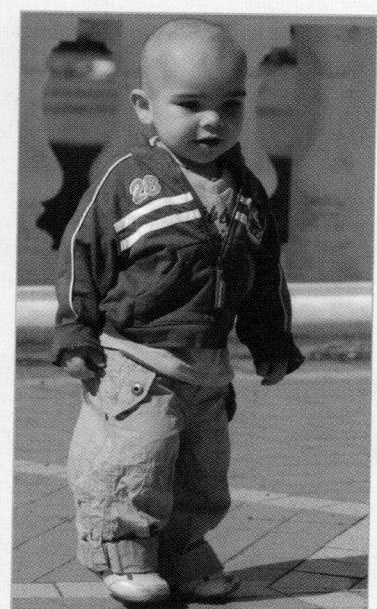

Figure 9-6 A toddler.

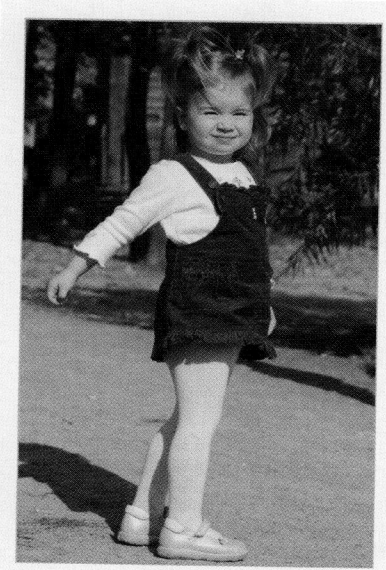

Figure 9-7 A preschooler.

more time around play-mates and classmates, they acquire their own immunity as the body is exposed to various viruses and germs.

Neuromuscular growth also makes considerable progress at this age. Toddlers and preschoolers spend a great deal of time finding out exactly how to use their expansive nervous system and the muscles it controls by walking, running, jumping, and playing catch **Figure 9-8 ▶** . This stage also includes the continued development of the renal system and of elimination patterns (ie, toilet training).

Other developments that occur during this time frame include the emergence of "baby" teeth. Teething (ie, "breaking teeth" through the gums) can be painful and accompanied by fever. In addition, parents and toddlers are enthralled with sensory development—for example, tickling.

Psychosocial Changes

This period of development is often exciting for parents. The toddler or preschooler is learning to speak and express himself or herself, thereby taking a major step toward independence. By the age of 3 or 4 years,

most children can use and understand full sentences. As they progress through this stage of their life, they will go from using language to communicate what they want, to using language creatively and playfully.

This is also the time when toddlers begin to interact with other play-mates and start to play games. Playing games teaches control, following of rules, and even competitiveness. A lot of learning and development takes place by the child watching his or her peers during group outings, such as "play dates" with other children. Of course, behavior observed on television and computers can also be learned, which is why some parents limit their children's viewing choices or the amount of time they devote to these activities. During this phase of development, children also learn to recognize sexual differences by observing their role models.

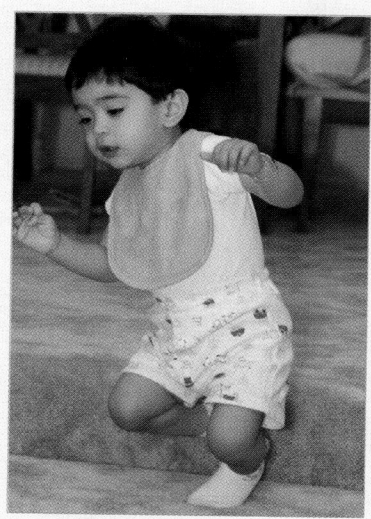

Figure 9-8 Toddlers learn to walk, one of the major milestones in life.

School-Age Children

Physical Changes

From ages 6 to 12 years, a school-age child's vital signs and body gradually approach those observed in adulthood **Figure 9-9 ▶** . Obvious physical traits and body function changes become apparent as most children grow about 4 lb (2 kg) and 2½" (6 cm) each year. Their permanent teeth also come in during this period.

Psychosocial Changes

Children are engaged in a lot of psychosocial growing up during the school years. Parents as a whole do not devote as much time to their

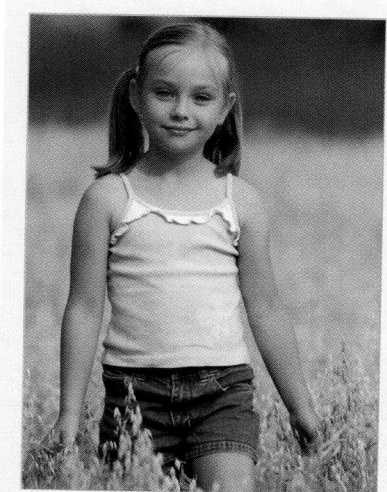

Figure 9-9 A school-age child.

In the Field

With toddlers and preschoolers, you might try to "break the ice" by giving them a teddy bear and explaining what you are going to do by showing them on the teddy bear. Such children may be able to understand by show-and-tell more clearly than using only a verbal description.

children during this phase. Nevertheless, it is at this critical time in human development that children learn various types of reasoning. In preconventional reasoning, children act almost purely to avoid punishment and to get what they want. In conventional reasoning, they look for approval from their peers and society. In postconventional reasoning, children make decisions guided by their conscience.

During this stage, children begin to develop their self-concept and self-esteem. Self-concept is our perception of ourselves; self-esteem is how we feel about ourselves and how we "fit in" with our peers.

Adolescents (Teenagers)

Physical Changes

The vital signs of adolescents (ages 12 to 18 years Figure 9-10 ▾) begin to level off within the adult ranges, with

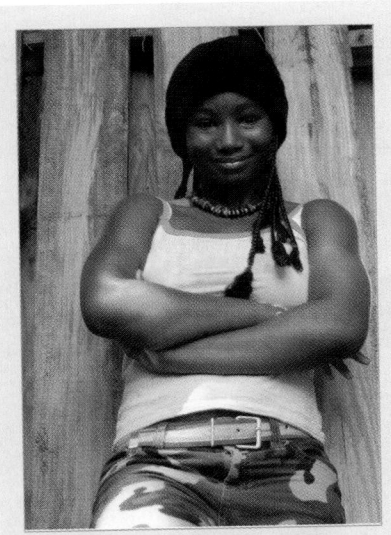

Figure 9-10 An adolescent.

a systolic blood pressure generally between 90 and 110 mm Hg, a pulse rate between 60 and 100 beats/min, and respirations in the range of 12 to 16 breaths/min. Adolescence is also the time of life when humans experience a growth spurt (ie, an increase in muscle and bone growth) and blood changes. As a whole, boys experience this stage of development later in life than girls do. When this period of growth has finished, however, boys are generally taller and stronger than girls.

One of the more subtle changes during this phase of life is the maturation of the human reproductive system. Secondary sexual development begins, along with enlargement of the external sex organs. Pubic hair and axillary hair begin to appear. Voices start to change in range and depth. In females, the breasts and thighs increase in size as adipose tissue is deposited there. Menstruation begins during this time; menarche is starting to occur at increasingly younger ages, however, so it is not uncommon to begin menstruation prior to becoming a teenager. Another key development in female teenagers is the release of follicle-stimulating hormone and luteinizing hormone, both of which increase estrogen and progesterone production. In contrast, the hormone gonadotropin is secreted in males and results in the production of testosterone. Acne can occur due to hormonal changes.

Psychosocial Changes

Adolescents and their families often deal with conflict as teenagers try to gain control of their lives from their parents. Privacy becomes an issue among adolescents, their siblings, and their parents. Adolescents may struggle to create their own identity—to define who they are Figure 9-11 ▾ . They may also show greater interest in sexual relations. Many adolescents

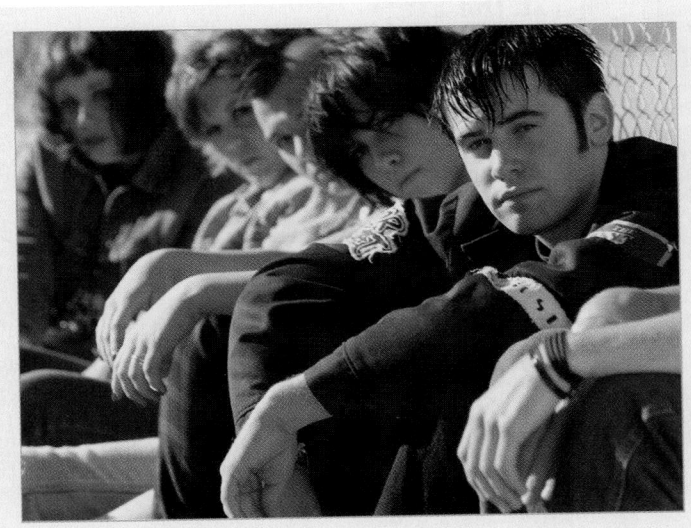

Figure 9-11 Adolescents want to fit in and may struggle to create an identity.

You are the Provider Part 3

You and your partner load your frightened patient into the back of your ambulance and begin the 20-minute transport to the local hospital. You asked the father to ride in the cab of the ambulance, telling him that he'd be safer there.

Once you are in the back of the ambulance, you ask the patient again about her sexual activity and the possibility of pregnancy, reminding her that it is important to her health that you know the truth. She confides in you that she is sexually active and that she missed taking a couple of her birth control pills in the past few months. She says, "I'm freaking out. I think I'm pregnant and my dad's going to kill me!" You try to calm the patient and continue to provide care, including the initiation of an IV line. At the hospital, you give your report to the emergency department nurse and your partner shows the patient's father to the waiting area.

7. What is your primary differential diagnosis now?

8. Did this diagnosis alter your care?

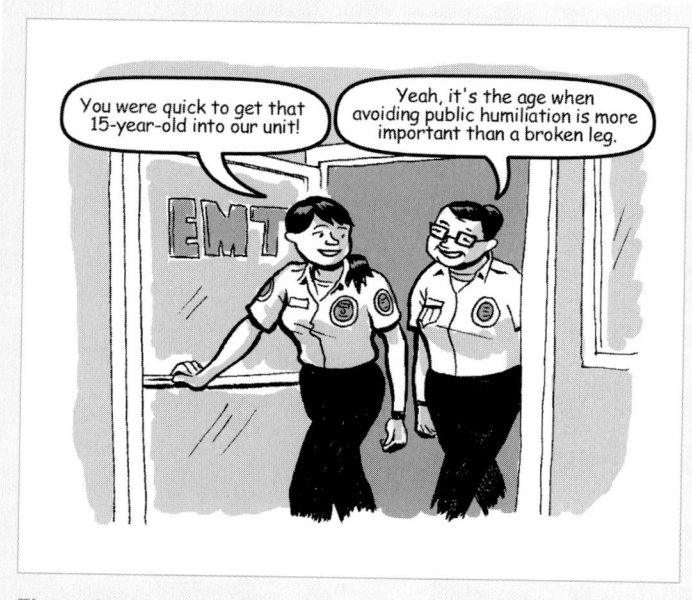

You were quick to get that 15-year-old into our unit!

Yeah, it's the age when avoiding public humiliation is more important than a broken leg.

Figure 9-12

In the Field

When you interview adolescents in the presence of their family, they may not tell you the complete truth so as to protect their privacy or image. It is best to ask these patients certain questions in total privacy, where they feel they can answer without constraint.

are fixated on their public image and are terrified of being embarrassed **Figure 9-12 ▲**. At this age, a code of personal ethics is developed, based partly on parents' ethics and values and partly on the influence of the teenager's environment. At this tumultuous time, teenagers are at a higher risk than other populations for suicide and depression.

■ Early Adults

Physical Changes

Early adults range in age from 19 to 40 years **Figure 9-13 ▶**. Their vital signs do not vary greatly from those seen throughout adulthood. Ideally, the human heart rate will stay around 70 beats/min, the respiratory rate will stay in the range of 12 to 20 breaths/min, and the systolic blood pressure will be approximately 120/80 mm Hg.

From age 19 years to just a little after 25 years, the human body should be functioning at its optimal level. After this point, the disks in the spine begin to settle, and height can sometimes be affected, causing a "shrinking." Fatty tissue increases, which leads to weight gain. Muscle strength

decreases, and the reflexes slow. For all these reasons, accidents are common causes of death in this age group.

Psychosocial Changes

Three words best describe a human's world during this stage of life: work, family, stress. During this period, humans strive to create a place for themselves in the world, and many do everything they can to "settle down." Along with this natural tendency to settle comes

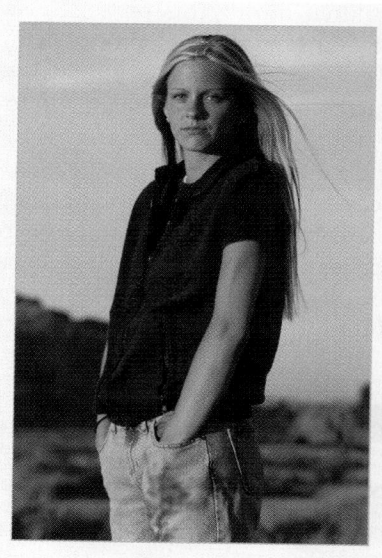

Figure 9-13 An early adult.

love and childbirth. Despite all of this stress and change, this age group enjoys one of the more stable periods of life.

■ Middle Adults

Physical Changes

Middle adults are ages 41 to 60 years **Figure 9-14 ▼**. This group is vulnerable to vision and hearing loss. Cardiovascular health also becomes an issue in many of these individuals, as does the greater incidence of cancer. In women, menopause— the cessation of menstruation—begins in the late 40s or early 50s.

Psychosocial Changes

Middle adults tend to focus on achieving their life's goals, as they realize that they are approaching the halfway point in human life expectancy. At this point, many parents must cope with becoming a married couple

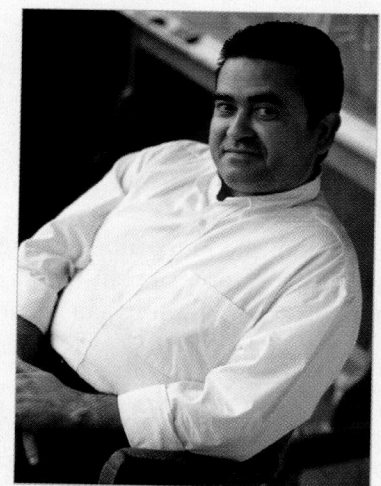

Figure 9-14 A middle adult.

again and reprioritize their lives as their children leave the home, creating "empty nest" syndrome. Finances may become a worrisome issue, as people look forward to retirement and experience small crisis moments. The term *mid-life crisis* describes a person who makes a dramatic gesture in a bid to

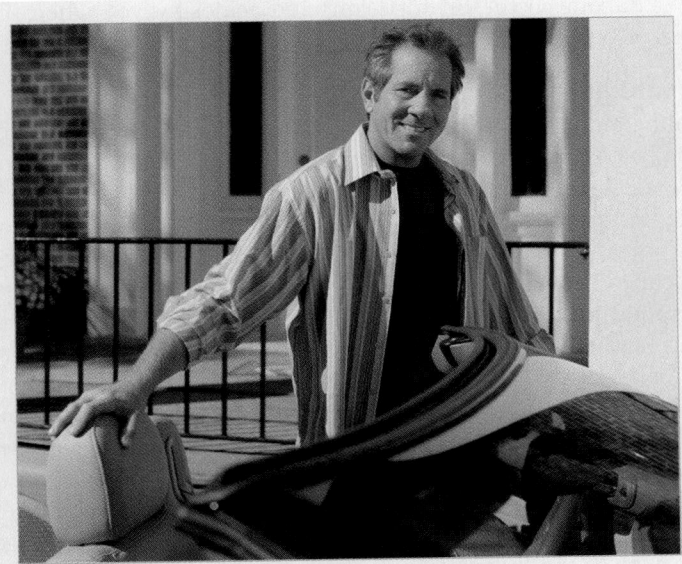

Figure 9-15 The classic example of the mid-life crisis is the middle-age man who buys a fancy, expensive sports car!

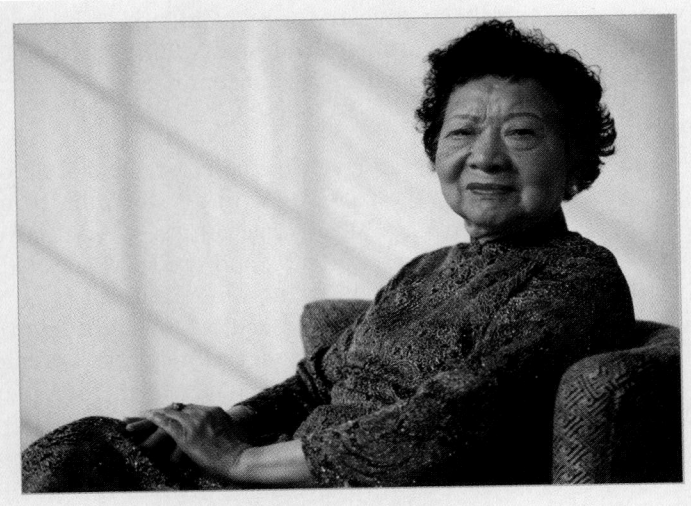

Figure 9-16 A late adult.

reclaim his or her youth. The classic example is the 45-year-old father of three who buys a bright red, two-seat convertible sports car Figure 9-15 ▲ .

Late Adults

Physical Changes

Late adults include those ages 61 and older Figure 9-16 ▲ . Life expectancy is constantly changing. When the first edition of this text was printed in 1979, life expectancy was about 73 years. It is approximately 77 years at this time, with maximum life expectancy estimated at 120 years.

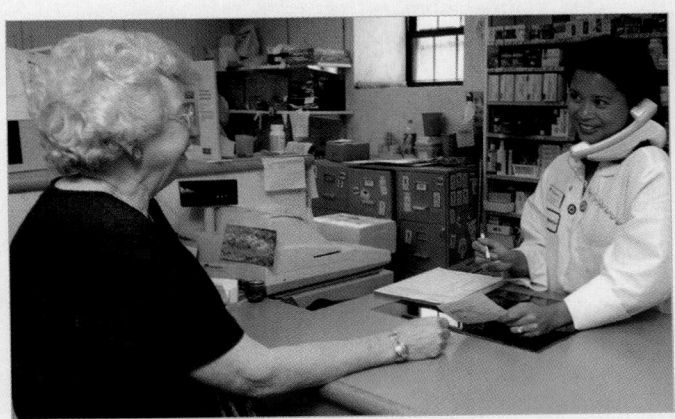

Figure 9-17 Older people are often on multiple medications to help them stay active.

Later in life, the vital signs depend on the patient's overall health, medical conditions, and medications taken. Today's late adults are staying active longer than their ancestors. Thanks to medical advances, they are often able to overcome numerous medical problems, but may need multiple medications to do so Figure 9-17 ▲ .

Cardiovascular System

Cardiac function declines with age consequent to anatomic and physiologic changes that are largely related to atherosclerosis. In this disorder, which most commonly affects coronary vessels, cholesterol and calcium build up inside the walls of blood vessels, forming plaque. The accumulation of plaque eventually leads to partial or complete blockage of blood flow. Atherosclerosis can also contribute to development of an aneurysm, or weakening and bulging of the blood vessel wall; an aneurysm may potentially rupture if it is subjected to high stretching forces. More than 60% of people older than age 65 have atherosclerotic disease.

Other age-related changes typically include a decrease in heart rate, a decline in cardiac output (the amount of blood circulated each minute), and the inability to elevate cardiac output to match the demands of the body. The vascular system also becomes stiff. For example, the pressure of systole increases with age. The left ventricle must then work harder, so it becomes thicker, losing its elasticity in this process. The thickening and stiffening of this muscle hinders filling in the ventricle, thereby decreasing cardiac output. Similar stiffening occurs in the heart valves, which may impede normal blood flow into and out of the heart. As the blood passes through these stiffened valves, a heart murmur may be heard, even in the absence of disease. Decreases in elastin and collagen in blood vessel walls, in turn, reduce the elasticity of the peripheral vessels by as much as 70%. Compensation for blood pressure changes will be hampered because these vessels are less able to distend and contract.

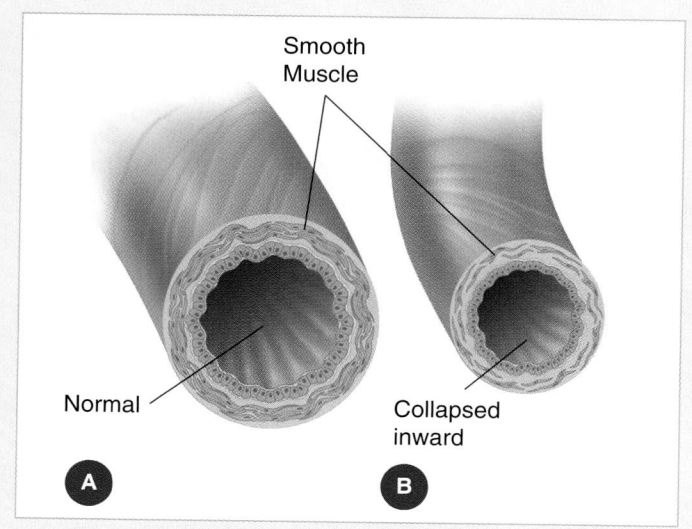

Figure 9-18 A. Healthy muscle in a younger patient's airway helps maintain the open airway during the pressures of inhalation. **B.** Muscle weakening with age can lead to airway collapse that may produce wheezing.

Respiratory System

In late adults, the size of the airway increases and the surface area of the alveoli decreases. The natural elasticity of the lungs also decreases, forcing them to use their intercostal muscles more to breathe. In addition, the chest becomes more rigid because of calcification of the ribs to the sternum, which adds to the difficulty breathing.

The loss of the mechanisms that protect the upper airway can include a decreased ability to clear secretions as well as decreased cough and gag reflexes. The cilia that line the airways diminish with age, while the innervation of the structures in the airway provides increasingly less sensation. Without the ability to maintain the upper airway, aspiration and obstruction become more likely.

When a younger patient inhales, the airway maintains its shape, allowing air to enter. As the smooth muscles of the lower airway weaken with age, strong inhalation can make the walls of the airway collapse inward and cause inspiratory wheezing (**Figure 9-18 ▲**). The collapsing airways result in low flow rates, because less air can move through the smaller airways, and air trapping, because air does not completely exit the alveoli (incomplete expiration).

By age 75 years, the vital capacity (the volume of air moved during the deepest inspiration and expiration) may amount to only 50% of the vital capacity noted in young adulthood. Factors contributing to this decline include loss of respiratory muscle mass, increased stiffness of the thoracic cage, and decreased surface area available for the exchange of air.

Physiologically, vital capacity decreases and residual volume (the amount of air left in the lungs after expiration of the maximum possible amount of air) increases with age. As a consequence, stagnant air remains in the alveoli and hampers gas exchange. This effect can produce hypercarbia (increased car-

bon dioxide in the bloodstream) and acidosis, even when the person is at rest.

Renal and Gastric Systems

In the kidneys, both structural and functional changes occur in the late adult. The filtration function of these organs, for example, declines by 50% between the ages of 20 and 90 years. Kidney mass decreases by 20% over the same span. The number of nephrons—the basic filtering units in the kidneys—also declines between the ages of 30 and 80 years. Aging kidneys respond less efficiently to hemodynamic stress (ie, stress relating to the circulation of blood) and to fluid and electrolyte imbalances.

Changes in gastric and intestinal function may inhibit nutritional intake and utilization in older adults. For example, taste bud sensitivity to salty and sweet sensations decreases. Saliva secretion decreases, which reduces the body's ability to process complex carbohydrates. Gastric motility slows with age because of the loss of intestinal tract neurons, which can lead older adults to feel constipated or not hungry. Likewise, gastric acid secretion diminishes. Blood flow in the mesenteries (membranes that connect organs to the abdominal wall) may drop by as much as 50%, decreasing the ability of the intestines to extract nutrients from digested food. Gallstones become increasingly common with age, and anal sphincter changes reduce elasticity and can produce fecal incontinence.

Nervous System

Nervous system changes can result in the most debilitating of age-related ailments. In the central nervous system, the brain weight may shrink 10% to 20% by age 80 years. A selective loss of 5% to 50% of neurons occurs, and the surviving neurons shrink in size. The frontal lobe may lose as much as 20% of its synapses (the junctions between neurons) over the course of a person's life. Motor and sensory neural networks become slower and less responsive. The metabolic rate in the older brain does not change, however, and oxygen consumption remains constant throughout life.

The brain, which is surrounded by the meninges, takes up almost all of the space in the skull. Cerebrospinal fluid protects the brain inside these membranes. Unfortunately, age-related shrinkage creates a void between the brain and the outermost layer of the meninges, which provides room for the brain to move when stressed. This shrinkage also stretches the bridging veins that return blood from inside the brain to the dura mater. If trauma moves the brain forcibly, the bridging veins can tear and bleed (**Figure 9-19 ▶**). Bleeding can empty into this void, resulting in a subdural hematoma, which may go unnoticed for some time. Increased intracranial pressure is required for signs of head trauma to be present; the intracranial pressure will not rise—and, therefore, its signs will not be present—until the void has been filled and pressurized. (For more information, see Chapter 21.)

Functioning of the peripheral nervous system also slows with age. Sensation becomes diminished and misinterpreted. The resulting slowdown in reflexes may contribute to the incidence of trauma. Nerve endings deteriorate, and the ability of

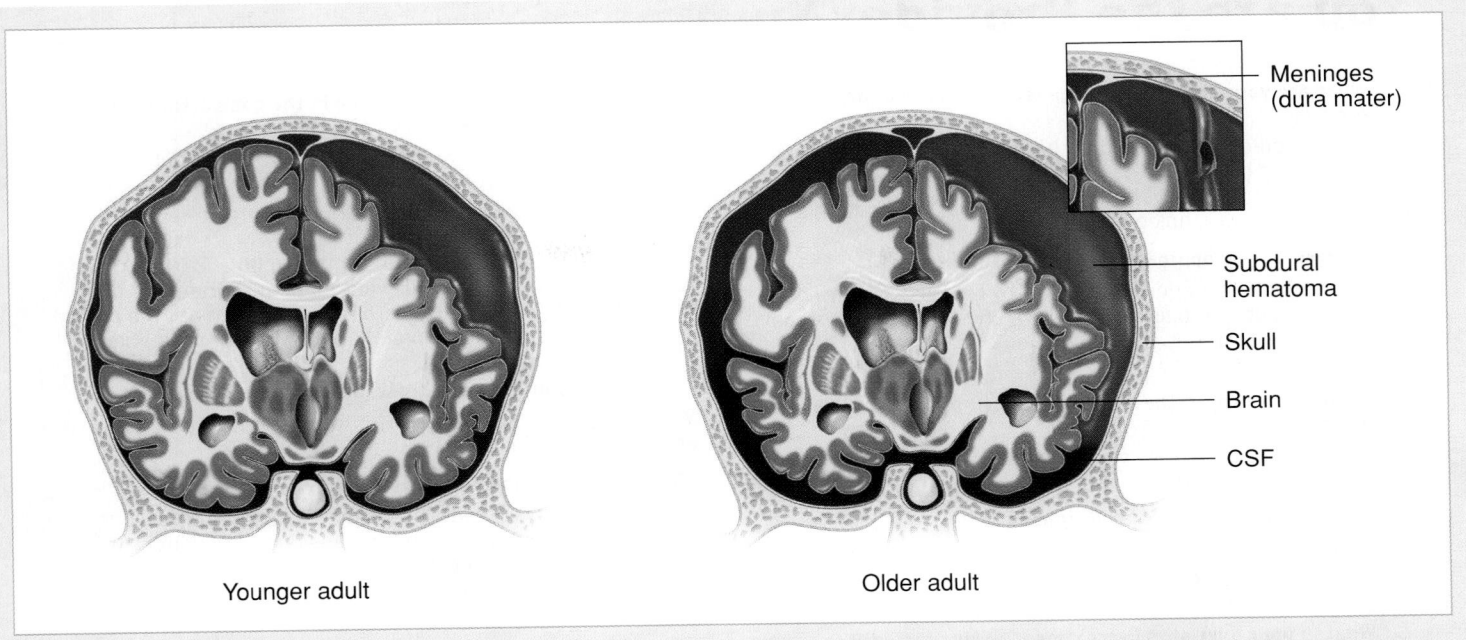

Meninges (dura mater)

Subdural hematoma

Skull

Brain

CSF

Younger adult

Older adult

Figure 9-19 Brain atrophy with age can make tearing of the bridging veins more likely with trauma. It may also create a space into which bleeding can occur without producing immediate signs of increased intracranial pressure.

the skin to sense the surroundings becomes hindered. Hot, cold, sharp, and wet items can all create dangerous situations because the body cannot sense them quickly enough.

Sensory Changes

Pupillary reaction and ocular movements become more restricted with age. The pupils are generally smaller in older patients, and the opacity of the eye's lens diminishes visual acuity and makes the pupils sluggish when responding to light. Visual distortions are also common in older people. Thickening of the lens makes it harder for the eye to focus, especially at close range. Peripheral fields of vision become narrower, and a greater sensitivity to glare constricts the visual field.

Hearing loss is about four times more common than loss of vision in late adults. Changes in several hearing-related structures may lead to a loss of high-frequency hearing, or even deafness.

Psychosocial Changes

Paramedics should treasure their opportunities to spend time with and communicate with late adults. Many of them have amazing stories and experiences to share with us, yet we often take them for granted. Our elderly share with us a great amount of wisdom, and we need to remind them of their self-worth. Indeed, until about 5 years before death, most late-stage adults retain high brain function. In the 5 years preceding death, however, mental function is presumed to decline, a theory referred to as the terminal drop hypothesis.

As the elderly population continues to grow, we have the responsibility to seek out unique ways to accommodate their needs during their last 20 to 40 years of life. While many older adults refuse to give up the independence of having their own home, the number of assisted-living communities is growing

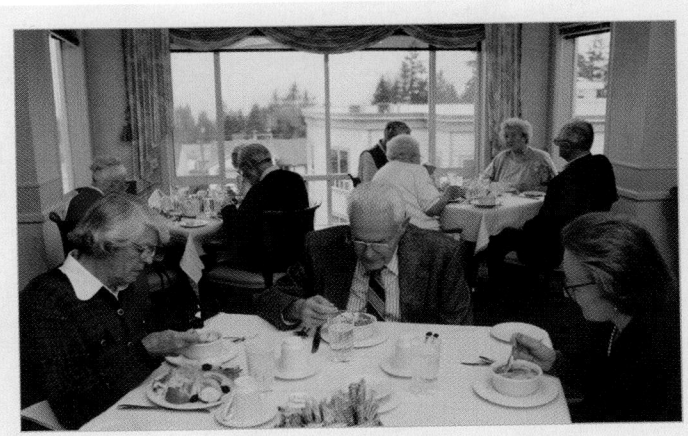

Figure 9-20 Many older adults live in assisted-living facilities.

across the nation. These facilities allow older adults to live in campus-based communities with people in their own age group, while enjoying the privacy of their own apartment and the security of nursing care, maintenance, and food preparation, if desired Figure 9-20 ▲. Unfortunately, these facilities can be expensive.

Most people need to deal with financial issues throughout their lives. Few things in life produce more worry and stress than money problems. Late adults, in particular, may constantly worry about rising costs of health care and are often forced to make decisions such as whether to pay for groceries or their medication. Modern families often take less responsibility for their elderly family members than earlier generations did. Today, more than 50% of all single women in the United States who are 60 years of age or older are living at or below the poverty level. This problem remains to be resolved.

You are the Provider Summary

1. What are your differential diagnoses given the information provided?

Differential diagnoses should include, but are not limited to, ovarian cysts, influenza, gastroenteritis, appendicitis, pregnancy, ectopic pregnancy, hernia, menstrual cramps, abdominal aortic aneurysm, psychological emergency, and nephritis.

2. How would you approach your patient interview?

In approaching this patient, you need to remember that she is very much capable of being a woman in physical terms, but may still be a teenage girl at a social and emotional level. Treat her with respect and privacy.

3. What could explain the slightly elevated patient respirations and pulse?

A response to pain and/or anxiety can increase the pulse, blood pressure, and respirations.

4. What are your differential diagnoses now?

At this point, you cannot rule out any differential diagnosis. Nevertheless, you should maintain a high index of suspicion for ectopic pregnancy.

5. What is your next step in treatment of this patient?

The paramedic should initiate IV access and draw blood samples while keeping the patient in the best position for comfort and repeated reassessment of her condition.

6. Do you allow the parent to ride in the compartment of the ambulance along with the patient?

The parent should ride in the front seat of the ambulance on the way to the hospital for two very important reasons:

- The parent is safer when wearing a seatbelt in the passenger seat in the cab.
- With the parent in the front of the ambulance, he or she can still be near the child without being in range of the paramedic's voice. The paramedic can then ask the patient questions and ensure patient privacy while promoting forthright answers.

7. What is your primary differential diagnosis now?

Your primary diagnosis at this point should be to rule out ectopic pregnancy.

8. Did this diagnosis alter your care?

The possibility of ectopic pregnancy shouldn't alter your care, but it will better prepare you for transition of patient care at the hospital. You will also be able to provide better comfort for your extremely anxious patient.

Ready for Review

- While each developmental stage is marked by different changes and characteristics, infants (1 month to 1 year) develop at a startling rate.
- The vital signs of toddlers (ages 1 to 3 years) and preschoolers (ages 3 to 6 years) differ somewhat from those of an infant.
- From ages 6 to 12 years, the school-age child's vital signs and body gradually approach those observed in adulthood.
- The vital signs of adolescents (ages 12 to 18 years) begin to level off within the adult ranges.
- Early adults are those who are age 19 to 40 years.
- Middle adults are those who are age 41 to 60 years.
- Late adults are those who are age 61 years and older.
- Vital signs do not vary greatly through adulthood.

Vital Vocabulary

adolescents Persons who are 12 to 18 years of age.

aneurysm A swelling or enlargement of part of a blood vessel, resulting from weakening of the vessel wall.

anxious avoidant attachment A bond between an infant and his or her parent or caregiver in which the infant is repeatedly rejected and develops an isolated lifestyle that does not depend upon the support and care of others.

atherosclerosis A disorder in which cholesterol and calcium build up inside the walls of the blood vessels, forming plaque, which eventually leads to partial or complete blockage of blood flow.

barotrauma Injury resulting from pressure disequilibrium across body surfaces, for example from too much pressure in the lungs.

bonding The formation of a close, personal relationship.

conventional reasoning A type of reasoning in which a child looks for approval from peers and society.

ductus arteriosus A duct that is present before birth that connects the pulmonary artery to the aorta in order to move unoxygenated blood back to the placenta.

ductus venosus A duct that is present before birth that connects the placenta to the heart in order to move oxygenated blood to the fetus.

early adults Persons who are 19 to 40 years of age.

fontanelles Areas where the infant's skull has not fused together; usually disappear at approximately 18 months of age.

foramen ovale An opening in the septum of the heart before birth, and which closes after birth.

growth plates Structures located on either end of an infant's bone, which aid in lengthening bones as the child grows.

hypercarbia Increased carbon dioxide levels in the bloodstream.

infants Persons who are from 1 month to 1 year of age.

late adults Persons who are 61 years old or older.

life expectancy The average amount of years a person can be expected to live.

mesenteries The membranes that connect organs to the abdominal wall.

middle adults Persons who are 41 to 60 years of age.

moro reflex An infant reflex in which, when an infant is caught off guard, the infant opens his or her arms wide, spreads the fingers, and seems to grab at things.

nephrons The basic filtering units in the kidneys.

palmar grasp An infant reflex that occurs when something is placed in the infant's palm; the infant grasps the object.

postconventional reasoning A type of reasoning in which a child bases decisions upon his or her conscience.

preconventional reasoning A type of reasoning in which a child acts almost purely to avoid punishment to get what he or she wants.

preschoolers Persons who are 3 to 6 years of age.

rooting reflex An infant reflex that occurs when something touches an infant's cheek, and the infant instinctively turns his head toward the touch.

school age A person who is 6 to 12 years of age.

secure attachment A bond between an infant and his or her parent or caregiver, in which the infant understands that his parents or caregivers will be responsive to his needs and take care of him when he needs help.

sucking reflex An infant reflex in which the infant starts sucking when his or her lips are stroked.

terminal drop hypothesis The theory that a person's mental function declines in the last 5 years of life.

toddlers Persons who are 1 to 3 years of age.

trust and mistrust A phrase that refers to a stage of development from birth to approximately 18 months of age, during which infants gain trust of their parents or caregivers if their world is planned, organized, and routine.

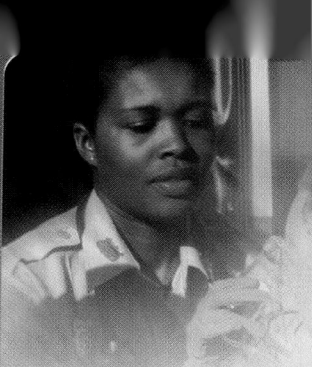

Assessment in Action

Your unit has arrived on the scene of an accident in which a minivan has rear-ended another vehicle at a fairly low speed. The minivan's airbag did not deploy. Inside the minivan you have four patients. The driver of the vehicle is a 38-year-old woman who was wearing a seatbelt. In the passenger seat is a 70-year-old woman who was also wearing a seatbelt. In the back seat are an infant who is restrained in a car seat and a toddler who has freed himself from his car booster seat.

1. **Which of your patients will be most prone to having airway occlusion problems?**
   A. Infant
   B. Adolescent
   C. Early adult
   D. Late adult

2. **When you assess the infant's vital signs, what should a normal respiratory rate be?**
   A. 12 to 20 breaths/min
   B. 18 to 24 breaths/min
   C. 30 to 60 breaths/min
   D. 26 to 40 breaths/min

3. **When you assess the infant's respiratory rate, you notice that the infant's chest is not moving but his abdomen is moving with his respirations. Is this a normal finding?**
   A. No, there is obviously an injury to the infant's chest.
   B. No, loosen the car seat straps and see if that makes a difference.
   C. No, remove the infant from the car seat immediately.
   D. Yes, infants are normally "belly breathers."

4. **The toddler in the vehicle is withdrawing from your attempts at a hands-on assessment. How will you continue to assess this toddler?**
   A. Reason with him.
   B. Explain what you want to do.
   C. Show the child what you are going to do using a prop.
   D. Let a family member continue the assessment.

5. **When doing your assessment on the 70-year-old patient, you attempt to check the pulse, motor function, and sensation on her lower extremities. The pulse is very hard to locate, and sensation appears to be nonexistent. You see no signs of trauma to the patient's lower extremities. To what source can you attribute this loss of sensation?**
   A. Peripheral nerve function slows with aging.
   B. You must be missing a traumatic injury.
   C. There is no change to nerve function but there is with circulation.
   D. The patient is cold and does not adjust well.

6. **The female patient in the driver's seat is approximately 38 years old. What would you expect her normal vital signs to be if she had not been involved in this accident?**
   A. P = 70, R = 30, BP = 180/90
   B. P = 70, R = 16, BP = 120/80
   C. P = 100, R = 30, BP = 180/90
   D. P = 100, R = 16, BP = 120/80

Challenging Question

You have notified your dispatcher that you will need a second ambulance to respond to this location due to the number of patients. All of the patients appear to have nonemergent injuries, which allows you to choose which patients will travel together.

7. **How will you use your knowledge of human development to make this decision?**

Points to Ponder

You are about to transport a toddler to the hospital for a minor laceration that will need a few stitches. The toddler will not lie down on the stretcher and fights your attempts to calm him down. The mother of the child is willing to ride with you to the hospital.

Where will you have her ride—in the front passenger seat or in the treatment compartment in visual contact with the child?

Issues: Physical and Psychological Changes in Human Development, Stranger Anxiety.

10 Patient Communication

Objectives

Cognitive

1-9.1   Define communication. (p 10.4)

1-9.2   Identify internal and external factors that affect a patient/bystander interview conducted by a paramedic. (p 10.3)

1-9.3   Restate the strategies for developing patient rapport. (p 10.5)

1-9.4   Provide examples of open-ended and closed or direct questions. (p 10.8)

1-9.5   Discuss common errors made by paramedics when interviewing patients. (p 10.9)

1-9.6   Identify the nonverbal skills that are used in patient interviewing. (p 10.10)

1-9.7   Restate the strategies to obtain information from the patient. (p 10.8)

1-9.8   Summarize the methods to assess mental status based on interview techniques. (p 10.11)

1-9.9   Discuss the strategies for interviewing a patient who is unmotivated to talk. (p 10.12)

1-9.10   Differentiate the strategies a paramedic uses when interviewing a patient who is hostile compared to one who is cooperative. (p 10.12)

1-9.11   Summarize developmental considerations of various age groups that influence patient interviewing. (p 10.12)

1-9.12   Restate unique interviewing techniques necessary to employ with patients who have special needs. (p 10.13)

1-9.13   Discuss interviewing considerations used by paramedics in cross-cultural communications. (p 10.13)

Affective

1-9.14   Serve as a model for an effective communication process. (p 10.4)

1-9.15   Advocate the importance of external factors of communication. (p 10.3)

1-9.16   Promote proper responses to patient communication. (p 10.5)

1-9.17   Exhibit professional nonverbal behaviors. (p 10.10)

1-9.18   Advocate development of proper patient rapport. (p 10.5)

1-9.19   Value strategies to obtain patient information. (p 10.8)

1-9.20   Exhibit professional behaviors in communicating with patients in special situations. (p 10.11)

1-9.21   Exhibit professional behaviors in communication with patients from different cultures. (p 10.13)

Psychomotor

None

Introduction

The scenario with the Kellars in *You are the Provider Part 1* illustrates the importance of something we all need to remember throughout our careers. However well-intentioned we may be, some of us see people not as people but as their medical problems. That's a shallow approach to emergency medicine in the field. It always begins with something else that's hard to teach, and which most of us never hear much about. The following pages are intended to guide you through the art and skills of communicating with people on the worst days of their lives.

People are not just medical puzzles for you to solve, and they're certainly not just nuisances or interruptions. They're the reason paramedics exist. They elect the officials who give you your certificates. And they deserve your best efforts at service—what that "S" in EMS stands for.

Being a good paramedic requires a major talent for multitasking. When you're kneeling in front of Mr. Kellar, who is sitting there on his couch and denying his symptoms, you should also be aware that Mrs. Kellar, seated right there next to him, is scared to death that she could lose him. More than that, you have to *feel* something for both of them. These are abilities you would not expect to find, and probably wouldn't need, in most other jobs. These abilities are the gifts of caregivers.

Internal Factors for Effective Communication

You need to be able to *naturally like people* (which is difficult for some people). You don't have to like them all, and you don't have to like them every day. But liking them has to be real for you, and it has to come easily. Why? Because when they defecate in your ambulance, vomit on your shoes, or bleed all over your clean uniform, you have to be able to toler-

ate that without so much as a syllable of protest. These events are all part of a paramedic's job.

This chapter is based on the presumption that you like people, you care about them, and you honestly want to serve them. You'd better. Because if you don't, they will pick up your true feelings and poor attitude in the blink of an eye—and so will their families. And if you don't like people, you're pretty much guaranteed to hate doing what paramedics do every day: serving people, in their own time and on their own terms. As a paramedic you may see people looking their worst. They may smell like urine, vomit, digested blood, stale perspiration, feces, or worse. But that's how real people really are, especially when they're sick. If you go into the field expecting anything else, the mistake will be all yours and your patients will pay for it in the marginal care they may get from you. And you'll pay for it by having a really short career.

At least half of the calls you will run as a paramedic will take you into people's homes, day and night and in the most private moments of their lives. Try to see every invitation into the home of someone else as a personal honor in a time and place where no one else would be welcome ▶ Figure 10-1 ▶. You will be there when a lot of people are born, and you will be there when a lot of people die. In many cultures, people believe that God is present in times like these. Whether you subscribe to that belief or not, try hard to sense the privilege of being invited. It can make your career a lasting and fulfilling experience, instead of a source of drudgery.

External Factors for Effective Communication

A paramedic who looks the part of a professional inspires a lot more confidence in patients, in family members, and in the public than one who pays no attention to his or her appearance

You are the Provider Part 1

Mary and Bill Kellar have been married for 44 years. Their four children have all moved away, and the two of them share a quiet suburban home in southern California. Late one evening while watching TV, Mary notices that one side of her husband's face appears flaccid. When she asks him if he is all right, he says he's fine, but his words are slurred and difficult to understand. She waits only a few more minutes before announcing that she is going to call for help, and she dials 9-1-1 despite his protests. The paramedics who arrive a few minutes later are obviously tired from running calls.

Initial Assessment	Recording Time: 0 Minutes
Appearance	Flaccid and weak muscles on left side of patient's face
Level of consciousness	A (Alert to person, place, and day)
Airway	Open
Breathing	Normal rate; adequate depth
Circulation	Radial pulse present

1. What communication difficulties do you immediately anticipate in this scenario?

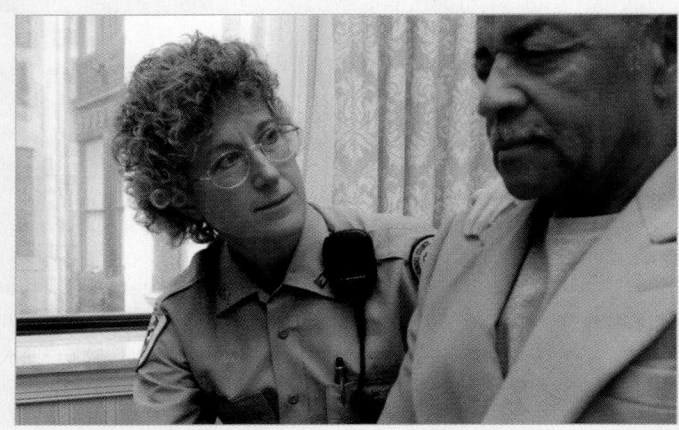

Figure 10-1 Think of it as an honor to be asked into a patient's home. Be respectful, and always be kind.

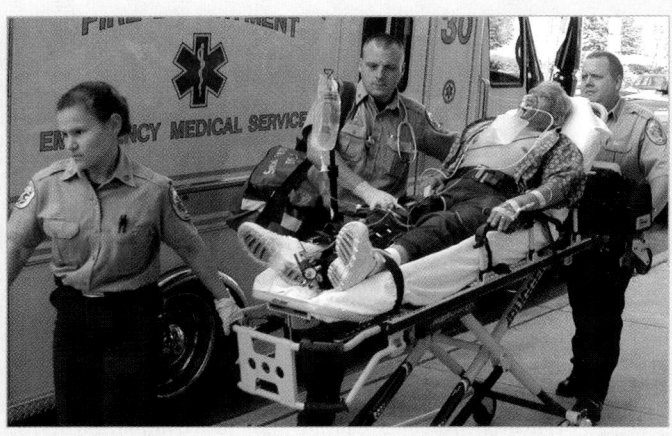

Figure 10-2 One way to comfort patients is to look as though you can help them, to look in charge. Be sure that your uniform is clean and that your shoes are clean, in good shape, and polished.

Figure 10-2 ▸ . You've heard this in other chapters but listen to this advice once again: polish your leather shoes and iron your shirt before you show up for work. Make it easy for others to read your first name and at least your last initial, as well as your level of certification. Learn the principles of professional etiquette, and make sure your overall behavior inspires respect in people you don't know. That's more than making nice; it's what a professional does.

In the Field

Patients will pick up on how you treat or are treated by other EMS officials at the scene. If you are treated with respect, and if you treat the other EMS officials with respect, the patient will see this and have more confidence in you as well.

If you want people to tell you about their problems, convince them you want to hear what they have to say. Communication is the act of transmitting information to another person—and, for paramedics, it can be verbal or through body language. Give patients your undivided attention; don't treat them like nuisances. There's nothing worse than talking about someone in his or her presence, as though he or she is an inanimate object—or worse, as though the person doesn't even exist. And it's unforgivable to ask someone a question you're just going to repeat later because you didn't pay attention to the answer the first time. Jot it down. When it's time to communicate, *communicate.* That means listen, don't just talk. Listening is part of communicating too, because it transmits information as well.

An excellent way to convince someone that you're really listening to him or her is a technique called "active listening." Almost all professional interviewers use it routinely. Active listening is repeating the key parts of a patient's responses to

You are the Provider Part 2

Mary gets the impression from the paramedics' demeanor that they would prefer to be somewhere else. Twice she asks them what they think is happening to Bill, but they don't reply. Instead, they focus on applying oxygen, starting an IV, attaching electrodes, and performing various other skills and assessments. They don't talk to the patient except to ask questions, and they don't seem to appreciate or address the fact that Mary is terrified.

Vital Signs	Recording Time: 3 Minutes
Skin	Pale and cool; perspiring
Pulse	88 beats/min, irregular
Blood pressure	184/94 mm Hg
Respirations	18 breaths/min
Sao$_2$	97% on 15 L/min via nonrebreathing mask

2. Describe what the phrase "total patient care" means to you.

questions. Especially when you're taking notes at the same time, it helps you to convince patients that you really want to hear what they're saying. Active listening also helps confirm the information patients are providing. This ensures there is no misunderstanding between you and your patients.

Some specific expressions that are helpful are:

- When patients thank you, say, "You're very welcome!" (not "No problem." "No problem" implies, "That's OK; you aren't too much of a nuisance." It's definitely not as nice as saying, "You're welcome.")
- When patients apologize to you because they're incontinent or vomiting or because you have to carry them down a flight of stairs, tell them something like, "It's OK; you don't need to be sorry. This is what we do, *and we're here because we want to be.*"

If you like serving people, these kinds of expressions will feel natural to you, and no doubt you will find your colleagues imitating you after only a short time.

Try hard not to shout. Some scenes are very noisy. But even so, when you shout, so does everyone else. And when people are shouting, they tend to get excited. If you're answering a call in a noisy place such as a bar, ask the bartender to help by turning off the music, turning up the lights, and keeping an eye on the other patrons. (In this type of situation, get your patient out of there as soon as you can.) Move the patient to your "office"—the back of the ambulance. If you must use a compressor or run a noisy diesel on the scene, shut it off as soon as you can to cut down on the noise level. Meanwhile, try to talk close to your patient's ears in a calm voice. It lets him or her know that you have your emotions under control, which helps him or her stay calm as well. Try managing your history-taking all at one time. Taking the patient's medical and health history helps you stay organized and encourages people to take your questions seriously.

If you want reliable answers to personal questions, try to manage your scene so you can ask these kinds of questions quietly and in private. Even if you do earn a patient's trust, there are things people just don't want to talk about in front of others. Don't forget to ask a few payoff questions—questions that don't fall under the category of routine medical history but that, time after time, will net you information that's critical to a presumptive diagnosis. Some payoff questions are listed and explained later in this chapter.

Some scenes are easy to manage. But paramedics very often work in bizarre, noisy, chaotic, and sometimes dangerous environments that are challenging at best **Figure 10-3 ▶**. Under these circumstances, communicating with patients (and their family members) is especially critical to the skills of assessment and the art of bringing about calm (and therefore healing).

Developing Rapport

When you find yourself standing at someone's bedside in the middle of the night, if you really don't want to be there, if you

Special Considerations
Do not assume that all elderly patients are hard of hearing. You will be put in your place if you begin by talking loudly or too slowly to an older patient only to be told by the patient, "I'm not deaf."

really don't care how he or she feels, and if you just want to get back to bed, he or she will get the message, *whether you intended to send it or not.* Nothing you pretend, say, or do will fool your patient. If you really *do* want to be there, you really *do* care, and you really *don't* mind being awakened, your patient will get that message too.

People in crisis are highly perceptive, and there is no greater crisis than being scared to death that you're about to lose someone you love more than anyone in the whole world.

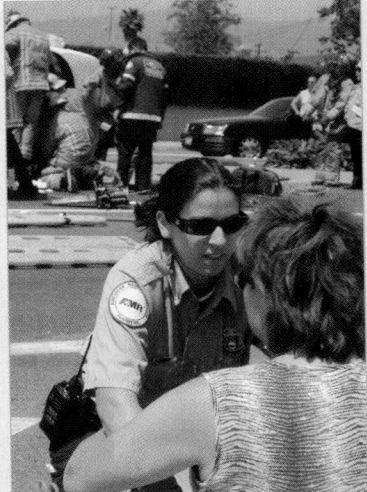

Figure 10-3 Even in the most chaotic conditions, try to create a safe zone for your patient. Shut out everything else the best you can, and focus on helping this one person.

Your most essential challenge as a therapeutic communicator is to convey calm, unmistakable, genuine concern for someone you've never met. People in crisis do much better if someone like you can relieve their fear and help them to harness their own internal healing power.

Watch Your Inflection

Your voice is just as important in communication as your words. You know what someone's voice sounds like when he or she is really concerned for you. Think about how the voice of someone who cares for you sounds when you are hurt or upset. Use that calm and steady tone of reassurance to reinforce your interest in and concern for the patient.

Respond to the Patient

There is probably nothing as insulting to a patient as asking or telling a caregiver something and receiving no response at all. Regardless of what the patient says, acknowledge what he or she said. If you are not comfortable responding, simply nod or restate what the patient said, without providing a definitive answer right away. If you later figure out how you can give more information, you may tell the patient at that point.

Tell People Who You Are

Once you break that initial ice with someone, tell him or her who you are. That's just common courtesy, but it is often overlooked by medical professionals. Tell them something more too. Tell them you're a paramedic. Remember, they're about to entrust their privacy and their medical well-being to someone they didn't know a moment ago. They deserve to know what you know (and what you don't). By introducing yourself, you are also saying, "You are, no matter what the indignities of treatment, in charge of your health care, and you can communicate with me as an equal."

Use the Patient's Name

Most of us use the same few words to greet our patients, both in the field and in the hospital: "Hi. What's the problem?" That's OK for an amateur, but it doesn't say much for a professional. Why? Because people's names are important to them and to their families. Your name is the first thing you receive after birth, and it's the only thing you keep when you die (think about every gravestone you've ever seen). As a caregiver, use the importance of a person's name like a tool.

Don't just start your patient contact with a question about the medical problem. Introduce yourself, and then ask patients their name. That simple practice tells them their discomfort is important, but it also opens a window through which you can quickly assess a lot. Think about that for a few moments.

When you address patients with an expression like, "Hi. My name is Lee Jones and I'm a paramedic. What's your name?" what do they have to be able to do in order to answer appropriately? They have to go through a very specific sequence of physical and mental processes, which amounts to a mini-mental status examination. Consider the following:

- They have to hear your words.
- They have to locate the source of your voice and meet your gaze.
- They have to process the meaning of your words (in your common language).
- They have to formulate a meaningful, accurate response from memory.
- They have to put their response into coherent speech.
- They have to be able to do all of that within about 1 second.

During that second, if you're close enough to see the size of their pupils, you can assess their mental state and the function of at least six pairs of cranial nerves. That's a fair amount of assessment.

In addition, you've communicated something very important to the patient and his or her family just by asking that question—your respect. Part of your respectful behavior is to introduce yourself with your full name and your profession. You've told him or her (and family members), "Mr. or Mrs. Edwards, you may be about to lose your dignity and possibly your shorts, but you're going to be able to keep your name." Finally, using the names of people is good for us and for our colleagues. It reminds us that we're not just dealing with broken brains and broken livers and broken hearts day after day. Instead, we're dealing with *people*. It also lets the patient establish the level of formality they are comfortable with. If they say, "You can call me Joey," then do so, but if they say, "I am Mr. Jones," do not call them Joey, Buddy, or any other pet name.

Anticipate and Deal With Fear

Usually, after a few weeks of ambulance calls, you will be impressed with the fact that most patients are scared to death of the situation. If the patient isn't afraid, consider that one or more of his or her loved ones may be absolutely terrified **Figure 10-4 ▸**. Reassurance may be one of the most important treatments you can provide.

You are the Provider Part 3

As the paramedics assess Mr. Kellar, his wife hears them casually discussing the likelihood of stroke. This is her worst nightmare as their physician had warned Bill about the risks of his high blood pressure and high cholesterol. After repeated attempts to communicate with the paramedics have failed, she becomes so frustrated that she screams, "Why do you keep ignoring me?"

Reassessment	Recording Time: 7 Minutes
Level of consciousness	A (Alert to person, place, and day)
Skin	Pale and cool; perspiring
Pulse	88 beats/min, irregular
Blood pressure	184/98 mm Hg
Respirations	18 breaths/min
SaO_2	96% on 15 L/min via nonrebreathing mask
ECG	Atrial fibrillation

3. Although the paramedics in this scenario are attending to the patient's medical needs, could the wife have a valid complaint regarding their caregiving?
4. How can your introductions (or lack thereof) and general demeanor affect your ability to communicate with your patients as well as with their friends and family members?

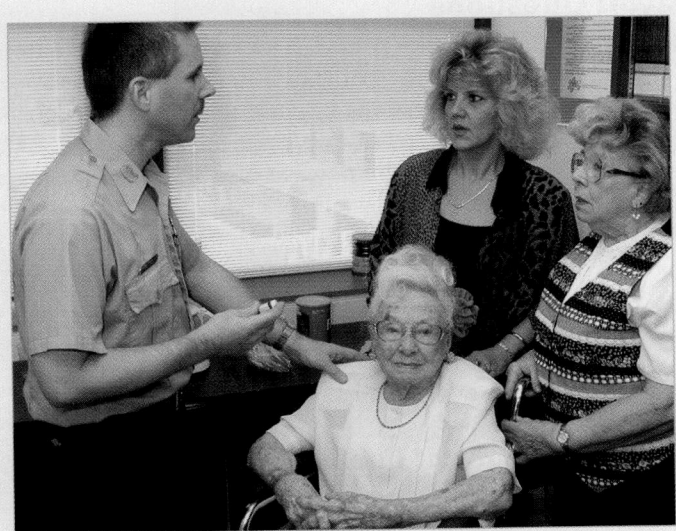

Figure 10-4 As soon as possible, you or your partner should explain to the patient's family members what is happening and what they can do. This information can help them deal with their fear and worry.

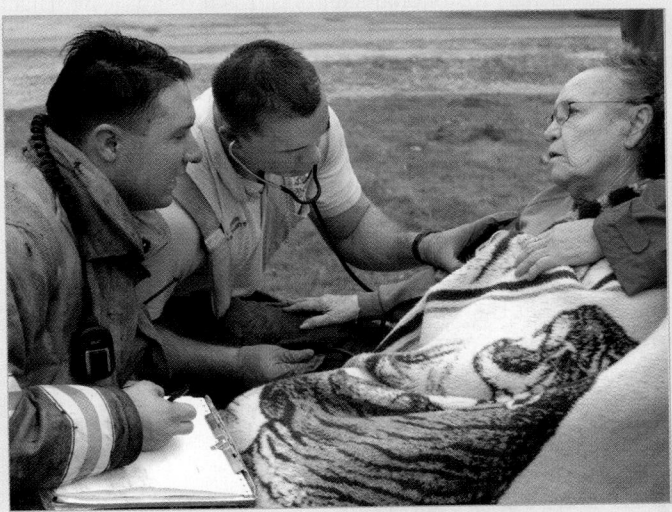

Figure 10-5 Show your patient the same respect you'd want others to show your father or brother or your mother or sister. Protect modesty with a blanket or towel.

How do you control fear? First, by your own sense of competence and professional calm. Second, by honestly caring about someone (a fact that, like kindness, patients and family members alike can easily detect). Third, by giving people information. When someone wakes up in the middle of the night with a dull, crushing chest pain, that person doesn't want to be treated like a child or someone who cannot understand what is happening. Tell your patients what you think is happening. Show patients what their ECG reveals, tell them their blood pressure, explain how you're planning to make them better, and let them know how they're doing. There is no better way to harness a patient's own power to self-heal, nor is there a better way to harness the healing power of loved ones, while at the same time stabilizing their emotions.

Documentation and Communication

In Spanish, "Yo voy a cuidar muy bien de usted" means "I will take good care of you."

Respect the Importance of Pain

When someone tells you he or she is in pain, let that person know you grasp and appreciate the situation, and then do something about it. One of the most grievous offenses by caregivers (in and out of hospitals) is ignoring pain. People deserve to have their pain relieved as completely as possible, then and there—with a medical consultation if necessary. Don't make them wait. You wouldn't want your loved ones to wait for pain relief. A patient should never have to be patient about any pain you can alleviate, whether in the field or in the hospital.

Respect and Protect People's Modesty

Modesty matters—no matter how acute the medical condition. It's especially important to the very old, adolescents, and sometimes, the very young. If the patient is not personally sensitive to modesty (because of an impaired mental state, for example), family members most certainly are Figure 10-5 ▲.

Help, Don't Judge

When you become a paramedic, you will need to know a person's medical history in order to help him or her. For example, you will need to use naloxone to treat an opiate addict. Sadly, drug and alcohol addicts support their addictions by lying. Few addicts will admit to drinking more than two beers, let alone to taking an opiate. Here's where your own moral code has to take a backseat to professional ethics. Try to avoid judging patients because the causes of addiction can be very complex. We can't pretend to know why people make the choices they make; we, as health care providers, see only the results of these choices.

When you ask someone an uncomplicated question in plain, simple English, and he or she responds with an unnecessarily complicated or inappropriate response, one of the things you should probably consider is the possibility that the patient is lying. Of course, that's not always true. Also, one of the most common strategies people develop to cope with stress is lying. Plenty of people who are not addicted lie too. Patients may also be mentally impaired (by chemicals, hypoxia, psychiatric disorders, or other causes of disorganized thinking). But lying does happen often enough, so you should anticipate it.

Whatever you do, don't appoint yourself judge. Instead, merely consider this individual a poor historian and move on with your interview. One of the things that can happen to you over time if you allow yourself to judge people is that you can become cynical. Professional skepticism is a useful tool; it facilitates sound, clinical decision-making. But cynicism is skepticism gone wild and is unproductive to you and your patients.

Conducting the Interview

The reason we question people is to find out how they're feeling, what happened that may have made them sick or hurt them, and what their lives have been like. But to quote the old expression about computers: "Garbage in, garbage out." If we're not careful about what questions we ask, we may not obtain the information we need. Following are three techniques that can make your questioning more productive.

Open-Ended Questions

When you need to know how someone feels, first try asking a question that makes the patient do the thinking. This is an open-ended question—a question that does not have a yes or no answer, and which does not give the patient specific options to choose from. For instance, if you ask patients to describe their own chest pain, don't suggest qualities like sharpness, dullness, or pressure. Instead, let them think of a word that describes how the pain feels; their own words will probably more accurately describe what they are feeling. Some examples of open-ended questions are:

- How have you been feeling lately?
- Do you have an idea of what is causing this?
- Do you have any other concerns about your health?
- Is there anything else you would like to discuss?

Closed-Ended Questions

Sometimes (for example, when you're trying to find out about a patient's medical history) you need answers to specific questions. In these cases, try a direct, or closed-ended question. In fact, it's a good idea to develop a standard set of questions concerning medical history that you ask almost all patients. Avoid talking down to them (that's insulting), but avoid using medical terms. Instead, try using words that people without medical training can understand. Your standard questions may include the following:

- Have you ever had any heart problems?
- Any lung problems?
- Any high or low blood pressure?
- Diabetes?
- Seizures?
- Fainting spells?
- Any prior head injury?
- Do you have both lungs and both kidneys?

If the patient is female and of childbearing age (generally, 12 to 50 years old), be sure to ask about her history of pregnancies, deliveries, and abortions, when her last menstrual period was and if it was normal, and if she has had any gynecologic surgeries.

Payoff Questions

Most seasoned paramedics have developed their own repertoire of additional questions for patients in specific circumstances. We call them payoff questions because they're like icebergs—tiny questions that can reveal huge subsurface issues. Sometimes these issues are the hidden reason we've been called to help someone. Some examples of payoff questions are:

- Have you ever felt like this before?
- Have you been upset about anything lately?
- Are you afraid of someone? (Save this one for the privacy of the ambulance.)
- Have you been thinking about hurting yourself?
- What happened the last time you felt this way?

Strategies to Elicit Useful Responses to Questions

To get the right answers, it's not always enough just to ask the right questions. Why? Because when people are in crisis, some of them are terrible communicators. It can be almost impossible to think and organize your thoughts when you are terrified. Fortunately, good interviewers also have the following tools to use to get answers.

Facilitate the Response

If patients hesitate to answer questions completely, encourage them to provide you with more information. One useful expression is simply, "Please say more." Another is, "Please feel welcome to tell me about that."

Be Quiet

If you sense that patients are trying to put something into words but are having trouble expressing themselves, try this famous tip "Never miss a good opportunity to shut up." Be patient. Don't say anything at all for a few seconds. Let them talk.

Documentation and Communication

If you must stop patients from talking to get an urgent task done, explain to them why they need to be quiet and that they will be able to talk to you when you finish your task.

Clarify the Response

If you don't understand what patients have told you, ask them to explain what they mean. This communicates that you are listening and taking their comments seriously. It may also help you understand what they are trying to tell you.

Redirect the Response

Sometimes patients will mention something in passing or will avoid answering a specific question. You can politely redirect their attention to that question (several times, if necessary) until you get them to answer it.

Chapter 10 Patient Communication

Interpret the Response

If you've tried clarification and you're still not sure what patients are trying to tell you, sometimes it helps to vocalize what you think they've said and invite them to correct you.

Simplify and Summarize the Response

Some patients have a hard time speaking plainly, no matter how hard they try. It can be difficult to communicate with people who have psychiatric problems, who fabricate their diseases, and who are afraid or upset. If patients give you a confusing or disorganized response, try putting their comments into simpler terms and see if they agree with your synopsis. It can help them focus their thoughts and help you as an interviewer.

▌Common Interviewing Errors

None of us are perfect, and all of us have made errors in the course of questioning patients. Learn to improve your interviewing skills by observing what other paramedics have done:

Assume Nothing!

Most mistakes caregivers make have happened as the result of assuming things. Assuming that a patient is faking unconsciousness or seizures, assuming that a companion is a spouse, assuming that a fight victim is a member of a gang, or assuming that a patient is inebriated are very common mistakes. Try hard to become a careful observer and to keep your mind open to a wide range of possibilities. Remember that when we assume, sometimes it makes an "ass" out of "u" and "me."

Giving Medical Advice

Patients and their families often ask their paramedics and EMTs for medical advice, in much the same way as they would con- sult a physician. That's an honor because it conveys their trust. Patients may even ask you to comment on a decision by their physician. Don't fall for that one (however well-intentioned the question may be). Instead, suggest they obtain their medical advice from a doctor.

Providing False Hope

Try not to overencourage patients or their family members if a patient is very ill. You can't possibly see in advance what's going to happen to someone. But remember that the question, "Am I going to die?" is a lot different than the statement, "I think I'm going to die." Lots of patients whose status seems very stable will ask you if they're going to die. A good answer to that one is, "Some day—but you look pretty good to us today." Another option is "I don't know, but I sure hope not. What do you think?" As for the latter case, patients who look you right in the eye and tell you they feel they're going to die are probably right. People in cardiogenic shock or who have end-stage chronic obstructive pulmonary disease do that with uncanny regularity. Invite their family members to give them a kiss before taking them to the emergency department. It may be their last oppor- tunity, and they will treasure that memory forever.

If the patient or a family member asks you if the patient is going to die, and the patient is not in stable condition, you could say, "We think he (or she) is very sick, but we're doing everything we possibly can to help."

Assuming Excessive Authority

Just as we're not qualified to judge people, it's important to remember that we're not police officers either. Adopting the no-nonsense demeanor of a law officer can frighten your patient, and make your job of caring for that patient nearly impossible. (How do *you* feel when you are pulled over, even for expired tags, by a law officer?)

You are the Provider Part 4

Upon seeing his wife so distraught, Mr. Kellar becomes upset as well. He tries to explain that she has recently had a heart attack, but his words are garbled and the paramedics are unable to understand him, in spite of his best efforts, so his message goes undelivered.

Reassessment	Recording Time: 10 Minutes
Level of consciousness	A (Alert to person, place, and day)
Skin	Pale, cool, and moist
Pulse	98 beats/min, irregular
Blood pressure	190/104 mm Hg
Respirations	18 breaths/min
Sao$_2$	96% on 15 L/min via nonrebreathing mask
ECG	Atrial fibrillation
Blood glucose	100 mg/dL

5. How has this crew's lack of people skills affected this call?

6. Can this situation be mended?

Sidestepping the Truth

Patients deserve to know what their blood pressure is, and what their ECG reveals about them. Their blood sugar (blood glucose level) isn't a secret you need to keep from them, nor is your presumptive diagnosis. When patients ask you what you think is wrong, remember that you're serving them. Remind them that you don't have definitive answers and that you're not a physician, but tell them what you think may be going on. Be honest and sincere about what you're telling them, but never harsh.

Distancing Yourself From Patients as People

Another Western medical technique for maintaining the relationship between physicians and patients is professional distancing—that is, avoiding contact with patients as people. This can take the form of using lots of big, complicated medical words you hope they won't understand, and answering patients' questions with half-truths. No matter who uses these techniques, do not adopt them as your own. They will not serve your own or your patients' well-being in the long run.

Nonverbal Skills

People in crisis are still people, and you can use many of the same methods that other professional interviewers use to get them to tell you things. Following are a few of those skills or tools.

Eye Contact

Direct eye contact is something you avoid with animals; they perceive it as a sign of aggression. But people expect brief, frequent, direct eye contact, especially when they need reassurance. "Seeing eye-to-eye" with people generally communicates honesty and concern and is considered a baseline necessity of sincere communication of any kind   Figure 10-6 ▶ . Think about that when you start to interview a patient with your mirrored sunglasses on.

You won't always have time to simply visit with some patients, especially if they're very sick. But try to remember that when a patient's status is subacute, your busy hands may correlate to you engaging in less (or no) eye contact. If the patient needs someone to talk to, take the time to listen when you can.

Touch

Some people don't like to be touched at all; to others, it's a valuable assurance that someone cares about them. You should try gently touching patients on a neutral part of the body, such as a shoulder or arm, especially when you're trying to reassure them or mitigate their fear   Figure 10-7 ▶ . But watch how they react. If they pull away from you, chances are that touch in this instance won't be a valuable strategy. If they react positively (for instance, by leaning toward you or seeming to relax), than touch as a form of reassurance will work with them.

Gentleness

Being gentle is actually a quality of touch (mentioned above). You can use it even with a patient who prefers not to be

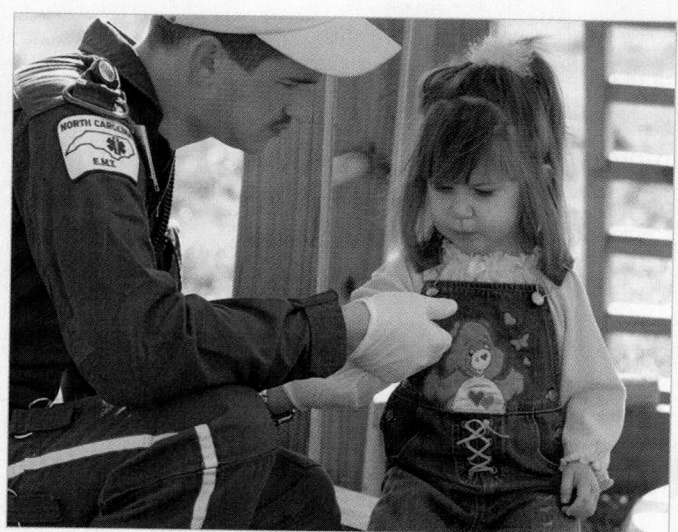

Figure 10-6 Whenever possible, put yourself at eye level with your patient. This is especially important when you're treating a child or an adult who is bedridden or wheelchair bound.

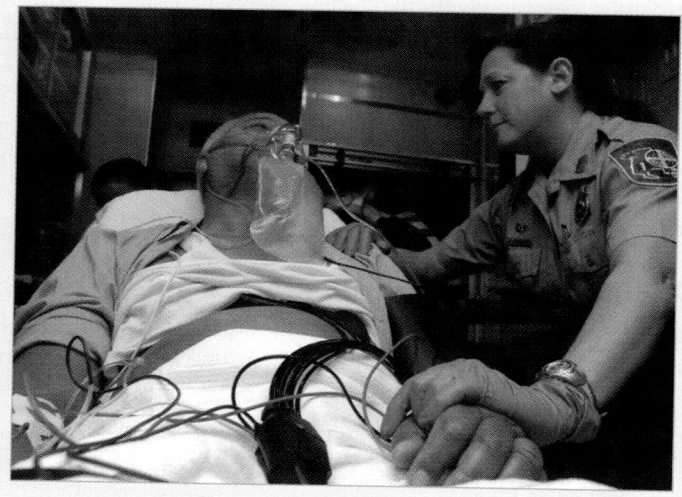

Figure 10-7 A gentle touch on the hand, arm, or shoulder can comfort someone who is sick or hurt and very scared.

touched. Gentleness can be the easy way you place the head of your stethoscope against the patient's chest or the way you apply a blood pressure cuff or blanket.

Posture

When you're dealing with patients who are terrified, don't stand in front of them with your arms folded across your chest. That conveys confrontation, not concern. Instead, try to position yourself at the same level as (or below the level of) their eyes. Sit or kneel at an angle that would not encroach on their personal space. For instance, lots of paramedics squat on the floor or ground in front of people who are seated in a car or on a bus bench or couch. Some choose to sit on the drug box.

Demeanor

A pleasant demeanor comes easily to people who like people. To others, it doesn't come at all; and it's one of the reasons we emphasized liking people earlier in this chapter. It's absolutely necessary when you're dealing with people in crisis, because they need to see you as someone who is safe to be with, who does not pose a threat, and who honestly cares. With that comes the belief that you are going to handle the crisis.

Therapeutic Smile

Anyone who has dealt with even a few scared people can tell you that a smile can greatly help relieve stress. Think back to a time when you were troubled by something and someone's smile told you that everything was going to be OK. Your ability to smile can be just as valuable when you're dealing with people in crisis.

Assessing Mental Status

Excellent communication is vital in assessing how alert and oriented your patients are. There are many useful techniques for assessing mental status, and most of them are simple and based on plain old common sense. We have already discussed the most versatile first step ever invented: asking a patient for his or her name. Beyond that, consider the patient's ability to express himself or herself in the following ways.

Appropriate Humor

The highest form of mental function is the spontaneous expression of appropriate humor. To generate that degree of mental status, a person has to possess a high degree of cognitive function and an intact memory. People who aren't thinking clearly don't have the neuronal function to invest in spontaneous humor.

Timing of Responses to Questions

Assess how long it takes a patient to respond appropriately to your questions. A patient who is thinking clearly should be able to answer simple questions that make sense within 1 second.

Memory (Person, Place, Day, and Event)

Patients should be able to tell you quickly and accurately who they are and who you are, where they are, what day of the week it is, and what happened that necessitated your being called. Incorrect responses to any of these constitute a memory dysfunction and therefore decreased blood flow to the brain.

Ability to Obey Simple Commands

Any disruption in a patient's ability to comply with requests in the preceding steps indicates a brain dysfunction in the cerebrum or possibly the cerebellum. The dysfunction may be acute and could even be preexisting.

Special Interview Situations

There are situations in paramedic practice that may require special communication techniques. Some of these may include uncommunicative patients, hostile patients, very old or very young patients, and patients with special needs. Stereotyping any of these groups of patients, however, will only work

You are the Provider Part 5

The paramedics attempt to calm Mrs. Kellar and apologize to her. She is now crying uncontrollably, and says she's experiencing chest pain and shortness of breath. She sits down next to her husband and self-administers a nitroglycerin tablet under her tongue. An IV of normal saline has been established at a keep vein open rate.

Reassessment	Recording Time: 15 Minutes
Level of consciousness	A (Alert to person, place, and day)
Skin	Pale and cool; perspiring
Pulse	118 beats/min, irregular
Blood pressure	188/102 mm Hg
Respirations	18 breaths/min
Sao_2	98% on 15 L/min via nonrebreathing mask
ECG	Atrial fibrillation

7. What would be the best course of action in this situation?
8. What are the different forms of communication and how do they impact patient care?

against effective communication. A good paramedic is never judgmental about his or her patients. No one calls you to judge them or their circumstances; they call for your medical care! But you can and should try the following techniques when you find yourself *not* communicating well with some patients.

People Who Are Unmotivated to Talk

There's nothing wrong with a little quiet; in fact, people who talk too much can be fairly irritating. When patients refuse to talk and you're not seeing signs of decreased mental status, there's no need to force the issue. Instead, make lots of eye contact, express your concern in every way possible, explain everything you are doing, invite them repeatedly to answer questions, and let them know it's all right if they don't wish to talk. This strategy of accepting them as they are can be very effective at breaking down barriers.

People Who Are Hostile

You are guaranteed to receive some unpleasant insults from people who are in crisis, and the insults will probably happen quite frequently. It's especially predictable when you're dealing with people who are chemically impaired. Discipline yourself never to respond in kind. Nothing escalates a situation faster than trading insults. Very often, when it involves a patient or bystanders, there are plenty of witnesses. It makes no sense and it can be very dangerous, especially when you're on their turf (about which you know nothing and they know everything). Remember, you're a helper. Remember, just as you can't fix everybody medically, you can't fix everybody emotionally either. Consider the possibility that you may not be able to defuse someone's anger. If the situation gets out of control, you may have to defer to police.

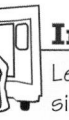

In the Field

Learn to look for aggressive body language that signals increased anger and a possible attack such as clenched fists, intense staring directed at you, and breathing heavily through clenched teeth.

People Who Are Very Old or Very Young

Try not to presume that older people are any harder to communicate with than anyone else just because they're older. Their illnesses may tend to be more complex than the illnesses of younger people because they may have more than one disease or disorder and they may be taking more kinds of medicines concurrently. You may note individual differences among the geriatric population related to hearing, eyesight, mental status, and mobility; you need to adapt to them. The fact remains, older people are individuals and their differences are individual.

Children can be difficult patients because they pose communication challenges, even to the best paramedic. They tend to protest pain vigorously, they may be afraid of strangers (like

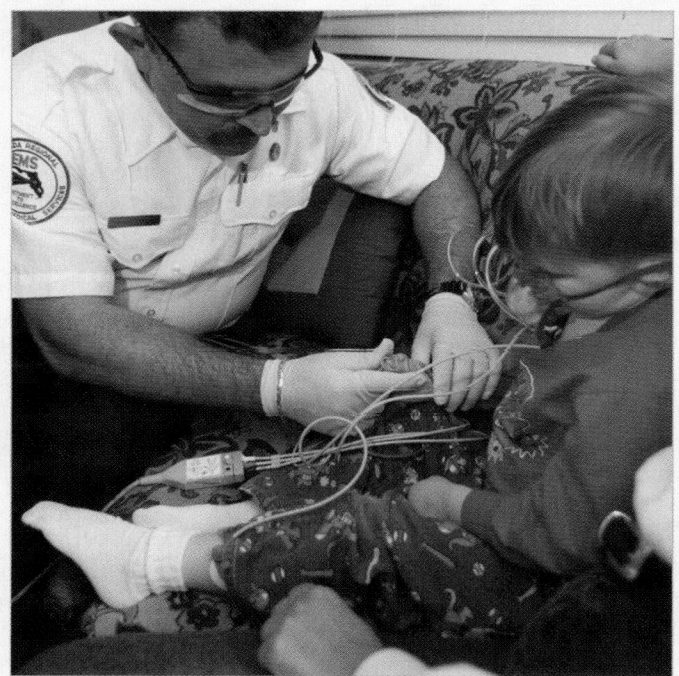

Figure 10-8 When you're examining a very young child, involve the parents. Have the father hold the child on his lap, or ask the mother to keep the toddler occupied while you work.

you), they may panic when separated from their parents, and their bodies may not be as familiar to many of us as are the bodies of adults. With a little practice, we can become comfortable treating them too.

Equipment (such as stethoscopes or needles) is not as important early in our contact with children as are friendly eye contact, smiles, and calm, subdued explanations, geared to match each child's age. Discipline yourself to minimize your movements, lower your voice, and touch as gently as you can. Try placing yourself at or below the child's eye level, for instance by sitting on the floor and placing the child on the cot or on a parent's lap **Figure 10-8 ▲**. If possible, involve a parent in the hands-on care of a conscious small child (for instance, by holding an extremity while you insert an IV). This is much less helpful when treating older children but is more important with infants and toddlers.

When parents are not available, toys are very useful for bridging the emotional gap between paramedics and some kids. Many crews stock their ambulances with teddy bears for toddlers. Short of those, you can make a serviceable chicken out of an exam glove by inflating the glove and marking its eyes with a felt marker **Figure 10-9 ▶**. You are more likely to connect with the child if you do this right in front of the child rather than if you ask someone else to do it.

Adolescents (beginning at about age 12) may not want their parents present at all during questioning or examination. In fact, an adult who insists on monitoring your conversation

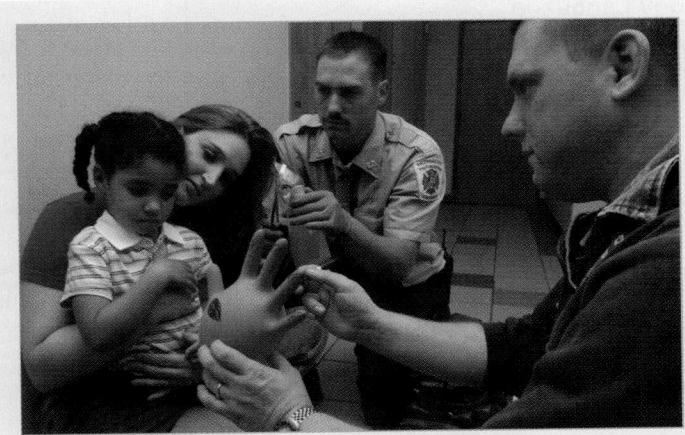

Figure 10-9 An exam-glove chicken can put a youngster at ease.

with an adolescent should raise questions in your mind. Don't refuse the prerogative of a parent, but be sure you communicate the situation to the emergency department physician, and chart it accurately. Generally, it's a good idea to deal with adolescents as adults. You gain better cooperation from them by offering them options and honoring their choices. (Hint: Never offer an option you know you can't honor.) Make special efforts to protect the modesty of adolescents in particular. They are, for the most part, obsessed with their image and what others think of them.

People Who Live With Special Challenges

It would be a mistake to overlook the needs of people who have speech, hearing, sight, or other kinds of communication disorders. Many caregivers enroll in sign-language or lip-reading classes to facilitate communication with these patients.

When you encounter a patient who has trouble communicating, remember that family members or primary caregivers who know these patients well can facilitate your efforts. Just as importantly, they can also help you to alleviate fear.

Many caregivers find that touch and eye contact are helpful bridging mechanisms when dealing with these patients. For example, a light touch on a patient's shoulder can convey kindness, while a firm grasp can express reassurance. Some patients respond well to brief, one-armed hugging. In still other situations, you can grasp a patient's face between your hands and use your eyes to convey concern or to calm him or her down.

Documentation and Communication

Many hospitals and 9-1-1 dispatch centers have interpreter capabilities and are a good resource for communicating with patients who speak a language that is different from yours. Know what resources are available for patients who use sign language as a means of communication as well.

Cross-Cultural Communication

To effectively communicate to save lives, you must strive to understand the differences inherent in all peoples, then you can adjust your efforts to accommodate and overcome cultural barriers. The most common barriers to communication include the barriers of race, ethnicity, age, gender, language, education, religion, geography, and even economic status. The combination of all these groups can be defined as "culture." No matter who we are, or where we come from, or how open-minded we think ourselves to be, we *all* have some level of prejudice we must be conscious of. You cannot treat your patients effectively if you use your own culture as your only reference—it is much like imposing your own morality on patients. While understanding other cultures is not necessarily an ethical issue, it still is best not to have preconceived ideas about how you should communicate when you care for a patient.

Cultural sensitivity and cultural diversity have become important buzzwords in business today. There are literally thousands of classes and seminars on how to deal with cultural differences of both employees and business contacts. What do all these classes and seminars actually teach? In a word, "respect."

Sounds simple enough in theory, but in practice? Many people fall short of giving even basic respect in everyday interactions, let alone in a health care environment. In the United States, emphasis falls on getting the job done, and many people seem to be too hurried and busy, and too self-absorbed, to be really concerned about how we are viewed. We can offend with the abruptness of our behavior. In other cultures, appearance and manners mean everything and lack of respect is unforgivable.

While the social practices, mannerisms, etiquette, and idiosyncrasies of all cultures are too numerous to list in one book, let alone in a chapter, it is highly important that you be open to educating yourself. It is the responsibility of the individual paramedic to research what cultural groups, ethnic groups, or religious groups are prevalent in his or her area of practice and learn how to deal with each culture accordingly. You may not get everything right when you encounter a representative from one of these groups, but your efforts at communicating will translate the idea of respect and that makes all the difference in the world.

Manners

Manners are also important. American culture has come to a place where many young people no longer have even a rudimentary understanding of good manners. Pop culture has destroyed many concepts of appropriateness in dress and behavior. Take for instance, the ubiquitous baseball cap in the United States. Not too long ago, it was considered rude for a man to wear a hat indoors, when a woman walked by, or even in a bar. Today we wear baseball caps with our paramedic uniforms. We wear them inside, outside, backwards, and sideways. Some people wear them with remarks or pictures on them that are designed to shock. While wearing a baseball cap has become accepted practice in some places in the United

States, many people are offended if they see a hat worn indoors. However, in another culture, covering your head by wearing a hat at all times is considered a demonstration of your faithfulness to God. It is important for the paramedic to know the difference.

Additionally, many of the polite forms of address have fallen by the wayside. Patients have been referred to as "dude," "mac," "man," and even "bubba." Responses to patient's questions have included "naw," "yep," "yeah," and "nuh uh." This is slang, it is lazy, and it is not professional. Get used to saying "Yes sir," "No ma'am," "Thank you," and "Please." You would be amazed at how far such niceties go in instilling confidence and establishing a professional relationship with your patient.

"Would you . . . ," "Could you . . . ," and "May I . . ." are equally important. Most people like to give permission before being touched. Lack of address and assumption of permission is particularly demeaning to an elderly person in a nursing home. You are nonverbally communicating, "You are not important enough or mentally competent enough to be asked for permission."

Manners are also important in the area of involuntary bodily functions, which often have the embarrassing tendency to erupt while performing a patient examination. Simply say, "Excuse me," and the embarrassment should be temporary.

Hand Gestures

Another American usage that may be looked upon with disfavor is our use of hand gestures. The thumbs-up sign that Americans use to indicate "everything is OK" or "ready to go" is actually the equivalent of an extended middle finger in many Arabic and some Latin countries.

The OK sign, made with thumb and index finger circled, and the other three fingers extended, is standard American for "good to go." In Latin countries, it is a reference to a circular orifice located posteriorly. It also has this meaning in Germany, Italy, and Russia. In France, the gesture means zero and can be used to indicate something is worthless. In other cultures, it represents the evil eye. In Japan, it indicates that money is needed, or that coins are preferred.

The extended middle finger is probably the rudest gesture in the American gesture catalog. In Japan, the middle digit is used as the index finger and has the same significance as pointing. Please remember this fact when providing care to a Japanese family, and they seem to "flip you off" when you ask to be shown where it hurts.

Body Language

Body language and gestures are common the world over, but an innocent gesture in one country may be a serious insult in another. Perhaps the most cross-cultural gesture, and the easiest to remember, is the simple smile. A smile is readily received by most every culture on earth and has the tendency to convey good will and acceptance. Practice it often when dealing with patients.

Every culture in the world has its own peculiarities and social and religious practices that are unique. The list below is by no means all-inclusive, but illustrates some of the differences you may see when providing cross-cultural care:

- **Bowing.** Shows rank and status in Japan. The deeper the bow, the more respect is communicated.
- **Touching the head.** Many Asians do not touch the head. The head is considered the most sacred part of the body and is the residence of the soul. Touching the head may put the soul in jeopardy.
- **Touching with the left hand.** Islamic and Hindu cultures avoid touching with the left hand, as traditionally this hand was used for unclean functions. It is considered rude and offensive to offer the left hand in greeting.
- **Feet.** Showing the bottom of the feet is considered offensive in Muslim nations, as well as most of Thailand. To point the soles of your shoes or the soles of your feet at someone is to say "you are beneath my feet" or "you are worth less than dirt."
- **Slouching.** Considered rude in Japan and in Northern European areas.
- **Hands in pockets.** A gesture of disrespect in Turkey.
- **Sitting with legs crossed.** Disrespectful in Turkey and Ghana.
- **Hands on hips.** Sign of hostility in Mexico and Argentina.
- **Eye contact.** Avoid direct eye contact to show respect in most Asian, African, Latin American, and Caribbean cultures (Somalian and Brazilian cultures are exceptions). Prolonged eye contact is acceptable in Arab, Somalian, and Brazilian cultures; in these cultures, it is believed prolonged eye contact communicates honesty and interest in the recipient.
- **Nodding.** Indian and Arabic people may signal agreement by moving the head from side-to-side (the Western "no" gesture). They may indicate no by tipping the head back, and clicking the tongue against the roof of the mouth.

You are the Provider Summary

Your ability to communicate compassion, care, and understanding can be just as important as your ability to start IVs and perform other advanced life-support skills. If you rebel against acquiring the emotional intelligence that will help you communicate effectively, you will likely experience a bumpy road as an EMS provider. Possessing a high emotional intelligence quotient will positively affect your relationships with subordinates, peers, and superiors, as well as with your patients. Possessing an understanding of the human side of EMS is essential to becoming an outstanding EMS provider.

1. What communication difficulties do you immediately anticipate in this scenario?

Patients experiencing a stroke can have difficulties understanding and communicating language. You should immediately be concerned with communication when you suspect your patient is experiencing a stroke. As you can imagine, it would be very frustrating and frightening to understand speech but be unable to respond (or vice versa). If normal methods of communication fail, think outside the box to effectively communicate with your patient.

2. Describe what the phrase "total patient care" means to you.

Total patient care involves caring for all of the patient's needs, including his or her physical, mental, and emotional needs. To ignore any of these is not caring for the entire patient and is therefore considered incomplete care. To ignore a patient's pain, for instance, is not only poor patient care but can also be considered grounds for a lawsuit if you have the ability to medicate or otherwise ease the patient's pain and fail to do so.

3. Although the paramedics in this scenario are attending to the patient's medical needs, could the wife have a valid complaint regarding their caregiving?

Yes! Although the paramedics are tired, they should not ignore questions from the wife, nor should they treat the patient as though he is a manikin. It's important to remember that EMS personnel exist to care for life-threatening conditions. Your care needs to include an education and communication component. If you choose not to work on your people skills or to learn the qualities needed for emotional intelligence, you will likely experience difficulties in communicating and caring for your patients.

4. How can your introductions (or lack thereof) and general demeanor affect your ability to communicate with your patients as well as with their friends and family members?

Failing to establish a connection with your patients will likely cause problems with your patients right from the start. You need to quickly establish a bond of trust between yourself and your patient. It can be difficult if you are tired, hungry, or otherwise having a bad day, but failing to do so will translate these feelings to your patients who may respond negatively to them.

5. How has this crew's lack of people skills affected this call?

Their failure to address the softer aspects of patient care really made this call more difficult than it needed to be. Total patient care should also encompass the needs of family members or other loved ones. Failure to address their questions or concerns can directly and negatively affect patient care and, in some instances, can exacerbate a patient's medical condition. If you don't have time to address every issue, at minimum, acknowledge questions and explain that you will address their questions after you have finished with the task at hand.

6. Can this situation be mended?

It is very difficult to undo a situation such as this one. One bad PR move can cost an EMS or fire agency and its personnel in many ways. It is very important to keep and maintain the public's trust, and one incident can destroy years of good relations between members of the public and an EMS agency.

7. What would be the best course of action in this situation?

Calling an additional crew to diffuse the situation (as well as to transport Mrs Kellar to the hospital for her chest pain) would be the best course of action. Consider the possibilities of what would happen if her condition suddenly worsened (for example, if she had an acute myocardial infarction and had a cardiac arrest). Obviously, offering a sincere apology is ideal, although it may not be enough in this situation. Requesting an additional crew to interject new faces may be required to calm both patients as well as to provide the required medical care they both need.

8. What are the different forms of communication and how do they impact patient care?

Much of how we communicate as people is done without the use of words. Body language is very powerful and can send a very different message than what is being communicated through words. Be mindful of your facial expressions, stance, and tone of voice as these will communicate your true intention or message beyond your words. Sometimes it's not what you say but how you say it that has the biggest impact on what is communicated between you and your patient.

Prep Kit

Ready for Review

- People are not just medical puzzles for us to solve; they are the reason we as paramedics exist.
- Most of the people you will meet during responses will be in crisis, and having the worst days of their lives.
- At least half of the calls you will run as a paramedic will take you into people's homes, day and night, and in the most private moments of their lives. Try to see every invitation into the home of someone else as a personal honor in a time and place where no one else would be welcome.
- If you want people to tell you about their problems, convince them you want to hear what they have to say. Give them your undivided attention.
- Active listening is repeating the key parts of a patient's responses to questions. It helps confirm the information the patient is providing. This assures there is no misunderstanding.
- Your most essential challenge as a therapeutic communicator is to convey calm, unmistakable, genuine concern for someone you've never met.
- When you first meet your patients, introduce yourself and ask them for their name. By doing so, you communicate your respect for them.
- Even if you're not convinced that patients are in real trouble, consider the possibility that they're scared to death.
- When patients tell you they're in pain, let them know you grasp and appreciate their situation, and then do something about it.
- Modesty matters, no matter how acute the medical condition. If the patient is not personally sensitive to it, family members most certainly are.
- When you need to know how patients feel, try asking open-ended questions—questions that do not have a yes or no answer, and which do not give them specific options to choose from.
- When you're trying to find out about facts (for example, a medical history), use the closed-ended, or direct, question.
- If you sense that patients are trying to put something into words, but are having trouble, be patient. Don't say anything at all for a few seconds. Let them talk.
- Never assume. Try hard to become a careful observer and to keep your mind open to a wide range of possibilities.
- Nonverbal communication can be as powerful as words.
- Direct eye contact generally communicates honesty and concern.
- Posture is important. Try to position your eyes at the same level or below the level of the patient's eyes.

- A smile can greatly help relieve a stressful situation. Your ability to smile can be valuable when you're dealing with people in crisis.
- The highest form of mental function is the spontaneous expression of appropriate humor.
- Assess how long it takes for a patient to respond appropriately to your questions. Patients who are thinking clearly should be able to answer simple questions within 1 second.
- Patients should be able to tell you accurately who they are and who you are, where they are, what time of day it is, and what happened that necessitated your being called.
- When you ask patients to perform a simple task, they should be able to do the task correctly within about 1 second.
- When a patient refuses to talk and you're not seeing signs of decreased mental status, there's no need to force the issue. Instead, make lots of eye contact, express your concern in every way possible, explain everything you are doing, invite them repeatedly to answer questions, and let them know it's all right if they don't wish to talk.
- Try not to presume that older people are any harder to communicate with than anyone else, just because they're older.
- Children can pose treatment and communication challenges even to the best of us. Minimize your movements, lower your voice, and touch them as gently as you can—possibly without gloves at first. Try keeping your eye level at or below the child's, by sitting on the floor and placing the child on the cot or on a parent's lap.
- When you encounter a patient who has trouble communicating, remember that family members or primary caregivers who know these patients well can facilitate your efforts. Just as importantly, they can also help you alleviate fear.
- Dealing with people of cultures different from your own can be challenging. It's always considered a mark of your respect if you make an effort to learn about their language and culture.

Vital Vocabulary

closed-ended question A question that is specific and focused, either demanding a yes or no answer, or an answer chosen from specific options.

communication The transmission of information to another person—whether it be verbal or through body language.

open-ended question A question that does not have a yes or no answer, and which does not give the patient specific options to choose from.

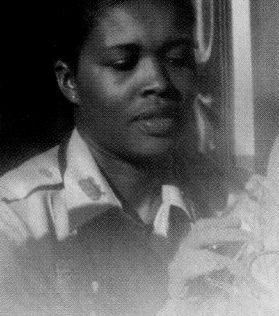

Assessment in Action

Your crew gets a call to the home of an older couple. The man has been sick with a cough and fever and is now vomiting. His wife is extremely concerned. She is also lonely and happy for the chance to talk to anyone at all. When you arrive, she takes her time telling you how his illness started, how he is doing now, and then starts talking about how long they've been married, their children, and so on. In this situation, how would you answer the following questions?

1. **The act of communicating involves:**
   - **A.** talking as much as listening.
   - **B.** listening as much as talking.
   - **C.** listening only.
   - **D.** talking only.

2. **If the man or woman in this scenario were hard of hearing, how would you handle it?**
   - **A.** Scream at him or her at the top of your lungs.
   - **B.** Get closer to him or her, but try not to be exceptionally loud.
   - **C.** Tell him or her to turn up his or her hearing aid.
   - **D.** Do whatever it takes to get the information you need, including talking loudly or writing notes.

3. If the woman in this scenario were a person who calls paramedics for every ache and pain and, as much as you like people, she drives you crazy, how would you react?
   A. Let your impatience show, hoping she will get to the point of the visit so you can do your job.
   B. Ignore her and concentrate on talking to her ill husband since he is the patient.
   C. Be patient and redirect her when she gets off track, without letting your impatience show.
   D. Listen to her whole story, picking out what's needed, and thinking about what job you'd like to switch to when you're done with that shift.

4. Just in case your patient has chest pain or cardiac issues, you need to ask if he's taking any erectile dysfunction medication. Since this couple is older, how would you go about this?
   A. Explain that you need to know some personal information in case of any cardiac issues, and explain the possible interaction with nitroglycerin or other cardiac medications.
   B. Ask her directly, making a joke out of it to make her more comfortable.
   C. Ask him instead, elbowing him jokingly and referring to "keeping her happy."
   D. Ask them both very professionally, and see who answers.

5. With this older couple, would you call them by their first names or use their last names with Mr and Mrs?
   A. Call them whatever you want, you are in charge and they are the patients.
   B. Call them by their first name to let them know you remember who they are and are on a very personal level with them.
   C. Call them pet names like "honey" and "sugar."
   D. Call them by their last names preceded by Mr and Mrs unless they say otherwise.

6. What if the woman in this scenario were so scared for her husband that she was having trouble staying calm and answering questions?
   A. Tell her to calm down and that she's doing him no good acting like that.
   B. Keep your voice calm and even. Get close enough to him so that you can do some assessments while you try to calm her down with your own calm demeanor.
   C. Have your partner take her out of the room so she isn't a distraction, and try to get the information that you need from her husband.
   D. Let your partner try to talk to her about her family while you try to talk with the patient.

7. After examining the man in this scenario, you have no idea what may be wrong with him, or if taking him to the hospital will make any difference. His wife asks you what you think. What is your best option?
   A. Tell her the truth; you have no idea, he's just sick.
   B. Talk in big medical terms she won't understand, and get busy transporting him so she can't ask for clarification.
   C. Tell her that she must face that they're both getting old and they will be more and more ill as time goes on, she should just get used to it.
   D. Tell her that you have some ideas, but it's best to let the doctor check him out. He'll be taken care of by you and the hospital staff.

Challenging Questions

An older woman fell in the shower and hurt her hip badly. You are told she has a history of osteoporosis. When you arrive, she is still lying in the bathtub with a towel covering her; her family didn't want to move her. You can see and sense that she is very modest and doesn't want that towel moved so that you can assess her injury.

8. What is the best way to handle this situation?

You have been called to the home of a 14-year-old girl who has severe cramps and heavy vaginal bleeding. You need to ask her about her sexual activity, and if there is any chance that she may be pregnant. Her parents are standing right there.

9. What should you do?

■ Points to Ponder

You are called to the scene of a car crash in which the driver of one car has significant leg injuries. He is conscious and alert, and is also deaf.

How would you best communicate with this patient?

Issues: Communicating With Patients in Special Situations, Alternative Strategies for Communication.

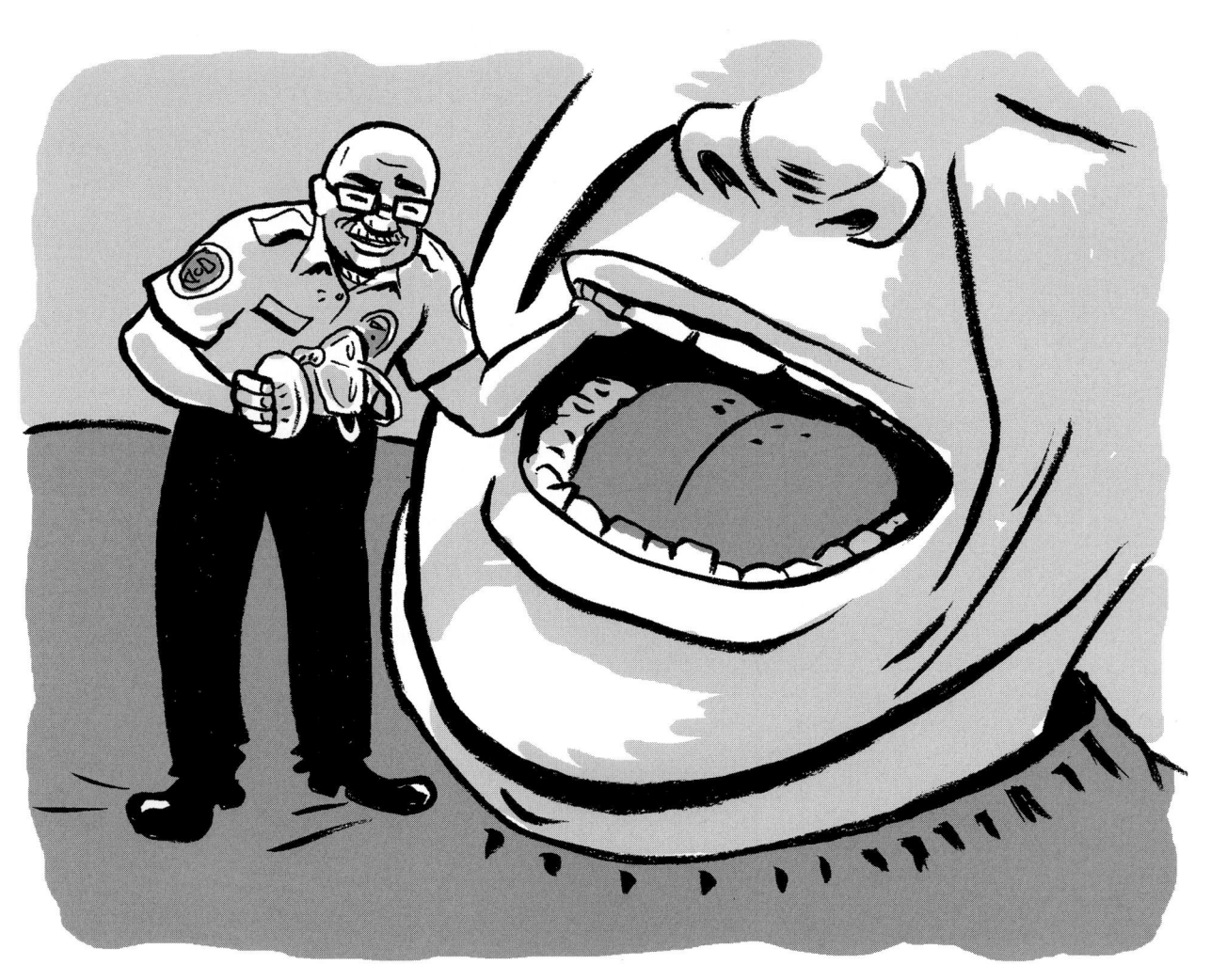

My five rules of airway management are pretty simple. 1. Blue is bad. 2. Oxygen is good. 3. Air should go in and out. 4. Noisy breathing is obstructed breathing. 5. Bare the chest!"

—Ronald D. Stewart, OC, MD, FRCPC, DSc

Airway

Section Editor: Stephen J. Rahm, NREMT-P

2

Section

11 Airway Management and Ventilation

Objectives

Cognitive

2-1.57 Differentiate endotracheal intubation from other methods of advanced airway management. (p 11.49)

2-1.58 Describe the indications, contraindications, advantages, disadvantages and complications of endotracheal intubation. (p 11.52)

2-1.59 Describe laryngoscopy for the removal of a foreign body airway obstruction. (p 11.27)

2-1.60 Describe the indications, contraindications, advantages, disadvantages, complications, equipment, and technique for direct laryngoscopy. (p 11.54)

2-1.61 Describe visual landmarks for direct laryngoscopy. (p 11.57)

2-1.62 Describe use of cricoid pressure during intubation. (p 11.96)

2-1.63 Describe indications, contraindications, advantages, disadvantages, complications, equipment and technique for digital endotracheal intubation. (p 11.68)

2-1.64 Describe the indications, contraindications, advantages, disadvantages, complications, equipment and technique for using a dual lumen airway. (p 11.84)

2-1.65 Describe the indications, contraindications, advantages, disadvantages, complications and equipment for rapid sequence intubation with neuromuscular blockade. (p 11.95)

2-1.66 Identify neuromuscular blocking drugs and other agents used in rapid sequence intubation. (p 11.94)

2-1.67 Describe the indications, contraindications, advantages, disadvantages, complications and equipment for sedation during intubation. (p 11.91)

2-1.68 Identify sedative agents used in airway management. (p 11.91)

2-1.69 Describe the indications, contraindications, advantages, disadvantages, complications, equipment and technique for nasotracheal intubation. (p 11.64)

2-1.70 Describe the indications, contraindications, advantages, disadvantages and complications for performing an open cricothyrotomy. (p 11.98)

2-1.71 Describe the equipment and technique for performing an open cricothyrotomy. (p 11.99)

2-1.72 Describe the indications, contraindications, advantages, disadvantages, complications, equipment and technique for translaryngeal catheter ventilation (needle cricothyrotomy). (p 11.101)

2-1.73 Describe methods of assessment for confirming correct placement of an endotracheal tube. (p 11.59)

2-1.74 Describe methods for securing an endotracheal tube. (p 11.61)

2-1.75 Describe the indications, contraindications, advantages, disadvantages, complications, equipment and technique for extubation. (p 11.75)

2-1.76 Describe methods of endotracheal intubation in the pediatric patient. (p 11.77, 11.83)

Affective

2-1.77 Defend the need to oxygenate and ventilate a patient. (p 11.11)

2-1.78 Defend the necessity of establishing and/or maintaining patency of a patient's airway. (p 11.15)

2-1.79 Comply with standard precautions to defend against infectious and communicable diseases. (p 11.30)

Psychomotor

2-1.80 Perform body substance isolation (BSI) procedures during basic airway management, advanced airway management, and ventilation. (p 11.54)

2-1.81 Perform pulse oximetry. (p 11.19)

2-1.82 Perform end-tidal CO_2 detection. (p 11.61)

2-1.83 Perform peak expiratory flow testing. (p 11.19, 11.20)

2-1.84 Perform manual airway maneuvers, including:
a. Opening the mouth
b. Head tilt-chin lift maneuver
c. Jaw-thrust without head-tilt maneuver
d. Modified jaw-thrust maneuver (p 11.20–11.23)

2-1.85 Perform manual airway maneuvers for pediatric patients, including:
a. Opening the mouth
b. Head tilt-chin lift maneuver
c. Jaw-thrust without head-tilt maneuver
d. Modified jaw-thrust maneuver (p 11.26)

2-1.86 Perform the Sellick maneuver (cricoid pressure). (p 11.48)

2-1.87 Perform complete airway obstruction maneuvers, including:
a. Heimlich maneuver
b. Finger sweep
c. Chest thrusts
d. Removal with Magill forceps (p 11.25–11.28)

2-1.88 Demonstrate suctioning the upper airway by selecting a suction device, catheter and technique. (p 11.30, 11.31)

2-1.89 Perform tracheobronchial suctioning in the intubated patient by selecting a suction device, catheter and technique. (p 11.78)

2-1.90 Demonstrate insertion of a nasogastric tube. (p 11.50)

2-1.91 Demonstrate insertion of an orogastric tube. (p 11.51)

2-1.92 Perform gastric decompression by selecting a suction device, catheter and technique. (p 11.48)

2-1.93 Demonstrate insertion of an oropharyngeal airway. (p 11.32, 11.33)

2-1.94 Demonstrate insertion of a nasopharyngeal airway. (p 11.34)

2-1.95 Demonstrate ventilating a patient by the following techniques:
a. Mouth-to-mask ventilation
b. One person bag-valve-mask
c. Two person bag-valve-mask
d. Three person bag-valve-mask
e. Flow-restricted, oxygen-powered ventilation device
f. Automatic transport ventilator
g. Mouth-to-stoma
h. Bag-valve-mask-to-stoma ventilation (p 11.41–11.43, 11.45, 11.46, 11.106, 11.107)

2-1.96 Ventilate a pediatric patient using the one and two person techniques. (p 11.46)

2-1.97 Perform ventilation with a bag-valve-mask with an in-line small-volume nebulizer. (p 11.39)

2-1.98 Perform oxygen delivery from a cylinder and regulator with an oxygen delivery device. (p 11.36, 11.37)

2-1.99 Perform oxygen delivery with an oxygen humidifier. (p 11.39)

2-1.100 Deliver supplemental oxygen to a breathing patient using the following devices: nasal cannula, simple face mask, partial rebreather mask, non-rebreather mask, and Venturi mask. (p 11.38)

2-1.101 Perform stoma suctioning. (p 11.103)

2-1.102 Perform retrieval of foreign bodies from the upper airway. (p 11.25)

2-1.103 Perform assessment to confirm correct placement of the endotracheal tube. (p 11.59)

2-1.104 Intubate the trachea by the following methods:
a. Orotracheal intubation
b. Nasotracheal intubation
c. Multi-lumen airways
d. Digital intubation
e. Transillumination
f. Open cricothyrotomy (p 11.65, 11.68, 11.70, 11.72, 11.76, 11.86, 11.87, 11.100)

2-1.105 Adequately secure an endotracheal tube. (p 11.61–11.63)

2-1.106 Perform endotracheal intubation in the pediatric patient. (p 11.80)

2-1.107 Perform transtracheal catheter ventilation (needle cricothyrotomy). (p 11.101)

2-1.108 Perform extubation. (p 11.79)

2-1.109 Perform replacement of a tracheostomy tube through a stoma. (p 11.108)

Maintaining a Patent Airway: A Critical Concern

Establishing and maintaining a patent (open) airway and ensuring effective oxygenation and ventilation are vital aspects of effective patient care. Attempting to stabilize a patient whose airway is compromised is futile. No airway, no patient—it's that simple! The human body needs a constant supply of oxygen to carry out the physiologic processes necessary to sustain life; the airway is where it all begins. Few situations will cause such acute deterioration and death more rapidly than airway and ventilation compromise. Therefore, the patient's airway must remain patent at all times.

The function of the respiratory system is quite simple: It brings in oxygen and eliminates carbon dioxide (the primary waste product of oxygen metabolism). If this process is interrupted, vital organs of the body will not function properly. For example, the brain can survive for only 6 minutes or so without oxygen before permanent brain damage is virtually assured.

Failure to manage the airway or inappropriate management of the airway is a major cause of preventable death in the prehospital setting. Unfortunately, basic techniques to secure a patent airway are commonly neglected or performed improperly in the rush to proceed to advanced interventions. Poor technique (eg, improper bag-mask seal, improper airway positioning) and failure to reassess the patient's condition merely serve to increase mortality and morbidity.

Health care providers must understand the importance of early detection of airway problems, rapid and effective intervention, and continual reassessment of a patient with airway or breathing compromise.

This chapter examines the airway in detail, beginning with a review of the anatomy and physiology of the respiratory system. It follows a "basic-to-advanced" approach, just as airway management should be performed in the field. The chapter describes the various techniques of opening and maintaining a patent airway, recognizing and treating airway obstructions, assessing a patient's ventilation status, administering supplemental oxygen, and providing ventilatory assistance. Advanced techniques, including advanced airway devices and procedures, are then discussed in detail.

Anatomy of the Upper Airway

The upper airway consists of all anatomic airway structures above the level of the vocal cords. Its major functions are to warm, filter, and humidify air as it enters the body through the nose and mouth. The first portion of the upper airway, the pharynx (throat), is a muscular tube that extends from the nose and mouth to the level of the esophagus and trachea. The pharynx is composed of the nasopharynx, oropharynx, and laryngopharynx (also called the hypopharynx). The laryngopharynx is the lowest portion of the pharynx; it opens into the larynx anteriorly and the esophagus posteriorly **Figure 11-1 ▼** .

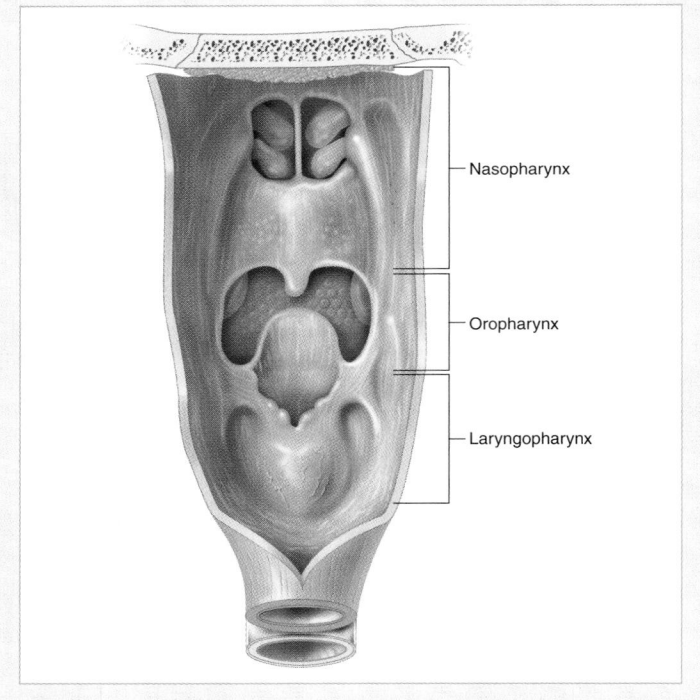

Figure 11-1 The pharynx.

You are the Provider Part 1

You are dispatched to a grocery store for a 50-year-old man with difficulty breathing. You and your paramedic partner reach the scene in approximately 5 minutes. Upon arrival, you find the patient sitting on a bench in front of the store. He is conscious, alert, and in mild respiratory distress. He tells you, in complete sentences, that he suddenly began having trouble breathing while inside the store.

1. Is this patient's airway patent?
2. How will you proceed with your assessment of this patient?

Nasopharynx

On inhalation, air normally enters the body through the nose and passes into the nasopharynx, which is formed by the union of the facial bones.

The entire nasal cavity is lined with a ciliated mucous membrane that keeps contaminants such as dust and other small particles out of the respiratory tract. In illness, the body produces additional mucus to trap potentially infectious agents. This mucous membrane is extremely delicate and has a rich blood supply. Any trauma to the nasal passages, such as improper or overly aggressive placement of airway devices, may result in profuse bleeding from the posterior nasal cavity. Bleeding from this area cannot be controlled by direct pressure. Extrinsic factors (eg, cocaine use) can also damage the delicate nasal passages or the septum, which separates the two nares.

Three bony shelves, called turbinates, protrude from the lateral walls of the nasal cavity and extend into the nasal passageway, parallel to the nasal floor. The turbinates serve to increase the surface area of the nasal mucosa, thereby improving the processes of warming, filtering, and humidification of inhaled air.

The nasopharynx is divided into two passages by the nasal septum, a rigid partition composed of bone and cartilage. Normally, the nasal septum is in the midline of the nose. In some people the septum may be deviated to one side or the other—a condition that becomes important when contemplating insertion of a nasal airway.

The sinuses are cavities formed by the cranial bones. Fractures of these bones may cause cerebrospinal fluid (CSF) to leak from the nose (cerebrospinal rhinorrhea) or the ears (cerebrospinal otorrhea). The sinuses prevent contaminants from entering the respiratory tract and act as tributaries for fluid to and from the eustachian tubes and tear ducts.

Oropharynx

The oropharynx forms the posterior portion of the oral cavity, which is bordered superiorly by the hard and soft palates, laterally by the cheeks, and inferiorly by the tongue **Figure 11-2 ▾**. The 32 adult teeth are embedded in the gums in such a manner that significant force is required to dislodge them. However, trauma of lesser severity may result in fracture or avulsion of the teeth, potentially obstructing the upper airway or causing aspiration of tooth fragments into the lungs.

The tongue is a large muscle attached to the mandible and the hyoid bone—a small, horseshoe-shaped bone to which the jaw, epiglottis, and thyroid cartilage attach as well. From an airway perspective, the most important anatomical consideration regarding the tongue is its tendency to fall back and occlude the posterior pharynx when the mandible relaxes. In fact, the tongue is the most common cause of anatomic upper airway obstruction, especially in patients with a decreased level of consciousness.

The palate forms the roof of the mouth and separates the oropharynx and nasopharynx. Its anterior portion, which is formed by the maxilla and palatine bones, is called the hard palate. The soft palate is posterior to the hard palate.

The adenoids, which are located on the posterior nasopharyngeal wall, are lymphatic tissue that filters bacteria. The tonsils, which are also made of lymphatic tissue, are located in posterior pharynx; they help to trap bacteria. The adenoids and

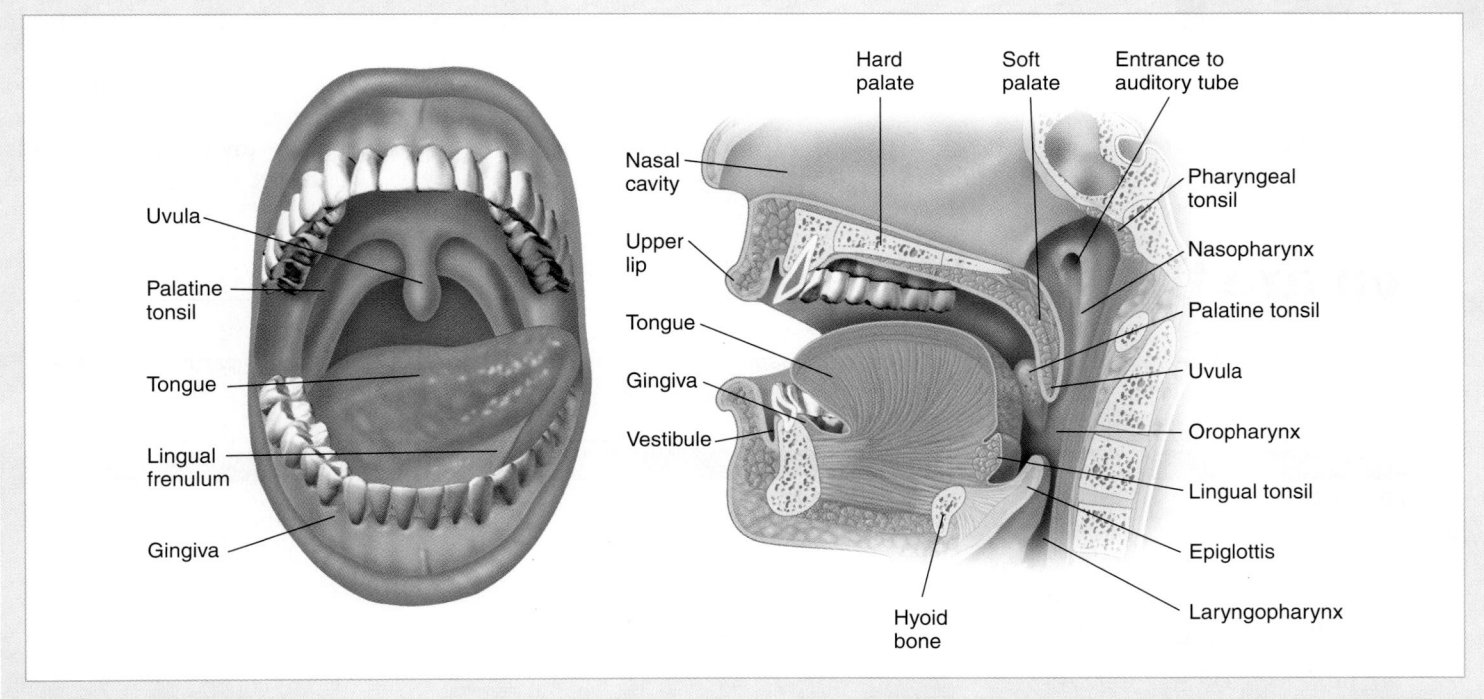

Figure 11-2 The oral cavity.

tonsils often become swollen and infected. Severe swelling of the tonsils can potentially cause obstruction of the upper airway.

The uvula, a soft-tissue structure that resembles a punching bag, is located in the posterior aspect of the oral cavity, at the base of the tongue.

The superior border of the glottic opening is the epiglottis. This leaf-shaped cartilaginous flap prevents food and liquid from entering the larynx during swallowing.

The vallecula is an anatomic space, or "pocket," located between the base of the tongue and the epiglottis. It is an important landmark for endotracheal intubation.

Larynx

The larynx is a complex structure formed by many independent cartilaginous structures (Figure 11-3 ▾). It marks where the upper airway ends and the lower airway begins.

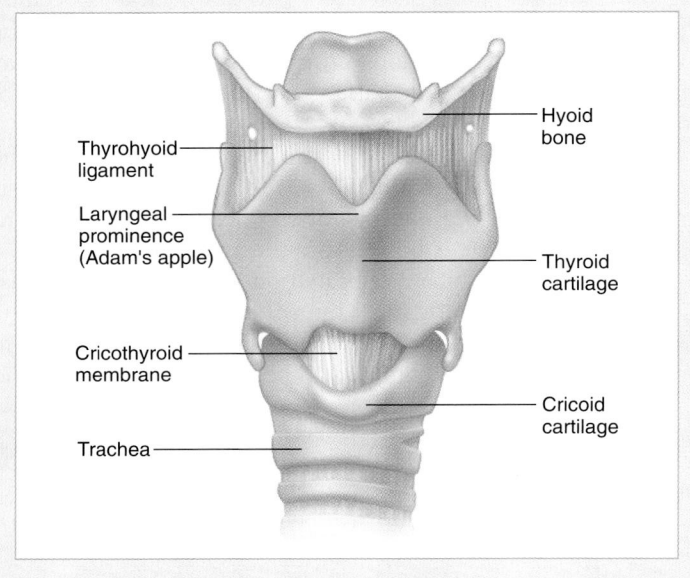

Figure 11-3 The larynx.

The thyroid cartilage is a shield-shaped structure formed by two plates that join in a "V" shape anteriorly to form the laryngeal prominence known as the Adam's apple. The thyroid cartilage is suspended in place by the thyroid ligament and is directly anterior to the glottic opening.

The cricoid cartilage, or cricoid ring, lies inferiorly to the thyroid cartilage; it forms the lowest portion of the larynx. The cricoid cartilage is the first ring of the trachea and the only upper airway structure that forms a complete ring.

Between the thyroid and cricoid cartilages is the cricothyroid membrane, which is a site for emergency surgical and nonsurgical access to the airway (cricothyrotomy). Because it is bordered laterally and inferiorly by the highly vascular thyroid gland, EMS personnel must locate the anatomic landmarks carefully when accessing the airway via this site.

The glottis, also called the glottic opening, is the space in between the vocal cords and the narrowest portion of the adult's airway (Figure 11-4 ▸). Airway patency in this area is heavily dependent on adequate muscle tone. The lateral borders of the glottis are the vocal cords. At rest, these white bands of tough tissue are partially separated (ie, the glottis is partially open). During forceful inhalation, the vocal cords open widely to provide minimum resistance to air flow.

The arytenoid cartilages are pyramid-like cartilaginous structures that form the posterior attachment of the vocal cords; they are valuable guides for endotracheal intubation. As the arytenoid cartilages pivot, the vocal cords open and close, which regulates the passage of air through the larynx and controls the production of sound; hence, the larynx is sometimes called the "voice box."

The pyriform fossae are two pockets of tissue on the lateral borders of the larynx. Airway devices are occasionally inadvertently inserted into these pockets, resulting in a tenting of the skin under the jaw.

When the airway is stimulated (eg, during aspiration of foreign material or submersion incident), defensive reflexes cause a laryngospasm—spasmodic closure of the vocal cords, which seals off the airway. This reflex normally lasts a few

You are the Provider Part 2

Closer examination of the patient reveals that he has mild accessory muscle use and intercostal retractions. As your partner opens the jump kit, you perform an initial assessment and note the following:

Initial Assessment	Recording Time: 0 Minutes
Appearance	Obvious respiratory distress; anxious; pale
Level of consciousness	A (Alert to person, place, and day)
Airway	Open and clear
Breathing	Increased respiratory rate, labored breathing with adequate tidal volume
Circulation	Skin, pale and diaphoretic; radial pulse, rapid and bounding

3. What immediate management is indicated for this patient?

4. What questions would be pertinent to ask this patient?

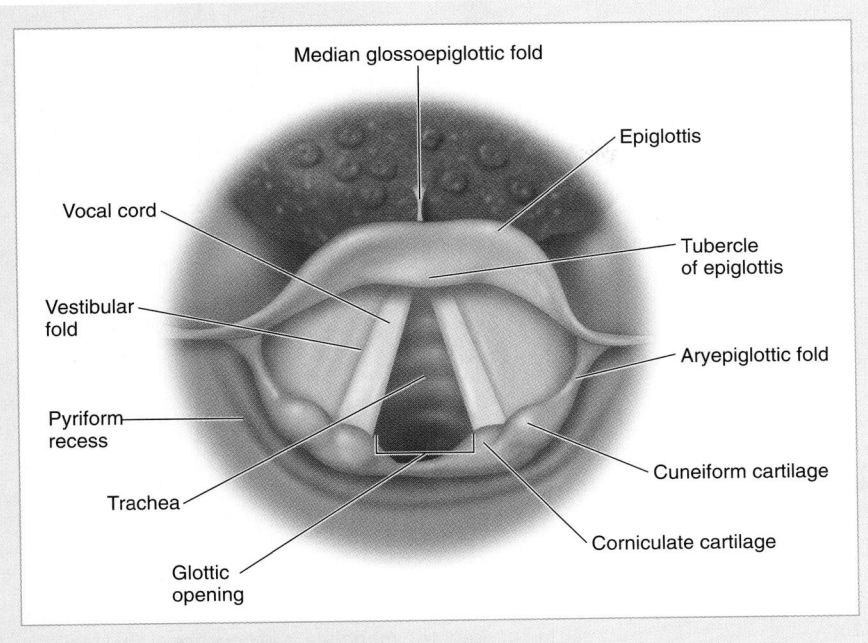

Figure 11-4 The glottis and surrounding structures.

seconds. Persistent laryngospasm can threaten the airway by preventing ventilation altogether.

Anatomy of the Lower Airway

The function of the lower airway is to exchange oxygen and carbon dioxide. Externally, it extends from the fourth cervical vertebra to the xiphoid process. Internally, it spans the glottis to the pulmonary capillary membrane.

The trachea, or windpipe, is the conduit for air entry into the lungs. This tubular structure is approximately 10 to 12 cm in length and consists of a series of C-shaped cartilaginous rings. The trachea begins immediately below the cricoid cartilage and descends anteriorly down the midline of the neck and chest to the level of the fifth or sixth thoracic vertebra. It divides into the right and left mainstem bronchi at the level of the carina. These bronchi are lined with mucus-producing cells and beta-2 receptors that, when stimulated, result in bronchodilation.

The right bronchus is somewhat shorter and straighter than the left bronchus. Thus an endotracheal tube that is inserted too far will often come to lie in the right mainstem bronchus.

All of the blood vessels and the bronchi enter each lung at the hilum. The lungs consist of the entire mass of tissue that includes the smaller bronchi, bronchioles, and alveoli **Figure 11-5 ▶**. In total, the lungs can hold approximately 6 L of air.

The right lung has three lobes and the left lung has two lobes, which are covered with a thin, slippery outer lining called the visceral pleura. The parietal pleura lines the inside of the thoracic cavity. A small amount of fluid is found between the pleurae, which decreases friction during breathing.

Upon entering the lungs, each bronchus divides into increasingly smaller bronchi, which in turn subdivide into bronchioles. The bronchioles, which are made of smooth muscle, dilate or constrict in response to various stimuli. The smaller bronchioles branch into alveolar ducts that end at the alveolar sacs.

The balloon-like clusters of single-layer air sacs known as alveoli are the functional site for the exchange of oxygen and carbon dioxide. This exchange occurs by simple diffusion between the alveoli and the pulmonary capillaries.

The alveoli are lined with a proteinaceous substance called surfactant, which decreases surface tension on the alveolar walls and keeps them expanded. If the amount of pulmonary surfactant is decreased or the alveoli are not inflated, they will collapse—a condition called atelectasis.

Lung and Respiratory Volumes

The total lung capacity in the average adult male is approximately 6 L, but only a fraction of this capacity is used during normal breathing. While a small amount of gas exchange occurs in the alveolar ducts and terminal bronchioles, most of the gas exchange occurs in the alveoli.

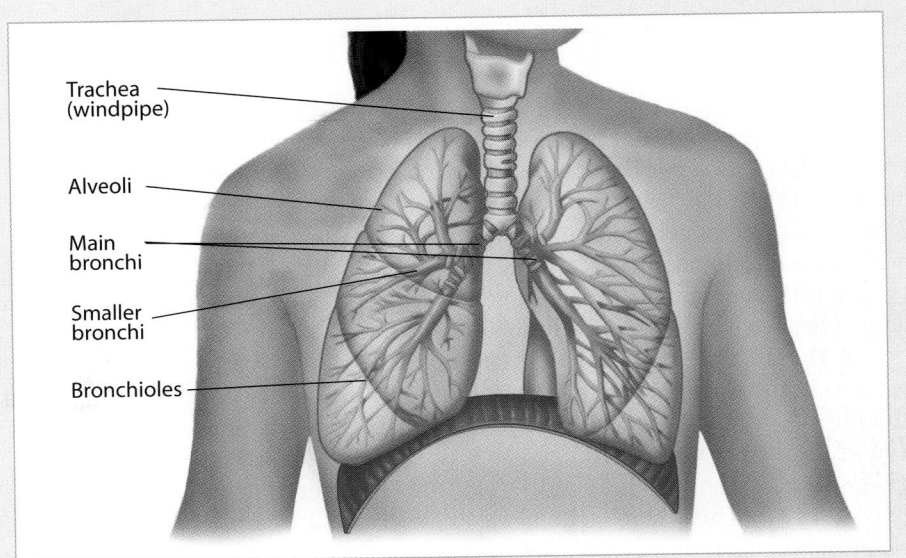

Figure 11-5 The trachea and the lungs (lower airway structures).

Special Considerations

Although the maneuvers, techniques, and indications for airway management are essentially the same in children as they are in adults, several anatomic differences in the child make mastery of these techniques critical.

Infants and small children have a proportionately larger occiput, which causes the head to flex when the child lies supine; this position itself can cause an airway obstruction. When positioning the airway of an infant or child, you should place a folded towel under his or her shoulders to maintain a neutral position of the head.

Compared to adults, children have a proportionately smaller mandible and a proportionately larger tongue **Figure 11-6 ▸**. Both factors increase the incidence of airway obstruction in children.

The child's epiglottis is more floppy and omega-shaped than an adult's. As a consequence, it must be lifted out of the way to visualize the vocal cords for intubation **Figure 11-7 ▸**.

In general, the infant's and child's airway is smaller and narrower at all levels. The larynx lies more superior and anterior than in an adult—an important consideration when visualizing the vocal cords for intubation. The larynx is also funnel-shaped due to the narrow, underdeveloped cricoid cartilage. In children younger than 10 years, the narrowest portion of the airway is at the cricoid ring. Further narrowing of the child's inherently narrow airway, such as that caused by soft-tissue swelling or foreign body aspiration, can result in a major decrease in airway resistance and breathing inadequacy.

Children do not have well-developed chest musculature, and their ribs and cartilage are softer and more pliable than an adult's. As a result, the thoracic cavity cannot optimally contribute to lung expansion. Children rely heavily on their diaphragm for breathing, which moves their abdomen in and out. For this reason, infants and children are commonly referred to as "belly breathers."

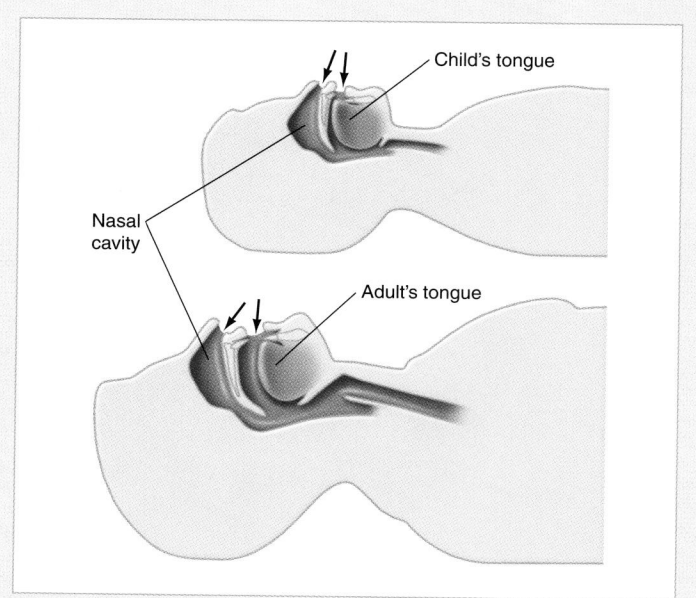

Figure 11-6 In children, the mandible is proportionately smaller and the tongue is proportionately larger than in an adult.

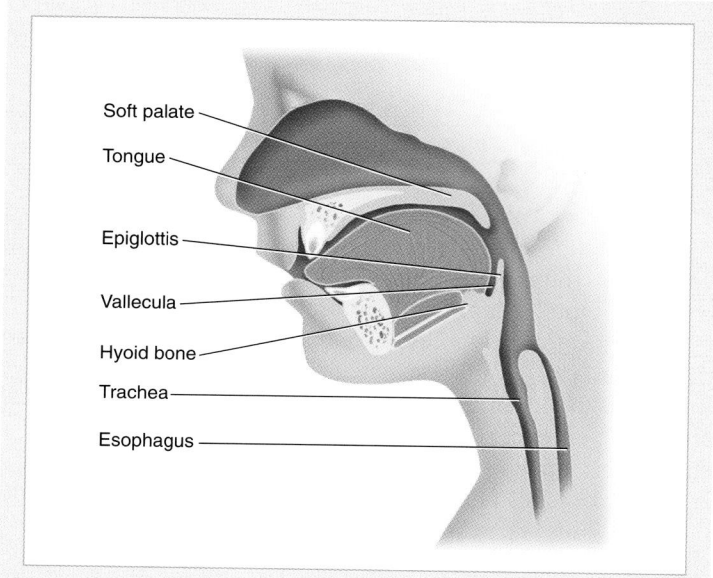

Figure 11-7 The child's epiglottis and surrounding structures.

Tidal volume (V_T), a measure of the depth of breathing, is the volume of air that is inhaled or exhaled during a single respiratory cycle. Normal tidal volume in the average adult male is 5 to 7 mL/kg (approximately 500 mL). In infants and children, normal tidal volume is approximately 6 to 8 mL/kg. Inspiratory reserve volume is the amount of air that can be inhaled in addition to the normal tidal volume; it is normally about 3,000 mL.

In the adult, about 30% of the normal tidal volume remains in the upper airway passages; this so-called dead space volume (V_D) is approximately 150 mL. Dead space is any portion of the airway where air lingers, but does not participate in gas exchange. The anatomic dead space includes the trachea and larger bronchi, where residual gas may remain at the end of inhalation. Certain respiratory diseases increase dead space by creating intrapulmonary obstructions or atelectasis; these areas are called physiologic dead space.

The remaining volume of inhaled air, which does reach the alveoli and therefore does participate in gas exchange, is called alveolar volume. Alveolar volume is equal to tidal volume minus dead space volume; it is approximately 350 mL in the average adult male.

It is important to understand the concepts of minute volume (V_M) and minute alveolar volume (V_A). Minute volume is simply the amount of air that moves in and out of the respiratory tract per minute; it is determined by multiplying the tidal volume by the respiratory rate ($V_M = V_T \times RR$). Minute alveolar volume (V_A) is the amount of air that actually reaches the alveoli per minute and participates in gas exchange; it is determined by multiplying the tidal volume (minus dead space volume) by the respiratory rate. For example:

$$(500 \text{ mL } [V_T] - 150 \text{ mL } [V_D]) \times 16 \text{ breaths/min} = 5,600 \text{ mL } (V_A)$$

Minute volume will increase if the tidal volume, respiratory rate, or both, increases. Conversely, minute volume will decrease if the tidal volume, respiratory rate, or both, decreases. As the respirations become faster, however, they typically become more shallow (reduced tidal volume). When respirations are too rapid *and* too shallow, the inhaled air may reach only the anatomic dead space before it is promptly exhaled, resulting in decreased minute alveolar volume.

Table 11-1 ▶ demonstrates how tidal volume and respiratory rate can influence a patient's minute alveolar volume and, therefore, overall breathing adequacy. This information will prove useful for assessing a patient's breathing adequacy and identifying patients who require assisted ventilation.

Following an optimal inspiration, the amount of air that can be forced from the lungs in a single exhalation is called the functional reserve capacity. The amount of air that you can exhale following normal (relaxed) exhalation is called the expiratory reserve volume; this amount is about 1,200 mL. Even if you exhale forcefully, however, you cannot completely empty your lungs of air. Residual volume is the air that remains in the

Table 11-1	How Tidal Volume and Respiratory Rate Affect Minute Alveolar Volume
Example 1: Normal tidal volume and respiratory rate $(500 \text{ mL } [V_T] - 150 \text{ mL } [V_D]) \times 16 \text{ breaths/min} = \textbf{5,600 mL } (V_A)$ *Good!*	
Example 2: Reduced tidal volume and a normal respiratory rate $(250 \text{ mL } [V_T] - 150 \text{ mL } [V_D]) \times 14 \text{ breaths/min} = \textbf{1,400 mL } (V_A)$ *Not good!*	
Example 3: Reduced tidal volume and a slow respiratory rate $(350 \text{ mL } [V_T] - 150 \text{ mL } [V_D]) \times 6 \text{ breaths/min} = \textbf{1,200 mL } (V_A)$ *Not good!*	
Example 4: Reduced tidal volume and a fast respiratory rate $(200 \text{ mL } [V_T] - 150 \text{ mL } [V_D]) \times 40 \text{ breaths/min} = \textbf{2,000 mL } (V_A)$ *Not good!*	

lungs after maximal expiration; it is also about 1,200 mL in the average adult male.

The fraction of inspired oxygen (FIO_2) is the percentage of oxygen in inhaled air. FIO_2 increases when supplemental oxygen is given to a patient and is commonly documented as a decimal point.

Ventilation

Ventilation is the process of moving air into and out of the lungs. If a patient is not breathing or is breathing inadequately, he or she no longer has an effective mechanism to intake oxygen and eliminate carbon dioxide. Therefore, ensuring adequate ventilation is one of the highest priorities in treating any patient.

Ventilation consists of two phases:

- **Inspiration** (inhalation) is the process of moving air into the lungs.
- **Expiration** (exhalation) is the process of moving air out of the lungs.

Documentation and Communication

A person breathing room air, which contains 21% oxygen, would be documented as having an FIO_2 of 0.21. A nonrebreathing mask, which delivers about 90% oxygen, would be documented as delivering an FIO_2 of 0.90 to an adequately breathing patient.

You are the Provider Part 3

Your partner applies a nonrebreathing mask on the patient and sets the flow rate at 15 L/min as you perform a focused history and physical examination. The patient tells you that he has congestive heart failure. The following baseline vital signs are obtained:

Vital Signs	Recording Time: 2 Minutes
Respirations	28 breaths/min, labored, adequate depth
Pulse	120 beats/min, regular and bounding
Skin	Pale and diaphoretic
Blood pressure	144/94 mm Hg
Sao_2	95% while receiving 100% oxygen via nonrebreathing mask

5. Is this patient breathing adequately? Why or why not?

6. What are the signs of inadequate ventilation?

One ventilation cycle consists of one inspiration, which occupies approximately one third of the ventilation cycle, and one expiration, which occupies the remaining two thirds.

Regulation of Ventilation

The body's need for oxygen is dynamic; it is constantly changing. The respiratory system must be able to accommodate those changes in oxygen demand by altering the rate and depth of ventilation. These changes are regulated primarily by the pH of the CSF, which is directly related to the amount of carbon dioxide dissolved in the plasma portion of the blood (Pa_{CO_2}). The regulation of ventilation involves a complex series of receptors and feedback loops that sense gas concentrations in the body fluids and send messages to the respiratory center in the brain to adjust the rate and depth of ventilation accordingly.

Neural Control of Ventilation

Neural (nervous system) control of breathing can be traced to the medulla. The involuntary control of breathing originates in the brain stem—specifically, in the pons and the medulla. The impulses for automatic breathing descend through the spinal cord and can be overridden (to a point) by voluntary control, such as when you talk or hold your breath.

Two types of motor nerves affect breathing. The phrenic nerves innervate the diaphragm. The intercostal nerves innervate the external intercostal muscles between the ribs.

The respiratory center in the medulla is divided into three regions: the respiratory rhythmicity center, the apneustic center, and the pneumotaxic center. The respiratory rhythmicity center sets the respiratory rate. During normal, quiet breathing, it gradually increases the stimulation for inhalation over 2 seconds and then relaxes for 3 seconds, allowing passive exhalation, and then repeats the cycle. This results in a resting respiratory rate.

As the chest expands, mechanical (stretch) receptors in the chest wall and bronchioles send a signal to the apneustic center via the vagus nerve to inhibit the inspiratory center, and expiration occurs. This feedback loop, which combines neural and mechanical control, is called the Hering-Breuer reflex. It is a protective mechanism that terminates inhalation, thus preventing overexpansion of the lungs.

The apneustic center influences the respiratory rate by increasing the number of inspirations per minute. Its activity is countered by the functioning of the pneumotaxic center, which inhibits inspiration. In times of increased demand, the pneumotaxic center decreases its influence, thereby increasing the respiratory rate.

Chemical Control of Ventilation

The respiratory system must keep the blood's concentrations of oxygen and carbon dioxide and its acid-base balance within a very narrow range. The body has a number of chemoreceptors that monitor the levels of O_2, CO_2, and the pH of the CSF and provide feedback to the respiratory centers to modify the rate and depth of breathing based on the body's needs at any given time **Figure 11-8 ▶** .

The chemoreceptors that monitor the carbon dioxide content in arterial blood are located in the carotid bodies and the

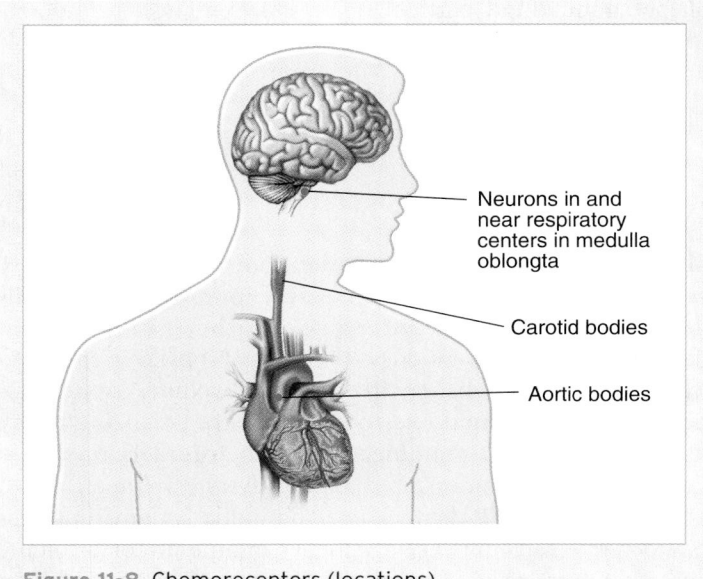

Figure 11-8 Chemoreceptors (locations).

Neurons in and near respiratory centers in medulla oblongta

Carotid bodies

Aortic bodies

aortic arch. These receptors sense minute changes in the Pa_{CO_2} and send signals to the respiratory centers via the glossopharyngeal nerve (ninth cranial nerve) and the vagus nerve (tenth cranial nerve).

Central chemoreceptors, which monitor the pH of the CSF, are located adjacent to the respiratory centers in the medulla. An increase in the acidity (decreased pH) of the CSF triggers these chemoreceptors to increase the rate and depth of breathing. These receptors are very sensitive to small changes in pH and provide for "fine-tuning" of the body's acid-base balance.

Under normal circumstances, fluctuations in Pa_{CO_2} and pH of the CSF are the dominant influence on respiration, and the primary respiratory drive derives from the body's attempt to regulate the Pa_{CO_2} within normal limits. However, some patients with chronic respiratory diseases are unable to take in O_2 and eliminate CO_2 effectively, so their respiratory centers have gradually accommodated to high Pa_{CO_2} levels.

In such cases, the body uses a "backup system" to control breathing. Although the primary control of breathing is based on the Pa_{CO_2} and the pH of the CSF, the chemoreceptors in the carotid bodies and aortic arch also respond to decreased levels of oxygen dissolved in the plasma (Pa_{O_2}). In this scenario, the chemoreceptors send messages to the respiratory center to increase the rate and depth of breathing. This secondary control of breathing is called the hypoxic drive. Usually only end-stage COPD patients are on hypoxic drive.

Control of Ventilation by Other Factors

Numerous factors other than changes in the pH and Pa_{CO_2} can influence ventilation. As the body temperature rises (ie, in the case of fever), respirations increase in response to the increased metabolic activity. Certain medications cause respirations to increase or decrease, depending on their physiologic action. For example, amphetamines (eg, Ritalin, Adderall), which produce a sympathomimetic effect, would cause an increase in

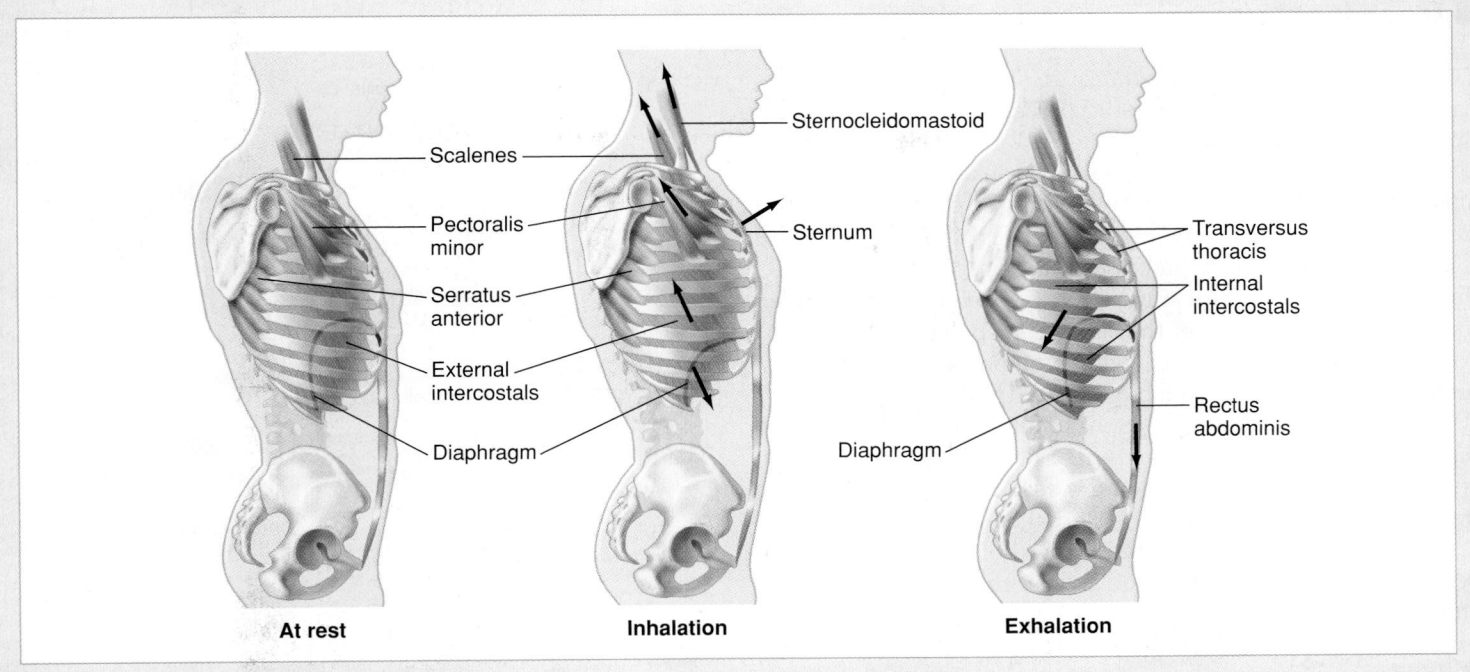

Figure 11-9 The mechanics of breathing.

respirations, whereas narcotic analgesics (eg, morphine, Demerol) would cause a decrease in respirations due to their central nervous system depressant effects. Pain and strong emotions can also increase respirations.

Hypoxia is a powerful stimulus to breathe, and would result in increased respirations in an effort to bring more oxygen into the body. Conversely, acidosis increases respirations as a compensatory response to promote the elimination of excess carbon dioxide produced by the body.

A person's metabolic rate also influences the rate of breathing. When the metabolic rate is high (eg, during exercise), respirations increase to eliminate the excess carbon dioxide produced. Conversely, when the metabolic rate is low (eg, during sleep), respirations slow.

The Mechanics of Ventilation

Ventilation is accomplished through pressure changes in the lungs, which in turn are brought about by contraction and relaxation of the intercostal muscles and diaphragm. The diaphragm, which is the major muscle of breathing, is the anatomic point of separation between the thoracic cavity and the abdominal cavity.

Inhalation is an active process that is initiated by contraction of the respiratory muscles. As the diaphragm contracts after receiving impulses from the phrenic nerves it flattens out, increasing the vertical dimensions of the thorax. At the same time, the intercostal muscles contract after receiving impulses from the intercostal nerves, causing the ribs and sternum to move upward and outward, increasing the horizontal dimensions of the chest cavity. The net effect is to increase the volume

of the chest. The lungs, being highly elastic and "glued" via the visceral pleura to the chest wall, undergo a comparable increase in volume. The air in the lungs now suddenly occupies a larger space, so the pressure within the lungs drops rapidly. As the air pressure inside the chest falls below that of the outside atmosphere, air begins to flow from the region of higher pressure (outside the body) to the region of lower pressure (the lungs)—a process called negative-pressure ventilation. When the pressures inside and outside the lungs are equalized, inhalation stops. Oxygen and carbon dioxide then diffuse across the alveolar-capillary membrane in the lungs.

In contrast to inhalation, exhalation is a passive process. At the end of inhalation, the respiratory muscles relax. The natural elasticity (recoil) of the lungs passively exhales the air. **Figure 11-9 ▲** illustrates the processes of inhalation and exhalation.

In the Field

Normal breathing involves negative intrathoracic pressure and the pulling of air into the lungs.

With ineffective chest movement (eg, reduced tidal volume) or no chest movement (eg, apnea), negative intrathoracic pressure cannot be created. The only way to move air into the lungs is then by positive-pressure ventilation, the forcing of air into the lungs. Positive pressure can be created with a bag-mask device, pocket face mask, or a mechanical ventilation device.

Respiration

Every living cell in the body requires an uninterrupted supply of oxygen to carry out its metabolic processes. The cells of the brain and heart, for example, can tolerate only very short periods of oxygen deprivation—usually less than about 6 minutes—after which they will die. Once brain cells or myocardial (heart muscle) cells have died, they can never be replaced.

The same metabolic processes that consume oxygen produce carbon dioxide as a waste product. This carbon dioxide must be carried away from the cell and disposed of, or it may accumulate to toxic levels. Therefore, the body needs a mechanism to eliminate the carbon dioxide produced by metabolism.

As it happens, the body very economically uses the same mechanism—respiration—to ensure a constant oxygen supply and to remove the excess carbon dioxide. Two types of respiration occur in the human body: external and internal. External respiration (pulmonary respiration) is the exchange of gases between the lungs and the blood cells in the pulmonary capillaries. Internal respiration (cellular respiration) is the exchange of gases between the blood cells and the tissues **Figure 11-10 ▶**.

Gas exchange in the body occurs by diffusion, a process in which a gas moves from an area of higher concentration to an area of lower concentration. Both oxygen and carbon dioxide pass through the alveolar membrane by diffusion.

Dissolved oxygen crosses the pulmonary capillary membrane and binds to the hemoglobin molecule of the red blood cell. Without hemoglobin, oxygen transport is not possible. Consequently, replacing large amounts of lost blood with isotonic crystalloid solutions (eg, normal saline, lactated Ringer's), which lack hemoglobin, will be not be as effective as replacing lost blood with whole blood or packed red blood cells.

Approximately 97% of the body's total oxygen is bound to hemoglobin; the remainder is dissolved in the plasma portion of the blood. A pulse oximeter reads the percentage of hemoglobin that is saturated with oxygen (Sao_2), which is normally greater than 95%. The remaining oxygen that is dissolved in the plasma makes up the partial pressure of oxygen (Pao_2 or Po_2).

The majority of carbon dioxide is transported in the blood in the form of bicarbonate ions, with about 33% being bound to the hemoglobin. As O_2 crosses from the alveoli into the blood, CO_2 diffuses from the blood into the alveoli. The carbon dioxide dissolved in the plasma makes up the partial pressure of CO_2 ($Paco_2$ or Pco_2).

Causes of Decreased Oxygen Concentrations in the Blood

Numerous conditions can result in decreased blood-oxygen concentrations. A lower partial pressure of atmospheric oxygen, such as an environment rich in carbon monoxide (CO), decreases the available amount of oxygen. CO has a much greater affinity for hemoglobin than oxygen (250 times more). Severe bleeding decreases the hemoglobin levels in the blood,

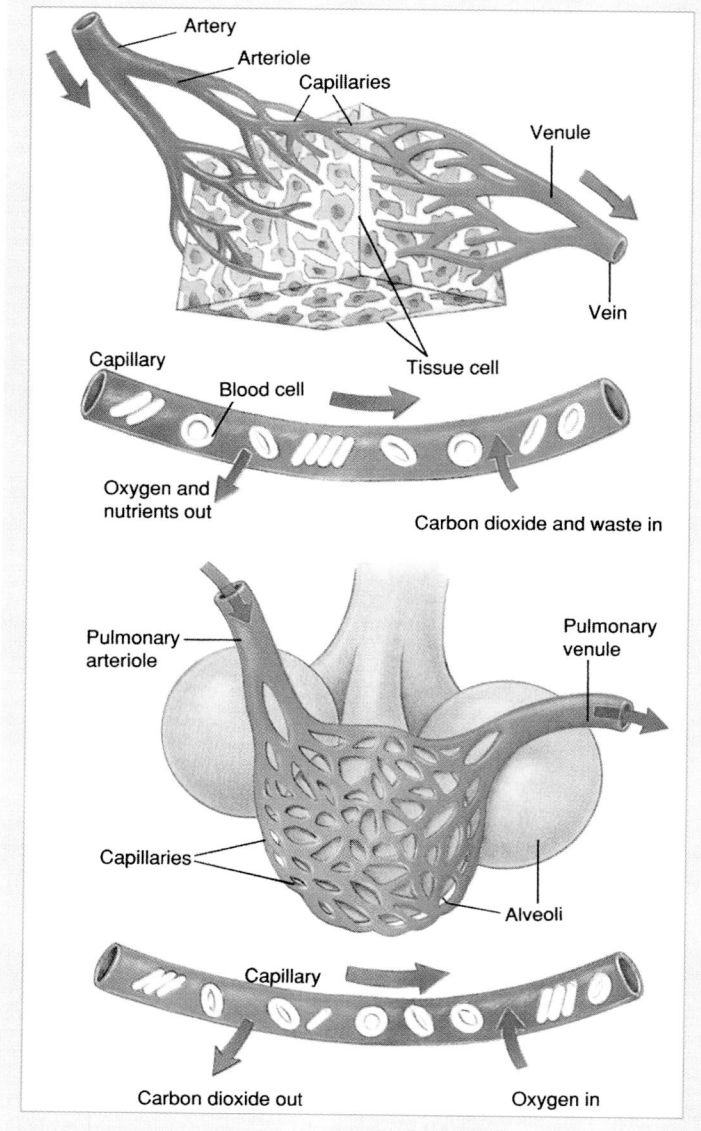

Figure 11-10 Internal and external respiration.

thereby decreasing the oxygen-carrying capability of the blood and, in turn, decreasing the amount of oxygen available to the cells. Anemia, a deficiency of red blood cells, results in a chronically decreased ability of the blood to carry oxygen. Without sufficient circulating red blood cells, there is nothing for the hemoglobin molecule to unite with.

Conditions that reduce the surface area for gas exchange also decrease the body's available oxygen supply—for example flail chest, diaphragmatic injury, simple or tension pneumothorax, open pneumothorax (sucking chest wound), hemothorax, and hemopneumothorax.

Decreased mechanical effort also decreases the availability of oxygen for respiration. Patients experiencing severe chest pain secondary to trauma or a medical condition tend to breathe as shallowly as possible in an effort to reduce chest wall movement and alleviate the pain; this is called "respiratory splinting." Traumatic asphyxia, an injury caused by severe compression of the chest, and hypoventilation from any cause also result in decreased oxygen levels in the blood.

Medical conditions such as pneumonia, pulmonary edema, and chronic obstructive pulmonary disease (COPD) may also result in decreased blood-oxygen levels. These conditions decrease the surface area of the alveoli either by damaging the alveoli or by leading to an accumulation of fluid in the lungs. Nonfunctional alveoli inhibit the diffusion of oxygen and carbon dioxide. As a result, blood entering the lungs from the right side of the heart will bypass the alveoli and will return to the left side of the heart in an unoxygenated state, a condition called intrapulmonary shunting.

Causes of Abnormal Carbon Dioxide Concentrations in the Blood

The $Paco_2$ in the arterial blood represents a balance between the CO_2 produced in metabolism and the CO_2 eliminated during ventilation. The amount of CO_2 produced normally remains relatively constant. As the metabolic rate goes up (eg, fever), however, more CO_2 is produced. As the metabolic rate falls (eg, hypothermia), the production of CO_2 declines. The type of metabolism also influences CO_2 production, with any metabolic process that results in the formation of acids increasing the amount of CO_2 in the blood. For example, excess lactic acid in the blood (caused by anaerobic metabolism) or excess ketoacids in the blood (caused by fat metabolism due to absent cellular glucose) will increase the circulating levels of CO_2.

If CO_2 production exceeds the body's ability to eliminate it by ventilation, the level of $Paco_2$ rises to produce hypoventilation. Theoretically, hypoventilation can occur in two ways: CO_2 production can exceed the body's ability to eliminate it, or CO_2 elimination can be depressed to the extent that it no longer keeps up with normal metabolism.

At the other extreme is hyperventilation, which occurs when CO_2 elimination exceeds CO_2 production. For example,

Table 11-2	Carbon Dioxide Balance	
	Hypoventilation	Hyperventilation
Minute volume	↓	↑
CO_2 elimination	↓	↑
$Paco_2$	↑ (hypercarbia)	↓ (hypocarbia)

patients experiencing an anxiety attack tend to breathe very deep and very fast (eg, minute volume is increased), so they eliminate CO_2 at a rate faster than their body produces it. The level of CO_2 in their blood then falls below normal and they experience symptoms such as dizziness and numbness/tingling in the face and extremities.

Given a steady rate of CO_2 production and CO_2 elimination, $Paco_2$ is directly proportional to minute volume Table 11-2 ▲. Decrease the minute volume, and you decrease CO_2 elimination, so CO_2 builds up in the blood (hypercarbia). Increase the minute volume, and you increase carbon dioxide elimination, so the level of CO_2 in the blood falls (hypocarbia).

The Measurement of Gases

Dalton's law of partial pressure states that the total pressure of a gas is the sum of the partial pressure of the components of that gas, or the pressure exerted by a specific atmospheric gas. The major components of air are nitrogen (78.62%); oxygen (20.84%); CO_2 (0.04%); and water vapor (0.50%).

▋Airway Evaluation

The importance of carefully assessing a patient's airway and ventilatory status cannot be overemphasized. In the field, you will encounter patients with a variety of airway problems—some of these problems are easily corrected, others require aggressive

You are the Provider Part 4

As you continue with your focused history and physical examination of the patient, you note that his level of consciousness has diminished and that cyanosis is developing around his mouth. You perform an immediate reassessment.

Reassessment	Recording Time: 5 Minutes
Level of consciousness	V (Responsive to verbal stimuli); confused
Respirations	32 breaths/min, shallow
Pulse	130 beats/min, weak and regular
Skin	Pale and diaphoretic, developing perioral cyanosis
Blood pressure	130/78 mm Hg
Sao_2	82% while breathing 100% oxygen via nonrebreathing mask

7. How should you adjust your treatment for this patient? Why?

management. *The care you provide to a patient with an airway or breathing problem is only as good as the assessment you perform.*

Essential Parameters

Breathing at rest should appear effortless, not labored. If you can see or hear a patient breathing, there is usually a problem. Normally, an adult at rest should have a respiratory rate between 12 and 20 breaths/min ◀ Table 11-3 ▾ ▶. The respirations should be of adequate depth (tidal volume) and follow a regular pattern of inhalation and exhalation.

Patients experiencing respiratory distress often attempt to compensate with preferential positioning, such as an upright tripod position (elbows out), or a semi-Fowler's (semi-sitting) position. Obviously, patients with respiratory distress will avoid a supine position.

Recognition of Airway Problems

A patient who is conscious, alert, and able to speak to you in complete sentences has no immediate airway or breathing problems. Nonetheless, you must still closely monitor a patient's airway and breathing status and be prepared to intervene should his or her condition deteriorate. Changes in respiratory rate, depth, and regularity may be subtle. If these subtleties are overlooked, and the appropriate care is not provided, the patient's outcome may be less than desirable. In case of inadequate breathing, it is critical to intervene immediately with some form of positive-pressure ventilation and 100% oxygen.

The adult patient with an abnormal respiratory rate must be evaluated for other signs of inadequate ventilation ◀ Table 11-4 ▾ ▶. Causes of inadequate ventilation include severe infection (sepsis), trauma, brain stem insult, a noxious or oxygen-poor atmosphere, and renal failure, to name a few. In addition to inadequate ventilation, causes of respiratory distress may include upper and/or lower airway obstructions, impairment of the respiratory muscles (eg, spinal cord injury), or impairment of the nervous system (eg, head injury, drug overdose).

Table 11-3	Normal Respiration Rate Ranges
Adults	12 to 20 breaths/min
Children	15 to 30 breaths/min
Infants	25 to 50 breaths/min

Note: These ranges are per the 2002 Airway Management supplement to the US DOT 1994 EMT-Basic National Standard Curriculum. Ranges presented in other courses or texts may vary.

Table 11-4	Signs of Inadequate Breathing

- Slow (< 12 breaths/min) or fast (> 20 breaths/min) respirations
- Shallow breathing (reduced tidal volume)
- Adventitious (abnormal) breath sounds
- Altered mental status
- Cyanosis (blue or purple skin; indicates low blood oxygen content)

Dyspnea is defined as any difficulty in respiratory rate, regularity, or effort. It may result from hypoxemia, a decrease in arterial oxygen levels. If left untreated, hypoxemia will progress to hypoxia, a lack of oxygen to the body's cells and tissues. Untreated hypoxia will lead to anoxia, an absence of oxygen that results in cellular and tissue death.

If a patient's airway is not patent, or if breathing is absent or inadequate, all therapies that you may attempt will prove futile. Proper airway management involves opening the airway, clearing the airway, assessing breathing, and providing the appropriate intervention(s)—in that order.

Evaluation of the airway includes the techniques of look, listen, and feel. Visual techniques should be used at first sight of the patient. The following questions must be answered when assessing the patient with respiratory distress:

- How is the patient positioned?
  - Is he or she in a tripod position?
  - Is the patient experiencing orthopnea (positional dyspnea)?
- Is rise and fall of the chest adequate (eg, adequate tidal volume)?
- Is the patient gasping for air (air hunger)?
- What is the skin color?
- Is there flaring of the nostrils?
- Is the patient breathing through pursed lips?
- Do you note any retractions (skin pulling in between and around the ribs during inhalation):
  - Intercostal?
  - At the suprasternal notch?
  - At the supraclavicular fossa?
  - Subcostal?
- Is the patient using accessory muscles to breathe? (Accessory muscles, which are not normally used during normal breathing, include the sternocleidomastoid muscles of the neck.)
- Is the patient's chest wall moving symmetrically? (Asymmetric chest wall movement, when one side of the chest moves less than the other, indicates that airflow into one lung is decreased.)

Listen for air movement at the patient's nose and mouth. Is the patient taking a series of quick breaths, followed by a prolonged exhalation phase? If so, this is a sign of inadequate ventilation.

Auscultate breath sounds with a stethoscope. Breath sounds should be clear and equal on both sides of the chest (bilateral), anteriorly and posteriorly. Compare each apex (top) of the lung to the opposite apex and each base (bottom) of the lung to the opposite base ◀ Figure 11-11 ▶ ▶.

If you are ventilating the patient with a bag-mask device, note any resistance or change in ventilatory compliance. Increased compliance (decreased resistance) means that air can be forced into the lungs with relative ease; decreased compliance (increased resistance) suggests an upper or lower airway obstruction.

Assess for pulsus paradoxus (paradoxical pulse), which occurs when the systolic blood pressure drops more than

10 mm Hg during inhalation. A change in pulse quality, or even the disappearance of a pulse during inhalation, may also be detected. Pulsus paradoxus is typically seen in patients with decompensating COPD, severe pericardial tamponade, or other conditions that increase intrathoracic pressure (eg, tension pneumothorax, severe asthma attack).

A history of the patient's present illness is a vital part of your assessment of the patient with respiratory distress. You should ask questions to determine the evolution of the current problem:

- Was the onset of the problem sudden or gradual over time?
  - Some people may perceive respiratory distress that occurred 2 days prior as arising gradually, when, in fact, the onset was sudden; the patient may have simply waited 2 days before calling for help.
- Is there any known cause or "trigger" of the event?
  - Asthma is commonly exacerbated by stress or cold weather. A foreign body airway obstruction is commonly preceded by a sudden onset of difficulty in breathing during a meal or, in children, while playing with small toys or other objects.
- What is the duration (is it constant or recurrent)?
- Does anything alleviate or exacerbate the problem?
- Are there any other associated symptoms, such as a productive cough, chest pain or pressure, or fever?
- Were any interventions attempted prior to EMS arrival?
- Has the patient been evaluated by a physician or admitted to the hospital for this condition in the past?
  - Determine specifically whether the patient was hospitalized or merely seen in the emergency department and then released. If the patient was hospitalized, ask whether he or she was admitted to an intensive care unit (ICU) or a regular, unmonitored floor. A condition that warranted an ICU admission is clinically significant.
- Is the patient currently taking any medications?
  - Don't simply ask which medications were taken today. Instead, determine the *overall* compliance by asking whether the patient has been taking the medications as prescribed. Verify this information by looking at the prescription date on the medication bottle(s), reading the prescription directions, and counting the pills remaining in the bottle.
  - Ask whether the patient has had any changes in his or her current prescription, such as a new medication or changes in the prescribing directions of an existing medication.

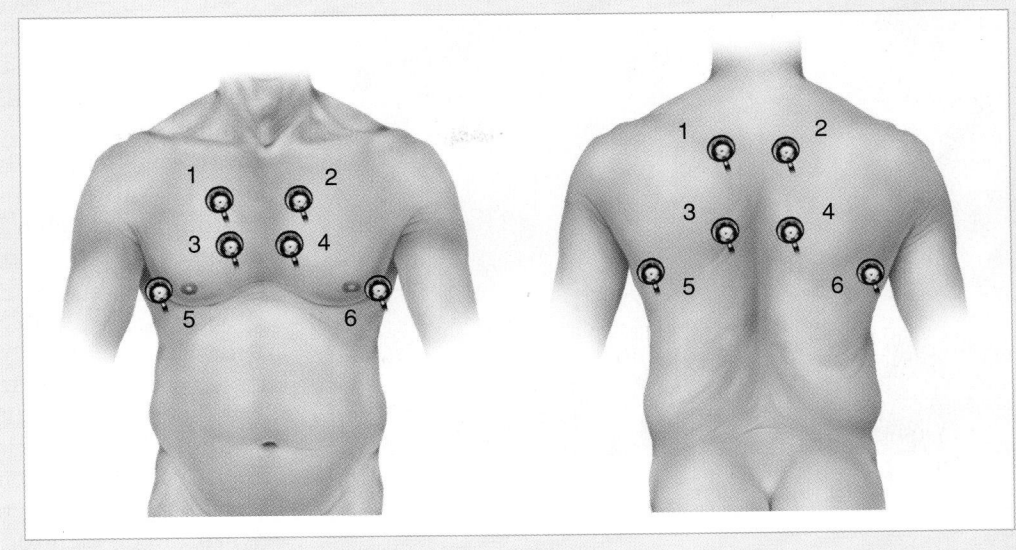

Figure 11-11 Auscultation of breath sounds (1 to 6).

- Does the patient have any risk factors that could cause or exacerbate his or her condition, such as alcohol or illicit drug use, cigarette smoking, or a poor diet?

Evaluate the patient for any modified forms of respiration. Protective reflexes of the airway include coughing, sneezing, and gagging. Coughing is a forceful exhalation produced with a greater than normal volume of breath. The patient whose cough mechanism is suppressed—whether by drugs, by pain, by trauma, or by any other cause—is at serious risk of aspirating foreign material.

Sneezing is also a sudden, forceful exhalation, but in this instance air is expelled through the nose rather than through the mouth. Sneezing is usually elicited by irritation of the nose.

Gagging is a forceful muscular contraction of the pharyngeal muscles and the glottis. This reaction is automatic when something touches an area deep in the oral cavity. The gag reflex helps protect the lower airway from aspiration, or entry of fluids or solids into the trachea, bronchi, and lungs. The eyelash reflex is a fairly reliable indicator of the presence or absence of an intact gag reflex (Figure 11-12 ▶). If the patient's lower eyelid contracts when you gently stroke the upper eyelashes, he or she probably has an intact gag reflex.

In the Field

A critical question to ask the patient with respiratory distress is if he or she has ever been intubated for the same problem. A condition serious enough to warrant intubation—especially a lengthy intubation—requires urgent attention to prevent a repeated occurrence. Also, determine whether other interventions (eg, defibrillation, transcutaneous pacing) were required to treat the same problem in the past. This information will increase your index of suspicion and prepare you for a potential rapid deterioration in the patient's condition.

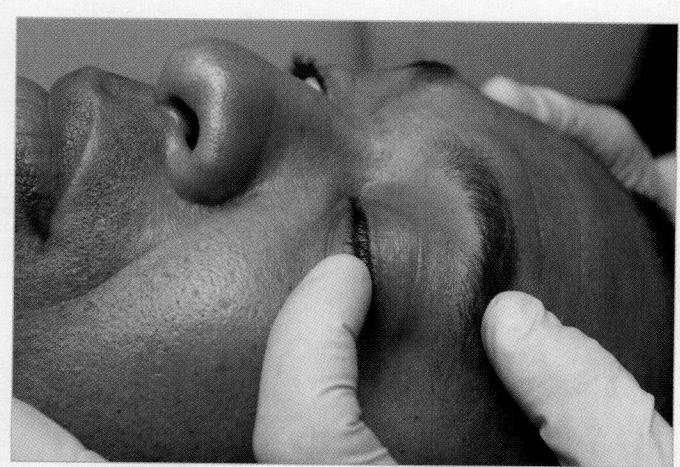

Figure 11-12 The eyelash reflex.

Table 11-5	Abnormal Respiratory Patterns
Cheyne-Stokes respirations	Gradually increasing rate and depth of respirations followed by gradual decrease of respirations with intermittent periods of apnea; associated with brain stem insult.
Kussmaul respirations	Deep, gasping respirations; common in diabetic coma (ketoacidosis).
Biot respirations	Irregular pattern, rate, and depth with intermittent periods of apnea; results from increased intracranial pressure.
Agonal respirations	Slow, shallow, irregular respirations or occasional gasps; results from cerebral anoxia; may be seen briefly after the heart has stopped as the brain continues to send signals to the respiratory muscles.

Sighing is a slow, deep inhalation followed by a prolonged and sometimes quite audible exhalation. Sighing periodically hyperinflates the lungs, thereby reexpanding atelectatic (collapsed) alveoli. The average person sighs about once per minute.

Hiccuping is a sudden inhalation, due to spasmodic contraction of the diaphragm, cut short by closure of the glottis. Hiccuping serves no physiologic purpose, although persistent hiccups may be clinically significant.

Patients with serious injuries or illness may present with changes in their respiratory pattern. Table 11-5 ▲ shows various abnormal respiratory patterns and their causes.

Diagnostic Testing

In addition to your hands-on assessment of the patient with an airway or breathing problem, several methods and devices are used to quantify oxygenation and ventilation. Pulse oximetry is a simple, rapid, safe, and noninvasive method of measuring—minute by minute—how well a person's hemoglobin is saturated.

A pulse oximeter Figure 11-13 ▶ measures the percentage of hemoglobin in the arterial blood that is saturated. Under normal circumstances, hemoglobin is saturated with oxygen. When carbon monoxide is available, hemoglobin will bind to it rather than

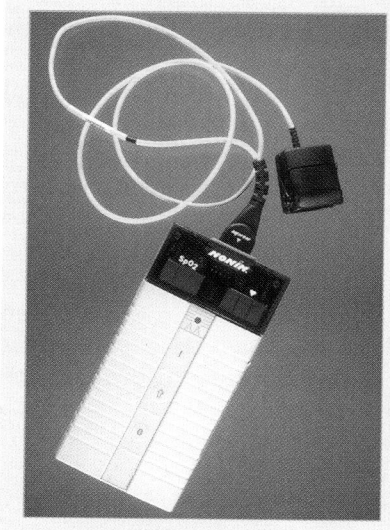

Figure 11-13 A pulse oximeter.

oxygen, and can "fool" the oximeter. A sensor probe, clipped to the patient's finger or ear lobe, uses a light-emitting diode (LED) to transmit light through the vascular bed to a light-sensing detector. The amount of light transmitted across the vascular bed depends on the proportion of hemoglobin that is saturated with oxygen. To ensure that the instrument is measuring arterial and not venous oxygen saturation, pulse oximeters are designed to assess only pulsating blood vessels. As a consequence, they also measure the patient's pulse. One way to check the functioning of a pulse oximeter is to compare the pulse reading it provides with your own measurement of the patient's pulse by palpation.

A normally oxygenated, normally perfused person should have an Sao_2 between 95% and 99%. Any reading below 95% indicates respiratory compromise; a reading below 90% signals a need for aggressive oxygen therapy.

Situations in which pulse oximeters may be useful in prehospital emergency care include the following:

- **Monitoring the oxygenation of a patient during an intubation attempt or during suctioning.** The low-saturation alarm on the pulse oximeter can signal that the paramedic should abort the intubation attempt and ventilate the patient.
- **Identifying deterioration in a trauma victim.** In the patient with multiple trauma, the signs of a developing tension pneumothorax, for instance, may not be evident until the problem is quite advanced. A declining Sao_2 level can alert the paramedic that something bad is happening and prompt a search for the cause of the problem.
- **Identifying deterioration in the cardiac patient.** Pulse oximetry may enable early identification of patients who are experiencing congestive heart failure in the wake of a myocardial infarction.
- **Identifying high-risk patients with respiratory problems.** For example, pulse oximetry may identify patients with asthma who are having serious attacks or patients with emphysema who are in severe decompensation.

■ **Assessing vascular status in orthopaedic trauma.** Pulse oximetry is routine practice in assessing a fractured extremity to evaluate the pulse distal to the fracture. Loss of a pulse means that the limb is in jeopardy and may require urgent action in the field if transport time is long. A pulse oximeter clipped to a finger or toe on a broken limb might provide critical information about the ongoing circulation to the limb.

The usefulness of a pulse oximeter depends on its ability to provide accurate information. A pulse oximeter that gives a reading of 99% when the patient is actually severely hypoxemic will not be much help to anyone. Be aware of circumstances that might produce erroneous readings:

■ **Bright ambient light** may enter the spectrophotometer of the pulse oximeter and create an incorrect reading. Protect the sensor clip by covering it with a towel or aluminum foil.

■ **Patient motion** can confuse the pulse oximeter, as it may mistake motion for arterial pulsation and read the oxygen saturation from a vein rather than an artery.

■ **Poor perfusion** makes it difficult for the oximeter to sense a pulse and therefore to generate a reading. Poor perfusion occurs in states such as shock, cardiac arrest, and cold exposure. If the patient's limbs are vasoconstricted and cold, it may be necessary to place the pulse oximeter clip on the ear lobe or nose.

■ **Nail polish** will prevent the sensor from working properly. Carry disposable acetone (nail polish remover) swabs to quickly remove nail polish.

■ **Venous pulsations** may occur in some patients with right-sided heart failure. If a vein is pulsating, the oximeter may regard it as an artery and measure venous oxygen saturation.

■ **Abnormal hemoglobin** may produce a falsely high SaO_2. Carboxyhemoglobin, for example, is formed by the attachment of CO to the hemoglobin molecule. Because the pulse oximeter cannot distinguish between oxyhemoglobin (hemoglobin that is occupied by oxygen) and carboxyhemoglobin, it may give a high SaO_2 reading for a patient who is severely hypoxemic from CO poisoning. The results of pulse oximetry should therefore be interpreted cautiously in victims of smoke inhalation or other circumstances likely to have produced CO poisoning.

When in Doubt, Look at the Patient!

Always weigh the information provided by pulse oximetry (or any other device) against clinical observations. If the patient is turning blue and struggling to breathe, you may ignore the pulse oximeter reading that says the patient is adequately oxygenated.

The steps for performing pulse oximetry are listed here and shown in Skill Drill 11-1 ▾.

1. Clean the patient's finger and remove nail polish as needed. Place the index or middle finger into the pulse oximeter probe. Turn on the pulse oximeter and note LED reading of the SaO_2 Step 1.

2. Palpate the radial pulse to ensure that it correlates with the LED display on the pulse oximeter Step 2.

In patients with certain reactive airway diseases (eg, asthma), bronchoconstriction can be evaluated by measuring the peak rate of a forceful exhalation with a peak expiratory flow monitor. An increasing peak expiratory flow suggests that the patient is responding to treatment (eg, inhaled bronchodilators). A decreasing peak expiratory flow may be an early indication that the patient's condition is deteriorating.

Peak expiratory flow varies based on sex, height, and age. Normal adults have a peak expiratory flow rate of 350 to 750 mL.

The steps for performing peak expiratory flow measurement are listed here and shown in Skill Drill 11-2 ▸.

1. Place the patient in a seated position with the legs dangling. Assemble the flowmeter and make sure that it reads zero Step 1.

Skill Drill 11-1:
Performing Pulse Oximetry

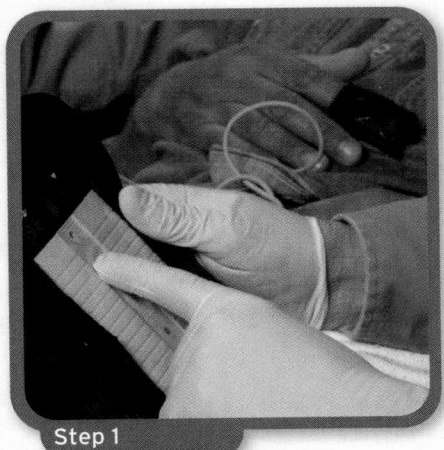

Step 1

Clean the patient's finger and place his or her finger in the pulse oximeter probe. Turn on the pulse oximeter and note the LED display of the SaO_2.

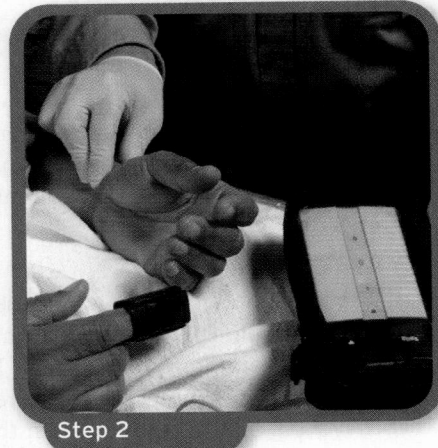

Step 2

Palpate the radial pulse to ensure that it correlates with the LED display on the pulse oximeter.

Skill Drill 11-2: Peak Expiratory Flow Measurement

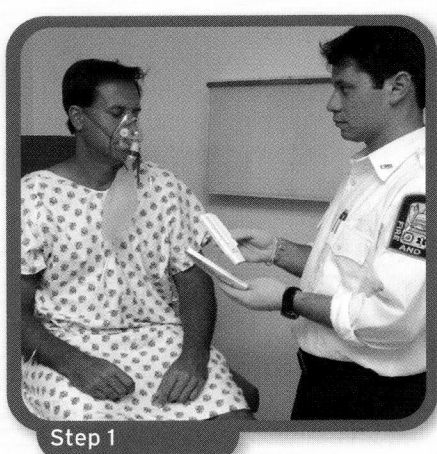

Step 1

Assemble the flowmeter and make sure it reads zero.

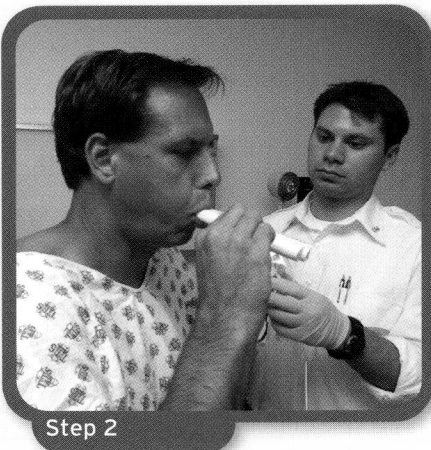

Step 2

Ask the patient to take a deep breath, place the mouthpiece in his or her mouth, and ask the patient to exhale as forcefully as possible. Make sure no air leaks around the device or comes from the patient's nose.

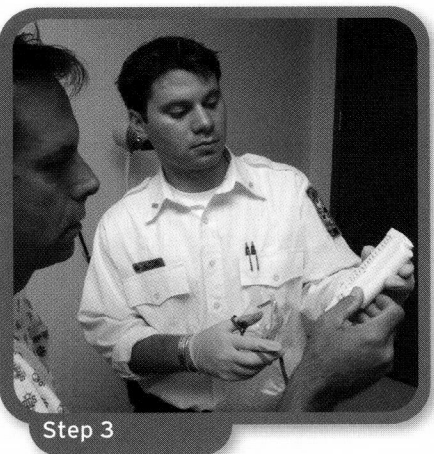

Step 3

Perform the test three times, and take the best rate of the three readings.

---

2. Ask the patient to take a deep breath, place the mouthpiece in his or her mouth, and ask the patient to exhale as forcefully as possible. Make sure no air leaks around the device or comes from the patient's nose (Step 2).

3. Perform the test three times, and take the best rate of the three readings (Step 3).

▮ Airway Management

Clearly, a patient who is conscious and is talking, screaming, or crying has a patent airway. In a patient with an altered LOC, however, the airway is often not patent and manual maneuvers will be required to open it. In addition, artificial airway adjuncts may be needed to assist in maintaining the airway

Positioning the Patient

In a perfect world, all patients would present in a supine position, so that you could quickly open the airway, assess breathing, and intervene without moving them. If patients are found unconscious and in a prone position, however, you must position them properly so that you can open the airway, assess respirations, and provide ventilation or CPR if needed.

To move a patient to a supine position, log roll the individual as a unit. Once the patient is in a supine position, open his or her airway and assess breathing status. The recovery position, which involves placing the patient in a left lateral recumbent position, should be used in all nontrauma patients with a

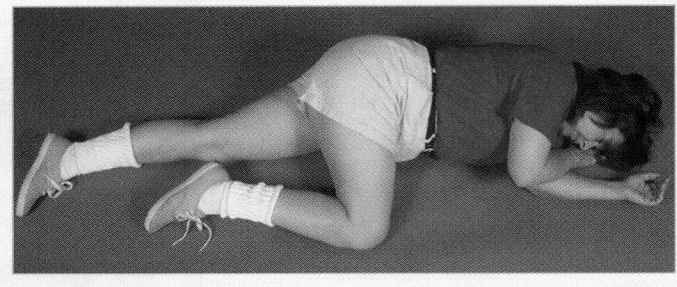

Figure 11-14 The recovery position.

decreased LOC who are able to maintain their own airway spontaneously and are breathing adequately (Figure 11-14 ▲).

Manual Airway Maneuvers

In the unresponsive patient, the most common cause of airway obstruction is the patient's tongue (Figure 11-15 ▶). To correct this problem, manually maneuver the patient's head to propel the tongue forward and open the airway. Techniques used to accomplish this include the head tilt–chin lift maneuver and the jaw-thrust maneuver (with or without head tilt).

Head Tilt–Chin Lift Maneuver

Opening the airway to relieve an obstruction can often be done quickly and easily by simply tilting the patient's head back and lifting the chin. This head tilt–chin lift maneuver is the preferred technique for opening the airway of a patient

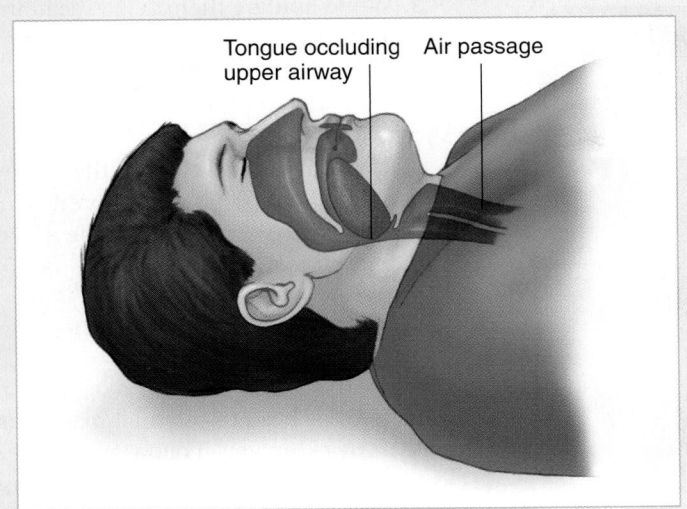

Tongue occluding upper airway   Air passage

Figure 11-15 When the tongue falls back and occludes the posterior pharynx, it may obstruct the airway.

Perform the head tilt–chin lift maneuver in the following manner **Skill Drill 11-3 ▶**.

1. With the patient in a supine position, position yourself beside the patient's head **Step 1**.
2. Place one hand on the patient's forehead, and apply firm backward pressure with your palm to tilt the patient's head back **Step 2**. This extension of the neck will propel the tongue forward, away from the posterior pharynx and clear the airway.
3. Place the tips of your fingers of your other hand under the lower jaw near the bony part of the chin **Step 3**. Do not compress the soft tissue under the chin, as this may block the airway.
4. Lift the chin upward, bringing the entire lower jaw with it, helping to tilt the head back **Step 4**. Do not use your thumb to lift the chin. Lift so that the teeth are nearly brought together, but avoid closing the mouth completely. Continue to hold the forehead to maintain backward tilt of the head.

Jaw-Thrust Maneuver

If you suspect that the patient has experienced a cervical spine injury, open his or her airway with the jaw-thrust maneuver. In this technique, you open the airway by placing your fingers behind the angle of the jaw and lifting the jaw forward. The jaw is displaced forward at the mandibular angle. You can easily seal a mask around the patient's nose and mouth while performing this maneuver. Following are some considerations when using the jaw-thrust maneuver:

- **Indications.** An unresponsive patient, possible cervical spine injury, or a patient who is unable to protect his or her own airway.
- **Contraindications.** A responsive patient with resistance to opening the mouth. The jaw-thrust maneuver may be needed in the responsive patient who has sustained a jaw fracture to keep the tongue away from the back of the throat.

who has not sustained trauma. Occasionally, this simple maneuver is all that is required for the patient to resume breathing. Following are some considerations when using the head tilt–chin lift maneuver:

- **Indications.** An unresponsive patient, no mechanism for cervical spine injury, or a patient who is unable to protect his or her own airway.
- **Contraindications.** A responsive patient or a possible cervical spine injury.
- **Advantages.** No equipment is required, and the technique is simple, safe, and noninvasive.
- **Disadvantages.** It is thought to be hazardous to patients with spinal injury and does not protect from aspiration.

You are the Provider Part 5

You are now assisting the patient's breathing with a bag-mask device and 100% oxygen. You radio dispatch and ask for an engine company to respond for manpower assistance. Your partner quickly reassesses the patient and notes the following:

Reassessment	Recording Time: 8 Minutes
Level of consciousness	P (Responsive to painful stimuli)
Respirations	36 breaths/min, shallow (baseline); you are assisting ventilations with a bag-mask device and 100% oxygen
Pulse	150 beats/min, regular and weak
Skin	Pale and diaphoretic extremities and trunk; facial cyanosis
Blood pressure	118/70 mm Hg
Sa_{O_2}	86% while being ventilated with a bag-mask device and 100% oxygen

8. Why is your patient's condition not improving with assisted ventilation?
9. What must you do to correct the situation?

Skill Drill 11-3: Head Tilt–Chin Lift Maneuver

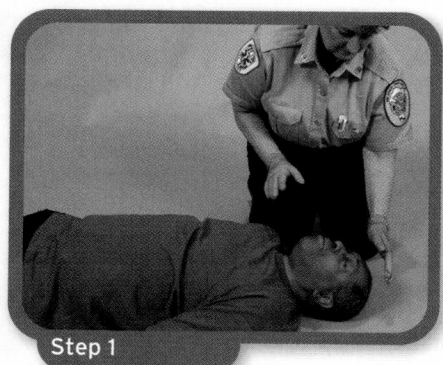

Step 1

Position yourself at the side of the supine patient.

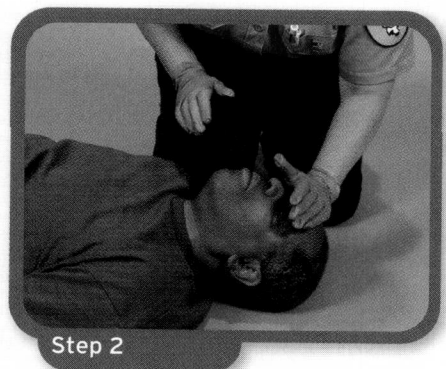

Step 2

Place your hand closest to the patient's head on the forehead.

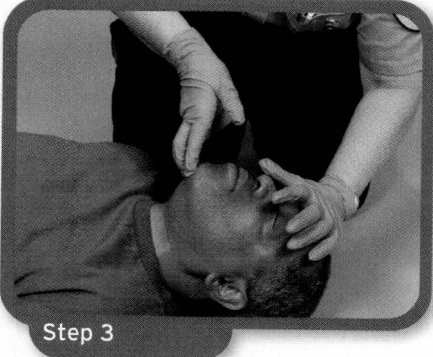

Step 3

With your other hand, place two fingers on the underside of the patient's chin.

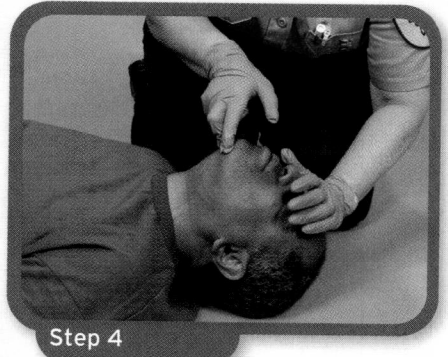

Step 4

Simultaneously apply backward and downward pressure to the patient's forehead and lift the jaw straight up. Do not depress the soft tissue below the chin.

- **Advantages.** May be used in patients with cervical spine injury, may use with cervical collar in place, and does not require special equipment.
- **Disadvantages.** Cannot maintain if patient becomes responsive or combative, difficult to maintain for an extended period of time, very difficult to use in conjunction with bag-mask ventilation, thumb must remain in place to maintain jaw displacement, requires second rescuer for bag-mask ventilation, and does not protect against aspiration. Perform the jaw-thrust maneuver in the following manner ▶ **Skill Drill 11-4 ▶** .

1. Position yourself at the top of the supine patient's head (**Step 1**).
2. Place the meaty portion of the base of your thumbs on the zygomatic arches and hook the tips of your index fingers under the angle of the mandible, in the indent below each ear (**Step 2**).

3. While holding the patient's head in a neutral inline position, displace the jaw upward and open the patient's mouth with the tips of your thumbs (**Step 3**).

If you are unable to open the airway with the jaw-thrust maneuver, you should carefully perform the head tilt–chin lift maneuver.

Jaw-Thrust Maneuver With Head Tilt

The jaw-thrust maneuver with head tilt is similar to the head tilt–chin lift maneuver, with a few exceptions. Following are some considerations when using the jaw-thrust maneuver with head tilt:

- **Indications.** An unresponsive patient or a patient unable to protect his or her own airway.
- **Contraindications.** A responsive patient or a patient with a possible cervical spine injury.
- **Advantages.** It is noninvasive and does not require special equipment.
- **Disadvantages.** It is difficult to maintain, requires a second rescuer for bag-mask ventilation, and does not protect against aspiration.

Perform the jaw-thrust maneuver with head tilt in the following manner **Skill Drill 11-5 ▶** .

1. Position yourself at the top of the patient's head (**Step 1**).
2. Place the meaty portion of the base of your thumbs on the zygomatic arches, and hook the tips of your index fingers under the angle of the mandible, in the middle indent below the patient's ear (**Step 2**).
3. Displace the jaw upward and tilt the head back (**Step 3**).

Tongue-Jaw Lift Maneuver

The tongue-jaw lift maneuver is used more commonly to open a patient's airway for the purpose of suctioning or inserting an oropharyngeal airway. It cannot be used to ventilate a patient, because it will not allow for an adequate mask seal on the patient's face. Perform the tongue-jaw lift in the following manner **Skill Drill 11-6 ▶** .

1. Position yourself at the side of the patient (**Step 1**).
2. Place the hand closest to the patient's head on the forehead (**Step 2**).
3. With the other hand, reach into the patient's mouth and hook your first knuckle under the incisors or gum line. While holding the patient's head and maintaining the hand on the forehead, lift the jaw straight up (**Step 3**).

Skill Drill 11-4: Jaw-Thrust Maneuver

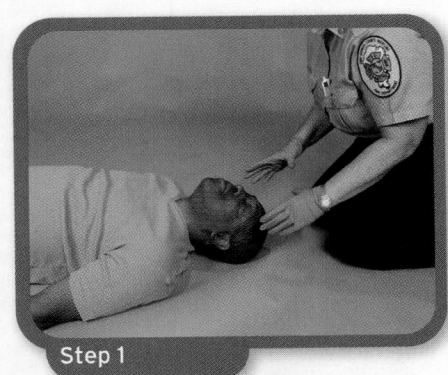

Step 1

Position yourself at the top of the patient's head.

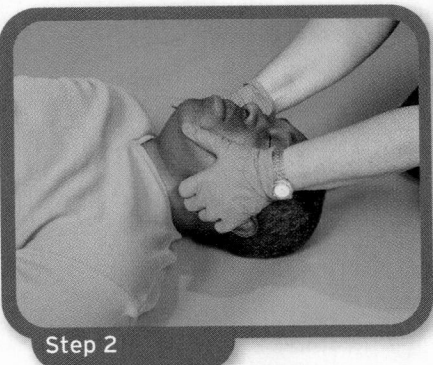

Step 2

Place the meaty portion of the base of your thumbs on the zygomatic arches, and hook the tips of your index fingers under the angle of the mandible, in the indent below each ear.

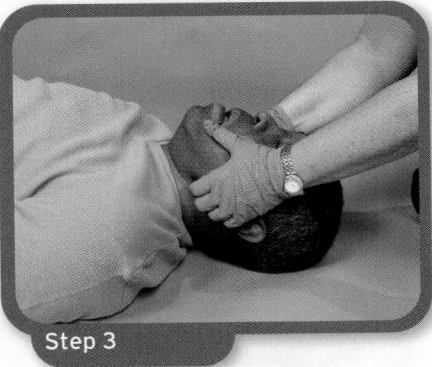

Step 3

While holding the patient's head still, displace the jaw upward and open the patient's mouth with your thumb tips.

Skill Drill 11-5: Jaw-Thrust Maneuver With Head Tilt

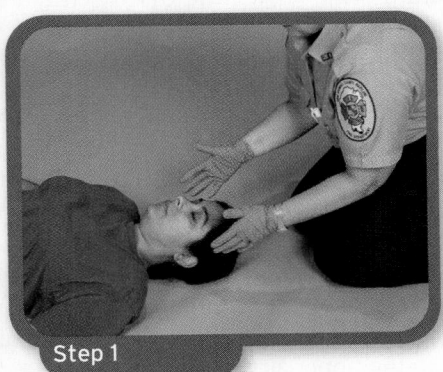

Step 1

Position yourself at the top of the patient's head.

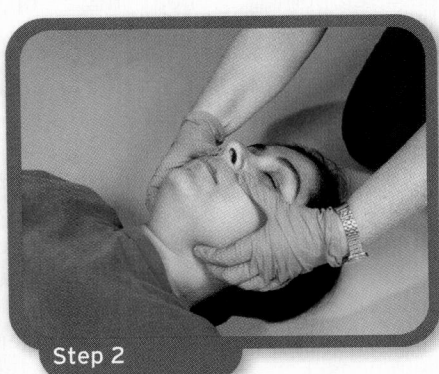

Step 2

Place the meaty portion of the base of your thumbs on the zygomatic arches, and hook the tips of your index fingers under the angle of the mandible, in the middle indent below each ear.

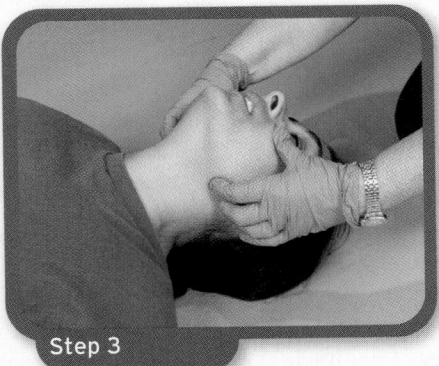

Step 3

Displace the jaw upward and tilt the head back.

▌Airway Obstructions

The airway connects the body to the life-giving oxygen in the atmosphere. If it becomes obstructed, this lifeline is cut and the patient dies—often within minutes. The paramedic must recognize the signs of an obstructed airway and immediately take corrective action.

Causes of Airway Obstruction

In an adult, sudden foreign body airway obstruction usually occurs during a meal. In children, it typically occurs while eating or playing with small toys. An otherwise healthy child who presents with a sudden onset of difficulty breathing—especially in the absence of fever—should be suspected of having a foreign body airway obstruction. A multitude of other conditions

Skill Drill 11-6: Tongue-Jaw Lift Maneuver

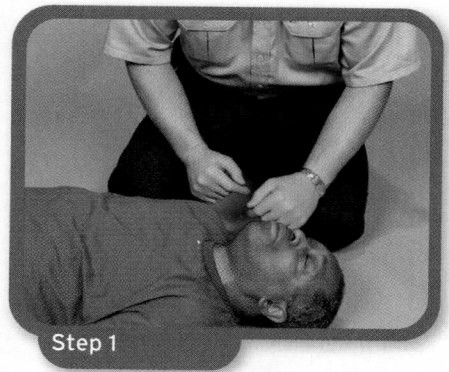

Step 1

Position yourself at the patient's side.

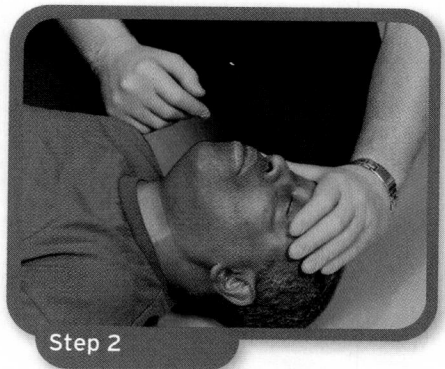

Step 2

Place the hand closest to the patient's head on the forehead.

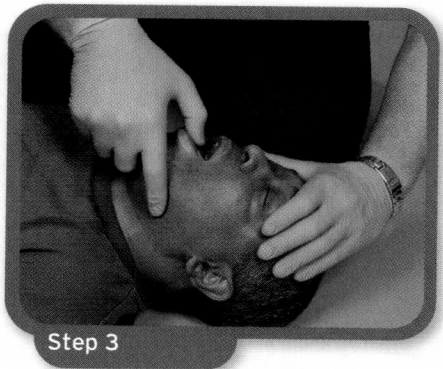

Step 3

With your other hand, reach into the patient's mouth and hook your first knuckle under the incisors or gum line. While holding the patient's head and maintaining the hand on the forehead, lift the jaw straight up.

can cause an airway obstruction, however, including the tongue, laryngeal edema, laryngeal spasm (laryngospasm), trauma, and aspiration.

When the airway is obstructed secondary to an infectious process or a severe allergic reaction, repeated attempts to clear the airway as if it were obstructed by a foreign body will be unsuccessful and potentially harmful. These patients require specific management (discussed in the appropriate chapters of this book) and prompt transport to an appropriate medical facility.

Tongue

In the patient with an altered LOC, the jaw relaxes and the tongue tends to fall back against the posterior wall of the pharynx, closing off the airway. A patient with partial obstruction from the tongue will have snoring respirations; a patient whose airway is completely obstructed will have no respirations. Fortunately, obstruction of the airway by the tongue is simple to correct using a manual maneuver (eg, head tilt–chin lift, or jaw-thrust).

Foreign Body

A significant number of people die from foreign body airway obstructions each year, often as the result of choking on a piece of food. The typical victim is middle-aged or older and wears dentures. He or she has usually had a few alcoholic drinks, which depresses protective reflexes and adversely affects a person's judgment regarding how large a piece of food can be prudently placed in the mouth. Additionally, patients with conditions that decrease their airway reflexes (eg, stroke) are at an increased risk for a foreign body airway obstruction. A foreign body may cause a mild or severe airway obstruction, depending on the size of the object and its location in the airway.

Signs may include choking, gagging, stridor, dyspnea, aphonia (inability to speak), and dysphonia (difficulty speaking). Treatment for the patient depends on whether he or she is effectively moving air. Techniques for foreign body airway obstruction removal will be discussed later in this chapter.

Laryngeal Spasm and Edema

A laryngeal spasm (laryngospasm) results in spasmodic closure of the vocal cords, completely occluding the airway. It is often caused by trauma during an overly aggressive intubation attempt or immediately upon extubation, especially when the patient has an altered LOC.

Laryngeal edema causes the glottic opening to become extremely narrow or totally closed. Conditions that commonly cause this problem include epiglottitis, anaphylaxis, or inhalation injury (eg, burns to the upper airway).

Airway obstructions caused by laryngeal spasm or edema may be relieved by aggressive ventilation to force air past the narrowed airway or a forceful upward pull of the jaw in an attempt to reposition the airway. In certain cases, muscle relaxant medications may be effective in relieving laryngeal spasm. Do not let your guard down after the laryngospasm has appeared to have resolved; resolution of the crisis does not mean that laryngospasm will not recur. The patient should be transported to the hospital for evaluation.

Fractured Larynx

Airway patency depends on good muscle tone to keep the trachea open. Fracture of the larynx increases airway resistance by decreasing airway size secondary to decreased muscle tone, laryngeal edema, and ventilatory effort. An advanced airway may be required to maintain a patent airway.

Aspiration

Aspiration of blood or other fluid significantly increases mortality. In addition to potentially obstructing the airway, aspiration destroys delicate bronchiolar tissue, introduces pathogens into the lungs, and decreases the patient's ability to ventilate (or be ventilated).

Suction should be readily available for any patient who is unable to maintain his or her own airway. Patients requiring emergency care should always be assumed to have a full stomach.

Recognition of an Airway Obstruction

A foreign body lodged in the upper airway can cause a mild (partial) or severe (complete) airway obstruction. A rapid but careful assessment is required to determine the seriousness of the obstruction, as the differences in managing mild versus severe cases are significant.

A patient with a mild airway obstruction is conscious and able to exchange air, but may show varying degrees of respiratory distress. The patient will usually have noisy respirations and may be coughing. He or she may wheeze between coughs but does not become cyanotic. *Patients with a mild airway obstruction should be left alone! A forceful cough is the most effective means of dislodging the obstruction.* Attempts to manually remove the object could force it farther down into the airway and cause a severe obstruction. Closely monitor the patient's condition and be prepared to intervene if you see signs of severe airway obstruction.

A patient with a severe airway obstruction typically experiences a sudden inability to breathe, talk, or cough—classically during a meal. The patient may grasp at his or her throat (universal sign of choking), begin to turn cyanotic, and make frantic, exaggerated attempts to move air **Figure 11-16 ▶**. Patients with a severe airway obstruction have a weak, ineffective, or absent cough and are in marked respiratory distress; weak inspiratory stridor and cyanosis are often present.

Emergency Medical Care for Foreign Body Airway Obstruction

If the patient with a suspected airway obstruction is conscious, ask, "Are you choking?" If the patient nods "yes," begin treatment immediately. If the obstruction is not promptly cleared, the amount of oxygen in the blood will decrease dramatically, resulting in severe hypoxia and death.

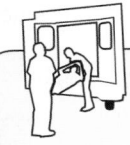

In the Field

Causes of Airway Obstruction

- Relaxation of the tongue in an unresponsive patient
- Foreign objects—food, small toys, dentures
- Blood clots, broken teeth, or damaged oral tissue following trauma
- Airway tissue swelling—infection, allergic reaction
- Aspirated vomitus (stomach contents)

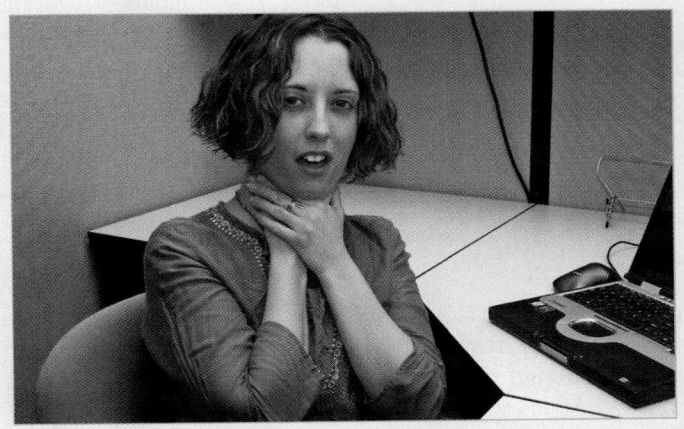

Figure 11-16 The universal sign of choking.

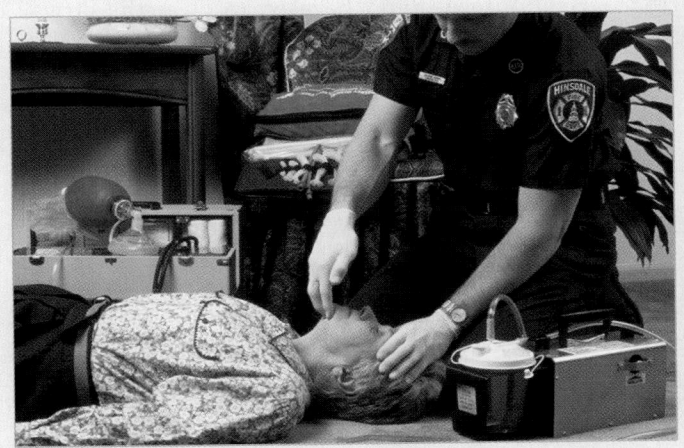

Figure 11-17 Securing and maintaining a patent airway and ensuring adequate ventilation are among the most important steps in caring for an unconscious patient.

Manage any unresponsive person as if he or she has a compromised airway. Open and maintain the airway with the appropriate manual maneuver (eg, head tilt–chin lift for nontrauma patients, jaw-thrust for trauma patients), assess for breathing, and provide artificial ventilation if necessary **Figure 11-17 ▲**.

If, after opening the airway, you are unable to ventilate the patient (no chest rise and fall) or you feel resistance when ventilating (poor lung compliance), reopen the airway and again attempt to ventilate the patient. Lung compliance is the ability of the alveoli to expand when air is drawn into the lungs, either during negative-pressure ventilation or positive-pressure ventilation. Poor lung compliance is characterized by increased resistance during ventilation attempts.

If large pieces of vomitus, mucus, loose dentures, or blood clots are found in the airway, sweep them forward and out of the mouth with your gloved index finger. *Blind finger sweeps of*

Notes from Nancy

Blind insertion of any instrument, whether improvised or specially designed, into a patient's pharynx is extremely dangerous. Don't do it!

the mouth—*regardless of the patient's age—are not recommended and may cause further harm; only attempt to remove foreign bodies that you can see and easily retrieve.* After the patient's airway is open, insert your index finger down along the inside of the patient's cheek and into his or her throat at the base of the tongue, then try to hook the foreign body to dislodge it and maneuver it into the mouth. Take care not to force the foreign body deeper into the airway. Do *not* blindly insert any object other than your finger into the patient's mouth to remove a foreign body, as an instrument jammed into the throat can damage the delicate structures of the pharynx and compound the obstruction with hemorrhage. Suctioning should be used to clear the airway of secretions as needed.

Special Considerations

According to current Emergency Cardiovascular Care (ECC) guidelines, a child is defined as a patient from 1 year of age to the onset of puberty (12 to 14 years of age).

The steps for managing a severe airway obstruction in a conscious adult or child are listed here and shown in Skill Drill 11-7 ▾ .

1. Determine whether the patient is choking by asking, "Are you choking?" If the patient nods "yes," then help is needed (Step 1).

2. Perform the Heimlich maneuver until the object is expelled or the patient becomes unresponsive (Step 2).

The steps for managing a severe airway obstruction in an unconscious adult or child are listed here and shown in Skill Drill 11-8 ▸ .

1. Open the airway with the head tilt–chin lift maneuver and look in the patient's mouth (Step 1). If you see the object, carefully remove it from the patient's mouth.

2. Attempt to ventilate the patient (Step 2). If unsuccessful, reopen the airway and again attempt ventilation.

3. Perform chest compressions (Step 3). Perform 30 chest compressions if you are by yourself or if the patient is an adult; perform 15 chest compressions if two rescuers are present or if the patient is a child. In the child, chest compressions can be performed with one or two hands, depending on the size of the child.

4. Open the airway with the head tilt–chin lift maneuver and look in the patient's mouth (Step 4). If you see the object, carefully remove it from the patient's mouth. Repeat steps 2 through 4 until successful or until help arrives.

The steps for managing a severe airway obstruction in a conscious infant are listed here and shown in Skill Drill 11-9 ▸ .

1. Perform five back blows (slaps) (Step 1).

2. Perform five chest thrusts (Step 2). Repeat steps 1 and 2 until the object is expelled or the infant becomes unresponsive.

The steps for managing a severe airway obstruction in an unconscious infant are listed here and shown in Skill Drill 11-10 ▸ .

1. Open the infant's airway with slight extension of the neck and look in the mouth (Step 1). If you see the object, carefully remove it from the infant's mouth.

2. Attempt to ventilate (Step 2). If unsuccessful, reopen the airway and again attempt ventilation.

3. Perform chest compressions (Step 3). Perform 30 chest compressions if you are by yourself; perform 15 chest compressions if two rescuers are present.

4. Open the infant's airway with slight extension of the neck and look in the mouth (Step 4). If you see the object, carefully remove it from the infant's mouth. Repeat steps 2 through 4 until successful or until help arrives.

Skill Drill 11-7: Managing Severe Airway Obstruction in a Conscious Adult or Child

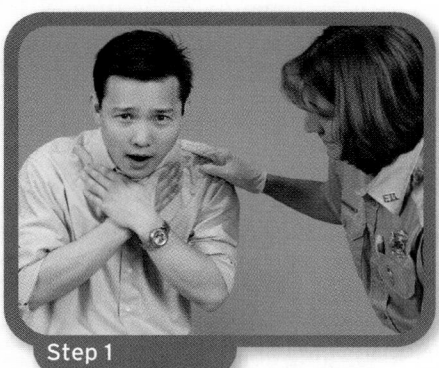

Step 1

Determine whether the patient is choking by asking, "Are you choking?" If the patient nods "yes," then help is needed.

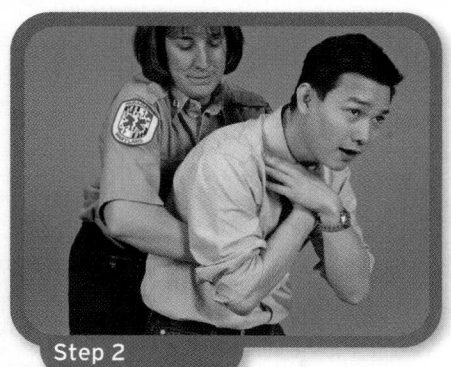

Step 2

Perform the Heimlich maneuver until the object is expelled or the patient becomes unresponsive.

Skill Drill 11-8: Managing Severe Airway Obstruction in an Unconscious Adult or Child

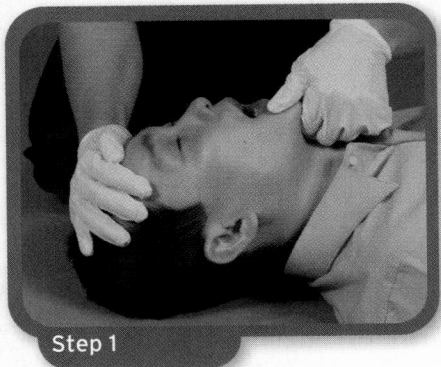

Step 1

Open the airway and look in the mouth. If you see the object, carefully remove it from the patient's mouth.

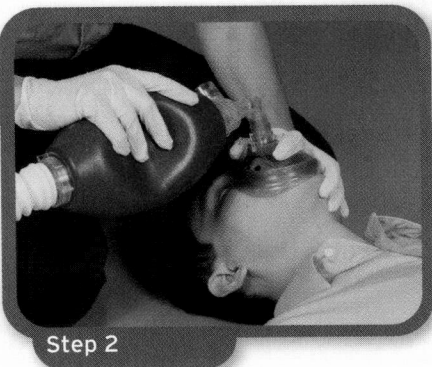

Step 2

Attempt to ventilate the patient. If unsuccessful, reopen the airway and again attempt ventilation.

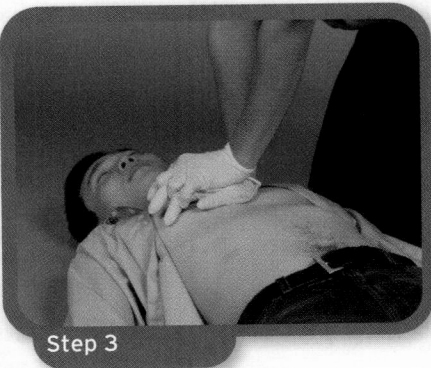

Step 3

Perform chest compressions.

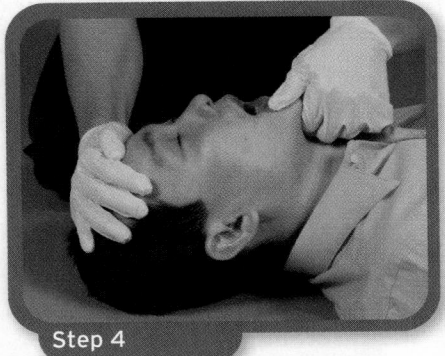

Step 4

Open the airway and look in the mouth. If you see the object, carefully remove it from the patient's mouth. Repeat steps 2 through 4 until successful or until help arrives.

Skill Drill 11-9: Managing Severe Airway Obstruction in a Conscious Infant

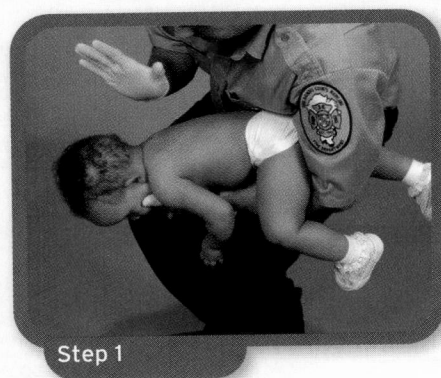

Step 1

Perform five back blows (slaps).

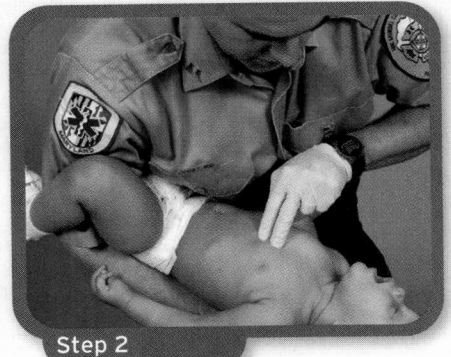

Step 2

Perform five chest thrusts. Repeat steps 1 and 2 until the object is expelled or the infant becomes unresponsive.

The Heimlich maneuver (abdominal thrusts) is the most effective method of dislodging and forcing an object out of the airway. It aims to create an artificial cough by forcing residual air out of the victim's lungs, thereby expelling the object. You should perform the Heimlich maneuver on any conscious child or adult with a severe airway obstruction until the obstructing object is expelled or until the patient becomes unresponsive. If the conscious patient with a severe airway obstruction is in the advanced stages of pregnancy or is morbidly obese, perform chest thrusts instead of abdominal thrusts.

If you are unable to relieve a severe airway obstruction in an unconscious patient with the basic techniques previously discussed, you should proceed with direct laryngoscopy (visualization of the airway with a laryngoscope) for the removal of the foreign body in unresponsive patients. Insert the laryngoscope blade into the patient's mouth. If you see the foreign body, carefully remove it from the upper airway with Magill forceps, a special type of curved forceps Figure 11-18 ▸. The steps for removal of an upper airway obstruction with Magill forceps are listed here and shown in Skill Drill 11-11 ▸.

1. With the patient's head in the sniffing position, open the patient's mouth and insert the laryngoscope blade Step 1.
2. Visualize the obstruction, and retrieve the object with the Magill forceps Step 2.
3. Remove the object with the Magill forceps Step 3.
4. Attempt to ventilate the patient Step 4.

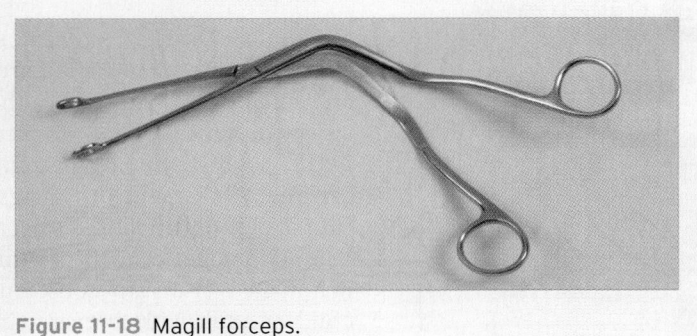

Figure 11-18 Magill forceps.

In the Field

A patient with a severe upper airway obstruction has very little time before severe hypoxia develops. If several attempts to relieve the obstruction with conventional BLS methods fail, you should proceed with direct laryngoscopy without delay. As you are performing BLS maneuvers, your partner should be preparing the laryngoscope handle and blade.

■ Suctioning

When the patient's mouth or throat becomes filled with vomitus, blood, or secretions, a suction apparatus enables you to remove the liquid material quickly and efficiently, thereby allowing you to ventilate the patient. Ventilating a patient with secretions in his or her mouth will force material into the lungs, resulting in an upper airway obstruction or aspiration. Therefore, clearing the patient's airway with suction, if needed, is your next priority after opening the patient's airway. *If you hear gurgling, the patient needs suctioning!*

Suctioning Equipment

Ambulances should carry both a fixed suction unit (which operates off a vacuum from the engine manifold) and a portable suction unit (battery operated or hand powered) **Figure 11-19 ▶**. Regardless of your location—in the patient's residence, the middle of a field, or in the back of the ambulance—you must have quick access to suction. It is essential for resuscitation.

Hand-operated suctioning units with disposable cannisters are reliable, effective, and relatively inexpensive; they can easily

Skill Drill 11-10: Managing Severe Airway Obstruction in an Unconscious Infant

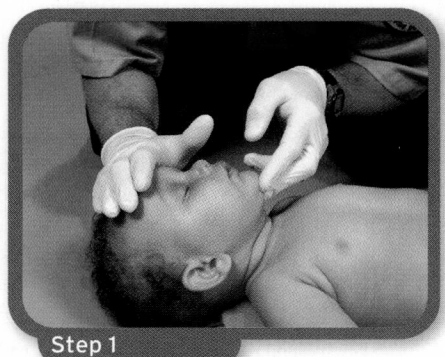

Step 1

Open the infant's airway and look in the mouth. If you see the object, carefully remove it from the infant's mouth.

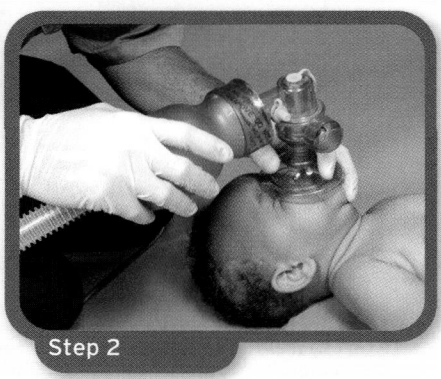

Step 2

Attempt to ventilate. If unsuccessful, reopen the airway and again attempt ventilation.

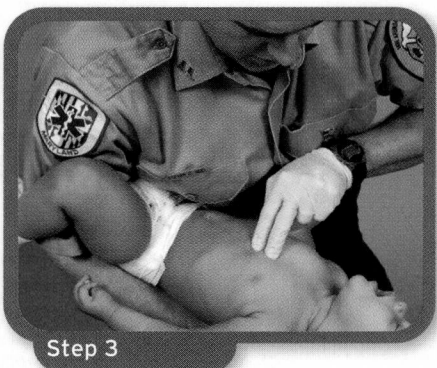

Step 3

Perform chest compressions.

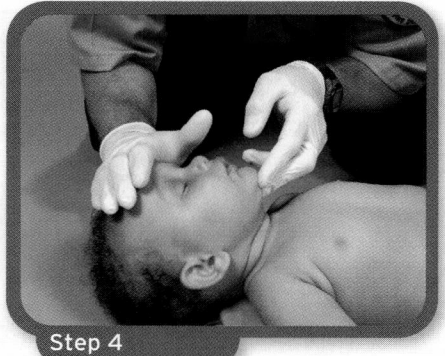

Step 4

Open the infant's airway and look in the mouth. If you see the object, carefully remove it from the infant's mouth. Repeat steps 2 through 4 until successful or until help arrives.

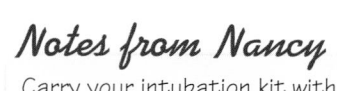

Notes from Nancy

Carry your intubation kit with you whenever you respond to a call in a restaurant.

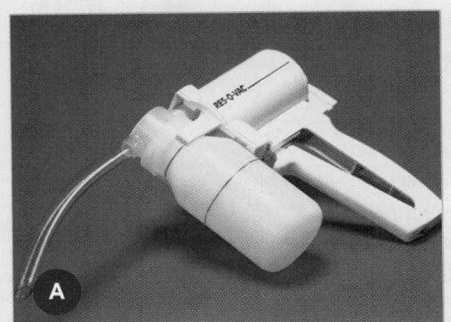 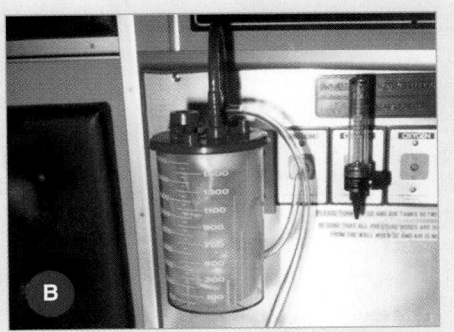 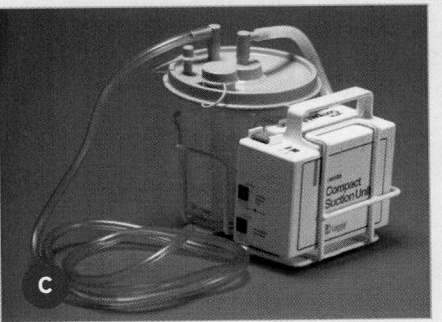

Figure 11-19 Suctioning equipment is essential for good airway management. **A.** Hand-operated device. **B.** Fixed unit. **C.** Portable unit.

Skill Drill 11-11: Removal of an Upper Airway Obstruction With Magill Forceps

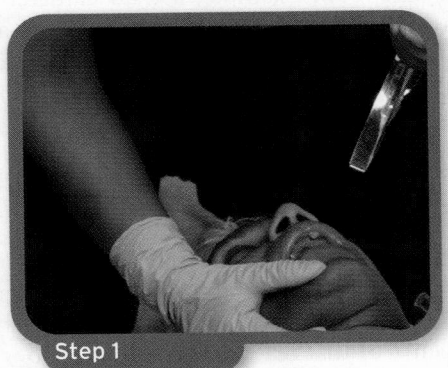

Step 1

With the patient's head in the sniffing position, open the patient's mouth and insert the laryngoscope blade.

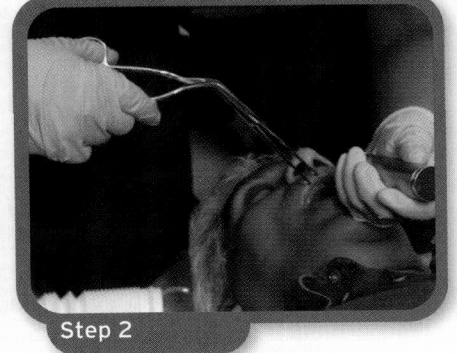

Step 2

Visualize the obstruction, and retrieve the object with the Magill forceps.

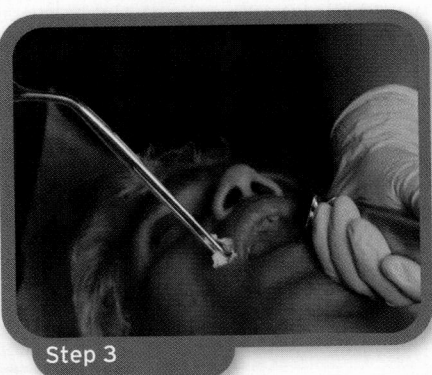

Step 3

Remove the object with the Magill forceps.

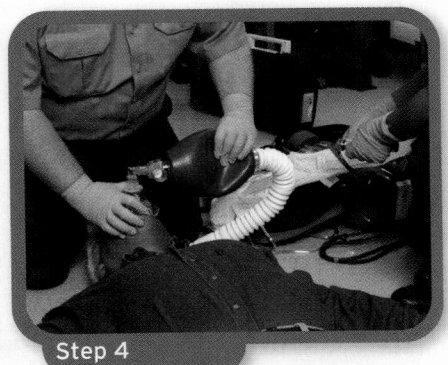

Step 4

Attempt to ventilate the patient.

the beginning of every shift by turning on the device, clamping the tubing, and making sure the pressure gauge registers 300 mm Hg. Ensure that all battery-charged units have fully charged batteries. **Table 11-6 ▶** lists the advantages and disadvantages of the most common types of suction devices.

Regardless of which type of suction unit you are using, the device must be able to generate enough vacuum pressure to adequately suction the patient's mouth and oropharynx. In addition to the suctioning unit, the following supplies should be readily accessible at the patient's head:

- Wide-bore, thick-walled, nonkinking tubing
- Soft and rigid suction catheters
- A nonbreakable, disposable collection bottle
- A supply of water for rinsing the catheters

A suction catheter is a hollow, cylindrical device that is used to remove fluids and secretions from the patient's airway. A Yankauer catheter (<u>tonsil-tip catheter</u>) is a good option for suctioning the pharynx in adults and the preferred device for infants and children. These plastic-tip catheters have a large diameter and are rigid, so they do not collapse. Rigid catheters are capable of suctioning large volumes of fluid rapidly. Tips with a curved contour allow for easy, rapid placement in the pharynx **Figure 11-20 ▶**.

fit into your first in bag. Mechanical or vacuum-powered suction units should be capable of generating a vacuum of 300 mm Hg within 4 seconds of clamping off the tubing. The amount of suction should be adjustable for use in children and intubated patients. Check the vacuum on the mechanical suction unit at

Table 11-6	Suction Devices	
Suction Device	**Advantages**	**Disadvantages**
Hand powered	• Lightweight • Portable • Mechanically simple • Inexpensive	• Limited volume • Manually powered • Fluid contact • Components not disposable
Oxygen-powered portable	• Lightweight • Small	• Limited suction power • Uses a lot of oxygen for limited suctioning power
Battery-operated portable	• Lightweight • Portable • Excellent suction power • May "field troubleshoot" most problems with the device	• More complicated mechanics • May lose battery integrity over time • Some fluid contact • Components not disposable
Mounted vacuum powered	• Extremely strong vacuum • Adjustable vacuum power • Components disposable	• Not portable • Fluid contact • Cannot "field service" or substitute power source

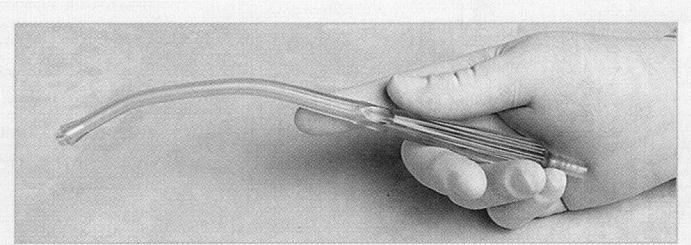

Figure 11-20 Tonsil-tip catheters are a good choice for suctioning the oropharynx because they have wide-diameter tips and are rigid.

Soft plastic, nonrigid catheters, sometimes called French or whistle-tip catheters, can be placed in the oropharynx or nasopharynx or down an endotracheal (ET) tube. They come in various sizes and have a smaller diameter than hard-tip catheters. Soft catheters are used to suction the nose and liquid secretions in the back of the mouth and in situations in which you cannot use a rigid catheter, such as for a patient with a stoma Figure 11-21 ▸ . For example, a rigid catheter could break a tooth in a patient with clenched teeth, whereas a flexible catheter may be worked along the cheeks without causing injury. Suction tubing without the attached catheter facilitates suctioning of large debris in the oropharynx and allows access to the back of the pharynx in a patient with clenched teeth.

Suctioning Techniques

Mortality increases significantly if a patient aspirates; therefore, suctioning the upper airway is critical to avoid this potentially fatal event. Suctioning removes not only liquids from the airway, but also oxygen. For that reason, any patient who is to be suctioned should be adequately preoxygenated first; this will provide a small oxygen reserve that can be drawn upon while you are suctioning. Even so, each suctioning attempt must be limited to a maximum of 15 seconds in the adult (less in infants and children). Be careful not to stimulate the back of

You are the Provider Part 6

The patient's airway has been cleared appropriately and bag-mask ventilations with 100% oxygen are continued. The engine arrives and two fire fighters assist you in loading the patient into the ambulance, where you attach a cardiac monitor, start an IV, and perform a reassessment. The closest appropriate hospital is approximately 40 miles away.

Reassessment	Recording Time: 11 Minutes
Level of consciousness	V (Responsive to verbal stimuli)
Respirations	28 breaths/min, shallow (baseline); you are assisting ventilations with a bag-mask device and 100% oxygen
Pulse	120 beats/min, regular and weak
Skin	Remains pale and diaphoretic; facial cyanosis is improving
Blood pressure	114/72 mm Hg
Sao_2	95% while receiving assisted ventilations with a bag-mask device and 100% oxygen

10. What is your most appropriate action at this point?

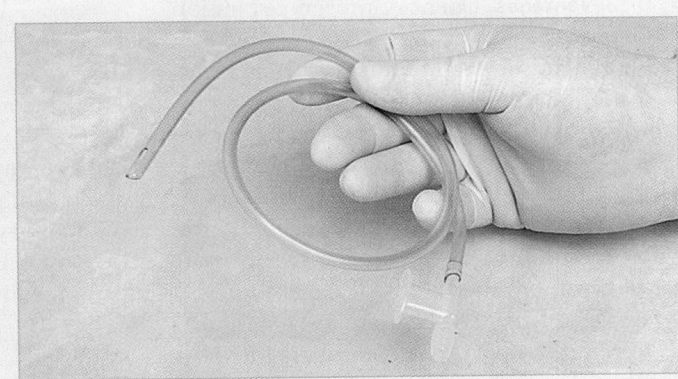

Figure 11-21 French (whistle-tip) catheters are used in situations in which rigid catheters cannot be used, such as when a patient has a stoma or if the patient's teeth are clenched.

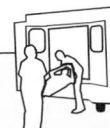

In the Field

Suctioning Time Limits

Adult	15 seconds
Child	10 seconds
Infant	5 seconds

4. Apply suction in a circular motion as you withdraw the catheter. Do not suction an adult for more than 15 seconds (Step 4).

Airway Adjuncts

The first step in the initial management of an unconscious patient is to open the airway, initially by manual methods (eg, head tilt–chin lift, jaw-thrust). If the patient has an altered LOC, an artificial airway may then be needed to help maintain

the throat of a young child or infant as the vagal stimulus can cause the heart rate to drop. After the patient has been suctioned, continue ventilation and oxygenation.

Soft-tip catheters must be lubricated when suctioning the nasopharynx and used through an ET tube. The catheter is inserted, and suction is applied during extraction of the catheter to clear the airway. After the patient has been suctioned, reevaluate the patency of his or her airway, and continue to ventilate and oxygenate as needed.

Before inserting any suction catheter into a patient, make sure you measure for the proper size, going from the corner of the mouth to the earlobe. Never insert a catheter past the base of the tongue, as it may cause the patient to gag or vomit.

The steps for properly suctioning a patient's airway are listed here and shown in (Skill Drill 11-12 ▶).

1. Turn on the assembled suction unit (Step 1).
2. Measure the catheter from the corner of the mouth to the earlobe (Step 2).
3. Before applying suction, open the patient's mouth by using the crossfinger technique or tongue-jaw lift, and insert the tip of the catheter to the predetermined depth. Do not suction while inserting the catheter (Step 3).

Skill Drill 11-12: Suctioning a Patient's Airway

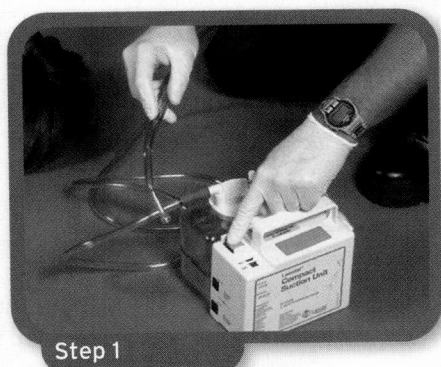

Step 1
Make sure the suctioning unit is properly assembled, and turn on the suction unit.

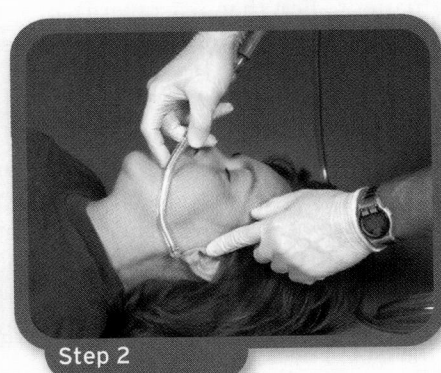

Step 2
Measure the catheter from the corner of the mouth to the earlobe.

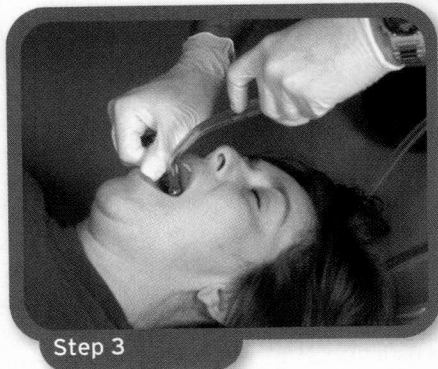

Step 3
Open the patient's mouth, and insert the catheter to the predetermined depth without suctioning.

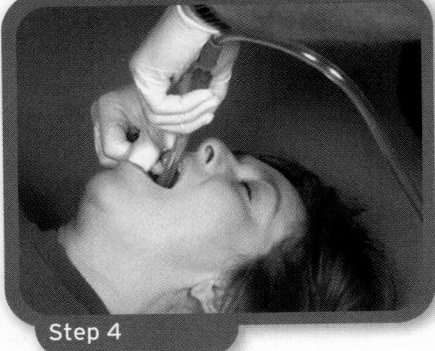

Step 4
Apply suction in a circular motion as you withdraw the catheter. Do not suction an adult for more than 15 seconds.

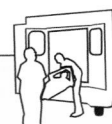

In the Field

Wear a mask and protective eyewear whenever you are managing a patient's airway. Body fluids can become aerosolized, and the mucous membranes of the paramedic's mouth, nose, and eyes can easily come in contact with these contaminants.

an open air passage. *An artificial airway is not a substitute for proper head positioning.* Even after an airway adjunct has been inserted, the appropriate manual position of the head must be maintained.

Oropharyngeal Airway

The oropharyngeal (oral) airway is a curved, hard plastic device that fits over the back of the tongue with the tip in the posterior pharynx **Figure 11-22 ▼**. It is designed to hold the tongue away from the posterior pharyngeal wall, and its use makes it much easier to ventilate patients with a bag-mask device. The oral airway can also serve as an effective bite-block, preventing an intubated patient from chomping down on the ET tube.

An oral airway should be inserted promptly in unresponsive patients—breathing or not—who have no gag reflex. Because its distal end sits in the back of the throat, this device will stimulate gagging and retching in a conscious or semiconscious patient. For that reason, the oropharyngeal airway should be used only in unconscious, unresponsive patients without a gag reflex. To assess a patient's gag reflex, use the eyelash reflex (discussed earlier in this chapter). *If the patient gags during insertion of the oral airway, remove the device immediately and be prepared to suction the oropharynx.* Following are some considerations when using an oropharyngeal airway:

- **Indications.** Unresponsive patients, absent gag reflex.
- **Contraindications.** Conscious patients, patients with a gag reflex.
- **Advantages.** Noninvasive, easily placed, prevents blockage of the glottis by the tongue.

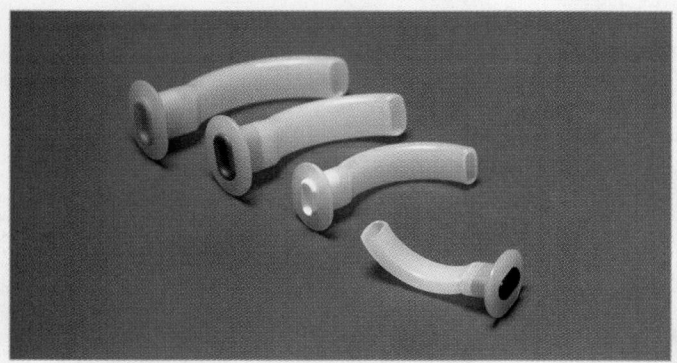

Figure 11-22 An oral airway is used for unconscious patients who have no gag reflex. It helps to keep the tongue from blocking the airway.

- **Disadvantages.** Does not prevent aspiration.
- **Complications.** Unexpected gag may cause vomiting, pharyngeal or dental trauma with poor technique.

If the oral airway is improperly sized or is inserted incorrectly, it could actually push the tongue back into the pharynx, creating an airway obstruction. Rough insertion of the airway can injure the hard palate, resulting in oral bleeding and creating a risk of vomiting or aspiration. Prior to inserting an oral airway, suction the oropharynx as needed to ensure that the mouth is clear of blood or other fluids. The steps for inserting an oral airway are listed here and shown in **Skill Drill 11-13 ▶**.

1. To select the proper size, measure the distance from the patient's earlobe to the corner of the mouth **Step 1**.
2. Open the patient's mouth with the crossfinger technique or tongue-jaw lift. Hold the airway upside down with your other hand. Insert the airway with the tip facing the roof of the mouth **Step 2**.
3. Rotate the airway 180°, flipping it over the tongue. When inserted properly, the airway will rest in the mouth, with the curvature of the airway following the contour of the teeth. The flange should rest against the lips, with the distal end in the posterior pharynx **Step 3**.

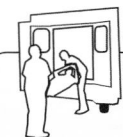

In the Field

An easy way to insert an oral airway is to use the "hard palate, soft palate, rotate" technique. As the airway is gliding across the hard palate, you should feel a slight bump as the airway reaches the soft palate. Because the soft palate is just above the curvature of the tongue, you should rotate the airway 180° as soon as you feel the bump; this will allow the airway to catch the base of the tongue and propel it forward.

If you encounter difficulty while inserting the oral airway, try this alternative technique **Skill Drill 11-14 ▶**.

1. Use a tongue blade to depress the tongue, ensuring that the tongue remains forward **Step 1**.
2. Insert the oral airway sideways from the corner of the mouth, until the flange reaches the lips **Step 2**.
3. Rotate the oral airway 90°, removing the tongue blade as you exert gentle backward pressure on the oral airway, until the flange rests securely in place against the lips **Step 3**.

Special Considerations

In children, using a tongue blade to hold the tongue down while inserting an oral airway is the preferred method. Because the airways of children are less developed than those of adults, rotating the oral airway in the posterior pharynx may cause damage.

Skill Drill 11-13: Inserting an Oral Airway

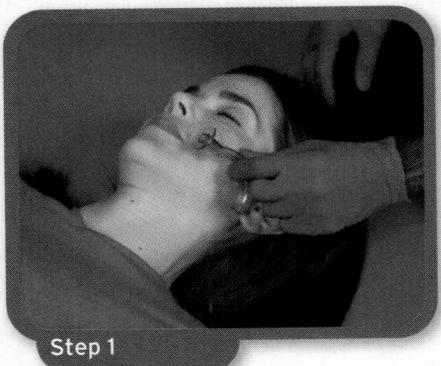

Step 1

Determine the size of the airway by measuring the distance from the patient's earlobe to the corner of the mouth.

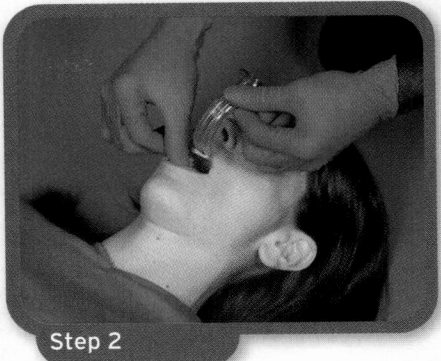

Step 2

Open the patient's mouth with the crossfinger technique or tongue-jaw lift. Hold the airway upside down with your other hand. Insert the airway with the tip facing the roof of the mouth and slide it in until it touches the roof of the mouth.

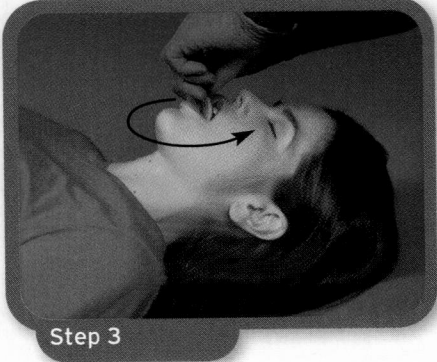

Step 3

Rotate the airway 180°, flipping it over the tongue. Insert the airway until the flange rests on the patient's lips. In this position, the airway will hold the tongue away from the posterior pharynx.

Skill Drill 11-14: Inserting an Oral Airway With a 90° Rotation

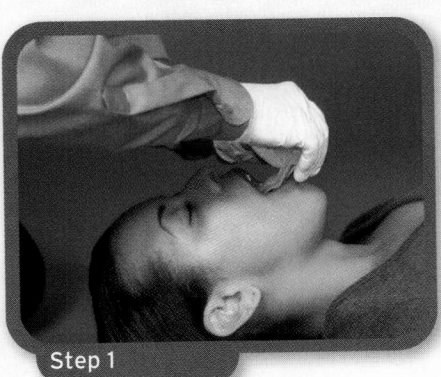

Step 1

Depress the tongue with a tongue blade so the tongue remains forward.

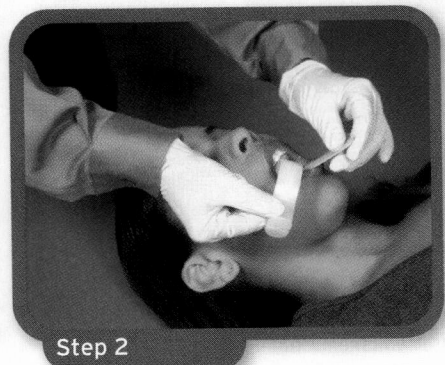

Step 2

Insert the oral airway sideways from the corner of the mouth, until the flange reaches the lips.

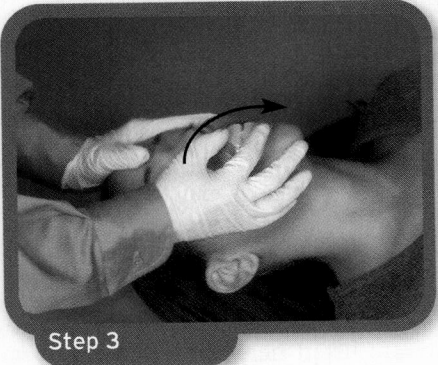

Step 3

Rotate the oral airway 90°, and remove the tongue blade as you exert gentle backward pressure on the oral airway until the flange rests securely in place against the lips.

Nasopharyngeal Airway

The <u>nasopharyngeal (nasal) airway</u> is a 6″-long, soft, rubber tube that is inserted through the nose into the posterior pharynx behind the tongue, thereby allowing passage of air from the nose to the lower airway. The nasal airway is much better tolerated than an oral airway in patients who have an intact gag reflex yet an altered LOC **Figure 11-23 ▶**. Do not use this device when is the patient has experienced trauma to the nose or you have reason to suspect a skull fracture (eg, CSF leakage from the nose). Inserting the airway in such cases may cause it to enter the brain through the hole caused by the fracture.

The nasopharyngeal airway must be inserted gently to avoid precipitating epistaxis (nosebleed). Lubricate the airway generously with a water-soluble jelly, preferably one that contains local anesthetic, and slide it gently, tip downward, into one nostril. *Do not try to force it.* If you meet resistance, try to

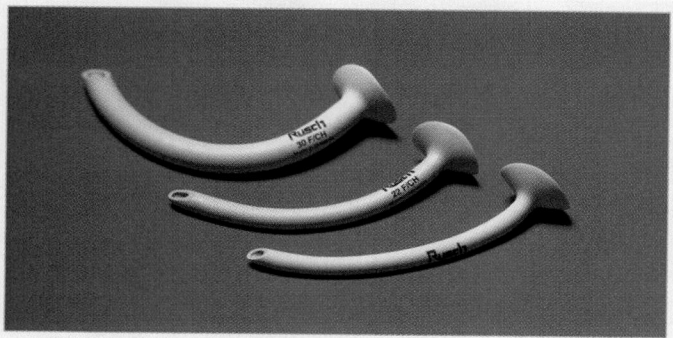

Figure 11-23 A nasal airway is better tolerated by patients who have an intact gag reflex.

pass the airway down the other nostril. Following are considerations when using a nasopharyngeal airway:

- **Indications.** Unresponsive patients, patients with an altered mental status who have an intact gag reflex.
- **Contraindications.** Patient intolerance, caution in the presence of facial fracture or skull fracture.
- **Advantages.** Can be suctioned through, provides a patent airway, can be tolerated by awake patients, can be safely placed "blindly," does not require the mouth to be open.
- **Disadvantages.** Poor technique may result in severe bleeding (resulting epistaxis may be extremely difficult to control), does not protect from aspiration.

The steps for inserting a nasal airway are listed here and shown in **Skill Drill 11-15 ▶**.

1. Before inserting the airway, make sure you have selected the proper size. Measure the distance from the tip of the nostril to the earlobe. In almost all individuals, one nostril is larger than the other. The diameter should be roughly equal to the patient's little finger **Step 1**.
2. After lubricating the nasal airway with a water-soluble gel, place the airway in the larger nostril, with the curvature of the device

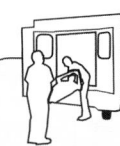
In the Field
Oxygen is one of the most powerful drugs for saving lives that you will carry in your ambulance. Don't be afraid to use it!

following the curve of the floor of the nose and the bevel facing the septum **Step 2**.

3. Place the bevel toward the septum and insert it gently along the nasal floor, parallel to the mouth. *Do not force the airway* **Step 3**.
4. When completely inserted, the flange should rest against the nostril. The distal end of the airway will open into the posterior pharynx **Step 4**.

As an alternative, the proper size of nasal airway can be determined by measuring from the tip of the nostril to the angle

Skill Drill 11-15:
Inserting a Nasal Airway

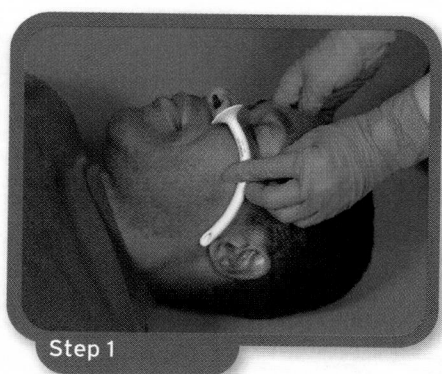

Step 1

Determine the size of the airway by measuring the distance from the tip of the nose to the patient's earlobe. Coat the tip with a water-soluble lubricant.

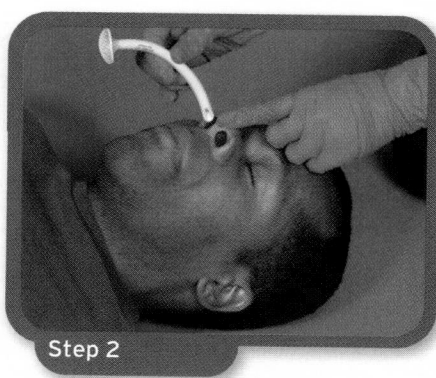

Step 2

Insert the lubricated airway into the larger nostril, with the curvature following the floor of the nose and the bevel facing the septum.

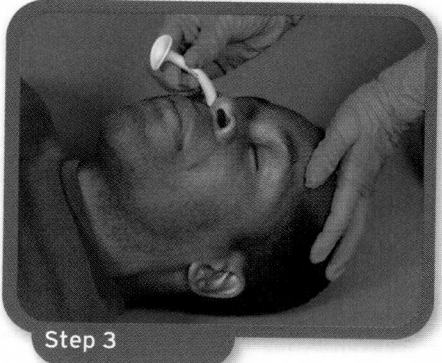

Step 3

Gently advance the airway. If using the left nostril, insert the nasal airway until it meets with resistance, then rotate the airway 180° into position. *This rotation is not required if you are using the right nostril.*

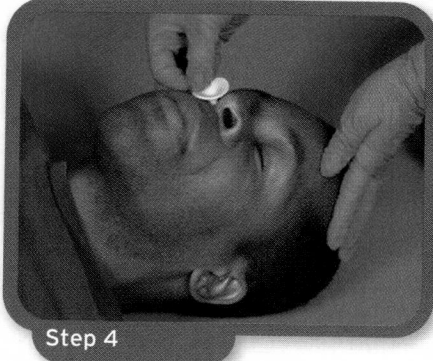

Step 4

Continue until the flange rests against the nostril. If you feel any resistance or obstruction, remove the airway and insert it into the other nostril.

of the jaw rather than the earlobe. If the nasal airway is too long, it may obstruct the patient's airway. If the patient becomes intolerant of the nasal airway, gently remove it from the nasal passage. Although the nasal airway is not as likely to cause vomiting as the oral airway, you should still have suction readily available.

Supplemental Oxygen Therapy

Supplemental oxygen should be administered to any patient with potential hypoxia, regardless of his or her clinical appearance. In some conditions, a part of the patient's body does not receive enough oxygen, *even though the oxygen supply to the body as a whole is entirely adequate.* For example, when a patient experiences an acute myocardial infarction (heart attack), a portion of the myocardium is hypoxic, *even though the rest of the body is well oxygenated.* Increasing the available oxygen supply also enhances the body's compensatory mechanisms during shock and other distressed states.

The oxygen-delivery method must be appropriate for the patient's ventilatory status and should be reassessed frequently and adjusted accordingly based on the patient's clinical condition and breathing adequacy. When a patient needs oxygen, the paramedic's first priority is to provide that oxygen quickly.

Oxygen Sources

Pure (100%) oxygen is stored in seamless steel or aluminum cylinders, whose colors may vary from silver, to chrome, to green, or some combination thereof. Make sure that the cylinder is labeled "medical oxygen." Also, look for letters and numbers stamped on the collar of the cylinder Figure 11-24 . Of particular importance are the month and year stamps, which indicate when the cylinder was last hydrostat tested.

Oxygen cylinders are available in various sizes. You will most often use the D cylinder, which contains 350 L of oxygen and is typically carried from the ambulance to the patient, and the M cylinder, which contains 3,450 L of oxygen and remains on board the ambulance as a main supply tank. The E (or super/jumbo) cylinder, another common size, holds 625 L of oxygen.

Oxygen delivery is measured in terms of liters per minute (L/min). As a precaution against running out at an inconvenient moment, you should replace an oxygen cylinder with a full one when the pressure falls to 200 psi or below. That level is called the safe residual pressure, indicating that it is *unsafe* to continue using the oxygen cylinder. On the basis of the pressure in the oxygen cylinder and the flow rate of oxygen delivery, you can calculate how long the supply of oxygen in the cylinder will last—that is, the tank life Table 11-7 .

Liquid Oxygen

Liquid oxygen is oxygen that is cooled to its aqueous state. It converts to a gaseous state when warmed. Although much larger volumes of gaseous oxygen can be stored in the aqueous state, units for liquid oxygen generally require upright storage

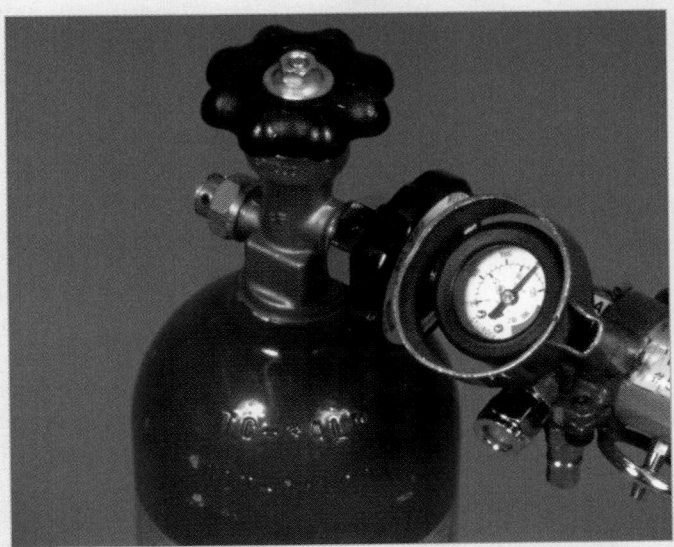

Figure 11-24 Oxygen cylinders for medical use have a series of letters and numbers stamped into the metal on the collar of the cylinder.

Table 11-7	Oxygen Cylinders: Duration of Flow
Formula	
$\dfrac{\text{Tank pressure in psi} - 200\ \text{psi (the safe residual pressure)} \times \text{cylinder constant}}{\text{Flow rate in L/min}}$	= Duration of flow in minutes

Cylinder Constant

D = 0.16	G = 2.41
E = 0.28	H = 3.14
M = 1.56	K = 3.14

Calculation

Determine the life of a D cylinder that has a pressure of 2,000 psi and a flow rate of 15 L/min.

$$\frac{(2{,}000\ [\text{psi}] - 200\ [\text{safe residual pressure}] \times 0.16\ [\text{cylinder constant}])}{15} = \frac{288}{15\ (\text{L/min})} = 19.2\ (19)\ \text{min}$$

Note: psi indicates pounds per square inch.

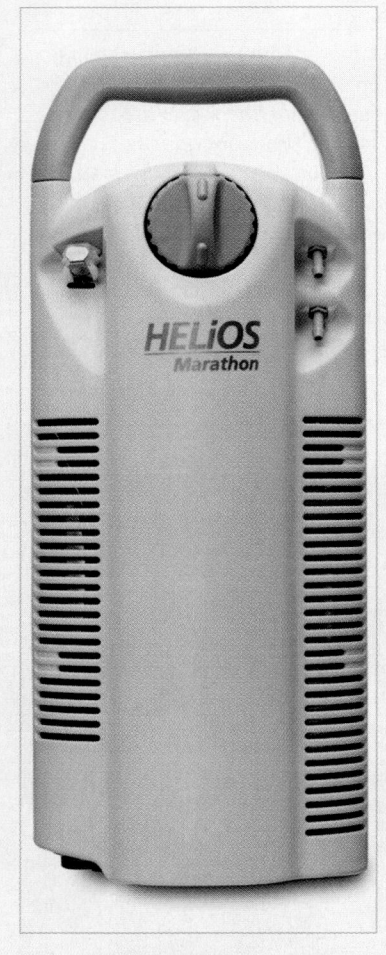

Figure 11-25 Liquid oxygen converts to a gas when warmed. It must be stored upright.

Figure 11-25 ◄ . Additionally, there are special requirements for large volume storage and cylinder transfer.

Oxygen Regulators and Flowmeters

High-pressure regulators are attached to the cylinder stem to deliver cylinder gas under high pressure. These regulators are used to transfer cylinder gas from tank to tank, such as when you are refilling a portable oxygen cylinder.

The pressure of gas in a full oxygen cylinder is approximately 2,000 psi. Clearly, this is far too much pressure to deliver directly into a patient's airway. Instead, gas flow from an oxygen cylinder to the patient is controlled by a therapy regulator, which attaches to the stem of the oxygen cylinder and reduces the high pressure of gas to a safe range (about 50 psi).

Flowmeters, which are usually permanently attached to the therapy regulator, allow the oxygen delivered to the patient to be adjusted within a range of 1 to 25 L/min. The two types of flowmeters most commonly used are the pressure-compensated flowmeter and the Bourdon-gauge flowmeter.

A pressure-compensated flowmeter incorporates a float ball within a tapered calibrated tube; this float rises or falls based on the gas flow in the tube. The gas flow is controlled by a needle valve located downstream from the float ball. Because this type of flowmeter is affected by gravity, it must remain in an upright position to obtain an accurate flow reading Figure 11-26 ▶ .

By contrast, the Bourdon-gauge flowmeter is not affected by gravity and can be placed in any position. This pressure gauge is calibrated to record the flow rate Figure 11-27 ▶ . The major disadvantage of this type of flowmeter is that it does not compensate for backpressure. As a result, it will usually record a higher flow rate when there is any obstruction to gas flow downstream.

Preparing an Oxygen Cylinder for Use

Prior to administering supplemental oxygen to your patient, you must prepare the oxygen cylinder and therapy regulator. To place an oxygen cylinder into service, follow these steps Skill Drill 11-16 ▶ .

1. Inspect the cylinder and its markings. Remove the plastic seal covering the valve stem opening (if commercially filled). Inspect the opening to ensure that it is free of dirt or other debris. With the tank facing away from yourself and others, use an oxygen wrench to "crack" the cylinder— quickly opening and closing the valve to ensure that dirt particles and other contaminants do not enter the oxygen flow Step 1 .

2. Attach the regulator/flowmeter to the valve stem, ensuring that the pin-index system is correctly aligned. A metal or plastic O-ring is placed around the oxygen port to optimize the airtight seal between the collar of the regulator and the valve stem Step 2 .

3. Place the regulator collar over the cylinder valve, with the oxygen port and pin-indexing pins on the side of

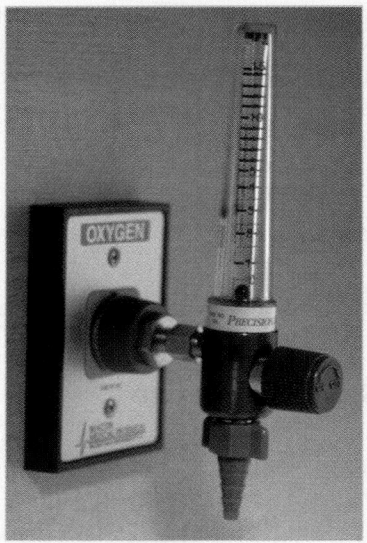

Figure 11-26 Pressure-compensated flowmeters contain a float ball that rises or falls based on the gas flow in the tube. It must remain in an upright position for an accurate flow reading.

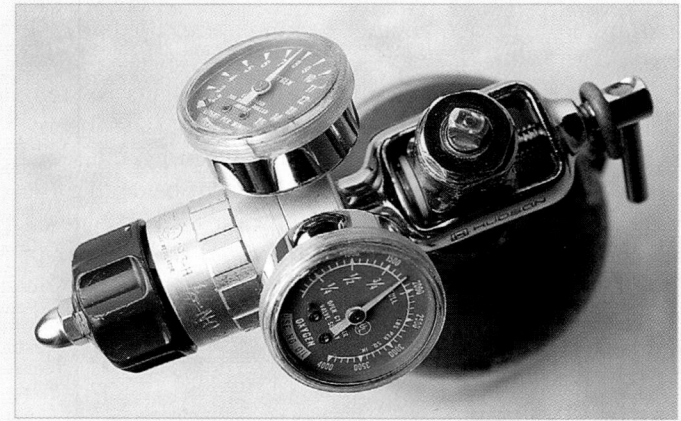

Figure 11-27 The Bourdon-gauge flowmeter is not affected by gravity and can be placed in any position.

Skill Drill 11-16: Placing an Oxygen Cylinder Into Service

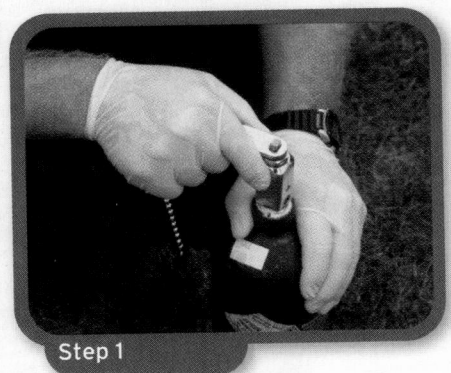

Step 1

Using an oxygen wrench, turn the valve counterclockwise to "crack" the cylinder.

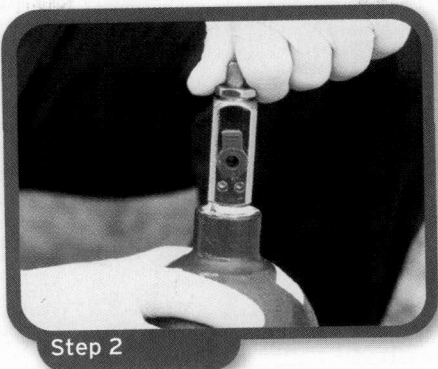

Step 2

Attach the regulator/flowmeter to the valve stem using the two pin-indexing holes, and make sure that the O-ring is in place over the larger hole.

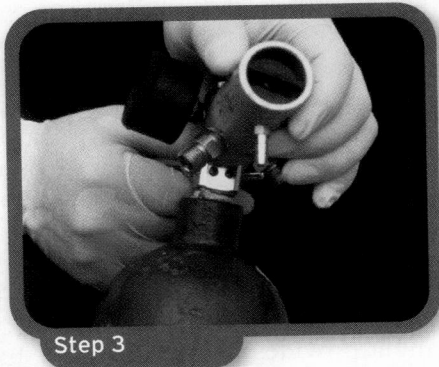

Step 3

Align the regulator so that the pins fit snugly into the correct holes on the valve stem and hand-tighten the regulator.

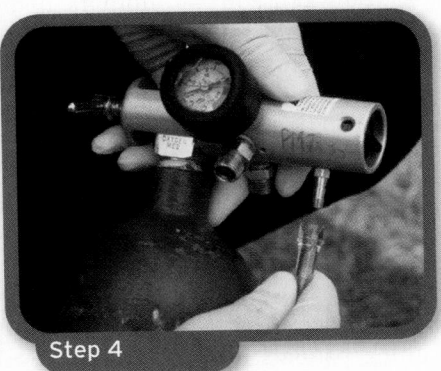

Step 4

Attach the oxygen connective tubing to the flowmeter.

flowmeter and select the oxygen flow rate that is appropriate for your patient's condition (Step 4).

Safety Considerations

Any cylinder containing compressed gas under high pressure has the potential, under the right conditions (actually, the *wrong* conditions!), to assume the properties of a rocket. Furthermore, oxygen presents the additional hazard of fire, because it supports the combustion process. For these reasons, safety precautions are necessary when you are handling oxygen cylinders:

- Keep combustible materials, such as oil or grease, away from contact with the cylinder itself, the regulators, fittings, valves, or tubing.
- Do not permit smoking in any area where oxygen cylinders are in use or on standby.
- Store oxygen cylinders in a cool, well-ventilated area. Do not subject the cylinders to temperatures above 125°F (approximately 50°C).
- Use an oxygen cylinder only with a safe, properly fitting regulator valve. Regulator valves for one gas should never be modified for use with another gas.
- Close all valves when the cylinder is not in use, even if the tank is empty.
- Secure cylinders so that they will not topple over. In transit, keep them in a proper carrier or rack, or strap them onto the stretcher with the patient.
- When working with an oxygen cylinder, always position yourself to its side. Never place any part of your body over the cylinder valve! A loosely fitting regulator can be blown off the cylinder with sufficient force to demolish any object in its path.
- Have the cylinder hydrostat tested every 10 years, to make sure it can still sustain the high pressures required. The original test date is stamped onto the cylinder together with its serial number.

the valve stem that has three holes. Align the regulator so that the oxygen port and the pins fit into the correct holes on the valve stem; align the screw bolt on the opposite side with the dimpled depression. Tighten the screw bolt until the regulator is firmly attached to the cylinder. At this point, you should not see any space between the sides of the valve stem and the interior walls of the collar (Step 3).

4. With the regulator firmly attached, open the cylinder and read the pressure level on the regulator gauge. Follow your local protocols regarding minimum cylinder pressures.

5. A second gauge or a selector dial on the flowmeter indicates the oxygen flow rate. Attach the oxygen connective tubing to the "Christmas tree" nipple on the

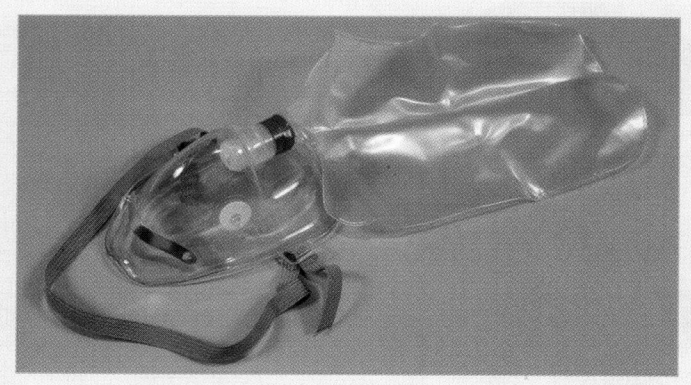
Figure 11-28 Nonrebreathing mask.

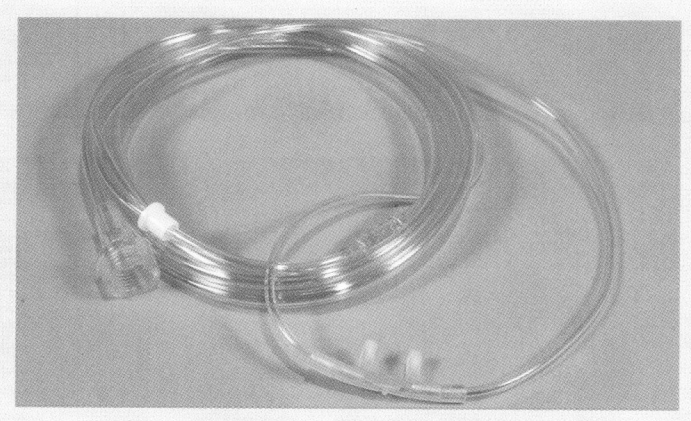
Figure 11-29 Nasal cannula.

Supplemental Oxygen-Delivery Devices

The most common oxygen-delivery devices that you will use in the prehospital setting are the nonrebreathing mask, nasal cannula, and bag-mask device. However, if your EMS system performs interfacility transfers, you may encounter other oxygen-delivery devices, such as the simple face mask, partial rebreathing mask, and Venturi mask. Small-volume nebulizers, which are typically used to deliver aerosolized medications, may also be used to administer supplemental oxygen.

Nonrebreathing Mask

The nonrebreathing mask is the preferred device for delivering supplemental oxygen to spontaneously breathing patients in the prehospital setting. With a good mask-to-face seal and a flow rate of 15 L/min, it is capable of delivering between 90% and 100% inspired oxygen.

The nonrebreathing mask is a combination mask and reservoir bag system. Oxygen fills a reservoir bag that is attached to the mask by a one-way valve. This permits the patient to inhale from the reservoir bag but not to exhale back into it. The only gas that can enter the reservoir, therefore, is 100% oxygen piped in from the oxygen cylinder. Exhaled gas escapes through one-way flapper valves located on the side of the mask (Figure 11-28 ▲).

Prior to administering oxygen to a patient with a nonrebreathing mask, you must ensure that the reservoir bag is completely filled. The oxygen flow rate is adjusted from 12 to 15 L/min to prevent collapse of the bag during inhalation. Use a pediatric nonrebreathing mask, which has a smaller reservoir bag, for infants and small children; they inhale smaller volumes of air.

The nonrebreathing mask is indicated for spontaneously breathing patients who require high-flow oxygen concentrations (eg, shock, hypoxia from any cause) and have adequate tidal volume (ie, good chest rise). Contraindications include apnea and poor respiratory effort. Because the nonrebreathing mask delivers oxygen passively, the patient's respirations must be of adequate depth to open the one-way valve and draw air from the reservoir bag into the lungs. A patient with reduced tidal volume (shallow breathing) will benefit very little, if any, from the nonrebreathing mask.

Nasal Cannula

The nasal cannula delivers oxygen via two small prongs that fit into the patient's nostrils (Figure 11-29 ▲). With an oxygen flow rate of 1 to 6 L/min, the nasal cannula can deliver an oxygen concentration of 24% to 44%. Higher flow rates will merely irritate the nasal mucosa without increasing the delivered oxygen concentration. An oxygen humidifier should be used when delivering oxygen via nasal cannula for a prolonged period of time, as it will help prevent mucosal drying and irritation.

The nasal cannula provides low to moderate oxygen enrichment and is most beneficial to patients who require long-term oxygen therapy (eg, for COPD). It is ineffective if the patient is apneic, has poor respiratory effort, is severely hypoxic, or is a mouth-breather. In the prehospital setting, the nasal cannula is primarily used when patients who need oxygen cannot tolerate a nonrebreathing mask.

The nasal cannula is generally well tolerated, especially in patients who are claustrophobic and intolerant of an oxygen mask over their face. However, it does not deliver high volumes or concentrations of oxygen.

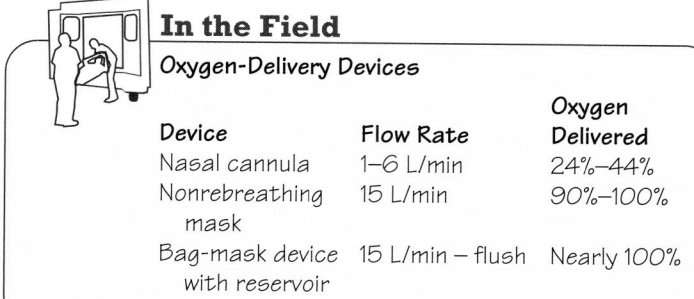

In the Field

Oxygen-Delivery Devices

Device	Flow Rate	Oxygen Delivered
Nasal cannula	1–6 L/min	24%–44%
Nonrebreathing mask	15 L/min	90%–100%
Bag-mask device with reservoir	15 L/min – flush	Nearly 100%

2. The second paramedic squeezes the bag completely with both hands over 1 second, observing for visible chest rise (Step 2).

Three-Person Bag-Mask Ventilation

The one-person, two-person, and three-person bag-mask techniques can be understood in terms of progressive difficulty. If you cannot ventilate a patient effectively with one person, use two. If you cannot ventilate effectively with two, use three. With this approach, there are very few patients that you cannot ventilate.

The three-person bag-mask technique is indicated for apneic patients, patients who are breathing inadequately, patients who cannot be ventilated by one or two rescuers, and patients with a possible spinal injury. It is contraindicated in patients who are intolerant of the device.

The major disadvantage is that this technique requires additional personnel. Furthermore, the area around the patient's head can become very crowded when he or she is being ventilated by three rescuers.

Complications associated with the three-person bag-mask technique are the same as those for the one-person and two-person techniques—hyperinflation of the patient's lungs and gastric distention. Therefore, the patient must be continually

monitored for adequate chest rise and ventilation compliance. If the patient's chest does not rise and fall during ventilations, you may need to reposition the head, insert an airway adjunct, or apply cricoid pressure.

The steps for performing the three-person bag-mask ventilation technique are listed here and shown in Skill Drill 11-20 ▾ .

1. The first paramedic maintains a mask seal by the most appropriate method (Step 1).
2. The second paramedic squeezes the bag completely with both hands over 1 second (Step 2).
3. The third paramedic applies cricoid pressure (Step 3).

Skill Drill 11-19: Two-Person Bag-Mask Ventilation

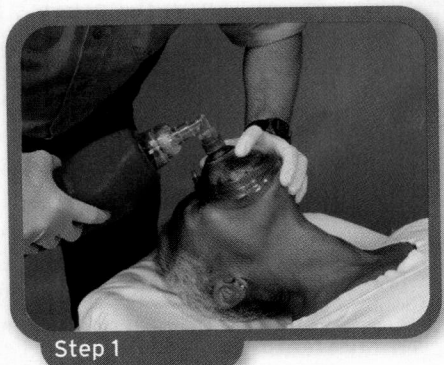

Step 1

The first paramedic maintains the mask seal by the most appropriate method.

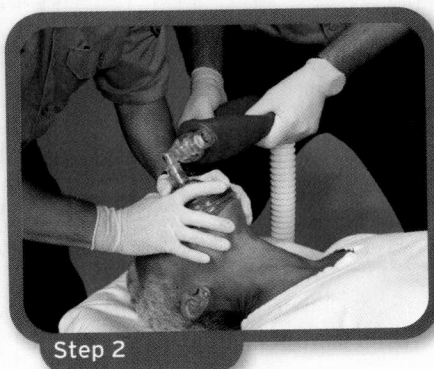

Step 2

The second paramedic squeezes the bag completely over 1 second to provide visible chest rise.

Skill Drill 11-20: Three-Person Bag-Mask Ventilation

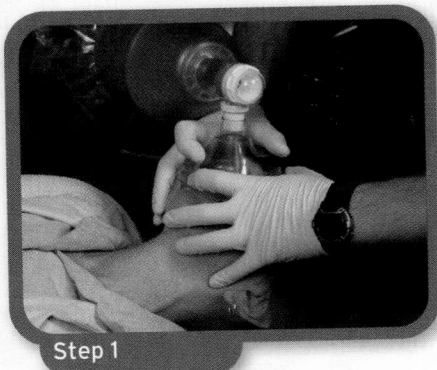

Step 1

The first paramedic maintains a mask seal by the most appropriate method.

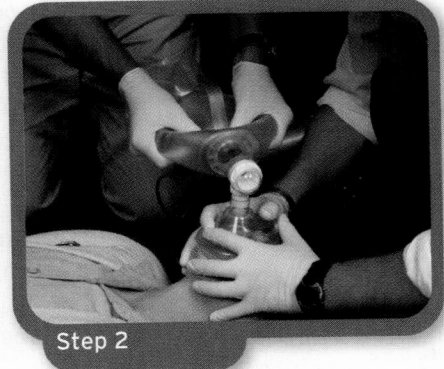

Step 2

The second paramedic squeezes the bag over 1 second to achieve visible chest rise.

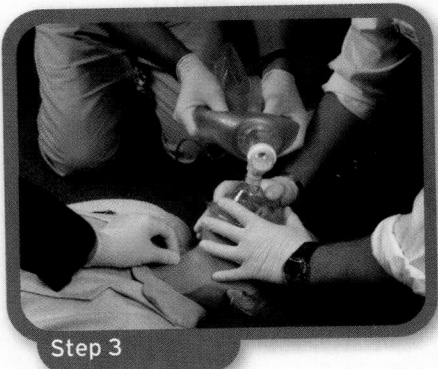

Step 3

The third paramedic applies cricoid pressure.

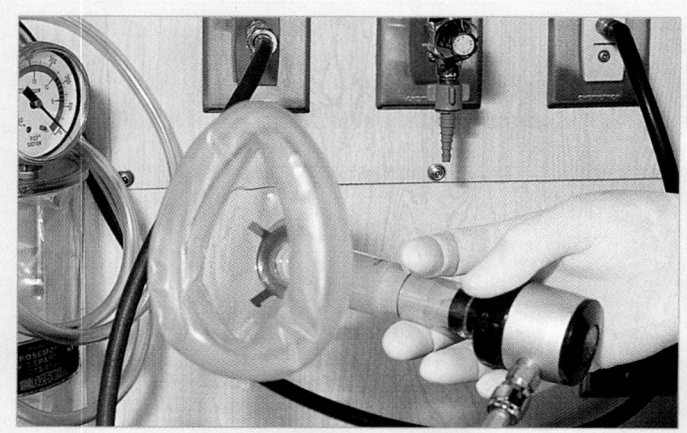

Figure 11-36 Flow-restricted, oxygen-powered ventilation device.

The bag-mask device may also be used in conjunction with an ET tube or with other advanced airway devices such as the Combitube and the laryngeal mask airway (LMA).

Flow-Restricted, Oxygen-Powered Ventilation Device

A third potential source for artificial ventilation is the flow-restricted, oxygen-powered ventilation device (FROPVD), also referred to as a manually triggered ventilator or demand valve **Figure 11-36 ▲** . The FROPVD can be used to ventilate apneic patients or to administer supplemental oxygen to spontaneously breathing patients. Its plastic housing includes a 15/22-mm adapter designed to fit onto standard ventilation masks as well as advanced airways (eg, ET tube, Combitube).

The FROPVD has a demand valve that is triggered by the negative pressure generated during inhalation. This valve automatically delivers 100% oxygen as the spontaneously breathing patient begins to inhale and stops the flow of gas at

the end of inhalation. Generally, patients find it most comfortable if they hold the mask to their face themselves. The FROPVD delivers only the volume needed by the patient during inhalation, rather than wasting oxygen by providing a constant flow. Because the FROPVD makes an airtight seal with the patient's face, the patient inhales almost 100% oxygen. If the patient is conscious, he or she must have adequate tidal volume to be able to self-administer oxygen via the FROPVD. Do not use this device if the spontaneously breathing patient has an altered level of consciousness or is intolerant of the FROPVD.

For ventilation of apneic patients, a pushbutton on top of the FROPVD can control the flow of oxygen. When the button is depressed, 100% oxygen streams out at a fixed flow rate of 40 L/min. This flow continues until the operator takes his or her finger off the button or the pop-off valve releases when the device reaches the preset pressure limit of 30 cm H_2O.

The valve opening pressure at the cardiac sphincter (opening into the stomach) is also about 30 cm H_2O. As a consequence, the FROPVD may reduce (but not eliminate) gastric distention, compared with bag-mask ventilation. This limited pressure is a disadvantage for certain patients who need greater pressure to overcome increased airway resistance, including those with COPD or an airway obstruction. Therefore, whenever you are ventilating patients with a FROPVD, ensure that they are receiving enough volume by observing the chest for adequate rise.

Unlike a bag-mask device or pocket mask, the FROPVD requires an oxygen source to function—a potential disadvantage. In addition, the operator cannot feel whether the patient is being adequately ventilated with this device. Changes in compliance can be an important early indication of an impending problem. You must closely monitor the patient being ventilated mechanically and remain vigilant for changes in his or her condition.

The FROPVD has been used in EMS for several years; however, recent findings suggest that they should not be used routinely because of the high incidence of gastric distention and damage to intrathoracic structures caused by barotrauma. This device *should not* be used when ventilating infants or children or for patients with possible cervical spine or chest injury. *Cricoid pressure must be maintained whenever FROPVDs are used to ventilate nonintubated patients.* This will help to reduce the incidence of gastric distention.

The steps for ventilating an apneic patient with the FROPVD are listed here and shown in **Skill Drill 11-21 ▶** .

1. Choose the proper mask size to seat the mask from the bridge of the nose to the chin **Step 1** .
2. Position the mask on the patient's face by the most appropriate method **Step 2** .
3. Open the patient's airway and hold the mask in place with one hand, maintaining an adequate mask-to-face seal **Step 3** .
4. Press the ventilation button until you see visible chest rise **Step 4** .
5. Allow the patient to exhale passively **Step 5** .

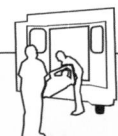

In the Field

Indications That Artificial Ventilation Is Adequate*

- Adequate and equal chest rise and fall with ventilation
- Ventilations are delivered at the appropriate rate:
  - 10 to 12 breaths/min for adults
  - 12 to 20 breaths/min for infants and children
- Heart rate returns to a normal range

Indications That Artificial Ventilation Is Inadequate

- Minimal or no chest rise and fall
- Ventilations delivered too fast or too slow for patient's age
- Heart rate does not return to a normal range

*In patients who are apneic with a pulse (ie, not in cardiac arrest).

Skill Drill 11-21: Flow-Restricted, Oxygen-Powered Ventilation for Apneic Patients

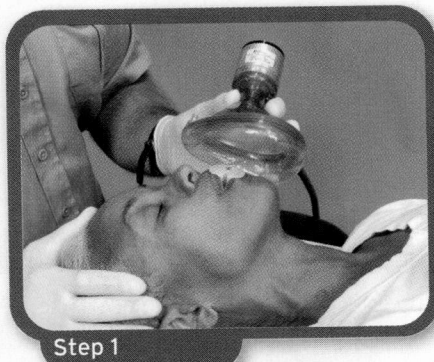

Step 1

Choose the proper mask size to seat the mask from the bridge of the nose to the chin.

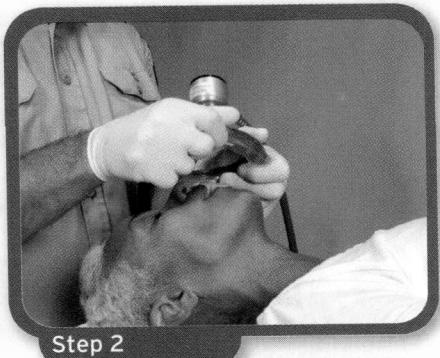

Step 2

Position the mask on the patient's face by the most appropriate method.

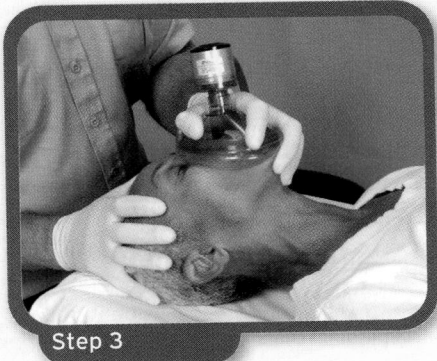

Step 3

Open the patient's airway and hold the mask with one hand.

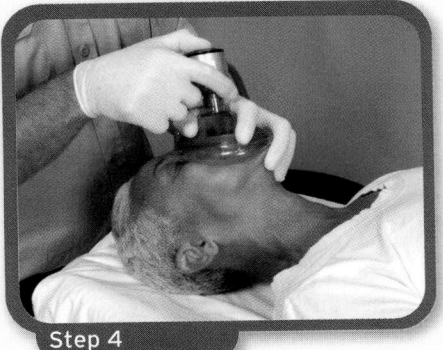

Step 4

Press the ventilation button until you achieve visible chest rise.

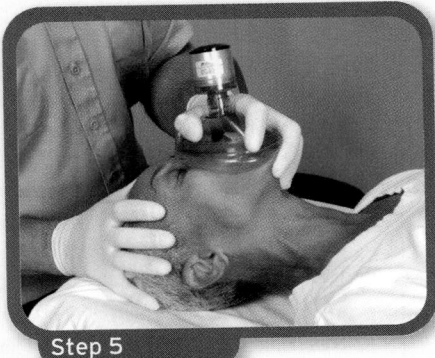

Step 5

Allow the patient to exhale passively.

The steps for administering supplemental oxygen to a spontaneously breathing patient with the FROPVD are listed here and shown in (Skill Drill 11-22 ▸).

1. Prepare your equipment by attaching the appropriate-sized mask to the FROPVD and ensuring that it is connected to an oxygen source (Step 1).

2. Whenever possible, have the patient hold the mask to his or her own face to maintain a good seal (Step 2).

3. When the patient inhales, the negative pressure created will trigger the valve within the FROPVD and deliver 100% oxygen (Step 3).

Automatic Transport Ventilators

The automatic transport ventilator (ATV) is basically a FROPVD attached to a control box in which the variables of ventilation—tidal volume and respiratory rate—can be set, thus allowing accurate regulation of a patient's minute volume (Figure 11-37 ▸). The ATV is used for intubated patients who need extended periods of ventilation.

Most ATVs are small and compact. The mechanical simplicity, durability, and portability of the ATV make it a valuable prehospital ventilation device. It frees up your hands to tend to other non-airway-related tasks.

The respiratory rate on the ATV is usually set at the midpoint or average for the patient's age. Tidal volume is usually set between 6 and 7 mL/kg, but can be adjusted based on the patient's chest rise and clinical response.

Like the FROPVD, the ATV is dependent on an oxygen source. It also has a pressure relief valve, which can lead to unrecognized hypoventilation in patients with poor lung compliance (eg, COPD, CHF), increased airway resistance (eg, asthma), or airway obstruction. (Table 11-10 ▸) describes the steps for using an ATV.

Continuous Positive Airway Pressure

Continuous positive airway pressure (CPAP) delivers positive pressure to the airways of a spontaneously breathing patient during the respiratory cycle. With CPAP, the patient exhales

Skill Drill 11-22: Flow-Restricted, Oxygen-Powered Ventilation Device for Conscious, Spontaneously Breathing Patients

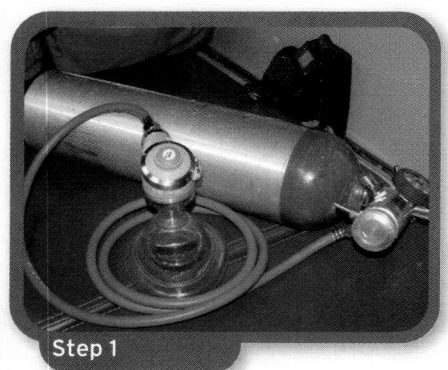

Step 1

Prepare your equipment.

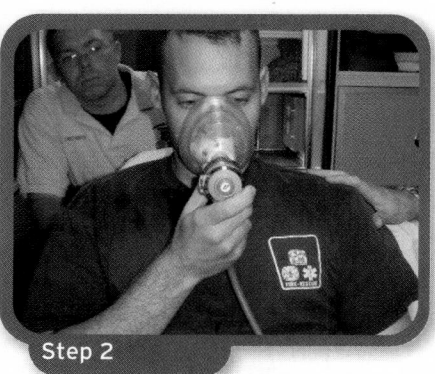

Step 2

Whenever possible, have the patient hold the mask to his or her own face to maintain a good seal.

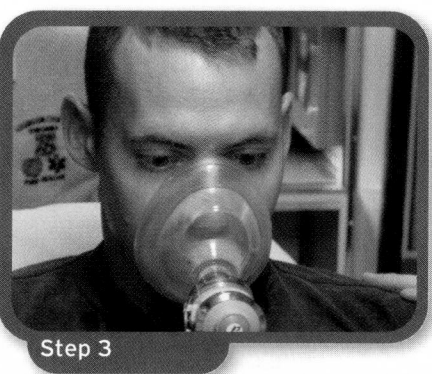

Step 3

When the patient inhales, the negative pressure created will trigger the valve within the FROPVD and deliver 100% oxygen.

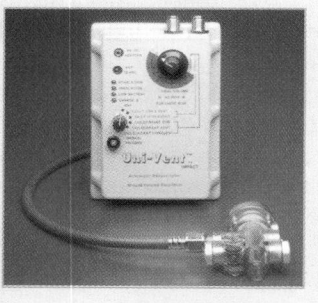

Figure 11-37 Automatic transport ventilator.

against positive pressure (positive end-expiratory pressure [PEEP]); this prevents atelectasis, forces fluid from the alveoli, and improves pulmonary respiration. CPAP is an effective treatment for patients with pulmonary edema (ie, CHF), and has been shown to reduce the need for intubation when used in conjunction with drug therapy. CPAP has also proven useful for patients with acute bronchospasm (ie, asthma) and obstructive lung disease.

CPAP is delivered through a tight-fitting face mask that is attached to an oxygen source; the amount of PEEP can be adjusted between 2.5 and 10 cm H_2O. Patient anxiety is common during initial CPAP therapy; coaching and reassurance are often needed to facilitate compliance. After applying the CPAP device, observe for signs of clinical improvement, which include decreased work of breathing, increased ease in speaking, decreases in respiratory and heart rate, and increased SaO_2.

Table 11-10	Ventilating a Patient With an Automatic Transport Ventilator

1. Attach the ATV to the wall-mounted oxygen source.
2. Set the tidal volume and ventilatory rate on the ATV as appropriate for the patient's age and clinical condition.
3. Connect the ATV to the 15/22-mm fitting on the ET tube.
4. Auscultate the patient's breath sounds and observe for chest rise to ensure adequate ventilation.

Special Considerations

Artificial Ventilation of the Pediatric Patient

The flat nasal bridge of the pediatric patient makes achieving an effective mask-to-face seal more difficult in children than in adults. Furthermore, compressing the mask against the face to improve mask seal may result in obstruction. The best mask seal is achieved by the two-person bag-mask ventilation technique with jaw displacement, although current standards support either the one- or two-rescuer technique.

A pediatric bag-mask device with a minimum tidal volume of 450 mL should be used for full-term neonates and infants. In children (1 year of age to the onset of puberty [12 to 14 years of age]), consider the size of the child when determining bag size. An adult bag with a 1,500-mL volume may be used, but a pediatric bag-mask is preferred. Children older than 12 to 14 years of age require the adult-sized bag-mask for adequate ventilation. Choose a size to ensure a proper mask fit. The mask should reach from the bridge of the nose to the cleft of the chin. A length-based resuscitation tape may also be used to determine the most appropriate-sized bag-mask device for pediatric patients who weigh up to 75 lb (34 kg).

When you are ventilating a pediatric patient, ensure that there is a proper mask seal by using the EC-clamp technique 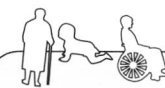. Place the mask over the mouth and nose, avoiding compression of the eyes. With one hand, place your thumb on the mask at the apex (over the nose) and your index finger on the mask at the chin to form a "C." With gentle pressure, push down on the mask to establish an adequate seal. Maintain the airway by lifting the bony prominence of the chin with your remaining fingers, forming an "E." Avoid placing pressure on the soft area under the chin, as this may cause an airway obstruction.

(continued on next page)

(continued)

Say, "Squeeze," as you compress the bag as a guide for squeezing. Provide just enough volume to initiate chest rise. Do not overinflate. Obtain adequate chest rise with each ventilation. Pause to allow adequate time for exhalation. Begin releasing the bag and say, "Release, release," to allow time for air to escape. Continue ventilations using the "squeeze, release, release" method.

During ventilation, look for adequate chest rise. Listen for bilateral lung sounds at the third intercostal space on the midaxillary line. Also assess the patient for improvement in skin color and heart rate.

If needed, apply cricoid pressure to minimize gastric distention and passive regurgitation. Locate the cricoid ring by palpating the trachea for a prominent horizontal band inferior to the thyroid cartilage and the cricothyroid membrane. Apply gentle downward pressure using one fingertip in infants and the thumb and index finger in children. Avoid excessive pressure, as it may cause tracheal compression and obstruction in infants.

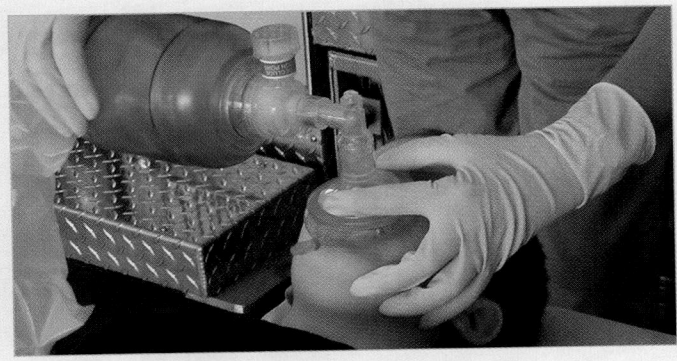

Figure 11-38 The EC-clamp technique will facilitate proper hand placement to maintain a good mask-to-face seal.

Cricoid Pressure (Sellick Maneuver)

When ventilating any patient who is not intubated, you must be alert for gastric distention. This problem can be partially prevented or alleviated by using the Sellick maneuver, also called cricoid pressure. When performed properly, this noninvasive procedure can also help prevent passive regurgitation with aspiration during positive-pressure ventilation.

When you apply posterior pressure to the cricoid cartilage, the esophagus is partially occluded between the cricoid ring and the cervical vertebrae, providing more air delivery into the lungs and less air delivery into the stomach Figure 11-39 ▶. Cricoid pressure is indicated only in unconscious patients who cannot protect their own airway and are at imminent risk for vomiting (or if vomiting is occurring). This technique can also be used during endotracheal intubation to move the larynx posteriorly and facilitate an adequate view of the vocal cords.

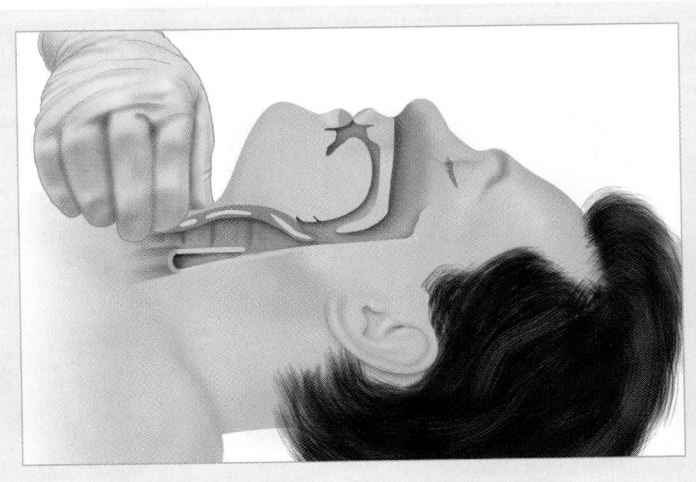

Figure 11-39 Cricoid pressure, or the Sellick maneuver.

Disadvantages of this technique include extreme or a large quantity of emesis if pressure is removed; therefore, cricoid pressure should be maintained until the patient is intubated. In addition, the procedure requires two rescuers or providers. If a cervical spine injury is present, cricoid pressure may cause further injury, so this technique is contraindicated in these patients. Potential complications associated with cricoid pressure include trauma to the larynx if excessive force is used, esophageal rupture from unrelieved high gastric pressures, and obstruction of the trachea when the technique is used in small children.

The steps for performing cricoid pressure are listed here and shown in Skill Drill 11-23 ▶.

1. Visualize the cricoid cartilage Step 1.
2. Palpate the cricoid cartilage to confirm its location—inferior to the thyroid cartilage Step 2.
3. Apply firm pressure on the cricoid ring with your thumb and index finger on either side of the midline. Maintain pressure until the patient is intubated Step 3.

Gastric Distention

Any form of artificial ventilation that blows air into the patient's mouth—as opposed to blowing air directly into the trachea via an endotracheal tube—may lead to inflation of the patient's stomach with air. Gastric distention is especially likely to occur when excessive pressure is used to inflate the lungs, when ventilations are performed too fast, or when the airway is partially obstructed during ventilation attempts. The pressure in the airway forces open the esophagus, and air flows into the stomach. Gastric distention occurs most often in children but is common in adults as well.

A distended stomach is harmful to the patient for at least two reasons. First, it promotes regurgitation of stomach contents, and vomitus creeping up the back of the throat rapidly finds its way into the patient's lungs (aspiration). Second, a distended stomach pushes the diaphragm upward into the chest, reducing the amount of space in which the lungs can expand.

Skill Drill 11-23: Cricoid Pressure (Sellick Maneuver)

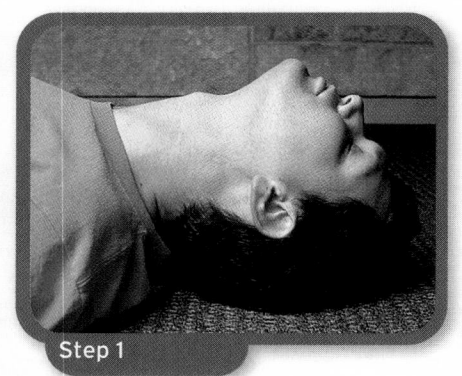

Step 1

Visualize the cricoid cartilage.

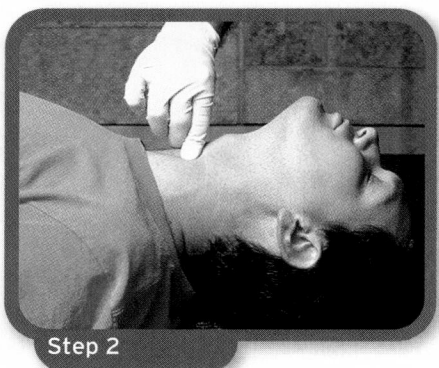

Step 2

Palpate to confirm its location.

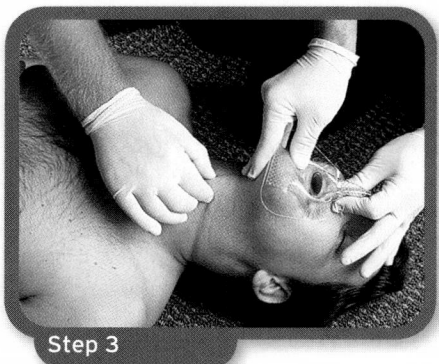

Step 3

Apply firm pressure with your thumb and index finger on either side of the midline.

Signs of gastric distention include an increase in the diameter of the stomach, an increasingly distended abdomen, and increased resistance to bag-mask ventilations. If these signs are noted, you should reassess and reposition the airway as needed, apply cricoid pressure, and observe the chest for adequate rise and fall as you continue ventilating. In addition, limit ventilation times to 1 second or the time needed to produce adequate chest rise.

Invasive Gastric Decompression

Invasive gastric decompression involves inserting a gastric tube into the stomach and then removing the contents with suction. The gastric tube is a very effective tool for removing air and liquid from the stomach, as it decreases the pressure on the diaphragm and virtually eliminates the risk of regurgitation and aspiration.

The gastric tube can be inserted into the stomach through the mouth (orogastric [OG] tube) or through the nose (nasogastric [NG] tube). It should be considered for any patient who will need positive-pressure ventilation for an extended period of time, especially if he or she is not intubated. An NG or OG tube should also be inserted when gastric distention interferes with ventilations—for example, when children are receiving positive-pressure ventilation or have swallowed large volumes of air secondary to increased work of breathing.

NG and OG tubes must be used with extreme caution in any patient with known esophageal disease (eg, tumors or varices). They should never be used in a patient whose esophagus is not patent. After insertion, make sure that the tube has been placed into the stomach. Occasionally it may remain in the esophagus without actually entering the stomach (supragastric placement) or may have been inadvertently placed into the trachea.

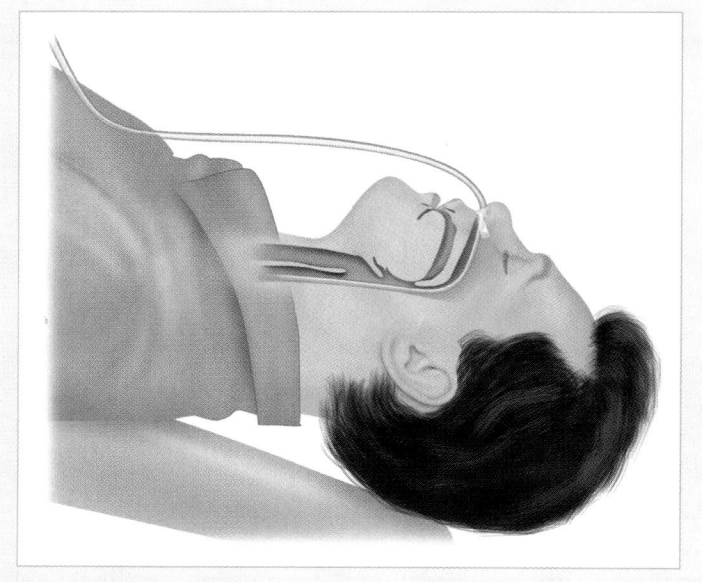

Figure 11-40 Nasogastric tube.

Nasogastric Tube

An NG tube is inserted through the nose, into the nasopharynx, through the esophagus, and into the stomach **Figure 11-40 ▲**. In airway management and ventilation, it decompresses the stomach, thereby decreasing pressure on the diaphragm and limiting the risk of regurgitation. The NG tube is also used to perform gastric lavage—a procedure in which the stomach is decontaminated following a toxic ingestion.

The NG tube is relatively well tolerated, even by patients who are awake. Patients can still talk with an NG tube in place, and, after a few hours, most get used to it. For these reasons, the NG route of insertion is generally preferred for conscious patients.

During the insertion of an NG tube, most patients who are awake will gag and may vomit, even if their gag reflex is suppressed. In a patient with a decreased level of consciousness, vomiting can seriously threaten the airway.

Insertion of an NG tube in patients with severe facial injuries, particularly midface fractures and skull fractures, is contraindicated. In such patients, the NG tube may be inadvertently inserted through the fracture and into the cranial vault. For patients with these conditions, use the OG route of insertion.

Poor technique during NG tube insertion can cause trauma to the nasal passageways, esophagus, or gastric lining; therefore, you must use caution and be gentle when inserting the tube.

Use of the NG tube in patients who are not intubated interferes with the mask seal of the bag-mask device. If you cannot effectively ventilate a patient because of severe gastric distention, however, you must balance the benefit of gastric decompression against the risk of a poor mask seal and determine which has a higher priority. Of course, if the patient is unconscious and requires endotracheal intubation, you can easily pass the ET tube around the NG tube.

The steps of NG tube insertion are listed here and shown in **Skill Drill 11-24 ▶**.

1. Explain the procedure to the patient, and oxygenate him or her, if necessary and possible. Ensure that the patient's head is in a neutral position. Suppress the gag reflex with a topical anesthetic spray (Step 1).
2. Constrict the blood vessels in the nares with a topical alpha agonist (Step 2).
3. Measure the tube for the correct depth of insertion (nose to ear to xiphoid process) (Step 3).
4. Lubricate the tube with a water-soluble gel (Step 4).
5. Advance the tube gently along the nasal floor (Step 5).
6. Encourage the patient to swallow or drink to facilitate passage of the tube into the esophagus (Step 6).
7. Advance the tube into the stomach (Step 7).
8. Confirm proper placement: auscultate over the epigastrium while injecting 30 to 50 mL of air into the tube and/or observe for gastric contents in the tube (Step 8).
9. Apply suction to the tube to aspirate the stomach contents, and secure the tube in place (Step 9).

Orogastric Tube

An OG tube serves the same purpose as an NG tube but is inserted through the mouth instead of the nose **Figure 11-41 ▶**. The advantages and disadvantages of the OG tube are essentially the same as they are for the NG tube. The major differences are that the OG tube carries no risk of nasal bleeding and is safer in patients with severe facial trauma. Additionally, you can use larger tubes, which is helpful if the patient requires aggressive gastric lavage.

The OG tube, however, is less comfortable for conscious patients, causing gagging much more often, and increases the

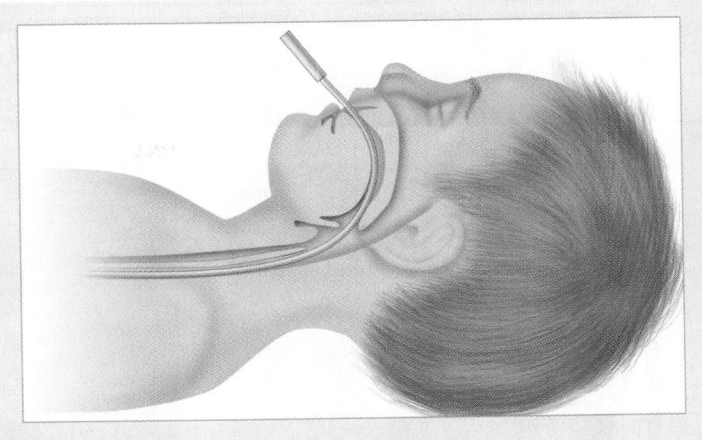

Figure 11-41 Orogastric tube.

possibility of vomiting. Conscious patients also tend to bite the tube as it is passed orally.

The OG route is generally preferred for patients who are unconscious without a gag reflex. Because these patients need aggressive airway management, the OG tube is almost always inserted *after* the patient's airway is protected with an ET tube; insertion of the OG tube before intubating the patient may obscure your view of the vocal cords.

The steps of OG tube insertion are listed here and shown in **Skill Drill 11-25 ▶**.

1. Position the patient's head in a neutral or flexed position (Step 1).
2. Measure the tube for the correct depth of insertion (mouth to ear to xiphoid process) (Step 2).
3. Lubricate the tube with a water-soluble gel (Step 3).
4. Introduce the tube at the midline, and advance it gently into the oropharynx (Step 4).
5. Advance the tube into the stomach (Step 5).
6. Confirm proper placement: Auscultate over the epigastrium while injecting 30 to 50 mL of air and/or observe for gastric contents in the tube. There should be no reflux around the tube (Step 6).
7. Apply suction to the tube to aspirate the stomach contents, and secure the tube in place (Step 7).

Advanced Airway Management

One of the most common mistakes in the situation of respiratory or cardiac arrest is to proceed with advanced airway management too early, forsaking the basic techniques of establishing and maintaining a patent airway in a patient who is already hypoxemic. *Never abandon the basics of airway management and immediately proceed with advanced techniques simply because you can!*

Endotracheal Intubation

Endotracheal intubation is defined as passing an endotracheal (ET) tube through the glottic opening and sealing the tube

Skill Drill 11-24: Nasogastric Tube Insertion in a Conscious Patient

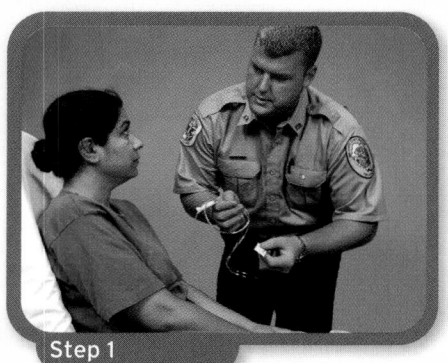

Step 1

Explain the procedure to the patient, and oxygenate the patient if necessary. Ensure that the patient's head is in a neutral position and suppress the gag reflex with a topical anesthetic spray.

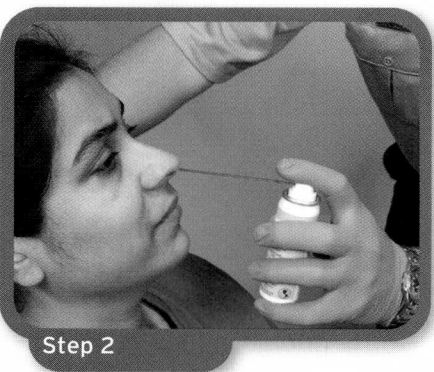

Step 2

Constrict the blood vessels in the nares with a topical alpha agonist.

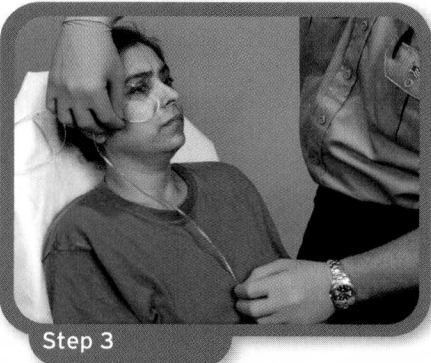

Step 3

Measure the tube for the correct depth of insertion (nose to ear to xiphoid process).

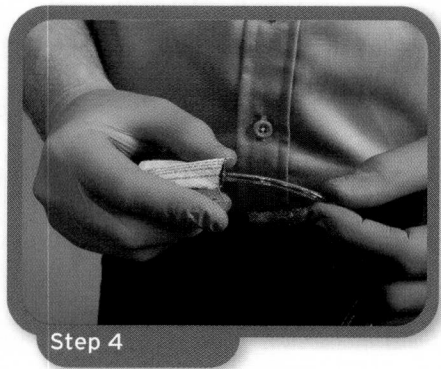

Step 4

Lubricate the tube with a water-soluble gel.

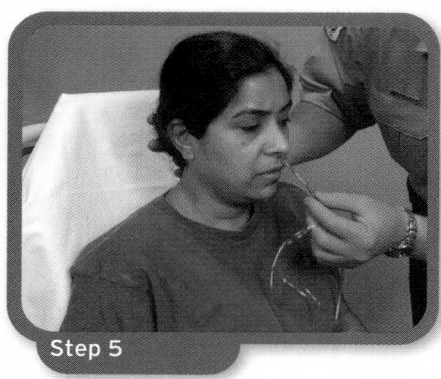

Step 5

Advance the tube gently along the nasal floor.

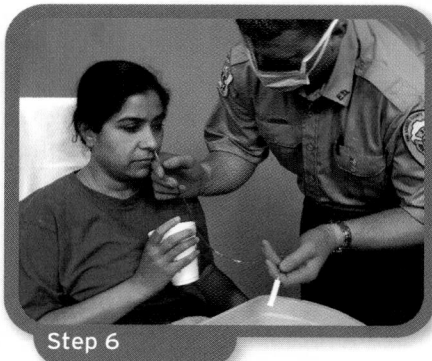

Step 6

Encourage the patient to swallow or drink to facilitate passage of the tube.

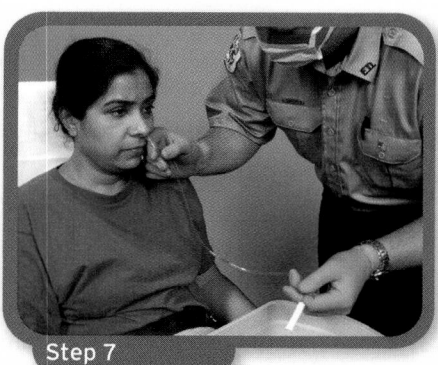

Step 7

Advance the tube into the stomach.

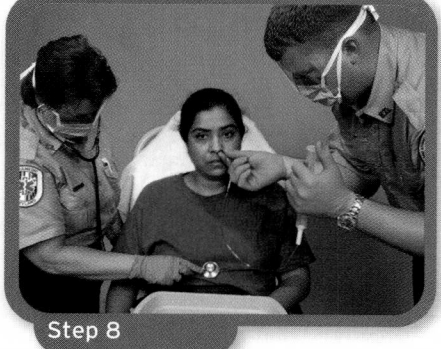

Step 8

Confirm proper placement: auscultate over the epigastrium while injecting 30 to 50 mL of air and/or observe for gastric contents in the tube. There should be no reflux around the tube.

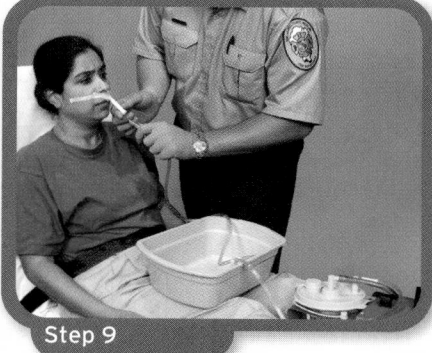

Step 9

Apply suction to the tube to aspirate the gastric contents, and secure the tube in place.

Skill Drill 11-25: Orogastric Tube Insertion

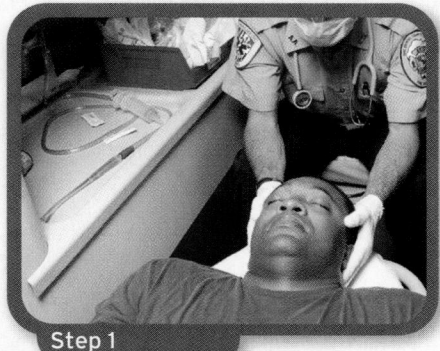

Step 1

Position the patient's head in a neutral or flexed position.

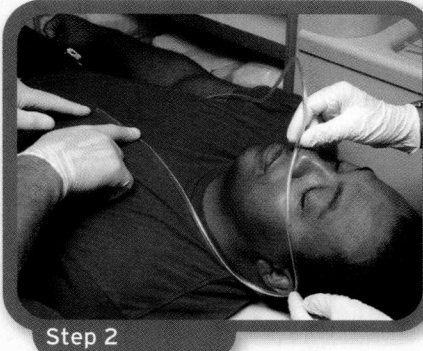

Step 2

Measure the tube for the correct depth of insertion (mouth to ear to xiphoid process).

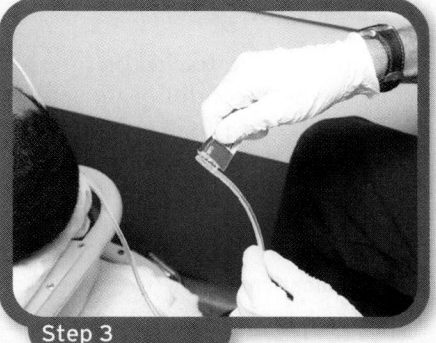

Step 3

Lubricate the tube with a water-soluble gel.

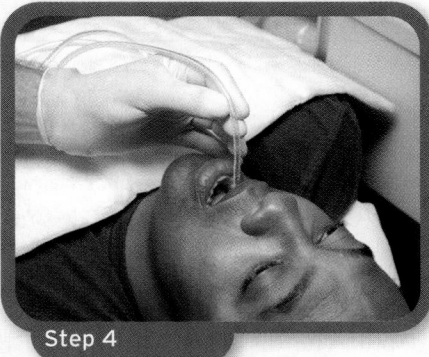

Step 4

Introduce the tube at the midline, and advance it gently into the oropharynx.

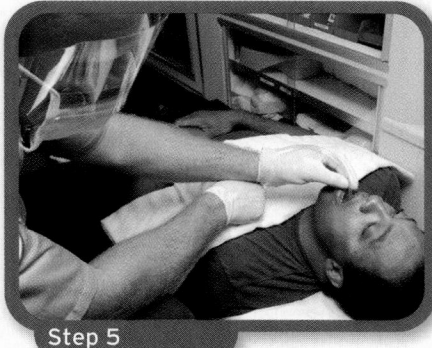

Step 5

Advance the tube into the stomach.

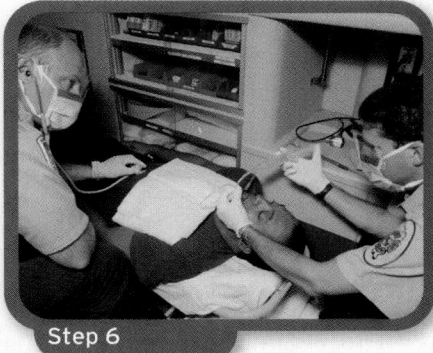

Step 6

Confirm proper placement: auscultate over the epigastrium while injecting 30 to 50 mL of air and/or observe for gastric contents in the tube. There should be no reflux around the tube.

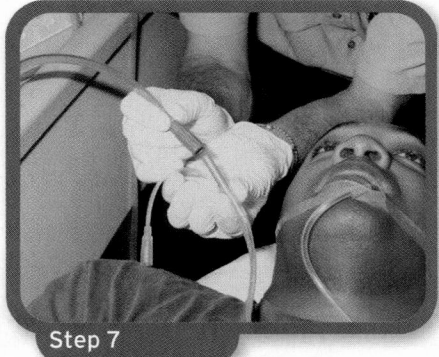

Step 7

Apply suction to the tube to aspirate the stomach contents, and secure the tube in place.

with a cuff inflated against the tracheal wall. When the tube is passed into the trachea through the mouth, the procedure is called <u>orotracheal intubation</u>. When the tube is passed into the trachea through the nose, the procedure is called <u>nasotracheal intubation</u>.

Intubation of the trachea is the *most* definitive means of achieving complete control of the airway. A solid understanding of the basics of this technique is needed when making urgent decisions about when to intubate a patient. Following are considerations when performing endotracheal intubation:

- **Indications.** Present or impending respiratory failure, apnea, inability of the patient to protect own airway.
- **Contraindications.** None in emergency situations. However with inexperienced personnel, other advanced airways (eg, Combitube or LMA) may be easier and equivalent.
- **Advantages.** Provides a secure airway, protects against aspiration, provides an alternate route to IV/IO for certain medications (as a last resort).
- **Disadvantages.** Requires special equipment, bypasses physiologic functions of the upper airway (warming, filtering, humidifying).
- **Complications.** Bleeding, hypoxia, laryngeal swelling, laryngospasm, vocal cord damage, mucosal necrosis, barotrauma.

The basic structure of an <u>endotracheal (ET) tube</u> **Figure 11-42 ▶** 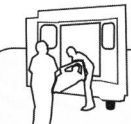 includes the proximal end, the tube itself, the cuff and pilot balloon, and the distal tip. The proximal end is equipped with a standard 15/22-mm adapter that allows it to be attached to any ventilation device. It also includes an inflation port with a pilot balloon; the distal cuff is inflated with a syringe attached to the inflation port, which has a one-way valve. The pilot balloon indicates whether the distal cuff is inflated or deflated once the tube has been inserted into the mouth.

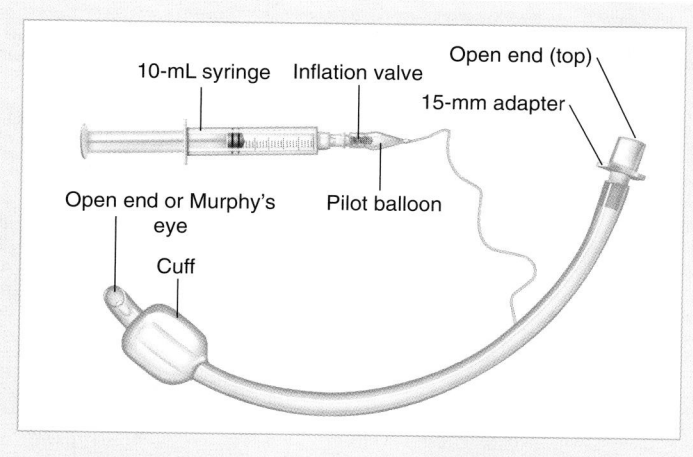

Figure 11-42 Endotracheal tube.

In the Field

Perform ventilations with a bag-mask device and 100% oxygen for *at least 2 to 3 minutes* prior to attempting intubation. The patient needs an oxygen reserve to tolerate the period of time without ventilation that will occur during insertion of an advanced airway. You also need the time to check your equipment properly.

Centimeter markings along the length of the tube provide a measurement of its depth. The distal end of the tube has a beveled tip to facilitate insertion and an opening on the side called <u>Murphy's eye</u>, which enables ventilation to occur even if the tip becomes occluded by blood, mucus, or the tracheal wall.

Endotracheal tubes range in size from 2.5 to 9.0 mm inside diameter, and their length ranges from 12 to 32 cm

You are the Provider Part 7

One of the fire fighters drives your ambulance to the hospital so that your partner can assist you with bag-mask ventilation using 100% oxygen en route to the hospital. You find that you are having difficulty maintaining an adequate mask-to-face seal with the bag-mask device; the patient looks worse. You tell the fire fighter to stop the ambulance so that you and your partner can safely assess and treat the problem. Reassessment of the patient reveals the following:

Reassessment	Recording Time: 16 Minutes
Level of consciousness	U (Unresponsive)
Respirations	30 breaths/min and shallow (baseline); you are having difficulty maintaining an adequate mask-to-face seal with the bag-mask device
Pulse	160 beats/min, regular and weak
Skin	Severe facial cyanosis
Blood pressure	98/58 mm Hg
Sao_2	83% while receiving assisted ventilations with a bag-mask device and 100% oxygen

11. What are the signs of inadequate artificial ventilation?

12. What management is required to prevent further deterioration of this patient's condition?

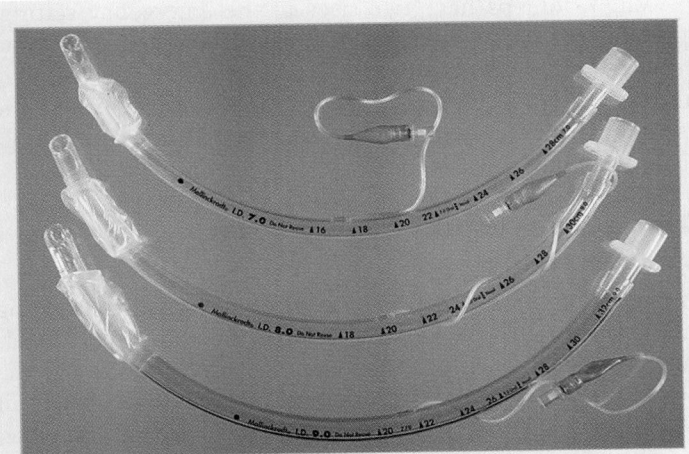

Figure 11-43 Endotracheal tubes are available in a variety of sizes.

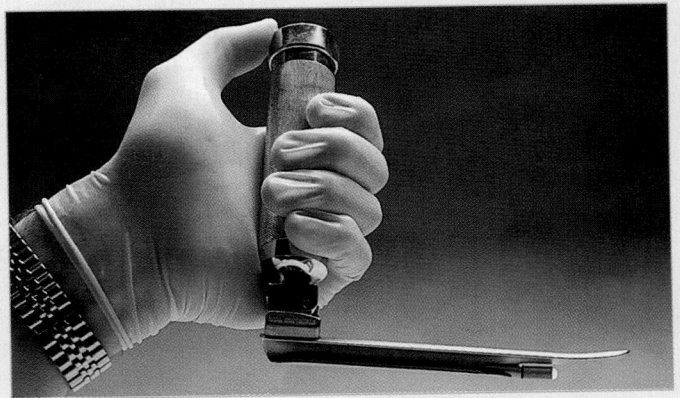

Figure 11-44 A laryngoscope with a straight blade.

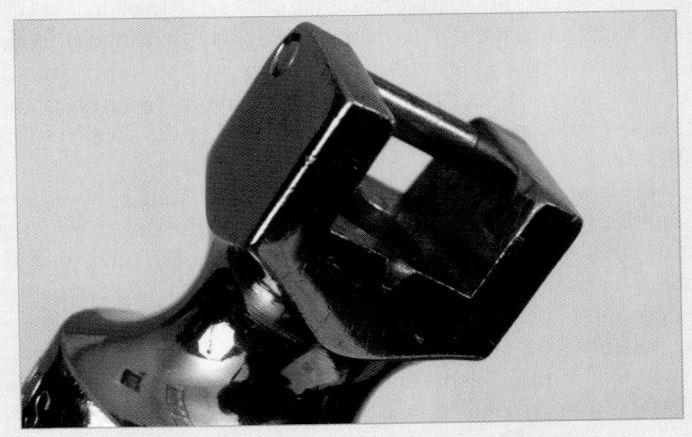

Figure 11-45 The laryngoscope's handle has a bar designed to connect with a notch on the blade.

Figure 11-43 ▲ . Sizes ranging from 5.0 to 9.0 mm are equipped with a distal cuff that, when inflated, makes an airtight seal with the tracheal wall. A tube that is too small for the patient will lead to an increased resistance to airflow and difficulty in ventilating. A tube that is too large can be difficult to insert and may cause trauma. Normally, an adult female will require a 7.0- to 8.0-mm tube, while an adult male will require a 7.5- to 8.5-mm tube.

ET tubes ranging from 2.5 to 4.5 mm are used in pediatric patients. In children the funnel-shaped cricoid ring (the narrowest portion of the pediatric airway) forms an anatomic seal with the ET tube, eliminating the need for a distal cuff in most cases. There are limited situations where a cuffed pediatric tube may be used in the hospital setting. The proximal end of the tube still has a 15/22-mm adapter for use with standard ventilation devices, and the distal end has a beveled tip with distal end markings. However, because it lacks a balloon cuff, there is no pilot balloon.

A number of anatomic clues can help determine the proper size of ET tube for adults and children. The internal diameter of the nostril is a good approximation of the diameter of the glottic opening. The diameter of the little finger or the size of the thumbnail is also a good approximation of airway size. Because all attempts to predict the tube size required for a given patient are estimates, however, you should always have *three* ET tubes ready: one tube of the size you *think* will be appropriate, one a size larger, and one a size smaller.

The laryngoscope and blade are required to perform orotracheal intubation by direct laryngoscopy—a procedure in which the vocal cords are directly visualized for placement of the ET tube. The laryngoscope consists of a handle and interchangeable blades Figure 11-44 ▶ . The handle contains the power source for the light on the laryngoscope blade. Most laryngoscopes run on batteries, but some are rechargeable. The handle has a bar designed to connect with a notch on the blade Figure 11-45 ▶ . When the blade is moved into the perpendi-

cular position, the bright light shines near the tip of the blade.

The two most common types of laryngoscope blades are the straight (Miller) blade and the curved (Macintosh) blade. The straight laryngoscope blade is designed so that its tip will extend beneath the epiglottis and lift it up Figure 11-46 ▶ —a particularly useful feature in infants and small children, who often have a long, floppy epiglottis that is difficult to elevate out of the way with a curved blade. In the adult, use of a straight blade requires great care; if used improperly and levered across

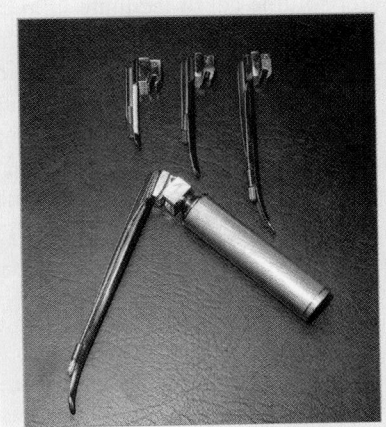

Figure 11-46 A straight (Miller) blade with three additional size blades shown.

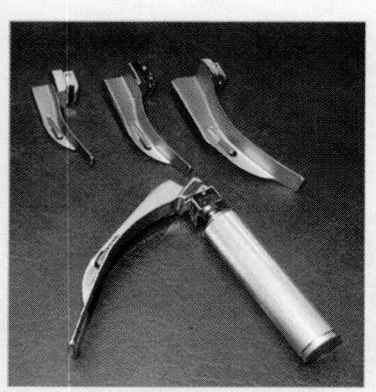

Figure 11-47 A laryngoscope and an assortment of curved (Macintosh) blades.

the upper jaw, the straight blade is more likely to damage the patient's teeth. The curved laryngoscope blade is less likely to be levered against the teeth by an inexperienced paramedic and is usually preferred by beginners Figure 11-47 ◀ . The direction of the curve conforms to that of the tongue and pharynx, so the blade follows the outline of the pharynx with relative ease. The tip of the curved blade is placed in the vallecula (the space between the epiglottis and the base of the tongue) rather than beneath the epiglottis; it indirectly lifts the epiglottis to expose the vocal cords. You should have *both* curved and straight blades readily available during an orotracheal intubation attempt.

Blade sizes range from 0 to 4. Sizes 0, 1, and 2 are appropriate for infants and children, whereas 3 and 4 are considered adult sizes. For pediatric patients, blade sizes are often recommended based on the child's age or height. Most paramedics choose the blade for adults based on experience and the size of the patient (3 for average-sized adults and 4 for larger persons).

It is common, especially in emergency situations, to be unable to obtain a full view of the glottic opening. The stylet, a semirigid wire that is inserted into the ET tube to mold and maintain the shape of the tube, enables you to guide the tip of the tube over the arytenoid cartilage, even if you cannot see the entire glottic opening. This device should be lubricated with a water-soluble gel to facilitate its removal, and its end should be bent to form a gentle "hockey stick" curve. The end of the stylet should rest at least ½″ back from the end of the ET tube; if the stylet protrudes beyond the end of the tube, it may damage the vocal cords and surrounding structures. Bend the other end of the stylet over the proximal tube connector, so that the stylet cannot slip farther into the tube.

Controversies

If you cannot obtain vascular access (eg, IV, IO), your protocol may allow you to administer certain resuscitative medications via the ET tube. This is a last resort.

These medications should be administered in a dose that is 2 to 2.5 times the standard IV/IO dose. The LEAN mnemonic will help you remember which drugs can be delivered via the ET route:

- Lidocaine
- Epinephrine
- Atropine
- Narcan

Magill forceps have two uses in the emergency setting. First, they are used to remove airway obstructions under direct visualization, as discussed earlier in this chapter. Second, they are used to guide the tip of the ET tube through the glottic opening if you are unable to get the proper angle with simple manipulation of the tube.

Orotracheal Intubation by Direct Laryngoscopy

Orotracheal intubation by direct laryngoscopy involves inserting an ET tube through the mouth and into the trachea while visualizing the glottic opening with a laryngoscope; it is by far the most common method of performing endotracheal intubation in the emergency setting. Following are some considerations when performing orotracheal intubation by direct laryngoscopy:

- **Indications.** Apnea, hypoxia, poor respiratory effort, suppression or absence of a gag reflex.
- **Contraindications.** Caution in an unsuppressed gag reflex.
- **Advantages.** Direct visualization of anatomy and tube placement, ideal method for confirming placement, may be performed in breathing or apneic patients.
- **Disadvantages.** Requires special equipment.
- **Complications.** Dental trauma, laryngeal trauma, misplacement (right main stem bronchus, esophagus).

Table 11-11 ▶ summarizes the equipment and preparation required prior to performing orotracheal intubation. Make a copy of this table and tack it to your intubation kit, so that you can check the kit systematically at the beginning of every shift.

Body Substance Isolation

Intubation may expose you to blood or other body fluids, so take proper precautions when performing this procedure. In addition to gloves, wear a mask that covers your *entire* face, which will be relatively close to the patient's mouth and nose, and that will protect you if the patient vomits or coughs during intubation.

Preoxygenation

Adequate preoxygenation with a bag-mask device and 100% oxygen is a critical step prior to intubating a patient. You should mildly hyperoxygenate (approximately 24 breaths/min) the apneic or hypoventilating patient for 2 to 3 minutes. During the intubation attempt, the patient will undergo a period of forced apnea when he or she will not be ventilated. The goal of preoxygenation is to prevent hypoxia from occurring during this time. Unfortunately, you will be unable to perform an extensive preintubation evaluation of the patient (eg, obtaining hemoglobin and hematocrit levels), and patients who are intubated in the prehospital setting are usually physiologically unstable.

You should monitor the patient's Sao_2 and achieve as close to 100% saturation as possible during the 2- to 3-minute period of preoxygenation. During the intubation attempt itself, you must continually monitor the Sao_2. Do not let it fall below 95%.

The consequences of even brief periods of hypoxia can be disastrous. Do not rely solely on pulse oximetry to quantify a patient's oxygenation status; it can produce falsely high

Table 11-11	Preparing Equipment for Intubation
Equipment	**What to Check, Prepare, and Assemble**
Ventilation equipment	Have an assistant ventilate the patient while you are assembling, checking, and preparing your equipment. Ensure that the patient is being ventilated with 100% oxygen and that the pulse oximeter reading is greater than 95%.
Endotracheal tube	Select the proper size ET tube (7.0- to 8.0-mm for an adult female; 7.5- to 8.5-mm for an adult male). Inject 10 mL of air into the cuff, and ensure that the cuff holds air. Confirm that the 15/22-mm adapter is firmly inserted into the tube. Insert the stylet, and ensure that the tip is proximal to Murphy's eye. Bend the tube/stylet into a "hockey stick" configuration. Increase the angle of the bend if you anticipate a difficult intubation.
Laryngoscope and blades	It is best to have an assortment of blades available because some patients are easier to intubate with one than with another. Confirm the blade that you plan to use is free of any nicks (which could easily cause soft-tissue trauma). Check the bulb to ensure that the light is "bright, white, steady, and tight." The light should be bright enough so that it is uncomfortable to look at directly. It should be white, not yellow or dim. The light should not flicker, especially as the blade is moved on the handle. Most important, the bulb must be tightly screwed into the blade to prevent it from being aspirated into the airway.
Towels	Towels are needed to position the patient's head.
Suction	Suction may be needed to clear the airway of secretions to obtain an adequate laryngoscopic view of the glottic opening.
Magill forceps	Have Magill forceps available should you need to guide the ET tube into the trachea or if you encounter a foreign body obstruction during laryngoscopy.
Confirmation devices	Stethoscope and an end-tidal carbon dioxide (ET_{CO_2}) detector or an esophageal detector device (EDD).
ET tube securing device	Have the appropriate device readily available to secure the tube (eg, tape or a commercial ET tube securing device).

In the Field

Ideally, the patient should have an Sa_{O_2} of 100% (or as close to it as possible) prior to the intubation attempt. If you are unable to obtain an Sa_{O_2} reading, however, you should moderately hyperoxygenate (24 breaths/min) the patient for at least 2 minutes before attempting to intubate. If you are attempting to preoxygenate the patient, and the Sa_{O_2} continues to drop despite your best efforts at manual airway management and ventilation, it is best to proceed with intubation without delay.

In the Field

If the patient has experienced a possible neck injury, his or her head must be placed in a neutral in-line position. *Do not use the sniffing position or extend the patient's head in any way.* Intubation of the trauma patient is most effectively performed by two paramedics.

readings, even if the patient is severely hypoxic. Although some sequelae of hypoxia are dramatic and occur immediately, most are subtle and occur gradually. Clearly, some of the poor neurologic outcomes following aggressive airway management result from intubation-induced hypoxia.

Positioning the Patient

Successful laryngoscopy will be extremely difficult—if not impossible—to perform without proper positioning of the patient's head. The airway has three axes: the mouth, the pharynx, and the larynx. When the head is in a neutral position, these axes are at acute angles, facilitating entry of food into the esophagus rather than into the trachea Figure 11-48A . Although this positioning is advantageous to the conscious, spontaneously breathing patient, the angles of these axes make laryngoscopy difficult.

To facilitate visualization of the airway, the three axes must be aligned to the greatest extent possible. This is most effec-

tively achieved by placing the patient in the "sniffing" position (the position of the head when intentionally sniffing). The position involves approximately a 20° extension of the atlanto-occipital joint and a 30° flexion of the neck at C6 and C7 for patients with short necks and/or no chins, increasing the angle even further will help improve visualization. The Sellick maneuver further improves the ability to see the vocal cords 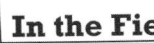 .

In most supine patients, the sniffing position can be achieved by extending the head and elevating the occiput 2.5 to 5 cm. Elevate the head and/or neck with folded towels until the ear is at the level of the sternum Figure 11-49 . When you are using towels, their thickness can easily be adjusted by changing the number of folds. With obese patients, padding under the head alone may not result in the sniffing position; you may need to add padding under the shoulders and neck as well. To determine whether the patient is in a true sniffing position, view the person from the side to evaluate the adequacy of his or her head position.

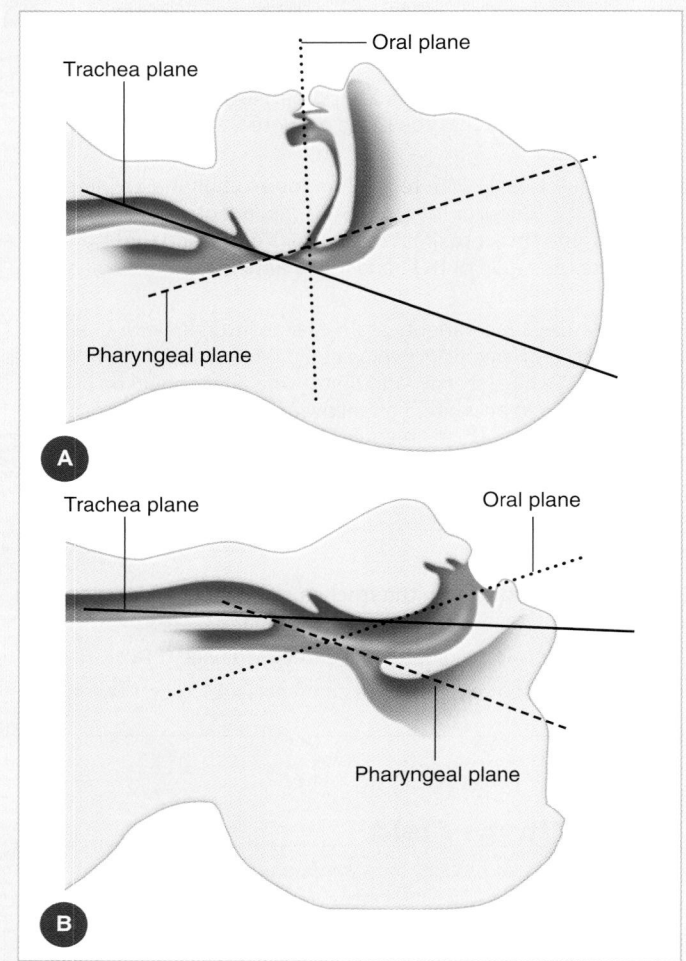

Figure 11-48 Three axes of the airway: oral, pharyngeal, and tracheal. **A.** Neutral position. **B.** Sniffing position.

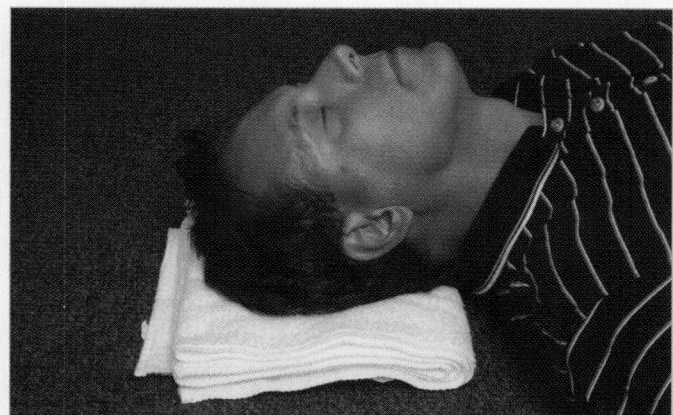

Figure 11-49 Head elevation is best achieved with folded towels positioned under the head.

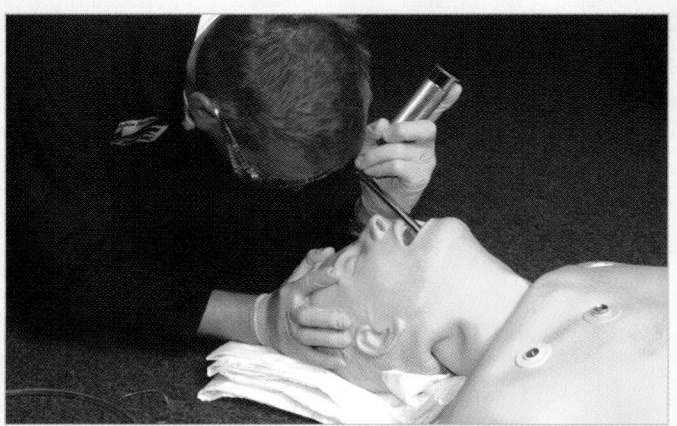

Figure 11-50 If the patient is on the floor or ground, you may need to kneel and lean forward or lie on the floor to get into the proper position.

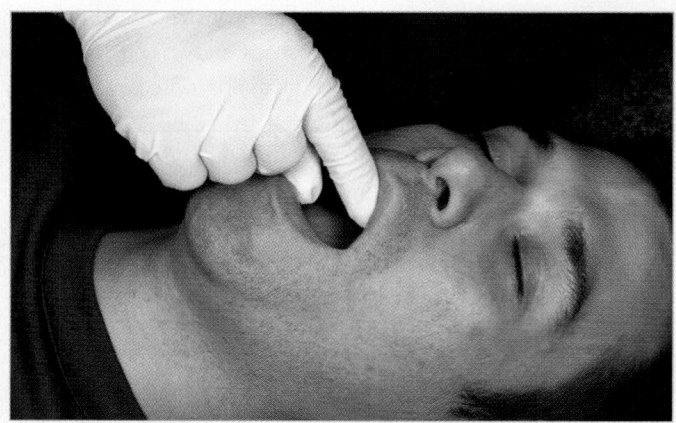

Figure 11-51 Place the side of your right-hand thumb just below the bottom lip and push the mouth open, or scissor your thumb and index finger between the molars.

Blade Insertion

After you have properly positioned the patient's head and provided preoxygenation, direct your partner to stop ventilating. Position yourself at the top of the patient's head. If the patient is on a stretcher, you can squat to put your head at the level of the patient's face. If the patient is on the floor or ground, you may need to kneel and lean forward or lie down to get into the proper position (Figure 11-50 ▲).

Grasp the laryngoscope with your left hand and hold it as low down on the handle as possible. If the patient's mouth is not open, place the side of your right-hand thumb just below the bottom lip and push the mouth open, or "scissor" your thumb and index finger between the molars (Figure 11-51 ▲).

Insert the blade into the *right* side of the patient's mouth. Use the flange of the blade to sweep the tongue gently to the left side of the mouth while moving the blade into the midline. Take care not to catch the patient's lips between the laryngoscope

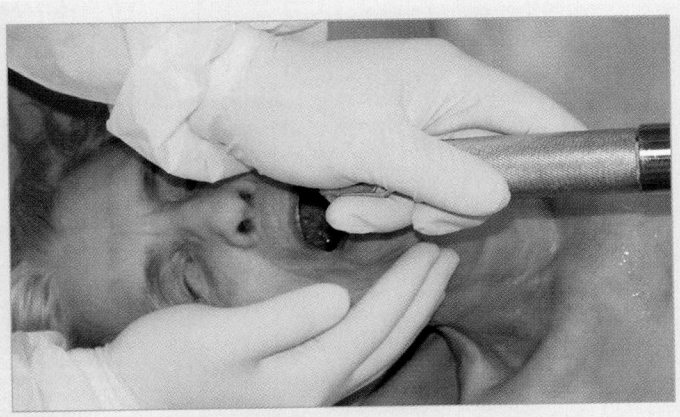

Figure 11-52 The tongue is a sticky, amorphous structure that can be a major hindrance to visualizing the airway. Proper use of the laryngoscope is critical to controlling the tongue.

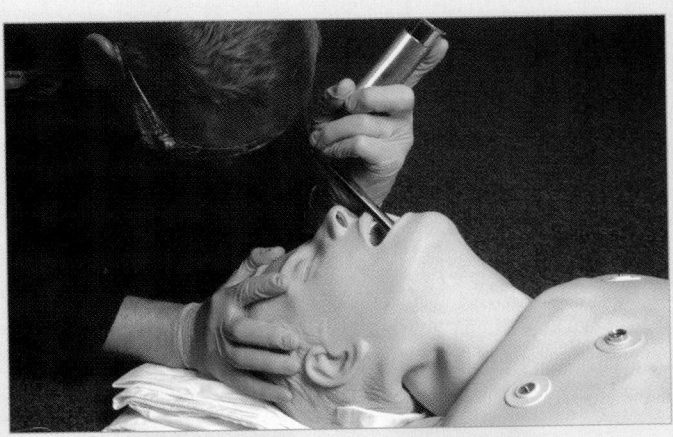

Figure 11-54 Keep your back and your left arm straight as you pull upward. This allows you to use the strength of your shoulders to lift the patient's jaw.

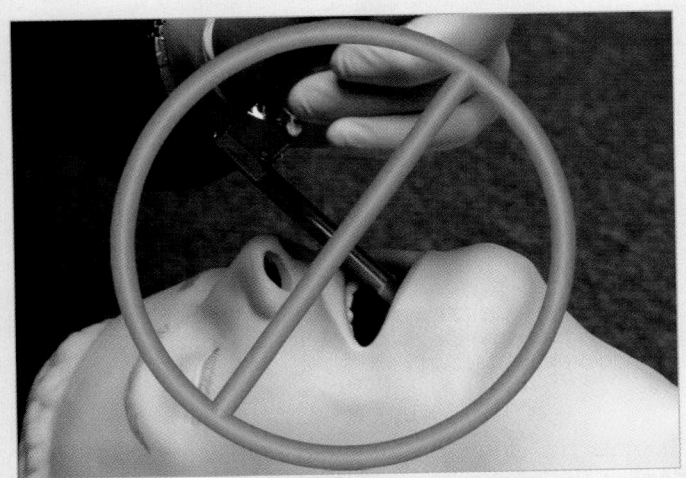

Figure 11-53 Prying against the upper teeth with the laryngoscope can result in breaking and potential aspiration of the teeth. Don't do it!

Visualization of the Glottic Opening

Continue lifting the laryngoscope as you look down the blade. You should see some familiar anatomic landmarks—the epiglottis or the arytenoid cartilage. Identifying these structures enables to you make small adjustments in the position of the blade to aid in visualization of the glottic opening.

With the curved blade, walk the blade down the tongue because you know that the vallecula and the epiglottis lie at the base of the tongue. With the straight blade, insert the blade straight back until the tip touches the posterior pharyngeal wall.

As you continue to work the tip of the blade into position (lifting the epiglottis with the straight blade or the vallecula with the curved blade), the glottic opening should come into full view. The vocal cords are the white fibrous bands that lie vertically within the glottic opening; they should be slightly open Figure 11-55 ▶ .

If you are having difficulty seeing the glottic opening, take your right hand and locate the lower third of the thyroid cartilage. By applying Backward, Upward, and Rightward Pressure (the BURP maneuver), you can often move the larynx into view

blade and the teeth. Moving the tongue from right to left is a critical step. If you simply insert the blade in the midline, the tongue will hang over both sides of the blade and all you will see is the tongue Figure 11-52 ▲ .

Slowly advance the blade—the curved blade into the vallecula or the straight blade beneath the epiglottis—while sweeping the tongue to the left. Exert *gentle* traction at a 45° angle to the floor as you lift the patient's jaw. *Do not "pry" back on the laryngoscope;* this will cause you to use the patient's upper teeth as a fulcrum, resulting in breaking and potential aspiration of teeth Figure 11-53 ▲ . Keeping your back and your left arm straight as you pull upward allows you to use the strength of your shoulders to lift the patient's jaw and decreases the likelihood of levering the laryngoscope blade against the patient's teeth Figure 11-54 ▶ . The correct motion is similar to holding a wine glass and offering a toast.

In the Field

Improving Your Laryngoscopic View: The Sellick Maneuver and the BURP Maneuver

When the angle of the pharynx and the larynx is particularly acute, it is often difficult to see the entire glottic opening. You can do two things to increase the percentage of the glottic opening that you can see: the Sellick maneuver or the BURP maneuver. The Sellick maneuver, which reduces the incidence of gastric distention during positive-pressure ventilation, also moves the larynx more posteriorly. If applied by an assistant during direct laryngoscopy, it reduces the acuity of the angle between the pharynx and larynx and can improve your laryngoscopic view.

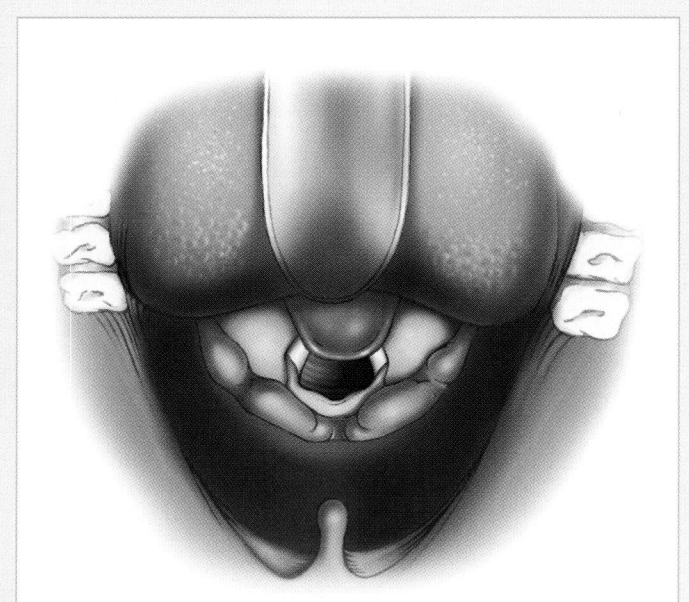

Figure 11-55 Laryngoscopic view of the vocal cords (white fibrous bands).

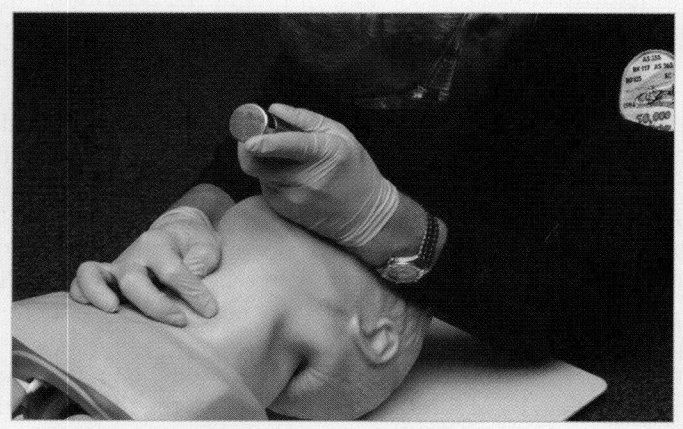

Figure 11-56 BURP maneuver.

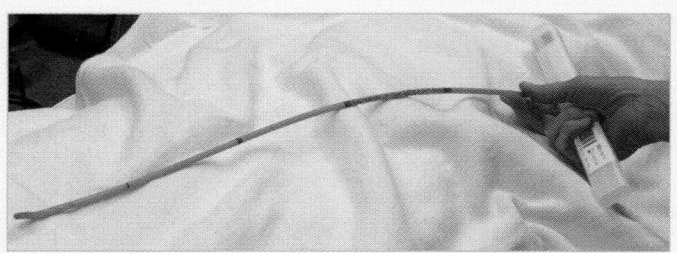

Figure 11-57 The gum bougie device.

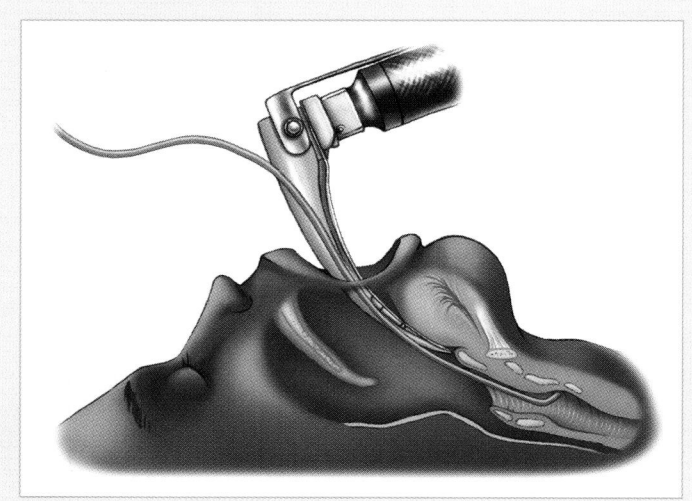

Figure 11-58 The angle at the distal tip of the gum bougie facilitates entry into the glottic opening and enables you to feel the ridges of the tracheal wall.

Figure 11-56 ▲ . Unfortunately, sometimes when you let go to pass the tube with your right hand, you will lose view of the vocal cords. If possible, have an assistant hold the larynx in position as you pass the tube. The BURP maneuver can also be applied to the cricoid ring or the hyoid bone.

The elastic gum bougie, also called the Eschmann stylet, is a flexible device that is approximately 1 cm in diameter and 60 cm long **Figure 11-57 ▶** . It can make intubation possible in some difficult situations, especially when your view of the glottic opening is limited. The gum bougie is rigid enough that it can be easily directed through the glottic opening, yet flexible enough that it does not cause damage to the tracheal walls.

The gum bougie is inserted through the glottic opening under direct laryngoscopy. The angle at its distal tip facilitates

entry into the glottic opening and enables you to "feel" the ridges of the tracheal wall **Figure 11-58 ▲** . Once the gum bougie is placed deeply into the trachea, it becomes a guide for the ET tube. Simply slide the tube over the gum bougie and into the trachea. Remove the gum bougie, ventilate, and confirm proper ET tube placement.

Tube Insertion
Once you have visualized the glottic opening, pick up the preselected endotracheal tube in your right hand, holding it near the connector as you would hold a pencil. Under direct vision, insert the tube from the right corner of the patient's mouth through the vocal cords. Continue to insert the tube until the proximal end of the cuff is 1 to 2 cm past the vocal cords. *You must see the tip of the ET tube pass through the vocal cords. If you cannot see the vocal cords, do not insert the tube!* An ET tube shoved blindly down the throat will often come to rest in the esophagus, not in the trachea; the only way to be certain that the tube has passed through the vocal cords is to *see* it pass through the vocal cords. If you take your eye off the tip of the tube (and the vocal cords), even for a second, you significantly increase the likelihood of allowing the tube to slip into the esophagus.

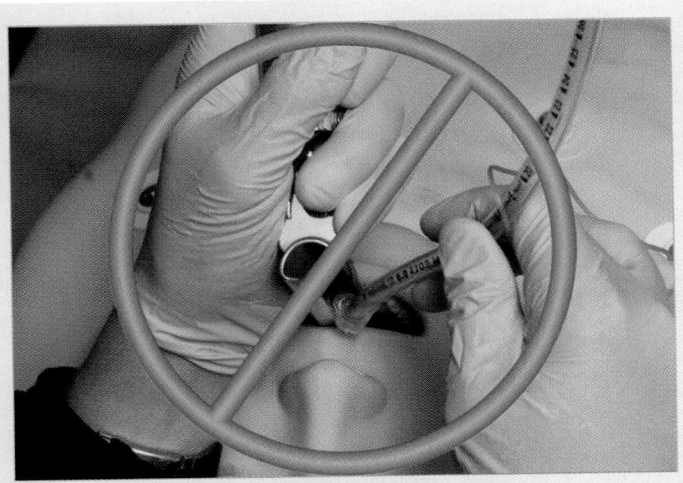

Figure 11-59 Placing a tube down the barrel of the blade obscures your view of the glottic opening.

In the Field

An intubation attempt should not take more than 30 seconds. If you are unable to intubate the patient within 30 seconds, abort the attempt and reoxygenate the patient for at least 30 seconds to 1 minute with 100% oxygen before attempting intubation again.

Multiple intubation attempts, provided that you perform appropriate oxygenation and ventilation in between attempts, will generally not harm your patient; however, prolonged individual attempts will. During CPR, compressions should not be stopped for more than 10 seconds.

A major mistake of beginners is to try to pass the tube down the barrel of the laryngoscope blade—especially when using a straight blade. The laryngoscope blade is not designed as a guide for the tube; it is a tool used only to visualize the glottic opening. Placing the tube down the barrel of the blade will obscure your view of the glottic opening **Figure 11-59 ▲**.

Ventilation

After you have seen the cuff of the ET tube pass roughly ½ inch beyond the vocal cords, gently remove the blade, hold the tube securely in place with your right hand, and remove the stylet from the tube. Inflate the distal cuff with 5 to 10 mL of air and then detach the syringe from the inflation port. If the syringe is not removed immediately following inflation of the distal cuff, air from the cuff may leak back into the syringe, resulting in a loss of an adequate seal between the cuff and the tracheal wall. Avoid inflating the distal cuff with excess pressure as this may cause tissue necrosis of the tracheal wall.

Have your assistant attach the bag-mask device to the ET tube and continue ventilation. As the first ventilations are delivered, look at the patient's chest to ensure that it rises with each

ventilation. At the same time, listen with a stethoscope to both lungs at both the apices and bases and to the stomach over the epigastrium. If the tube is properly positioned, you will hear equal breath sounds bilaterally and a quiet epigastrium. Epigastric sounds may be transmitted to the lungs in obese patients or those with significant gastric distention, however, leading you to believe that you have inadvertently intubated the esophagus.

Ventilation should continue as dictated by the patient's age and clinical condition. It would be prudent to slightly hyperventilate the patient for 30 seconds to 1 minute immediately after intubation to eliminate any accumulated carbon dioxide.

Confirmation of Tube Placement

Visualizing the ET tube passing in between the vocal cords is your first (and most reliable) method of confirming that the tube has entered the trachea; however, you must continue gathering information to assess the location of the tube. A misplaced tube that goes undetected is a fatal error. You *must* incorporate multiple assessment findings into the determination of where the tube is located.

Auscultation is the first step in confirming proper tube placement. Unequal or absent breath sounds suggest esophageal placement, right mainstem placement, pneumothorax, or bronchial obstruction.

Bilaterally absent breath sounds or gurgling over the epigastrium when auscultating during ventilation indicates that you have intubated the esophagus rather than the trachea. In that case, you must *immediately* remove the ET tube and be prepared to vigorously suction the patient's airway. If gastric distention is present, the likelihood of emesis is increased. After clearing the airway with suction (if needed), ventilate the patient with 100% oxygen for 30 seconds to 1 minute before you make another attempt at intubation.

If breath sounds are heard only on the right side of the chest, the tube has likely been advanced too far and entered the right mainstem bronchus. Follow these steps to reposition the tube:

1. Loosen or remove the tube securing device.
2. Deflate the distal cuff.
3. Place your stethoscope over the left side of the chest.
4. While ventilation continues, *slowly* retract the tube while simultaneously listening for breath sounds over the left side of the chest.
5. Stop as soon as bilaterally equal breath sounds are heard.
6. Note the depth of the tube (in cm) at the patient's teeth.
7. Reinflate the distal cuff.
8. Secure the tube.
9. Resume ventilations.

If the ET tube has been properly positioned in the trachea, the bag-mask device should be easy to compress and you should see corresponding chest expansion. Increased resistance (decreased ventilation compliance) during ventilations may indicate gastric distention, esophageal intubation, or tension pneumothorax. Any of these conditions warrant immediate reassessment and corrective action.

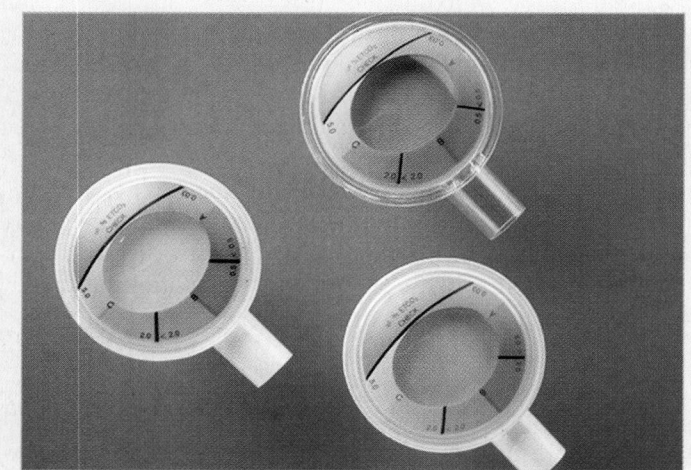

Figure 11-60 Colorimetric capnographers.

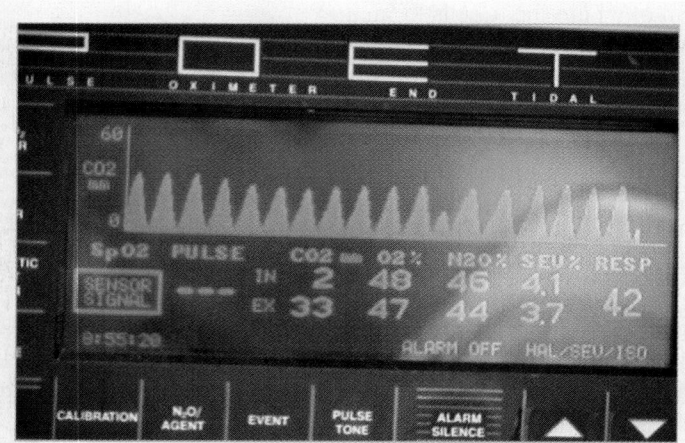

Figure 11-61 A capnometer.

End-tidal carbon dioxide (ETco_2) detectors detect the presence of carbon dioxide in exhaled air. Because carbon dioxide is not present in the esophagus, use of the ETco_2 detector is a reliable method for confirming proper tube placement. ETco_2 detectors may be colorimetric, digital, or digital/waveform. A capnographer attaches in between the ET tube and bag-mask device. It contains colorimetric paper, which should turn yellow during exhalation, indicating proper tube placement Figure 11-60 ▲ . A capnometer performs the same function and attaches in the same way as a capnographer, but provides an LED readout of the patient's exhaled carbon dioxide Figure 11-61 ▲ . Ongoing assessment with digital capnometry is an excellent indicator of continued correct placement of the ET tube, especially in the back of a moving ambulance, where breath sounds are often difficult to hear. If the patient's ETco_2 begins to fall (less than 30 mm Hg), it should alert you that a problem exists, such as inadvertent ET tube displacement or inadequate ventilation. Note that capnography may be inaccu-

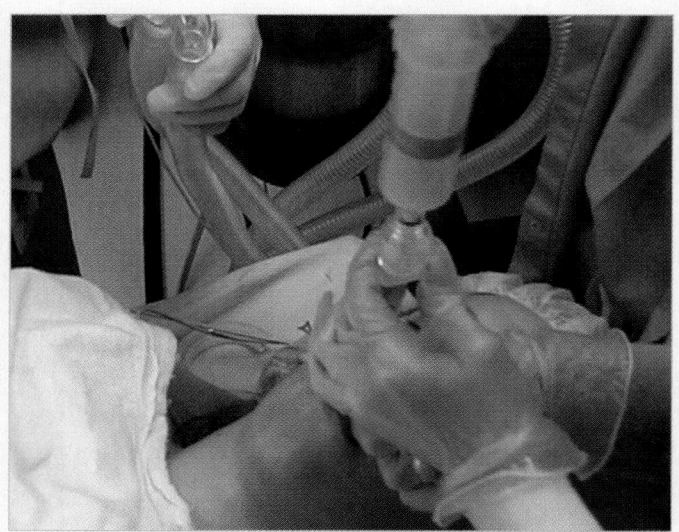

Figure 11-62 With the esophageal detector device syringe, the ability to freely withdraw air indicates placement of the tube in the trachea.

rate in patients with cardiac arrest, who are severely acidotic and only eliminating minimal carbon dioxide.

The steps for performing ETco_2 detection are listed here and shown in Skill Drill 11-26 ▶ .

1. Detach the ventilation device from the ET tube Step 1 .
2. Attach an in-line capnographer or capnometer to the proximal adapter of the ET tube Step 2 .
3. Reattach the ventilation device to the ET tube, and resume ventilations Step 3 .
4. Monitor the capnographer or capnometer for appropriate reading (appropriate color change or digital reading) Step 4 .

The esophageal detector device (EDD) is yet another method of confirming proper ET tube placement. The EDD is a bulb or syringe with a 15/22-mm adapter. With the syringe model, the syringe is attached to the end of the ET tube and the plunger is withdrawn, creating negative pressure Figure 11-62 ▲ . If the tube is in the trachea (which has rigid, noncollapsible walls), air is easily drawn into the syringe and the plunger does not move when released. Unlike the trachea, however, the esophagus is a flaccid, easily collapsible tube. Thus, if the tube is in the esophagus, a vacuum is created as the EDD's plunger is withdrawn and the plunger moves back toward zero when released.

With the bulb model, the bulb is squeezed and then attached to the end of the ET tube. If it remains collapsed or inflates slowly, the esophageal wall has occluded the distal tip of the tube, indicating that esophageal intubation has likely occurred. If the bulb briskly expands, the tube is properly positioned in the trachea Figure 11-63 ▶ .

After confirming proper tube placement, note and mark the ET tube with an ink line or piece of tape at the point where

Skill Drill 11-26: Using Colorimetric Capnography for Carbon Dioxide Detection

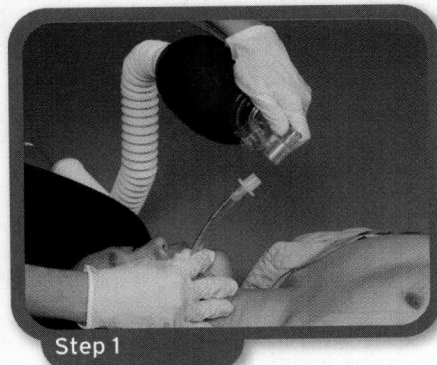

Step 1

Detach the ventilation device from the ET tube.

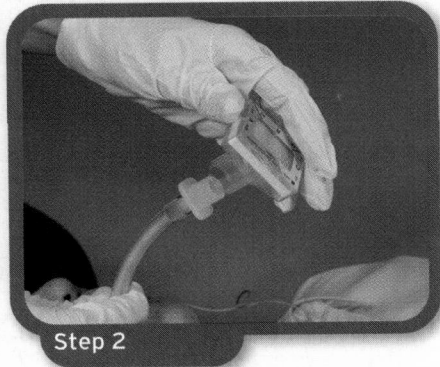

Step 2

Attach an in-line colorimetric capnographer or capnometer to the proximal adapter of the ET tube.

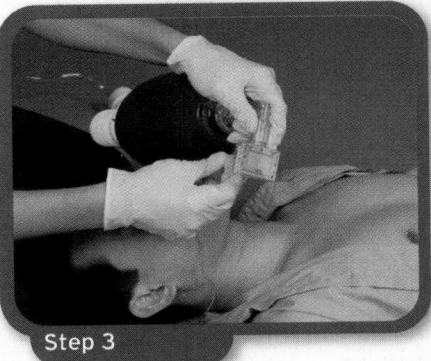

Step 3

Reattach the ventilation device to the ET tube, and resume ventilations.

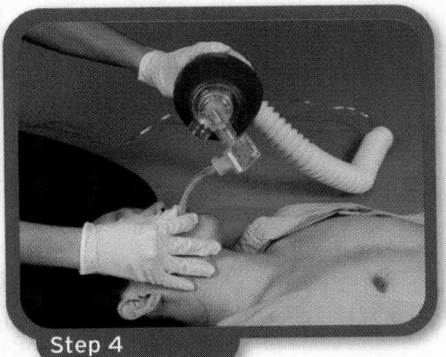

Step 4

Monitor the device for appropriate reading (appropriate color change or digital reading).

it emerges from the patient's mouth; this will enable medical personnel involved in the subsequent care of the patient to determine whether the tube has slipped in or out. The average depth for adult patients is 21 to 25 cm.

Securing the Tube

The last, and very important step, is to secure the ET tube. Inadvertent extubation caused by the patient or someone else is relatively common and can be very traumatic to the patient. There are few things more discouraging than to accomplish a difficult intubation, only to have the tube slip out of the trachea. Reintubation will almost certainly be even more difficult. *Never take your hand off the ET tube before it has been secured with tape or a commercial device!* Even then, it is a good idea to support the tube manually while you ventilate the patient to avoid a sudden jolt from the bag-mask device that yanks the tube from the trachea.

Many commercial tube-securing devices are available. You should be familiar with the specific device used by your EMS system. Every paramedic should also know how to secure a tube using tape, because it is almost always available. The steps for securing an ET tube with tape are listed here and shown in **Skill Drill 11-27 ▶**.

1. Note the centimeter marking on the tube at the level of the patient's teeth **Step 1**.
2. Remove the bag-mask device from the ET tube **Step 2**.
3. Move the ET tube to the corner of the patient's mouth **Step 3**.

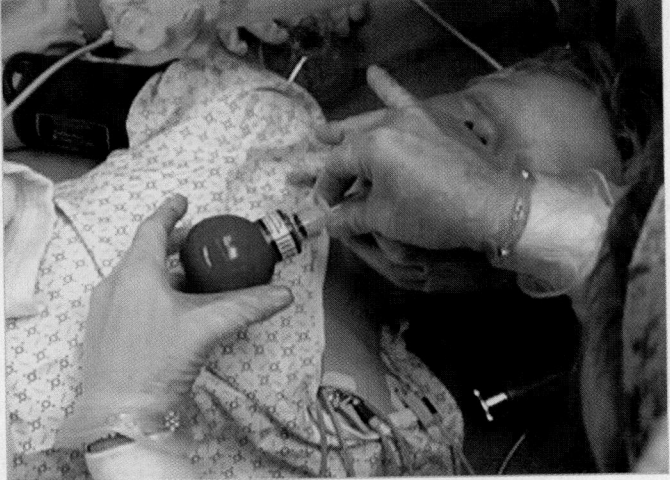

Figure 11-63 If the ET tube is in the trachea, the EDD bulb should briskly fill with air.

In the Field

The presence of condensation (vapor mist) in the ET tube during exhalation is a fairly reliable indicator that the ET tube is in the trachea. However, this finding by itself should not be used for definitive confirmation of proper tube placement. Instead, use multiple methods to confirm proper tube placement.

Skill Drill 11-27: Securing an Endotracheal Tube With Tape

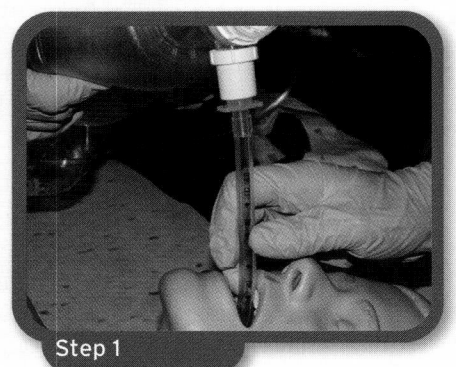

Step 1

Note the centimeter marking on the tube at the level of the patient's teeth.

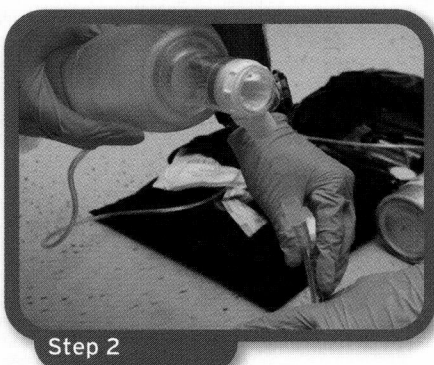

Step 2

Remove the bag-mask device from the ET tube.

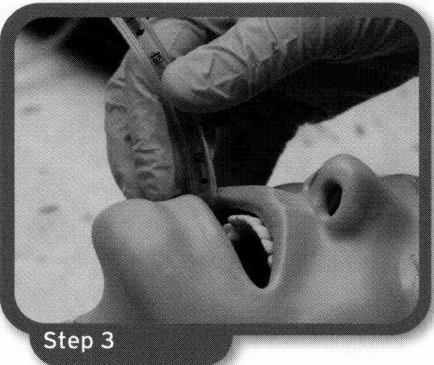

Step 3

Move the ET tube to the corner of the patient's mouth.

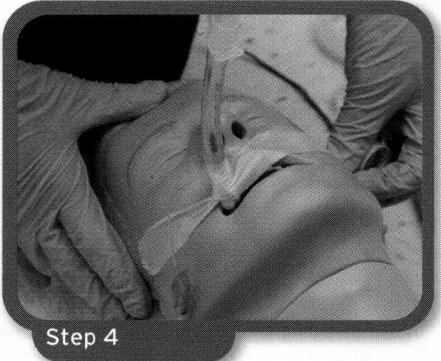

Step 4

Encircle the ET tube with tape, and secure the tape to the patient's maxilla (using tincture of benzoin to facilitate tape adhesion).

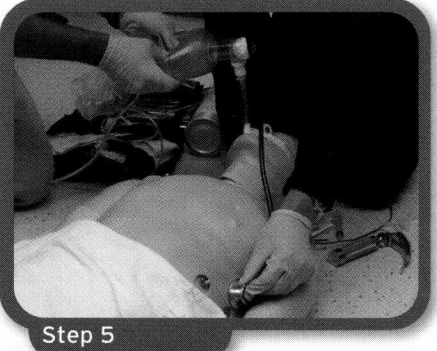

Step 5

Reattach the bag-mask device, and auscultate again over the apices and bases of the lungs and over the epigastrium.

---

4. Encircle the ET tube with tape, and secure the tape to the patient's maxilla (using tincture of benzoin to facilitate tape adhesion) **Step 4**.

5. Reattach the bag-mask device, and auscultate again over the apices and bases of the lungs and over the epigastrium **Step 5**.

The steps for securing an ET tube with a commercial device are listed here and shown in **Skill Drill 11-28 ▸**.

1. Note the centimeter marking on the tube at the level of the patient's teeth **Step 1**.

2. Remove the bag-mask device from the ET tube **Step 2**.

3. Position the ET tube in the center of the patient's mouth **Step 3**.

4. Place the commercial device over the ET tube. Tighten the screw to secure it in place **Step 4**. Fasten the strap.

5. Reattach the bag-mask device, and auscultate again over the apices and bases of the lungs and over the epigastrium **Step 5**.

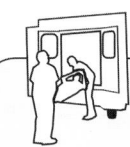

In the Field

No *single* test for correct ET tube placement is 100% accurate. Always use *at least* two methods of tube placement confirmation.

If the patient bites the tube or experiences a seizure, the ET tube may become occluded; therefore, after properly securing the tube, insert a bite block or oral airway in between the patient's molars. Many commercially manufactured ET tube-securing devices feature a built-in bite block for this purpose.

It is also important to minimize head movement in the intubated patient. With a firmly secured tube, the tip can move as much as 5 cm during head flexion and extension. Consider applying a cervical collar, placing the patient on a long backboard, and stabilizing the patient's head with lateral immobilization blocks to reduce the likelihood of tube dislodgement during transport.

Skill Drill 11-28: Securing an Endotracheal Tube With a Commercial Device

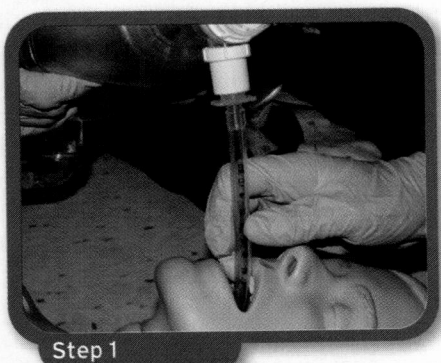

Step 1

Note the centimeter marking on the tube at the level of the patient's teeth.

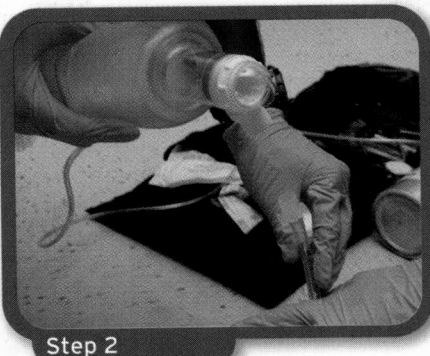

Step 2

Remove the bag-mask device from the ET tube.

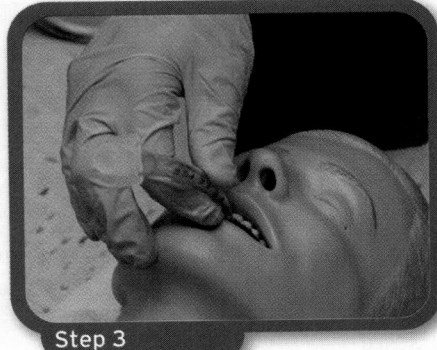

Step 3

Position the ET tube in the center of the patient's mouth.

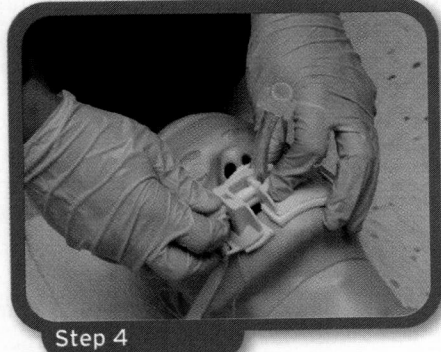

Step 4

Place the commercial device over the ET tube. Tighten the screw and fasten the strap to secure.

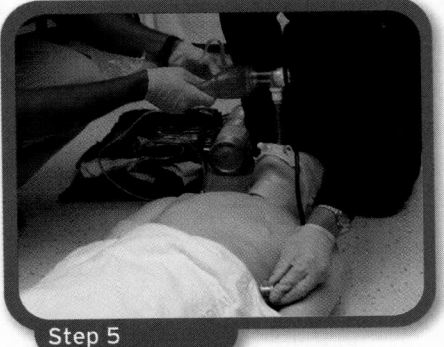

Step 5

Reattach the bag-mask device, and auscultate again over the apices and bases of the lungs and over the epigastrium.

You are the Provider Part 8

After definitively securing the patient's airway, you attach an automatic transport ventilator (ATV) and continue transport. En route, you note marked improvement in his condition. Your reassessment reveals the following:

Reassessment	Recording Time: 22 Minutes
Level of consciousness	P (Responsive to painful stimuli); improving, patient is becoming resistant to the ET tube
Respirations	Ventilated with an ATV and 100% oxygen at a rate of 12 breaths/min
Pulse	118 beats/min, regular and stronger
Skin	Cyanosis is dissipating; skin is cool and dry
Blood pressure	118/70 mm Hg
Sao$_2$	97% while being ventilated with an ATV and 100% oxygen

13. Should you extubate this patient? Why or why not?

14. Are any pharmacologic interventions required?

The steps for orotracheal intubation by direct laryngoscopy are summarized here and shown in **Skill Drill 11-29 ▶**.

1. Use BSI precautions (gloves and face shield) **Step 1**.
2. Preoxygenate the patient for 2 to 3 minutes with a bag-mask device and 100% oxygen **Step 2**.
3. Check, prepare, and assemble your equipment **Step 3**.
4. Place the patient's head in the sniffing position **Step 4**.
5. Insert the blade into the right side of the patient's mouth, and displace the tongue to the left **Step 5**.
6. Gently lift the long axis of the laryngoscope handle until you can visualize the glottic opening and the vocal cords **Step 6**.
7. Insert the ET tube through the right corner of the mouth, and visualize its entry between the vocal cords **Step 7**.
8. Remove the laryngoscope from the patient's mouth **Step 8**.
9. Remove the stylet from the ET tube **Step 9**.
10. Inflate the distal cuff of the ET tube with 5 to 10 mL of air, and detach the syringe from the inflation port **Step 10**.
11. Attach an end-tidal carbon dioxide detector to the ET tube **Step 11**.
12. Attach the bag-mask device, ventilate, and auscultate over the apices and bases of both lungs and over the epigastrium **Step 12**.
13. Secure the ET tube **Step 13**.
14. Place a bite block in the patient's mouth **Step 14**.

Nasotracheal Intubation

Nasotracheal intubation is the insertion of a tube into the trachea through the nose. In the prehospital setting, it is usually performed without directly visualizing the vocal cords—hence the term "blind" nasotracheal intubation.

Blind nasotracheal intubation is an excellent technique for establishing control over the airway in situations where it is either difficult or hazardous to perform laryngoscopy. Because the procedure must be performed on patients with spontaneous breathing, it is less likely to result in hypoxia.

Indications and Contraindications

Nasotracheal intubation is indicated for patients who are breathing spontaneously, but require definitive airway management to prevent further deterioration of their condition. Con-

Documentation and Communication

On the patient care report, document the means of assessing placement of the ET tube, such as breath sounds, visualization, and capnography or capnometry findings. The depth of the tube, as noted by the centimeter marking at the patient's teeth, should also be documented. Additionally, indicate when correct placement was confirmed: at the time the ET tube was placed, when the patient was moved into the ambulance, and upon arrival at the hospital.

scious patients or patients with an altered mental status and with an intact gag reflex, who are in respiratory failure secondary to conditions such as COPD, asthma, or pulmonary edema, are excellent candidates for nasotracheal intubation.

Nasotracheal intubation is contraindicated in apneic patients (eg, in respiratory or cardiac arrest); such patients should receive orotracheal intubation. This procedure is also contraindicated in patients with head trauma and possible midface fractures, as evidenced by CSF drainage from the nose following a head injury. In these patients, a nasally inserted ET tube may enter the cranial vault and penetrate the brain. Other contraindications to nasotracheal intubation include anatomic abnormalities, such as in patients with a deviated septum, patients with nasal polyps, or patients who frequently use cocaine. Nasal insertion of an ET tube in these patients may result in severe epistaxis.

Likewise, you should avoid nasotracheal intubation, if possible, in patients with blood-clotting abnormalities or in those who take anticoagulation medications (eg, Coumadin). These conditions also increase the likelihood and severity of epistaxis following insertion of anything in the nose.

Advantages and Disadvantages

The primary advantage of blind nasotracheal intubation is that it can be performed on patients who are awake and breathing. This procedure does not require that you place anything in the mouth (eg, laryngoscope), so the nasotracheal route is associated with much less retching and a lower risk of vomiting in patients with an intact gag reflex.

Another major advantage of nasotracheal intubation is that there is no need for a laryngoscope, which eliminates the risk of trauma to the teeth or soft tissues of the mouth. Because the patient's mouth does not need to be opened, this technique is better suited to patients with limited temporomandibular joint mobility, such as those with mandibular wiring, mandibular fractures, seizures, or clenched teeth (trismus).

Nasotracheal intubation does not require the patient to be placed in a sniffing position, which makes it an ideal technique for intubating patients with a possible spinal injury, unless a midface fracture is suspected. Finally, because the tube is inserted through the nose, the patient cannot bite the tube. Furthermore, it can be secured more easily than a tube that is inserted orally because the nose generally has fewer secretions than the mouth.

On the downside, because nasotracheal intubation is a blind technique, the paramedic cannot use one of the major tube confirmation methods—visualizing the tube passing through the vocal cords. Confirming proper tube position is important, regardless of which intubation method is employed; however, the paramedic should be even more diligent when confirming tube placement following nasotracheal intubation.

Complications

Bleeding is the most common complication associated with nasotracheal intubation. If intubation is successful, the airway is protected and the risk of aspiration is eliminated. However,

Skill Drill 11-29: Intubation of the Trachea Using Direct Laryngoscopy

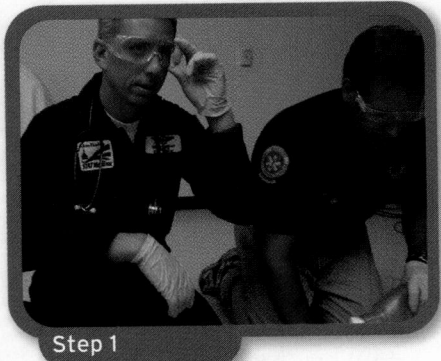

Step 1

Use BSI precautions (gloves and face shield).

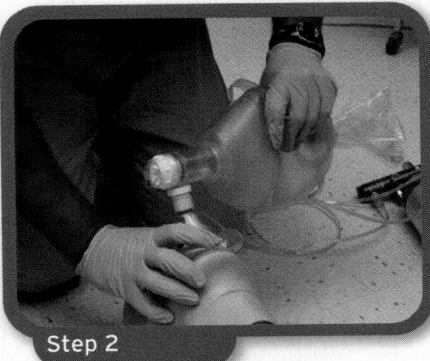

Step 2

Preoxygenate the patient for 2 to 3 minutes with a bag-mask device and 100% oxygen.

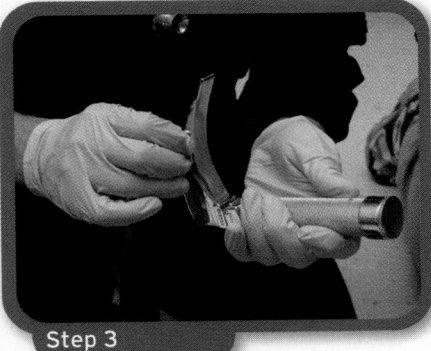

Step 3

Check, prepare, and assemble your equipment.

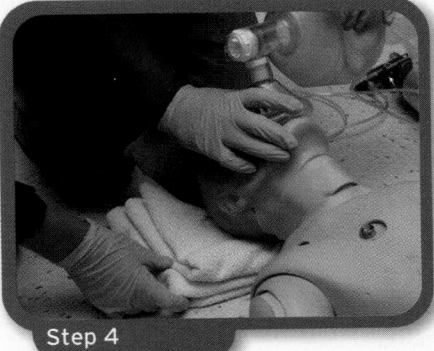

Step 4

Place the patient's head in the sniffing position.

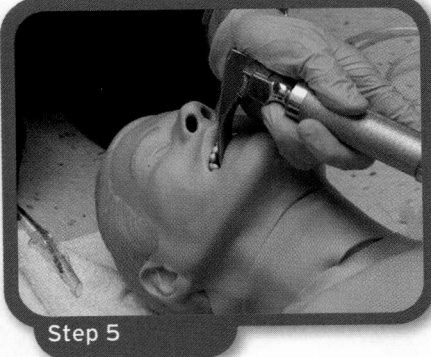

Step 5

Insert the blade into the right side of the patient's mouth, and displace the tongue to the left.

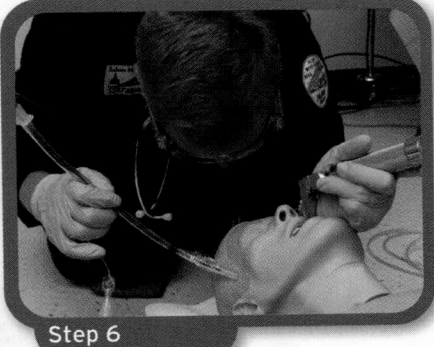

Step 6

Gently lift the long axis of the laryngoscope handle until you can visualize the glottic opening and the vocal cords.

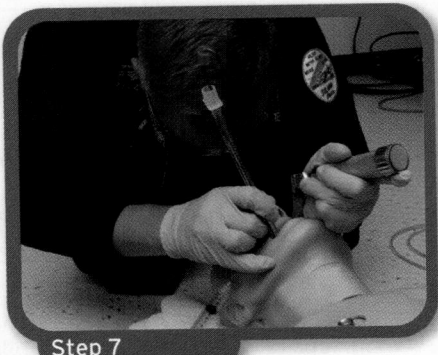

Step 7

Insert the ET tube through the right corner of the mouth, and visualize its entry between the vocal cords.

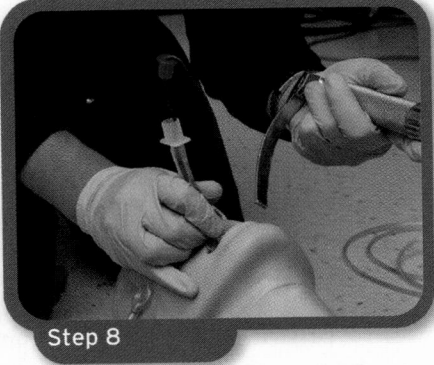

Step 8

Remove the laryngoscope from the patient's mouth.

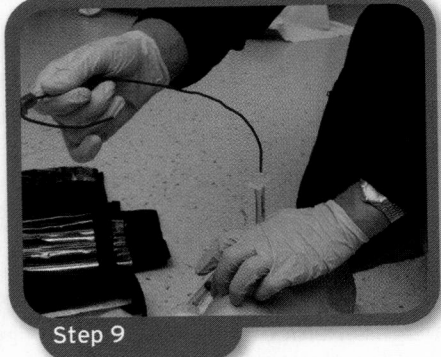

Step 9

Remove the stylet from the ET tube.

Skill Drill 11-29: Intubation of the Trachea Using Direct Laryngoscopy (*continued*)

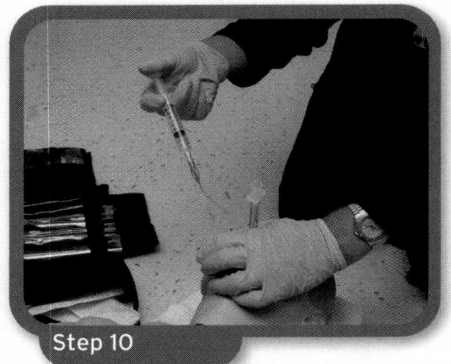

Step 10
Inflate the distal cuff of the ET tube with 5 to 10 mL of air, and detach the syringe from the inflation port.

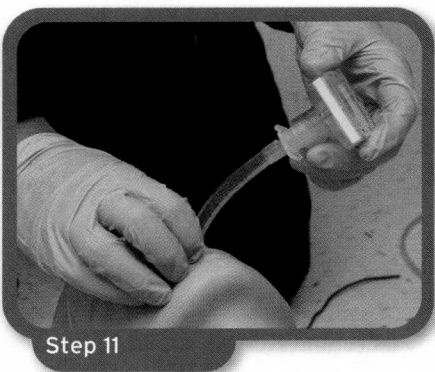

Step 11
Attach the end-tidal carbon dioxide detector to the ET tube.

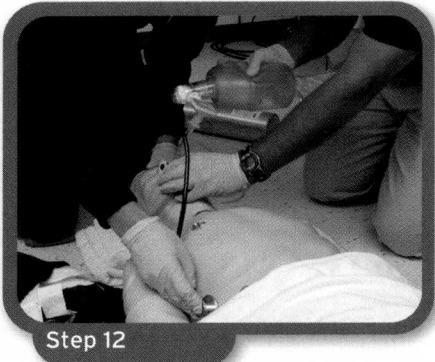

Step 12
Attach the bag-mask device, ventilate, and auscultate over the apices and bases of both lungs and over the epigastrium.

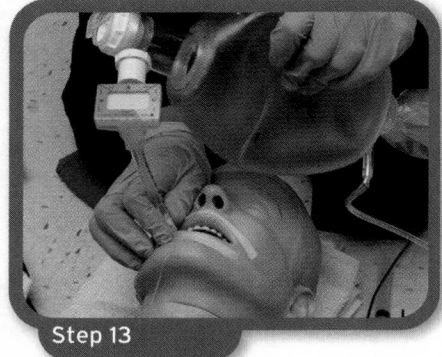

Step 13
Confirm placement and then secure the ET tube.

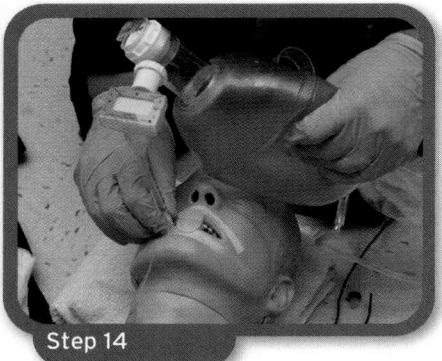

Step 14
Place a bite block in the patient's mouth.

---

severe bleeding can occur, especially with rough technique, posing an additional threat to an already compromised airway as the swallowing of blood greatly increases the likelihood of vomiting and subsequent aspiration.

The incidence of bleeding associated with nasotracheal intubation can be reduced by being very gentle when inserting the tube into the nostril and by lubricating the tip with a water-soluble gel. If available, an anesthetic lubricant containing a vasoconstrictive agent (eg, phenylephrine hydrochloride [Neo-Synephrine]) will reduce the amount of patient discomfort as well as the likelihood and severity of nasal bleeding.

Equipment

The same equipment used for orotracheal intubation—minus the laryngoscope and stylet—is used for blind nasotracheal intubation. Standard ET tubes can be used for both orotracheal and nasotracheal intubation, although they should be 1.0 to 1.5 mm smaller when inserted nasally. When choosing the size of tube, select one that is slightly smaller than the nostril in which it will be inserted.

Some ET tubes have been designed specifically for blind nasotracheal intubation. For example, the Endotrol tube **Figure 11-64 ▶** is slightly more flexible than a standard ET tube and is equipped with a "trigger" that is attached to a piece of line, which is itself attached to the tip of the tube. Pulling the trigger moves the tip of the tube anteriorly and increases the tube's overall curvature. This feature replaces the function of the stylet.

The movement of air through the ET tube helps determine proper tube placement following nasotracheal intubation. A number of devices have been developed to allow the paramedic to confirm successful nasotracheal intubation without the need to place his or her face next to the tube and thus risk contact with contaminants in the patient's exhaled breath **Table 11-12 ▶**.

Technique for Nasotracheal Intubation

When you perform blind nasotracheal intubation, you use the patient's spontaneous respirations to guide the ET tube into the

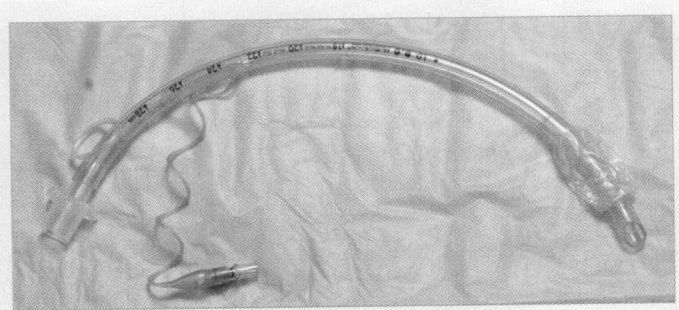

Figure 11-64 The Endotrol tube makes the nasotracheal procedure safer, easier, and more efficient.

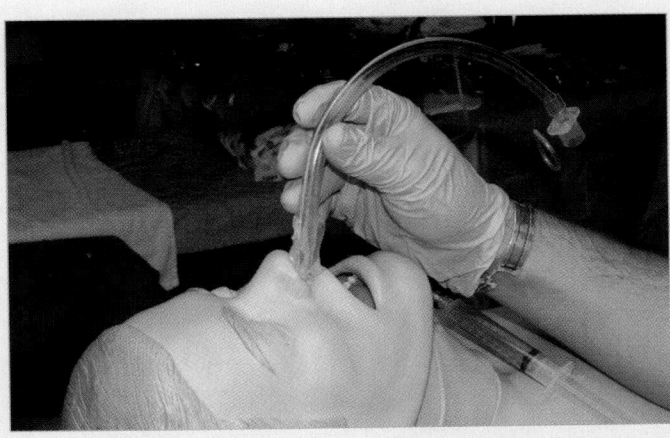

Figure 11-65 Aim the tip of the tube straight back toward the ear.

Table 11-12	Devices Used to Determine Maximum Airflow Through the Tube During Nasotracheal Intubation	
Humid-Vent 1	Device that attaches to the 15/22-mm adapter at the end of the ET tube to prevent secretions from being expelled from the tube.
BAAM® (Beck Airway Airflow Monitor)	A small whistle that attaches to the 15/22-mm adapter and emits a high-pitched sound as air moves in and out of the tube.
Stethoscope with head removed	Stethoscope tubing placed in the proximal 2 to 3 cm of the ET tube enables the paramedic to hear air movement without placing his or her face next to the tube.
IV tubing attached to an earpiece	The tubing in the proximal 2 to 3 cm of the ET tube enables the intubator to hear air movement without placing his or her face next to the tube.

trachea and confirm proper placement. The tube is advanced as the patient inhales, at which point the vocal cords are open at their widest, which facilitates placement of the tube into the trachea.

After preparing your equipment and preoxygenating the patient, insert the tube into the nostril with the bevel facing toward the nasal septum. The right nostril is typically used because the curvature of the tube is in the correct orientation in relation to the bevel. If the right nostril is obstructed or if significant resistance is met, insert the tube into the left nostril, but rotate the tube 180° as its tip enters the nasopharynx.

The angle of insertion is critical when performing nasotracheal intubation. Aim the tip of the tube straight back toward the ear **Figure 11-65** . The goal is to follow the floor of the nasal cavity until the tube enters the nasopharynx. *Do not* insert the tube with the tip aimed upward toward the eye, as this can damage the turbinates and cause significant bleeding.

As the tube is advanced into the nasopharynx, you will begin to hear air rushing in and out of the tube as the patient breathes. Your goal is to position the tube just above the glottic opening so that the patient will draw the tube into the trachea when he or she inhales deeply. Manipulate the patient's head to control the position of the tip of the tube. Cup your left hand (if the tube is inserted in the right nostril) under the patient's occiput. Move the patient's head until you find the position that offers the maximum amount of air moving through the tube. At this point, the tube should be positioned just above the glottic opening.

As the patient inhales, the negative pressure created by inhalation facilitates movement of the tube through the glottic opening. Instruct the patient to take a deep breath, and *gently* advance the tube with the inhalation. Placement of the tube in the trachea will be evidenced by an increase in air movement through the tube.

If you see a soft-tissue bulge on either side of the airway, the tube has probably been inserted into the pyriform fossa. Hold the patient's head still and slightly withdraw the tube. Once maximum airflow is detected, advance the tube on inhalation. If you do not see a soft-tissue bulge and no air is moving through the tube, the tube has entered the esophagus. Withdraw the tube until you detect airflow, and then extend the head.

Once the tube has been properly positioned, inflate the distal cuff with the minimum amount of air necessary to achieve an airtight seal. Attach a bag-mask device to the tube and ventilate the patient according to his or her clinical condition. Because you do not have the benefit of visualizing the tube passing in between the vocal cords, confirmation (by multiple techniques) and continuous monitoring of proper tube position is more important following blind nasotracheal intubation than with any other intubation technique. Although the movement of air in and out of the tube during breathing is a good indicator that the tube is in the trachea, it is not foolproof. In many cases, only the tip of the ET tube has passed through the glottic opening; even slight patient movement may dislodge the tube, potentially unrecognized, into the esophagus. Movement of the tube can also result in right mainstem placement.

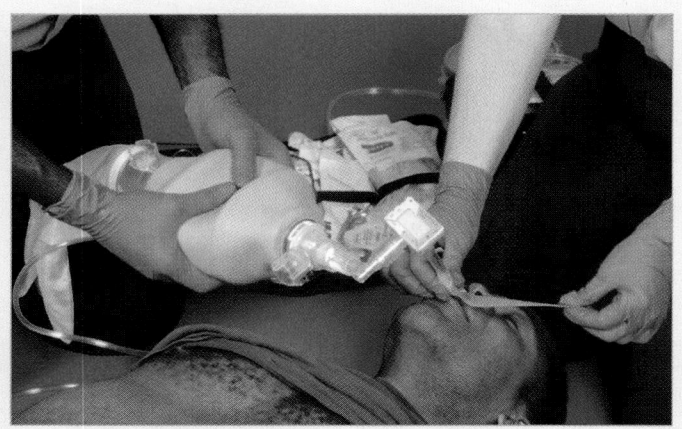

Figure 11-66 Clean up any secretions or excess lubricant and secure the tube with tape.

Clean up any secretions or excess lubricant and secure the tube with tape **Figure 11-66 ▲** . Document the depth of insertion at the nostril and monitor it frequently to detect movement of the tube.

The steps for performing blind nasotracheal intubation are listed here and shown in **Skill Drill 11-30 ▶** .

1. Use BSI precautions (gloves and face shield) (Step 1).
2. Preoxygenate the patient whenever possible with a bag-mask device and 100% oxygen (Step 2).
3. Check, prepare, and assemble your equipment (Step 3).
4. Place the patient's head in a neutral position (Step 4).
5. Pre-form the ET tube by bending it in a circle (Step 5).
6. Lubricate the tip of the tube with a water-soluble gel (Step 6).
7. Gently insert the ET tube into the most compliant nostril with the bevel facing toward the nasal septum and advance the tube along the nasal floor (Step 7).
8. Advance the ET tube through the vocal cords as the patient inhales (Step 8).
9. Inflate the distal cuff with 5 to 10 mL of air and detach the syringe (Step 9).
10. Attach an end-tidal carbon dioxide detector to the ET tube (Step 10).
11. Attach the bag-mask device, ventilate, and auscultate over the apices and bases of both lungs and over the epigastrium (Step 11).
12. Secure the ET tube (Step 12).

Digital Intubation

Suppose you are in the midst of attempting to intubate your patient and suddenly the light on your laryngoscope sputters out. You must have a contingency plan for these kinds of unexpected events, including a set of fresh batteries and a back-up laryngoscope handle.

Fortunately, there *is* a way to intubate the trachea without a laryngoscope. Digital intubation (also referred to as "blind" or

"tactile" intubation) involves directly palpating the glottic structures and elevating the epiglottis with your middle finger while guiding the ET tube into the trachea by feel. Being adept at digital intubation provides you with an option in some extreme circumstances, such as equipment failure when attempting to intubate an apneic patient, who, because of his or her apnea, is not a candidate for blind nasotracheal intubation.

Indications and Contraindications

Digital intubation may be used in the following exceptional circumstances:

- A laryngoscope is not available or has malfunctioned.
- Other techniques to intubate the patient have failed.
- The patient is in a confined space.
- The patient is extremely obese or has a short neck.
- Copious secretions obscure your view of the airway.
- The head cannot be moved due to trauma or immobilization equipment interferes with direct laryngoscopy.
- Massive airway trauma has made visualization of the intubation landmarks impossible.

Although digital intubation can be performed in pediatric patients, the size of the paramedic's fingers (it takes two fingers) relative to the size of the child's mouth usually makes the technique impossible. Also, digital intubation is absolutely contraindicated if your patient is breathing, is not deeply unconscious, or has an intact gag reflex.

Advantages and Disadvantages

Because digital intubation does not require a laryngoscope, this technique is most advantageous in the event of equipment failure. It is also ideal in situations in which your view of the vocal cords is obscured by copious, uncontrollable oral secretions. Because digital intubation does not require the patient's head to be in a sniffing position, it can be performed on trauma patients and patients whose heads cannot be placed in a sniffing position (eg, obese or short-necked patients).

The major disadvantage of digital intubation is that it requires you to place your fingers in the patient's mouth, thus posing a risk of being accidentally bitten. Digital intubation should therefore be performed only in patients who are deeply unresponsive and apneic, *and* who have a bite block in their mouth to prevent closure. There is also a potential risk of exposure to an infectious disease. The patient's teeth could easily tear through a paramedic's gloves and cut his or her fingers, especially if the teeth are sharp or broken.

Skill Drill 11-30: Blind Nasotracheal Intubation

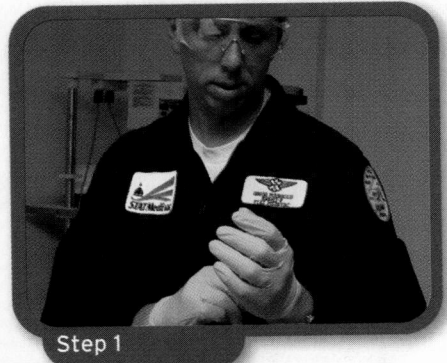

Step 1

Use BSI precautions (gloves and face shield).

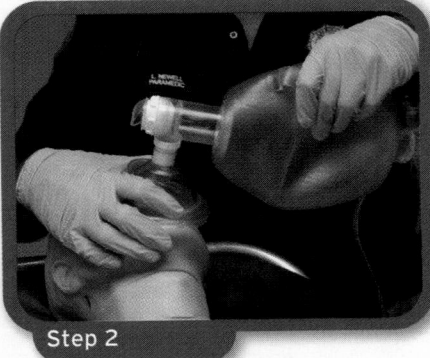

Step 2

Preoxygenate the patient whenever possible with a bag-mask device and 100% oxygen.

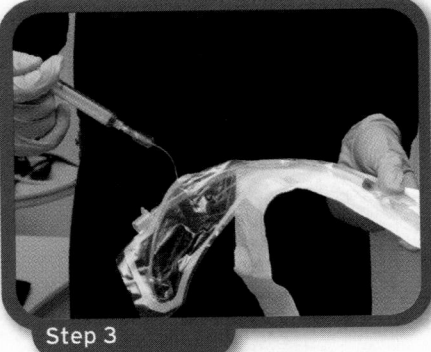

Step 3

Check, prepare, and assemble your equipment.

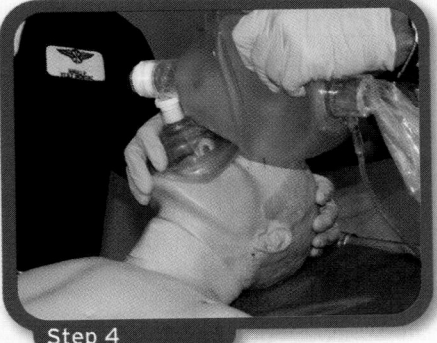

Step 4

Place the patient's head in a neutral position.

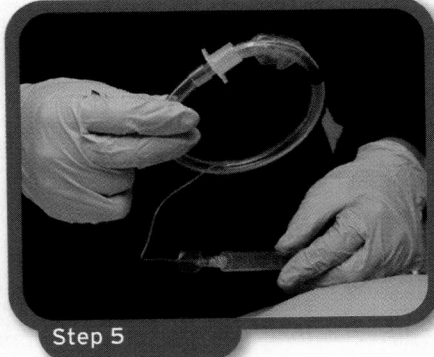

Step 5

Pre-form the ET tube by bending it in a circle.

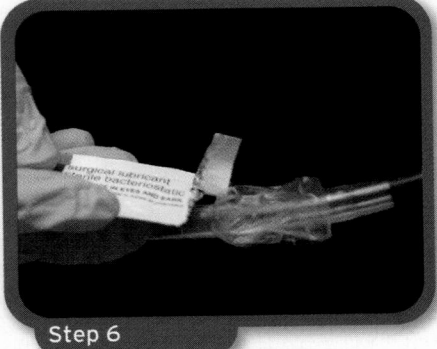

Step 6

Lubricate the tip of the tube with a water-soluble gel.

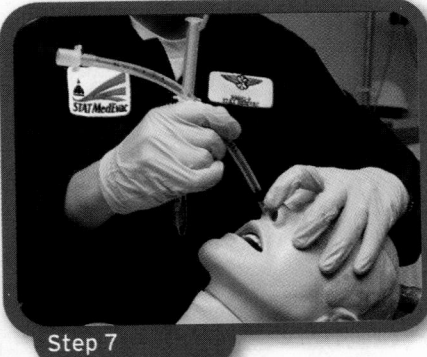

Step 7

Gently insert the ET tube into the most compliant nostril, with the bevel facing toward the nasal septum and advance the tube along the nasal floor.

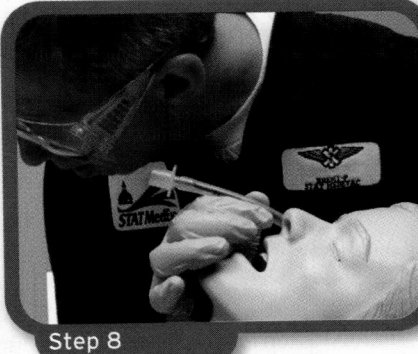

Step 8

Advance the ET tube through the vocal cords as the patient inhales. The BAAM® device can be helpful in this step.

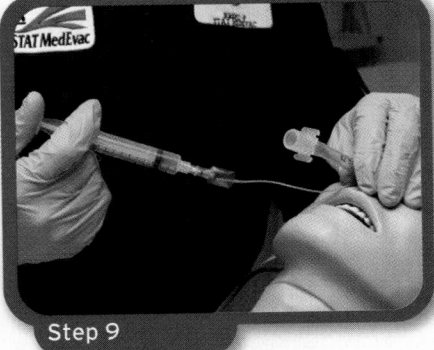

Step 9

Inflate the distal cuff with 5 to 10 mL of air and detach the syringe.

Skill Drill 11-30: Blind Nasotracheal Intubation (*continued*)

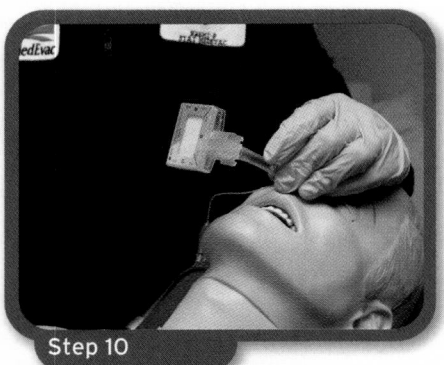

Step 10

Attach an end-tidal carbon dioxide detector to the ET tube.

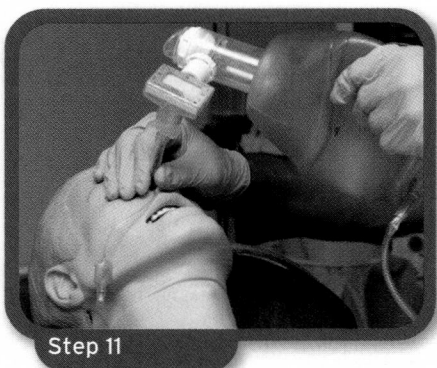

Step 11

Attach the bag-mask device, ventilate, and auscultate over the apices and bases of both lungs and over the epigastrium.

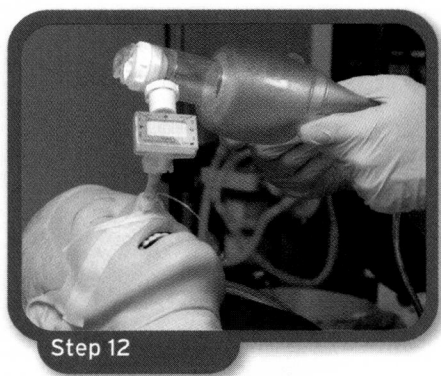

Step 12

Confirm placement and then secure the ET tube.

In the Field

Always check your intubation equipment at the beginning of each shift to ensure that it is fully functional. Failure to do so increases the risk of equipment breakdown when it is needed the most. Digital intubation, although an acceptable technique, is clearly the least desirable option. Having functional equipment when you need it will avoid the need to stick your fingers down the patient's throat to place the ET tube.

Successful placement of the ET tube via digital intubation depends on frequency of practice, experience, manual dexterity, and the size and length of the paramedic's fingers. Paramedics with short fingers or fingers that are large in diameter will have greater difficulty performing digital intubation.

Complications

Misplacement of the ET tube is the major complication of digital intubation. Although the intubation is tactilely guided, it is easy to misdirect the tip of the tube during insertion. Therefore, diligent attention to tube confirmation is absolutely essential with this technique.

Because it does not require the use of a laryngoscope, digital intubation is associated with a much lower incidence of dental trauma; however, the insertion of a bite block or dental prod can cause lip trauma, tooth damage, or both. Additionally, vigorous attempts at insertion or improper technique can cause airway trauma or swelling.

Any intubation attempt, regardless of the technique used, can result in hypoxia. Therefore, you must carefully monitor the patient's clinical condition (eg, pulse oximetry, skin color, heart rate) during the technique, limit your intubation attempts to 30 seconds, and ventilate the patient appropriately in between attempts.

Equipment

Less equipment is needed for digital intubation. In fact, you will usually attempt the digital technique because you have limited (or malfunctioning) equipment. Except for the laryngoscope, you will essentially use the same equipment required for orotracheal intubation, plus your fingers. That is, you will need traditional intubation equipment and supplies—a stylet, $ETco_2$ detector or EDD, and an appropriate device to adequately secure the tube.

Technique for Digital Intubation

Today, because of the variety of alternative airway devices available (eg, Combitube, PtL, LMA), digital intubation is rarely performed. Nonetheless, you should work, through frequent practice, to become just as skilled and competent with digital intubation as you are with more common advanced airway management techniques.

Prepare your equipment for the digital intubation as your assistant is ventilating the patient with a bag-mask device and 100% oxygen. Select an ET tube that is one half to a full size smaller than that used for intubation with direct laryngoscopy. In this technique, the tip of the tube is guided into the trachea while using your index finger as a leverage point. A stylet provides the tube with the rigidity necessary to make the bend in the tube. Two configurations are recommended; you should practice with both to determine which you prefer.

- In an "open J" configuration, the stylet is inserted and a large J shape is made in the distal end of the tube.
- In the "U-handle" configuration, the tube is bent into a U shape and the proximal half of the tube is bent into a 90° handle toward your dominant hand Figure 11-67 ▶.

Because a sniffing position is not required to perform digital intubation, the paramedic can be positioned at the patient's left side facing toward the head. This position facilitates digital intubation if the patient is trapped in a seated or standing position Figure 11-68 ▶.

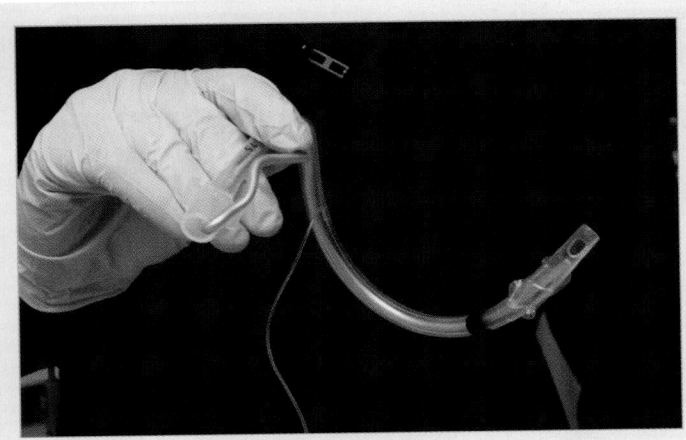

Figure 11-67 The U-handle configuration.

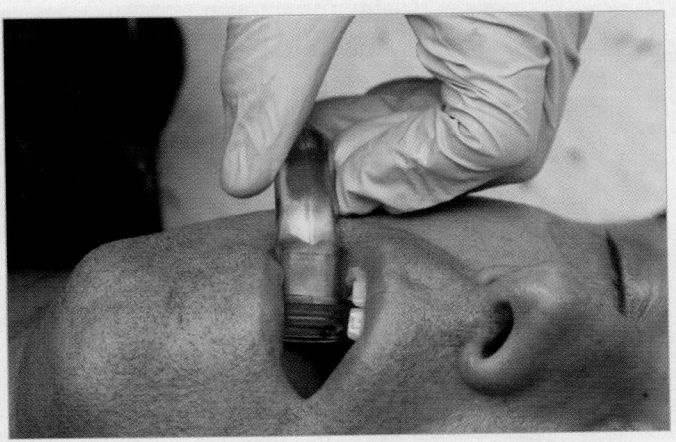

Figure 11-69 The flange of an oral airway can be inserted into the mouth and turned sideways to act as a bite block.

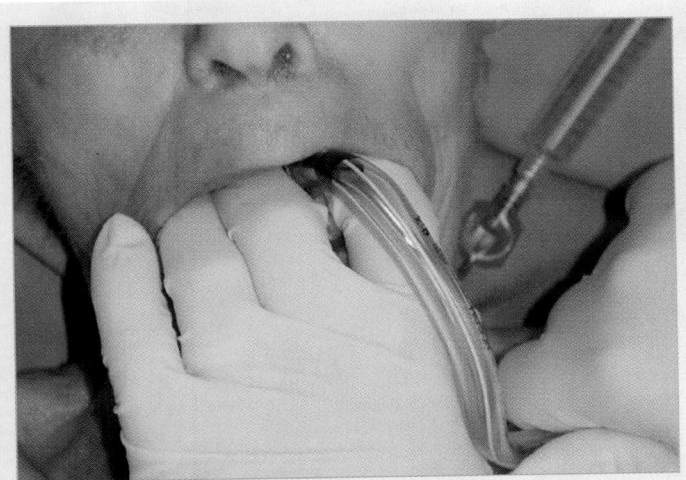

Figure 11-68 If the patient is trapped in a seated or standing position, digital intubation can be performed from a position facing the patient.

Before even considering placing your fingers in the patient's mouth, insert a bite block or the flange of an oral airway, turned sideways, between the patient's molars **Figure 11-69 ▶**. This will prevent complete closure of the patient's mouth, affording protection for your fingers in the event of a sudden change in consciousness or seizure.

Insert the index and middle fingers of your left hand into the right side of the patient's mouth. Press down against the tongue as you slide your fingers along the midline of the tongue until you can feel the epiglottis. Then pull the epiglottis forward with your middle finger.

Hold the endotracheal tube in your right hand, as you would hold a pencil, and insert it into the left side of the patient's mouth. Advance the tube along the outer surface of your left index finger or between your middle and index fingers, and guide its tip toward the glottis. Once you feel the cuff of the tube pass about 2 inches beyond the tip of your finger, stabilize the tube with your right hand while

you gently withdraw your two left fingers from the patient's mouth.

After the tube has been positioned and stabilized manually, carefully remove the stylet and inflate the distal cuff with 5 to 10 mL of air (don't forget to detach the syringe from the inflation port). Attach the bag-mask device to the ET tube—with an ETCO$_2$ detector between the bag and tube—and ventilate the patient while observing for visible chest rise.

Because digital intubation is truly a blind technique, rigorous tube confirmation protocol must be followed. Auscultate both lungs and over the epigastrium, monitor ETCO$_2$, and properly secure the tube in place. Continue ventilations according to the patient's clinical condition.

The steps for performing digital intubation are listed here and shown in **Skill Drill 11-31 ▶**.

1. Take BSI precautions (gloves and face shield) **Step 1**.
2. Preoxygenate the patient for 2 to 3 minutes with a bag-mask device and 100% oxygen **Step 2**.
3. Check, prepare, and assemble your equipment **Step 3**.
4. Bend the ET tube by placing a slight curve at its distal end (like a hockey stick) **Step 4**.
5. Place the patient's head in a neutral position **Step 5**.
6. Place a bite block in between the patient's molars to prevent the patient from biting your fingers **Step 6**.
7. Insert your left middle and index fingers into the patient's mouth and shift the patient's tongue forward as you advance your fingers toward the patient's larynx **Step 7**.
8. Palpate and lift the epiglottis with your left middle finger **Step 8**.
9. Advance the tube with your right hand and guide it in between the vocal cords with your index finger **Step 9**.
10. Remove the stylet from the ET tube **Step 10**.
11. Inflate the distal cuff of the ET tube with 5 to 10 mL of air and detach the syringe **Step 11**.

Skill Drill 11-31: Digital Intubation

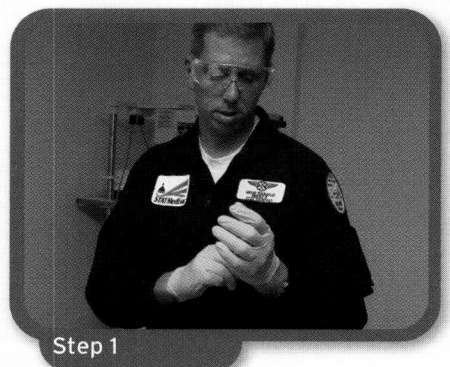

Step 1

Take BSI precautions (gloves and face shield).

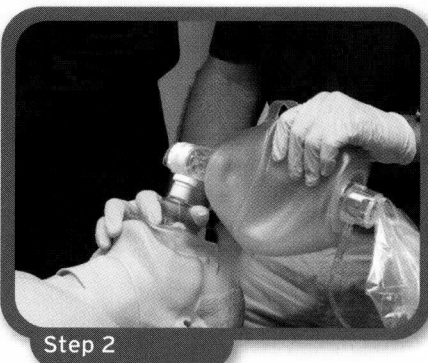

Step 2

Preoxygenate the patient for 2 to 3 minutes with a bag-mask device and 100% oxygen.

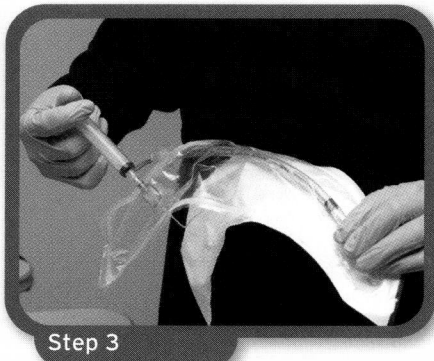

Step 3

Check, prepare, and assemble your equipment.

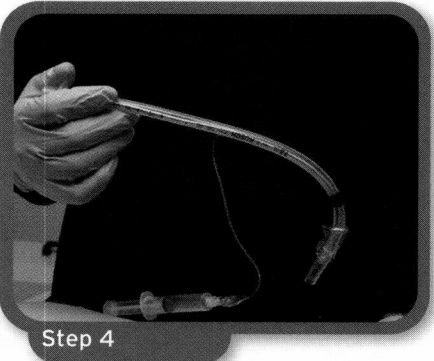

Step 4

Bend the ET tube by placing a slight curve at its distal end (like a hockey stick).

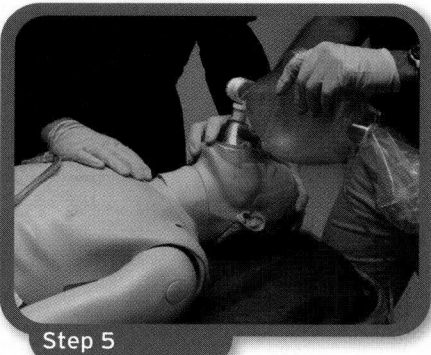

Step 5

Place the patient's head in a neutral position.

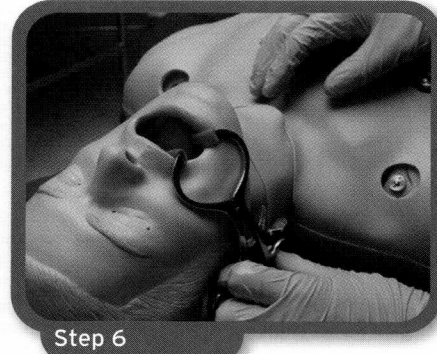

Step 6

Place a bite block in between the patient's molars to prevent the patient from biting your fingers.

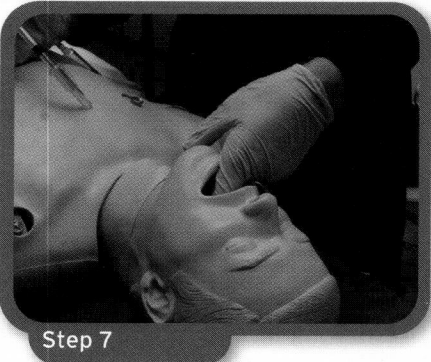

Step 7

Insert your left middle and index fingers into the patient's mouth and shift the patient's tongue forward as you advance your fingers toward the larynx.

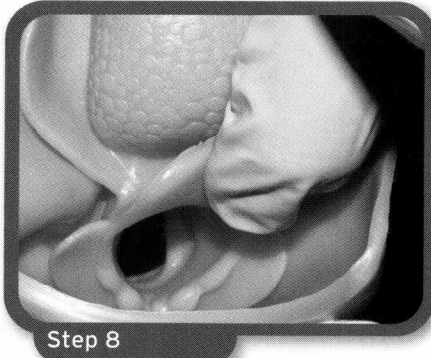

Step 8

Palpate and lift the epiglottis with your left middle finger.

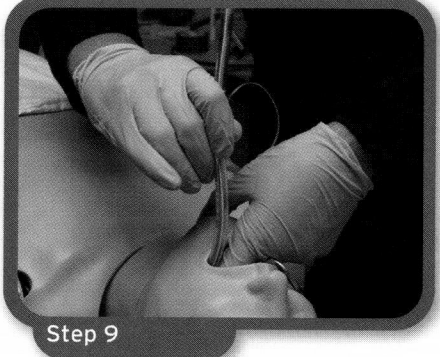

Step 9

Advance the tube with your right hand and guide it in between the vocal cords with your left index finger.

12. Attach the $ETCO_2$ detector to the ET tube (Step 12).

13. Attach the bag-mask device, ventilate, and auscultate over the apices and bases of both lungs and over the epigastrium (Step 13).

14. Secure the ET tube (Step 14).

Transillumination Techniques for Intubation

Transillumination intubation, like digital intubation, is rarely considered a first-line technique to definitively secure the airway, but it may prove valuable in some situations. The tissue that overlies the trachea is relatively thin. Therefore, a bright

Skill Drill 11-32: Transillumination Intubation (continued)

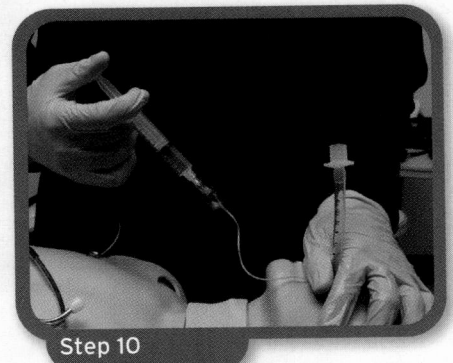

Step 10

Inflate the distal cuff of the ET tube with 5 to 10 mL of air and detach the syringe.

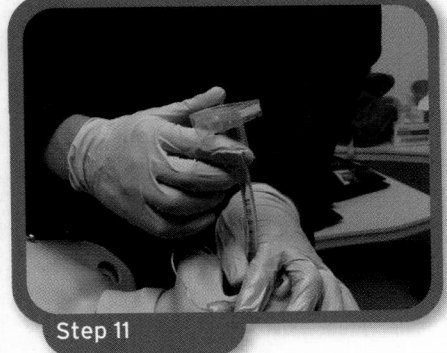

Step 11

Attach the ETco₂ detector to the ET tube.

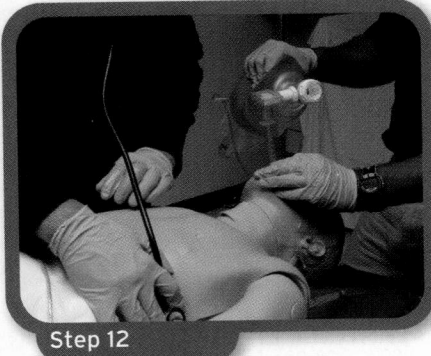

Step 12

Attach the bag-mask device, ventilate, and auscultate over the apices and bases of both lungs and over the epigastrium.

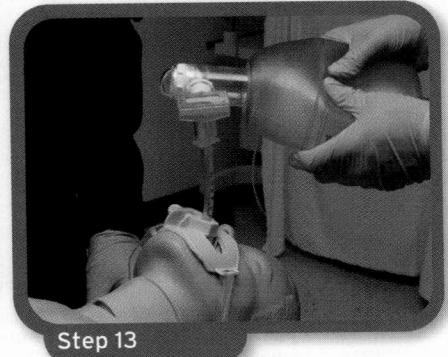

Step 13

Secure the ET tube and recheck breath sounds.

If field extubation is indicated, you must first hyperoxygenate the patient. Discuss the procedure with the patient, and explain what you plan to do. If possible, have the patient sit up or lean slightly forward; this will place him or her in a safe position should vomiting occur after extubation. Assemble and have available all equipment to suction, ventilate, and reintubate, if necessary. After confirming that the patient remains responsive enough to protect his or her own airway, suction the oropharynx to remove any secretions or debris that may threaten the airway once the tube has been removed. Deflate the distal cuff on the ET tube as the patient begins to exhale so that any accumulated secretions proximal to the cuff are not aspirated into the lungs. On the next exhalation, *remove the tube in one steady motion,* following the curvature of the airway. Consider placing a towel or emesis basin in front of the patient's mouth in case vomiting occurs.

The steps for performing extubation are listed here and shown in Skill Drill 11-34 ▶.

1. Hyperoxygenate the patient Step 1.
2. Ensure that ventilation and suction equipment are immediately available Step 2.
3. Confirm patient responsiveness Step 3.
4. Lean the patient forward Step 4.
5. Suction the oropharynx Step 5.
6. Deflate the distal cuff of the ET tube Step 6.
7. Remove the ET tube as the patient coughs or begins to exhale Step 7.

Prior to considering field extubation, you should contact medical control or follow locally established protocols.

The most obvious risk associated with extubation is overestimation of the patient's ability to protect his or her own airway. Additionally, when extubation is performed on conscious patients, there is a high risk of laryngospasm, and most patients experience some degree of upper airway swelling because of the trauma of having the tube in the trachea. These two facts, along with the ever-present potential for vomiting, make successful reintubation challenging, if not impossible. If you are not *absolutely* sure that you can reintubate the patient, do not remove the tube! In most cases, this involves sedating the patient with a benzodiazepine or possibly even using a paralytic for RSI. Field extubation is absolutely contraindicated if there is *any* risk of recurrent respiratory failure or if you are uncertain that the patient can maintain his or her own airway spontaneously.

Pediatric Endotracheal Intubation

Although endotracheal intubation has been considered the means for definitive prehospital airway management in adults, recent studies suggest that effective bag-mask ventilations in the pediatric patient can be as effective as intubation for EMS systems that have short transport times. However, if bag-mask

Skill Drill 11-33: Performing Tracheobronchial Suctioning

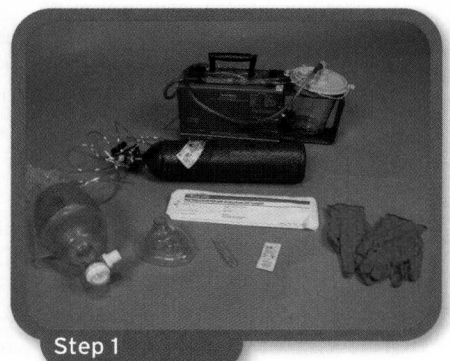

Step 1

Check, prepare, and assemble your equipment.

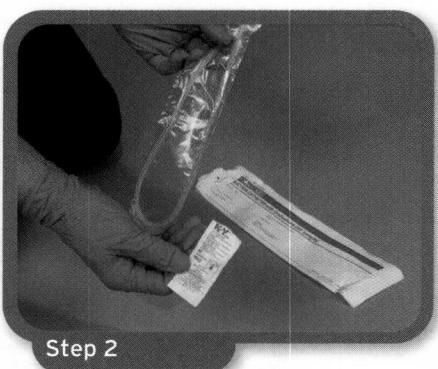

Step 2

Lubricate the suction catheter.

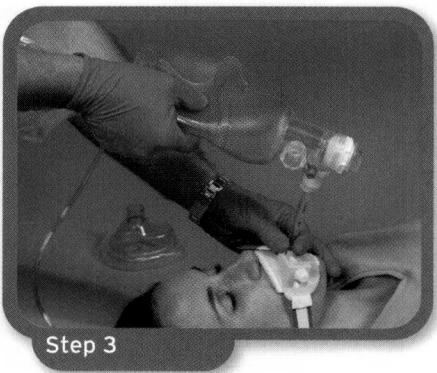

Step 3

Preoxygenate the patient.

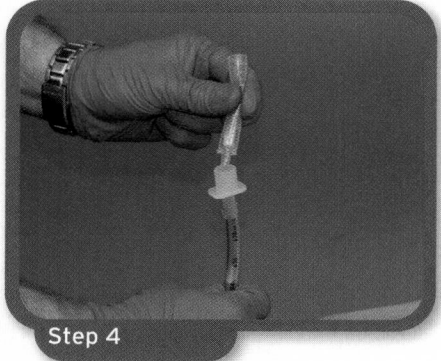

Step 4

Detach the bag-mask device and inject 3 to 5 mL of sterile water down the ET tube.

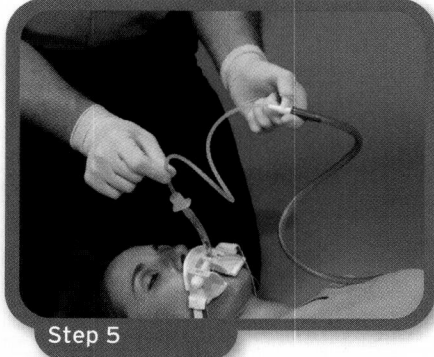

Step 5

Gently insert the catheter into the ET tube until resistance is felt.

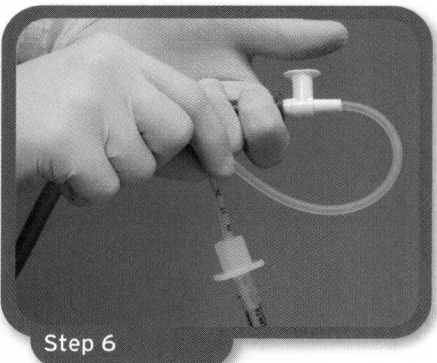

Step 6

Suction in a rotating motion while withdrawing the catheter. Monitor the patient's cardiac rhythm and oxygen saturation during the procedure.

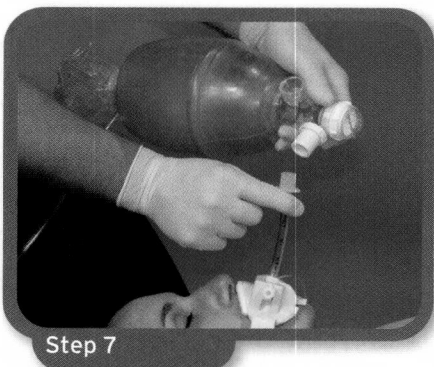

Step 7

Reattach the bag-mask device and resume ventilation and oxygenation.

Skill Drill 11-34: Performing Extubation

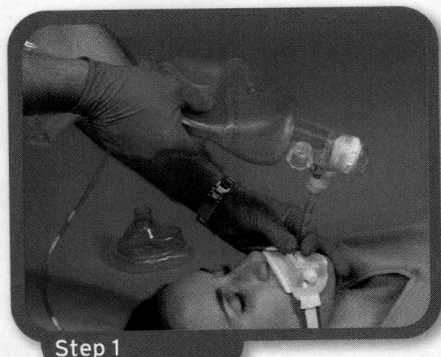
Step 1
Hyperoxygenate the patient.

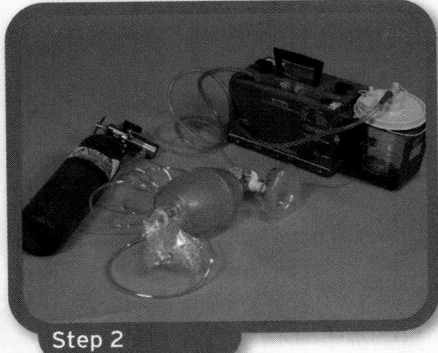
Step 2
Ensure that ventilation and suction equipment are immediately available.

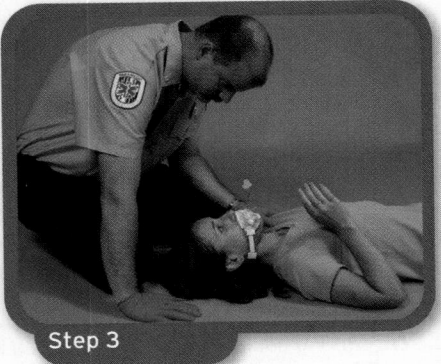
Step 3
Confirm patient responsiveness.

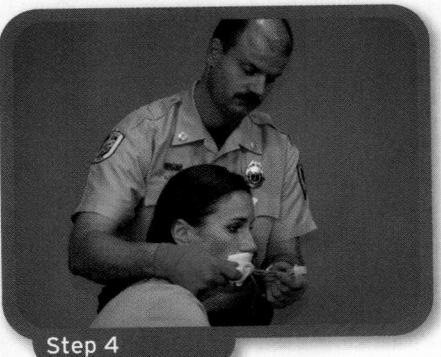
Step 4
Lean the patient forward.

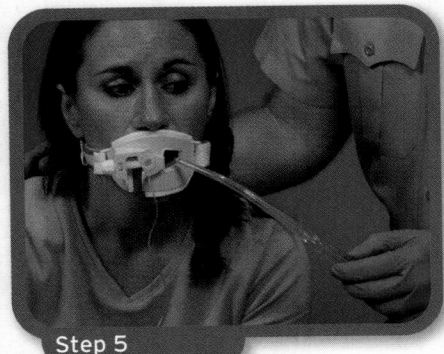
Step 5
Suction the oropharynx.

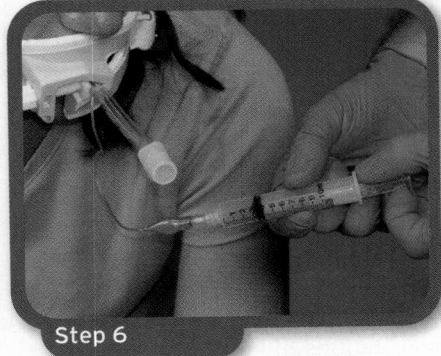
Step 6
Deflate the distal cuff of the ET tube.

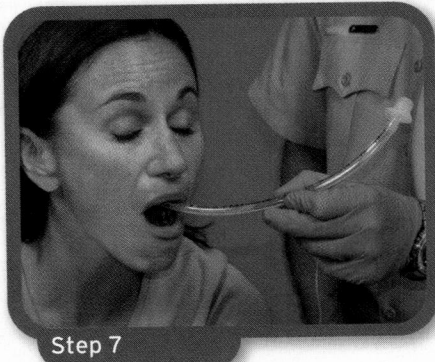
Step 7
Remove the ET tube as the patient coughs or begins to exhale.

Table 11-13	Differences in the Pediatric Airway

- Infants have a larger, rounder occiput, which causes the head of an infant or small child who lies supine to be in a flexed position.
- In children, the tongue is proportionately larger and the mandible is proportionately smaller—differences that increase children's propensity for airway obstruction.
- The epiglottis in a child is more floppy and omega-shaped, so it must be lifted, or positioned, out of the way to visualize the vocal cords.
- The trachea in a child is smaller, shorter, and narrower than an adult's, and it is positioned more anteriorly and superiorly.
- The narrowest portion of the child's airway is the cricoid ring, which is below the vocal cords (subglottic), and the anatomy below the vocal cords is funnel-shaped. This makes a cuff less necessary for occluding the trachea; the developing cartilage of the cricoid ring could potentially be injured by inflation of a cuffed ET tube.

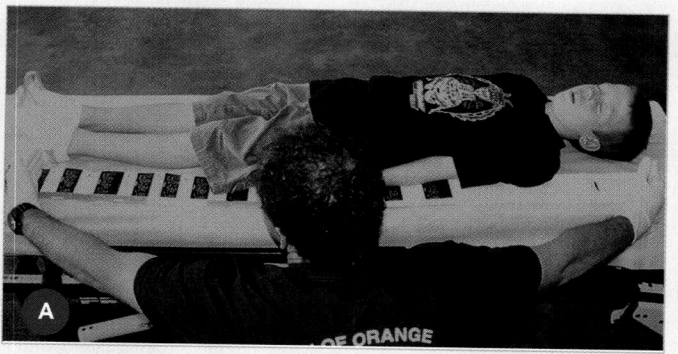

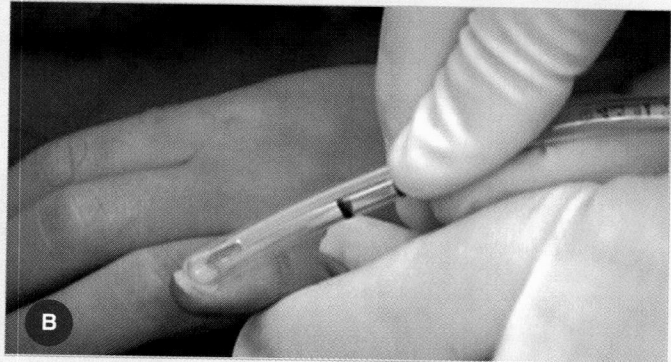

Figure 11-70 A. A length-based resuscitation tape can help estimate a child's ET tube size. **B.** The width of the child's small fingernail can be used to estimate ET tube size.

ventilations are not producing adequate ventilation and oxygenation, the infant or child should be intubated. Indications for endotracheal intubation in pediatric patients are the same as those in adults:

- Cardiopulmonary arrest
- Respiratory failure/arrest
- Traumatic brain injury
- Unresponsiveness
- Inability to maintain a patent airway
- Need for prolonged ventilation
- Need for endotracheal administration of resuscitative medications (if no IV or IO)

Certain anatomic differences between children and adults Table 11-13 ▲ play a key role in performing a successful intubation, as proper airway positioning is critical.

Laryngoscope and Blades

Although any laryngoscope handle can be used to intubate a child, most paramedics prefer the thinner pediatric handles. Straight blades facilitate lifting of the floppy epiglottis. If a curved blade is used, the tip of the blade is positioned in the vallecula to lift the jaw and epiglottis to visualize the vocal cords.

The blade should extend from the child's mouth to the tragus of the ear. Acceptable means of measuring this length include use of a length-based resuscitation tape measure or using the following general guidelines:

- Premature newborn: size 0 straight blade
- Full-term newborn to 1 year of age: size 1 straight blade
- 2 years of age to adolescent: size 2 straight blade
- Adolescent and older: size 3 straight or curved blade

Endotracheal Tubes

ET tube size can be selected by using a length-based resuscitation tape measure Figure 11-70A ▶ . For children older than 1 year of age, *either* of the following formulae can be used:

- Age (in years) ÷ 4 + 4
  - A 4-year-old child would need a 5.0-mm tube (4 [age in years] ÷ 4 + 4 = 5.0)

Table 11-14	Guidelines for Selecting Pediatric Endotracheal Tubes	
Age	**ET Tube (mm)**	**Insertion Depth (cm)**
Premature infant	2.5–3.0 uncuffed	8.0
Full-term infant	3.0–3.5 uncuffed	8.0–9.5
Infant to 1 year	3.5–4.0 uncuffed	9.5–11.0
Toddler	4.0–5.0 uncuffed	11.0–12.5
Preschool	5.0–5.5 uncuffed	12.5–14.0
School age	5.5–6.5 uncuffed	14.0–20.0
Adolescent	7.0–8.0 cuffed	20.0–23.0

- Age (in years) + 16 ÷ 4
  - A 2-year-old child would need a 4.5-mm tube (2 [age in years] + 16 ÷ 4 = 4.5)

Certain anatomic clues, such as the nares or the width of the child's small fingernail Figure 11-70B ▲ can be used to estimate tube size, or you can follow general guidelines based on the child's age Table 11-14 ▲ .

Uncuffed ET tubes should be used in the field until the child is 8 to 10 years of age. A cuff at the cricoid ring is unnecessary to obtain a seal in children in this age range. Furthermore, a cuff can cause ischemia and damage the tracheal mucosa at the level of the cricoid ring. When selecting the appropriate size ET tube, you should have a tube one size smaller as well as one size larger than expected for situations in which there is variability in the child's upper airway diameter.

The appropriate depth of insertion of the ET tube is 2 to 3 cm beyond the vocal cords. After the tube has been inserted, the depth at the corner of the child's mouth should be recorded and monitored. For uncuffed tubes, a black band—the vocal cord guide—often encircles the tube at its distal end. When you see this band at the level of the vocal cords, stop. Cuffed tubes should be inserted until the cuff is just below the level of the vocal cords. Another guideline is to insert the tube to a depth equal to three times the inside diameter (mm) of the ET tube. For example, a 4.0-mm tube should be inserted to a depth of 12.0 cm (12.0 = three times 4 mm).

Pediatric Stylet

The use of a stylet, for the most part, is a matter of personal preference when intubating the pediatric patient. If a stylet is used, insert it into the ET tube, stopping at least 1 cm from the end of the tube. Pediatric stylets will fit into tubes of size 3.0 to 6.0 mm, whereas the adult stylets are used for tubes of size 6.0 mm and larger. After inserting the stylet into the ET tube, bend the tube into a gentle upward curve. In some cases, bending the tube into the shape of a hockey stick is beneficial.

Preoxygenation

Adequate preoxygenation with a bag-mask device and 100% oxygen for at least 30 seconds prior to attempting intubation cannot be overemphasized—respiratory failure or arrest is the most common cause of cardiac arrest in the pediatric population. While preoxygenating the child, you must also ensure that the child's head is in the proper position; this is the neutral position for patients with suspected trauma or the sniffing position otherwise. If needed, insert an airway adjunct; in conjunction with proper manual positioning of the head, it will maintain airway patency and facilitate effective ventilation.

Additional Preparation

Stimulation of the parasympathetic nervous system with resultant bradycardia can occur during intubation in children; therefore, you should apply a cardiac monitor, if available. A pulse oximeter should be used throughout the intubation attempt to monitor the child's heart rate and oxygen saturation. In addition, suction should be readily available to clear oral secretions from the child's airway. In some situations, atropine sulfate in a dose of 0.02 mg/kg may be administered to prevent vagal-induced bradycardia secondary to parasympathetic stimulation.

Intubation Technique

With the child's head in a sniffing position, open his or her mouth by applying thumb pressure on the chin. Some children may require use of the crossfinger technique: use your thumb and index finger or thumb and middle finger to push the upper and lower teeth apart. If an oral airway has been inserted, remove it. If needed, suction the child's mouth and pharynx to remove any secretions.

Hold the laryngoscope handle in your left hand, using your thumb, index finger, and middle finger to hold the handle (the "trigger finger" position). Insert the laryngoscope blade in the right side of the child's mouth, sweeping the tongue to the left side and keeping it under the blade. Advance the blade straight along the tongue, while applying gentle traction upward along the axis of the laryngoscope handle at a 45° angle. *Never use the teeth or gums as a fulcrum for the blade.* A child's teeth could easily be loosened or cracked during a traumatic intubation attempt.

When the blade passes the epiglottis, gently lift the epiglottis if you are using a straight blade. If you are using a curved blade, place the tip of the blade in the vallecula, and lift the jaw, tongue, and blade gently at a 45° angle.

Identify the vocal cords and other normal anatomic landmarks. If they are not visible, have your partner gently apply cricoid pressure. Additional gentle suctioning may be needed to facilitate your view of the vocal cords.

Hold the ET tube in your right hand, and insert the tube from the right-side corner of the child's mouth. Do not pass the tube through the channel of the laryngoscope blade, as you will lose sight of the vocal cords. Guide the tube through the vocal cords, and advance the tube until the glottic/vocal cord mark (black band) is positioned just beyond the vocal cords (approximately 2 to 3 cm). Record the depth of the tube as measured at the right-side corner of the child's mouth, and remove the laryngoscope blade.

Carefully remove the stylet if one was used, while holding the tube securely in place. Next, recheck the tube depth to ensure that it did not become displaced during removal of the stylet. If you are using a cuffed ET tube, inflate the cuff until the pilot balloon is full. Suction the tracheal tube if fluid is present. Attach the tube to a bag-mask device and 100% oxygen. Release cricoid pressure, if used.

Confirm proper ET tube placement by using one or more techniques. Observe the patient for bilateral chest rise during ventilation. Auscultate the lungs bilaterally at the midaxillary line at the third intercostal space, listening for two breaths in each location. If breath sounds are decreased on the left side, the tube may be positioned too deep and aimed toward or in the right mainstem bronchus. To correct this problem, listen to the left side of the chest while ventilating and *carefully* withdrawing the tube, until breath sounds are equal on both sides of the chest. Re-record the depth of the tube.

Breath sounds travel easily in a child because of a child's small chest size. Auscultate over the epigastrium to ensure that no bubbling or gurgling sounds are present. These sounds indicate esophageal intubation, mandating immediate removal of the tube, suctioning as needed, and ventilation with a bag-mask device and 100% oxygen prior to reattempting intubation.

Additional clinical methods to confirm proper ET tube placement include improvement in the child's skin color, pulse rate, and oxygen saturation, as well as use of an ET_{CO_2} detector or esophageal detector device. When using these devices in children, remember two important points: (1) The adult colorimetric $ETCO_2$ detector cannot be used in children weighing less than 15 kg; and (2) the esophageal bulb or syringe cannot be used in children weighing less than 20 kg.

After you confirm proper tube placement, hold the ET tube firmly in place and secure it with tape or a commercially available device. Although several methods for securing an ET tube exist, no single method is foolproof. One person should always hold the tube in place while another properly secures it.

It is important to reconfirm tube placement not only after securing the tube but also following any patient movement (eg, onto the stretcher or into the ambulance), because tubes can easily become dislodged. To do so, auscultate for bilateral breath sounds and epigastric sounds. Once tube position has been confirmed, resume ventilations with 100% oxygen at the appropriate rate.

If you realize the tube is too large or you cannot identify the vocal cords and glottic landmarks, abort the intubation attempt and ventilate the child with the bag-mask device and 100% oxygen. Modify your equipment selection accordingly, and start the procedure from the beginning. If intubation cannot be accomplished after two attempts, discontinue attempts, and resume bag-mask ventilation for the remainder of the transport.

The steps for performing pediatric endotracheal intubation are listed here and shown in Skill Drill 11-35 ▶.

1. Take BSI precautions (gloves and face shield) (Step 1).
2. Check, prepare, and assemble your equipment (Step 2).
3. Manually open the child's airway and insert an adjunct if needed (Step 3).
4. Preoxygenate the child with a bag-mask device and 100% oxygen for at least 30 seconds (Step 4).
5. Insert the laryngoscope in the right side of the mouth and sweep the tongue to the left. Lift the tongue with firm,

gentle pressure. Avoid using the teeth or gums as a fulcrum (Step 5).
6. Identify the vocal cords. If the cords are not yet visible, instruct your partner to apply cricoid pressure (Step 6).
7. Introduce the ET tube in the right corner of the child's mouth (Step 7).
8. Pass the ET tube through the vocal cords to approximately 2 to 3 cm below the vocal cords. Inflate the cuff if a cuffed tube is used (Step 8).
9. Attach an $ETCO_2$ detector (Step 9).
10. Attach the bag-mask device, and auscultate for equal breath sounds over each lateral chest wall high in the axillae. Ensure absence of breath sounds over the epigastrium (Step 10).
11. Secure the ET tube, noting the placement of the distance marker at the child's teeth or gums and reconfirm tube placement (Step 11).

If an intubated child's condition acutely deteriorates, you must take immediate action to identify and correct the underlying problem. The DOPE mnemonic (Displacement, Obstruction, Pneumothorax, and Equipment failure) can be used to recall the common causes of acute deterioration in the intubated child (Table 11-15 ▼).

Complications of Endotracheal Intubation

Complications associated with endotracheal intubation in the pediatric patient are essentially the same as those for adult patients:

- **Unrecognized esophageal intubation.** *Frequently* monitor the position of the tube, especially after *any* major patient move.
- **Induction of emesis and possible aspiration.** *Always* have a suctioning device immediately available.
- **Hypoxia resulting from prolonged intubation attempts.** Limit pediatric intubation attempts to *20 seconds.* Monitor the child's cardiac rhythm and oxygen saturation during intubation.
- **Damage to teeth, soft tissues, and intraoral structures.** Technique, technique, technique!

Table 11-15	Troubleshooting Acute Deterioration With the DOPE Mnemonic in the Intubated Child
Displacement	■ Reauscultate breath sounds and over the epigastrium ■ If breath sounds are stronger on the right, slowly withdraw the tube until they are equal bilaterally ■ If breath sounds are absent and you hear epigastric gurgling, immediately remove the ET tube, suction as needed, and ventilate with a bag-mask device and 100% oxygen
Obstruction	■ If thick pulmonary secretions are interfering with your ability to effectively ventilate the intubated child, perform tracheobronchial suctioning ■ Consider tube obstruction if ventilation compliance is decreased (eg, it is hard to squeeze the bag)
Pneumothorax	■ Suspect a pneumothorax if breath sounds are stronger on the *left* and decreased or absent on the right; such findings are not consistent with right mainstem intubation ■ Ventilation compliance may also be decreased in a child with a pneumothorax ■ Prepare to perform needle decompression
Equipment failure	■ Ensure that you are delivering 100% oxygen ■ Check the reservoir bag on the bag-mask device for tears, ensure that the device is attached to a 100% oxygen source, and check the bag itself for tears ■ Immediately replace defective or damaged equipment

Skill Drill 11-35: Performing Pediatric Endotracheal Intubation

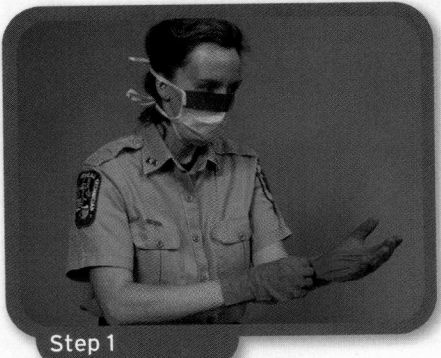

Step 1

Take BSI precautions (gloves and face shield).

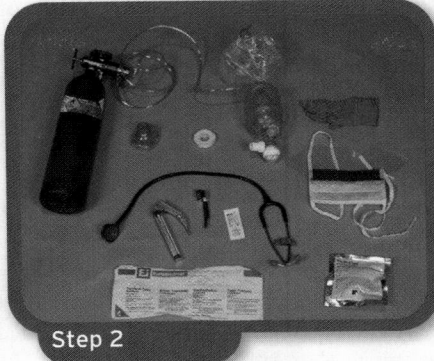

Step 2

Check, prepare, and assemble your equipment.

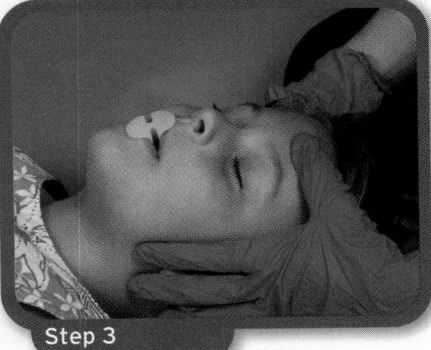

Step 3

Manually open the child's airway and insert an adjunct if needed.

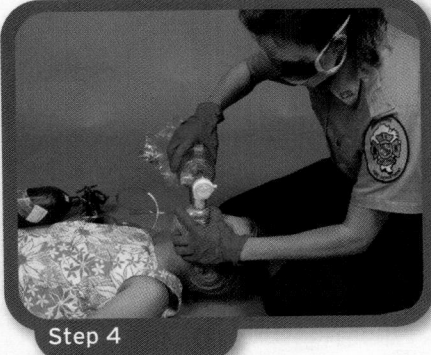

Step 4

Preoxygenate the child with a bag-mask device and 100% oxygen for at least 30 seconds.

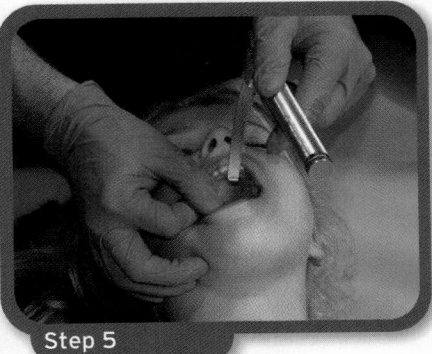

Step 5

Insert the laryngoscope in the right side of the mouth and sweep the tongue to the left. Lift the tongue with firm, gentle pressure. Avoid using the teeth or gums as a fulcrum.

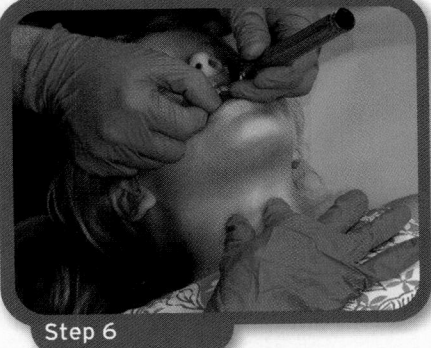

Step 6

Identify the vocal cords. If the cords are not yet visible, instruct your partner to apply cricoid pressure.

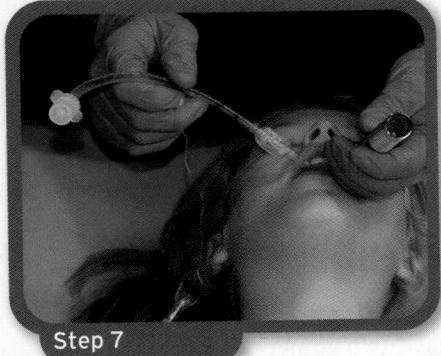

Step 7

Introduce the ET tube in the right corner of the child's mouth.

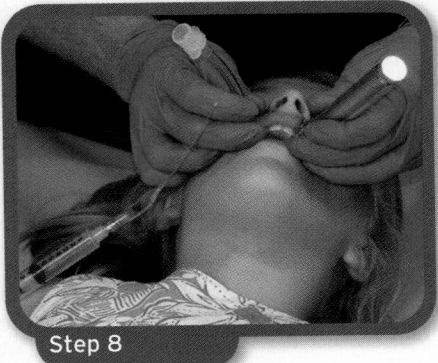

Step 8

Pass the ET tube through the vocal cords to approximately 2 to 3 cm below the vocal cords. Inflate the cuff if a cuffed tube is used.

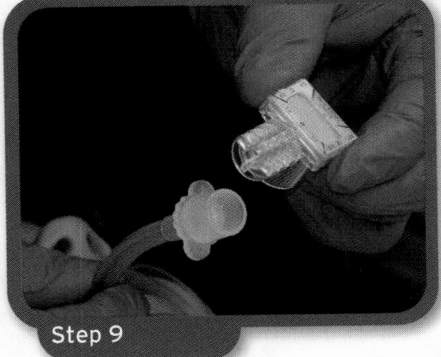

Step 9

Attach an ET$_{CO_2}$ detector.

Skill Drill 11-35: Performing Pediatric Endotracheal Intubation (*continued*)

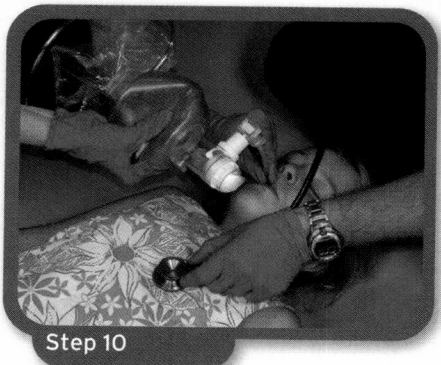

Step 10

Attach the bag-mask device, and auscultate for equal breath sounds over each lateral chest wall high in the axillae. Ensure absence of breath sounds over the epigastrium.

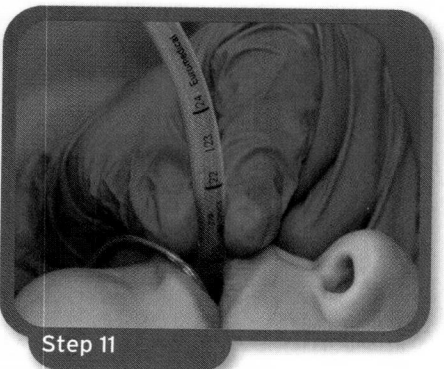

Step 11

Secure the ET tube, noting the placement of the distance marker at the child's teeth or gums and reconfirm tube placement.

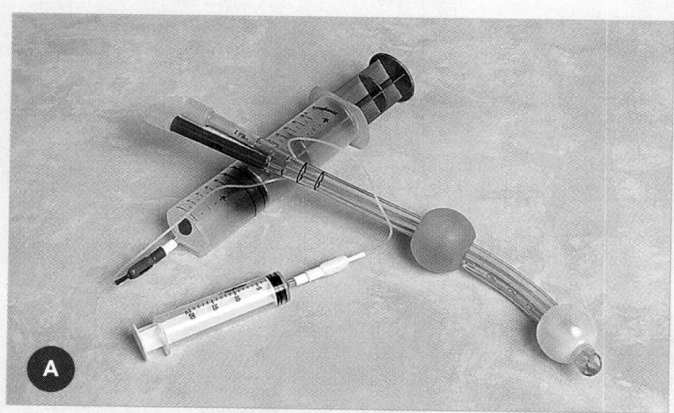

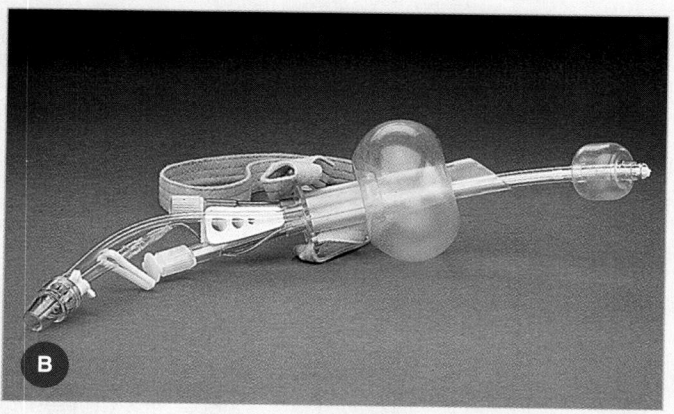

Figure 11-71 A. Combitube. **B.** Pharyngeotracheal lumen airway.

In the Field

A single pediatric intubation attempt should not exceed 20 seconds. If intubation cannot be performed within this time frame, abort the attempt and resume bag-mask ventilations with 100% oxygen.

Multilumen Airways

Compared with esophageal airways, the Combitube and the pharyngeotracheal lumen airway (PtL) have shown to provide better airway management and ventilation Figure 11-71 ▲ . Both devices have a long tube that is blindly inserted into the airway. This tube can be used for either esophageal obturation or endotracheal intubation; as a result, ventilation is possible regardless of whether the tube is placed into the esophagus or the trachea. The presence of an oropharyngeal balloon also eliminates the need for a mask seal.

These devices have two lumens, each with a 15/22-mm ventilation adapter. The proper port for ventilation depends on where the tube is positioned during insertion. Both types of multilumen airways have a proximal cuff, which is inflated in the oropharynx to eliminate the need for a face mask.

Indications and Contraindications

Multilumen airways are indicated only for use in deeply unresponsive, apneic patients without a gag reflex. If the patient regains consciousness, the device must be removed.

These devices are contraindicated in pediatric patients, and they should be used only for patients between 5 and 7 feet tall.

While there is only one size PtL, a smaller version of the Combitube, called the Combitube SA (small adult), can be used on adults taller than 4 feet. Because the tube is typically inserted into the esophagus, neither the PtL nor the Combitube should be used in patients with esophageal trauma, known esophageal diseases (eg, cancer, varices), or in those who have ingested a caustic substance.

Advantages and Disadvantages

The major advantage of the multilumen airway is that, in effect, it cannot be improperly placed; effective ventilation is possible if the tube enters the esophagus or the trachea. Insertion of the multilumen airway is also technically easier than endotracheal intubation. Furthermore, because insertion of the airway is performed with the patient's head in the neutral position, cervical spine movement is kept to a minimum. Additionally, no mask seal is required to ventilate with the Combitube or PtL.

Multilumen airways also provide some patency to the airway. If the tube is placed in the trachea, it functions exactly like an ET tube, and no upper airway positioning is required. If the tube is placed in the esophagus, the pharyngeal balloon creates an airtight seal in the oropharynx, making the tongue position less of a factor in the maintenance of a patent airway. A jaw-thrust maneuver should easily alleviate any ventilatory difficulty if the epiglottis partially obstructs the airway.

Use of a multilumen airway requires strict attention and good assessment skills because ventilation in the wrong port results in no pulmonary ventilation. These devices are usually considered temporary airways and should be replaced as soon as possible. The pharyngeal balloon mitigates, but does not completely eliminate, the risk of aspiration. Additionally, intubating the trachea via direct laryngoscopy with a multilumen airway in place, although possible, can be extremely challenging.

Complications

The most significant complication associated with the use of multilumen airways is unrecognized displacement of the tube into the esophagus. Good assessment skills are essential to properly confirm tube placement, and multiple confirmation techniques should be employed following insertion of the device.

Laryngospasm, vomiting, and possible hypoventilation may occur during insertion of a multilumen airway. Additionally, pharyngeal or esophageal trauma may result secondary to poor technique.

Ventilation may be difficult if the pharyngeal balloon pushes the epiglottis over the glottic opening. A few cases of difficult ventilation have occurred with multilumen airways. However, in all cases, ventilation became easier when the device was withdrawn 2 to 4 cm.

Equipment

The PtL consists of two tubes and two cuffs. The longer tube passes through the shorter, wider tube. The longer tube is 31 cm long and 8 mm in diameter and usually is inserted into the esophagus. This tube is open at its distal tip and has a balloon at its distal end. A semirigid stylet maintains the curvature and

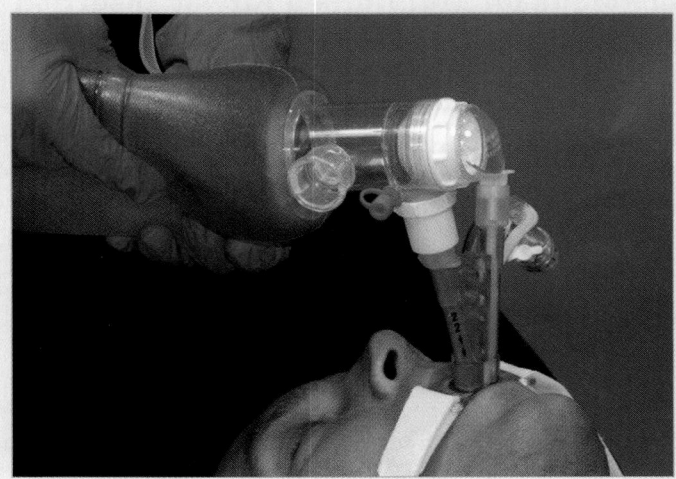

Figure 11-72 Ventilation with a PtL in place.

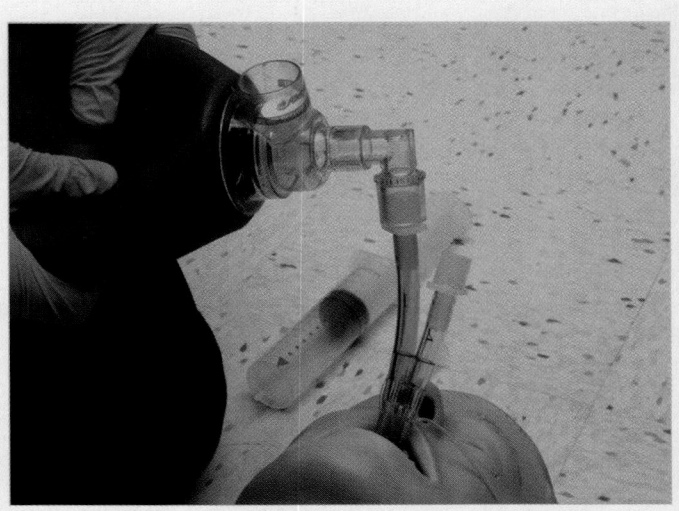

Figure 11-73 Ventilation with a Combitube in place.

rigidity of the long tube and occludes the tip. The shorter tube is 21 cm long and is designed to come to rest with its distal tip deep in the oropharynx. A large low-pressure cuff is inflated proximal to the tip of the shorter tube. Both cuffs are inflated simultaneously with an in-series valve system that can be inflated with a bag-mask device. The short tube is made of hard plastic to resist damage from biting, and a strap goes around the head to secure the device Figure 11-72 ▲.

The Combitube consists of a single tube with two lumens, two balloons, and two ventilation ports. One lumen is open at its distal end; the other is closed. The closed lumen has side holes distal to the pharyngeal balloon. The proximal balloon is designed to be inflated with 100 mL of air and provides a pharyngeal seal. The distal balloon is inflated with 15 mL of air and makes an airtight seal with the walls of the trachea (if placed in the trachea) or leads to esophageal obturation (if placed in the esophagus) Figure 11-73 ▲.

Technique for Multilumen Airway Insertion

While multilumen airways can be used to ventilate regardless of whether the tube is placed into the esophagus or the trachea, this flexibility makes confirmation of ventilation extremely important. If you use the wrong port, the patient will not receive any pulmonary ventilation. Confirmation of ventilation is, therefore, a critical part of the procedure for using multilumen airways.

Procedures Before and During Insertion

Check and prepare all your equipment. Check both cuffs to ensure that they hold air. The patient should be preoxygenated with a bag-mask device and 100% oxygen before insertion. *Ventilation should not be interrupted for longer than 30 seconds to accomplish airway placement.* For both PtL and Combitube insertion, the patient's head should be placed in a neutral position.

- *Forwardly displace the jaw.* With the patient's head in a neutral position, insert the thumb of your gloved nondominant hand into the patient's mouth and lift the jaw. This action lifts the hyoid bone and pulls the base of the tongue off the posterior pharyngeal wall.
- *Insert the device.* Following the curvature of the tube, insert the device blindly into the posterior pharynx. Insert the Combitube until the incisors are between the two black lines printed on the tube. Insert the PtL until the flange comes to rest on the teeth. Be gentle, and stop advancing the tube if you meet resistance.
- *Inflate the cuffs.* In the PtL, the cuffs inflate together through an in-line valve system. Attach a bag-mask device to the inflation adapter, and inflate the cuffs until the pilot balloon is firm. Close the clamp to prevent air leakage. In the Combitube, two independent inflation valves must be inflated sequentially. The first inflation valve goes to the pharyngeal balloon and is inflated with 100 mL of air. The second inflation valve inflates the distal balloon and is filled with 15 mL of air.

Procedures After Insertion

After you inflate the balloons, begin to ventilate the patient. With the PtL, first ventilate through the short tube (the tube without the stylet); with the Combitube, ventilate through the longer (blue) tube. Confirm adequate chest rise and the presence of breath sounds. If there are no breath sounds and the chest does not rise during ventilation, switch immediately to the other ventilation port. Be sure to continuously monitor ventilation. Both multilumen airways are generally secure in the airway owing to the large pharyngeal balloons. Nevertheless, the head strap of the PtL should be attached because inadvertent removal of a multilumen airway would be traumatic.

The steps for insertion of a PtL are listed here and shown in **Skill Drill 11-36 ▶**.

1. Take BSI precautions (gloves and face shield) (Step 1).
2. Preoxygenate the patient with a bag-mask device and 100% oxygen (Step 2).

3. Place the patient's head in a neutral position (Step 3).
4. Open the patient's mouth with the tongue-jaw lift maneuver, and insert the PtL in the midline of the patient's mouth (Step 4).
5. Inflate the proximal and distal cuffs (Step 5).
6. Ventilate the patient through the pharyngeal (green) tube first. If the chest rises, continue to ventilate through the green tube (Step 6).
7. If the chest does not rise, remove the stylet from the clear tube and ventilate through the clear tube (Step 7).
8. Confirm placement by auscultating for breath sounds over the lungs and gastric sounds over the abdomen (Step 8).

The steps for insertion of a Combitube are listed here and shown in **Skill Drill 11-37 ▶**.

1. Take BSI precautions (gloves and face shield) (Step 1).
2. Preoxygenate the patient with a bag-mask device and 100% oxygen (Step 2).
3. Gather your equipment (Step 3).
4. Place the patient's head in a neutral position (Step 4).
5. Open the patient's mouth with the tongue-jaw lift maneuver, and insert the Combitube in the midline of the patient's mouth. Insert the tube until the incisors lie between the two reference marks (Step 5).
6. Inflate the pharyngeal cuff with 100 mL of air (Step 6).
7. Inflate the distal cuff with 15 mL of air (Step 7).
8. Ventilate the patient through the pharyngeal (blue) tube first. Chest rise indicates esophageal placement of distal tip; continue to ventilate (Step 8).
9. No chest rise indicates tracheal placement; switch ports and ventilate (Step 9).
10. Confirm placement by auscultating for breath sounds over the lungs and gastric sounds over the abdomen (Step 10).

▌ The Laryngeal Mask Airway

The laryngeal mask airway (LMA) was originally developed for use in the operating room as an alternative to bag-mask ventilation, which is commonly used during short surgical procedures, and endotracheal intubation, during which longer periods of anesthesia are required **Figure 11-74 ▶**. The LMA was not designed for emergency use, and, although it is not a replacement for endotracheal intubation, it may have a role in emergency situations if intubation is not possible, multilumen airways (eg, PtL, Combitube) are not available, and the only viable option is mask ventilation.

The LMA is designed to provide a conduit from the glottic opening to the ventilation device. It surrounds the opening of the larynx with an inflatable silicone cuff positioned in the hypopharynx. When properly inserted, the opening of the LMA is positioned at the glottic opening, and the tip is inserted into the proximal esophagus, the lateral portions in the pyriform fossae, and the upper border at the base of the tongue.

Skill Drill 11-36: Insertion of the PtL

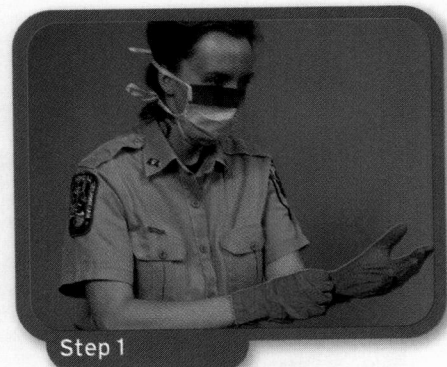

Step 1

Take BSI precautions (gloves and face shield).

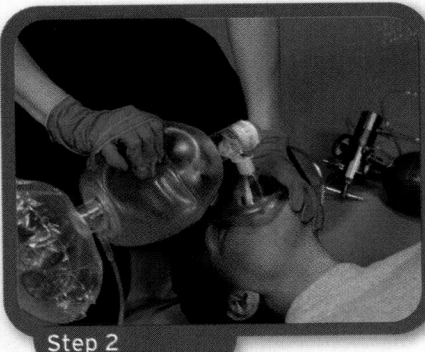

Step 2

Preoxygenate the patient with a bag-mask device and 100% oxygen.

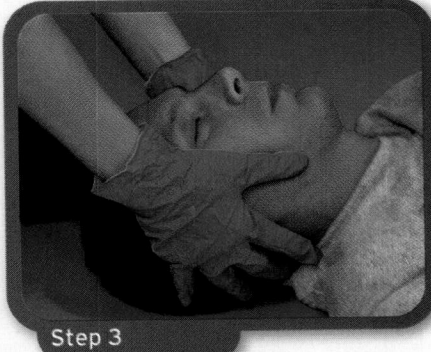

Step 3

Place the patient's head in a neutral position.

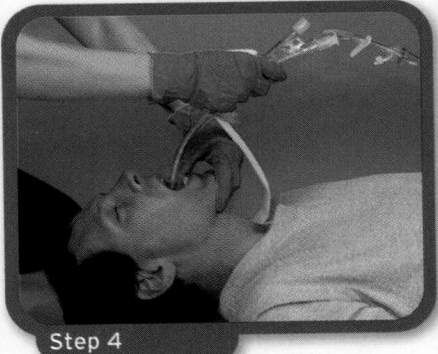

Step 4

Open the patient's mouth with the tongue-jaw lift maneuver, and insert the PtL in the midline of the patient's mouth.

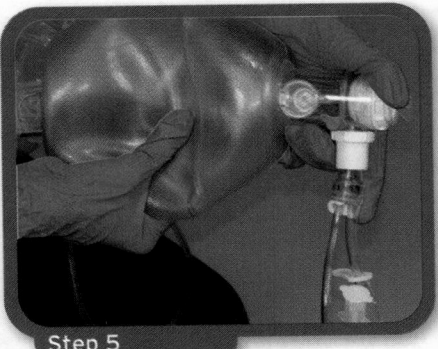

Step 5

Inflate the proximal and distal cuffs.

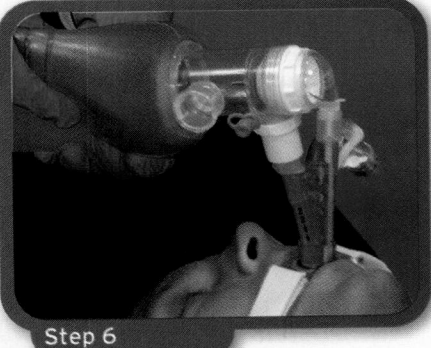

Step 6

Ventilate the patient through the pharyngeal (green) tube first. If the chest rises, continue to ventilate through the green tube.

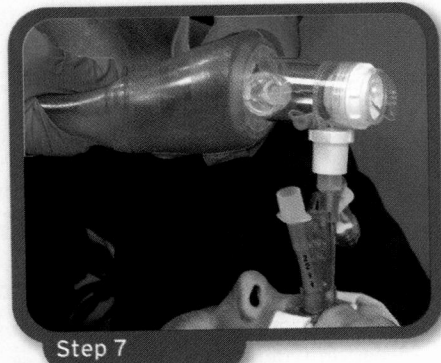

Step 7

If the chest does not rise, remove the stylet from the clear tube and ventilate through the clear tube.

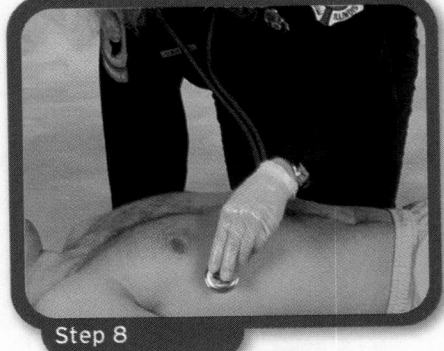

Step 8

Confirm placement by auscultating for breath sounds over the lungs and gastric sounds over the abdomen.

Skill Drill 11-37: Insertion of the Combitube

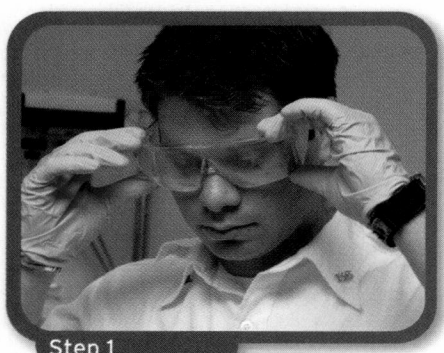

Step 1

Take BSI precautions (gloves and face shield).

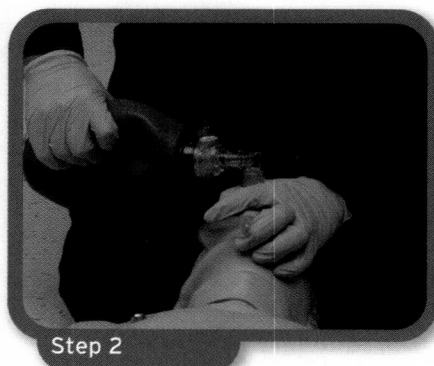

Step 2

Preoxygenate the patient with a bag-mask device and 100% oxygen.

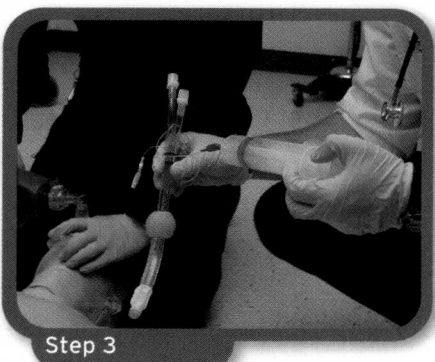

Step 3

Gather your equipment.

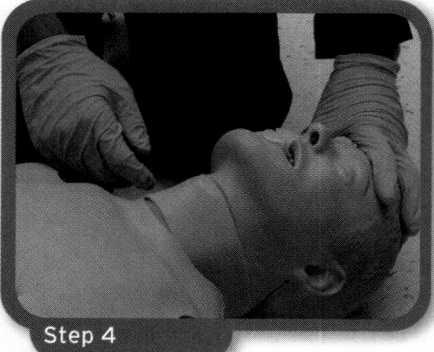

Step 4

Place the patient's head in a neutral position.

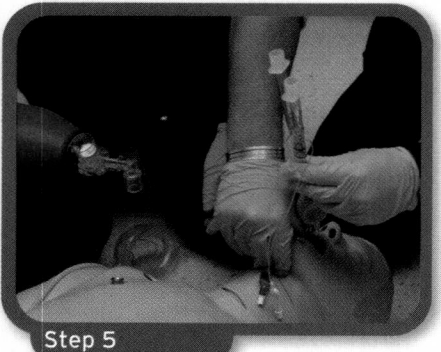

Step 5

Open the patient's mouth with the tongue-jaw lift maneuver, and insert the Combitube in the midline of the patient's mouth. Insert the tube until the incisors lie between the two reference marks.

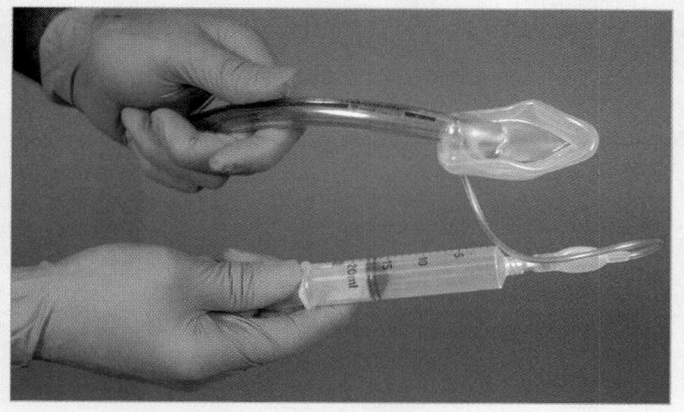

Figure 11-74 The laryngeal mask airway.

The inflatable cuff conforms to the contours of the airway and forms a relatively airtight seal **Figure 11-75 ▶**.

Indications and Contraindications

The LMA should be considered as an alternative to bag-mask ventilation when the patient cannot be intubated.

The product literature states that the LMA should be used only in patients who are fasting. Unfortunately, this would eliminate all emergency patients, who should always be presumed to have full stomachs. You must weigh the risk of aspiration against the risk of hypoventilation with bag-mask ventilation in the context of the clinical scenario.

The LMA is less effective in obese patients and should not be used in morbidly obese patients. Pregnant patients and patients with a hiatal hernia are at an increased risk for regurgitation and must be evaluated carefully if LMA use is considered.

Skill Drill 11-37: Insertion of the Combitube (*continued*)

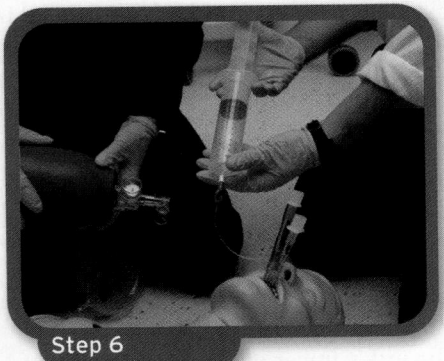

Step 6
Inflate the pharyngeal cuff with 100 mL of air.

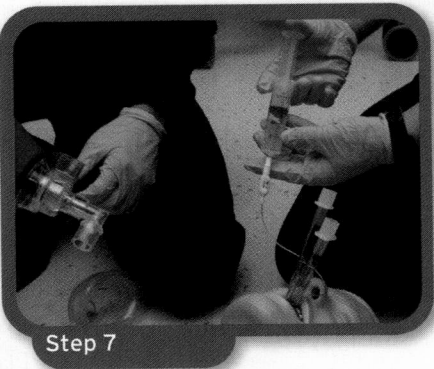

Step 7
Inflate the distal cuff with 15 mL of air.

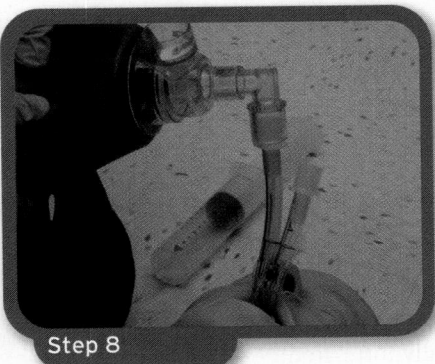

Step 8
Ventilate the patient through the pharyngeal (blue) tube first. Chest rise indicates esophageal placement of distal tip; continue to ventilate.

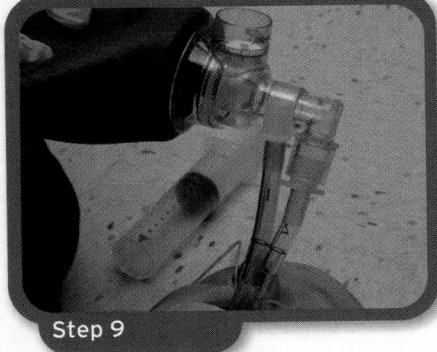

Step 9
No chest rise indicates tracheal placement; switch ports and ventilate.

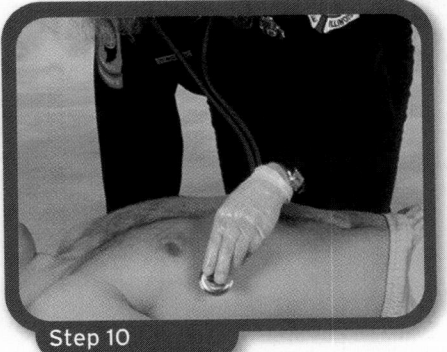

Step 10
Confirm placement by auscultating for breath sounds over the lungs and gastric sounds over the abdomen.

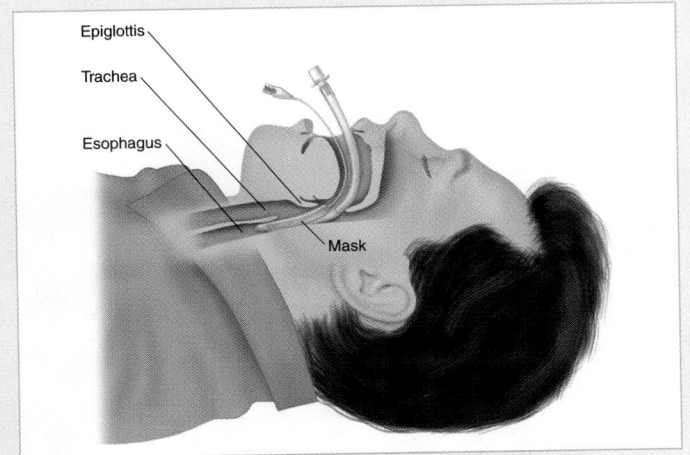

Figure 11-75 The opening of the LMA is positioned at the glottic opening, the tip at the entrance of the esophagus, the lateral portions in the pyriform fossae, and the upper border at the base of the tongue.

The LMA is ineffective for the ventilation of patients requiring high pulmonary pressures (eg, COPD, congestive heart failure).

Advantages and Disadvantages

The LMA has been shown to provide better oxygenation than bag-mask ventilation with an oral airway. Furthermore, ventilation with the LMA does not require the continual maintenance of a mask seal. Compared to endotracheal intubation, LMA insertion is easier and does not require laryngoscopy. There is also significantly less risk of trauma to soft tissue, vocal cords, the tracheal wall, and teeth. The LMA provides protection from upper airway secretions, and the tip of the LMA wedged into the proximal esophagus may provide some obturation.

The main disadvantage of the LMA, especially in emergencies, is that it does not provide protection against aspiration. In fact, the LMA actually increases the risk of aspiration if the patient regurgitates because his or her stomach contents would most likely be directed into the trachea. During prolonged LMA ventilation, some air may be insufflated into the stomach because the seal made in the airway is not airtight. Because of this risk of aspiration, the LMA is unlikely to replace endotracheal intubation in prehospital emergency airway management. *The LMA should not be considered a primary airway device for emergency patients.* It should, however, be considered superior to bag-mask ventilation in patients who cannot be endotracheally intubated.

Complications

The most significant complications associated with use of the LMA involve regurgitation and subsequent aspiration. The incidence of LMA misplacement in the operating room is relatively low and appears to decrease with experience. Nonetheless, the paramedic should observe the patient for clinical indications of inadequate ventilation (eg, chest rise, breath sounds) during LMA ventilation. Hypoventilation of patients who require high ventilatory pressures can also occur. A few cases of upper airway swelling have been reported.

Equipment

The LMA comes in five sizes, with the selection of a size being based on the patient's weight. The device consists of an inflatable cuff attached to an obliquely cut tube. The cuff provides a collar that positions the opening of the tube at the glottic opening when inflated. Two vertical bars at the opening of the tube prevent occlusion. The proximal end of the tube is fitted with a standard 15/22-mm adapter that is compatible with any ventilation device. The cuff has a one-way valve assembly and should be inflated with a predetermined volume of air (based on the size of the airway) **Figure 11-76 ▾** .

Technique for Laryngeal Mask Airway Insertion

Procedures Before and During Insertion

Check and prepare all equipment. Check the cuff of the LMA by inflating it with 50% more air than is required for that size airway. Next, deflate the cuff so that no folds appear near the tip. Deflation is best accomplished by pressing the device, cuff down, on a flat surface **Figure 11-77 ▾** . Lubricate the base of the device.

Preoxygenate the patient with a bag-mask device and 100% oxygen prior to inserting the LMA. Ventilation should not be interrupted for more than 30 seconds to accomplish placement of the LMA. Place the patient's head in a sniffing position.

- *Insert your finger between the cuff and the tube.* Proper insertion of the LMA depends on holding the device properly. Place the index finger of your dominant hand in the notch between the tube and the cuff. Open the patient's mouth.
- *Insert the LMA along the roof of the mouth.* The key to proper insertion is to slide the convex surface of the LMA along the roof of the mouth. Use your finger to push the airway against the hard palate. Once it slides past the tongue, the LMA will move easily into position.
- *Inflate the cuff.* Inflate the cuff of the LMA with the amount of air indicated for that size airway. If the LMA is properly positioned, it will move out of the airway slightly (1 to 2 cm) as it seats into position.

Procedures After Insertion

Following inflation of the cuff, attach the bag-mask device and begin to ventilate the patient. Confirm chest rise and the presence of breath sounds. Continuously and closely monitor for regurgitation in the tube. Carefully reassess the airway during any patient movement, and be prepared to ventilate with a bag-mask device and 100% oxygen if the LMA becomes dislodged.

A 6.0-mm ET tube can be passed through a size 3 or 4 LMA, allowing for intubation. The vertical bars are designed to allow a well-lubricated tube to pass straight through, and research in the operating room found a high success rate of

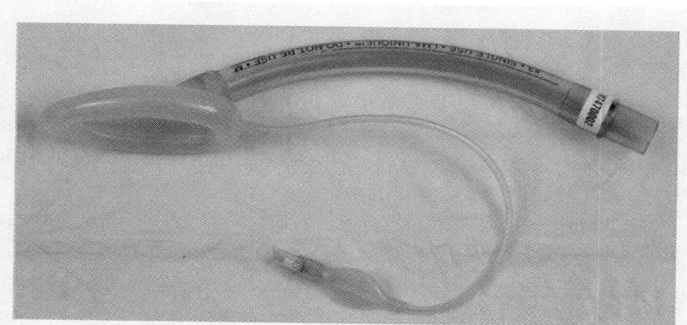

Figure 11-76 The LMA with the cuff inflated.

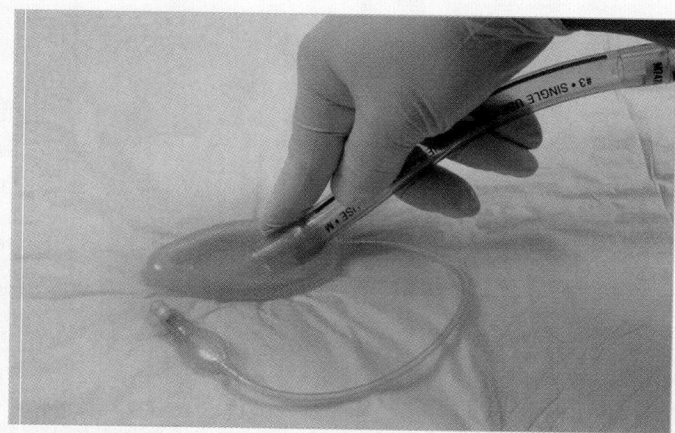

Figure 11-77 Press the LMA, cuff down, against a flat surface to remove all wrinkles from the cuff.

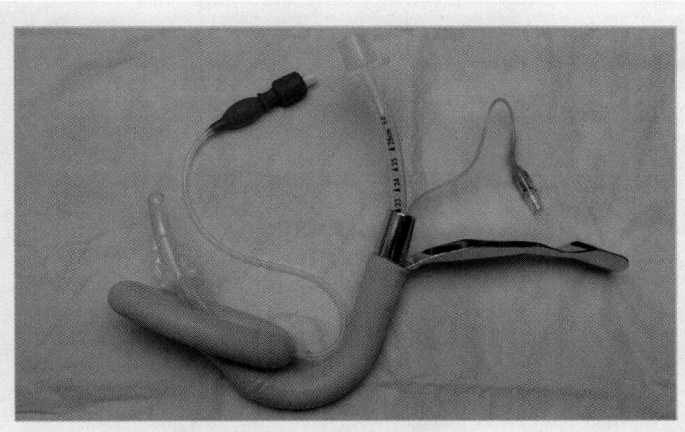

Figure 11-78 The Fasttrach LMA with a 6.0-mm ET tube.

endotracheal intubation following this technique. The Fast-trach LMA is designed to guide an ET tube into the trachea and may prove to be a viable alternative to direct laryngoscopy Figure 11-78 ▲ .

The steps for inserting an LMA are summarized here and shown in Skill Drill 11-38 ▶ .

1. Check the cuff of the LMA by inflating it with 50% more air than is required for that size airway. Then deflate the cuff completely Step 1 .
2. Lubricate the base of the device Step 2 .
3. Preoxygenate the patient with a bag-mask device and 100% oxygen. Ventilation should not be interrupted for more than 30 seconds to accomplish LMA placement. Place the patient's head in the sniffing position Step 3 .
4. Insert your finger between the cuff and the tube. Place the index finger of your dominant hand in the notch between the tube and the cuff. Open the patient's mouth Step 4 .
5. Insert the LMA along the roof of the mouth. Use your finger to push the airway against the hard palate Step 5 .

6. Inflate the cuff with the amount of air indicated for that sized airway Step 6 .
7. Attach the bag-mask device and begin to ventilate the patient. Confirm chest rise and the presence of breath sounds. Continuously and closely monitor the patient Step 7 .

Pharmacologic Adjuncts to Airway Management and Ventilation

Pharmacologic agents in airway management are used to decrease the discomfort of intubation, decrease the incidence of complications associated with laryngoscopy and intubation, and make aggressive airway management possible for patients who need it but who are too conscious or combative to cooperate.

Sedation in Emergency Intubation

Sedation is used in airway management to reduce the patient's anxiety, induce amnesia, and to decrease the gag reflex. It is useful for anxious, combative, or agitated patients, as well as for patients who need aggressive airway management but who are too conscious to tolerate intubation. If used properly, and under the correct circumstances, sedation effectively increases patient compliance, thus making definitive airway management easier and safer to perform. If used improperly, however, it can cause further harm.

The complications associated with sedation in airway management are related primarily to undersedation or oversedation. Undersedation can result in poor patient cooperation, the complications of gagging (eg, trauma, tachycardia, hypertension, vomiting, or aspiration), and incomplete amnesia of the event. Oversedation can result in uncontrolled general anesthesia, loss of protective airway reflexes, respiratory depression, complete airway collapse, and hypotension.

You are the Provider Part 10

Your patient's condition has now stabilized. He is delivered to the emergency department, where you give your verbal report to the attending physician. The patient is admitted with a diagnosis of acute exacerbation of congestive heart failure.

Reassessment	Recording Time: 35 Minutes
Level of consciousness	Sedated
Respirations	Ventilated with an ATV and 100% oxygen at a rate of 12 breaths/min
Pulse	100 beats/min, strong and regular
Skin	Pink and moist
Blood pressure	130/80 mm Hg
Sao_2	98% while being ventilated with an ATV and 100% oxygen

17. What treatment would have been appropriate had this clinically unstable patient been too conscious or combative to intubate?

Skill Drill 11-38: LMA Insertion

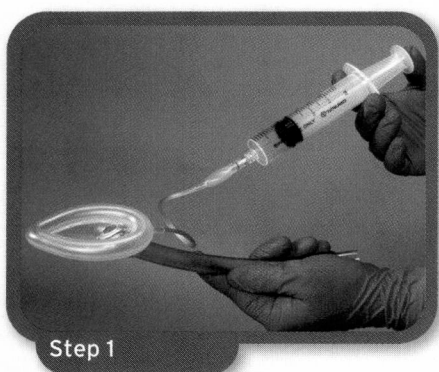

Step 1

Check the cuff of the LMA by inflating it with 50% more air than is required for that size airway. Then deflate the cuff completely.

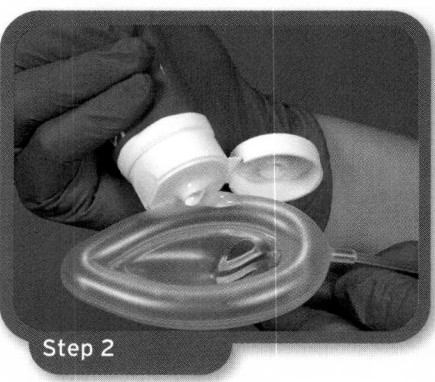

Step 2

Lubricate the base of the device.

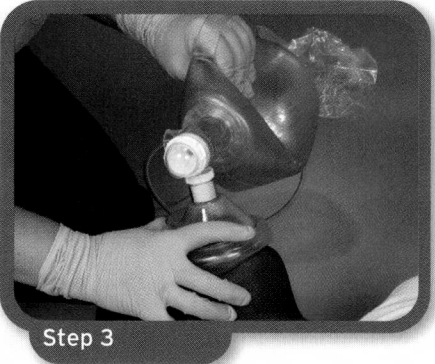

Step 3

Preoxygenate the patient with a bag-mask device and 100% oxygen. Ventilation should not be interrupted for more than 30 seconds to accomplish LMA placement. Place the patient's head in the sniffing position.

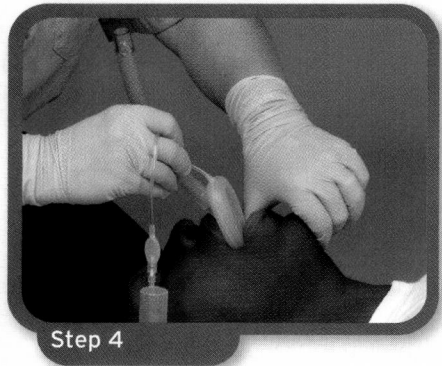

Step 4

Insert your finger between the cuff and the tube. Place the index finger of your dominant hand in the notch between the tube and the cuff. Open the patient's mouth.

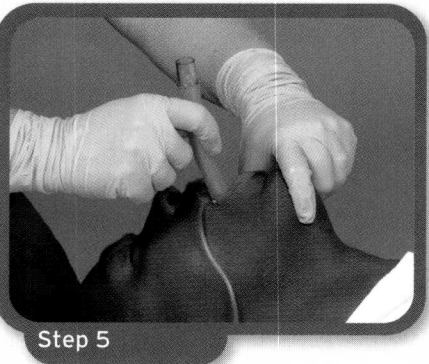

Step 5

Insert the LMA along the roof of the mouth. Use your finger to push the airway against the hard palate.

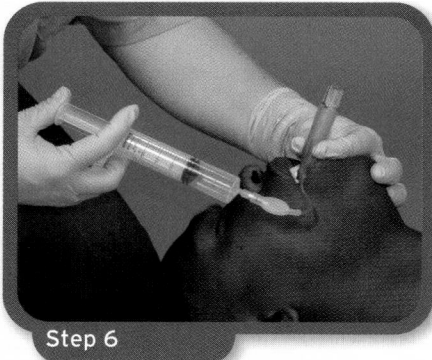

Step 6

Inflate the cuff with the amount of air indicated for that size airway.

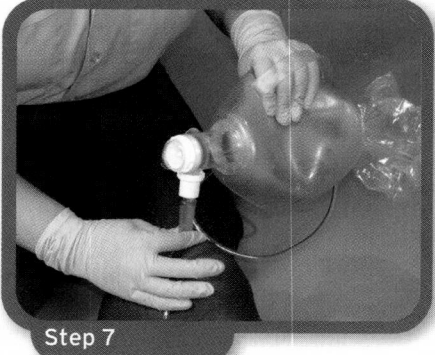

Step 7

Attach the bag-mask device and begin to ventilate the patient. Confirm chest rise and the presence of breath sounds. Continuously and closely monitor the patient.

Table 11-16	Sedatives Used in Airway Management	
Drug Type	**Examples**
Butyrophenones: sedative	Haloperidol (Haldol) Droperidol (Inapsine)
Benzodiazepines: sedative-hypnotic	Diazepam (Valium) Midazolam (Versed)
Barbiturates: sedative-hypnotic	Thiopental (Pentothal) Methohexital (Brevital)
Narcotics (opioids): sedative-analgesic	Fentanyl (Sublimaze) Alfentanil (Alfenta)
Etomidate (Amidate): sedative-hypnotic	
Ketamine (Ketalar): sedative-analgesic-hypnotic	

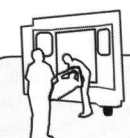

In the Field

Hypersensitivity to sedative medications is the primary contraindication to the use of these drugs. Obtain an accurate medical history prior to giving any drug to any patient.

The level of sedation desired dictates the amount of the medication administered. The patient's response to sedatives is dose dependent. The paramedic should follow local protocol or should contact medical control regarding the appropriate dose for a given patient.

Two major classes of sedatives are commonly used in airway management: analgesics and sedative-hypnotics **Table 11-16 ▲**. Analgesics decrease the perception of pain. Sedative-hypnotics induce sleep and decrease anxiety; they do not reduce pain.

Butyrophenones

Butyrophenones are potent, effective sedatives. Two of these drugs, haloperidol (Haldol) and droperidol (Inapsine), are frequently used in emergency situations for anxiolysis, the relief of anxiety. These medications are effective for calming agitated patients, trauma patients who are combative, patients who are experiencing alcohol withdrawal, and patients with acute psychoses. They do not produce apnea and have little effect on the cardiovascular system. Droperidol is faster acting than haloperidol and is generally preferred in emergency situations. Butyrophenones are not recommended for induction of anesthesia.

Benzodiazepines

Benzodiazepines are sedative-hypnotic drugs. Diazepam (Valium) and midazolam (Versed) provide muscle relaxation and mild sedation and are used extensively as anxiolytic and anticonvulsant medications. They also provide antegrade amnesia, which is beneficial when you are performing invasive or uncomfortable procedures; the patient will not be able to recall the event.

Midazolam is two to four times as potent as diazepam, is faster acting, and has a shorter duration of action. Because large doses of midazolam are necessary to achieve the desired

effect, it should not be used as an induction agent. Some clinicians use midazolam to induce general anesthesia prior to intubation; however, the likelihood of complications increases because of the large dose necessary to induce muscle relaxation. In general, the use of neuromuscular blockers (paralytics) to achieve muscle relaxation is preferred because they require smaller doses to achieve the desired effect.

Respiratory depression and slight hypotension are potential side effects of benzodiazepine administration. Flumazenil (Romazicon) is a benzodiazepine antagonist that can reverse the effects of diazepam and midazolam.

Barbiturates

Barbiturates are sedative-hypnotic medications that have a long history of use. Thiopental (Pentothal) is short acting and causes a rapid onset of profound sedation. Methohexital (Brevital) is ultra-short acting and twice as potent as thiopental. Barbiturates can cause significant respiratory depression and a drop in blood pressure of approximately 10% in normovolemic patients. This drop in blood pressure can be profound and potentially irreversible in hypovolemic patients.

Opioids/Narcotics

Opioids are potent analgesics with sedative properties. Narcotics are used in emergency airway management as a premedication, during induction, and in maintenance of sedation/amnesia. The two most commonly used narcotics for airway management are fentanyl (Sublimaze) and alfentanil (Alfenta). Fentanyl is 70 to 150 times more potent than morphine. It has a short onset of action and a relatively short duration of action. Alfentanil is less potent than fentanyl but has a faster onset of action and a shorter duration of action. It is also eliminated from the body faster.

Opioids can cause profound respiratory and central nervous system depression and produce severe hypotension and bradycardia, especially in hemodynamically unstable patients. These negative effects can be reversed with naloxone (Narcan), a narcotic antagonist.

Etomidate

Etomidate (Amidate) is a nonnarcotic, nonbarbiturate hypnotic-sedative drug. It is a fast-acting agent of short duration. This drug has little effect on heart rate, blood pressure, and intracranial pressure, and does not cause the histamine release and bronchoconstriction that may occur with other agents. However, a high incidence of uncomfortable myoclonic muscle movement is associated with its use. Etomidate is a useful induction agent in patients with coronary artery disease, increased intracranial pressure, or borderline hypotension/hypovolemia.

Ketamine

Ketamine (Ketalar) is a drug with sedative, analgesic, and hypnotic properties. It was created in the laboratory from phencyclidine (PCP). Ketamine is not commonly used in emergency situations involving adults because of the incidence of nightmares, referred to as emergence phenomenon. In children, these emergence phenomena are less common; therefore, ketamine is used as a supplemental sedative, analgesic, hypnotic agent in the pediatric population. Ketamine has potent sedative, analgesic, and hypnotic properties. Protective airway reflexes are maintained, and there is little respiratory depression following administration. Ketamine is not frequently used in the prehospital setting for airway management.

Neuromuscular Blockade in Emergency Intubation

Cerebral hypoxia can make an ordinarily docile person combative, aggressive, belligerent, and uncooperative. This can make for a very difficult and potentially dangerous situation—both for the patient and for the paramedics. The patient with cerebral hypoxia must be treated with aggressive oxygenation and ventilation, but his or her combativeness often makes this a difficult, if not impossible, task to perform. Clenching of the patient's teeth due to spasm of the jaw muscles (trismus) and vocal cords spasm (laryngospasm) can also hamper your efforts to obtain a definitive airway.

In the past, it was common practice to physically restrain the patient to obtain a definitive airway. A safer, more effective approach is to "chemically paralyze" the patient with neuromuscular blocking agents (paralytics). With the patient chemically paralyzed and sedated, his or her protective airway reflexes are lost; you can effectively perform oxygenation and ventilation, and the patient will not gag during insertion of an ET tube.

Neuromuscular Blocking Agents

Although sedatives alone can be used to facilitate intubation, the incidence of complications and side effects is unacceptably high. It is much more effective to administer a drug specifically designed to induce paralysis. Paralytic drugs affect every skeletal muscle in the body, including the diaphragm and the intercostal muscles. Within about a minute of receiving an IV dose of a paralytic, a patient will become *totally* paralyzed. That is, the patient will stop breathing; his or her jaw muscles will go slack, and the base of the tongue will flop back against the posterior pharynx and obstruct the airway. Put bluntly, paralytics convert a breathing patient with a marginal airway into an apneic patient with no airway. Before you bring about such a change, you must be *absolutely* sure that you can place an ET tube into the patient's trachea within the next 30 seconds. Once a patient is paralyzed, you are completely responsible for that patient's breathing and well-being. Fortunately, paralytic agents do not affect cardiac or smooth muscle.

A paralyzed patient will *appear* to be asleep or unconscious, but is not! Paralytic agents, unlike sedatives, have no effect on level of consciousness. The patient is fully aware and can hear, feel, and think.

Pharmacology of Neuromuscular Blocking Agents

To understand how medications induce paralysis, recall how skeletal muscles contract. All skeletal (striated) muscles are voluntary and require input from the somatic nervous system to initiate contraction. As an impulse to contract reaches the terminal end of a motor nerve, acetylcholine (ACh) is released into the synaptic cleft (the junction between the nerve cell and the muscle cell). This neurotransmitter diffuses across the short distance of the synaptic cleft and binds to receptor sites on the motor end plate. Acetylcholine occupying the receptor sites triggers changes in electrical properties of the muscle fiber, a process called depolarization. When enough motor end plates have been depolarized, a threshold is reached and the muscle fiber contracts. Depolarization lasts for only a few milliseconds because of the presence of acetylcholinesterase, an enzyme that quickly removes acetylcholine from the synaptic cleft and from the receptors on the motor end plate.

Paralytic medications all function at the neuromuscular junction and relax the muscle by impeding the action of acetylcholine. Collectively, all paralytics are referred to as neuromuscular blocking agents. They are classified into two categories: depolarizing and nondepolarizing agents. **Table 11-17 ▸** lists the standard dosages for these agents used in the prehospital setting.

Depolarizing Neuromuscular Blocking Agents

Depolarizing neuromuscular blockers competitively bind with the acetylcholine receptor sites but are not affected as quickly by acetylcholinesterase. Therefore, they cause depolarization of the muscle and prevent future signals for depolarization from having an effect because all of the acetylcholine receptor sites are already occupied.

Succinylcholine chloride (Anectine) is the only depolarizing neuromuscular blocking agent. Because succinylcholine causes depolarization, fasciculations—characterized by brief, uncoordinated twitching of small muscle groups in the face, neck, trunk, and extremities—can be observed during its

Table 11-17	Neuromuscular Blocking Drug Dosages
Drug	**Dosage**
Succinylcholine (depolarizing)	1.5 to 2.0 mg/kg via IV push (initial dose) - Repeat doses can be given based on the patient's response
Vecuronium bromide* (nondepolarizing)	0.1 mg/kg via IV push (initial dose for adults and children older than 10 years of age) - 0.01 to 0.015 mg/kg can be given 25 to 40 minutes after the initial dose
Pancuronium bromide* (nondepolarizing)	0.06 to 0.1 mg/kg via IV push (initial dose for adults and children older than 1 month of age) - Can repeat at 0.01 mg/kg every 20 to 60 minutes as needed
Rocuronium	1.2 mg/kg

*Administer 10% of the initial dose (defasciculating dose) prior to administering succinylcholine.

In the Field

If you administer only a depolarizing paralytic (eg, succinylcholine) to your patient, you will have to give the medication by continuous infusion or administer a bolus every 5 minutes. This significantly increases the risk of complications.

administration (Figure 11-79). These fasciculations tend to cause generalized muscle pain at the termination of paralysis (when the succinylcholine wears off).

Depolarizing neuromuscular blockers are characterized by a very rapid onset (60 to 90 seconds) of total paralysis and a relatively short duration of action (5 to 10 minutes). For this reason, succinylcholine is often used as an initial paralytic. With this drug, if you are unable to secure the patient's airway, you have to support ventilation for only a short period of time before the patient can breathe again on his or her own.

Succinylcholine should be used with caution in patients with burns, crush injuries, and blunt trauma—that is, conditions that can result in hyperkalemia.

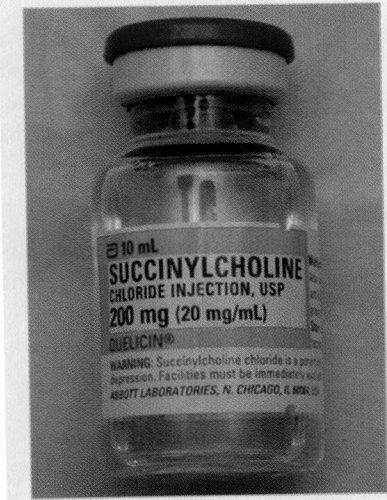
Figure 11-79 Succinylcholine.

Additionally, because its chemical structure is similar to that of acetylcholine, succinylcholine can cause bradycardia, especially in pediatric patients. Premedication with atropine, which prevents succinylcholine-induced bradycardia, should precede the administration of succinylcholine in pediatric patients if at all possible.

Nondepolarizing Neuromuscular Blocking Agents

Nondepolarizing neuromuscular blockers also bind to acetylcholine receptor sites; however, unlike depolarizing neuromuscular blockers, they do not cause depolarization of the muscle fiber. When given in sufficient quantity, the amount of nondepolarizing medication exceeds the amount of acetylcholine in the synaptic cleft, and the critical threshold of depolarization cannot be achieved. Thus, when nondepolarizing paralytics are administered in small quantities prior to administering a depolarizing paralytic, they prevent fasciculations. The defasciculating dose is typically 10% of the normal dose; it does not induce paralysis, but does cause weakness.

The most commonly used nondepolarizing neuromuscular blockers are vecuronium bromide (Norcuron) and pancuronium bromide (Pavulon). Vecuronium (Figure 11-80) has a rapid onset of action (2 minutes), but a longer duration of action (45 minutes). Pancuronium (Figure 11-81) also has a rapid onset of action (3 to 5 minutes), and a slightly longer duration of action (1 hour).

Nondepolarizing neuromuscular blockers, because of their longer duration of action, are ideal when the patient requires extended periods of paralysis, such as when there is a prolonged transport time or when the patient's airway has been secured and you need to manage other injuries or conditions. However, these agents should not be given before the patient's airway has been secured.

Rapid-Sequence Intubation

Rapid-sequence intubation (RSI) represents a culmination and integration of all of your

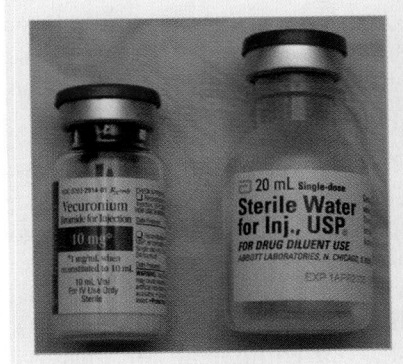
Figure 11-80 Vecuronium.

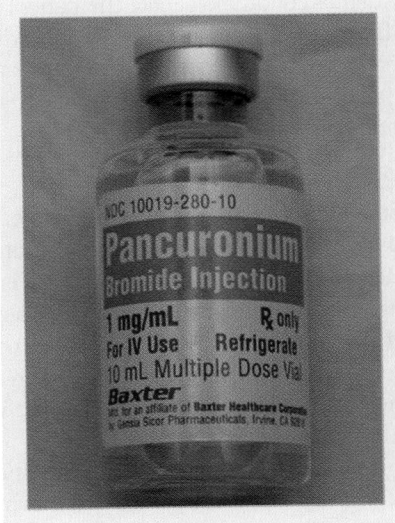
Figure 11-81 Pancuronium.

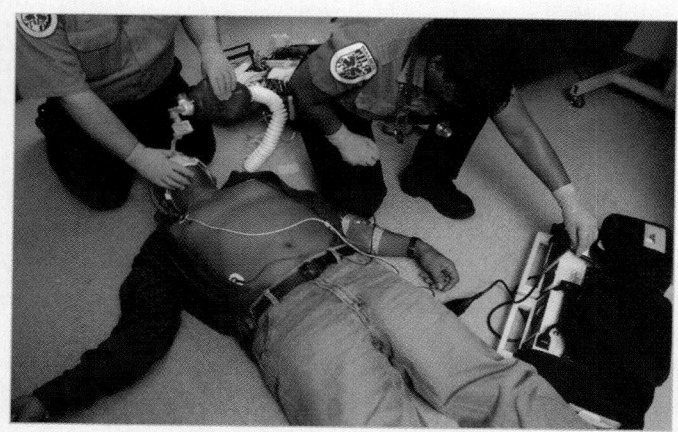

Figure 11-82 Preoxygenate the patient prior to performing rapid-sequence intubation.

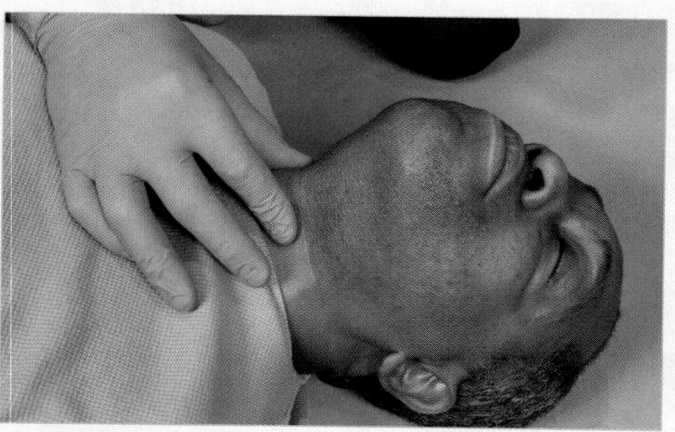

Figure 11-83 A second paramedic should apply posterior cricoid pressure to reduce the risk of regurgitation.

airway, problem-solving, and decision-making skills into one procedure. It includes the safe, smooth, and rapid induction of sedation and paralysis followed immediately by intubation. Although RSI has been successfully performed in the operating room for years, its use in the prehospital setting is relatively new. It is generally used for conscious or combative patients who need to be intubated but who are unable or unwilling to cooperate.

Preparation of the Patient and Equipment

The experience of being intubated is frightening for patients, so you must explain what you are going to do and reassure the patient that he or she will be asleep during the procedure and will not feel or remember anything. Place the patient on a cardiac monitor and pulse oximeter. Check, prepare, and assemble your equipment and ensure that it is in good working order. In particular, have suction *immediately* available.

Preoxygenation

Adequately preoxygenate the patient with 100% oxygen to ensure that positive-pressure ventilation will not be necessary until the patient has been successfully intubated Figure 11-82 ▲ . If the patient is not ventilating adequately, you will need to assist ventilations during the procedure itself.

Premedication

Stimulation of the glottis associated with intubation can cause dysrhythmias and a substantial increase in intracranial pressure (ICP)—a particularly problematic issue for patients with closed head injuries or other conditions associated with increased ICP. If you are performing RSI on a patient with closed head trauma, administer 1 to 1.5 mg/kg of lidocaine to decrease the risk of dysrhythmias and the spike in ICP associated with stimulation of the upper airway.

As previously discussed, you should administer a defasciculating dose (typically 10% of a normal dose) of a nondepolarizing paralytic, if time permits. Atropine sulfate should also be administered to decrease the incidence of bradycardia associ-

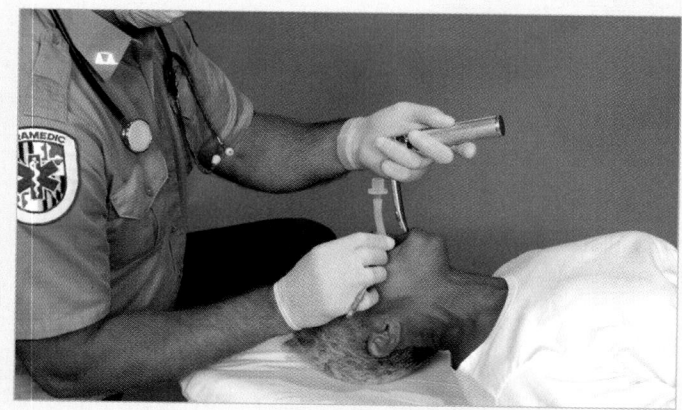

Figure 11-84 Intubate the trachea.

ated with the administration of succinylcholine. The usual dose for the adult is 0.5 mg and 0.02 mg/kg for infants and children.

Sedation and Paralysis

As long as the patient is hemodynamically stable (systolic BP > 90 mm Hg), administer a sedative agent to induce sedation and amnesia. Immediately thereafter, administer succinylcholine. Paralysis will begin in 30 seconds and will be complete within 2 minutes.

Posterior Cricoid Pressure

Immediately after the patient is sedated and paralyzed (as evidenced by the loss of the eyelash reflex), have an assistant apply posterior cricoid pressure Figure 11-83 ▲ . As long as the patient's oxygen saturation is maintained, do not provide positive-pressure ventilation, as this will significantly increase the risk of regurgitation and aspiration.

Intubation

Intubate the trachea as carefully as possible Figure 11-84 ▲ . If you cannot accomplish the intubation within 30 seconds, stop and ventilate the patient for 30 seconds to 1 minute with a bag-mask

In the Field

Rapid-sequence intubation should be attempted only if you have confidence that you will be able to intubate and ventilate the patient, or ventilate the patient without intubation, if necessary. Otherwise, a patient who has been sedated and paralyzed will die. Above all else, *do no harm!*

Table 11-18	Sample Protocols for Rapid-Sequence Intubation

For hemodynamically stable patients

1. Prepare patient and equipment.
2. Preoxygenate with 100% oxygen for at least 2 to 3 minutes.
3. Consider a defasciculating dose of nondepolarizing paralytic, lidocaine, or atropine.
4. Sedate.
5. Administer succinylcholine.
6. Apply cricoid pressure.
7. Intubate, verify tube placement, and release cricoid pressure.
8. Administer a nondepolarizing paralytic and maintain adequate sedation.

For hemodynamically unstable patients

1. Prepare patient and equipment.
2. Preoxygenate and ventilate as necessary.
3. Consider sedation.
4. Administer succinylcholine.
5. Apply cricoid pressure.
6. Intubate, verify tube placement, and release cricoid pressure.
7. Administer a nondepolarizing paralytic.

device and 100% oxygen before trying again. *If you must ventilate the patient with a bag mask, do so slowly (1 second per breath [enough to produce visible chest rise]) while maintaining cricoid pressure to minimize the risk of regurgitation.* If the patient is inadequately paralyzed, you may give a second dose of succinylcholine.

Once the tube is in the trachea, inflate the cuff, remove the stylet, verify correct position of the ET tube, and release cricoid pressure. Secure the tube in place as normal and continue ventilations at the appropriate rate.

Maintenance of Paralysis and Sedation

When you are *absolutely* sure that you have successfully intubated the trachea, administer a nondepolarizing blocker (eg, Norcuron, Pavulon) to maintain long-term paralysis. Continue to administer a sedative if the patient's blood pressure is adequate. Monitor the patient's heart rate and blood pressure to ensure that sedation is not wearing off.

While the general steps of RSI are the same for all patients, some modification is necessary for unstable patients. If the patient's oxygen saturation drops at any point, you have no choice except to ventilate (just do it slowly). If the patient is hemodynamically unstable, you must judge whether sedation is appropriate or whether the risk of profound hypotension is too great to sedate the patient prior to inducing paralysis. **Table 11-18 ▶** lists sample protocols for RSI in hemodynamically stable and unstable patients.

Surgical and Nonsurgical Airways

In most cases, the paramedic is able to secure a patent airway with relative ease using either basic (bag-mask device with oral airway) or advanced (endotracheal intubation) methods. In some situations, however, the patient's condition or other factors preclude the use of conventional airway techniques, and a more aggressive and invasive approach must be taken to secure the airway and maximize survival.

Two methods of securing a patent airway can be used when conventional techniques and methods fail: the open

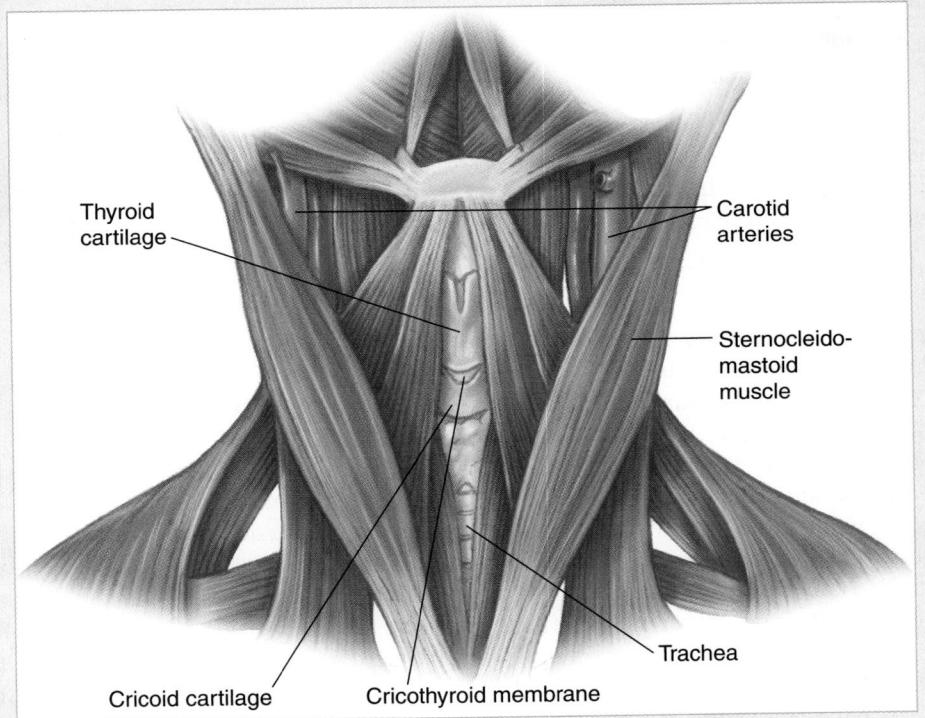

Figure 11-85 Anatomy of the anterior part of the neck.

Thyroid cartilage — Carotid arteries — Sternocleidomastoid muscle — Cricoid cartilage — Cricothyroid membrane — Trachea

(surgical) cricothyrotomy and translaryngeal catheter ventilation (nonsurgical, or needle cricothyrotomy). To perform these procedures, you must be familiar with the key anatomic landmarks that lie in the anterior aspect of the neck **Figure 11-85 ▲** .

In addition, you must be familiar with the important blood vessels in this area. The superior cricothyroid vessels run at a transverse angle across the upper third of the cricothyroid membrane. The external jugular veins run vertically and are located lateral to the cricothyroid membrane. If the cricothyroid membrane is incised vertically when performing a cricothyrotomy, the jugular veins can be avoided altogether.

When performing cricothyrotomy, you should expect to encounter some minor bleeding from the subcutaneous and small skin vessels as you incise the cricothyroid membrane. This bleeding should be easily controlled with light pressure after the tube has been inserted into the trachea.

Open Cricothyrotomy

Open cricothyrotomy (surgical cricothyrotomy) involves incising the cricothyroid membrane with a scalpel and inserting an endotracheal or tracheostomy tube **Figure 11-86 ▾** directly into the subglottic area (below the vocal cords) of the trachea. The

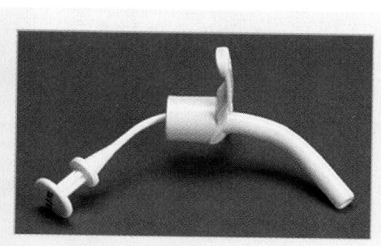

Figure 11-86 Tracheostomy tube.

cricothyroid membrane is the ideal site for making a surgical opening into the trachea because no important structures lie between the skin and the airway. The airway at this level lies relatively close to the skin and is easy to enter through the thin cricothyroid membrane. The posterior wall of the airway at this level is formed by the tough cricoid cartilage, which helps prevent accidental perforation through the back of the airway into the esophagus.

Indications and Contraindications

Open cricothyrotomy is indicated when you are unable to secure a patent airway with more conventional means. *It is not the preferred means of initially securing a patient's airway.* For example, if you are unable to intubate a patient but can provide effective bag-mask ventilations, cricothyrotomy would not be appropriate.

Situations that may preclude conventional airway management include severe foreign body upper airway obstructions that cannot be extracted with Magill forceps and direct laryngoscopy, airway obstructions from swelling (eg, epiglottitis, anaphylaxis, upper airway burns), massive maxillofacial trauma, and the inability to open the patient's mouth. Patients with massive maxillofacial trauma **Figure 11-87 ▸** often have associated mandibular fractures, which makes it extremely difficult to maintain an effective mask-to-face seal with a bag-mask device. Intubation in these patients would also be extremely difficult due to posterior tongue lacerations with profuse bleeding. In such cases, frequent suctioning to prevent aspiration would delay intubation and increase patient hypoxia.

Patients with head injuries and trismus (clenched teeth) may require cricothyrotomy, especially if you do not have the

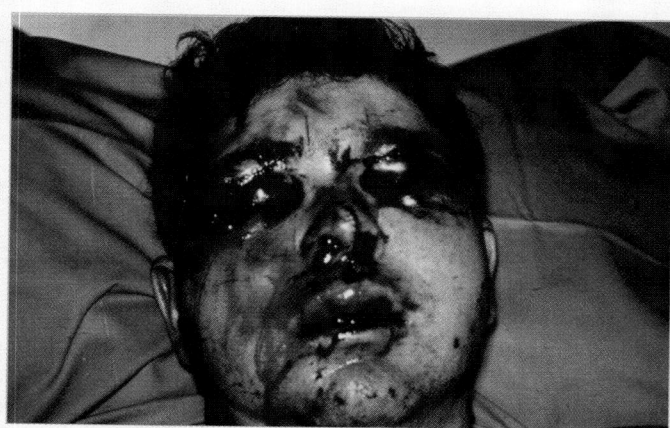

Figure 11-87 Patients with massive maxillofacial trauma often have mandibular fractures or profuse oral bleeding, both of which can make bag-mask ventilations or intubation extremely difficult, if not impossible, to perform.

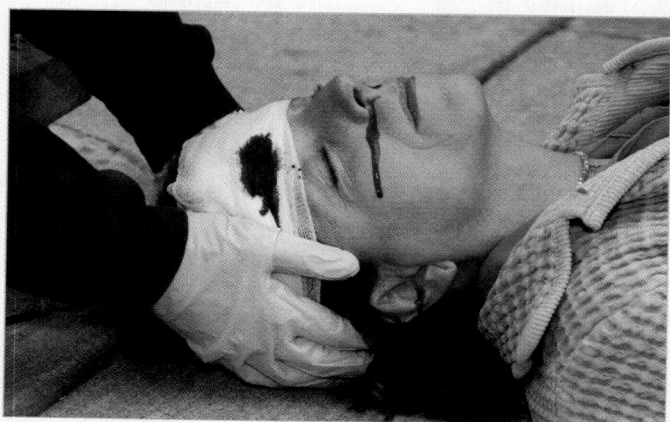

Figure 11-88 Endotracheal intubation may not be possible in patients with a head injury and trismus. Nasotracheal intubation is contraindicated in patients with head injury and fluid drainage from the ears or nose.

resources or protocols to perform RSI. Furthermore, head injury, which is commonly accompanied by facial trauma, is a contraindication for nasotracheal intubation or placement of a nasopharyngeal airway, especially if fluid is draining from the patient's ears or nose **Figure 11-88 ▴** . If this fluid is CSF, it indicates either a basilar skull fracture or a fracture of the cribriform plate. If nasotracheal intubation is attempted in these patients, the ET tube or nasal airway may be inadvertently placed into the cranial vault.

As noted earlier, the main contraindication for open cricothyrotomy is the ability to secure a patent airway by less invasive means. Other contraindications include inability to identify the correct anatomic landmarks (cricothyroid membrane), crushing injuries to the larynx and tracheal transection, underlying anatomic abnormalities (eg, trauma, tumors, or subglottic stenosis), and age younger than 8 years. The larynx of a small child is generally unable to support a tube large enough to produce effective ventilation without causing damage to the larynx; you would be safer performing a needle cricothyrotomy (discussed later in this chapter) in young children.

In situations where cricothyrotomy is contraindicated, the paramedic must rapidly transport the patient to the closest appropriate facility, where an emergency tracheostomy can be performed.

Advantages and Disadvantages

Open cricothyrotomy can be performed quickly, is technically easier than performing a tracheostomy, and can be performed without manipulating the cervical spine. The latter characteristic is especially advantageous because many cricothyrotomies involve patients with massive facial trauma.

Disadvantages of cricothyrotomy include difficulty in performing the procedure in children (younger than 8 years) and in patients with short, muscular, or fat necks. In contrast to needle cricothyrotomy, an open cricothyrotomy is more difficult to perform; however, inserting a large-bore tube (eg, an ET tube or tracheostomy tube) enables you to achieve greater tidal volume, which facilitates more effective oxygenation and ventilation.

Complications

You should expect some minor bleeding when performing an open cricothyrotomy. More severe bleeding is usually the result of inadvertent laceration of the external jugular vein. Incising the cricothyroid membrane vertically, instead of horizontally, will minimize this potential complication. It will also minimize the risk of damaging the highly vascular thyroid gland. After the incision has been made, *gently* inserting the tube will minimize the risk of perforating the esophagus or damaging the laryngeal nerves.

An open cricothyrotomy must be performed quickly. Taking too long to complete a cricothyrotomy will result in unnecessary hypoxia to the patient, which may result in cardiac arrhythmias, permanent brain injury, or cardiac arrest.

> ### In the Field
>
> Frequent practice on a cadaver, if available, or a special cricothyrotomy manikin, will maximize your ability to perform cricothyrotomy quickly. In general, skills that are not frequently performed in the field should be routinely practiced to maintain proficiency and competence.

Tube misplacement should be suspected when subcutaneous emphysema is encountered after performing a cricothyrotomy. Subcutaneous emphysema occurs when air infiltrates the subcutaneous (fatty) layers of the skin, and is characterized by a "crackling" sensation when palpated.

Any invasive procedure performed in the prehospital setting carries the risk of infection to the patient. Therefore, you should make all attempts to maintain aseptic technique when performing an open cricothyrotomy.

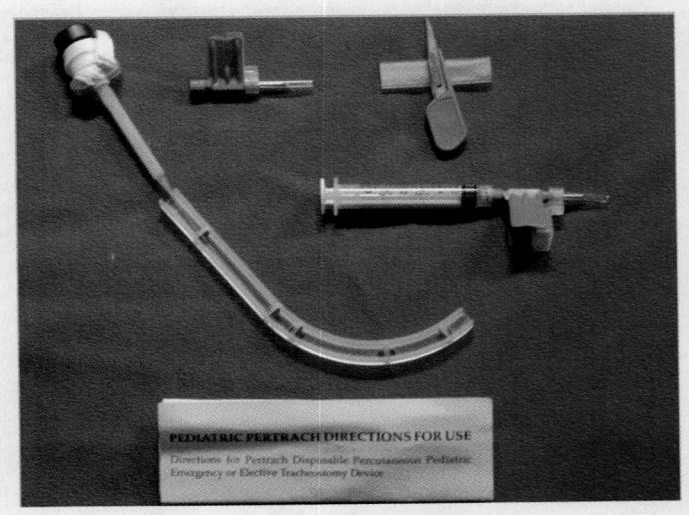

Figure 11-89 Cricothyrotomy kit.

Equipment

Commercially manufactured cricothyrotomy kits are available **Figure 11-89 ▲**. If such a kit is not available, however, you must prepare the following equipment and supplies:

- Scalpel
- ET tube or tracheostomy tube (6.0 mm minimum)
- Commercial device (or tape) for securing the tube
- Curved hemostats
- Suction apparatus
- Sterile gauze pads for minor bleeding control
- Bag-mask device attached to 100% oxygen

Technique for Performing Open Cricothyrotomy

Once you determine that an open cricothyrotomy is needed, you must proceed rapidly, yet cautiously. Identify the cricothyroid membrane by palpating for the V notch of the thyroid cartilage, which feels like a high, sharp bump. Stabilize the larynx between your thumb and middle fingers while you palpate with your index finger. When you have located the V notch, slide your index finger down into the depression between the thyroid and cricoid cartilage; that is the cricothyroid membrane.

While you are locating and preparing the site, your partner should be preparing your equipment as well as ensuring that the cardiac monitor and pulse oximeter are attached to the patient.

Maintain aseptic technique as you cleanse the area with iodine; avoid touching the area once cleansed. While stabilizing the larynx with one hand, make a 1- to 2-cm vertical incision over the cricothyroid membrane. Some advocate making an additional 1-cm incision horizontally across the membrane to facilitate easier placement of the tube. If you elect to do so, remember that the thyroid gland and external jugular veins are lateral to the area and can be damaged if the horizontal incision is too long. Once the incision has been made, insert the curved hemostats into the opening and spread it apart. Your partner should be readily available to control any bleeding that might occur.

Skill Drill 11-39: Performing an Open Cricothyrotomy

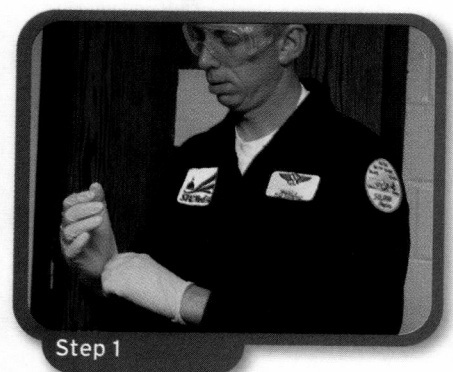

Step 1

Take BSI precautions (gloves and face shield).

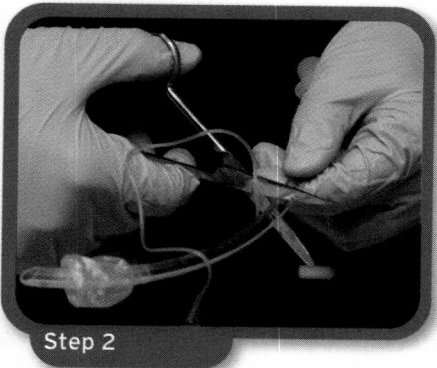

Step 2

Check, assemble, and prepare the equipment.

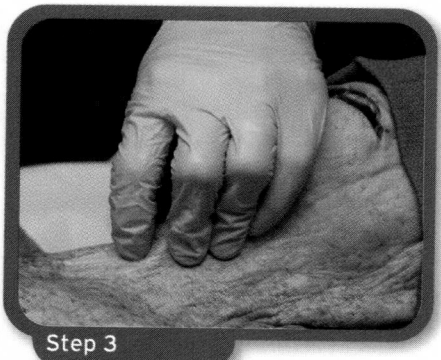

Step 3

With the patient's head in a neutral position, palpate for and locate the cricothyroid membrane.

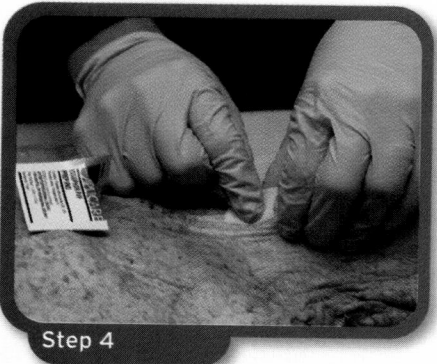

Step 4

Cleanse the area with an iodine-containing solution.

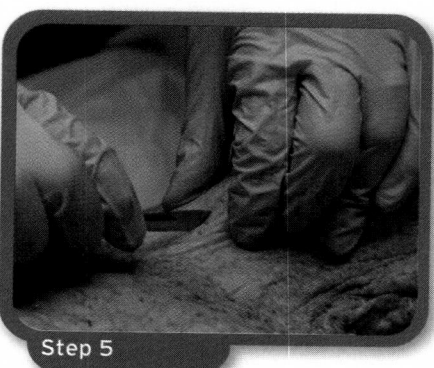

Step 5

Stabilize the larynx and make a 1- to 2-cm vertical incision over the cricothyroid membrane.

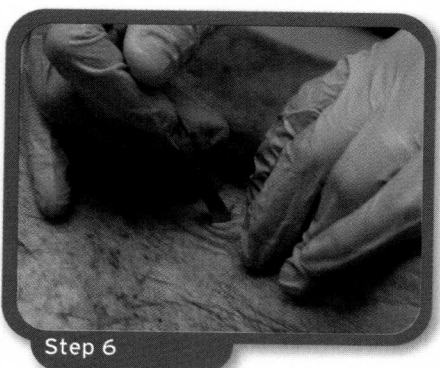

Step 6

Puncture the cricothyroid membrane and make a horizontal cut 1 cm in each direction from the midline.

With the trachea exposed, gently insert a 6.0-mm cuffed ET tube or a 6.0 tracheostomy (Shiley) tube and direct it into the trachea. Once the tube is in place, inflate the distal cuff with the appropriate volume of air—typically 5 to 10 mL. Attach the bag-mask device to the standard 15/22-mm adapter on the tube and ventilate the patient while your partner auscultates to ensure the presence of bilaterally clear breath sounds as well as the absence of epigastric sounds. If epigastric sounds are heard, you have likely perforated and inadvertently inserted the tube into the esophagus.

Additional confirmation of correct tube placement can be accomplished by attaching an $ETCO_2$ detector in between the tube and bag-mask device. After confirming proper tube placement, ensure that any minor bleeding has been controlled, properly secure the tube, and continue to ventilate the patient at the appropriate rate.

The steps for performing an open cricothyrotomy are listed here and shown in **Skill Drill 11-39 ▲**.

1. Take BSI precautions (gloves and face shield) **Step 1**.
2. Check, assemble, and prepare the equipment **Step 2**.

3. With the patient's head in a neutral position, palpate for and locate the cricothyroid membrane **Step 3**.
4. Cleanse the area with an iodine-containing solution **Step 4**.
5. Stabilize the larynx and make a 1- to 2-cm vertical incision over the cricothyroid membrane **Step 5**.
6. Puncture the cricothyroid membrane and make a horizontal cut 1 cm in each direction from the midline **Step 6**.
7. Spread the incision apart with curved hemostats **Step 7**.
8. Insert the tube into the trachea **Step 8**.
9. Inflate the distal cuff of the tube **Step 9**.
10. Attach an $ETCO_2$ detector in between the tube and the bag-mask device **Step 10**.
11. Ventilate the patient and confirm correct tube placement by auscultating the apices and bases of both lungs and over the epigastrium **Step 11**.
12. Secure the tube with a commercial device or tape. Reconfirm correct tube placement and resume ventilations at the appropriate rate **Step 12**.

Skill Drill 11-39: Performing an Open Cricothyrotomy (*continued*)

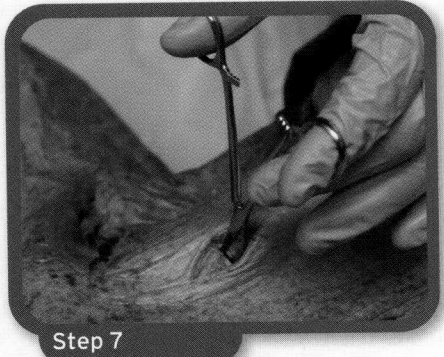

Step 7

Spread the incision apart with curved hemostats.

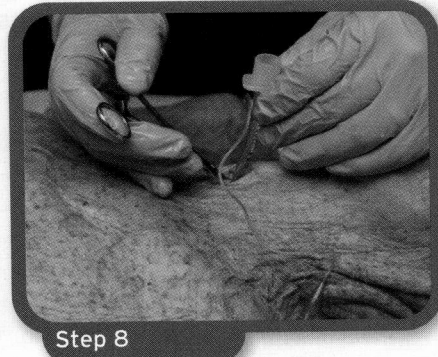

Step 8

Insert the tube into the trachea.

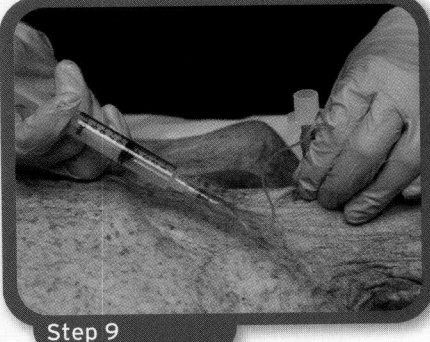

Step 9

Inflate the distal cuff of the tube.

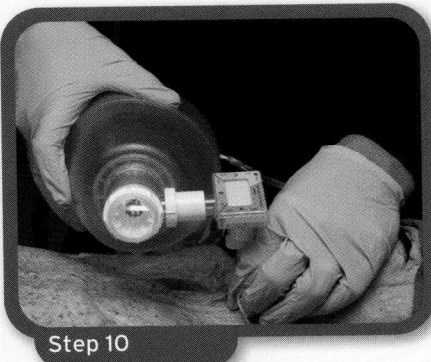

Step 10

Attach an ETco₂ detector in between the tube and the bag-mask device.

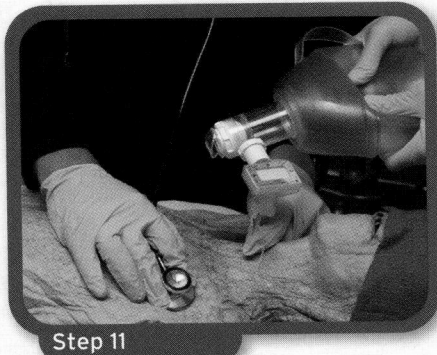

Step 11

Ventilate the patient and confirm correct tube placement by auscultating the apices and bases of both lungs and over the epigastrium.

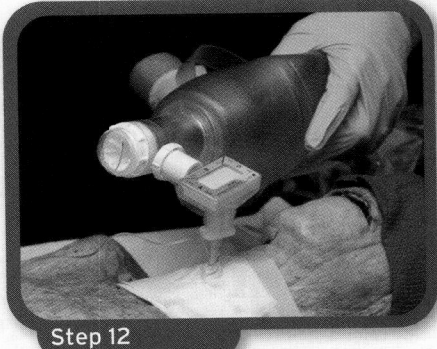

Step 12

Secure the tube with a commercial device or tape. Reconfirm correct tube placement and resume ventilations at the appropriate rate.

Needle Cricothyrotomy

Needle cricothyrotomy also uses the cricothyroid membrane as an entry point into the airway. In this procedure, a 14- to 16-gauge over-the-needle IV catheter (angiocath) is inserted through the cricothyroid membrane and into the trachea. Adequate oxygenation and ventilation are then achieved by attaching a high-pressure jet ventilator **Figure 11-90 ▸** to the hub of the catheter. Known as translaryngeal catheter ventilation, this procedure is commonly used as a temporary measure until a more definitive airway can be obtained (eg, via open cricothyrotomy or tracheostomy).

Indications and Contraindications

The indications for needle cricothyrotomy and translaryngeal catheter ventilation are essentially the same as for the open cricothyrotomy—the inability to ventilate the patient by other, less invasive techniques; massive maxillofacial trauma; inability to open the patient's mouth; and uncontrolled oropharyngeal bleeding.

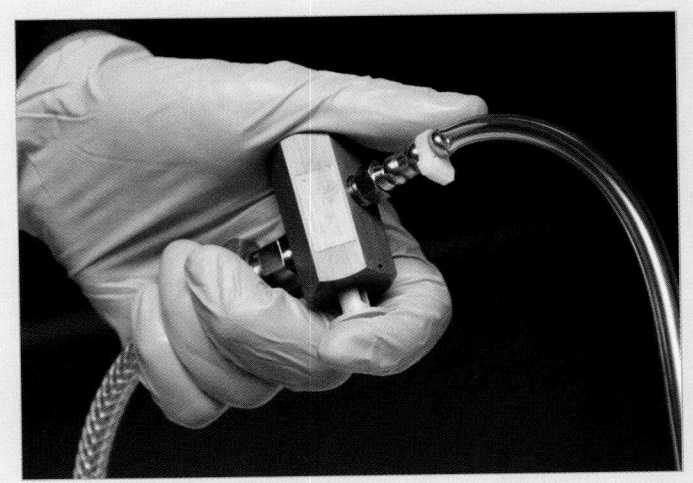

Figure 11-90 High-pressure jet ventilator.

Needle cricothyrotomy is contraindicated in patients who have a severe airway obstruction above the site of catheter insertion. Exhalation is not as effective using a small-bore catheter when compared with a large-bore tube (eg, ET tube, tracheostomy tube). Additionally, exhalation via the glottic opening is not possible because the airway is completely obstructed superior to the catheter insertion site. As the result of minimal and ineffective exhalation, hypercarbia as well as hypoxia may occur. The high-pressure ventilator used with needle cricothyrotomy would cause an increase in intrathoracic pressure, resulting in barotrauma and a potential pneumothorax. Barotrauma can also be caused by overinflation of the lungs with the jet ventilator, so take care to open the release valve only until the patient's chest adequately rises.

If the equipment necessary to perform translaryngeal catheter ventilation is not immediately available, you should opt to perform an open cricothyrotomy.

Advantages and Disadvantages

Compared with an open cricothyrotomy, needle cricothyrotomy is faster and technically easier to perform. In particular, it is associated with a lower risk of causing damage to adjacent structures because you are puncturing the cricothyroid membrane with an IV catheter—not incising it with a scalpel. Needle cricothyrotomy also allows for subsequent intubation attempts because it uses a small-bore catheter, thus allowing an ET tube to easily pass beside it. This could be particularly beneficial if you do not have the equipment or protocols to perform an open cricothyrotomy. In addition, this procedure does not require manipulation of the patient's cervical spine.

There are, however, some disadvantages to performing a needle cricothyrotomy. Using a smaller-bore tube (angiocath) to ventilate the patient does not provide protection from aspiration as an ET tube or tracheostomy tube would during an open cricothyrotomy. (A larger-bore tube, combined with the distal cuff, would fill the diameter of the trachea, protecting it from esophageal regurgitation.) Also, this technique requires a

In the Field

If you do not have the protocols to perform an open cricothyrotomy and/or you do not have a jet ventilator on your ambulance, there is an alternative—albeit less effective—method of ventilating the patient via needle cricothyrotomy. Attach a 7- to 7.5-mm ET tube adapter into the barrel of a 10-mL syringe. Next, connect the syringe to the IV catheter that has been inserted into the cricothyroid membrane. Connect the bag-mask device to the ET tube adapter and begin ventilations. Although you will not be able to deliver nearly the tidal volume as would be possible with a jet ventilator, this approach may be your only alternative to provide some oxygenation and ventilation until a more definitive airway can be achieved at the emergency department.

specialized, high-pressure jet ventilator to deliver adequate tidal volume. This jet ventilator will expend high volumes of oxygen very rapidly.

Complications

Improper catheter placement can result in severe bleeding secondary to damage of adjacent structures. Even if the catheter is correctly placed, excessive air leakage around the insertion site can cause subcutaneous emphysema, especially if the patient has undetected laryngeal trauma. If too much air infiltrates into the subcutaneous space, compression of the trachea and subsequent obstruction may occur.

Extreme care must be exercised when ventilating the patient with a jet ventilator. The release valve should be opened just long enough for adequate chest rise to occur. Overinflation of the lungs can result in barotrauma, which carries the risk of pneumothorax. Conversely, opening the release valve for too short a period of time could cause hypoventilation, resulting in inadequate oxygenation and ventilation.

Equipment

The following pieces of equipment are needed to perform needle cricothyrotomy and translaryngeal catheter ventilation:

- Large-bore IV catheter (14 to 16 gauge)
- 10-mL syringe
- 3 mL of sterile water or saline
- Oxygen source (50 psi)
- High-pressure jet ventilator device and oxygen tubing

Technique for Performing Needle Cricothyrotomy

In preparing your equipment, draw up approximately 3 mL of sterile water or saline into a 10-mL syringe and attach the syringe to the IV catheter. Next, place the patient's head in a neutral position and locate the cricothyroid membrane. If time permits, cleanse the area with an iodine-containing solution.

While you are stabilizing the patient's larynx, carefully insert the needle into the midline of the cricothyroid membrane at a 45° angle toward the feet (caudally). You should feel a pop as the needle penetrates the membrane. After the pop is felt, insert the needle approximately 1 cm farther, and then aspirate with the syringe. If the catheter has been correctly placed, you should be able to easily aspirate air and see the saline or water bubbling within the syringe. If blood is aspirated or if you meet resistance, you should reevaluate catheter placement because it is likely outside the trachea.

After confirming correct placement, advance the catheter over the needle until the catheter hub is flush with the skin, then withdraw the needle and place it in a puncture-proof biohazard container. Next, attach one end of the oxygen tubing to the catheter and the other end to the jet ventilator.

Begin ventilations by opening the release valve on the jet ventilator and observing for adequate chest rise. Auscultation of breath and epigastric sounds will further confirm correct catheter placement. To prevent overexpansion of the lungs and subsequent barotrauma, turn the release valve off as soon as you see the chest rise. Exhalation will occur passively via the glottis. Ventilate the patient as dictated by his or her clinical condition.

Secure the catheter by placing a folded 4″ × 4″ gauze pad under the catheter and taping it in place. Continue ventilations while frequently reassessing the patient for adequacy of ventilations as well as for potential complications (eg, subcutaneous emphysema from incorrect placement).

The steps for performing needle cricothyrotomy with translaryngeal catheter ventilation are listed here and shown in Skill Drill 11-40 ▶ .

1. Take BSI precautions (gloves and face shield) (Step 1).
2. Attach a 14- to 16-gauge IV catheter to a 10-mL syringe containing approximately 3 mL of sterile saline or water (Step 2).
3. With the patient's head in a neutral position, palpate for and locate the cricothyroid membrane (Step 3).
4. Cleanse the area with an iodine-containing solution (Step 4).
5. Stabilize the larynx and insert the needle into the cricothyroid membrane at a 45° angle toward the feet (Step 5).
6. Aspirate with the syringe to determine correct catheter placement (Step 6).
7. Slide the catheter off of the needle until the hub of the catheter is flush with the patient's skin (Step 7).
8. Place the syringe and needle in a puncture-proof container (Step 8).
9. Connect one end of the oxygen tubing to the catheter and the other end to the jet ventilator (Step 9).
10. Open the release valve on the jet ventilator and adjust the pressure accordingly to provide adequate chest rise (Step 10).
11. Auscultate the apices and bases of both lungs and over the epigastrium to confirm correct catheter placement (Step 11).
12. Secure the catheter with a 4″ × 4″ gauze pad and tape. Continue ventilations while frequently reassessing for adequate ventilations and any potential complications (Step 12).

▌Special Patient Considerations

Laryngectomy, Tracheostomy, Stoma, and Tracheostomy Tubes

A laryngectomy is a surgical procedure in which the larynx is removed. This procedure is performed by making a tracheostomy (surgical opening into the trachea), thus creating a stoma, an orifice that connects the trachea to the outside air. The tracheal stoma is located in the midline of the anterior part of the neck. Surgical removal of the entire larynx is called total laryngectomy. A person who has had this procedure is a laryngectomee, or "neck breather"—he or she breathes through the hole in his or her neck. Because there is no longer any connection between the patient's pharynx and lower airway, you cannot ventilate such a patient by the mouth-to-mouth or mouth-to-nose technique. The

air blown into the mouth or nose can only go down the esophagus into the stomach; it will not reach the lower airway.

A partial laryngectomy entails surgical removal of a portion of the larynx. People who have had this procedure are called "partial neck breathers"—they breathe through both the stoma and the nose or mouth. In practice, you may not be able to tell if an apneic laryngectomee is a neck breather or only a partial neck breather until you attempt artificial ventilation.

Suctioning of a Stoma

You may encounter patients who require suctioning of thick secretions from the stoma. Failure to recognize and identify these patients could result in hypoxia. It is not uncommon for a patient's stoma to become occluded with mucous plugs. Patients with laryngectomies possess a less efficient cough; therefore, they will have difficulty spontaneously clearing the stoma by themselves.

Suctioning of the patient's stoma must be performed with extreme care, especially if laryngeal swelling is suspected. Even the slightest irritation of the tracheal wall can result in a violent laryngospasm and complete airway closure. Limit suctioning of the stoma to 10 seconds.

The steps for suctioning a stoma are listed here and shown in Skill Drill 11-41 ▶ .

1. Take BSI precautions (gloves and face shield) (Step 1).
2. Preoxygenate the patient with a bag-mask device and 100% oxygen (Step 2).
3. Inject 3 mL of sterile saline through the stoma and into the trachea (Step 3).
4. Instruct the patient to exhale, and insert the catheter (without providing suction) until resistance is felt (no more than 12 cm) (Step 4).
5. Suction while withdrawing the catheter as you instruct the patient to cough or exhale (Step 5).
6. Resume oxygenating the patient with a bag-mask device and 100% oxygen (Step 6).

Ventilation of Stoma Patients

Neither the head tilt–chin lift nor the jaw-thrust maneuver is required for ventilating a patient with a stoma. If the patient has a stoma and no tracheostomy tube in place, ventilations can be performed using the mouth-to-stoma (with a resuscitation mask) technique or with a bag-mask device. Regardless of the technique used, you should use an infant- or child-size mask to make an adequate seal over the stoma. Seal the patient's nose and mouth with one hand to prevent the leakage of air up the trachea. Release the seal of the patient's mouth and nose following each ventilation, allowing exhalation to occur through the upper airway. Obviously, two rescuers will be needed to perform bag-mask device-to-stoma ventilations: one to seal the nose and mouth and the other to squeeze the bag-mask device. If you are unable to ventilate a patient who has a stoma, try suctioning the stoma and mouth with a French or soft-tip catheter before providing artificial ventilation through the nose and mouth. If you seal the stoma during ventilation, the ability to

Skill Drill 11-40: Performing Needle Cricothyrotomy and Translaryngeal Catheter Ventilation

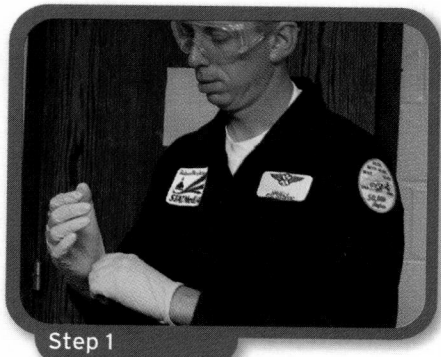

Step 1

Take BSI precautions (gloves and face shield).

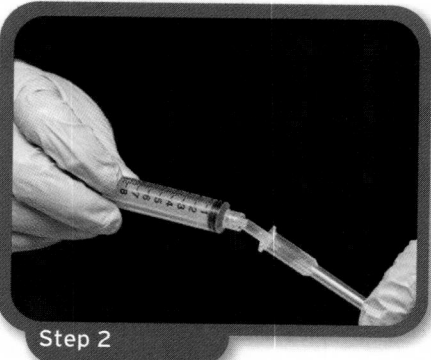

Step 2

Attach a 14- to 16-gauge IV catheter to a 10-mL syringe containing approximately 3 mL of sterile saline or water.

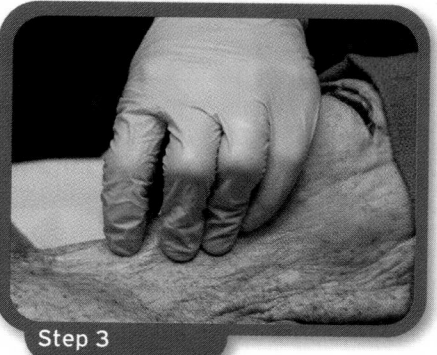

Step 3

With the patient's head in a neutral position, palpate for and locate the cricothyroid membrane.

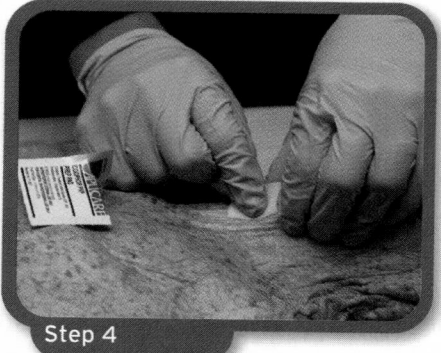

Step 4

Cleanse the area with an iodine-containing solution.

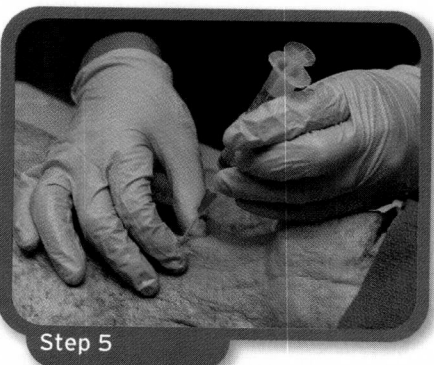

Step 5

Stabilize the larynx and insert the needle into the cricothyroid membrane at a 45° angle toward the feet.

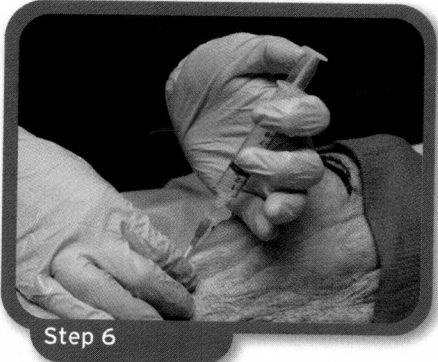

Step 6

Aspirate with the syringe to determine correct catheter placement.

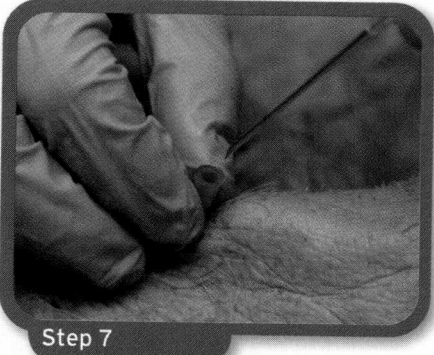

Step 7

Slide the catheter off of the needle until the hub of the catheter is flush with the patient's skin.

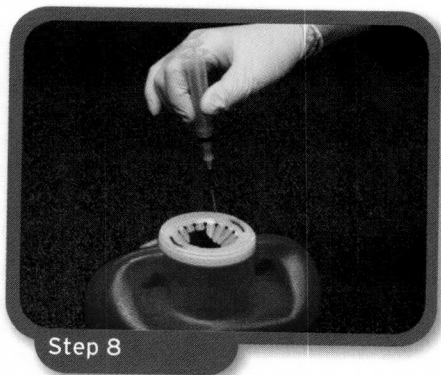

Step 8

Place the syringe and needle in a puncture-proof container.

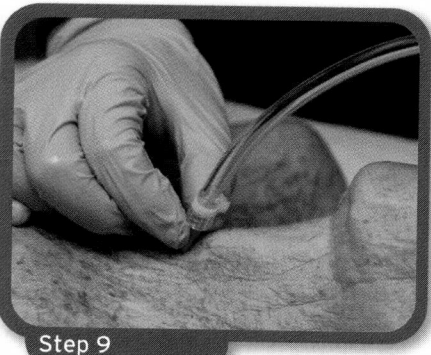

Step 9

Connect one end of the oxygen tubing to the catheter and the other end to the jet ventilator.

Skill Drill 11-40: Performing Needle Cricothyrotomy and Translaryngeal Catheter Ventilation (*continued*)

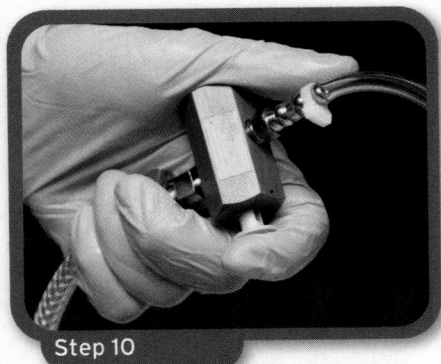

Step 10

Open the release valve on the jet ventilator and adjust the pressure accordingly to provide adequate chest rise.

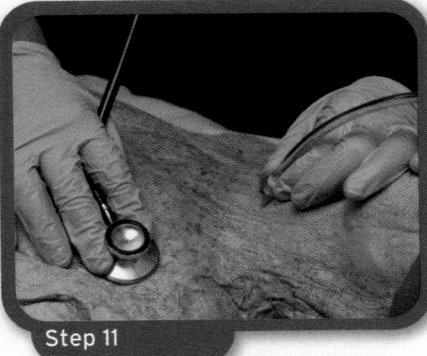

Step 11

Auscultate the apices and bases of both lungs and over the epigastrium to confirm correct catheter placement.

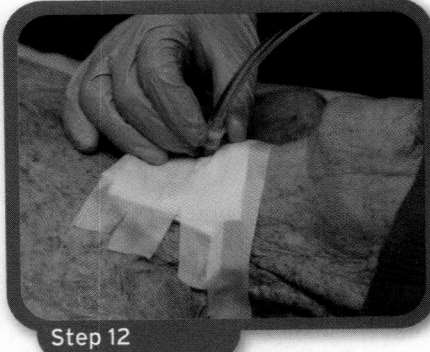

Step 12

Secure the catheter with a 4″ × 4″ gauze pad and tape. Continue ventilations while frequently reassessing for adequate ventilations and any potential complications.

Skill Drill 11-41: Suctioning of a Stoma

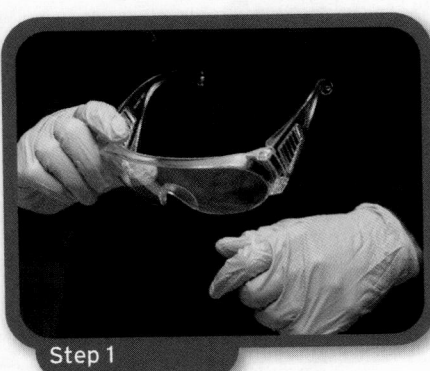

Step 1

Take BSI precautions (gloves and face shield).

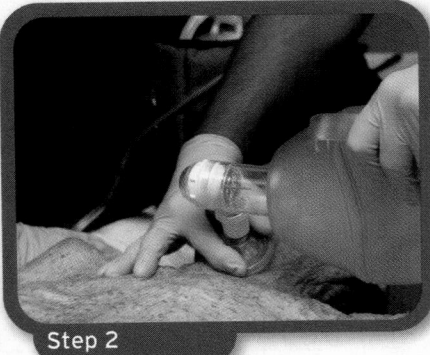

Step 2

Preoxygenate the patient with a bag-mask device and 100% oxygen.

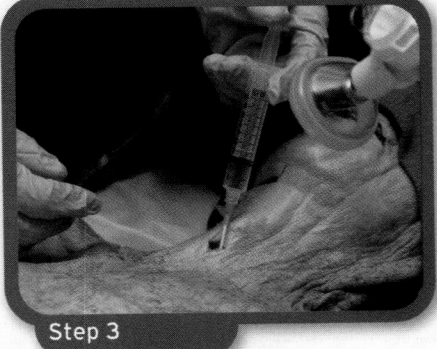

Step 3

Inject 3 mL of saline through the stoma and into the trachea.

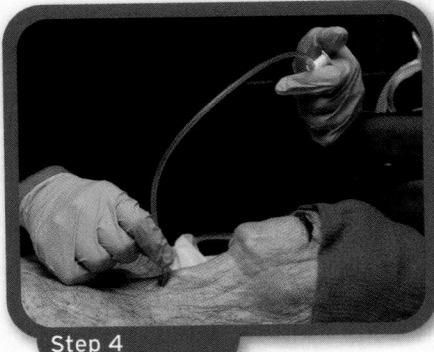

Step 4

Instruct the patient to exhale, and insert the catheter (without providing suction) until resistance is felt (no more than 12 cm).

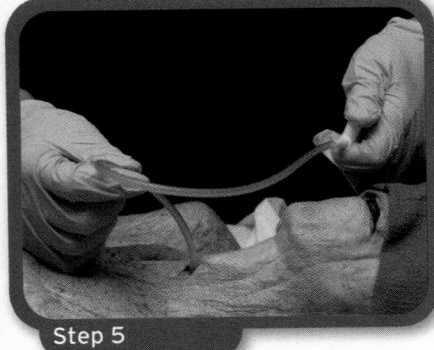

Step 5

Suction while withdrawing the catheter as you instruct the patient to cough or exhale.

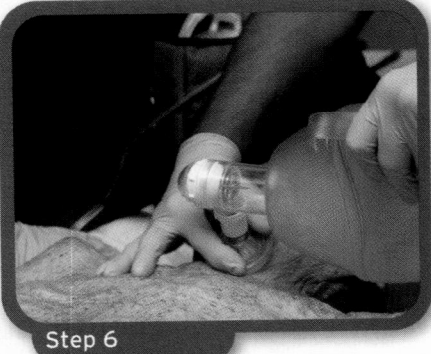

Step 6

Resume oxygenating the patient with a bag-mask device and 100% oxygen.

Skill Drill 11-42: Mouth-to-Stoma Ventilation (Using a Resuscitation Mask)

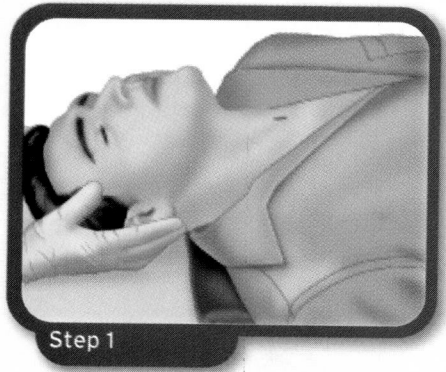

Step 1

Position the patient's head in a neutral position with the shoulders slightly elevated.

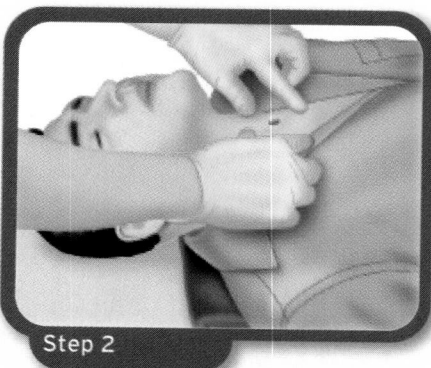

Step 2

Locate and expose the stoma site.

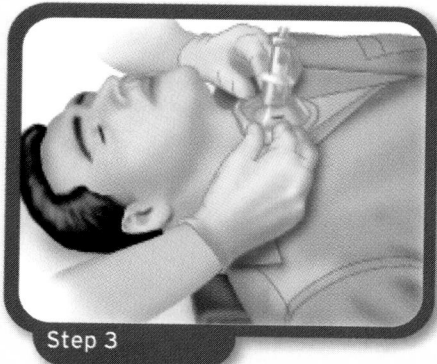

Step 3

Place the resuscitation mask (pediatric mask preferred) over the stoma, and ensure an adequate seal.

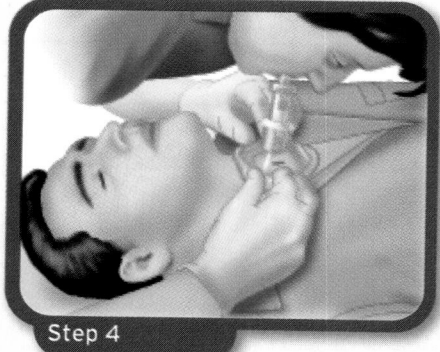

Step 4

Maintain the patient's neutral head position, and ventilate the patient by exhaling directly into the resuscitation mask.
Assess the patient for adequate ventilation by observing his or her chest rise and feeling for air leaks around the mask.

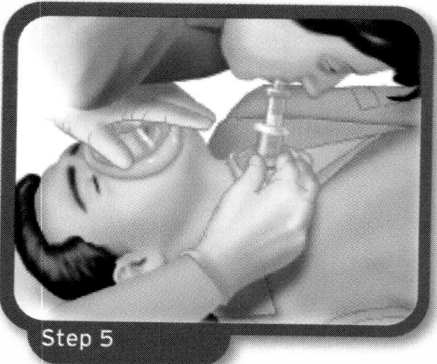

Step 5

If air leakage is evident, seal the patient's mouth and nose and ventilate.

artificially ventilate the patient in this way may be improved, or it may help to clear any obstructions.

The steps for performing mouth-to-stoma ventilation with a resuscitation mask are listed here and shown in **Skill Drill 11-42 ▲**.

1. Position the patient's head in a neutral position with the shoulders slightly elevated (Step 1).
2. Locate and expose the stoma site (Step 2).
3. Place the resuscitation mask (pediatric mask preferred) over the stoma, and ensure an adequate seal (Step 3).
4. Maintain the patient's neutral head position, and ventilate the patient by exhaling directly into the resuscitation mask.
5. Assess the patient for adequate ventilation by observing his or her chest rise and feeling for air leaks around the mask (Step 4)

6. If air leakage is evident, seal the patient's mouth and nose and ventilate (Step 5).

The steps for performing bag-mask device-to-stoma ventilation are listed here and shown in **Skill Drill 11-43 ▶**.

1. With the patient's head in a neutral position, locate and expose the stoma (Step 1).
2. Place the bag-mask device over the stoma and ensure an adequate seal (Step 2).
3. Ventilate the patient by squeezing the bag-mask device, and assess for adequate ventilation by observing chest rise and feeling for air leaks when using a mask. Seal the mouth and nose if an air leak is evident from the upper airway (Step 3).
4. Auscultate over the lungs to confirm adequate ventilation (Step 4).

Skill Drill 11-43: Bag-Mask Device-to-Stoma Ventilation

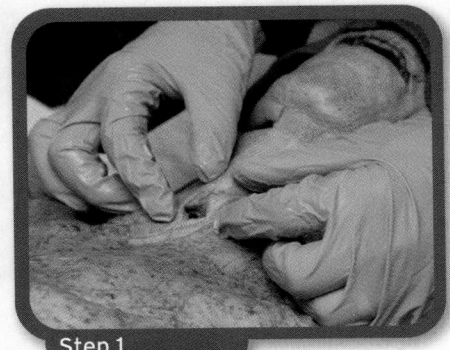

Step 1

With the patient's head in a neutral position, locate and expose the stoma.

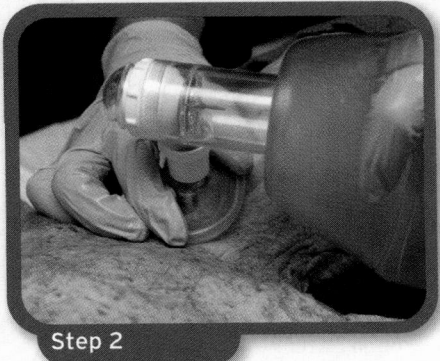

Step 2

Place the bag-mask device over the stoma and ensure an adequate seal.

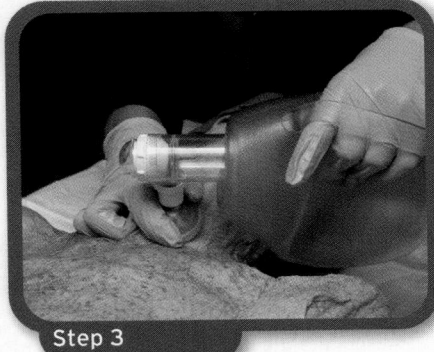

Step 3

Ventilate the patient by squeezing the bag-mask device, and assess for adequate ventilation by observing chest rise.

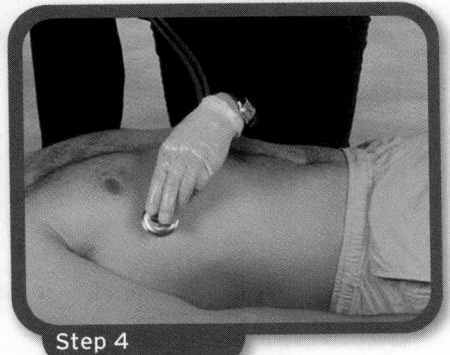

Step 4

Auscultate over the lungs to confirm adequate ventilation.

may have to insert an ET tube into the stoma before it becomes totally occluded. Because the patient with the stoma already has a significant medical problem (eg, brain injury, chronic respiratory insufficiency), he or she may be less tolerant of even brief periods of hypoxia.

The steps for replacing a dislodged tracheostomy tube are listed here and shown in **Skill Drill 11-44 ▸**.

1. Take BSI precautions (gloves and face shield) **Step 1**.
2. Lubricate the same-sized tracheostomy tube or an ET tube (at least 5.0 mm) **Step 2**.
3. Instruct the patient to exhale, and gently insert the tube approximately 1 to 2 cm beyond the balloon cuff **Step 3**.
4. Inflate the balloon cuff **Step 4**.
5. Ensure that the patient is comfortable, and confirm patency and proper placement of the tube by listening for air movement from the tube and noting the patient's clinical status. Ensure that a false lumen was not created **Step 5**.
6. Auscultate the lungs to confirm correct tube placement **Step 6**.

Tracheostomy Tubes

A <u>tracheostomy tube</u> is a plastic tube placed within the tracheostomy site (stoma) **Figure 11-91 ▸**. It requires a 15/22-mm adapter to be compatible with ventilatory devices, such as a mechanical ventilator or bag-mask device. Patients with a tracheostomy tube may receive supplemental oxygen via tubing designed to fit over the tube or by placing an oxygen mask over the tube. Ventilation is accomplished by simply attaching the bag-mask device to the tracheostomy tube.

Patients with a tracheostomy tube who experience sudden dyspnea often have thick secretions in the tube. In this case, perform suctioning through the tracheostomy tube as you would through a stoma.

When a tracheostomy tube becomes dislodged, <u>stenosis</u> (narrowing) of the stoma may occur. Stenosis is potentially life-threatening because soft-tissue swelling decreases the stoma's diameter and impairs the patient's ventilatory ability. In such cases, you may not be able to replace the tracheostomy tube itself and

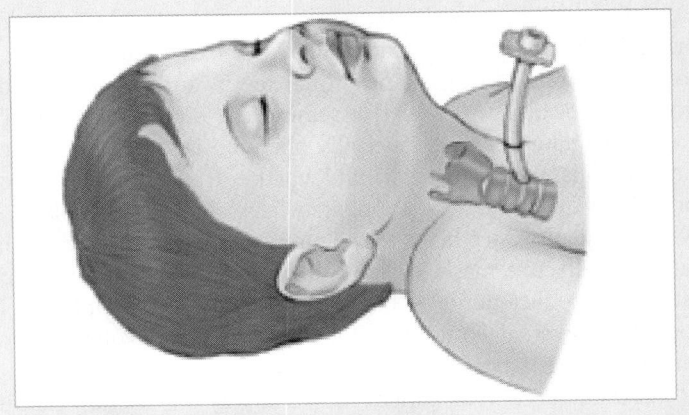

Figure 11-91 A tracheostomy tube.

Skill Drill 11-44: Replacing a Dislodged Tracheostomy Tube

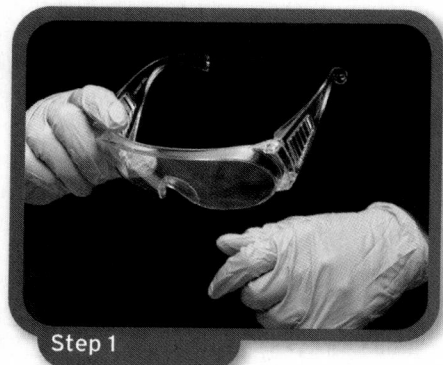

Step 1

Take BSI precautions (gloves and face shield).

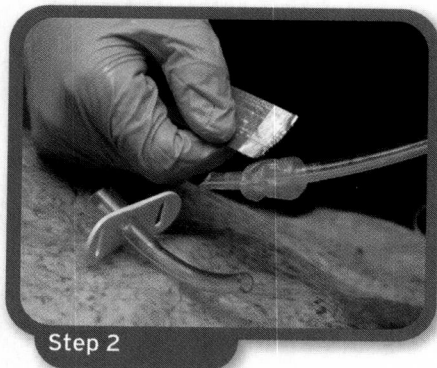

Step 2

Lubricate the same-sized tracheostomy tube or an ET tube (at least 5.0 mm).

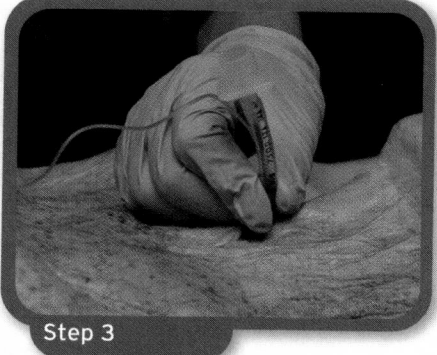

Step 3

Instruct the patient to exhale, and gently insert the tube approximately 1 to 2 cm beyond the balloon cuff.

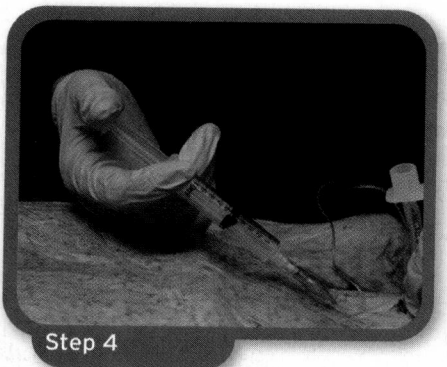

Step 4

Inflate the balloon cuff.

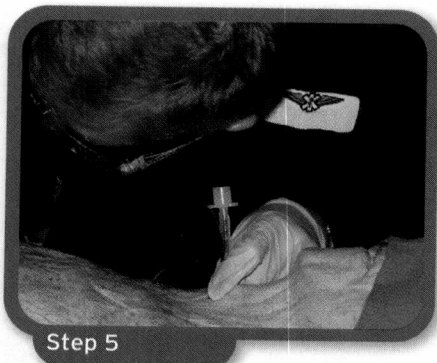

Step 5

Ensure that the patient is comfortable, and confirm patency and proper placement of the tube by listening for air movement from the tube and noting the patient's clinical status. Ensure that a false lumen was not created.

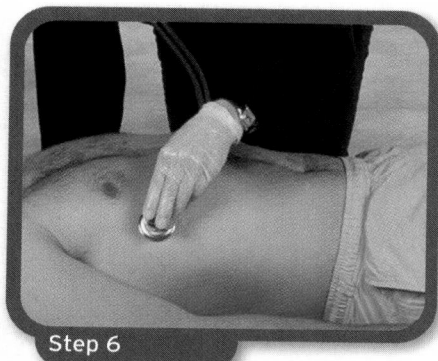

Step 6

Auscultate the lungs to confirm correct tube placement.

Dental Appliances

Dental appliances, which are frequently encountered in the elderly population, can take many different forms: dentures (upper, lower, or both), bridges, individual teeth, and braces (in the younger population). When assessing the airway of a patient with a dental appliance, especially one who is semiconscious or unconscious, you must determine whether the appliance is loose or fitting well. If the dental appliance fits well, leave it in place. A well-fitting appliance helps to maintain the face's structure, facilitating an effective mask-to-face seal if the patient requires ventilation via pocket mask or bag-mask device. If the appliance is loose, however, it could easily become an airway obstruction, and should be removed.

If the unconscious patient has an airway obstruction caused by a dental appliance, perform the usual steps in clearing an obstruction, such as chest compressions, direct laryngoscopy,

and use of the Magill forceps. Great care must be taken if the obstruction is caused by a bridge; these devices often contain sharp metal ends that can easily lacerate the posterior pharynx or larynx.

Often it is not the dental appliance itself that hinders the paramedic's ability to perform a safe and effective intubation, but rather attempts to identify and remove the device. The paramedic may become overly concerned with the presence of the dental appliance rather than concentrating on performing the intubation. Additionally, the oropharyngeal anatomy may be somewhat distorted by the presence of a dental appliance.

In general, it is best to remove dental appliances before intubating a patient. Once the ET tube is in place and has been secured, removal of the dental appliance will be extremely difficult and dangerous, as it may cause dislodgement of the tube or inflict unnecessary oropharyngeal trauma.

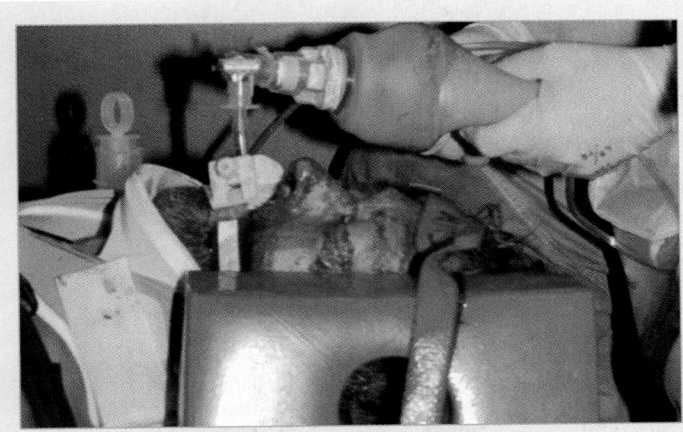

Figure 11-92 Airway management can be especially challenging in patients with facial injuries.

Facial Trauma

It can be especially challenging to effectively manage the airway of a patient with facial injuries Figure 11-92 ▲ . Because the face is highly vascular, facial trauma can result in severe tissue swelling and bleeding into the airway. Control bleeding with direct pressure and suction the airway as needed. You may encounter a patient with severe facial trauma who is breathing inadequately *and* has severe oropharyngeal bleeding—both problems are life-threatening. This situation is most effectively managed by suctioning the patient's airway for 15 seconds (less in infants and children) and then providing positive-pressure ventilation for 2 minutes. This alternating pattern of suctioning and ventilating should continue until the oral secretions have been cleared or the patient has been intubated.

Facial injuries should also increase your index of suspicion for a cervical spine injury. Therefore, when managing the airway, use the jaw-thrust maneuver and keep the patient's head in a neutral in-line position. Endotracheal intubation of the trauma patient is most effectively performed by two paramedics—one who maintains neutral in-line stabilization of the patient's head and the other who performs the intubation. An alternative technique, especially if you are the only paramedic managing the patient's airway, is to stabilize the patient's head in a neutral in-line position with your thighs and then perform the intubation.

When ventilating the patient with facial injuries, stay alert for changes in ventilation compliance or sounds that may indicate laryngeal edema (eg, stridor). If you are unable to effectively ventilate or orally intubate the patient with severe facial injuries, perform a cricothyrotomy (surgical or needle).

You are the Provider Summary

1. Is this patient's airway patent?

Although the patient is experiencing respiratory distress, he is conscious, alert, and talking in complete sentences. Therefore, his airway appears to be patent *at this time.*

2. How will you proceed with your assessment of this patient?

You have already formed a general impression of the patient as you approached him. You must now perform an initial assessment of the patient to determine if he has any problems with airway, breathing, or circulation that require immediate treatment.

3. What immediate management is indicated for this patient?

Immediate management for this patient includes administering 100% supplemental oxygen via nonrebreathing mask. He is experiencing signs and symptoms of hypoxemia, such as pallor, diaphoresis, tachypnea, and tachycardia. You must closely monitor his respiratory effort and be prepared to assist ventilations if his breathing becomes inadequate (eg, a reduced tidal volume, profoundly labored breathing).

4. What questions would be pertinent to ask this patient?

During your focused history and physical exam of the patient, you should use the OPQRST mnemonic to question the patient regarding his present illness. Pertinent questions for a patient complaining of dyspnea include the pattern of the problem (acute or chronic), factors that provoke or palliate his respiratory distress (Can he lie flat?), the patient's perception of the severity of his respiratory distress, and the time of onset. Also determine whether the patient has any medical problems that could be causing (or be exacerbated by) his respiratory distress—for example, congestive heart failure, asthma, COPD, or recent pneumonia.

5. Is this patient breathing adequately? Why or why not?

Although his respirations are tachypneic (28 breaths/min) and labored, his respirations are producing adequate tidal volume at the present time, which suggests that his respiratory effort is adequate. Close monitoring for signs of inadequate breathing is essential, however. You must be prepared to assist ventilations if needed.

6. What are the signs of inadequate ventilation?

Signs of inadequate ventilation include a slow (< 12 breaths/min) or fast (> 20 breaths/min) respiratory rate, reduced tidal volume (shallow breaths), an irregular pattern of inhalation and exhalation, cyanosis, and a decreased mental status.

7. How should you adjust your treatment for this patient? Why?

This patient's respiratory effort is no longer adequate. His level of consciousness has decreased, his heart rate has increased, his respirations have become shallow (reduced tidal volume), and cyanosis is developing around his lips. Additionally, his oxygen saturation is falling despite 100% oxygen via nonrebreathing mask. Therefore, you must begin assisting his ventilations with a bag-mask device and 100% oxygen. Because of his decreased mental status, a nasopharyngeal airway should be inserted to assist in maintaining airway patency.

8. Why is your patient's condition not improving with assisted ventilation?

As evidenced by the patient's gurgling respirations, oral secretions are impairing your ability to effectively ventilate him. Patients with congestive heart failure, especially during periods of exacerbation, frequently cough up pink, frothy sputum. These secretions must be cleared from the airway to allow effective oxygenation and ventilation.

9. What must you do to correct the situation?

When you hear gurgling, think suction! This patient's oropharynx must be suctioned to clear the secretions from his airway, thus improving your ability to effectively oxygenate and ventilate him. This suctioning should not exceed 15 seconds.

If the patient continues to produce oral secretions, you have two problems to manage: aspiration of secretions and inadequate respiratory effort. This is most effectively managed by suctioning the oropharynx for 15 seconds and providing positive-pressure ventilation for 2 minutes. This alternating pattern of suctioning and ventilating should continue until the oral secretions have been removed or the patient's airway has been definitively secured with an ET tube.

10. What is your most appropriate action at this point?

Suctioning the patient's airway has improved his condition (eg, increased Sao_2, improved mentation, decreased heart rate), but he is still in need of ventilatory assistance and the closest hospital is 40 miles away. Immediate transport, with further management en route, is an appropriate intervention. Another option, given this patient's progressive deterioration, would be to proceed with intubation prior to transport rather than trying to manage an unstable airway through a lengthy transport.

11. What are the signs of inadequate artificial ventilation?

Signs of inadequate artificial ventilation include minimal or absent rise of the chest, a heart rate that does not improve, persistent or worsening cyanosis, and a decreasing Sao_2 despite ventilations. Remember, it can be very difficult to ventilate an adult patient with a bag-mask device by yourself, especially if you don't do so on a regular basis. The one-person bag-mask technique takes practice and experience. This is why it is so important to ensure that two providers are available to ride in the patient care compartment en route to the hospital for a patient with an unstable airway.

12. What management is required to prevent further deterioration of this patient's condition?

This patient's clinical condition has deteriorated significantly: He is unresponsive, his respirations have slowed, and he is profoundly cyanotic. Your bag-mask ventilations are not effective because of an ineffective mask-to-face seal (a common complication). This patient's airway needs to be definitively secured with an ET tube, before his condition further deteriorates to respiratory or cardiac arrest.

13. Should you extubate this patient? Why or why not?

Absolutely not! The improvement in this patient's clinical condition is the result of your intubation and providing him with 100% oxygen directly into his lungs. There is no guarantee that he will be able to maintain his own airway or you will be able to reintubate him.

14. Are any pharmacologic interventions required?

Instead of extubating a patient and facing the potential risks associated with removal of the tube (eg, laryngospasm, regurgitation with aspiration), it is *safer* and more efficient to sedate the patient. A variety of sedative-hypnotic drugs can be used for this purpose, including midazolam (Versed) and diazepam (Valium). Follow your locally established protocols regarding sedation agents and dosages.

15. What has most likely caused this patient's increased heart rate and decreased Sao_2?

Acute deterioration in the condition of an intubated patient is usually caused by one of the following: tube dislodgement, obstruction of the tube with secretions, pneumothorax, or equipment failure. Although you hear gurgling in the ET tube, you have already reconfirmed proper placement of the ET tube by auscultation and capnography. The ET tube is probably partially occluded with pulmonary secretions—most likely secondary to the patient's congestive heart failure.

16. How will you remedy the situation?

Occlusion of the ET tube can interfere with effective oxygenation and ventilation of the intubated patient, and must be treated by suctioning the tracheobronchial tree. Preoxygenate the patient for 30 seconds to 1 minute. Inject 3 to 5 mL of sterile saline or water down the ET tube to loosen the secretions, and insert a soft-tip catheter down the ET tube until you meet resistance. Suction in a circular motion while withdrawing the catheter. *Do not exceed 15 seconds during any one suction attempt.* Because suctioning can result in hypoxia, you should closely monitor the patient's cardiac rhythm and oxygen saturation.

17. What treatment would have been appropriate had this clinically unstable patient been too conscious or combative to intubate?

Patients who require intubation, but who are too conscious or combative to tolerate laryngoscopy and tube placement, are candidates for rapid-sequence intubation (RSI), especially if your transport time to the hospital will be lengthy. RSI involves sedating the patient to induce amnesia and suppress the gag reflex. A neuromuscular blocking drug (paralytic) is then given to induce paralysis, facilitating placement of the ET tube. After the patient has been intubated, sedation and paralysis are maintained as needed. RSI is not without risk: You must be absolutely certain that you will be able to intubate the patient once he or she is paralyzed. Follow locally established protocols and/or consult with medical control as needed regarding RSI.

Prep Kit

◼ Ready for Review

- The upper airway consists of all structures above the vocal cords—the larynx, oropharynx, nasopharynx, and tongue. Its functions include warming, filtering, and humification of inhaled air.
- The lower airway consists of all structures below the vocal cords—the trachea, mainstem bronchi, bronchioles, pulmonary capillaries, and alveoli. Pulmonary gas exchange takes place at the alveolar level in the lungs.
- The diaphragm is the major muscle of breathing; it is innervated by the phrenic nerves. The intercostal muscles, the muscles between the ribs, are innervated by the intercostal nerves. Accessory muscles, which are used during times of respiratory distress, include the sternocleidomastoid muscles of the neck.
- The primary breathing stimulus in a healthy patient is based on increasing arterial carbon dioxide levels. The hypoxic drive—a backup system to breathe—is based on decreasing arterial oxygen levels.
- Ventilation is the movement of air into and out of the lungs. Negative-pressure ventilation is the drawing of air into the lungs due to changes in intrathoracic pressure. Positive-pressure ventilation is the forcing of air into the lungs and is provided via bag-mask device, pocket mask, or mechanical ventilation device to patients who are not breathing (apneic) or are breathing inadequately.
- Manual airway maneuvers include the head tilt–chin lift, jaw-thrust (with and without head tilt), and the tongue-jaw lift.
- Regardless of the patient's condition, his or her airway must remain patent at all times. Clearing the airway means removing obstructing material; maintaining the airway means keeping it open, manually or with adjunctive devices.
- Airway obstruction can be caused by choking on food (or, in children, on toys), epiglottitis, inhalation injuries, airway trauma with swelling, and anaphylaxis. It is critical to differentiate between a mild (partial) airway obstruction and a severe (complete) airway obstruction.
- Chest compressions, finger sweeps (only if the object can be seen and easily retrieved), manual removal of the object, and attempts to ventilate is the recommended sequence of events to attempt to remove a foreign body airway obstruction in the unconscious adult. Abdominal thrusts should be performed continuously in the conscious adult or child with an airway obstruction until the obstruction is relieved or he or she becomes unresponsive.
- Back slaps and chest thrusts are performed to relieve a severe airway obstruction in conscious infants. Chest compressions are performed in unconscious infants with a severe airway obstruction.
- Patients with a mild airway obstruction should be closely monitored and transported. Encourage the patient who is coughing forcefully to continue coughing, as it is the most effective way of clearing the airway.
- If conventional methods of airway obstruction removal fail, perform direct laryngoscopy and attempt to retrieve the object with Magill forceps.
- Basic airway adjuncts include the oropharyngeal (oral) airway and the nasopharyngeal (nasal) airway. The oral airway keeps the tongue off of the posterior pharynx; it is used only in unresponsive patients without a gag reflex. The nasal airway is better tolerated in patients with altered mental status who have an intact gag reflex.
- Oropharyngeal suctioning may be required after opening a patient's airway. Rigid (tonsil-tip) catheters are preferred when suctioning the pharynx. Soft, plastic (whistle-tip) catheters are used to suction secretions from the nose, and can be passed down the endotracheal tube to suction pulmonary secretions.
- Oropharyngeal suction should be limited to 15 seconds in the adult, 10 seconds in the child, and 5 seconds in the infant.
- The recovery position involves placing the patient in a left lateral recumbent position. It is the preferred position to maintain the airway of unconscious patients without traumatic injuries, who are breathing adequately.
- Adequate breathing features a respiratory rate between 12 and 20 breaths/min, adequate depth (tidal volume), a regular pattern of inhalation and exhalation, symmetrical chest rise, and bilaterally clear and equal breath sounds.
- Inadequate breathing features a rate that is too slow (< 12 breaths/min) or too fast (> 20 breaths/min), a shallow depth of breathing (reduced tidal volume), an irregular pattern of inhalation and exhalation, asymmetrical chest movement, adventitious airway sounds, cyanosis, and an altered mental status.
- The nonrebreathing mask is the preferred device for delivering oxygen to adequately breathing patients in the prehospital setting; it can deliver up to 90% oxygen when the flow rate is set at 15 L/min. The nasal cannula should be used if the patient cannot tolerate the nonrebreathing mask; it can deliver oxygen concentrations of 24% to 44% when the flowmeter is set at 1 to 6 L/min. Other types of oxygen delivery devices include the simple face mask, partial rebreathing mask, and Venturi mask.
- The pulse oximeter measures the percentage of blood that is saturated with oxygen (Sao_2). This type of measurement depends on adequate perfusion to the capillary beds and can be inaccurate when the patient is cold, is in shock, or has been exposed to carbon monoxide.
- Peak expiratory flow is a fairly reliable assessment of the severity of a patient's bronchoconstriction. It is also used to gauge the effectiveness of treatment, such as inhaled beta-2 agonists (eg, Albuterol).
- Patients with inadequate breathing require some form of positive-pressure ventilation; patients with adequate breathing who are suspected of being hypoxemic require 100% supplemental oxygen via nonrebreathing mask. Never withhold oxygen from any patient suspected of being hypoxemic.
- Unrecognized inadequate breathing will lead to hypoxia, a dangerous condition in which the body's cells and tissues do not receive adequate oxygen.
- The methods of providing artificial ventilation—in order of preference—include the mouth-to-mask technique; the two-person bag-mask technique; the flow-restricted, oxygen-powered ventilation device (FROPVD); and the one-person bag-mask technique. Use extreme caution with the FROPVD and never use this device in children and those with cervical spine or thoracic injuries.
- Combined with your own exhaled breath, mouth-to-mask ventilation with supplemental oxygen attached will deliver approximately 55% oxygen to the patient. A bag-mask device with supplemental oxygen, a reservoir, and an adequate mask-to-face seal can deliver almost 100% oxygen.
- Ventilating too forcefully or too fast can cause gastric distention, which can cause regurgitation and aspiration. Delivering ventilations over 1 second and the use of posterior cricoid pressure (Sellick maneuver) will reduce the incidence of gastric distention and the associated risk of regurgitation/aspiration.
- Invasive gastric decompression involves the insertion of a gastric tube into the stomach. A nasogastric (NG) tube is inserted into the stomach via the nose; an orogastric (OG) tube is inserted into the stomach via the mouth.
- Unresponsive patients or patients who cannot maintain their own airway should be considered candidates for endotracheal intubation, the insertion of an endotracheal (ET) tube into the trachea. In orotracheal intubation, the ET tube is inserted into the trachea via the mouth; in nasotracheal intubation (a blind technique), the ET tube is inserted into the trachea via the nose. Other methods

of endotracheal intubation include digital (or tactile) intubation and intubation with the use of a lighted stylet (transillumination).

- Tracheobronchial suctioning is indicated if the condition of the intubated patient deteriorates due to pulmonary secretions in the ET tube.
- Extubation should not be performed in the prehospital setting unless the patient is unreasonably intolerant of the tube. It is generally best to sedate the intubated patient who is becoming intolerant of the ET tube.
- Alternative airway devices, which may be used if endotracheal intubation is not possible or is unsuccessful, include the Combitube, pharyngeotracheal lumen airway (PtL), and the laryngeal mask airway (LMA).
- Pediatric endotracheal intubation involves the same technique as for adult patients, but with smaller equipment.
- Patients with a tracheal stoma or tracheostomy tube may require ventilation, suctioning, or tube replacement. Ventilation through a tracheostomy tube involves attaching the bag-mask device to the 15/22-mm adapter on the tube; ventilation of the patient with a stoma and no tracheostomy tube can be performed with a pocket mask or bag-mask device. Use pediatric-size masks when ventilating a patient through his or her stoma.
- Open (surgical) cricothyrotomy involves incising the cricothyroid membrane, inserting a tracheostomy tube or ET tube into the trachea, and ventilating the patient with a bag-mask device. Needle cricothyrotomy involves inserting a 14- to 16-gauge over-the-needle catheter through the cricothyroid membrane and ventilating the patient with a high-pressure jet ventilation device.
- Rapid-sequence intubation (RSI) involves using pharmacologic agents to sedate and paralyze the patient to facilitate placement of an ET tube. It should be considered when a conscious or combative patient requires intubation but cannot tolerate laryngoscopy.
- Drugs used for RSI include sedatives, such as diazepam (Valium) and midazolam (Versed), and neuromuscular blocking agents (paralytics) to induce complete paralysis. The latter agents are classified into depolarizing paralytics (eg, succinylcholine) and nondepolarizing paralytics (eg, vecuronium, pancuronium).
- Check for loose dental appliances in a patient before providing artificial ventilation. Loose dental appliances should be removed to prevent them from obstructing the airway; tight-fitting dental appliances should be left in place during artificial ventilation.
- Dental appliances should be removed before intubating a patient. Removing them after the patient has been intubated may result in inadvertent extubation.
- Patients with massive maxillofacial trauma are at high risk for airway compromise due to oral bleeding. Assist ventilations and provide oral suctioning as needed.

Vital Vocabulary

accessory muscles Muscles not normally used during normal breathing; includes the sternocleidomastoid muscles of the neck.

acetylcholine (ACh) Chemical neurotransmitter of the parasympathetic nervous system.

adenoids Lymphatic tissues located on the posterior nasopharyngeal wall that filter bacteria.

adventitious Abnormal.

agonal respirations Slow, shallow, irregular respirations or occasional gasping breaths; results from cerebral anoxia.

alveolar volume Volume of inhaled air that reaches the alveoli and participates in gas exchange; equal to tidal volume minus dead space volume and is approximately 350 mL in the average adult.

alveoli Balloon-like clusters of single-layer air sacs that are the functional site for the exchange of oxygen and carbon dioxide in the lungs.

anatomic dead space Includes the trachea and larger bronchi. The air remaining in these areas is the result of residual gas in the upper airway at the end of inhalation.

anoxia An absence of oxygen.

antegrade amnesia Inability to remember from this point in time forward.

anxiolysis Relief of anxiety.

aphonia Inability to speak.

apneustic center Portion of the brain stem that influences the respiratory rate by increasing the number of inspirations per minute.

arytenoid cartilages Pyramid-like cartilaginous structures that form the posterior attachment of the vocal cords.

aspiration Entry of fluids or solids into the trachea, bronchi, and lungs.

asymmetric chest wall movement When one side of the chest moves less than the other; indicates decreased airflow into one lung.

atelectasis Collapsing of the alveoli.

atlanto-occipital joint Joint formed at the articulation of the atlas of the vertebral column and the occipital bone of the skull.

automatic transport ventilator (ATV) Portable mechanical ventilator attached to a control box that allows the variables of ventilation (eg, rate, tidal volume) to be set.

bag-mask device Manual ventilation device that consists of a bag, mask, reservoir, and oxygen inlet; capable of delivering up to 100% oxygen.

barbiturates Sedative-hypnotic medications; includes drugs such as thiopental (Pentothal) and methohexital (Brevital).

barotrauma Trauma resulting from excessive pressure.

benzodiazepines Sedative-hypnotic drugs that provide muscle relaxation and mild sedation; includes drugs such as diazepam (Valium) and midazolam (Versed).

Biot respirations Irregular pattern, rate, and depth with intermittent periods of apnea; results from increased intracranial pressure.

Bourdon-gauge flowmeter An oxygen flowmeter that is commonly used because it is not affected by gravity and can be placed in any position.

bronchioles Subdivision of the smaller bronchi in the lungs; made of smooth muscle and dilate or constrict in response to various stimuli.

BURP maneuver Acronym for Backward, Upward, Rightward Pressure.

butrophenones Potent, effective sedatives; includes drugs such as haloperidol (Haldol) and droperidol (Inapsine).

capnographer Device that attaches in between the endotracheal tube and bag-mask device; contains colorimetric paper, which should turn yellow during exhalation, indicating proper tube placement.

capnometer Device that attaches in the same way as a capnographer, but provides a light-emitting diode (LED) readout of the patient's exhaled carbon dioxide.

carboxyhemoglobin Abnormal hemoglobin that is formed by the attachment of carbon monoxide to the hemoglobin molecule.

carina Point at which the trachea bifurcates (divides) into the left and right mainstem bronchi.

cerebrospinal otorrhea Cerebrospinal fluid drainage from the ears.

cerebrospinal rhinorrhea Cerebrospinal fluid drainage from the nose.

chemoreceptors Monitor the levels of O_2, CO_2, and the pH of the CSF and then provide feedback to the respiratory centers to modify the rate and depth of breathing based on the body's needs at any given time.

Cheyne-Stokes respirations Gradually increasing rate and depth followed by a gradual decrease with intermittent periods of apnea; associated with brain stem insult.

Combitube Multilumen airway device that consists of a single tube with two lumens, two balloons, and two ventilation ports; an alternative device if endotracheal intubation is not possible or has failed.

continuous positive airway pressure (CPAP) A form of noninvasive ventilation in which the patient exhales against positive-pressure via a tight-fitting face mask; used to treat patients with pulmonary edema and severe bronchospasm.

cricoid cartilage Forms the lowest portion of the larynx; also referred to as the cricoid ring; the first ring of the trachea and is the only upper airway structure that forms a complete ring.

cricoid pressure The application of posterior pressure to the cricoid cartilage to reduce the risk of regurgitation during positive-pressure ventilation; also called the Sellick maneuver.

cricothyroid membrane A thin, superficial membrane located between the thyroid and cricoid cartilages that is relatively avascular and contains few nerves; the site for emergency surgical and nonsurgical access to the airway.

curved laryngoscope blade Also called the Macintosh blade; designed to fit into the vallecula, indirectly lifting the epiglottis and exposing the vocal cords.

cyanosis Blue or purple skin; indicates inadequate oxygen in the blood.

dead space Any portion of the airway that does not contain air and cannot participate in gas exchange.

depolarizing neuromuscular blockers Competitively bind with the acetylcholine receptor sites but are not affected as quickly by acetylcholinesterase; includes drugs such as succinylcholine.

diaphragm The major muscle of breathing. It is the anatomic point of separation between the thoracic cavity and the abdominal cavity.

diffusion Movement of a gas from an area of higher concentration to an area of lower concentration.

digital intubation Method of intubation that involves directly palpating the glottic structures and elevating the epiglottis with your middle finger while guiding the ET tube into the trachea by feel.

direct laryngoscopy Visualization of the airway with a laryngoscope.

dysphonia Difficulty speaking.

dyspnea Any difficulty in respiratory rate, regularity, or effort.

emergence phenomenon Nightmares associated with the use of ketamine.

endotracheal intubation Passing an endotracheal (ET) tube through the glottic opening and sealing the tube with a cuff inflated against the tracheal wall.

endotracheal (ET) tube Tube that is inserted into the trachea; equipped with a distal cuff, proximal inflation port, a 15/22-mm adapter, and cm markings on the side.

end-tidal carbon dioxide ($ETco_2$) detectors Device that detects the presence of carbon dioxide in exhaled air.

epiglottis Leaf-shaped cartilaginous structure that closes over the trachea during swallowing.

esophageal detector device (EDD) Bulb or syringe that is attached to the proximal end of the ET tube; a device used to confirm proper ET tube placement.

etomidate A nonnarcotic, nonbarbiturate hypnotic-sedative drug; also called Amidate.

exhalation Passive movement of air out of the lungs; also called expiration.

expiration Passive movement of air out of the lungs; also called exhalation.

expiratory reserve volume The amount of air that you can exhale following a normal exhalation; average volume is about 1,200 mL.

external respiration The exchange of gases between the lungs and the blood cells in the pulmonary capillaries; also called pulmonary respiration.

extubation The process of removing the tube from an intubated patient.

eyelash reflex Contraction of the patient's lower eyelid when it is gently stroked; fairly reliable indicator of the presence or absence of an intact gag reflex.

fasciculations Characterized by brief, uncoordinated twitching of small muscle groups in the face, neck, trunk, and extremities; caused by the administration of depolarizing neuromuscular blocking agents (eg, succinylcholine).

flow-restricted, oxygen-powered ventilation device (FROPVD) Also referred to as a manually triggered ventilator or demand valve. Can be used to ventilate apneic or to administer supplemental oxygen to spontaneously breathing patients.

fraction of inspired oxygen (Fio_2) The percentage of oxygen in inhaled air.

functional reserve capacity The amount of air that can be forced from the lungs in a single exhalation.

gag reflex Automatic reaction when something touches an area deep in the oral cavity; helps protect the lower airway from aspiration.

gastric distention Inflation of the patient's stomach with air.

gastric tube A tube that is inserted into the stomach to remove its contents.

glottis The space in between the vocal cords that is the narrowest portion of the adult's airway; also called the glottic opening.

gum bougie Also called the Eschmann stylet; a flexible device that is inserted in between the glottis under direct laryngoscopy. The ET tube is then threaded over the device, facilitating its entry into the trachea.

head tilt-chin lift maneuver Manual airway maneuver that involves tilting the head back while lifting up on the chin; used to open the airway of a semiconscious or unconscious nontrauma patient.

Heimlich maneuver Abdominal thrusts performed to relieve a foreign body airway obstruction.

hemoglobin An iron-containing protein within red blood cells that has the ability to combine with oxygen.

Hering-Breuer reflex A protective mechanism that terminates inhalation, thus preventing overexpansion of the lungs.

hilum Point of entry of all of the blood vessels and the bronchi into each lung.

hyoid bone A small, horseshoe-shaped bone to which the jaw, tongue, epiglottis, and thyroid cartilage attach.

hypercarbia Increased CO_2 content in arterial blood.

hyperventilation Occurs when CO_2 elimination exceeds CO_2 production.

hypocarbia Decreased CO_2 content in arterial blood.

hypoventilation Occurs when CO_2 production exceeds the body's ability to eliminate it by ventilation.

hypoxemia A decrease in arterial oxygen levels.

hypoxia A lack of oxygen to the body's cells and tissues.

hypoxic drive Secondary control of breathing that stimulates breathing based on decreased PaO_2 levels.

inspiration The active process of moving air into the lungs; also called inhalation.

inspiratory reserve volume The amount of air that can be inhaled after a normal inhalation; the amount of air that can be inhaled in addition to the normal tidal volume.

intercostal nerves Nerves that innervate the external intercostal muscles, the muscles between the ribs.

internal respiration The exchange of gases between the blood cells and the tissues; also called cellular respiration.

intrapulmonary shunting Bypassing of oxygen-poor blood past non-functional alveoli.

jaw-thrust maneuver Manual airway maneuver that involves stabilizing the patient's head and thrusting the jaw forward; the preferred method of opening the airway of a semiconscious or unconscious trauma patient.

jaw-thrust maneuver with head tilt Manual airway maneuver that involves thrusting the jaw forward while tilting back on the head.

ketamine A drug with sedative, analgesic, and hypnotic properties; created in the laboratory from phencyclidine (PCP).

Kussmaul respirations Deep, gasping respirations; common in diabetic coma (ketoacidosis).

laryngeal mask airway (LMA) Device that surrounds the opening of the larynx with an inflatable silicone cuff positioned in the hypopharynx; an alternative device to bag-mask ventilation.

laryngectomy A surgical procedure in which the larynx is removed.

laryngoscope Device that is used in conjunction with a laryngoscope blade in order to perform direct laryngoscopy.

laryngospasm Spasmodic closure of the vocal cords.

larynx A complex structure formed by many independent cartilaginous structures that all work together; where the upper airway ends and the lower airway begins.

lung compliance The ability of the alveoli to expand when air is drawn into the lungs, either during negative-pressure ventilation or positive-pressure ventilation.

Magill forceps A special type of forcep that is curved, thus allowing the paramedic to maneuver it in the airway.

minute alveolar volume The amount of air that actually reaches the alveoli per minute and participates in gas exchange.

minute volume The amount of air that moves in and out of the respiratory tract per minute.

Murphy's eye An opening on the side of an endotracheal tube at its distal tip that enables ventilation to occur even if the tip becomes occluded by blood, mucus, or the tracheal wall.

nasal cannula Delivers oxygen via two small prongs that fit into the patient's nostrils. With an oxygen flow rate of 1 to 6 L/min, the nasal cannula can deliver an oxygen concentration of 24% to 44%.

nasal septum A rigid partition composed of bone and cartilage; divides the nasopharynx into two passages.

nasogastric (NG) tube Gastric tube is inserted into the stomach through the nose.

nasopharyngeal (nasal) airway A soft rubber tube about 6″ long that is inserted through the nose into the posterior pharynx behind the tongue, thereby allowing passage of air from the nose to the lower airway.

nasopharynx The nasal cavity; formed by the union of the facial bones.

nasotracheal intubation Insertion of an endotracheal tube into the trachea through the nose.

nebulizer Device used primarily to deliver aerosolized medications. Oxygen enters an aerosol chamber that contains 3 to 5 mL of fluid. The pressurized oxygen in this chamber aerosolizes the medication for inhalation.

needle cricothyrotomy Insertion of a 14- to 16-gauge over-the-needle IV catheter (angiocath) through the cricothyroid membrane and into the trachea.

negative-pressure ventilation Drawing of air into the lungs; airflow from a region of higher pressure (outside the body) to a region of lower pressure (the lungs); occurs during normal (unassisted breathing).

nondepolarizing neuromuscular blockers Binds to acetylcholine receptor sites; however, unlike depolarizing neuromuscular blockers, they do not cause depolarization of the muscle fiber; includes drugs such as vecuronium (Norcuron) and pancuronium (Pavulon).

nonrebreathing mask A combination mask and reservoir bag system. Oxygen fills a reservoir bag that is attached to the mask by a one-way valve. This permits the patient to inhale from the reservoir bag but not to exhale back into it. With a good mask-to-face seal and a flow rate of 15 L/min, it is capable of delivering up to 90% inspired oxygen.

open cricothyrotomy Also referred to as a surgical cricothyrotomy; an emergent procedure that involves incising the cricothyroid membrane with a scalpel and inserting an endotracheal or tracheostomy tube directly into the subglottic area of the trachea.

opioids Also called narcotics; potent analgesics with sedative properties; includes drugs such as fentanyl (Sublimaze) and alfentanil (Alfenta).

orogastric (OG) tube Gastric tube inserted into the stomach through the mouth.

oropharyngeal (oral) airway A hard plastic device that is curved in such a way that it fits over the back of the tongue with the tip in the posterior pharynx.

oropharynx Forms the posterior portion of the oral cavity, which is bordered superiorly by the hard and soft palates, laterally by the cheeks, and inferiorly by the tongue.

orotracheal intubation Insertion of an endotracheal tube into the trachea through the mouth.

orthopnea Positional dyspnea.

oxygen humidifier Small bottle of water through which the oxygen leaving the cylinder is moisturized before it reaches the patient.

oxyhemoglobin Hemoglobin that is occupied by oxygen.

palate Forms the roof of the mouth and separates the oropharynx and nasopharynx.

pancuronium A nondepolarizing neuromuscular blocking agent; used to maintain paralysis following succinylcholine-facilitated intubation; also called Pavulon.

paralytics Also called neuromuscular blocking agents; paralyzes skeletal muscles; used in an emergency situation to facilitate intubation.

parietal pleura Thin membrane that lines the chest cavity.

partial laryngectomy Surgical removal of a portion of the larynx.

partial rebreathing mask Similar to the nonrebreathing mask except that there is no one-way valve between the mask and the reservoir. Room air is not entrained with inspiration; however, residual expired air is mixed in the mask and rebreathed.

patent Open.

peak expiratory flow An approximation of the extent of bronchoconstriction; used to determine whether patients are improving with therapy (eg, inhaled bronchodilators).

pharyngeotracheal lumen airway (PtL) Multilumen airway device that consists of two tubes and two cuffs; an alternative device if endotracheal intubation is not possible or has failed.

pharynx Throat.

phrenic nerves Nerves that innervate the diaphragm.

physiologic dead space Additional dead space created by intrapulmonary obstructions or atelectasis.

pneumotaxic center Area of the brain stem that has an inhibitory influence on inspiration.

positive-pressure ventilation Forcing of air into the lungs.

pressure-compensated flowmeter An oxygen flowmeter that incorporates a float ball within a tapered calibrated tube. The float rises or falls according to the gas flow within the tube. Because this type of flowmeter is affected by gravity, it must remain in an upright position to obtain an accurate flow reading.

primary respiratory drive Normal stimulus to breathe; based on fluctuations in $Paco_2$ and pH of the CSF.

pulse oximeter Device that measures oxygen saturation.

pulsus paradoxus A drop in the systolic BP of 10 mm Hg or more; commonly seen in patients with pericardial tamponade or severe asthma.

pyriform fossae Two pockets of tissue on the lateral borders of the larynx.

rapid-sequence intubation (RSI) A specific set of procedures, combined in rapid succession, to induce sedation and paralysis and intubate a patient quickly.

recovery position Left-lateral recumbent position; used in all semiconscious and unconscious nontrauma patients, who are able to maintain their own airway spontaneously and are breathing adequately.

residual volume The air that remains in the lungs after maximal expiration.

respiration The exchange of gases between a living organism and its environment.

retractions Skin pulling in between and around the ribs during inhalation.

safe residual pressure A term that implies that it is *unsafe* to continue using an oxygen cylinder with a pressure of less than 200 psi.

sedation Reduction of a patient's anxiety, induction of amnesia, and suppression of the gag reflex.

Sellick maneuver The application of posterior pressure to the cricoid cartilage to minimize the risk of regurgitation during positive-pressure ventilation; also referred to as cricoid pressure.

Shiley A type of tracheostomy tube.

simple face mask A full mask enclosure with open side ports. Room air is drawn in through the side ports on inhalation, diluting the concentration of inspired oxygen. Exhaled air is vented through holes on each side of the mask. The simple face mask will deliver between 40% and 60% oxygen at 10 L/min.

sinuses Cavities formed by the cranial bones that trap contaminants from entering the respiratory tract and act as tributaries for fluid to and from the eustachian tubes and tear ducts.

stenosis Narrowing.

stoma The resultant orifice of a tracheostomy that connects the trachea to the outside air; located in the midline of the anterior neck.

straight laryngoscope blade Also called the Miller blade; designed to lift the epiglottis and expose the vocal cords.

stylet A semirigid wire that is inserted into the ET tube to mold and maintain the shape of the tube.

succinylcholine chloride A depolarizing neuromuscular blocker frequently used as the initial paralytic during rapid-sequence intubation; causes muscle fasciculations; also referred to as Anectine.

surfactant A proteinaceous substance that lines the alveoli; decreases alveolar surface tension and keeps the alveoli expanded.

therapy regulator Attaches to the stem of the oxygen cylinder, and reduces the high pressure of gas to a safe range (about 50 psi).

thyroid cartilage The main supporting cartilage of the larynx; a shield-shaped structure formed by two plates that join in a "V" shape anteriorly to form the laryngeal prominence known as the Adam's apple.

tidal volume A measure of the depth of breathing; the volume of air that is inhaled or exhaled during a single respiratory cycle.

tongue-jaw lift maneuver A manual maneuver that involves grasping the tongue and jaw and lifting; commonly used to suction the airway and to place certain airway devices.

tonsils Lymphatic tissues that are located in the posterior pharynx; they help to trap bacteria.

tonsil-tip catheter A hard or rigid suction catheter; also called a Yankauer catheter.

total laryngectomy Surgical removal of the entire larynx.

total lung capacity The total volume of air that the lungs can hold; approximately 6 L in the average adult male.

trachea The conduit for all entry into the lungs; a tubular structure that is approximately 10 to 12 cm in length and is composed of a series of C-shaped cartilaginous rings; also called the windpipe.

tracheobronchial suctioning Passing a suction catheter into the endotracheal tube to remove pulmonary secretions.

tracheostomy Surgical opening into the trachea.

tracheostomy tube Plastic tube placed within the tracheostomy site (stoma).

transillumination intubation Method of intubation that uses a lighted stylet to guide the endotracheal tube into the trachea.

translaryngeal catheter ventilation Used in conjunction with needle cricothyrotomy to ventilate a patient; requires a high-pressure jet ventilator.

trismus Clenched teeth caused by spasms of the jaw muscles.

turbinates Three bony shelves that protrude from the lateral walls of the nasal cavity and extend into the nasal passageway, parallel to the nasal floor; serve to increase the surface area of the nasal mucosa, thereby improving the processes of warming, filtering, and humidification of inhaled air.

upper airway Consists of all anatomic airway structures above the level of the vocal cords.

uvula A soft-tissue structure that resembles a punching bag; located in the posterior aspect of the oral cavity, at the base of the tongue.

vallecula An anatomic space, or "pocket," located between the base of the tongue and the epiglottis; an important anatomic landmark for endotracheal intubation.

vecuronium A nondepolarizing neuromuscular blocking agent; used to maintain paralysis following succinylcholine-facilitated intubation; also called Norcuron.

ventilation The process of moving air into and out of the lungs.

Venturi mask A mask that has a number of interchangeable adapters that draws room air into the mask along with the oxygen flow; allows for the administration of highly specific oxygen concentrations.

visceral pleura Thin membrane that lines the lungs.

vocal cords White bands of tough tissue that are the lateral borders of the glottis.

whistle-tip catheters Soft plastic, nonrigid catheters; also called French catheters.

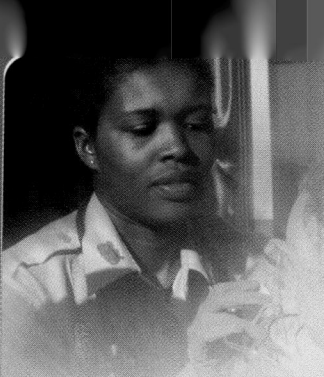

Assessment in Action

You are dispatched to a residence for an "unconscious male." You arrive at the scene 6 minutes after being dispatched and are met at the door of the residence by a frantic woman.

Your initial assessment reveals that the man is unresponsive. His respirations are slow and shallow, and his pulse is rapid and weak. Further assessment reveals facial cyanosis and vomitus around his mouth. The patient's wife tells you that she thinks her husband has had a stroke. You and your partner begin immediate treatment; a second paramedic unit is dispatched to the scene to provide assistance.

1. **Vomitus that has been aspirated into the lungs will:**
   A. cause a rapid, fatal infection.
   B. impair pulmonary diffusion.
   C. increase ventilation compliance.
   D. require deep tracheal suctioning.

2. **The goal of providing assisted ventilation to a hypoventilating patient is to:**
   A. minimize hypocarbia.
   B. reduce gastric distention.
   C. improve cardiac output.
   D. maintain minute volume.

3. **Signs of adequate ventilation in the adult include:**
   A. pink mucous membranes.
   B. a prolonged exhalation phase.
   C. a shallow depth of breathing.
   D. respirations of 30 breaths/min.

4. **Positive-pressure ventilation is defined as:**
   A. forcing air into the lungs.
   B. drawing air into the lungs.
   C. deep spontaneous breathing.
   D. a reduction in tidal volume.

5. **Which of the following oxygen delivery devices is MOST appropriate for a patient with suspected hypoxemia and adequate tidal volume?**
   A. Nasal cannula
   B. Simple face mask
   C. Nonrebreathing mask
   D. Bag-mask device with reservoir

6. **Negative-pressure ventilation occurs when:**
   A. the diaphragm relaxes and ascends.
   B. pressure within the thoracic cavity decreases.
   C. air is blown into the lungs with a bag-mask device.
   D. a patient is ventilated with a demand valve.

7. **The volume of air moved into and out of the lungs per breath is called:**
   A. tidal volume.
   B. stroke volume.
   C. minute volume.
   D. alveolar volume.

8. **The primary respiratory drive in a healthy individual is based on:**
   A. decreasing Pao_2 levels.
   B. the pH of venous blood.
   C. progressive hypocarbia.
   D. increasing Pco_2 levels.

9. **In contrast to hypoxia, hypoxemia is defined as:**
   A. a complete lack of oxygen to the brain.
   B. a deficiency of oxygen in the arterial blood.
   C. decreased oxygen to the body's tissues and cells.
   D. an insufficient supply of oxygen to the myocardium.

10. **What is the MOST commonly encountered problem when ventilating a patient with the one-person bag-mask technique?**
    A. Inability to squeeze the bag
    B. Forgetting to attach the reservoir
    C. Difficulty maintaining a mask seal
    D. Not manually positioning the head

11. **The phrenic nerves innervate the:**
    A. diaphragm.
    B. intercostal muscles.
    C. accessory muscles.
    D. pons and medulla.

12. **Physiologic dead space would increase with:**
    A. atelectatic alveoli.
    B. increased tidal volume.
    C. reduced minute volume.
    D. gastric distention.

13. **Alveolar surface tension would increase with:**
    A. positive-pressure ventilation.
    B. inadvertent esophageal intubation.
    C. increased ventilatory compliance.
    D. a deficiency of pulmonary surfactant.

14. **What is the usual anatomic dead space volume in the average adult male?**
    A. 70 mL
    B. 150 mL
    C. 200 mL
    D. 350 mL

15. **The exchange of gases between a living organism and its environment is called:**
    A. ventilation.
    B. respiration.
    C. expiration.
    D. inhalation.

16. **If performed properly, the Sellick maneuver will minimize the risk of:**
    A. shallow breathing.
    B. excessive tidal volume.
    C. gastric distention.
    D. tracheal intubation.

17. **The volume of air that remains in the lungs after maximal expiration is called:**
    A. residual volume.
    B. expiratory reserve volume.
    C. inspiratory reserve volume.
    D. functional reserve capacity.

18. **A patient who has an altered mental status and has shallow respirations should be treated initially with:**
    A. immediate endotracheal intubation.
    B. a nonrebreathing mask at 15 L/min.
    C. insertion of a laryngeal mask airway.
    D. some form of positive-pressure ventilation.

19. **Which of the following MOST accurately describes pulsus paradoxus?**
    A. An increase in the heart rate during inhalation
    B. A decrease in systolic BP during inhalation
    C. An increase in diastolic BP during exhalation
    D. A decrease in the heart rate during exhalation

20. **Which of the following respiratory patterns is characterized by occasional, irregular, shallow breaths?**
    A. Biot breathing
    B. Agonal breathing
    C. Cheyne-Stokes breathing
    D. Kussmaul breathing

21. **Immediately after inserting an endotracheal tube through the vocal cords, the paramedic should:**
    A. begin ventilations.
    B. attach an ETco_2 detector.
    C. inflate the distal cuff.
    D. auscultate for breath sounds.

22. **To properly align the three airway axes prior to endotracheal intubation, the patient's head should be placed in what position?**
    A. Sniffing
    B. Flexed
    C. Extended
    D. Neutral

23. **Multilumen airway devices are not intended to be used in patients who:**
    A. are deeply unconscious.
    B. weigh more than 75 kg.
    C. have an esophageal disease.
    D. are in cardiopulmonary arrest.

24. **Following a needle cricothyrotomy, ventilations are MOST effectively performed with which of the following devices?**
    A. Bag-mask device and 100% oxygen
    B. Flow-restricted oxygen-powered device
    C. ET tube adapter and a 10-mL syringe
    D. High-pressure jet ventilation device

25. **Medications used during rapid-sequence intubation (RSI) include which of the following?**
    A. Epinephrine
    B. Norcuron
    C. Amiodarone
    D. Furosemide

Challenging Question

You and your partner are caring for a 67-year-old man with congestive heart failure. The patient is extremely restless and agitated, and is laboring to breathe. Your repeated attempts to provide 100% oxygen via nonrebreathing mask have failed; the patient keeps pulling the mask away from his face. He is becoming physically exhausted; however, he is still agitated and noncompliant with your treatment. He has cyanosis to his face, an oxygen saturation of 78%, an end-tidal carbon dioxide reading of 15 mm Hg per capnometry, and a weak pulse at 120 beats/min. The closest appropriate medical facility is 25 miles away.

26. **What measures must be taken to prevent this patient from developing cardiac arrest?**

▇▇ Points to Ponder

Your partner is attempting to perform endotracheal intubation on a middle-aged unconscious, apneic man. The patient is attached to a cardiac monitor, which is displaying a normal sinus rhythm, and a pulse oximeter, which is reading 98%. Approximately 15 seconds into the intubation attempt, you note that the patient's heart rate has dropped approximately 30 beats/min and the pulse oximeter now reads 82%. You immediately advise your partner of the change in the patient's condition, to which he replies, "I still have 15 seconds left." He continues with the intubation attempt, which is successful. As you are in the process of securing the ET tube in place, the patient experiences cardiac arrest. Despite aggressive management and prompt transport to the hospital, the patient dies.

Why did this patient experience cardiac arrest? What could have been done to prevent it?

Issues: Knowing When to Abort an Intubation Attempt, Understanding the Importance of Adequate Oxygenation and Ventilation, Working Effectively as a Team.

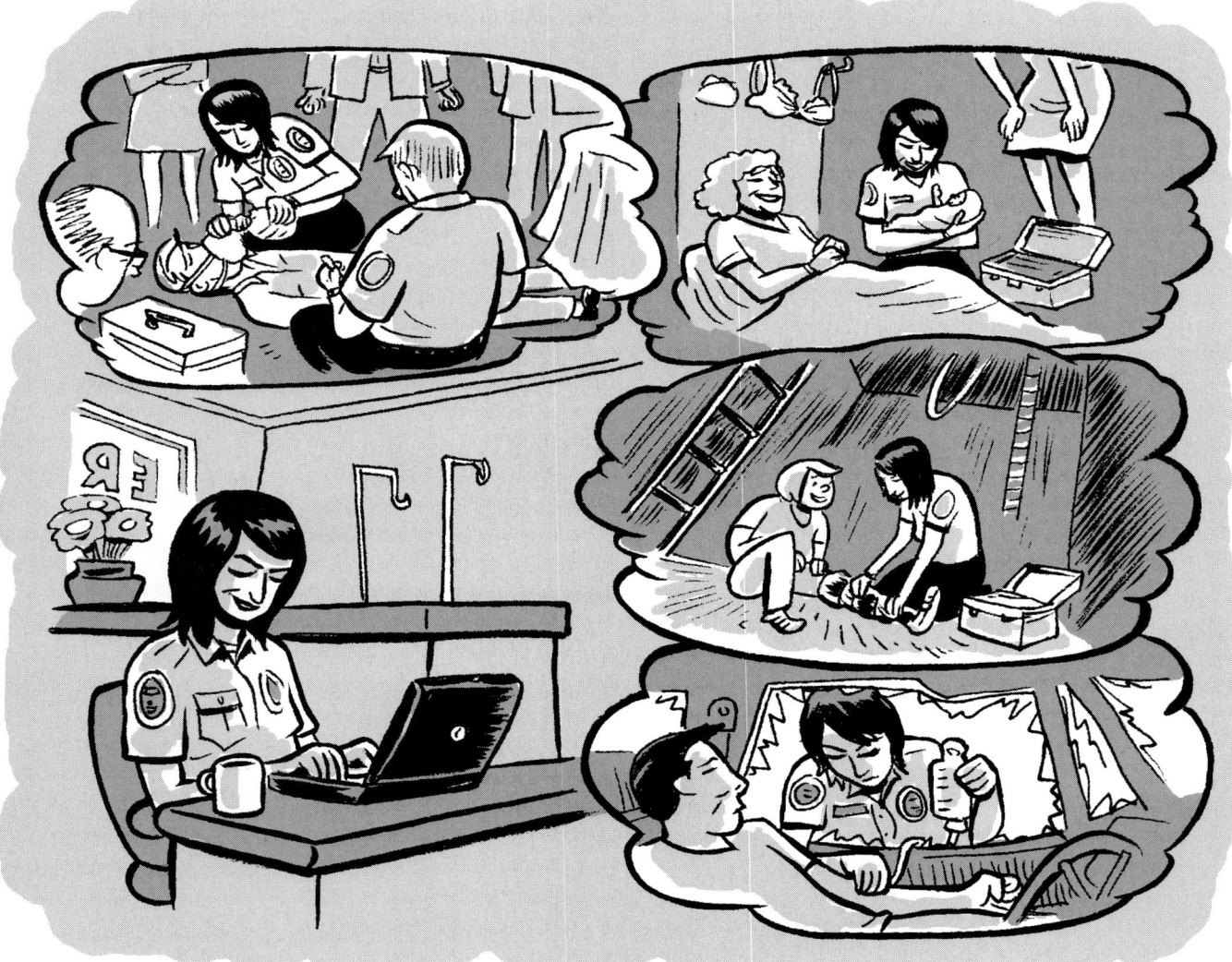

"

I learned the special stresses and constraints of rendering care outside the controlled conditions of a hospital: CPR in a crowded restaurant, childbirth in the lingerie section of a department store, splinting at the bottom of an elevator shaft, intravenous infusions inside a wrecked automobile."

—Nancy L. Caroline, MD

Patient Assessment

3

Section

Section Editor: Mike Smith, BS, MICP

12 Patient History

Objectives

Cognitive

3-1.1   Describe the techniques of history taking. (p 12.7)

3-1.2   Discuss the importance of using open ended questions. (p 12.8)

3-1.3   Describe the use of facilitation, reflection, clarification, empathetic responses, confrontation, and interpretation. (p 12.11–12.13)

3-1.4   Differentiate between facilitation, reflection, clarification, sympathetic responses, confrontation, and interpretation. (p 12.11–12.13)

3-1.5   Describe the structure and purpose of a health history. (p 12.7)

3-1.6   Describe how to obtain a comprehensive health history. (p 12.9)

3-1.7   List the components of a comprehensive history of an adult patient. (p 12.7–12.10)

Affective

3-1.8   Demonstrate the importance of empathy when obtaining a health history. (p 12.12)

3-1.9   Demonstrate the importance of confidentiality when obtaining a health history. (p 12.9)

Psychomotor

None

Introduction

Most practicing EMTs, paramedics, nurses, and physicians quickly learn that patient assessment is one of the most important parts of their job. Assessment combines a number steps—assessing the scene, getting your patient's chief complaint, taking care of life-threatening problems, taking your patient's medical history, and doing a physical examination. One of the most unique things about your patient assessment skills is that *there is no limit to how good they can be.* With a positive attitude and a commitment to excellence, you will have the opportunity to continue to polish and improve these critical skills throughout your career as a paramedic.

Paramedics often work with seriously ill or injured patients without the input of specialized resources, like clinical laboratories and x-ray departments Figure 12-1 ▸ . However, you can be confident in a good field diagnosis if you learn excellent history-taking skills. Many physicians say that hospital tests more often than not confirm a diagnosis the physician arrived at *by taking a patient history.*

To the patient, the entire assessment process should appear to be a seamless process. To the provider, it is most often a blend of questions and answers with a physical examination. What varies from patient to patient is the number and types of questions that must be asked and to what extent the patient should be examined before a working diagnosis is reached. Never forget that the entire patient assessment process should be organized and systematic, but, at the same time, be reasonably flexible.

Aside from performing the initial assessment, which focuses on the identification and correction of any life threats to the patient, virtually all of the remaining history-gathering and physical examination components come with a lot of latitude as to when each is sequenced into the patient assessment process. In other words, you can do the majority of your assessment and examination in the order that is in the best interest of patient care, *once the initial assessment and correction of life threats is completed.*

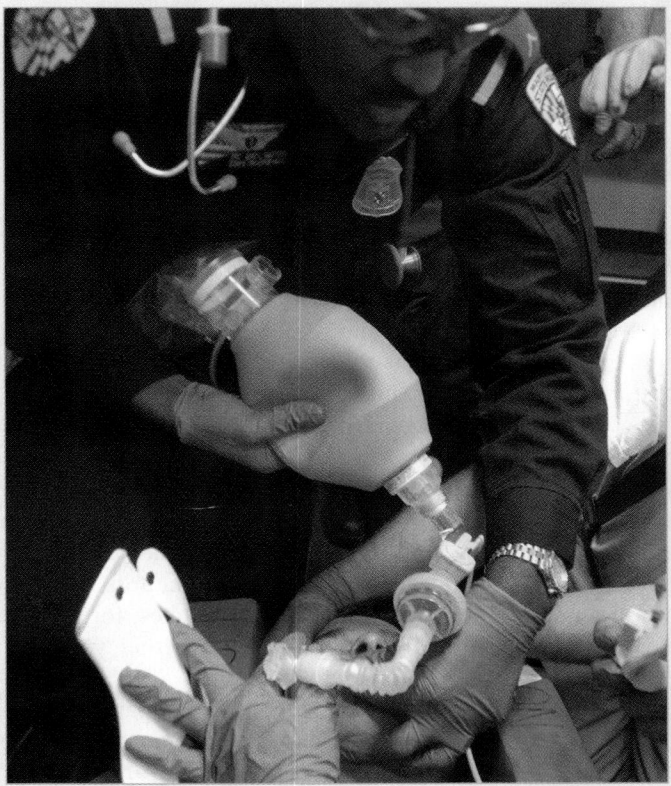

Figure 12-1 As a paramedic, you will work with seriously ill or injured patients.

You are the Provider Part 1

You are dispatched to 3401 Webberville Road for a 65-year-old man who has "passed out." En route to the scene, dispatch informs you that your patient is now conscious and alert and reportedly was stung by a bee.

As you arrive on the scene, someone waves for you from the backyard of the residence. As you approach, you see a man seated at a picnic table surrounded by an obviously concerned group of people. There are a few large bowls of food placed in the middle of the table, and several insects are flying around them. You introduce yourself to the group, and they introduce you to your patient, Lawrence Smith. Your patient's adult daughter tells you that they were all eating dinner when the patient was stung by a bee. He is complaining of itching at the sting site and dizziness.

Initial Assessment	Recording Time: 0 Minutes
Appearance	Eyes open, talking with family members
Level of consciousness	A (Alert to person, place, and day)
Airway	Patent
Breathing	Adequate rate and tidal volume
Circulation	Radial pulse present

1. What are your immediate concerns?
2. At this point, what would you want to know about his medical history?

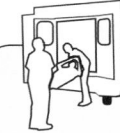

In the Field

For peak efficiency, communicate your patient assessment findings with your partner(s) and share with them the patient care plan.

Most EMS teams are made up of two people working in tandem to quickly identify and address the patient's needs. The EMS team may be composed of two paramedics, or, it may be a split team, with one paramedic and an EMT-B or an EMT-I. In either case, with the limited physical resources of a two-person team, working in the dynamic, often unstable field environment, providing quality patient care can be quite a challenge.

A key part of making your practice of prehospital care successful is for you to develop and cultivate your own style of assessment and an overall strategy for evaluating and providing care for the patients you will encounter in the unique and varied circumstances in the field setting. You will have to work within the parameters of the published standards of care in your system, adding your own personal touches, for example, what gear you take in on a given call or whether you like to kneel or sit while you interview the patient.

Always remember that your overall job as a paramedic is to quickly identify your patient's problem(s), set your care priorities, develop a patient care plan, and quickly and efficiently execute the patient care plan.

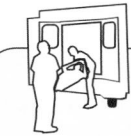

In the Field

In prehospital emergency care, the priorities of evaluation and treatment are based on the degree of threat to the patient's life.

Sick Versus Not Sick

The most important assessment skill for a paramedic to acquire, and one that comes only from lots of experience, is quickly determining whether the patient is *sick* or *not sick*. This quick visual assessment is based on the chief complaint, respirations, pulse, mental status, and skin signs and color. For trauma patients, the mechanism of injury and obvious trauma should be factored in as well. These items together reflect the overall performance of the respiratory, cardiovascular, and neurologic systems and can quickly provide you with a sound medical basis for determining whether a patient is in stable or unstable condition. Abnormalities in any of these areas could indicate a life-threatening condition.

If the patient is sick, the next step is to determine "how sick." On one end of the sick scale is a patient with a miserable sinus infection. Is the patient sick? Yes. Is this a life-threatening event? Probably not. On the other end of the scale is a patient who is a dusky gray, struggling to answer your questions, and so short of breath that only one- or two-word bursts are possible. Is the patient sick? Yes. Is this a life-threatening event? Unlike the previous scenario, the answer is yes.

Documentation and Communication

One key to getting a good patient history is to develop rapport with your patient—even though you spend only a short time with him or her.

Every time you assess a patient, you have to *qualify* whether your patient is sick or not sick, and then you must *quantify* how sick the patient is. Once this has been accomplished, you are in a position to decide what, if any, care needs to be provided at the scene versus in the ambulance, en route to the hospital.

Making Your Field Diagnosis

More often than not, you will make your field diagnosis based on the *patient history* and the *chief complaint.* Your ability to obtain quality information from patients with differing educational, cultural, and ethnic backgrounds; patients with various levels of cognitive ability; and patients impaired by alcohol or drugs is no small challenge. In addition, you still have to ask the right questions to get the information needed to make the best decisions for your patient.

For the most part, being good at patient assessment is a lot like being a good detective. As you interview your patient, you will sift through the information you obtain, and throughout that process, you will continuously glean clues **Figure 12-2 ▾** . On the basis of clues, you will ask more questions to seek information relevant to the patient's chief complaint. You may pursue one line of questioning about current medications that yields nothing important, yet the next line of questioning about medical history is a goldmine.

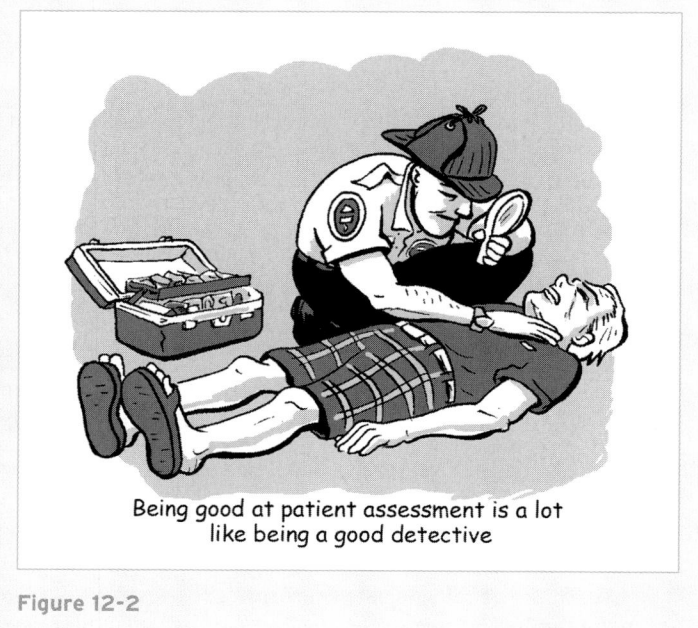

Being good at patient assessment is a lot like being a good detective

Figure 12-2

Controversies

There is much controversy about paramedics making a "diagnosis" in the field. However, a "field diagnosis" must be made to understand which treatment protocol to use.

Just as the veteran detective methodically collects and analyzes clues to ultimately "solve the case," so must you use a similar process to best meet your patient's needs.

In time, every paramedic develops his or her own *style* of patient assessment. As you work at developing this most important job skill, it is critical that you to think of patient assessment as a "fluid" process. The overall assessment process must be organized and systematic but still flexible enough to allow you to maximize your information gathering. As the patient interview unfolds, you need be able to change the sequence of your questioning as the situation or patient's condition dictates. You must know when to expand your questioning to elicit more information and when to focus your questioning to ascertain the most relevant facts.

Medical Versus Trauma

Last, keep in mind that there are two basic categories of patient problems: medical and trauma. For patients with medical problems, identifying their chief complaint and sifting carefully through their medical history will allow you to provide the quality care the patients need.

Unlike medical emergencies, trauma calls are generally the result of unexpected events. When trauma is the primary culprit, the patient's medical history often has little or no impact on your care plan. Because of that, trauma cases require a modified approach to assessment. That will be covered in more detail in Chapter 13.

That said, it is important to never forget that medical events can cause trauma; for example, a person with diabetes takes insulin, forgets to eat breakfast, the blood glucose level drops, and, as a result, the person falls down the steps. By comparison, traumatic events can produce medical problems; for example, a person with asthma wrecks a new car and the stress of the event results in an asthma attack. Keep your mind open to the varied patient care scenarios you may encounter in your practice so you are mentally ready to respond to your patient's needs.

Evaluation of the Emergency Scene

Regardless of when and where you respond to an emergency call, the *very first* step, *before patient care is initiated,* is to *take a look around* and evaluate the overall safety and stability of the emergency scene for any risks to you or any other member of the rescue team, the patient, and any friends, family, and bystanders Figure 12-3 ▸ .

If you do not take a few moments to evaluate the scene and address safety issues, you may find that you and/or your partner have joined the list of casualties. An injured paramedic simply adds to the list of injured and subtracts from the list of rescue resources, making more work for the rest of the rescue team.

Notes from Nancy

Dead heroes can't save lives. Injured heroes are a nuisance. So check the scene for hazards before you lurch in.

Content of the Patient History

Patient Information

There are a number of components that collectively make up the patient history. On most runs, the two most important pieces of patient history information that you need to obtain are the patient's name and the chief complaint. After that, you can obtain the rest of the patient history in whatever order is most conducive to good patient care and most convenient.

Your first step in approaching your patient is to introduce yourself and to explain that you are a paramedic. Then you can ask your patient his or her name and why he or she asked for your help (the chief complaint). Along with the patient's *name,* you need to ask about the *date, time, location,* and *events* surrounding the current situation. This is important information and gives you the chance to quickly determine if the patient is alert to person, place, time, and events. Your EMS system may require you to collect some additional identifying data such as age, sex, race, address, marital status, and occupation. You will

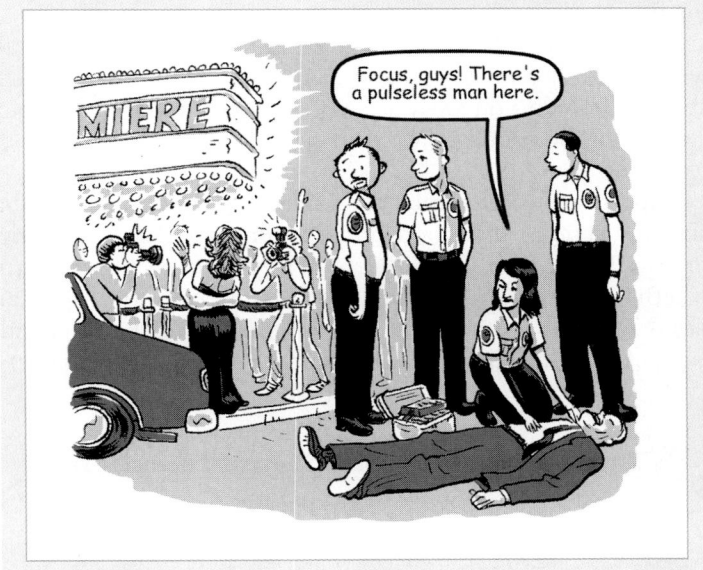

Figure 12-3

also want to know who called 9-1-1; did the patient place the call for help, or was it a friend, family member, or bystander who placed the call?

If first responders are already on the scene, find out the information they have already obtained and the results of any care they provided. This information saves time by avoiding your having to ask the same questions again, which in turn, keeps the patient from getting frustrated. Is bleeding controlled? Was oxygen administered?

Learning About the Present Illness

Once the meet-and-greet phase is over, start gathering information. Again, take a moment to make sure the patient is as comfortable as possible before you start—warm or cool enough, privacy ensured—and that you have gained the patient's confidence and trust.

The history of the present illness starts with one of the most open-ended of all medical questions: "What's going on today that made you call 9-1-1?" An open-ended question cannot be answered with a "yes" or "no." This or a similar question gets the ball rolling. More often than not, the answer you get involves some problem(s) with the person being in pain or discomfort. If your patient's behavior is inappropriate, consider the possibility that it might be a psychiatric emergency.

Sometimes patients will have multiple complaints. Let's say a 64-year-old man tells you, "I'm really weak, and it feels like there are butterflies in my chest." You will need to figure out whether these symptoms are related. If you believe that they are related, to provide appropriate care, you need to identify the *origin of the problem*. In this case, you may want to ask, "Have you had this problem before?"

On the other hand, let's say your patient is complaining of "being dizzy and having pain in her left ankle." You can ask a couple of questions and may determine, for example, that the two complaints are not related. You must then decide which of the two is your priority.

Once you've established the chief complaint(s), you will want to flesh out the history of the present illness, which should provide you with a clear sequence and chronologic account of the patient's signs and symptoms, that is, *what happened* and *when*.

You need to ask about the patient's *general state of health* and any serious childhood or adult illnesses. Ask about any mental health problems the patient might be having and whether he or she has ever been hospitalized for a mental health problem. Although it is often difficult for patients and families to admit to mental health problems, if you are matter-of-fact and dignified in asking the question, you can get a "straight" answer.

You will also need to ask about any accidents or injuries the patient had within the last month or so and about any operations or hospitalizations within the last 6 months or so.

One of the more challenging aspects of the history-taking process is that of pulling together the patient's *current health status,* because it is made up of many unrelated pieces of information. However, it often ties together some of the past history with the history of the current event, so it has definite value to the assessment process. The simple fact of the matter is, you don't need to obtain each and every piece of information on the following list for every patient. It takes time and practice and a certain amount of common sense for you to know the right questions to ask each patient.

Questions that will be most helpful in getting a useful history include the following:

- What prescription medicines are you currently taking? How much and how often? (Patients can and do confuse when and how to take their medications—and if your patient has, you could be witnessing a drug reaction. Also, as you gain paramedic experience, your familiarity with the drugs will give you an idea of the patient's illness. Medications will also give you a clue about mental health problems or dementia without your needlessly antagonizing a reluctant patient.)
- Do you take any over-the-counter medication like aspirin, herbs, or vitamins?
- Are you allergic to any medicines or other substances?
- Do you smoke? How much? Do you drink beer, wine, or cocktails? How often?
- Have you been smoking or taking drugs other than cigarettes? Assure your patient of confidentiality.
- What did you have to eat yesterday and today?
- Ask about screening tests that are appropriate. For example, for difficulty breathing ask: "Have you had a chest x-ray lately?"
- Are your immunizations up-to-date? How about a flu shot or pneumococcal vaccine? Ask about children's immunizations, too.
- Have you been getting a good night's sleep? Look for maladaptive sleep patterns.
- Do you like to exercise? How much?
- What kinds of chemical cleaners do you have in your house? Do you have any strong chemicals where you work? You might need to probe for environmental hazards.
- Does the family use seatbelts and car seats for the children? Do you have baby gates? Are medicines locked away (if it seems necessary)?
- Do you have a history of any specific diseases in your family?
- Where do you live? What do you like to do at home? Is there anyone in your life that you might be afraid of? You might need to assess a difficult home situation.
- How do you spend your time during the day?

Documentation and Communication

The history of present illness should always be documented clearly and accurately. This is often the most important information, medically and legally.

- Do you have anything in your religion that would prevent me from administering treatment?
- Are you an optimistic person? You might feel it important to get your patient's overall outlook on life.

Special Considerations

In some cases, a patient's religious beliefs may be relevant, for example if the beliefs pertain directly to medical care. If your patient indicates that such beliefs are important, this information should be passed along to emergency department staff.

You have to decide which of the listed items you want to explore and which you do not. For a really sick patient with immediate life threats, you may have no time to explore any of them. For a patient in stable condition who appears to be in no apparent distress, you may have time and decide to explore all relevant topics.

Last, you'll want to do a quick check on the body systems. A great way to gain insight is to ask, "Has your doctor ever told you that you have a heart, lung, or brain problem?" After that, you can ask about things like bowel movements, and so on, which tend to be non–life threatening.

Techniques for History Taking

Setting the Stage for Quality Patient Care

Every time you care for a patient, you must first establish a professional relationship. In most cases, this is a *short-term* relationship, less than 2 hours' duration, until you provide your hand-off report and turn the patient over to the emergency department staff.

Your Demeanor and Appearance

Although time is short, you will want to have a positive patient outcome in the care you provide and the communication you establish with all involved. When you first meet your patient, they should be looking at a clean, neat, health care provider. You should have good personal hygiene and grooming and attire that is professional, clean, and pressed Figure 12-4 ►. If you look professional, your patient will likely develop a good first impression of you.

Along with your appearance, there is the matter of your demeanor. On every call, your attitude is always on display. If you are unhappy, a look of unhappiness is almost certainly on your face. Your facial expression and body language can send powerful messages. If you have come to believe that calls to 9-1-1 need to meet *your* expectations, *you are wrong*. If patients think a problem is serious enough to merit a call to 9-1-1, you have an obligation to treat patients and their complaints accordingly—professionally and to the best of your ability.

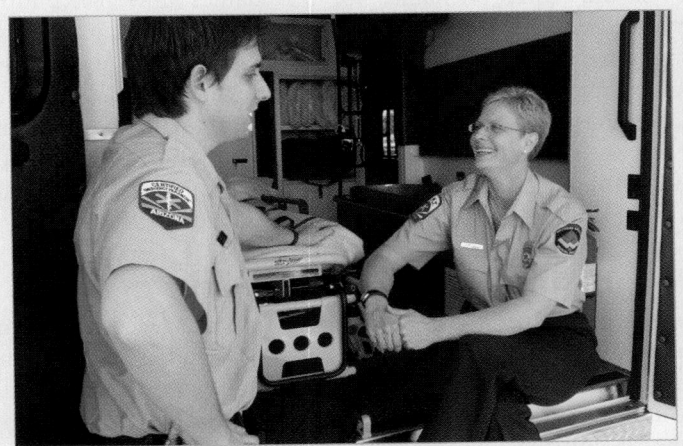

Figure 12-4 Your appearance should be professional and your demeanor positive and friendly.

Introduce yourself to your patient and tell him or her the name of your service and your certification level. Introduce your partner as well.

Try to interview the patient in a private setting. Don't hesitate to ask any nonessential personnel to leave the room or to at least step back because you will frequently find yourself asking your patients personal or intimate questions. Most people do not want to admit some bad habits (for example, cigarettes) that have a negative impact on their health. But you need to know. If the setting makes the patient uncomfortable, the patient may choose to not answer your questions or to answer inaccurately. Working to ensure the patient's privacy, confidentiality, and comfort level goes a long way toward establishing positive patient rapport and encourages more honest, open communication.

Confidentiality

As discussed in Chapter 4, it is your duty to maintain confidentiality of the patient's information. The Health Information Portability and Accountability Act, or HIPAA, and state laws govern the disclosure of patient information. You need to be familiar with the relevant laws. Also, showing the patient that you respect the confidentiality of his or her medical information helps build rapport and contributes to total patient care.

How to Address the Patient

After introducing yourself, ask the patient his or her name and how he or she would like to be addressed. Err on the side of formality, using Mr., Miss, Mrs., or Ms. There is a world of difference in Mr. John Markham (formal), John (more casual), or Johnnie (really casual). Your patient will say, "Call me John" if that is what he prefers. Calling patients by the name of their choosing is professional, but assuming formality will help establish more rapport than being too familiar.

Avoid "catch-all names" or "pet names" like pal, buddy, sport, dude, friend, honey, sweetie, cutie, and darling. You can bog down the process of obtaining a history by demeaning the patient and treating the patient unprofessionally. Using casual nicknames also can be problematic when there are cultural differences. Some terms have negative connotation in some cultures. You need to be familiar with the cultural groups in your area and with issues that could lead to misunderstanding.

Note Taking

As you get ready to start the assessment process, let the patient know that you are going to be asking a number of questions and that while he or she is answering, you or your partner will be taking notes. This lets patients know they aren't being ignored and that the information being provided is important enough to write down Figure 12-5 ▶ .

Too often, EMS providers read off a list of questions to patients to fill in all the blanks on the run report. With this approach comes the problem of making little to no eye contact with the patient. Don't bury your nose in the clipboard! If possible, position yourself at the eye level of your patient.

Reviewing the Medical History and Information Reliability

Frequently, you will obtain information not just from your patient but also from other sources. It is important that you document the source of this information in your record. Family members are commonly involved at emergency scenes, as are friends. Law enforcement personnel and bystanders also can be valuable sources of information.

A large number of the patient contacts in day-to-day EMS are routine patient transfers from assisted living or extended care facilities to the hospital and back. Take a few moments to review the transfer paperwork. You need to know the medical history of the patient so you are prepared to provide care should your planned routine transfer suddenly turn unroutine.

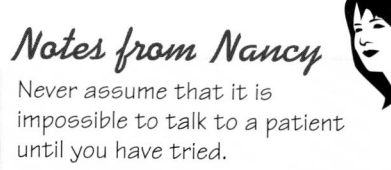

Notes from Nancy

Never assume that it is impossible to talk to a patient until you have tried.

Keep in mind the importance of evaluating your sources of information for reliability. Although the medical records in the transfer packet from an extended care facility should be assumed to be reasonably accurate, individual performances of caregivers vary. When all is said and done, you are responsible for patient care decisions, so make sure you work with information that is as accurate as possible.

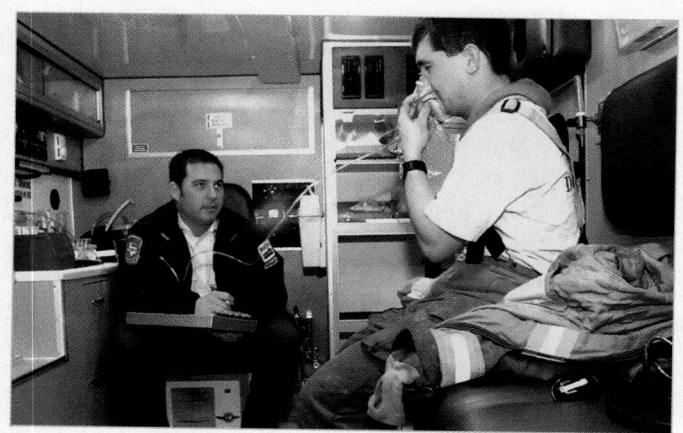

Figure 12-5 You may want to take notes during the patient history.

You are the Provider Part 2

After moving the bowls of food out of the immediate area and asking the other members of the family to give you and your patient some privacy, you notice localized swelling and redness at the sting site and a venom sac embedded in his skin. You scrape the stinger away with a tongue depressor, obtain vital signs, give the patient high-flow supplemental oxygen, and insert an 18-gauge intravenous (IV) catheter in the right antecubital vein to give normal saline to keep the vein open. The patient denies having shortness of breath and any history of severe allergic reactions. He also denies carrying or using an EpiPen or having taken any antihistamines before your arrival. When you ask about his medical history, he says he has occasional chest pain with exertion and that his only medication is nitroglycerin. He has no allergies to medication. He tells you that currently he has no chest pain.

Vital Signs	Recording Time: 3 Minutes
Skin	Localized redness and swelling at the sting site and hives on the abdomen
Pulse	98 beats/min, regular
Blood pressure	108/58 mm Hg
Respirations	24 breaths/min
Sao$_2$	100% with oxygen at 12 to 15 L/min via nonrebreathing mask

3. What medication(s) would you administer to this patient?

4. What other assessment tools would you like to use?

Communication Techniques

Encourage Dialog

On the basis of the questions asked and answers received, you will make patient care decisions. A number of approaches and conversation techniques can help to improve the volume and quality of information you obtain during the patient interview.

Facilitation

A dictionary definition of facilitation is to "make easy or easier." Facilitation in communication means using techniques that permit your patient to feel open to giving you some of the most delicate information he or she can share. Patients of all ages are hesitant to share private or embarrassing information. Your job is to make your patients feel so secure with you that they will give you the information you need.

The most important thing you can do to facilitate the information exchange is pay attention. Good eye contact is essential. It's hard to believe that someone who never makes eye contact is really listening. Use phrases that encourage the patient to share more information such as, "That's helpful," "Anything else you can think of?" or "Please go on." Nodding your head and using an appropriately placed, "Okay," every now and then lets the patient know you are getting the message.

> **Documentation and Communication**
>
> Do not put ideas into the patient's head, such as, "Is the pain in your chest a dull ache that is behind your sternum and radiates into your jaw?"

Another helpful facilitation technique is repeating key information from the patient's answers.

Patient: *"I've been feeling weird since I got up, and my chest just aches bad. It never felt like this before."*
Paramedic: *"Your chest aches?"*
Patient: *"Real bad. I've never had it ache like this."*
Paramedic: *"You've had chest pain before?"*
Patient: *"Yeah, I've been seeing a heart doctor pretty regularly for going on 5 years now. Used to be I would get kind of a squeezing feeling in my chest, I'd take a nitro, and it would go away. Well, this is nothing like that! I took two nitro right away, and I'll bet it's been close to an hour and a half, and nothing has changed."*

In this case, with just two short questions, you greatly expanded what you knew about the patient. You now know that the patient:

- Has a history of heart disease.
- Has been seeing a cardiologist for 5 years.
- Is having pain today that is different from and more serious than pain in the past.
- Is having pain today that is the worst it has ever been.

- Has taken nitroglycerin for symptom relief in the past.
- Took two nitroglycerin doses today that failed to relieve the symptoms.

Reflection

Reflection is the *repetition* of a word or phrase that a patient has used to encourage more detail.

Your patient might say: *"I couldn't catch my breath."*
You could respond: *"You couldn't catch your breath, Mrs. Slocum?"*
Your patient might elaborate: *"I don't know. I recall my heart just all of a sudden seemed to start beating really fast, and then I got scared, and all of a sudden I was breathing superfast but not getting enough air."*

Reflection is a powerful tool for getting a good patient history for two reasons: (1) Reflection usually does not break the flow or your patient's thoughts. It helps you both stay focused. (2) The information you will obtain is not biased by "leading" the patient. You are using the words the patient used, not your own description, which is very important in good histories.

Clarification

Clarification is the technique of asking your patients for more information when some aspect of the history is vague or unclear to you **Figure 12-6 ▼**. The clearer you are about your patient's condition, the more helpful and appropriate your care will be. On the other hand, if you are unsure about your patient's problem, the more likely your care is based on guesswork and happenstance.

Paramedic: *"What's going on today, Mrs. Hendrickson?"*
Patient: *"Oh I don't know. I'm just . . . well I'm just not feeling like myself."*
Paramedic: *"I'm sorry. Could you try to be a little more specific? If you could do that, it will help me figure out what's going on with you today."*
Patient: *"I'm always full of energy first thing in the morning, but I'm so weak right now that I couldn't even take Princess out to do her business."*

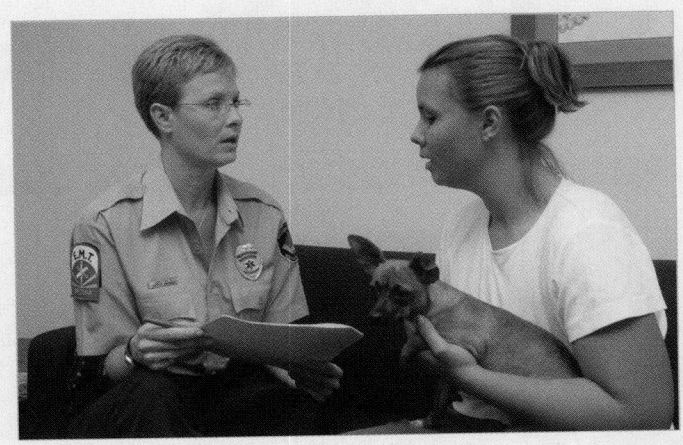

Figure 12-6 Use clarification to gain more information about the patient's chief complaint.

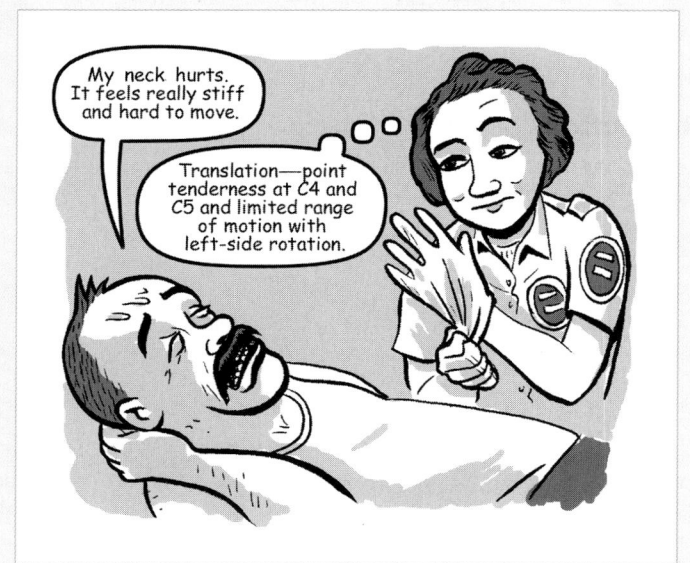

Figure 12-7

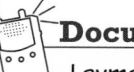

Documentation and Communication

Layman's Lingo	EMS Lingo
My sugars	I'm a diabetic
Fell out	Had a syncopal episode
Has the fits	History of seizures
Water pills	Furosemide (Lasix)

With this example, having identified the chief complaint as "weakness" is medically clearer than the complaint of "not feeling like myself."

Clarification is one of the more frequently used interview techniques in EMS. By the nature of your job, you may want to speak and listen to the language of medicine, but the average layperson has a limited medical vocabulary. Patients will generally use nonmedical terms to answer your assessment questions **Figure 12-7 ◄**. You will need to clarify what they mean.

Empathetic Response

Empathy is often described as one step further than sympathy; empathy is a psychological gift that allows you to feel what your patient is feeling—putting yourself into his or her shoes. At times, you will hear sad and tragic information from your patients. Do not hesitate to communicate your feelings and address the emotional impact of what has been said **Figure 12-8 ▶**.

Paramedic: *"What is the reason you called for help today, Mr. Ortiz?"*
Patient: *"I've just been horribly depressed."*
Paramedic: *"And why is that, Mr. Ortiz?"*
Patient: *"My wife and two kids were hit and killed by a drunk driver 6 months ago, and I just can't get over it."*
Paramedic: *"I am so sorry to hear that, Mr. Ortiz. That seems so wrong to me."*

Mr. Ortiz, the man who has lost his entire family, might not have an overt medical problem, but certainly you should consider the possibility that he might be so depressed that some kind of mental health referral is needed.

You are the Provider Part 3

With your patient's blood pressure low, his pulse rate elevated, and the presence of hives, you consider epinephrine administration. With his heart history and lack of breathing difficulty, epinephrine should be administered with caution. You decide that the subcutaneous route of 0.3 to 0.5 mg 1:1,000 is appropriate, and your partner begins preparing the equipment and site. You also choose to administer diphenhydramine (Benadryl) IV, but just as you move your patient to the gurney, you see a small, open pill bottle lying on his chair.

Reassessment	Recording Time: 5 Minutes
Skin	Slightly moist, pale, and warm
Pulse	100 beats/min, regular
Blood pressure	108/58 mm Hg
Respirations	24 breaths/min
Sao_2	100% with oxygen at 12 to 15 L/min via nonrebreathing mask
ECG	Sinus rhythm with no ectopy

5. What could be another reason for his low blood pressure and elevated pulse rate?
6. What should you immediately ask your patient?
7. Should you consider rethinking your diagnosis and treatment plans now?

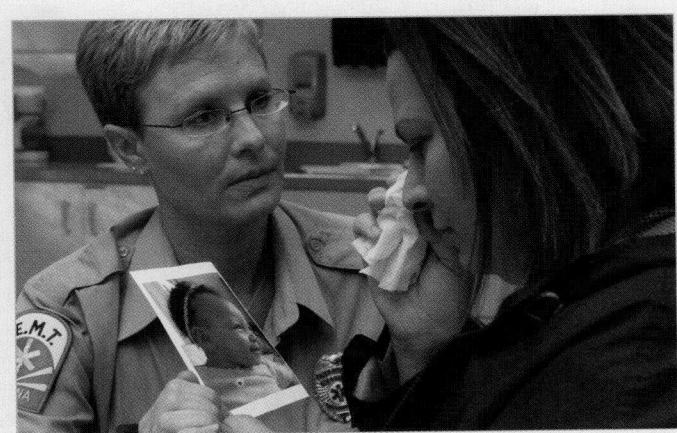

Figure 12-8 Be empathetic when the patient conveys sad or tragic information.

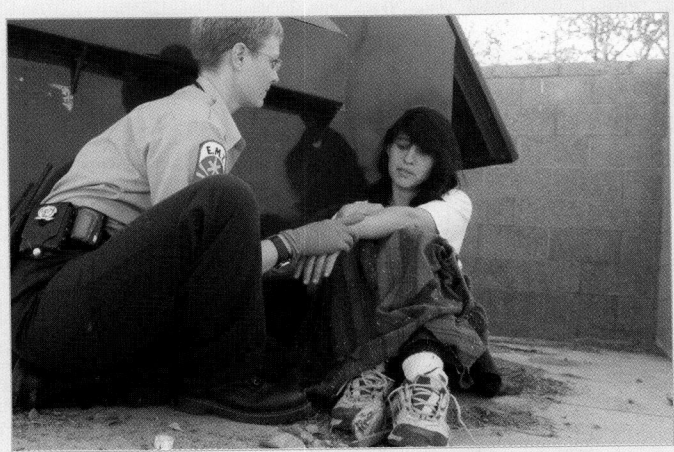

Figure 12-9 Use a nonjudgmental approach when confronting a patient.

Paramedics, unlike most other health care providers, see people when the illness or trauma just occurred. Your patients are uniquely vulnerable and uniquely demanding. Try your best to develop empathy for your patients.

Remember that in earlier chapters we discussed being active in your community to keep yourself aware of other sources of help for your patients. Empathy can help you set your patient on a path to healing—no matter what the diagnosis.

Confrontation

Confrontation is making your patients aware that you perceive something that is not consistent with their behavior, the actual scene, or the information the patient is giving you. Nevertheless, avoiding confrontations with your patients is a good practice. If you must confront a patient, for example about using illegal drugs or alcohol, a professional approach can help you get medically appropriate information. Sometimes patients want a chance to deal with their problems. The key is to remain professional and nonjudgmental Figure 12-9 ▶ .

Patient: *"My life just sucks. I don't why I even go on living."*
Paramedic: *"Are you considering suicide?"*
Patient: *"I'm thinking that might just be the best thing."*
Paramedic: *"Have you made plans on how you are going to do it?"*
Patient: *"I don't know, I haven't given it that much thought."*

This patient's response clearly points toward possible suicide. Use a direct approach and ask the patient about whether he is contemplating suicide and if so, if he has a plan. This information helps you assess how distressed the patient is so that you can decide how to best ensure safe transport of the patient.

Interpretation

If your patient refuses to give you information, you need to infer what could be causing the distress and then ask the patient if you are right. (In the preceding situation, the para-

medic, who spoke with a clearly distressed patient used interpretation about whether the patient was suicidal.)

The skill of interpretation demands that paramedics use their best diplomatic skills. One of the best phrases with which to begin an inference is the ever-reliable, "So, if I understand you correctly . . ."

Asking About Feelings

Asking about feelings is one of the most difficult roles of a paramedic. But as part of a good health history, you will need to ask if a patient is tired, depressed, or any number of feelings that are most easily dealt with by denial. (You will even need to ask these questions of a colleague if you see the symptoms.)

Try to keep possible unpleasant sights, sounds, and smells from your patient who is feeling badly. You can also validate feelings. "This is a tough situation." That's empathy in action. Do your best to attend to psychological needs at the scene. It is a tough job, but these needs profoundly affect physical health.

Be effective. Do not ask, "Are you okay?" This is the most tempting of all questions (and it *can* be answered with a yes or no!). Instead, ask for facts first, then follow up. Even with someone you know quite well, you need to establish rapport to ask a question about how he or she is feeling. Most of us would deny that we are exhausted, frazzled, scared, or depressed. Your patients met you only a few minutes ago. Establish that you are a caring health professional during a series of "safe" questions about physical health.

Getting More Information

You've gotten a lot of information from your patient, but in many cases, you need to refine your thinking to come up with a valid diagnosis. Let's say you were exploring a particular symptom such as "abdominal pain" with your patient. (As you will soon learn, abdominal pain can suggest a startlingly large number of diagnoses.) Some possible questions you might ask the patient about the *region* or location of the pain include the following:

- Where exactly does it hurt?
- Does it hurt in one particular spot or in a general area?
- Can you point to where it hurts with one finger?
- Does the pain stay right there, or does it move or radiate anywhere else?
- If your pain does move or radiate, where does it go?

Questions you may ask about the *quality* of the abdominal pain include the following:

- What type of pain is it: a sharp pain or more of a dull ache?
- Does the pain come and go, or is it constant?
- If you wanted me to feel the same feeling that you do, what would you do to me to make me feel that way?

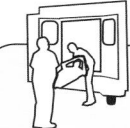

In the Field

Letting patients describe their pain in their own words will be very helpful for your assessment.

Questions you may ask about the *severity* of the abdominal pain include the following:

- In your opinion, how bad is this pain?
- Is it more of an uncomfortable feeling or a feeling of hurt?
- Would you say the pain is similar to or worse than with previous episodes?
- On a scale of 1 to 10, with 10 being the *worst* pain you've ever felt and 1 being very minor, how would you rate your pain?

The questions in these lists are not exhaustive or all-inclusive. Add and modify questions to the patient interview as you need to. Subtract questions if time is of the essence. Use open-ended questions whenever you can **Figure 12-10 ▾**. Pin your patient down

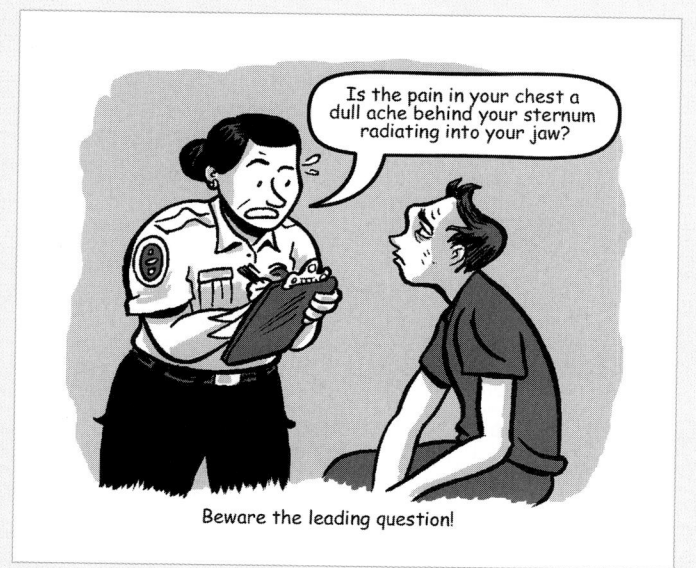

Is the pain in your chest a dull ache behind your sternum radiating into your jaw?

Beware the leading question!

Figure 12-10

with a close-ended question if that's what the situation requires.

Try to be *orderly* and *systematic* in your information gathering and assessment, while at the same time *flexible* in your approach. Being flexible in an emergency is a lot harder than it sounds, but it is attainable with practice—lots and lots of practice.

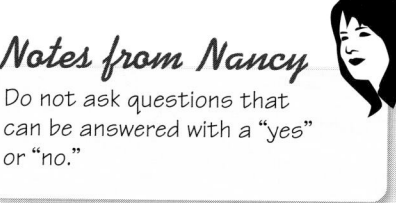

Notes from Nancy

Do not ask questions that can be answered with a "yes" or "no."

You could probably use some help in remembering what to cover. The mnemonic OPQRST offers an easy-to-remember approach to analyzing a patient's chief complaint that is simple and effective.

- **Onset.** When did you start to feel pain?
- **Provocation.** What do you think brought on your pain?
  - Did the pain start all of a sudden or come on over a period of time?
  - Does anything make the pain go away or feel better or feel worse?
- **Quality.** If you were trying to make me feel the way you do, what would you do to me to give me that same feeling?
- **Region/Radiation/Referral.**
  - Can you point to the place where it hurts with one finger?
  - Does the pain stay there, or does it go somewhere else?
- **Severity.** On a scale of 1 to 10, with 1 being very minor and 10 the worst pain you've ever felt, how would you rank this?
- **Time.** How long have you felt this way?

Documentation and Communication

Documenting pain severity ratings is important. Also note how distressed the patient appears: mild, moderate, or severe.

Clinical Reasoning

The results of your questions should expand your thinking about problems and other body systems that are associated with the symptoms your patient has mentioned. In Chapter 15, you will learn the details of critical thinking. Critical thinking consists of (1) concept formation, (2) data interpretation, (3) application of principles (guidelines or algorithms), (4) reflection in action (being willing to change course as you interpret your patient's condition), and (5) reflection on action (doing honest and thorough postrun critiques to benefit learning).

Being able to think and perform well under pressure is a big part of being able to be good paramedic. In many ways, critical thinking and decision making are just two more skills you will need to work on, not just while you are a student, but for the rest of your career as a practicing paramedic.

One of the most important elements of the interview process is for you to be a *great listener,* and a big part of being a great listener is also being a *patient listener.* For a number of reasons, patients can be slow to respond. Maybe they didn't hear your question. Maybe they didn't understand you. Maybe they are afraid to answer. There are many possible explanations. Ask, then wait, and give your patients time to gather their thoughts so they can answer you.

Communicate with your patients by using terminology matched to their knowledge and understanding. For example, a patient who is an emergency department nurse or a retired surgeon will understand medical terminology. On the other hand, a patient who speaks little English needs simple and focused communication.

Throughout the assessment process, look for nonverbal communication, such as changes in facial expression, heavy sighs, or aggressive gestures (finger pointing), any of which can impact your information processing.

Direct Questions

To complete the history, direct questions could be required. Patients might not be giving you easy-to-digest facts about themselves, and if you need a date, time, or other specific information, you should ask for it.

Getting a History on Sensitive Topics

As a paramedic, you will be privileged to care for people who depend on you during some of the worst moments of their lives. You represent hope and comfort no matter how difficult, even horrific, your patient's situation might be.

Some sensitive factors like drug and alcohol abuse can stand in the way of your best efforts for the health of your patients. Here are some ways that can help you be the paramedic you want to be, no matter how sensitive the situation.

Alcohol and Drug Abuse

People who regularly abuse drugs or alcohol become adept at hiding the signs and symptoms from their friends, family, and workplace associates and denying there is a problem. Such denial can go on for years, and the signs and symptoms can be hidden even from people closest to the patient.

If asked how much alcohol or drug has been consumed, the amount is often understated. Some experienced paramedics say the standard answer to the question about how many drinks is "two," when the behavior indicates many more. Slightly *fewer* than half of all motor vehicle crashes involve alcohol. Just *more* than half of all motor vehicle crashes that result in fatalities involve alcohol **Figure 12-11 ▶**.

It is probable that an alcohol-impaired patient will give an unreliable history. Do not assume that all that you are told is completely accurate. Keep in mind that alcohol can mask any number of signs and symptoms. When a patient who experienced a significant traumatic event denies neck or back pain, if

you smell what you believe to be alcohol on the patient's breath or behavior raises your suspicion of alcohol or drug use, take precautions to restrict spinal motion.

Alcohol is a legal drug. If your patient is using other substances to "get high," using them is most likely illegal. The fear of punishment for illegal use of drugs might lead patients to deny their use. Let your patient know that you are a medical person and anything that he or she tells you will be kept in confidence. Do your best to win your patient's trust because you need the information to provide proper treatment.

Keep your best professional attitude as you work with patients you suspect of using drugs or alcohol. Paramedics should never judge their patients by appearances or behavior. An unkempt homeless person might be in desperate need of assessment for head trauma, not alcoholism. A suburban executive might have hit his head during a crash, but drinking alcohol might be the cause of the accident.

Physical Abuse and Domestic Violence

As a paramedic, you are required to report a case if you have reason to suspect physical abuse or domestic violence. Although it is inappropriate for you to accuse someone of abuse at the scene, never hesitate to call for law enforcement personnel if you have reason to believe that abuse has occurred. They will help stabilize the scene and provide another set of professional eyes.

A number of clues may lead you to suspect domestic violence. Injuries inconsistent with the information you are being given are common, as are multiple injuries in various stages of healing. Unspoken messages can be given by the family's behavior. Maybe it's the cowering posture of the woman at the kitchen table as her husband or significant other towers over her and answers your questions for her. If the injured family member does not give you the information but waits for someone else to speak up, that's a clue that the injured family member is being repressed. You can suggest that the significant other who is doing all the talking go to the

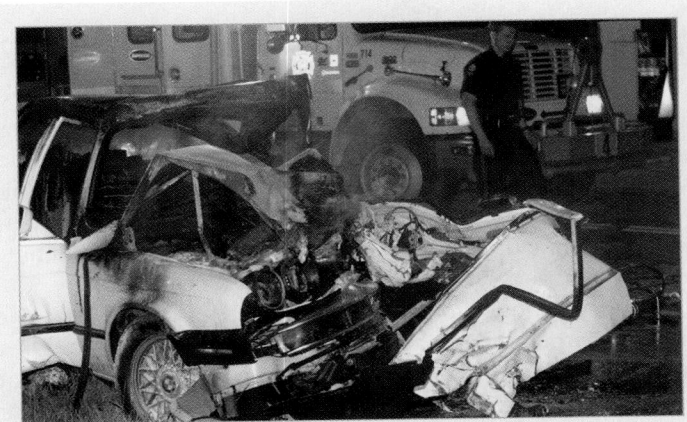

Figure 12-11 Many crashes involve alcohol. In these cases, the patient history may not be reliable.

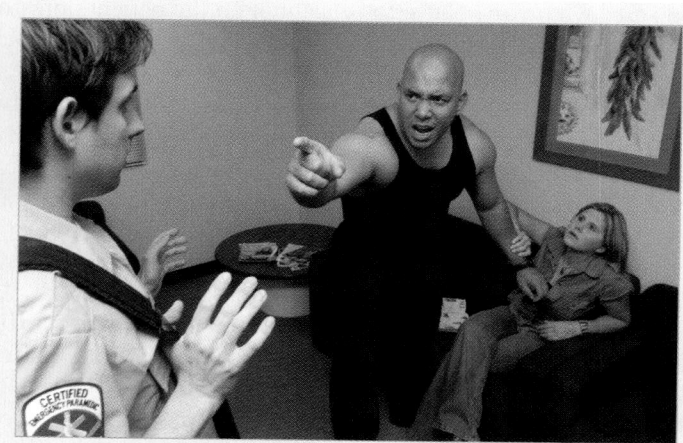

Figure 12-12 Do not handle potentially violent calls alone. Summon law enforcement personnel.

In the Field

If you find yourself suddenly in a potentially dangerous position and your partners are not aware of it, use a predetermined code word to alert them. One inconspicuous code is to use the trade name of something in your ambulance—"could you get the Ferno cot?" Your partners should know that it means there is danger and that they should summon law enforcement personnel.

rig to help with the gurney. The moment the door shuts, you may receive valuable information, such as, "My husband is beating me and I'm scared to death. You've got to get me out of here before he kills me or one of the kids." *Immediately* request law enforcement personnel if this or if anything close to this happens.

Emergency scenes involving domestic violence are some of the most dangerous for EMS and law enforcement professionals alike Figure 12-12 ▲ . Don't even think of handling them without law enforcement personnel on hand.

Sexual History

A number of factors may influence a patient about being less than forthcoming about sexual history. Religious upbringing, cultural or societal mores, and exotic or bizarre sexual tastes may inhibit a patient from sharing sexual history because this is truly one of the most private and personal aspects of a person's life. When the topic is someone's sexual history, obtaining the history in as private a setting as possible is essential.

Keep your questions focused and on task. For a female patient complaining of acute abdominal pain, foul smelling vaginal discharge, pain on urination, genital lesions, or similar complaints, you will need to know such things as when your patient last had a period and when she last had sexual intercourse. You will also need to find out if there is vaginal bleeding, whether she has had multiple sex partners, the

Special Considerations

Some younger teens may be confused when asked about sexual issues. Be direct and avoid using questions like, "Are you sexually active?" because they may think active means often.

characteristics of the vaginal discharge, and whether she uses a birth control method.

Male patients with complaints of pain on urination, discharge from the penis, genital lesions, and so forth, need to be asked about their most recent sexual encounter, whether they use condoms, the characteristics of their discharge and lesions, and so forth.

You may need to ask female and male patients if they have ever been tested for HIV, AIDS, or hepatitis. Do not interject any opinions or biases about sexual choices or behavior. Their choices aren't your choices, just as your choices are not theirs. Every patient you care for deserves to be treated with compassion and respect.

Special Assessment Challenges

Simply put, it is impossible to address every scenario you may encounter in your work as a paramedic, but there are a number of special assessment challenges that occur often enough to be worth talking about.

Silence

When you are on a mission to obtain your patient's history in a timely manner, a period of silence on the part of your patient can make you uneasy. Don't let it. Your patient may be simply trying to gather his or her thoughts, trying to recall possibly distant details relative to the questions(s) you just asked, or trying to decide if he or she trusts you enough to answer your question(s) truthfully or at all. In any case, be patient.

Keep your antenna extended for nonverbal signs of distress. Pain, psychological distress, or fear often register in body movements and facial expression.

As you work in the field while you are a student, you will learn how to read the many nonverbal cues that patients give. The paramedics you work with will help, as will working with experienced caregivers in the emergency department and the hospital. Although paramedics work outside the hospital, you will still find help in learning to read nonverbal cues from everyone you work with.

Another pair of essential skills you can learn from these seasoned veterans are how to time your questions and how to be patient. Learn to ask questions and then *wait*. What seems like an eternity to you is but 1 or 2 seconds to your patients, as they think, retrieve facts, or assess your trustworthiness.

5. **You must ask the patient what medication he is taking. This is important because medications can suggest past and present illnesses. To best determine medications that are being taken, you should:**
   A. review his pharmacy receipts.
   B. call his physician.
   C. consult his relatives.
   D. ask him what medications, including prescription, over-the-counter, and herbal supplements he is taking.

6. **The posture of the patient's wife stiffens, and she begins to look angry. She starts yelling at you and your partner, telling you to hurry up and do something. You should:**
   A. have your partner take her aside and calmly explain what you are doing.
   B. call for back up at the first opportunity.
   C. have police stand by during the history taking.
   D. ignore her.

7. **You smell alcohol on the patient's breath. You wonder if he might be intoxicated. Problems encountered with intoxicated patients include which of the following?**
   A. Intoxicated patients may not understand what you are trying to say, making effective communications difficult or impossible.
   B. Intoxication may mask symptoms, making treatment decisions difficult.
   C. Intoxicated patients can present potentially violent situations.
   D. All of the above.

Challenging Questions

8. **You are dispatched to an unknown injury. You and your partner arrive on scene and hear loud noises and yelling from inside the residence. You then hear the sound of glass breaking. What should you do?**

9. **You arrive on scene at the home of a patient with hearing difficulty. What can you do to better enable effective communications?**

▇ Points to Ponder

You respond to a medical call involving a 46-year-old man. On arrival you recognize the patient as a teacher at the local middle school. You ask why you were called today and the patient tells you that he has been experiencing serious anxiety. You inquire about medical history, and your patient tells you that he checked himself into a psychiatric hospital during the summer break to get treatment for paranoia.

After shift, you are eating dinner at a popular restaurant with your partner and two other paramedics from your service. They ask if any-thing interesting happened today. You begin to tell them about the teacher, and your eyes meet those of your partner. You realize that this is not appropriate.

Why is this not appropriate, and what should you do now?

Issues: Confidentiality, History Taking.

13

Physical Examination

Objectives

Cognitive

3-2.1 Define the terms inspection, palpation, percussion, auscultation. (p 13.4)

3-2.2 Describe the techniques of inspection, palpation, percussion, and auscultation. (p 13.4)

3-2.3 Describe the evaluation of mental status. (p 13.10)

3-2.4 Evaluate the importance of a general survey. (p 13.10)

3-2.5 Describe the examination of skin, hair, and nails. (p 13.11)

3-2.6 Differentiate normal and abnormal findings of the assessment of the skin. (p 13.11)

3-2.7 Distinguish the importance of abnormal findings of the assessment of the skin. (p 13.11)

3-2.8 Describe the examination of the head and neck. (p 13.13)

3-2.9 Differentiate normal and abnormal findings of the scalp examination. (p 13.13)

3-2.10 Describe the normal and abnormal assessment findings of the skull. (p 13.13)

3-2.11 Describe the assessment of visual acuity. (p 13.13)

3-2.12 Explain the rationale for the use of an ophthalmoscope. (p 13.9)

3-2.13 Describe the examination of the eyes. (p 13.15)

3-2.14 Distinguish between normal and abnormal assessment findings of the eyes. (p 13.15)

3-2.15 Explain the rationale for the use of an otoscope. (p 13.9)

3-2.16 Describe the examination of the ears. (p 13.17)

3-2.17 Differentiate normal and abnormal assessment findings of the ears. (p 13.17)

3-2.18 Describe the examination of the nose. (p 13.18)

3-2.19 Differentiate normal and abnormal assessment findings of the nose. (p 13.18)

3-2.20 Describe the examination of the mouth and pharynx. (p 13.18)

3-2.21 Differentiate normal and abnormal assessment findings of the mouth and pharynx. (p 13.19)

3-2.22 Describe the examination of the neck. (p 13.19)

3-2.23 Differentiate normal and abnormal assessment findings of the neck. (p 13.19)

3-2.24 Describe the survey of the thorax and respiration. (p 13.20)

3-2.25 Describe the examination of the posterior chest. (p 13.21)

3-2.26 Describe percussion of the chest. (p 13.21)

3-2.27 Differentiate the percussion notes and their characteristics. (p 13.21)

3-2.28 Differentiate the characteristics of breath sounds. (p 13.22)

3-2.29 Describe the examination of the anterior chest. (p 13.21)

3-2.30 Differentiate normal and abnormal assessment findings of the chest examination. (p 13.21)

3-2.31 Describe special examination techniques related to the assessment of the chest. (p 13.21)

3-2.32 Describe the examination of the arterial pulse including rate, rhythm, and amplitude. (p 13.26)

3-2.33 Distinguish normal and abnormal findings of arterial pulse. (p 13.26)

3-2.34 Describe the assessment of jugular venous pressure and pulsations. (p 13.26)

3-2.35 Distinguish normal and abnormal examination findings of jugular venous pressure and pulsations. (p 13.26)

3-2.36 Describe the examination of the heart and blood vessels. (p 13.25)

3-2.37 Differentiate normal and abnormal assessment findings of the heart and blood vessels. (p 13.25)

3-2.38 Describe the auscultation of the heart. (p 13.21, 13.22)

3-2.39 Differentiate the characteristics of normal and abnormal findings associated with the auscultation of the heart. (p 13.22)

3-2.40 Describe special examination techniques of the cardiovascular examination. (p 13.25, 13.26)

3-2.41 Describe the examination of the abdomen. (p 13.27, 13.28)

3-2.42 Differentiate normal and abnormal assessment findings of the abdomen. (p 13.29)

3-2.43 Describe auscultation of the abdomen. (p 13.29)

3-2.44 Distinguish normal and abnormal findings of the auscultation of the abdomen. (p 13.29)

3-2.45 Describe the examination of the female genitalia. (p 13.30)

3-2.46 Differentiate normal and abnormal assessment findings of the female genitalia. (p 13.30)

3-2.47 Describe the examination of the male genitalia. (p 13.30)

3-2.48 Differentiate normal and abnormal findings of the male genitalia. (p 13.30)

3-2.49 Describe the examination of the anus and rectum. (p 13.31)

3-2.50 Distinguish between normal and abnormal findings of the anus and rectum. (p 13.31)

3-2.51 Describe the examination of the peripheral vascular system. (p 13.35)

3-2.52 Differentiate normal and abnormal findings of the peripheral vascular system. (p 13.35)

3-2.53 Describe the examination of the musculoskeletal system. (p 13.31)

3-2.54 Differentiate normal and abnormal findings of the musculoskeletal system. (p 13.31)

3-2.55 Describe the examination of the nervous system. (p 13.40)

3-2.56 Differentiate normal and abnormal findings of the nervous system. (p 13.43)

3-2.57 Describe the assessment of the cranial nerves. (p 13.41)

3-2.58 Differentiate normal and abnormal findings of the cranial nerves. (p 13.41)

3-2.59 Describe the general guidelines of recording examination information. (p 13.45)

3-2.60 Discuss the considerations of examination of an infant or child. (p 13.44)

Affective

3-2.61 Demonstrate a caring attitude when performing physical examination skills. (p 13.4)

3-2.62 Discuss the importance of a professional appearance and demeanor when performing physical examination skills. (p 13.4)

3-2.63 Appreciate the limitations of conducting a physical exam in the out-of-hospital environment. (p 13.45)

Psychomotor

3-2.64 Demonstrate the examination of skin, hair, and nails. (p 13.11)

3-2.65 Demonstrate the examination of the head and neck. (p 13.13)

3-2.66 Demonstrate the examination of the eyes. (p 13.15)

3-2.67 Demonstrate the examination of the ears. (p 13.17)

3-2.68 Demonstrate the assessment of visual acuity. (p 13.14)

3-2.69 Demonstrate the examination of the nose. (p 13.18)

3-2.70 Demonstrate the examination of the mouth and pharynx. (p 13.18)

3-2.71 Demonstrate the examination of the neck. (p 13.19)

3-2.72 Demonstrate the examination of the thorax and ventilation. (p 13.20)

3-2.73 Demonstrate the examination of the posterior chest. (p 13.21)

3-2.74 Demonstrate auscultation of the chest. (p 13.21)

3-2.75 Demonstrate percussion of the chest. (p 13.21)

3-2.76 Demonstrate the examination of the anterior chest. (p 13.21)

3-2.77 Demonstrate special examination techniques related to the assessment of the chest. (p 13.21)

3-2.78 Demonstrate the examination of the arterial pulse including location, rate, rhythm, and amplitude. (p 13.26)

3-2.79 Demonstrate the assessment of jugular venous pressure and pulsations. (p 13.26)

3-2.80 Demonstrate the examination of the heart and blood vessels. (p 13.27)

3-2.81 Demonstrate special examination techniques of the cardiovascular examination. (p 13.27)

3-2.82 Demonstrate the examination of the abdomen. (p 13.28)

3-2.83 Demonstrate auscultation of the abdomen. (p 13.29)

3-2.84 Demonstrate the external visual examination of the female genitalia. (p 13.30)

3-2.85 Demonstrate the examination of the male genitalia. (p 13.30)

3-2.86 Demonstrate the examination of the peripheral vascular system. (p 13.35)

3-2.87 Demonstrate the examination of the musculoskeletal system. (p 13.31)

3-2.88 Demonstrate the examination of the nervous system. (p 13.40)

Introduction

Physical examination is the process by which quantifiable, objective (based on fact or observable) information is obtained from a patient about his or her overall state of health. This information is compared with subjective (observed or perceived by the patient), historical information that is obtained from the patient. Armed with these two types of information, you can make a comprehensive assessment of the patient. While performing an assessment, you may see the patient's condition as a clinical manifestation; however, a caring and empathetic approach will yield better results and a more accurate evaluation. Likewise, a professional appearance and demeanor will instill trust and confidence in the abilities of the care provider.

The physical examination consists of two elements—obtaining vital signs that measure overall body function, and performing a head-to-toe survey that evaluates the workings of specific body organ systems. This survey is done in a sequential manner, ensuring that every aspect of the body's function is evaluated. Of course, the conditions in the prehospital setting may determine precisely how the physical examination is performed. Sometimes, the physical exam may be condensed. For example, for an unresponsive medical patient or a trauma patient with a significant mechanism of injury (MOI), a rapid trauma/medical assessment can be performed.

The overall patient assessment is intended to determine whether a problem exists, so that actions can be taken to manage that problem. Before you can appreciate abnormalities on examination, you must understand the wide variety of normal presentations. This is something that can be learned only through direct hands-on experience and interaction with patients. Thus every patient encounter represents an opportunity for you to gain experience about the normal human condition.

Exam Techniques

The techniques of inspection, palpation, percussion, and auscultation allow you to use your physical senses to obtain physical information and to understand the normal (versus abnormal) functions of a patient's body. Inspection involves looking at the patient, either in general or at a specific area (ie, a patient's overall appearance from the doorway versus looking specifically at the chest wall for abnormalities/deformities) **Figure 13-1 ▼**. Palpation is physical touching for the purpose of obtaining information—for example, tenderness (elicited pain), deformity, crepitance, mass effect, pulse quality, and abnormal organ enlargement **Figure 13-2 ▶**.

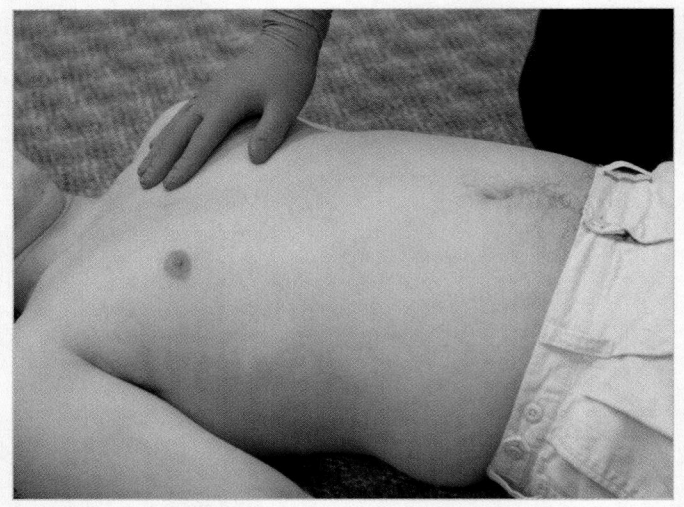

Figure 13-1 Inspection.

You are the Provider Part 1

You and your partner brave the harsh winter winds as you leave the protective warmth of the emergency department and race to your truck. It is one of the coldest days of the season and, unfortunately, one of the busiest. Just as you manage to get the truck heated, you and your partner are dispatched to a doctor's office for a patient complaining of shortness of breath. When you arrive, you are immediately brought to an examination room where you find a 75-year-old man in acute respiratory distress.

Initial Assessment	Recording Time: 0 Minutes
Appearance	Patient is leaning forward in tripod position
Level of consciousness	A (Alert to person, place, and day)
Airway	Open
Breathing	Rapid and shallow, visible retractions and audible wheezes, pursed lip breathing
Circulation	Strong radial pulses; pale, warm skin with cyanotic lips and nail beds

1. What is your general impression of the patient? Is he sick or not sick?
2. What do you think is the most valuable assessment tool at your disposal?

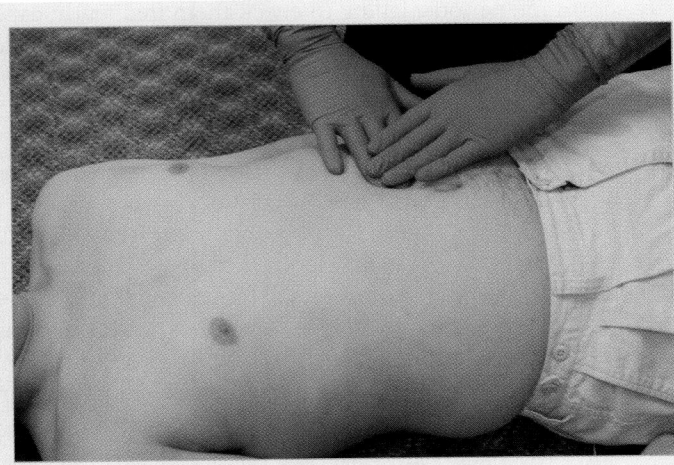
Figure 13-2 Palpation.

Percussion is a skill that requires a lot of practice to perfect. Follow the steps in Skill Drill 13-1 ▾:

1. Place your nondominant hand lightly against the surface to be examined Step 1.
2. Hyperextend the middle finger and apply firm pressure to the surface to be percussed Step 2.
3. Directly strike the middle phalanx of the middle finger with one or two fingertips of the other hand Step 3.
4. Apply the same force over each area of the body to accurately compare the sounds produced by percussion.

Auscultation involves listening with a stethoscope Figure 13-3 ▸. The body generates a variety of high- and low-frequency sounds—both normal and abnormal—that can be detected via auscultation. Bowel sounds can be assessed via auscultation, as can lung sounds. Appreciating the presence of and differences in auscultated sounds requires keen attention.

In the Field

When done properly, palpation should never cause harm. Deep palpation requires practice and knowing when to stop.

Vital Signs

Vital signs consist of a measurement of pulse rate, rhythm, and quality; respiratory rate, rhythm, and quality; blood pressure; temperature; and pulse oximetry. Other than overall patient

In the Field

There are important differences between the bell and diaphragm of the stethoscope. The bell is cup-shaped and is used to listen for deep and low-pitched sounds (heart sounds). It is placed very lightly on the skin, just enough to make a seal. The diaphragm is flat-shaped and is used to listen for high-pitched sounds (breath, bowel, and normal heart sounds); it is placed firmly on the skin.

Percussion entails gently striking the surface of the body, typically where it overlies various body cavities. This technique allows the paramedic to detect changes in the densities of the underlying structures. For example, percussion of a normal lung will yield medium to loud, low-pitched, resonant sounds. Percussion sounds over muscle and bone should be soft, high-pitched, and flat. Percussion sounds over hollow organs such as the intestines are often described as loud, high-pitched, and tympanic (like a drum).

Skill Drill 13-1: Percussion

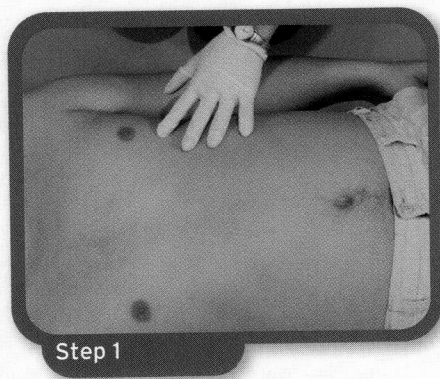
Step 1
Place your hand lightly against the surface to be examined.

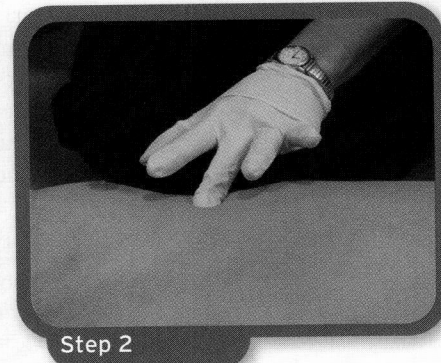
Step 2
Hyperextend the middle finger and apply firm pressure.

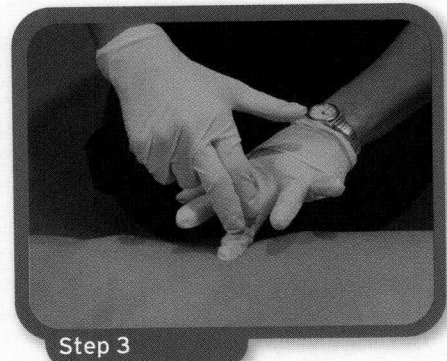
Step 3
Strike the middle finger with one or two fingertips of the other hand.

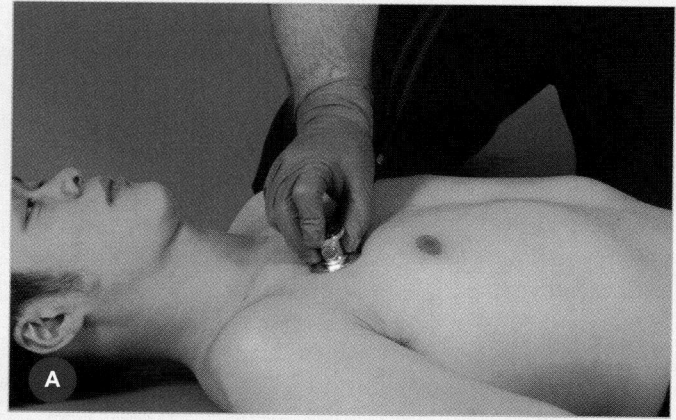

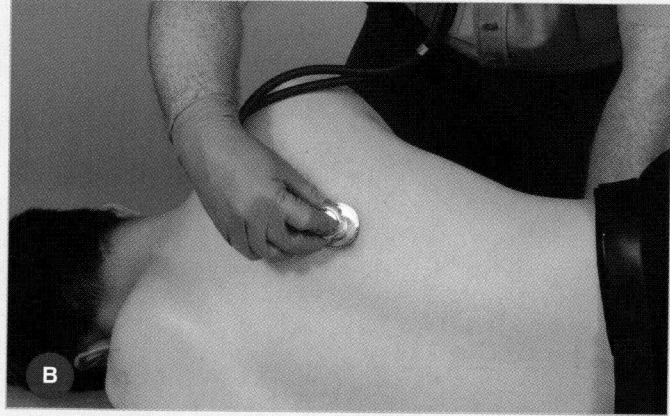

Figure 13-3 Auscultation of the (**A**) anterior chest and the (**B**) posterior chest.

In the Field

Be aware that the patient's age, underlying physical and mental conditions, and current medications can affect the patient's vital signs. Like any other assessment tool, consider the vital signs but devote your attention to the patient.

appearance, vital signs are the most basic objective data for determining patient status. Their measurement requires the paramedic to use the techniques of auscultation, palpation, and inspection.

Vital signs are aptly named; strict attention should be paid to the assessment of these critically important parameters. Normal limits can vary depending on several factors, including age and medication use, and vital signs should be interpreted with those factors in mind. Vital signs should be obtained both accurately and serially to help determine overall stability of the patient. Because vital signs can change dramatically over rela-

Notes from Nancy
Measure vital signs frequently.

tively short time periods, failing to check them frequently, especially in the context of a significantly ill or injured patient, can lead to faulty patient care.

Blood Pressure

Blood pressure is the measurement of the force exerted against the walls of the blood vessels. It is commonly measured in a peripheral artery, although it can be obtained essentially anywhere in the circulatory system. Blood pressure is the product of cardiac output and peripheral vascular resistance, so it includes two components: systolic pressure and diastolic pressure. Systolic pressure is created by the left ventricle while it is contracting (ie, in systole). Diastolic pressure is the result of residual pressure in the system while the left ventricle is relaxing (ie, in diastole). Normally, diastolic pressure should not go to zero, because peripheral vascular resistance in the arteriolar side of the circulatory system should continually provide for a diastolic pressure. The coronary arteries receive blood flow by this mechanism, so lower diastolic pressure means less myocardial perfusion.

In the Field

Many patients exhibit an increase in blood pressure due to anxiety and the stress of an acute injury or illness. Look at your patient as well as trends in vital signs before concluding that the blood pressure is truly abnormal.

Blood pressure must be measured using a cuff that is appropriate to the patient's size and habitus (physique or body build). Too small or tight a cuff will yield an artificially high pressure; too large or loose a cuff will give inappropriately low results. Although blood pressure ideally will be auscultated, it can be palpated to estimate the systolic pressure. Periodic inspection of the blood pressure cuff's gauge is important, as it can lose accuracy and require recalibration.

Pulse

Pulse measurements should assess the rate, presence, location, quality, and rhythm of the pulses. To palpate the pulse, gently compress an artery against a bony prominence, which allows you to feel the pressure wave generated by the heart's contraction. Pulses can be obtained at several points in the body, including the radial, brachial, femoral, and carotid arteries **Figure 13-4 ▶**. When formally counting the pulse rate, time the pulses for a minimum of 15 seconds and then multiply by 4 to obtain the rate

In the Field

Whenever possible, avoid taking a blood pressure on a painful/injured extremity, an arm with an arteriovenous shunt or fistula, or on a postmastectomy side. This can cause pain and/or result in inaccurate readings.

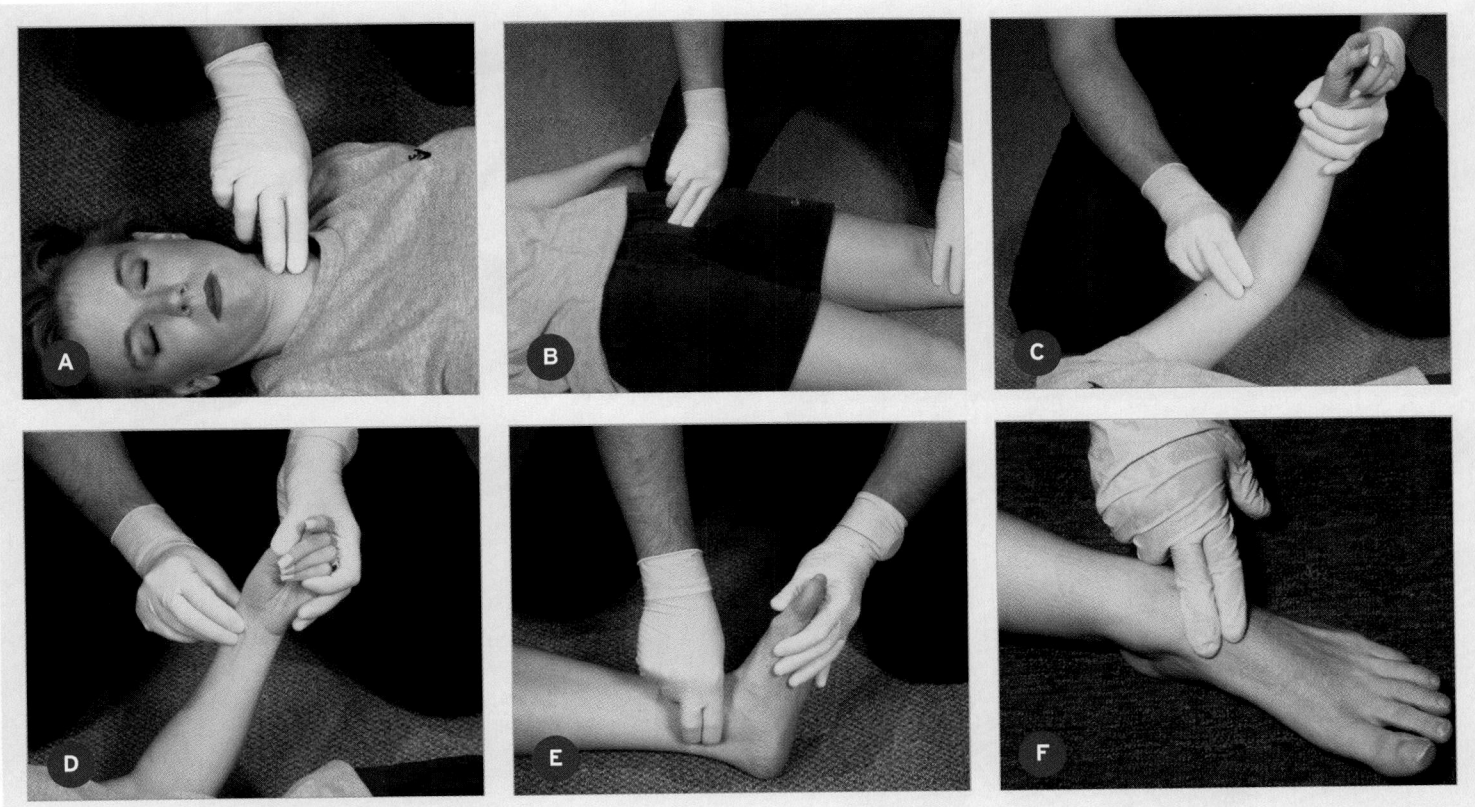

Figure 13-4 Common pulse points. **A.** Carotid pulse. **B.** Femoral pulse. **C.** Brachial pulse. **D.** Radial pulse. **E.** Posterior tibial pulse. **F.** Dorsalis pedis pulse.

Special Considerations

Palpating the pulse in an infant may present a problem. Because an infant's neck is often very short and fat, and its pulse is often quite fast, you may have a hard time finding the carotid pulse. Therefore, in infants younger than 1 year, you should palpate the brachial artery to assess the pulse.

per minute. Palpating a pulse is a basic way to evaluate perfusion and cardiac output. EMS providers should compare proximal and distal pulses during patient evaluations.

Although it is appropriate to check for the presence of a central pulse in an unresponsive patient, the actual pulse rate should be counted in the most peripheral location that can be palpated, to aid with rapid estimation of the blood pressure. In the responsive patient, you may want to determine respiratory rate while you appear to be checking the pulse; this may decrease patients' tendency to inadvertently alter their breathing pattern or rate when they become aware of being evaluated.

Respiration

The respiratory rate is typically measured by inspection of the patient's chest, but respiratory movements can also be assessed by visualizing portions of the abdominal wall, neck, face, and

overall accessory muscle use. Although the absolute respiratory rate is important, the quality of the respiratory effort should be evaluated as well. In particular, you should learn to recognize pathologic respiratory patterns or rhythms (eg, tachypnea, Kussmaul, Cheyne-Stokes, and Biot breathing). Similarly, you should recognize breathing difficulties when patients exhibit tripod positioning, accessory muscle use, or retractions. This information is especially helpful in the assessment of pediatric patients. Respiratory rate should be measured for a minimum of 30 seconds, and then multiplied by 2 to obtain the rate per minute.

Temperature

Many methods can be used to evaluate body temperature. If you use a tympanic device for obtaining a patient's body temperature, however, be aware of extrinsic factors that may increase or decrease the temperature reading.

In the Field

The accuracy of tympanic membrane temperatures has been called into question by some data, especially in patients with severe infections. If your patient looks sick, feels warm, and the tympanic membrane temperature is "normal," consider using a different type of thermometer.

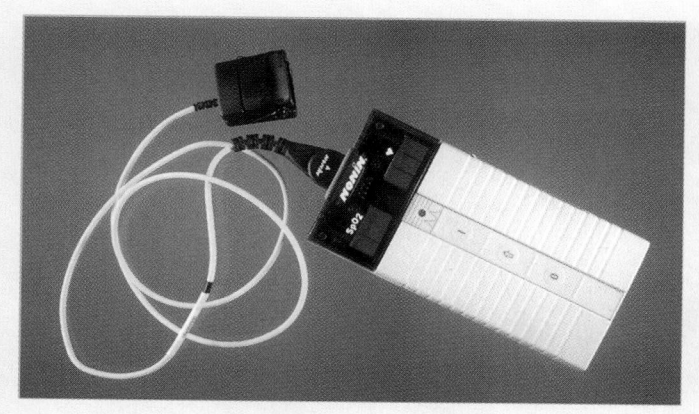

Figure 13-5 A pulse oximeter.

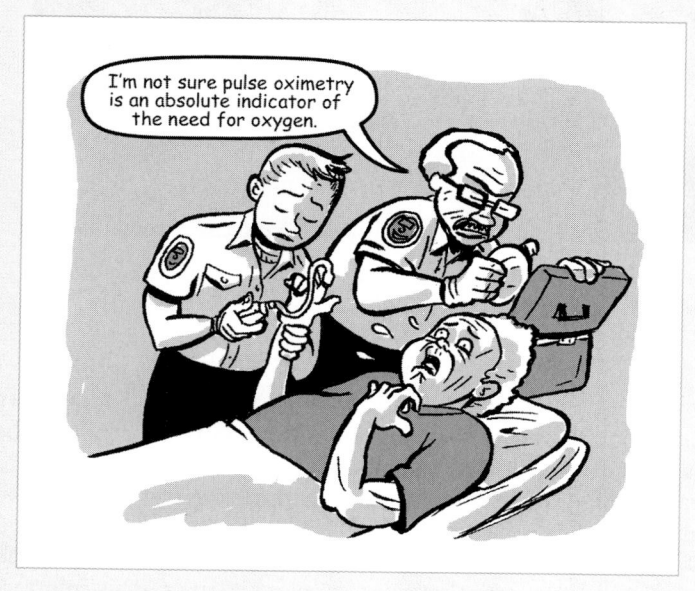

Figure 13-6

Pulse Oximetry

Arterial oxygen saturation determination made via pulse oximetry has earned a place in emergency health care as part of regular vital signs monitoring Figure 13-5 ▲ . Although pulse oximetry is a valuable tool, it should never be used as an absolute indicator of the need for oxygen therapies. Pulse oximetry measures the percentage of hemoglobin saturation and can provide inaccurate information in certain situations. EMS providers need to understand potential complications with pulse oximetry in order to appropriately process the information it provides Figure 13-6 ▲ . Inaccurate readings may be obtained for a variety of reasons—a hypotensive or cold patient, carbon monoxide poisoning, abnormal hemoglobin (ie, sickle-cell disease), vascular dyes, patient motion, and incorrect placement.

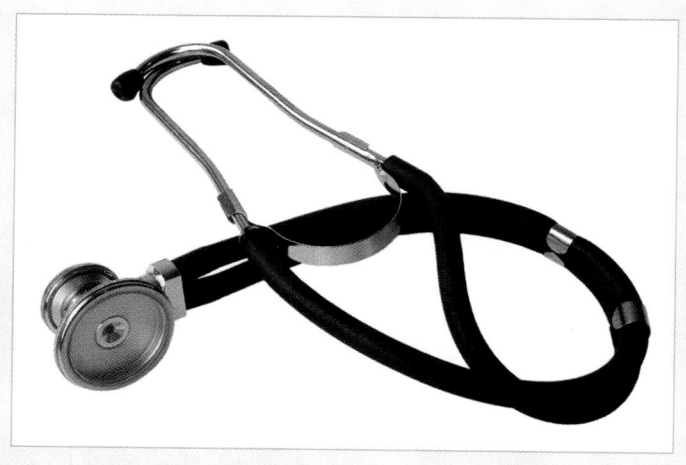

Figure 13-7 Stethoscope.

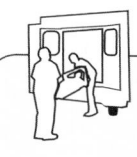

In the Field

Remember to look at your patient, not the "number." If the patient looks sick, and the pulse oximetry reading is "normal," then the patient is still sick.

Equipment Used in the Physical Examination

Equipment used to perform the physical examination includes a stethoscope, blood pressure cuff (sphygmomanometer), ophthalmoscope, otoscope, scissors, a reliable light source, gloves, and a sheet or blanket.

Stethoscopes Figure 13-7 ▲ are available in two forms: acoustic and electronic. Today's acoustic stethoscope, which is the most commonly seen in the prehospital setting, consists of two earpieces attached to an air-filled tube that connects to a chest piece. The chest piece has two sides—a diaphragm (plastic disk) and a bell (hollow cup)—that can be placed against the patient to sense sounds. The diaphragm is vibrated by the sounds of the body, which are then transmitted up to the stethoscope's earpieces; thus the diaphragm side is used to pick up higher-frequency sounds. The bell, which usually transmits lower-frequency sounds, senses the sounds directly off the skin of the patient.

The acoustic stethoscope doesn't amplify sounds; rather, it simply blocks out ambient noises, allowing the paramedic to hear and appreciate the sounds of the body. In contrast, the electronic stethoscope converts the acoustic sound waves into an electronic signal that is then amplified.

The sphygmomanometer, or blood pressure cuff, is used in the measurement of the patient's blood pressure Figure 13-8 ▶ . This device consists of an inflatable cuff, which occludes blood flow, and a manometer (pressure meter),

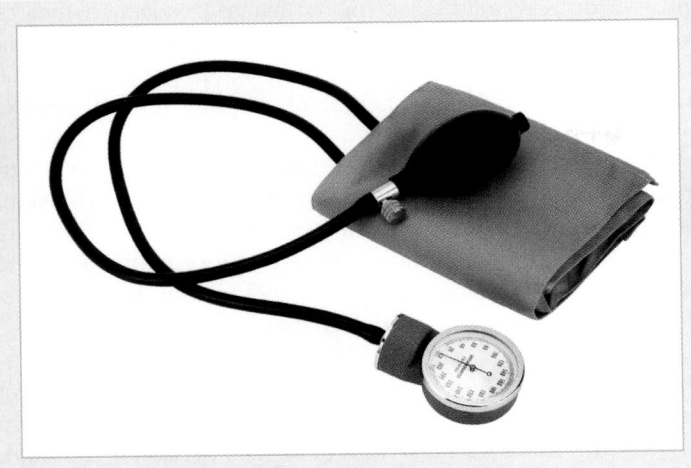

Figure 13-8 Sphygmomanometer.

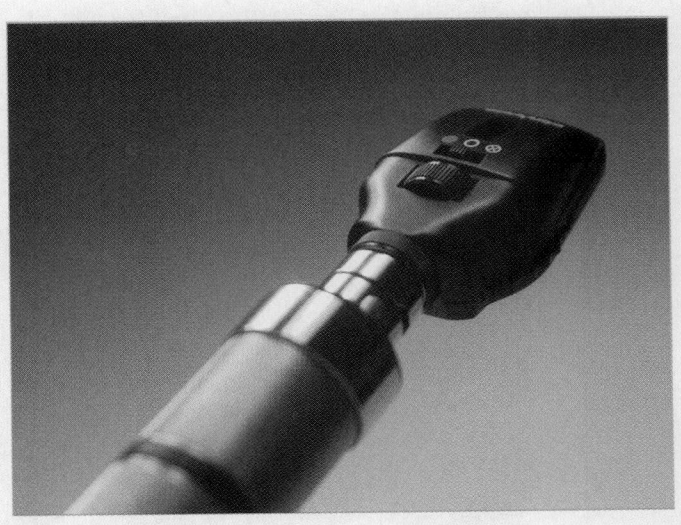

Figure 13-9 Ophthalmoscope.

which is used to determine the pressure in the artery at various points in the physical exam. These two components are connected via tubing. In manual cuffs, a separate tube connects to an inflation bulb.

Many sizes of blood pressure cuffs are available, and using the appropriate size for the patient is essential to obtain an accurate reading. The cuff should be one half to two thirds the size of the upper arm. The blood pressure measurement is separated into systolic and diastolic pressures and is reported in millimeters of mercury (mm Hg).

The ophthalmoscope allows you to look into a patient's eyes and view the retina and aqueous fluid. This tool consists of a concave mirror and a battery-powered light, which is usu-

ally contained in the device's handle   Figure 13-9 ▲ . The care provider looks through a monocular eyepiece that is usually equipped with a rotating disk of lenses; selection of a lens allows for adjustment of the depth and magnification. Use of the ophthalmoscope is usually reserved for hospital and physician's office examination, because effective evaluation requires dilation of the patient's pupils with medication.

The otoscope is used to evaluate the ears of a patient. This instrument consists of a head and a handle. The head contains an electric light source and a low-power magnifying lens. The front of the headpiece has an attachment for a disposable plastic

You are the Provider Part 2

Your partner starts to obtain the patient's vital signs and you begin your patient assessment. The medical assistant tells you that the patient made an emergency appointment this morning for increasing shortness of breath that began last night around 10:00 PM. He presented in severe respiratory distress with an increased work of breathing and audible wheezes. He was administered a nebulizer treatment with 0.25 mg of salbutamol (Ventolin) 20 minutes prior to EMS being called. Your examination reveals that the patient is still experiencing severe respiratory distress. He has a barrel-shaped chest with marked intercostal and supraclavicular retractions, pursed lipped breathing, audible inspiratory and expiratory wheezes, and can only speak in one- or two-word sentences. You also observe cyanosis around his mouth and nail beds with clubbing of the fingers. The medical assistant also provides you with the patient's medical history, which is significant for a 60-year smoking habit, emphysema, and hypertension. He is prescribed nebulizer treatments with 2.5 mg of Ventolin/normal saline four times a day, two puffs of budesonide (Pulmicort) inhaler twice a day, 200 mg of metoprolol (Toprol XL) once a day, and home oxygen at 3 L/min. He has an allergy to iodine and penicillin.

Vital Signs	Recording Time: 5 Minutes
Skin	Pale, warm, with cyanotic lips and nail beds
Pulse	130 beats/min, regular; strong radial
Blood pressure	168/82 mm Hg
Respirations	40 breaths/min, labored, audible wheezes
Sao_2	70% on nasal cannula at 4 L/min

3. Which signs and symptoms are acute? Which are chronic?
4. Which interventions should you consider at this point?

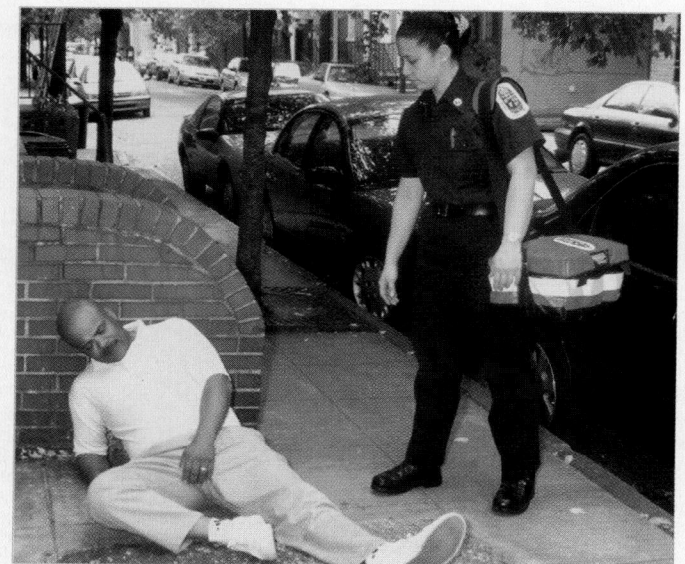

Figure 13-10 Get a general impression of the overall situation as you approach the patient.

earpiece (speculum). The examiner inserts the speculum into the ear and looks through a lens on the rear of the headpiece. Some otoscopes include a sliding rear window that allows for the insertion of an additional instrument (eg, to remove ear wax). Most have an insertion point for a bulb that is used to push air into the ear canal, allowing the examiner to visualize the movement of the tympanic membrane. The batteries are located in the handle unless it is a wall-mounted unit, such as those found in a physician's office.

The General Impression

The general impression begins as you approach the scene, simultaneously sizing up the situation and the patient's overall presentation **Figure 13-10 ▲** . A quick look at the environment in which the patient is found and the general appearance of the patient provides a substantial amount of information before you ask the first question. An important skill that many paramedics develop is a sense as to when a patient is seriously ill, based primarily on his or her initial appearance. The expression "sick or not sick?" sums up this approach.

Look for signs of significant distress such as mental status changes, anxiousness, labored breathing, difficulty speaking, diaphoresis, obvious pain, obvious deformity, and guarding or splinting of a painful area. It is not uncommon for persons experiencing substantial and incapacitating pain to present with a quiet and still affect.

Other aspects that may be readily apparent and worth noting as you develop a general impression include dress, hygiene, expression, overall size, posture, untoward odors, and overall state of health. When characterizing the overall state of the patient, be sure to use appropriate terms to describe degree of distress: no

apparent distress, mild (slight or not harsh), moderate (small or average), acute (very great or bad), and severe (dangerous or difficult to endure). Other acceptable terms to describe the general state of a patient's health include chronically ill, frail, feeble, robust, and vigorous.

Perhaps the quickest and most reliable initial way to evaluate a patient's overall degree of distress is to look at the skin. Relatively subtle but serious changes in overall perfusion are usually manifested early on in the skin's appearance. Evaluate the skin's color, relative moisture, and relative temperature. Note any obvious lesions or deformities.

Pallor is present when red blood cell perfusion to the capillary beds of the skin is poor. You may also be able to detect pallor by looking at the patient's lips or eye conjunctiva. Cyanosis indicates a relative lack of oxygen perfusion, although the number of red blood cells may be adequate to carry any available oxygen. Cyanosis correlates extremely well with low arterial oxygen saturation. It can be visualized generally in the skin, but more specifically in the fingernail beds, face, and lips.

Ecchymosis is localized bruising or blood collection within or under the skin. Evaluate large ecchymoses for the possibility of serious underlying soft-tissue, bony, or organ injury. Serious wounds to the head, neck, and torso should also be noted, as well as any evidence of a potential hemorrhage.

▌The Physical Exam

The physical examination of a patient in the prehospital setting is the most important skill a health care provider can master. This ability is first developed as an EMT-B and should be refined as an advanced practitioner. Starting intravenous access, pushing medications, and performing endotracheal intubation are simply mechanical skills that require only practice to achieve proficiency. The skills of patient assessment and interpreting the findings of a physical exam, by comparison, truly separate the accomplished paramedic from the basic provider. The physical exam consists of a comprehensive review of systems to determine the nature and extent of the patient's illness or injury.

Mental Status

Evaluation of a patient's mental status involves assessing cognitive function (ie, ability to use reasoning or perception). At a minimum, evaluate the patient's degree of alertness. This assessment is accomplished by using the AO × 4 method, which means the patient is alert to person, place, time, and events leading up to this particular moment. The AVPU scale is a rapid method of assessing the patient's level of consciousness using one of the following four designations:

  A *Alert* (oriented to person, place, and day)
  V Responds to *Verbal* stimuli
  P Responds to *Painful* stimuli
  U *Unresponsive*

When classifying the response to stimuli, grade the patient according to the best response you can elicit. For example, a patient passed out on the street who moans in response to a loud shout from the paramedic would score a V on the AVPU scale. Response to tactile stimuli (eg, pinching the nail bed, twisting the skin of the forearm) would earn a P. No response to verbal or tactile stimuli would be classified as U.

Skin, Hair, and Nails

Skin

The skin, which is the largest organ system in the body, serves three major functions: It regulates the temperature of the body, transmits information from the environment to the brain, and protects the body in the environment.

The skin is the major organ governing the body's thermoregulation. In a cold environment, constriction of the blood vessels shunts blood away from the skin to decrease the amount of heat radiated from the body surface (observed as pale skin). When the outside environment is hot, the vessels in the skin dilate, the skin becomes flushed or red, and heat radiates from the body surface. Also, in a hot environment, sweat is secreted to the skin surface from the sweat glands. Energy, in the form of body heat, is lost during the evaporation process, which causes body temperature to fall.

Information from the environment is carried to the brain through a rich supply of sensory nerves that originate in the skin. Nerve endings that lie in the skin are adapted to perceive and transmit information about heat, cold, external pressure, pain, and the position of the body in space. In this way, the skin recognizes changes in the environment. It also reacts to pressure, pain, and pleasurable stimuli.

The skin is composed of two layers: the epidermis and the dermis Figure 13-11 ▶ . The epidermis, or outermost layer, is the body's first line of defense. It serves as the principal barrier against water, dust, microorganisms, and mechanical stress.

Underlying the epidermis is the dermis—a tough, highly elastic layer of connective tissues. This complex material is composed chiefly of collagen fibers, elastic fibers, and a mucopolysaccharide gel. Numerous fibroblasts (cells that secrete collagen, elastin, and ground substance) are found within the dermis as well.

The dermis is subdivided into the papillary dermis and a reticular layer. The vasculature inside the papillary dermis serves two functions—it provides nutrients to the epidermis, and aids in thermoregulation. Dilation of these vessels increases blood flow to the skin, allowing heat to dissipate. Conversely, blood vessel constriction results in retention of heat. The reticular layer consists of dense, irregular connective tissue, which provides both strength and elasticity. With age, the skin undergoes significant changes, including loss of the collagen connective tissues and diminished capillary supply.

Examination of the skin involves both inspection and palpation. Pay careful attention to the skin color, moisture, temperature, texture, turgor, and any significant lesions. Look for evidence of diminished perfusion, evaluate for pallor and cyanosis, and be wary of diaphoresis. Reddened or pink skin can be seen in a variety of normal states, but it is also evident in states of relative vasodilatation (flushing). Flushed skin is usually apparent in patients with fever, and it may be seen in patients experiencing an allergic process. Reddened skin should also be considered in the context of superficial burns.

Examining the skin for changes in perfusion is usually best accomplished in areas where the epidermis is thinnest, such as the fingernails, lips, and conjunctivae. It is sometimes useful to examine the palms and soles as well. Pale skin is a relatively common finding in the seriously ill patient and may indicate severe vasoconstriction, as seen in profound anemia, acute cardiovascular events, other shock-like states, and hypothermia. Local areas of blanched, cool, white skin are typical of frostbite.

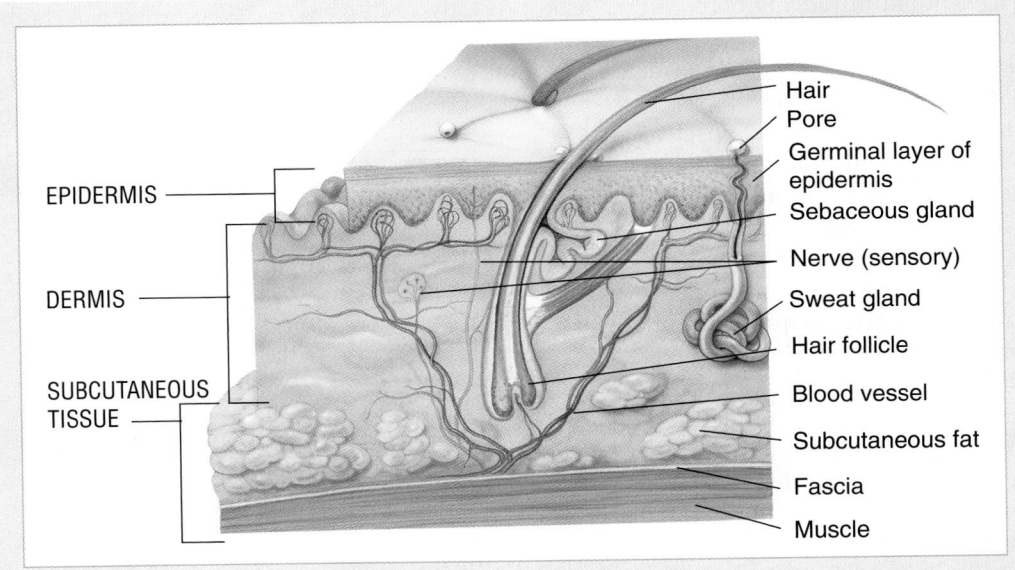

Figure 13-11 The skin is composed of a tough external layer (the epidermis) and a vascular inner layer (the dermis).

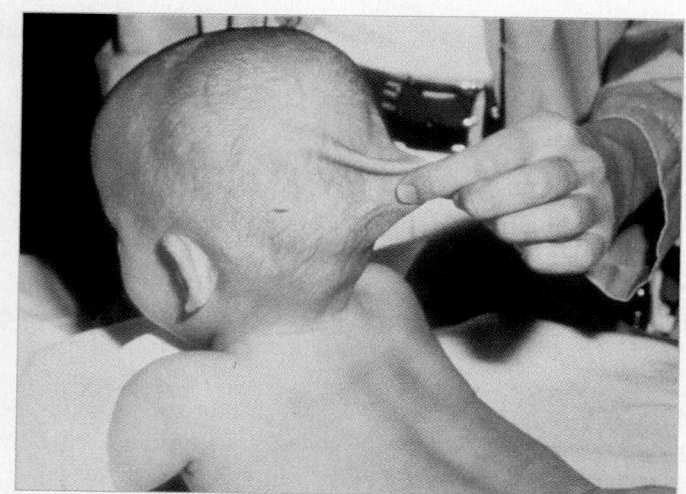

Figure 13-12 Tenting is evident with extreme dehydration.

Special Considerations

When assessing skin turgor in an older patient, use the skin of the upper chest. This is a much more reliable indicator than the extremities.

Although cyanotic skin is commonly seen in states of oxygen desaturation, it can also be a function of hypothermia, especially in very young patients. Mottling is a typical finding in states of severe protracted hypoperfusion and shock and is readily evident in pediatric patients.

It takes practice to accurately gauge patients' relative perfusion and hydration status. Becoming familiar with the abnormal findings of the skin and mucous membranes is an excellent aid in judging both. Turgor relates directly to hydration. Poor skin turgidity is an expression of poorly hydrated skin, with associated tenting evident in extreme cases, particularly in young children Figure 13-12 ▲ . Because of normal changes in elastin and connective tissues with advanced age, skin turgor is an insignificant indicator in geriatric patients, as is skin that is abnormally dry to the touch. Paying attention to skin temperature can sometimes prove useful when trying to determine the etiologies of different problems (eg, respiratory distress). Sometimes making a clinical distinction between congestive heart failure with pulmonary edema versus pneumonia is a function of the patient's temperature, which may be readily apparent from tactile examination of the skin.

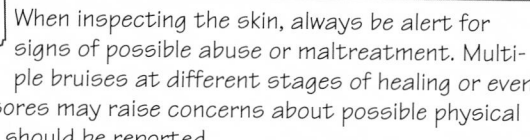

In the Field

When inspecting the skin, always be alert for signs of possible abuse or maltreatment. Multiple bruises at different stages of healing or even pressure sores may raise concerns about possible physical abuse and should be reported.

Skin lesions may sometimes be the only external evidence of a serious internal injury. Take note of any large areas of ecchymosis, palpable crepitus (palpable fractures), and open wounds. Devastating internal injuries can result from wounds whose only external signs are relatively benign-appearing penetrations. Be aware of any body areas that are hidden by clothing or by devices such as a backboard and head immobilizer. Always visually inspect and manually palpate the patient's back and expose body parts. Likewise, evaluation for rashes is usually best accomplished by discreetly examining areas of skin otherwise hidden by clothing.

Hair

Examination of the hair is done by inspection and palpation. In this survey, note the quantity, distribution, and texture of the hair. Recent changes in the growth or loss of hair can indicate an underlying endocrine disorder, such as diabetes, or may result from treatment modalities for disease processes (eg, chemotherapy or radiation treatment of cancer). Although the recent loss of hair may be related to a disease process, the thinning and loss of hair can also be a normal finding in the older patient.

Nails

The examination of the fingernails and toenails can reveal many subtle findings Table 13-1 ▼ . The color, shape, texture, and presence or absence of lesions should all be assessed. The normal nail should be firm and smooth on palpation. Normal changes to the nails with aging include the development of striations and a change in color (yellowish tint) related to the reduction in body calcium.

Table 13-1	Abnormal Findings in the Nails	
Condition	**Findings**	**Possible Cause**
Beau's lines	Transverse depressions in the nail inhibiting growth	Systemic illness, severe infection, or nail injury
Clubbing	The angle between the nail and the nail base approaches or exceeds 180°	Flattening and enlargement of the fingertips is associated with chronic respiratory disease
Psoriasis	Pitting, discoloration, and subungual thickening of the nail	
Splinter hemorrhages	Red or brown linear streaks in the nail bed	Bacterial endocarditis or trichinosis
Terry's nails	Transverse white bands that cover the nail except for the distal tip	Cirrhosis

Head, Ears, Eyes, Nose, and Throat

The head, ears, eyes, nose, and throat (HEENT) exam consists of a comprehensive evaluation of the head and related structures. It is crucial because the head contains the brain, numerous important sensory organs, and all of the upper airway anatomy. The eyes are a nervous system structure that involves both motor pathways (lids, extraocular muscles, pupilary constrictors, corneal blink reflex) and sensory pathways. The ears provide for both hearing and balance control. The nose is a sensory organ involved with the senses of smell and taste; it also plays an important role in assisting with breathing. The throat consists of the mouth and posterior pharynx, and all the structures intrinsic to them. This complicated organ simultaneously coordinates many motor and sensory functions, while also coordinating the initial activities of both the respiratory and digestive systems.

Head

The head is divided into two parts: the cranium and the face. The cranium, or skull, contains the brain. The brain connects to the spinal cord through the foramen magnum, a large opening at the base of the skull. The most posterior portion of the cranium is the occiput. On each side of the cranium, the lateral portions are called the temples or temporal regions. Between the temporal regions and the occiput lie the parietal regions. The forehead is called the frontal region. Just anterior to the ear, in the temporal region, you can feel the pulse of the superficial temporal artery. A layer of muscle fascia covers the skull. The thick skin covering the cranium, which usually bears hair, is called the scalp.

Within the skull lie the meninges, three distinct layers of tissue that suspend the brain and the spinal cord within the skull and the spinal canal. The dura mater is the tough, fibrous, outer layer that resembles leather. It forms a sac that contains the central nervous system (CNS), with small openings through which the peripheral nerves exit. The inner two layers of the meninges, called the arachnoid and the pia mater, are much thinner than the dura mater. They contain the blood vessels that nourish the brain and spinal cord. Cerebrospinal fluid (CSF) is produced in a chamber inside the brain, called the third ventricle. CSF fills the space between the meninges and acts as shock absorber.

When you are examining the head, you should both feel it and inspect it visually. This step is important in the management of potential trauma patients and with patients who have altered mental status or are unresponsive. If you find evidence of external bleeding, attempt to separate the hair manually and irrigate the clot; this should allow you to identify the source of

Special Considerations

Always inspect the fontanelle in infants.
Bulging = Increased intracranial pressure in a quiet child
Sunken = Dehydration

bleeding. Evaluate the skull for any deformity, step-off, or tenderness. Observe the general shape and contour of the skull.

In children younger than 18 months, routinely palpate the anterior fontanelle (the "soft spot"). Prior to its normal physiologic closure, it can serve as an excellent relative indicator of hydration and intracranial pressure. The fontanelle is usually characterized as open and flat (the normal state), bulging (common while crying, pathologic when observed in a quiet child), and sunken (in severe dehydration).

When you are evaluating the face, observe the color and moisture of the skin, as well as expression, symmetry, and contour of the face itself. Also pay attention to any swelling or apparent areas of injury, and note any signs of respiratory distress. Use the mnemonic DCAP-BTLS—Deformities, Contusions, Abrasions, Punctures/penetrations, Burns, Tenderness, Lacerations, and Swelling—to assist you during the physical exam. Follow the steps in **Skill Drill 13-2 ▶** to assess the head:

1. Visually inspect the head, looking for any obvious DCAP-BTLS (Step 1).
2. Palpate the top and back of the head to locate any subtle abnormalities (Step 2). Use a systematic approach, going from front to back, to ensure that nothing is missed.
3. Part the hair in several places to examine the condition of the scalp. Identify any lesions under the hair (Step 3).
4. Note any pain during the process (this exam should not cause the patient any pain).
5. Palpate the structure of the face noting any DCAP-BTLS. Pay attention to the condition of the skin, hair distribution, and shape of the face (Step 4).

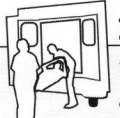

In the Field

Protecting fragile CNS structures from further damage is vital to the patient's prospects for living a normal life. Lean toward caution and overprotection in assessing and treating possible brain and spinal cord injuries.

Eyes

The eyes are a tremendously complex sensory organ **Figure 13-13 ▶**. They process light stimuli for the brain, so that the brain is able to decode light impulses presenting to the eyes and form a visual image. The eyes are a critical link to the CNS, and as such they allow the examiner to more precisely assess the functions of the CNS.

Each eye consists of an anterior chamber and a posterior chamber, which are always assessed in a standardized fashion (ie, from "front to back"). The outer aspects of the eye are checked first, with deeper structures subsequently evaluated. General issues to ask about include any pain or redness, loss of vision, diplopia (double vision), photophobia, blurring, discharge, and corrective lens use.

After addressing these general questions, assess for visual acuity (VA)—that is, the ability or inability to see, and how

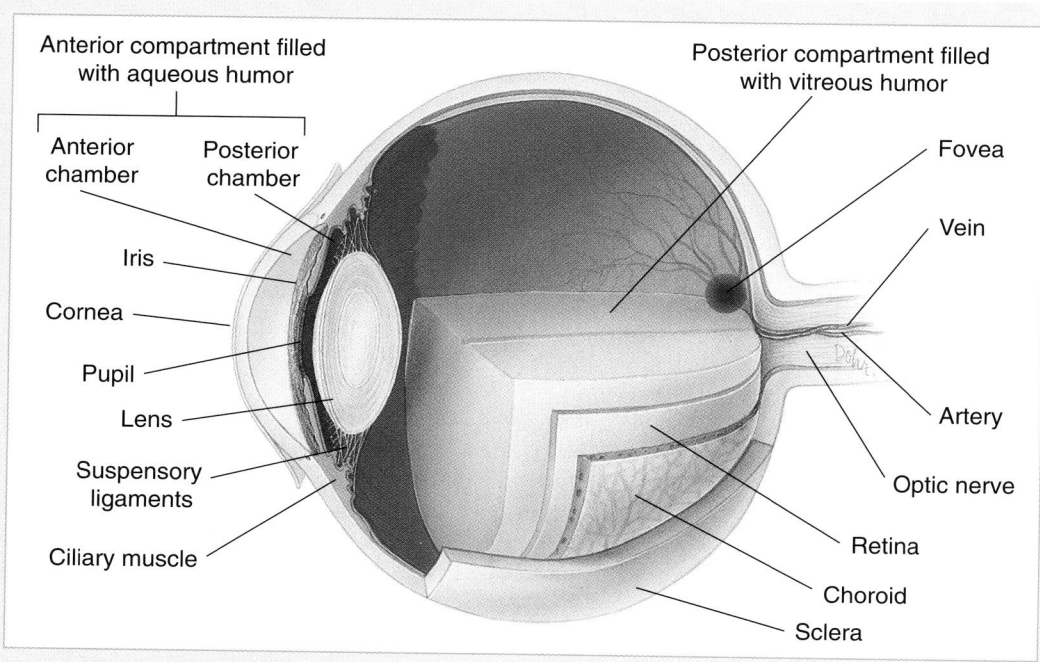

Figure 13-13 The structure of the eye.

Anterior compartment filled with aqueous humor

- Anterior chamber
- Posterior chamber
- Iris
- Cornea
- Pupil
- Lens
- Suspensory ligaments
- Ciliary muscle

Posterior compartment filled with vitreous humor

- Fovea
- Vein
- Artery
- Optic nerve
- Retina
- Choroid
- Sclera

Skill Drill 13-2: Assessing the Head

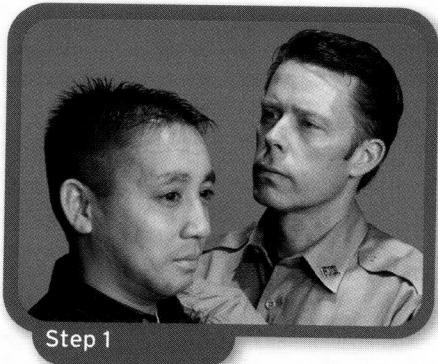

Step 1

Visually inspect the head, looking for any obvious DCAP-BTLS.

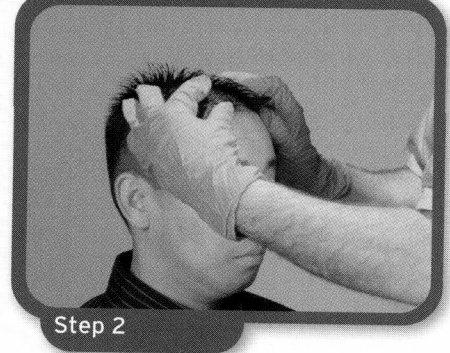

Step 2

Palpate the top and back of the head to locate any subtle abnormalities.

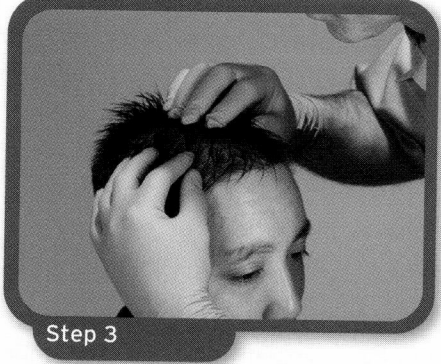

Step 3

Part the hair in several places to examine the condition of the scalp.

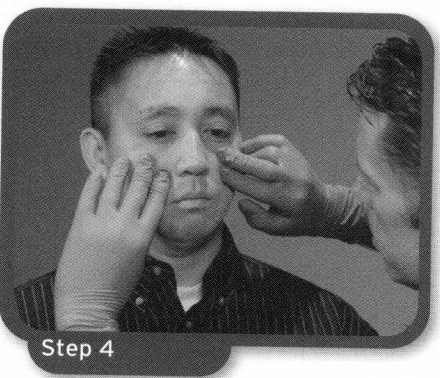

Step 4

Palpate the structure of the face, noting any DCAP-BTLS.

well the patient can see. Check VA by examining each eye in isolation. If corrective lenses are normally worn, check VA with the correction in place. The standard device for checking VA is the Snellen ("E") chart Figure 13-14 ▸ , although it is not an appropriate tool in the prehospital setting. More appropriate tools in this environment include simple tests such as light/dark discrimination and finger counting. Finger counting should be done from a noted distance, typically 6′, 3′, and 1′. Reporting on VA must include the distance from which finger counting was measured.

The pupil is a circular opening in the center of the pigmented iris of the eye. The diameter and reactivity of the patient's pupil to light reflect the status of the brain's perfusion, oxygenation, and condition. The pupils are normally round and of approximately equal size; they serve as optical diaphragms, adjusting their size depending on the available light. In normal room light, the pupils appear to be midsized. With less light, they dilate to allow more light to enter the eye, making it possible to see even in dim light. With high light levels or when a bright light is suddenly introduced, the pupils instantly constrict, allowing less light to enter and protecting the sensitive receptors in the inner eye from damage. When a brighter light is introduced into one eye (or higher levels of light enter one eye only), both pupils should constrict equally to the appropriate size for the pupil receiving the most light.

In the absence of any light, the pupils will become fully relaxed and dilated. When light is introduced, each eye sends sensory signals to the brain, indicating the level of light

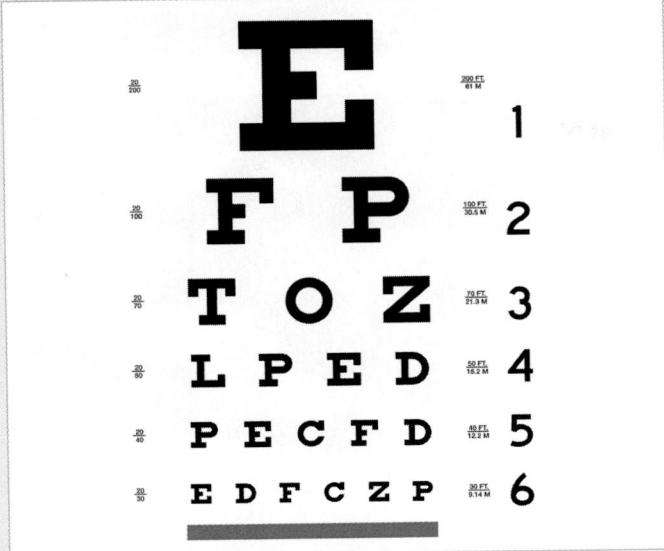

Figure 13-14 Due to its size and complexity, the Snellen chart is not a good prehospital tool.

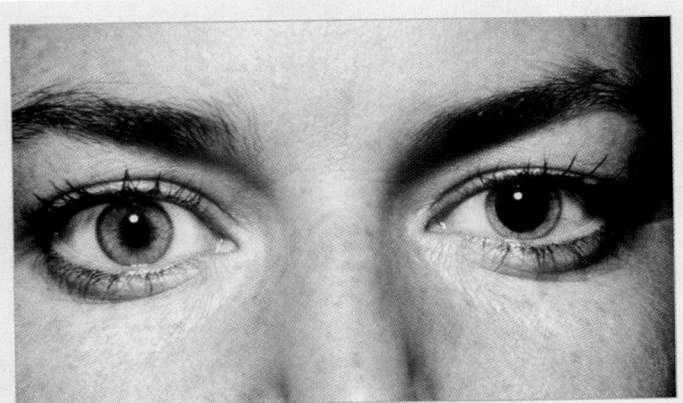

Figure 13-15 Asymmetric pupils may be normal or may signify a severe brain injury.

received. Pupil size is regulated by a series of continuous motor commands that the brain automatically sends through the oculomotor nerves (third cranial nerve) to each eye. Normally, pupil size changes instantly to any change in light level.

When assessing the pupils, check for size (in millimeters), shape, and symmetry. Also check for a reaction to light shined on them, performing this assessment in as darkened an environment as possible. Asymmetric pupils (anisocoria, which can be found in 20% of the population) may indicate significant ocular or neurologic pathology, but must be correlated with the patient's overall presentation Figure 13-15 ▲. Topical applications of certain medicines and substances can also provoke pupilary changes.

Muscles are responsible for physically moving the eyes from side to side and up and down, which allows for seamless binocular vision. When asked to follow a finger moved in a "Z" or "H" pattern, the eyes should move smoothly and symmetrically with the finger. Visual field examination assesses the

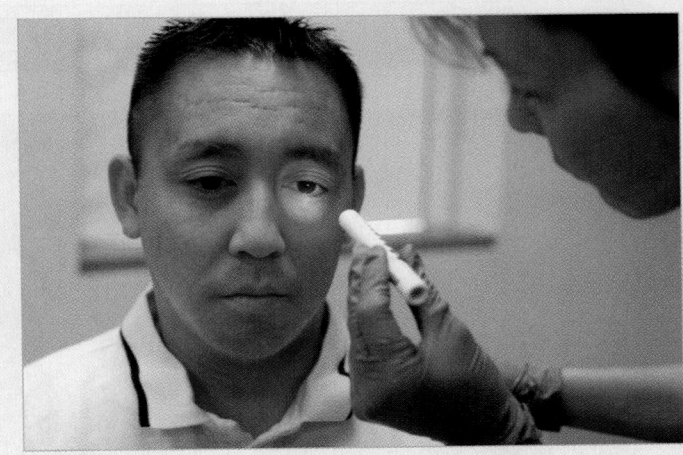

Figure 13-16 Pen light exam of the eye.

retina's (and therefore the optic nerve's) ability to perceive light. This is done by checking the patient's peripheral vision, examining each eye in isolation.

Following the general eye exam, a more precise pen light exam is typically undertaken Figure 13-16 ▲. Check the lids, lashes, and tear ducts. Look for foreign bodies, evidence of wounds and trauma, and discharge. Turn up the lids to look for foreign bodies, and inspect the conjunctivae and sclera. The sclera ought to be white, not jaundiced or injected (red). Painless subconjunctival hemorrhage is a common but benign presentation. The conjunctivae ought to be pink—not cyanotic, pale, or overly reddened. The cornea and lens will be difficult to examine without additional assessment tools—although in a trauma situation, you should note whether the globe is patent. Next, examine the anterior chamber and iris for clarity, noting any cloudiness or bleeding. Finally, examine the posterior chamber and retina; however, this exam is more useful after chemical dilation of the pupil and appropriate use of an ophthalmoscope. Follow the steps in Skill Drill 13-3 ▶ and Skill Drill 13-4 ▶ :

1. Examine the exterior portion of the eye. Look for any obvious trauma or deformity Step 1 .
2. Ask the patient about any pain, altered vision (eg, blurred or double vision), discharge, or sensitivity to light.
3. Measure visual acuity by having the patient count the number of fingers you are holding up at varying distances (usually 6′, 3′, and 1′ away from the patient). Perform this exam on each eye independently of the other Step 2 .
4. Exam the pupils for size, shape, and symmetry. They should be equal.
5. Test the pupils for their reaction to light. Both pupils should constrict when exposed to light, and they should be equal in their response Step 3 .
6. Test for cranial nerve function by asking the patient to follow your fingers in a "Z" or "H" pattern. Note any abnormal movement of the eyes Step 4 .
7. Inspect the eyelids, lashes, and tear ducts for evidence of trauma, foreign bodies, or discharge Step 5 .

Skill Drill 13-3: Examining the Eye

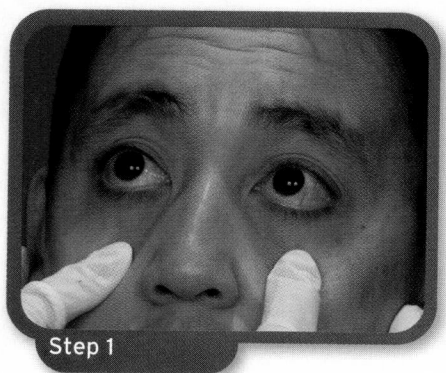

Step 1

Examine the exterior portion of the eye.

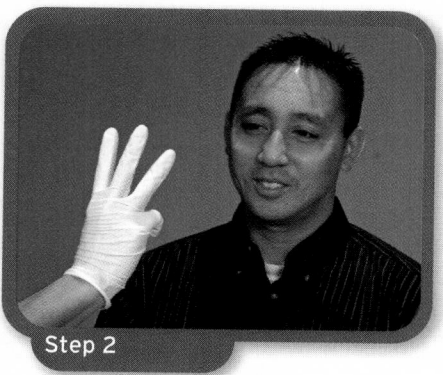

Step 2

Measure visual acuity by having the patient count the number of fingers you are holding up at varying distances.

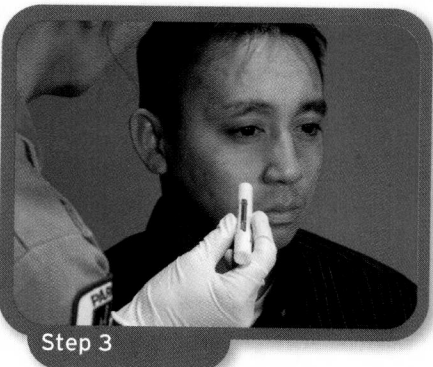

Step 3

Test the pupils for their reaction to light.

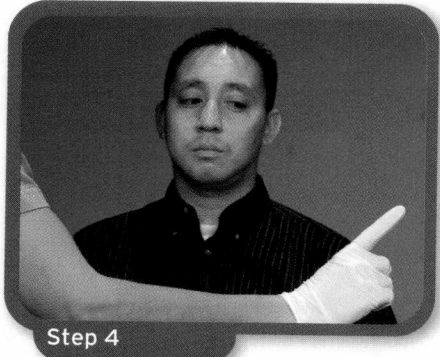

Step 4

Test for cranial nerve function by asking the patient to follow your fingers in a "Z" or "H" pattern.

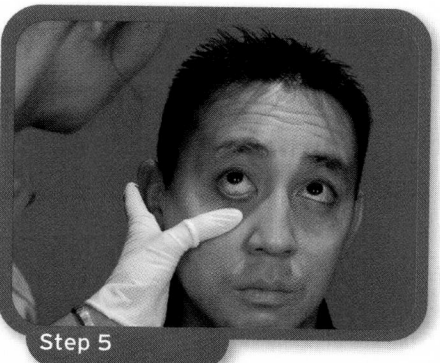

Step 5

Inspect the eyelids, lashes, and tear ducts.

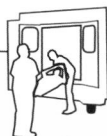

In the Field

Eye movement is not parallel. Failure to follow in a certain direction indicates weakness of an extraocular muscle or dysfunction of a cranial nerve innervating it.

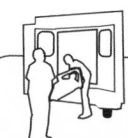

In the Field

Cataracts appear as opaque black areas against the red reflex.

1. Darken the environment as much as possible.
2. Ask the patient to look straight ahead and focus on a distant object (Step 1).
3. Set the light on the ophthalmoscope to a setting no brighter than necessary and the lens to 0 unless another setting works better for your eyes.
4. Use your right hand and eye to examine the patient's right eye; use your left hand and eye to examine the patient's left eye (Step 2).
5. Place the scope to your eye and look into the patient's pupil from 10″ to 20″ away at a 45° angle to the eye. You

should see the retina as a "red reflex" or a bright orange glow (Step 3).

6. Slowly move toward the patient to appreciate the structures of the fundus. Adjust the lens as needed to improve the focus. Locate a blood vessel and follow it back to the disk. Use this blood vessel as a point of reference.
7. Inspect for the size, color, and clarity of the disk. Note the integrity of the blood vessels and any lesions present on the retina. Move nasally to observe the macula (Step 4).
8. Repeat the process with the other eye.

Skill Drill 13-4: Eye Examination With an Ophthalmoscope

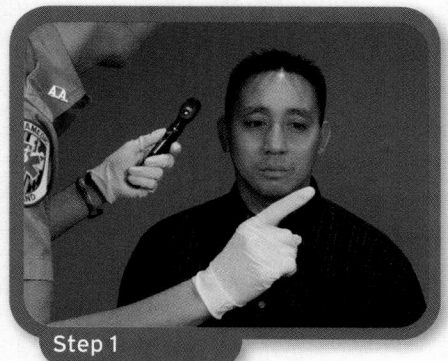

Step 1

Ask the patient to look straight ahead and focus on a distant object.

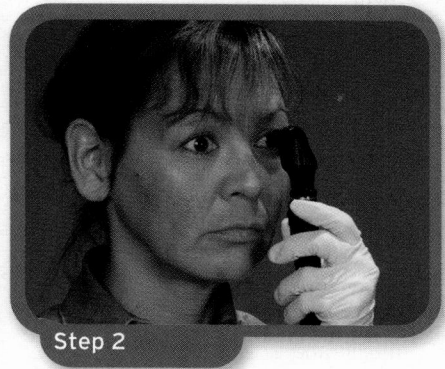

Step 2

Use your right hand and eye to examine the patient's right eye; use your left hand and eye to examine the patient's left eye.

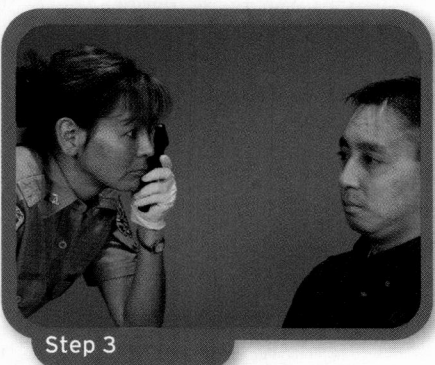

Step 3

Place the scope to your eye and look into the patient's pupil from 10″ to 20″ away at a 45° angle to the eye.

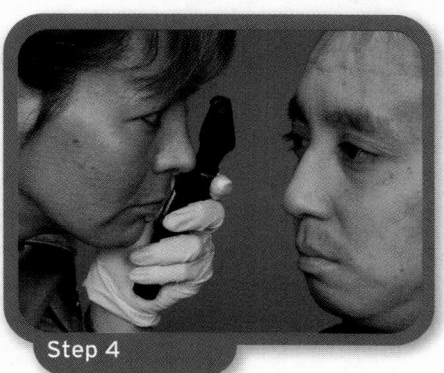

Step 4

Inspect for the size, color, and clarity of the disk.

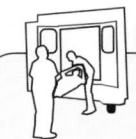

In the Field

Use of the ophthalmoscope requires frequent practice. It is not routinely used in prehospital care.

Ears

The ear is a sensory organ that is chiefly involved with hearing and sound perception but is also intimately involved with balance control. The ear consists of an outer portion, a middle portion, and an inner portion **Figure 13-17 ▶** .

The external ear consists of the pinna, or auricle (the part lying outside of the head), and the external auditory canal, which leads in toward the tympanic membrane, or eardrum.

The middle ear contains three small bones (hammer, anvil, and stirrup) that move in response to sound waves hitting the tympanic membrane. This mechanism controls how we hear and differentiate sounds. The middle ear is connected to the nasal cavity by the Eustachian tube, or internal auditory canal. This connection permits equalization of pressure in the middle ear when external atmospheric pressure changes.

The inner ear consists of bony chambers filled with fluid. As the head moves, so does the fluid. In response, fine nerve endings within the fluid send impulses to the brain, indicating the position of the head and the rate of change of position.

Assessing the ears essentially involves checking for new aberrations in hearing perception plus inspecting and palpating for wounds, swelling, or drainage (pus, blood, CSF). Often the mastoid process of the skull, which is palpated immediately posterior to the auricle, is assessed for discoloration and tenderness (Battle's sign). Abnormalities of the external canal and tympanic membrane are visualized by use of an otoscope. Follow the steps in **Skill Drill 13-5 ▶** :

1. Select an appropriately sized speculum. Dim the lights as much as possible.
2. Ensure that the ear is free of foreign bodies.
3. Place your hand firmly against the patient's head and gently grasp the patient's auricle. Move the ear to best visualize the canal, usually upward and back in the adult patient **Step 1** .
4. Instruct the patient not to move during the exam to avoid damaging the ear.
5. Turn on the otoscope and insert the speculum into the ear **Step 2** . Insertion toward the patient's nose usually provides the best view. Don't insert the speculum deeply into the canal.

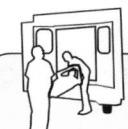

In the Field

When looking for a foreign body, don't advance an otoscope tip blindly; you may accidentally push the foreign body in further.

6. Inspect the canal for any lesions or discharge. A small amount of cerumen (ear wax) is normal (Step 3).

7. Visualize the tympanic membrane (eardrum), and inspect it for integrity and color. It should be translucent or a pearly gray color. Note any signs of inflammation, including swelling or discoloration (pink or redness in the canal or tympanic membrane).

Nose

The nose is a sensory organ involved with smell and taste; it is also part of the respiratory system. In assessing injuries involving the nose, it helps to picture the inside of the nose itself (**Figure 13-18** ▶). The nasal cavity is divided into two sections or chambers by the nasal septum, which is made of cartilage. Each nasal chamber contains three layers of bone (the turbinates) that are covered with a moist lining. Both chambers have superior, middle, and inferior turbinates. During nasal breathing, the air moves through the nasal chambers and is humidified as it passes over the turbinates.

When checking the nose, assess it both anteriorly and inferiorly. Look for evidence of asymmetry, deformity, wounds, foreign bodies, discharge or bleeding, and tenderness. Note any evidence of respiratory distress, such as flaring of the nostrils. Inspect the exterior of the nose, looking for color changes, symmetry, and structural abnormalities. The nose should be firm and the nares clear of obstruction. Examine the column of the nose; it should be midline with the face. Inspect the septum for any deviation from midline. The nares should be symmetrical. Slight deviation or asymmetry of the nares, septum, and column are normal findings; however, gross abnormalities should be noted. Note any drainage or discharge. Small amounts of mucosal discharge are normal, but large amounts of mucus and any blood or CSF fluid are serious findings.

Throat

Assessment of the throat should include an evaluation of the

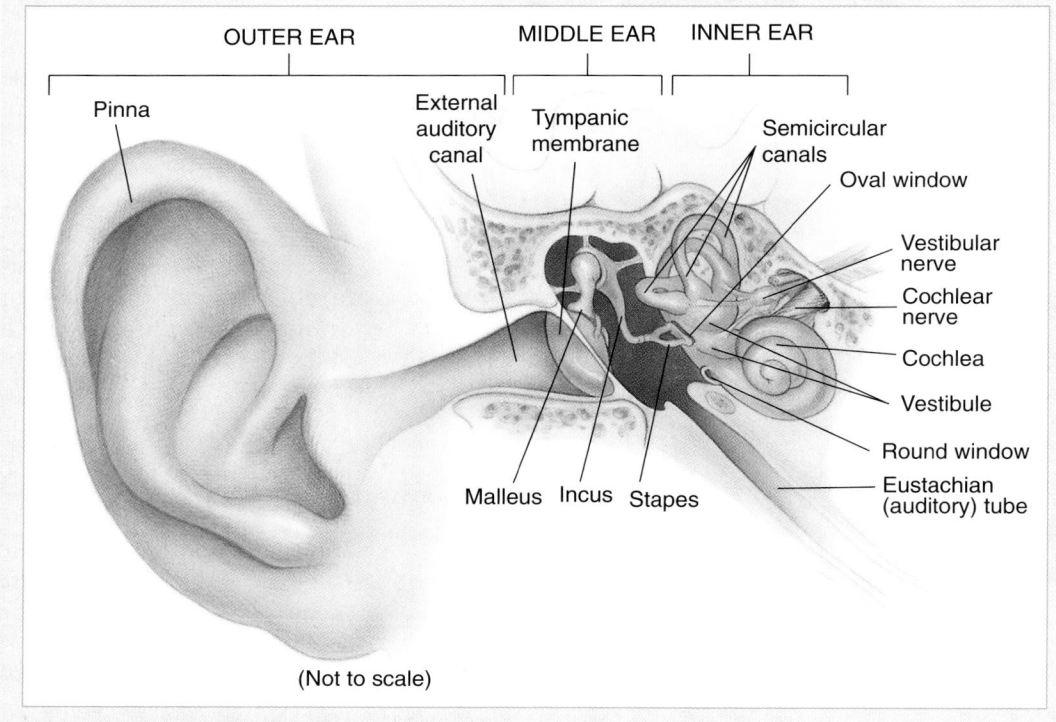

Figure 13-17 The structure of the outer, middle, and inner ear.

Skill Drill 13-5: Examining the Ear With an Otoscope

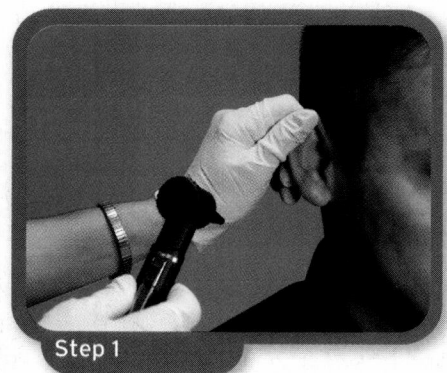

Step 1

Place your hand firmly against the patient's head and gently grasp the patient's auricle.

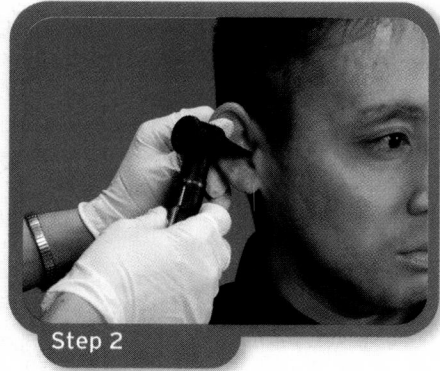

Step 2

Turn on the otoscope and insert the speculum into the ear.

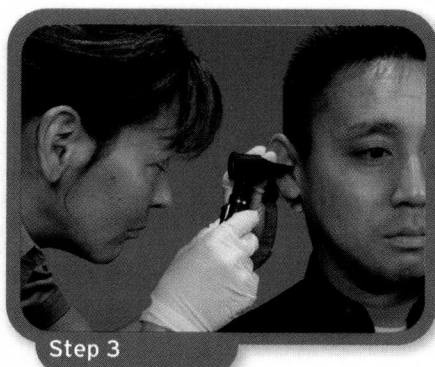

Step 3

Inspect the canal for any lesions or discharge.

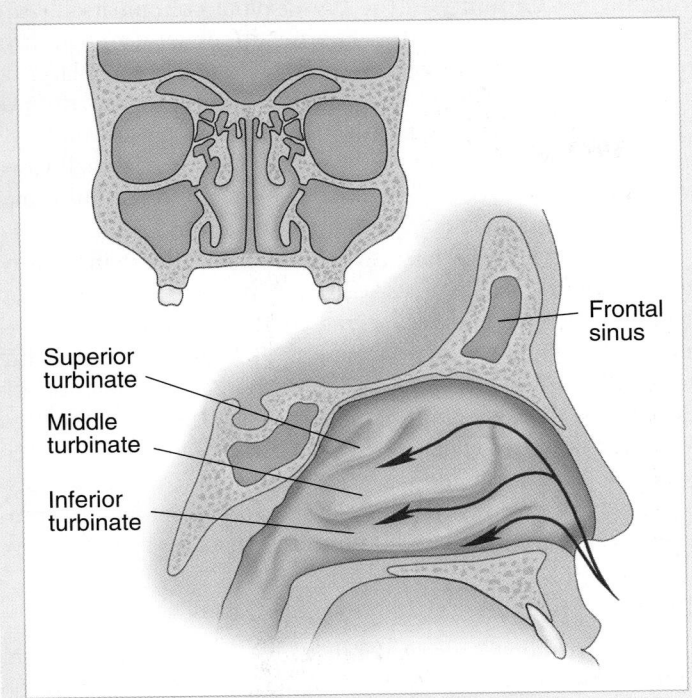

Figure 13-18 The nose has two chambers, divided by the septum. Each chamber is composed of layers of bone called turbinates. Above the nose are the frontal sinuses. On either side of the nose are the orbits of the eyes.

Labels: Frontal sinus; Superior turbinate; Middle turbinate; Inferior turbinate

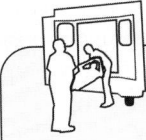

In the Field

Frank blood or clear, watery drainage (CSF) from the ears or nose following trauma suggests a basilar skull fracture.

mouth, the pharynx, and sometimes the neck. The throat is a conduit for both respiration and digestion, and it's in close proximity to numerous vital neurovascular structures.

As part of the assessment of overall hydration status, pay close attention to the lips, teeth, oral mucosa, and tongue. In patients who present with markedly altered mental status, you'll need to rapidly determine upper airway status; prompt assessment of the throat and upper airway structures is mandatory. Depending on the situation, assess for the presence of a foreign body or aspiration in either the throat or lower airway structures. Situations requiring removal of foreign bodies, secretions, or blood can manifest in many types of emergency cases. Always be prepared to assist with clearing the pharynx using manual techniques and suction.

The examination of the mouth begins with the lips, which should be pink and free of edema or surface irregularities. Confirm that the mouth is symmetrical. The gums should be pink, with no lesions or edema. Inspect the airway to ensure that it's free of obstructions. Visualize the tongue, noting its color, size, and moisture. The tongue should be located at midline, without swelling, and moist. Examine the oropharynx, identifying any discoloration or pustules that might indicate an infection. Note

any unusual odors on the breath, as they can indicate certain illnesses. Inspect the uvula for edema and redness.

The neck is an extraordinarily muscular region, through which many vital structures pass. External anatomy includes the jaw, cricothyroid membrane, external jugular veins, thyroid cartilage, suprasternal notch, and cervical spinous processes. When assessing the neck, take the time to look for any abnormalities, including those related to symmetry, masses, and venous distention. When noting venous distention, consider the patient's body position relative to lying flat (0°). Describe how far up the neck the distention tracks (from the base of the neck to the angle of the jaw), using either an approximate or centimeter scale. Palpate the carotid pulses and note relative strength of impulse. Look for any pulsating or expanding mass near the carotid pulse point. Palpate the suprasternal notch in an effort to identify any tracheal deviation. Have the patient open and close the jaws while you palpate over the temporomandibular joint during your examination of the jaw. To examine the neck, follow the steps in **Skill Drill 13-6 ▶**:

1. If trauma is suspected, take precautions to protect the cervical spine (Step 1).
2. Assess for the usage of accessory muscles during respiration.
3. Palpate the neck to find any structural abnormalities or subcutaneous air, and to ensure the trachea is midline. Begin at the suprasternal notch and work your way toward the head (Step 2). Be careful about applying pressure to the area of the carotid arteries, as it may stimulate a vagal response.
4. Assess the lymph nodes and note any swelling, which may indicate infection (Step 3).
5. Assess the jugular veins for distention; it may indicate a problem with blood returning to the heart (Step 4).

Cervical Spine

The cervical spine is the pathway by which the spinal cord makes its way out of the brain and into the torso, enabling the spinal nerves to emanate to and innervate the rest of the body **Figure 13-19 ▶**. It is also the point at which the head connects to the body. The spine is supported by a large mass of muscle, as well as multiple tendinous and ligamentous supports. Cervical injury can present in a variety of ways, and the assessment for such injury must be conducted in a careful manner.

Evaluate the patient first for the MOI and then for the presence of pain. Does the patient have an altered mental status, or did a loss of consciousness occur at the time of the event? Is there a significant MOI, or do multiple or serious distracting injuries make assessment of the cervical spine difficult? Is the patient under the influence of any intoxicating substances? Being able to confidently answer all of those questions will allow you to decide which patients may (or may not) require further treatment of a potential cervical spine injury.

When examining the cervical spine, inspect and palpate it, looking for evidence of tenderness and deformity. Midline posterior tenderness involving the bony spinous processes should always raise concerns. Palpable discomfort over the lateral aspects of the neck usually signals a muscular or ligamentous

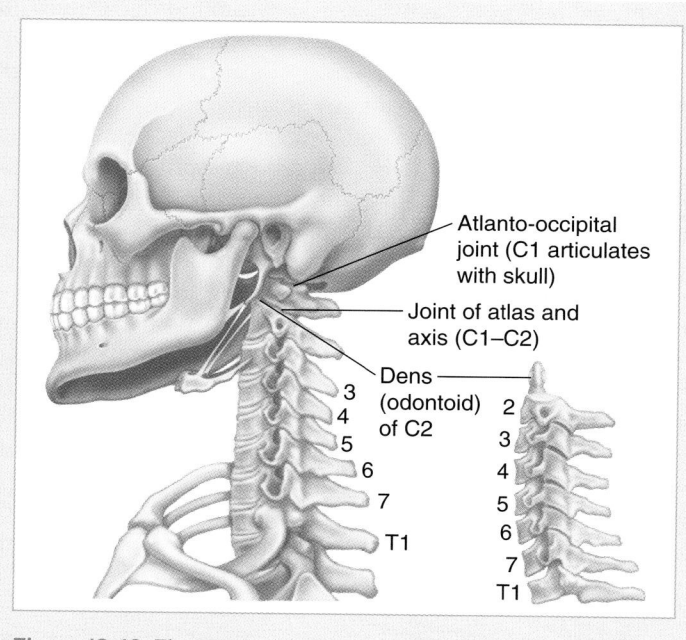

Atlanto-occipital
joint (C1 articulates
with skull)

Joint of atlas and
axis (C1–C2)

Dens
(odontoid)
of C2

3
4
5
6
7
T1

2
3
4
5
6
7
T1

Figure 13-19 The cervical vertebrae.

problem, not an injury to the bony spinal column itself. Any manipulations that result in pain, tenderness, or tingling should prompt you to stop the exam *immediately* and place the patient into a properly sized collar. With any complaints of neck pain in patients who have suffered a significant MOI, immediate stabilization of the head and neck is essential. Continued assessment of a patient's range of motion should take place only when there is no potential for serious injury.

When ranging the neck to assess for an underlying injury, first perform the activity in a passive manner, in which you are in control of the head and neck. Next, conduct the exam actively—that is, with the patient performing the directed maneuvers but being cautioned to stop if he or she experiences any pain or tingling. When checking range of motion, first slowly rotate the head from shoulder to shoulder. Then extend the head back, followed by flexing of the head and neck, touching chin to chest. Any discomfort elicited by these maneuvers should prompt you to terminate the exam immediately and protect the patient's spine.

Chest

The chest (or thorax) consists of the superior aspect of the torso, from the base of the neck to the diaphragm as delineated by the costal arch Figure 13-20 ▶. The chest wall is divided into anterior and posterior portions—literally, the patient's front and back. The back of the chest extends down the patient's back, to the level of the diaphragm posteriorly, which tends to move up and down with breathing. The chest contains many vital structures, including the lungs and mediastinal elements (heart, great vessels). The chest wall serves as a protective covering for the internal components. It consists of numerous musculoskeletal, vascular, nervous, connective, and lining structures.

Typically, the chest exam proceeds in three phases. The chest wall is checked, a pulmonary evaluation is conducted, and finally the cardiovascular assessment is performed. The chest must be inspected to assess for deformities in wall patency as well as to look for external clues of respiratory distress. Expose the chest and then begin its assessment, using the techniques of inspection, palpation, percussion, and auscultation. The examination of the posterior chest is the

Skill Drill 13-6: Examining the Neck

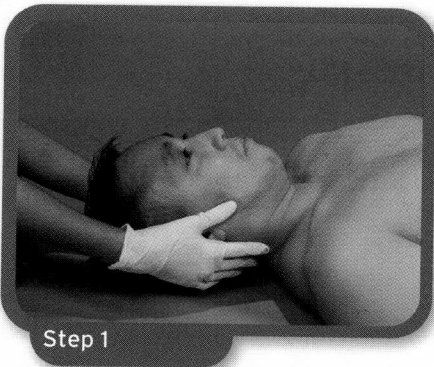

Step 1

If trauma is suspected, take precautions to protect the cervical spine.

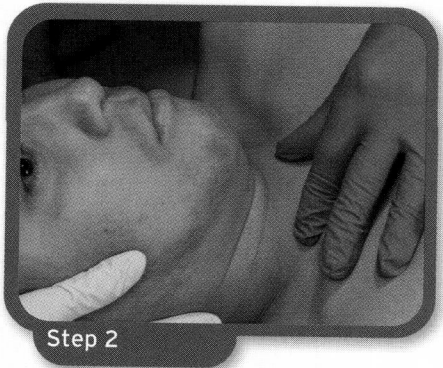

Step 2

Palpate the neck to find any structural abnormalities or subcutaneous air, and to ensure the trachea is midline. Begin at the suprasternal notch and work your way toward the head.

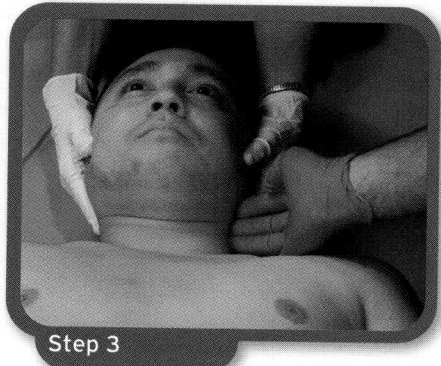

Step 3

Assess the lymph nodes.

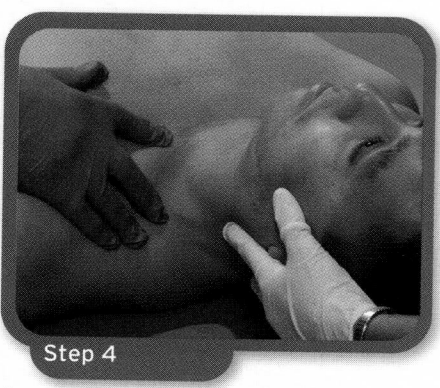

Step 4

Assess the jugular veins for distention.

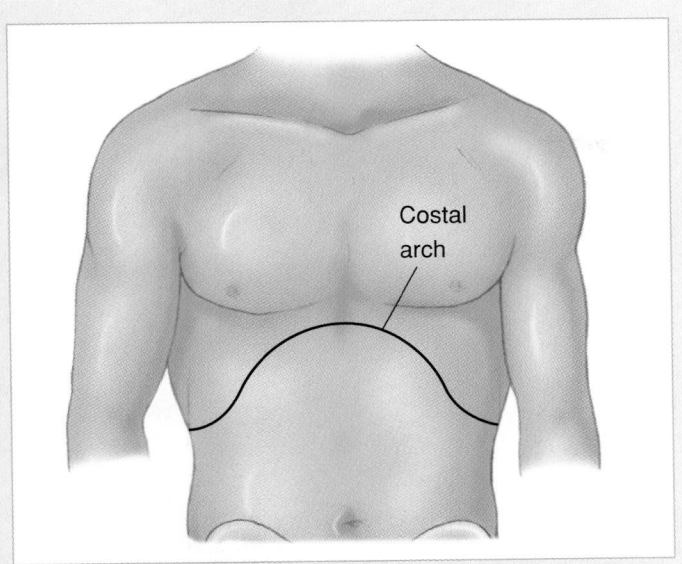

Figure 13-20 The chest (thorax) consists of the superior aspect of the torso, from the base of the neck to the diaphragm as delineated by the costal arch.

chest wall for respiratory effort, and document the respiratory rate, depth, and rhythm. Listen to the patient's breathing, and note the general shape of the chest wall. Pay close attention to any signs of abnormal breathing movements (paradox, accessory muscle use, impaired or diminished breathing movement) and retractions (suprasternal, sternal, intercostal, and subcostal). The presence of retractions is an important indicator of pulmonary issues, especially in children. Note any chest deformities, such as barrel chest (chronic obstructive pulmonary disease [COPD]), flail segments/subcutaneous air (trauma), kyphoscoliosis of the spine (compression fractures, COPD), significant bruising, and any suspicious wounds.

When palpating the chest wall, note any tenderness or crepitance/crepitus. Be sure to palpate areas that were initially noted to be abnormal on inspection. Palpation will also enable you to better appreciate respiratory symmetry and expansion. Although often impractical in the prehospital environment, percussion of the chest wall can allow for enhanced evaluation of the underlying chest cavity by distinguishing either dullness or hyperresonance versus normal resonance.

Auscultate the breath sounds Figure 13-21 ▶ . The lungs consist of five discrete lobes: The right side contains the right upper, right middle, and right lower lobes; the left side contains the left upper and left lower lobes, as well as the lingual

same as the examination of the anterior chest. Follow the steps in Skill Drill 13-7 ▶ :

1. Ensure the patient's privacy as best you can.
2. Inspect the chest for any obvious DCAP-BTLS Step 1 .
3. If you find any open wounds, dress them appropriately.
4. Note the shape of the patient's chest—it can give you clues to many underlying medical conditions (eg, emphysema or bronchitis) Step 2 .
5. Look for any surgical scars that may be a result of pacer implantation or a midline scar (a "zipper") that indicates previous cardiac surgery. Palpation of the chest may also reveal air under the skin (ie, subcutaneous emphysema).
6. Auscultate the lung fields, noting any abnormal lung sounds Step 3 .
7. Use percussion to detect any abnormalities Step 4 .
8. Auscultate for heart tones.
9. Repeat the appropriate portions of the examination for the posterior aspect of the thorax.

Compare the two sides of the chest for symmetry. Observe the

Skill Drill 13-7: Examining the Chest

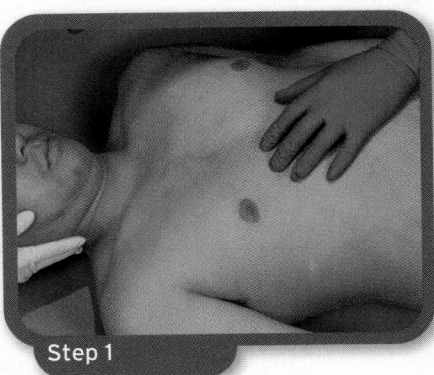

Step 1
Inspect the chest for any obvious DCAP-BTLS.

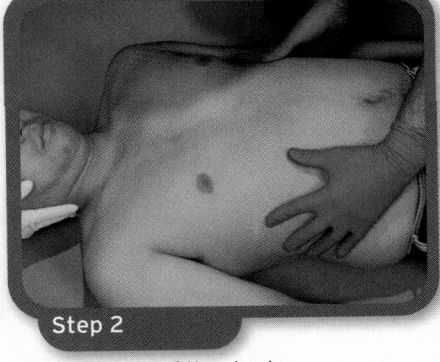

Step 2
Note the shape of the chest.

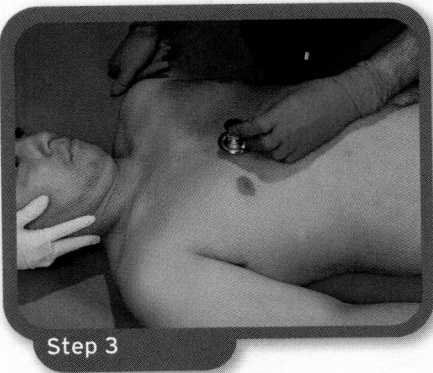

Step 3
Auscultate the lung fields, noting any abnormal lung sounds.

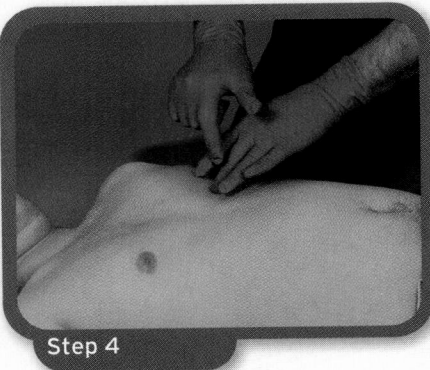

Step 4
Percuss the chest to detect any abnormalities.

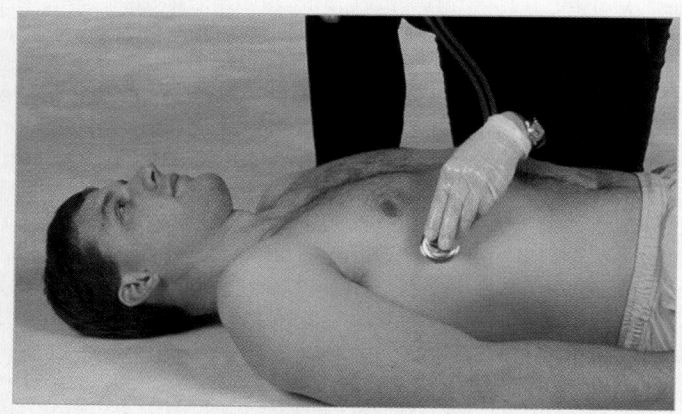

Figure 13-21 Auscultate the breath sounds on both sides of the chest.

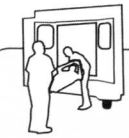
In the Field

Lungs are hyperinflated with chronic emphysema, resulting in hyperresonance where you would expect cardiac dullness.

Figure 13-22 ▸). During your examination, listen over each lobe, both anteriorly and posteriorly. Have the patient take as deep a breath as he or she can via an open mouth to facilitate your auscultatory assessment. Listen to as many portions of the lungs as possible, preferably avoiding any bony prominences, attached medical equipment, or clothing. Always use the best stethoscope available.

Normal lung sounds include bronchial, vesicular, and bronchovesicular sounds. They are a function of the particular pul-

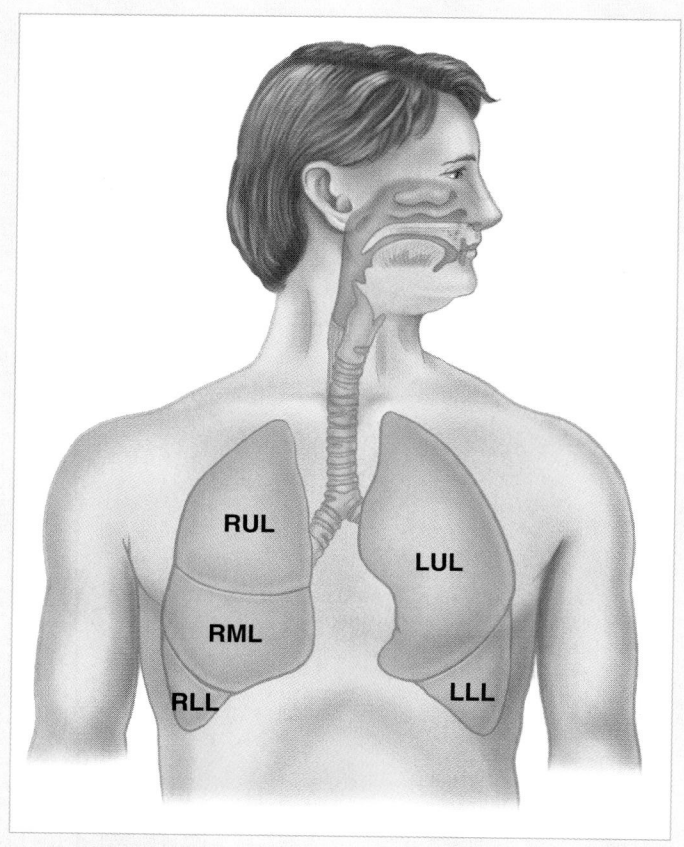

Figure 13-22 The five lobes of the lungs.

monary structure that air is passing through. Pathologic or adventitious (added) breath sounds include wheezes, rales (or crackles), and rhonchi (or low wheezes). They are indications of lung tissue consolidation, atelectasis, edema, mucus collection,

You are the Provider Part 3

You administer another nebulizer treatment with 2.5 mg of Ventolin/normal saline via face mask as you prepare him to be moved to the ambulance. Once you have your patient safely in the back you establish an IV of normal saline in his left antecubital vein with an 18-gauge needle. Upon reassessment of the patient following the breathing treatment, you find that he still has audible inspiratory and expiratory wheezes and increased work of breathing evidenced by intercostal and supraclavicular retractions. The patient states that he does not feel any relief and asks if there is anything else you can do. You administer a second breathing treatment with 2.5 mg of Ventolin/normal saline and contact medical control for additional orders.

Reassessment	Recording Time: 12 Minutes
Skin	Pale, warm, and dry with cyanotic nail beds and lips
Pulse	138 beats/min, regular, strong distal pulses
ECG	Sinus tachycardia
Blood pressure	164/82 mm Hg
Respirations	38 breaths/min, labored
Sa$_{O_2}$	78% on a nebulizer at 8 L/min
Pupils	Equal and reactive to light

5. Would an increased work of breathing be present upon reassessment of the patient if your treatment was effective?

6. How should your patient management progress?

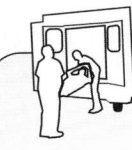

and hemorrhage. Stridor is an abnormal respiratory sound of
the upper airway that is often apparent on general examination,
but can also be auscultated in more subtle presentations. Rubs
can be heard emanating from either the lungs or the heart. A
rub is produced by a partial loss of intrapleural integrity, when
an abnormal collection of fluid has accumulated between a portion of the visceral and parietal pleura, resulting in "pleuritic"
pain and a perceived rub on auscultation.

One of the most important—and perhaps most often overlooked—aspects of pulmonary assessment is appreciating
when breath sounds are diminished or absent. You can't be
aware of this phenomenon without first developing an appreciation of the wide spectrum of normal presentations that exist.
Before going out into the field, you should spend many hours
listening to normal breath sounds, in order to develop an
understanding of what constitutes the many variations of normal breathing. After that, you'll spend time listening to patients
with respiratory difficulty, preferably alongside an experienced
individual who can point out the significant variations in the
presenting abnormalities.

Decreased breath sounds can be localized to a portion of
one lung, or they can encompass the entire chest. When
hypoventilation is suspected, you must take immediate action.
Decreased breath sounds typically signal a lack of respiratory
excursion or decreased tidal volume. Numerous problems can
cause decreased breath sounds, including pneumothorax,
hemothorax, pleural effusion, pulmonary edema,
atelectasis/consolidation, exacerbated COPD, status asthmaticus, opiate intoxication, pneumonia, bronchitis, and altered
mental status.

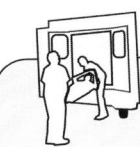
In the Field

Normal breathing should be quiet and not
grossly evident to you. If you can see or hear the
patient breathe, there's a problem.

Cardiovascular System

The cardiovascular system circulates blood throughout the
body, an activity that maintains perfusion of the body's tissues
Figure 13-23 ▶. The cardiovascular system comprises a
pump (the heart), a set of pipes (the blood vessels), and a liquid transported within those pipes (blood).

Blood consists of plasma, red blood cells, white blood
cells, and platelets. Plasma is essentially a mild saline solution,
but it also contains blood-clotting factors and particles that
play important roles in the body's immune response.

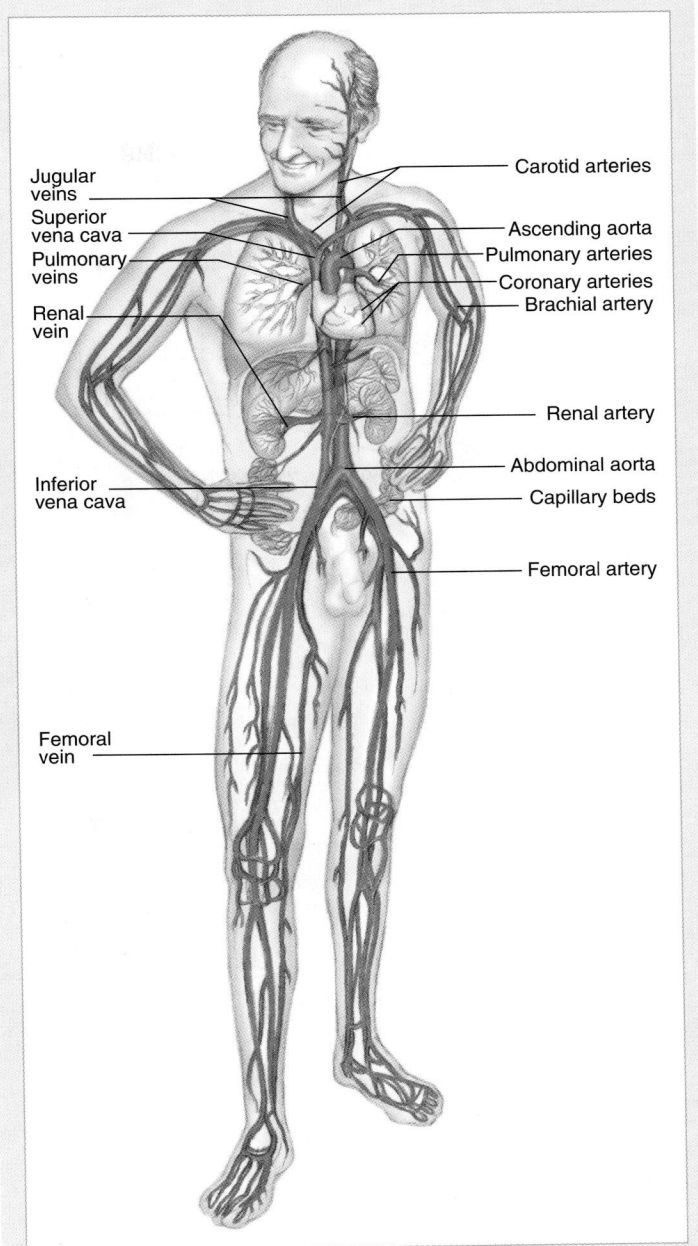
Figure 13-23 The cardiovascular system.

The complex arrangement of connected tubes in the circulatory system includes the arteries, arterioles, capillaries,
venules, and veins. This system is entirely closed, with capillaries connecting the arterioles and the venules.

Blood flows through two circuits in this system: the systemic circulation in the body and the pulmonary circulation in
the lungs. The systemic circulation carries oxygen-rich blood
from the left ventricle through the body and back to the right
atrium. As this blood passes through the tissues and organs, it
gives up oxygen and nutrients and absorbs cellular wastes and
carbon dioxide. The cellular wastes are, in turn, eliminated
as the blood flows through the liver and the kidneys. The

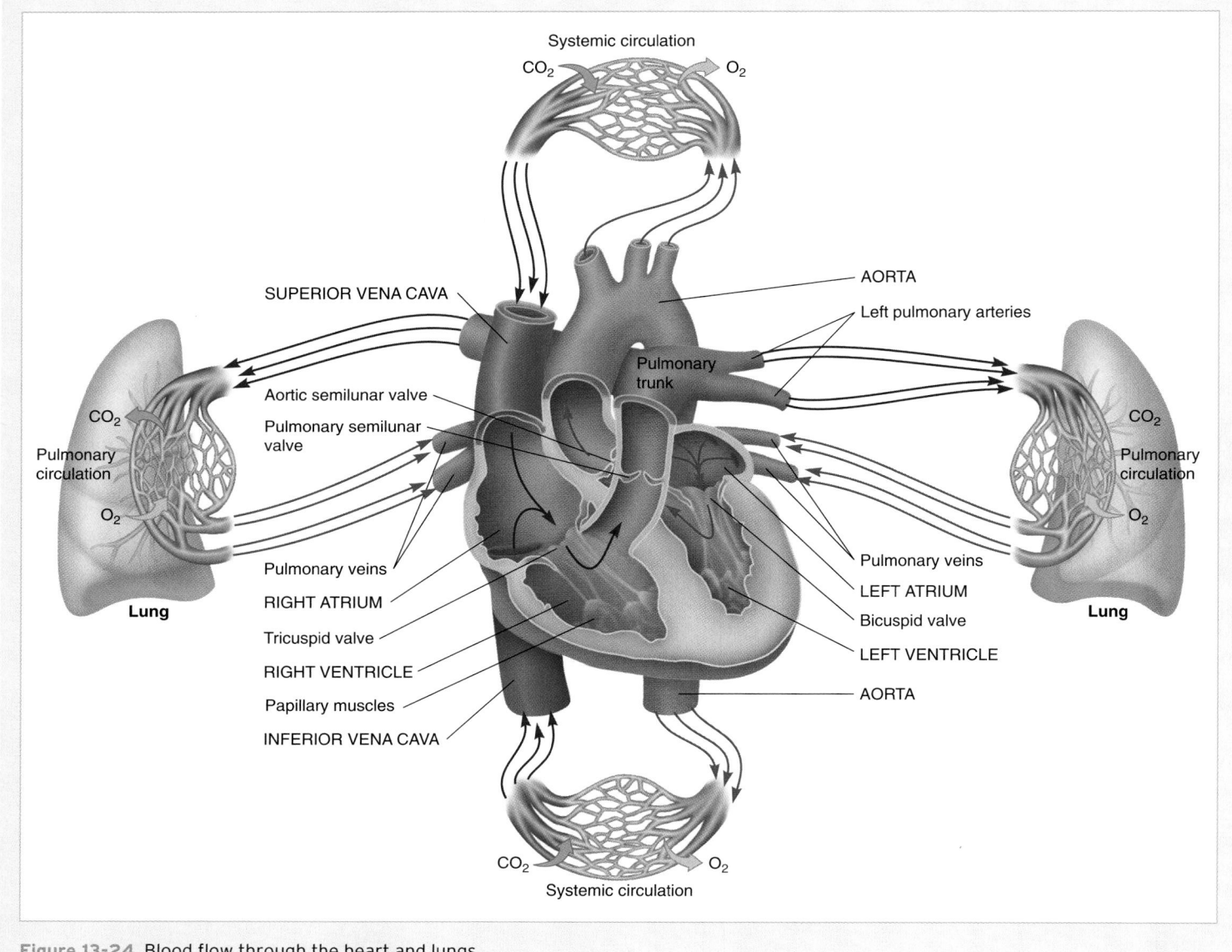

Figure 13-24 Blood flow through the heart and lungs.

pulmonary circulation carries oxygen-poor blood from the right ventricle through the lungs and back into the left atrium.

The cardiac cycle involves the events of cardiac relaxation (diastole), filling, and contraction (systole). These mechanical events are coordinated electrically with the heart's pacing and conduction system. The heart consists of four chambers: two atria (upper chambers) and two ventricles (lower chambers). Each side of the heart contains one atrium and one ventricle. The interatrial septum (membrane) separates the two atria; a thicker wall, the interventricular septum, separates the right and left ventricles. Each atrium receives blood that is returned to the heart from other parts of the body; each ventricle pumps blood out of the heart. The upper and lower portions of the heart are separated by the atrioventricular valves, which prevent backward flow of blood. The semilunar valves, which are

located between the ventricles and the arteries into which they pump blood, serve a similar function **Figure 13-24** ▲.

Blood enters the right atrium via the superior and inferior vena cavae and the coronary sinus, which consists of veins that collect blood returning from the walls of the heart. Blood from four pulmonary veins enters the left atrium. Between the right and left atria is the fossa ovalis, a depression that represents the former location of the foramen ovale, an opening between the two atria that is present in the fetus.

The cardiac cycle coordinates the movement of blood between the chambers of the heart. The atria always relax and contract together, as do the ventricles. While the atria are contracting (and filling the ventricles), the ventricles are relaxing. Conversely, when the ventricles are contracting, the atria are relaxing, being filled by either the vena cava or the pulmonary veins.

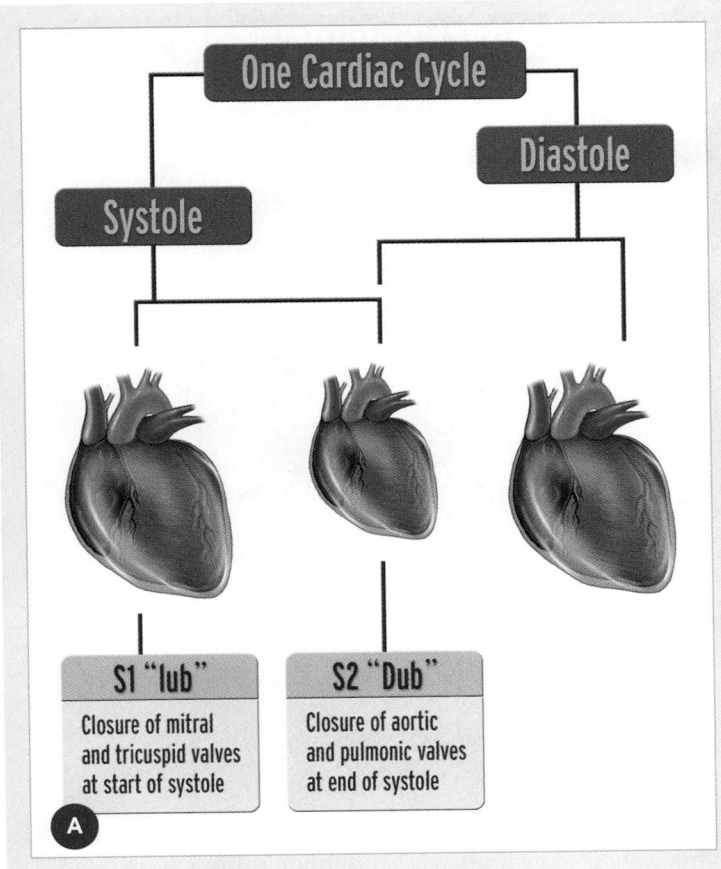

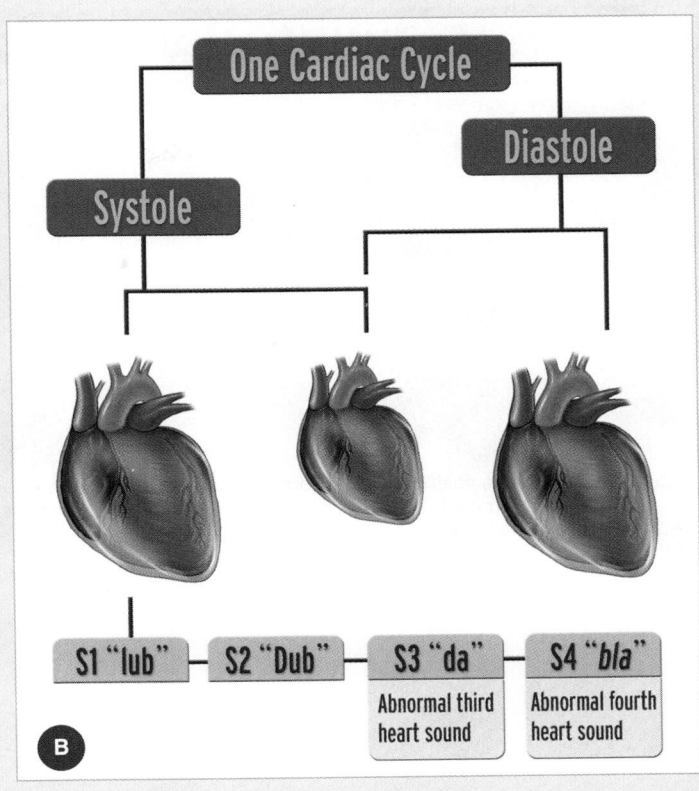

Figure 13-25 Heart sounds. **A.** The normal S_1 and S_2 heart sounds. **B.** The abnormal S_3 and S_4 heart sounds.

The contraction and relaxation of the heart, combined with the flow of blood, generates characteristic heart sounds during auscultation with a stethoscope. The normal pattern sounds much like this: "lub-DUB lub-DUB, lub-DUB . . ." The "lub" is referred to as the first heart sound or S_1, and the "DUB" (emphasized because it is often louder) as the second heart sound or S_2. Pathologic heart sounds include S_3 and S_4 Figure 13-25 ▲ . The S_3 or third heart sound is a soft, low-pitched heart sound that occurs about one third of the way through diastole. Although S_3 is sometimes present in healthy young people, it most commonly is associated with abnormally increased filling pressures in the atria secondary to moderate to severe heart failure. S_4, which is considered a "gallop" rhythm, is a moderately pitched sound that occurs immediately before the normal S_1 sound; it's always abnormal. The S_4 sound represents either decreased stretching (compliance) of the left ventricle or increased pressure in the atria.

Heart sounds can be appreciated by listening to the chest wall in the parasternal areas superiorly and inferiorly as well as in the region superior to the left nipple. Follow the steps in Skill Drill 13-8 ▶ :

1. Place the patient in one of these positions, to bring the heart closer to the left anterior chest wall:
   - Sitting up and leaning slightly forward Step 1
   - Supine
   - Left lateral recumbent position
2. Place your stethoscope at the fifth intercostal space over the apex of the heart Step 2 .
3. To appreciate the S_1 sound, ask the patient to breathe normally and hold the breath on expiration.
4. To appreciate the S_2 sound, ask the patient to breathe normally and hold the breath on inhalation Step 3 .
5. Auscultate the area above the left nipple to listen for S_3 and S_4 heart sounds.

Korotkoff sounds are detected while listening to a patient's blood pressure. A bruit is an abnormal "whoosh"-like sound that indicates turbulent blood flow moving through a narrowed artery (most significant in the carotid arteries). A murmur is an abnormal whoosh-like sound heard over the heart that indicates turbulent blood flow around a cardiac valve. Murmurs are graded as a range of intensity from 1 (softest) to 6 (loudest). Many people have normal, physiologic murmurs. In some patients, they can represent a degree of pathology, depending on the nature of the underlying problem and the specific anatomy

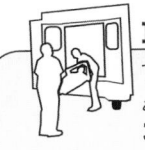

In the Field

The S_3 sound is associated with heart failure and is always abnormal in patients over 35 years of age.

Skill Drill 13-8: Auscultation of Heart Sounds

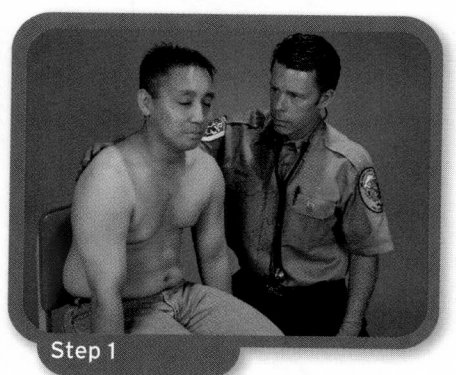

Step 1

Place the patient in a position that will bring the heart closer to the left anterior chest wall, such as sitting up and leaning slightly forward.

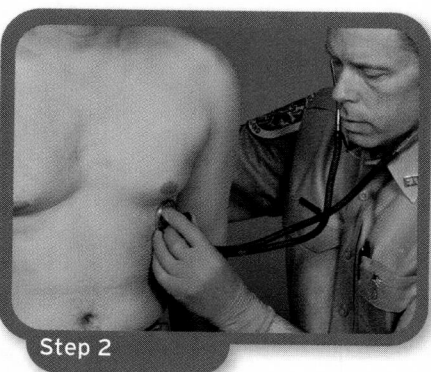

Step 2

Place your stethoscope at the fifth intercostal space over the apex of the heart.

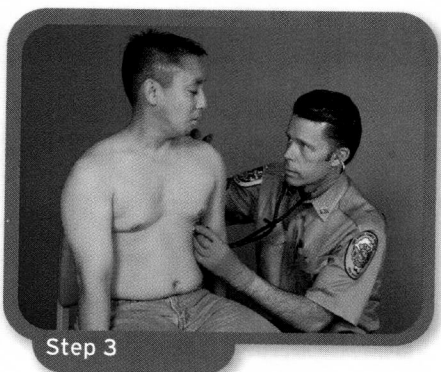

Step 3

Ask the patient to breathe normally and hold the breath on inhalation.

of the valve involved. To fully appreciate the nature and quality of normal heart sounds and murmurs, you must thoroughly practice your listening skills using excellent equipment.

Arterial pulses are a physical expression of systolic blood pressure. They are caused when contraction of the left ventricle and ejection of blood into the systemic circulation generate a pressure wave, which then travels throughout the arterial system. Arterial pulses are palpable wherever an artery crosses a bony prominence.

Venous pressure tends to be very low. In fact, in the normal setting, the pressure in the vena cava just before blood is received into the right atrium is close to zero. Veins are relatively nonmuscular, thin-walled vessels that have no effect on systemic vascular resistance and do not assist in promoting systemic blood pressure. Blood flows through the venous system and returns to the heart in part because it is propelled from behind in a continuous fashion, draining the capillary network. Most venous return of blood is a function of the respiratory cycle, generated by negative intrathoracic pressure that is developed at inspiration during normal breathing.

Occasionally, you can estimate the capacity of the venous system by observing a patient's jugular venous pressure, also known as jugular venous distention (JVD). In right-sided heart failure, blood tends not to be readily accepted into the right atrium. Venous capacitance increases in an effort to compensate for this failure, which in turn results in elevated pressures and corresponding JVD. JVD can be most readily observed by evaluating the anterolateral aspects of the neck; it can also be provoked in a normal person by having the person lie supine

and elevate the legs. While examining a patient for JVD, it is important to note how much distention is present, measured in terms of centimeters of distention from the origin of the jugular vein at the base of the neck. Note the angle of the patient relative to 0° (flat) while making the observation.

In situations involving hypotension, there may be no evidence of JVD, even while the patient is supine. Hypotensive patients with JVD must be carefully assessed as to the nature of their condition, however. Depending on the clinical situation, patients with JVD may be experiencing cardiogenic shock or have a ruptured cardiac valve. In the setting of chest trauma, neck vein distention and hypotension may symbolize a tension pneumothorax or pericardial tamponade.

The ability of the circulatory system to constrict and dilate can diminish markedly as a person ages. Although this limitation may vary considerably from patient to patient, an older patient's ability to compensate for cardiovascular insults may be profoundly curtailed by age-related changes, especially arterial atherosclerosis and diabetes. In addition, many medications that older persons routinely use to manage problems such as high blood pressure can negatively affect the body's ability to handle sudden changes in the demand for blood supply. By contrast, children and young adults have an enhanced ability to vasoconstrict and increase the pulse rate to compensate for a vascular insult; this compensation mechanism can fool paramedics into believing that young patients are "less sick" than they actually are.

When you are examining the cardiovascular system, pay attention to arterial pulses, noting their location, rate, rhythm,

5. Because of the large number of organs within the abdomen, the _____ serves as a central reference point.
   A. lower rib cage
   B. pelvic girdle
   C. xyphoid process
   D. umbilicus

6. The above patient is complaining of pain near her gallbladder. This would be located in the_____.
   A. RUQ
   B. LUQ
   C. RLQ
   D. LLQ

7. When a patient is contracting his or her abdominal muscles, this is called_____.
   A. rigidity
   B. guarding
   C. soft
   D. nontender

Challenging Question

8. Are there any special considerations you should take based on your patient's gender?

▬ Points to Ponder

You are dispatched to the home of a 65-year-old woman who is complaining of a feeling of general malaise that began about 4 days ago. When you arrive on scene, the patient appears to be in no distress. You introduce yourself and begin your physical exam. The patient denies having any chest pain, shortness of breath, nausea, or vomiting. Her vital signs are as follows: respiratory rate, 18 breaths/min; pulse oximetry reading, 99% on room air; blood pressure, 110/70 mm Hg; and pulse rate, 75 beats/min with a normal sinus rhythm on the monitor. The patient states that she "hasn't felt right" for a few days and she called now because she had no way to get to the doctor.

Where should you begin your examination?

Issues: Understanding the Importance of a Complete Physical Exam, Understanding the Need for a Caring Attitude When Performing a Physical Exam, Understanding the Importance of a Professional Appearance and Demeanor When Performing a Physical Exam.

14 Patient Assessment

Objectives

Cognitive

3-3.1   Recognize hazards/potential hazards. (p 14.7)

3-3.2   Describe common hazards found at the scene of a trauma and a medical patient. (p 14.7)

3-3.3   Determine hazards found at the scene of a medical or trauma patient. (p 14.7)

3-3.4   Differentiate safe from unsafe scenes. (p 14.7)

3-3.5   Describe methods to making an unsafe scene safe. (p 14.8)

3-3.6   Discuss common mechanisms of injury/nature of illness. (p 14.9)

3-3.7   Predict patterns of injury based on mechanism of injury. (p 14.9)

3-3.8   Discuss the reason for identifying the total number of patients at the scene. (p 14.9)

3-3.9   Organize the management of a scene following size-up. (p 14.8)

3-3.10   Explain the reasons for identifying the need for additional help or assistance. (p 14.9)

3-3.11   Summarize the reasons for forming a general impression of the patient. (p 14.11)

3-3.12   Discuss methods of assessing mental status. (p 14.11)

3-3.13   Categorize levels of consciousness in the adult, infant and child. (p 14.11)

3-3.14   Differentiate between assessing the altered mental status in the adult, child and infant patient. (p 14.11)

3-3.15   Discuss methods of assessing the airway in the adult, child and infant patient. (p 14.12)

3-3.16   State reasons for management of the cervical spine once the patient has been determined to be a trauma patient. (p 14.12)

3-3.17   Analyze a scene to determine if spinal precautions are required. (p 14.12)

3-3.18   Describe methods used for assessing if a patient is breathing. (p 14.13)

3-3.19   Differentiate between a patient with adequate and inadequate minute ventilation. (p 14.12)

3-3.20   Distinguish between methods of assessing breathing in the adult, child and infant patient. (p 14.12)

3-3.21   Compare the methods of providing airway care to the adult, child and infant patient. (p 14.12)

3-3.22   Describe the methods used to locate and assess a pulse. (p 14.13)

3-3.23   Differentiate between locating and assessing a pulse in an adult, child and infant patient. (p 14.13)

3-3.24   Discuss the need for assessing the patient for external bleeding. (p 14.14)

3-3.25   Describe normal and abnormal findings when assessing skin color. (p 14.13)

3-3.26   Describe normal and abnormal findings when assessing skin temperature. (p 14.13)

3-3.27   Describe normal and abnormal findings when assessing skin condition. (p 14.13)

3-3.28   Explain the reason for prioritizing a patient for care and transport. (p 14.14)

3-3.29   Identify patients who require expeditious transport. (p 14.14)

3-3.30   Describe the evaluation of patient's perfusion status based on findings in the initial assessment. (p 14.13)

3-3.31   Describe orthostatic vital signs and evaluate their usefulness in assessing a patient in shock. (p 14.13)

3-3.32   Apply the techniques of physical examination to the medical patient. (p 14.16)

3-3.33   Differentiate between the assessment that is performed for a patient who is unresponsive or has an altered mental status and other medical patients requiring assessment. (p 14.18)

3-3.34   Discuss the reasons for reconsidering the mechanism of injury. (p 14.18)

3-3.35   State the reasons for performing a rapid trauma assessment. (p 14.21)

3-3.36   Recite examples and explain why patients should receive a rapid trauma assessment. (p 14.21)

3-3.37   Apply the techniques of physical examination to the trauma patient. (p 14.21)

3-3.38   Describe the areas included in the rapid trauma assessment and discuss what should be evaluated. (p 14.28)

3-3.39   Differentiate cases when the rapid assessment may be altered in order to provide patient care. (p 14.21)

3-3.40   Discuss the reason for performing a focused history and physical exam. (p 14.27)

3-3.41   Describe when and why a detailed physical examination is necessary. (p 14.27)

3-3.42   Discuss the components of the detailed physical exam in relation to the techniques of examination. (p 14.27)

3-3.43   State the areas of the body that are evaluated during the detailed physical exam. (p 14.27)

3-3.44   Explain what additional care should be provided while performing the detailed physical exam. (p 14.27)

3-3.45   Distinguish between the detailed physical exam that is performed on a trauma patient and that of the medical patient. (p 14.27)

3-3.46   Differentiate patients requiring a detailed physical exam from those who do not. (p 14.25)

3-3.47   Discuss the reasons for repeating the initial assessment as part of the on-going assessment. (p 14.31)

3-3.48   Describe the components of the on-going assessment. (p 14.31)

3-3.49   Describe trending of assessment components. (p 14.31)

3-3.50   Discuss medical identification devices/systems. (p 14.16)

Affective

3-3.51   Explain the rationale for crew members to evaluate scene safety prior to entering. (p 14.7)

3-3.52   Serve as a model for others explaining how patient situations affect your evaluation of mechanism of injury or illness. (p 14.9)

3-3.53   Explain the importance of forming a general impression of the patient. (p 14.14)

3-3.54   Explain the value of performing an initial assessment. (p 14.11)

3-3.55 Demonstrate a caring attitude when performing an initial assessment. (p 14.18)

3-3.56 Attend to the feelings that patients with medical conditions might be experiencing. (p 14.16)

3-3.57 Value the need for maintaining a professional caring attitude when performing a focused history and physical examination. (p 14.27)

3-3.58 Explain the rationale for the feelings that these patients might be experiencing. (p 14.27)

3-3.59 Demonstrate a caring attitude when performing a detailed physical examination. (p 14.27)

3-3.60 Explain the value of performing an on-going assessment. (p 14.31)

3-3.61 Recognize and respect the feelings that patients might experience during assessment. (p 14.11)

3-3.62 Explain the value of trending assessment components to other health professionals who assume care of the patient. (p 14.31)

Psychomotor

3-3.63 Observe various scenarios and identify potential hazards. (p 14.7)

3-3.64 Demonstrate the scene size-up. (p 14.7)

3-3.65 Demonstrate the techniques for assessing mental status. (p 14.11)

3-3.66 Demonstrate the techniques for assessing the airway. (p 14.12)

3-3.67 Demonstrate the techniques for assessing if the patient is breathing. (p 14.12)

3-3.68 Demonstrate the techniques for assessing if the patient has a pulse. (p 14.13)

3-3.69 Demonstrate the techniques for assessing the patient for external bleeding. (p 14.21, 14.22)

3-3.70 Demonstrate the techniques for assessing the patient's skin color, temperature, and condition. (p 14.13)

3-3.71 Demonstrate the ability to prioritize patients. (p 14.14)

3-3.72 Using the techniques of examination, demonstrate the assessment of a medical patient. (p 14.11)

3-3.73 Demonstrate the patient care skills that should be used to assist with a patient who is responsive with no known history. (p 14.16)

3-3.74 Demonstrate the patient care skills that should be used to assist with a patient who is unresponsive or has an altered mental status. (p 14.18)

3-3.75 Perform a rapid medical assessment. (p 14.21)

3-3.76 Perform a focused history and physical exam of the medical patient. (p 14.16)

3-3.77 Using the techniques of physical examination, demonstrate the assessment of a trauma patient. (p 14.21)

3-3.78 Demonstrate the rapid trauma assessment used to assess a patient based on mechanism of injury. (p 14.18)

3-3.79 Perform a focused history and physical exam on a non-critically injured patient. (p 14.25)

3-3.80 Perform a focused history and physical exam on a patient with life-threatening injuries. (p 14.18)

3-3.81 Perform a detailed physical examination. (p 14.27)

3-3.82 Demonstrate the skills involved in performing the on-going assessment. (p 14.31)

Patient Assessment

Scene Size-up

Body Substance Isolation
Scene Safety
Consider Mechanism of Injury/Nature of Illness
Determine the Number of Patients
Consider Additional Resources
Consider C-Spine Immobilization

Initial Assessment

Approach and Form a General Impression
Assess Mental Status
Assess the Airway
Assess Breathing
Assess Circulation
Identify Priority Patients and Make Transport
  Decisions

Trauma Patients   Medical Patients

Focused History and Physical Exam

Reconsider Mechanism of Injury

Significant Mechanism of Injury	No Significant Mechanism of Injury
Rapid Trauma Assessment	Focused Trauma Assessment Based on Chief Complaint
Baseline Vital Signs	Baseline Vital Signs
SAMPLE History	SAMPLE History
Reevaluate Transport Decision	Reevaluate Transport Decision

Focused History and Physical Exam

Evaluate Responsiveness

Responsive	Unresponsive
History of Illness	Rapid Medical Assessment
SAMPLE History	Baseline Vital Signs
Focused Medical Assessment Based on Chief Complaint	SAMPLE History
Baseline Vital Signs	Reevaluate Transport Decision
Reevaluate Transport Decision	

Detailed Physical Exam

Perform the Detailed Physical Exam
Reassess Vital Signs

Ongoing Assessment

Repeat the Initial Assessment
Reassess and Record Vital Signs
Repeat the Focused Assessment
Check Interventions

Introduction

Patient assessment is the platform on which quality prehospital care is built and the single most important skill you bring to bear on patient care. Patient assessment is a complex skill made up of two primary components: information gathering and physical examination. In the first component, called history-taking, you try to determine the nature of the patient's problems by asking questions, listening to and analyzing answers, and observing the way the patient presents and the setting in which he or she is found. In the second component, called physical assessment, you perform a hands-on evaluation of the patient to further explore the chief complaint(s) and to detect injuries or signs of illness.

This chapter describes the skill of patient assessment, focusing primarily on the *what* aspects of patient assessment (that is, what needs to done as part of an organized, systematic assessment). Chapters 12 and 13 presented the *how* aspects of the patient assessment in more detail. Now you will learn how to pull everything together. Please note that pediatric assessment in covered in detail in Chapter 41: *Pediatrics*.

The information gleaned during the patient assessment process helps you make key patient care decisions. The first and most important question during the initial assessment is always "Does my patient have any life-threatening conditions?" If life threats are present, you must quickly decide how to address them. Patient findings obtained early in the assessment process often dictate whether the patient needs to be transported by ground or by air ambulance and to which facility. For these reasons, your patient assessment skills are the single most important tools in your EMS toolbox. While *some* of your patients may need spinal immobilization and *others* may need a breathing treatment, *all of your patients* need excellent patient assessment.

The fundamental components of your job are to identify problems (the chief complaint, or why someone called 9-1-1), set priorities (rank the problems from most to least serious), develop a care plan (address the problems), and execute the plan (provide care for the patient). As you gain field experience and run more calls, however, the breadth and depth of your knowledge base should increase and you should see a corresponding increase in your assessment skills. Patient assessment is a skill that you should hone *throughout your entire EMS career.*

The Elements of Patient Assessment

Several elements make up the skill of patient assessment, with each being used in some way to gather information. The primary source of information during your assessment is usually the patient, but you will also gather information from sources such as the patient's family or friends or eyewitnesses to the emergency event. That information is then added to information gathered from the emergency scene itself, along with the data you obtain from your diagnostic tools and tests (such as cardiac monitor, glucometer, pulse oximetry, and capnography).

Care in the prehospital setting is very similar to the process used in solving a "whodunit" murder mystery. In this case, however, you are the detective, and the mystery is finding out what is wrong with your patient and what you can do about it. To solve the mystery, you gather "clues" about your patient's problem, sift through the clues, and analyze the data. Missed clues resulting from a weak, disorganized, or incomplete patient assessment may keep you from solving the mystery, which in the real world of patient care equates with your patient getting less than optimal care.

You are the Provider Part 1

You are dispatched to a local high school football practice for a "player down." Upon arrival, you find a 17-year-old youth lying on the sidelines, unconscious. His teammates tell you that they were participating in a no-contact, warm-up drill when Mike suddenly collapsed. They also state that Mike had no complaints just before the event and seemed to be "just fine."

In your initial assessment, the patient responds only to deep, painful stimuli, and you find no obvious signs of trauma. The team's coach isn't sure if Mike has any medical conditions, and he can't provide any further information.

Initial Assessment	Recording Time: 0 Minutes
Appearance	Wearing full protective gear; supine
Level of consciousness	P (Responsive to painful stimuli)
Airway	Patent
Breathing	Slightly fast but adequate
Circulation	Strong, full radial pulse

1. What is the best method of airway assessment and management for a patient who is wearing a football helmet and shoulder pads?
2. Although other players deny the occurrence of any trauma, should you immobilize this patient?

Patient Assessment

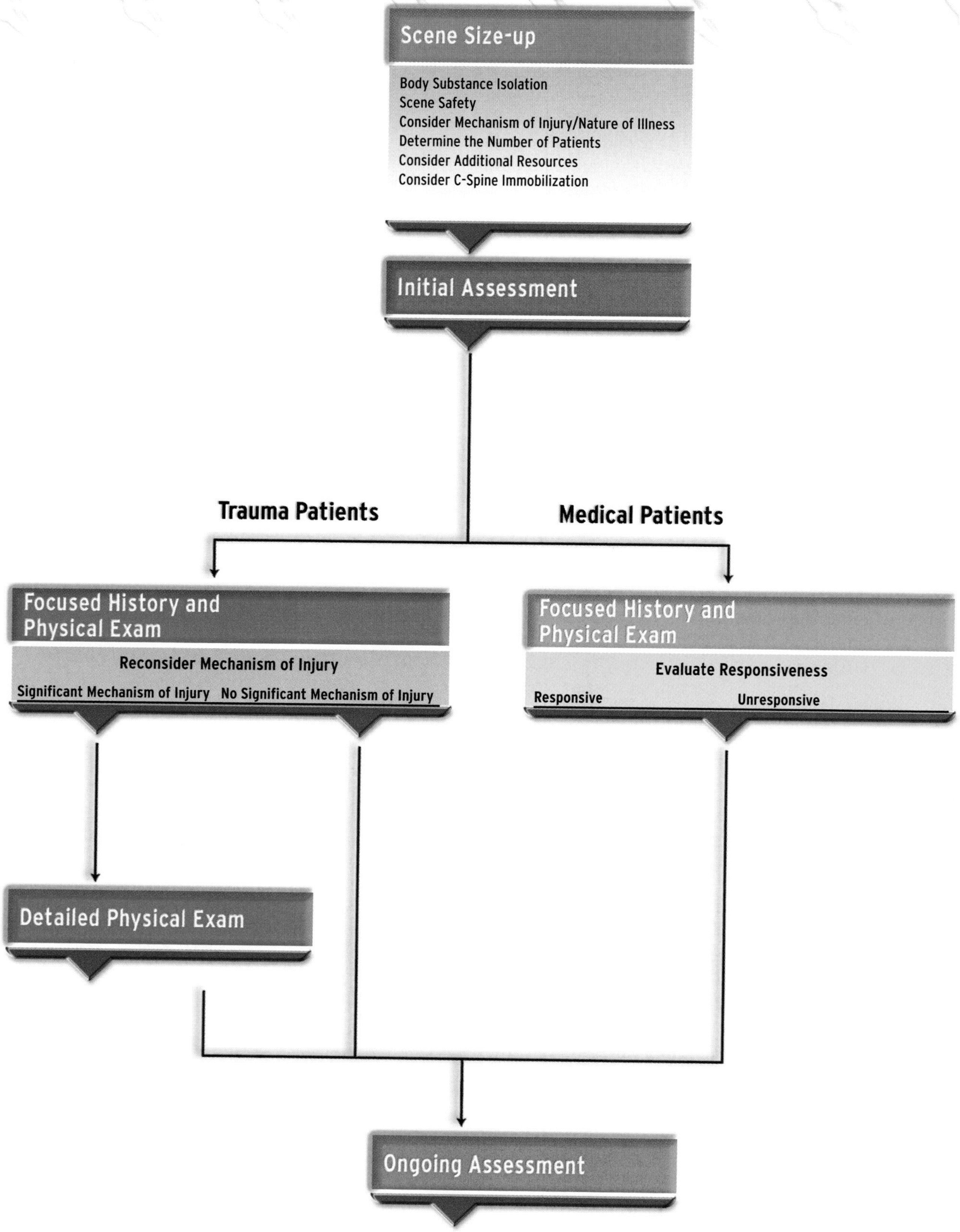

Scene Size-up

Scene Size-up

Body Substance Isolation
Scene Safety
Consider Mechanism of Injury/Nature of Illness
Determine the Number of Patients
Consider Additional Resources
Consider C-Spine Immobilization

Initial Assessment

Trauma Patients

Medical Patients

Focused History and Physical Exam

Reconsider Mechanism of Injury

Significant Mechanism of Injury   No Significant Mechanism of Injury

Focused History and Physical Exam

Evaluate Responsiveness

Responsive   Unresponsive

Detailed Physical Exam

Ongoing Assessment

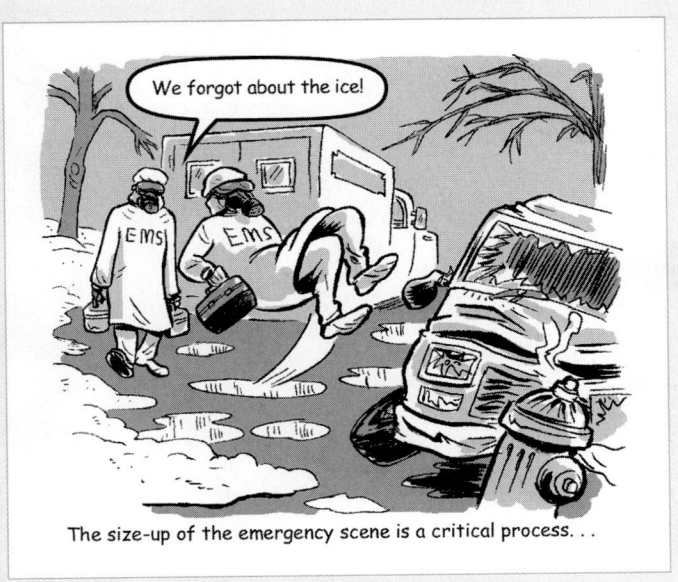

We forgot about the ice!

The size-up of the emergency scene is a critical process...

Figure 14-1

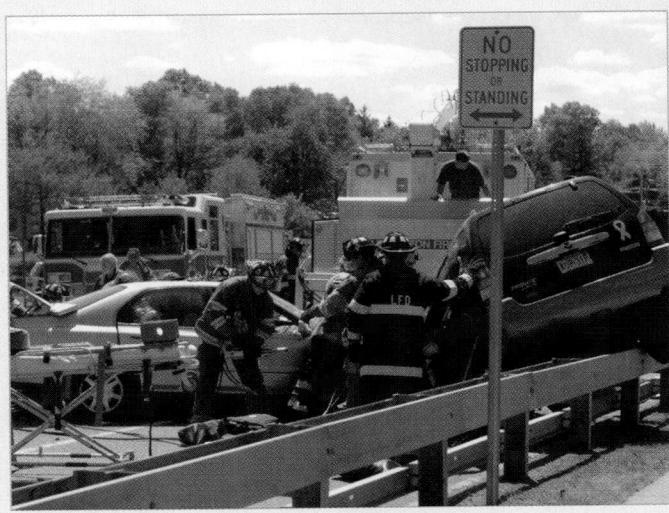

Figure 14-2 Crash scenes have many risks to you, your partners, and the patient.

Scene Size-up and Evaluation

Body Substance Isolation and Standard Precautions

The first step of the patient assessment process is the scene size-up. Your first and foremost concern on any call is ensuring your own safety and the safety of the other EMS team members Figure 14-1 ▲ . You are of no value to the patient if you get injured and can't provide care. Suppose you get an infectious disease because you neglected to follow standard precautions and body substance isolation (BSI) procedures; you may then miss time from work because you are sick. In the worst-case scenario, you might contract a career-ending or life-threatening disease, all because you chose to ignore a simple but important set of rules—the rules of BSI and the standard precautions.

You should wear properly sized gloves on every call. If blood or other fluids could potentially splash or spray, wear eye protection. When inhaled particles are a risk factor, wear a properly sized and fitted mask (HEPA or N95). In rare cases, a gown is also indicated. Always take the steps necessary to protect yourself on calls. When in doubt about the nature of the threat, it's always better to err on the side of caution and protect yourself too much rather than too little. Infection control is covered in depth in Chapters 2 and 36.

Scene Safety

In the assessment and evaluation of the emergency scene, the main focus is to ensure the safety and well-being of the EMS team and any other emergency responders. Ask yourself, "Is it safe for me and my team to enter this scene and to approach the patient?" To answer that question, you need to use a "wide-angle lens" thought process when you assess and evaluate the scene. Some of the issues you might encounter in particular scenes are described next.

Crash and rescue scenes often include multiple risks, such as unstable vehicles, moving traffic, jagged metal and broken glass, fire or explosion hazards, downed power lines, and, possibly, hazardous materials Figure 14-2 ▲ .

Toxic substances are found at many scenes. From the lawn and garden chemicals found in almost every home to the countless chemicals used in industry and manufacturing, you should always be alert for the presence of toxic substances. You should also be wary of working in toxic environments (that is, the atmosphere itself). Smoke is the by-product of incomplete combustion and can contain many toxins, pathogens, and carcinogens. In these cases, having proper body and respiratory protection is a must before entering the scene and initiating patient care Figure 14-3 ▶ .

Don't just think of crime scenes in the past tense because there is always the possibility that more violence may occur. Under ideal circumstances, when dispatched to a potential crime scene, law enforcement personnel should enter and secure the scene first. All too frequently, however, the EMS team arrives first

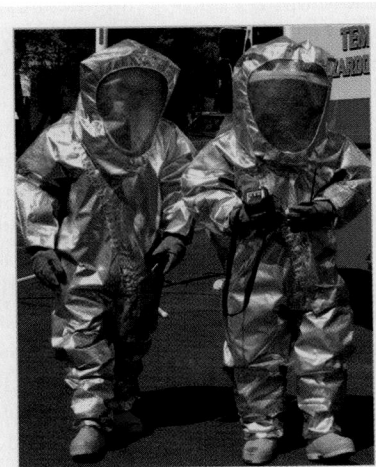

Figure 14-3 Scenes involving toxic substances may require specially trained rescuers with extra protective equipment.

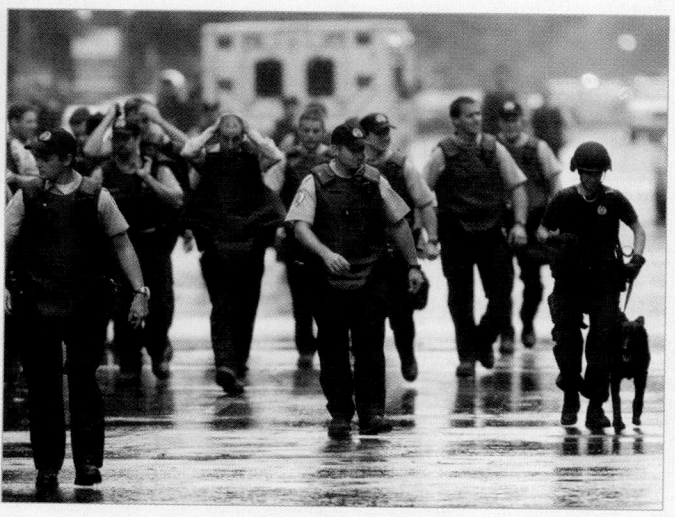

Figure 14-4 If the scene is unsafe, request law enforcement support, and wait in your vehicle at a safe distance.

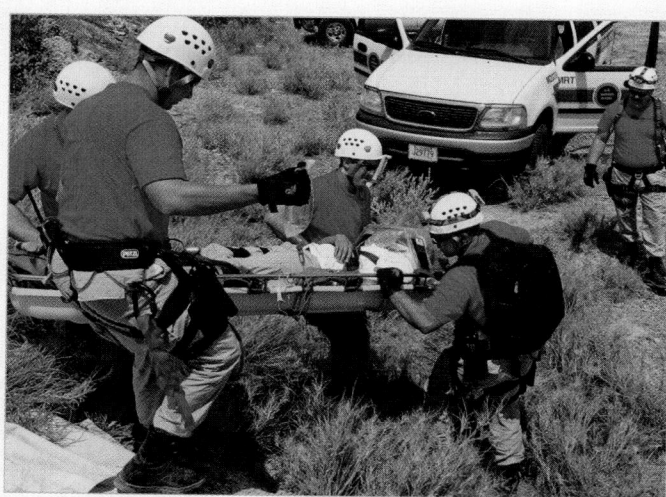

Figure 14-5 At times you may need a team to carry patients out of areas with unstable terrain.

and unknowingly enters a crime scene. For example, dispatch might receive a call for a "man down"; on arrival, the EMS team might discover that the patient has been stabbed three times in the chest. Law enforcement personnel should be requested immediately in such cases because it is nearly impossible for you and your partner to control the scene and care for the patient at the same time **Figure 14-4 ▲**—and because the perpetrator could return with more firepower.

When faced with a currently unstable scene or a scene that begins deteriorating (for example, people become progressively louder or more unruly or make aggressive gestures or threats), consider retreating to the rig until the scene is secured and deemed safe. If you believe that you can pull it off safely, remove the patient from the scene with you, but making such an attempt is clearly a judgment call on your part.

Unstable surfaces are everyday occurrences in the field. In some parts of the United States, snow- or ice-covered surfaces can persist for 3 or 4 months out of the year. In the Northwest, it typically rains from November to May. Most of the United States has terrain issues ranging from minor hills to mountains to sandy beaches. Thus, working on unstable surfaces is an inevitable part of prehospital medicine **Figure 14-5 ▶**. Take the time to make all of your patient lifts and moves as safe and controlled as possible. Just making a mental commitment to focus on this aspect of your practice will go a long way toward helping prevent a fall and a possible injury. Also, consider investing in a good pair of boots that will serve to keep your feet comfortable and to provide good traction, which helps to avoid surprise slips.

Behavioral emergencies are common and challenging calls, and they always present with the possibility of some sort of violent outbreak occurring. With the continued increase in the

manufacture and abuse of methamphetamine, EMS workers are seeing a growing number of patients who are on the tail end of multiple sleepless days fueled by methamphetamine. The people are often paranoid, emotionally unstable, and almost always armed, making them far more a threat than an average patient with a non–drug-induced behavioral emergency. In addition, methamphetamine and crack users are at high risk of experiencing excited or agitated delirium, such that they may present in a blind rage and are almost uncontrollable. In one case, the patient was shot with a TASER device by law enforcement personnel *14 times in fewer than 5 minutes*; despite this barrage, it still took six people to secure the patient in handcuffs and place him on the stretcher. There is a clear message here: Never hesitate to call for law enforcement assistance when managing any patient who has the potential for becoming violent.

While protecting the emergency response team is clearly a priority, so is protecting the patient and bystanders. Establishing a perimeter around an emergency scene may prevent bystanders from entering a dangerous scene and potentially becoming patients themselves. Environmental issues can also influence scene safety and the patient care process. The longer a patient is exposed to wind and rain, the more likely hypothermia will become a factor. Of course, leaving a patient lying on a hot asphalt highway as the midday sun beats down is not good medicine either. When the environment is unfriendly, perform the initial assessment, address life threats, and get the patient into the controlled environment of the ambulance as quickly as possible.

Mechanism of Injury/Nature of Illness

Most calls to 9-1-1 will be for a medical emergency or some form of trauma. A generic-sounding call such as a "sick man" in no way guarantees that a sick, hypoglycemic patient didn't also fall and injure himself as a result of a low blood glucose level. Or, a trauma patient may have crashed her car when she passed out because of an abnormal heart rhythm. Prudent paramedics keep their minds open to multiple possibilities when trying to figure out just what's going on with patients. The mechanism of injury (MOI) is the way in which traumatic injuries occur—the forces that act on the body to cause damage. Assessing and evaluating the MOI can help you predict the likelihood of certain injuries having occurred and estimate their severity. (The patterns of injuries sustained in traumatic events are discussed in detail in Chapter 17.)

On purely medical calls, you should quickly determine from the patient (or family, friends, or bystanders) why EMS

services were requested. The nature of illness (NOI) is the general type of illness a patient is experiencing.

At this point, if there is more than one patient or the patient is obese, you can call for additional resources. If multiple patients are present and have similar symptoms or complaints, you might consider carbon monoxide poisoning (or contact with some other noxious agent) or food poisoning as prime candidates. Irrespective of the cause of the problem, the presence of multiple patients means that they must be triaged to determine which additional resources you need and how you will allocate the resources.

Likewise, when you have multiple patients at a trauma scene, you must triage all patients. Once you have identified the total number of patients and estimated the severity of their injuries, you should request any additional resources—for example, fire, police, rescue, public utilities, or hazardous materials personnel—needed to support the efforts of first responders already on the scene.

The process of scene size-up is completed in a very short time. Once you have digested the dispatch information, evaluated the overall scene and safety, determined the MOI or NOI, and summoned additional help, you are ready to manage patient care. By contrast, if the responding crew can manage the situation without further assistance, you should assess the need for spinal motion restriction and continue with patient care. Based on the scene size-up and MOI, EMS providers must ensure that spinal motion restriction takes place on reaching the patient. Indications for spinal motion restriction will be covered further in Chapter 22.

In the Field

Assessing the safety of a scene before entering may be the single most important way in which emergency responders can attend to their own well-being. Subtle signs of danger not immediately recognized and neutralized—or avoided—at this point can become more threatening without being noticed once you shift your attention to patient assessment and care. Initial scene assessment often allows you to distinguish between a manageably safe scene and one that could spin dangerously out of control without further warning.

You are the Provider Part 2

As you gain access to the patient's airway, your partner applies a pulse oximeter and obtains vital signs. High-flow supplemental oxygen is applied, venous access is established, and the patient is readied for transport.

Vital Signs	Recording Time: 5 Minutes
Level of consciousness	V (Responsive to verbal stimuli) with a Glasgow Coma Scale score of 7
Skin	Pink, warm, and moist
Pulse	70 beats/min, regular
Blood pressure	104/68 mm Hg
Respirations	24 breaths/min
Sao$_2$	100% while breathing room air

3. Because this patient is a minor, what are some important considerations for treatment and transport?
4. Of all your differential diagnoses, which ones should be considered a diagnosis of exclusion?

Patient Assessment

Initial Assessment

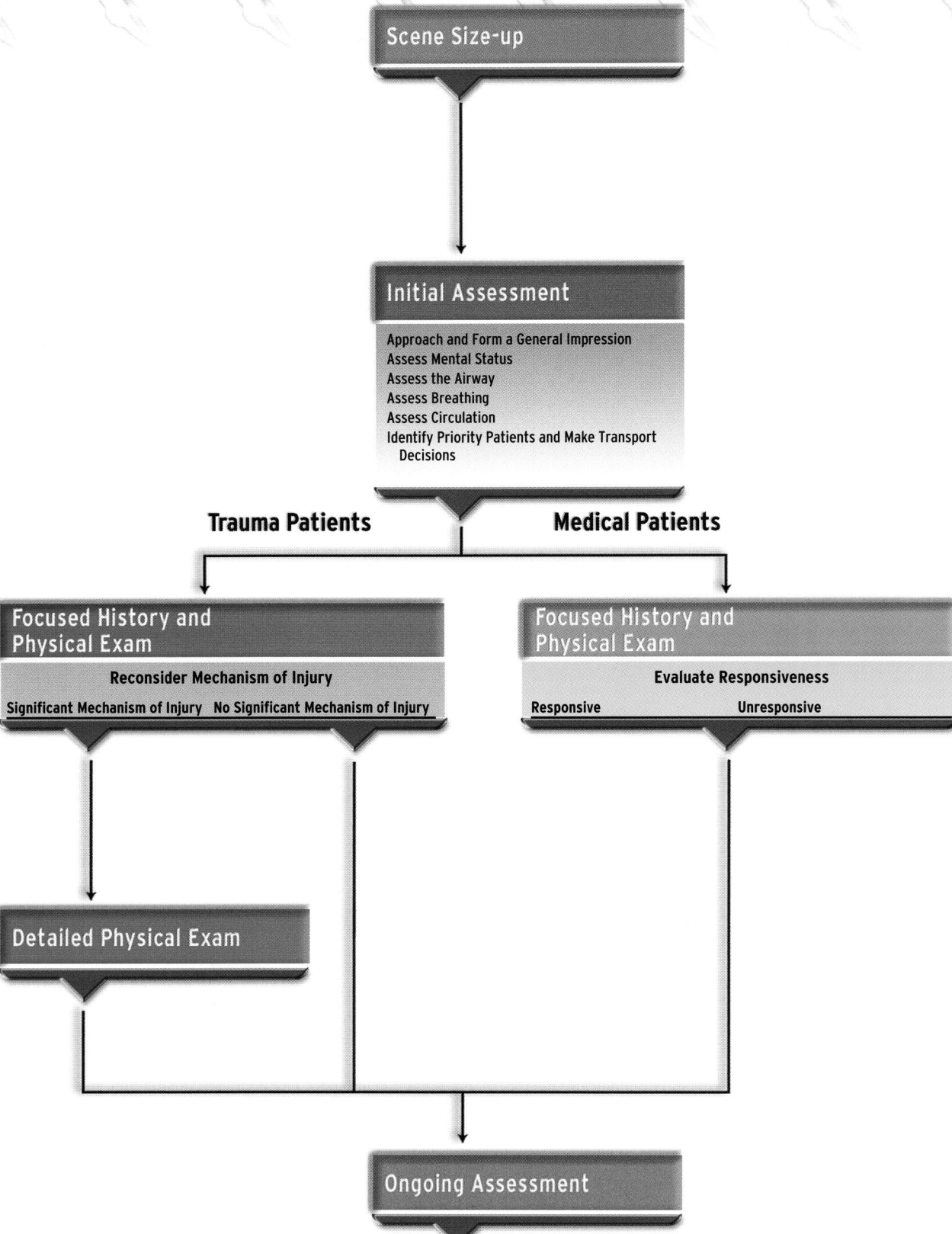

Scene Size-up

Initial Assessment

Approach and Form a General Impression
Assess Mental Status
Assess the Airway
Assess Breathing
Assess Circulation
Identify Priority Patients and Make Transport
  Decisions

Trauma Patients   **Medical Patients**

Focused History and Physical Exam

Reconsider Mechanism of Injury

Significant Mechanism of Injury   No Significant Mechanism of Injury

Focused History and Physical Exam

Evaluate Responsiveness

Responsive   Unresponsive

Detailed Physical Exam

Ongoing Assessment

The Initial Assessment

The initial assessment is the most time-intensive portion of the assessment process because it focuses on the identification and management of life-threatening problems. In the first 60 to 90 seconds, as you look at, talk with, and touch your patient, you should be able to identify threats to the ABCs. More often than not, you will form the general impression of your patient based almost solely on the initial presentation and chief complaint.

Each of us, without even trying or being conscious of doing so, makes dozens of observations about the appearance of another person during the first few seconds of an encounter—for example, whether the other person is sitting or standing, overweight or thin, smiling or frowning, dressed neatly or sloppily. In assessing a patient, we must make similar observations, but in a much more conscious, objective, and systematic manner, looking for specific clues to give us an immediate sense of the seriousness of the situation. A complaint of "I just can't catch my breath" that comes to you in one- or two-word bursts clearly points to a very sick patient. A patient complaining of "chest pain" after being stabbed in the chest is an even more obvious example of a priority.

You are trying to answer two questions: Is my patient sick? If so, how sick is he or she? In the case of trauma, the questions take a slightly different form: Is my patient hurt? If so, how badly hurt is he or she?

Whether it is medical or trauma, the first question is a qualification and the second is a quantification. "Is my patient sick?" has a yes or no answer, whereas "How sick is my patient?" attempts to rate the event's severity. With time and experience, you should be able to answer both questions in that 60- to 90-second window, forming your general impression.

Once these questions are answered, you can move forward with determining your priorities of care, developing a care plan, and putting the care plan into action. If the primary problem seems to be a traumatic injury, identify and evaluate the MOI. If the primary problem seems to be medical, identify the NOI. As you mentally move through this process, keep in mind that an injured patient might have a medical component to his or her problem, just as a patient with a medical emergency might have a trauma component to his or her problem.

You will also need to identify the age and sex of your patient because each can change how your patient presents. For example, an older woman having a heart attack may have an atypical presentation (no chest pain) compared with the more traditional presentation seen with an older man with the same condition. Likewise, a girl of middle school age will often be more emotionally mature than a boy of the same age, changing how each answers your questions and reacts to the emergency itself.

The information gleaned from the initial assessment is crucial to the overall outcome for your patient. Treat life threats as you find them, but also decide what additional care is needed, what needs to be done on scene versus en route, when to initi-

ate transport, and which facility is most appropriate given your patient's needs.

Documentation and Communication

Be aware of how your body language and physical presence might affect a frightened patient. Standing over and looking down on a patient can be intimidating. In such a case, try to get even with the patient's eye level so that you present a more "equal" impression of communication.

Assess the Patient's Mental Status and Neurologic Function

The patient's mental status is often one of the prime indicators of how sick the patient really is. Changes in the state of consciousness may provide the first clue to an alteration in the patient's condition, so establish a baseline as soon as you encounter the patient. At the same time you are assessing mental status, if trauma is involved, you need to decide whether you will implement spinal motion restriction procedures.

The quickest and simplest way to assess the patient's mental status or level of consciousness (LOC) is to use the AVPU process:

A *Alert* to person, place, and day
V Responsive to *Verbal* stimuli
P Responsive to *Pain*
U *Unresponsive*

You can further assess mental status by considering whether the patient is alert and oriented (A × O) in four areas: person, place, day, and the event itself. Assessing whether the patient can recall his or her name and the day tests long-term memory, whereas assessing whether the patient knows where he or she is and what happened tests short-term memory.

The most reliable and consistent method of assessing mental status and neurologic function is the Glasgow Coma Scale (GCS), which assigns a point value (score) for eye opening, verbal response, and motor response; these values are totaled for a total score **Table 14-1 ▶**. While it may take slightly longer to perform than the AVPU, the GCS provides much greater insight into the patient's overall neurologic function.

Let's work through a scenario. You encounter an older man who tracks you with his eyes as you enter his room. As you

In the Field

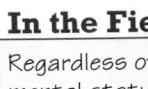

Regardless of the method you use to evaluate mental status, avoid using phrases such as "semiconscious," "lethargic," and "obtunded." These terms are too vague to be useful from a clinical perspective.

Table 14-1	Glasgow Coma Scale						
Eye Opening			**Best Verbal Response**			**Best Motor Response**	
Spontaneous	4		Oriented and converses	5		Follows commands	6
To verbal command	3		Disoriented conversation	4		Localizes pain	5
To pain	2		Speaking but nonsensical	3		Withdraws to pain	4
No response	1		Moans or makes unintelligible sounds	2		Decorticate flexion	3
			No response	1		Decerebrate extension	2
						No response	1

Scores:
14–15: Mild dysfunction
11–13: Moderate to severe dysfunction
10 or less: Severe dysfunction (The lowest possible score is 3.)

speak with the man, you note that his verbal response is disoriented, even though he follows your commands. His GCS values would be 4, 4, and 6, for a total score of 14. By comparison, if the patient opened his eyes only to pain, moaned as the only verbal response, and withdrew to pain, he would be assigned GCS values of 2, 2, and 4, for a total score of 8. Clearly, a child or infant will respond differently than an adult. A modified assessment should be used for these patients. This is addressed in Chapter 41.

Assess the Patient's Airway Status

Assessment of the patient's airway status focuses on two questions: Is the airway open and patent? Is it likely to remain so? For air to be drawn into the lungs, the airway has to be properly positioned and not obstructed (open from an anatomic perspective). If you hear sonorous (snoring respirations), think "position problem"—the sounds you are hearing are most likely from the tongue partially obstructing the airway. If you hear gurgling or bubbling sounds, think "suction"—there are most likely fluids such as blood, mucus, or vomit in the mouth or posterior pharynx.

When approaching airway management, think from the simple to the complex. The easiest problem to solve is one of position. Its resolution requires no equipment and can be done quickly. The possibility of a spine injury (or lack thereof) drives the decision of which technique to use to open the airway (head tilt–chin lift or jaw-thrust maneuver). In the case of obstruction, such as by food, BLS procedures to clear the obstruction require no equipment and can be done quickly.

Assessment of a patient's airway is completed in the same way regardless of the patient's age. In responsive patients of any age, talking or crying will give clues about the adequacy of the airway. For all unconscious patients, you must establish responsiveness and look, listen, and feel for breathing. If breathing is ineffective or absent, you must open the airway with a head tilt–chin lift (in nontrauma patients) or jaw thrust (in trauma patients).

When performing the head tilt–chin lift maneuver, remember the anatomic differences in the various age groups and make sure that you do not create an airway obstruction with an improper position of the head. Infants and young children do not have the developed tracheal rings that provide support, which means the trachea is easily collapsed or occluded when the head position changes.

Suctioning takes longer (because of the need to set up and use the equipment) and is a more complicated procedure than positioning. If you suction the patient for too long, you create a new problem: hypoxia.

If a mechanical means is required to keep the airway open and patent, you must choose an airway adjunct. If you opt to place an oropharyngeal or nasopharyngeal airway, you must retrieve the equipment, choose the right size for the specific patient, and then place the airway. This procedure takes considerable time.

If you determine that the patient cannot maintain his or her airway and you cannot maintain it by any other means, you need to use a more invasive technique, such as endotracheal intubation. This invasive procedure involves several pieces of equipment: a laryngoscope handle, a laryngoscope blade, a properly sized endotracheal tube, a syringe, a stylet, an OPA, an end-tidal carbon dioxide detector, a bag-mask device, and a method to secure the tube once it is placed. Obviously, gathering the equipment, preparing the patient, and performing the intubation procedure is more time-intensive than previously mentioned interventions.

Other advanced airway management options include use of a multilumen airway (Combitube), laryngeal mask airway, or surgical airway (discussed in Chapter 11).

Assess the Patient's Breathing

Breathing is proportional and related to airway adequacy. The assessment of breathing likewise focuses on two questions: First, is the patient breathing? If not, then you have to breathe for the patient. Second, if the patient is breathing, is breathing adequate?

Recall from Chapter 11 that the respiratory rate multiplied by the tidal volume inspired with each breath equals the minute volume. For example, a patient breathing slowly and deeply at 10 breaths/min and 500 mL/breath has a minute volume of 5,000 mL. By comparison, a patient breathing faster and shallower at a rate of 24 breaths/min and 200 mL/breath would have a minute volume of 4,800 mL. On a per-minute basis, the volumes of the two patients are virtually identical, even though the second patient is breathing more than twice as fast as the first patient. Always keep in mind that the amount of air actually moved in and out of the lungs each minute is the best measure of breathing adequacy. Besides the assessment of tidal volume, note the patient's breathing rate, effort of breathing (accessory muscle use), breath sounds, skin color, and LOC or mental status as part of the breathing assessment.

The techniques used to assess a patient's breathing status are not new: Look, listen, and feel. Look for chest rise and fall, noting symmetry of the chest wall and depth of respirations. Listen for breath sounds by using your sense of hearing or by auscultation with a stethoscope. Note adventitious lung sounds, and treat the patient accordingly. Finally, feel for air movement by placing your cheek or the palm of your hand near the patient's mouth.

Assess the Patient's Circulation

Assessing the pulse gives a rapid check of the patient's cardiovascular status and provides information about the rate, strength, and regularity of the heartbeat. In adults and children, the pulse is best palpated over the radial (responsive) and carotid or femoral (unresponsive) artery by using the tips of your index and middle fingers. In responsive or unresponsive infants, palpate the pulse over the brachial artery. First measure the pulse rate by counting the number of beats during 15 seconds; then multiply by 4. If the pulse is irregular or slow, it is best to count for a full minute.

As you count the pulse rate, note the force of the pulse. A normal pulse feels "full," as if a strong wave has passed beneath your fingertips. When there is severe vasoconstriction or in the case of hypotension with a fast pulse, the pulse may feel weak or "thready." By comparison, a patient who is hypertensive will produce a pulse that is more forceful than usual—a "bounding" pulse.

Finally, note the rhythm of the pulse. A normal rhythm is regular, like the ticking of a clock. If some beats come early or late or are skipped, the pulse is irregular. Although many cardiac dysrhythmias are not life threatening, in the case of heart blocks, an irregular pulse can indicate a serious condition. As such, consider all patients with an irregular pulse at risk until proven otherwise.

Report your findings by describing the rate, force, and rhythm of the pulse. For example, state that "The patient's pulse was 72, full, and regular," or "The pulse was 138, thready, and regular."

As part of this phase of the initial assessment, assess the patient's skin for color, temperature, and moisture. Collectively, these criteria provide insight into the patient's overall perfusion. Use the back of your hand to assess the warmth and moisture of the patient's skin because it tends be more sensitive than your palm Figure 14-6 ▶ .

The color of the skin Table 14-2 ▶ , especially in light-skinned patients, reflects the status of the circulation immediately underlying the skin, including the oxygen saturation of the blood. In people of color, changes may not be readily evi-

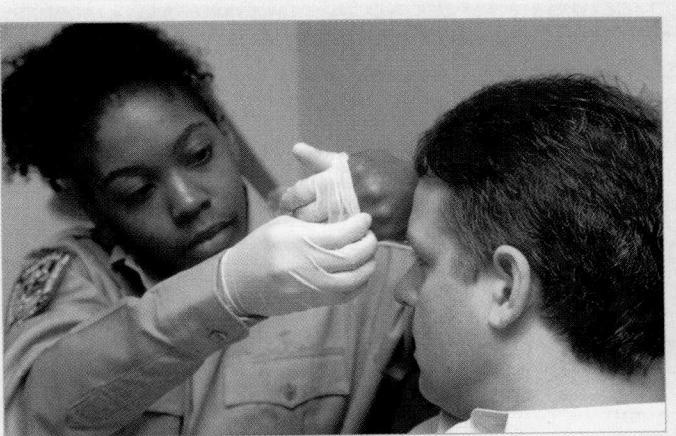
Figure 14-6 Assessing the skin condition. Use the back of the hand to assess the temperature and moisture of the skin.

Table 14-2	Inspection of the Skin
Skin Color	**Possible Cause**
Red	Fever Hypertension Allergic reactions Carbon monoxide poisoning (late sign)
White (pallor)	Excessive blood loss Fright
Blue (cyanosis)	Hypoxemia
Mottled	Cardiovascular embarrassment (as in shock)

dent in the skin but may be assessed by examining the mucous membranes (such as the lips or conjunctivae). When the blood vessels supplying the skin are fully dilated, the skin becomes warm and pink. When the blood vessels supplying the skin constrict or the cardiac output drops, the skin becomes pale or mottled and cool. If the patient does not get enough oxygen, as in the case of a narcotic overdose where the patient is breathing four times per minute, the blood will desaturate as the oxygen level drops; the skin will turn a dusky gray or blue (cyanosis). Pallor occurs if arterial blood flow ceases to part of the body, as in the case of a blood clot or massive bleeding. Hypothermia will also result in pallor as the body shunts blood to the core and away from the extremities.

Skin temperature rises as peripheral blood vessels dilate; it falls as blood vessels constrict. Fever and high environmental temperatures usually stimulate vasodilation, whereas shock elicits vasoconstriction. Normal skin is moderately warm and dry. The dryness or moisture of the skin is largely determined by the sympathetic nervous system. Stimulation of the sympathetic nervous system, as in shock or any other severe stress, causes sweating. Depression of the sympathetic nervous system, as in an injury to the thoracic or lumbar spine, can cause the skin in the affected area to become abnormally dry and cool Table 14-3 ▶ .

Table 14-3	Palpation of the Skin
Skin Condition	**Possible Cause**
Hot, dry	Excessive body heat (heat stroke)
Hot, wet	Reaction to increased internal or external temperature
Cool, dry	Exposure to cold
Cool, wet	Shock

Identify Priority Patients

Early in the assessment process, you need to identify priority patients who will benefit from limited time at the scene and rapid transport, as in the case of a patient with internal bleeding from trauma. Such a patient needs to see a surgeon who will sew up the holes and replace the lost blood, neither of which can be accomplished in the field setting.

When you have a priority patient, you need to expedite transport, doing only what is absolutely necessary at the scene and handling everything else en route, including the appropriate focused history and physical examination. Determining a priority patient requires that you think through a variety of possibilities:

- **Poor general impression.** The patient is in obvious distress and does not "look well."
- **Unresponsive patients.** Unresponsiveness is never a good sign and typically points to a patient in serious or critical condition.

- **Responsive but does not or cannot follow commands.** Altered mentation is another bad sign; the question you need to answer is "How bad?"
- **Difficulty breathing.** Breathing problems are one of the most common chief complaints in prehospital care. Patients who have difficulty breathing are in trouble; those who are "working to breathe" are in serious trouble.
- **Hypoperfusion or shock.** Without question, hypoperfusion or shock is an obvious sign of a high-risk patient. Weak or absent peripheral pulse, sustained tachycardia, and pale, cool, wet skin all point to serious consequences.
- **Complicated childbirth.** Anything that presents from the birth canal other than the newborn's head represents a situation not likely to be managed in the field setting.
- **Chest pain with a systolic blood pressure less than 100 mm Hg.** Especially in the context of tachycardia, this sign indicates cardiac compromise and a high-risk patient in unstable condition.
- **Uncontrolled bleeding.** Whether internal or external, such bleeding is a serious life threat.
- **Severe pain anywhere.** Any person with severe pain, especially enough to wake the person up in the middle of the night, should be considered a priority patient.
- **Multiple injuries.** While a patient may have multiple minor injuries that by themselves aren't serious, several small problems can add up to one big problem.

You are the Provider Part 3

The patient's mother is contacted at work. She reports that, other than mild scoliosis identified during his freshman year, Mike's health history is unremarkable. She further states that her son has a 4.0 GPA and no history of problems at school. When asked, she denies Mike having any recent history of significant trauma and drug use beyond "sneaking a few beers with friends."

Reassessment	Recording Time: 15 Minutes
Level of consciousness	V (Responsive to verbal stimuli) with a Glasgow Coma Scale score of 7
Skin	Pink, warm, and moist
Pulse	72 beats/min, regular
Blood pressure	106/70 mm Hg
Respirations	24 breaths/min with adequate depth
Sao_2	100% on room air
Temperature	99°F
Pupils	3 mm/PEARRL
Blood glucose	104 mg/dL

5. Does this patient need high-flow supplemental oxygen? Why or why not?
6. Should this patient be intubated? Why or why not?

Focused History and Physical Exam

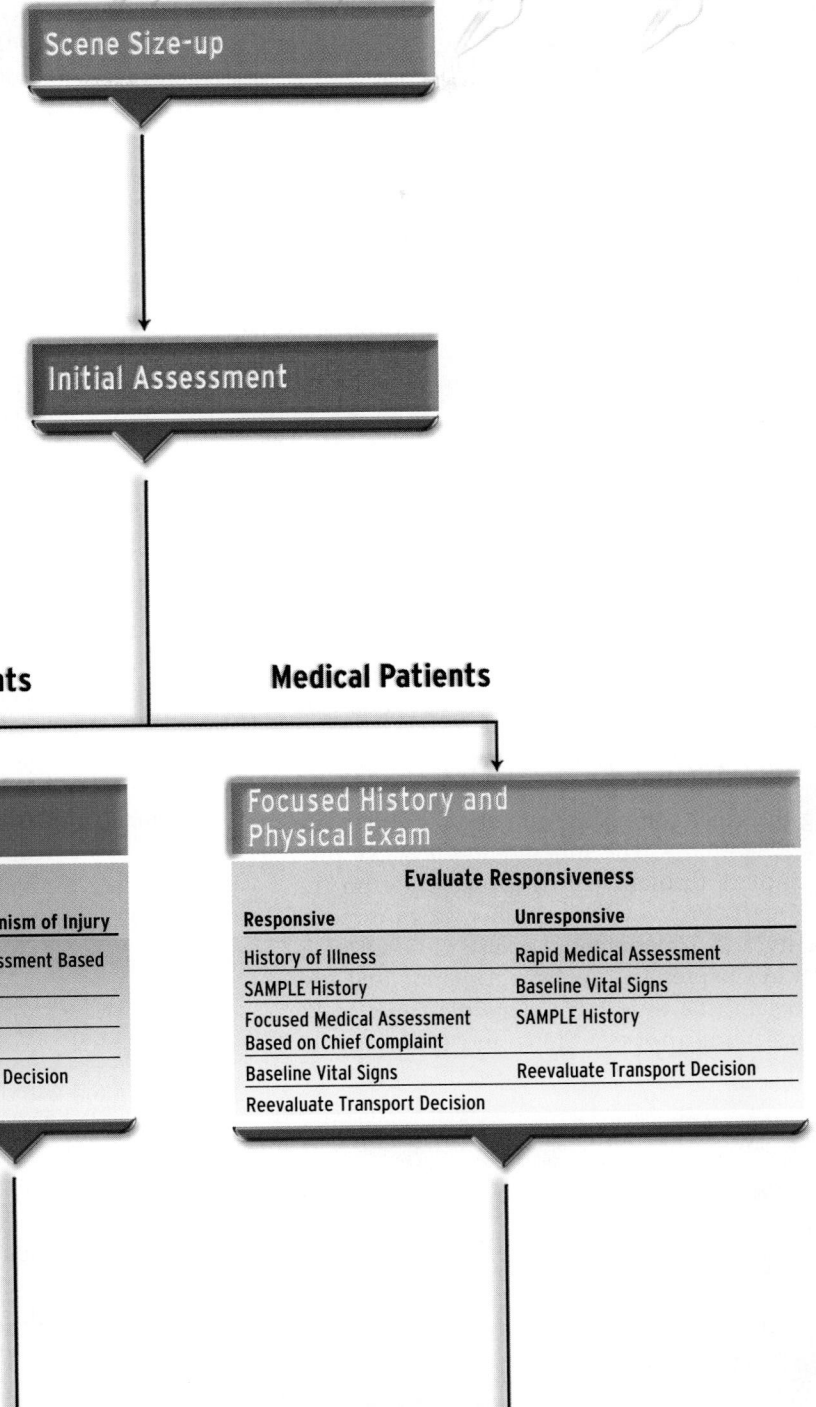

The Focused History and Physical Examination

Once the initial assessment is complete and all life threats have been addressed, you can move into the focused history and physical exam phase of patient assessment. Although the problems of many patients—especially older ones—will have medical and traumatic aspects, we will look at medical and trauma patients separately in this section.

Responsive Medical Patients

For a responsive patient with a medical problem, you will usually form your working field diagnosis based on information gathered during the history-taking process. The focused physical exam and any diagnostic tests you perform after taking the history will help further pinpoint the problem.

With a responsive medical patient, you must first identify the chief complaint. In most cases, some type of pain, discomfort, or body dysfunction (such as hasn't had a bowel movement in 4 days) prompts the call for help. In some cases, the complaint may be vague (such as "I just don't feel right today"). Vague complaints are common in older people. They challenge you to ask the right questions and be a patient listener as you work to obtain the information you need to make good care decisions Figure 14-7 ▾.

History of the Present Illness

After determining the chief complaint, you should obtain the history of the present illness. The mnemonic OPQRST provides a helpful template through which to elaborate on the chief complaint: Onset, Provocation, Quality, Region/radiation/referral, Severity, and Timeframe. (The use of OPQRST is explained in detail in Chapter 12.) As part of the focused history and physical exam, the SAMPLE mnemonic can also be useful in the interviewing process: Signs and symptoms of current complaint; Allergies; Medications; Pertinent past history; Last oral intake; and Events that led to the current injury or illness.

While taking the history, look for a medical information tag or card. Medical identification devices may take the form of a bracelet, necklace, or wallet card. Such a device is used to identify patients with a history of allergies, certain medical conditions (such as diabetes, cardiac conditions, hypertension, renal disease), and other conditions that may need to be addressed in the treatment of the patient.

Past Medical History

The past medical history is frequently linked to the patient's current problem. For example, people with diabetes who don't manage their blood glucose levels experience progressively worsening problems with their peripheral circulation, eyesight, and kidney function. Also, stable angina frequently transitions into unstable angina; at some point, the patient's condition may worsen and the patient may have a heart attack.

Components of the past medical history include the patient's general state of health, childhood and adult diseases, surgeries and hospitalizations, psychiatric or mental health illness, and traumatic injuries. As you inquire about the patient's past medical history, take the time to explore how some of his or her problems were solved (for example, "It took a couple of breathing treatments before I felt better" or "After my last asthma attack, I had to be intubated and was in the hospital on a ventilator for a week").

Equally important is the case in which the patient presents with a problem he or she has never experienced. An acute presentation of a new problem or condition is best considered serious until proven otherwise.

Current Health Status

The patient's current health status is a composite picture that includes numerous factors in the patient's life. To some degree, each of these items may have contributed to the problem you are confronted with today:

- Dietary habits
- Current medications (including prescription, over-the-counter, herbal, and recreational drugs)
- Allergies (environmental and medication)
- Exercise (or lack thereof)
- Alcohol or tobacco use
- Recreational drug use (if the patient is forthcoming)
- Sleep patterns and disorders
- Immunizations (such as flu shots, tetanus)

Focused Physical Exam

The focused physical exam should be driven by the information you gathered during the initial assessment and the history-taking phase. For a patient who tells you, "I just can't catch my breath," assessment of breath sounds early on is a must. If the patient tells you, "My leg feels numb," assessment of pulse, motor function, and sensation in the affected and unaffected extremities is indicated. You need to exercise good judgment to

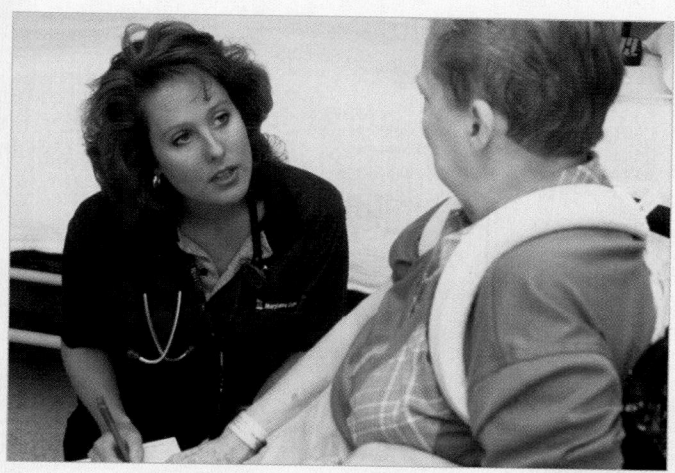

Figure 14-7 Be patient when obtaining information about a vague complaint.

make the best use of your time. Don't waste time palpating a patient's abdomen or auscultating heart sounds if the person complains of a stiff neck. In general, the care you provide for a responsive medical patient will be driven by your local protocols in conjunction with your consultation with the base station physician.

The most common complaints from a responsive medical patient will involve the head, heart, lungs, or abdomen, individually or in combination.

For patients with a "head" problem (confusion, headache, altered mentation), you should assess and palpate the head looking for signs of trauma. Check for facial asymmetry, such as facial droop or other signs of a suspected stroke. Dilated or constricted pupils may point to recreational drug use, whereas red conjunctiva may suggest drug or alcohol use. Elevated blood pressure often accompanies a headache, possibly secondary to hypertension.

For a suspected heart problem, assess the pulse for regularity and examine the skin for signs of hypoperfusion (pallor, cool, wet) or oxygen desaturation (cyanosis). Listen to breath sounds—many cardiac problems are associated with respiratory problems (such as rales secondary to pulmonary edema). Obtain baseline vital signs. Serious hypotension with sustained or progressive tachycardia is common in cardiogenic shock; stay alert for this condition because its mortality rate is more than 80%. Check for jugular venous distension (JVD) because it can indicate heart failure or pneumothorax. Examine the extremities for signs of peripheral edema that may result from right-sided heart failure.

For patients with respiratory complaints, assess breath sounds early and often. Possible findings or problems include the following:

- Lung fields with absent breath sounds: pneumothorax
- Silent breath sounds: status asthmaticus
- Lung fields with areas of consolidation: pneumonia
- Wheezing (localized or diffuse): asthma or bronchoconstriction
- Rales (wet lung sounds): pulmonary edema, heart failure, toxic inhalation, submersion

For any patient with a respiratory complaint, be alert for the appearance of accessory muscle use or retractions, both of which are signs of increased work of breathing. Also, keep an eye out for the signs of ventilatory fatigue, such as decreased mentation or a tired, worn-out appearance that often precedes ventilatory failure and, frequently, respiratory or cardiac arrest. Watch for the appearance of JVD with respiratory patients because it may point to pneumothorax or heart failure.

One of the most challenging complaints in the field setting is that of abdominal pain because it can result from multiple causes and often presents with little or no external signs. Three basic mechanisms produce abdominal pain:

- *Visceral pain* results when hollow organs are obstructed, thereby stretching the smooth muscle wall, which in turn produces cramping and more diffuse, widespread pain.
- *Inflammation* or irritation of the somatic pain fibers located in the skin, the abdominal wall, and the musculature may

produce sharp, localized pain, as in the case of pelvic inflammatory disease or appendicitis. If gastric contents, blood, or urine enters the peritoneum, it will also produce somatic pain, albeit usually much less localized and more diffuse.

- *Referred pain* has its origin in a particular organ but is described by the patient as pain in a different location. Examples include flank pain associated with kidney stones, inner thigh pain from appendicitis or pelvic inflammatory disease, scapular pain from cholecystitis, and groin pain (waves of pain) from renal colic.

Inspection and palpation of the abdomen can provide valuable information, although it is often general. Tightness or guarding can result from internal bleeding, an inflamed organ, and many other causes. With upper left quadrant pain, possible sources include a ruptured spleen from a sickle cell crisis and mononucleosis. Patients with lower left abdominal pain, especially if they have a history of constipation, nausea, vomiting, and fever, should be suspected of having diverticulitis. With lower right abdominal pain, appendicitis is a likely culprit. Generalized abdominal pain in women of childbearing age can be the result of an ectopic pregnancy, a ruptured ovarian cyst, or some other obstetric or gynecologic problem.

During the focused physical exam, along with history taking, obtain a full set of vital signs, including an auscultated blood pressure, accurate pulse and respiratory rates, and the patient's temperature. Use other diagnostic tools as indicated.

Baseline vital signs are an integral part of any focused history and physical exam. Clues provided will help you determine the seriousness of the patient's condition and the function of internal organs. Remember that shock, whether medical or trauma-related, is seen in different stages. Changes in a patient's blood pressure may be the last piece of evidence providers see when shock changes from one level to the next. Keep in mind that blood pressure must be sufficient to maintain adequate end-organ perfusion.

Orthostatic vital signs and the tilt test are measurements of a patient's blood pressure and pulse that are taken in the supine and sitting or standing positions. The results of such a test can help you determine the extent of volume depletion. The tilt test is generally used for patients with complaints of nausea, vomiting, diarrhea, syncope, and potential gastrointestinal problems; it indicates whether the patient needs fluid replacement. Normally, baroreceptors in the body sense changes in the blood pressure and volume and stimulate a catecholamine and renin-aldosterone response. This, in turn, causes peripheral vasoconstriction, increased heart rate, and fluid retention, which puts more blood into core circulation and increases volume. In patients who are volume-depleted, there is not enough circulating blood to push into the core circulation, especially when they move from a supine position to sitting or standing.

In some studies, a tilt test or orthostatic change is considered positive when the patient's blood pressure shows a decrease in systolic pressure (up to 20 mm Hg), an increase in

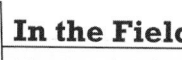

In the Field

Many technological devices are available to EMS to aid in patient assessment. While they are excellent equipment, always remember that you are assessing a patient—not a machine. Take the time to explain what your tools are and why you are using them. This simple action may help lessen patient anxiety.

diastolic pressure of 10 mm Hg (a narrowing pulse pressure), and an increase in heart rate by 20 beats/min. Vital signs should be taken at 1-minute intervals between moving a patient to a new position, and the cuff should be placed on the same arm in the same location. Documentation should include whether the pulse was regular, if the patient is being monitored and there is an attached strip, and whether the patient is experiencing other symptoms. If fluid replacement is given, providers should repeat the orthostatic assessment.

An Unresponsive Medical Patient

With an unresponsive medical patient, you start at a disadvantage in your assessment because your most reliable source of information—the patient—can't answer your questions. Owing to this serious limitation, assessment of an unresponsive medical patient looks much like a trauma assessment. You must rely on a thorough head-to-toe physical examination plus the normal diagnostic tools (pulse oximetry, capnography, cardiac monitor, and glucometer) to acquire the information needed to care for your patient. If family or friends are present, they may be able to provide information about the chief complaint, history of the present illness, past medical history, and possibly current health status. Nevertheless, the information they offer is almost never as good as that provided directly by the patient.

After completing the initial assessment, and assuming you have ruled out trauma, position unresponsive medical patients in the recovery position (left lateral recumbent position) to facilitate drainage of vomit, blood, or other fluids and to help prevent aspiration. If trauma is a factor, position the patient in neutral alignment, place a properly sized and fitted rigid cervical collar, and implement spinal motion restriction procedures as per the local protocol.

Perform a thorough assessment of the head, neck, chest, abdomen, pelvis, posterior body, and extremities, looking for signs of illness such as rash or urticaria, fever, unusual or excessive bruising, pulmonary or peripheral edema, and irregular pulse. Follow up your examination with at least two sets of vital signs—one taken now and another taken a few minutes after you've started your initial interventions (such as supplemental oxygen and IV therapy). The first set establishes a baseline (baseline vital signs); the second and additional sets (serial vital signs) provide comparative data to help you evaluate whether the patient's condition is improving, status quo, or worsening. If time allows, additional sets of vital signs add further data, allowing you to map trends (such as a progressively

increasing pulse rate). Make sure the vital signs include an auscultated blood pressure, accurate pulse and respiratory rates, and the patient's temperature. A recheck of breath sounds is always a prudent choice as well.

Unconscious, unresponsive medical patients should always be considered in unstable condition and at high risk, so rapid transport to the appropriate facility is indicated. Throughout transport, perform ongoing assessment, which includes rechecking the ABCs and reassessing anything associated with the patient's chief complaint.

Trauma Patients
Focused History and Physical Examination

Trauma patients may be classified into two major groups: patients with an isolated injury and patients with multisystem trauma. The biggest difference from an assessment perspective is that an isolated injury allows you to immediately focus on the main problem. In contrast, with multisystem trauma, you must first find all (or as many as you can reasonably find) of the various problems (for example, a hematoma on the forehead, a fractured arm, and neck and lower back pain). Then you need to prioritize the injuries by severity and the order in which you plan to address them. During the assessment, you must continually think about how each injury or condition relates to the others. For example, the mortality rate for a patient with a serious traumatic brain injury who has just a single episode of hypotension doubles. In such a case, not recognizing and addressing the hypotension and the lack of adequate perfusion pressure has a huge impact—in some cases, a fatal impact.

Another important consideration is the "high visibility factor" of many injuries, which sometimes creates a visual distraction. A compound fracture of the lower leg and ankle, with the foot twisted sideways and jammed under the brake pedal in a car, is not a pretty sight— but it is not a life-threatening injury. Because of the visual distraction, you might

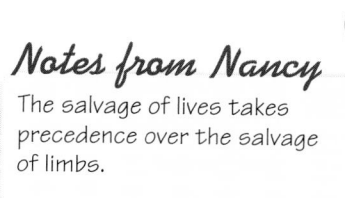

Notes from Nancy

The salvage of lives takes precedence over the salvage of limbs.

focus on the grossly deformed ankle and miss the early signs and symptoms of shock caused by the internal injuries and bleeding that you can't see.

As you move into the focused history and physical exam of a trauma patient, quickly revisit all of the information from your initial assessment, including reconsidering the mechanism of injury. Collectively, these data may help you identify patients who need to be priority transports to the trauma center.

A number of mechanisms have the potential to produce life-threatening injuries **Figure 14-8 ▶**:

- Ejection from *any* vehicle (car, motorcycle, or all-terrain vehicle)
- Death of another patient in the same passenger compartment

Skill Drill 14-1: The Rapid Trauma Assessment (*continued*)

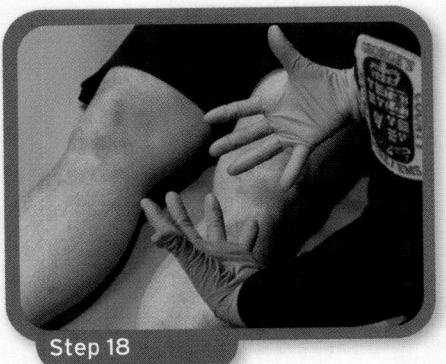

Step 18

Check your gloves for blood.

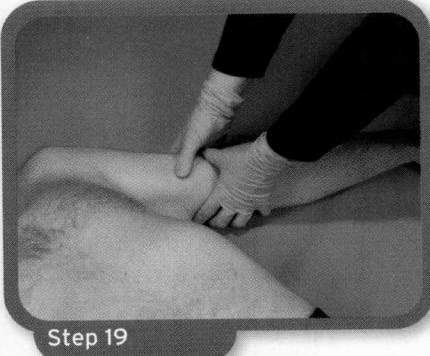

Step 19

Inspect and palpate the arms, and assess pulse, motor function, and sensation.

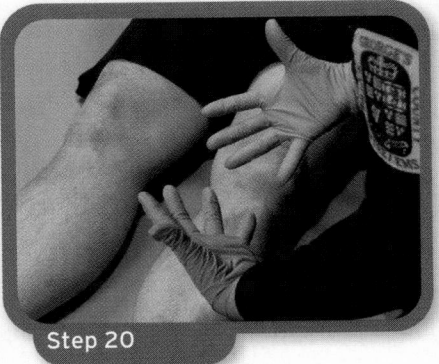

Step 20

Check your gloves for blood.

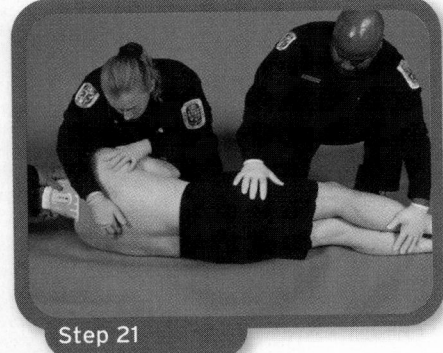

Step 21

Inspect and palpate the back.

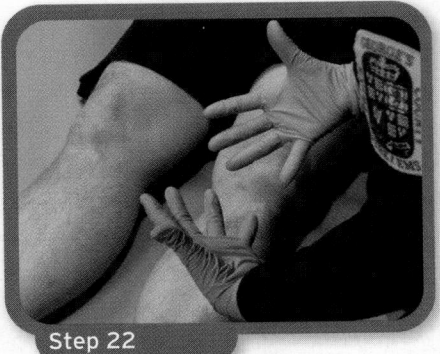

Step 22

Check your gloves for blood.

In the Field

It may be difficult to assess the stability of a large patient's chest for paradoxical motion. Try fanning out the fingers of both of your hands as wide as possible; then assess the up-and-down motion of the patient's breathing. This will give you a better assessment of equality and movement of the chest with respiration.

Patients With Minor Injuries or No Significant Mechanism of Injury

Most trauma calls involve patients with a single, isolated injury or, on occasion, several minor injuries. In almost all of these cases, the lack of serious or critical injuries is consistent with the lack of a significant mechanism of injury: A collision on the basketball court results in a sprained ankle; a skater crashes and ends up with a Colles fracture; a loose piece of metal spins off a lathe in the machine shop, lacerating the machinist's forearm. Patients should not show any signs of systemic involvement (hypotension). If they do, there is more going on than an isolated injury. You need to continue with your assessment with the goal of finding the more serious problem.

Focused History and Physical Exam

Detailed Physical Exam

Patient Assessment

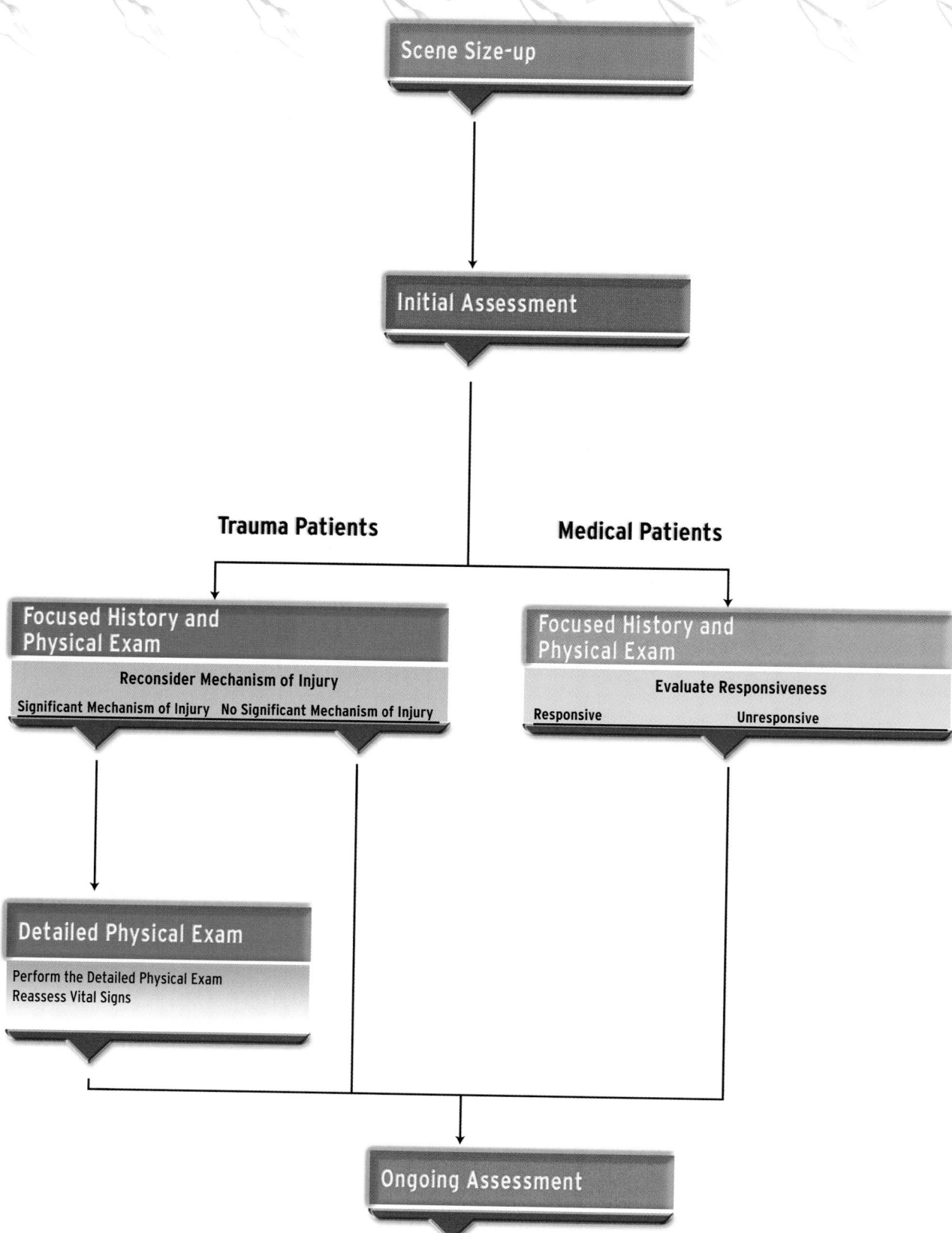

Scene Size-up

Initial Assessment

Trauma Patients

Focused History and Physical Exam

Reconsider Mechanism of Injury

Significant Mechanism of Injury   No Significant Mechanism of Injury

Medical Patients

Focused History and Physical Exam

Evaluate Responsiveness

Responsive   Unresponsive

Detailed Physical Exam

Perform the Detailed Physical Exam
Reassess Vital Signs

Ongoing Assessment

The Detailed Physical Exam

The detailed physical exam is another specialized form of patient assessment. In many cases, you won't need to do this assessment (such as for a finger laceration) or won't have time (such as when you have a patient in serious or critical condition). The detailed physical exam can take 15 minutes or more to gather a more detailed and comprehensive history and perform a detailed and thorough physical examination (such as checking range of motion [ROM]).

In the majority of cases when you perform a detailed physical exam, it will be done on a trauma patient en route when you have extended transport time (usually more than 15 minutes). Frequently, you will find yourself modifying the exam based on the patient's chief complaint. Use this tool as you see fit—or not at all, if you don't think it will provide meaningful information.

The detailed physical exam can be stressful and produce anxiety in patients because you are asking them to divulge personal information to a paramedic they have known for 10 minutes, and they would normally share such information only with their personal physician, whom they may have known for 10 years. Be respectful of patients' privacy, and maintain your most professional demeanor as you perform a detailed physical exam.

As you prepare to perform this exam, you will want to review the patient data gathered when you identified the chief complaint and performed the initial assessment. Add in the history of the present illness, the medical history, and the current health status. Keeping this information in mind will help keep you focused and on task as you delve into your patient's problem(s).

A detailed physical exam seeks to define complaints or problems that were not identified in the focused history and physical exam. During this process, providers reevaluate any treatment that is under way, based on new information gathered. New treatments are also started to deal with problems found during the detailed physical exam. In addition, providers reevaluate the patient's vital signs and assess trends in any changes.

Begin your detailed physical exam by evaluating the patient's mental status:

- Is the patient's appearance and behavior appropriate?
- How is the patient's posture and general motor behavior?
- Evaluate the patient's speech and language by listening to what the patient says and how he or she says it.
- Pay attention to the patient's thought process and perceptions.
- Assess the insights the patient does or does not have, along with the judgments the patient makes. (The patient is really sick but doesn't want to go to the hospital today ". . . but maybe tomorrow.")
- Assess memory and attention in the remote and the recent domains. For example, ask about memorable past birthdays, then about the events of the day.
- Evaluate new learning ability. For example, give the patient a simple phrase to remember (such as "You can't teach an old dog new tricks" or "Jack and Jill went up the hill") and explain that you plan to ask the patient about the phrase in a little while. Wait 5 minutes and do just that.

After you complete the mental status exam, begin the general survey of the patient. Assess the patient's LOC and compare it with baseline data. Has the LOC changed? If so, how? What is the skin color? Are there any visible lesions? Look carefully at the patient's facial expression. Does the patient show obvious signs of anxiety or distress, or does the patient look pale and lethargic as if he or she might be in end-stage shock? Assess the patient's apparent state of health and ask yourself that all-important question: "Sick or not sick?" (In the case of trauma, this question becomes "Hurt or not hurt?")

Other considerations covered in the detailed physical exam include the following:

- The patient's height and weight (Are they proportional to the patient's build?)
- Dress, grooming, and personal hygiene
- General posture, gait, and motor activity
- Unusual breath or body odors
- Skin color, temperature, moisture, and turgor

Head and Face

Start your hands-on assessment at the patient's head. Inspect and feel the entire cranium for signs of deformity or asymmetry, being careful not to palpate any depressions, lest you push bone fragments into the cranial vault or the brain Figure 14-12 ▾. Note any warm, wet areas; they usually represent blood, CSF, or a combination of the two.

Carefully inspect and palpate the upper and lower orbits, starting at the nose and working toward the lateral edge. Assess the eyes for shape and symmetry, and check the pupils for size and reactivity (fixed, dilated, sluggish). Evaluate whether the eyes move in harmony (conjugate gaze) and whether they can track in all fields (up, down, left, right, across). Note periorbital ecchymosis (raccoon's eyes).

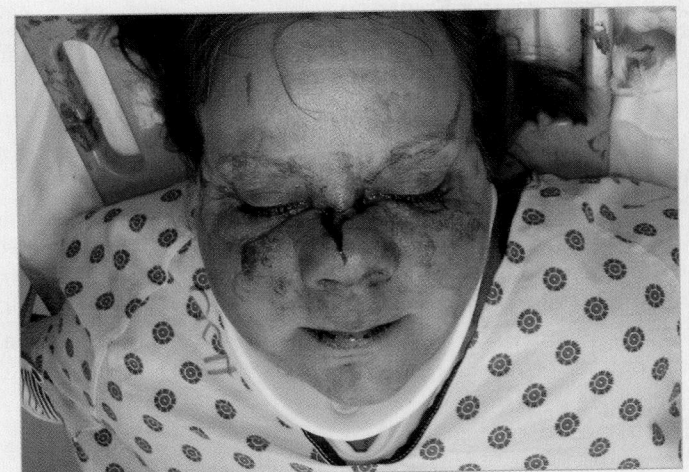

Figure 14-12 Do not palpate any depressions in the skin; you could push bone fragments into the cranial vault or brain.

Inspect and palpate the nose for structural integrity, and look inside for signs of trauma and fluids that may need suctioning. If there is drainage, determine whether it is bloody or clear (in which case, it could be mucus or CSF). Inspect and palpate the maxilla and the mandible, assessing the integrity and symmetry of both structures. Open the mouth, and look for signs of trauma (such as cracked or missing teeth, missing crowns or on-lays). Check the bite for fit. Be alert for any unusual odors on the patient's breath (such as alcohol or ketones). Check the posterior pharynx for fluids that may need to be suctioned.

Check in, around, and behind the ears for fluids or bruising (Battle's sign). Look carefully into the ear canal, and examine the structure of the ear for signs of trauma. Inspect the anterior part of the neck, assessing for JVD, swelling, and other signs of trauma. Assess for midline placement of the trachea.

Chest and Lungs

Before starting the physical examination of the chest, look at the overall symmetry, then assess for equal rise and fall, and finally look for retractions, accessory muscle use, and other signs of increased work of breathing. Remember—flail segments may not have paradoxical movement early on due to the splinting effect of muscle spasms. When you reassess lung sounds later, look for signs of flail segments that may just be presenting.

Inspect and palpate the clavicles from the suprasternal notch out to the shoulder girdles. Assess the ROM of the acromioclavicular joint. Confirm that the sternum is structurally intact. By using the flat surface of your palms, barrel-hoop the rib cage, feeling for asymmetry, deformities, and unstable segments, and evaluate the overall integrity of the chest wall. If the environment is quiet enough, percuss the chest for hyperresonance (pneumothorax, asthma, chronic obstructive pulmonary disease) and hyporesonance (hemothorax). Finally, assess breath sounds in a minimum of six fields.

Cardiovascular System

Check and compare distal pulses. Reassess the skin condition for pallor and diaphoresis (signs of sympathetic discharge). Be alert for patients with sustained bradycardia (which lowers blood pressure and may decrease the patient's mental state) or tachycardia (increases cardiac workload and may lower blood pressure). Run a 3-lead ECG for all patients with a cardiac history. If the patient has a significant heart history and you have the time, acquire a 12-lead ECG. It would be tragic to miss an evolving MI due to hypotension caused by trauma. If the environment is quiet enough, consider auscultating for abnormal heart sounds.

Abdomen

Start your assessment of the abdomen by inspecting the entire area for signs of swelling or bruising. Bluish discoloration in the periumbilical area (Cullen's sign) is indicative of intraperitoneal hemorrhage, with two of the more common causes being ruptured ectopic pregnancy and acute pancreatitis. Look for a rash or other signs of an allergic reaction. Take note of scars from previous trauma or surgeries.

Palpate each quadrant gently but firmly, and recognize that the patient may respond in many ways. A moan, a guarding posture or withdrawing, or a facial grimace all send the same message: You have touched something or somewhere that causes pain or discomfort. That information is worth pursuing with your assessment. Consider any signs or symptoms of abdominal injury as serious and indicative of a high-priority patient in unstable condition.

Rebound tenderness checks are rarely done in the field setting primarily because they can be painful for the patient as you slowly push down and then rapidly release sections of the abdomen. A positive sign (the patient cries out or withdraws) indicates peritoneal irritation.

Genitalia

Unless the patient complains of pain or discomfort or of feeling that he or she is bleeding, there is no reason to examine the genitalia. If you note wetness or bleeding during your exam, you should examine the genitalia because these vascular organs can bleed extensively when injured. Take note of priapism in male patients; a prolonged erection is usually the result of a spinal cord injury.

In cases of sexual assault or rape, handle all clothing per local protocol and bag it with any other evidence (no biodegradable garbage bags). Sexual assault and rape have huge psychological impacts. Be as supportive, caring, and nonjudgmental as possible throughout your care for the patient. It is almost always helpful to have a member of the EMS who is the same sex as the patient involved in care. If that is not possible, however, do not delay care of the patient because of it.

Anus and Rectum

Unless the patient has a history or indication of trauma to the anus or rectum, there is generally no reason to examine this area. With a positive history or signs or symptoms of trauma, examine the area to assess for the need of bleeding control or another intervention (such as treatment for shock, care of eviscerated parts).

Peripheral Vascular System

Moving from the upper extremities to the lower limbs, inspect the extremities for asymmetry and any skin signs, such as bruising, pallor, mottling, or other signs of trauma. Check skin temperature and moisture. When you assess pulses in the extremities, do both sides simultaneously so that you can compare pulse strength, rate, and regularity from side to side. A significant variation in pulse strength in one extremity, especially when associated with pallor or cyanosis, points to vascular compromise.

Musculoskeletal System

Start your assessment of the musculoskeletal system by performing a global inspection of the patient. Do all extremities appear to be properly positioned and functioning normally? If the patient is standing or seated, assess his or her posture for signs of scoliosis or the telltale lean of a suspected stroke. Look for redness or inflammation at the joints (signs of arthritis). Stay alert for red, swollen areas on the extremities, especially those that are warm to the touch (signs of a clot or thrombus).

Check the ROM. First, have patients move the extremities by themselves; significantly decreased ROM in this setting may be attributed to joint-related problems. Next, have patients work their extremities through a normal ROM, only this time with you providing resistance against their movements. Decreased or diminished ROM under these circumstances usually points to muscular weakness or atrophy or possibly problems with innervation. Assess for equality of grips.

Nervous System

The check of the nervous system is one of the most time-consuming elements of the detailed physical exam, mainly because it involves five separate miniassessments: mental status, motor response, cranial nerve function, reflexes, and sensory response.

The mental status examination essentially repeats the exam done in the rapid trauma assessment. Think of it as checking "mental vital signs." Assess the patient's LOC, and compare it with your baseline and any other LOC checks during other parts of your assessment. A handy mnemonic to guide you through the mental status exam is the mnemonic COASTMAP:

- **Consciousness.** Along with LOC, note the patient's ability to pay attention and concentrate. Is the patient easily distracted?
- **Orientation.** Ask about the year, season, month, day, and date. Have the patient identify the present location—that is, state, town, and specific location. Can the patient recall and describe the event(s) currently going on?
- **Activity.** Does the patient appear anxious or restless? Is he or she sitting very still, scarcely moving at all? Is he or she making any strange or repetitive motions (possibly because of methamphetamine use)?
- **Speech.** Note the rate, volume, articulation, and intonation of the patient's speech. Does it sound pressured? Does the speech have a flat, monotone delivery consistent with depression? Is the speech garbled or slurred (dysarthria)? Garbled or slurred speech may have many causes,

including alcohol or drug impairment, stroke, and head injury.

- **Thought.** Listen to the patient's story. What's on his or her mind? Is the patient making sense? Is there anything unusual about his or her reasoning? Is the patient expressing apparently false ideas (delusions)? Are voices telling the patient what to do or think (psychotic)? Does the patient report that people are "out to get me" (paranoia)?
- **Memory.** You can usually form an impression of the patient's memory by listening to his or her reconstruction of events. A more precise assessment requires asking a few questions. Ask the patient if you may test his or her memory. If the patient assents, slowly say the names of three unrelated subjects (such as apple, bicycle, sewing machine). Now ask the patient to repeat those words; that will test registration. A few minutes later, ask the patient if he or she can remember the three words you named before; that tests retention and memory.
- **Affect.** The patient's affect (mood) may be most apparent in his or her body language. The patient sitting with shoulders drooping and head bent, for example, conveys depression. Note whether the affect—the expression of inner feelings—seems appropriate to the situation.
- **Perception.** Detecting disorders of perception may be difficult because patients are often hesitant to answer questions about hallucinations. Sometimes it is helpful to ask the patient, "Do you ever hear things that other people can't hear?"

It is also helpful to assess the following:

- **Cranial nerves.** Quickly assess the cranial nerves, as described in Chapter 13.
- **Motor system.** Take an overall look at how the patient moves. Are his or her movements smooth or jerky? Note unusual or repetitive movements. Check for muscle strength by assessing bilateral grips.
- **Reflexes.** By using a reflex hammer, evaluate the patient's deep tendon reflexes in the knees and elbows for diminished or heightened responses. Additional reflex checks are probably not warranted in the field.
- **Sensory system.** By using the appropriate tools, test the patient for pain (dull versus sharp), sensation, position, and vibration. Compare distal sensation and proximal sensation and one side with the other as you assess the dermatomes.

After completing this assessment, make certain that all assessment findings have been accurately recorded, take one more set of vital signs, and recheck breath sounds.

Ongoing Assessment

Patient Assessment

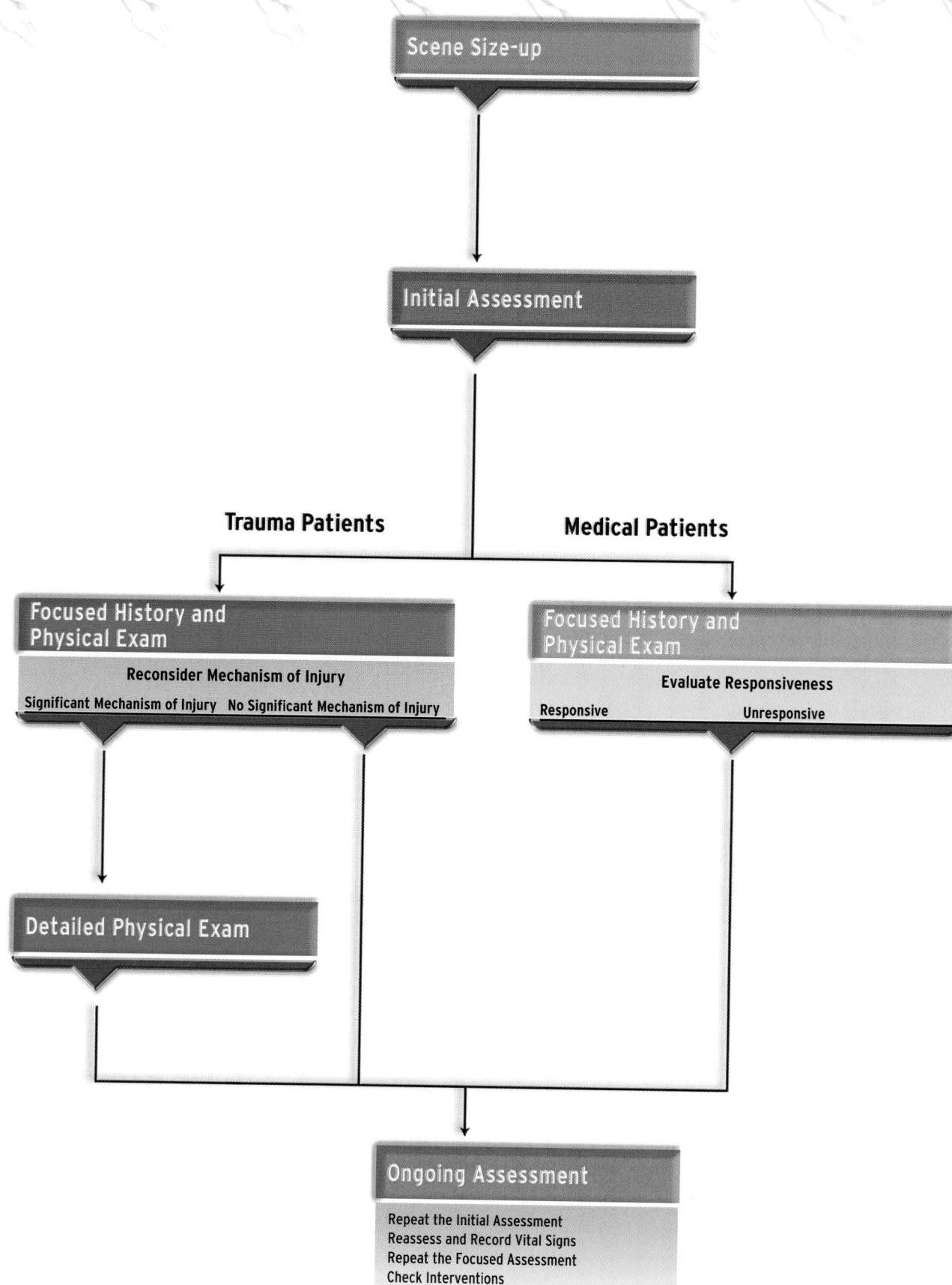

Scene Size-up

Initial Assessment

Trauma Patients

Focused History and Physical Exam

Reconsider Mechanism of Injury

Significant Mechanism of Injury   No Significant Mechanism of Injury

Detailed Physical Exam

Medical Patients

Focused History and Physical Exam

Evaluate Responsiveness

Responsive   Unresponsive

Ongoing Assessment

Repeat the Initial Assessment
Reassess and Record Vital Signs
Repeat the Focused Assessment
Check Interventions

The Ongoing Assessment

After the initial assessment, the <u>ongoing assessment</u> is the single most important assessment process you will perform. It represents a continuous, yet cyclical, process that you perform throughout transport, right up to the time you turn patient care over to the emergency department staff. For patients in stable condition, you should do an ongoing assessment every 15 minutes or so. For patients in unstable condition, you need to make a concerted effort to repeat the ongoing assessment every 5 minutes.

Reassessment of Mental Status and the ABCs

The ongoing assessment combines repetition of the initial assessment, reassessment of vital signs and breath sounds, and repetition of the focused assessment. During the ongoing assessment, you continue to evaluate and reevaluate the patient's status and any treatments already administered. Trends in the patient's current condition may give clues about the effectiveness of treatments: Have they improved the patient's condition? Are identified problems better or worse? This information indicates which changes have occurred and which critical conditions have been addressed and corrected.

First, compare the patient's LOC with your baseline assessment. Is the LOC changing? If so, how? If mentation is decreasing, can the patient still protect the airway? If you have doubts, consider inserting an advanced airway.

Second, review the patient's airway. Is it patent? Swelling, bleeding, or just a change of position can obstruct the airway in the blink of an eye, so make certain that the airway is properly positioned and dry. Always be prepared to suction, and don't delay if you hear gurgling in the upper airway. It's far better to prevent aspiration than to treat it later. If the airway needs to be secured, *do it immediately,* and intubate the patient. Once intubation is accomplished, recheck lung sounds and perform oximetry and capnography periodically to confirm that the tube is properly placed.

Third, reassess breathing. Is the patient breathing adequately? If not, figure out why and fix the problem. For hypoventilation, assist breathing with oxygen and a bag-mask device. Correct hypoxia with high-concentration oxygen therapy. For patients with diminished or absent breath sounds, JVD, and progressive dyspnea (signs of pneumothorax), decompress the chest.

Stay alert for signs that the patient is experiencing ventilatory fatigue (for example, decreasing pulse oximetry reading, looks increasingly tired). Be especially alert for this possibility in children because it a classic sign that precedes disaster for the patient. Patients of any age who are going into ventilatory fatigue need to have their airway managed for them.

Finally, reassess the patient's circulation. Assess overall skin color as an initial measure of cardiovascular function and hemodynamic status. With pale, cool, wet skin, think shock; with cyanosis, think oxygen desaturation; with mottling, think end-stage shock.

Make certain that all bleeding is controlled. If you find blood-soaked dressings, add more fresh dressings to the stack and rebandage in place. Reassess the blood pressure, watching closely for signs that the patient is beginning to decompensate.

Reassess the pulse, including its rate, strength, and regularity. Progressive tachycardia may indicate that the patient is still bleeding, is hypoxic, or is developing cardiogenic shock. In contrast, sustained or progressively worsening bradycardia may reflect rising intracranial pressure (from trauma or a stroke) or end-stage shock.

Reassessment of Patient Care and Transport Priorities

After repeating the initial assessment as part of your ongoing assessment, think about your present care plan. Have you addressed all life threats? Based on what you now know, do you need to revise your priority list? If so, make the change and get on with patient care. In contrast, if your plan is working well and you've addressed most or all of the patient's complaints, there is no need to revise the care plan.

While you are reevaluating your patient care priorities, you should reassess the transport plan as well. Should routine transport be stepped up to priority? Is the patient's condition worsening to the point that you need to consider diverting to a closer facility? Do you need to set up a rendezvous with an air ambulance and fly the patient to the health care facility? If your patient's condition has improved and stabilized, you should step down from priority and transport the patient as a routine case, the clearly safer choice.

Get another complete set of vital signs, and compare them with the expected outcomes from your therapies. For example, if you administered a 500-mL bolus of normal saline to a patient with gastrointestinal bleeding, you usually would expect a rise in blood pressure and a decrease in pulse rate. With any priority patient, you should have, at a minimum, three sets of vital signs—and that would be if you had a short transport. With most priority patients, you will have four or five sets of vital signs. Thus, you can look for trends or patterns such as a slowing pulse, rising blood pressure, and erratic respiratory patterns that represent the <u>Cushing's reflex</u>, a grave sign for patients with head trauma. Alternatively, narrowed pulse pressure, muffled heart tones, and JVD are associated with cardiac tamponade (<u>Beck's triad</u>), usually secondary to penetrating chest trauma.

The last element of the ongoing assessment is to revisit the patient's complaints (from the focused history), along with your interventions. Have any complaints improved or resolved? Has the 9 over 10 chest pain improved with the nitroglycerin you administered? Did the second albuterol treatment ease the patient's breathing? Which situations remain unresolved? Situations that are worsening are especially concerning because they could mean an unseen problem or ineffective interventions. If you have not reached the receiving facility, get ready to do the ongoing assessment again—that's why it's called the ongoing assessment.

Ongoing Assessment

You are the Provider Summary

1. What is the best method of airway assessment and management for a patient who is wearing a football helmet and shoulder pads?

The quickest way to access this patient's airway is to remove the helmet's face guard rather than the entire helmet. This technique addresses two issues, airway assessment and management, and keeps the spine in a neutral position should the patient require spinal immobilization. (Spinal immobilization is covered in Chapter 22.)

2. Although the players deny any trauma, should you immobilize this patient?

There is no evidence to suggest that this patient requires spinal precautions. When in doubt, err on the side of caution and immobilize the patient. This will be a determination for you to make in accordance with your local protocols.

3. Because this patient is a minor, what are some important considerations for treatment and transport?

Most high schools require an updated student file that includes current phone numbers for parents in case of an emergency. If the parents are unavailable, this patient would be treated and transported under the rules of implied consent.

4. Of all your differential diagnoses, which ones should be considered a diagnosis of exclusion?

Although at some point during the course of your career you will likely encounter patients who exaggerate signs or falsify symptoms (including feigning unconsciousness), this should be the last thing you suspect, even in patients who have a history of malingering. Consider this possibility only after you've carefully reviewed all other potential causes. Doing otherwise will likely cause a misdiagnosis and/or delay of essential care and prompt transport.

5. Does this patient need high-flow supplemental oxygen? Why or why not?

The adage, "Never withhold oxygen," is good advice. It is appropriate to apply high-flow oxygen because the patient is unconscious and can benefit from supplemental oxygen therapy. Be ever mindful of what you're doing and why, especially when administering drugs, including oxygen. Note that pulse oximetry is not always accurate, even when it provides a reading. Patients with carbon monoxide poisoning may have an acceptable or even a 100% oximetry reading. Patients who have cold hands or who wear nail polish may initially have a lower pulse oximetry reading but, in fact, are better oxygenated than their carbon monoxide–poisoned counterparts.

6. Should this patient be intubated? Why or why not?

It can be argued that because this patient is unconscious, he cannot maintain his airway and should, therefore, be intubated via rapid-sequence induction (RSI; "Less than 8, intubate!"). If an airway cannot be kept patent with basic techniques, insert an endotracheal tube. Before making this decision, look at the patient's vital signs, oximetry and capnography readings, and other signs. Is the patient ventilating and oxygenating adequately? All information in this scenario would suggest that the answer to this question is "yes." Obviously, local protocols dictate the when, how, why, and where of RSI, but you will find in your career that gray areas exist. This patient can be managed effectively without taking the risks of RSI.

7. If no field diagnosis is possible, what should your patient care goals be?

As a paramedic, your goals are to assess and treat any life-threatening conditions, monitor ABCs, provide supportive measures, and continue to search for underlying causes of the patient's signs and symptoms.

8. Under normal circumstances, when an abrupt loss of consciousness occurs, which four primary probabilities should you consider as part of your rule-out diagnosis?

Any sudden change in mentation should make you question the presence of underlying illnesses or injuries related to the neurovascular system as well as hypoglycemia, drug toxicity, and cardiac arrhythmias.

Prep Kit

■ Ready for Review

- Patient assessment is the platform on which quality prehospital care is built and the single most important skill you bring to bear on patient care.
- Patient assessment is a complex skill made up of two primary components: information gathering and physical exam.
- Several elements make up the skill of patient assessment, with each being used in some way to gather information.
- The first step of the patient assessment process is the scene size-up because your first and foremost concern on any call is ensuring your own safety and the safety of the other EMS team members.
- During the initial assessment, in the first 60 to 90 seconds, as you look at, talk with, and touch your patient, you should be able to identify threats to the ABCs.
- Once the initial assessment is complete and all life threats have been addressed, you can move into the focused history and physical exam phase of patient assessment.
- The detailed physical examination can take 15 minutes or more for a more detailed and comprehensive history and a more detailed and thorough physical exam (such as checking ROM).
- After the initial assessment, the ongoing assessment is the single most important assessment process you will perform.

■ Vital Vocabulary

alert and oriented (A × O) A determination made when assessing mental status by looking at whether the patient is oriented to four elements: person, place, time, and the event itself. Each element provides information about different aspects of the patient's memory.

AVPU A method of assessing mental status by determining whether a patient is Awake and alert, responsive to Verbal stimuli or Pain, or Unresponsive; used principally in the initial assessment.

Beck's triad The combination of a narrowed pulse pressure, muffled heart tones, and JVD associated with cardiac tamponade; usually resulting from penetrating chest trauma.

current health status A composite picture of a number of factors in a patient's life, such as dietary habits, current medications, allergies, exercise, alcohol or tobacco use, recreational drug use, sleep patterns and disorders, and immunizations.

Cushing's reflex The combination of a slowing pulse, rising blood pressure, and erratic respiratory patterns; a grave sign for patients with head trauma.

detailed physical exam The part of the assessment process in which a detailed area-by-area exam is performed on patients whose problems cannot be readily identified or when more specific information is needed about problems identified in the focused history and physical exam.

focused history and physical exam The part of the assessment process in which the patient's major complaints or any problems that are immediately evident are further and more specifically evaluated.

focused physical exam The exam done on a responsive medical patient, driven by the information gathered during the initial assessment and the history-taking phase.

general impression The overall initial impression that determines the priority for patient care; based on the patient's surroundings, the mechanism of injury, signs and symptoms, and the chief complaint.

Glasgow Coma Scale (GCS) An evaluation tool used to determine level of consciousness, which evaluates and assigns point values (scores) for eye opening, verbal response, and motor response, which are then totaled; effective in helping predict patient outcomes.

history of the present illness Information about the chief complaint, obtained using the OPQRST mnemonic.

initial assessment The part of the assessment process that helps you identify immediately or potentially life-threatening conditions so that you can initiate lifesaving care.

mechanism of injury (MOI) The way in which traumatic injuries occur; the forces that act on the body to cause damage.

nature of illness (NOI) The general type of illness a patient is experiencing.

ongoing assessment The part of the assessment process in which problems are reevaluated and responses to treatment are assessed.

past medical history Information obtained during the patient history, such as the patient's general state of health, childhood and adult diseases, surgeries and hospitalizations, psychiatric and mental illnesses, or traumatic injuries, which may relate to the patient's current problem.

rapid trauma assessment A unique and specialized assessment performed between the initial assessment and the focused physical exam of a trauma patient, usually on patients with a significant mechanism of injury, assessing specific parts of the entire body.

scene size-up A quick assessment of the scene and its surroundings made to provide information about scene safety and the mechanism of injury or nature of illness, before you enter and begin patient care.

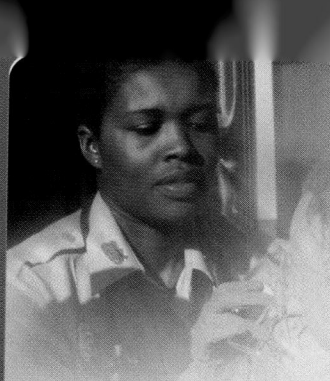

Assessment in Action

Your unit has been dispatched to a motor vehicle crash in which a small car has struck a utility pole. Dispatch has advised you that there appears to be one patient in the vehicle. As you arrive on the scene, you notice that the wooden utility pole is leaning at a 45° angle toward the car, and the utility wires are hanging low over the vehicle but not touching it. Without leaving the unit, you see a person sitting in the driver's seat who appears to be leaning over the steering wheel but is not moving. You are not sure, but you believe you see the top of a child's car seat in the rear of the car. No traffic or crowd control has been started, and you do not see a utility crew on the scene.

1. **What is the first step in your patient assessment?**
   A. Assess the patient's chief complaint.
   B. Perform a detailed physical exam to determine the extent of the condition.
   C. Perform a scene size-up.
   D. Assess AVPU.

2. **What is the first and foremost concern during your scene size-up?**
   A. The patient's level of consciousness
   B. The patient's breathing
   C. The safety of you and the rest of your team members
   D. The safety of the patient and their family members

3. **What best describes the term mechanism of injury?**
   A. The forces that act on the body to cause damage
   B. The internal forces of the human body
   C. The way an accident happened
   D. The external circumstances that caused an accident to happen

4. **How long should your initial assessment take?**
   A. 10 to 20 seconds
   B. 30 to 40 seconds
   C. 60 to 90 seconds
   D. More than 90 seconds

5. **A rapid trauma assessment be should performed on any trauma patient with a(n):**
   A. fracture.
   B. significant MOI.
   C. significant medical history.
   D. significant NOI.

6. **When should a detailed physical exam be done?**
   A. For every patient encounter
   B. When you have time on scene to complete it
   C. While you are transporting the patient to the hospital
   D. During the scene size-up

Challenging Questions

You arrive at a construction site where a worker fell approximately 20′ from a ladder and landed on his left side. Your initial assessment does not reveal threats to the ABCs. The patient, who is conscious and alert, complains of pain to the left side of his body; he denies having chest pain and shortness of breath and states that he did not lose consciousness. Other than some minor abrasions to the patient's left arm and lateral thigh, the remainder of your exam is unremarkable. Your partner reports the following vital signs: blood pressure, 126/76 mm Hg; pulse rate, 86 beats/min and regular; and respirations, 14 breaths/min and unlabored.

7. **Does this patient require transport to a trauma center?**

8. **Could you defend a transport mode of code 3 for this patient?**

■ Points to Ponder

You and your partner have been dispatched to a call for "chest pain." When the dispatcher provides an update, he states that the patient is a 70-year-old woman who started having chest pain about 2 hours ago. The patient has a cardiac history, but the extent of the history is unclear because of a language barrier. The dispatcher also states that there is an 8-year-old child with the patient.

Upon arrival, you find the patient sitting upright in a chair. She is leaning slightly forward, with her arms folded across her chest. You introduce yourself and ask her for information about her chief complaint. She looks up at you and says, "No English," in a heavy accent that you do not recognize. You have already formed your initial impression of the patient and have determined that she is in considerable distress.

How do you proceed with your physical assessment given that this patient does not speak English and you do not speak her native language? Would you consider using the 8-year-old as an interpreter? How will you address a time delay in your assessment progression?

Issues: Assessing Persons of Differing Cultures, Communications Barriers, Time Delay During Assessment.

Critical Thinking and Clinical Decision Making

Objectives

Cognitive

3-4.1   Compare the factors influencing medical care in the out-of-hospital environment to other medical settings. (p 15.5)

3-4.2   Differentiate between critical life-threatening, potentially life-threatening, and non-life-threatening patient presentations. (p 15.6)

3-4.3   Evaluate the benefits and shortfalls of protocols, standing orders and patient care algorithms. (p 15.5)

3-4.4   Define the components, stages and sequences of the critical thinking process for paramedics. (p 15.6)

3-4.5   Apply the fundamental elements of critical thinking for paramedics. (p 15.10)

3-4.6   Describe the effects of the "fight or flight" response and the positive and negative effects on a paramedic's decision making. (p 15.10)

3-4.7   Summarize the "six Rs" of putting it all together: Read the patient, Read the scene, React, Reevaluate, Revise the management plan, Review performance. (p 15.11)

Affective

3-4.8   Defend the position that clinical decision making is the cornerstone of effective paramedic practice. (p 15.3)

3-4.9   Practice facilitating behaviors when thinking under pressure. (p 15.5)

Psychomotor

None

Introduction

The most fundamental description of what a paramedic does on a day-to-day basis is as follows: identify problems, set patient care priorities, develop a care plan, and, finally, execute that plan. If you were to say that looks like cookbook medicine, you would be right. However, effective cookbook medicine requires the provider be a *thinking cook*, as often patients do not present exactly as those described in a textbook. To complicate matters further, the prehospital environment is constantly changing, which can affect the stability of any scene Figure 15-1 ▾ . Some paramedics who have worked in hospital emergency departments say that the chaos of the emergency department cannot be compared with the dynamics of the streets. Still, a paramedic is expected to work in this environment and provide *quality* patient care.

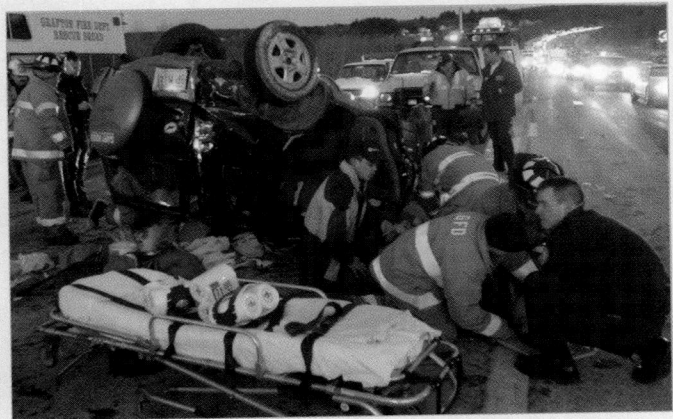

Figure 15-1 Your work as a paramedic will rarely be done in a quiet, stress-free place. You will have to learn the skill of making decisions in a chaotic environment.

This chapter is divided into two parts: first, an explanation of critical thinking, and second, how you can apply critical thinking skills in the streets. Initially, you will learn about *the science of thinking*. Then comes the practical subject matter: how to use this knowledge and *take it to the streets*. To master critical thinking, you will need to know the cornerstone thinking processes and terms.

The Cornerstones of Effective Paramedic Practice

Gathering, Evaluating, and Synthesizing

The first cornerstone of your practice is having the ability to *gather, evaluate,* and *synthesize* information. Every day, call by call, you will find yourself challenged as you try to obtain information from patients of different age groups and educational backgrounds, with varying abilities to communicate. Many times, alcohol or other drug use will impair a patient's ability to respond to your questions, which will further complicate your information gathering.

Once you have gathered the information, you must assess and evaluate it to formulate a care plan. You must check out the validity of the information—often relying on your own judgment and communication skills. For example, let's say you encounter a patient with a minor sprained ankle who immediately asks you for morphine for pain. Your first thought might be that this person is an illicit drug user. Another consideration, however, is that your patient is a health care professional or knowledgeable in medicine and has a low tolerance for pain. If morphine is not the first-line drug for a sprained ankle, you will need to explain this to your patient. The thinking paramedic must consider both possibilities to be as objective as possible in the decision-making process.

You are the Provider Part 1

During the past two weeks, the cold and flu season has hit and has affected many members of the community, including some of your coworkers. As you sip your morning coffee and listen to the shift captain relay the plan for the day's events, you hear dispatch tones.

You are dispatched to 1611 Lynne Lane for a 65-year-old woman complaining of weakness, fatigue, and dizziness. A family member requested no lights or siren. As you arrive on the scene, you are met by the patient's daughter, who called 9-1-1 after speaking to her mother on the phone. She explains that her mom believes "she just has a cold." Her daughter is concerned it might be something more.

Initial Assessment	Recording Time: 0 Minutes
Appearance	Eyes open, flat affect
Level of consciousness	A (Alert to person, place, and day)
Airway	Patent
Breathing	Rapid with adequate tidal volume
Circulation	Radial pulse present, fast

1. When do you begin patient assessment?
2. What are the benefits and the risks of diagnosing based on dispatch?

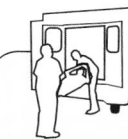

In the Field

Remember, your professional ethics demand that you consider all the possibilities when communicating with a patient. You must not judge. You must figure out: what does your patient need?

In the Field

Hypercarbia means an excess of carbon dioxide (CO_2) in the blood, as indicated by an elevated PCO_2 level.

Once you have evaluated the information you obtained from the scene, the patient, or a bystander, and determined which information is valid or invalid, you need to process—or *synthesize*—this information.

For example, consider a patient, a 64-year-old man having chest pains, who has had type 1 diabetes since childhood, started smoking in high school, and has had chronic obstructive pulmonary disease (COPD) since his 50s. Synthesis requires that you look at each of those three facts about your patient, any of which may or may not be life threatening. Your job is to paint a mental picture of how each fact affects the other   Figure 15-2 ▾ .

In this scenario, we know that diabetes is a metabolic dysfunction that includes a disorder of circulation. While an extremely low level of blood glucose may kill someone or result in brain damage quickly, a chronic, higher-than-normal blood glucose level takes its toll on every organ and every system. Think about how many long-term diabetics you encounter with vision problems or amputated fingers or toes. The patient's COPD, which is primarily a disease of gas exchange, at some point results in some combination of hypoxia (low levels of oxygen in the blood) and hypercarbia (high levels of carbon dioxide in the blood). You need to assess the new onset of chest pains. It is likely that coronary artery disease has caused one or more of the vessels of the heart muscle to become blocked, in turn causing the part of the heart to begin to necrose or die. Taking all of the information you have gathered and synthesizing it would basically work something like this: "I have a patient with diseases of both circulation and gas exchange. There is a good chance that part of the patient's heart is dying because vessels are unable to deliver oxygenated blood to a portion of the

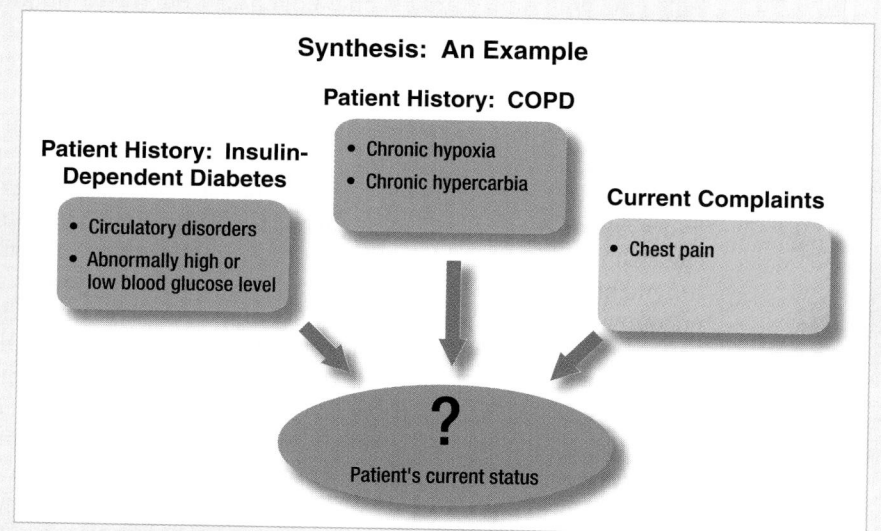

Figure 15-2 When you synthesize patient information you have gathered, you will assess the relative importance of the patient's medical history (blue boxes) and his or her current complaints (yellow box). These factors all affect each other.

You are the Provider Part 2

The patient tells you that she's sorry her daughter has bothered you. She tells you that she asked her daughter to bring over some food and cold medicine, not for her to call an ambulance. She says it's true that she hasn't been feeling well since early this morning, but she doesn't think it's anything major. She apologizes to you again and says, "I'm sure you have better things to do."

Vital Signs	Recording Time: 10 Minutes
Skin	Slightly moist, slightly pale, and warm
Pulse	110 beats/min, regular
Blood pressure	130/82 mm Hg
Respirations	36 breaths/min
Sao_2	95% on room air

3. What are pertinent negatives?

4. What information is missing from the above assessment?

heart muscle." You must treat the combined effect of your patient's disease processes to prevent the unperfused section of heart from dying, which may cause the death of your patient. That is synthesis—taking conditions and assessing their potential for having life-threatening impact. In the end, the patient could be having a heart attack, a life-threatening problem.

Developing and Implementing a Patient Care Plan

The second cornerstone of your practice is the *development and implementation of a patient care plan*. This is actually much simpler than analyzing the validity of the information you've gathered. Once you've determined the patient's primary problem by identifying the chief complaint and establishing a working diagnosis, your care plan is almost always defined by the patient care protocols or standing orders in the EMS system where you work. Protocols, or standing orders, define the essential standard of care for patients with certain injuries, illnesses, or behavioral conditions. They further specify your performance parameters, which define what you can or cannot do without direct medical control, as well as when you need to contact medical control before providing care. Collectively, standing orders and protocols promote both a standard approach and a standard of quality care as defined by regional, state, or national standards.

Unfortunately, protocols, standing orders, and patient care algorithms only address classic patient care presentations. They frequently don't address vague patient complaints that don't fit into a neat clinical description—nor do they address patients with multiple disease etiologies (remember synthesis?) and/or those patients who will require multiple treatment modalities as part of the care plan.

So, your next step is to figure out what you should do in your patient's best interest.

Judgment and Independent Decision Making

The third cornerstone is *judgment and making independent decisions* **Figure 15-3** ▸ . Let's say that you encounter a machinist who has had an incident in which one of the parts of a machine has seriously gashed the upper part of his leg. You can see significant amounts of blood gushing from the area of his femoral artery with every contraction of his heart. You realize that you do not have time to make radio or cell phone contact with a base station doctor, identify your unit and yourself, present the patient problem, get directions for patient care, and *then* take action before the patient may die. Even under the best circumstances, your patient would have died long before your "call the doc" process was completed. To save the patient, you immediately recognize the severed artery as an immediate life threat and apply continuous direct pressure, possibly combined with use of a pressure point to control the bleeding.

Another scenario you may encounter—a patient in cardiac arrest on their front porch. With your resource hospital only a

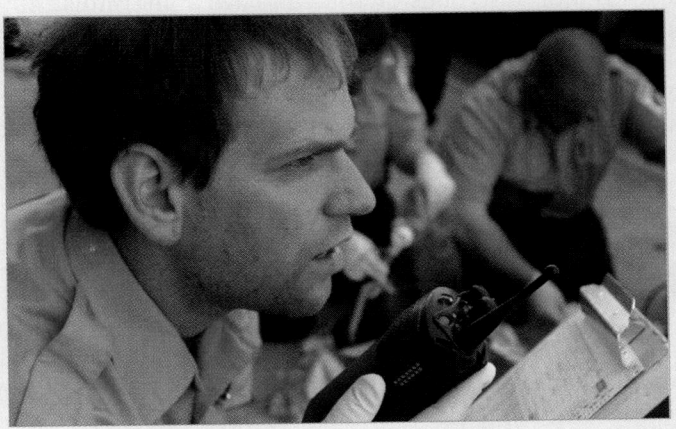

Figure 15-3 Each run that you make will have its own unique circumstances and challenges. Much of your skill rests with the use of careful, nonjudgmental decision making.

few blocks away, you choose to shock any shockable rhythm (as you will learn in Chapter 27), secure the airway and administer oxygen, and get an IV line established. At that point you decide to load the patient and initiate transport, performing CPR and administering medication while en route. Put that same patient in a third-story attic apartment with a small, almost useless stairway access, and you may find yourself dealing with outcomes ranging from the patient being either fully resuscitated and viable or pronounced dead. Because of the restrictive physical requirement, you realize it is impossible to quickly and efficiently get the patient out of the house and en route to the care facility. As such, you manage the patient to one end point or another. Either the resuscitation gets called off, or you get the patient back and stabilized before you attempt to package and transport. As circumstances change, so may your patient care plan. However that will only happen if you are using your critical thinking and decision-making skills to the best of your abilities.

Documentation and Communication

Documenting difficulties such as darkness, limited access, and unruly crowds that you encounter while caring for a patient will help to justify your decisions made for patient care.

Thinking Under Pressure

The fourth and final cornerstone of your practice is your ability to *think and work under pressure*. Imagine ringing the doorbell at the address to which you have been dispatched and having the door open, at which point a hysterical mother hands you her cyanotic, apneic 2-year-old who she just dragged out of the bottom of the bathtub. Your critical thinking faculties should tell you to get that child breathing in the next handful of seconds or you will have a full cardiac arrest on your hands, diminishing the likelihood of saving the child's life. Only a combination of excellent knowledge coupled with excellent psychomotor clinical skills will allow you to avert a patient care disaster: the death of a child. To accomplish that, you must be able to work under extreme pressure and be able to perform both quickly and effectively.

The Range of Patient Conditions

One of the key elements of your practice is to be able to quickly determine if your patient is *sick or not sick*. For patients who are sick, you must further be able to quantify *how sick they are*. That will, in turn, allow you to make good choices as to what care you must provide at the scene and what care you should provide in the back of the ambulance while en route.

Special Considerations

The best way to recognize "sick" infants and small children is to know what "not sick" infants and small children act like according to their age. To improve your ability to recognize this difference, take every continuing education pediatrics course and read every article you can.

Clear thinking in a chaotic emergency starts with a triage model. Critical patients need immediate care to survive. Serious patients need care within the next few minutes to possibly the next half hour (or they become critical patients) to have a positive outcome **Figure 15-4 ▶**. The two groups of patients that are left are the mortally wounded or dead, and those often termed the walking wounded or minimally injured. For the sake of discussion, we will combine both these groups under the heading of non-life threats.

Examples of patients with *critical life threats* would include those with:

- Major multisystem trauma
- Devastating single-system trauma
- End-stage disease presentations
- Acute presentations of chronic conditions

Examples of patients in *serious condition* would include those with:

- Serious multisystem trauma
- Acute presentations of "first-time" medical events
- Multiple disease etiologies

Examples of patients who are "walking wounded" or have *minimal, non-life-threatening injuries* would include those with:

- Simple abrasions
- Partial-thickness burns of an extremity of less than 5% body surface area
- Small lacerations with only capillary bleeding

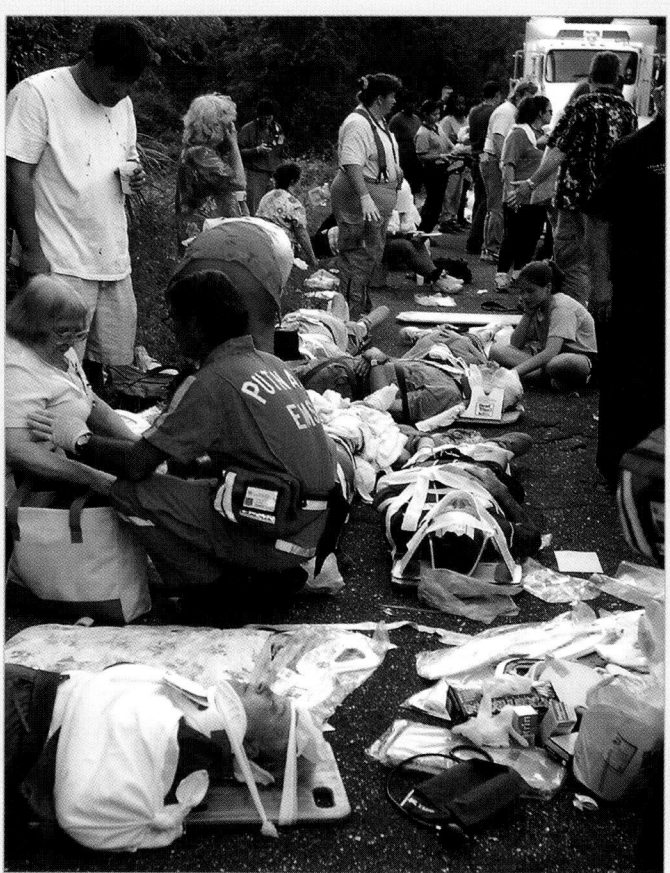

Figure 15-4 With multiple patients, you must quickly assess and prioritize the urgency of each person's condition. After a size-up of the scene, call for additional help.

Critical Thinking and Clinical Decision Making

It is important for you to have a command of the vocabulary for the process psychologists and philosophers call *thinking* and *decision making*. By having a better understanding of how your thoughts are formed and processed, you can make the best decisions possible in caring for your patients **Figure 15-5 ▶**.

Concept Formation

The first stage of the thought process in prehospital care is that of gathering information—things you see, hear, smell, or feel. This process is concept formation. In EMS, you will form your concepts on several variables, including your initial assessment of your patient's condition, your general impression including assessment of your patient's affect, the patient's vital signs, and actual measurements from your other diagnostic EMS tools.

The process starts as you arrive at the scene and evaluate it from a safety perspective for both the EMS team and your patient. You need to evaluate the mechanism of injury for

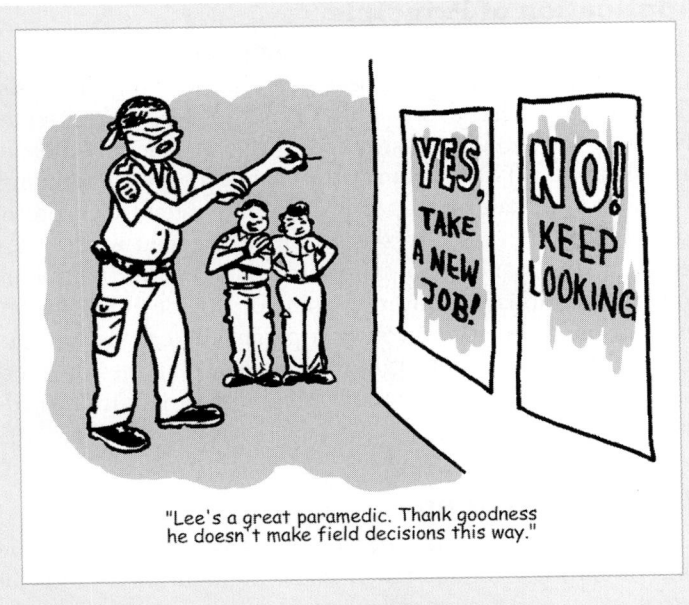

"Lee's a great paramedic. Thank goodness he doesn't make field decisions this way."

Figure 15-5

trauma, or for medical calls, the nature of the present illness. How does your patient present? Does the patient appear uncomfortable, or frightened, or deathly ill? You need to assess the patient's level of consciousness (LOC), in part to determine whether the person can provide you with reliable information to act on. This initial evaluation of their LOC will also establish a baseline for you to refer to later as the call progresses and the patient's condition changes.

In the Field

Observe family members for clues also. Do they seem worried or nervous? Does calling 9-1-1 seem "routine" for them? Are they huddled in a corner crying or are they trying to watch television during your assessment? Be alert for situations that are not what they seem to be.

You move further into the information gathering process as you perform your initial assessment, focusing on the identification of any serious threats to your patient's life that you need to immediately address. You continue on as you perform an appropriate physical examination. As you examine your patient, identify the patient's chief complaint, and get a pertinent medical history, including any medications the patient is taking: prescription, over-the-counter, illicit, or possibly herbal.

One of the most important observations you need to judge is your patient's affect—or emotional state reflected in physical behavior 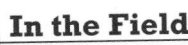 **Figure 15-6 ▶**. The affect might not tally with what patients tell you. For example, suppose you have a patient who presents with the hyper-kind-of-manic behavior

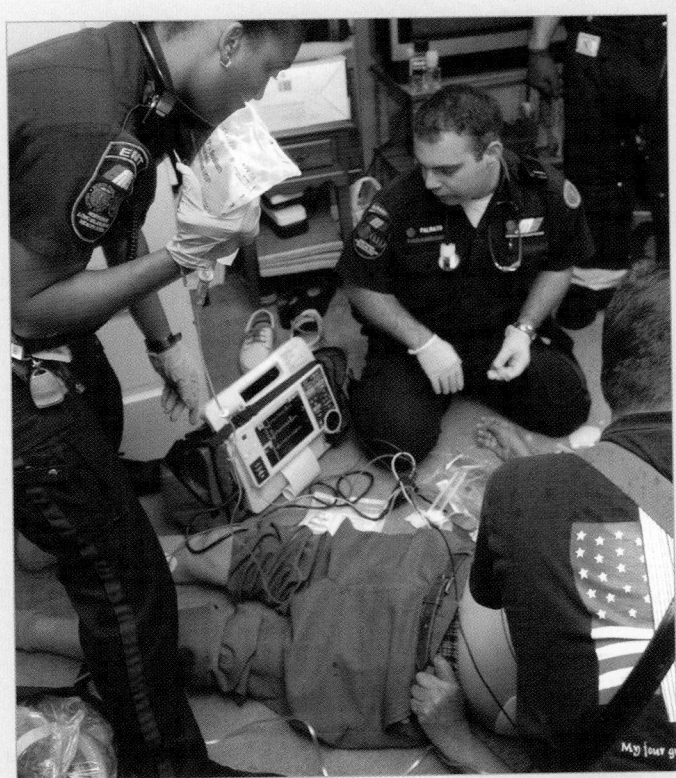

Figure 15-6 Take in clues not only from your patient's status, but also from his or her surroundings. Assess the entire environment to make sure that you fully understand how it may impact your patient's condition.

associated with amphetamine abuse, yet denies any drug use. You might even see drug paraphernalia. You must balance the story you are getting with the patient's affect—there should be a match. If there isn't a reasonable match, you need to ask yourself why.

Last on your information-gathering quest is obtaining the patient's vital signs by using your primary diagnostic tools: the glucometer, pulse oximeter, capnometer, cardiac monitor, blood pressure cuff, and your stethoscope.

Data Interpretation

During the second stage of the critical thinking process, you must evaluate all the information that you have gathered, which is called data interpretation. You will need a good background in anatomy and physiology as well as pathophysiology so you understand both how the body works, and when problems arise, how it responds to those problems. Another key element is your experience. If you have come to the paramedic program with lots of experience as an EMT-B, you will have an excellent platform to build on.

How you think and form conclusions is affected not only by the attitudes of patients, but by your attitude as a provider. This means, for example, you should never consider a call a

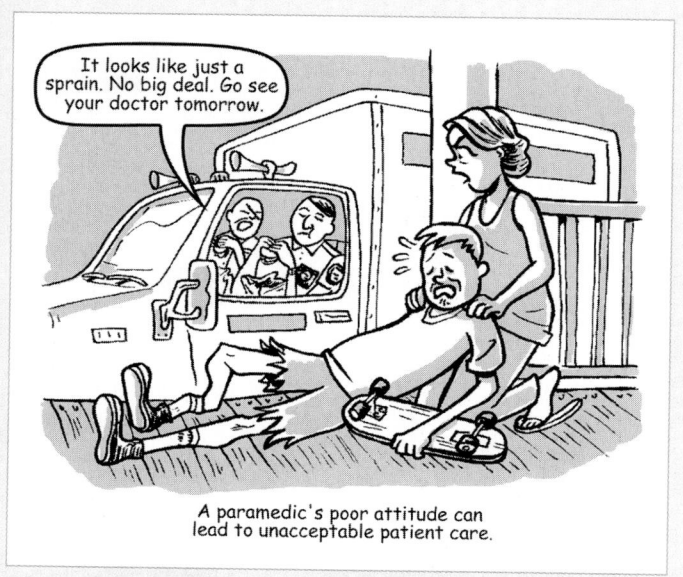

A paramedic's poor attitude can lead to unacceptable patient care.

Figure 15-7

waste of your time or talent. Furthermore, unprofessional comments such as "I can't believe you called us for THIS!" show a lack of compassion and interest in providing the best possible care Figure 15-7 ▲ .

Having a negative attitude about any patient or patient care situation will almost guarantee that the care you provide will be suboptimal. To maintain the standards set by your profession, you must provide the best care you can for every patient you encounter. Period.

Application of Principle

The next stage of the critical thinking process in EMS comes when your field impression becomes your working diagnosis. The key word here is "working." Think of it as being "tentative." It is what you feel is at the root of your patient's problem, and what you will focus your patient care efforts on correcting.

Now, your care plan is driven by the patient care protocols or standing orders in the system where you work. They represent the standard of care and describe the treatments and interventions you are expected to provide. In addition, they further define what you as a paramedic can do without contacting medical control, as well as what therapies or interventions you cannot do without obtaining orders from medical control.

Reflection in Action

You are now actively treating your patient while at the same time monitoring the effects of your interventions. Think of *reflection in action* as simply *thinking while doing*.

Let's say your patient was complaining of having "difficulty breathing." You apply a nonrebreathing mask with oxygen flowing at 15 L/min. After a few minutes you ask, "Is it getting any easier for you to breathe?" Too often, paramedics get caught up in thinking they must do one thing after another, frequently forgetting to periodically check and see whether what they are doing is actually solving the problem and making the patient feel better. If you ask your patient how your treatment is working, you will also be reassessing your patient Figure 15-8 ▶ . Reassessment is an important and continuous part of your patient care.

You are the Provider Part 3

The patient denies having a recent history of productive cough, fever, chills, body aches, nausea, or vomiting, but does admit she's felt quite tired and a bit short of breath since she woke around 6 AM.

Your partner asks her if she wishes to be transported to the hospital, and she asks, "Do I really need to go?" You tell her since her daughter was concerned enough to call 9-1-1 coupled with her feeling of shortness of breath, these are both good reasons to be transported to the hospital for further evaluation. After hearing this explanation, she agrees to treatment and to transport. You place her on oxygen, start an 18-gauge IV of normal saline in her right hand to keep the vein open, and place her on the cardiac monitor.

Reassessment	Recording Time: 15 Minutes
Skin	Slightly moist, pale, and warm
Pulse	102 beats/min, regular
Blood pressure	130/74 mm Hg
Respirations	30 breaths/min
Sao_2	98% on 4 L/min via nasal cannula
Temperature	98.6°F (37°C)
ECG	Sinus rhythm

5. How can a patient's opinion affect treatment and transport decisions?
6. Can men and women have different symptoms of acute illness?

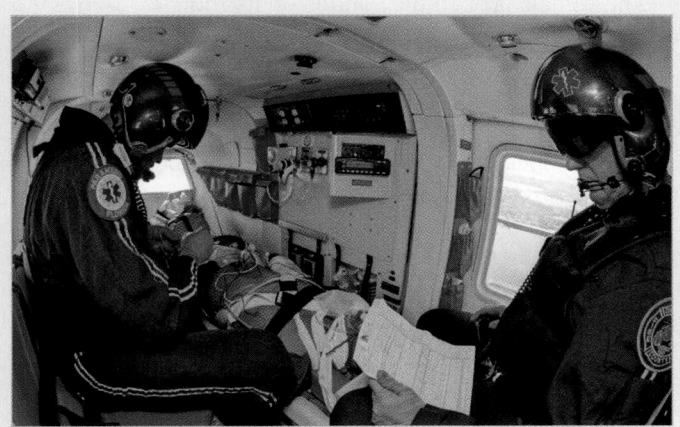

Figure 15-8 A patient's condition can change rapidly—especially if he or she is critically ill or injured. Monitor any changes to a patient's condition.

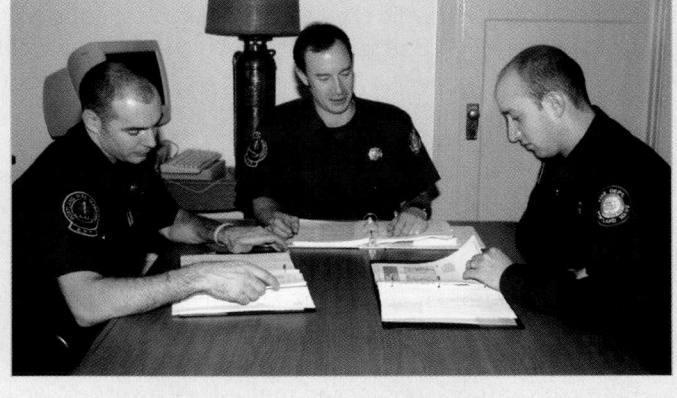

Figure 15-9 A formal review, or audit, of your performance can seem intimidating. However, it is also an opportunity for you to gain important feedback and improve yourself professionally.

Documentation and Communication

It is important not only to document procedures done and medications given but also what effect the procedure or medication had, if any.

In another scenario, let's say you are treating a 58-year-old man who experienced chest pain while moving some rocks to landscape his yard. Although he has no previous cardiac history, he is in the right age group for a heart problem to appear. When you ask him if he can pinpoint where the pain seems to be, he points to a spot on his chest directly over his heart. You continue down the same care plan.

Then you ask if anything makes the pain better or worse and the patient explains that if he holds his left arm still, the pain goes away. However, upon movement it hurts terribly in the area over his heart. This is key information, because you know that *the pain associated with a heart attack is not relieved by simply sitting still and not moving.* You now *revise your impression,* and focus your assessment on the possibility of a musculoskeletal injury, and your treatment plan and interventions change accordingly.

Instead of giving the patient aspirin, nitroglycerin, and high-flow oxygen to improve delivery of oxygen to a potentially infarcting heart, you now provide nitrous oxide for pain relief for an isolated musculoskeletal injury.

One of the key elements of this stage of the critical thinking process is to avoid *tunnel vision* and always keep your mind

In the Field

Tunnel vision, ie, seeing little and missing a lot—the demise of many paramedics.

open to all the possible causes of your patient's current condition. Your patient might be having a heart attack that presents in a way that is not in the textbooks. Reassess constantly.

Reflection on Action

The last stage in the critical thinking process occurs after the call is over and is commonly associated with run review or run critiques. This is the time when you look back at the total call and reflect on how you processed the signs and symptoms and reached the decisions that you did. One of the most difficult aspects of this stage is learning to say either, "I was wrong" or "I made a mistake." Both are difficult phrases for any health care provider to say, because none of us wants to make mistakes or ever be wrong. However, there is not a single health care provider who doesn't make a mistake every now and then.

In truth, you will periodically encounter patients with atypical presentations, or in other words, patients who just don't follow the textbook. For example, you may see a patient with a neck fracture who has no pain. Even though pain is the single best predictor of a possible spine injury, it is not an absolute predictor 100% of the time. To make an accurate diagnosis, you must also bring into play all that you have learned about communication and the ethical treatment of patients—your patient might come from a culture that denies having pain.

Reflection gives you the chance to continuously improve your thinking and decision making, and, in turn, your patient care as you modify your experience base. Always having a "learning attitude" makes every run you go on, every class you take, and every run review you attend an opportunity to improve yourself to provide better care for your patients **Figure 15-9 ▲**. When your call gets selected for a continuous quality improvement audit, look at it as an opportunity to have an outside reviewer look at your work in hopes that you continue to grow and improve in your practice. See it as a growth opportunity. Growth won't happen if you can't admit to your mistakes or if you are unwilling to learn. Never *ever* forget that the successful completion of the paramedic class is really just the starting point in your career as an ALS provider. To provide the best possible care requires that you make a commitment to a lifetime of learning. The most important trait for a lifetime career is a true desire to become better and better as a paramedic.

Let's review the fundamental elements of the critical thinking and decision-making process. As you look over each item on the following list, ask yourself, *"Do I have this quality already or do I need to develop it?"*

- Adequate fund of knowledge in anatomy and pathophysiology
- Ability to gather and organize data and form concepts
- Ability to focus on specific and multiple elements of data
- Ability to identify and deal with <u>medical ambiguity</u>— uncertainty regarding the specific cause of the patient's condition; few calls follow the scripts in your protocols
- Able to differentiate between relevant and irrelevant data
- Capable of analyzing and comparing similar situations
- Capable of analyzing and comparing contrary situations
- Ability to articulate your reasoning and construct arguments

From Theory to Practical Application

A number of factors come into play with every call, making each one unique to a certain degree. Consider the following:

You are dispatched to a "car off the road" involving a single car with four passengers that has spun off into a ditch at an estimated speed of 35 miles per hour. Think about how each of the following variables might change the call and how you might manage it:

- None of the passengers had on a seatbelt.
- The car was traveling at 65 miles per hour.

- The vehicle flipped over and is on its roof.
- It's 20°F outside and the crash was not discovered for at least an hour.

As you can see from the list, each variable change creates dozens of possible "new" outcomes, and as those possibilities increase, so does your challenge as a paramedic to manage the call and patient care properly.

Still in all, few of the calls you respond to on a day-to-day basis represent true life-threatening emergencies. That doesn't in any way imply that they are less important; just that they are less challenging.

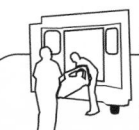

In the Field

Never be fooled by patients who initially appear uninjured or healthy. Never hesitate to do a thorough history and physical exam.

To focus yourself even further consider this:

- Minor medical and traumatic events require very little critical thinking, and as such, decision making is relatively easy.
- Patients with obvious life-threats pose limited critical thinking challenges, and again, simple decision making.
- Patients whose conditions fall somewhere around the midpoint on the spectrum between "no-big-deal" minor and "oh-my-gosh" serious pose the greatest critical thinking and decision-making challenges to you as a paramedic.

As we transition into the street application of this material, keep in mind that behind your patch you are just a person like anybody else, and because of that, you too have to deal with the impact of the "fight or flight" response when you are confronted with extreme cases that push *your* buttons (sensory overload).

You are the Provider Part 4

You are writing your patient care report when you hear the emergency department physician say, "Mrs. Jones, it appears that you are having a heart attack." Your heart drops as you realize you've made a big mistake. As the doctor passes by, he tells you the news and lets you know your call will be brought up in your department's monthly quality assurance/quality improvement review.

Reassessment	Recording Time: 20 Minutes
Skin	Slightly moist, pink, and warm
Pulse	94 beats/min, regular
Blood pressure	130/80 mm Hg
Respirations	30 breaths/min
Temperature	98.6°F (37°C)
ECG	Sinus rhythm

7. Do good paramedics make mistakes like this one?

8. How can a paramedic's attitude affect patient care?

9. What was done right in this call?

10. How could this mistake have been avoided?

The hormonal response has an impact on you both positively and negatively. On the positive side, you may have enhanced visual and auditory acuity as well as improved reflexes and muscle strength. On the negative side, you may have impaired critical thinking skills and diminished concentration and assessment abilities. One way to counter these negative effects is to improve your mental conditioning. Practice your skills until you can do them almost instinctively and can perform them on command, almost flawlessly, in the skills lab setting. Once you reach that level, you can draw on these skills in a real-life setting, allowing you to better focus on patient assessment or other decision-making areas.

Facilitate better thinking under pressure by memorizing the following mental checklist for all calls:

1. Take a moment to *scan the situation.*
2. Take another moment to *stop and think.*
3. *Make decisions and act* on behalf of the patient.
4. *Stay calm,* and maintain clear, concise *mental control.*
5. Plan to regularly and continually *reevaluate the patient.*

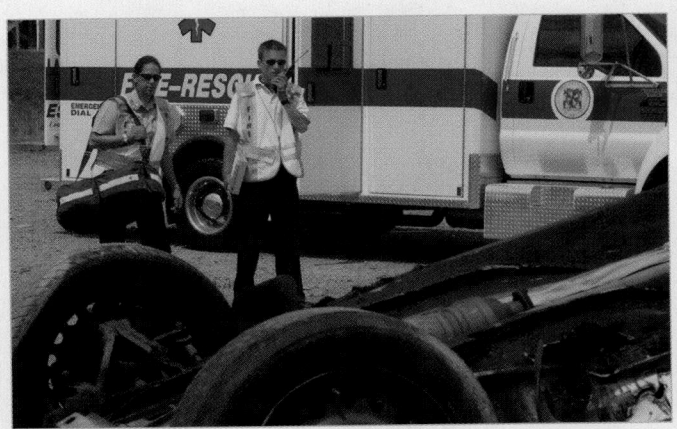

Figure 15-10 Although you need to focus on treating patients as soon as possible, always take a moment to register important information about the scene. What has happened that will help you assess each patient's condition?

Taking It to the Streets

Having now looked at the science side of critical thinking, let's transition to the practical side. When you are out on a call, critical thinking can be summed up with the *Six Rs.*

1. Read the Scene

The emergency scene is a relative goldmine of information readily available to you, if you are wise enough to mine it. Equally important to consider is that this information is *only* available at the scene and becomes unavailable once you initiate transport to the hospital. Some of the primary elements involved in reading the scene are: evaluating the overall safety of the situation, the environmental conditions, the immediate surroundings, access and exit issues, and finally evaluating the mechanism of injury Figure 15-10 ▶ . In particular, when you are looking at the mechanism of injury, take time to evaluate all aspects. For example, with a car crash look at the length of the skid marks or

> ### Notes from Nancy
> If you do not take a few moments to survey the scene . . . , you are very likely to become one of the casualties yourself. And a paramedic who is injured because he or she rocketed out of the ambulance without taking a good look around, will be of no benefit to the patient(s). Indeed, an injured paramedic just increases the number of victims that the remaining rescue personnel have to care for, and that will very likely detract from the care given to the other patients. The moral is: *Dead heroes can't save lives. Injured heroes are a nuisance,* so check the scene for hazards before you lurch in.

note whether there are none, what the vehicle struck, how much intrusion there is into the passenger compartment, and whether seatbelts were worn. In another example, the case of a fall, you would look for the height of a fall, how the patient landed, and what the patient landed on.

Other issues when you "read the scene" include assessing the environment in which the patient was found. Was it hot, cold, wet? Also, are there eyewitnesses or friends or family to provide additional information?

2. Read the Patient

Probably one of the greatest skills you can develop is learning to read a patient quickly. As you approach the patient, does the patient see you and track you with his or her eyes? Offer the patient your hand to shake, and introduce yourself and ask why 9-1-1 was called. If the patient takes your hand and answers you appropriately, you have just determined that the patient has a Glasgow Coma Scale score of 15 (spontaneous eye opening, follows commands, appropriate verbal response). Other components of effectively reading a patient include:

- **Observe** the patient. What's the patient's LOC and level of comfort or discomfort? Skin color? Position? Work of breathing? Any obvious deformity or asymmetry? Figure 15-11 ▶
- **Talk** to the patient. Determine the chief complaint. Is this a new problem or the worsening of a preexisting condition? Obtain the medical history and the history of the present problem.
- **Touch** the patient. What's the skin temperature and moisture level like? Assess the pulse rate, regularity, and strength.
- **Auscultate** lungs sounds. Confirm the adequacy or inadequacy of respirations and reassess the patency of the airway.
- **Identify** life threats. Correct any life threats relative to airway, breathing, and circulation in the order you find them.

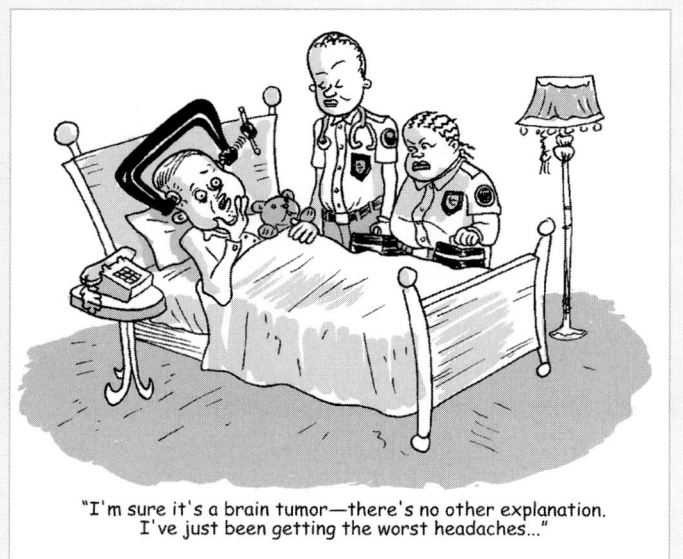

"I'm sure it's a brain tumor—there's no other explanation. I've just been getting the worst headaches..."

Figure 15-11

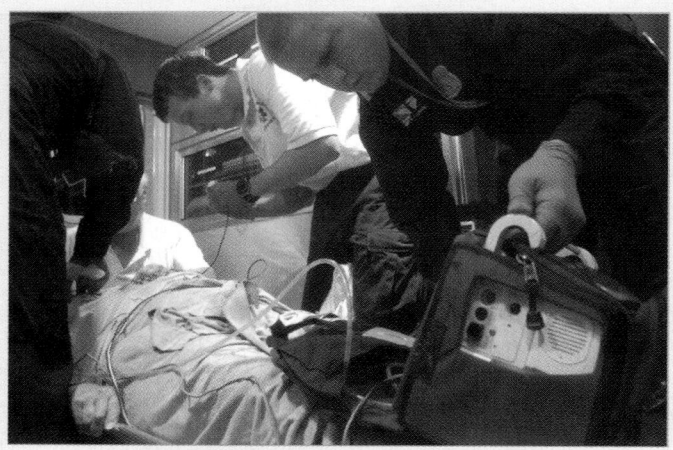

Figure 15-12 The more accurate your patient readings, the more reliable your diagnosis will be. Take the time to collect a set of baseline vital signs on every patient.

■ **Obtain** complete and accurate vital signs (Figure 15-12 ▲). For every patient, even for transfer patients, a baseline set of vital signs is a must. For patients with serious problems, two sets of vital signs provide comparative data. With critical patients, three or more sets of vital signs allow you to assess trends and to reassess whether the patient's condition is stabilizing, getting better, or getting worse. If your patient's condition is getting worse, multiple sets of vital signs provide some indication of how fast the patient's condition is deteriorating.

3. React

You must begin patient care by addressing life threats in the order you find them. Next, consider the worst-case scenario that

could be causing your patient's symptoms, and either rule it out or rule it in. After that, your primary focus should be to determine the most common and statistically probable cause for the patient's current condition. By addressing the worst-case scenario, you can try to avoid any catastrophes in patient care and then can take the time to look for less lethal problems.

If, at the end of your assessment, you haven't been able to develop a working diagnosis, it is acceptable to provide care based on the presenting signs and symptoms. If your patient is having difficulty breathing, you administer high-flow oxygen and place the patient in a position of comfort. For symptoms of shock, you elevate the feet, provide a cover for warmth, administer high-flow oxygen, and establish a large-bore IV line while you continue to try to search for the cause of the condition. When you put the limited physical and technical resources of the field up against the number of possible diagnoses a patient might have, you will find that you will regularly be treating patients who cannot be diagnosed until they reach the hospital. In some cases, the diagnosis may elude the doctor as well, so this is nothing to be ashamed of or worried about. It is simply a reality of medicine and has to be dealt with in a professional fashion.

4. Reevaluate

As patient care is continuing, another key element of good care is to make certain that you follow up on any interventions. See whether the splint you applied has eased the pain in your patient's injured leg. If you are treating frequent PVCs (premature ventricular contractions) with an antidysrhythmic medication, check the monitor to see whether the contractions have resolved. On challenging calls, once paramedics get into the treatment mode, they too often just focus on *doing things* and forget to see whether the *things they are doing* are actually improving the patient's situation.

As you reassess your patient, take the time to add any information you may have gathered from the detailed or focused physical examination and add it to the information you found in the initial assessment. Say you find that your patient has no breath sounds in the upper right lobes secondary to a fractured rib that caused a small pneumothorax. By itself, the small pneumothorax is not an immediate life threat to a relatively healthy individual. But let's say the patient also has bilateral fractured femurs, significant blood loss, and a minor head injury. Under those circumstances, a small pneumothorax may complicate matters far more than if it were the only condition. When you encounter patients, especially trauma patients, with multiple pathophysiologies, it is up to you to add them up as

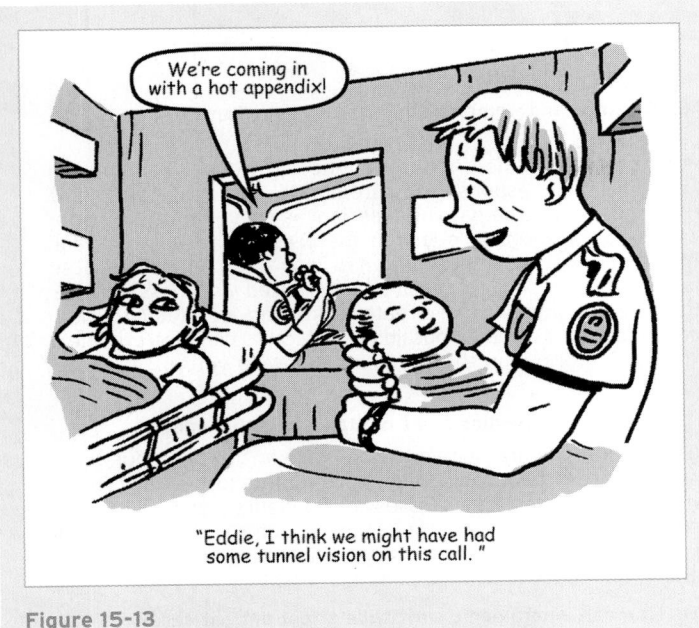

Figure 15-13

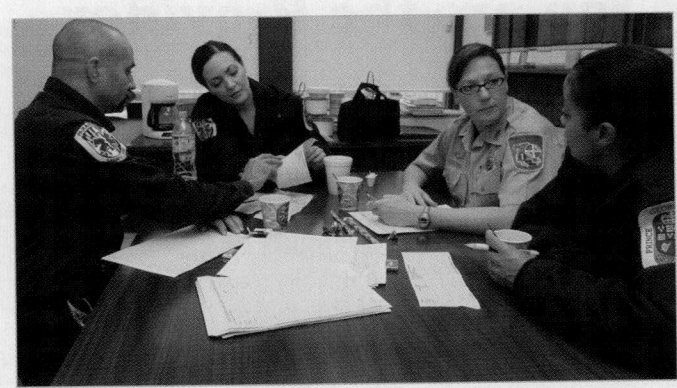

Figure 15-14 You will learn something new with every patient run. One of the best ways to review your performance—and to learn—is to talk it over with peers.

you develop your care plan to make sure nothing is overlooked that can be addressed in the field setting.

5. Revise the Plan

As you continue to care for your patient, you may get indications that what you once thought was a head injury is a problem secondary to glue sniffing; two very different causes. The thinking paramedic, no matter how sure he or she is of the working diagnosis, always keeps part of the thought process open to other possibilities Figure 15-13 ▲ . As other information becomes available as the call unfolds, you should always be prepared to change directions as necessary. By remaining mentally "light on your feet," you position yourself to be receptive to changing presentations or circumstances, which in turn helps you avoid tunnel vision.

6. Review Your Performance

Again, once a call is over, you as a provider have the opportunity to look back and reexamine your work Figure 15-14 ▶ . Whether this review is in the formal setting of a continuous

quality improvement (CQI) meeting or just back at the station reviewing the call with your partner, taking the time to critically look at your work allows you real growth opportunities. This is particularly true when you have made a mistake. While success is satisfying and certainly feels good, there is little growth opportunity to be had. However, when you make a mistake, take the time to analyze the call so that you can avoid repeating your behavior and making the same mistake. Mistakes will only change if you want to find out what they were, and why they recurred. Excellence in prehospital care is the gradual result of you as a provider constantly striving to improve your practice, which requires that you *always* have an attitude that is open to learning.

Being a thinking paramedic will only happen if you choose to work on your critical thinking skills throughout your career. As you continue to improve the way you think and make decisions, your patient care will improve as well. Your reward will be excellence in your practice—the ultimate job satisfaction.

You are the Provider Summary

1. When do you begin patient assessment?

Most people consider patient assessment to begin as early as the dispatch, but some would argue there is one step even before the dispatch. Fire departments are well-versed in the aspect of preplanning. They regularly inspect buildings in their response area to identify life, fire, and special hazards related to that structure. Good EMS providers know their primary service areas, and can use this information to add even further understanding to information that dispatchers provide regarding their patients. As a good paramedic, your antenna would go up when dispatched to a local orchard for difficulty breathing. Could your patient be suffering from anaphylaxis related to a bee sting or a respiratory emergency related to the inhalation of a pesticide?

2. What are the benefits and the risks of diagnosing based on dispatch?

Dispatchers are adept at gathering and distilling information from 9-1-1 callers. Dispatchers not only gather information, but calm callers, provide instructions, and send appropriate resources to a caller's location. Despite the dispatcher's best efforts, the information gained from callers may or may not be accurate. Oftentimes, this information gives you a good list of possible causes related to a patient's chief complaint, but it is very important to refrain from making a diagnosis. Information provided by the dispatcher should be used to see the big picture, where you can begin to determine whether other resources are likely to be necessary and discuss en route to the scene what role you and the other provider will play. The bottom line—generate a list of possible causes, but be flexible!

3. What are pertinent negatives?

Pertinent negatives are findings you would expect to see in a medical condition, but do not. If a paramedic suspects an infection, you would ask questions about the recent history of a productive cough, fever, or chills—all indicators of infection. If your patient denies having any of these signs and symptoms, you are faced with a pertinent negative—it is possible that your patient does not have an infection.

4. What information is missing from the above assessment?

Temperature can yield a wealth of information, particularly in this case. The presence or lack of fever can aid you in narrowing down your list of possible causes. All of your assessment tools aid you in narrowing your list of differential diagnoses.

5. How can a patient's opinion affect treatment and transport decisions?

Patients sometimes self-diagnose, although they are not trained to see what you can. Don't let a patient talk you into a different diagnosis. Of course, you will consider your patient's feelings and opinions but only in conjunction with your physical findings. Patients' feelings and opinions are important, but you make the final determination about treatment based on your training.

6. Can men and women have different symptoms of acute illness?

More and more is learned about the differences of men and women in their response to acute illness. In most classic heart attack scenarios, the patient experiences chest pain. This symptom is not required to question the presence of a myocardial infarction. Postmenopausal women may have only associated complaints of a sudden onset of generalized weakness, fatigue, dizziness, or shortness of breath. Obtaining an adequate medical history to include all possible risk factors can also provide a wealth of information to aid you in narrowing your list of possible causes.

7. Do good paramedics make mistakes like this one?

Yes. Because we are human, we all make mistakes. In our work, mistakes are not welcomed and may result in loss of life. This is why we must assess and reassess our patients and why we must strive to maintain our skills and improve our knowledge. The key is to learn from mistakes (both your mistakes and mistakes by others) and to try to avoid repeating them.

8. How can a paramedic's attitude affect patient care?

Because we are human, we can allow our personal feelings to affect patient care. This is not always a bad thing, but our personal attitudes should never have a negative impact on patient care. Being tired, hungry, or otherwise distracted is not your patient's concern. Your patient's needs come first, and second only to the safety of yourself and your crew.

9. What was done right in this call?

You erred on the side of the patient. Although you failed to adequately gather data about your patient's condition, you encouraged her to seek evaluation by a physician. Being genuinely concerned for the patient's well-being will oftentimes prevent poor patient care or outcomes. You also provided oxygen, established an IV, and placed her on the cardiac monitor. Your assessment and care, albeit incomplete, did have a positive effect. When reviewing calls, it is important to note what you do right as well as what you can improve on.

10. How could this mistake have been avoided?

For all calls, you should have a list of possible causes. Always be suspicious for serious, life-threatening conditions. Rule out the worst possible scenario. Don't make assumptions or be complacent or lazy. Every patient deserves a thorough assessment regardless of time of day or if your needs are or aren't being met at the time. It's also important to continue to read the latest in medical research. Medicine is an evolving field, and each year more is learned about the human body and its response to various treatments.

Prep Kit

■ Ready for Review

- The first cornerstone of your practice as a paramedic is having the ability to *gather, evaluate,* and *synthesize* information.
- Once you have gathered information, you must assess and evaluate this information as to its validity and the impact it will have on the patient care plan you are developing.
- Once you have evaluated the information you obtained from the scene, the patient, or any bystanders and determined what information is valid, then you need to process—or *synthesize*—that information.
- The second cornerstone of your practice is the *development and implementation of patient care plans*.
- Your care plan is almost always defined by the patient care protocols or standing orders in the EMS system where you work.
- The third cornerstone is *judgment and making independent decisions*.
- The fourth and final cornerstone of your practice is your ability to *think and work under pressure*.
- The first stage of the thought process in prehospital care is gathering information—things you see, hear, smell, or feel. This is *concept formation*.
- The second stage of the critical thinking process is data interpretation—evaluating the information you have gathered.
- The last stage in the critical thinking process occurs after the call is over and is commonly associated with run review or run critiques. Look back at the total call and reflect on how you processed the signs and symptoms and reached the decisions that you did.

- The *Six Rs* can be used to summarize what must be done on a call:
  - Read the scene
  - Read the patient
  - React
  - Reevaluate
  - Revise the plan
  - Review your performance
- Excellence in prehospital care results from a constant striving to improve your practice, which requires that you ALWAYS have an attitude that is open to learning.

■ Vital Vocabulary

concept formation Pattern of understanding based on initially obtained information.

cookbook medicine Treatment based on a protocol or algorithm without adequate knowledge of the patient being treated.

data interpretation The process of formulating a conclusion based on comparing the patient's condition with information from your training, education, and past experiences.

medical ambiguity Uncertainty regarding the specific cause of the patient's condition.

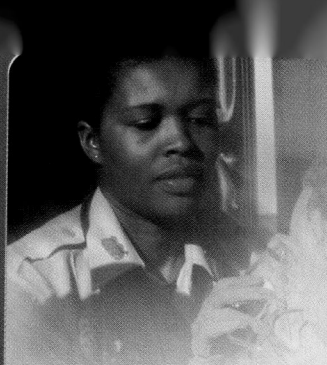

Assessment in Action

You are called to a scene where a 16-year-old male has had a seizure, is vomiting, and isn't making much sense to his family. By the time you get there, he is making a little more sense, and is no longer actively vomiting. The family tells you he came home from a party, began vomiting almost immediately, and had a mild seizure that lasted about a minute. He has not answered any of their questions, and they have no idea what he may have eaten or taken at the party.

1. **You introduce yourself to the family and the patient, and ask him how he is feeling. He doesn't answer. You tell him you'd really like to help him feel better, and need for him to answer your questions and be honest. You can see that his pupils are very dilated, he is sweating, and his face is very pale. He doesn't want to answer any of your questions, but does shake his head "no" when you ask if he drank or took any kind of drugs at the party. What do you do?**
   A. Continue with your evaluation as you normally would, in front of his family, despite his denial of having drunk alcohol or taken any drugs.
   B. Tell him you know he's lying based on what his body is telling you, and be confrontational until he tells you what he drank or took.
   C. Try to embarrass him in front of his family so he will tell you the truth.
   D. Continue your evaluation as normal, until you can get him in a private setting so that he may be more inclined to be honest because he is not in front of his family.

2. **In the back of your ambulance, the teen still denies having taken or drank anything. The symptoms he is experiencing tell you otherwise. What do you do?**
   A. Try to scare him by telling him that he will get much worse, and could even die, if he is not honest so you can treat him appropriately.
   B. Call medical control, give them all known information, and ask what you should do.
   C. Treat him based on what you *think* he may have taken, without confirmation from the patient himself.
   D. Take him to the hospital and let the doctor deal with him.

3. **In the back of the ambulance, the teenager admits to drinking some beer at the party. He says he is not on any medications, has no known allergies, has never had any type of seizure previously, and has never taken drugs. His pupils are still dilated, he is still somewhat confused, he is sweating and pale, and he is developing stomach cramps. He begins vomiting again, but does not smell like beer at all. He seems to be getting worse. He does not want to go to the hospital, and begs you not to tell his parents about the beer. What do you do?**
   A. Tell his parents you believe he may have a stomach virus, keeping his secret for him. After all, you were a teenager once too and have had your share of partying days.
   B. Tell his parents the truth—that you believe he has taken some kind of drug and that he needs to be taken to the emergency department for treatment, asking their permission to take him against his will for treatment.
   C. Honor the teenager's request to deny treatment, tell him what risks he is facing, and that you will be happy to return and take him to the emergency department if he changes his mind.
   D. Tell his parents nothing except that you are taking him to the hospital for evaluation and that he cannot refuse treatment because he has an altered mental status.

4. **While in the ambulance, your partner suggests the possibility that the teenager, based on his symptoms, is experiencing some kind of blood glucose issue. What do you do?**
   A. Consider this possibility and check the teenager's blood glucose level.
   B. Tell your partner that you are in charge, you've already made up your mind about what is wrong with the teenager, and that is that.
   C. Call medical control and ask if you should even consider any possibility of blood glucose issues.
   D. Tell your partner when he has the experience and knowledge that you have, he can make the decision.

5. **The patient's family is impatiently waiting outside your ambulance. His mother begins knocking on the door, then banging on it, insisting she know exactly what is being said and done to her son. She begins yelling and swearing that you are not doing your job right, she doesn't trust you, and she no longer wants you to treat her son. What do you do?**
   A. Send your partner out to calm her down, explaining that you are evaluating her son and doing what is best for him.
   B. Ignore her and continue to evaluate and treat her son.
   C. Explain to her how sick her son is, and that he must be treated based on his altered mental status, with or without her consent.
   D. Let her into the ambulance, apologize, explain what you are doing, what you believe is wrong, what you think will happen if he is not treated at all, and ask that she give her consent.

6. **If the young man mentioned in the above scenario had a rapidly deteriorating mental status (confusion that got worse and worse in a short amount of time) and other signs such as his breathing rate also deteriorated, how would this affect your evaluation and treatment?**
   A. It would not affect it; you would evaluate and treat him as you would in other questions listed above.
   B. You would panic, tell his parents the outlook was not good, and take him to the emergency department as quickly as possible.
   C. You would tell his parents that their son's condition was his own fault for drinking alcohol while under age or taking drugs, and he should have known better.
   D. You would consider it an ALS call, and treat all symptoms as they occurred on your way to the emergency department.

7. **What if the patient in the scenario became combative, stubborn, and mean, and insisted that you give him narcotic pain medication before you do anything else? What if he would not allow you to examine or otherwise treat him unless you did this first? You know he needs to go to the hospital, and that he has more problems than just the pain he is dealing with. What would you do?**
   A. Give him the pain medication to make him more cooperative, and to make your assessment, diagnosis, and treatment easier.
   B. Bribe him—tell him if he's cooperative for the evaluation and treatment, you will give him what he wants (even if you have no intention of doing so).
   C. Tell him that you work under a physician and have certain rules you must follow, which do not allow you to give him the pain medication he wants unless you do a full exam and diagnosis and your medical director allows it.
   D. Tell him that if he does not cooperate and let you do your job, you will tell his parents that you believe he has taken drugs, and may even get the police involved.

Challenging Questions

You are called to the home of an older man whose neighbors saw him walking around his house and yard late in the evening in his underwear, seeming confused. When you arrive, he does not answer his open front door. You walk in, calling his name, and take note of some small insulin syringes lying on the kitchen counter. You find him standing in the backyard, looking confused. When you introduce yourself and question him, he says he has no idea why he's in the backyard and had no idea he wasn't dressed. You note that he is also wearing a medical ID bracelet, but it does not have a condition listed on it. He asks you at least four times who you are, and why you're there. You ask him how he's feeling; he says he's fine. You ask him about his medical history, asking specifically if he is diabetic. He tells you he is not. But you know from neighbors that he lives alone. He is extremely confused and irrational.

8. **Do you listen to your patient's answers and put faith into them, assuming he knows what he is talking about, and try to assess and diagnose him based on that information? Or do you take into account his behavior and what you have seen (insulin syringes, medical ID bracelet), heard, and observed?**

9. **If the patient in this scenario were naked and began saying inappropriate things to your young female partner, how would you (and your partner) handle it?**

▬ Points to Ponder

You are dispatched to a "two-vehicle crash that occurred at a slow speed; minor or no injuries reported by bystander."

How should you prioritize this call?

Issues: Preparation, Priorities, Response Time to Scene.

16 Communications and Documentation

Objectives

Cognitive

3-5.1   Identify the importance of communications when providing EMS. (p 16.4)

3-5.2   Identify the role of verbal, written, and electronic communications in the provision of EMS. (p 16.4)

3-5.3   Describe the phases of communications necessary to complete a typical EMS event. (p 16.5)

3-5.4   Identify the importance of proper terminology when communicating during an EMS event. (p 16.4)

3-5.5   Identify the importance of proper verbal communications during an EMS event. (p 16.5)

3-5.6   List factors that impede effective verbal communications. (p 16.11, 16.16)

3-5.7   List factors which enhance verbal communications. (p 16.11)

3-5.8   Identify the importance of proper written communications during an EMS event. (p 16.17)

3-5.9   List factors which impede effective written communications. (p 16.20)

3-5.10   List factors which enhance written communications. (p 16.20)

3-5.11   Recognize the legal status of written communications related to an EMS event. (p 16.4)

3-5.12   State the importance of data collection during an EMS event. (p 16.5)

3-5.13   Identify technology used to collect and exchange patient and/or scene information electronically. (p 16.6)

3-5.14   Recognize the legal status of patient medical information exchanged electronically. (p 16.11, 16.12)

3-5.15   Identify the components of the local EMS communications system and describe their function and use. (p 16.6)

3-5.16   Identify and differentiate among the following communications systems:
  a. Simplex
  b. Multiplex
  c. Duplex
  d. Trunked
  e. Digital communications
  f. Cellular telephone
  g. Facsimile
  h. Computer (p 16.5, 16.7–16.9)

3-5.17   Identify the components of the local dispatch communications system and describe their function and use. (p 16.9)

3-5.18   Describe the functions and responsibilities of the Federal Communications Commission. (p 16.7, 16.10)

3-5.19   Describe how an EMS dispatcher functions as an integral part of the EMS team. (p 16.14)

3-5.20   List appropriate information to be gathered by the Emergency Medical Dispatcher. (p 16.15)

3-5.21   Identify the role of Emergency Medical Dispatch in a typical EMS event. (p 16.5)

3-5.22   Identify the importance of pre-arrival instructions in a typical EMS event. (p 16.5)

3-5.23   Describe the purpose of verbal communication of patient information to the hospital. (p 16.13)

3-5.24   Describe information that should be included in patient assessment information verbally reported to medical direction. (p 16.14)

3-5.25   Diagram a basic model of communications. (p 16.10)

3-5.26   Organize a list of patient assessment information in the correct order for electronic transmission to medical direction according to the format used locally. (p 16.14)

3-6.1   Identify the general principles regarding the importance of EMS documentation and ways in which documents are used. (p 16.17)

3-6.2   Identify and use medical terminology correctly. (p 16.18)

3-6.3   Recite appropriate and accurate medical abbreviations and acronyms. (p 16.19)

3-6.4   Record all pertinent administrative information. (p 16.19)

3-6.5   Explain the role of documentation in agency reimbursement. (p 16.18)

3-6.6   Analyze the documentation for accuracy and completeness, including spelling. (p 16.17)

3-6.7   Identify and eliminate extraneous or nonprofessional information. (p 16.11, 16.12)

3-6.8   Describe the differences between subjective and objective elements of documentation. (p 16.4)

3-6.9   Evaluate a finished document for errors and omissions. (p 16.19, 16.20)

3-6.10   Evaluate a finished document for proper use and spelling of abbreviations and acronyms. (p 16.19, 16.20)

3-6.11   Evaluate the confidential nature of an EMS report. (p 16.20)

3-6.12   Describe the potential consequences of illegible, incomplete, or inaccurate documentation. (p 16.20, 16.22)

3-6.13   Describe the special considerations concerning patient refusal of transport. (p 16.20, 16.21)

3-6.14   Record pertinent information using a consistent narrative format. (p 16.19)

3-6.15   Explain how to properly record direct patient or bystander comments. (p 16.20)

3-6.16   Describe the special considerations concerning mass casualty incident documentation. (p 16.21)

3-6.17   Apply the principles of documentation to computer charting, as access to this technology becomes available. (p 16.22)

3-6.18   Identify and record the pertinent, reportable clinical data of each patient interaction. (p 16.19)

3-6.19   Note and record "pertinent negative" clinical findings. (p 16.20)

3-6.20   Correct errors and omissions, using proper procedures as defined under local protocol. (p 16.21)

3-6.21   Revise documents, when necessary, using locally approved procedures. (p 16.21)

3-6.22   Assume responsibility for self-assessment of all documentation. (p 16.20)

3-6.23   Demonstrate proper completion of an EMS event record used locally. (p 16.20)

Affective

3-5.27   Show appreciation for proper terminology when describing a patient or patient condition. (p 16.18)

3-6.24   Advocate among peers the relevance and importance of properly completed documentation. (p 16.17)

3-6.25   Resolve the common negative attitudes toward the task of documentation. (p 16.20)

Psychomotor

3-5.28   Demonstrate the ability to use the local dispatch communications system. (p 16.5)

3-5.29   Demonstrate the ability to use a radio. (p 16.6)

3-5.30   Demonstrate the ability to use the biotelemetry equipment used locally. (p 16.7)

Introduction

In EMS communication, relaying information from one person to another becomes extremely urgent in the short time that you will have to care for a patient. That information needs to move rapidly, efficiently, and effectively. As a paramedic, you must be able to effectively communicate verbally and in writing with many other people.

You need to know what constitutes an EMS communications system, who needs to be able to talk with whom, what technical resources are available to you to make those conversations possible, and what you can do to make communications as efficient as possible. You also need to understand the crucial role of the emergency medical dispatcher (EMD) in facilitating all phases of EMS communications. You need to know how to organize patient information into a brief, orderly verbal report that can be transmitted by radio or by telephone.

Written communication in the form of reports or documentation is as vital to your patient care as following local medical protocols. Learning to write effectively and accurately with only the absolutely necessary subjective information is an important paramedic skill. Subjective information includes the symptoms patients describe—the degree of pain, for example. Objective information includes the measurable signs that you observe and record, such as blood pressure. You must record subjective *and* objective information and the details of patient care for every call in a written or computer-based report, and in some cases, both. This report needs to be complete, accurate, and legible because it can provide the basis of defense in legal proceedings and is of vital importance to your service or agency for many other reasons as well, including facilitation of quality care, continuity, and billing insurance. Your written report should "paint a picture" of the entire call that is clear and accurate to the reader.

Phases of Communication

Communication during an emergency call has several phases that are essential to appropriate patient care and transportation. You will be exchanging information with many people, including the patient, bystanders with valuable information, the patient's family, medical control, the receiving medical facility staff, your dispatch center, law enforcement officials, and other members of the EMS team. One paramount responsibility in an emergency is communication with your partner. Staying in constant touch will keep each of you on top of your responsibilities and working effectively as a team while caring for your patient.

Each phase of the communication process requires using terminology understood by the people you are communicating with. Patients might need you to explain their medical condition in terms they know and understand. When you relay information to the receiving medical facility, you can use the medical terminology you have learned to make your radio report clear. The old saying, "When in Rome, do as the Romans do," applies in EMS. Using medical terminology and avoiding slang terms shows your professionalism and respect for everyone you work with.

Although you might not think of yourself as a "number-crunching" scholar, collecting information and data is essential to EMS. You can help gather the data, analyze it, and determine what changes are necessary by writing clear, accurate, and easy-to-read reports. Although data collection may

You are the Provider Part 1

It is a beautiful summer day when you and your partner are dispatched to a bicycle collision at 1277 Cochran Mill Road. On arrival, you are greeted by a bystander who tells you that during his usual afternoon walk he found a woman lying next to the trail. He said he was worried she had been hit by a car or was otherwise injured, so he didn't move her and immediately called 9-1-1.

You find a 45-year-old woman lying on the ground and unresponsive. Her bike is lying on top of her, and she is wearing a helmet, bike shorts, and a T-shirt.

Initial Assessment	Recording Time: 0 Minutes
Appearance	Pale, obviously diaphoretic
Level of consciousness	U (Unresponsive)
Airway	Open; secretions present
Breathing	Noisy breathing present; secretions present
Circulation	Rapid radial pulse present

1. Why did the dispatcher supply very little information for this call?
2. What immediate challenges do you foresee regarding this call?
3. How does the initial information you're given from dispatchers, family, bystanders, or other responders impact your decisions regarding patient care?

seem time-consuming, ensure that the information you record and report to your EMS agency is accurate for data collection, billing, and reporting purposes. Even in cases of multiple-casualty incidents (MCIs), collecting data is especially essential for determining patient care totals, severity of injuries, outcomes, and mass care procedures.

Who Needs to Communicate With Whom?

For the EMS system to work, a number of people have to be able to contact a number of other people. Let's follow an emergency call from its inception to its conclusion to see who needs to reach whom.

The first stage of the EMS response is notification, that is, someone has to tell EMS that an emergency exists. Usually notification is carried out by telephone or cellular phone, and the person requesting help communicates with the emergency medical dispatcher (EMD). A universal emergency telephone number—9-1-1 in the United States—and the availability of telephones and cellular phones in most places has greatly helped notification. Notification may, less frequently, come by radio, when the emergency is detected by a law enforcement or other public vehicle.

The next step is dispatch, communicating from the service headquarters with the responding paramedic team. The person who directs that team to the scene of the emergency is called the dispatcher Figure 16-1 ▾ . Dispatch may be accomplished by telephone, pager, fax, or two-way radio that may include push-to-talk technology. Push-to-talk devices can include mobile phones or walkie-talkies known as half-duplex devices. These allow the voice to be transmitted when a button is pushed and allow the listener to hear if the button is released. Most telecommunications equipment today uses digital technology rather than direct or analogue transmission and radio tubes. Digital technology offers many advantages in terms of speed, privacy, programmability, and the global positioning system, or GPS. Many dispatch centers use computer-aided

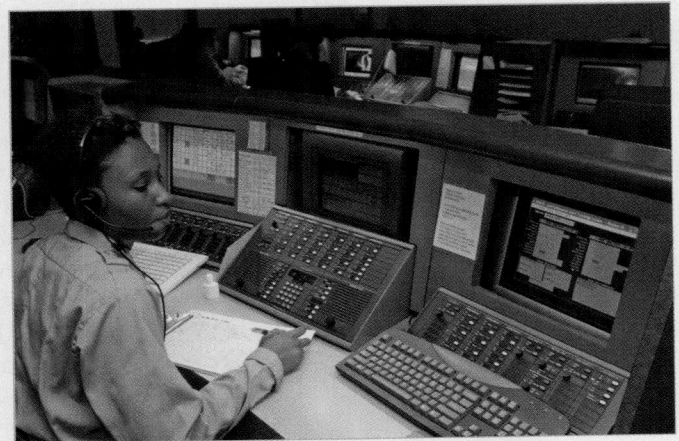

Figure 16-1 The dispatcher receives the call to 9-1-1 and dispatches EMS to the scene.

dispatch systems, automated computer systems that process the information received and assist dispatchers with multiple functions and tasks.

Your dispatcher may have to speak with you en route to give you additional information about the call. You may need to request other resources, such as police, fire, hazardous materials, or another specialty rescue unit. Communications between you and the dispatcher are usually carried out by mobile (in the vehicle) or portable (in your hand) radios. Cellular telephones may also be used for that purpose provided coverage is available.

Your service might require special training in emergency medical dispatch procedures, which means your dispatchers may be able to provide basic medical instructions to callers who are able to provide basic first aid steps while you are on your way. Some dispatch centers have trained EMS providers to relay basic medical instructions to callers when needed. Such prearrival instructions give your service what many in EMS call "zero response time," providing immediate aid and assistance, which can be vital in saving a life. Simple but lifesaving acts such as clearing an obstructed airway, performing chest compressions, or reassuring the patient can be carried out by a layperson under the instructions of a good dispatcher. In many cases, these prearrival instructions may bring a sense of emotional support to a caller in a time of great need, reassuring people close to the patient that everything that can be done is being done and actively getting the caller to perform lifesaving tasks.

Your dispatcher can give you prearrival information that will keep you on top of events as they are unfolding, with updates on the situation and your patient while you are en route.

Once you are at the scene, communications among you, the receiving facility, and your medical control are necessary to allow physician orders for invasive procedures to be transmitted and to coordinate the care of your patient. Your medical control physician can receive any required telemetry for patient assessment. In the early years, it was a common practice for paramedics to send electrocardiograms (ECGs) to medical control. For a time, the transmission of a lead II ECG was discontinued in most communities because of competition for the air waves, and medical control physicians let paramedics work under more expanded standing orders. Since the American Heart Association recommendation in the year 2000 that a 12-lead ECG be taken and transmitted to the receiving facility for all patients with potential acute coronary syndrome, the use of telemetry has returned. In some services, a facsimile or fax of the ECG is transmitted directly by cellular phone to the coronary catheterization laboratory to help the staff determine the best treatment, preparing for fibrinolytic therapy or a catheterization procedure.

Communication with the physician in charge, whether by voice or telemetry, can require two-way radios, a telephone patch (telephone-to-radio connection), cellular telephones, or facsimile capabilities.

Once your patient is ready to be moved, you must communicate with the receiving facility to let the hospital know what to

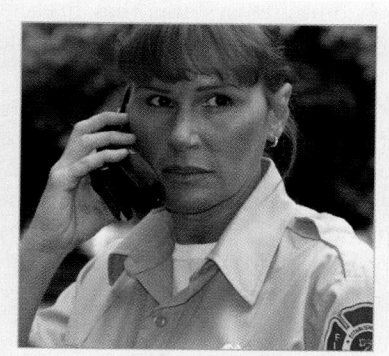

Figure 16-2 Use of cellular phones is becoming more common in EMS communications systems.

expect. Once again, most ambulance-to-hospital communications are by radio, but cellular telephones also have an increasingly important role Figure 16-2 ◂ . Computer-based transmissions are also becoming more widely used. Some services have wireless systems that transmit the data in the prehospital care report (PCR) to the emergency department (ED) as the ambulance is pulling into the hospital's parking lot. Once back at their station, these lucky paramedics transmit the billing and patient profile to the service's computer as the ambulance pulls into the garage. The bill is sent to the insurance company before the crew actually steps out of the ambulance!

These communications links are essential to ensure an efficient response to an emergency call. However, a complete EMS communications system requires a few other components as well:

- It is highly desirable to link all area hospitals into the communications network. In case of a disaster, multiple casualties may be appropriately distributed and hospitals may be informed of the number of patients they will be receiving. Interhospital communications can be carried out by telephone networks, by radio, or through computer-based programs. Some hospitals now participate in regional programs that allow hospital bed availability to be displayed on a computer screen and shared in case of diversion and overcrowding issues.
- Other agencies that may be involved in an emergency response (police, fire, public utilities, helicopter services, poison centers) should be able to communicate with one another. Cellular technology has made such communications much more accessible, but a backup radio network is still desirable in case telephone lines and frequencies become overloaded during an MCI. Satellite phones, which often work when the cellular system is down, are an additional tool an EMS provider may have available to assist in communicating during a disaster. Coordination of such systems should be done well in advance of a disaster and tested periodically to ensure the system will work.
- Finally, it is important, especially in disasters, to be aware of other broadcast systems that may be recruited to assist in communications within the community:
  1. The Amateur Radio Public Service Corps (ARPSC) may be available in your community. If so, it should be involved in planning for disaster communications. The Radio Amateur Civil Emergency Services (RACES) is another group that can be of assistance.

  2. Even in areas where there is no organized amateur radio service, it is useful for the EMS dispatcher to monitor channel 9 on the Citizen's Band (CB) frequency, the channel reserved for emergency communications (or other channels, such as channel 15 for marine emergencies, where applicable).
  3. Finally, managers of commercial broadcast services (radio and television) should be assigned specific communications responsibilities in the event of a disaster.

■ Components of an EMS Communications System

Even though the digital revolution will improve communications, most EMS communications systems today are based on the use of radios, so you need to learn about what radio signals are and what equipment is available for sending and receiving radio signals.

Radio Communications and Telemetry

Radio transmits signals by electromagnetic waves. Remember, energy can be emitted in the form of waves or particles. When energy is emitted in the form of waves, the energy can be characterized by the length of the waves it produces. Energy of a relatively long wavelength produces audible sound; energy of shorter wavelength is in the infrared light spectrum. Between sound and infrared light are the wavelengths for radio transmission. Radio wavelengths are used for tuning by adjusting your radio to the proper frequency—how frequently the wave recurs in a given time (usually 1 second). Short wavelengths are repeated more often—with higher frequency—than longer wavelengths. Radio frequencies are designated by their cycles per second, or hertz (Hz) (named for the man who first described the propagation of electromagnetic waves). The following abbreviations are commonly used:

- hertz (Hz)—cycles per second
- kilohertz (kHz)—1,000 cycles per second
- megahertz (MHz)—1 million cycles per second
- gigahertz (GHz)—1 billion cycles per second

Radio waves are confined to the part of the electromagnetic frequency spectrum extending from 3 kHz to about 3,000 GHz. A normal voice channel requires a minimum of 3 kHz. Frequency bands are portions of the radio frequency spectrum assigned for specific uses. The most commonly used bands for medical communications are the very high frequency (VHF) band and the ultrahigh frequency (UHF) band. The VHF band extends from roughly 30 to 175 MHz and has been arbitrarily divided into a low band (30 to 50 MHz) and a high band (150 to 175 MHz). The low-band frequencies may have ranges up to 2,000 miles but are unpredictable because changes in ionospheric conditions may cause "skip interference," with patchy losses in communication. The high-band frequencies are almost wholly free of skip interference, but at a price—a much shorter transmission range. The most commonly used of the VHF high-band frequencies for emergency medical purposes are in the 150 to 160 MHz range. The UHF band extends from 300 to 3,000 MHz, with most medical communications occurring around 450 to 470 MHz. At these frequencies, communications are entirely free of skip interference and have minimal noise (signal distortion). The UHF band has better penetration in dense metropolitan areas, and UHF reception is usually quite adequate inside buildings. The UHF band, however, has a shorter range than the VHF band, and energy at UHF is more readily absorbed by rain and environmental objects, such as trees and brush.

Radios that operate at 800 MHz are common in EMS systems. This frequency offers excellent penetration of buildings and has minimal interference and reduced channel noise. Because of this, it works quite well in metropolitan areas; 800 MHz also allows for trunking, in which multiple agencies or systems can share frequencies. An 800-MHz radio can also be linked to a computer system to transmit voiceless communications. The use of trunked systems has allowed the dispatcher to reprogram the radios so that agencies that do not routinely talk to each other can easily do so at the scene of a mass-casualty incident, a rescue, a hazardous materials incident, or other special operations.

The Federal Communications Commission (FCC), which controls frequency allocation in the United States, has set aside medical VHF band assignments for general emergency radio communications and UHF band assignments for ambulance-to-hospital telemetry systems, especially where communications from physicians to rescue personnel are needed to consult or direct patient care activities. Those band assignments will be given to you by your EMS system.

Biotelemetry

Biotelemetry (usually called simply telemetry) is the capability of measuring vital life signs and transmitting them to a distant terminal. Biotelemetry started out with ECGs but often is used for other measurements. Even the United States space program uses telemetry to send the pulse and respiratory rate of astronauts from space to a receiving station on earth.

The term *biotelemetry* in emergency medical care is usually shortened to *telemetry*. Most often, telemetry is a short way of saying you are transmitting an ECG signal from your patient to a distant receiving station. The standard ECG is composed of low-frequency signals (100 Hz or less), which would be filtered out by a voice communications system. To make sure voice communication doesn't filter the ECG out, the ECG signal must be encoded if it is to be sent over the same radio channels used to transmit voice. The ECG signal is encoded by using a reference audio tone, for example at 1,000 Hz, which is made to vary with the voltage generated by the electric events in the heart. The reference tone, or calibration, of a varying 1,000-Hz tone is used to modulate the frequency of the transmitter to ensure that all signals are being transmitted. When the ECG signal is received at the distant terminal at the receiving hospital or medical control, it is amplified and decoded to produce a voltage that is an exact replica of the original. That voltage is then converted to the graphic plot seen on the oscilloscope or printout.

ECG telemetry over UHF frequencies is confined to one lead of a 12-lead ECG, so it can be used to interpret cardiac rhythms. For a more complete diagnosis of an ECG, such as in the case of examining the ECG of a patient with suspected acute coronary syndrome, one must examine all 12 leads of the ECG. Some EMS systems use facsimile technology to allow transmission of ECGs, including 12-lead ECGs, to receiving hospitals before the arrival of the ambulance at the facility.

Distortion of the ECG signal by extraneous spikes and waves is known as noise and may arise from a variety of sources:

- Muscle tremor
- Loose ECG electrodes
- Sources of 60-cycle alternating current (AC), such as transformers, power lines, and electric equipment
- Attenuation (reduction) of transmitter power, caused by weak batteries or transmission beyond the range of the transmitter

ECG telemetry, begun in Miami, Florida, by Eugene Nagel, MD, during the early 1970s, had a very important role in establishing the paramedic profession—it made it possible for doctors in the hospital to supervise paramedics caring for patients in the field. It was the technical feasibility of such supervision that convinced the medical community and the public to accept the idea of paramedics carrying out procedures such as defibrillation and administration of cardiac drugs, and many states made it mandatory for all ALS units to have telemetry capabilities.

In the past several years, as paramedics have become more and more skilled in dysrhythmia recognition, the trend has been to make less and less use of ECG telemetry; rather, most systems rely solely on the paramedic's assessment of the patient's cardiac rhythm and rarely require confirmation of the assessment by a physician. Just as ECG telemetry seemed headed for the fate of the horse-drawn ambulance, however, two developments occurred to bring about a reassessment of prehospital ECG telemetry. First, conclusive research on the use of fibrinolytic agents indicated that the earlier the agents were given during an acute myocardial infarction, the better the chances of myocardial reperfusion. Second, cellular telephone and facsimile technology made it possible to transmit a 12-lead ECG from a moving ambulance to a hospital and, therefore, to diagnose myocardial infarction before the patient reaches the hospital. At the least, such early diagnosis enables the hospital to gear up for administration of fibrinolytic therapy immediately as the patient arrives; and in some EMS systems, the fibrinolytics are actually administered in the prehospital setting. Because technology can facilitate assessment and treatment in the prehospital setting, it is probable that telemetry in one form or another will remain a part of emergency care for some time. Information other than ECGs may also be transmitted to the receiving hospital before the patient arrives. Because advancements in technology are occurring rapidly, EMS systems must keep up with the technology that will allow better methods for communication of patient information.

Cellular Telephones

Cellular telephones operate on 3 W of power or less. Mobile antennas are much closer to the ground than base station antennas, so communications from the unit are typically limited to 10 to 15 miles over average terrain. Base station antennas are usually located on high sites to increase the coverage area.

Cellular telephones are becoming more common in EMS communications systems. These telephones are simply low-power portable radios that communicate through a series of interconnected repeater stations called "cells" (hence the name "cellular"). Cells are linked by a sophisticated computer system and connected to the telephone network. Cellular telephones are also popular with other public safety agencies, particularly as more cell sites are constructed in rural areas.

Cell phones have advantages that radio does not: (1) The public is encouraged to make use of the free service for 9-1-1 or other emergency numbers. (2) Cell phone technology incorporates GPS to let emergency responders know where the patient is.

Many cellular systems make equipment and air time available to EMS services at little or no cost as a public service. The public is often able to call 9-1-1 or other emergency numbers on a cellular telephone free of charge. However, this easy access may result in overloading and jamming of cellular systems in MCI and disaster situations, and you should have a backup communications plan in your service to circumvent these overloads.

Most newer cell phones have GPSs built in specifically for emergencies. (It is possible to turn off GPS in a cellular phone but not for EMS). The so-called enhanced 9-1-1 helps the EMS operator know exactly where the cell call is being placed from. In the past, when a cell phone call was made by a patient who drove off the road, rescuers would need to search blindly because many patients became unconscious or did not know their location. Many vehicles also have vehicle locator and navigation systems that notify emergency services when a collision has occurred. These, too, are based on GPS technology. Typically, these cell phone calls for emergency services may go through a routing center rather than directly to the local dispatch center. The 9-1-1 cellular calls often go through a regional or statewide agency such as the state police. The National Emergency Number Association estimates that more than 75% of the nation's population resides in areas where wireless 9-1-1 services deliver the caller's call-back number and location to the appropriate public safety answering point.

▋Modes of Radio Operation

Assigned radio frequencies may be used in a variety of systems. In a simplex system, portable units can transmit only in one mode (voice or telemetry) or receive (voice) at any given time. A simplex system requires only a single radio frequency. A network that uses two different frequencies at the same time, to permit simultaneous transmission and reception (like a telephone), is referred to as duplex. Another alternative is to combine, or multiplex, two or more signals—such as the paramedic's voice and the patient's ECG—for simultaneous transmission on one frequency.

You are the Provider Part 2

You see that additional assistance will be required to extricate the patient from her bike, and you request it. An engine crew is dispatched from a nearby fire station. You and your partner err on the side of caution and initiate spinal precautions. Your partner controls the patient's cervical spine while you manage the airway.

Fire fighters quickly arrive and extricate the patient and place her on the backboard. You next insert an intravenous (IV) line, and, per local protocol, perform a blood glucose check. No trauma is noted beyond a few minor abrasions to her right arm, shoulder, and leg.

Vital Signs	Recording Time: 5 Minutes
Level of consciousness	Unresponsive, with a Glasgow Coma Scale score of 5
Skin	Pale, cool, and diaphoretic
Pulse	128 beats/min, strong and regular
Blood pressure	132/86 mm Hg
Respirations	22 breaths/min
Sao$_2$	92% ambient air

4. How did this call change from dispatch to arrival?

5. Given her level of consciousness, what concerns do you have regarding her airway?

6. What are your top priorities at the moment?

Suppose that an ambulance service wanted the possibility of voice communications and continuous telemetry. There are at least four ways to design the communications system to meet those requirements:

- The ambulance could transmit on two frequencies of a UHF-frequency pair (channel) allocated for telemetry (duplex). One frequency would transmit the voice signal and the other, the telemetry signal. Such a system requires that the ambulance have two UHF transmitters (one for voice, one for telemetry) and one receiver (voice).
- The ambulance service could multiplex (combine) telemetry and voice on one frequency of the allocated UHF pair and receive voice communications on the other frequency of the pair. That requires only one UHF transmitter on the vehicle, but the base station must be fitted with demultiplexing equipment to separate the two signals coming in on one frequency.
- The ambulance could transmit telemetry data on one frequency of the allocated telemetry pair and transmit voice data on a VHF frequency. That requires a UHF and a VHF transmitter on the vehicle (two simplex systems).
- As noted, there is an increasing trend toward using cellular telephones for ECG telemetry. Cellular phones have full duplex capability, a multitude of available channels, a very high-quality signal that is unlikely to degrade over distance, and a much lower capital and maintenance cost.

Building Blocks of a Communications System

Although EMS communications systems vary considerably among one another, most systems serving moderate to large populations are constructed of the following components.

Base Stations

The base station is a collection of radio equipment consisting, at minimum, of a transmitter, receiver, and antenna. The base station serves as a dispatch and coordination area and ideally should be in contact with all other elements of the system. Base stations generally use relatively high power output (45 to 275 W); the maximum allowable power is determined by the FCC and printed on the station's license.

The base station must be equipped with an antenna sited in suitable terrain, preferably on a hill or high building, close to the base. The antenna system has a vital part in transmission and reception efficiency. A good antenna system can compensate for FCC limits on power output and human-made signal distortion in the area.

Mobile Transmitter/Receivers (Transceivers)

A mobile transmitter/receiver, or mobile transceiver, is a two-way radio mounted in a vehicle. Mobile transmitter/receivers come in a variety of power ranges, and the power output largely determines the distance over which the signal can be effectively transmitted. A transmitter in the 7.5 W range, for example, will transmit for distances of 10 to 12 miles over

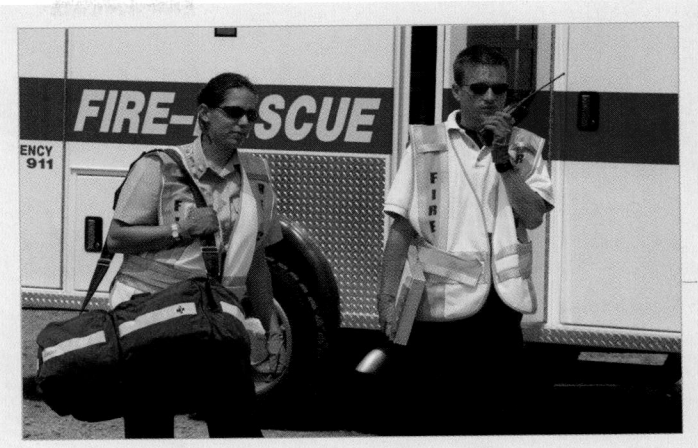

Figure 16-3 A portable radio is essential if you need to communicate with the dispatcher or medical control when you are away from the ambulance.

slightly hilly terrain. Transmission distances are greater over water or flat terrain and reduced in mountainous areas or where there are many tall buildings. Mobile transmitters with higher outputs have proportionally greater transmission ranges. Today, the typical mobile transmitter operates at between 20 and 50 W.

Portable Transmitter/Receivers

Portable, hand-held radios are useful when paramedics must work at a distance from their vehicle but need to stay in communication with the base or with one another Figure 16-3. Portable units may also be used by physician consultants when not stationed at the hospital. Portable units usually have power outputs of up to 5 W and, thus, have limited range by themselves, although the signal of a hand-held transmitter can be boosted by retransmission through the vehicle.

Repeaters

A repeater is a miniature base station used to extend the transmitting and receiving range of a telemetry or voice communications system Figure 16-4. Repeaters may be stationary in one location (fixed repeaters) or carried in emergency vehicles (mobile repeaters). A repeater picks up a weak signal and retransmits it at a higher power on another frequency, so it extends the range of low-power portables and allows more members of the system to hear one another. This is how the trooper on the side of the state highway can talk to a supervisor on the other end of the state.

Remote Consoles

A remote console, usually located in the ED of a hospital, is a terminal that receives transmissions of telemetry and voice from the field and transmits messages back, usually through the base station. Remote consoles are connected to the base station by dedicated telephone lines, microwave, or radio. They contain an amplifier and speaker for incoming voice reception, a decoder

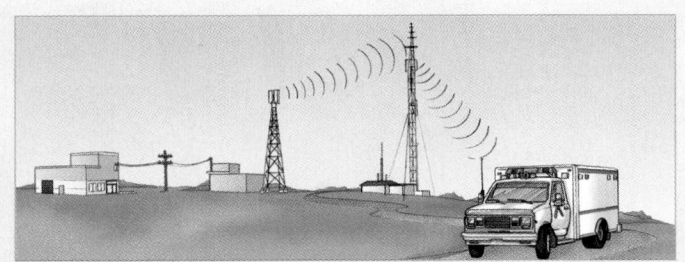

Figure 16-4 A message is sent from the control center by a landline to the transmitter. The radio carrier wave is picked up by the repeater for rebroadcast to outlying units. Return radio traffic is picked up by the repeater and rebroadcast to the control center.

for translating the telemetry signal into an oscilloscope tracing or printout, and a microphone for voice transmission.

Backup Communications Systems

In addition to radio communications, most systems use land-line (telephone) backup to link various fixed components of the system, such as hospitals, public safety services, and poison control. Telephones may also be patched into radio transmissions through the base station, enabling, for example, communication between paramedics using radios in the field and a physician using his or her telephone at home. Finally, as mentioned earlier, cellular telephones are becoming an increasingly important part of EMS communications, overcoming many of the problems of overcrowded EMS radio frequencies. Cellular phones are cheaper than radios and generally give a much clearer signal. Furthermore, they enable a paramedic in the field to communicate with anyone who has a telephone—the patient's family physician, an injured child's parent, an expert in another state who can advise on a hazardous materials situation. The possibilities are as varied as the listings in the telephone directory.

▌Communicating by Radio

The effectiveness of an EMS communications network depends on the technical hardware and on the people who use it. Communicating effectively by radio under emergency conditions requires skill and experience. Some paramedics "freeze" at the microphone, whereas others find themselves acting out their latent ambitions as disk jockeys with unlimited streams of patter. Neither behavior is appropriate or useful. Effective radio communication in EMS requires knowledge of the rules that govern the communications and an understanding of conven-

Notes from Nancy
The purpose of talking on the radio is to transmit pertinent information.

tions for transmitting medical information by radio. It is not complicated if you bear in mind that the purpose of talking on the radio is to transmit pertinent information. Keep communications simple, brief, and direct.

You should practice effective communications skills and be familiar with all of the various methods of communication that will be required through your radio. As part of your job, you will need to demonstrate how to communicate effectively with your dispatcher for the call, from call receipt to call end. In addition, you must be able to effectively communicate with the receiving medical facility and deliver a precise and direct radio report in an organized and systematic manner.

FCC Regulations

As mentioned earlier, the FCC is the agency of the US government assigned to regulate all radio and television communications in the United States. For radio, the FCC issues licenses, allocates frequencies, establishes technical standards, and establishes and enforces rules and regulations for the operation of radio equipment. FCC officials monitor transmissions on various frequencies and conduct spot checks of base stations to ensure that they are properly licensed. Fines can be imposed for failing to follow the FCC rules and regulations.

The FCC requires that communications over frequencies allocated for emergency medical use be confined to that use. According to the FCC, "Except for test transmissions, stations licensed to ambulance operators or rescue squads may be used only for the transmission of messages pertaining to the safety of life or property and urgent messages necessary for the rendition of an efficient ambulance or emergency rescue service." The use of obscenity and the transmission of messages unrelated to provision of medical services are forbidden. When it is necessary to communicate a personal message to a paramedic in the field, it is best simply to notify her or him by radio to contact the base by phone. Similarly, a paramedic with a personal request of the dispatcher should use a telephone, not a two-way radio to communicate that message **Figure 16-5 ▶**.

All EMS radio communications are regulated by the Special Emergency Radio Service provisions of the FCC Rules and Regulations, Part 90, and a copy of the Part 90 regulations should be available for reference at every base station.

Clarity of Transmission

The basic model of communication, whether by radio, intercom, telephone, or face-to-face involves a *sender,* a clear message, a *receiver,* and a *feedback loop* to ensure that the exact message that was sent is received and interpreted properly by the receiver. The purpose of communications equipment is to permit communication. That sounds obvious, yet it is often forgotten. Simply blurting something into a microphone is not communicating. For communication to occur, someone at the other end of the radio has to be able to hear and understand what you say. The first principle of communicating by radio is clarity.

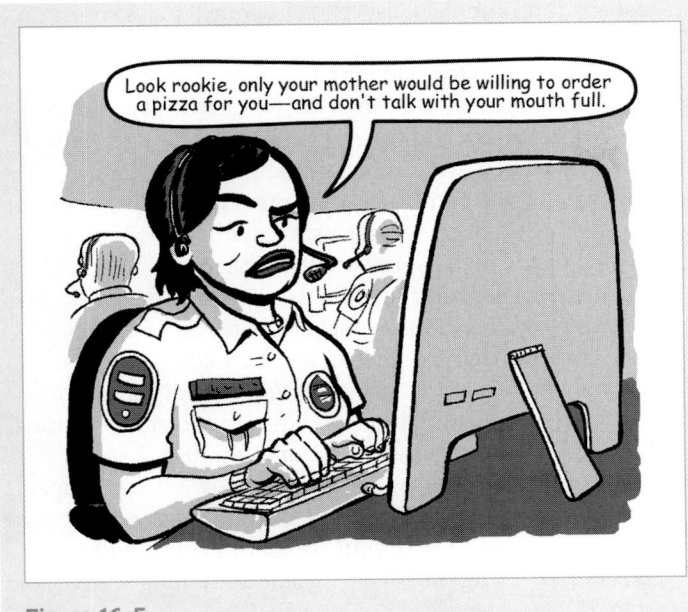

Figure 16-5

Table 16-1	International Phonetic Alphabet	
A Alpha	**J** Juliette	**S** Sierra
B Bravo	**K** Kilo	**T** Tango
C Charlie	**L** Lima	**U** Uniform
D Delta	**M** Mike	**V** Victor
E Echo	**N** November	**W** Whiskey
F Foxtrot	**O** Oscar	**X** X-ray
G Golf	**P** Papa	**Y** Yankee
H Hotel	**Q** Quebec	**Z** Zebra (or Zulu)
I India	**R** Romeo	

A number of guidelines can help you improve the clarity of transmissions:

- Before you begin to transmit, listen to make sure the channel is clear. If another radio transmission is in progress, wait until the parties have finished transmitting before you try to get on the air. Cutting in on someone else's transmission will only ensure that neither of you will be adequately heard.
- Once the channel is quiet, press the transmit key for at least 1 second before you start speaking to ensure that the beginning of your message is not lost.
- Start your transmission with the identifying information: give the number or the name of the unit being called first, then your own identification (for example, "Williamsburg Hospital, this is Medic 3"). That way, the unit being called is alerted immediately and will be listening when you give your own identification, so they can reply at once, "Go ahead, Medic 3." If you do say, for example, "Medic 3 calling Williamsburg Hospital", the recipients might listen only when you've mentioned their identification and, therefore, will miss your identification. So what inevitably happens then is, "This is Williamsburg Hospital. What unit is calling?" That extra transmission is a waste of time.
- Keep your mouth close to the microphone, but not too close. About 2 to 3 inches is usually ideal.
- Speak clearly and distinctly, pronouncing each word carefully.
- Don't shout! Shouting distorts the signal. Speak in a normal pitch; very high- and low-pitched sounds do not transmit well. Whispering is not effective for transmitting.
- Don't talk with your mouth full. It muffles transmission.
- Keep calm and keep your voice free from emotion. You don't have to imitate a talking computer; a normal conversational tone is fine. Just keep your voice and mind free of panic, anger, excitement, and other feelings that can distort your transmission and your judgment.
- Keep your transmissions brief. Air time is precious, and emergency medical frequencies are not the place for long philosophic dialogues. Try having your radio reports taped at some point to critique your own transmissions and perfect your style.
- If you have a long message to transmit, break up the message into 30-second segments, checking at the end of each segment to determine whether it was received and understood.
- Don't waste air time with unnecessary phrases, such as "be advised." Also bear in mind that courtesy is taken for granted; there is no need to use air time for social graces such as "please," "thank you," and "how nice to hear your voice."
- When speaking a word or name that might be misunderstood, spell it out, using the international phonetic alphabet 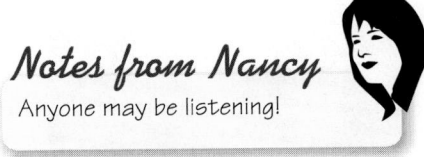 or a similar system. Suppose, for example, you are asking the hospital to notify the patient's family doctor whose name might be mistaken for that of another doctor on the staff; you might say, "Notify Dr. Wilby. That's Dr. WHISKEY-INDIA-LIMA-BRAVO-YANKEE, Wilby."
- When presenting numbers that might be misunderstood, transmit the number as a whole, then digit by digit. For example, if the respirations are 16, you would say, "The respirations are sixteen, that is, one-six."

Notes from Nancy
Anyone may be listening!

Content of Transmissions

Radio transmissions for emergency medical services should be brief, to the point, and professional in tone Figure 16-6 ▶.

Here are some guidelines about what should and should not be included in EMS radio communications:

■ The first thing to remember when you get "on the air" is that your words are, quite literally, in the air, floating around for anyone to hear. Remember, anyone may be listening ◖**Figure 16-7 ▾**◗.

The medical staff at the local ED, a patient signing in at the front desk of another ED, a 12-year-old radio buff playing with his scanner at home . . . any of them may be listening with great attention to your transmission. Therefore, it is essential to protect the privacy of the patient at all times. Do not use the patient's name on the air, and do not transmit personal information about the patient. It is an issue with Health Information Portability and Accountability Act (HIPAA) guidelines on confidentiality. Also, check local laws applicable to your EMS systems. Certain types of cases, such as rape or psychiatric problems, confidential communicable disease history (such as HIV status), are best identified on the air by an established code or given in face-to-face communications when you arrive in the ED.

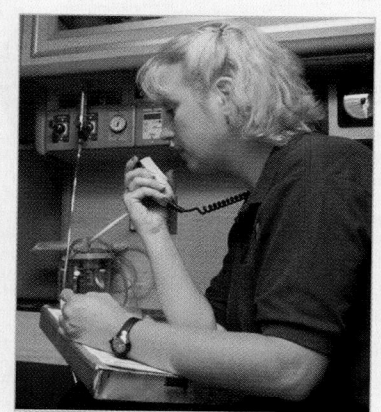

Figure 16-6 The patient report should be given in an objective, accurate, professional manner.

Don't assume that your cellular telephone offers you protected conversations. There are scanners on the market that can tune into the local cellular frequencies. So don't say anything on the radio or the cellular phone that you don't want everyone in town to hear.

■ Be impersonal. Use "we," not "I," to refer to yourself, and use proper names and titles ("Sergeant York," not "Billy") to refer to others when necessary.

■ Don't try to be a comedian or a critic. There is no place for unprofessional behavior, sarcasm, or other poor conduct on emergency medical radio frequencies.

■ Don't use profane language on the air. Aside from the reflection on your professional character, the FCC might issue civil monetary penalties, revoke a license, or deny a renewal application. In addition, violators of the law, if convicted in a federal district court, are subject to criminal fines and/or imprisonment for not more than 2 years.

■ Use professional language, but don't show off. Once again, remember that the object of the exercise is to communicate information, not to stun your listener into awe and admiration. Using proper medical terminology is advisable when done correctly.

■ Avoid using words that are difficult to hear. The word "yes," for example, is easily lost in transmission; use "affirmative" instead. Similarly, use "negative" instead of "no."

■ Use standard formats agreed on by your EMS service for transmission of information. The patient's history, for example, should always be presented in the same order. When the listeners know what they are listening for, they are less likely to miss parts of the transmission.

■ When you finish transmitting, obtain confirmation that the transmission was received. When you receive instructions by radio from the dispatcher or from medical control, echo the order back to make certain you have understood it correctly. Thus, for example, if the physician instructs you to administer 75 mg of lidocaine slowly IV, you would respond, "That is lidocaine, 75 milligrams, repeat, 75 milligrams, slowly IV. Is that confirmed?"

■ Question any orders you did not hear clearly or did not understand.

■ Use EMS frequencies only for emergency medical communications.

Codes

Some ambulance services still use radio codes; most do not. Codes were used for several reasons:

■ To maintain security of communication
■ To keep air time as brief as possible
■ To diminish the likelihood of misunderstanding or noise
■ To prevent the patient, family, and bystanders from understanding what is being said

The last-mentioned reason is particularly important when the information you need to convey to the dispatcher or physician could alarm the patient. Suppose that you want to tell the physician that your patient is probably having an acute myocardial infarction and is in very serious condition. It is preferable that the patient not be privy to that assessment because it could

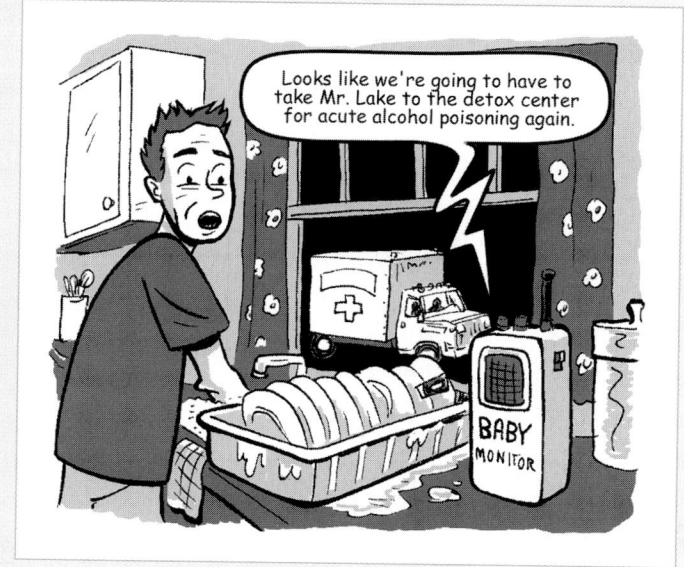

Figure 16-7

increase anxiety and possibly worsen the patient's condition. In fact, it is best not to be sitting right next to the patient when transmitting your report to the emergency department.

For a code to be of any use, everyone using the radio must know the meaning of the code words. When codes are used, therefore, they should be simple and standardized within a given region, and a copy of the code should be posted at every radio terminal.

The ten-code system, once commonly used has been phased out in many EMS systems, and use is not recommended in the National Incident Management System (NIMS), which is discussed further in Chapter 47. If codes are still used in your agency, be sure to learn the code system used.

Documentation and Communication

In 2003, the president directed the secretary of Homeland Security to develop and administer the NIMS. This system is intended to provide a consistent nationwide template to enable federal, state, and local governments and private-sector and nongovernmental organizations to work together effectively and efficiently to prepare for, prevent, respond to, and recover from domestic incidents, regardless of cause, size, or complexity, including acts of catastrophic terrorism.

One area addressed by NIMS is communication and documentation. Collection, tracking, and reporting of incident information and incident resources are included in the concepts, principles, terminology, and technologies addressed by NIMS. Effective communications, information management, and information and intelligence sharing are critical aspects of domestic incident management. The NIMS communications and information systems enable the essential functions needed to provide a common operating picture and interoperability for incident management at all levels.

When and if you use codes, remember that one of their main purposes is to shorten air time.

Whenever codes are used, they should be kept simple and reserved for cases in which they are really needed. During MCIs, when personnel unfamiliar with the codes may be staffing radios and when everyone is apt to be anxious, it is usually best to abandon codes and use words that all understand. Most services use standard terms rather than codes for regular day-to-day operations as well.

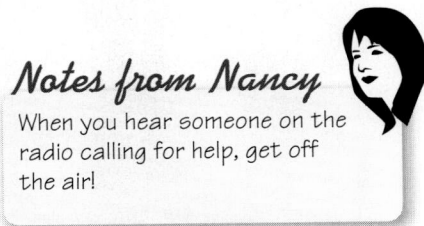

Notes from Nancy

When you hear someone on the radio calling for help, get off the air!

Relaying Information to Medical Control

Radio communications between paramedics in the field and their medical control physician need to be concise and accurate. A standard format for communicating patient information over the radio will ensure that significant information is relayed in a consistent manner and that nothing is omitted **Figure 16-8** ▸.

When relaying medical information in person, such as when a bedside transfer of patient care occurs, be mindful of the information you are supplying, many times in the presence of the patient **Figure 16-9** ▸. At times, it may be more practical to step outside the patient care room or to speak in a softer tone to provide the history and transferring information to the receiving medical practitioner. In addition, be brief. At this time, additional information should be shared that may not have been given in the radio report to the receiving facility. Ensure you are providing this information in person to a medical practitioner of an equal or a higher level of care to avoid abandonment and confidentiality issues and to ensure continuity of care. In many

You are the Provider Part 3

The glucometer reads "29." You immediately tell your partner, who assembles a preload of D_{50}. As you give the dextrose, your patient's level of consciousness begins to improve. The patient no longer needs ventilatory assistance. She remains somewhat confused but can provide her name and states that she has type 2 diabetes. You provide supplemental oxygen at 15 L/min via nonrebreathing mask, and her ECG indicates sinus tachycardia.

Reassessment	Recording Time: 10 Minutes
Level of consciousness	Alert, with a Glasgow Coma Scale score of 14
Skin	Pale, warm, slightly diaphoretic
Pulse	120 beats/min, strong and regular
Blood pressure	128/86 mm Hg
Respirations	20 breaths/min
Sao_2	95%
Blood glucose	29 mg/dL

7. As your patient's level of consciousness improves, what issues do you foresee?

8. How does your ability to effectively communicate impact patient care?

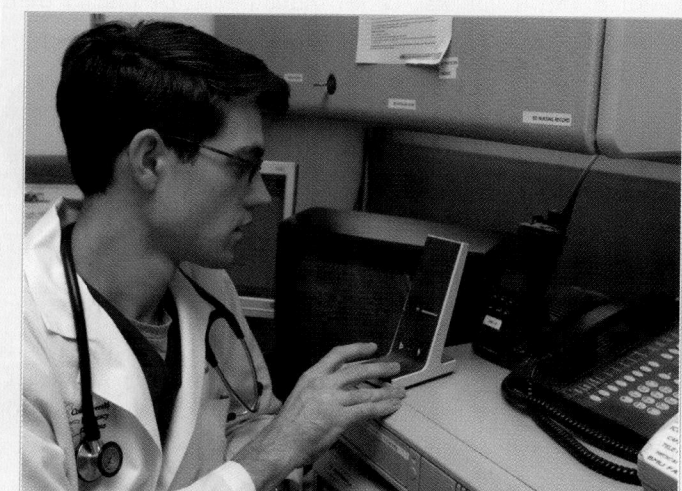

Figure 16-8 Use a standard format for communicating patient information to medical control.

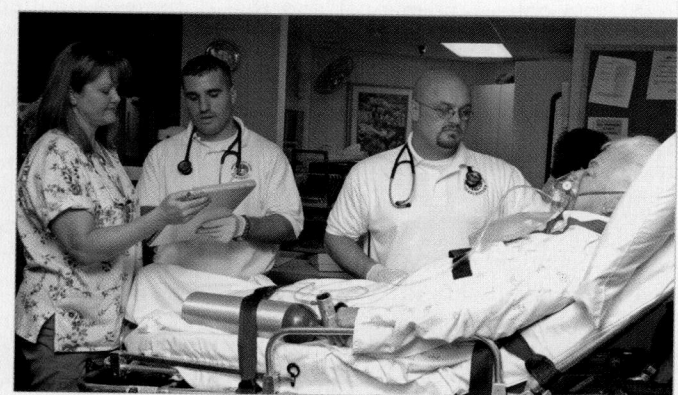

Figure 16-9 Be mindful of how you provide your report when the patient is present.

cases, a copy of the written report will be given to the receiving facility before you leave. Be sure to follow local protocols on providing patient care reports, or PCRs.

Format for Reporting Medical Information

The following list shows the items that should be included when reporting medical information:

- The patient's age and sex
- The patient's chief complaint
- A brief, pertinent history of the present illness or injury
- Anything the physician needs to know about the patient's other medical history relative to the current situation, including major underlying medical conditions, medications, and important allergies
- The patient's level of consciousness and degree of distress
- The vital signs

- The pertinent physical findings in head-to-toe order
- ECG findings
- Treatment given so far and response to treatment

For example, here is a transmission regarding a patient in congestive heart failure: "We have a 53-year-old man complaining of severe shortness of breath, which wakened him from sleep and is worse when he is lying down. He has a history of hypertension and takes Diuril. He is alert but in significant respiratory distress, with a pulse of 130 and regular, respirations 36 and labored, and BP 190/120. Physical exam reveals no JVD but crackles and wheezes in both lung fields. He has 2+ pitting ankle edema. We are sending you an ECG."

The preceding transmission can be relayed in less than 30 seconds, and any physician hearing that information will immediately recognize that this is a hypertensive patient in moderately severe left-sided heart failure.

When paramedics call in without a standard reporting format, the physician might have to waste time gleaning the information needed to know what is going on. Consider the following dialogue:

Paramedic: *We have a patient with a pulse of 130, a blood pressure of 190/120, and respirations of 30. We're sending you a strip.*

Physician: *Fine, but what's his problem?*

Paramedic: *He's short of breath.*

Physician: *How long has this been going on?*

Paramedic: *Just a minute (pause). He says it woke him up from sleep about an hour ago.*

Physician: *Does he have any underlying medical problems?*

Paramedic: *He takes medicine for hypertension.*

Physician: *Is he in any distress?*

Paramedic: *Yeah, he's having a hard time breathing.*

Physician: *What do his lungs sound like?*

Paramedic: *He has crackles and wheezes all over.*

Clearly, disorganized and incomplete communication is not efficient. It is a waste of time and causes frustration. The physician might respond to transport him immediately rather than try to get complete information. To avoid ineffective dialogues, gather your information thoroughly at the scene, organize it clearly in your mind, and only then get on the air to the physician. Because even the best of us can be rattled under pressure, it's a good idea to write the reporting format on a card and affix the card to your hand-held transmitter or the dashboard of the ambulance so you may refer to it while reporting in.

Dispatching

The verb "to dispatch" means "to send out on a mission," but the EMD does a lot more than just send ambulances out to emergencies. The EMD functions as a vital part of the paramedic team who obtains as much information as possible about the emergency, then directs the appropriate vehicle to the scene, and provides the caller with whatever advice may be needed to manage the situation until help arrives. The EMD also monitors and coordinates communication with the field and maintains written records pertaining to the response to the call.

Let us consider the EMD's tasks in each phase of the call.

Receipt of the Call for Help

Whenever someone telephones for an ambulance, the EMD has to assume that the caller needs help, even if the caller is too upset to be clear about the nature of the problem. The EMD, therefore, has to be able to put himself or herself in the caller's place and understand the caller's distress. That means the EMD must:

- *Answer the telephone promptly*, within two or three rings; each ring may seem like an eternity to a panicky person.
- *Identify himself or herself and the agency*. The caller needs immediate confirmation of having reached the right number.
- *Speak directly into the mouthpiece*, clearly and without mumbling.
- *Observe telephone courtesy*. The EMD must be calm and professional, informing the caller exactly what is being done and how soon assistance can be expected. As mentioned earlier, in some cases, EMDs provide prearrival instructions such as in the form of emergency medical dispatching—the EMD relays vital first aid information to the caller who can then apply the aid techniques while waiting for the ambulance to arrive.
- *Take charge of the conversation*. Once the EMD has identified the ambulance service, he or she must start asking the caller questions to which immediate answers are needed. Questions pertaining to safety issues are a priority. Additional useful information may also be obtained, such as specific situations the EMS crew might encounter: Is the residence door locked? What pets does the patient have? These nuggets of information are invaluable in the field.

Information Gathering

The method used to gather information from a caller is most often a series of short questions asked by the EMD. When a call for EMS comes in, the EMD should elicit the following minimum information:

- The exact location of the patient (s), including the street name and number; the proper geographic designation (such as whether the street is East Maple or West Maple) and the name of the community (adjacent towns may have streets by the same name). If the call comes from a rural area, the dispatcher should try to establish landmarks (such as the nearest cross-street or business establishment, water tower, or antenna).
- The telephone number (call-back number) of the caller, in case the call is disconnected or there is a need to phone the caller back for more information. It is not uncommon for paramedics not to be able to find the address and to ask for help from the original caller. Asking for the caller's telephone number also helps discourage nuisance calls to EMS because prank callers are reluctant to supply their phone numbers. Finally, the caller's telephone exchange may help to pinpoint his or her location if the caller is unfamiliar with the region, as is often the case of a traveler calling from the road. In services equipped with an enhanced 9-1-1 system, a lot of the information mentioned—such as the phone number and location of the caller—is recorded automatically through sophisticated telephone technology, and the EMD need only confirm the information on the screen.

- The caller's perception of the nature of his or her or the patient's problem.
- Specific information concerning the patient's condition that will help evaluate the urgency of the situation and the EMD's need to provide the caller with prearrival instructions by phone. The EMD should ask specifically:
  - Is the patient conscious?
  - If not, is the patient breathing?
  - Is the patient bleeding badly?
- If the emergency is a motor vehicle collision, further important information should be obtained:
  - The kinds of vehicles involved (that is, cars, trucks, motorcycles, buses). If a truck is involved, is there any indication of the cargo it is carrying? A truck carrying dynamite requires a different approach from one carrying bananas!
  - The number of persons injured and an estimate of the extent of injuries. This information will enable the EMD to estimate the magnitude of the problem.
  - Apparent hazards at the scene, such as heavy traffic, downed power lines, fire, spilled chemicals, and peculiar odors.

Information about such hazards enables the EMD to contact other agencies that may have to be involved, such as utility workers to take care of downed wires or an engine company to deal with spilled fuel. In most modern dispatch centers, the EMD has visual prompts with the key questions to ask on the computer screen.

Dispatch

At the point when your EMD has obtained the address of the emergency, the telephone number of the caller, and the apparent problem, the EMD should ask the caller to wait on the line. The EMD must then decide, assuming the call is a medical emergency within the service's jurisdiction, which crew(s) and vehicle(s) will be dispatched. That decision will be governed by the nature and location of the call and the availability of various units at the time. The appropriate crew is contacted and informed of the nature of the call and its exact location ("Medic 5, possible heart attack at 573 East Main Street, that's five-seven-three East Main Street with Jones Drive on the cross"). Once the ambulance is dispatched, the EMD may return to the telephone to obtain the rest of the information previously outlined. Further questioning may reveal special conditions that might affect your travel to the scene or your actions at the scene. If so, that information should be relayed to you while you are en route, for two reasons:

- So that you may know if the response requires travel under emergency conditions, using emergency warning devices
- So that while en route you may anticipate and prepare for tasks to be performed at the scene: assembling the

equipment to deliver a baby or transmitting cardiac information to the receiving hospital

The EMD might also remind you to buckle up en route to the scene because this is usually the most dangerous part of the call!

Advice to the Caller

After directing you and any rescue crew(s) to the scene and alerting all of you to any special conditions, your EMD should return to the telephone and tell the caller what is being done ("An ambulance is on the way and should be there in about 5 minutes."). If your EMD suspects your patient has a life-threatening emergency, your EMD should also provide instructions to the caller in very simple terms about emergency care techniques (such as airway maintenance, Heimlich maneuver, CPR, hemorrhage control). The caller is likely to be in an agitated state, so instructions must be clear and simple.

Excellent protocols have been developed for giving such instructions by telephone, and all EMDs should undergo training in those procedures. Most often, this training will be based on the original medical priority dispatch system designed by Jeff Clawson, MD in Salt Lake City, Utah, in the early 1980s. The system is used throughout the world.

Ongoing Communications With the Field

It is important for your EMD to monitor the communications of the ambulance and to be aware of what is occurring in the field. Your EMD must coordinate communications between the ambulance and medical control and contact any other agencies (such as fire and police) whose presence may be required at the scene. The EMD should also receive and record communications from you when you are in the field regarding the following:

- The time the ambulance departed for the scene
- The time the ambulance arrived at the scene
- The time the crew made contact with the patient
- The time the ambulance left the scene
- The time the ambulance arrived at the hospital
- The time the ambulance went back in service

Paramedics involved in giving emergency care simply don't have time to keep looking at their watches and recording the moment each of those events occurred. The times cited, along with the time the call was received, must be recorded accurately at the communications center **Figure 16-10 ▶**. The easiest way to accomplish that is to have paramedics radio in at each time indicated (for example, "En route to hospital") and for the EMD to record the times. Your record of the times permits a gamut of medical, administrative, and academic evaluations. Your supervising medical personnel can evaluate the appropriateness of the time emergency personnel spend with a patient, and managers can assess how long it takes a team to get back in service after a call.

The phases of the EMD's work are summarized in **Table 16-2 ▶**.

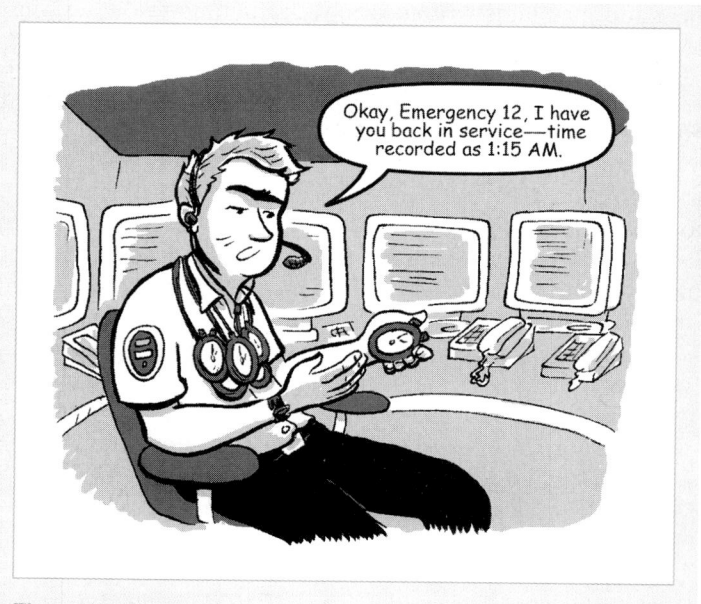

Figure 16-10

Table 16-2	Phases of Dispatch
Information Gathered	**Dispatcher Action**
Answers telephone promptly Identifies agency Address of incident Call-back number Perceived problem Patient's name	Dispatches (first) ambulance

Patient's condition
For road accident:
   Number of vehicles
   Kinds of vehicles
   Number of victims
	Gives patient care instructions
	  by phone if required

Hazards at the scene	Notifies responding ambulances
	  of special situations
	Dispatches additional
	  ambulances as needed
	Contacts other agencies
	  as needed
	Monitors communications
	  from the field

Documenting Times

In general, it is routine practice to use standard military time when documenting times for calls. Most dispatchers use this format when providing times over the radio as well. **Table 16-3 ▶** shows how military time relates to standard AM and PM time.

Factors That May Affect Communications

In communication, many things may go wrong, and not all of them are equipment failures. You need to be prepared for

Table 16-3	Military Times		
Regular Time	Military Time	Regular Time	Military Time
Midnight	0000	Noon	1200
1:00 AM	0100	1:00 PM	1300
2:00 AM	0200	2:00 PM	1400
3:00 AM	0300	3:00 PM	1500
4:00 AM	0400	4:00 PM	1600
5:00 AM	0500	5:00 PM	1700
6:00 AM	0600	6:00 PM	1800
7:00 AM	0700	7:00 PM	1900
8:00 AM	0800	8:00 PM	2000
9:00 AM	0900	9:00 PM	2100
10:00 AM	1000	10:00 PM	2200
11:00 AM	1100	11:00 PM	2300

such situations. Radio communication is very technical and technology-driven. At times, systems may have problems, such as radio tower issues, computer crashes, and audio problems, and you may have to adapt to necessary changes. Follow your local protocols regarding radio failure.

You have learned how important communication skills are in previous chapters. You can be faced with a number of problems, including patients who do not speak your primary language or patients with communication disorders. Ask "those in the know" about telephone interpreters, people on your service who speak more than one language, and learn what you can do before you see your patients. Review your patient assessment skills for patients with impaired hearing.

Documentation and Communication

Cultural diversity is found in EMS every day. If you are not familiar with the various cultures present in your community, consider a training session in which leaders from various cultural organizations in your community are invited to meet your organization members. This could open up dialogue for both groups and could create an avenue for growth and development to reduce communication barriers in EMS calls. In addition, training members of your EMS organization to speak other languages that are spoken in your area may also be of significant benefit to your community.

Documentation

What do you call the report in your agency or EMS setting? Here is a list of different terms used to describe the written documentation or report for calls for service:

- Patient care report (PCR)
- Prehospital patient report (PPR)
- Ambulance call report (ACR)
- Call report
- Trip sheet
- Run sheet
- Run report
- Ambulance trip sheet

Whatever you call it, do you know and understand the importance of it? The adage, "No job is finished until the paperwork is done" is very true in EMS. Your written report, most commonly referred to as the PCR (prehospital/patient care report), is the only written record of the events that transpired during the call for service. It needs to be one of the most important skills you learn as a paramedic. It will be the legal record for the call and a part of the patient's medical record and the hospital's ED chart. The PCR provides for a continuum of patient care on arrival at the receiving facility. Time will not allow you to relay all of the information obtained through patient assessment and findings in a radio report or the verbal report on arrival. Your verbal report should be a brief summary of the assessment findings and the event, but your written report should be a more detailed account from the very moment the call began until it concluded. The written report should accurately reflect, or paint a picture, of the events of the call.

Although you may include subjective information from the patient, such as statements from him or her about symptoms, no bias or personal opinions (subjectivity) of yours should be contained within your written report. Poorly written, inappropriately documented PCRs could have adverse implications for patient care and for your career. Omissions or errors in your report could lead to further errors in care. Improper and inadequate reports also could result in litigation, loss of job or position, a negative reflection on one's reputation as an EMS professional, and more.

No matter your particular writing style, your report should be complete, well-written, legible, professional, and your sole source of information about the call. Your report may also be used in legal proceedings. In some cases, it may be your only defense against a complaint about a call—if you document what happened, you will have solid evidence of your conduct and what transpired on the call. Your memory may not serve you well 5 years from now, but your written report will remain the same. If it is well written, it will jog your memory and should provide a picture of the events of the call to all who read it. As a health care professional, it is important that you use proper spelling, proper grammar, and accurate terminology in your report. Do not attempt to use medical terms and abbreviations if you do not fully understand their meaning. Never make up your own abbreviations because they will only be meaningful to you and could confuse others. Doing so could result in patient care errors and leave your professional character at stake if the report is called into question.

In addition, you should write every PCR as if your medical director were reading it, such as in a quality assurance review. Your report is the only record (unless your medical director was on the call with you) of why you performed a certain procedure or why you administered a particular medication to a patient. Reports that your medical director and EMS agency can read and understand will help them evaluate your performance accurately.

On occasion, EMS reports may be requested for medical audits and other educational settings. Run reviews, or sessions in which peers and other medical professionals review care reports for adherence to local protocols, quality assurance, and quality monitoring, may occur. Your written and computer-based reports may be used to calculate the number of times you have performed a specific skill, such as medication administration or oral intubation. Always accurately document all skills attempted and performed with patient care.

Billing and administration are significant reasons why PCR writing needs to be accurate and complete. Most EMS agencies now need to bill for services to recover the costs of providing patient care. For complete and accurate revenue recovery, you must ensure that all procedures performed are documented, insurance codes obtained, and the appropriate medical necessity signature obtained (where required). You need to document why a patient may have needed emergency care, especially in the case of private or scheduled transports, to ensure your service's billing information will result in payment from the responsible insurer, agency, or private payer. You will often be trained by your agency and its billing company about what additional forms you need to complete as a part of each EMS response. EMS providers may grumble about these tasks, but you must understand that it is a necessary portion of the call to complete billing paperwork and to supply the most accurate and defensible information to the EMS agency. Just as billing has become necessary in EMS, so has research. Proper documentation done by all EMS providers often justifies innovative, lifesaving techniques when data are

put together by researchers. Many states now require EMS agencies to submit data to their state EMS office to verify call volumes and skills used. These data may include the number of calls an agency responds to, the types of calls, care provided, and patient outcomes. Such patient care data collection can lead to improvement of the EMS system as a whole.

Do you know if the procedures you are performing are making a difference in your patient's outcome? Your careful documentation of procedures is the basis of research and evaluation of their effectiveness. Research is very difficult to do without accurate data and information. The data come from your written report.

At the national level, the National Highway Traffic Safety Administration has supported the National Emergency Medical Services Information System, or NEMSIS, as the repository to store the EMS data for each of the states. This effort will help to assist the states in collecting comparable data elements so the entire nation can benefit from research and use the trends for future curricula development.

Medical Terminology

Using medical terminology correctly is essential to EMS communications. You should learn the established and accepted medical terms and abbreviations for your EMS operations. Some EMS systems have specific approved lists of medical abbreviations and terms that must be used.

Medical terminology may seem to be a foreign language. Well, it is! Most terminology comes from the ancient Roman language, Latin. In addition, some common words used in EMS such as "packaging a patient for transport" or "bagging the patient during airway management" might be used. Be sure to know acceptable terms and words used in your EMS agency. An ongoing

You are the Provider Part 4

As your patient becomes alert and oriented, she tells you that she was riding her bike home from work when she became shaky. She says that she thought she had some candy in her backpack but was unable to find it. She decided to continue home, and the next thing she remembered she was lying on the ground surrounded by strangers.

Reassessment	Recording Time: 15 Minutes
Level of consciousness	Alert, with a Glasgow Coma Scale score of 15
Skin	Pale, warm, slightly diaphoretic
Pulse	110 beats/min, strong and regular
Blood pressure	126/82 mm Hg
Respirations	18 breaths/min
Sao_2	98%
Blood glucose	120 mg/dL

9. How do body language and tone of voice communicate as much or more than words?

10. How does total patient care enter into this scenario?

11. What is the purpose of documentation?

12. Who is your documentation audience?

8. **When a PCR is inappropriate or care is inadequately documented, it can be presumed that:**
   - **A.** the paramedic had a bad day.
   - **B.** the paramedic was not trained properly.
   - **C.** others may question the care given to the patient.
   - **D.** the paramedic forgot to include something.

9. **The documentation of starting IVs in the field should include all of the following, EXCEPT:**
   - **A.** the size of the catheter used.
   - **B.** the site of the IV.
   - **C.** multiple attempts if not successful on the first try.
   - **D.** who adjusted the drip.

Challenging Questions

You are dispatched for a motor vehicle collision. When you arrive, you find a male patient, unknown age, unconscious, and unresponsive in the street. He appears to have a significant head injury; as you examine him, you notice brain matter on the road. His injuries are incompatible with life. The ECG shows asystole in all three leads. You call your medical control physician, who pronounces the patient dead. There are two other vehicles involved in this crash with a total of three patients who have minor injuries.

10. **How do you properly document this call?**

11. **Why is accurate documentation important?**

Points to Ponder

You are dispatched to a private residence for a person having a seizure. While responding, you are informed by your dispatcher that the call has been upgraded to a cardiac arrest. You arrive at the home and are unable to gain access. You advise your dispatch center. The dispatcher uses the call-back number received with the 9-1-1 call. Someone runs from next door and tells you that the call is at another house. You go over, treat the patient, and transport to the hospital. After the call, you find out you received the wrong address—the 9-1-1 call originated at the house you were sent to because the person in need did not have a phone.

What information could have helped you en route to the call? How do you document the delay in patient contact, especially because this was a cardiac arrest and seconds matter?

Issues: Understanding the Role of Your Dispatch Center, Advocating Among Peers, Completing Documentation, Resolving the Negative Attitude Toward Documentation.

www.Paramedic.EMSzone.com

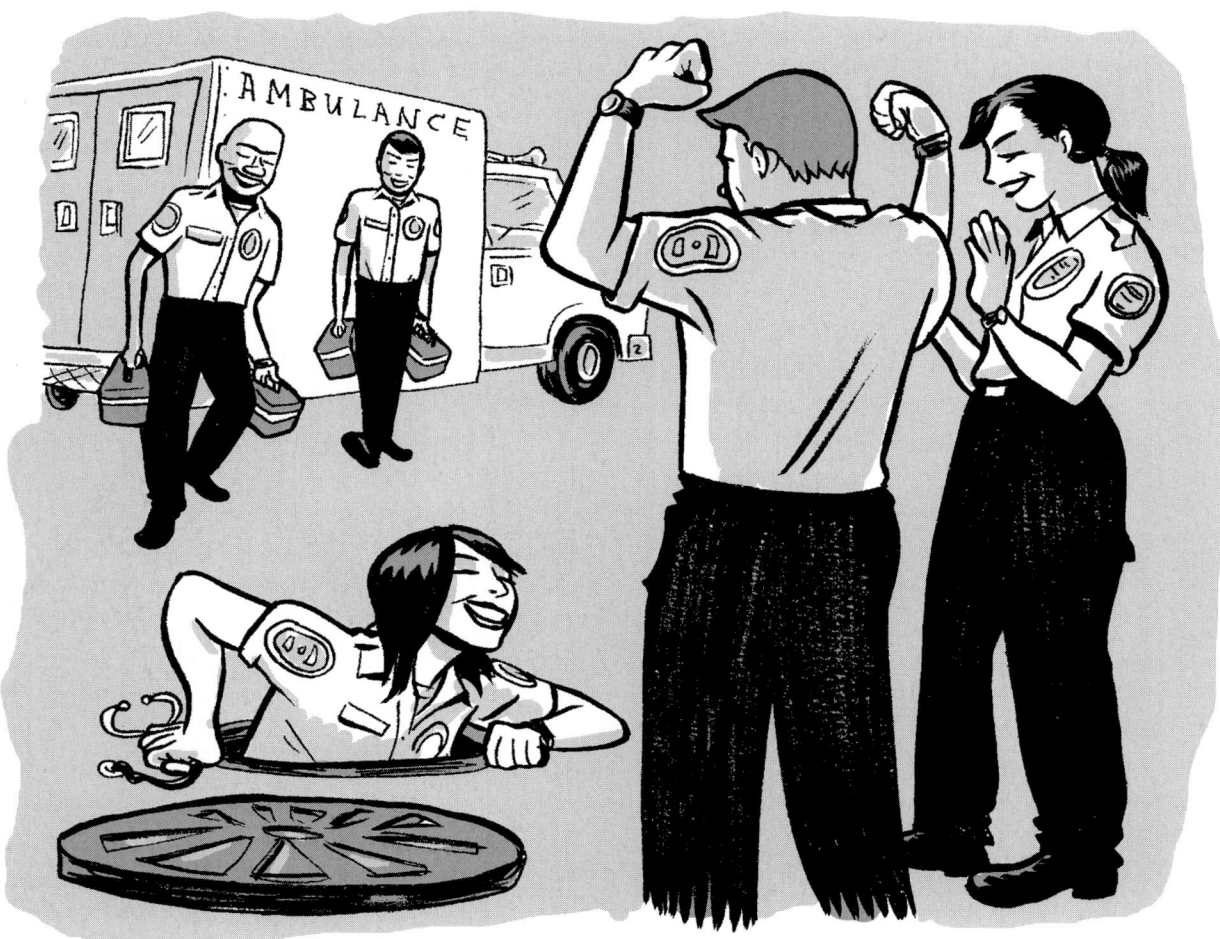

"

The first time I climbed into a sewer to do a resuscitation, I realized there were lots of things they never told me in medical school."

—Nancy L. Caroline, MD

Trauma

4

Section

Section Editors: Bob Elling, MPA, NREMT-P
Connie J. Mattera, RN, MS, TNS, EMT-P

17

Trauma Systems and Mechanism of Injury

Objectives

Cognitive

4-1.1   List and describe the components of a comprehensive trauma system. (p 17.6)

4-1.2   Describe the role of and differences between levels of trauma centers. (p 17.8)

4-1.3   Describe the criteria for transport to a trauma center. (p 17.7)

4-1.4   Describe the criteria and procedure for air medical transport. (p 17.8)

4-1.5   Define energy and force as they relate to trauma. (p 17.9)

4-1.6   Define laws of motion and energy and understand the role that increased speed has on injuries. (p 17.11)

4-1.7   Describe each type of impact and its effect on unrestrained victims (e.g., "down and under," "up and over," compression, deceleration). (p 17.14)

4-1.8   Describe the pathophysiology of the head, spine, thorax, and abdomen that result from the above forces. (p 17.15)

4-1.9   List specific injuries and their causes as related to interior and exterior vehicle damage. (p 17.18)

4-1.10 Describe the kinematics of penetrating injuries. (p 17.22)

4-1.11 List the motion and energy considerations of mechanisms other than motor vehicle crashes. (p 17.21)

4-1.12 Define the role of kinematics as an additional tool for patient assessment. (p 17.14)

Affective

None

Psychomotor

None

Introduction

Trauma has emerged to become the primary cause of death and disability in people 1 to 34 years of age. With improvements in health care and management of chronic diseases, death rates due to conditions such as heart disease, neoplasms, cerebrovascular events, and respiratory illnesses have decreased significantly in younger age groups. During the last 40 years, unintentional trauma, which excludes suicide, was the fifth leading cause of death in all age groups, accounting for 106,742 deaths reported in the United States in 2002.

Basic concepts of the mechanics and biomechanics of trauma will help you analyze and manage your patient's injuries. Analyzing a trauma scene is a vital skill because you are the eyes and ears of the emergency department physicians at the scene of the trauma. Your paramedic-written patient history is the *only* source for physicians and surgeons to understand the events and mechanisms that led to your trauma patient's chief complaint. Your information is critical as a foundation to visualize and search for injuries that may not be apparent on physical examination.

Trauma, Energy, Biomechanics, and Kinematics

Trauma is the acute physiologic and structural change (injury) that occurs in a patient's body when an external source of

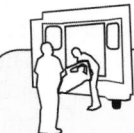

In the Field

The top five causes of trauma death are motor vehicle crashes, falls, poisonings, burns, and drownings.

energy dissipates faster than the body's ability to sustain and dissipate it   Figure 17-1 ▾ .

If a body in an automobile—your patient's body—smashes into a wall, the energy delivered by an external source—the moving automobile—is released when the car is stopped by the wall. Your patient's body is moving at the same rate of speed as the automobile, and his or her body does not have bumpers to absorb the energy from stopping. If the energy is not absorbed in other ways, the patient's body absorbs it, often with bones that break and internal organs that rupture—what you see as trauma injuries.

Different forms of energy produce different kinds of trauma. These external energy sources can be mechanical, chemical, thermal, electrical, and barometric.

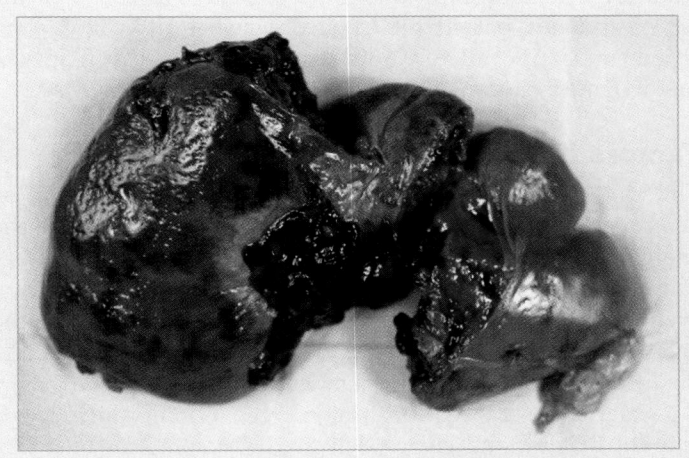

Figure 17-1 Traumatic injury occurs when the body's tissues are exposed to energy levels beyond their tolerance. Some traumatic injuries may not be visible. This photo shows a ruptured spleen.

You are the Provider Part 1

You are dispatched to 1601 South Main Street for "man fallen from a roof." This address is located in the business district of your service area. En route to the call, you learn that this man had been running from police and had come from a building in the downtown area. The patient is in police custody, and the scene is considered safe.

You arrive but are unable to assess much because the patient is combative and unwilling to answer your questions. You can see that his skin is slightly moist and a bit pale.

Initial Assessment	Recording Time: 0 Minutes
Appearance	Grimacing, screaming, punching
Level of consciousness	A (Alert to person, place, and day)
Airway	Patent
Breathing	Rapid and deep
Circulation	Unable to assess due to patient combativeness

1. What initial information about the fall gives rise for concern?
2. How does knowing your primary service area impact your understanding of potential patient injuries?
3. Given the location, what other conditions are you worried about?

Mechanical energy is energy from motion (kinetic energy ie, a moving vehicle) or energy stored in an object (potential energy—a concrete bridge abutment). Kinetic energy would be found in two moving vehicles colliding. Potential energy would be present in a fall from a height. In that case, gravity would be the *potential* source of energy that can cause the object to fall. Chemical energy can be found in an explosive or an acid or even from a reaction to an ingested or medically delivered agent or drug. Electrical energy comes in the form of high voltage electrocution or a lightning strike. Barometric energy can result from sudden and radical changes in pressure, often occurring during diving or flying.

Biomechanics is the study of the physiology and mechanics of a living organism using the tools of mechanical engineering. Biomechanics provides a way of analyzing the mechanisms and results of trauma sustained by the human body. Kinetics studies the relationships among speed, mass, direction of the force, and, for paramedics, the physical injury caused by speed, mass, and force. Knowledge of kinetics can help you predict injury patterns found in a patient.

Factors Affecting Types of Injury

The kind of injury resulting after trauma is sustained will be determined by the ability of the patient's body to disperse the energy delivered by the traumatic event. Some patients' bodies can stretch and bend to absorb the energy of the traumatic event. But other patients' bone and tissue cannot absorb the energy. A healthy football player can absorb a "hit" on the playing field better than an older man with diminished bone mass.

External factors that determine types of injury include the amount of *force* and *energy* delivered. The amount of injury your patient sustains varies with the size (or mass) of the objects delivering the force and energy, with the change in velocity (how fast your patient is traveling), with acceleration or deceleration (how much the object or your patient speeds up or slows down), and with the body area of the application of force. The primary reasons for the extent of trauma your patients sustain are the amount of energy in the object and the mechanism by which the object is delivered to the body. The body receives wider-spread trauma from a cannon ball (more energy inside) than it does from a bullet, although both are often lethal. (Proving, if proof were needed, that size does matter.)

Duration and *direction* of the force of application are also important. In vehicle collisions, paramedics learn to recognize the directional patterns in injuries from front-end, side, and rear-end collisions. The larger the area of force dissipation, the more pressure is reduced to a specific spot on the body, often without making a visible cut. Bullet impact is less if the energy in the bullet is dissipated over the ceramic plate inside a bulletproof vest than if all the force of the bullet is applied at a small location on the skin.

In trauma medicine, this spreading of impact is described as *blunt trauma*. EMS providers at all levels quickly learn in the field that blunt trauma is difficult to diagnose because there is often little external damage. Paramedics study kinetics to find this lethal, but almost invisible trauma.

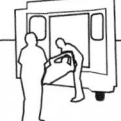

In the Field

Suspect a spinal injury when you see a cracked windshield, steering wheel or dashboard damage, intrusion into a vehicle, or fractured feet or ankles after a fall. It will make a difference in how you handle the ABCs.

The *rate of force application* affects trauma because rapidly applied amounts of energy are less tolerated than a similar amount of energy delivered over a longer period. Rapidly delivered energy causes broken wrists, whereas longer term energy delivery might show up as repetitive stress injuries—even though the amount of force ultimately might be exactly the same.

The position of the trauma victim—how he or she is positioned—at the time of the event is an external factor. Seatbelts have done a great deal to effect the reduction in lethal injuries by keeping occupants in positions less likely to cause fatal injuries.

Internal injuries sustained when the break point of an organ is exceeded are easier to diagnose. In the skin, they include contusions, abrasions, lacerations, punctures, and degloving injuries. Bones will fracture or buckle. The viscera covering structures of internal organs will have ruptures, or disruptions.

The *impact resistance of body parts* will also have a bearing on types of tissue disruption. Impact resistance is often determined by what is inside your patient's organs: gas, liquid, or solid.

Biomechanical engineers would measure the *densities of tissues* that are traumatized. Paramedics need to know that organs that have gas inside, such as in the lungs and intestinal tract, will scatter energy more than liquid or solid boundaries. This means that the organ around the gas will be easily compressed, so look for lung and intestinal trauma first. Water-bearing organs include the vascular system, the liver, spleen, and muscle. Water-bearing tissues are less compressible than gas-containing tissues. Solid density interfaces occur mostly in bones such as in the cranium, spine, and long bones.

Because many injuries are not obvious on first presentation, understanding the effects of forces and energy transfer patterns will help in the assessment of the *mechanism of injury* (MOI), which in turn can help predict the most likely type of injuries you will see when you are in the field **Figure 17-2 ▶**. Paramedic students need to learn to have a *high index of suspicion* for injuries that otherwise might be undetected for several hours. Anticipate the possibility of specific types of injury: you will help your patient and the trauma team who will need your assessment of the scene. Sometimes, you will find you need to be aggressive with your initial assessment ABC interventions to prevent further problems for your patient.

■ Trauma Centers

Paramedics need a good working knowledge of the hospital resources with a reasonable idea of how long transport will

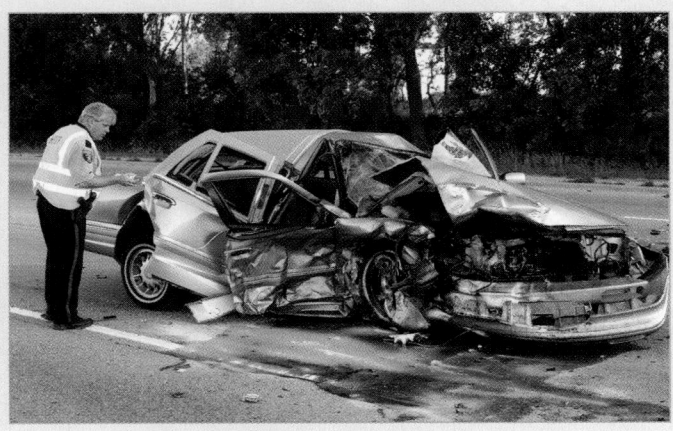

Figure 17-2 The appearance of the car can provide you with critical information about the severity of the crash and the possible injuries to the occupants.

Documentation and Communication

So much emphasis is placed on the MOI because obtaining a complete and accurate history of the incident can help identify as many as 95% of the injuries present. After ensuring your personal safety and maintaining the ABCs, the mechanism of injury is key information to obtain from the trauma scene. You must relay what you suspect as the MOIs by radio and by written report to the receiving trauma center. You are the eyes and ears of the trauma team in the emergency department.

take. Frequently, you will be the decision maker about where your patient should be transported. Before you even get to the scene, you should know what is available in your area.

The Committee on Trauma (COT) of the American College of Surgeons is the governing body responsible for the designation of trauma centers. There are four separate categories of verification in the COT's program (Level I, II, III, and IV). The guidelines in **Table 17-1** ▶ are an overview of the COT's verification criteria.

Criteria for Referral to a Trauma Center

Paramedics are responsible for determining whether a patient should go to a trauma center—and at what level. You might even have to determine whether air transport is required to a Level I center. *The criteria for transport to a trauma center vary from system to system.* However, the criteria for transport to a trauma center as defined by the American College of Surgeons in its ATLS protocols are summarized below:

1. If one of the following is present, the patient should be referred to a trauma center:
   - GCS (Glasgow Coma Scale score) < 14
   - RR (respiratory rate) < 10 or > 29
   - SBP (systolic blood pressure) < 90
   - RTS (revised trauma score) < 11
   - PTS (pediatric trauma score) < 9

In the Field

The Trauma Registry is a reporting system designed to collect trauma-related data in an effort to improve the quality and cost-effectiveness of care and to aid in outcome research. Two software programs produced by the American College of Surgeons are National Tracs and the National Trauma Data Bank. Your contribution as a paramedic is the record of what you found *at the scene.*

2. If one of the following is diagnosed in the field, the trauma center is a more appropriate triage endpoint:
   - Flail chest
   - Two or more proximal long bone fractures
   - Amputation proximal to wrist or ankle
   - All penetrating trauma to head, neck, torso, or extremities proximal to elbow or knee
   - Any limb paralysis
   - Pelvic fractures
   - Combination of trauma with burns
   - Open and depressed skull fractures
   - Major burns
3. Evaluate at this point the MOI and examine the trauma scene for evidence of high-energy trauma. If one of the following is present, refer to a trauma center:
   - Ejection from automobile
   - Death in same passenger compartment
   - Pedestrian thrown or run over or auto-pedestrian injury at > 5 mph
   - High-speed auto crash (> 40 mph)
   - Intrusion into passenger compartment of > 12″
   - Major auto deformity > 20″
   - Vehicle rollover with unrestrained passenger
   - Extrication time > 20 minutes
   - Falls > 20′
   - Motorcycle crash at > 20 mph or with separation of rider and bike
4. If none of the above criteria are met, then consider transfer to trauma center if:
   - Patient of age < 5 or > 55 years
   - Patient is pregnant
   - Known immunosuppressed patients
   - Known cardiac disease or respiratory disease comorbidity
   - Type 1 diabetes, cirrhosis, morbid obesity, or coagulopathy

In the Field

In addition to being trauma centers, some hospitals specialize in neurology, burns, pediatric trauma, cardiac care (centers for heart transplantation, coronary catheter labs), microsurgery (hand and limb reimplantation), or hyperbaric therapy. When you work with a service, you must know this information for your patient's sake.

Table 17-1	Key Elements for Trauma Centers

Level	Definition	Key Elements
Level I	A comprehensive regional resource that is a tertiary care facility. Capable of providing total care for every aspect of injury—from prevention through rehabilitation.	1. 24-hour in-house coverage by general surgeons 2. Availability of care in specialties such as orthopaedic surgery, neurosurgery, anesthesiology, emergency medicine, radiology, internal medicine, and critical care 3. Should also include cardiac, hand, pediatric, and microvascular surgery and hemodialysis 4. Provides leadership in prevention, public education, and continuing education of trauma team members 5. Committed to continued improvement through a comprehensive quality assessment program and organized research to help direct new innovations in trauma care
Level II	Able to initiate definitive care for all injured patients.	1. 24-hour immediate coverage by general surgeons 2. Availability of orthopaedic surgery, neurosurgery, anesthesiology, emergency medicine, radiology, and critical care 3. Tertiary care needs such as cardiac surgery, hemodialysis, and microvascular surgery may be referred to a Level I trauma center 4. Committed to trauma prevention and continuing education of trauma team members 5. Provides continued improvement in trauma care through a comprehensive quality assessment program
Level III	Has demonstrated the ability to provide prompt assessment, resuscitation, and stabilization of injured patients and emergency operations.	1. 24-hour immediate coverage by emergency medicine physicians and prompt availability of general surgeons and anesthesiologists 2. Program dedicated to continued improvement in trauma care through a comprehensive quality assessment program 3. Has developed transfer agreements for patients requiring more comprehensive care at a Level I or Level II trauma center 4. Committed to continuing education of nursing and allied health personnel or the trauma team 5. Must be involved with prevention and have an active outreach program for its referring communities 6. Also dedicated to improving trauma care through a comprehensive quality assessment program
Level IV	Has demonstrated the ability to provide Advanced Trauma Life Support (ATLS) before transfer of patients to a higher level trauma center.	1. Include basic emergency department facilities to implement ATLS protocols and 24-hour laboratory coverage 2. Transfer to higher level trauma centers follows the guidelines outlined in formal transfer agreements 3. Committed to continued improvement of these trauma care activities through a formal quality assessment program 4. Involved in prevention, outreach, and education within its community

The prehospital assessment of trauma patients is key to the management of and transport to the appropriate definitive care facility.

Transport Considerations

When making a decision to transport a patient, several options must be considered. What are the needs of the patient? What is the level of the receiving facility? The patient should be transported to the closest, most appropriate facility to receive optimal care. You must also decide on the mode of transport that will offer the greatest benefit. Should you call for air transport, or is ground transport sufficient?

When making the decision to transport by ground, several factors should be taken into consideration. Can the appropriate facility be reached within a reasonable timeframe by ground? What is the extent of injuries? If in a congested area, can the patient be transported to a more accessible landing zone for air medical transport?

Air transport must be considered in several situations: (1) when there is extended transport time by ground, (2) when there are multiple casualties, (3) when extrication times are prolonged and patients are critically injured, and (4) when there are long distances to an appropriate facility as opposed to the closest emergency department. There also may be other

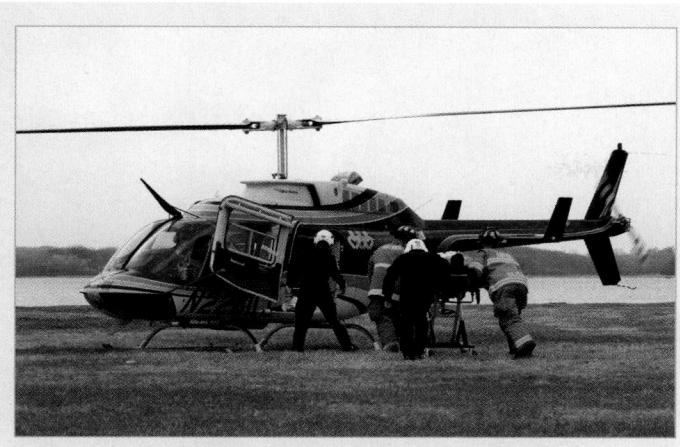

Figure 17-3 A helicopter may be used to transport patients quickly to the proper trauma center.

In the Field

The Platinum Ten Minutes refers to the goal of the maximum time spent at a scene for a critical trauma patient. Scene times should be limited as much as possible to get the patient to more definitive care at a trauma center. Trauma, more often than not, means that onsite stabilization is a questionable paramedic procedure. However, other problems may be better handled by onsite paramedic stabilization. One of your major tasks as a student paramedic is to learn the difference between the two.

times that air transport is appropriate **Figure 17-3 ▲** . If the patient can be transported to definitive care within a reasonable amount of time by ground, there is no need to call for air transport. Take into consideration the time it will take for the aircraft to lift off, travel, and land, just to reach the scene. By weighing the timeframe against transport by ground, you will be able to make an informed decision. Also take into account the terrain. Is there a safe area for landing? If not, how far will the patient need to be transported to reach a secure landing zone? If there is a great distance, ground transport may be a more reasonable option. Once the decision is made to call for air medical transport, contact your dispatcher to request a unit, or follow local protocols regarding contacting air support.

Helicopter Triage Criteria

All levels of prehospital providers should recognize the need for and criteria used in making the decision to use aeromedical

transport in their service area. The key to success is recognizing the need for the aeromedical transport of patients and activating the service as early as possible. The trauma triage guidelines in this chapter should be used as a guideline.

▌ A Little Physics

Although drivers of motor vehicles might not obey the community's traffic laws, they must—whether they want to or not—obey the laws of physics that govern all objects on our planet. A little familiarity with these laws will help you understand more about the mechanisms of trauma.

Velocity (V) is the distance an object travels per unit time. The difference between velocity and speed is that velocity is also defined by moving in a specific direction. Acceleration (a) of an object is the rate of change of velocity that an object is subjected to, whether speeding up or slowing down. Gravity (g) is the downward acceleration that is imparted to any object on earth by the effect of the earth's mass. During each second of a fall, the velocity or speed of the falling object increases by 9.8 m/sec^2.

You are the Provider Part 2

The police officers advise you that the patient was probably under the influence of PCP (phencyclidine hydrochloride), and in his attempts to avoid arrest, he climbed up a fire escape and fell. He landed on his hands and feet, stumbled for a few steps, and continued to try to run away unsuccessfully.

Vital Signs	Recording Time: 5 Minutes
Level of consciousness	V (Responsive to verbal stimuli)
Skin	Slightly moist, slightly pale, and cool
Pulse	Carotid (unable to access radial pulses because patient is being restrained); rapid (142 beats/min)
Blood pressure	168 by palpation
Respirations	60 breaths/min
Sao_2	99% while breathing room air

4. Given commonalities of fire escape locations, what other information do you have?
5. How does your patient's condition hinder your assessment techniques?
6. How do you compensate for this hindrance?

Controversies

Some situations may have contraindications or relative contraindications for aeromedical transport. These situations include traumatic cardiac arrest, inclement weather conditions, extremely combative patients, morbidly obese patients, patients with barotrauma (diving injuries may necessitate lower flying altitudes), and situations in which ground transport and appropriate level of care are available and would permit quicker care.

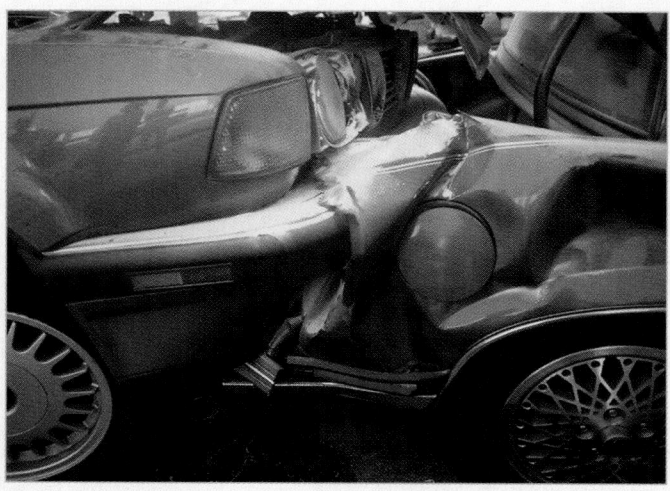

Figure 17-5 The kinetic energy of a speeding car is converted into the work of stopping the car, usually by crushing the car's exterior.

The kinetic energy (KE) of an object is the energy associated with that object in motion. It reflects the relationship between the weight (mass) of the object and the velocity at which it is traveling and is expressed mathematically as:

$$\text{Kinetic energy} = \frac{\text{Mass}}{2} \times \text{Velocity}^2$$

$$\text{or, KE} = \frac{m}{2} \times v^2$$

Thus, velocity has a much greater effect on KE than weight because it is squared (**Figure 17-4 ▾**).

In other words, an object increases its kinetic energy more by increasing its velocity than by increasing its mass. The kinetic energy of an object involved in a collision must be *dissipated* as the object comes to rest. The kinetic energy of a car in motion that stops suddenly must be somewhere (**Figure 17-5 ▸**). In a car, kinetic energy can be dissipated by braking, transforming to heat (another form of energy). If all the energy is not transformed into heat, however, the KE is transformed into deformed metal (potential energy), which results in damage to the car and its occupants. The mechanics of dissipation can result in injury. For example, a car traveling at 35 mph hits a wall, which stops the car, but the driver is still traveling at 35 mph until stopped by the seatbelts or the air bag, or, if not wearing a seatbelt, the steering wheel, dashboard, or windshield.

Speed kills exponentially: look what happens when velocity increases 10 mph versus when the person weighs in at 10 lb heavier.

- 150-lb person at 10 mph = 7,500 KE units
- 150-lb person at 20 mph = 30,000 KE units
- 150-lb person at 30 mph = 67,500 KE units
- 150-lb person at 40 mph = 120,000 KE units
- 160-lb person at 40 mph = 128,000 KE units
- 150-lb person at 55 mph = 226,875 KE units
- 150-lb person at 65 mph = 316,875 KE units

Note that when weight increases by 10 lb but velocity remains the same, there is not much change in the kinetic energy. However, when the velocity increases from 55 to 65 mph (a difference of only 10 mph), the KE (remember, that's energy in motion!) increases by 90,000 KE units!

Modern cars are designed to have crumple zones to maximize the amount of energy dissipated by deformation before the passenger compartment is involved. Because the automobile damage so often shows just how fast the car was going, the amount of damage provides information to help in your decision about transferring your patient to a trauma center.

In addition to the velocity at which the car (and its passengers) are traveling, the vehicle's angle of impact (front collision versus side impact, or how your patient hit the inside of an automobile), the differences in the sizes of the two vehicles, and the restraint status and protective gear of the occupants will affect the amount of energy dissipation that affects your patients in a crash.

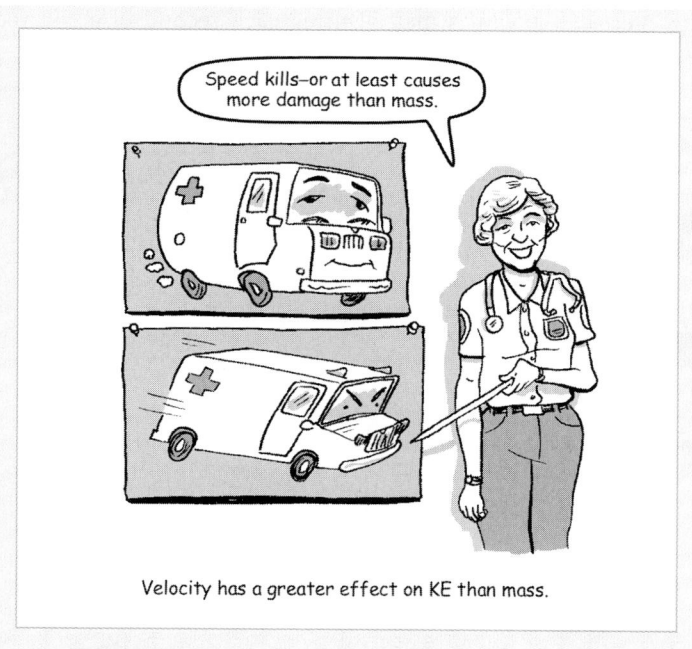

Velocity has a greater effect on KE than mass.

Figure 17-4

Remember the laws of physics that no driver can break? Here's a quick review in physics-ese. The law of conservation of energy states that energy can be neither created nor destroyed, it can only change form. Energy generated from a sudden stop or start must be transformed to one of the following energy forms: thermal, electrical, chemical, radiant, or mechanical (as discussed earlier).

Energy dissipation, as you know, is the process by which KE is transformed into one of these forms of mechanical energy. When a car stops slowly, its KE is converted to thermal energy—heat—by friction of the braking action. If the car crashes, KE is also dissipated into mechanical energy as the car body crumples in a collision. Mechanical energy is further dissipated in the form of injury as the occupants sustain fractures or other bodily harm.

Protective devices such as seatbelts, air bags, and helmets are designed to *manipulate* the way in which energy is dissipated into injury. For example, a seatbelt converts kinetic energy of the occupants into a seatbelt–to-body pressure force rather than into a steering wheel deformation against the torso or a windshield shattering against the head.

Newton's first law of motion states that a body at rest will remain at rest unless acted on by an outside force. Similarly, a body in motion tends to remain in motion at a constant velocity, traveling in a straight line, unless acted on by an outside force. Most bodies in motion (without the assistance of a motor or other propulsion device) tend to eventually stop owing to the action of forces of friction, wind resistance, or other force resulting in deceleration.

Newton's second law of motion states that the force that an object can exert is the product of its mass times its acceleration:

$$\text{Force} = \text{Mass (Weight)} \times \text{Acceleration (or Deceleration)}$$

The higher an object's mass and acceleration, the higher the *force* that needs to be applied to make a change of course or stop the object. Remember our cartoon? Force equals mass × acceleration or deceleration. Deceleration is slowing to a stop. Rapid deceleration, as may occur in a collision, dissipates tremendous forces and, therefore, major injuries. Deceleration and acceleration can also be measured in numbers of *g* forces. One *g* force is the normal acceleration of gravity. A two or three *g* acceleration or deceleration force is, logically enough, two or three times the force associated with the acceleration of gravity. A two *g* deceleration would make you feel like you are twice as heavy as you are at rest. Three *g* acceleration would make you feel three times heavier. High-speed collisions can generate decelerations in *hundreds* of *g*'s. The human limit to deceleration is about 30 *g*.

In a *head-on collision* with two vehicles traveling in opposite directions along a straight line, transferred energy is represented in part as the sum of both their speeds. If a car strikes an immovable object, forces generated come from the speed of the only moving object. In a *rear impact* of two vehicles traveling along the same line, the energy potential is lessened because it is the difference in speed between them, also known as the *closing speed.*

It is important to have an understanding of these laws of physics because they help define the types and patterns of trauma you will see in the field. You are the most important witness the hospital trauma team has—the information you learn from physics will affect the outcome of your patient's life.

Types of Trauma

Injuries are generally described as the consequence of blunt or penetrating trauma. Blunt trauma refers to injuries in which the tissues are not penetrated by an external object **Figure 17-6 ▾**. Blunt trauma commonly occurs in motor vehicle crashes, in pedestrians hit by a vehicle, in motorcycle crashes, in falls from heights, in serious sports injures, and in blasts when no shrapnel is involved and the pressure wave is the primary cause of the injuries.

Penetrating trauma results when tissues are penetrated by single or multiple objects **Figure 17-7 ▸**. Penetrating trauma results from gunshot wounds caused by a single or multiple projectiles, stab wounds, and blasts with shrapnel or secondary projectiles. Penetrating trauma may also occur in combination with blunt injuries such as in implement injuries during a motor vehicle crash or a fall out of a tree and onto a fence.

In the Field

As a general rule, the entrance wound is always smaller than the exit wound. Assume that cavitation involves internal structures that are not readily visible on your clinical exam.

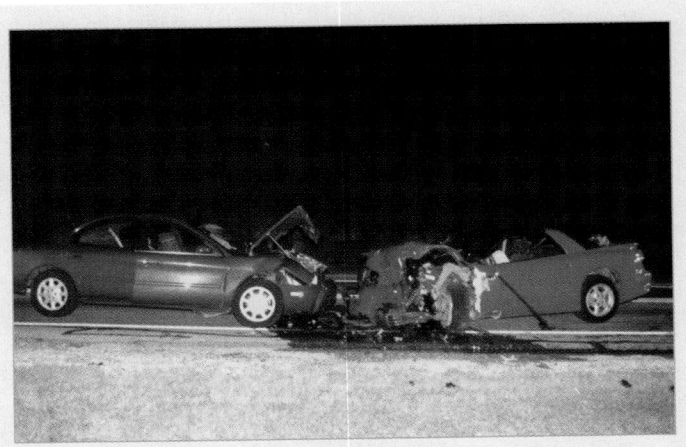

Figure 17-6 Blunt trauma typically occurs in motor vehicle crashes.

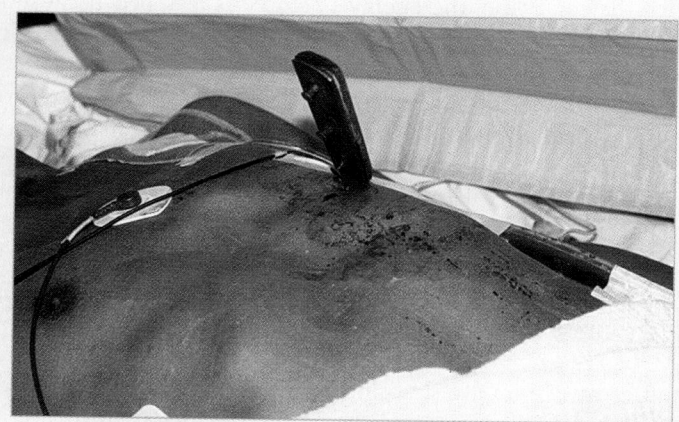

Figure 17-7 Injuries from low-energy penetrations, such as a stab wound, are caused by the sharp edges of the object moving through the body.

Injuries Caused by Deceleration

Abrupt deceleration injuries are produced by a sudden stop of a body's forward motion. Whether from a fall, shaking a baby, or a high-speed vehicle crash, decelerating forces can induce shearing, avulsing, or rupturing of organs and their restraining fascia, vasculature, nerves, and other soft tissues. These injuries are often invisible during examination, so every paramedic needs to understand how such injuries are sustained.

The head is particularly vulnerable to deceleration injuries. The brain is a fairly heavy organ that lies in fluid inside the skull. Any trauma that will jerk the patient's head causes the brain to hit the inside of the skull, causing bleeding, bruising, tearing, and crush injuries. All of these injuries are extremely dangerous and might not show up on a cursory examination.

Your paramedic index of suspicion should be on high alert for these injuries.

The chest is vulnerable to aorta injury. The *aorta*, the largest blood vessel in the body, is the most common site of deceleration injury in the chest. The aorta is often torn away from its points of fixation in the body. Shearing of the aorta can result in rapid loss of all the body's blood and immediate death.

Abdominal blunt trauma results as the forward motion of the body stops and internal organs continue their forward motion, resulting in tearing at their points of attachment, in shearing injuries, and tearing in abdominal walls. Organs that can be affected include the liver, kidneys, small intestine, large intestine, pancreas, and spleen.

Kidneys are injured as forward motion produces tears to the organ or to points of attachment with the abdominal aorta or through the renal arteries. Also, as forward motion is restrained by the large bowel, the small bowel can tear and result in free air in the abdomen. Trauma can also do damage without tearing by causing an insufficient supply of blood to the bowel. The spleen can also be torn, sometimes resulting in left upper quadrant pain and life-threatening internal bleeding.

Injuries Caused by External Forces

Crush and compression injuries are the result of forces applied to the body by things external to the body at the time of impact. Crush and compression injuries occur *at* the time of impact, unlike deceleration injuries, which occur *before* impact. Crush and compression injuries are often caused by dashboards, windshields, the floor, and heavy objects falling on the body.

Compression head injuries, which may result in skull fractures, often are associated with cervical spine injury. Therefore, you need to assume spinal cord injuries and severe injury to the brain. Brain tissue does not compress; it swells within the

You are the Provider Part 3

The police officers restrain the patient so that you can perform your initial assessment and a rapid trauma assessment, all while taking spinal precautions. You are able to apply a cervical collar and minimize his movement on a backboard. During your rapid trauma assessment, you find that he has deformity of both legs below the knees. He also has some abrasions to both hands and arms. It appears as though the majority of force was absorbed by the legs during the fall.

Reassessment	Recording Time: 10 Minutes
Level of consciousness	V (Responsive to verbal stimuli)
Skin	Slightly moist, slightly pale, and cool
Pulse	Carotid (unable to access radial pulses as patient is being restrained); rapid
Blood pressure	168 by palpation
Respirations	60 breaths/min
Sao$_2$	98% while breathing room air; patient noncompliant with nonrebreathing mask

7. Given this information, what other injuries do you suspect?

8. How can a patient who is under the influence of drugs be difficult to manage?

9. In addition to trauma, what other medical emergencies can ensue from the use of PCP?

In the Field

- According to 2003 National Highway Transportation Safety Administration (NHTSA) statistics, the overall traffic fatality rate dropped to a record low of 1.48 fatalities per 100 million vehicle miles traveled in 2003.
  - This still represents a total of 6.3 million crashes, of which 38,252 involved a fatality.
- In 2003 alone, 42,643 people were killed: 33,471 were vehicle occupants, 3,661 were motorcycle riders, and 5,511 were nonmotorists.
  - There were 2,889,000 injured.
  - Of the 42,643 killed, 40% involved alcohol-related crashes.
  - Of drivers killed, males accounted for 74.5% and females for 25.5%.
  - Of passengers killed, 51.8% were males and 48.1% were females.
  - Of occupants injured, 49.6% were males and 50.4% were females.
- The age group with the most fatalities was 16- to 20-year-olds, accounting for 27.54 fatalities per 100,000 population.
- The next age group in number of fatalities was 21- to 24-year-olds with 24.51 fatalities per 100,000 population, followed by people older than 74 years with 18.77 per 100,000.

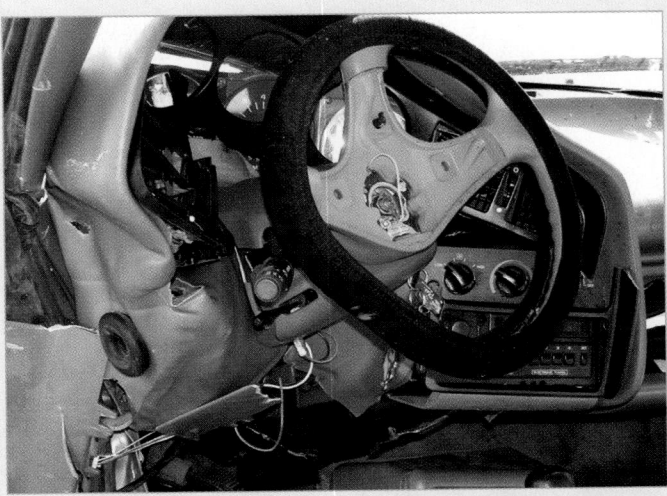

Figure 17-8 Deceleration of the occupant starts during sudden braking and continues during impact and collision. The appearance of the interior of the car can provide you with information about the severity of the patient's injuries.

enclosed area of the skull. As the brain swells inside the skull, it is crushed, causing a catastrophic injury.

Compression injuries of the chest may produce *fractured ribs*, which can lead to internal injuries of the lungs and heart. One of the signs of a lung injury is a *flail chest*, a condition in which the chest wall moves paradoxically with respirations (moves opposite of normal). Fractured ribs may also cause blood or air to seep into the chest space, which would require decompression and placement of a chest tube. Blunt cardiac injury can compress the heart between bones in the chest, causing arrhythmias and direct injury to the heart muscle. If the lungs are compressed, acute respiratory distress syndrome (ARDS) can require intubation to maintain your patient's breathing.

Almost all abdominal organs can be affected by hitting an external object. Organs often injured are the pancreas, spleen, liver, and, occasionally, kidneys. Compression against the seatbelt may result in *bowel rupture, bladder rupture, diaphragm tearing,* and *spinal injuries.* The abdomen has its own large blood-carrying vessel called the aorta. A common injury is the rupture of a valve in this vessel, caused by blood going the wrong way in the abdominal aorta.

Pelvic fractures also result from external compressive trauma, potentially injuring the bladder, vagina, rectum, lumbar plexus, and pelvic floor and leading to severe bleeding in the large arteries near the hip bones.

Motor Vehicle Crashes

When a motor vehicle collides with another object, trauma in the collision is composed of *five phases* tied to the affects of progressive deceleration. The first phase, *deceleration of the vehicle,* occurs when the vehicle strikes another object and is brought to an abrupt stop. The forward motion of the car continues until its KE is dissipated in the form of mechanical deformation and damage to the vehicle and occupant or until the restraining force of the object is removed (for example, sheared off pole, yielding of a guard rail) and the vehicle motion continues until its KE is gently dissipated by drag or continued braking. The second phase is *deceleration of the occupant,* which starts during sudden braking and continues during impact and collision. This results in deceleration, compression, and shear trauma to the occupants **Figure 17-8 ▲**. The effects on vehicle occupants will vary depending on the mass of each occupant, protective mechanisms in the vehicle such as restraints and air bags, body parts involved, and points of impact. The third phase, *deceleration of internal organs,* involves the body's supporting structures (skull, sternum, ribs, spine, and pelvis) and movable organs (brain, heart, liver, spleen, and intestine) that continue their forward momentum until stopped by anatomic restraints **Figure 17-9 ▶**. Energy is dissipated by internal organs as they are injured. Movement of fixed and nonfixed parts may result in tears and shearing injuries. The fourth phase is the result of *secondary collisions,* which occur when a vehicle occupant is hit by objects moving within the auto such as packages, animals, or other passengers. These objects may continue to travel at the auto's initial speed and then hit a passenger who has come to rest. These types of collisions have been known to cause severe spine and head trauma. The final phase is the result of *additional impacts* that the vehicle may receive, as when it is hit and deflected into another vehicle, tree, or another object. This

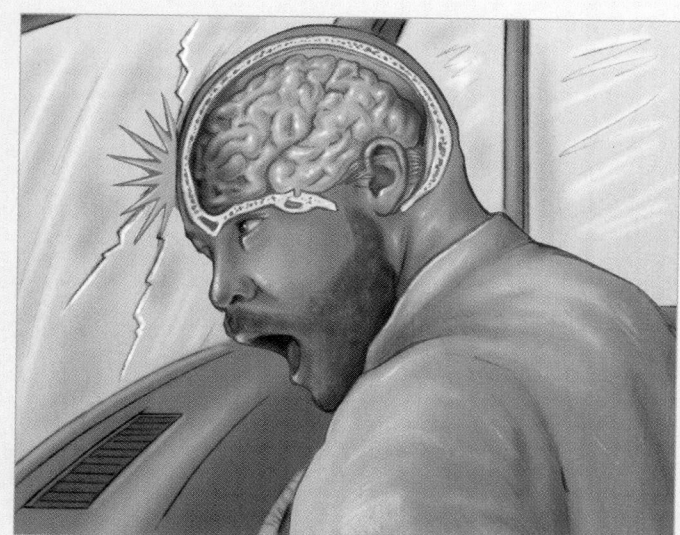

Figure 17-9 Deceleration of internal organs involves the body's supporting structures and movable organs that continue their forward momentum until stopped by anatomic restraints. In this illustration, the brain continues its forward motion and strikes the inside of the skull, resulting in a compression injury to the anterior portion of the brain and stretching of the posterior portion.

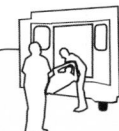

In the Field

Don't forget that the collision of internal organs striking against the body can result in severe damage, though this may not always be obvious.

Notes from Nancy

When the windshield is cracked or broken, the front seat occupant has a cervical spine injury until proved otherwise.

may increase the seriousness of original injuries or cause further injury. For example, a frontal collision may cause a posterior hip dislocation and an acetabular fracture via a dashboard mechanism and a subsequent side impact from another vehicle may add a lateral compression pelvic ring injury, resulting in complex pelvic and acetabular trauma. **Table 17-2 ▶** shows the structural clues, body clues, and resulting injuries for different types of collisions.

Predicting Types of Injury by Examining the Scene

Important clues to predict injury types can be obtained by paying attention to the history of the collision and by an examination of the scene. Using your new-found knowledge of the physics of trauma, you can make a good estimate of how hurt your patients might be by looking at the amount of damage around the scene. How dented and deformed the vehicle looks is a clear indication of the forces involved and of the degree of deceleration sustained by your patient. Dents and deformities on the inside of the vehicle will show you the point of impact on the patient. Do a quick check for injury types visible on your patient: head injury or seat-belt marks show what parts of the body may have been involved in energy absorption. Tire skid marks at the scene indicate whether significant energy was dissipated by braking before collision. Debris along the course of the crash may indicate multiple collisions and different force vectors acting on the patient along the course of the collision.

There are primarily *five types of impact patterns*: Frontal or head on, lateral or side impact, rear impact, rotational, and rollover. In *frontal and head-on crashes,* the front end of the car distorts as it dissipates kinetic energy and decelerates its forward motion. Passengers decelerate at the same rate as the vehicle. At a 30-mph collision, the front end of an average American car will crush 2 ft at the rough estimate of 1" of deformity for each 1 mph. The forces applied to the driver will differ based on car design, materials, and safety features of the vehicle. The interior will also suggest possible injuries by the damage your patient's body has done to the dash, windshield, or steering wheel, for example.

Position at the precise time of impact is very important in determining an occupant's movements and injuries during a collision. Unrestrained occupants usually follow one of two trajectories, a *down-and-under pathway,* or an *up-and-over pathway.*

The down-and-under pathway is traveled by an occupant who slides under the steering column **Figure 17-10 ▶**. As the vehicle is decelerating, the occupant continues to travel downward and forward into the dashboard or steering column, led by the knees. The knees hit the dashboard, transmitting the energy of the deceleration up the femurs to the pelvis. With knees locked in the dash and hips in the seat, force vectors go down the tibia and along the femur. If the feet are not locked by folding floorboards or brake pedals, energy along the tibia will be transferred to the lower leg, with no immediate injury. If the feet are locked in place, midshaft femur fracture can occur. In some cases, the heads of the femurs will dislocate. If the occupant's knees hit the dashboard, look for a fracture-dislocation of the knee or other injuries. Look also for hip and pelvic fractures or hip dislocation. Your patient's torso can twist in such a way that his or her head hits the steering column. Always look for spinal injuries.

The upper torso continues forward until it impacts the car, be it the steering wheel or the seatbelt and air bag protection system. Look for rib fractures or pulmonary or cardiac injuries caused by internal striking and compressing. When your patient is a child, assume that there will be

Notes from Nancy

When there is damage to the steering assembly, there is critical injury to the driver until proved otherwise.

Table 17-2	MOI: Motor Vehicle Crash		
Structural Clues	**Body Clues**	**Look for These Injuries**	
Head-on collision			
Deformed front end Cracked windshield	Bruised or lacerated head or face	• Brain injury • Scalp, facial cuts • Cervical spine injury • Tracheal injury	
Deformed steering column	Bruised neck Bruised chest	• Sternal or rib fracture • Flail chest • Myocardial contusion • Pericardial tamponade • Pneumothorax or hemothorax • Exsanguination from aortic tear	
Deformed dashboard	Bruised abdomen Bruised knee, misplaced kneecap	• Ruptured spleen, liver, bowel, diaphragm • Fractured patella • Dislocated knee • Femoral fracture • Dislocated hip	
Lateral collision			
Deformed side of car	Bruised shoulder	• Clavicular fracture • Fractured humerus • Multiple rib fractures	
Door smashed in	Bruised shoulder or pelvis	• Fractured hip • Fractured iliac wing • Fractured clavicle or ribs	
"B" pillar deformed	Bruised temple	• Brain injury • Cervical spine fracture	
Broken door or window handles	Bruised or deformed arms	• Contusions	
Broken window glass	Dicing lacerations	• Multiple lacerations	
Rear-end collision			
Posterior deformity of the auto Headrest not adjusted	Secondary anterior injuries, especially if the patient was unrestrained	• "Whiplash" injuries • Deceleration injuries of a head-on collision	

pulmonary or cardiac injuries—children have more flexible ribs but often sustain compression injuries. Remember how gas-containing organs absorb more of the energy of the crash?

In the up-and-over pathway, the lead point is the head. In this sequence, rotation occurs around the ankles with the torso moving in an upward and forward direction. The head takes a higher trajectory, impacting the windshield, roof, mirror, or dashboard, causing compression and deceleration injuries in your patient that can include significant head and cervical spine trauma. The anterior part of the neck may strike the steering wheel, causing laryngeal fracture, serious lacerations, and other soft-tissue injury.

Ejection is possible if the windshield does not stop the body from projecting through it. This leads to second-impact injuries when the body contacts the ground or objects outside of the car. These injuries can be as severe as initial-impact injuries, and they increase the likelihood of great vessel damage and death. The spine absorbs energy as it is compressed between the stationary head and the moving torso, which leads to injury.

A dangerous lung injury may occur if your patient reflexively takes a deep breath just before impact, hyperinflating the lungs and closing the glottis. The impact of the steering wheel can injure the lungs via generation of pressures beyond the capabilities of lung tissue, like a "paper bag being exploded" (60% to 70% of pneumothoraces may occur this way) **Figure 17-11 ▶**.

The abdomen, pelvis, or upper thigh contacts the lower aspect of the steering wheel or dash, and lower leg fractures

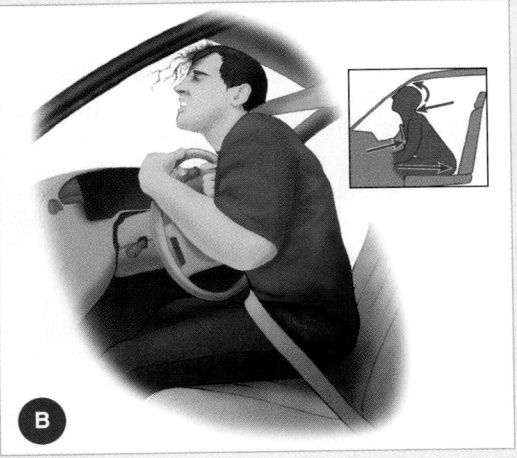

Figure 17-10 **A.** The down-and-under pathway. **B.** The up-and-over pathway.

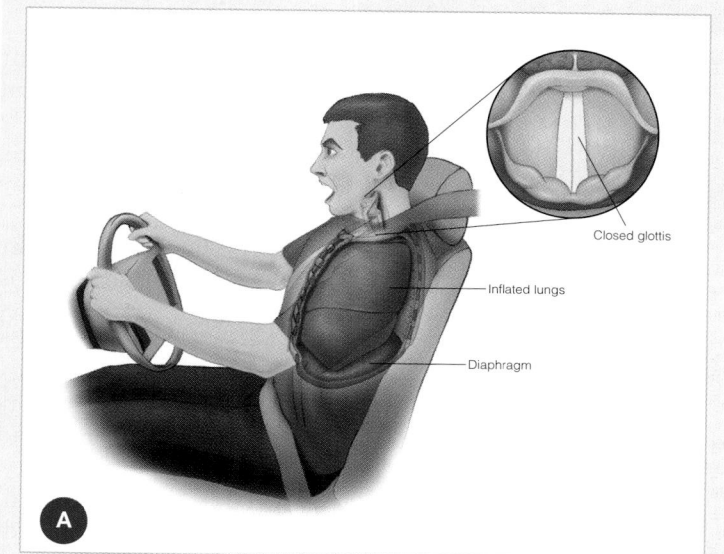

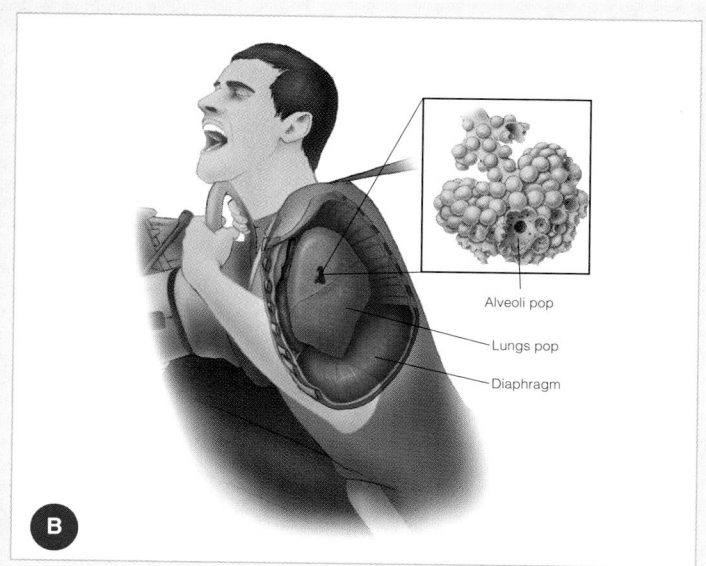

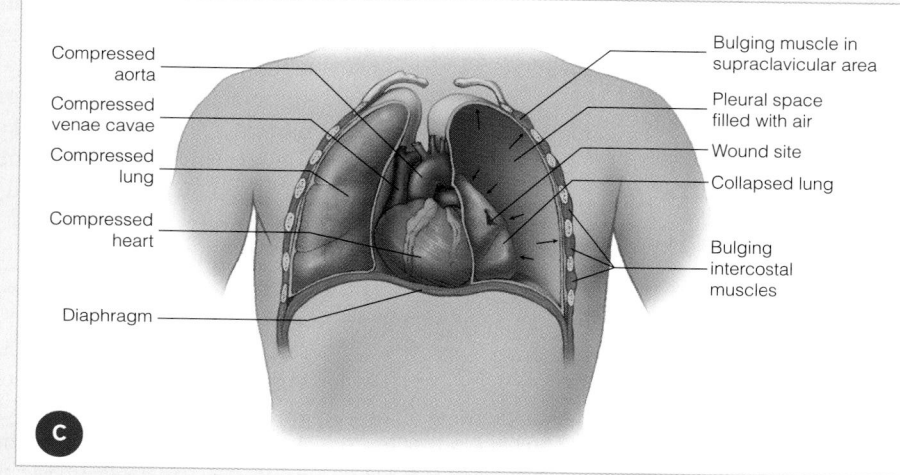

Figure 17-11 The paper-bag syndrome. **A.** The occupant takes a deep breath just before crashing, closing the glottis and filling the lungs with air. **B.** The occupant's chest hits the steering wheel, popping the alveoli in the lungs. **C.** A pneumothorax results.

could be present. Table 17-3 ▶ lists the "ring" of chest injuries that can occur from impacting the steering wheel or the dashboard.

Lateral impact, "T"-bone, and *side collisions* impart energy to the near-side occupant almost directly to the pelvis and chest Figure 17-12 ▶ . Unrestrained occupants will remain almost motionless, literally having the car pushed out from under them. Seatbelts do little to protect these passengers because they are designed to limit forward hinging injuries, not side impacts. As one vehicle makes contact with the side of the other vehicle, the occupant nearest the impact is hit by the door of the car as the passenger compartment begins to deform and collapse. The head can strike the hood of the impacting vehicle or object. Injury results from direct trauma to the affected side and to tension developed on the far side. Older vehicles may not have safety glass on the side windows. Upper extremity trauma depends on the spatial orientation of the arm at impact. The shoulder frequently rotates outward and

Table 17-3	"Ring" of Chest Injuries From Impacting the Steering Wheel or Dashboard

- Facial injuries
- Soft-tissue neck trauma
- Larynx and tracheal trauma
- Fractured sternum
- Myocardial contusion
- Pericardial tamponade
- Pulmonary contusion
- Hemothorax, rib fractures
- Flail chest
- Ruptured aorta
- Intra-abdominal injuries

posteriorly, exposing the chest and ribs to injury. Forces transmitted to the chest cause rib fractures, lateral flail chest, and lung contusions. If the humerus remains between the door and chest, the clavicle may absorb side motion and fracture. As the body of the occupant is pushed in one direction, the head

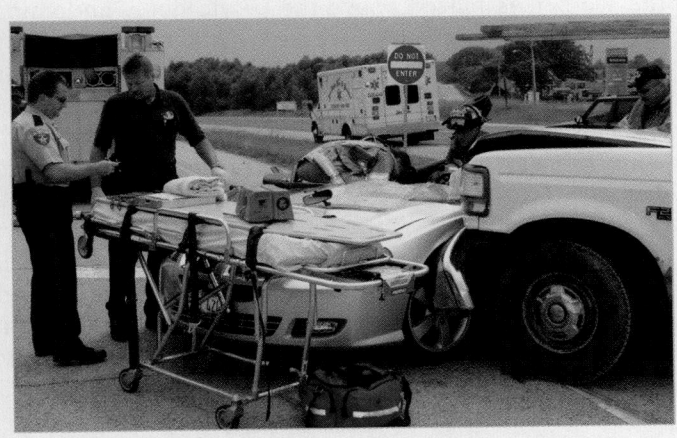

Figure 17-12 In a lateral collision, the car may be struck above its center of gravity and begins to rock away from the side of impact. This causes a type of lateral whiplash in which the passenger's shoulders and head whip toward the intruding vehicle.

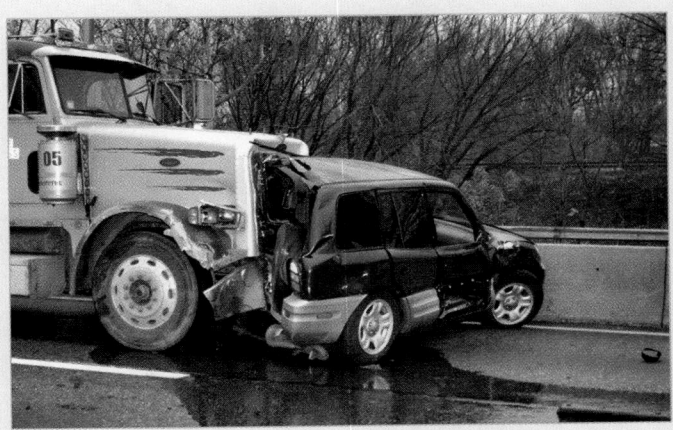

Figure 17-13 Rear-end impacts often cause whiplash-type injuries, particularly when the head and/or neck is not restrained by a headrest.

moves toward the impacting object, creating a line of tension along the contralateral side. This may result in ligamentous disruption and dislocation of the spine on the opposite side of the impact. The far-side occupant, if properly restrained, has the advantage of "riding down" with the car, thereby receiving considerably less force. If unrestrained, he or she may move in a direction parallel but opposite to the impact. This passenger receives forces similar to any unrestrained occupant. Furthermore, because both passengers travel in a direction parallel to impact but in opposite directions, they collide with each other, causing additional injury.

In a lateral collision, if the greater trochanter of the femur is impacted and transmits forces to the pelvis, sometimes it may be driven through the acetabulum into the pelvis. If the force reaches the ilium, the pelvis may also fracture. The typical pattern of pelvic injury that occurs in this scenario is a lateral compression injury that trauma surgeons call pelvic ring disruption. Lateral compression injuries are less serious than anterior compression injuries. Death in lateral collisions is usually the result of associated torso or head injuries.

Rear-impact collisions have the most survivors, if the driver and passengers are properly restrained **Figure 17-13 ▶** . If the vehicle coming from the rear is traveling at excessive speed, however, most bets on survivability are off. Most often in this kind of crash, a stationary (or slower moving) vehicle is struck from behind and the impact energy is transmitted as a sudden forward accelerating force. The neck hyperextends as the body moves forward relative to the head. The head does not move forward with the body unless a headrest is in the proper position; if the headrest is not in proper position, the head is snapped back and then forward. Because most seats have some degree of elasticity after the sudden forward acceleration has ended, the stored potential energy in the seat is converted to an energy of forward motion, which can aggravate the hyperextension trauma to the neck and then follow with some rebound

forward flexion of the head on the chest resulting in hyperflexion. A third episode of extension may occur as the chest moves forward. This is the so-called whiplash injury.

In a rear-impact collision, energy is imparted to the front vehicle, which accelerates rapidly, while frontal impact energy to the rear driver is reduced because energy is being transferred to the front car. One concern with rear-impact collisions is the frequency with which seat backs collapse, causing unrestrained occupants to be propelled into the back seat. Head restraints developed to prevent the head and torso from moving separately are not always adjusted correctly. Many are placed too low and act as a fulcrum that may actually facilitate the extension injury. They need to be adjusted so they are behind the head and not behind the neck.

A *rotational* or *quarter-panel impact* occurs when the collision is off center. In this case, rotation occurs as part of the car continues to move and part of the car comes to a stop. The vehicle stops at the point of impact, but the opposite side continues in rotational motion around the impact point. The point of greatest speed loss of the vehicle is the site where the greatest damage to the occupant will occur. The resultant forces act along a vector oblique to the direction of travel. For example, in a ten o'clock impact with twelve o'clock being frontal, the driver would initially move forward and then diagonally as the auto rotates, striking the A pillar, the support for the windshield. The front-seat passenger would strike the rearview mirror area. The point of greatest deceleration becomes the location of the most severely injured patients. Occupants tend to receive a combination of frontal and lateral injuries. Because rigid objects may be in line with vector forces, head injuries may result. Three-point belts are effective in preventing injury in angled collisions of up to 45°.

Rollover scenarios have the greatest potential to cause lethal injuries. Injuries will be serious even if seatbelts are worn. However, if your patients did not wear seatbelts, they may be ejected, and they will have been struck hard with each change

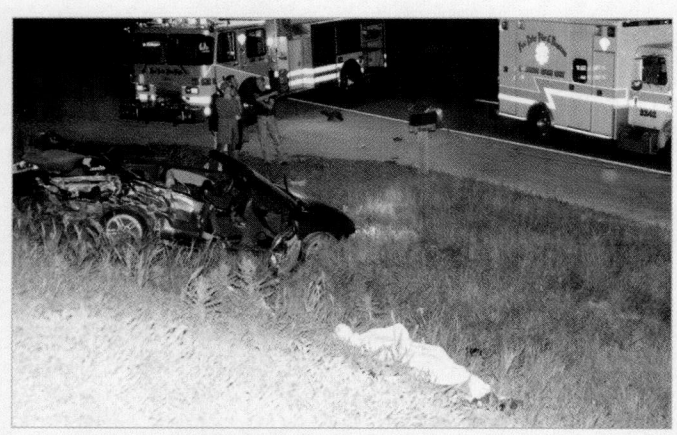

Figure 17-14 Occupants who have been ejected or partially ejected may have struck the interior of the car many times before ejection.

in direction the car makes with the rollover. Even a restrained occupant's head and neck will change direction with each change in the vehicle's position.

Ejection of the patient from the vehicle increases the chance of death by 25 times Figure 17-14 ▲ . One of three ejected victims will sustain a cervical-spine fracture. A partial ejection can result in an arm or leg injured by being caught between the vehicle and the ground.

Restrained Versus Unrestrained Occupants

Seatbelts are highly effective because they stop the motion of any automobile occupant who will otherwise travel at the same speed as the vehicle, until stopped. The seatbelt, although capable of delivering some injury at high speeds, will prevent the serious-to-fatal injuries of being unrestrained in the car and being ejected from the car. One of every 13 victims of ejection sustains major and permanent cervical spine damage. Restrained victims "ride down" the deceleration with belt elasticity and crush time of the car, with a nearly 45% reduction in fatalities. Restraints limit the contact of the occupants with the interior of the vehicle, prevent ejection, distribute deceleration energy over a greater surface, and prevent the occupants from violently contacting each other. As a result, all types of injuries are decreased, including head, facial, spine, thoracic, intra-abdominal, pelvic, and lower extremities, and ejection is also limited.

All arguments against seatbelt use are unfounded. Every unrestrained passenger poses a hazard to themselves and to other occupants in the vehicle, especially for front seat passengers who are at double risk for injury in a front-end collision if the back seat occupants are unrestrained.

Specific injuries associated with seatbelt use include cervical fractures due to flexion stresses and neck sprains due to deceleration and hyperextension. Most serious injuries occur because the patient did not use the seatbelt correctly. If the occupant does not use the lap strap, severe upper body injuries, including spinal injuries and decapitation, can occur.

If the seatbelt is placed above the pelvic bone, abdominal injuries and lumbar spine injuries result.

Air bags were another great step up for patient safety. NHTSA has estimated that air bags have reduced deaths in direct frontal crashes by about 30%. Front air bags will not activate in side impact collisions or impacts to the front quarter panel, and without the use of a seatbelt, they are insufficient to prevent ejection. They are self-deflating and function only for a first impact, not the secondary ones. The rapidly inflating bag can also result in secondary injuries from direct contact with the air bag or from the chemicals used to inflate it. Common injuries include abrasions and burns to the face, chest, and arms; minor corrosive toxic effects, chemical keratitis, conjunctivitis, or corneal abrasion, and inhalation injuries Figure 17-15 ▼ .

Small children can be severely injured or killed if air bags inflate while they are in the front seat. That is why all EMS providers are encouraged to participate in teaching parents how to properly place and secure children's car seats.

Unique Patient Populations

Increased morbidity and mortality, especially chest trauma, is more common in *geriatric patients,* particularly rib and sternal fractures. Fatalities also increase if *child* restraint devices are improperly installed or used. Children who have outgrown a

> ### Special Considerations
>
> The different mechanisms of injury in children and the unique anatomic features of children together produce predictable patterns of injury. Because penetrating injuries are uncommon and because the head (compared with the rest of the body) is larger in childhood, injured children often have blunt injuries primarily involving the head. If the energy impact is severe and involves the entire body, the child may have a pattern involving the head, chest, abdomen, and long bones.

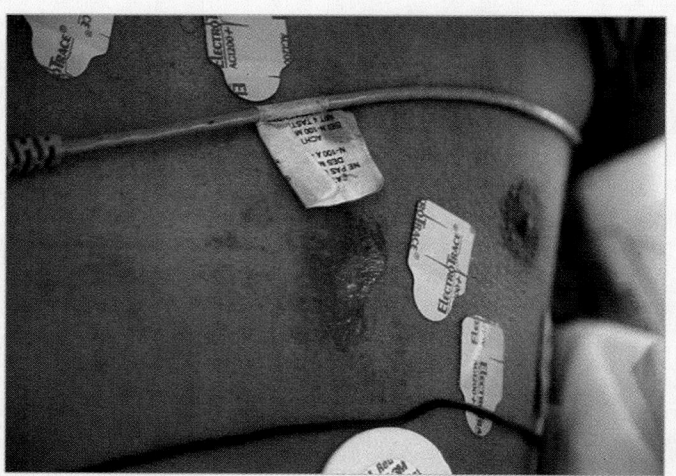

Figure 17-15 Air bags can cause abrasions to the face, chest, and arms.

car seat but are too small to be restrained by belts designed for adults are at risk for hyperflexion and abdominal injury.

Pregnant women in general wear seatbelts less frequently than do nonpregnant women owing to the unproven concern that the seatbelt may increase damage to the unborn child in the case of a crash. However, no study has reported that seatbelts increase fetal mortality. If lap belts are worn alone and too high, they allow enough forward flexion and subsequent compression to rupture the uterus because deceleration forces are transmitted directly to the uterus. Lap belts with shoulder harnesses are essential to provide equal distribution of forces and to prevent forward flexion of the mother. Without the shoulder harness, the protuberant uterus will also receive the impact of the steering wheel or dashboard. Steering wheel or dashboard injuries sustained because seatbelts were not worn or worn improperly are associated with a 50% fetal death rate.

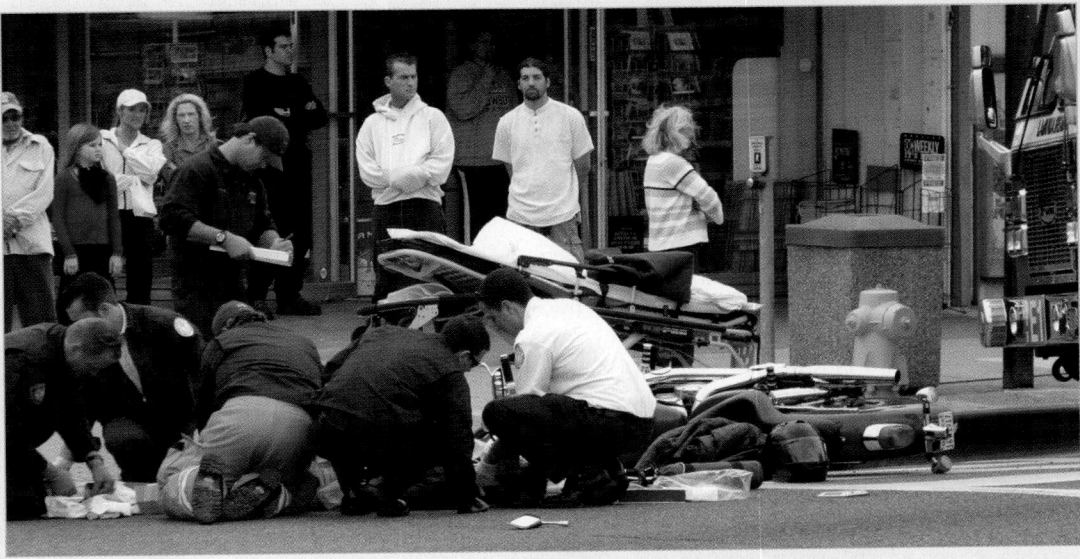

Figure 17-16 At a motorcycle crash scene, attention should be given to the deformity of the motorcycle, the side of most damage, the distance of skid in the road, the deformity of stationary objects or other vehicles, and the extent and location of deformity in the helmet.

Motorcycle Crashes

NHTSA data for 2003 shows that motorcycle-related deaths are 70% higher than they were in 1997. In 2003, 3,661 motorcycle riders were killed, accounting for about 8.5% of all deaths in vehicular crashes. Of interest is that while motorcycle-related deaths increased in all age groups, the highest increase in absolute number of victims was in the 50-year-old and older group. However, deaths in the 21-year-old and younger group increased by 21%. The increase in number of deaths parallels an increase in engine capacity of production motorcycles.

In a motorcycle crash, any structural protection afforded to the victims is not derived from a steel cage, as is the case in an automobile, but from protective devices worn by the rider, that is, helmet, leather or abrasion-resistant clothing, and boots. While helmets are designed to protect against impact forces to the head, they transmit any impact into the cervical spine, and as such, do not protect against severe cervical injury. Leather and synthetic gear worn over the body was initially designed to protect professional riders in competition, where falls tend to be controlled and result in long sliding mechanisms on hard surfaces rather than multiple collisions against road objects and other vehicles. Leather clothing will protect mostly against road abrasion but offers no protection against blunt trauma from secondary impacts. In a street crash, collisions occur usually against other larger vehicles or stationary objects.

When you are assessing the scene of a motorcycle crash, attention should be given to the deformity of the motorcycle, the side of most damage, the distance of skid in the road, the deformity of stationary objects or other vehicles, and the extent and location of deformity in the helmet **Figure 17-16 ▲**. These findings can be helpful in estimating the extent of trauma in a patient.

There are *four types of motorcycle impacts.* In a *head-on collision,* the motorcycle strikes another object and stops its forward motion while the rider and parts of the motorcycle that are broken off continue their forward motion until stopped by an outside force, such as drag from the road or another opposing force from a secondary collision. Because the motorcycle's center of gravity is above the front axle, there is a forward and upward motion at the point of the collision, causing the rider to go over the handle bars. If the rider's feet remain on the pegs or pedals, the forward and upward motion of the upper torso is restrained by femurs and tibias, producing bilateral femur or tibia fractures and severe foot injuries.

For motorcycles with a low riding seat below the level of the gas tank, such as Japanese racing bikes or Italian transalpine style motorcycles, the tank can act as a wedge on the pelvis during the initial phase of the collision resulting in severe APC (anterior-posterior compression) injuries to the pelvis, often resulting in severe neurovascular compromise.

> **Special Considerations**
>
> Changes in vision, hearing, posture, and motor ability predispose older people to a greater risk of being struck by a vehicle.

Open pelvic fractures are also common, resulting in severe perineal injuries with loss of the pelvic floor. Mortality associated with open pelvic fractures approaches 50%.

In an *angular collision,* the motorcycle strikes an object or another vehicle at an angle so that the rider sustains direct crushing injuries to the lower extremity between the object and the motorcycle. This usually results in severe open and comminuted lower extremity injuries with severe neurovascular compromise, often requiring surgical amputation.

Traumatic amputations are also common high-speed injuries. After the initial crush injury to the lower extremity, mechanisms such as a described in the head-on collision also apply. Often the rider is propelled over the hood of the colliding vehicle. Because the collision is at an angle, severe thoracoabdominal torsion and lateral bending spine injuries can result, in addition to head injury and pelvic trauma.

An *ejected* rider will travel at high speed until stopped by a stationary object, another vehicle, or by road drag. Severe abrasion injuries (road rash) down to bone can occur with drag. An unpredictable combination of blunt injuries can occur from secondary collisions.

A technique used to separate the rider from the body of the motorcycle and the object to be hit is referred to as *laying the bike down.* It was developed by motorcycle racers and adapted by street bikers as a means of achieving a controlled crash. As a collision approaches, the motorcycle is turned flat and tipped sideways at 90° to the direction of travel so that one leg is dropped to the grass or asphalt. This slows the occupant faster than the motorcycle, allowing for the rider to become separated from the motorcycle. If properly protected with leather or synthetic abrasion-resistant gear, injuries should be limited to those sustained by rolling over the pavement and any secondary collision that may occur. When executed properly, this maneuver prevents the rider from being trapped between the bike and the object. However, a rider unable to clear the bike will continue into the vehicle, often with devastating results.

With any type of crash, the helmet should remain on unless airway management techniques cannot be performed with the helmet in place or the helmet does not fit snuggly to the head. Dents and abrasions must be assumed to have caused c-spine fractures until proven otherwise by an x-ray. Precautions should be taken to remove the helmet, which should be cut if it cannot be removed without introducing further deformation to the neck.

Pedestrian Injuries

Of the 42,643 traffic fatalities recorded in the United States in 2003, 4,749 involved pedestrians. In addition, another 70,000 pedestrians were injured; 68% were male, and 32% were female. The largest number of pedestrians killed was in the 35- to 44-year-old age group (18%); children younger than 9 years accounted for about 5% of the deaths. Most deaths (25%) occurred between 6:00 and 9:00 PM, and an additional 21% died between 9:00 PM and midnight. Of all deaths, 78% occurred in areas other than intersections, and 22% occurred

at intersections. In 2003, 622 deaths were a result of bicycles being hit by a vehicle.

More than 85% of pedestrians are struck by the vehicle's front end, sustaining a predictable pattern of injuries starting with those caused by direct impact with the bumper. Adult injuries are generally lateral and posterior because adults tend to turn to the side or away from impact, whereas children will face forward into the oncoming vehicle.

There are *three predominant mechanisms of injury.* When the auto strikes an adult body with its bumpers, it creates lower extremity injuries, particularly to the knee and leg. These are in the form of various patterns of tibia-fibula fractures, often open knee dislocations and tibial plateau fractures. Usually the tibia is fractured on the side of impact; the impact potentially fractures the other leg as well. Knee dislocations are common with severe multiligamentous injury.

In the field, a dislocated knee should be splinted in the position found if the patient has good distal PMS—pulse, and motor and sensory function. It is key to remember that if the knee reduces spontaneously, you must communicate this to the trauma team verbally and in your report. Spontaneous reduction is an indication of possible vascular injury that can be missed by the trauma team if you do not report the spontaneous reduction.

A *second impact* occurs as the adult is thrown on the hood and/or grill, resulting in head, pelvis, chest, and coup-contrecoup traumatic brain injuries. Lateral compression pelvic fractures are common in this mechanism and can cause open fractures with bony punctures of the vagina in women and in other viscera. A *third impact* occurs when the body strikes the ground or some other object after it has been subjected to a sudden acceleration by the colliding vehicle.

Pediatric patterns of pedestrian injury are different from patterns in adults. Small children are shorter, so the car bumper is more likely to strike them in the pelvis or torso, causing severe injuries from direct impact **Figure 17-17 ▾** . Although they are less likely than adults to fly over the hood of the car, they are more likely to be run over by the vehicle as they are propelled to

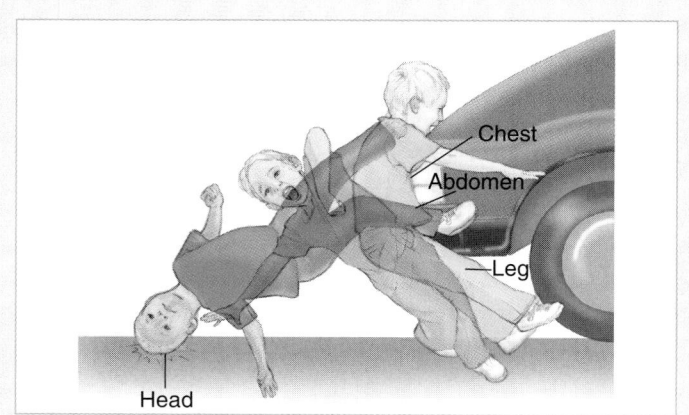

Figure 17-17 In car versus pedestrian crashes, children frequently sustain multisystem injuries involving the head, chest, abdomen, and long bones.

the ground by the impact. Multiple extremity and pelvic fractures and abdominal and thoracic crush injuries are to be expected. Closed head trauma often kills young patients.

The Waddell triad refers to the pattern of automobile pedestrian injuries in children and people of short stature: (1) The bumper hits the pelvis and femur instead of the knees and tibias. (2) The chest and abdomen hit the grille or low on the hood of the car (sternal and rib fractures). (3) The head strikes the vehicle and then the ground (skull and facial fractures, facial abrasions, and closed head injury).

Falls From Heights

High falls most commonly involve children younger than 5 years of age who are left unsupervised near a high window (more than 10′) or on a porch higher than 10′ with inadequate railings. Adult falls from heights usually occur in the context of criminal activity, attempted suicide, or intoxication such as in alcohol, narcotic, or hallucinogen use, especially PCP.

Remember that a fall produces acceleration downward at 9.8 m/sec^2. On contact with the floor or ground, an instantaneous deceleration occurs that decelerates the victim from whatever velocity had been achieved at the end of the fall to zero velocity. If a person falls for 2 seconds, the speed at impact nearly 20 m/sec.

The severity of injuries you can expect to find in your patient will depend on a number of factors, all of which will be important in your patient assessment:

- **Height.** The height from which the patient has fallen will determine the *velocity* of the fall. A person falling one story (12′) onto concrete, for example, will fall at about 28 feet per second (fps) and experience an impact force of about 48 g. A person falling from the second story (24′) will reach a velocity of 39 fps and experience an impact force of 95 g on the same surface. Height plus stopping distance predicts the magnitude of deceleration forces. A fall greater than 15′ or 2.5 to 3 times the height of the patient will have a greater incidence of morbidity and mortality, although it is usually assumed that a fall from four stories may be survivable. At five stories, survival is questionable; at six stories, survival is unlikely, and a fall from seven stories or higher is rarely survivable.
- **Position.** The position or orientation of the body at the moment of impact will also be a determinant of type of injuries sustained and their survivability. Children tend to fall headfirst, owing to the relatively greater mass of a child's head, so head injuries are common in children, as are injuries to the wrists and upper extremities when the child attempts to break his fall with outstretched arms. Adults, on the other hand, usually try, when not intoxicated, to land on their feet, thus controlling their fall. However, they often tilt backward, landing on their buttocks and outstretched hands. The group of potential injuries from a vertical fall to a standing position is commonly referred to as the *Don Juan syndrome* or *lover's*

leap pattern of injuries **Figure 17-18 ▶**. Injuries include foot and lower extremity fractures, along with hip, acetabular, and pelvic ring and sacral fractures. Lumbar spine axial loading also results in vertebral compression and burst fractures particularly of T12-L1 and L2. Vertical deceleration forces to organs (liver, spleen, and aorta) and fractures of the forearm and wrist (Colles' fracture) are also common.

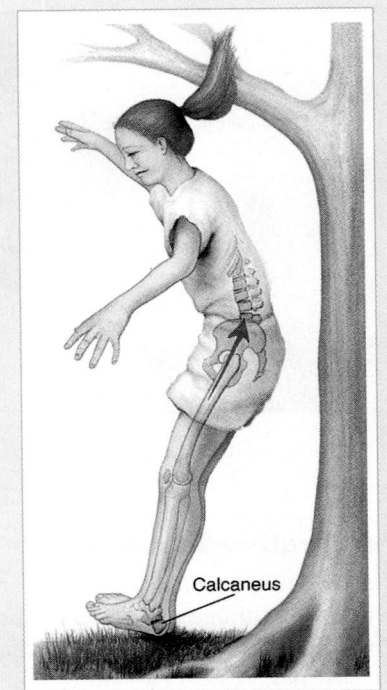

Figure 17-18 When an adult jumps or falls and lands on his or her feet, the energy is transmitted to the spine, sometimes producing a spinal injury in addition to injuries to the legs and pelvis.

Calcaneus

- **Area.** The area over which the impact is distributed—the larger the area of contact at the time of impact, the greater the dissipation of the force and the lesser the peak pressures generated.
- **Surface.** The surface onto which the person has fallen and the degree to which that surface can deform (degree of plasticity) under the force of the falling body can help dissipate the forces of sudden deceleration. Deep snow, for example, has a relatively large capacity to deform, whereas concrete has scarcely any plasticity. Also, contrary to what may be expected, water also has very little plasticity at high-speed impacts. The surface of contact may also present hazards in the form of irregularities or protruding structures; it is far more dangerous to fall onto a wrought-iron picket fence, for example, than onto the grass beside it. If the surface does not conform, the unprotected body will.
- **Physical condition.** The physical condition of the patient in the form of preexisting medical conditions may also influence the injuries sustained. Most notably is the case of older patients with osteoporosis, a condition that predisposes to fractures even with minimal falls. Patients with hematologic conditions resulting in an enlarged spleen may also be more prone to ruptured spleen in a fall. Children younger than 3 years of age have fewer injuries from falls greater than three stories than do older children and adults, most likely because of the more elastic nature of their tissues and less ossification.

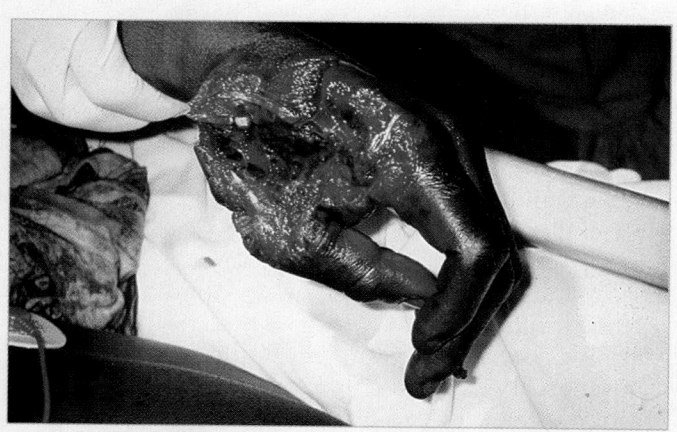

Figure 17-19 Guns are a common cause of penetrating trauma, as shown in this case.

Penetrating Trauma

Unlike blunt trauma, which can involve a large surface area, penetrating trauma involves a disruption of the skin and underlying tissues in a small, focused area. Although a variety of objects may cause penetrating injuries in a variety of settings, penetrating trauma is usually interpreted as being more specific to injuries caused by firearms, knives, and other devices used as a means to cause intentional or accidental harm.

In the United States, the most common sources of penetrating injuries are firearms **Figure 17-19 ▲** . In 2001, 29,573 people died by gunfire in the United States according to US Department of Justice statistics. The 29,573 deaths in 2001, while a staggering number, actually represent a 25% decline in firearm-associated deaths from a peak in 1993 of 39,595 deaths. Of the gun-related deaths in 2001, 57% were suicides, 39% were homicides (including justified shootings by law enforcement personnel and gun owners), 3% were unintentional, and 1% are unclassified. Of the deaths in 2001, 2,937

victims (9.9%) were younger than 19 years. Of those, 32% were suicides and 39% were homicides, with 414 of the patients younger than 14 years, or 1.4% of all firearm-related deaths.

Stab Wounds

The severity of a stab wound depends on the anatomic area involved, depth of penetration, blade length, and angle of penetration. A stab wound may also involve a cutting- or hacking-type force such as in machete wounds, which not only can result in laceration, but also can cause fractures and blunt injury to underlying soft tissues and bone and potentially amputation.

Neck wounds can involve critical anatomic structures such as the carotid arteries, subclavian vessels, apices of the lung, the upper mediastinum, trachea, esophagus, and thoracic duct. Deep neck wounds of sufficient energy can result in spinal cord involvement and cervical fracture.

Lower chest or upper abdominal wounds have the potential of involving the thoracic and abdominal cavities, depending on the location of the diaphragm at the time of injury, that is, whether the person was taking a breath or exhaling.

The pattern of stab wounds closely relates to the mechanism involved and should be documented in detail because your records may be needed in criminal proceedings. Be sure to record the directions of the stab wounds. Wounds delivered to the back are generally downward, whereas stab wounds from the front are generally upward.

Gunshot Wounds

Firearms are the primary mechanism resulting in penetrating trauma. The amount of damage a firearm can cause will depend on a number of factors, including the type of firearm (rifle, shotgun, or handgun), velocity of the projectile, physical design of the projectile, the distance to the target from the muzzle of the firearm, and the type of tissue that is struck.

You are the Provider Part 4

After the patient is placed on the backboard, you decide to load the patient into the ambulance where you reattempt splinting of injured extremities, establish vascular access, and administer a 500-mL bolus of normal saline en route to the hospital. You alert the hospital staff of the need for security personnel on your arrival to the emergency department.

Reassessment	Recording Time: 15 Minutes
Level of consciousness	V (Responsive to verbal stimuli)
Skin	Slightly moist, slightly pale, and cool
Pulse	136 beats/min
Blood pressure	160/88 mm Hg
Respirations	34 breaths/min
Sao₂	98% while breathing room air; patient noncompliant with nonrebreathing mask
ECG	Sinus tachycardia with occasional unifocal premature ventricular contractions

10. What will remain a concern throughout this call?

There are hundreds if not thousands of firearm models and designs. However, they can be classified primarily into three types: shotguns, rifles, and handguns.

Shotguns fire round pellets (referred to as "shot"), from about half a dozen to several dozen at a time, depending on the type of load used. The load denominated 00 or 000 "buckshot" is the larger pellets, and smaller shot such as No. 7 is a common fowl hunting shot or "birdshot." At short range, even the smaller shot can cause devastating injuries. Shotgun shells can also be loaded with a single large and heavy projectile called a sabot, which can cause even worse harm. A shotgun typically has a smooth bore, and its numerous projectiles are not stabilized in flight by spin, as is the single projectile fired from a rifle barrel. The pellets, therefore, leave the barrel and immediately start dispersing so that the shot density (that is, the separation between any two pellets) at the time of impact on a target will be determined by the distance traveled.

At very close range (less than 10 yards), a shotgun can induce destructive injuries. Entrance and exit wounds can be very large, with shotgun wadding, bits of clothing, skin, and hair driven into the wound that can cause massive contamination, leading to increased infection potential should the patient survive the initial trauma.

Rifles are firearms firing a single projectile at very high velocity through a grooved barrel that imparts a spin to the projectile that stabilizes the projectile's flight for accuracy.

Handguns are of two types: revolvers and pistols. Revolvers have a cylinder holding from 6 to 10 rounds of ammunition, and pistols have a separate magazine holding as many as 17 rounds of ammunition in some models. Handguns also have rifled barrels to impart spin to a bullet, but their accuracy is more limited than a rifle's because their barrels (and sight radius) are shorter. The ammunition handguns fire is also, in general, less powerful than ammunition fired from rifles, and handguns fire at lower velocities.

The most important factor for the seriousness of a gunshot wound is the *type of tissue* through which the projectile passes. Tissue of high elasticity like muscle, for example, is better able to tolerate stretch (temporary cavitation) than tissue of low elasticity, like the liver. A high-velocity bullet fired through a fleshy part of the leg may do much less damage than a relatively low-velocity bullet that punctures the aorta or the liver. Many bullet wounds of the extremities that are found to have caused no fracture or neurovascular compromise will be treated by the trauma team with splinting and a single dose of antibiotic without a need for wound exploration or bullet retrieval.

An entry wound is characterized by the effects of initial contact and implosion. Skin and subcutaneous tissues are pushed in, cut, or abraded externally as missile fragments pass and heat is transferred to the tissues. At close range, tattoo marks from powder burns can occur. At extremely close ranges, burns can occur from muzzle blast. Heavy wound contamination results from negative pressure generated behind the traveling projectile, which sucks surrounding elements such as clothing into the wound, greatly increasing infection potential.

Deformation and tissue destruction sustained in soft tissues and bone is based on a combination of factors, including density, compressibility, missile velocity, and missile fragmentation. The initial path of tissue destruction is caused by the projectile crushing the tissue during penetration. This creates a permanent cavity that may be a straight line or an irregular pathway as the bullet is deflected into a number of angles after initial penetration. Pathway expansion refers to the tissue displacement that occurs as the result of low-displacement shock waves (sonic pressure waves) that travel at the speed of sound in tissue (four times the speed of sound in air). These shock waves push tissues in front of and lateral to the projectile and may not necessarily increase the wound size or cause permanent injury, but they result in cavitation (cavity formation). Tissue is compressed and accelerated away, causing injury. The waves of tissue are similar to throwing a rock into a pond. The rock creates a hole in the pond that quickly refills while waves emanate from the penetrating "wound," or hole in the pond.

Bowel, muscle, and lung are relatively elastic, resulting in fewer permanent effects of temporary cavitation. Liver, spleen, and brain are relatively inelastic, and the temporary cavity may become a permanent defect. Missile fragmentation is a major cause of tissue damage as the projectile sends off fragments that create their own separate paths through tissues. Secondary missiles can also be generated by pieces of bone, teeth, buttons, or other objects encountered in the projectile's path as it enters the body. Exit wounds occur when the projectile has sufficient energy that is not entirely dissipated along its trajectory through the body. The projectile then exits the patient and can injure other bystanders as well.

The size of the exit wound depends on the energy dissipated and the degree of cavitation at the point of exit. Exit wounds usually have irregular edges and may be larger than the entry wound **Figure 17-20 ▾** . There may be multiple

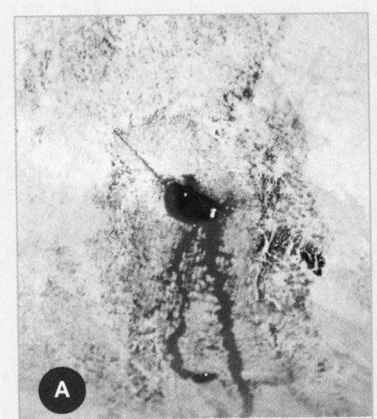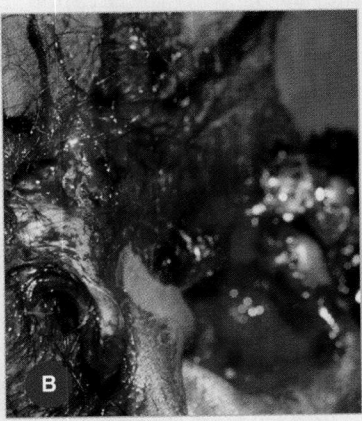

Figure 17-20 A. Entrance wound from a gunshot. **B.** Exit wound from a gunshot.

exit wounds in the case of fragmentation. The number of exit wounds and the extent of tissue damage encountered must be assessed and carefully documented.

Shotgun wounds are the result of tissue impacted by numerous projectiles. As described earlier, the greater the distance from the muzzle to the target, the more dispersion the multiple projectiles will have and the more KE that will be lost before impact. Thus, shotguns are most lethal when used as short-range weapons. Also, the velocity of each pellet is less than the velocity of any bullet fired from a rifle.

Wounding potential from an injury sustained from a shotgun depends on the powder charge, the size and number of pellets, and the dispersion of the pellets. Dispersion is in turn determined by the range at which the weapon was fired, the barrel length (shorter barrels have more scatter), and the type of choke at the end of the barrel.

To give the trauma team at the hospital as much information as possible, try to obtain the following information:

- *What kind of weapon* was used (handgun, rifle, or shotgun; type and caliber, if known)?
- At *what range* was it fired?
- *What kind of bullet* was used? (Ideally, see if the police can find an unfired cartridge.)

What to look for:

- Powder residue around the wound
- Entrance and exit wounds (the exit wound is usually larger and more ragged)

In the real world, the assailant is usually gone, along with the weapon, and patient care is the first goal of paramedics, a far more pressing matter than obtaining answers to the previous questions.

Blast Injuries

Although most commonly associated with military conflict, blast injuries are also seen in civilian practice in mines, shipyards, chemical plants, and, increasingly, in association with terrorist activities. People who are injured in explosions may be injured by any of four different mechanisms **Figure 17-21 ▶** :

- **Primary blast injuries.** These are due entirely to the blast itself, that is, damage to the body caused by the pressure wave generated by the explosion.

- **Secondary blast injuries.** Damage results from being struck by flying debris, such as shrapnel from the device or from glass or splinters, that has been set in motion by the explosion. Objects are propelled by the force of the blast and strike the victim, causing injury. These objects can travel great distances and be propelled at tremendous speeds, up to nearly 3,000 mph for conventional military explosives.
- **Tertiary blast injuries.** These occur when the patient is hurled by the force of the explosion against a stationary object. A "blast wind" also causes the patient's body to be hurled or thrown, causing further injury. In some cases, wind injuries can amputate limbs.
- **Miscellaneous blast injuries.** These include burns from hot gases or fires started by the blast, respiratory injury from inhaling toxic gases, and crush injury from the collapse of buildings, among others.

The vast majority of patients who survive an explosion will have some combination of the four types of injury mentioned. We will confine our discussion here to primary blast injuries because they are the most easily overlooked.

The Physics of an Explosion

When a substance is detonated, a solid or liquid is chemically converted into large volumes of gas under pressure with resultant energy release. Propellants, like gunpowder, are explosives

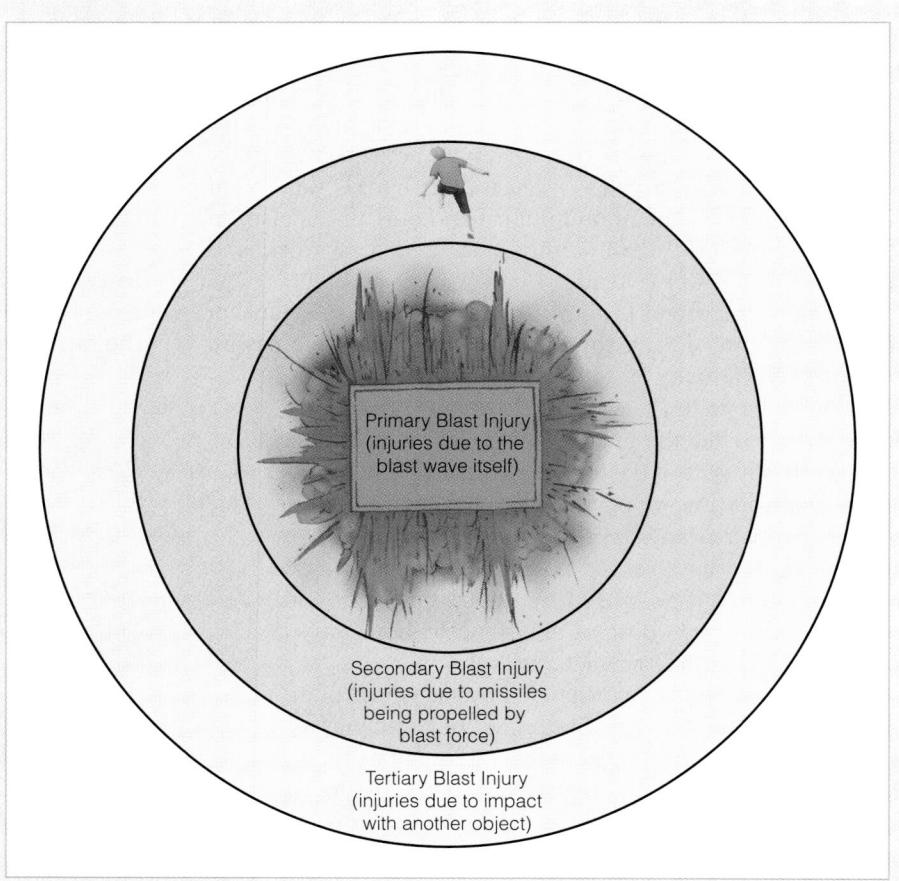

Figure 17-21 The mechanisms of blast injuries.

designed to release energy relatively slowly compared with high explosives (for example, trinitrotoluene), which are designed to detonate very quickly. Composition C4 can create initial pressures of more than 4 million pounds per square inch. This generates a pressure pulse in the shape of a spherical blast wave that expands in all directions from the point of explosion. Flying debris and high winds commonly cause conventional blunt and penetrating trauma.

Components of Blast Shock Wave
The leading edge of the shock wave is called the blast front. A positive wave pulse refers to the phase of the explosion in which there is a pressure front higher than atmospheric pressure. The peak magnitude of the wave experienced by a patient becomes lessened the farther the person is from the center of the explosion. The increase in pressure from a blast can be so abrupt that high-explosive blast waves are also referred to as "shock waves." Shock waves possess a characteristic, brisance, that describes the shattering effect of the wave and its ability to cause disruption of tissues as well as structures. Tissue damage is dependent on the magnitude of the pressure spike and the duration of force application. The negative wave pulse refers to the phase in which pressure is less than atmospheric; it may last 10 times as long as the positive wave pulse. It occurs as air displaced by the positive wave pulse returns to fill the space of the explosion. It can lead to massive movements of air resulting in high-velocity winds.

The speed, duration, and pressure of the shock wave are affected by the following:

- The *size* of the explosive charge. The larger the explosion, the faster the shock waves and the longer they will last.
- The nature of the *surrounding medium.* Pressure waves travel much more rapidly in water, for example, and are effective at greater distances in water than in air.
- The *distance* from the explosion. The farther one is from the explosion, the slower the shock wave velocity and the longer its duration.
- The presence or absence of *reflecting surfaces.* If the pressure wave is reflected off a solid object, its pressure may be multiplied several times. For example, a shock wave that might cause minimal injury in the open can cause devastating trauma if the patient is standing beside a wall or similar solid object.

The changes in pressure produced by the shock wave are accompanied by transient *winds,* sometimes of very high velocity, that can accelerate small objects to speeds of hundreds of feet per second. A missile traveling at 50 fps can easily penetrate human skin; at 400 fps, a missile can enter any of the major body cavities and cause serious internal injury. Blast winds can also send the human body flying against larger, more stationary objects, or as mentioned previously, amputate limbs.

In an *underwater explosion,* a shock wave travels at greater velocity than in open air, thereby making it possible to receive injuries at three times the distance that would normally be required to receive such injuries. This is because positive pressures are higher and there are no negative pressures or high-

velocity wind. Blast fragments and gases move shorter distances in water.

An explosion is significantly more damaging in *closed spaces* because of a limited dissipation environment for the forces involved and for the generation of toxic gasses and smoke. The blast wave is magnified when it comes into contact with a solid surface such as a wall, causing patients near a wall to be hit with significantly higher pressure, resulting in increased risk of injury and death.

Remember the discussion of the types of tissue and the effect of trauma on tissues that contain air, water, or hard bone? Blast pressures cause destruction at the interface between tissues of different densities or the interface between tissues and trapped air. When the shock wave passes from a higher to lower density medium, a severe pressure disturbance develops at the interface of the denser medium. The result is fragmentation of the heavier medium, or spalling. When the shock wave contacts small gas bubbles, the bubbles are compressed and high local pressures are created, called implosion. The bubbles can then reexpand and cause further damage. *Acceleration and deceleration* of organs at their fixation points will occur in a manner similar to that in blunt trauma.

Tissues at Risk
Air-containing organs such as the middle ear, lung, and gastrointestinal tract are most susceptible to pressure changes. Junction between tissues of different densities and exposed tissues such as head and neck are prone to injury as well. The ear is the organ system most sensitive to blast injuries. The tympanic membrane evolved to detect minor changes in pressure and will rupture at pressures of 5 to 7 pounds per square inch above atmospheric pressure. Thus, the tympanic membranes are a sensitive indicator of the possible presence of other blast injuries. The patient may complain of ringing in the ears, pain in the ears, or some loss of hearing, and blood

Notes from Nancy
When there is evidence of ear problems after an explosion, look for serious injury to the lungs.

may be visible in the ear canal. Dislocation of structural components of the ear, such as the ossicles conforming the inner ear, may occur. Permanent hearing loss is possible.

Primary pulmonary blast injuries occur as contusions and hemorrhages. When the explosion occurs in an open space, the side toward the explosion is usually injured, but the injury can be bilateral when the victim is located in a confined space. The patient may complain of tightness or pain in the chest and may cough up blood and have tachypnea or other signs of respiratory distress. Subcutaneous emphysema (crackling under the skin) over the chest can be palpated, indicating air in the thorax. Pneumothorax is common and may require emergency decompression (which will be covered in the chapter on pulmonary injuries) in the field for your patient to survive. Pulmonary edema may ensue rapidly. If there is *any* reason to suspect lung injury in a blast victim (even just the presence of a ruptured eardrum), administer oxygen. Avoid giving oxygen under positive pressure, however (that is, by demand valve) because that may simply increase the damage to the lung. Be cautious as well with intravenous fluids, which may be poorly tolerated in patients with this lung injury and result in pulmonary edema.

One of the most concerning pulmonary blast injuries is arterial air embolism, which occurs on alveolar disruption with subsequent air embolization into the pulmonary vasculature. Even small air bubbles can enter a coronary artery and cause myocardial injury. Air embolisms to the cerebrovascular system can produce disturbances in vision, changes in behavior, changes in state of consciousness, and a variety of other neurologic signs.

Notes from Nancy

If the victim of a blast injury has any neurologic abnormalities, notify the base physician at once!

Solid organs are relatively protected from shock wave injury but may be injured by secondary missiles or a hurled body. Hollow organs, however, may be injured by similar mechanisms as for lung tissue. Petechiae, or pinpoint hemorrhages that show up on the skin, to large hematomas are the dominant form of pathology. Perforation or rupture of the bowel and colon is a risk. Underwater explosions result in the most severe abdominal injuries.

Neurologic injuries and *head trauma* are the most common causes of death from blast injuries. Subarachnoid (beneath the arachnoid layer covering the brain) and subdural (beneath the outermost covering of the brain) hematomas are often seen. Permanent or transient neurologic deficits may be secondary to concussion, intracerebral bleeding, or air embolism. Instant but transient unconsciousness, with or without retrograde amnesia, may be initiated not only by head trauma, but also by cardiovascular problems. Bradycardia and hypotension are common after an intense pressure wave from an explosion. This is a vagal nerve–mediated form of cardiogenic shock without compensatory vasoconstriction (for example, vasovagal syncope).

Extremity injuries, including traumatic amputations, are common. Other injuries are often associated with tertiary blasts. Patients with traumatic amputation by postblast wind are likely to sustain fatal injuries secondary to the blast. In present combat, improved body armor has increased the number of survivors of blast injuries from shrapnel wounds to the torso. The number of severe orthopaedic and extremity injuries, however, has increased. In addition, while body armor may limit or prevent shrapnel from entering the body, it also "catches" more energy from the blast wave, possibly resulting in the victim being thrown backward, thus increasing potential spine and spinal cord injury.

Although blast injuries have usually been the domain of military surgeons, they often occur in industrial settings and are, unfortunately, more common today owing to the increased use of explosives as a tool for urban terrorism and, in the US, from methamphetamine lab explosions. Although civilian blast injuries in an industrial or mining setting used to be mostly characterized by blast injuries and burns, terrorist bombs often have shrapnel. Modern EMS and trauma services personnel should be fully educated and aware of what to expect in these scenarios.

You are the Provider Summary

1. What initial information about the fall gives rise for concern?

The height of buildings without occupants and drug-related nature of the incident create concern about safety issues for yourself, your partner, the police, and the general public at large.

2. How does knowing your primary service area impact your understanding of potential patient injuries?

Being familiar with various aspects of your response area can aid you in understanding potential hazards or general conditions of an area. In this case, because it is a nonresidential area with buildings much higher than a typical single-family residence, you begin to wonder about the height of the fall and extent of the patient's injuries.

3. Given the location, what other conditions are you worried about?

This is a business location where the ground will be asphalt or concrete. Surfaces that an individual lands on relay much information about the forces placed on the body. Residential areas have more areas with grass, dirt, or gravel, which can absorb energy as a result of the impact of a fall.

4. Given commonalities of fire escape locations, what other information do you have?

If the fire escape is located in an alley, the patient can become entangled in lines or wires of various uses and can land on objects such as parked cars, dumpsters, or other people.

5. How does your patient's condition hinder your assessment techniques?

Patients under the influence of drugs can be unwilling or unable to provide reliable information about their injuries because their mentation and ability to perceive pain can be greatly diminished. When a patient not under the influence would guard an injury or self-splint a fracture, patients under the influence have lost these safety mechanisms and can fail to provide feedback that could aid you in determining the extent of their injuries.

6. How do you compensate for this hindrance?

You must rely on the information given to you by the mechanism of injury, any available witnesses, and your assessment techniques to determine the location and nature of the patient's injuries. Understanding the forces placed on the body in common traumatic injuries will aid you in treating obvious and not obvious injuries.

7. Given this information, what other injuries do you suspect?

Given the height of the fall and his position upon landing, you would also suspect lumbar spine fractures. The force of landing on pavement will travel up the heels, legs, and into pelvis and spine.

8. How can a patient who is under the influence of drugs be difficult to manage?

These patients will fail to comply with simple commands or treatment, and you may find it extremely difficult to provide necessary treatment. Depending on their reaction to the drugs, they can remove intravenous lines and otherwise fail to remain still despite obvious injuries.

9. What other medical emergencies can ensue from the use of PCP?

Depending on the amount and route of administration, PCP can result in hallucinations, paranoia, psychosis, cardiac arrhythmias, seizures, hyperthermia, kidney failure, and death. Sedation may be required, especially if the patient cannot be restrained by other means. Any patient who requires restraints must be continually monitored, particularly if chemical restraints must be used.

10. What will remain a concern throughout this call?

When dealing with a patient who is under the influence of drugs or alcohol and who exhibits combative behavior, you must remain diligent regarding scene safety. These patients can be very unpredictable, and law enforcement personnel should accompany you in the ambulance during transport.

Prep Kit

■ Ready for Review

- Trauma is the primary cause of death and disability in people 1 to 34 years old.
- The amount of force and energy delivered are factors in the extent of trauma sustained. Duration and direction of the force of application are also important.
- Understanding the effects of forces and energy will help in developing a high index of suspicion for the mechanism of injury and the likely types of injuries.
- There are four categories of trauma centers. Your EMS system may include a Level I, which is the highest level trauma center.
- Situations in which there is extended transport time by ground, mass casualties, prolonged extrication times, and critically injured patients, or when there is a long distance to an appropriate facility may warrant transporting a patient via air medical transport.
- Kinetic energy (KE) of an object is the energy associated with that object in motion. It reflects the relationship between the weight (mass) of the object and the velocity at which it is traveling.
- In a motor vehicle collision, the angle of impact, mechanical characteristics of the vehicle, and the occupant's position at the time of impact will determine types of injury.
- The law of conservation of energy states that energy can be neither created nor destroyed, it can only change form.
- Trauma in a collision is composed of five phases representing the effects of progressive deceleration: deceleration of the vehicle, deceleration of the occupant, deceleration of internal organs, secondary collisions, and additional impacts.
- There are five primary types of impacts: frontal or head on, lateral or side, rear, rotational, and rollover.
- The front seat occupants of vehicles during a frontal or head-on collision usually follow one of two trajectories, a down-and-under pathway or an up-and-over pathway.
- Protective devices such as seatbelts, air bags, and helmets are designed to manipulate the way in which energy is dissipated into injury.
- Adult pedestrians involved in a collision experience three predominant mechanisms of injury: lower extremity injuries from the initial hit, second impact injuries from being thrown onto the hood or grill, and third impact injuries when the body strikes the ground or another object.
- The severity of injuries from falls from heights depends on the height, position, and orientation of the body at the moment of impact; the area over which the impact is distributed; the surface onto which the person falls; and the physical condition of the patient.
- The severity of a stab wound depends on the anatomic area involved, depth of penetration, blade length, and angle of penetration. Document the pattern of a stab wound; this is closely related to the mechanism.
- Firearms are the primary mechanism resulting in penetrating trauma. The magnitude of tissue damage depends on the projectile's velocity, the orientation of the projectile as it entered the body, the distance from which the weapon was fired, the design of the projectile, and the type of tissue through which the projectile passed.
- Blast injuries include primary, secondary, tertiary, and miscellaneous injuries.

■ Vital Vocabulary

acceleration The rate of change in velocity.

acute respiratory distress syndrome (ARDS) A respiratory syndrome characterized by respiratory insufficiency and hypoxemia.

angle of impact The angle at which an object hits another; this characterizes the force vectors involved and has a bearing on patterns of energy dissipation.

arterial air embolism Air bubbles in the arterial blood vessels.

avulsing A tearing away or forcible separation.

barometric energy The energy that results from sudden changes in pressure as may occur in a diving accident or sudden decompression in an airplane.

biomechanics The study of the physiology and mechanics of a living organism using the tools of mechanical engineering.

blast front The leading edge of the shock wave.

blunt cardiac injury Contusion as the heart is compressed between the sternum and the spine.

blunt trauma An impact on the body by objects that cause injury without penetrating soft tissues or internal organs and cavities.

brisance The shattering effect of a shock wave and its ability to cause disruption of tissues and structures.

cavitation Cavity formation; shock waves that push tissues in front of and lateral to the projectile and may not necessarily increase the wound size or cause permanent injury but can result in cavitation.

chemical energy The energy released as a result of a chemical reaction.

deceleration A negative acceleration, that is, slowing down.

electrical energy The energy delivered in the form of high voltage.

entry wound The point at which a penetrating object enters the body.

exit wound The point at which a penetrating object leaves the body, which may or may not be in a straight line from the entry wound.

gravity The acceleration of a body by the attraction of the earth's gravitational force, normally 32.2 ft/sec^2.

implosion A bursting inward.

kinetic energy The energy associated with bodies in motion, expressed mathematically as half the mass times the square of the velocity.

kinetics The study of the relationship among speed, mass, vector direction, and physical injury.

law of conservation of energy The principle that energy can be neither created nor destroyed, it can only change form.

mechanical energy The energy that results from motion (kinetic energy) or that is stored in an object (potential energy).

missile fragmentation A primary mechanism of tissue disruption from certain rifles in which pieces of the projectile break apart, allowing the pieces to create their own separate paths through tissues.

negative wave pulse The phase of an explosion in which pressure from the blast is less than atmospheric pressure.

Newton's first law of motion The principle that a body at rest will remain at rest unless acted on by an outside force.

Newton's second law of motion The principle that the force that an object can exert is the product of its mass times its acceleration.

pathway expansion The tissue displacement that occurs as a result of low-displacement shock waves that travel at the speed of sound in tissue.

penetrating trauma Injury caused by objects that pierce the surface of the body, such as knives and bullets, and damage internal tissues and organs.

permanent cavity The path of crushed tissue produced by a missile traversing part of the body.

positive wave pulse The phase of the explosion in which there is a pressure front with a pressure higher than atmospheric pressure.

potential energy The amount of energy stored in an object, the product of mass, gravity, and height, that is converted into kinetic energy and results in injury, such as from a fall.

pulmonary blast injuries Pulmonary trauma resulting from short-range exposure to the detonation of high explosives.

shearing An applied force or pressure exerted against the surface and layers of the skin as tissues slide in opposite but parallel planes.

spalling Delaminating or breaking off into chips and pieces.

trauma Acute physiologic and structural change that occurs in a victim as a result of the rapid dissipation of energy delivered by an external force.

tympanic membrane The eardrum; a thin, semitransparent membrane in the middle ear that transmits sound vibrations to the internal ear by means of the auditory ossicles.

velocity The speed of an object in a given direction.

Waddell triad A pattern of automobile-pedestrian injuries in children and people of short stature in which (1) the bumper hits pelvis and femur, (2) the chest and abdomen hit the grille or low hood, and (3) the head strikes the ground.

whiplash An injury to the cervical vertebrae or their supporting ligaments and muscles, usually resulting from sudden acceleration or deceleration.

■ Points to Ponder

You and your partner are dispatched as a second paramedic unit to assist in a two-car motor vehicle collision. You arrive on scene and are directed to a vehicle approximately 100 yards from the initial impact. Witnesses state that this vehicle was struck on the passenger side at a high rate of speed and slid out of control through a metal fence and the driver's side is now resting against a large tree. You are told that the other vehicle involved in the collision drove through a red light, driving approximately 50 mph. The passenger side has an intrusion of more than 2′. There are two women inside the van. They are conscious, alert, and orientated and very upset, crying hysterically. The fire department is extricating the patients from the vehicle.

What is the mechanism(s) of injury to the vehicle? What type of injuries would you suspect the patients may have? What are major concerns and thoughts you must have during your assessment and treatment of these trauma patients? What level trauma hospital would you take these patients to?

Issues: Understanding Kinematics of Trauma, Predicting Injury Patterns, Examining the Scene and Patients, Knowledge of Trauma Center Levels.

Assessment in Action

You are dispatched for a single motor vehicle collision and encounter a wet, slippery road. The driver of the vehicle is slumped in the driver compartment. Witnesses tell you that she was driving and then suddenly lost control of her vehicle, struck a mail box, and then drove head on into a telephone pole.

1. **What is Newton's first law of motion?**
   A. The force that an object can exert is the product of its mass times its acceleration.
   B. A body at rest will remain at rest and a body in motion will remain in motion unless acted on by an outside force.
   C. Energy cannot be created or destroyed but can be changed in form.
   D. Kinetic energy is a function of an object's weight and speed.

2. **Trauma in a collision is composed of how many phases, which represent the effects of progressive deceleration?**
   A. 2
   B. 3
   C. 4
   D. 5

3. **A patient's ability to dissipate the energy determines the pattern of injury.**
   A. True
   B. False

4. **What type of impact would you suspect in the preceding scenario?**
   A. Lateral
   B. Rear
   C. Frontal
   D. Rotational

5. **Injuries are generally categorized as:**
   A. head and spinal trauma.
   B. extremity and body trauma.
   C. blunt and penetrating trauma.
   D. closed and open trauma.

6. **The role of air bags is to:**
   A. cushion forward movement of the occupant.
   B. protect the occupant from ejection.
   C. accelerate the occupant away from the point of impact.
   D. block the occupant's view of the impact.

Challenging Questions

You are dispatched to a woman who has fallen. On arrival, you find a 38-year-old woman supine on the ground. Initially, she is responsive to deep painful stimuli.

7. **The severity of injuries will depend on a number of factors that will be important in assessing the patient. List these factors.**

18 Bleeding and Shock

Objectives

Cognitive

4-2.1   Describe the epidemiology, including the morbidity/mortality and prevention strategies, for shock and hemorrhage. (p 18.4, 18.8)

4-2.2   Discuss the anatomy and physiology of the cardiovascular system. (p 18.4)

4-2.3   Predict shock and hemorrhage based on mechanism of injury. (p 18.9, 18.22)

4-2.4   Discuss the various types and degrees of shock and hemorrhage. (p 18.8, 18.17)

4-2.5   Discuss the pathophysiology of hemorrhage and shock. (p 18.8, 18.15)

4-2.6   Discuss the assessment findings associated with hemorrhage and shock. (p 18.9, 18.15)

4-2.7   Identify the need for intervention and transport of the patient with hemorrhage or shock. (p 18.11, 18.14)

4-2.8   Discuss the treatment plan and management of hemorrhage and shock. (p 18.11, 18.24)

4-2.9   Discuss the management of external hemorrhage. (p 18.11)

4-2.10   Differentiate between controlled and uncontrolled hemorrhage. (p 18.8)

4-2.11   Differentiate between the administration rate and amount of IV fluid in a patient with controlled versus uncontrolled hemorrhage. (p 18.8, 18.25)

4-2.12   Relate internal hemorrhage to the pathophysiology of compensated and decompensated hemorrhagic shock. (p 18.21)

4-2.13   Relate internal hemorrhage to the assessment findings of compensated and decompensated hemorrhagic shock. (p 18.21)

4-2.14   Discuss the management of internal hemorrhage. (p 18.14)

4-2.15   Define shock based on aerobic and anaerobic metabolism. (p 18.17, 18.19)

4-2.16   Describe the incidence, morbidity, and mortality of shock. (p 18.19)

4-2.17   Describe the body's physiologic response to changes in perfusion. (p 18.16)

4-2.18   Describe the effects of decreased perfusion at the capillary level. (p 18.16)

4-2.19   Discuss the cellular ischemic phase related to hemorrhagic shock. (p 18.19)

4-2.20   Discuss the capillary stagnation phase related to hemorrhagic shock. (p 18.20)

4-2.21   Discuss the capillary washout phase related to hemorrhagic shock. (p 18.20)

4-2.22   Discuss the assessment findings of hemorrhagic shock. (p 18.9)

4-2.23   Relate pulse pressure changes to perfusion status. (p 18.7)

4-2.24   Relate orthostatic vital sign changes to perfusion status. (p 18.22)

4-2.25   Define compensated and decompensated hemorrhagic shock. (p 18.21, 18.22)

4-2.26   Discuss the pathophysiological changes associated with compensated shock. (p 18.21)

4-2.27   Discuss the assessment findings associated with compensated shock. (p 18.21)

4-2.28   Identify the need for intervention and transport of the patient with compensated shock. (p 18.28)

4-2.29   Discuss the treatment plan and management of compensated shock. (p 18.24)

4-2.30   Discuss the pathophysiological changes associated with decompensated shock. (p 18.22)

4-2.31   Discuss the assessment findings associated with decompensated shock. (p 18.22)

4-2.32   Identify the need for intervention and transport of the patient with decompensated shock. (p 18.28)

4-2.33   Discuss the treatment plan and management of the patient with decompensated shock. (p 18.24)

4-2.34   Differentiate between compensated and decompensated shock. (p 18.21)

4-2.35   Relate external hemorrhage to the pathophysiology of compensated and decompensated hemorrhagic shock. (p 18.8, 18.9)

4-2.36   Relate external hemorrhage to the assessment findings of compensated and decompensated hemorrhagic shock. (p 18.27)

4-2.37   Differentiate between the normotensive, hypotensive, or profoundly hypotensive patient. (p 18.26)

4-2.38   Differentiate between the administration of fluid in the normotensive, hypotensive, or profoundly hypotensive patient. (p 18.26)

4-2.39   Discuss the physiologic changes associated with the pneumatic anti-shock garment or military anti-shock trousers (PASG/MAST). (p 18.12)

4-2.40   Discuss the indications and contraindications for the application and inflation of the PASG/MAST. (p 18.12)

4-2.41   Apply epidemiology to develop prevention strategies for hemorrhage and shock. (p 18.28)

4-2.42   Integrate the pathophysiological principles to the assessment of a patient with hemorrhage or shock. (p 18.22)

4-2.43   Synthesize assessment findings and patient history information to form a field impression for the patient with hemorrhage or shock. (p 18.22)

4-2.44   Develop, execute and evaluate a treatment plan based on the field impression for the hemorrhage or shock patient. (p 18.24)

Affective

None

Psychomotor

4-2.45   Demonstrate the assessment of a patient with signs and symptoms of hemorrhagic shock. (p 18.22)

4-2.46   Demonstrate the management of a patient with signs and symptoms of hemorrhagic shock. (p 18.24, 18.27)

4-2.47   Demonstrate the assessment of a patient with signs and symptoms of compensated hemorrhagic shock. (p 18.22)

4-2.48   Demonstrate the management of a patient with signs and symptoms of compensated hemorrhagic shock. (p 18.24, 18.27)

4-2.49   Demonstrate the assessment of a patient with signs and symptoms of decompensated hemorrhagic shock. (p 18.27)

4-2.50   Demonstrate the management of a patient with signs and symptoms of decompensated hemorrhagic shock. (p 18.27)

4-2.51   Demonstrate the assessment of a patient with signs and symptoms of external hemorrhage. (p 18.9)

4-2.52   Demonstrate the management of a patient with signs and symptoms of external hemorrhage. (p 18.11)

4-2.53   Demonstrate the assessment of a patient with signs and symptoms of internal hemorrhage. (p 18.9)

4-2.54   Demonstrate the management of a patient with signs and symptoms of internal hemorrhage. (p 18.14)

Introduction

After managing the airway, recognizing bleeding and understanding how it affects the body are perhaps the most important skills you will learn as a paramedic. Any kind of bleeding is potentially dangerous because it may first cause weakness and then lead to shock. Uncontrolled bleeding may eventually lead to serious injury and, ultimately, death.

Bleeding is also the most common cause of shock. As used in this chapter, shock describes a state of collapse and failure of the cardiovascular system in which blood circulation slows and eventually ceases. Shock is actually a normal compensatory mechanism used by the body to maintain systolic blood pressure (BP) and brain perfusion during times of distress. This response can accompany a broad spectrum of events, ranging from heart attacks to falls to allergic reactions to automobile crashes. If not treated promptly, shock will injure the body's vital organs and ultimately lead to death. Your early and rapid actions can help significantly reduce the morbidity and mortality rates from bleeding and shock.

Anatomy and Physiology of the Cardiovascular System

The cardiovascular system is designed to carry out one crucial job: keep blood flowing between the lungs and the peripheral tissues. In the lungs, blood dumps the gaseous waste products of metabolism—chiefly carbon dioxide—and picks up life-sustaining oxygen. In the peripheral tissues, the process is reversed: Blood unloads oxygen and picks up wastes. If blood flow were to stop or slow significantly, the results would be catastrophic. The cells of the brain, heart, and other organs of the body would have nowhere to eliminate their wastes and would be rapidly engulfed by the toxic by-products of their own metabolism. Oxygen delivery to the tissues also would be disrupted. For a few minutes, the cells could switch to an emergency metabolic system—one that does not require oxygen (anaerobic metabolism), but that form of metabolism produces even more acids and toxic wastes. Within a few minutes of circulatory failure, cells throughout the body would begin to suffocate and die, leading to the state known as *shock*.

To keep the blood moving continuously through the body, the circulatory system requires three intact components Figure 18-1 ▶ :

- A functioning pump: the heart
- Adequate fluid volume: the blood and body fluids
- An intact system of tubing capable of reflex adjustments (constriction and dilatation) in response to changes in pump output and fluid volume: the blood vessels

All three components must interact effectively to maintain life. If any one becomes damaged or is deficient, the whole system is in jeopardy.

Structures of the Heart

The heart is a muscular, cone-shaped organ whose function is to pump blood throughout the body. Located behind the

You are the Provider Part 1

You and your partner have just finished dinner on what has been a quiet night shift. Suddenly, chatter erupts on the police scanner and you are called to a shooting at a local gas station/minimarket. The dispatcher alerts you that police on the scene are requesting "a rush on the bus."

As you park in front of the store, you notice a crowd gathering on the sidewalk. Police officers are establishing a perimeter. You grab your initial assessment bag and head inside as your partner pulls out the stretcher with the help of a police officer.

As you enter the store, a detective informs you, "There was a robbery; the clerk was shot and the perpetrator has left the scene." You observe a 22-year-old man sitting on the floor behind the counter and leaning against the wall. He is holding his left upper quadrant with his bloody hand. The patient appears to weigh about 150 lb. Although he is conscious, alert, and in obvious pain, he tells you that the shooting occurred just as the clock struck 11:00 PM. It is now 11:10, and you hit the elapsed time counter on your digital watch as you don your personal protective equipment (PPE). As you begin to talk to the patient, you reach down to palpate his radial pulse but cannot feel it.

Initial Assessment	Recording Time: 0 Minutes
Appearance	Awake and anxious
Level of consciousness	A (Alert to person, place, and day)
Airway	Open and clear
Breathing	Rapid, shallow, and labored
Circulation	Unpalpable radial pulse

1. Do the lack of significant visible bleeding and the fact that he is alert indicate that this patient is not bleeding seriously?
2. What is the significance of time in this type of incident?

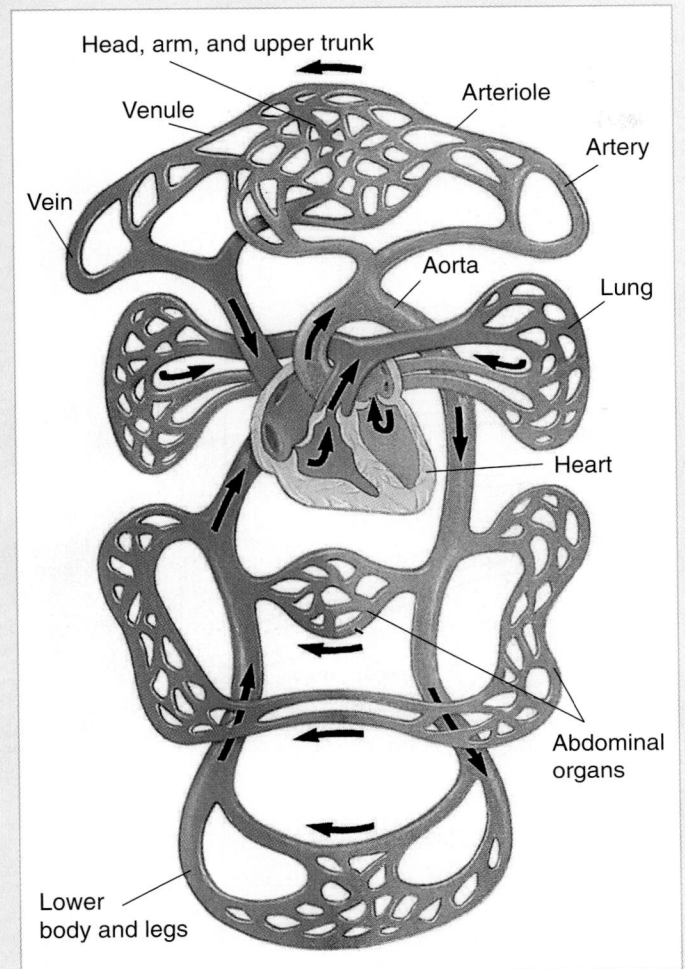

Figure 18-1 The circulatory system requires continuous operation of its three components: the heart, the blood and body fluids, and the blood vessels.

Labels: Head, arm, and upper trunk; Venule; Vein; Arteriole; Artery; Aorta; Lung; Heart; Abdominal organs; Lower body and legs

Blood Flow Within the Heart

Two large veins, the superior vena cava and the inferior vena cava, return deoxygenated blood from the body to the right atrium **Figure 18-2 ▶**. Blood from the upper part of the body returns to the heart through the superior vena cava; blood from the lower part of the body returns through the inferior vena cava (the larger of the two veins). From the right atrium, blood passes through the tricuspid valve into the right ventricle. The right ventricle then pumps the blood through the pulmonic valve into the pulmonary artery and then to the lungs.

In the lungs, oxygen is returned to the blood and carbon dioxide and other waste products are removed from it. The freshly oxygenated blood returns to the left atrium through the pulmonary veins. Blood then flows through the mitral valve into the left ventricle, which pumps the oxygenated blood through the aortic valve, into the aorta (the body's largest artery), and then to the entire body.

The Cardiac Cycle

The cardiac cycle is the repetitive pumping process that begins with the onset of cardiac muscle contraction and ends with the beginning of the next contraction. Myocardial contraction results in pressure changes within the cardiac chambers, causing the blood to move from areas of high pressure to areas of low pressure.

The pressure in the aorta against which the left ventricle must pump blood is called the afterload. The greater the afterload, the harder it is for the ventricle to eject blood into the aorta. A higher afterload, therefore, reduces the stroke volume, or the amount of blood ejected per contraction.

The amount of blood pumped through the circulatory system in 1 minute is referred to as the cardiac output (CO). CO is expressed in liters per minute (L/min). The cardiac output equals the pulse rate multiplied by the stroke volume:

Cardiac Output = Stroke Volume × Pulse Rate

Factors that influence the pulse rate, the stroke volume, or both will affect CO and, therefore, oxygen delivery (perfusion) to the tissues.

Increased venous return to the heart stretches the ventricles somewhat, resulting in increased cardiac contractility. This relationship, which was first described by the British physiologist Ernest Henry Starling, is known as the Starling law of the heart. Starling noted that if a muscle is stretched slightly before it is stimulated to contract, it would contract with greater force. Thus, if the heart is stretched, the muscle contracts more forcefully.

Although the amount of blood returning to the right atrium varies somewhat from minute to minute, a normal heart continues to pump the same percentage of blood returned, a measure called the ejection fraction. If more blood returns to the heart, the stretched heart pumps harder rather than allowing the blood to back up into the veins. As a result, more blood

sternum, the heart is about the size of a closed fist—roughly 5″ long, 3″ wide, and 2½″ thick. It weighs 10 to 12 oz in men and 8 to 10 oz in women. Roughly two thirds of the heart lies in the left part of the mediastinum, the area between the lungs that also contains the great vessels.

The human heart consists of four chambers: two atria (upper chambers) and two ventricles (lower chambers). Each atrium receives blood that is returned to the heart from other parts of the body; each ventricle pumps blood out of the heart. The upper and lower portions of the heart are separated by the atrioventricular valves, which prevent backward flow of blood. The semilunar valves, which serve a similar function, are located between the ventricles and the arteries into which they pump blood. Blood enters the right atrium via the superior and inferior venae cavae and the coronary sinus, which consists of veins that collect blood returning from the walls of the heart. Blood from four pulmonary veins enters the left atrium.

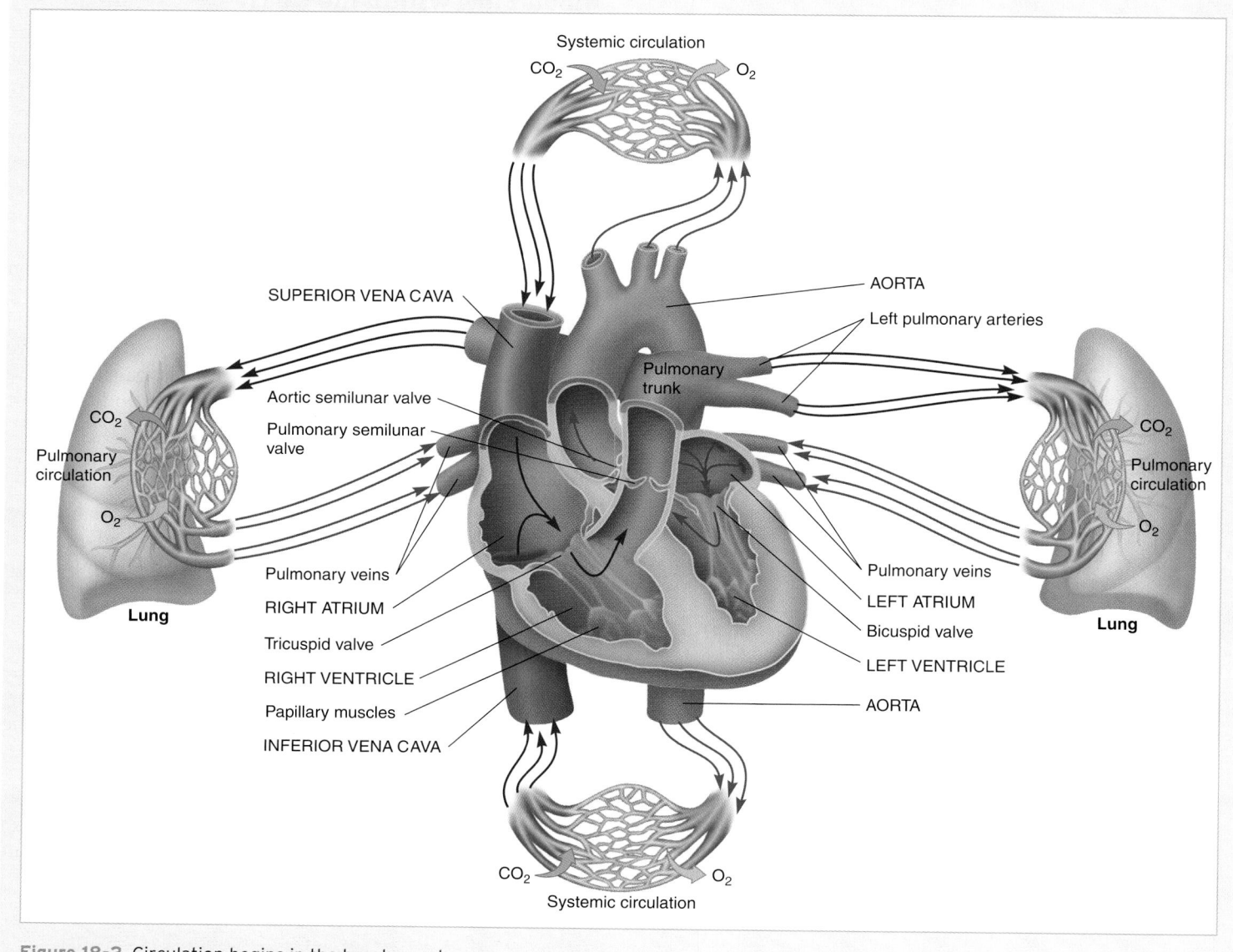

Figure 18-2 Circulation begins in the heart muscle.

is pumped with each contraction, yet the ejection fraction remains unchanged: The amount of blood that is pumped increases, but so does the amount of blood returned. This relationship maintains normal cardiac function when a person changes positions, coughs, breathes, or moves.

Blood and Its Components

Blood consists of plasma and formed elements or cells that are suspended in the plasma. These cells include red blood cells (RBCs), white blood cells (WBCs), and platelets. The purpose of blood is to carry oxygen and nutrients to the tissues and cellular waste products away from the tissues. In addition, the formed elements serve as the mainstay of numerous other body functions, such as fighting infections and controlling bleeding.

Plasma is a watery, straw-colored fluid that accounts for more than half of the total blood volume. It consists of 92% water and 8% dissolved substances such as chemicals, minerals, and nutrients. Water enters the plasma from the digestive tract, from fluids between cells, and as a by-product of metabolism.

The disk-shaped RBCs (erythrocytes) are the most numerous of the formed elements. Erythrocytes are unable to move on their own; instead, the flowing plasma passively propels them to their destinations. RBCs contain hemoglobin, a protein that gives them their reddish color. Hemoglobin binds oxygen that is absorbed in the lungs and transports it to the tissues where it is needed.

Several types of WBCs (leukocytes) exist, each of which has a different function. The primary function of all WBCs is to fight infection. Antibodies to fight infection may be produced, or leukocytes may directly attack and kill bacterial invaders.

Platelets are small cells in the blood that are essential for clot formation. The blood clotting (coagulation) process is a complex series of events involving platelets, clotting proteins in the plasma (clotting factors), other proteins, and calcium. During coagulation, platelets aggregate in a clump and form much of the foundation of a blood clot. Clotting proteins produced by the liver solidify the remainder of the clot, which eventually includes red and white blood cells.

Blood Circulation and Perfusion

Arteries are blood vessels that carry blood away from the heart. Veins are blood vessels that transport blood back to the heart. As arteries get farther from the heart, they become smaller. Eventually, they branch into many small arterioles, which themselves divide into even smaller capillaries (microscopic, thin-walled blood vessels). Oxygen and nutrients pass out of the capillaries and into the cells, and carbon dioxide and waste products pass from the cells and into the capillaries in a process called diffusion. To return deoxygenated blood to the heart, groups of capillaries gradually enlarge to form venules. Venules then merge together, forming larger veins that eventually empty into the heart.

Perfusion is the circulation of blood within an organ or tissue in adequate amounts to meet the cells' current needs for oxygen, nutrients, and waste removal. Blood must pass through the cardiovascular system at a speed that is fast enough to maintain adequate circulation throughout the body, yet slow enough to allow each cell time to exchange oxygen and nutrients for carbon dioxide and other waste products. Although some tissues, such as the lungs and kidneys, never rest and require a constant blood supply, most tissues require circulating blood only intermittently, but especially when they are active. Muscles, for example, are at rest and require a minimal blood supply when you sleep. In contrast, during exercise, muscles need a large blood supply. As another example, the gastrointestinal (GI) tract requires a high flow of blood after a meal. After digestion is completed, it can do quite well with a small fraction of that flow.

The autonomic nervous system monitors the body's needs from moment to moment, adjusting the blood flow as required. During emergencies, it automatically redirects blood away from other organs and toward the heart, brain, lungs, and kidneys. Thus, the cardiovascular system is dynamic, constantly adapting to changing conditions. Sometimes, however, it fails to provide sufficient circulation for every body part to perform its function, resulting in hypoperfusion or shock.

The heart requires constant perfusion, or it will not function properly. The brain and spinal cord cannot go for more than 4 to 6 minutes without perfusion, or the nerve cells will be permanently damaged—recall that cells of the central nervous system do not have the capacity to regenerate. The kidneys will be permanently damaged after 45 minutes of inadequate perfusion. Skeletal muscles cannot tolerate more than 2 hours of inadequate perfusion. The GI tract can exist with limited (but not absent) perfusion for several hours. These times are based on a normal body temperature (98.6°F [37.0°C]). An organ or tissue that is considerably colder is better able to resist damage from hypoperfusion because of the slowing of the body's metabolism.

You are the Provider Part 2

Additional help arrives on the scene as you complete your initial assessment. Your partner has brought in the stretcher and is beginning to administer supplemental oxygen via a nonrebreathing mask at 15 L/min. Police inform you that the robber's weapon may have been a "sawed-off shotgun" that was fired at a fairly close range. The patient tells you a single shot was fired after he told the robber that he would not open the safe.

You give the patient some gauze and tell him to hold it firmly against the wound. When you complete your initial assessment of the patient, you decide to perform the rapid physical exam in the back of the ambulance and the SAMPLE history as you have time, given the higher priorities and need for rapid transport.

Initial Assessment	Recording Time: 3 Minutes
Breathing	Rapid, labored, but no obstructions to breathing process (flail segment, punctures, or impaled objects). Oxygen has been started.
Circulation	A rapid, weak carotid pulse can be felt, the external bleeding is easily controlled with direct pressure and gauze. The skin is pale, cool, and moist.

3. On the basis of the information you have so far, and remembering that the patient weighs approximately 150 lb, how much blood did he have before the incident? How much could he have lost so far?

4. What phase or stage of shock is this patient in?

5. Which BLS and ALS interventions would be most appropriate for this patient at this time? Should you insert an intravenous (IV) line at the scene?

Pathophysiology of Hemorrhage

Hemorrhage simply means bleeding. Bleeding can range from a "nick" to a capillary while shaving, to a severely spurting artery from a deep slash with a knife, to a ruptured spleen from striking the steering column during a car crash. External bleeding (visible hemorrhage) can usually be easily controlled by using direct pressure or a pressure bandage. Internal bleeding (hemorrhage that is not visible) is usually not controlled until a surgeon locates the source and sutures it closed. Because internal bleeding is not as obvious, you must rely on signs and symptoms to determine the extent and severity of the hemorrhage.

External Hemorrhage

External bleeding is usually due to a break in the skin. Its extent or severity is often a function of the type of wound and the types of blood vessels that have been injured. (Wound types are discussed in detail in Chapter 19.) Bleeding from a capillary usually oozes, bleeding from a vein flows, and bleeding from an artery spurts.

These descriptions are not infallible. For example, considerable oozing from capillaries is possible when a patient gets a very large abrasion (such as the road rash when a cyclist slides along the pavement without protective clothing). Likewise, varicose veins on the leg can produce copious bleeding.

Arteries may spurt initially, but as the patient's BP decreases, often the blood simply flows. In addition, an artery that is incised directly across or in a transverse manner will often recoil and attempt to slow its own bleeding. By contrast, if the artery is cut on a bias, it does not recoil and continues to bleed.

Some injuries that you might expect to be accompanied by considerable external bleeding do not always have serious hemorrhaging. For example, a person who falls off the platform at the train station and is run over by a train may have amputations of one or more extremities, yet experience little bleeding because the wound was cauterized by the heat of the train's wheels on the rail. Conversely, a person who pulled over on the shoulder of the road and was removing the jack from his car's trunk when another motorist slammed into the rear of the car, pinning him between the two vehicles, may have severely crushed legs. In such a case, bleeding may be severe, with the only effective means of bleeding control being two tourniquets.

Internal Hemorrhage

Internal bleeding as a result of trauma may appear in any portion of the body. A fracture of a small bone (such as humerus, ankle, or tibia) produces a somewhat controlled environment in which a relatively small amount of bleeding can occur. By contrast, bleeding into the trunk (that is, thorax, abdomen, or pelvis), because of its much larger space, tends to be severe and uncontrolled. Nontraumatic internal hemorrhage usually occurs in cases of GI bleeding from the upper or lower GI tract, ruptured ectopic pregnancies, ruptured aneurysms, or other conditions.

Any internal bleeding must be treated promptly. The signs of internal hemorrhage (such as discoloration, hematoma) do not always develop quickly, so you must rely on other signs and symptoms and an evaluation of the MOI to make this diagnosis. Pay close attention to patient complaints of pain or tenderness, development of tachycardia, and pallor. In addition to evaluating the MOI, be alert for the development of shock when you suspect internal bleeding.

Management of a patient with internal hemorrhaging focuses on the treatment of shock, minimizing movement of the injured or bleeding part or region, and rapid transport. Eventually, the patient will likely need a surgical procedure to stop the bleeding. In recent years, ultrasound has been used to locate bleeding in the emergency department (ED) before moving the patient to the surgical suite for the ultimate resolution of the problem.

Controlled Versus Uncontrolled Hemorrhage

Bleeding that you can control (such as external bleeding that responds to a pressure bandage) and bleeding that you cannot control (such as a bleeding peptic ulcer) are serious emergencies. As a consequence, the initial assessment of the patient includes a search for life-threatening bleeding. If found, the hemorrhage must be controlled; if the hemorrhage cannot be controlled in the field, all of your efforts should concentrate on attempting to control the bleeding as you rapidly transport the patient to the ED.

Most external bleeding can be managed with direct pressure, although arterial bleeding may take 5 or more minutes of direct pressure to form a clot. (Remember this if you accidentally cannulate the brachial artery instead of the vein in the arm!) Military experience has shown that the use of pressure points is not as effective as previously thought and is difficult to manage while trying to rapidly evacuate a person from the battlefield. For this reason, most military medical training calls for use of a tourniquet for external bleeding to an extremity that cannot be controlled with direct pressure and a pressure bandage.

Because most cases of internal bleeding are rarely fully controlled in the prehospital setting, a patient with this type of injury needs rapid transport to the ED. Some strategies may be effective in the field depending on the cause of the bleeding. For example, the external circumferential pressure of the pneumatic antishock garment/military antishock trousers (PASG/MAST) may help control the massive bleeding that accompanies a pelvic fracture.

The Significance of Bleeding

When patients have serious external hemorrhage, it is often difficult to determine the amount of blood loss. Blood looks different on different surfaces, such as when it is absorbed in clothing versus when it has been diluted by being mixed in water. Although you should attempt to determine the amount of external blood loss, the patient's presentation and your assessment will ultimately direct your care and treatment plan.

In the Field

Not every person has the same amount of blood, so you must be able to estimate the patient's blood volume *before* the trauma occurred. Blood volume is relative to weight—it accounts for 6% to 8% of the total body weight. One pint of blood weighs approximately 1 lb.

Human adult male bodies contain approximately 70 mL of blood per kilogram of body weight, whereas adult female bodies contain approximately 65 mL/kg. For a typical adult weighing 80 kg (176 lb), the total blood volume is approximately 6 L (10 to 12 units). The body cannot tolerate an acute blood loss of more than 20% of this total blood volume. Thus, if the typical adult loses more than 1 L (approximately 2 units) of blood, significant changes in vital signs will occur, including increasing heart and respiratory rates and decreasing BP. An isolated femur fracture, for example, can easily result in the loss of 1 L or more of blood in the soft tissues of the thigh.

Because infants and children have less blood volume than their adult counterparts, they may experience the same effect with smaller amounts of blood loss. For example, a 1-year-old child has a total blood volume of about 800 mL, so significant symptoms of blood loss may occur after only 100 to 200 mL of blood loss. To put this in perspective, remember that a soft drink can holds roughly 345 mL of liquid Figure 18-3 ▼.

How well people compensate for blood loss is related to how rapidly they bleed. A healthy adult can comfortably donate one unit (500 mL) of blood in a period of 15 to 20 minutes without having ill effects from this decrease in blood volume. If a similar blood loss occurs in a much shorter period, hypovolemic shock, a condition in which low blood volume results in inadequate perfusion and even death, may rapidly develop.

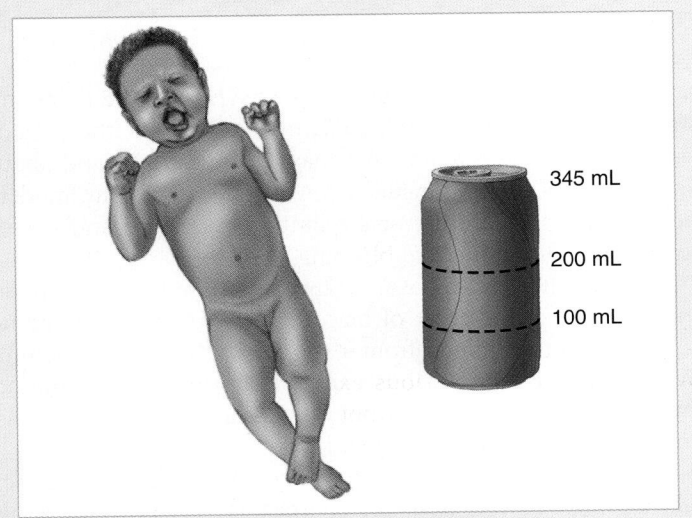

Figure 18-3 A soft drink can holds roughly 345 mL of liquid.

345 mL

200 mL

100 mL

Consider bleeding to be serious if any of the following conditions are present:

- A significant MOI, especially when the MOI suggests that severe forces affected the abdomen or chest
- Poor general appearance of the patient
- Signs and symptoms of shock
- Significant amount of blood loss
- Rapid blood loss
- Uncontrollable bleeding

Physiologic Response to Hemorrhage

Typically, bleeding from an open artery is bright red (because of the high oxygen content) and spurts in time with the pulse. The pressure that causes the blood to spurt also makes this type of bleeding difficult to control. As the amount of blood circulating in the body drops, so does the patient's BP and, eventually, the arterial spurting diminishes.

Blood from an open vein is much darker (low oxygen content) and flows steadily. Because it is under less pressure, most venous blood does not spurt and is easier to manage. Bleeding from damaged capillary vessels is dark red and oozes from a wound steadily but slowly. Venous and capillary bleeding is more likely to clot spontaneously than arterial bleeding.

On its own, bleeding tends to stop rather quickly, within about 10 minutes, in response to internal clotting mechanisms and exposure to air. When vessels are lacerated, blood flows rapidly from the open vessel. The open ends of the vessel then begin to narrow (vasoconstrict), which reduces the amount of bleeding. Platelets aggregate at the site, plugging the hole and sealing the injured portions of the vessel, a process called hemostasis. Bleeding will not stop if a clot does not form, unless the injured vessel is completely cut off from the main blood supply. Direct contact with body tissues and fluids or the external environment commonly triggers the blood's clotting factors.

Despite the efficiency of this system, it may fail in certain situations. A number of medications, including anticoagulants such as aspirin and prescription blood thinners, interfere with normal clotting. With a severe injury, the damage to the vessel may be so extensive that a clot cannot completely block the hole. Sometimes, only part of the vessel wall is cut, preventing it from constricting. In these cases, bleeding will continue unless it is stopped by external means. In a case involving acute blood loss, the patient might die before the body's hemostatic defenses of vasoconstriction and of clotting can help.

Assessment of a Bleeding Patient

The assessment of any patient begins with a good scene size-up and proceeds to your general impression and initial assessment. Once the scene is deemed safe to enter, you will need to take the appropriate level of BSI precautions. Depending on the severity of bleeding and your general impression, this will entail gloves, mask, eyeshield, and, when the patient is very bloody or blood is spurting, a gown Figure 18-4 ▶.

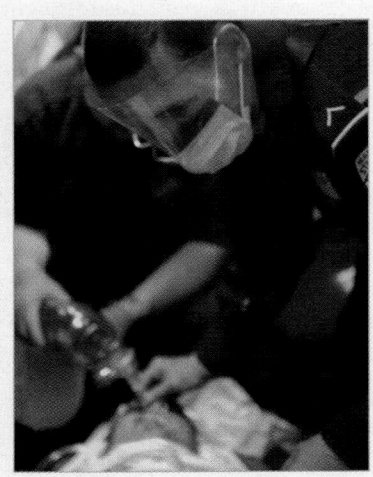

Figure 18-4 Depending on the severity of bleeding and your general impression, BSI precautions will entail gloves, mask, eyeshield, and, in some cases, a gown.

During the initial assessment, after determining the patient's mental status with AVPU, you must locate and manage immediate threats to life involving the airway, breathing, and circulation. Ensure that the patient has a patent airway. If you observe bleeding from the mouth or facial areas, keep the suction unit within reach.

If the patient has minor external bleeding, you can note it and move on with the initial assessment; management of this problem can wait until the patient has been properly assessed and prioritized. Do not get sidetracked by applying dressings and bandages to a patient who has much more serious problems. If major external bleeding is present, you should deal with it during the initial assessment. If you suspect internal bleeding, begin management by keeping the patient warm and administering supplemental oxygen by a nonrebreathing mask at 15 L/min.

In the Field

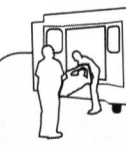

When you are dealing with a bleeding patient, be sure to take necessary precautions to protect yourself from splashing or splattering. Wear appropriate PPE, including gloves, gown, mask, and eye protection. This is especially essential when arterial bleeding is present. Also remember that frequent, thorough handwashing between patients and after every run is a simple yet important protective measure.

Carefully assess the MOI in trauma patients because it may be your best indicator that the patient has sustained an internal injury and may be bleeding. **Table 18-1 ▶** lists some MOIs that can give clues about internal bleeding.

During your focused history, elaborate on the patient's chief complaint using the OPQRST mnemonic, and obtain a history of the present illness using SAMPLE. Ask the patient if

In the Field

Consider any patient exhibiting signs and symptoms of shock without obvious injury to have probable internal bleeding, usually in the abdominal cavity.

Table 18-1	The MOI: Indicators of Internal Bleeding
Mechanism of Injury	**Potential Internal Bleeding Sources**
Fall from a ladder striking head	Head injury or hematoma
Fall from a ladder striking extremities	Possible fractures; consider chest injury
Child struck by car (Waddel triad)	Head trauma, chest and abdomen injuries, leg fractures
Fall on outstretched arm	Possible broken bone or joint injury
Child thrown or falls from height	Children usually have a head-first impact, causing head injury
Unrestrained driver in head-on collision (up-and-over route)	Head and neck, chest, abdomen injuries
Unrestrained driver in head-on collision (down-and-under route)	Knees, femur, hip, and pelvis injuries
Unrestrained front-seat passenger, side impact collision with intrusion into vehicle	Humerus broken exposing the chest wall (possible flail chest); pelvis and acetabulum injuries
Unrestrained driver crushed against steering column	Chest and abdomen injuries, ruptured spleen, neck trauma
Road bike or mountain bike (over the handlebars)	Fractured clavicle, road rash, head trauma if no helmet
Abrupt motorcycle stop, causing rider to catapult over the handlebars	Fractured femurs, head and neck injuries
Diving into the shallow end of a swimming pool	Head and neck injuries
Assault or fight	Punching or kicking injury to chest and abdomen and the face
Blast or explosion	Injury from direct strike with debris; indirect and pressure wave in enclosed space

he or she experiences any dizziness or syncope. Are there any signs and symptoms of hypovolemic shock? Ask the patient about current medications that may thin the blood and about any history of clotting insufficiency. Is there any pain, tenderness, bruising, guarding, or swelling? These signs and symptoms may indicate internal bleeding.

During the physical exam (rapid or focused, depending on the MOI), note the color of bleeding and try to determine its source. Bright red blood from a wound or the mouth, rectum, or other orifice indicates fresh arterial bleeding. Coffee-ground emesis is a sign of upper GI bleeding; this kind of blood is old and looks like used coffee grounds.

Melena, the passage of dark, tarry stools, indicates lower GI bleeding. Hematochezia, by contrast, is the passage of stools containing bright red blood and may indicate bleeding near the external opening of the colon. Hemorrhoids in the lower colon

Special Considerations

In older patients, dizziness, syncope, or weakness may be the first sign of nontraumatic internal hemorrhage.

tend to cause hematochezia. Hematuria (blood in the urine) may suggest serious renal injury or illness. Nonmenstrual vaginal bleeding is always significant as well.

Management of a Bleeding Patient

Always take BSI precautions when treating bleeding patients. As with all patient care, ensure that the patient has an open airway and is breathing adequately. Provide high-flow supplemental oxygen, and assist ventilation if needed, paying special attention to cervical spine control in trauma patients.

Managing External Hemorrhage

To control external hemorrhaging, follow these steps:
1. Apply direct pressure over the wound.
2. Elevate the injury above the level of the heart if no fracture is suspected.
3. Apply a pressure dressing.
4. Apply pressure at the appropriate pressure point while maintaining direct pressure.

A tourniquet is generally used only as a last resort, when it may be necessary to sacrifice the limb to save the life.

Bleeding From the Nose, Ears, and Mouth

Bleeding from the nose (epistaxis) or bleeding from the ears following a head injury may indicate a skull fracture. In such a case, you should not attempt to stop the blood flow. Applying excessive pressure to the injury may force the blood leaking through the ear or nose to collect within the head, ultimately increasing intracranial pressure and possibly causing permanent damage. If you suspect a skull fracture, cover the bleeding site loosely with a sterile gauze pad to collect the blood and help keep contaminants away from the site—there is always a risk of infection to the brain with a skull fracture. Apply light compression by wrapping the dressing loosely around the head. If blood or drainage contains cerebrospinal fluid, the dressing will show a characteristic staining of the dressing that resembles a bull's-eye target.

Bleeding From Other Areas

With bleeding from other areas of the body, control bleeding through use of direct pressure and elevation, if appropriate. Apply pressure dressings, especially at pressure points for the upper and lower extremities. In addition, use splints (or air splints) as necessary, always following your local protocols. Pack large, gaping wounds with sterile dressings. Consider

applying the PASG/MAST per your local protocol, but reserve the tourniquet for use as a last resort.

Once bleeding is controlled and a sterile dressing and pressure bandage have been applied, keep the patient warm and in the appropriate position. Allow the patient's condition to dictate the mode of transport.

Special Management Techniques for External Hemorrhage

Much of the bleeding associated with broken bones occurs because the sharp ends of the bones lacerate vessels, muscles, and other tissues. As long as a fracture remains unstable, the bone ends will move and continue to damage tissues and vessels. They may also break up clots that have partially formed, resulting in ongoing bleeding. For these reasons, immobilizing a fracture is a priority in the prompt control of bleeding. Often, simple splints will quickly control the bleeding associated with a fracture. If not, you may need to use another splinting device.

Air Splints

Air splints can control the bleeding associated with severe soft-tissue injuries, such as massive or complex lacerations, or with fractures. They also stabilize the fracture itself. An air splint acts like a pressure dressing applied to an entire extremity rather than to a small, local area.

Once you have applied an air splint, monitor circulation in the distal extremity. Because an air splint is typically inflated to approximately 50 mm Hg (so you can still dent the splint with your fingertips), it would not be appropriate to use on arterial bleeding because the splint would not actually control the bleeding until the patient's systolic BP dropped to the pressure of the splint. Use only BSI-approved, clean or disposable valve stems when orally inflating air splints.

Hemostats

Hemostats may be helpful when a vessel has been severed, especially if it has retracted into the surrounding tissue. Simply apply hemostats to the ends of the vessel. Be sure to check your local protocols about the use of hemostats in your area.

Tourniquets

The tourniquet is useful if a patient is bleeding severely from a partial or complete amputation and other methods of bleeding control have proved ineffective. The paramedic should realize that its application can cause permanent damage to nerves, muscles, and blood vessels, resulting in the loss of an extremity. The procedure for tourniquet application is shown in Skill Drill 19-2 in Chapter 19. Whenever applying a tourniquet, make sure you observe the following precautions:
- Do not apply a tourniquet directly over any joint. Keep it as close to the injury as possible.
- Use the widest bandage possible. Make sure that it is tightened securely.
- Never use wire, rope, a belt, or any other narrow material as the tourniquet; it could cut into the skin.
- Use wide padding under the tourniquet, if possible, to protect the tissues and help with arterial compression.

- Never cover a tourniquet with a bandage. Leave it open and in full view.
- Do not loosen the tourniquet after you have applied it. Hospital personnel will loosen it once they are prepared to manage the bleeding.

Pneumatic Antishock Garment/Military Antishock Trousers

MAST, also known as PASG, is an inflatable garment that surrounds the legs and abdomen of a patient to provide circumferential pressure. It is by far one of the most controversial pieces of equipment used in the prehospital setting. This device is primarily used for controlling blood loss and is not designed for resuscitation, except with authorization of local medical control in a few situations of extreme hypotension.

The idea of a pneumatic pressure suit is not new. In 1903, George Crile reported on "the resuscitation of the apparently dead and a demonstration of the pneumatic blood pressure." That early work led Crile to develop the G suit for the US Army Air Corps in 1942. In the 1960s, a US Army researcher, Dr. Burt Kaplan, modified the G suit for medical use. A prototype of the PASG/MAST was tested by the US Army in the Vietnam conflict, with apparently favorable results. The device made its civilian debut with the Miami Fire Department in the early 1970s. By 1977, experience with the device had been so favorable that the Committee on Trauma of the American College of Surgeons included the PASG/MAST in its list of essential equipment for ambulances **Figure 18-5 ▾** .

In the 1980s, researchers began to question whether this device, and IV fluid infusion, were really effective in the treatment of shock. At the time of this writing, it is still not possible to state with certainty what the device can and cannot accomplish **Figure 18-6 ▸** .

By applying uniform pressure to sources of bleeding, the PASG/MAST, when pumped up to the point where the Velcro crackles (60 to 80 mm Hg), seems to control bleeding and promote hemostasis. Its benefits derive from the same principle cited when applying pressure over a wound to control hemorrhage manually. The circumferential pressure also compresses the tissue and vessels and, ultimately, results in a decrease in the vascular container size under the suit. With this increase in the systemic vascular resistance (SVR), it has been theorized that a small amount of blood (approximately 200 mL) is autotransfused back to the torso and the mean arterial pressure (MAP) increases. These effects seem to increase the patient's CO.

The PASG/MAST raises the BP of a patient in shock. Whether elevating the BP is beneficial has not been proved. Some researchers believe that raising the BP before bleeding has been controlled may have harmful effects. In addition, raising the patient's BP can be useful to *paramedics,* because veins that were collapsed and invisible may "pop up" after the device has been inflated, making the job of inserting IV lines easier.

The inflated device provides a good splint for a fractured pelvis and does a marginal job splinting fractures of the lower extremities. Ideally, fractures of the femur should be traction-splinted in conjunction with the application of the PASG/MAST.

As yet, we do not know whether the PASG/MAST improves the overall outcome for seriously injured patients. Recent research at Baylor College of Medicine suggests that, at least in certain types of injuries, the device does not improve chances of survival and may adversely affect the outcome. Medical directors of local EMS systems should stay abreast of the research in this area and make their decisions regarding deployment of the device accordingly.

In EMS systems that continue to use the PASG/MAST, use is appropriate in patients with shock from blood loss (hemorrhagic shock) in the following circumstances:

- To stabilize suspected pelvic fractures with hypotension
- To begin to control severe hypotension (systolic BP < 50 to 60 mm Hg)

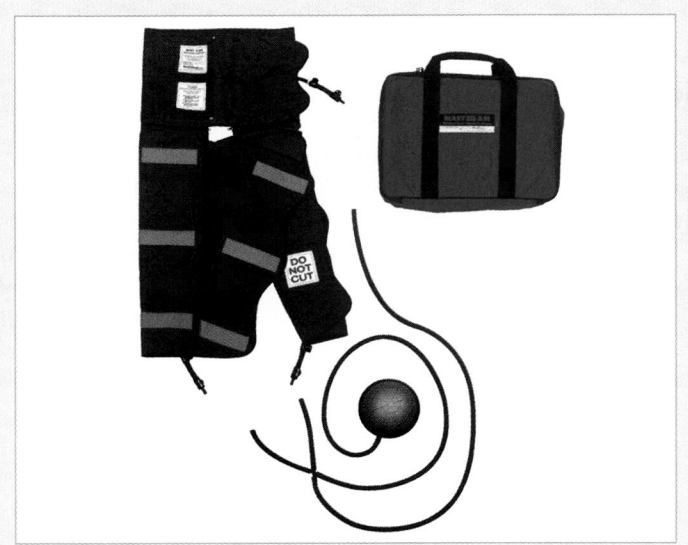

Figure 18-5 PASG/MAST device.

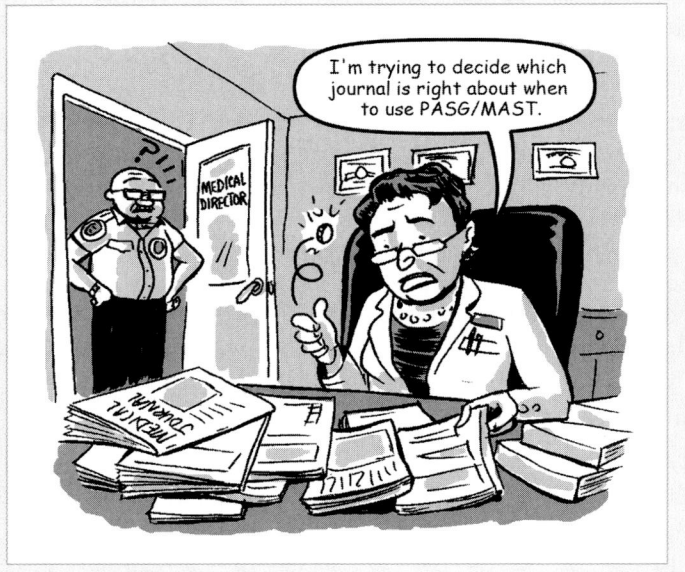

Figure 18-6

- To begin to control suspected intraperitoneal bleeding with hypotension (solid organs such as the liver and spleen, mesenteric vessels)
- To begin to control retroperitoneal bleeding with hypotension (such as in kidneys, aorta, and vena cavae)

Current contraindications to use of the PASG/MAST include the following:

- Penetrating thoracic trauma
- Splinting of the lower extremities in the absence of hypotension. The PASG/MAST is not a good splint and has been known to cause compartment syndrome of the calf when fractures were present.
- Evisceration of abdominal organs
- Impaled objects of the abdomen
- Pregnancy
- Acute pulmonary edema
- Traumatic cardiac arrest
- Major head injuries

The steps in applying the device are described here and shown in Skill Drill 18-1 ▾ :

1. Rapidly expose and examine the areas to be covered by the PASG/MAST. Pad any exposed bone ends to prevent puncture of the garment as it is inflated.
2. Apply the garment. If you will immobilize or move the patient on a backboard, lay the device out on the board before rolling the patient onto it. Position the top of the abdominal section of the PASG/MAST below the lowest rib to ensure that it does not compromise chest expansion Step 1 .
3. Close and fasten both leg compartments and the abdominal compartment Step 2 .
4. Open the stopcocks (valves) to the compartments you are preparing to inflate, ensuring that the other compartments are closed off.
5. Auscultate breath sounds for pulmonary edema before inflation Step 3 .

Skill Drill 18-1: Applying PASG/MAST

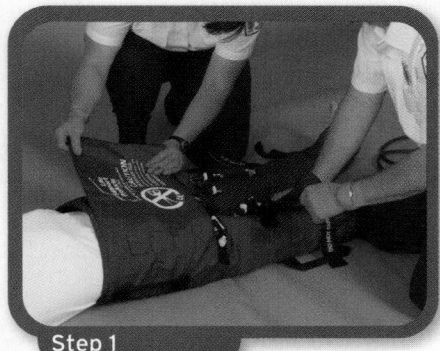

Step 1

Rapidly expose and examine the areas to be covered by the device. Pad any exposed bone ends. Apply the garment so that the top is below the lowest rib.

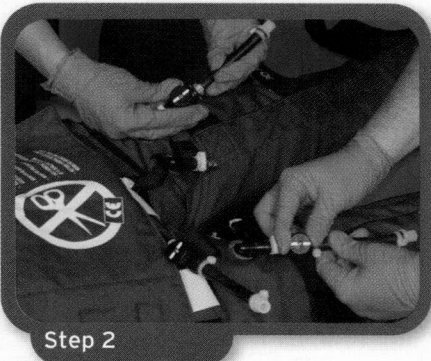

Step 2

Close and fasten both leg compartments and the abdominal compartment.

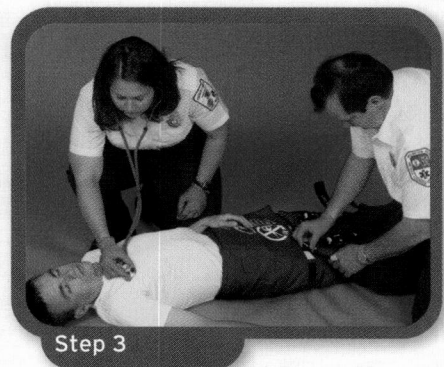

Step 3

Open the three stopcocks (valves). Auscultate breath sounds for pulmonary edema before inflation.

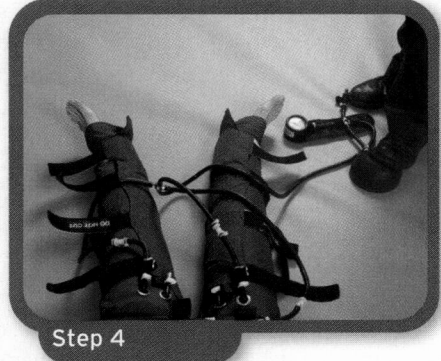

Step 4

Inflate with the foot pump until the Velcro crackles (approximately 60 to 80 mm Hg).

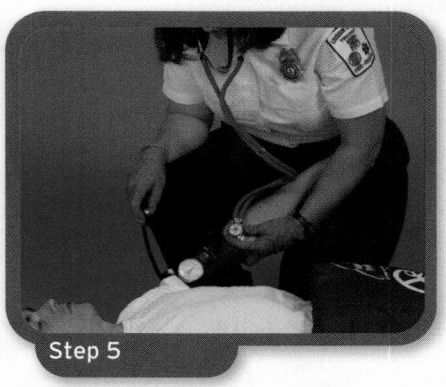

Step 5

Check the patient's BP again, and begin transport if not already in the transport mode.

6. Inflate the compartments with the foot pump until the Velcro crackles. Turn off compartment valves after inflation to maintain pressure in the garment. When using the device to stabilize a pelvic fracture, apply pressure only until the garment is firm to the touch. Overinflation may cause the bones to shift, creating further injury and bleeding. Higher inflation pressures may cause local tissue damage and/or compartment syndrome (Step 4).

7. Check the patient's BP. Continue to monitor serial vital signs at least every 5 minutes because a patient who is subjected to this intervention is considered unstable. Remember that the pressure gauges on the device measure the air pressure in the device—not the patient's BP. Be aware of temperature extremes or external pressure changes that might significantly affect the pressure exerted by the PASG/MAST, thus requiring frequent monitoring and adjustment (Step 5).

The simplest rule to remember regarding deflation of the PASG/MAST is this: Do not deflate the device in the field. To the extent that the device supports the BP and provides hemostasis, the effects will be reversed when the PASG/MAST is deflated. An extreme case in which it might be necessary to deflate the device in the field—albeit with medical control's permission—would be for a suspected ruptured diaphragm (causing abdominal contents to herniate into the chest cavity immediately after inflation of the device). It is desirable, therefore, to have restored at least some of the patient's circulating blood volume before releasing the pressure provided by the PASG/MAST. Remember that the patient's container size will have been decreased and deflation will increase the container, potentially leading to dramatic declines in the SVR, preload (venous return), and CO.

Before the PASG/MAST is deflated in the hospital setting, the patient should have at least two large-bore IV infusions running, with typed and cross-matched blood on standby. If the patient's serial vital signs are relatively stable and the ED physician so instructs, cautious deflation of the PASG/MAST may proceed as follows:

1. Record the patient's pulse and BP.
2. Slowly deflate the abdominal section *only*.
3. Recheck the patient's serial vital signs for 5 to 10 minutes. If the BP drops by 5 mm Hg or more, infuse 100 to 200 mL of fluid until the BP restabilizes.
4. When the patient's vital signs are again stable, slowly deflate one leg section.
5. Recheck the vital signs for 5 to 10 minutes. If there is another BP drop, again infuse volume until the BP comes back up.
6. If vital signs are stable, deflate the other leg section—again slowly, with careful monitoring of BP every few minutes.

In severely injured patients, this deflation procedure, which can take between 20 and 60 minutes, will usually not be feasible. Instead, the patient must be taken straight to the operating room with the PASG/MAST still on and inflated.

Managing Internal Hemorrhage

The definitive management of a patient with internal hemorrhage occurs in the hospital. Prehospital management of suspected internal bleeding involves treating for shock and splinting injured extremities:

1. Keep the patient supine, open the airway, and check breathing and pulse.
2. Administer high-flow supplemental oxygen and assist ventilation if needed.
3. Splint broken bones or joint injuries. If a pelvic fracture is suspected, you may consider use of the PASG/MAST per your local protocols.
4. Place blankets under and over the patient to maintain body heat.
5. If no fractures are suspected, elevate the legs 12″. Insert a large-bore (14- or 16-gauge) IV catheter, and administer a fluid challenge of 250 mL (provided the lungs are clear) en route to the ED. Insert an IV line at the scene only if transport is delayed (such as if the patient is pinned). Whenever possible, use warm IV fluids to prevent the patient from becoming chilled.
6. Consider giving pain medication if the vital signs are stable and after consultation with medical control.
7. Monitor the serial vital signs, and watch diligently for developing shock.

If the patient shows any signs of shock (hypoperfusion), transport rapidly while providing aggressive management en route. Because a patient in shock is usually emotionally upset, you should provide psychological support as well.

▌Transportation of Patients With Hemorrhage

In case of hemorrhage, the issue is not whether the patient will be transported, but rather how fast the transport decision should be made and where the patient should be taken for definitive care. There are a few exceptions to this rule—for example, if you are standing by at a sporting event or concert and are asked by a "walk-in" to evaluate a minor wound that has been bleeding. The decision to transport a patient with even a relatively minor wound should take into consideration factors such as the need for stitches, whether the patient has had a tetanus shot in the past 10 years, and whether the patient or his or her companion is reliable and will follow up properly. (Wounds are discussed in more detail in Chapter 19.)

Most patients with internal or external hemorrhage will need to be transported to a hospital for further care. Consideration for the priority of the patient and the availability of a regional trauma center should be your concerns when making a transport decision in such cases. Patients who have severe internal or external bleeding, especially if uncontrolled, will usually be candidates for surgical interventions and should be transported to a facility with those capabilities. Patients with specific causes of bleeding such as major trauma or specific devastating wounds (such as leg amputation, glove avulsion) should be taken to a facility that is fully prepared to care for the patient. In EMS systems with helicopters available, it may be appropriate to consider this method of transportation for a patient with suspected severe internal or uncontrollable external bleeding.

Pathophysiology of Shock

Hypoperfusion occurs when the level of tissue perfusion decreases below normal. Early decreased tissue perfusion may result in subtle changes, such as aberrant mental status, long before a patient's vital signs (blood pressure, pulse, respiratory rate) appear abnormal. Shock refers to a state of collapse and failure of the cardiovascular system that leads to inadequate circulation, creating inadequate tissue perfusion. Like internal bleeding, shock cannot be seen. It is not a specific disease or injury, but rather a dangerous condition that results in inadequate flow of blood to the body's cells and failure to rid the body of metabolic wastes.

Notes from Nancy

Don't wait until the BP falls before you suspect shock and begin treatment!

Evaluation of a patient's level of organ perfusion is important in diagnosing shock. If the conditions causing shock are not promptly addressed, the patient will soon die. When the body senses tissue hypoperfusion, compensatory mechanisms are set into action. In some cases, this is enough to stabilize the patient's condition. In other cases, the severity of disease or injury overwhelms the normal compensatory mechanisms, leading to progressive deterioration in the patient's condition. Perfusion depends on CO, SVR, and transport of oxygen:

Cardiac Output = Pulse Rate × Stroke Volume

Blood Pressure = Cardiac Output × Systemic Vascular Resistance

Because the heart cannot pump out what is not in its holding chambers, BP varies directly with CO, SVR, and blood volume. Hypoperfusion, therefore, can result from inadequate CO, decreased SVR, or the inability of RBCs to deliver oxygen to tissues.

In the Field

Remember that BP may be the last measurable factor to change in shock. The body has several automatic mechanisms to compensate for initial blood loss and to help maintain BP. Thus, by the time you detect a drop in BP, shock is well developed. This is particularly true in infants and children, who can maintain their BP until they have lost close to half their blood volume.

Mechanisms of Shock

Recall that normal tissue perfusion requires three intact mechanisms: a pump (heart), fluid volume (blood and body fluids), and tubing capable of reflex adjustments (constriction and dilatation) in response to changes in pump output and fluid volume (blood vessels). If any one of those mechanisms is damaged, tissue perfusion may be disrupted, and shock will ensue.

When shock arises because of failure of the heart, it is called cardiogenic shock (*cardio* = heart + *genic* = causing). Cardiac arrest is the most drastic form of cardiogenic shock, but not the only form. Cardiogenic shock may occur secondary to myocardial infarction, cardiac arrhythmias, pulmonary embolism, severe acidosis, or a variety of other conditions. All of these conditions have one thing in common: They interfere with the heart's ability to pump normally.

Shock may also occur because of a loss of fluid volume; perfusion cannot take place if there isn't enough fluid to propel through the system. When shock comes about because of inadequate volume, it is termed hypovolemic shock (*hypo* = deficient + *vol* = volume + *emia* = in the blood). Volume can be lost as blood (hemorrhagic shock), plasma (as in burns), or electrolyte solution (as in vomiting, diarrhea, sweating). Suspect a hypovolemic component of shock in any patient with unexplained shock, and treat the patient for hypovolemia first.

Notes from Nancy

Suspect a hypovolemic component of shock in any patient with unexplained shock, and treat for hypovolemia first.

Failure of vasoconstriction (that is, a decrease in the peripheral vascular resistance [PVR]) may lead to neurogenic shock, so called because the sympathetic nervous system ordinarily controls the dilatation and constriction of blood vessels. In a healthy person, the caliber of the blood vessels constantly changes in response to signals from the nervous system, allowing the body to adapt to changes in position, fluid volume, and so forth. When you stand up, for example, blood vessels in your legs reflexively constrict to divert the circulation toward more vital areas, like the brain. Similarly, when you donate a pint of blood or sweat a liter of fluid, your blood vessels constrict to accommodate a smaller fluid volume. In certain situations, nervous system control over the caliber of blood vessels becomes deranged—for example, after spinal cord injury or in some cases of pulmonary embolism or gastric overdistention—and the blood vessels lose their tone and dilate. A given blood volume then has to be accommodated quite suddenly in a much larger container. The net effect is a relative hypovolemia (the volume in the container is now inadequate relative to the increased size of the container), which the body experiences as shock.

More than one component of the circulatory system may be affected in case of shock. For example, a patient in shock after a myocardial infarction is likely to have an element of cardiogenic shock, because the damaged heart can no longer pump efficiently, and an element of hypovolemic shock, if the patient has been vomiting, sweating, or too nauseated to take in fluids. Some types of shock always result from combined deficits from both fluid leakage into the interstitial space as well as vasodilatation.

Certain categories of patients are at high risk to develop shock. They include patients known to have had trauma or bleeding; elderly people, but especially elderly men with urinary tract infections; patients with massive myocardial infarction; pregnant women; and patients with a possible source for septic shock (such as burned patients and people with diabetes or cancer).

Compensation for Decreased Perfusion

Central among the homeostatic mechanisms that regulate cardiovascular dynamics are those that maintain BP. When any event results in decreased perfusion (such as in blood loss, myocardial infarction, loss of vasomotor tone, or tension pneumothorax), the body must respond immediately to preserve the vital organs. Baroreceptors located in the aortic arch and carotid sinuses sense the decreased blood flow and activate the vasomotor center, which oversees changes in the diameter of blood vessels, to begin constriction of the vessels.

Stimulation typically occurs when the systolic pressure is between 60 and 80 mm Hg in adults or even lower in children. A decrease in systolic pressure to less than 80 mm Hg stimulates the vasomotor center to increase arterial pressure by constricting vessels. The drop in arterial pressure decreases the stretching of the arterial walls, thereby decreasing baroreceptor stimulation. Normally, baroreceptor stimulation inhibits the vasoconstrictor center of the medulla and excites the vagal center, leading to vasodilatation in the peripheral circulatory system and a decrease in pulse rate and contractility, causing a concomitant decrease in arterial pressure. The sympathetic nervous system is also stimulated as the body recognizes a potential catastrophic event.

In response to hypoperfusion, the renin-angiotensin-aldosterone system is activated and antidiuretic hormone is released from the pituitary gland. Together, these mechanisms trigger salt and water retention and peripheral vasoconstriction. The result is an increase in the patient's BP and CO. Depending on the severity of the insult, variable amounts of fluid will shift from the interstitial tissues into the vascular compartment. The spleen also releases some RBCs that are normally sequestered there to augment the blood's oxygen-carrying capacity. The overall response of the initial compensatory mechanisms is to increase the preload, stroke volume, and pulse rate, which usually results in an increase in CO.

As hypoperfusion persists, the myocardial oxygen demand continues to increase. Eventually, the accelerated compensatory mechanisms are no longer able to keep up with the body's demand. Myocardial function then worsens, with decreased CO and ejection fraction. Tissue perfusion decreases, leading to impaired cell metabolism. Often, the systolic BP decreases, especially in progressive hypoperfusion or "decompensated" shock. Fluid may leak from the blood vessels, causing systemic and pulmonary edema. Other signs of hypoperfusion may also be present, such as dusky skin color, oliguria, and impaired mentation.

The body produces its own "medicines," epinephrine and norepinephrine, in the adrenal glands in response to hypoperfusion. These substances are released by the body as part of the global compensatory state. Epinephrine is also administered by caregivers in cases of anaphylaxis, severe airway disease, and cardiac arrest.

You are the Provider Part 3

You decide that the patient does not have spinal involvement. He reports that he was not blown to the ground, but rather felt dizzy and sat down on his own. You and your partner decide to quickly pick the patient up and load him onto the stretcher, rather than spending the time for spinal immobilization to a long backboard. You also decide to insert the IV line en route to the regional trauma center.

The patient is starting to become confused as you place him into Trendelenburg position and head out the door. He states that he is nauseated and thirsty and asks your partner, "Am I going to die?" When closing the back of the ambulance, you note on your watch that 7 minutes have elapsed on the scene. Your plan for the next few minutes is to redo the initial assessment, get IV fluids running, notify the ED, do the rapid trauma assessment and SAMPLE history, and consider PASG/MAST.

Vital Signs	Recording Time: 5 Minutes
Mental status	V (Responsive to verbal stimuli), confused about place and day
Respirations	26 breaths/min, shallow and labored
Pulse	120 beats/min, thready (core, only not peripheral)
Blood pressure	106 mm Hg by palpation
Skin	Pale, cool, and moist
Sao$_2$	95% on nonrebreathing mask at 15 L/min of supplemental oxygen
ECG	Sinus tachycardia with no ectopy

6. For this patient, is the Sao$_2$ a helpful indicator?

7. Why weren't the baseline vital signs taken on the scene?

Release of epinephrine improves CO by increasing the pulse rate and strength. The alpha-1 response to its release includes vasoconstriction, increased peripheral vascular resistance, and increased afterload from the arteriolar constriction. Alpha-2 effects ensure a regulated release of alpha-1. Beta responses from the release of epinephrine primarily affect the heart and lungs. Increases in pulse rate, contractility, conductivity, and automaticity occur in tandem with bronchodilation.

Effects of norepinephrine are primarily alpha-1 and alpha-2 in nature and center on vasoconstriction and increasing PVR. This vasoconstriction allows the body to shunt blood from areas of lesser need to areas of greater need; that is, it serves to keep the brain and other vital organs perfused in the early phases of shock. In an effort to maintain circulation to the brain, the body will shunt blood away from the following tissues, in this order: placenta, skin, muscles, gut, kidneys, liver, heart, lungs. The skin and muscles can survive with minimal blood flow from vasoconstriction for a much longer period than can major organs such as the kidneys, liver, heart, and lungs. If the blood supply is inadequate to the major organs for more than 60 minutes, they often develop complications that will lead to death, such as renal failure and shock lung. This concept has been traditionally referred to as the "golden hour of trauma," and it explains why it is so important to address the cause of the shock in as timely a manner as possible.

Failure of compensatory mechanisms to preserve perfusion leads to decreases in preload and CO. Myocardial blood supply and oxygenation decrease, reducing myocardial perfusion. As CO further decreases, coronary artery perfusion also decreases, leading to myocardial ischemia.

Types of Shock

The inadequate oxygen and nutrient delivery to the metabolic apparatus of the cell experienced in shock results in impaired cellular metabolism. Once a certain level of tissue hypoperfusion is reached, cell damage proceeds in a similar manner, regardless of the type of initial insult. Impairment of cellular metabolism results in the inability to properly use oxygen and glucose at the cellular level. The cell converts to anaerobic metabolism, which causes increased lactic acid production and metabolic acidosis, decreased oxygen affinity for hemoglobin, decreased adenosine triphosphate (ATP) production, changes in cellular electrolytes, cellular edema, and release of lysosomal enzymes. Glucose impairment leads to an elevated blood glucose level due to release of catecholamines and cortisol. In addition, fat breakdown (lipolysis) with ketone formation may occur.

Shock can occur due to inadequacy of the central circulation (the heart and great vessels) or the peripheral circulation (the remaining vessels and the microscopic circulation, such as arterioles, venules, and capillaries). The Weil-Shubin classification considers shock from a mechanistic point of view. From this perspective, two types of shock are distinguished: central shock, which consists of cardiogenic shock and obstructive shock, and peripheral shock, which includes hypovolemic shock and distributive shock.

Regardless of type, shock is characterized by reduced CO, circulatory insufficiency, and rapid heartbeat. Most types of shock also include pallor, except for spinal shock and sepsis. The patient's mental status may be altered. Low BP, although classically associated with shock, is a late sign, especially in children.

Cardiogenic Shock

Cardiogenic shock occurs when the heart is unable to circulate sufficient blood to maintain adequate peripheral oxygen delivery. Circulation of blood throughout the vascular system requires the constant pumping action of a normal and vigorous heart muscle. Many diseases can cause destruction or inflammation of this muscle. Within certain limits, the heart can adapt to these problems. If too much muscular damage occurs, however, the heart no longer functions effectively. Filling is impaired because of a lack of pressure to return blood to the heart (preload), or outflow is obstructed by a lack of pumping function. In either case, direct pump failure is the cause of shock. In the case of ischemic heart disease, pump failure is generally due to a loss of 40% or more of the functioning myocardium.

The most common cause of cardiogenic shock is extensive infarction of the left ventricle, diffuse ischemia, or decompensated congestive heart failure resulting in primary pump failure. The heart damage may be due to a single massive event or result from cumulative damage. Other forms of cardiac dysfunction may result in cardiogenic shock as well—for example, large ventricular septal defect, cardiomyopathy, or hemodynamic significant arrhythmias.

Patients have a poor prognosis when more than 40% of the left ventricle is destroyed. Historically, in about 7.5% of patients with acute myocardial infarction, cardiogenic shock develops, and mortality rates range as high as 80%, even with appropriate therapy.

Obstructive Shock

Obstructive shock occurs when blood flow in the heart or great vessels becomes blocked. In pericardial tamponade, diastolic filling of the right ventricle is impaired, leading to a decrease in CO. Aortic dissection leads to a false lumen (aortic opening) with loss of normal blood flow. A left atrial tumor may obstruct flow between the atrium and ventricle, thereby decreasing CO. Obstruction of the superior or inferior vena cava (such as vena cava syndrome as in third-trimester pregnancy) decreases CO by decreasing venous return. A large pulmonary embolus or tension pneumothorax may prevent adequate blood flow to the lungs, resulting in inadequate venous return to the left side of the heart.

Hypovolemic Shock

Hypovolemic shock occurs when the circulating blood volume does not deliver adequate oxygen and nutrients to the body. It is subdivided into two types, exogenous and endogenous, depending on where the fluid loss occurs.

The most common cause of exogenous hypovolemic shock is external bleeding. Hemorrhage is most prevalent in trauma patients due to blunt or penetrating injuries to vessels or organs, long bone or pelvic fractures, major vascular injuries (as in traumatic amputation), and multisystem injury. The organs and organ systems with a high incidence of exsanguination from penetrating injuries include the heart, thoracic vascular system, abdominal vascular system (such as abdominal aorta, superior mesenteric artery), venous system (such as inferior vena cava or portal vein), and liver.

Endogenous hypovolemic shock occurs when the fluid loss is contained within the body, as in dehydration, burn injury, crush injury, and anaphylaxis. With severe thermal burns, for example, intravascular plasma leaks from the circulatory system into the burned tissues that lie adjacent to the injury. By comparison, crushing injuries may result in the loss of blood and plasma from damaged vessels into injured tissues.

Abnormal losses of fluids and electrolytes (that is, dehydration) may occur through a variety of mechanisms:

- GI losses, especially through vomiting and diarrhea
- Increased loss as a consequence of fever, hyperventilation, or high environmental temperatures (through the lungs)
- Increased sweating
- Internal losses ("third-space" losses), as in peritonitis, pancreatitis, and ileus
- Plasma losses from burns, drains, and granulating wounds

Other causes of body fluid deficits include ascites, diabetes insipidus, acute renal failure, and osmotic diuresis secondary to hyperosmolar states (such as diabetic ketoacidosis).

In each case, the fluid lost has a unique electrolyte composition, and long-term therapy aims to restore the deficient body chemicals. For treatment in the field, however, all excessive fluid losses can be considered to lead to dehydration.

Symptoms of dehydration include loss of appetite (anorexia), nausea, vomiting, and sometimes fainting when standing up (postural syncope). Physical examination of a dehydrated patient reveals poor skin turgor (the skin over the forehead or sternum will "tent" when pinched); a shrunken, furrowed tongue; and sunken eyes. The pulse will be weak and rapid, rising more than 15 beats/min when the patient is raised from a recumbent to a sitting position (a maneuver that may cause the patient to feel faint). When fluid and electrolyte depletion are severe, shock and coma may be present.

A dehydrated patient needs replacement of fluid and electrolytes and should be given an IV infusion of normal saline or lactated Ringer's solution at a rate of 100 to 200 mL/h for an adult, depending on the circumstances. Keep the patient flat to optimize circulation to the brain.

Distributive Shock

Distributive shock occurs when there is widespread dilation of the resistance vessels (small arterioles), the capacitance vessels (small venules), or both. As a result, the circulating blood volume pools in the expanded vascular beds and tissue perfusion decreases. The three most common types of distributive shock are septic shock, neurogenic shock, and anaphylactic shock.

Septic Shock

Sepsis comes from the Greek word meaning "to putrefy." Septic shock is defined as the presence of sepsis syndrome plus a systolic BP of less than 90 mm Hg or a decrease from the baseline BP of more than 40 mm Hg.

Sepsis occurs as a result of widespread infection, usually due to gram-negative bacterial organisms; gram-positive bacteria, fungi, viruses, and rickettsia can also be causative agents. Complex interactions occur between the pathogen and the body's defense systems. Initially, the body's defense mechanisms may keep the infection at bay. The infection activates the inflammatory-immune response, which invokes humoral, cellular, and biochemical pathways. This response results in increased microvascular permeability (leaky capillaries), vasodilation, third-space fluid shifts, and microthrombi formation. In some patients, an uncontrolled and unregulated inflammatory-immune response occurs, resulting in hypoperfusion to the cells owing to opening of AV shunts, tissue destruction, and organ death. Left untreated, the result is multiple-organ dysfunction syndrome and, often, death.

Septic shock is a complex problem. First, there is an insufficient volume of fluid in the container, because much of the blood has leaked out of the vascular system (hypovolemia). Second, the fluid that leaks out often collects in the respiratory system, interfering with ventilation. Third, a larger-than-normal vascular bed is asked to contain the smaller-than-normal volume of intravascular fluid.

Neurogenic Shock

Neurogenic shock usually results from spinal cord injury. Less commonly, it may derive from medical causes such as brain conditions, tumors, pressure on the spinal cord, or spina bifida. The effect of these conditions is loss of normal sympathetic nervous system tone and vasodilation.

In neurogenic shock, the muscles in the walls of the blood vessels are cut off from the nerve impulses that cause them to contract. As a consequence, all vessels below the level of the spinal injury dilate widely, increasing the size and capacity of the vascular system and causing blood to pool. The available 5 to 6 L of blood in the body can no longer fill this enlarged vascular system. Perfusion of organs and tissues becomes inadequate, even though no blood or fluid has been lost, and shock occurs. The patient experiences relative hypovolemia, which leads to hypotension (systolic BP usually between 80 and 100 mm Hg). In addition, relative bradycardia occurs because the sympathetic nervous system is not stimulated to release catecholamines. The skin is pink, warm, and dry because of cutaneous vasodilation. There is no release of epinephrine and norepinephrine, which would otherwise produce the classic sign of pale, cool, diaphoretic skin. Instead, a characteristic sign of neurogenic shock is the absence of sweating below the level of injury.

The term *spinal shock* refers to the local neurologic condition that occurs immediately after a spinal injury produces motor and sensory losses (which may not be permanent).

▣ Points to Ponder

You respond to the scene of a single motor vehicle collision in which a 45-year-old woman is walking around the scene. It is obvious from the spiderlike crack in the windshield and her forehead laceration that she struck the glass with her head. She is nervous that she will get in trouble and states she was wearing a seatbelt and did not hit the windshield. You also note the smell of alcohol on her breath, and she denies any medical history. She allowed you to feel her weak rapid radial pulse but now is refusing to let you do any further assessment. Her head lacerations are no longer bleeding, although she has plenty of blood on her white blouse. She is refusing to go to the hospital, stating there is nothing wrong with her. The police officer, who has been dealing with the traffic congestion, states he is going to administer a breathalyzer test.

How should you deal with this patient's refusal to go to the hospital?

Issues: MOI for Internal Injury, Recognition of Shock, Estimating Phases of Shock, Compensation Versus Decompensation During Shock, Treatment Plan for a Patient With Suspected Shock, and Patient Refusal.

19 Soft-Tissue Injury

Objectives

Cognitive

4-3.1 Describe the incidence, morbidity, and mortality of soft tissue injuries. (p 19.4)

4-3.2 Describe the layers of the skin, specifically:
a. Epidermis and dermis (cutaneous)
b. Superficial fascia (subcutaneous)
c. Deep fascia (p 19.5, 19.6)

4-3.3 Identify the major functions of the integumentary system. (p 19.4)

4-3.4 Identify the skin tension lines of the body. (p 19.6)

4-3.5 Predict soft tissue injuries based on mechanism of injury. (p 19.14)

4-3.6 Discuss the pathophysiology of wound healing, including:
a. Hemostasis
b. Inflammation phase
c. Epithelialization
d. Neovascularization
e. Collagen synthesis (p 19.6, 19.7)

4-3.7 Discuss the pathophysiology of soft tissue injuries. (p 19.6)

4-3.8 Differentiate between the following types of closed soft tissue injuries:
a. Contusion
b. Hematoma
c. Crush injuries (p 19.9, 19.11)

4-3.9 Discuss the assessment findings associated with closed soft tissue injuries. (p 19.14)

4-3.10 Discuss the management of a patient with closed soft tissue injuries. (p 19.17)

4-3.11 Discuss the pathophysiology of open soft tissue injuries. (p 19.9)

4-3.12 Differentiate between the following types of open soft tissue injuries:
a. Abrasions
b. Lacerations
c. Major arterial lacerations
d. Avulsions
e. Impaled objects
f. Amputations
g. Incisions
h. Crush injuries
i. Blast injuries
j. Penetrations/punctures (p 19.9–19.13)

4-3.13 Discuss the incidence, morbidity, and mortality of blast injuries. (p 19.12)

4-3.14 Predict blast injuries based on mechanism of injury, including:
a. Primary
b. Secondary
c. Tertiary (p 19.12–19.14)

4-3.15 Discuss types of trauma including:
a. Blunt
b. Penetrating
c. Barotrauma
d. Burns (p 19.4)

4-3.16 Discuss the pathophysiology associated with blast injuries. (p 19.12)

4-3.17 Discuss the effects of an explosion within an enclosed space on a patient. (p 19.14)

4-3.18 Discuss the assessment findings associated with blast injuries. (p 19.26)

4-3.19 Identify the need for rapid intervention and transport of the patient with a blast injury. (p 19.26)

4-3.20 Discuss the management of a patient with a blast injury. (p 19.26)

4-3.21 Discuss the incidence, morbidity, and mortality of crush injuries. (p 19.11)

4-3.22 Define the following conditions:
a. Crush injury
b. Crush syndrome
c. Compartment syndrome (p 19.11, 19.12)

4-3.23 Discuss the mechanisms of injury in a crush injury. (p 19.11)

4-3.24 Discuss the effects of reperfusion and rhabdomyolysis on the body. (p 19.12)

4-3.25 Discuss the assessment findings associated with crush injuries. (p 19.11)

4-3.26 Identify the need for rapid intervention and transport of the patient with a crush injury. (p 19.25)

4-3.27 Discuss the management of a patient with a crush injury. (p 19.25)

4-3.28 Discuss the pathophysiology of hemorrhage associated with soft tissue injuries, including:
a. Capillary
b. Venous
c. Arterial (p 19.18, 19.19)

4-3.29 Discuss the assessment findings associated with open soft tissue injuries. (p 19.14)

4-3.30 Discuss the assessment of hemorrhage associated with open soft tissue injuries. (p 19.17)

4-3.31 Differentiate between the various management techniques for hemorrhage control of open soft tissue injuries, including:
a. Direct pressure
b. Elevation
c. Pressure dressing
d. Pressure point
e. Tourniquet application (p 19.19–19.21)

4-3.32 Differentiate between the types of injuries requiring the use of an occlusive versus non-occlusive dressing. (p 19.17)

4-3.33 Identify the need for rapid assessment, intervention and appropriate transport for the patient with a soft tissue injury. (p 19.17)

4-3.34 Discuss the management of the soft tissue injury patient. (p 19.17)

4-3.35 Define and discuss the following:
  a. Dressings
    1. Sterile
    2. Non-sterile
    3. Occlusive
    4. Non-occlusive
    5. Adherent
    6. Non-adherent
    7. Absorbent
    8. Non-absorbent
    9. Wet
    10. Dry
  b. Bandages
    1. Absorbent
    2. Non-absorbent
    3. Adherent
    4. Non-adherent
  c. Tourniquet (p 19.17, 19.18)
4-3.36 Predict the possible complications of an improperly applied dressing, bandage, or tourniquet. (p 19.18)
4-3.37 Discuss the assessment of wound healing. (p 19.17)
4-3.38 Discuss the management of wound healing. (p 19.23)
4-3.39 Discuss the pathophysiology of wound infection. (p 19.17)
4-3.40 Discuss the assessment of wound infection. (p 19.17)
4-3.41 Discuss the management of wound infection. (p 19.23)
4-3.42 Integrate pathophysiological principles to the assessment of a patient with a soft tissue injury. (p 19.15)
4-3.43 Formulate treatment priorities for patients with soft tissue injuries in conjunction with:
  a. Airway/face/neck trauma
  b. Thoracic trauma (open/closed)
  c. Abdominal trauma (p 19.26, 19.27)
4-3.44 Synthesize assessment findings and patient history information to form a field impression for the patient with soft tissue trauma. (p 19.16)
4-3.45 Develop, execute, and evaluate a treatment plan based on the field impression for the patient with soft tissue trauma. (p 19.17)

Affective

4-3.46 Defend the rationale explaining why immediate life-threats must take priority over wound closure. (p 19.15)
4-3.47 Defend the management regimens for various soft tissue injuries. (p 19.17)
4-3.48 Defend why immediate life-threatening conditions take priority over soft tissue management. (p 19.15)
4-3.49 Value the importance of a thorough assessment for patients with soft tissue injuries. (p 19.14)
4-3.50 Attend to the feelings that the patient with a soft tissue injury may experience. (p 19.17, 19.23)
4-3.51 Appreciate the importance of good follow-up care for patients receiving sutures. (p 19.23)
4-3.52 Understand the value of the written report for soft tissue injuries, in the continuum of patient care. (p 19.27)

Psychomotor

4-3.53 Demonstrate the assessment and management of a patient with signs and symptoms of soft tissue injury, including:
  a. Contusion
  b. Hematoma
  c. Crushing
  d. Abrasion
  e. Laceration
  f. Avulsion
  g. Amputation
  h. Impaled object
  i. Penetration/puncture
  j. Blast (p 19.9–19.13, 19.22)

Introduction

The skin is the largest organ of the human body and serves as the interface between the body and outside world. For that reason, injuries involving the skin are common. Injuries to the skin are often the most immediately obvious of a person's injuries, although not necessarily the most serious. An inexperienced EMS provider is apt to be distracted by dramatic external wounds and neglect to check for higher-priority problems, such as an obstructed airway or significant hypotension. Paramedics can avoid making this critical mistake by ensuring that they have a thorough understanding of the anatomy and physiology of the skin.

This chapter describes each layer of this vital organ along with its function. It also describes soft-tissue injuries along with factors that inhibit normal healing. Finally, it looks at how to assess and manage crush injuries.

Incidence, Mortality, and Morbidity

The soft tissues of the body can be injured through a variety of mechanisms. A blunt injury occurs when the energy exchange between the patient and an object is more than the tissues can tolerate, as can happen in an automobile collision that leads to the person striking the steering wheel. A penetrating injury occurs when an object, such as a bullet or knife, breaks through the skin and enters the body. Barotrauma injuries occur from sudden or extreme changes in air pressure, such as can occur during a scuba diving emergency. Burns may also result in soft-tissue injuries.

Soft-tissue trauma is the leading form of injury. Open wounds account for approximately 6.5 million emergency department (ED) visits, and nearly 5 million patients present with contusions. In fact, wound care is one of the most frequently performed procedures in EDs across the United States. Most of these injuries require basic interventions such as wound irrigation, dressing, bandaging, and limited suturing.

Death due to soft-tissue injury is often related to hemorrhage or infection. Uncontrolled hemorrhage can quickly lead to shock and death. When the skin barrier is breached, invading pathogens—bacteria, fungi, and viruses—can cause local or systemic infection. Infection can be life or limb threatening, especially in people with diabetes. Preventing soft-tissue injuries and their associated complications involves simple protective actions. The use of gloves when working with abrasive materials, for example, can prevent skin injuries. Workplace safety measures to reduce injury include use of safety devices to prevent interaction between machine parts and body parts. Teaching children to avoid using sharp objects also helps prevent injury. Plastic scissors, plastic knives, and plastic drinking cups are all designed to reduce the risk of cuts and other skin injuries among children.

Structure and Function of the Skin

The human skin is much more than a wrapping. Rather, skin, or integument, is a complex organ with a crucial role in maintaining the constancy of the internal environment (homeostasis):

- The skin protects the underlying tissue from injury, including that caused by extremes of temperature, ultraviolet radiation, mechanical forces, toxic chemicals, and invading microorganisms.
- The skin aids in temperature regulation, preventing heat loss when the core body temperature starts to fall and facilitating heat loss when core temperature rises.
- As a watertight seal, the skin prevents excessive loss of water from the body and drying of tissues, thereby helping

You are the Provider Part 1

While standing by at a high school football game, you and your partner witness a running back injure his right leg after a linebacker fell on him during a tackle. The patient, a 16-year-old male, has an open deformity to his right leg. The injury is actively bleeding and a bone is protruding through the skin. With the appropriate BSI precautions in place, your partner stabilizes the injury site and applies direct pressure to control the bleeding. You perform an initial assessment.

Initial Assessment	Recording Time: 0 Minutes
Appearance	In severe pain
Level of consciousness	A (Alert to person, place, and day)
Airway	Patent; clear of secretions
Breathing	Increased respirations; adequate depth
Circulation	Open injury to leg (bleeding controlled); pulse, rapid and strong; skin, pink and diaphoretic

1. Does this patient require spinal motion restriction precautions? Why or why not?
2. What are your main concerns regarding this patient's injury?

maintain the chemical stability of the internal environment.

- The skin serves as a sense organ, keeping the brain informed about the external environment. Changes in temperature, touch, and body position and sensations of pain are mediated through the sense receptors in the skin.

Significant damage to the skin may make the body vulnerable to bacterial invasion, temperature instability, and major disturbances of fluid balance—precisely what happens when an injury results in an opening in the skin.

Epidermis

The skin is composed of two layers: the epidermis and the dermis (Figure 19-1 ▾). The epidermis, or outermost layer, is the body's first line of defense, the principal barrier against water, dust, microorganisms, and mechanical stress. It consists of five layers: an outermost layer (stratum corneum) of hardened, non-living cells, which are continuously shed through a process called desquamation; and four inner layers of living cells that constantly divide to give rise to the cells of the stratum corneum.

The deeper layers of the epidermis also contain variable numbers of cells bearing melanin granules; these cells are known as melanocytes. The darkness of a person's skin is directly proportional to the amount of melanin present.

Dermis

Underlying the epidermis is a tough, highly elastic layer of connective tissues called the dermis. This complex material is composed chiefly of collagen fibers, elastic fibers, and a mucopolysaccharide gel. Numerous fibroblasts—cells that secrete collagen, elastin, and ground substance—are found within the dermis as well. Collagen, a fibrous protein with a high tensile strength, gives the skin high resistance to breakage under mechanical stress. Elastin, as the name implies, imparts elasticity to the skin, allowing the skin to spring back to its usual contours. Ground substance, which is found in connective tissues in differing amounts, is a transparent mucopolysaccharide gel that gives the skin resistance to compression.

The dermis is subdivided into the papillary dermis and a reticular layer. The vasculature inside the papillary dermis serves two functions: It provides nutrients to the epidermis, and it aids in thermoregulation. Dilation of these vessels increases blood flow to the skin, allowing heat to dissipate. Conversely, blood vessel constriction results in retention of heat. The reticular layer is made of dense, irregular connective tissue, which provides strength and elasticity.

Macrophages and lymphocytes are also found within the dermal layer. Both are part of the inflammatory process and are responsible for combating microorganisms that breach the epidermal layer. Once a pathogen enters the dermis, macrophages and lymphocytes destroy the invading microorganism and signal other cells to migrate into the area. Physical injury will trigger mast cells to degranulate and synthesize special chemical mediators. The result is increased blood flow to the affected area, manifested as redness and warmth.

Several specialized structures can be identified in the dermis:

- **Nerve endings**—mediate the senses of touch, temperature, pressure, and pain.
- **Blood vessels**—carry oxygen and nutrients to the skin and remove carbon dioxide and metabolic waste products. Cutaneous blood vessels also have a crucial role in regulating body temperature by regulating the volume of blood that flows from the body's warm core to its cooler surface.
- **Sweat glands**—produce sweat and discharge it through ducts passing to the surface of the skin. Sweat consists of water and salts, and sweating is regulated through the action of the sympathetic nervous system. The average volume of sweat lost during 24 hours under normal conditions ranges from 500 to 1,000 mL; during strenuous exercise, however, sweat glands may secrete as much as

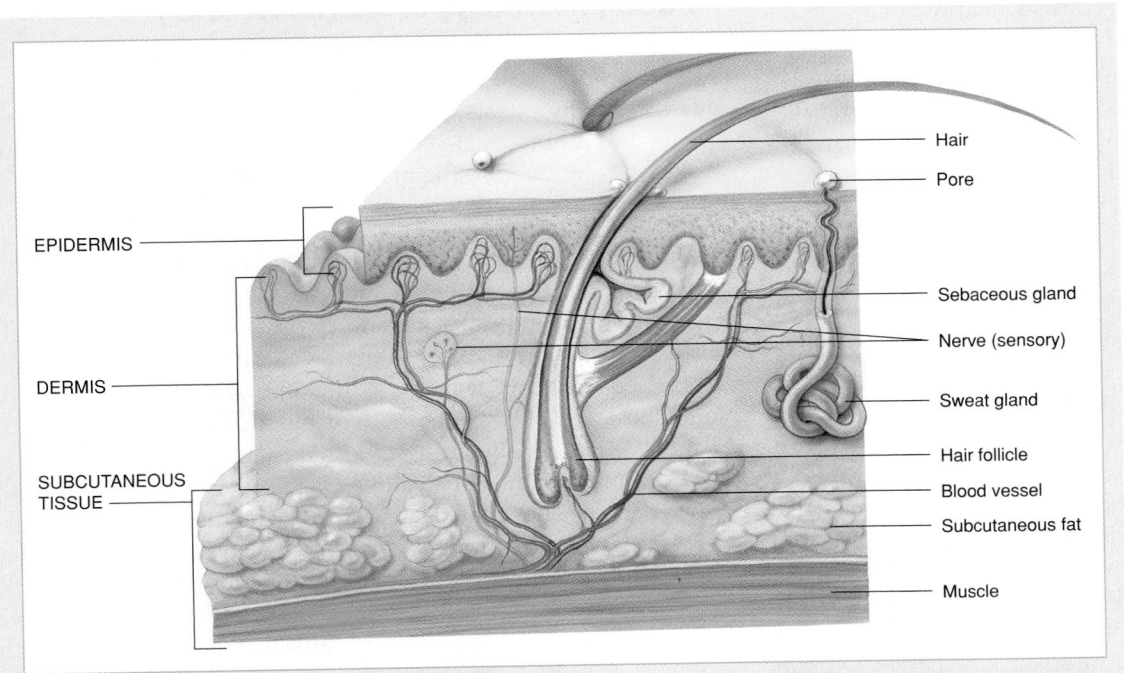

EPIDERMIS

DERMIS

SUBCUTANEOUS TISSUE

Hair
Pore
Sebaceous gland
Nerve (sensory)
Sweat gland
Hair follicle
Blood vessel
Subcutaneous fat
Muscle

Figure 19-1 The skin is composed of a tough external layer called the epidermis and a vascular inner layer called the dermis.

1,000 mL in an hour. This evaporation of water from the skin surface is one of the body's major mechanisms for shedding excess heat.

- **Hair follicles**—produce hair and enclose the hair roots. Each follicle contains a single hair. Attached to the hair follicle is a small muscle that, on contraction, causes the follicle to assume a more vertical position. Hairs in each part of the body have definite periods of growth, after which they are shed and replaced; scalp hair, for example, has a life span of 2 to 5 years and grows 1.5 to 3.9 mm per week.
- **Sebaceous gland**—located at the neck of each hair follicle, is a specialized secretory mechanism that produces an oily substance called sebum. The secretions of the sebaceous glands empty into the hair follicles and from there reach the surface of the skin. The precise function of sebum is not well understood, although it may keep the skin supple so that it doesn't crack.

Notes from Nancy

Sensations such as cold and fright stimulate the autonomic nervous system, which in turn brings about contraction of those muscles; the result is the appearance of the skin called "gooseflesh."

Subcutaneous Tissue

The layer of tissue beneath the dermis—that is, the subcutaneous layer (superficial fascia)—consists mainly of adipose tissue (fat). Blood vessels, lymph vessels, and hair follicle roots are also found in this layer. Subcutaneous fat insulates the underlying tissues from extremes of heat and cold. It also provides a cushion for underlying structures and an energy reserve for the body.

Deep Fascia

Below the subcutaneous tissue is a thick, dense layer of fibrous tissue known as the deep fascia. The deep fascia is composed of tough bands of tissue that ensheath muscles and other internal structures. It supports and protects underlying structures from injury. Muscles and bones are found below this layer.

Skin Tension Lines

The skin is arranged over the body structures in a manner that provides tension. This tautness varies by body region but occurs in patterns known as tension lines. Static tension develops over areas that have limited movement, such as the scalp. Lacerations occurring parallel to the skin tension lines may remain closed with little or no intervention. Larger wounds may be pulled open by the normal tension and require closure with sutures, staples, or a biodegradable "glue." Even small lacerations that lie perpendicular to the tension lines result in a

wound that remains open. Healing occurs more slowly in an open wound, and abnormal scar formation is more likely.

Dynamic tension is found in areas that lie over muscle. The tension varies according to the contraction of the underlying muscle and subsequent movement of the skin. Open injuries to dynamic tension lines interfere with healing because they disrupt the clotting process and the tissue repair cycle, resulting in slowed healing and a tendency toward abnormal scar formation.

An abnormal scar may prompt the patient to seek scar revision—surgery to improve its appearance. The surgeon takes skin tension into account when determining the best procedure for revision. This factor must also be considered when wound debridement is necessary or when hospital personnel must remove an impaled object.

Wound Healing

A wound is any injury to the soft tissues—that is, an injury to the skin with or without involvement of the subcutaneous tissues and muscle. Most soft-tissue wounds are relatively low-priority injuries. Although they may be the most obvious and dramatic injuries, they are seldom the most serious of the patient's problems unless they compromise the airway or are associated with massive bleeding. Always search systematically and thoroughly for other injuries or life-threatening conditions before tending to soft-tissue trauma. *Don't let dramatic soft-tissue injuries distract you from thorough initial assessment!*

Pathophysiology of Wound Healing

Healing of wounds is a natural process that involves several overlapping stages, all directed toward the larger goal of maintaining homeostasis. Ultimately, the goal is for the body to return to a functional state, although the injured area may not always be restored to the preinjury condition.

Hemostasis

Among the primary concerns in wound healing is the cessation of bleeding. Loss of blood, internal or external, hinders the provision of vital nutrients and oxygen to the affected area. It also impairs the tissue's ability to eliminate wastes. The end result is abnormal or absent function, which interferes with homeostasis. To stop the flow of blood, the vessels, platelets, and clotting cascade must work in unison.

Injury to soft tissue causes chemicals in the vessel wall to be released. These chemicals constrict the blood vessels, resulting in less space through which blood can flow. The muscular layer in the arteries, arterioles, and some veins constricts to reduce the size of the lumen. Skeletal muscles also have a role in the constriction process. Because capillaries lack smooth muscle, bleeding continues, albeit at a slower rate.

Platelets are also activated by the release of these chemicals. Activated platelets adhere to the affected area and to other platelets. This aggregation of platelets forms a platelet plug.

Although not the permanent repair, the plug temporarily stops the blood loss and is the beginning of blood clot formation.

Inflammation

In inflammation (the next stage of wound healing), additional cells move into the damaged area to begin repair. White blood cells migrate to the area to combat pathogens that have invaded exposed tissue. Chemicals and proteins known as chemotactic factors are released and call repairing cells into the area. Granulocytes and macrophages, among the first restoration cells to arrive, engulf bacteria through phagocytosis, which involves ingestion of damaged cellular parts. Foreign products and bacteria can also be removed from the body by phagocytosis. Similarly, lymphocytes (a type of white blood cell) destroy bacteria and other pathogens.

Mast cells release histamine as part of the body's response in the early stages of inflammation. Histamine causes dilation of blood vessels, increasing blood flow to the injured area and resulting in a reddened, warm area immediately around the site. Histamine makes capillaries more permeable, and swelling may occur as fluid seeps out of these "leaky" capillaries.

Inflammation ultimately leads to the removal of foreign material, damaged cellular parts, and invading microorganisms from the wound site. Reconstruction of the injured region through epithelialization, neovascularization, and collagen synthesis can then begin.

Epithelialization

In the outer layer of skin, epithelial cells are stacked in layers. To replace the area damaged in a soft-tissue injury, a new layer of epithelial cells must be moved into this region—a process known as epithelialization. Cells from the stratum germinativum quickly multiply and redevelop across the edges of the wound. Except in cases of clean incisions, the appearance of the restructured area seldom returns to the preinjury state. For example, large wounds or injuries that result in significant disruption of the skin will often have incomplete epithelialization.

In persons with lightly pigmented skin, a pink line of scar tissue may signal the presence of collagen, a structural protein that has reinforced the damaged tissue. Despite the changed appearance, the function of the area may be restored to near normal.

Neovascularization

In neovascularization, new blood vessels form as the body attempts to bring oxygen and nutrients to the injured tissue. New capillaries bud from intact capillaries that lie adjacent to the damaged skin. These vessels provide a conduit for oxygen and nutrients and serve as a pathway for waste removal. Because they are new and delicate, bleeding might result from a very minor injury. It may take weeks to months for the new capillaries to be as stable as preexisting vessels.

Collagen Synthesis

Collagen is a tough, fibrous protein found in scar tissue, hair, bones, and connective tissue. This vital structural repair unit is synthesized by fibroblasts, repair cells that migrate into damaged tissue. In wound healing, collagen provides stability to the damaged tissue and joins wound borders, thereby closing the open tissue. Unfortunately, collagen cannot restore the damaged tissue to its original strength.

Alterations of Wound Healing

Wound healing does not always follow the pattern described previously. Infection or an abnormal scar may develop, excessive bleeding may occur, or healing may be slow. This section discusses altered wound healing and potential complications.

Anatomic Factors

Areas of the body subjected to repeated motion throughout the day, such as the fingers, tend to heal slowly. One strategy used to speed healing in such cases is to splint the affected part, preventing movement. The arrangement of an open wound in relation to skin tension lines also affects how the wound will heal and determines whether an abnormal scar will form.

You are the Provider Part 2

After bandaging and splinting the patient's leg, you assess pulse, motor, and sensory functions; they are grossly intact. The remainder of your focused physical exam is unremarkable. After placing the patient onto the stretcher and loading him into the ambulance, your partner gathers SAMPLE history information from the patient while you obtain a set of baseline vital signs.

Vital Signs	Recording Time: 8 Minutes
Skin	Pink and diaphoretic
Pulse	120 beats/min; strong and regular at the radial artery
Blood pressure	148/88 mm Hg
Respirations	24 breaths/min; adequate depth
Sao2	98% on room air
Pain scale	10 on a scale of 0 to 10

3. Is this patient in shock?

4. What additional care should you provide to this patient?

Some medications can delay healing—namely, corticosteroids, nonsteroidal anti-inflammatory drugs, penicillin, colchicine, anticoagulants, and antineoplastic agents. Likewise, a variety of medical conditions may interfere with normal healing—advanced age, severe alcoholism, acute uremia, diabetes, hypoxia, severe anemia, peripheral vascular disease, malnutrition, advanced cancer, hepatic failure, and cardiovascular disease.

High-Risk Wounds

Wounds that carry a high risk for developing infection include human and animal bites. Because the mouth is warm and constantly moist, it offers a hospitable environment for growth of bacteria. Injection of human saliva into tissue can result in significant infection. In particular, rabies is a serious infection that can develop from the bite of an infected animal (such as wild raccoons, dogs, and cats).

Cases in which a foreign body or organic matter is embedded in an open wound are considered high-risk injuries because of the likelihood that the material involved is impregnated with microorganisms. Once the material breaches the skin barrier, the pathogen has easy entry into the rest of the body. A foreign body that remains in place on evaluation should be left in place because a lacerated blood vessel may not be bleeding freely because of the foreign body's position. *Do not remove an impaled object in the field unless it interferes with the airway.*

Other high-risk wounds include injection wounds, wounds with significant devitalized tissue, crush wounds, wounds in immunocompromised patients, and injuries to patients with poor peripheral circulation.

Abnormal Scar Formation

Excessive collagen formation can occur if the healing process is not balanced between the building up and breaking down phases of healing. A hypertrophic or keloid scar may develop from the excess protein. Hypertrophic scar formation occurs in areas subject to high tissue stress, such as the elbow and knee. Such a scar does not extend past the borders of the wound margins and tends to form in people with lightly pigmented skin. In contrast, a keloid scar typically develops in people with darkly pigmented skin. It grows over the wound margins and can become larger than the wound area. Keloid scars tend to form on the ears, upper extremities, lower abdomen, and sternum.

Pressure Injuries

Pressure injuries may occur when a patient is bedridden or when pressure is applied for a prolonged period in an unconscious patient or a patient immobilized on a backboard. The involved tissues are deprived of oxygen, which leads to localized hypoxia and cell deterioration. Prevention involves determining the risk and providing a mechanism to reduce or release the pressure on the skin.

Wounds Requiring Closure

Many open wounds heal without intervention from caregivers, but some require closure with sutures, staples, or medical glue (octyl-2-cyanoacrylate). Closure involves bringing the wound edges together to allow for optimal healing. Open injuries that require closure include those that affect cosmetic areas, such as the lips, face, or eyebrows. Such injuries should be considered for closure because scarring often has psychological implications. Gaping wounds and those over tension lines also require closure. Degloving injuries require substantial irrigation and debridement before closing by an emergency practitioner. Closure is also indicated for ring injuries and skin tears.

Open injuries should be closed within 6 to 8 hours in most cases, although there is some variation based on body region. Initial hospital management for open wounds involves assessment for foreign material followed by irrigation. The practitioner can then determine appropriate wound closing options.

Three types of wound closure are performed: primary closure, secondary intention, and tertiary closure. In primary closure, the wound margins are brought together as neatly and evenly as possible. Secondary intention entails dressing high-risk wounds and allowing them to heal through normal body processes. Tertiary closure, also known as delayed primary closure, is applied to wounds that would have a poor cosmetic appearance if treated by secondary intention.

Patients who receive sutures need appropriate follow-up care to determine whether healing is normal or abnormal. Serious complications, including localized or systemic infection, can arise without adequate follow-up care. In some cases, sutures may need to be removed early to allow a wound to drain infectious material.

Infection

Because the skin serves as an initial barrier against microorganisms, any break can lead to infection. Larger openings and deeper penetrations result in a higher level of risk for developing an infection. Not only will there be a delay in healing from the infection, but additional complications or systemic infection can result.

Once in the body tissues, pathogens begin to grow and multiply, although clinical signs of infection may not appear for several days. Visible clues of infection include erythema, pus, warmth, edema, and local discomfort. Red streaks adjacent to the wound indicate that the patient has developed lymphangitis, an inflammation of the lymph channels. More serious infections can cause systemic signs, such as fever, shaking, chills, joint pain, and hypotension.

Gangrene

Approximately 3,000 cases of gangrene occur in the United States each year, of which 60% result from trauma and 25% end in the patient's death. *Clostridium perfringens* is an anaerobic, toxin-producing bacterium that leads to the development of gangrene. Once it enters deeply into tissue, it causes the production of a foul-smelling gas. If the gangrene is not treated, the skin will become necrotic and the infection may lead to sepsis. Prompt recognition and early, aggressive hospital therapy offer the best chance for reducing morbidity and mortality.

Tetanus

Tetanus is caused by infection with an anaerobic bacterium, *Clostridium tetani* (a member of the same family that causes gangrene). This bacterium causes the body to produce a potent toxin, which results in painful muscle contractions that are strong enough to fracture bones. Muscle stiffness may be noted first in the jaw ("lockjaw") and neck, with progression down the remainder of the body. Early recognition is important because conventional therapy does not result in rapid recovery.

Tetanus has become rare, thanks to the availability of a vaccine. In the United States, vaccination against tetanus is part of childhood immunization programs. A booster is needed every 10 years, although an inoculation is typically provided to patients who are injured and have not been immunized in the last 5 years. Given the severity of tetanus, you should ask injured patients about the last time they received a tetanus booster.

Necrotizing Fasciitis

Necrotizing fasciitis involves the death of tissue from bacterial infection. This disease is caused by more than one infecting organism—most commonly, *Staphylococcus aureus* and hemolytic streptococci. Although necrotizing fasciitis is rare, the mortality rate ranges from 70% to 80%. Antibiotic therapy and surgical debridement are among the available treatments.

Closed Versus Open Wounds

Closed Wounds

In a closed wound, soft tissues beneath the skin surface are damaged, but there is no break in the epidermis. The characteristic closed wound is a contusion Figure 19-2 ▾. In a contusion (bruise), the skin is intact, but damage has occurred beneath the epidermis. Trauma to the nerve endings produces pain, and leakage of fluid into spaces between the damaged cells produces swelling (edema). If small blood vessels in the dermis are disrupted, a black-and-blue mark (ecchymosis) will cover the injured area; if large blood vessels are torn beneath the contused area, a hematoma—a collection of blood beneath the skin—will be evident as a lump with a bluish discoloration Figure 19-3 ▸ .

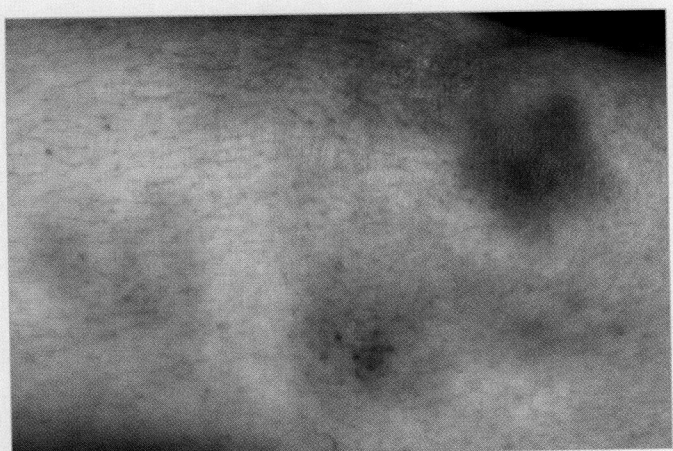

Figure 19-2 A contusion, or bruise, produces characteristic black-and-blue discoloration (ecchymosis).

Open Wounds

An open wound is characterized by a disruption in the skin. Open wounds are potentially much more serious than closed wounds for two reasons. First, they are vulnerable to infection. An open wound is contaminated—that is, microorganisms enter it. Whether the contamination produces infection depends in large measure on how the wound is managed. Second, open wounds have a greater potential for serious blood loss. When the skin is unbroken, bleeding from a disrupted blood vessel is limited. Although a significant volume of blood—up to about 2 units—can be lost into the soft tissues of the leg, eventually the increasing pressure within the leg will prevent further bleeding. In an open wound, the patient's entire blood volume may be lost.

Certain wounds should always be evaluated by a physician. The injuries in Table 19-1 ▾ require transport, even if they appear minor.

Abrasions

An abrasion Figure 19-4 ▸ is a superficial wound that occurs when the skin is rubbed or scraped over a rough surface and part of the epidermis is lost. So-called brush burns or mat burns are good examples. Abrasions typically ooze small amounts of blood and may be quite painful. They may also be contaminated with dirt and debris—for example, from "road rash" caused by sliding on the pavement in a motorcycle crash. Because the skin has been disrupted, infection is a danger.

Don't try to clean an abrasion in the field; you don't have the means to do so properly. If you feel compelled to do *something,* cover the wound lightly with a sterile dressing.

Lacerations

A laceration Figure 19-5 ▸ is a cut inflicted by a sharp instrument, such as a knife or razor blade, that produces a clean or jagged incision through the skin surface and underlying structures. Sometimes the word *laceration* is reserved for jagged or irregular cuts, and incision is used to refer to a clean (linear) cut. Incisions tend to heal better than lacerations because of their relatively even

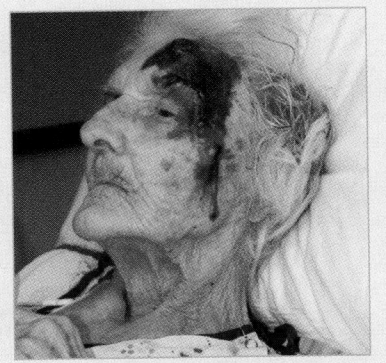

Figure 19-3 A hematoma.

Table 19-1	Conditions That Require Transport

- Compromise of:
  - Nerves
  - Vessels
  - Muscles
  - Tendons or ligaments
- Foreign body or cosmetic complications
- Heavy contamination

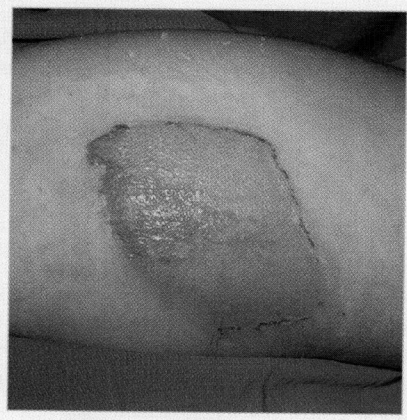
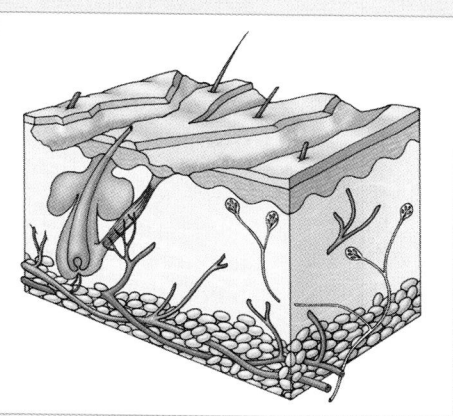

Figure 19-4 Abrasions usually do not penetrate completely through the dermis, but blood may ooze from the capillaries. These wounds are typically superficial and result from rubbing or scraping across a hard, rough surface.

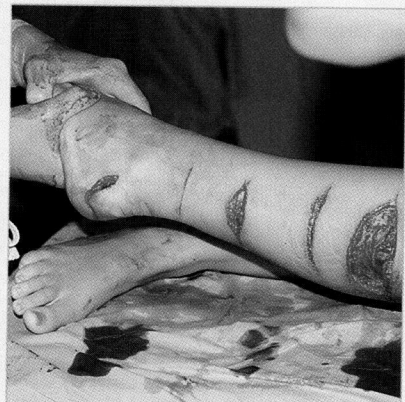
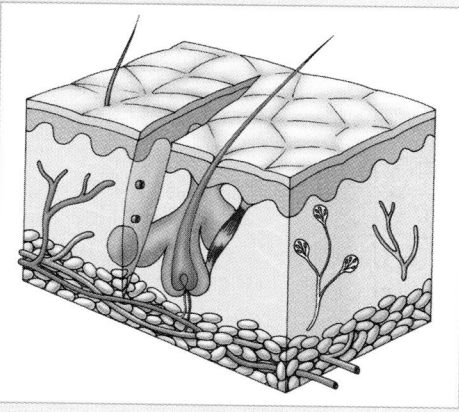

Figure 19-5 Lacerations can vary in depth and can extend through the skin and subcutaneous tissue to the underlying muscles, nerves, and blood vessels. These wounds can be smooth or jagged as a result of a cut by a sharp object or a blunt force that tears the tissue.

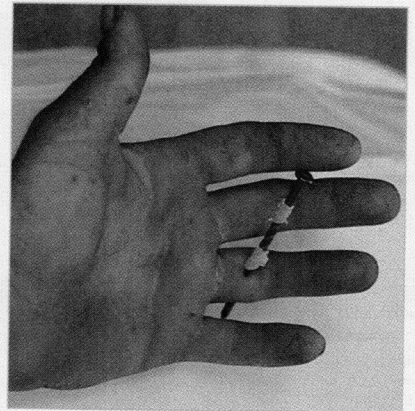
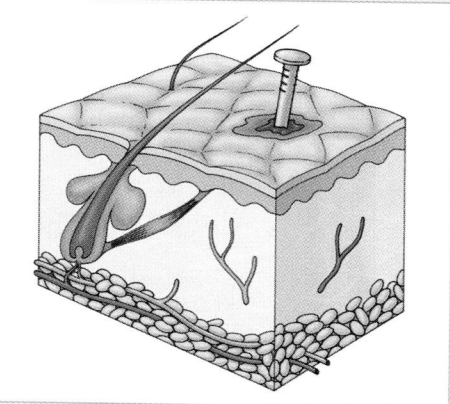

Figure 19-6 Penetrating wounds may cause very little external bleeding but can damage structures deep in the body.

wound margins. The seriousness of a laceration will depend on its depth and the structures that have been damaged. Lacerations may be the source of significant bleeding if they disrupt the wall of a blood vessel, particularly in regions of the body where major arteries lie close to the surface (as in the wrist). The first priority in treating a laceration is to control bleeding, initially by applying direct manual pressure over the wound. Laceration of a major artery can be fatal due to the severe bleeding that can occur.

Puncture Wounds

A puncture wound ` Figure 19-6 ◂ ` is a stab from a pointed object, such as a nail or a knife. Technically speaking, a bullet wound is a puncture wound. Most puncture wounds do not cause significant external bleeding, but they may produce extensive—even fatal—internal bleeding and wreak other havoc that cannot be seen from the outside of the body.

A special case of the puncture wound is the impaled foreign object ` Figure 19-7 ▸ `. When the instrument that caused the injury remains embedded in the wound, immobilize the object, and transport the patient.

Avulsions

An avulsion occurs when a flap of skin is torn loose, partially ` Figure 19-8 ▸ ` or completely. Depending on where the avulsion occurs, it may or may not be accompanied by profuse bleeding. The principal danger in this type of injury—besides blood loss and contamination—is loss of the blood supply to the avulsed flap. If the part of the flap that connects it to the body (the pedicle) is folded back or kinked, circulation to the flap will be compromised and that piece of skin will die if the circulation is not restored quickly.

Amputations

An amputation is an avulsion involving the complete loss of a body part, typically one or more of the extremities. If the amputation was produced by a sharp object, blood loss is often much less than expected because the blood vessels retain the ability to constrict. In contrast, a crushing or tearing amputation can result in exsanguination (excessive blood loss due to hemorrhage) if the provider does not intervene rapidly.

Wound edges in an amputation are commonly jagged, and sharp bone edges may protrude ` Figure 19-9 ▸ `. During wound

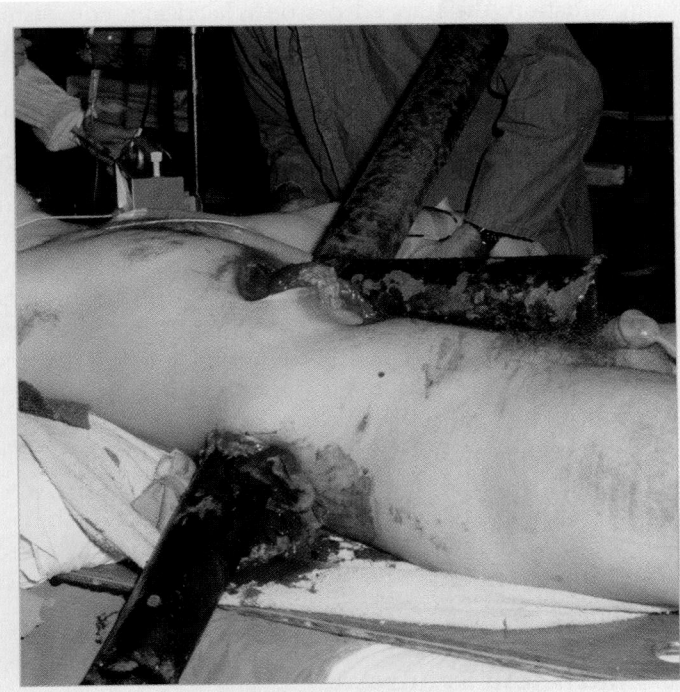

Figure 19-7 An impaled object remains embedded in the wound.

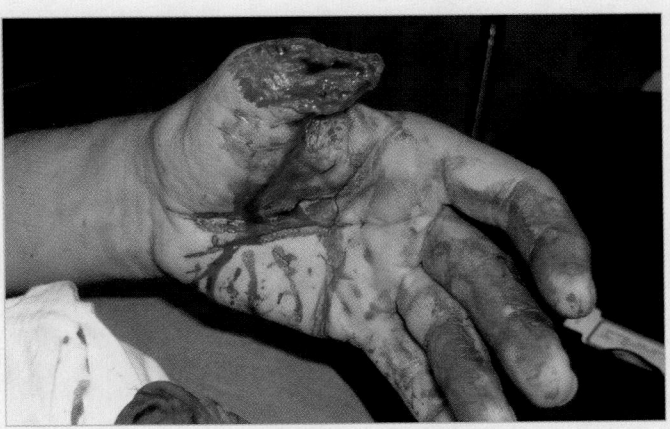

Figure 19-9 An amputation involving the thumb.

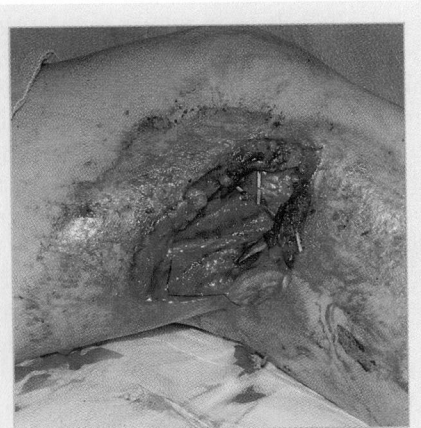
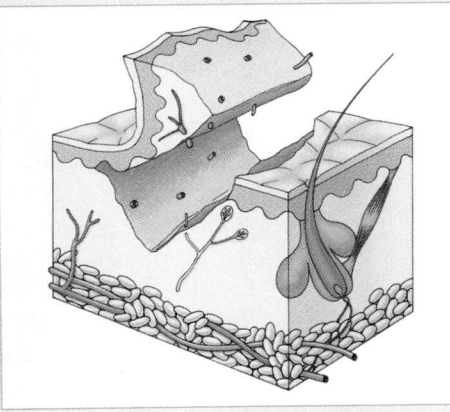

Figure 19-8 Avulsions are characterized by complete separation of tissue or tissue hanging as a flap. Significant bleeding is common.

care, be aware of any sharp bone protrusions that may lead to an exposure. Large, thick dressings should be used to cover the site. In some cases, the body part will be completely detached. In a partial amputation, soft tissues remain attached. A degloving injury is a specific form of amputation that involves unraveling of skin from the hand, much like partial removal of a glove.

Crush Injuries

When a body part is crushed between two solid objects, a crush injury may occur to the underlying soft tissues and bones Figure 19-10 ▶. Such injuries range from an innocuous finger injury to a life-threatening entrapment of the torso. The latter is likely to be encountered in cases involving structural collapse (such as in collapse of masonry or steel structures, earthquakes, tornadoes, construction accidents, mudslides, motor vehicle collisions, warfare injuries, and industrial accidents). A crush injury can also occur when an unconscious patient has an upper extremity pinned between the body and the floor. Likewise, a crush injury may develop when a pneumatic antishock garment (PASG) is left in place for an excessive period or a cast is applied too tightly.

The forces involved in a crush injury may be great enough to rupture internal organs. You must rapidly assess the mechanism of injury and determine the likelihood for massive internal trauma. Also, note that the longer an injured area remains compressed, the greater the chance for systemic complications.

In a crush injury, the external appearance may not adequately represent the level of internal damage. An upper extremity that merely appears swollen may, in fact, have enough muscle destruction to cause systemic problems, especially if the extremity has been trapped for longer than 4 hours, which is enough time to develop crush syndrome. In other cases, the injured region may be mangled beyond recognition. Remember that grotesque injuries may not necessarily be the primary problem. Always concentrate on threats to life before addressing injured extremities, no matter how bad the initial appearance.

One of the body's first responses to a vessel injury is localized vasoconstriction that reduces the flow of blood. When vessels are crushed and torn, they often lose the ability to constrict, resulting in a free flow of blood from any unnatural opening. Crush injuries tend to result in hemorrhage

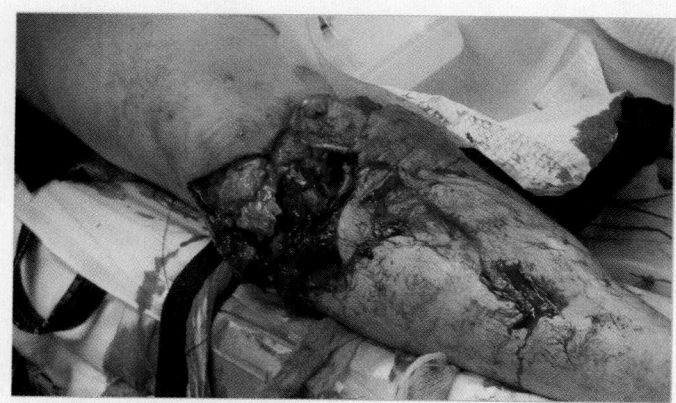

Figure 19-10 A crush injury is characterized by extensive tissue damage and deformity that is often accompanied by swelling and extreme pain.

Table 19-2	The Progression of Crush Syndrome

1. A body part is trapped for more than 4 hours.
2. Rhabdomyolysis occurs.
3. The trapped body part is freed.
4. By-products of metabolism and harmful products from tissue destruction are released, possibly resulting in cardiac arrest, dysrhythmias, kidney damage, hyperkalemia, and hyperphosphatemia.

that cannot easily be controlled by standard methods. Inability to precisely locate bleeding or massive extremity trauma may also lead to difficulty in controlling hemorrhage.

Crush Syndrome

When an area of the body is trapped for longer than 4 hours and arterial blood flow is compromised, crush syndrome can develop (Table 19-2 ▲). When muscles are crushed beyond repair, tissue necrosis develops and leads to release of harmful products, a process known as rhabdomyolysis. As muscle cells are destroyed, they experience an influx of water, sodium chloride, and calcium from extracellular fluid. In addition, the body develops an efflux of potassium, purines (from disintegrating nuclei), phosphate, lactic acid, myoglobin, thromboplastin, creatine, and creatine kinase. The oppressing force prevents the return of blood from the injured body part, so the release of these products into the systemic circulation does not occur until *after* the limb is freed from entrapment. For this reason, rescuers must intervene *before* lifting the crushing object off the body.

Freeing the limb or other body part from entrapment not only results in release of by-products of metabolism and harmful products of tissue destruction, but also involves the potential for cardiac arrest. In prolonged entrapment, "smiling death" may occur if providers do not take proactive measures.

In this situation, the trapped person is alert and conversing with rescuers; however, when the entrapped body part is freed, cardiac arrest is almost instantaneous.

Renal failure is another serious complication that may develop after release of the crushing force. Glomerular filtration can be impaired when the kidneys do not receive enough blood, such as when hypotension develops from bleeding. In addition, the release of large quantities of myoglobin into the central circulation can clog the filtering tubules. The high levels of acids and phosphates can directly damage the kidneys. This problem is compounded by the development of oxygen free radicals. These products travel throughout the affected area, scavenging oxygen molecules and damaging and destroying cells that might otherwise survive the initial injury.

Life-threatening dysrhythmias may also develop from increased blood potassium levels (hyperkalemia). Hyperphosphatemia can lead to calcifications that can interfere with normal blood flow and normal nervous tissue function. Increased levels of uric acid, lactic acid, and potassium may also cause metabolic acidosis.

Compartment Syndrome

Compartment syndrome develops when edema and swelling result in increased pressure within soft tissues. Because the skin can stretch only so far, pressure begins to increase within the compartment, which in turn leads to compromised circulation. Compartment syndrome commonly develops in the extremities and may occur in conjunction with open or closed injuries (although it is more likely with closed injuries due to the buildup of pressure inside the body). As pressure develops, delivery of nutrients and oxygen is impaired and by-products of normal metabolism accumulate. The longer this situation persists, the greater the chance for tissue necrosis.

Compartment syndrome presents with the six Ps: Pain, Paresthesia, Paresis, Pressure, Passive stretch pain, and Pulselessness. Many of these signs may be delayed or nonspecific. Distal perfusion, sensation, and motor function may be intact.

Compartment syndrome that persists for more than 8 hours carries a serious risk for death of local tissues. In such cases, disfiguring wound debridement that can leave visible and psychologic scars is required. There is also a risk of sepsis. In-hospital intervention includes fasciotomy, or incision of the skin and underlying soft tissue with a scalpel. This limb-saving procedure also prevents a Volkmann contracture—a deformity of the hand, fingers, and wrist resulting from damage to forearm muscles—and preserves cutaneous sensation. In some cases, medical direction may authorize field caregivers to perform a fasciotomy.

Blast Injuries

From 1983 to 2002, there were a reported 36,000 bombings in the United States that caused nearly 6,000 injuries and almost 700 deaths. When the Alfred P. Murrah Building in Oklahoma

City was turned to rubble, hundreds of people were killed and injured Figure 19-11 ▶ . Although this attack clearly illustrated the devastating power of an explosive force, many other circumstances can lead to an explosion—dust buildup in grain silos, sawdust in wood factories, and explosive products transported by rail, sea, or air. You must be mentally and physically prepared to respond to an incident involving an explosion.

Blast injuries occur in four phases: primary, secondary, tertiary, and quaternary.

Primary Phase

When an explosion occurs, a pressure wave rapidly develops; this tremendous but concentrated pressure results from air displacement and heat originating from the center of the blast. The pressure wave damages air-filled cavities (such as the ears and lungs). Burns may occur.

All origins of the pressure wave carry a high risk of injury or death. Explosions from a bomb start at the center and move outward, so persons closer to the device will be affected to a greater extent. Explosions from fumes or dust involve an entire area, so there is no "safe" region. Underwater blasts have a three times greater range because of the near incompressibility of water. Explosions that occur within a confined space result in more force applied to the body.

Secondary Phase

A blast wind occurs as combustible gases move across the affected area. Although less forceful than the pressure wave, the blast wind is longer lasting. Projectiles also present serious hazards—flying debris may cause blunt and penetrating injuries. With bombs, the casing fragments rip apart with monumental force, spreading in all directions. Structural elements can break apart and travel at high rates of speed. Nails,

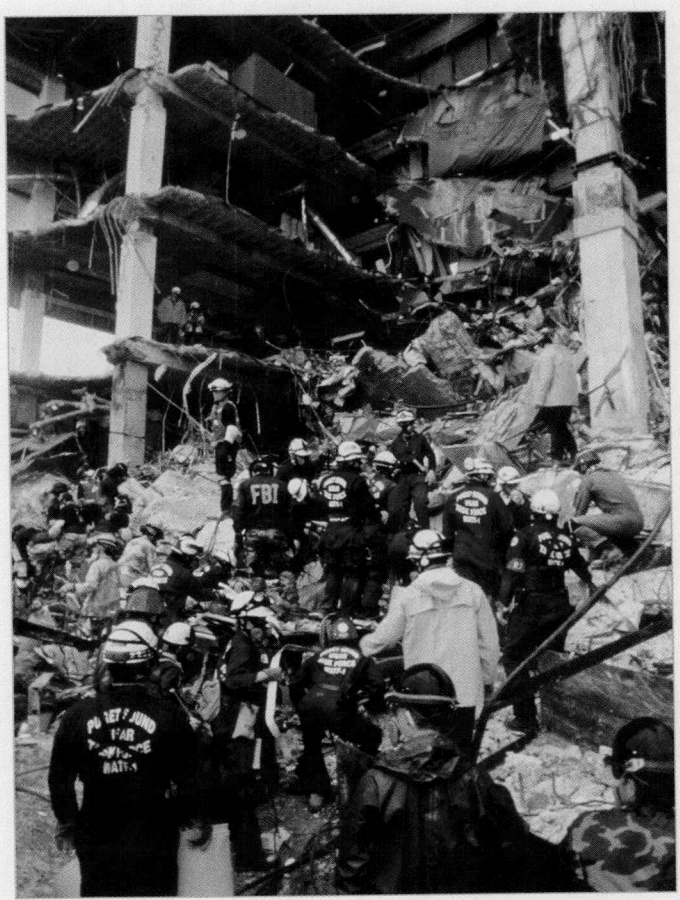

Figure 19-11 The Alfred P. Murrah building's destruction in Oklahoma City killed hundreds.

You are the Provider Part 3

After establishing an IV line of normal saline and administering further treatment, you begin transport to a hospital located approximately 15 miles away. The patient remains conscious and alert and states that his pain is not as severe as it was initially. With an estimated time of arrival at the hospital of 10 minutes, you reassess the patient.

Reassessment	Recording Time: 15 Minutes
Skin	Pink and diaphoretic
Pulse	94 beats/min; strong and regular at the radial artery
Blood pressure	122/68 mm Hg
Respirations	18 breaths/min; adequate depth
Sao$_2$	99% on room air
Pain scale	5 on a scale of 0 to 10

5. What is compartment syndrome and is this patient at risk for it?

6. What are the signs and symptoms of compartment syndrome?

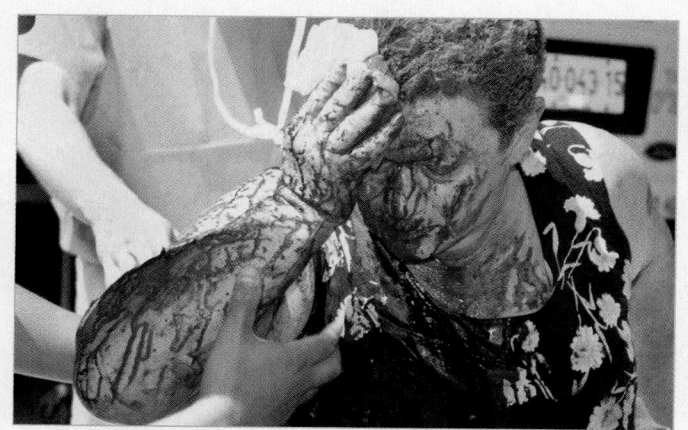

Figure 19-12 Nails, wood splinters, and glass shards can impale victims of a blast explosion.

wood splinters, and glass shards can impale victims located in the area of the blast (Figure 19-12 ▲).

Tertiary Phase

Victims may be injured from displacement away from the blast site or from collapse of the surrounding structure. Displacement occurs when a person is in proximity to the explosion; survival in this circumstance is highly unlikely. Falling structural beams, walls, and other heavy items may lead to crush injuries that compound the conditions already present. Injuries develop when the person is thrown against rigid surfaces, such as the ground, walls, or other rigid objects. There is also a risk for entrapment that can be prolonged for days. In addition, there may be multiple victims (as in the Alfred P. Murrah and World Trade Center bombings).

Quaternary Phase

Injuries result from the miscellaneous events that occur during an explosion. For example, the heat generated during an explosion may cause burns, ranging from superficial flash burns to full-thickness burns involving the entire or large areas of the body.

■ Assessment of Soft-Tissue Injuries

Although skin trauma is often dramatic, it rarely is immediately life threatening. It is important to stay focused on the assessment format used throughout this book to first identify threats to you and your crew using the scene size-up and then identify life threats to the patient using the initial assessment.

The skin is more than just a wrapper; it performs important functions that are altered by trauma. When conducting your initial assessment, you need to determine the nature and mechanism of the injury. The severity of the injury may not be initially apparent, but it will be revealed as you do your rapid trauma assessment or focused physical exam.

Scene Safety and Size-up

The first aspect to address in any scenario is safety. If you are responding to a vehicle collision, ensure that traffic is controlled and personnel are operating with protective measures in place. When responding to a reported explosion, wait for police personnel to secure the scene and declare it safe before you approach any victims. When a blast seems to be intentional, look for possible secondary devices. Responders have been injured and killed by other explosive devices planted away from the original detonation site.

Once you have determined that the scene is safe, begin evaluating the mechanism of injury. Maintain a high index of suspicion whenever a significant mechanism of injury is present, even if external injuries appear minor. Carefully consider the forces involved as you determine the likelihood of internal damage.

Next, determine how many patients are involved. Diligently search for ejected patients in the case of a significant vehicle collision.

As a part of your scene size-up, be aware that skin injuries typically result in a risk of exposure to blood and other bodily fluids. Significant exposures include contact with body fluids through open wounds or mucous membranes. Less worrisome exposures include body fluid contact with intact skin. Be sure to protect yourself and the patient, and review Chapters 2 and 36 regarding infection control procedures.

Initial Assessment

When the scene has been secured and body substance isolation measures have been taken, rapidly determine whether threats to life are present. First, note your general impression as you approach the patient. Much information can be obtained from simply looking at the patient and the immediate surroundings. For example, a patient who is lying prone on the ground in a large pool of blood is clearly in worse shape than a patient who meets you at the door with a cut finger.

Many patients have potential injuries to the neck or spine. In such cases, you should assign a crew member to manually immobilize the head and neck. This is an important step because it will determine which maneuvers are used to open the airway.

Evaluation of the patient's initial level of consciousness is also important. Determine whether the patient is alert, responsive to verbal stimuli, responsive to painful stimuli, or completely unresponsive. This assessment may reveal a potential brain injury even when the patient has a seemingly innocuous soft-tissue injury to the head.

Assess the airway as soon as you arrive at the patient's side. Determine whether air is moving from the nose, mouth, or stoma. When present, immediately suction blood, vomit, or any other product from the airway. If direct airway trauma is present, it may severely compromise the airway. Soft-tissue injuries that result in a flow of blood into the airway can also

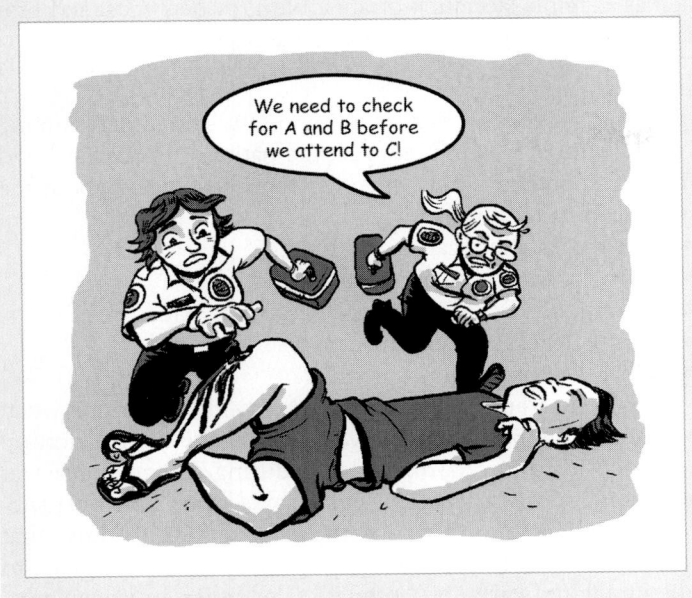

Figure 19-13

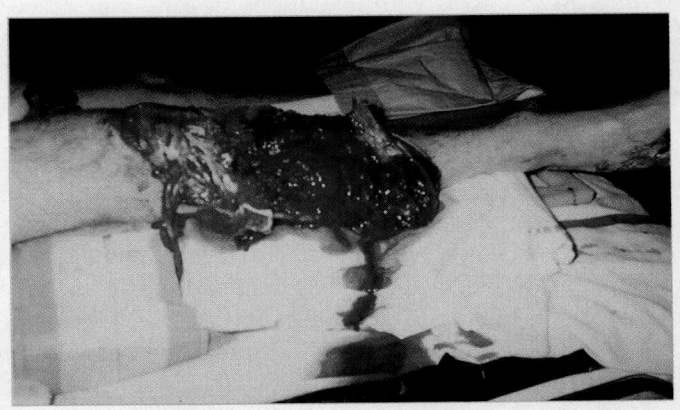

Figure 19-14 A high-velocity gunshot wound to the leg.

prove extremely challenging. Immediately correct anything that interferes with airway patency; failure to provide a patent airway can quickly lead to the patient's death (Figure 19-13 ▲).

Assess the patient's breathing. During the initial assessment, it is not important to obtain an exact rate—just determine whether the patient's breathing is abnormally slow or rapid or excessively deep or shallow. Address a significant alteration in breathing by using a nonrebreathing mask with oxygen at 15 L/min or a bag-mask device and supplementary oxygen. An inadequate depth or rate that results in compromised breathing should prompt you to take immediate action.

Assessment of circulatory status involves palpating a pulse and checking the skin signs. In an unresponsive adult, assess the carotid pulse; in a conscious patient, assess the radial pulse. If no pulse is present, take resuscitative measures (see Appendix A). When a pulse is palpated, determine whether it is abnormally fast or slow (an exact rate will be calculated later). The goal at this step is to determine if immediate intervention is necessary.

Palpate and inspect the skin (CTC—Color, Temperature, and Condition). Pale or ashen skin points to inadequate perfusion. Cool, moist skin is an early indicator of shock. When present, determine if the skin is cool and moist only in the extremities or over the entire body.

Ensure that the patient is adequately exposed during the initial assessment. Sometimes, you need to look at only the chest area. On more serious calls, the patient may need to be completely exposed from head to toe. Gunshot wounds and stab wounds, for example, warrant complete removal of the patient's clothing (Figure 19-14 ▶).

Once the initial assessment has been completed, you will need to make a priority decision to rapidly package and trans-

port or to stabilize and treat on scene. Patients with significant trauma (significant mechanism of injury [MOI]) should be rapidly transported in accordance with the "golden hour" principle. Patients with isolated injuries (no significant MOI) are often better managed by carefully treating the injuries on scene.

Focused History and Physical Exam
Physical Examination

Patients are stratified into two categories: patients with a significant MOI and patients with no significant MOI. When serious trauma is present, soft-tissue injuries take a lower priority than airway control, breathing inadequacy, and bleeding. *Do not let soft-tissue injuries distract you from life threats that may not be readily apparent.* Patients with less serious injuries will need an exam focused on the specific body part and its function but probably will not need a detailed physical exam.

Significant MOI

Serious trauma is indicated by an altered level of consciousness, lack of airway protection or lack of patency, inadequate breathing, uncontrolled bleeding, and a significant MOI. If any are present or your analysis points to a possibility for serious injury, perform a rapid trauma assessment. Life threats should have been addressed during the initial assessment; if additional life threats are found now, manage them immediately. For example, if examination of the chest reveals absent breath sounds on one side, the chest may need ventilation, sealing with an occlusive dressing, and decompression if there is a tension pneumothorax. Interventions can occur simultaneously during the initial assessment of the patient.

The rapid trauma assessment involves a head-to-toe assessment that focuses on detecting serious injury to major body compartments. Rapidly assess the head, neck, chest, abdomen, pelvis, lower extremities, upper extremities, and posterior. Identify deformities, discolorations, impaled objects, open injuries, and other trauma that demands immediate attention. The mnemonic DCAP-BTLS is a useful reminder of what to look at: Deformities, Contusions, Abrasions, Punctures or penetrations, Burns, Tenderness, Lacerations, and

Swelling. Assess areas with alterations in sensation, uneven temperature, or abnormal muscle tone. Note if any blood appears on your gloves. For example, hair can conceal hemorrhage, but if you find blood on your gloves during your exam of the head, you have identified an injury.

Address airway compromises, breathing inadequacies, and uncontrolled hemorrhage that may have been missed in the initial assessment. Trauma patients are often critically injured, and life threats evolve over time, so reassessments may reveal problems not found in the initial examination. Airway takes priority over breathing issues, and both take precedence over active bleeding. In practice, you will work as a part of a team to manage each issue as it is found rather than addressing each life threat sequentially. For example, the paramedic positioned at the head can manage the airway while another provider performs bleeding control. Prioritize the injuries that need to be addressed first. Remember that optimal on-scene time is less than 10 minutes, and any intervention that can be done en route should be delayed until in the ambulance.

Once the head and neck have been assessed, you can apply a cervical collar to limit motion and prevent secondary injury. Collars are designed to allow assessment of the front of the neck while in place but do not offer a means to assess the back of the neck without their removal. Completely assess the neck before applying a cervical collar. Once it is in position, a rescuer must continue to stabilize the neck until the patient's torso and head are properly fixed to a long backboard. Be diligent about ensuring that the airway stays open and clear. If the collar is in the way, you may need to resort to manual immobilization of the neck while maintaining an open airway with a jaw-thrust maneuver.

At the conclusion of the rapid trauma assessment, you must decide whether to rapidly transport or remain on scene for more detailed care. The detailed physical exam, which is conducted on trauma patients with a significant MOI, is typically performed en route to the ED. Completion of the rapid trauma assessment should prompt you to reconsider or reconfirm the initial transport priority. A complete set of baseline vital signs and the SAMPLE history should also be obtained on concluding this assessment.

No Significant MOI

A complete head-to-toe examination is not always warranted. Patients with isolated extremity trauma do not require a full body evaluation. If you are unsure whether a significant MOI exists, conduct a complete rapid trauma assessment and then perform a detailed physical exam en route to the ED. In all other cases, direct your attention to assessing the chief complaint and area with outward signs of injury.

When local protocols allow, some patients can be treated on scene and released. For example, a patient at a rock concert with a minor laceration; good distal pulses, motor response, and sensation; and recent history of a tetanus shot might be able to be released to a sober adult. Some systems have established a means for referring the patient for further medical care at a local emergency clinic or other suitable medical facility. Release or referral may be preferred for a patient with relatively minor injuries, such as a simple laceration or abrasion. Providers must still provide basic care, such as dressing and bandaging.

History

Gathering information is also an important step in determining how the patient was injured. Ask the patient (if conscious and able to respond) or family members and bystanders about the events leading to injury:

- Was the patient wearing a seatbelt?
- How fast was the vehicle traveling?
- How high is the location from which the patient fell?
- Was there a loss of consciousness?
- What type of weapon was used?

When time and patient condition permit, determine when the last tetanus booster was given. Record the information on the patient care record, and relay it during patient transfer at the hospital. Ask the patient about prescribed and over-the-counter medications, paying particular attention to those that interfere with hemostasis. A higher priority should be given to patients taking warfarin (Coumadin) or other anticoagulants. Other medications that can lead to continued bleeding include aspirin, ticlodipine (Ticlid), and clopidogrel bisulfate (Plavix). To obtain a complete history, use the mnemonic SAMPLE described in previous chapters.

Detailed Physical Examination

After the focused history and physical exam is complete, a more thorough examination should generally be conducted en route when there is a significant MOI and adequate time and the patient is in stable condition. This detailed assessment examines every anatomic region, looking for hidden injuries and clinical signs. A detailed physical examination is an excellent way to gather information but should never delay transport of a patient in critical condition. In most cases, this assessment is completed while traveling to the ED.

Documentation and Communication

Most people charged with shooting another person end up in court at some point, and you may be called to testify. In cases of gunshot wounds, it is even more important than usual that you carefully document the circumstances surrounding the scene, the injury, the patient's condition, and the treatment you give.

Ongoing Assessment

Frequent reassessments of the patient's conditions should be made en route to the hospital and in conjunction with any necessary interventions. A patient in stable condition should be reassessed every 15 minutes; a more serious condition warrants reexamination every 5 minutes. As part of this assessment, vital signs should be obtained and evaluated, any interventions checked, and the patient monitored. Document all findings, and track trends in the patient's condition.

Management of Soft-Tissue Injuries

Management of soft-tissue trauma varies according to the injury present; however, some basic management principles apply to nearly every scenario. Although attending to clinical issues is important, providers must also tend to the patient's feelings about the injury. Be empathetic, because the injury may be perceived very differently in the patient's eyes. From a clinical standpoint, bleeding is controlled using direct pressure, elevation, pressure points, and, occasionally, a tourniquet. Irrigate wounds to reduce the risk of infection. Immobilization of an injury site can also be helpful in caring for soft-tissue damage. Once all assessments and interventions are complete and patient care has been transferred, thoroughly document any care provided.

Treatment of Closed Wounds

Small contusions do not require any special treatment. When an extensive closed injury is present, however, bleeding beneath the skin may reach significant proportions, and swelling may compromise vital structures. In such cases, take steps to minimize the bleeding and swelling by following the ICES mnemonic:

I   Apply *Ice* or cold packs to the injured area. Cold will stimulate blood vessels to constrict, slowing the bleeding.

C   Apply firm *Compression* over the injured area to decrease bleeding. Compression may be manual initially, but is most effectively applied with an air splint thereafter.

E   *Elevate* the injured part to a level above the heart, to encourage drainage and decrease swelling.

S   Apply a *Splint* to an injured extremity. By preventing motion, a splint decreases bleeding. An air splint gives a double benefit—splinting *and* compression.

Treatment of Open Wounds: General Principles

Two general principles govern the treatment of all open wounds:

- Control bleeding by whatever method is most effective.
- Keep the wound as clean as possible. Cut away clothing covering the wound. Wash away loose dirt and debris by pouring sterile water or tap water over the area. Do *not* try to pick out foreign matter embedded in a wound. Simply irrigate the site copiously, and then cover the wound with a dry, sterile dressing.

Determine the magnitude of the injury and relay the findings to the receiving facility. If bleeding is present, determine the color of the blood, amount lost, and site of origin. Obtaining an accurate history is important when bleeding has stopped before EMS arrival. Ask the patient to describe the bleeding in terms of color and type of flow.

For wounds already in the healing stage, examine the edges to determine if the wound is closing properly or if the edges are separating. Inspect the area to identify signs of infection, such as redness, swelling, and pain. Discolored pus may also be present. Signs of systemic infection—fever, general malaise, and altered mental status—warrant transport to a hospital for further examination.

Bandaging and Dressing Wounds

Dressing and bandage materials are used to cover the wound, control bleeding, and limit motion. Simple application of a dressing over an open wound will help prevent infection by providing an artificial barrier against microorganisms. Using bleeding control techniques with dressings will stop all but the most serious active blood loss. Correct application of bandage material will limit motion of the affected area, helping the body to recover from the insult.

A variety of materials are used to dress and bandage wounds. A dressing directly covers a wound and controls bleeding, whereas a bandage keeps the dressing in place. When properly applied, both keep pathogens from entering the open injury.

Sterile and Nonsterile Dressings

Sterile dressings are completely free of microorganisms. These materials are used when a high probability of infection is present, particularly in cases of large open wounds. Each such dressing comes individually wrapped and is marked as being sterile. Because sterility is lost when the package is opened, it is important to quickly dress open wounds when using sterile dressings.

Nonsterile dressings are used when there is a lower risk of infection. Although they are not completely devoid of microorganisms, they are packaged in a clean manner. Nonsterile dressings often come packaged as one large unit without the individual wrapping found in sterile packaging. The field caregiver would first dress the wound with a sterile dressing and then apply multiple nonsterile dressings to increase the ability to absorb blood.

Occlusive and Nonocclusive Dressings

Occlusive dressings are used when it is important to keep air from passing through the material—for example, with open wounds to the neck or thorax where negative pressure would draw air into lacerated blood vessels or the pleural cavity. When an occlusive dressing is applied to an open wound in the thorax, it should be sealed on three sides to allow air to escape. Allowing one corner to remain open helps prevent development of a tension pneumothorax. Because most open wounds do not present a risk for air entering the body, the majority of dressing materials are nonocclusive.

Adherent and Nonadherent Dressings

Adherent dressings allow exudate from the wound to mesh with dressing material. This action facilitates clotting and aids in bleeding control. Because the material becomes bound to exudates, removal of the dressing is painful and may precipitate bleeding.

Nonadherent dressings allow the products of wound repair to pass through the material. This design allows for easy removal of dressing material but does not aid in clot formation. A nonadherent dressing would be applied after a wound closure.

Wet and Dry Dressings

Dry dressings are the most commonly used options in prehospital care. Because wet dressings provide a medium for bacteria and other pathogens to grow, their use is limited in the field. Moist dressings can be of benefit for burn care, although commercial burn dressings (Water-Jel) made with a water-based gel better facilitate pain relief. This sterile form of wet dressing does not stick to open wounds.

Roller and Gauze Bandages

Bandage material is often self-adherent (for example, Kling or Kerlix). As a consequence, when you roll the bandage material over the dressing, the overlapping material will adhere to it and keep the bandage in place. A roller bandage is ideal for wrapping extremity injuries. It is available in a variety of sizes, although the 1″ and 6″ versions are the most popular.

A gauze bandage also works well for wrapping dressings into place but is a nonadherent bandage. Although it does not remain in position as readily as roller gauze, it is still an effective means to secure a dressing. This material does not offer much stretch, which can result in excess pressure to areas that begin to swell.

Roller and gauze bandages are considered absorbent bandage materials. Nonabsorbent bandages, which do not absorb fluid but prevent leaking, are also commercially available.

Absorbent Gauze Sponges

When heavy bleeding is present, a thicker, bulkier dressing is needed. An absorbent gauze sponge assists in controlling hemorrhage while providing a dressing. Sponges are available in a variety of sizes and may be sterile or nonsterile.

Elastic Bandages

Elastic bandage material stretches to allow some pressure to be applied. This characteristic is useful to control bleeding. Elastic bandages are also used in musculoskeletal trauma to facilitate healing of damaged tendons and ligaments. Be careful to avoid applying excessive pressure with such bandages because blood flow may be compromised.

Triangular Bandages

Triangular bandages (cravats) are an ideal shape for making slings and swathes. They are typically made of cotton and come packaged with safety pins. Because they do not stretch, there is little conformance to body contours, which is not ideal if pressure must be applied. These bandages can be wrapped into a thin strip to be used as a tourniquet.

Taping

A dressing may be secured with tape alone or in conjunction with bandage material. Several types of medical tape are available, ranging in size from a 1″ to a 4″ roll. Be cautious when using tape on patients with skin conditions that might lead to damage upon the tape's removal (such as older patients, who often have very thin skin).

Complications of Improperly Applied Dressings

Improper application of dressing and bandage material can result in significant complications. It is important to learn how to properly dress a wound in the laboratory, clinical, and field settings to avoid causing harm.

Although it is not always possible to use sterile technique, make every effort to avoid further wound contamination. Irrigate open wounds with normal saline to flush out contaminants. If available, apply antibiotic ointment to smaller open wounds to help speed healing and avoid infection. Large open injuries should not have ointment applied but should be irrigated. Once the wound is irrigated, apply a dressing over the site. Clean blood around the dressing site, and neatly wrap a bandage over the dressing.

Hemodynamic complications include the possibility for continued bleeding. Once a dressing has been placed, it should not be removed because of the risk of disrupting clot formation. If a wound continues to bleed, additional dressings should be applied in conjunction with bleeding control interventions. Frequent reassessments will help prevent unchecked blood loss and hemodynamic complications. Exsanguination is a possibility when a pressure dressing does not stop blood loss; the same is true for an improperly applied tourniquet. If a tourniquet occludes only venous flow, bleeding may actually increase. A properly applied dressing in conjunction with direct pressure is often sufficient to stop blood loss. Conversely, a dressing applied too tightly can occlude distal flow when blood loss is not a concern.

Structural elements—blood vessels, nerves, tendons, muscles, skin, and internal organs—can be damaged, particularly when dressings are excessively tight. Prevention of damage entails assessing and readjusting the dressing and bandage as necessary. Distal pulses, motor, and sensation should be assessed when extremity dressings are in place. Tight dressings may cause pain in a patient who already has an injury.

Control of External Bleeding

External bleeding is bleeding that can be seen coming from a wound when the integrity of the skin has been violated. Bleeding can be characterized according to the type of blood vessel that has been damaged. Arterial bleeding occurs in spurts, and the blood is usually bright red because of the fully saturated hemoglobin. Venous bleeding is more likely to be slow and steady, and the color of the blood is darker because it is relatively deoxygenated. In reality, most open wounds show a combination of arterial and venous bleeding. Capillary bleeding is characterized by a slow, even flow of bright or dark red blood and is present in minor injuries, such as abrasions or superficial lacerations.

Five methods are used in the field to control external bleeding: direct pressure, elevation, pressure point control, immobilization, and a tourniquet.

Direct Pressure

Application of pressure over a bleeding wound stops blood from flowing into the damaged vessels, allowing the platelets to seal the vascular walls.

Notes from Nancy

Steady, direct pressure against the bleeding site is the most effective means to control bleeding.

If possible, use a sterile dressing to exert pressure, and then use your gloved hand to apply pressure over the bleeding site. The steps for controlling bleeding are shown in :

1. Apply a dry, sterile dressing over the entire wound. Apply pressure to the dressing with your gloved hand (Step 1).
2. Maintain the pressure, and secure the dressing with a roller bandage (Step 2).
3. If bleeding continues or recurs, leave the original dressing in place. Apply a second dressing on top of the first, and secure it with another roller bandage (Step 3).
4. Splint the extremity to stabilize the injury, even if there is no suspected fracture, which helps to minimize movement, further control the bleeding, and keep the dressing in place (Step 4).

To maintain pressure, apply a pressure dressing over the site. On an extremity, one effective way of maintaining uniform pressure on a bleeding site is to apply an air splint over the

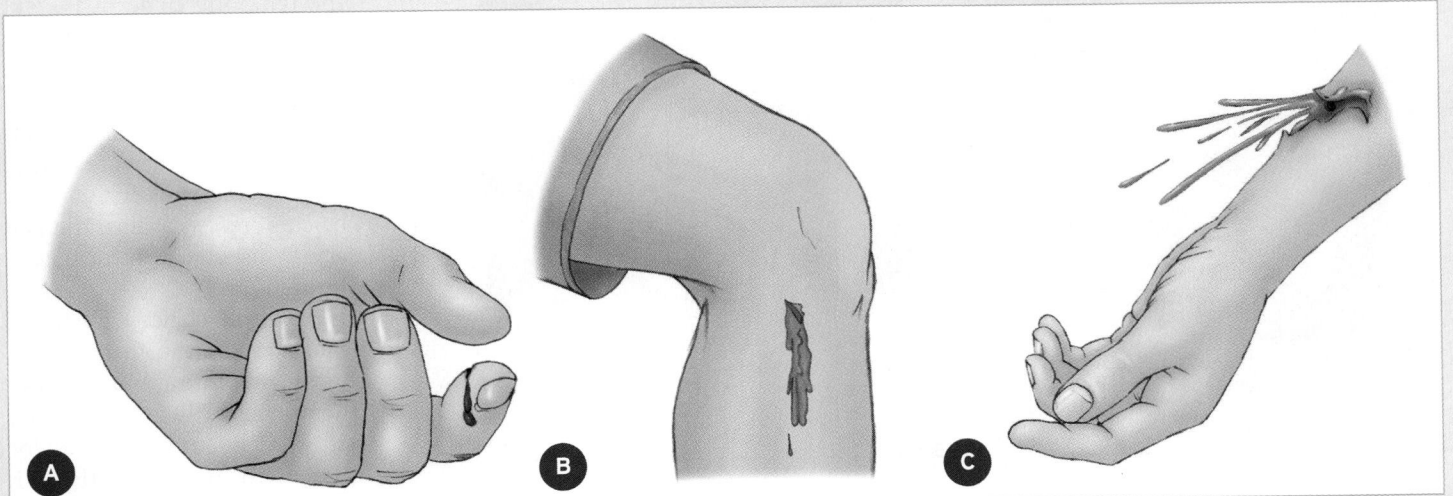

Figure 19-15 **A.** Capillary bleeding is dark red and oozes from the wound slowly but steadily. **B.** Venous bleeding is darker than arterial bleeding and flows steadily. **C.** Arterial bleeding is characteristically brighter red and spurts in time with the pulse.

You are the Provider Part 4

The patient remains hemodynamically stable throughout transport; however, he tells you that his leg is still hurting. You reassess his vital signs and consider the need for additional treatment. Your estimated time of arrival at the hospital is 5 minutes.

Reassessment	Recording Time: 20 Minutes
Skin	Pink and diaphoretic
Pulse	100 beats/min; strong and regular at the radial artery
Blood pressure	124/70 mm Hg
Respirations	18 breaths/min; adequate depth
SaO_2	98% on room air
Pain scale	5 on a scale of 0 to 10

7. Is further treatment indicated for this patient?
8. Are there any special considerations regarding the treatment you have provided to this patient?

Skill Drill 19-1: Controlling Bleeding From a Soft-Tissue Injury

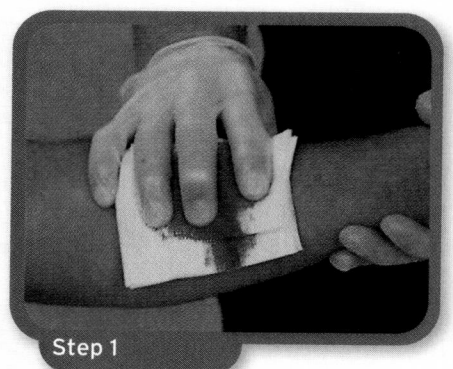

Step 1

Apply direct pressure with a sterile bandage.

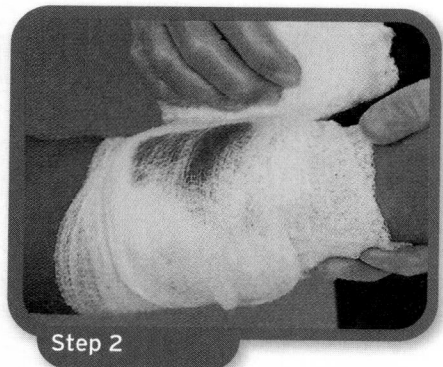

Step 2

Maintain pressure with a roller bandage.

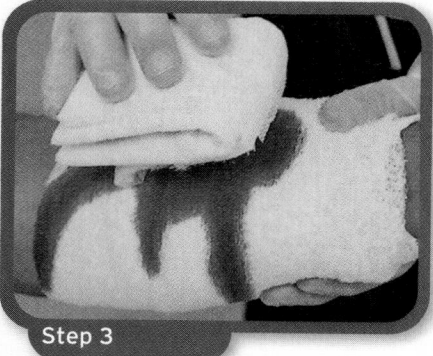

Step 3

If bleeding continues, apply a second dressing and roller bandage over the first.

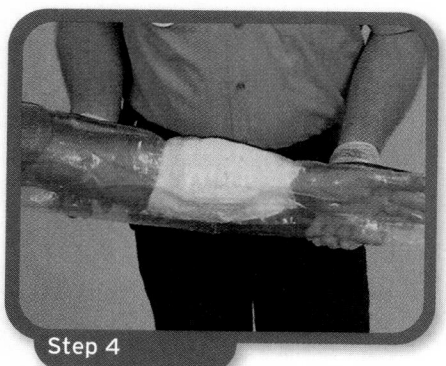

Step 4

Splint the extremity.

dressed wound. If one or both of the lower extremities are bleeding, you can use the PASG to apply pressure, as discussed in Chapter 18. Maintain pressure over the bleeding site until the bleeding stops or until the patient reaches the hospital and other personnel take responsibility for care.

Some commercially available pressure dressings allow for simultaneous dressing of the wound and application of pressure. If one of these products is not available, standard dressing material may be used in conjunction with triangular bandages to create localized pressure. This type of dressing will often allow you to focus on other tasks while pressure is applied. Always assess distal circulation before and after you apply a pressure dressing. Adjust the dressing as needed in case of a complication, such as loss of distal pulse, diminished sensation, or change in skin color and temperature distal to the dressing.

Elevation

In cases of venous bleeding from an extremity, the rate of bleeding can be substantially slowed by elevating the extremity above

the level of the heart. This measure alone will not control bleeding, but it may be helpful in conjunction with other measures, such as direct pressure.

Pressure Point Control

When direct pressure is not sufficient to control bleeding or when the same artery is associated with a number of bleeding points, pressure point control may help slow the bleeding. The artery chosen must be fairly superficial and overlie a hard structure against which it can be compressed. Three pressure points are typically used: (1) the temporal artery, which overlies the temporal bone of the skull and is used to control bleeding from the scalp; (2) the brachial artery, which overlies the humerus and is used to control bleeding from the forearm; and (3) the femoral artery, which can be compressed against the pelvis and is used to control bleeding from the leg.

Recent studies have brought into question the effectiveness of using pressure points in severe hemorrhage. It is acceptable, if allowed by protocol and local policy, to move directly to the use of a tourniquet without attempting pressure point control. If a tourniquet is deemed necessary, it should be applied quickly and not released in the prehospital setting.

Immobilization

Any movement of an extremity, even an uninjured extremity, promotes blood flow within that extremity. When the extremity is also injured, motion may disrupt the clotting process and lacerate more blood vessels. It follows that preventing motion of an injured extremity will have the opposite effects. Advise the patient to make

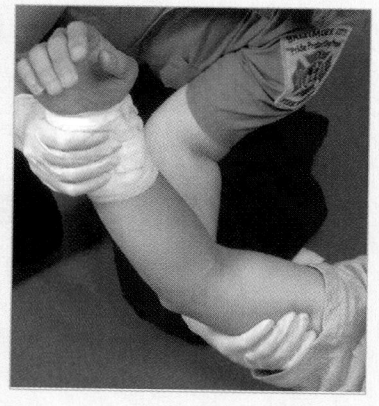

Figure 19-16 Applying pressure at the appropriate pressure point while holding direct pressure may slow difficult-to-control bleeding.

every effort to minimize movement. If that is not possible and conditions warrant, apply a splint to prevent motion.

An air splint or padded board works well to keep an upper or lower extremity immobilized. Use of an air splint gives a double benefit—splinting and direct pressure. Remember to assess distal pulses, motor function, and sensation distal to the splint before and after application.

Tourniquet

In the civilian setting, it is rarely necessary to use a tourniquet for control of external hemorrhage. Bleeding control can almost always be achieved by one or more of the four methods already described. Furthermore, use of a tourniquet has been associated with potential hazards, including damage to nerves and blood vessels and, when the tourniquet is in place for an extended period, loss of the distal extremity. A tourniquet applied too loosely, by contrast, may increase bleeding if it occludes venous return without hampering arterial outflow.

In military settings, application of a tourniquet would occur more often owing to the nature of injuries experienced during battle. In addition, rapid transport to a medical facility is typically more difficult on the battlefield than in civilian situations. In such a scenario, a tourniquet may be lifesaving, particularly in patients with a traumatic partial amputation of a limb.

Some tourniquets can be applied with one arm Figure 19-17 ▾ , although you may not have access to them. If a tourniquet is required, observe the following application guidelines Skill Drill 19-2 ▸ :

1. Use wide, flat materials, such as a cravat or folded handkerchief. Never use rope, wire, or other narrow materials that might cut into the skin and damage underlying tissues. A blood pressure cuff inflated above the systolic reading works well for upper extremities.

2. Apply a pad over the artery to be compressed.

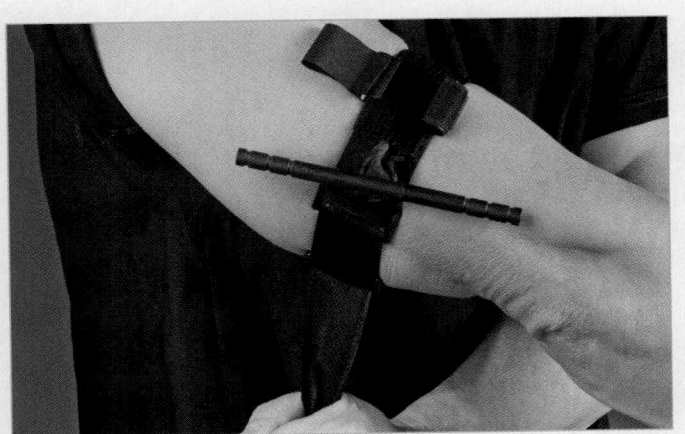

Figure 19-17 A tourniquet that can be applied using only one arm has been developed.

3. Wrap the tourniquet twice around the extremity, at a point about 4 inches distal to the axilla or groin, and tie a half-knot Step 1 .

4. Place a stick, pencil, or similar object on top of the half knot, and complete the square knot above the stick Step 2 .

5. Twist the stick to tighten the tourniquet just until the bleeding stops Step 3 .

6. Secure the stick in that position so that it will not unwind. Never cover a tourniquet with a bandage or anything else, lest it escape notice when the patient arrives at the hospital. To make doubly sure that the tourniquet is not overlooked, write "TK" and the exact time you applied the tourniquet on a piece of adhesive tape, and fasten the tape to the patient's forehead Step 4 .

7. Do not remove a tourniquet because removal can result in release of an embolus, significant rebleeding, or tourniquet shock.

8. Record on the patient care report the time at which the tourniquet was applied.

Pain Control

Application of a cold compress will help reduce pain and diminish blood flow to an open wound. Once the dressing is in place, apply the cold pack. Avoid placing the compress directly on the site because excessively cold temperature may do further harm. A pressure dressing may alleviate pain and minimize swelling.

If basic life support measures fail to relieve pain, consider administering morphine sulfate or other agents as allowed by protocol. The common dosage for morphine is .05 mg/kg intravenously every 5 minutes to a maximum of 10 mg. As with all medications, carefully assess the patient for allergies, and document pertinent information.

Managing an Avulsion

In treating a partially avulsed piece of skin, quickly irrigate any dirt or debris out of the wound and then gently fold the skin flap back onto the wound so that it is more or less normally aligned. Hold the flap in place with a dry, sterile compression dressing.

Preservation of Amputated Parts

When a part of the body is completely avulsed (torn off) or amputated (cut off)—whether a section of skin or an entire limb—it is important to try to preserve the amputated part in optimal condition to maximize the chances of its being successfully reimplanted. Once the patient's injuries have been stabilized, turn your attention to the amputated part, which will also require meticulous care. Follow these guidelines:

- Rinse the amputated part free of debris with cool, sterile saline.
- Wrap the part loosely in saline-moistened sterile gauze.

Skill Drill 19-2: Applying a Tourniquet

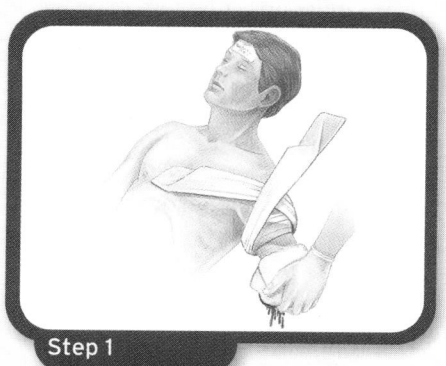

Step 1

Create a 4″, multilayered bandage. Wrap the bandage twice around the extremity, just above the bleeding site, and tie a half-knot.

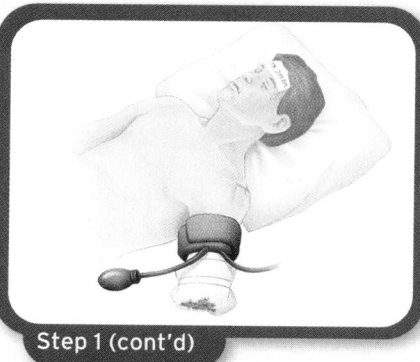

Step 1 (cont'd)

You can also use a blood pressure cuff as an effective tourniquet.

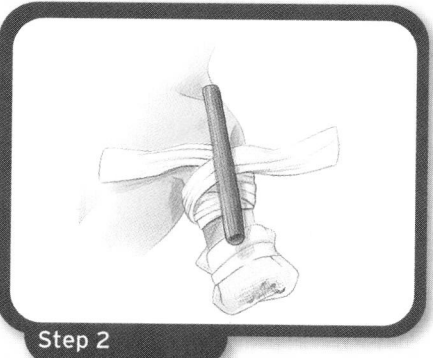

Step 2

Place a stick on top of the half-knot and tie a square knot over the stick.

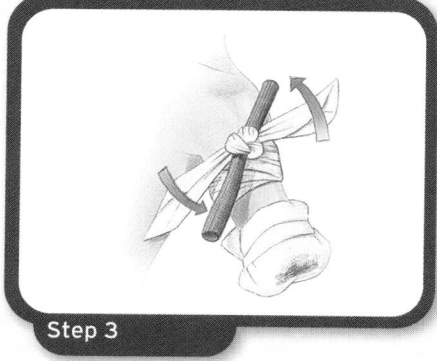

Step 3

Twist the stick until the bleeding stops.

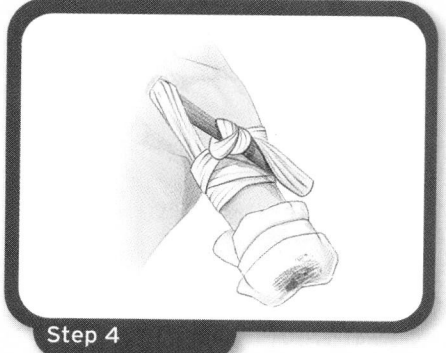

Step 4

Secure the stick so that it will not unwind. Write "TK" and the exact time you applied the tourniquet on a piece of adhesive tape, fasten the tape to the patient's forehead, and notify hospital personnel on arrival.

- Seal the amputated part inside a plastic bag, and place it in a cool container (such as a Styrofoam cooler). Keep it cold, but do not allow it to freeze.
- Never warm an amputated part.
- Never place an amputated part in water.
- Never place an amputated part directly on ice.
- Never use dry ice to cool an amputated part.

Transport the patient and the amputated part as expeditiously as possible. When the amputated part is a limb or part of

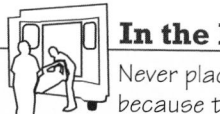

In the Field

Never place an amputated part directly on ice because this may cause frostbite and prevent reattachment.

a limb, notify emergency department staff in advance of the type of case you are transporting and your estimated time of arrival so that a surgical team can be mobilized while you are en route.

Managing Impaled Objects

The following are basic points regarding management of an impaled object:

- Do not try to remove an impaled object. Efforts to do so may precipitate uncontrolled internal hemorrhage, which may lead to exsanguination or further injury to underlying structures.
- Control hemorrhage by direct compression, but do not apply pressure on the impaled object itself or on immediately adjacent tissues.
- Do not try to shorten an impaled object unless it is extremely cumbersome (such as a fence post impaled in

the chest); any motion of the object may damage surrounding tissues.

■ Stabilize the object in place with a bulky dressing, and immobilize the extremity (if the object is impaled in an extremity) with a splint to prevent motion.

The goal for prehospital care is to limit motion of the impaled object as soon as possible to minimize additional damage. One technique that is effective for thin objects is to use gauze pads cut midway through the center. Stack several pads vertically, and arrange the cut portions so that each stack of pads overlaps. Once it is determined that enough pads are in place for stabilizing, tape or bandage them securely. This technique has the dual benefits of providing stabilization and aiding in bleeding control. Larger objects that are impaled in the body can be secured with rolled towels or splinting materials.

Impaled objects in the eye can be managed using gauze pads, a paper or Styrofoam cup, and bandage material. Do not apply pressure to the eye because pressure may cause vital fluids (the vitreous humor) to leak out. First, stabilize the object by hand. Once that is accomplished, use gauze pads cut midway into the center as outlined previously. Place the cup on top of the stacked pads after the height is sufficient. Bandage or tape the cup into place. It is important to cover both eyes because consensual movement may cause additional damage Figure 19-18 . In such cases, it is particularly important to continually provide reassurance to the patient, who may be anxious because of the object and the blocked vision.

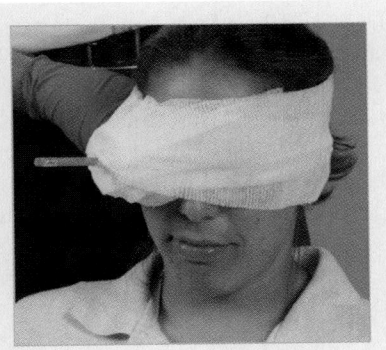

Figure 19-18 Stabilize an object impaled in the eye using gauze pads, a paper or Styrofoam cup, and bandage material.

Whatever presentation you may encounter, it is important to avoid causing additional harm. Secure the object as best as possible, and be creative in using securing materials. Provide reassurance to the patient and family. Constantly assess the risk for developing threats to life, such as airway compromise, breathing inadequacy, and uncontrolled hemorrhage.

On rare occasions, removal of an impaled object may be the best course of action. If the object directly interferes with airway control and the patient's condition is deteriorating rapidly, medical direction may authorize removal. It may also be necessary to remove an object that interferes with chest compressions in a patient who is in cardiac arrest and deemed viable. In severe cases, it may be impossible to leave the object in place, such as when the patient is impaled on an immovable object. Establish direct contact with medical control immediately in such cases, and ask for guidance.

Managing Wound Healing and Infection

In the prehospital setting, management of altered wound healing and infection entails basic measures. Wounds that are not healing properly or show signs of infection should be dressed and bandaged appropriately. In severe cases, pain control measures may be indicated.

Dressing Specific Anatomic Sites

Dressing and bandaging wounds is not the same for every part of the body. This section describes the various factors that need to be considered for a given body region.

Scalp Dressings

Scalp injuries tend to bleed profusely owing to their rich blood supply. When bleeding is present, application of direct pressure is often effective owing to the rigid skull that lies under the scalp. Be careful to accurately determine the extent of the injury because significant trauma may lead to skull damage. In that case, control of bleeding must be balanced against the issue of not causing additional damage. When the skull has been compromised and bleeding must be controlled, apply pressure to the areas around the break. Use a bulky dressing that assists in stopping blood loss and helps prevent excessive direct pressure on the already fractured cranium.

The shape of the skull is a consideration when dressing wounds that involve the scalp. Improperly applied dressings can easily slide up or down the scalp, becoming ineffective. In addition, hair may interfere with securing dressings in place.

Facial Dressings

Facial injuries tend to cause significant anxiety for patients and family. While tending to the clinical needs, take the time to reassure the patient. Application of direct pressure is an effective means to control bleeding from soft-tissue disruption along the face. If an avulsed piece of tissue is present, attempt to replace the pedicle to its normal anatomic location as closely as possible. Note that bleeding tends to be quite heavy owing to the rich blood supply in this area.

Assess the patient for the presence of or potential for airway compromise early in your encounter. Blood pouring into an unprotected airway is a recipe for disaster. Be prepared to suction and position the patient to facilitate drainage. Do not allow a gruesome facial injury to distract you from attending to life threats.

Ear or Mastoid Dressings

Trauma to the ear is commonly external, although internal injury is a possibility. Never place a dressing in the ear canal, but loosely apply it along the entire length of the external ear. Gauze sponges work well to aid in stopping blood loss. If blood is flowing from the ear canal, do not attempt to control it directly. Cerebrospinal fluid may be leaking, and halting the blood flow may increase pressure within the skull. Place a bulky dressing to the external ear, and transport the patient rapidly.

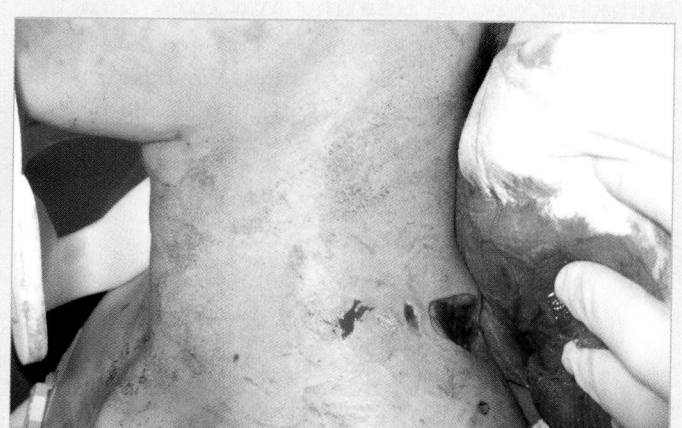

Figure 19-19 Neck wounds can lead to other serious situations such as air embolism and airway problems. Seal with an occlusive dressing right away.

Neck Dressings

Important anatomic structures in the neck include large blood vessels, the airway, and the cervical spine. There is little room for error when trauma is present in this area. A minor neck laceration can lead to an air embolism, a small puncture can penetrate the spinal canal, and an anterior open wound can disrupt the airway Figure 19-19 ▲ . Pay close attention to the clinical signs that accompany the external trauma.

Open injuries to the neck require use of an occlusive dressing to prevent the drawing of air into the circulatory system. Apply dressings carefully so that they do not interfere with blood flow or movement of air through the trachea.

Shoulder Dressings

The shoulder is relatively easy to dress and bandage. Apply direct pressure to control external hemorrhage in this region. If immobilization is indicated, a sling and swathe will prevent motion of the shoulder girdle.

Truncal Dressings

Injuries to the torso require vigilant assessment for underlying internal trauma. A seemingly innocuous hole may be the only indication that a gunshot wound is present. Cover open wounds with an occlusive dressing that is taped on three sides. Assessment of breath sounds becomes a high priority when you find an open chest wound because a pneumothorax or hemothorax may develop from penetrating trauma to the thorax. Continually reassess a patient with thoracic soft-tissue injuries.

The best choice for securing a truncal dressing in place is medical tape. Wrapping the entire torso may interfere with air movement.

Groin and Hip Dressings

Soft-tissue injuries to the groin and hip do not present a significant challenge to paramedics. Typically, application of a dressing and bandage in combination with direct pressure work well to control blood loss in this region. Injuries to the genitalia are best managed by a provider of the same sex, whenever feasible.

In many cases, it is possible to provide the patient with a dressing and allow self-directed care. This makes an uncomfortable scenario easier for patient and provider. If proper care cannot be accomplished by working directly with the patient, you must be exceedingly professional and respect the patient's modesty in all but the most serious of cases.

Hand, Wrist, and Finger Dressings

The hands, wrists, and fingers are among the easiest sites to properly dress and bandage. A dressing is applied over any open wound, and bandage material is wrapped completely around the affected area. When possible, the hand should be placed in the position of function. This is accomplished by placing a roll of gauze in the patient's hand Figure 19-20 ▶ . If limited motion is necessary, the hand and wrist can be easily splinted.

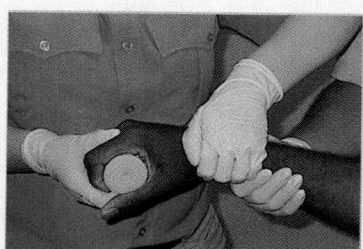

Figure 19-20 The position of function for the hand.

Elbow and Knee Dressings

Joints are not difficult to dress and bandage, but movement may cause the materials to shift from their original position. It is a good practice to provide immobilization of the elbow or the knee when a larger wound is present. Even smaller wounds may be difficult to manage because of skin tension lines and high tissue stress in these areas. When either of these joints is injured, it becomes very important to assess distal neurovascular status. Elbow injuries have a higher risk for neurovascular compromise because of the limited space available for blood vessels and nerves.

Ankle and Foot Dressings

The ankle and foot are simple to dress and bandage. Control of bleeding is accomplished by direct pressure and may be augmented by elevation and pressure points in cases involving significant bleeding. Application of a bandage must not be so tight that it interferes with circulation or sensation. Always assess distal neurovascular function before and after caring for the wound.

Crush Syndrome Management

Crush syndrome has been widely studied in recent years. In January 1995, a massive earthquake shook the southern part of Hyogo Prefecture, Japan, producing 41,000 casualties and 5,500 deaths. When researchers evaluated 372 patients who were diagnosed with crush syndrome, they found that most had lower extremity injuries that led to development of crush syndrome. Upper extremity injuries and trunk entrapment also caused some cases of crush syndrome, albeit to a much lesser extent.

openings yet produce internal damage that can quickly lead to death. It is important to determine the MOI while conducting the initial assessment to detect life threats.

Assessment includes four steps: inspection, palpation, auscultation, and percussion. Examine the entire chest for signs of visible injury. Listen to breath sounds in at least two sites on each side of the chest. If breath sounds are diminished or absent on one side, suspect a pneumothorax. Palpate the entire chest wall, noting any abnormalities. Subcutaneous emphysema is indicative of a disruption in the tracheobronchial tree. Percussion along the chest wall can help you differentiate between a pneumothorax and a hemothorax—either of which can lead to the patient's death.

Open wounds to the thorax require the application of an occlusive dressing to prevent a pneumothorax or at least stop its progression. Tape the dressing on only three sides to allow air to escape. Failure to provide a small opening for relief of pressure can result in a tension pneumothorax, which can be fatal.

Abdomen

Abdominal injuries range from minor abrasions to evisceration. Inspect the abdomen for visible signs of injuries. Palpate the area to identify pain, rigidity, and distention. Cover open wounds that are higher on the abdominal wall with an occlusive dressing to accommodate diaphragmatic movement. As the diaphragm travels downward during inspiration, the relative sizes of the thoracic and abdominal cavities change. This process increases the risk of drawing air into the pleural space when an open wound is present.

Maintain a high index of suspicion when an abdominal injury is readily evident. Blunt or penetrating trauma can lead to fracture of solid organs or rupture of hollow organs. Solid organs tend to bleed profusely, whereas hollow organs spill their contents into the peritoneum. Either can be fatal.

Documentation

Written documentation must be completed for every patient contact. When filling out the patient care report, include all relevant scene findings, such as a severely damaged vehicle or caliber of weapon used. Also record patient findings, including patency of airway, ventilation, and circulation, and any interventions administered. Describe the patient's presentation on your arrival at the scene, and note the body position on arrival (for example, prone or supine).

Note specific injuries. Describe wounds in terms of size, location, depth, and associated complications. Note your assessment findings for distal neurovascular status, range of motion, and presence or absence of infection. Obtain patient demographic information, such as age, date of birth, and home address. Include the patient's medical history, medications, and allergies.

If you performed an intervention, record it on the patient care report. Note how the patient responded to therapy (ie, the same, better, or worse condition). Also document the patient's level of understanding for each intervention. Finally, note which provider attended to the patient en route to the receiving facility.

You are the Provider Summary

1. Does this patient require spinal motion restriction precautions? Why or why not?

The mechanism of injury—an isolated injury to the leg—does not suggest a high potential for a spinal injury; therefore, spinal motion restriction precautions are likely not necessary. However, it is important to conduct a careful assessment of the patient to determine if any other injuries are present. Football is arguably one of the roughest organized sports; players may experience injuries to multiple parts of their body, especially during a rough tackle.

2. What are your main concerns regarding this patient's injury?

Your patient has an open fracture of his leg, which should raise concern for several potential problems. First, you must control the external bleeding. The fractured bone may have damaged a large blood vessel in the patient's leg and may make bleeding difficult to control—especially if an artery is involved. Second, the bone has broken through the skin, which has placed this patient at risk for infection of the bone and adjacent muscle (osteomyelitis). Although this will not present acutely in the field, preventing further contamination (ie, covering the wound with sterile dressings) will certainly reduce the risk of infection.

3. Is this patient in shock?

On the basis of the mechanism of injury, the patient's vital signs—tachycardia, tachypnea, and hypertension—represent pain, not shock. Isolated distal long bone fractures (open or closed) typically do not cause shock in adolescent and adult patients unless they are associated with prolonged uncontrolled bleeding. Nonetheless, careful patient assessment and close monitoring remain essential elements in the overall care of the patient. As noted earlier, football is a rough sport; occult injury cannot be ruled out in the prehospital setting.

4. What additional care should you provide to this patient?

Primary treatment for an open fracture consists of controlling external bleeding, preventing further contamination, and splinting the injury. However, you must not overlook the aspect of pain relief in patients with such injuries. Your patient is in severe pain (10/10); to overlook this would be inappropriate (and inhumane), especially considering the fact that he is hemodynamically stable. Therefore, a narcotic analgesic is clearly indicated. Morphine and fentanyl are the two most commonly administered medications for this purpose. Follow local protocols regarding the appropriate doses of these medications.

5. What is compartment syndrome and is this patient at risk for it?

Compartment syndrome is seen commonly when a part of the body is entrapped for a lengthy period of time—usually greater than 4 hours. However, it can also occur as the result of a fracture. Compartment syndrome can occur following open or closed fractures.

Compartment syndrome develops when hemorrhage and edema cause increased pressure within the osteofascial compartment. Increased compartment pressure results in ischemia and further tissue swelling. As pressure increases, venous return is compromised first, followed by arterial inflow. This causes two significant problems: cellular and tissue damage within the injured compartment and the accumulation of metabolic waste products (ie, lactic acid). Left untreated, compartment syndrome can result in permanent muscle and tissue damage and necrosis of the muscles within the affected compartment.

6. What are the signs and symptoms of compartment syndrome?

Signs and symptoms of compartment syndrome include pain that is disproportionate to the injury, firmness of the area around the injury, a feeling of "pressure" expressed by the patient, and pain when the affected muscles are passively stretched. Later signs include parasthesia, pallor, and loss of the pulse distal to the injury.

7. Is further treatment indicated for this patient?

Your patient remains hemodynamically stable, yet because he is still in pain (5/10), it would not be unreasonable to administer a second dose of a narcotic analgesic (eg, fentanyl, morphine). Again, follow locally established protocols regarding initial and repeat dosing of these medications.

8. Are there any special considerations regarding the treatment you have provided to this patient?

As noted earlier, you should monitor this patient for signs of compartment syndrome and circulatory compromise distal to the injury (just as you would any patient who you have bandaged and splinted). Additionally, because you have administered a narcotic analgesic, it would be prudent to have naloxone (Narcan)—a narcotic antagonist—readily available in the event that the patient experiences central nervous system (CNS) depression (ie, hypotension, bradycardia, hypoventilation). If signs of CNS depression become apparent, administer an appropriate dose of naloxone—usually 0.4 to 2 mg via slow IV push. If IV access is not available, you can administer naloxone intramuscularly.

Ready for Review

- The skin is a complex organ that fulfills several crucial roles, including maintaining homeostasis, protecting tissue from injury, and regulating temperature.
- The main layers of the skin are the epidermis and the dermis. The epidermis, the outer layer, serves as the principal barrier. The dermis, the inner layer, includes collagen, elastin, and ground substance, which contribute to the skin's strength. It also contains nerve endings, blood vessels, sweat glands, hair follicles, and sebaceous glands.
- The subcutaneous layer lies beneath the dermis and contains adipose tissue. Below the subcutaneous layer is the deep fascia, which offers support and protection to underlying structures such as muscle and bone.
- The skin is arranged in patterns of tautness known as tension lines. Wounds that occur parallel to skin tension lines may remain closed. Wounds that run perpendicular to tension lines may remain open.
- Soft-tissue injuries may be dramatic but are seldom the most serious. Don't let them distract you from thorough initial assessment!
- The first stage of wound healing is cessation of bleeding. The body uses several mechanisms to control bleeding, such as constricting the size of vessels and releasing platelets to form a blood clot.
- The second stage of healing is inflammation, in which additional cells enter the damaged area in an effort to repair it. Epithelialization (creation of a new layer of epithelial cells) occurs, followed by neovascularization (formation of new vessels).
- Wound healing is affected by factors such as the amount of movement the part is subjected to, medications, and medical conditions. A wound is more likely to become infected if it is caused by a human or an animal bite or if a foreign body has been impaled. Pressure injuries can develop when a patient is bedridden or remains on a backboard for too long.
- Signs of infection include redness, pus, warmth, edema, and local discomfort. Gangrene, tetanus, and necrotizing fasciitis are serious infection-related conditions that must be recognized early.
- In a closed wound, the skin is not broken but soft tissues beneath the skin are damaged. An example is a bruise. A hematoma (collection of blood beneath the skin) can also form.
- In an open wound, the skin is broken. Such an injury can become infected and can result in serious blood loss. Open wounds include abrasions, lacerations, puncture wounds, avulsions, and amputations.
- In a crush injury, a body part is crushed between two solid objects, resulting in damage to soft tissues and bone. The patient's external appearance may not adequately represent the level of internal damage.
- Crush syndrome may develop after a body part has been trapped for more than 4 hours. Necrosis occurs in crushed muscles, and harmful products are released in a process called rhabdomyolysis. Freeing the trapped body part can cause these harmful products to be released into the circulation, which can prove fatal. Kidney damage, cardiac arrest, and arrhythmias can also result.
- Compartment syndrome results when pressure increases in the injured area. Tissue necrosis and sepsis may then develop. Patients present with the six Ps: Pain, Paresthesia, Paresis, Pressure, Passive stretch pain, and Pulselessness.
- Blasts (explosions) can result in soft-tissue injuries. A blast wind from the gases released can be very forceful, and projectiles can impale victims; both cause injuries. Falling structures can injure patients, and burns can also occur.
- Observe scene safety before assessing patients with soft-tissue injuries; hazards that caused the injury may still be present. Regardless of the grotesqueness of the injury, assess the ABCs first.
- While taking the history, ask about the event that caused the injury, such as whether a weapon was used or whether the patient lost consciousness. Find out when the patient last had a tetanus booster. Pay attention to whether the patient is taking any medications that may affect hemostasis.
- Depending on whether the mechanism of injury is significant or not, complete your physical exam en route or at the scene, respectively. Direct your attention to the chief complaint and area of injury, and perform frequent reassessments.
- Be empathetic to patients with soft-tissue injuries.
- Managing soft-tissue injuries includes controlling bleeding. With closed injuries, follow the ICES mnemonic: Ice, Compression, Elevation, and Splinting.
- When managing open wounds, control bleeding and keep the wound as clean as possible by irrigating and using sterile dressings. Try to determine the color and type of bleeding and the amount of blood the patient has lost.
- Dressings and bandages are used to cover the wound, control bleeding, and limit motion. Types of dressings include sterile and nonsterile, occlusive and nonocclusive, adherent and nonadherent, and wet and dry. Types of bandages include roller and gauze, absorbent gauze sponges, elastic, and triangular bandages.
- Medical tape may be used to secure a bandage in place, except for patients with thin skin such as older patients because it can cause damage on removal. Do not apply dressings too tightly.
- Methods of bleeding control include direct pressure, elevation, pressure point control, immobilization, and tourniquets. Cold compresses may help reduce pain. IV medications may be administered if basic measures do not relieve pain.
- Tourniquets are rarely needed in the civilian setting but may be used as a last resort. They can damage nerves and blood vessels and lead to loss of an extremity.
- Management of an avulsion includes irrigation, gently folding the flap back onto the wound, and applying a dry, sterile compression dressing. If the wound is an amputation, preserve the amputated part and transport it.
- Do not remove impaled objects in the field. Instead, stabilize the object in place with a bulky dressing. Control bleeding with direct compression, but do not apply pressure on the object or on the immediately adjacent tissues.
- Dressing and bandaging techniques vary for different parts of the body. For example, the shape of the skull and the presence of hair make dressing the scalp challenging.
- Trapped patients must be managed before being freed from the crushing object because this approach improves their chances of survival after experiencing crush syndrome. Aggressive fluid therapy can help prevent kidney failure. Normal saline should be infused. Administration of sodium bicarbonate may help prevent an efflux of potassium. Rapidly transport the patient once freed.
- Blast injuries can include pulmonary damage such as tension pneumothorax and pulmonary contusion, abdominal trauma such as ruptured organs and internal hemorrhage, damage to the ears, and penetrating wounds. Use the DCAP-BTLS guideline to assess the patient rapidly.
- Soft-tissue injuries of the face, neck, thorax, and abdomen deserve special attention because these areas contain vital structures. Do not underestimate the seriousness of these injuries, and maintain a high index of suspicion.
- Document scene findings, including vehicle damage or the caliber of weapon used and patient presentation and position; size, location, depth, and complications of injuries; assessment findings; and interventions.

◼ Vital Vocabulary

abrasion An injury in which a portion of the body is denuded of epidermis by scraping or rubbing.

adipose Referring to fat tissue.

amputation An injury in which part of the body is completely severed.

avulsion An injury that leaves a piece of skin or other tissue partially or completely torn away from the body.

bandage Material used to secure a dressing in place.

chemotactic factors The factors that cause cells to migrate into an area.

closed wound An injury in which damage occurs beneath the skin or mucous membrane but the surface remains intact.

collagen Protein that gives tensile strength to the connective tissues of the body.

compartment syndrome A condition that develops when edema and swelling result in increased pressure within soft tissues, causing circulation to be compromised, possibly resulting in tissue necrosis.

contaminated Containing microorganisms.

contusion A bruise; an injury that causes bleeding beneath the skin but does not break the skin.

crush injury An injury in which the body or part of the body is crushed, preventing tissue function and, possibly, resulting in permanent tissue damage.

crush syndrome Significant metabolic derangement that can lead to renal failure and death. It develops when crushed extremities or other body parts remain trapped for prolonged periods.

deep fascia A dense layer of fibrous tissue below the subcutaneous tissue; composed of tough bands of tissue that ensheath muscles and other internal structures.

degloving A traumatic injury that results in the soft tissue of the hand being drawn downward like a glove being removed.

degranulate To release granules into the surrounding tissue.

dermis The inner layer of skin, containing hair follicle roots, glands, blood vessels, and nerves.

dressing Material used to directly cover a wound.

ecchymosis Extravasation of blood under the skin to produce a "black-and-blue" mark.

elastin A protein that gives the skin its elasticity.

epidermis The outermost layer of the skin.

epithelialization The formation of fresh epithelial tissue to heal a wound.

erythema Reddening of the skin.

fasciotomy A surgical procedure that cuts away fascia to relieve pressure.

gangrene An infection commonly caused by *C perfringens*. The result is tissue destruction and gas production that may lead to death.

glomerular filtration The first step in the formation of urine; calculated to determine renal function.

granulocytes Cells that contain granules.

ground substance Material between cells.

hematoma A localized collection of blood in the soft tissues as a result of injury or a broken blood vessel.

homeostasis The tendency to constancy or stability in the body's internal environment.

hyperkalemia An increased level of potassium in the blood.

hyperphosphatemia An increased level of phosphate in the blood.

hypertrophic scar An abnormal scar with excess collagen that does not extend over the wound margins.

impaled object An object that has caused a puncture wound and remains embedded in the wound.

incision A wound usually made deliberately, as in surgery; a clean cut, as opposed to a laceration.

integument The skin.

keloid scar An abnormal scar commonly found in people with darkly pigmented skin. It extends over the wound margins.

laceration A wound made by tearing or cutting tissues.

lymphangitis Inflammation of a lymph channel.

lymphocytes White blood cells that function to remove invading pathogens.

macrophages Cells that are responsible for protecting the body against infection.

melanin The pigment that gives skin its color.

mucopolysaccharide gel A key component of ground substance that is a polysaccharide that forms complexes with proteins.

myoglobin A protein found in muscle that is released into the circulation after crush injury or other muscle damage and whose presence in the circulation may produce kidney damage.

neovascularization Development of vessels to aid in healing an injured soft tissue.

open wound An injury in which there is a break in the surface of the skin or the mucous membrane, exposing deeper tissue to potential contamination.

pedicle A narrow strip of tissue by which an avulsed piece of tissue remains connected to the body.

puncture wound A stab injury from a pointed object, such as a nail or a knife.

rhabdomyolysis The destruction of muscle tissue leading to a release of potassium and myoglobin.

scar revision A surgical procedure to improve the appearance of a scar, reestablish function, or correct disfigurement from soft-tissue damage, surgical incision, or lesion.

sebaceous gland The gland located in the dermis that secretes sebum.

sebum An oily substance secreted by the sebaceous glands.

subcutaneous Beneath the skin.

tension lines The pattern of tautness of the skin, which is arranged over body structures and affects how well wounds heal.

Volkmann contracture Deformity of the hand, fingers, and wrist resulting from damage to forearm muscles; develops from muscle ischemia and is associated with compartment syndrome.

◼ Points to Ponder

You are dispatched to the site of a motorcycle crash on the off ramp of a major highway. When you arrive on scene, you see a man lying on his right side. You've carried your backboard and cervical collar with you, so you begin to provide full cervical-spine stabilization. You note a tremendous amount of "road rash" and numerous lacerations. While you are placing the board and collar on this patient, your partner begins to attend to the obvious wounds. After you log roll the patient onto the backboard, you note copious amounts of blood in the patient's airway and determine that he has agonal respirations at about 8 breaths/min. You do not feel a radial pulse; however, you are able to obtain a weak and thready carotid pulse at about 110 beats/min. The patient is nonverbal. Your partner is cleaning the patient's arm of debris and glass.

What are your priorities supposed to be in this situation? What do you need to do for this patient?

Issues: Priorities Regarding Life-Threatening Injuries and Wound Closure, The Value of the Written Report.

Assessment in Action

You are dispatched to the outside of a private residence for a dog bite. When you arrive, you notice that the patient is sitting upright, speaking in full sentences. She is conscious, alert, oriented, and complaining of pain in both of her arms and head. The family has wrapped towels over both arms and one over her head.

When you unwrap the right arm, you note two large lacerations greater than 4″ long and multiple puncture wounds. When you examine the upper arm, you notice white material that looks like muscle fascia. You control the bleeding with bandages. The left arm is not as bad, but it is bleeding. When you begin to check out the head, you notice that a piece of the scalp is missing. The family hands you a plastic bag with the missing piece.

1. **A "wound" is defined as:**
   A. any injury to the soft tissues, with or without involvement of the subcutaneous tissues and muscle beneath.
   B. any injury to the soft tissues that requires special care to stop the bleeding.
   C. any injury to the soft tissues, with involvement of the subcutaneous tissues and muscle beneath.
   D. any injury to the soft tissues that extends into the bone.

2. **What are the two types of wound classifications?**
   A. Open wounds and lacerations
   B. Lacerations and incisions
   C. Contusions and closed wounds
   D. Closed and open wounds

3. **A laceration is defined as:**
   A. a superficial wound that occurs when the skin is rubbed or scraped over a rough surface so that part of the epidermis is lost.
   B. a cut inflicted by a sharp instrument, such as a knife or razor blade, that produces a clean or jagged incision through the skin surface and underlying structure.
   C. a clean (linear) cut.
   D. a stab from a pointed object, such as a nail or a knife.

4. **A puncture wound is defined as:**
   A. a superficial wound that occurs when the skin is rubbed or scraped over a rough surface so that part of the epidermis is lost.
   B. a cut inflicted by a sharp instrument, such as a knife or razor blade, that produces a clean or jagged incision through the skin surface and underlying structure.
   C. a clean (linear) cut.
   D. a stab from a pointed object, such as a nail or a knife.

5. **An avulsion is defined as:**
   A. a superficial wound that occurs when the skin is rubbed or scraped over a rough surface so that part of the epidermis is lost.
   B. a cut inflicted by a sharp instrument, such as a knife or razor blade, that produces a clean or jagged incision through the skin surface and underlying structure.
   C. a flap of skin that has been torn loose, partially or completely.
   D. a complete loss of a body part, typically involving the extremities.

6. **Evaluation of the skin involves:**
   A. inspection and auscultation.
   B. auscultation and circulation.
   C. inspection and palpation.
   D. palpation and auscultation.

7. **Bleeding may be controlled by using:**
   A. direct pressure.
   B. elevation.
   C. pressure point control.
   D. all of the above.

8. **It is important to preserve the amputated part because this:**
   A. maximizes the chances of its being successfully reimplanted.
   B. allows it to be donated.
   C. minimizes the chances of it being unsuccessfully reimplanted.
   D. all of the above.

9. **Scalp injuries tend to bleed more because:**
   A. there is no blood supply to this area.
   B. there is a rich blood supply in this area.
   C. there is an excessive number of veins in the scalp.
   D. these are life-threatening injuries.

10. **Written documentation must be completed for every patient contact. It should include all of the following, EXCEPT:**
    A. ABCs.
    B. relevant scene findings.
    C. interventions and how the patient responded to them.
    D. paraphrasing of the patient's statements.

Challenging Questions

You are dispatched to a scene involving a man caught between a car and a low-end loader. When you arrive, you see that the man is pinned between the two vehicles. He complains of pain in his lower abdomen and pelvic region.

11. **What type of injury is this?**

12. **What treatment do you need to administer?**

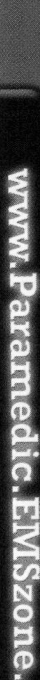

20 Burns

Objectives

Cognitive

4-4.1   Describe the anatomy and physiology pertinent to burn injuries. (p 20.4)

4-4.2   Describe the epidemiology, including incidence, mortality/morbidity, risk factors, and prevention strategies for the patient with a burn injury. (p 20.4)

4-4.3   Describe the pathophysiologic complications and systemic complications of a burn injury. (p 20.6)

4-4.4   Identify and describe types of burn injuries, including a thermal burn, an inhalation burn, a chemical burn, an electrical burn, and a radiation exposure. (p 20.7)

4-4.5   Identify and describe the depth classifications of burn injuries, including a superficial burn, a partial-thickness burn, a full-thickness burn, and other depth classifications described by local protocol. (p 20.16)

4-4.6   Identify and describe methods for determining body surface area percentage of a burn injury including the "rule of nines," the "rule of palms," and other methods described by local protocol. (p 20.16)

4-4.7   Identify and describe the severity of a burn including a minor burn, a moderate burn, a severe burn, and other severity classifications described by local protocol. (p 20.15)

4-4.8   Differentiate criteria for determining the severity of a burn injury between a pediatric patient and an adult patient. (p 20.16)

4-4.9   Describe special considerations for a pediatric patient with a burn injury. (p 20.27)

4-4.10   Discuss considerations which impact management and prognosis of the burn injured patient. (p 20.19, 20.20)

4-4.11   Discuss mechanisms of burn injuries. (p 20.14)

4-4.12   Discuss conditions associated with burn injuries, including trauma, blast injuries, airway compromise, respiratory compromise, and child abuse. (p 20.7)

4-4.13   Describe the management of a burn injury, including airway and ventilation, circulation, pharmacological, non-pharmacological, transport considerations, psychological support/communication strategies, and other management described by local protocol. (p 20.20)

4-4.14   Describe the epidemiology of a thermal burn injury. (p 20.7)

4-4.15   Describe the specific anatomy and physiology pertinent to a thermal burn injury. (p 20.7)

4-4.16   Describe the pathophysiology of a thermal burn injury. (p 20.7)

4-4.17   Identify and describe the depth classifications of a thermal burn injury. (p 20.16)

4-4.18   Identify and describe the severity of a thermal burn injury. (p 20.15)

4-4.19   Describe considerations which impact management and prognosis of the patient with a thermal burn injury. (p 20.19, 20.20)

4-4.20   Discuss mechanisms of burn injury and conditions associated with a thermal burn injury. (p 20.7)

4-4.21   Describe the management of a thermal burn injury, including airway and ventilation, circulation, pharmacological, non-pharmacological, transport considerations, and psychological support/communication strategies. (p 20.20)

4-4.22   Describe the epidemiology of an inhalation burn injury. (p 20.8)

4-4.23   Describe the specific anatomy and physiology pertinent to an inhalation burn injury. (p 20.8)

4-4.24   Describe the pathophysiology of an inhalation burn injury. (p 20.8)

4-4.25   Differentiate between supraglottic and infraglottic inhalation injuries. (p 20.8)

4-4.26   Identify and describe the depth classifications of an inhalation burn injury. (p 20.8)

4-4.27   Identify and describe the severity of an inhalation burn injury. (p 20.8)

4-4.28   Describe considerations which impact management and prognosis of the patient with an inhalation burn injury. (p 20.20)

4-4.29   Discuss mechanisms of burn injury and conditions associated with an inhalation burn injury. (p 20.8)

4-4.30   Describe the management of an inhalation burn injury, including airway and ventilation, circulation, pharmacological, non-pharmacological, transport considerations, and psychological support/communication strategies. (p 20.20)

4-4.31   Describe the epidemiology of a chemical burn injury and a chemical burn injury to the eye. (p 20.9)

4-4.32   Describe the specific anatomy and physiology pertinent to a chemical burn injury and a chemical burn injury to the eye. (p 20.9)

4-4.33   Describe the pathophysiology of a chemical burn injury, including types of chemicals and their burning processes and a chemical burn injury to the eye. (p 20.10)

4-4.34   Identify and describe the depth classifications of a chemical burn injury. (p 20.10)

4-4.35   Identify and describe the severity of a chemical burn injury. (p 20.10)

4-4.36   Describe considerations which impact management and prognosis of the patient with a chemical burn injury and a chemical burn injury to the eye. (p 20.23)

4-4.37   Discuss mechanisms of burn injury and conditions associated with a chemical burn injury. (p 20.9)

4-4.38   Describe the management of a chemical burn injury and a chemical burn injury to the eye, including airway and ventilation, circulation, pharmacological, non-pharmacological, transport considerations, and psychological support/communication strategies. (p 20.23)

4-4.39   Describe the epidemiology of an electrical burn injury. (p 20.11)

4-4.40   Describe the specific anatomy and physiology pertinent to an electrical burn injury. (p 20.11)

4-4.41   Describe the pathophysiology of an electrical burn injury. (p 20.11)

4-4.42   Identify and describe the depth classifications of an electrical burn injury. (p 20.11)

4-4.43 Identify and describe the severity of an electrical burn injury. (p 20.11)

4-4.44 Describe considerations which impact management and prognosis of the patient with an electrical burn injury. (p 20.24)

4-4.45 Discuss mechanisms of burn injury and conditions associated with an electrical burn injury. (p 20.11)

4-4.46 Describe the management of an electrical burn injury, including airway and ventilation, circulation, pharmacological, non-pharmacological, transport considerations, and psychological support/communication strategies. (p 20.25)

4-4.47 Describe the epidemiology of a radiation exposure. (p 20.13)

4-4.48 Describe the specific anatomy and physiology pertinent to a radiation exposure. (p 20.13)

4-4.49 Describe the pathophysiology of a radiation exposure, including the types and characteristics of ionizing radiation. (p 20.13)

4-4.50 Identify and describe the depth classifications of a radiation exposure. (p 20.13)

4-4.51 Identify and describe the severity of a radiation exposure. (p 20.13)

4-4.52 Describe considerations which impact management and prognosis of the patient with a radiation exposure. (p 20.26)

4-4.53 Discuss mechanisms of burn injury associated with a radiation exposure. (p 20.13)

4-4.54 Discuss conditions associated with a radiation exposure. (p 20.13)

4-4.55 Describe the management of a radiation exposure, including airway and ventilation, circulation, pharmacological, non-pharmacological, transport considerations, and psychological support/communication strategies. (p 20.26)

4-4.56 Integrate pathophysiological principles to the assessment of a patient with a thermal burn injury. (p 20.15)

4-4.57 Integrate pathophysiological principles to the assessment of a patient with an inhalation burn injury. (p 20.15)

4-4.58 Integrate pathophysiological principles to the assessment of a patient with a chemical burn injury. (p 20.15)

4-4.59 Integrate pathophysiological principles to the assessment of a patient with an electrical burn injury. (p 20.15)

4-4.60 Integrate pathophysiological principles to the assessment of a patient with a radiation exposure. (p 20.15)

4-4.61 Synthesize patient history information and assessment findings to form a field impression for the patient with a thermal burn injury. (p 20.16)

4-4.62 Synthesize patient history information and assessment findings to form a field impression for the patient with an inhalation burn injury. (p 20.16)

4-4.63 Synthesize patient history information and assessment findings to form a field impression for the patient with a chemical burn injury. (p 20.16)

4-4.64 Synthesize patient history information and assessment findings to form a field impression for the patient with an electrical burn injury. (p 20.16)

4-4.65 Synthesize patient history information and assessment findings to form a field impression for the patient with a radiation exposure. (p 20.16)

4-4.66 Develop, execute and evaluate a management plan based on the field impression for the patient with a thermal burn injury. (p 20.19, 20.20)

4-4.67 Develop, execute and evaluate a management plan based on the field impression for the patient with an inhalation burn injury. (p 20.20)

4-4.68 Develop, execute and evaluate a management plan based on the field impression for the patient with a chemical burn injury. (p 20.23)

4-4.69 Develop, execute and evaluate a management plan based on the field impression for the patient with an electrical burn injury. (p 20.24)

4-4.70 Develop, execute and evaluate a management plan based on the field impression for the patient with a radiation exposure. (p 20.24)

Affective

4-4.71 Value the changes of a patient's self-image associated with a burn injury. (p 20.20)

4-4.72 Value the impact of managing a burn injured patient. (p 20.27)

4-4.73 Advocate empathy for a burn injured patient. (p 20.15)

4-4.74 Assess safety at a burn injury incident. (p 20.14)

4-4.75 Characterize mortality and morbidity based on the pathophysiology and assessment findings of a patient with a burn injury. (p 20.15)

4-4.76 Value and defend the sense of urgency in burn injuries. (p 20.15)

4-4.77 Serve as a model for universal precautions and body substance isolation (BSI). (p 20.14)

Psychomotor

4-4.78 Take body substance isolation procedures during assessment and management of patients with a burn injury. (p 20.14)

4-4.79 Perform assessment of a patient with a burn injury. (p 20.15)

4-4.80 Perform management of a thermal burn injury, including airway and ventilation, circulation, pharmacological, non-pharmacological, transport considerations, psychological support/communication strategies, and other management described by local protocol. (p 20.20)

4-4.81 Perform management of an inhalation burn injury, including airway and ventilation, circulation, pharmacological, non-pharmacological, transport considerations, psychological support/communication strategies, and other management described by local protocol. (p 20.20)

4-4.82 Perform management of a chemical burn injury, including airway and ventilation, circulation, pharmacological, non-pharmacological, transport considerations, psychological support/communication strategies, and other management described by local protocol. (p 20.23)

4-4.83 Perform management of an electrical burn injury, including airway and ventilation, circulation, pharmacological, non-pharmacological, transport considerations, psychological support/communication strategies, and other management described by local protocol. (p 20.25)

4-4.84 Perform management of a radiation exposure, including airway and ventilation, circulation, pharmacological, non-pharmacological, transport considerations, psychological support/communication strategies, and other management described by local protocol. (p 20.26)

Introduction

Approximately 82% of all civilian fire-related deaths occur in residential constructions Figure 20-1 ▼ . The incidence of burn injuries and death in the United States has decreased somewhat with the advent of stricter building codes and widespread use of smoke detectors. Other effective burn prevention techniques include reducing domestic water heater temperatures to 120°F to prevent severe scalds and making disposable lighters child-safe. Unfortunately, some 4,000 people still die of fire-related causes each year. Children younger than 5 years and elderly people are at particularly high risk of dying in fires.

Just as code enforcement and smoke detectors have decreased fire-related deaths, our ability to treat large burns effectively has steadily improved. Before the medical advances of the 20th century, death was "almost inevitable" when more than one third of the body was burned. Now, however, better

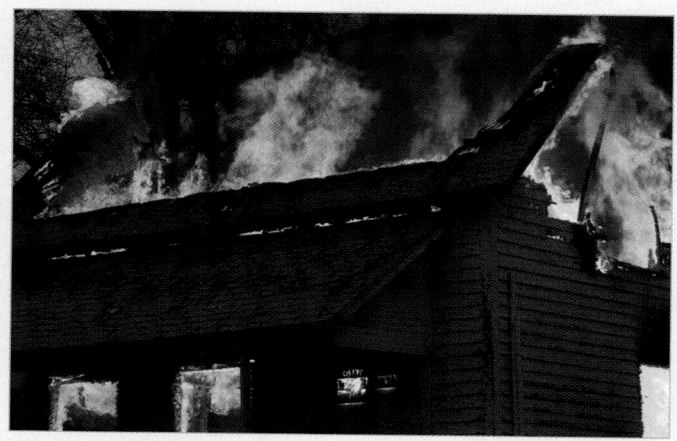

Figure 20-1 Of all civilian fire fatalities, 82% occur in the home.

understanding of "burn shock," advances in the use of fluid therapy and antibiotics, improved ability to excise dead tissue, and the use of biologic dressings to aid early wound closure have vastly improved burn care. The formation of specialized teams to resuscitate patients from burn shock, delay infection, and achieve wound closure has resulted in impressive gains in survival rates.

Deaths and serious injuries also occur from electrical and chemical burns. As a consequence, numerous public safety campaigns have focused on the use of smoke detectors and the dangers that surround the use of flammable liquids, petroleum products, solvents, propane, and fireworks.

Although you probably won't see moderate or severe burns on a daily basis, you will encounter some serious burn injuries during your career, and you might encounter serious electrical, chemical, and radiation injuries as well. Accurate recognition of the severity of burn injuries can dramatically enhance the care of burned patients by allowing you to institute proper emergency care and notify the receiving facility so personnel can be better prepared to care for the patient and by allowing triage to or consultation with a specialized burn center.

Anatomy and Function of the Skin

The human skin is much more than a wrapping that keeps the inside of the body from falling out. The skin, also known as the integument, is the largest and one of the most complex organs in the body. It has a crucial role in maintaining homeostasis (balance) within the body. The skin is durable, flexible, and usually able to repair itself. It varies in thickness from almost 1 cm on the heel to 1 mm on the eye's surface. The skin has four functions:

- It acts as an all-purpose fortress to protect the underlying tissue from injury and exposure from extremes of

You are the Provider Part 1

You are dispatched to assist the fire department with a structure fire at 9116 East Leesburg Way. Within a few minutes, you hear radio traffic from an interior crew indicating they have found a fire victim. The crew members announce which side of the structure they will exit, and you take your equipment and wait for them there.

Within a few moments, the fire fighters emerge with a child who appears to be approximately 8 years old. She is crying, coughing, and holding up her forearm. As you approach, you can see that the young girl has what seems to be a partial-thickness burn to her right arm.

Initial Assessment	Recording Time: 0 Minutes
Appearance	Tearful and upset
Level of consciousness	A (Alert to person, place, and day)
Airway	Patent, loud crying
Breathing	Tachypneic but with good tidal volume
Circulation	Not yet assessed, skin covered with soot

1. What are your patient care priorities?
2. What are patient care concerns when dealing with structure fire victims?

temperature, ultraviolet radiation, mechanical forces, toxic chemicals, and invading microorganisms.

- The skin aids in temperature regulation (thermoregulation), preventing heat loss when the core body temperature starts to fall and facilitating heat loss when core temperature rises.
- As a watertight seal, the skin prevents excessive loss of water from the body and drying of tissues, thereby helping maintain the chemical stability of the internal environment. Without skin, a person would become water-logged after the first rain and would resemble a prune after the first hot day of summer.
- The skin serves as a sense organ, keeping the brain informed about the external environment. Changes in temperature and sensations of pain are mediated through skin sense receptors.

Significant damage to the skin may make the body vulnerable to bacterial invasion, temperature instability, and major disturbances of fluid balance. People who survive serious burns must live with the ramifications of the damage to large portions of the integument:

- Difficulty with thermoregulation
- Inability to sweat from the scarred portions of the skin
- Impaired vasoconstriction and vasodilation in the areas of severe damage
- Little or no melanin (pigment) in the scar tissue, which makes the skin susceptible to sunburn
- Inability to grow hair on the injured site and little or no sensation in the scarred areas

All of these factors may restrict a person's ability to function even many years after the burn trauma has healed (Figure 20-2 ▶). Patients who survive serious burns also have a high rate of depression.

Underlying the epidermis is a tough, highly elastic layer of connective tissues called the dermis. The dermis is a complex material composed chiefly of collagen fibers, elastin fibers, and a mucopolysaccharide gel. Collagen is a fibrous protein with a very high tensile strength, so it gives the skin high resistance to breakage under mechanical stress. Elastin imparts elasticity to the skin, allowing it to spring back to its usual contours. The mucopolysaccharide gel gives the skin resistance to compression.

Enclosed within the dermis are several specialized skin structures. Nerve endings mediate the senses of touch, temperature, pressure, and pain, for example. Blood vessels carry oxygen and nutrients to the skin and remove the carbon dioxide and metabolic waste products. Cutaneous blood vessels also

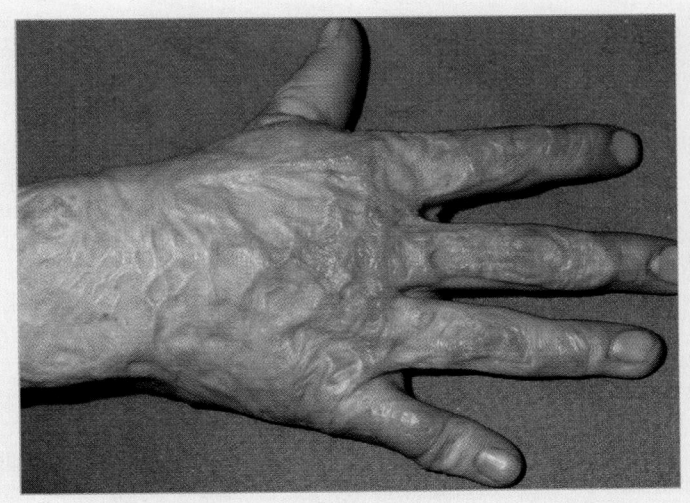

Figure 20-2 People who survive serious burns must live with the ramifications of their injury.

Layers of the Skin

To carry out its functions, the skin needs a specialized structure (Figure 20-3 ▶). The skin is composed of two principal layers: the epidermis and the dermis.

The epidermis, or outermost layer, is the body's first line of defense, constituting the major barrier against water, dust, microorganisms, and mechanical stress. The epidermis is itself composed of several layers: an outermost layer of hardened, nonliving cells, which are continuously shed through a process called desquamation, and three inner layers of living cells that constantly divide to give rise to new "dead layer" skin cells. The deeper layers of the epidermis also contain variable numbers of cells bearing melanin granules. The darkness of a person's skin is directly proportional to the amount of melanin present.

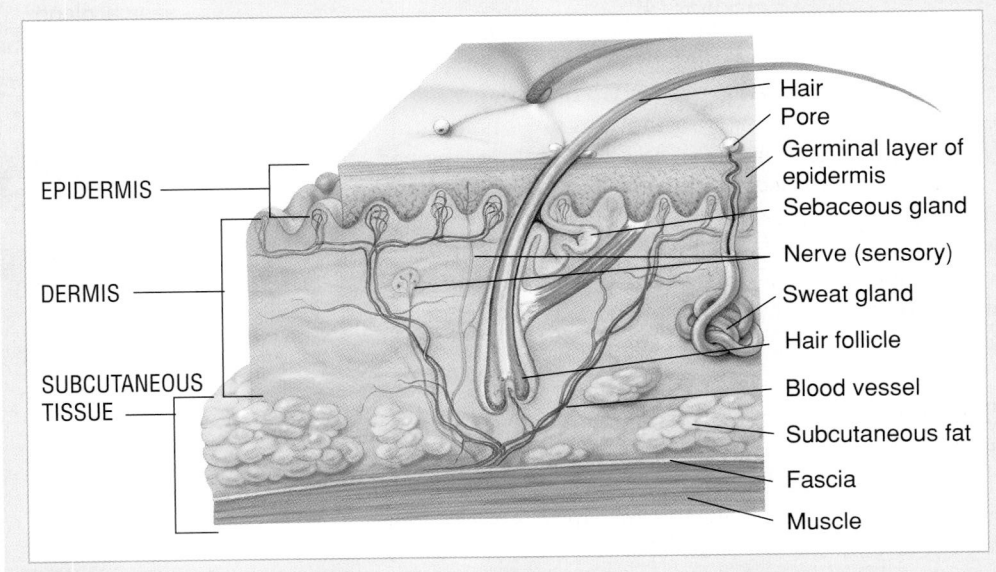

EPIDERMIS

DERMIS

SUBCUTANEOUS TISSUE

Hair
Pore
Germinal layer of epidermis
Sebaceous gland
Nerve (sensory)
Sweat gland
Hair follicle
Blood vessel
Subcutaneous fat
Fascia
Muscle

Figure 20-3 The skin has two principal layers: the epidermis and the dermis.

serve a crucial role in regulating body temperature by regulating the volume of blood that flows from the body's warm core to its cooler surface.

Also in the dermis, sweat glands produce sweat and discharge it through ducts passing to the surface of the skin in a process regulated by the sympathetic nervous system. Sweat consists of water and salts. The average volume of sweat lost during 24 hours under normal conditions ranges from 500 to 1,000 mL. During strenuous exercise, sweat glands may secrete as much as 1,000 mL in an hour. Evaporation of water from the skin surface is one of the body's major mechanisms for shedding excess heat.

Hair follicles are structures that produce hair and enclose the hair roots. Each follicle contains a single hair. Attached to the hair follicle is a small muscle that, on contraction, causes the follicle to assume a more vertical position. Sensations such as cold and fright stimulate the autonomic nervous system, which in turn brings about contraction of those muscles and results in "gooseflesh." Hairs in each part of the body have definite periods of growth, after which they are shed and replaced; scalp hair, for example, has a life span of 2 to 5 years and grows at an average rate of 1.5 to 3.9 mm per week. Hair melts when it burns, yet sometimes appears to remain on the patient. When you brush your hand over it, you may find that what you thought was a mustache is now simply a streak of ash. Closely observe nasal hair, eyebrows, and eyelashes in burn patients because damage to them may indicate airway injury. When hair on the arms or legs "falls out" or can be removed without pain, deeper skin structures have been damaged.

At the neck of each hair follicle is a sebaceous gland that produces an oily substance called sebum. The secretions of the sebaceous glands empty into the hair follicles and ultimately reach the surface of the skin. Sebum is believed to keep the skin supple so it doesn't dry out and crack. When sebaceous glands become obstructed, a hard comedo forms, which may serve as the base of an acne pimple.

The tissue beneath the dermis, called the subcutaneous layer, consists mainly of adipose tissue (fat). Subcutaneous fat insulates the underlying tissues from extremes of heat and cold. It also provides a substantial cushion for underlying structures, while serving as an energy reserve for the body.

Finally, beneath the subcutaneous layer are the muscles, tendons, bones, and vital organs. Muscles have thick, fibrous capsules that are prone to hypoxia and anaerobic metabolism in a burn state. Bones are living tissue that can be severely affected by burn injury. Vital organs may also be damaged by thermal, chemical, or electrical energy.

The Eye

The specific anatomy and physiology of the eye are covered in Chapter 21. Clearly, the eyes are sensitive to burn injuries—from a flame, superheated gases, light source (such as a welder's torch), or chemicals. The tear ducts and eyelids combine to constantly lubricate the surface of the eyes Figure 20-4 ▶ . Unfortunately, intense heat, light, or chemi-

cal reactions on the surface of the eye can quickly burn the thin membrane or skin covering the surface of the eye. Ocular damage is a common result of alkali (base) injury: The higher the pH of the substance, the more severe the damage to the eye. When a patient gets a substance like lime in the eyes, the damage is worsened by repeatedly rubbing the eyes as opposed to initiating copious irrigation and essential treatment in the emergency department (ED).

Pathophysiology

Burns are diffuse soft-tissue injuries created by destructive energy transfer via radiation, thermal, or electrical energy. Thermal burns can occur when skin is exposed to temperatures higher than 111°F (44°C). In general, the severity of a thermal injury correlates directly with temperature, concentration, or amount of heat energy possessed by the object or substance and the duration of exposure. For example, solids generally have higher heat content than gases, so exposure to a hot solid (such as the rack inside an oven) typically causes a more significant burn than exposure to hot gases (such as those coming out of an oven). Burns are a progressive process: The greater the heat energy, the deeper the wound.

Exposure time is another important factor. Thermal injury can occur to unresponsive or paralyzed patients from seemingly innocuous heat sources such as heating pads, transcutaneous oxygen sensors, and heat lamps left unattended for long periods.

It may be difficult to evaluate the amount of heat energy or the amount of exposure time in many cases. The temperature of a fire may vary tremendously from the floor to the ceiling.

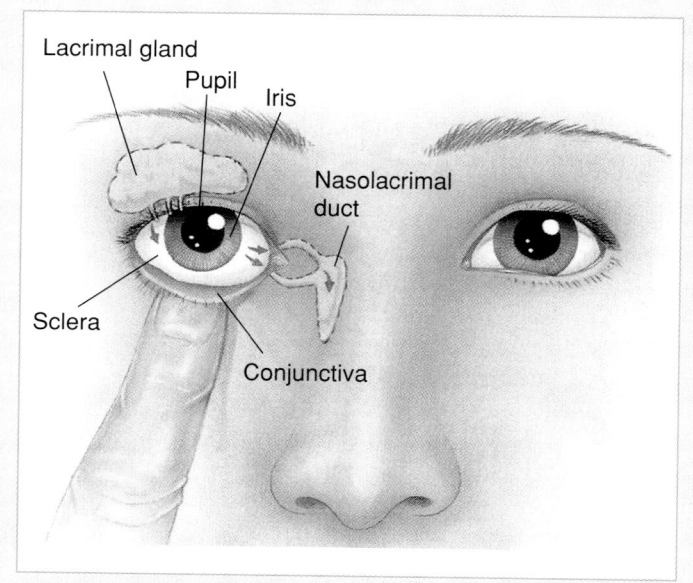

Figure 20-4 Tears act as lubricants and keep the front of the eye protected.

Although most people reflexively limit the amount of time exposed to such heat, if clothing is on fire or the person is trapped or unconscious, exposure time will be longer.

Thermal Burns

A thermal burn is sometimes called trauma by fire Figure 20-5 ▾ . However, heat energy can be transmitted in a variety of ways in addition to fire. Although these burns are all caused by heat (as opposed to electricity, chemicals, or radiation), many different situations can cause thermal burns and pose a safety hazard to responding paramedics.

Flame Burns

Most commonly, thermal burns are caused by open flame. A flame burn is very often a deep burn, especially if a person's clothing catches fire Figure 20-6 ▸ . The fire is fanned by running—hence the adage "stop, drop, and roll" that is taught in the schools. Flame burns may also be associated with inhalation injuries.

Scald Burns

Hot liquids produce scald injuries. A scald burn is most commonly seen in children and handicapped adults but can happen to anyone, particularly while cooking. Scald burns often cover large surface areas because liquids can spread quickly. Hot liquids can soak into clothing and continue to burn until the clothing is removed. Some hot liquids, such as oil and grease, adhere to the skin, causing particularly deep scald injuries. Scalds are sometimes associated with child abuse Figure 20-7 ▸ .

About 100,000 scald burns result annually from spilled food and beverages. A child may pull a pot or other container of hot liquid off the stove or counter, a toddler may bump into an adult carrying or holding a hot beverage or food, or a toddler may pull the tablecloth, spilling a hot food or beverage off the table.

Contact Burns

Coming in contact with hot objects produces a contact burn. Ordinarily, reflexes protect a person from prolonged exposure to a very hot object, so contact burns are rarely deep unless the patient was prevented from drawing away from the hot object (for example, unconscious, intoxicated, restrained, or impaired). Prolonged contact with something that is just moderately hot can eventually result in a severe burn, however. A patient who has a stroke and falls against a household radiator, for example, may end up with severe burns.

Burns in children, older people, and people with disabilities may be signs of abuse. Burns with formed shapes or unusual patterns and burns in atypical places such as the genitalia, buttocks, and thighs are often consistent with abuse.

Steam Burns

A steam burn can produce a topical (scald) burn. Minor steam burns are common when microwaving food covered with plastic wrap. When the plastic is peeled away, hot steam escapes directly onto the hand of the hungry chef. Steam (that is, gaseous water) is also notorious for causing airway burns.

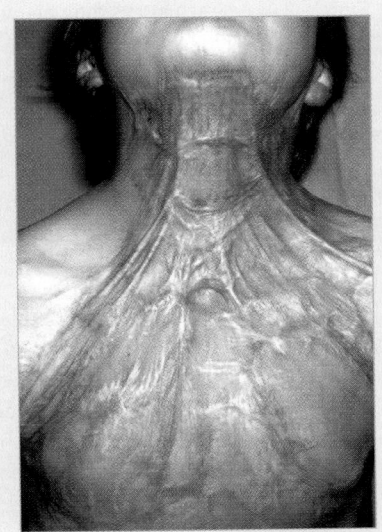
Figure 20-6 Flame burns are often very deep burns.

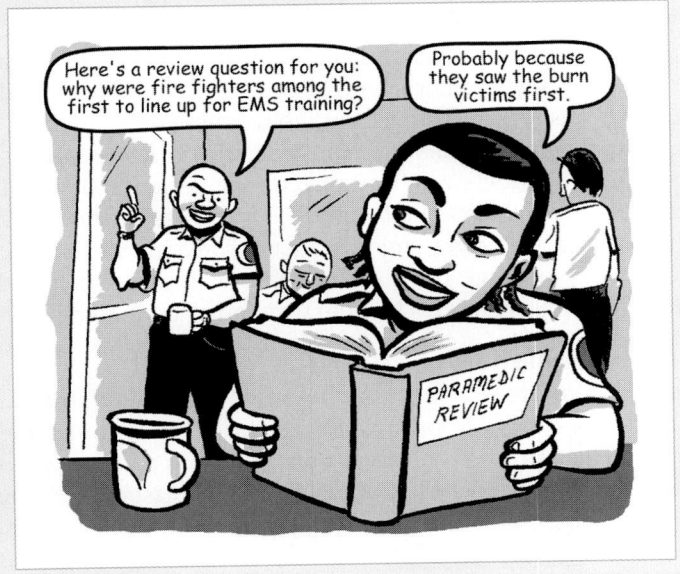
Figure 20-5

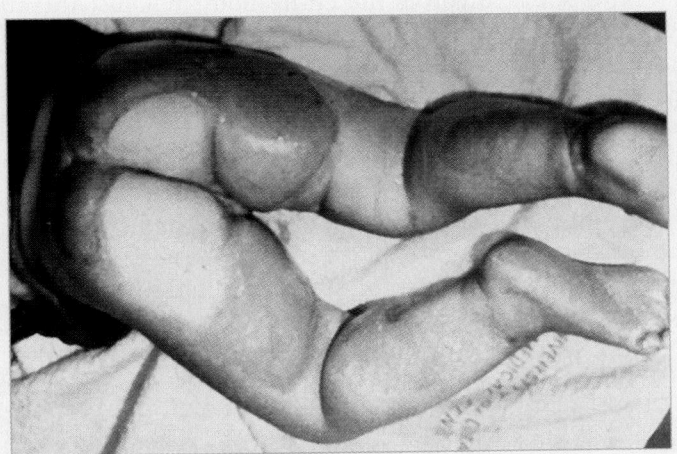
Figure 20-7 Scalds are sometimes associated with child abuse.

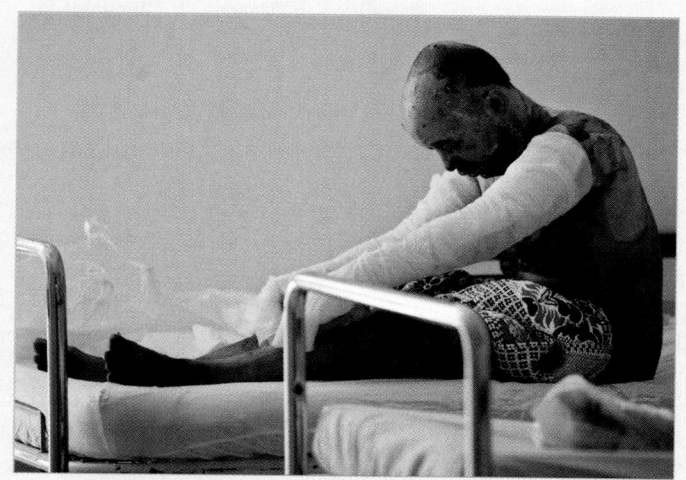

Figure 20-8 Flash burns may be minor compared with the additional trauma inflicted by an explosion.

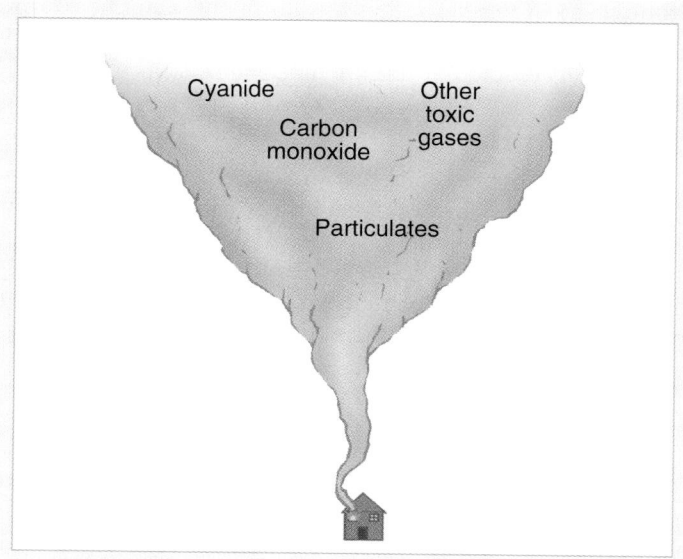

Figure 20-9 Smoke from fires contains many toxins.

Inhalation of other hot gases may cause supraglottic (upper airway) trauma but rarely leads to burns in the lower airway. Steam is unique because the minute particles of hot water *can* cause significant injury to the lower airway.

Flash Burns

A relatively rare source of thermal burns is the flash produced by an explosion, which may briefly expose a person to very intense heat. Lightning strikes can also cause a flash burn. These injuries are usually minor compared with the potential for trauma from whatever caused the flash Figure 20-8 ▲ .

Burn Shock

Burn shock occurs because of two types of injury: fluid loss across damaged skin and a series of volume shifts within the rest of the body. Capillaries become leaky, so intravascular volume oozes out of the circulation and into the interstitial spaces. The cells of normal tissues then take in increased amounts of salt and water from the fluid around them.

Burn shock involves the entire body, not just the area burned. You may have experienced sunburn over a reasonably large surface area, like your back. In addition to the skin-related discomfort from the sunburn, you may have developed chills and nausea and felt "real sick" as a result of the fluid shifts and electrolyte disturbances. This is a mild form of burn shock. Just as in other forms of shock, these changes limit the effective distribution of oxygen and glucose to the tissues and hamper the circulation's ability to remove waste products from healthy and damaged tissues. Adequate fluid resuscitation is essential to avoid the devastating consequences of burn shock.

Burn shock sets in during a 6- to 8-hour period, so you will not typically witness it in the field. Therefore, if an acutely burned patient is in shock in the prehospital phase, look for another injury as the source of shock. People who are caught in fires may fall through floors, jump out of windows, and have things fall on them. There are ample opportunities for trau-

matic injuries at fire and explosion scenes, so you must be diligent in your assessment.

Airway Burns

Inhalation burns can cause rapid and serious airway compromise. Heat can be an irritant to the lungs and the airway, causing coughing, wheezing, and swelling of the upper airway tissues, often evidenced by stridor. Infraglottic (vocal cords and larynx) and lower airway damage is more often associated with the inhalation of steam or hot particulate matter. Supraglottic (upper airway) damage is more often associated with the inhalation of superheated gases. In rare cases, you may encounter severe upper airway swelling, requiring intervention immediately after a severe burn, although this problem may not manifest itself until transport. Application of cool mist or aerosol therapy may help reduce some minor edema. Because most ambulances do not carry misters, apply an ice pack to the throat.

More aggressive airway management may be necessary if supraglottic tissue swelling threatens the patient's airway. In addition, heat inhalation may produce laryngospasm and bronchospasm in the lower airway. Patients sometimes experience pulmonary damage from direct thermal injury. Later pulmonary involvement may be from toxic inhalation injury.

Smoke Inhalation

According to the National Fire Protection Association, the vast majority of deaths from fires are not from burns, but rather from inhalation of toxic gases, upper airway compromise, or pulmonary injury. When materials such as plastic, polyvinyl chloride pipes, and synthetic carpets burn, they release toxic chemicals Figure 20-9 ▲ . Fire fighters routinely protect themselves from these toxins by wearing self-contained breathing apparatus. Anyone who is exposed to smoke from a fire,

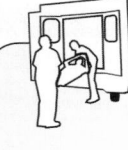

In the Field

Many fires generate toxic compounds such as cyanides (thiocyanate), which are produced as a result of the combustion of synthetic fabrics and furniture.

however, may experience thermal burns to the airway, hypoxia from lack of oxygen (oxygen is consumed by the burning process), and tissue damage and toxic effects caused by chemicals in the smoke. Such problems are particularly common when a person is caught in a burning building, stands up, and breathes in superheated gases.

Carbon Monoxide Intoxication

The combustion process produces a variety of toxic gases. The less efficient the combustion process, the more toxic the gases—such as carbon monoxide (CO) and carbon dioxide (CO_2)—that may be created. When furnaces, kerosene heaters, and other heating devices are in poor repair, they may emit unsafe levels of these toxic gases. Internal combustion engines may emit many of the same gases and, consequently, should always have their exhaust vented to the outdoors. A common cause of CO exposure is running a small engine in an enclosed space like a garage or basement. For this reason, many ambulance services and fire departments have added CO detectors to their garages or ambulance bays. Fire fighters who are performing an overhaul after a fire may be exposed to high levels of CO, as may people who are exposed to large amounts of car exhaust (such as toll takers and auto mechanics). Methylene chloride (found in some paint removers) may also produce CO gas.

CO intoxication should be considered whenever a group of people in the same place all complain of headache or nausea (a malfunctioning furnace or car exhaust being sucked into the air-handling system can cause CO intoxication in groups of people). Similarly, you should be suspicious when people complain of feeling sick at home but not when they go to work or school.

CO can displace oxygen from the alveolar air and the blood hemoglobin. Because CO binds to receptor sites on hemoglobin at least 250 times more easily than oxygen (O_2), the patient's hemoglobin may become saturated with the wrong chemical. Being exposed to relatively small concentrations of CO (such as in cigarette smoke) will result in progressively higher blood levels of CO. Most people have approximately 2% CO attached to their hemoglobin, but these levels may be as high as 4% to 8% in heavy smokers. Levels of 50% or higher may be fatal.

Traditional wisdom tells us that patients with CO intoxication will appear "cherry red." Most practitioners agree that this cherry red skin is most commonly seen in people who have died, not living people. So, never rule out CO intoxication because the patient's skin isn't cherry red.

Patients with severe CO intoxication usually present with an O_2 saturation of normal or better. For this reason, you should never trust a pulse oximeter when dealing with a sus-

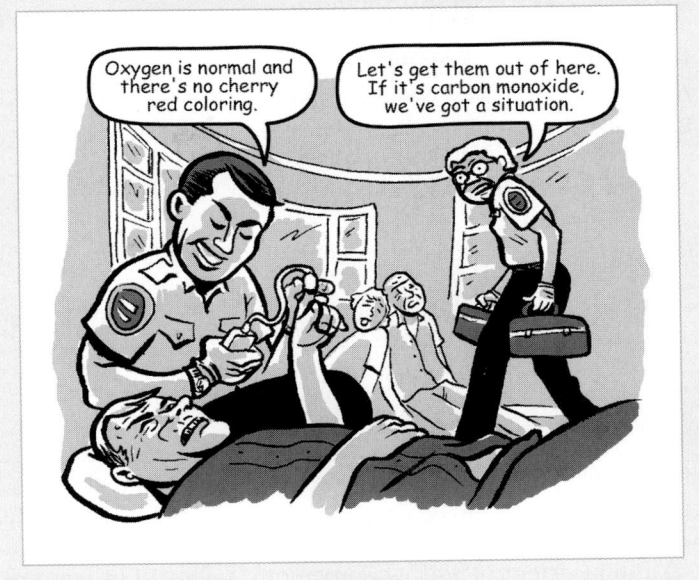

Figure 20-10

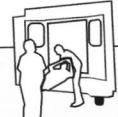

In the Field

Regardless of the cause, hyperbaric oxygen therapy for CO inhalation may be beneficial because it decreases the time it takes for hemoglobin to become saturated with oxygen. The treatment of patients with fairly low levels of CO may also be helpful.

pected CO poisoning case **Figure 20-10 ▲**. New devices that can measure CO levels will soon be common in prehospital care; they will allow us to find and treat low-level CO intoxication far more readily than we can today.

Chemical Burns

Chemical burns occur when the skin comes in contact with strong acids, alkalis or bases, or other corrosive materials **Table 20-1 ▶**. The burn progresses as long as the corrosive substance remains in contact with the skin. The cornerstone of therapy is, therefore, removal of the chemical from contact with the patient's body.

Skin destruction is determined by the chemical's concentration and duration of contact. Systemic toxicity is determined by the degree of absorption. Immediately removing the patient's clothing will often remove the majority of the chemical from skin contact. Most chemicals are most efficiently removed by washing with copious amounts of low-pressure water (such as in a shower, sink, or eye-wash station). Have the patient bend over when washing the hair and head to avoid having residual chemicals run over the rest of the body. Chemicals can collect in skin folds, where they remain in contact with the tissue and continue to cause more severe damage. Care

Table 20-1 Chemical Burns		
Chemical Type	**Examples**	**Injury**
Acids	Battery acid (sulfuric acid), hydrochloric acid, hydrofluoric acid	Coagulative necrosis
Bases and alkalis	Potassium hydroxide, sodium hydroxide, lime, drain cleaner, oven cleaner, lye	Liquefactive necrosis
Oxidizing agents	Hydrogen peroxide, sodium chlorate	Exothermic (heat) reaction in addition to tissue destruction; could cause systemic poisoning
Phosphorus	White phosphorus, tracer ammunition, fireworks	Burns when exposed to air; could cause systemic poisoning
Vesicants	Lewisite, sulfur mustard (mustard gas), phosgene oxime	Blister agents; respiratory compromise if inhaled

must be taken to meticulously wash the skin folds at joints and between fingers and toes. Once you think washing is complete, wash the body again. Some chemicals may adhere to the skin, and a mild detergent (dishwashing liquid) will aid in removal. Rinse and wash gently to avoid abrading the skin and exacerbating the injury or absorption of the chemical.

Some chemicals react violently with water, which obviously precludes irrigation. Such chemicals are usually powders, so it is reasonable to brush off as much dry powder as possible before irrigating any chemical exposure.

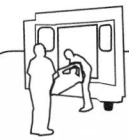

In the Field

Continue the irrigation until the patient experiences absence of or a significant decrease in pain or burning in the wound.

Injuries From Chemical Burns

Six mechanisms of injury may damage the body's tissues in case of chemical burns:

- **Reduction.** Protein denaturation caused by the reduction of the amide linkages following exposure to a reducing agent (such as alkyl mercuric compounds, diborane, lithium aluminum hydride and other metallic hydrides)
- **Oxidation.** Caused when a chemical inserts oxygen, sulfur, or a halogen (such as chlorine) atoms (such as from sodium hypochlorite, potassium permanganate, peroxides, chromic acid) into the body's proteins
- **Corrosion.** Chemicals that corrode the skin and cause massive protein denaturing (such as phenols, hydroxides, sodium, potassium, ammonium, and calcium)
- **Protoplasmic poisons.** Chemicals that form esters with proteins (such as formic acid and acetic acid) or that bind or inhibit the inorganic ions needed for the body's normal functions (such as oxalic acid and hydrofluoric acid)
- **Desecration.** Desiccants that damage the body by extracting water from tissues (such as concentrated or fuming

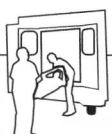

In the Field

Hydrofluoric acid is a corrosive, inorganic acid used in the manufacture of plastics, pottery glazing, and rust removers. Pain and erythema at the site of exposure are the symptoms of exposure to this chemical. After irrigation, some providers apply topical calcium gluconate gel or inject it subcutaneously to neutralize the acid.

sulfuric acid); reaction often causes heat (exothermic), which adds insult to the injury
- **Vesication.** Vesicants rapidly produce cutaneous blisters and typically are referred to as chemical warfare agents or weapons of mass destruction (such as mustard gas).

With a chemical burn injury, it is difficult to estimate the extent of the burn—it may have penetrated deep into the body's tissues. By using the rule of nines, estimate the body surface area affected, but be aware that the extent of the injury may be much more severe. Do not underestimate the power of a small quantity of chemical. Chemicals such as phenols and highly corrosive acids can cause considerable damage to the skin and its underlying tissues very quickly. Flush, flush, and then flush some more!

When contacting medical control for advice on handling specific chemical substances, you will need to identify the chemical and estimate the depth (superficial, partial thickness, or full thickness) of the chemical burn injury.

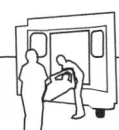

In the Field

Prolonged contact with petroleum products such as gasoline or diesel fuel may produce a chemical injury to the skin that is actually a full-thickness burn but initially appears to be only a partial-thickness injury. Sufficient absorption of the hydrocarbon may cause organ failure and even death.

Typically, chemical burns react with the skin and tissues quickly. In some cases, however, the injury may take time to develop, as in a person who is exposed to cement (calcium oxide). Cement tends to penetrate through clothing and can react with sweat on the surface of the skin. Hours later, the patient may notice that a burn injury has occurred.

Considerations that influence the management and affect the prognosis of a patient with a chemical burn injury include the specific chemical involved, the duration and amount of exposure, and the delay in neutralizing the chemical or decontaminating the patient. This is especially important when considering an injury that may have occurred to the patient's eyes.

Chemical Burns of the Eye

Chemicals known to cause burning injuries to the eyes include acids (such as concentrated liquid chlorine), alkalis (such as cement powder or a strong cleaning agent), dry chemicals (such as lye or lime), and phenols. Always wear eye protection when working with chemicals!

Electricity-Related Injuries
Electricity-Related Burns

Electricity can cause three types of burns Figure 20-11 ▶ , designated as I, II, and III. The most common is the type I burn, or contact burn. In this true electrical injury, the current is most intense at the entrance and exit sites. At those points, you may see a characteristic bull's-eye lesion, with a central, charred zone of full-thickness burns; a middle zone of cold, gray, dry tissue; and an outer, red zone of coagulation necrosis. The contact burn, while usually not in itself very serious, may signal devastating injury inside the body.

The type II burn, or flash burn, is an electrothermal injury caused by the arcing of electric current. A person who passes close enough to a source of high-voltage current will reach a point where the resistance of the air between the cur-

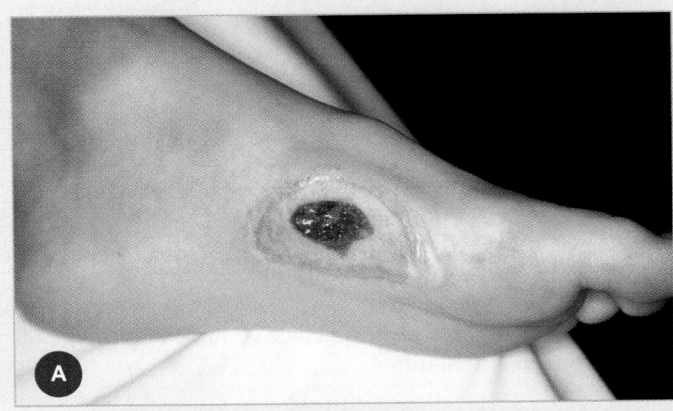
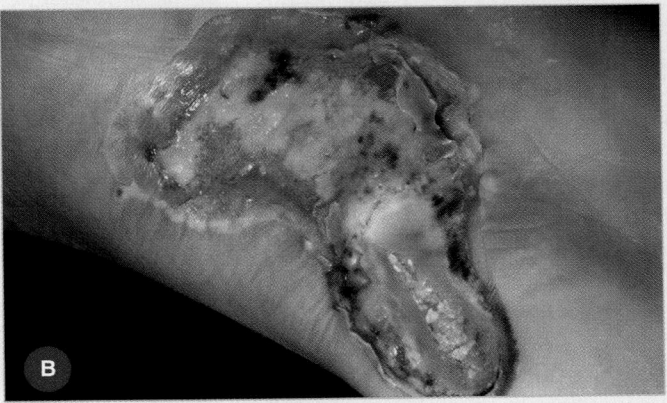

Figure 20-11 Electrical burns have entrance and exit wounds. **A.** The entrance wound is often quite small. **B.** The exit wound can be extensive and deep.

rent source and the person is sufficiently low that current arcs through the air, from the current source to the passerby. This arc has a temperature from 3,000°C to 20,000°C—high enough to produce significant charring. Victims standing near an object that was struck by lightning, for example, may get "splashed" and have areas of burns that resemble a fine red rash.

The type III electrical burn, or flame burn, is another thermal injury. It occurs when electricity ignites a person's clothing or surroundings.

Before beginning your assessment and management of an electrical burn, first and foremost you must size up the scene and ensure that it is safe. If the power could still be on and the patient still energized (such as lying on a live wire), do not approach the patient. Instead, call the power company to turn off all power and make the scene safe.

Electrical burns are most often classified as critical burns because there is a strong possibility of severe internal injury between the point of entry and the point of exit from the body. In some cases, the electricity may have flowed across the chest, potentially injuring the cardiac conduction system.

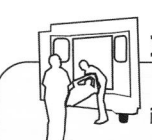

In the Field

Many electrical injuries are obvious. Even so, you should always consider the possibility of an "occult" electrical exposure in patients with findings suggesting injury and no obvious mechanism of injury.

Nonburn Injuries From Electricity

Burns may be only one of the problems experienced by a patient who has come in contact with an electrical source—and not necessarily the most serious. The two most common causes of death from electrical injury are asphyxia and cardiac arrest.

Asphyxia may occur when prolonged contact with alternating current induces tetanic contractions of the respiratory muscle. It may also result from current passing through the respiratory center in the brain and knocking out the impulse to breathe.

Cardiac arrest may occur secondarily, from hypoxia, or as a direct result of the electrical shock. Even currents as small as 0.1 ampere (amp) can trigger ventricular fibrillation if they pass directly through the heart, as when current travels across the body from hand to hand. When cardiac arrest does not occur, cardiac damage may still be manifest in various rhythm disturbances on the electrocardiogram tracing.

A host of neurologic complications have been reported in connection with electrical injury, including seizures, delirium, confusion, coma, and temporary quadriplegia. Damage to the kidneys after electrical injury resembles the syndrome seen after a crush injury, which occurs when the breakdown products of damaged muscle (myoglobin) are liberated into the circulation.

Severe, tetanic muscle spasms may lead to fractures and dislocations, which are often overlooked because of the preoccupation with the electrical injury. Posterior dislocation of the shoulder and fracture of the scapula—otherwise rare injuries—have been reported in several cases of electrocution. And don't forget the cervical spine, especially in a worker who has fallen from a utility pole.

All of these potential injuries conspire to make the victim of an electrical contact a very complex assessment challenge. Never let obvious injuries distract you from a complete assessment, including the neurologic, respiratory, cardiac, and musculoskeletal systems. In dealing with a patient who has an electrical injury, the usual priorities apply.

In the Field

Dysrhythmias commonly seen with electrical injury include atrial fibrillation and atrial flutter.

Injuries From Lightning

One special case of electrical injury deserves specific mention—the injury sustained from lightning. Approximately 500 people are injured by lightning in the United States each year, and about 100 of them die of their injuries.

Lightning strikes when a massive discharge of electricity occurs between two bodies that have different charges—for example, between a thundercloud and the ground. The stream of current travels from its origin to its destination and directly to the ground. If any object projects above the surface of the earth that is a better conductor of electricity than the air—such as a building, a light pole, an antenna, a flagpole, or a tree—that object will "attract" the lightning bolt.

A person need not sustain a direct hit from lightning to be injured; in fact, most victims are not struck directly. Much more commonly, the victim is splashed by lightning striking a nearby tree or other projecting object. Ground current produced by lightning striking the ground near the victim can also cause severe injury and accounts for incidents in which there are multiple casualties in an extended area, such as on a golf course.

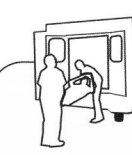

In the Field

A "stride potential" develops if a person is standing with the legs apart and the current enters the leg closest to the strike, travels up the trunk, and exits through the opposite leg.

The best treatment for lightning injuries is prevention, and all health care professionals have a responsibility to educate the public in preventive measures. Clearly, the most effective precaution is to come in out of the rain, but that is not always possible. Bear in mind that a lightning strike may happen before or after the actual storm has passed, and it can strike up to 10 miles away from the storm. Lightning tends to strike the tallest objects that are good conductors. The following rules can help avoid lightning injuries:

Rule 1. *Don't be the tallest object that is a good conductor.* Stay away from the middle of fields, lakes, golf courses, and other large, open areas. If you are stuck in the middle of an open area, try to be as small as you can. Don't hold up an umbrella, golf club, or lightning rod. Don't fly a kite.

Rule 2. *Don't stand under or near the tallest object that is a good conductor.* Although you don't want to be in the middle of the field, you also do not want to be under the tallest tree, radio antenna, or golf umbrella.

Rule 3. *Take shelter in the most substantial structure that you can to remain safe if it is hit by lightning.* A large building with a lightning suppression system is the best choice. An enclosed building is better than an open one (shed, lean-to). Close the shelter as much as possible. If in a car, keep the windows rolled up. Lightning tends to flash over the outside of objects (and people). It can travel substantial distances through conductors, however.

Rule 4. *Avoid touching good conductors during a lightning storm.* Examples of good conductors include plumbing fixtures, fences, and electrical appliances, particularly those connected to wires outside (such as the telephone, TV, and computer).

Lightning carries enormous electrical power—its energy can reach 100 *million* volts, and peak currents can be in the range of 200,000 amps. Unlike other high-voltage electric current, it is *direct*—not alternating—current, and the duration of exposure is measured in milliseconds. Thus, lightning injuries tend to resemble blast injuries more than they do high-voltage injuries, with damage to the tympanic membranes of the ears and air-containing internal organs. Many reports of lightning strikes indicate victims' clothes were "blown off" of their bodies. Muscle damage may occur, and the release of myoglobin from injured muscle may jeopardize the kidneys.

For the cardiovascular system, lightning acts as a cosmic defibrillator, delivering a massive direct-current countershock that depolarizes the entire heart. The heart may resume beating spontaneously shortly after the shock or after 5 cycles (30:2) or approximately 2 minutes of CPR that is started immediately. Because respiratory arrest is apt to persist in patients who have been struck by lightning, continued ventilatory support may be required. The phenomenon of someone regaining a pulse after a lightning strike and having respiratory arrest is known to lead to a secondary cardiac arrest if left untreated. The central nervous system is almost invariably affected by a lightning strike. At least 70% of victims will lose consciousness for some period, and nearly 90% will have some confusion or amnesia (loss of memory). Temporary paralysis of the legs has occurred, and permanent paralysis and quadriplegia have been reported in a few cases.

A lightning burn may have a feathery or zigzag appearance caused by the splash effect. Despite its unique appearance, the immediate threats to life caused by a lightning strike are the same as those caused by a high-voltage power line injury: airway obstruction, respiratory arrest, and cardiac arrest.

Radiation Burns

Acute radiation exposure has become more than a theoretical issue as use of radioactive materials increases in industry and medicine, and you must understand it to function effectively in the prehospital arena. Since 1944, there have been more than 400 radiation accidents involving significant radiation exposure to more than 3,000 people. Potential threats include incidents related to the use and transportation of radioactive isotopes and intentionally released radioactivity in terrorist attacks. To be effective, you must first suspect radiation and attempt to determine whether ongoing exposure exists. Increasingly, special response units are equipped with pager-sized radiation detectors, or such detection may be provided by other public safety services.

There are three types of ionizing radiation: alpha, beta, and gamma **Figure 20-12 ▶**. Alpha particles have little penetrating energy and are easily stopped by the skin. Beta particles have greater penetrating power and can travel much farther in air than alpha particles. They can penetrate the skin but can be blocked by simple protective clothing designed for this purpose. The threat from gamma radiation is directly proportional to its wavelength. This type of radiation is very penetrating and easily passes through the body and solid materials.

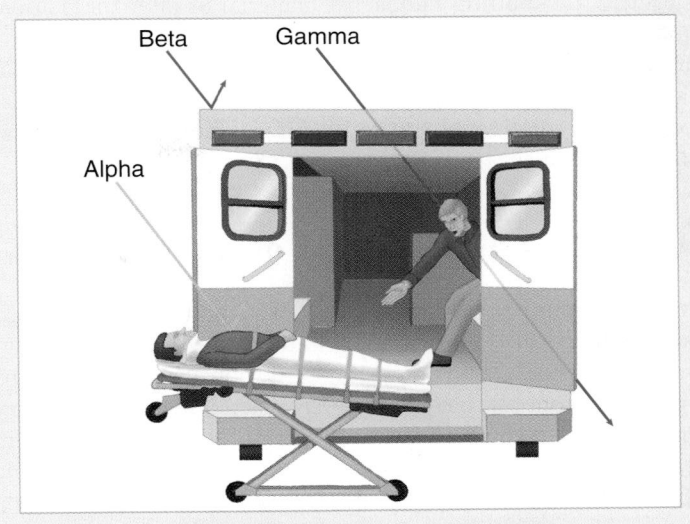

Figure 20-12 Alpha, beta, and gamma radiation shielding.

Radiation is measured in units of radiation absorbed dose (rad) or radiation equivalent in man (rem): 100 rad = 1 gray (Gy). Small amounts of everyday background radiation are measured in rad; the amount of radiation released in a major incident may be measured in gray. The average human exposure from background radiation is 0.36 rem per year. Mild radiation sickness can be expected with exposures of 1 to 2 Gy (100 to 200 rad), moderate sickness at 2 to 5 Gy, and severe sickness at 4 to 6 Gy. Exposure to more than 8 Gy is immediately fatal.

The vast majority of ionizing radiation accidents involve gamma radiation, or x-rays. People who have suffered a radiation exposure generally pose no risk to the people around them. However, in some types of incidents—particularly those involving explosions—patients may be contaminated with radioactive particulate matter. It is speculated that after a nuclear explosion, most patients will have sustained some type of trauma in addition to the radiation exposure.

Acute Radiation Syndrome

Acute radiation syndrome causes hematologic, central nervous system, and gastrointestinal changes. Many of these changes occur over time and so will not be apparent during contact with EMS providers. Patients who are rendered unconscious by radiation or who manifest vomiting within 10 minutes of exposure will not survive. Those who manifest vomiting in less than an hour have severe exposure and 30% to 80% survival rate. Many people with moderate exposure will vomit within 1 to 2 hours and have a 95% to 100% survival rate. Clearly, the onset of vomiting soon after exposure is a predictor of poor outcomes. Consider this fact when triaging patients or considering the risks of entering a high-radiation environment to attempt rescue.

Radiation Contact Burns

A person who handles a radioactive source briefly may sustain a local soft-tissue injury without a lot of total body irradiation. This scenario might arise, for example, in a collision involving a vehicle transporting radioactive material or after the detonation of a "dirty bomb." The injury could resemble anything from superficial sunburn to a chemical burn. Although chemical burns usually become apparent almost immediately after exposure, radiation burns could appear hours or even days after exposure.

General Assessment of Burns

Burns can fool paramedics, because we expect critically injured patients to act sick. Most severely injured and dying cardiac and trauma patients are hypotensive, unresponsive, or in obvious distress. In contrast, patients with an isolated severe burn injury may walk up to you on a scene. The chief complaint may be "I'm terribly cold," and the severity of the injuries may not become apparent until you complete your assessment and realize that the person fits criteria for transfer to a burn center. Many paramedics have been surprised to find that the moderately burned patient they delivered to the hospital was intubated and transferred to a burn center within a few hours of arrival.

In other cases, burns may occur in remote locations, and you may not meet the patient until hours after the traumatic burn event. Such patients may present with an entirely different spectrum of problems than you are used to dealing with. Sometimes the patient doesn't realize the ramifications of a burn injury until hours later. Some patients will have additional traumatic injuries from falling debris, explosions, or their attempts to get away from the source of the burn. Seriously burned patients may need to be transferred from tertiary facilities to larger burn centers, and you may need to deal with complex issues such as an escharotomy, a surgical cut through the burned tissue to allow swelling, and advanced fluid management during the transport.

The many types of burns, coupled with the many possible presentations of burn patients, can challenge your assessment skills. As with any trauma patient, it is important to address burned patients in a consistent, efficient, and systematic manner so you don't develop tunnel vision for the major burn trauma and miss other occult injuries that could affect the patient's outcome.

Scene Size-up

Should you run into a burning building to save a patient? Not if you are not a trained and properly equipped fire fighter. Be wary of entering closed spaces if you see evidence of a recent fire. Toxic gases are often present, even if the fire is out. Never enter a burning building—there is the danger of flashover, when the contents of a room rise in temperature to the point where they all ignite at once. Remember also that plastics contain cyanide, which may be released when they burn.

With modern building construction, be concerned about structural damage to the building. Burning (or recently burned) buildings are notoriously dangerous places; the floors, roofs, beams, and walls may collapse at any time. Electrical wires, gas lines, and plumbing and heating systems can be

unstable and dangerous. Look for placards indicating hazardous materials or other signs that hazardous materials may be present. Never enter an area that may contain hazardous materials—only properly trained and protected personnel should enter such areas.

Safety is a primary concern whenever you are operating near a fire scene. Stage yourself and others in a place where it is safe to provide patient care—this distancing allows you to stay far enough from the scene to keep a global focus. Remember that your role may include treating victims of the fire and providing rehabilitation for fire fighters and other emergency personnel. When EMS providers are too close to the hot zone, it is detrimental to their own safety, the care they provide, and the overall medical response to the situation.

When a recently burned patient comes before you, your initial actions must include extinguishing the flame and cooling the burn. That step may seem obvious, but it is remarkable how many patients arrive by ambulance at hospital emergency departments with clothes still smoldering. A person whose clothing is on fire should not be permitted to run because running fans the flames; nor should the person remain standing because inhaling flame and igniting hair are more likely in the upright position. Rather, have the patient stop, drop to the ground, and roll. If the patient cannot roll, lower the patient to the ground, cover with a blanket, and pat the fire out.

Remove all smoldering clothing and any articles that may retain heat. Watchbands, zippers, and rings not only can retain enough heat to continue burning the patient, but also can melt through your gloves and burn you as well. Make sure that any jewelry on a patient has been cooled appropriately. If the person's hands are burned, they will swell considerably and rings may become tourniquets if not removed quickly enough. If bits of smoldering cloth adhere to the skin, do not pull them off, but rather

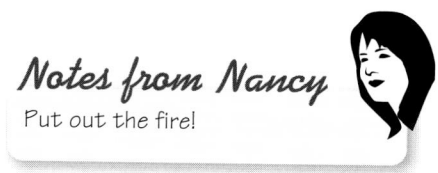

Notes from Nancy
Put out the fire!

cut them away. Let burn center or hospital personnel deal with materials that are melted to the flesh.

If possible, determine the mechanism of injury. As mentioned earlier, patients who have been burned also often have sustained other trauma. Consider and examine other mechanisms associated with the burn: Did the patient jump from a high window to escape flames? Does the patient have musculoskeletal trauma from tetanic spasms after an electrical burn? Was the patient trapped in an enclosed space? Did the patient lose consciousness?

As a part of your scene size-up, do not forget to wear the most appropriate personal protective equipment, perhaps including gloves and a combination mask/eye shield. The burned patient may be "leaking" body fluids and is highly susceptible to infection. Use the most appropriate body substance isolation precautions to ensure that you are not exposed and the patient is not exposed to you!

Initial Assessment

As you approach a burn trauma patient, simple clues may help identify how serious the injuries are and how quickly you need to assess and treat the patient. If the patient greets you with a hoarse voice and a chief complaint of "trouble breathing," your general impression might be that the patient has a potential airway and/or breathing problem. In the absence of hypoxia or other trauma, a patient with a severe burn may be conscious and is often able to hold a conversation. Although burns are often painful, the more serious burns may present with little or no pain. Indeed, the chief complaint is often "I'm cold." What may first appear to be tattered clothing could turn out to be sheets of the patient's own skin hanging from his burned limbs. Recently burned patients may appear dazed or disconnected from events around them.

Despite what the injuries may look or smell like, you must use compassion when approaching the patient. Burns are obviously traumatic for the patient; if the person survives, he or she may face significant hospitalization and years of rehabilitation. But burns are also traumatic for you, the provider. Focusing on the basic principles of emergency care—the ABCs—can help you perform properly in this chaotic situation.

Evaluate Mental Status

Patients with a burn injury may demonstrate varied mental status responses. Combative patients should be considered hypoxic until proven otherwise. Because partial-thickness burns are extremely painful, a patient with this type of injury may be awake and in pain. Even patients with excessive burns will often be awake and attempting to communicate. Isolated burns do not cause unconsciousness (although toxic inhalations can). Unresponsive burn patients must be carefully assessed for the presence of other deadly injuries.

Ensure an Open Airway

As in any other seriously ill or injured patient, airway management is a priority in a patient with a burn. The airway may be in particular jeopardy because the same heat and flames that caused the external burn may have produced potentially life-threatening damage to the airway.

Although rare, laryngeal edema can develop with alarming speed in burn patients, especially in infants and children. Early endotracheal intubation—before the airway has closed off—could be lifesaving in such cases and should be performed by the most experienced paramedic on your team. To intervene early, however, you need to spot the problem early. Airway management is discussed in greater detail later in this chapter.

Assess for Adequate Breathing

Listen to lung sounds, with special attention to stridor, which may be a sign of impending upper airway compromise. Note that patients with preexisting lung disease may have bronchospasm after even relatively minor exposure to smoke; they may respond well to inhaled beta-2 agonists.

Anyone suspected of having a burn to the upper airway may benefit from humidified, cool oxygen. If you do not carry a high-output humidifier (a "bubble humidifier" is *not* a high-output humidifier), consider using an aerosol nebulizer to administer nebulized normal saline. This approach will not provide a high concentration of oxygen, so you will need to balance the need for a high O_2 concentration against the desire for cool humidity. Keep in mind that the patient's oxygen saturation may be suspect if there is the possibility of CO intoxication.

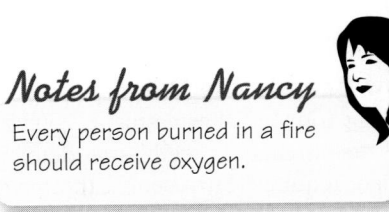

Notes from Nancy

Every person burned in a fire should receive oxygen.

Ensure Adequate Circulation

During the first 24 to 48 hours of a patient's burn care, a great deal of emphasis is placed on fluid resuscitation to prevent burn shock. Burn shock is caused by fluid shifts that typically occur 6 to 8 hours after the burn. Severely burned patients will ultimately require large volumes of fluid, but they don't need it during the first minutes of prehospital care unless their burn injury occurred some time ago. Most patients will ultimately require central venous access, and most intravenous (IV) lines placed in the prehospital setting will be removed owing to tissue swelling and infection risk. If the patient is not grossly hypotensive, do not delay transport by making multiple attempts at vascular access. Of course, if the patient has an obvious peripheral vessel, your early vascular access will be put to good use by hospital or burn center staff for fluid replacement and pain management.

Patients with other trauma may require immediate vascular access just like any other trauma patient. Although it is preferable to avoid starting IV lines through burned tissue, it isn't frankly contraindicated. Burn patients may challenge your vascular access skills. New options for intraosseous access may provide you with more choices than were available to your predecessors.

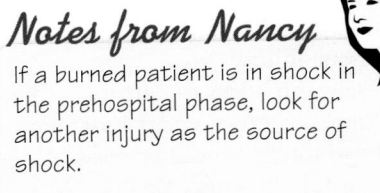

Notes from Nancy

If a burned patient is in shock in the prehospital phase, look for another injury as the source of shock.

Burn Severity

The burn wound is categorized by the degree of injury. Historically, such an injury has been described by three pathologic progressions or zones, which radiate from the central zone of greatest damage. Skin nearest the heat source suffers the most profound cellular changes. The central area of the skin, which suffers the most damage, is called the zone of coagulation. There is little or no blood flow to the injured tissue in this area. The peripheral area surrounding the zone of coagulation has decreased blood flow and inflammation; it is known as the zone of stasis. This area may undergo necrosis within 24 to

48 hours after the injury, particularly if perfusion is compromised by burn shock. Last, the zone of hyperemia is the area least affected by the thermal injury. In this area, cells will typically recover in 7 to 10 days.

How Deep Is the Burn?

During your initial assessment, your goal is to identify and manage life threats, as well as to determine the level of care the patient requires (burn center, trauma center, local hospital). This means you will need to get an idea of the burn's size and severity to report to the receiving facility. The nature of the patient's burns will evolve during the next 24 hours, and estimations of their size and severity will inevitably change, so little is to be gained by conducting a comprehensive and time-consuming evaluation of every inch of the patient's body in the field. Nevertheless, a reasonably accurate estimation of the scope of the patient's injuries is helpful for determining the appropriate care.

The traditional labels given to burns were first, second, and third degree. Many centers have expanded that concept, describing burns as fourth, fifth, and sixth degree as tissue destruction goes into the deeper tissues, muscle, and bone. Paramedics should limit their assessment to partial- versus full-thickness burns (described later) to simplify the process and avoid confusion and miscommunication. Multiple providers may disagree on the extent of a given burn in the field, and reaching a consensus isn't important enough to justify spending time on the discussion. The hospital staff need to know, for example, that they are getting an x-year old male with approximately x% full-thickness and x% mixed partial-thickness burns with possible airway decompensation.

Quickly assess the burns while considering the presence or absence of pain, swelling, skin color, capillary refill time, moisture and blisters, the appearance of the wound edges, the presence of foreign bodies, debris and contaminants, bleeding, and circulatory adequacy. Make sure you assess for concomitant soft-tissue injury.

Determination of burn depth is a subjective assessment that depends on provider judgment. Based on this assessment, the burn injury should be classified as superficial, partial thickness, or full thickness Figure 20-13 ▸ .

A superficial burn (first-degree burn) involves the epidermis only. The skin is red and, when touched, the color will blanch and return. Usually blisters are not present. Patients will experience pain because nerve endings are exposed to the air. Such a burn will heal spontaneously in 3 to 7 days. The most common example is a sunburn.

A partial-thickness burn (second-degree burn) involves the epidermis and varying degrees of the dermis. This category can be subdivided into superficial partial-thickness and deep partial-thickness burns. With a *superficial partial-thickness burn,* the skin is red; when touched, the color will blanch and return. Usually there are blisters or moisture present, and the patient may experience extreme pain. Hair follicles remain intact. A superficial partial-thickness burn will heal spontaneously but may scar or have a changed appearance. In contrast, a *deep partial-thickness*

burn extends into the dermis, damaging the hair follicle and sweat and sebaceous glands. Hot liquids, steam, or grease are often to blame for these injuries. In the out-of-hospital setting, the delineation between deep partial thickness and full thickness may be difficult to determine.

A full-thickness burn (third-degree burn) involves destruction of both layers of the skin, including the basement membrane of dermis that produces new skin cells. In such an injury, the skin is white and pale, brown and leathery, or charred. Dry and leathery skin is referred to as eschar. No capillary refill occurs with this type of burn because the capillaries have been destroyed. Sensory nerves are destroyed as well, so there may be no pain in the full-thickness section. Because patients usually have mixed depths of burns, they will often experience significant pain in the areas surrounding the full-thickness burns. Treatment of a full-thickness burn will usually require skin grafting because the dermis has been destroyed.

How Much Surface Area Is Burned?

While evaluating the patient's burns, you must approximate the total body surface area (TBSA) burned. Most practitioners advocate counting only the areas of partial- and full-thickness burns (ignoring the areas of superficial burns). The most universal mechanism of calculating the area burned is the rule of nines, which is based on dividing the body into 9% segments. The provider adds the portions of the body to obtain a total of the body area affected by the burn injury. Because our proportions change as we grow, different rules of nines apply to infants, children, and adults Figure 20-14 ▸ .

Another mechanism of assessing the TBSA is the rule of palm. This assessment uses the size of the patient's palm (excluding the fingers) to represent about 1% of the patient's body surface area. This calculation is helpful when the burn covers less than 10% of the body surface area or is irregularly shaped. The Lund and Browder chart is an even more specific method used to estimate the burned area by dividing the body into even smaller and more specific regions Figure 20-15 ▸ .

You must balance the need for accuracy against the time required to make an estimate of the TBSA. The out-of-hospital estimation is used to guide the patient to the correct place for treatment. The ED estimation of burned area may be used to initiate fluid therapy. The burn center's estimation of injured area will undoubtedly be more accurate and specific.

Focused History and Physical Exam

With burn patients, proceed through the steps of physical assessment in the usual sequence, starting with the general appearance and moving on to the vital signs. Obtaining vital signs may be challenging if the patient has extensive burns on the arms. Nevertheless, you should try to document vital signs accurately because the management of shock, airway compromise, and pain control depends on them to some degree.

When you have finished your brief inspection of the patient's skin, you have only just begun the head-to-toe exam. The detailed physical exam is intended to make sure that no

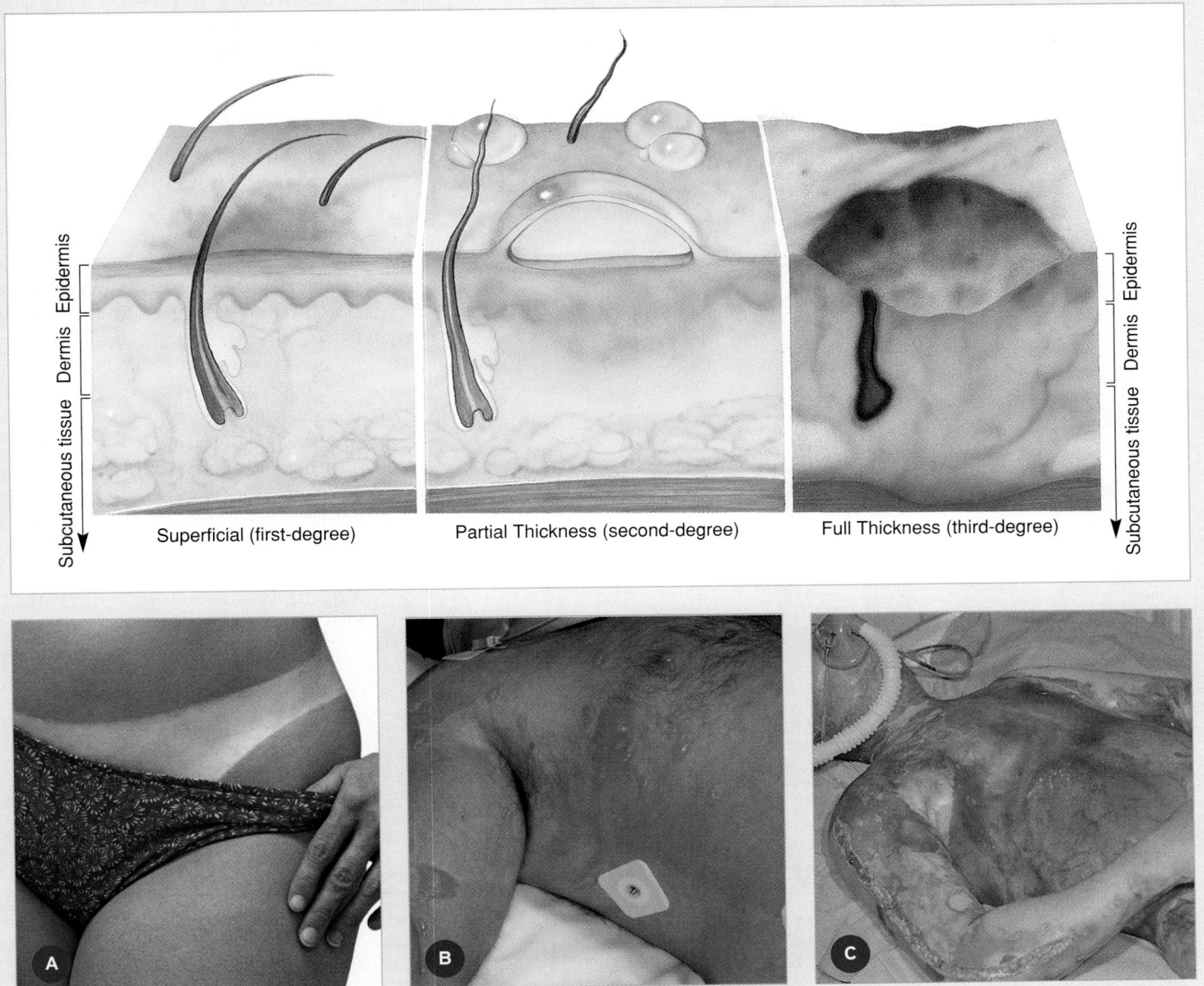

Epidermis / Dermis / Subcutaneous tissue

Superficial (first-degree)   Partial Thickness (second-degree)   Full Thickness (third-degree)

Epidermis / Dermis / Subcutaneous tissue

A   **B**   **C**

Figure 20-13 Classification of burns. **A.** Superficial (first-degree) burns involve only the epidermis. **B.** Partial-thickness (second-degree) burns involve some of the dermis but do not destroy the entire thickness of the skin. The skin is mottled, white to red, and often blistered. **C.** Full-thickness (third-degree) burns extend through all layers of the skin and may involve subcutaneous tissue and muscle. The skin is dry, leathery, and often white or charred.

other injuries have higher priority for treatment. Often such injuries may be obscured by the burn itself, so you need to pay attention to the circumstances of the burn and the possible mechanisms of injury. If the patient jumped from a second-story window, for example, there may be fractures beneath the obvious burns on the legs.

Look for injuries to the eyes, and cover injured eyes with moist, sterile pads. Check the neck, chest, and extremities for <u>circumferential burns</u>. Progressive edema beneath a

In the Field

Signs and symptoms of vascular compromise in a burned extremity that may necessitate an escharotomy include cyanosis, pallor, deep tissue pain, progressive paresthesia, progressive decrease or absence of the pulse, or sensation of a cold extremity.

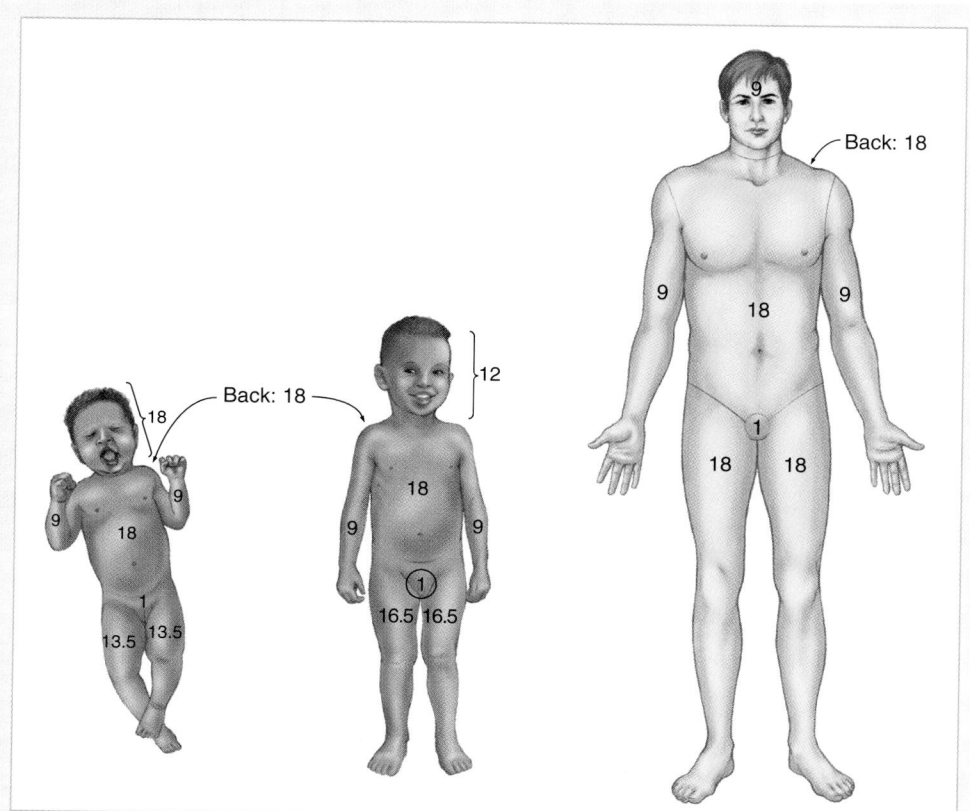

circumferential burn—especially when the burned skin has become leathery and unyielding—may act as a tourniquet. In the neck, a circumferential burn may obstruct the airway; in the chest, it may restrict respiratory excursion; and in an extremity, it may cut off the circulation and put the extremity in jeopardy. Patients with circumferential burns must reach a medical facility quickly because it may be necessary to make an incision into the burned area to decompress it. Check and document the distal pulses in burned extremities often.

To the degree possible, get a brief history from the patient. Patients with preexisting diseases, such as chronic obstructive pulmonary disease or acute coronary syndromes, may be triaged as critical burns even if the burn injury is small. As in any other trauma, allergies, medications, and other pertinent medical history may influence the patient's care plan.

Figure 20-14 The rule of nines is a quick way to estimate the amount of surface area that has been burned. It divides the body into sections, each representing approximately 9% of the total body surface area. The proportions differ for infants, children, and adults.

You are the Provider Part 2

You immediately begin treating your patient, who tells you her name is Pamela. When you ask what happened, the patient says that she was playing with gasoline and matches with her older brother (who escaped the house unharmed and now is with police officers). As she reached to light a pile of gasoline-soaked rags, the vapors flashed, and she burned her right arm. She is able to talk without difficulty, and there is no indication of burns to her face or airway. She has no other apparent injuries.

By using the rule of palm, you estimate the size of Pamela's burn to be approximately 4% to 5% involving her right arm and hand. You administer supplemental oxygen. Your partner initiates an IV line in the unburned arm while you irrigate the area with cool, sterile saline and assess the right arm. Pulse and motor and sensory functions are present.

Vital Signs	Recording Time: 5 Minutes
Level of consciousness	Alert, with a Glasgow Coma Scale score of 15
Skin	Warm, pink, dry with some soot on skin and clothing
Pulse	Radial pulse, 120 beats/min, strong and regular
Blood pressure	116 by palpation
Respirations	36 to 42 breaths/min, clear and equal breath sounds bilaterally
Sao_2	100% while breathing room air

3. Why is pulse oximetry unreliable in these circumstances?

4. Are your transport considerations affected by the location of her burn?

5. What are common complications of burns?

Region	%
Head	
Neck	
Ant. Trunk	
Post. Trunk	
Right arm	
Left arm	
Buttocks	
Genitalia	
Right leg	
Left leg	
Total burn	

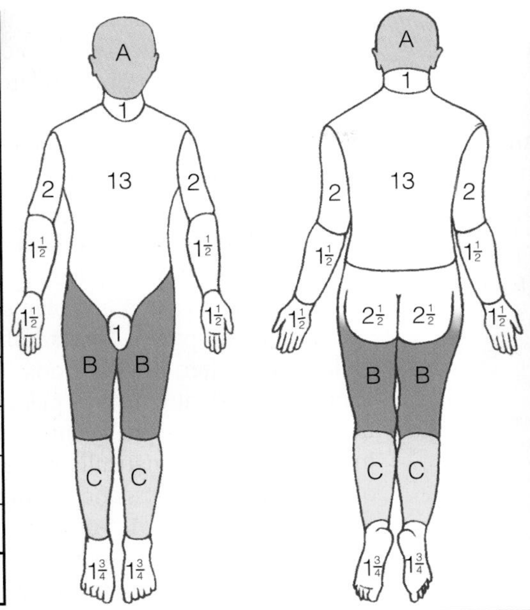

Relative percentages of body surface area affected by growth

Age (years)	A ($\frac{1}{2}$ of head)	B ($\frac{1}{2}$ of one thigh)	C ($\frac{1}{2}$ of one leg)
0	$9\frac{1}{2}$	$2\frac{3}{4}$	$2\frac{1}{2}$
1	$8\frac{1}{2}$	$3\frac{1}{4}$	$2\frac{1}{2}$
5	$6\frac{1}{2}$	4	$2\frac{3}{4}$
10	$5\frac{1}{2}$	$4\frac{1}{4}$	3
15	$4\frac{1}{2}$	$4\frac{1}{2}$	$3\frac{1}{4}$
Adult	$3\frac{1}{2}$	$4\frac{3}{4}$	3

Figure 20-15 The Lund and Browder chart.

In the Field

Heat loss is a critical problem for burn patients. Take immediate steps to prevent hypothermia, such as heating the ambulance until it's uncomfortable for the crew and using warm blankets and fluids.

Detailed Physical Exam and Ongoing Assessment

If the patient is considered to have a significant mechanism of injury, en route to the ED, you should perform a detailed physical exam and the ongoing assessment (see Chapters 13 and 14). Reassessment of vital signs to establish trends is done every 5 minutes for critical patients and every 15 minutes for lower priority patients (in stable condition).

Assessment of Radiation Burns

First and foremost, the assessment of a patient who may have been exposed to radiation involves a scene size-up to determine if the scene is safe for rescuers to enter. In some cases, it may be appropriate to contact the hazardous materials response team so they may determine the appropriate precautions, including exposure-limiting suits, and the most appropriate ED for the patient's treatment. Not all EDs are set up to handle a patient who has been exposed to radiation, so learn the capabilities of your hospitals before an incident occurs! EMS agencies that operate in an area where there is a nuclear power plant or other research facility typically have additional training offered by the facility and regularly practice responding to radiation-related emergencies.

Once the scene is deemed safe, you may proceed with your initial assessment of the patient. Assess the patient's mental status and ABCs, and then prioritize the patient's care. Unfortunately, patients who have sustained a significant radiation exposure and a major burn are unlikely to survive, even with major resources expended to keep them alive (a burn of > 70% of the TBSA is probably fatal by itself; a burn and radiation of > 30% of the TBSA are probably fatal). When confronted with large numbers of patients who have been exposed to radiation and simultaneously received thermal burns, keep the 30% rule in mind when triaging and making transport decisions. Of course, you should also consult with medical control in these complicated cases. In the field, it is difficult to determine the extent of the patient's internal injuries because radiation can "cook from the inside out" (like the microwave ovens we are all too familiar with).

Management of Burns

Definitive burn care can be divided into four phases. While paramedics will be most heavily involved in the first phase, it is important to appreciate the magnitude of care that a patient with a severe, or even moderate, burn must receive. Early actions of the paramedic may dramatically affect the patient's long-term outcome. Paramedics may also find themselves transporting patients to specialty or rehabilitation facilities at later stages of their care.

Unlike many emergencies you will encounter, burn patient care is measured in weeks, not hours. Burns are devastating multisystem traumatic injuries that dramatically alter a person's life. You should recognize not only the massive physical trauma caused by burns, but also the emotional, psychological, and financial burdens these horrific injuries impose. Once these costs are appreciated, it is easy to understand the importance of teaching injury prevention strategies to the people we serve.

General Management

Management of a burned patient begins with the steps taken during the scene size-up and initial assessment to extinguish the fire and ensure adequate ABCs. Only when the ABCs are under control should you turn your attention to the burn itself. It is important to have all resuscitative equipment ready for use when treating a burn patient, including advanced airway equipment and heart monitors.

Immediate Management

Stop the burning. When a person burns a hand on a hot oven rack at 450°F, the person will usually stick the hand under cool running water for a few seconds. Is that long enough to cool the tissues and stop the burning? Usually not. It often takes several minutes to completely cool the burned area and achieve some pain relief. The fire needs to be put out, and the burned areas need to be cooled. All jewelry, metal buttons, zippers, and hooks should be cool to the touch as well. Of course, never use ice on a burn.

After cooling the burns, *keep the patient warm.* This seems like a contradiction, because it is. The trick is to put out the fire without making the patient hypothermic. Remember, people with large burned areas have lost their primary mechanism for thermoregulation. Keep the patient covered and move him or her into the ambulance as soon as possible to minimize hypothermic stress.

Don't forget other injuries. If the patient is at risk for spinal trauma from a fall or explosion, address this injury the same way you would in any other trauma patient. The same is true for gross bleeding and other traumatic injuries. Burns can also exacerbate a patient's underlying medical conditions, such as chronic obstructive pulmonary disease, asthma, and cardiac conditions. Follow the same priorities for these emergencies as you would for any other patient.

Airway Management

Many burn patients will ultimately require intubation, even though they were talking to you and in no distress in the field. Although it is obviously preferable to have such patients intubated in a controlled environment with a full complement of anesthesia agents, a few patients will absolutely require an emergency advanced airway in the field. Burn patients fall into four general categories for airway management.

1. **The patient with an acutely decompensating airway who requires field intubation.** This group includes burn patients who are in cardiac or respiratory arrest and conscious patients whose airways are swelling before your eyes. In these chaotic and difficult situations, you need to plan for the possibility that you cannot intubate. Supraglottic swelling or complete obstruction can occur in some burn scenarios. Surgical airways or rescue devices may be necessary if intubation is not possible and bag-mask ventilation fails.

2. **The patient with a deteriorating airway from burns and toxic inhalations who might require intubation.** It is obviously better for the patient to defer treatment of this airway problem to hospital teams with anesthesia, surgery, specialized equipment, and a fully stocked pharmacy. Patients will often be conscious and may become combative with attempts to place them supine, let alone intubate them. "Awake" techniques, such as nasal intubation, are dramatically more complicated in victims of upper airway burns and should be avoided. Attempt to intubate only if left with no other choice. If the patient's airway continues to swell and intubation will become impossible if you wait for arrival at the hospital, you have little choice but to attempt intubation. Try to consult medical control for advice.

Intubation of an awake, scared patient in the field is difficult, and considerable damage may be inflicted on the airway if the patient continues to struggle. If intubation becomes necessary under such circumstances, explain carefully to the patient what is to be done, why it is necessary, and how he or she can best cooperate. Have all equipment set up at your side so that intubation, once begun, can proceed rapidly and smoothly. Serious consideration should be made toward performing rapid-sequence intubation if you have been trained in this procedure, carry the appropriate medications, and have medical control authorization. The procedure for rapid-sequence intubation is discussed in Chapter 11. It is also advised that the "most experienced" intubator perform this procedure because the swelling can make for a difficult intubation.

An airway compromised by advancing edema represents another classic scenario in which administering a neuromuscular blocker to provide respiratory paralysis may be extremely dangerous. It places the paramedic in the dangerous position of having a patient with no gag reflex or ability to breathe and an airway you may be unable to control.

The choice of endotracheal (ET) tube may present another conundrum. It would obviously be beneficial to use the largest tube possible. Sometimes the ET tube will clog with soot from the patient's airway, causing complete occlusion. At the same time, a smaller than usual ET tube may be necessary owing to airway edema. Select the largest ET tube that will not cause additional trauma during insertion. Never cut the ET tube down to make it shorter.

Edema of the face can actually cause ET tube dislodgment on postburn day 2 or 3.

3. **The patient whose airway is currently patent but who has a history consistent with risk factors for eventual airway compromise.** Cool, humidified oxygen from a high-output nebulizer (not a bubble humidifier) is appropriate. Alternatively, you may use an aerosol nebulizer with saline. The patient will probably *not* require acute interventions in the field, but make sure you report the patient's history to hospital personnel. Many patients will ultimately undergo elective intubation.

4. **The patient with no signs of or risk factors for airway compromise who is in no distress.** It is reasonable to provide supplemental oxygen to burn patients, even if they are not in distress. It is safe to oxygenate until you are comfortable with the situation surrounding the burn and have completed a full assessment.

Fluid Resuscitation

An IV line may be inserted in the field to administer fluids and/or pain medications. A large-bore IV catheter should be inserted as early as possible in any patient who has been severely burned. Do not delay transport to do so, but try to get a large-bore IV catheter into a large vein, and give lactated Ringer's solution or normal saline. You can use the burned extremity for the IV site if you cannot find another site—an IV line in a burned upper extremity is still preferable to an IV line in a lower extremity.

Approximate the amount of fluid the burned patient will need by using the Parkland formula, which states that *during the first 24 hours,* the burned patient will need:

4 mL × body weight (in kg) × percentage of body surface burned

Half of that amount needs to be given during the first 8 hours. For example, if a 70-kg man has sustained burns to 30% of his body, his fluid needs during the first 24 hours will be:

4 mL × 70 kg × 30 = 8,400 mL

Half of the 8,400 mL—that is, 4,200 mL—should be administered during the first 8 hours.

As aggressive as the Parkland formula may seem, current trends actually lean toward delivering *more* fluid than the Parkland formula indicates **Table 20-2 ▾**. Of course, you do not need to attempt to deliver the entire initial amount in the field. Most seriously burned patients will need central venous access, and IV lines placed in the prehospital setting will most often be lost as peripheral swelling begins.

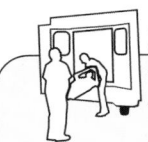

In the Field

The adequacy of resuscitation is based on monitoring the vital signs, the patient's mentation, and the urine output.

Pain Management

With any patient with burns, you should provide aggressive pain management. Assess the patient's pain before administering any analgesia. Reassessment should be completed using the same scale (for example, 1 to 10) every 5 minutes.

Burn patients may require higher than usual doses of pain medications to achieve relief. Their metabolism rates are accelerated, which creates the need for higher than normal doses of analgesics. Consult your protocols or contact medical control for guidance in administering analgesics.

Table 20-2	Parkland Formula Chart									
% Burn	10 kg	20 kg	30 kg	40 kg	50 kg	60 kg	70 kg	80 kg	90 kg	100 kg
10	25	50	75	100	125	150	175	200	225	250
20	50	100	150	200	250	300	350	400	450	500
30	75	150	225	300	375	450	525	600	675	750
40	100	200	300	400	500	600	700	800	900	1,000
50	125	250	375	500	625	750	875	1,000	1,125	1,250
60	150	300	450	600	750	900	1,050	1,200	1,350	1,500
70	175	350	525	700	875	1,050	1,225	1,400	1,575	1,750
80	200	400	600	800	1,000	1,200	1,400	1,600	1,800	2,000
90	225	450	675	900	1,125	1,350	1,575	1,800	2,025	2,250
20 mL/kg	200	400	600	800	1,000	1,200	1,400	1,600	1,800	2,000

This table represents the fluid recommended in the *first hour* (⅛ of the initial 8-hour dose) by the Parkland formula. The final row represents the amount of a 20-mL/kg bolus.

Management of Superficial Burns

Although superficial burns can be very painful, they rarely pose a threat to life unless they involve nearly the entire surface of the body. If you reach a patient with superficial burns within the first hour after the injury occurred, immerse the burned area in cool water or apply cold compresses to the burn. Burned hands or feet may be soaked directly in cool water; and towels soaked in cold water may be applied to burns of the face or trunk.

The objectives of this exercise are twofold: stop the burning process and relieve pain. Commercial products are available that meet both objectives Figure 20-16 ▶ . However you cool the burn, take care not to cool the whole body—don't let the patient become chilled. A dry sheet or blanket applied over the wet dressings will help prevent systemic heat loss.

Do not use salves, ointments, creams, sprays, or any similar materials on any type of burn. They will just have to be scrubbed off in the ED or burn unit, causing the patient further pain. Never apply ice to burns because it can exacerbate the tissue injury.

No further treatment should be necessary in the field for an uncomplicated, superficial burn. Simply transport the patient in a comfortable position to the hospital.

Management of Partial-Thickness Burns

Treatment of partial-thickness burns in the field is similar to that of superficial burns. Cooling the burned area with water or application of wet or Water-Jel dressings within the first

In the Field

Pain medication is best given via the IV route. Owing to changes in fluid volume and tissue blood flow, absorption of any intramuscular or subcutaneous drug is unpredictable. Accurately measure and assess the patient's pain, and continuously monitor response to pain medication.

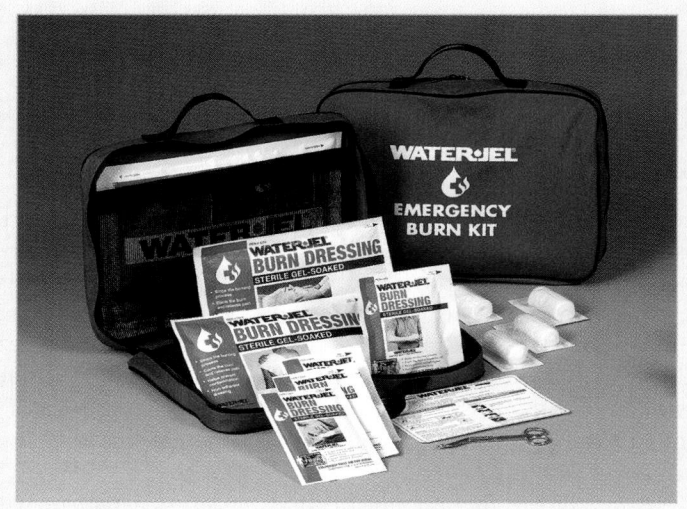

Figure 20-16 Burn dressing (Water-Jel) kits.

You are the Provider Part 3

As you are en route to the appropriate facility, your partner works with the local police department in an attempt to contact the patient's parents. One relative is found—the patient's grandmother, who consents to Pamela's treatment and transport and adds that she is a normally healthy child with no medications or allergies. You address the patient's pain by providing an analgesic (morphine sulfate, 3.5 mg via slow IV push), elevate her arm with pillows, cover her with a blanket, and place her in a comfortable position. You also reassess the affected extremity for the presence of pulse and motor and sensory functions throughout transport.

Reassessment	Recording Time: 10 Minutes
Level of consciousness	Alert, with a Glasgow Coma Scale score of 15
Skin	Warm, pink, and dry
Pulse	Radial pulse, 118 beats/min, strong and regular
Blood pressure	116 by palpation
Respirations	28 to 36 breaths/min
Sao_2	100%
Blood glucose	90 mg/dL
ECG	Sinus tachycardia without further ectopy

6. What is appropriate fluid resuscitation for a pediatric patient?
7. Given the nature of burns, what is another important consideration regarding burn care?

hour can diminish edema and provide significant pain relief. Burned extremities should be elevated to minimize edema formation.

Do not attempt to rupture blisters over the burn; they initially act as a physiologic burn dressing. Establish IV fluids with lactated Ringer's solution or normal saline as dictated by local protocol. Pain in partial-thickness burns may be severe, so complete a pain assessment and administer pain medication as allowed by your protocols.

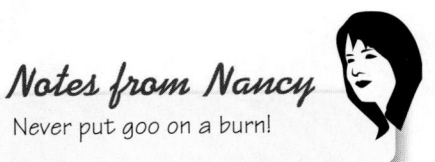

Notes from Nancy

Never put goo on a burn!

Management of Full-Thickness Burns

Although full-thickness burns may not cause pain, most patients will have varying degrees of burns within the affected region of injury. For this reason, a pain assessment should be completed and pain medication should be administered as described earlier. Usually, dry dressings are used after the fire is out. Check with your burn center or medical center on their view on wet dressings or analgesia.

Management of Chemical Burns

Speed is essential when treating chemical burns. Begin flushing the exposed area of the patient's body immediately with copious quantities of water Figure 20-17 . If the patient is in or near the home, the shower or a garden hose is ideal. In an industrial setting, use the decontamination shower or a hose. While flushing, rapidly remove the patient's clothing, especially shoes and socks that may have become contaminated with the offending agent, taking care not to get any of the hazardous chemicals on your own clothing or skin.

Do not waste time looking for specific antidotes; copious flushing with water is more effective and more immediately available Figure 20-18 . Flushing is preferable for 30 minutes before moving the patient; for chemical burns caused by strong alkalis (such as oven and drain cleaners), 1 to 2 *hours* of flushing has been recommended. Paramedics must weigh the realities of flushing on the scene for long periods against the benefits of transport and their ability to continue flushing en route. After flushing, limit hypothermia by keeping the patient covered and warm.

Special Cases of Chemical Burns

If you do not know the identity of the chemical that caused the burn, assume it is *not* a special case, and flush the burn wound with copious water as described.

In alkali burns caused by dry lime, combination with water will produce a highly corrosive substance. For that reason, when a patient has been in contact with dry lime, *first* remove the patient's clothing and *brush* as much lime as you can from the skin (wear gloves!). *Then* start flushing copiously with a garden hose or shower. Your intention is to completely

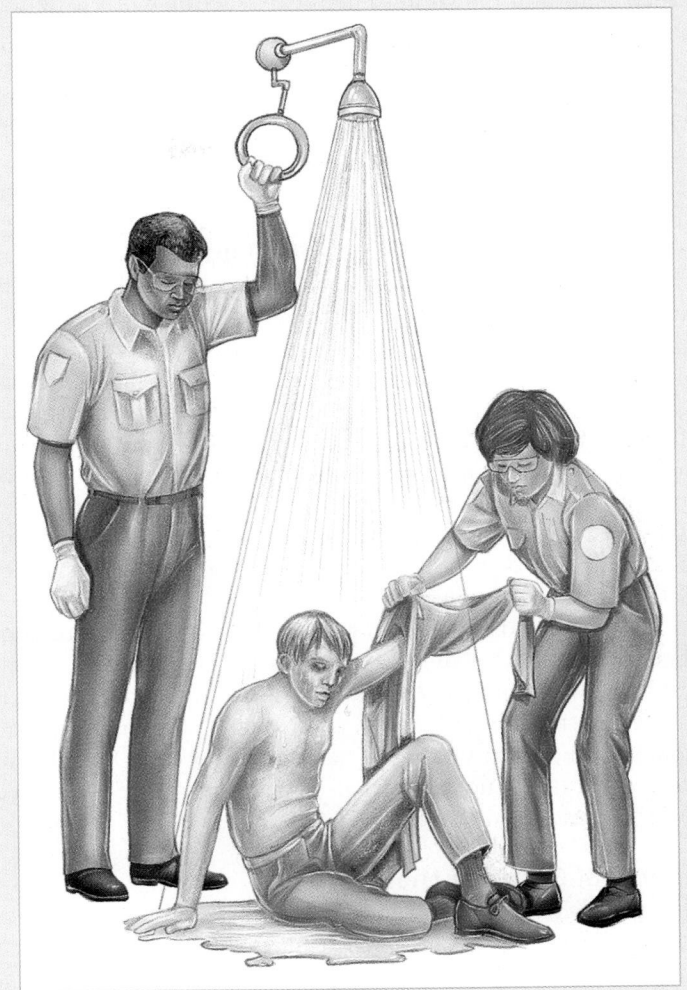

Figure 20-17 Flush the burned area with large amounts of water.

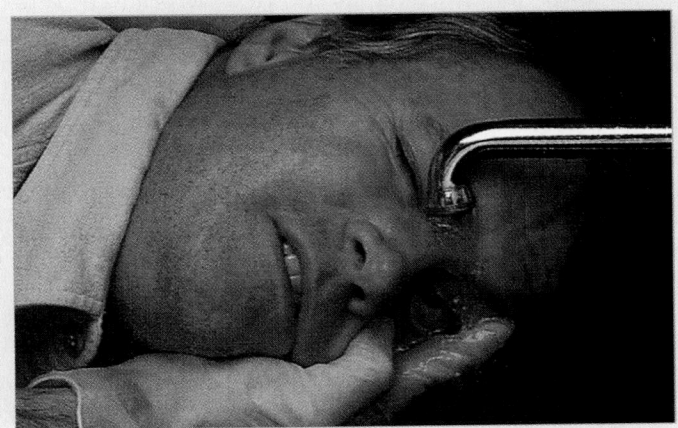

Figure 20-18 Flood the affected eye with a gentle stream of water. Hold the eyelids open—a challenging task because the patient's reflex is to keep the eye shut. Take care to prevent the chemical from getting into the other eye during the flushing.

overwhelm any damaging chemical reaction with a deluge of water.

Sodium metals produce considerable heat when mixed with water and may explode. Cover this type of burn with oil, which will stop the reaction by preventing the sodium from coming in contact with the atmosphere.

Hydrofluoric (HF) acid is used in drain cleaners in the home and for etching glass and plastic in industrial settings. HF acid burns that exceed 3% to 5% of the TBSA can be fatal. The patient will complain bitterly of pain (caused by the HF acid sucking calcium out of the body), and the pain will not improve even with continuous flushing—a sign that the process of tissue destruction is ongoing. Calcium chloride (CaCl) jelly may be available in an industrial setting that uses HF acid; this jelly is placed on small-area HF acid burns (small burns from splashing or pinholes in gloves) to help reduce continued pain and injury. An ampule of CaCl (10 mL of a 10% CaCl solution) can be mixed with a water-based lubricant to make CaCl jelly in an emergency. Medical control may order IV CaCl for HF acid burns.

Hot tar burns are, strictly speaking, thermal burns, not chemical burns, although they tend to be classified with chemical burns. The most important step in the prehospital phase is to immerse the affected area in cold water to dissipate the heat from the tar and speed up the hardening process. Once the tar has cooled, it will not do further damage, and there is no need to try to remove it in the field.

Chemical Burns of the Eye

If chemicals have splashed into the patient's eyes, flush the eyes with copious amounts of water. It may be most expeditious to simply support the patient's head under a faucet or at an eye-wash station, directing a steady stream of lukewarm tap water into the affected eye (Figure 20-18). If the patient wears contact lenses and the stream of water does not flush them out, pause after a minute or two of irrigation to allow the patient to remove the contact lenses—if they remain in place, they will prevent water from reaching the cornea underneath. Be sure to irrigate well underneath the eyelids.

Never use chemical antidotes (such as vinegar or baking soda) in the eyes. Irrigate with water only. After irrigating, patch the patient's eyes with lightly applied dressings and begin transport to the hospital for evaluation.

Eye irrigation is extremely important whenever a chemical has gotten into the eye **Figure 20-19** . It may be uncomfortable and inefficient to attempt to irrigate an eye by prying it open and rinsing with a standard normal saline IV set.

Another option is the Morgan lens, which may makes eye irrigation more comfortable, efficient, and effective. It is essentially a plastic contact lens with IV tubing attached to it, which allows IV fluids to flow directly over the surface of the eye. Ocular anesthetic drops are preferable, but care must be taken when the eye is "numb" to keep the patient from scratching or rubbing it. It is important to keep fluid running through the Morgan lens during insertion and removal. Suc-

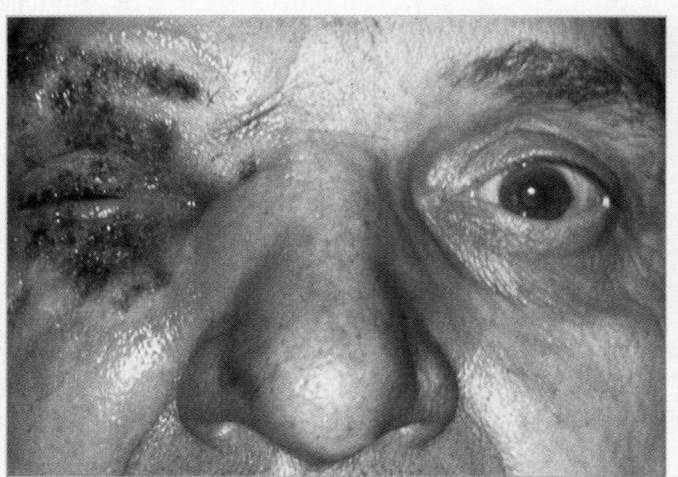

Figure 20-19 The eyes are particularly vulnerable to chemical burns.

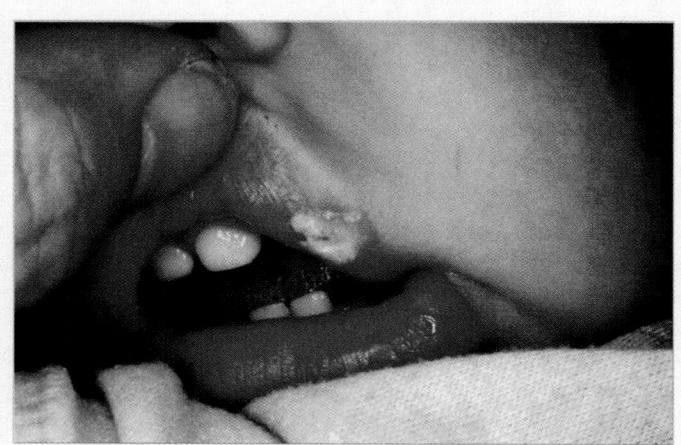

Figure 20-20 Children often sustain electrical burns from chewing on electrical cords.

tion can occur between the lens and the eye if the fluid flow is stopped before removal.

Management of Electrical Burns

One of every five construction deaths is caused by electrical contact. Statistics from the National Institute of Occupational Safety and Health indicate that electrocution is the fifth leading cause of death in the workplace, causing more than 400 deaths per year (more than one per day). Children are involved in the majority of electrocutions in the home **Figure 20-20** .

The first priority at the scene of an electrical injury is to protect yourself and bystanders from becoming the next victims. Do *not* use a rope, wooden pole, or any other object to try to dislodge the patient from the current source. Do *not* try to cut the wire. Do *not* go anywhere near a high-tension line.

Many parts of the electrical grid are protected by automatically resetting breakers. When the wind blows a branch into wires or a rambunctious squirrel bridges the gap between two wires, it is desirable to have the breaker reset after a few moments to avoid power outages. As a consequence, a downed wire that "looks dead" can jump back to life, perhaps several times. There is only one safe way to deal with a downed high-tension wire: Call the electric company. Wait until a qualified person has shut off the power before you approach the patient. This can be a traumatic event for paramedics, who will feel helpless waiting for the power to be shut down while a possibly critical patient lies on the ground nearby. But remember—*rescuers die in these situations.* You can help the greatest number of people by being cautious and safe in this circumstance.

Once the electric hazard has been neutralized, proceed to the ABCs. Open the airway using the jaw-thrust maneuver, keeping in mind the possibility of cervical spine injury. Start CPR as indicated, and attach the monitor to identify ventricular fibrillation. If the patient is not in cardiac arrest, dysrhythmias remain a risk, and cardiac monitoring is indicated for 24 hours after the injury.

Make careful note of the patient's state of consciousness, and record his or her vital signs. Try to determine the path the current has taken through the body by looking for entrance and exit wounds and by carefully palpating the skin and soft tissues. When deep tissues have been seriously damaged by heat, the surrounding muscle may swell and become rock-hard. Thus, a rigid abdomen or rigid extremity may indicate a serious internal injury. Be alert for fractures or dislocations, and check the distal pulses in all four extremities.

Electrical burns may produce devastating internal injuries with little external evidence. The degree of tissue injury is related to the resistance of the body tissues, the intensity of current that passes through the victim, and the duration of exposure.

When a person comes in contact with an electrical source, the amount of current delivered to the inside of the body depends to some extent on the resistance of the skin. Wet, thin, clean skin offers less resistance than dry, thick, dirty skin; thus a moist inner surface of the forearm will have much less resistance than a dry, callused palm.

As electric current travels from the contact site into the body, it is converted to heat, which follows the current flow—usually along blood vessels and nerves—causing extensive damage to the tissues in its path. The greater the current flow, the greater the heat generated. When the voltage is low (< 1,000 volts, as in household sources), current follows the path of least resistance, generally along blood vessels, nerves, and muscles. When the voltage is high (as from high-tension lines), current takes the shortest path.

Alternating current is considerably more dangerous than direct current because the alternations cause repetitive muscle contractions, which may "freeze" the victim to the conductor until the current source is turned off. Furthermore, alternating current is more likely than direct current to induce ventricular fibrillation. The direction of current flow is also significant. Current moving from one hand to the other is particularly dangerous because current may then flow across the heart; a current of only 0.1 amp to the heart can provoke ventricular fibrillation.

Management of an electrical burn injury includes initial assessment focusing on the mental status and ABCs and prioritizing care of the patient. If the patient has life-threatening injuries, begin related care and prepare to transport the patient as soon as practical. Generally, aside from the fluid therapy for the care of a burn injury, no specific pharmacologic interventions are indicated, other than the normal medications used to manage a cardiac dysrhythmia or extreme pain (if authorized by medical control). Early oxygen therapy is helpful, as is managing the patient for impending shock. Transport decisions should be made early and take into consideration the regional resources for the care of a patient with a severe (electrical) burn. Contact medical control for advice in making a transport decision or regarding the need to use aeromedical evacuation directly to the burn center. The patients will be very anxious and scared, so be sure to talk with them calmly and explain what you are doing and how you plan to obtain the best care for them.

Management of Lightning-Related Injuries

When you reach the scene of a lightning strike, all the usual priorities apply, but there are two special considerations to keep in mind.

First, if the electrical storm is still going on, your first priority is to get any patients and rescuers to a safe place, preferably indoors, or at least inside the ambulance. Lightning *can* strike twice in the same place. There is, however, no hazard in touching the victim of a lightning strike—contrary to what your grandmother may have told you, electricity does not remain within the body of a person who has been hit by lightning.

Second, be aware that a lightning strike is apt to injure more than one person. Therefore, the first thing you need to do on arrival at the scene—before you leave the safety of the ambulance—is a rapid size-up of the entire scene to determine the number of patients.

Carry out the initial assessment as usual, and start CPR when necessary. When establishing an airway, bear in mind the possibility of cervical spine injury, and do not hyperextend the neck; use the jaw-thrust maneuver.

Patients with cardiac arrest caused by a lightning strike deserve aggressive, continuing CPR. The chances of a successful resuscitation in such a case are good, even when the patient appears beyond help initially and even when there is a long

Notes from Nancy

In a lightning strike with multiple victims, priority goes to the victims who are not breathing.

delay in the return of spontaneous breathing. Minimize the interruption in compressions, and push hard and fast with full chest recoil!

Treatment of lightning injuries is similar to that of injuries sustained from high-voltage lines:

- Make sure the scene is safe. Move the victim to a safer location if necessary.
- Priority for treatment goes to patients who are not breathing.
- Establish an airway, with cervical spine precautions. Perform CPR as needed.
- Administer supplemental oxygen.
- Monitor cardiac rhythm.
- Insert a large-bore IV catheter and run in normal saline solution wide open to keep the kidneys flushed out.
- Cover any surface burns with dry, sterile dressings.
- Splint fractures.
- If the patient has fallen, immobilize the cervical spine.

Management of Radiation Burns

Patients with radiation burns may be contaminated with radioactive material, so they should be decontaminated before transport. The majority of contaminants can be removed by simply disrobing the patient.

Irrigate open wounds. Washing should be gentle to avoid further damage to the skin, which could result in additional internal radiation absorption. The head and scalp should be irrigated the same way. The ED should be notified as soon as practical if you are transporting a potentially contaminated patient. In contrast with other types of contamination, radioactive particulate matter probably poses a relatively small risk to the rescuer. Consider providing basic care to the patient before decontamination if you are wearing protective clothing.

Radiation injury follows the "inverse square law": Exposure drops exponentially as distance is increased. Increasing your (and your patient's) distance from the source by even a few feet may dramatically decrease your exposure, so it is important to identify the radioactive source and the length of the patient's exposure to it. You must try to limit your duration of exposure, increase your distance from the source, and attempt to place shielding between yourself and sources of gamma radiation.

With contact radiation burns, decontaminate the wound as if it were a chemical burn to remove any radioactive particulate matter. You may then treat it as a burn.

Many radioactive isotopes are used in medicine and industry, some of which can be absorbed or have their toxic effects blunted by another substance. Like their radioactive effects, the toxic effects of these isotopes vary. Antidotes may help bind an isotope, enhance its elimination from the body, or reduce the toxic effects on other organs. Such antidotal therapy should be considered only under the guidance of a knowledgeable physician or public health agency.

Potassium iodide is distributed to people who live near a nuclear power plant and may help protect the thyroid gland if taken within 6 hours of exposure. Contrary to popular belief, however, it is effective only for radionuclides released from fission products from nuclear power plants and would be of little value for exposure to medical radiation.

You are the Provider Part 4

As you arrive at the hospital, the patient seems much more comfortable. She is no longer crying as vigorously and occasionally gives you a glimpse of a smile. The grandmother meets you at the hospital and informs you that Pamela's mother is nowhere to be found. You provide a report including the history of events (including the home situation) to the ED staff.

Reassessment	Recording Time: 20 Minutes
Level of consciousness	Alert, with a Glasgow Coma Scale score of 15
Skin	Warm, pink, and dry
Pulse	Radial pulse, 98 beats/min, strong and regular
Blood pressure	108/58 mm Hg
Respirations	24 breaths/min
Sao$_2$	100%
Temperature	98.6°F (37°C)
ECG	Normal sinus rhythm without ectopy

8. What is burn shock, and how does it relate to the prehospital setting?
9. What other considerations must be made when dealing with a pediatric burn patient?

Management of Burns in Pediatric Patients

Escaping from a fire can be difficult for children. More than half of the fire-related deaths and injuries in children involve preschoolers. Research suggests that young children are not as effectively awakened by smoke detectors, and they are often disoriented immediately after waking. The "reliable waking rate" in children younger than 15 years may be as low as 6%. Young children are also more likely to sustain severe scald injuries. Children's thin skin and delicate respiratory structures are more easily damaged by thermal insults than are those of older children and adults.

In children, fluid resuscitation may be more challenging because of their increased body surface/weight ratio. As a consequence, children may require more fluid per kilogram than adults. You may start with the Parkland formula in children, only to find that medical control orders additional fluids for severe burns. Also, because of poor glycogen stores, children may require dextrose-containing solutions earlier than adults. Blood glucose monitoring should be routinely performed in seriously ill children.

Burns may raise the suspicion of child abuse. Pay careful attention to the mechanism of injury, and relay this information to the hospital staff.

Management of Burns in Geriatric Patients

Approximately 1,200 older adults die of fire-related causes each year, making it the sixth leading cause of death in this population. Some 13% of older adults smoke, and smoking is the leading cause of fires that lead to death of elderly people. Burns from fires caused by smoking while wearing supplementary oxygen are the leading sentinel event in home care. Cooking fires represent another distinct hazard to elderly people, who may be less able to smell a gas leak or a fire in the kitchen. Elderly patients are also particularly sensitive to respiratory insults. Relatively small fires can produce toxic fumes before detection or suppression devices are activated.

Geriatric patients may also have poor glycogen stores, so their blood glucose levels should be checked to assess for hypoglycemia. Cardiac monitoring should, of course, be implemented. Although fluid resuscitation is important, pulmonary edema is more likely to develop in geriatric patients. Routinely assess lung sounds.

Transfer to a Burn Specialty Center

According to the referral criteria identified by the American Burn Association, patients with the following injuries should be transferred to a burn specialty center:
- Partial-thickness burns of more than 10% of the body surface area
- Burns that involve the face, hands, feet, genitalia, perineum, or major joints
- Full-thickness burns in any age group
- Electrical burns, including lightning
- Chemical burns
- Inhalation burns
- Burn injuries in conjunction with preexisting medical conditions that could complicate management, prolong recovery, or affect mortality
- Burns and concomitant trauma in which the burn injury poses the greatest risk of morbidity or mortality
- Burn injury that requires special social, emotional, or long-term rehabilitation

The American Burn Association has also published burn severity classifications:
- **Minor burns**
  - Superficial—body surface area less than 50% (such as sunburns)
  - Partial thickness—body surface area less than 15%
  - Full thickness—body surface area less than 2%
- **Moderate burns**
  - Superficial—body surface area greater than 50%
  - Partial thickness—body surface area less than 30%
  - Full thickness—body surface area less than 10%
- **Critical burns**
  - Partial thickness—body surface area greater than 30%
  - Full thickness—body surface area greater than 10%
  - Inhalation injury
  - Partial- or full-thickness burns involving hands, feet, joints, face, or genitalia

All critical burns should be transported to a specialty burn center.

Consequences of Burns

The Patient

Serious burn injuries are devastating events that leave patients with long-term physical and psychological challenges. People with major injuries average about 1 day of inpatient treatment for each 1% of the TBSA burned. Extensive rehabilitation may also be necessary to regain function. Survivors of serious burns are left with a host of long-term consequences, including problems with thermoregulation, motor function, and sensory function. Although tremendous improvements in the care of critical burn patients have made long-term survival possible for many who would have died of their injuries a decade ago, large surface area burns remain a critical care challenge on par with other forms of severe multisystem trauma.

The Provider

Caring for patients with severe burn emergencies can be one of the most horrifying tasks undertaken by paramedics. Fire scenes are chaotic and dangerous. Patients are often in severe pain. The smell of burned hair and flesh permeates your clothes and equipment. Sheets of tissue may peel off the patient when you perform simple tasks like attempting to take vital signs or moving the patient. Despite the traumatic circumstances, with the proper training and the right mix of confidence and courage, you can make a tremendous impact in the treatment and overall survival of burn patients.

You are the Provider Summary

1. What are your patient care priorities?

Your patient care priorities, after ensuring the safety of the scene, are the ABCs. For fire victims, issues of maintaining a patent airway with good ventilation and oxygenation can present a particular challenge for prehospital providers.

2. What are patient care concerns when dealing with structure fire victims?

Superheated gases and by-products of combustion can cause airway irritation and severe edema. It is essential to act quickly if you believe your patient has inhalation burns—time is of the essence in obtaining and maintaining a patent airway. The presence of soot or burns around the nose or mouth, singed facial hair, wheezing, and stridor are ominous signs. Be prepared to provide advanced airway management.

3. Why is pulse oximetry unreliable in these circumstances?

By-products of incomplete combustion include noxious gases such as CO, formaldehyde, sulfur dioxide, nitrogen dioxide, hydrogen sulfide, cyanide, and particulates. Inhalation of these gases (particularly CO) can be deadly because hemoglobin's affinity for CO is roughly 240 times greater than its affinity for oxygen. The excess CO causes severe tissue hypoxia despite the possibility of acceptable or somewhat normal readings on the pulse oximeter.

4. Are your transport considerations affected by the location of her burn?

Yes. This child should be taken to a burn center because her right hand is burned. Accepted criteria for transport to a burn center include partial-thickness burns on greater than 10% of the TBSA; any full-thickness burns; burns involving the hands, feet, face, major joints, or groin; burns involving the airway; circumferential burns (especially involving the chest or neck); electrical burns (including lightning and high-voltage electricity injuries); chemical burns; underlying medical conditions and/or traumatic injuries that could be exacerbated; or the lack of facilities capable of appropriately treating burn patients.

5. What are common complications of burns?

Depending on the area affected (usually when an area greater than 10% of the TBSA is involved) and the thickness of the burn, patients may experience difficulties with thermoregulation. For this reason, you should take steps to preserve body temperature.

6. What is appropriate fluid resuscitation for a pediatric patient?

The Parkland formula provides guidelines for fluid resuscitation of burn patients. During the first 24 hours, the burn patient will receive 4 × body weight (in kilograms) × percentage of body surface burned. Half of that amount needs to be given during the first 8 hours. However, pediatric patients may need more fluids than their adult counterparts, so be prepared to make adjustments accordingly.

7. Given the nature of burns, what is another important consideration regarding burn care?

Beyond estimating the extent of the burn and cooling and covering the area, be aware that burns are extremely painful. As health care professionals, we must be prepared to provide appropriate pain management. Morphine sulfate is highly effective at 0.1 to 0.2 mg/kg, with repeated doses as needed.

8. What is burn shock, and how does it relate to the prehospital setting?

Burn shock occurs because of fluid loss through the damaged skin and a series of volume shifts within the body. Capillaries become leaky, so intravascular fluid oozes out of the circulation and into the interstitial spaces. Meanwhile, cells of normal tissues take in increased amounts of salt and water from the fluid around them. This process occurs during a 6- to 8-hour period. Therefore, if a burned patient is in shock in the prehospital phase, look for another injury as the source of shock. In particular, make sure that you auscultate lung sounds before administration of fluid therapy.

9. What other considerations must be made when dealing with a pediatric burn patient?

Monitor the patient's blood glucose level, and be prepared to administer dextrose as needed. Also, when dealing with minors or older people, be aware of the potential for child or elder abuse. It is your responsibility to report suspected abuse or neglect to the proper authorities.

Prep Kit

Ready for Review

- Although you probably won't see moderate or severe burns on a daily basis, you will encounter some serious burn injuries during your career.
- The skin has four functions:
  - Protect the underlying tissue from injury and exposure
  - Regulate temperature
  - Prevent excessive loss of water from the body
  - Act as a sense organ
- Significant damage to the skin may make the body vulnerable to bacterial invasion, temperature instability, and major disturbances of fluid balance.
- Burns are diffuse soft-tissue injuries created from destructive energy transferred via radiation, thermal, or electrical energy.
- The many types of burns, coupled with the many possible presentations of burn patients, can challenge your assessment skills. Address a burned patient in a consistent, efficient, and systematic manner so you don't develop tunnel vision for the major burn trauma and miss other occult injuries that could affect the patient's outcome.
- Although you will be most heavily involved in the first phase of burn care, it is important to appreciate the magnitude of care that a patient with a severe or even moderate burn must receive. Early actions of paramedics may dramatically affect the patient's long-term outcome.
- Serious burn injuries are devastating events that leave patients with long-term physical and psychological challenges.

Vital Vocabulary

acute radiation syndrome The clinical course that usually begins within hours of exposure to a radiation source. Symptoms include nausea, vomiting, diarrhea, fatigue, fever, and headache. The long-term symptoms are dose-related and are hematopoietic and gastrointestinal.

adipose tissue Fat tissue.

anaerobic metabolism The metabolism that takes place in the absence of oxygen; the principal product is lactic acid.

burn shock The shock or hypoperfusion caused by a burn injury and the tremendous loss of fluids.

circumferential burns Burns on the neck or chest that may compress the airway or on an extremity that might act like a tourniquet.

collagen A protein that gives tensile strength to the connective tissues of the body.

comedo A noninflammatory acne lesion.

contact burn A burn produced by touching a hot object.

cutaneous Pertaining to the skin.

dermis The inner layer of skin containing hair follicle roots, glands, blood vessels, and nerves.

desquamation The continuous shedding of the dead cells on the surface of the skin.

elastin A protein that gives the skin its elasticity.

epidermis The outermost layer of the skin.

escharotomy A surgical cut through the eschar or leathery covering of a burn injury to allow for swelling and minimize the potential for development of compartment syndrome in a circumferentially burned limb or the thorax.

flame burn A thermal burn caused by flames touching the skin.

flash burn An electrothermal injury caused by arcing of electric current.

full-thickness burn A burn that extends through the epidermis and dermis into the subcutaneous tissues beneath; previously called a third-degree burn.

homeostasis A tendency to constancy or stability in the body's internal environment.

integument The skin.

Lund and Browder chart A detailed version of the rule of nines chart that takes into consideration the changes in body surface area brought on by growth.

melanin The pigment that gives skin its color.

mucopolysaccharide gel One of the complex materials found, along with the collagen fibers and elastin fibers, in the dermis of the skin.

Parkland formula A formula that recommends giving 4 mL of normal saline for each kilogram of body weight, multiplied by the percentage of body surface area burned; sometimes used to calculate fluid needs during lengthy transport times.

partial-thickness burn A burn that involves the epidermis and part of the dermis, characterized by pain and blistering; previously called a second-degree burn.

rule of nines A system that assigns percentages to sections of the body, allowing calculation of the amount of skin surface involved in the burn area.

rule of palm A system that estimates total body surface area burned by comparing the affected area with the size of the patient's palm, which is roughly equal to 1% of the patient's total body surface area.

scald burn A burn produced by hot liquids.

sebaceous gland A gland located in the dermis that secretes sebum.

sebum An oily substance secreted by sebaceous glands.

steam burn A burn that has been caused by direct exposure to hot steam exhaust, as from a broken pipe.

subcutaneous layer Beneath the skin.

superficial burn A burn involving only the epidermis, producing very red, painful skin; previously called a first-degree burn.

supraglottic Located above the glottic opening, as in the upper airway structures.

thermal burn An injury caused by radiation or direct contact with a heat source on the skin.

thermoregulation The ability of the body to maintain temperature through a combination of heat gain by metabolic processes and muscular movement and heat loss through respiration, evaporation, conduction, convection, and perspiration.

total body surface area (TBSA) Used in the calculation of a burn injury to determine the percentage of the surface of the patient's body that has been injured. This is commonly estimated by using the rule of palm or the rule of nines.

zone of coagulation The reddened area surrounding the leathery and sometimes charred tissue that has sustained a full-thickness burn.

zone of hyperemia In a thermal burn, the area that is least affected by the burn injury.

zone of stasis The peripheral area surrounding the zone of coagulation that has decreased blood flow and inflammation. This area can undergo necrosis within 24 to 48 hours after the injury, particularly if perfusion is compromised due to burn shock.

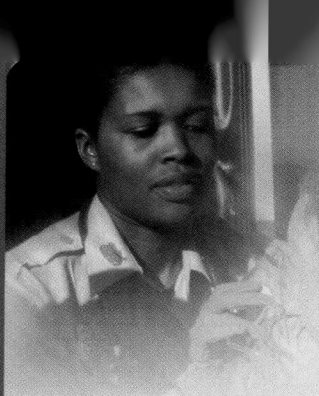

Assessment in Action

You are dispatched to a private residence to care for an unconscious victim with possible smoke inhalation. You arrive on scene to find an 81-year-old woman outside being attended to by fire department personnel. The fire fighters report that the patient was found on the floor in the kitchen by her grandson. The kitchen was full of smoke, and the grandson carried her outside. The patient is conscious but combative and asking repetitive questions. The fire fighters transfer the patient to the ambulance, where you begin your assessment.

The patient's blood pressure is 150/90 mm Hg, respirations are 18 breaths/min, heart rate is 110 beats/min, and pulse oximetry is 95% while breathing room air. You notice a significant amount of soot around the patient's face, especially in the nostrils, mouth, and oral airway. The patient remains conscious but does not recognize her family and continues to ask repetitive questions. You insert an IV line, give lactated Ringer's solution, and begin your transport to the local burn center, which is approximately 25 minutes away.

En route to the hospital, you sedate the patient and successfully intubate her with a 7.0 ET tube. You notice a significant amount of soot around the vocal cords. You transfer the patient to the emergency department. When doing your follow-up at the end of your shift, you are told the patient was admitted to the intensive care unit for respiratory failure secondary to an inhalation injury.

1. **What type of burn is described in this scenario?**
   A. Thermal burn
   B. Scald burn
   C. Contact burn
   D. Airway burn

2. **Anyone exposed to smoke from a fire may have _____ burns.**
   A. thermal
   B. scald
   C. contact
   D. radiation

3. **_____ airway damage is more often associated with the inhalation of superheated gases.**
   A. Upper airway
   B. Lower airway
   C. Upper and lower airway
   D. None of these

4. **In the lower airway, _____ and _____ may result from heat inhalation.**
   A. laryngospasm, pulmonary damage
   B. pulmonary damage, bronchospasm
   C. laryngospasm, bronchospasm
   D. mild, severe damage

5. **True or false? If your patient greets you with a hoarse voice and a chief complaint of "trouble breathing," your general impression should be that there is probably nothing wrong with this patient.**
   A. True
   B. False

6. **Combative patients should be considered:**
   A. as having head trauma.
   B. intoxicated.
   C. diabetic.
   D. hypoxic.

7. **_____ can develop with alarming speed in burn patients, especially in infants and children.**
   A. Laryngeal edema
   B. A pulmonary injury
   C. An inhalation burn
   D. Bronchial edema

8. **After listening to lung sounds, you hear _____. This may be a sign of impending upper airway compromise.**
   A. wheezing
   B. stridor
   C. rhonchi
   D. rales

9. **Burn patients fall into several general categories for airway management. They include:**
   A. the patient with the acutely decompensating airway who requires field intubation.
   B. the patient with the deteriorating airway from burns and toxic inhalations.
   C. the patient with no signs of or risk factors for airway compromise who is in no distress.
   D. all of the above.

10. **Approximately _____ older adults die of fire-related causes each year, making it the sixth leading cause of death in this population group.**
    A. 1,200
    B. 1,000
    C. 200
    D. 1,100

Challenging Questions

It is 2:00 AM and you are sent to a "structure fire." On arrival, you hear the members of the fire department calling your name, stating they have a victim. The patient was inside the burning house and was standing on the roof when the fire fighters arrived. Fire fighters had the patient drop and roll. The patient is still smoldering and is in a great deal of pain. You call for a medical helicopter and transfer the patient to the landing zone. You estimate that the burn involves 30% of the TBSA.

11. **What is your treatment while you are driving to the landing zone?**

12. **How do you assess the TBSA burned?**

13. **How much fluid will this patient require?**

Points to Ponder

You and your crew are called to the scene of a large apartment fire in which two to three units are involved. When you arrive, you find three other patients being treated by fire fighters for minor inhalation injuries. The patient in the worst condition seems to be a man in his mid 30s. He has dark, discolored patches of skin on his chest, lower right arm, and lower back. He also has a circumferential burn on his left upper arm. His voice is slightly hoarse, and twice he coughs up dark-colored sputum. However, he denies having difficulty breathing or having much pain. He is sitting up at the scene, watching all that is going on around him.

Why is this patient of particular concern? What must you make sure to do in treating this patient?

Issues: The Impact of Managing a Burn-Injured Patient, Mortality and Morbidity Based on Pathophysiology and Assessment Findings.

21 Head and Face Injuries

Objectives

Cognitive

4-5.1 Describe the incidence, morbidity, and mortality of facial injuries. (p 21.29)

4-5.2 Explain facial anatomy and relate physiology to facial injuries. (p 21.4)

4-5.3 Predict facial injuries based on mechanism of injury. (p 21.16)

4-5.4 Predict other injuries commonly associated with facial injuries based on mechanism of injury. (p 21.16)

4-5.5 Differentiate between the following types of facial injuries, highlighting the defining characteristics of each:
  a. Eye
  b. Ear
  c. Nose
  d. Throat
  e. Mouth (p 21.16–21.29)

4-5.6 Integrate pathophysiological principles to the assessment of a patient with a facial injury. (p 21.16)

4-5.7 Differentiate between facial injuries based on the assessment and history. (p. 21.17)

4-5.8 Formulate a field impression for a patient with a facial injury based on the assessment findings. (p 21.16)

4-5.9 Develop a patient management plan for a patient with a facial injury based on the field impression. (p 21.21)

4-5.10 Explain the pathophysiology of eye injuries. (p 21.17)

4-5.11 Relate assessment findings associated with eye injuries to pathophysiology. (p 21.18)

4-5.12 Integrate pathophysiological principles to the assessment of a patient with an eye injury. (p 21.21)

4-5.13 Formulate a field impression for a patient with an eye injury based on the assessment findings. (p 21.21)

4-5.14 Develop a patient management plan for a patient with an eye injury based on the field impression. (p 21.21)

4-5.15 Explain the pathophysiology of ear injuries. (p 21.23)

4-5.16 Relate assessment findings associated with ear injuries to pathophysiology. (p 21.24)

4-5.17 Integrate pathophysiological principles to the assessment of a patient with an ear injury. (p 21.25)

4-5.18 Formulate a field impression for a patient with an ear injury based on the assessment findings. (p 21.25)

4-5.19 Develop a patient management plan for a patient with an ear injury based on the field impression. (p 21.25)

4-5.20 Explain the pathophysiology of nose injuries. (p 21.7)

4-5.21 Relate assessment findings associated with nose injuries to pathophysiology. (p 21.15)

4-5.22 Integrate pathophysiological principles to the assessment of a patient with a nose injury. (p 21.17)

4-5.23 Formulate a field impression for a patient with a nose injury based on the assessment findings. (p 21.17)

4-5.24 Develop a patient management plan for a patient with a nose injury based on the field impression. (p 21.17)

4-5.25 Explain the pathophysiology of throat injuries. (p 21.26)

4-5.26 Relate assessment findings associated with throat injuries to pathophysiology. (p 21.27)

4-5.27 Integrate pathophysiological principles to the assessment of a patient with a throat injury. (p 21.28)

4-5.28 Formulate a field impression for a patient with a throat injury based on the assessment findings. (p 21.28)

4-5.29 Develop a patient management plan for a patient with a throat injury based on the field impression. (p 21.28)

4-5.30 Explain the pathophysiology of mouth injuries. (p 21.25)

4-5.31 Relate assessment findings associated with mouth injuries to pathophysiology. (p 21.25)

4-5.32 Integrate pathophysiological principles to the assessment of a patient with a mouth injury. (p 21.26)

4-5.33 Formulate a field impression for a patient with a mouth injury based on the assessment findings. (p 21.25)

4-5.34 Develop a patient management plan for a patient with a mouth injury based on the field impression. (p 21.26)

4-5.35 Describe the incidence, morbidity, and mortality of head injuries. (p 21.29)

4-5.36 Explain anatomy and relate physiology of the CNS to head injuries. (p 21.11, 21.30)

4-5.37 Predict head injuries based on mechanism of injury. (p 21.29)

4-5.38 Distinguish between head injury and brain injury. (p 21.31)

4-5.39 Explain the pathophysiology of head/brain injuries. (p 21.30)

4-5.40 Explain the concept of increasing intracranial pressure (ICP). (p 21.32)

4-5.41 Explain the effect of increased and decreased carbon dioxide on ICP. (p 21.38)

4-5.42 Define and explain the process involved with each of the levels of increasing ICP. (p 21.32)

4-5.43 Relate assessment findings associated with head/brain injuries to the pathophysiologic process. (p 21.36)

4-5.44 Classify head injuries (mild, moderate, severe) according to assessment findings. (p 21.34)

4-5.45 Identify the need for rapid intervention and transport of the patient with a head/brain injury. (p 21.40)

4-5.46 Describe and explain the general management of the head/brain injury patient, including pharmacological and non-pharmacological treatment. (p 21.40)

4-5.47 Analyze the relationship between carbon dioxide concentration in the blood and management of the airway in the head/brain injured patient. (p 21.38)

4-5.48 Explain the pathophysiology of diffuse axonal injury. (p 21.33)

4-5.49 Relate assessment findings associated with concussion, moderate and severe diffuse axonal injury to pathophysiology. (p 21.33)

4-5.50 Develop a management plan for a patient with a moderate and severe diffuse axonal injury. (p 21.36)

4-5.51 Explain the pathophysiology of skull fracture. (p 21.30)

4-5.52 Relate assessment findings associated with skull fracture to pathophysiology. (p 21.30)

4-5.53	Develop a management plan for a patient with a skull fracture. (p 21.38)
4-5.54	Explain the pathophysiology of cerebral contusion. (p 21.33)
4-5.55	Relate assessment findings associated with cerebral contusion to pathophysiology. (p 21.33)
4-5.56	Develop a management plan for a patient with a cerebral contusion. (p 21.36)
4-5.57	Explain the pathophysiology of intracranial hemorrhage, including:

    a. Epidural
    b. Subdural
    c. Intracerebral
    d. Subarachnoid (p 21.34, 21.35)

| 4-5.58 | Relate assessment findings associated with intracranial hemorrhage to pathophysiology, including: |

    a. Epidural
    b. Subdural
    c. Intracerebral
    d. Subarachnoid (p 21.34, 21.35)

| 4-5.59 | Develop a management plan for a patient with an intracranial hemorrhage, including: |

    a. Epidural
    b. Subdural
    c. Intracerebral
    d. Subarachnoid (p 21.36)

4-5.60	Describe the various types of helmets and their purposes. (p 22.24, 22.25)
4-5.61	Relate priorities of care to factors determining the need for helmet removal in various field situations including sports related incidents. (p 22.24, 22.25)
4-5.62	Develop a management plan for the removal of a helmet for a head injured patient. (p 22.24, 22.25)
4-5.63	Integrate the pathophysiological principles to the assessment of a patient with head/brain injury. (p 21.36)
4-5.64	Differentiate between the types of head/brain injuries based on the assessment and history. (p 21.36)
4-5.65	Formulate a field impression for a patient with a head/brain injury based on the assessment findings. (p 21.38)
4-5.66	Develop a patient management plan for a patient with a head/brain injury based on the field impression. (p 21.38)

Affective

None

Psychomotor

None

Head and Face Injuries

As a paramedic, you will commonly encounter patients with injuries to the head, neck, and face, ranging in severity from a broken nose to traumatic brain injury. The first part of this chapter provides a detailed review of the anatomy and physiology of the head and face. The second part discusses head and face injuries, including their respective signs and symptoms and appropriate prehospital care: maxillofacial injuries, eye and ear injuries, oral and dental injuries, injuries to the anterior part of the neck, and head and traumatic brain injuries.

The Skull and Facial Bones

The Scalp

The brain—the most important organ in the body—requires maximum protection from injury. The human body ensures that it receives this protection by housing the brain within several layers of soft and hard wrappings.

Starting from the outside and proceeding inward toward the brain, the first protective layer is the scalp, which consists of the following layers, given in descending order:

- Skin, with hair
- Subcutaneous tissue, which contains major scalp veins that bleed profusely when lacerated.
- Galea aponeurotica, a tendon expansion that connects the frontal and occipital muscles of the cranium
- Loose connective tissue (alveolar tissue), which is easily stripped from the layer beneath in "scalping" injuries. The looseness of the alveolar layer also provides room for blood to accumulate after blunt trauma between the scalp and skull bone (subgaleal hematoma).
- Periosteum, the dense fibrous membrane covering the surface of bones

The Skull

At the top of the axial skeleton is the skull, which consists of 28 bones in three anatomic groups: the auditory ossicles, the cranium, and the face. The six auditory ossicles function in hearing and are located, three on each side of the head, deep

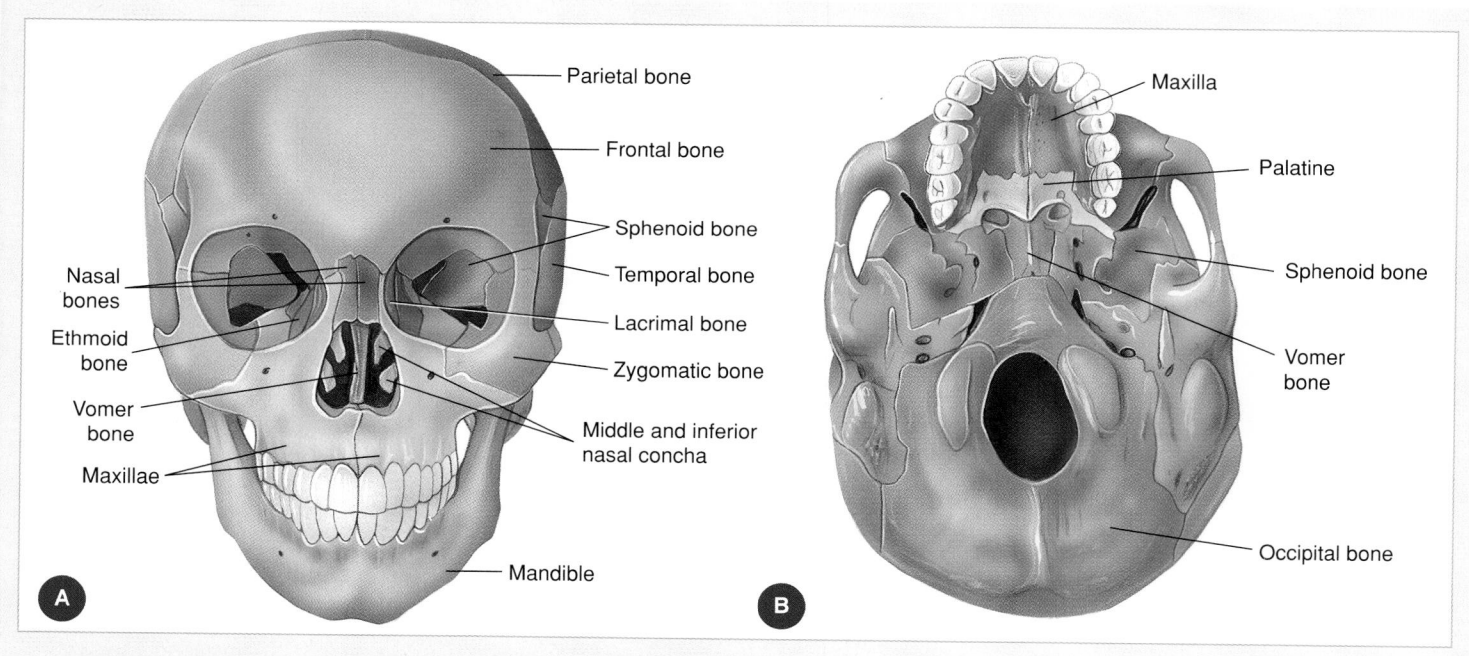

Figure 21-1 The skull and its components. **A.** Front view. **B.** Bottom view.

A
Parietal bone
Frontal bone
Sphenoid bone
Temporal bone
Lacrimal bone
Zygomatic bone
Middle and inferior nasal concha
Mandible
Nasal bones
Ethmoid bone
Vomer bone
Maxillae

B
Maxilla
Palatine
Sphenoid bone
Vomer bone
Occipital bone

You are the Provider Part 1

You respond to the scene of a motorcycle crash. The patient, a young male, was ejected from his motorcycle when it struck a tree; he was not wearing a helmet. The scene is safe, and two police officers are at the scene directing the flow of traffic. As you approach the patient, you note that he is lying in a supine position. His eyes are closed, and he is not moving.

1. What should be your initial concern about this patient?
2. How should you direct your initial care of this patient?

within the cavities of the temporal bone. The remaining 22 bones constitute the cranium and the face (**Figure 21-1** ◂).

The cranial vault consists of eight bones that encase and protect the brain: the parietal, temporal, frontal, occipital, sphenoid, and ethmoid bones. The brain connects to the spinal cord through a large opening at the base of the skull called the foramen magnum.

The bones of the skull are connected at special joints known as sutures (**Figure 21-2** ▾). The paired parietal bones

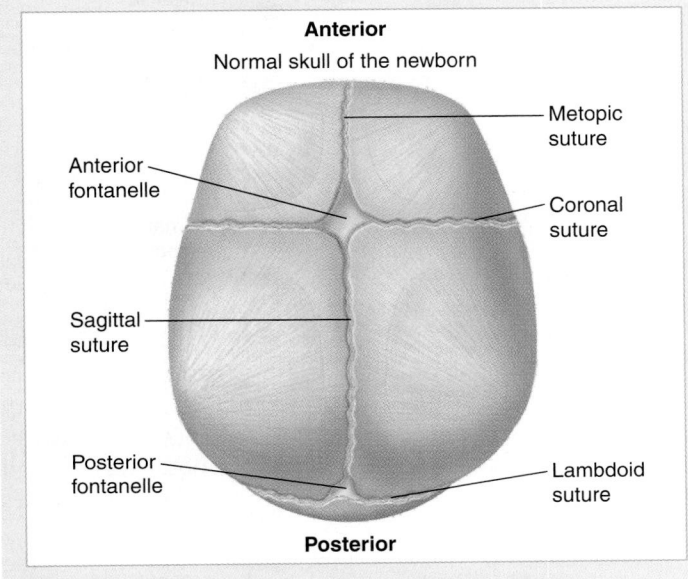

Figure 21-2 The sutures of the skull in a newborn.

join together at the sagittal suture. The parietal bones abut the frontal bone at the coronal suture. The occipital bone attaches to the parietal bones at the lambdoid suture. Fibrous tissues called fontanelles, which are soft in infants, link the sutures. The tissues felt through the fontanelles are layers of the scalp and thick membranes overlying the brain. Under normal conditions, the brain may not be felt through the fontanelles. By the time a child is 18 months old, the sutures should have solidified and the fontanelles closed.

At the base of each temporal bone is a cone-shaped section of bone known as the mastoid process. This area is an important site for attachment of various muscles. In addition, a portion of the mastoid process contains hollow mastoid air cells (**Figure 21-3** ▾).

The Floor of the Cranial Vault
Viewed from above, the floor of the cranial vault is divided into three compartments: the anterior fossa, middle fossa, and posterior fossa (**Figure 21-4** ▸). The crista galli forms a prominent bony ridge in the center of the anterior fossa and is the point of attachment of the meninges, the three layers of membranes that surround the brain and spinal cord. On the other side of the crista galli is the cribriform plate of the ethmoid bone, a horizontal bone that is perforated with numerous openings (foramina) allowing the passage of the olfactory nerve filaments from the nasal cavity. The olfactory nerves, the cranial nerves for smell, send projections through the foramina in the cribriform plate and into the nasal cavity, the chamber inside the nose that lies between the floor of the cranium and the roof of the mouth.

The Base of the Skull
When the mandible is removed, the base of the skull appears amazingly complex, with numerous foramina visible (**Figure 21-5** ▸). The occipital condyles on the occipital bone, which are the points of articulation between the skull and the vertebral column, lie on either side of the foramen magnum. Portions of the maxilla and the palatine bone, the irregularly shaped bone in the posterior nasal cavity, form the hard palate, which is the bony anterior part of the palate, or roof, of the mouth. The zygomatic arch is the bone that extends along the front of the skull below the orbit.

The Facial Bones
The frontal and ethmoid bones are part of the cranial vault and the face. The

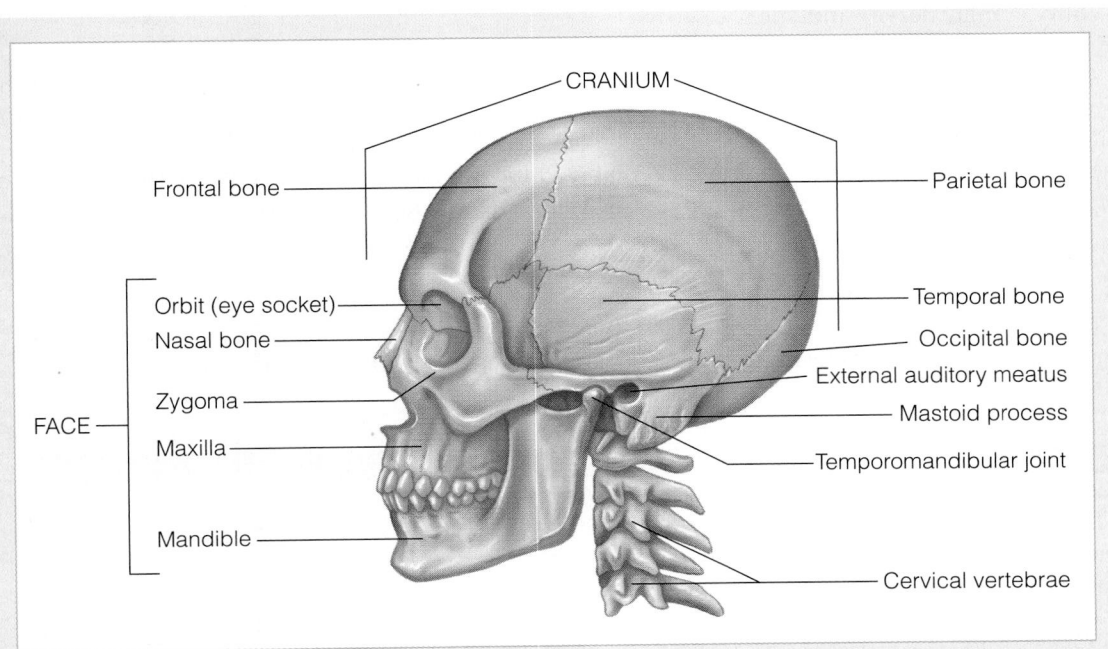

Figure 21-3 The mastoid air cells are located in the mastoid process. Just anterior to the mastoid is the external auditory meatus, which is associated with the ear canal.

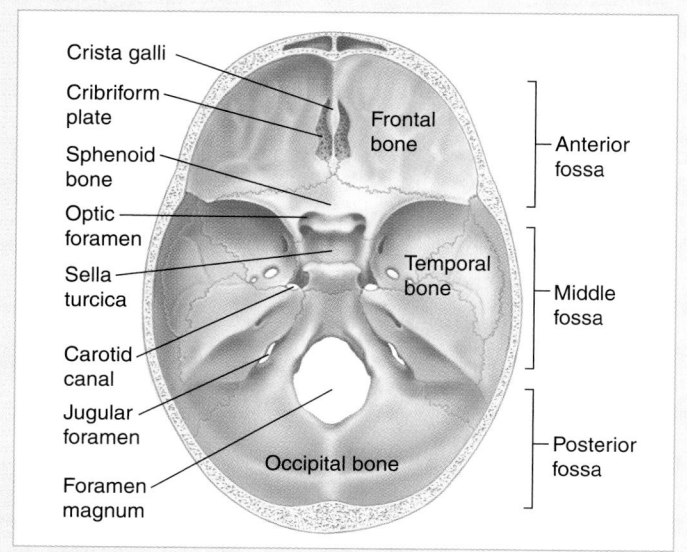

Figure 21-4 The floor of the cranial vault and its anatomy.

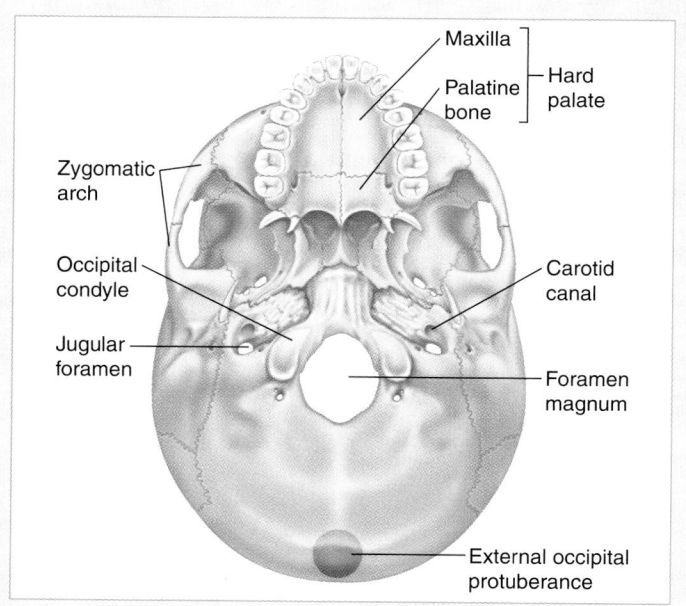

Figure 21-5 The base of the skull from below.

14 facial bones form the structure of the face, without contributing to the cranial vault. They include the maxillae, vomer, inferior nasal concha, and the zygomatic, palatine, nasal, and lacrimal bones (see Figure 21-1A).

The facial bones protect the eyes, nose, and tongue; they also provide attachment points for the muscles that allow chewing. The zygomatic process of the temporal bone and the temporal process of the zygomatic bone form the zygomatic arch (Figure 21-6 ▶), which lends shape to the cheeks.

Two major nerves provide sensory and motor control to the face: the trigeminal nerve (fifth cranial nerve) and the facial nerve (seventh cranial nerve). The trigeminal nerve branches into the ophthalmic nerve, maxillary nerve, and mandibular nerve. The ophthalmic nerve (a sensory nerve) supplies the skin of the forehead, upper eyelid, and conjunctiva. The maxillary nerve (another sensory nerve) supplies the skin on the posterior part of the side of the nose, lower eye-

lid, cheek, and upper lip. The mandibular nerve (a sensory and motor nerve) supplies the muscles of chewing (mastication) and skin of the lower lip, chin, temporal region, and part of the external ear. The facial nerve supplies the muscles of facial expression.

Blood supply to the face is provided primarily through the external carotid artery, which branches into the temporal, mandibular, and maxillary arteries. Because the face is highly vascular, it tends to bleed heavily when injured.

The Orbits
The orbits are cone-shaped fossae that enclose and protect the eyes. In addition to the eyeball and muscles that move it, the orbit contains blood vessels, nerves, and fat.

A blow to the eye may result in fracture of the orbital floor because the bone is extremely thin and breaks easily. A

You are the Provider Part 2

As your partner maintains manual stabilization of the patient's head and simultaneously opens his airway with the jaw-thrust maneuver, you perform an initial assessment.

Initial Assessment	Recording Time: 0 Minutes
Appearance	Supine, not moving, massive facial trauma
Level of consciousness	P (Responsive to painful stimuli)
Airway	Blood is draining from the patient's mouth
Breathing	Respirations are gurgling, slow, and irregular
Circulation	Radial pulses are rapid and bounding; bleeding from the mouth; no other gross bleeding

3. How will you manage this patient's airway?
4. Would it be appropriate to intubate this patient? If so, when?

blowout fracture (**Figure 21-7** ▾) results in transmission of forces away from the eyeball itself to the bone. Blood and fat then leak into the maxillary sinus.

The Nose

The nose is one of the two primary entry points for oxygen-rich air to enter the body. The nasal septum—the separation between the nostrils—is located in the midline. Often, it bulges slightly to one side or the other. The external portion of the nose is formed mostly of cartilage.

Several bones associated with the nose contain cavities known as the paranasal sinuses (**Figure 21-8** ▸). These hollowed sections of bone, which are lined with mucous membranes, decrease the weight of the skull and provide resonance for the voice. The contents of the sinuses drain into the nasal cavity.

The Mandible and Temporomandibular Joint

The mandible is the large movable bone forming the lower jaw and containing the lower teeth. Numerous muscles of chewing attach to the mandible and its rami. The posterior condyle of the mandible articulates with the temporal bone at the temporomandibular joint (TMJ), allowing movement of the mandible (see Figure 21-3).

The Hyoid Bone

The hyoid bone "floats" in the superior aspect of the neck just below the mandible. While it is not actually part of the skull, it supports the tongue and serves as a point of attachment for many important neck and tongue muscles.

The Eyes, Ears, Teeth, and Mouth

The Eye

The globe, or eyeball, is a spherical structure measuring about 1 inch in diameter that is housed within the eye socket, or orbit. The eyes are held in place by loose connective tissue and several muscles. These muscles also control eye movements. The oculomotor nerve (third cranial nerve) innervates the muscles that cause motion of the eyeballs and upper eyelids. It also carries parasympathetic nerve fibers that cause constriction of the pupil and accommodation of the lens. The optic nerve (second cranial nerve) provides the sense of vision (**Figure 21-9** ▸).

The structures of the eye (**Figure 21-10** ▸) include the following:

- The sclera ("white of the eye") is a tough, fibrous coat that helps maintain the shape of the eye and protect the contents of the eye. In some illnesses, such as hepatitis, the sclera become yellow (icteric) from staining by bile pigments.
- The cornea is the transparent anterior portion of the eye that overlies the iris and pupil. Clouding of the cornea during aging results in a condition known as cataract.
- The conjunctiva is a delicate mucous membrane that covers the sclera and internal surfaces of the eyelids but not the iris. Cyanosis can be detected in the conjunctiva when it is not easily assessed on the skin of dark-skinned patients.

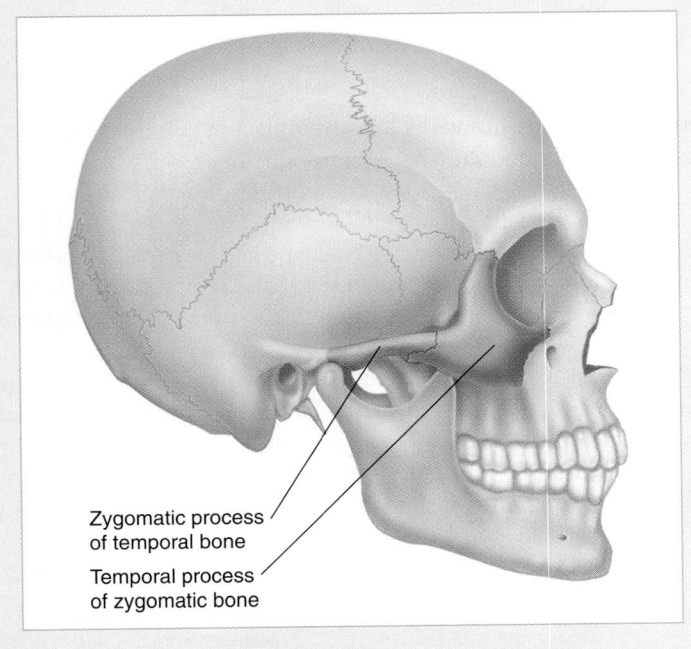

Zygomatic process of temporal bone

Temporal process of zygomatic bone

Figure 21-6 The zygomatic arch.

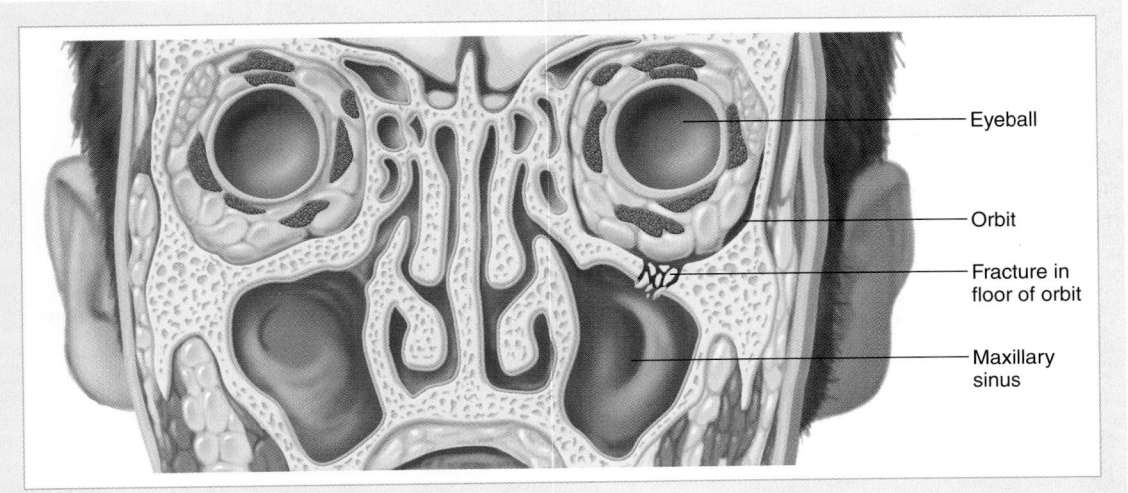

Eyeball

Orbit

Fracture in floor of orbit

Maxillary sinus

Figure 21-7 A blowout fracture of the left orbit.

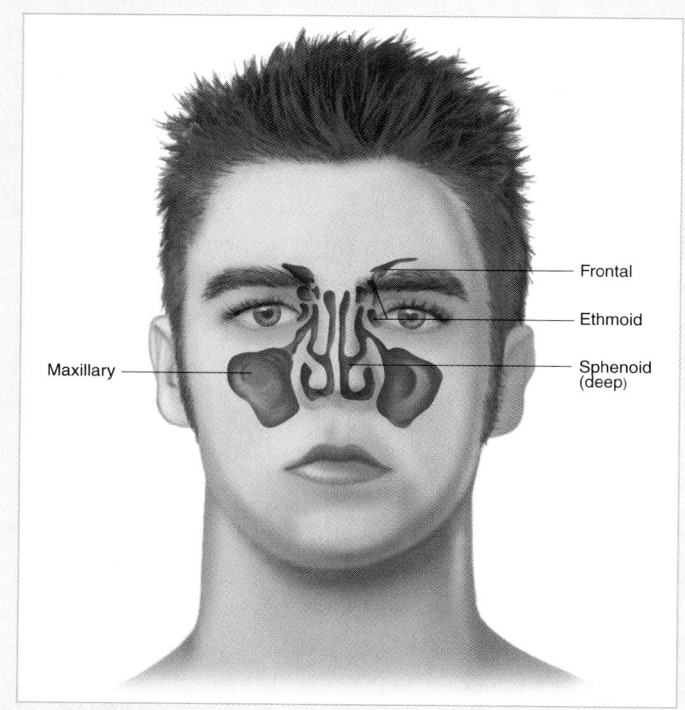

Figure 21-8 The paranasal sinuses.

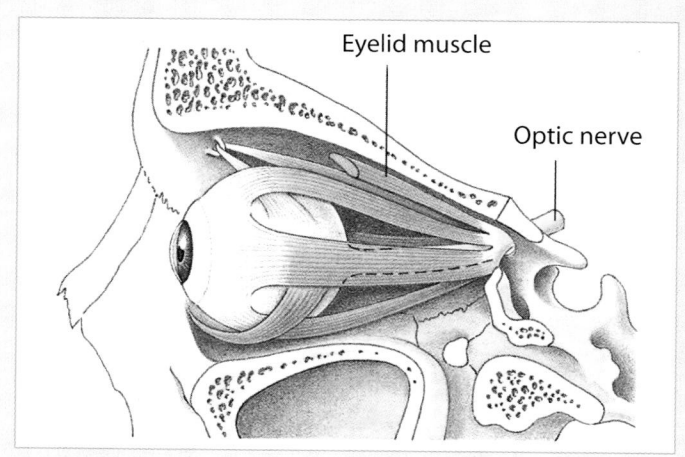

Figure 21-9 The optic nerve.

- The iris is the pigmented part of the eye that surrounds the pupil. It consists of muscles and blood vessels that contract and expand to regulate the size of the pupil.
- The pupil is the circular adjustable opening within the iris through which light passes to the lens. A normal pupil dilates in dim light to permit more light to enter the eye and constricts in bright light to decrease the light entering the eye.
- Behind the pupil and iris is the lens, a transparent structure that can alter its thickness to focus light on the retina at the back of the eye.
- The retina, which lies in the posterior aspect of the interior globe, is a delicate, 10-layered structure of nervous tissue that extends from the optic nerve. It receives light impulses and converts them to nerve signals that are conducted to the brain by the optic nerve and interpreted as vision.

The anterior chamber is the portion of the globe between the lens and the cornea. It is filled with aqueous humor, a clear watery fluid. If aqueous humor is lost through a penetrating injury to the eye, it will gradually be replenished.

The posterior chamber is the portion of the globe between the iris and the lens which is filled with vitreous humor, a jelly-like substance that maintains the shape of the globe. If vitreous humor is lost, it cannot be replenished, and blindness may result.

Light rays enter the eyes through the pupil and are focused by the lens. The image formed by the lens is cast on the retina, where sensitive nerve fibers form the optic nerve. The optic nerve transmits the image to the brain, where it is converted into conscious images in the visual cortex.

There are two types of vision: central and peripheral. Central vision, facilitates visualization of objects directly in front

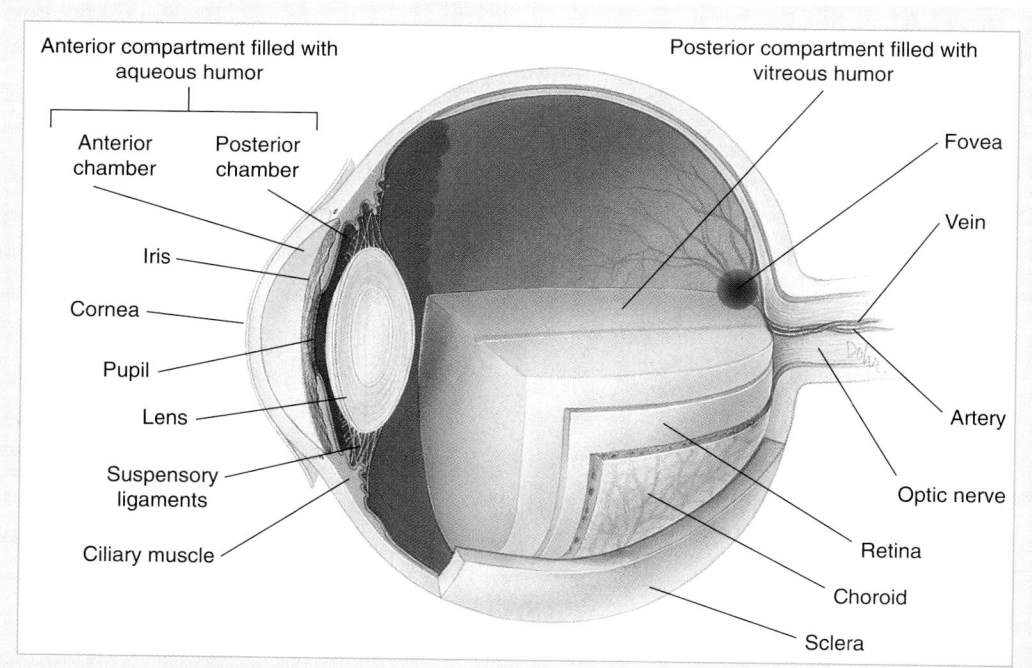

Figure 21-10 The structures of the eye.

of you, and is processed by the macula, the central portion of the retina. The remainder of the retina processes peripheral vision, which gives us visualization of lateral objects while looking forward.

The lacrimal apparatus secretes and drains tears from the eye. Tears produced in the lacrimal gland drain into lacrimal ducts, then into lacrimal sacs that pass into the nasal cavity via the nasolacrimal duct. Tears moisten the conjunctivae Figure 21-11 ▼ .

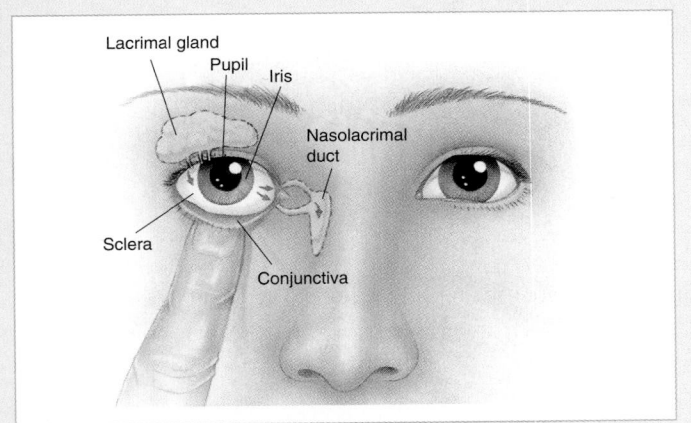

Figure 21-11 The lacrimal system consists of tear glands and ducts. Tears act as lubricants and keep the anterior part of the eye from drying.

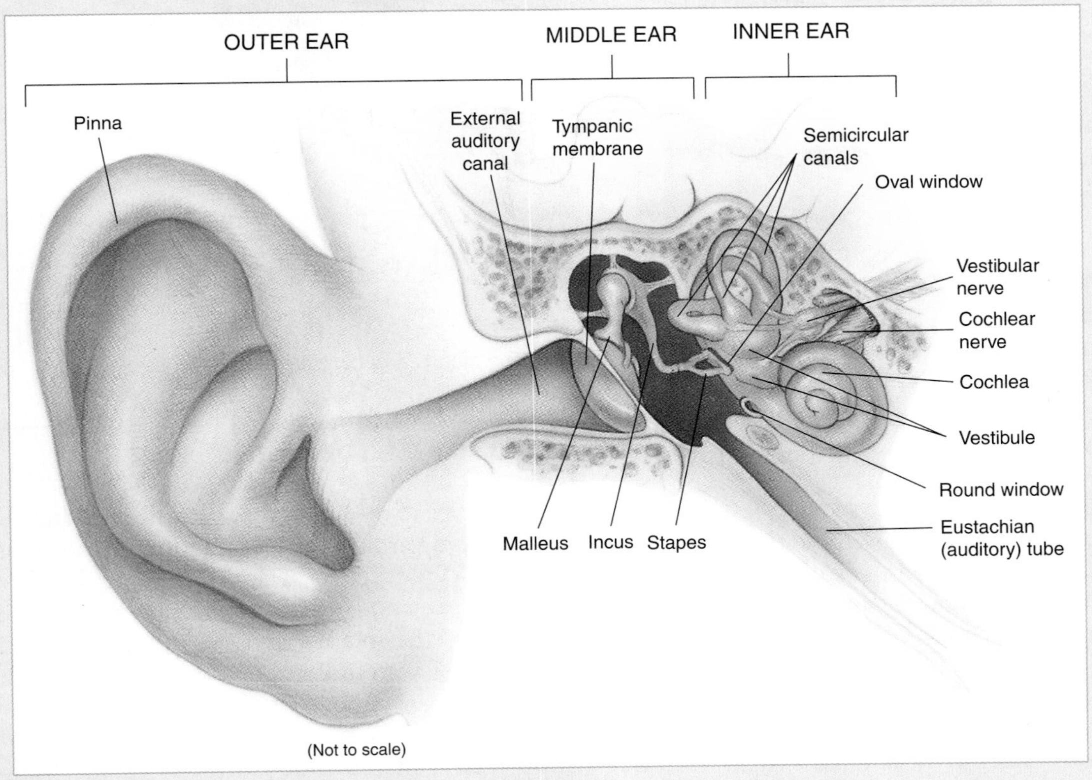

Figure 21-12 The structures of the ear.

The Ear

The ear is divided into three anatomic parts: external, middle, and inner Figure 21-12 ▼ . The external ear consists of the pinna, external auditory canal, and the exterior portion of the tympanic membrane or what is commonly known as the eardrum. The middle ear consists of the inner portion of the tympanic membrane and the ossicles while the inner ear consists of the cochlea and semicircular canals.

Sound waves enter the ear through the auricle, or pinna, the large cartilaginous external portion of the ear. They then travel through the external auditory canal to the tympanic membrane. Vibration of sound waves against the tympanic membrane sets up vibration in the ossicles, the three small bones on the inner side of the tympanic membrane. These vibrations are transmitted to the cochlear duct at the oval window, the opening between the middle ear and the vestibule. Movement of the oval window causes fluid within the cochlea, a shell-shaped structure in the inner ear, to vibrate. Within the cochlea at the organ of Corti, vibration stimulates hair movements that form nerve impulses that travel to the brain via the auditory nerve. The brain then converts these impulses into sound.

The Teeth

The normal adult mouth contains 32 permanent teeth. The primary or deciduous teeth are lost during childhood. Adult teeth are distributed about the maxillary and mandibular arches. The teeth on each side of the arch are mirror images of each other and form four quadrants: right upper, left upper, right lower, and left lower. Each quadrant contains one central incisor, one lateral incisor, one canine, two premolars, and three molars Figure 21-13A ▶ . The third molars or what are called wisdom teeth (which have nothing to do with wisdom) do not appear until late adolescence.

The top portion of the tooth, external to the gum, is the crown, containing one or more cusps. Below the crown lie the neck and the root. The pulp cavity fills the center of the tooth and contains blood vessels, nerves, and specialized connective tissue, called pulp. Dentin and enamel surround the pulp cavity and protect the tooth from damage. Dentin,

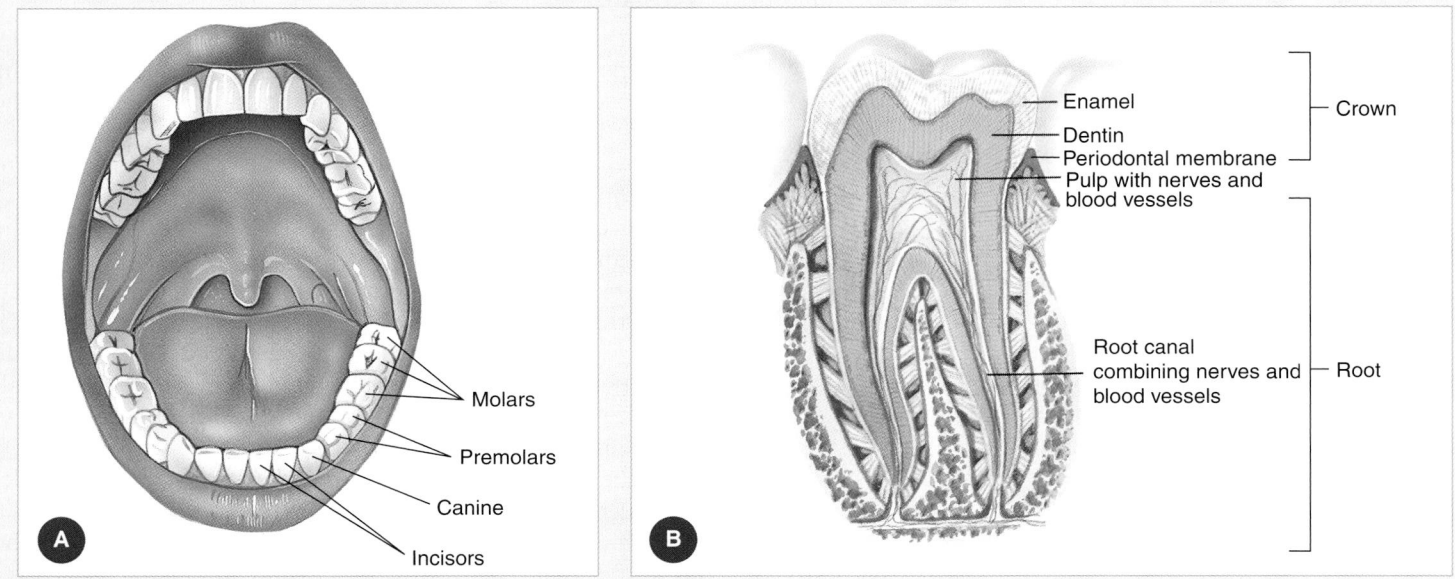

Figure 21-13 The teeth of the adult mouth. **A.** The incisors are used for biting. Canines are used for tearing food. The premolars and molars are used for grinding and crushing. **B.** Each tooth contains nerves and blood vessels.

which forms the principal mass of the tooth, is much denser and stronger than bone. The bony sockets for the teeth that reside in the mandible and maxilla are called alveoli. The ridges between the teeth, the alveolar ridges, are covered by the gingiva, or gums, which are thickened connective tissue and epithelium. Teeth are attached to the alveolar bone by a periodontal membrane (Figure 21-13B ▲).

The Mouth

Digestion begins in the mouth with mastication, or the chewing of food by the teeth. During mastication, food is mixed with secretions from the salivary glands.

The tongue, a muscular process in the floor of the mouth, is the primary organ of taste; it is also important in the formation of speech and in chewing and swallowing of food. The tongue is attached at the mandible and hyoid bone, is covered by a mucous membrane, and extends from the back of the mouth upward and forward to the lips (Figure 21-14 ▶).

The hypoglossal, glossopharyngeal, trigeminal, and facial nerves supply the mouth and its structures. The hypoglossal nerve (12th cranial nerve) provides motor function to the muscles of the tongue. The glossopharyngeal nerve (ninth cranial nerve) provides taste sensation to the posterior portions of the tongue and carries parasympathetic fibers to the salivary glands on each side of the face. The mandibular branch of the trigeminal nerve (fifth cranial nerve) provides motor innervation to the muscles of mastication. The facial nerve (seventh cranial nerve), in addition to supplying motor activity to all muscles of facial expression, provides the sense of taste to the anterior two thirds of the tongue and cutaneous sensations to the tongue and palate.

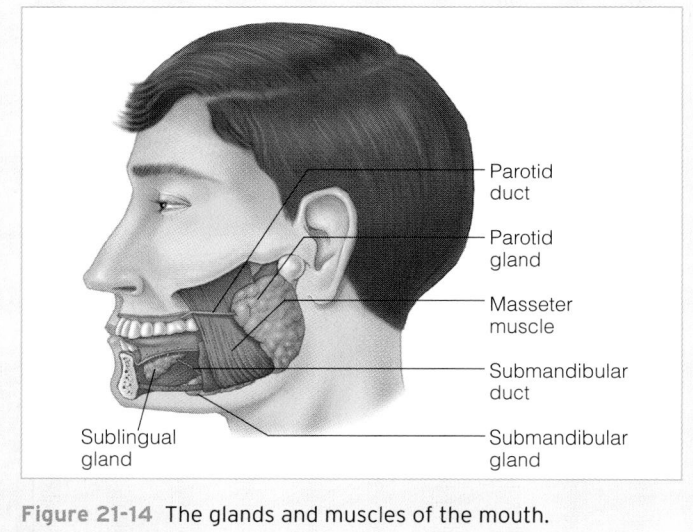

Figure 21-14 The glands and muscles of the mouth.

The Anterior Part of the Neck

The principal structures of the anterior part of the neck include the thyroid and cricoid cartilage, trachea, and numerous muscles and nerves (Figure 21-15 ▶). The major blood vessels in this area are the internal and external carotid arteries (Figure 21-16 ▶) and the internal and external jugular veins (Figure 21-17 ▶). The vertebral arteries run laterally to the cervical vertebrae in the posterior part of the neck.

The major arteries of the neck—the carotid and vertebral arteries—supply oxygenated blood directly to the brain. Therefore, in addition to causing massive bleeding and hemorrhagic shock, injury to any of these major vessels can produce

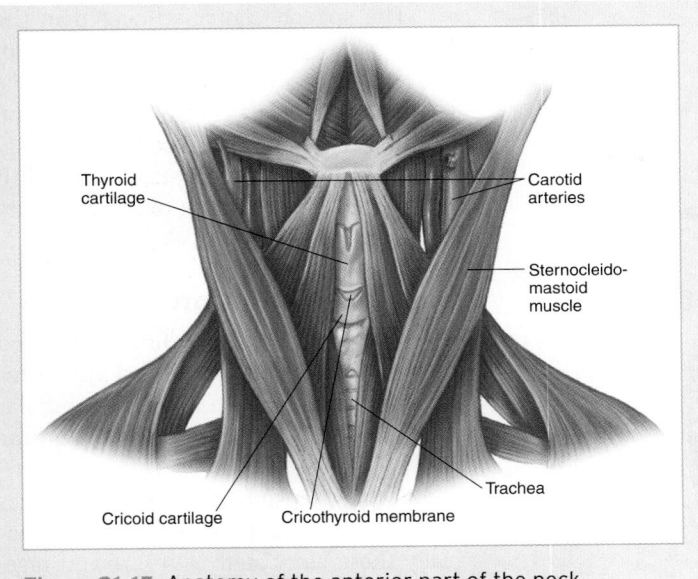

Figure 21-15 Anatomy of the anterior part of the neck.

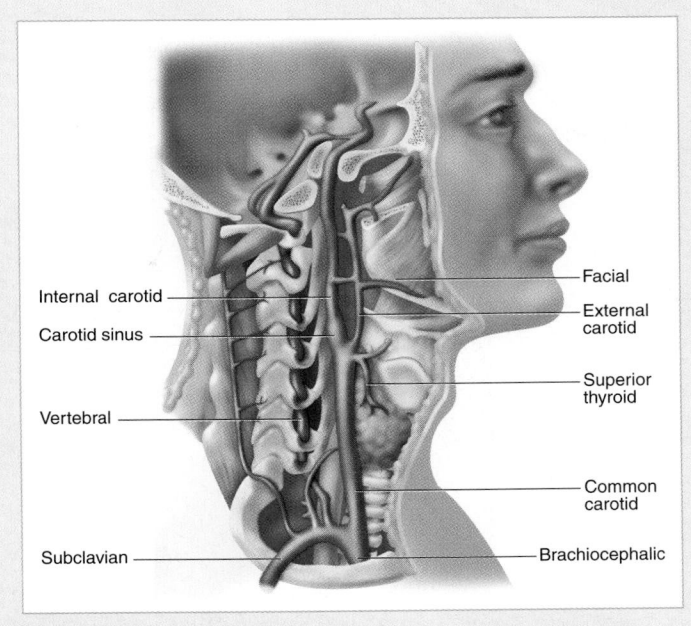

Figure 21-16 The arteries of the neck.

cerebral hypoxia, infarct, air embolism and/or permanent neurologic impairment.

Other key structures of the anterior part of the neck that may sustain injury from blunt or penetrating mechanisms include the vagus nerves, thoracic duct, esophagus, thyroid and parathyroid glands, lower cranial nerves, brachial plexus (which is responsible for function of the lower arm and hand), soft tissue and fascia, and various muscles.

The Brain

The brain, which occupies 80% of the cranial vault, contains billions of neurons (nerve cells) that serve a variety of vital functions Figure 21-18 ▶ . The major regions of the brain are the cerebrum, diencephalon (thalamus and hypothalamus), brain stem (medulla, pons, midbrain [mesencephalon]), and the cerebellum. The remaining intracranial contents include cerebral blood (12%) and cerebrospinal fluid (8%).

The brain accounts for only 2% of the total body weight, yet it is the most metabolically active and perfusion-sensitive organ in the body. The brain metabolizes 25% of the body's glucose, burning approximately 60 mg/min, and consumes 20% of the total body oxygen (45 to 50 L/min). Because the brain has no storage mechanism for oxygen or glucose, it is totally dependent on a constant source of both fuels via cerebral blood flow provided by the carotid and vertebral arteries. As such, the brain will continually manipulate the physiology

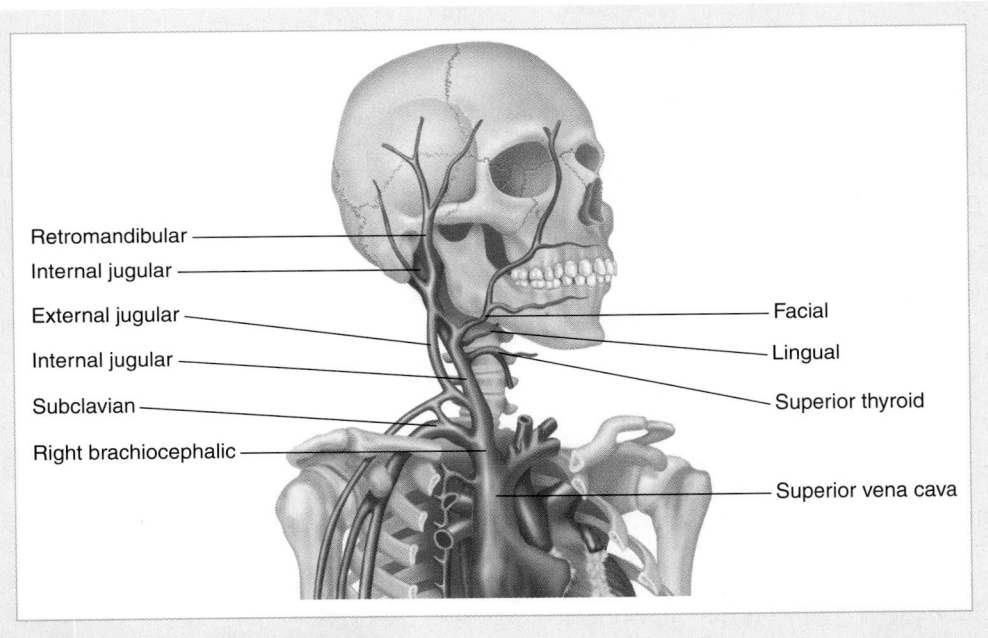

Figure 21-17 The veins of the neck.

as needed to guarantee that a ready supply of oxygen and glucose are available.

The Cerebrum

The largest portion of the brain is the cerebrum, which is responsible for higher functions, such as reasoning. The cerebrum is divided into right and left hemispheres by a longitudinal fissure. The hemispheres of the cerebrum are not entirely equivalent functionally. In a right-handed person, for example,

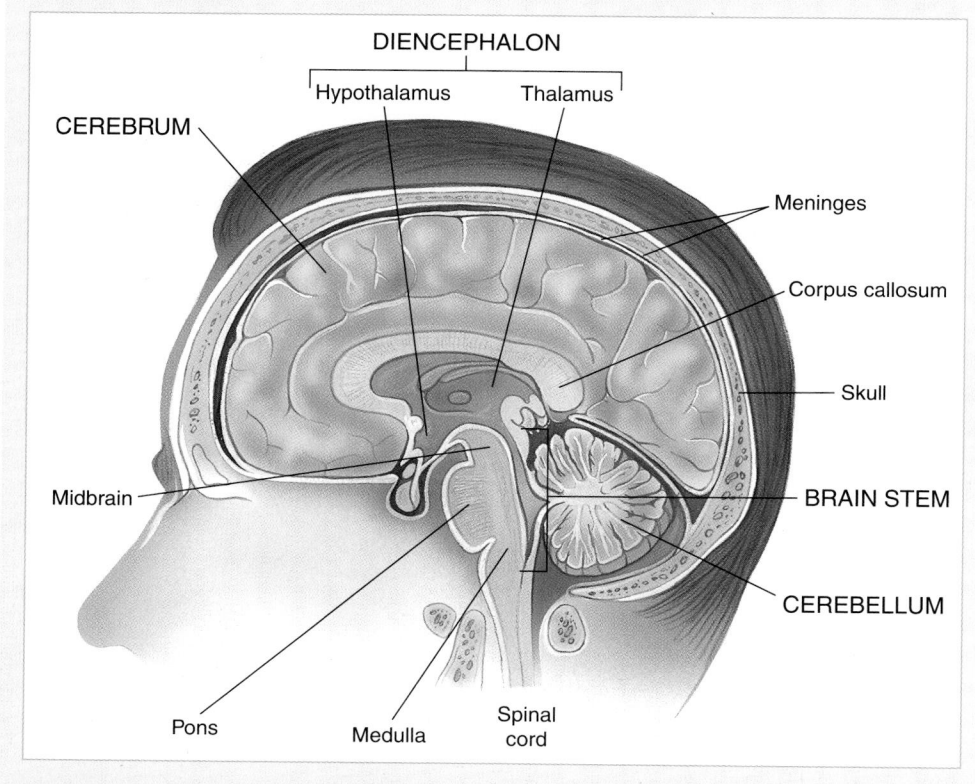

Figure 21-18 The major regions of the brain.

The speech center is located in the temporal lobe. In approximately 85% of the population, the speech center is located on the left side of the temporal lobe. The temporal lobe also controls long-term memory, hearing, taste, and smell. It is separated from the rest of the cerebrum by a lateral fissure.

The Diencephalon

The diencephalon, which is located between the brain stem and the cerebrum, includes the thalamus, subthalamus, hypothalamus, and epithalamus Figure 21-20 ▸ . The thalamus processes most sensory input and influences mood and general body movements, especially those associated with fear and rage. The subthalamus controls motor functions. The functions of the epithalamus are unclear. The most inferior portion of the diencephalon, the hypothalamus, is vital in the control of many body functions, including heart rate, digestion, sexual development, temperature regulation, emotion, hunger, thirst, vomiting, and regulation of the sleep cycle.

The Cerebellum

The cerebellum is located beneath the cerebral hemispheres in the inferoposterior part of the brain. It is sometimes called the "athlete's brain" because it is responsible for the maintenance

the speech center is usually located in the left cerebral hemisphere, which is then said to be the dominant hemisphere.

The largest portion of the cerebrum is the cerebral cortex, which regulates voluntary skeletal movement and the level of awareness. Injury to the cerebral cortex may result in paresthesia, weakness, and paralysis of the extremities.

Each cerebral hemisphere is divided functionally into specialized areas called lobes Figure 21-19 ▸ . The frontal lobe is important for voluntary motor action and personality traits. Injury to the frontal lobe may result in seizures or placid reactions (flat affect). The parietal lobe controls the somatic or voluntary sensory and motor functions for the opposite (contralateral) side of the body, as well as memory and emotions; it is separated from the frontal lobe by the central sulcus. Posteriorly, the occipital lobe, from which the optic nerve originates, is responsible for processing visual information. After a blow to the back of the head, a person may "see stars" which results when the occipital poles of the brain (the vision centers) bang against the back of the skull.

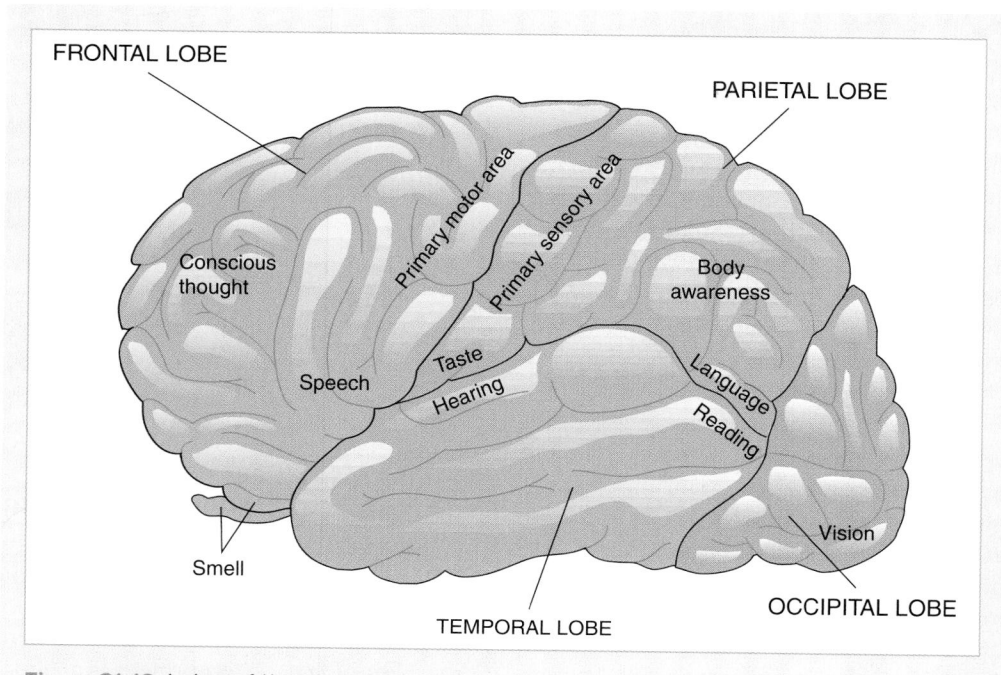

Figure 21-19 Lobes of the cerebrum.

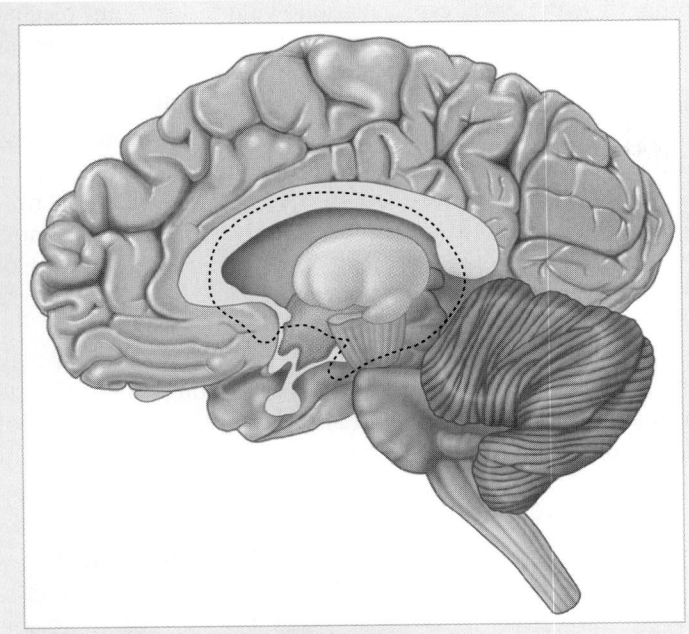

Figure 21-20 The diencephalon.

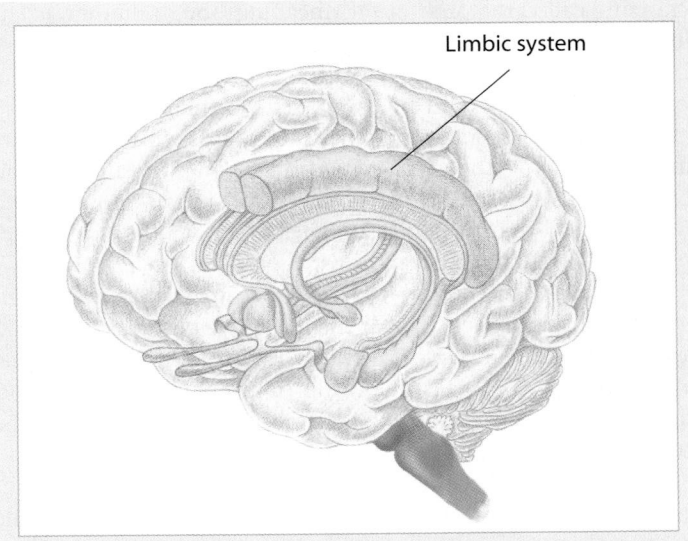

Figure 21-21 The limbic system is the seat of emotions, instincts, and other functions.

of posture and equilibrium and the coordination of skilled movements.

The Brain Stem

The brain stem consists of the midbrain, pons, and the medulla. It is located at the base of the brain and connects the spinal cord to the remainder of the brain. The brain stem houses many structures that are critical to the maintenance of vital functions. High in the brain stem, for example, is the reticular activating system (RAS), which is responsible for maintenance of consciousness, specifically one's level of arousal. The centers that control basic but critical functions—heart rate, blood pressure, and respiration—are located in the lower part of the brain stem. Damage to this area can easily result in cardiovascular derangement, respiratory arrest, or death.

The midbrain lies immediately below the diencephalon and is the smallest region of the brain stem. Deep within the cerebrum, diencephalon, and midbrain are the basal ganglia, which have an important role in coordination of motor movements and posture. Portions of the cerebrum and diencephalon constitute the limbic system, which influences emotions, motivation, mood, and sensations of pain and pleasure Figure 21-21 ▶ .

The oculomotor nerve (third cranial nerve) originates from the midbrain; it controls pupillary size and reactivity.

The pons, which lies below the midbrain and above the medulla, contains numerous important nerve fibers, including those for sleep, respiration, and the medullary respiratory center.

The inferior portion of the midbrain, the medulla, is continuous inferiorly with the spinal cord (see Figure 21-18). It serves as a conduction pathway for ascending and descending nerve tracts. It also coordinates heart rate, blood vessel diameter, breathing, swallowing, vomiting, coughing, and sneezing. The vagus nerve (tenth cranial nerve), a bundle of nerves that primarily innervates the parasympathetic nervous system, originates from the medulla.

The Meninges

The meninges are protective layers that surround and enfold the entire central nervous system—specifically the brain and spinal cord Figure 21-22 ▾ . The outermost layer is a strong, fibrous

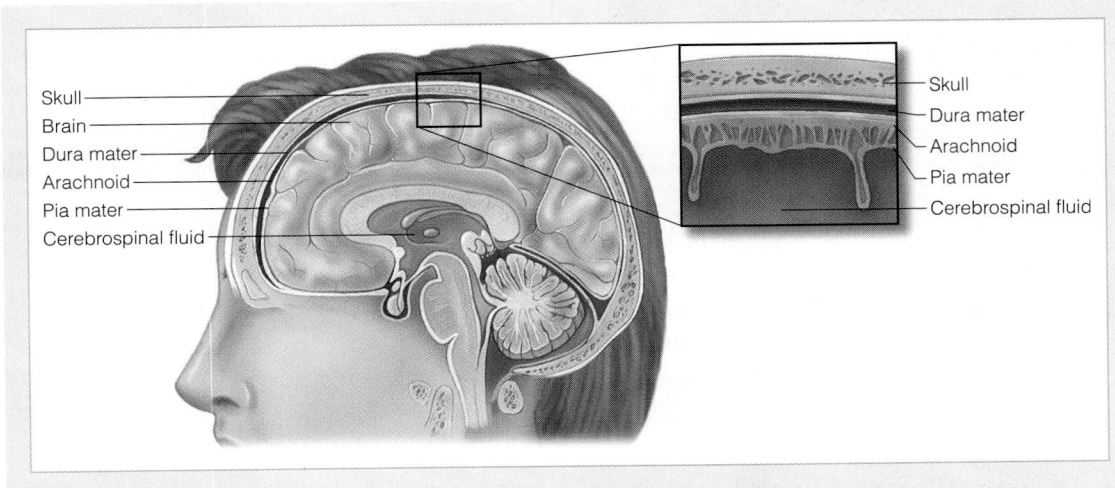

Skull
Brain
Dura mater
Arachnoid
Pia mater
Cerebrospinal fluid

Skull
Dura mater
Arachnoid
Pia mater
Cerebrospinal fluid

Figure 21-22 The meninges.

wrapping called the dura mater (meaning "tough mother"). The dura mater covers the entire brain, folding in to form the tentorium, a structure that separates the cerebral hemispheres from the cerebellum and brain stem. The dura mater is firmly attached to the internal wall of the skull. Just beneath the suture lines of the skull the dura mater splits into two surfaces and forms venous sinuses. When those venous sinuses are disrupted during a head injury, blood can collect beneath the dura mater to form a subdural hematoma.

The second meningeal layer is a delicate, transparent membrane called the arachnoid. It is so named because the blood vessels it contains resemble a spider web. The third meningeal layer, the pia mater ("soft mother"), is a thin, translucent, highly vascular membrane that firmly adheres directly to the surface of the brain.

The meningeal arteries are located between the dura mater and the skull. When one of these arteries (usually the middle meningeal artery) is disrupted, bleeding occurs above the dura mater, resulting in an epidural hematoma.

The meninges float in cerebrospinal fluid (CSF), which is manufactured in the ventricles of the brain. CSF flows in the subarachnoid space, located between the pia mater and the arachnoid.

CSF is manufactured by cells within the choroid plexus in the ventricles, hollow storage areas in the brain. These areas normally are interconnected, and CSF flows freely between them. CSF is similar in composition to plasma. The meninges and CSF form a fluid-filled sac that cushions and protects the brain and spinal cord.

Face Injuries

Soft-Tissue Injuries

Although open soft-tissue injuries to the face—lacerations, abrasions, and avulsions—by themselves are rarely life threat-

ening, their presence, especially following a significant mechanism of injury, suggests the potential for more severe injuries (eg, closed head injury, cervical spine injury). Furthermore, massive soft-tissue injuries to the face, especially if associated with oropharyngeal trauma and bleeding, can compromise the patient's airway and lead to ventilatory inadequacy.

Maintain a high index of suspicion when a patient presents with closed soft-tissue injuries to the face, such as contusions and hematomas **Figure 21-23 ▾** . These indicators of blunt force trauma suggest the potential for more severe underlying injuries.

Impaled objects in the soft tissues or bones of the face may occur in association with facial trauma. Although these objects can damage facial nerves, the risk of airway compromise is of far greater consequence. This is especially true when an

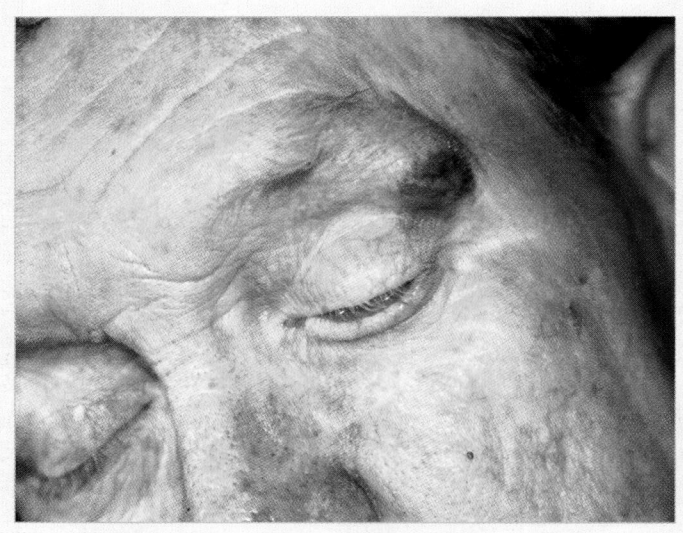

Figure 21-23 Closed soft-tissue injuries to the face may indicate more severe underlying injuries.

You are the Provider Part 3

Your partner is appropriately managing the patient's airway. You perform a rapid trauma assessment, which reveals a hematoma to the patient's forehead, massive soft-tissue trauma to the face, unstable facial bones, and bilaterally angulated femurs.

Vital Signs	Recording Time: 5 Minutes
Level of consciousness	Glasgow Coma Scale score of 6
Respirations	6 breaths/min and irregular (baseline); your partner is providing bag-mask ventilation at a rate of 10 breaths/min and 100% oxygen
Pulse	110 beats/min; regular and bounding
Skin	Warm and dry
Blood pressure	140/90 mm Hg
Sao_2	96% (with assisted ventilation and 100% oxygen)

5. How can facial trauma complicate airway management?
6. Is this patient in hypovolemic shock? Why or why not?

impaled object penetrates the cheek, because massive oropharyngeal bleeding can result in airway obstruction, aspiration, and ventilatory inadequacy. In addition, blood is a gastric irritant. For many people, just swallowing a couple of tablespoons of blood can make them vomit, further increasing the likelihood of aspiration.

Maxillofacial Fractures

Maxillofacial fractures commonly occur when the facial bones absorb the energy of a strong impact. The forces involved may be massive. For example, a force up to 150g (g = acceleration of the body due to gravity) is required to fracture the maxilla; a force of that magnitude will likely produce closed head injuries and cervical spine injuries as well. Therefore, when assessing a patient with a suspected maxillofacial fracture, you should protect the cervical spine and monitor the patient's neurologic signs, specifically their level of consciousness.

The first clue to the presence of a maxillofacial fracture is usually ecchymosis, so a black-and-blue mark on the face should alert you to this possibility. A deep facial laceration should likewise increase your index of suspicion that the underlying bone may have been fractured, and pain over a bone tends to support the suspicion of fracture. General signs and symptoms of maxillofacial fractures include ecchymosis, swelling, pain to palpation, crepitus, dental malocclusion, facial deformities or asymmetry, instability of the facial bones, impaired ocular movement, and visual disturbances.

Nasal Fractures

Because the nasal bones are not as structurally sound as the other bones of the face, nasal fractures are the most common facial fracture. These fractures are characterized by swelling, tenderness, and crepitus when the nasal bone is palpated. Deformity of the nose, if present, usually appears as lateral displacement of the nasal bone from its normal midline position.

Nasal fractures, like any maxillofacial fracture, are often complicated by the presence of an anterior or a posterior nosebleed (epistaxis), which can compromise the patient's airway.

Mandibular Fractures and Dislocations

Second only to nasal fractures in frequency, fractures of the mandible typically result from massive blunt force trauma to the lower third of the face; they are particularly common following an assault injury. Because significant force is required to fracture the mandible, this structure may be fractured in more than one place and, therefore, unstable to palpation. The fracture site itself is most commonly located at the angle of the jaw.

Mandibular fractures should be suspected in patients with a history of blunt force trauma to the lower third of the face who present with dental malocclusion (misalignment of the teeth), numbness of the chin, and inability to open the mouth. There will likely be swelling and ecchymosis over the fracture site, and teeth may be partially or completely avulsed.

Although temporomandibular joint (TMJ) dislocations may occur as the result of blunt force trauma to the lower third of the face, this outcome is rare. Mandibular dislocations are most often the result of yawning extravagantly or otherwise opening the mouth very widely. The patient commonly feels a "pop" and then cannot close his or her mouth; it is locked in a wide-open position. The jaw muscles eventually go into spasm, causing severe pain.

Maxillary Fractures

Maxillary fractures to the midface area are most commonly associated with mechanisms that produce massive blunt facial trauma, such as motor vehicle crashes, falls, and assaults. They produce massive facial swelling, instability of the midfacial bones, malocclusion, and an elongated appearance of the patient's face. Midfacial structures include the maxilla, zygoma, orbital floor, and nose.

Le Fort fractures **Figure 21-24 ▾** are classified into three categories:

- **Le Fort I fracture.** A horizontal fracture of the maxilla that involves the hard palate and inferior maxilla
- **Le Fort II fracture.** A pyramidal fracture involving the nasal bone and inferior maxilla
- **Le Fort III fracture** (craniofacial disjunction). A fracture of all midfacial bones, separating the entire midface from the cranium.

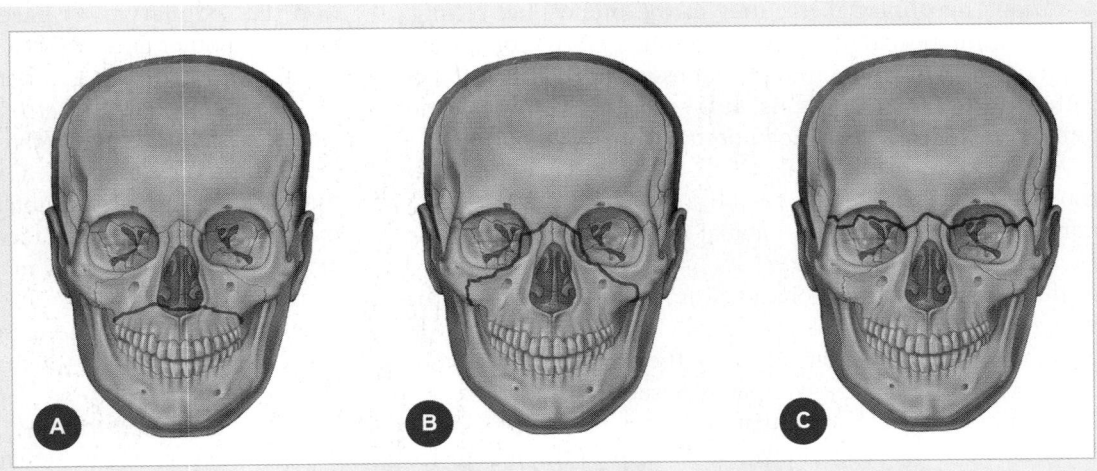

Figure 21-24 Le Fort fractures. **A.** Le Fort I. **B.** Le Fort II. **C.** Le Fort III.

Le Fort fractures can occur as isolated fractures (Le Fort I) or in combination (Le Fort I and II), depending on the location of impact and the amount of trauma.

Orbital Fractures

The patient with an orbital fracture (such as a blowout fracture [see Figure 21-7]) may complain of double vision (<u>diplopia</u>) and lose sensation above the eyebrow or over the cheek secondary to associated nerve damage. Massive nasal discharge may occur, and vision is often impaired. Fractures of the inferior orbit are the most common type and can cause paralysis of upward gaze (the patient's injured eye will not be able to follow your finger *above* the midline).

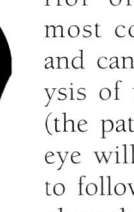

Notes from Nancy

Check eye movements in all planes in the patient with possible facial fractures.

Zygomatic Fractures

Fractures of the zygomatic bone (cheek bone) commonly result from blunt trauma secondary to motor vehicle crashes and assaults. When the zygomatic bone is fractured, that side of the patient's face appears flattened, and there is loss of sensation over the cheek, nose, and upper lip; paralysis of upward gaze may also be present. Other injuries commonly associated with zygomatic fractures include orbital fractures, ocular injury, and epistaxis.

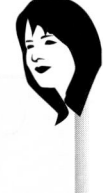

Notes from Nancy

Any patient with significant head injury also has cervical spine injury until proved otherwise.

◼ Assessment and Management of Face Injuries

Table 21-1 ▶ summarizes the characteristics of various maxillofacial fractures. It is not important to distinguish among the various maxillofacial fractures in the prehospital setting; this determination requires radiographic evaluation in the emergency department. Rapid patient assessment, management of life-threatening conditions, full spinal precautions, and prompt transport are far more important considerations.

Management of the patient with facial trauma begins by protecting the cervical spine. Because many severe facial injuries are complicated by a spinal injury, you must assume that one exists.

If the patient is semiconscious or unconscious, open the airway with the jaw-thrust maneuver while simultaneously maintaining manual stabilization of the head in the neutral position unless the patient complains of severe pain or discomfort upon movement. Should that occur, the head/neck should be immobilized in the position found. Inspect the mouth for fragments of teeth, dentures, or any other foreign bodies that

Table 21-1	Summary of Maxillofacial Fractures
Injury	**Signs and Symptoms**
Multiple facial bone fractures	• Massive facial swelling • Dental malocclusion • Palpable deformities • Anterior or posterior epistaxis
Zygomatic and orbital fractures	• Loss of sensation below the orbit • Flattening of the patient's cheek • Paralysis of upward gaze
Nasal fractures	• Crepitus and instability • Swelling, tenderness, lateral displacement • Anterior or posterior epistaxis
Maxillary (Le Fort) fractures	• Mobility of the facial skeleton • Dental malocclusion • Facial swelling
Mandibular fractures	• Dental malocclusion • Mandibular instability

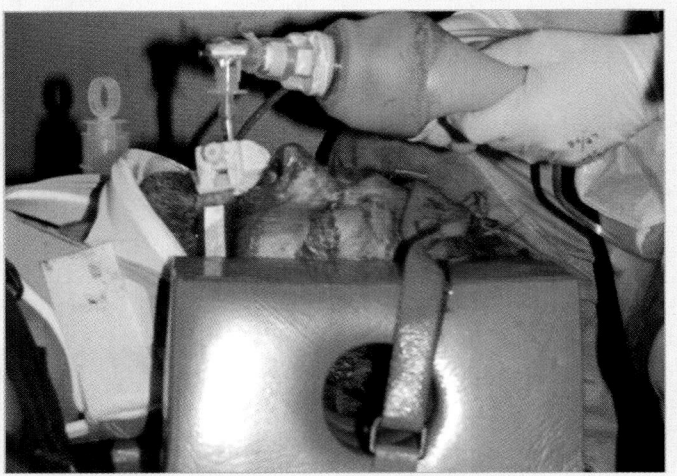

Figure 21-25 Airway management can be especially challenging in patients with massive facial injuries.

could obstruct the airway, and remove them immediately. Suction the oropharynx as needed to keep the airway clear of blood and other liquids.

Insert an airway adjunct as needed to maintain airway patency. However, *do not insert a nasopharyngeal airway or attempt nasotracheal intubation in any patient with suspected nasal fractures or in patients with CSF or blood leakage from the nose.* After establishing and maintaining a patent airway, assess the patient's breathing and intervene appropriately. Apply 100% oxygen via nonrebreathing mask if the patient is breathing adequately. Patients who are breathing inadequately (ie, fast or slow rate, reduced tidal volume [shallow breathing], irregular pattern of inhalation and exhalation) should receive bag-mask ventilation with 100% oxygen. Maintain the patient's oxygen saturation at greater than 95%.

Airway management can be especially challenging in patients with massive facial injuries **Figure 21-25 ▲**.

In the Field

Blood or CSF drainage from the nose (cerebrospinal rhinorrhea) suggests a skull fracture. Do not make any attempt to control this bleeding; doing so may increase intracranial pressure (ICP) if the patient has a concomitant brain injury. Furthermore, the insertion of nasal airway adjuncts and nasotracheal intubation should be avoided in patients with suspected nasal fractures, especially if rhinorrhea is present. A nasally inserted airway device could enter the cranial vault through an occult fracture (such as a cribriform plate fracture) and penetrate the brain further worsening the situation.

Oropharyngeal bleeding poses an immediate threat to the airway, and unstable facial bones can hinder your ability to maintain an effective mask-to-face seal for bag-mask ventilation. Therefore, perform tracheal intubation of patients with facial trauma, especially those who are unconscious, to protect their airway from aspiration and to ensure adequate oxygenation and ventilation. Cricothyrotomy (surgical or needle) may be required for patients with extensive maxillofacial injuries when endotracheal intubation is extremely difficult or impossible to perform (ie, in cases of unstable facial bones, massive swelling, severe oral bleeding).

Treat facial lacerations and avulsions as you would any other soft-tissue injury. Control all bleeding with direct pressure, and apply sterile dressings. If you suspect an underlying facial fracture, apply just enough pressure to control the bleeding. Leave impaled objects in the face in place and appropriately stabilize them, unless they pose a threat to the airway (such as an object impaled through the cheek). When removing an object from the cheek, carefully remove it from the same side that it entered. Next, pack the inside of the cheek with sterile gauze and apply counterpressure with a dressing and bandage firmly secured over the outside of the wound. If profuse bleeding continues, position the patient on his or her side—while maintaining stabilization of the cervical spine—to facilitate drainage of secretions from the mouth and suction the airway as needed.

For severe oropharyngeal bleeding in patients with inadequate ventilation, suction the airway for 15 seconds and provide ventilatory assistance for 2 minutes; continue this alternating pattern of suctioning and ventilating until the airway is cleared of blood or secured with an endotracheal (ET) tube. Monitoring the pulse oximeter during this process can further serve to keep the patient from becoming hypoxic.

Epistaxis following facial trauma can be severe and is most effectively controlled by applying direct pressure to the nares. If the patient is conscious and spinal injury is not suspected, instruct the patient to sit up and lean forward as you pinch the nares together. Unconscious patients should be positioned on their side, unless contraindicated by a spinal injury. Proper positioning of the patient with epistaxis is important to prevent blood from draining down the throat and compromising the airway either by occlusion or by vomiting and then aspirating

gastric contents. If the conscious patient with severe epistaxis is immobilized on a backboard, you should consider pharmacologically assisted intubation (eg, rapid-sequence intubation [RSI]) to gain definitive control of the airway.

Although facial lacerations and avulsions can contribute to hemorrhagic shock, they are rarely the sole cause of this condition in adults. Severe epistaxis, however, can result in significant blood loss. To counter this problem, you should carefully assess the patient for signs of hemorrhagic shock and administer intravenous (IV) crystalloid fluid boluses as needed to maintain adequate perfusion.

If the facial fracture is associated with swelling and ecchymosis, cold compresses may help minimize further swelling and alleviate pain. Do not apply a compress to the eyeball (globe) if you suspect that it has been injured following an orbital fracture; doing so may increase the intraocular pressure (IOP) and further damage the eye. Other than protecting the airway, little can be done to treat facial instabilities; however, firmly applying a self-adhering roller bandage (such as Kerlix or Kling) can stabilize the mandible. Make sure that you do not compromise the airway when stabilizing the mandible.

After addressing all life-threatening injuries and conditions, you should attempt to ascertain the events that preceded the injury and determine whether the patient has any significant medical problems. The incident that caused the injury may have been preceded by exacerbation of an underlying medical condition (such as acute hypoglycemia, cardiac dysrhythmia, seizure). For unconscious patients, medications that the patient is taking may provide information about his or her medical history. Determine the approximate time that the injury occurred, and ask about any drug allergies and the last oral intake during your SAMPLE history **Figure 21-26 ▶**.

Special Considerations

Relative to younger, healthy adults, elderly patients are at high risk for severe epistaxis following even minor facial injuries, especially in those with a history of hypertension or anticoagulant medication use (such as warfarin [Coumadin]). This bleeding often originates in the posterior nasopharynx and may not be grossly evident during your assessment.

Eye Injuries

Approximately 1.5 million eye injuries occur in the United States each year, of which 50,000 result in some degree of visual loss. Because trauma to the eyes is so common and the potential consequences are so serious, you must know how to assess and manage ocular injuries.

Eye injuries are frequently caused by blunt trauma, penetrating trauma, or burns. Blunt mechanisms of injury may

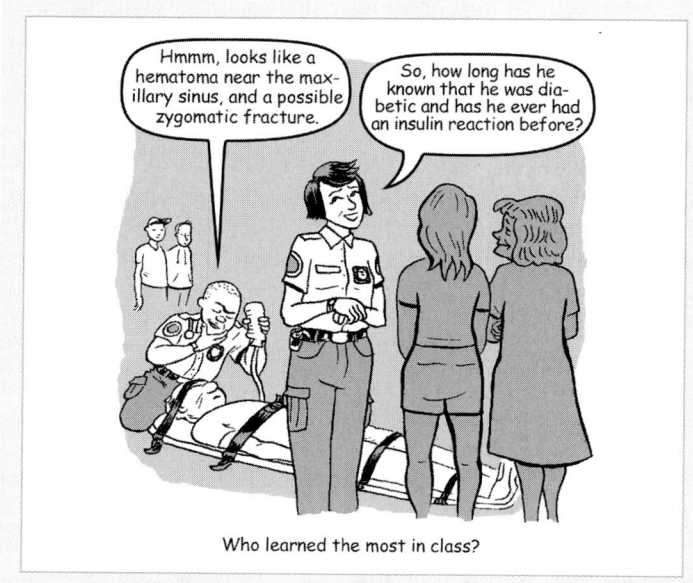

Figure 21-26

include motor vehicle crashes, motorcycles crashes, falls, and assaults. Penetrating injuries are often secondary to foreign bodies on the surface of the eye (such as sand) or an object impaled in the globe. Burns to the eye can result from a variety of corrosive chemicals or during industrial accidents (such as welding burns).

Lacerations, Foreign Bodies, and Impaled Objects

Lacerations of the eyelids require meticulous repair to restore appearance and function. Bleeding may be heavy, but it usually can be controlled by gentle, manual pressure. *If there is a laceration to the globe itself, apply no pressure to the eye;* compression can interfere with the blood supply to the back of the eye and result in loss of vision from damage to the retina. Furthermore, pressure may squeeze the vitreous humor, iris, lens, or even the retina out of the eye and cause irreparable damage or blindness Figure 21-27 ▶ .

The protective orbit prevents large objects from penetrating the eye. However, moderately sized and smaller foreign objects can still enter the eye and, when lying on the surface of the eye, produce severe irritation Figure 21-28 ▶ . The conjunctiva becomes inflamed and red—a condition known as conjunctivitis—almost immediately, and the eye begins to produce tears in an attempt to flush out the object Figure 21-29 ▶ . Irritation of the cornea or conjunctiva causes intense pain. The patient may have difficulty keeping the eyelids open, because the irritation is further aggravated by bright light.

Foreign bodies ranging in size from a pencil to a sliver of metal may be impaled in the eye Figure 21-30 ▶ . Clearly, these objects must be removed by a physician. Prehospital care involves stabilizing the object and preparing the patient for

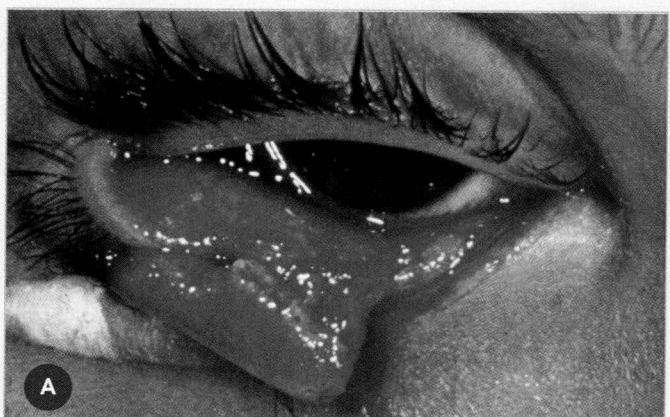

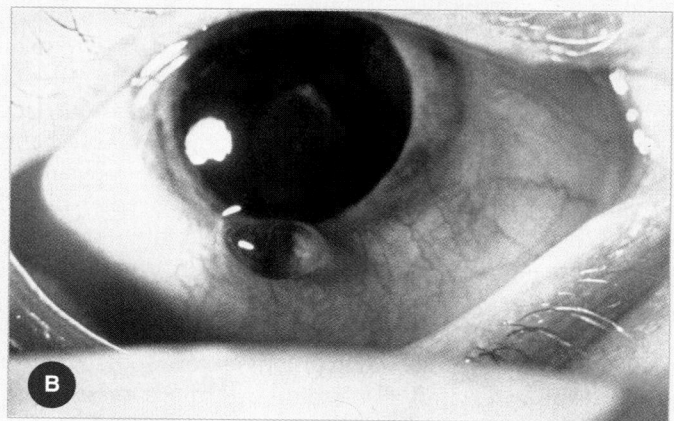

Figure 21-27 Eye lacerations are serious injuries that require prompt transport. **A.** Although bleeding can be heavy, never exert pressure on the eye. **B.** Pressure may squeeze the vitreous humor, iris, lens, or retina out of the eye.

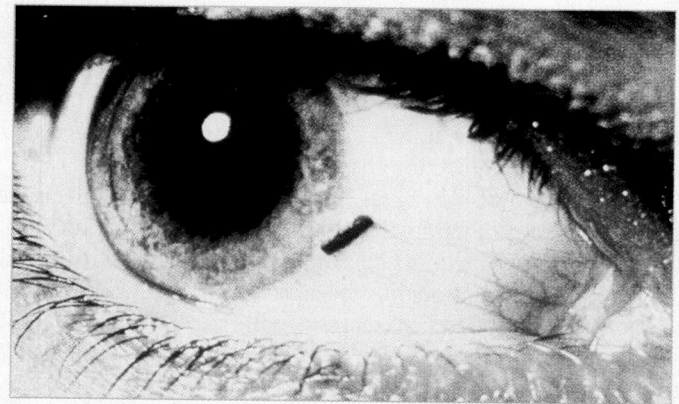

Figure 21-28 A foreign object on the surface of the eye.

transport. The greater the length of the foreign object sticking out of the eye, the more important stabilization becomes in avoiding further damage. Whenever possible, cover both eyes to limit unnecessary movement as the patient tries to use the uninjured eye to compensate for the loss or limited vision of the injured eye.

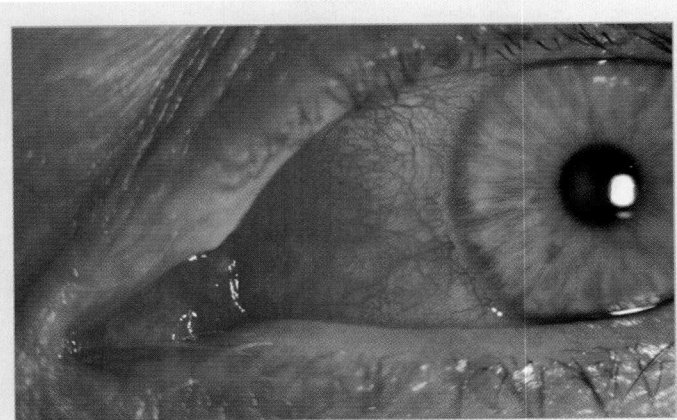

Figure 21-29 Conjunctivitis is often associated with the presence of a foreign object in the eye.

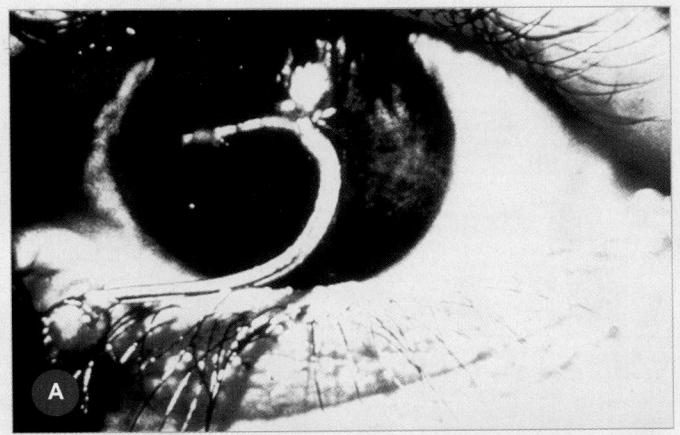

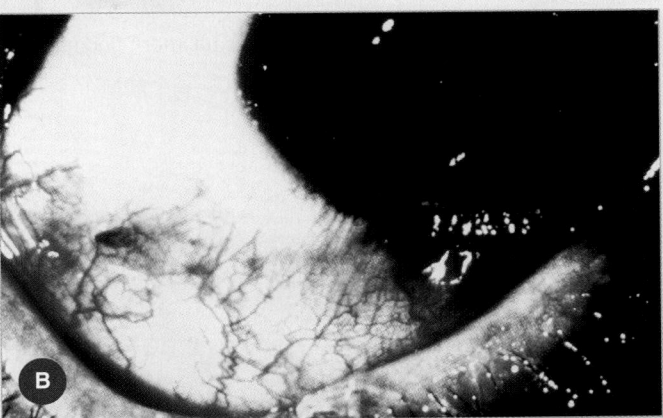

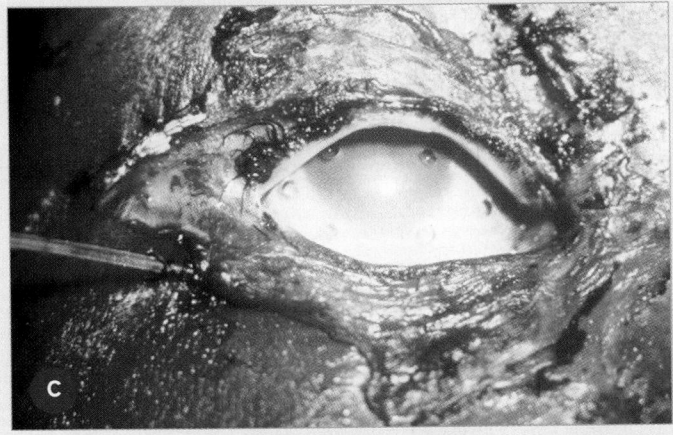

Figure 21-30 Any number of objects can be impaled in the eye. **A.** Fishhook. **B.** Sharp, metal sliver. **C.** Knife blade.

In the Field

Large and small foreign bodies, particularly small metal fragments, can become completely embedded in the globe. The patient may not even be aware of the cause of the problem. Suspect such an injury when the history includes metal work (such as hammering, exposure to splinters, grinding, vigorous filing) and when you observe signs of ocular injury (such as redness, irritation, inflammation).

Blunt Eye Injuries

Blunt trauma can cause serious eye injuries, ranging from swelling and ecchymosis Figure 21-31 ▶ to rupture of the globe. Hyphema is bleeding into the anterior chamber of the eye that obscures vision, partially or completely Figure 21-32 ▶ . It often follows blunt trauma and may seriously impair vision. Approximately 25% of hyphemas are associated with globe injuries.

In orbital blowout fractures, the fragments of fractured bone can entrap some of the muscles that control eye movement, causing double vision (diplopia) Figure 21-33 ▶ . Any patient who reports pain, double vision, or decreased vision following a blunt injury about the eye should be assumed to have a blowout fracture and should be promptly transported to an appropriate medical facility.

Another potential result of blunt eye trauma is retinal detachment, or separation of the inner layers of the retina from the underlying choroid (the vascular membrane that nourishes the retina). Retinal detachment is often seen in sports injuries, especially boxing. This painless condition produces flashing lights, specks, or "floaters" in the field of vision and a cloud or shade over the patient's vision. Because it can cause devastating damage to vision, retinal detachment is an ocular emergency and requires *immediate* medical attention.

Burns of the Eye

Chemicals, heat, and light rays can all burn the delicate tissues of the eye, often causing permanent damage. Your role is to stop the burning process and prevent further damage.

Chemical burns, which are usually caused by acid or alkali solutions, require immediate emergency care Figure 21-34 ▶ . Flush the eye with water or a sterile saline

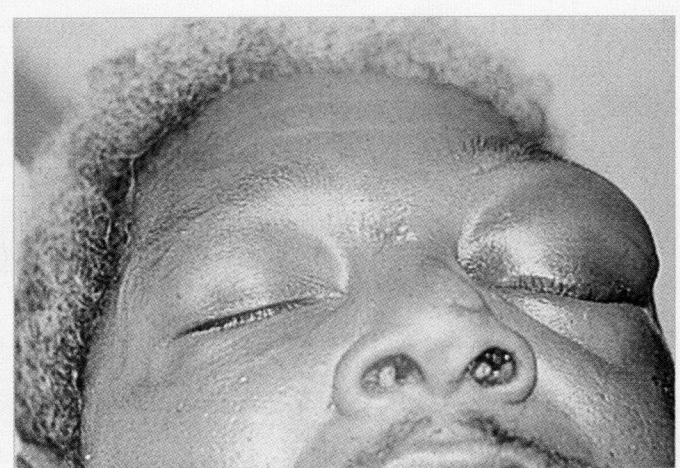

Figure 21-31 Swelling and ecchymosis are hallmark findings associated with blunt trauma to the eye.

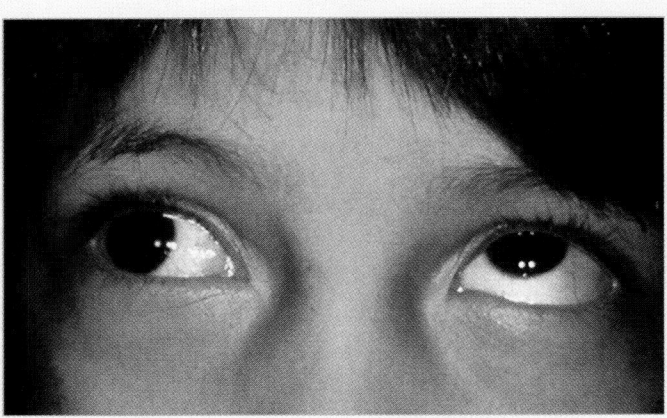

Figure 21-33 In a patient with a blowout fracture, the eyes may not move together because of muscle entrapment, so the patient sees double images of any object.

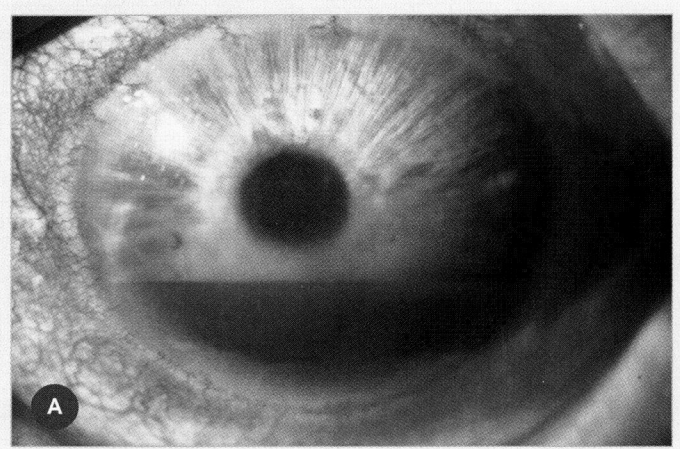

A

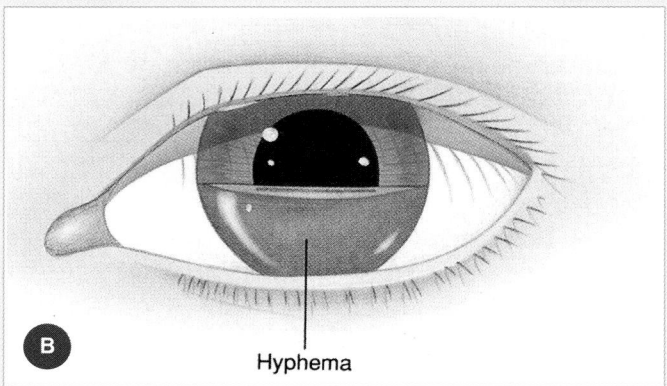

B Hyphema

Figure 21-32 A hyphema, characterized by bleeding into the anterior chamber of the eye, can occur following blunt trauma to the eye. This condition should be considered a sight-threatening emergency. **A.** Actual hyphema. **B.** Illustration.

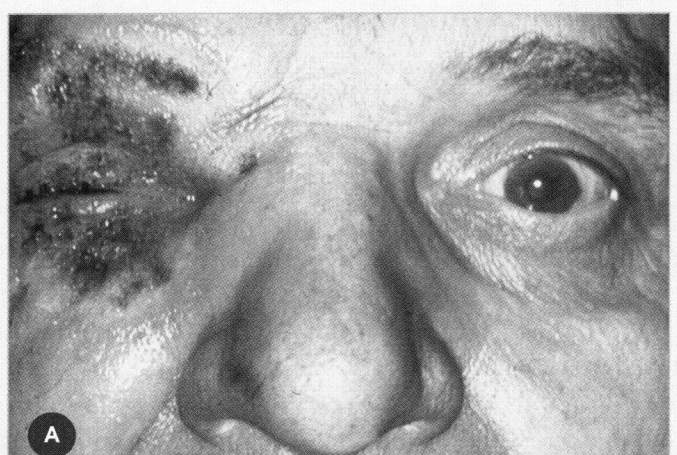

A

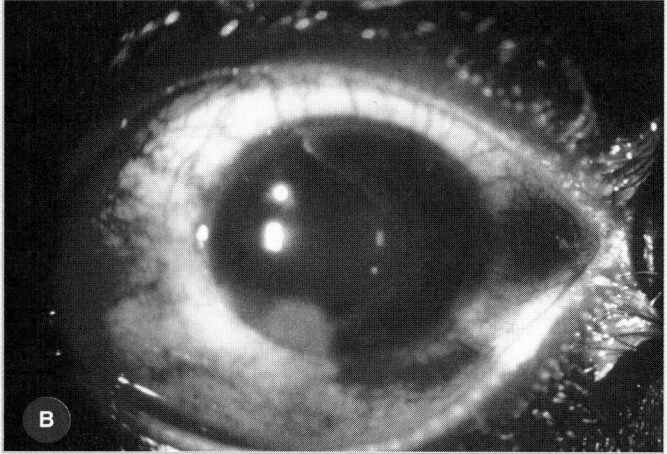

B

Figure 21-34 **A.** Chemical burns typically occur when an acid or alkali is splashed into the eye. **B.** A chemical burn from lye, an alkaline solution.

reticular activating system (RAS) Located in the upper brain stem; responsible for maintenance of consciousness, specifically one's level of arousal.

retina A delicate 10-layered structure of nervous tissue located in the rear of the interior of the globe that receives light and generates nerve signals that are transmitted to the brain through the optic nerve.

retinal detachment Separation of the inner layers of the retina from the underlying choroid, the vascular membrane that nourishes the retina.

retrograde amnesia Loss of memory relating to events that occurred before the injury.

sagittal suture The point of the skull where the parietal bones join.

sclera The white part of the eye.

secondary brain injury The "after effects" of the primary injury; includes abnormal processes such as cerebral edema, increased intracranial pressure, cerebral ischemia and hypoxia, and infection; onset is often delayed following the primary brain injury.

skull The structure at the top of the axial skeleton that houses the brain and consists of 28 bones that comprise the auditory ossicles, the cranium, and the face.

subarachnoid hemorrhage Bleeding into the subarachnoid space, where the cerebrospinal fluid (CSF) circulates.

subarachnoid space The space located between the pia mater and the arachnoid mater.

subdural hematoma An accumulation of blood beneath the dura but outside the brain.

subthalamus The part of the diencephalon that is involved in controlling motor functions.

sympathetic eye movement The movement of both eyes in unison.

temporal lobe The portion of the brain that has an important role in hearing and memory.

temporomandibular joint (TMJ) The joint between the temporal bone and the posterior condyle that allows for movements of the mandible.

tentorium A structure that separates the cerebral hemispheres from the cerebellum and brain stem.

thalamus The part of the diencephalon that processes most sensory input and influences mood and general body movements, especially those associated with fear or rage.

tracheal transection Traumatic separation of the trachea from the larynx.

traumatic brain injury (TBI) A traumatic insult to the brain capable of producing physical, intellectual, emotional, social, and vocational changes.

trigeminal nerve Fifth cranial nerve; supplies sensation to the scalp, forehead, face, and lower jaw and innervates the muscles of mastication, the throat, and the inner ear.

trismus Clenching of the teeth owing to spasm of the jaw muscles.

tympanic membrane A thin membrane that separates the middle ear from the inner ear and sets up vibrations in the ossicles; also called the eardrum.

ventricles Specialized hollow areas in the brain.

visual cortex The area in the brain where signals from the optic nerve are converted into visual images.

vitreous humor A jellylike substance found in the posterior compartment of the eye between the lens and the retina.

zygomatic arch The bone that extends along the front of the skull below the orbit.

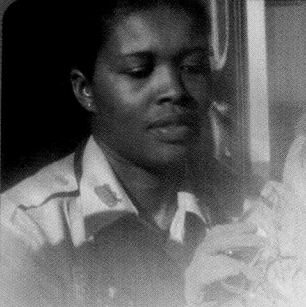

Assessment in Action

Your unit is dispatched to a residence for an assault. An on-scene police officer advises you that the scene is safe to enter. Your response time to the scene is approximately 7 minutes. When you arrive, a police officer escorts you to the patient, a man in his late 30s. According to witnesses, the patient was struck in the side of the head with a steel pipe during an altercation with his neighbor. As you approach the patient, you note that he is lying in a supine position and is not moving; there is no gross bleeding. The neighbor is in police custody.

1. **After your partner manually stabilizes the patient's cervical spine, you should:**
   A. vigorously shake the patient to determine his level of consciousness.
   B. open his airway with the head tilt–chin lift maneuver or tongue jaw lift.
   C. suction his oropharynx for 30 seconds to ensure that it is clear of blood.
   D. determine his level of consciousness, and ensure that his airway is clear.

2. **Your initial assessment reveals that the patient is unconscious and unresponsive. You insert an oropharyngeal airway and assess his respirations, which are slow and shallow. His radial pulses are slow and bounding. What must you do next?**
   A. Perform immediate endotracheal intubation.
   B. Provide bag-mask ventilation and 100% oxygen.
   C. Apply a nonrebreathing mask, and reassess him.
   D. Start an IV line and administer atropine sulfate.

3. **The patient's BP is 170/100 mm Hg, his pulse rate is 50 beats/min and bounding, and his baseline respirations are 6 breaths/min and have now become irregular. What is the pathophysiology of this patient's vital signs?**
   A. An increase in mean arterial pressure, cerebral vasodilation, and pressure on the brain stem
   B. Cerebral vasoconstriction, shunting of blood from the brain, and complete brain stem herniation
   C. A decrease in mean arterial pressure, cerebral vasodilation, and a decrease in cerebral perfusion pressure
   D. Cerebral vasodilation, a decrease in cerebral blood flow, and increased parasympathetic tone

4. **All of the following are clinical signs of pressure on the upper brain stem, EXCEPT:**
   A. Cheyne-Stokes respirations.
   B. an increase in the patient's BP.
   C. a marked increase in heart rate.
   D. bilaterally fixed and dilated pupils.

5. **Which of the following are indications for hyperventilation of a brain-injured patient?**
   A. A systolic BP that exceeds 200 mm Hg
   B. Bilaterally dilated and slowly reactive pupils
   C. An absent motor response to painful stimuli
   D. Withdrawal from pain with flexor posturing

6. **Your patient has been intubated and ventilations are continuing. Further assessment reveals that the patient is unresponsive to all stimuli, has unequal pupils, and shows extensor posturing. How many ventilations per minute should this patient receive?**
   A. 10
   B. 20
   C. 25
   D. 30

7. **Which of the following is the most appropriate IV fluid regimen for a head-injured patient with a BP of 70/50 mm Hg?**
   A. An amount sufficient to maintain a systolic BP of at least 90 mm Hg
   B. 1,000 mL to 2,000 mL followed by a reassessment of the patient's BP
   C. A crystalloid solution infusion set to run at approximately 120 mL/h
   D. Set the IV line(s) to keep the vein open because fluids will worsen cerebral edema

8. **Which of the following drugs would you be *least* likely to use when treating a patient with a severe head injury?**
   A. Lorazepam (Ativan)
   B. Lidocaine
   C. 50% dextrose
   D. Normal saline

9. **Which of the following parameters does the Glasgow Coma Scale (GCS) measure?**
   A. Pupil size, eye opening, verbal response
   B. Eye opening, motor response, heart rate
   C. Verbal response, pupil size, motor response
   D. Eye opening, verbal response, motor response

10. **You have arrived at the hospital and have transferred patient care to the attending physician. You later learn that the patient had bleeding between the outer meningeal layer and the skull. This is called a(n):**
    A. subdural hematoma.
    B. epidural hematoma.
    C. subarachnoid hemorrhage.
    D. intraparenchymal hematoma.

Challenging Questions

A 27-year-old highly intoxicated male was riding in the back of a pickup truck, when he fell out and struck his head on the pavement. Your assessment reveals that the patient is unconscious and unresponsive. His respirations are slow and irregular and his pulse rate is slow and bounding. The only visible injuries are a non-bleeding laceration to his right temporal region and blood draining from his right ear. Your partner manually stabilizes the patient's c-spine and begins ventilation assistance with a bag-mask device and 100% oxygen. Suddenly, the patient begins regurgitating massive amounts of liquid.

11. **What is the most effective way to initially manage this patient's airway?**

12. **What is the pathophysiology of the patient's vital signs? What would you expect his blood pressure to be?**

Points to Ponder

You are transporting a 30-year-old woman with blunt head trauma. She is conscious but persistently confused. You have applied 100% oxygen via nonrebreathing mask, started an IV line of normal saline and set the flow rate to keep vein open, and applied the cardiac monitor. Because of the mechanism of injury, full spinal motion restriction precautions have been applied. The patient's BP is 138/88 mm Hg, pulse rate is 100 beats/min, and respirations are 20 breaths/min and regular. As you are conversing with the patient, you note that her level of consciousness is progressively decreasing. You reassess her airway, which is still patent, but her respirations are now slow. The patient's pupils have increased in size but are still equal and reactive to light. She responds to pain by pushing your hand away. Noting these changes, you insert an airway adjunct and begin hyperventilating by bag-mask ventilation at a rate of 24 breaths/min and continue to do so until you arrive at the hospital 20 minutes later. After delivering the patient to the hospital and returning to service, you learn that the patient experienced an anoxic brain injury.

Why did this occur? Could you have done something to prevent it?

Issues: Recognizing Clinical Signs of the Different Levels of Intracranial Pressure, Knowing the Appropriate Ventilation Rates for Head-Injured Patients, Understanding the Importance of Maintaining Cerebral Perfusion Pressure.

22 Spine Injuries

Objectives

Cognitive

4-6.1 Describe the incidence, morbidity, and mortality of spinal injuries in the trauma patient. (p 22.3)

4-6.2 Describe the anatomy and physiology of structures related to spinal injuries.
- a. Cervical
- b. Thoracic
- c. Lumbar
- d. Sacrum
- e. Coccyx
- f. Head (p 21.4)
- g. Brain
- h. Spinal cord
- i. Nerve tract(s)
- j. Dermatomes (p 22.4–22.6, 22.15)

4-6.3 Predict spinal injuries based on mechanism of injury. (p 22.10)

4-6.4 Describe the pathophysiology of spinal injuries. (p 22.7)

4-6.5 Explain traumatic and non-traumatic spinal injuries. (p 22.26)

4-6.6 Describe the assessment findings associated with spinal injuries. (p 22.11)

4-6.7 Describe the management of spinal injuries. (p 22.17)

4-6.8 Identify the need for rapid intervention and transport of the patient with spinal injuries. (p 22.12)

4-6.9 Integrate the pathophysiological principles to the assessment of a patient with a spinal injury. (p 22.13)

4-6.10 Differentiate between spinal injuries based on the assessment and history. (p 22.12)

4-6.11 Formulate a field impression based on the assessment findings. (p 22.12)

4-6.12 Develop a patient management plan based on the field impression. (p 22.17)

4-6.13 Describe the pathophysiology of traumatic spinal injury related to:
- a. Spinal shock
- b. Spinal neurogenic shock
- c. Quadriplegia/paraplegia
- d. Incomplete cord injury/cord syndromes:
  1. Central cord syndrome
  2. Anterior cord syndrome
  3. Brown-Sequard syndrome (p 22.9)

4-6.14 Describe the assessment findings associated with traumatic spinal injuries. (p 22.13)

4-6.15 Describe the management of traumatic spinal injuries. (p 22.17)

4-6.16 Integrate pathophysiological principles to the assessment of a patient with a traumatic spinal injury. (p 22.13)

4-6.17 Differentiate between traumatic and non-traumatic spinal injuries based on the assessment and history. (p 22.12)

4-6.18 Formulate a field impression for traumatic spinal injury based on the assessment findings. (p 22.13)

4-6.19 Develop a patient management plan for traumatic spinal injury based on the field impression. (p 22.17)

4-6.20 Describe the pathophysiology of non-traumatic spinal injury, including:
- a. Low back pain
- b. Herniated intervertebral disk
- c. Spinal cord tumors (p 22.7–22.8, 22.26–22.27)

4-6.21 Describe the assessment findings associated with non-traumatic spinal injuries. (p 22.26)

4-6.22 Describe the management of non-traumatic spinal injuries. (p 22.27)

4-6.23 Integrate pathophysiological principles to the assessment of a patient with non-traumatic spinal injury. (p 22.26)

4-6.24 Differentiate between traumatic and non-traumatic spinal injuries based on the assessment and history. (p 22.26)

4-6.25 Formulate a field impression for non-traumatic spinal injury based on the assessment findings. (p 22.26)

4-6.26 Develop a patient management plan for non-traumatic spinal injury based on the field impression. (p 22.27)

Affective

4-6.27 Advocate the use of a thorough assessment when determining the proper management modality for spine injuries. (p 22.9)

4-6.28 Value the implications of failing to properly immobilize a spine injured patient. (p 22.17)

Psychomotor

4-6.29 Demonstrate a clinical assessment to determine the proper management modality for a patient with a suspected traumatic spinal injury. (p 22.9)

4-6.30 Demonstrate a clinical assessment to determine the proper management modality for a patient with a suspected non-traumatic spinal injury. (p 22.11)

4-6.31 Demonstrate immobilization of the urgent and non-urgent patient with assessment findings of spinal injury from the following presentations:
- a. Supine
- b. Prone
- c. Semi-prone
- d. Sitting
- e. Standing (p 22.17, 22.19, 22.23)

4-6.32 Demonstrate documentation of suspected spinal cord injury to include:
- a. General area of spinal cord involved
- b. Sensation
- c. Dermatomes
- d. Motor function
- e. Area(s) of weakness (p 22.11)

4-6.33 Demonstrate preferred methods for stabilization of a helmet from a potentially spine injured patient. (p 22.24, 22.25)

4-6.34 Demonstrate helmet removal techniques. (p 22.24, 22.25)

4-6.35 Demonstrate alternative methods for stabilization of a helmet from a potentially spine injured patient. (p 22.24, 22.25)

4-6.36 Demonstrate documentation of assessment before spinal immobilization. (p 22.13)

4-6.37 Demonstrate documentation of assessment during spinal immobilization. (p 22.13)

4-6.38 Demonstrate documentation of assessment after spinal immobilization. (p 22.13)

Introduction

Spinal cord injury (SCI) is one of the most devastating injuries encountered by prehospital providers. Unfortunately, treatment options for SCIs are currently limited, with therapy relying heavily on rehabilitation over acute intervention. Preventive measures directed toward reducing the incidence of primary and secondary SCIs are the health care provider's best option for decreasing the morbidity and mortality associated with SCI.

In the United States, an estimated 11,000 new cases of SCI occur each year. The prevalence (existing cases) of SCI in the United States is 183,000 to 230,000 individuals. The average age at the time of injury is 32.1 years; 80% of patients are younger than 40 years old and 55% are between the ages of 16 and 30. The National Spinal Cord Injury Database recognizes 38 separate causes of injury, which are classified into five major categories: motor vehicle crashes (35%–40%); acts of violence (24.5%); falls, especially in the elderly (21.8%); recreational/athletic activities, especially diving (7.2%); and other causes, including diseases such as polio, spina bifida, and Friedreich's ataxia.

The overall in-hospital mortality rate is 7% for isolated SCI. In the first few months after injury, the mortality is as high as 20%, a rate that increases with age. The leading causes of death for SCI patients who are discharged from the hospital are pneumonia, pulmonary embolism, and septicemia.

In the Field

Patients with SCI face dramatic changes in lifestyle. A simple walk in the park, a trip to the shopping mall, or the commute to work becomes much more difficult. Caring for the SCI patient also brings significant financial costs.

Anatomy and Physiology

An understanding of the form and function of spinal anatomy coupled with a high level of suspicion for SCI is required to decipher the often subtle findings associated with a possible SCI.

The Spine

The spine consists of 33 irregular bones (vertebrae) articulating to form the vertebral column, which is the major structural component of the axial skeleton   Figure 22-1 ▶ . These skeletal components are stabilized by both ligaments and muscle. Together these components support and protect neural elements while allowing for fluid movement and erect stature.

Vertebrae are identified according to their location as cervical, thoracic, lumbar, sacral, or coccyx. The vertebral body, the anterior weight-bearing structure, is made of bone that provides support and stability. Components of the vertebra include the lamina, pedicles, and spinous processes   Figure 22-2 ▶ . Each vertebra is unique in appearance and, with the exception of the atlas and axis (C1 and C2)   Figure 22-3 ▶ , shares basic structural characteristics.

The inferior border of each pedicle contains a notch forming the intervertebral foramen. This space in the middle of the vertebra allows the exit of a peripheral nerve root and spinal vein as well as the entrance of a spinal artery on both sides at each vertebral junction.

You are the Provider Part 1

On your first day of work as a paramedic, you are dispatched to 9121 Floyd Trail for an "aircraft crash." En route to the scene, dispatch informs you that a witness saw a single-passenger gyrocopter fly into some power lines, then plummet to the ground.

You arrive to find a small rotary wing aircraft that has crashed in the middle of a large field of tall grass. You see power lines lying across the craft and an entrapped occupant who appears pale. A technician from the power company determines that the power lines are not energized so you approach the patient.

Initial Assessment	Recording Time: 0 Minutes
Appearance	Eyes open, anxious, holding lower back
Level of consciousness	A (Alert to person, place, and day)
Airway	Patent; calling for help
Breathing	Rapid and deep
Circulation	Fast, regular radial pulse

1. What is your primary concern?
2. What additional resources (if any) would you request and when?
3. How can you immediately assess and communicate with this patient in a safe manner?

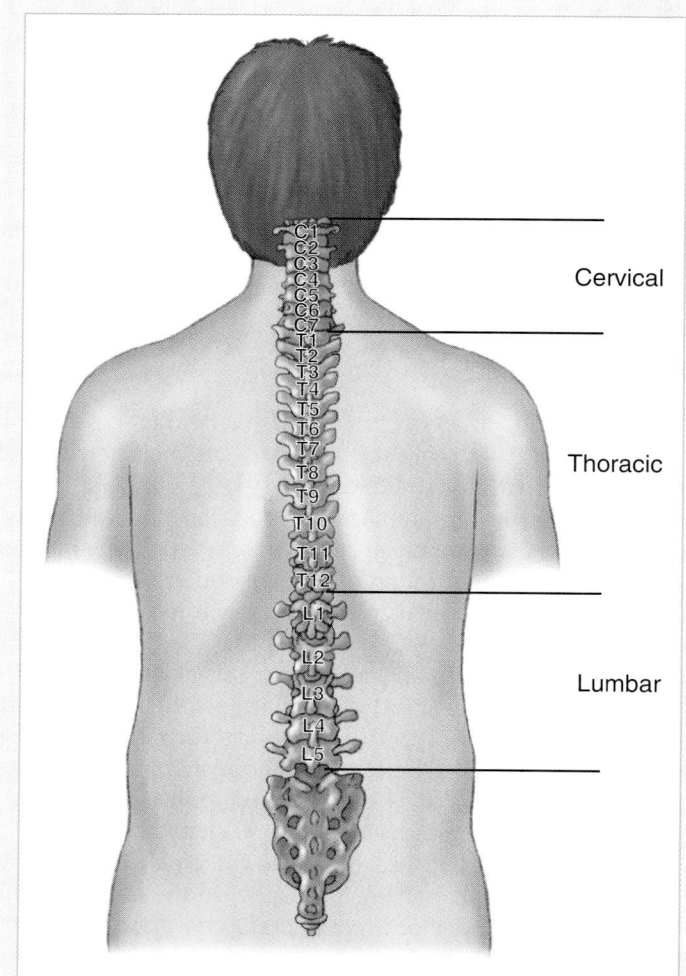

Figure 22-1 The spinal column consists of 33 bones divided into five sections. Each vertebra is numbered and referred to by a letter corresponding to the section of the spine where it is located plus its number. For example, the fifth thoracic vertebra is referred to as T5.

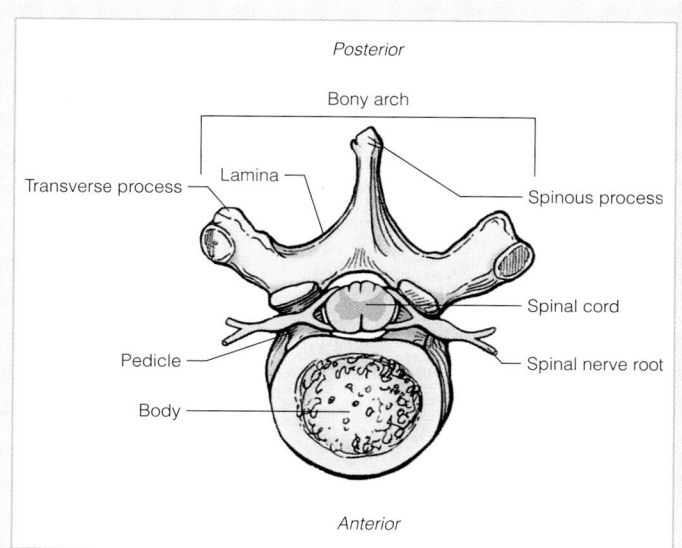

Figure 22-2 The human vertebra. Vertebrae in different sections of the spinal column vary in shape; this is a general representation. The space through which the spinal cord passes is called the canal, and the space through which a nerve root passes is called a foramen.

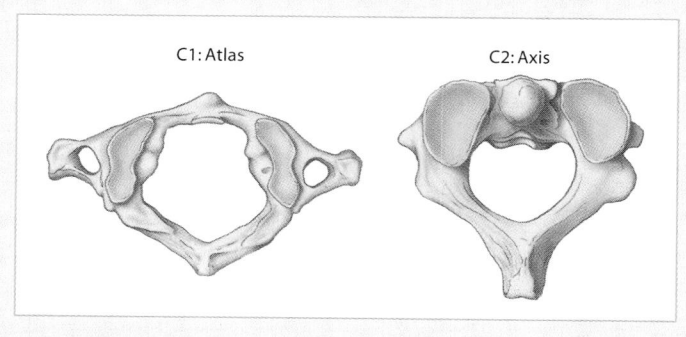

Figure 22-3 Structure of the atlas and axis.

The transverse spinous processes comprise the junction of each pedicle and lamina on each side of a vertebra. They project laterally and posteriorly and form points of attachments for muscles and ligaments. The posterior spinous process is formed by the fusion of the posterior lamina and serves as an attachment site for muscles and ligaments.

The cervical spine includes the first seven bones of the vertebral column and its supporting structures. In addition to protecting the vital cervical spinal cord, the cervical spine supports the weight of the head and permits a high degree of mobility in multiple planes. The atlas (C1) and axis (C2) are uniquely suited to allow for rotational movement of the skull.

The thoracic spine consists of 12 vertebrae in addition to the supporting muscles and ligaments found in the vertebral column; the thoracic spine is further stabilized by the rib attachments. The spinous processes are slightly larger, reflecting their role as attachment points for muscles that hold the

upper body erect and assist with the movement of the thoracic cavity during respiration.

The lumbar spine includes the five largest bones in the vertebral column, and is integral in carrying a large portion of the upper body weight. The lumbar spine is especially susceptible to injury because of this weight-bearing capacity.

The sacrum is composed of five fused vertebrae that form the posterior plate of the pelvis. The coccyx is made up of three to five small fused vertebrae. Coccyx injuries, although often extremely painful, are typically clinically insignificant.

Each vertebra is separated and cushioned by intervertebral disks that limit bone wear and act as shock absorbers. As the body ages, these disks lose water content and become thinner, causing the height loss associated with aging. Stress on the vertebral column may cause a disk to herniate into the spinal canal, resulting in a spinal cord or nerve root injury **Figure 22-4 ▸** .

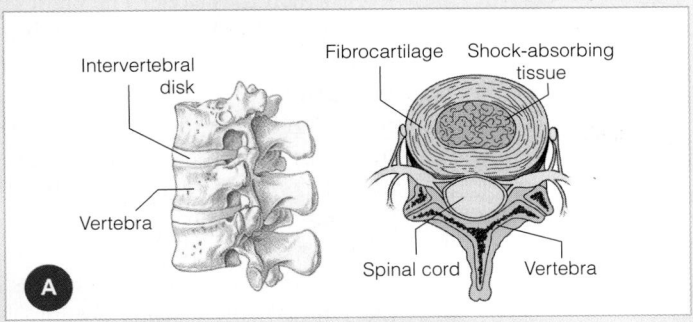 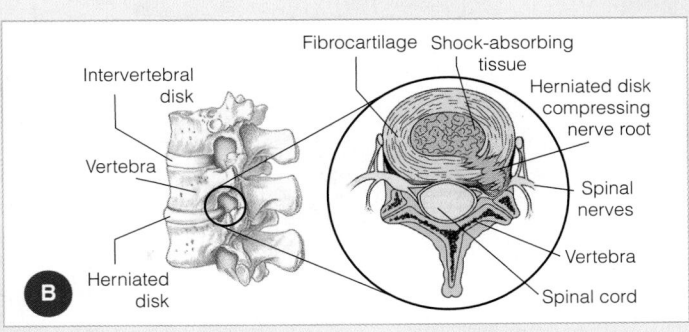

Figure 22-4 **A.** Normal, uninjured vertebral disk. **B.** Herniated disk.

In the Field

The lumbar spine is a common site of injury. Many of these injuries involve muscle spasm and do not threaten the integrity of the spinal cord and its roots. Nonetheless, low back pain is a common problem, as well as a major cause of impairment and disability.

The muscles, tendons, and ligaments that connect the vertebrae allow the spinal column a degree of flexion and extension, limited to an extent by the stabilization they must provide to the spinal column. The vertebral column can sustain normal flexion and extension of 60% to 70% without stressing the spinal cord. Flexion or extension beyond those limits may damage structural ligaments and allow excess vertebral movement that could expose the spinal cord to injury.

The Brain and Meninges

The central nervous system (CNS) consists of the brain and the spinal cord, both of which are encased in and protected by

bone. The brain, located within the cranial cavity, is the largest component of the CNS. It contains billions of neurons that serve a variety of vital functions.

The brain stem, which consists of the medulla, pons, and midbrain, connects the spinal cord to the remainder of the brain. The brain stem is vital for numerous basic body functions. Damage to this critical structure can easily result in death. All but two of the 12 cranial nerves exit from the brain stem.

The entire CNS is enclosed by a set of three membranes collectively known as the meninges **Figure 22-5 ▶**. The outer membrane, called the dura mater, is tough and fibrous. The middle layer, called the arachnoid, contains blood vessels that give it the appearance of a spider web. The innermost layer, resting directly on the brain or spinal cord, is the pia mater. The meninges float in cerebrospinal fluid (CSF). The meninges and CSF form a fluid-filled cushion that protects the brain and spinal cord.

The Spinal Cord

The spinal cord transmits nerve impulses between the brain and the rest of the body. Located at the base of the brain, it

You are the Provider Part 2

You request additional resources to aid you in safely treating and transporting the patient. After the known hazards have been addressed, you approach the patient, who says her name is Lynn Chase, to begin your hands-on assessment. As you near her, you notice a strong odor of gasoline and the patient says, "I stink! I have gasoline all over me!"

Reassessment	Recording Time: 10 Minutes
Level of consciousness	A (Alert to person, place, and day)
Skin	Cool, slightly pale, and dry
Pulse	110 beats/min, strong and regular
Blood pressure	140/74 mm Hg
Respirations	36 breaths/min
Sao₂	98% on 15 L/min via nonrebreathing mask

4. Given the information your patient has provided, have your priorities changed?
5. Given the mechanism of injury and other factors, what injuries do you suspect?

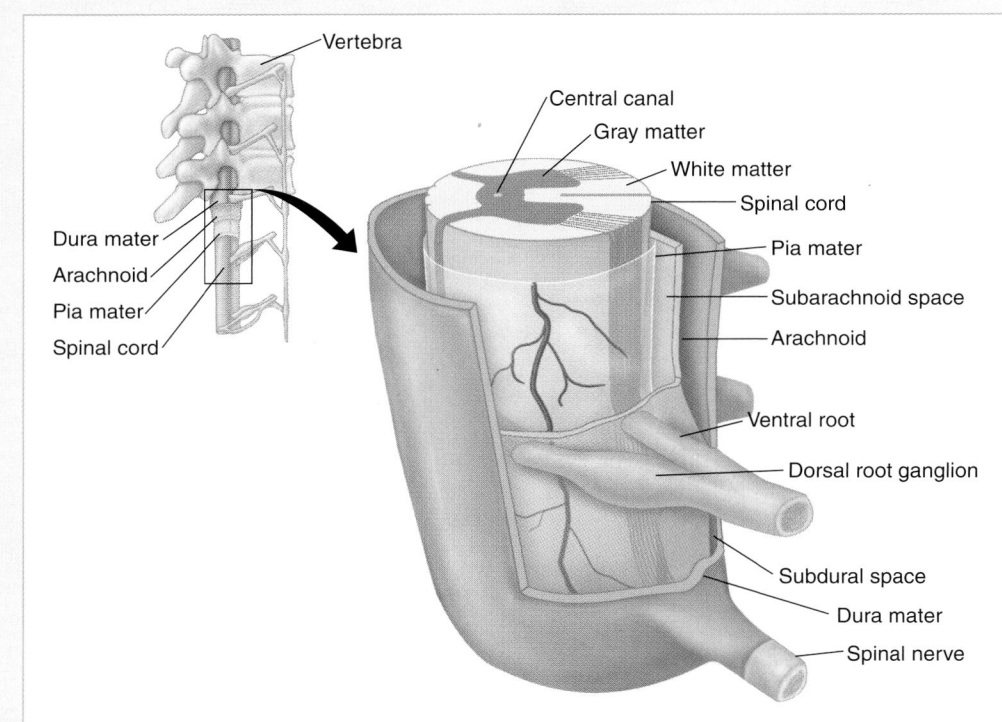

Figure 22-5 The spinal cord and its layers. The meninges enclose the brain and spinal cord.

represents the continuation of the CNS. This bundle of nerve fibers leaves the skull through a large opening at its base called the foramen magnum. The spinal cord extends from the base of the skull to L2; here it separates into the cauda equina, a collection of individual nerve roots. Thirty-one pairs of spinal nerves arise from the different segments of the spinal cord; each pair is named according to its corresponding segment.

A cross-section of the spinal cord (see Figure 22-5) reveals a butterfly-shaped central core of gray matter that is composed of neural cell bodies and synapses. This gray matter is divided into posterior (dorsal) horns, which carry sensory input, and anterior (ventral) horns, which innervate the motor nerve of that segment. Surrounding the gray matter on each side are three columns of peripheral white matter composed of myelinated ascending and descending fiber pathways. Messages are relayed to and from the brain through these spinal tracts.

Specific groups of nerves are named based on their source of origin and point of termination. Ascending tracts carry information to the brain, and descending tracts carry information to the rest of the body Table 22-1 ▶ .

Spinal Nerves
The 31 pairs of spinal nerves emerge from each side of the spinal cord and are named for the vertebral region and level

from which they arise. The eight cervical roots perform different functions in the scalp, neck, shoulders, and arms. The 12 thoracic nerve roots have varying functions; the upper thoracic nerves supply muscles of the chest that help in breathing and coughing, while the lower thoracic nerves provide abdominal muscle control and contain nerves of the sympathetic nervous system. The five lumbar nerve roots supply hip flexors and leg muscles, as well as provide sensation to the anterior legs. The five sacral nerves provide for bowel and bladder control, sexual function, and sensation in the posterior legs and rectum. The coccyx has a single nerve root.

Nerve roots occasionally converge in a cluster called a plexus that permits peripheral nerve roots to rejoin and function as a group Figure 22-6 ▶ . For example, the cervical plexus includes C1 through C5; the phrenic nerve (C3–C5) arises from this plexus and innervates the diaphragm. The brachial plexus (C5–T1) joins nerves controlling the upper extremities; the main nerves arising from this plexus are the axillary, median, musculocutaneous, radial, and ulnar. The lumbar plexus (L1–L4) supplies the skin and muscles of the abdominal wall, external genitalia, and part of the lower limbs. The sacral plexus (L4–S4) gives rise to the pudendal

Table 22-1	Major Spinal Tracts
Anterior Spinal Tracts	
Anterior spinothalamic tracts (ascending)	Carry sensation of crude touch and pressure sensation to the brain
Lateral spinothalamic tracts (ascending)	Carry pain and temperature
Spinocerebellar tracts (ascending)	Coordinate impulses necessary for muscular movements by carrying impulses from muscles in the legs and trunk to the cerebellum
Corticospinal tracts (descending)	Voluntary motor commands
Reticulospinal tracts (descending)	Muscle tone and sweat gland activity
Rubrospinal tracts (descending)	Muscle tone
Posterior Spinal Tracts	
Fasciculus gracilis and cuneatus	Proprioception, vibration, light touch, deep pressure, two-point discrimination, and stereognosis

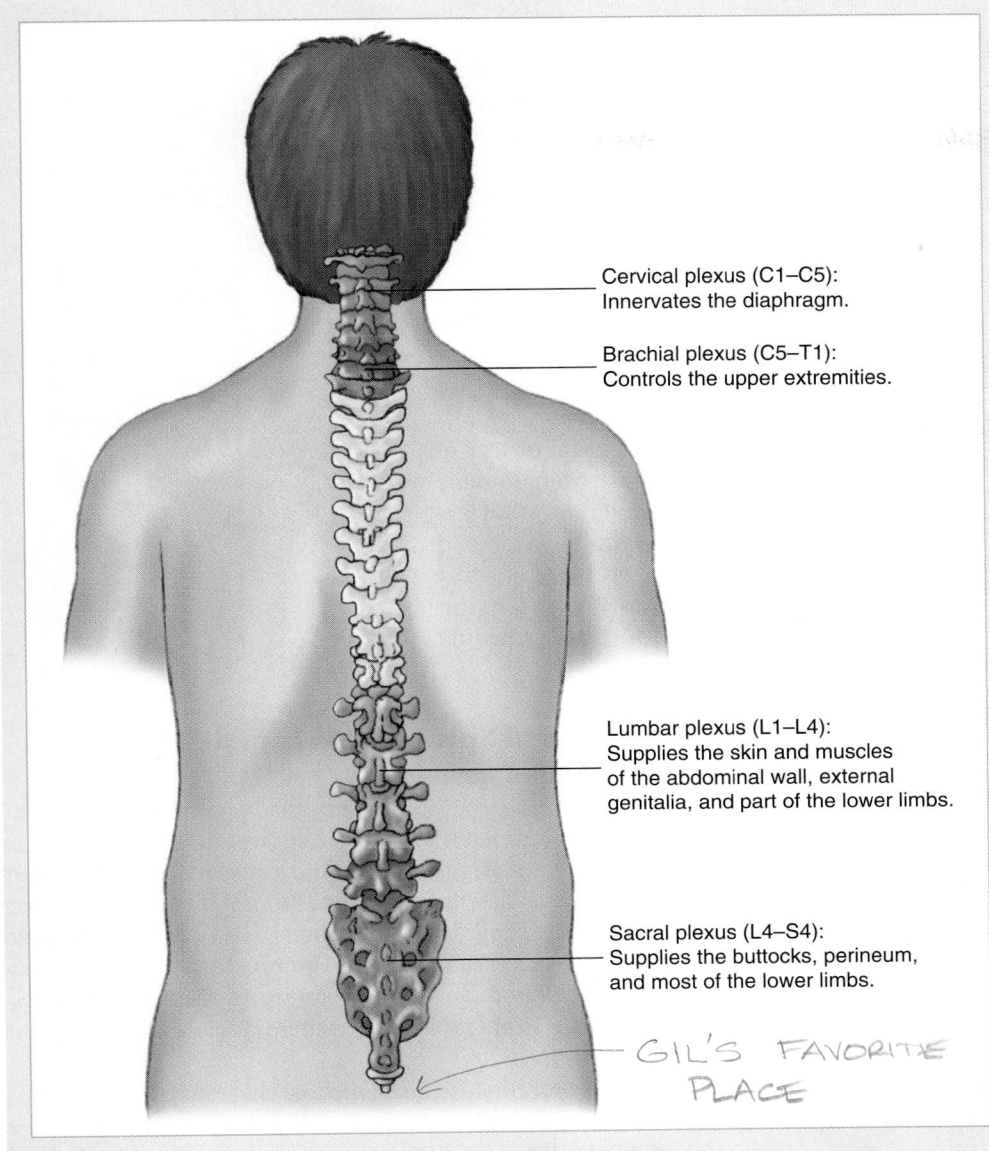

Figure 22-6 Nerve roots converge in plexuses, allowing them to function as a group.

Cervical plexus (C1–C5): Innervates the diaphragm.

Brachial plexus (C5–T1): Controls the upper extremities.

Lumbar plexus (L1–L4): Supplies the skin and muscles of the abdominal wall, external genitalia, and part of the lower limbs.

Sacral plexus (L4–S4): Supplies the buttocks, perineum, and most of the lower limbs.

GIL'S FAVORITE PLACE

cles in blood vessels and bronchioles, and have chronotropic and inotrophic effects on myocardial cells. The sympathetic nervous system is also responsible for sweating, pupil dilation, and temperature regulation, as well as the shunting of blood from the periphery to the core—the "flight or fight" responses.

A spinal cord injury at or above the level of T6 may disrupt the flow of sympathetic communication. Loss of sympathetic stimulation can disrupt homeostasis and leave the body poorly equipped to deal with changes in its environment. Stimulation of sympathetic nerves without parasympathetic input can cause sympathetic overdrive, resulting in autonomic dysreflexia; this complication of SCI is discussed later in this chapter.

The Parasympathetic Nervous System

The parasympathetic nervous system includes fibers arising from the brain stem and upper spinal cord that carry signals to organs of the abdomen, heart, lungs, and the skin above the waist. The vagus nerve travels from its origins outside of the medulla to the heart via the carotid arteries, thus vagal tone remains intact following a spine injury. When the sympathetic nerves are stimulated and produce autonomic dysreflexia, the parasympathetic nerves attempt to control the rapidly increasing blood pressure by slowing the heart rate. Parasympathetic nerves that supply the reproductive organs, pelvis, and leg begin at the sacral level (S2–S4). Disruption of the lower parasympathetic nerves in the sacrum results in the loss of bowel/bladder tone and sexual function.

and sciatic nerves and supplies the buttocks, perineum, and most of the lower limbs.

The Sympathetic Nervous System

The sensory (afferent) and motor (efferent) nerves are responsible for the somatic functions of the spinal cord and often overshadow the role of the spinal cord in the involuntary autonomic nervous system. The sympathetic nervous system is controlled by the brain's hypothalamus. Information from the brain is transmitted through the brain stem and the cervical spinal cord and then exits at the thoracic and lumbar levels of the spine to reach target structures. The thoracolumbar system provides sympathetic stimulation to the periphery largely through alpha and beta receptors. Alpha receptor stimulation induces smooth muscle contraction in blood vessels and bronchioles. Beta receptors respond with relaxation of smooth mus-

Pathophysiology

Mechanism of Injury

Acute injuries of the spine are classified according to the associated mechanism, location, and stability of the injury. Vertebral fractures can occur with or without associated SCI. Because stable fractures do not involve the posterior column, they pose less risk to the spinal cord. Unstable injuries involve the posterior column of the spinal cord and typically include damage to portions of the vertebrae and ligaments that directly protect the spinal cord and nerve roots. Unstable injuries carry a higher risk of complicating SCI and progression of injury without appropriate treatment.

Flexion Injuries

Flexion injuries result from forward movement of the head, typically as the result of rapid deceleration (eg, in a car crash) or from a direct blow to the occiput. At the level of C1–C2, these forces can produce an unstable dislocation with or without an associated fracture. Farther down the spinal column, flexion forces are transmitted anteriorly through the vertebral bodies and can result in an anterior wedge fracture. Depending on their severity, anterior wedge fractures can be stable or unstable. Loss of more than half the original size of the vertebral body or multiple levels of injury suggest involvement of the posterior column.

Hyperflexion injuries of greater force can result in teardrop fractures—avulsion fractures of the anterior-inferior border of the vertebral body. The injuries to ligaments associated with teardrop fractures raise concern for possible SCI and qualify as unstable fractures. Severe flexion can also result in a potentially unstable dislocation of vertebral joints. This situation does not involve fracture but can severely injure the ligaments. Strong forces can result in the anterior displacement of facet joints. A bilateral facet dislocation is an extremely unstable fracture.

Rotation with Flexion

The only area of the spine that allows for significant rotation is C1–C2. Injuries to this area are considered unstable due to its high cervical location and scant bony and soft-tissue support. Rotation-flexion injuries often result from high acceleration forces. Rotation with abrupt flexion can produce a stable dislocation in the cervical spine. In the thoracolumbar spine, rotation-flexion forces typically cause fracture rather than dislocation.

Vertical Compression

Vertical compression forces are transmitted through vertebral bodies and directed either inferiorly through the skull or superiorly through the pelvis or feet. They typically result from a direct blow to the crown (parietal region) of the skull or rapid deceleration from a fall through the feet, legs, and pelvis. Forces transmitted through the vertebral body cause fractures, ultimately shattering and producing a "burst" or compression fracture without associated SCI **Figure 22-7 ▶**. Compression forces can cause the herniation of disks, subsequent compression on the spinal cord and nerve roots, and fragmentation into the canal.

Although most fractures resulting from these injuries are stable, primary SCI can occur when the vertebral body is shattered and fragments of bone become embedded in the cord. Some compression injuries may be associated with significant retropharyngeal edema, and serious airway compromise is a consideration.

Hyperextension

Hyperextension of the head and neck can result in fractures and ligamentous injury of variable stability. The hangman's fracture

(C2), or distraction, results from hyperextension due to rapid deceleration of the skull, atlas, and axis as a unit. The resulting bilateral pedicle fracture of C2 is an unstable fracture but is rarely associated with SCI. A teardrop fracture of the anterior-inferior edge of the vertebral body results from hyperextension, resulting in rupture or tear of the anterior longitudinal ligament. The injury is stable with the head and neck in flexion, but unstable in extension due to loss of structural support.

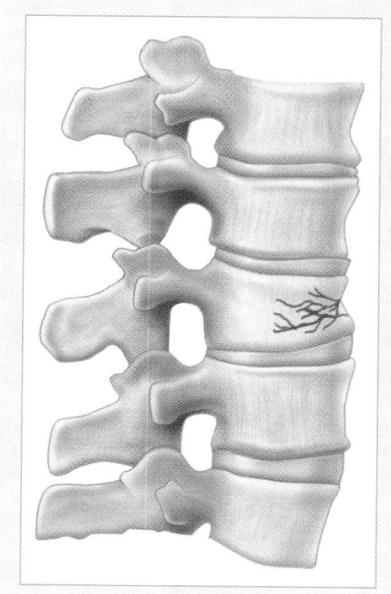

Figure 22-7 A compression fracture.

Categories of Spinal Cord Injuries

Primary Spinal Cord Injury

Primary spinal cord injury is injury that occurs at the moment of impact. Penetrating trauma typically results in transection of nonregenerative neural elements and complete injuries. Blunt trauma may displace ligaments and bone fragments, resulting in compression of points of the spinal cord or an incomplete dislocation of the vertebral body. Hypoperfusion and ischemia may also result from this type of injury to the spinal vasculature. Necrosis from prolonged ischemia leads to permanent loss of function.

Spinal cord concussion, which is characterized by a temporary dysfunction that lasts from 24 to 48 hours, accounts for 3% to 4% of all SCIs. Cord concussion is considered an incomplete injury and may present in patients with simple compression fractures or in those without radiologic evidence of a fracture. The temporary dysfunction may be due to a short-duration shock or pressure wave within the cord.

Spinal cord contusions are caused by fracture, dislocation, or direct trauma. They are associated with edema, tissue damage, and vascular leakage. Hemorrhagic disruption may cause temporary to permanent loss of function despite normal radiographs.

Cord laceration usually occurs when a projectile or bone enters the spinal canal. Such an injury is likely to result in hemorrhage into the cord tissue, swelling, and disruption of some portion of the cord and its associated communication pathways.

Secondary Spinal Cord Injury

Secondary spinal cord injury occurs when multiple factors permit a progression of the primary SCI; the ensuing cascade of inflammatory responses may result in further deterioration. These effects can be exacerbated by exposing neural elements to further hypoxemia, hypoglycemia, and hypothermia. Although some SCI may be unavoidable, the prehospital provider should minimize further injury through stabilization—that is, through spinal motion restriction and neutral alignment. In addition, minimizing heat loss and maintaining oxygenation and perfusion are key elements in the care of a patient with a possible SCI.

Regardless of the mechanism of injury, all SCIs are classified as complete or incomplete depending on the degree of damage. Complete spinal cord injury involves complete disruption of all tracts of the spinal cord, with permanent loss of all cord-mediated functions below the level of transection. When the injury affects the patient high in the cervical spine, quadriplegia results. A similar injury in the high thoracic area would result in paraplegia. In an incomplete spinal cord injury, the patient retains some degree of cord-mediated function. The degree of SCI is best determined 24 hours after the initial injury; the initial dysfunction may be temporary, and there is some potential for recovery.

Anterior cord syndrome results from the displacement of bony fragments into the anterior portion of the spinal cord, often due to flexion injuries or fractures. The anterior spinal artery provides blood to the anterior two thirds of the spinal cord; disruption of this flow will present as an anterior cord syndrome. Physical findings include paralysis below the level of the insult with loss of sensation to pain, temperature, and touch.

In central cord syndrome, hyperextension injuries to the cervical area present with hemorrhage or edema to the central cervical segments. This type of damage is rarely associated with fractures or bone disruption but more often occurs in conjunction with tears to the anterior longitudinal ligament. Central cord syndrome is frequently seen in older patients, who may already have a significant degree of cervical spondylosis and stenosis due to arthritic changes. A brief episode of hyperextension can exert pressure on the spinal cord within the relatively diminished spinal canal. Within the central cord, motor (efferent) fibers are distributed in a unique fashion, with more cervical and thoracic motor and sensory tracts than in the periphery of the cord. The patient with central cord syndrome will present with greater loss of function in the upper extremities than in the lower extremities, with variable loss of sensation to pain and temperature. The patient may also have some bowel and bladder dysfunction. The prognosis for central cord syndrome is typically good; many patients regain all motor function or have only some residual weakness in the hands.

Posterior cord syndrome is associated with extension injuries. This relatively rare syndrome produces dysfunction of the dorsal columns, presenting as decreased sensation to light touch, proprioception (the ability to perceive the position and movement of one's body), and vibration, while most other motor and sensory functions remain intact. Recovery of function is less prevalent than with central cord syndrome, but the overall prognosis remains good with therapy and rehabilitation.

Brown-Sequard syndrome occurs when penetrating trauma is accompanied by hemisection of the cord and complete damage to all spinal tracts on the involved side. Injury to the corticospinal motor tracts causes motor loss on the same side as the injury, but below the lesion. Damage to the dorsal column causes loss of sensation to light touch, proprioception, and vibration on the same side as the injury (below it). Disruption of the spinothalamic tracts causes loss of sensation to pain and temperature on the opposite side of injury, below the lesion.

Spinal shock refers to the temporary local neurologic condition that occurs immediately after spinal trauma. Swelling and edema of the cord begin within 30 minutes of the initial insult and can lead to a physiologic transection, mechanically disrupting all nerve conduction distal to the injury. The patient may present with variable degrees of acute spinal injury, potentially with flaccid paralysis, flaccid sphincters, and absent reflexes. Sensory function below the level of injury will be impaired, as will thermoregulation and visceral sensation below the lesion, resulting in bowel distention from a loss of peristalsis. Spinal shock usually subsides in hours to weeks, depending on the severity of injury.

Neurogenic shock results from the temporary loss of autonomic function, which controls cardiovascular function, at the level of injury. Marked hemodynamic and systemic effects are seen: hypotension occurs due to absent or impaired peripheral vascular tone with the loss of alpha receptor stimulation; blood pools in the enlarged vascular space, causing a relative hypovolemia and making the patient extremely sensitive to sudden position changes; and cardiac preload decreases, resulting in decreased stroke volume and cardiac output. Bradycardia results as well. The adrenal gland loses its sympathetic stimulation and does not produce epinephrine or norepinephrine. Hypothermia and absence of sweating are also seen because of the loss of sympathetic stimulation. The classic case of neurogenic shock is a hypotensive, bradycardic patient whose skin is warm, flushed, and dry below the level of the spinal lesion.

Patient Assessment

Limiting the progression of secondary SCI is a major goal of prehospital management of SCI. You should be familiar with the circumstances that commonly produce SCI and try to determine, through history-taking and examination of the scene, whether any of these circumstances exist.

Special Considerations

Spinal cord injury without radiographic abnormalities (SCIWORA) can occur in children because their vertebrae lie flatter on top of each other Figure 22-8 ▸ : in adults, the vertebrae are more curved. A child's vertebrae can easily dislocate and quickly relocate back into their normal positions. The radiograph of a child who has experienced SCIWORA may have no evidence of fracture and will show a perfectly aligned vertebral column, yet the cord itself has been compressed or transected. SCIWORA cannot be diagnosed in the prehospital setting. Even in the emergency department, sophisticated studies such as MRI may be required.

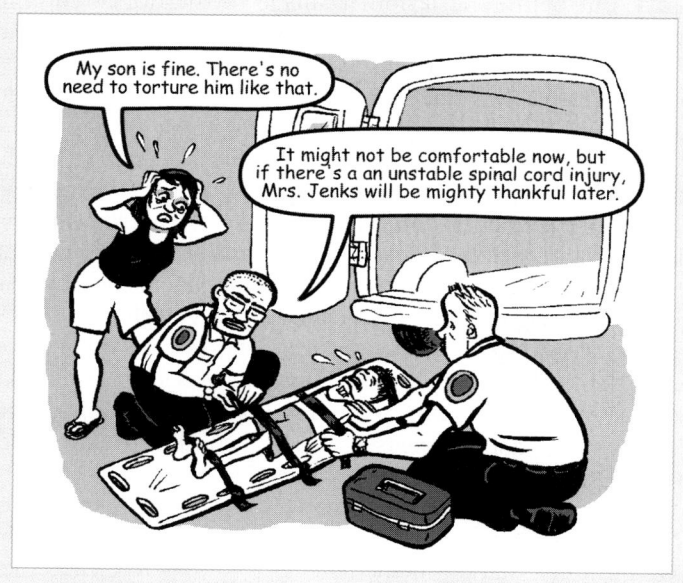

Figure 22-8

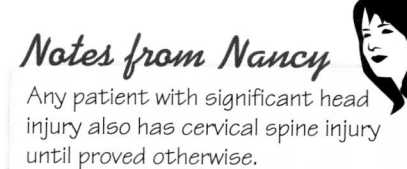

Notes from Nancy

Any patient with significant head injury also has cervical spine injury until proved otherwise.

The following high-risk mechanisms of injury strongly suggest spine injury and require full spine immobilization regardless of the physical exam findings:

- High-velocity crash (> 40 mph) with severe vehicle damage
- Unrestrained occupant of moderate- to high-speed motor vehicle crash
- Vehicular damage with compartmental intrusion (12″) into the patient's seating space
- Fall from three times the patient's height
- Penetrating trauma near the spine
- Ejection from a moving vehicle
- Motorcycle crash > 20 mph with separation of rider from vehicle
- Diving injury
- Auto-pedestrian or auto-bicycle crash > 5 mph
- Death of occupant in the same passenger compartment
- Rollover crash (unrestrained)

Mechanisms of uncertain risk for spine injury include the following events:

- Moderate- to low-velocity motor vehicle crash (< 40 mph)
- Patient involved in a motor vehicle crash has an isolated injury without positive assessment findings for SCI
- Isolated minor head injury without positive mechanism for spine injury
- Syncopal event in which the patient was already seated or supine
- Syncopal event in which the patient was assisted to a supine position by a bystander

When to Suspect a Spinal Cord Injury

The history of present illness typically provides most of the information necessary to reach a diagnosis. Maintain a high index of suspicion in any case for which the mechanism of injury suggests the possibility of SCI. Associated injuries, especially those that reflect involvement of massive forces, may also provide clues of the presence of SCI. Treat all patients who experience multiple trauma or those who are found unconscious after trauma as if a spine injury exists, because the majority of cervical spine injuries are associated with head injury. Patients with evidence of major trauma above the clavicle should be considered at risk for an associated spine injury.

You are the Provider Part 3

Fire fighters aid you in decontaminating the patient as well as applying spinal precautions. She finds it difficult to lie flat on the board, and tells you that her back hurts a lot. She reports, "It feels better if I hold it." She denies any weakness, numbness, or tingling in her extremities.

Reassessment	Recording Time: 15 Minutes
Level of consciousness	A (Alert to person, place, and day)
Skin	Cool, slightly pale, and dry
Pulse	110 beats/min, strong and regular
Blood pressure	142/76 mm Hg
Respirations	36 breaths/min
Sao2	100% on 15 L/min via nonrebreathing mask

6. What other factors can impact a patient's ability to handle the stress of trauma?
7. What other information beyond the history of events should you obtain from your patient?
8. If you must decontaminate a patient in the open, how can you preserve patient modesty?

Determine as precisely as possible the circumstances of the incident and types of energy imparted to the patient, including the degree of force and the speed and trajectory of impact. Was there blunt or penetrating trauma? Was it a flexion injury, such as the classic diving accident? Was there torsion on the neck? In the case of a fall, estimate the height of the fall and determine whether anything was struck on the way down, how the patient landed, and what the patient landed on. In vehicular collisions, note the use and positioning of restraints, the patient's position in the vehicle, and the degree of damage to the vehicle. Find out the exact time of the initial injury and record any times and changes in the patient's presentation throughout the prehospital phase.

Special Considerations

The indications for long backboard spinal immobilization of infants and toddlers are unknown. Infants and young children cannot verbally communicate symptoms such as weakness, numbness, or pain, so the threshold for immobilization must be lower than for older children and adults. However, restraining a conscious child on a long backboard will cause pain and agitation in a short time. Reassure nervous children that the immobilization is necessary but only temporary. Try distraction techniques.

Modify the physical examination of any patient with suspected SCI based on the patient's level of consciousness, reliability as a historian, and mechanism of injury. In cases of high- or intermediate-risk mechanisms, whenever possible complete the physical exam with the patient in a neutral position without any movement of the spine. Apply manual stabilization while asking the patient not to move unless specifically asked to do so. The neck and trunk must not be flexed, extended, or rotated. Frequent reassessments are necessary to determine whether the patient is stabilizing, improving, or deteriorating. Also, be sure to document suspected spinal cord injury, noting the area involved, sensation, dermatomes (discussed in the next section), motor function, and areas of weakness.

Controversies

Several states and EMS systems have instituted field spinal clearance protocols with good initial results. Ask your service's medical director how he or she feels about this issue. Always follow your local protocols and medical direction.

Scene Size-up

After donning BSI, the initial step of any assessment should be a determination of scene safety and the need for any additional resources. Decide whether the trauma system should be activated (eg, air evacuation of the patient to a Level I trauma center). Note the general age and gender of the patient. Observe the position in which the patient is found and determine if the patient's condition

is life-threatening. While maintaining the head and neck in a neutral position through manual stabilization, determine the level of consciousness, using AVPU initially and then the Glasgow Coma Scale (GCS score—a standardized method of relaying information regarding a patient's overall level of consciousness) as time allows. A cervical collar may be applied as soon as the assessment of the airway and neck are complete. Sedation or rapid sequence intubation (RSI) procedures, depending on local protocols, may be required for a combative patient to ensure the patient's protection and spine stabilization.

Notes from Nancy

The most important single sign in the evaluation of a head-injured patient is a changing state of consciousness.

Initial Assessment
Airway

After confirming that the scene is safe and determining the patient's mental status, the next priority is to ensure an open airway. Sonorous respirations usually indicate a positional problem, while gurgling respirations often indicate a need for suction. The oropharynx may become occluded by the tongue, secretions, blood, vomitus, foreign bodies, or improperly inserted airways. A retropharyngeal hematoma associated with injury of the upper cervical spine (C2) may also compromise the airway.

While maintaining the head and neck in neutral alignment, clear the mouth and carefully but quickly suction if necessary. Use a jaw-thrust maneuver to open the airway; if this technique is successful, insert an oropharyngeal airway or a nasopharyngeal airway as appropriate. An intact gag reflex is a contraindication for an oropharyngeal airway, because vomiting will increase the likelihood of airway compromise and increase the risk of aspiration. Facial fractures and physical findings or suspicion for a basilar skull fracture are relative contraindications for a nasopharyngeal airway.

A definitive airway with in-line orotracheal intubation should follow the placement of any temporary airway device. If the patient is awake with an impaired airway or has a deteriorating GCS score (8 or less), consider drug-assisted orotracheal intubation with in-line stabilization (ie, RSI). Turn the patient to the side to allow gravity to assist in evacuation of the airway while secured to a long backboard or while you maintain manual in-line stabilization of the head and neck. Follow up with suction to remove the secretions. Local protocols may include sedation or RSI.

Breathing

Evaluate the patient's breathing, noting the rate, depth, and symmetry of each respiration. The diaphragm is innervated by the phrenic nerve (C3–C5). Lesions occurring at or above C3–C4, may consequently lead to diaphragmatic paralysis, which is seen clinically as abdominal breathing with use of the accessory muscles of the neck. An injury involving the lower cervical or upper thoracic spinal cord (T2) may result in paralysis of the intercostal muscles, leaving the patient dependent on the diaphragm and accessory muscles of the neck for breathing. Inadequate respirations with or without evidence of decreased oxygenation will require assisted ventilation with a bag-mask device with 12 to 15 L/min of supplementary oxygen flowing, at 10 to 12 breaths/min. If a head injury is suspected, use ET_{CO_2} monitoring to maintain CO_2 levels at 35 to 45 mm Hg.

Circulation

To assess perfusion, compare the radial and carotid pulses for their presence, rate, quality, regularity, and equality, and examine the patient's skin color, temperature, and moisture. Patients with significant sensory loss from SCI may equilibrate to the surrounding environmental temperature due to the lack of input from the periphery for temperature control. In neurogenic shock, the skin is usually warm, dry, and flushed due to vasodilation and the absence of sweating. These findings should be correlated with the patient's mental status.

In the absence of a pulse, immediately initiate CPR. Control any external bleeding with direct pressure or pressure dressings. Volume resuscitation may be necessary in patients with absent or diminished pulses, especially in the setting of multisystem trauma with hypovolemic shock. Patients with SCI in pure neurogenic shock may not require large amounts of volume resuscitation but may need vagolytic drugs (eg, atropine) and vasopressors (such as dopamine) to reverse the uninhibited vagal stimulation and alpha receptor blockade associated with this type of shock.

Transport Decision

Early on in the initial assessment, you must decide whether to complete the focused history and physical exam on scene or to transport the patient immediately with interventions en route. The unstable or potentially unstable patient should be transported as soon as possible to the most appropriate hospital per local trauma guidelines or online medical control instruction.

Focused History and Physical Exam

An accurate history and physical examination are critical for directing management of patients with potential SCIs. A patient's reliability as a historian must always be assessed before performing a focused or detailed assessment. The patient should appear calm, cooperative, nonimpaired, and able to perform cognitive functions appropriately. Patients who present with an acute stress reaction, distracting injuries (eg, long-bone fractures, rib fractures, pelvic fractures, or clinically significant abdominal pain), or an alteration in mental status due to brain injury or intoxication from drugs and/or alcohol must be considered unreliable in terms of the neurologic exam. These patients should have continuous spine protection until the presence of an injury can be excluded radiographically at the receiving hospital.

The focused physical examination should begin with baseline vital signs and a SAMPLE history. In case of potential spine injuries, the exam includes rapid inspection and palpation of the head, neck, chest, abdomen, pelvis, extremities, and back for injuries. Use the mnemonic DCAP-BTLS—Deformity, Contusion, Abrasion, Puncture/penetration wounds, Bruising, Tenderness, Laceration, and Swelling—to help you remember specific points. An evaluation of neurovascular integrity should include distal PMS (pulse, motor, and sensory function) for all four extremities. Any deficits in the neurologic examination must be noted and monitored.

In addition to evaluating responsiveness with AVPU during your initial assessment, also obtain a GCS score because it

You are the Provider Part 4

As soon as your patient is packaged, you begin transport. You establish vascular access, apply the cardiac monitor, and reassess your patient. Her mental status and vital signs remain stable throughout transport, and you transfer patient care to the hospital staff without incident.

Reassessment	Recording Time: 20 Minutes
Level of consciousness	A (Alert to person, place, and day)
Skin	Warm, pink, and dry
Pulse	106 beats/min, strong and regular
Blood pressure	138/70 mm Hg
Respirations	30 breaths/min
Sao₂	100% on 15 L/min via nonrebreathing mask
ECG	Sinus tachycardia

The patient experienced compression fractures of her lumbar spine, but no spinal cord damage. She underwent surgery and made a recovery that did not limit her quality of life, including her ability to function as a pilot.

9. What is the standard for maximum on-scene time for any significant trauma patient?

10. How does prompt, appropriate care affect the patient beyond immediate survival of the injuries sustained?

provides more specific clinical information. Assess the pupils for their size, shape, equality, and reactivity to light. If possible, obtain a glucose level in patients who show evidence of alterations in sensation. Perform a brief motor and sensory exam, including PMS in all four extremities, in patients with potential SCI.

You will need to expose the patient for your examination. Cut away the clothes to minimize motion of the spine during examination or treatment. Directly observe the back to assess for penetrating trauma. Palpate the spine to assess for deformity or displacement (step off) of vertebral bodies. Once the exam is completed, recover the patient with a blanket to maintain normal body temperature. Hypothermia will impair the patient's ability to unbind oxygen from hemoglobin and increase the risk of mortality and morbidity. In colder climates, move the patient to a warmer environment, such as the ambulance, as quickly as possible without compromising the spine further.

Placement on the Backboard

Before you immobilize a patient, be sure you have documented your assessment thus far. It will also be important to document your findings after the patient has been immobilized.

Most patients can be log rolled with visualization for deformity or injury as well as palpation over each posterior spinous process for pain, deformity, or step off. The absence of pain or tenderness along the spine, coupled with a normal neurologic exam and low-risk mechanism of injury, may eliminate the need for manual in-line spinal immobilization. In contrast, paralyzed limbs should always be protected with appropriate backboard and stretcher immobilization.

Patients in severe pain may require an alternative method of transfer to a long backboard. Use of a scoop stretcher often results in less movement of the patient. Once the scoop is in place, another paramedic or EMT can slide the backboard or air mattress underneath the patient. Although the patient can still be palpated with this method, inability to conduct visual inspection of the area is a disadvantage of this procedure.

Time on a backboard should be kept to a minimum because skin breakdown can be a major complication of SCI Figure 22-9 ▶ . This problem occurs as a result of excessive pressure over the bones of the buttocks, the scapular ridges, and the base of the occiput. These five areas are the primary points supporting the patient's weight. The initial stages of pressure lesions may occur in a matter of hours; 32% of patients with SCI develop a skin lesion within 24 hours of injury. Blood distribution shifts to the skin and subcutaneous tissues, and decreased muscle tone and sensation predispose the SCI patient to these injuries.

Several new devices have been developed to enhance patient comfort. The Back Raft takes pressure off specific areas of the back and fills voids that may otherwise allow patient movement. This low-profile air mattress fits under the patient from the shoulders to the waist Figure 22-10 ▶ . Slightly flexing the knees with towel rolls or a blanket and slightly separating the legs with a pillow or blanket increases patient com-

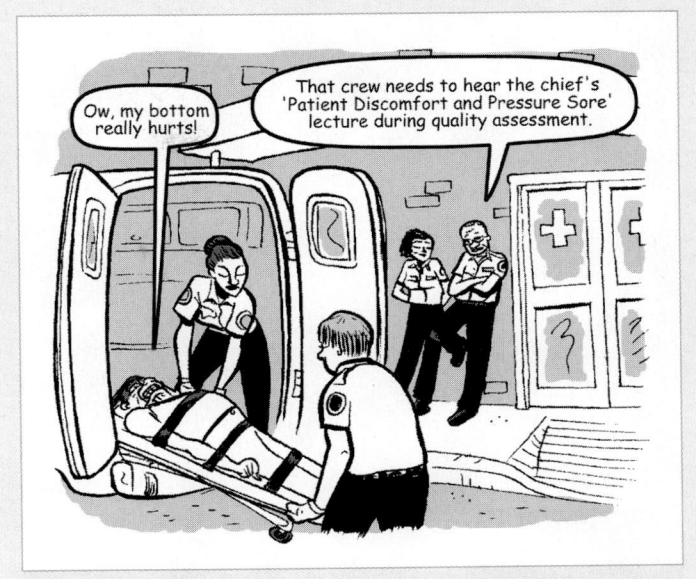

Figure 22-9

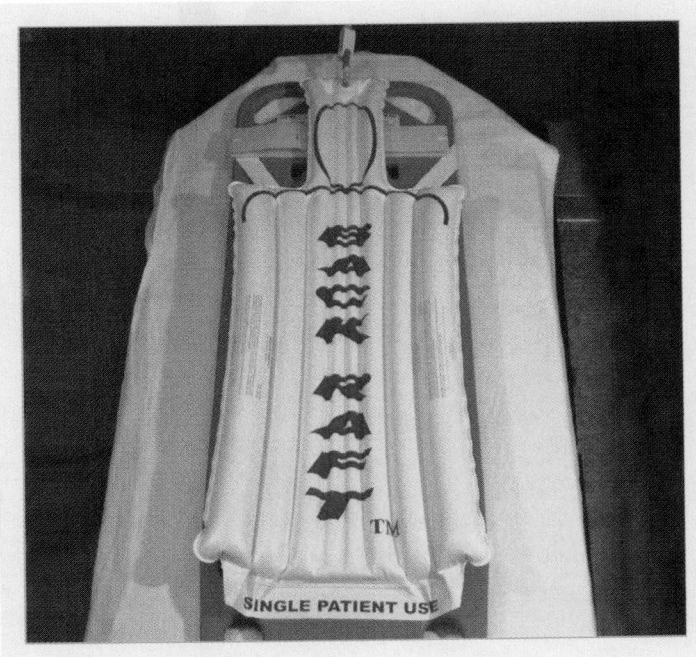

Figure 22-10 The Back Raft.

fort and decreases the likelihood of postimmobilization problems, yet still provides adequate immobilization of the patient Figure 22-11 ▶ . Concave backboards also conform more closely to a patient's anatomy than do flat boards. Spider straps should be used to properly immobilize a patient.

Detailed Physical Exam

A detailed physical exam for a trauma patient with a significant MOI should take place while en route to the hospital. Closely

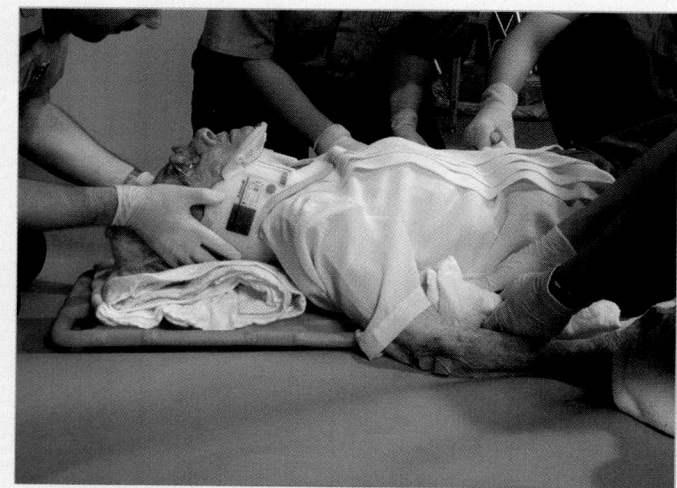

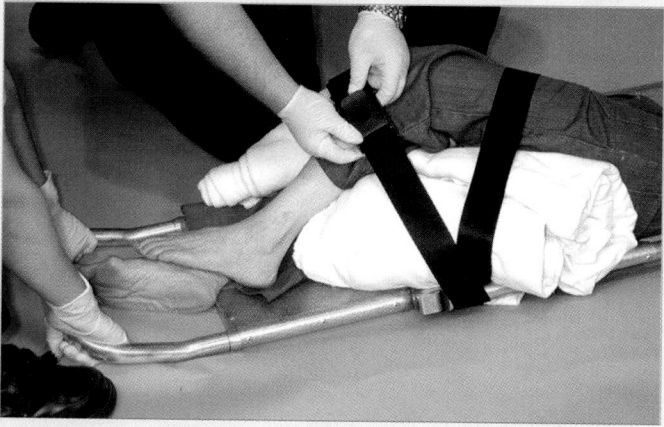

Figure 22-11 Using towel rolls or blankets to pad the backboard will increase patient comfort and can minimize problems resulting from immobilization of the older patient.

In the Field

Always palpate over the spinous process before concluding that a patient "has no neck pain." Some providers simply ask the patient and never perform a physical exam.

examine the head, neck, chest, abdomen, pelvis, extremities, back, and buttocks. A detailed head-to-toe exam can often reveal significant findings, especially in patients with questionable reliability, unclear mechanisms, or multisystem trauma.

Thoroughly assess the head and neck, as many SCI patients will have associated head and facial injuries; a complaint of pain is most predictive of a spine injury. Examination of the neck should include gentle palpation of the cervical spine for pain, deformity, or dislocation (step off).

Evaluate the chest and abdomen for both internal and external injuries. Fractures of the ribs, sternum, clavicle, scapula, or pelvis are often associated with SCI in patients with

multisystem trauma. Visualization and palpation are the mainstays of this evaluation. Bear in mind that the physical exam in the SCI patient may be skewed due to potentially decreased sensation below the level of the spine injury. Assess the chest wall visually for symmetry of chest wall movement, work of breathing, and use of accessory muscles. Auscultation to assess breath sounds may reveal a shortened inspiratory phase. Inadequate ventilation, accessory muscle use, or paradoxical respirations may indicate diaphragmatic impairment due to SCI.

Continually monitor the cardiovascular system for signs of shock. Neurogenic shock may require pharmacologic management, volume replacement, and/or transcutaneous pacing.

Examination of the gastrointestinal system may be unreliable in the presence of a neurologic deficit. First, inspect the abdomen for evidence of trauma, noting its contour. Severe gastric distention may impair respiration and lead to airway compromise due to vomiting. Palpate all four quadrants for tenderness, guarding, or rigidity, but remember that patients may be insensitive to pain and may not develop a rigid abdomen because of absence of muscle tone. Lower abdominal distention with or without suprapubic tenderness may be due to urinary retention. In men, assess the ureteral meatus for evidence of blood, scrotal swelling, and scrotal ecchymosis, which may be present with pelvic fractures. Assess for priapism as well.

Inspect all extremities for deformity, contusion, abrasions, punctures, lacerations, and edema. Palpate for deformity, tenderness, instability, or crepitus. Look for any abnormal posturing, and assess the patient for potential long bone or other significantly distracting painful injuries that may mask a potential spine or cord injury.

Notes from Nancy

A normal neurologic examination does not rule out the possibility of spinal cord injury.

Neurologic Exam

The focused neurologic evaluation in the field is intended to establish a baseline level of the lesion for later comparison—that is, to determine the completeness of the lesion and to identify cord syndromes if the lesion is incomplete. A normal neurologic examination does not rule out the possibility of SCI. Patients who experienced vehicular trauma have been known to walk away from the crash only to become totally paralyzed hours later, when a casual nod of the head squeezed an unstable vertebral column down against the spinal cord. Accordingly, when the mechanism of injury indicates that the patient could have sustained SCI, treat the individual as having a spine injury regardless of the neurologic findings. The neurologic assessment is intended not only to determine whether the patient should be immobilized, but also to furnish data to the hospital about the precise initial presentation of the patient so that personnel there may evaluate any changes in condition and determine if immediate surgery is necessary.

The initial step of any neurologic assessment is a determination of the level of consciousness. First note the patient's AVPU in the initial assessment, and then address the GCS level

Table 22-2	Landmark Myotomes		
Nerve Root	**Muscle Group**	**Nerve Root**	**Muscle Group**
C3-C5	Diaphragm	L2	Hip flexors: iliopsoas
C5	Elbow flexors: biceps, brachialis, brachioradialis	L3	Knee extensors: quadriceps
C6	Wrist extensors	L4	Ankle dorsiflexors: tibialis anterior
C7	Elbow extensors: triceps	L5	Long toe extensors: extensor hallucis longus
C8	Finger flexors: flexor digitorum profundus to middle finger	S1	Ankle plantar flexors (gastronemius, soleus)
T1	Hand intrinsics: interossei, small finger abductors	S4-S5	Anus, bowel, bladder
T2-T7	Intercostal muscles		

Table 22-3	Landmark Dermatomes		
Nerve Root	**Anatomic Location**	**Nerve Root**	**Anatomic Location**
C2	Occipital protuberance	T10	Umbilicus
C3	Supraclavicular fossa	L1	Inguinal line
C5	Lateral side of antecubital fossa	L2	Mid anterior thigh
C6	Thumb and medial index finger (6-shooter)	L3	Medial aspect of the knee
C7	Middle finger	L5	Dorsum of the foot
C8	Little finger	S1-S3	Back of leg
T2	Apex of axilla	S4-S5	Perianal area
T4	Nipple line		

during further assessment. When assigning the GCS, do not score the patient as having no motor response if limbs are paralyzed. Ask the patient to blink or move some facial muscles that would be innervated by a cranial nerve. Remember that an unconscious patient is always at risk for having a spinal injury.

Motor components of spinal nerves innervate discrete tissues and muscles of the body in regions called myotomes Table 22-2 ▲ . The examination of these myotomes should take place in the typical head-to-toe fashion, starting with an assessment of the cranial nerves. Cranial nerve assessment is especially important in circumstances suggestive of a high cervical injury. Observe the patient for drooping of the upper eyelid and a small pupil (Horner's syndrome) that would indicate an injury to C3.

Bilaterally assess each major motor group from the top down to identify the lowest spinal segment associated with normal voluntary motor function. Because of the possibility of incomplete spinal cord lesions, it is important to determine the extent of function in segments below this level. Monitor for possible ascending lesions, paying special attention to alterations in respiratory patterns with cervical lesions.

Ask the patient to flex (C5) and extend (C7) both elbows and then both wrists (C6). Have the patient abduct the fingers and keep them open against resistance, and then adduct the fingers and attempt to close them against resistance (T1) Figure 22-12 ▶ . As an alternative maneuver, have the patient curl all four fingers while the examiner applies opposing pull with his or her fingers to determine strength against resistance. This will test the finger flexors (C8).

To evaluate the lower extremities, ask the patient to bend and extend the knees. Next ask the patient to plantar flex the feet and ankles as if pressing down on the gas pedal of a car (S1–S2) and to dorsiflex the toes to gravity and against resistance (L5) Figure 22-13 ▶ .

Assessment of motor integrity in an unconscious patient is largely based on the patient's response to a painful stimulus. Spine injury with loss of motor function is likely if an unconscious patient grimaces, vocalizes, or opens his or her eyes to a painful response above the level of the neurologic deficit but does not move the limbs. Pain responses should be tested at several locations before assuming an absence of response. If the motor exam cannot be completed due to local injury, the exam is considered unreliable and spine motion restriction is necessary.

Sensor components of spinal nerves innervate specific and discrete areas of the body surface called dermatomes Table 22-3 ▲ . In addition to testing a general loss of sensation, ask the patient about abnormal sensations in these areas such as "pins and needles," electric shock, or hyperacute pain to touch (hyperesthesia). As with the motor exam, sensory integrity must be assessed bilaterally but from the feet up. Determine the lowest level of normal sensation and any areas of intact or "spared" sensation below this level. In the conscious patient, a thorough evaluation will include perception of light touch, temperature, and position (proprioception).

Reflexes are usually not assessed in the field but can provide valuable information regarding sensory input, especially in the unconscious patient. In significant SCIs, reflexes are usually absent but return several hours to several weeks after injury. If reflexes are intact, the preservation of motor and sensory activity in the same spinal cord segments is likely. A positive Babinski reflex occurs when the toes move upward in response to stimulation of the sole of the foot. Under normal circumstances, the toes move downward.

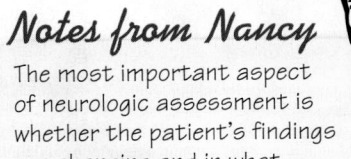

Notes from Nancy

The most important aspect of neurologic assessment is whether the patient's findings are changing and in what direction.

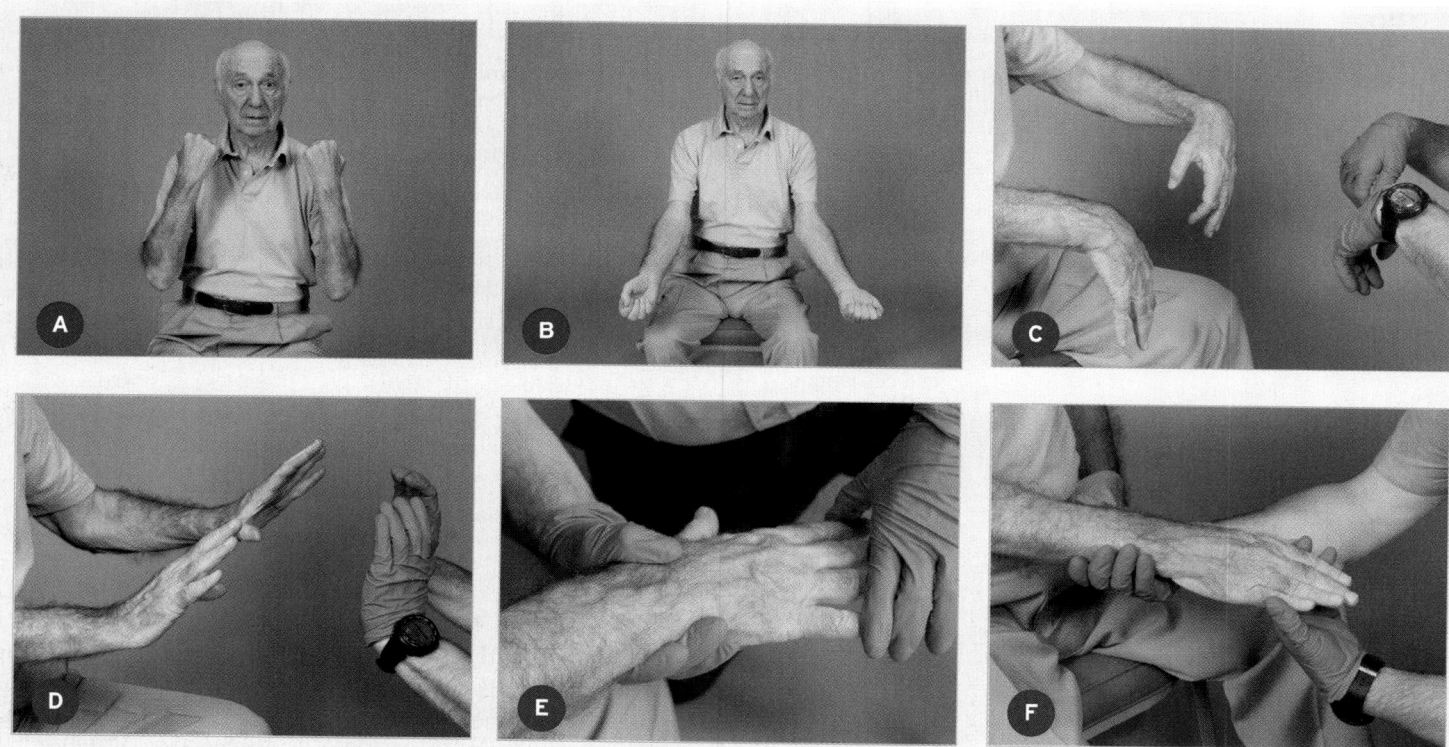

Figure 22-12 Neurologic evaluation of the upper extremities. Ask the patient to flex (**A**) and then extend (**B**) both elbows. Ask the patient to flex (**C**) and then extend (**D**) both wrists. Have the patient abduct the fingers and keep them open against resistance (**E**). Have the patient adduct the fingers and attempt to close them against resistance (**F**).

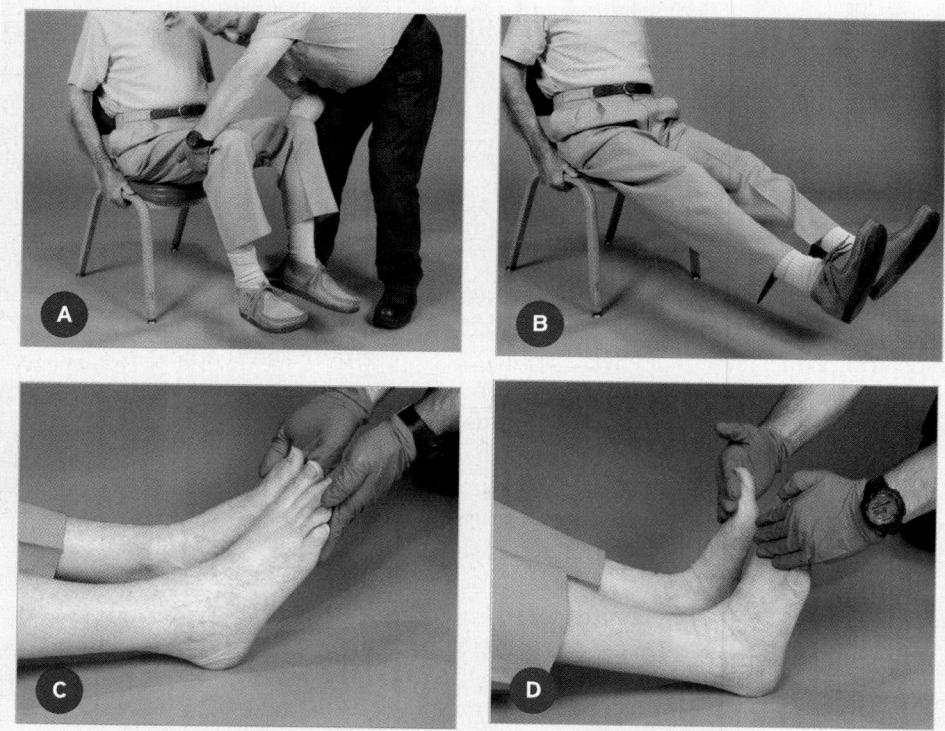

Figure 22-13 Neurologic evaluation of the lower extremities. Ask the patient to bend (**A**) and extend (**B**) the knees. Ask the patient to flex the feet and ankles downward (**C**) and flex the toes upward (**D**).

Ongoing Assessment

Vital signs should be monitored every 5 minutes (unstable patients) to 15 minutes (stable patients), with special attention to the patient's cardiovascular status. Be alert for hypotension without other signs of shock. The combination of hypotension with a normal or slow pulse and warm skin is highly suggestive of neurogenic shock. The SCI responsible for neurogenic shock also generally produces a flaccid paralysis and complete loss of sensation below the level of the injury. In contrast to neurogenic shock, hypovolemic shock is associated with pale, cold, clammy skin and tachycardia.

Check interventions such as oxygen flow and spinal immobilization to ensure that they are still effective. Some EMS systems may administer an antiemetic or corticosteroid per medical control. Repeat the physical exam and reprioritize the patient as necessary.

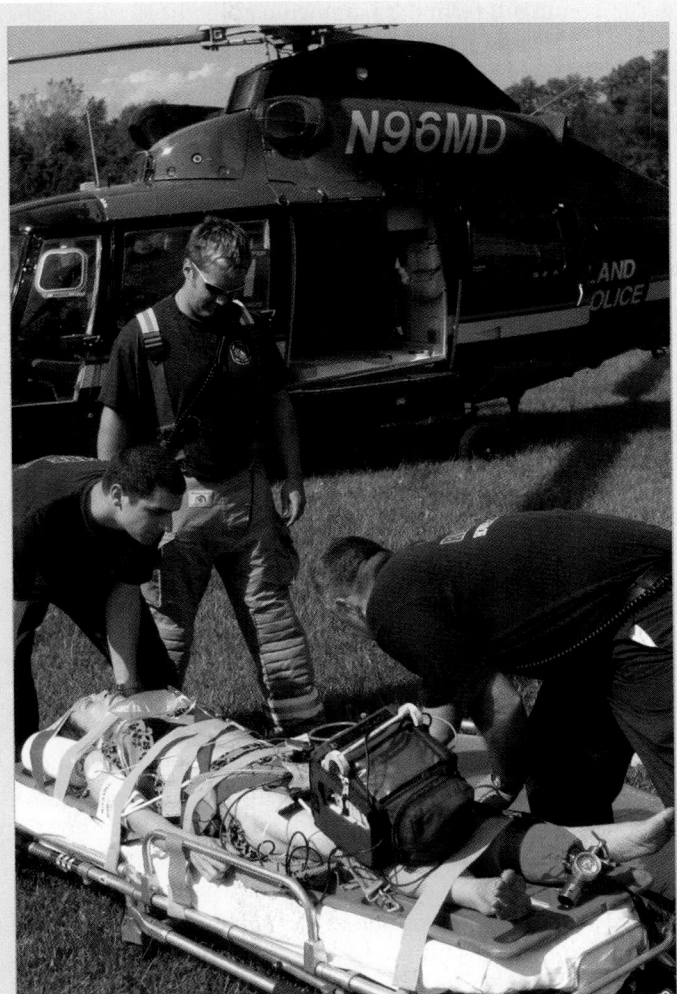

Figure 22-14 Spend no more than 10 minutes on scene unless lengthy extrication is underway or you are waiting for air evacuation.

Management

Current principles of spine trauma management include recognition of potential or actual injury, appropriate immobilization (ie, spinal motion restriction), and reduction or prevention of the incidence of secondary injury. The primary goal of spinal immobilization is to prevent further injuries. Unfortunately, studies have shown that complete spinal immobilization can be painful, especially at pressure points of the occiput and lumbrosacral areas, and can produce a restriction on ventilation. Spinal motion restriction also increases the risk for aspiration. Rigid cervical collars have been implicated as contributing to elevated intracranial pressure. Prolonged scene times can also be an issue, as with any trauma patient. The goal of all EMS providers, no matter what level, should be to spend no more than 10 minutes on the scene before the patient is transported to the most appropriate facility unless lengthy extrication is taking place or the team is awaiting air evacuation **Figure 22-14 ▲**.

Special Considerations

When immobilizing pregnant patients, tilt the backboard 15° to 20° to the left using a pillow or blankets. If this is not possible, manually displace the uterus to the left side.

Although a definitive prehospital clinical spine clearance protocol has not yet been established, current practices reflect the principles of hospital-based models. Specific criteria to determine whether complete immobilization is necessary should be reviewed by medical directors for efficacy. If the patient has no neurologic deficit; is not under the influence of alcohol, drugs, or medications; has no distracting injuries; has no motor or sensory deficit; and has no pain or tenderness upon movement or palpation, then he or she may not require immobilization. If there is any doubt, the patient should be immobilized. As always, follow local protocols as determined by the medical director.

Spinal Splinting Procedures

For splinting purposes, the spine should be considered one long bone articulating with the head and the pelvis at either end. Thus the paramedic cannot isolate and splint at only one level of the spinal column; there is simply *no such thing as partial spinal immobilization.*

Special Considerations

In most instances, a toddler can be immobilized in a child seat. If the child and seat need to be placed in a supine position, the child must be extricated from the car seat to avoid placing extra pressure on the abdomen and reducing the lung expansion.

Supine Patients

A supine patient can be effectively immobilized by securing him or her to a long backboard. The preferred procedure for moving a patient from the ground to a backboard is the four-person log roll; this method is recommended whenever you suspect a spinal injury. In other cases, you may choose to slide the patient onto a backboard or use a scoop stretcher. The patient's condition, the scene, and available resources will dictate which method you choose. Ideally, the patient should be log rolled away from the side of injury. Another technique that limits movement of the spine is the use of a scoop stretcher to lift a patient a few inches off the floor or ground while another paramedic or EMT slides a long backboard under the patient.

Your job is to ensure that the head, torso, and pelvis move as a unit, with your teammates controlling the movement of the body. If necessary, you may recruit bystanders to the team, but instruct them fully before moving the patient.

To immobilize a patient on a backboard, follow these steps:

1. *Take BSI precautions, and then begin manual in-line stabilization* from a kneeling position at the patient's head. Hold the head firmly with both hands. The paramedic at the head directs all patient movement.

2. *Support the lower jaw with your index and long fingers, and support the head with your palms.* If the patient's head is not facing forward, gently move it until the patient's eyes are looking straight ahead and the head and torso are in line (neutral alignment). Never twist, flex, or extend the head or neck excessively. Do not remove your hands from the patient's head until the patient is properly secured to a backboard and the head is immobilized.

3. *Assess distal PMS function in each extremity.*

4. *Apply an appropriately sized cervical collar.* A cervical collar is used in addition to—not instead of—manual in-line cervical spine (also called c-spine) immobilization. Select the collar based on the manufacturer's specifications, and make sure it fits correctly. An improperly sized immobilization device could cause further injury. If you do not have the correct size, use a rolled towel; tape it to the backboard around the patient's head, and provide continuous manual support **Figure 22-15 ▾**. Place the chin support snugly underneath the chin. While maintaining manual in-line stabilization, wrap the collar around the neck and secure the collar to the far side of the chin support. Recheck that the patient is in a neutral in-line position.

5. The other team members should *position the immobilization device* (backboard) and place their hands on the far side of the patient to increase their leverage. Instruct them to use their body weight and their shoulder and back muscles to ensure a smooth, coordinated pull, concentrating their pull on the heavier portions of the patient's body **Figure 22-16A ▸**.

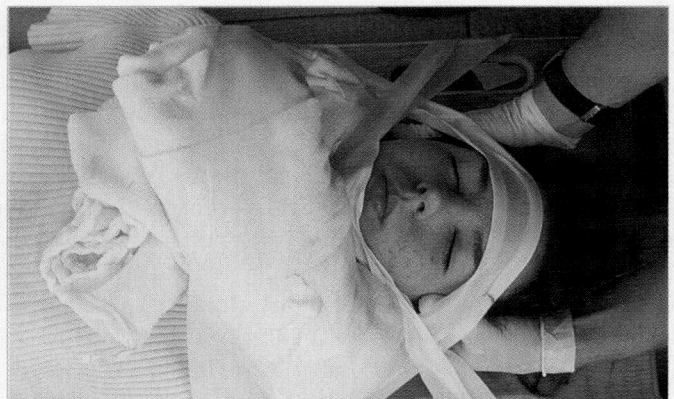

Figure 22-15 If you don't have an appropriately sized cervical collar, use a rolled towel. Tape it to the backboard around the patient's head and provide continuous manual support.

6. On command from the paramedic at the head, the rescuers should *roll the patient* toward themselves. One rescuer should then quickly examine the back while the patient is rolled on the side, then slide the backboard behind and under the patient. The team should then roll the patient back onto the board, avoiding rotation of the head, shoulders, and pelvis **Figure 22-16B ▸**.

7. *Make sure the patient is centered on the board.*

8. *Secure the upper torso* to the board once the patient is centered on the backboard **Figure 22-16C ▸**.

9. *Secure the pelvis and upper legs*, using padding as needed. For the pelvis, use straps over the iliac crests and/or groin loops (leg straps).

10. *Immobilize the head* to the board by positioning a commercial immobilization device or towel rolls. Secure the head to the board only after spider straps or something comparable have secured the torso. If the head is secured first and the body shifts, the spine may be compromised. Securing the majority of the body weight first provides better protection.

11. *Secure the head* by taping the head-immobilization device across the forehead. To prevent airway problems and maintain access to the airway, do not tape over the throat or chin. Instead, tape across the cervical collar just under the chin without covering the opening **Figure 22-16D ▸**.

12. *Check and readjust straps* as needed to ensure that the entire body is snugly secured and will not slide during movement of the board or patient transport.

13. *Reassess distal PMS function* in each extremity, and continue to do so periodically.

Do not force the head into a neutral, in-line position if the patient has muscle spasms in the neck; increased pain with movement (ie, interlocked facets); numbness, tingling, or weakness; or a compromised airway or ventilation. In these situations, immobilize the patient in the position in which you found him or her.

The patient should be maintained in the neutral position unless pain or resistance to movement prevent it, in which case you should maintain the patient in the position found. Neutral positioning provides the most space for the spinal cord and may reduce cord hypoxia and excess pressure on the tissue. Do not place pillows under the patient's head. MRI studies, however, have revealed that the adult cervical spinal canal is anatomically aligned if the head is elevated by padding under the occiput with a folded towel or pad. About 80% of adult

Special Considerations

Do not accept the labeled sizes ("pediatric" or "infant") for cervical collars. Measure each patient individually. Never place tape across the child's neck; it may obstruct the airway. Also, remember to add padding so that the child is as wide as the board.

patients placed flat on a long backboard will be in extension and will require ½″ to 2″ of padding to achieve neutral positioning. Pediatric patients have relatively larger heads, so they need padding under the torso to maintain alignment and prevent neck flexion if immobilized on an adult backboard. Newer pediatric backboards include a recessed portion that accommodates the head or torso padding.

Patients who are found in a prone position or on their side should be log rolled into the supine position with the head and neck manually stabilized in the position in which they were found, and then immobilized as described earlier. One rescuer should take control of the cervical spine using a crossed-hand position to roll the patient. The second rescuer should be positioned at the torso, with any additional help at the pelvis and legs. The rescuer at the head counts, and the patient is rolled as a unit into a supine position. Assessment and immobilization should then continue as usual.

An unconscious patient whose head and neck are passively rotated to one side should be maintained in this position unless respiration is compromised. In case of respiratory distress, attempt to bring the head into axial alignment with gentle traction. A conscious and reliable patient can be asked to turn the head if there are no overt signs of injury or neurologic deficit. If the patient experiences neck pain or nervous system complaints, this movement should be halted and the patient should be transported in the position of comfort.

Seated Patients

Patients found in a sitting position (eg, after a motor vehicle crash) who are without cardiorespiratory compromise but require spine immobilization should also be approached with manual stabilization of the head and neck. A rigid cervical collar should be measured and placed appropriately, and a vest-type extrication device should be used to facilitate the transfer of the patient onto a long backboard. Exceptions to this rule include the following situations in which you do not have time to first secure the patient to the short board:

- You or the patient is in danger.
- You need to gain immediate access to other patients.
- The patient's injuries justify urgent removal.

In these situations, your team should lower the patient directly onto a long backboard, using the rapid extrication technique discussed later in this chapter. Provide manual stabilization of the cervical spine as you move the patient. Rapid

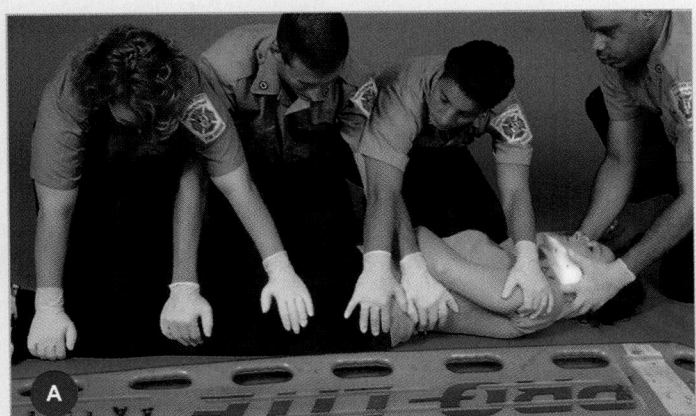
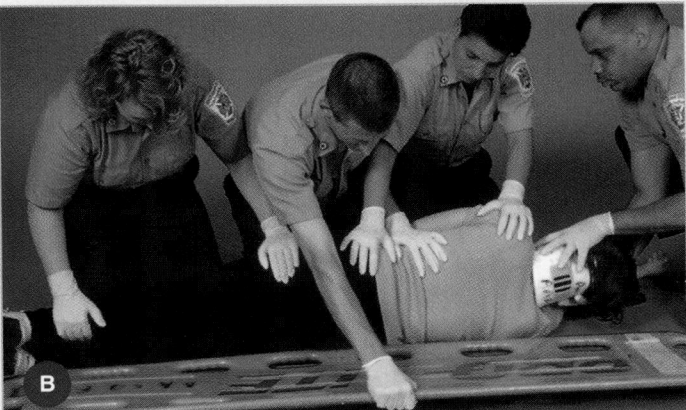
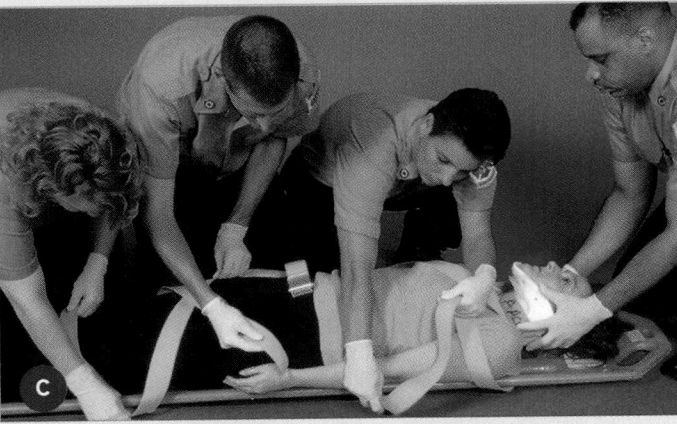
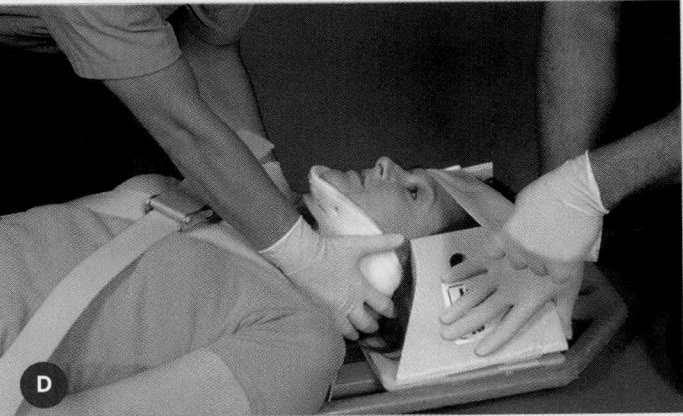

Figure 22-16 Immobilizing a patient to a long backboard. **A.** Placing hands on the far side of the patient. **B.** Rolling the patient and examining the back. **C.** Securing the upper and lower torso. **D.** Securing the head.

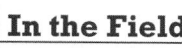

In the Field

Never release manual in-line neck stabilization until the entire spine is properly immobilized. A patient's cervical spine is not properly immobilized until lateral immobilization is securely in place. Cervical collars will not eliminate neck movement entirely. The collar simply reminds both the patient and the EMS provider that there is a potential vertebral or spinal problem and to take special caution.

extrication is indicated only in cases of life- or limb-threatening injury. In all other cases, follow these steps to immobilize a sitting patient:

1. *Stabilize the head and then maintain manual in-line stabilization* until the patient is secured to the long backboard.

2. *Assess distal PMS function* in each extremity.

3. *Apply the rigid cervical collar.* Because the cervical collar does not provide complete stabilization of the cervical spine, continue manual stabilization of the patient's head and neck until the patient is fully immobilized on a backboard.

4. *Insert a short spine immobilization device* between the patient's upper back and the seat back.

5. *Open the board's side flaps* (if present) and position them around the patient's torso, snug to the armpits Figure 22-17A ▾ .

6. Once the device is properly positioned, *secure the upper torso straps.*

7. *Position and fasten both groin loops* (leg straps). Pad the groin as needed. Check all torso straps and make sure they are secure. Make any adjustments necessary without excessive movement of the patient.

8. *Pad any space* between the patient's head and the device.

9. *Secure the forehead* strap or tape the head securely, then fasten the lower head strap around the rigid cervical collar Figure 22-17B ▾ .

10. *Place the long backboard* next to the patient's buttocks, perpendicular to the trunk.

11. *Turn the patient* parallel to the long board, and slowly lower him or her onto it.

12. *Lift the patient* and the vest-type device together as a unit (without rotating the patient), and slip the long backboard under the patient and device Figure 22-17C ▾ .

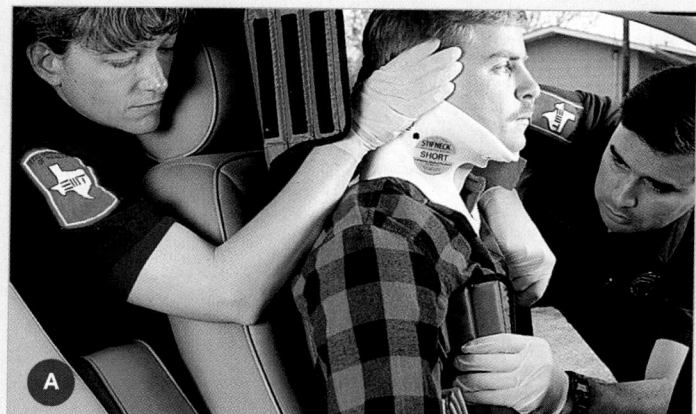

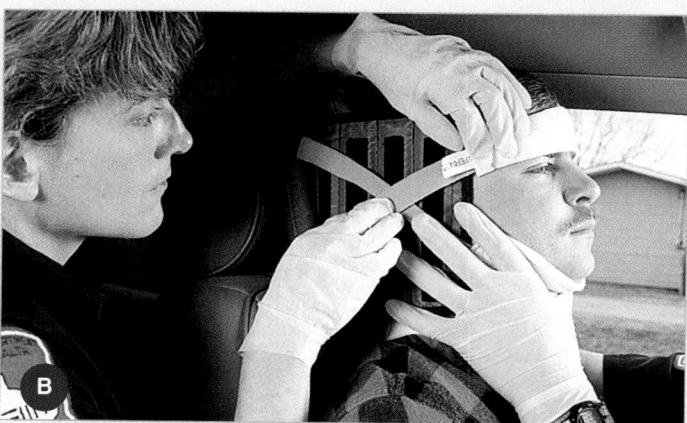

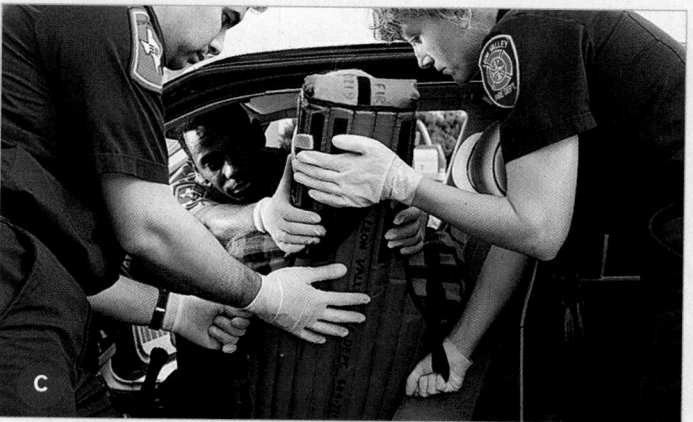

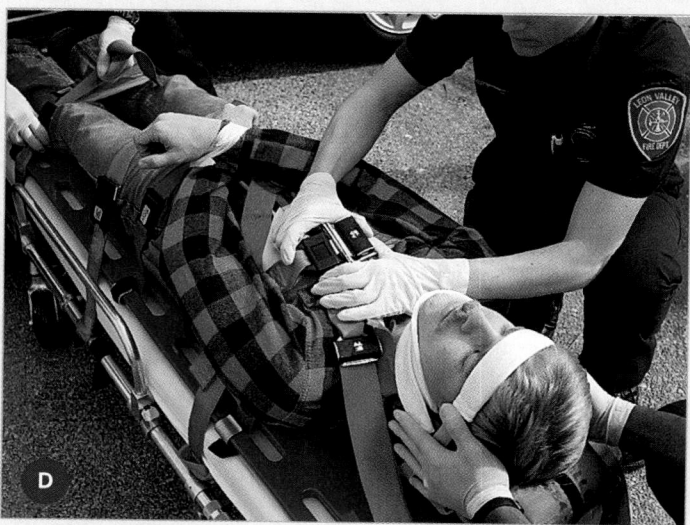

Figure 22-17 Immobilizing a patient found in a sitting position. **A.** Positioning around the patient's torso. **B.** Securing the head straps. **C.** Lowering the patient onto the backboard. **D.** Securing immobilization devices.

Osteoporosis in the thoracic and lumbar spine contributes to a high rate of injury in older patients. Three types of fractures are commonly encountered in these individuals:

- **Compression fractures**—stable injuries that often result from minimal trauma, eg, simply bending over, rising from a chair, or sitting down forcefully.
- **Burst fractures**—unstable fractures that typically result from a high-energy mechanism of injury such as a motor vehicle crash or a fall from substantial height. They may lead to neurologic injury secondary to shifting of the vertebrae with damage to the spinal cord.
- **Seatbelt-type fractures**—involve flexion and cause a fracture through the entire vertebral body and bony arch. These injuries typically result from an ejection or in individuals who are wearing only a lap belt without a shoulder harness.

13. *Release the leg straps* and loosen the chest strap to allow the legs to straighten and give the chest room to fully expand.

14. *Secure the short device and long backboard together*. Do not remove the vest-type device from the patient.

15. *Reassess distal PMS function* in all four extremities. Note your findings on the patient care report, and prepare for transport Figure 22-17D ◄ .

Rapid Extrication

With the rapid extrication technique, the patient can be moved from sitting in a car to lying supine on a backboard in approximately 2 minutes. You should use the rapid extrication technique in the following situations:

- The vehicle or scene is unsafe.
- The patient cannot be properly assessed before being removed from the car.
- The patient needs immediate intervention that requires a supine position.
- The patient's condition requires immediate transport to the hospital.
- The patient blocks the paramedic's access to another seriously injured patient.

In such cases, the delay that results from applying an extrication-type vest or half-board is contraindicated and unacceptable. Unfortunately, the manual support and immobi-

To immobilize kyphotic patients, several blankets and pillows or vacuum splints may be required to provide support to the head and upper back. Make sure that the empty spaces under the patient's knees or lumbar spine are padded as well.

lization that you provide when using the rapid extrication technique carry a greater risk of spine movement. You should not use the rapid extrication technique if no urgency exists.

The rapid extrication technique requires a team of three providers who are knowledgeable and practiced in the procedure. Follow these steps:

1. The first rescuer provides manual in-line stabilization of the patient's head and cervical spine from behind. Support may be applied from the side, if necessary, by reaching through the driver's door.

2. The second rescuer serves as a team leader and gives the commands to coordinate the team's moves until the patient is supine on the backboard. Because the second rescuer lifts and turns the patient's torso, he or she must be physically capable of moving the patient. The second rescuer works from the driver's doorway. If the first rescuer is also working from that doorway, the second rescuer should stand closer to the door hinges toward the front of the vehicle. The second rescuer applies a rigid cervical collar and performs an initial assessment.

3. The second rescuer provides continuous support of the patient's torso until the patient is supine on the backboard. Once the second rescuer takes control of the torso, usually in the form of a body hug, he or she should not let go of the patient for any reason. Some type of cross-chest shoulder hug usually works well, but you must decide which method will work best for any given patient. You cannot simply reach into the car and grab the patient, because this will twist the patient's torso. You must rotate the patient as a unit.

4. The third rescuer works from the front passenger seat and rotates the patient's legs and feet as the torso is turned, ensuring that they are free of the pedals and any other obstruction. The third rescuer should first carefully move the patient's nearer leg laterally, without rotating the patient's pelvis and lower spine. The pelvis and lower spine rotate only as the third rescuer moves the second leg during the next step. Moving the nearer leg first makes it much easier to move the second leg in concert with the rest of the body. Once the third rescuer moves the legs together, they should be moved as a unit Figure 22-18A ► .

5. The patient is rotated 90° so that the back faces out the driver's door and the feet are on the front passenger's seat. This coordinated movement is done in three or four short, quick, one eighth to one quarter turns. The second rescuer coordinates the sequence of moves and the first rescuer directs each quick turn by saying, "Ready, turn" or "Ready, move." Hand position changes should be made between moves.

6. In most cases, the first rescuer will be working from the back seat. At some point, either because the doorpost is in the way or because he or she cannot reach farther from the back seat, the first rescuer will be unable to follow the torso rotation. At that time, the third rescuer should assume temporary manual in-line stabilization of the head and neck until the first rescuer can regain control of the

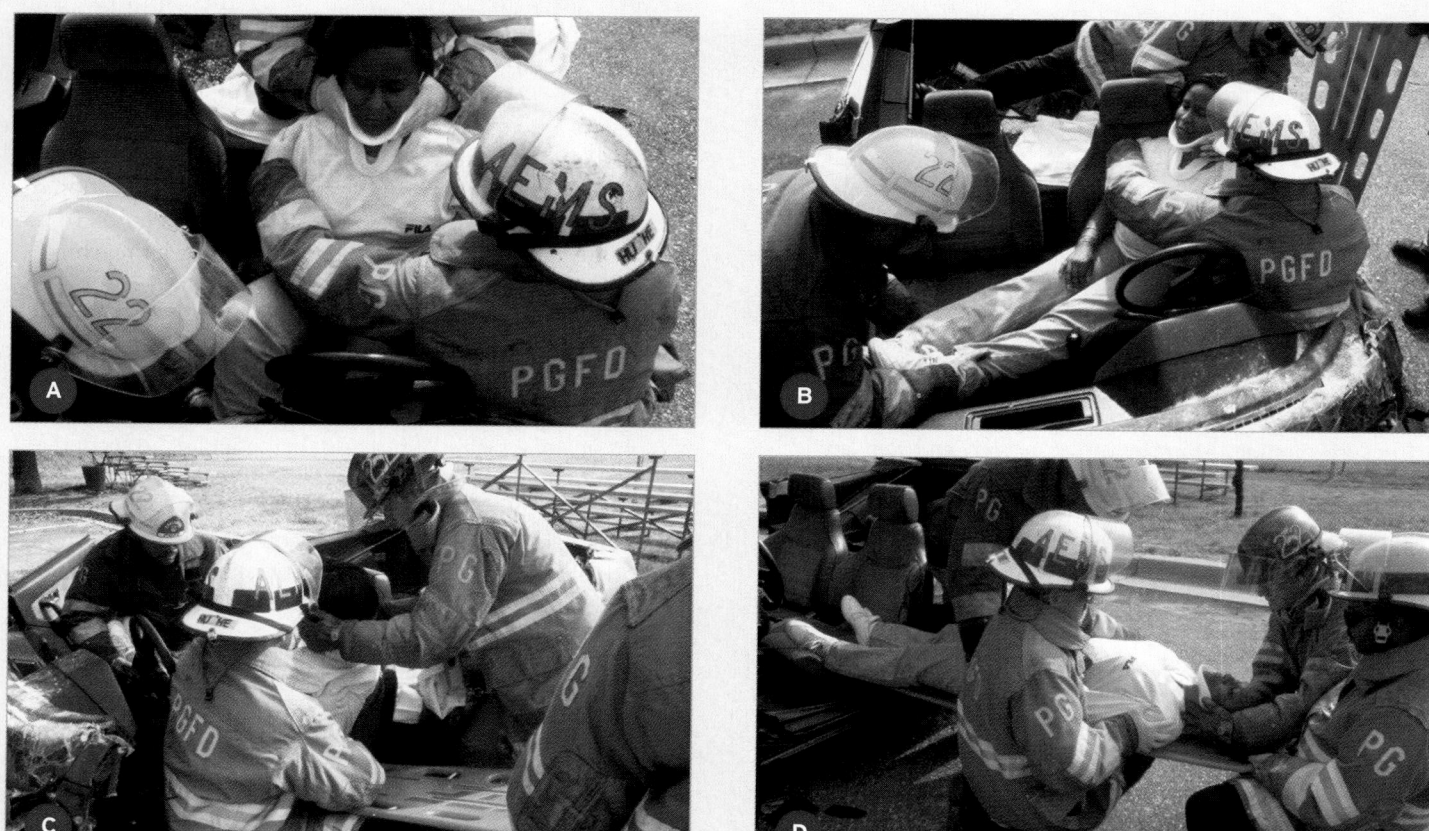

Figure 22-18 Rapid extrication technique. **A.** Moving the patient's legs without moving the pelvis or spine. **B.** Rotating the patient as a unit. **C.** Placing the backboard on the seat. **D.** Sliding the patient onto the board.

head from outside the vehicle. If a fourth rescuer is present, the fourth rescuer stands next to the second rescuer. The fourth rescuer takes control of the head and neck from outside the vehicle without involving the third rescuer. As soon as the change has been made, the rotation can continue Figure 22-18B.

7. Once the patient has been fully rotated, the backboard is placed against the patient's buttocks on the seat. Do not try to wedge the backboard under the patient. If only three rescuers are present, place the backboard within arm's reach of the driver's door before the move so that the board can be pulled into place when needed; the far end of the board can be left on the ground. When a fourth rescuer is available, the first rescuer exits the rear seat of the car, places the backboard against the patient's buttocks, and maintains pressure in toward the vehicle from the far end of the board. When the door opening allows, some rescuers prefer to insert the backboard onto the car seat before the patient is rotated.

8. As soon as the patient has been rotated and the backboard is in place, the second and third rescuers lower the patient onto the board while supporting the head and torso so that neutral alignment is maintained. The first rescuer holds the backboard until the patient is secured Figure 22-18C.

9. The third rescuer moves across the front seat to be in position at the patient's hips. If the third rescuer stays at the patient's knees or feet, he or she will be ineffective in helping to move the body's weight. The knees and feet follow the hips.

10. The fourth rescuer maintains in-line support of the head and takes over giving the commands. If a fourth rescuer is not present, you can direct a volunteer to assist you. The second rescuer maintains direction of the extrication; this rescuer stands with his or her back to the door, facing the rear of the vehicle. The backboard should be immediately in front of the third rescuer. The second rescuer grasps the patient's shoulders or armpits. On command, the second and third rescuers slide the patient 8″ to 12″ along the backboard, repeating this slide until the patient's hips are firmly on the backboard.

11. The third rescuer gets out of the vehicle and moves to the opposite side of the backboard, across from the second rescuer. The third rescuer takes control at the shoulders, and the second rescuer moves back to take control of the hips. On command, these two rescuers move the patient along the board in 8″ to 12″ slides until the patient is completely on the board Figure 22-18D.

12. The first (or fourth) rescuer continues to maintain manual in-line support of the head. The second and third rescuers

grasp their side of the board, and then carry it and the patient away from the vehicle onto the prepared cot nearby.

In some cases, you will be able to rest the head end of the backboard on the cot while the patient is moved onto the backboard; in others, you will not. Once the backboard and patient have been placed on the cot, you should begin lifesaving treatment immediately. If you used the rapid extrication technique because the scene was dangerous, you and your team should immediately move the cot a safe distance away from the vehicle before you assess or treat the patient.

The steps of the rapid extrication technique must be considered a general procedure to be adapted as needed. Every situation will be different—a different car, a different size and priority patient, and a different crew. Your resourcefulness and ability to adapt are necessary elements of a successful rapid extrication.

Standing Patients

Ambulatory patients found on the scene may require immobilization after examination and determination of mechanism and reliability. If you suspect underlying head, neck, or spine injuries, carefully take down the patient using the standing takedown (described below), then immobilize the patient to a long backboard. This will require a minimum of three rescuers, undertaking the following steps:

1. Establish manual, in-line stabilization, apply a rigid cervical collar, and instruct the patient to remain still.
2. Position the board upright, directly behind the patient.
3. Two rescuers stand on either side of the patient; the third is directly behind the patient, maintaining immobilization.
4. The two rescuers grasp the handholds at shoulder level or slightly above by reaching under the patient's arms while standing at either side   Figure 22-19A ▶ .
5. Prepare to lower the patient to the ground   Figure 22-19B ▶ .

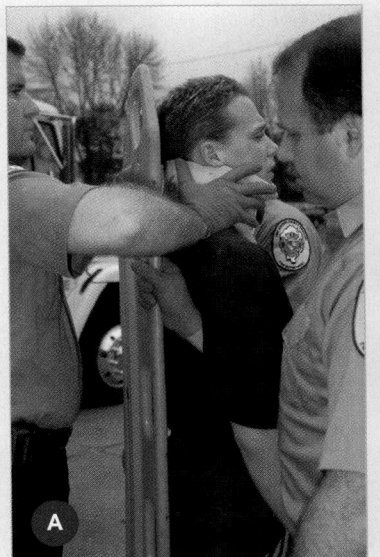
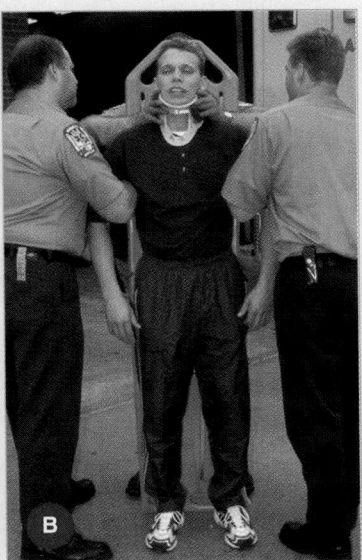
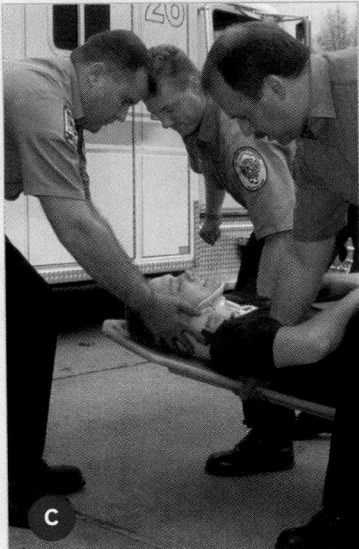

Figure 22-19 Immobilizing a patient found in a standing position. **A.** Positioning rescuers at the sides of the backboard. **B.** Preparing to lower the patient. **C.** Lowering the patient to the ground. Once the patient's head is on the board, do not lift it off the board!

6. Carefully lower the patient as a unit under the direction of the rescuer at the head. The rescuer at the head must make sure the head stays against the board and carefully rotate his or her hands while the patient is being lowered to maintain in-line stabilization   Figure 22-19C ▲ .

Packaging and Removal of Injured Patients From the Water

Whatever the type of accident, the principles of packaging and removal are the same: Keep the head, neck, and trunk in alignment. When the patient may have sustained a spine injury in a confirmed diving accident, spinal immobilization must be initiated even before the patient is removed from the water. If respiratory arrest is suspected, ventilation can be done while still in the water; in case of cardiac arrest, however, the rescuer should quickly evaluate the mechanism of injury. If a spine injury is not obvious, immediately remove the patient from the water and

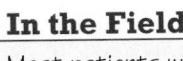

In the Field

Most patients who have just sustained a potential spine injury and are standing up at a collision scene still need to be immobilized. Use of the standing takedown technique is strongly recommended. They are not backboarded in the standing position because many of these patients will not stand still for the amount of time it takes to complete the immobilization. Some may be dizzy, weak, or intoxicated. Patients who have sustained head trauma may have a head injury. Also, if the backboard is applied and the patient is then placed in the supine position, the straps and padding may loosen as the patient lies down.

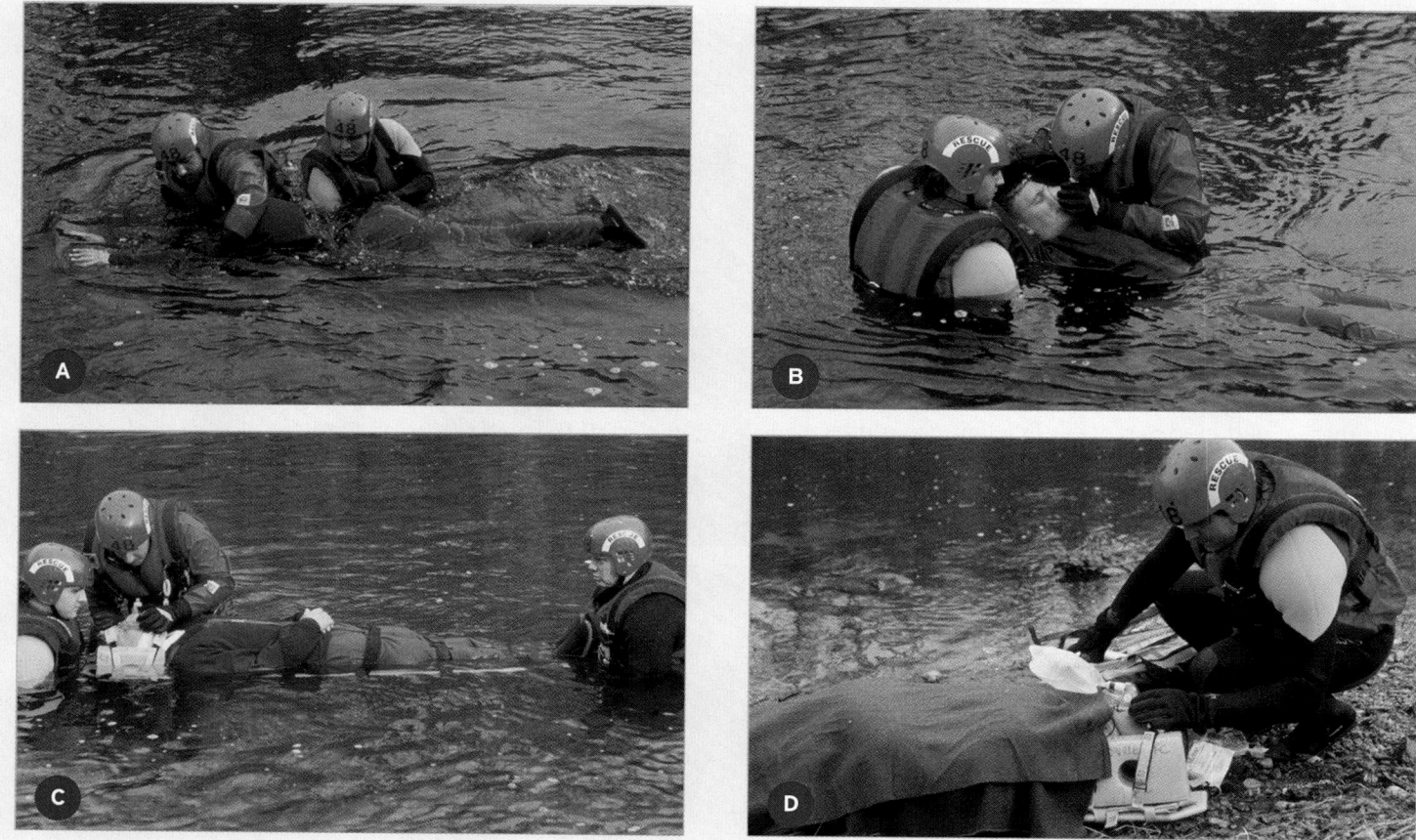

Figure 22-20 Stabilizing a suspected spine injury in the water. **A.** Turning the patient to a supine position in the water. **B.** Providing artificial ventilation. **C.** Securing the patient to a backboard. **D.** Providing care once out of the water.

begin CPR. However, if there is any indication of a spine injury, follow these steps to stabilize the patient in the water:

1. If the patient is prone in the water, *approach the individual from the top of the head*, and place one arm under the body so that the head is supported on your arm and the chest on your hand. Place your other arm across the head and back to splint the head and neck between your arms. Continuing to support the patient's head and neck in that fashion, take a step backward and smoothly turn the patient to the supine position **Figure 22-20A ▲** . Two rescuers are usually required to turn the patient safely, but in some cases one rescuer will suffice. Always rotate the entire upper half of the patient's body as a single unit. Twisting only the head, for example, may aggravate any injury to the cervical spine.

2. *Open the airway and begin ventilation.* Immediate ventilation is the primary treatment of all drowning and submersion patients. As soon as the patient is face up in the water, use a pocket mask if it is available. Have the other rescuer support the head and trunk as a unit while you open the airway and begin artificial ventilation **Figure 22-20B ▲** .

3. *Float a buoyant backboard under the patient* as you continue ventilation.

4. *Secure the head and trunk* to the backboard to eliminate motion of the cervical spine. Do not remove the patient from the water until this step is complete **Figure 22-20C ▲** .

5. *Remove the patient from the water*, on the backboard.

6. *Remove wet clothes*, and cover the patient with a blanket. Give supplementary oxygen if the patient is breathing adequately; give positive-pressure ventilation if the patient is apneic or breathing inadequately. Begin CPR if there is no pulse. Effective chest compressions cannot be performed when the patient is still in the water **Figure 22-20D ▲** .

7. *Consider using an advanced airway device* to maintain the airway if needed. Place the patient on a cardiac monitor and treat dysrhythmias according to the ACLS algorithms (discussed in other chapters).

Patients Wearing Helmets

Helmets are a relatively common finding in motor vehicle and sports-related injuries. The use of helmets has been shown to reduce both the incidence and the severity of brain injuries associated with trauma, and their use is widely encouraged. Most helmets consist of an inner foam layer surrounded by a durable plastic shell. Helmets can inhibit full exposure of the patient and could hinder the provider's efforts at airway management and spinal stabilization. Unfortunately, the removal of most types of helmets can result in some spinal motion even under the best circumstances. However, a securely fitting helmet can provide a degree of stabilization and under the proper circumstances can actually assist in maintaining the spine in a neutral position.

The Inter-Association Task Force for the Appropriate Care of the Spine-Injured Athlete (convened in 1999) recommended helmet removal in the following situations:

- The helmet and chin strap fail to hold the head securely, as with a loose-fitting helmet.
- The helmet and chin strap design prevent adequate airway control, even after the removal of a face mask.
- A helmet with a face mask cannot be removed after a reasonable amount of time.
- The helmet prevents proper immobilization for transport.

Only providers who are familiar with the procedure should attempt helmet removal. A single rescuer should not attempt helmet removal, because the maneuver requires two providers:

1. *Kneel at the patient's head.* Leave enough room between your knees and the helmet so that you can remove the helmet. Your partner should kneel on one side of the patient, at the shoulder area.

2. *Stabilize the helmet* by placing your hands on either side of it, with your fingers on the patient's lower jaw to prevent movement of the head. Once your hands are in position, your partner can loosen the face strap.

3. Your partner should open the face shield, if there is one, and *assess the patient's airway and breathing.* Remove eyeglasses if the patient is wearing them.

4. Once the strap is loosened, your partner should place one hand on the patient's lower jaw at the angle of the jaw and the other behind the head at the back of the helmet. You may then pull the sides of the helmet away from the patient's head   Figure 22-21A ▶ .

5. *Gently slip the helmet partly off the patient's head*, stopping when the helmet reaches the halfway point.

6. Your partner then slides his or her hand from the back of the helmet to the occiput, preventing the head from falling back once the helmet is completely removed   Figure 22-21B ▶ .

7. Once your partner's hand is in place, remove the helmet and provide manual in-line cervical spine stabilization.

8. *Apply a rigid cervical collar* and secure the patient to the backboard.

Controversies

Considerable controversy exists regarding whether to remove helmets in the field. The key considerations boil down to the urgency of airway management, the fit of the helmet, and the best-trained hands to take it off.

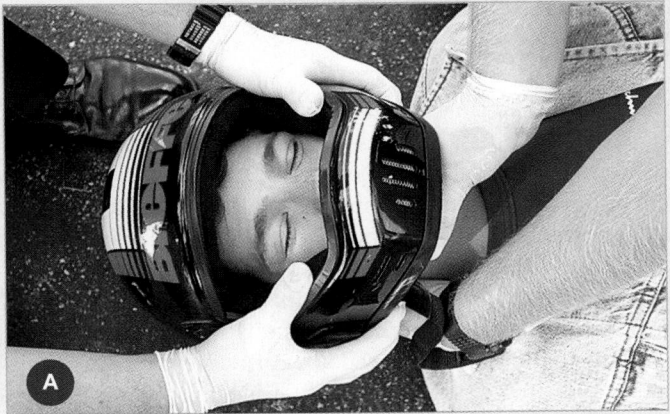
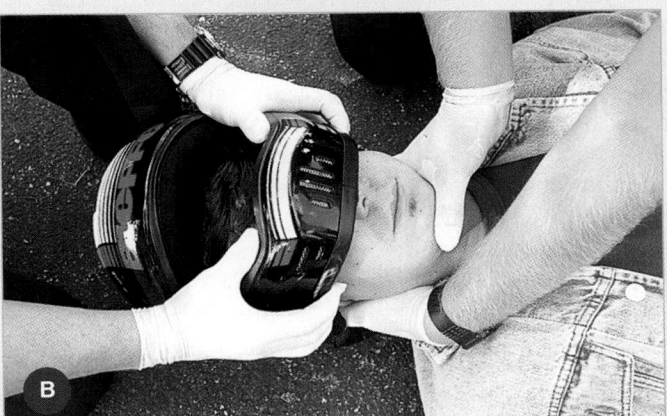
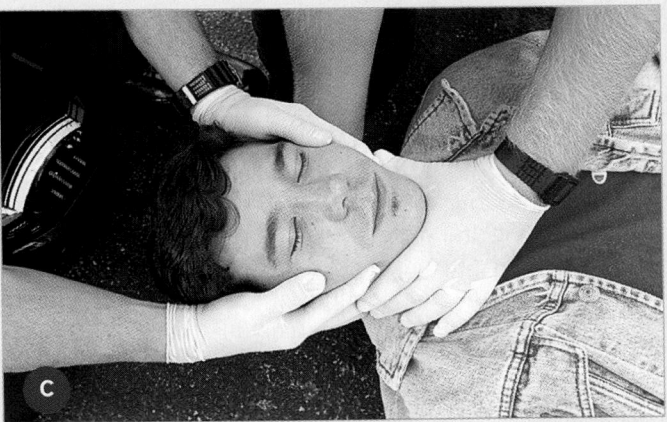

Figure 22-21 Removing a helmet. **A.** Hand positioning for removing a helmet. **B.** Supporting the occiput. **C.** Removing the helmet while stabilizing the head.

9. With large helmets or small patients, you may need to add padding under the shoulders to prevent flexion of the neck. If the patient is wearing shoulder pads or a heavy jacket, you may need to pad behind the head to prevent extension of the neck   Figure 22-21C ▲ .

You do not need to remove a helmet if you can access the patient's airway, the head is snug inside the helmet, and the helmet can be secured to an immobilization device.

Pharmacotherapy of Spinal Cord Injury

Short-acting, reversible sedatives are recommended for the acute agitated patient after a correctible cause of agitation (eg, hypoxia) has been excluded. The risk of secondary injury due to movements from acute agitation must be balanced with potential airway and ventilatory compromise as well as a reliable neurologic exam. Pain medication may also be necessary.

The use of corticosteroids in the acute phase of SCI remains controversial yet the practice is relatively widespread. Recommendations for intravenous corticosteroids vary from a one-time loading dose of dexamethasone at 1 mg/kg IV immediately after injury to the widely accepted methylprednisolone sodium succinate guidelines developed as a result of the National Acute Spinal Cord Injury Study II and III, which call for use of methylprednisolone in acute nonpenetrating SCI less than 3 hours after injury. The latter regimen includes a 30-mg/kg bolus of methylprednisolone over 15 minutes. After a 45-minute interval following infusion, a drip of 5.4 mg/kg/h continues over the next 23 hours. If treatment with methylprednisolone begins within 3 to 8 hours after injury, the drip is typically continued for 48 hours.

Complications of Spinal Cord Injury

The complications of SCI are a consistent cause of the high morbidity and mortality—and high financial cost—associated with this type of injury. Many of the acute-phase complications of SCI have already been addressed in this chapter, such as the potential for aspiration or respiratory arrest, especially with high cervical injuries. Lower cervical lesions may preserve the diaphragm, but the loss of intercostal muscles ultimately impairs coughing and deep breathing, predisposing the patient to atelectasis and pneumonia. Deep-vein thrombosis and pulmonary embolism are late complications that may result from immobility and can become potentially life-threatening.

Autonomic dysreflexia, also called autonomic hyperreflexia, is typically a late complication of SCI but can occur acutely. This potentially life-threatening emergency most commonly occurs with injuries above T4–T6 and results from the loss of parasympathetic stimulation. Patients present clinically with evidence of a massive, uninhibited, uncompensated cardiovascular response due to some stimulation of the sympathetic nervous system below the level of injury **Table 22-4 ▶**. The irritated area sends a signal that is not able to reach the brain, and unabated sympathetic nervous system stimulation results in vasoconstriction as evidenced by cool, pale extremities, systolic blood pressures greater than 200 mm Hg, and diastolic blood pressures of 130 mm Hg or greater. Hypertension leads to parasympathetic stimulation from activation of the vasomotor center in the medulla. Vagal compensation causes bradycardia and vasodilation of peripheral and visceral vessels above the

Table 22-4	Signs and Symptoms of Autonomic Dysreflexia	
■ Hypertension	■ Rebound hypotension	
■ Headache	■ Flushing and sweating above SCI	
■ Nasal congestion	■ Erect hairs above SCI	
■ Dilation of the pupils	■ Chills without fever	
■ Anxiety	■ Bronchospasm	
■ Bradycardia	■ Seizures, stroke, and death	

level of the lesion, although vessels below the SCI remain constricted. Selective vasodilation results in flushed, diaphoretic skin and nasopharyngeal vessel congestion.

Autonomic dysreflexia can be precipitated by any noxious stimuli below the level of a cervical or high thoracic SCI. Common precipitators include skin lesions such as insect bites, constrictive clothing, or sharp objects compressing the skin. Sharp objects should be removed from pockets or seat cushions. Localized wounds such as lacerations, abrasions, decubitus ulcerations, or ingrown toenails are often the source of stimulation. Irritation from skin lesions should be minimized with cold packs. Distention of the bladder due to obstructed urine outflow from spasm or kinked Foley catheters as well as bladder infection, constipation, or bowel impaction must be suspected. Catheters should be irrigated and obstructions removed. In men, tight condom catheters can pinch genitalia and should be checked and removed if necessary. In women, menstrual cramps or pregnancy can be a source of the stimulation.

Management of autonomic dysreflexia is usually not a prehospital intervention. If the source cannot be found or minimized to an effective extent, it may be necessary to reduce blood pressure with vasodilators.

Nontraumatic Spinal Conditions

Back pain is one of the most common physical complaints in emergency departments throughout the United States. An estimated 60% to 90% of the US population is afflicted with some form of low back pain. Expenses related to back pain are high due to the extensive costs of therapy and lost wages from missed work days. Upright posture brings a significant amount of weight to bear on the lumbar spine—specifically at L4–L5, where the natural bend in the spine's curvature changes. As a consequence, most people are susceptible to injury or degenerative disease. Spinal tumors can also be a cause of pain and debilitation. Occupations that require repetitive lifting, exposure to vibrations from vehicles or industrial machinery, and comorbid diseases such as osteoporosis are all risks for developing low back pain.

Most cases of low back pain are idiopathic, and making a precise diagnosis can be difficult. When evaluating nontraumatic back pain, it is important to consider disease processes that can result in significantly debilitating lesions, including SCI **Table 22-5 ▶**. In the absence of trauma, the patient

Table 22-5	Common Causes of Low Back Pain
■ Muscle or ligament strains ■ Fractures ■ Osteomyelitis—bone infection ■ Degenerative joint/disk disease	■ Spondylolysis ■ Bursitis/synovitis ■ Disk herniation ■ Tumor

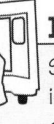

In the Field

Spondylolysis is a structural defect of the spine involving the lamina or vertebral arch. It usually occurs between the superior and inferior articulating facets. In most people, it is congenital and may be hereditary. A radiograph is necessary to confirm spondylolysis.

who presents with the complaint of lower back pain must be assessed with the anatomy and neurophysiology of the spine and spinal cord in mind. Pay particular attention to the medications the patient is taking, because patients with chronic back pain and tumors may require very high levels of narcotics to control the intense pain.

Pain may result from strain or sprain of paravertebral muscles and supporting ligamentous structures without significant injury to nerve elements. Older patients (especially women) with a history of osteoporosis are at high risk for spontaneous compression fractures of the spine; these typically stable frac-

Controversies

Classic education holds that intervertebral disks have no sensory nerve fibers. In reality, sensory nerves extend into the disk over at least one third the radius of the outer rim, the anulus fibrosis. In the clinical setting, it is impossible to tell whether low back pain is coming solely from the irritation of these nerves. However, this etiology is always a possibility, even if MRI and CT show no damage. Injury to these nerves occurs at a microscopic level that is undetectable on standard tests.

tures are not associated with SCI. Furthermore, tumors in the spine from a variety of metastatic carcinomas can cause pathologic spine fractures, with extension of bone fragments or the tumor itself into the spinal canal causing SCI.

Degenerative disk disease is a common entity in patients older than age 50 years. Over time, biomechanical alterations of the intervertebral disk will result in loss of height and reduce the shock-absorbing effect of the disk. Significant narrowing may result in variable segment stability.

Disk herniation is usually caused by some degree of trauma in patients with preexisting disk degeneration. It typically affects men between the ages of 30 and 50 years, and often results from poor lifting technique. Herniation most commonly occurs at L4–L5 and L5–S1 but may also occur in C5–C6 and C6–C7. Patients will present with pain, usually with straining; they may have tenderness of the spine and often have limited range of motion. Alterations in sensation and motor functions may exist as well. Cervical herniations may present with upper extremity pain or paresthesias that worsen with neck motion. Motor weakness may also occur due to spinal cord compression.

Definitive diagnosis of back pain may require multiple modalities of radiographic imaging. Prehospital management of low back pain in the absence of trauma is primarily palliative, directed at decreasing any pain or discomfort with movement. Patients who experience significant pain with movement or have neurologic deficits may benefit from spinal immobilization for greater comfort and to prevent irritation of neural elements.

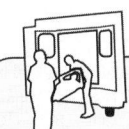

In the Field

Some patients with acute low back spasm are literally paralyzed with pain. To move them, use a "scoop-type" metal stretcher that fits under the patient. Administration of IV diazepam may be extremely helpful in relieving severe muscle spasm.

You are the Provider Summary

1. What is your primary concern?

Scene safety is always your primary concern. Many factors can create an unsafe scene when dealing with downed aircraft. You must address those concerns before undertaking patient care. To do otherwise can result in injury or death of yourself, your fellow responders, or the patients in your care.

2. What additional resources (if any) would you request and when?

Unless you are cross-trained as a fire fighter and are responding with other fire department apparatus, you must request fire department personnel. This scene may potentially involve fire (including the aircraft, grass, and other structures), extrication, and hazardous materials. You also need to request assistance from the utility companies. Until the power has been shut off, it is unsafe to engage in patient care.

3. How can you immediately assess and communicate with this patient in a safe manner?

You can assess your patient using binoculars at a safe distance. You should attempt to gain as much information regarding her overall condition, taking note if she is alert, shows signs of distress through either posture or facial expression, or has a visible skin condition. Communication with your patient is possible with a vehicle-mounted loudspeaker system or bullhorn. If these are not available, hand signals can be used to communicate the need for the patient to stay inside the craft or vehicle.

4. Given the information your patient has provided, have your priorities changed?

Again, you face a safety issue. You must take steps to decontaminate the patient to prevent the possibility of ignition and serious burns.

5. Given the mechanism of injury and other factors, what injuries do you suspect?

You can obtain a wealth of information from the patient's posture, guarding, and facial expression. This patient has a mechanism of injury consistent with a spinal column compression fracture. She is also attempting to stabilize her lumbar spine through her posture and her use of self-splinting. This is the body's natural response to prevent further pain and injury.

6. What other factors can impact a patient's ability to handle the stress of trauma?

Many factors can play a role in the patient's ability to compensate for the stressors of trauma: extremes of age, diseases, certain medications, and environmental conditions. For example, a patient who has a previous history of myocardial infarction and suffers significant blood loss will lack the compensatory mechanisms or "cardiac reserves" that a young, healthy adult will possess. These patients may succumb to the effects of trauma more quickly, and their injuries may be masked.

7. What other information beyond the history of events should you obtain from your patient?

Obtaining a SAMPLE history is important even when caring for trauma patients. Pertinent past medical history will give you an overall sense of your patient and his or her ability to compensate in the presence of blood loss and injury.

8. If you must decontaminate a patient in the open, how can you preserve patient modesty?

If you cannot move a patient to a private location to decontaminate or perform assessments that require visualization of injuries, you can create a visual barrier by using sheets and other responders (facing outward). Consider creating such a visual barrier whenever your exam may compromise patient modesty.

9. What is the standard for maximum on-scene time for any significant trauma patient?

Most responders know about the "golden hour" and its impact on caring for the trauma patient. To significantly lessen morbidity and mortality rates, patients with significant trauma require the definitive care of the trauma surgeon and trauma surgical suite available at trauma centers. This equates to the "platinum 10 minutes" for EMS providers: Ideally, no more than 10 minutes should be spent on-scene preparing a patient for transport. Every effort should be made to adhere to this time standard. If you must deviate from it, then detailed documentation is required.

10. How does prompt, appropriate care affect the patient beyond immediate survival of the injuries sustained?

For emergency medical personnel, it is sometimes difficult to think beyond the acute situation at hand. It is important, however, to realize how responders' actions (or lack thereof) can affect the patient and his or her quality of life beyond the short span of the field encounter. If they are treated inappropriately, patients may need weeks or even months in the ICU to recover. Responders should be concerned with their patients' ability to return to the quality of life they are accustomed to. Beyond focusing on prevention measures, responders cannot change what has happened to patients; however, they can review the care in terms of how it affected the patient over the long term.

Prep Kit

Ready for Review

- SCIs are among the most devastating injuries encountered by prehospital providers.
- In order to decipher the often subtle findings associated with SCI, you need to understand the form and function of spinal anatomy.
- Acute injuries of the spine are classified according to the associated mechanism, location, and stability of injury.
- Vertebral factures can occur with or without associated SCI.
- Stable fractures do not involve the posterior column and pose lower risk to the spinal cord.
- Unstable injuries involve the posterior column of the spinal cord and typically include damage to portions of the vertebrae and ligaments that directly protect the spinal cord and nerve roots.
- Primary SCI occurs at the moment of impact.
- Secondary SCI occurs when multiple factors permit a progression of the primary SCI. The ensuing cascade of inflammatory responses may result in further deterioration.
- Limiting the progression of secondary SCI is a major goal of prehospital management of SCI.
- Current principles of spine trauma management include recognition of potential or actual injury, appropriate immobilization, and reduction or prevention of the incidence of secondary injury.
- Short-acting, reversible sedatives are recommended for the acute patient after a correctible cause of agitation has been excluded.
- The use of corticosteroids in the acute phase of SCI remains controversial yet is relatively widespread.
- The complications of SCI are a consistent cause of the high morbidity and mortality associated with this type of injury.
- Back pain is one of the most common physical complaints to present to emergency departments throughout the United States. Most cases of low back pain are idiopathic and difficult to precisely diagnose.

Vital Vocabulary

anterior cord syndrome A condition that occurs with flexion injuries or fractures resulting in the displacement of bony fragments into the anterior portion of the spinal cord; findings include paralysis below the level of the insult and loss of pain, temperature, and touch sensation.

arachnoid The middle membrane of the three meninges that enclose the brain and spinal cord.

autonomic dysreflexia A potentially life-threatening late complication of spinal cord injury in which massive, uninhibited uncompensated cardiovascular response occurs due to stimulation of the sympathetic nervous system below the level of injury. Also known as autonomic hyperreflexia.

Babinski reflex When the toe(s) moves upward in response to stimulation to the sole of the foot. Under normal circumstances, the toe(s) moves downward.

brain Part of the central nervous system, located within the cranium and containing billions of neurons that serve a variety of vital functions.

brain stem The portion of the brain that connects the spinal cord to the rest of the brain, and contains the medulla, pons, and midbrain.

Brown-Sequard syndrome A condition associated with penetrating trauma with hemisection of the spinal cord and complete damage to all spinal tracts on the involved side.

cauda equina The location where the spinal cord separates, composed of nerve roots.

central cord syndrome A condition resulting from hyperextension injuries to the cervical area that cause damage with hemorrhage or edema to the central cervical segments; findings include greater loss of function in the upper extremities with variable sensory loss of pain and temperature.

central nervous system (CNS) The system containing the brain and spinal cord.

cerebrospinal fluid (CSF) Fluid produced in the ventricles of the brain that flows in the subarachnoid space and bathes the meninges.

complete spinal cord injury Total disruption of all tracts of the spinal cord, with all cord mediated functions below the level of transection lost permanently.

dermatomes Areas of the body innervated by sensor components of spinal nerves.

dura mater The outermost of the three meninges that enclose the brain and spinal cord, it is the toughest membrane.

facet joint The joint on which each vertebra articulates with adjacent vertebrae.

flexion injury A type of injury that results from forward movement of the head, typically as the result of rapid deceleration, such as in a car crash, or with a direct blow to the occiput.

foramen magnum A large opening at the base of the skull through which the spinal cord exits the brain.

hyperesthesia Hyperacute pain to touch.

hyperextension Extension of a limb of other body part beyond its usual range of motion.

incomplete spinal cord injury Spinal cord injury in which there is some degree of cord-mediated function; initial dysfunction may be temporary and there may be potential for recovery.

lamina Arise from the posterior pedicles and fuse to form the posterior spinous processes.

myotomes Regions of the body innervated by the motor components of spinal nerves.

neurogenic shock Shock caused by massive vasodilation and pooling of blood in the peripheral vessels to the extent that adequate perfusion cannot be maintained.

parasympathetic nervous system Subdivision of the autonomic nervous system, involved in control of involuntary, vegetative functions, mediated largely by the vagus nerve through the chemical acetylcholine.

pedicles Thick lateral bony struts that connect the vertebral body with spinous and transverse processes and make up the lateral and posterior portions of the spinal foramen.

pia mater The innermost of the three meninges that enclose the brain and spinal cord, it rests directly on the brain and spinal cord.

plexus A cluster of nerve roots that permits peripheral nerve roots to rejoin and function as a group.

posterior cord syndrome A condition associated with extension injuries with isolated injury to the dorsal column; presents as decreased sensation to light touch, proprioception, and vibration while leaving most other motor and sensory functions intact.

posterior spinous process Formed by the fusion of the posterior lamina, this is an attachment site for muscles and ligaments.

primary spinal cord injury Injury to the spinal cord that is a direct result of trauma, for example transection of the spinal cord from penetrating trauma or displacement of ligaments and bone fragments, resulting in compression of the spinal cord.

proprioception The ability to perceive the position and movement of one's body or limbs.

rotation-flexion injury A type of injury typically resulting from high acceleration forces; can result in a stable unilateral facet dislocation in the cervical spine.

secondary spinal cord injury Injury to the spinal cord, thought to be the result of multiple factors that result in a progression of inflammatory responses from primary spinal cord injury.

spinal cord The part of the central nervous system that extends downward from the brain through the foramen magnum and is protected by the spine.

spinal shock The temporary local neurologic condition that occurs immediately after spinal trauma; swelling and edema of the spinal cord begin immediately after injury, with severe pain and potential paralysis.

sympathetic nervous system Subdivision of the autonomic nervous system that governs the body's fight-or-flight reactions by inducing smooth muscle contraction or relaxation of the blood vessels and bronchioles.

transverse spinous process The junction of each pedicle and lamina on each side of a vertebra; these project laterally and posteriorly and form points of attachment for muscles and ligaments.

vertebral body Anterior weight-bearing structure in the spine made of cancellous bone and surrounded by a layer of hard, compact bone that provides support and stability.

vertical compression A type of injury typically resulting from a direct blow to the crown of the skull or rapid deceleration from a fall through the feet, legs, and pelvis, possibly causing a burst fracture or disk herniation.

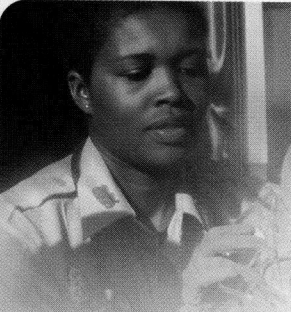

Assessment in Action

You and your partner respond to a patient who has fallen. On arrival, you find a 42-year-old man lying conscious and supine on the ground outside a home. A ladder is lying beside him, with paint spilled on the lawn. Neighbors say the patient fell at least 25' while painting the second-floor windows. On initial assessment, he complains of pain in his neck area and lower back. His respirations are 22 breaths/min; pulse, 58 beats/min; and blood pressure, 94/58 mm Hg. The skin is warm, red, and dry. He has no sensation below the navel. He cannot move his lower extremities and has no reflexes below the hip.

1. **After the initial assessment reveals adequate ABCs, you should:**
   A. inquire about history.
   B. notify the local hospital.
   C. apply manual in-line cervical spine immobilization.
   D. perform a neurologic exam.

2. **You apply oxygen and apply a long backboard and rigid cervical collar. Now you must decide whether to treat on scene or transport. Which factor should you base your decision on?**
   A. Distance of fall
   B. Patient preference
   C. Vital signs
   D. Mechanism of injury

3. **You are beginning the transport. Where should the patient be transported to?**
   A. The closest hospital
   B. A trauma center
   C. A local medical center
   D. None of the above

4. **What is the maximum scene time for this patient?**
   A. 5 minutes
   B. 10 minutes
   C. 15 minutes
   D. However long it takes to immobilize the patient safely

5. **Based on the vital signs and mechanism, what should you suspect is causing the hypotension?**
   A. Blood loss
   B. Head injury
   C. Neurogenic shock
   D. All of the above

6. **What should your treatment actions be?**
   A. Continue assessment and seek out other injuries.
   B. Determine the Glasgow Coma Scale score.
   C. Initiate IV therapy.
   D. All of the above

7. **Based on the level of sensation, what area of the spine may be injured?**
   A. C7
   B. L3
   C. T10
   D. S1

Challenging Questions

You respond to a motor vehicle crash. The vehicle struck a bridge abutment on the interstate, resulting in substantial damage to the car. The driver is unconscious and slumped over the steering wheel. He is breathing with difficulty. You suspect partial airway obstruction by his tongue. Smoke is coming from the car's engine compartment.

8. **What should you do?**

■ Points to Ponder

You respond to a call about a fall. On arrival, you find the patient at the foot of a staircase at the local community college. The patient reports that he slipped while running up the steps, and fell backward from the top to the bottom. The patient is conscious, alert, and oriented, complaining only of pain in his left leg. He has several bruises on the head, legs, and arms. No serious bleeding is noted, and the patient denies loss of consciousness. You immediately secure the cervical spine and begin a neurologic assessment. The patient's pupils are equal and reactive. He has good pulse, motor, and sensation in all extremities, and his reflexes are normal. You find no neurologic abnormalities.

Should you immobilize this patient?

Issues: Thorough Assessment, Proper Management of Spine Injuries.

Objectives

Cognitive

4-7.1 Describe the incidence, morbidity, and mortality of thoracic injuries in the trauma patient. (p 23.3)

4-7.2 Discuss the anatomy and physiology of the organs and structures related to thoracic injuries. (p 23.3)

4-7.3 Predict thoracic injuries based on mechanism of injury. (p 23.6)

4-7.4 Discuss the types of thoracic injuries. (p 23.7)

4-7.5 Discuss the pathophysiology of thoracic injuries. (p 23.6)

4-7.6 Discuss the assessment findings associated with thoracic injuries. (p 23.14)

4-7.7 Discuss the management of thoracic injuries. (p 23.16)

4-7.8 Identify the need for rapid intervention and transport of the patient with thoracic injuries. (p 23.17)

4-7.9 Discuss the pathophysiology of specific chest wall injuries, including:
a. Rib fracture
b. Flail segment
c. Sternal fracture (p 23.7, 23.8)

4-7.10 Discuss the assessment findings associated with chest wall injuries. (p 23.17)

4-7.11 Identify the need for rapid intervention and transport of the patient with chest wall injuries. (p 23.17)

4-7.12 Discuss the management of chest wall injuries. (p 23.17)

4-7.13 Discuss the pathophysiology of injury to the lung, including:
a. Simple pneumothorax
b. Open pneumothorax
c. Tension pneumothorax
d. Hemothorax
e. Hemopneumothorax
f. Pulmonary contusion (p 23.8–23.10)

4-7.14 Discuss the assessment findings associated with lung injuries. (p 23.18)

4-7.15 Discuss the management of lung injuries. (p 23.18)

4-7.16 Identify the need for rapid intervention and transport of the patient with lung injuries. (p 23.17)

4-7.17 Discuss the pathophysiology of myocardial injuries, including:
a. Pericardial tamponade
b. Myocardial contusion
c. Myocardial rupture (p 23.10, 23.11)

4-7.18 Discuss the assessment findings associated with myocardial injuries. (p 23.22)

4-7.19 Discuss the management of myocardial injuries. (p 23.22)

4-7.20 Identify the need for rapid intervention and transport of the patient with myocardial injuries. (p 23.23)

4-7.21 Discuss the pathophysiology of vascular injuries, including injuries to:
a. Aorta
b. Vena cava
c. Pulmonary arteries/veins (p 23.12)

4-7.22 Discuss the assessment findings associated with vascular injuries. (p 23.23)

4-7.23 Discuss the management of vascular injuries. (p 23.23)

4-7.24 Identify the need for rapid intervention and transport of the patient with vascular injuries. (p 23.23)

4-7.25 Discuss the pathophysiology of diaphragmatic injuries. (p 23.12)

4-7.26 Discuss the assessment findings associated with diaphragmatic injuries. (p 23.24)

4-7.27 Discuss the management of diaphragmatic injuries. (p 23.24)

4-7.28 Identify the need for rapid intervention and transport of the patient with diaphragmatic injuries. (p 23.24)

4-7.29 Discuss the pathophysiology of esophageal injuries. (p 23.13)

4-7.30 Discuss the assessment findings associated with esophageal injuries. (p 23.25)

4-7.31 Discuss the management of esophageal injuries. (p 23.25)

4-7.32 Identify the need for rapid intervention and transport of the patient with esophageal injuries. (p 23.25)

4-7.33 Discuss the pathophysiology of tracheo-bronchial injuries. (p 23.13)

4-7.34 Discuss the assessment findings associated with tracheo-bronchial injuries. (p 23.25)

4-7.35 Discuss the management of tracheo-bronchial injuries. (p 23.25)

4-7.36 Identify the need for rapid intervention and transport of the patient with tracheo-bronchial injuries. (p 23.17)

4-7.37 Discuss the pathophysiology of traumatic asphyxia. (p 23.13)

4-7.38 Discuss the assessment findings associated with traumatic asphyxia. (p 23.25)

4-7.39 Discuss the management of traumatic asphyxia. (p 23.25)

4-7.40 Identify the need for rapid intervention and transport of the patient with traumatic asphyxia. (p 23.25)

4-7.41 Integrate the pathophysiological principles to the assessment of a patient with thoracic injury. (p 23.14)

4-7.42 Differentiate between thoracic injuries based on the assessment and history. (p 23.16)

4-7.43 Formulate a field impression based on the assessment findings. (p 23.14)

4-7.44 Develop a patient management plan based on the field impression. (p 23.16)

Affective

4-7.45 Advocate the use of a thorough assessment to determine a differential diagnosis and treatment plan for thoracic trauma. (p 23.14)

4-7.46 Advocate the use of a thorough scene survey to determine the forces involved in thoracic trauma. (p 23.14)

4-7.47 Value the implications of failing to properly diagnose thoracic trauma. (p 23.14)

4-7.48 Value the implications of failing to initiate timely interventions to patients with thoracic trauma. (p 23.17)

Psychomotor

4-7.49 Demonstrate a clinical assessment for a patient with suspected thoracic trauma. (p 23.14)

4-7.50 Demonstrate the following techniques of management for thoracic injuries:
a. Needle decompression
b. Fracture stabilization
c. Elective intubation
d. ECG monitoring
e. Oxygenation and ventilation (p 23.6–23.18, 23.20, 23.22)

Introduction

Thoracic (chest) trauma is not a disease of modern society. For as long as humans have been capable of falling or injuring one another, damage to the thoracic cavity has been a significant concern in the management of the trauma patient Figure 23-1 ▾ . As more rapid forms of transportation and more lethal weapons continue to evolve, the incidence and severity of thoracic trauma is not likely to diminish, nor is the need for its rapid assessment and treatment.

Today, thoracic trauma accounts for a significant number of serious injuries and fatalities each year. According to the Centers for Disease Control and Prevention (CDC), thoracic trauma causes more than 700,000 emergency department visits and more than 18,000 deaths in the United States annually.

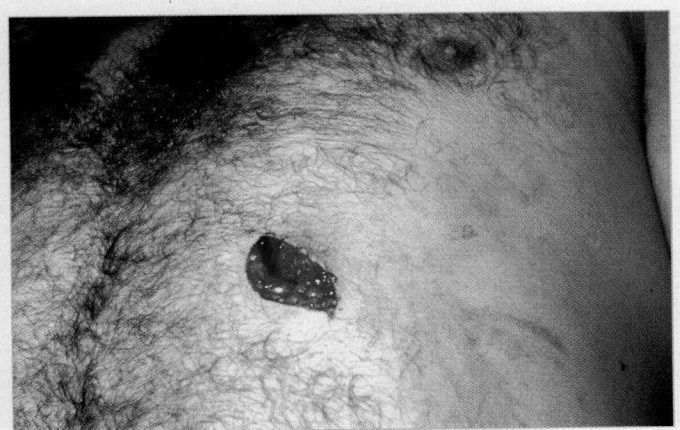

Figure 23-1 Thoracic trauma is a significant concern in the management of the trauma patient.

Only head trauma and traumatic brain injuries account for more deaths among trauma victims. An estimated one in four trauma deaths is directly due to thoracic injuries, and thoracic trauma is a contributing factor in another 25% of trauma patients who die of their injuries.

Given the specific organs that are housed within the thoracic cavity, it is not surprising that these injuries can be so deadly. In addition, the mechanism producing these injuries often involves a great deal of force transmitted to the body, with motor vehicle crashes accounting for seven of every ten patients with blunt thoracic trauma.

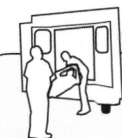

In the Field

Thoracic injuries, whether severe or seemingly minor, often give rise to elusive findings that are overshadowed by associated injuries.

Anatomy

The thorax consists of a bony cage overlying some of the most vital organs in the human body. The dimensions of the thorax are defined posteriorly by the thoracic vertebrae and ribs, inferiorly by the diaphragm, anteriorly and laterally by the ribs, and superiorly by the thoracic inlet Figure 23-2 ▸ .

The dimensions of this area of the body are of great importance in the physical assessment of the patient. Although the thoracic cavity extends to the 12th rib posteriorly, the diaphragm inserts into the anterior thoracic cage just below the fourth or fifth rib. With the movement of the diaphragm during respiration, the size and dimensions of the thoracic cavity

You are the Provider Part 1

While you are working as a paramedic for a local aeromedical service, your helicopter is requested by a nearby township to assist with a motor vehicle crash. After lifting off from the helipad, you are informed that you are en route to a head-on collision on a major highway. Two people have already been pronounced dead at the scene.

You arrive to find an 18-year-old male passenger who was partially ejected from the vehicle; he was not wearing a seatbelt. Fire department personnel have extricated the patient from the vehicle, applied full spinal precautions, and are currently assisting his ventilations with a bag-mask device.

Initial Assessment	Recording Time: 0 Minutes
Appearance	Secured to a long backboard
Level of consciousness	U (Unresponsive)
Airway	Patent with an oropharyngeal airway inserted
Breathing	Assisted ventilations with 100% supplemental oxygen
Circulation	Pale skin, with a fast, regular radial pulse

1. What will your initial priorities be when assessing and managing this patient?
2. Given the mechanism of injury for an unrestrained passenger in a car and this patient's vital signs, what kinds of injuries should you think about during your assessment?

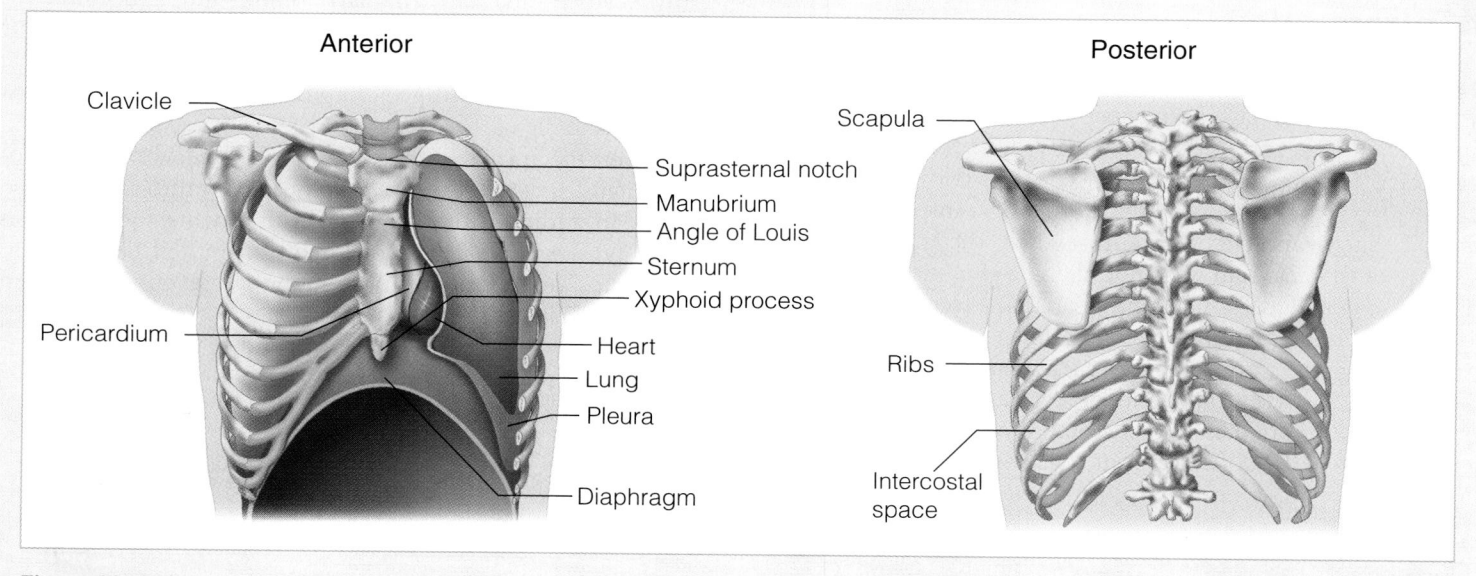

Figure 23-2 The thorax, front and back views.

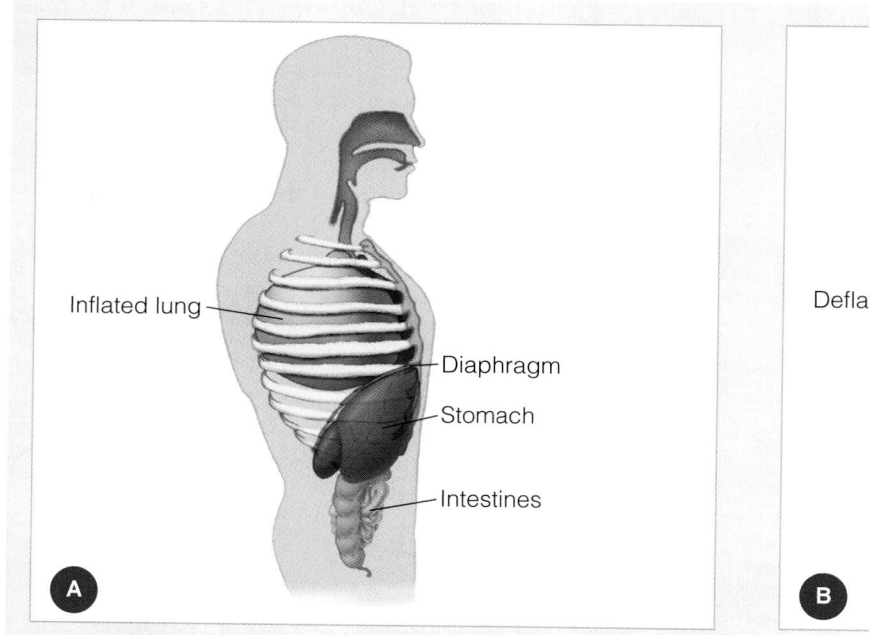

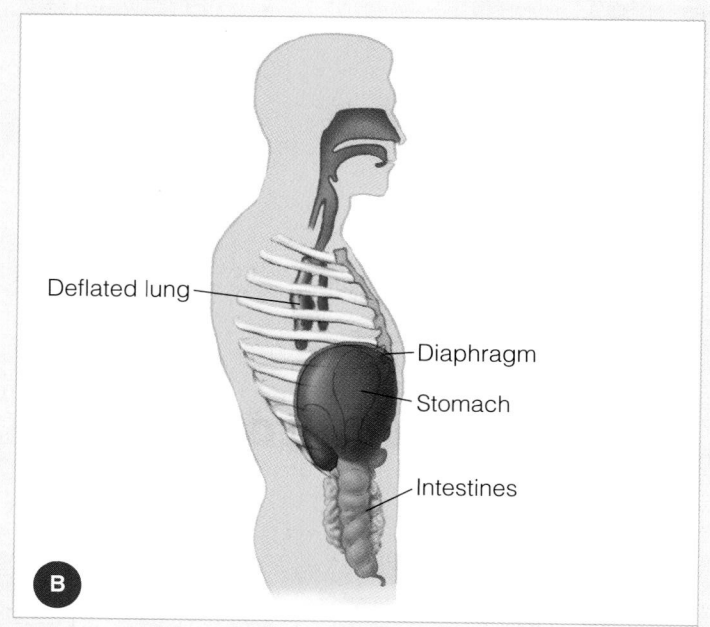

Figure 23-3 The anatomy of the thoracic cavity during inspiration (**A**) and expiration (**B**).

will vary (**Figure 23-3** ▲), which could in turn affect the organs or cavities (thoracic versus abdominal) in case of blunt or penetrating injury.

The bony structures of the thorax include the sternum, clavicle, scapula, thoracic vertebrae, and 12 pairs of ribs. The sternum consists of three separate portions: the superior manubrium, the central sternal body, and the inferior xyphoid process. The space superior to the manubrium is termed the suprasternal notch; the junction of the manubrium and sternal body is referred to as the angle of Louis.

The clavicle is an elongated, S-shaped bone that connects to the manubrium medially and overlies the first rib as it proceeds laterally toward the shoulder. Beneath the clavicle lies the subclavian artery and vein. Laterally, the clavicle connects to the acromion process of the scapula, the triangular bone that overlies the posterior aspect of the upper thoracic cage.

Each of the 12 matched pairs of ribs attach posteriorly to the 12 thoracic vertebrae. Anteriorly, the first seven pairs of ribs attach directly to the sternum via the costal cartilage. The costal cartilage then continues inferiorly from the seventh ribs and provides an indirect connection between the anterior portions of the eighth, ninth, and tenth ribs and the sternum. The eleventh and twelfth ribs have no anterior connection and, therefore, are known as the "floating ribs."

Between each rib lies an intercostal space. These spaces are numbered according to the rib superior to the space (ie, the space between the second and third ribs is the second intercostal space). These spaces house the intercostal muscles and the neurovascular bundle, which consists of an artery, vein, and nerve.

The central region of the thorax is the mediastinum, which contains the heart, great vessels, esophagus, lymphatic channels, trachea, mainstem bronchi, and paired vagus and phrenic nerves. The heart resides within a tough fibrous sac called the pericardium. Much like the pleura, the pericardium has two surfaces—the inner visceral layer, which adheres to the heart and forms the epicardium, and the outer parietal layer, which comprises the sac itself. The pericardium that covers the inferior aspect of the heart is directly attached to the diaphragm. The heart is positioned so that the most anterior portion is the right ventricle, which has relatively thin chamber walls. The pressure within the right ventricle is approximately one fourth of the pressure within the left ventricle. Most of the heart is protected anteriorly by the sternum. With each beat, the apex of the heart can be felt in the fifth intercostal space along the midclavicular line, a phenomenon known as cardiac impulse. The average cardiac output for an adult (heart rate times the stroke volume) is $70 \times 70 = 4,900$ mL/min, though it varies depending on the patient's size.

The aorta is the largest artery in the body. As it exits the left ventricle, it ascends toward the right shoulder before turning to the left and proceeding inferiorly toward the abdomen. This artery has three points of attachment—the anulus at its origin from the aortic valve, the ligamentum arteriosum, and the aortic hiatus. These attachments represent sites of potential injury when the vessel is subject to significant shearing forces, such as those seen during sudden deceleration mechanisms.

The lungs occupy most of the space within the thoracic cavity. Like the pericardium, the lungs are lined with a dual layer of connective tissue known as the pleura. The parietal pleura lines the interior of each side of the thoracic cavity. The visceral pleura lines the exterior of each lung.

A small amount of viscous fluid separates the two layers of pleura. This fluid allows the two layers of connective tissue to move against each other without friction or pain. It creates a surface tension that holds the layers together, thereby keeping the lung from collapsing away from the thoracic cage on exhalation. If this space becomes filled with air, blood, or other fluids, the surface tension is lost and the lung collapses.

The diaphragm, the primary muscle of breathing, forms a barrier between the thoracic and abdominal cavities. It works in conjunction with the intercostal muscles to increase the size of the thoracic cavity during inspiration, creating the negative pressure that pulls air in via the trachea. In times of distress, this breathing effort can be aided by other accessory muscles of the thoracic cavity, including the trapezius, latissmus dorsi, rhomboids, pectoralis, and sternocleidomastoid Figure 23-4 ▶.

You are the Provider Part 2

As you assume patient care, you begin by reassessing the patient's airway. As the bag-mask ventilations continue, you find the patient has a patent airway. His mental status remains unresponsive with a Glasgow Coma Scale score of 5 and some decorticate posturing. You and your partner decide to manage the patient's airway with endotracheal intubation, while still maintaining manual in-line immobilization of the cervical spine.

The patient is intubated without difficulty, the placement of the endotracheal tube is confirmed by multiple methods, and assisted ventilation is continued. You prepare for transport, as your partner starts an IV to administer a fluid bolus of lactated Ringer's solution. After moving the patient, you reassess his ventilation and note that his breath sounds are absent on the right side. His neck reveals jugular vein distention, and you're not really sure if the trachea is deviated to the left side.

Vital Signs	Recording Time: 10 Minutes
Level of consciousness	Unresponsive, with a Glasgow Coma Scale score of 5
Pulse	Radial pulse, 128 beats/min
Blood pressure	70/38 mm Hg
Respirations	Intubated; ventilating with 100% supplemental oxygen
Skin	Cool, pale, and diaphoretic
Sao$_2$	88% on room air

3. Why does the patient remain hypoxic despite confirmed airway patency and the effective delivery of high-concentration oxygen?
4. Do his vital signs and physical examination suggest any threats to his breathing that may be correctable?

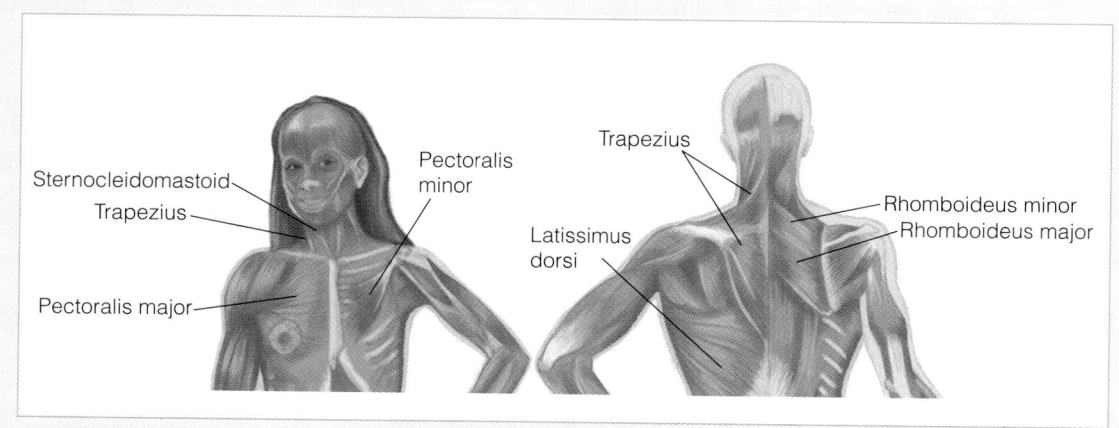

Figure 23-4 The muscles of the thoracic cavity include the trapezius, latissimus dorsi, rhomboid, pectoralis, and sternocleidomastoid muscles.

Physiology

The primary physiologic functions of the thorax and its contents are to maintain oxygenation and ventilation and (via the heart) to maintain circulation.

The process of breathing includes both the delivery of oxygen to the body and the elimination of carbon dioxide from the body. While these processes are often accomplished simultaneously, they are, in fact, different aspects of the breathing process.

First, however, the brain must stimulate the person to breathe. This stimulation occurs via chemoreceptors that are located in the carotid sinus and aortic arch. These receptors are in essence "little chemists" that analyze the arterial blood. When the level of carbon dioxide gets too high, the receptors send a message to the brain, which responds by increasing the respiratory rate in an effort to "blow off the CO_2." Some patients with end-stage chronic obstructive pulmonary disease (COPD) may employ a secondary mechanism called hypoxic drive for this function because they retain excess CO_2 on a chronic basis.

As the diaphragm contracts downward, the intercostal and accessory muscles pull the chest wall out and away from the center of the body. The resulting negative pressure within the thoracic cavity draws air in through the mouth and nose, down the trachea, passing through smaller and smaller bronchioles until finally it reaches the alveolar spaces. The new air both mixes with and replaces the air contained within the alveoli.

While respiration is occurring, blood is being delivered via the pulmonary circulation to the capillaries that lie adjacent to the alveoli. This blood has returned to the heart after traversing the body, having delivered its oxygen to the cells and removed the cellular waste products such as CO_2. As a result, the blood entering the capillaries adjacent to the alveoli has a low O_2 concentration and a high CO_2 concentration.

The process of oxygenation includes the delivery of oxygen from the air to the blood, where it is carried to cells and tissues throughout the body. Because the air entering the alveoli contains a higher concentration of O_2 (ranging from 21% in room air to as much as 100% in a nonrebreathing mask or bag mask under ideal circumstances) than the blood in the nearby capillaries, the oxygen will follow its concentration gradient and enter the blood. Most of the oxygen binds to hemoglobin within the red blood cells, and the oxygen returns to the heart with the blood, where it is then pumped throughout the body.

Ventilation is the process by which CO_2 is removed from the body. The air in our environment contains very little CO_2 (0.033%). As a result, when air enters the alveoli, it contains very little CO_2 compared to the blood in the nearby capillaries. The CO_2 diffuses down its concentration gradient, leaving the blood and entering the air within the alveoli.

As the diaphragm and the chest wall relax, positive pressure is created within the thorax. The air from which oxygen has been absorbed and into which carbon dioxide has been diffused is then exhaled. With each subsequent respiration (inhalation and exhalation), the process is repeated.

Proper functioning of the heart is essential to the delivery of blood to the body's tissues. As blood returns from the body via the inferior and superior vena cavae, it's pumped from the right side of the heart to the lungs, where the processes of oxygenation and ventilation take place. As oxygenated blood returns from the lungs, it enters the left side of the heart and is then pumped out to the body.

The ability to pump blood depends on having a functional pump (the heart), an adequate volume of blood to be pumped, and a lack of resistance to the pumping mechanism (afterload)—properties that are collectively known as cardiac output. Cardiac output is the volume of blood delivered to the body in 1 minute. The volume is identified by counting the number of times the heart beats in a minute (heart rate) and determining the amount of blood delivered to the body with each beat (stroke volume). Thus cardiac output equals the heart rate (beats/min) multiplied by the stroke volume (milliliters of blood per beat). Any injury that limits the heart's pumping ability, the delivery of blood to the heart, the blood's ability to leave the heart, or the heart rate will affect cardiac output.

Pathophysiology of Thoracic Injuries

Traumatic injury to the thoracic cavity presents the possibility of compromise of ventilation, oxygenation, or circulation. Accordingly, the assessment of the thoracic cavity becomes an integral part of the overall assessment of the patient's ABCs, the initial assessment, and the continuing assessment. These injuries, if missed or inappropriately treated, could contribute significantly to the patient's morbidity or even cause death.

The patient's ventilation may be affected by both mechanical and functional impairments. Air or blood entering the pleural space may result in the loss of airspace in which ventilation normally occurs. Similarly, injuries to the chest wall or diaphragm may limit the movement of the thorax, thereby constraining the patient's ability to ventilate. Finally, ventilation may be affected simply by a painful injury that limits the patient's ability or willingness to fully ventilate his or her lung tissue with each breath.

Within the lung itself, loss of alveolar space may result in the inability to exchange gases such as oxygen, ultimately leading to clinical hypoxemia. This problem may be caused by alveolar collapse (atelectasis) due to incomplete chest wall and lung expansion, hemorrhage into the lung tissue itself, or airway obstruction.

Within the cardiovascular structures of the thoracic cavity, acute blood loss from vascular injury may result in systemic hypoperfusion. In such a case, localized blood loss within the pericardium may result in immediate cardiovascular collapse.

Chest Wall Injuries
Flail Chest

Flail chest Figure 23-5 , a major injury to the chest wall, may result from a variety of blunt force mechanisms such as falls, motor vehicle crashes, assaults, and even birth trauma. It occurs in as many as 20% of admitted trauma patients. The associated mortality rates range from 50% in some series to even higher rates in patients older than age 60. Mortality rates are directly related to the underlying and associated injuries. Patients are more likely to suffer a mortal injury if they are elderly, have seven or more rib fractures or three or more associated injuries, present with shock, or have associated head trauma.

A flail segment is defined as two or more adjacent ribs that are fractured in two or more places. The segment between those two fracture sites becomes separated from the surrounding chest wall, leaving it free to succumb to the underlying pressures—hence the name "free-floating segment." Both the location and the size of the segment can affect the degree to which the flail segment impairs chest wall motion and subsequent air movement. In a flail sternum (the most extreme case), the sternum is completely separated from the ribs because of fractures or ruptured costal cartilage. This type of injury results in mechanical dysfunction of both sides of the chest and more severe respiratory impairment.

Once a flail segment has occurred, the underlying physiologic pressures cause paradoxical movement of the segment when compared to the rest of the chest wall. Expansion of the chest wall on inspiration results in negative pressure within the thoracic cavity, which in turn draws the flail segment in toward the center of the chest. As the chest relaxes or is actively contracted (depending on the degree of dyspnea), the resulting positive pressure forces air from the lungs and also forces the flail segment out away from the thoracic cavity. Because of these movements, the lung tissue beneath the flail segment is not adequately ventilated. Clearly, a flail segment can quickly become life-threatening, which explains why it is managed in the initial assessment of the patient. Typical management involves pressing down on the segment as the patient exhales so that the free-floating segment conforms with the rest of the chest wall. Some providers still use a bulky dressing to stabilize the segment; 3″ adhesive tape can also be used as a functional binder to tape the ribs so that they move in tandem.

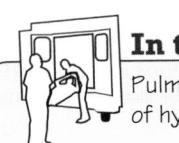
In the Field
Pulmonary contusion is the main cause of hypoxemia seen with flail chest injuries.

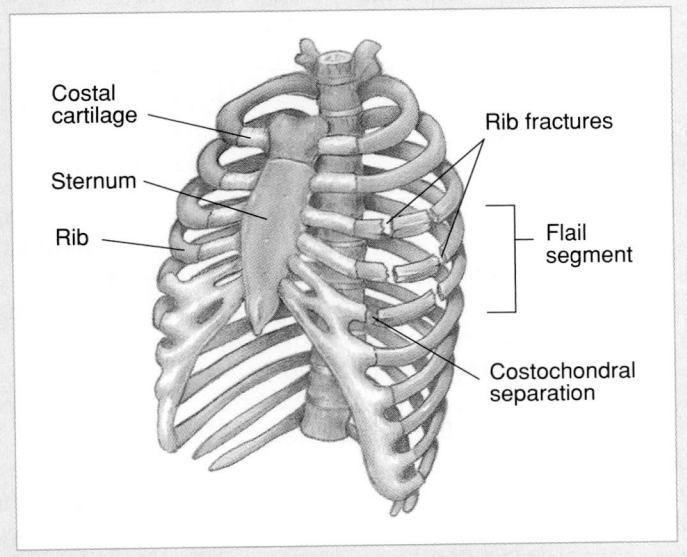
Figure 23-5 In flail chest injuries, two or more adjacent ribs are fractured in two or more places. A flail segment will move paradoxically when the patient breathes.

The blunt force trauma that causes the flail segment can also produce a pulmonary contusion Figure 23-6 , an injury to the underlying lung tissue that inhibits the normal diffusion of oxygen and carbon dioxide. Three physics principles contribute to the formation of a pulmonary contusion: the Spalding effect, inertial effects, and implosion. With the Spalding effect, the pressure waves generated by either penetrating or blunt trauma disrupt the capillary-alveolar membrane, resulting in hemorrhage. Inertial effects are created by tissue density differences between the alveoli and the larger bronchioles. These tissues accelerate and decelerate at different rates, causing them to tear and hemorrhage. Finally, the positive pressure created by the trauma compresses the gases within the lung, which quickly re-expand.

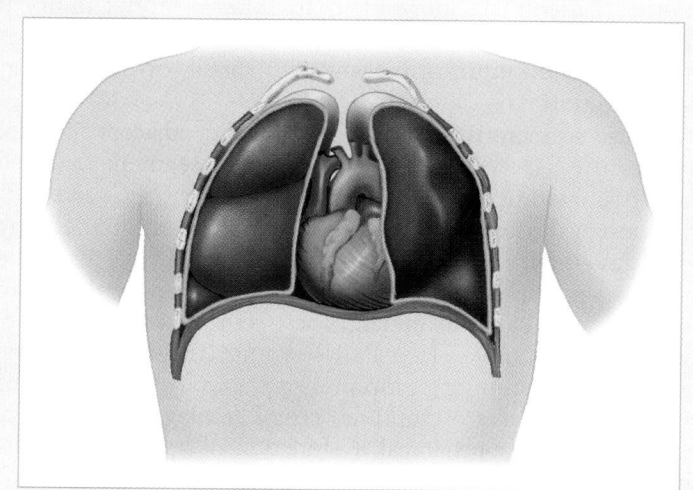

Figure 23-6 Pulmonary contusion.

If this re-expansion is too great, the lung tissue will suffer an implosion injury.

If the blunt force that fractures the ribs drives those bone fragments farther into the body, a pneumothorax or hemothorax may result. In addition, the pain associated with the fractures may prevent the patient from taking in adequate tidal volume because he or she is consciously trying to minimize the movement of that segment of the chest. This "self-splinting" action uses the intercostal muscles and purposefully limited chest wall movement to minimize pain. Unfortunately, it further limits the pulmonary system's ability to compensate for the injury.

Rib Fractures

Rib fractures—the most common thoracic injuries—are seen in more than half of all thoracic trauma patients. Even when the patient experiences no underlying or associated injury, the pain produced by the broken ribs can result in significant morbidity as it contributes to inadequate ventilation, self-splinting, atelectasis, and the possibility of infection (pneumonia) due to inadequate respiration.

When you are examining the chest of a patient who has sustained either blunt or penetrating injury, palpate for subcutaneous emphysema (air under the skin), which can indicate a potential pneumothorax. It has been described as a "snap, crackle, pop" sensation under the skin or a feeling like popping the plastic bubbles in the wrap used to protect fragile items during shipping.

Special Considerations

The incidence of rib fractures varies with age. The ribs of children are pliable, so they may injure underlying structures without being fractured. In older patients, the frail nature of the bones makes the ribs more likely to fracture.

In blunt trauma, the force applied to the thoracic cage results in a fracture of the rib in one of three areas: the point of impact, the edge of the object, or the posterior angle of the rib (weak point). Because they are less well protected by other bony and muscular structures, ribs 4 through 9 are the most commonly fractured.

The ribs are part of a ring that helps to expand and contract the thoracic cavity. Because a fracture of one or more ribs destroys the integrity of this ring, the patient's ability to adequately ventilate is diminished. Just as importantly, the patient will attempt to limit the pain caused by these injuries by using shallow breathing. This tendency results in atelectasis and may lead to hypoxia or pneumonia.

The presence of rib fractures is also suspicious for other associated injuries. When the clinical examination suggests a fracture of ribs 4 through 9, you should be concerned about associated aortic injury, tracheobronchial injury, pneumothorax, vascular injury, or other more serious injuries. Similarly, fractures of the lower ribs (9 through 11) should raise your concern for an associated intra-abdominal injury.

Sternal Fractures

Approximately one in 20 patients with blunt thoracic trauma will suffer a sternal fracture. Although this injury is of little consequence by itself, it is associated with other injuries that cause more than one fourth of patients with this fracture to die. Specifically, findings of myocardial contusions, flail sternum, pulmonary contusions, head injuries, intra-abdominal injuries, and myocardial rupture increase the likelihood of death.

In the Field

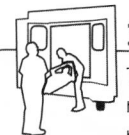

The sternum is a very thick bone. If the thorax receives enough force to fracture the sternum, you must assume that the same force was transmitted to the heart, great vessels, lungs, and diaphragm.

Lung Injuries
Simple Pneumothorax

Small pneumothoraces that are not under tension are a frequent occurrence in the blunt trauma patient, occurring in almost half of patients with thoracic trauma. Patients with penetrating trauma to the chest almost always have a pneumothorax—that is, the accumulation of air or gas in the pleural cavity.

Injuries may result in pneumothoraces either by direct injury to the lung (ie, rib fracture, gunshot, stabbing) or through barotrauma. In the latter case, pressure (eg, from the steering wheel during a motor vehicle collision) is applied to the chest at a time when the patient has inhaled and closed the glottis in anticipation of the trauma and/or pain. This increased pressure is translated to the intrathoracic cavity, where it results in rupture of the lung. In both direct injury and barotrauma, air is allowed to escape into the pleural space, causing a pneumothorax Figure 23-7 ▶.

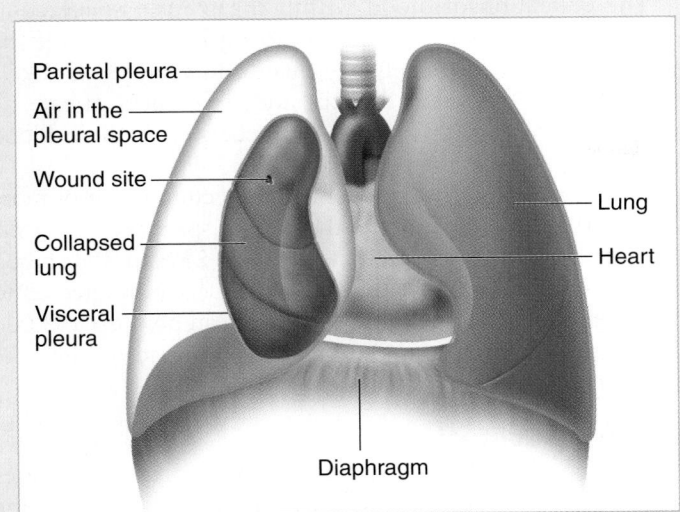

Figure 23-7 Pneumothorax occurs when air leaks into the space between the pleural surfaces from an opening in the chest or the surface of the lung. The lung collapses as air fills the pleural space.

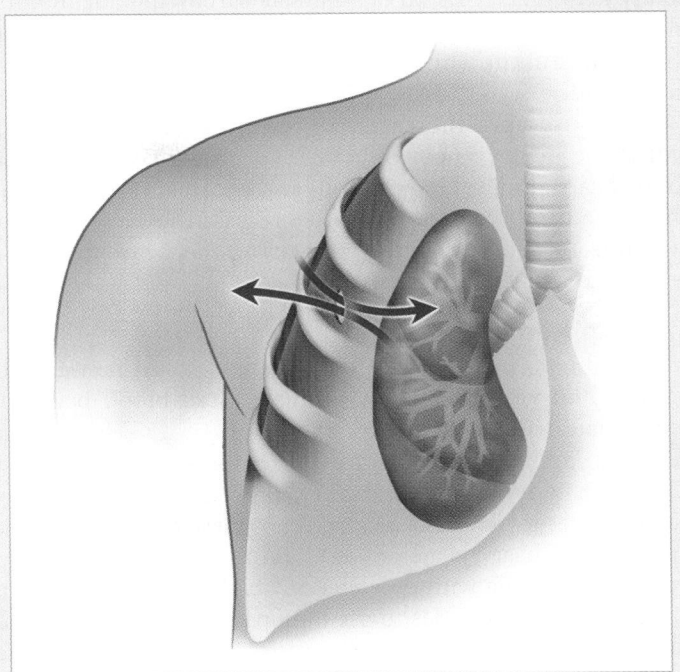

Figure 23-8 With a sucking chest wound, air passes from the outside into the pleural space and back out with each breath, creating a sucking sound. The size of the defect does not need to be large to compromise ventilation.

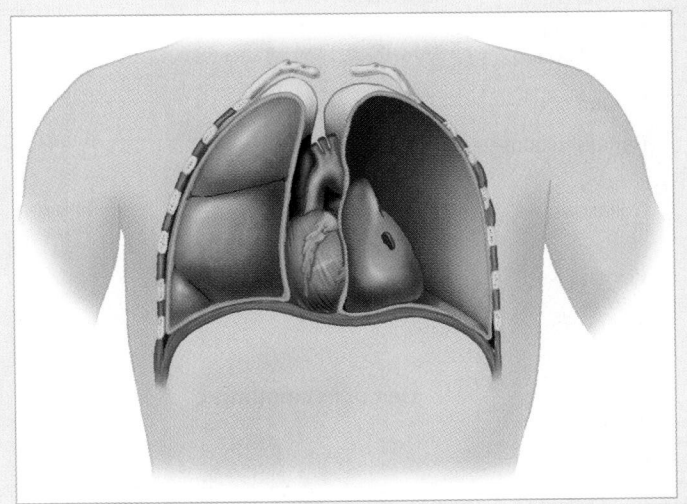

Figure 23-9 In a tension pneumothorax, air accumulates in the pleural space, eventually causing compression of the heart and great vessels.

Open Pneumothorax

An open pneumothorax occurs when a defect in the chest wall allows air to enter the thoracic space. It results from penetrating chest trauma—for example, gunshot/knife wounds or other impaled objects. The penetrating injury creates a link between the external environment and the pleural space. With each inspiration, the negative pressure created within the thoracic cavity draws more air into the pleural space, resulting in a pneumothorax. As the pneumothorax increases in size, the lung on the involved side loses its ability to expand. Also, if the "hole" is larger than the glottic opening, the air is more likely to enter the chest wall rather than entering via the trachea. As a consequence, the respiratory effort moves air in through the chest wound rather than through the lung, creating the "sucking chest wound" **Figure 23-8 ▸** .

The collapse of the involved lung creates a mismatch between ventilation and perfusion. If you assume that the pulmonary vasculature on the involved side remains intact, the heart will continue to perfuse the involved lung while the pneumothorax prevents adequate ventilation. The result is an inability to deliver oxygen to the involved lung (hypoxia) and an inability to eliminate carbon dioxide (hypercarbia).

Tension Pneumothorax

A tension pneumothorax **Figure 23-9 ▸** is a life-threatening condition that results from continued air accumulation within the intrapleural space. Air may enter the pleural space from an open thoracic injury, an injury to the lung parenchyma due to blunt trauma (the most common cause of tension pneumothorax), barotrauma due to positive-pressure ventilation, or tracheobronchial injuries due to shearing forces. Although the exact incidence of this injury is unknown, it has been estimated that 10% to 30% of patients transported to level 1 regional trauma centers receive emergent treatment for this condition.

An injury to the lung can cause a one-way valve to develop, allowing air to move into the pleural space but not to exit from it. As it continues to accumulate, the air exerts increasing pressure against the surrounding tissues. This growing pressure compresses the involved lung, diminishing its ability to oxygenate blood or eliminate carbon dioxide from the blood. Eventually, the lung will both collapse and push toward the mediastinum, shifting the mediastinum away from the injured side.

This pressure increase may even exceed the pressure within the major venous structures, decreasing venous return to the heart, diminishing preload, and eventually resulting in a shock state. As venous return decreases, the patient's body attempts to compensate by increasing the heart rate in an attempt to maintain cardiac output.

Massive Hemothorax

A hemothorax occurs when the potential space between the parietal and visceral pleura is violated and blood begins to accumulate within this space (Figure 23-10 ▾). Hemothorax occurs in approximately 25% of patients with chest trauma. Although it is most commonly caused by tears of lung parenchyma, it may also result from penetrating wounds that puncture the heart or major vessels within the mediastinum or from blunt trauma with deceleration shearing of major vessels. Rib fractures and injuries to the lung parenchyma are the most common sources of injury in the case of a hemothorax. Other causes include injury to the liver, spleen, aorta, intercostal arteries (which can lose up to 50 mL of blood per minute), and other intrathoracic vessels.

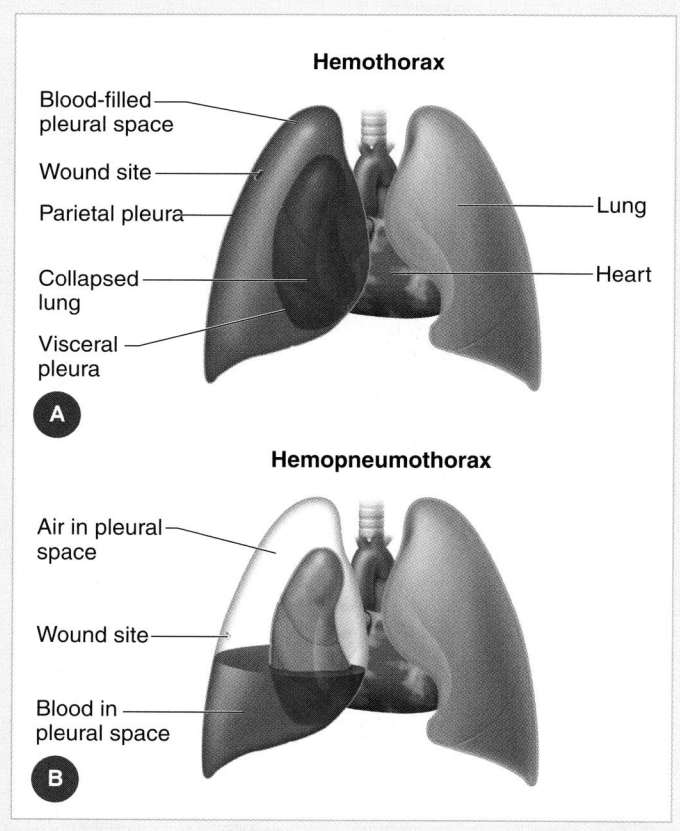

Hemothorax

- Blood-filled pleural space
- Wound site
- Parietal pleura
- Collapsed lung
- Visceral pleura
- Lung
- Heart

A

Hemopneumothorax

- Air in pleural space
- Wound site
- Blood in pleural space

B

Figure 23-10 **A.** A hemothorax is a collection of blood in the pleural space produced by bleeding within the chest. **B.** In a hemopneumothorax, both blood and air are present.

The collection of blood within the pleural space compresses and displaces the surrounding lung, limiting the patient's ability to adequately oxygenate and ventilate. Unlike a pneumothorax, this injury has the added potential of causing hypovolemia. A hemopneumothorax occurs when both blood and air are present in the pleural space.

A massive hemothorax is defined as accumulation of more than 1,500 mL of blood within the pleural space. For the average adult, this amount represents a nearly 25% to 30% blood volume loss, meaning that the patient will have progressed to decompensated shock. Because each lung can hold up to 3,000 mL, it is possible for a patient to completely bleed out into the thoracic cavity.

Pulmonary Contusion

The position of the lungs just beneath the thoracic cage places them at increased risk for injury with thoracic trauma. As the lung tissue is compressed against the chest wall by force or by the positive pressure within the chest during a thoracic injury, alveolar and capillary damage results. It leads immediately to a loss of fluid and blood into the involved tissues, followed by white blood cell migration into the area, and, eventually, local tissue edema.

This local tissue injury and edema dilute the local surfactant in the alveoli, diminishing their compliance and causing alveolar collapse (atelectasis). The edema also reduces the delivery of oxygen across the capillary-alveolar interface, resulting in hypoxia. The hypoxia then worsens the situation by thickening the mucus produced, which may in turn lead to bronchiolar obstruction and further atelectasis.

If the contusion is large, the body compensates by vasoconstricting pulmonary blood flow and increasing cardiac output. This is an attempt to shunt blood from the injured area and increase its delivery to pulmonary tissue that may be able to oxygenate the blood. This pulmonary shunting decreases the functional reserve capacity and leads to mixed venous blood being returned to the heart, further worsening the hypoxemia.

Myocardial Injuries

Pericardial Tamponade

Pericardial tamponade (Figure 23-11 ▸) is defined as excessive fluid in the pericardial sac, causing compression of the heart and decreased cardiac output. The hemodynamic effects of cardiac tamponade are determined by the size of the perforation in the pericardium, the rate of hemorrhage from the cardiac wound, and the chamber of the heart involved. The injury may be caused by a blunt or (more commonly) penetrating mechanism. Very few patients with blunt thoracic trauma experience pericardial tamponade, whereas almost all patients with cardiac stab wounds develop this condition.

The mortality associated with tamponade varies, with high-velocity injuries (gunshots) carrying a higher risk of death than low-velocity injuries (stabbings). If pericardial tamponade is the only injury, mortality is greatly reduced.

Pericardial tamponade can occur in both medical and trauma patients. In the medical setting, inflammatory processes (ie, pericarditis, uremia, myocardial infarction) lead to the slow collection of fluid within the pericardial sac and the gradual distention of the parietal pericardium. Through this process, 1,000 to 1,500 mL of fluid may accumulate in the pericardial sac. Conversely, the bleeding in the trauma patient is rapid, with blood loss from the coronary vasculature or the myocardium itself quickly collecting between the visceral and parietal pericardium. Because the parietal pericardium is not able to stretch in such a case, as little as 50 mL of blood may lead to pericardial tamponade.

As the pericardium fills, the continued bleeding increases the pressure within the pericardium. The more pliable structures within the pericardium—namely, the atria and the vena cavae—become compressed, which drastically reduces the preload being delivered to the heart and thereby diminishes stroke volume. The heart initially attempts to compensate for this reduction in preload by increasing the heart rate. This attempt to maintain cardiac output is only temporary, as the continued bleeding will further restrict preload and diastolic filling. The pressure within the pericardial sac will also reduce the perfusion in the myocardium, resulting in global myocardial dysfunction. The combination of these two processes leads to the development of hypotension.

Myocardial Contusion

The heart's anterior and unprotected position just behind the sternum puts it in a potentially precarious position during a blunt force mechanism. At speeds of greater than 20 to 35 miles per hour, the sudden deceleration of the chest wall may cause the heart to move forward until it collides with the posterior aspect of the sternum, leading to the blunt cardiac injury known as myocardial contusion. This type of injury is characterized by local tissue contusion and hemorrhage, edema, and cellular damage within the involved myocardium. Direct damage to the epicardial vessels (coronary arteries and veins) may compromise the blood flow to the heart. Damage to the myocardium tissue at a cellular level may result in ectopic activity, re-entry pathways, and dysrhythmias.

Complications of myocardial contusions are similar to the complications seen in patients who experience a myocardial infarction. Dysrhythmias may occur (although they are uncommon in children) due to cellular membrane injury and changes in the myocardial action potential. Structural changes may include the development of a ventricular septal defect, myocardial rupture or aneurysm formation, and coronary artery occlusion.

Myocardial Rupture

Myocardial rupture is an acute perforation of the ventricles, atria, intraventricular septum, intra-atrial septum, chordae, papillary muscles, or valves. The application of severe blunt force to the chest compresses the heart between the sternum and the vertebrae, which can rupture the myocardium. In penetrating trauma, a foreign object or bony fragment may be propelled into the heart, resulting in a laceration of the myocardial wall. Whether it occurs from a penetrating injury or blunt trauma, a ruptured myocardium is a life-threatening condition that accounts for 15% of fatal chest injuries.

Commotio Cordis

If the thorax receives a direct blow during the critical portion of the heart's repolarization period, the result may be immediate cardiac arrest. This phenomenon, termed commotio cordis, has been documented to have occurred after patients were struck with softballs, baseballs, bats, snowballs, fists, and

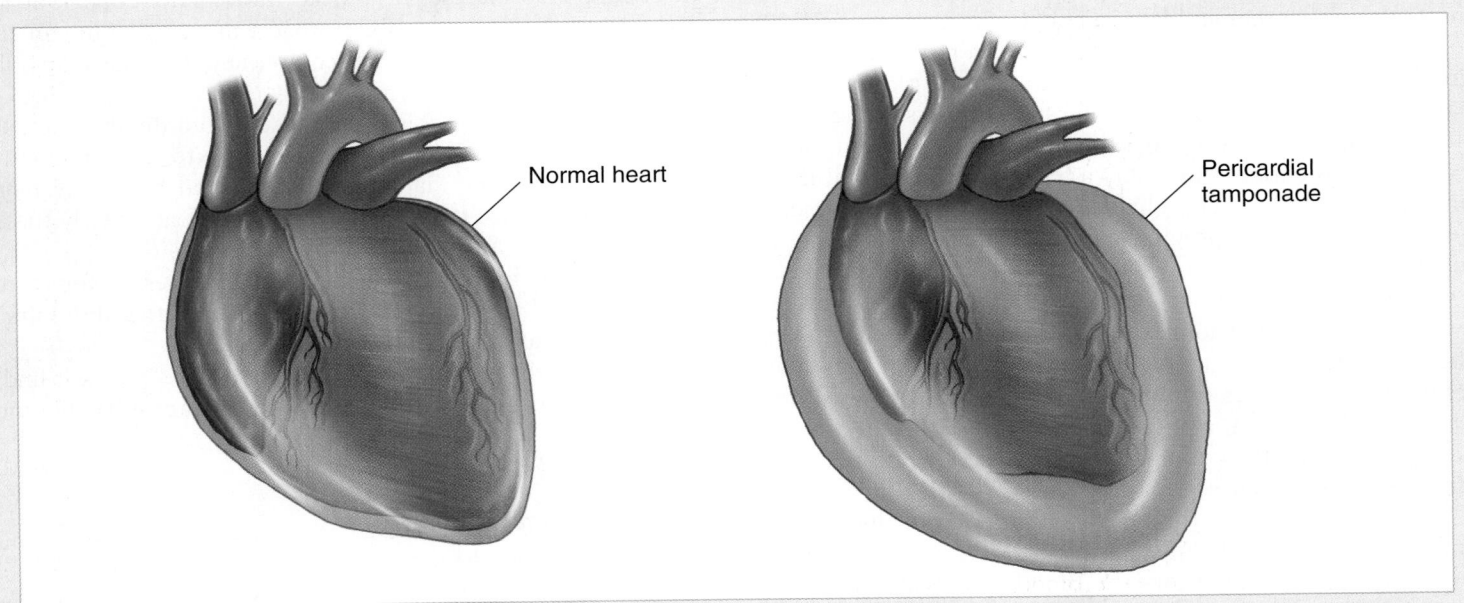

Figure 23-11 Pericardial tamponade is a potentially fatal condition in which fluid builds up within the pericardial sac, compressing the heart's chambers and dramatically impairing its ability to pump blood.

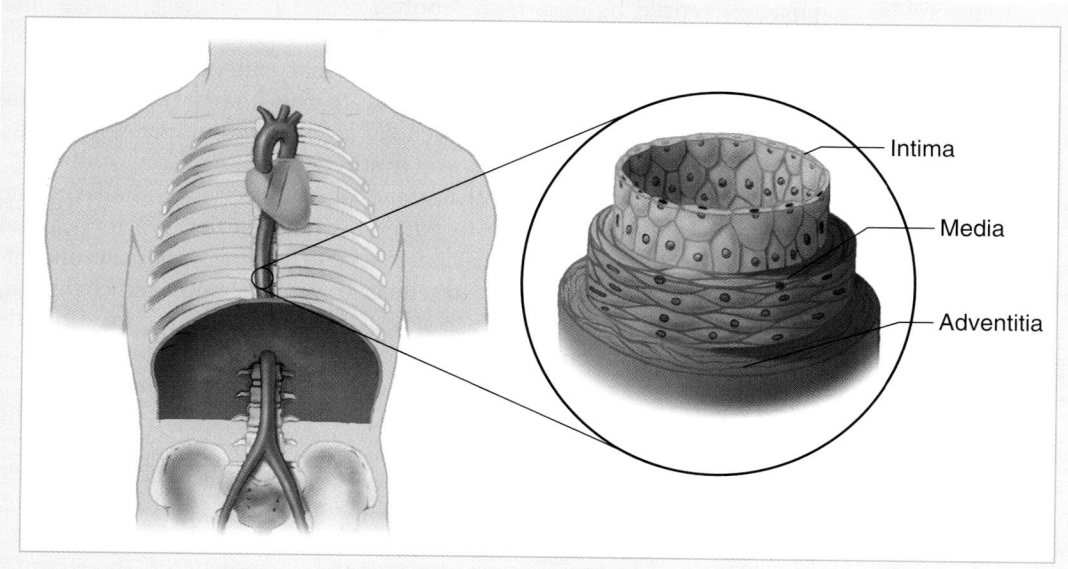

Figure 23-12 The aortic arch, descending aorta, and layers of the aorta.

even kicks during kickboxing. Such a patient may present with ventricular fibrillation that responds positively to early defibrillation if provided within the first 2 minutes. For this reason, public access to defibrillators in schools and sports venues is essential.

Vascular Injuries
Thoracic Aortic Dissection/Transection
One in every five deaths due to blunt trauma includes a transection of the aorta; the most common causes are high-speed motor vehicle crashes and falls from a height. Each year, 5,000 to 8,000 people in the United States die as a result of aortic or great vessel rupture. Given that the body's entire blood volume passes through this vessel, the high mortality associated with such an injury comes as no surprise. Of those patients who experience an aortic injury, only a few will survive until EMS units arrive; most of the individuals reached by EMS personnel can survive with prompt management including surgical intervention.

The most widely accepted theory of how this injury evolves holds that the aorta is injured at its fixed points due to shearing forces. The high-velocity, high-energy impacts that result in these injuries cause the aortic arch to swing forward. The resulting tension, along with rotation and torque on the area, causes the descending aorta to rupture at its point of attachment to the posterior thoracic wall **Figure 23-12 ▲** .

The aorta includes three layers—the intima, the media, and the adventitia. If the injury tears the intima, the high pressure within the aorta allows the blood to dissect along the media. More severe injuries damage all three layers of the aorta, allowing blood to leak from the aorta into the surrounding tissues. If these tissues can't stop the bleeding, the patient

may survive with prompt intervention. Otherwise, the injury will be fatal.

Great Vessel Injury
With the exception of the aorta, the great vessels are located in areas that offer protection from adjacent bony structures and other tissues. As a consequence, injury to these vessels is much more likely with penetrating trauma. In rare instances, blunt trauma may damage the overlying structures or produce a severe rotational injury (such as that caused by machinery).

Some great vessel injuries may result in occlusion or spasm of the involved artery. These injuries will present with ischemic changes (pain, pallor, paresthesias, pulselessness, paralysis) in the area with a blood supply coming from the involved artery.

Other Thoracic Injuries
Diaphragmatic Injuries
Diaphragmatic injury occurs in a relatively small percentage of all trauma patients, yet the potential for this injury has prompted a change in the management of penetrating trauma in recent years. For example, some surgeons manage penetrating trauma between the midaxillary lines, below the clavicle, and above the iliac crests by undertaking surgical exploration to ensure that the diaphragm is intact. This conservative approach reflects the possibility that a missed diaphragmatic injury may result in significant complications in the years following the injury.

Injury to the diaphragm may result from direct penetrating injury or blunt force trauma leading to diaphragmatic rupture. Because the diaphragm is protected by the liver on the right side, most diaphragmatic injuries (particularly those due to blunt trauma) occur on the left side. Once the diaphragm has been injured, the healing process is inhibited by the natural pressure differences between the abdominal and thoracic cavities.

Injury to the diaphragm and the associated physical findings have been separated into three phases: acute, latent, and

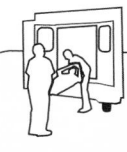

In the Field

Blunt disruptions of the diaphragm are usually associated with herniation of all or part of the liver into the right side of the chest and the stomach into the left side of the chest.

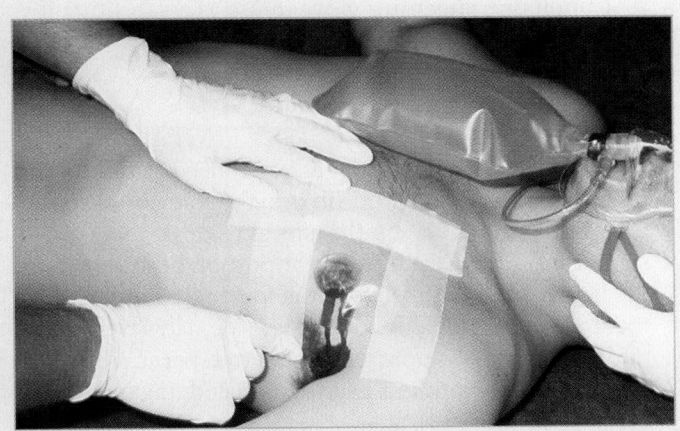

Figure 23-16 A sucking chest wound should be covered with a large occlusive dressing that seals on three sides with the fourth left open as a flutter valve.

may use sedation or neuromuscular blockade to facilitate this process, depending on your local protocols.

An open pneumothorax rarely progresses to a tension pneumothorax. If it does, you should remove the patient's occlusive dressing to allow the pneumothorax to "vent" through the opening in the thoracic cavity. If this measure does not relieve this life-threatening condition, treatment should progress as described in the next section.

Tension Pneumothorax

The classic signs of a tension pneumothorax are an absence of breath sounds on the affected side, tachycardia, jugular vein distention, and tracheal deviation. While tachycardia may not be a unique finding in the trauma patient, tension pneumothorax induces this change—not because of a hypovolemic state, but rather because of the inability of blood to easily return to the heart from the venous system. The increasing pressure within the thoracic cavity leads to the accumulation of blood within the great vessels just outside the thoracic cavity. As the pressure is translated into the most superficial of these veins—the jugular veins—they become distended with blood. Such jugular vein distention is usually a late sign of tension pneumothorax.

The jugular veins, which exit the thoracic cavity from beneath the clavicles and cross over the sternocleidomastoid muscles as they move superiorly, are considered to be distended when they are engorged to a level 1 to 2 cm above the clavicle. This assessment is properly done with the patient in a 45° Fowler's position, however—something that can't be accomplished during the initial assessment of the patient in the field.

Because of the mediastinal shift caused by the increasing pressure, palpation or visualization of the trachea may manifest

You are the Provider Part 4

An assessment of the patient's circulation reveals no evidence of muffled heart tones, jugular vein distention, dullness to chest percussion, or evidence of traumatic asphyxia. After loading the patient into the helicopter, you complete a detailed physical exam, establish a second IV line, and continue fluid resuscitation.

Your physical assessment reveals crepitus and palpable deformity over the ninth and tenth ribs on the left, as well as a rigid abdomen. Deformity of the left lower leg is evident, and the patient has multiple soft-tissue injuries on all extremities.

Reassessment	Recording Time: 20 Minutes
Skin	Pale, cool extremities with a pink core
Pulse	108 beats/min
Blood pressure	104/58 mm Hg
Respirations	Intubated; ventilating with 100% supplemental oxygen
Sao$_2$	98%
ECG	Sinus tachycardia without further ectopy

7. What additional injuries might your physical findings suggest?

8. What additional treatments may be needed for this patient?

in a deviation of the trachea away from the affected side. Nevertheless, this late finding in a tension pneumothorax may not be present despite the rapid decompensation of the patient's clinical status. For this reason, you must be vigilant in watching for the cardiopulmonary findings associated with a tension pneumothorax and not rely on the presence of all the classic physical findings in making the diagnosis.

The accumulation of air within the pleural space decreases the lung volume and diminishes the breath sounds on the affected side when you auscultate the chest. Because air causes the loss of breath sounds on that side, the chest will be resonant (like a bell) when percussed, as opposed to the dull sensation expected with fluid or blood.

Due to the injury and the collapsing lung, a patient with a tension pneumothorax often complains of pleuritic chest pain and dyspnea. The resulting hypoxia may cause the patient to become anxious, tachycardic, tachypneic, and even cyanotic.

Hypotension, as a late finding of tension pneumothorax, should not be used to either confirm or exclude the possibility of a tension pneumothorax. Its presence may suggest that the pneumothorax has produced such significant pressure as to severely impede preload, or it may represent a simultaneous shock state due to other injuries. Normal blood pressure suggests that, when other signs of a tension pneumothorax are present, the heart is adequately compensating for the diminished venous return.

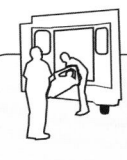

In the Field

Shock (a late sign), decreased breath sounds, and hyperresonance to percussion on the same side of the chest mean a tension pneumothorax until proven otherwise.

All patients presenting with signs of a tension pneumothorax should immediately be placed on high-flow supplemental oxygen (12 to 15 L/min) via a nonrebreathing mask. Immediate relief of the elevated pressures must then be accomplished through a needle decompression, also referred to as a "needle thoracentesis." The steps for performing a needle decompression are described below (**Skill Drill 23-1 ▸**):

1. Assess the patient to ensure that the presentation matches that of a tension pneumothorax (Step 1):
   - Difficult ventilation despite an open airway
   - Jugular vein distention (may not be present with associated hemorrhage)
   - Absent or decreased breath sounds on the affected side
   - Hyperresonance to percussion on the affected side
   - Tracheal deviation away from the affected side (this late sign is not always present)
2. Prepare and assemble the necessary equipment (Step 2):
   - Large-bore IV catheter, preferably 10- to 14-gauge and at least 2″ long
   - Alcohol or povidone iodine (Betadine) preps

   - Cut off one finger of a glove to use as a substitute if you don't have a commercial device or condom available.
   - Adhesive tape
3. Obtain orders from medical control.
4. Locate the appropriate site (**Figure 23-17 ▾**) (Step 3). Find the second or third rib, as you'll need to insert the needle just above the third rib into the intercostal space at the midclavicular line on the affected side. If there is significant trauma to the anterior portion of the chest, use the intercostal space between the fourth and fifth ribs at the midaxillary line on the affected side. However, the midclavicular line approach is preferred because it's usually easier to access with less chance of dislodging the needle.
5. Cleanse the appropriate area using aseptic technique (Step 4).
6. Make a one-way valve, or flutter valve, by inserting the catheter through the end of a condom or use a commercially prepared device or the finger of a medical glove, cut off from the glove (Step 5).
7. Insert the needle at a 90° angle, and listen for the release of air (Step 6). Insert the needle just superior to the third rib, midclavicular, or just above the sixth rib, midaxillary. (The nerves, arteries, and veins run along the inferior borders of each rib.)
8. Advance the catheter over the needle, and place the needle in the sharps container (Step 7).

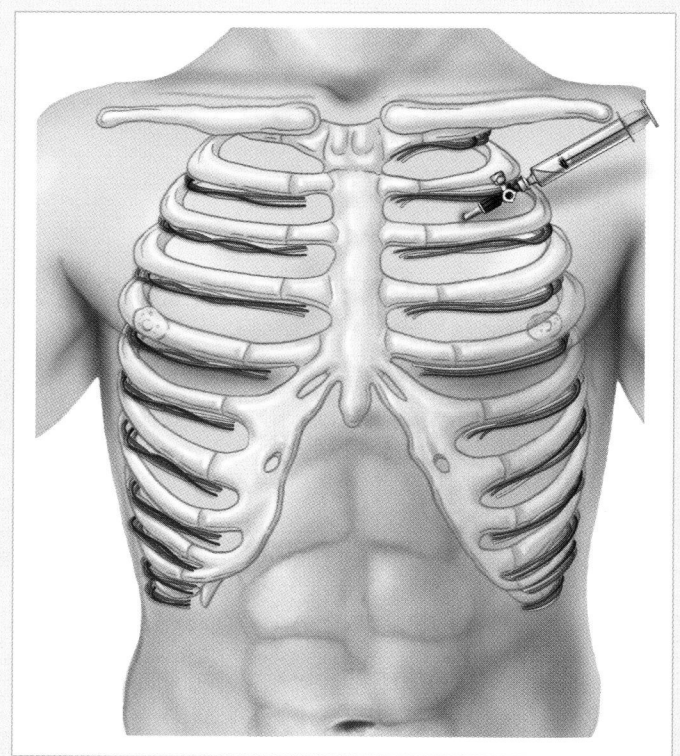

Figure 23-17 Correct placement of needle for decompression. The position of nerves, arteries, and veins are shown in relation to the ribs.

Skill Drill 23-1: Needle Decompression (Thoracentesis) of a Tension Pneumothorax

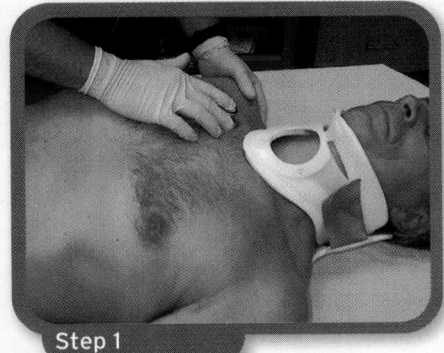

Step 1

Assess the patient.

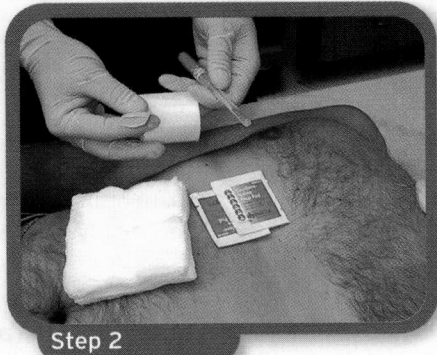

Step 2

Prepare and assemble all necessary equipment. Obtain orders from medical control.

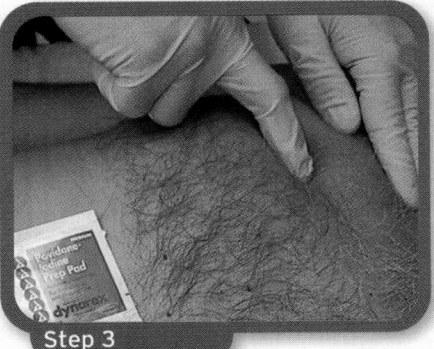

Step 3

Locate the appropriate site between the second and third rib.

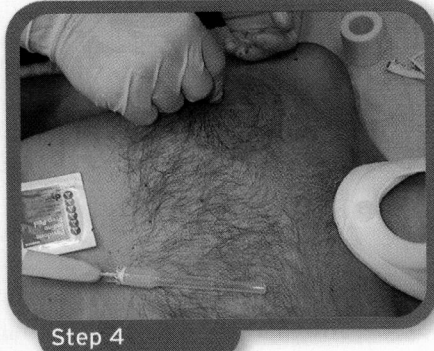

Step 4

Cleanse the appropriate area using aseptic technique.

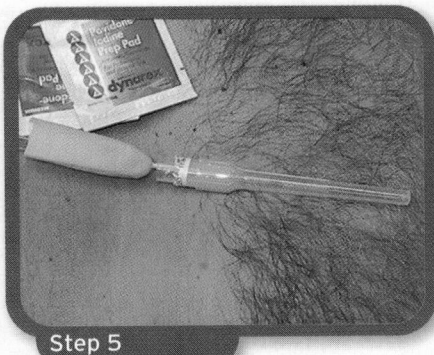

Step 5

Make a one-way valve or flutter valve.

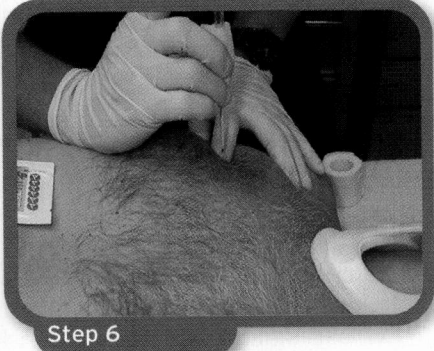

Step 6

Insert the needle at a 90° angle.

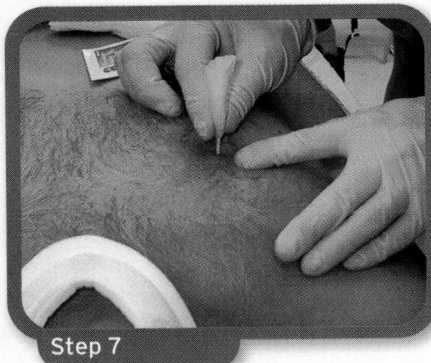

Step 7

Remove the needle and listen for release of air. Properly dispose of the needle in the sharps container.

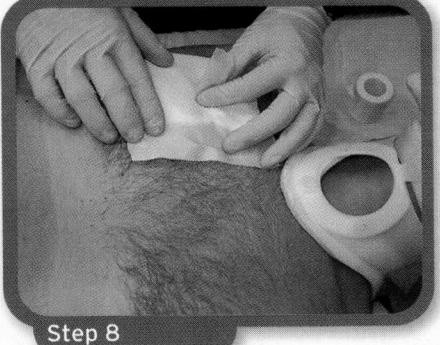

Step 8

Secure the catheter in place. Monitor the patient closely for recurrence of the tension pneumothorax.

9. Secure the catheter in place in the same manner you would use to secure an impaled object (Step 8).

10. Monitor the patient closely for recurrence of the tension pneumothorax. This procedure may need to be repeated several times before arrival at the emergency department.

The performance of a needle decompression is not without risk. If the needle is improperly placed (ie, not inserted over the top of the rib), injury to the intercostal vessels may result in significant hemorrhage. Similarly, passing the needle into the chest may injure the lung parenchyma. Failure to treat this condition will cause the patient to progress to pulseless electrical activity and cardiopulmonary arrest.

Massive Hemothorax

Physical assessment of the massive hemothorax will reveal signs of both ventilatory insufficiency (hypoxia, agitation, anxiety, tachypnea, dyspnea) and hypovolemic shock (tachycardia, hypotension, pale and clammy skin). The physical findings that help to differentiate this hemothorax from other injuries include the lack of jugular vein distention, the lack of tracheal deviation, possible bloody sputum (hemoptysis), and dullness that may be noted on percussion of the affected side of the chest.

The prehospital management of a suspected hemothorax is supportive. If the airway does not require intervention, place the patient on high-flow supplemental oxygen via a nonrebreathing mask. Initiate two large-bore peripheral IVs, with fluid resuscitation being guided by local protocols and directed at limiting the duration of hypotension. Hypovolemic shock with hypotension that persists for more than 30 minutes raises the mortality from one in ten patients to as high as one in two. For individuals older than age 65, that risk jumps dramatically, to nine out of ten patients.

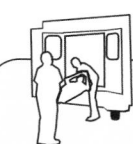

In the Field

The major problem following a massive hemothorax is the development of hypovolemic shock and respiratory compromise.

Pulmonary Contusion

The assessment of the patient with a pulmonary contusion may not initially reveal the presence or severity of the injury as it may take 24 hours before the severity of the injury becomes clinically evident. Because not every trauma patient presents immediately (eg, cases involving domestic violence, assaults, injuries that occur while intoxicated, patients in remote areas who are not immediately located, or search and rescue operations), it is important to be familiar with the clinical presentation of this injury.

Hypoxia and carbon dioxide retention lead to respiratory distress, dyspnea, tachypnea, agitation, and restlessness. Due to the capillary injury and the hemorrhage into the pulmonary parenchyma, the patient may present with hemoptysis (coughing up blood). Evidence of overlying injury may include contu-

sions, tenderness, crepitus, or paradoxical motion. Auscultation may reveal wheezes, crackles or rales, or diminished lung sounds in the affected area. In severe cases, cyanosis and low oxygen saturations may be found.

The treatment of pulmonary contusion begins with the assessment and, as needed, management of the patient's airway. Both high-concentration oxygen and positive-pressure ventilation may be used to overcome the pathologic changes described earlier. Because edema may exacerbate the injury, use caution when administering IV fluids. In some cases, the administration of small amounts of analgesics may aid the patient in maximizing ventilatory function without suppressing ventilatory drive.

Myocardial Injuries
Pericardial Tamponade

Beck's triad is the classic combination of physical findings in patients with pericardial tamponade: muffled heart tones, narrowed pulse pressures, and jugular vein distention. Even so, this triad is seen in only 30% of patients diagnosed with cardiac tamponade.

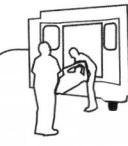

In the Field

Hypotension and distended neck veins in the presence of normal lung sounds (which rules out pneumothorax), combined with an appropriate history, suggest cardiac tamponade.

Another classic finding in pericardial tamponade (albeit one that is not always present) is the ECG finding of electrical alternans. As fluid accumulates within the pericardial sac, the heart begins to oscillate with each beat. As the heart swings back and forth within the pericardium, its electrical axis changes. Electrical alternans is not commonly seen in acute pericardial tamponade and must be differentiated from bigeminal ectopy, but it is a classic sign of pericardial tamponade.

The reduced cardiac output, hypoperfusion, and hypotension observed in pericardial tamponade produce the findings typical of a patient in shock: weak or absent peripheral pulses, diaphoresis, dyspnea, cyanosis, altered mental status, tachycardia, tachypnea, and agitation. Although these symptoms by themselves do not suggest or exclude the presence of pericardial tamponade, identifying them can flesh out the physical assessment.

Physical findings in a patient with pericardial tamponade are not significantly different than those of a tension pneumothorax—namely, hypotension, jugular vein distention, tachycardia, altered mental status, and signs of tissue hypoperfusion. Table 23-2 ▸ compares the physical findings of these two emergencies.

The treatment of the patient with pericardial tamponade begins by ensuring adequate oxygen delivery and establishing intravenous access. Giving IV fluids might appear to slow the

Table 23-2	Physical Findings of Pericardial Tamponade Versus Tension Pneumothorax	
Physical Finding	**Pericardial Tamponade**	**Tension Pneumothorax**
Presenting sign/ symptom	Shock	Respiratory distress
Neck veins	Distended	Distended
Trachea	Midline	Deviated
Breath sounds	Equal on both sides	Decreased or absent on side of injury
Chest percussion	Normal	Hyperresonant on side of injury
Heart sounds	Muffled	Normal

patient's deterioration by momentarily increasing preload. The patient with a pericardial tamponade should be transported rapidly to a trauma center for a pericardiocentesis—a procedure in which blood is removed from the pericardial sac via an intracardiac needle inserted through the chest wall. Definitive management occurs in the operating department, in the hands of a cardiothoracic surgeon.

Myocardial Contusion

Sharp, retrosternal chest pain is the most common complaint among patients with myocardial contusion. Inspection of the area may reveal soft-tissue or bony injury in the area. Crackles or rales (due to pulmonary edema from left ventricular dysfunction) may be heard on auscultation.

In the Field

Many patients with myocardial contusion are relatively asymptomatic, at least initially. Accompanying injuries may present more dramatically. Helpful signs are ECG changes, and persistent sinus tachycardia without obvious hypovolemia.

The ECG in a patient with a myocardial contusion is often abnormal. Sinus tachycardia is the most common ECG abnormality seen in cardiac contusion patients. Additional ECG changes may include atrial fibrillation or flutter, premature atrial contractions (PACs) or premature ventricular contractions (PVCs), a new right bundle branch block, AV blocks, nonspecific ST-segment and T-wave changes, and ventricular tachycardia or fibrillation. In the event of a coronary artery injury (likely the right coronary artery), ischemic changes consistent with those seen in myocardial infarction may also occur.

The treatment of patients with possible myocardial contusion begins with nonspecific, supportive care, including oxygen administration, frequent assessment of vital signs, cardiac monitoring, and establishing IV access. Fluid resuscitation should be instituted as needed to maintain the patient's blood pressure. Unless allowed by local protocols, consultation with online medical control should precede the administration of antiarrhythmic agents to trauma patients.

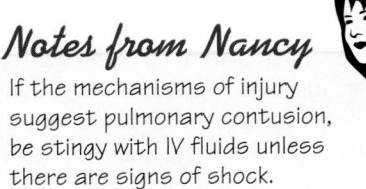

Notes from Nancy

If the mechanisms of injury suggest pulmonary contusion, be stingy with IV fluids unless there are signs of shock.

Myocardial Rupture

Remember that myocardial rupture is life-threatening. Patients may present with acute pulmonary edema or signs of cardiac tamponade. Unless the latter is present and a pericardiocentesis can be done, patients with myocardial rupture should receive supportive care and be rapidly transported to a facility where a thoracotomy can be performed.

Vascular Injuries
Thoracic Aortic Dissection/Transection

Depending on the exact nature of the injury, the symptoms and physical exam in cases of thoracic aortic dissection or transection will vary from an unstable patient to one with no physical

You are the Provider Part 5

The patient's vital signs are monitored en route to the hospital with no further deterioration. You administer IV fluids to maintain perfusion. You and your partner care for the patient's injuries en route to the trauma center.

When you arrive at the trauma center, the trauma team takes over the patient's care. You and your partner provide a concise, complete report to the team, including the mechanism of injury, the deaths of two other passengers, your initial physical assessment, the interventions you performed, and the patient's response to those treatments.

During the emergency department evaluation, the patient is found to have a right-sided pneumothorax, a left-sided pulmonary contusion, fractures of left ribs 8 through 11, a lacerated spleen, a fractured left tibia and fibula, and multiple soft-tissue injuries. A tube thoracotomy is performed in the emergency department. The patient is taken to surgery for repair of his abdominal and orthopaedic injuries and, after a 15-day hospitalization, is discharged home with no permanent disability.

complaints. However, most patients will have a complaint of pain behind the sternum or in the scapula. Other findings may include signs of hypovolemic shock, dyspnea, and altered mental status. If a hematoma forms in the area of the esophagus, trachea, or larynx, the patient may present with dysphagia, stridor, and hoarseness, respectively. A harsh murmur may be noted due to the turbulence created as the blood passes the site of the injury to the intima in the aorta.

Assessment of the patient's pulses in all extremities is an important key to the identification of these injuries. As the dissection or rupture compresses the aorta and progresses along its branch vessels, blood flow to the extremities may be compromised. This phenomenon results in diminished pulses compared to those closer to the injury. On exam, you will note a stronger pulse (and higher blood pressure) in the right arm than in the left arm or the lower extremities.

Because of the high energy involved with aortic injuries, associated injuries are to be expected. They may include multiple rib fractures, flail segment, sternal or scapular fracture, pericardial tamponade, hemothorax or pneumothorax, and clavicle fracture.

Controversies

It has long been taught that first or second rib fractures (which are often a radiographic finding rather than a physical exam finding) are indicative of aortic injuries, but this association has lately come into question.

The prehospital management of potential aortic injuries is symptomatic. After assessment and management of the ABCs, the patient should receive gradual IV hydration for the treatment of hypotension. Aggressive fluid administration may result in sudden changes in the intra-aortic pressure that could worsen the injury. Expedited transport to a trauma center with an available cardiothoracic surgeon is essential.

Notes from Nancy

Suspect aortic rupture in any accident involving powerful deceleration forces.

Great Vessel Injury

If the vessel is not injured in such a way that bleeding is prevented, the patient will present with signs and symptoms of hypovolemic shock, hemothorax, or cardiac tamponade. If the bleeding results in formation of a hematoma, the compression of adjacent structures (ie, esophagus, trachea) may produce additional signs and symptoms.

The management of potential injuries to the great vessels is no different from the management of any other form of acute blood loss. Establish IV hydration en route to the emergency department, and treat pericardial tamponade immediately if it

is found. Don't use a pneumatic antishock garment, as it will increase the pressures within the involved vessels and may contribute to greater blood loss.

Other Thoracic Injuries

Diaphragmatic Injuries

Although diaphragmatic injuries are not likely to be identified in the prehospital setting, you should still maintain clinical suspicion for such injuries 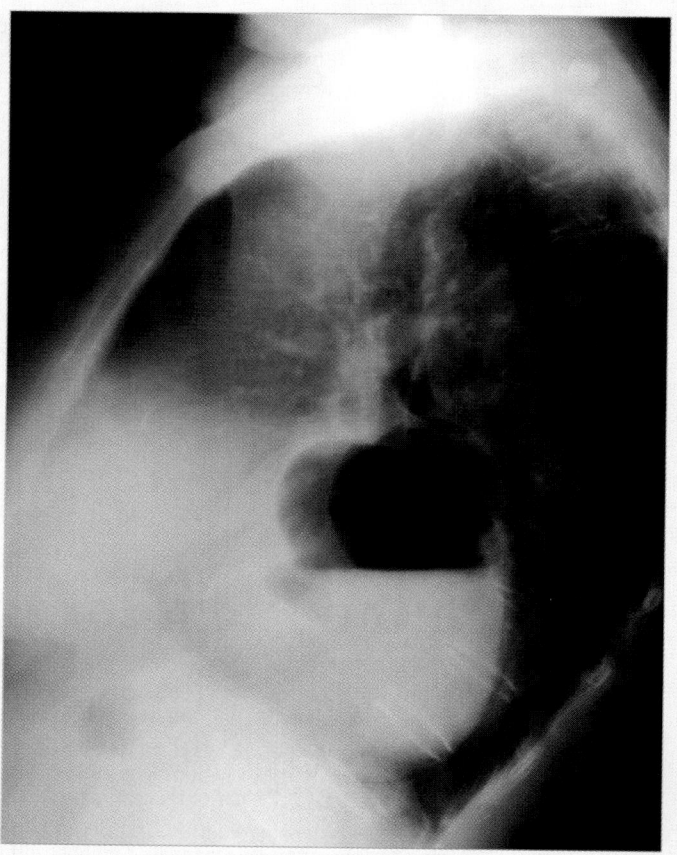 Figure 23-18 ▾ . You are most likely to care for the patient during the acute phase, but delayed presentations in the obstructive phase are also possible.

In the acute phase, the patient may present with hypotension, tachypnea, bowel sounds in the chest, chest pain, or absence of breath sounds on the affected side. These signs indicate a large diaphragmatic injury that may be followed by herniation of the abdominal contents into the thoracic cavity.

In the obstructive phase, as the blood supply to the herniated organs becomes compromised, symptoms will include nausea, vomiting, abdominal pain, constipation, dyspnea, and abdominal distention. In many cases, these symptoms are severe and unrelenting. The most severe findings may be consistent with a tension gastrothorax.

In both the acute and obstructive phases, management of diaphragmatic injury focuses on maintaining adequate oxy-

Figure 23-18 Radiograph of a diaphragmatic rupture.

pubis to the xiphoid process and the horizontal axis extending to both flanks, this would create four quadrants. These four regions are as follows: the right upper quadrant (RUQ), the right lower quadrant (RLQ), the left lower quadrant (LLQ), and the left upper quadrant (LUQ). The area around the umbilicus is referred to as the periumbilical area.

The abdominal cavity is lined with a membrane called the peritoneum, which is similar to the pleura that line the thoracic cavity. The mesentery is a membranous double fold of tissue in the abdomen that attaches various organs to the body wall. The internal abdomen is structurally divided into three regions: the peritoneal space, the retroperitoneal space, and the pelvis **Figure 24-3 ▸**. Intraperitoneal structures, encased in the peritoneum, include the liver, spleen, stomach, small bowel, colon, gallbladder, and, in women, the female reproductive organs. The retroperitoneal space contains the aorta, vena cava, pancreas, kidneys, ureters, and portions of the duodenum and large intestine. The rectum, ureters, pelvic vascular plexus, major vascular structures, pelvic skeletal structures, and reproductive organs lie in the pelvis.

Abdominal Organs

The abdomen contains many organs, including those that belong to many organ systems such as the digestive system.

The liver is a solid organ and is the largest organ in the abdomen. It lies in the right upper quadrant (extending to the epigastrium), superior and anterior to the gallbladder and the hepatic and cystic ducts. Among its many functions, the liver detoxifies the blood and produces bile (which is necessary to break down ingested fats) that drains into the small intestines.

Like the liver, the spleen is a solid organ in the peritoneum. This highly vascular organ lies in the left upper quadrant and is partially protected by the left lower rib cage. It functions to clear bloodborne bacteria.

The gallbladder is a saclike organ located on the lower surface of the liver that acts as a reservoir for bile, one of the digestive enzymes produced by the liver. The liver continually secretes bile, and the gallbladder stores it until it is released through the cystic duct during the digestive process.

The pancreas is an organ located in the retroperitoneal space in the middle of the abdomen. It secretes enzymes into the bowel that aid in digestion. The pancreas also secretes the hormone insulin, which is responsible for helping glucose enter the cells.

The stomach is an intraperitoneal hollow organ that lies in the left upper quadrant and epigastric region. The esophagus passes through the diaphragm and opens into the stomach. The stomach secretes an acid that assists in the digestive process.

The small and large intestines run from the end of the stomach to the anus. The majority of the intestines are in the intraperitoneal area. They digest and absorb water and nutrients. The first part of the small intestine, the duodenum, is retroperitoneal. As contents pass through the stomach, they move through the pylorus, a circumferential muscle at the end of the stomach that acts as a valve between the stomach and

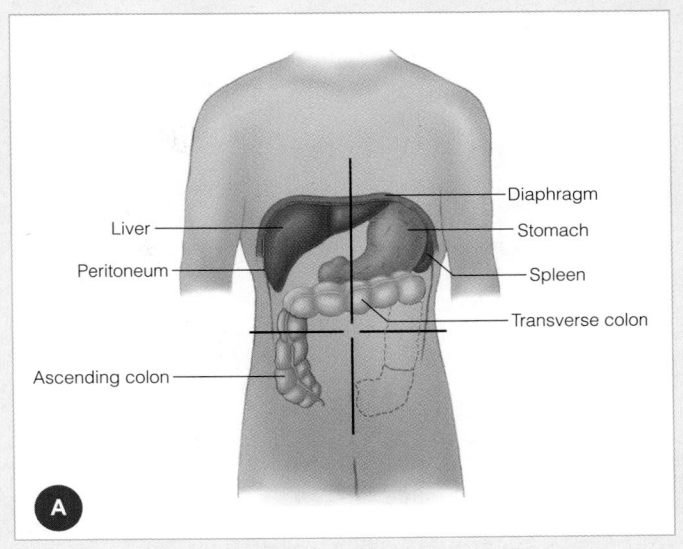

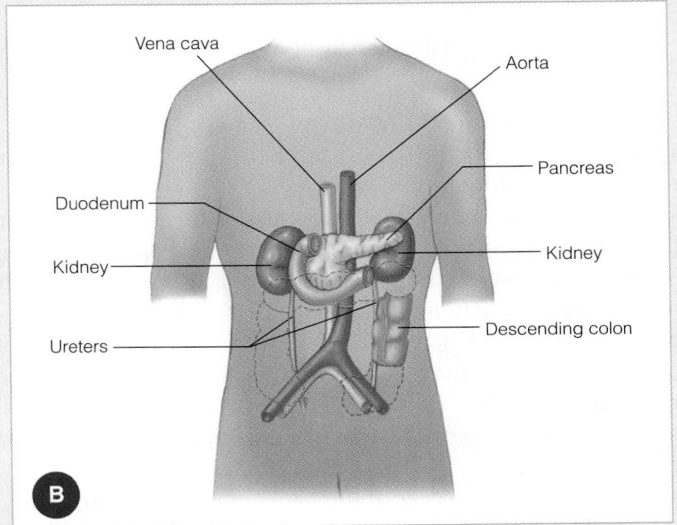

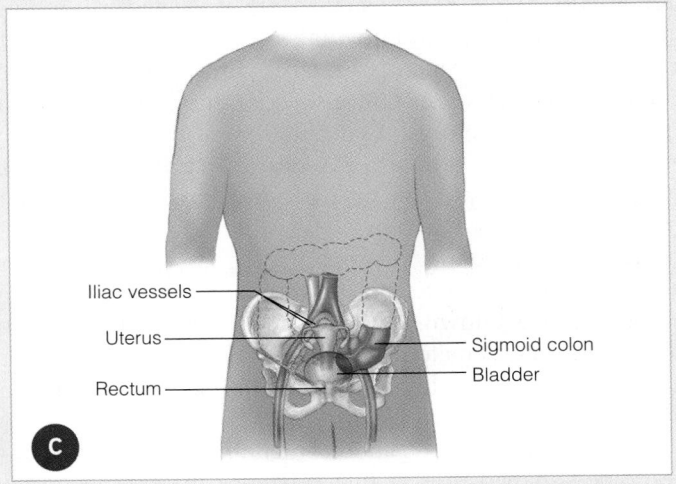

Figure 24-3 Different organs of the abdomen are contained in the peritoneum (**A**), the retroperitoneal space (**B**), and the pelvis (**C**).

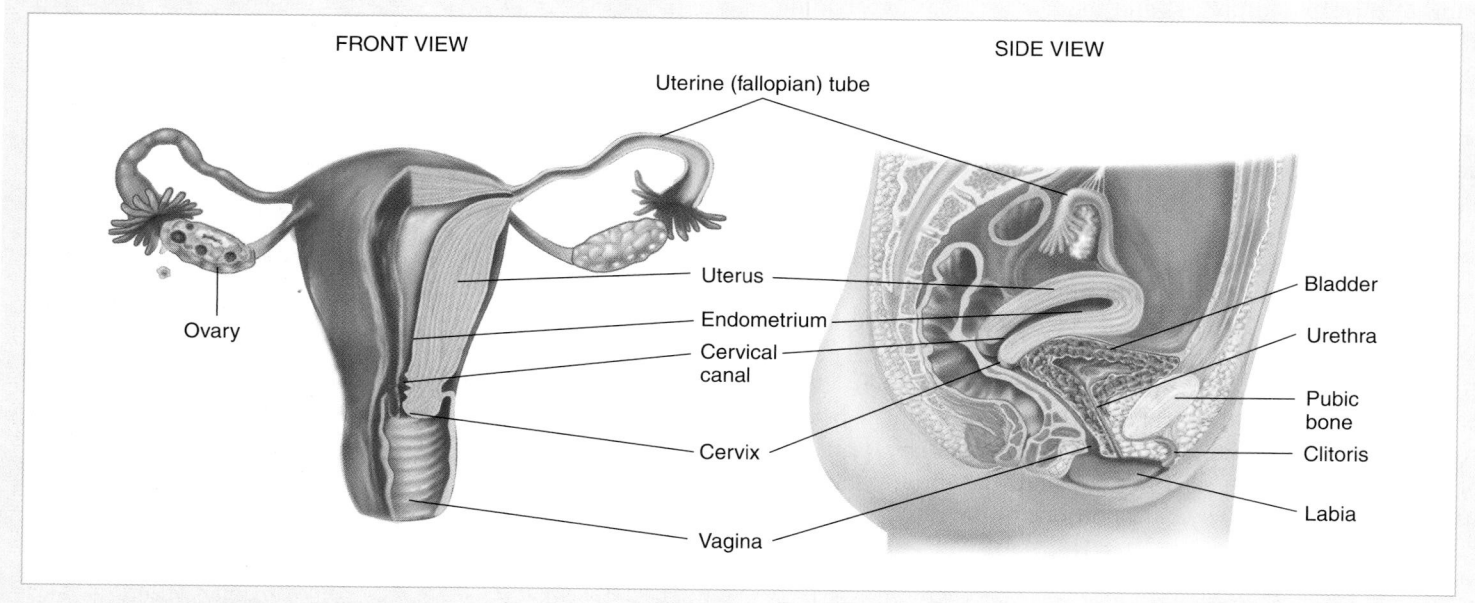

FRONT VIEW   SIDE VIEW

Uterine (fallopian) tube

Ovary

Uterus

Endometrium

Cervical canal

Cervix

Vagina

Bladder

Urethra

Pubic bone

Clitoris

Labia

Figure 24-4 The female reproductive system.

the duodenum. Finally, stool passes through the rectum and out of the body through the anus.

The abdomen also contains organs of the urinary system. The kidneys are located in the retroperitoneal space. They filter blood and excrete body wastes in the form of urine. The kidneys will be discussed in greater detail in Chapter 32, *Renal and Urologic Emergencies.* The urinary bladder is a hollow, muscular sac situated in the pelvis along the midline that stores urine until it is excreted. The ureters are a pair of thick-walled, hollow tubes that carry urine from the kidneys to the urinary bladder.

The abdomen also contains organs of the reproductive system. The female reproductive system ⟨ **Figure 24-4 ▲** ⟩ contains the uterus, a pear-shaped organ located in the midline of the lower abdomen that allows the implantation, growth, and nourishment of a fetus during pregnancy. The female reproductive system also contains the ovaries (the female reproductive organs), located one on each side of the lower abdominal quadrants. The ovaries produce the precursors to mature eggs, and produce hormones that regulate female reproductive function.

The male reproductive system ⟨ **Figure 24-5 ▶** ⟩ contains the penis, the male external reproductive organ, as well as the testes, also known as the testicles. The testes produce sperm and secrete male hormones such as testosterone. The scrotum is the pouch of skin and muscle that contains the testes.

Last but not least, the abdomen contains the diaphragm—the domed-shaped muscle that separates the thoracic cavity from the abdominal cavity. It curves from its point of attachment in the flanks at the twelfth rib and peaks in the center at the fourth intercostal space.

▌**Physiology Review**

When abdominal trauma occurs, the places where enough blood can be lost to cause shock include the abdomen, retroperitoneal space, and muscle compartments of the proximal lower extremities, (as well as a bed, floor, or street, as a result of bleeding from open wounds) ⟨ **Figure 24-6 ▶** ⟩. Because the abdomen and retroperitoneum can accommodate large amounts of blood, the bleeding may produce few signs and symptoms of the trauma. Even the patient's vital signs and physical exam may not indicate the bleeding.

The organs that are most frequently injured after a blunt trauma are the spleen (in approximately 50% of the cases), followed by the liver (in approximately 30%). Because of its size, the liver is the organ that is most frequently injured in penetrating trauma. Solid organs, such as the liver or spleen, can easily be crushed by external blunt trauma. They both have a large blood supply and can bleed profusely. If a trauma patient has unexplained symptoms of shock, you should suspect abdominal trauma.

Hollow organs are more resilient to blunt trauma and less likely to be injured by trauma unless they are full. When a hollow organ is full, it is likely to be injured and can burst in the same way a chemical cold pack breaks when you apply pressure to the outer bag. The danger of bursting hollow organs is that they hold toxins (such as urine, bile, or stomach acids) that can spill out into the abdominal cavity. This spillage can cause <u>peritonitis</u>, an inflammation of the lining of the abdomen (the peritoneum). Peritonitis is a life-threatening infection.

The management of trauma in the hospital has changed substantially in the past few years, with more than 95% of patients receiving nonoperative management. You must have a

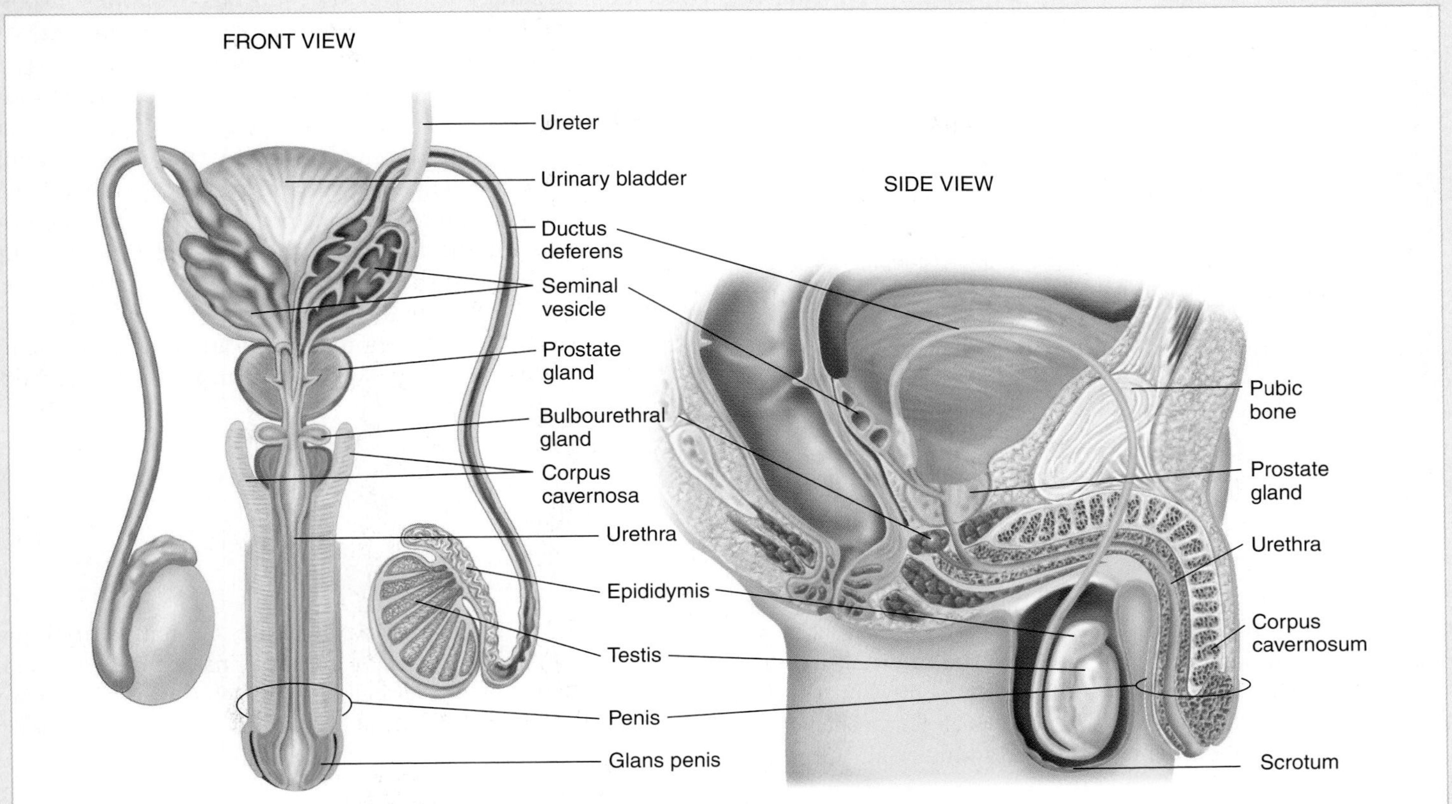

FRONT VIEW

Ureter
Urinary bladder
Ductus deferens
Seminal vesicle
Prostate gland
Bulbourethral gland
Corpus cavernosa
Urethra
Epididymis
Testis
Penis
Glans penis

SIDE VIEW

Pubic bone
Prostate gland
Urethra
Corpus cavernosum
Scrotum

Figure 24-5 The male reproductive system.

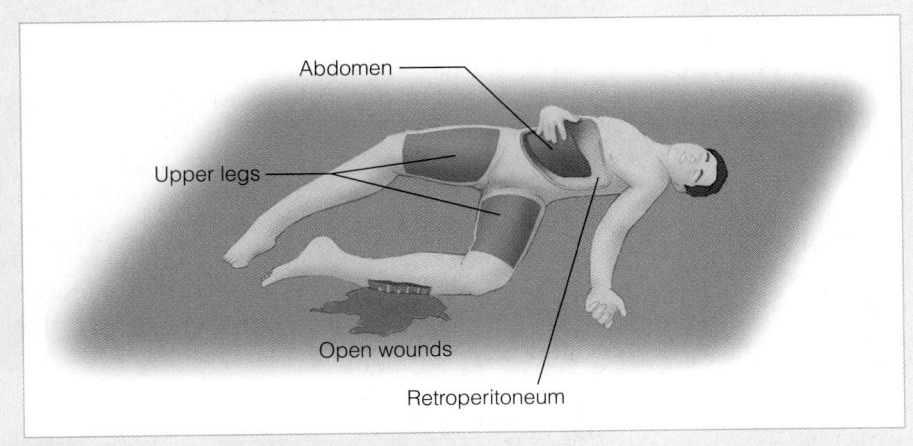

Abdomen
Upper legs
Open wounds
Retroperitoneum

Figure 24-6 The places where enough blood can be lost to cause shock.

high index of suspicion and a clear understanding of the mechanism of injury (MOI) your trauma patient was exposed to.

Mechanism of Injury

Trauma is a significant cause of death in adults and is the leading cause of death in patients 1 to 44 years of age. About 80% of all significant trauma involves the abdomen; however, the exact definition of the term "significant" is not clear in the literature, with most of the trauma statistics coming from regional trauma centers. Unrecognized abdominal trauma is the leading cause of unexpected deaths because it results in a delay in surgical intervention. Other causes of trauma include injuries from not wearing vehicle restraints or from wearing them improperly, crush injuries to the chest and abdomen from the steering column, injuries to pedestrians from being struck by a motor vehicle, and assaults.

Blunt Trauma

At least two thirds of all abdominal injuries involve blunt trauma, most of which occur during motor vehicle collisions **Figure 24-7 ▶**, with a resulting mortality of about 5%. Blunt trauma to the abdomen results from compression or deceleration forces and can often lead to a closed abdominal injury—one in which soft-tissue damage occurs inside the body, but the skin remains intact. When assessing the abdominal cavity in a patient who has received blunt trauma, consider three common mechanisms of injury:

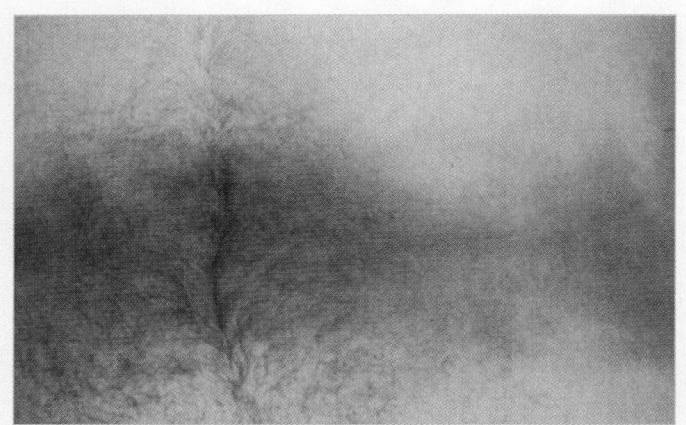

Figure 24-7 Blunt trauma occurs most frequently in vehicle collisions, and typically leads to closed abdominal injury—the internal organs are injured, but the skin remains intact.

shearing, crushing, and compression. In the rapid deceleration of a patient during a motor vehicle crash or fall from a height, a shearing force can be created as the internal organs continue their forward motion. This will cause hollow, solid, and visceral organs and vascular structures to tear, especially at their points of attachment to the abdominal wall. Organs that shear or tear would include the liver, kidneys, small and large intestines, and spleen. In motor vehicle collisions, this MOI has been described as the third collision (such as the car into the wall, the patient into the steering column, or the internal organs into the patient's inner rib cage).

Crush injuries are the result of external factors at the time of impact; they differ from decelerating injuries occurring before impact. When abdominal contents are crushed between the anterior abdominal wall and the spinal column (or other structures in the rear), crushing occurs. Solid organs like the kidneys, liver, and spleen are at the greatest risk of injury from this mechanism. Direct application of crushing forces to the abdomen would come from things like the dashboard or the front hood of a car (in a vehicle collision) or from falling objects. Additionally, these injuries can be caused by a restraining device that has not been properly attached or worn or by the steering wheel striking the abdominal cavity of an unrestrained driver as the person is propelled forward.

The last MOI to consider is compression injury resulting from a direct blow or external compression from a fixed object (such as a lap belt or air bag). These compression forces will deform hollow organs, increasing the pressure within the abdominal cavity. This dramatic change in abdominal pressure can cause a rupture of the small intestine or diaphragm. Rupture of organs can lead to uncontrollable hemorrhage and peritonitis.

Penetrating Trauma

Penetrating trauma results most commonly from low-velocity (< 200′ per second) gunshot or stab wounds. Penetrating trauma causes an open abdominal injury—one in which a

break in the surface of the skin or mucous membrane exposes deeper tissue to potential contamination. In general, gunshot wounds cause more injury than stab wounds because bullets travel deep into the body and have more kinetic energy. Gunshot wounds most commonly involve injury to the small bowel, colon, liver, and vascular structures; the extent of injury is less predictable than the injury caused by stab wounds because gunshot wounds depend mostly on the characteristics of the weapon and the characteristics of the bullet. In penetrating trauma from stab wounds, the liver, small bowel, diaphragm, and colon are the organs most frequently injured.

The extent of damage from a penetrating injury is often a function of the energy that has been imparted to the body. Remember:

$$\text{Kinetic energy} = \frac{\text{Mass}}{2} \times \text{Velocity}^2$$

$$\text{or, KE} = \frac{m}{2} \times v^2$$

Thus the permanent injury as well as the temporary injury from the tract of the projectile can be considerable with high-velocity penetrations. The velocity delivered during penetrating trauma is typically divided into three levels. Low velocity (< 200′ per second) such as from a knife, ice pick, or handgun; medium velocity (200 to 2,000′ per second) such as from a 9-mm gun or shotgun; and high velocity (> 2,000′ per second) such as from a high-powered sporting rifle or military weapon. The trajectory or direction the projectile traveled and the distance it had to travel, as well as the profile of the bullet, can contribute considerably to the extent of the injury.

Motor Vehicle Collisions

In motor vehicle crashes there are five typical patterns of impact (frontal, lateral, rear, rotational, and rollover), which are discussed in depth in Chapter 17. Each of these different mechanisms, with the exception of the rear impact, has the potential to cause significant injury to abdominal organs. In a rear impact collision, the patient is less likely to have an injury to his or her abdomen if he or she has been restrained properly. However, if restraints are improperly worn or not used at all, all bets are off—the potential for injury is great.

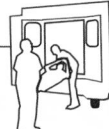 **In the Field**

Always remember the concept of associated injuries. On the basis of the MOI, some of the following syndromes are common:

- Fractures of the lower rib cage → suspect spleen and/or liver injuries
- Upper abdominal injuries → suspect chest trauma
- Pelvic fractures → suspect intra-abdominal trauma (bladder laceration)
- Penetrating wounds at the nipple line → suspect intra-abdominal injury

Rollover impacts present the greatest potential to inflict lethal injuries. Unrestrained occupants may change direction several times with an increased risk of ejection from the vehicle. The occupants involved in a rollover may collide with each other as well as with the vehicle interior, producing a wide range of probable injuries.

Motorcycle Falls or Collisions

With the popularity of motorcycles and the production of high-performance racing bikes that are most attractive to younger and inexperienced riders, motorcycle collisions continue to increase. In a motorcycle crash, any structural protection from a steel cage, as is the case in an automobile, does not exist. The motorcyclist's only protection are those protective devices worn by the rider, such as the helmet and abrasion-resistant or leather pants, gloves, jacket, and boots. Although helmets are designed to protect against impact to the head, they transmit any impact to the cervical spine so they do not protect against severe cervical injury.

Falls From Heights

When an adult falls from a height, the fall usually occurs in the context of criminal activity, attempted suicide, or intoxication. The position or orientation of the body at the moment of impact will help determine the type of injuries sustained and their survivability. The surface onto which the person has fallen, and the degree to which that surface can deform (plasticity) under the force of the falling body can help in dissipating the forces of sudden deceleration.

Blast Injuries

Although most commonly associated with military conflict, blast injuries are also seen in civilian practice in mines, shipyards, chemical plants, and increasingly in association with terrorist activities. Blast injuries, particularly those from weapons designed specifically for antipersonnel effects (such as mines or grenades) can generate fragments traveling at velocities of 4,500′ per second. This is nearly double the velocity of a projectile from a high-speed rifle. Any energy transmitted from a blast fragment will cause extensive and disruptive damage to tissue. People who are injured in explosions may be injured by any of four different mechanisms. The primary blast injury is an injury from the pressure wave. The secondary blast injury is caused by debris or fragments from the explosion. The tertiary blast injury is produced when a victim is propelled through the air and strikes another object. There are also injuries called miscellaneous blast injuries that include burns and respiratory injuries from hot gases or chemicals.

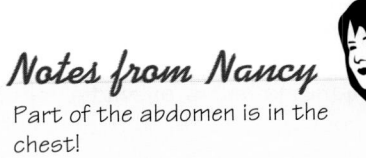

Notes from Nancy

Part of the abdomen is in the chest!

Pathophysiology

Hemorrhage is a major concern in abdominal trauma. It can occur when there is external or internal blood loss. When we

You are the Provider Part 2

The child's parents are alerted, and he is escorted to his school bus. Police officers quickly arrive and stand ready to assist you if necessary. The patient tells you he's unsure exactly how he ended up in the alleyway, but remembers having an argument with a friend. In fact, he cannot tell you where he is other than the name of the town. He does not know the current day, month, or year. In your past experience with him, this is very unusual.

Before moving your patient, you perform an initial assessment and a rapid trauma exam from head-to-toe and find that he is guarding his abdomen. You see bruising from his right upper quadrant, extending from his anterior axillary line across his left upper quadrant, midclavicular line. He also has noticeable swelling and deformity of his left ankle.

Reassessment	Recording Time: 5 Minutes
Level of consciousness	Verbal, oriented only to person and place
Skin	Cool, pale, and slightly moist
Pulse	130 beats/min; weak and regular
Blood pressure	102/60 mm Hg
Respirations	40 breaths/min
Sao$_2$	96% while receiving 15 L/min oxygen via nonrebreathing mask

4. What do these signs indicate to you?
5. What does abdominal guarding usually indicate?
6. Is this condition an early or late finding?

deal with abdominal trauma, especially blunt abdominal trauma, the estimation of the volume of blood lost is difficult. Signs and symptoms will vary greatly depending on the volume of blood lost and the rate at which the body is losing blood. Key indicators of hemorrhagic shock will become apparent with the assessment of the neurologic and cardiovascular systems.

As hypovolemia increases, the patient will have initial agitation and confusion. The heart compensates early for this loss by an increase in heart rate (tachycardia) and stroke volume. As hypoperfusion continues, the coronary arteries can no longer meet the increased demands of the myocardium, which leads to ischemia and heart failure. The symptoms of cardiac dysfunction are demonstrated by the presence of chest pain, tachypnea with adventitious (abnormal) lung sounds, and dysrhythmias. If left untreated, hypoperfusion will result in anaerobic metabolism and acidosis.

Injuries to hollow or solid organs can result in the spillage of their contents into the abdominal cavity. When the enzymes, acids, or bacteria leak from hollow organs into the peritoneal or retroperitoneal space, they cause irritation of the nerve endings. These nerve ending are found in the fascia of the surrounding tissues. As the inflammation affects deeper nerve endings (such as the endings of the afferent nerves), localized pain will result. Pain is localized if the extent of the contamination is confined; pain becomes generalized if the entire peritoneal cavity is involved.

Injuries to Solid Abdominal Organs

The solid organs in the abdomen include the liver, spleen, kidneys, and pancreas. When a solid organ in the abdomen is injured during blunt or penetrating trauma, the organ releases blood into the peritoneal cavity. This can cause nonspecific signs such as tachycardia and hypotension. Because these signs may not develop until a patient has lost a significant volume of blood, normal vital signs do not rule out the possibility that there has been a significant intra-abdominal injury. Bleeding into the peritoneal cavity from solid organ injuries can also produce abdominal tenderness or distention even though the distention may not be evident until the patient has lost nearly all the blood in the abdomen. Palpation of the abdomen may reveal localized or generalized tenderness, rigidity, or rebound tenderness, all of which suggest a peritoneal injury. (Kidney injuries are discussed in Chapter 32.)

Liver Injuries

The superior border of the liver can be as high as the patient's nipples, so a liver injury must be suspected in all patients who have right-sided chest trauma as well as abdominal trauma. When injured, the liver releases blood and bile into the peritoneal cavity. The blood loss can be massive, resulting in abdominal distention, hypotension, tachycardia, shock, and even death. In addition, the release of bile into the peritoneum can produce abdominal pain and peritonitis.

Spleen Injuries

Falls and motor vehicle crashes can injure the spleen. However, less obvious injury patterns in activities such as sports

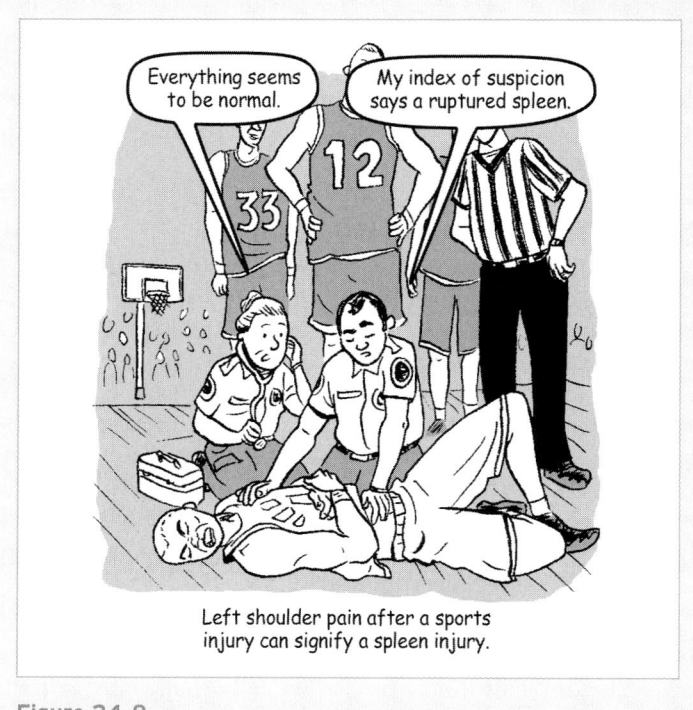

Left shoulder pain after a sports injury can signify a spleen injury.

Figure 24-8

(for instance, tackling in football or checking in lacrosse) can also cause injury to the spleen. There are case reports of patients who have ruptured spleens even though the contact was relatively minor. This is especially true if the spleen is enlarged from mononucleosis or other underlying disease. When the spleen ruptures, blood spills into the peritoneum, which can ultimately cause shock and death. As with other intra-abdominal organ injuries, the signs and symptoms of splenic rupture are nonspecific, and as many as 40% of patients have no symptoms. Some patients report only pain in the left shoulder (Kehr's sign) because of referred pain from diaphragmatic irritation 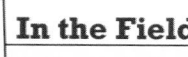 .

Pancreas Injuries

Pancreatic injury occurs in less than 5% of all major abdominal trauma. Because of the anatomical position of the pancreas in

In the Field

In the past, the complete removal of the spleen (splenectomy) was routine for any splenic injury. The surgical approach has changed radically in recent years. The spleen provides an important immune function; without it, people are susceptible to life-threatening infections from organisms that would otherwise not be a problem. Surgeons have devised numerous methods of salvaging the spleen, ranging from simply suturing lacerations to grinding up residual splenic tissue and re-implanting it into the omentum (splenosis). Both splenic preservation techniques limit the risk of sepsis (overwhelming infection).

the retroperitoneum, it is relatively well protected. It typically takes a high-energy force to damage the pancreas. These high-energy forces are most commonly produced by penetrating trauma (for example, from a bullet) but can also be caused by blunt trauma (such as from a motor vehicle crash). In blunt trauma, an unrestrained driver who hits the steering column or a bicyclist who hits the handlebars is at risk of pancreatic injury.

Injuries to the pancreas have subtle or absent signs and symptoms initially and should be suspected in any rapid decelerating injury. Over the course of hours to days, pancreatic injuries result in the spillage of enzymes into the retroperitoneal space, which can damage surrounding structures and lead to infection and retroperitoneal abscess. Injury should be suspected after a localized blow to the midabdomen. These patients usually experience a vague upper and midabdominal pain that radiates to the back. Peritoneal signs may develop several hours after the injury. Patients have been known to develop a form of diabetes after a severe injury to the pancreas.

Diaphragm Injuries

The diaphragm plays the primary role in a patient's ventilatory process. Any injury to the diaphragm will cause signs and symptoms of ventilatory compromise. Diaphragmatic injuries or ruptures are not isolated incidents; patients often have associated thoracic, abdominal, head, and extremity injuries.

Injuries to the diaphragm are rare, and result from both blunt trauma (typically high-speed motor vehicle crashes) and from penetrating trauma. A lateral impact during a motor vehicle crash is most likely to cause a diaphragmatic rupture because of the twisting or distortion of the chest wall that may shear or tear the diaphragm. In frontal motor vehicle crashes, the patient may strike the steering wheel or column. This may cause a significant change in abdominal pressure, which may also tear the diaphragm.

Injuries to Hollow Intraperitoneal Organs

The hollow organs of the abdomen include the stomach, small and large intestines, and bladder. Hollow visceral injuries produce most of their symptoms from peritoneal contamination. When a hollow organ such as the stomach or bowel is injured, it releases its contents into the abdomen. These contents may irritate the abdomen, producing symptoms. When the patient has the seatbelt sign—a contusion or abrasion across the lower abdomen—this usually means that he or she also has intraperitoneal injuries.

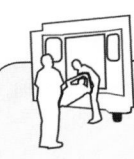
In the Field

The best way to prevent hollow organs (such as the intestines or bladder) from bursting during a car crash is to empty them before you get in the car!

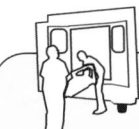
In the Field

During a collision, lap belts cause compression, potentially resulting in the rupture of the small intestine, large intestine, or bladder.

Injuries to the Small and Large Intestines

The intestines are commonly injured from penetrating trauma, although they can be injured from severe blunt trauma as well. When ruptured, the intestines spill their contents (which contain fecal matter and a large amount of bacteria) into the peritoneal or retroperitoneal cavities, resulting in peritonitis.

Stomach Injuries

Most injuries to the stomach result from penetrating trauma; the stomach is rarely injured from blunt trauma. When rupture of the stomach does occur after blunt trauma, it is usually associated with a recent meal or inappropriate use of a seatbelt. Trauma to the stomach fre-

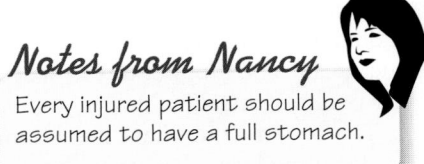
Notes from Nancy

Every injured patient should be assumed to have a full stomach.

quently results in the spillage of acidic material into the peritoneal space, creating a chemical irritation that produces abdominal pain and peritoneal signs relatively quickly, although patients taking antacid medications may have delayed symptoms.

Bladder Injuries

Bladder injuries occur as a result of penetrating and blunt abdominal trauma. The likelihood of a bladder injury varies by the severity of the mechanism, but also by the degree of the bladder distention. The fuller the bladder, the greater the opportunity for injury. Bladder injuries are usually associated with pelvic injuries from motor vehicle crashes, falls from heights, and physical assaults to the lower abdomen. These MOI may cause a pelvic fracture to perforate the bladder.

The signs and symptoms of bladder injuries are generally nonspecific but may present as gross hematuria, suprapubic pain and tenderness, difficulty voiding, and abdominal distention, guarding, or rebound tenderness. The presence of signs of peritoneal irritation may also indicate the possibility of an intraperitoneal bladder rupture.

Retroperitoneal Injuries

Structures contained within the retroperitoneal cavity are the pancreas, kidneys, vascular structures, and part of the small intestine. Injuries confined to the retroperitoneum can be very difficult to diagnose because, in general, they produce few visible signs or symptoms. Because the blood or other contaminants are held in the retroperitoneal space, they do not frequently cause abdominal pain, peritoneal signs, or abdominal distention. Occasionally, retroperitoneal bleeding can lead to ecchymosis of the flanks

(Grey Turner's sign) or around the umbilicus (Cullen's sign). This ecchymosis is usually delayed hours to days, however, and is unreliable in the prehospital setting.

Vascular Injuries

Besides the kidneys, the vascular structures found in the retroperitoneal space include the descending aorta (and its

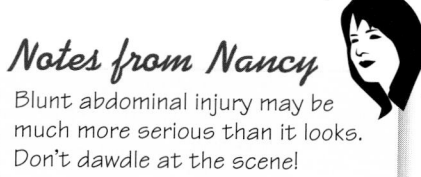

Notes from Nancy
Blunt abdominal injury may be much more serious than it looks. Don't dawdle at the scene!

branches), the superior phrenic artery, the inferior phrenic artery, the inferior vena cava, and the mesenteric vessels. Injuries to these structures occur with both blunt and penetrating trauma, but penetrating trauma is the major cause. Penetrating trauma that causes injury to the great vessels of the abdomen will also be associated with injuries to multiple intra-abdominal organs. Blunt trauma can cause injuries to vascular structures in the intraperitoneal space as they are sheared from their points of attachment.

The patient could have an abdominal aortic aneurysm that has developed and become worse as a result of abdominal trauma. The specifics on abdominal aortic aneurysm are discussed in Chapter 27.

Assessment findings in a patient with vascular injuries depend on whether or not the bleeding is contained (a hematoma) or there is active hemorrhage. In active hemorrhage, the patient will present with significant hypotension, tachycardia, and shock.

Duodenal Injuries

In abdominal trauma, the duodenum can rupture, spilling its contents into the retroperitoneum, usually because of high-speed deceleration injuries **Figure 24-9**. Contamination of the retroperitoneum with duodenal contents may ultimately produce abdominal pain or fever, although symptoms will not likely develop for hours to days. Abdominal pain, nausea, and vomiting may develop, although belatedly. Because of the delayed presentation and variable symptoms, a high degree of suspicion for duodenal injury must be maintained in any abdominal trauma, but especially in high-speed deceleration crashes.

Assessment

During the evaluation of the abdominal cavity, you must look for evidence of hemorrhage (shock) or spillage of bowel contents (pain or tenderness) into the abdominal space. Have a high index of suspicion and understand that intra-abdominal injuries are likely with trauma to the chest or abdomen. Priorities in resuscitation begin with providing adequate tissue perfusion and oxygen delivery. In 10% of mortalities after trauma, the abdominal injury proves to be the primary cause of death; however, in a substantial number of cases, the exact cause of death is not clear.

The evaluation of a patient who has abdominal trauma must be systematic, keeping the entire patient in mind and prioritizing injuries accordingly. Approximately 20% of all patients with significant hemoperitoneum—collection of blood in the abdominal cavity—have a benign abdominal exam upon

You are the Provider Part 3

Given the unclear events surrounding this situation, you take spinal precautions with the patient, apply high-flow supplemental oxygen, and establish a large-bore IV en route to the emergency department.

You are very concerned about internal bleeding and organ damage associated with this apparent blunt trauma and initiate immediate transport to the local trauma center. En route to the hospital, you start a second large-bore IV and splint his left ankle. You administer normal saline wide open with frequent reassessment. You place him on a cardiac monitor. His chief complaint remains pain in his left leg.

Reassessment	Recording Time: 10 Minutes
Level of consciousness	Verbal, still oriented only to person and place
Skin	Cool, pale, and slightly moist
Pulse	130 beats/min, weak and regular
Blood pressure	102/60 mm Hg
Respirations	42 breaths/min
Sao2	96% while receiving 15 L/min via nonrebreathing mask
ECG	Sinus tachycardia

7. Why is it important to provide rapid transport and interventions such as IVs en route to the hospital?
8. Are patients' chief complaints and primary problems always identical?
9. Which organs are at risk of injury given the apparent location of this patient's injury?

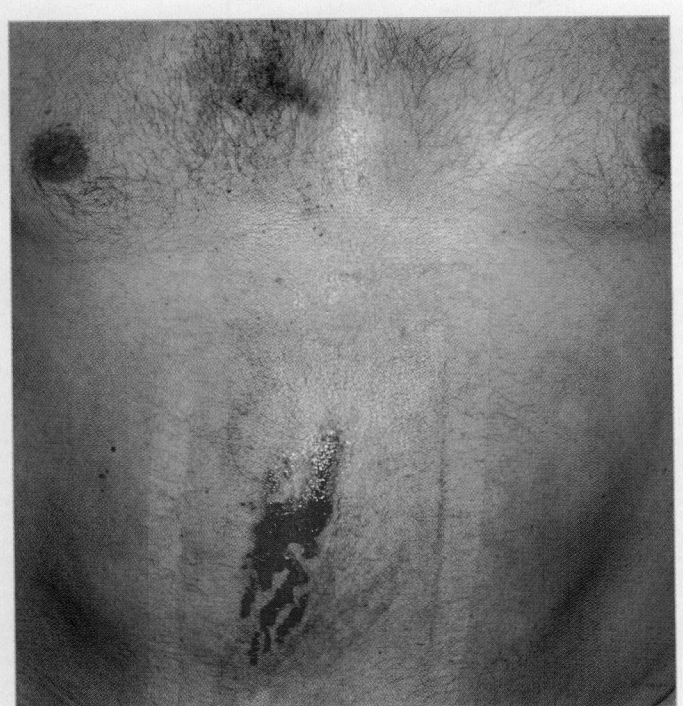

Figure 24-9 Remember that abdominal injury can be severe even in the absence of symptoms. Contamination of the intra-abdominal space may not produce pain or fever for hours or even days.

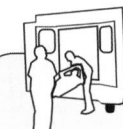

In the Field

All trauma patients should be assumed to have a full stomach, even if they deny recent ingestion of food or liquids.

tizing the patient. Many of these patients live through the initial assessment; their more subtle signs and symptoms are uncovered in the focused history and physical exam.

Focused History and Physical Exam

The first step in the focus history and physical exam is inspection of the abdomen. This means you will need to expose the abdomen and inspect for signs of trauma (such as DCAP-BTLS). Often the injury to the abdomen involves ecchymosis, abrasions, or lacerations.

Blood, gastrointestinal contents, and urine that have spilled into the peritoneum may produce peritonitis that could result in decreased or absent abdominal sounds, but auscultation of bowel sounds is not a useful assessment tool in the prehospital setting. The next steps in the abdominal exam are percussion and palpation. With these maneuvers, look for tenderness and signs of peritonitis (such as the patient guarding his or her abdomen or experiencing pain while being gently moved to the stretcher). Carefully palpate the entire abdomen while assessing the patient's response and noting abdominal masses and deformities.

Controversies

Listening to bowel sounds in the field may not be helpful. To properly auscultate bowel sounds, it is necessary to listen for several minutes. This is not practical in the field, and the ambient noise may be too great to determine the presence or absence of bowel sounds.

A common misconception is that patients without abdominal pain or abnormal vital signs are unlikely to have serious intra-abdominal injuries. Keep in mind that peritonitis can take hours to days to develop. Similarly, nonspecific symptoms such as hypotension, tachycardia, and confusion may not develop until the patient has lost more than 40% of his or her circulating blood volume. Always maintain a high index of suspicion in any patient who has a mechanism of injury consistent with abdominal trauma, regardless of the examination findings.

Special Considerations

Because older people usually have a more flaccid abdominal wall (containing less muscle and more fat) than younger people, apply increased pressure when palpating the abdomen to assess for injury. You should suspect that any older trauma patient who complains of abdominal pain has an internal organ injury.

initial assessment. The abdomen should be examined closely for bruising, road rash, localized swelling, lacerations, distention, or pain. Clues to intra-abdominal trauma will include symptoms of shock not proportional to obvious external evidence or estimated blood loss. Retroperitoneal hemorrhage may be present because of damaged muscle, lacerated or avulsed kidneys, and injuries to the vessels of the supporting mesentery. All abdominal organs have a generous blood supply, making them susceptible to significant bleeding as a result of blunt forces causing a shearing-type injury. An injury to the abdomen can be fatal primarily because of hemorrhage. The injury can be slow to develop, and may be subtle and difficult to locate and assess.

Scene Size-up

As with all other aspects of prehospital care, scene safety remains the priority before providing any patient care. It is always important to remember that if a patient has penetrating or blunt trauma, some external force caused this injury (such as a gun, knife, or the baseball bat in the corner of the room!). These cases could also potentially be dangerous to the paramedic.

Initial Assessment

Once you have sized up the scene and determined that it is safe, the first patient priorities are those of the initial assessment: mental status, airway, breathing, circulation, and priori-

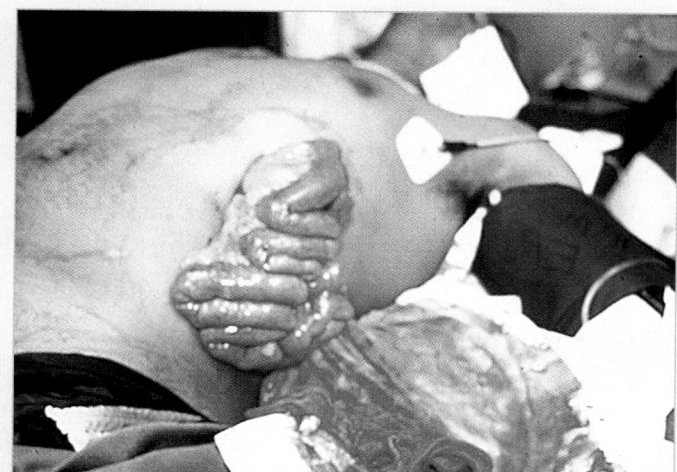

Figure 24-10 An abdominal evisceration is an open abdominal wound from which internal organs or fat protrude.

Abdominal distention is a late indication of abdominal trauma. Patients must have a significant volume of blood enter the abdominal cavity to fill it and produce distention.

Try to obtain as many details about an injury as possible, keeping in mind that trauma patients should be transported to the hospital quickly. In other words, in addition to getting information about the patient (such as the SAMPLE history), it is important to obtain details on how the injury occurred, whether from the patient, witnesses, police, or other EMS providers.

In blunt trauma caused by a motor vehicle collision, determine the types of vehicles involved, the speed at which they were traveling, and how the cars collided. You should also try to find out other information about the event, such as the use of seatbelts, the deployment of air bags, and the patient's position in the vehicle.

In penetrating trauma, it's helpful to identify the type of weapon used. However, this is often impossible because assailants usually leave with their weapon. In a gunshot case, determine the type of gun and the number of shots, if possible. Providers should try to ascertain an estimated distance between the victim and the assailant whenever possible. In stab wounds, determine the type of knife, possible angle of the entrance wound, and number of stab wounds.

As part of the focused history and physical exam of a trauma patient, you may be faced with a number of challenges associated with abdominal trauma. You may discover the presence of an abdominal eviceration—displacement of an organ outside the body **Figure 24-10 ▲**. This is where the abdominal organs are found protruding through a wound in the abdominal wall. Generally, little pain is associated with this type of injury; do not apply any material that will adhere to the abdominal structures. Providers may also be confronted with impaled objects **Figure 24-11 ▶**. Impaled objects are stabilized and transported in the position they were found. Stabilization of impaled objects can be impractical under some field conditions, but effective stabilization and safe transportation

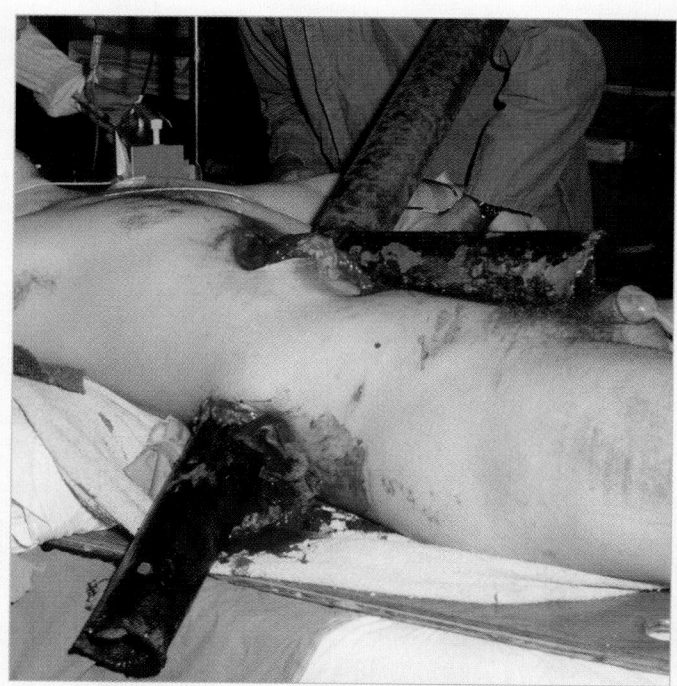

Figure 24-11 An object impaled in the abdomen.

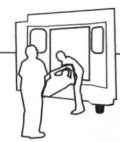 **In the Field**

Always examine the back of the patient as carefully as you examine the front. Gunshot wounds or stab wounds can easily be missed in creases of the body, especially if the patient is obese or has large quantities of body hair.

can help reduce serious tissue damage. Additionally, significant infection often develops in this type of wound, so early intervention with sterile techniques should be employed.

If you suspect injury to the diaphragm, focus on the airway, breathing, and circulatory status of the patient. Remember that the diaphragm plays a large role in the mechanical process of breathing. Examine the patient's neck and chest, paying particular attention to the trachea (tracheal deviation due to mediastinal shift), symmetry of the chest during expansion, and absence of breath sounds.

In the Field

Cullen's sign is a black-and-blue discoloration (ecchymosis) in the umbilical region caused by peritoneal bleeding. Grey Turner's sign includes ecchymosis present in the lower abdominal and flank regions. They are both caused by intra-abdominal bleeding found 12 to 24 hours after the initial injury. The presence of these signs is helpful, but their absence does not rule out life-threatening abdominal hemorrhage.

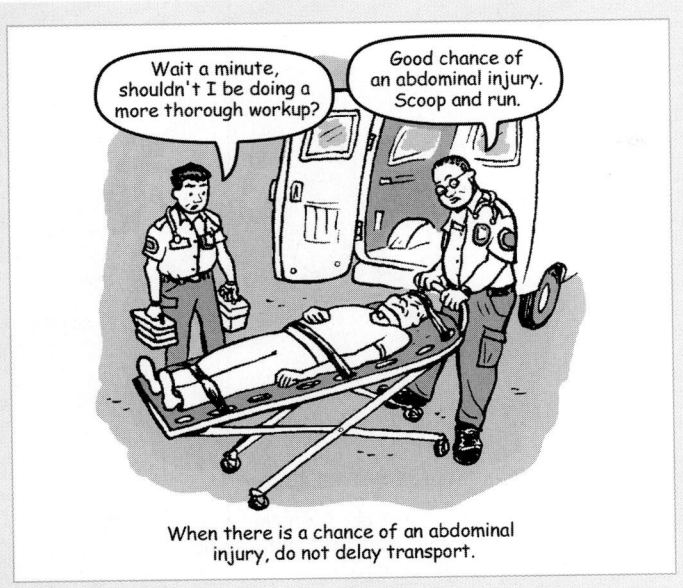

When there is a chance of an abdominal injury, do not delay transport.

Figure 24-12

Detailed Physical Exam

Perform a detailed physical exam on a patient who has abdominal trauma and was found to have a significant MOI. Because, at this point, you will have completed the initial assessment as well as the rapid trauma exam, the detailed physical exam should be conducted en route to the emergency department to avoid any unnecessary delays **Figure 24-12 ▲**. Basically, the detailed physical exam assesses the same structures as the rapid trauma exam, except

Notes from Nancy

An injury to the chest anywhere below the nipples is also an injury to the abdomen.

Documentation and Communication

Pertinent field documentation of the abdominal trauma assessment should include the following: whether or not seatbelts were worn, which type, and their position on the patient; the location, intensity, and quality of pain; whether or not nausea or vomiting is present; the contour of the abdomen; any ecchymosis or open areas present on the soft-tissue inspection; the presence or absence of rebound tenderness, guarding, rigidity, spasm, or localized pain; any changes in the level of consciousness and serial vital signs; other injuries found; the presence or absence of alcohol, narcotics, or any type of analgesic; and the results of your ongoing assessment.

more methodically. Close examination may uncover additional findings that were either not picked up during the rapid trauma exam or are only now starting to develop (such as hematoma, bruises, or tender areas). As long as you can ensure that the problems found in the initial assessment have been attended to, and there is time en route, perform a very thorough detailed physical exam on your patient.

Ongoing Assessment

The ongoing assessment includes reassessment of the initial assessment as well as retaking vital signs and checking interventions on the patient.

▌Management Overview

In general, the prehospital management of patients who have abdominal trauma is straightforward. As always, ensuring an open airway while taking spinal precautions is the first step. Administer high-concentration oxygen to the patient via a nonrebreathing mask. Establish IV access with two large-bore lines, and start replacing fluid with lactated Ringer's solution or normal saline (lactated Ringer's solution is the preferred crystalloid). Do not delay transport to initiate IV therapy; establish IV lines whenever possible during transport. Minimize external hemorrhage by applying pressure dressings. Apply a cardiac monitor. Transport the patient to the appropriate hospital or regional trauma center, depending on your local transport protocols. Note that the assessment should also not delay patient care and transport. Repeated abdominal examinations are the key to discovering a patient's worsening condition before vital signs change. Perform your exams en route during the ongoing assessment.

In some cases of penetrating injury, part of an abdominal organ may protrude outside of the body (evisceration). If this occurs, do not attempt to place the organ back into the body. Rather, cover it with a sterile dressing moistened with saline, and protect the organ from damage during transport.

Administering pain medication is somewhat controversial as it may mask symptoms and often is contraindicated because of the patient's hypotension. In most instances, it may be appropriate to consult with medical direction en route to the hospital to discuss analgesia.

Notes from Nancy

A distended, tender abdomen after injury means internal bleeding. Treat for shock and transport immediately.

▌Pelvic Fractures

The pelvis is best thought of as a ring, with its sacral, iliac, ischial, and pubic bones held together by ligaments. Large

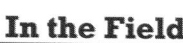

In the Field

There is an old medical school scenario of a patient who was shot in the head who is hypotensive. The puzzle is, "What's wrong with the patient?" The answer, as we have learned in this chapter, is that the patient was probably shot in the belly with a second bullet! Always remember that hemorrhaging will continue until controlled in the operating room under "bright lights and cold steel." Survival may be determined by the length of time from the injury to definitive surgical control of the hemorrhage. Delays in the field may negatively impact the patient's long-term survival. So, if you are not the solution to this patient's problem, don't add to the problem. Get the patient to the trauma center!

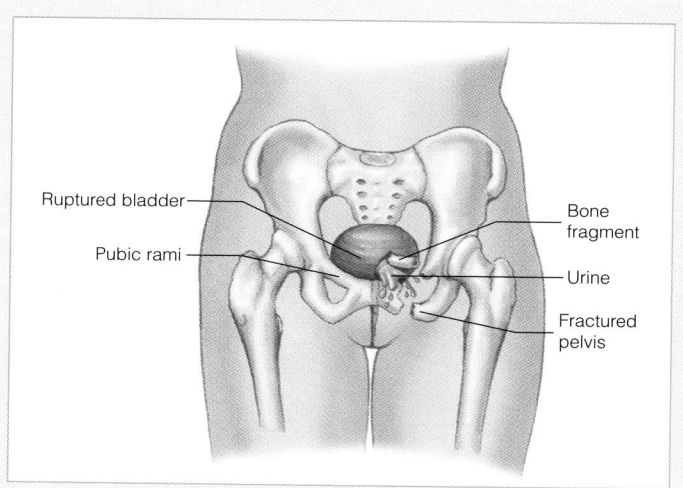

Figure 24-13 Pelvic fractures occasionally cause laceration of the bladder as a result of penetration by bony fragments. Externally, pelvic fractures can cause severe bruising and swelling.

forces are required to damage this ring. The majority of pelvic fractures are a result of blunt trauma from motor vehicle collision or from vehicles striking pedestrians.

Because of the forces required to break the pelvis, suspect multisystem trauma if your patient has a pelvic injury (until proven otherwise). Commonly associated injuries are urethral disruptions, bladder rupture, and abdominal, thoracic, and head trauma **Figure 24-13 ▶**. Signs and symptoms of blunt trauma to the pelvis include pain in the pelvis, groin, or hips; hematomas or contusions to the pelvic region; obvious external bleeding; or hypotension without obvious external bleeding.

Special Considerations

Pediatric trauma patients are less likely to have pelvic fractures than adults.

Anteroposterior compression, which can result from a head-on collision, may lead to an "open-book" pelvic fracture in which the pubic symphysis spreads apart. The subsequent increase in volume of the pelvis means a patient with internal pelvic bleeding may lose a much larger amount of blood than someone without an open-book fracture. Such patients will require IV fluids with lactated Ringer's solution or normal saline but may still remain hypotensive in the field.

Lateral compression of the pelvis results from a side impact. It generally does not result in an unstable pelvis.

Because the volume in the pelvis is reduced, not increased, life-threatening hemorrhage is less of a concern in such cases.

Vertical shear is seen in falls from heights. It results in one side of the pelvis moving superiorly or inferiorly compared to the other, disrupting the bony or ligamentous structures. This unstable fracture results in an increased pelvic volume.

Saddle injuries result from falling on an object. They may result in fractures of the bones that are directly under the female and male genitalia (pubic rami fractures).

Although penetrating trauma to the pelvis may result in bony fractures, the more worrisome injury is to the major vascular structures, which can cause life-threatening hemorrhage. Open fractures (not to be confused with open-book fractures) may result from either penetrating or blunt trauma and frequently result in chronic pain and disability that persist for years after the initial injury.

Assessment and Management

Properly evaluating and treating the patient is more important than identifying the specific type of pelvic fracture. A search for entry and exit wounds for a penetrating trauma is helpful but an extended search should never delay quick transport and treatment of hypotension. In both blunt and penetrating

You are the Provider Part 4

Upon your arrival at the hospital, the patient's condition is immediately evaluated and he is taken to surgery. You later learn that he had significant blood loss from liver lacerations and a ruptured spleen. He also had multiple fractures of his left distal tibia and fibula as a result of several blows from a baseball bat.

10. How can age and medical problems make traumatic injuries worse?

Controversies

Anecdotal cases of the successful use of the pneumatic antishock garment (PASG) in the treatment of ruptured aortic aneurysms and ectopic pregnancy abound, especially in areas with prolonged transport times. Always follow your local protocols.

trauma, the presence of thoracic trauma may result in a life-threatening tension pneumothorax. In addition, if you suspect an open-book pelvic fracture in a patient with hypotension, tie a sheet around the patient's hips at the level of the superior anterior iliac crests, thereby decreasing the pelvic volume.

There are several devices specific to the management of this type of injury that provide superior immobilization and are faster to apply. One device, the SAM Sling, has a patented "autostop" buckle to provide the correct circumferential force to close and stabilize open-book pelvic fractures.

The pneumatic antishock garment (PASG) is a controversial treatment that can be used to stabilize the pelvis during rapid transports. It can potentially decrease pain by causing less movement of the fractured bones and decrease bleeding by reducing pelvic volume, although some emergency medicine specialists believe that the PASG may increase bleeding by putting pressure on pelvic vessels. For a review of this skill, see Chapter 18.

You are the Provider Summary

1. What are your immediate concerns?

Your first priority is always scene safety. Given your previous exposure to the patient and your knowledge of his history of drugs, alcohol, and assaultive behavior, you should discretely request police response as well as ask one of your department members to locate the child's parents. If the child's parents are not available, he should be moved to a safe location (possibly to school) until his parents or his legal guardian can be contacted.

2. What about this patient immediately grabs your attention?

The patient's location, his level of consciousness, and his body position are immediate causes for concern. Given the time of day, question how long he has been lying in this location. You should also wonder about the possibilities of alcohol and/or drug use and their effects in limiting your patient's ability to accurately perceive pain and injury.

3. At this point, what are your treatment priorities?

Assessing and managing life-threatening conditions is always your top priority. A patient who exhibits a decreased level of consciousness, tachycardia, and tachypnea should be treated swiftly and appropriately.

4. What do these signs indicate to you?

Given the patient's decreased level of consciousness, skin signs, tachycardia, and hypotension in the presence of abdominal guarding, he has likely lost a significant amount of blood.

5. What does abdominal guarding usually indicate?

Abdominal guarding usually indicates peritonitis, an inflammation of the lining of the abdomen that results from either blood or hollow organ contents spilling into the abdominal cavity.

6. Is this condition an early or late finding?

Peritonitis is a late finding: It can take hours or even days to develop. Blood loss significant enough to produce signs and symptoms of shock may not develop until 60% or more of the patient's blood volume is lost. For this reason, you should be highly suspicious of injuries resulting from significant blunt or penetrating trauma. Patients with these injuries can appear to have normal vital signs in the presence of significant injuries in the early stages.

7. Why is it important to provide rapid transport and interventions such as IVs en route to the hospital?

Definitive care for the trauma patient is available at the nearest appropriate trauma center. To delay transport so as to initiate IVs, splint fractures, and the like would delay the care the patient ultimately needs. Be aware of scene times, striving to keep these to 10 minutes or less. Obviously, if extra time has to be spent on the scene for issues such as extrication, provide interventions as required and document the reasons for the delayed transport.

8. Are patients' chief complaints and primary problems always identical?

Your patients may or may not complain of pain or discomfort associated with the source of their primary problem. In this scenario, the patient is more concerned about his leg and ankle pain; you should be more concerned about the internal bleeding in his abdomen. This is an important lesson for any paramedic—don't allow yourself to become consumed with the outward, most obvious injuries, as they may or may not be life threatening.

9. Which organs are at risk of injury given the apparent location of this patient's injury?

You should be worried that the liver and spleen could have significant damage given the patient's skin condition and vital signs. Injury to one or both of these organs can produce significant bleeding. The liver can suffer lacerations as well as contusions in blunt trauma, and the spleen is at great risk of rupture.

10. How can age and medical problems make traumatic injuries worse?

Geriatric and pediatric patients do not have the same compensatory mechanisms that healthy young and middle-aged adults possess. Extremes of age (and disease processes such as diabetes, heart conditions, and high blood pressure, along with their accompanying medicines) can mask signs and symptoms in otherwise healthy patients. Also, mechanisms of injury and their associated damage can change with age. Children who are struck by cars have different injury patterns than those of adults. Older patients on beta-blockers are not able to compensate for blood loss with increased heart rates in the same way that younger patients can. For this reason, whenever possible, you should obtain a trauma patient's medical history, including medications and allergies.

Prep Kit

Ready for Review

- Unrecognized abdominal trauma is the leading cause of unexpected death in trauma patients. Recognizing abdominal injuries and providing rapid transport is one of the best contributions you can make to a patient who has these injuries.
- The abdomen contains many vital organs and structures, including the kidneys, liver, spleen, pancreas, diaphragm, small and large intestines, stomach, bladder, and several great vessels.
- The quadrant system is generally used to describe a location in the abdomen. These are the right upper quadrant (RUQ), the right lower quadrant (RLQ), the left lower quadrant (LLQ), and the left upper quadrant (LUQ).
- The peritoneum is a membrane that lines the abdominal cavity. Abdominal trauma can lead to peritonitis, an inflammation of the peritoneum that results from either blood or hollow organ contents spilling into the abdominal cavity. This is a life-threatening infection.
- The retroperitoneal space is the area behind the peritoneum and contains the aorta, vena cava, pancreas, kidneys, ureters, and portions of the duodenum and large intestine.
- When a patient has experienced trauma to the chest or abdomen, suspect that he or she also has additional internal abdominal injuries. Also suspect abdominal trauma in patients who have unexplained symptoms of shock.
- Injury to the abdomen can be slow to develop, and can be fatal. An injury may be subtle and difficult to locate and assess.
- Solid organs such as the liver and spleen have a large blood supply and can easily be crushed by blunt trauma. The abdomen and retroperitoneum can accommodate large amounts of blood but produce few signs and symptoms.
- Injury to hollow organs can cause the release of toxins such as urine, bile, or stomach acid into the abdominal cavity, causing major peritonitis.
- At least two thirds of all abdominal injuries involve blunt trauma, occurring mostly during motor vehicle collisions. Blunt trauma can often lead to a closed abdominal injury.
- Penetrating trauma most commonly results from stab wounds or low-velocity gunshot wounds. Penetrating trauma causes open abdominal injury.
- During the assessment, try to obtain as many details about an injury as possible. Also note the use of seatbelts, deployment of air bags, and the patient's position in the vehicle. If a weapon was involved, note the type of weapon if this information is available.
- Peritonitis can take hours to days to develop. Shock, tachycardia, and confusion may not develop until the patient has lost a significant amount of blood. Maintain a high index of suspicion for a patient who has a mechanism of injury consistent with abdominal trauma, regardless of vital signs and other findings.
- Generally, management of patients with abdominal trauma is straightforward:
  - Ensure a secure airway.
  - Establish intravenous access and fluid replacement without delaying transport.
  - Minimize hemorrhaging with pressure dressings.
  - Apply a cardiac monitor and oxygen therapy, and then transport.
- Assessment should never delay patient care and transport!
- Pelvic fractures can result in damage to the major vascular structures, which can cause life-threatening hemorrhage.
- Because of the forces required to break the pelvis, if the patient has a pelvic fracture, suspect multisystem trauma.

Vital Vocabulary

blunt trauma Injury resulting from compression or deceleration forces, potentially crushing an organ or causing it to rupture.

closed abdominal injury An injury in which there is soft-tissue damage inside the body, but the skin remains intact.

duodenum The first part of the small intestine.

evisceration Displacement of an organ outside the body.

hemoperitoneum The presence of extravasated blood in the peritoneal cavity.

Kehr's sign Left shoulder pain that may indicate a ruptured spleen.

mesentery A membranous double fold of tissue in the abdomen that attaches various organs to the body wall.

open abdominal injury An injury in which there is a break in the surface of the skin or mucous membrane, exposing deeper tissue to potential contamination.

penetrating trauma An injury in which the skin is broken; direct contact results in laceration of the structure.

peritoneum A membrane in the abdomen encasing the liver, spleen, diaphragm, stomach, and transverse colon.

peritonitis Inflammation of the peritoneum (the lining around the abdominal cavity) that results from either blood or hollow organ contents spilling into the abdominal cavity.

periumbilical Pertaining to the area around the umbilicus.

pylorus A circumferential muscle at the end of the stomach that acts as a valve between the stomach and duodenum.

retroperitoneal space The area in the abdomen containing the aorta, vena cava, pancreas, kidneys, ureters, and portions of the duodenum and large intestine.

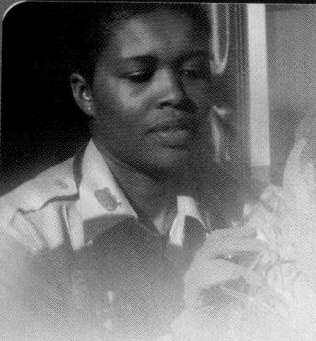

Assessment in Action

You are dispatched to a motor vehicle collision at an intersection. When you arrive, you find two vehicles, one which is broadsided on the driver's side. The driver is still in the vehicle and the fire department is in the process of extricating her. You notice that the damage to the driver's side door is significant with extensive damage to the B post. There is approximately an 18″ intrusion.

The driver is conscious, alert, and oriented. She is complaining only of pain in the left upper quadrant of her abdomen, just below her rib cage. Her vital signs are: respirations, 20 breaths/min; pulse, 130 beats/min; blood pressure, 100/60 mm Hg; and pulse oximetry, 98% on room air. The patient's c-spine is immobilized and she is removed from the vehicle. In the ambulance, you perform a complete assessment. Everything is unremarkable except she has pain on palpation to her left upper quadrant and pain in her left shoulder. Her abdomen is soft, and she is not guarding it. You initiate two large-bore IVs, apply oxygen, and transport the patient to the nearest trauma-designated hospital.

1. **What type of injury should you suspect?**
   - A. Lacerated liver
   - B. Ruptured spleen
   - C. Contusion of the heart
   - D. Ruptured appendix

2. **What type of impact did this patient receive?**
   - A. Frontal impact
   - B. Rear impact
   - C. Lateral or side impact
   - D. Rotational impact

3. **Which are solid organs of the abdomen?**
   - A. Liver, spleen, kidneys, and pancreas
   - B. Liver, spleen, and pancreas
   - C. Large intestine, small intestine, and kidneys
   - D. Liver, spleen, kidneys, and intestines

4. **On-scene care of a patient who has signs of shock from abdominal injury should include which of the following?**
   - A. Comprehensive physical exam
   - B. Initiation of IV fluid therapy
   - C. Ongoing assessment
   - D. Oxygen administration

5. **When the spleen ruptures, blood spills into the:**
   - A. duodenum.
   - B. peritoneum.
   - C. stomach.
   - D. pylorus.

6. **Some patients who have a splenic injury may report only left shoulder pain. This is called:**
   - A. Cullen's sign.
   - B. Grey Turner's sign.
   - C. Peritoneal's sign.
   - D. Kehr's sign.

7. **The abdominal cavity is lined with a membrane called the:**
   - A. retroperitoneal space.
   - B. pylorus.
   - C. peritoneum.
   - D. periumbilical.

8. **The spleen is a highly vascular organ that lies in the _____ quadrant.**
   - A. right upper
   - B. left lower
   - C. left upper
   - D. right lower

9. **Rupture of an organ can lead to hemorrhage and:**
   - A. peritoneum.
   - B. peritonitis.
   - C. hemoperitoneum.
   - D. internal bleeding.

10. **True or false? Patients without abdominal pain or abnormal vital signs are unlikely to have serious intra-abdominal injuries.**
    - A. True
    - B. False

Challenging Questions

You are dispatched to the local bar for an assault victim. On arrival you find a 38-year-old man on the ground, conscious, and alert and orientated to person, place, and time. He is in the right lateral recumbent position. You notice a large pool of blood under him. He has a weak radial pulse and his skin is cool, pale, and diaphoretic. His vital signs are: respirations, 40 breaths/min; pulse, 120 beats/min with sinus tachycardia on the monitor; systolic blood pressure, 80 mm Hg; and pulse oximetry, 92% on room air. He is complaining of pain to his stomach and is becoming very agitated. There is a 12″ knife lying next to him. You check his back for wounds and then quickly log roll him onto a backboard and provide c-spine precautions. On examination of the abdomen, you see a stab wound to the upper right quadrant. You immediately move the patient to your ambulance.

11. **What type of injury should you suspect?**

12. **What are the major complications of a lacerated liver?**

13. **What is your further treatment for this patient?**

■ Points to Ponder

You are called to the scene of a minor car collision in which a car has hit a telephone pole. When you arrive, you immediately notice that the driver is not inside the car. The air bag has deployed, but the windshield appears intact. The steering wheel appears slightly deformed. Bystanders say the car was not traveling very fast when it hit the pole. They do not think the driver was wearing a seatbelt.

You approach the driver to ask him about the crash. He is sitting on the grass, with no apparent external injuries. Even though it is early afternoon, you smell what you think is alcohol as you speak with him. He tells you he doesn't know how the crash happened, but he insists he is fine and doesn't want to be examined or questioned. Though you can see no injuries, he is guarding his abdomen, and grimaces as though he's in pain as you're speaking. The more you try to encourage him to be examined by either you or a doctor, the more defensive and angry he gets. You tell him the risks of not being examined, and tell him he can sign a consent form to not be treated. He agrees to let you take his vital signs and then signs the consent form to refuse treatment. His blood pressure is 80/60 mm Hg; pulse, 130 beats/min; and respirations, 27 breaths/min.

When you find this, what do you do?

Issues: Thorough Scene Size-up, Thorough Assessment, Patient Refusal of Treatment.

25 Musculoskeletal Injuries

Objectives

Cognitive

4-9.1 Describe the incidence, morbidity, and mortality of musculoskeletal injuries. (p 25.3)

4-9.2 Discuss the anatomy and physiology of the musculoskeletal system. (p 25.3)

4-9.3 Predict injuries based on the mechanism of injury, including:
- a. Direct
- b. Indirect
- c. Pathologic (p 25.12)

4-9.4 Discuss the types of musculoskeletal injuries:
- a. Fracture (open and closed)
- b. Dislocation/fracture
- c. Sprain
- d. Strain (p 25.14–25.17)

4-9.5 Discuss the pathophysiology of musculoskeletal injuries. (p 25.12)

4-9.6 Discuss the assessment findings associated with musculoskeletal injuries. (p 25.19)

4-9.7 List the six "P"s of musculoskeletal injury assessment. (p 25.19)

4-9.8 List the primary signs and symptoms of extremity trauma. (p 25.19)

4-9.9 List other signs and symptoms that can indicate less obvious extremity injury. (p 25.19)

4-9.10 Discuss the need for assessment of pulses, motor and sensation before and after splinting. (p 25.24)

4-9.11 Identify the need for rapid intervention and transport when dealing with musculoskeletal injuries. (p 25.23)

4-9.12 Discuss the management of musculoskeletal injuries. (p 25.23)

4-9.13 Discuss the general guidelines for splinting. (p 25.23)

4-9.14 Explain the benefits of cold application for musculoskeletal injury. (p 25.23)

4-9.15 Explain the benefits of heat application for musculoskeletal injury. (p 25.23)

4-9.16 Describe age associated changes in the bones. (p 25.7)

4-9.17 Discuss the pathophysiology of open and closed fractures. (p 25.14)

4-9.18 Discuss the relationship between volume of hemorrhage and open or closed fractures. (p 25.18)

4-9.19 Discuss the assessment findings associated with fractures. (p 25.18)

4-9.20 Discuss the management of fractures. (p 25.23)

4-9.21 Discuss the usefulness of the pneumatic anti-shock garment (PASG) in the management of fractures. (p 25.25)

4-9.22 Describe the special considerations involved in femur fracture management. (p 25.27)

4-9.23 Discuss the pathophysiology of dislocations. (p 25.16)

4-9.24 Discuss the assessment findings of dislocations. (p 25.16)

4-9.25 Discuss the out-of-hospital management of dislocation/fractures, including splinting and realignment. (p 25.36)

4-9.26 Explain the importance of manipulating a knee dislocation/fracture with an absent distal pulse. (p 25.37)

4-9.27 Describe the procedure for reduction of a shoulder, finger or ankle dislocation/ fracture. (p 25.36)

4-9.28 Discuss the pathophysiology of sprains. (p 25.16)

4-9.29 Discuss the assessment findings of sprains. (p 25.16)

4-9.30 Discuss the management of sprains. (p 25.17)

4-9.31 Discuss the pathophysiology of strains. (p 25.17)

4-9.32 Discuss the assessment findings of strains. (p 25.17)

4-9.33 Discuss the management of strains. (p 25.17)

4-9.34 Discuss the pathophysiology of a tendon injury. (p 25.17)

4-9.35 Discuss the assessment findings of tendon injury. (p 25.17)

4-9.36 Discuss the management of a tendon injury. (p 25.17)

4-9.37 Integrate the pathophysiological principles to the assessment of a patient with a musculoskeletal injury. (p 25.18)

4-9.38 Differentiate between musculoskeletal injuries based on the assessment findings and history. (p 25.18)

4-9.39 Formulate a field impression of a musculoskeletal injury based on the assessment findings. (p 25.20)

4-9.40 Develop a patient management plan for the musculoskeletal injury based on the field impression. (p 25.23)

Affective

4-9.41 Advocate the use of a thorough assessment to determine a working diagnosis and treatment plan for musculoskeletal injuries. (p 25.19)

4-9.42 Advocate for the use of pain management in the treatment of musculoskeletal injuries. (p 25.23)

Psychomotor

4-9.43 Demonstrate a clinical assessment to determine the proper treatment plan for a patient with a suspected musculoskeletal injury. (p 25.19)

4-9.44 Demonstrate the proper use of fixation, soft and traction splints for a patient with a suspected fracture. (p 25.27)

Introduction

Musculoskeletal injuries are one of the most common reasons that patients seek medical attention. Complaints related to the musculoskeletal system lead to almost 60 million visits to physicians annually in the United States, more than for any other reason. Approximately 1 in 7 Americans will experience some type of musculoskeletal impairment, leading to millions of missed days of work or school and costing hundreds of billions of dollars yearly. An estimated 70% to 80% of all patients with multiple system trauma have one or more musculoskeletal injuries. Some areas of public policy, legislative changes, and public education have been effective in reducing the injury problem. For example, efforts related to cell phone use by drivers, child safety seat use and availability, and falls in older people have had positive impacts.

Injuries related to the musculoskeletal system are usually easily identifiable because of the associated pain, swelling, and deformity. Although these injuries are rarely fatal, they often result in short- or long-term disability. By providing prompt temporary measures, such as splinting and analgesia, paramedics may help reduce the period during which patients are disabled. However, despite the sometimes dramatic appearance of these injuries, you should not focus on the musculoskeletal injury without first determining that no life-threatening injury exists. *Never forget the ABCs!*

Anatomy and Physiology of the Musculoskeletal System

The musculoskeletal system gives the body its shape and allows for its movement. It is essential that you understand its basic anatomy and physiology.

Functions of the Musculoskeletal System

The musculoskeletal system performs many important functions within the body. Bones help *support* the soft tissues of the body and form a framework that gives the human body its shape and allows it to maintain an erect posture. *Movement* is generated because muscles are attached to bones by tendons. (Reminder: Muscles-To-Bones [MTB] means Muscles–Tendons–Bones.) When a muscle contracts, the force generated by the muscle is transferred to a bone on the opposite side of the joint from the muscle, leading to motion. Bones also offer *protection* to the more fragile organs and structures beneath them—for example, the skull's protection of the brain, the rib cage's protection of the heart and lungs, and the spinal column's protection of the spinal cord.

Another important function of the musculoskeletal system is hematopoiesis—the process of generating blood cells. In adults, it most commonly occurs in the red bone marrow of the sternum, ribs, vertebral bodies, pelvis, and the proximal portions of the femur and humerus. Each day, the body produces new red blood cells, white blood cells, and platelets from the stem cells that are present in the bone marrow, thereby replacing those that have been lost or that are no longer functional.

The Body's Scaffolding: The Skeleton

The integrated structure formed by the 206 bones of the body is called the skeleton. It may be divided into two distinct portions: the axial skeleton and the appendicular skeleton. The axial skeleton is composed of the bones of the central part, or axis, of the body; its divisions include the vertebral column, skull, ribs, and sternum. The skull is composed of the cranium, basilar skull, face, and inner ear Figure 25-1 ▶ .

The spine is composed of 33 spinal vertebrae: 7 cervical, 12 thoracic, 5 lumbar, 5 sacral, and 4 coccygeal. Moving anteriorly, the thorax is formed by the sternum and 12 pairs of

You are the Provider Part 1

You are dispatched to a private residence for a man who has fallen off a ladder. En route to the scene, dispatch advises you that a neighbor witnessed the incident and estimated the fall to be 15′ to 20′. The witness also reports the man appears to be awake and breathing and looks to be in great pain.

On arrival, you find a 63-year-old man on the ground next to a ladder that is leaning against the house. He complains of pain in his left leg and left wrist, is slow to respond to your questions, but remembers what happened.

Initial Assessment	Recording Time: 0 Minutes
Appearance	Wincing and holding his left arm
Level of consciousness	A (Alert to person, place, and day)
Airway	Patent
Breathing	Rapid with adequate tidal volume
Circulation	Blood-soaked left sleeve, rapid radial pulse

1. What are your initial assessment and treatment priorities?
2. What other information should be obtained about the patient and the incident?

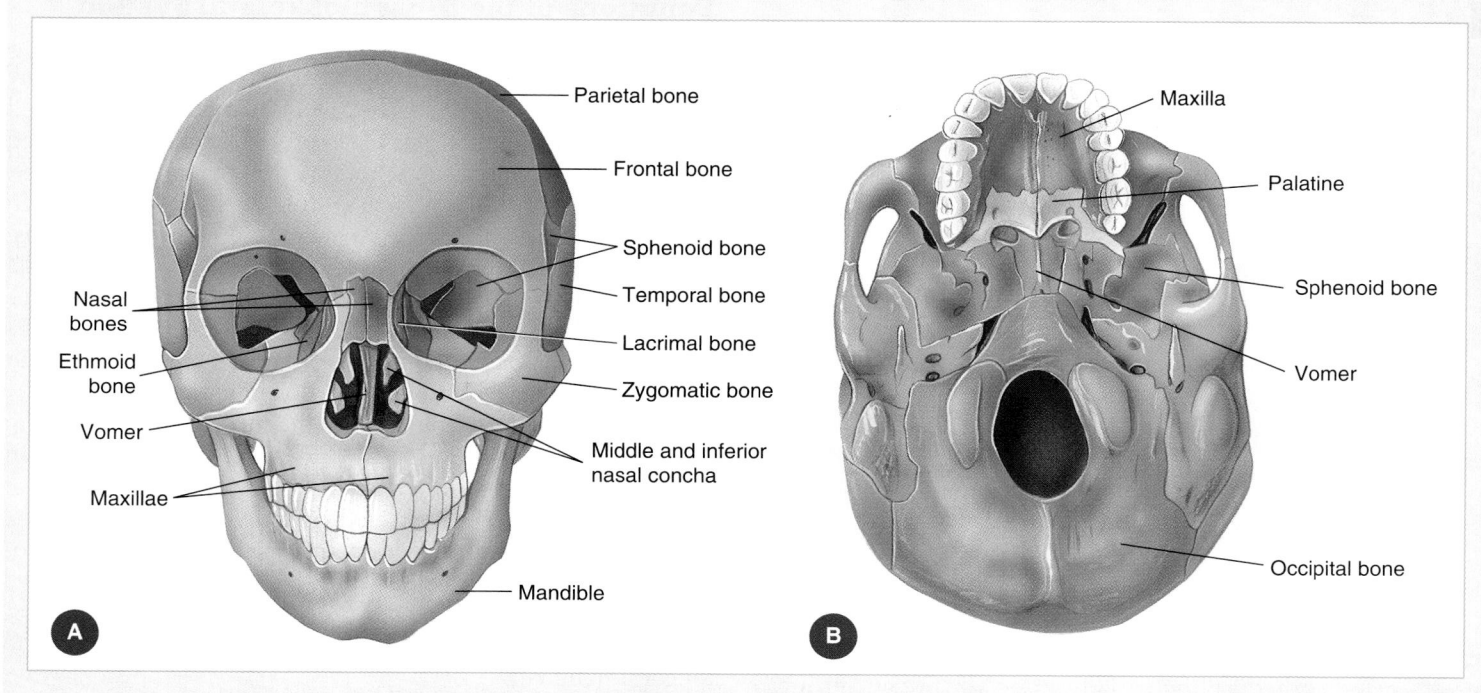

Figure 25-1 The skull and its components. **A.** Front view. **B.** Bottom view.

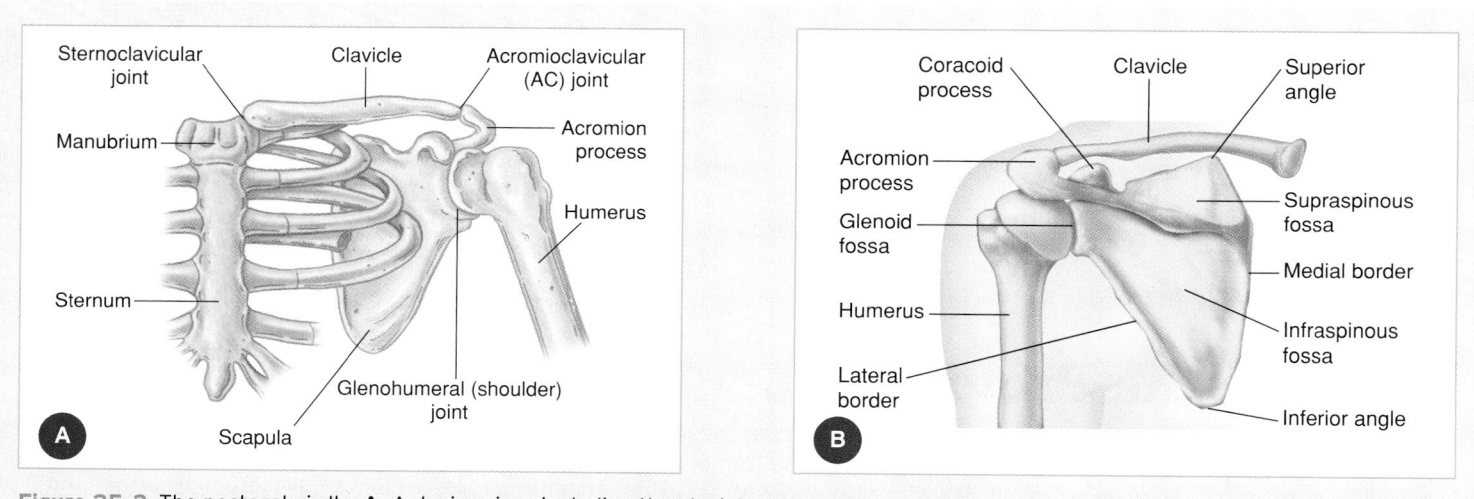

Figure 25-2 The pectoral girdle. **A.** Anterior view, including the clavicle. **B.** Posterior view, including the scapula.

ribs. The appendicular skeleton is divided into the pectoral girdle, the pelvic girdle, and the bones of the upper and lower extremities.

Shoulder and Upper Extremities

The pectoral girdle (Figure 25-2 ▲), also referred to as the shoulder girdle, consists of two scapulae and two clavicles. The scapula (shoulder blade) is a flat, triangular bone held to the rib cage posteriorly by powerful muscles that buffer it against injury. The clavicle (collarbone) is a slender, S-shaped bone attached by ligaments at the medial end to the sternum and at the lateral end to the raised tip of the scapula, called the acromion. The clavicle acts as a strut to keep the shoulder propped up; however, because it is slender and very exposed, this bone is vulnerable to injury.

The upper extremity (Figure 25-3 ▶) joins the shoulder girdle at the glenohumeral joint. The proximal portion contains the humerus, a bone that articulates proximally with the scapula and distally with bones of the forearm—the radius and ulna—to form the hinged elbow joint.

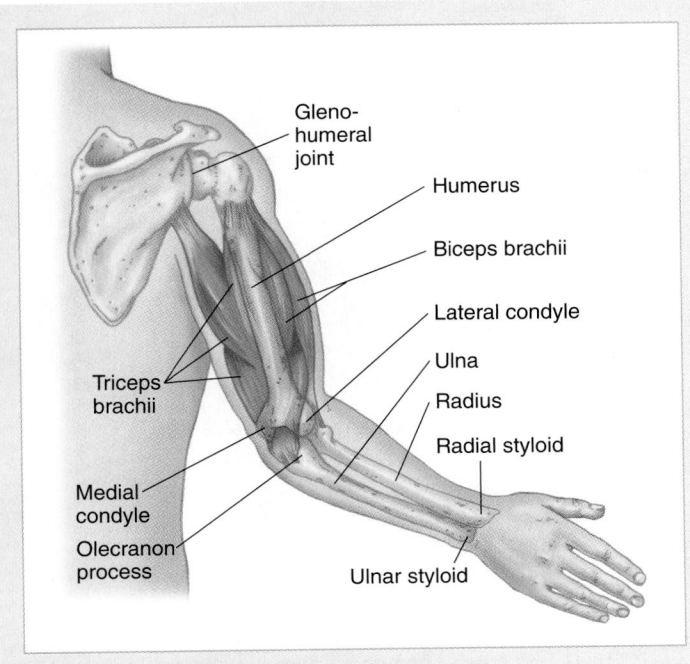

Figure 25-3 The anatomy of the arm.

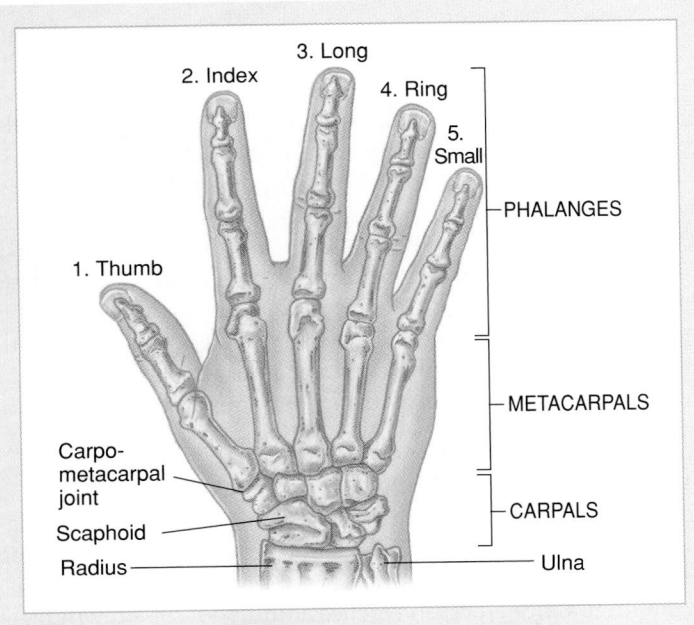

Figure 25-4 The anatomy of the wrist and hand.

The radius and ulna make up the forearm. The radius, the larger of the two forearm bones, lies on the *thumb* side of the forearm. Distally, the ulna is narrow and is on the little-finger side of the forearm. It serves as the pivot around which the radius turns at the wrist to rotate the palm upward (supination) or downward (pronation). Because the radius and the ulna are arranged in parallel, when one is broken, the other is often broken as well.

The hand (Figure 25-4 ▲) contains three sets of bones: wrist bones (carpals), hand bones (metacarpals), and finger

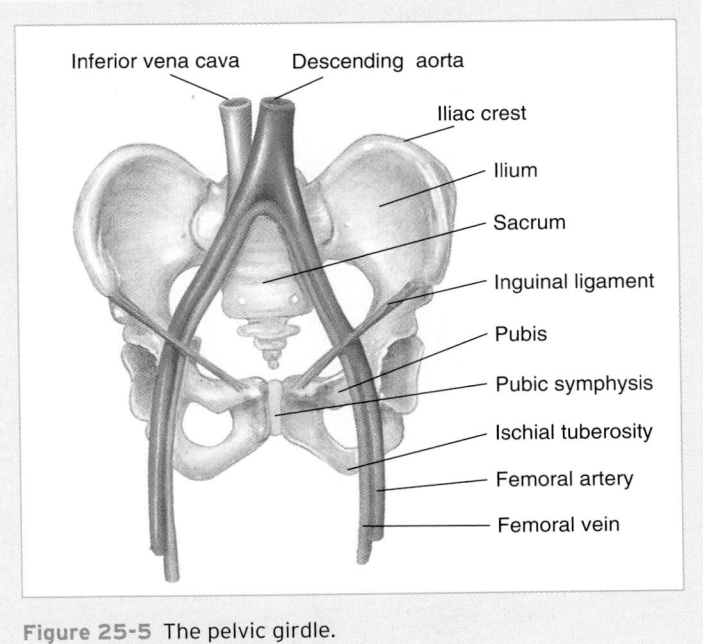

Figure 25-5 The pelvic girdle.

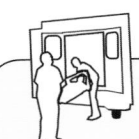

In the Field

To remember the difference between supination and pronation, think of soup. The SUPinated hand can hold a cup of SOUP.

bones (phalanges). The carpals, especially the scaphoid, are vulnerable to fracture when a person falls on an outstretched hand. Phalanges are more apt to be injured by a crushing injury, such as being slammed in a car door.

Pelvis and Lower Extremities

The pelvic girdle (Figure 25-5 ▲) is actually three separate bones—the ischium, ilium, and pubis—fused together to form the innominate bone. The two iliac bones are joined posteriorly by tough ligaments to the sacrum at the sacroiliac joints; the two pubic bones are connected anteriorly by equally tough ligaments to one another at the pubic symphysis. These joints allow very little motion, so the pelvic ring is strong and stable.

The lower extremity consists of the bones of the thigh, leg, and foot (Figure 25-6 ▶). The femur (thigh bone) is a long, powerful bone that articulates proximally in the ball-and-socket joint of the pelvis and distally in the hinge joint of the knee. The head of the femur is the ball-shaped part that fits into the acetabulum. It is connected to the *shaft,* or long tubular portion of the femur, by the femoral *neck.* The femoral neck is a common site for fractures, generally referred to as hip fractures, especially in the older population.

The lower leg consists of two bones, the tibia and the fibula. The tibia (shin bone) forms the inferior component of the knee joint. Anterior to this joint is the patella (kneecap), a bone that is important for knee extension. The tibia runs down the front of

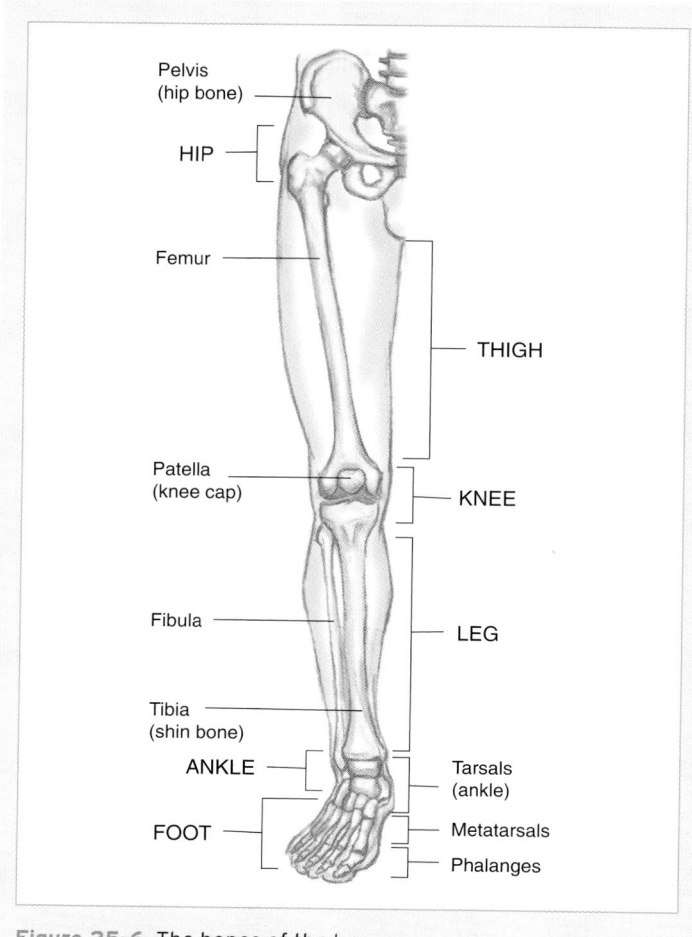

Figure 25-6 The bones of the leg.

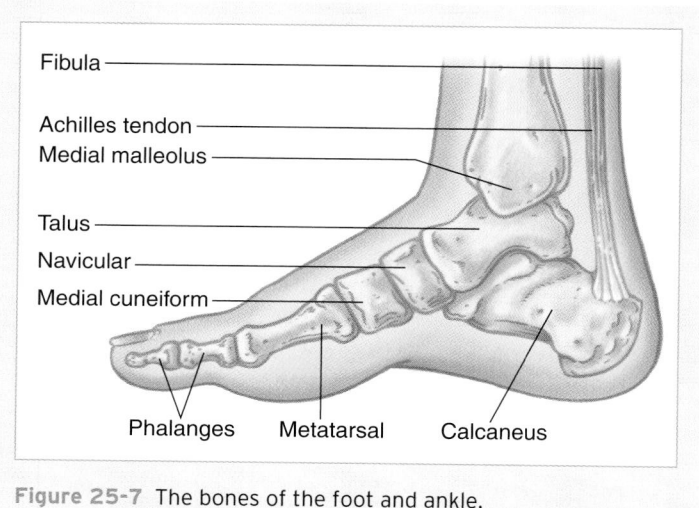

Figure 25-7 The bones of the foot and ankle.

In the Field

Here's a tip to help remember which bones are carpal (hand bones) and which bones are tarsal (foot bones): "I steer my CAR (pal) with hands and walk through TAR (sal) with my feet."

In the Field

Fractures that occur through the growth plate in a bone of a child may affect the future growth of that bone.

the lower leg, where it is vulnerable to direct blows, and can be felt just beneath the skin. The much smaller fibula runs posteriorly and laterally to the tibia. The fibula is not a component of the knee joint, but it does make up the lateral knob of the ankle joint (lateral malleolus) at its distal articulation.

The foot consists of three classes of bones: *ankle bones* (tarsals), *foot bones* (metatarsals), and *toe bones* (phalanges) 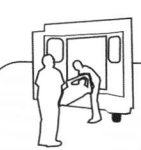 . The largest of the tarsal bones is the heel bone, or calcaneus, which is subject to injury when a person jumps from a height and lands on the feet.

Characteristics and Composition of Bone
Bone Shapes

Bones may be classified based on their shape. Long bones are longer than they are wide; examples include the femur,

humerus, tibia, fibula, radius, and ulna. Short bones are nearly as wide as they are long; they include the phalanges, metacarpals, and metatarsals. Flat bones are thin, broad bones; they include the sternum, ribs, scapulae, and skull. Irregular bones do not fit into one of the other categories but rather have a shape that is designed to perform a specific function, such as the bones of the vertebral column and the mandible. Round bones are generally found in proximity to a joint and help with movement. They are often referred to as sesamoid bones because of their location within a tendon. The patella is the largest of these bones.

Typical Long Bone Architecture

Long bones have several distinct regions and anatomical features Figure 25-8 ▸ . These bones can grow to such long lengths because of the presence of the growth plate, or physis, in children. Once a person reaches adulthood, the growth plate closes and the mature adult bone is complete. The long bone is divided into three regions: the diaphysis, the epiphysis, and the metaphysis.

The articular surfaces of a long bone come in contact with other bones to form articulations (joints). These regions of the bone are covered by articular cartilage, a substance that acts as a cushion to protect the bone from damage and wear.

The portion of bone that is not covered by articular cartilage is, instead, covered by the periosteum. This dense, fibrous membrane contains capillaries and cells that are important for bone repair and maintenance. In the inner portion of the long bone, blood comes from the nutrient artery of the bone. Once

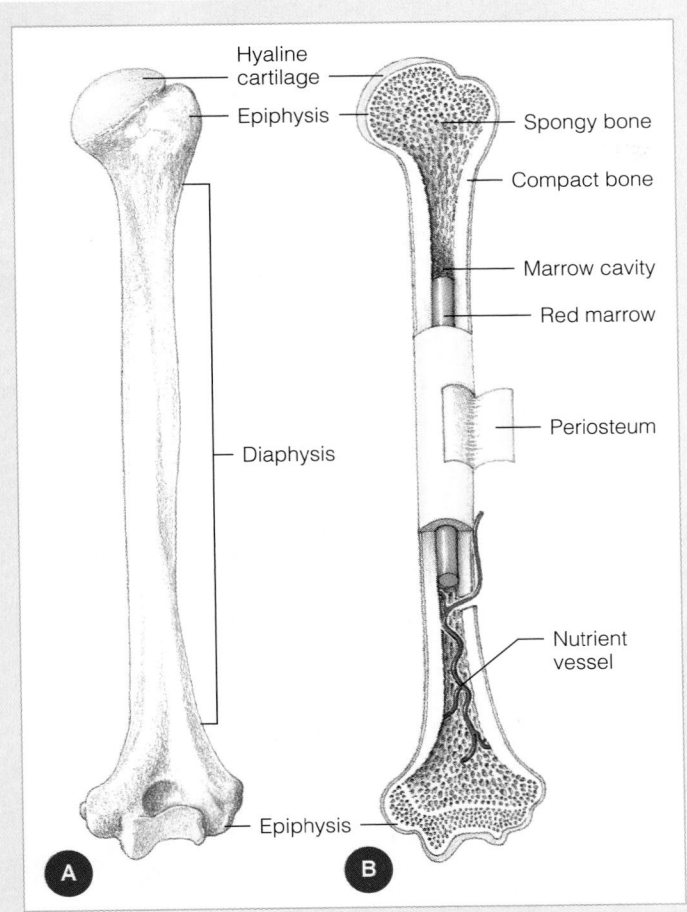

Figure 25-8 Anatomy of the long bone. **A.** The humerus. Notice the long shaft and dilated ends. **B.** Longitudinal section of the humerus showing compact bone, spongy bone, and marrow.

Labels (Figure 25-8):
Hyaline cartilage — Epiphysis — Spongy bone — Compact bone — Marrow cavity — Red marrow — Diaphysis — Periosteum — Nutrient vessel — Epiphysis — **A** — **B**

Special Considerations

Splinting an injured extremity (for example, a fractured forearm) is most optimally performed with the extremity in a straightened position. In some older patients, however, straightening the injured extremity may not be possible and may cause further injury. This is particularly true in patients with arthritis—a degenerative condition that causes a reduced range of motion in the joints. If, while attempting to straighten the extremity, the patient complains of increasing joint pain or you feel resistance, stop and splint the injured limb in the position in which it is resting.

decreases, increasing the risk of disk herniation. In some joints, the cartilage may become degraded, leading to arthritis and pain; in others, the cartilage becomes calcified, leading to restricted motion.

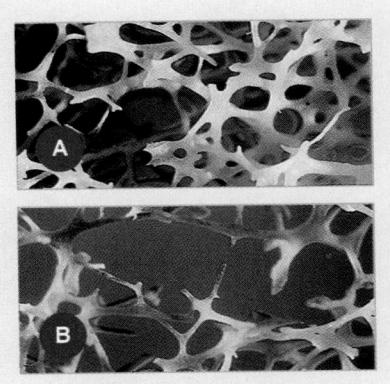

Figure 25-9 The structural difference between normal and osteoporotic bone. **A.** Normal bone in a 29-year-old woman. **B.** Osteoporotic bone in a 92-year-old-woman.

it penetrates the bone's outer cortex, the artery enters the medullary canal, the hollow inner portion of the shaft that is lined by the endosteum (similar to the periosteum, but on the inside) and contains yellow (fatty) marrow in adults.

Age-Associated Changes in Bone

Bone ages just like any other tissue of the body, decreasing in density after the age of 35 years, leading to a loss of height, and producing changes in facial structure. In women, this decrease in density is further accelerated once menopause is reached because of the loss of estrogen, a hormone that helps promote bone formation. A significant decrease in bone density, called osteoporosis (Figure 25-9 ▶), is associated with a higher risk of fracture. People with osteoporosis are at risk for incurring a fracture, especially in the hip, spine, and wrist.

Other changes associated with aging of bone include aging of muscles, cartilage, and other connective tissues that may also lead to degradation of joints and disk herniation. For example, the water content of the intervertebral disks

Joints

When two bones come together, they articulate with one another to form a joint. Some joints are fused and allow for no motion, such as the joints of the skull. Other joints allow for motion by permitting movement between the two bones, typically within a certain plane of motion that is defined by the structure of the bones that form it. The various motions that a joint may allow include flexion, extension, abduction, adduction, rotation, circumduction, pronation, and supination (Figure 25-10 ▶).

Types of Joints

The three general types of joints are fibrous, cartilaginous, and synovial (Figure 25-11 ▶). Fibrous joints, also referred to as synarthroses or fused joints, contain dense fibrous tissue that does not allow for movement. Examples include the bones of the skull and the distal tibiofibular joint.

Cartilaginous joints, also called amphiarthroses, allow for very minimal movement between the bones. The pubic symphysis and the joints connecting the ribs to the sternum are examples of this type of joint.

Synovial joints, or diarthroses, are the most mobile joints of the body. They are surrounded by an extension of the periosteum called the joint capsule, with the bones that form them being held in place by very strong ligaments. Within the joint are the articular cartilage and the synovial membrane, which secretes synovial fluid into the joint cavity to lubricate it.

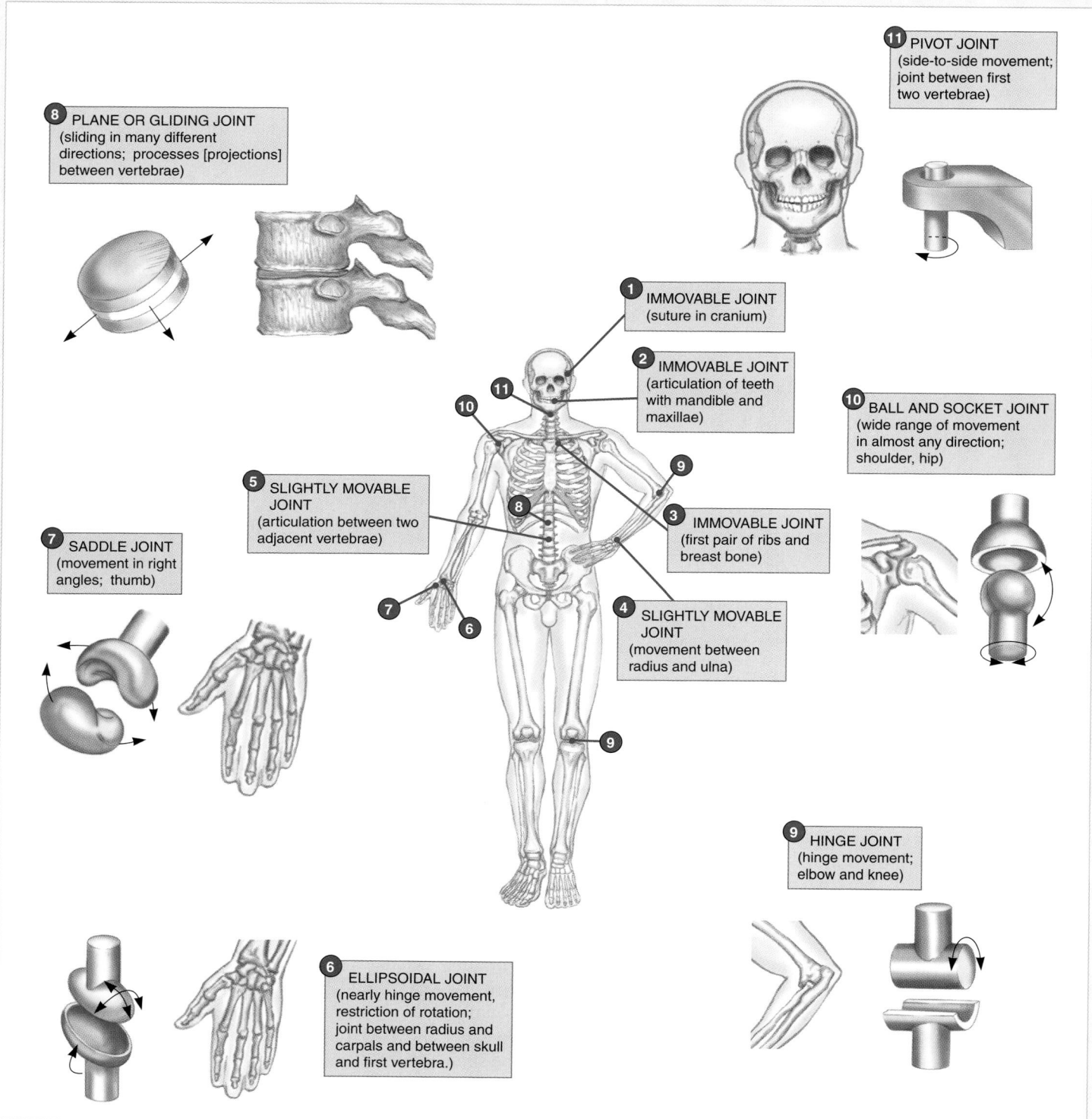

Figure 25-10 Joints in the body.

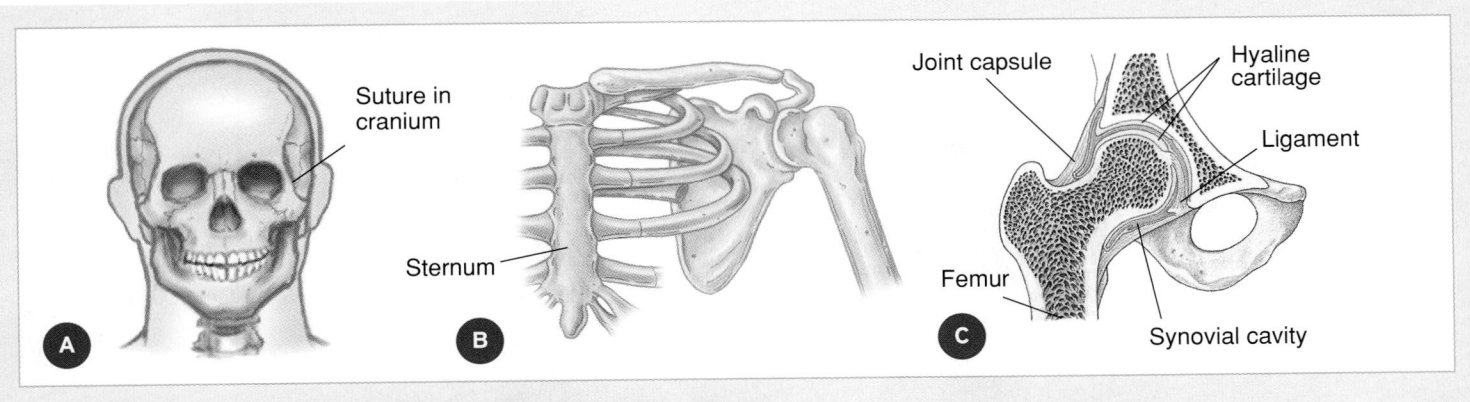

Figure 25-11 Types of joints. **A.** Fibrous. **B.** Cartilaginous. **C.** Synovial.

Bursa

A <u>bursa</u> is a padlike sac or cavity located within the connective tissue, usually in proximity to a joint. It may be lined with a synovial membrane and typically contains fluid that helps reduce the amount of friction between a tendon and a bone or between a tendon and a ligament. Examples include the olecranon bursa of the elbow and the prepatellar bursa of the knee. Bursitis is inflammation of a bursa.

Skeletal Connecting and Supporting Structures

Tendons connect muscle to bone. These flat or cordlike bands of connective tissue are white and have a glistening appearance.

Ligaments connect bone to bone and help maintain the stability of joints and determine the degree of joint motion. These inelastic bands of connective tissue have a structure similar to that of tendons.

Cartilage consists of fibers of collagen embedded in a gelatinous substance. This flexible connective tissue forms the smooth surface over bone ends where they articulate, provides cushioning between vertebrae, gives structure to the nose and external ear, forms the framework of the larynx and trachea, and serves as the model for the formation of the skeleton in children. Cartilage has a very limited neurovascular supply—it receives nutrients through diffusion from the outer covering of the cartilage or from the synovial fluid—so it does not heal well if it is injured.

The Moving Forces: Muscles

Muscles are composed of specialized cells that contract (shorten) when stimulated to exert a force on a part of the body. Three types of muscle are found in the body: smooth muscle, cardiac muscle, and skeletal muscle ⟨ **Figure 25-12** ▸ ⟩ .

Skeletal Muscle

<u>Skeletal muscle</u> ⟨ **Figure 25-13** ▸ ⟩ is also called <u>voluntary muscle</u>, because its contractions are largely under voluntary control, or <u>striated muscle</u>, because striations can be seen in it during microscopic examination. Skeletal muscle includes all

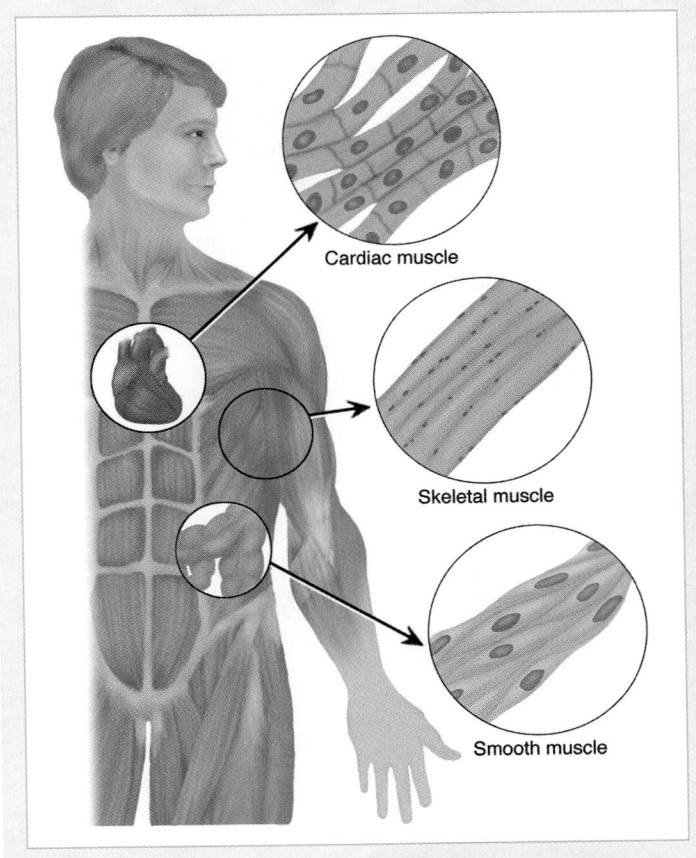

Figure 25-12 The three types of muscle are skeletal, smooth, and cardiac.

of the muscles attached to the skeleton and forms the bulk of the tissue of the arms and legs. It is also found along the spine and buttocks. By maintaining a state of partial contraction, this type of muscle allows the body to maintain its posture and to sit or stand. It varies greatly in size and shape, from thin strands to the large muscles of the thigh and back. It also constitutes the muscles of the tongue, soft palate, scalp, pharynx, upper esophagus, and eye. About 40% to 50% of normal body

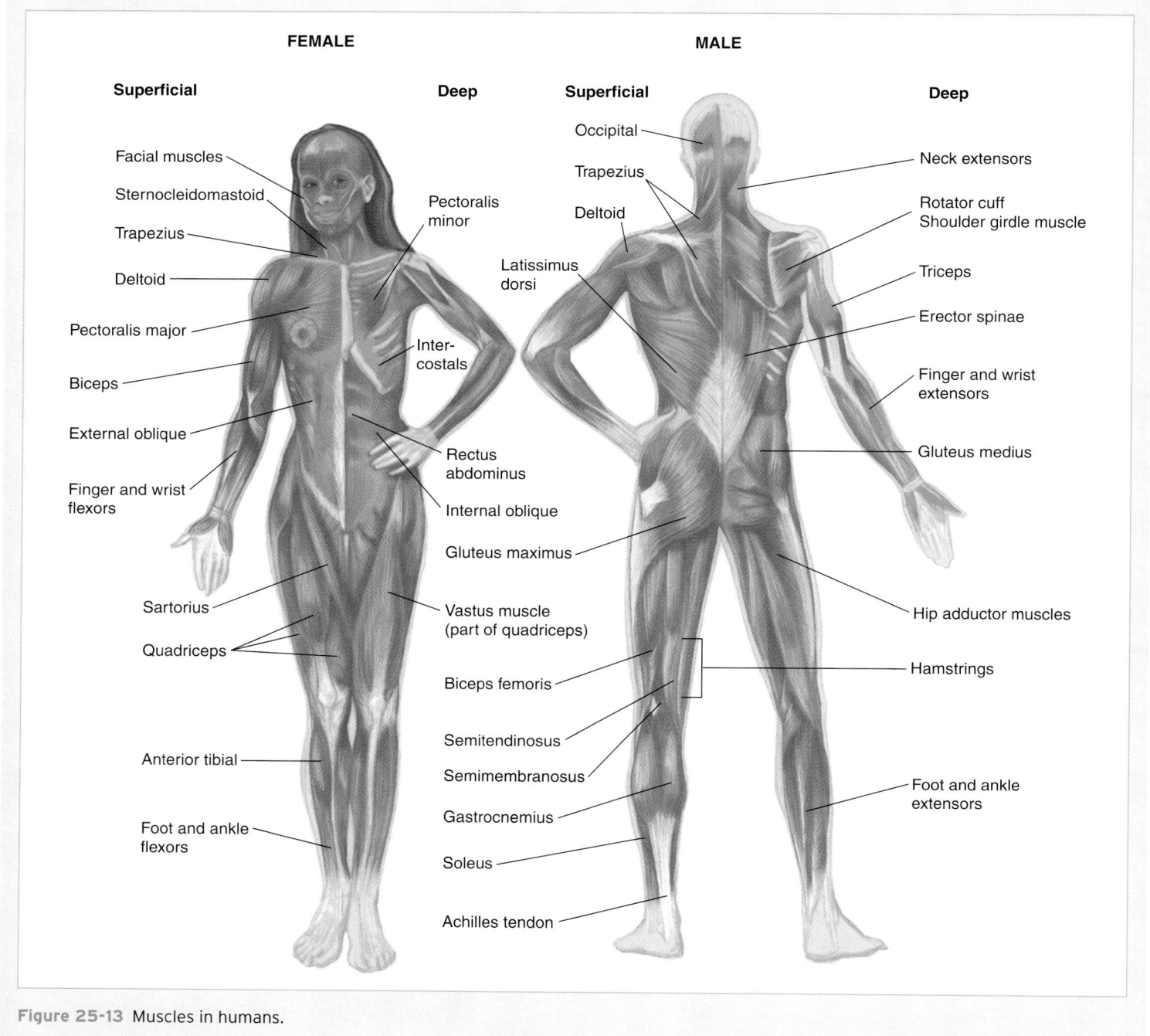

FEMALE

Superficial   Deep

- Facial muscles
- Sternocleidomastoid
- Trapezius
- Deltoid
- Pectoralis major
- Biceps
- External oblique
- Finger and wrist flexors
- Pectoralis minor
- Inter-costals
- Rectus abdominus
- Internal oblique
- Gluteus maximus
- Sartorius
- Quadriceps
- Vastus muscle (part of quadriceps)
- Biceps femoris
- Semitendinosus
- Semimembranosus
- Gastrocnemius
- Soleus
- Anterior tibial
- Foot and ankle flexors
- Achilles tendon

MALE

Superficial   Deep

- Occipital
- Trapezius
- Deltoid
- Latissimus dorsi
- Neck extensors
- Rotator cuff Shoulder girdle muscle
- Triceps
- Erector spinae
- Finger and wrist extensors
- Gluteus medius
- Hip adductor muscles
- Hamstrings
- Foot and ankle extensors

Figure 25-13 Muscles in humans.

weight is skeletal muscle, as it has a high water content. In addition, because of its high metabolic rate and demand for energy and oxygen, skeletal muscle has a very rich blood supply, which causes it to bleed significantly when injured.

Skeletal muscles are profoundly affected by the amount of training and work to which they are subjected. Unused muscles tend to atrophy (shrink or waste away), whereas physical training promotes hypertrophy (increase in size).

Skeletal muscles are attached to bones by tendons. Tendons cross joints to create a pulling force between two bones

when a muscle contracts. The biceps muscle, for example, has its origin on the scapula; the biceps tendon passes over the head of the humerus, where it fuses with the body of the biceps muscle; at the distal end of the biceps, a tendon passes over the anterior surface of the elbow and inserts on the radius. Thus, when the biceps muscle contracts, the force causes the elbow to bend (flex).

Muscle contraction requires energy. This energy is derived from the metabolism of glucose and results in the production of lactic acid (lactate). Lactic acid, in turn, must be converted

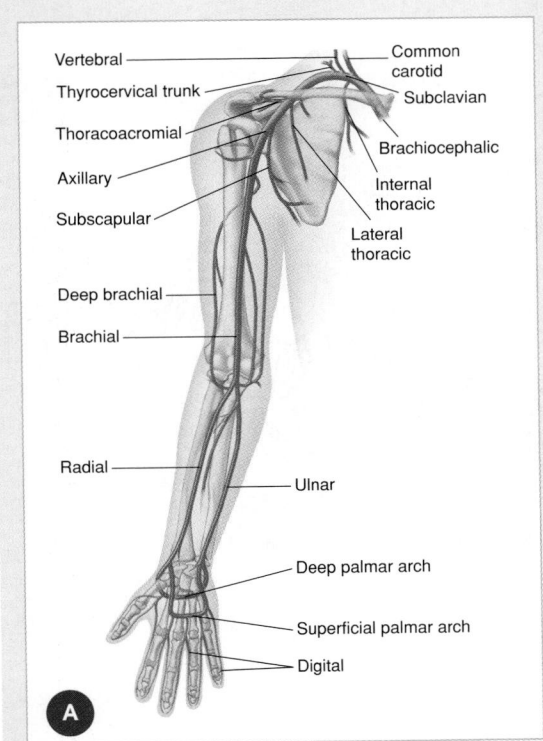 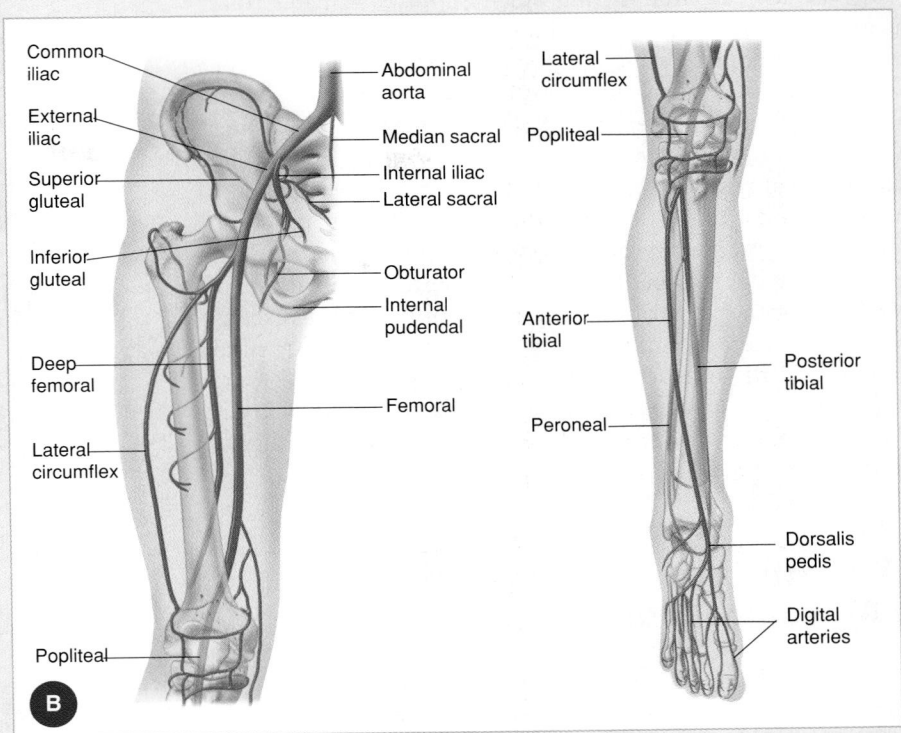

Figure 25-14 The arterial supply of the extremities. **A.** Upper extremities. **B.** Lower extremities.

into carbon dioxide and water, a process that requires oxygen. For that reason, vigorous muscular activity is often followed by an increased respiratory rate, which increases oxygen delivery to and carbon dioxide removal from the tissues.

The sensation of muscle fatigue occurs when the energy supply to the muscle is inadequate to meet the energy demands. If muscle fatigue occurs as a result of excessive muscular activity, rest produces quick recovery. If it occurs from a lack of oxygen or essential nutrients or electrolytes (such as sodium or calcium), however, rest will not lead to such a quick recovery.

Muscle Innervation

Skeletal muscle is innervated by somatic motor neurons. These neurons transmit electrical stimuli to a muscle that cause it to contract. The combination of the muscle and the neuron that innervates it constitutes a motor unit. A motor unit that receives a signal to contract responds as forcefully as possible or does not contract at all: It is an all-or-nothing response. To generate a more forceful contraction, more neurons need to signal more muscle cells to contract, a process called recruitment.

Innervation of the upper extremities arises from the brachial plexus. The brachial plexus is formed by a network of nerves that originate from the spinal cord at the C5–T1 levels.

After the fibers of these nerves network with one another, five distinct nerves are formed: the axillary, radial, musculocutaneous, ulnar, and median. Innervation of the lower extremities is provided by the lumbar and lumbosacral plexuses, which are formed by the spinal nerves that originate from L1–S4. The networking of nerves within these two plexuses leads to the formation of multiple distinct nerves, including the sciatic nerve, which branches in the popliteal fossa to form the peroneal and tibial nerves, and the femoral nerve.

Musculoskeletal Blood Supply

When a person has a musculoskeletal injury, the arteries that supply the injured region may also be damaged. Therefore, it is important to realize which arteries are present in each part of the extremity **Figure 25-14 ▲**.

The upper extremity's blood supply originates from the subclavian artery. When the subclavian artery reaches the axilla, it is referred to as the axillary artery. After giving off several branches that supply the shoulder region with blood, the artery leaves the axilla and becomes the brachial artery. After the brachial artery passes through the elbow, it divides into the radial artery and ulnar artery. In the hand, the radial and ulnar arteries form superficial and deep arcades of blood vessels that branch to form the arteries of each finger, the digital arteries.

In the lower extremity, the blood supply originates from the external iliac artery. When the external iliac artery reaches the leg, it becomes the femoral artery. When it reaches the knee, the femoral artery turns posteriorly and laterally and is referred to as the popliteal artery. The popliteal artery divides into the anterior tibial artery and posterior tibial artery. The anterior tibial artery travels along the anterior and lateral surface of the tibia until it reaches the ankle, where it proceeds along the dorsal surface of the foot toward the great toe and becomes the dorsalis pedis artery. The posterior tibial artery travels along the posterior aspect of the tibia until it reaches the ankle, where it follows a path just behind the medial malleolus until it reaches the plantar aspect of the foot. Within the foot, arcades of arteries supply the various structures with blood and give off branches that form the digital arteries of the toes.

Patterns and Mechanisms of Musculoskeletal Injury

Skeletal injuries result from blunt and penetrating trauma. In some cases, a force that might not generally cause harm to normal healthy bone produces a fracture. Such a pathologic fracture occurs when a medical condition causes the bone to become abnormally weak. In adults and children, motor vehicle crashes, falls, and athletic activities are common causes of injury. Among children, intentional trauma or abuse is a common cause of fractures and musculoskeletal injuries.

Sports account for a significant number of musculoskeletal injuries Figure 25-15 ▸.

Injury Forces and Motions
Direct Force
An object that strikes a person will transfer its energy to its point of impact. This energy is first absorbed by the soft tissues in the region of the impact. When the amount of force is so great that the soft tissues cannot fully dissipate it, a fracture occurs.

Penetrating injuries may also lead to a fracture or other musculoskeletal injury. A high-velocity injury, such as that caused by a high-power rifle, typically shatters bone and causes extensive soft-tissue damage.

An impalement injury commonly causes a soft-tissue injury similar to that seen in a low-velocity penetrating injury. If the impaled object happens to strike a bone, it may cause a fracture. In any case of impalement, it is essential to stabilize the object to protect the soft tissues from further injury.

Indirect Force
An indirect injury occurs when a force is applied to one region of the body but causes an injury in another region of the body. In this type of injury, the force is transmitted through the skeleton until, at some point, it reaches an area that is structurally

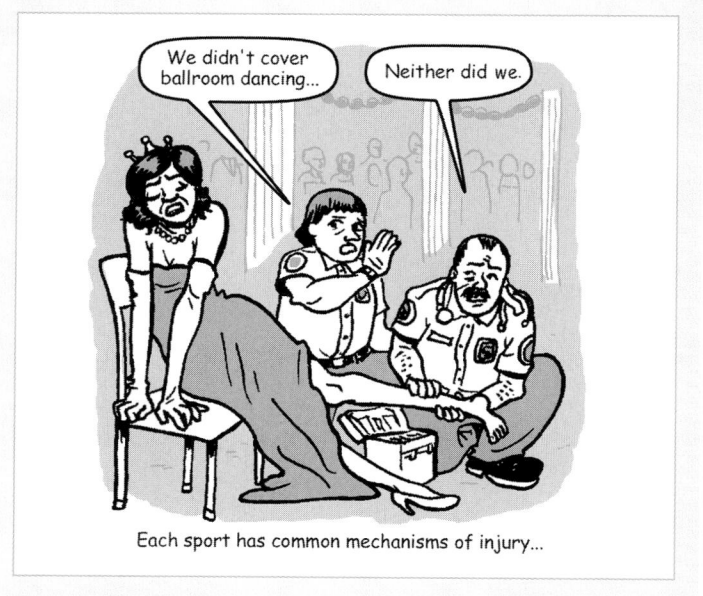

Figure 25-15

weak in comparison with the other parts of the musculoskeletal system through which the force has traveled.

For example, a hip fracture may occur when a person's knee strikes the dashboard during a motor vehicle crash. In this case, the force is applied to the knee and travels proximally along the femur. When this force reaches the femoral neck, it causes the femoral neck to fracture.

Forces may be transmitted along the entire length of a bone or through several bones in series and may cause an injury anywhere along the way. Thus, a person falling on an outstretched hand may have one or more injuries as the result of forces transmitted proximally from the point of impact: (1) fracture of the scaphoid bone of the hand (direct blow); (2) fracture of the distal ulna and radius (Colles fracture Figure 25-16 ▸); (3) fracture-dislocation of the elbow; (4) fracture-dislocation of the shoulder; or (5) fracture of the clavicle.

Twisting injuries, like those that commonly occur in football or skiing, result in fractures, sprains, and dislocations. Typically, the distal part of the limb remains fixed, as when cleats or a ski holds the foot to the ground, while torsion develops in the proximal section of the limb; the resulting force causes tearing of tendons and ligaments and spiral fractures of bone. Fatigue fractures, also called march fractures, are caused by repetitive stress and most commonly occur in the feet after prolonged walking.

Pathologic fractures are seen in patients with diseases that weaken areas of bone, such as metastatic cancer, and may occur with minimal force. Older people, particularly those with osteoporosis, also have weaker, more brittle bones and are more susceptible to fractures than younger people.

Some injuries are commonly encountered together because of the way the causative forces are transmitted; thus, if you find one, look for the others (Table 25-1 ▸). Pain and swelling over the scaphoid (navicular) bone of the wrist, for example, means that the patient fell hard against an outstretched hand, so he or she may have other injuries anywhere along the axis from the hand to the shoulder.

Fractures

A fracture is a break in the continuity of a bone. Fractures occur when the magnitude of the force applied to a bone (a single

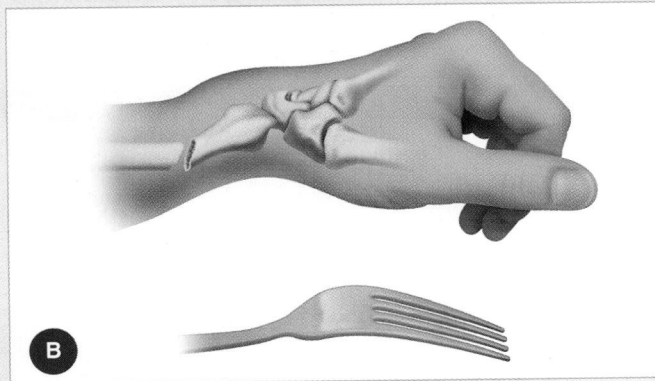

Figure 25-16 **A.** Fractures of the distal radius produce a characteristic Colles fracture (silver fork deformity). **B.** An artist's illustration of the injury.

Documentation and Communication

Some services take digital or Polaroid pictures at crash scenes to include in reports to the receiving hospital. These images allow emergency department staff to better understand the forces involved.

Table 25-1	Musculoskeletal Injuries That Commonly Occur Together
If You Find	**Look For**
Scapular fracture	Rib fracture, pulmonary contusions, pneumothorax
Scaphoid fracture	Wrist, elbow, or shoulder fracture
Pelvic fracture	Lumbosacral spine and other long bone fractures, intra-abdominal or genitourinary injury
Hip dislocation	Fracture of the acetabulum or femoral head
Femoral fracture	Dislocation of ipsilateral hip
Patellar fracture	Fracture-dislocation of ipsilateral hip
Knee dislocation	Tibial fracture; distal pulse may be absent
Calcaneal fracture	Fracture of the ankle, leg, hip, pelvis, spine, and the other calcaneus

You are the Provider Part 2

As you continue your initial assessment, an engine company arrives and assists with application of spinal precautions and high-flow supplemental oxygen. Soon afterward, the neighbor approaches and identifies himself. He says that the patient seemed to have lost his balance while painting and may have struck the air conditioner during his fall. On further assessment, you note that the patient appears to have an open fracture of his left arm, which is bleeding significantly.

Vital Signs	Recording Time: 2 Minutes
Level of consciousness	A (Alert to person, place, and day)
Skin	Pink, warm, and slightly moist
Pulse	110 beats/min, full and regular
Blood pressure	144/90 mm Hg
Respirations	42 breaths/min
Sao₂	96% with 15 L/min via nonrebreathing mask

3. What are the potential complications of an open fracture?

4. Why are open fractures prone to bleeding more than closed fractures?

5. Would your treatment priorities change if the patient complained of abdominal pain in the presence of hypotension?

application or an accumulation of repetitive applications) overcomes the strength of the bone. The strength of a bone is affected by age, osteoporosis, nutritional status, and disease processes.

Fracture Classification
Fracture Type
A fracture may be classified based on the direction that the fracture line travels through a bone, number of fractures on the bone, or number of cortices involved **Table 25-2 ▾**.

Special Considerations

Children with fractures may not want you to see, touch, or splint the injured extremity. You should always be honest with children about what you are doing and whether it will hurt. In particular, splinting is a necessary and sometimes painful intervention for a child with a fracture. Once the splint is in place, cold is applied, and analgesia is considered, the child will likely have less pain because the fracture is stabilized.

Fracture Classification Based on Displacement
Fractures may be classified based on the type of displacement **Table 25-3 ▸**.

Angulation of a fracture means that each end of the fracture is not aligned in a straight line and that an angle has formed between them. Angulation may occur in the frontal plane, sagittal plane, or both.

Open Versus Closed Fractures
In an open fracture **Figure 25-18 ▸**, sometimes called a compound fracture, a break in the overlying skin allows the fracture to communicate with the outside environment. In a closed fracture, the skin over the fracture site remains intact.

In addition to having a higher risk of infection, open fractures have the potential for more blood loss than a closed fracture for two reasons. First, open fractures usually result from high-energy injuries, so they typically involve more soft-tissue damage. Second, in most fractures, the periosteal vessels and the vessels supplying the surrounding soft tissues are disrupted, leading to the formation of a hematoma. In a closed

---

Table 25-2 Fracture Classification Based on Fracture Type

Type of Fracture	Description	Common Causes
Direction the Fracture Line Travels Through a Bone **Figure 25-17 ▸**		
Linear fracture	Parallel to the long axis of the bone	Low-energy stress injuries
Transverse fracture	Straight across a bone at right angles to each cortex	Direct, low-energy blow
Oblique fracture	At an angle across the bone	Direct or twisting force
Spiral fracture	Encircles the bone	Twisting injury
Impacted fracture	End of one bone becomes wedged into another bone	Fall from a significant height
Number of Fractures on One Bone		
Comminuted fracture	> 2 fracture fragments located in one area of the bone	High-energy injury (such as crush injury)
Segmental fracture	> 2 fracture fragments, but breaks occur in different parts of the bone	High-energy injury
Number of Cortices Injured		
Complete fracture	Break through both cortices	High-energy injury
Incomplete fracture	Break through one cortex	Low-energy injury
■ Greenstick fracture	Typically occurs in the proximal metaphysis or diaphysis of the tibia, radius, or, when this fracture occurs in the shaft, the cortex on the convex side of the deformity is broken, but the cortex on the concave side remains intact	Usually occurs in children
■ Buckle fracture (torus fracture)	Occurs in the metaphysis of long bones in response to excessive compression loading on one side of the bone; the compressed cortex buckles, and the opposite cortex is pulled away from the physis	Unique to children; most commonly seen in the distal radius, usually resulting from a fall on an outstretched hand
■ Bowing fracture	When a compression force is applied to a bone, numerous small fractures on the compressed side of the bone cause it to bend	Often occurs in children and young adults; most commonly affects the radius, ulna, tibia, fibula, or clavicle
■ Fatigue fracture (stress fracture)	Occurs when the muscle develops faster than the bone and places exaggerated stress on the less developed bone; may also be due to repetitive small injuries that eventually lead to bone failure	Usually occurs in the legs or feet of people who engage in strenuous, repetitive activities (such as dancers, joggers, military recruits)

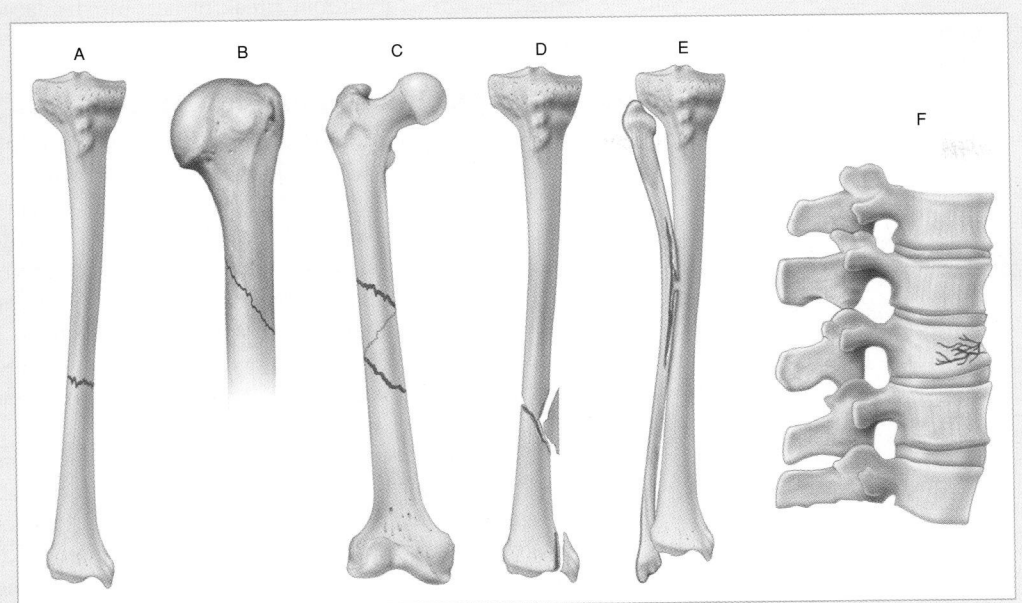

Figure 25-17 Types of fractures. **A.** Transverse fracture of the tibia. **B.** Oblique fracture of the humerus. **C.** Spiral fracture of the femur. **D.** Comminuted fracture of the tibia. **E.** Greenstick fracture of the fibula. **F.** Compression fracture of a vertebral body.

fracture, the increased interstitial pressure within the hematoma compresses the blood vessels, limiting the size of the hematoma. In a closed femur fracture, the blood loss may exceed 1 L before enough pressure develops to tamponade the bleeding. In contrast, open fractures allow much of the blood to escape, so tamponade does not occur as readily or at all.

Signs and Symptoms of a Fracture

The primary symptom of a fracture is *pain* that is usually well localized to the fracture site. In addition, the patient may report hearing a snap or feeling a break. Signs of fracture detected on physical examination include the following:

- *Deformity* is one of the most reliable signs of a fracture. The limb may be found in an unnatural position or show motion at a place where there is no joint. Compare the deformed limb with the extremity on the other side Figure 25-19 ▸ .
- *Shortening* occurs in fractures when the broken ends of a bone override one another. It is characteristic of femur fractures, for example, because the broken femur can no longer serve as a strut to oppose spasm in the powerful thigh muscles.

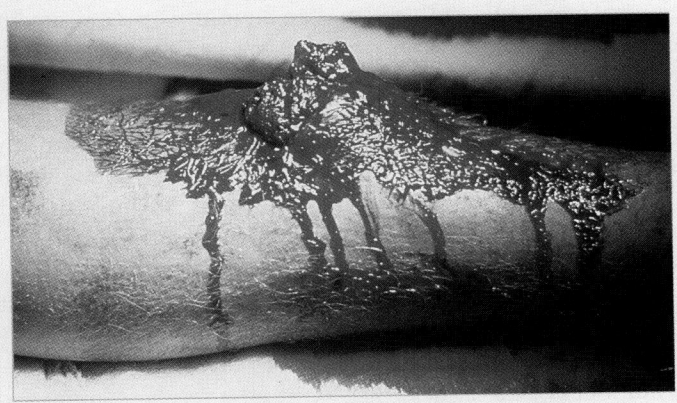

Figure 25-18 An open fracture.

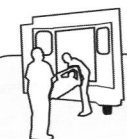

In the Field

The ends of a fractured bone are sharp. Use caution whenever bone ends are exposed to prevent a puncture injury to yourself, your crew, or the splint.

Table 25-3	Fracture Classification Based on Displacement	
Type of Fracture	**Description**	**Common Causes**
Nondisplaced fracture	Bone remains aligned in its normal position, despite the fracture.	Low-energy injury
Displaced fracture	Ends of the fracture move from their normal positions.	High-energy injury
▪ Overriding	Muscles pull the distal fracture fragment alongside the proximal one, leading them to overlap; the limb becomes shortened.	Only occurs when a fracture is fully displaced and there is no bone contact
▪ Distraction injury	A powerful tensile force is rapidly applied to a bone, causing it to fracture—the bone ends are pulled apart.	Industrial equipment, machinery
▪ Impacted fracture (impaction injury)	A massive compressive force is applied to a bone, causing it to become wedged into another bone.	More likely to happen in cancellous bone
▪ Avulsion fracture	A powerful muscle contraction causes the insertion site of the muscle to be fractured off of the bone.	Sudden "jerking" of a body part
▪ Depression fracture	Blunt trauma to a flat bone (such as the skull) causes the bone to be pushed inward.	Blunt injury

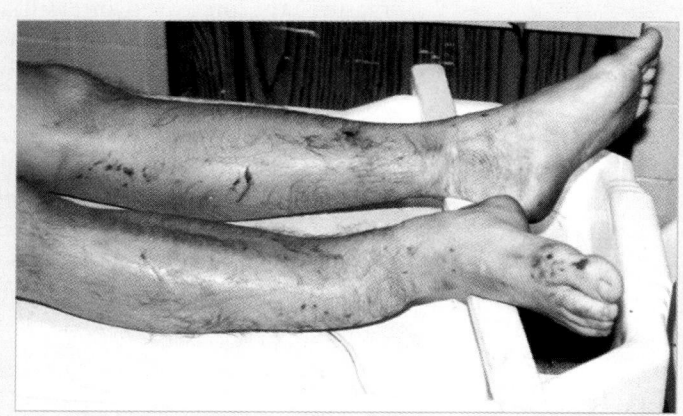

Figure 25-19 Obvious deformity is a sign of bone fracture.

- Visual inspection will usually reveal *swelling* at the fracture site due to bleeding from the broken bone and the accumulation of fluid. As blood infiltrates the tissues around the broken bone ends, *ecchymosis* will become apparent.
- *Guarding* and *loss of use* characterize most fractures. The patient will try to keep a fractured bone still and will avoid putting any stress on it. Sometimes the measures a patient takes to protect a fractured bone from movement are so characteristic that one can almost diagnose the fracture without examining the extremity. A patient who walks to the ambulance holding the dorsum of one wrist in the other hand, for example, almost certainly has a Colles fracture. A patient standing with the head cocked toward a "knocked-down shoulder" probably has a fracture of the clavicle on the side to which the head is leaning.
- A fractured bone is almost invariably *tender to palpation* over the fracture site.
- Palpation may reveal crepitus, a grating sensation, over the broken bone ends. Crepitus may be noted as an incidental finding during splinting attempts. Do *not* try to elicit this sign, because your efforts may result in further injury to the bone and surrounding soft tissues, not to mention severe pain.
- In an open fracture, *exposed bone ends* may be visible in the wound.

Notes from Nancy

The best way to detect deformity or any other abnormality in an extremity is to compare it to the extremity on the other side.

Ligament Injuries and Dislocations

The shapes of the bones that form a joint and the tightness of the ligaments that hold them in place are key factors in determining a joint's range of motion. When forced beyond their normal limit, the bones that form a joint may break or become displaced and the supporting ligaments and joint capsule may tear.

Dislocations, Subluxations, and Diastases

In a dislocation, a bone is totally displaced from the joint. Typically, at least part of the supporting joint capsule and some of the joint's ligaments are disrupted. Dislocations occur when a body part moves beyond its normal range of motion and the articular surfaces are no longer intact. The dislocated bones are then locked in place by muscle spasms. Evaluation of the patient usually reveals an obvious and significant deformity, a significant decrease in the joint's range of motion (ROM), and severe pain. In all cases of a dislocation, a fracture should be suspected until ruled out by radiographs.

The partial dislocation of a joint is a subluxation. In this type of injury, the articular surfaces of the bones that form the joint are no longer completely in contact. In some cases, part of the joint capsule and supporting ligaments may be damaged. Despite the subluxation, the patient may be able to move the joint to some degree. Failure to recognize and treat a subluxation may lead to persistent joint instability and pain.

When the ligaments that hold two bones in a fixed position with respect to one another are disrupted and the space between them increases, a situation known as a diastasis occurs. An example of this would be an injury to the ligaments that hold the pubic symphysis together, causing the width of the joint to increase (diastasis of the pubic symphysis).

The principal symptom of a dislocation is pain or a feeling of pressure over the involved joint, plus loss of motion of the joint. A patient with a posterior dislocation of the shoulder, for example, is unable to raise the arm but holds it against the side instead. Sometimes the joint will seem "frozen." The principal sign of dislocation is deformity.

A dislocation is considered an urgent injury because of its potential to cause neurovascular compromise distal to the site of injury. If the dislocated bone presses on a nerve, there may be numbness or weakness distally; if an artery is compressed, there may be absent distal pulses (such as in a knee dislocation). For these reasons, you should always assess the patient's neurovascular status distal to the site of dislocation (check pulse and motor and sensory functions [PMS]).

Sprains

Sprains are injuries in which ligaments are stretched or torn. They usually result from a sudden twisting of a joint beyond its normal range of motion that also causes a temporary subluxation. The majority of sprains involve the ankle or the knee because most occur after a person misjudges a step or landing. Evasive moves, like those done during a sporting event, commonly cause sprains in athletes. Sprains are typically characterized by pain, swelling, and discoloration over the injured joint and unwillingness to use the limb. In contrast with fractures and dislocations, sprains usually do not involve deformity and joint mobility is usually limited by pain, not by joint incongruity.

Because it may be difficult to differentiate among the various types of injuries in the field, it is best to err on the side of

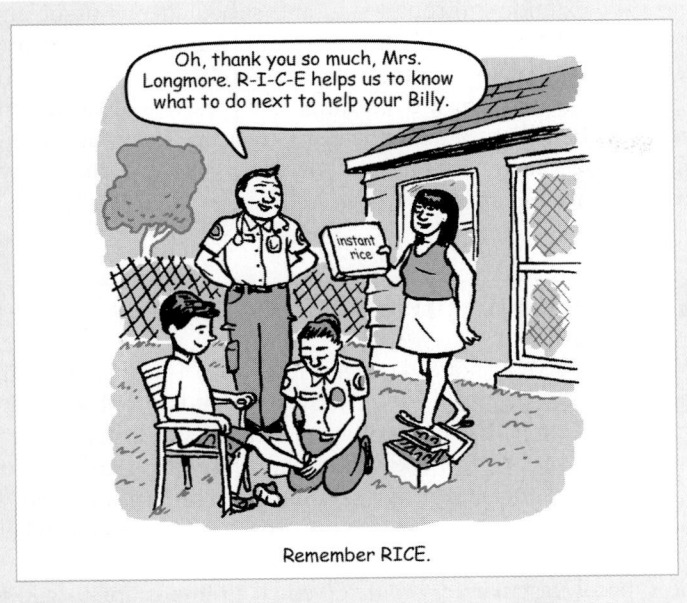

Figure 25-20

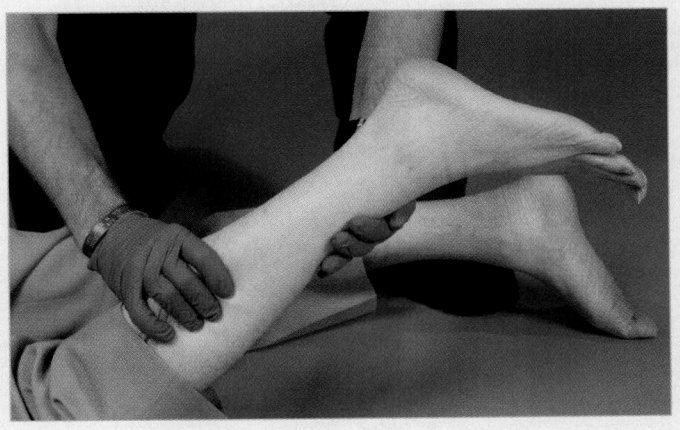

Figure 25-21 The Thompson test.

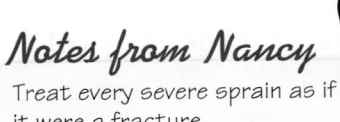

Notes from Nancy

Treat every severe sprain as if it were a fracture.

caution and treat every severe sprain as if it were a fracture. General treatment of sprains is similar to that of fractures and includes the following (numbers 1 through 4 form the mnemonic RICE) **Figure 25-20 ▲**):

1. **Rest**. Immobilize or splint injured area
2. **Ice** or cold pack over the injury
3. **Compression** with an elastic bandage (usually applied at the hospital once radiography rules out a fracture)
4. **Elevation**
5. Reduced or protected weight bearing
6. Pain management as soon as practical

■ Muscle and Tendon Injuries

Strains

A strain (pulled muscle) is an injury to a muscle and/or tendon that results from a violent muscle contraction or from excessive stretching. Often no deformity is present and only minor swelling is noted at the site of injury. Some patients may complain of increased pain with passive movement of the injured extremity.

Achilles Tendon Rupture

A rupture of the Achilles tendon usually occurs in athletes older than 30 years who are involved in start-and-stop sports such as basketball or football. The most immediate indications are pain from the heel to the calf and a sudden inability for plantar flexion of the foot. As time passes, the calf muscles begin to con-

tract proximally and a deformity within the calf may develop. The Thompson test can be performed in the field to identify an Achilles tendon rupture. To perform this test, have the patient assume a prone position and then squeeze the calf muscles of the injured leg **Figure 25-21 ▲** . If the foot plantar flexes while squeezing, the tendon is most likely intact. If there is no movement of the foot, the Achilles tendon has likely been torn. Management of an Achilles tendon injury includes RICE and pain control. These injuries are treated with surgery or multiple casts and can require up to 6 months for recovery.

Inflammatory Processes

When a muscle is subjected to frequent and repetitive use, its tendon or nearby bursa are at risk for becoming inflamed. When inflammation of the tendon causes pain, the patient is said to have tendinitis. There will typically be point tenderness on the inflamed tendon with pain often increasing if the person performs the movement that led to the inflammation. When a bursa becomes painful and inflamed, it is called bursitis. Patients with bursitis often complain of pain in the region of the inflamed bursa, especially with motions that cause the space where the bursa sits to become smaller. Examination of the site may reveal tenderness, swelling, erythema, and warmth. Tendinitis and bursitis are treated with RICE, pain relievers, and, in many cases, steroid injections.

■ Arthritis

Arthritis means inflammation of a joint. The three most common types of arthritis are osteoarthritis, rheumatoid arthritis, and gouty arthritis.

Osteoarthritis (OA) is a disease of the joints that occurs as they age and begin to wear. It is characterized by pain and stiffness, which typically get worse with use, and "cracking" or "crunching" of the affected joints. The spine, hands, knees, and hips are the most commonly affected sites. In general, the risk of developing OA increases with age, but other factors also increase the risk, such as obesity and prior joint injury. Treatment of OA involves low-impact physical therapy, pain control, anti-inflammatory medications, joint injections, and, in severe cases, joint replacement surgery.

Rheumatoid arthritis (RA) is a systemic inflammatory disease that affects joints and other body systems. In RA, significant bone erosion at the affected joints makes them more susceptible to fractures and dislocations. Of particular concern is the cervical spine, which is at high risk of subluxating following trauma or during intubation. Give extra attention to the cervical spine of a patient with RA to prevent further injury.

Gout is a condition in which the body has difficulty eliminating uric acid. When the concentration of uric acid in the blood becomes too great, the uric acid may crystallize within a joint. The patient will then have a hot, red, swollen joint with decreased range of motion. Prehospital treatment involves immobilization, pain relief, and transportation to an emergency department (ED) where the fluid in the joint can be aspirated to search for the characteristic crystals of gouty arthritis.

Injuries That May Signify Fractures

Amputations

An amputation is the separation of a limb or other body part from the remainder of the body **Figure 25-22 ▾**. The amputation may be incomplete, leaving only a small segment of tissue connecting the part, or it may be complete, causing the part to be fully separated. Hemorrhage from complete or incomplete amputations can be severe and life threatening. Fractures may also be present with amputations. Amputations are discussed in more detail in Chapter 19.

Lacerations

A laceration is a smooth or jagged cut caused by a sharp object or a blunt force that tears the tissue. The depth of the injury

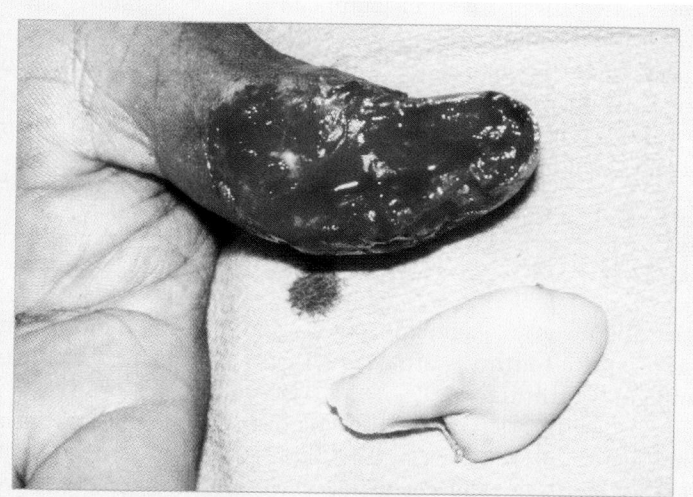

Figure 25-22 A partial avulsion involving the thumb.

can vary, extending through skin and subcutaneous tissue and even into the underlying muscles and adjacent nerves and blood vessels. Lacerations involved in damaged arteries or veins may result in severe bleeding. The presence of lacerations may also be a sign of an underlying fracture. Deep lacerations may injure the muscle nerves, or vasculture, so distal PMS functions should always be evaluated.

Vascular Injuries

When blood vessels are damaged following a musculoskeletal injury, devascularization of the body part that is supplied by the vessel may occur. The types of injuries that a vessel may sustain include a contusion of the vessel wall, laceration, kinking or bending, and formation of pseudoaneurysms. In addition, a blood vessel may thrombose (become occluded by a clot) when the injury causes blood flow to become very slow. Regardless of the type of vascular injury involved, it is important to assess and reassess pulses, control bleeding, and maintain adequate intravascular volume by using intravenous (IV) fluid.

General Principles of Assessment and Management

When assessing an injured patient, *do not be distracted by visually impressive injuries!* It is essential to complete the initial assessment of the patient before focusing on the extremities. In cases of musculoskeletal injuries, patients may be classified based on the presence or absence of associated injuries:

- Life- or limb-threatening injury or condition, including life- or limb-threatening musculoskeletal trauma
- Life-threatening injuries and only simple musculoskeletal trauma
- Life- or limb-threatening musculoskeletal trauma and no other life-threatening injuries
- Isolated, non–life- or non–limb-threatening injuries

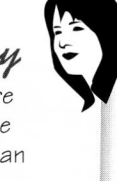

Notes from Nancy
Musculoskeletal injuries are rarely, if ever, an immediate threat to life. A fracture can wait. The airway cannot.

Volume Deficit Due to Musculoskeletal Injuries

Fractures may lead to significant blood loss from damage to vessels within the bone and musculature around the bone and, in some cases, from damage to large blood vessels in the region of the fracture. When caring for patients with fractures, undertake interventions such as applying direct pressure, splinting,

Table 25-4	Potential Blood Loss from Fracture Sites
Fracture Site	**Potential Blood Loss (mL)**
Pelvis	1,500–3,000
Femur	1,000–1,500
Humerus	250–500
Tibia or fibula	250–500
Ankle	250–500
Elbow	250–500
Radius or ulna	150–250

and administering IV fluids to prevent hypotension and unstable condition of the patient. **Table 25-4 ▲** lists the potential blood loss from various fracture sites and may serve as a guideline for estimating the amount of resuscitation required. The goal of prehospital management should be to keep the patient's volume, vital signs, and mental status normal.

Principles of Assessment

As with all patients, you should conduct a scene size-up, focusing on safety and body substance isolation precautions and then proceed to an initial assessment focusing on the patient's mental status, ABCs, and priority. If the initial assessment indicates that the patient has no immediately life-threatening condition and only localized musculoskeletal trauma, continue with a focused history and physical exam. If the patient has a significant mechanism of injury, complete a rapid trauma assessment and perform a detailed physical exam en route to the ED. The priorities throughout the assessment and management of musculoskeletal injuries should include identifying the injuries, preventing further harm or damage to the injured structures and surrounding tissues, supporting the injured area, and administering pain medication if necessary.

History of Present Injury

Obtain information about the incident that led to the injury from the patient and any bystanders who witnessed it. In particular, determine the condition of the patient immediately before the incident, the details of the incident, and the patient's position after the incident. Also, ask the patient for a subjective description of the injury: How did this happen? Did you hear a pop? Do you have pain? What functional limitations do you now have?

Medical History

Obtain the patient's medical history using the standard SAMPLE format. This history should also identify any preexisting musculoskeletal disorders and attempt to learn more about the injury. Some information obtained will be very relevant to the injury (such as the patient is taking anticoagulant medications).

Examination

When examining the patient, obtain a baseline set of vital signs. The focus can then shift to evaluating the injured extremity. One of the simplest ways to assess an extremity is to compare one side with the other, noting any discrepancy in length, position, or skin color. Next, complete an exam noting DCAP-BTLS (Deformity, Contusions, Abrasions, Penetrating injury–Burns, Tenderness, Lacerations, Swelling) as you observe and palpate the soft tissue from head to toe and assess the patient for limitations, such as inability to move a joint. While performing the exam, be sure to cover the 6 Ps of musculoskeletal assessment: Pain, Paralysis, Paresthesias (numbness or tingling), Pulselessness, Pallor (pale or delayed capillary refill in children), and Pressure.

Pain

A person experiences acute pain when peripheral pain receptors (nocioceptors) convert painful stimuli into electrical impulses that are transmitted via the peripheral nerve fibers to the spinal cord. The signal ascends along the spinal cord to the pain-sensing region of the brain. When a tissue is injured, various chemical mediators are released that facilitate the conduction of the painful stimulus to the brain.

When assessing a patient's pain, remember the OPQRST mnemonic: Onset of the pain; Provoking or Palliating factors; Quality of the pain (such as sharp, pressure, crampy); Region of the pain, including its primary location and areas where pain radiates or refers; Severity of the pain; and the Time (duration) that the patient has been experiencing pain. It is also useful to have the patient quantify the severity of the pain by using a scale of 1 to 10 or with visual images such as faces that appear to be happy or in pain.

Inspection

When inspecting an injured extremity, always evaluate the joint above and the joint below the site of injury because the injuring force may have affected these sites as well. In particular, compare the injured side with the uninjured side. While inspecting a patient's injuries, look for the following signs:

- Deformity, including asymmetry, angulation, shortening, and rotation
- Skin changes, including contusions, abrasions, avulsions, punctures, burns, lacerations, and bone ends
- Swelling
- Muscle spasms
- Abnormal limb positioning
- Increased or decreased range of motion
- Color changes, including pallor and cyanosis
- Bleeding, including estimating the amount of blood loss

Palpation

Palpation of an injured extremity should include the injury site and the regions above and below it. Regions of point tenderness should be identified. Reassess any tender areas frequently to determine whether there are changes in the location or severity of the pain or tenderness. Note that while point tenderness is one of the best indicators of an injury, it may be absent in patients who are intoxicated or who have an injury to the spinal cord.

When palpating an injured site, attempt to identify instability, deformity, abnormal joint or bone continuity, and displaced bones. Feel for crepitus, which is commonly found at the site of a fracture. Palpate distal pulses on all extremities, with special attention to comparing the strength of the pulses in the injured extremity with those in a normal one.

On occasion, an arterial injury may be identified while palpating an extremity. Signs of an arterial injury include a pulsatile expanding hematoma, diminished distal pulses, a palpable thrill (vibration) over the site of injury that correlates with the patient's heartbeat, and difficult-to-control bleeding.

The purpose of palpating the pelvis is to identify instability and point tenderness. Apply pressure over the pubic symphysis to evaluate for tenderness and crepitus. Next, press the iliac wings toward the midline and then posteriorly. Any gross instability found during this examination should be reported to hospital personnel because it may indicate a severe pelvic injury. Do not repeatedly examine the pelvis if instability is found because the manipulation may disrupt blood clots and cause further bleeding.

The upper and lower extremity exam should include palpation of the entire length of each arm and leg to identify any sites of injury. The most efficient way to accomplish this is to place your hands around the extremity and squeeze. Repeat this procedure every few centimeters until you reach the end of the extremity. When evaluating the upper extremities, always examine the cervical spine and shoulder because complaints within the arm may be caused by a more proximal disorder. Likewise, with the lower extremities, always conduct an exam of the pelvis and hip if the patient complains of pain in the leg.

Motor Function and Sensory Exam

It is essential to assess a patient's distal pulse, as well as motor and sensory function, in the case of a musculoskeletal injury. A motor function exam should be performed whenever a patient has an injury to an extremity, provided the patient does not also have a life-threatening injury. When assessing motor function, consider the preinjury level of function. In some cases, weakness or motor deficits may be due to prior injuries or medical problems. For this reason, you should perform a careful review of the patient's history whenever a patient complains of being weak or unable to move an extremity.

While performing a motor exam, carry out each test with and without resistance because some patients may be too weak to overcome any outside resistance. Also, perform the test on both sides of the body simultaneously so that each extremity can be compared.

A sensory exam should be performed on all patients who have an injury or complaint related to an extremity, assuming that it does not take attention away from a potentially fatal condition. The sensory exam and history should attempt to identify any pre-existing deficits in function or other disorders, including diabetes and nerve disorders that may cause changes in sensation. It is important to assess not only for the presence or absence of sensation, but also for the quality and symmetry of sensation.

To perform a sensory exam, first ask the patient if he or she feels any abnormal sensations, such as numbness, tingling, or burning. Next, conduct a gross sensory exam by lightly touching the injured extremity and the unaffected side simultaneously; have the patient report whether the two sides feel the same or different. In some cases, a patient may complain of an abnormally severe sensation of pain when just lightly touched. Such hyperesthesia may be a sign of an injury to the spinal cord.

To perform a motor function and sensory exam, follow the steps shown in **Skill Drill 25-1 ▶**:

1. Have the patient abduct his or her arms at the elbow to test axillary nerve motor function (Step 1).
2. Evaluate the patient's ability to extend the arms at the elbow to test musculocutaneous nerve motor function (Step 2).
3. Have the patient extend the thumbs (thumbs up) to test radial nerve motor function (Step 3).
4. Assess the patient's ability to make an "okay" sign to test median nerve motor function (Step 4).
5. Check the patient's ability to spread his or her fingers apart to test ulnar nerve motor function (Step 5).
6. Instruct the patient to extend his or her legs at the knee to test femoral nerve motor function (Step 6).
7. Have the patient plantarflex his or her feet to test tibial nerve motor function (Step 7).
8. Assess the patient's ability to dorsiflex the feet to test peroneal nerve motor function (Step 8).
9. Check light touch over the lateral surface of the shoulder (over the deltoid) to test axillary nerve sensory function (Step 9).
10. Evaluate light touch on the anterolateral surface of the forearm to test musculocutaneous nerve sensory function (Step 10).
11. Assess light touch on the dorsal surface of the web space of the thumb to test radial nerve sensory function (Step 11).
12. Lightly touch the volar surface of the distal thumb, index, and middle fingers to test median nerve sensory function (Step 12).
13. Lightly touch the distal volar surface of the small finger to test ulnar nerve sensory function (Step 13).
14. Examine the patient's sense of light touch over the anteromedial surface of the thigh to test femoral nerve sensory function (Step 14).
15. Evaluate light touch on the plantar surface of the toes to test tibial nerve sensory function (Step 15).
16. Assess light touch in the web space between the great toe and the second toe to test peroneal nerve sensory function (Step 16).

Documentation and Communication

Always document the findings of a neurovascular exam, even if they are normal. When an abnormality is identified, document the specific deficit—for example, the patient was unable to extend the thumb or the wrist.

Skill Drill 25-1: Performing a Motor Function and Sensory Exam

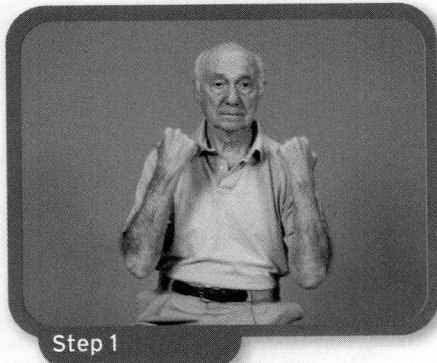

Step 1

Have the patient flex his or her arms at the elbow.

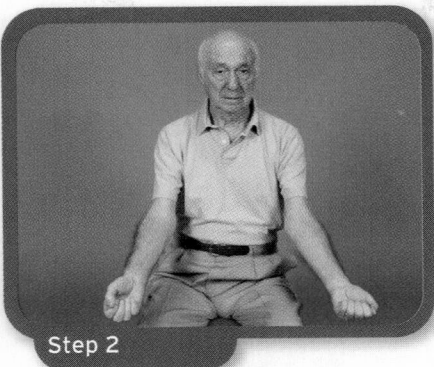

Step 2

Have the patient extend the arms at the elbow.

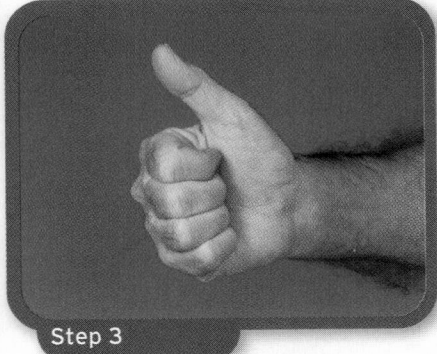

Step 3

Have the patient extend the thumbs (thumbs up).

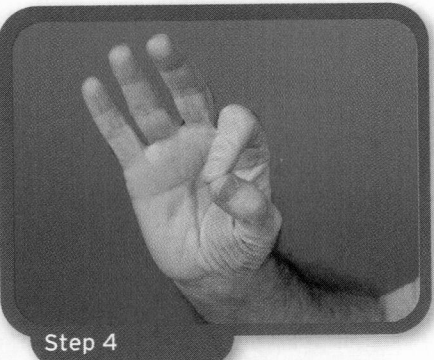

Step 4

Have the patient make an "okay" sign.

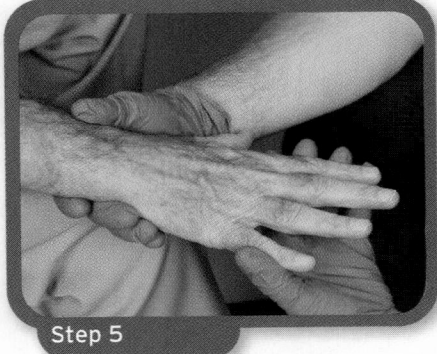

Step 5

Have the patient spread his or her fingers apart.

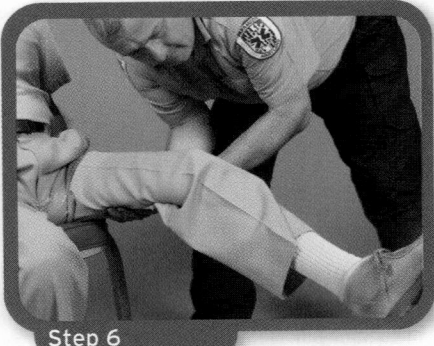

Step 6

Instruct the patient to extend his or her leg at the knee.

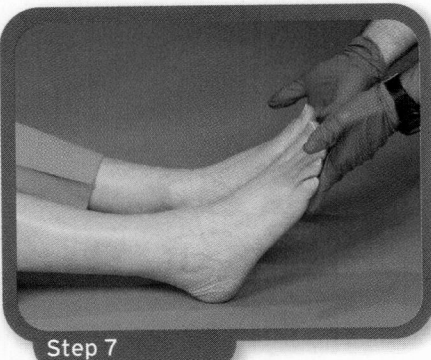

Step 7

Have the patient flex his or her feet and ankles downward.

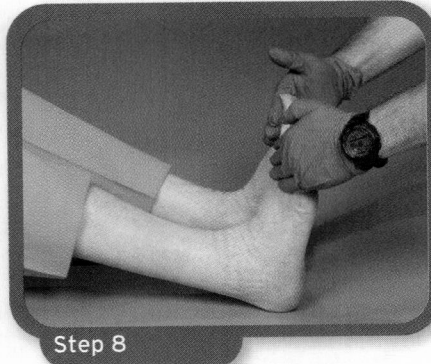

Step 8

Instruct the patient to flex the ankles upward.

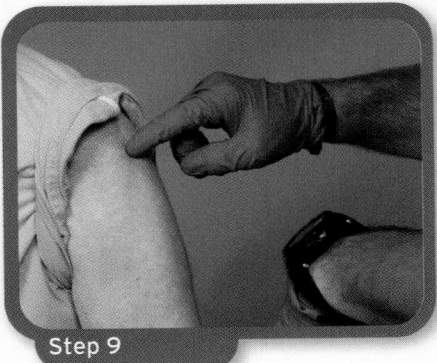

Step 9

Check light touch over the lateral surface of the shoulder (over the deltoid).

Skill Drill 25-1: Performing a Motor Function and Sensory Exam (*continued*)

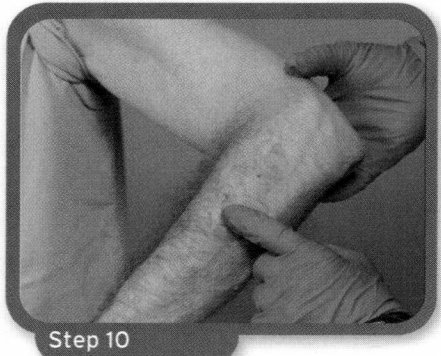

Step 10

Evaluate light touch on the anterolateral surface of the forearm.

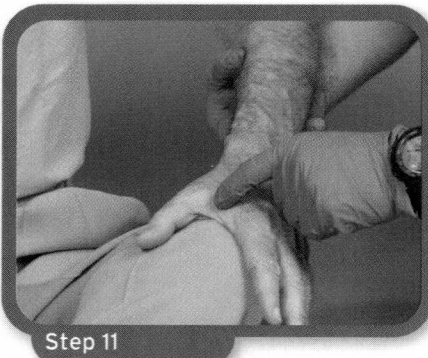

Step 11

Assess light touch on the dorsal surface of the web space of the thumb.

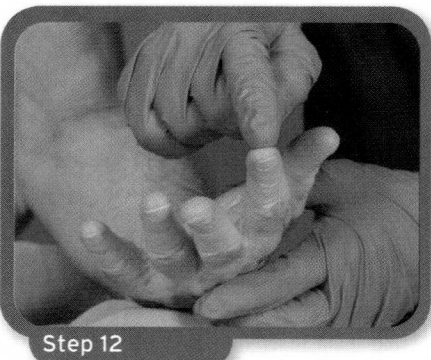

Step 12

Lightly touch the volar surface of the distal thumb, index, and middle fingers.

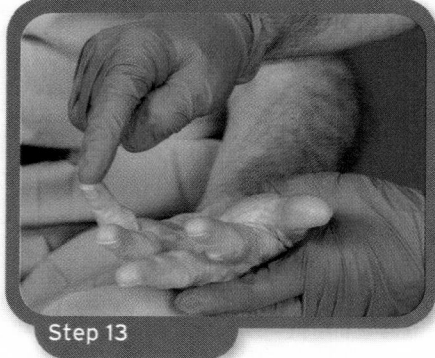

Step 13

Lightly touch the distal volar surface of the small finger.

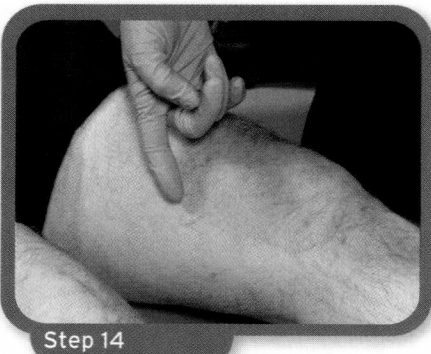

Step 14

Examine the patient's sense of light touch over the anteromedial surface of the thigh.

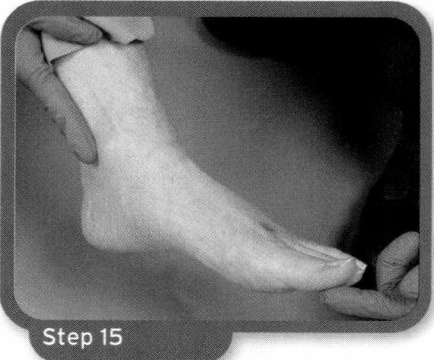

Step 15

Evaluate light touch on the plantar surface of the toes.

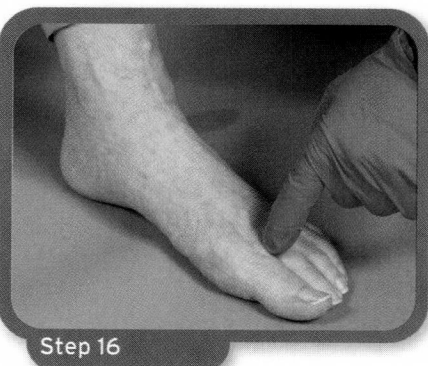

Step 16

Assess light touch in the web space between the great toe and the second toe.

that are used to secure it to the extremity, this step is not required.) Leave the fingers or toes out of the bandage so that distal circulation can be monitored.

Sling and Swath

An arm sling may be fashioned from a triangular bandage and is useful to immobilize injuries that involve the shoulder or as an adjunct to a rigid splint of the upper extremity. The sling holds the injured part against the chest wall and takes some of the weight off the injured area.

To apply a sling, place the splinted extremity in a comfortable position across the chest and lay the long edge of a triangular bandage along the patient's side opposite the injury. Bring the bottom edge of the bandage up and over the forearm, and tie it *at the side* of the neck to the other end. Tie or pin the pointed end of the sling, at the elbow, to form a cradle. Secure the sling so that the hand is carried higher than the elbow and the fingers are visible for checking peripheral circulation **Figure 25-25 ▾** .

An arm that is splinted with a sling can be further immobilized by adding a swath. Create a swath by using one or more triangular bandages to secure the arm firmly to the chest wall. This technique is particularly useful for injuries to the clavicle and for anterior dislocations of the shoulder. Do not use a sling if the patient has a neck injury.

Pneumatic Splints

Pneumatic splints (also known as air splints or inflatable splints) are useful for immobilizing fractures involving the lower leg or forearm. They are not effective for angulated fractures or for fractures that involve a joint because they will forcefully attempt to straighten the fracture or joint. Likewise, air splints should not be used on open fractures in which the bone ends are exposed.

Air splints offer two distinct advantages: They can help slow bleeding and minimize swelling by applying pressure over fracture sites to decrease small-vessel bleeding. For injuries involving the pelvis or femur, the pneumatic antishock garment (PASG) may be used as an air splint and can potentially tamponade bleeding from larger vessels. If a PASG is used for this purpose, it is necessary to use high pressure in the device (106 mm Hg or until the pop-off valves for the compartments blow off).

The method of application for an air splint depends on whether it is equipped with a zipper. If it is not, gather the splint on your own arm so that its proximal edge is just above your wrist. Grasp the patient's hand or foot while an assistant maintains proximal countertraction, then slide the air splint over your hand and onto the patient's extremity. Position the air splint so that it is free of wrinkles. Then, while you continue to maintain traction, instruct your assistant to inflate the splint with a commercially available device that is compatible with the splint system—do *not* use a compressed air tank to inflate an air splint. If the air splint has a zipper, apply it to the injured area while an assistant maintains traction proximally and distally; then zip it up and inflate **Figure 25-26 ▾** . In either case, inflate the splint just to the point at which finger pressure will make a slight dent in the splint's surface.

You must watch air splints carefully to ensure that they do not lose pressure or become overinflated. Overinflation is particularly

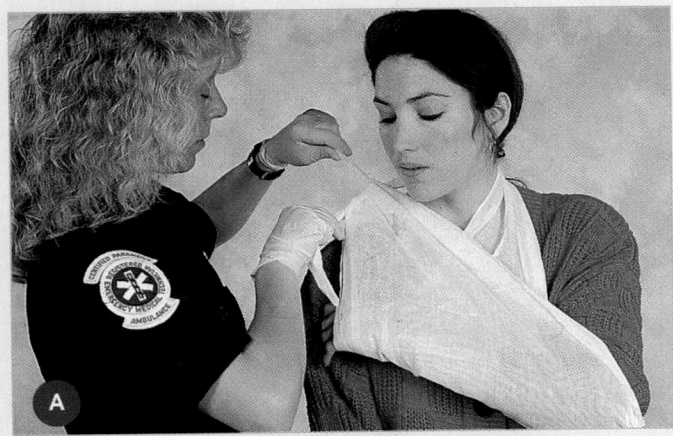

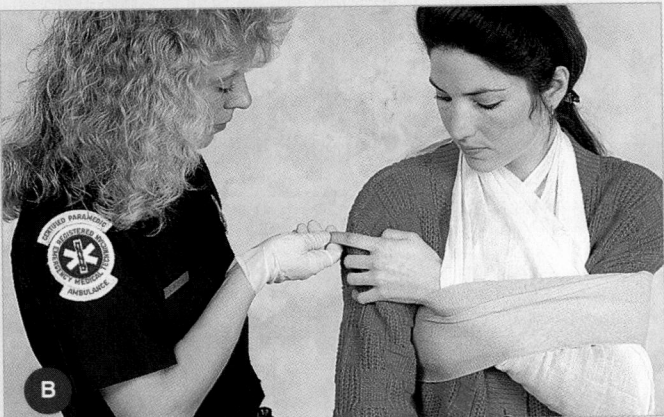

Figure 25-25 A. Apply the sling so that the knot is tied at one side of the neck. **B.** Secure the sling. Leave the fingers exposed to allow for circulation checks.

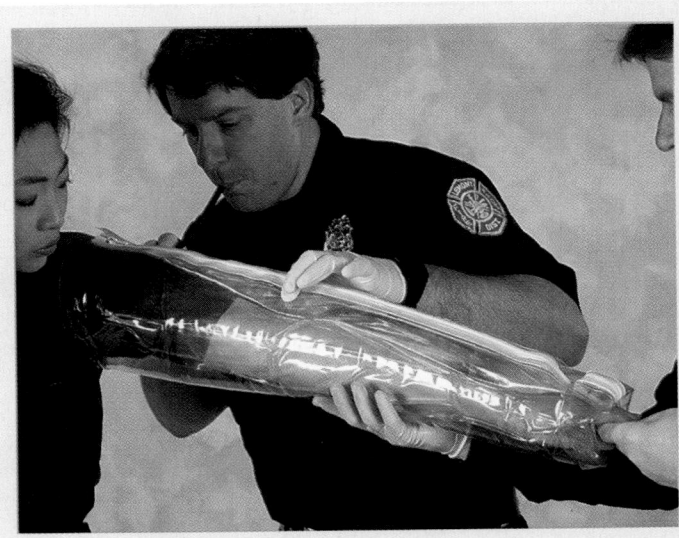

Figure 25-26 Positioning an air splint that features a zipper.

likely when the splint is applied in a cold area and the patient is subsequently moved to a warmer area because the air inside the splint will expand as it gets warmer. Air splints will also expand when going to a higher altitude if the patient compartment is unpressurized, a factor that must be considered when patients are transported by air ambulance.

Vacuum Splints

A vacuum splint consists of a sealed mattress that is filled with air and thousands of small plastic beads. The mattress is laid out on the stretcher, and the patient is placed on top of it and allowed to settle into a comfortable position. A suction pump attached to the mattress is then used to evacuate the air from inside the mattress. The resulting vacuum inside the mattress compresses the beads in such a way that the whole splint becomes rigid, much like a plaster cast that has been molded to conform to the contours of the patient's entire posterior surface.

The vacuum mattress is an excellent splint, but there are a few factors that may limit its broad appeal. The splint is quite bulky, so it not only takes up a lot of storage room in the vehicle, but also can be difficult to work with in cramped quarters. Furthermore, like all vacuum splints, it requires a mechanical suction pump, yet another piece of equipment to grab.

A smaller vacuum splint is available to splint individual limbs. This type of splint is applied by positioning the injured limb on the splint and then evacuating the air from inside of it. The result is a splint that is molded to the extremity   Figure 25-27 ▸ . This type of vacuum splint requires less space than a mattress-style vacuum splint but is still relatively expensive compared with standard rigid splints.

Pillow Splints

A pillow is an effective means to immobilize an injured foot or ankle. Simply mold an ordinary pillow around the affected foot and ankle in a position of comfort, then secure the pillow in place with several cravats. Pillows can also be molded around an injured knee or elbow and are invaluable for padding backboards when they are used to immobilize patients with dislocated hips.

Special Considerations

Because vacuum mattresses conform to the body, they may be the best choice to immobilize older patients who have abnormal curvatures of the spine and are suspected of having spinal column injuries.

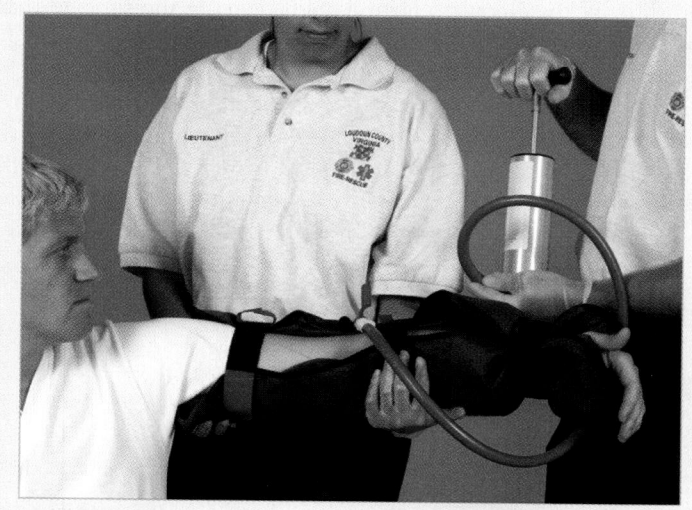

Figure 25-27 Applying a vacuum splint to a limb.

You are the Provider Part 3

You have assessed the patient's airway, breathing, and circulation and have controlled significant bleeding found on the left arm. During this time, your partner has inserted a large-bore IV catheter in the right arm. She has also noted that the patient's lung sounds are clear and initiated a bolus of 200 mL normal saline.

As you continue your rapid trauma exam, you find that the left pedal pulse is absent. When you expose the leg, you see significant deformity of the knee consistent with a posterior dislocation. The patient has difficulty feeling his foot and moving his toes. This is a true emergency. With your patient immobilized on the backboard, you decide to move him to the ambulance as per your local protocols.

Reassessment	Recording Time: 7 Minutes
Skin	Pink, warm, and slightly moist; pale and cool left foot
Pulse	110 beats/min, full and regular
Blood pressure	144/92 mm Hg
Respirations	40 breaths/min
Sao₂	100% on 15 L/min via nonrebreathing mask
ECG	Sinus tachycardia with no ectopy

6. Why would this dislocation be considered a true emergency?

7. What is an important consideration before manipulating a dislocation?

Traction Splints

Following a femur fracture, the strong muscles of the thigh go into spasm and often lead to significant pain and deformity. Traction splints provide constant pull on a fractured femur, thereby preventing the broken bone ends from overriding as a result of unopposed muscle contraction. In addition, these splints help maintain alignment of the fracture pieces and provide effective immobilization of the fracture site. As a result, patients are likely to experience less pain.

Traction splints also reduce blood loss. Normally, the thigh is shaped like a cylinder. In a femur fracture, the thigh is shortened and becomes spherical. The volume of a sphere can be substantially greater than that of a cylinder, so a person with an untreated femur fracture can accumulate more blood in the thigh than a person whose thigh is pulled out to length by a traction splint.

Traction splints are indicated for the treatment of most femur fractures. They should not be used when the patient has an additional fracture below the knee on the same extremity. The most commonly used traction splints are the Sager and the Hare traction splints. The basic principles of application are the same for both. After assessing the injured extremity for distal PMS functions, place the splint next to the uninjured leg to determine the proper length. The traction splint should extend 6″ to 10″ beyond the foot.

Support and stabilize the leg to minimize movement while another rescuer applies the ankle hitch. When the hitch is secure, the second rescuer will apply gentle longitudinal traction using enough force to realign the extremity. The initial rescuer can then place the splint into position and connect the upper attachment point of the splint and then the ankle hitch **Figure 25-28 ▼**. After applying the splint, reassess PMS functions before securing the patient and splint for transport.

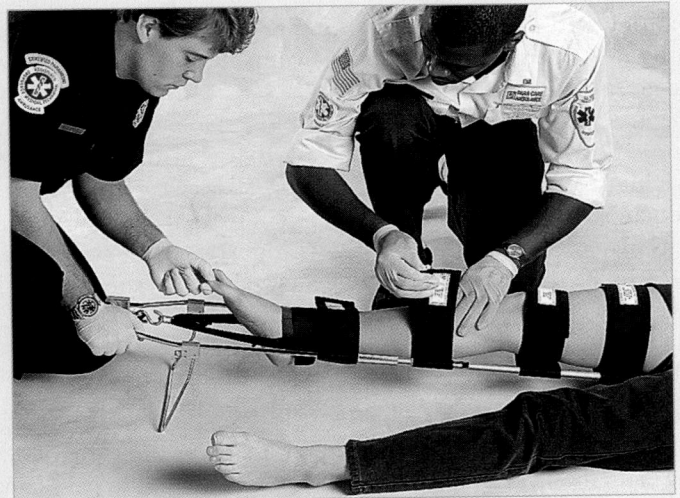

Figure 25-28 A Hare traction splint is shown here. One rescuer connects the straps and another checks distal pulse, motor function, and sensation.

Buddy Splinting

Buddy splinting is used to splint injuries that involve the fingers or toes. With this technique, an adjacent uninjured finger or toe serves as a splint to the injured one. To buddy splint, tape the injured digit to an uninjured one. Place a gauze pad between the digits that are taped together, and ensure that the tape does not pass over joints.

Complications of Musculoskeletal Injuries

Musculoskeletal injuries can lead to numerous complications—not just those involving the musculoskeletal system, but also systemic changes or illness. It is essential to not focus all of your attention on the musculoskeletal injury: Keep in mind that there is a patient attached to the injured extremity!

The likelihood of having a complication is often related to the strength of the force that caused the injury, the injury's location, and the patient's overall health. Any injury to a bone, muscle, or other musculoskeletal structure is likely to be accompanied by bleeding. In general, the greater the force that caused the injury, the greater the hemorrhage that will be associated with it.

Following a fracture, the sharp ends of the bone may damage muscles, blood vessels, arteries, and nerves, or the ends may penetrate the skin and produce an open fracture. A significant loss of tissue may occur at the fracture site if the muscle is severely damaged or if the bone's penetration of the skin causes a large defect. To prevent infection following an open fracture, you should brush away any obvious debris on the skin surrounding an open fracture before applying a dressing. Do not enter or probe the open fracture site in an attempt to retrieve debris because this may lead to further contamination.

Long-term disability is one of the most devastating consequences of a musculoskeletal injury. In many cases, a severely injured limb can be repaired and made to look almost normal. Unfortunately, many patients cannot return to work for long periods because of the extensive rehabilitation required and because of chronic pain. Paramedics have a critical role in mitigating the risk of long-term disability. By preventing further injury, reducing the risk of wound infection, minimizing pain by the use of cold and analgesia, and transporting patients with musculoskeletal injuries to an appropriate medical facility, they help reduce the risk or duration of long-term disability.

Neurovascular Injuries

The skeletal system normally protects the neurovascular structures within the limbs from injury. These critical structures typically lie deep within the limb and close to the skeleton. For example, the brachial plexus is situated within the axilla and the inner aspect of the arm, shielded from injury by the shoulder girdle. When the shoulder girdle or proximal humerus is fractured, displaced fracture fragments may lacerate or impale the nerves of the plexus, leading to a neurologic deficit. Neurovascular injuries are also likely to occur following a joint dislocation because the nerves and vessels in the region of a joint tend to be more securely tethered to the soft tissues and are less likely to escape injury.

Compartment Syndrome

Within a limb, groups of muscles are surrounded by an inelastic membrane called fascia. Thus, the muscles are confined to an enclosed space, or compartment, that can accommodate only a limited amount of swelling. When bleeding or swelling occurs within a compartment as the result of a fracture or severe soft-tissue injury, the pressure within it rises. Too-high pressure may impair circulation and lead to pain, sensory changes, and progressive muscle death. This condition, known as compartment syndrome, is one of the most devastating consequences of a musculoskeletal injury.

External and internal factors can lead to the development of compartment syndrome. External factors include bandages, splints, casts, and a PASG that are applied too tightly and restrict circulation. A number of internal factors can also increase the amount of material within a compartment. For example, bleeding within a compartment may occur because of a fracture, dislocation, crush injury, vascular injury, soft-tissue injury, or bleeding disorder. Alternatively, fluid leakage or edema may occur secondary to ischemia, excessive exercise, trauma, burns, or any condition associated with the leakage of proteins and fluid from vessels into the interstitial space. A common misconception is that open fractures are safe from compartment syndrome—a notion that is not true.

Signs and symptoms of compartment syndrome include early and late findings. Typically, the first complaint will be of a searing or burning *pain* that is localized to the involved compartment and out of proportion to the injury. This pain is often severe and typically not relieved with pain medication, including narcotics. When examining the patient, passive stretching of an ischemic muscle will result in severe pain. In the lower extremities, test for this condition by flexing and extending the great toe and by dorsiflexion and plantar flexion of the foot. In the upper extremity, use finger and hand flexion and extension.

During examination of the patient, the affected area may feel very firm and there may be skin pallor. Typical neurologic changes include paresthesias, such as a burning sensation, numbness, or tingling, and paralysis of the involved muscles, which occurs late in the condition. Another late sign of compartment syndrome is pulselessness. By the time the pressure within the compartment reaches the point where it totally occludes the artery passing through it, significant muscle necrosis has probably occurred.

The goal of prehospital care is to deliver the patient to an emergency facility before the extremity is pulseless. Thus, management should include elevating the extremity to heart level (*not above!*), placing ice packs over the extremity, and opening or loosening constrictive clothing and splint material.

Crush Syndrome

Crush syndrome occurs because of a prolonged compressive force that impairs muscle metabolism and circulation—actually, following the extrication or release of an entrapped limb. This condition happens not only in trauma patients, but also in patients who have been lying on an extremity for an extended period (4–6 hours of compression)—for example, when a drug overdose or stroke victim is not found for an extended period.

After a muscle is compressed for 4 to 6 hours, the muscle cells begin to die and release their contents into the localized vasculature. When the force compressing the region is released, blood flow is reestablished and the material from the cells that was released into the local vasculature quickly returns to the systemic vasculature. The primary substances that are of concern are lactic acid, potassium, and myoglobin. In particular, the return of myoglobin is likely to result in decreased blood pH, hyperkalemia, and renal dysfunction.

Treatment of crush syndrome, which aims to prevent complications due to toxin release, should always be performed with medical direction. A number of steps must be taken *before* releasing the compressing force. As with all patients, assess the ABCs in case of suspected crush syndrome. Ensure that the patient is being given high-flow supplemental oxygen, and then administer a bolus of crystalloid solution to increase the intravascular volume and to protect the kidneys from the forthcoming myoglobin load. Establish cardiac monitoring to evaluate for electrocardiographic (ECG) changes related to hyperkalemia (such as peaked T waves, widening QRS complex, prolonged P-R interval, dysrhythmia). To protect against the surge of potassium, a nebulizer treatment with albuterol may be given during extrication (beta-2 agonists promote the movement of potassium into cells). Once the patient is freed, if the ECG shows changes consistent with hyperkalemia, administer calcium to stabilize the myocardium; also give sodium bicarbonate to promote the intracellular shift of potassium. Insulin may also be given intravenously with dextrose, in the hospital, to facilitate the intracellular movement of potassium. Compressive devices such as a PASG should not be applied.

Thromboembolic Disease

Thromboembolic disease, including deep vein thrombosis (DVT) and pulmonary embolism, is a significant cause of death following musculoskeletal injuries, especially injuries to the pelvis and lower extremities that lead to prolonged immobilization.

Signs and symptoms of DVT include disproportionate swelling of an extremity, discomfort in an extremity that worsens with use, and warmth and erythema of the extremity.

In the Field

A patient who shows evidence of compartment syndrome must be transported on an emergency basis to the hospital. There is no treatment for this syndrome other than surgery—do not delay transport.

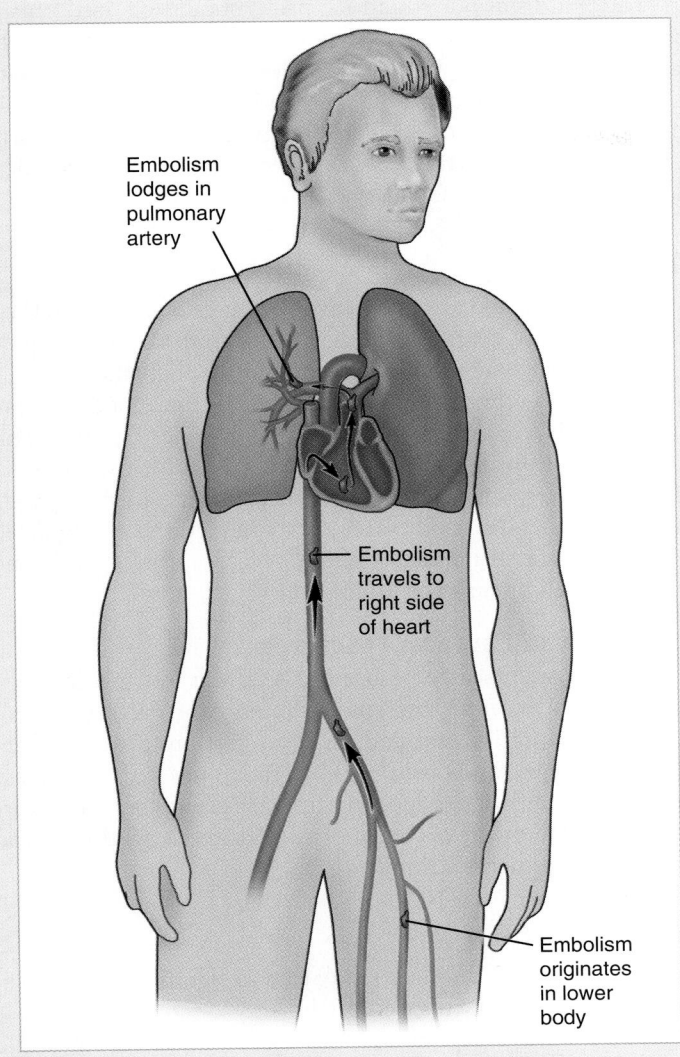

Figure 25-29 When a portion of a DVT dislodges, it may travel to the pulmonary arteries and inhibit blood flow from the heart to the lungs.

Embolism lodges in pulmonary artery

Embolism travels to right side of heart

Embolism originates in lower body

When a DVT dislodges, it may cause a pulmonary embolism—a blood clot that occludes a portion or all of the pulmonary arteries **Figure 25-29 ▲**. Signs and symptoms of a pulmonary embolism include a sudden onset of dyspnea, pleuritic chest pain, dyspnea, tachypnea, tachycardia, right-sided heart failure, shock, and, in some cases, cardiac arrest.

In addition to the risk of DVT, patients with long bone or pelvic fractures are at risk for developing a fat embolism. In this condition, fat droplets become lodged in the vasculature of the lungs. Affected patients have inflammation of the vasculature of the lungs and other blood vessels where fat is deposited. Generally, symptoms begin within 12 to 72 hours of injury; they include tachycardia, dyspnea, tachypnea, pulmonary congestion, fever, petechiae, change in mental status, and organ dysfunction.

Treatment for thromboembolic disease in the field is limited to maintaining an airway, adequate oxygenation, and intravascular volume and rapid transportation to an ED.

Specific Fractures

Shoulder Girdle

The shoulder girdle consists of the clavicle, shoulder, and scapula.

Clavicle

Clavicle fractures are very common and often occur in children. In most cases, the clavicle fractures in the middle third of the bone, typically from a fall onto an outstretched hand or from direct lateral trauma to the shoulder (as in contact sports, snowboarding, and cycling). Patients have pain in the region of the shoulder, swelling, unwillingness to raise the arm, and tilting of the head toward the injured side.

Shoulder

Fractures of the shoulder include those that involve the glenoid fossa of the scapula, the humeral head, and the humeral neck. Most shoulder fractures are caused by a fall onto an outstretched hand and usually occur in elderly patients (younger patients tend to dislocate the shoulder because they have stronger bones). Patients with a shoulder fracture rarely have evidence of a significant deformity, but instead have considerable swelling, ecchymosis, and pain with movement of the arm. In some cases, an associated injury to the brachial plexus may be identified during the neurologic examination.

Scapula

Injuries to the scapula usually result from violent, direct trauma. Therefore, when a scapular injury is suspected, it is essential to look for associated injuries—particularly intrathoracic injuries, such as pneumothorax, hemothorax, and fractured ribs. Signs and symptoms of a scapular fracture include pain that increases with arm abduction and swelling in the region of the scapula. Potential complications include axillary artery or nerve injury, brachial plexus injury, pulmonary contusion, and clavicle fractures.

Treatment of Shoulder Girdle Fractures

Fractures in the shoulder region may usually be treated by using a sling and swath. These bindings should be applied to maintain the extremity in the position of comfort, often keeping the arm against the chest wall to allow the body to act as a splint. In cases of suspected scapula fractures, full spinal immobilization is usually warranted given the amount of force required to cause a fracture.

Midshaft Humerus

Fractures of the shaft of the humerus usually occur in younger patients secondary to high-energy injuries, such as motor vehicle crashes. Unlike fractures that occur more proximally, these injuries typically have substantial deformity. Examination of the extremity usually reveals a significant amount of swelling, ecchymosis, gross instability of the region, and crepitus. If the force that caused the injury is severe enough, the nerves and blood vessels in the upper arm may also be damaged. Of particular concern is the radial nerve, which may be injured by the force itself or could become entrapped within the fracture site. The classic sign of a radial nerve injury is wrist drop.

Treatment of Midshaft Humerus Fractures

If the fracture is angulated, longitudinal traction may be applied to correct the deformity, but efforts should be halted if the patient's pain is too severe or if neurovascular status worsens. Once the extremity is in the desired position, apply a rigid splint that extends from the axilla to the elbow. Next, apply a sling and swath to immobilize the arm to the chest wall, and place cold packs over the fracture site to decrease the patient's pain and swelling.

Elbow
Distal Humerus

Supracondylar fractures of the humerus occur most often in children. The typical mechanism is a fall onto an outstretched hand with the elbow in extension, thereby breaking the distal humerus; as a result, the distal fragment of the humerus is pushed posteriorly and the humeral shaft is pulled anteriorly, where it compresses the brachial artery and the radial and median nerves. If the brachial artery is compromised, the patient could develop compartment syndrome in the forearm. When this complication occurs, the patient is at risk for a Volkmann ischemic contracture, a condition in which muscles of the forearm degenerate from prolonged ischemia. The patient's muscles that allow for movement of the fingers become contracted and nonfunctional, and the patient loses the ability to use the hand. Patients with a distal humerus fracture will complain of pain in the area of the elbow and typically have a significant degree of swelling and ecchymosis.

Proximal Radius and Ulna

Radial head fractures may result from a fall onto an outstretched hand or from a direct blow to the bone. This injury causes the patient to have significant pain when he or she attempts supination or pronation. In either case, the patient is likely to have pain and ecchymosis in the region of the injury. Similar to distal humerus fractures, these injuries may lead to an injury of the nerves or blood vessels in proximity to the fracture site. Therefore, a careful neurovascular examination should be performed.

Treatment of Elbow Fractures

Treatment of injuries in the region of the elbow is the same regardless of the exact location of the injury. The injured extremity must be repeatedly assessed for evidence of compartment syndrome. Before splinting the extremity, it is mandatory to document a neurovascular exam. The injured extremity should be splinted in the position that it is found if the patient

has a strong distal pulse, and ice packs should be used only if there is no evidence of compartment syndrome. If the patient has an absent distal pulse or neurologic deficits, consult with the appropriate medical facility to determine whether you should attempt fracture reduction. In any event, the patient must be transported urgently to the closest appropriate medical facility for definitive treatment.

Forearm

Fractures of the forearm may involve the radius, the ulna, or, more commonly, both. Injury may result from a direct blow to the bone, the classic example of which is the nightstick fracture of the ulna. In other cases, injury occurs because of a fall onto an outstretched hand, as in the case of a Colles fracture. This fracture typically occurs in older patients with osteoporosis who have fallen but may be found in younger patients as well. A patient with a Colles fracture usually has a dorsally angulated deformity of the distal forearm (the "silver fork deformity") and pain and swelling near the injured site.

Treatment of Forearm Fractures

A variety of splints may be used to secure a forearm fracture. Regardless of the type, the splint should provide immobilization of the entire forearm and, in cases of more proximal fractures, the elbow. Apply cold packs to the injury site to decrease pain and swelling. Frequent neurovascular exams are warranted to monitor for evidence of compartment syndrome and acute carpal tunnel syndrome.

Wrist and Hand

Injuries to the wrist and hand may lead to significant long-term disability, especially in people who rely on the use of their hands to earn a living. Sometimes these injuries occur while working at the job or at home; in other cases they result from a fall or during a sporting event. Careful splinting of the injured site is essential to help reduce the risk of long-term disability.

Scaphoid

The scaphoid, also called the carpal navicular, is located just distal to the radius. It may be injured from a fall onto an outstretched hand, for which the classic finding is pain and tenderness in the anatomic snuffbox. To identify the anatomic snuffbox on yourself, extend your thumb. Two tendons will be visible at the base of the thumb on the radial aspect of the wrist. The region between these two tendons is the snuffbox **Figure 25-30 ▶**. The major complication of a scaphoid fracture is avascular necrosis of the bone, or poor fracture healing because of the limited blood supply to this bone.

Boxer's Fracture

A boxer's fracture is a fracture of the neck of the fifth metacarpal (small finger). It commonly occurs after punching a hard object, such as a wall or a door. The patient typically has pain over the ulnar aspect of the hand and may have noticeable swelling.

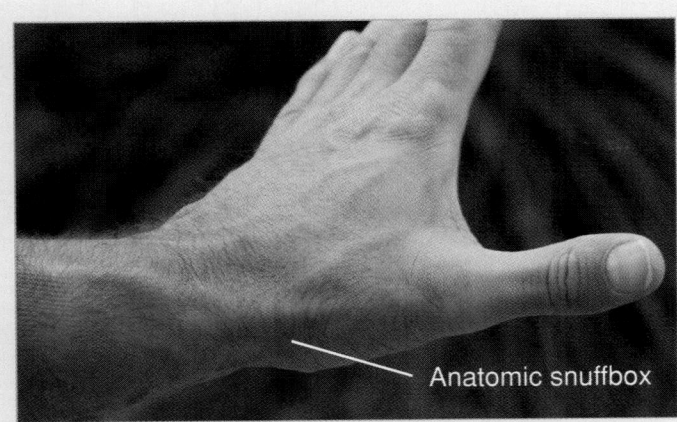

Figure 25-30 The region between the two tendons shown is the anatomic snuffbox.

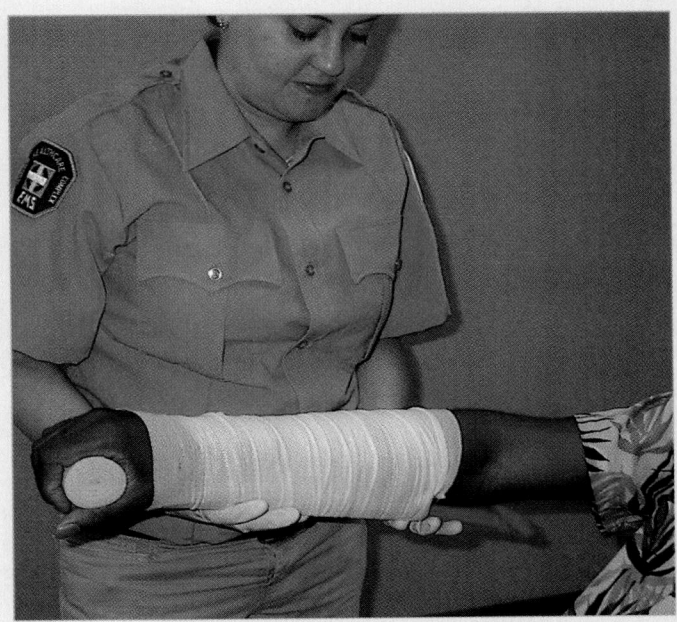

Figure 25-31 Splinting the hand and wrist.

Metacarpal Shaft

Fractures of the metacarpals may result from a crush injury or from direct trauma. Assessment of the injured hand may reveal abnormal rotation or alignment of the fingers, swelling of the palm, and pain and tenderness in the region of injury. You should assess the neurovascular function of the hand and fingers following a crush injury, because development of compartment syndrome is possible within the hand.

Mallet Finger (Baseball Fracture)

A mallet finger occurs when a finger is jammed into an object, such as a baseball or basketball, resulting in an avulsion fracture of the extensor tendon. The patient will not be able to extend the distal phalynx of the finger and will maintain it in a flexed position.

Treatment of Wrist and Hand Fractures

Splint the injured hand in the position of function by placing the wrist in about 30° of dorsiflexion with fingers slightly flexed (a roll of gauze approximately 2″ to 3″ in diameter accomplishes this nicely). Next, secure the extremity to an armboard or other rigid splint that extends proximally to the elbow and is slightly elevated to help reduce swelling **Figure 25-31 ▶**. For injuries that are isolated to the digits, use a foam-padded flexible aluminum splint to splint the injured digit, if available. In the case of penetrating injuries, regardless of whether a fracture is present, apply bulky dressings to the site of injury and splint the injured hand in the position of function.

Pelvis

Pelvic fractures are relatively uncommon injuries, accounting for fewer than 3% of all fractures. Despite their low incidence, these injuries are responsible for a significant number of deaths in blunt trauma patients. The risk of death following a pelvic fracture ranges from 8% to 50%, depending on the severity of the injury; when the fracture is open, the mortality rate rises to 25% to 50%. Death after a pelvic fracture commonly results from massive hemorrhage caused by damage to the arteries and veins of the pelvis.

Disruptions of the pelvic ring occur secondary to high-energy trauma such as crush injuries, motorcycle crashes, and falls from a significant height. A number of structures within the pelvis are at risk for injury when it is fractured—the bladder, urethra, rectum, vagina, and sacral nerve plexus. The blood vessels that are most prone to damage are the veins within the pelvis, but there may be damage to the internal or external iliac and arteries in the lumbar region. The nerves at greatest risk of injury are those in the lumbar and sacral regions and the sciatic and femoral nerves.

Patients with pelvic ring disruptions who have a stable injury, such as a minimal lateral compression injury, may complain of pain in the pelvis and difficulty bearing weight. Patients with a more severe injury may show evidence of profound shock, gross pelvic instability, and diffuse pelvic and lower abdominal pain. There may also be bruising or lacerations in the perineum, scrotum, groin, suprapubic region, and flank and hematuria (blood in the urine) or blood coming from the meatus of the penis, vagina, or rectum.

Lateral Compression Pelvic Ring Disruptions

Lateral compression injuries result from an impact on the side of the body (such as being struck by a car from the side or falling from a significant height and landing on one side of the body). The side of the pelvis that sustains the impact becomes internally rotated around the sacrum, and the actual volume within the pelvis decreases **Figure 25-32 ▶**. Although this injury is not commonly associated with massive hemorrhage into the pelvis, it is often associated with injuries in other regions of the body.

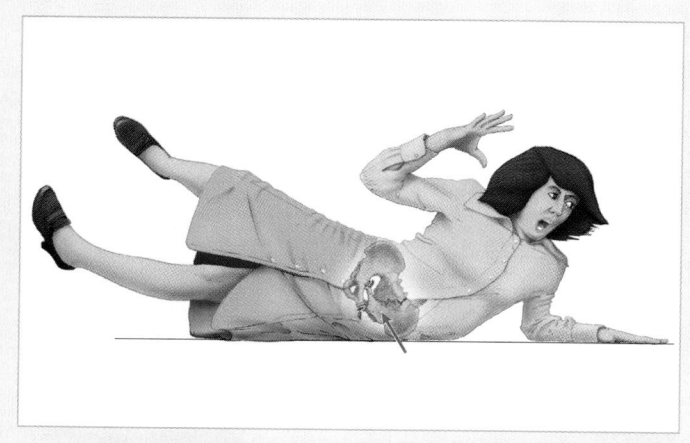

Figure 25-32 A lateral compression injury to the pelvis.

Anterior-Posterior Compression Pelvic Ring Disruptions

These injuries may occur following a head-on motor vehicle crash, motorcycle crash, or fall or in a pedestrian who is struck head-on by a vehicle. The force of the impact compresses the pelvis in the anterior-to-posterior direction, causing the pubic symphysis and posterior supporting ligaments to be disrupted and tear apart. The pelvis then spreads apart and opens like a book—hence the name open book pelvic fracture. Such an injury has the potential for massive blood loss because the volume of the pelvis is greatly increased.

Vertical Shear

Vertical shear injuries occur when a major force is applied to the pelvis from above or below, such as when a person falls from a significant height and lands on the feet. On landing, the force is transmitted through the legs to the pelvis, leading to the complete displacement of one or both sides of the pelvis toward the head. Thus, this kind of injury has anterior and posterior components. The anterior component involves a fracture of the rami or disruption of the symphysis pubis. The posterior component involves a fracture of the ilium or sacrum or a disruption of the sacroiliac joint. The patient is likely to have significant shortening of the limb on the affected side and is at risk for massive hemorrhage into the pelvis.

Straddle Fracture

A straddle fracture occurs after a fall when a person lands in the region of the perineum and sustains bilateral fractures of the inferior and superior rami. This injury does not interfere with weightbearing, but it does carry a risk owing to its associated complications, particularly those of the lower genitourinary system.

Open Pelvic Fractures

Open pelvic fractures are life-threatening injuries. Such an injury is defined by the presence of a laceration of the skin in the pelvic region, vagina, or rectum. This uncommon fracture

In the Field

Controlling bleeding from a severely injured pelvis is a major challenge, even to the most experienced trauma surgeon. Nevertheless, reducing the volume of an unstable pelvis can decrease bleeding and be a lifesaving intervention. This may be accomplished by using a PASG, applying a commercially made pelvic binder, or applying a sheet. When a sheet or pelvic binder is used, place it around the iliac wings and secure it while a provider on each side of the patient applies medially directed pressure. Emergency workers often make the mistake of placing this device too low on the pelvis, which decreases its effectiveness in reducing the pelvic volume.

is caused by a high-velocity injury with subsequent massive hemorrhage and has a mortality rate of 25% to 50%. Even small amounts of blood found during a vaginal or rectal exam should raise your suspicion for an open fracture.

Treatment of Pelvic Fractures

Assessment of the patient with a possible pelvic fracture should begin as in any other trauma patient—with an initial assessment of the mental status and ABCs, taking spinal precautions. During the rapid trauma exam of the patient, you should search for injuries typically associated with pelvic fractures. Assess the pelvis for bleeding, lacerations, bruising, and instability. To assess for instability, apply pressure over the iliac wings in a medial direction and in a posterior direction. Once instability of the pelvis is identified, the pelvis should not be reassessed for instability to avoid causing increased bleeding.

Treatment should include careful monitoring of the ABCs, spinal immobilization, and IV access with at least one (if not two) large-bore catheters. Management of the pelvic injury is aimed at reducing the amount of bleeding and decreasing the degree of instability. It is often appropriate to seek medical direction for the management of these patients, especially for determining how to best stabilize the pelvis. Methods used to accomplish this may include application of a PASG or pelvic binder or simply tying a sheet around the pelvis. Applying pressure to the iliac wings and forcing them to shift toward the midline reduces the potential space within the pelvis, which may allow for tamponade of the bleeding vessels. Once packaged, the patient should be rapidly transported to a trauma center, and IV fluid should be administered to maintain adequate tissue perfusion but avoiding hypertension.

Hip

A hip fracture involves a fracture of the femoral head, femoral neck, intertrochanteric region, or proximal femoral shaft. Fractures of the femoral head are uncommon injuries that are usually associated with a hip dislocation. Femoral neck and intertrochanteric fractures typically occur in older patients with osteoporosis who have fallen and sustained direct trauma to the hip. They may occur in younger patients with healthy

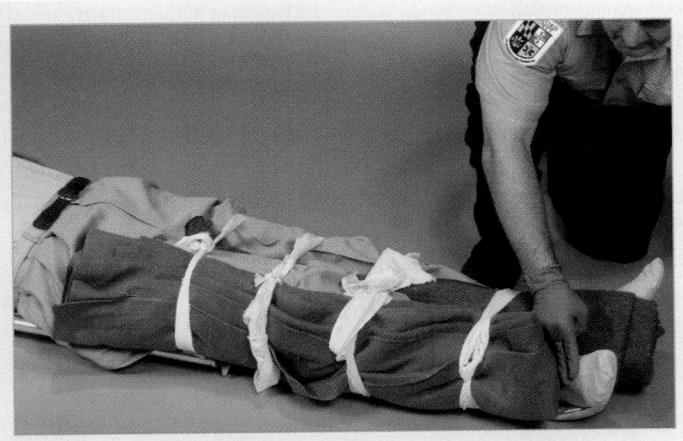

Figure 25-33 An acceptable method for splinting a hip fracture.

bone, typically as the result of a high-energy mechanism. Proximal femoral shaft fractures can occur in patients of any age and result from a high-energy mechanism.

Patients with a hip fracture will complain of pain in the affected hip, especially with attempts at movement, and report an inability to bear weight. They may also report hearing or feeling something snap. If the fracture is displaced, the patient almost always has an externally rotated and shortened leg. If there is no displacement, the leg may appear normal. Examination of the injury site usually finds tenderness to palpation, and there may be noticeable swelling, deformity, or ecchymosis.

Treatment of Hip Fractures

The treatment of hip fractures depends on the mechanism of injury. Hip fractures in older patients who sustained a low-energy injury, such as a fall from a standing position, do not require traction splints. Treat these injuries by supporting the injured extremity in the position in which it is found. This may be accomplished by placing pillows or blankets under the affected extremity and securing them in place Figure 25-33 ▲ .

In younger patients and in those with high-energy injuries, place the injured extremity in a traction splint to reduce the amount of bleeding. For patients who have multiple lower extremity injuries, use a PASG. In either case, treat the patient as you would any other trauma patient: Fully immobilize the patient, establish vascular access, monitor for shock, and transport to a trauma center.

Special Considerations

A hip fracture in an elderly patient can be a debilitating and life-altering injury. In many cases, these injuries occur in the home after slipping on a throw rug, tripping over an object that extends into the walkway, or stumbling because of poor lighting. To help prevent this injury and other fall-related problems, you should point out any safety hazards in the home to the patient or a family member. It takes only a minute, and most patients and families appreciate the advice.

Definitive treatment of a hip fracture almost always requires surgery. If possible, the bone is repaired with plates, rods, or screws. Sometimes, however, the hip must be replaced.

Femoral Shaft

Femoral shaft fractures occur following high-energy impacts. Thus, the presence of a fracture of the femoral shaft should alert you to the risk of other injuries. Patients with femoral shaft fractures will complain of severe pain. The fracture may be severely angulated or lead to significant limb shortening, or it may be open. Examination may identify significant thigh edema, bruising, crepitus, and muscle spasm.

There is often significant blood loss (perhaps 500–1,500 mL) at the fracture site. In addition, damage to the neurovascular structures of the thigh is possible. Femoral shaft fractures also place the patient at risk for fat emboli.

Treatment of Femoral Shaft Fractures

Management of femoral shaft fractures includes monitoring for evidence of shock, full spinal immobilization, and establishing vascular access. Place the injured extremity in a traction splint, and use a PASG, if necessary, for further stability and hemorrhage control. Because these injuries may be extremely painful, consider the administration of pain medication.

Knee

Fractures of the knee may involve the distal femur, proximal tibia, or patella. An injury to this region may result from a direct blow to the knee, an axial load of the leg, or powerful contractions of the quadriceps. Assessment of the patient generally reveals significant pain in the knee, decreased range of motion, pain with movement and weightbearing, ecchymosis, swelling, and, in the case of displaced fractures, deformity.

Treatment of Knee Fractures

Management of knee fractures depends on the position of the leg and the status of distal pulses. If the patient has a good distal pulse, splint the extremity in the position that it is found. If there is no distal pulse, seek medical consultation to determine whether you should attempt manipulation before transportation. In all cases, elevate the leg to the heart level and apply cold packs. Frequent neurovascular checks are mandatory, given the high incidence of compartment syndrome and neurovascular injury in cases of knee fracture.

Notes from Nancy

When you find a knee injury in the victim of a motor vehicle crash, look for posterior dislocation of the hip.

Tibia and Fibula

Fractures of the tibia and/or fibula may result from direct trauma to the lower leg or from application of rotational or compressive forces. These injuries often present with significant deformity and soft-tissue injury. Complications may include compartment syndrome, neurovascular injury, infection, poor healing, and chronic pain.

Treatment of Tibia and Fibula Fractures

Apply a rigid, long leg splint, and administer pain medication as necessary. If there is gross angulation, attempt to align the leg after giving pain medication, documenting the premanipulation and postmanipulation neurovascular status. Monitor the patient for evidence of compartment syndrome, elevate the extremity to heart level, and apply cold packs.

Ankle

Fractures of the ankle (**Figure 25-34 ▶**) usually result from sudden and forceful movements of the foot that damage the malleoli and sometimes produce dislocation (called a fracture-dislocation). In other cases, an axial load is transmitted through the foot and causes the talus (the bone of the foot that articulates with the tibia) to impact the distal tibia, leading to a fracture. Signs and symptoms of an ankle fracture include pain, deformity, and swelling. Ankle fractures may lead to damage of the nerves and blood vessels that supply the foot, the development of compartment syndrome, and chronic ankle pain and arthritis.

Treatment of Ankle Fractures

All ankle fractures should be immobilized using a commercially available splint or a pillow splint. The toes should be exposed to allow for frequent checks of distal neurovascular function. Elevate the extremity to the heart level, and apply cold packs to reduce swelling.

If an ankle fracture-dislocation is associated with a pulseless foot, medical direction may recommend that you

attempt reduction. To reduce a fracture-dislocation of the ankle, first relax the calf muscles to allow the foot to move more freely by flexing the patient's leg at the knee. With the leg flexed, grasp the heel and the foot just proximal to the toes and apply gentle traction. Next, rotate the foot back into its normal position without forcing it. If this procedure is successful, reassess the distal neurovascular status and splint the extremity in the reduced position, using care not to allow the ankle to dislocate again. If the fracture-dislocation cannot be reduced, notify medical control and expedite

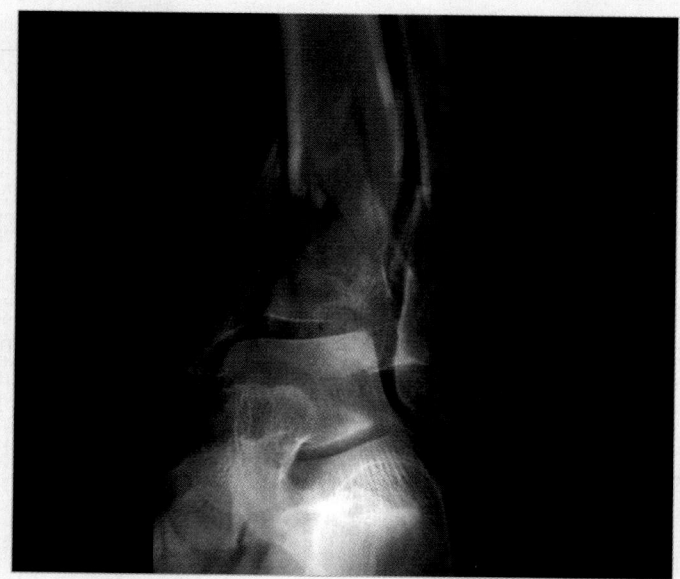

Figure 25-34 A severe fracture of the ankle.

You are the Provider Part 4

You have set the IV of normal saline at a "keep vein open" rate. After consulting with medical direction, you receive an order to administer 0.5 mg of midazolam (Versed) and 50 μg of fentanyl to take the edge off the pain and permission to carefully attempt manipulation of the knee to restore its circulation. After movement of the tibia, PMS functions are restored distal to the knee. You carefully splint the leg and notice improvement of local skin signs. You reassess the splint on the left arm and note no changes. The patient tells you his pain is much less, and he thanks you for taking care of him. You place blankets on the patient and continue to monitor him throughout transport.

Reassessment	Recording Time: 15 Minutes
Skin	Pink, warm, and dry
Pulse	90 beats/min, full and regular
Blood pressure	134/76 mm Hg
Respirations	28 breaths/min
Sao₂	100% while breathing 10 L/min via nonrebreathing mask
ECG	Sinus rhythm with no ectopy

8. Why should a joint that has just been manipulated be splinted immediately?

9. What facts should be relayed to the emergency department staff in your radio report?

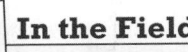

In the Field

Whenever an open fracture is reduced, there is a risk that blood will be splashed. Always wear safety glasses and a gown, in addition to gloves, when splinting or manipulating an open fracture.

transportation after splinting the ankle in the position in which it was found.

Calcaneus

The calcaneus may be fractured when a patient jumps from a height and lands on the feet or when a powerful force is applied directly to the heel. These injuries present with foot pain, swelling, and ecchymosis and should alert providers to the possibility of injuries in the knee, pelvis, and spine.

Treatment of Calcaneus Fractures

When a calcaneus fracture is suspected, splint the injured extremity with a pillow and apply ice packs to help decrease swelling. Any patient with a suspected calcaneus fracture requires spinal immobilization given the high risk of an associated spine injury.

Joint Injuries and Dislocations

Shoulder Girdle Injuries and Dislocations

Acromioclavicular Joint Separation

Separation of the acromioclavicular (AC) joint **Figure 25-35** usually occurs from a direct blow to the superior aspect or point of the shoulder, as may happen during contact sports and falls. Patients generally complain of pain and tenderness in the region of the AC joint, and the prominence of the distal clavicle may lead to a noticeable protrusion.

Posterior Sternoclavicular Joint Dislocation

Posterior dislocation of the clavicle at its junction with the sternum most often occurs as a result of a direct blow to the clavicle but is sometimes seen after strong pressure is applied to the posterior shoulder (as when a football player ends up at the bottom of a pile-up). This injury is rarely difficult to identify because there is pain and swelling at the sternoclavicular joint. What makes this a potentially dangerous and even potentially fatal injury is not the dislocation itself, but the possible damage to underlying structures—specifically, the trachea, esophagus, jugular vein, subclavian vein and artery, carotid artery, and other vascular structures. Any symptoms that suggest such underlying injury—such as *dyspnea, pain on swallowing, a sensation of choking, loss of pulses,* or a *sensory deficit* in the upper extremity on the same side—are *danger signals* and should prompt rapid transport of the patient to the hospital.

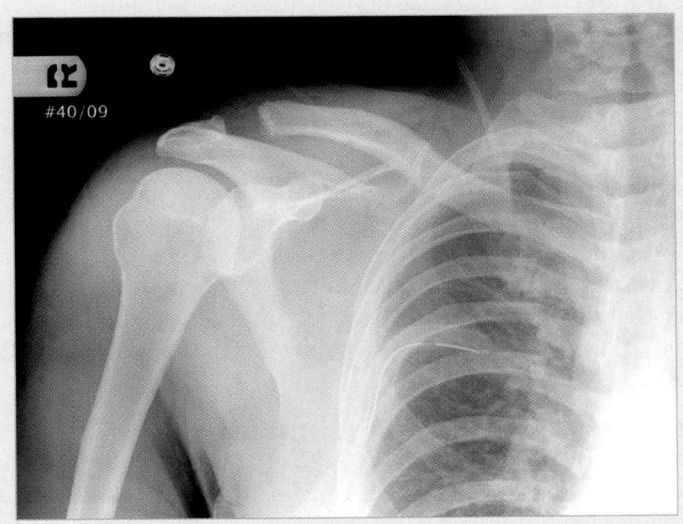

Figure 25-35 Separation of the AC joint. This space is wider than it should normally be.

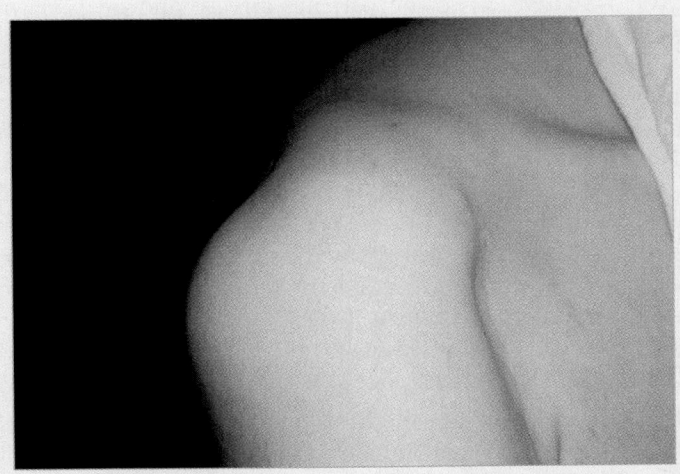

Figure 25-36 The typical appearance of an anterior shoulder dislocation.

Shoulder Dislocation

Roughly 90% of shoulder dislocations are anterior dislocations. Usually, anterior shoulder dislocations are caused by a fall onto an outstretched arm that is abducted and externally rotated. Patients complain of severe pain and have significantly decreased range of motion at the shoulder. The arm is usually abducted and externally rotated, and any efforts at moving it result in extreme pain **Figure 25-36**. A prominent bulge from the acromion is often noted on the anterior surface of the shoulder, the humeral head may be palpable, and the patient may experience frequent and painful muscle spasms.

Posterior shoulder dislocations are much less common and are often caused by massive muscle contractions such as those seen with electrical shocks and seizures. These injuries present with the same complaints of pain and limited motion, but the arm is maintained in internal rotation and adduction.

In some patients, a shoulder dislocation will produce a tear of the rotator cuff or a fracture of the glenoid. Some patients may have a concomitant injury to the brachial plexus, axillary artery, or axillary vein. The axillary nerve is also prone to injury during a shoulder dislocation; assess sensation over the deltoid muscle to determine whether there is a sensory deficit in the distribution of this nerve. Patients with a shoulder dislocation are also at risk for future dislocations, especially during the first 2 years following the injury and if the patient is young.

Treatment of Joint Injuries Involving the Shoulder Girdle

In cases of an AC joint separation, a sling and swath will often provide significant pain relief. In case of a posterior sternoclavicular joint dislocation, position the patient supine with the arm on the affected side abducted and place a rolled towel under the shoulder blade, a position that may take some of the pressure off the structures beneath the sternoclavicular joint. Pay close attention to the patient's airway, and keep airway equipment readily available.

For a dislocated shoulder, splint the injured extremity in the position in which it was found by using blankets, pillows, and, when possible, a sling and swath. When applying the swath, it may be necessary to connect two cravats together so as to encircle the patient's body, extremity, and pillows or blankets. Given the likelihood of muscle spasm and pain, use of pain medication and antispasmodic agents may be necessary. Perform neurovascular assessments frequently to monitor for changes in function.

Elbow Dislocation

Elbow dislocations are medical emergencies because of the high risk of neurovascular injury. The vast majority of elbow dislocations are posterior injuries that result from a fall onto an outstretched hand or from hyperextension of the elbow joint. Patients usually complain of significant pain in the region of the elbow and may have a large degree of swelling and ecchymosis. A palpable deformity may be present at the elbow from the prominence of the <u>olecranon</u> process **Figure 25-37 ▶**, and there is typically locking or resistance to movement of the joint. Major complications of an elbow dislocation include an associated fracture in the region of the joint, brachial artery injury, median nerve injury, and injury to the ulnar nerve.

Notes from Nancy

When there is injury to a joint, splint the extremity in the position in which it is found.

Radial Head Subluxation

Subluxation of the radial head is also referred to as <u>nursemaid's elbow</u>. It commonly occurs in children younger than 6 years

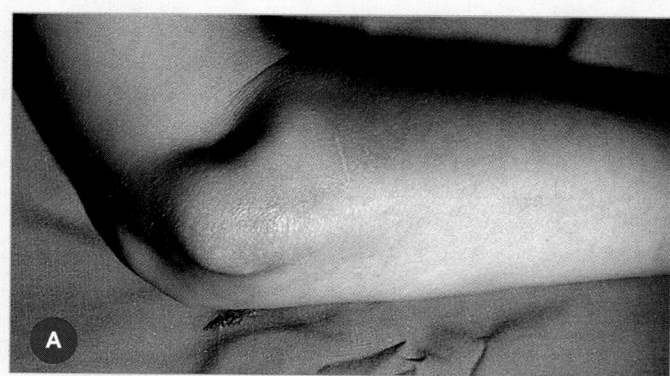
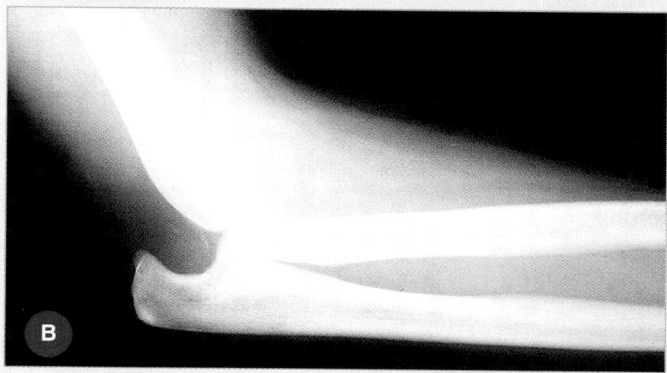

Figure 25-37 A posteriorly dislocated elbow. **A.** The clinical appearance of an elbow dislocation. **B.** Radiographic appearance of the same elbow.

and is caused by a sudden pull on the child's arm. Clinically, the injured arm is held in flexion and the child will often refuse to move the hand or elbow on the injured side. In general, there is only mild swelling in the region of the elbow.

Treatment of Elbow Dislocation

When you suspect a dislocation or subluxation in the elbow, splint the injured extremity in the position in which it was found. A sling and swath may be applied to provide additional stabilization to the injured elbow.

Finger Dislocation

Finger dislocations are caused by a sudden "jamming" force or from extension of the fingers beyond the normal range of motion. There is generally pain and deformity at the affected joint, and there may be compromise of the neurovascular structures of the digit, leading to paresthesias.

Treatment of Finger Dislocation

Manage the dislocated finger by splinting the entire hand in the position of function and using soft dressings as needed to support the digit. Do not attempt to relocate the injured digit in the field unless you are directed to do so by medical control. To reduce a dislocated digit, if the digit is dislocated to the dorsal side, extend the digit; if it is dislocated to the volar side, flex the digit. Next, use gentle longitudinal traction to bring the digit back into its normal position. It may be helpful to apply pressure at the dislocated joint to push the distal part into position. Following reduction, the neurovascular status of the digit should be reassessed and the digit should be fully immobilized to prevent it from dislocating again.

Hip Dislocation

More than 90% of all hip dislocations involve posterior dislocation. The majority of these occur due to deceleration injuries, in which a flexed knee strikes an immobile object with a great degree of force Figure 25-38 ▼ . When a patient has a posterior hip dislocation, the leg of the affected side is typically found in flexion, adduction, and internal rotation, and it is noticeably shorter. Patients complain of severe pain and inability to move the leg, and significant soft-tissue swelling may be evident. Complications arising from such injuries include sciatic nerve injury, avascular necrosis of the hip, and associated fractures of the acetabulum.

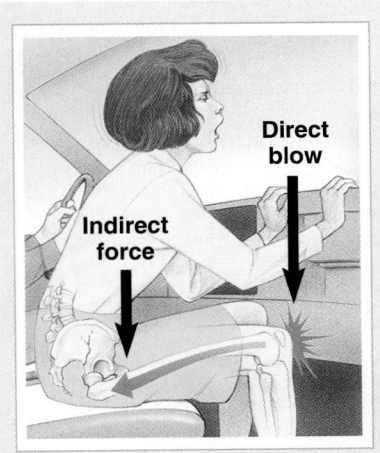

Figure 25-38 When a flexed knee strikes a dashboard, the force may be transmitted to the femur causing it to be driven posteriorly. The hip may dislocate, and the acetabulum may fracture.

Anterior hip dislocations usually follow a forceful spreading injury that occurs while the hip is flexed. The affected leg is usually flexed, abducted, and externally rotated, and the patient complains of severe pain. Major complications of this type of injury include injury to the femoral artery or nerve and avascular necrosis of the hip.

Treatment of Hip Dislocation

Because the majority of hip dislocations are associated with a high-energy mechanism, a full trauma assessment should be conducted and the patient fully immobilized. Splint the injured extremity in the position in which it is found by using blankets and pillows. Perform and document frequent neurovascular checks on your PCR. Once at the hospital, the patient generally requires sedation and muscle relaxants to allow the hip to be reduced.

Knee Dislocation

Dislocations of the knee are true emergencies that may threaten the limb. When the knee is dislocated, the ligaments that provide support to it may be damaged or torn. The knee may be dislocated by high-energy trauma (as in motor vehicle crashes), or it may dislocate secondary to powerful twisting forces (as when athletes attempt to avoid another player). In most cases, the knee will spontaneously reduce following the injury and there may be no obvious evidence of injury.

The direction of dislocation refers to the position of the tibia with respect to the femur. Anterior knee dislocations, which result from extreme hyperextension of the knee, are the most common, occurring in almost half of all cases. Commonly, the anterior and posterior cruciate ligaments are damaged, but there is also a high risk of injury to the popliteal artery.

In posterior dislocations, a direct blow to the knee forces the tibia to shift posteriorly. There is also the possibility of damage to the cruciate ligaments and injury to the popliteal artery.

Medial dislocations result from a direct blow to the lateral part of the leg. Because the deforming force causes the medial aspect of the knee to stretch apart, there is a high likelihood of injury to the medial collateral and cruciate ligaments. When the force is applied from the medial direction, a lateral dislocation occurs and the lateral part of the knee is stretched apart, injuring the lateral collateral ligament. Lateral and medial dislocations happen less commonly and have a lesser risk of injuring the popliteal artery.

Patients with a knee dislocation will typically complain of pain in the knee and report that the knee "gave out." If the knee did not spontaneously reduce, there may be evidence of significant deformity and decreased range of motion. Complications may include limb-threatening popliteal artery disruption; injuries to the popliteal, peroneal, and tibial nerves; and joint instability. Do not confuse this injury with a relatively minor patella dislocation.

Treatment of Knee Dislocation

In all cases of knee dislocation, distal neurovascular function must be assessed frequently and will often guide the management. If a pulse is palpable in the foot, splint the knee in the position in which it is found. If there is no palpable pulse, you may need to reduce the knee to restore circulation. A number of factors, including time to the hospital and duration of dislocation, will affect this decision, so you should always seek medical direction before reducing a dislocated knee.

To reduce a dislocated knee, apply longitudinal traction to the tibia in the direction of the foot. While the first rescuer is applying traction, a second provider should apply pressure to the distal femur and proximal tibia. If the knee is dislocated anteriorly, apply pressure to the femur in the anterior direction and to the tibia in the opposite direction. In the case of a posterior dislocation, apply pressure in the opposite manner, with the tibia pressed anteriorly and the femur pressed posteriorly. Once the reduction has been accomplished, check the patient's neurovascular status and splint the leg securely. If the attempt at reduction fails, splint the knee in the position in which it is found and undertake rapid transportation to an appropriate facility.

You are the Provider Summary

1. What are your initial assessment and treatment priorities?

As with any trauma patient, after assuring that the scene is safe, the initial assessment priorities for this patient are the mental status, the ABCs, and prioritizing the patient. Then proceed with a rapid trauma exam to identify the patient's injuries. Because this patient fell from a significant height, it is also important to protect his spine. During the initial assessment, you note that he has a site of bleeding from his arm; this bleeding should be controlled. Once this is accomplished, IV access should be obtained and the assessment should continue in a systematic and orderly manner.

2. What other information should be obtained about the patient and the incident?

Obtain information about the events that led the patient to fall, such as how he felt before falling and why he thought he fell. It is also important to learn details about the fall, such as how his extremities were positioned when he landed or whether he struck any other objects while falling. Obtain any other information related to the patient's status after the fall, such as loss of consciousness, mental status, and movement of extremities, from the patient or anyone who witnessed the fall. Also obtain information about any allergies the patient may know he has, any medication he takes, and the last time he had anything to eat or drink.

3. What are the potential complications of an open fracture?

One of the most significant complications following an open fracture is infection of the bone or soft tissues. To reduce the risk of infection, do not probe open fractures, brush away any debris on the surface of the skin, and cover the wound with a sterile dressing. Other complications of open fractures include poor healing of the fracture, soft-tissue loss, neurovascular injury, and long-term disability.

4. Why are open fractures prone to bleeding more than closed fractures?

In general, open fractures are higher-energy injuries than closed fractures, so they are likely to have more soft-tissue damage and, hence, more bleeding. Also, because the fracture is open, the blood that would normally accumulate within the closed fracture site is allowed to escape, so there is no tamponade of the bleeding vessels.

5. Would your treatment priorities change if the patient complained of abdominal pain in the presence of hypotension?

If the patient were found to be in unstable condition with evidence of an intra-abdominal injury, immediate and rapid transportation to a trauma center would be warranted. For a trauma patient in unstable condition who has a fracture, place the patient on a long backboard and fully immobilize the patient. While immobilizing the spine, the injured extremities may be immobilized as well by securing them to the board. The result is a compromise: The injured extremity is secured in place and protected from further movement without dedicating precious time to applying a formal splint.

6. Why would this dislocation be considered a true emergency?

When a patient with a dislocated knee has a pulseless foot, medical direction should be obtained and consideration should be given to manipulating the dislocation. Some paramedics may have a standing order to deal with this type of situation. Factors that will influence this decision include the duration of the dislocation, time to the hospital, the patient's vital signs, and the patient's overall condition.

7. What is an important consideration before manipulating a dislocation?

If the patient has no contraindications (such as hypotension), sedation should be considered before attempting manipulation of the extremity. This can be a very painful procedure, and without determining the appropriateness of analgesics such as morphine, you will not be addressing an important patient care issue—comfort.

8. Why should a joint that has just been manipulated be splinted immediately?

A dislocation is often associated with damage to the ligaments and capsule that support the affected joint, making it susceptible to recurrent dislocations. Once a dislocated joint has been manipulated, it should be splinted to prevent movements that may allow for it to once again dislocate.

9. What facts should be relayed to the emergency department staff in your radio report?

The presence of a dislocation and/or fracture with compromised neurovascular status should be relayed immediately to the receiving facility. Any attempts to correct the impairment should be explained, along with any changes or responses to treatment. Paint a clear picture of the mechanism of injury and the patient's condition. Remember, the only information the emergency department staff have to plan for your arrival is based on your brief radio report.

Prep Kit

Ready for Review

- Injuries and complaints related to the musculoskeletal system are one of the most common reasons that patients seek medical attention.
- Musculoskeletal injuries are sometimes very dramatic, but attention should not be focused on them until life-threatening conditions have been excluded.
- You have a vital role in reducing the complications associated with musculoskeletal injuries by promptly and effectively splinting injured extremities.
- Assume the existence of a fracture whenever a patient who complains of a musculoskeletal injury has deformity, bruising, decreased range of motion, or swelling.
- Always perform and record an accurate neurovascular examination before and after splinting an injured extremity.
- When a dislocation is associated with absent distal pulses, obtain medical direction to determine whether the injury should be reduced.
- Look for injuries to the chest and abdomen, and fully immobilize the spine when patients have evidence of a high-energy injury, such as a femoral shaft or scapular fracture.
- Because fractures may be associated with significant blood loss, resuscitation with IV fluid may be necessary.
- Pelvic fractures are potentially lethal injuries owing to the massive potential for blood loss.
- *Never forget the ABCs!* Do not become distracted; the fracture can wait, if airway, breathing, or circulation problems are noted.

Vital Vocabulary

6 Ps of musculoskeletal assessment Pain, Paralysis, Parasthesias, Pulselessness, Pallor, and Pressure.

abduction Movement *away* from the midline of the body.

acetabulum The cup-shaped cavity in which the rounded head of the femur rotates.

acromion Lateral extension of the scapula that forms the highest point of the shoulder.

adduction Movement *toward* the midline of the body.

amputation Severing of a part of the body.

angulation The presence of an abnormal angle or bend in an extremity.

anterior tibial artery The artery that travels through the anterior muscles of the leg and continues to the foot as the dorsalis pedis.

appendicular skeleton The part of the skeleton comprising the upper and lower extremities.

arthritis Inflammation of the joints.

articulations The locations where two or more bones meet; *joints*.

atrophy Wasting away of a tissue.

avascular necrosis Tissue death resulting from the loss of blood supply.

avulsion fracture A fracture that occurs when a piece of bone is torn free at the site of attachment of a tendon or ligament.

axial skeleton The part of the skeleton comprising the skull, spinal column, and rib cage.

axilla The armpit.

axillary artery The artery that runs through the axilla, connecting the subclavian artery to the brachial artery.

bowing fracture An incomplete fracture typically occurring in children in which the bone becomes bent as the result of a compressive force.

boxer's fracture A fracture of the head of the fifth metacarpal that usually results from striking an object with a clenched fist.

brachial artery The artery that runs through the arm and branches into the radial and ulnar arteries.

buckle fracture A common incomplete fracture in children in which the cortex of the bone fractures from an excessive compression force.

buddy splinting Securing an injured digit to an adjacent uninjured one to allow the intact digit to act as a splint.

bursa A fluid-filled sac located adjacent to joints that reduces the amount of friction between moving structures.

bursitis Inflammation of a bursa.

calcaneus The heel bone; the largest of the tarsal bones.

cancellous bone Trabecular or spongy bone.

carpals The eight small bones of the wrist.

cartilage Tough, elastic substance that covers opposable surfaces of moveable joints and forms part of the skeleton.

cartilaginous joints Joints that are spanned completely by cartilage and allow for minimal motion.

clavicle The collar bone.

closed fracture A fracture in which the skin is not broken.

comminuted fracture A fracture in which the bone is broken into three or more pieces.

compartment syndrome An increase in tissue pressure in a closed fascial space or compartment that compromises the circulation to the nerves and muscles within the involved compartment.

complete fracture A fracture in which the bone is broken into two or more completely separate pieces.

compound fracture An open fracture; a fracture beneath an open wound.

crepitus A grating sensation felt when moving the ends of a broken bone.

crush syndrome A condition that arises after a body part that has been compressed for a significant period is released, leading to the entry of potassium and other metabolic toxins into the systemic circulation.

deep vein thrombosis (DVT) The formation of a blood clot within the larger veins of an extremity, typically following a period of prolonged immobilization.

depression fracture A fracture in which the broken region of the bone is pushed deeper into the body than the remaining intact bone.

devascularization The loss of blood to a part of the body.

diaphysis The shaft of a long bone.

diastasis An increase in the distance between the two sides of a joint.

digital arteries The arteries that supply blood to the fingers and toes.

dislocation The displacement of a bone from its normal position within a joint.

distraction injury An injury that results from a force that tries to increase the length of a body part or separate one body part from another.

dorsal Referring to the back or posterior side of the body or an organ.

dorsiflex To bend the foot or hand backward.

endosteum The inner lining of a hollow bone.

fascia A strong, fibrous membrane that covers, supports, and separates muscles.

fatigue fractures Fractures that result from multiple compressive loads.

femoral artery The main artery supplying the thigh and leg.

femoral shaft fractures A break in the diaphysis of the femur.

femur The proximal bone of the leg that extends from the pelvis to the knee.

fibrous joints The joints that contain dense fibrous tissue and allow for no motion.

fibula The smaller of the two bones of the lower leg.

flat bones Bones that are thin and broad, such as the scapula.

fracture A break or rupture in the bone.

glenoid fossa Socket in the scapula in which the head of the humerus rotates.

gout A painful disorder characterized by the crystallization of uric acid within a joint.

greenstick fracture A type of fracture occurring most frequently in children in which there is incomplete breakage of the bone.

hematopoiesis The generation of blood cells.

humerus The bone of the upper arm.

hypertrophy An increase in size.

ilium The broad, uppermost bone of the pelvis.

impacted fracture A broken bone in which the end of one bone becomes wedged into another bone, as could be the case in a fall from a significant height.

incomplete fracture A fracture in which the bone does not fully break.

indirect injury An injury that results from a force that is applied to one region of the body but leads to an injury in another area.

intertrochanteric fractures Fractures that occur in the region between the lesser and greater trochanters.

irregular bones Bones with unique shapes that allow them to perform a specific function and that do not fit into the other categories based on shape.

ischium The lowermost dorsal bone of the pelvis.

joint The point at which two or more bones articulate, or come together.

joint capsule A saclike envelope that encloses the cavity of a synovial joint.

lactic acid A metabolic end product of the breakdown of glucose that accumulates when metabolism proceeds in the absence of oxygen.

lateral compression A force that is directed from the side toward the midline of the body.

ligaments Tough bands of tissue that connect bone to bone around a joint or support internal organs within the body.

linear fracture A fracture that runs parallel to the long axis of a bone.

long bones Bones that are longer than they are wide.

malleolus The large, rounded bony protuberance on either side of the ankle joint.

mallet finger An avulsion fracture of the extensor tendon of the distal phalynx caused by jamming a finger into an object.

march fractures *See* fatigue fractures.

medullary canal The hollow center portion of a long bone.

metacarpals The five bones that form the palm and back of the hand.

metaphysis The region of the long bone between the epiphysis and diaphysis.

metatarsals The five long bones extending from the tarsus to the phalanges of the foot.

muscle fatigue The condition that arises when a muscle depletes its supply of energy.

neurovascular compromise The loss of the nerve supply, blood supply, or both to a region of the body, typically distal to a site of injury; characterized by alterations in sensation, including numbness and tingling, or by a loss or decrease of motor function; vascular compromise is indicated by weak or absent pulses, poor skin color, and cool skin.

nondisplaced fracture A break in which the bone remains aligned in its normal position.

nursemaid's elbow The subluxation of the radial head that often results from pulling on an outstretched arm.

oblique fracture A fracture that travels diagonally from one side of the bone to the other.

olecranon The proximal bony projection of the *ulna* at the elbow; the part of the ulna that constitutes the "funny bone."

open book pelvic fracture A life-threatening fracture of the pelvis caused by a force that displaces one or both sides of the pelvis laterally and posteriorly.

open fracture Any break in a bone in which the overlying skin has been damaged.

osteoarthritis (OA) The degeneration of a joint surface caused by wear and tear that leads to pain and stiffness.

osteoporosis A condition characterized by decreased bone density and increased susceptibility to fractures.

overriding The overlap of a bone that occurs from the muscle spasm that follows a fracture, leading to a decrease in the length of the bone.

paresthesias Abnormal sensations such as burning, numbness, or tingling.

patella The kneecap.

pathologic fracture A fracture that occurs in an area of abnormally weakened bone.

pectoral girdle The shoulder girdle.

pelvic girdle The large bone that arises in the area of the last nine vertebrae and sweeps around to form a complete ring.

periosteum The fibrous tissue that covers bone.

phalanges The bones of the fingers or toes.

physis The growth plate in long bones.

plantar Referring to the sole of the foot.

plantar flexion Bending of the foot toward the ground.

point tenderness The tenderness that is sharply localized at the site of the injury, found by gently palpating along the bone with the tip of one finger.

popliteal artery The artery in the area or space behind the knee joint.

posterior tibial artery The artery that travels through the calf muscles to the plantar aspect of the foot.

pronation The act of turning the palm of the hand backward or downward, performed by internal rotation of the forearm.

pubic symphysis The midline articulation of the pubic bones.

pubis One of two bones that form the anterior portion of the pelvic ring.

pulmonary embolism Obstruction of a pulmonary artery or arteries by solid, liquid, or gaseous material swept through the right side of the heart into the lungs.

radial artery The artery pertaining to the wrist.

radius The bone on the thumb side of the forearm.

range of motion (ROM) The arc of movement of an extremity at a joint in a particular direction.

recruitment The process of signaling additional muscle fibers to contract to create a more forceful contraction.

rheumatoid arthritis (RA) An inflammatory disorder that affects the entire body and leads to degeneration and deformation of joints.

round bones The small bones that are found adjacent to joints that assist with motion.

sacroiliac joints The points of attachment of the *ilium* to the sacrum.

scaphoid The wrist bone that is found just beyond that most distal portion of the radius.

scapula The shoulder blade.

segmental fracture A bone that is broken in more than one place.

short bones The bones that are nearly as wide as they are long.

silver fork deformity The dorsal deformity of the forearm that results from a Colles fracture.

skeletal muscle Muscle that is attached to bones and usually crosses at least one joint; striated or voluntary muscle.

snuffbox The region at the base of the thumb where the scaphoid may be palpated.

somatic motor neurons The nerve fibers that transmit impulses to a muscle.

spiral fracture A break in a bone that appears like a spring on a radiograph.

sprains Injuries, including a stretch or a tear, to the ligaments of a joint that commonly lead to pain and swelling.

straddle fracture A fracture of the pelvis that results from landing on the perineal region.

strain Stretching or tearing of a muscle by excessive stretching or overuse.

stress fracture A fracture that results from exaggerated stress on the bone caused by unusually rapid muscle development.

striated muscle Skeletal muscle that is under voluntary control.

subclavian artery The artery that travels from the aorta to each upper extremity.

subluxation A partial or incomplete dislocation.

supination To turn the forearm laterally so that the palm faces forward (if standing) or upward (if lying supine).

supracondylar fractures Fractures of the distal humerus that occur just proximal to the elbow.

synovial joints Joints that permit movement of the component bones.

synovial membrane The lining of a joint that secretes synovial fluid into the joint space.

talus The bone of the foot that articulates with the tibia.

tarsals The ankle bones.

tendinitis Inflammation of a tendon that most commonly results from overuse.

tendons The fibrous portions of muscle that attach to bone.

Thompson test Squeezing of the calf muscle to evaluate for plantar flexion of the foot to determine whether the Achilles tendon is intact.

thromboembolic disease The condition in which a patient has a DVT or pulmonary embolism.

tibia The shin bone.

torus fracture See buckle fracture.

transverse fracture A fracture that runs in a straight line from one edge of the bone to the other and that is perpendicular to each edge.

twisting injuries Injuries that commonly occur during athletic activities in which an extremity rotates around a planted foot or hand.

ulna The larger bone of the forearm, on the side opposite the thumb.

ulnar artery The artery of the forearm that travels along its medial aspect.

vertical shear The type of pelvic fracture that occurs when a massive force displaces the pelvis superiorly.

volar Pertaining to the palm or sole; referring to the flexor surfaces of the forearm, wrist, or hand.

Volkmann ischemic contracture Contraction of the fingers and, sometimes, the wrist, with loss of muscular power, that sets in rapidly after severe injury around the elbow joint.

voluntary muscle Muscle that can be controlled by a person.

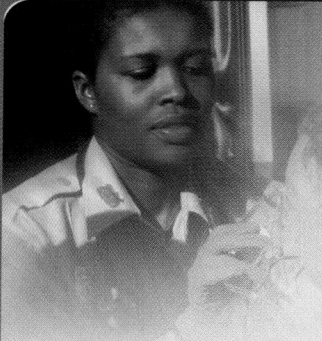

Assessment in Action

You are dispatched to the home of a 13-year-old boy with pain in his foot. When you arrive, the boy is sitting in his mother's car complaining of severe pain in his left foot, ankle, and leg. On assessment, he has a distal pulse; his foot is cold and has limited range of motion. There is swelling noted in ankle region. There is no discoloration or obvious deformity. The remainder of his vital signs are within normal limits.

He tells you that he was in the mountains and was snowboarding. He went down a hill when suddenly, a tree was in the way. He struck the tree with the bottom of his left foot (traveling approximately 20 mph). He felt immediate pain in his foot and then began to feel a burning sensation up his left leg. His mother drove him back to their house, approximately 45 minutes away. He had no pain while traveling, but when he attempted to step out of the vehicle, the pain soared through him. You provide comfort care for the young man and transport him to the hospital. He tells you that his pain is about 7 on a 1 to 10 scale. You follow-up at the hospital and are told that he has a comminuted fracture in his heel and a fractured ankle.

1. **What type of injury force did this young man sustain?**
   A. Tapping injury force
   B. Crush injury force
   C. Penetrating injury force
   D. Indirect injury force

2. **With the complaint of pain in his left leg, what other type of injury should have been suspected?**
   A. Indirect injury
   B. Direct injury
   C. Twisting injury
   D. March fracture

3. **The foot consists of three classes of bones. Which are they?**
   A. Tarsals, metatarsals, and calcaneus
   B. Tarsals, metatarsals, and phalanges
   C. Tarsals, calcaneus, and tibia
   D. Tibia, fibula, and malleolus

4. **Signs and symptoms of extremity trauma that have a high urgency include which of the following?**
   A. Absent distal pulses
   B. Crepitus
   C. Decreased range of motion
   D. Swelling and deformity

5. **Flexion, extension, abduction, and circumduction are all movements allowed by what type of joint?**
   A. Hinge
   B. Synovial
   C. Saddle
   D. Ball and socket

6. **Muscles are composed of specialized cells that contract when stimulated to exert a force on a part of the body. Three types of muscles found in the body are:**
   A. smooth, cardiac, and skeletal.
   B. smooth, cardiac, and striated.
   C. ligaments, cartilage, and smooth.
   D. cardiac, skeletal, and cartilage.

7. **When a person sustains a musculoskeletal injury, the arteries that supply the injured region may be damaged as well. What arteries supply the ankle and the foot?**
   A. Tibial artery; anterior tibial artery
   B. Popliteal artery; anterior tibial artery
   C. Anterior tibial artery; posterior tibial artery
   D. Popliteal artery; posterior tibial artery

8. **What is the *primary* symptom of a fracture?**
   A. Pain
   B. Deformity
   C. Shortening
   D. Loss of use

9. **When assessing the patient's pain, you should use the mnemonic:**
   A. PQRST.
   B. OPRST.
   C. OPQRST.
   D. OPRST.

Challenging Questions

You are dispatched to the home of a 60-year-old man found by neighbors. On your arrival, you find the man in a right lateral recumbent position and he is moaning. You're not sure how long he has been on the ground, but there is 4 days worth of mail in the mailbox. You apply a backboard and cervical collar because you are not sure of the reason the patient is on the ground. His blood pressure is 100/60 mm Hg and the heart rate is 120 beats/min with sinus tachycardia, he has strong radial pulses, and his respirations are 12 breaths/min. He is verbally responsive by moaning. He is unable to tell you what happened or if anything hurts.

You provide supportive and comfort care en route to the hospital. His body is very stiff and you have difficulty manipulating his extremities. When you perform an assessment, you note that there is a nickel embedded in his head. There are large areas of ecchymosis along his right pelvic area and his right leg. His right shoulder has open wounds. He is incontinent of urine and feces. This man was admitted to the intensive care unit with a diagnosis of acute sepsis and crush syndrome.

10. **What signs and symptoms would you recognize for the crush syndrome?**

11. **How would you treat this type of injury?**

12. **What will be the concerns of the hospital staff for this patient?**

■ Points to Ponder

You are responding to a call at an assisted care facility for an older woman who has fallen out of bed while attempting to get up. When you arrive, the woman is still on the floor next to her bed. She tells you that her left leg and back hurt, but she is mentally alert and denies any other symptoms. She is sitting up, and it does not seem that she has bumped her head or injured herself in any other way besides the fall. Your physical exam reveals tenderness and pain in her left leg and crepitus and instability in her left hip. The staff tells you that the woman has osteoporosis but no other major medical problems.

How would you best treat this patient?

Issues: Thorough Assessment of Musculoskeletal Injuries, Pain Management.

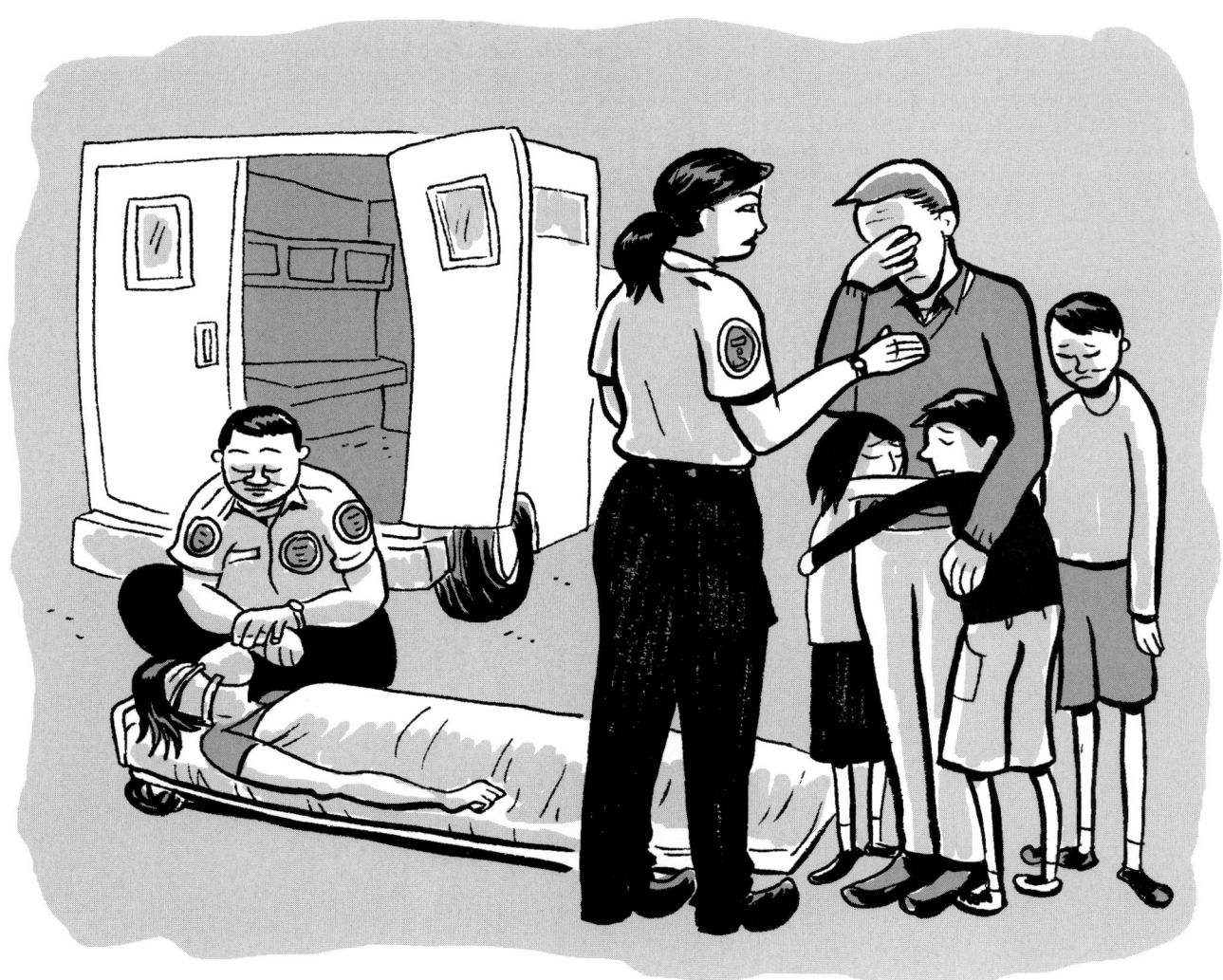

“

Remember, behind every medical emergency is a person.”

—Mickey Eisenberg, MD, PhD

Medical

Section Editor: Bob Elling, MPA, NREMT-P

26 Respiratory Emergencies

Objectives

Cognitive

5-1.1 Discuss the epidemiology of pulmonary diseases and conditions. (p 26.15)

5-1.2 Identify and describe the function of the structures located in the upper and lower airway. (p 26.5–26.9)

5-1.3 Discuss the physiology of ventilation and respiration. (p 26.12–26.15)

5-1.4 Identify common pathological events that affect the pulmonary system. (p 26.6)

5-1.5 Discuss abnormal assessment findings associated with pulmonary diseases and conditions. (p 26.16)

5-1.6 Compare various airway and ventilation techniques used in the management of pulmonary diseases. (p 26.44)

5-1.7 Review the pharmacological preparations that paramedics use for management of respiratory diseases and conditions. (p 26.40)

5-1.8 Review the pharmacological preparations used in managing patients with respiratory diseases that may be prescribed by physicians. (p 26.40–26.44)

5-1.9 Review the use of equipment used during the physical examination of patients with complaints associated with respiratory diseases and conditions. (p 26.20, 26.23)

5-1.10 Identify the epidemiology, anatomy, physiology, pathophysiology, assessment findings, and management for the following respiratory diseases and conditions:
   a. Adult respiratory distress syndrome
   b. Bronchial asthma
   c. Chronic bronchitis
   d. Emphysema
   e. Pneumonia
   f. Pulmonary edema
   g. Pulmonary thromboembolism
   h. Neoplasms of the lung
   i. Upper respiratory infections
   j. Spontaneous pneumothorax
   k. Hyperventilation syndrome (p 26.28–26.37)

Affective

5-1.11 Recognize and value the assessment and treatment of patients with respiratory diseases. (p 26.16)

5-1.12 Indicate appreciation for the critical nature of accurate field impressions of patients with respiratory diseases and conditions. (p 26.16)

Psychomotor

5-1.13 Demonstrate proper use of airway and ventilation devices. (p 26.23–26.25)

5-1.14 Conduct a history and patient assessment for patients with pulmonary diseases and conditions. (p 26.16, 26.18)

5-1.15 Demonstrate the application of a CPAP/BiPAP unit. (p 26.44)

Introduction

There are few incentives to dial 9-1-1 more powerful than the feeling of being unable to breathe (dyspnea). In the majority of cases, that distressing feeling is caused by a problem in the respiratory system itself. In this chapter, we examine some of the respiratory problems that produce dyspnea. We begin by reviewing the anatomy and physiology of the respiratory system. We next consider the assessment of a patient whose chief complaint is dyspnea—namely, which aspects to emphasize in taking the history and carrying out the physical examination. Then we look at some of the problems that may assault each component of the respiratory system—from the respiratory control centers in the brain to the alveolus, the smallest functional unit of respiration in the lung.

Review of Respiratory Anatomy and Function

The primary components of the respiratory system are often compared to an inverted tree, with the trachea representing the tree's trunk and the alveoli resembling the tree's leaves. That is a nice analogy to get things started, but in reality a respiratory tree would have to branch 24 times and have nearly a billion leaves   Figure 26-1 ▾ . Imagine attempting to pull fluid from the ground into those leaves by exerting a negative pressure at the leaf ends, and you may begin to appreciate the complexities of breathing.

The Upper Airway

Air enters the upper airway primarily through the nares (nostrils) of the nose. Nares are lined with nasal hairs. The hairs serve as filters that catch particulate matter in the air we breathe. The external nares are separated by the nasal septum.

At any given time, one nostril is usually more open than the other and would be the better choice for the insertion of a nasogastric (NG) tube, a nasopharyngeal airway, or to use for nasotracheal intubation. Occlude one nostril and have the patient inhale, and repeat the procedure with the other nostril. It is usually easy to tell which one is less obstructed.

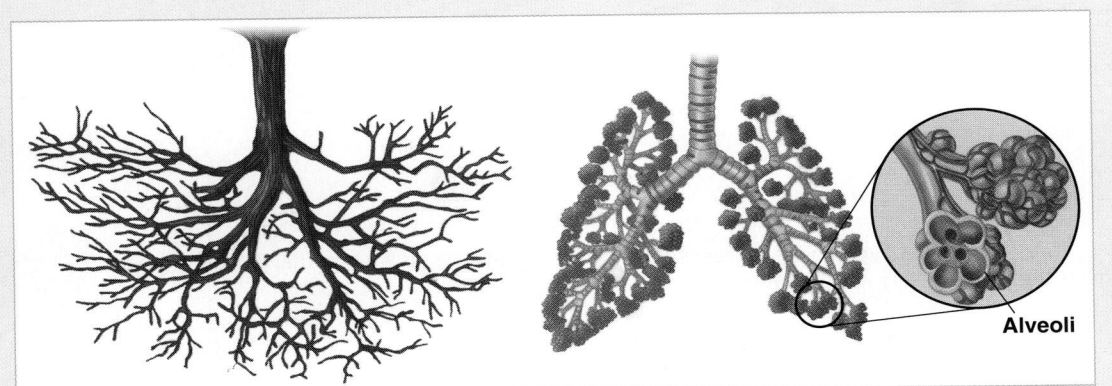

Alveoli

Figure 26-1 The tracheobronchial tree branches in much the same way as a tree, except that even the most branched tree has only half as many branchings as those inside the lung.

You are the Provider Part 1

You are dispatched to 275 Thomas Lane to help an older man who is having difficulty breathing. You arrive to find a 65-year-old man sitting in the tripod position at his kitchen table. As you speak with him, you notice that he is struggling to breathe and can give you only one- or two-word responses. His extremities are pale and his face is flushed. As you attempt to obtain more information regarding his medical history, the patient grabs your arm and says, "I'm so tired!"

Initial Assessment	Recording Time: 0 Minutes
Appearance	Anxious, tired
Level of consciousness	V (Responsive to verbal stimuli)
Airway	Open; accessory muscle use
Breathing	Rapid and labored
Circulation	Weak radial pulse

1. What about this patient's presentation gives you cause for concern?
2. What are your assessment and treatment priorities?
3. If you are unable to gather much information from your patient about his medical history, what other ways can you obtain this information?

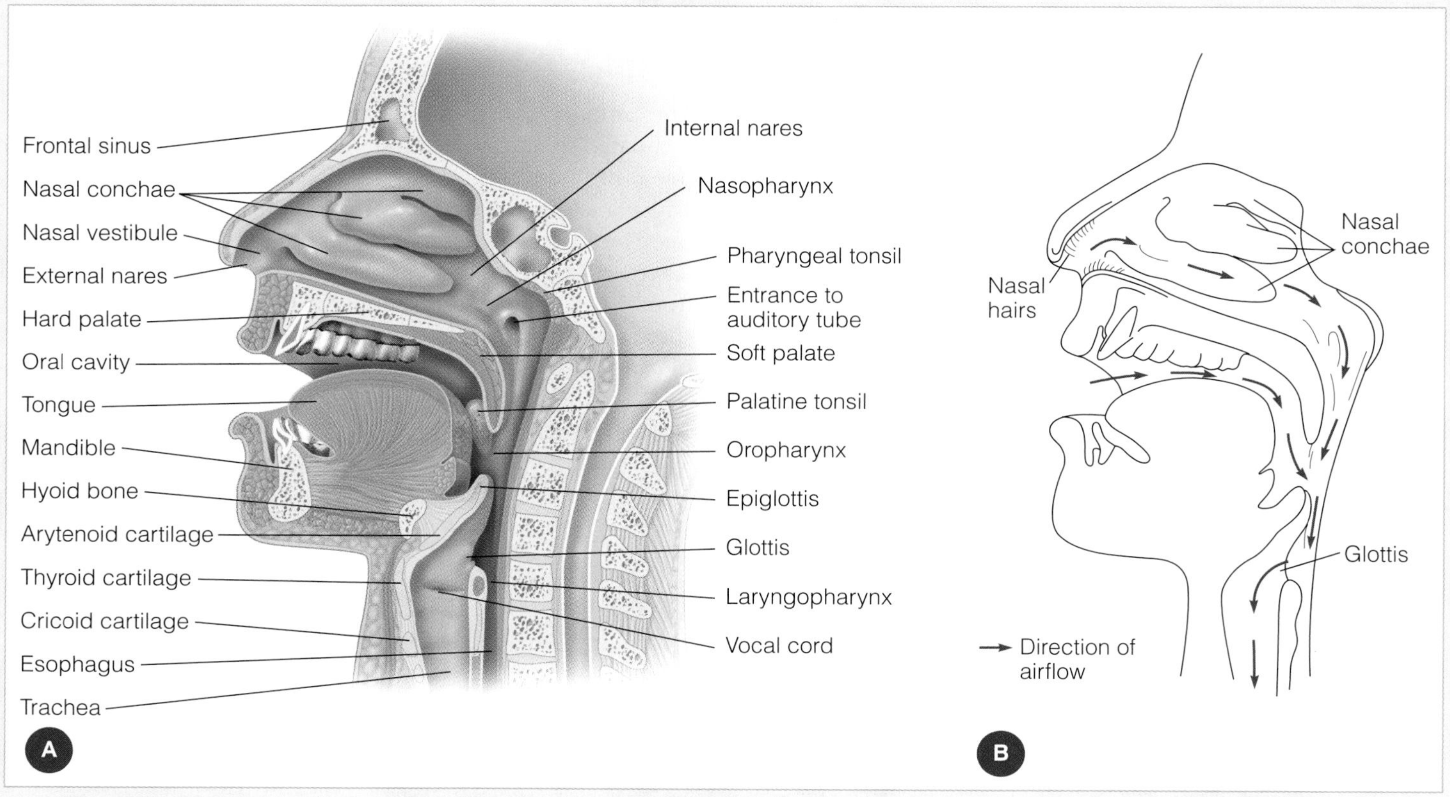

Figure 26-2 **A.** The upper airway contains many blood vessels and serves to heat and humidify the air we breathe. **B.** Note that an important filter is lost when we bypass the upper airway via intubation.

After passing through the nares, air is pulled over the turbinates. These ridges of tissue are covered with a mucous membrane and contain many blood vessels. The mucous membrane traps more particulate matter, and the large surface area of the turbinates warms and humidifies the air we breathe as the air passes over it. Processes such as intubation or a tracheostomy allow inhaled air to skip this trip through the nose, bypassing the humidification and filtering. Because the turbinates contain many blood vessels, they easily swell (causing a stuffy nose) or bleed (epistaxis).

Anyone with hay fever can attest to the severe swelling that can occur in the nasal cavity. In children, foreign bodies such as pencil erasers, candy, and beans frequently obstruct a nostril. These items often sit in the nose for a day or two before the child presents with pain and a foul-smelling nasal discharge. Don't try to remove the obstruction yourself. Emergency departments are skilled in performing "beanectomies."

Quiet breathing typically allows air to flow through the nose **Figure 26-2 ▲** . Even people who breathe through their mouth usually have some nasal airflow. It is typically not necessary to tell patients that they must breathe through their nose when you apply a nasal cannula. Unless the nasal passages are actually swollen shut from edema or trauma, the cannula will function well.

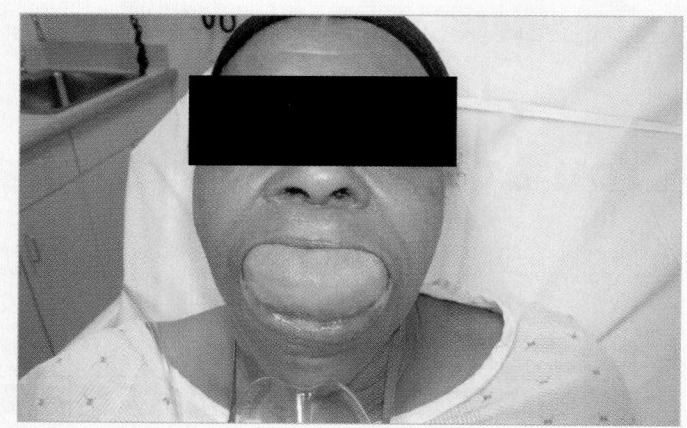

Figure 26-3 Angioedema is an acute swelling, usually of the lips and tongue, secondary to an allergic reaction. Some medications cause angioedema after the first or second dose.

The mouth and oropharynx also contain many blood vessels and are covered by a mucous membrane. Swelling can be extreme, and potentially dangerous. Bee stings to the lips or tongue can cause profound swelling. Angioedema **Figure 26-3 ▲** is an allergic reaction that may cause severe swelling of the tongue and lips. Always ask patients who may be experiencing an allergic reaction if their tongue "feels thick." Monitor their speech for symptoms (such as low volume or a raspy voice) of oral or laryngeal swelling.

The oropharynx and nasopharynx meet in the back of the throat at the hypopharynx (sometimes called the posterior pharynx). The gag reflex is most profound in this area. Triggering the gag reflex, on purpose or by accident, can cause vagal bradycardia (a slow heartbeat caused by stimulation of the vagus nerve), vomiting, and increased intracranial pressure. A strong gag reflex may make the use of many airway devices difficult or inappropriate **Figure 26-4 ▶**. Conversely, patients with a diminished or absent gag reflex may require endotracheal intubation to help isolate and protect the airway from foreign materials.

The <u>larynx</u> (voicebox) **Figure 26-5 ▼** and <u>glottis</u> (opening at the top of the trachea) are typically considered the dividing line between the upper airway and the sterile lower airway. The thyroid cartilage is the most obvious external landmark of the larynx. The glottis and vocal cords are found in the middle of the thyroid's cartilaginous structure.

Several cartilages that may be visible when intubating the patient support the vocal cords. The <u>arytenoid cartilages</u> appear as two pearly white lumps at the distal end of each vocal cord. In some people, the cuneiform and corniculate cartilages may also be visible during laryngoscopy. On either side of the glottis, tissue forms a pocket called the <u>piriform fossa</u> **Figure 26-6 ▶**. Sometimes NG tubes or endotracheal (ET) tubes will get stuck here during placement, causing "tenting" that is visible externally on the neck. Any device stuck in a piriform fossa must be withdrawn a few inches and reinserted.

The glottic opening is covered by the epiglottis. Most of us were taught that the epiglottis covers the glottis like a trap door when we swallow, keeping food and liquid from entering the trachea. In reality, many people aspirate around their epiglottis, but others seem to swallow just fine even after their epiglottis has been surgically removed. Because the epiglottis can make it difficult to see the vocal cords, one of your primary tasks during endotracheal intubation is to identify the epiglottis and use

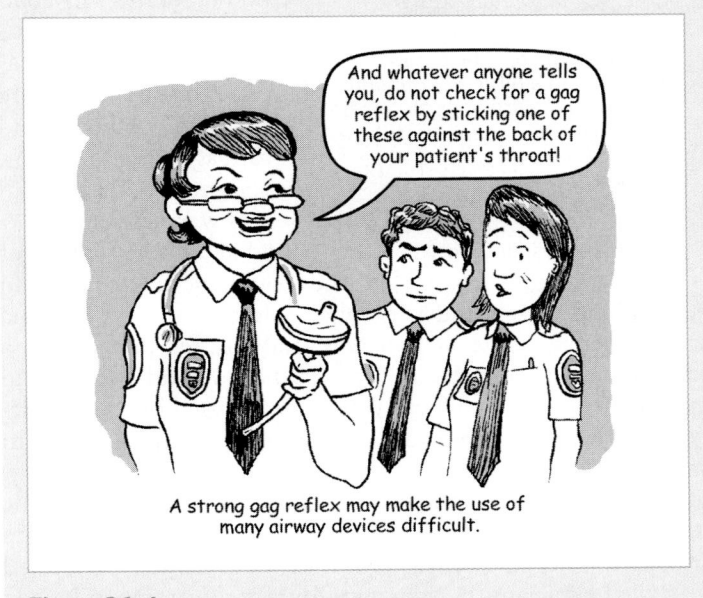

And whatever anyone tells you, do not check for a gag reflex by sticking one of these against the back of your patient's throat!

A strong gag reflex may make the use of many airway devices difficult.

Figure 26-4

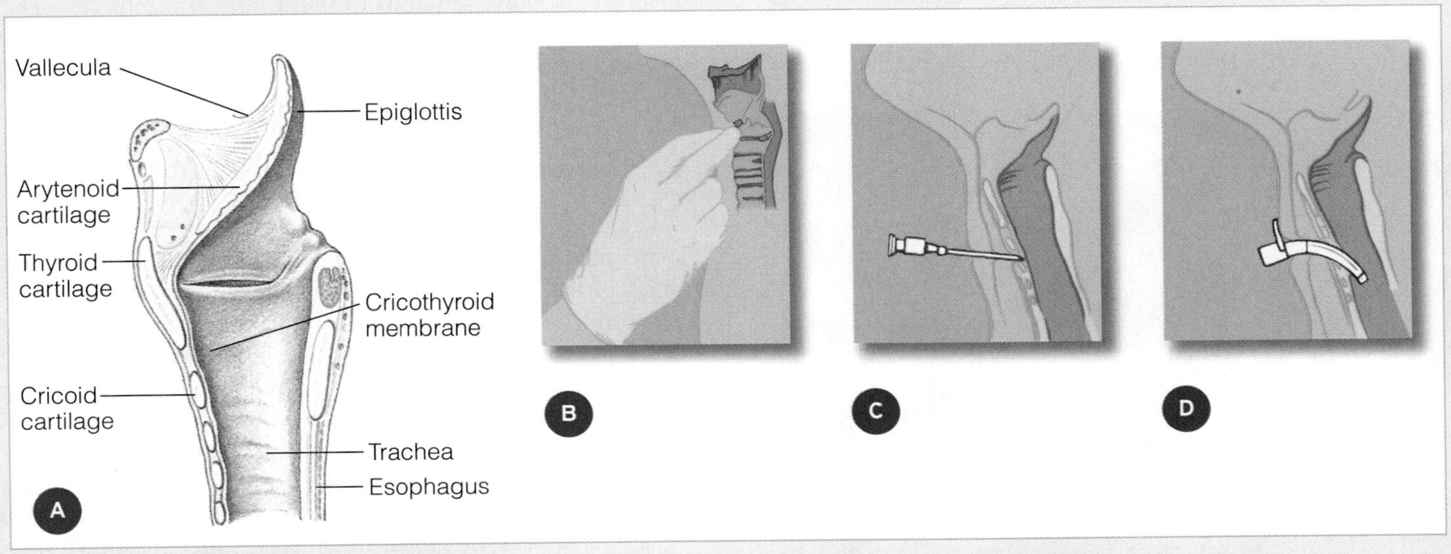

Vallecula
Epiglottis
Arytenoid cartilage
Thyroid cartilage
Cricothyroid membrane
Cricoid cartilage
Trachea
Esophagus

A
B
C
D

Figure 26-5 It is imperative that you completely understand the anatomy of the larynx in order to perform a number of airway management skills. **A.** Anatomy of the larynx. **B.** Applying pressure to the cricoid cartilage, which compresses the esophagus while keeping the trachea open (Sellick maneuver). **C.** An IV cannula is inserted into the cricothyroid membrane. **D.** A tracheostomy tube is inserted below the cricoid cartilage.

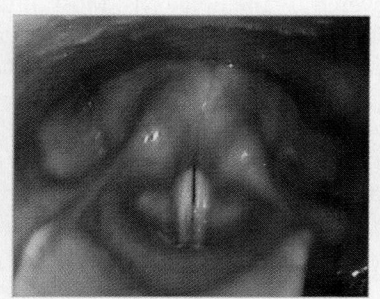

Figure 26-6 The arytenoid cartilages and piriform fossae are sometimes the only landmarks visible during a difficult intubation. The arytenoid cartilages are a pair of small pyramid-shaped cartilages to which the vocal cords are attached.

the laryngoscope to move it out of the way.

The cricoid cartilage can be palpated just below the thyroid cartilage in the neck. It forms a complete ring and maintains the trachea in an open position. Pressing on the anterior portion of this ring compresses the esophagus while keeping the trachea open. Applying pressure to the cricoid cartilage (Sellick maneuver) may be helpful in airway maintenance.

The small space between the thyroid and cricoid cartilages is the cricothyroid membrane. The membrane doesn't contain many blood vessels and is covered only by skin and minimal subcutaneous tissue. It is a potential site for performing a cricothyrotomy (an incision through the skin and cricothyroid membrane to relieve difficulty breathing caused by an obstruction in the airway) if you are unable to secure the airway with an advanced airway device. The rest of the neck contains large blood vessels, important nerves, and other critical anatomic structures that you must avoid cutting when performing a cricothyrotomy. Cricothyrotomies look easy when performed by skilled clinicians, but this procedure can turn into a bloody disaster if you aren't absolutely certain of anatomic landmarks, or have poor technique.

Trauma or swelling of any of the laryngeal structures can create a life-threatening airway obstruction **Figure 26-7** . In the worst-case scenario, this entire anatomic region may be

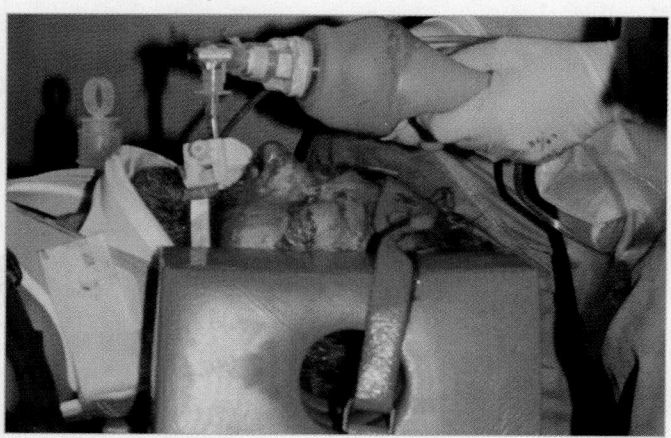

Figure 26-7 Trauma to the head and neck can completely obscure your view of the anatomy of the airway. You must be comfortable enough with airway anatomy to manage the airway, even when it has been significantly altered.

bypassed by a tracheostomy (a surgical opening into the trachea). By their very nature, traumatic injuries may alter the typical anatomy of the upper airway. Procedures such as a cricothyrotomy can prove highly challenging when the airway is filled with blood and vomit, and the anatomic landmarks are obscured by swelling or subcutaneous air.

The Lower Airway

Inspired gas is distributed to the millions of alveoli by a network of conducting airways. Gas in these tubes does not come into close contact with capillaries, so it does not participate in ventilation. This wasted ventilation is called anatomic dead space. Typically, anatomic dead space is about 1 mL per pound of ideal body weight (a 150-lb person has about 150 mL of anatomic dead space). This dead space remains relatively constant. If a 150-lb patient took an average breath (tidal volume [V_T]) of 700 mL, about 550 mL would participate in ventilation at the alveolar level; the other 150 mL would fill the tubes and would never be exposed to blood flow. If the same patient were to drop his or her V_T to 500 mL, only 350 mL would participate in ventilation, because 150 mL would be stuck in the tubes.

The trunk of these tubes—the tracheobronchial tree—is the trachea. It is about 10 to 13 cm long and extends from the level of the sixth cervical vertebra to its point of bifurcation (carina) at roughly the fifth thoracic vertebra (approximately nipple level) **Figure 26-8** . At this point, it forks into the right and left mainstem bronchi. In adults, the right mainstem bronchus typically branches at a less acute angle than the left. Thus, if you advance an ET tube too far into an adult, it almost always goes down the right mainstem bronchus. Similarly, aspirated foreign bodies often end up in the right mainstem bronchus.

The mainstem bronchi branch into lobar bronchi, segmental bronchi, subsegmental bronchi, and bronchioles. These structures account for approximately 15 branchings of the airway and are lined with ciliated epithelium. Cilia are little hairlike structures that rhythmically wave in a pattern that helps move particulate matter up and out of the airway **Figure 26-9** . If a particle gets deeper into the lungs than level 15, there is no mechanism to get it back out.

Goblet cells are also found in the lining of these airways. These cells produce a blanket of mucus that covers the entire lining of the conducting airways. The mucus covers the cilia and forms a two-layered blanket that is thick at the surface (gel layer) and thin and watery next to the cilia (sol layer). The gel layer of the mucous blanket is thick and floats over the sol layer. Cilia constantly push the gel layer up and out of the airway in the healthy individual. As the cilia beat, they reach out into the gel layer, pushing it up and toward the glottis. On the return stroke, the cilia collapse into the sol layer, so that they don't pull the gel layer back down. In this manner, the cilia slowly move the entire gel layer up and out of the tracheobronchial tree, where it is either swallowed or expectorated.

If a person is dehydrated, or if he or she has taken medications such as antihistamines that dry the normal secretions, the sol layer will begin to dry up, and the cilia will not be able to effectively move secretions. The same is true if the patient is overhydrated: the cilia will wave meaninglessly in a deep watery layer without ever affecting the thick gel layer.

Smooth muscle surrounds the conducting airways down to the subsegmental level. Bronchoconstriction occurs when the smooth muscle constricts around these larger airways. Below this level, bronchodilator medications have little effect upon the airways. Wheezing that is resolved with bronchodilator medication was probably caused by constriction of the smooth muscles. Wheezing that is not resolved with these medications may be caused by a variety of pathologic conditions deeper in the tracheobronchial tree.

The terminal airways and alveoli include branches 16 through 24 of the tracheobronchial tree, the so-called terminal bronchioles. The tracheobronchial tree ends with the alveoli, but the transfer of oxygen and carbon dioxide can nevertheless take

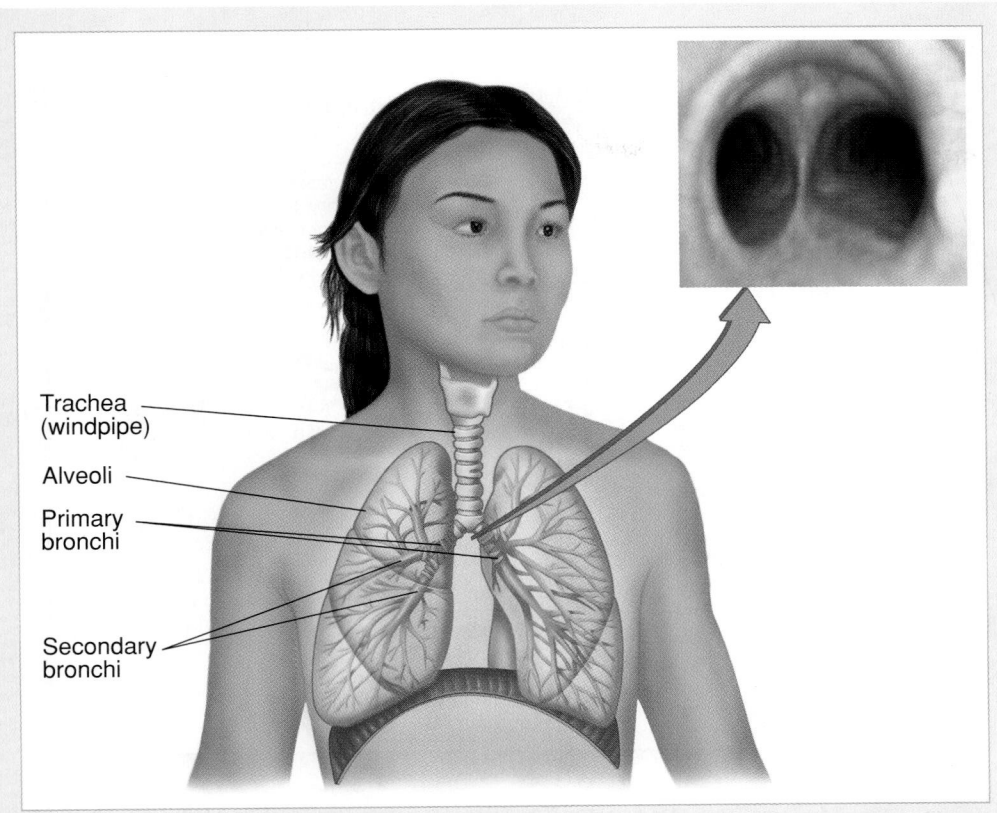

Trachea (windpipe)
Alveoli
Primary bronchi
Secondary bronchi

Figure 26-8 The carina is the point of bifurcation of the right and left mainstem bronchi. In an adult, it is located at roughly the fifth intercostal space.

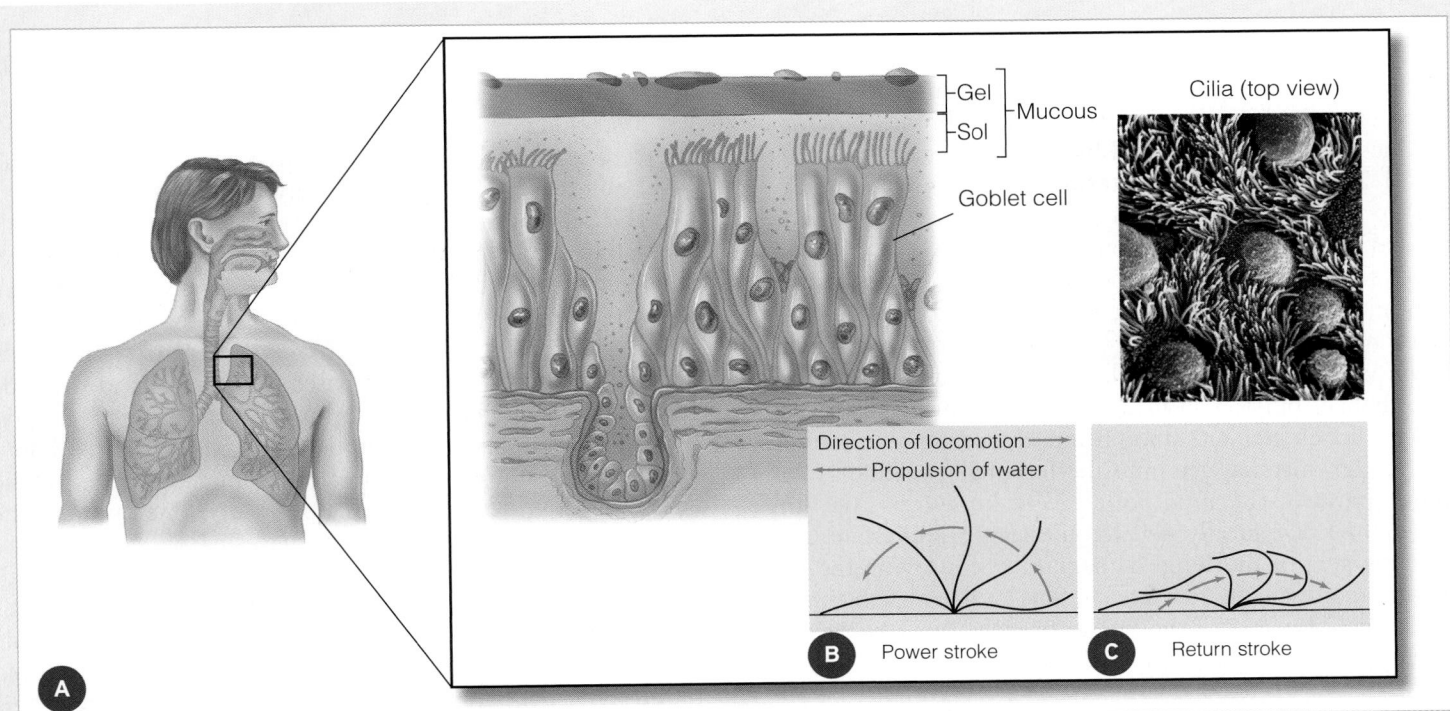

Gel
Sol
Mucous
Cilia (top view)
Goblet cell
Direction of locomotion
Propulsion of water
B Power stroke
C Return stroke
A

Figure 26-9 Cilia line the larger airways of the respiratory tract (**A**). Their regular pattern of movement between the gel and sol layers of mucus helps move foreign material out of the tracheobronchial tree (**B** and **C**).

Inset photo: © Dr. Kessel & Dr. Kardon/Tissue & Organs/Visuals Unlimited

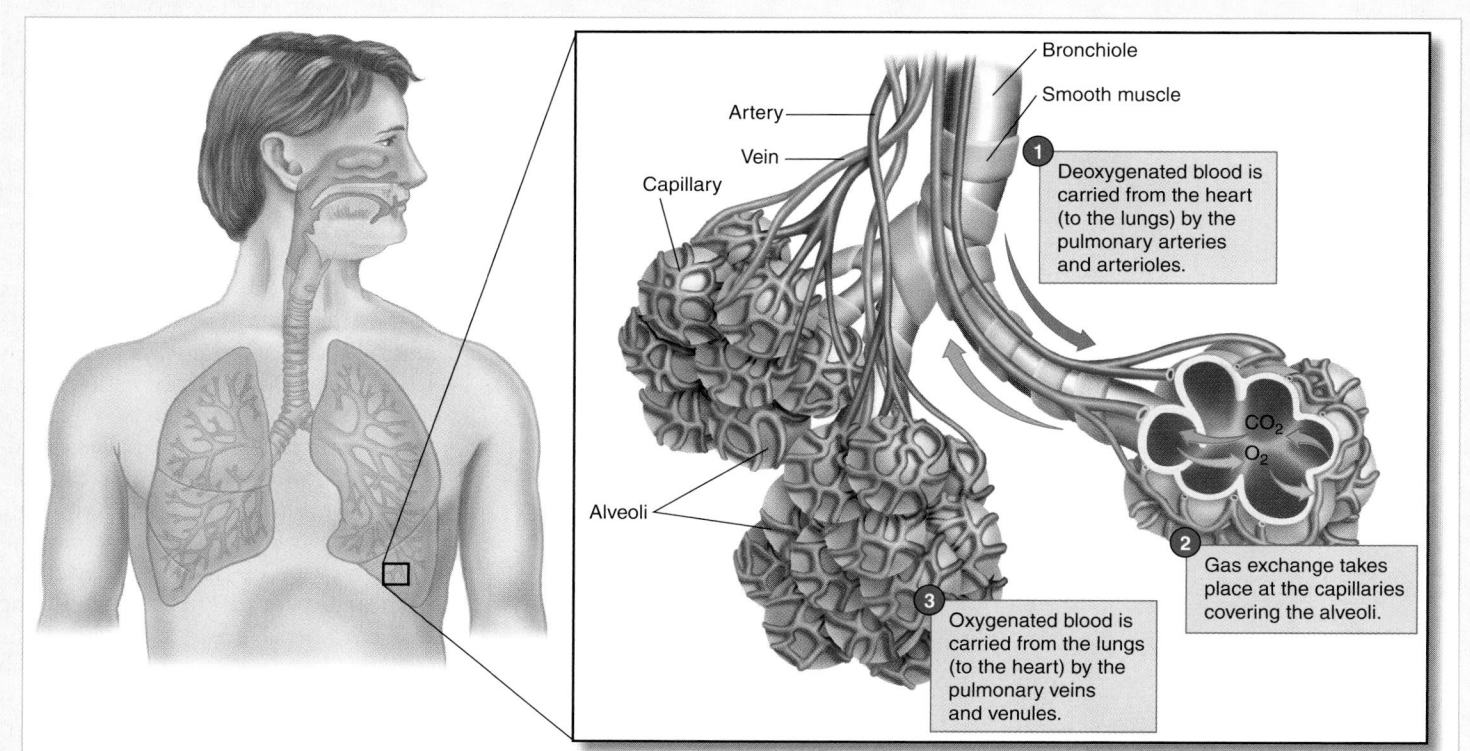

Figure 26-10 The respiratory bronchioles, sometimes called terminal bronchioles, include the alveoli and the last several branches of the tracheobronchial tree. Gas exchange occurs over this entire area, not just the alveoli.

place across both the alveoli and the terminal bronchioles. It is often helpful to think of alveoli as little balloons at the end of a straw. Alveoli cluster around the terminal bronchioles, and capillaries cover the alveoli and bronchial tubes from level 16 to level 24. The alveoli and terminal bronchioles actually make up the majority of the lung mass. This tissue feels more like solid tissue than it does an air-filled sponge.

Gas transfer is probably most efficient in the alveoli, but a significant amount of gas is also exchanged across the respiratory bronchioles **Figure 26-10 ▲**. These terminal bronchioles are very thin and have little structure. This is helpful for gas exchange, but it also means that these bronchioles lack cilia, a mucous blanket, smooth muscle, or rigid structures. Once foreign material gets into the terminal bronchioles and alveoli (parts of the lung collectively known as the lung parenchyma), it typically never comes out. Emphysema may affect this area of the lung, damaging or destroying the few structural components that are present. When that happens, the terminal branches of the tracheobronchial tree become so weak that they collapse during exhalation, and trap air in the alveoli.

The alveoli are lined with a substance known as surfactant, which reduces surface tension and helps keep the alveoli expanded. If the amount of surfactant is decreased or the alveoli

are not inflated, the alveoli collapse, which results in a condition known as atelectasis.

If smoking or disease destroys certain types of cells in an alveolus, it cannot repair itself. Conversely, alveoli can repair significant damage if certain cells survive an illness.

The pulmonary circulation begins at the right ventricle where the pulmonary artery (the only artery that usually carries deoxygenated blood) branches into increasingly smaller vessels until the pulmonary capillary bed surrounds the alveoli and terminal bronchioles **Figure 26-11 ▶**. There is significantly more circulation to the lung bases than there is to the lung apices. Unfortunately, because humans are upright, gravity-dependent creatures, most infections and pathologic conditions affect the bases of our lungs. It is uncommon for a person who isn't bedridden to experience upper lobe pneumonia. The appearance of upper lobe lesions is suggestive of cancer.

Like all the capillaries in the body, the pulmonary capillaries are very narrow, and typically allow only red blood cells to pass through in single-file fashion. People with chronic lung disease and chronic hypoxia often make a surplus of red blood cells over time (polycythemia), which makes their blood thick. Pushing this thicker-than-normal blood through the tiny pulmonary capillaries can put a significant strain on the right side of the heart. When alveoli are distended by

COPD, they push against the capillary bed, further narrowing the capillaries and straining the right side of the heart. Right heart failure secondary to chronic lung disease is known as cor pulmonale.

Airway Problems Versus Breathing Problems

From your first cardiopulmonary resuscitation (CPR) class, the differences between maintaining the airway and breathing for the patient are highlighted. Unfortunately, a paramedic can still easily become confused between pathologic conditions that affect one versus the other. Many patients present with an airway that can use a little assistance. No one should be snoring, gurgling, squeaking, or using accessory muscles to inhale. You must remain vigilant that secretions, soft tissue, blood, or

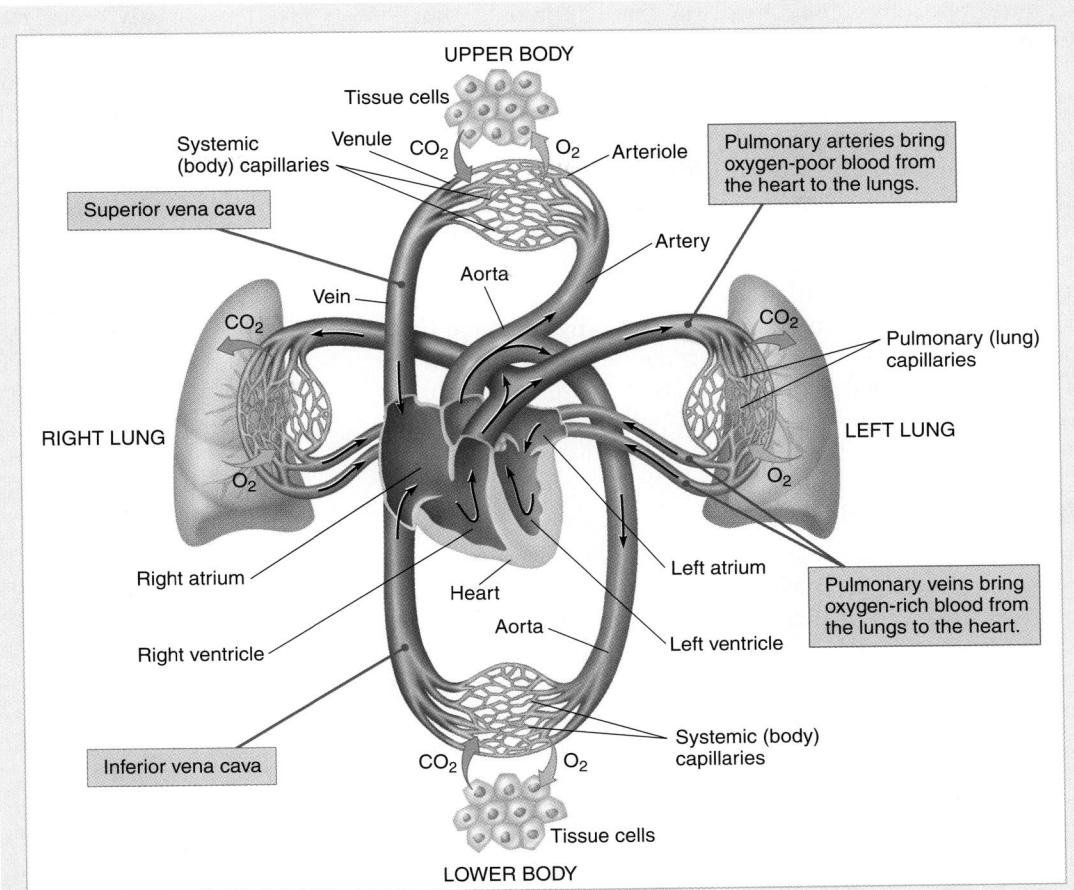

Figure 26-11 Pulmonary circulation begins as blood leaves the right ventricle via the pulmonary artery. The pulmonary capillary bed brings red blood cells very close to the terminal bronchioles. There is more perfusion to the bases of the lungs than to the apices. After picking up oxygen, the blood returns to the left atrium via the pulmonary veins.

You are the Provider Part 2

As you apply oxygen and obtain vital signs, you notice that the nail beds and oral mucosa of your patient are bluish (cyanosis). You adjust the sensor location of the pulse oximeter and obtain a reading. The patient's wife tells you that her husband has been running a fever, has experienced progressive weakness, and has had a productive cough (with thick, yellowish green sputum) for the past 4 to 5 days. She also tells you that her husband has been up all night struggling to breathe. He also has COPD and has smoked two packs of cigarettes a day since he was 15 years old. On auscultation of the chest, you note rhonchi in all lung fields on both inspiration and expiration.

Vital Signs	Recording Time: 5 Minutes
Level of consciousness	A (Alert to person, place, and day)
Skin	Pale, cool extremities, diaphoretic
Pulse	110 beats/min, weak; occasionally irregular
Blood pressure	108/54 mm Hg
Sao_2	75% (receiving 100% oxygen via nonrebreathing mask)
Temperature	102°F (reported by wife)
ECG	Sinus tachycardia with occasional premature ventricular contractions

4. Given the patient's presentation, which assessment tools should you use to obtain a greater understanding of the patient's medical condition?
5. What was likely the initial problem with obtaining a pulse oximetry reading?

vomit do not compromise an airway that you initially thought was open.

At the same time, an open airway does not ensure that an adequate volume of gas is moving in and out of the lungs. Proper ventilation is necessary to provide adequate oxygen to the bloodstream and to remove carbon dioxide. Increasing the amount of available oxygen ensures that even a patient who is not moving adequate volumes of gas (eg, hypoventilating) can still maintain adequate oxygen saturation. Unfortunately, if ventilation remains inadequate, carbon dioxide levels will increase. Hypoventilating patients become hypercapnic (have too much carbon dioxide in their blood) and acidotic (the pH of their arterial blood falls too low). Both conditions can interrupt important body systems and, if uncorrected over a period of time, can result in death.

Ventilation Revisited

Many airway problems can be bypassed by inserting an ET tube. By contrast, alterations in breathing can be much more complex. They can involve problems with the conducting airways (branches), such as asthma or bronchitis; difficulties at the alveolar level, such as pneumonia or emphysema; problems with the muscles and nerves that make breathing work, as in Guillain-Barré syndrome or spinal cord injury; or problems with the rigid structure of the thorax that allows the pressure changes that make breathing work, such as flail chest.

We are usually negative-pressure breathers (air suckers). Think about a vacuum cleaner at the base of the lungs sucking in air as you inhale. This air is pulled in through the mouth and the nose, over the turbinates, and around the complex terrain of the epiglottis and glottis. Air typically does not enter the esophagus and stomach because it is preferentially sucked into the trachea (Figure 26-12 ▾).

This negative-pressure vacuum effect occurs because the thorax is essentially an airtight box with a flexible diaphragm (the major muscle of breathing) at the bottom and an open tube (the trachea) at the top. During quiet breathing, when the diaphragm flattens, the overall size of the container increases, and air is sucked in through the tube at the top to fill the increasing space inside the thorax. You can increase the amount of air you move each minute (minute ventilation) by dropping the diaphragm more aggressively (deep breathing, or hyperpnea) or by breathing more rapidly (tachypnea). To breathe even more deeply, you can use additional muscles to pull the ribs up and out, further increasing both the size of the thoracic cavity as well as increasing the negative-pressure environment and moving larger volumes of air. Clearly, disruptions of the thoracic cage will hinder your ability to move air by this mechanism.

Holes in the thorax provide another place for air to be sucked in, resulting in a sucking chest wound (Figure 26-13 ▾). When multiple ribs are broken in more than one place (flail chest), free-floating sections of the thorax get pulled in when you breathe, limiting the amount of air that can be sucked in through the trachea. Infants and small children have a lot of elastic cartilage in their chest wall; when they use a lot of muscle to breathe, the sternum or ribs often collapse, causing retractions.

When you ventilate someone with positive-pressure (ie, with a pocket mask or bag-mask ventilation), air is forced into the upper airway and flows into both the trachea and esophagus unless steps are taken to help direct it into the trachea (Figure 26-14 ▸). Indeed, positive-pressure ventilation with bag-mask ventilation or a pocket mask is physiologically the opposite of normal (negative-pressure) ventilation.

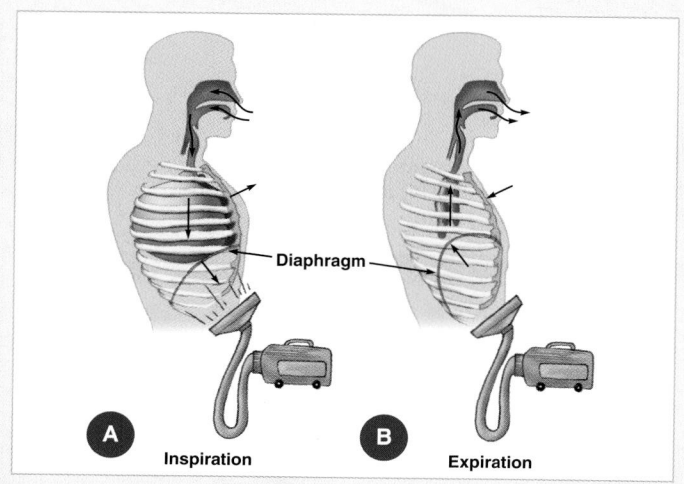

Figure 26-12 Normal ventilation is negative-pressure ventilation, meaning that we suck air into our lungs, much as a vacuum cleaner sucks in air. The negative pressure pulls down the diaphragm, causing the lungs to fill (**A**). When the pressure is released, the diaphragm relaxes and the lungs empty (**B**). Compare with positive-pressure ventilation, shown in Figure 26-14.

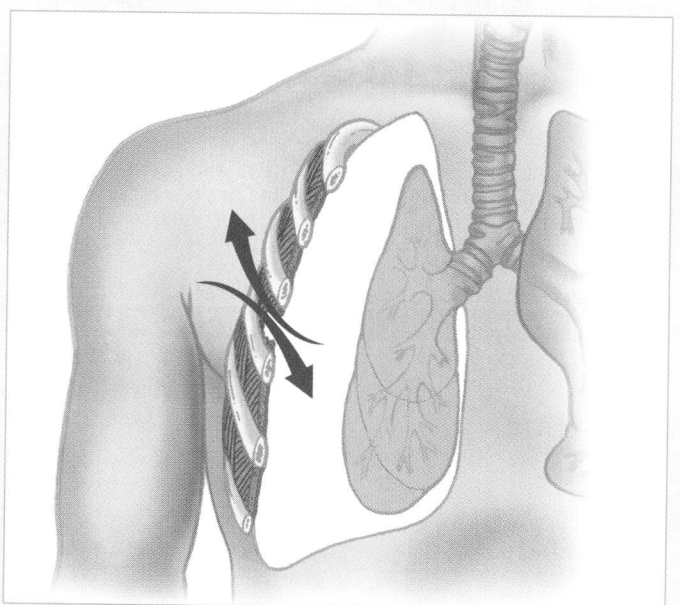

Figure 26-13 A sucking chest wound reduces ventilation by allowing air to enter the thorax during the inspiratory or negative-pressure phase of ventilation.

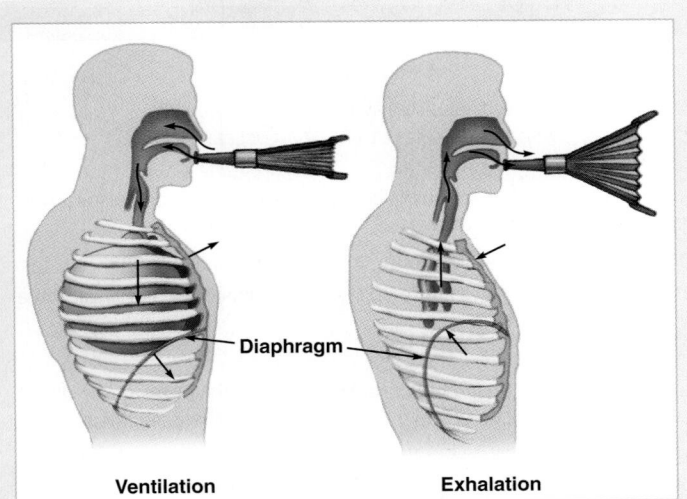

Figure 26-14 Positive-pressure ventilation is physiologically the opposite of normal ventilation. Air is pushed into the respiratory tract with bag-mask ventilation and can go into the esophagus and stomach unless careful technique is applied. Compare with negative-pressure ventilation, shown in Figure 26-12.

brain injuries may exhibit bizarre respiratory patterns when one or more of these respiratory centers are damaged or deprived of adequate blood flow. Table 26-1 ▶ summarizes the various breathing patterns.

Most of these respiratory centers are in and around the brain stem Figure 26-15 ▼. Patients who suffer serious trauma to the upper cerebral hemispheres (such as from a gunshot wound) are often still breathing despite mortal wounds. Apneustic breathing results from damage to the apneustic center in the brain, which regulates inspiratory pause. A patient exhibiting apneustic respirations will have a short, brisk inhalation with a long pause before exhalation. This pattern is indicative of severe pressure within the cranium or direct trauma to the brain. Similarly, Biot respirations are seen when the center that controls breathing rhythm is damaged. This respiratory pattern is grossly irregular, sometimes with lengthy apneic periods.

Cheyne-Stokes respirations are more of a high-brain function. Many deep sleepers or intoxicated people will exhibit this type of respiratory pattern. The depth of breathing (or volume of snoring) gradually increases, then decreases (crescendo-decrescendo), followed by an apneic period. The apneic period is usually brief in the relatively healthy patient. Exaggerated Cheyne-Stokes respirations may be seen in patients who have a severe brain injury, where the crescendo-decrescendo is much more prominent. The apneic period may last 30 to 60 seconds.

Exhalation is usually a passive process. After the size of the thorax has increased during inhalation, the components of the respiratory system return to their original places, and air is pushed out of the trachea under positive pressure. When a patient has trouble exhaling, for example, in asthma, reactive airway disease, or COPD, he or she may need to use the abdominal muscles to push air out. When this occurs, exhalation is no longer a passive process. Watch your patient work as he or she breathes. Is the patient having trouble pulling air in or pushing air out? Difficulty in exhalation usually indicates obstructive disease; difficulty in inhalation may indicate upper airway obstruction.

The neurologic control of respiration is complex. At least four parts of the brain are responsible for the smooth, rhythmic respirations that we take for granted—one area helps control rate, another depth, another inspiratory pause, and yet another rhythmicity. Patients with traumatic

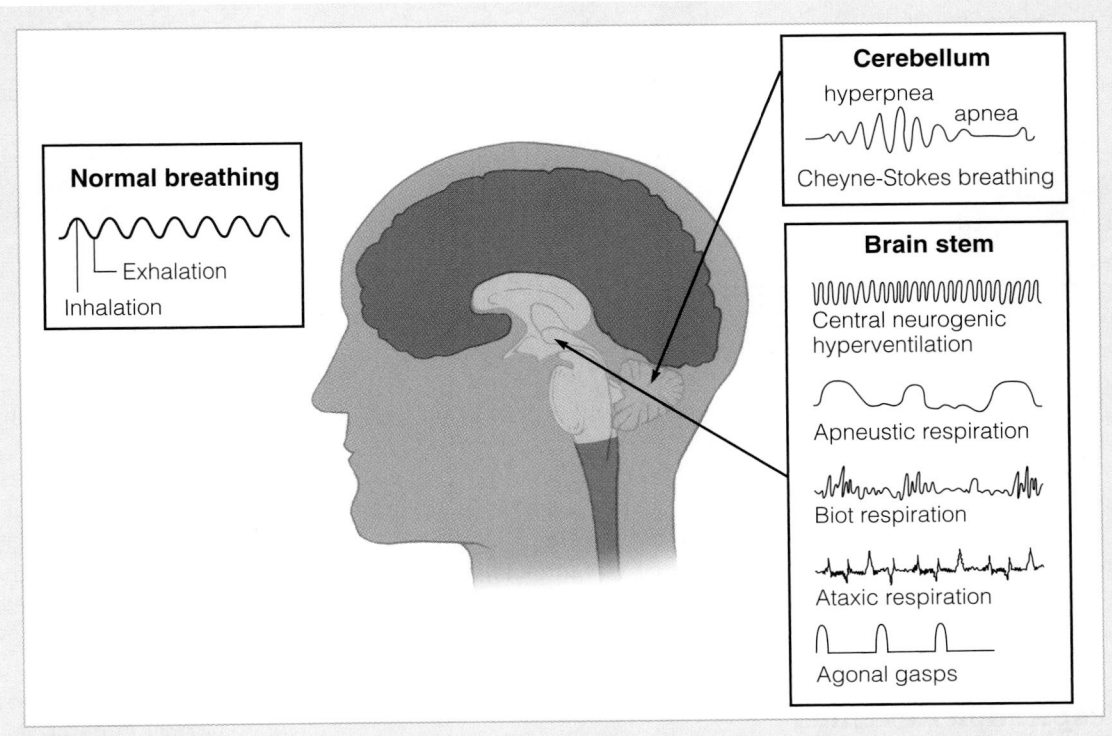

Figure 26-15 The neurologic control of respiration is complex, and many variations in the respiratory pattern may be noted in the scenario of brain injury. The respiratory patterns shown—each recorded for 1 minute—have been documented using an end-tidal carbon dioxide detector. Note that most irregular breathing patterns are controlled by the brain stem.

Table 26-1	Breathing Patterns
Pattern	**Comments**
Agonal	Irregular gasps that are few and far between. Usually represent stray neurologic impulses in the dying patient. It is not unusual for patients who are pulseless to have an occasional agonal gasp.
Apneustic	When the pneumotaxic center in the brain is damaged, the apneustic center causes a prolonged inspiratory hold (fish breathing). This ominous sign indicates severe brain injury.
Ataxic	Completely irregular respirations that indicate severe brain injury or brain-stem herniation.
Biot respirations	Respirations with an irregular pattern, rate, and depth with intermittent patterns of apnea. Indicative of severe brain injury or brain-stem herniation.
Bradypnea	Unusually slow respirations.
Central neurogenic hyperventilation	Tachypneic hyperpnea. Rapid and deep respirations caused by increased intracranial pressure or direct brain injury. Drives carbon dioxide levels down and pH levels up, resulting in respiratory alkalosis.
Cheyne-Stokes respirations	Crescendo-decrescendo breathing with a period of apnea between each cycle. It is not considered ominous unless grossly exaggerated or in the context of a patient who has brain trauma.
Cough	Forced exhalation against a closed glottis; an airway-clearing maneuver. Also seen when foreign substances irritate the airways. Controlled by the cough center in the brain. Antitussive medications work on the cough center to reduce this sometimes-annoying physiologic response.
Eupnea	Normal breathing.
Hiccup	Spasmodic contraction of the diaphragm causing short exhalations with a characteristic sound. Sometimes seen in cases of diaphragmatic (or phrenic nerve) irritation from acute myocardial infarction, ulcer disease, or endotracheal intubation.
Hyperpnea	Unusually deep breathing. Seen in various neurologic or chemical disorders. Certain drugs may stimulate this type of breathing in patients who have overdosed. It does not reflect respiratory rate—only respiratory depth.
Hypopnea	Unusually shallow respirations.
Kussmaul respirations	The same pattern as central neurogenic hyperventilation, but caused by the body's response to metabolic acidosis; the body is trying to rid itself of blood acetone via the lungs. Kussmaul respirations are seen in patients who have diabetic ketoacidosis, and are accompanied by a fruity (acetone) breath odor. The mouth and lips are usually cracked and dry.
Sighing	Periodically taking a very deep breath (about twice the normal volume). Sighing forces open alveoli that close in the course of day-to-day events.
Tachypnea	Unusually rapid breathing. This term does not reflect depth of respiration, nor does it mean that the patient is hyperventilating (lowering the carbon dioxide level by breathing too fast and too deep). In fact, patients who breathe very rapidly frequently move only small volumes of air and are *hypo*ventilating (much like a panting dog).
Yawning	Yawning seems to be beneficial in the same manner that sighing is. It also appears to be contagious!

Stretch receptors in the lungs are responsible for the Hering-Breuer reflex, which causes you to cough if you take too deep a breath. Prehospital providers become accustomed to ventilating unresponsive patients. When called upon to assist a conscious patient's respirations, as may happen when a patient is breathing shallowly, many paramedics give breaths that are too large, causing repeated coughing and discomfort to the patient. Assisting the spontaneously breathing patient with bag-mask ventilation can be a complex skill, requiring practice.

Respiration Revisited

Respiration is the process by which oxygen is taken into the body, distributed to the cells, and used by the cells to make energy. Respiration takes place in each cell. It involves using oxygen and glucose to make energy that allows the cell to do

its work. The oxygen must be supplied by the lungs and circulatory systems. The primary byproduct of this process is carbon dioxide.

The respiratory system is involved in the delivery of the oxygen to the bloodstream and the removal of the waste carbon dioxide from the body. If the lungs are not functioning appropriately, both of these vital functions may be impaired. Failure to deliver oxygen efficiently results in cellular hypoxia. Hypoxia kills cells by making it impossible for them to make enough energy to do their work; it also causes acidosis. We can often help the patient with hypoxia by providing additional oxygen.

Under normal circumstances, the carbon dioxide evolved during cellular respiration is returned to the lungs by the circulatory system, where it is exhaled during ventilation. When the lungs are not working adequately, carbon dioxide is not efficiently disposed of and accumulates in the blood. This carbon dioxide combines with water to form bicarbonate ions and hydrogen (H^+) ions, also known as acid (pH is an expression of how many free H^+ ions are in a solution). The result is acidosis. By contrast, in hyperventilation, the person breathes too effectively and blows off more carbon dioxide than usual, resulting in alkalosis.

A Systems Approach to Respiratory Emergencies

Evaluation of the respiratory organs is clearly an important component of assessing respiratory emergencies. However, the job performed by the respiratory system so dramatically impacts other body systems that a thorough respiratory assessment includes much more than listening to the patient's lungs.

Neurologic Status

The brain is very sensitive to reduced levels of oxygen. For this reason, any alteration in level of consciousness could represent a degree of respiratory compromise. Anxiety can be an early sign of hypoxia, while confusion, lethargy, and coma are typically later signs. A brief seizure often accompanies a hypoxic event or cardiac arrest. Dizziness and tingling extremities could signify hyperventilation. Major neurologic insults may also manifest themselves with some altered respiratory pattern.

Brain trauma or anything else that disturbs the function of the brain may depress the respiratory control centers in the medulla. For example, the increasing intracranial pressure in closed head trauma may literally put the squeeze on the medulla to produce a variety of respiratory abnormalities, including apnea. A stroke may have a similar effect by depriving portions of the brain of circulation (see Chapter 28). Overdose with drugs that depress the central nervous system (such as narcotics or barbiturates) may also severely depress the activity of the respiratory center.

Injury high in the spinal cord may paralyze the intercostal muscles and even the diaphragm. Polio attacks the nerves that supply the respiratory muscles, but certain chronic illnesses, such as myasthenia gravis, weaken the respiratory muscles themselves. The net effect of these conditions is the inability of the respiratory muscles to function normally in response to the respiratory drive. As a consequence, the tidal volume is shallow, and the minute volume is correspondingly decreased. Patients with such conditions often need assisted ventilation to increase the tidal volume and, thus, minute volume.

Cardiovascular Status

Think of the lungs as lying between the right and left sides of the heart (in terms of function). Although an anatomic drawing may not depict the lungs in this way, the description is a very accurate concept when reviewing blood flow through the body. The right side of the heart pumps blood to the lungs, while the left side of the heart receives blood from the lungs and then pumps it around the body. Any major change in the function of the lungs, right side of the heart, or left side of the heart almost always affects the other components. The body's immediate response to mild hypoxemia is to increase the heart rate (tachycardia). Severe hypoxia often causes bradycardia. Any uncorrected hypoxic insult may result in lethal cardiac arrhythmias, such as ventricular fibrillation or ventricular tachycardia. Changes in fluid balance, right-heart pumping pressures, or left-heart pumping pressures can cause various forms of congestive heart failure. A thorough evaluation of the cardiovascular system is requisite in the evaluation of the respiratory patient.

Muscles and Mechanics

Muscles have to work to allow you to breathe under normal circumstances, and they have to work a lot harder when you are in respiratory distress. This extra work comes at a cost. People who have asthma, for instance, can often compensate for their respiratory distress by devoting lots of energy to their breathing. They can maintain their oxygen and carbon dioxide levels in an acceptable range as long as they continue to apply their muscles to this effort. The tremendous workload causes them to use tremendous amounts of energy, which requires even more oxygen and ventilation. Such patients are typically not in a position to eat and drink normally, so they continue to get more dehydrated, more malnourished, and more tired. At some point they will tire out and be unable to continue doing the necessary work of breathing; they will then look sleepy, the rate and depth of their respirations will slowly drop, and they will experience decompensation (respiratory failure).

Other things may interfere with the mechanics of breathing. Placing a patient in the Trendelenburg position, or even laying the patient flat, especially if the patient is overweight, causes the abdominal organs to push up against the diaphragm. With each breath, the patient must move the abdominal contents out of the way to expand the thorax and breathe. This explains why most people seek a sitting position when they are short of breath (orthopnea). If the abdomen is distended with air or blood, the situation is compounded. Things that bind the chest or abdomen (such as tight clothing or undergarments, a pneumatic antishock garment, or backboard straps) can also make it very difficult to breathe. Diseases that cause muscle weakness (such as botulism, amyotrophic lateral sclerosis, or Guillain-Barré syndrome) are often fatal when they render the patient unable to breathe.

Renal Status

Fluid balance, acid-base balance, and blood pressure are controlled, in part, by the kidneys. Each of these factors also affects the pulmonary mechanics and hence the delivery of oxygen to the tissues. Patients with severe renal disease often present with respiratory signs and symptoms, so the paramedic should always note signs of severe renal disease when evaluating the conditions of such patients. The conditions of patients who have congestive heart failure secondary to renal disease can be difficult to manage because diuresis may be difficult or impossible for them. Patients who have renal disease may also have acid-base disturbances that cause them to hyperventilate and that are sometimes mistaken for respiratory disorders. Often, a patient's need for emergency dialysis may influence your transport decisions and options.

Assessment of the Patient With Dyspnea

As always, remember that recognizing and treating life threats is the priority in the initial assessment, and throughout care.

Initial Assessment

Your first glance at a patient may identify a body type associated with a particular pathologic condition. The classic presentation of a patient with emphysema includes a barrel chest (a chest that is bigger in the front-to-back dimension than in the side-to-side dimension, from years of having air trapped in the thorax), muscle wasting (the patient has cannibalized his or her own body mass for energy), and pursed-lip breathing (because of the obstructive disease). Such patients are often tachypneic and do not typically present with profound hypoxia and cyanosis—hence the term pink puffer.

Patients who have chronic bronchitis tend to be more sedentary and thus may be obese. These patients are often encountered in a chair or recliner, where they sleep in an upright position. They may be surrounded by a wastebasket overflowing with tissues, a cup into which they spit their copious secretions, a urinal to avoid frequent trips to the bathroom, and an overflowing ashtray. The table next to their chair may have several medications, inhalers, or an aerosol nebulizer. Such a scene can disclose volumes of information about the patient and his or her history long before the paramedic ever places a stethoscope on the chest.

Severely ill patients with end-stage diseases, cancer, or immune system disorders are often easy to spot, as are the sickly appearance, rigors, and chills of a patient with pneumonia. Tall, thin young adults are predisposed to spontaneous pneumothorax, and women who smoke and take birth-control pills are predisposed to pulmonary embolus. Clues to a variety of pathologic conditions may be evident from your very first impression of a patient, but keep in mind that they are only clues. Avoid making a hasty field impression based on minimal information. The patient's presentation may make you suspicious about a particular condition, but make sure you confirm your suspicions with a thorough assessment.

Position and Degree of Distress

Patients in respiratory distress tend to seek the sitting position. The tripod position involves leaning forward and rotating the scapulae outward by placing the arms on a table or by placing the hands on the knees **Figure 26-16 ▶**. This opens up a little more space in the lung apices for airflow, as well as dropping the abdominal structures away from the diaphragm. Because there is considerably more perfusion to the lung bases than to

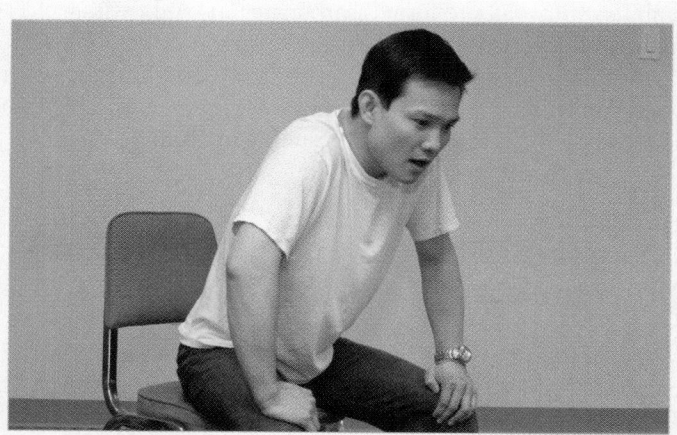

Figure 26-16 The tripod position (elbows out) allows better diaphragmatic movement by getting the abdomen out of the way, as well as a little more airflow to the apices, by rotating the scapulae laterally. This takes work, which requires more oxygen.

the apices, this maneuver may use more energy than it gains in oxygenation. Beware of the patient in respiratory distress who is willing to lie flat; this could be a sign of sudden deterioration.

Purposeful hyperextension occurs when a patient maximizes airflow through the upper airway. Such patients essentially hold their heads in the head tilt–chin lift or "sniffing" position. This position may indicate upper airway swelling, but it is also commonly seen in patients who are trying to maximize airflow. Maintaining this position uses up valuable energy. As a patient who is severely ill with respiratory disease begins to feel fatigue, he or she may hold the head up in this position only during inhalation, letting it fall into flexion during exhalation. This head bobbing is a very ominous sign, signaling the potential for imminent decompensation. Head bobbing is frequently preterminal behavior!

Work of Breathing

Patients who are using lots of muscles to breathe are in danger of tiring out, so it is important to note the use of accessory muscles. Is the patient using the muscles of the abdomen to push air out (as in asthma or COPD), or is the patient using muscles in the chest and neck to pull air in? Patients who are using a lot of extra muscles to breathe may cause dramatic pressure changes within the thorax and exhibit the following signs and symptoms:

- **Bony retractions.** These are most common in infants and small children, where the rigid structure of the thorax is still flexible. On inhalation, the child may pull (or retract) the sternum or ribs into the chest, causing a visible deformity with each breath **Figure 26-17 ▶**.
- **Soft-tissue retractions.** In most patients, the bones are rigid and don't move, but the soft tissue is pulled in around the bones. Dramatic retractions can be seen during inhalation in the supraclavicular, intercostal, and subxiphoid areas.

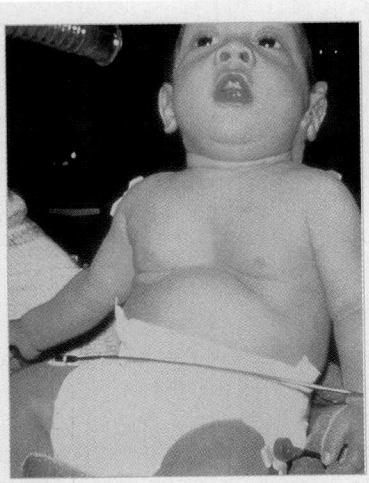

Figure 26-17 Bony retractions are not only a sign of severe distress and increased work of breathing, they also contribute to respiratory failure. With inhalation, the lower sternum is pulled into the lungs. Every cubic centimeter of space displaced by the retraction is a cubic centimeter of air that cannot get into the chest.

- **Nasal flaring.** The nostrils are pulled wide open on inhalation.
- **Tracheal tugging.** The thyroid cartilage is pulled upward and the area just above the sternal notch is sucked inward with inhalation.
- **Paradoxical respiratory movement.** The epigastrium is pulled in with inhalation while the abdomen pushes out, creating a see-saw appearance as the two move in opposing directions.
- **Pulsus paradoxus.** Profound intrathoracic pressure changes cause the peripheral pulses to weaken (or disappear!) on inspiration; these pulses are easier to palpate during exhalation. This is rare.

Assessing breathing for rate and depth is an obvious component of a respiratory assessment, but one that is often not accurately determined. Respiratory rate may be a commonly "guessed" vital sign, but respiratory depth is even more commonly misjudged. A patient with an adequate rate but a low volume will still have a pitifully low minute volume (respiratory rate × tidal volume = minute volume). While assessing the respirations, note their pattern (see Table 26-1) and the inspiratory-to-expiratory (I:E) ratio. Is the patient working hard to inhale, to exhale, or both? Does the breath have a peculiar odor (such as the acetone breath odor associated with diabetic ketoacidosis)? Are there any audible abnormal respiratory noises? As a general rule, *any* respiratory noises that you can hear without a stethoscope are abnormal noises.

Notes from Nancy

Noisy breathing is obstructed breathing.

Snoring indicates partial obstruction of the upper airway by the tongue—a form of obstruction that is easily corrected by head tilt maneuvers. Gurgling signals the presence of fluid in the upper airway. Stridor, a harsh, high-pitched sound heard on inhalation, indicates narrowing, usually as a result of swelling (laryngeal edema).

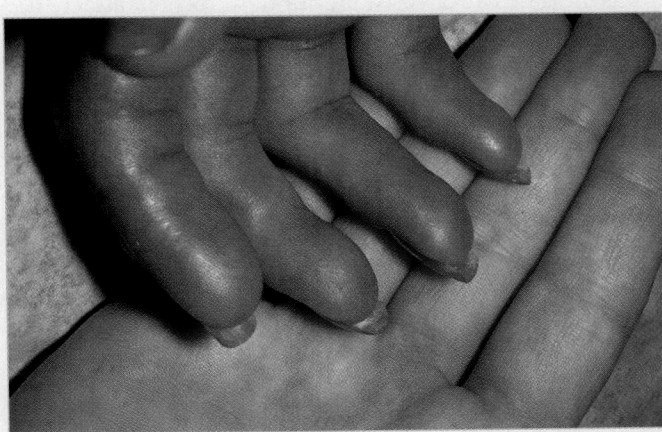

Figure 26-18 Skin color can provide an early, fast indication of several disease processes. Cyanosis (shown here) presents as bluish skin and indicates at least 5 g/dL of unoxygenated hemoglobin. Carbon monoxide intoxication can present as cherry-red skin, though this is a very late sign. When making any preliminary diagnosis, allow for the wide variation in patients' skin color and tone.

Quiet breathing should also be of interest. The patient with tachypnea who has crystal-clear breath sounds may have hyperventilation syndrome but may also be breathing fast because of acidosis. Quiet tachypnea should prompt you to consider shock. Paramedics occasionally mistake tachypnea caused by pain, anxiety, or metabolic disorders as the patient's primary problem, and administer aerosol treatments for diabetic crisis or sepsis. Obviously, aerosol bronchodilators don't help those conditions.

Neurologic Assessment

Assessing the level of consciousness is enormously important in patients with dyspnea. Although you cannot measure the patient's arterial blood gases in the field, the patient's brain is constantly doing precisely that. Any decline in Pao_2 (hypoxemia) will manifest initially as restlessness, confusion, and in worst case scenarios, as combative behavior. An increase in $Paco_2$, by contrast, usually has sedative effects, making the patient sleepy and hard to rouse.

Skin Color

Assessing skin color is a fast way to begin forming an early impression of the patient's condition **Figure 26-18 ▲**. While it is obviously important to note the generalized cyanosis of oxygen desaturation or the profound pallor of shock, more subtle information can be gained by assessing the patient's mucous membranes. The tissue inside the mouth, under the eyelids, and even under the nail beds is usually the same pink color in all healthy patients. A few notable variations are described below:

- **Cyanosis.** Healthy adults have a hemoglobin level of 12 to 14 g/dL. Under those conditions, a person will begin to exhibit the blue discoloration of cyanosis when about

5 g/dL is desaturated (does not have oxygen attached). That means their oxygen saturation would be roughly 65%! If a person's hemoglobin level were only 10 g/dL, 50% of it (5 of the 10 g/dL) would have to be desaturated before the patient would look cyanotic. Some patients in cardiac arrest are a deep blue, while others are simply pale. Similarly, patients with high hemoglobin levels (those who have chronic respiratory disease) may develop cyanosis earlier than patients who have normal hemoglobin levels. Of course, there are slight variations in what is considered normal. Also, some patients who have chronic respiratory conditions who have an artificially low oxygen saturation may also have a low level of chronic cyanosis (which explains the use of the term blue bloater to describe patients who have chronic bronchitis).

- **Chocolate brown skin.** High levels of methemoglobin derived from nitrates and some toxic exposures may turn the mucous membranes brown. This transformation is typically more evident in the patient's venous blood than in the skin and mucous membranes.
- **Pale skin.** Pale skin and mucous membranes are caused by a reduction of blood flow to the small vessels near the surface of the skin. The source of this condition could be hypoxia, shock, catecholamine release, such as from epinephrine or norepinephrine, or a cold environment.

While you are noting the color of the mucous membranes, also note their moistness. Dehydration can be seen in the mucous membranes of the mouth and eyes. Dry, cracked lips; a dry, furrowed tongue; and dry, sunken eyes point to obvious dehydration. The skin of an older patient may always look dry with poor turgor, so skin assessment may be of less value in some older people.

The Focused History: Elaboration on the Chief Complaint

One challenge in assessing respiratory patients is that they may not be able to talk to you because of having difficulty breathing. While it is usually best to ask open-ended questions and allow patients to tell their own stories, dyspneic patients may be able to speak only in short sentences, or may be reduced to nodding in response to a series of yes-or-no questions. In some cases, the bulk of your history-taking may have to be hastily obtained from a family member, or gleaned from the few clues (such as medications) immediately available. You often have to institute basic therapy (such as oxygen or aerosol therapy) before getting the complete story from patients. Sometimes, you must immediately intubate patients, which will eliminate your ability to get a history from them from that point on.

When it is possible to discuss the history of the present illness with patients, several lines of questioning can provide important data. Utilizing the OPQRST mnemonic can help you elaborate on the chief complaint.

Reason for Calling for Help

Have patients explain in their own words what they are feeling. Many patients will identify their problem and tell you the best way to treat it without you having to dig for the information. Patients who have chronic respiratory conditions are often knowledgeable about their disease or disorder and may have tried several potential treatment options already. If they have been intubated and placed on a ventilator in past episodes, that is important information for you to have.

Onset and Duration

The speed with which the patient's distress has worsened is an important consideration in determining the underlying cause. Rapid-onset dyspnea may be caused by acute bronchospasm, anaphylaxis, pulmonary embolism, or pneumothorax. Left heart failure typically progresses much faster than right heart failure. Right heart failure may slowly worsen over many days, whereas left heart failure resulting from a massive AMI can kill a patient in a matter of minutes! Infectious diseases sometimes present very rapidly, but at other times may occur at the end of a lengthy battle with a low-grade infection. Did this problem arise suddenly, or did it get worse over time? How long has it been this bad?

Paroxysmal nocturnal dyspnea—dyspnea that comes on suddenly in the middle of the night is an ominous sign. It may signal left heart failure, worsening of COPD, or both. It occurs because of accumulation of fluid in the alveoli or pooling of secretions in the bronchi during sleep.

The position of comfort and difficulty speaking may also help you gauge the degree of distress. A patient who is comfortable while lying flat and speaking in full sentences can be deemed to be in little distress. A patient who is sitting in a Fowler's position and speaking only in two- or three-word statements is probably in considerable distress, possibly even life-threatening distress.

History of the Problem

Asthma attack, congestive heart failure, pneumonia in immunocompromised patients, and even spontaneous pneumothorax are often repeating pathologic conditions. If the patient has some experience with these types of events, they can serve as a baseline to assess the current condition. Ask these questions: Do you feel better or worse than last time? How often does this happen to you? What did the doctor tell you it was? What helped you or what happened last time?

Attempts at Treatment

When respiratory disorders are chronic or recurring, patients may already have strategies to manage their crises. Determine what the patient may have already tried, and whether it had any effect (positive or negative). By following this simple line of questioning, you can determine which medications the patient is supposed to be taking (which often gives valuable clues to other problems) and whether the patient is taking those medications correctly. Patients also often know exactly what caused their problems.

Associated Symptoms

Respiratory difficulty must always be evaluated in light of the patient's cardiovascular and renal status. Many acute myocardial infarctions present as congestive heart failure, as do renal crises. Tachypnea can signal anxiety, diabetes, or shock. In addition, the vast majority of chronically ill patients have a respiratory component to their disease. A whole host of pathologic conditions can masquerade as respiratory distress, especially in patients who have underlying respiratory disease. Don't be too quick to conclude that your patient's *only* problem is a relatively straightforward respiratory issue. Always dig deeper to determine what else may be triggering or worsening the patient's respiratory distress.

The Focused Physical Examination

By the time you have elicited the history of a patient who has respiratory complaints, you should already have some important information about the patient's physical signs. In particular, you should have observed the patient's level of consciousness, position, degree of distress, and so forth. This section presents the components of the physical exam in sequence, noting at each step the points of particular relevance to the dyspneic patient.

Neck Exam

In the neck, look for jugular venous distention when a patient is in a semi-sitting position. Jugular venous distention is a condition in which the jugular veins are engorged with blood. It is common all of the time in patients who have an obstructive lung disease such as asthma or COPD. Healthy young adults often demonstrate jugular venous distention when they are supine (lying on their back), and it is common to see gross jugular venous distention when people are laughing or singing 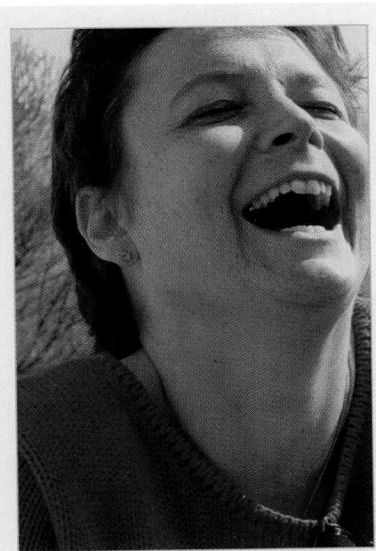 Figure 26-19 ◄ . When jugular venous distention is present in patients who are sitting upright, it can provide a rough measure of the pressure in the right atrium of the heart. Distended neck veins may implicate cardiac failure as the source of the patient's dyspnea. Jugular venous distention may also indicate high pressure in the thorax, which keeps the blood from draining out of the head and neck. Cardiac tamponade, pneumothorax, heart failure, and COPD can all cause jugular venous distention. Hepatojugular reflux occurs when mild pressure on the patient's liver causes the jugular veins to engorge further. This is a specific sign of right heart failure.

Obviously, jugular venous distention must be interpreted in light of the patient's position and other vital signs. The trauma patient who demonstrates grossly distended jugular veins despite a blood pressure of 80/40 mm Hg should cause considerable concern. A healthy 20 year old who has jugular venous distention when lying flat (but not while sitting) is of little concern.

While looking at the neck, note the trachea. Tracheal deviation is a classic—albeit late—sign of a tension pneumothorax Figure 26-20 ▾ . Tension pneumothorax is very difficult to

Figure 26-19 Jugular venous distention may be a normal finding in a healthy young adult who is supine or laughing. But in an adult who is sitting upright, it may indicate blood backing up as it tries to enter the thorax or the right atrium.

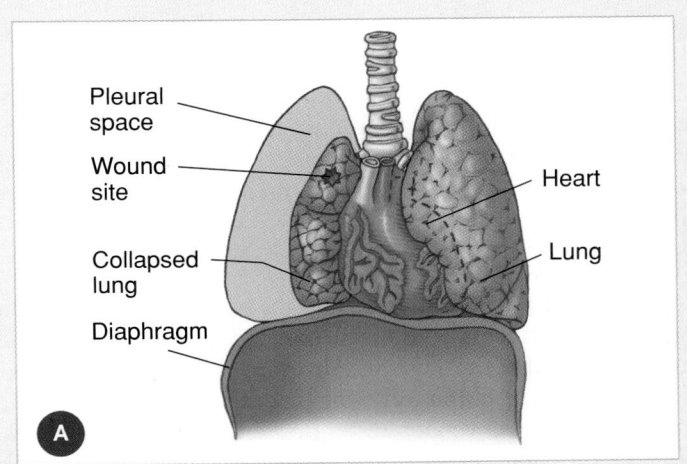

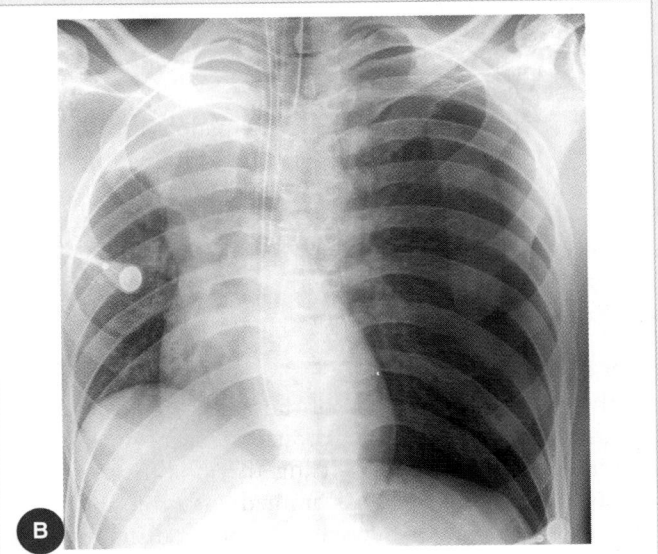

Figure 26-20 A pneumothorax occurs when air leaks into the pleural space between the lung and the chest wall (**A**). The radiograph (**B**) shows a collapsed lung on the right, which appears darker.

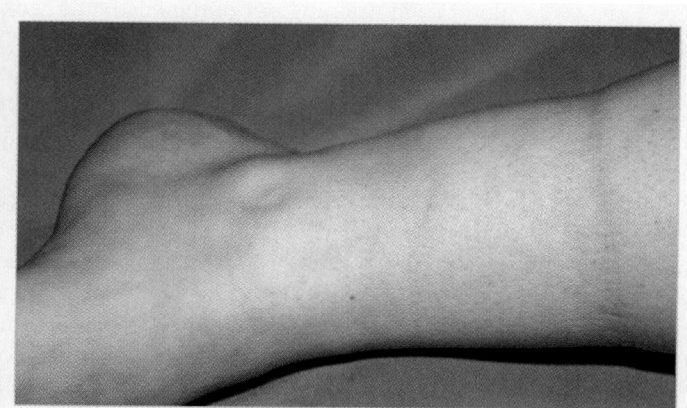

Figure 26-21 Pitting edema is present when you palpate the area, and your fingers leave temporary depressions in the tissue.

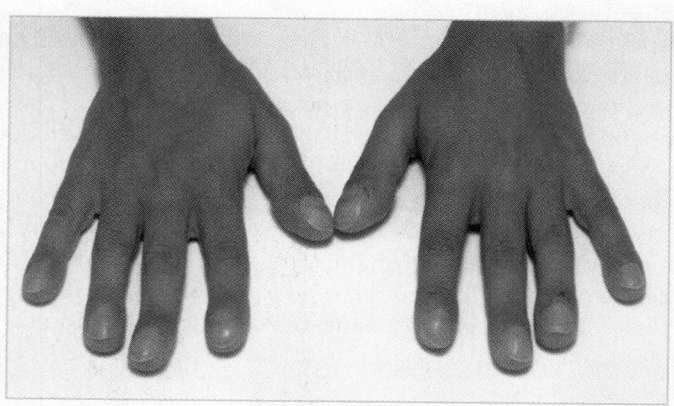

Figure 26-22 Digital clubbing is a sign of chronic hypoxia. It is seen in young people who have congenital heart disease and in older people who have severe chronic lung disease.

see except in extreme cases. On a radiograph, the trachea can clearly be seen deviating because of a tension pneumothorax. The deviation occurs behind the sternum, so it may not be seen or even felt. Consider palpating the trachea at the suprasternal notch. When the trachea does deviate, it often does so at a point behind the sternum, so it may not be palpable or visible.

Chest and Abdominal Exam

Hepatojugular reflux is specific to right heart failure. When the right ventricle is not pumping effectively, blood backs up, making it difficult for the jugular veins and the large reservoir of blood in the liver to drain into the thorax. As a result, the combination of jugular venous distention and hepatomegaly (distended liver) may present in right heart failure. If you gently press on the liver, the blood you squeeze out will further engorge the jugular veins. When a patient in respiratory distress is sitting up in a semi-Fowler's (45°) position, it is easy to check for hepatojugular reflux.

Feel the chest for vibrations as the patient breathes (tactile fremitus); secretions in the large airways are usually easy to feel and to hear. Some people recommend percussing the chest. With experience, you can tell the difference between a normal chest and a bad pneumothorax, but this remains a difficult procedure to perform in the field setting because of ambient noise around you and the patient.

Exam of the Extremities

Does the patient have edema of the ankles or lower back? If so, does it pit, and leave a depression, when you push your finger into the edema Figure 26-21 ▲ ? Is there peripheral cyanosis? Check the pulse. Is the patient profoundly tachycardic (from exertion or hypoxia)? Is there pulsus paradoxus? Also note the patient's skin temperature. Does the patient have an obvious fever, or is he or she cool and clammy from shock? Is there distal clubbing (from chronic hypoxia) Figure 26-22 ▶ ?

Data Collection

As appropriate to your patient care plan, attach any monitors that are immediately available to you. Repeated vital signs, ECG, and pulse oximetry readings are the data most commonly collected. In some situations, depending on available equipment, you might also record peak expiratory flow, end-tidal carbon dioxide, or even transcutaneous carbon monoxide levels. (Monitoring devices are discussed later in the chapter.)

The Stethoscope

As far as stethoscopes go, the following guideline applies: the longer the tubing, the more extraneous the noise you will probably hear. Avoid overly long stethoscopes. Higher-quality stethoscopes have a tubing-within-the-tubing design that limits its external noise interference. Although the Sprague-Rappaport design is popular Figure 26-23 ▶ , its two parallel tubes often bang against each other while moving, which can create extra noise.

Practically speaking, your stethoscope is the single most important investment you will make as a paramedic. Buy the best you can afford and take good care of it. Periodically check to make sure the

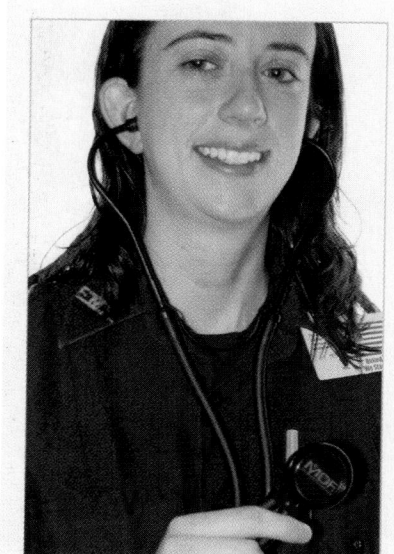

Figure 26-23 Earpieces should follow the normal (forward) slant of your ear canals. Note the Sprague-Rappaport–style stethoscope.

earpieces are clean and clear of earwax. On a regular basis, wipe down the length of the main tubing with an all-purpose cleaner. This helps slow the breakdown of the tube from the oils it picks up when you place it around your neck.

The diaphragm of the stethoscope is for high-pitched sounds (breath sounds); the bell (if present) is for low-pitched sounds (some heart tones). If you press the bell firmly against the skin, it stretches the skin beneath it and makes it act like a diaphragm. Hence, the bell should be placed lightly against the skin if you hope to hear the lower-pitched sounds. Some newer stethoscopes take advantage of this principle, allowing a single head to help transmit high- and low-pitched sounds based upon the pressure exerted by the operator. In older style stethoscopes, the bell rotates, allowing you to better hear the sounds you are trying to assess.

Your ear canals tend to point anteriorly in your skull (toward your eyes). You may wish to tilt the earpieces on your scope more forward for a better fit. But be careful: you may hear little or nothing if you accidentally place your scope in your ears backward, causing the earpieces to hit the sides of your ear canal.

Auscultation

Whenever possible, auscultate the lungs systematically. While we tend to compare the left and right sides, the lungs are not symmetrical. The right lung has three lobes: right upper lobe (RUL), right middle lobe (RML), and right lower lobe (RLL). The left lung has only two lobes: left upper lobe (LUL) and left lower lobe (LLL). Understand where you must listen to hear the various lobes Figure 26-24 ▸ . Some of the pathologic conditions you will listen for are gravity-dependent, meaning most pneumonias and congestive heart failure will tend to be found in the lung bases. In the case of wheezing, it may be diffuse and spread throughout the lung fields. The bases are almost exclusively heard by listening to the patient's back. The upper lobes, which rarely have abnormalities, are heard by listening to the anterior part of the chest. The right middle lobe can best be heard by listening just beneath, or lateral to, the right breast. The best left-right differentiation can be appreciated in the midaxillary line; this is the best place to listen for ET tube placement. If you listen to the anterior part of the chest, you are very close to the noise-maker (the endotracheal tube), whether it is in the trachea or the esophagus.

Specific Breath Sounds

The breath sounds you hear are made by turbulent flow in the large airways as they are transmitted through the chest to your stethoscope. Tracheal breath sounds are not commonly auscultated, but note how harsh and tubular they sound. Bronchial breath sounds are also quite loud, but note that exhalation predominates. Moving farther toward the periphery, bronchovesicular sounds are softer, and have equal inspiratory and expiratory sides. Finally, the most commonly heard breath sounds are the soft, breezy vesicular sounds heard in the periphery. They have a much more obvious inspiratory compo-

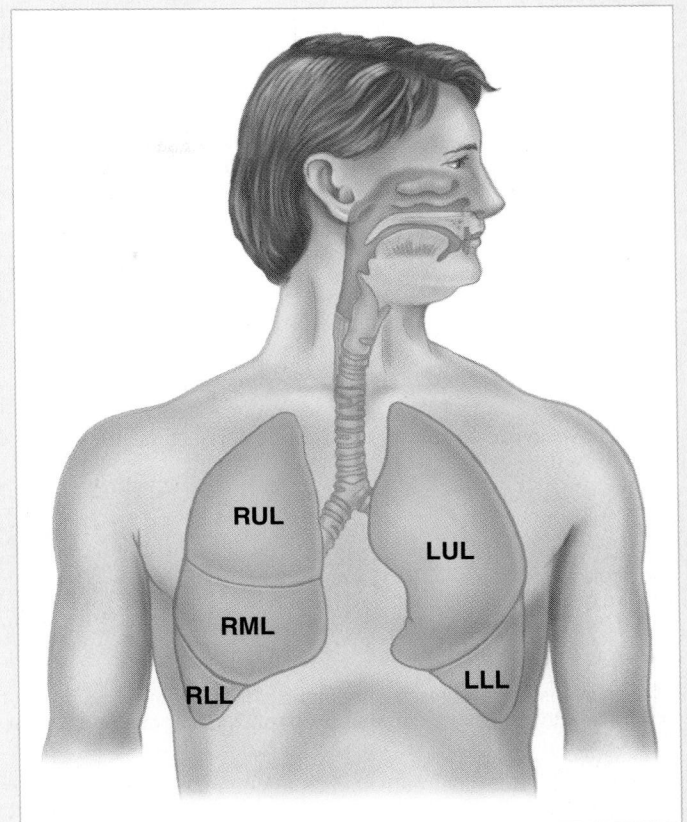

Figure 26-24 The lungs are not symmetrical. Most acute pathologic conditions are best heard in the lung bases, requiring you to listen to the patient's back. The right middle lobe is best heard beneath the right breast, or just lateral to it. LUL, left upper lobe; LLL, left lower lobe; RUL, right upper lobe; RML, right middle lobe; RLL, right lower lobe.

nent. You will want to listen to a large number of healthy lungs to become familiar with the four different sounds Figure 26-25 ▸ . Pathologic conditions may cause you to hear some normal breath sounds in abnormal places!

Sound moves better through fluid than it does through air. Thus, the more air that is present in a patient's chest (as in COPD or asthma), the more distant, diminished, or absent the breath sounds will be in the periphery. Conversely, the more "wet" the patient's lungs are (as in pneumonia; consolidation, when fluid causes the lungs to become firm; or congestive heart failure), the louder the sounds will be in the periphery. If a patient has pneumonia in the right middle lobe, you may hear bronchovesicular (equal inspiration and expiration) or even bronchial (greater expiration than inspiration) in the periphery, instead of the expected vesicular sounds (greater inspiration than expiration).

The quality of the breath sounds also depends on the amount of extra tissue you must listen through and the patient's respiratory effort. For this reason, it is often helpful to

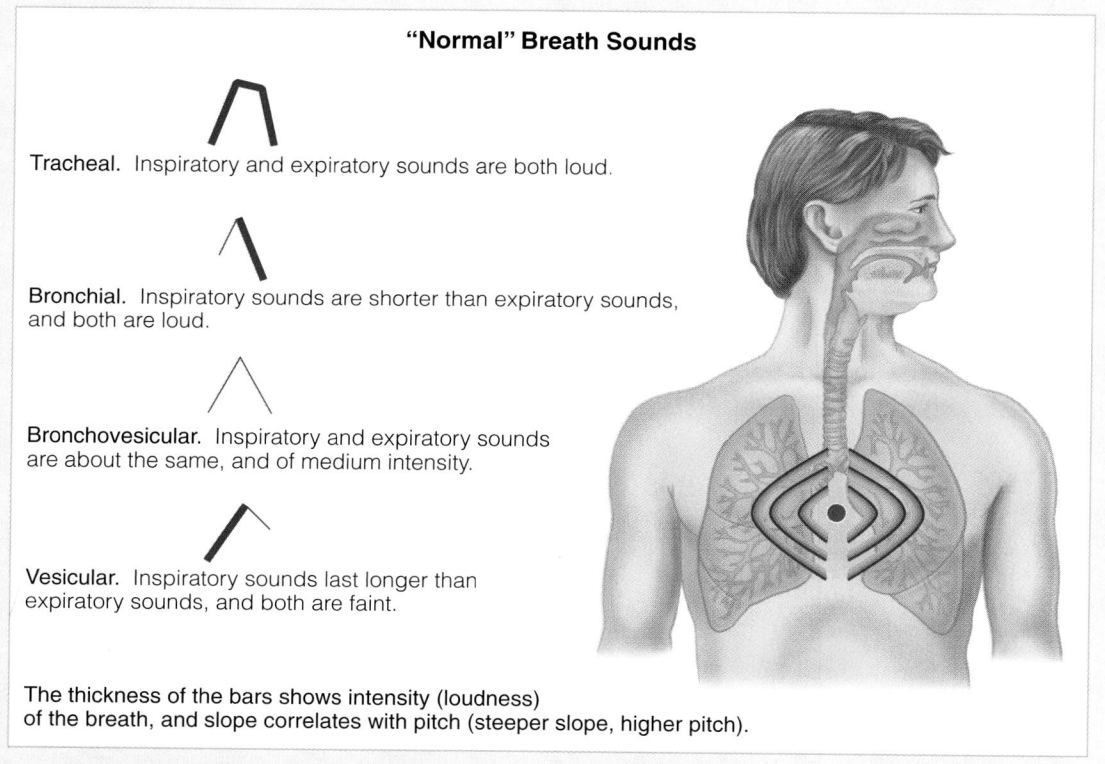

"Normal" Breath Sounds

Tracheal. Inspiratory and expiratory sounds are both loud.

Bronchial. Inspiratory sounds are shorter than expiratory sounds, and both are loud.

Bronchovesicular. Inspiratory and expiratory sounds are about the same, and of medium intensity.

Vesicular. Inspiratory sounds last longer than expiratory sounds, and both are faint.

The thickness of the bars shows intensity (loudness) of the breath, and slope correlates with pitch (steeper slope, higher pitch).

Figure 26-25 Normal breath sounds are heard over different parts of the chest. As you move away from the largest airways, breath sounds will become softer. The character of inspiration versus exhalation also changes.

compare breath sounds on the right versus the left. The breath sounds of a patient who has a one-sided pathologic condition (such as pneumonia) will sound *louder* over the side with the abnormality than they will over the healthy side.

Both breath sounds and vocalizations travel more efficiently through a firm, fluid-filled lung than through a healthy lung, but travel poorly through a hyperinflated lung. If a patient speaks while you are auscultating the chest, you cannot usually understand what he or she is saying through your stethoscope. If you can, it may mean consolidation from pneumonia or atelectasis. You will likely hear these sounds directly only over the consolidated lobe. **Table 26-2 ▶** lists tests that indicate consolidation.

Adventitious (abnormal) breath sounds are the extra noises that you may hear on top of the breath sounds described previously. Continuous sounds (for example, a wheeze) can be heard across some portion of each breath. Discontinuous sounds are the instantaneous pops, snaps, and clicks that we often identify as crackles **Figure 26-26 ▶**.

Wheezes are high-pitched, whistling sounds made by air being forced through narrowed airways, which makes them vibrate, much like the reed in a musical instrument. Wheezing may be diffuse, as in asthma and congestive heart failure, or localized, as when a foreign body obstructs a bronchus. Pathologic conditions such as asthma rarely cause one-sided wheez-

ing. Have the patient cough and listen again if you hear a sound on only one side; it could be caused by the movement of secretions. If a single bronchus is vibrating, the wheeze will be a single note (monophonic); if many bronchi are vibrating, the wheeze may have many notes, like a bagpipe (polyphonic). A wheeze may begin at the start of exhalation and continue until the end of exhalation.

Crackles are any discontinuous noises heard on auscultation of the lungs and are caused by the popping open of air spaces. They are usually associated with increased fluid in the lungs. These sounds are often referred to as crackles (rales) or rhonchi. A rhonchus is classically defined as a low-pitched continuous sound (such as a low wheeze or death rattle), but the term is sometimes used to mean a low-pitched crackle (thick secretions in the large airways).

The most ominous breath sounds are no breath sounds at all. They mean the patient is not moving enough air to ventilate the lungs. *Silence means danger!*

Sputum

It is probably not productive to discuss specific pathologic conditions suggested by various sputum colors, but it is appropriate to note whether the patient is coughing up colorful sputum **Table 26-3 ▶**. Many smokers or patients who have chronic respiratory diseases cough up sputum every day (especially

Table 26-2	**Signs of Consolidation**
Sign	**Test**
Bronchophony	When the patient says "99" repeatedly, it sounds like a hum through the normal lung. Through the consolidated lung, you can understand the words "99."
Egophony	The patient says "eeeeee" while you are auscultating, and you hear "aaaaaa." The sound may be heard particularly well over a pleural effusion.
Whispered pectoriloquy	The patient whispers while you are auscultating, and you can understand what is said.

Table 26-3	Classic Sputum Types
Type of Sputum	**Causes**
Frothy, sometimes with a pink tinge	Congestive heart failure
Thick	Dehydration or antihistamine use
Purulent	Infectious process (because the pus contains dead white blood cells)
Yellow, green, brown	Older secretions in various stages of decomposition
Clear or white	Bronchitis
Blood streaked	Tumor, tuberculosis, pulmonary edema, or trauma from coughing

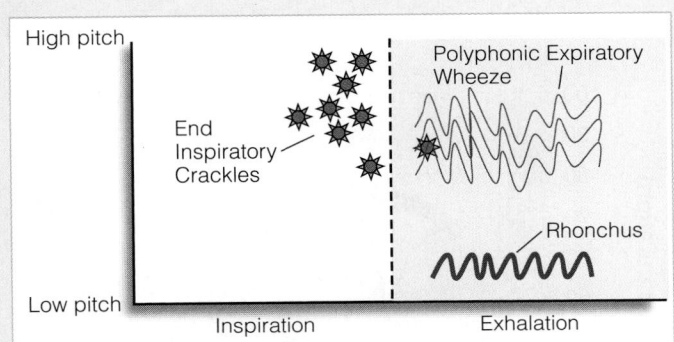

Figure 26-26 Adventitious sounds can be described as either continuous (wheezes and rhonchi) or discontinuous (crackles). They can also be characterized by their pitch (such as high or low), by where they are in the respiratory cycle (end inspiration or forced exhalation), and by their complexity (monophonic versus polyphonic).

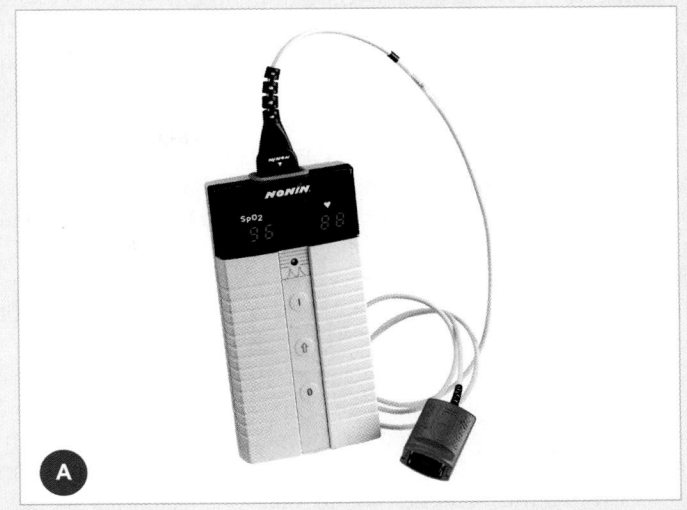

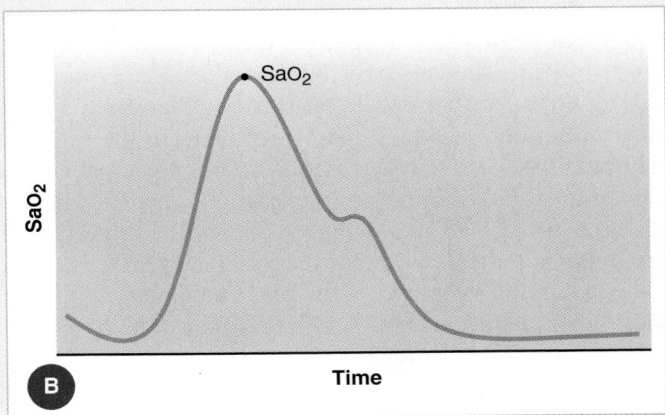

Figure 26-27 Pulse oximeters come in many sizes and, increasingly, are built into cardiac monitors (**A**). Some oximeters provide a waveform (**B**), which should demonstrate this characteristic shape when the oximeter is properly sensing.

first thing in the morning), so determine if the color or amount of this sputum has changed. Many patients don't spit their sputum out, whereas others will keep a cup or emesis basin next to their chair to spit in. Blood-tinged sputum may be a warning sign of tuberculosis or pulmonary edema, or it may mean the patient has been coughing forcefully and broken small blood vessels in the airway. Also note if mucus is purulent (puslike). Ask the patient these questions: Have you been coughing up anything colorful? Is that different for you?

Monitoring Devices

Pulse Oximetry

Under normal circumstances, a pulse oximeter is a noninvasive device that tells us what percentage of the patient's hemoglobin has oxygen attached to it **Figure 26-27**. For example, an oxygen saturation of 97% indicates that 97% of the patient's hemoglobin has oxygen attached to it. An oxygen saturation greater than 95% is considered normal. Most healthy people would feel short of breath at a saturation rate of less than 90%.

A pulse oximeter must "see" a pulsatile capillary bed to read properly. If the patient is wearing nail polish, you may need to remove it with an acetone nail polish remover before

obtaining a reading (although some research indicates that if you are getting a consistent reading through nail polish, the reading is probably accurate). Poor peripheral perfusion, cold extremities, or patient movement (tremors or shivering) can make the reading inaccurate. Most pulse oximeters also display the patient's heart rate; this reading should match the patient's palpated heart rate.

If the patient's hemoglobin level is low (as happens after trauma or hemorrhage), the pulse oximetry will be correspondingly high. If you have only 6 g/dL of hemoglobin (normal = 14 g/dL), ideally all of them will have oxygen attached (100%).

If the patient has an abnormally high hemoglobin level, as is common in someone who is chronically hypoxic, as in the case of COPD, or who lives at a high altitude, such as in Denver, Colorado, the oxygen saturation will be correspondingly low. For example, a patient with a combination of moderate hypoxia and polycythemia (excess red blood cell production) may have a normal oxygen saturation level as low as 89% to 90%.

Pulse oximetry does not recognize the difference between an oxygen molecule attached to hemoglobin and a carbon monoxide molecule attached to hemoglobin. From living in an industrialized society, most of us have a 1% to 2% carbon monoxide level all of the time. Smokers may have a 3% to 4% level. Thus a 97% pulse oximetry reading may actually consist of 95% oxygen + 2% carbon monoxide. Patients who have toxic or even fatal levels of carbon monoxide may show normal or high pulse oximetry values. Portable devices that specifically measure carbon monoxide levels are poised to become important tools, enabling us to readily assess for carbon monoxide poisoning in the field **Figure 26-28 ▾**.

The oxyhemoglobin dissociation curve **Figure 26-29 ▸** describes the relationship between oxygen saturation and the amount of oxygen dissolved in the plasma (Pao_2). It demonstrates that when present at very low levels, oxygen molecules bind easily to the hemoglobin, so that small changes in Pao_2 result in relatively large changes in oxygen saturation. As the hemoglobin begins to fill up with oxygen molecules, larger changes in Pao_2 (shown on the horizontal axis) are required to produce changes in oxygen saturation. Placing a healthy patient on a nonrebreathing mask may increase the saturation level from 96% to 99%, whereas placing a hypoxic patient on a nasal cannula at 2 L/min may increase the oxygen saturation from 80% to 92% (a much bigger change). Conversely, the more hypoxic patients become, the faster they will desaturate as they fall off the steep part of the oxyhemoglobin dissociation curve. Other factors, such as acid-base balance, body temperature, and amount of hemoglobin, can also affect the entire system and shift the entire curve to the left or the right.

End-Tidal Carbon Dioxide Detector

Carbon dioxide is returned to the lungs in the venous blood, where it is exhaled during ventilation. We can measure this exhaled carbon dioxide by various methods.

Colorimetric end-tidal carbon dioxide ($ETCO_2$) detecting does not measure the exact amount of carbon dioxide exhaled,

but it does indicate whether carbon dioxide is present in *reasonable* amounts in the exhaled breath of the patient **Figure 26-30 ▾**. This type of monitoring helps in identifying placement of an ET tube. Air exhaled through an ET tube that has been properly placed in the trachea of a normally perfused patient should contain 4% to 5% carbon dioxide (a yellow reading on the colorimetric device). If the tube has been mistakenly placed in the esophagus, less than 0.5% carbon dioxide will be present in the exhaled gas (a purple reading). Note that the monitor might be fooled if the patient has carbon dioxide trapped in the stomach from the ingestion of carbonated beverages, so confirm the reading over at least six breaths to be certain it isn't a false positive.

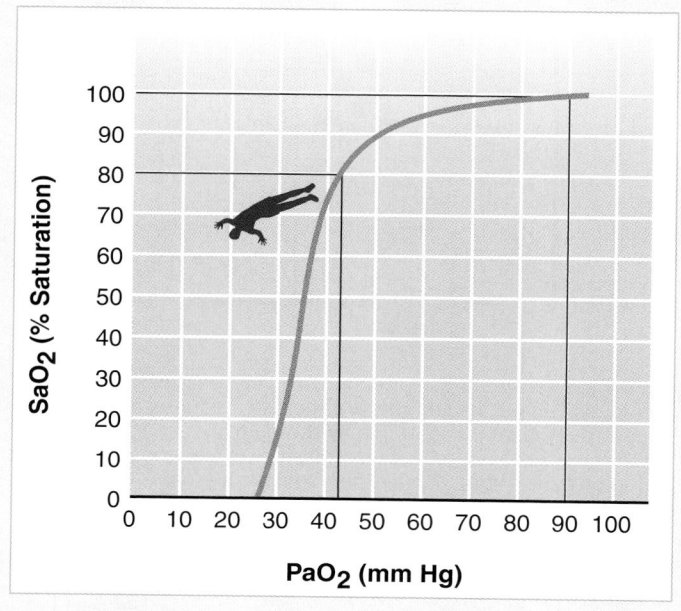

Figure 26-29 The oxyhemoglobin dissociation curve. As patients become increasingly hypoxic (lower percentage of Sao_2), they may "fall off" the curve and drop their saturation rapidly.

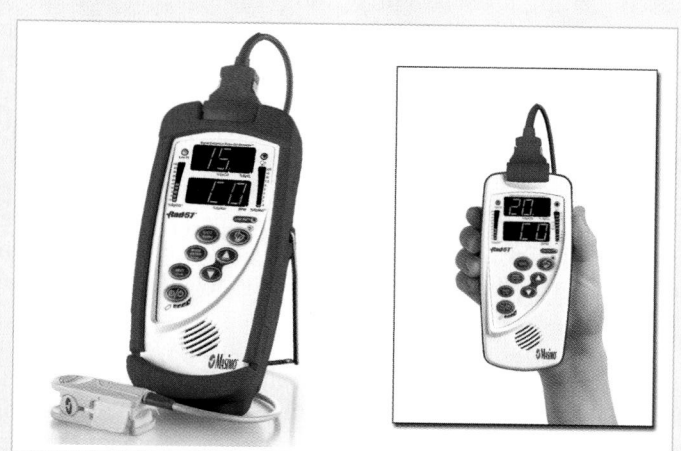

Figure 26-28 Devices are becoming available that can measure oxygen saturation as well as carbon monoxide levels.

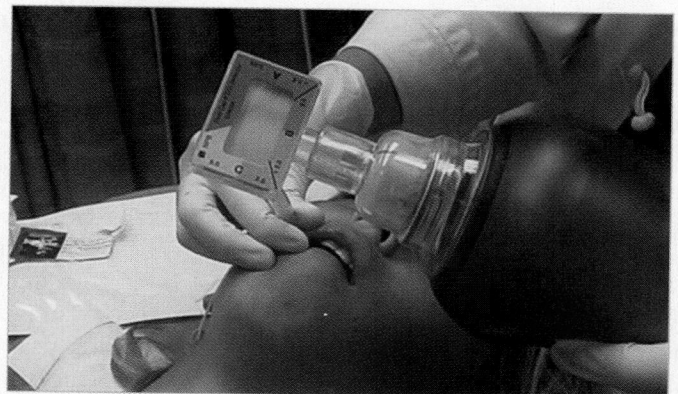

Figure 26-30 Carbon dioxide detectors are common devices used to help confirm endotracheal placement.

The exact percentage of carbon dioxide contained in the last few milliliters of the patient's exhaled air can be measured by a special sensor. For example, some electronic end-tidal carbon dioxide detectors use a photoelectric sensor that relies on absorption of infrared light by carbon dioxide to provide this measurement. The sensor can evaluate $ETCO_2$ in the spontaneously breathing patient via a specialized nasal cannula–type device, or it can be attached to the end of an ET tube. These devices typically display a waveform **Figure 26-31 ▾** that can give additional data about the patient's respiratory status. In addition, such monitors serve as alarms that can alert paramedics to changes in respiratory rate or depth.

Peak Expiratory Flow

The peak flow is the maximum flow rate at which the patient can expel air from the lungs. (Skill Drill 11-1 in Chapter 11 describes the use of a peak expiratory flowmeter.) A lower value indicates that the patient's larger airways are narrowed by bronchial constriction or bronchial edema. Many patients who have pulmonary disease check their peak flow twice per day and chart the results. They may present this chart to you upon your arrival. Normal peak flow values vary by age, sex, and height, but generally run from about 350 to 700 L/min, while a peak flow below 150 L/min is considered very low and signals significant distress. Some people with chronic asthma have a peak flow that never exceeds 100!

■ Upper Airway Obstruction

Anatomic Obstruction

The most common cause of upper airway obstruction in the semiconscious or unconscious patient is the tongue. Indeed, this problem results in the death of some trauma patients, diabetics,

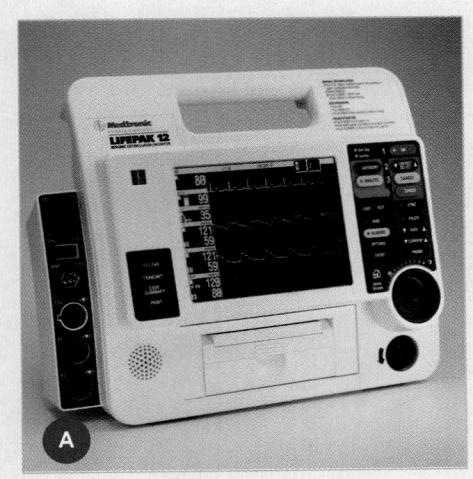

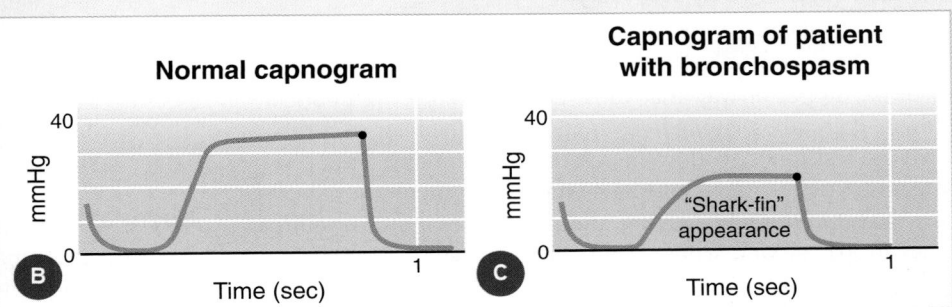

Figure 26-31 The waveform supplied by end-tidal carbon dioxide detectors (**A**) provides important data in addition to the actual $ETCO_2$ value. Variations in waveform shape—normal is shown in graph (**B**) may help identify air-trapping disorders such as asthma (**C**) and COPD. It may also document altered respiratory patterns and serve as an alarm for apnea, bradypnea, or tachypnea.

You are the Provider Part 3

Your patient is not interacting with you, but rather stares blankly around the room and only responds by withdrawing from painful stimuli. His pulse oximetry reading continues to fall, and he is unable to sit upright without assistance. The patient readily accepts a nasal airway, but still has a gag reflex. You begin to provide ventilations with a bag-mask ventilation device and 100% supplemental oxygen, but the patient's condition continues to worsen rapidly. You establish an 18-gauge IV of normal saline in the right antecubital vein and run it at a rate to keep the vein open.

Reassessment	Recording Time: 10 Minutes
Level of consciousness	Responsive to pain, with a Glasgow Coma Scale score of 9
Skin	Pale, cool, perspiring
Pulse	106 beats/min; weak; occasionally irregular
Blood pressure	102 mm Hg by palpation
Respirations	30 breaths/min; shallow
Sao₂	72% via bag-mask ventilation and 100% supplemental oxygen
Capnography	65 mm Hg
ECG	Sinus tachycardia with occasional premature ventricular contractions

6. Do you believe that your patient is able to maintain his airway?

7. What options do you have available to maintain this patient's airway?

patients who have had a seizure, or intoxicated patients every year. There seems to be an inherent urge on the part of bystanders to place a pillow behind the head of an unresponsive individual, which merely exacerbates this problem. If the patient is snoring, take away the pillow and reposition the patient's airway!

Excess soft tissue in the airway is one cause of obstructive sleep apnea, and some people go so far as to have tissue surgically removed from their pharynx to limit this anatomic obstruction. Fortunately, you can manually displace the soft tissue of the upper airway with a variety of simple maneuvers; these maneuvers were discussed in Chapter 11. Also, whenever you do not have a concern for spinal motion restriction, unconscious patients may be positioned on their side (the recovery position) to avoid blocking the airway. Many postseizure, intoxicated, or hypoglycemic patients can be transported most safely on their side, which also reduces the risk of aspiration if they vomit.

The Hot (Infected) Airway

A variety of infections can cause swelling in the upper airway. The most common is probably croup, a distressing viral infection of the upper airway that most commonly occurs in small children. Poiseuille's law tells us that, as the diameter of a tube decreases, resistance to flow increases exponentially. This phenomenon explains why children—who have inherently narrow airways—get croup when a viral infection causes a little swelling in their upper airway, while adults with the same virus do not
Figure 26-32 ▾. In recent decades, many deadly upper air-

way infections have become very rare as a result of immunization efforts. Unfortunately, the rate of childhood immunizations has begun to decline as the general public becomes complacent about these diseases, so paramedics must remain vigilant for these pathologic conditions. **Table 26-4 ▸** lists infections that can impair the upper airway.

Croup and tonsillitis are common, especially in children, but the other conditions are rare. When these pathologic conditions do occur, they are critical emergencies, because the airway could swell shut with little warning, making orotracheal intubation extremely difficult or impossible. *Avoid manipulating the airway* in these patients unless absolutely necessary. It is usually possible to ventilate such patients with bag-mask ventilation by paying careful attention to technique. If intubation is essential because of an inability to effectively ventilate the patient with bag-mask ventilation, you may find that the airway is entirely obscured by the swelling, and your attempts at laryngoscopy may merely make the swelling worse. Try to have a partner press on the patient's chest while you look for a stream of bubbles coming from the airway (use an ET tube at least two full sizes smaller than what you would typically choose for that patient). If this effort fails after a single attempt, a needle or surgical cricothyrotomy will be necessary.

Aspiration

Aspirating stomach contents into the lungs carries a significantly high mortality rate. It is a common but profoundly dangerous complication in patients who have had a cardiac arrest or in unresponsive patients who have had trauma or who overdosed. Follow these guidelines when treating such patients:

1. Aggressively reduce the risk of aspiration by avoiding gastric distention when ventilating and by decompressing the stomach with an NG tube whenever appropriate.

2. Aggressively monitor the patient's ability to protect his or her own airway, and seek to protect the patient's airway with an advanced airway if this is impossible.

3. Aggressively treat aspiration with suction and airway control if steps 1 and 2 fail!

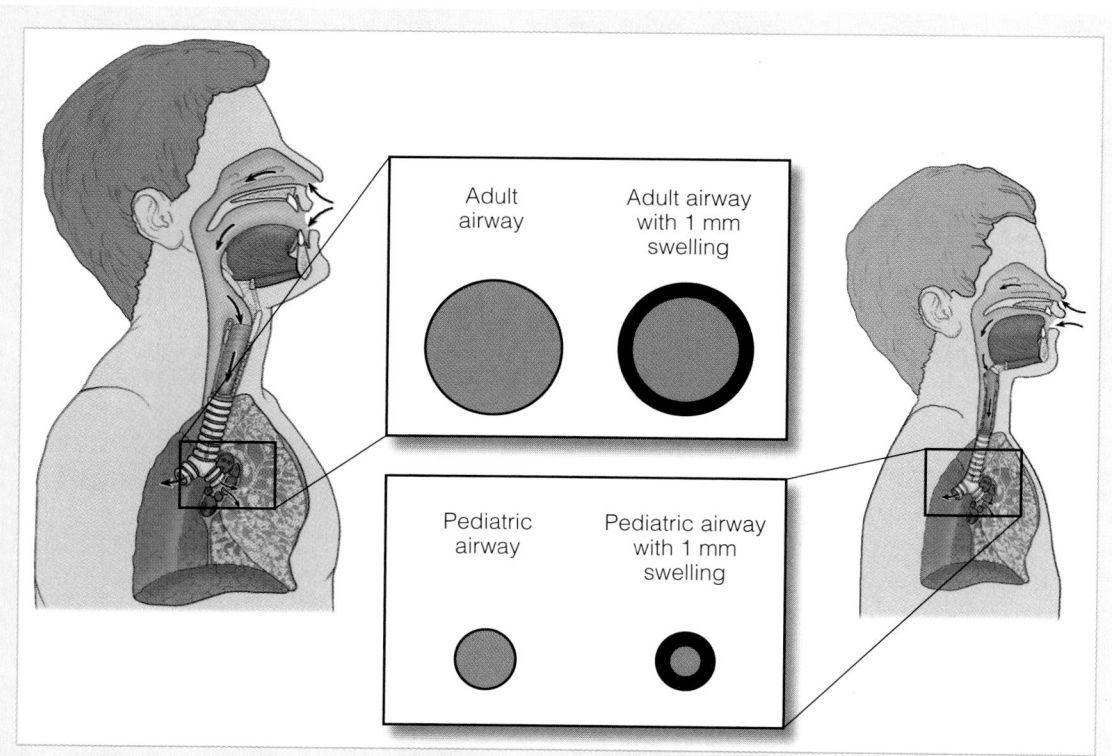

Figure 26-32 Any constriction of an airway (caused by a condition such as asthma) can cause a severe reduction in the volume of airflow, especially in children. Pouiselle's law explains conditions such as croup and presents implications for the choice of the size of an endotracheal tube.

Adult airway

Adult airway with 1 mm swelling

Pediatric airway

Pediatric airway with 1 mm swelling

Table 26-4	Infections That Can Impair the Upper Airway
Infection	**Comments**
Croup	Viral infection of area around glottis. Most common in children between 6 months and 3 years of age. Most commonly occurs in middle of night when air gets cool (in spring and fall). Child has classic seal-bark cough. May be distressing but is not typically fatal. Also called laryngotracheobronchitis. Do not manipulate the airway.
Epiglottitis	Severe, rapidly progressive infection of epiglottis and surrounding tissues that may be fatal because of sudden respiratory obstruction. Most common infectious organism is *Haemophilus influenzea* type b. Vaccination has helped make acute epiglottitis rare. Unlike croup, patients may present at any age and at any time of year. Patients typically drool and have a fever, hoarse voice, and purposeful hyperextension. Epiglottitis is a true emergency. Do not manipulate airway.
Peritonsillar abscess	Uncommon in children (more common in young adults). Abscess forms behind pharyngeal tonsil on one side. Patient has fever and sore throat. May be mistaken for epiglottitis until you look in throat and see lateral abscess (instead of enlarged epiglottis). Do not manipulate the airway.
Retropharyngeal abscess	Most common in children, in whom infections from retropharyngeal lymph nodes can flourish. May also be caused by direct trauma to pharynx. Patient may have fever and sudden stridor. May be mistaken for epiglottitis until laryngoscope examination reveals huge retropharyngeal pus sack (instead of cherry-red epiglottis). Do not manipulate the airway.
Diphtheria	Causative bacterium attacks and kills layer of epithelial tissue, creating pseudomembrane that is often seen in tonsillar area. Membrane (and swelling of upper airway caused by disease) can obstruct upper airway. Most children receive diphtheria, tetanus, and pertussis (DTP) immunization and receive boosters. Do not manipulate the airway.
Enormous tonsils	Palatine tonsils can swell excessively, resulting in fever, difficulty swallowing, and throat pain. Tonsils can grow to golf-ball size in some individuals. Severely swollen tonsils rarely compromise the airway but can cause snoring or stridor. Do not manipulate the airway.

If basic life-support maneuvers fail to clear an obstructed airway, use laryngoscopy and Magill forceps and, if necessary, perform a needle or surgical cricothyrotomy.

Aspiration could also refer to foreign body airway obstruction. Remember that most adults choke when they are intoxicated or traumatized or have a reduced gag reflex from stroke or aging. Chronic aspiration of food is also a common cause of pneumonitis in older patients. Make sure you don't make the situation worse by allowing these patients to eat when they are having difficulty breathing.

Obstructive Airway Diseases

Obstructive airway diseases are characterized by diffuse obstruction to airflow within the lungs. The most common obstructive airway diseases are emphysema and chronic bronchitis (chronic diseases), and asthma (an acutely episodic syndrome); these three conditions collectively affect as many as 10% to 20% of adults in the United States. Emphysema and chronic bronchitis are collectively classified as COPD because the changes in pulmonary structure and function are chronic, progressive, and irreversible. Asthma is considered a separate entity because—at least in its early stages—it is a condition of *reversible* airway narrowing.

Obstructive disease occurs when the positive pressure of exhalation causes the small airways to pinch shut, trapping gas in the alveoli. The harder the patient tries to push air out, the more it gets trapped in the alveoli Figure 26-33 ▶ . Hence, patients with obstructive disease end up with large amounts of gas trapped in their lungs that they can't effectively expel. Patients with obstructive disease learn that if they push the gas out slowly at a low pressure, they can exhale more than if they try to push it out hard and fast.

Patients with obstructive airway disease may demonstrate a variety of physical findings that can alert you to the nature of their disease:

- **Pursed-lip breathing.** Breathing in this way allows patients to push a breath out slowly under controlled pressure.
- **Increased inspiratory-to-expiratory (I:E) ratio.** The I:E ratio is typically 1:2 in healthy people breathing quietly (it takes about twice as long to exhale as it does to inhale). Patients who are very sick with obstructive disease may have an I:E ratio of 1:6 or 1:8.
- **Abdominal muscle use.** We use abdominal muscles to push air out (exhalation). Patients with obstructive disease must work to push air out with every breath. Patients who have asthma often complain of abdominal pain after an attack. They do the equivalent of hundreds of sit-ups as they force each exhalation.
- **Jugular venous distention.** The trapped air creates a higher pressure in the thorax. Blood draining into the superior vena cava from the head and neck can back up in the jugular veins, causing jugular venous distention.

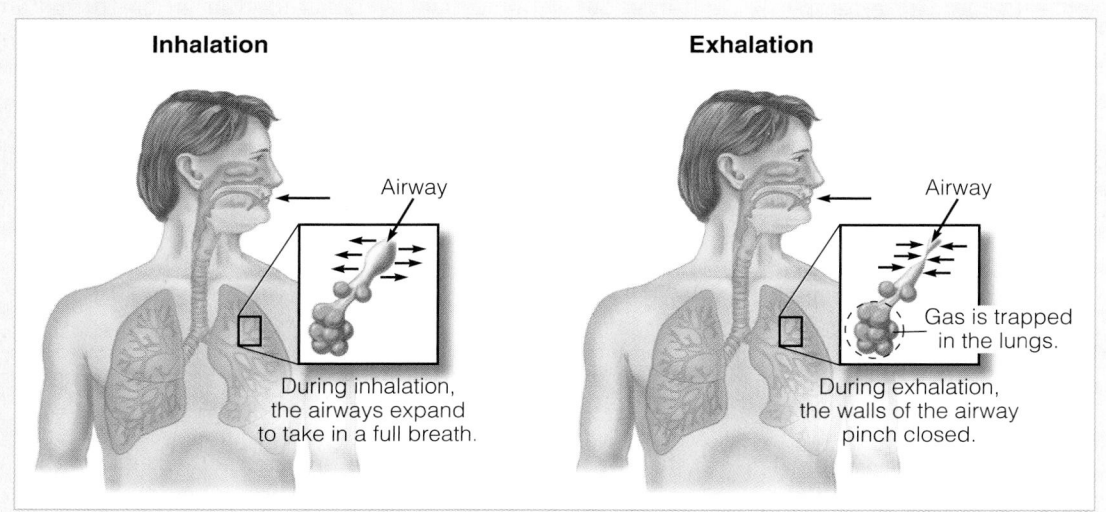

Figure 26-33 Obstructive disease involves changes to the smaller airways that cause them to pinch closed during exhalation, trapping air inside the patient's lungs. Healthy airways narrow during exhalation but not to the extent that causes obstruction or air trapping.

The death rates from asthma are increasing across the United States, although not equally across all populations. The fastest-growing asthma rates are observed in children younger than 5 years. Overall death rates from asthma are also higher in those under 35 years. Asthma is more common in males but tends to be more severe in females. African Americans, especially those living in large urban centers, are three times more likely to be diagnosed with asthma and have death rates that are five times higher than those observed in whites.

Asthma

The name asthma (from Greek, meaning "panting") was first given to this disease by the second-century Greek physician Aretaeus "because in the paroxysms, the patients also pant for breath." Bronchial asthma is characterized by an increased reactivity of the trachea, bronchi, and bronchioles to a variety of stimuli. That hyperreactivity results in widespread, reversible narrowing of the airways, or bronchospasm **Figure 26-34 ▸** . Sometimes we refer to this condition as reactive airway disease to indicate that the patient experiences bronchospasm when exposed to certain triggers, such as dust, cold, or smoke. In addition, edema (swelling, or inflammation) of the airways and increased mucous production can cause significant airway obstruction.

Asthma characteristically occurs in acute attacks of variable duration. Between attacks, the patient may be relatively asymptomatic.

More than 14 million people in the United States reported having asthma in 1995, and the incidence appears to be increasing. Each year, 2 million people will visit the emergency department because of asthma, and one quarter of them will be admitted to the hospital. Approximately 5,000 people (1 in 100 admissions) will die because of asthma. The overall mortality rate for this disease is 5%.

In the Field

Asthma is a term describing a triad of airway problems: acute air trapping, increased work of breathing, and ultimately fatigue. It may present differently in different people, but it is a very common pathologic condition.

Bronchospasm

Bronchospasm is caused by the constriction of smooth muscle that surrounds the larger bronchi in the lungs **Figure 26-35 ▸** . This may occur because of stimulation by an allergen or irritants such as dust, perfume, cat dander, or cold temperatures or by other stimuli such as exercise or stress. When air is forced through the constricted tubes, it causes them to vibrate, which creates wheezing. Bronchospasm can also reduce the peak expiratory flow caused by a turbulent airflow. The primary treatment of bronchospasm is

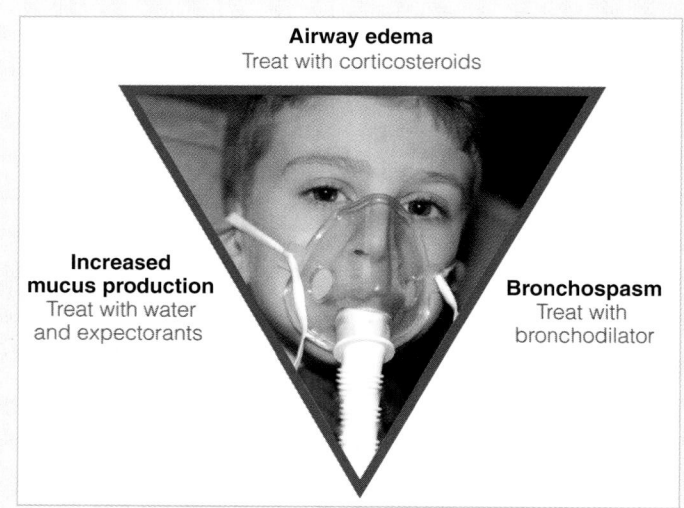

Figure 26-34 The asthma triad demonstrates the three primary components of asthma, and the corresponding treatments for each component. Asthma presents differently in different people, so individual treatments will need to vary as well.

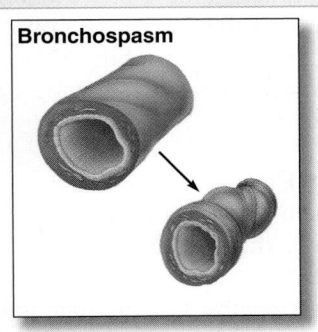
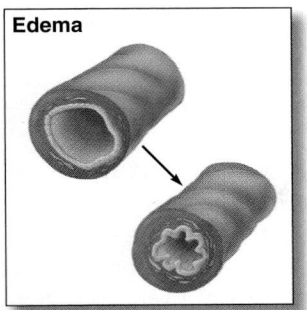

Bronchospasm

Edema

With bronchospasm, the muscle contracts, causing the entire tube to narrow.

With edema, the wall of the tube swells, causing only the lumen to narrow.

Figure 26-35 Bronchospasm is a constriction (narrowing) of the entire airway, whereas bronchial edema is a swelling of the airway wall. Both cause the functional diameter of airways to be reduced.

a breathing treatment for the administration of bronchodilator medication.

Bronchial Edema

Swelling of the bronchioles also creates turbulent airflow, wheezing, and air trapping. Bronchodilator medications do little to reduce bronchial edema. If a patient takes such a medication and the peak flow does not dramatically improve, you should suspect some degree of bronchial edema. The primary treatment of bronchial edema is corticosteroids, which may or may not be administered in the field setting. Unlike a breathing treatment which can improve breathing immediately, steroids take a few hours to reduce inflammation.

Increased Mucous Production

Thick secretions may plug the distal airways and contribute to air trapping. People who have asthma may be significantly dehydrated because of their increased fluid loss from tachypnea and their often-poor fluid intake. Dehydration makes secretions even thicker, further worsening the air trapping event. Taking antihistamine medications may further thicken secretions. The primary approach to dealing with secretions in asthma is to improve hydration. Mucolytics (which break down thick mucus) or expectorants (which loosen thick secretions so they can be coughed out) are also sometimes used, most often in the hospital setting.

Most people who have asthma have a combination of these three pathologic conditions, although their predominance varies in individual patients. The condition of a person who has asthma whose primary issue is bronchoconstriction would respond very well to aerosol bronchodilators. The condition of a person who has asthma whose primary issue is bronchial edema would respond much less to aerosol bronchodilators, and probably would not show significant improvement until administered corticosteroids have taken effect (typically several hours after their administration).

Status asthmaticus is a severe, prolonged asthmatic attack that cannot be broken with conventional treatment. It is a dire medical emergency. Just as the patient with COPD ordinarily does not call for an ambulance unless there has been a marked change in his condition, so too the average asthmatic does not dial 9-1-1 unless the attack is much worse than those he usually has to deal with. So it is a reasonably safe assumption that *any asthmatic who feels sick enough to call an ambulance is in status asthmaticus until proved otherwise.*

On examining the patient in status asthmaticus, you will find him fighting desperately to move air through his obstructed airways, with prominent use of accessory muscles of respiration. The chest is maximally hyperinflated. Breath sounds and wheezes may be entirely inaudible because air movement is negligible, and the patient is usually exhausted, severely acidotic, and dehydrated.

Table 26-5	Potentially Fatal Asthma

- Previous intubation for respiratory failure or respiratory arrest
- Respiratory acidosis
- Two or more admissions to the hospital despite oral corticosteroid use
- Two or more episodes of pneumothorax

Potentially Fatal Asthma

Patients who have potentially fatal asthma often have severely compromised ventilation all of the time. Such patients are at serious risk if something triggers acute bronchospasm or if they get an infection. A patient who has asthma is at high risk of respiratory arrest if he or she has a history consistent with any of the factors in Table 26-5 . Medication noncompliance and severe psychiatric disorders also predispose a patient to asthma.

COPD

COPD comprises at least two distinct clinical entities: emphysema and chronic bronchitis.

Emphysema

Emphysema is a chronic weakening and destruction of the walls of the terminal bronchioles and alveoli. Some people have emphysema caused by a congenital enzyme deficiency (alpha$_1$-antitrypsin deficiency), but the most common cause of emphysema in the United States is cigarette smoking. More than 3 million people in the United States have symptomatic emphysema.

In pure emphysema, the breakdown of the connective tissue structure of the terminal airways results in groups of alveoli

Notes from Nancy

All that wheezes is not asthma.

Among the other causes of diffuse wheezing are acute left heart failure ("cardiac asthma"), smoke inhalation, chronic bronchitis, and acute pulmonary embolism. Localized wheezing reflects an obstruction, by foreign body or tumor, in a specific area. Only a careful history and physical examination will enable you to reach the correct diagnosis. It is particularly important to distinguish the wheezing of asthma from that caused by left heart failure, because the treatment of the two conditions is markedly different.

In the acute asthmatic attack, silence is not golden—it's deadly!

merging into large blebs or bullae, which are far less efficient and collapse far more easily (causing obstruction) than does normal lung tissue. Although little can be done in the field to help this condition, many patients have associated bronchospasm, edema, fluid, or infections that can be relieved, helping improve the patient's overall situation. Many patients who have emphysema have a barrel chest caused by chronic lung hyperinflation. These patients are often tachypneic, as they attempt to maintain a normal carbon dioxide level despite their dysfunctional lungs. They often use extreme amounts of energy attempting to breathe, cannibalizing their own muscle mass in the process.

Chronic Bronchitis

Chronic bronchitis is officially defined as sputum production most days of the month for 3 or more months out of the year for more than 2 years. The hallmark of this disease is excessive mucous production in the bronchial tree, which is nearly always accompanied by a chronic or recurrent productive cough (a cough that produces phlegm). The typical patient who has chronic bronchitis is almost invariably a heavy cigarette smoker. He or she is usually somewhat obese, congested, and sometimes has a bluish complexion. His or her blood gases tend to be abnormal, with elevated $PaCO_2$ (hypercapnia) and decreased PaO_2 (hypoxemia) levels. Often he or she has associated heart disease and right heart failure (cor pulmonale).

Notes from Nancy

Patients with COPD ordinarily come to some sort of modus vivendi with their disease. Over the years, they learn how much exertion they can tolerate, in what position sleep is possible, and so forth. So when a patient with COPD calls for an ambulance, it nearly always means that something has changed— and changed for the worse.

The pink puffer (emphysema) and blue bloater (chronic bronchitis) represent two extremes of the COPD spectrum. In reality, as the disease progresses, most patients with COPD fall somewhere between these two clinical extremes, showing signs and symptoms of both disease processes.

Typical Presentations of COPD

Patients who have COPD are often very sick people, with little or no respiratory reserves to help them deal with any additional respiratory insults. You must actively search for what has pushed them over the edge from a relatively stable state to the insufficiency that caused them to call 9-1-1. The following are some common issues that conspire to cause the patient who has COPD to decompensate.

COPD With Pneumonia

Because they are chronically ill, have poor secretion clearance, and sometimes have excessive mucous production (which acts like a culture medium for nasty bugs), these patients often get infections in their bronchi and lungs. Do they have a fever? Has the color or amount of their sputum production changed? Do they have other signs of infection (such as body aches, general malaise, or pain when breathing)? Are auscultated breath sounds (such as localized rhonchi) consistent with pneumonia?

COPD With Right Heart Failure

It is very difficult for the right side of the heart to push the patient's thick blood—thick because of polycythemia—through capillaries that are being squashed by hyperinflated alveoli. This commonly causes right heart failure secondary to the patient's lung disease (cor pulmonale). If patients take in too much salt or fluid, or if they do not get rid of fluid (because of renal failure or insufficient diuretic use), they may have an episode of congestive heart failure. Do they have peripheral edema? Jugular venous distention with hepatojugular reflux? End inspiratory crackles? (It may be difficult to tell the difference between the crackles of congestive heart failure and the crackles that these patients always have secondary to their COPD.) Do they say they have had a progressive increase in dyspnea over several days? Have they taken in more fluid than usual, or run out of their diuretics?

COPD With Left Heart Failure

Patients with COPD are at high risk of having a sudden cardiac event. Any sudden left ventricular dysfunction such as an AMI or cardiac rhythm disturbance (dysrhythmia) can cause them to have sudden-onset left heart failure. Don't allow your initial impression of COPD to prevent you from identifying the patient who is also having an acute myocardial infarction!

Acute Exacerbation of COPD

In the acute exacerbation, no co-pathologic condition such as congestive heart failure or pneumonia clearly accounts for the patient's sudden decompensation. Instead, the patient's condition suddenly becomes worse, often because of some environmental change such as weather, humidity, or sudden activation of the heating or cooling system. An acute exacerbation can also be prompted by the inhalation of trigger substances. Did your patient decide to go through some old boxes today? Did a neighbor just visit with a cat? Is someone painting in the next room?

End-Stage COPD

Patients with severe COPD will eventually reach a point when their lungs simply cannot support oxygenation and ventilation any longer. You may come to know these patients well as their calls to 9-1-1 become more frequent. Some will be in hospice care. In the end stages of the disease, it can be difficult to determine whether a patient has an exacerbation that can be resolved or if he or she has reached the end of the disease process. Unfortunately, endotracheal intubation may result in a situation where the patient cannot make his or her wishes known. In addition, the more frequently the patient has to be intubated and placed on a ventilator, the more difficult it becomes to wean the patient off the ventilator. Having this knowledge increases the anxiety level of the patient, thus increasing his or her cardiac workload and cardiac oxygen consumption—a potentially lethal combination for the end-stage COPD patient.

All EMS systems have their own ways of dealing with do-not-resuscitate orders. It is important to secure documentation of the patient's wishes as the terminal phase of the disease begins. Follow local protocol or contact medical control as needed regarding such issues.

Hypoxic Drive

Hypoxic drive is a rare phenomenon that affects only a very small percentage of patients who have the most chronic forms of pulmonary disease in the end stage of their disease. As a paramedic, you will routinely care for the sickest of the sick, so you should understand this concept. You will likely encounter patients whose respiratory drive can be decreased by high levels of oxygen. However, 100% supplemental oxygen is foundational therapy for most patients, so it makes no sense to withhold oxygen from anyone who needs it for fear of decreasing the respiratory drive of those few individuals who might have this complication.

When a patient has chronic hypoventilation, bicarbonate (HCO_3) ions migrate into the cerebrospinal fluid, fooling the brain into thinking that acid and base are in balance. The patient might then switch to a hypoxic drive, meaning that the primary stimulus to breathe comes from decreased levels of oxygen, *not* increased levels of carbon dioxide. This places the paramedic in the position of having to decide whether the administration of oxygen is appropriate. In making this decision, consider the following points:

1. Only a small subset of patients with COPD breathe because of hypoxic drive, but you cannot tell who they are just by looking at them.
2. Such patients do not suddenly become apneic after a whiff of oxygen. High levels of oxygen slowly depress their

respiratory drive, and their respiratory rate slowly declines. They become sleepy and, eventually, their respiratory rate falls into the single digits before they become apneic. Although the paramedic is likely to be close enough to the patient to recognize this phenomenon, the real concern is the in-hospital patient who receives 100% supplemental oxygen but then is left by himself or herself for a prolonged period.
3. You can encourage breathing with verbal and physical stimulation. If the respiratory rate begins to drop, gently shake the patient and yell "Breathe!" This technique works well in the early stages.
4. If a patient becomes apneic because of increased oxygenation, his or her skin may still appear perfused.
5. If the patient becomes apneic, provide artificial ventilation and consider intubation.

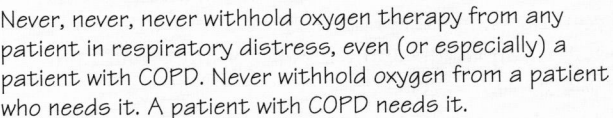

Notes from Nancy

Never, never, never withhold oxygen therapy from any patient in respiratory distress, even (or especially) a patient with COPD. Never withhold oxygen from a patient who needs it. A patient with COPD needs it.

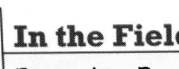

In the Field

Bagged to Death

Not everyone should be ventilated the same way. If you are ventilating a patient who has severe obstructive disease such as those with either decompensated asthma or COPD, remember that *these patients have difficulty exhaling.* If each breath is not allowed to come back out before the delivery of the next, then pressures in the thorax will continually go up. This phenomenon, which is called auto-PEEP (positive end-expiratory pressure), can eventually cause a pneumothorax or cardiac arrest. If the pressure in the chest exceeds the pressure of blood returning to the heart, thus limiting venous return, cardiac arrest may occur.

Such patients should be ventilated as little as four to six breaths per minute to avoid "bagging them to death." This is very difficult to do when your partner, bystanders, the BLS crew, and your own epinephrine release are all telling you to hyperventilate the patient, but it is an absolute necessity if you hope to avoid the dire consequences of raising the thoracic pressure more with each breath. Seek guidance from your medical director and local protocols when you encounter patients who have severe COPD or asthma who are in cardiac arrest or near-arrest. However, also remember that the standard ventilation rate for adults is only 10 to 12 breaths/min.

In the Field

Tuberculosis Presentation

The classic presentation of tuberculosis (TB) includes sudden weight loss, night sweats, fever, and cough with blood-tinged sputum. This clinical presentation should raise a red flag. The best protection against TB is good airflow through your environment. Don't let the patient cough in your face, and keep the rear windows of the ambulance open, weather permitting. Consider using an oxygen mask on the patient instead of a nasal cannula. You can deliver the same FIO_2 while limiting the spread of droplets when the patient coughs. Also, you should wear a high-efficiency particulate air (HEPA) filter mask that meets NIOSH N95 or Occupational Safety and Health Administration (OSHA) criteria (ie, a TB or duckbill mask).

6. These patients are poor candidates for intubation. If you intubate these patients, you may doom them to live what is left of their life on a ventilator.

7. While oxygen saturation (SaO_2) may be a valuable adjunct to your decision, SaO_2 numbers are a little different for patients with COPD and tell you nothing about their carbon dioxide levels.

Common Respiratory Presentations

Asthma With Fever

When patients with reactive airways begin wheezing, their inhalers usually will help for only a little while before their symptoms return. The typical asthma attack that responds to treatment but occurs again in a few hours is sometimes caused by an underlying infection (such as pneumonia or bronchitis) that continually triggers the asthmalike symptoms. The asthma attack won't go away until the patient receives treatment of the trigger. Does your patient have a fever or chills? Is he or she coughing up colorful sputum?

Failure of a Metered-Dose Inhaler

Metered-dose inhalers indicate how many actuations (puffs) they are designed to deliver, but most patients don't keep track of their usage very well. Often the medication may be exhausted even though some propellant remains in the canister. The patient may have been sucking nothing but propellant for days, which explains why their wheezing isn't getting better. Similar problems can occur when patients use grossly outdated medications or medications that have been overheated (left in a hot automobile or similar environment). In this case, your bronchodilator may work well, even though theirs has failed. Another problem that can occur is that patients who do not fully understand how to use the device do not inhale at an appropriate point and then end up spraying the medicine on the inside of their mouths. This is one reason why physicians often prescribe a spacer device to be added to the metered-dose inhaler for children and for adults who have difficulty using the device.

Travel-Related Problems

Some patients present with significant pulmonary edema after a lengthy journey. The culprit: they didn't want to take their diuretics while traveling. Who wants to have to look for a bathroom every half hour while on the road? Don't forget to ask the obvious: "What medications do you use?" Which should always be followed by: "And did you take them today?"

Dyspnea Triggers

Just because someone knows that their reactive airways are triggered by cats, perfume, cigarette smoke, cold, or pollen doesn't mean that they can always avoid these triggers. Sometimes a social or family situation is important enough that patients are willing to risk experiencing an episode of dyspnea. Sometimes people who are allergic to cats will hold a cat, and people who are on strict fluid restriction will drink like a fish.

Seasonal Issues

Many ugly things grow in heating ducts and air conditioners during their off-seasons. When the weather suddenly changes, and heating systems or air conditioners begin turning on in houses all over your district, you can expect an increase in calls from chronically ill respiratory patients. Excessive heat, humidity, cold, pollen, dust, and smog can all conspire to push someone over the edge and experience a flare-up of respiratory disease.

Noncompliance With Therapy

Many patients who have chronic respiratory disease will rebel against their therapy as a means of seeming to regain some control over their lives. Sometimes, the long-term nature of their therapy isn't fully understood, and they attempt to wean themselves off of their medications, oxygen, or respiratory support devices. Unfortunately, this may cause them to have a crisis.

Many patients have been prescribed home oxygen, aerosol therapy, continuous positive airway pressure (CPAP), bilevel positive airway pressure (BiPAP), and a variety of medications that they refuse to use or use only sporadically. Some medications, such as oral corticosteroids, can cause dangerous complications if their use is terminated abruptly.

Failure of Technology/Running Out of Medicine

Advances in technology have allowed patients who have chronic respiratory disease much more freedom to get out of the house and to travel. This creates the risk that you will be called to assist someone whose oxygen tank has run dry, whose portable ventilator has suddenly malfunctioned, or whose medications were left behind.

Clots may also form when patients are immobile for long periods of time. Sudden pulmonary embolisms sometimes occur in people after long car trips or lengthy airplane flights. Bedridden patients are often prescribed anticoagulants or wear special stockings or other devices to reduce the formation of blood clots in the legs. Especially for patients with a history of deep venous thrombosis, a Greenfield filter may be inserted. This device, which opens like a mesh umbrella in the main vein that returns blood to the heart, is intended to catch any clots that break loose and travel from the legs.

Very large pulmonary emboli can lodge at the bifurcation of the right and left pulmonary arteries. These are called a saddle embolus and may be immediately fatal. Cardiac arrest caused by a large pulmonary embolus is a very difficult situation that few patients survive. You may note cape cyanosis—deep cyanasis of the face, neck, chest, and back—despite good-quality CPR and ventilation with 100% supplemental oxygen in this scenario.

Disorders of Ventilation

Ventilation is the movement of air in and out of the lungs. With the use of supplemental oxygen, reasonable and even high oxygen levels are easy to maintain in patients who have healthy lungs, even if ventilation is severely compromised. The best measurement of ventilation, however, is the carbon dioxide level. Under normal circumstances, the volume of ventilation (minute volume) is regulated by the need to maintain the Pa_{CO_2} in the range of 35 to 45 mm Hg. In a person at rest, that goal is usually accomplished by breathing a tidal volume of around 500 mL at a rate of 12 to 16 breaths/min—that is, with a minute volume in the range of 6 to 8 L. During deep sleep, a smaller minute volume may suffice, while the muscular exertion associated with exercise may require a larger minute volume. As long as the Pa_{CO_2} remains in the normal range, ventilation is considered normal.

The carbon dioxide level is also directly related to pH (acid-base balance). Patients who are hypoventilating usually have respiratory acidosis. As their carbon dioxide level goes up, their pH level goes down. Patients who are hyperventilating are usually in respiratory alkalosis. As their carbon dioxide level goes down, their pH level goes up.

Respiratory Failure Resulting From Hypoventilation

Many different problems can cause patients to hypoventilate:
- Conditions that impair lung function
- Conditions that impair the mechanics of breathing
- Conditions that impair the neuromuscular apparatus
- Conditions that reduce respiratory drive

In these circumstances, you must often provide aggressive treatment to help the patient's respiratory efforts.

Conditions That Impair Lung Function
When the patient is breathing but gas exchange is impaired, carbon dioxide levels rise. This can happen in severe cases of atelectasis, pneumonia, pulmonary edema, asthma, or COPD.

Conditions That Impair the Mechanics of Breathing
A high cervical fracture, flail chest, diaphragmatic rupture, severe retractions, an abdomen full of air or blood, abdominal or chest binding (using a pneumatic antishock garment or immobilization straps), or anything else that impairs the pressure changes that allow breathing can result in reduced gas flow.

Pickwickian syndrome is the name given to respiratory compromise secondary to extreme obesity. One of the earliest descriptions of the combination of obesity, respiratory compromise, and sleep apnea can be found in the character of "Joe the fat boy" in Charles Dickens's *Pickwick Papers*. Poor Joe would fall asleep in midsentence, snore loudly, and generally exhibit signs of hypercapnia. This syndrome does not seem to be on the decline in today's society given the almost constant media coverage of obesity.

Conditions That Impair the Neuromuscular Apparatus
Patients who have had head trauma, intracranial infections, or brain tumors may have damage to the respiratory centers of the brain, which in turn may compromise ventilation. Serious injury to the spinal cord (above C5) may block the nerve impulses that cause breathing to occur. Guillain-Barré syndrome causes progressive muscle weakness and paralysis that moves up the body from the feet. If the paralysis reaches the diaphragm, the patient will be unable to breathe effectively. Amyotrophic lateral sclerosis also causes progressive muscle weakness. This disease is fatal, with death usually coming from respiratory failure as the muscles of respiration become unable to maintain adequate ventilation. Botulism is caused by the bacterium *Clostridium botulinum*. Though somewhat rare, it is usually the result of food poisoning or from an unknowing mother giving her infant or young child raw honey. Botulism can cause muscle paralysis and is typically fatal when it reaches the muscles of respiration.

Conditions That Reduce Respiratory Drive
Perhaps the most common hypoventilation crisis seen by EMS systems is the acute heroin overdose. Intoxication with alcohol, narcotics, and a host of other drugs or toxins can reduce the respiratory drive. Head injury, hypoxic drive, or asphyxia can all present with grossly low respiratory rates and volumes. Of course, the ultimate expression of hypoventilation is respiratory and then cardiac arrest.

Hyperventilation
Hyperventilation occurs when people breathe in excess of metabolic need. This typically occurs when they breathe so much by either increasing the rate at which they breathe, the depth they breathe, or both, that their carbon dioxide level begins to fall. Interestingly, a falling carbon dioxide level may make the patient feel short of breath, so they tend to become anxious and breathe even more rapidly and deeply. In acute hyperventilation syndrome, patients usually feel as if they cannot breathe at all. The continued fall in their carbon dioxide level leads to a rise in their pH level, which results in

respiratory alkalosis that in turn causes numbness or tingling in the hands and feet and around the mouth. If this continues, patients may complain of chest pain and will ultimately experience carpopedal spasm, during which the hands and feet lock up in a clawlike position. These symptoms frighten the patient even further, and usually make him or her hyperventilate even more. The hysterical hyperventilator may eventually lose consciousness, but not before undergoing extreme distress. If the patient doesn't calm down and stop hyperventilating upon awakening, the process could repeat itself.

The traditional therapy for hyperventilation called for patients to rebreathe their own carbon dioxide by breathing into a paper bag, or by applying a partial rebreather mask at 21% oxygen. This a very dangerous practice for important reasons:

- Patients quickly exhaust the oxygen in the gas they are breathing (and rebreathing). Remember, hyperventilation does not mean that the patient has too much oxygen, but rather that he or she is blowing off too much carbon dioxide. Do not cause the patient to become hypoxic while trying to stop a relatively benign hyperventilation episode.
- Any patient who is acidotic might be hyperventilating in an attempt to drive their pH level down to normal levels. In diabetic ketoacidosis, for example, the patient's body is making too much acid because of inadequate glucose metabolism, so the body attempts to compensate for the acidosis by hyperventilating (Kussmaul respirations). It would be a grave error to force such a patient to breathe into a paper bag. A variety of overdoses, toxic exposures, and metabolic abnormalities can also result in acidosis and compensatory hyperventilation, and none of them have the kind of hyperventilation that should be treated by

rebreathing carbon dioxide. You should never come to the conclusion that your patient is just hyperventilating until you have ruled out all other potential causes for their presentation, which would be very difficult if not impossible to do in the field.

Ultimately, treatment may include sedating the truly hysterical hyperventilator, but that rarely occurs in the field. Frequently, hyperventilation will follow some emotional stressor, ie, after a family fight, finding out about an unexpected pregnancy in a teen, or being notified that you are having an IRS audit. More often than not, a variety of psychological support techniques will help. Probably the single most important part of your patient care is to make the patient understand that if the behavior that precipitated the hyperventilation is repeated, almost without fail, they will hyperventilate again. Contacting social services or a teen pregnancy counselor will provide the patient with confidence to confront the situation. Other techniques include breathing *with* the patient, having the patient count to two between each breath (increasing to higher numbers as he or she is successful), and various distraction techniques (such as asking the patient to recite his or her life stories). Hyperventilation that is not caused by some metabolic crisis is usually self-limiting. At the very least, try not to feed into the patient's anxieties and make things worse, and don't let them do that either.

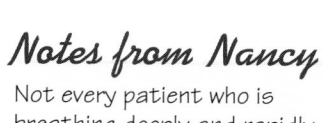

Notes from Nancy

Not every patient who is breathing deeply and rapidly is hyperventilating.

You are the Provider Part 4

Your protocols allow for rapid sequence induction, and you choose to perform this procedure on your patient. You successfully place the airway and administer 1 mg of midazolam (Versed), 50 µg of fentanyl, and 120 mg of succinylcholine (Anectine). Approximately 10 minutes later you give 8 mg of rocuronium. You also note that you have infused a total of 350 mL normal saline. You notice marked improvement in his pulse oximetry and skin signs throughout your transport to the hospital.

Reassessment	Recording Time: 20 Minutes
Level of consciousness	Sedated, pharmacologically paralyzed
Skin	Improving in color; pinker, no cyanosis noted in mucosa or nail beds
Pulse	98 beats/min, regular
Blood pressure	110/60 mm Hg
Respirations	Intubated; ventilated at 15 breaths/min
Sao_2	92% with bag-mask ventilation and 100% supplemental oxygen
Capnography	45 mm Hg
ECG	Sinus rhythm

8. Beyond inadequate ventilation and oxygenation, what must you take into consideration before attempting intubation?
9. If capnography, pulse oximetry, and other similar pieces of assessment equipment are unavailable, how can you determine whether your interventions are improving the patient's condition?
10. What other techniques can you use to improve ventilation and oxygenation?

Managing the Patient Who Has Dyspnea

The paramedic has a relatively short list of tools to treat respiratory compromise. At the most basic level, we provide supportive care, administer high-concentration supplemental oxygen therapy, and provide monitoring and transport for many patients. In actuality, there is little we can do in the field to alter their pathologic conditions (such as COPD, pneumonia, or pulmonary contusion).

The primary exception is the treatment of bronchoconstriction. A whole host of bronchodilators are available to help relax bronchial smooth muscle. This therapy can be extremely helpful if the patient's primary problem is bronchial muscle spasm resulting from anaphylaxis or asthma. Bronchodilator therapy may be somewhat helpful to many other patients as well.

At the other end of the spectrum of care are the patients who are in overt respiratory failure. The primary approach to this population is to take over the work of breathing completely by intubating them and manually ventilating them.

Ensure an Adequate Airway

The first part of assessing and managing any respiratory problem is to ensure an open and maintainable airway. Get rid of any food, gum, chewing tobacco, or like items out of the patient's mouth. Suction if necessary, and keep the airway in the optimal position, which typically is the position that makes the patient most comfortable.

Decrease the Work of Breathing

Remove constricting clothing (such as belts or tight collars). Reduce the patient's breathing workload. Help the patient sit up if they feel that position is more comfortable. *Don't make the person walk.* Don't let a big abdomen get in the way of the diaphragm. Relieve gastric distention (perhaps with a nasogastric tube). Don't bind the chest or make the patient lie on the good lung.

Provide Supplemental Oxygen

It is essential to deliver supplemental oxygen to any patient who needs it. If the patient is breathing adequately, administer 100% oxygen via a nonrebreathing mask. Patients who are not breathing adequately should receive bag-mask ventilation and 100% oxygen. Closely reassess the patient's breathing status and adjust your treatment accordingly.

Bronchodilate

Many patients who have respiratory distress can benefit a little from bronchodilation, and some patients can benefit a lot. Today's aerosol bronchodilators rarely hurt patients, so we tend to use them aggressively in the field. Patients who do not have bronchospasm will probably benefit only a little from aerosol bronchodilators, and you may have to drop their delivered

oxygen concentration during a typical aerosol treatment. In these circumstances, the nonrebreathing mask trumps the aerosol treatment. Follow local protocol.

Consider Fluid Balance

Rehydration is supplemental therapy for patients with respiratory problems who are dehydrated (for example, some patients who have pneumonia or asthma). It is common practice to give a fluid bolus to younger patients in these scenarios. Any elderly patient or patient who has a cardiac dysfunction could be pushed into pulmonary edema by too much fluid. Always assess breath sounds *before* and *after* giving a fluid bolus to make certain you have not overhydrated the patient. Of course, patients who have respiratory problems can become very sick in a hurry, and you will almost always want to have an IV lifeline in place, just in case.

Provide Diuresis

Many patients who have respiratory disease have a component of congestive heart failure and could benefit from a loop diuretic such as furosemide (Lasix). Of course, not every patient who has crackles has pulmonary edema. Giving diuretics to patients who have pneumonia or asthma may actually worsen their overall condition by drying them out and causing their secretions to further plug smaller airways. As always, careful assessment and interpretation must lead you to a correct diagnosis. If transport time is short and the patient's condition is not dire, perhaps the emergency department can make a better decision after seeing a radiograph and some labwork.

Support/Assist Ventilation

If the patient becomes fatigued, you may need to support breathing in a more aggressive fashion. Therapy with CPAP and BiPAP is becoming increasingly common and can allow you to avoid intubation in many patients. Some patients may simply require bag-mask ventilation for a short period to reoxygenate, improve their hemoglobin saturation, and reduce $Paco_2$ levels.

You must be confident in your bag-mask ventilation technique so that you don't make a patient's condition worse. Trying to breathe for a patient who is *already breathing on his or her own* is one of the most difficult interventions to pull off. Gastric distention and vomiting from overaggressive ventilation do not help an already worsening situation. As always, *do no harm.* The same is true when providing sedation to anxious and possibly combative patients. The need to control them must be balanced against the possibility of depressing their respirations further. It is almost always a bad idea to sedate someone in the field because they are wild from dyspnea.

Take Over Ventilation

Ultimately, you may need to intubate and ventilate patients who are in respiratory failure. Intubation can be lifesaving, and many patients can be extubated within a day or two and go on to have excellent outcomes. However, there are some issues to consider when intubating a patient. The paramedic must weigh these issues along with the protocols, medical direction, and any expression of the patient's wishes. Keep these issues in mind:

- Intubation should be the last option for patients who have severe asthma. These patients are extremely difficult to ventilate and are prone to pneumothoraces.
- Be proactive; ventilate patients *before* cardiac arrest occurs. When in doubt, attempt to ventilate. If they fight you, they may not be ready for intubation. If they allow you to bag them, they probably are ready for intubation. Patients who are conscious, however, yet still in respiratory distress, will require sedation and neuromuscular blocking medications (through rapid sequence intubation) to facilitate intubation.
- Patients who have had a stroke or who are severely intoxicated may have little or no gag reflex. This is a very dangerous situation if they vomit. You may consider intubating these patients to protect the airway, even if they have adequate ventilation.
- Some patients who have diabetes or have overdosed present with an obvious need for intubation. However, if an ampule of 50% dextrose or naloxone (Narcan) is likely to completely change that picture, it might be better to use bag-mask ventilation for a few minutes to monitor the effect of the initial therapy, assuming you can do so without causing gastric distention and vomiting. Remember to ventilate slowly (over 1 second), and use only enough ventilation to produce visible chest rise.

Respiratory Pharmacology

Medication Delivery

Pharmaceutical therapy for respiratory problems is delivered via a variety of methods, some of which are discussed here.

Metered-Dose Inhalers

When properly used, the metered-dose inhaler should deliver the same amount of medication as an aerosol treatment. This device is small, easy for the patient to carry and use, and convenient. Because it does not require additional equipment (such as a nebulizer or air compressor), it is usually the delivery method of choice for both bronchodilators and corticosteroids in the home setting **Figure 26-39**.

Metered-dose inhalers do have some drawbacks. First, using such a device requires a cooperative patient who is able (and willing) to perform the maneuver correctly. Because the entire dose is delivered in one or two breaths, improper technique may result in little or no medication actually getting into the lungs. Also, patients may not realize when they are using an empty inhaler, ie, some propellant remains but there is no medication.

The metered-dose inhalers that you carry on the ambulance should ideally be equipped with spacers. A spacer is a device that collects the medication as it is released from the canister, allowing more to be delivered to the lungs and less to

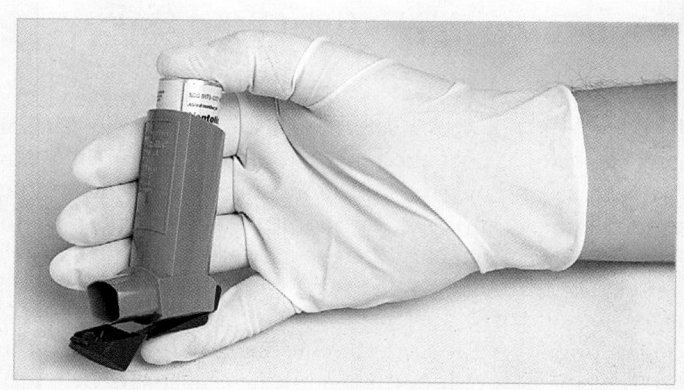

Figure 26-39 Metered-dose inhalers are a common delivery platform for respiratory medications. Their effectiveness is greatly increased by the use of a spacer, which regulates the release of medication into the inhaler.

be lost to the environment. Remember, the mist you see coming out of the inhaler isn't what reaches the patient's alveoli; rather, the 5-μm particles, which stay suspended in the spacer for several minutes, are pulled deep into the lungs by smooth laminar flow. When a spacer is used, the patient does not have to worry about timing the inhalation to coincide with the discharge of the inhaler. Spacers also reduce deposition of the drug into the mouth and oropharynx, which is a problem with the inexperienced user.

Achieving the proper technique when using a metered-dose inhaler isn't difficult, but it requires constant reinforcement. The steps for administering medication with a metered-dose inhaler are demonstrated in Chapter 8.

Following are some tips on common errors when using or administering a metered-dose inhaler, and how to avoid them:

- The mist from the metered-dose inhaler isn't breath spray. Patients need to deeply inhale as they discharge the inhaler to suck the medication deep into their lungs. Placing the inhaler directly into the patient's mouth (without a spacer) often causes much of the medication to fall on the posterior pharynx, from where it is swallowed and digested, thus negating its intended effect.
- Some patients mistakenly blow into the spacer. Tell them to think of the spacer as a big straw, and they should try to suck the medication out of the bottom.
- Many spacers will make a harmonica-like sound if the patient sucks too hard. The best particle deposition comes from smooth, low-pressure, laminar flow. Sucking too hard causes turbulent flow, which makes a lot of the particles stick to the trachea and large bronchi, where they aren't as effective.
- Patients should try to inhale the medication deeply, and then hold their breath for a few seconds. This is a lot to ask of someone who is dyspneic, and it isn't always possible. Sometimes the inhaler causes the patient to cough immediately after inhaling the medication, which also doesn't result in the best delivery, but may be unavoidable.

- In asthma camp, kids learn to take a puff of their bronchodilator inhaler, turn over a sandglass egg timer, and wait a full minute or two before taking the next puff. Let the first puff open up the airways a little, so the second puff gets in deeper.
- Give the bronchodilator first. Many patients have multiple inhalers. A common package might include a rapid-acting beta-2 agonist (rescue inhaler), a corticosteroid, and a slow-acting bronchodilator. Always use the rescue inhaler first. It will dilate the bronchi so that subsequent medications are more effective. In an emergency situation, the other medications will not have any immediate effect, so they would not be given.
- After using a corticosteroid inhaler, patients are encouraged to rinse out their mouth with water or mouthwash. Residual corticosteroid in the pharynx can predispose the patient to thrush, an annoying fungal infection in the pharynx or mouth.
- Make sure the inhaler contains medication. Most inhalers list the number of puffs of medication in the canister on the label. Patients should be encouraged to keep track of how many times they have used the inhaler, and to discard it when they reach the recommended number of uses. Just because you can hear fluid in the canister when you shake it does not mean that there is medication left.
- Keep the spacer and canister holder clean. The spacer and canister holder should occasionally be rinsed off. Aggressively inhaling pocket fuzz and dust bunnies is never a good thing. Always dry respiratory devices after cleaning them. Most evil respiratory bugs love to grow in water, so it is just as important to keep respiratory devices dry as it is to keep them clean.

Aerosol Therapy

Aerosol nebulizers deliver liquid medications in the form of a fine mist Figure 26-40 ▶ . Recall that 5-μm or smaller particles ride laminar airflow into the lower respiratory tract. Larger particles rain out in the mouth and pharynx and get swallowed, so they have little ultimate effect. To generate the optimal particle size, most nebulizers need to have gas flow of at least 6 L/min. Running the gas more slowly generates particles that are too large; running it significantly faster makes the treatment go faster, with the potential of less medication delivery.

In the home, most people run their aerosol treatments off of a small air compressor; in the ambulance, we typically run this therapy off of either our tanked oxygen or off a wall unit attached to the main oxygen supply. As a result, you might be giving only 35% to 40% oxygen via an aerosol treatment, which is still more than the 21% oxygen contained in room air.

A nebulizer can be attached to a mouthpiece (pipe), a face mask, a tracheostomy collar, or simply held in front of the patient's face (blow-by technique). The less the patient breathes in the mist, the less medication he or she actually receives. Blow-by and mouthpiece treatments are not very effective if patients keep turning their head or removing the mouthpiece to answer your questions. As such, once the decision is made

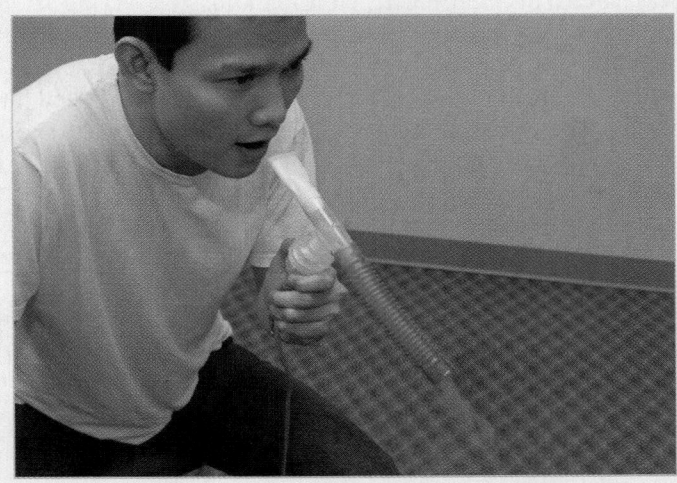

Figure 26-40 Aerosol nebulizers are often used to deliver medications directly to the respiratory tract. Unfortunately, they may give only 35% oxygen during a treatment. Flow rate is an important factor in how much medication makes it into the lungs.

to deliver a breathing treatment, try to stop the conversation and let the patient focus on breathing in the medication.

Always remember that aerosol treatment is a simple method of drug delivery. Just because a patient is wearing a face mask and is a smoker, it doesn't mean the person uses a bronchodilator. Although bronchodilators are the drugs most commonly delivered by this method, corticosteroids, anesthetic agents, antitussives, and mucolytics can all be dispersed through an aerosol. Aerosol lidocaine is an extremely effective method of numbing the upper airway before procedures, and aerosol fentanyl is used to reduce chronic coughing in patients who are terminally ill with lung cancer.

Aerosols also deliver significant humidity to the airway. A quick way to provide a cooling mist to the swollen upper airway of a burn patient or child with croup is to give an aerosol treatment of saline solution. (Chapter 20 describes burns of the upper airway in more detail.) Check with medical command or your local protocols to learn more about these less common uses of aerosol therapy.

The newer aerosol bronchodilators cause far less tachycardia than the older, less beta-2 specific ones. As a result, it has become possible to give repeated treatments to patients with bronchospasm. Continuous nebulizers are available that hold up to 10 times the usual medication dosages, and run for an hour or more. The steps for administering medications via small-volume nebulizer were demonstrated in Chapter 8.

Dry Powder Inhalers

Some respiratory medications are most stable in the form of a very fine powder. Such medications are often placed inside a plastic device that the patient places in his or her mouth and from which he or she inhales deeply. These devices are reasonably convenient and easy to use, but they are rarely used during emergency care.

Several common corticosteroids and slow-acting bronchodilators are routinely packaged in a disc-like device, which holds about 1 month's medication. Each time the device is opened, the small plastic blister that holds a dose is rotated into position. The patient then pushes a small lever to puncture the blister and sucks the powder out of the device. The device is then closed. The device is used to deliver reasonably expensive medications, so be careful not to open and close it repeatedly; you would be wasting several days' worth of medication as the blisters rotate into, and then past, their turn to be punctured.

Other devices require the patient to insert a capsule of powdered medication, which is then pierced when the patient compresses a button or lever on the device. The patient sucks the powder out in a similar fashion to that described above.

Subcutaneous Injections

Drug administration methods that require the patient to inhale the medication may become unreliable or ineffective when the patient's breathing effort is inadequate (reduced tidal volume). In some circumstances, it may be beneficial to attempt beta-2 stimulation the old way—that is, by delivering subcutaneous terbutaline or epinephrine. These medications are not as beta-2 specific as their aerosol cousins but, when the patient's airways are severely closed, they are sometimes the more effective approach.

Direct Instillation

Under certain circumstances, such as cardiac arrest when prompt vascular access is delayed, the administration of select drugs via the endotracheal tube is an option. The dose usually 2 to 2½ times the usual dose, because much of the drug sticks to the inside of the ET tube or drains onto the carina. Newer devices "mist" the drug into the tube, allowing this process to occur without interrupting CPR. While research has shown that this is clearly an inferior delivery model for medications, it is still an option to consider if all else fails.

Fast-Acting Bronchodilators

The most commonly used and fastest-acting bronchodilators work by stimulating the beta-2 receptors in the lungs—part of the sympathetic nervous system. These so-called rescue inhalers provide almost instant relief, a property that sometimes leads to their misuse. Present-day bronchodilators are very beta-2 specific, meaning that they stimulate only beta-2 receptors without acting on other parts of the body, but many patients still use older, less specific medications. Albuterol (Proventil, Ventolin), which is currently the most common beta-2 agonist, is routinely given every 4 hours, but more frequent treatments, and even continuous therapy for hours at a time, is often used without tachycardia.

Anticholinergics

In general, the sympathetic and parasympathetic nervous systems act as opposites. In terms of heart rate and bronchodilation, it is reasonable to think of them as the gas (sympathetic stimulation speeds up heart rate [beta-1] and produces bronchodilation

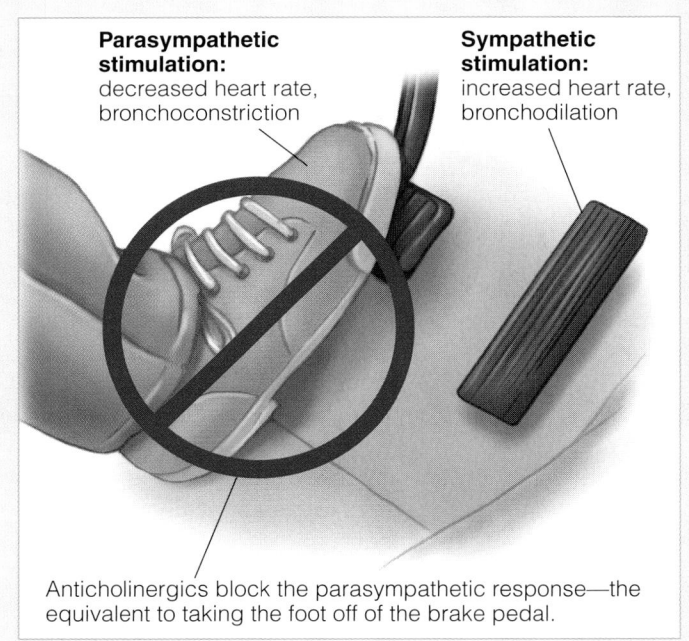

Figure 26-41 Blocking the parasympathetic nervous system (the anticholinergic effect) is like pulling your foot off the brake pedal, whereas giving sympathetic nervous system stimulators is like stepping on the gas.

[beta-2]) and the brake (parasympathetic stimulation slows heart rate and causes bronchoconstriction). Anticholinergic medications block the parasympathetic response, so they are like taking the foot off the brake. Just as it is hard to drive your car if someone has constant pressure on the brake pedal, so we can see how bronchodilation can be enhanced by specifically blocking the bronchoconstriction mechanism **Figure 26-41 ▲**.

In the past, the strategy was to disperse atropine (the most common parasympathetic blocker) through an aerosol. Today, we have a medication specifically designed for aerosol use, ipratropium; also available in a metered-dose inhaler). The combination of albuterol (beta-2 agonist) and ipratropium (anticholinergic) is also available as a pre-mixed cocktail, marketed as an aerosol or a metered-dose inhaler.

Anticholinergics have emerged as a very important component in the management of COPD. Tiotropium, a once-a-day anticholinergic for this indication, is taken via a type of dry powder inhaler. Patients taking tiotropium would not typically also use aerosol ipratropium.

Slow-Acting Bronchodilators

A variety of bronchodilators exist that work by mechanisms other than beta-2 stimulation. Although most of these medications do not provide immediate relief of symptoms, if taken daily they can reduce the frequency and severity of asthma attacks. Patients who are used to the immediate change in their symptoms after using beta-2 agonists often complain that these agents don't work and have to be encouraged to take them as prescribed until they note the long-term benefits.

Popular long-acting bronchodilators include salmeterol (Serevent) and cromolyn (Intal, NasalCrom). Such agents have dramatically improved the quality of life for many patients who have respiratory illness and who use the drugs correctly.

Leukotriene Modifiers

Some patients release bronchoconstricting chemicals called leukotrienes, particularly during an allergic response. Such patients often benefit from a leukotriene blocker such as montelukast (Singulair), which is usually taken via a dry powder inhaler.

Methylxanthines

Methylxanthines, which include aminophylline and theophylline, were once the mainstay of asthma and COPD therapy. Their popularity has declined in recent years because their adverse effects (particularly cardiac effects) are more onerous compared to the many new drugs available. Some patients who have long-term COPD, however, still take aminophylline or theophylline. These drugs can be administered orally (in tablet form or in sprinkles that are placed in food); they can also be given intravenously. Overdose with these agents may cause cardiac dysrhythmias and hypotension, and the level of the drugs in the bloodstream must be closely monitored.

Electrolytes

Some studies indicate that magnesium plays a role in bronchodilation, although this link remains controversial. In very serious asthma attacks, some physicians give 0.5 to 2 g of magnesium sulfate intravenously as a last-ditch effort before intubating. Consult with medical control or follow local protocols regarding this therapy.

Corticosteroids

Corticosteroids are used to reduce bronchial swelling (edema). Although these are not the anabolic corticosteroids that may be abused by athletes, the corticosteroids used in respiratory medicine do have a variety of adverse effects. Long-term corticosteroid use can cause Cushing's syndrome, which is characterized by the classic moon face and generalized edema. Corticosteroids also make blood glucose go haywire, and can blunt the immune system, allowing any infection to suddenly flourish. Patients taking corticosteroids such as prednisone must taper their use gradually. Because of these long-term adverse effects, patients are usually prescribed a course of corticosteroid therapy that lasts 1 or 2 weeks, with a particular end date in mind in an attempt to avoid long-term use.

Inhaled Corticosteroids

Fortunately, inhaled corticosteroids do not appear to have the same adverse effects as their oral counterparts. For that reason, inhaled corticosteroids are becoming very common adjuncts to the treatment of asthma and COPD. Reviewing the asthma triad, you can see how a slow-acting bronchodilator can reduce bronchial constriction, while an inhaled corticosteroid can reduce bronchial swelling.

IV Corticosteroids

In an emergency, it is reasonably common to give corticosteroids intravenously. A single bolus of IV corticosteroids does not appear to cause any negative long-term consequences and is reasonably safe. Methylprednisolone and hydrocortisone are both IV corticosteroid preparations given as an IV bolus, usually for acute exacerbations of COPD or acute asthma attacks. Their onset of action takes hours, so you will not see any results in the field. As always, consult your local protocols and medical direction before administering these agents.

Expectorants

Expectorants thin secretions so that they can be coughed out. Most common expectorants can be purchased in over-the-counter products. Unfortunately, many products mix expectorants with antitussives or antihistamines. These combinations are often at odds with each other. Patients with increased secretions should avoid antihistamine products, taking only products that contain guaifenesin (a type of expectorant).

Antitussives

Antitussives are designed to stop a cough. Coughs can be very annoying, particularly if they interrupt the patient's sleep. However, the need for comfort must be weighed against the need to get rid of excess secretions. Overuse of antitussives can sedate the patient, reduce respiratory drive, and cause excessive plugging of secretions. Many over-the-counter cough syrups also contain antihistamines that can cause problems if not used appropriately.

Aerosol fentanyl is sometimes used to stop the severe coughing associated with tracheobronchial cancers. Because fentanyl is very addictive, it is typically used only in end-of-life scenarios.

Diuretics

Diuretics are used to help reduce blood pressure and to maintain fluid balance in patients who have heart failure. Patients who present with pulmonary edema may benefit from diuretics to remove excess fluid from the circulation, which ultimately keeps it out of the lungs. Loop diuretics (Bumex and Lasix) are the most commonly used agents in emergent situations. Thiazide diuretics are also commonly taken orally to treat high blood pressure or heart failure. Many diuretics cause the patient to lose not only fluid but also potassium. Patients who do not take their potassium supplements may have low potassium levels, and a subsequent predisposition to cardiac dysrhythmias and chronic muscle cramping.

Don't give diuretics to patients who have pneumonia or to patients who are already dry—try to reserve them for those who clearly have pulmonary edema. In fact, some EMS systems reserve furosemide (Lasix, a diuretic) on standing orders for patients with wet lungs and peripheral edema. Patients who have some degree of renal failure may require very large doses of diuretics, or they may be completely unresponsive to diuretics. If your patient requires dialysis for renal failure, trying to induce diuresis is unlikely to be an effective strategy.

Vasodilators

Another common treatment of pulmonary edema is morphine, which dilates the vascular bed, reducing cardiac preload along with allowing fluid to leave the lungs and return to the bloodstream. Morphine, a strong narcotic, also reduces pain and anxiety, which can be very helpful in the scenario of respiratory distress. Too much morphine, however, can decrease respiratory drive and cause a drop in blood pressure. Use morphine carefully, titrating it based on blood pressure and respiratory status.

▌Assisted Ventilation

Continuous Positive Airway Pressure

Continuous positive airway pressure (CPAP) is used in two distinctly different ways.

Many people who have been diagnosed with obstructive sleep apnea wear a CPAP unit at night to maintain their airways while they sleep. This type of CPAP may be applied via nasal pillows, a nasal mask, a face mask that resembles a typical mask used for bag-mask ventilation, or a mask that covers the entire face. Note that this is *not* the type of CPAP that you will apply to the critically ill patient. The positive pressure delivered maintains the stability of the posterior pharynx, thereby preventing obstruction of the upper airway when the person sleeps. This limits both hypoxic episodes and snoring.

The CPAP used as therapy for respiratory failure is almost always delivered via a face mask that is held to the head with some type of strapping system. You should ensure that there is a good seal with minimal leakage ⬤ **Figure 26-42 ▸** . In the field, 100% supplemental oxygen is the most common driving gas for the positive pressure. Be vigilant about monitoring your gas supply—depending on the flow and the patient's respiratory rate, some CPAP units may empty a D cylinder in as little as 5 to 10 minutes. The mask is fitted with a pressure-relief valve that determines the amount of pressure delivered (such as 5 cm H_2O). The end effect is similar to having a gale-force wind blowing in your face (high inspiratory flow) and having to push a pressure valve open with exhalation. This would appear to require a great deal of effort, and to tire out the already-decompensating patient who is in respiratory failure. Miraculously, many patients who appear

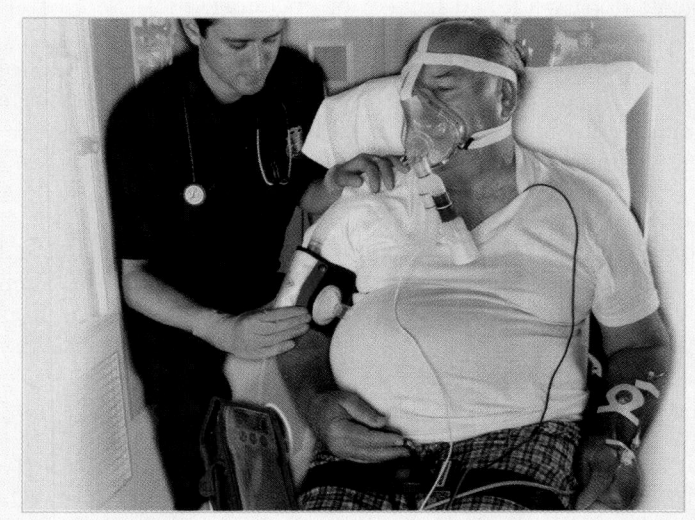

Figure 26-42 The CPAP used in the acute setting is usually administered via face mask, which must make a tight seal to function properly.

to be preparing to take their last breath will make a dramatic turnaround when CPAP is applied.

Some patients find the CPAP mask claustrophobic, and will fight its application. You will be able to talk some of these patients through the process with good results, but other patients simply cannot tolerate the mask. Do not fight with your patient if he or she is unwilling to apply the mask, as you will only increase the patient's anxiety, cardiac workload, and cardiac oxygen consumption. That is a bad trade off. When CPAP works as planned, it can provide dramatic relief and avoid intubation. When CPAP fails, you need to recognize if the patient's condition is deteriorating and be prepared to move to the next step (usually intubation). Within several minutes of application, the patient's oxygen saturation should increase, and the respiratory rate should decrease. The success of CPAP is grossly related to the patient's respiratory rate soon after its application. If this rate *increases*, the therapy is likely to fail; if this rate *decreases*, then the therapy is likely to succeed.

Administering CPAP increases pressure in the chest. If the patient's blood pressure is already low, too much CPAP can stop venous return to the heart and make the patient's blood pressure suddenly drop. This isn't common with lower levels of CPAP, but blood pressure should be carefully monitored whenever CPAP is applied (especially at levels above 10 cm H_2O). Keep in mind that CPAP can turn a simple pneumothorax into a tension pneumothorax in a few breaths.

Bilevel Positive Airway Pressure

Bilevel positive airway pressure (BiPAP) is just CPAP with IPAP and EPAP: it can deliver one pressure during inspiration (inspiratory positive airway pressure [IPAP]) and a different pressure during exhalation (expiratory positive airway pressure [EPAP]). Instead of delivering 20 cm H_2O of CPAP, you might set the BiPAP at 20/8 (20 cm H_2O pressure on inhalation, 8 cm H_2O pressure during exhalation). Because this type of positive airway pressure is a little more like normal breathing, it is often more comfortable for the patient. It causes a pressure variation in the chest, which allows for more normal blood flow. It is also a more complex and expensive device, and one that is not commonly used in the field.

Automated Transport Ventilators

Automated transport ventilators are essentially flow-restricted oxygen-powered ventilation devices (FROPVDs) with timers on them. They can be set to deliver a particular volume at a particular rate, which can be very helpful when you need an extra pair of hands Figure 26-43 ▸ . They are particularly good for replacing the role of bag-mask ventilation when the patient is in cardiac or respiratory arrest. Basic automated transport ventilators may lack any alarms, the ability to control flow rate, or the ability to provide various modes of ventilatory support. They are *not* little ventilators and are *not* intended to ventilate patients without direct observation and attention by a skilled paramedic.

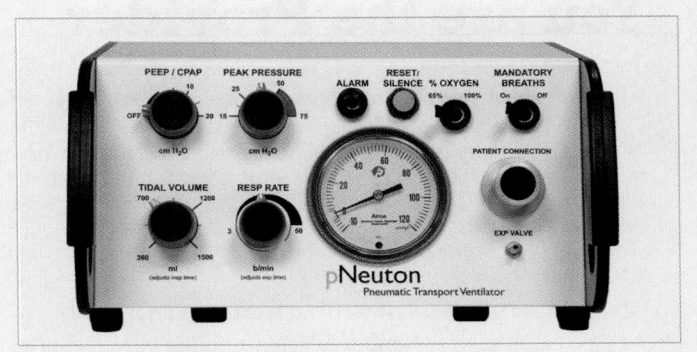

Figure 26-43 Automated transport ventilators are flow-restricted oxygen-powered ventilation devices. They can be very helpful during a cardiac arrest, but the preset flow of 40 L/min is not appropriate for conscious patients.

Conscious patients require up to 150 L/min of flow to comfortably breathe. Most automated transport ventilators are permanently set to deliver 40 L/min, which would be extremely uncomfortable for the spontaneously breathing patient. Both FROPVDs and automated transport ventilators are preset to 40 L/min, which is the optimal flow for ventilating a patient who has had a cardiac arrest—via face mask, and without causing gastric distention.

You are the Provider Summary

1. What about this patient's presentation gives you cause for concern?

The patient's body position, facial expression, increased work of breathing, accessory muscle use, and cries for help are very worrisome. All of these signs point to a patient who is in severe respiratory distress. This patient will need appropriate, aggressive care to prevent his condition from significantly and rapidly worsening.

2. What are your assessment and treatment priorities?

As always, assessment and treatment priorities involve airway, breathing, and circulation. These priorities are learned in EMT-Basic (or sooner). No matter how advanced you become in your certifications and knowledge as a medical professional, you must always remember that the fundamentals of emergency medicine are built upon the principles of basic life support—that is, assessment and treatment of life-threatening illness and injury inherently related to a problem with airway, breathing, and circulation.

3. If you are unable to gather much information from your patient about his medical history, in what other ways can you obtain this information?

Utilize the scene or—better yet—the patient's family members or friends. Significant others are usually highly aware of acute changes in the patient's condition. They may be the first to offer information that can clarify the patient's condition or provide new insight that the patient had not noticed. If no family member is available, you should look for medical identification tags or bracelets and prescription bottles, and assess the scene to gain a better understanding of your patient's medical history. Use resources wisely to avoid delaying lifesaving patient care by searching throughout the home.

4. Given the patient's presentation, which assessment tools should you use to obtain a greater understanding of the patient's medical condition?

Listening to lung sounds is a given and, as a well-trained medical professional, you will likely have many other assessment tools at your disposal. It is critical that you understand when and how to use tools such as tactile fremitus, egophony, bronchophony, whispered pectoriloquy, and percussion. It is not always wise to spend precious minutes using these assessment tools on a patient whose condition is deteriorating rapidly. As a paramedic, you must determine how to best use your time and your resources in accordance with your patient's condition. For example, to delay transport to check the function of all 12 cranial nerves in the presence of an obvious cerebrovascular accident is inappropriate and could cost the patient his or her life.

5. What was likely the initial problem with obtaining a pulse oximetry reading?

In cases of shock, the body shunts blood away from the extremities and directs it to the vital organs. Therefore, when the body is poorly perfused or when the extremities are cold, this will affect the oximeter's ability to obtain a reading. Choose alternative sites in which to place the sensor, such as the ear or the bridge of the nose.

6. Do you believe that your patient is able to maintain his airway?

Given the information regarding his level of consciousness; his respiratory rate, depth, and quality; his skin signs; and the oximetry reading, it is obvious that this patient is not ventilating or oxygenating adequately.

7. What options do you have available to maintain this patient's airway?

The most important skills for successfully maintaining a patient's airway are basic life support measures—specifically, bag-mask ventilation and use of airway adjuncts. The importance of these skills becomes painfully obvious in the event of failed intubations or failure of alternative airways.

Controversy exists in the medical community regarding the appropriateness of prehospital rapid sequence induction. The medical director must determine whether his or her EMS providers should use this advanced airway management tool. If the medical director has decided that rapid sequence induction is an appropriate skill for his or her personnel, you must commit to maintaining the knowledge and skills required to safely and successfully perform this procedure.

For those agencies that do not have the capabilities to perform rapid sequence induction or intubation, nasal airways can be an appropriate choice, assuming your patient has not had head trauma. If you are unable to manage the airway with either of these procedures, and the patient continues to have an intact gag reflex, then laryngeal mask airways and Combitubes will not be an option. In these cases, use nasogastric or orogastric tubes to remove the stomach contents, ventilate the patient using bag-mask ventilation and 100% oxygen, and continually monitor the airway for the need to suction secretions.

8. Beyond inadequate ventilation and oxygenation, what must you take into consideration before attempting intubation?

You must always consider the patient's anatomy and your ability to place the ET tube correctly. Patients with small mouths or short necks or who are obese can be quite difficult to intubate.

9. If capnography, pulse oximetry, and other similar pieces of assessment equipment are unavailable, how can you determine whether your interventions are improving the patient's condition?

Almost anyone who has worked with a seasoned partner has likely heard that new medics are too dependent on gadgets. Some of this disdain could be rooted in fear of change, but it still makes a valid point. Field providers can become overly dependent on equipment to provide information that can and should be validated in the patient's signs and symptoms. Reassess the patient for signs of improvement.

10. What other techniques can you use to improve ventilation and oxygenation?

Another advantage of obtaining a definitive airway is your ability to provide tracheal suctioning. This patient definitely would benefit from the removal of secretions.

Prep Kit

Ready for Review

- The primary components of the respiratory system are like an inverted tree, with the trachea representing the tree's trunk and the alveoli resembling the tree's leaves.
- The mouth and oropharynx are very vascular and are covered by a mucous blanket. Swelling can be profound and potentially dangerous.
- The larynx and glottis are typically considered the dividing line between the upper airway and the lower airway. The thyroid cartilage is the most obvious external landmark of the larynx. The glottis and vocal cords are found in the middle of the thyroid cartilage.
- The cricoid cartilage can be palpated just below the thyroid cartilage in the neck. It forms a complete ring and maintains the trachea in an open position. Applying cricoid pressure or Sellick maneuver may be helpful with intubation.
- The small space between the thyroid and cricoid cartilages is the cricothyroid membrane. It is a good choice for inserting a large IV catheter or a small breathing tube.
- Cilia line the larger airways and help move foreign material out of the tracheobronchial tree. If a patient is dehydrated or has taken medications that dry secretions (such as antihistamines), the cilia will not be able to effectively move secretions. The same is true if the patient is overhydrated.
- Pulmonary circulation begins at the right ventricle, where the pulmonary artery branches into increasingly smaller vessels until it reaches the pulmonary capillary bed, which surrounds the alveoli and terminal bronchioles.
- Patients who have traumatic brain injuries may exhibit bizarre respiratory patterns, including agonal gasps; apneustic and ataxic patterns; and Biot, Cheyne-Stokes, and Kussmaul respirations; as well as central neurogenic hyperventilation, bradypnea, hyperpnea, hypopnea, and tachypnea.
- The respiratory system delivers oxygen to the body and removes the primary waste product of metabolism, carbon dioxide. If the lungs are not functioning appropriately, both of these vital functions may be impaired. Hypoxia, cell death, and acidosis can then occur.
- The brain is very sensitive to reduced levels of oxygen. It requires a regular supply of both oxygen and glucose to function, but can store neither. Alteration in level of consciousness could represent respiratory compromise.
- A patient who has respiratory disease may not be able to talk because he or she is having difficulty breathing. You may have to obtain the history from a family member or from only a few clues.
- It is critical to evaluate how hard your patient is working to breathe. Patients in respiratory distress may be able to compensate at first, but will eventually become sleepy, have a decreased respiratory rate and depth, and then, decompensate.
- Patients who have chronic respiratory disease are often knowledgeable about their disease and may have tried several potential treatment options already. Ask them about these efforts and what results, if any, they produced.
- Onset and duration of distress are important considerations in determining the underlying cause. Find out if the problem happened suddenly or gradually worsened over time.
- Assessing the patient's position of comfort and difficulty speaking may help you gauge the patient's degree of distress. A patient sitting in a Fowler's position and speaking only in two- or three-word statements is probably in considerable distress.
- Patients in respiratory distress tend to seek the tripod position. The condition of a patient in respiratory distress who is willing to lay flat may be quickly deteriorating. Head bobbing is also an ominous sign.
- Find out if the patient's condition is a recurrence of a past condition. If so, compare the current situation with other episodes.
- Note any audible abnormal respiratory noises. Noisy breathing is obstructed breathing.
- Snoring indicates partial obstruction of the upper airway by the tongue. Stridor indicates narrowing of the upper airway, usually as a result of swelling (laryngeal edema).
- Assessing the level of consciousness is enormously important in dyspneic patients.
- Assess the patient's mucous membranes for cyanosis (a bluish or dusky color), pallor, and moisture.
- Look for jugular venous distention in the neck, with the patient in a semi-sitting position. Distended neck veins may be caused by cardiac failure.
- Feel the chest for vibrations as the patient breathes. Check for edema of the ankles or lower back. Check for peripheral cyanosis. Check the pulse and note the patient's skin temperature. Attach any available monitors.
- Auscultate the lungs whenever possible. Adventitious breath sounds are the extra noises that you may hear; they include wheezing or crackles.
- Crackles are any discontinuous noises heard on auscultation of the lungs. They are caused by the popping open of air spaces and are usually associated with increased fluid in the lungs.
- Wheezes are high-pitched, whistling sounds made by air being forced through narrowed airways, which makes them vibrate. Wheezing may be diffuse in conditions such as asthma and congestive heart failure or localized when caused by a foreign body obstructing a bronchus.
- *Silence means danger!* If you don't hear anything with your stethoscope, the patient is not moving enough air to ventilate the lungs.
- Note whether the patient is coughing up colorful sputum, if the color or amount of sputum has changed, and if it contains blood or pus.
- A pulse oximeter indicates what percentage of the patient's hemoglobin has oxygen attached to it. An oxygen saturation level greater than 95% is considered normal.
- The peak flow is the maximum flow rate at which the patient can expel air from the lungs. Normal peak flows run from about 350 to 700 L/min. A peak flow of less than 150 L/min is very low and signals significant distress.
- A variety of infections can cause swelling in the upper airway. Croup is one of the most common, though it usually occurs only in small children.
- Pulmonary aspiration of stomach contents is very dangerous. Avoid causing gastric distention when bagging the patient, and monitor the patient's ability to protect his or her airway. If you determine that the patient can't protect his or her airway, one of your primary jobs is to protect it for them, and that means intubation.
- Common obstructive airway diseases include emphysema, chronic bronchitis, and asthma. Emphysema and chronic bronchitis are collectively classified as COPD.
- Asthma is caused by allergens or irritants and is characterized by widespread, reversible narrowing of the airways (bronchospasm), edema of the airways, and increased mucous production. It can cause significant airway obstruction.
- Primary treatment of bronchospasm is bronchodilator medication. Primary treatment of bronchial edema is corticosteroids, which may or may not be administered in the field setting.

- Status asthmaticus is a severe, prolonged asthmatic attack that cannot be broken with conventional treatment. It is a dire medical emergency. Any person with asthma who feels sick enough to call an ambulance is in status asthmaticus until proved otherwise.
- When a patient has recurring asthma attacks, his or her inhaler could be empty or the medication could no longer be effective. Try administering a new bronchodilator.
- Emphysema is a chronic weakening and destruction of the walls of the terminal bronchioles and alveoli. A patient with emphysema classically has a barrel chest, muscle wasting, and pursed-lip breathing. Such patients are often tachypneic.
- Chronic bronchitis is characterized by excessive mucous production in the bronchial tree, nearly always accompanied by a chronic or recurrent productive cough. A patient with chronic bronchitis tends to be sedentary and obese, sleep in an upright position, use many tissues, have copious secretions, and be cyanotic.
- In assessing patients who have COPD, search for what pushed them over the edge. Look for signs of infection, peripheral edema, jugular venous distention with hepatojugular reflux, and crackles. Find out if the onset of dyspnea was sudden or gradual.
- Not everyone should be ventilated the same way. Allow each breath to come back out before the delivery of the next breath. If you don't, pressures in the thorax will rise, eventually causing pneumothorax or cardiac arrest. Patients with severe obstructive diseases should be ventilated as little as 4 to 6 breaths/min.
- Noncompliance could trigger an asthma attack. Ask what the patient was doing when the asthma attack began. Ask if the patient took his or her medications today. Ask if movement worsens the dyspnea.
- Pneumonia may be caused by a variety of bacterial, viral, and fungal agents. The patient with pneumonia usually reports weakness, productive cough, fever, and sometimes chest pain that worsens with coughing. Supportive care includes oxygenation, suctioning, and transport to an appropriate facility.
- Pulmonary edema occurs when fluid migrates into the lungs. The patient expectorating pink and foamy secretions probably has severe pulmonary edema.
- When a patient has a pneumothorax, air collects between the visceral pleura and the parietal pleura. Administer supplemental oxygen and monitor the patient's respiratory status closely.
- Pleural effusion will make the patient dyspneic. Supportive care, including proper positioning and aggressive oxygen administration, should be given.
- A pulmonary embolism occurs when a blood clot breaks off in the circulation and travels to the lungs, blocking blood flow and nutrient exchange. Bedridden patients and people with thrombophlebitis are at risk of pulmonary embolism. The hallmark of pulmonary embolus is cyanosis that does not resolve with oxygen therapy.
- Respiratory failure, or insufficient ventilation, can occur from a multitude of pathologic conditions, from injuries to the lungs, heart, and neurologic system to overdoses. Care includes providing supplemental oxygen.
- In hyperventilation syndrome, ventilation is excessive. If it continues, the patient may experience chest pain and carpopedal spasm. Psychological support techniques such as counting breaths, and distraction work best and help calm the patient.
- In managing the condition of a patient who is in respiratory distress, begin by ensuring that there is an open and maintainable airway. Suction if necessary and keep the airway optimally posi-

tioned. Remove constricting clothing. Reduce the patient's effort to breathe.
- Patients in respiratory failure may ultimately need to be intubated. There are major drawbacks and risks to intubating in the field, but it can also be lifesaving. Weigh these issues along with protocols, medical direction, and the patient's wishes.
- Metered-dose inhalers deliver medication as an aerosol treatment. They are usually the delivery method of choice for both bronchodilators and corticosteroids in the home setting. Improper technique may result in little or no medication actually getting into the lungs.
- Aerosol nebulizers deliver liquid medications in the form of a fine mist to the respiratory tract. Weigh the potential benefits of aerosol therapy against the lower FIO_2 delivered during the treatment.
- Drug administration methods that require the patient to inhale the medication may become unreliable or ineffective when the patient's airways are severely compromised. Some cases may warrant delivering medications subcutaneously instead.
- Medications can be instilled directly into the tracheobronchial tree when patients are intubated or have a tracheotomy. Stop CPR compressions for a moment when you instill the medication.
- Continuous positive airway pressure (CPAP) is used as therapy for respiratory failure. Within several minutes of application, the patient's oxygen saturation should increase, and the respiratory rate should decrease.
- Bilevel positive airway pressure (BiPAP) is CPAP that delivers one pressure during inspiration and a different pressure during exhalation. It is more like normal breathing and is often more comfortable for the patient.
- Automated transport ventilators are essentially flow-restricted oxygen-powered breathing devices with timers on them. They are particularly good choices for filling the role of the bag-mask ventilator when the patient is in cardiac or respiratory arrest, but are not intended to ventilate patients without direct observation and attention from a skilled practitioner.

■ Vital Vocabulary

abscess A collection of pus in a sac, formed by necrotic tissues and an accumulation of white blood cells.

adventitious A type of breath sound that occurs in addition to the normal breath sounds; examples are crackles and wheezes.

alveoli Sac-like units at the end of the bronchioles where gas exchange takes place (singular: alveolus).

angioedema An allergic reaction that may cause profound swelling of the tongue and lips.

arytenoid cartilages One of the paired, pitcher-shaped cartilages at the back of the larynx, at the upper border of the cricoid cartilage.

atelectasis Collapse of the alveolar air spaces of the lungs.

beta-2 agonists Pharmacologic agents that stimulate the beta-2 receptor sites found in smooth muscle; include common bronchodilators like albuterol and levalbuterol.

botulism Poisoning from eating food containing botulinum toxin.

bronchospasm Severe constriction of the bronchial tree.

cape cyanosis Deep cyanosis of the face and neck and across the chest and back; associated with little or no blood flow; it is particularly ominous.

carina Point at which the trachea bifurcates into the right and left mainstem bronchi.

carpopedal spasm Contorted position of the hand in which the fingers flex in a clawlike attitude and the thumb curls toward the palm.

chronic bronchitis Chronic inflammatory condition affecting the bronchi that is associated with excess mucous production that results from overgrowth of the mucous glands in the airways.

cilia Hairlike microtubule projections on the surface of a cell that can move materials over the cell surface.

cor pulmonale Heart disease that develops secondary to a chronic lung disease, usually affecting primarily the right side of the heart.

crackles Abnormal breath sounds that have a fine, crackling quality; previously called rales.

cricoid cartilage Ringlike cartilage forming the lower and back part of the larynx.

cricothyroid membrane Membrane between the cricoid and thyroid cartilages of the larynx.

croup Common disease of childhood characterized by spasm of the larynx and resulting upper airway obstruction.

dead space The portion of the tidal volume that does not reach the alveoli and thus does not participate in gas exchange.

diuresis Secretion of large amounts of urine by the kidney.

edema A condition in which excess fluid accumulates in tissues, manifested by swelling.

emphysema Infiltration of any tissue by air or gas; a chronic obstructive pulmonary disease characterized by distention of the alveoli and destructive changes in the lung parenchyma.

end-tidal carbon dioxide The numeric percentage of carbon dioxide contained in the last few milliliters of the patient's exhaled air.

epistaxis Nosebleed.

Fowler's position A sitting position with the head elevated to 90° (sitting straight upright).

glottis Opening between the vocal cords.

goblet cells Cells that produce a protective mucous lining.

Greenfield filter A mesh filter placed in the inferior vena cava to catch blood clots in patients who are at high risk of pulmonary embolus.

Guillain-Barré syndrome A disease of unknown etiology that causes paralysis that progresses from the feet to the head (ascending paralysis). If the paralysis reaches the diaphragm, the patient may require respiratory support.

hemoglobin Oxygen-carrying pigment of the red blood cells. When hemoglobin has absorbed oxygen in the lungs, it is bright red and is called oxyhemoglobin. After hemoglobin has given up its oxygen in the tissues, it is purple and is called reduced hemoglobin.

hemoptysis Coughing up blood.

Hering-Breuer reflex The nervous system mechanism that terminates inhalation and prevents lung overexpansion.

hypoventilate To not move adequate volumes of gas; underventilate.

hypoxic drive A situation in which a person's stimulus to breathe comes from a fall in Pao_2 rather than the normal stimulus, a rise in $Paco_2$.

jugular venous distention The visible bulging of the jugular veins when the patient is in semi-Fowler's or full Fowler's position. This is indicative of inadequate blood movement through the heart and/or lungs.

Kussmaul respirations A respiratory pattern characteristic of the person with diabetes who is in ketoacidosis, with marked hyperpnea and tachypnea.

larynx The organ of voice production.

metastasis Change in location of a disease from one organ or part of the body to another. Often used to describe a cancer that has migrated to other parts of the body.

monophonic The sound of one note during wheezing, caused by the vibration of a single bronchus.

oropharynx The area behind the base of the tongue between the soft palate and the upper portion of the epiglottis.

orthopnea Severe dyspnea experienced when recumbent and relieved by sitting or standing up.

palatine tonsils One of three sets of lymphatic organs that comprise the tonsils; located in the back of the throat, on each side of the posterior opening of the oral cavity; help protect the body from bacteria introduced into the mouth and nose.

parenchyma The substance of a gland or solid organ.

paroxysmal nocturnal dyspnea Severe shortness of breath occurring at night after several hours of recumbency, during which fluid pools in the lungs.

piriform fossa Hollow pockets on the lateral sides of the glottic opening.

pleural effusion Excessive accumulation of fluid in the pleural space.

pneumonitis Inflammation of the lung. Implies lung inflammation from an irritant such as a chemical, dust, or radiation, or from aspiration. When lung inflammation is caused by an infectious agent, it would typically be called pneumonia.

polycythemia The production of more red blood cells over time, making the blood thick; a characteristic of people who have chronic lung disease and chronic hypoxia.

polyphonic The sound of multiple notes during wheezing, caused by the vibrations of many bronchi.

pseudomembrane A false membrane formed by a dead tissue layer. Seen in the posterior pharynx of patients with diphtheria.

pulsus paradoxus Weakening or loss of a palpable pulse during inhalation, characteristic of cardiac tamponade and severe asthma.

purulent Full of pus; having the character of pus.

rales Old terminology for abnormal breath sounds that have a fine, crackling quality; now called crackles.

reactive airway disease A term used to describe any condition that causes hyperreactive bronchioles and bronchospasm.

retraction Drawing in the intercostal muscles and the muscles above the clavicles in respiratory distress.

rhonchus A coarse, low-pitched breath sound heard in patients who have chronic mucus in the airways (plural: rhonchi).

Sellick maneuver Pressure applied over the cricoid to seal off the esophagus and prevent reflux of gastric contents.

shunt Situation in which a portion of the output of the right side of the heart reaches the left side of the heart without being oxygenated in the lungs; may be caused by atelectasis, pulmonary edema, or a variety of other conditions. In hemodialysis, an anastomosis between a peripheral artery and vein.

smooth muscle Nonstriated involuntary muscle found in vessel walls, glands, and the gastrointestinal tract.

snoring Noise made on inhalation when the upper airway is partially obstructed by the tongue.

spacer A device that collects medication as it is released from the canister of a metered-dose inhaler, allowing more to be delivered to the lungs and less to be lost to the environment.

status asthmaticus A severe, prolonged asthma attack that cannot be broken with epinephrine.

stridor Harsh, high-pitched sound associated with severe upper airway obstruction, such as that caused by laryngeal edema.

surfactant A liquid protein substance that coats the alveoli in the lungs.

tactile fremitus Vibrations in the chest as the patient breathes.

tidal volume The amount of air inhaled or exhaled during one breath.

tracheostomy Surgically opening the trachea to create an airway.

tuberculosis A chronic bacterial disease caused by *Mycobacterium tuberculosis* that usually affects the lungs but can also affect other organs such as the brain or kidneys.

turbinates A set of bony convolutions formed by the conchae in the nasopharynx that help to maintain smooth airflow.

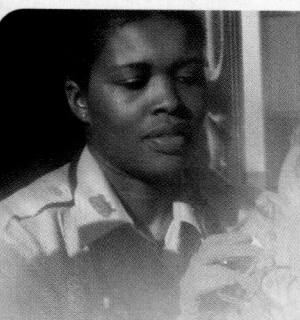

Assessment in Action

You arrive on the scene and find a 63-year-old woman in moderate respiratory distress. She is in the tripod position, using some accessory muscles, and is speaking in three- to four-word sentences. The patient is conscious, alert, and orientated to person, place, and time. Her blood pressure is 134/70 mm Hg; heart rate is 118 beats/min and regular; and her respiratory rate is 28 breaths/min. The pulse oximeter reads 90%. The patient's skin is warm and her nail beds are slightly cyanotic. She has been taking her albuterol inhaler all day and it hasn't worked. She states this all began 2 days ago and has not gotten any better. She is wheezing in all lung fields.

1. **Which of the following is essential for normal ventilations to occur?**
   A. Functional diaphragm and intercostal muscles
   B. Interstitial space that is not filled with fluid
   C. Adequate blood volume
   D. Pulmonary capillaries that are not occluded

2. **What is chronic obstructive pulmonary disease?**
   A. A recurring condition of partially reversible airflow obstruction
   B. An acute inflammation of the lungs
   C. An absence of breath sounds on one side
   D. A progressive and irreversible disease of the airway

3. **What might bring about an exacerbation in an underlying respiratory condition?**
   A. Stress and infections
   B. Cigarette smoking
   C. Exercising
   D. All of the above

4. **What are important questions to ask this patient?**
   A. Has this happened before?
   B. Have you ever been intubated in the past?
   C. Is breathing uncomfortable when you lie down (more comfortable when you are sitting up or standing)?
   D. All of the above.

5. **What is usually the most reliable indicator of the patient's severity of respiratory distress?**
   A. One-word sentences
   B. Gross diaphoresis and pale color
   C. Patient's description of respiratory distress
   D. Tachycardia

6. **What are wheezes?**
   A. High-pitched, whistling sounds
   B. Noises heard on auscultation of lungs, caused by popping open of air spaces
   C. Absent breath sounds
   D. Bubbling sounds heard at bases of the lungs

7. **What is emphysema?**
   A. Reversible narrowing of the airways
   B. Chronic weakening and destruction of the walls of the terminal bronchioles and alveoli
   C. An acute inflammatory condition of the lungs
   D. The leading cause of respiratory illnesses in children

8. **What is the hypoxic drive?**
   A. To not move adequate volumes of gas
   B. A respiratory pattern characterized by ketoacidosis
   C. A situation in which a person's stimulus to breathe comes from a fall in Pao_2 rather than the normal stimulus, a rise in $Paco_2$
   D. The portion of tidal volume that does not reach the alveoli

9. **True or false? You should withhold oxygen from a patient who has been diagnosed with COPD.**
   A. True
   B. False

10. **What is peak expiratory flow?**
    A. Maximum flow rate at which patients can expel air from their lungs
    B. Partial obstruction of the upper airway by the tongue
    C. Adventitious breath sounds when auscultating the lungs
    D. Silent lung fields

Challenging Questions

You are dispatched to the train station. Arriving on the scene, you find a 54-year-old man in respiratory distress. Upon auscultation of his lungs, you note wheezing in all lung fields. The patient is unable to talk to you.

11. **Is this patient having an asthma attack?**

■■ Points to Ponder

Your shift is just beginning and you are dispatched to the home of a 90-year-old man who has respiratory problems. It's a cold winter evening and the BLS crew is about ready to bring him to the ambulance. You enter the house and immediately hear audible crackles coming from the next room. The crew has the patient on 100% oxygen via nonrebreathing mask. The patient is conscious, alert, and orientated to person, place, and time. Blood pressure is 220/110 mm Hg, respiratory rate is 40 breaths/min, heart rate is 85 beats/min, pulse oximetry is 91%. The patient has jugular venous distention and peripheral edema.

The patient appears to be in severe respiratory distress, using accessory muscles, speaking in one-word sentences, and grossly diaphoretic. Family states that this all began while he was watching TV approximately 45 minutes ago, and has gotten progressively worse. The patient's medications include metoprolol (Toprol), pravastatin (Pravachol), furosemide (Lasix), potassium, and digoxin. The family cannot tell you much about his medical history.

What do you know about this patient, based on his presentation and medications?

Issues: Recognizing a Respiratory Emergency, Timely and Correct Treatment, Determining Medical History Based on Medications.

27 Cardiovascular Emergencies

Objectives

Cognitive

5-2.1 Describe the incidence, morbidity and mortality of cardiovascular disease. (p 27.6)

5-2.2 Discuss prevention strategies that may reduce the morbidity and mortality of cardiovascular disease. (p 27.6)

5-2.3 Identify the risk factors most predisposing to coronary artery disease. (p 27.6)

5-2.4 Describe the anatomy of the heart, including the position in the thoracic cavity, layers of the heart, chambers of the heart, and location and function of cardiac valves. (p 27.6–27.8)

5-2.5 Identify the major structures of the vascular system. (p 27.7)

5-2.6 Identify the factors affecting venous return. (p 27.8)

5-2.7 Identify and define the components of cardiac output. (p 27.13)

5-2.8 Identify phases of the cardiac cycle. (p 27.9)

5-2.9 Identify the arterial blood supply to any given area of the myocardium. (p 27.9)

5-2.10 Compare and contrast the coronary arterial distribution to the major portions of the cardiac conduction system. (p 27.9, 27.10)

5-2.11 Identify the structure and course of all divisions and subdivisions of the cardiac conduction system. (p 27.13)

5-2.12 Identify and describe how the heart's pacemaking control, rate, and rhythm are determined. (p 27.13–27.16)

5-2.13 Explain the physiological basis of conduction delay in the AV node. (p 27.14)

5-2.14 Define the functional properties of cardiac muscle. (p 27.13)

5-2.15 Define the events comprising electrical potential. (p 27.14–27.16)

5-2.16 List the most important ions involved in myocardial action potential and their primary function in this process. (p 27.14, 27.15)

5-2.17 Describe the events involved in the steps from excitation to contraction of cardiac muscle fibers. (p 27.14–27.16)

5-2.18 Describe the clinical significance of Starling's law. (p 27.13)

5-2.19 Identify the structures of the autonomic nervous system (ANS). (p 27.16–27.19)

5-2.20 Identify the effect of the ANS on heart rate, rhythm and contractility. (p 27.16–27.19)

5-2.21 Define and give examples of positive and negative inotropism, chronotropism and dromotropism. (p 27.19)

5-2.22 Discuss the pathophysiology of cardiac disease and injury. (p 27.27)

5-2.23 Identify and describe the details of inspection, auscultation, and palpation specific to the cardiovascular system. (p 27.25)

5-2.24 Define pulse deficit, pulsus paradoxus, and pulsus alternans. (p 27.25)

5-2.25 Identify the normal characteristics of the point of maximal impulse (PMI). (p 27.7)

5-2.26 Identify and define the heart sounds. (p 27.8, 27.9)

5-2.27 Relate heart sounds to hemodynamic events in the cardiac cycle. (p 27.8, 27.9)

5-2.28 Describe the differences between normal and abnormal heart sounds. (p 27.9)

5-2.29 Identify and describe the components of the focused history as it relates to the patient with cardiovascular compromise. (p 27.23, 27.24)

5-2.30 Explain the purpose of ECG monitoring. (p 27.41)

5-2.31 Describe how ECG wave forms are produced. (p 27.43)

5-2.32 Correlate the electrophysiological and hemodynamic events occurring throughout the entire cardiac cycle with the various ECG wave forms, segments and intervals. (p 27.43)

5-2.33 Identify how heart rates, durations, and amplitudes may be determined from ECG recordings. (p 27.43)

5-2.34 Relate the cardiac surfaces or areas represented by the ECG leads. (p 27.65)

5-2.35 Given an ECG, identify the arrhythmia. (p 27.47)

5-2.36 Identify the limitations to the ECG. (p 27.70)

5-2.37 Differentiate among the primary mechanisms responsible for producing cardiac arrhythmias. (p 27.47)

5-2.38 Describe a systematic approach to the analysis and interpretation of cardiac arrhythmias. (p 27.45–27.47)

5-2.39 Describe the arrhythmias originating in the sinus node, the AV junction, the atria, and the ventricles. (p 27.47, 27.49, 27.52)

5-2.40 Describe the arrhythmias originating or sustained in the AV junction. (p 27.47)

5-2.41 Describe the abnormalities originating within the bundle branch system. (p 27.56)

5-2.42 Describe the process of differentiating wide QRS complex tachycardias. (p 27.55–27.57)

5-2.43 Recognize the pitfalls in the differentiation of wide QRS complex tachycardias. (p 27.56)

5-2.44 Describe the conditions of pulseless electrical activity. (p 27.59, 27.75)

5-2.45 Describe the phenomena of reentry, aberration and accessory pathways. (p 27.13–27.16)

5-2.46 Identify the ECG changes characteristically produced by electrolyte imbalances and specify the clinical implications. (p 27.61)

5-2.47 Identify patient situations where ECG rhythm analysis is indicated. (p 27.68)

5-2.48 Recognize the changes on the ECG that may reflect evidence of myocardial ischemia and injury. (p 27.68)

5-2.49 Recognize the limitations of the ECG in reflecting evidence of myocardial ischemia and injury. (p 27.70)

5-2.50 Correlate abnormal ECG findings with clinical interpretation. (p 27.70)

5-2.51 Identify the major therapeutic objectives in the treatment of the patient with any arrhythmia. (p 27.41)

5-2.52 Identify the major mechanical, pharmacological and electrical therapeutic interventions. (p 27.31)

5-2.53 Based on field impressions, identify the need for rapid intervention for the patient in cardiovascular compromise. (p 27.23)

5-2.54 Describe the incidence, morbidity and mortality associated with myocardial conduction defects. (p 27.6)

5-2.55 Identify the clinical indications for transcutaneous and permanent artificial cardiac pacing. (p 27.83)

5-2.56 Describe the components and the functions of a transcutaneous pacing system. (p 27.83)

5-2.57 Explain what each setting and indicator on a transcutaneous pacing system represents and how the settings may be adjusted. (p 27.84)

5-2.58 Describe the techniques of applying a transcutaneous pacing system. (p 27.84)

5-2.59 Describe the characteristics of an implanted pacemaking system. (p 27.60)

5-2.60 Describe artifacts that may cause confusion when evaluating the ECG of a patient with a pacemaker. (p 27.60)

5-2.61 List the possible complications of pacing. (p 27.60)

5-2.62 List the causes and implications of pacemaker failure. (p 27.60)

5-2.63 Identify additional hazards that interfere with artificial pacemaker function. (p 27.60)

5-2.64 Recognize the complications of artificial pacemakers as evidenced on ECG. (p 27.60)

5-2.65 Describe the epidemiology, morbidity and mortality, and pathophysiology of angina pectoris. (p 27.28)

5-2.66 List and describe the assessment parameters to be evaluated in a patient with angina pectoris. (p 27.29)

5-2.67 Identify what is meant by the OPQRST of chest pain assessment. (p 27.23)

5-2.68 List other clinical conditions that may mimic signs and symptoms of coronary artery disease and angina pectoris. (p 27.29)

5-2.69 Identify the ECG findings in patients with angina pectoris. (p 27.28)

5-2.70 Identify the paramedic responsibilities associated with management of the patient with angina pectoris. (p 27.29)

5-2.71 Based on the pathophysiology and clinical evaluation of the patient with chest pain, list the anticipated clinical problems according to their life-threatening potential. (p 27.29)

5-2.72 Describe the epidemiology, morbidity and mortality of myocardial infarction. (p 27.29)

5-2.73 List the mechanisms by which an MI may be produced by traumatic and non-traumatic events. (p 27.29)

5-2.74 Identify the primary hemodynamic changes produced in myocardial infarction. (p 27.29)

5-2.75 List and describe the assessment parameters to be evaluated in a patient with a suspected myocardial infarction. (p 27.30)

5-2.76 Identify the anticipated clinical presentation of a patient with a suspected acute myocardial infarction. (p 27.31)

5-2.77 Differentiate the characteristics of the pain/discomfort occurring in angina pectoris and acute myocardial infarction. (p 27.29)

5-2.78 Identify the ECG changes characteristically seen during evolution of an acute myocardial infarction. (p 27.32)

5-2.79 Identify the most common complications of an acute myocardial infarction. (p 27.31)

5-2.80 List the characteristics of a patient eligible for fibrinolytic therapy. (p 27.34)

5-2.81 Describe the "window of opportunity" as it pertains to reperfusion of a myocardial injury or infarction. (p 27.33)

5-2.82 Based on the pathophysiology and clinical evaluation of the patient with a suspected acute myocardial infarction, list the anticipated clinical problems according to their life-threatening potential. (p 27.31)

5-2.83 Specify the measures that may be taken to prevent or minimize complications in the patient suspected of myocardial infarction. (p 27.31)

5-2.84 Describe the most commonly used cardiac drugs in terms of therapeutic effect and dosages, routes of administration, side effects and toxic effects. (p 27.84)

5-2.85 Describe the epidemiology, morbidity and mortality of heart failure. (p 27.34)

5-2.86 Define the principle causes and terminology associated with heart failure. (p 27.34)

5-2.87 Identify the factors that may precipitate or aggravate heart failure. (p 27.34)

5-2.88 Describe the physiological effects of heart failure. (p 27.34)

5-2.89 Define the term "acute pulmonary edema" and describe its relationship to left ventricular failure. (p 27.34)

5-2.90 Define preload, afterload and left ventricular end-diastolic pressure and relate each to the pathophysiology of heart failure. (p 27.35)

5-2.91 Differentiate between early and late signs and symptoms of left ventricular failure and those of right ventricular failure. (p 27.35)

5-2.92 Explain the clinical significance of paroxysmal nocturnal dyspnea. (p 27.23)

5-2.93 Explain the clinical significance of edema of the extremities and sacrum. (p 27.36)

5-2.94 List the interventions prescribed for the patient in acute congestive heart failure. (p 27.36)

5-2.95 Describe the most commonly used pharmacological agents in the management of congestive heart failure in terms of therapeutic effect, dosages, routes of administration, side effects and toxic effects. (p 27.36)

5-2.96 Define the term "cardiac tamponade." (p 27.36)

5-2.97 List the mechanisms by which cardiac tamponade may be produced by traumatic and non-traumatic events. (p 27.37)

5-2.98 Identify the limiting factor of pericardial anatomy that determines intrapericardiac pressure. (p 27.37)

5-2.99 Identify the clinical criteria specific to cardiac tamponade. (p 27.37)

5-2.100 Describe how to determine if pulsus paradoxus, pulsus alternans or electrical alternans is present. (p 27.25, 27.37)

5-2.101 Identify the paramedic responsibilities associated with management of a patient with cardiac tamponade. (p 27.37)

5-2.102 Describe the incidence, morbidity and mortality of hypertensive emergencies. (p 27.40)

5-2.103 Define the term "hypertensive emergency." (p 27.40)

5-2.104 Identify the characteristics of the patient population at risk for developing a hypertensive emergency. (p 27.40)

5-2.105 Explain the essential pathophysiological defect of hypertension in terms of Starling's law of the heart. (p 27.40)

5-2.106 Identify the progressive vascular changes associated with sustained hypertension. (p 27.40)

5-2.107 Describe the clinical features of the patient in a hypertensive emergency. (p 27.40)

5-2.108 Rank the clinical problems of patients in hypertensive emergencies according to their sense of urgency. (p 27.40)

5-2.109 From the priority of clinical problems identified, state the management responsibilities for the patient with a hypertensive emergency. (p 27.40)

5-2.110 Identify the drugs of choice for hypertensive emergencies, rationale for use, clinical precautions and disadvantages of selected antihypertensive agents. (p 27.41)

5-2.111 Correlate abnormal findings with clinical interpretation of the patient with a hypertensive emergency. (p 27.40)

5-2.112 Define the term "cardiogenic shock." (p 27.37)

5-2.113 Describe the major systemic effects of reduced tissue perfusion caused by cardiogenic shock. (p 27.37)

5-2.114 Explain the primary mechanisms by which the heart may compensate for a diminished cardiac output and describe their efficiency in cardiogenic shock. (p 27.37)

5-2.115 Differentiate progressive stages of cardiogenic shock. (p 27.37)

5-2.116 Identify the clinical criteria for cardiogenic shock. (p 27.37)

5-2.117 Describe the characteristics of patients most likely to develop cardiogenic shock. (p 27.37)

5-2.118 Describe the most commonly used pharmacological agents in the management of cardiogenic shock in terms of therapeutic effects, dosages, routes of administration, side effects and toxic effects. (p 27.38)

5-2.119 Correlate abnormal findings with clinical assessment of the patient in cardiogenic shock. (p 27.37)

5-2.120 Identify the paramedic responsibilities associated with management of a patient in cardiogenic shock. (p 27.38)

5-2.121 Define the term "cardiac arrest." (p 27.72)

5-2.122 Identify the characteristics of patient population at risk for developing cardiac arrest from cardiac causes. (p 27.72)

5-2.123 Identify non-cardiac causes of cardiac arrest. (p 27.72)

5-2.124 Describe the arrhythmias seen in cardiac arrest. (p 27.59)

5-2.125 Identify the critical actions necessary in caring for the patient with cardiac arrest. (p 27.73)

5-2.126 Explain how to confirm asystole using the 3-lead ECG. (p 27.59)

5-2.127 Define the terms defibrillation and synchronized cardioversion. (p 27.80, 27.83)

5-2.128 Specify the methods of supporting the patient with a suspected ineffective implanted defibrillation device. (p 27.61)

5-2.129 Describe the most commonly used pharmacological agents in the managements of cardiac arrest in terms of therapeutic effects. (p 27.84)

5-2.130 Identify resuscitation. (p 27.73)

5-2.131 Identify circumstances and situations where resuscitation efforts would not be initiated. (p 27.77, 27.78)

5-2.132 Identify and list the inclusion and exclusion criteria for termination of resuscitation efforts. (p 27.77, 27.78)

5-2.133 Identify communication and documentation protocols with medical direction and law enforcement used for termination of resuscitation efforts. (p 27.77, 27.78)

5-2.134 Describe the incidence, morbidity and mortality of vascular disorders. (p 27.28)

5-2.135 Describe the pathophysiology of vascular disorders. (p 27.28)

5-2.136 List the traumatic and non-traumatic causes of vascular disorders. (p 27.28)

5-2.137 Define the terms "aneurysm," "claudication," and "phlebitis." (p 27.28)

5-2.138 Identify the peripheral arteries most commonly affected by occlusive disease. (p 27.28)

5-2.139 Identify the major factors involved in the pathophysiology of aortic aneurysm. (p 27.38)

5-2.140 Recognize the usual order of signs and symptoms that develop following peripheral artery occlusion. (p 27.28)

5-2.141 Identify the clinical significance of claudication and presence of arterial bruits in a patient with peripheral vascular disorders. (p 27.28)

5-2.142 Describe the clinical significance of unequal arterial blood pressure readings in the arms. (p 27.25)

5-2.143 Recognize and describe the signs and symptoms of dissecting thoracic or abdominal aneurysm. (p 27.38)

5-2.144 Describe the significant elements of the patient history in a patient with vascular disease. (p 27.28)

5-2.145 Identify the hemodynamic effects of vascular disorders. (p 27.28)

5-2.146 Identify the complications of vascular disorders. (p 27.27)

5-2.147 Identify the Paramedic's responsibilities associated with management of patients with vascular disorders. (p 27.31)

5-2.148 Develop, execute and evaluate a treatment plan based on the field impression for the patient with vascular disorders. (p 27.31)

5-2.149 Differentiate between signs and symptoms of cardiac tamponade, hypertensive emergencies, cardiogenic shock, and cardiac arrest. (p 27.36–27.41)

5-2.150 Based on the pathophysiology and clinical evaluation of the patient with chest pain, characterize the clinical problems according to their life-threatening potential. (p 27.29)

5-2.151 Apply knowledge of the epidemiology of cardiovascular disease to develop prevention strategies. (p 27.6)

5-2.152 Integrate pathophysiological principles into the assessment of a patient with cardiovascular disease. (p 27.27)

5-2.153 Apply knowledge of the epidemiology of cardiovascular disease to develop prevention strategies. (p 27.27)

5-2.154 Integrate pathophysiological principles into the assessment of a patient with cardiovascular disease. (p 27.23)

5-2.155 Synthesize patient history, assessment findings and ECG analysis to form a field impression for the patient with cardiovascular disease. (p 27.27)

5-2.156 Integrate pathophysiological principles to the assessment of a patient in need of a pacemaker. (p 27.60)

5-2.157 Synthesize patient history, assessment findings and ECG analysis to form a field impression for the patient in need of a pacemaker. (p 27.60, 27.61)

5-2.158 Develop, execute, and evaluate a treatment plan based on field impression for the patient in need of a pacemaker. (p 27.61)

5-2.159 Based on the pathophysiology and clinical evaluation of the patient with chest pain, characterize the clinical problems according to their life-threatening potential. (p 27.29)

5-2.160 Integrate pathophysiological principles to the assessment of a patient with chest pain. (p 27.27)

5-2.161 Synthesize patient history, assessment findings and ECG analysis to form a field impression for the patient with angina pectoris. (p 27.28)

5-2.162 Develop, execute and evaluate a treatment plan based on the field impression for the patient with chest pain. (p 27.29)

5-2.163 Integrate pathophysiological principles to the assessment of a patient with a suspected myocardial infarction. (p 27.29)

5-2.164 Synthesize patient history, assessment findings and ECG analysis to form a field impression for the patient with a suspected myocardial infarction. (p 27.29)

5-2.165 Develop, execute and evaluate a treatment plan based on the field impression for the suspected myocardial infarction patient. (p 27.31)

5-2.166 Integrate pathophysiological principles to the assessment of the patient with heart failure. (p 27.34)

5-2.167 Synthesize assessment findings and patient history information to form a field impression of the patient with heart failure. (p 27.36)

5-2.168 Develop, execute, and evaluate a treatment plan based on the field impression for the heart failure patient. (p 27.36)

5-2.169 Integrate pathophysiological principles to the assessment of a patient with cardiac tamponade. (p 27.31)

5-2.170 Synthesize assessment findings and patient history information to form a field impression of the patient with cardiac tamponade. (p 27.31)

5-2.171 Develop, execute and evaluate a treatment plan based on the field impression for the patient with cardiac tamponade. (p 27.37)

5-2.172 Integrate pathophysiological principles to the assessment of the patient with a hypertensive emergency. (p 27.40)

5-2.173 Synthesize assessment findings and patient history information to form a field impression of the patient with a hypertensive emergency. (p 27.40)

5-2.174 Develop, execute and evaluate a treatment plan based on the field impression for the patient with a hypertensive emergency. (p 27.40)

5-2.175 Integrate pathophysiological principles to the assessment of the patient with cardiogenic shock. (p 27.37)

5-2.176 Synthesize assessment findings and patient history information to form a field impression of the patient with cardiogenic shock. (p 27.37)

5-2.177 Develop, execute, and evaluate a treatment plan based on the field impression for the patient with cardiogenic shock. (p 27.37)

5-2.178 Integrate the pathophysiological principles to the assessment of the patient with cardiac arrest. (p 27.72)

5-2.179 Synthesize assessment findings to formulate a rapid intervention for a patient in cardiac arrest. (p 27.73)

5-2.180 Synthesize assessment findings to formulate the termination of resuscitative efforts for a patient in cardiac arrest. (p 27.77, 27.78)

5-2.181 Integrate pathophysiological principles to the assessment of a patient with vascular disorders. (p 27.28)

5-2.182 Synthesize assessment findings and patient history to form a field impression for the patient with vascular disorders. (p 27.28)

5-2.183 Integrate pathophysiological principles to the assessment and field management of a patient with chest pain. (p 27.31)

Affective

5-2.184 Value the sense of urgency for initial assessment and intervention in the patient with cardiac compromise. (p 27.23)

5-2.185 Value and defend the sense of urgency necessary to protect the window of opportunity for reperfusion in the patient with suspected myocardial infarction. (p 27.33)

5-2.186 Defend patient situations where ECG rhythm analysis is indicated. (p 27.41)

5-2.187 Value and defend the application of transcutaneous pacing system. (p 27.83)

5-2.188 Value and defend the urgency in identifying pacemaker malfunction. (p 27.61)

5-2.189 Based on the pathophysiology and clinical evaluation of the patient with acute myocardial infarction, characterize the clinical problems according to their life-threatening potential. (p 27.30)

5-2.190 Defend the measures that may be taken to prevent or minimize complications in the patient with a suspected myocardial infarction. (p 27.31)

5-2.191 Defend the urgency based on the severity of the patient's clinical problems in a hypertensive emergency. (p 27.40)

5-2.192 From the priority of clinical problems identified, state the management responsibilities for the patient with a hypertensive emergency. (p 27.40)

5-2.193 Value and defend the urgency in rapid determination of and rapid intervention of patients in cardiac arrest. (p 27.73)

5-2.194 Value and defend the possibility of termination of resuscitative efforts in the out-of-hospital setting. (p 27.77)

5-2.195 Based on the pathophysiology and clinical evaluation of the patient with vascular disorders, characterize the clinical problems according to their life-threatening potential. (p 27.27)

5-2.196 Value and defend the sense of urgency in identifying peripheral vascular occlusion. (p 27.28)

5-2.197 Value and defend the sense of urgency in recognizing signs of aortic aneurysm. (p 27.38)

Psychomotor

5-2.198 Demonstrate how to set and adjust the ECG monitor settings to varying patient situations. (p 27.42)

5-2.199 Demonstrate a working knowledge of various ECG lead systems. (p 27.65)

5-2.200 Demonstrate how to record an ECG. (p 27.42)

5-2.201 Perform, document and communicate a cardiovascular assessment. (p 27.23)

5-2.202 Set up and apply a transcutaneous pacing system. (p 27.83)

5-2.203 Given the model of a patient with signs and symptoms of heart failure, position the patient to afford comfort and relief. (p 27.36)

5-2.204 Demonstrate how to determine if pulsus paradoxus, pulsus alternans or electrical alternans is present. (p 27.25)

5-2.205 Demonstrate satisfactory performance of psychomotor skills of basic and advanced life support techniques according to the current American Heart Association Standards and Guidelines, including:
   a. Cardiopulmonary resuscitation
   b. Defibrillation
   c. Synchronized cardioversion
   d. Transcutaneous pacing (p 27.83, App A)

5-2.206 Complete a communication patch with medical direction and law enforcement used for termination of resuscitation efforts. (p 27.77)

5-2.207 Demonstrate how to evaluate major peripheral arterial pulses. (p 27.28)

Introduction

Cardiovascular disease (CVD) has been the number one killer in the United States almost every year since 1900. It was for the purpose of providing early, definitive treatment for patients with acute myocardial infarction (AMI) that the job of paramedic first came into being more than 30 years ago. Even with paramedic availability, more than 600,000 Americans die every year of coronary heart disease; approximately half die in an emergency department (ED) or before reaching a hospital, during the first minutes and hours after the onset of symptoms. It is easy to see why the recognition and management of cardiovascular emergencies continue to receive strong emphasis in paramedic education.

This chapter is intended to prepare you to integrate pathophysiologic principles and assessment findings to formulate a field impression and implement the treatment plan for patients with CVD. We begin by looking at the epidemiology of CVD in terms of its prevalence, mortality and morbidity, risk factors, and prevention strategies. After reviewing the anatomy and function of the cardiovascular system, we examine some of the clinical manifestations of CVD. Considerable emphasis is given to the interpretation of cardiac arrhythmias and their management within the context of the patient's overall clinical condition. Finally, we examine the pharmacologic and other treatment modalities that make up advanced cardiac life support (ACLS).

Epidemiology

According to the American Heart Association (AHA), CVD was the cause of about 37% of all US deaths. The many risk factors for coronary artery disease (CAD) include age, family history, hypertension, elevated cholesterol level, smoking, and carbohydrate intolerance. It was previously thought that CAD was a man's disease, but we now realize that more women die of a cardiac event than men. Other factors contributing to CAD include diet, obesity, oral contraceptive use, sedentary lifestyle, stress, and personality type.

A healthy lifestyle may be all a person with a low risk needs to ward off CAD. High-risk people may be treated by using a combination of drug and nondrug therapies. This aggressive approach can reduce the risk of heart attack by 50% according to data presented by Scott Grundy, MD, PhD, of the Center for Human Nutrition in Dallas, Texas. Patients classified as being at intermediate risk may benefit from further testing for signs of atherosclerosis, which is an indicator of heart disease.

Education and early recognition are also important prevention strategies. Making people aware of the risk factors and signs and symptoms of CVD may decrease its prevalence. This is an area of interest for EMS providers who are involved in community heath promotion. **Table 27-1 ▾** lists goals for decreasing CVD risks.

Cardiovascular Anatomy and Physiology

Structure and Function

The cardiovascular system is composed of the heart and blood vessels. Its primary function is to deliver oxygenated blood and nutrients to every cell in the body. It is also responsible for

Table 27-1	Goals for Decreasing CVD Risks
■ Quit smoking	
■ Lower and control blood pressure	
■ Lower total cholesterol level	
■ Lower LDL cholesterol level	
■ Increase HDL cholesterol level	
■ Lower weight, if overweight	
■ Increase aerobic exercise	

LDL indicates low-density lipoprotein; and HDL, high-density lipoprotein.

You are the Provider Part 1

You and your partner are enjoying the rare treat of a quiet Sunday shift. You are watching television, and your partner is studying for final exams. You are about to drift off when the pager disrupts the tranquility. You are dispatched to the medical school library for an unknown medical emergency. On arrival you and your partner are led to the third floor stacks where you find a 22-year-old man complaining of palpitations.

Initial Assessment	Recording Time: 0 Minutes
Appearance	Young, well-nourished man; appears anxious and nervous
Level of consciousness	A (Alert to person, place, and day)
Airway	Open
Breathing	Normal rate, adequate volume
Circulation	Strong and rapid radial pulses with pink, warm, diaphoretic skin

1. What are some potential causes of palpitations?
2. What questions would you like to ask your patient at this time?

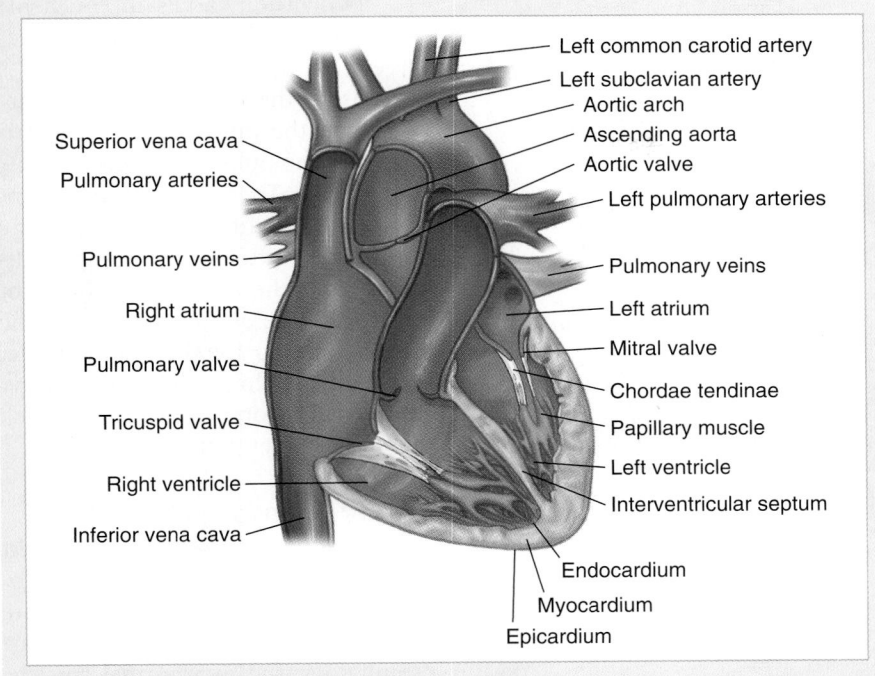

Figure 27-1 Anatomy of the heart.

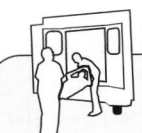

In the Field

Three components are required to have adequate tissue perfusion: pump (heart), container (vessels) and fluid (blood).

delivering chemical messages (hormones) within the body and for transporting the waste products of metabolism from the cells to sites of recycling or waste disposal.

The Heart

The driving force behind this extensive pickup and delivery service is the heart Figure 27-1, a remarkable little pump that sits in the chest, above the diaphragm, behind and slightly to the left of the lower sternum (retrosternal). The heart is not much larger than a man's fist and weighs only 250 to 300 g (about 9 oz). Despite its relatively small size, it is big and strong enough to move 7,000 to 9,000 L of blood around the body every day of our lives!

On visualization of the chest, one may be able to see the apical thrust or point of maximal impulse (PMI). The PMI is normally located on the left anterior part of chest, in the midclavicular line, at the fifth intercostal space. This thrust occurs when the heart's apex rotates forward with systole, gently beating against the chest wall and producing a pulsation.

Surrounding the heart is a tough, fibrous sac called the pericardium. The pericardium normally contains about 30 mL of serous fluid, which serves as a lubricant—that is, it enables the heart muscle, as it contracts and relaxes, to slide easily within the pericardial sac. The pericardium does not stretch readily, so it cannot accommodate sudden accumulations of fluid.

The wall of the heart consists of three layers:
- The epicardium, the outermost surface layer, is a thin serous membrane.
- The endocardium is the innermost smooth layer of connective tissue.
- The myocardium is the muscular layer of the cardiac wall found between the epicardium and endocardium.

Like all cells in the body, myocardial cells require an uninterrupted supply of oxygen and nutrients. Indeed, the cardiac demand for oxygen is particularly unremitting because the heart never stops to rest (not without catastrophic consequences), so it is essential that the heart have an absolutely reliable blood supply. Oxygenated blood reaches the heart through the coronary arteries Figure 27-2 ▶, which branch off the aorta at the coronary ostia, just above the leaflets of the aortic valve. There are two main coronary arteries—left and right. The left main coronary artery subdivides into the left anterior descending and circumflex coronary arteries, both of which branch widely to supply the more muscular left ventricle of the heart along with the interventricular septum and part of the right ventricle. The right coronary artery (RCA) supplies the right atrium and ventricle and part of the left ventricle. The numerous connections (anastomoses) between the arterioles of the various coronary arteries allow for the development of alternative routes of blood flow (collateral circulation) in case of blockage. Unfortunately, the coronary arteries are also vulnerable to narrowing in atherosclerotic heart disease. When the lumen (channel) of one of those arteries becomes so narrowed that blood flow through it is impeded, the symptoms of angina occur.

The arteries and the main coronary vein cross the heart in a groove, called the coronary sulcus, that separates the atria from the ventricles. Venous blood empties into the coronary sinus, a large vessel in the posterior part of the coronary sulcus, which in turn ends in the right atrium of the heart.

Structurally, the heart consists of four chambers (see Figure 27-2). The upper chambers of the heart, or atria, are separated from their respective lower chambers, or ventricles, by atrioventricular (AV) valves, which prevent backflow during ventricular contraction. The tricuspid valve separates the right atrium from the right ventricle; the mitral valve separates the left atrium from the left ventricle. Anatomic guide wires, called chordae tendineae, attached to papillary muscles within the heart anchor those two valves and keep them from inverting (prolapsing) during ventricular contraction. Injury or disease, however, may disrupt the chordae tendineae and permit a valve leaflet to prolapse, allowing blood to regurgitate from the ventricle into the atrium.

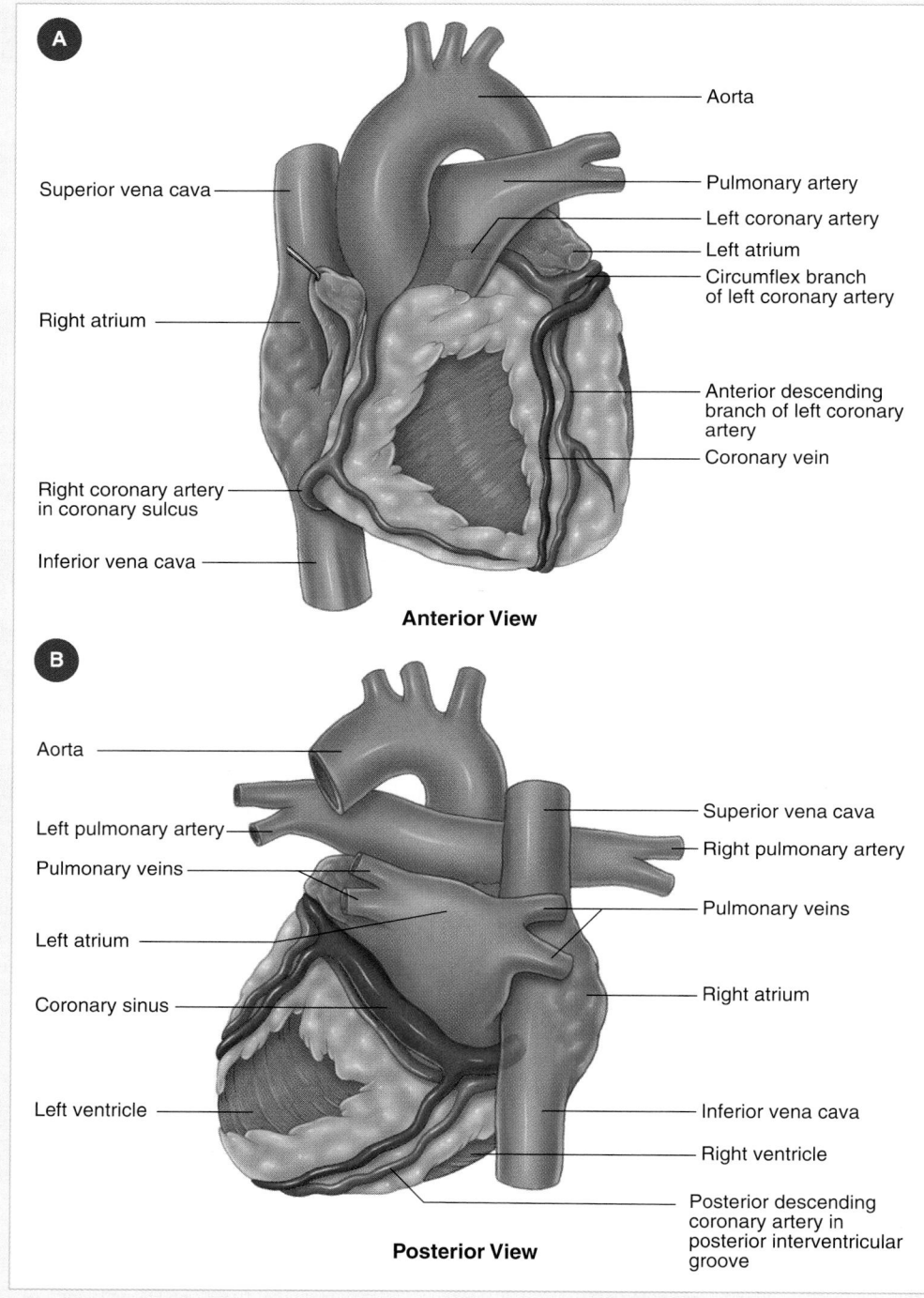

A

Aorta

Superior vena cava

Pulmonary artery

Left coronary artery

Left atrium

Circumflex branch
of left coronary artery

Right atrium

Anterior descending
branch of left coronary
artery

Coronary vein

Right coronary artery
in coronary sulcus

Inferior vena cava

Anterior View

B

Aorta

Left pulmonary artery

Pulmonary veins

Left atrium

Coronary sinus

Left ventricle

Superior vena cava

Right pulmonary artery

Pulmonary veins

Right atrium

Inferior vena cava

Right ventricle

Posterior descending
coronary artery in
posterior interventricular
groove

Posterior View

Figure 27-2 Coronary arteries. **A.** Anterior view, showing takeoff point of left and right main coronary arteries from the aorta. **B.** View from below and behind, showing the coronary sinus.

In the Field

The mitral valve is on the left side of the heart. The left side has higher pressure than the right. Because the mitral valve is involved in the higher pressure side, remember it as the "mighty" valve.

Two other valves in the heart **Figure 27-3 ▸**, which are collectively known as semilunar valves because of their half-moon shape, are found at the junction of the ventricles and the pulmonary and systemic circulation. The pulmonic valve separates the right ventricle from the pulmonary artery, preventing backflow from the artery into the right ventricle. The aortic valve serves the same function for the left ventricle, preventing blood that has already entered the aorta from flowing back into the left ventricle.

Heart Sounds

The purpose of listening to heart sounds is to identify the "lub-dub" that indicates the cardiac valves are operating properly. The major heart sounds are the two normal sounds, S_1 and S_2 **Figure 27-4 ▸**, and the two abnormal sounds, S_3 and S_4 **Figure 27-5 ▸**.

S_1 occurs near the beginning of ventricular contraction (systole), when the tricuspid and mitral valves close. The closing of these two valves should occur simultaneously as the pressure within the ventricles increases. Any delay in the closing of these two valves, heard as a split sound, is considered abnormal.

S_2 occurs near the end of ventricular contraction (systole), when the pulmonary and aortic valves close. As the ventricles relax, these valves close because of backward flow in the pulmonary artery and aorta. The two valves can close simultaneously or with a slight delay between them under normal physiologic circumstances.

S_3 is the result of the end of the rapid filling period of the ventricle during the beginning of diastole. An S_3 sound should occur 120 to 170 milliseconds (ms) after S_2, if it is heard at all. S_3 is generally heard in children and young adults. When it is heard in older adults, it often signifies heart failure.

S_4, if heard, coincides with atrial contraction at the end of ventricular diastole. If heard at any other time, it usually occurs in patients who have resistance to ventricular filling, as in a weak left ventricle.

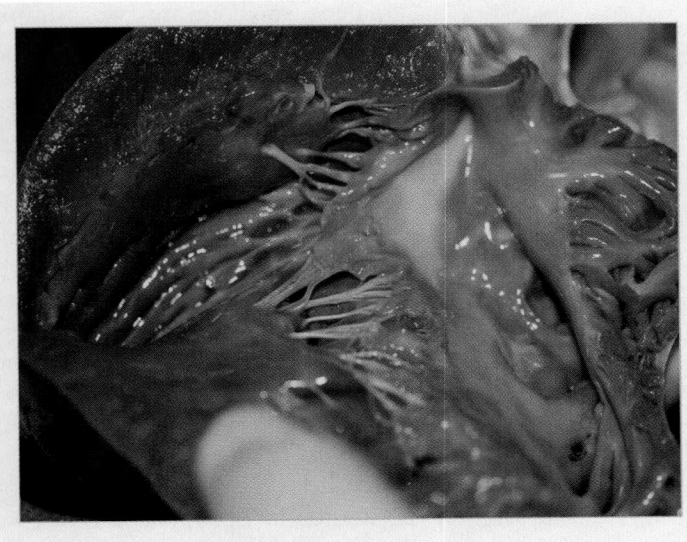

Figure 27-3 Heart valves.

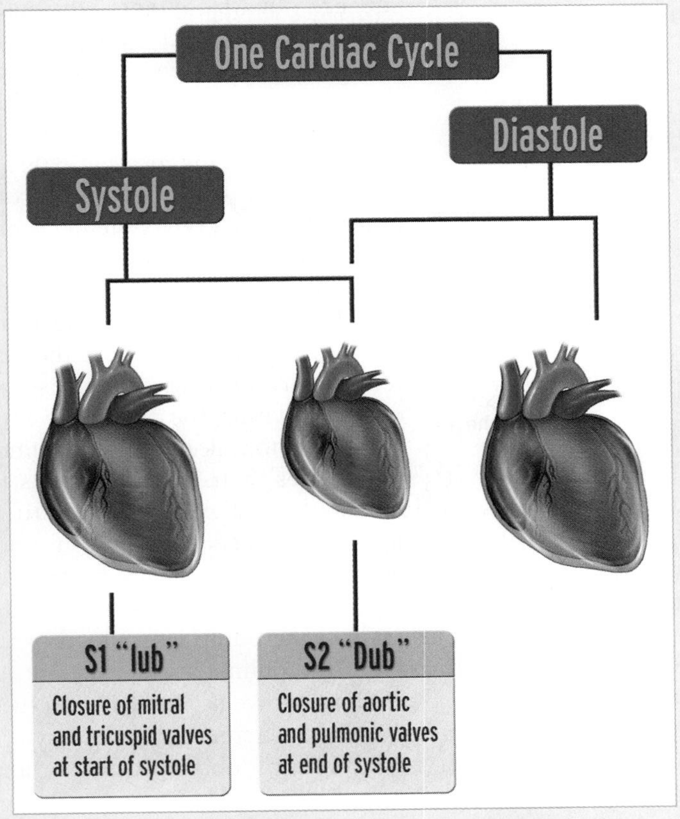

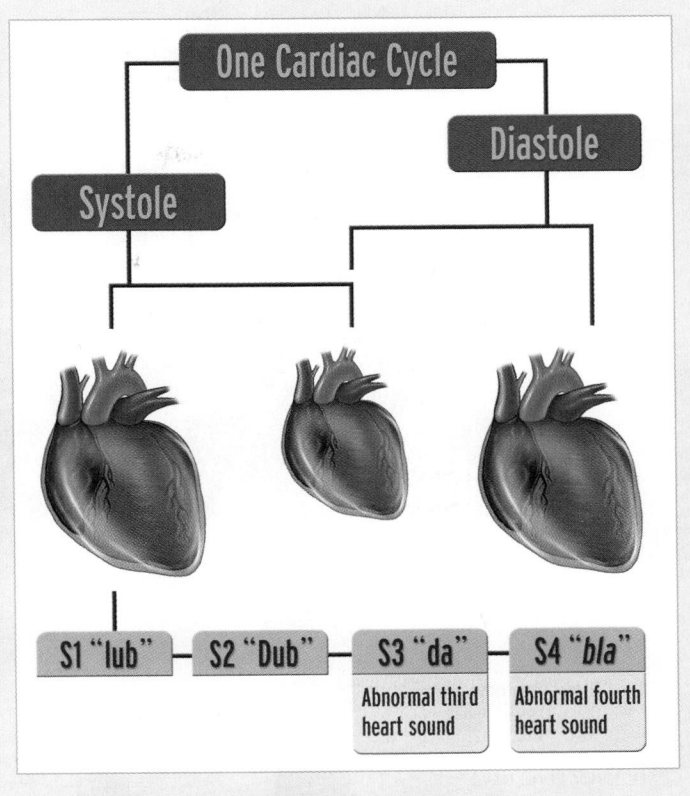

Figure 27-5 The abnormal S₃ and S₄ heart sounds.

In the Field

Atrial kick describes approximately 20% of blood flow that comes from the atria to the ventricles by contraction. The other 80% gets from the atria to the ventricles passively via gravity.

One Cardiac Cycle — Systole — Diastole

S1 "lub" — S2 "Dub"

S1 "lub"
Closure of mitral and tricuspid valves at start of systole

S2 "Dub"
Closure of aortic and pulmonic valves at end of systole

Figure 27-4 The normal S₁ and S₂ heart sounds.

The Cardiac Cycle

The cardiac cycle comprises one complete phase of atrial and ventricular relaxation (diastole), followed by one atrial and ventricular contraction (systole).

During the relatively longer relaxation phase (normally 0.52 second [s]), the left atrium fills passively with blood, under the influence of venous pressure. Approximately 80% of ventricular filling also occurs during this time as blood flows through the open tricuspid and mitral valves.

With atrial contraction (normally both atria contract at the same time), the contents of each atrium are squeezed into the respective ventricle to complete ventricular filling. The contribution to ventricular filling made by contraction of the atrium is referred to as atrial kick—it is the amount of blood "kicked in" by the atrium. At the beginning of ventricular contraction, the AV valves snap shut, the two ventricles contract (ventricular systole), and the semilunar valves are forced open. Blood squeezed out of the right ventricle moves forward, through the pulmonic valve, and into the pulmonary arteries. Blood from the left ventricle is pushed through the aortic valve and out into the aorta. Systole is usually accomplished in a little more than half the time it takes to fill the ventricles, about 0.28 s.

Two Pumps in One

Although we called the heart a pump, that description is not entirely accurate. Functionally, the heart is actually *two*

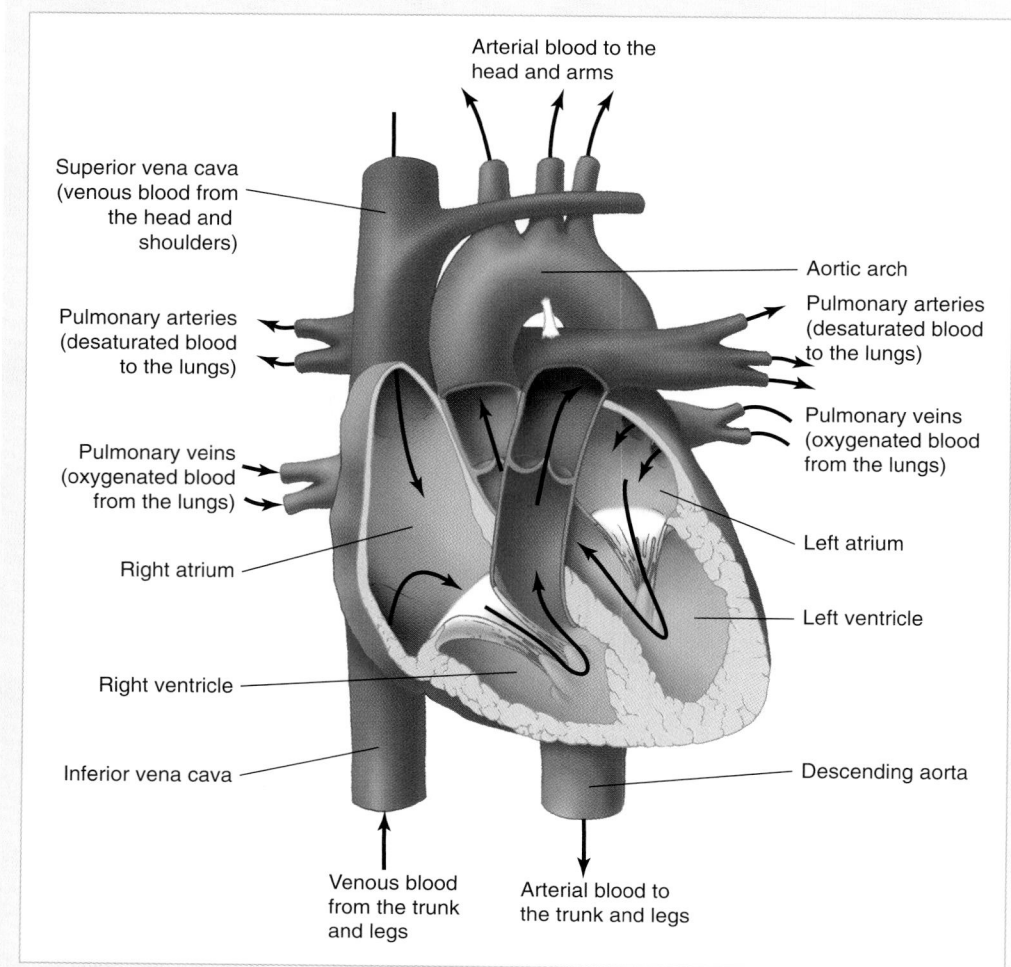

Arterial blood to the head and arms

Superior vena cava (venous blood from the head and shoulders)

Aortic arch

Pulmonary arteries (desaturated blood to the lungs)

Pulmonary arteries (desaturated blood to the lungs)

Pulmonary veins (oxygenated blood from the lungs)

Pulmonary veins (oxygenated blood from the lungs)

Left atrium

Right atrium

Left ventricle

Right ventricle

Inferior vena cava

Descending aorta

Venous blood from the trunk and legs

Arterial blood to the trunk and legs

Figure 27-6 Blood flow through the heart. Desaturated blood enters the right atrium from the venae cavae, proceeds to the right ventricle, and from there moves via the pulmonary arteries to the lungs. Oxygenated blood enters the left atrium from the pulmonary veins, proceeds to the left ventricle, and then goes out to the body via the aorta.

pumps—a right pump and a left pump, separated by a thin wall (the interventricular septum)—that just happen, for purposes of efficiency, to be housed in one organ and to work in parallel **Figure 27-6 ▲** .

The right side of the heart, which is composed of the right atrium and right ventricle, is a *low-pressure* pump: It pumps against the relatively low resistance of the pulmonary circulation. The right atrium collects oxygen-poor venous blood from the venae cavae and the coronary sinus and pumps it into the right ventricle, which pumps the blood into the pulmonary artery for distribution to the alveoli and oxygenation.

The pulmonary veins collect the now oxygen-rich blood and return it to the left side of the heart—specifically, to the left atrium, which pumps it into the powerful left ventricle. The left side of the heart is a *high-pressure* pump: It drives blood out of the heart against the relatively high resistance of the systemic arteries.

Because there are two pumps, there must be two sets of tubing into which the pumps empty. Thus, the human body, in effect, has two circulations. The systemic circulation **Figure 27-7A ▸** consists of all blood vessels beyond the left ventricle up to the right atrium, which receive the output of the left side of the heart. The pulmonary circulation **Figure 27-7B ▸** comprises the blood vessels between the right ventricle and left atrium, which receive the output of the right side of the heart.

At any given time, a major proportion of the body's blood flow may be shunted into one of these two circulations. If, for example, the right side of the pump fails and cannot squeeze out its contents efficiently, blood will back up behind the right atrium into the systemic veins, which then become engorged and distended. The most readily visible of the systemic veins are the external jugular veins, which reflect the condition of all the other systemic veins. Distention of the external jugular veins signals that there is considerable back pressure from the right side of the heart throughout the systemic circulation. As pressure increases within the systemic veins, fluid starts to leak into the surrounding tissues, causing the tissues to swell. When enough fluid has leaked into the interstitial spaces, that swelling becomes visible as edema in the subcutaneous tissues; it is less readily visible, but equally present, in the liver, walls of the intestine, and other internal tissues.

By contrast, if the left side of the pump fails, blood backs up behind the left atrium into the pulmonary circulation. As pressure builds up in the pulmonary veins, fluid is squeezed into the alveoli, producing the characteristic signs and symptoms of pulmonary edema: dyspnea, bubbling crackles, and frothy sputum.

The Blood Vessels

Besides the "cardio" component (the heart), the cardiovascular system includes a second, "vascular" component—that is, the blood vessels. There are two principal types of blood vessels in the human body—arteries and veins—both of which share a common structure **Figure 27-8 ▸** . A protective outer layer of fibrous tissue, the tunica adventitia, provides blood vessels with the strength needed to withstand high pressure against their

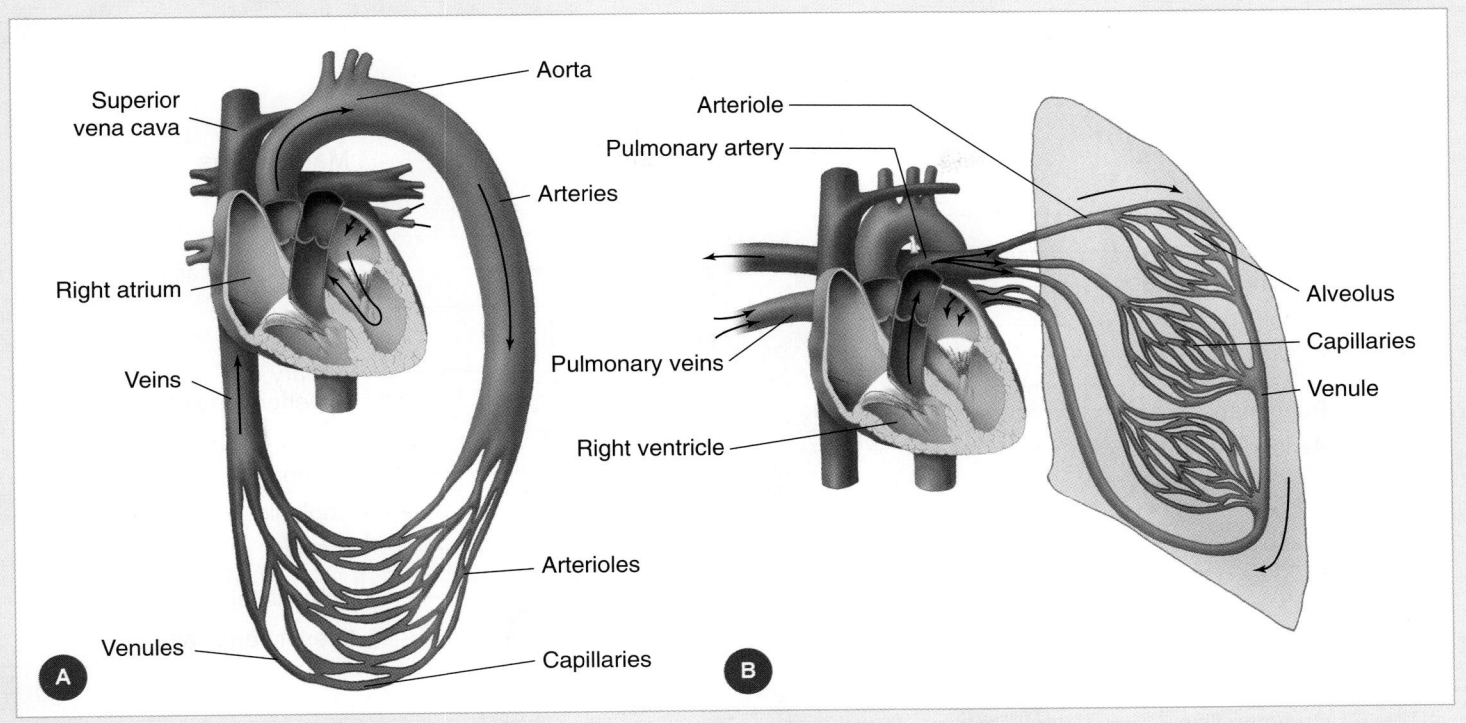

Figure 27-7 Dual human circulation. **A.** The systemic circulation consists of all blood vessels distal to the left ventricle. **B.** The pulmonary circulation consists of all blood vessels between the right ventricle and the left atrium.

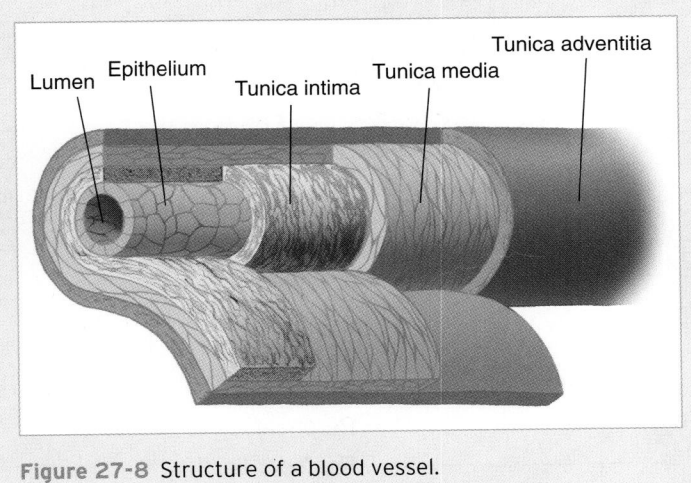

Figure 27-8 Structure of a blood vessel.

walls. A middle layer of elastic fibers and muscle, the tunica media, gives strength and contractility to blood vessels. This medial layer is much thicker and more powerful in arteries than in veins. The innermost layer of the blood vessel, the tunica intima, is a smooth inner lining that is only one cell thick. The opening within the blood vessel is referred to as the lumen.

Arteries are thick-walled, muscular vessels—befitting pipes operating in a high-pressure system—that carry blood away from the heart. Usually, arteries carry *oxygenated* blood; the only exceptions are the pulmonary arteries, which carry

oxygen-depleted blood from the right ventricle to the lungs (they carry blood away from the heart). Arteries range in size from the largest artery in the body, the aorta, to the tiniest arterial branch, or arteriole. **Figure 27-9** ▶ depicts the major arteries in the body.

Arterial walls are highly sensitive to stimulation from the autonomic nervous system. Indeed, in response to that stimulation, their diameter may change significantly as the arteries contract and relax. In that manner, the arteries help to regulate blood pressure—that is, the pressure exerted by the blood against the arterial walls. Blood pressure is generated by repeated forceful contractions of the left ventricle, which keep blood flowing through the body. The magnitude of the blood pressure is influenced not only by the output of the heart and the volume of blood present in the system, but also by the relative constriction or dilatation of arteries.

Veins, which operate on the low-pressure side of the system, have thinner walls than arteries and, consequently, less capacity to decrease their diameter. The thinner walls also make the veins much more likely to distend when exposed to small increases in "backpressure." Veins carry blood to the heart—as a rule, oxygen-poor blood. The only exceptions are the pulmonary veins, which carry oxygenated blood to the left side of the heart. The smallest veins, or venules, gradually empty into larger and larger veins, terminating in the two largest veins of the body, the inferior and superior venae cavae. Veins also contain valves (which are unnecessary in arteries); these valves keep the blood flowing in the forward direction only.

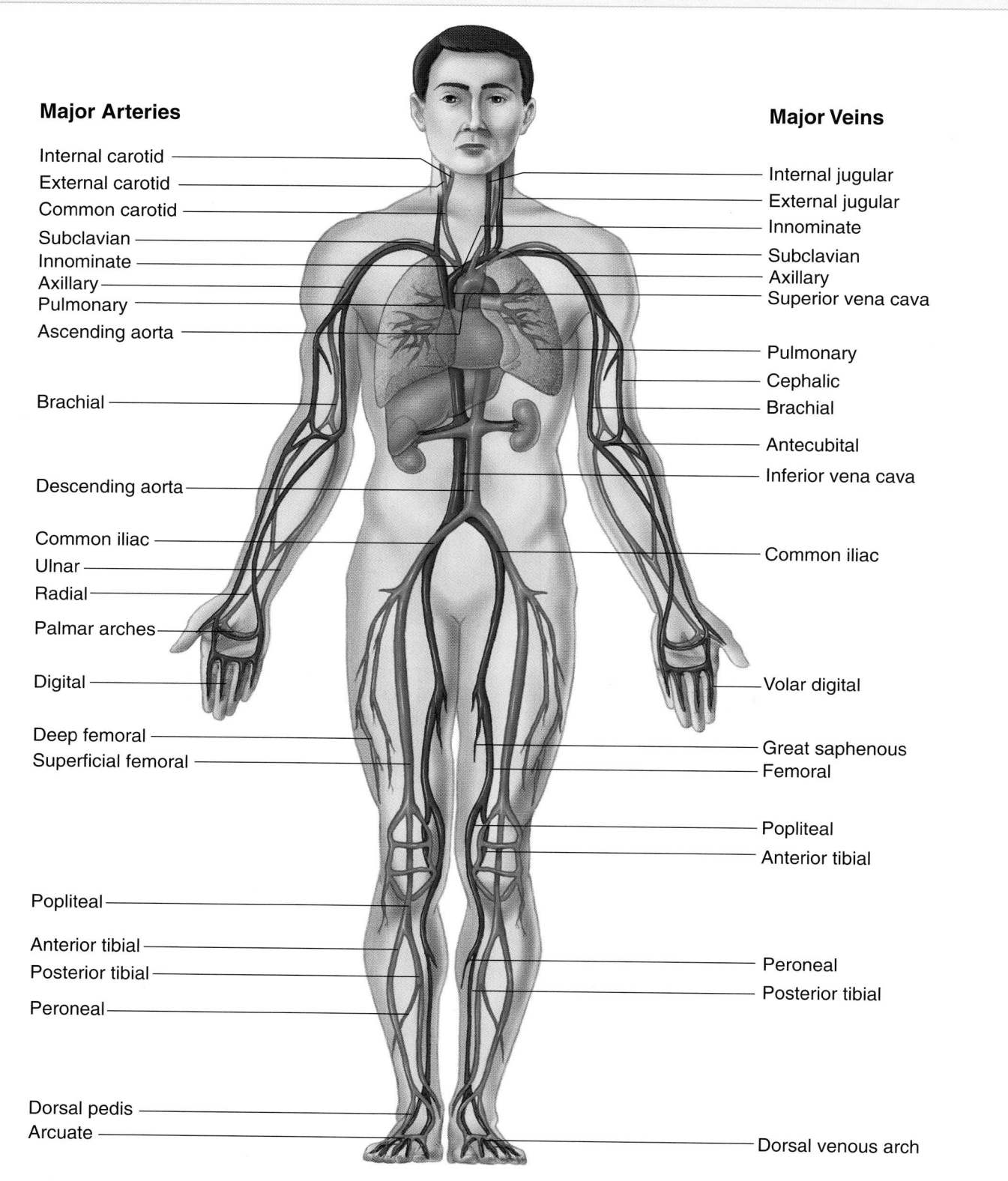

Major Arteries

Internal carotid
External carotid
Common carotid
Subclavian
Innominate
Axillary
Pulmonary
Ascending aorta

Brachial

Descending aorta

Common iliac
Ulnar
Radial
Palmar arches

Digital

Deep femoral
Superficial femoral

Popliteal

Anterior tibial
Posterior tibial
Peroneal

Dorsal pedis
Arcuate

Major Veins

Internal jugular
External jugular
Innominate
Subclavian
Axillary
Superior vena cava

Pulmonary
Cephalic
Brachial

Antecubital
Inferior vena cava

Common iliac

Volar digital

Great saphenous
Femoral

Popliteal
Anterior tibial

Peroneal

Posterior tibial

Dorsal venous arch

Figure 27-9 The major arteries and veins.

Between the tiny arterioles and venules at the tissue level is a network of microscopic blood vessels called capillaries. The walls of capillaries are extremely thin—only one cell thick—enabling the exchange of gases and nutrients across them; the capillary diameter is so small that red blood cells must pass through them single file.

The Pump at Work

To understand how the heart functions as a pump, it is necessary to learn some technical terms:

- **Cardiac output (CO).** The amount of blood that is pumped out by either ventricle. The left and right ventricles are approximately equal in interior size, so the two ventricles have relatively equivalent outputs. Normal CO for an average adult is 5 to 6 L/min.
- **Stroke volume (SV).** The amount of blood pumped out by either ventricle in a single contraction (heartbeat). Normally, the SV is 60 to 100 mL, but the healthy heart has considerable spare capacity and can easily increase SV by at least 50%.
- **Heart rate (HR).** The number of cardiac contractions (heartbeats) per minute—in other words, the pulse rate. The normal HR for adults is 60 to 100 beats/min.

The volume of blood that either ventricle pumps out per minute equals the volume of blood it pumps out in a single contraction times the number of contractions per minute:

$$CO = SV \times HR$$

To meet changing demands, the heart must be able to increase its output several times over in response to the body's increased demand for oxygen—for example, during exercise. The CO equation tells us that the heart can increase its output by increasing its SV, increasing its rate, or both.

In a mechanical piston pump, the SV is a fixed quantity related to the distance traveled by the piston and the size of the cylinder. The heart, by contrast, has several ways of increasing SV. One characteristic of cardiac muscle is that, when it is stretched, it contracts with greater force to a limit—a property called the Frank-Starling mechanism. If an increased volume of blood is returned from the systemic veins to the right side of the heart or from the pulmonary veins to the left side of the heart, the muscle surrounding the cardiac chambers must stretch to accommodate the larger volume. The more the cardiac muscle stretches, the greater the force of its contraction, the more completely it empties, and, therefore, the greater the SV. From the CO equation, it is clear that any increase in SV, with the HR held constant, will cause an increase in the overall CO.

The pressure under which a ventricle fills is called the preload and is influenced by the volume of blood returned by the veins to the heart. In situations of increased oxygen demand, the body returns more blood to the heart (preload increases), and CO consequently increases through the Frank-Starling mechanism. In a diseased heart, the same mechanism is used

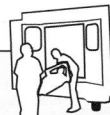

In the Field

The Frank-Starling mechanism is named after the two men who first described it. In the late 19th century, Otto Frank discovered that in the frog heart, the strength of ventricular contraction was increased when the ventricle was stretched before contraction. In the 20th century, Ernest Starling expounded on this information with studies finding that increasing venous return, and, therefore, the filling pressure of the ventricle, led to increased SV in dogs.

to achieve a normal resting CO (which explains why some diseased hearts become enlarged).

The heart can also vary the degree of contraction of its muscle *without* changing the stretch on the muscle—a property called contractility. Changes in contractility may be induced by medications that have a positive or negative inotropic effect. The ventricles are never completely emptied of blood with any single beat. However, if the heart squeezes into a tighter ball when it contracts, a larger percentage of the ventricular blood will be ejected, thereby increasing SV and overall CO. Nervous controls regulate the contractility of the heart from beat to beat. When the body requires increased CO, nervous signals increase myocardial contractility, thereby augmenting SV.

The heart can also increase its CO, given a constant SV, by increasing the number of contractions per minute—that is, by increasing the HR (positive chronotropic effect). As an example, consider a heart that has a resting SV of 70 mL/beat and a resting rate of 70 beats/min:

$$CO = 70\ mL \times 70\ beats/min = 4,900\ mL$$

Suppose that the owner of that heart begins to exercise. Oxygen demand increases, and nervous mechanisms stimulate the heart to increase its rate. If, for example, the HR increases to 110 beats/min without any change in the SV, the CO would increase as follows:

The Frank-Starling mechanism is an intrinsic property of heart muscle—that is, it is not under nervous system control. By contrast, contractility and changes in HR are regulated by the nervous system.

$$CO = 70\ mL/beat \times 110\ beats/min = 7,700\ mL/min$$

The Electrical Conduction System of the Heart

Heart muscle is unique among body tissues because it can generate its own electric impulses without stimulation from nerves, a property known as automaticity. In addition, the heart is endowed with specialized conduction tissue that can rapidly propagate electrical impulses to the muscular tissue of the heart. The area of conduction tissue in which the electrical activity arises at any given time is called the pacemaker, because it sets the pace (that is, rate) for cardiac contraction. This system as a whole is termed the electrical conduction system.

The Dominant Pacemaker: The Sinoatrial Node

Theoretically, any cell within the heart's electrical conduction system can act as a pacemaker. In the normal heart, however, the dominant pacemaker is the sinoatrial (SA) node, which is located in the right atrium, near the inlet of the superior vena cava (Figure 27-10 ▼). The SA node receives blood from the

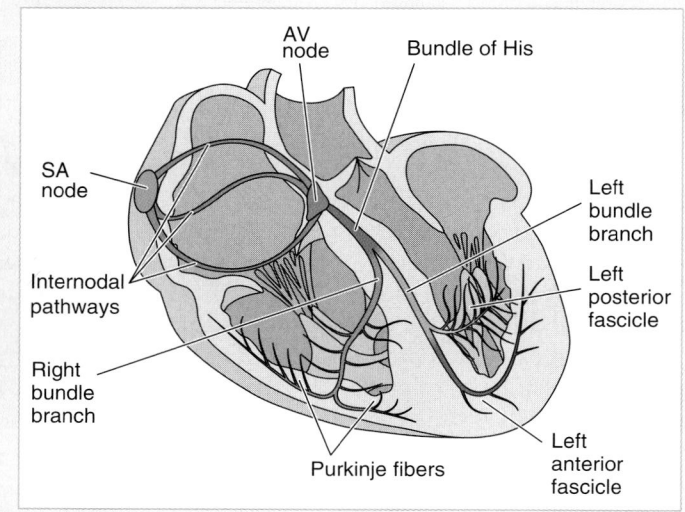

Figure 27-10 Electrical conduction system of the heart. Impulses that originate in the SA node spread through the atria and along the internodal pathways to the AV node. From the AV node, they travel down the bundle of His and right and left bundle branches and into the Purkinje network of the ventricles.

RCA. If the RCA is occluded, as in a myocardial infarction (MI), the SA node will become ischemic. The subsequent death of the conduction cells will prevent the SA node from firing.

The SA node is the fastest pacemaker in the heart. Electric impulses generated in this node spread across the two atria through internodal pathways (including the Bachman bundle) in the atrial wall in about 0.08 s, causing the atrial tissue to depolarize as they pass. From there, they move to the atrioventricular (AV) node in the region of the AV junction (which includes the AV node and its surrounding tissue along with the bundle of His). The AV node serves as a "gatekeeper" to the ventricles. In 85% to 90% of humans, its blood supply comes from a branch of the RCA; in 10% to 15%, it comes from a branch of the left circumflex artery. The conduction of the impulse is delayed in the AV node for about 0.12 s so that the atria can empty into the ventricles. Approximately 70% to 90% of the blood in the atria fills the ventricles by gravity; the remaining 10% to 30% comes from atrial contraction (atrial kick).

When the atrial rate becomes very rapid, not all atrial impulses can get through the AV junction. Normally, however, impulses pass through it into the bundle of His and then move rapidly into the right and left bundle branches located on either side of the interventricular septum. Next, they spread into the Purkinje fibers, thousands of fibrils distributed through the ventricular muscle. It takes about 0.08 s for an electric impulse to spread across the ventricles, during which time the ventricles contract simultaneously. The effect on the velocity of conduction is referred to as the dromotropic effect.

Depolarization and Repolarization

Depolarization—the process by which muscle fibers are stimulated to contract—comes about through changes in the concentration of electrolytes across cell membranes (Figure 27-11A ▶). Myocardial cells, like all cells in the body, are bathed in an electrolyte solution. Chemical pumps inside the cell maintain the concentrations of ions within the cell, in the process creating an electric gradient across the cell wall. As a consequence, a resting

You are the Provider Part 2

You ask your partner to obtain an initial set of vital signs while you begin your patient assessment. When asked about the palpitations, the patient tells you that they began about 45 minutes ago while he was studying for finals. He is a first-year medical student and needs to do well on finals to avoid being placed on academic probation. He admits to being awake for the past 36 hours with the help of "Monster" energy drinks and caffeine pills. His last oral intake was pizza last night around 11:00 PM. He denies any medical history or allergies and emphatically denies the use of any drugs other than the caffeine pills.

Vital Signs	Recording Time: 5 Minutes
Skin	Pink, warm, and diaphoretic
Pulse	210 beats/min, regular; strong radial pulses
Blood pressure	104/62 mm Hg
Respirations	20 breaths/min, nonlabored
Sao_2	95% on room air

3. What are some of your concerns based on this information?
4. Which interventions should you consider at this point?

(polarized) cell normally has a net charge of –90 millivolts (mV) with respect to the outside of the cell (Figure 27-11, part A1). When the myocardial cell receives a stimulus from the conduction system (Figure 27-11, part A2), the permeability of the cell wall changes through opening of specialized channels in such a way that sodium ions (Na⁺) rush into the cell, causing the inside of the cell to become more positive. Calcium ions (Ca⁺⁺) also enter the cell—albeit more slowly and through a different set of specialized channels—helping maintain the depolarized state of the cell membrane and supplying calcium ions for use in contraction of the cardiac muscle tissue. This reversal of electric charge—depolarization—starts at one spot in the cell and spreads in a wave along the cell until the cell is completely depolarized (Figure 27-11, part A3). As the cell depolarizes and calcium ions enter, mechanical contraction occurs.

If the cell were to remain depolarized, it could never contract again! Fortunately, the cell is able to recover from depolarization through a process called repolarization **Figure 27-11B ▾**. Repolarization starts with the closing of the sodium and calcium channels, which stops the rapid inflow of these ions. Next, special potassium channels open, allowing a rapid escape of potassium ions (K⁺) from the cell. This helps restore the inside of the cell to its negative charge; the proper electrolyte distribution is then reestablished by pumping sodium ions out of the cell and potassium ions back in. After the potassium channels close, this sodium-potassium pump helps move sodium and potassium ions back to their respective locations. For every three sodium ions this pump moves out of the cell, it moves two potassium ions into the cell, thereby maintaining the polarity of the cell membrane. To accomplish this task, the sodium-potassium pump moves ions against the

natural gradient by a process called active transport, which requires the expenditure of energy.

Table 27-2 ▾ summarizes the roles of the various electrolytes in cardiac function.

A myocardial cell cannot respond to an electric stimulus from the conduction system normally unless it is fully polarized. The period when the cell is depolarized or in the process

Table 27-2	Role of Electrolytes in Cardiac Function
Electrolyte	**Role in Cardiac Function**
Sodium (Na⁺)	Flows into the cell to initiate depolarization
Potassium (K⁺)	Flows out of the cell to initiate repolarization *Hypokalemia* → increased myocardial irritability *Hyperkalemia* → decreased automaticity/conduction
Calcium (Ca⁺⁺)	Has a major role in the depolarization of pacemaker cells (maintains depolarization) and in myocardial contractility (involved in contraction of heart muscle tissue) *Hypocalcemia* → decreased contractility and increased myocardial irritability *Hypercalcemia* → increased contractility
Magnesium (Mg⁺⁺)	Stabilizes the cell membrane; acts in concert with potassium, and opposes the actions of calcium *Hypomagnesemia* → decreased conduction *Hypermagnesemia* → increased myocardial irritability

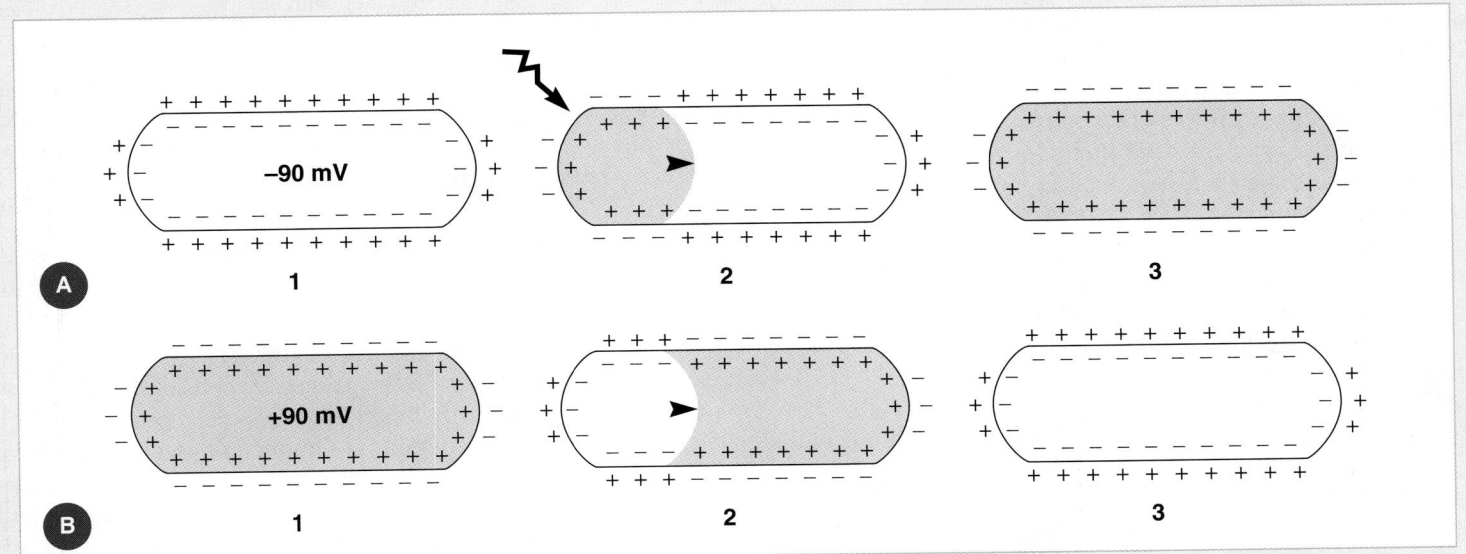

Figure 27-11 Movement of ions to produce a net current flow. **A.** Depolarization. (1) At rest, the cellular interior has a net charge of –90 mV. (2) The wave of depolarization begins as sodium ions pour into the cell. (3) Depolarized cell. **B.** Repolarization. (1) Depolarized cell. (2) The wave of repolarization begins as potassium ions leave the cell. (3) Repolarized cell.

Table 27-3	Pacemaker Rates
Pacemaker	**Rate (beats/min)**
SA node	60 to 100
AV junction	40 to 60
Purkinje	20 to 40

of repolarizing—the so-called refractory period—consists of two phases. In the absolute refractory period, the heart muscle has been drained of energy and needs to recharge; it will not contract during this period. In the relative refractory period, the heart is partially charged, albeit not strongly enough to create a full contraction.

Secondary Pacemakers

The SA node normally has the most rapid intrinsic rate of firing (60 to 100 times/min), so it will literally outpace any slower conduction tissue. If it becomes damaged or is suppressed, any component of the conduction system may act as a secondary pacemaker. The farther removed the conduction tissue is from the SA node, the slower its intrinsic rate of firing. Thus, the AV junction will spontaneously fire 40 to 60 times/min, whereas the ventricular Purkinje system, which is farther removed from the SA node, will spontaneously fire only 20 to 40 times/min.

Suppose that the SA node is damaged by ischemia (tissue injury caused by hypoxemia) and does not fire. When it fails to receive impulses from the SA node, the AV junction might then begin firing at its own rate; thus, an electrocardiogram (ECG) would show a "junctional rhythm" at a rate of 40 to 60 beats/min. If both nodes fail to initiate an impulse, the Purkinje fibers will initiate an impulse, resulting in a "ventricular rhythm" at a rate of 20 to 40 beats/min Table 27-3 ▲ .

Measuring the Heart's Electrical Conduction Activity

The electrical conduction events in the heart can be recorded on an ECG as a series of waves and complexes Figure 27-12 ▶ . The depolarization of the atria produces the P wave. It is followed by a brief pause as conduction is momentarily slowed through the AV junction. Next, the QRS complex occurs, representing depolarization of the ventricles. Repolarization of the atria and ventricles produces T waves; however, the atrial repolarization wave is small and is buried within the QRS complex, so it isn't seen Table 27-4 ▶ . The larger, ventricular T wave follows the QRS complex.

The intervals between waves and complexes also have names. The P-R interval is the distance from the beginning of the P wave to the beginning of the QRS complex. It represents the time required for an impulse to traverse the atria and AV junction and is normally 0.12 to 0.20 s (three to five boxes on ECG paper). The ST segment is the line from the end of the QRS complex to the beginning of the T wave (the beginning of which is referred to as the J-point). The ST segment should normally be at the same level as the baseline (isoelectric line). An elevated or

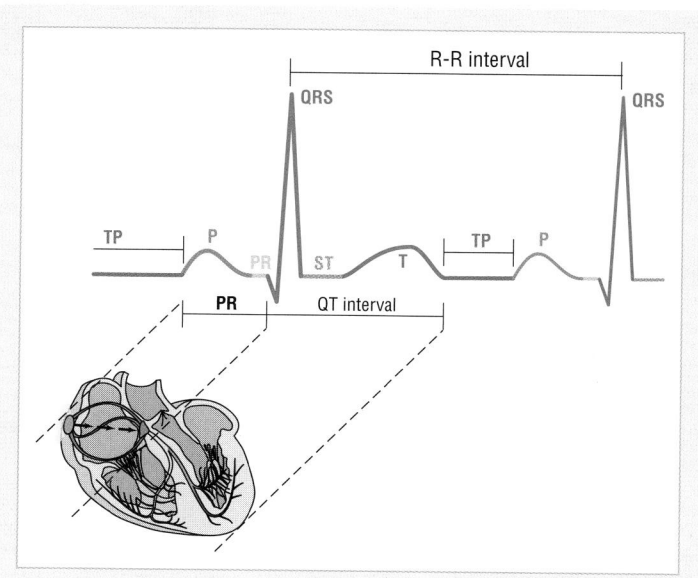

Figure 27-12 The ECG and cardiac events.

Table 27-4	Components of the ECG
ECG Representation	**Cardiac Event**
P wave	Depolarization of the atria
P-R interval	Depolarization of the atria and delay at the AV junction
QRS complex	Depolarization of the ventricles
ST segment	Period between ventricular depolarization and beginning of repolarization
T wave	Repolarization of the ventricles
R-R interval	Time between two ventricular depolarizations

depressed ST segment may indicate myocardial ischemia or injury. The R-R interval is the time between two successive QRS complexes. It represents the interval between two ventricular depolarizations and gives an indication of the HR.

The Autonomic Nervous System and the Heart

The autonomic nervous system is the part of the human nervous system that controls automatic (that is, involuntary) actions. Its importance can be gauged by considering the alternative: Suppose all body functions were solely under voluntary control. Sixty times a minute, 24 hours a day, you would have to remind your heart to beat. Twelve times a minute, 24 hours a day, you would be required to order your lungs to inflate and relax. You would have to warn your stomach that food was on the way, tell your pancreas and gallbladder to step up their activities, and urge your gut to speed up or slow down as necessary. Whenever you changed your level of activity—for example, during exercise—you would be forced to issue a

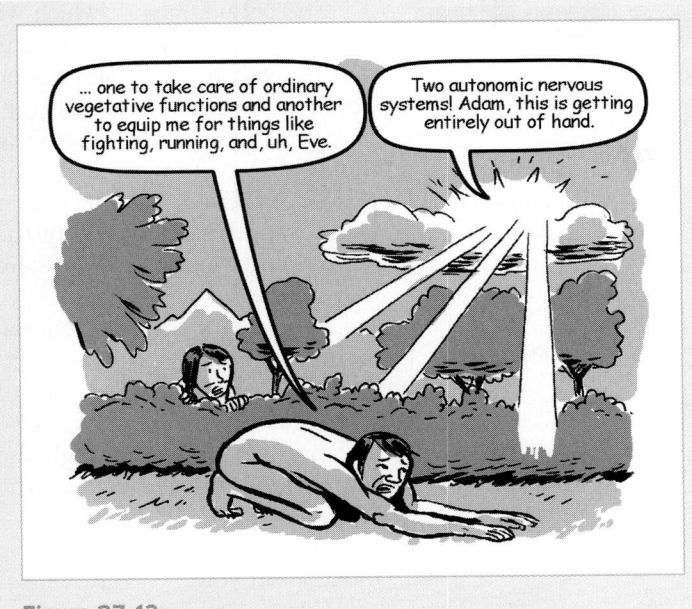

Figure 27-13

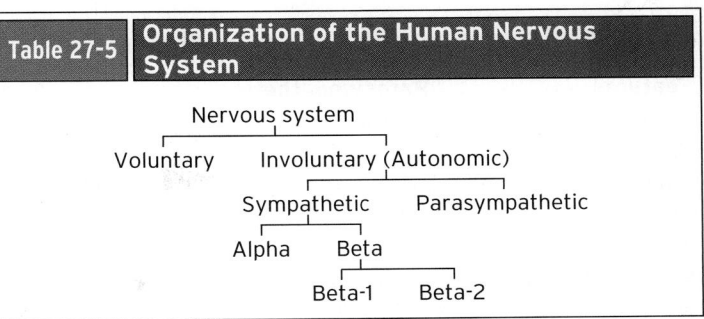

Table 27-5	Organization of the Human Nervous System

Nervous system
- Voluntary
- Involuntary (Autonomic)
  - Sympathetic
    - Alpha
    - Beta
      - Beta-1
      - Beta-2
  - Parasympathetic

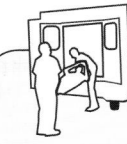

In the Field

The parasympathetic nervous system is your "brake pedal," and the sympathetic nervous system is your "gas pedal."

complex series of orders to your cardiovascular system to ensure that CO increased sufficiently to meet increased metabolic demands.

Fortunately, this administrative work is accomplished for us, without conscious effort on our part. It happened more or less like this:

In the beginning, when God was working out the circuitry for humans, Adam persuaded Him to include an autonomic nervous system (Figure 27-13 ▲). "Look," said Adam, "I don't want to spend all my time thinking about my CO and ventilation and digestion. I want to think great philosophic thoughts and maybe have a little fun on the side."

"I'll see what I can do," said God.

After some debate, they worked out a compromise. "I tell you what I'll do for you, Adam. I'll give you *two* nervous systems. One will be fully automatic—an autonomic nervous system—so that your body functions can proceed without your having to bother yourself about them. The other will be voluntary, so that you can consciously control the movement of your muscles."

That seemed reasonable, and Adam agreed. So it came to pass that humans have two nervous systems.

One day God noticed that Adam was looking sad.

"What's the matter, Adam?" asked God.

"It's my autonomic nervous system," said Adam. "It's not quite right yet."

"What do you mean, it's not quite right? I designed it according to our agreement, didn't I?"

"I know. But I've noticed that my life is divided into two kinds of activity. I do a lot of rather vegetative things, like sleeping and digesting my food, during which my heart needs to slow down. But I also do really exciting things—especially since Eve arrived—during which my heart needs to speed up. What I really need are two autonomic nervous systems—one

to take care of ordinary vegetative functions and another to equip me for things like fighting, running, and, uh, Eve."

"*Two* autonomic nervous systems! Adam, this is getting entirely out of hand."

"This is supposed to be Eden, isn't it? And everything's supposed to be perfect, isn't it? If You were really concerned about my welfare, You'd give me two autonomic nervous systems like it says in the medical textbooks."

"All right, all right," said God. "I'll see what I can do."

The next day, God said to Adam, "I've got everything fixed up. From now on, you'll have a voluntary nervous system and *two* autonomic nervous systems. One of them will be called the parasympathetic nervous system, and it will regulate your vegetative functions: It will slow your HR, help you digest your food, and all that stuff. The other will be called the sympathetic nervous system: It will speed up your heart, constrict your blood vessels, dilate your bronchi and pupils, and so forth."

"Why do they have to have such funny names?" asked Adam.

"Because I said so," said God, "and I'm still Boss around here, in case you've forgotten."

Thus, the human nervous system consists of a voluntary and an involuntary system. The latter, also called the autonomic nervous system, is further divided into the sympathetic and parasympathetic systems, as shown in (Table 27-5 ▲). (Table 27-6 ▶) provides a review of the properties of the autonomic nervous system.

The Parasympathetic Nervous System

The parasympathetic nervous system is concerned primarily with vegetative functions and sends its messages mainly through the vagus nerve. Think of it as the "rest and digest" nervous system. The vagus can be stimulated in a number of ways, including pressure on the carotid sinus, straining against a closed glottis (Valsalva maneuver), and distention of a hollow organ (such as the bladder or stomach).

Suppose that the brain decided the heart should slow a little; perhaps someone applied pressure over the carotid or

Table 27-6	Autonomic Nervous System	
Features	**Parasympathetic**	**Sympathetic**
Other name	Cholinergic; "rest and digest"	Adrenergic; "fight or flight"
Natural chemical mediator	Acetylcholine	Norepinephrine, epinephrine
Primary nerve(s)	Vagus	Nerves from the thoracic and lumbar ganglia of the spinal cord
Effect of stimulation	Decreases contractility (negative inotropic effect) Slows conduction velocity (negative dromotropic effect) Slows the heart* (negative chronotropic effect) Constricts pupils Increases salivation Increases gut motility	Increases contractility (positive inotropic effect) Speeds conduction velocity (positive dromotropic effect) Speeds the heart (positive chronotropic effect) Dilates pupils Constricts blood vessels Slows the gut Dilates the bronchi
Stimulating drugs	Neostigmine, reserpine	Alpha: phenylephrine Beta: isoproterenol Beta-2: albuterol Alpha + beta: norepinephrine, epinephrine, dopamine
Blocking drugs	Atropine	Alpha: chlorpromazine, phentolamine Beta: propranolol, metoprolol, labetalol, atenolol

* Slowing occurs mostly in the atria.

strained during a bowel movement. A message in the form of an electric impulse would go barreling down the vagus nerve to the place where this nerve abuts on the SA node of the heart. There, the electric impulse would cause the release of a naturally occurring chemical, acetylcholine (ACh). (The parasympathetic nervous system derives its other name, the *cholinergic* nervous system, from this chemical.) The ACh would cross over to the SA node of the heart and say, "Listen, SA node, the brain says you ought to slow down; I just heard it from the vagus." Just to be on the safe side, another ACh molecule would wander down to talk to the AV node of the heart: "We've just instructed the SA node to slow down; just in case, it didn't get the message, we want you to make sure that no extra impulses get through to the ventricles, understand?"

"Sure thing," says the AV node, which is more sensitive to criticism from the vagus nerve. "They shall not pass."

"Okay," says the ACh, as it is escorted away by cholinesterase. (Cholinesterase is a naturally occurring chemical that causes ACh to be released from the receptors to which it has attached.)

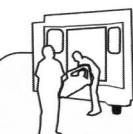

In the Field

Atropine is also referred to as an "anticholinergic" drug with "vagolytic" properties.

The only drug with which we shall be concerned that interacts directly with the parasympathetic nervous system is atropine. Atropine is a parasympathetic blocker; that is, it opposes the action of ACh on the heart and elsewhere, thereby allowing the body's natural sympathetic system to increase the HR.

Suppose the heart is plodding along at a rate of 50 beats/min, and you administer 0.5 mg of atropine intravenously. The atropine will travel through the bloodstream until it reaches the SA node.

"You're firing a little slowly today, aren't you?" says atropine.

"Just following orders," says the SA node. "The vagus told me to take it easy."

"The vagus, the vagus—that's all I ever hear. Why do you want to listen to that old stick-in-the-mud? Listen, stick with me, and I'll add a little excitement to your life."

"No kidding?"

"No kidding."

So the SA node speeds up. Meanwhile, the atropine reaches the AV node. "How are you doing, AV?" asks the atropine.

"Oh, it's kind of slow lately. The vagus ordered me to close down two lanes southbound."

"The vagus again. Listen, AV node, if you keep paying attention to the vagus, before you know it, that nerve will close down the entire highway to the ventricles, and they'll go off merrily on their own."

"Gee whiz," says the AV node. "What should I do?"

"Take my advice, bud, and open the gates wide. Let all the impulses through."

"Are you sure that's a good idea? The vagus said . . ."

"Forget about the vagus. He's just an old obstructionist."

"Okay," says the AV node, always eager to please when atropine is around. And he opens all southbound lanes.

The Sympathetic Nervous System

The sympathetic nervous system prepares the body to respond to various stresses; it is the fight-or-flight system mentioned earlier. The parasympathetic nervous system works well for routine activities such as keeping the heart beating during rest or coordinating digestion, but it provides no mechanism for the body to adapt to changing demands. By contrast, the sympathetic nervous system increases the HR, strengthens the force of cardiac muscle contractions, and provides other adaptive responses to ensure that the tissues' increased oxygen demands are satisfied with increased CO.

Suppose you start running to catch a bus. After a few seconds, your muscles will have used up all the oxygen and nutrients immediately on hand. "It's getting awfully stuffy down here," says one muscle to another.

"You said it!"

"I wish the heart would increase the delivery of oxygen."

So the muscles send a message to the brain: "HELP! We can't breathe!"

In response to their pleas, the brain sends a message through sympathetic nerves, passing through the thoracic and lumbar ganglia, ultimately arriving at the heart. Whereas the vagus nerve releases ACh, sympathetic nerves convey their commands through release of norepinephrine. Norepinephrine travels to the SA node, AV node, and ventricles, spreading the command from the sympathetic nerves: "Let's speed this operation up," says norepinephrine. "The muscles are suffocating and threatening to bomb the circulation with lactic acid if they don't get more oxygen." So the heart speeds up, increasing CO and, therefore, delivering more oxygen and nutrients throughout the body.

When intense stimulation of the sympathetic nervous system occurs, a special hormone—epinephrine—may be mobilized to spread the alarm and command the heart to speed up. Epinephrine is produced in the adrenal gland and is also called adrenaline, leading to the other name of the sympathetic system—the *adrenergic* system.

Drugs That Act on the Sympathetic Nervous System

Drugs that influence the sympathetic nervous system are classified according to the receptors with which they interact. A drug receptor can be visualized as analogous to the ignition switch in a car. When the proper key is inserted into the car's ignition and turned, a predictable sequence of events follows: The battery sends a current to the starter and the spark plugs, which fire; combustion of gasoline and air occurs; and the engine starts. Although many keys may fit into a specific car's ignition, not every key that fits will turn and start the car—but all that do turn cause the same reaction. Likewise, the organs of the body have a number of "ignition switches." In the sympathetic nervous system, those switches, or receptors, are labeled alpha and beta. Whenever one of those switches is activated by a "key" (a drug or hormone), a predictable sequence of responses will occur Table 27-7 ▸ .

The heart has only one ignition switch for a beta agent. Any beta agent will have the same effect on the heart—that is, it will increase the heart's rate, force, and automaticity. The arteries, by contrast, have receptors for alpha and beta agents. An alpha drug will turn on the switch that

causes vasoconstriction; a beta agent will activate the switch that causes vasodilation. Similarly, the lungs have alpha and beta receptors. Alpha agents don't have much effect on the lungs; at most, they cause minor bronchoconstriction. By contrast, beta agents (such as drugs used to treat asthma) trigger significant bronchodilation. Figure 27-14 ▾ represents these concepts schematically.

Drugs that have alpha or beta sympathetic properties are called sympathomimetic drugs because they imitate (mimic) the actions of naturally occurring sympathetic chemicals. If we know whether a sympathomimetic drug is an alpha or beta agent, we can predict the response by the heart, lungs, and arteries.

Consider isoproterenol (Isuprel). It is a pure beta agent. Armed with this knowledge, we can immediately recognize that isoproterenol acts in the manner shown in Figure 27-15 ▸ —it stimulates the heart, dilates the bronchi, and dilates the arteries.

In the Field

To remember the difference between beta-1 and beta-2, ask yourself, "How many hearts do I have?" One heart—beta-1. "How many lungs do I have?" Two lungs—beta-2.

Table 27-7	Responses to Sympathetic Stimulation
Organ	**Sympathetic Stimulation**
Heart	Increased HR (positive chronotropic effect) (beta-1)
	Increased force of contraction (positive inotropic effect) (beta-1)
	Increased conduction velocity (positive dromotropic effect) (beta-1)
Arteries	Constriction (alpha)
Lungs	Bronchial muscle relaxation (beta-2)

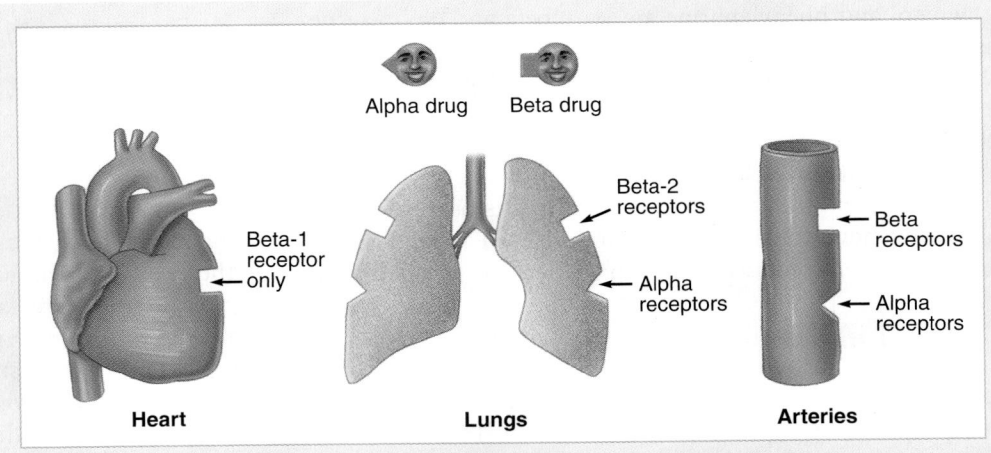

Figure 27-14 Receptor sites of the sympathetic nervous system in the heart, lungs, and arteries.

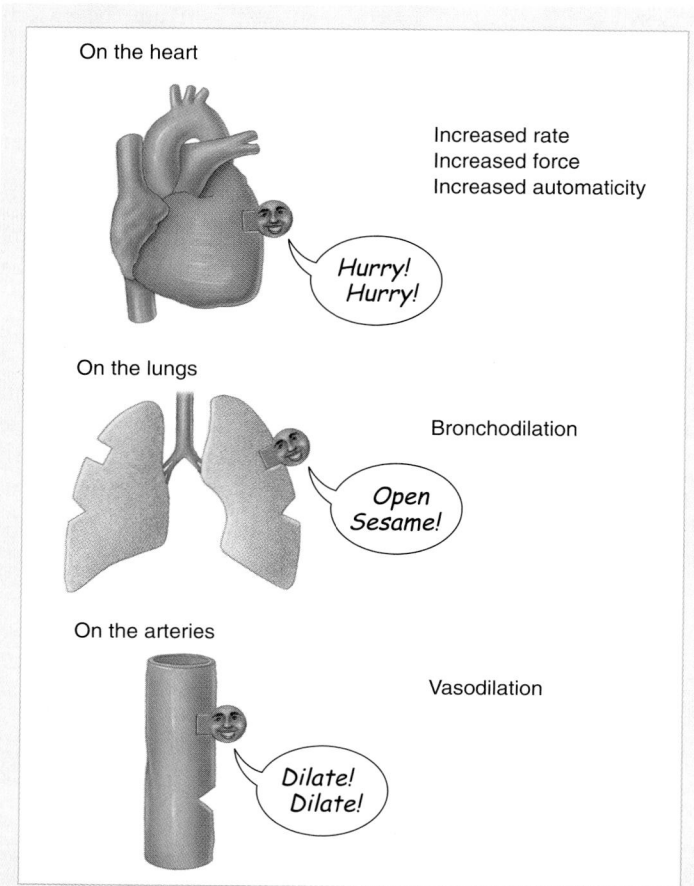

Figure 27-15 Beta sympathetic agents increase the rate, force, and automaticity of the heart; dilate the bronchi; and dilate peripheral arteries.

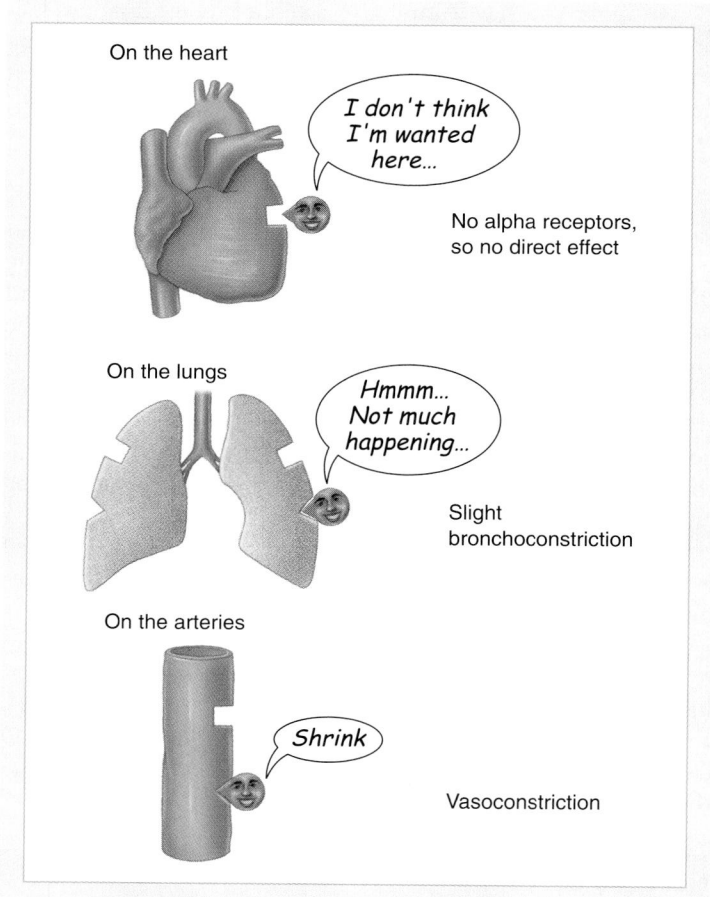

Figure 27-16 Alpha agents have no direct effect on the heart; they cause slight bronchoconstriction and marked vasoconstriction.

Phenylephrine (Neo-Synephrine), by contrast, is a pure alpha agent. It has no direct effect on the heart but causes slight bronchoconstriction and marked vasoconstriction **Figure 27-16 ▸** .

In reality, things are not always so simple. Although isoproterenol and phenylephrine are pure beta and alpha agents, respectively, most other sympathomimetic drugs have varying degrees of alpha and beta activity **Figure 27-17 ▸** . Norepinephrine (Levophed) is chiefly an alpha agent, and its alpha effects predominate; because it also has some beta activity, however, it will have effects on the heart. Conversely, epinephrine (Adrenalin) is chiefly a beta agent, and its beta effects predominate; nevertheless, when administered in high doses, epinephrine will produce some alpha effects, especially on the arteries.

Table 27-8 ▸ lists several sympathomimetic agents that are commonly encountered in the field. Two of the drugs, norepinephrine and epinephrine, are also naturally occurring chemicals of the sympathetic nervous system. Their actions are the same whether they are produced in the body and released from the nervous system or manufactured in a factory and injected.

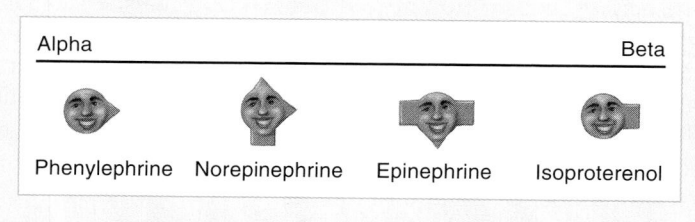

Figure 27-17 Many sympathomimetic agents have alpha and beta properties.

Beta sympathetic agents can be classified into two groups based on the subtle differences between the beta receptors in the heart and the lungs. Drugs that act primarily on cardiac beta receptors are called beta-1; those that act chiefly on pulmonary beta receptors are called beta-2. Some newer bronchodilators—such as albuterol, isoetharine, and terbutaline—are selective beta-2 agents, so they provide effective bronchodilation with far fewer cardiac side effects.

Another class of drugs that acts on the sympathetic nervous system comprises the sympatholytic or sympathetic blockers. As their name implies, they block the action of sym-

Table 27-8	Common Sympathomimetic Agents
Alpha	Phenylephrine (Neo-Synephrine)
Alpha ↓ Beta	Norepinephrine bitartrate (Levophed) Dopamine Epinephrine
Beta	Albuterol (Proventil; beta-2-specific) Isoproterenol (Isuprel; pure beta-specific)

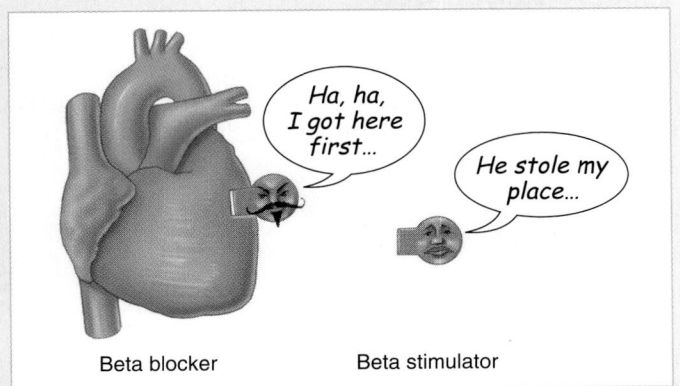

Ha, ha, I got here first...

He stole my place...

Beta blocker   Beta stimulator

Figure 27-18 A sympathetic blocker occupies the receptor site for the stimulating drug, thereby preventing the stimulating drug from exerting its usual effect.

pathetic agents by beating them to the receptor sites and preventing these agents from turning on the ignition. The receptor sites, which aren't very smart, cannot distinguish a blocker from a stimulator until it is too late. With the blocker occupying the receptor site, the stimulating agent cannot get in to turn on the switch Figure 27-18 .

Beta blockers occupy beta receptors in the heart, lungs, and arteries, as well as elsewhere in the body Figure 27-19 . Thus beta agents, whether released from sympathetic nerve endings or given intravenously, cannot exert their full effects when a beta blocker such as propranolol has been administered previously Figure 27-20 .

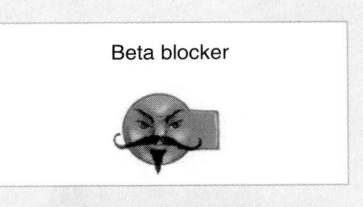

Beta blocker

Figure 27-19 A beta blocker is a sympathetic blocking agent.

The indications for the major autonomic stimulating and blocking agents can be deduced once we know the properties of the drugs and the manner in which they interact with the autonomic nervous system:

- **Atropine.** Parasympathetic blocker, opposing the vagus nerve. It is used to speed the heart when excessive vagal firing has caused bradycardia.
- **Norepinephrine.** Sympathetic agent (primarily alpha), causing vasoconstriction. It is used to increase the blood pressure when hypotension is caused by vasodilation (as in neurogenic shock).
- **Isoproterenol.** Sympathetic agent (almost pure beta), causing a strong increase in HR and dilation of bronchi. It is used in extreme cases to increase CO and to dilate bronchi in asthma.
- **Epinephrine.** Sympathetic agent (predominantly beta), with actions similar to those of isoproterenol, but having an additional, primarily peripheral vasoconstrictor effect. Indications for epinephrine are similar to those for isoproterenol, but also include asystole, pulseless electrical activity (PEA), and ventricular fibrillation (to increase the

You are the Provider Part 3

Your partner has applied the cardiac monitor and is giving oxygen at 4 L/min via nasal cannula. The cardiac monitor displays a narrow complex tachycardia at a rate of 212 beats/min. While looking for a site to insert an intravenous (IV) line, you ask the patient to bear down hard as if he were having a bowel movement. There is no change in his rate and rhythm. You insert an 18-gauge IV catheter in his right forearm and prepare to administer 6 mg of adenosine (Adenocard). You rapidly administer the 6 mg of adenosine, followed by a 20-mL fluid bolus. The monitor showed a transient decrease in the HR to 165 beats/min, which quickly picked back up to a rate of 206 beats/min. Anthony tells you that he experienced "the strangest sensation" in his chest when you gave him the medication and asks what you gave him.

Reassessment	Recording Time: 11 Minutes
Skin	Pink, warm, and diaphoretic
Pulse	206 beats/min, regular; strong distal pulses
ECG	Supraventricular tachycardia
Blood pressure	102/64 mm Hg
Respirations	20 breaths/min, nonlabored
SaO₂	99% on nasal cannula at 4 L/min of oxygen
Pupils	Equal and reactive to light

5. How does adenosine work?

6. What should you tell your patient before you administer adenosine?

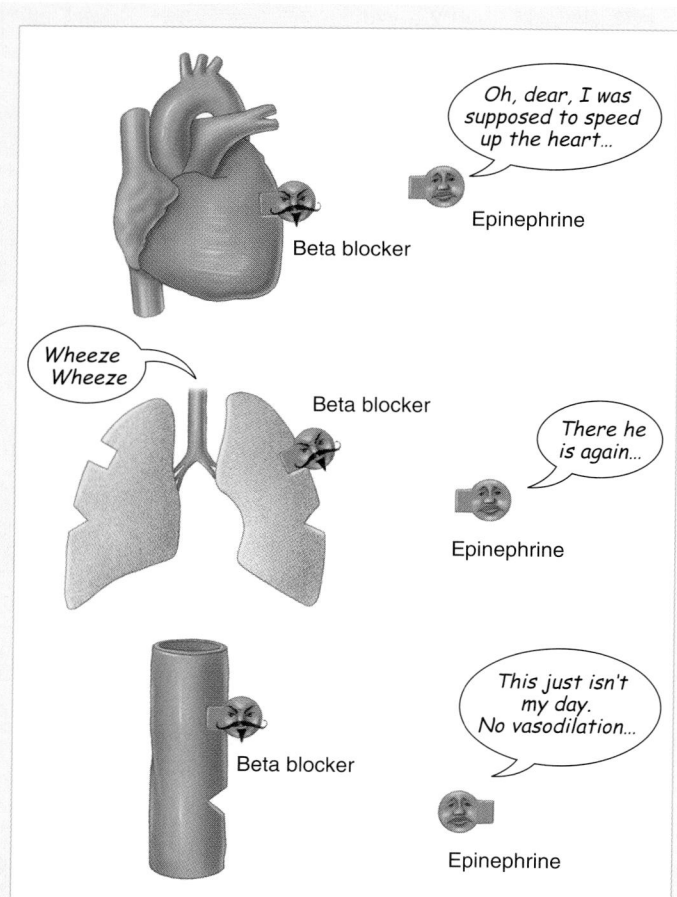

Figure 27-20 By occupying beta receptor sites, the beta blocker prevents epinephrine from exerting its usual effects on the heart, lungs, and blood vessels.

automaticity of the heart and vasoconstriction); and anaphylactic shock (for all of its effects—bronchodilation, vasoconstriction, increased CO).

- **Dopamine.** Sympathetic agent, used at low (beta) doses to increase the force of cardiac contractions in cardiogenic shock. Its dilation (beta) effects on renal and mesenteric arteries mean that dopamine may help maintain urine flow and good perfusion to abdominal organs.
- **Albuterol, isoetharine, terbutaline.** Sympathetic beta-2 agents that act on the lungs. These agents are used to induce bronchodilation in asthma, chronic obstructive pulmonary disease, and other bronchospastic conditions.

- **Propranolol.** Sympathetic beta blocker, opposing the actions of beta-stimulating agents. It is used clinically to slow the HR in certain tachyarrhythmias, to decrease the pain of chronic angina (by decreasing the work of the heart), and to depress irritability in the heart (by decreasing the tendency of the heart to fire automatically). Its use is contraindicated in asthma.

The Sympathetic Nervous System and Blood Pressure Regulation

The body attempts to maintain a fairly constant blood pressure to ensure perfusion of vital organs. At any given moment, the blood pressure is influenced by the CO and the resistance (degree of constriction) of the arterioles:

$$Blood\ Pressure = CO \times Peripheral\ Resistance$$

Thus, the blood pressure can be increased by increasing the CO, the peripheral resistance, or both.

Under normal circumstances, the body balances flow and resistance to maintain a stable blood pressure. That is, alterations in one variable bring about compensatory changes in the other variable to restore blood pressure toward normal. Consider, for example, a situation in which CO decreases suddenly, as in hemorrhage. The fall in CO will inevitably lead to a fall in blood pressure unless the peripheral resistance is altered. The falling CO activates the sympathetic nervous system, however, which in turn causes the arterioles to constrict. Vasoconstriction increases the peripheral resistance, thereby tending to restore the blood pressure back toward normal.

The resistance against which the ventricle contracts is termed the afterload. The greater the afterload, the harder the ventricle must work to pump the blood. In conditions of chronically high afterload, such as arteriosclerosis-induced high blood pressure, the left ventricle may eventually grow exhausted from the extra work and cease pumping efficiently or even fail.

Patient Assessment

Patients experience a variety of symptoms when they have a cardiovascular problem. The most common complaints are chest pain, dyspnea, fainting, palpitations, and fatigue. If the patient is pulseless or breathless, basic life support (BLS) measures may be used. In some cases, ACLS procedures may be necessary. This section reviews the organized approach to assessing patients by focusing on their cardiac and pulmonary systems. For this assessment, we will assume the patient is conscious and breathing and has a pulse.

Scene Size-up

The initial assessment begins with sizing up the scene and ensuring scene safety. In addition, you should try to anticipate the need for other resources such as extra personnel.

Initial Assessment

Observe the patient's general appearance as you approach him or her, and assess for apparent life threats. The initial assessment is fairly consistent for all patients, but this discussion has a cardiac focus. Sometimes assessing the ABCs can be accomplished easily by merely greeting the patient and introducing yourself, assuming that the patient can answer you, is conscious, has an open airway, is breathing, and has a pulse. Determine the patient's level of consciousness (LOC) based on his or her response to your greeting, and use the AVPU scale.

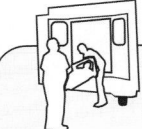

In the Field

Just by shaking someone's hand and introducing yourself, you can learn a lot about the patient.

Determine the patency of the patient's airway. If the patient is talking to you, airway is patent. The patient may be able to maintain an open airway or, depending on the LOC, may need help with clearing obstructions (debris, blood, or teeth) by your properly positioning the head and/or placing an airway adjunct. Note the rate, quality, and effort of the breathing, and consider initiating oxygen therapy at this time.

Assessment of circulation is done primarily by checking the patient's pulse. For a conscious patient, you will typically check the radial pulse; if the patient is unconscious, check the carotid pulse. While checking the pulse, note the rate, regularity, and overall quality. Is it weak, bounding, or irregular?

While holding the patient's hand in yours, assess the skin color and condition. The skin is the largest organ of the body, so a good indication that the rest of the body is getting adequate circulation is that the skin and mucous membranes are pink and the skin is warm and dry. Is there edema, poor turgor, or skin "tenting"?

The initial assessment ends with making a transport decision for your patient. Based on your findings to this point, you should be able to determine whether the patient requires immediate transport. If you are unsure, continue with the focused assessment, and the correct decision may become more apparent.

Focused History and Physical Exam

During the focused history and physical exam, you will perform a focused assessment. This inquiry into the patient's medical history and a physical exam are based on the patient's chief complaint; the inquiry is also referred to as the history of present illness. The SAMPLE history is included in this assessment. In patients with acute coronary syndromes (ACSs), the most common chief complaints are chest pain, dyspnea, fainting, palpitations, and fatigue.

Symptoms

Chest pain is often the presenting symptom of an AMI. The patient's description of the pain is important for assessing its significance. The OPQRST format can be used to elaborate on the patient's chief complaint:

- **O** What is the *Onset* or origin of the pain—that is, how did it begin (suddenly or gradually)? Has anything like this ever happened before?
- **P** What *Provoked* the pain—that is, what, if anything, brought it on? Is it exertional or nonexertional? What was the patient doing at the time? Sitting in a chair? Changing a tire? Having an argument with the boss? Does anything make it worse? What palliates the pain—that is, does anything make it better? Patients with chronic CAD may take nitroglycerin for episodes of chest pain. Ask whether the patient did so and, if so, whether it helped.
- **Q** What is the *Quality* of the pain—that is, what does it feel like? Get the patient's narrative description. Dull? Sharp? Crushing? Heavy? Squeezing? Note the exact words the patient uses to describe the pain, and observe the patient's body language as he or she does so. Try not to lead the patient's description unless he or she is unable to describe the pain. In such cases, try to give alternatives, such as "Is it sharp or dull?"
- **R** Does the pain *Radiate*? From where to where? To the jaw? Down the left arm? Into the back?
- **S** What is the *Severity* of the pain—that is, how bad is it? Use the pain scale of 1 to 10, with 10 being the worst. If the patient has chronic angina, ask him or her to compare the pain with the usual angina pain.
- **T** What was the *Timing* of the attack—that is, when did it start? How long did it last? What time did it get worse or better? Was it continuous or intermittent?

Another chief complaint among patients with an ACS is dyspnea. In the context of ACSs, dyspnea may be the first clue to failure of the left side of the heart. To explore this possibility, ask the following questions:

- When did the dyspnea start? Did it awaken the patient from sleep? Paroxysmal nocturnal dyspnea (PND) is an acute episode of shortness of breath in which the patient suddenly awakens from sleep with a feeling of suffocation. Often the patient will report going to a window to get "more air" or will move from the bed to a recliner. PND is one of the classic signs of left-sided heart failure, although it may also occur in chronic lung diseases.
- Did the dyspnea come on gradually or suddenly?
- Is it continuous or intermittent?
- Does it happen during activity or while at rest?

- Does any position make the dyspnea better or worse? The dyspnea of pulmonary edema usually worsens when the patient is lying down (orthopnea), because blood pools in the lungs when the body is horizontal. Patients with significant orthopnea will often sleep with several pillows, or even sitting in a recliner, to maintain a semiupright position.
- Has the patient ever had dyspnea like this before? If so, under what circumstances?
- Does the patient have a cough? Is it dry or productive?
- Were there any associated symptoms?

Fainting (syncope) occurs when CO suddenly declines, leading to a reduction in cerebral perfusion. Cardiac causes of syncope include arrhythmias, increased vagal tone, and heart lesions. There are also numerous noncardiac causes of syncope (discussed in Chapter 28). As part of taking a history from someone who has fainted, try to sort out whether the patient fainted from cardiac or noncardiac causes:

- Under what circumstances did the syncopal episode occur? What was the patient doing at the time? A 20-year-old who faints at the sight of blood is unlikely to have significant underlying cardiac disease; a 60-year-old who faints after feeling some "fluttering" in the chest may have a dangerous cardiac arrhythmia.
- Were there any warning feelings before the episode, or did the fainting spell occur suddenly and unexpectedly?
- What position was the patient in when he or she fainted? Standing? Sitting? Lying down? Losing consciousness while sitting or lying down has more ominous implications than fainting while standing up.
- Has the patient fainted before? If so, under what circumstances?
- Were there any associated symptoms, such as nausea, vomiting, urinary incontinence, or seizures?

Finally, patients with cardiac problems may present with a chief complaint of palpitations. Palpitations refer to the sensation of an abnormally fast or irregular heartbeat—except after extreme exertion, a person normally remains blissfully unaware of his or her heartbeat. The cause of palpitations is often a cardiac arrhythmia, such as premature ventricular contractions (PVCs) or paroxysmal supraventricular tachycardia (PSVT). The patient may not use the word "palpitations" but may report feeling the heart "skip a beat" or use words to that effect. In such a case, inquire about the onset, frequency, and duration of this symptom and previous episodes of palpitations. Also ask about the presence of associated symptoms (such as chest pain, dizziness, and dyspnea).

Patients may report a variety of other related symptoms as you explore their history of present illness. They may have a "feeling of impending doom" or a sense that they will soon experience a life-changing event. Some patients relate feeling nauseous or having vomited. Listen carefully for indications that trauma may be involved or that their activity has been limited as a result of their condition. Observe their faces as you listen to them tell their stories. Do you see a look of fear or anguish? Are they holding their chest? Most of the other associated complaints your patients may have are related to hypoxia or poor perfusion resulting from inadequate CO—for example, decreased LOC, diaphoresis, restlessness and anxiety, fatigue, headache, behavioral changes, and syncope.

After exploring the patient's chief complaint, inquire briefly about pertinent aspects of the patient's other medical history:

- Is the patient under treatment for any serious illnesses or conditions? Ask specifically whether he or she has ever been diagnosed with any of the following:
  - Coronary artery disease
  - Atherosclerotic heart disease: angina, previous MI, hypertension, congestive heart failure (CHF)
  - Valvular disease
  - Aneurysm
  - Pulmonary disease
  - Diabetes
  - Renal disease
  - Vascular disease
  - Inflammatory cardiac disease
  - Previous cardiac surgery (such as coronary artery bypass graft or valve replacement)
  - Congenital anomalies
- Is the patient taking any medications regularly? The focused history is a great opportunity to ask about which drugs have been prescribed and whether the patient is taking them as instructed. Be sure to ask when the patient took the medications last. Is he or she taking medications that were prescribed for someone else (borrowed)? Also ask about any over-the-counter medications or any herbal supplements the patient uses. It may be appropriate to ask about recreational drug use. Take particular note of the groups of medications prescribed for the treatment of cardiac problems listed in **Table 27-9 ▸**. If you are unfamiliar with any medication, ask the patient what it was prescribed for. It is also a good idea to ask if the patient takes any medication for each medical condition he or she reports as part of the history and to verify these medical conditions match the medications the patient is actually taking.
- Does the patient have known allergies to foods or medications? If so, ask what kind of reaction the patient has with each one.
- Ask the patient when he or she last had anything to eat or drink, and note the time that occurred. This information will prove helpful later in many situations.
- If you haven't asked already, find out the history of the current event. Get any extra information about what was happening when the problem started and what was done before your arrival.

Vital Signs
Pulse

When you take the vital signs, make a careful assessment of the patient's pulse. Is it regular or irregular? Abnormally fast or

Table 27-9	Medicines Prescribed to Treat or Prevent Heart Disease
Category	**Drug**
Angiotensin-converting enzyme inhibitors	Captopril (Capoten); enalapril (Vasotec); lisinopril (Prinivil, Zestril); benazepril (Lotensin); fosinopril (Monopril); ramipril (Altace); quinapril (Accupril); perindopril (Aceon); trandolapril (Mavik); moexipril (Univasc)
Calcium channel blockers	Amlodipine (Norvasc); felodipine (Plendil); diltiazem (Cardizem, Cardizem CD, Cardizem SR, Dilacor XR, Diltiazem XT, Tiazac); verapamil (Calan, Calan SR, Covera-HS, Isoptin, Isoptin SR, Verelan, VerelanPM); nifedipine (Adalat, Adalat CC, Procardia, Procardia XL); nicardipine (Cardene, Cardene SR); nisoldipine (Sular); bepridil (Vascor)
Angiotensin II receptor blockers	Losartan (Cozaar); valsartan (Diovan); irbesartan (Avapro); candesartan (Atacand)
Cholesterol-lowering drugs	Statins: lovastatin (Altacor, Mevacor); fluvastatin (Lescol); pravastatin (Pravachol); atorvastatin (Lipitor); simvastatin (Zocor) Niacins: nicotinic acid (Niacor); extended-release niacin (Niaspan) Bile acid resins: colestipol (Colestid); cholestyramine (Questran); cholesevelam (Welchol) Fibrates: clofibrate (Atromid); gemfibrozil (Lopid); fenofibrate (Tricor)
Antiarrhythmics	Amiodarone (Cordarone); sotalol (Betapace)
Cardiac glycoside	Digoxin (Lanoxin, Lanoxi-caps)
Antiplatelet agents	Clopidogrel (Plavix); ticlopidine (Ticlid); aspirin
Diuretics	Furosemide (Lasix); bumetanide (Bumex); torsemide (Demadex); hydrochlorothiazide (Esidrix); metolazone (Zaroxolyn); spironolactone (Aldactone)
Beta blockers	Acebutolol (Sectral); bisoprolol (Zebeta); esmolol (Brevibloc); propranolol (Inderal); atenolol (Tenormin); labetalol (Normodyne, Trandate); carvedilol (Coreg); metoprolol (Lopressor, Toprol-XL)
Vasodilators	Isosorbide dinitrate* (Dilatrate-SR, Iso-Bid, Isonate, Isorbid, Isordil, Isotrate, Sorbitrate); isosorbide mononitrate (Imdur); hydralazine* (Apresoline)
Coumarin anticoagulant	Warfarin (Coumadin)

*Isosorbide dinitrate and hydralazine are given together.

slow? Strong or weak? An irregular pulse signals a disturbance in cardiac rhythm. A very rapid pulse (tachycardia) may simply indicate anxiety, but it can also occur secondary to severe pain, CHF, or a cardiac arrhythmia. A weak, thready pulse suggests a reduction in CO.

You should be familiar with the potentially abnormal pulse findings. For example, the patient may have a pulse deficit. A deficit occurs when the palpated radial pulse rate is less than the apical pulse rate; it is reported numerically as the difference between the two. To assess for a deficit, check the peripheral radial pulse while listening to an apical pulse.

Another abnormal pulse finding is pulsus paradoxus. Pulsus paradoxus is an excessive drop (> 10 mm Hg) in the systolic blood pressure with each inspired breath. Pulsus paradoxus can sometimes be palpated as a decrease in the amplitude of the pulse waveform, which makes the affected pulse beats feel weaker than the others. This observation can best be made when the rhythm is regular. If the variation is slight, it can be detected only by use of a blood pressure cuff and stethoscope.

Finally, you might recognize pulsus alternans. This pulse alternates in strength from one beat to the next.

Blood Pressure
In patients older than 50 years, a systolic blood pressure of more than 140 mm Hg is a much more important risk factor for CVD than the diastolic pressure. Patients with a systolic blood pressure of 120 to 139 mm Hg or a diastolic blood pressure of 80 to 89 mm Hg are considered "prehypertensive" and need to adopt a healthier lifestyle to prevent CVD.

In emergency situations, an elevated blood pressure may reflect the patient's anxiety or pain. A systolic blood pressure of less than 90 mm Hg might suggest serious hypotension and shock, depending on the patient's overall condition and chief complaint. The pulse pressure (the difference between the systolic and diastolic pressures) gives a rough indication of the elasticity of the arterial walls and the SV. In patients with arteriosclerosis, the arterial walls are stiffened, and the pulse pressure is increased. In cardiogenic shock or cardiac tamponade, the SV is reduced because the heart cannot pump effectively, so the pulse pressure is narrowed accordingly.

It may be beneficial to take the blood pressure in both arms and compare the readings. Some conditions such as stroke or aortic aneurysm may cause blood pressures to vary from the right to the left side.

Respirations
Note the rate and quality of the patient's respirations. Is the respiratory rate abnormally rapid (tachypnea)? Is the patient laboring to breathe? Respiratory distress in a cardiac patient suggests the possibility of CHF, with fluid in the lungs. Remember the old saying, "Look, listen, and feel"? In this physical exam, it is called inspection, auscultation, and palpation.

Cardiac Monitoring and Pulse Oximetry
As part of taking the vital signs, attach the cardiac monitor and pulse oximeter if you have not done so already. Use the ECG

interpretation and oxygen saturation measurement just as you do other vital signs—that is, as tools to help you in your assessment and not as the only guide to treatment (treat the patient, not the monitor). When caring for a patient in relatively stable condition who does not require rapid assessment, the physical exam may be done at this point.

Focused Physical Exam

The focused physical exam is similar for many medical patients. Nevertheless, certain aspects warrant greater emphasis in the patient whose chief complaint suggests a cardiac problem.

When observing the patient's general appearance, pay particular attention to the LOC, which is an excellent indicator of the adequacy of cerebral perfusion. If a patient is alert and oriented, the brain is getting enough oxygen, which in turn means the heart is doing its job as a pump. Conversely, stupor or confusion may indicate poor CO, which may be the result of myocardial damage or dysfunction. Skin color and temperature are also valuable indicators of the state of the patient's circulation: The cold, sweaty skin of many patients with MI reflects massive peripheral vasoconstriction.

Physical Exam

In continuing the physical exam, begin by inspecting the neck and tracheal position. Is the trachea midline and mobile to gentle manipulation? Press down with your finger in the patient's suprasternal notch to verify that the trachea is midline.

What about the adjacent structures such as the neck veins? The external jugular veins reflect the pressure within the patient's systemic circulation. Normally, they are collapsed when a person is sitting or standing. If the function of the right side of the heart is compromised, however, blood will back up into the systemic veins behind the right side of the heart and distend those veins. To estimate the patient's venous pressure, place the patient in a semisitting position (45° angle) with the

head slightly rotated away from the jugular vein you are examining; observe the height of the distended fluid column within the vein, and note how far up the distention extends above the sternal angle.

Continue the assessment by inspecting and palpating the chest. Look for surgical scars that might indicate previous cardiac surgery. Is there a nitroglycerin patch on the patient's skin? Is there a bulge under the patient's skin indicating a pacemaker or an automated implanted cardioverter defibrillator (AICD)? These devices are implanted just below the right or left clavicle and are about the size of a half-dollar Figure 27-21 ▾ . Is the

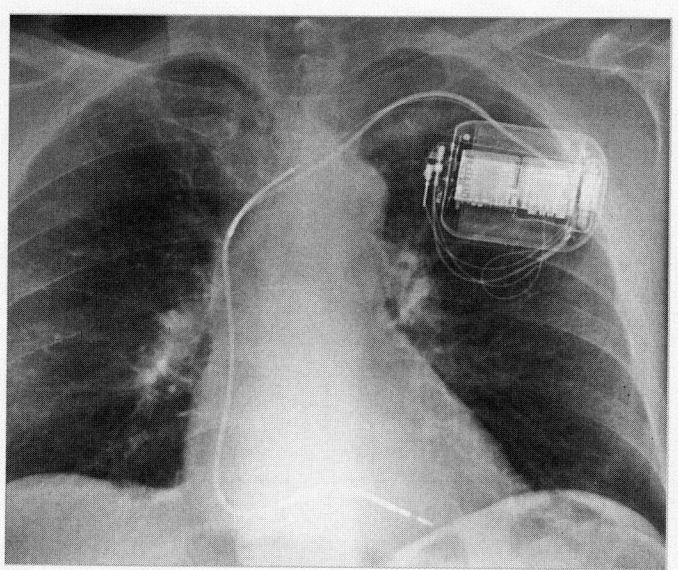

Figure 27-21 An AICD is attached directly to the heart and continuously monitors heart rhythm, delivering shocks as needed. The electricity from the AICD is so low that it has no effect on rescuers.

You are the Provider Part 4

Since the initial dose of adenosine caused a transient drop in the HR, you decide to administer 12 mg of adenosine after 2 minutes has passed. This time, you let Anthony know that you will be administering the medication and give it followed by a 20-mL flush. The monitor showed a 3-second period of asystole followed by a gradual increase in the HR to approximately 210 beats/min. After waiting 2 minutes, you administer another 12 mg of adenosine, the third and final dose, with similar results.

Reassessment	Recording Time: 17 Minutes
Skin	Pink, warm, and diaphoretic
Pulse	210 beats/min; regular, with strong distal pulses
ECG	Supraventricular tachycardia
Blood pressure	104/66 mm Hg
Respirations	18 breaths/min, nonlabored
Sao_2	99% on nasal cannula at 4 L/min of oxygen
Pupils	Equal and reactive to light

7. How should your treatment proceed?

anterior-posterior diameter of the chest enlarged, as in a barrel-chested patient with COPD? On palpation, do you observe any sign of crepitus?

Listen carefully to the chest with your stethoscope. Crackles or wheezes may be suggestive of left-sided heart failure with pulmonary edema. Listen for a third heart sound ("lub da-da" instead of "lub-dub"), known as an S₃ gallop, which again gives evidence of CHF. Examine the extremities and back for edema, a sign of failure of the right side of the heart.

Ongoing Assessment

Once the history and vital signs have been taken and the physical exam has been completed, treatment of the patient should be continued and transportation initiated. The ongoing assessment is accomplished en route to the hospital. It begins with a repeated initial assessment (LOC and ABCs). The vital signs should be taken every 5 to 15 minutes during this time as well. A repeated physical exam should be accomplished to see if any changes have occurred or if any conditions were missed in the initial physical exam. Finally, all the effectiveness of interventions implemented should be assessed. For example, is the IV fluid still flowing or has the pain diminished after nitroglycerin administration?

Pathophysiology and Management of Cardiovascular Problems

CAD and Angina

Coronary artery disease (CAD) is the most common form of heart disease and the leading cause of death in US adults. The coronary arteries supply oxygen and nutrients to the myocardium. If one of these blood vessels becomes blocked, the muscle it supplies will be deprived of oxygen (ischemia). If this oxygen supply is not quickly restored, the ischemic area of heart muscle will eventually die (undergo infarction).

Atherosclerosis is of particular concern because it affects the inner lining of the aorta and cerebral and coronary blood vessels, leading to the narrowing of those vessels and reduction of blood flow through them. The atherosclerotic process begins, probably in childhood, when small amounts of fatty material are deposited along the inner wall (intima) of arteries, usually at points of turbulent blood flow (such as where the arteries bifurcate or where the arterial wall has been damaged). As the streak of fat enlarges, it becomes a mass of fatty tissue, an atheroma, which gradually calcifies and hardens into a plaque. The atheromatous plaque infiltrates the arterial wall and decreases its elasticity. At the same time, it narrows the arterial lumen and interferes with blood flow through the lumen. The narrowed, roughened area of the arterial intima provides a locus for the formation of a fixed blood clot, or thrombus, which may then obstruct the artery altogether (when in a coronary artery is known as a coronary thrombosis). In addition, calcium may precipitate from the bloodstream

into the arterial walls, causing arteriosclerosis, which greatly reduces the elasticity of the arteries.

Risk Factors for Atherosclerosis

Although atherosclerosis is widespread in industrialized countries, certain factors increase the risk of developing atherosclerosis and CAD: hypertension (high blood pressure), cigarette smoking, diabetes, high serum cholesterol levels (which may be related to a high dietary intake of saturated fats and calories), lack of exercise, obesity, family history of heart disease or stroke, and male sex. Clearly, these risk factors include some things we can't do anything about (other than thank our parents). We cannot, for example, select our parents and grandparents or choose to be born female. Nevertheless, we can do something about nearly half the risk factors for CAD, which are, therefore, called modifiable risk factors:

- Cigarette smoking is the most significant cause of preventable death in the United States, and a smoker's chances of sudden death are several times greater than those of a nonsmoker. The good news is that smokers who quit return very rapidly to the same risk level as nonsmokers.
- Hypertension cannot be prevented or cured, but it can be controlled with changes in diet and with medications. A person with uncontrolled hypertension has two to three times the risk of CAD as a person with normal blood pressure.
- The levels of serum cholesterol are at least in part a consequence of dietary intake of saturated fats. In populations with low fat intake, the incidence of CAD is also low. Furthermore, lowering the serum cholesterol levels has been shown to reduce the incidence of heart attacks and other dangerous cardiac events. Cholesterol may also be controlled with medications, if necessary.
- One behavior that may have a role in elevating serum cholesterol is lack of exercise, which also has a variety of other untoward effects on the body. Exercise improves overall fitness, cardiac reserve, and collateral coronary circulation.
- Obesity may go hand in hand with several other risk factors (such as diabetes and hypertension). But obesity by itself also may contribute to an increased risk of CAD. Weight reduction, through consumption of a sensible diet and increased physical exercise, can reap several lifelong and life-extending benefits. Normalizing body weight will lower elevated blood pressure, elevated serum cholesterol levels, elevated blood glucose levels, and the risk of CAD.

Data suggest that risk factor modification can make a difference in the impact of CAD. According to the AHA, from 1993 to 2003, mortality from CAD declined 22% in the United States   Figure 27-22 ▸ . Although we cannot say precisely what caused that decline (we would like to think that paramedic-staffed ambulances had a significant role!), reduction in smoking, better control of hypertension, changes in dietary habits, and an upsurge of interest in fitness undoubtedly made substantial contributions to this trend.

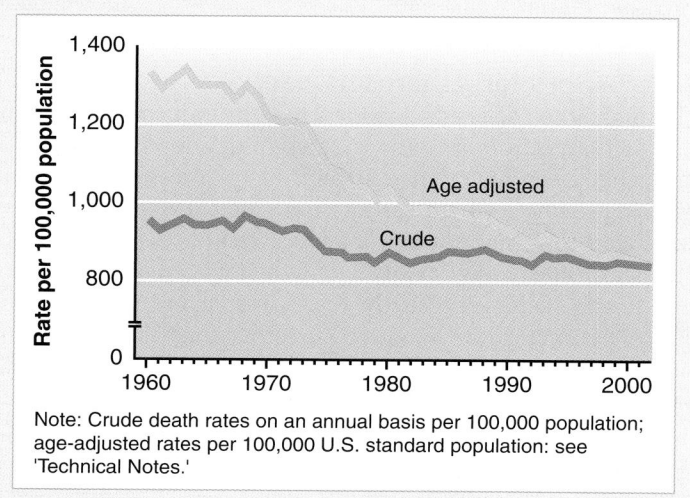

Note: Crude death rates on an annual basis per 100,000 population; age-adjusted rates per 100,000 U.S. standard population: see 'Technical Notes.'

Figure 27-22 Crude and age-adjusted death rates, United States, 1960–2002.

Source: Centers for Disease Control and Prevention.

Peripheral Vascular Disorders

Although atherosclerosis is rarely the primary cause of medical emergencies, it is a major contributor to other conditions that may become medical emergencies. For example, arterial bruits or "swishing" sounds (heard with a stethoscope placed over the carotid arteries) signal the presence of atherosclerosis and contraindicate the use of carotid sinus massage. Atherosclerosis can also contribute to claudication, a severe pain in the calf muscle caused by narrowing of the arteries in this muscle and leading to a painful limp. Finally, atherosclerosis may be associated with phlebitis—swelling and pain along the veins that can lead to the formation of blood clots (thrombophlebitis). If dislodged, these thrombi become emboli that could travel to the heart and through its right side, lodging in the pulmonary arterial tree and causing a pulmonary embolism.

An estimated 5 to 20 million Americans are affected by significant peripheral vascular disorders annually. The most dangerous complication of these disorders is pulmonary embolism, which causes approximately 200,000 deaths each year. Risk factors for peripheral vascular disorders include age, oral contraceptive use, smoking, recent surgery, recreational IV drug use, trauma, and extended immobilization. Identification of these risk factors has a significant role in diagnosing peripheral vascular occlusions. Signs of peripheral vascular occlusion may include pain, redness, swelling, warmth, and tenderness in the extremity; these signs are present in only about half of all cases, however. The presence of claudication indicates a significant narrowing of the peripheral arteries associated with peripheral vascular disorders. Arterial bruits are another sign of vascular narrowing that can contribute to ischemia or stroke.

Because peripheral vascular disorders can have serious consequences, such as pulmonary embolism or loss of limb through arterial occlusions, you must be familiar with the signs, symptoms, and risk factors for these conditions. Unfortunately, prehospital treatment of peripheral vascular conditions is limited. Beyond supplementary oxygen, IV access, and, possibly, aspirin administration, little can be done in the field if you suspect a peripheral vascular disorder.

Acute Coronary Syndrome

Acute coronary syndrome (ACS) is the term used to describe any group of clinical symptoms consistent with acute myocardial ischemia. Acute myocardial ischemia typically presents as chest pain due to insufficient blood supply to the heart muscle, which itself is a result of CAD. The life-threatening ACS disorders are responsible for much of the emergency medical care and hospitalization in the United States.

Patients experiencing symptomatic, acute myocardial ischemia should receive a 12-lead ECG to determine whether they have an ST-segment elevation. Most patients whose ECG displays ST-segment elevation will ultimately develop a "Q-wave AMI" (heart attack), also known as STEMI (ST-elevation myocardial infarction. Patients who have ischemic discomfort (chest pain) without an ST-segment elevation are having unstable angina or a non–ST-segment elevation MI that usually leads to a non–Q-wave MI; these conditions are collectively known as UA/NSTEMI (unstable angina/non–ST-elevation myocardial infarction). Patients who experience angina may also present with ST-segment depression. Finally, some patients experiencing angina or MI may have *no* changes indicated by the ECG.

Angina Pectoris

The principal symptom of CAD is angina pectoris (literally "choking in the chest"). Angina occurs when the supply of oxygen to the myocardium is insufficient to meet the demand. As a result, the cardiac muscle becomes ischemic, and a switch to anaerobic metabolism leads to the accumulation of lactic acid and carbon dioxide. The concept of "supply and demand" is critical here. When at rest, a person with heart disease may have an adequate supply of oxygen to the heart to meet these sedentary needs, despite some narrowing of the coronary arteries. When the same person exercises or experiences some other stress, however, the blood flow to the myocardium may not be able to satisfy the heart's increased demand for oxygen; in that case, angina will result. Clearly, the patient who experiences angina at rest, when oxygen needs are minimal, has more severe CAD than a person who experiences angina only with vigorous exercise.

When taking the history from a patient with chest pain, it is important to distinguish between stable angina and unstable angina. Stable angina follows a recurrent pattern: A person with stable angina experiences pain after a certain, predictable amount of exertion, such as climbing one flight of stairs or walking for three blocks. The pain also has a predictable location, intensity, and duration. The patient may report, for example, "Every time I walk up the hill to the bus stop, I get a squeezing pain under my breast bone, and I have to sit down for 2 or 3 minutes until it goes away."

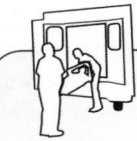

In the Field

Other names for unstable angina include pre-infarction angina, crescendo angina, and ACS.

Patients with chronic, stable angina often take nitroglycerin or some other form of "nitrate" for relief of anginal pain. In its usual formulation, nitroglycerin is supplied as a white tablet, which is placed under the tongue (sublingual) and allowed to dissolve there, or in a spray form that is sprayed under the tongue. It may also be given as sustained-release capsules taken two or three times a day, as a cream rubbed into the skin (topical), or as a patch worn on the skin. Regardless of which form is used, nitroglycerin will have a predictable effect in stable angina, producing relief of symptoms within a few minutes.

Unstable angina is much more serious than stable angina and indicates a greater degree of obstruction of the coronary arteries. It is characterized by noticeable changes in the frequency, severity, and duration of pain and often occurs without predictable stress. The patient may report that the anginal attacks have grown more frequent and severe during the past several days or weeks or that they awaken him or her from sleep or occur when otherwise at rest. Such attacks are often warning signs of an impending MI.

Management Considerations

Of course, not all chest pain is caused by cardiac ischemia or injury. Many other conditions—such as pulmonary embolism, pneumothorax, pneumonia, pericarditis, aortic dissection, indigestion, and peptic ulcer—may cause chest pain that can be mistaken for angina or an MI. It is important to perform a thorough physical exam, including a focused history, to determine whether the cause of the complaint is likely cardiac in origin.

Notes from Nancy

When a patient with chest pain calls for an ambulance, it means that the patient never had chest pain before or that his or her chronic chest pain has changed. Either way, it's serious.

As a general rule, it is safe to assume that any patient who has called for an ambulance because of chest pain has, at the least, unstable angina and perhaps an evolving AMI. Patients with chronic, stable angina rarely call for help unless something has changed—often dramatically—for the worse. Because it is difficult and sometimes impossible to differentiate between angina and an MI in the field, the treatment of angina should be the same as for an MI. It is far better to overtreat angina as an MI than to undertreat an MI by assuming it is angina.

Acute Myocardial Infarction

An acute myocardial infarction (AMI), or heart attack, occurs when a portion of the cardiac muscle is deprived of coronary blood flow long enough that portions of the muscle die (undergoes necrosis, or infarcts). Several things can diminish flow through coronary vessels, especially if the vessels are already narrowed by atherosclerotic disease: occlusion of a coronary artery by a blood clot (thrombus), spasm of a coronary artery, or reduction of overall blood flow from any cause (such as shock, arrhythmias, or pulmonary embolism).

The location and size of a myocardial infarct depend on which coronary artery is blocked and where along its course the blockage occurred. The majority of infarcts involve the left ventricle. When the anterior, lateral, or septal walls of the left ventricle are infarcted, the source is usually occlusion of the left coronary artery or one of its branches. Inferior wall infarcts are usually the result of RCA occlusion. When the ischemic process affects only the inner layer of muscle, the infarct is referred to as subendocardial. When the infarct extends through the entire wall of the ventricle, it is a transmural MI. The infarcted tissue is invariably surrounded by a ring of ischemic tissue—an area that is relatively deprived of oxygen but still viable. That ischemic tissue tends to be electrically unstable and is often the source of cardiac arrhythmias.

Notes from Nancy

For purposes of treatment outside the hospital, the patient with chest pain must be assumed to be suffering an acute myocardial infarction until proven otherwise and should therefore be treated as any other patient with a suspected AMI.

Acute myocardial infarction is the leading cause of death in the United States, accounting for more than 500,000 deaths per year; of those deaths, 60% to 70% occur outside the hospital, during the first 2 to 3 hours after the onset of symptoms. Of all deaths from AMI, 90% are due to arrhythmias, usually ventricular fibrillation, which typically occur during the early hours of the infarct. Arrhythmias can be prevented or treated, so *most deaths from AMI are preventable.*

Symptoms of AMI

Although there is no "typical AMI patient," when most Americans think about the symptoms of an AMI, they envision the classic pain presentation usually associated with men. In fact, AMIs can occur in younger and older people and in men and women. The patient may be slightly overweight and may have recently overindulged at the dinner table or perhaps on the tennis court. Nevertheless, many heart attacks occur at rest or just after arising in the morning.

The most common symptom of AMI is chest pain. This pain is similar to that of angina but can be much more severe and last more than 15 minutes. A patient with chronic angina will be aware that something very different from previous anginal attacks is happening. The pain of AMI is typically felt just beneath the sternum and is variously described as heavy, squeezing, crushing, or tight. Often the patient unconsciously clenches a fist when describing the pain (Levine sign) to convey in body language the squeezing nature of the pain. In 25% of cases, the pain radiates to the arms (most often the left arm) and into the fingers; it may also radiate to the neck, jaw, upper back, or epigastrium. Occasionally, a patient will mistake the pain of AMI for indigestion and may take antacids in an attempt to relieve the discomfort. The pain of AMI is not influenced by coughing, deep breathing, or other body movements.

Not every AMI patient has chest pain, however. In fact, 10% to 20% of patients with AMI *do not experience any chest pain.* Diabetics, older people, and heart transplant patients, for example, generally do not present with chest pain, a condition referred to as "silent MI." Instead, these patients may present with symptoms related to a drop in CO. It is not unusual for them to develop sudden dyspnea, progressing rapidly to pulmonary edema, a sudden loss of consciousness, an unexplained drop in blood pressure, an apparent stroke, or simply confusion.

Women with an AMI may present differently from men with the same condition. Women may experience nausea, lightheadedness, epigastric burning, or sudden onset of weakness or unexplained tiredness. Because they are not experiencing the typical chest pain expected with an AMI, many women ignore their symptoms. Unfortunately, CVD is the number one cause of death for US women.

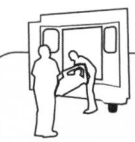

In the Field

More men have heart disease, but more women die of heart disease, in part because their symptoms are less clear-cut.

When obtaining the history from a patient whose chief complaint is chest pain, ask the usual OPQRST questions to elaborate on the chief complaint, but also ask whether the patient has taken anything for the pain and, if so, whether it helped. If the patient reports having taken nitroglycerin without relief, it is important to establish *why* the patient did not obtain relief.

Two reasons might explain this failure. One possibility is that the patient is, indeed, having an AMI, for which nitroglycerin would not provide complete pain relief. The other possibility is that the nitroglycerin has simply gone stale. To retain its potency, nitroglycerin must be stored in a dark, airtight container; if it is left out in the open for any period (for example, if the patient stores the medicine on the window sill above the kitchen sink), it loses its therapeutic effectiveness. To distinguish between the two explanations, ask the patient whether he or she noticed the usual effects of the nitroglycerin. Nitroglycerin tablets that are therapeutically active cause a slight burning under the tongue, may make the patient feel flushed,

Notes from Nancy

Start treatment immediately for any patient with chest pain.

or may give the patient a transient throbbing headache. If the patient confirms that he or she felt one of those effects but the chest pain still wouldn't go away, then you know there was nothing wrong with the nitroglycerin but there may be something very wrong with the patient.

As soon as you have elicited a chief complaint of a cardiac nature, you will need to start treatment of the patient; obtaining a focused history and physical examination can wait. For purposes of discussion, though, we shall continue here to proceed through the history and physical examination. Besides pain (or, sometimes, instead of pain), a number of other symptoms are associated with AMI:

- Diaphoresis (sweating), often profuse, is principally the result of massive discharge by the autonomic nervous system. The patient may soak through his or her clothing and complain of a cold sweat.
- Dyspnea may be a warning of impending left-sided heart failure.
- Anorexia (loss of appetite), nausea, vomiting, or belching frequently accompanies MI. Hiccups may occasionally occur as well, due to irritation of the diaphragm by an inferior wall MI.
- Weakness may be profound, and the patient may describe this feeling with phrases such as "a limp rag."
- If CO is significantly diminished, dizziness may reflect the reduced circulation to the brain.
- Palpitations are sometimes experienced by patients with cardiac arrhythmias as a sensation that the heart has skipped a beat.
- A feeling of impending doom is common among patients having an MI. The patient is frightened, looks frightened, and expresses his or her fear to other people—all of which adds to a general atmosphere of panic and dread.

Signs of AMI

Although patients with AMI often have abnormalities in the physical exam, many have relatively normal physical exam findings, and the diagnosis in the field (and, indeed, in the ED) depends chiefly on the history. Nevertheless, it is important to take note of a few specific things during the physical exam to detect the development of complications to AMI, such as heart failure or cardiogenic shock.

- Pay attention to the patient's general appearance. Does the patient appear anxious? Frightened? In obvious pain?
- What is the patient's state of consciousness? Is he or she fully alert? Confused? Remember: Poor perfusion creates confusion. If the patient does not seem "all there," it may be because the heart is giving out and not enough oxygenated blood is reaching the brain.
- Is the skin pale, cold, and clammy?
- Assess the patient's vital signs. Is the pulse strong or weak? Regular or irregular? Is the respiratory rate abnormally rapid? Is the blood pressure abnormally high or low?
- Are there signs of left-sided heart failure (wheezes or crackles)? Signs of right-sided heart failure (distended neck veins, pedal or presacral edema)?

A typical patient with an AMI is very apprehensive, with an ashen-gray pallor and cold, wet skin. He or she *looks* scared. The pulse may be rapid unless heart block has occurred. The blood pressure may be decreased, reflecting decreased CO from the damaged heart, or it may be elevated from pain and anxiety.

Management of ACSs in the Field

On your arrival at the scene, start treatment at once for any middle-aged or older patient with chest pain, even before you complete the history and physical exam. The longest delay in treatment seems to be the phase from onset of symptoms to patient recognition, so your care must begin immediately. The goals of treatment are to limit the size of the infarct, to decrease the patient's fear and pain, and to prevent the development of serious cardiac arrhythmias.

Place the Patient at Physical and Emotional Rest

The stress response causes the adrenal glands to squeeze out a surge of catecholamines (epinephrine and norepinephrine), which in turn can send the damaged heart racing. At the same time, the massive discharge throughout the fight-or-flight system puts the peripheral circulation in a state of severe vasoconstriction; thus, not only is the heart being flogged to go faster and faster, but it also has to work harder and harder against the increased afterload. The heart's need for oxygen, therefore, soars precisely when it is already in a state of marked oxygen deprivation. This cycle can lead quickly to arrhythmias and death. Prehospital deaths are related to arrhythmias (often ventricular fibrillation), and most occur during the first 4 hours after onset of symptoms. Nevertheless, this deadly cycle can be interrupted by community education programs designed to assist citizens in early recognition of symptoms, early activation of EMS, and, if needed, CPR and early access to an automated external defibrillator (AED).

To begin your treatment, put the patient physically at ease. Recall that one goal of treatment is to try to limit the size of the infarct; one way to do so is to decrease the amount of work that the heart must do, which will begin to decrease the patient's myocardial oxygen requirements immediately. The position in which cardiac work is minimal is the semi-Fowler's position—that is, reclining on the stretcher with the back of the stretcher raised about 30°. Of course, the patient has to get to the stretcher and must not be permitted to do so alone. From the time you arrive, the patient must not do anything, including walking to the ambulance.

Administer Oxygen and Aspirin

The mnemonic MONA is used to help remember the supportive treatments of Morphine, Oxygen, Nitroglycerin, and Aspirin for a patient with an ACS—but these treatments are not to be given in that order. MONA is administered in the following order, provided these measures are not contraindicated by hypotension: (1) oxygen, (2) aspirin, (3) nitroglycerin, and (4) morphine.

Oxygen may limit ischemic myocardial injury and reduce the amount of ST-segment elevation. Its effects on morbidity

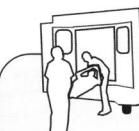

In the Field
Oxygen is the first drug in the treatment of AMI.

and mortality in acute infarction are unknown. The recommendation is to initiate oxygen at a rate of 4 to 6 L/min via nasal cannula, although a nonrebreathing mask that provides oxygen at a rate of 12 to 15 L/min is also acceptable. Monitor the Sao_2 and titrate until the patient is in stable condition or the hypoxemia is corrected (that is, $Sao_2 > 90\%$).

In most EMS systems, as long as the patient has no aspirin allergy or gastrointestinal bleeding, dispatchers may advise patients to chew baby aspirin (160 to 325 mg). If this has not been done before your arrival or the patient has not already taken aspirin on his or her own, then give the patient 160 to 325 mg of non–enteric-coated aspirin to chew.

Provide Pain Relief

Some form of pain relief must be provided because the pain of AMI is very severe and places enormous stress on the patient's autonomic nervous system—stress that may contribute to complications. Nitroglycerin is a good place to start, but make sure the patient's blood pressure is adequate before its administration. In particular, before giving this medication, it is imperative that you ascertain whether the patient is taking phosphodiesterase-5 (PDE-5) inhibitors for erectile dysfunction **Table 27-10 ▾**. These drugs may worsen certain medical conditions and interact with a number of drugs, especially nitrate medications (such as nitroglycerin) prescribed to prevent or treat acute angina. Both types of medication dilate blood vessels, and their combined effects can cause dizziness, low blood pressure, and loss of consciousness.

Place a 0.4-mg tablet (or spray) of nitroglycerin under the patient's tongue. If the patient is experiencing an AMI and not simply angina, this medication is unlikely to relieve his or her pain, but it may help to reduce the size of the infarction. Do *not* give nitroglycerin if there is hypotension or bradycardia, and do *not* give it to patients having epigastric symptoms ("indigestion") or hiccups. Nitroglycerin may be repeated every 3 to 5 minutes, up to a total of three doses as long as the patient's condition remains stable.

If nitroglycerin provides no relief of pain and if authorized by medical command, morphine sulfate may be titrated in IV doses according to local protocols. Give this medication in 2- to 4-mg IV doses as needed for pain, being sure to reassess

Table 27-10	PDE-5 Inhibitors	
Brand Name	**Generic Name**	**Duration of Effect**
Viagra	Sildenafil citrate	Up to 4 h
Levitra	Vardenafil	Up to 4 h
Cialis	Tadalfil	24 to 36 h

the patient's blood pressure, pulse, and respiratory rate after each dose, until the patient experiences relief of pain or experiences a drop in pulse or blood pressure. If bradycardia occurs, notify the physician immediately. Remember that morphine should *not* be given to patients with low blood pressure (less than about 100 mm Hg systolic or according to local protocol), dehydrated patients, or patients suspected of having an AMI involving the inferior wall of the heart. At least half of all patients with MI of the inferior wall will also experience a right ventricular infarction; as a consequence, they may already be hypotensive or the administration of nitroglycerin and morphine may cause hypotension.

In some EMS medical protocols, fentanyl is favored over morphine for pain not relieved with nitroglycerin because of its rapid onset and relatively short duration. Fentanyl also has fewer side effects than morphine.

Perform Cardiac Monitoring

Apply the ECG monitor, and run a strip to document the initial rhythm. As long as you are applying electrodes to the chest, also place your anterior chest leads in anticipation of doing a 12-lead ECG. Ideally, your monitor should have an audible tone that beeps with each QRS complex (also called systole beep), so that you can keep track of the patient's cardiac rhythm even when you have to take your gaze from the monitor to do other things. The ear, in any case, is far more sensitive than the eye to slight irregularities in rhythm, so the chances are that you will *hear* the beginning of a cardiac arrhythmia much sooner than you will see it on the monitor. Keep the other cardiac drugs that you carry close at hand so you can reach them quickly if a cardiac arrhythmia develops.

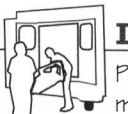

In the Field

Patients may not be forthcoming about taking medications. They may omit something from their list of home medications if they do not take the medicine daily. Be sure to ask.

Record the Vital Signs

Obtain vital signs, including pulse, respirations, blood pressure, and oxygen saturation. Measure the blood pressure, and repeat that measurement at least every 5 minutes. Measure the pulse. The ECG monitor provides information only about the electrical activity of the heart; it gives no information about the strength of the heartbeat (muscular activity) or even about whether the heart is beating at all! It is, therefore, necessary to monitor the patient's pulse to assess peripheral blood flow, especially during transport, when blood pressure measurements are difficult and unreliable.

Perform a Detailed History and Physical Exam

After you have completed the preceding steps (as appropriate), you should obtain a more detailed history and perform a physical exam. Find out if the patient has a history of cardiac disease; takes any heart medications, such as beta-blockers, angiotensin-converting enzyme inhibitors, diuretics, or nitroglycerin (nitrates); or has had a previous heart attack or any heart surgery (such as coronary artery bypass graft). Also obtain a more complete description of the present symptoms, especially regarding their onset. Gathering that information should not, however, delay transport to the hospital. Once you have taken

You are the Provider Part 5

The adenosine did not work, and your patient continues to be in hemodynamically stable condition, which gives you the opportunity to continue treating Anthony pharmacologically. In accordance with department protocols you reach into the drug box, grab a prefilled syringe of diltiazem, and wipe the sweat off of your brow. Before administering the diltiazem, you recheck the protocol book and confirm the dose as 25 mg by IV push. You hold your breath as you administer the diltiazem, knowing that at any time Anthony's condition can become unstable. After about a minute passes, you note that the HR on the cardiac monitor begins to steadily decrease, finally stabilizing at 94 beats/min. Both you and Anthony can breathe a sigh of relief. You contact the receiving ED, give your report, and receive no further orders.

On arrival at the ED, a diltiazem drip is started. He is admitted overnight for observation on the telemetry floor. After an uneventful night, Anthony is discharged home with strong suggestions not to overindulge in energy drinks and caffeine pills and to find healthier study habits!

Reassessment	Recording Time: 25 Minutes
Skin	Pink, warm, and dry
Pulse	94 beats/min, regular; strong distal pulses
ECG	Normal sinus rhythm
Blood pressure	124/76 mm Hg
Respirations	18 breaths/min, nonlabored
Sao$_2$	99% on nasal cannula at 4 L/min of oxygen
Pupils	Equal and reactive to light

8. What type of medication is diltiazem?

9. How does diltiazem work?

the necessary precautions to stabilize the patient's condition (aspirin, oxygen, IV saline lock, monitor/12-lead ECG, analgesia), there is no reason to remain any longer at the scene unless a cardiac arrest or arrhythmia requires immediate treatment. Take the rest of the history en route to the hospital. Remember that "time is muscle": Heart cells are being destroyed during the infarction before reperfusion is started in the hospital.

Transport the Patient

Once the patient is in stable condition, transport him or her to an appropriate hospital in a semi-Fowler position (unless the patient is in shock, in which case he or she should be supine). Do all you can to ensure that the patient is as relaxed and as comfortable as possible. En route, some additional treatment measures may be worthwhile, especially when transport will take a long time.

Safe and appropriate transport is the name of the game. *Do not rush* and *do not use sirens* when transporting the patient to the hospital. High speed and sirens send two clear messages to the patient: (1) Something is terribly wrong. (2) The personnel on the ambulance don't feel capable of dealing with the situation. Those are *not* the messages you want to convey to a frightened patient with a damaged heart! The patient needs to feel confident that those caring for him or her are in control of the situation.

If a serious arrhythmia occurs during transport, consider stopping the vehicle, institute treatment immediately, and notify medical control. Except under unusual circumstances, treatment of life-threatening situations should not be attempted in a moving ambulance. Whenever possible, the driver should pull over to the side of the road and go to the back of the vehicle to help the other provider.

Reperfusion Techniques for ACSs

The majority of AMIs occur as a result of thrombus (fixed blood clot) formation at the site of a preexisting atherosclerotic plaque. The thrombus occludes the coronary artery, preventing further blood flow through it. Thus, it seems reasonable to try to restore circulation through the occluded coronary artery, thereby restoring perfusion to the ischemic myocardium. Simply put, that is reperfusion.

The most immediate forms of reperfusion are fibrinolytic therapy and percutaneous intervention (PCI). All paramedics should be alert for patients who are good candidates for reperfusion, should know which hospitals in their area carry out fibrinolytic therapy and/or PCI, and should provide early notification (along with 12-lead ECG results) to the ED that a candidate for such therapy is en route.

Fibrinolysis

One way in which to reperfuse the blocked coronary artery is to try to dissolve the occluding blood clot, thereby restoring circulation to the ischemic heart. That idea is the essence of fibrinolytic therapy.

In fact, this concept is not altogether new. Attempts to use fibrinolytic agents in the treatment of AMI were reported at least 40 years ago, albeit without success. In retrospect, we realize that one reason the early attempts failed was that fibrinolytic therapy was started too late, after irreversible damage to the myocardium had already occurred. With that realization came the concept that "time is myocardium": The longer a segment of myocardium remains unperfused, the smaller the chances of salvaging that tissue and restoring its normal function. The obvious corollary is that the sooner fibrinolytic therapy can begin with respect to the onset of the blockage, the better the chances for saving the affected distal myocardium. Indeed, fibrinolytic treatment given within 30 to 60 minutes of the onset of symptoms can sometimes abort the MI altogether.

In the 1980s, providers began to start fibrinolytic treatment as soon as possible after the patient with an AMI reached the ED, rather than waiting until he or she was admitted to the coronary care unit. Inevitably, applying the doctrine that time is myocardium led to the idea of starting fibrinolytic treatment even earlier, in the prehospital phase of care.

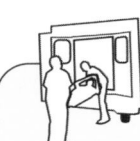

In the Field

Time is muscle (myocardium)!

Recent clinical trials have shown the benefit of starting fibrinolysis as soon as possible after the onset of ischemic-type chest pain in patients with STEMI or new or presumably new left bundle branch block. Several prospective studies have also documented reduced time to administration of fibrinolytics and decreased mortality rates when out-of-hospital fibrinolytics were given to patients with STEMI and no contraindications to fibrinolytics. Some EMS systems may opt to start fibrinolytic treatment in the field, and in rural areas with very long transport times, prehospital initiation of fibrinolytic therapy may make a lot of sense. Even in EMS systems in which paramedics do not give fibrinolytic therapy, their ability to identify candidates for such therapy has a decisive role in helping ED personnel administer fibrinolytic therapy early enough to make a difference. For these reasons, all paramedics should thoroughly understand the principles of fibrinolytic therapy for AMI.

Fibrinolytic therapy seeks to administer, during the early hours of AMI, an agent that will activate the body's own internal system for dissolving clots, the fibrinolytic system. Once activated, that system can begin to dissolve the clot that has formed within the coronary artery, thereby reopening the artery (recanalization) and allowing the resumption of blood flow through it (reperfusion). Unfortunately, if an agent capable of promoting clot dissolution is given intravenously, its effects cannot be limited to the clot in the coronary artery; it can also act anywhere else in the body where clots are being formed and, therefore, may lead to bleeding. Thus, the benefit of fibrinolytic therapy—the possible salvage of myocardium—must always be weighed against its risks—principally, the risk of bleeding.

To determine the appropriate candidates for fibrinolytic agents, we need to be as certain as possible that we are really

Table 27-11	ST-Segment Elevation or New or Presumably New LBBB: Evaluation for Reperfusion

Step 1: Assess time and risk

- Time since onset of symptoms
- Risk of STEMI
- Risk of fibrinolysis
- Time required to transport to skilled PCI catheterization suite

Step 2: Select reperfusion (fibrinolysis or invasive) strategy

Note: If presentation < 3 hours and no delay for PCI, then no preference for either strategy.

Fibrinolysis is generally preferred if:

- Early presentation (≤ 3 hours from symptom onset)
- Invasive strategy is not an option (eg, lack of access to skilled PCI facility or difficult vascular access) or would be delayed
  —Medical contact-to-balloon or door-balloon > 90 min
  —(Door-to-balloon) minus (door-to-needle) is > 1 hour
- No contraindications to fibrinolysis

An invasive strategy is generally preferred if:

- Late presentation (symptom onset > 3 hours ago)
- Skilled PCI facility available with surgical backup
- Medical contact-to-balloon or door-balloon < 90 min
- (Door-to-balloon) minus (door-to-needle) is < 1 hour
- Contraindications to fibrinolysis, including increased risk of bleeding and ICH
- High risk from STEMI (CHF, Killip class is ≥ 3)
- Diagnosis of STEMI is in doubt

Modified from ACC/AHA 2004 Update Recommendations.

dealing with a patient who is having an AMI. A patient having chest pain from another source would receive no potential benefit from fibrinolytic therapy—so he or she would be subjected to this therapy's risks for no reason. Although it is difficult in the early hours of an AMI to be certain of the diagnosis, inclusion criteria have been established to help select patients most likely to be having an AMI. At the same time, exclusion criteria are used to identify patients for whom the risk of fibrinolytic therapy is unacceptably high—for example, patients most likely to experience hemorrhagic complications. **Table 27-11 ▲** summarizes the inclusion and exclusion criteria for fibrinolytic therapy.

Most treatment regimens for fibrinolysis include one of three agents: alteplase (Activase; a tissue plasminogen activator), streptokinase (Streptase), or reteplase (Retavase; recombinant tissue). All of them work by converting, in one way or another, the body's own clot-dissolving enzyme from its inactive form, plasminogen, to its active form, plasmin.

According to the AHA's 2005 guidelines, the key to realizing the benefits of fibrinolysis is to start early. A prehospital fibrinolytic program is recommended only in systems with well-established protocols, checklists, experience in ACLS, ability to communicate with the receiving institution, and a medical director with training and experience in the management of STEMI.

Percutaneous Intervention

As an alternative to fibrinolysis, many institutions perform a PCI. Patients with complex, multivessel disease or ACSs may benefit from PCI. In this therapy, balloons, stents, or other devices are passed through a 2-mm-diameter catheter via a peripheral artery to recanalize and keep the blocked coronary artery open. The success rate is high, and the risks are low. PCI is often used for patients who are not candidates for fibrinolytic therapy.

Congestive Heart Failure

Congestive heart failure (also known as chronic heart failure) occurs when the heart is unable, for any reason, to pump powerfully enough or fast enough to empty its chambers; as a result, blood backs up into the systemic circuit, the pulmonary circuit, or both. Although CHF may develop in situations other than AMI—for example, in a patient with chronic high blood pressure—the basic principles of diagnosis and treatment are similar, whatever the precipitating factors.

More than 2 million people in the United States have CHF, and an additional 500,00 cases are diagnosed each year. Nearly half of the patients with CHF classified as severe die within 1 year of diagnosis.

Left-Sided Heart Failure

The left ventricle is most commonly damaged during an AMI. Likewise, in chronic hypertension, the left ventricle tends to suffer the long-term effects of having to pump against an increased afterload (constricted peripheral arteries). In both cases, the right side of the heart continues to pump relatively normally and to deliver normal volumes of blood to the pulmonary circulation. By comparison, the left side of the heart may no longer be able to pump the blood being delivered from the pulmonary vessels. As a result, blood backs up behind the left ventricle, and the pressure in the left atrium and pulmonary veins increases. As the pulmonary veins become engorged with blood, serum is forced out of the pulmonary capillaries and into the alveoli. The serum mixes with air in the alveoli to produce foam (pulmonary edema).

When fluid occupies the alveoli, oxygenation is impaired. The patient experiences that impairment as shortness of breath (dyspnea), particularly in the recumbent position (orthopnea). If left ventricular failure is the result of chronic overload (as opposed to AMI), the patient is likely to give a history of a

Table 27-12	Differentiation and Treatment of Asthma and Left-Sided Heart Failure	
	Asthma	**Left-Sided Heart Failure**
History	Often a younger patient May have allergic history or family history of allergy Previous attacks of acute, episodic dyspnea May have had recent respiratory infection Unproductive cough Medications may include: ■ Inhalers: Isoproterenol (Medihaler), albuterol (Vaponefrin), epinephrine (microNEFRIN), isoetharine (Bronkosol), isoproterenol (Isuprel) ■ Pills: calcium carb/glycine chew (Tedrol), pseudoephedrine (Sudafed), theophylline and guaifenesin (Quibron), triprolidine and pseudoephedrine (Actifed), theophylline/ephedrine/hydroxyaine-oral (Marax)	Often an older patient May have history of heart problems, hypertension Dyspnea worse when lying down (orthopnea) Recent rapid weight gain Cough with watery or foamy sputum Medications may include: ■ Digitalis glycosides: digoxin (Lanoxin), digitoxin ■ Diuretics: chlorothiazide (Diuril), furosemide (Lasix), hydrochlorothiazide (Esidrix), ethacrynic acid (Edecrin), trichlormethiazide (Metahydrin, Naqua)
Possible physical findings	Wheezing Chest hyperinflated and hyperresonant Use of accessory muscles to breathe If bronchospasm severe, chest may be silent	Wheezing Crackles S_3 gallop Distended neck veins Pedal or presacral edema
Treatment	Oxygen (humidified) Intermittent positive-pressure breathing Monitor IV: normal saline Selective beta-2 adrenergic medications Sometimes bicarbonate (morphine and diuretics contraindicated)	Oxygen Intermittent positive-pressure breathing Monitor IV: normal saline to keep open or saline lock (adrenergics and bicarbonate usually contraindicated) Morphine Diuretics (furosemide) Nitroglycerin

week or two of PND. To compensate for the impairment in oxygenation, the patient's respiratory rate increases (tachypnea); even so, if the patient's condition is advanced enough, cyanosis may become evident. In some patients with pulmonary edema, especially elderly patients, Cheyne-Stokes respirations may be present.

Fluid from the pulmonary vessels also leaks into the interstitial spaces in the lungs, and increasing interstitial pressure causes narrowing of the bronchioles. Air passing through the narrowed bronchioles creates wheezing noises, whereas air bubbling through the fluid-filled alveoli produces crackles. Furthermore, the patient may cough up the edema fluid in the form of foamy, blood-tinged sputum. As the airways narrow and the lungs grow heavier from the accumulation of fluid, the work of breathing increases, which puts an even greater strain on the already floundering heart. Dyspnea and hypoxemia produce a state of panic, which induces the release of epinephrine from the adrenals. The heart is pushed even harder, and its oxygen demand is increased precisely when fluid in the alveoli is reducing the amount of oxygen available.

To make matters worse, the sympathetic nervous system response produces peripheral vasoconstriction: Peripheral resistance (afterload) increases, and the weakened, hypoxic heart finds itself trying to push blood out into smaller and smaller pipes. Clinically, peripheral vasoconstriction is apparent as pallor and elevated blood pressure. The massive sympathetic discharge also produces sweating of the pale, cold skin.

It is not unusual for a patient with left-sided heart failure to become frantic from air hunger. He or she may pace or thrash about or may even be combative and struggle with the rescue team. Furthermore, hypoxemia results in inadequate oxygen supply to the brain, often manifested as confusion or disorientation. If hypoxemia is severe, cardiac arrest may follow quickly.

Signs and Symptoms of Left-Sided Heart Failure

The signs and symptoms of left-sided heart failure include extreme restlessness and agitation, confusion, severe dyspnea and tachypnea, tachycardia, elevated blood pressure, crackles and possibly wheezes, and frothy, pink sputum. Sometimes, it may be difficult to distinguish the wheezing of asthma from that of left-sided heart failure. Table 27-12 ▲ presents some of the features that can help you differentiate the two conditions.

Management of Left-Sided Heart Failure

Prehospital treatment of left-sided heart failure is aimed at improving oxygenation, decreasing the workload of the heart (by reducing preload), and forcing fluid from the alveoli.

Continuous positive airway pressure (CPAP) is an effective treatment for patients with left-sided heart failure and pulmonary edema. Through the use of positive end-expiratory pressure (PEEP), CPAP drives fluid out of the alveoli, thus improving pulmonary respiration. In conjunction with drug therapy, CPAP has shown to reduce the need for intubation. If the patient will not tolerate CPAP, give 100% oxygen via nonrebreathing mask. Monitor the patient's end-tidal CO_2 and oxygen saturation.

Sit the patient up, with the feet dangling. That position encourages venous pooling in the legs, thereby reducing venous return to the heart. The sitting position also makes breathing easier for a patient in respiratory distress.

Start a saline lock or an IV with normal saline at a keep-vein-open rate. Also, attach monitoring electrodes because patients in CHF are prone to arrhythmias.

Pharmacologic therapy of left-sided heart failure may vary slightly from place to place, but the mainstays of drug therapy include the drugs mentioned below (in order of the author's preference). Refer to your usual protocols, and have the appropriate medications drawn up and ready, pending the physician's order to administer them. Remember to constantly monitor the blood pressure because many of these medications lower it.

Nitroglycerin, 0.4 mg sublingually, may be ordered as a vasodilator to create venous pooling, thereby reducing the volume of blood returned from the periphery to the heart. Before ordering this medication, the physician will want to know how much, if any, nitroglycerin the patient has already taken. The initial dose of 0.4 mg may be repeated at 5-minute intervals up to a total of 1.2 mg (three doses).

Furosemide (Lasix) is a diuretic that has two positive effects in left-sided heart failure. Initially (within the first 5 to 10 minutes), it has a venodilating effect, increasing peripheral pooling of blood. Subsequently, it removes excess fluid from the body by promoting its excretion by the kidneys. If ordered, furosemide is given in a dose of 20 to 40 mg or 0.5 to 1 mg/kg by IV bolus. If the patient already takes furosemide, the higher dose should be used. Furosemide should *not* be given to older patients in the prehospital phase of management.

Morphine sulfate has long been part of the standard treatment of cardiogenic pulmonary edema. Like nitroglycerin, morphine works as a vasodilator, increasing the pooling of blood in the periphery, but it also has a substantial calming effect on a frantic patient. If morphine is ordered, first check the patient's blood pressure (do not give morphine if the patient is hypotensive). Then give approximately 3 mg slowly by IV bolus, and recheck the blood pressure. If the blood pressure remains stable, another 3 mg may be given. Proceed in that manner until the total dose ordered by the physician has been administered.

The presence of wheezing indicates that bronchoconstriction has developed from the excessive fluid. In such a case, bronchodilator drugs such as albuterol (Proventil, Ventolin, HFA, Volmax), metaproterenol sulfate (Alupent), or ipratropium (Atrovent) may be ordered.

If transport will be prolonged and the patient is hypotensive, medical control may order an inotropic agent, such as dopamine, in order to increase cardiac output and improve blood pressure.

Transport the patient to the hospital in a sitting position, with legs dangling down.

Right-Sided Heart Failure

Right-sided heart failure most commonly occurs as a result of left-sided heart failure. As blood backs up from the left side of the heart into the lungs, the right side has to work increasingly harder to pump blood into the engorged pulmonary vessels. Eventually, the right side of the heart is unable to keep up with the increased workload, and it, too, fails. Right-sided heart failure may also occur as a result of pulmonary embolism or long-standing COPD, especially chronic bronchitis.

When right-sided heart failure occurs, blood backs up behind the right ventricle and increases the pressure in the systemic veins, causing them to become engorged. Distention can be seen in the veins visible on the surface of the body, such as the external jugular veins. Over time, as the pressure within the systemic veins increases, serum is forced out of the veins and into the surrounding tissues, producing edema. Edema is most likely to be visible in dependent parts of the body, such as the feet in a person who is sitting or standing or the lower back in a bedridden patient. Edema is also present in parts of the body that are *not* visible; a painful liver easily palpable in the right upper quadrant, for example, signals engorgement and swelling within that organ (hepatomegaly).

The development of right-sided heart failure can actually improve left-sided heart failure because the failing right side of the heart can no longer pump as much blood into the lungs. The decrease in output from the right side, in essence, amounts to a decrease in preload for the left side of the heart and may lessen pulmonary congestion.

Right-sided heart failure, by itself, is seldom a life-threatening emergency. Usually it develops gradually over days to weeks; likewise, it requires days to weeks to reverse the process by slowly ridding the body of excess salt and water. Treatment in the field of a patient with right-sided heart failure, therefore, is simply to make the patient comfortable, preferably in the semi-Fowler's position. Monitoring is always indicated in any patient with significant cardiac disease. If signs of associated left-sided heart failure are present, treat them as outlined in the previous section.

Cardiac Tamponade

The pericardium is a tough, fibrous membrane with the ability to stretch only up to a point. Normally, a small amount of pericardial fluid separates the pericardium and the outer surface of the heart. Cardiac tamponade occurs when excessive fluid accumulates within the pericardium, limiting the heart's ability to expand fully after each contraction and resulting in reduced CO. If unrecognized and untreated, this condition will reduce cardiac filling to the point that the heart is unable to circulate the blood.

Signs and Symptoms of Cardiac Tamponade
Cardiac tamponade can occur as a result of tumors, pericarditis, or trauma to the chest. Pericarditis, for example, can cause excessive amounts of fluid to accumulate in the pericardial space. Blunt or penetrating trauma can cause bleeding from blood vessels on the surface of the heart, allowing accumulation of blood in the pericardial space.

Signs and symptoms of cardiac tamponade vary depending on its cause. If the onset is gradual (as with pericarditis), the initial complaints might be dyspnea and weakness. If the cause is traumatic, the chief complaint might be chest pain. As the volume of fluid increases in the pericardium, the SV decreases, causing an initial drop in the systolic blood pressure. Eventually, the diastolic pressure will slowly rise, resulting in the classic symptom of narrowing pulse pressure. The initial drop in blood pressure is usually followed by an increase in HR, which leads to tachycardia. The heart sounds may be muffled or quieter than usual owing to the buildup of fluid, although this sign may be difficult to identify in the field. The patient may experience jugular vein distention as well, owing to the backup of blood from the right side of the heart. The combination of narrowing pulse pressure (hypotension) along with jugular vein distention and muffled heart sounds is commonly known as the Beck's triad.

The ECG is of limited value in identifying cardiac tamponade. Aside from tachycardia, you might see electrical alternans (alternating small- and large-amplitude QRS complexes). In addition, you might identify pulsus alternans (alternating strong and weak pulses). Pulsus paradoxus—a drop in systolic blood pressure of more than 10 mm Hg with the patient's inhalation that may be associated with a weakening pulse during inhalation—may also be present.

Identification of cardiac tamponade requires a thorough assessment. Changes in blood pressure can be recognized only after at least three values have been obtained, usually 5 to 10 minutes apart. Muffled heart sounds, pulsus alternans, electrical alternans, and pulsus paradoxus are not common signs and so may be easily overlooked. Occasionally, you may have difficulty distinguishing between cardiac tamponade and tension pneumothorax. One way to differentiate between the two is to remember that in cardiac tamponade, the breath sounds will be equal and the trachea will be midline because the lungs are not affected.

Management of Cardiac Tamponade
The ultimate treatment for cardiac tamponade is pericardiocentesis, which involves inserting a needle attached to a syringe into the chest far enough to penetrate the pericardium and then withdrawing fluid. Often, withdrawal of as little as 50 mL of fluid will result in significant improvement in the patient's condition. This technique is risky, however, and medical direction rarely allows it to be performed by paramedics. If pericardiocentesis is not allowed, the one treatment that will significantly enhance the patient's survival is rapid transport to a facility that can perform this procedure.

Supporting the patient's airway, breathing, and oxygenation during transport are essential. An IV fluid bolus of 500 mL of saline might be ordered by medical direction. When reporting to medical control, make sure that you identify all signs and symptoms that led you to believe the patient has cardiac tamponade so that the receiving hospital will be prepared to perform the pericardiocentesis.

Cardiogenic Shock
Cardiogenic shock occurs when the heart is so severely damaged that it can no longer pump a volume of blood sufficient to maintain tissue perfusion. An AMI nearly always produces some impairment of left ventricular function. When 25% of the left ventricular myocardium is involved in the AMI, left-sided heart failure usually develops. When 40% or more of the left ventricle has been infarcted, cardiogenic shock occurs. Thus, cardiogenic shock indicates extensive injury to the myocardium; accordingly, there is a high mortality rate. Transient cardiogenic shock can occur after resuscitation. Patients recovering from defibrillation for V-fib, for example, often have signs of cardiogenic shock.

Signs and Symptoms of Cardiogenic Shock
The signs and symptoms of cardiogenic shock are similar to those of most other kinds of shock. Because of the reduced cerebral perfusion, the patient is often confused or even comatose; if awake, he or she is likely to be restless and anxious. Massive peripheral vasoconstriction results in pale, cold skin, and poor renal perfusion is reflected in minimal or absent urine output. Respirations are rapid and shallow, with a possibility of adventitious breath sounds, and the pulse is racing and thready.

As these compensatory mechanisms begin to fail, the blood pressure will fall, sometimes to less than 90 mm Hg systolic. This vital sign may be deceptive, however: In patients with preexisting hypertension, systolic pressures higher than 90 mm Hg may still be associated with cardiogenic shock. The goal in treatment of cardiogenic shock is to identify and support the patient before the blood pressure drops to the point where the shock becomes irreversible.

Management of Cardiogenic Shock
Treatment of cardiogenic shock focuses on improving oxygenation and peripheral perfusion without adding to the work of the heart. Secure the patient's airway, and administer 100% supplemental oxygen by mask or bag-mask device. An advanced airway (that is, endotracheal tube, laryngeal mask airway, or Combitube) will be necessary if the patient is comatose. Place the patient in a supine position unless pulmonary edema is present; in that case, the patient should be placed in the semi-Fowler's position.

Table 27-13	Vasopressor Agents			
Drug	Preparation	Concentration (μg/mL)		Rate
Dopamine (Intropin)	400 mg in 250 mL normal saline	1,600		5 to 20 μg/kg/min For 70-kg man: 350 μg/min (13 microdrops/min)
Norepinephrine (Levophed)	4 mg in 250 mL D_5W	16		0.5 to 1.0 μg/min (2–4 microdrops/min)
Epinephrine (Adrenalin)	1 mL (1 mg) in 250 mL normal saline	4		2 to 10 μg/min (30–150 microdrops/min)

Start an IV with normal saline at a keep-vein-open rate. The physician may order a trial of fluids to determine whether the shock includes a hypovolemic component. If so, rapidly infuse 100 to 200 mL of saline, and closely monitor the patient's pulse, blood pressure, and LOC. Report those observations to the physician.

Apply monitoring electrodes and obtain a 12-lead ECG. Arrhythmias may bring about hypotension by causing severe disturbances in CO; thus, until major arrhythmias are corrected, you cannot be certain that the patient's hypotension is due to cardiogenic shock.

Depending on the distance to the hospital and local protocols, you may be asked to administer a vasopressor drug, such as one of those listed in **Table 27-13 ▲** . Dopamine might be preferred because, at beta doses, it maintains renal perfusion better than the other agents listed. To prepare a dopamine infusion, add 400 mg of dopamine to a 250-mL bag of normal saline, to yield a concentration of 1,600 μg/mL. The infusion rate will depend on the patient's weight and response, but it is usually initiated at 5 μg/kg/min. The administration of dopamine or any other vasopressor drug requires careful titration and frequent monitoring of the blood pressure. Measure the blood pressure at least every 5 minutes. Slow the infusion if the systolic pressure rises to more than 90 or 100 mm Hg; speed up the infusion if the systolic pressure falls below 70 mm Hg.

Transport the patient expeditiously to the hospital. Except for the correction of life-threatening arrhythmias, there are no measures that can stabilize the condition of a patient in cardiogenic shock in the field. Thus, there is nothing to be gained by tarrying at the scene.

Aortic Aneurysm

The word aneurysm comes from a Greek word meaning a widening; it refers to the dilatation or outpouching of a blood vessel. The aneurysms of greatest concern to you are those that involve the aorta, particularly acute dissecting aneurysms of the thoracic aorta and expanding or ruptured aneurysms of the abdominal aorta.

Acute Dissecting Aneurysm of the Aorta

The proximal aorta is subject to enormous hemodynamic forces. Anywhere from 60 to 100 times a minute, 60 minutes an hour, 24 hours a day—that is, around 40 million times a year—pulsatile waves of blood come pounding out of the left ventricle against the aortic walls. Over the years, that pounding takes its toll, producing degenerative changes in the media (the middle layer) of the aorta, especially the ascending aorta (the part of the aorta that rises from the heart toward the aortic arch). The degenerative changes are more pronounced with advancing age and in people with chronic high blood pressure, and their effect is to "unglue" the layers of the aortic wall from one another.

Eventually, the degenerative changes in the aortic media may lead to a disruption of the underlying intima (innermost layer of the artery). Tearing of the intima is most likely to occur in the portions of the thoracic aorta that are under the greatest stress—specifically, the ascending aorta just distal to the aortic valve (approximately 65% of cases) and the descending aorta just beyond the takeoff point of the left subclavian artery.

Once the intima is torn, the process of dissection, or separation of the arterial wall, often begins. With each ventricular systole, a jet of blood is forced into the torn arterial wall, creating a false channel between the intimal and medial layers of the wall. This channel is propagated distally and sometimes proximally along the length of the wall. If the dissection progresses back into the aortic valve, it may prevent the valve from closing, so that blood regurgitates back from the aorta into the left ventricle during systole. Recall that the coronary arteries branch off from the aorta just above the leaflets of the aortic valve; thus, if the valve is affected, coronary blood flow will likely be affected as well. If the dissection involves the takeoff point of the innominate, left common carotid, or left subclavian artery, blood flow through the affected artery or arteries will be compromised.

Signs and Symptoms of Acute Dissecting Aneurysm of the Aorta

The typical patient with a dissecting aneurysm is a middle-aged or older man with chronic hypertension, although dissection may occur during pregnancy and in younger patients with Marfan syndrome. By far, the most common chief complaint is chest pain, which is usually described as "the worst pain I have ever experienced," or as "ripping," "tearing," "sharp," or "like a knife." This pain comes on very suddenly and is located in the anterior part of the chest or in the back between the shoulder blades.

On the basis of the patient's description, it may be difficult to differentiate the chest pain of a dissecting aneurysm from that of an AMI, but a number of distinctive features may help. The pain of an AMI is often preceded by other symptoms—nausea, "indigestion," weakness, and sweating—and tends to come on gradually, getting more severe with time and often being described as "pressure" rather than "stabbing." By contrast, the pain of a dissecting aneurysm usually comes on full

Table 27-14	AMI Versus Dissecting Aortic Aneurysm	
	AMI	**Dissecting Aneurysm**
Onset of pain	Gradual, with prodromal symptoms	Abrupt, without prodromal symptoms
Severity of pain	Increases with time	Maximal from the outset
Timing of pain	May wax and wane	Does not abate once it has started
Location of pain	Substernal; back is rarely involved	Back is often involved, between the shoulder blades
Clinical signs	Peripheral pulses equal	Blood pressure discrepancy between arms or decrease in a femoral or carotid pulse

force from one minute to the next, without prodromal symptoms. Table 27-14 summarizes the differences in the clinical presentations of AMI and dissecting aortic aneurysm.

Other signs and symptoms of dissecting aneurysm will depend on the site of the intimal tear and the extent of the dissection. In dissections of the ascending aorta, which tend to occur in younger patients previously in good health, one or more of the vessels of the aortic arch are usually compromised. Disruption of flow through the innominate artery, for example, is likely to produce a difference in blood pressure between the two arms. (If you don't routinely check the blood pressure in both arms, you'll never pick up that sign!) You may also find that one femoral or carotid pulse is missing or weak. Disruption of blood flow into the left common carotid artery may produce signs and symptoms of a stroke. When the dissection extends proximally to the ostia of the coronary arteries, coronary blood flow is apt to be compromised, and ECG changes of myocardial ischemia are likely. Death from dissection of the ascending aorta is nearly always a result of aortic rupture into the pericardium and resultant cardiac tamponade. In such a case, you will see the characteristic signs of cardiac tamponade: distended neck veins, hypotension, narrow pulse pressure, and muffled heart sounds.

Dissection of the descending aorta occurs more commonly in older patients, especially those with a history of hypertension. The pain is apt to be somewhat less severe when the descending aorta is involved; indeed, the patient may wait a few days before seeking help. The dissection usually proceeds distally, so the aortic arch is spared, which means that blood pressure discrepancies between the two arms are not part of the picture. The pulses in the lower extremities, however, may be affected.

Management of Acute Dissecting Aneurysm of the Aorta

The goal of prehospital management in a suspected dissecting aneurysm is primarily to provide adequate pain relief. In the hospital setting, medications will be given to lower the patient's blood pressure and reduce myocardial contractility to take some of the hemodynamic load off the aorta. Only in very unusual circumstances would such therapy be started in the field, however, because it requires careful monitoring of intra-arterial pressure.

The steps of prehospital management in suspected dissecting aneurysm are as follows:
- Calm and reassure the patient.
- Administer 100% supplemental oxygen by nonrebreathing mask.
- Insert an IV, and give a crystalloid solution.
- Apply monitoring electrodes and obtain an ECG rhythm strip.
- If the patient is not hypotensive, administer IV morphine sulfate, 2 mg at a time, up to a total dose of 10 mg during 10 to 15 minutes.
- Transport without delay. Nothing can be done to stabilize the patient's condition in the field. He or she will need aggressive therapy in the intensive care unit and possibly surgery, so don't dawdle!

Expanding and Ruptured Abdominal Aortic Aneurysms

Abdominal aortic aneurysms (AAAs) affect approximately 2% of the US population older than 50 years and account for 15,000 deaths each year. Most commonly, the aneurysm is located just distal to the renal arteries. An expanding aneurysm is, as the name implies, an aneurysm that is getting larger and producing symptoms by compressing on adjacent structures, although the aortic wall remains intact. When an aneurysm starts expanding and producing symptoms, one can assume that rupture is imminent.

Signs and Symptoms of Expanding and Ruptured AAAs

The typical patient with an AAA is a man in his late 50s or 60s. So long as the aneurysm is stable, the patient will usually be asymptomatic. When the aneurysm starts to expand, however, the patient becomes symptomatic, with the sudden onset of abdominal or back pain. When the pain is principally in the abdomen, it tends to center on the umbilicus. Often, the pain may be located solely in the lower back, leading the patient to think he or she has "pulled a muscle" or otherwise injured the back. The pain is constant and moderate to severe; it cannot be relieved by changes in position. It tends to radiate into the thigh and groin. If the aneurysm is leaking blood into the retroperitoneal space, the patient may complain of an urge to defecate. In some patients, an episode of syncope heralds the onset of symptoms.

The most characteristic physical finding in an AAA is a pulsatile mass palpable in the abdomen. The patient is likely to be normotensive when first seen, but signs of shock, with or without hypotension, may develop rapidly if the aneurysm has ruptured.

Management of Expanding and Ruptured AAAs

Prehospital management of an expanding or ruptured aortic aneurysm is aimed at getting the patient to the hospital as expeditiously as possible because the definitive treatment requires urgent surgery. The key is to maintain a high index of suspicion whenever a middle-aged or older man presents with sudden back pain and a pulsatile abdominal mass. The more likely problem in the field in a conscious patient is a leaking aneurysm that has yet to rupture.

The steps of prehospital management in expanding or ruptured aortic aneurysm are as follows:

- Administer supplemental oxygen.
- Consider applying (but do not inflate) the pneumatic antishock garment (PASG)/military antishock trousers (MAST) if available.
- Transport without delay.
- Insert an IV line en route, and give normal saline or lactated Ringer's. Use a large-gauge catheter, but maintain the flow to keep the vein open unless signs of shock appear. If there are signs of shock, treat as for any other case of shock, with IV fluids, and consult the physician for orders to inflate the PASG/MAST.

Hypertensive Emergencies

Hypertension (high blood pressure) afflicts nearly 60 million Americans and is directly responsible for more than 30,000 deaths per year. In addition, it is a major contributing cause in many cases of MI, CHF, and stroke. Most hypertension is the result of advanced atherosclerosis or arteriosclerosis, which decreases the lumen of the arteries and reduces their elasticity. The resulting high afterload on the heart leads to an increase in filling volume and stimulates the Frank-Starling reflex, which raises the pressure behind the blood leaving the heart.

Hypertension is present when the blood pressure at rest is consistently greater than about 140/90 mm Hg. Many conditions, such as anxiety or pain, can transiently elevate a person's blood pressure (especially the systolic blood pressure), so a single blood pressure measurement taken during an emergency scarcely constitutes adequate grounds for telling a patient that he or she is hypertensive. Instead, one may say something like this: "Sir, your blood pressure is a little high right now. That may be because of the stress you are under and may not have any real significance. To be safe, you should have your blood pressure rechecked a couple of times in the next few months under less stressful circumstances."

Persistent elevation of the diastolic pressure, by contrast, is indicative of hypertensive disease. If left untreated, hypertension significantly shortens the life span and predisposes the patient to a variety of other medical problems. The most common complications of hypertension include renal damage, stroke, and heart failure—the last a result of the left ventricle having to pump for years against a markedly increased afterload.

Signs and Symptoms of Hypertensive Disease

In the majority of cases, hypertension is entirely asymptomatic and is detected by chance during routine examination. By the time symptoms start to occur, hypertension is already in a more advanced stage and has probably produced at least some damage to organs such as the heart, kidneys, and brain.

The symptoms that occur in advanced hypertensive disease may be related to the elevated blood pressure or to secondary complications. Headache is the most common symptom directly related to blood pressure elevation; hypertensive headache is usually localized to the occipital region of the head and occurs when the patient first awakens in the morning, then subsides gradually over the next few hours. Other symptoms of moderately severe hypertension include dizziness, weakness, epistaxis, and blurring of vision. Often a patient with these hypertension-related signs and symptoms has already been prescribed medication for hypertension but is not taking it as prescribed.

Management of Hypertensive Diseases

Hypertensive emergencies occur in about 1% of all hypertensive patients. A hypertensive emergency is defined as an acute elevation of blood pressure with evidence of end-organ damage. That last phrase is important, because it is the evidence of end-organ dysfunction that determines the urgency of the situation, not the reading on the sphygmomanometer. Two end-organ emergencies that may result from uncontrolled hypertension were discussed earlier in this chapter: left-sided heart failure and dissecting aortic aneurysm. A rare but much more devastating complication of hypertension is hypertensive encephalopathy.

Hypertensive encephalopathy (also known as acute hypertensive crisis) may complicate any form of hypertension. Hypertensive crisis is usually signaled by a sudden, marked rise in blood pressure to levels greater than 200/130 mm Hg. The determining factor for hypertensive encephalopathy is usually the mean arterial pressure (MAP). The MAP is calculated by adding one third of the difference between the systolic blood pressure (SBP) and diastolic blood pressure (DBP) to the diastolic pressure.

$$MAP = DBP + \frac{1}{3}(SBP - DBP)$$

When the MAP exceeds 150 mm Hg, the pressure breaches the blood-brain barrier and fluid leaks out, increasing intracranial pressure. Usually the first symptoms noticed are severe headache, nausea, and vomiting. They are followed by seizures and alternations in mental status (that is, confusion to unresponsiveness). Sometimes patients may show focal neurologic signs, such as sudden blindness, aphasia (disturbances in speech production or comprehension), or hemiparesis. Widespread neuromuscular irritability may be signaled by muscle twitching.

The goal of treatment in hypertensive encephalopathy is to lower the blood pressure in a gradual, controlled manner during a 30- to 60-minute period so that cerebral blood flow is restored to normal. That is best accomplished under controlled conditions in a hospital. Thus, if you are within 20 to 30 minutes of the nearest hospital, provide supportive treatment only:

- Secure the airway, and administer supplemental oxygen by nasal cannula or nonrebreathing mask.
- Establish an IV with normal saline at a keep-vein-open rate.
- Apply monitoring electrodes, and run an ECG rhythm strip (consider running a 12-lead ECG en route to the ED).
- Transport without delay. Be prepared to deal with seizures en route, and have diazepam (Valium) ready.

Paramedics working in rural areas or other circumstances where long transport times to the hospital are unavoidable may have to initiate drug therapy of hypertensive encephalopathy in the field. One widely accepted drug for this purpose is labetalol (Normodyne, Trandate), which has alpha- and beta-blocking properties. As an alpha blocker, it prevents vasoconstriction, thereby decreasing the overall peripheral vascular resistance. Meanwhile, its beta-blocking actions prevent the reflex tachycardia that would otherwise occur in response to a drop in blood pressure. As a beta blocker, however, labetalol is relatively contraindicated in patients with asthma and COPD.

Labetalol can be given initially by slow IV push at 20 mg, repeated in 10 minutes as necessary, or an IV drip can be started. To administer a labetalol drip, add 250 mg to 250 mL of normal saline, yielding a concentration of 1 mg/mL. Start the infusion at a rate of 2 mg/min (2 mL/min), and watch the infusion like a hawk! A runaway IV could prove disastrous. Monitor the patient's blood pressure every 2 to 3 minutes. When the blood pressure has fallen to the target level specified by the physician, stop the infusion.

The other drug that may be ordered to lower a dangerously high blood pressure is nitroglycerin, 0.4 mg sublingual. This drug is not the first choice for this indication, but its use is acceptable if labetalol is not available.

Whenever you give a drug to lower a patient's blood pressure, keep the patient supine, and measure his or her blood pressure at least every 3 to 5 minutes. Record each measurement on a flowchart.

Cardiac Arrhythmias

Cardiac rhythm disturbances or arrhythmias Table 27-15 ▶ may arise from a variety of causes; they are not solely caused by AMI. A cardiac arrhythmia is simply a disturbance in the normal cardiac rhythm, which may or may not be clinically significant. Sometimes arrhythmias are caused by ischemia, electrolyte imbalances, disturbances or damage in the electrical conduction system resulting in escape beats, circus reentry, or enhanced automaticity. Thus, it is always necessary to evaluate the arrhythmia in the context of the patient's overall clinical condition. Indeed, it is the patient's clinical condition—not the lines and squiggles on a piece of paper—that should ultimately determine whether treatment is necessary. Treat the patient, not the monitor!

One of the most important tasks in the prehospital care of a patient with an AMI is to anticipate, recognize, and treat life-

Table 27-15	Causes of Cardiac Arrhythmias
■ Myocardial ischemia or infarction ■ Other forms of heart disease ■ Rheumatic heart disease ■ Cor pulmonale ■ Generalized hypoxemia from any cause ■ Autonomic nervous system imbalance ■ Increased vagal tone ■ Increased sympathetic output ■ Distention of cardiac chambers (as in heart failure) ■ Electrolyte disturbances, especially those involving	potassium, calcium, or magnesium ■ Drug toxicity ■ Certain poisons (such as organophosphate insecticides) ■ Central nervous system damage ■ Hypothermia ■ Metabolic imbalance ■ Normal variations ■ Trauma (such as cardiac contusions)

threatening arrhythmias. Arrhythmias develop after an AMI for two principal reasons. First, irritability of the ischemic heart muscle surrounding the infarct may cause the damaged muscle to generate abnormal currents of electricity that cause abnormal cardiac contractions. When the arrhythmia arises from irritable spots in the myocardium (ectopic foci), it is usually a rapid arrhythmia (tachyarrhythmia), such as (V-tach), premature atrial contractions, or PVCs. Second, arrhythmias may occur after an AMI because the infarct damages the conduction tissues. In such a case, the abnormal rhythm is usually a block or a bradyarrhythmia.

Very slow HRs (< 40 to 50 beats/min) lead to inadequate CO and often precede electrical instability of the heart. Furthermore, when the sinus rate becomes very slow, ectopic pacemakers in the AV node or ventricles may fire and produce escape beats to assist in maintaining CO.

Conversely, very rapid HRs (> 120 to 140/min) increase the work of the heart, causing further myocardial ischemia and damage. Tachycardias may also be associated with decreased CO secondary to decreased SV because the ventricles have less time to fill between beats. Hypoxia, metabolic alkalosis, hypokalemia, and hypocalcemia can lead to electrical instability; cells with no automaticity property may then begin to fire impulses. This kind of enhanced automaticity may occur with the use of drugs such as digitalis or atropine and is manifested by ectopic beats anywhere in the heart. The result is the potential for tachycardias, flutters, and fibrillations in the atria or ventricles, heralding grave rhythms such as V-tach and V-fib. Circus reentry can also be a serious problem Figure 27-23 ▶ . The AV node may be bombarded by more than one impulse—potentially blocking the pathway for one impulse and allowing the other to stimulate cardiac cells that have already depolarized. The danger here comes when these impulses get "stuck" in a pattern of repetition, causing multiple ectopic beats or V-fib.

ECG analysis is indicated in any patient who might have a cardiac-related condition. Any patient with a chest pain should certainly undergo ECG analysis, but this monitoring should also be instituted for any patient with a history of heart problems.

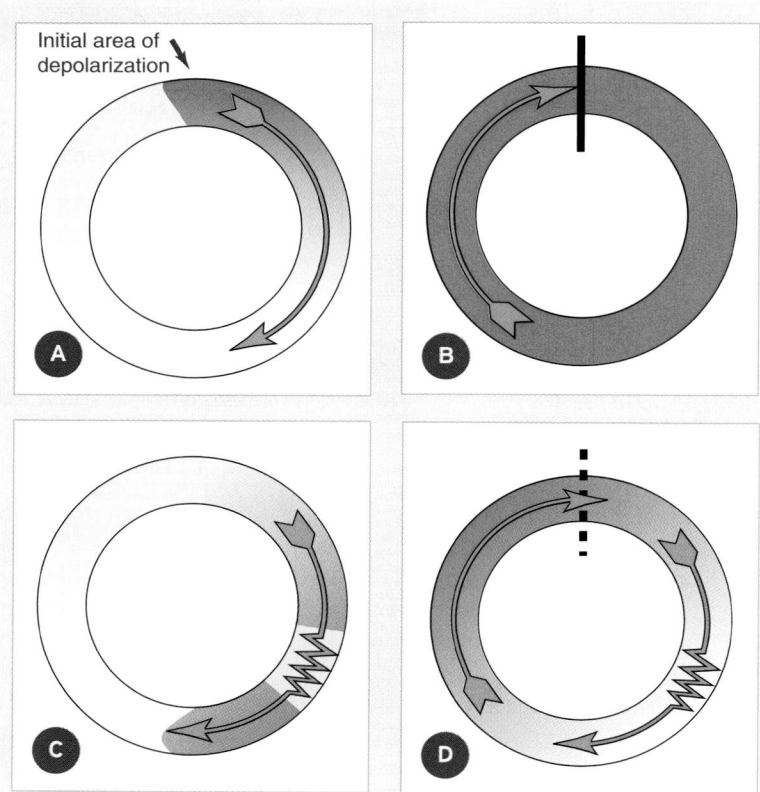

Figure 27-23 A. The original impulse site fires and triggers a depolarization wave that spreads throughout the rest of the cells in the direction shown. **B.** By the time the depolarization wave reaches the original site (represented by the black line) the original site is still refractory and cannot accept the new impulse. The depolarization wave essentially dies at this point. **C.** The area in yellow represents an area of slow conduction. The depolarization wave slows down as it traverses this area. **D.** By the time the depolarization wave reaches the original site (represented by the dotted black line) the original site is now ready to receive a new impulse. The result is a circus movement that is self-perpetuating.

Given that age is a contributing factor to heart disease, ECG analysis is appropriate for elderly patients in many situations. Indeed, the ECG should be thought of as another vital sign, similar to the blood pressure or pulse oximetry.

ECG Monitoring: Placement of Leads and Electrodes

How reliable would ECG tracings or 12 leads be if the electrodes were placed anywhere on the patient? To maintain consistency in monitoring and obtaining a useful ECG, there are predetermined locations to place electrodes and leads.

Electrodes used in the prehospital setting are generally adhesive and have a gel center to aid in skin contact. Some manufacturers offer a "diaphoretic" electrode that sticks to a sweating patient more effectively. Whichever type is used, certain basic principles should be followed to achieve the best skin contact and minimize artifact in the signal:

- To maintain the correct lead placement, it may be necessary to shave body hair from the electrode site. Don't

be fooled by a hairy chest. It may appear that you have great skin contact initially, but the electrode will rise off the skin and stick to the hair. Shaving should also be done when using hands-free adhesive defibrillation pads.

- To remove oils and dead tissues from the surface of the skin, rub the electrode site briskly with an alcohol swab before application. Wait for the alcohol to dry before electrode application or dry it with a quick wipe of a 4″ × 4″ gauze pad.
- Another trick of the trade to provide excellent skin contact is to gently scrape the electrode site with the disposable plastic backing of the electrode to "rough up" the skin cells before application.
- Attach the electrodes to the ECG cables before placement. Confirm that the appropriate electrode is attached to the appropriate cable (each cable is marked and color coded as to the correct location for placement).
- Once all electrodes are in place, switch on the monitor, and print a sample rhythm strip. If the strip shows any "interference" (artifact), verify that the electrodes are firmly applied to the skin and the monitor cable is plugged in correctly.

Artifact on the monitor can be tricky. A straight-line ECG in an alert, communicative patient indicates a loose or disconnected lead, not asystole (flat line). Similarly, a wavy baseline resembling V-fib may be caused by patient movement or muscle tremor. Before you lunge for the defibrillator paddles, look at the patient! If he or she is alert and in no obvious distress, recheck the leads and equipment.

Although acquisition of a 12-lead ECG in the prehospital setting has become a standard of care, you will still need to monitor the patient's heart rhythm using one of three leads. A lead offers an electrical snapshot of certain parts of the heart. The standard is to use one of the "bipolar" leads for monitoring purposes—that is, lead I, II, or III. Generally, lead II will give the best overall view of the PQRST complexes. Bipolar leads (that is, "limb leads") consist of two electrodes, one positive and one negative, that are placed on two different limbs. When using bipolar leads, any impulse in the body moving to a positive electrode will cause a positive deflection on the ECG. Conversely, if an impulse is moving toward a negative electrode, it will result in a negative deflection on the ECG tracing. A lack of electrical impulse will produce an isolectric or flat line. If the impulse moves perpendicular to the lead, the result will be a "biphasic" waveform, which is above and below the isoelectric baseline.

In the Field

Here are two easy ways to remember cable placement: "White is on the right, smoke (black) is over fire (red)" (on the left) or (starting on the right) "salt (white), pepper (black), ketchup (red)."

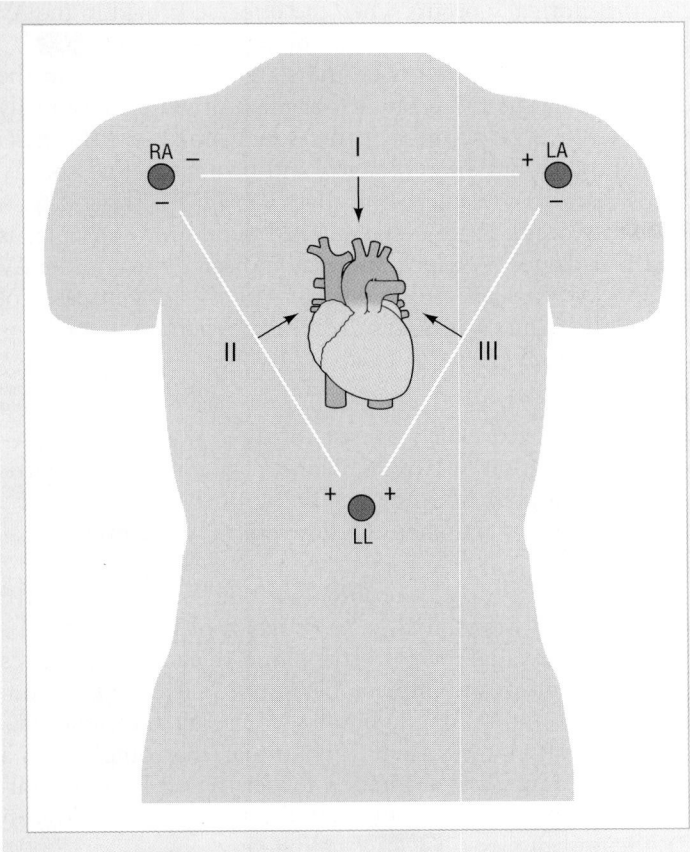

Figure 27-24 The Einthoven triangle.

When correctly positioned on the chest, these leads form a triangle around the heart, called the Einthoven triangle **Figure 27-24 ◄** . Today, it is not necessary to change the electrical poles of the electrodes to get a different lead. ECG monitors have the ability to change the polarity of the leads so that we can view leads I, II, and III by turning a knob or pressing a soft key.

Reading an ECG Rhythm Strip

The most reliable method of analyzing a rhythm strip is to use a systematic approach and examine every strip the same way. By using such an approach, you will find in most cases that even the most complex-appearing arrhythmias can be reduced to simple terms and correctly identified.

ECGs are recorded on standardized graph paper, which is moved past a stylus at a standardized speed (25 mm/s). Thus, a given distance on the graph paper represents a given time. Specifically, one small (1 mm) box is equivalent to 0.04 second (1/25th of a second), and one large box (which consists of five small boxes) is equivalent to 0.20 second (0.04 × 5 = 0.20) **Figure 27-25 ▼** .

Components of an ECG Complex

Let's break down the ECG waveforms into their individual components.

P Wave

The P wave is normally a small, upright waveform (in leads I and II). It immediately precedes the QRS. The P wave is formed as the impulse is generated by the SA node in the right atrium and spreads over the atria, causing depolarization.

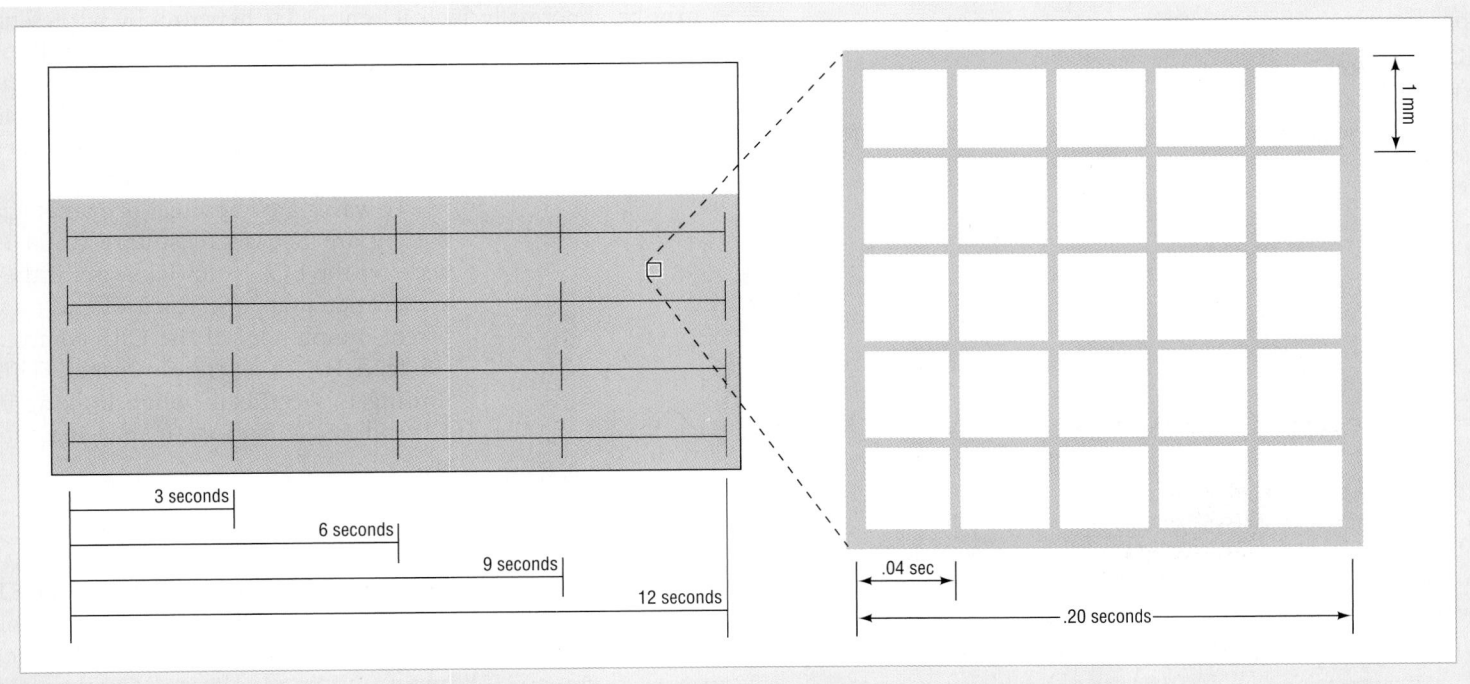

Figure 27-25 ECG paper. Height (amplitude) is measured in millimeters (mm) and width in milliseconds (ms).

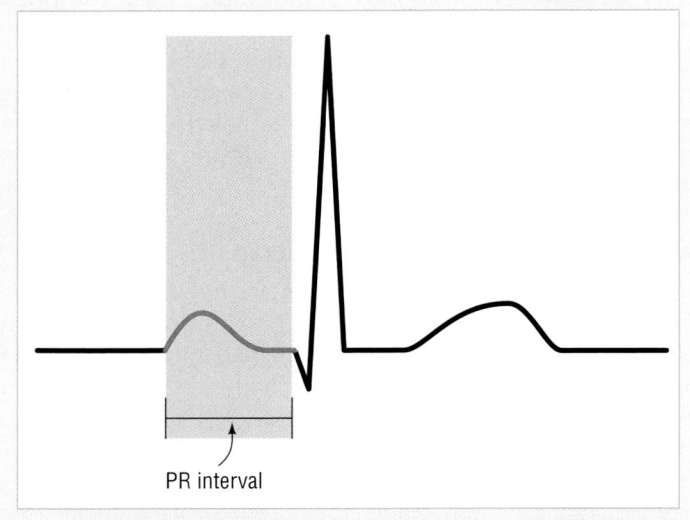

Figure 27-26 The normal P-R interval is 0.12 to 0.20 s.

Lasting only 0.06 to 0.11 s, P waves can give clues to the pacemaker site if they are missing or do not have a uniform appearance.

If there are no P waves, the pacemaker for the heart is not in the SA node, and one must consider the possibility of atrial fibrillation or a junctional or ventricular rhythm. If a QRS complex is not preceded by a P wave, the pacemaker site for that beat is not in the SA node, but rather in some ectopic focus (a location other than the SA node). If a P wave is present but not followed by a QRS complex, a block is present somewhere in the AV junction or below and is preventing conduction from the atria to the ventricles. P waves that vary in size and configuration mean that there are several pacemaker sites at different locations throughout the atria.

P-R Interval
The PRI includes atrial depolarization and the conduction of the impulse through the AV junction. It includes the slight

delay that normally occurs when the impulse is held in the AV node, allowing time for ventricular filling Figure 27-26 ◄ .

The PRI is measured from the start of the P wave to the point at which the QRS complex begins. Although it normally lasts 0.12 to 0.20 s (three to five small boxes on the ECG strip), the PRI may be prolonged and give clues that the AV node is diseased or damaged, as in an MI Figure 27-27 ▼ . A PRI that exceeds 0.20 s (five small boxes), for example, is called first-degree AV block and may indicate injury to the AV junction. A PRI may also be shorter than 0.12 s in cases of Wolff-Parkinson-White syndrome, when the AV node is bypassed altogether.

QRS Complex
The QRS complex, which consists of three waveforms, represents depolarization of two simultaneously contracting ventricles. It is measured from the beginning of the Q wave to the end of the S wave and should follow each P wave in a consistent manner.

In healthy people, the QRS complex is narrow, with sharply pointed waves, and has a duration of less than 0.12 s (three small boxes on the ECG strip). Such a complex indicates that conduction of the impulse has proceeded normally from the AV junction, through the bundle of His, left and right bundles, and the Purkinje system. If abnormal, the complex has a bizarre appearance and a duration longer than 0.12 s. It signifies some abnormality in conduction through the ventricle as in a bundle branch block Figure 27-28 ► .

The first downward deflection in the QRS is called a Q wave; this wave represents conduction through the ventricular septum. The electricity spreads from right to left through the septum. The first upward deflection of the QRS is referred to as the R wave. Most of both ventricles are depolarized during the R wave. The R wave may be wide if the ventricle is enlarged and may be abnormally high if ventricular hypertrophy is present. The S wave is any downward deflection after the R wave. If the S wave is abnormally large, it may indicate hypertrophy of the ventricles. If there is a second upward deflection, it is called an R-prime (R′) wave. R-prime waves are never normal, and they indicate trouble in the conduction system of the ventricle.

Q waves are abnormal or pathologic if they are one small square (0.04 s) wide on the ECG strip. Likewise, if they are deeper than one third of the total height (amplitude) of the QRS complex (in lead II), they are abnormal. This finding is significant when looking at 12-lead ECGs because it may indicate an AMI.

J Point
The J point is the point in the ECG where the QRS complex ends and the ST segment begins. Thus, it represents the end of depolarization and the apparent beginning of repolarization. In some

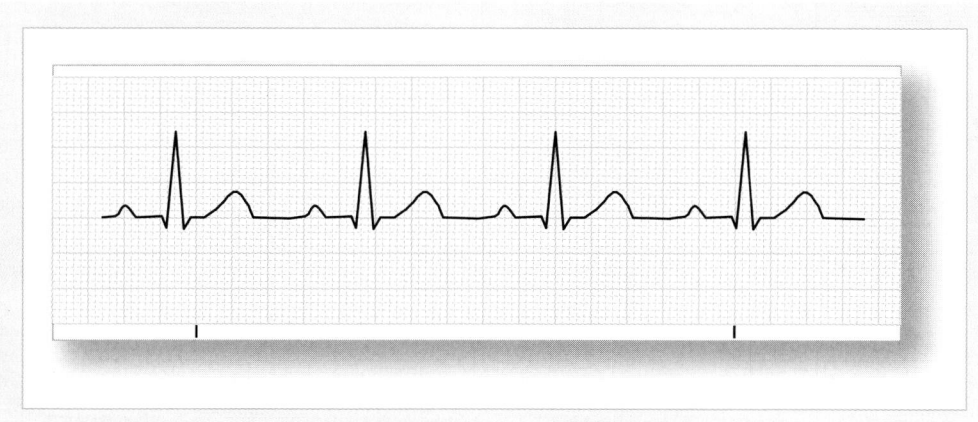

Figure 27-27 A P-R interval greater than 0.20 s is considered prolonged.

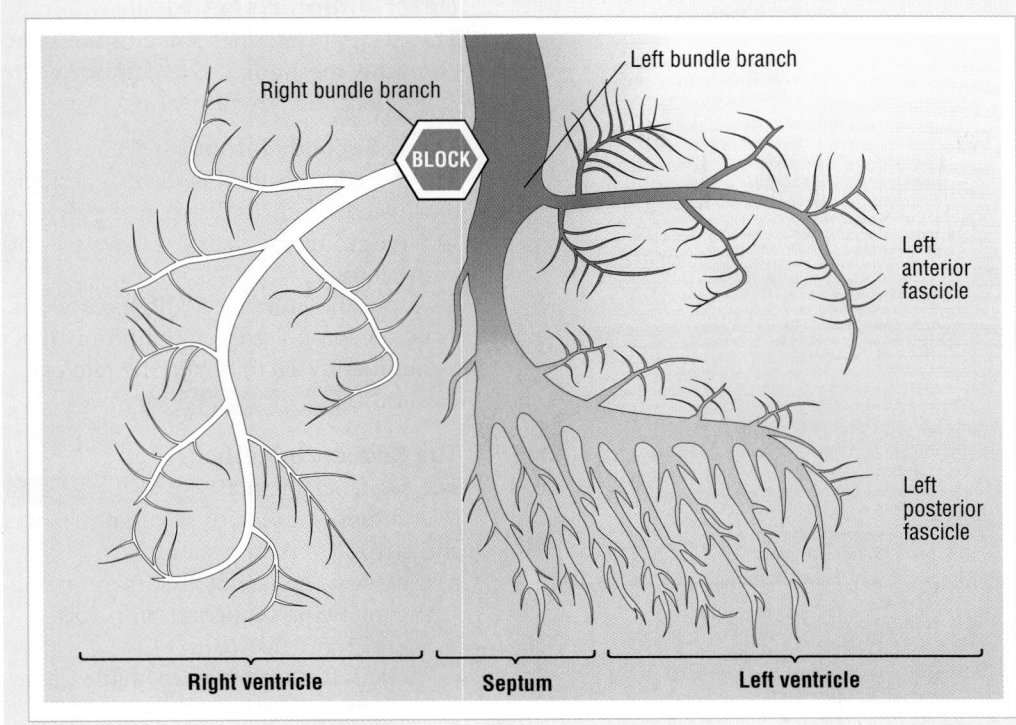

Figure 27-28 Bundle branch block.

cases, the J point may be easier to locate than the ST segment when you are looking for elevation (another clue to an AMI).

ST Segment

The ST segment, which is the line between the QRS complex and the beginning of the T wave, is normally isoelectric. An ST segment that is significantly (> 1 mm or one small box) above or below the isoelectric line is highly suggestive of myocardial ischemia or injury, although a full 12-lead ECG is required to determine the precise significance of ST segment elevation or depression.

T Wave

A T wave represents ventricular repolarization, but may also show abnormalities such as those found with electrolyte disturbances. In hyperkalemia, for example, the T wave may be tall and sharply peaked.

For the most part, the T wave remains in a state of relative refractoriness, which means that the cells are partially repolarized. Early in the T wave, the cells will not accept another impulse. However, on the down slope (the vulnerable period), a strong impulse could cause depolarization, overpowering the primary pacemaker to take over the pacemaker control. The supernormal phase is the time near the end of the T wave (the last one third), just before the cells become completely repolarized. During this period, a stimulus weaker than normally required can cause depolarization, resulting in a dangerous heart rhythm.

This behavior of the T wave is the main reason there are "synch" (synchronize) buttons on monitors and defibrillators.

When using the cardioversion technique on a rhythm that has regular T waves, you must press the synch button so that the shock will be delivered during the safest period of the ECG.

Q-T Interval

The Q-T interval includes all activity that occurs during the QRS complex and T wave (that is, ventricular depolarization and repolarization). It begins with the onset of the Q wave and ends with the T wave as it comes back to the isoelectric line. If there is no Q wave, measurements begin with the R wave.

The Q-T interval normally lasts 0.36 to 0.44 s. A prolonged Q-T interval (long Q-T syndrome) indicates that the heart is experiencing an extended refractory period, making the ventricle more vulnerable to arrhythmias. Such prolongation may occur with administration of some drugs, hypocalcemia, an AMI, or pericarditis. Conversely, the Q-T interval may be shortened in hypercalcemia and in patients taking digitalis.

Regular or Irregular: That Is the Question!

What makes a rhythm irregular? How much variability is allowed within R-R intervals? The distinction between regular and irregular rhythms is not always clear-cut. It is acceptable to have less than 0.12 s (three small boxes) variance between the shortest and longest R-R interval to be able to call a rhythm regular Figure 27-29 ▼ . If there is a gap of 0.12 s or more between the shortest and longest R-R intervals, however, the rhythm is considered irregular Figure 27-30 ▶ .

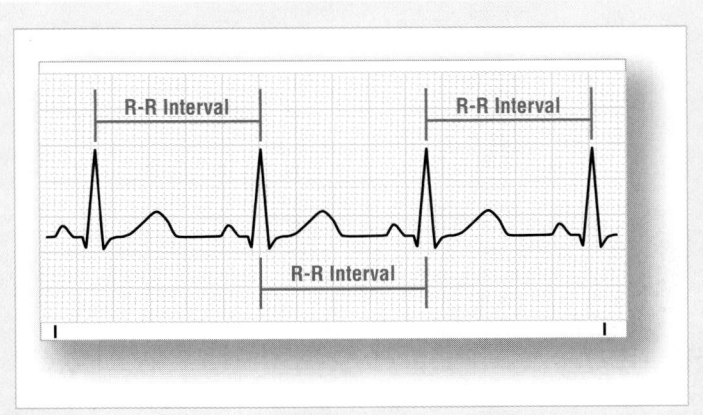

Figure 27-29 When the rhythm is regular, the R-R intervals are the same.

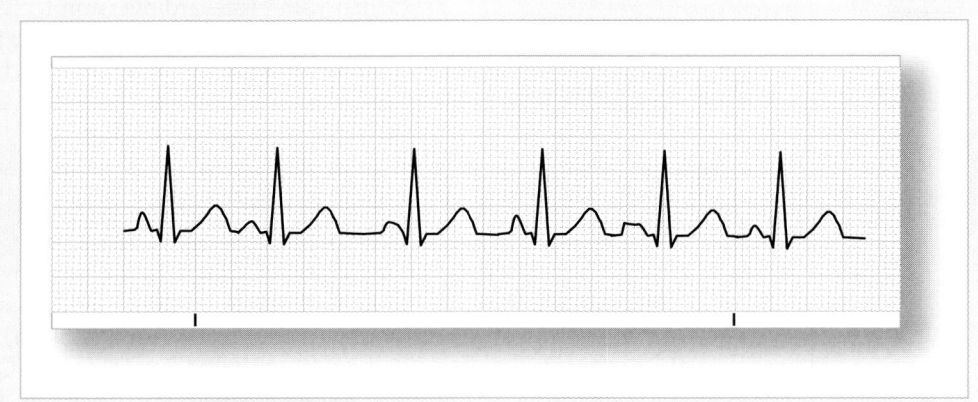

Figure 27-30 In an irregular rhythm, not all R-R intervals are the same.

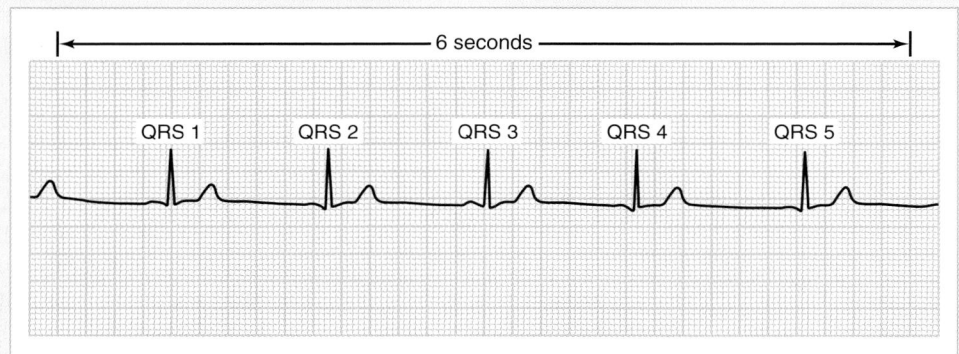

Figure 27-31 Calculation of rate. To calculate the rate, multiply the number of QRS complexes in a 6-second strip by 10.

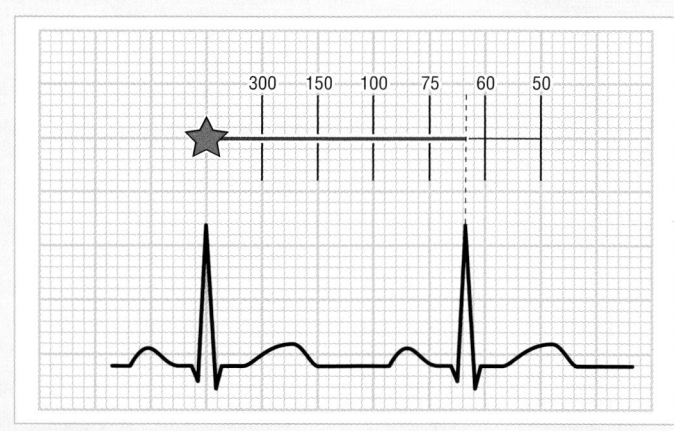

Figure 27-32 The sequence method.

Determining Heart Rate

This section describes some of the more common methods of determining the rate of a cardiac rhythm strip.

The 6-Second Method

The 6-second method is the simplest and most accurate method when the rhythm is irregular or very slow (< 60 beats/min):

- Count the number of QRS complexes in a 6-second strip, and multiply that number by 10 to obtain the rate per minute **Figure 27-31** ◄.

The Sequence Method

The sequence method **Figure 27-32** ◄ is commonly used for regular rhythms and strips less than 6 s long:

- Calculate the rate by first memorizing the following sequence: 300, 150, 100, 75, 60, 50.
- Find an R wave on a heavy line (large box), and count off "300, 150, 100, 75, 60, 50" for each large box you land on until you reach the next R wave. (Estimate the rate if the second R wave doesn't fall exactly on a heavy black line.)
- If the R-R interval spans fewer than three large boxes, the rate is greater than 100 (tachycardia). If it covers more than five large boxes, the rate is less than 60 (bradycardia).

The Grid Method

The grid method is completely accurate only when the rhythm is absolutely regular:

- Calculate the rate by counting the number of large boxes between any two QRS complexes (the R-R interval), and then divide that number into 300.
- In Figure 27-33, for example, there are approximately 5.6 large boxes between two successive QRS complexes; 300/5.6 = 54, so the rate would be about 54 beats/min.

Systematic Analysis of the ECG Rhythm Strip

So, now we are to the point of using a systematic approach to the ECG and examining every strip the same way. When examining the rhythm strip, proceed in the following, stepwise manner:

1. Are QRS complexes present? Are they normal or abnormal in shape and duration (or width)? Are they all the same?
2. Are there P waves? Is there a P wave before every QRS complex and a QRS complex after every P wave? Do all of the P waves look the same? Based on the information on P and QRS waves, what is the pacemaker site?
3. What is the PRI? Is it prolonged? Shortened? Does it vary?

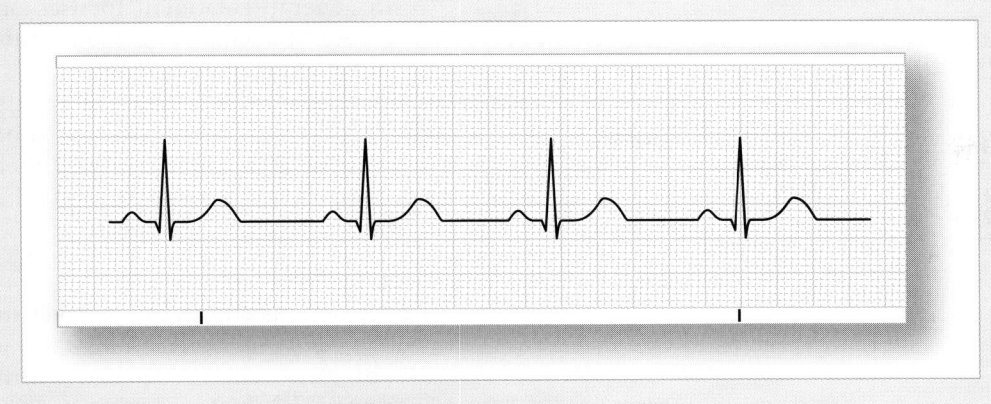

Figure 27-33 A HR less than 60 beats/min is considered bradycardia.

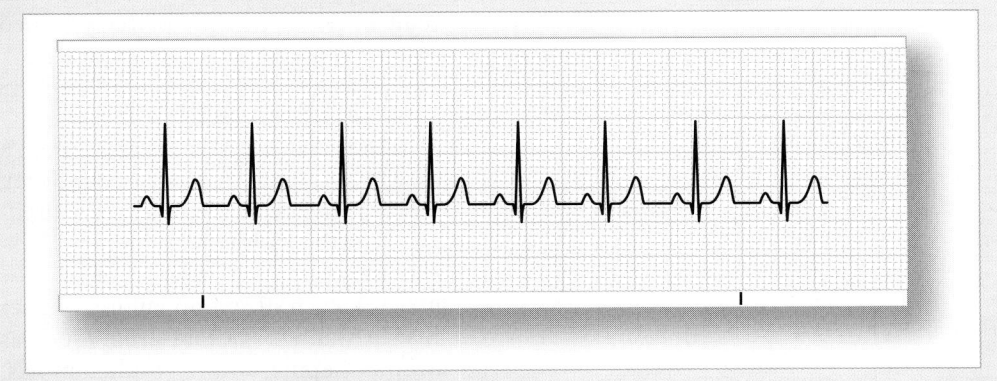

Figure 27-34 A HR greater than 100 beats/min is considered tachycardia.

4. Is the rhythm regular or irregular? Are the R-R intervals equal? Often one can determine whether the rhythm is irregular at a casual glance, but sometimes it will be necessary to measure the R-R intervals and compare them (special ECG calipers are available for that purpose).

5. What is the rate? The normal HR is considered to be between 60 and 100 beats/min. Rates less than 60 per minute are generally called bradycardia Figure 27-33 ▲; rates greater than 100 per minute are called tachycardia Figure 27-34 ▲.

In the Field

Systematic Analysis of the ECG Rhythm: Five Things to Look for in Every Rhythm Strip
- Are QRS complexes present and normal or abnormal in shape and duration?
- Are there P waves? Is there a P wave before every QRS complex and a QRS complex after every P wave? Do all of the P waves look the same?
- What is the PRI? Is it prolonged? Shortened? Does it vary?
- Is the rhythm regular or irregular?
- What is the rate?

By the time you have answered those questions, you should have a good idea of the identity of the arrhythmia in question.

Specific Cardiac Arrhythmias

Cardiac arrhythmias can be induced by a variety of events. Many can be traced to ischemia in the heart, especially in areas related to the cardiac conduction system. Often ischemia will cause a particular area of the heart to spontaneously depolarize, resulting in a premature complex. These premature complexes interfere with the normal conduction of impulses and produce arrhythmias. In other situations, the ischemia occurs within the conduction system itself, causing it to malfunction directly.

It is difficult to estimate the number of people affected by cardiac arrhythmias because many arrhythmias are well tolerated and cause no serious effects. It is well documented, however, that cardiac arrhythmias are the most common cause of cardiac arrest.

There are nearly as many systems for classifying cardiac arrhythmias as there are cardiologists who have written books on the subject. Arrhythmias may, for example, be categorized according to whether they are disturbances of automaticity or disturbances of conduction, whether they are tachyarrhythmias or bradyarrhythmias, or whether they are life threatening or non–life threatening. In this text, we will study the cardiac arrhythmias based on the site from which they arise (and as they appear in lead II). After looking at a normal sinus rhythm for comparison, we will consider the arrhythmias that arise in the SA node, those that arise in the atrial tissue, those that arise in the AV junction, and so on, down the conduction pathway.

Rhythms of the SA Node

Normal Sinus Rhythm

The SA node is the primary pacemaker for the heart. A normal sinus rhythm Figure 27-35 ▶ has an intrinsic rate of 60 to 100 beats/min. The rhythm is regular, with minimal variation between R-R intervals. The P wave is present, is upright, and precedes each QRS complex. The PRI will measure 0.12 to 0.20 s. The QRS complex will measure 0.04 to 0.12 s.

Sinus Bradycardia

In sinus bradycardia, the pacemaker is still the SA node, but with a rate of less than 60 beats/min Figure 27-36 ▶. The rhythm is regular, and P waves are present and upright, preceding every QRS complex. The PRI is 0.12 to 0.20 s. The QRS complex is 0.04 to 0.12 s.

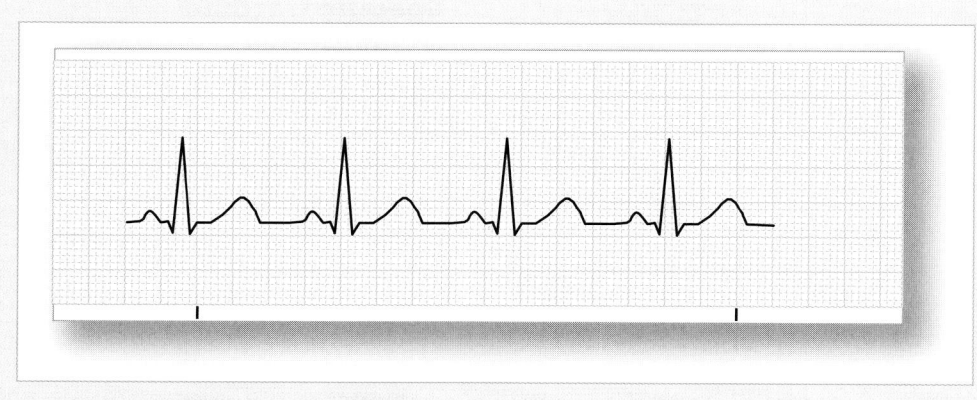

Figure 27-35 Normal sinus rhythm.

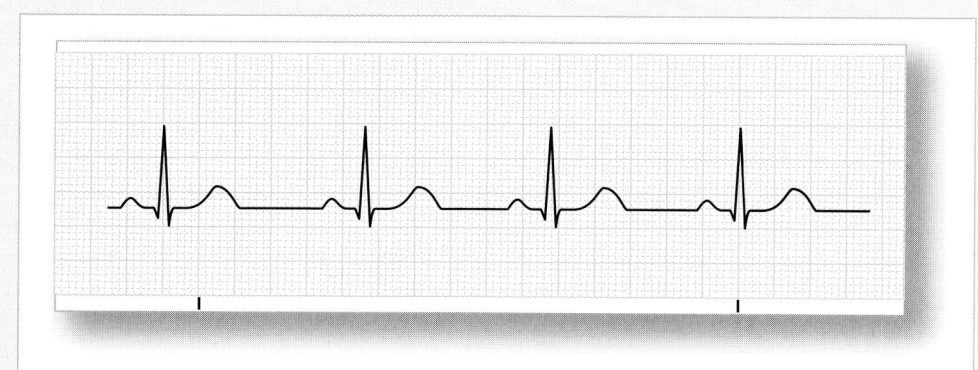

Figure 27-36 Sinus bradycardia.

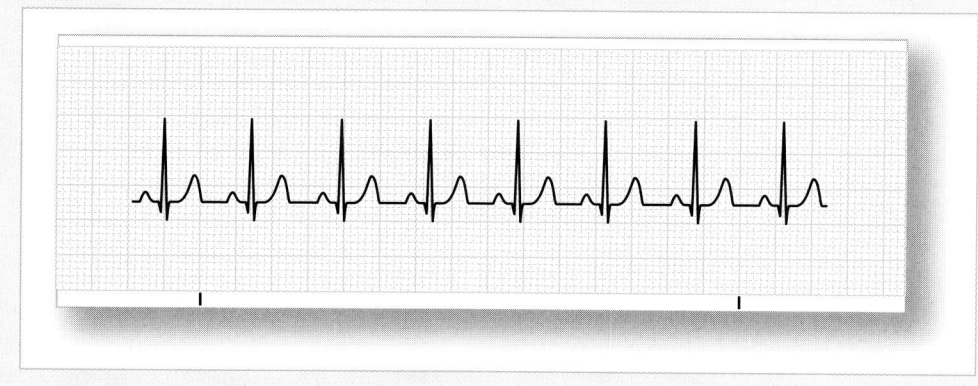

Figure 27-37 Sinus tachycardia.

In general, treatment focuses on the patient's tolerance to the bradycardia and looking for causative factors. Atropine may be necessary. Patients who are symptomatic and do not respond to atropine may require a transcutaneous pacemaker to assist the heart in increasing its ventricular rate.

Sinus Tachycardia

The SA node is still the pacemaker in sinus tachycardia but demonstrates a rate of more than 100 beats/min Figure 27-37 ◄ . The rhythm is regular, and P waves are present and upright, preceding every QRS complex (although they may occasionally be difficult to see if they are partially buried in the T wave of the beat before them). The PRI is 0.12 to 0.20 s. The QRS complex is 0.04 to 0.12 s.

Sinus tachycardia may result from a variety of causes, including pain, fever, hypoxia, hypovolemia, exercise, stimulation of the sympathetic nervous system (such as by stress, fright, or anxiety), an AMI, pump failure, or anemia. In addition, certain drugs (such as atropine, epinephrine, amphetamines, and cocaine), caffeine, nicotine, and alcohol can cause tachycardia.

Prolonged tachycardia will increase the work of the heart, leading to further ischemia and infarction during an AMI. In addition, CO may be significantly reduced when the HR exceeds 120 to 140 beats/min because the ventricles do not have enough time between contractions to fill completely with blood. The treatment of sinus tachycardia is related to the underlying cause.

Sinus Arrhythmia

Sinus arrhythmia is defined as a slight variation in cycling of a sinus rhythm, usually one that exceeds 0.12 s between the longest and shortest cycles Figure 27-38 ► . The SA node is still the pacemaker; P waves are present and upright, preceding every QRS complex; and a PRI of 0.12 to 0.20 s still exists. The QRS complex is 0.04 to 0.12 s.

Sinus arrhythmia is often somewhat more prominent with fluctuation in the respiratory cycle because the HR accelerates with inspiration and slows with expiration. Increased filling pressures of the heart during inspiration stimulate the Bainbridge reflex, which increases the HR and is partially responsi-

Sinus bradycardia can be an asymptomatic phenomenon in healthy adults and conditioned athletes and may be exhibited during sleep. More serious causes include hypothermia; SA node disease; AMI, which may stimulate vagal tone (parasympathetic stimulation); increased intracranial pressure; and use of beta blockers, calcium channel blockers, morphine, quinidine (including interactions between quinidine and some calcium channel blockers), or digitalis.

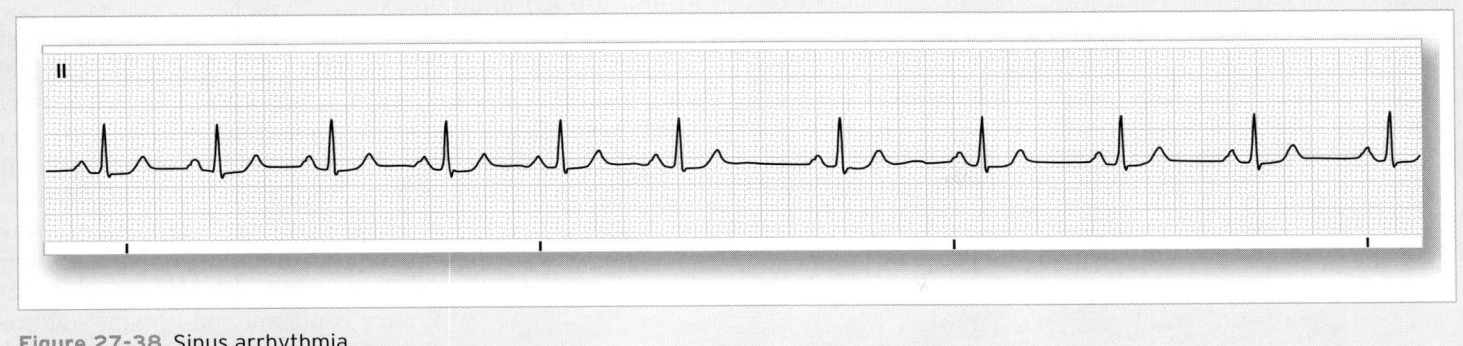

Figure 27-38 Sinus arrhythmia.

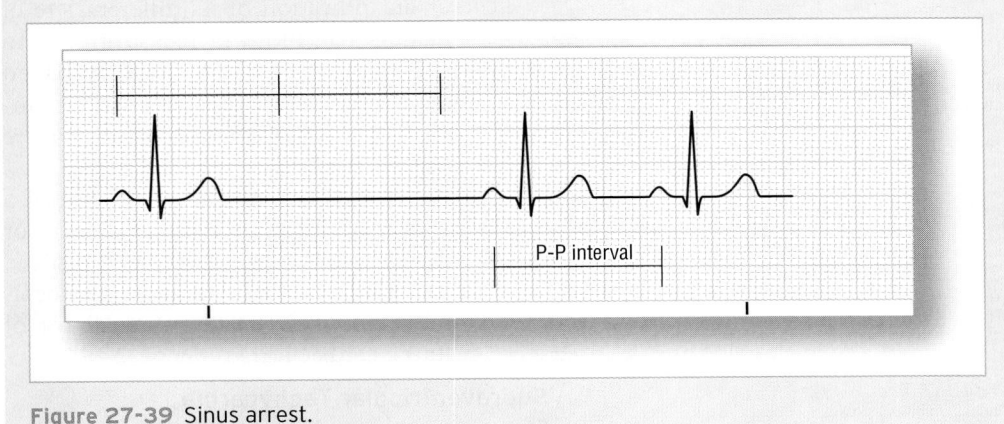

P-P interval

Figure 27-39 Sinus arrest.

ble for respiratory sinus arrhythmia. The increased filling pressure on the heart increases SV (remember the Frank-Starling mechanism) and blood pressure. The increase in blood pressure stimulates the baroreceptor reflex (baroreflex), which attempts to block the rate increase caused by the Bainbridge reflex. In this way, the baroreflex inhibits the respiratory sinus arrhythmia.

Sinus arrhythmia is often a normal finding in children and young adults and tends to diminish or disappear with age.

Sinus Arrest

Sinus arrest occurs when the SA node fails to initiate an impulse, eliminating the P wave, QRS complex, or/and T wave for one cardiac cycle (Figure 27-39 ▲). After this missed set of complexes, the SA node resumes normal functioning just as if nothing ever happened. In sinus arrest, the atrial and ventricular rates are usually within normal limits and the rhythm is regular except for the absent complexes. P waves are present and upright, preceding every QRS complex, and the PRI, when present, is 0.12 to 0.20 s. The QRS complex, when present, is 0.04 to 0.12 s.

Common causes of sinus arrest include ischemia of the SA node, increased vagal tone, carotid sinus massage, and use of drugs such as digitalis and quinidine. Occasional episodes of sinus arrest are not significant; however, if the HR drops below

30 to 50 beats/min, the CO may fall and an ectopic focus from the ventricles may take over. In such a case, treatment is based on the overall HR and tolerance by the patient and may include a temporary pacemaker (a transvenous pacer in the field) or a permanent pacemaker once the patient is admitted to the hospital.

Sick Sinus Syndrome

Sick sinus syndrome (SSS) encompasses a variety of rhythms that involve a poorly functioning SA node and is common in elderly patients. On an ECG, SSS announces itself in many ways, including sinus bradycardia, sinus arrest, SA block, and alternating patterns of extreme bradycardia and tachycardia (bradycardia-tachycardia syndrome). As a result of SSS, some patients may experience a syncopal or near-syncopal episode, dizziness, and palpitations. Other patients remain asymptomatic.

Rhythms of the Atria

Although the SA node is normally the pacemaker for the heart, any area in the atria may originate an impulse, thereby usurping the pacemaking authority of the SA node within the body's electrical conduction system. Rhythms originating from the atria will have upright P waves that precede each QRS complex but that are not as well rounded as those coming from the SA node. Atrial rhythms generally result in HRs of 60 to 100 beats/min.

Wandering Atrial Pacemaker

In wandering atrial pacemaker, as the name suggests, the pacemaker of the heart (Figure 27-40 ▶) moves from the SA node to various areas within the atria. Wandering atrial pacemaker usually has a rate of 60 to 100 beats/min. The rhythm is slightly irregular, with variations between R-R intervals based on the site of the pacemaker for that particular complex. The P wave is present and upright and precedes each QRS complex; however, the shapes of the P waves vary as an indication of their different sites of origin. The definition of wandering atrial pacemaker depends on having at least three different shapes of P waves within one ECG strip. The PRI will measure 0.12 to 0.20 s, but will also vary slightly based on the origin of the particular complex. The QRS complex will measure 0.04 to 0.12 s.

Wandering atrial pacemaker is most commonly seen in patients with significant lung disease. Treatment is usually not indicated in the prehospital setting, although the rhythm is an indication of likely future cardiac complications.

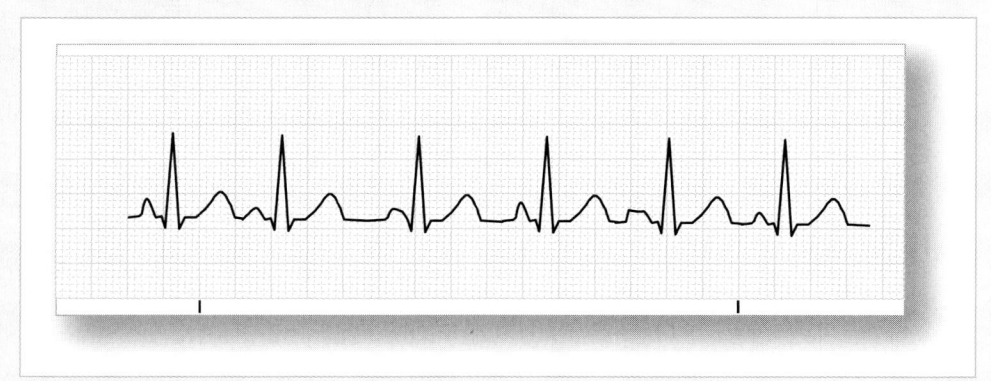

Figure 27-40 Wandering atrial pacemaker.

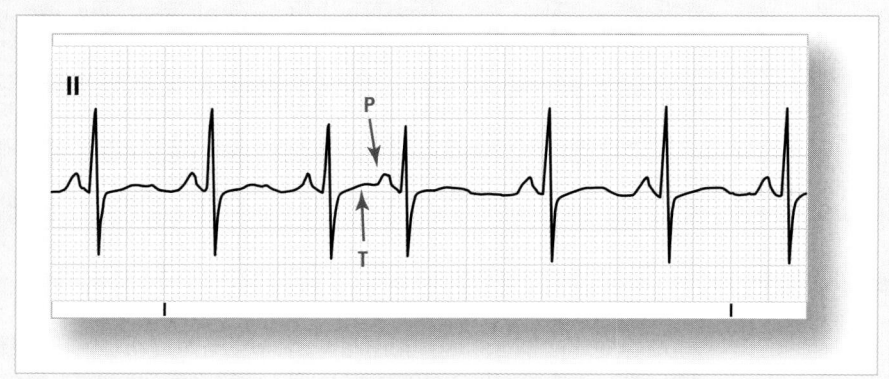

Figure 27-41 Premature atrial complex.

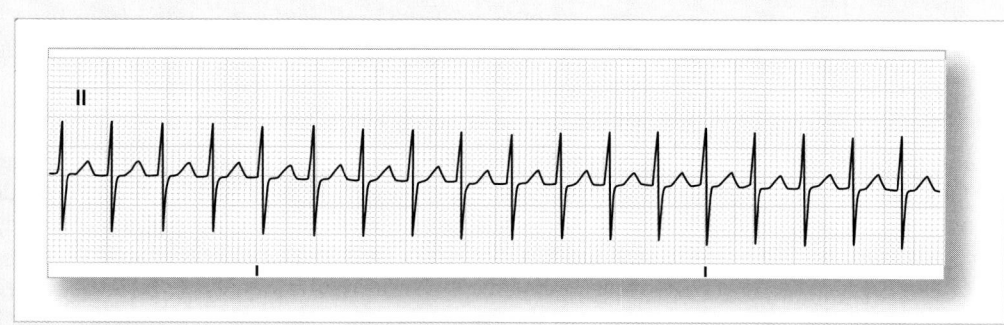

Figure 27-42 Supraventricular tachycardia.

Premature Atrial Complex

A premature atrial complex (PAC) is not, strictly speaking, an arrhythmia, but rather the existence of a particular complex within another rhythm (Figure 27-41 ▾). Premature atrial complexes are also known as ectopic complexes, meaning that they occur out of the normal location. A PAC occurs earlier in time than the next expected sinus complex, leading to an abnormally short R-R interval between it and the previous complex. Because the HR depends on the underlying rhythm, the presence of a PAC will make the rhythm irregular. The P wave is present and upright and precedes each QRS complex; however, its shape differs from the shapes of the P waves originating from the SA node, as an indication of its different site of origin. The PRI will measure 0.12 to 0.20 s but may vary slightly based on the origin of the premature complex. The QRS complex will measure 0.04 to 0.12 s.

A PAC can be caused by use of a variety of drugs (including caffeine), or it may result from organic heart disease. It is not usually treated in the prehospital setting but may be a predictor of future cardiac arrhythmias.

Supraventricular Tachycardia

Supraventricular tachycardia (SVT) is defined as a tachycardic rhythm originating from a pacemaker above the ventricles (Figure 27-42 ▾). Once called atrial tachycardia, it occurs when the true origin of a tachycardia is unknown (which is why the name was changed).

When tachycardias reach 150 to 180 beats/min, the P waves (if present) tend to be completely obscured by the T wave of the preceding beat. At lower HRs, P waves can be identified; thus, to be considered SVT, a rhythm should have a rate exceeding 150 beats/min. The rhythm is regular, with essentially no variation between R-R intervals. SVT is known to originate from a point above the ventricles because the QRS complexes are of normal width. The PRI is not measurable because the P wave is obscured. The QRS complex will measure 0.04 to 0.12 s.

Very often SVT is referred to as PSVT, reflecting its tendency to begin and end abruptly (*paroxysmal* means "occurring in spasms"). Technically, to call this arrhythmia a PSVT, you would need to witness the rhythm speed up on the ECG.

The most up-to-date terminology, which is used in the AHA algorithms, is reentry SVT.

When the ventricular rate exceeds 150 beats/min, the ventricular filling time is greatly diminished, which will in turn greatly reduce the CO. For this reason, SVT should be treated promptly. The treatment, which is discussed later in this chapter, includes using medication or electrical therapy to slow the HR.

Multifocal Atrial Tachycardia

In multifocal atrial tachycardia (MAT), the pacemaker of the heart moves within various areas of the atria (Figure 27-43 ▾). Multifocal atrial tachycardia is characterized by a rate of more than 100 beats/min and is, in effect, a tachycardic wandering atrial pacemaker. The rhythm is irregular, with variation between R-R intervals based on the site of the pacemaker for that particular complex. The P wave is present and upright and precedes each QRS complex; however, the shapes of the P waves vary as an indication of their different sites of origin. The PRI will measure 0.12 to 0.20 s, but also varies slightly based on the origin of the particular complex. If the MAT increases to a rate exceeding 150 beats/min, the P waves may no longer be visible; thus, the only indication of the rhythm may be the irregularity associated with the varying sites of origin within the atria. The QRS complex will measure 0.04 to 0.12 s.

Like a wandering atrial pacemaker, MAT is most commonly seen in patients with significant lung disease. Treatment is usually not attempted in the prehospital setting, and therapies aimed at correcting SVT are usually ineffective with MAT.

Atrial Flutter

Atrial flutter is a rhythm in which the atria contract at a rate much too rapid for the ventricles to match (Figure 27-44 ▾). The atrial complexes in atrial flutter are known as flutter or F waves rather than P waves. F waves have a distinctive shape, resembling a sawtooth or picket fence.

In atrial flutter, one or more of the F waves is blocked by the AV node, resulting in several flutter waves before each QRS complex. The rhythm may be regular (most common), with a constant (usually 2:1) conduction, or irregular if the conduction of impulses to the ventricles varies. The PRI will measure 0.12 to 0.20 s for conducted complexes. The QRS complex will measure 0.04 to 0.12 s.

Atrial flutter is usually a sign of a serious heart problem. In many cases, it is a transient rhythm that degenerates into atrial fibrillation. Treatment generally consists of medication or electrical cardioversion, although neither of these measures is usually attempted in the field unless the patient's condition is very critical and transport time is long.

Atrial Fibrillation

Atrial fibrillation is a rhythm in which the atria no longer contract but rather fibrillate or quiver without any organized contraction (Figure 27-45 ▸). It occurs when many different cells in the atria depolarize independently rather than in response to an impulse from the SA node. The result of this random depolarization, which occurs throughout the atria, is a fibrillating or chaotic baseline.

In atrial fibrillation, there are usually no visible P waves on the ECG strip and, hence, no PRI to measure. Instead, one of the keys to identifying this condition is its "irregularly irregular" appearance. Because the AV node is bombarded with impulses from the fibrillating atria, it allows impulses to pass on to the ventricles in a random manner, which results in the highly irregular ventricular rhythm. The QRS complex will measure 0.04 to 0.12 s.

Atrial fibrillation is usually a sign of a serious heart problem and is a fairly

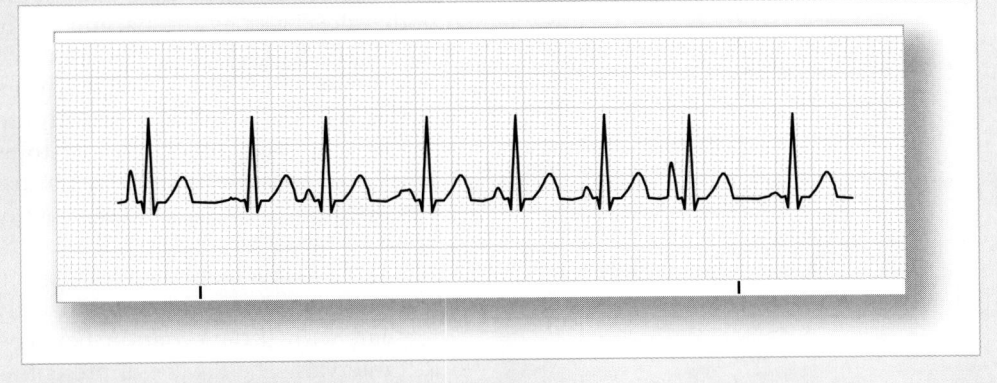

Figure 27-43 Multifocal atrial tachycardia.

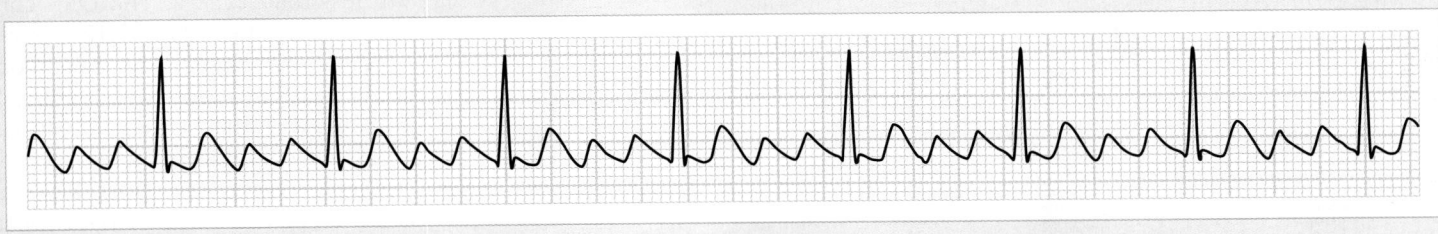

Figure 27-44 Atrial flutter.

common rhythm among elderly patients. One of the main hazards associated with this arrhythmia is that the blood moving through the fibrillating atria has a tendency to form small clots, which may then become emboli and block circulation elsewhere in the body. Because of this risk, many elderly patients whose normal rhythm is atrial fibrillation take an anticoagulant medication such as warfarin (Coumadin), as well as other medications, such as digitalis, to regulate the rate of ventricular response. Prehospital treatment of atrial fibrillation is rare because of the risks involved. If required, it consists of electrical cardioversion when the patient's condition is very critical and transport time is long.

Rhythms of the AV Node or AV Junction

If the SA node—the body's dominant pacemaker—fails to initiate an impulse, the AV node will take over as pacemaker of the heart. Rhythms originating from the AV node are commonly referred to as "junctional" rhythms owing to the proximity of the AV node to the junction of the atria and ventricles. Junctional rhythms feature inverted or missing P waves but normal QRS complexes.

When an impulse is generated in the AV node, it travels down through the conduction system into the ventricles as if it had come from the SA node, resulting in normal QRS complexes. At the same time, the impulse travels upward through the atria and the internodal pathways toward the SA node. There are then three possible cases, none of which includes an upright P wave, but in which the QRS complex appears normal:

- If the impulse begins moving upward through the atria before the other part of it enters the ventricles, an upside-down P wave will be visible (upside down because the impulse is traveling in the opposite direction from that which causes normal upright P waves). This P wave is usually followed immediately by the QRS complex, without any pause between the two.
- If the impulse moving through the atria occurs at the exact same time as the impulse is traveling through the ventricles, the smaller inverted P wave will be buried within the larger QRS complex. This will give the appearance of a missing P wave—that is, the baseline remains flat until the beginning of a normal QRS complex.
- The impulse may start late through the atria and result in an inverted P wave appearing after the QRS complex.

Because the intrinsic rate of the AV node is 40 to 60, junctional rhythms normally present with rates of 40 to 60 beats/min.

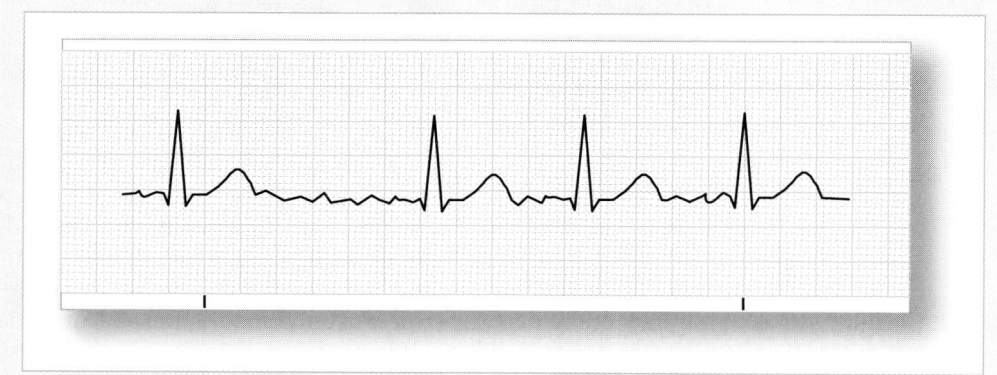

Figure 27-45 Atrial fibrillation.

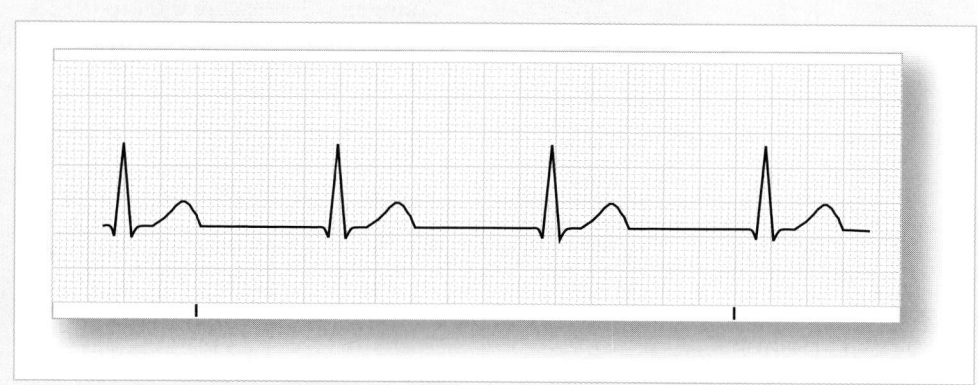

Figure 27-46 Junctional rhythm.

Junctional (Escape) Rhythm

A junctional rhythm occurs when the SA node ceases functioning and the AV node takes over as the pacemaker of the heart **Figure 27-46 ▾**. Because this allows the heart to "escape" from stopping completely, junctional rhythms are sometimes referred to as junctional escape rhythms. A normal junctional escape rhythm has a rate of 40 to 60 beats/min owing to the intrinsic rate of the AV node as a pacemaker. A junctional escape rhythm is usually regular, with little variation between R-R intervals. The P wave, if present, is inverted or upside down but may appear to be absent. The PRI, if an inverted P wave is present, will measure less than 0.12 s. The QRS complex will measure 0.04 to 0.12 s.

Junctional rhythms are most commonly seen in patients with significant problems with the SA node. Treatment usually consists of a surgically implanted pacemaker. Thus, little can be done in the field other than to institute transcutaneous pacing (TCP) if the patient's condition is severely compromised.

Accelerated Junctional Rhythm

Occasionally, a junctional rhythm will present with a rate that exceeds its normal upper rate of 60 beats/min but remains less than 100 beats/min. Because the rhythm is greater than 60 beats/min, it cannot be considered a "normal" junctional rhythm; because it is less than 100 beats/min, it cannot be called tachycardia either. In this case, the name given the rhythm is accelerated junctional rhythm.

An accelerated junctional rhythm is also regular, with little variation between R-R intervals Figure 27-47 ▾ . The P wave, if present, is inverted or upside down but may appear to be absent. The PRI, if an inverted P wave is present, will measure less than 0.12 s. The QRS complex will measure 0.04 to 0.12 s.

Accelerated junctional rhythms are serious, but they seldom require treatment in the prehospital setting because the rate is usually fast enough to maintain a reasonable CO.

Junctional Tachycardia

Occasionally, a junctional rhythm will present with a rate that exceeds 100 beats/min. Any rhythm that results in a ventricular rate greater than 100 beats/min is referred to as tachycardia. In this case, the rhythm is termed junctional tachycardia.

Junctional tachycardia is also regular, with little variation between R-R intervals Figure 27-48 ▾ . The P wave, if present, is inverted or upside down but may appear to be absent. The PRI, if an inverted P wave is present, will measure less than 0.12 s. The QRS complex will measure 0.04 to 0.12 s.

Junctional tachycardia is serious, but it seldom requires treatment in the prehospital setting because the rate is usually fast enough to maintain a reasonable CO. If the rate exceeds 150 beats/min, however, the CO could suffer. In such a case, the rhythm is rarely junctional and is referred to as SVT.

Premature Junctional Complex

Premature junctional complex (PJC) is not, strictly speaking, an arrhythmia (just as PAC is not), but rather the existence of a particular complex within another rhythm Figure 27-49 ▸ . Premature junctional complexes are also known as ectopic complexes, meaning that they occur out of the normal location. A PJC also occurs earlier in time than the next expected sinus complex, causing the R-R interval to be less between it and the previous complex.

The rate depends on the underlying rhythm, and the PJC will make the rhythm irregular. The P wave, if present, will be inverted or upside down, and it may precede or follow the QRS complex. The PRI, if present, will measure less than 0.12 s. The QRS complex will measure 0.04 to 0.12 s.

Premature junctional complexes can be caused by many of the same problems that cause premature atrial contractions. They are rarely treated in the prehospital setting but may be a predictor of future cardiac arrhythmias.

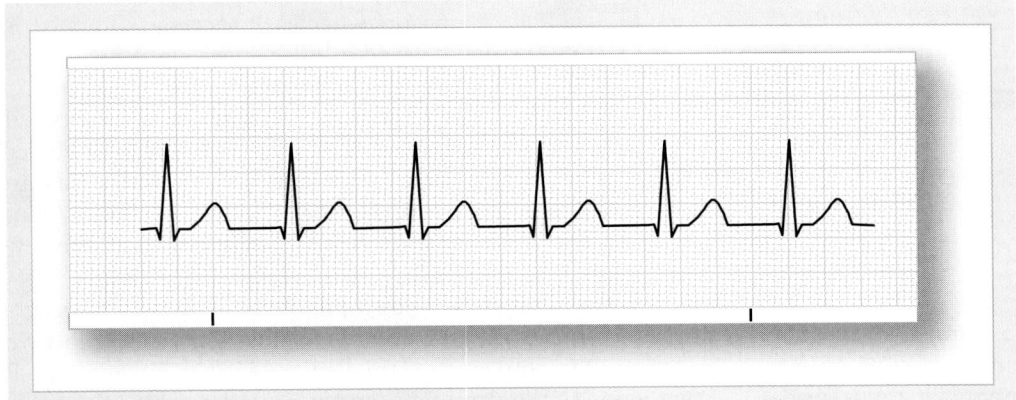

Figure 27-47 Accelerated junctional rhythm.

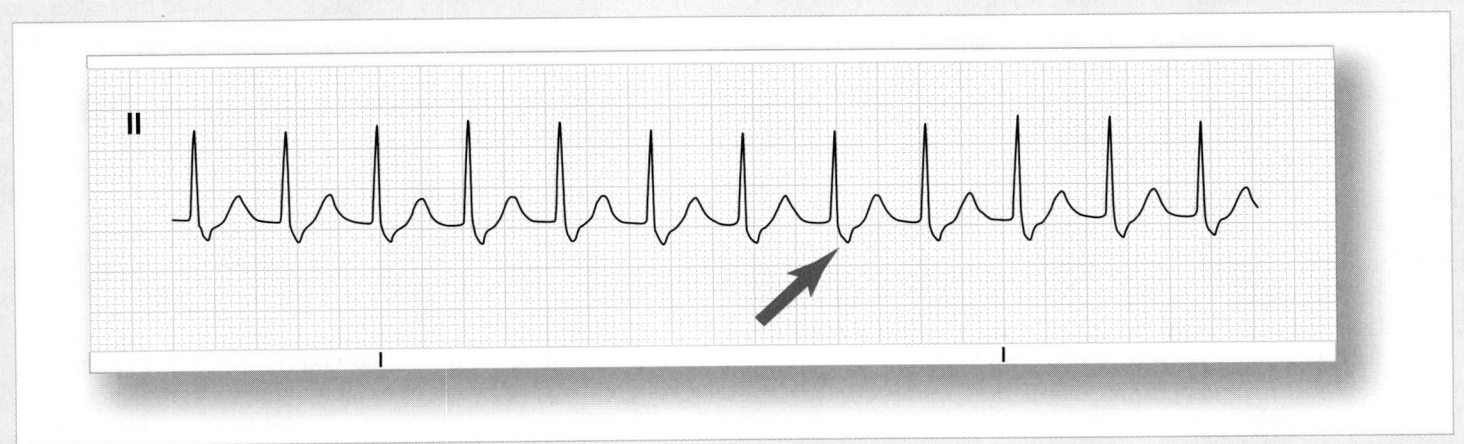

Figure 27-48 Junctional tachycardia. The blue arrow points to an inverted P wave after the QRS wave.

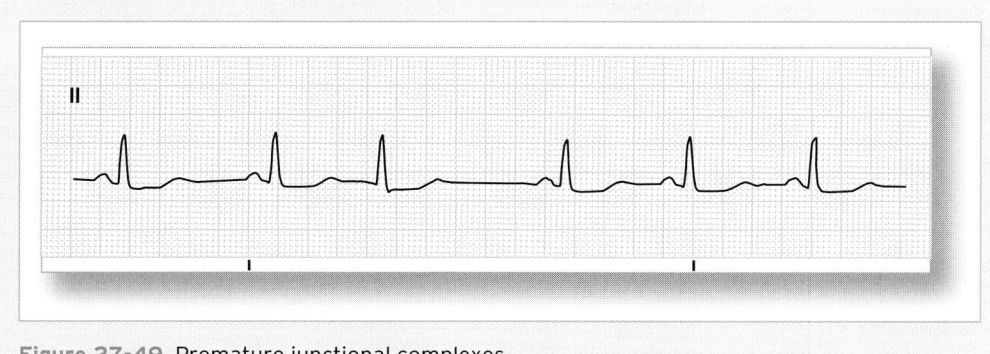

Figure 27-49 Premature junctional complexes.

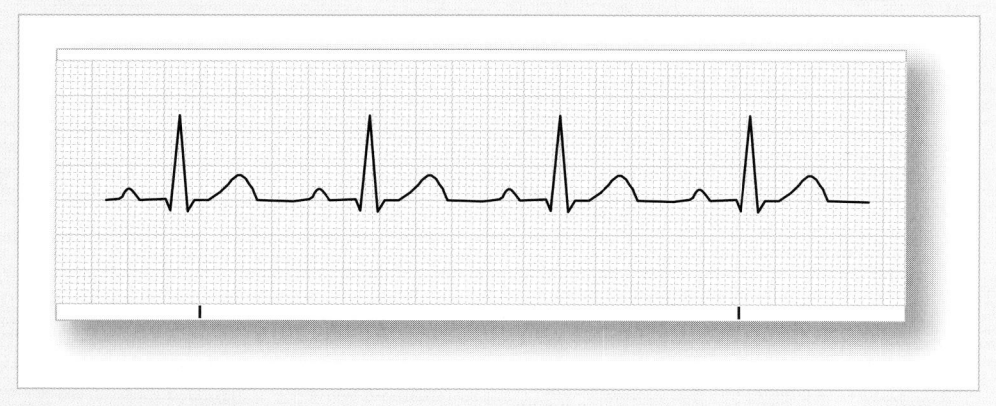

Figure 27-50 First-degree heart block.

Heart Blocks

After the SA node initiates impulses, the impulses proceed through the atria and ventricles and result in contraction of the heart. When they reach the AV node, the impulses are delayed to allow the atria to contract and fill the ventricle. This delay is a normal function of the AV node and usually causes no problems. Occasionally, however, the impulses traveling through the AV node are delayed more than usual, resulting in heart blocks.

Heart blocks are classified into different degrees based on the seriousness of the block and the amount of myocardial damage. The least serious heart block is a first-degree heart block; the most serious is a third-degree block. In between are two types of second-degree block.

First-Degree Heart Block

A first-degree heart block occurs when each impulse reaching the AV node is delayed slightly longer than is expected and results in a PRI greater than 0.20 s. Because each impulse eventually passes through the AV node and causes a QRS complex, this block is considered the least serious. Nevertheless, it is often the first indication of damage that has occurred to the AV node.

Because it originates from the normal pacemaker of the heart, first-degree heart block usually has an intrinsic rate of 60 to 100 beats/min, although it typically occurs at the low end of

this range Figure 27-50 ▾ . The rhythm is regular, with minimal variation between R-R intervals. The P wave is present and upright, and it precedes each QRS complex. The PRI will measure greater than 0.20 s. The QRS complex will measure 0.04 to 0.12 s. The only difference between first-degree heart block and normal sinus rhythm is the prolonged PRI.

First-degree heart block is rarely treated in the prehospital setting unless it is associated with bradycardia that results in significantly reduced CO.

Second-Degree Heart Block: Mobitz Type I (Wenckebach)

A second-degree heart block occurs when an impulse reaching the AV node is occasionally prevented from proceeding to the ventricles and causing a QRS complex. Second-degree heart block, Mobitz type I (Wenckebach), occurs when each successive impulse is delayed a little longer, until finally one impulse is not allowed to continue.

Because it begins from the normal pacemaker of the heart, second-degree heart block, type I, usually has an intrinsic rate of 60 to 100 beats/min, although it typically occurs at the low end of this range Figure 27-51 ▸ . The rhythm is irregular, with a prolonged R-R interval occurring between the last QRS complex before the blocked P wave and the QRS complex after the first unblocked P wave. The P wave is present and upright, and it precedes most QRS complexes. The PRI starts out within the normal limits of 0.12 to 0.20 s but, with each successive P wave, grows longer. It finally results in a P wave that is followed not by a QRS complex, but by another P wave; this P wave is then followed by a QRS complex with a normal PRI. This pattern repeats over and over in the rhythm. The QRS complex will measure 0.04 to 0.12 s.

The key to identification of second-degree type I heart block is the recognition of the increasing PRI followed by the P wave without a QRS complex. This rhythm is always irregular, and you can often easily see the wide R-R interval with the "extra" P wave located there.

Second-degree type I heart blocks are treated in the prehospital setting only if they are associated with bradycardia that results in significantly reduced CO.

Second-Degree Heart Block: Mobitz Type II (Classical)

Second-degree heart block, Mobitz type II, occurs when several impulses are not allowed to continue. It is sometimes called classical because it was well known before the Wenckebach heart block was discovered.

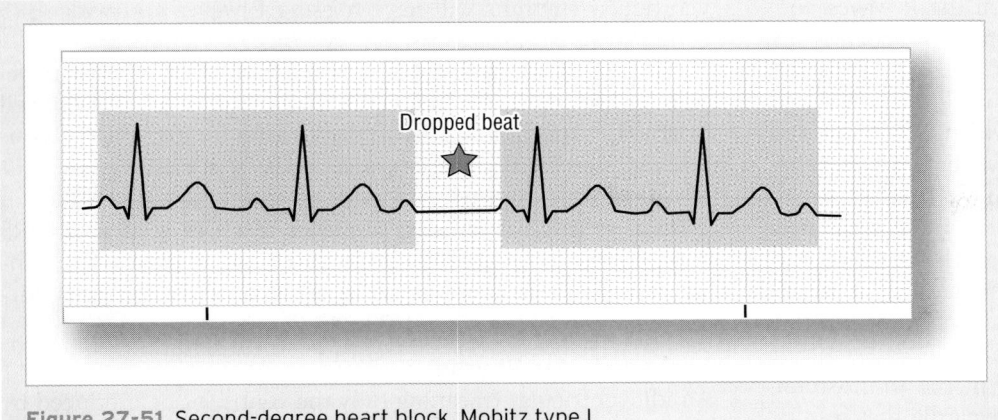

Figure 27-51 Second-degree heart block, Mobitz type I.

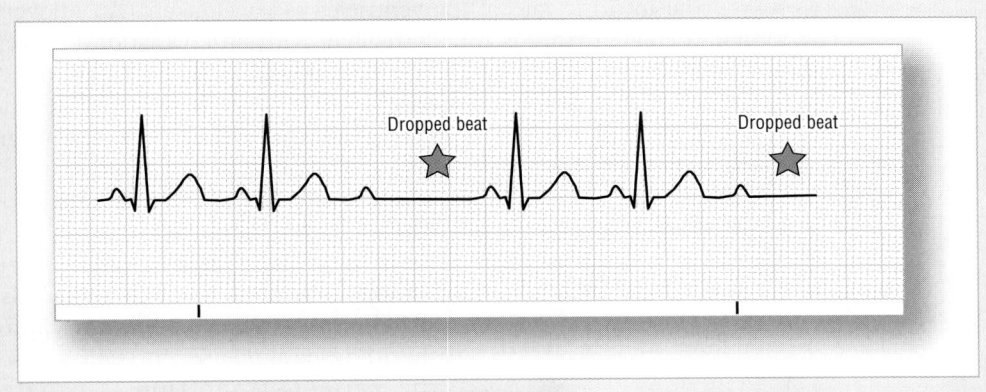

Figure 27-52 Second-degree heart block, Mobitz type II.

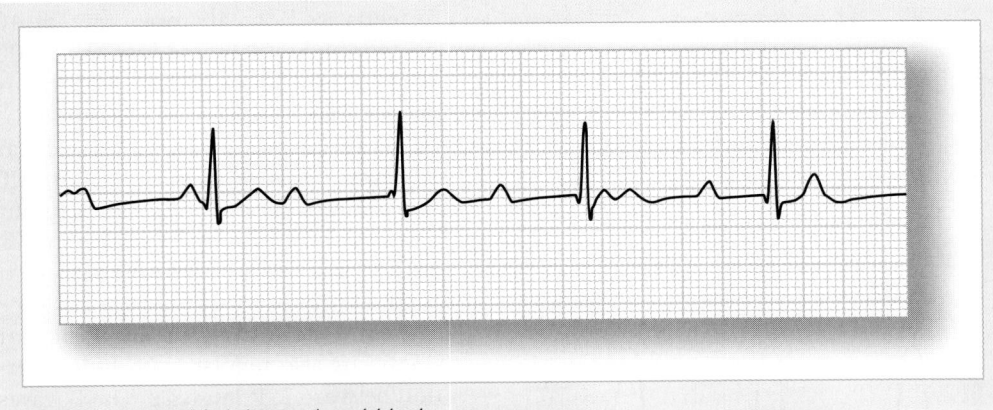

Figure 27-53 Third-degree heart block.

unblocked P wave. The P wave is present and upright, and it precedes some QRS complexes. The PRI is always constant. In fact, this is the easiest way to identify a second-degree type II heart block. If you see a rhythm with some nonconducted P waves, but the PRI is constant among all conducted P waves and their corresponding QRS complexes, you have identified a second-degree type II heart block.

It is important to remember that this block can be regular or irregular. Sometimes several normal beats will occur without a nonconducted P wave; sometimes two or more nonconducted P waves may appear before one P wave is conducted. In other situations, a pattern develops that consists of one conducted P wave followed by one nonconducted P wave.

Second-degree type II heart blocks are treated in the prehospital setting only if they are associated with bradycardia that results in significantly reduced CO.

Third-Degree Heart Block (Complete Heart Block)

A third-degree heart block occurs when all impulses reaching the AV node are prevented from proceeding to the ventricles and causing a QRS complex. Unlike in first- and second-degree heart blocks, in a third-degree heart block *all* impulses from the atria are prevented from traveling to the ventricles. As a consequence, this block is also known as a complete heart block. Because all impulses from the atria are blocked, the ventricles will develop their own pacemaker to continue circulation of blood, albeit at a greatly reduced rate.

Because it originates from the normal pacemaker of the heart, third-degree heart block usually has an intrinsic atrial rate of 60 to 100 beats/min, but the ventricular rate—which depends on the activity of a ventricular pacemaker—is less than 60 beats/min **Figure 27-53 ▲**. The rhythm is usually regular, with the P-P and R-R intervals being consistent. The P wave is present and upright. The PRI in this type of heart block is nonexistent.

The classic way of identifying a third-degree heart block is to identify the presence of nonconducted P waves and then to

Because it originates from the normal pacemaker of the heart, second-degree heart block, type II, usually has an intrinsic rate of 60 to 100 beats/min, although it typically occurs at the low end of this range **Figure 27-52 ▲**. The rhythm may be regular, with every other P wave blocked, or irregular, with a prolonged R-R interval between the last QRS complex before the blocked P wave and the QRS complex after the first

be unable to identify a relationship between the P waves and the QRS complexes. Because the ventricular rate depends on the presence of a ventricular pacemaker, it is common to see the QRS complexes in a third-degree heart block that are wider than 0.12 s. When you see a rhythm with wide QRS complexes (and no narrow QRS complexes) along with P waves, you should suspect a third-degree heart block. If the rhythm is regular and the PRI is not constant, it is almost certainly a third-degree heart block. The major issue with looking for third-degree heart blocks to be regular is the fact that if a premature ventricular complex (described later) occurs within the block, it will make the block appear irregular.

Third-degree heart blocks are treated in the prehospital setting only if they are associated with bradycardia that results in significantly reduced CO. In such a case, the patient will require TCP.

Rhythms of the Ventricles

If the SA node fails to initiate an impulse, the AV node will usually take over as pacemaker. If the AV node cannot perform this duty, however, the ventricles may begin to originate their own impulses and become the pacemaker of the heart. Such

ventricular rhythms will have missing P waves and wide QRS complexes.

If an impulse is generated in the ventricles, it must travel through the ventricles in a cell-to-cell manner because the cell originating the impulse is unlikely to be located on the conduction system. Because impulses travel more slowly via cell-to-cell transmission than when they travel on the conduction system, ventricular-initiated impulses result in very wide QRS complexes—more than 0.12 s in duration. Because the intrinsic rate of the ventricles is 20 to 40, ventricular rhythms normally demonstrate rates of 20 to 40 beats/min.

Idioventricular Rhythm

An idioventricular (meaning only the ventricles or produced by the ventricles) rhythm occurs when the SA and AV nodes fail and the ventricles must takes over pacing the heart **Figure 27-54 ▾**. It has a rate of 20 to 40 beats/min owing to the intrinsic rate of the ventricles as pacemakers. An idioventricular rhythm is usually regular, with little variation between R-R intervals. P waves are absent owing to the failure of the SA and AV nodes. Because there is no P wave, there is no PRI. The QRS complex will measure greater than 0.12 s because it originates in the ventricles.

Idioventricular rhythms are serious and may or may not result in a palpable pulse. Treatment is geared toward improving the CO by increasing the rate and, if possible, treating the underlying cause. In such a case, the patient's condition is usually severely compromised.

Accelerated Idioventricular Rhythm

Occasionally, an idioventricular rhythm exceeds its normal upper rate of 40 beats/min but remains less than 100 beats/min. Because the rhythm is greater than 40 beats/min, it cannot be considered a "normal" ventricular rhythm; because it is less than 100 beats/min, it cannot be called tachycardia either. In this case, the rhythm is called accelerated idioventricular rhythm.

An accelerated idioventricular rhythm is also regular, with little variation between R-R intervals. The P waves are absent, so the PRI does not exist **Figure 27-55 ◂**. The QRS complex will measure greater than 0.12 s.

Accelerated idioventricular rhythms are serious, but they are seldom treated in the prehospital setting.

Ventricular Tachycardia

Ventricular rhythms occur when the SA and AV nodes fail as the pacemakers of

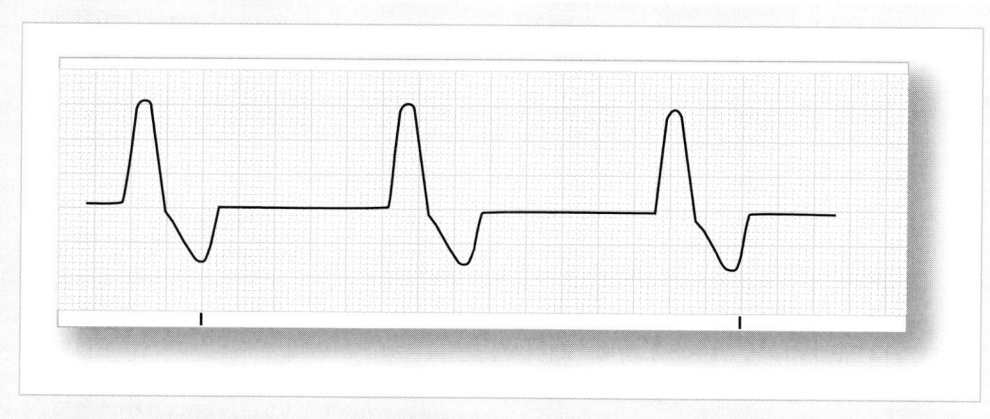

Figure 27-54 Idioventricular rhythm.

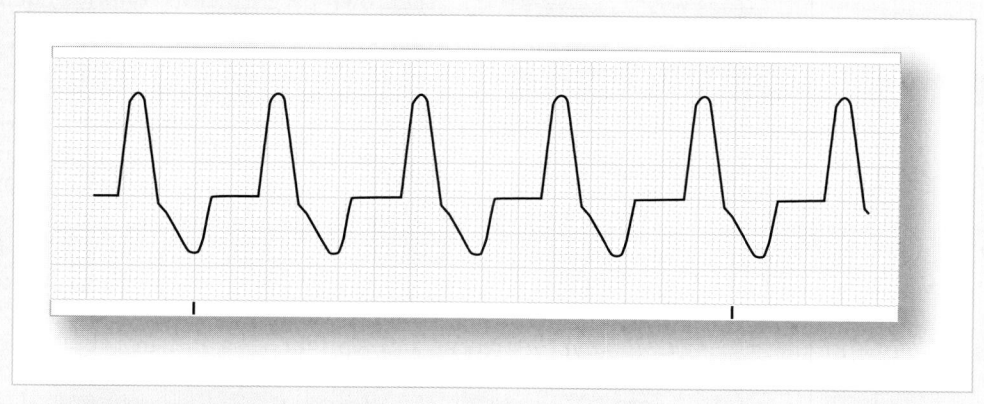

Figure 27-55 Accelerated idioventricular rhythm.

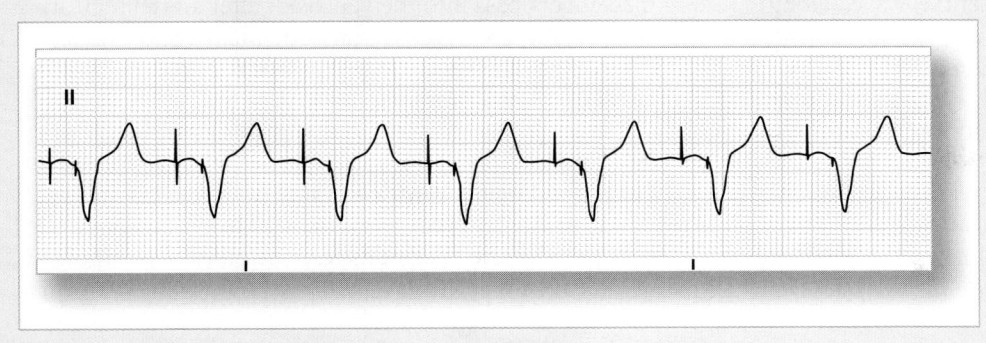

Figure 27-69 Artificial pacemaker rhythm (AV sequential).

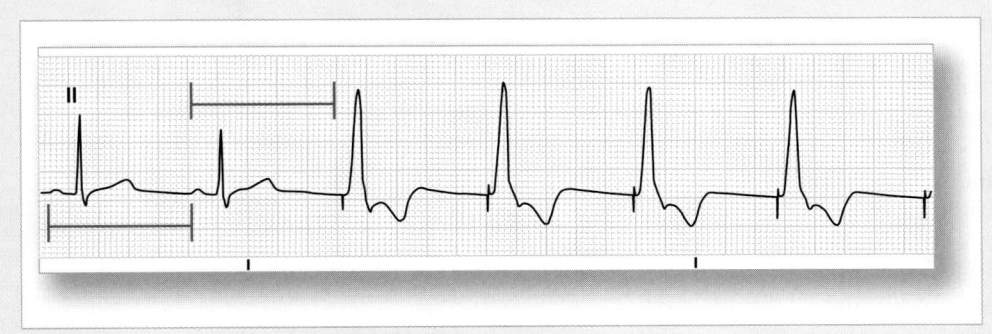

Figure 27-70 Artificial pacemaker rhythm (demand pacemaker).

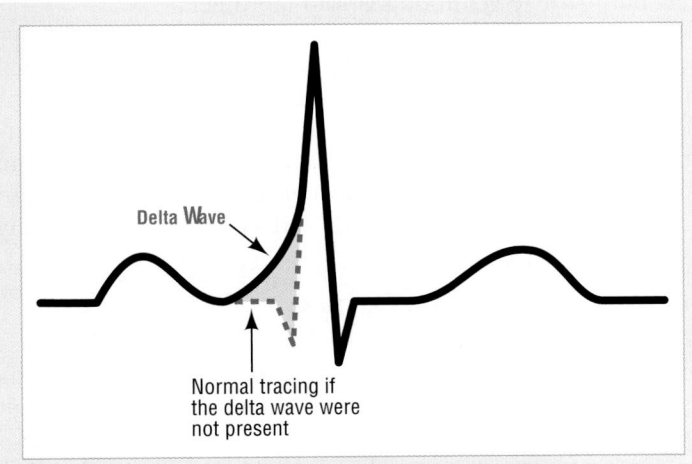

Figure 27-71 Delta wave: WPW syndrome.

Another type of pacemaker failure involves a "runaway" pacemaker. A runaway pacemaker presents as a very tachycardic pacemaker rhythm that must be slowed to preserve the patient's cardiac function. Usually a strong magnet placed over the pacemaker will "reset" a runaway pacemaker.

Other ECG Abnormalities

A few other ECG abnormalities are not identified as arrhythmias but are indicative of significant cardiac conditions. For example, a delta wave is an indication of Wolff-Parkinson-White (WPW) syndrome. Patients with WPW syndrome have an accessory pathway between the atria and the ventricles called the bundle of Kent. This bundle of conductive tissue bypasses the AV node and begins ventricular depolarization early, resulting in a rapid up slope to the R wave immediately after the end of the P wave Figure 27-71 ▼. This early up slope can be interpreted as a widened QRS complex (more than 0.12 s), which would seem to indicate a ventricular pacemaker. This situation, which is referred to as aberrant conduction, can lead to the misinterpretation of SVTs as ventricular in origin. Patients with WPW syndrome are highly susceptible to SVTs.

Another important abnormality is an Osborne, or J, wave. It occurs in cases of hypothermia and presents as what appears to be a P wave at the end of the QRS complex Figure 27-72 ▼. The J wave may also be accompanied by ST-segment depression and T-wave inversion. Generally, the more serious the hypothermia, the larger the J wave. Evidence of a J wave should be considered only an indication of hypothermia; it is not enough to make a definitive diagnosis.

Electrolyte imbalances can also cause changes in the ECG that are not arrhythmias but can be indicators of serious conditions. The two most common of these electrolyte imbalances are hyperkalemia and hypokalemia. Hyperkalemia often presents with very tall, pointed T waves; these T waves may be as tall or taller than the QRS complex Figure 27-73 ▶ . By contrast, hypokalemia

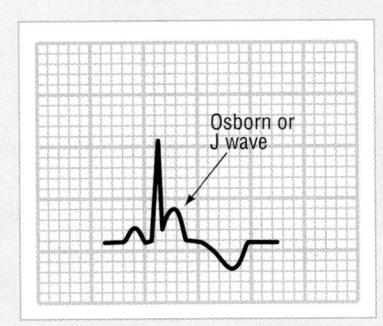

Figure 27-72 Osborne (J) wave.

but they will not be followed by a QRS complex. This loss of capture indicates the pacemaker is not operating properly. A loss of capture may also occur if the wire connecting the pacemaker to the patient's heart becomes dislodged. In either of these cases, the patient's heartbeat now depends on the natural pacemaker (usually the ventricles), resulting in greatly reduced CO. In such cases, patients need TCP instituted as quickly as possible.

usually presents with flat or apparently absent T waves along with the development of a U wave. The U wave is a small wave (smaller even than a P wave) that occurs after a T wave but before the next P wave. U waves are very uncommon and may often be mistaken for extra P waves or another unknown abnormality **Figure 27-74 ▾** .

Other electrolyte imbalances do not cause such obvious changes in the ECG. Hypercalcemia may cause a shortened Q-T interval, for example, whereas hypocalcemia may slightly lengthen the Q-T interval. These changes would likely not be obvious in the field.

Bedtime Stories: Tragic Tales of Arrhythmias

Cast

Sidney Sinus. Sidney, the SA node, is boss of the heart. He ordinarily dispatches messengers 70 to 80 times per minute; the messengers are supposed to dash down the atria, slip through the AV junction, and depolarize the ventricles. Sidney is not terribly bright but is usually conscientious and reliable.

Albert and Alice Atria. Albert and Alice are the right and left atria. These somewhat temperamental little pouches normally contract in response to the messages sent by Sidney and squeeze their blood into the ventricles, providing the ventricles with an atrial kick. Their contraction is represented on the ECG by the P wave.

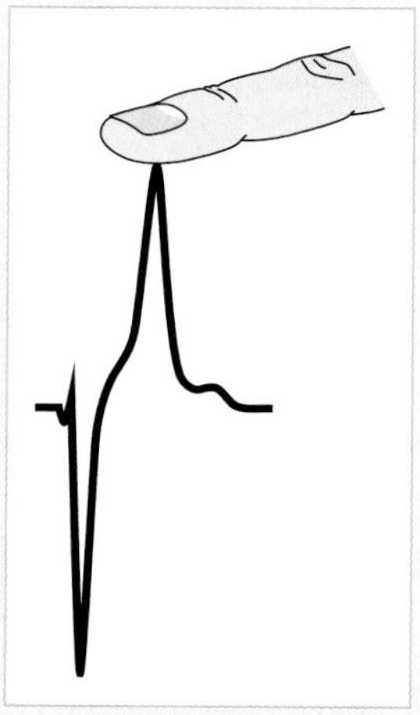

AV Abe. Abe, the AV node, is a lower-level pacemaker who secretly yearns to be boss of the heart. Unfortunately, because of his lower intrinsic rate, he rarely gets the opportunity to run the show. Abe stands at the threshold of the ventricles and checks out every messenger sent by Sidney Sinus. Normally, Abe lets the messengers pass into the ventricles after a brief security check (PRI). However, as the node in charge of traffic control into the ventricles, Abe does regulate the flow of messengers and occasionally closes a few southbound lanes, especially when the traffic gets very heavy or when he's not feeling well.

Vance and Virginia Ventricle. Vance and Virginia are big, tough, muscular types, also not very bright, who are charged with the enormous responsibility of pumping blood to the whole body. Normally, they take their orders from the messengers sent by Sidney Sinus, but sometimes the Ventricles grow irritable and contract without orders, especially when they run a little short on oxygen. They also tend to be impatient when they don't hear from Sidney on time; under that circumstance, they sometimes contract on their own.

Montgomery, Mimi, Mortimer, Millicent, et al. These messengers consist of tiny electric impulses. Earnest and dedicated, their job is to carry the orders for depolarization from Sidney's headquarters all the way to the ventricles.

First-Degree AV Block, or "The Little Messenger That Could"

One fine day, Sidney Sinus dispatched Mortimer Messenger with the usual order: "Depolarize the ventricles." Mortimer scampered down the atria without difficulty but arrived at the AV node to find a pile of debris blocking the entrance to the ventricles. "Sorry," said AV Abe, "we're closed for repairs."

"But I *have* to get through," said Mortimer.

"Impossible," said Abe.

But Mortimer was brave and determined. "I think I can. I think I can. I know I can," he said, gathering his few milliamps of strength. Finally, after a long struggle (prolonged PRI), Mortimer crashed through the AV junction into the ventricles and breathlessly issued the order to contract **Figure 27-75 ▸** . The ventricles were depolarized, and everyone lived happily ever after, until . . .

Second-Degree AV Block, Type I

When Montgomery Messenger left for work that day, there was no sign there would be trouble. He took his first set of orders from Sidney Sinus, whistled down the atria, zipped through the AV node, and smartly ordered the ventricles to depolarize.

On the next trip down, however, Montgomery felt just a bit tired and slowed slightly as he crossed the AV junction. "Why break my neck?" he thought. "So, the PRI will be a tiny bit prolonged. Who'll notice, anyway?"

On his third trip, Montgomery encountered several roadblocks in the region of the AV junction and had to pick his way around them. Glancing at his watch as he reached the ventricles, he scowled. "Nuts," he said, "0.24 s. Boy, is Sidney going to be mad."

Making his fourth trip from the SA node, Montgomery found the gates to the ventricles closed and locked. Frantically, he banged on the gates. "Come on, Abe, I know you're around

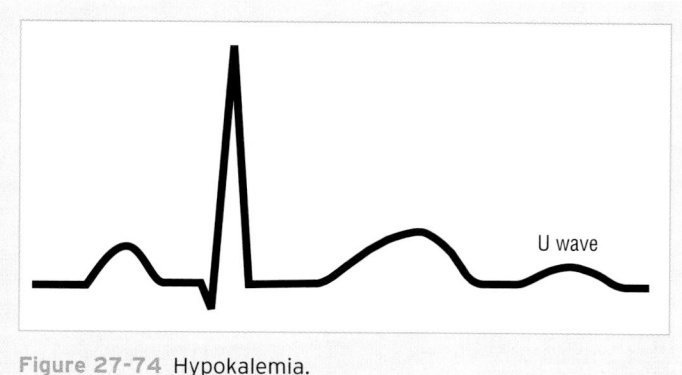

Figure 27-73 Hyperkalemia.

Figure 27-74 Hypokalemia.

somewhere. Let me through." To no avail. The gates remained tightly shut. Defeated, Montgomery returned to the SA node, leaving a lonely P wave to chronicle his struggle Figure 27-76 ▾.

"What do you mean, you couldn't get through?" Sidney Sinus demanded.

"I couldn't get through," Montgomery said. "I'm telling you the gates were locked tight."

"Okay," said Sid, "off to the showers. You've had it for the day." So Sidney called Mimi Messenger. "Now look," he told her, "I want you to go straight down to the ventricles and give them this message, and no fooling around at the AV junction, understand?"

"Oh, yes sir," said Mimi, always eager to please. So off Mimi went, sailing down the atria, through the AV junction, and into the ventricles. "Hmm, 0.14 s," she noted to herself. "Sid can't complain about that." On her second run, however, Mimi tripped over a shoelace and barely made it in under 0.2 s. On the third trip, some highway construction held her up for 0.24 s. But the fourth trip south was the worst, for she arrived at the AV junction to find that once again Abe had locked the gates. Mimi banged and banged on the gates. "Come on, Abe,

open up. I'm going to lose my job." No response. Crestfallen, Mimi returned to the SA node.

"And what happened to you?" Sid demanded.

"I couldn't get through to the ventricles this time."

"Couldn't get through? Did you get lost, maybe?"

"But at least I made a nice P wave," Mimi ventured.

"A nice P wave! A nice *P wave,* she says. What good's a P wave without a QRS complex? Do you think the atria are going to supply blood to the whole body? They're strictly small-time, sweetheart. The big guns are in the ventricles. That's why I sent you to depolarize them. Now you get to the showers."

And so it went. Messenger after messenger faltered at the AV junction, but the worst was yet to come.

Second-Degree AV Block, Type II

It just wasn't Montgomery's week. Reporting for work the next day, he received the usual order from Sidney to depolarize the ventricles. Montgomery set out full of confidence and vigor, traversing the atria without difficulty. But when he arrived at the threshold of the ventricles, he found his path blocked by AV Abe.

"Let me through," Montgomery said. "I have an important message for the ventricles."

"Get lost," said Abe, who was feeling rather dyspeptic that day.

"But I have to get through. I've already used up 0.19 s."

"Beat it, sonny. I'm the boss around here."

Montgomery returned to Sidney Sinus disgraced. "What happened to you?" Sidney wanted to know. "You were supposed to order the ventricles to contract."

"I couldn't get past Abe," Montgomery replied.

"What do you mean, you couldn't get past Abe? I just sent your friend, Mimi Messenger down there, and she got through without any problem."

"But he wouldn't let me pass," whimpered Montgomery.

"I don't want to hear any excuses. You just go right back down there and deliver your message to the ventricles. I can't tolerate weaklings on my staff."

So Montgomery squared his shoulders, sailed down the atria again, and arrived once more at the gate of the ventricles.

"Are you here again?" said Abe. "I thought I told you to beat it."

"Please," said Montgomery, "I have to get through. You don't know what Sid is like when he gets upset."

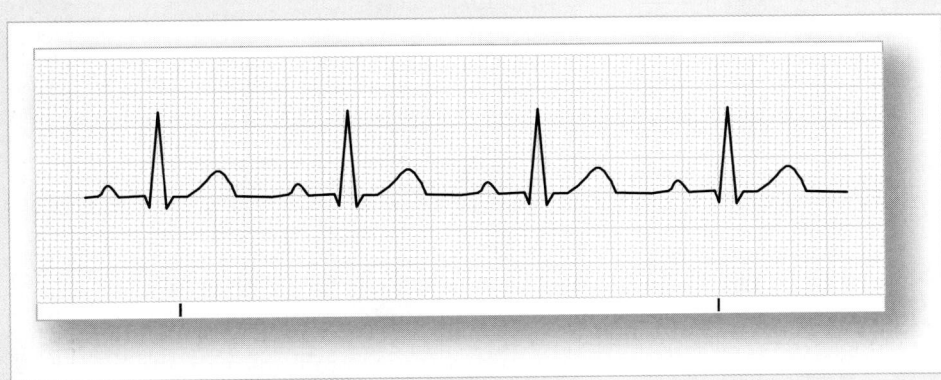

Figure 27-75 First-degree AV block. When there is trouble at the AV junction, it may take the messengers from the SA node longer to get through.

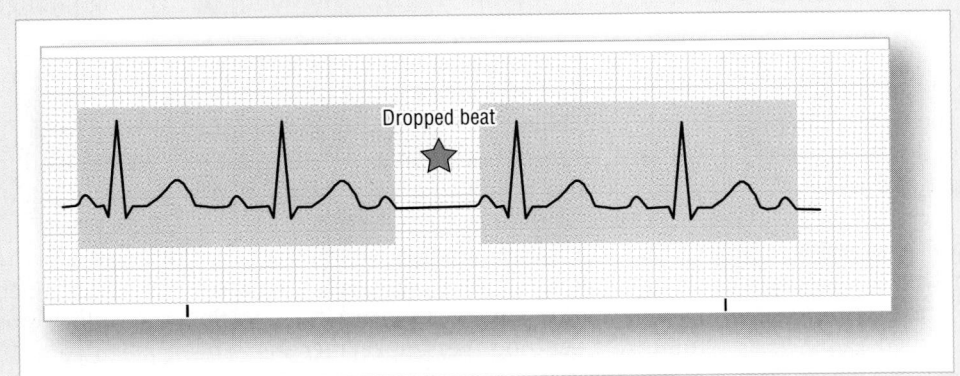

Figure 27-76 Second-degree AV block, type I (Wenckebach). Each transit through the AV junction is a bit slower, until finally the messenger cannot get through, and a beat is dropped.

"Sorry, sonny, I'm closed for lunch."

Montgomery returned to Sidney Sinus. "I couldn't make it," he said.

"Look, Montgomery," said Sidney, "Millicent Messenger just breezed by Abe right after you left. Now you march back down there and do your job."

"Yes, sir," said Montgomery.

Arriving again at the threshold of the ventricles, Montgomery once more found Abe blocking his path.

"Listen, Abe, I'm not kidding this time. If you don't let me through, I'm going to use some atropine and blast the gate open."

"Those are big words, sonny," said Abe, "but I'm not scared of a little atropine."

"The last time they used atropine, you were zonked for hours," Montgomery reminded him.

"I'll take my chances."

And so it went. Each time Montgomery reached the gate to the ventricle, AV Abe barred his path. Yet the messenger coming right after Montgomery kept getting through (2:1 block) **Figure 27-77** ▸.

"Montgomery," cautioned Sidney, "if this keeps up, they're going to put in a pacemaker, and we'll all be out of a job. Shape up."

But the worst was yet to come.

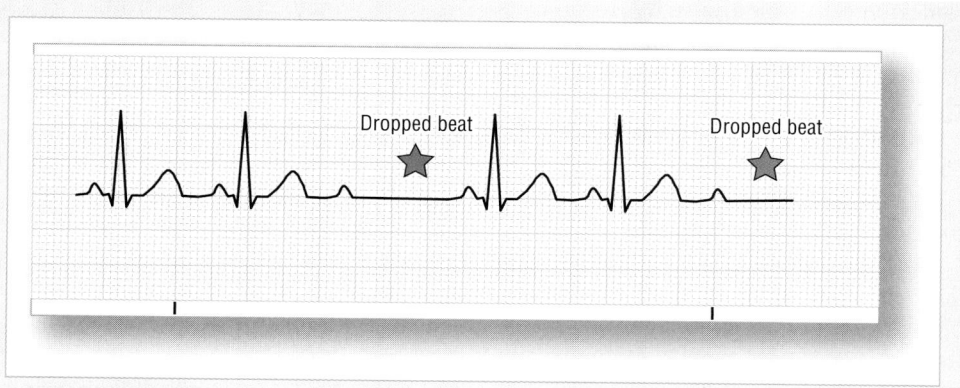

Figure 27-77 Second-degree AV block, type II. With this rhythm, impulses from the SA node are periodically blocked at the AV junction.

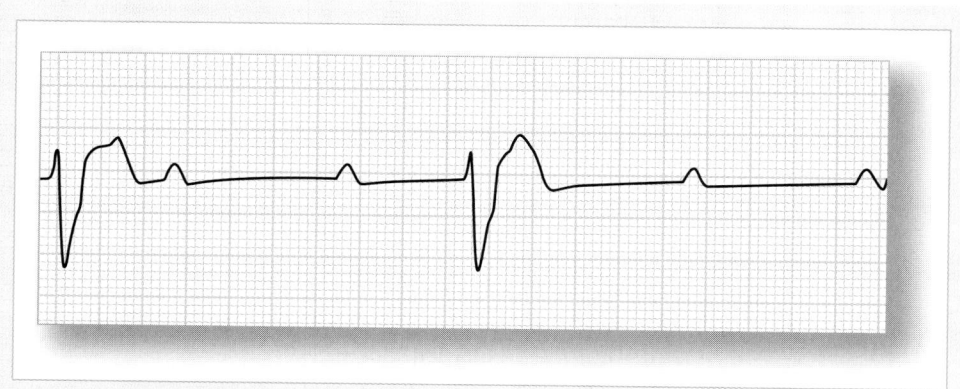

Figure 27-78 Third-degree AV block. The atria and ventricles are marching to the beat of different drummers.

Complete Heart Block (Third-Degree AV Block)

The next day was even worse for Sidney's operation. It was bad enough, Montgomery not getting through. "Every second P wave not followed by a QRS complex," wailed Sidney. "My reputation is being ruined!" But then, suddenly, the situation became even worse. Sidney had just sent Mildred Messenger down to the ventricles, and she arrived at the AV junction to find the gate shut and bolted. A sign tacked to the gate read: "Closed until further notice."

"That's impossible," said Sidney when he heard the story. "Abe can't do that to me." So he sent another messenger, Marvin, to depolarize the ventricles. Marvin charged down the atria and ran smack into the closed gate. He banged and shouted, but there was no response.

"Impossible," said Sidney. "Abe must be sleeping." So he dispatched Melvin Messenger. Again the door was bolted tight.

"Oh, what I'd give for a bolus of atropine," sighed Sidney.

Meanwhile, the ventricles were starting to get nervous, and Vance, the right ventricle, said to Virginia, the left ventricle, "Have you heard anything from the atria lately?"

"Not a thing."

"Funny. Those messengers are usually pretty prompt."

"Must have run into some problems with Abe."

"Yeah. Every time that guy has a little too much digitalis, he gets delusions of grandeur and starts hassling the messengers."

"How long do you suppose we ought to wait?"

"I don't know. It's already been more than a second, and the brain is starting to complain about not getting enough oxygen."

"The brain is always complaining about something."

"Yeah, but the kidneys don't sound very happy either."

"Okay, okay. Let's go ahead and contract. I hate to do it without authorization from above. The last time we decided to go ahead and fire on our own, some of that disgusting lidocaine came barreling down the pipes. I was sick for a week."

So Vance and Virginia set off on their own, contracting slowly (about 30 times per minute) so as not to attract much attention, little appreciating that back in the atria Sidney was frantically sending messenger after messenger, all in vain, to assault the closed gate **Figure 27-78** ▴.

"What's happened to Sidney?" Virginia said to Vance, as they plodded along slowly.

"I wish I knew," said Vance.

12-Lead ECGs

Up to now, we have considered ECG rhythm strips obtained from monitoring a single lead. For purposes of rhythm interpretation, a single lead (usually lead II) is usually sufficient. To localize the site of injury to heart muscle, however, we must be able to look at the heart from several angles. That is precisely the purpose of a 12-lead ECG.

What Is a 12-Lead ECG?

Suppose you wanted to check out the condition of a used car you were thinking of buying. If you needed to know only whether the motor was running, you could stand anywhere near the car and listen (just as you can use any one lead to monitor the cardiac rhythm). But if you wanted to know what kind of shape the car body is in, you would have to walk around the car and look at it from all sides. The driver's side might be in mint condition, but if you stroll around to the passenger's side, you might see that the entire door frame is caved in from a road accident.

Similarly, each ECG lead looks at the heart from a different angle. Although one lead may see a normal myocardium, another may be looking at major damage.

What Do ECG Leads Record?

What does a lead "see" when it looks at the heart? The word *lead,* as it is used in electrocardiography, can be somewhat confusing. Sometimes the word is used to refer to one of the cables and monitoring electrodes that connect the ECG machine to the patient (such as the "right arm lead"). A lead provides an electrical picture of the heart taken from a specified vantage point. Lead I, for example, "looks" at the heart from the left, so it "sees" the left side of the heart. Lead aVF looks up at the heart from the feet (F stands for "foot"), so it "sees" the bottom of the heart. In the standard ECG, we record 12 leads—that is, 12 different pictures of the electrical activity of the heart.

Six of the leads—I, II, III, aVR, aVL, and aVF—are called limb leads because the pictures taken by those leads are derived from attaching cables to the patient's limbs. The limb leads look at the heart from the sides and from the feet, in the vertical plane. **Figure 27-79 ▶** shows the viewpoint of each of the limb leads. For example, lead II has a direct view of the bottom of the heart (the inferior or diaphragmatic wall of the heart), whereas aVL (L stands for "left") looks at the heart from the vantage point of the left shoulder.

In addition to the limb leads, there are six precordial leads (V_1 to V_6), also called chest leads, anterior leads, or V leads. The six precordial leads are placed on the anterior and lateral chest walls, usually with adhesive electrodes, in the positions shown in **Figure 27-80 ▶**. These leads look at the heart in the horizontal plane (as shown in the inset to Figure 27-80), so they provide a picture of the heart taken from the front (anterior wall of the heart) and from the left side (anterolateral). More specifically, leads V_1 and V_2 look at the septum; V_3 and V_4 look at the anterior wall of the left ventricle; and V_5 and V_6 look at the lateral wall of the left ventricle.

12-Lead ECG Lead Placement

How reliable would 12-lead ECGs be if you could place the electrodes anywhere on the chest? When a 12-lead ECG is read, it is assumed that the person who performed the recording placed the electrodes correctly on the chest. Correct placement is important because the 12-lead ECGs are compared with previous ECGs. For the comparison to be reliable for identifying existing problems or highlighting the appearance of new problems (such as ST-segment elevation), the electrodes must be placed consistently. **Table 27-16 ▼** outlines where the different leads look.

When a current is moving toward a lead, it creates a positive (upright) deflection on the ECG tracing of that lead. Thus, in **Figure 27-81 ▶**, the current depolarizing the ventricles is moving toward lead II, so what we see in lead II is an upright QRS complex (recall that the QRS complex is produced by depolarization of the ventricles). If the depolarizing current is moving toward lead II, then it must be moving away from lead aVR, so we would expect to see a negative deflection in aVR. And, indeed, the QRS complex in aVR is a downward deflection. That makes intuitive sense. If you and a friend are standing facing each other at opposite ends of a football field, a ball thrown toward your friend will look bigger and bigger to the friend as it approaches; the same ball will meanwhile look

Table 27-16	Focus of ECG Leads			
Leads	Area of Damage	Coronary Artery Involved	Possible Complications	
II, III, and aVF	Inferior wall LV	RCA: posterior descending	Hypotension, LV dysfunction	
V_1 and V_2	Septum	LCA: LAD, septal	Infranodal blocks and BBBs	
V_3 and V_4	Anterior wall LV	LCA: LAD, diagonal	LV dysfunction, CHF, BBBs, complete heart block, PVCs	
V_5, V_6, I, and aVL	Lateral wall LV	LCA: circumflex	LV dysfunction, AV nodal block in some	
V_4R (II, III, aVF)	RV	RCA: proximal	Hypotension, supranodal and AV nodal blocks, atrial fibrillation, PACs	

LV indicates left ventricle; LAD, left anterior descending; BBB, bundle branch block; RV, right ventricle; RCA, right coronary artery; LCA, left coronary artery; PAC, premature atrial contraction; PVC, premature ventricular contraction.

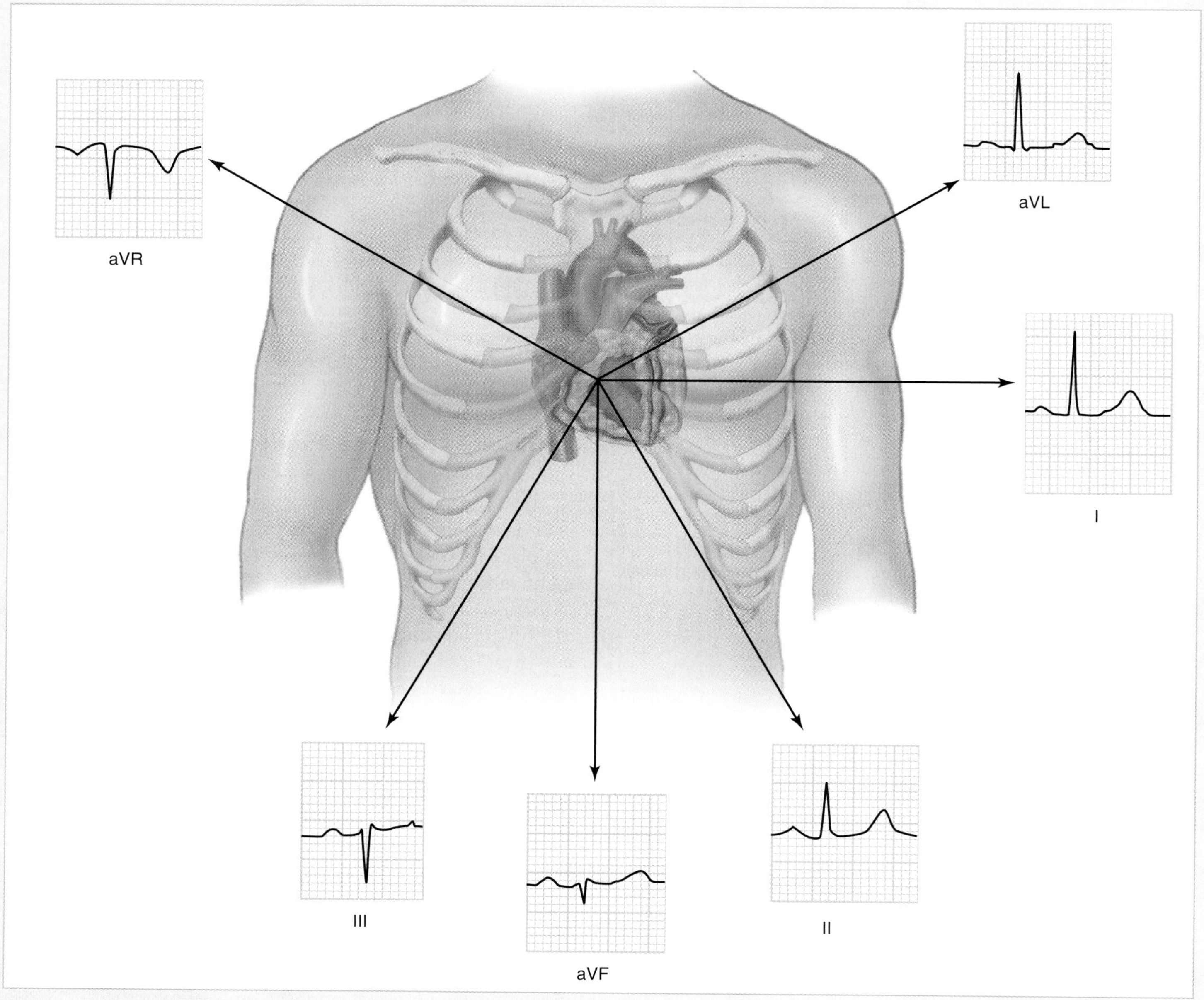

Figure 27-79 Limb leads look at the heart in the vertical plane. Leads II, III, and aVF give us a picture of the wall of the heart that rests on the diaphragm, the inferior wall.

smaller and smaller to you as it travels the same course. Similarly, leads II and aVR, being nearly opposite each other, will present nearly opposite pictures of the same wave of electrical depolarization. If a depolarizing wave is coming toward lead II, it will be going away from aVR.

The 12-Lead ECG in a Normal Heart

The gold standard for multilead ECGs is the 12-lead ECG. Cardiac catheterization laboratories, especially electrophysiology catheterization laboratories, may perform 15- or 18-lead ECGs! Any ECG that is recorded electronically always has the same layout on the paper, meaning that the leads will be plotted out in the same manner every time **Figure 27-82 ▶**

Each of the colors in **Figure 27-83A ▶** has a purpose; that is, each color represents the leads that look at a particular wall of the heart. Lead aVR is not used for this purpose, so no color is assigned to it.

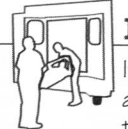 **In the Field**

If the PQRST configuration is upright in lead aVR, the limb leads are on wrong! Specifically, the red and white leads have been switched.

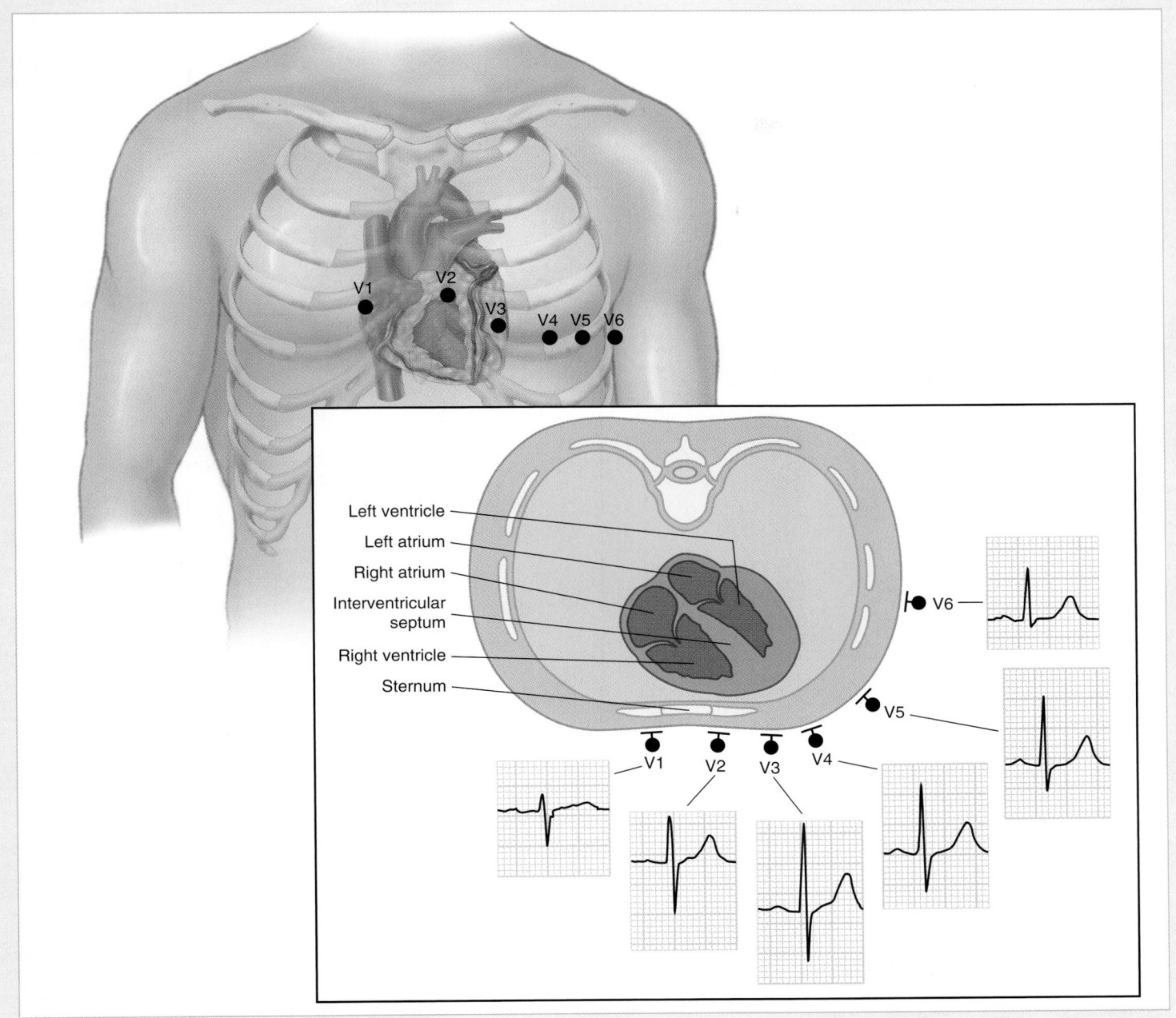

Figure 27-80 Precordial leads (chest leads) look at the heart in the horizontal plane. Inset: V_1 and V_2 look at the right ventricle. V_3 and V_4 "see" the interventricular septum. V_5 and V_6 see the anterior and lateral left ventricle.

Figure 27-83B ▶ depicts an ECG. (Some information has been added to help you out.) Notice that the specific wall of the left ventricle is listed along with the coronary artery that supplies that wall for each lead. The left ventricle is the stronger and more muscular of the two ventricles; it will be the first to let its owner know that it is not getting enough oxygen. If the left ventricle becomes damaged, in addition to pain, the patient may develop deadly arrhythmias such as ventricular fibrillation. Each wall requires 2 to 4 leads or views to see its image completely. Those leads are anatomically contiguous—that is, the leads look at the same general area of the heart. When we are looking for evidence of injury to the heart and we must see it in 2 or more contiguous leads, then the following information will be important:

Contiguous Inferior Leads
- Lead II is contiguous with lead III.
- Lead III is contiguous with leads II and aVF.
- Lead aVF is contiguous with lead III.

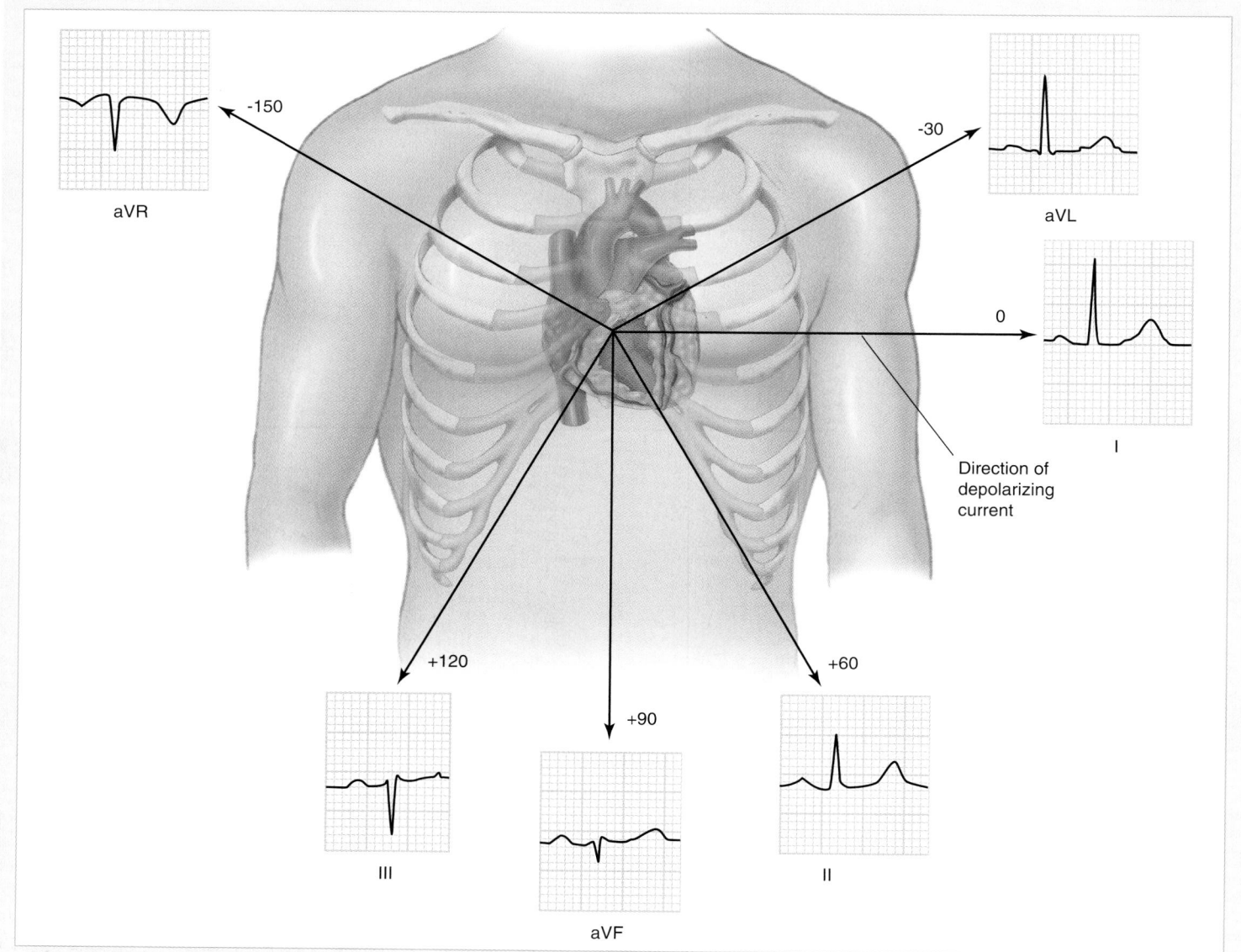

Figure 27-81 The morphology of QRS complexes varies based on the lead position and the direction of the electrical impulse movement within the heart. If the electrical impulses are moving primarily toward lead II, it will be upright as shown, while lead aVR will be inverted since the impulse is moving away from it.

Contiguous Septal-Anterior-Lateral Leads

- V_1 is contiguous with V_2.
- V_2 is contiguous with V_1 and V_3.
- V_3 is contiguous with V_2 and V_4.
- V_4 is contiguous with V_3 and V_5.
- V_5 is contiguous with V_4 and V_6.
- V_6 is contiguous with V_5 and lead I.
- Lead I is contiguous with V_6 and aVL
- aVL is contiguous with lead I.

The 12-Lead ECG in a Damaged Heart

The ECG tells the practitioner many things about a patient's heart. For our purposes in the field, we will keep it simple and look for any evidence that the patient is having an AMI. To do so, we must focus on three parts of the ECG: the ST segment, the Q wave, and the T wave.

Recall the sequence of events in an AMI. As the blood supply to the affected area of heart muscle slows to a trickle, the muscle no longer receives sufficient oxygen; that is, it becomes ischemic (deprived of blood). If ischemia persists more than a few minutes, it leads to actual injury to the heart muscle, which in turn will be followed by infarction (death of muscle) if the circulation to the area is not rapidly restored.

The ECG can provide a graphic record of that sequence of events **Table 27-17** . Ischemia commonly causes ST-segment depression and may also lead to T-wave inversion.

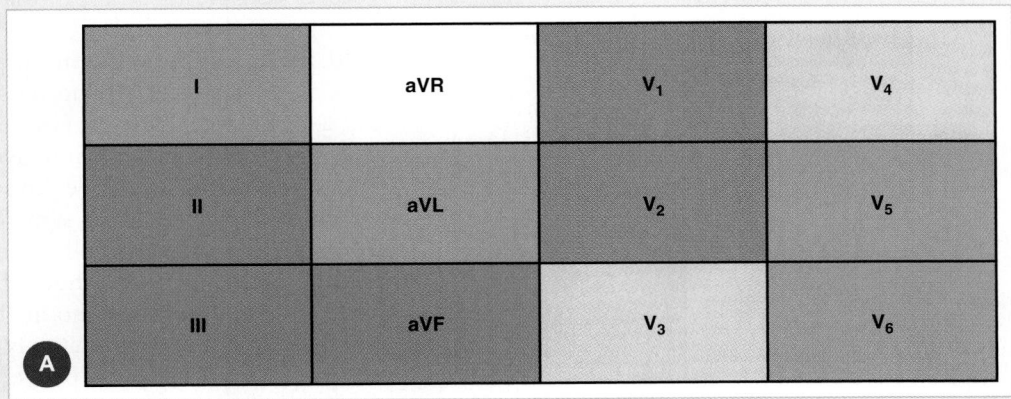

I	aVR	V₁	V₄
II	aVL	V₂	V₅
III	aVF	V₃	V₆

A

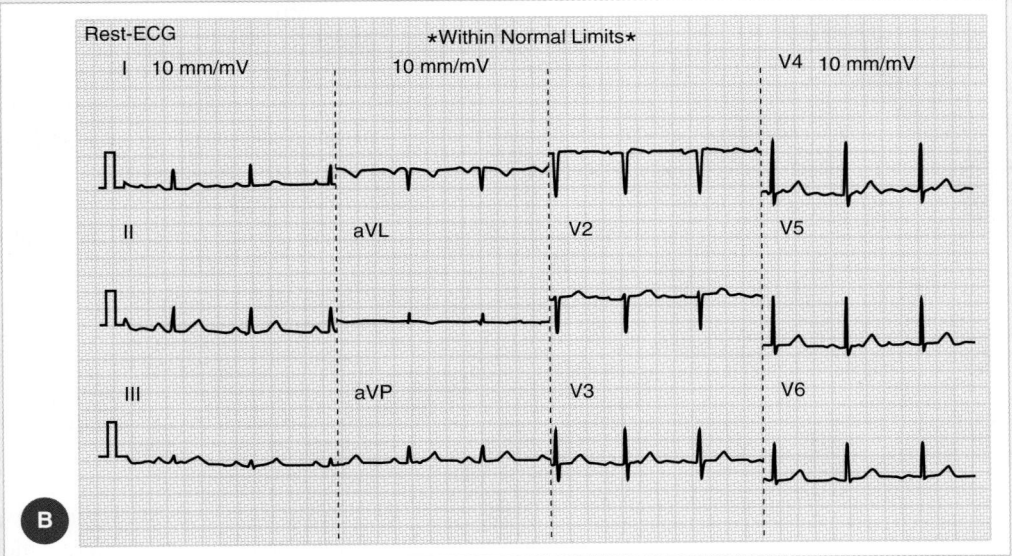

B

Figure 27-82 A. The areas on a 12-lead ECG correlate to different leads. **B.** A normal ECG with standard 12-lead format.

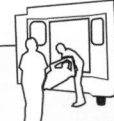

In the Field

When a doctor reads an ECG and sees pathologic Q waves, he or she will usually ask when the patient had his MI. These changes represent an evolved MI of unknown age.

erally indicates an infarction has happened at some time in the past Figure 27-84 ▶.

In 40% of patients who experience an inferior wall MI, a right ventricular MI will eventually develop as well. To verify this, an electrode can be placed in the fifth intercostal space at the midclavicular line on the right side of the chest (V₄R). Unsnap the original V₄ on the left side of the chest and snap it onto the new lead on the right side, leaving all the other electrodes in place. Now press "acquire" on the 12-lead ECG monitor. If you see ST-segment elevation of greater than 1 mm in the V₄R lead on this second ECG, there is a high likelihood that you have identified a right ventricular MI. Of course, the ECG monitor does not know that this V₄ is a right-sided one, so on printing this ECG tracing, you should add an "R" next to the "V₄," and circle the **V₄R** to make it stand out.

Patients who are experiencing an MI of the right ventricle may already be hypotensive or may become extremely hypotensive if nitroglycerin is given. For this reason, you are well advised to perform a V₄R (second ECG) every time you find a patient with an inferior wall MI. You may be ordered by the physician to give 1 to 2 L of saline IV before administering any nitroglycerin.

Figure 27-85 ▶ depicts an injury (ST-segment elevation) in the leads that look at the anterior wall of the heart, leads V₃ through V₅. Figure 27-86 ▶ shows the signs of ischemia (T-wave inversion) in the leads that look at the anterolateral wall of the heart, leads V₄ through V₆.

Sometimes, the ischemia or injury extends from one wall to the next. Such ischemia is evidenced by inverted (or flipped) T waves in leads V₃ through V₆.

Table 27-18 ▶ summarizes the leads corresponding to different locations of myocardial injury.

Table 27-17	Evolution of an AMI on the ECG	
Stage	**ECG Changes in Overlying Leads***	**Timing**
Ischemia	T-wave inversion	With the onset of ischemia
	ST-segment depression	
Injury	ST-segment elevation	Minutes to hours
Infarction	Q waves appear	Within several hours to several days

*Reciprocal changes will be seen in opposite leads.

Injury will cause ST-segment elevation; if left untreated, it will lead to infarction. Infarction (indicative of dead cardiac tissue) often results in the development of a pathologic Q wave. A Q wave that is wider than 0.04 s (one small box on the ECG strip) or deeper than one third of the height of the R wave that follows it and that is seen in two or more contiguous leads gen-

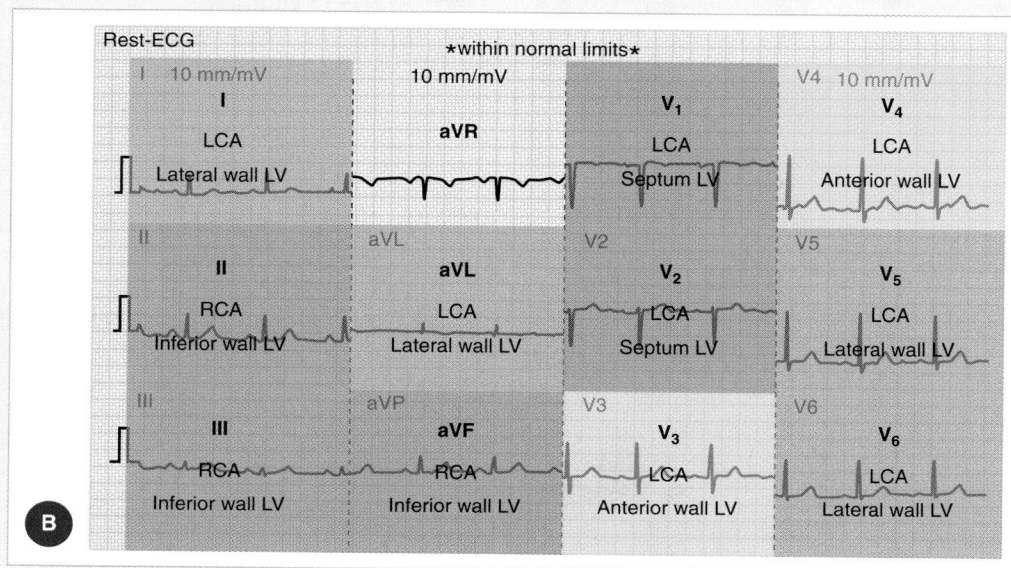

I	aVR	V₁	V₄
I LCA Lateral wall LV	**aVR**	**V₁** LCA Septum LV	**V₄** LCA Anterior wall LV
II RCA Inferior wall LV	**aVL** LCA Lateral wall LV	**V₂** LCA Septum LV	**V₅** LCA Lateral wall LV
III RCA Inferior wall LV	**aVF** RCA Inferior wall LV	**V₃** LCA Anterior wall LV	**V₆** LCA Lateral wall LV

A

B

Figure 27-83 A. A schematic representation of a 12-lead ECG. **B.** A normal ECG with standard 12-lead format.

Table 27-18 | Localization of AMI

Site of Infarction	Primary ECG Changes Seen in Leads
Inferior (diaphragmatic) wall	II, III, and aVF
Anteroseptal	V₁ to V₃
Anterolateral	V₄ to V₆
Extensive anterior wall	V₁ to V₆, I, and aVL
Posterior wall	V₁ to V₂ (tall R waves; reciprocal changes)

Benefits of Using 12-Lead ECGs

The most important 12-lead finding in the prehospital phase of care is simply the answer to the following question: Does this patient have ECG evidence of ischemia, injury, or infarction? This information will help the receiving hospital decide whether to mobilize its fibrinolytic therapy team. Meanwhile, the 12-lead ECG provides you with information that can help you choose the most appropriate emergency management in the field. For example, patients who have an inferior wall MI and possibly a right ventricular infarction will not respond well to nitroglycerin or morphine. If we know which leads to check for signs of injury to the inferior wall of the heart (and do a V₄R), we should be able to identify patients who might need a fluid bolus before nitroglycerin administration to prevent extreme hypotension.

Prehospital 12-lead ECGs and advanced notification to the receiving hospital can lead to faster diagnosis, decrease the time until fibrinolysis is administered, and, perhaps, decrease mortality rates. The time savings in door-to-perfusion therapy in most studies ranges from 10 to 60 minutes. Paramedics can efficiently acquire and transmit (or communicate their findings) diagnostic-quality ECGs to the ED with only a minimal increase (0.2 to 5.6 minutes) in their scene time. As we have learned, "Time is myocardium." The decision of where to transport patients with ACS should be based on current guidelines and recommendations from national groups such as the AHA and the American College of Cardiology. The 2005 AHA guidelines suggest that a checklist be used to assist in the triage of patients with ACS **Figure 27-87 ▸**.

The results of the 12-lead ECG should *not* be used to determine whether the patient should be treated in the field for AMI. That decision is made on clinical grounds alone! Remember—the absence of an MI on the ECG doesn't mean that the patient isn't having one. It may take hours for changes to appear in the ECG.

You should be equipped with portable ECG machines, monitors, and defibrillators that provide computerized ECG interpretation. Even if you're a whiz at reading 12-lead ECGs, computer ECG interpretations provide consistency and a high

Notes from Nancy

Every patient with a story of heavy, crushing, squeezing, or choking chest pain must be treated for AMI even if the ECG is perfectly normal.

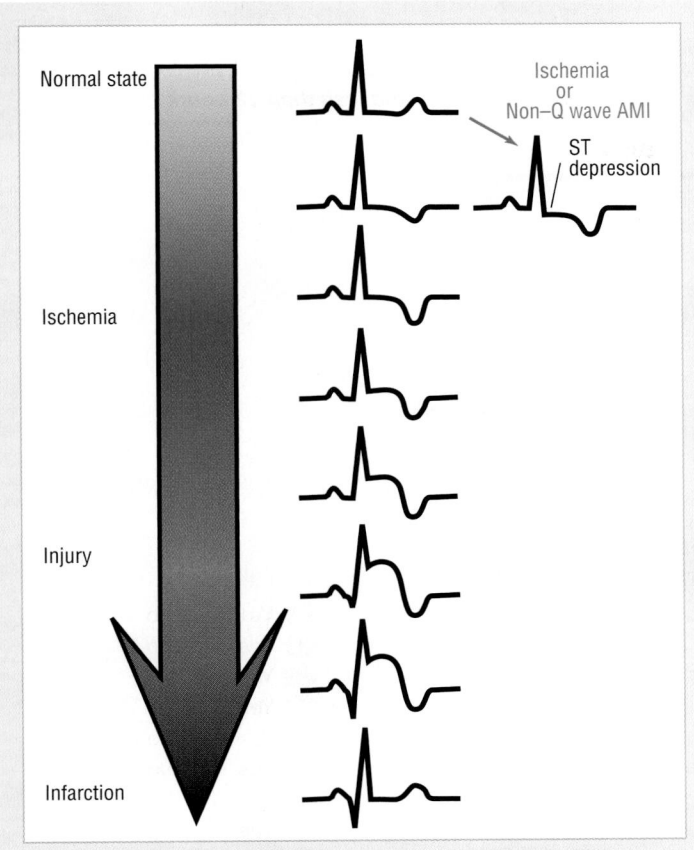

Figure 27-84 Evolutionary pattern or indicative changes of MI.

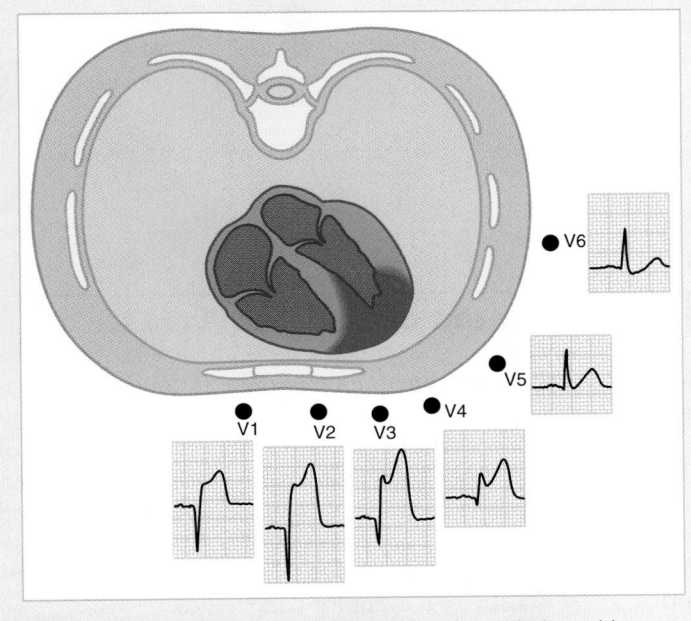

Figure 27-85 Anterior wall injury. (Question: What would *ischemia* in the anterior wall look like?)

degree of accuracy. (They also provide on-the-job refresher training in ECG interpretation!) As soon as you have the ECG printout, contact the receiving hospital and read the computer ECG interpretation to the emergency physician there. If you have something to add to what the computer says, by all means do so (briefly!). And, of course, provide details of the patient's history and the physical exam findings.

Guidelines for Taking a 12-Lead ECG

The only way to learn how to take a 12-lead ECG is to practice with the equipment itself. Here are some guidelines to help ensure that the ECGs you obtain are of the highest quality possible.

- The patient should be supine. If the patient feels short of breath in that position, you may elevate the back of the stretcher about 30°.
- Make sure the patient does not become chilled, because shivering will produce artifact in the ECG tracing. Note that 12-lead ECGs are more sensitive to artifact than 3-lead monitoring ECGs.
- Prepare the patient's skin as you would for placing monitoring electrodes.
- Connect the four limb electrodes. Double-check that the correct electrode is on each limb (the "LA" electrode on the left arm, the "RA" electrode on the right arm, and so on). Confirm that the limb electrodes are on the arms and legs and *not* on the trunk of the body, as sometimes is the case in a 3-lead ECG.
- Connect and apply the precordial leads as indicated in **Table 27-19** ▸.
- Record the ECG.

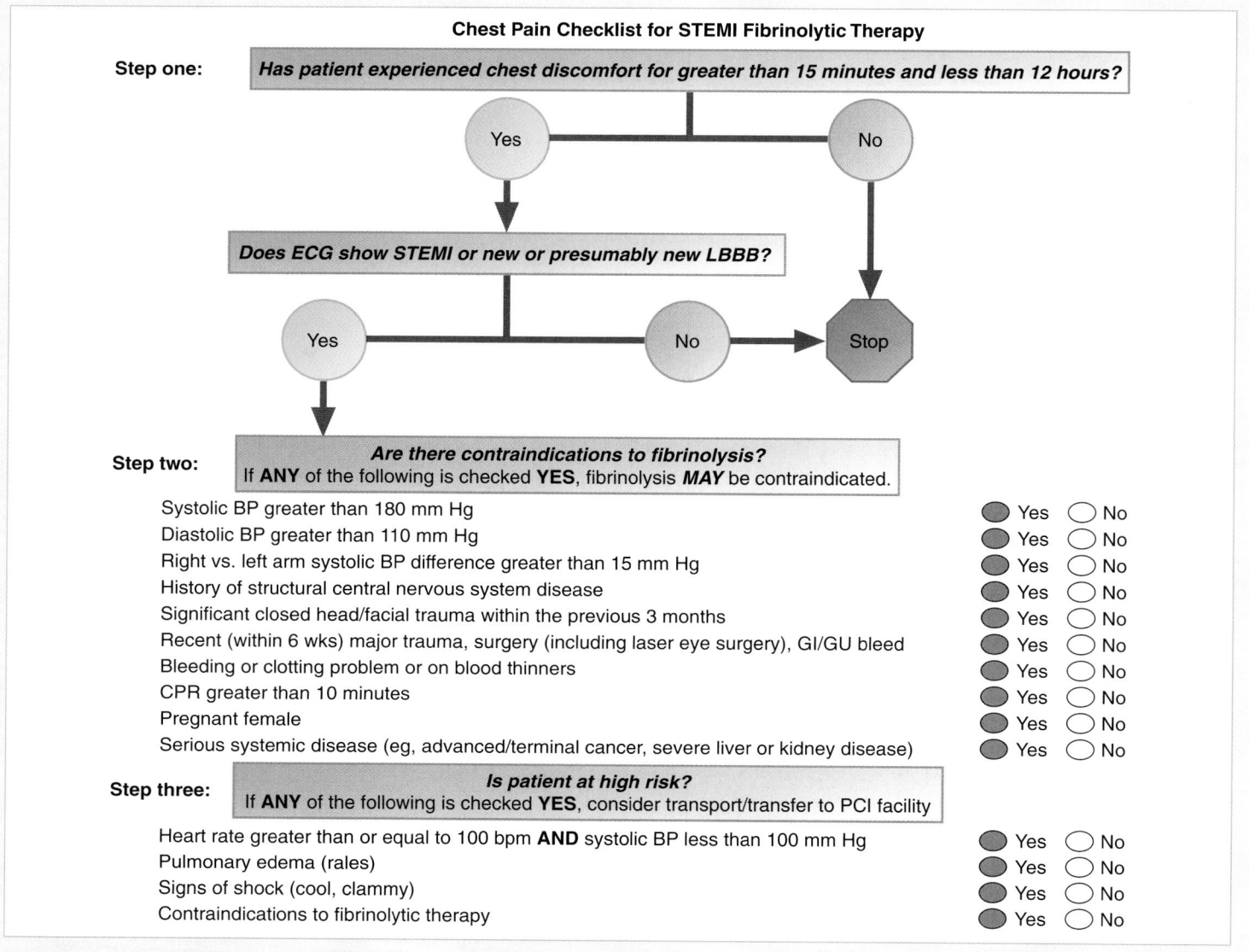

Chest Pain Checklist for STEMI Fibrinolytic Therapy

Step one: Has patient experienced chest discomfort for greater than 15 minutes and less than 12 hours?

Yes → Does ECG show STEMI or new or presumably new LBBB?

No → Stop

Does ECG show STEMI or new or presumably new LBBB?

Yes → Step two

No → Stop

Step two: Are there contraindications to fibrinolysis? If **ANY** of the following is checked **YES**, fibrinolysis **MAY** be contraindicated.

	Yes	No
Systolic BP greater than 180 mm Hg	● Yes	○ No
Diastolic BP greater than 110 mm Hg	● Yes	○ No
Right vs. left arm systolic BP difference greater than 15 mm Hg	● Yes	○ No
History of structural central nervous system disease	● Yes	○ No
Significant closed head/facial trauma within the previous 3 months	● Yes	○ No
Recent (within 6 wks) major trauma, surgery (including laser eye surgery), GI/GU bleed	● Yes	○ No
Bleeding or clotting problem or on blood thinners	● Yes	○ No
CPR greater than 10 minutes	● Yes	○ No
Pregnant female	● Yes	○ No
Serious systemic disease (eg, advanced/terminal cancer, severe liver or kidney disease)	● Yes	○ No

Step three: Is patient at high risk? If **ANY** of the following is checked **YES**, consider transport/transfer to PCI facility

	Yes	No
Heart rate greater than or equal to 100 bpm **AND** systolic BP less than 100 mm Hg	● Yes	○ No
Pulmonary edema (rales)	● Yes	○ No
Signs of shock (cool, clammy)	● Yes	○ No
Contraindications to fibrinolytic therapy	● Yes	○ No

Figure 27-87 Chest pain checklist.

Table 27-19	Applying the Precordial Leads
Lead	**Placement**
V_1	Fourth intercostal space at right sternal border
V_2	Fourth intercostal space at left sternal border
V_3	Equidistant between V_2 and V_4
V_4	Fifth intercostal space in left midclavicular line
V_5	Anterior axillary line (same horizontal plane as V_4)
V_6	Midaxillary line (same horizontal plane as V_4)

Management of Cardiac Arrest

Nothing gets the adrenaline pumping more furiously—in paramedics, even if not in the patient—than a "code," or cardiopulmonary arrest. Most cardiac arrest victims have evidence of atherosclerosis or other underlying cardiac disease. However, cardiac arrest can also occur after electrocution, drowning, and other types of trauma. Indeed, many cardiac arrest victims have no warning before the event occurs. No matter what the cause, cardiac arrest is a stressful event for paramedics.

Management of cardiac arrest requires you to deploy a great many of the advanced life support (ALS) skills that you have learned and to do so under very urgent circumstances in which minutes may mean the difference between life and death. It is very difficult to think clearly in such stressful circumstances, especially when there are likely to be other stressed and panicky people at the scene (the patient's family, for example). For these reasons, it is absolutely essential for you to follow an orderly, systematic approach to cardiac arrest emergencies. That approach needs to be rehearsed repeatedly, in a team setting, until it is nearly automatic, and must include the steps of BLS and ALS.

BLS: A Review

The techniques and sequences of BLS should be very familiar to all paramedic students. Here, we will simply review the guidelines for ensuring maximally effective (and minimally damaging) CPR to adults in cardiac arrest. For a complete review of this skill, see Appendix A.

- Concentrate on high-quality compressions (deep enough, fast enough, and with full chest recoil) with a minimum of interruptions.
- Avoid excessive inflation pressures in artificial ventilation. Inflate just enough to observe visible chest rise.
- Keep your compressions smooth, regular, and uninterrupted.
  1. Maintain each compression for at least half the compression-release cycle.
  2. Avoid bouncing or jerky compressions,
  3. Keep your shoulders directly over the patient's sternum, and keep your elbows straight.
  4. Maintain proper hand position: fingers off the chest, and hands coming up off the sternum slightly between compressions to allow for complete chest recoil.
- As a single rescuer for adults, give 30 compressions to two ventilations at a rate of 100 compressions per minute. Once an advanced airway is placed, compressions continue at a rate of 100/min uninterrupted with 8 to 10 ventilations given with 100% supplemental oxygen.
- Do not interrupt CPR compressions except for advanced airway placement, defibrillation, or moving the patient. In all cases, minimize the duration of the interruption to as close to 10 to 15 seconds as possible. Any stop in compressions also stops perfusion—and perfusion is what it is all about!

We shall now consider how to integrate these well-rehearsed steps of BLS into the sequences of ACLS.

Advanced Cardiac Life Support

We defined BLS as maintenance of the airway, breathing, and circulation—the ABCs—without adjunctive equipment. Basic life support is a holding action only and is unlikely to restore the heart to effective activity. You will be called on to deliver more definitive therapy as well, so the skills of ACLS must also become second nature, to be deployed swiftly and systematically in the event of cardiac arrest.

What Is ACLS?

The AHA has defined ACLS for a patient in cardiac arrest (or a patient at immediate risk of cardiac arrest) as consisting of the following elements:

- Effective and minimally interrupted chest compression (for cardiac arrest)
- Use of adjunctive equipment for ventilation and circulation
- Cardiac monitoring for arrhythmia recognition and control
- Establishment and maintenance of an IV infusion line
- Use of definitive therapy, including defibrillation and drug administration, to:
  1. Prevent cardiac arrest
  2. Aid in establishing an effective cardiac rhythm and circulation when cardiac arrest occurs
  3. Stabilize the patient's condition
- Transportation with continuous monitoring

We have already discussed the use of airway adjuncts and equipment for artificial ventilation. In this section, we focus on the sequence of actions in ACLS. The last section of the chapter will describe some of the specific techniques—such as defibrillation—for restoring an effective cardiac rhythm.

The Universal Algorithm

The approach to every patient in cardiac arrest will start with the same steps, which the AHA calls the *BLS Healthcare Provider Algorithm*. These basic steps are always deployed as soon as a person is found unresponsive and possibly in cardiac arrest. The BLS health care provider algorithm includes measures that bystanders should take before your arrival (such as "phone 9-1-1 or emergency number"), so we need to modify the universal algorithm a bit to make it applicable to emergency medical services personnel.

Whenever you are called for a case that might be a cardiac arrest (such as "man down," "unconscious woman," "choking," "stopped breathing"), carry the defibrillator with you on your first trip from the ambulance to the patient. You should also carry a portable oxygen cylinder and a "jump kit" that contains equipment for managing the airway. If you have enough help—for example, a three-person crew—by all means take the intubation kit, the IV equipment, and the drug box as well. But if you're shorthanded, don't spend the time carting every piece of equipment from the ambulance to the patient. You can send someone to the ambulance for other equipment later.

As soon as you reach the patient, one paramedic should ready the monitor-defibrillator while the other carries out the following steps:

1. **Assess responsiveness.** If the patient is *not* responsive:
   - *Open the airway and look, listen, and feel for breathing.* If the patient is *not* breathing:
   - *Give two slow breaths.* Use the bag-mask device or a barrier device.
2. **Assess the circulation.** *If there is no pulse, start CPR.* CPR should continue for 2 minutes or 5 cycles of 30 compressions and 2 ventilations. As CPR continues, the

second paramedic should attach the monitor-defibrillator. At the end of 2 minutes, pause CPR and:

3. **Check for a pulse, and check the rhythm on the monitor.**
   At this point, all you want to know is the answer to one question: Is V-fib or V-tach present?
   - *If V-fib or V-tach is present* on the monitor-defibrillator, follow the V-fib/V-tach arm of the algorithm.
   - *If V-fib or V-tach is not present* on the monitor-defibrillator, *resume CPR immediately.*

What you see on the monitor at this point will determine which side of the algorithm you will now follow. If the patient is still in cardiac arrest, he or she may be in any of the following situations:
- V-fib or pulseless V-tach
- PEA (that is, you can see an organized rhythm on the monitor, but there is no detectable pulse)
- Asystole

Each of these situations requires a different, specific approach (a different pathway down the pulseless arrest algorithm).

Treatment for V-fib or Pulseless V-tach

Managing V-fib or pulseless V-tach is probably the most important pathway down the algorithm for you to know because patients found in V-fib or V-tach are the most likely to be successfully resuscitated—*if* they receive timely and appropriate treatment. The steps in managing V-fib and pulseless V-tach are as follows:
- *Check the ABCs,* as described in the BLS algorithm (see Appendix A).
- *Perform CPR for 2 minutes while the defibrillator is being attached.*
- *Confirm V-fib or V-tach on the monitor-defibrillator.*
- *Confirm absence of a pulse* (in a maximum of 10 seconds). Other things besides V-fib and V-tach can make squiggly lines on a monitor, such as loose ECG leads or muscle tremor. Remember: Treat the patient, not the monitor.
- *Resume CPR while charging the defibrillator.*
- *Clear the patient and then defibrillate* the V-fib or V-tach:
  1. If using a biphasic defibrillator, set it to 120 to 200 joules (J). This energy level depends on the manufacturer's recommendation. If the recommendation is unknown and the defibrillator is biphasic, use 200 J as the default energy dose.
  2. If using a monophasic defibrillator, set it to 360 J.

As soon as the defibrillator discharges, resume CPR. It is important not to delay resuming CPR at this time to determine the rhythm. Continue CPR for 2 minutes or 5 cycles. Recent research indicates that even if an organized rhythm appears in the postresuscitation period, the presence of an immediate pulse is unlikely. It has also been shown that 2 minutes of postresuscitation CPR is unlikely to cause a return of V-fib. After 2 minutes or five cycles, stop CPR, and assess the patient's circulation and check the rhythm on the monitor.
- If a rhythm other than V-fib or V-tach appears on the monitor screen:
  1. *Identify the new rhythm.*
  2. If there is no pulse, move to the asystole-PEA pathway down the algorithm and resume CPR immediately.

3. If there is a pulse, move to the appropriate algorithm for the new rhythm.
- If the rhythm is persistent V-fib or V-tach, *resume CPR while charging the defibrillator.*
- *Clear the patient and then defibrillate* the V-fib or V-tach:
  1. Use the same energy setting as for the initial shock.
  2. *Resume CPR immediately,* and continue for 2 minutes after the shock. The CPR compressor and ventilator should change positions at the end of each 2-minute session of CPR (while the rhythm and pulse are being checked) to avoid fatigue, which can reduce the effectiveness of chest compressions.
  3. During this 2 minutes of CPR, you should *insert an advanced airway if the BLS airway is not adequate.* Advanced airways include the endotracheal tube, laryngeal mask airway, and Combitube. After intubation, verify placement using multiple methods and secure the tube. Once the patient has been intubated, it is no longer necessary to pause CPR compressions for ventilation to be administered. Ventilations should be administered at a rate of 8 to 10 breaths per minute (one breath every 6 to 8 seconds or one breath after each 10 to 12 compressions). The rate of compressions is 100/min.
  4. *Start an IV* with normal saline.
  5. *If unable to establish IV access, consider establishment of intraosseous (IO) access* via an adult IO access system. If IV access is not obtained but IO access is, all drugs and fluids that would normally be administered via IV should be administered via IO until IV assess is established.
  6. As soon as IV or IO has been established, *administer a vasopressor drug.* The two recommended vasopressor drugs are epinephrine and vasopressin. *Epinephrine (1:10,000) is given as 1 mg IV push;* this dose should be repeated every 3 to 5 minutes as long as a pulse is absent. *Vasopressin is given as 40 units IV push, one time only.* Vasopressin can be given in place of the first or second dose of epinephrine (but not both). Whenever you give a medication through a peripheral IV line during CPR, follow it immediately with a 20- to 30-mL bolus of IV fluid and then elevate the extremity to facilitate delivery of the medication to the central circulation (which may take 1 to 2 minutes).
- *At the end of 2 minutes of CPR, pause compressions to check for circulation and check the rhythm on the monitor.*
- If V-fib or V-tach is still present, *resume CPR while charging the defibrillator.*
- *Clear the patient and then defibrillate* the V-fib or V-tach:
  1. Use the same energy setting as before.
  2. Resume CPR immediately, and continue for 2 minutes after the shock. Remember to change CPR compressors after each rhythm check.
  3. During this 2 minutes of CPR, you should *consider the administration of an antiarrhythmic medication.* The preferred antiarrhythmic medication is *amiodarone,* which is given as a 300-mg bolus during CPR. Amiodarone may be repeated once at 150 mg in 3 to

Assessment in Action

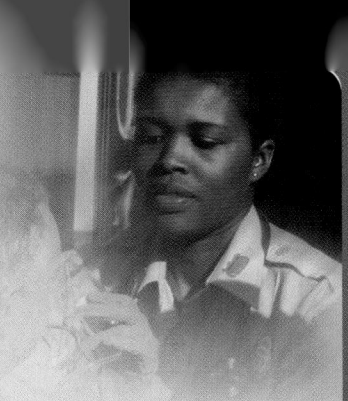

You are dispatched to the private residence of an 88-year-old man who is complaining of shortness of breath. When you arrive on scene, you find the patient in severe respiratory distress, speaking in two- to three-word sentences. He is grossly diaphoretic and complains of chest tightness. The patient tells you that he has no medical problems and does not take any medications. His vital signs are as follows: respiratory rate, 42 breaths/min with a room air pulse oximetry of 88%; blood pressure, 220/110 mm Hg; heart rate, 130 beats/min. The ECG monitor shows rapid atrial fibrillation.

1. **What differential diagnosis can you make?**
   A. Angina
   B. Angina pectoris
   C. Congestive heart failure
   D. Acute myocardial infarction

2. **Cardiac output is:**
   A. the amount of blood that is pumped out by either ventricle, measured in liters per minute.
   B. the pressure exerted by the blood against the arterial walls.
   C. the contribution to ventricular filling made by contraction of the atrium.
   D. one complete phase of atrial and ventricular relaxation.

3. **What is the most common form of heart disease and is the number one killer of men and women?**
   A. Angina
   B. Pulmonary edema
   C. Myocardial infarction
   D. Coronary artery disease

4. **What is the principal symptom of CAD?**
   A. Pulmonary edema
   B. Myocardial infarction
   C. Angina pectoris
   D. Unstable myocardium

5. **The term that describes when a portion of the cardiac muscle is deprived of coronary blood flow long enough that the muscle dies is:**
   A. unstable angina.
   B. stable angina.
   C. CAD.
   D. acute myocardial infarction.

6. **The mnemonic _____ is used to help remember the supportive treatments of a patient with acute coronary syndrome.**
   A. MONA
   B. MEMA
   C. NOMO
   D. OANE

7. **The most immediate methods of reperfusion for an AMI are:**
   A. nitroglycerin and oxygen.
   B. fibrinolytic therapy and percutaneous intervention.
   C. fibrinolytic therapy and intravenous therapy.
   D. percutaneous intervention alone.

8. **What term describes the situation when the heart is so severely damaged that it can no longer pump a volume of blood sufficient to maintain tissue perfusion?**
   A. Acute myocardial infarction
   B. Cardiogenic shock
   C. Unstable angina
   D. Pulmonary edema or congestive heart failure

Challenging Question

9. **Given the patient's age, are there any special considerations that you should keep in mind?**

Points to Ponder

You are dispatched to an assisted-living facility for a 78-year-old woman who is feeling weak, dizzy, and nauseous. When you arrive, you find the patient resting comfortably. She tells you that while she was trying to have a bowel movement, she suddenly became very dizzy. There was no diaphoresis or shortness of breath. Her vital signs are as follows: respiratory rate, 18 breaths/min with a room air pulse oximetry reading of 97%; blood pressure, 90/58 mm Hg; pulse rate, 40 beats/min. When you apply the ECG to monitor her pulse rate, you notice a third-degree block. The patient's medical history includes hypertension, congestive heart failure, and renal failure secondary to type 1 diabetes. Her medications consist of metoprolol, furosemide, potassium, digoxin, and insulin. She tells you that she has taken all of her medicines this morning as prescribed.

What steps should you take to manage this patient's condition?

Issues: Understanding the Importance of a Complete Physical Exam, Understanding the Importance of ECG Rhythm Analysis, Understanding When to Apply the Transcutaneous Pacer.

28 Neurologic Emergencies

Objectives

Cognitive

5-3.1 Describe the incidence, morbidity and mortality of neurological emergencies. (p 28.4)

5-3.2 Identify the risk factors most predisposing to the nervous system. (p 28.9)

5-3.3 Discuss the anatomy and physiology of the organs and structures related to the nervous system. (p 28.4)

5-3.4 Discuss the pathophysiology of non-traumatic neurologic emergencies. (p 28.9)

5-3.5 Discuss the assessment findings associated with non-traumatic neurologic emergencies. (p 28.14)

5-3.6 Identify the need for rapid intervention and the transport of the patient with non-traumatic emergencies. (p 28.15)

5-3.7 Discuss the management of non-traumatic neurological emergencies. (p 28.21)

5-3.8 Discuss the pathophysiology of coma and altered mental status. (p 28.29)

5-3.9 Discuss the assessment findings associated with coma and altered mental status. (p 28.29)

5-3.10 Discuss the management/treatment plan of coma and altered mental status. (p 28.29)

5-3.11 Describe the epidemiology, including the morbidity/mortality and prevention strategies, for seizures. (p 28.29)

5-3.12 Discuss the pathophysiology of seizures. (p 28.29)

5-3.13 Discuss the assessment findings associated with seizures. (p 28.29)

5-3.14 Define seizure. (p 28.29)

5-3.15 Describe and differentiate the major types of seizures. (p 28.29)

5-3.16 List the most common causes of seizures. (p 28.29)

5-3.17 Describe the phases of a generalized seizure. (p 28.29)

5-3.18 Discuss the pathophysiology of syncope. (p 28.31)

5-3.19 Discuss the assessment findings associated with syncope. (p 28.32)

5-3.20 Discuss the management/treatment plan of syncope. (p 28.32)

5-3.21 Discuss the pathophysiology of headache. (p 28.32)

5-3.22 Discuss the assessment findings associated with headache. (p 28.32)

5-3.23 Discuss the management/treatment plan of headache. (p 28.33)

5-3.24 Describe the epidemiology, including the morbidity/mortality and prevention strategies, for neoplasms. (p 28.33)

5-3.25 Discuss the pathophysiology of neoplasms. (p 28.33)

5-3.26 Describe the types of neoplasms. (p 28.33)

5-3.27 Discuss the assessment findings associated with neoplasms. (p 28.34)

5-3.28 Discuss the management/treatment plan of neoplasms. (p 28.34)

5-3.29 Define neoplasms. (p 28.33)

5-3.30 Recognize the signs and symptoms related to neoplasms. (p 28.34)

5-3.31 Correlate abnormal assessment findings with clinical significance in the patient with neoplasms. (p 28.34)

5-3.32 Differentiate among the various treatment and pharmacological interventions used in the management of neoplasms. (p 28.34)

5-3.33 Integrate the pathophysiological principles and the assessment findings to formulate a field impression and implement a treatment plan for the patient with neoplasms. (p 28.34)

5-3.34 Describe the epidemiology, including the morbidity/mortality and prevention strategies, for abscess. (p 28.33)

5-3.35 Discuss the pathophysiology of abscess. (p 28.33)

5-3.36 Discuss the assessment findings associated with abscess. (p 28.33)

5-3.37 Discuss the management/treatment plan of abscess. (p 28.33)

5-3.38 Define abscess. (p 28.33)

5-3.39 Recognize the signs and symptoms related to abscess. (p 28.33)

5-3.40 Correlate abnormal assessment findings with clinical significance in the patient with abscess. (p 28.33)

5-3.41 Differentiate among the various treatment and pharmacological interventions used in the management of abscess. (p 28.33)

5-3.42 Integrate the pathophysiological principles and the assessment findings to formulate a field impression and implement a treatment plan for the patient with abscess. (p 28.33)

5-3.43 Describe the epidemiology, including the morbidity/mortality and prevention strategies, for stroke and intracranial hemorrhage. (p 28.12)

5-3.44 Discuss the pathophysiology of stroke and intracranial hemorrhage. (p 28.12)

5-3.45 Describe the types of stroke and intracranial hemorrhage. (p 28.24)

5-3.46 Discuss the assessment findings associated with stroke and intracranial hemorrhage. (p 28.24)

5-3.47 Discuss the management/treatment plan of stroke and intracranial hemorrhage. (p 28.25)

5-3.48 Define stroke and intracranial hemorrhage. (p 28.24)

5-3.49 Recognize the signs and symptoms related to stroke and intracranial hemorrhage. (p 28.25)

5-3.50 Correlate abnormal assessment findings with clinical significance in the patient with stroke and intracranial hemorrhage. (p 28.24)

5-3.51 Differentiate among the various treatment and pharmacological interventions used in the management of stroke and intracranial hemorrhage. (p 28.25)

5-3.52 Integrate the pathophysiological principles and the assessment findings to formulate a field impression and implement a treatment plan for the patient with stroke and intracranial hemorrhage. (p 28.25)

5-3.53 Describe the epidemiology, including the morbidity/mortality and prevention strategies, for transient ischemic attack. (p 28.28)

5-3.54 Discuss the pathophysiology of transient ischemic attack. (p 28.28)

5-3.55 Discuss the assessment findings associated with transient ischemic attack. (p 28.28)

5-3.56 Discuss the management/treatment plan of transient ischemic attack. (p 28.28)

5-3.57 Define transient ischemic attack. (p 28.28)

5-3.58 Recognize the signs and symptoms related to transient ischemic attack. (p 28.28)

5-3.59 Correlate abnormal assessment findings with clinical significance in the patient with transient ischemic attack. (p 28.28)

5-3.60 Differentiate among the various treatment and pharmacological interventions used in the management of transient ischemic attack. (p 28.28)

5-3.61 Integrate the pathophysiological principles and the assessment findings to formulate a field impression and implement a treatment plan for the patient with transient ischemic attack. (p 28.28)

5-3.62 Describe the epidemiology, including the morbidity/mortality and prevention strategies, for degenerative neurological diseases. (p 28.10)

5-3.63 Discuss the pathophysiology of degenerative neurological diseases. (p 28.10)

5-3.64 Discuss the assessment findings associated with degenerative neurological diseases. (p 28.13)

5-3.65 Discuss the management/ treatment plan of degenerative neurological diseases. (p 28.21)

5-3.66 Define the following:
a. Muscular dystrophy
b. Multiple sclerosis
c. Dystonia
d. Parkinson's disease
e. Trigeminal neuralgia
f. Bell's palsy
g. Amyotrophic lateral sclerosis
h. Peripheral neuropathy
i. Myoclonus
j. Spina bifida
k. Poliomyelitis (p 28.19, 28.33–28.37)

5-3.67 Recognize the signs and symptoms related to degenerative neurological diseases. (p 28.16)

5-3.68 Correlate abnormal assessment findings with clinical significance in the patient with degenerative neurological diseases. (p 28.16)

5-3.69 Differentiate among the various treatment and pharmacological interventions used in the management of degenerative neurological diseases. (p 28.21)

5-3.70 Integrate the pathophysiological principles and the assessment findings to formulate a field impression and implement a treatment plan for the patient with degenerative neurological diseases. (p 28.21)

5-3.71 Integrate the pathophysiological principles of the patient with a neurological emergency. (p 28.9)

5-3.72 Differentiate between neurological emergencies based on assessment findings. (p 28.13)

5-3.73 Correlate abnormal assessment findings with the clinical significance in the patient with neurological complaints. (p 28.16)

5-3.74 Develop a patient management plan based on field impression in the patient with neurological emergencies. (p 28.21)

Affective

5-3.75 Characterize the feelings of a patient who regains consciousness among strangers. (p 28.22, 28.31)

5-3.76 Formulate means of conveying empathy to patients whose ability to communicate is limited by their condition. (p 28.18)

Psychomotor

5-3.77 Perform an appropriate assessment of a patient with coma or altered mental status. (p 28.14)

5-3.78 Perform a complete neurological examination as part of the comprehensive physical examination of a patient with coma or altered mental status. (p 28.15)

5-3.79 Appropriately manage a patient with coma or altered mental status, including the administration of oxygen, oral glucose, 50% dextrose and narcotic reversal agents. (p 28.21, 28.29)

5-3.80 Perform an appropriate assessment of a patient with syncope. (p 28.32)

5-3.81 Appropriately manage a patient with syncope. (p 28.32)

5-3.82 Perform an appropriate assessment of a patient with seizures. (p 28.29)

5-3.83 Appropriately manage a patient with seizures, including the administration of diazepam or lorazepam. (p 28.31)

5-3.84 Perform an appropriate assessment of a patient with stroke and intracranial hemorrhage or TIA. (p 28.25–28.29)

5-3.85 Appropriately manage a patient with stroke and intracranial hemorrhage or TIA. (p 28.25–28.29)

5-3.86 Demonstrate an appropriate assessment of a patient with a chief complaint of weakness. (p 28.16)

Introduction

Many paramedics love the challenge of trauma and the excitement of dealing with its sudden nature. Trauma injuries can be graphic and attract your attention easily. By contrast, the medical patient is an entirely different animal. These patients require a keen eye, sharp assessment skills, and—above all—critical thinking to determine the nature of the problem. Medical patients can be very challenging as they often have complaints that are not apparent.

According to the National Center for Health Statistics, 3 of the top 15 causes of death in the United States in 2003 were neurologic in nature. In this country, someone suffers a stroke every 45 seconds. **Table 28-1 ▸** shows the incidence of neurologic diseases throughout the United States. Clearly, the EMS provider will encounter many neurologic emergencies.

Neurologic patients can be extremely vulnerable or even helpless. Many of the reflexes that protect an awake person may not function when the nervous system is depressed. The eyelids don't blink away dust and irritants. The larynx doesn't gag and cough in reaction to secretions oozing down the airway. The body doesn't seek a more comfortable position in response to compression of a limb in an awkward position. The tongue goes slack. The airway is at risk.

In this chapter, the anatomy and physiology of the nervous system are reviewed first. Then the general pathology of neurologic conditions is explored, laying the proper foundation for discussion of their assessment and treatment.

Anatomy and Physiology

The nervous system is the most complex organ system within the human body. It consists of two major structures, the brain

Table 28-1	Approximated Occurrences of Neurologic Disorders in the United States*
Condition	**Estimated Incidence**
Abscess	1,500 cases
Acute polio	No new wild poliovirus cases since 1979
Alzheimer's disease	**4,500,000 cases**
Amyotrophic lateral sclerosis	20,000 cases
Bell's palsy	40,000 cases
Cerebral palsy	500,000 cases
Dystonia	300,000 cases
Guillain-Barré syndrome	2,700 cases
Headache	45,000,000 cases with chronic headaches
Multiple sclerosis	300,000 cases
Muscular dystrophy	40,000 cases combining all types
Myasthenia gravis	50,000 cases
Neoplasms	**40,000 cases**
Parkinson's disease	500,000 cases
Peripheral neuropathy	9,000,000 diabetics with neuropathy
Postpolio syndrome	100,000 cases
Seizures	2,500,000 cases
Spina bifida	1,500 new births per year
Stroke	**700,000 cases**
Syncope	3% of emergency department visits nationwide
Trigeminal neuralgia	11,000 cases

*Items in bold type fall into the top 10 causes of death according to the National Center for Health Statistics/National Vital Statistics System.
(Data from 2000–2003)

You are the Provider Part 1

You are dispatched to 16600 Courage Court for an older man who has fallen. You arrive to find Mr. Hishari, an 81-year-old man, lying on the floor. His two sons explain that they visited their father last night and left around 7:00 PM. When they returned this morning, they found the patient lying on the floor next to the chair in which he was sitting when they last saw him. He has been unable to explain what happened and, because he lives alone, no one is sure how long he's been on the floor.

The patient is awake and responding to his sons, but they say he is "not acting right." They describe him as "very sharp," but today he keeps getting their names confused. They say this only happens when his blood glucose level is low. The patient has type 2 diabetes.

Initial Assessment	Recording Time: 0 Minutes
Appearance	Lying on the floor, appears clean
Level of consciousness	V (Responsive to verbal stimuli), oriented to person and place, but not day
Airway	Patent
Breathing	Nonlabored
Circulation	Strong radial pulse

1. What do you suspect as the reason(s) why Mr. Hishari is on the floor?
2. How would you prioritize those reasons?

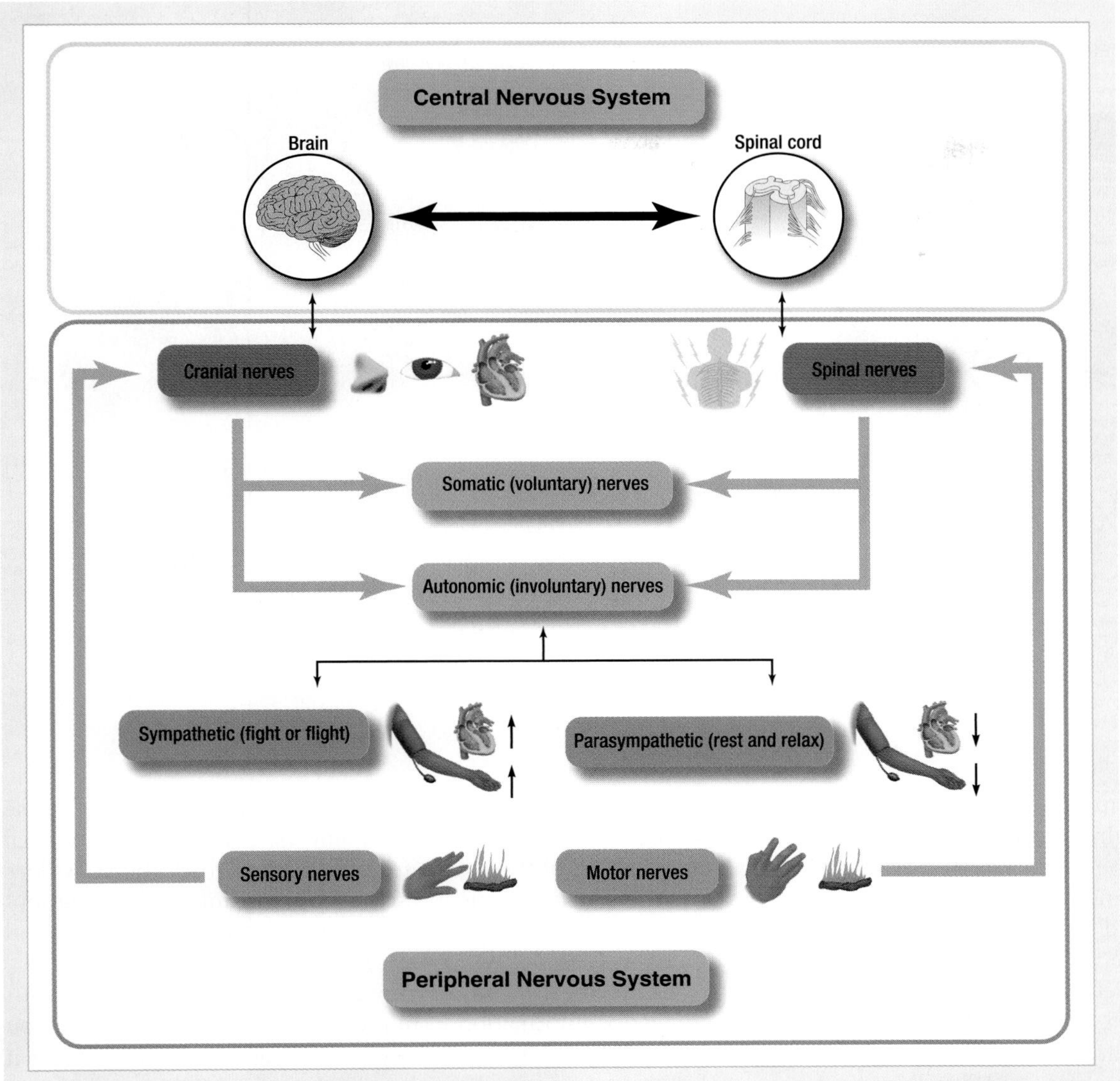

Central Nervous System

Brain ↔ Spinal cord

Cranial nerves

Spinal nerves

Somatic (voluntary) nerves

Autonomic (involuntary) nerves

Sympathetic (fight or flight)

Parasympathetic (rest and relax)

Sensory nerves

Motor nerves

Peripheral Nervous System

Figure 28-1 Organization of the nervous system.

Consider the case of Justin—a child riding a bicycle. This common and seemingly simple activity is rich with both conscious and unconscious functions. It's a beautiful summer morning, so Justin goes to the garage to get his bike. Already the brain is hard at work. As Justin enters the garage, the brain must determine which object is a bike. Justin scans the garage. The images produced by his eyes are transmitted via the optic nerve to the occipital lobe of the brain Figure 28-2 . There the image, which is transmitted upside down, is reoriented. The occipital lobe then pores through tens of thousands of stored images. Has this image been seen before?

Once the image is recognized, an existing pathway is accessed to the temporal lobe, where language and speech are stored. Now, as Justin walks through the garage, he is able to put names to what he sees—a car, a workbench, a bike. When Justin was learning to speak, he often became confused about the names of objects.

and spinal cord, plus thousands of nerves allowing every part of the body to communicate. This system is responsible for fundamental functions such as controlling breathing, heart rate, and blood pressure. But the real beauty of the nervous system is found in its higher level activity. Reading a good book (like this one), enjoying music, having a discussion with a friend, and even watching television require the brain to engage memory, understanding, and thought. Here is where the true complexity of this system can be seen.

Figure 28-1 ▲ shows the basic structure of the nervous system. The major structures are divided into two main categories: the central nervous system (CNS), which is responsible for thought, perception, feeling, and autonomic body functions; and the peripheral nervous system (PNS), which transmits commands from the brain to the body and receives feedback from the body.

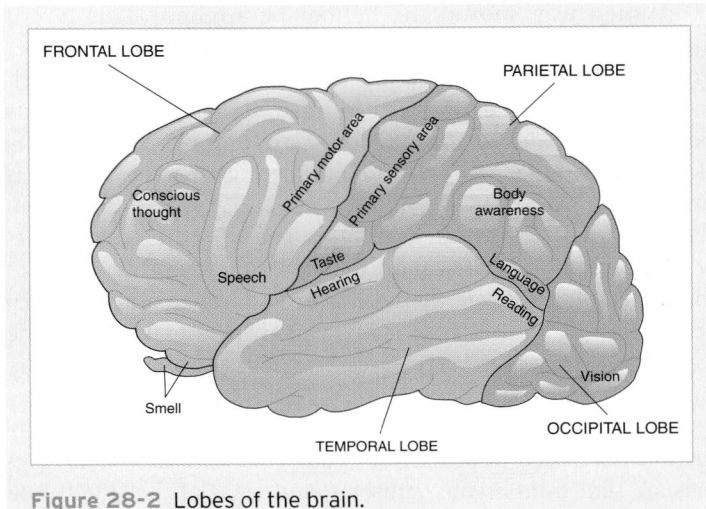

Figure 28-2 Lobes of the brain.

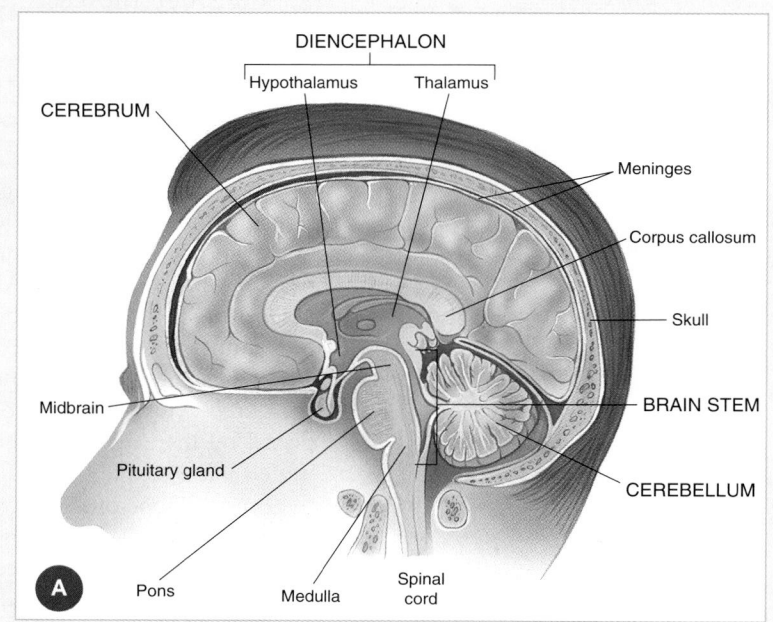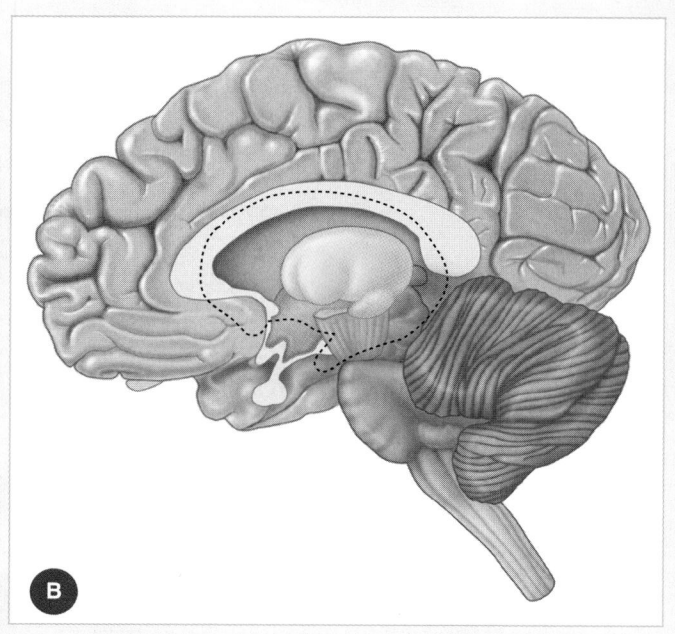

Figure 28-3 **A.** Areas of the brain, including the brain stem. **B.** The diencephalon.

As he practiced, he received reinforcement for the correct names and redirection for the incorrect names. In his brain, more pathways were established between the image of an object with two wheels, a seat, and pedals, which was stored in the occipital lobe, and the word for that object (bike), which was stored in the temporal lobe.

As Justin retrieves his helmet, the frontal lobe of his brain springs into action. The frontal lobe, which controls voluntary motion, sends signals out of the CNS along efferent nerves to the arms, shoulders, chest, and hands to perform the task of picking up the helmet. The efferent nerves leave the brain through the PNS and convey commands to other parts of the body.

Which way should the helmet be applied? This motor memory is stored in the frontal lobe; the brain stores memories in the areas that are initially stimulated. As he places the helmet on his head, Justin needs to make fine adjustments to its position. His brain is receiving impulses from nerves within the skull and muscles of his head, indicating that the helmet is uncomfortable. Justin senses pressure and possibly pain from the improperly positioned helmet. The afferent nerves (that send information to the brain) transmit signals of discomfort to the parietal lobe, where the body's sense of touch and pain perception are found. Signals sent from the parietal lobe to the frontal lobe make the body adjust the helmet until the pressure signals have stopped.

As you have been reading this tale, huge amounts of information have been pouring from your PNS into your CNS. Signals are sent from organs, muscles, and areas of the skin to the spinal cord until they reach the lower portions of the CNS. The

position of your legs, the distribution of your body weight, the sensation of the pages in your fingers, the state of your renal arteries—all of these data are being sent to the CNS. How does the brain manage this massive amount of information without confusion and misdirection? By using the diencephalon and brain stem **Figure 28-3 ▲**.

One major role of the diencephalon is to filter out unneeded information from the cerebral cortex. Imagine if you had to "think" about shifting your weight on a chair when it became uncomfortable. The signals of pressure or pain being sent via the peripheral nerves initially stop in the diencephalon. The body's administrative assistant then decides whether the big boss (the cerebral cortex) needs to be bothered with this information. In the case of an uncomfortable bottom, the diencephalon simply sends commands so that you move slightly. Unless you were concentrating on how you were sitting, you would never even know that you moved.

How did Justin know it was time to get up this morning? His internal alarm clock went off, of course. The midbrain (part of the brain stem) is responsible for regulating the level of consciousness (LOC). You often get tired at the same time each day due to the functions of the reticular activating system (RAS). Justin is wide awake and thinking clearly thanks to his RAS.

How are blood pressure, heart rate, respiratory rate, and breathing pattern controlled? Again, the brain stem is responsible. The pons **Figure 28-4 ▶**, which is located just inferior to the midbrain, regulates your respiratory pace and the depth at which you breathe. The medulla oblongata controls the blood pressure and heart rate. Of course, these functions need to occur constantly, but Justin couldn't ride his bike if he

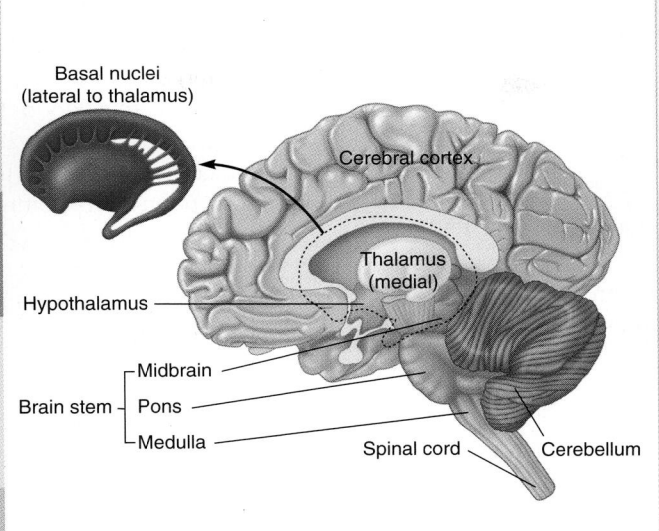

Cerebral cortex
- Receives sensory information from skin, muscles, glands, and organs
- Sends messages to move skeletal muscles
- Integrates incoming and outgoing nerve impulses
- Performs associative activities such as thinking, learning, and remembering

Basal nuclei
- Plays a role in the coordination of slow, sustained movements
- Suppresses useless patterns of movement

Thalamus
- Relays most sensory information from the spinal cord and certain parts of the brain to the cerebral cortex
- Interprets certain sensory messages such as those of pain, temperature, and pressure

Hypothalamus
- Controls various homeostatic functions such as body temperature, respiration, and heartbeat
- Directs hormone secretions of the pituitary

Cerebellum
- Coordinates subconscious movements of skeletal muscles
- Contributes to muscle tone, posture, balance, and equilibrium

Brain stem
- Origin of many cranial nerves
- Reflex center for movements of eyeballs, head, and trunk
- Regulates heartbeat and breathing
- Plays a role in consciousness
- Transmits impulses between brain and spinal cord

Basal nuclei (lateral to thalamus)
Cerebral cortex
Thalamus (medial)
Hypothalamus
Midbrain
Brain stem — Pons
Medulla
Spinal cord
Cerebellum

Figure 28-4 The pons.

(located in the posterior, inferior area of the skull) manages complex motor activity. When Justin first learned to ride a bike, he had to think about what to do, where to shift his weight, and how to hold his upper body. Eventually, the frontal lobe of the brain got tired of sending the same commands again and again, so this task was transferred to the cerebellum. This lobe keeps track of Justin's body position at all times and helps to manage activities such as walking, swimming, and riding a bike.

All of this wonderfully complex activity is made possible by the synapses. Nerve cells don't actually come in direct contact with one another. Instead, a slight gap separates the cells, which allows for a far greater level of fine control. The synapse, which is present wherever a nerve cell terminates, "connects" to the next cell via chemicals called neurotransmitters. A host of neurotransmitters are present in the brain and throughout the body. Dopamine, acetylcholine, epinephrine, and serotonin

needed to spend time and energy consciously controlling his pulse. The brain stem frees the cerebral cortex up to engage in higher level activities.

Justin now mounts his bike and begins to ride. The smile on his face reveals that he is having fun. Emotions come from two main areas within the brain: the limbic system Figure 28-5 ▶, where rage and anger are generated; and the hypothalamus (a part of the diencephalon), where pleasure, thirst, and hunger are found. All emotions are then mediated by the prefrontal cortex so people can choose how they are going to act in relation to how they feel.

Justin begins to pick up speed. As he approaches a corner, he must turn or risk crashing into a tree. The excitement increases his heart rate and blood pressure. The hypothalamus communicates to the pituitary gland, a member of the endocrine system. The pituitary gland, in turn, sends chemical commands to the adrenal glands to release epinephrine and norepinephrine. The release of these chemicals by the sympathetic nervous system gives Justin the increased strength and cardiovascular reserves that he needs to handle the bike in a tight turn. Just as quickly as these chemicals act, they are shut off to prevent the body from depleting its reserves. Too much epinephrine and norepinephrine can also be damaging over the long term.

Justin shifts his weight and makes the turn successfully, due in large part to his cerebellum. This lobe of the brain

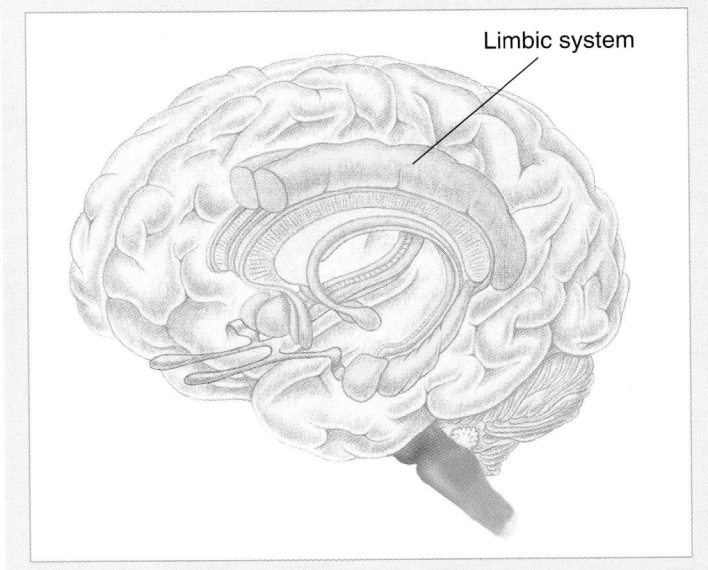

Limbic system

Figure 28-5 The limbic system is the seat of emotions, instincts, and other functions.

are all examples of neurotransmitters. These chemicals take the electrically conducted signal from one nerve cell (a neuron) and relay it to the next cell. Nerve cells respond to these signals in an "all or nothing" fashion: They either fire or they don't. A neuron can't fire weakly.

How do the neurotransmitters achieve a greater degree of control than that permitted by simply wiring the cells together? The answer lies in the connections made as the signal travels from the cell to the synapse (Figure 28-6 ▾).

1. The first neuron fires and sends a signal along its axon to the axon terminal.

2. The impulse reaches the axon terminal, where neurotransmitters are released and trickle across the synapse.

3. Dendrites detect these chemicals and are triggered to send the signal to the cell's nucleus, which then transmits it down that axon, and so on.

4. Dendrites release neurotransmitter deactivators so that one impulse from cell 1 generates one response from cell 2.

The complexity in the system derives from how the cells are connected. In Figure 28-6, each cell is connected in a straight-line fashion. Although this is a reliable method of getting a signal from point A to point B, gaining more control requires more complexity. In (Figure 28-7 ▾), three cells are brought together to connect with the same cell. Cell 4 will not respond unless it receives simultaneous stimulation from cells 1, 2, and 3. The same concept can be extended to the situation in which one cell sends signals to many different cells. In Figure 28-7, for example, cell 4 stimulates cells 5 and 6. As a consequence of this joint action, Justin is able to see his bike, recognize the object, know its name, instantly know how to use it, know how to make the muscles of his mouth say the word "bike," and appreciate how it will feel to ride the bike.

Neurons may or may not have myelin around their axons. Myelin is a type of "insulation" that allows the cell to consistently send its signal

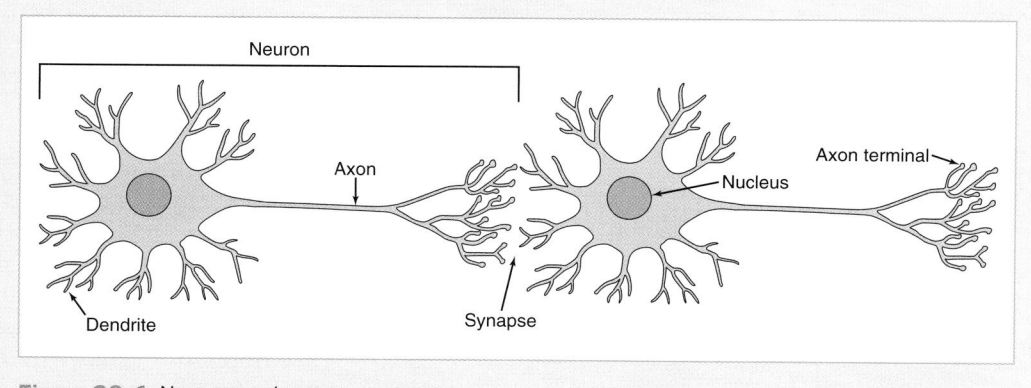

Figure 28-6 Neuron and synapse.

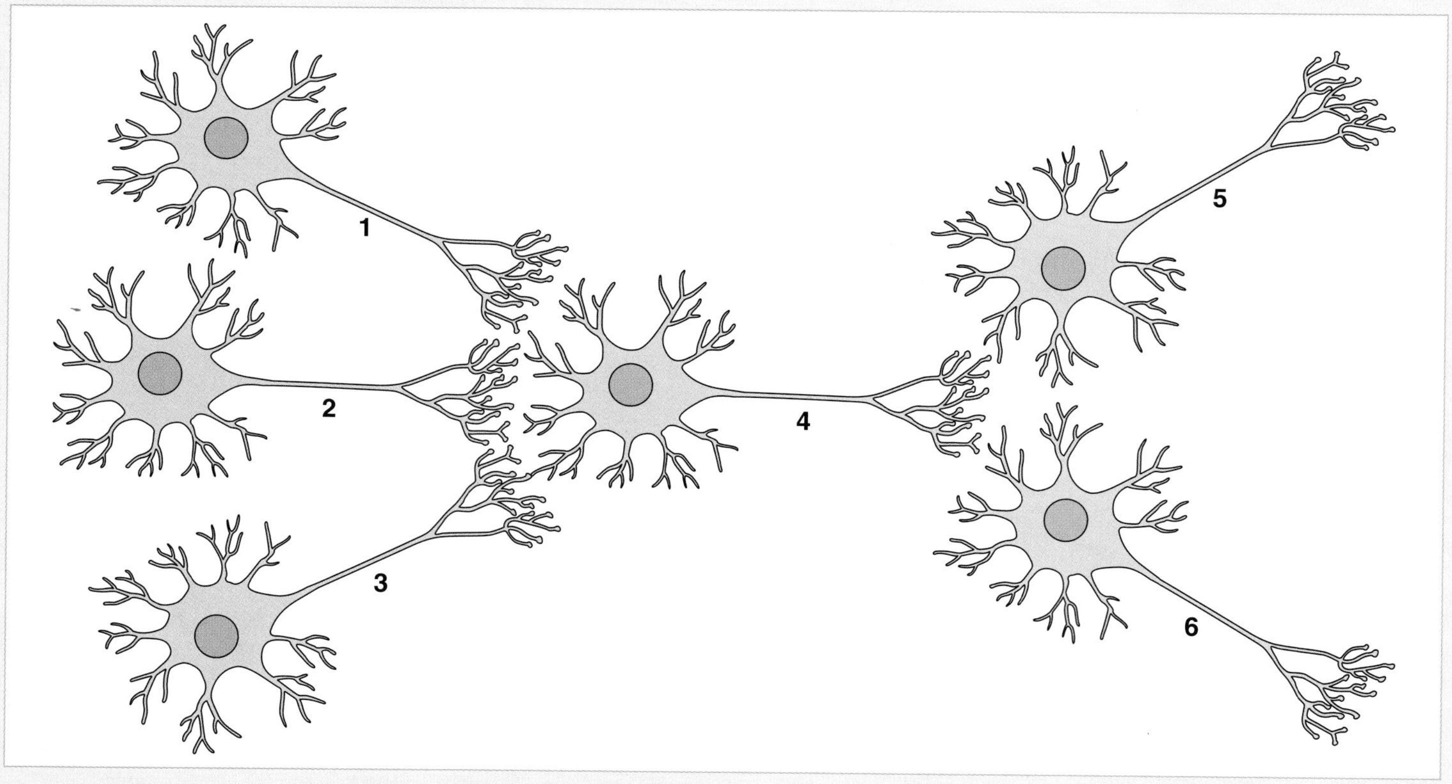

Figure 28-7 Complex synapse. Many cells (1, 2, 3) are brought together to connect with one cell (4). Cell 4 then connects with cells 5 and 6.

Table 28-2	Structures of the Nervous System and General Functions	
Major Structure	**Subdivision**	**General Function**
Central nervous system		
Brain	Occipital	Vision and storage of visual memories
	Parietal	Sense of touch and texture; storage of those memories
	Temporal	Hearing and smell; language; storage of sound and odor memories
	Frontal	Voluntary muscle control; storage of those memories
	Prefrontal	Judgment and predicting consequences of actions; abstract intellectual functions
	Limbic system	Basic emotions; basic reflexes (eg, chewing, swallowing)
	Diencephalon (thalamus)	Relay center; filters important signals from routine signals
	Diencephalon (hypothalamus)	Emotions; temperature control; interaction with endocrine system
Brain stem	Midbrain	LOC; RAS; muscle tone and posture
	Pons	Respiratory patterning and depth
	Medulla oblongata	Heart rate; blood pressure; respiratory rate
Spinal cord		Reflexes; relays information to and from body
Peripheral nervous system		
Cranial nerves		Brain to body part communication; special peripheral nerves that connect directly to body parts
Peripheral nerves		Brain to spinal cord to body part communication; receive stimuli from body; send commands to body

along the axon without "shorting out" or losing electricity to surrounding fluids and tissues. Myelin also increases the speed of conduction. Where speed is important, neurons have myelin. Where speed is less crucial, neurons don't have myelin. Most of the neurons within the body have myelin.

Table 28-2 ▲ summarizes the structures of the nervous system and their functions.

Pathophysiology

The pathophysiology of the nervous system can be examined from several angles. Discussion of cancerous, degenerative, developmental, infectious, vascular, and multifactorial causes of neurologic conditions will be followed by a review of increased intracranial pressure and its effects on the nervous system.

Neoplastic (Cancerous) Causes

Neoplasms (the medical term for new growth) are caused by errors that occur during cellular reproduction, especially during the unwinding and reproduction of the DNA during cell duplication. If the error is critical, the cell will not be able to survive; it will die, and the damaged DNA will die with it. If the error is subtler, however, the cell may survive. In this case, the daughter cell is not identical to the parent. The altered cell may then reproduce and copy the error to its daughter cells. The magnitude of the cancer depends on how effectively the altered cells get sufficient nutrients for their growth and reproduction.

Neoplasms can be categorized as either benign (noncancerous) or malignant (cancerous). Essentially, benign neoplasms are not very aggressive. They tend to remain within a capsule, so their growth is limited. In addition, these tumors are usually relatively easy to remove. By contrast, malignant neoplasms may forcefully take over blood supplies, grow unchecked, and move to other sites within the body (metastasis). They create finger-like projections into surrounding tissue, spreading and invading new areas. This growth without regard to other cells explains why many malignancies are fatal.

Degenerative Causes

Degenerative conditions result when a normal structure is altered over time. Such damage can occur in several ways—for example, due to wear and tear. Consider the effects of osteoarthritis on the knee joint. Every time a person falls on the knee, a small amount of damage is done to this joint. If the damage is not completely repaired, it may continue to accumulate until the patient experiences pain. With enough damage, the patient experiences limited mobility and pain to the joints.

Parkinson's disease is one neurologic condition that is influenced by wear and tear. If the portion of the brain that is responsible for production of dopamine becomes damaged or overused, Parkinson's disease can result.

Degenerative conditions may also occur through autoimmune effects. The body has the ability to determine which proteins are "self" and which are "nonself." This recognition enables the immune system to attack the bacteria in a cut yet

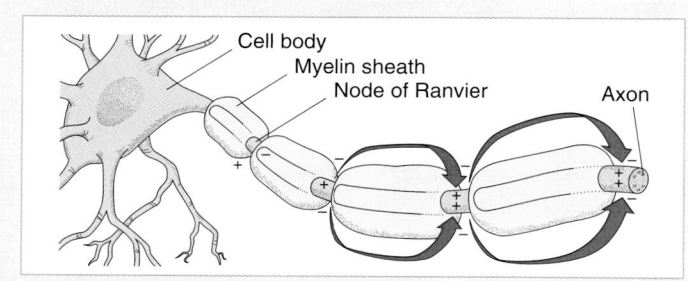

Figure 28-8 The myelin sheath normally allows impulses to jump from node to node, greatly accelerating the rate of transmission.

leave the surrounding skin cells alone. In autoimmune disorders, the body begins to attack its own cells. The immune system is no longer able to distinguish friend from foe.

Under normal conditions, myelin coats the axons of most nerve cells and allows for smooth transmission of signals to their target cell **Figure 28-8 ▲**. In multiple sclerosis (MS), however, the body believes that the proteins making up this insulation are foreign. It therefore attacks the myelin, creating gaps in the insulation that produce the signs and symptoms of MS.

Developmental Causes

Developmental conditions arise when portions of the nervous system are not formed correctly. Such an error can occur at any point in the development from embryo to fetus. The earlier the error occurs, the more severe the damage. In the case of spina bifida, embryonic growth does not proceed correctly.

Soon after conception, the fetus is a ball of cells—each cell identical to all the others. Within just 8 days, however, the once uniform ball of cells is ready to give rise to an embryo. One of the critical changes that must occur is the formation of the neural tube. Around days 15 to 20, a layer of cells will fold in and form a hollow tube that will eventually become the entire nervous system. In spina bifida, some cells do not fold correctly and remain outside the neural tube. This creates an outcropping of nervous system cells that expands as the embryo grows. The ultimate result is a child born with part of its nervous system outside the body.

Even if the fetus is formed correctly, other problems may occur. If an infection or chemical agent is able to gain access to the growing fetus, it may damage areas of the brain. Likewise, a temporary decrease in oxygen may lead to brain damage. These mechanisms are postulated as the causes of cerebral palsy.

Genetics appear to play a role in many diseases, which has implications for developmental causes of neurologic disorders. DNA provides the recipe for building every part of the body and outlining every process that should occur. If the recipe is perfect, then the body part will function normally. If the recipe is only slightly off, the final product may function

normally but may not be able to handle stress or wear and tear as easily. However, if the recipe is very wrong, a person has an obvious disease.

This concept helps to explain why some people seem to get diseases very easily while others do not. Consider a man who has been smoking for many years. Although smoking often leads to cardiovascular disease, this man lives to be 90 years old. Another man who eats correctly, exercises every day, and never smokes dies of a heart attack at age 45. Why?

Some of the answer lies in how their coronary arteries were created. Perhaps the smoker had larger, more resilient arteries than those of the 45-year-old heart attack victim. Even though the first man makes many unhealthy lifestyle choices, he benefits from the greater capacity of his coronary arteries, which prevents them from narrowing dramatically. The second man, even though he follows a much healthier lifestyle, has narrower arteries at the beginning, so even a small amount of narrowing has a more profound impact on coronary perfusion. This basic concept is becoming more important in understanding disease incidence and severity.

Infectious Causes

Infectious diseases result when bacteria, viruses, fungi, or prions (a certain type of protein) gain access to the body, where they reproduce and cause damage. These organisms have the same basic goal as humans do—to continue to live. When they begin to attack the body, they are simply looking for fuel so that they can create the next generation of bacteria, viruses, or other organisms. The damage that these invaders inflict occurs due to one of two mechanisms—the body's reaction to the infection or the activities of the attacking organisms.

The most common sign of infectious disease is the presence of a fever. Many organisms prefer to grow in a very narrow temperature range, so even a 2° or 3°F increase in body temperature can slow down the reproduction of some viruses or bacteria. This allows the immune system to get the upper hand. It also provides valuable time for neutrophils (the body's soldiers) to find and kill the invading organisms. Finally, it signals the rest of the body that an attack is under way. In response, more white blood cells are produced and chemical mediators are released to improve the body's effectiveness at finding and eliminating the organisms.

If the temperature of the body becomes too high, however, the brain can be affected. The increased temperature may make a person's thinking dull, make it difficult to concentrate, and lead to a headache. Neurons are highly sensitive to temperature changes. As the temperature rises, the effects on the neurons can become more profound. Eventually, a person may hallucinate, become delusional, or lose consciousness. The random firing of neurons might also produce a febrile seizure.

Infectious agents may also damage the body by destroying cells. These organisms may produce endotoxins or exotoxins that alter living cells. Endotoxins are proteins that are released by gram-negative bacteria when they die. Exotoxins

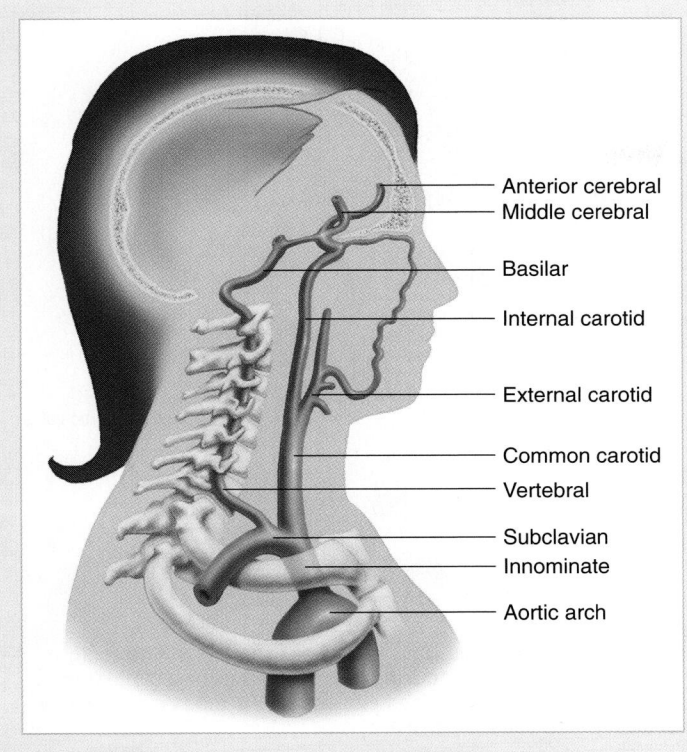

Figure 28-9 Blood supply to the brain.

Anterior cerebral
Middle cerebral
Basilar
Internal carotid
External carotid
Common carotid
Vertebral
Subclavian
Innominate
Aortic arch

and produces acidic by-products. If circulation is not restored quickly, the cell will not have enough fuel to survive.

Vascular emergencies may occur either suddenly or gradually over time. Sudden occurrences typically result from emboli or aneurysms. Emboli are insoluble objects that float in the bloodstream until they reach a point in the artery that is too narrow for them to pass through. Common types of emboli include pieces of a thrombus that have broken off or small clots that are produced by turbulent blood flow within the heart. Patients with atrial fibrillation, for example, need to have their heart rhythm controlled and take anticoagulants to prevent clots from forming in the heart and traveling to the brain, which could cause a stroke. Other types of emboli include globules of fat from long bone fractures, air bubbles infused from an IV, or a portion of an IV catheter that has been sheared off during insertion. These objects stop blood flow distal to the blockage, causing ischemia and necrosis of tissue Figure 28-10 ▶.

Artery walls consist of three layers of tissue. Aneurysms, which are weaknesses in those walls, occur in the following circumstances:

1. A small tear or defect occurs within the wall of an artery.
2. Blood penetrates between the layers of the artery.
3. Pressure builds up and the initial small tear increases in size.
4. If the buildup continues, the wall will become so damaged that it can no longer withstand the normal pressure of blood within it. A bulge may then develop. If the weakness is severe, the bulge may leak or fail catastrophically, causing an intracranial hemorrhage.

Gradual processes occur as plaque accumulates in blood vessels over the years. This buildup creates turbulence within the artery, allowing small clots (called thrombi) to form on its walls. The amount of plaque buildup reflects a combination of lifestyle choices (how we eat, exercise, and relieve stress) and family history (how we process food, manage fats, and the elasticity of our blood vessels). Over time, the buildup narrows the diameter of the arterial lumen. Eventually, the narrowing becomes so severe that blood flow is either diminished or cut off.

Even the blood vessel itself may cause difficulties for some patients. In trigeminal neuralgia, the normal functioning of facial blood vessels produces severe pain. As the blood vessels change in diameter to meet the needs of the surrounding tissue, their pulsations can irritate the trigeminal nerve. This nerve is responsible for receiving signals related to pain, temperature, and pressure on the face.

Multifactorial Causes

Most diseases or conditions are multifactorial, meaning that they have multiple causes. Just because a person gets an infection, that doesn't mean that the individual will experience

are proteins that are secreted by some bacteria or fungi to aid in the death and digestion of other cells. In poliomyelitis, for example, the virus responsible for the disease attacks the axons directly and destroys them. This virus shows a preference for motor axons—the neurons responsible for making muscles contract. Without these axons, the patient can experience weakness, paralysis, and respiratory arrest.

Vascular Causes

Blood vessels are needed to supply nutrients and oxygen to cells and to remove waste products Figure 28-9 ▲.

Notes from Nancy

Once brain cells are destroyed, from whatever cause, they cannot be regenerated. Clearly, then, it is of enormous importance to provide the brain with maximum protection from harm.

If a blood vessel suddenly becomes blocked, as in an embolism, the cells beyond the blockage may become ischemic. As oxygen and glucose levels drop, brain cells resort to anaerobic metabolism to stay alive. Unfortunately, this mechanism is only a stop-gap measure. Anaerobic metabolism creates minuscule amounts of energy for the cell

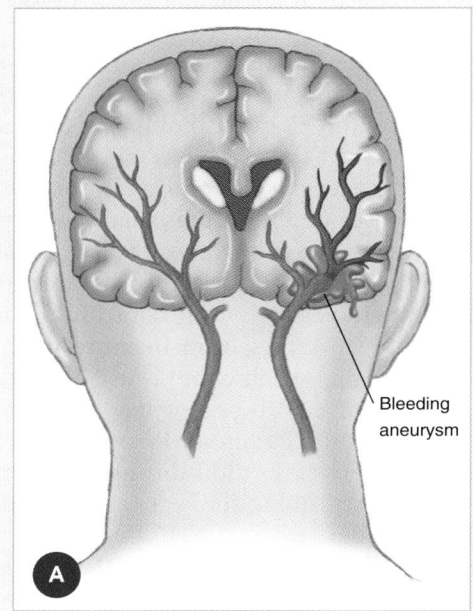 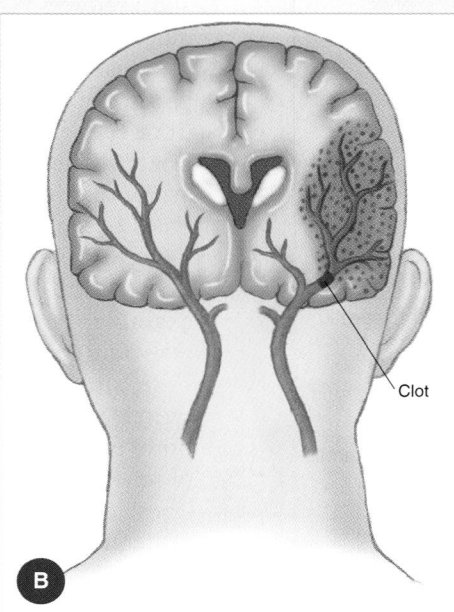 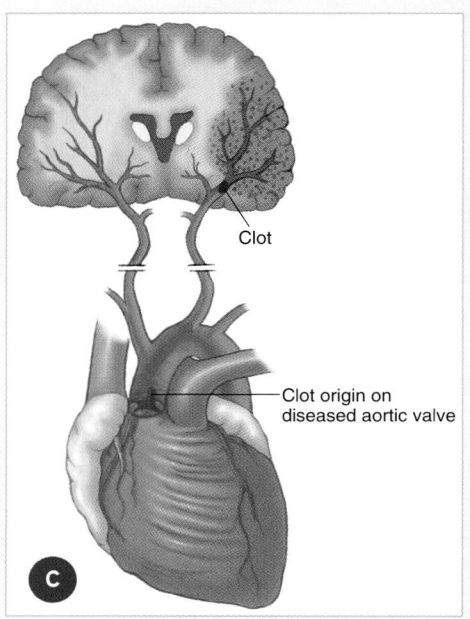

Figure 28-10 Vascular causes of neurologic conditions. **A.** Aneurysms are areas of weakness in the walls of arteries that can dilate (bulge out) and eventually rupture or leak. **B.** Atherosclerosis can damage the wall of a cerebral artery, producing narrowing and/or a clot. When the vessel is completely blocked, blood flow may be blocked and cells begin to die. **C.** An embolus, a blood clot usually formed on a diseased heart valve, can travel through the body's vascular system, lodge in a cerebral artery, and cause a stroke.

tissue damage. Just because someone eats unhealthy foods, it doesn't mean that his or her arteries will definitely become blocked. The following factors explain why many people get diseases:

- How well the body system was created during development as an embryo/fetus
- How effective the body's defense and repair mechanisms are
- How severe or prolonged the factors trying to damage the body are

Thus a health-conscious person may have a body that is less effective at repair and maintenance. In contrast, a person who smokes, drinks alcohol, and does not pursue a healthy lifestyle may have a body that is very effective at repair, which can help minimize the impact of those unhealthy activities.

Intracranial Pressure

Hemorrhagic strokes that cause bleeding into the brain place patients at risk for increased intracranial pressure (ICP). Treatment of these patients is directed at providing some degree of control over this potentially deadly effect.

The skull (cranial vault) is filled with three substances: brain, blood, and cerebrospinal fluid (CSF). These substances exert a pressure (ICP) against the skull, and the skull in turn exerts a reflected pressure. This balanced exchange allows the brain to fit snugly within the skull without permitting any voids. If the skull contained empty spaces, with head movement the brain would slam into the skull and cause damage.

When the pressure within the cranial vault begins to climb and remains high, it creates two major problems. The brain may either become ischemic due to lack of blood supply or herniate (push through the ligaments that compartmentalize the brain, such as the tentorium).

As ICP rises, the amount of blood available to the brain decreases. Cerebral perfusion pressure (CPP), the pressure of blood within the cranial vault, then begins to fall. CPP can be calculated by the following equation:

$$CPP = MAP - ICP$$

The mean arterial pressure (MAP) is the average (mean) pressure within the blood vessels. The average pressure is typically 80 to 90 mm Hg. Normal ICP usually ranges from 0 to 10 mm Hg. Normal CPP is, therefore, in the range of 70 to 80 mm Hg. The lower end of normal CPP is around 50 to 60 mm Hg. With CPP below 50 mm Hg, the brain begins to become ischemic.

ICP changes constantly. Coughing, vomiting, and bearing down, for example, will increase ICP. These momentary spikes in ICP are not harmful. By contrast, if there is blood, swelling, pus, or a tumor within the cranial vault, ICP will increase and remain high. Because the volume of the cranial vault is limited and inflexible, pressure increases as more substances squeeze into this space. As long as there is no significant drop in blood pressure or significant rise in ICP, the heart will still be able to get blood into the brain. However, if ICP rises sharply or blood pressure falls critically, patients may experience serious problems.

Consider a patient with meningitis (an infection of the membranes that cover the brain and spinal cord). The battle between the infecting organism and the immune system causes fluid to accumulate around the brain, which in turn causes ICP to climb. As long as the increase remains moderate, the brain will continue to receive adequate oxygen and nutrients. If the infection goes unchecked and travels to the general circulatory system, however, septicemia occurs. Then, as the organism continues to grow and feed, capillaries may begin to leak. Eventually, the blood pressure will decline and the MAP will fall. At a certain point, CPP may drop so low that the brain starts to become ischemic.

This concept dictates the priorities for treatment. Given how critical normal perfusion of the brain is, blood pressure must be closely monitored in any patient with a potential ICP problem. Frequent assessment becomes even more essential when a decrease in blood pressure is also present. For any patient at risk for ICP, the paramedic needs to ensure a blood pressure of at least 110 to 120 mm Hg systolic.

Another potential outcome of ICP is herniation, or displacement of the brain out of the cranial vault. Herniation results when pressure increases within the skull and the brain is pressed down through the foramen magnum (the "large hole" at the inferior portion of the skull where the spinal cord exits). Pressure on the medulla oblongata (located directly superior to the spinal cord) can result in rather bizarre vital signs and other findings, including slowed heart and respiratory rates.

Carbon dioxide and oxygen levels are important with increased ICP. Excessively high O_2 levels will cause vasoconstriction of cerebral arteries, which further impairs perfusion to the brain and causes cerebral hypoxia. Conversely, lowered CO_2 levels will decrease ICP, which yields a more suitable environment for brain perfusion. Thus hyperventilation will decrease CO_2 (thereby decreasing ICP) and increase O_2 (thereby decreasing brain perfusion)—a no-win situation for the paramedic. Prehospital treatment is simply not very effective at decreasing ICP.

Notes from Nancy

Always assume that the patient can understand what you are saying, even if he or she cannot talk.

General Assessment

The brain is the organ that is most sensitive to fluctuating levels of oxygen, glucose, and temperature; it responds to alterations in these levels with changes in its function. The difficulty for the paramedic is that the brain is relatively resilient to internal environmental changes: It doesn't simply shut down when oxygen levels fall. The key to identifying a neurologic problem is to look for both the gross or obvious changes and the subtle, sometimes hidden changes that can indicate disease.

This section reviews the assessment process for the neurologic patient. As with all patients, begin with the scene size-up.

Scene Size-up

Body substance isolation (BSI) precautions are taken for granted in many EMS systems. Its purpose is to protect the provider from exposure to potentially harmful organisms or

You are the Provider Part 2

You obtain the patient's vital signs. As your partner obtains his blood glucose level, you continue your assessment and determine that he is quite confused. He is alert and oriented to person and place, but is unsure as to what day it is and cannot describe the events leading up to your arrival.

The patient shows no signs of trauma. During your assessment of his pupils, however, he takes your penlight and tries to shave his face with it. He also seems to use inappropriate words for common, household objects and appears frustrated that you can't understand him.

Vital Signs	Recording Time: 5 Minutes
Level of consciousness	Verbal, oriented to person and place, but not day, with a Glasgow Coma Scale score of 14
Skin	Pale, warm, and dry
Pulse	90 beats/min and irregular
Blood pressure	142/86 mm Hg
Respirations	26 breaths/min
Sao₂	98% on 15 L/min via nonrebreathing mask
Blood glucose	100 mg/dL

3. Given the information you have now, what do you think could be this patient's underlying illness, injury, or condition?

4. Do your assessment and treatment priorities ever change?

5. What are appropriate interventions?

environments. Patients having grand mal seizures, for example, may be incontinent.

Some unconscious patients may be suffering from overdoses. With the use of illegal drugs, the presence of weapons, money, and crime increases. This potentially places the paramedic close to armed criminals.

Patients with altered levels of consciousness may not be able to walk, may be combative, or may be completely unresponsive. You may need additional assistance with lifting and moving these patients. Special circumstances can be overcome easier if additional resources—such as helicopter transportation, rescue equipment, or fire suppression—are requested early in the call.

Examine the scene to ascertain the number of patients. Clues can be obtained from the dispatch information. Also consider the mechanism of injury or history of present illness. Motor vehicle collisions typically involve more than one vehicle and, therefore, more than one patient. If many patients exhibit similar signs and symptoms, you should be very cautious. One patient with a headache does not stand out. If an entire family in the same house complains of a headache, then you should consider the possibility of carbon monoxide exposure. In such a case, the house may be an unsafe scene, so ensure that you have the correct personal protective equipment (PPE).

Weapons of mass destruction can follow similar patterns. If you encounter several patients who all exhibit the same signs and symptoms, all within the same general time frame and geographic location, you should consider immediate evacuation, donning appropriate PPE and contacting the dispatcher to begin a more in-depth investigation.

Initial Assessment

Begin assessing the neurologic patient as you would any other patient. Assess and secure the ABCs. Use the AVPU system to determine LOC. If the patient does not respond to verbal stimuli, consider whether he or she may be displaying some abnormal posturing; these unconscious movements may indicate severe brain dysfunction. There are two main abnormal postures that the patient may demonstrate with painful stimulation—decorticate and decerebrate. If you see either posture, you should immediately consider the patient to be critical.

In decorticate posturing, the patient flexes the arms and curls them toward the chest. At the same time, he or she points her toes. Finally, the wrists are flexed. This posture, which is also called abnormal flexion, may indicate damage to the area directly below the cerebral hemispheres **Figure 28-11 ▶** .

In decerebrate posturing, the patient again points the toes, but now extends the arms outward and rotates the lower arms in a palms-down manner (called pronation). The wrists are again flexed. This posture is a more severe finding than decorticate posturing, as the level of damage is within or near the brain stem (diencephalon/pons/midbrain) **Figure 28-12 ▶** .

Airway

The trigeminal, glossopharyngeal, vagus, and hypoglossal nerves are responsible for airway control. These nerves allow for

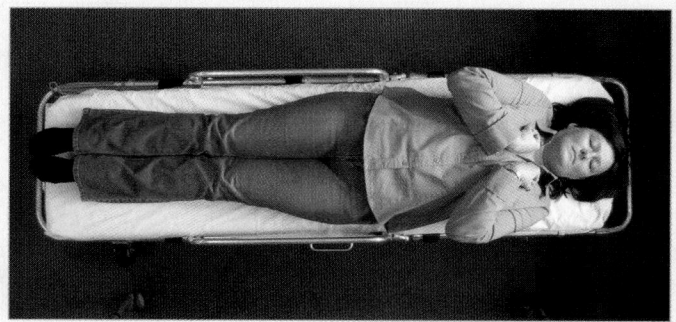

Figure 28-11 Decorticate posturing.

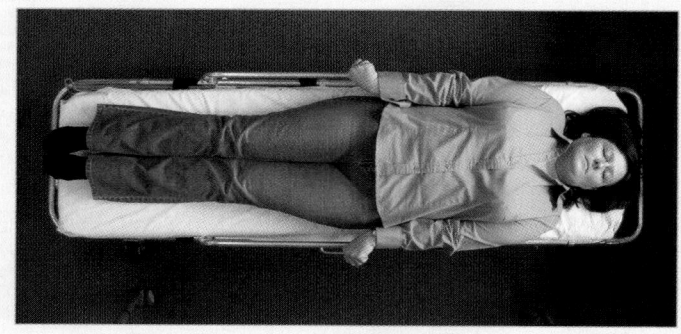

Figure 28-12 Decerebrate posturing.

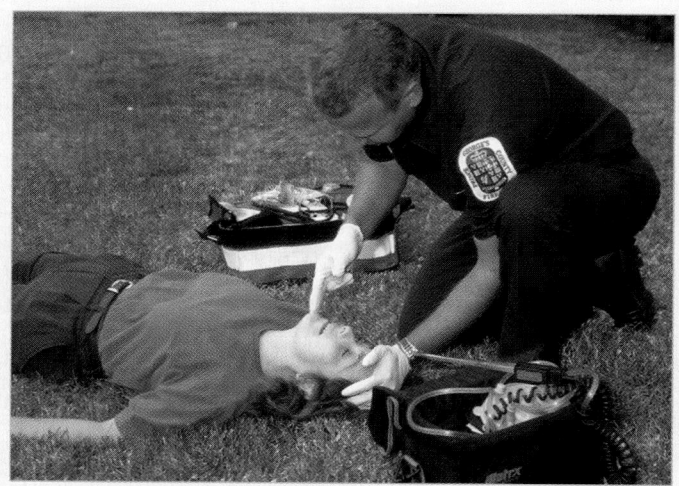

Figure 28-13 Securing and maintaining the airway in a patient who is unconscious is critical. Be sure to have suction readily available in the event that the patient vomits.

swallowing, controlling the tongue, and ensuring that the muscles in the hypopharnyx are slightly contracted. Alteration in the signals from these nerves can produce too much relaxation or too much constriction of the airway **Figure 28-13 ▲** .

Trismus, in which the teeth are clenched closed, can make managing the airway very difficult. Trismus can occur

| Table 28-3 | Vital Signs for Shock Versus Increased ICP |||||
	Heart Rate	Respiratory Rate	Blood Pressure	Pulse Pressure
Shock	↑	↑	↓	Narrowed
Increased ICP	↓	↓	↑	Widened

in conscious or unconscious patients. In an unconscious patient, it can indicate a seizure in progress, severe head injury, or cerebral hypoxia. The patient may need to be sedated or paralyzed to relax the clenched teeth and allow you to better control the airway.

Breathing

As part of your assessment of the neurologic patient, you need to check the rate and rhythm of breathing. Rhythms can have subtle changes or be dramatically different from normal. Generally, the greater the deviation from normal, the more severely the nervous system is affected.

Circulation

Evaluate the peripheral and central pulse pressures. Are they the same? The absence of a peripheral pulse with a central pulse present should cause the paramedic to suspect shock. What is the characteristic of the skin? Do you see evidence of gross bleeding? Is the pulse bounding? Remember, shock is rarely caused solely by a neurologic problem.

If a patient suffers from increased pressure within the cranium, the vital signs may provide evidence of this problem. Table 28-3 ▲ shows the vital signs associated with increased ICP. Notice how the blood pressure rises, the heart/respiratory rates fall, and the pulse pressure widens (systolic hypertension) in increased ICP. This set of conditions—known as Cushing's reflex—are the opposite of what is expected in shock.

As ICP rises, blood flow to the brain diminishes. To compensate, the medulla oblongata sends signals to the heart to increase the force of contraction. This causes systolic pressure to rise. If the ICP continues to increase, downward forces on the brain stem begin to damage the medulla's ability to send signals to the body. The diastolic blood pressure falls as the blood vessels relax or dilate, which in turn results in a widened pulse pressure. Finally, this pressure damages the ability to control respiratory and heart rate; consequently, both decrease.

Transport Decision

At this point in the examination, the paramedic may make a broad decision about whether to "load and go" or "stay and play." Critical patients—those with alterations in their initial assessment or significant mechanism of injury (MOI) and history of present illness—should be transported urgently to an emergency department. Defer gathering very detailed information about these patients; instead, focus on stabilizing and maintaining ABCs. With stable patients—those with normal initial assessments and minor MOI/history of present illness—

Special Considerations

When you are working with geriatric patients, take their past medical history into account. Patients with a history of dementia will be very complicated to manage. The primary question is: How much change has occurred in the patient's LOC? Don't assume that the patient's baseline LOC is what you would consider "normal"; speak to family, friends, or other caregivers to determine the patient's baseline LOC. Document that level clearly, using active language.

you have more time to gather detailed information at the scene. You can question family and bystanders to gain valuable insight into your patient's complaint.

Focused History and Physical Exam
Rapid Trauma Assessment

Once the initial assessment is complete, you need to decide how to proceed. Is the patient stable or unstable? Do you suspect a major problem just below the surface? How should you transport this patient? At this point, you have two choices:

- Complete a rapid assessment using a full head-to-toe approach
- Perform a focused history and physical exam (ie, evaluate only the area of patient complaint)

You should perform a rapid assessment for any patient who has an abnormal initial assessment, has a significant MOI/history of present illness, or whom you suspect may have a major problem. Examples would include individuals who are unconscious, are seizing, or experience a sudden loss of movement of the body. The focused history and physical exam is done on patients who are stable and have narrow complaints. These individuals have a completely normal initial assessment and a minor MOI/history of present illness, and you suspect a very local problem. Examples would include patients with headaches or nontraumatic back pain.

Be cautious. If a patient has a headache, stress may not be the cause. Stroke patients can also experience headaches. If you

Documentation and Communication

Avoid using terms that can have multiple meanings, such as "lethargic," "sleepy," "obtunded," or "out of it." Instead, describe the patient using active language.

Potentially confusing: "Arrive to find male patient who is out of it."

Better: "Arrive to find a male patient disoriented to place and day."

Potentially confusing: "Caring for a 43-year-old obtunded male."

Better: "Caring for a 43-year-old male who is very slow to respond to painful stimulation."

suspect a more complicated problem, perform a rapid assessment to ensure that you give the patient the best possible care.

History

History taking in the patient with a potential neurologic complaint should follow the same process followed for any other medical or trauma patient. For example, if weakness is a symptom found in a medical patient with no trauma, use the OPQRST mnemonic to elaborate on the complaint of general body weakness. The physical exam for this complaint should investigate potential cardiac, neurologic, respiratory, metabolic, or infectious causes. Appropriate tests and serial vital signs such as blood glucose levels, ECG, vital signs, lung sounds, and temperature will also help you rule out potential causes of the weakness.

Detailed Physical Exam

The detailed physical exam examines all of the areas covered within the rapid assessment, but looks at them more closely.

Head

The head is the area where you will spend the most time, gathering critical information on the functioning of the nervous system. Of course, you want to assess the head for trauma. Deformities, Contusion, Abrasions, Penetrations, Burns, Tenderness, Lacerations, and Swelling (DCAP-BTLS) are the trauma assessment components you should assess on every body area.

There are many shades of LOC and many ways to evaluate LOC. A patient may be interacting appropriately with the environment or not at all. **Figure 28-14 ▾** shows a continuum that ranges from what most would consider to be normal behavior to no response whatsoever. The point on the extreme right side of the continuum is coma, a state in which the patient does not respond to verbal or painful stimuli. The

Notes from Nancy

A patient in a coma is a patient in danger. Institute the ABCs immediately.

points in between (guide markings) are not intended to imply that every patient will stop at every point as his or her LOC increases or decreases, but rather illustrate the relationships between various levels of consciousness. While the extremes are easy to understand, the points in the middle (the shades of gray) can be more confusing.

One tool to assist with the consistent evaluation of LOC is the Glasgow Coma Scale (GCS) **Table 28-4 ▸**. This assessment

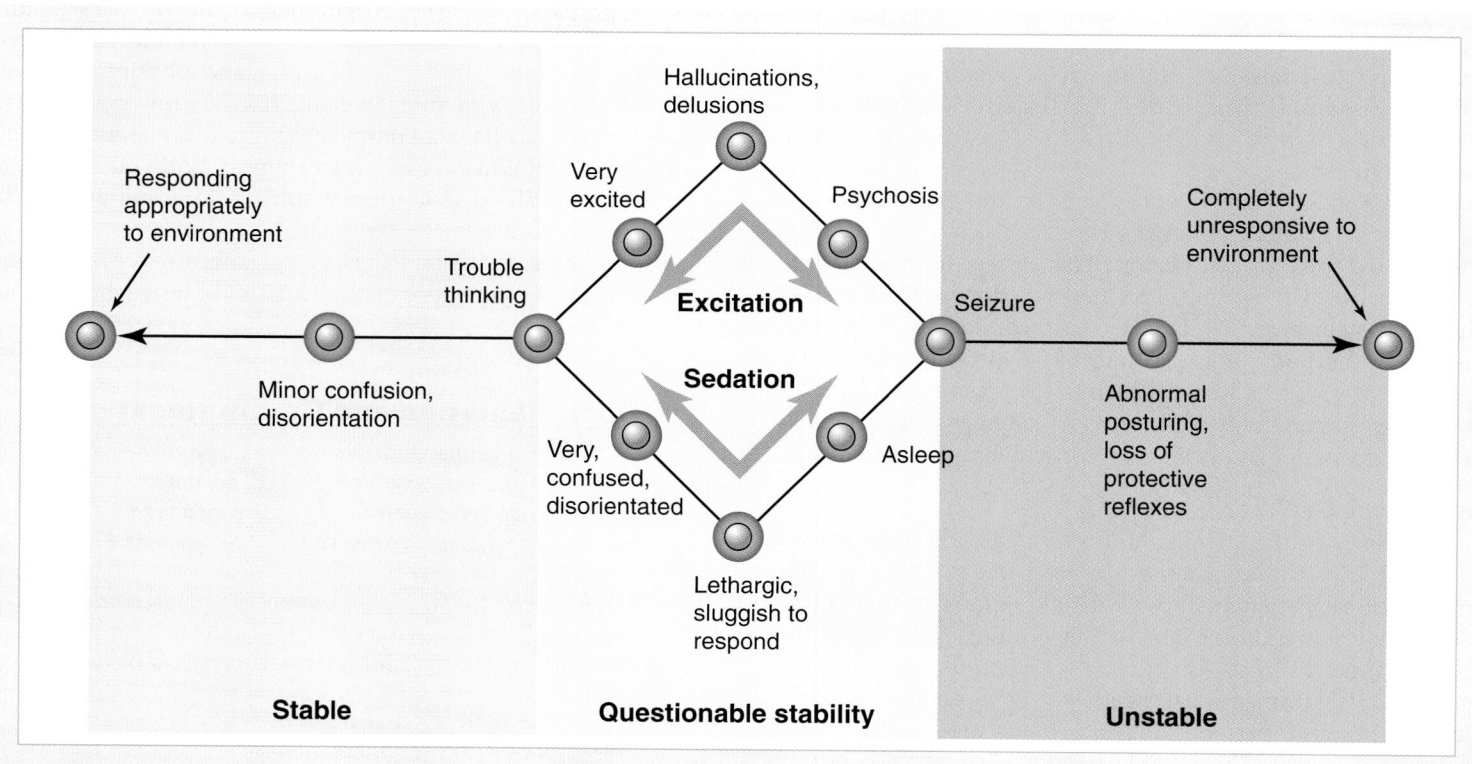

Figure 28-14 Level of consciousness continuum.

tool provides a basis to determine a patient's degree of illness or injury. It is used to determine the patient's LOC and evaluate responses to eye opening as well as verbal and motor skills **Figure 28-15** . To determine the GCS score, add the three numbers together from each of the subsections of the GCS.

The GCS score can provide information as to what care should be given and where the patient should be transported. **Table 28-5** provides general guidelines for using these scores. Patients with mild conditions need standard care; usu-

ally the paramedic can honor their request to be transported to a particular hospital. Patients with moderate conditions are very difficult to manage. They are not stable enough for you to relax, and not critical enough to completely get your attention. With this group, close assessment and transport to the nearest appropriate facility are prudent. Critical patients need airway management and rapid transport to the closest appropriate hospital.

Changes in the patient's mood or tempo of the nervous system should alert you to changes in neurologic status. Oxygen levels or blood pressure could be falling. Body temperature could be climbing. A psychiatric condition could be escalating. Blood glucose levels could be too high or too low. Regardless of the underlying cause, your observation of a change should prompt further evaluation to ensure the appropriate level of care. Mood or affect is another attribute that provides insight into the patient's condition. Ask the patient how he or she feels. Frustration, anger, or aggression can be caused by low glucose or oxygen levels.

Ask the patient how easy it is for him or her to think. Patients who have decreased blood glucose levels or who are taking narcotics can experience difficulty concentrating. Lower blood glucose levels and narcotics tend to produce sedation of the nervous system. In contrast, patients who are taking cocaine may experience difficulty concentrating due to excitement or mania. Cocaine, a sympathomimetic, increases nervous system activity, causing thoughts to come very quickly. If the speed of nervous system activity continues to increase, the patient may hallucinate or become delusional or psychotic.

Visual Findings

Perform the DCAP-BTLS assessment. Look at the symmetry of the face. Is there an obvious facial droop? Look at the eyes. Are the eyelids even bilaterally? Ptosis (drooping eyelids) can indicate Bell's palsy or a stroke. **Figure 28-16** demonstrates what happens when such a patient is asked to smile; weakness to one side of the face causes facial droop and slight ptosis.

Assess the cranial nerves, the peripheral nerves that control various portions of the body (see Chapter 13). Look for the ability to respond, strength of response, and symmetry. Patients with stroke, trigeminal neuralgia, myasthenia gravis, or other

Table 28-4	Glasgow Coma Scale	
	Adult	**Pediatric Patient (< 5 y)**
Eye opening	4. Spontaneous	4. Spontaneous
	3. Voice	3. To shout/voice
	2. Pain stimulation	2. Pain stimulation
	1. None	1. None
Verbal	5. Oriented	5. Cry, smile, coo, words correct for age
	4. Disoriented	4. Cries, inappropriate words for age
	3. Inappropriate words	3. Inappropriate scream or cry
	2. Incomprehensible	2. Grunts
	1. None	1. None
Motor	6. Obeys	6. Spontaneous
	5. Localizes pain	5. Localizes pain
	4. Withdraws from pain	4. Withdraws from pain
	3. Decorticate	3. Decorticate
	2. Decerebrate	2. Decerebrate
	1. None	1. None

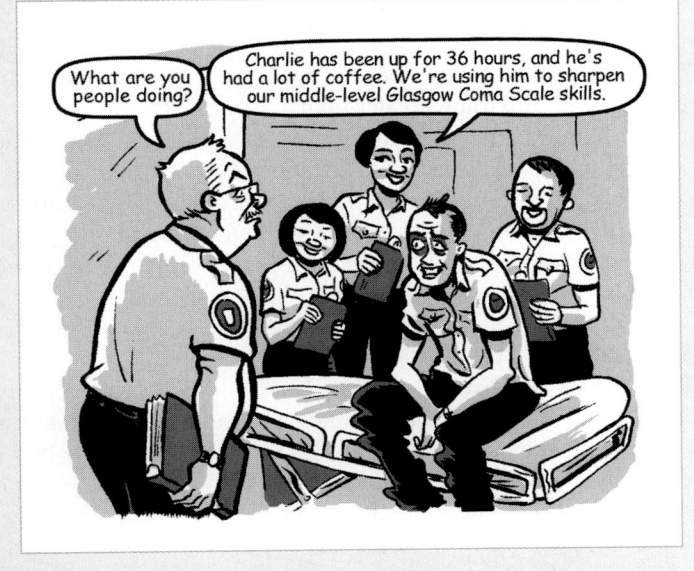

Figure 28-15

Table 28-5	Interpretations of Glasgow Coma Scale Scores		
GCS Score	Interpretation	Treatment	Facility
13–15	Mild	Standard care	Patient/family choice
9–12	Moderate	Close airway assessment, watch for decreasing consciousness	Closest appropriate facility
8 or less	Critical	Intubation, decrease scene time (less than 8, intubate)	Closest appropriate facility

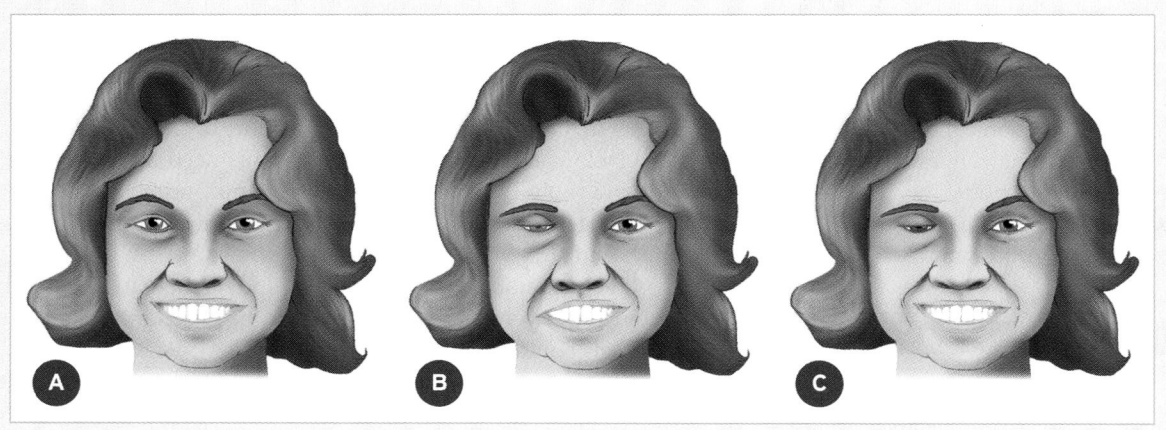

Figure 28-16 A. A normal smile. **B.** Facial droop, including a drooping eyelid (ptosis), which may or may not be present. **C.** A normal smile with ptosis present.

neurologic conditions may demonstrate abnormal cranial nerve functioning.

Speech

Listen to the quality of the speech. Is it slurred? Slurring is a classic finding with stroke. Is the speech appropriate? Focus on not only the quality of the words that are spoken, but also the appropriateness of those words. Sometimes speech may be clear but word choice is incorrect. Assess the patient's object recognition abilities.

Patients may be able to speak clearly, yet have subtle knowledge deficits. In agnosia (*a* = without, *gnosis* = knowledge), patients will be unable to name common objects because connections between visual interpretation of objects and the words that name them have become damaged. Apraxia (*a* = without, *praxia* = movement) refers to the inability to know how to use a common object.

To test for these signs, simply show the patient your pen, scissors, or a set of keys. Ask the patient to name the object. If the individual responds correctly, hand the object to the patient and ask him or her to demonstrate the object's use. The patient should write with the pen, cut with the scissors, and turn a lock with the keys. Patients may have one of these signs without the other. One is not a more severe finding than the other. They simply indicate that some degree of misfiring of neurons is occurring between the occipital lobe and the temporal lobe (agnosia) or between the temporal lobe and the frontal lobe (apraxia).

Language can be affected by injury or disease. In aphasia, speech is affected. There are three main forms of aphasia:

- **Receptive aphasia.** The patient cannot understand (receive) speech, but is able to speak clearly. This form of aphasia indicates damage to the temporal lobe. Ask patients questions to which both you and they know the answer: "Who is the president?" "What month is it?" Do not ask yes/no questions. If the patient speaks clearly but gives incorrect answers, he or she may have receptive aphasia.

- **Expressive aphasia.** The patient can't speak (express themselves) clearly, but is able to understand speech. This form of aphasia indicates damage to the frontal lobe, which controls the motor portion of speech. Ask patients to raise an arm. If they respond correctly, they can understand you. Ask patients their name. If they can't respond or their responses are slurred, they have expressive aphasia.

- **Global aphasia.** This form of aphasia is a combination of expressive and receptive aphasia. In this setting, the patient will not follow commands and can't answer your questions. Nevertheless, patients with global aphasia can often think clearly. They have needs, anxieties, and discomforts, but no way to express them. This can be incredibly frightening for patients who can't understand anything that you're saying and can't speak to you. Be sensitive to this state. Move slowly and purposely. Use therapeutic touch and good eye contact to reassure the patient.

Pupils

Pupillary shape can be changed by trauma, glaucoma, or increased ICP. Cocaine, methamphetamines, and hallucinogens tend to cause dilation of the pupils. Depressants usually lead to constriction of the pupils.

Equality of pupils is an important observation. Unequal pupils, called anisocoria, can be a sign of increased ICP **Figure 28-17 ▶**. Many people have a slight inequality in pupillary size. Anything greater than a 1-mm difference is worth noting, however. As pressure increases within the skull, the brain stem can be squeezed. This squeezing can interrupt signals to one pupil, resulting in dramatically different-size pupils.

Finally, determine whether the eyes are twitching. Nystagmus (the involuntary, rhythmic movement of the eyes) can be caused by seizures, vertigo, and MS.

Movement of the Body

Observe how the patient moves. Does the body move equally on both sides? Patients with strokes may suffer from weakness (hemiparesis) or paralysis (hemiplegia) of one side of the body. Sometimes you may discover patients with weakness on one side of their body but facial droop on the other side. This condition may be caused by decussation, in which nerves cross as they leave the cerebral cortex, move through the brain stem, and arrive at the spinal cord. Nerves that decussate start on one

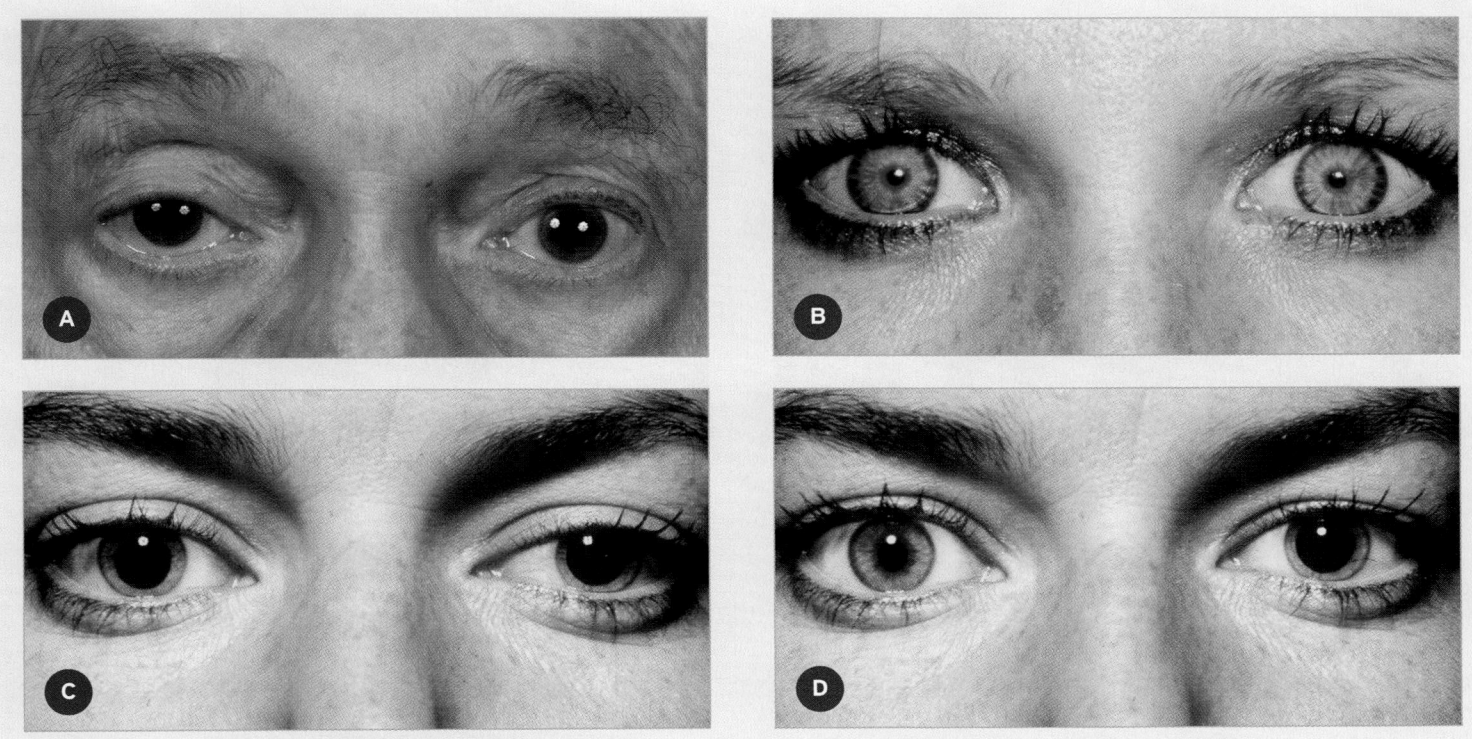

Figure 28-17 Pupil responses. **A.** Normal. **B.** Constricted (pinpoint). **C.** Dilated. **D.** Unequal.

side of the brain and then cross to control the opposite side of the body. Some nerves do not decussate—facial nerves, for example. The left side of the brain controls the right side of the body, but the left side of the face. A left cerebral stroke would therefore result in right-sided arm and leg weakness, but left-sided facial droop.

Examining the function of the cerebellum can also allow you to gather information about potential damage to the brain. Have the patient close his or her eyes and hold out the arms in front of the body at the same level. With the eyes closed, the patient's only way to tell where the arms are located is from the sensations being processed by the cerebellum. If the individual has suffered a stroke, one of the arms may drift away from the other   Figure 28-18 ▶ .

Have the patient walk for several steps (unless some medical reason rules the activity out). Assessing gait (walking patterns) is another way to test the activity of the cerebellum. Walking is really a controlled fall. As your center of gravity moves forward, you must move a leg forward to catch yourself. Once you learn how to walk, your cerebellum controls these mechanics, so you can focus on where you want to walk, not how to walk. Damage to the cerebellum may be manifested as erratic walking, stumbling, or even losing the ability to walk.

Several medical conditions cause alterations in the patient's gait. Ataxia is the term used to describe changes in a person's ability to perform coordinated motions like walking. Patients with Parkinson's disease exhibit a classic gait in which they place their feet very close together and shuffle. Their stride is short, and they have great difficulty changing direction. Such a patient will shuffle-walk in a straight line and, when asked to turn, will take very small steps until the turn is complete. With this kind of bradykinesia, routine motions may slow dramatically. In contrast, patients with cerebral palsy may walk with a scissors gait. In the spastic form of this disease, the person will point the toes inwardly, have a stiff gait, and nearly touch the knees together while walking.

In addition to the patient's gait, you should assess the posture. Have the individual stand straight. Place one hand on the patient's chest and the other hand behind the back (to catch the patient in the event that he or she can't do so), and then push on the chest. Normally, as you push backward, the patient will compensate quickly and take a step forward to prevent a fall. In Parkinson's disease, the patient's posture is so rigid that they can't compensate quickly enough and will fall over.

Bizarre movements may indicate a disruption within the nervous system. Myoclonus is a type of involuntary contraction of the muscles that is rapid and jerky in nature. Most people have suffered myoclonic jerks at some point. Have you ever seen a seated person who is very tired? As the person gets closer to falling sleep, the head will begin to sag. Often the

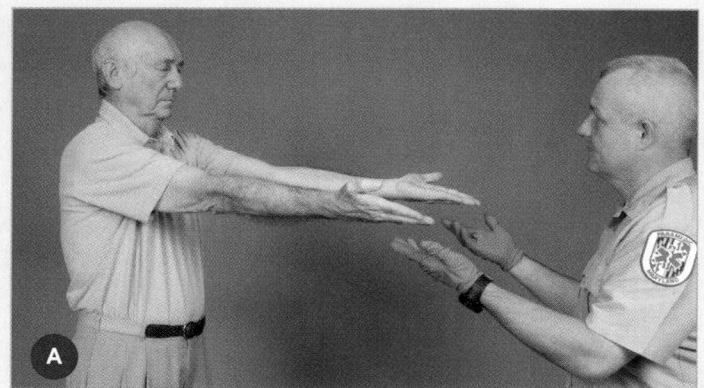 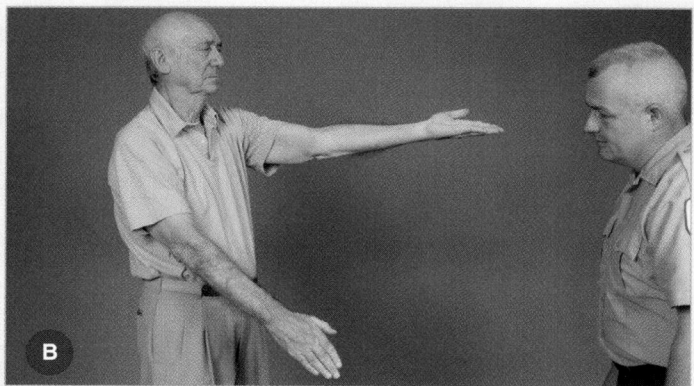

Figure 28-18 A. A person who has not experienced a stroke will be able to hold both hands in front of the body and maintain them there. **B.** If a person has had a suspected stroke, he or she may not be able to maintain this position. Instead, one arm will drift down and turn toward the body.

person will involuntarily jerk the head upward (myoclonic jerk) and wake up.

Another form of bizarre movement is dystonia, in which a part of the body contracts and remains contracted. A foot cramp where the great toe extends while the other toes curl under is an example of a common dystonia. Alternatively, the face may become extremely distorted as one side contracts. The head can twist to one side. An arm or leg can become frozen in a contracted position. Dystonia can be caused by brain injuries or medication reactions.

When you are watching the patient, does he or she move smoothly? This kind of motion requires proper functioning of the frontal lobe, cerebellum, brain stem, spinal cord, and peripheral nerves. When they are functioning correctly, muscle groups will alternately contract and relax, allowing the body to move smoothly. Patients with Parkinson's disease suffer from rigidity in which this fine balance is upset, so they move in fits and spurts.

Tremors are another potential alteration in smooth motion. These fine oscillating (back-and-forth) movements are usually found in the hands and head.

- **Rest tremors**—occur with the patient at rest and not in motion. They are common in Parkinson's disease.
- **Intension tremors**—occur when the patient tries to reach out and grab an object. These tremors may increase as the patient gets closer to the object to be grabbed. Intension tremors are common in MS.
- **Postural tremors**—occur when a body part is required to maintain the same position for a long period of time. Most people have experienced this type of tremor when they were working hard for a long time. As they tire, their worked body parts begin to shake. A postural tremor can also occur when a person is standing and the head oscillates back and forth. Patients with Parkinson's disease also experience these tremors.

Seizures may appear very similar to tremors. Generally, tremors are fine movements while seizures are larger, less

focused types of movement. There are two basic types of movements that patients can perform while seizing:

- **Tonic activity** is a very rigid, contracted body posture. The arms, legs, neck, and back can contract so tightly that the body part will shake slightly from the intensity of the contraction.
- **Clonic activity** is a rhythmic contraction and relaxation of muscle groups. It may appear as bizarre, nonpurposeful movements of any body part. Arms and legs may flail, teeth may clench, the head may bob, and the torso may move wildly.

Sensation

Many neurologic conditions can alter the ability to feel pain, temperature, pressure, or light touch. A sensation of numbness or tingling is called paresthesia. If the patient can feel nothing within a body part, the condition is called anesthesia.

Blood Glucose Level

Glucose is the fuel that runs the brain. The brain uses glucose faster than any other part of the body, but it has no means to store glucose. For this reason, all patients with a change in LOC should have their blood glucose level checked. A normal blood glucose reading is 60 to 120 mg/dL. As glucose levels fall below 60 mg/dL, LOC begins to decrease. LOC can also be affected by a high blood glucose level, although a significant increase is required before LOC is altered. Glucose levels below 10 mg/dL are incompatible with brain functioning and typically lethal. Generally, if levels are below 30 or above 300 mg/dL, confusion or unconsciousness will occur. Blood glucose monitoring is standard care for the patient with an altered LOC.

Chest

Evaluate the chest for DCAP-BTLS. Look for symmetry in its shape. Does the chest rise and fall equally? Apply the cardiac monitor and evaluate the ECG. Many cardiac dysrhythmias can cause neurologic disorders by decreasing the blood supply to the brain. Perform a 12-lead ECG in all patients with sudden loss of consciousness. How much effort must the patient make to breathe? Do you observe any degree of respiratory distress? Listen to lung sounds. Evaluate for the presence of adventitious sounds and equality of sounds. Determine the pulse oximeter reading, remembering that normal readings are 95% to 100% and that this number is affected by the amount of hemoglobin within the body and the presence of carbon monoxide.

Abdomen

Examine the abdomen for DCAP-BTLS. Do you note any masses? Are there any pulsations within the abdomen? Does the patient have any complaints related to the abdomen? Signs of nausea and vomiting are common with some neurologic conditions, such as headaches or increased ICP.

Pelvis

Examine the pelvis for DCAP-BTLS. Is it stable to stress? If the patient is able to walk without assistance, the pelvis should be stable. Does the patient have any incontinence? Urinary or fecal incontinence are common findings with seizures or syncope. Incontinence also serves as a relatively objective marker for the severity of the unconsciousness. When we sleep, we are not incontinent. Thus if incontinence is present, the LOC has decreased below that of sleep.

Extremities

Examine the limbs for DCAP-BTLS. Do you see any signs of edema? Look for venipuncture marks and note whether these marks are at various stages of healing. Such marks may indicate recent illegal drug use.

Ongoing Assessment

The ongoing assessment is intended to monitor patients for changes. Talk with them. Ask them how they're feeling. Ask about their children. Ask if they caught the game last night. Casual conversation will allow you to closely monitor brain functions. It also communicates a caring environment. If the patient is nonverbal, keep a close eye on respiratory patterns and eye and body movements, and monitor for seizure activity.

Routine monitoring should include heart rate, ECG, blood pressure, respiratory rate and pattern, pulse oximetry, and repeat glucose (if the level was low and sugar was given to the patient). Continue oxygenation and ventilation support. Monitor IVs closely to ensure that accidental fluid overload does not occur. If the patient's condition undergoes a sudden dramatic change,

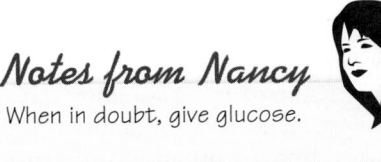

Notes from Nancy
When in doubt, give glucose.

repeat the rapid assessment and detailed physical exam as if this were a new patient. This will give you a chance to modify your care so as to manage the new development.

■ General Management

This management guideline should be followed with all patients who experience a change in LOC. The focus of care for neurologic patients is directed at ensuring that the body has an adequate internal environment to allow for optimal brain function. The three major elements that the brain needs to function are *oxygen, glucose,* and *normal temperature.* The general management techniques discussed in this section—the standard care—serve as the foundation on which additional care for specific neurologic problems is built.

As always, provide for BSI and scene safety. Ensure that you and your partner are safe and you have BSI precautions in place.

Evaluate the patient's airway and effectiveness of breathing. If necessary, secure the airway, and provide ventilatory support

You are the Provider Part 3

In the interest of time, you place your patient on the gurney, obtain IV access and administer normal saline TKO, draw blood, and perform an ECG. You also complete a fibrinolytic screen while en route to the hospital. You ask one of the patient's sons to accompany you and provide more information regarding his medical history. The patient's son tells you that his medical history includes atrial fibrillation (which you confirm on the monitor) and that the patient takes aspirin, diltiazem, Coumadin, and glucophage. The patient has no known drug allergies, has no recent history of illness, and has been compliant with his medications and diet.

Reassessment	Recording Time: 10 Minutes
Level of consciousness	Alert, with a Glasgow Coma Scale score of 14
Skin	Pale, warm, and dry
Pulse	92 beats/min, strong and irregular
Blood pressure	140/84 mm Hg
Respirations	24 breaths/min
Sao$_2$	100% on 15 L/min via nonrebreathing mask

6. Would you choose to place this patient in manual in-line spinal precautions?

7. What places this patient at greater risk for cerebrovascular accident?

Table 28-6	Hallmarks of Increased ICP	
Cushing's Reflex	**Other Signs**	
■ Bradycardia ■ Bradypnea ■ Widened pulse pressure (systolic hypertension)	■ Decorticate posturing ■ Decerebrate posturing ■ Anisocoria	■ Biot respirations ■ Apneustic respirations ■ Cheyne-Stokes respirations

to make sure oxygen saturation remains higher than 90%. Routine hyperventilation of neurologic patients can be harmful, so provide hyperventilation only to those patients with documented unconsciousness *and* signs of increased ICP.

Establish IV access, and then administer normal saline or lactated Ringer's solutions. Consider drawing blood samples for later analysis at the hospital. Don't use solutions containing dextrose. Check the patient's blood pressure and heart rate. Support hypotension to ensure adequate CPP; the target is a systolic blood pressure of 110 to 120 mm Hg.

Continuously monitor the patient on an ECG. Perform 12-lead ECG monitoring if permitted to do so.

Check the blood glucose level. If it's low, administer dextrose 50%, 25 g IVP. Be very cautious when you can't check the patient's blood glucose level. If the patient is unresponsive or has a decreased LOC and no blood glucose monitor is available, administer 12.5 g (½ syringe) and then reassess the response. Proceed with additional dextrose cautiously, based on responses to previous doses. Hyperglycemia can increase the morbidity rate among stroke patients.

Look for the hallmarks of increased ICP **Table 28-6 ▲** . In patients who are unconscious *and* demonstrate other signs of increased ICP, ensure a systolic blood pressure of 110 to 120 mm Hg. Administer fluids as needed. Unless you are concerned about possible cervical spine fracture, elevate the head 30°. Provide ventilatory support at 16 to 20 breaths/min. Don't increase the rate any higher than 30 breaths/min, as hyperventilation will cause vasoconstriction and decrease perfusion to the brain. Ensure that the airway is clear, but don't suction vigorously. Stimulating the cough and gag reflexes will increase ICP.

A patient with increased ICP may be bradycardic. Atropine and pacing are not indicated, however, due to the systolic hypertension that accompanies the bradycardia. The ICP is

Special Considerations

When assessing for ICP in infants, consider the quality of the cry. As ICP increases, the pitch of the cry will increase until a shriek similar to that of a cat can be heard. At the same time, the shape of the pupils can change from round to more oval. These two findings lead to the saying related to infants and ICP: "cats' eyes and cats' cries."

Documentation and Communication

You may be the only provider to witness some patient activity, so good documentation is critical to ensure continuity of care.

causing the bradycardia, not the reverse. Instead, notify the hospital and provide rapid transport.

Check for drug use. If the patient may have taken a narcotic, administer naloxone, 0.4 to 2 mg IVP. Watch for seizures. If the seizure is prolonged, administer diazepam or lorazepam.

Evaluate the patient's temperature. If it is low, cover the patient, turn on the heat, and prevent heat loss. If it is high, remove clothing, cover the naked patient in a sheet, and turn the heat off in the patient compartment.

Provide emotional support for the patient and family. Neurologic emergencies can produce confusion, fear, anger, and helplessness. Consider giving a therapeutic gentle touch on the shoulder. Touch can communicate compassion. Use a calm, reassuring voice to show that you're there to help. Try to reorient the patient, as confusion is often present in these cases.

Administration of Dextrose/Glucose

Consult your local protocol to determine whether the blood glucose reading is considered low. One guideline states that if the blood glucose level is below 60 mg/dL, then glucose is needed. Two medications are available for prehospital treatment of hypoglycemia: dextrose 50% (D_{50}) and glucagon. When administering D_{50}, you must establish an IV line. This access site should be within a large vessel (18-gauge or larger is preferred) because D_{50} is quite thick. Ensure that the IV is patent *before* you attempt to give the D_{50}. Extravasation of D_{50} into the interstitial space can cause severe damage to muscles, nerves, and skin or even death. The usual dose is 25 g of D_{50} or one full syringe. The effects from D_{50} typically begin in 30 seconds to 2 minutes. If no effect is apparent or the patient's blood glucose level remains low, ensure adequate IV access and administer a second dose of D_{50}.

You may need to give thiamine before administration of D_{50} begins. Patients who are severely malnourished, such as chronic alcoholics, may have insufficient supplies of vitamin B1 (thiamine) to adequately metabolize dextrose. Thiamine allows the body to convert its store of glycogen into glucose as part of the Krebs cycle. The typical dose in an emergent situation is 50 mg via slow IV bolus and 50 mg IM. Thiamine can cause hypotension if administered too quickly. If you cannot obtain vascular access, administer 0.5 to 1 mg of glucagon subcutaneously or IM. The LOC and blood glucose levels should increase within 20 minutes after administration. If the blood glucose levels remain low, repeat the glucagon in a maximum of three doses.

There is currently no safe way to lower high blood glucose levels in the field. Administration of insulin can be very problematic and can easily overshoot the mark, sending the patient into a hypoglycemic state. For these patients, provide standard care and ensure adequate blood pressure. Hyperglycemic patients are often dehydrated and usually need volume support.

Oral glucose administration is another option for the patients with a decreased LOC who can swallow safely. Assess these patients carefully, confirming that they are awake enough to follow commands. First give them a small amount of water to drink—say, 10 mL. If they can swallow that amount, then consider administering oral glucose 25 g (one tube). Alternatives to oral glucose include cake icing, a plain chocolate bar (without nuts), or orange juice with sugar added. Administration of sugar by mouth will take longer to raise blood glucose levels. Constantly supervise patients as they consume the sugar. Make sure they don't aspirate.

Airway Management

Sometimes patients may not be able to adequately protect the airway or ventilate themselves. The use of a bag mask, laryngeal mask airway, Combitube, or endotracheal intubation should be initiated to provide sufficient oxygen, ventilation, and airway protection in such cases. Endotracheal intubation is the most effective means by which you can isolate and protect the trachea from aspiration. Ensure that the pulse oximeter reading is higher than 90%. Provide oxygen via nasal cannula or mask as necessary. Provide ventilatory assistance as needed.

If the patient has trismus, determine how effectively the patient can be ventilated with a bag mask. If ventilation is poor or unsuccessful, you may attempt to place a nasotracheal airway. If this is unsuccessful, consider using a paralytic agent to relax the mouth and allow for airway management. If paralytics are not available or contraindicated and the patient can't be ventilated, transtracheal airway management is the only option to prevent hypoxia and death.

Administration of Naloxone

Naloxone is used for the treatment of unconscious/unknown patients or those with suspected narcotic overdose. The initial dose is 0.4 to 2.0 mg IVP. You may repeat this dose until you reach 10 mg. This narcotic antagonist will compete with any circulating narcotic, displacing it from its receptors and allowing the LOC to increase. Naloxone can have quite a dramatic effect: Patients with a GCS score of 3 can move to a score of 15 within 30 seconds. This rapid change in LOC may cause patients to become fearful and potentially angry or aggressive. Make sure that you have adequate resources to restrain the patient or that you have the ability to leave the scene quickly *before* you administer naloxone. It may be advisable to push the drug in small increments until an improvement in LOC or respiration is noted.

Airway management in relation to the narcotic overdose can also be tricky. Airway and ventilation are the focus of much of the care provided to unconscious patients. When you encounter a severely bradypneic, cyanotic patient, you reflexively want to establish an airway and intubate the patient quickly. When considering administering naloxone, however, a slightly different approach is recommended.

Ensure airway control and adequate ventilation but don't immediately intubate the patient. As you are oxygenating the patient, establish an IV and administer the naloxone carefully. Given the drug's quick onset of action and the potential for a dramatic response, an intubated patient may quickly wake up after the naloxone, grab the endotracheal tube, and yank it out. The result of this violent extubation may be vocal cord or tracheal trauma. If the medication doesn't produce a response, then intubation may be needed.

Temperature Assessment

The patient's temperature can be difficult to determine in the field. If you suspect hypothermia or hyperthermia, the standard of care is to use a thermometer to establish the patient's temperature. Oral, otic, transdermal, or rectal temperature can be measured. Avoid using the axillary method of measurement due to its inaccuracy.

Not all EMS systems have the ability to check a patient's temperature. In such a situation, you can still gather information about the history of present illness that can lead to a conclusion of temperature alteration. Was the patient in water for a long period of time? Has the patient been out in the snow? Did the patient fall and lie on the floor of a cold home, unable to get up for several days? In these cases, hypothermia should be considered. It would be reasonable to cover the patient in blankets and turn the heat up in the patient compartment.

Has the patient been out in the hot sun for several hours? Is the skin hot and dry? Is there a history of fever? In these cases, it would be prudent to remove the patient's clothing, place a sheet over the individual, and at least turn the heat off in the patient compartment.

▍ Assessment and Management of Specific Injuries and Illnesses

Table 28-7 ▶ will help you better classify specific neurologic conditions based first on the part of the nervous system they affect and then on the type of condition.

One way to manage these conditions is to try to create a patient profile that describes the circumstances that typically characterize a particular disease. How old is the typical patient? What sex and race is the patient? What are the common signs and symptoms of the condition? Are any unusual signs present that are uncommon in other conditions? How does the condition develop over time? If the patient profile indicates that men are most commonly affected by the condition, remember that females may also suffer from it.

The patient profile is intended to distill the condition down to its core elements. You can use this valuable system to

Table 28-7	Neurologic Disease by Type of Condition	
Major System	**Disease**	**Type of Condition**
Central nervous system	Neoplasm	Cancer (malignant or benign)
	Alzheimer's disease	Degenerative
	Amyotrophic lateral sclerosis	Degenerative
	Parkinson's disease	Degenerative
	Cerebral palsy	Developmental
	Spina bifida	Developmental
	Abscess	Infectious
	Poliomyelitis	Infectious
	Dystonia	Various causes
	Headaches	Various causes
	Seizures	Various causes
	Cerebral vascular accidents	Vascular
	Transient ischemic attacks	Vascular
Peripheral nervous system	Bell's palsy	Infectious
	Guillain-Barré syndrome	Degenerative
	MS	Degenerative
	Myasthenia gravis	Degenerative
	Trigeminal neuralgia	Various
Muscles	Muscular dystrophy	Degenerative

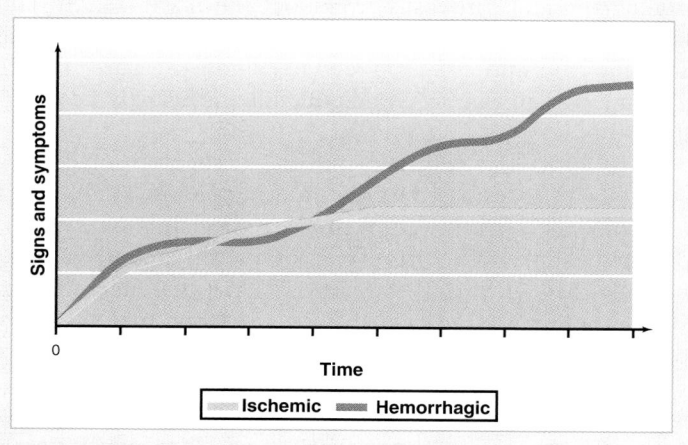

Figure 28-19 Symptom patterns for hemorrhagic versus ischemic CVA.

create flash cards that you can study. This summary of typical age, sex, race, history of present illness, signs and symptoms, and treatment will be provided for each condition discussed in the remainder of this chapter.

Stroke

Cerebrovascular accidents (CVAs) or strokes represent a serious medical condition in which the blood supply to areas of the brain becomes interrupted, resulting in ischemia. Today nearly half of all patients who suffer from brain attacks or strokes deny their symptoms. Many will not activate EMS and subsequently delay seeking care. The goal of treatment is early recognition and rapid, appropriate intervention. The longer the CVA continues without intervention, the less likely the patient will have a promising outcome. "Time is brain."

Two basic types of strokes are distinguished: ischemic and hemorrhagic. **Figure 28-19 ▶** provides some insight into the evolution of strokes.

The majority of the time (75%), strokes are ischemic rather than hemorrhagic. In ischemic stroke, a blood vessel is blocked, so the tissue distal to the blockage becomes ischemic. Eventually that tissue will die if blood flow is not restored. This pathology is self-limiting; only the tissue beyond the blockage

is affected, so the areas of the brain involved are limited. The signs and symptoms eventually stop increasing and then plateau, indicating that the area of the brain involved is no longer working. The extent and severity of the stroke will be dictated by which artery is involved and which portion of the brain is denied oxygen. An ischemic CVA to the brain stem is life-threatening.

In contrast, hemorrhagic CVAs tend to worsen over time due to bleeding within the cranium. This bleeding increases ICP and leads to herniation of the brain stem. One hallmark of a hemorrhagic CVA is the "worst headache of my life" complaint. If the patient complains of a very severe headache, later cannot speak, becomes difficult to arouse, and finally shows signs of increased ICP, you should strongly consider a diagnosis of hemorrhagic CVA.

Patients with a suspected stroke or transient ischemic attack (TIA; discussed in the next section) are usually older than age 65. Although men have more strokes, women die from them more often. African Americans experience double the rate of stroke than Caucasians.

Documentation and Communication

Patients with strokes can present a wide range of communication difficulties.
- Patients who are multilingual may lose understanding of only one language.
- Patients may be able to visually understand the written word but not the spoken word.
- Patients may not be able to understand any form of communication.
- Be open to trying various ways to communicate. Remember, communication problems do not indicate that the patient is not thinking, just that the patient can't get you to understand those thoughts.

Controversies

Health care in the United States is big business. The mission of hospitals is to provide high-quality patient care. But how can they provide quality care without seeing patients? Patients (or their insurers) provide the funding needed for hospitals to operate. In some systems, these two concepts—quality of care and number of patients served—can become entangled. The CVA patient provides an excellent example of this potential dilemma.

Suppose a 62-year-old woman is having a stroke. Your assessment reveals left-sided weakness, slurred speech, and an arm drift (she has a positive Cincinnati Prehospital Stroke Scale). These changes began around 8:15 AM. It's now 8:45 AM, and you are caring for the patient, who says that she has the worst headache of her life. She's getting very sleepy and becoming more difficult to arouse. You place the patient in the ambulance and begin transport to the local hospital, but the patient begins to have decorticate posturing. What should you do?

Appropriate care for this patient should include excellent airway management, initial hyperventilation, and rapid transport. But transport to where? Given the patient history, physical findings, and rapid deterioration of LOC, this patient appears to be suffering from a hemorrhagic CVA. If your field impression is correct, she will ultimately need a facility capable of neurosurgery. Her family wants her to go to the closest hospital, which is 15 minutes away but does not have neurosurgery capability. The closest facility with immediate neurosurgery capability is 30 minutes away. Which is better for the patient: immediate transfer to a facility that may not be able to completely manage the patient or a lengthened transport time?

Your main objective is to provide quality care, which includes acting as a patient advocate. One way to advocate for quality patient care is to engage in discussions with your ambulance service's medical director about the idea of triaging patients to appropriate hospitals. Before your discussion, you need to do your homework:

- Gather information about how different types of strokes present.
- Research hemorrhagic stroke and its care.
- Identify the capabilities of the local hospitals.
- Create a template guideline to be discussed with the medical director.

During the conversation with the medical director, control your emotions and be prepared to compromise. Speak from facts. Speak from good patient care. Whatever guideline or template you create, ensure that it leaves room for later modification. If you present yourself well, you'll pave the way for more responsibility as a paramedic and increased respect for the profession. You will also improve patient care.

Presentation

Patients with stroke can exhibit a variety of signs and symptoms. Language effects may include slurred speech, aphasia, agnosia, and apraxia. Movement effects—hemiparesis, hemiplegia, arm drifting, facial droop, ptosis, and ataxia—may be observed as well. Sensation effects may include headache (in hemorrhagic CVA), sudden blindness, and sudden unilateral paresthesia. Consciousness problems, such as decreasing LOC, difficulty thinking, seizures, and coma, may be noted. The patient may also develop hypertension.

When faced with a potential diagnosis of stroke, consider following the algorithm developed by the American Heart Association for management of patients with suspected stroke **Figure 28-20 ▶**. The hospital will take different paths of care for each type of stroke. In any event, speedy treatment is essential. For ischemic strokes, fibrinolytics must be administered within 3 hours of onset of symptoms. In hemorrhagic stroke, the more the patient bleeds into the cranium, the greater the potential for increased ICP and brain stem damage.

Prehospital Management

EMS providers need to be involved in educating the community about stroke signs and symptoms, the effects of strokes, and EMS. Too many patients deny their complaints or drive themselves to emergency departments. Reinforce with the public the common signs and symptoms of a stroke and how to activate the EMS system in their community.

Prehospital care of the stroke patient should begin with the standard care outlined previously. Ensure adequate ABCs and blood pressure. Establish the patient's oxygen and glucose level. Establish IV access in case fluids or medications are needed.

During the assessment phase, use a stroke assessment tool—either the Cincinnati Prehospital Stroke Scale **Table 28-8 ▶** or the Los Angeles Prehospital Stroke Screen **Table 28-9 ▶**—to increase the accuracy of your field impressions. Rapid identification is imperative.

Complete a fibrinolytic checklist. Focus on when the signs and symptoms started or when the patient was last seen without new complaints **Table 28-10 ▶**. In some cases, pinning down the exact time the stroke began can be very difficult, such as with patients who live alone. In those cases, ask family or care providers when the patient last seemed "normal." This checklist will allow you to gather information that the emergency department physician will need before fibrinolytics can be considered. Fibrinolytics need to be administered within 3 hours of stroke onset. Don't administer aspirin in the field; it

Documentation and Communication

Stroke documentation points:
- When did the patient last seem "normal"?
- When did the signs and symptoms begin?
- Was there any change in the patient during transport?
- Document the reason for the choice of hospital.

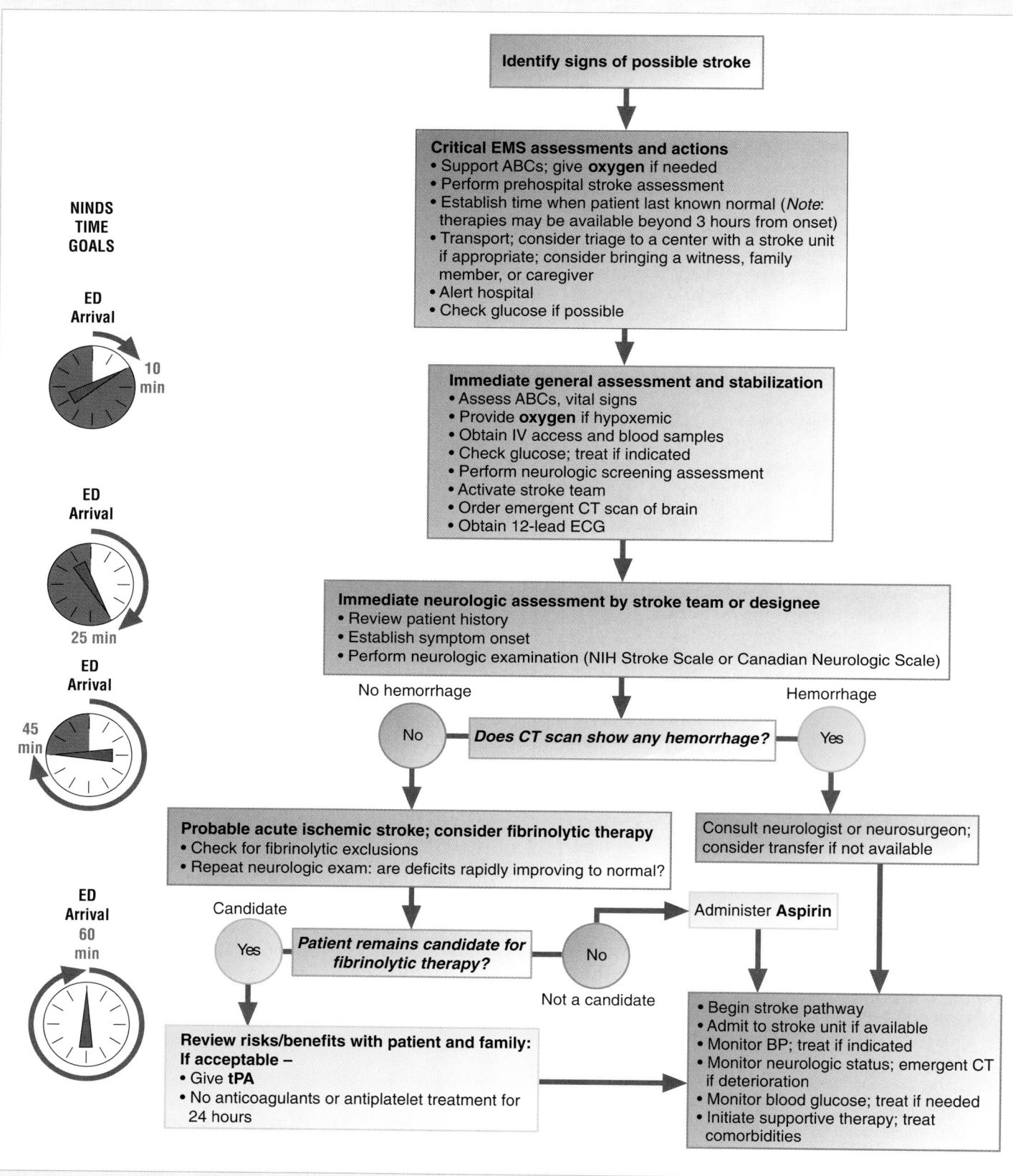

**NINDS
TIME
GOALS**

ED Arrival
10 min

ED Arrival
25 min

ED Arrival
45 min

ED Arrival
60 min

Identify signs of possible stroke

Critical EMS assessments and actions
- Support ABCs; give **oxygen** if needed
- Perform prehospital stroke assessment
- Establish time when patient last known normal (*Note*: therapies may be available beyond 3 hours from onset)
- Transport; consider triage to a center with a stroke unit if appropriate; consider bringing a witness, family member, or caregiver
- Alert hospital
- Check glucose if possible

Immediate general assessment and stabilization
- Assess ABCs, vital signs
- Provide **oxygen** if hypoxemic
- Obtain IV access and blood samples
- Check glucose; treat if indicated
- Perform neurologic screening assessment
- Activate stroke team
- Order emergent CT scan of brain
- Obtain 12-lead ECG

Immediate neurologic assessment by stroke team or designee
- Review patient history
- Establish symptom onset
- Perform neurologic examination (NIH Stroke Scale or Canadian Neurologic Scale)

No hemorrhage — **No** | ***Does CT scan show any hemorrhage?*** | Hemorrhage — **Yes**

Probable acute ischemic stroke; consider fibrinolytic therapy
- Check for fibrinolytic exclusions
- Repeat neurologic exam: are deficits rapidly improving to normal?

Consult neurologist or neurosurgeon; consider transfer if not available

Candidate — **Yes** | ***Patient remains candidate for fibrinolytic therapy?*** | **No** — Not a candidate

Administer **Aspirin**

Review risks/benefits with patient and family: If acceptable –
- Give **tPA**
- No anticoagulants or antiplatelet treatment for 24 hours

- Begin stroke pathway
- Admit to stroke unit if available
- Monitor BP; treat if indicated
- Monitor neurologic status; emergent CT if deterioration
- Monitor blood glucose; treat if needed
- Initiate supportive therapy; treat comorbidities

Figure 28-20 Algorithm for management of patients with suspected stroke.

Table 28-8 | Cincinnati Prehospital Stroke Scale

Assessment	Normal	Abnormal
Facial Droop. Ask the patient to smile and show the teeth.	Both sides of the face move equally well.	One side of the face does not move as well as the other.
Arm Drift. Ask the patient to close the eyes and hold the arms out with palms up for 10 seconds.	Both arms move the same, or both arms do not move.	One arm does not move, or one arm drifts down compared with the other.
Abnormal Speech. Ask the patient to say, "The sky is blue in Cincinnati" or "You can't teach an old dog new tricks."	The patient uses the correct words with no slurring.	The patient slurs words, uses inappropriate words, or is unable to speak.

Interpretation: If any assessment criterion is abnormal, the probability of a stroke is 72%.

Table 28-9 | Los Angeles Prehospital Stroke Screen

Criteria	Yes	Unknown	No
1. Age > 45	❑	❑	❑
2. History of seizures or epilepsy absent	❑	❑	❑
3. Symptoms < 24 hours	❑	❑	❑
4. At baseline, patient is not wheelchair-bound or bedridden	❑	❑	❑
5. Blood glucose between 60 and 400	❑	❑	❑
6. Obvious asymmetry (right versus left) in any of the following three exam categories (must be unilateral):	❑	❑	❑

	Equal	Right Weak	Left Weak
Facial smile/grimace	❑	❑ Droop	❑ Droop
Grip	❑	❑ Weak grip	❑ Weak grip
		❑ No grip	❑ No grip
Arm strength	❑	❑ Drifts down	❑ Drifts down
		❑ Falls rapidly	❑ Falls rapidly

Interpretation: If criteria 1–6 are marked yes, the probability of a stroke is 97%.

You are the Provider Part 4

During transport, the patient's condition did not change. You continue to monitor his mentation, vital signs, and deficits while en route to the hospital. You provide a prompt radio report to the receiving facility, and deliver your patient to the emergency department without incident.

Reassessment	Recording Time: 15 Minutes
Level of consciousness	Alert, with a Glasgow Coma Scale score of 14
Skin	Pale, warm, and dry
Pulse	88 beats/min, strong and irregular
Blood pressure	140 by palpation
Respirations	24 breaths/min
Sao$_2$	100% on 15 L/min via nonrebreathing mask

8. What other important considerations relate to total patient care?

Table 28-10	American Heart Association Fibrinolytic Checklist for Stroke

Use of tissue-type plasminogen activator (tPA) in a patient with acute ischemic stroke. All boxes must be checked before tPA can be given.

Note: The following checklist includes FDA-approved indications and contraindications for tPA administration for acute ischemic stroke. A physician with expertise in acute stroke care may modify this list.

Inclusion Criteria *(all Yes boxes in the section must be checked)*

Yes

❑ Age 18 years or older?
❑ Clinical diagnosis of ischemic stroke with a measurable neurologic deficit?
❑ Time of symptom onset (when patient was last seen normal) well established as < 180 minutes (3 hours) before treatment would begin?

Exclusion Criteria *(all No boxes in "Contraindications" section must be checked)*

Contraindications
No

❑ Evidence of intracranial hemorrhage on pretreatment noncontrast head CT?
❑ Clinical presentation suggestive of subarachnoid hemorrhage even with normal CT?
❑ CT shows multilobar infarction (hypodensity greater than one third cerebral hemisphere)?
❑ History of intracranial hemorrhage?
❑ Uncontrolled hypertension: At the time treatment should begin, systolic pressure remains > 185 mm Hg or diastolic pressure remains > 110 mm Hg despite repeated measurements?
❑ Known arteriovenous malformation, neoplasm, or aneurysm?
❑ Witnessed seizure at stroke onset?
❑ Active internal bleeding or acute trauma (fracture)?
❑ Active bleeding diathesis, including but not limited to
  · Platelet count < 100,000/mm³
  · Heparin received within 48 hours, resulting in an activated partial thromboplastin time (aPTT) that is greater than upper limit of normal for laboratory?
  · Current use of anticoagulant (eg, warfarin sodium) that has produced an elevated international normalized ratio (INR) > 1.7 or prothrombin time (PT) > 15 seconds.*
❑ Within 3 months of intracranial or intraspinal surgery, serious head trauma, or previous stroke?
❑ Arterial pressure at a noncompressible site within past 7 days?

Relative Contraindications/Precautions

Recent experience suggests that under some circumstances—with careful consideration and weighing of risk-benefit ratio—patients may receive fibrinolytic therapy despite one or more relative contraindications. Consider the pros and cons of tPA administration carefully if any of these relative contraindications is present.

  · Only minor or rapidly improving stroke symptoms (clearing spontaneously)
  · Within 14 days of major surgery or serious trauma
  · Recent gastrointestinal or urinary tract hemorrhage (within previous 21 days)
  · Recent acute myocardial infarction (within previous 3 months)
  · Postmyocardial infarction pericarditis
  · Abnormal blood glucose level (< 50 or > 400 mg/dL [< 2.8 or > 22.2 mmol/L])

*In patients without recent use of oral anticoagulants or heparin, treatment with tPA can be initiated before availability of the coagulation study results but should be discontinued if the INR > 1.7 or the partial thromboplastin time is elevated by local laboratory standards.

Source: Reproduced with permission, *2005 American Heart Association Guidelines for Cardiopulmonary Resuscitation and Emergency Cardiovascular Care.* © 2005, American Heart Association.

will help the ischemic CVA but hurt the hemorrhagic CVA. Aspirin should be administered only after a computed tomography (CT) scan or magnetic resonance imaging (MRI) has been completed in the hospital.

Protect any impaired limbs from injury. Patients may not be able to feel or move their arms or legs if they begin to get injured.

Identify an appropriate facility for transport—namely, a facility with a stroke team that's trained in the administration of fibrinolytics. Contact the facility to ensure that its CT/MRI scanner is operational. Some facilities will need to contact technicians to operate the scanners during night hours or weekends, so early hospital notification to the emergency department can

decrease the time until the patient gets scanned. If the patient is rapidly decompensating or you suspect a potential CVA, consider transport to a facility that can do neurosurgery.

Transient Ischemic Attack

Transient ischemic attacks (TIAs) are episodes of cerebral ischemia that do not inflict any permanent damage. Any of the typical presentations associated with a CVA can occur with TIAs, but the TIA signs and symptoms resolve within 24 hours without any residual damage to brain tissue. These ministrokes are often signs of a serious vascular problem that requires medical evaluation. More than one third of patients with TIAs will suffer a CVA soon afterward.

As with strokes, management of TIAs begins with standard care. Follow the same management guidelines as for CVA. Close neurologic assessment is needed. Patients may experience multiple TIAs in a short timeframe—coming and going.

Notes from Nancy
Just because the patient is a known alcoholic or because his breath smells of alcohol, it does not mean that he cannot be in a coma from other causes.

Strongly encourage the patient to be transported. If the individual refuses transportation, appeal to the patient's family for assistance. Encourage the patient to seek medical care very soon. It is important to reinforce the message that the TIA is a warning sign of a very serious and potentially deadly problem with the blood vessels within the brain. In fact, hypertension is the number one preventable cause of strokes and TIAs. Encourage the patient to talk with his or her doctor about blood pressure control and to take any antihypertensive medications prescribed.

Special Considerations
Many medications can alter LOC. Explore all medications that the patient is taking, including prescription, nonprescription, herbal, supplements, homeopathic substances, and illegal drugs. Geriatric patients may have many physicians, many conditions, and many medications. Combinations of medications can result in unexpected neurologic effects.

Altered Level of Consciousness/Coma

Altered mental status has many possible causes, so these calls are relatively common. One way to remember the most common causes is to use the mnemonic AEIOU-TIPS (Alcohol/acidosis, Epilepsy, Insulin, Overdose, Uremia, Trauma, Infection, Psychosis, and Stroke). As with most medical complaints, the history of present illness is vital to identifying the underlying cause of the patient's complaints. An easy approach is to determine when the patient was last seen functioning normally.

Presentation
Evaluate the speed of onset for the altered LOC; this may help distinguish its cause. It is very rare that a person would be absolutely healthy one minute and be unresponsive from infection the next, for example. By contrast, seizures can cause unresponsiveness almost instantly. The common signs and symptoms for altered LOC/coma are thought effects (decreasing LOC, confusion, hallucinations, delusions, psychosis, difficulty thinking, overly sleepy), speech effects (slurred speech, agnosia, apraxia, aphasia), movement effects (ataxia, seizures, posturing), and total unresponsiveness or coma.

Prehospital Management
In the case of altered LOC, care proceeds in two stages. First, the paramedic needs to support vital functions, including securing and maintaining ABCs. Second, the paramedic needs to gather information about the possible cause of the altered LOC. Determine past medical history, evaluate medications, look for signs of trauma, and determine the history of present illness. Does the patient have a medic alert tag? Was drug paraphernalia found near the patient? How was the patient acting before you were called?

In-hospital care will focus on supporting ABCs and attempting to discover the underlying problem. Patients will routinely need blood and urine specimens, radiographs, and CT/MRI scans.

Seizure

Seizures involve sudden, erratic firing of neurons. Patients who have epilepsy commonly have seizures, for example. Patients may experience a wide array of signs and symptoms when having seizures, ranging from one hand shaking or having a taste of pennies in the mouth to movement of every limb or the complete loss of consciousness. They may be aware of the seizure, or they may wake up afterward not knowing what happened.

The paramedic should try to determine the cause of the seizure. In particular, ask about medication compliance. Phenytoin, lorazepam, carbamezapine, and valproic acid are common anticonvulsant medications, but patients may be taking them in insufficient levels to prevent seizures. Patients may feel that they are cured because they haven't suffered a seizure in many months, and stop taking their medications. Children may outgrow their anticonvulsant dosage. Older patients may be unable to afford the medication.

Infants who have a fever may suffer a febrile seizure. Diabetics may have low blood glucose levels and consequently seize. Knowing the cause will help direct management. **Table 28-11** lists many of the causes of seizures.

Classification of Seizures
Seizures can be classified as generalized (affecting large portions of the brain) or partial (affecting a limited area of the brain). The classifications of seizures are outlined in **Table 28-12**.

Within the category of generalized seizures are the grand mal and petit mal types. Grand mal seizures, also called tonic/clonic seizures, present the paramedic with the most challenges. Most grand mal seizures follow a pattern, traveling

Table 28-11	Causes of Seizures	
▪ Abscess	▪ Idiopathic (no known cause)	
▪ AIDS	▪ Inappropriate medication dosage	
▪ Alcohol	▪ Organic brain syndromes	
▪ Birth defect	▪ Recreational drugs	
▪ Brain infections (meningitis, encephalitis)	▪ Stroke or TIA	
▪ Brain trauma	▪ Systemic infection	
▪ Diabetes mellitus	▪ Tumor	
▪ Fever	▪ Uremia (kidney failure)	

Table 28-12 Seizure Classifications	
Generalized Seizures	**Characteristics**
Petit mal (absence) seizure	■ Staring episodes or "absence spells," during which the patient's activity ceases; loss of motor control is uncommon, although eye blinking or lip smacking may occur. ■ Most common in children between 4 and 12 years of age; rarely occurs after age 20. ■ Typically lasts less than 15 seconds, after which the child's LOC immediately returns to normal.
Grand mal (tonic/clonic) seizure	■ Characterized by a loss of consciousness, followed by generalized (entire-body) muscle contraction (tonic phase) alternating with rhythmic "jerking" movements (clonic phase). ■ Often preceded by an aura—a strange taste, smell, or other abnormal sensation—that warns the patient of the impending seizure. ■ Can occur at any age. ■ Often lasts several minutes; may progress to status epilepticus—a prolonged seizure or two consecutive seizures without an intervening lucid interval. ■ Typically followed by a postictal phase, during which the patient is confused, appears sleepy, and may be agitated or combative.
Partial (Focal) Seizures	**Characteristics**
Simple partial seizure	■ Also referred to as focal motor or "Jacksonian March" seizures. ■ Characterized by tonic/clonic activity localized to one part of the body; may spread and progress to a generalized tonic/clonic seizure. ■ No aura or associated loss of consciousness.
Complex partial seizure	■ Also referred to as temporal lobe or psychomotor seizures. ■ Manifests as changes in behavior (mood changes, abrupt bouts of rage). ■ Often preceded by an aura. ■ Usually lasts less than 1 to 2 minutes, after which patient quickly regains normal mental status (no postictal phase).

through each of the following steps in order, although sometimes skipping a step:

1. **Aura.** A sensation the patient experiences before the seizure occurs (eg, muscle twitch, funny taste, seeing lights, hearing a high-pitched noise).
2. **Loss of consciousness.**
3. **Tonic phase.** Body-wide rigidity.
4. **Hypertonic phase.** Arched back and rigidity.
5. **Clonic phase.** Rhythmic contraction of major muscle groups. Arm, leg, head movement; lip smacking; biting; teeth clenching.
6. **Postseizure.** Major muscles relax, nystagmus may still be occurring. Eyes may be "rolled back."
7. **Postictal.** Reset period of the brain. This can take several minutes to hours before the patient gradually returns to the preseizure LOC **Figure 28-21 ▶**. During this time patients are often initially aphasic (unable to speak), confused or unable to follow commands, very emotional, and tired or sleeping. They may present with a headache. Gradually the brain will begin to function normally.

During the seizing process, respirations may become very erratic, loud, and obviously abnormal. Alternately, the patient may stop breathing and become cyanotic. These periods of apnea are usually very short-lived and do not require assistance. If the patient is apneic for more than 30 seconds, immediately begin ventilatory assistance. Another disconcerting aspect of seizures, particularly for the patient, is incontinence.

In contrast to grand mal seizures, petit mal or absence seizures present with little or any movement. The typical

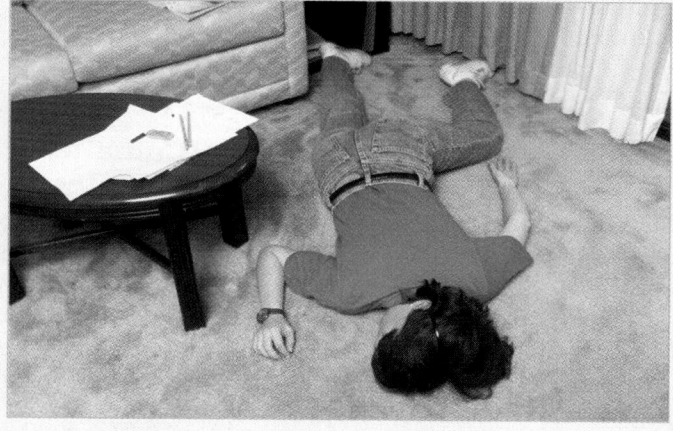

Figure 28-21 A patient who has had a seizure may be found in the postictal state when you arrive. In such a case, ask family members or bystanders to verify that a seizure has occurred and describe how the seizure developed.

patient with petit mal seizures is a child. Classically the child will simply stop moving; he or she may be walking and just stop, may be speaking and stop midsentence, or may be playing and freeze with a toy in the hand. The child will rarely fall. These seizures usually last no more than several seconds. There is no postictal period and no confusion. These may be brought on by flashing lights or hyperventilation.

Partial seizures may be classified as either simple partial or complex partial. Such seizures involve only a limited portion of the brain. They may be localized to just one spot within the brain or they may begin in one spot and move in wave-like fashion to other locations. Such a Jacksonian March wave is akin to the ripples that occur from dropping a pebble in a still pond.

Simple partial seizures involve either movement of one part of the body (frontal lobe) or altered sensations in one part of the body (parietal lobe). An example of a Jacksonian March in a simple partial seizure would be shaking of the left hand, which moves to the left arm, then to the shoulder, then to the head, then to the right arm, then to the right hand, and finally stops. Complex partial seizures involve subtle LOC changes. The patient may become confused, lose alertness, suffer hallucinations, or be unable to speak. The head or eyes may make small movements. Patients typically do not become unresponsive.

> ## Documentation and Communication
>
> Seizure documentation points:
> - Was any aura noted by the patient?
> - Which body parts were in motion?
> - Was the patient awake during the seizure?
> - How long did it last?
> - How was the patient after the seizure?
> - What was the response to your therapy?

Prehospital Management

Most seizures are self-limiting, so you simply need to monitor and protect patients from injuring themselves. Prehospital management of patients with seizure begins with standard care. Quickly determine whether trauma is a concern.

- Where was the patient before the seizure?
- What was the patient doing before the seizure?
- How did the patient get to the current position?
- If the situation is unclear or there is confirmed trauma, perform manual in-line immobilization.

Care during the seizure includes calmness on your part. Don't restrain the patient or try to stop the seizing movement. Prevent the patient from striking objects and becoming injured. Place nothing within the patient's mouth while the seizure is ongoing. If bystanders have placed objects (eg, spoons, butter knives) in the mouth, remove them.

Provide ventilatory assistance only if the seizure or apnea is prolonged. Ventilation of the actively seizing patient will be very difficult. Oral or nasotracheal intubation will be next to impossible during a seizure.

In the postseizure phase, emotional support is very important. Provide privacy. Speak calmly and slowly. Be prepared to repeat yourself. Reorient the patient to place and time. If a child is febrile, encourage parents to administer a drug for fever reduction (acetaminophen or ibuprofen).

Unless a clear and easily reversible cause for the seizure is found, all patients should be transported because seizures can be a warning sign of more serious nervous system problems. If the patient has a known history of seizures, he or she may not wish to go to the hospital. Advise the patient to follow up with the family doctor within 24 hours. The diabetic who is awak-

ened after glucose administration may not wish to be transported. Advise this patient to eat a good meal and follow up with the family doctor.

Any patient who you suspect could seize should have the following care.

- Establish IV access. Diazepam and lorazepam are the drugs of choice to stop seizures. In patients who are seizing and in whom IV access cannot be established, diazepam can be administered rectally at 0.2 mg/kg.
- Place blankets over the rails of the ambulance cot.
- Place blankets over hard surfaces near the patient.
- Ensure that the patient's cot straps are not too tight.

In-hospital management will seek to identify the cause of the seizure. Blood studies, including drug and blood glucose determinations, will be done. CT or MRI scans may be performed.

Status Epilepticus

Status epilepticus is a seizure that lasts for longer than 4 to 5 minutes or consecutive seizures that occur without consciousness returning between seizure episodes. This time frame is arbitrary, however, and some authors suggest that status epilepticus does not occur until 20 minutes of uninterrupted seizing. Refer to your local protocols for guidelines on how long a seizure can continue before you should intervene.

During a seizure, neurons are in a hypermetabolic state (using huge amounts of glucose and producing lactic acid). For a short period, this state does not produce long-term damage. If the seizure continues, however, the body can't remove the waste products effectively or ensure adequate glucose supplies. Such a hypermetabolic state can result in neurons being damaged or killed. The goal of prehospital care is to stop the seizure and ensure adequate ABCs.

Management of status epilepticus begins with standard care. Administer benzodiazepines (diazepam, 5.0 mg IV/IM, or lorazepam, 0.05 mg/kg [maximum 4 mg]). You may repeat diazepam every 10 to 15 minutes to a total dose of 30 mg. If you are unable to obtain IV access, you may give diazepam rectally. You may repeat the lorazepam dose in 10 to 15 minutes, with a maximum dose of 8 mg in 12 hours.

Be prepared to completely control airway and ventilation, as benzodiazepines can cause respiratory depression and arrest. Continue to use airway positioning and bag-mask ventilations until the seizure stops. If benzodiazepines do not quickly control the seizure and the patient can't be ventilated, paralytics may be needed to allow for adequate airway management.

Syncope

Syncope (fainting) is the sudden and temporary loss of consciousness with accompanying loss of postural tone. It affects mainly adults and accounts for nearly 3% of all emergency department visits. The brain uses glucose at a high rate and has no ability to store glucose, so even a 3- to 5-second interruption in blood flow can cause loss of consciousness. The question then becomes, What caused the sudden decrease in cerebral perfusion? **Table 28-13** ▶ lists the common causes of syncope.

Table 28-13	Causes of Syncope
Category	**Causes**
Cardiac rhythm	Bradycardia of any type Sick sinus syndrome Supraventricular tachycardia Torsade de pointes Transient asystole Transient ventricular fibrillation Ventricular tachycardia
Cardiac muscle	Cardiomyopathy Myocardial infarction
Others	Dehydration Hypoglycemia Vasovagal

Table 28-14	Differentiating Syncope from Seizure	
Characteristic	**Syncope**	**Seizure**
Position of patient before event	Standing	Any position
Prodromal signs and symptoms	Dizziness, visual changes, shortness of breath, weakness	Aura: funny taste, seeing lights, hearing sound, twitching
Activity during event	Relaxed	Generalized body movement
Response after event	Quick return of orientation	Slow return of orientation

Presentation

Classically, the patient with syncope is in a standing position when the event occurs. With young adults, the pattern is usually one of vasovagal syncope. The person will experience fear, emotional stress, or pain. Suddenly the room will seem to spin, and the individual will pass out. (This is why you should always seat a patient before drawing blood or starting an IV.) In older adults, cardiac dysrhythmia is a more typical cause of syncope. The patient experiences a sudden run of ventricular tachycardia, the blood pressure drops, and the person falls to the floor. The rhythm terminates, the blood pressure rises, and the individual regains consciousness. In either case, the whole process takes less than 60 seconds.

Patients with syncope usually experience prodrome, signs or symptoms that precede a disease or condition. For syncope, prodromal complaints include feelings of dizziness, weakness, shortness of breath, chest pain, headache, or visual disturbances. Incontinence is possible with syncope, though uncommon. Seizures and syncope can be difficult to differentiate; (Table 28-14 ▲) provides some guidelines for making this distinction.

Prehospital Management

Begin with standard care. Determine if the patient may have experienced trauma during the fall, and take cervical spine precautions as needed. Focus on blood glucose level and likely cardiac causes. Obtain orthostatic vital signs if possible.

Provide emotional support, as syncope can be very embarrassing. Transport the patient to the hospital. Syncope can be a sign of life-threatening cardiac dysrhythmias, stroke, or another serious medical condition.

Headache

Almost everyone has suffered a headache at one time or another. What exactly is hurting? The brain and skull don't have pain receptors. Headache pain originates from the nerves within the scalp, face, blood vessels, and muscles of the neck and head.

Several types of headaches may be identified. Muscle tension headaches—the most common type—are caused by life stress (tension) that results in residual muscle contractions within the face and head. The pain tends to occur on both sides of head and travels from back to front; it is a dull ache or squeezing in nature. The jaw, neck, or shoulders may be stiff or sore.

Migraine headaches are thought to be caused by changes in blood vessel size within the base of the brain. The patient may experience an aura (eg, seeing bright lights) and unilateral, focused pain that then spreads over time. The pain is throbbing, pounding, or pulsating in nature. Nausea or vomiting may be present. These patients prefer dark, quiet environments. Migraines can last several days.

Cluster headaches are rare vascular headaches that start in the face. They occur in groups or clusters. They last only 30 to 45 minutes, but a patient may have several each day. The headaches may recur for days and then stop entirely. They may return the next month. The pattern consists of minor pain around one eye, pain that quickly intensifies and spreads to one side of the face, and a feeling of anxiety.

Sinus headaches are caused by inflammation or infection within the sinus cavities of the face. The pain, which is located in the superior portions of the face, increases with bending the head forward. It's worse when first waking. The patient may have postnasal drip, a sore throat, and nasal discharge.

Other, rare types of headaches include those caused by tumors, inflammation of the temporal artery, strokes, CNS infections, or hypertension. Their presentations vary depending on the underlying cause.

Headaches can be frustrating calls for EMS providers. Many may feel that such calls are a waste of EMS resources—at least, until they experience a migraine of their own (Figure 28-22 ▶). One problem faced by paramedics is that the complaint is entirely subjective; there is no way to "prove" the person is or is not having a severe headache. Try to determine the patient's level of stress, possible infections, and history of headaches. The patient can have various locations and intensity of pain, and may have nausea, vomiting, or light and sound phobia.

The majority of patients have real pain and need assistance from EMS. Others, however, may be drug-seeking, addicted, or abusing medications. Here are some clues to drug-seeking behavior:

- Does the patient have a history of calling 9-1-1 for headaches?
- Do the patient's allergies limit him or her to a small number of narcotic medications?

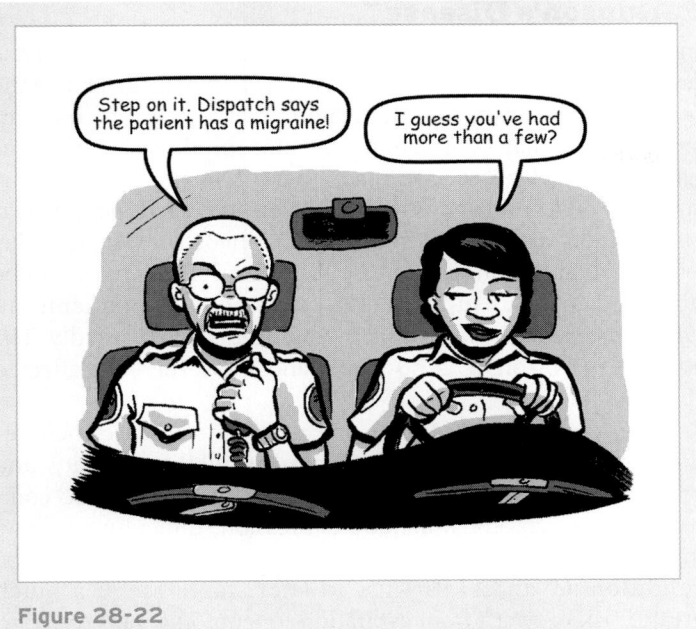

Figure 28-22

the continued destruction of tissue and the immune system's ongoing attempts to kill the agent, swelling can occur.

The underlying cause of an infection within the brain may be an infection of the sinuses, throat, gums, or ears that has spread. The organism can also be injected during trauma to the head. Such an infection has two major consequences: damage to the brain tissue and the presence of an abscess within the cranial vault that leads to increased ICP. These two factors may result in low- or high-grade fever, persistent headache (often localized), drowsiness, confusion, general or focal seizures, nausea and vomiting, focal motor or sensory impairments, and hemiparesis. Abscess usually occurs in people younger than 50 years of age and has a gradual onset.

Prehospital management starts with standard care. Although no specific care is available for the abscess patient in the prehospital setting, the paramedic needs to pay close attention for evidence of increased ICP. Look for changes in LOC, respiratory patterns, and posturing. If needed, begin hyperventilation. Notify the hospital of the critical nature of your patient. Take seizure precautions and be ready to administer diazepam if needed.

In-hospital management will likely involve antibiotics, seizure precautions, and potentially surgical removal of the abscess.

Multiple Sclerosis

Multiple sclerosis (MS) is an autoimmune condition in which the body attacks the myelin sheath of the neurons in the brain and spinal cord, leading to areas of scarring. This disease is more prevalent in temperate regions than in tropical regions. Some evidence suggests that an environmental trigger—perhaps a virus, although none have been identified—begins to focus the attention of the immune system on the myelin. MS typically affects people between the ages of 20 and 40.

The presentation of MS follows a pattern of attacks and remissions. The attacks can vary in intensity and the remissions can vary in length. Patients may recover or have long-term complaints. In the initial attack, double vision and blurred vision are common complaints. Other symptoms include muscle weakness; impairment of pain, temperature, and touch senses; pain (moderate to severe); ataxia; intension tremors; speech disturbances; vision disturbances; vertigo; bladder or bowel dysfunction; sexual dysfunction; depression; euphoria; cognitive abnormalities; and fatigue during attacks.

Prehospital management is supportive. Give standard care. In-hospital treatment will be directed at controlling the symptoms. Anti-inflammatory medications may be administered to decrease the length of the attack. There is currently no cure for MS.

Neoplasm

For the purposes of this chapter, a neoplasm is defined as cancer within the brain or spinal cord. Two basic types of cancer are identified: primary and metastatic. Primary neoplasms begin within the nervous system. Metastatic neoplasms begin in some other part of the body, gain access to the bloodstream

- Is the patient very reluctant to try other pain management options besides narcotics?
- Does the patient suddenly relax after being told that narcotics are on the way?

No single presentation characteristic should lead you to classify the patient as drug-seeking. Instead, consider the entire environment. What has the patient done to manage this headache? When did it start? How bad is it? Even if you suspect drug-seeking behavior, it would be inappropriate to withhold medication from the patient without first communicating with medical direction. Upon arrival at the hospital, relay your concerns to emergency department personnel in a fact-based conversation. Point out specifics of behavior, comments, history, and other factors that have led you to suspect possible drug-seeking.

Be cautious, as headaches can indicate a more serious problem. Give standard care. Consider stroke, abscess, tumor, hypertension, and CNS infections. Ask which medications the patient has taken. Many patients will appreciate a darkened, quiet environment, so don't use lights and sirens if transporting. Medications for pain management could include meperidine, morphine, and ketorolac. Also consider promethazine for nausea or vomiting. In-hospital management would include analgesics and ruling out serious medical problems.

Abscess

Abscesses result when an infectious agent invades the brain or spinal cord. The bacteria or fungi then attack brain cells and destroy tissue. In response, the immune system attempts to kill the infectious agent but fails to do so. To prevent the bacteria or fungi from spreading, the body erects a barrier around the area. The area within the barrier contains the infectious agent, dead or dying brain cells, dead white blood cells, and white blood cells that continue fighting the infection. Over time, with

or lymphatic system, and then take up residence within the nervous system. Lung and breast cancers are the cancers that most commonly metastasize to the CNS. Once mature, neurons no longer divide, so only rarely do they become cancerous. Primary CNS cancers are usually caused by mitosis errors in the support structures of the CNS.

Headache, nausea and vomiting, seizures, changes in mental status, and stroke-like signs and symptoms are common in cases of neoplasm. The rate and intensity of these signs and symptoms depend on the cancer's growth rate and location. Patients may have months of headaches, or suddenly experience a seizure without any prior complaints.

Prehospital management is supportive. Watch for status epilepticus and increased ICP. All patients with new-onset seizures or chronic headaches that cannot be managed need medical evaluation. In-hospital management is complex and depends on the type of cancer and location.

Dystonia

Dystonia are marked by severe, abnormal muscle spasms that cause bizarre contortions, repetitive motions, or postures. These movements are involuntary and often painful. The initial episode usually occurs before the patient is in his or her 40s. Sudden onset may be precipitated by stress or continuous use of a muscle group. Patients tend to have normal intelligence and no psychiatric medical history.

Dystonia is both a sign and a condition. Some patients who take antipsychotic medications may suffer a sudden onset of bizarre contortions of the face or body; this is considered a secondary dystonia. Primary dystonias occur for unknown reasons, although a defect in the body's ability to process neurotransmitters is thought to lie at the heart of this problem. Spasmodic torticollis is a primary dystonia in which the neck muscles contract, twisting the head to one side and pulling it forward or backward. The head then remains painfully frozen in that position.

Prehospital management should focus on ruling out other problems such as seizures, strokes, or psychiatric medication reaction. If you suspect a dystonic reaction to antipsychotics, diphenhydramine is the drug of choice to stop the contraction. Unfortunately, this medication is ineffective in primary dystonias. Give standard care. Regardless of the underlying cause, dystonias are socially upsetting as patients suddenly twist and writhe uncontrollably. Providing compassionate care is critical. In-hospital management involves a variety of medication options to control the condition. There currently is no cure for dystonia.

Parkinson's Disease

In Parkinson's disease, the substantia nigra (the portion of the brain that produces dopamine) becomes damaged. Dopamine is the neurotransmitter that, among other things, ensures smooth muscular contractions. Parkinson's disease symptoms have a gradual onset that spans months to years. The initial signs are often unilateral tremors. Over time, as dopamine levels fall, more areas of the body become involved. Genetics play an important role in this disease. Parkinson-like activity can be observed in head injuries and some overdose patients, in which progression of the symptoms occurs more rapidly. The average age of onset is 60 years, and more men are affected than women.

The classic presentation of Parkinson's disease includes four characteristics: tremor, postural instability, rigidity, and bradykinesia. Rest tremors and postural tremors are also common. Other symptoms include depression, difficulty swallowing, speech impairments, and fatigue. Prognosis is poor as the condition advances. Patients in later stages are at a much greater risk of death from aspiration, pneumonia, falls, or complications due to immobility.

Prehospital management involves standard care and emotional support. In-hospital management will include levodopa, which may temporarily restore dopamine levels. Other medications, surgery, and modification of diet and exercise are also options.

Trigeminal Neuralgia

Trigeminal neuralgia, also called tic douloureux, is an inflammation of the trigeminal nerve (fifth cranial nerve). The trigeminal nerve receives sensory information from the face. The usual cause of trigeminal neuralgia is irradiation by an artery lying too close to the nerve. Over time, as the artery changes diameter to meet blood supply needs, this motion grates the myelin sheath off the nerve. With its insulation gone, the nerve may "short out," causing pain without trauma to the area. Patients are usually older than age 50, and more women are affected than men.

Patients experience severe shock-like or stabbing pain, usually on one side of the face. These attacks can last for several minutes to several months. They may be triggered by touching the face, speaking, brushing the teeth, eating, putting on clothing, the wind—essentially any activity that stimulates the face. There is typically no loss of taste, hearing, or facial sensation with this condition. Likewise, there is no loss of motor control over the face, so facial droop, ptosis, and difficulty controlling the airway are very uncommon.

You are the Provider Part 5

A CT scan showed a mild stroke in the parietal lobe. The patient was not a candidate for fibrinolytics because the onset of his stroke couldn't be determined. He soon returned home with the support of his family and full-time nursing care. Because you rapidly recognized his stroke and transported him with the appropriate sense of urgency, the emergency department nurses and doctors were able to promptly confirm the type of stroke and begin appropriate care.

Although not life-threatening, this condition can be quite debilitating. Patients experience severe pain. Some will stay indoors, eat softer foods, or stop washing their faces in an effort to prevent an attack. These patients need compassion and understanding.

Prehospital care consists of standard care. Meperidine, morphine, or ketorolac may be indicated to help with pain management. Try to limit conversations to decrease facial movement. Administer oxygen if the patient is in respiratory distress or has a low pulse oximeter reading. Use of a nasal cannula or a nonrebreathing mask can instigate an attack. Even trying to administer blow-by oxygen could be painful to the patient. Long-term treatment for this condition is medication (carbamazepine or phenytoin) to calm the trigeminal nerve and sometimes surgery to place a barrier between the nerve and the artery.

Bell's Palsy

Bell's palsy is a temporary paralysis of the facial nerve (seventh cranial nerve). The facial nerve controls the muscles on each side of the face, including those used in eye blinking and facial expressions such as smiling and frowning. It also controls the tear glands and the saliva glands. Finally, the facial nerve transmits taste sensations from the tongue.

Patients typically experience a minor infection before Bell's palsy appears. The attack is very sudden and can easily be confused with a stroke. Signs and symptoms include ptosis, facial droop or weakness, drooling, and loss of the ability to taste. This condition strikes all races and both sexes equally. It is more common in middle-aged people (between 15 and 60 years old).

Bell's palsy will often resolve within 2 weeks. Prehospital management involves standard care. Make sure that these patients are not suffering from a stroke. Complete a full assessment. When in doubt, treat the case as if it were a stroke. In-hospital treatment for Bell's palsy includes corticosteroids (eg, prednisone) and acyclovir, which helps manage viral infections.

Amyotrophic Lateral Sclerosis

Amyotrophic lateral sclerosis (ALS), also known as Lou Gehrig's disease, is a disease that involves the death of voluntary motor neurons, for unclear reasons. One theory suggests that the body's immune system selectively attacks and kills these motor neurons. Some evidence indicates that genetics may play a role. ALS is more common in middle-aged males of any race.

Initially, this condition is rather subtle and progresses without drawing notice. Fatigue, general weakness of muscle groups, and difficulty performing routine activities such as eating, writing, and dressing are early signs. Patients may also experience difficulty speaking. As ALS progresses, the patient loses his or her ability to walk, move the arms, eat, and speak. The speed of progression differs for every patient. Because this condition affects only the motor neurons, patients remain completely aware of their surroundings.

The average person who is diagnosed with ALS will die within 3 to 5 years. As the destruction of motor neurons continues, eventually patients are unable to breathe effectively without ventilatory assistance. Patients die of respiratory infections or other complications related to immobility.

Prehospital treatment for these patients is standard care. Assess the ability to swallow, and monitor the airway closely. Patients may be surrounded by a variety of home medical technology, including feeding pumps, IV pumps, long-term IV access ports, and ventilators. Transportation becomes complicated by the management of this technology. General guidelines include asking for guidance from the family or home health care provider related to the operation of the technology. If necessary, disconnect the patient from the technology, after consulting medical direction, and transport.

In-hospital care for ALS is geared toward supporting vital functions. Patients will undergo physical therapy to help strengthen their remaining neurons and muscles. Medications can be given to assist with some of the symptoms; however, there is no cure for ALS.

Guillain-Barré Syndrome

Guillain-Barré syndrome is a rare condition that is rather scary for most patients. It begins as weakness and tingling sensations in the legs. This weakness moves up the legs and begins to affect the thorax and arms. It can quickly become severe and lead to paralysis. In fact, the transition from being able to walk and speak to needing a ventilator to breathe may take as little as several hours. Most patients will experience maximum muscle weakness and paralysis within 2 weeks.

The cause of this condition is unclear, although some degree of immune response appears to be present. Patients usually report having a minor respiratory or gastrointestinal infection prior to the onset of weakness. One theory is that the infectious agent creates a situation in which the body attacks its own neurons. This attack damages the myelin, thereby causing "shorting" of the signals traveling along the axon.

The reversal of this disease can be almost as dramatic as its onset. Some patients will have a complete recovery without residual weakness in as little as several weeks. About one third retain some degree of weakness after 3 years. Some patients will require ventilatory assistance for the remainder of their lives.

Prehospital management includes standard care and close assessment of the patient's ability to effectively protect the airway and ventilate. Because of the sheer terror that patients can experience, a comforting voice and use of therapeutic touch are important.

In-hospital management includes plasmapheresis (exchanging the plasma within the blood) and immunoglobulin injections. These therapies decrease the time until recovery.

Poliomyelitis

Poliomyelitis is a viral infection that is transmitted by the fecal-oral route. Its incidence in the United States peaked in the 1950s, after which a very effective vaccine was developed. No cases of spontaneous polio infection have been reported in the United States since 1979, and polio will likely be eradicated worldwide within 10 years. The vast majority of patients who contract the virus do not become ill. Polio can occur at any age, but very young and older patients are at greatest risk. Signs and symptoms may begin as soon as one week after infection. In the most severe cases, they include sore throat, nausea, vomiting, diarrhea, stiff neck, and weakness or paralysis of muscles.

Prehospital management consists of standard care. In severe cases, patients will need ventilatory assistance. In-hospital care for patients with the acute illness is directed at hydration, ventilation, and calorie support until the immune system gains control over the infection.

The way the virus damages the nervous system places patients at risk for problems decades after the initial infection. In the initial infection, the virus attacks motor neurons within the brain and brain stem, which causes the classic signs of weakness and paralysis. The remaining neurons then begin to send out new axons to try to compensate for this loss, which allows the patient to regain function. Over time, these neurons maintain their unusually high workload. When they begin to break down and die, the patient may develop postpolio syndrome. As a consequence, some patients who suffered polio in the early part of the 20th century (most are older than 60 years) are now having difficulty swallowing, weakness, fatigue, or breathing problems. Typically, wherever patients had symptoms when they were originally infected, they experience symptoms again, albeit in a milder form. Prehospital treatment is standard care, with emphasis on possible airway obstruction due to swallowing difficulties. In-hospital treatment includes physical therapy and experimental medications.

Cerebral Palsy

Cerebral palsy (CP) is a developmental condition in which damage is done to the brain (often the frontal lobe). Although it was believed that perinatal (around the time of birth) hypoxia was the primary cause, research has shown that this actually accounts for less than 10% of cases. Infections, jaundice, or Rh incompatibility also appear to be possible causes. The condition is self-limiting and does not worsen over time. Babies who are low birth weight, premature, delivered breech, or from multiple births (eg, twins or triplets) are at higher risk for CP.

The presentation of CP begins in infancy. Developmental milestones such as walking or crawling may be delayed. The type and extent of damage soon become apparent. In spastic CP (70% to 80% of cases), the muscles are in a near-constant state of contraction. If both lower legs are affected, patients will have a classic scissors walk in which the lower legs turn inward, with the legs remaining stiff and the knees almost touching. Other types of CP involve slow, uncontrolled writhing movements; tremors; or difficulties with coordination.

Prehospital management is supportive. Provide standard care. Patients may have ambulatory assistive devices (eg, wheelchairs, walkers, crutches, canes, leg braces) that will need to be transported along with them. In-hospital management is based on the particular set of symptoms. There is no cure or correction for the damage. Instead, care is directed at maximiz-

ing the child's abilities through surgery on affected limbs and physical/occupational therapy.

Spina Bifida

Spina bifida is a developmental condition resulting from a neural tube defect. Because the neural tube does not close (for unknown reasons), a portion of the spinal cord remains outside its normal location. The severity of the condition depends on where the defect lies on the cord and how much it is displaced from normal. In spina bifida occulta, one small section of vertebrae is malformed and slightly displaced. The mildest form of spina bifida, it rarely has any significant clinical features and patients may not even know the malformation is present. In the most severe form, known as myelomeningocele, a portion of the spinal cord remains completely outside the vertebral column and outside of the skin. There are also two intermediary forms of spina bifida.

Consequences of spina bifida can range from no complications to complete loss of motor and sensory functions below the defect. Patients may have muscle problems ranging from mild defects to paralysis, experience seizures, or have severe neurologic impairments. In the most severe forms, the defect interferes with normal movement of CSF. CSF is made within the brain, circulates, and is then reabsorbed. Hydrocephalus (water on the brain) is common in severe spina bifida because the CSF continues to be produced but cannot circulate effectively. Pressure builds within the brain, causing increased ICP problems and seizures.

EMS may be called for problems with spina bifida patients related to medical technology, seizures, trauma, or infections. Prehospital management is standard care. Be aware that many of these patients have latex allergies. In the most severe cases of spina bifida, children are in need of multiple types of medical technology, including feeding tubes, long-term IV access, ventilatory support, ambulatory assistive devices, and intraventricular shunts (designed to drain excess CSF from within the brain's ventricles). To avoid complications, consult with family and other home health care personnel when attempting to transport the patient. In-hospital management will be supportive. It is possible to reimplant the spinal cord, even while the fetus remains within the uterus, but the damage to the nerve tissue is permanent.

Myasthenia Gravis

Acetylcholine is an important neurotransmitter needed to allow for muscular contraction. In myasthenia gravis, the body creates antibodies against the acetylcholine receptors. The thymus gland (where T-cells mature) is believed to play a role in the production of these antibodies. As acetylcholine levels fall, muscle weakness begins. This weakness most commonly affects the eyes, eyelids, and facial muscles. Some patients will have difficulty swallowing or speaking, or leg or arm weakness. Patients suffer no sensory impairment. Myasthenia gravis usually affects women younger than 40 and men older than 60.

Myasthenia crisis is a sudden increase in the destruction of acetylcholine, resulting in weakness in the respiratory muscles. As a result, patients can become hypoxic. Infections, emotional stress, or reactions to medications can trigger this crisis.

Standard care will effectively manage these patients in the field. Be prepared to assist with ventilations in patients with crisis. In-hospital management includes removal of the thymus gland, medications to boost neurotransmitter levels, and immunosuppressants.

Alzheimer's Disease

Alzheimer's disease (discussed in more detail in Chapter 42) is the most common form of dementia. Dementia is a chronic deterioration of a person's personality, memory, and ability to think. Alzheimer's disease is a progressive organic condition in which neurons die; there is no definitive treatment for the destroyed neurons. Prehospital management is standard care.

Peripheral Neuropathy

Peripheral neuropathy comprises a group of conditions in which the nerves leaving the spinal cord become damaged. As a consequence, the signals moving to or from the brain become distorted. Causes of peripheral neuropathy include trauma, toxins, tumors, autoimmune attacks, and metabolic disorders. Trigeminal neuralgia and Guillain-Barré syndrome are examples. The remainder of this discussion focuses on the most common form, diabetic neuropathy. Diabetic neuropathy is frequently seen in diabetic patients older than age 50; more males than females are affected. Its onset is gradual, occurring over months and years.

As blood glucose levels rise, the peripheral nerves may become damaged, resulting in misfiring and shorting of signals. Affected individuals may then experience sensory or motor impairment. Loss of sensation, numbness, burning sensations, pain, paresthesia, and muscle weakness are common. Patients may eventually lose the ability to feel their feet or other areas.

Management in the prehospital setting is supportive. Provide standard care. In-hospital management will include pain medication. The use of antidepressants and anticonvulsants seems to have a positive effect on calming the peripheral nerves.

Muscular Dystrophy

Muscular dystrophy (MD) is a nonneurologic condition of genetic origin marked by the degeneration of muscular tissue. The defective DNA causes an error in muscle tissue, such that the malformed muscle cells rupture more easily. MD is diagnosed at age 2 to 5 years and occurs only in males. Its onset is gradual, with progression over months to years.

Several forms of MD exist, each distinguished by the involvement of a particular gene and a unique set of characteristics. Generally, MD presents with progressive muscle weakness, delayed development of muscle motor skills, ptosis, drooling, and poor muscle tone. The most common type of MD, Duchenne's, manifests itself in childhood and can include damage to the respiratory and cardiac muscles. These patients have a much shortened life expectancy, rarely living beyond their middle 20s. They often die from pneumonia or cardiogenic shock.

Standard care is effective in these patients. In severe cases, ventilatory support may be necessary. Blood pressure support may be required; fluids and dopamine may be needed to manage damaged heart muscle. These severely ill patients will have extensive use of home medical technology. In-hospital management is supportive, as there is no cure for MD.

Conclusion

Neurologic patients can present a major challenge to the paramedic. To avoid becoming overwhelmed, follow a methodical and systematic approach to the assessment and care of these patients. Use the same format for all of your physical exams. Focus your care on providing an environment that will facilitate optimal nervous system functioning. Reassess the patient after your interventions to note any changes. You are part of a health care team, so be aware of how your care will affect later activities within the emergency department. Know the material within this book. When you have mastered this information, you should be able to provide your patients with the highest level of care and your profession with an example of excellence.

You are the Provider Summary

1. **What do you suspect as the reason(s) why Mr. Hishari is on the floor?**

This patient could be on the floor for any number of reasons, including but not limited to a syncopal episode, loss of balance with a fall, sudden onset of weakness, or exacerbation of an underlying medical condition. At this point, there are many possibilities, which will require further investigation in both history-taking and physical assessment.

2. **How would you prioritize those reasons?**

As a paramedic, it's your job to recognize and treat life-threatening conditions. In some instances, definitive care can be provided; in other cases, treatment options are limited. With some underlying traumatic and medical emergencies, your job is to simply recognize the signs and symptoms, provide prompt transport to the nearest appropriate facility, and initiate supportive care without delay to definitive care.

3. **Given the information you have now, what do you think could be this patient's underlying illness, injury, or condition?**

Given the new information obtained, you believe the patient is experiencing a CVA. This life-threatening condition requires immediate recognition and prompt transport. There is no sure way of knowing what sort of stroke this patient is experiencing, so the goal of the paramedic is to ensure the fastest possible time to the hospital.

4. **Do your assessment and treatment priorities ever change?**

Although concern with ABCs is first, assessment and treatment priorities must be flexible to avoid tunnel vision and misappropriate field diagnosis. At first, the patient appeared to have confusion most likely as a result of a low blood glucose level. After you assessed his blood glucose level and found it to be within appropriate levels, your overall impression changed, causing you to consider other reasons for his decreased LOC.

5. **What are appropriate interventions?**

Appropriate care would include placing the patient on high-flow oxygen, obtaining an ECG, initiating at least one IV for the purposes of collecting blood samples and providing a port for administration of fibrinolytics if deemed necessary by emergency department staff, and completing a fibrinolytic checklist prior to arrival at the hospital.

6. **Would you choose to place this patient in manual in-line spinal precautions?**

Keeping in mind that "time is brain," you'll have to make the determination as to whether to place the patient in spinal precautions. If the mechanism of injury indicates risk for spinal fracture, if you are unsure, or if your local protocols dictate it, you should immobilize this patient. As with any intervention, you should consider whether this step is appropriate.

7. **What places this patient at greater risk for cerebrovascular accident?**

His history of atrial fibrillation places your patient at greater risk for ischemic stroke. Clots could develop in his atria and travel to the brain, resulting in stroke.

8. **What other important considerations relate to total patient care?**

For patients who are unable to communicate, this experience can be quite frustrating and frightening. If possible, use other forms of communication. If you are unable to obtain information or understand the patient, do everything you can to ease his or her anxiety and fear.

Prep Kit

▇ Ready for Review

- The nervous system is responsible for thought, judgment, personality, memory, emotions, voluntary motor activity, interpretation of sensory stimulation, and various autonomic activities within the body.
- Blood flow to the brain is described by the equation CPP = MAP − ICP.
- The nervous system is critical in maintaining airway control.
- Two abnormal postures that indicate brain damage in an unconscious patient are decorticate posturing (moving arms toward the core) and decerebrate posturing (moving arms away from body).
- Use the Glasgow Coma Scale to help determine a patient's level of consciousness, evaluate his or her responses to eye opening and verbal and motor skills, and guide care.
- Facial droop on one side of the face or a drooping eyelid can indicate a neurologic condition.
- Problems such as slurring or difficulty recognizing objects can signify a neurologic problem. Three forms of language problems are receptive aphasia, expressive aphasia, and global aphasia.
- Pupil shape, size, motion, and reactivity are indicators of nervous system functioning.
- Have the patient hold the arms out in front of the body and close the eyes. If one arm drifts away, the patient may have experienced a stroke.
- Abnormal, involuntary muscle contractions, such as tremors and seizures, can indicate a neurologic problem.
- Sensation can also be affected by nervous system conditions.
- The three major elements that the brain needs to function are oxygen, glucose, and normal temperature.
- Managing the neurologic patient includes administering IV solutions, monitoring the ECG, checking blood glucose levels, managing intracranial pressure, evaluating the patient's temperature, and providing emotional support.
- You may be able to administer dextrose or glucagon to treat low blood glucose levels, depending on your local protocol.
- Naloxone may be given to treat unconscious patients or those with suspected narcotic overdose.
- If you can't take the patient's temperature, use patient history to determine it. Don't actively warm or cool patients.
- Stroke is a serious medical condition in which blood supply to areas of the brain is interrupted. Ischemic stroke results from a blocked blood vessel. Hemorrhagic stroke results from bleeding within the brain.
- Patients with stroke can be affected in their language, movement, sensation, level of consciousness, and blood pressure.
- Time is essential in managing strokes. Fibrinolytics can be administered for ischemic strokes, but must be administered within 3 hours of stroke onset.
- Use the Cincinnati Prehospital Stroke Scale or Los Angeles Prehospital Stroke Screen during assessment of a potential stroke patient. You may also use a fibrinolytic checklist.
- Stroke patients should be transported to facilities trained in the administration of fibrinolytics, and to facilities with CT or MRI equipment.
- A TIA looks like a stroke but will resolve without damage; however, one third of patients with a TIA will eventually experience a stroke.
- Management of TIAs is the same as for stroke. Encourage the patient to be transported.
- Use the AEIOU-TIPS mnemonic to assess a patient with an altered level of consciousness. Evaluate the speed and onset. Common

effects of altered LOC are changes in thought, speech, and movement. Total unresponsiveness can also result.
- Care for a patient with an altered LOC includes the ABCs and gathering information about the possible cause.
- Seizures are the sudden erratic firing of neurons, generally characterized by involuntary shaking. They are classified as generalized (affecting large areas of the brain) or partial (affecting limited areas of the brain).
- Generalized seizures include grand mal and petit mal seizures. Grand mal seizures generally consist of an aura, loss of consciousness, tonic/clonic movement, and the postictal phase. Petit mal seizures involve little or no movement. Instead, the person—usually a child—simply "freezes."
- Partial seizures are categorized as simple or complex. Simple partial seizures involve movement or altered sensation in one part of the body. Complex partial seizures involve subtle changes in level of consciousness.
- When caring for a patient with a seizure, don't try to stop the seizing movement. Prevent the patient from injuring himself or herself. Once the seizure has ceased, provide care and emotional support.
- Status epilepticus is a seizure lasting more than 4 or 5 minutes or consecutive seizures without return of consciousness between events.
- Care for a patient with status epilepticus includes administration of benzodiazepines and management of airway and ventilation.
- Syncope (fainting) is the sudden loss of consciousness and postural tone. It can be caused by cardiac problems, dehydration, hypoglycemia, or a vasovagal reaction.
- Care for patient who experienced syncope includes standard care and emotional support.
- Types of headaches include muscle tension headaches, migraines, cluster headaches, sinus headaches, and headaches caused by a tumor, stroke, infections, hypertension, or inflammation of the temporal artery.
- Care for patients with headaches includes standard care, a thorough history, potentially medication administration, and providing a dark, quiet environment.
- An abscess is a walled-off infectious area within the cranial vault. Symptoms include a fever, persistent headache, drowsiness, confusion, general or focal seizures, nausea and vomiting, focal motor or sensory impairments, and hemiparesis. Provide standard care.
- Multiple sclerosis is an autoimmune disorder that damages myelin of the brain and spinal cord. Patients can experience attacks and remissions, muscle weakness, changes in sensation, pain, ataxia, intension tremors, and speech and vision changes. Prehospital management is supportive.
- Neoplasm, for the purposes of this chapter, is cancer in the brain or spinal cord. It can have a gradual or sudden onset. Symptoms include headaches, seizures, change in mental status, and stroke-like signs and symptoms. Prehospital care is supportive.
- Dystonia is the sudden onset of severe, sometimes painful, abnormal muscle contractions. Prehospital care involves ruling out other causes and administering diphenhydramine if you suspect the dystonia is a result of a reaction to antipsychotics.
- In Parkinson's disease, the brain cannot produce dopamine. These patients have tremors, bradykinesia, postural instability, and rigidity. Prehospital management is standard care.
- Trigeminal neuralgia is irritation of the trigeminal nerve. Patients experience severe electric shock-like pain in the face, which can be triggered by any activity that stimulates the face. Prehospital management is standard care.

- Bell's palsy is a temporary, sudden paralysis of the facial nerve triggered by an infection. The patient may have ptosis, facial droop, facial weakness, drooling, and loss of the ability to taste. Prehospital management is standard care.
- Amyotrophic lateral sclerosis is a disease in which the motor neurons die. It has a gradual onset with fatigue, weakness, ataxia, severe body-wide weakness, and eventual immobility. Prehospital management is standard care.
- Guillain-Barré syndrome is a rare condition characterized by a sudden onset of weakness and paresthesia ascending from the toes to the head. Patients usually have an infection prior to the attack. Prehospital management is standard care with airway management.
- Poliomyelitis is a viral infection that attacks the myelin of motor neurons in the brain and brain stem. Symptoms include a sore throat, nausea, vomiting, diarrhea, a stiff neck, and weakness or paralysis of muscles. Prehospital management is standard care with careful attention to the airway.
- Patients who had poliomyelitis in the past may develop postpolio syndrome later in life in which they experience the same symptoms as in the original infection, only milder.
- Cerebral palsy is a developmental condition in which the frontal lobe of the brain suffers damage. Infants may have developmental delays in walking and standing, muscles in constant contraction, a scissors walking gait, and tremors. Prehospital management is supportive.
- Spina bifida is a developmental condition in which the neural tube fails to close completely and part of the spinal cord or vertebrae are damaged and misplaced outside the normal position. Prehospital management is standard care.
- Myasthenia gravis is a condition in which the body creates antibodies against acetylcholine receptors, causing acetylcholine levels to fall. Symptoms include weakness of the face and eyes, difficulty swallowing, and leg weakness. Prehospital management is standard care.
- Peripheral neuropathy is a group of conditions characterized by damage to the peripheral nerves. Diabetic neuropathy occurs from high blood glucose levels. Patients may have paresthesia, burning sensation, and muscle weakness. Prehospital care is supportive.
- Muscular dystrophy is a group of nonneurologic conditions in which muscle tissue degenerates. It generally presents with progressive muscle weakness, delayed development of muscle motor skills, ptosis, drooling, and poor muscle tone. Prehospital management is standard care, possible with ventilatory support.

■■ Vital Vocabulary

abscesses Areas created as a result of infection within the brain or spinal cord, in which brain cells have been attacked and tissue destroyed. The immune system erects a wall to prevent spread of the infection, which results in a pus-filled area buried in tissue.

adrenal glands Endocrine glands located on top of the kidneys that release adrenaline when stimulated by the sympathetic nervous system.

agnosia Inability to connect an object with its correct name.

Alzheimer's disease A progressive organic condition in which neurons die, causing dementia.

amyotrophic lateral sclerosis (ALS) Also known as Lou Gehrig's disease, this disease strikes the voluntary motor neurons, causing their death. It is characterized by fatigue and general weakness of muscle groups; eventually, the patient will not be able to walk, eat, or speak.

anesthesia Lack of feeling within a body part.

anisocoria Unequal pupils (difference greater than 1 mm).

apraxia Inability to connect an object with its proper use.

ataxia Alteration in the ability to perform coordinated motions like walking.

aura Sensations experienced before an attack occurs. Common in seizures and migraine headaches.

axon A projection from a neuron that makes connections with adjacent cells.

Bell's palsy A temporary paralysis of the facial nerve (7th cranial nerve), which controls the muscles on each side of the face.

bradykinesia The slowing down of voluntary body movements. Found in Parkinson's disease.

brain stem The area of the brain between the spinal cord and cerebrum, surrounded by the cerebellum; controls functions that are necessary for life, such as respirations.

central nervous system (CNS) The brain and spinal cord.

cerebellum The region of the brain essential in coordinating muscle movements of the body.

cerebral palsy (CP) A developmental condition in which damage is done to the brain. It presents during infancy as delays in walking or crawling, and can take on a spastic form in which muscles are in a near constant state of contraction.

cerebrovascular accident (CVA) An interruption of blood flow to the brain that results in the loss of brain function.

clonic activity Type of seizure movement involving the contraction and relaxation of muscle groups.

coma A state in which one does not respond to verbal or painful stimuli.

decerebrate posturing Abnormal extension of the arms with rotation of the wrists along with toe pointing. This indicates brain stem damage.

decorticate posturing Abnormal flexion of the arms toward the chest with the toes pointed. This indicates lower cerebral damage.

decussation Movement of nerves from one side of the brain to the opposite side of the body.

dementia The slow onset of progressive disorientation, shortened attention span, and loss of cognitive function.

diencephalon The part of the brain between the brain stem and the cerebrum that includes the thalamus, the subthalamus, hypothalamus, and epithalamus.

dystonia Contractions of the body into a bizarre position.

endotoxin A toxin released by some bacteria when they die.

exotoxin A toxin that is secreted by living cells to aid in the death and digestion of other cells.

expressive aphasia Damage to or loss of the ability to speak.

gait Walking pattern.

Glasgow Coma Scale (GCS) Evaluation tool used to determine level of consciousness. Effective in determining patient outcomes.

global aphasia Damage to or loss of both the ability to speak and the ability to understand speech.

Guillain-Barré syndrome A rare condition that begins as weakness and tingling sensations in the legs and moves to the arms and thorax; it can lead to paralysis within 2 weeks.

hemiparesis Weakness of one side of the body.

hemiplegia Paralysis of one side of the body.

hemorrhagic One of the two main types of stroke; occurs as a result of bleeding inside the brain.

hypothalamus The most inferior portion of the diencephalon, it is responsible for control of many bodily functions, including heart rate, digestion, sexual development, temperature regulation, emotion, hunger, thirst, and regulation of the sleep cycle.

idiopathic Of no known cause.

intension tremors Tremors that occur when trying to accomplish a task.

ischemic One of the two main types of stroke; occurs when blood flow to a particular part of the brain is cut off by a blockage (eg, a clot) inside a blood vessel.

Jacksonian March The wave-like movement of a seizure from a point of focus to other areas of the brain.

limbic system Structures within the cerebrum and diencephalon that influence emotions, motivation, mood, and sensations of pain and pleasure.

medulla oblongata The inferior portion of the midbrain, which serves as a conduction pathway for both ascending and descending nerve tracts.

midbrain The part of the brain that is responsible for helping to regulate level of consciousness.

multiple sclerosis (MS) An autoimmune condition in which the body attacks the myelin of the brain and spinal cord, leading to gaps in the insulation normally provided by the myelin, causing scarring.

muscular dystrophy (MD) A nonneurologic condition of genetic origin in which defective DNA causes an error in the creation of muscle tissue, resulting in the degeneration of muscular tissue. This presents with progressive muscle weakness, delayed development of muscle motor skills, ptosis, drooling, and poor muscle tone.

myasthenia gravis A condition in which the body creates antibodies against the acetylcholine receptors, causing muscle weakness, often in the face.

myelin An insulating-type substance present in some neurons that allows the cell to consistently send its signal along the axon without "shorting out" or losing electricity to surrounding fluids and tissues.

myoclonus Jerking motions of the body.

neoplasms Tumors.

neurotransmitters Chemicals produced by the body that stimulate electrical reactions in adjacent neurons.

nystagmus The rhythmic shaking of the eyes.

paresthesia Sensation of tingling, numbness, or "pins and needles" in a body part.

Parkinson's disease A neurologic condition in which the portion of the brain responsible for production of dopamine is damaged or overused, resulting in tremors.

peripheral nervous system (PNS) The part of the nervous system that consists of 31 pairs of spinal nerves and 12 pairs of cranial nerves. These nerves may be sensory nerves, motor nerves, or connecting nerves.

peripheral neuropathy A group of conditions in which the nerves leaving the spinal cord are damaged, resulting in distortion of signals to or from the brain. One type is diabetic, in which the peripheral nerves are damaged as blood glucose levels rise, causing loss of sensation, numbness, burning, pain, paresthesia, and muscle weakness.

pituitary gland The gland that secretes hormones that regulate the function of many other glands in the body; also called the hypophysis.

poliomyelitis A viral infection that attacks the axons, especially motor axons, and destroys them, causing weakness, paralysis, and respiratory arrest. An effective vaccine has been developed and this disease is now rare.

pons The portion of the brain stem that lies below the midbrain and contains nerve fibers that affect sleep and respiration.

postictal The period of time after a seizure during which the brain is reorganizing activity.

postpolio syndrome A result of polio in which neurons break down and die, resulting in difficulty swallowing, weakness, fatigue, or breathing problems even after the patient has healed.

postural tremors Tremors that occur as the person holds a body part still.

prodrome The early signs and symptoms that occur before a disease or condition fully appear, eg, dizziness before fainting.

pronation Turning of the lower arms in a palm-downward manner.

psychosis Breaking with common reality and existing mainly within an internal world.

ptosis Drooping of an eyelid.

receptive aphasia Damage to or loss of the ability to understand speech.

rest tremors Tremors that occur when the body part is not in motion.

spina bifida A development defect in which a portion of the spinal cord or meninges may protrude outside of the vertebrae and possibly even outside of the body, usually at the lower third of the spine in the lumbar area.

status epilepticus A condition in which seizures recur every few minutes, or last more than 30 minutes.

synapses Gaps between nerve cells across which nervous stimuli are transmitted.

syncope Fainting spell or transient loss of consciousness.

tonic activity Type of seizure movement involving the constant contraction and trembling of muscle groups.

transient ischemic attack (TIA) A disorder of the brain in which brain cells temporarily stop working because of insufficient oxygen, causing stroke-like symptoms that resolve completely within 24 hours of onset.

trismus The involuntary contraction of the mouth resulting in clenched teeth. Occurs during seizures and head injuries.

uremia Severe kidney failure resulting in the buildup of waste products within the blood. Eventually brain functions will be impaired.

Assessment in Action

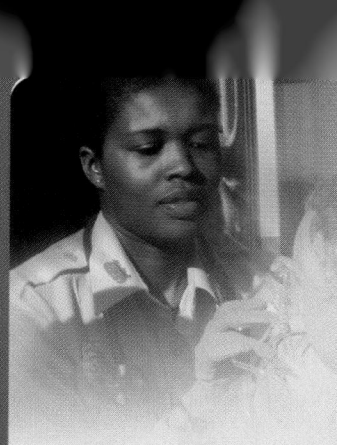

You're just walking in the door to start your shift when you are sent to a diabetic emergency. En route to the call, the fire department delivers an update: The patient is a 78-year-old man who is unconscious and unresponsive. On arrival, you find the patient supine on his bed. The fire department is preparing to move him to the ambulance. You notice that he has sonorous respirations; his skin is warm, dry, and normal in color; blood pressure is 240/140 mm Hg; respirations are 24 breaths/min and shallow; pulse oximetry is 95% on room air; and heart rate is 78 beats/min. The patient has a left-side eye gaze and doesn't respond to painful or verbal stimuli.

When you interview the family, they report that the patient woke up today with no complaints and took a shower. After the shower, he collapsed onto the bed. They called 9-1-1 at approximately 8:00 AM. The patient has type 2 diabetes. You immediately perform a blood glucose check, which comes back as 191 mg/dL. The patient is unable to control his airway; however, his mouth is clenched shut and you are unable to insert an oral airway. While the patient is being transferred to the ambulance, his respiratory rate decreases, allowing you to insert an oral airway. You prepare to intubate the patient and ventilate him with 100% oxygen via a bag-mask device. En route to the hospital, you successfully intubate and secure the endotracheal tube.

Arriving at the hospital, you give your report to the emergency department. When you do your end-of-shift report, you are told the patient had a "huge cerebellum bleed." His prognosis is poor and the emergency department staff is speaking with the family about removing him from the ventilator.

1. _____ is a serious medical condition in which blood supply to areas of the brain is interrupted, resulting in ischemia.
   A. Myocardial infarction
   B. Pulmonary embolism
   C. Cerebrovascular accident
   D. Bell's palsy

2. The two basic types of strokes are ischemic and:
   A. neurologic.
   B. hemorrhagic.
   C. pathologic.
   D. neoplasm.

3. A hallmark of a hemorrhagic CVA is the:
   A. "worst headache of my life."
   B. "worst chest pain of my life."
   C. "worst blurred vision of my life."
   D. "worst weakness of my life."

4. The nervous system is the most complex organ in the human body. It consists of two major structures—the_____ and_____—and thousands of nerves allowing every part of the body to communicate.
   A. brain, myocardium
   B. pulmonary, embolism
   C. brain, spinal cord
   D. spinal cord, myocardium

5. The major structures are divided into two main categories: the central nervous system and the:
   A. parasympathetic nervous system.
   B. sympathetic nervous system.
   C. peripheral nervous system.
   D. autonomic nervous system.

6. Weakness on one side of the body is called:
   A. hemiplegia.
   B. decussation.
   C. nystagmus.
   D. hemiparesis.

7. The _____ is located in the posterior, inferior area of the skull.
   A. medulla oblongata
   B. cerebellum
   C. midbrain
   D. cerebrum

8. The synapse, which is present wherever a nerve cell terminates, connects to the next cell through chemicals called:
   A. synapse.
   B. dendrites.
   C. neurotransmitters.
   D. axon terminals.

9. A hallmark of increased ICP is Cushing's reflex, which means:
   A. bradycardia, bradypnea, and widened pulse pressure.
   B. tachycardia, tachypnea, and narrowing pulse pressure.
   C. bradycardia, tachypnea, and widened pulse pressure.
   D. tachycardia, bradypnea, and widened pulse pressure.

10. Time is essential in treating either kind of stroke. The American Heart Association states:
    A. Time is muscle.
    B. Time is brain.
    C. Time is essential.
    D. Time doesn't matter.

Challenging Questions

You're dispatched to an assisted living home for an 83-year-old woman with an altered mental status. When you arrive and the patient is speaking to you, she appears confused and repeats her statements. Her vital signs are all within normal limits: blood pressure, 130/70 mm Hg; heart rate, 84 beats/min; respiratory rate, 18 breaths/min; and pulse oximetry, 99% on room air. The staff taking care of her reports that she "hasn't been right all day." The paperwork provided to you by the staff is incomplete; however, the medication list is there and you see Aricept.

11. What type of medical history do you suspect based on this medication?

12. How should you care for this patient?

Points to Ponder

You and your partner are dispatched to a private residence for a seizure. When you arrive on scene, you find a 24-year-old man who is responsive to verbal stimuli but is nonverbal. The family reports that the patient had a seizure, which lasted approximately 3 minutes. It was a full-body, normal seizure for the patient. He is in his normal postictal state as well. There is positive incontinence to urine and no tongue laceration. His blood pressure is 130/90 mm Hg; heart rate is 93 beats/min; respiratory rate is 16 breaths/min; and pulse oximetry is 98% on room air.

During transport to the hospital, the patient slowly becomes more responsive. He appears scared and keeps asking, "What happened?"

You explain that he apparently had a seizure. You keep reassuring him throughout the transport to the hospital. On arrival, he is less apprehensive and you give your report to the emergency department. During your follow-up, you find out he was treated and released from the hospital. The patient apparently did not take his Dilantin for several days.

How can you narrow down the cause of a seizure in the field? What benefits does this provide for patient care?

Issues: Understanding and Implementing Treatment of a Patient Who Experienced a Seizure, Empathy for the Patient Who Regains Consciousness Among Strangers.

29 Endocrine Emergencies

Objectives

Cognitive

5-4.1 Describe the incidence, morbidity and mortality of endocrinologic emergencies. (p 29.10)

5-4.2 Identify the risk factors most predisposing to endocrinologic disease. (p 29.9)

5-4.3 Discuss the anatomy and physiology of organs and structures related to endocrinologic diseases. (p 29.4)

5-4.4 Review the pathophysiology of endocrinologic emergencies. (p 29.9)

5-4.5 Discuss the general assessment findings associated with endocrinologic emergencies. (p 29.19)

5-4.6 Identify the need for rapid intervention of the patient with endocrinologic emergencies. (p 29.12)

5-4.7 Discuss the management of endocrinologic emergencies. (p 29.20)

5-4.8 Describe osmotic diuresis and its relationship to diabetes. (p 29.13)

5-4.9 Describe the pathophysiology of adult onset diabetes mellitus. (p 29.11)

5-4.10 Describe the pathophysiology of juvenile onset diabetes mellitus. (p 29.10)

5-4.11 Describe the effects of decreased levels of insulin on the body. (p 29.9)

5-4.12 Correlate abnormal findings in assessment with clinical significance in the patient with a diabetic emergency. (p 29.12)

5-4.13 Discuss the management of diabetic emergencies. (p 29.13)

5-4.14 Integrate the pathophysiological principles and the assessment findings to formulate a field impression and implement a treatment plan for the patient with a diabetic emergency. (p 29.12)

5-4.15 Differentiate between the pathophysiology of normal glucose metabolism and diabetic glucose metabolism. (p 29.11)

5-4.16 Describe the mechanism of ketone body formation and its relationship to ketoacidosis. (p 29.13)

5-4.17 Discuss the physiology of the excretion of potassium and ketone bodies by the kidneys. (p 29.13)

5-4.18 Describe the relationship of insulin to serum glucose levels. (p 29.8)

5-4.19 Describe the effects of decreased levels of insulin on the body. (p 29.9)

5-4.20 Describe the effects of increased serum glucose levels on the body. (p 29.9)

5-4.21 Discuss the pathophysiology of hypoglycemia. (p 29.12)

5-4.22 Discuss the utilization of glycogen by the human body as it relates to the pathophysiology of hypoglycemia. (p 29.11)

5-4.23 Describe the actions of epinephrine as it relates to the pathophysiology of hypoglycemia. (p 29.11)

5-4.24 Recognize the signs and symptoms of the patient with hypoglycemia. (p 29.11)

5-4.25 Describe the compensatory mechanisms utilized by the body to promote homeostasis relative to hypoglycemia. (p 29.11)

5-4.26 Describe the management of a responsive hypoglycemic patient. (p 29.12)

5-4.27 Correlate abnormal findings in assessment with clinical significance in the patient with hypoglycemia. (p 29.12)

5-4.28 Discuss the management of the hypoglycemic patient. (p 29.12)

5-4.29 Integrate the pathophysiological principles and the assessment findings to formulate a field impression and implement a treatment plan for the patient with hypoglycemia. (p 29.12)

5-4.30 Discuss the pathophysiology of hyperglycemia. (p 29.13)

5-4.31 Recognize the signs and symptoms of the patient with hyperglycemia. (p 29.14)

5-4.32 Describe the management of hyperglycemia. (p 29.14)

5-4.33 Correlate abnormal findings in assessment with clinical significance in the patient with hyperglycemia. (p 29.14)

5-4.34 Discuss the management of the patient with hyperglycemia. (p 29.14)

5-4.35 Integrate the pathophysiological principles and the assessment findings to formulate a field impression and implement a treatment plan for the patient with hyperglycemia. (p 29.14)

5-4.36 Discuss the pathophysiology of nonketotic hyperosmolar coma. (p 29.14)

5-4.37 Recognize the signs and symptoms of the patient with nonketotic hyperosmolar coma. (p 29.14)

5-4.38 Describe the management of nonketotic hyperosmolar coma. (p 29.15)

5-4.39 Correlate abnormal findings in assessment with clinical significance in the patient with nonketotic hyperosmolar coma. (p 29.15)

5-4.40 Integrate the pathophysiological principles and the assessment findings to formulate a field impression and implement a treatment plan for the patient with nonketotic hyperosmolar coma. (p 29.15)

5-4.41 Discuss the management of the patient with hyperglycemia. (p 29.14)

5-4.42 Integrate the pathophysiological principles and the assessment findings to formulate a field impression and implement a treatment plan for the patient with hyperglycemia. (p 29.13)

5-4.43 Discuss the pathophysiology of diabetic ketoacidosis. (p 29.13)

5-4.44 Recognize the signs and symptoms of the patient with diabetic ketoacidosis. (p 29.14)

5-4.45 Describe the management of diabetic ketoacidosis. (p 29.14)

5-4.46 Correlate abnormal findings in assessment with clinical significance in the patient with diabetic ketoacidosis. (p 29.14)

5-4.47 Discuss the management of the patient with diabetic ketoacidosis. (p 29.14)

5-4.48 Integrate the pathophysiological principles and the assessment findings to formulate a field impression and implement a treatment plan for the patient with diabetic ketoacidosis. (p 29.14)

5-4.49 Discuss the pathophysiology of thyrotoxicosis. (p 29.19)

5-4.50 Recognize signs and symptoms of the patient with thyrotoxicosis. (p 29.19)

5-4.51 Describe the management of thyrotoxicosis. (p 29.19)

5-4.52 Correlate abnormal findings in assessment with clinical significance in the patient with thyrotoxicosis. (p 29.19)

5-4.53 Discuss the management of the patient with thyrotoxicosis. (p 29.19)

5-4.54 Integrate the pathophysiological principles and the assessment findings to formulate a field impression and implement a treatment plan for the patient with thyrotoxicosis. (p 29.19)

5-4.55 Discuss the pathophysiology of myxedema. (p 29.18)

5-4.56 Recognize signs and symptoms of the patient with myxedema. (p 29.18)

5-4.57 Describe the management of myxedema. (p 29.18)

5-4.58 Correlate abnormal findings in assessment with clinical significance in the patient with myxedema. (p 29.18)

5-4.59 Discuss the management of the patient with myxedema. (p 29.18)

5-4.60 Integrate the pathophysiological principles and the assessment findings to formulate a field impression and implement a treatment plan for the patient with myxedema. (p 29.18)

5-4.61 Discuss the pathophysiology of Cushing's syndrome. (p 29.17)

5-4.62 Recognize signs and symptoms of the patient with Cushing's syndrome. (p 29.17)

5-4.63 Describe the management of Cushing's syndrome. (p 29.17)

5-4.64 Correlate abnormal findings in assessment with clinical significance in the patient with Cushing's syndrome. (p 29.17)

5-4.65 Discuss the management of the patient with Cushing's syndrome. (p 29.17)

5-4.66 Integrate the pathophysiological principles and the assessment findings to formulate a field impression and implement a treatment plan for the patient with Cushing's syndrome. (p 29.17)

5-4.67 Discuss the pathophysiology of adrenal insufficiency. (p 29.16)

5-4.68 Recognize signs and symptoms of the patient with adrenal insufficiency. (p 29.16)

5-4.69 Describe the management of adrenal insufficiency. (p 29.16)

5-4.70 Correlate abnormal findings in assessment with clinical significance in the patient with adrenal insufficiency. (p 29.16)

5-4.71 Discuss the management of the patient with adrenal insufficiency. (p 29.16)

5-4.72 Integrate the pathophysiological principles and the assessment findings to formulate a field impression and implement a treatment plan for the patient with adrenal insufficiency. (p 29.16)

5-4.73 Integrate the pathophysiological principles to the assessment of a patient with an endocrinologic emergency. (p 29.19)

5-4.74 Differentiate between endocrine emergencies based on assessment and history. (p 29.19)

5-4.75 Correlate abnormal findings in the assessment with clinical significance in the patient with endocrinologic emergencies. (p 29.20)

5-4.76 Develop a patient management plan based on field impression in the patient with an endocrinologic emergency. (p 29.20)

Affective

None

Psychomotor

None

Introduction

Few other systems in the body share the level of responsibility assigned to the endocrine system. This system directly or indirectly influences almost every cell, organ, and function of the body. Consequently, patients with an endocrine disorder often present with a multitude of signs and symptoms that require a thorough assessment and immediate treatment to interrupt life-threatening emergencies.

Anatomy and Physiology

The endocrine system comprises a network of glands that produce and secrete chemical messengers called hormones. The main function of the endocrine system and its hormone messengers is to maintain homeostasis and promote permanent structural changes. Maintaining homeostasis requires a response to any change in the body, such as low glucose or calcium levels in the blood.

Exocrine glands (*exo* means "outside") excrete chemicals for elimination. These glands have ducts that carry their secretions to the surface of the skin or into a body cavity. Sweat glands, salivary glands, and the liver are examples of exocrine glands.

Endocrine glands (*endo* means "inside") secrete or release chemicals that are used inside the body. These glands lack ducts, so they release hormones directly into the surrounding tissue and blood. Hormones act on the body's cells by increasing or decreasing the rate of cellular metabolism. They transfer information from one set of cells to another to coordinate bodily functions, such as the regulation of mood, growth and development, metabolism, tissue function, and sexual development and function.

Whereas the nervous system—the body's major controlling system—uses nerve impulses to activate and monitor the faster processes of the body, hormones of the endocrine system—considered the body's second great controlling system—are released directly into the bloodstream and act more slowly to achieve their effects. The hormones travel in the bloodstream to target tissues Figure 29-1 ▶ . Each target cell has specific receptor sites on the cell membrane, or inside the cell, to which the specific hormone can attach or bind. These receptors have two main functions: to recognize and bind to their particular hormones and to initiate an appropriate signal. Once the hormone has attached to the receptor site of the cell, the "message" to alter the cellular function is delivered.

Many cells contain multiple receptors and act as targets for several hormones—or for molecules introduced into the body as therapy. Agonists are molecules that bind to a cell's receptor and trigger a response by that cell; they produce some kind of action or biologic effect. Antagonists are molecules that bind to a cell's receptor and block the action of agonists. Hormone antagonists are widely used as drugs.

Hormonal Regulation Mechanism

Hormones operate within feedback systems (either positive or negative) to maintain an optimal internal operating environment in the body. Release of hormones is regulated by chemical

You are the Provider Part 1

You and your partner are among the millions of national television viewers watching the high-profile murder trial that's taking place in your city in which a physician is accused of murdering his wife. Currently on the stand is the medical examiner, explaining the autopsy protocol and describing photos from the crime scene and autopsy. In the middle of her testimony, the judge unexpectedly calls for a 15-minute recess and your pager goes off. You are dispatched to the county courthouse for an unknown medical emergency. As you and your partner approach the courthouse, a police escort meets you and guides you and your partner through a sea of news vehicles and reporters. You safely enter the building from a restricted back entrance. You are then met by a deputy, who escorts you to a judge's chambers where you find your patient.

Lying on the couch is a middle-aged, well-nourished female patient. She appears to be extremely lethargic, pale, and diaphoretic. A fellow member of the jury explains that as the photos of the autopsy were being shown, the woman, Ms. Engle, suddenly went pale and passed out. She was immediately brought to the judge's chambers and placed on the couch. It is estimated that she was unconscious for approximately 1 to 2 minutes.

Initial Assessment	Recording Time: 0 Minutes
Appearance	Looks ill
Level of consciousness	V (Responsive to verbal stimuli)
Airway	Open
Breathing	Adequate chest rise and volume
Circulation	Weak, rapid radial pulse

1. What are some potential differential diagnoses?
2. When do symptoms of hypoglycemia occur?

stops providing the critical negative feedback required to regulate function. Cell signaling is covered in more detail in Chapter 6.

The hypothalamic–pituitary system controls the function of multiple peripheral endocrine organs (eg, thyroid, adrenal cortex, gonads, breasts). It is often considered a part of the endocrine system, as it sends signals to the adrenal gland to release the hormones epinephrine and norepinephrine. It also produces its own hormones: antidiuretic hormone (ADH), oxytocin, and regulatory hormones. The regulatory hormones control the release of hormones by the pituitary gland.

Some of these hormones have pharmacologic effects that depend on their concentration. For example, if there is a low or physiologic level of ADH in the bloodstream, the renal tubules are stimulated to reabsorb sodium and water. At the same time, ADH acts as a vasopressor.

Components of the Endocrine System

The major components of the endocrine system are the hypothalamus, pituitary, thyroid, parathyroid, adrenals, and reproductive organs (gonads). The pancreas is also part of this system; it has a role in hormone production as well as in digestion.

Hypothalamus

The hypothalamus is a small region of the brain (not a gland) that contains several control centers for the body functions and emotions. It is the primary link between the endocrine system and the nervous system.

Pituitary Gland

The pituitary gland is often referred to as the "master gland" because its secretions control, or regulate, the secretions of other endocrine glands. It is located at the base of the brain and is about the size of a grape. The pituitary is attached to the hypothalamus by a very thin piece of tissue. This gland is

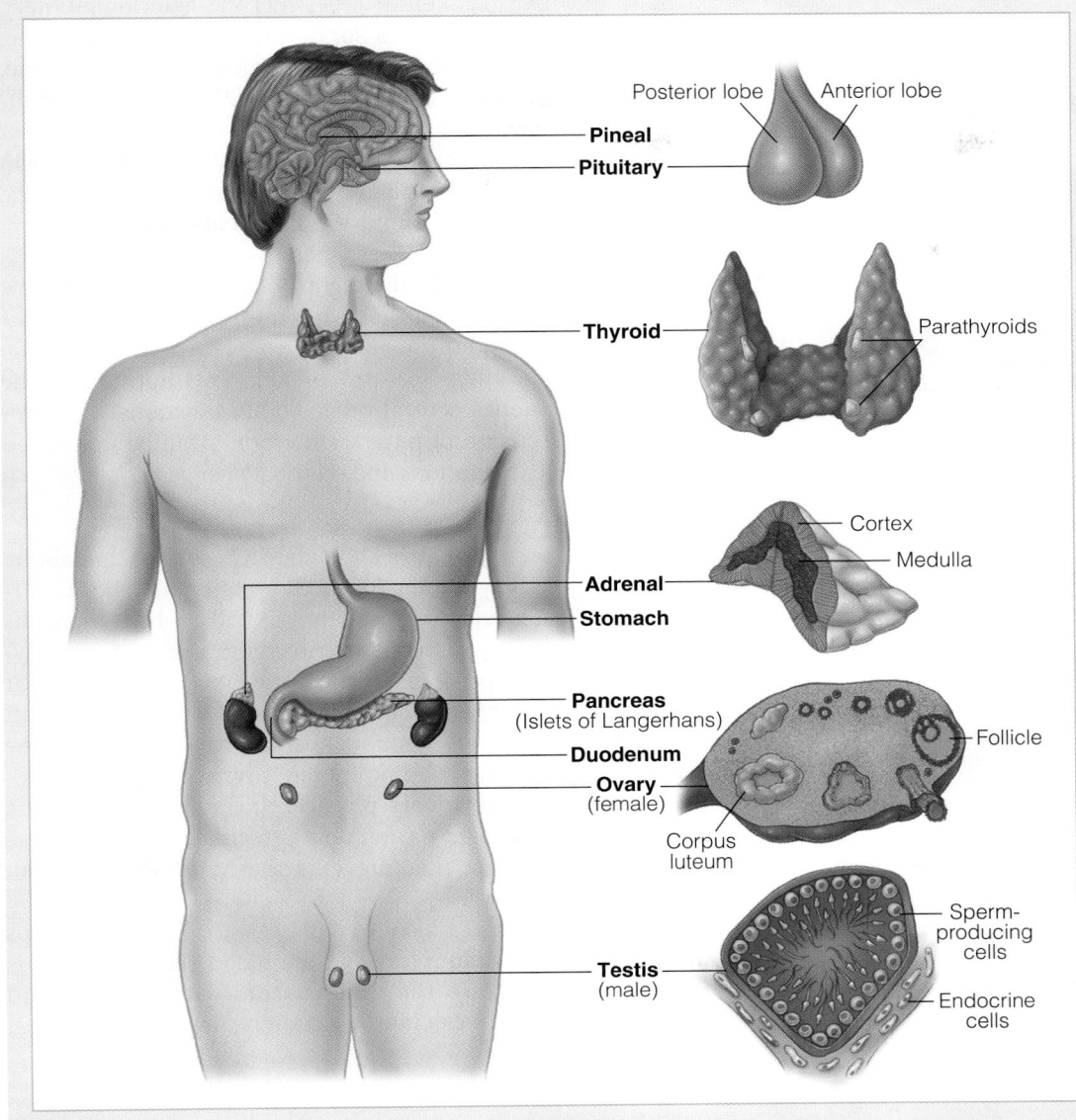

Figure 29-1 The endocrine system uses the various glands within the system to deliver chemical messages to organ systems throughout the body.

factors, other hormonal factors, and neural control. Endocrine regulation, through negative feedback, is the most important method by which hormonal secretion is maintained within a physiologic range.

One example of this negative feedback mechanism is the release of epinephrine from the adrenal medulla in response to stress. When stress stimulates the body's neural regulation (via the sympathetic nervous system), it releases epinephrine into the bloodstream from the adrenal medulla to assist the body's response to the stress stimuli. When the stress is removed, the nervous system stimulation decreases and less epinephrine is released **Figure 29-2 ▶**.

Disease occurs when normal cell signaling is interrupted and positive feedback is given. As a consequence, the system

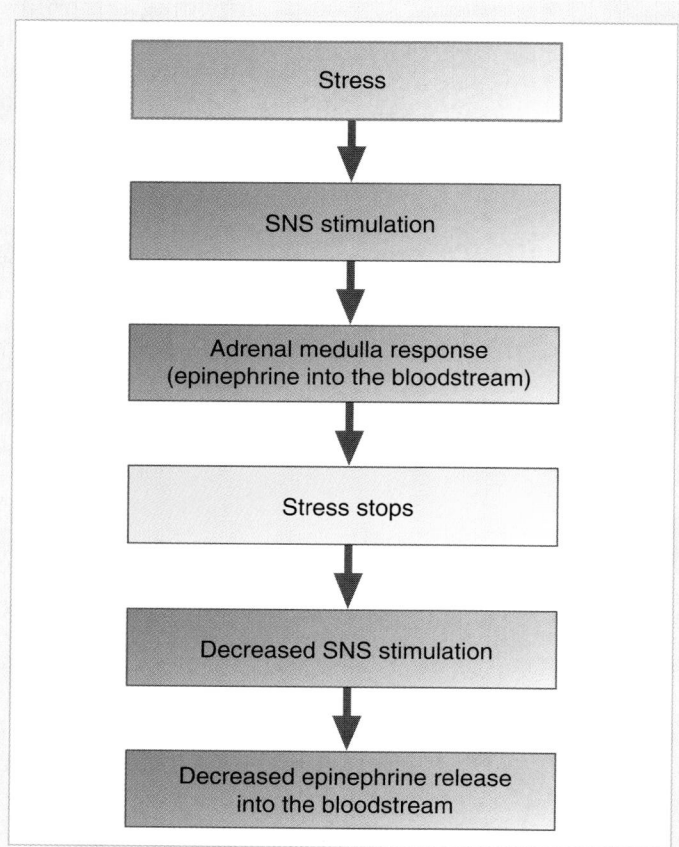

Figure 29-2 Stress stimulates the sympathetic nervous system (neural regulation) to signal the adrenal medulla to release epinephrine into the bloodstream to assist the body's "flight or fight" response. When the stimulus is eliminated, the neural regulating mechanism decreases its signals to the adrenal medulla and less epinephrine is released (negative feedback loop).

divided into two regions, or lobes: (1) the anterior pituitary, which produces and secretes six hormones (growth hormone, thyroid-stimulating hormone, adrenocorticotropin hormone, and three gonadotropic hormones); and (2) the posterior pituitary, which secretes two hormones (ADH and oxytocin) but does not produce them   Figure 29-3 ▶ . ADH and oxytocin are synthesized in hypothalamic neurons but are stored in the posterior pituitary gland until the hypothalamus sends nerve signals to the pituitary to release them.

Table 29-1 ▶ lists the eight hormones secreted by the pituitary gland. Six of these hormones stimulate other endocrine glands and are referred to as "tropic" (from the Greek *tropos,* meaning "to turn" or "change") hormones. The other two hormones control other bodily functions. The production and secretion of pituitary hormones can be influenced by factors such as emotions and seasonal changes.

Thyroid

The thyroid secretes thyroxine when the body's metabolic rate decreases. Thyroxine, the body's major metabolic hormone, stimulates energy production in cells, which increases the rate at which cells consume oxygen and use carbohydrates, fats, and proteins. When the body gets cold, for example, the increased cellular metabolism creates heat. Iodine is an important component of thyroxine. Without the proper level of dietary iodine intake, thyroxine can't be produced, and the individual's physical and mental growth are diminished. Thyroxine production is regulated by a negative feedback mechanism that prevents the hypothalamus from stimulating the thyroid.

The thyroid gland also secretes calcitonin, which helps maintain normal calcium levels in the blood. This hormone is secreted directly into the bloodstream when the thyroid detects high levels of calcium. Calcitonin travels to the bones,

You are the Provider Part 2

You ask your partner to obtain a set of vital signs and perform a blood glucose check while you begin your assessment of the patient. Your initial assessment reveals that she is responsive to verbal stimuli; however, she is unable to answer questions appropriately. The only other significant finding is a weak, rapid regular pulse. Your partner whispers to you that the blood glucose level came back at 27.

Vital Signs	Recording Time: 5 Minutes
Level of consciousness	Verbal
Pulse	130 beats/min, weak and regular
Blood pressure	122/68 mm Hg
Respirations	22 breaths/min, regular
Skin	Pale, cool, and diaphoretic
Sao$_2$	97% on room air

3. What are some of the causes of hypoglycemia?

4. How may a person with hypoglycemia present?

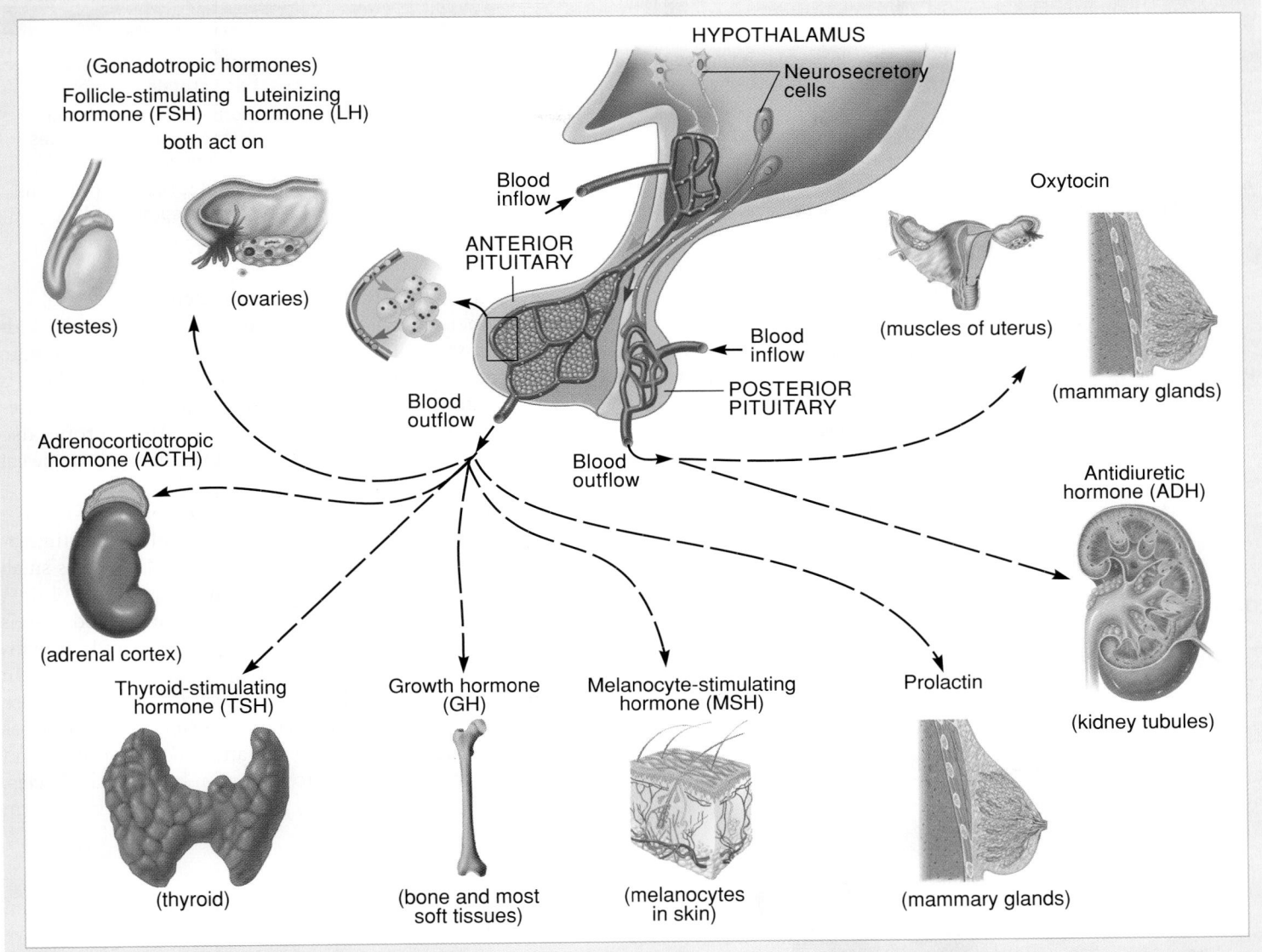

Figure 29-3 The pituitary gland secretes hormones from its two regions, the anterior pituitary lobe and the posterior pituitary lobe.

where it stimulates the bone-building cells to absorb the excess calcium. It also stimulates the kidneys to absorb and excrete excess calcium.

Parathyroid

The parathyroid gland also assists in the regulation of calcium. However, the parathyroid hormone (PTH), when secreted by the parathyroid, acts as an antagonist to calcitonin. PTH is secreted when calcium blood levels are low. It stimulates the bone-dissolving cells to break down bone and release calcium into the bloodstream. In the kidneys, PTH decreases the amount of calcium released in the urine. The secretion of PTH is regulated by the calcium level in the blood.

Adrenal Glands

The adrenal glands consist of two parts: an outer part, called the adrenal cortex, and an inner part, called the adrenal medulla Figure 29-4 ▸ . Both parts produce hormones Table 29-2 ▸ . The adrenal cortex produces hormones called corticosteroids, which regulate the body's metabolism, its balance of salt and water, the immune system, and sexual function. The adrenal medulla produces hormones called catecholamines (epinephrine and norepinephrine), which assist the body in coping with physical and emotional stress by increasing the heart and respiratory rates and the blood pressure.

During times of stress, the hypothalamus secretes a hormone that stimulates the anterior pituitary to release

Table 29-1	Hormones Secreted by the Pituitary Gland
Growth hormone (GH)	Regulates metabolic processes related to growth and adaptation to physical and emotional stressors
Thyroid-stimulating hormone (TSH)	Increases production and secretion of thyroid hormone
Adrenocorticotropic hormone (ACTH)	Stimulates the adrenal gland to secrete cortisol and adrenal proteins that contribute to the maintenance of the adrenal gland
Luteinizing hormone (LH)	In women: ovulation, progesterone production In men: regulates spermatogenesis, testosterone production
Follicle-stimulating hormone (FSH)	In women: follicle maturation, estrogen production In men: spermatogenesis
Prolactin	Milk production
Antidiuretic hormone (ADH)	Controls plasma osmolality; increases the permeability of the distal renal tubules and collecting ducts, which leads to an increase in water reabsorption
Oxytocin	Contracts the uterus during childbirth and stimulates milk production

Table 29-2	Hormones of the Adrenal Glands
Cortisol	Increases metabolic rate, using fat and protein for energy
Aldosterone	Reabsorbs sodium and water from the urine, and excretes excess potassium
Epinephrine/norepinephrine	Stimulates sympathetic nervous system receptors

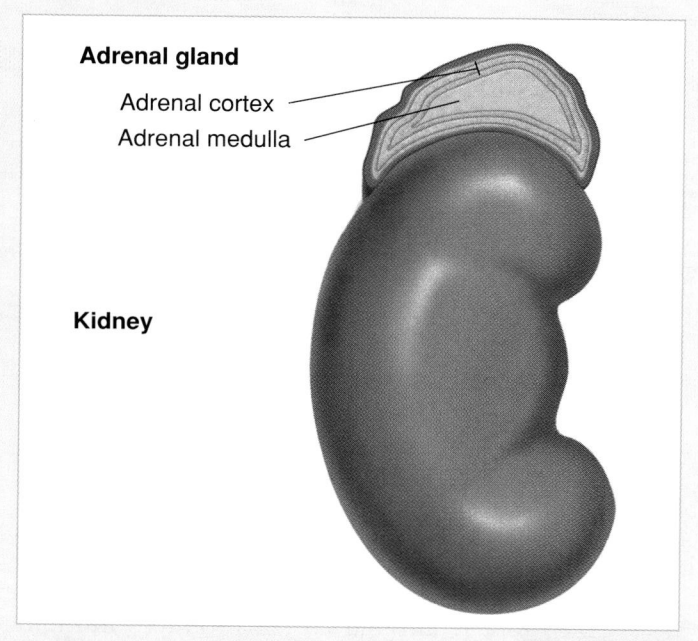

Figure 29-4 The adrenal glands, which sit on top of the kidney, consist of two parts—the adrenal cortex and the adrenal medulla.

adrenocorticotropic hormone (ACTH). ACTH targets the adrenal cortex and causes it to secrete cortisol (a glucocorticoid). Cortisol stimulates most body cells to increase their energy production.

If the body experiences a drop in blood pressure or volume, a decrease in sodium level, or an increase in the potas-

sium level, the adrenal cortex is stimulated to secrete aldosterone (a mineralocorticoid). Aldosterone stimulates the kidneys to reabsorb sodium from the urine and excrete potassium by altering the osmotic gradient in the blood. When sodium is reabsorbed into the blood, water follows; this action increases both blood volume and blood pressure. Aldosterone also reduces the amount of salt and water lost through the sweat and salivary glands.

The body's reaction to physical or emotional stress is referred to as the "fight or flight" response. Following stimulation from the hypothalamus, the adrenal medulla secretes small amounts of norepinephrine and large amounts of epinephrine. Norepinephrine raises blood pressure by causing blood vessels and skeletal muscles to constrict. Epinephrine stimulates sympathetic nervous system receptors throughout the body. In addition, it stimulates the liver to convert glycogen to glucose for use as energy in the cells. The action of both hormones results in increased levels of oxygen and glucose in the blood and faster circulation of blood to the brain, heart, and muscles, which in turn enables the body to respond to the short-term emergency situation.

Pancreas

The pancreas is a digestive gland that is considered both an endocrine gland and an exocrine gland. It secretes digestive enzymes into the duodenum through the pancreatic duct. The exocrine component is responsible for the secretion of the digestive enzymes. The endocrine component comprises the islets of Langerhans. These cell groups within the pancreas act like "an organ within an organ." The main hormones they secrete—glucagon and insulin—are responsible for the regulation of blood glucose levels **Figure 29-5 ▸** .

When the body's blood glucose level falls, such as between meals, glucagon (a starch form of the sugar glucose made up of thousands of glucose units) is secreted to raise the glucose level and bring the body's energy back to normal. When it enters the bloodstream, glucagon stimulates the liver to change glycogen into sugar and secrete it into the bloodstream, where cells can use it for energy.

Insulin is responsible for the removal of glucose from the blood for storage as glycogen, fats, and protein. When blood glucose levels are elevated, the islets of Langerhans secrete insulin, which is carried by the bloodstream to the cells. The cells then take in more glucose and use it to produce energy. Insulin also stimulates the liver to take in more glucose and

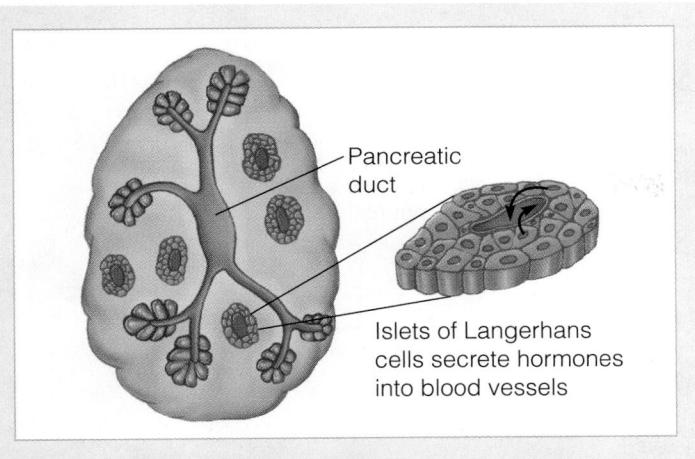

Figure 29-5 The islets of Langerhans secrete hormones into blood vessels.

In the Field

Although specific pathophysiology varies for each disease, endocrine emergencies are usually due to:
- Failure of normal hormone production
- Excessive hormone production
- Failure of feedback inhibition systems involving the hypothalamus, pituitary gland, endocrine gland, and the target organ

the menstrual cycle. At puberty, estrogen also supports development of the secondary sex characteristics: enlargement of the breasts, uterine enlargement, fat deposits in the hips and thighs, and development of hair under the arms and in the pubic area.

Pathophysiology

Endocrine disorders can be caused by either hypersecretion or insufficient secretion of a gland. Hypersecretion presents as overactivity of the target organ regulated by the gland. Insufficient secretion results in underactivity of the organ controlled by the gland.

The effects of a disturbance of endocrine gland function are determined by the degree of dysfunction of the gland, as well as by the age and sex of the patient. All degrees of glandular dysfunction are possible, ranging from barely detectable variations to extreme dysfunction.

In the Field

Despite their intricate pathophysiology, most clinically significant endocrine emergencies result in alterations of the ABCs, fluid balance, mental status, vital signs, and blood glucose level.

Table 29-3	Hormones of the Gonads
Male	
Testosterone	Main sex hormone in males Responsible for secondary sex characteristics: voice deepening, growth of facial hair, muscle development, pubic hair, growth spurts
Female	
Estrogen	Responsible for secondary sex characteristics: breast growth, fat accumulation at hips and thighs, pubic hair, growth spurts Involved in pregnancy Regulation of menstrual cycle
Progesterone	Involved in pregnancy Regulation of menstrual cycle Prevents maturation of additional egg during ovulation

store it as glycogen for later use by the body. Insulin is the *only* hormone that decreases the blood glucose levels. Insulin is essential in order for glucose to enter and nourish the cells. Once the blood glucose levels have returned to normal, the islets of Langerhans discontinue the secretion of insulin.

Gonads

The gonads are the main source of sex hormones
Table 29-3 ▲ . In men, the gonads, or testes, are located in the scrotum and produce hormones called androgens. The most important androgen in men is testosterone. Androgens regulate body changes associated with sexual development (puberty), including growth spurts, deepening of the voice, growth of facial and pubic hair, and muscle growth and strength.

In women, the gonads are the ovaries, which release the eggs and secrete the hormones estrogen and progesterone. Estrogen signals the anterior pituitary gland to secrete luteinizing hormone (LH) when an egg is developing in an ovarian follicle. Estrogen and progesterone also assist in the regulation of

Diabetes Mellitus

Medically, the term "diabetes" refers to a metabolic disorder in which the body's ability to metabolize simple carbohydrates (glucose) is impaired. It is characterized by the passage of large quantities of urine containing glucose, significant thirst, and deterioration of body function. Glucose (also known as dextrose) is one of the basic sugars in the body and, along with oxygen, is the primary fuel for cellular metabolism.

Diabetes mellitus means "sweet diabetes"—a reference to the presence of glucose in the urine. This disease is characterized by an inability to sufficiently metabolize glucose. It occurs either because the pancreas does not produce enough insulin or because the cells do not respond to the effects of the insulin that is produced. Both cases result in elevated glucose levels in the blood and glucose in the urine. Glucose builds up in the blood, overflows into the urine, and flows out of the body. Thus cells can starve even though the blood contains large amounts of glucose **Figure 29-6 ▶** .

The National Institute of Diabetes and Digestive and Kidney Diseases (NIDDK) estimates that the total prevalence of diabetes in the United States was 20.8 million people in 2005 (7% of the US population). Of those individuals, approximately 6.2 million are undiagnosed. According to the Centers for Disease Control and Prevention, diabetes was the sixth leading cause of death in 2002.

Left untreated, diabetes leads to wasting of body tissues and death. Even with medical care, some patients with particularly aggressive forms of diabetes will die relatively young from one or more complications of the disease. The severity of diabetic complications is related to how high the average blood glucose level is and how early in life the disease begins. Although most patients live a normal life span, they must be willing to adjust their lives to the demands of the disease, especially their eating habits and activities. There is no cure for the disease, so treatment focuses on maintaining blood glucose levels within the normal range.

Two forms of diabetes exist: type 1 and type 2. Both types are serious conditions that affect many tissues and functions other than the glucose-regulating mechanism, and both require life-long medical management.

Figure 29-6 Diabetes is defined as a lack of or ineffective action of insulin. Without insulin, cells begin to "starve" because insulin is needed to allow glucose to enter and nourish the cells.

Type 1 Diabetes Mellitus

Type 1 diabetes generally strikes children as opposed to adults, so it has been referred to as "juvenile diabetes." Although type 1 diabetes has a hereditary predisposition, it is now believed that environmental factors may be part of the cause—for example, an infection that triggers an autoimmune disorder (ie, antibodies destroy the islets of Langerhans).

In type 1 diabetes, most patients do not produce insulin at all. They require daily injections of supplementary, synthetic insulin throughout their lives to control blood glucose. In addition to daily insulin injections, strict diet control must be observed; this can be difficult with young children. Increased activity and alcohol consumption can lead to low blood glucose levels (alcohol depletes glycogen stores in the liver). It is important to consider low blood sugar as a cause of altered

In the Field

Macrovascular complications of diabetes include:
- Coronary artery disease/myocardial infarction (MI)
- Hypertension
- Dyslipidemia
- Peripheral vascular (foot ulcers/amputations)
- Cerebrovascular (stroke)

Microvascular complications of diabetes include:
- Retinopathy
- Nephropathy (end-stage renal disease)
- Neuropathy (paresthesias, sexual impotence, neurogenic bladder, constipation, diarrhea)

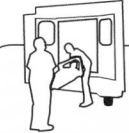

In the Field

The terms "juvenile onset" and "adult onset" diabetes have been replaced by type 1 and type 2 diabetes. The age of onset of the patient's symptoms is less important than whether or not the patient requires insulin to survive.

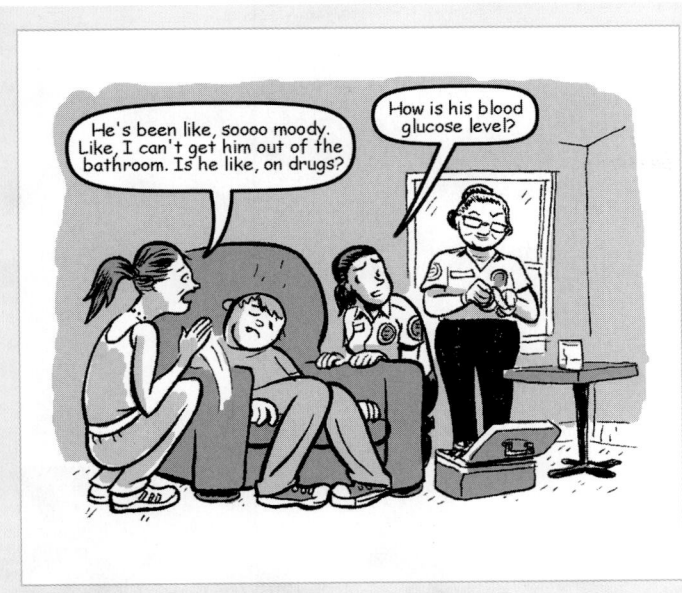

Figure 29-7

In the Field

You will likely encounter diabetic patients who use insulin pumps to treat their disease. These small devices consist of an infusion set, a reservoir for insulin, and the pump itself. A promising alternative to multiple daily injections of insulin, insulin pumps provide improved control of blood glucose levels for many diabetic patients.

mental status Figure 29-7 ▲ . Complications of diabetes include kidney problems, nerve damage, blindness (diabetes is the number one cause of blindness), heart disease, and stroke.

Type 2 Diabetes Mellitus

The most common form of diabetes is type 2 diabetes (sometimes called adult-onset diabetes), in which blood glucose levels are elevated. Approximately 90% of all diabetics in the United States suffer from type 2 diabetes, which typically develops later in life, usually when the patient is middle-aged, although the disease is becoming more common in younger people. Type 2 diabetes may be related to *metabolic syndrome*, a cluster of characteristics including excessive fat in the abdominal area, elevated blood pressure, and high levels of blood lipids. Risk factors for developing metabolic syndrome include excess weight, lack of physical activity, and genetic factors.

In many people with type 2 diabetes, the pancreas actually produces enough insulin; however, for reasons not fully understood, the body cannot effectively utilize it. This condition is known as insulin resistance. One possible explanation is that the insulin receptor cells located on the target cells have changed in some way and are no longer able to receive the

Special Considerations

New-onset weakness in a pre-existing diabetes patient may be considered an MI until proven otherwise. Many type 1 and type 2 diabetes patients have an acquired dysfunction in the peripheral nervous system (neuropathy). Also, increased insulin levels result in increased blood lipid levels. This combination often leads to an earlier onset of coronary artery disease. Diabetics don't always have typical clinical symptoms of acute coronary syndrome due to their alteration in sensation. They are more likely to present with general body weakness.

insulin when it arrives at the target cell. Type 2 diabetes can also be caused by a deficiency in insulin production.

Symptoms of type 2 diabetes may include fatigue; nausea; frequent urination; thirst; unexplained weight loss; blurred vision; frequent infections and slow healing of wounds; being cranky, confused, or shaky; unresponsiveness; and seizure. These symptoms tend to develop gradually and usually become noticeable in middle age. In fact, the onset of type 2 diabetes may be so insidious that patients may not realize they suffer from the disorder. In some instances, the symptoms can develop over several years in overweight adults older than 40 years. A small percentage of people do not display any symptoms.

Weight loss is an important factor in helping to control type 2 diabetes. Exercise and a well-balanced, nutritious diet are key components in combating the complications of diabetes. To maintain glucose levels within the normal range, food intake must be spread throughout an entire day in coordination with daily medications/insulin injections.

Hypoglycemia

Hypoglycemia in the insulin-dependent diabetic is often the result of having taken too much insulin, too little food, or both. Unlike other tissues, which can usually metabolize fat or protein in addition to sugar, the tissues of the central nervous system (including the brain) depend entirely on glucose as their source of energy. If the level of glucose in the blood drops dramatically, the brain is literally starved. The patient will experience trembling, a rapid heart rate, sweating, and a feeling of hunger—a result of the actions of epinephrine. These symptoms reflect both the disordered function of hungry brain cells and the alarm reaction (sympathetic nervous system discharge) set off by the brain's distress. If hypoglycemia persists, cerebral

In the Field

The longer a patient remains unconscious from hypoglycemia, the more likely there will be permanent brain damage! If more than 20 to 30 minutes go by, toxic compounds (free radicals) in the brain are produced that can cause permanent neuronal damage.

dysfunction progresses very quickly to permanent brain damage. Additional signs and symptoms associated with hypoglycemia include headache, mental confusion, memory loss, incoordination, slurred speech, irritability, dilated pupils, and seizures and coma in severe cases.

Normal blood glucose is approximately 80 to 120 mg/dL; hypoglycemia occurs when blood glucose drops to 45 mg/dL or less. Hypoglycemia develops *very rapidly,* from minutes to a few hours. It should be suspected in any patient with diabetes who presents with bizarre behavior, neurologic signs, or coma. Often the hypoglycemic patient appears intoxicated, because of slurred speech and lack of coordination, and may be paranoid, hostile, and aggressive.

Of course, diabetics are not the only individuals who are prone to episodes of hypoglycemia. Alcoholics, patients who have ingested certain poisons or overdosed with certain drugs (notably aspirin), and patients with certain cancers, liver disease, kidney disease, and some other conditions may also suffer hypoglycemic episodes. Don't discount the possibility of hypoglycemia in a comatose patient just because the individual is not known to have diabetes. Conversely, don't let a known diagnosis of diabetes prevent you from considering other causes of coma. Diabetics are not immune to head injury, stroke, seizures, meningitis, and other traumatic injuries or conditions. Keep an open mind and assess the patient thoroughly.

Whenever you suspect hypoglycemia, treat it *immediately:* A hungry brain is a very unhappy brain, and permanent cerebral damage may ensue if blood glucose levels are not restored rapidly. Measure the patient's blood sugar, especially if his or her age or clinical history suggests that the problem may be stroke—administration of concentrated glucose solutions in a suspected stroke situation may exacerbate cerebral damage **Figure 29-8 ▶** . When the comatose patient is older than 55 years or the family gives a history of recent transient ischemic attacks, perform a field glucose test (Dextrostix, Chemstrip BG) to rule out hypoglycemia.

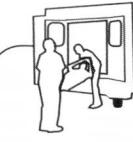 **In the Field**

If uncertain of a patient's blood glucose level, always err on the "low side" and assume that hypoglycemia is present. A period of hypoglycemia is more dangerous to the patient than an equivalent period of hyperglycemia.

If the patient is alert, is able to swallow, and has an intact gag reflex, administer sugar by mouth. Provide a candy bar, a glass of warm water to which a few teaspoons of sugar have been added, a nondiet cola drink—any of those should do the trick. Do *not* give anything by mouth to a patient whose level of consciousness is depressed!

If the patient is in a coma, treat him or her as any other comatose patient, with attention to the airway and supplemental oxygen. Hold off on use of an advanced airway (ie, endotracheal tube, Combitube, laryngeal mask airway), until you have

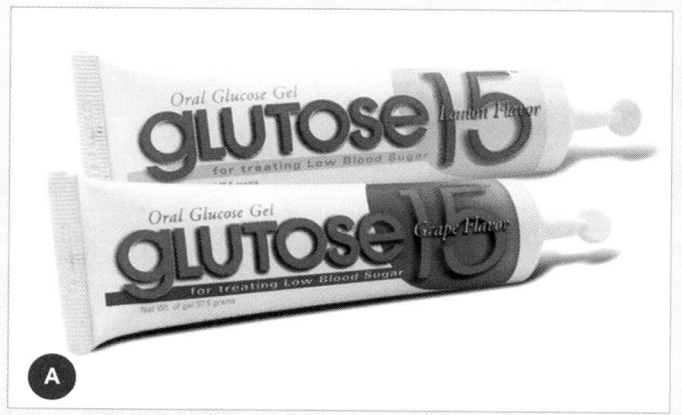
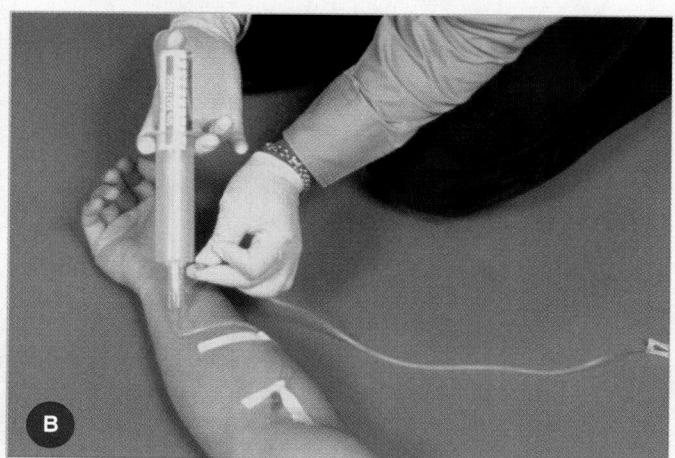

Figure 29-8 Administering glucose is appropriate in diabetic emergencies unless you have a reliable blood glucose measurement indicating normal or high blood glucose levels. Available forms include (**A**) oral glucose paste and (**B**) 50% glucose solution for IV administration.

In the Field

The exact value for the blood glucose is not extremely helpful. It's far more important to know the general range plus the patient's clinical presentation.

given the patient D_{50} (50% dextrose); if the D_{50} works, the patient will pull out the endotracheal tube as soon as he or she wakes up!

Start an IV with a *large-bore catheter* (no smaller than 18-gauge) in a *big vein,* and hook up a 0.9% normal saline (NS) infusion. Check the IV carefully to confirm that it's patent and flowing freely. Inject a test bolus of 10 to 20 mL of NS infusion fluid, making sure the IV is not prone to infiltration. Recheck its status by lowering the IV bag and looking for backflow of blood into the infusion set. D_{50} is both hypertonic and acidic, and it can do a lot of damage if it infiltrates out of the vein and enters the surrounding tissue.

Table 29-4	Characteristics of Hyperglycemia and Hypoglycemia	
	Hyperglycemia	**Hypoglycemia**
History		
Food intake	Excessive	Insufficient
Insulin dosage	Insufficient	Excessive
Onset	Gradual (hours to days)	Rapid, within minutes
Skin	Warm and dry	Pale and moist
Infection	Common	Uncommon
Gastrointestinal tract		
Thirst	Intense	Absent
Hunger	Absent	Intense
Vomiting	Common	Uncommon
Respiratory system		
Breathing	Rapid, deep (Kussmaul respirations)	Normal or rapid
Odor of breath	Sweet, fruity	Normal
Cardiovascular system		
Blood pressure	Normal to low	Low
Pulse	Normal or rapid and full	Rapid, weak
Nervous system		
Consciousness	Restless merging to coma	Irritability, confusion, seizure, or coma
Urine		
Sugar	Present	Absent
Acetone	Present	Absent
Treatment		
Response	Gradual, within 6 to 12 hours following medical treatment	Immediately after administration of glucose

Hyperglycemia occurs when levels of sugar in the blood exceed normal range (80 to 120 mg/dL). Doctors tend to try to keep the glucose levels of their diabetic patients at less than 160 mg/dL. Hyperglycemia can be caused by excessive food intake, insufficient insulin dosages, infection or illness, injury, surgery, and emotional stress. Onset may be rapid (within minutes) or gradual (hours to days), depending on the cause. For example, excessive food intake may cause blood glucose to rise quickly, whereas an infection or illness will result in hyperglycemia over the course of several days.

If left untreated, hyperglycemia will progress to diabetic ketoacidosis (DKA). A life-threatening condition, DKA occurs when certain acids accumulate in the body because insulin is not available Figure 29-9 ▶. Patients who suffer from this condition tend to be young—teenagers and young adults. In DKA, the deficiency of insulin prevents cells from taking up the extra sugar. From the viewpoint of the cells, famine is at hand, and a distress signal goes out over the sympathetic nervous system, causing the release of various stress hormones. Because the body can't utilize glucose, it turns instead to other sources of energy—principally, fat. The metabolism of fat generates *acids* and *ketones* as waste products. (The ketones give the characteristic fruity odor to the breath of a patent in DKA.) Because glucose must be excreted in the urine in solution, the body loses excessive amounts of water and electrolytes (sodium and potassium). This may lead to disturbances in water balance and acid–base balance. Disturbances in acid–base balance and the compensatory role of the kidneys are covered in more detail in Chapter 6.

Meanwhile, glucose continues to accumulate in the blood. As the blood sugar rises, the patient undergoes massive osmotic diuresis (passing large amounts of urine because of the high solute concentration of the blood); this, together with vomiting, causes dehydration and even shock.

These processes usually progress slowly, over a period of 12 to 48 hours, with the patient's level of consciousness deteriorating only gradually. Patients in DKA are seldom deeply comatose, so if the patient is totally unresponsive, look for another source of the coma, such as head injury, stroke, or drug overdose.

If you are certain the IV is reliable, open the IV wide (don't pinch it shut) and administer 25 g of D$_{50}$ *slowly,* over at least 3 minutes. To ensure the patency of the line, draw back on the D$_{50}$ syringe (eg, Bristojet) to observe a blood return. If the cause of coma is hypoglycemia, the patient will often waken with dramatic rapidity—although in cases of very severe hypoglycemia, another 25 g of D$_{50}$ may be required to restore a normal level of consciousness.

If vascular access is not available, glucagon, 1 mg by intramuscular injection, should be given.

Hyperglycemia and Diabetic Ketoacidosis

Hyperglycemia (high blood glucose level) is one of the classic symptoms of diabetes mellitus. Common early signs include frequent and excessive thirst, accompanied by frequent and excessive urination. A hyperglycemic condition without other classic symptoms is not dispositive of a diagnosis of diabetes mellitus, but hyperglycemia is also an independent medical condition with other causes. The signs and symptoms of hypoglycemia and hyperglycemia can be quite similar Table 29-4 ▲ .

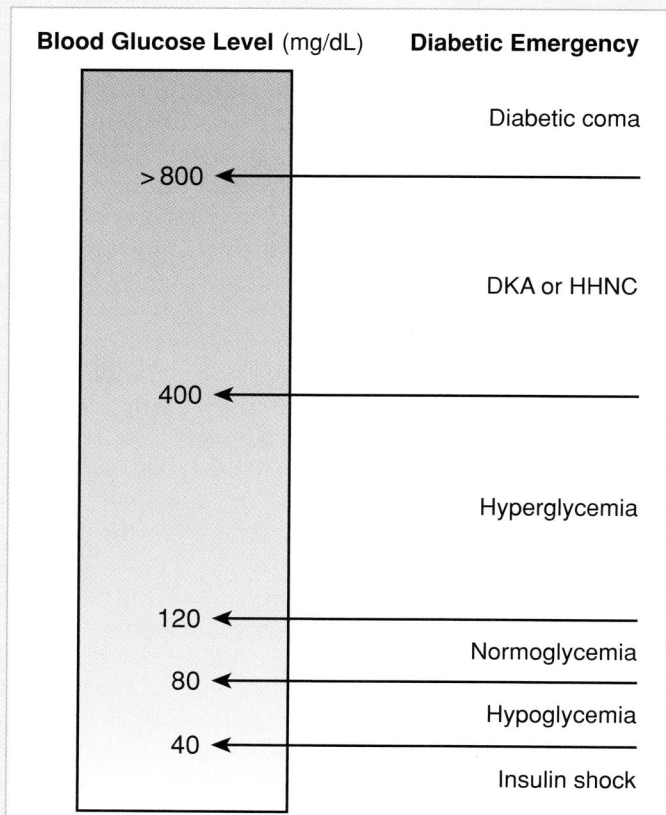

Blood Glucose Level (mg/dL)   **Diabetic Emergency**

Diabetic coma

> 800

DKA or HHNC

400

Hyperglycemia

120

Normoglycemia

80

Hypoglycemia

40

Insulin shock

Figure 29-9 The two most common diabetic emergencies, diabetic ketoacidosis and insulin shock, develop when the patient has too much or too little glucose in the blood, respectively.

In the Field

There is no predictable correlation between the increase in a patient's blood glucose level and the degree of ketoacidosis in the blood. Rely on the patient's clinical presentation rather than the "number."

The signs and symptoms of DKA are generally predictable from the underlying pathophysiology:

- Polyuria (excessive urine output), because of osmotic diuresis
- Polydipsia (excessive thirst), because of dehydration
- Polyphagia (excessive eating), probably related to inefficient utilization of nutrients
- Nausea and vomiting, the latter worsening dehydration
- Tachycardia as a consequence of dehydration
- Deep, rapid respirations (Kussmaul respirations)—the body's attempt to compensate for acidosis by blowing off carbon dioxide
- Warm, dry skin and dry mucous membranes, also reflecting dehydration
- Fruity odor of ketones on the breath
- Sometimes fever, abdominal pain, and hypotension

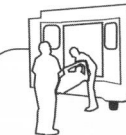

In the Field

Common causes of DKA include infection, injury, alcohol use, emotional discord, and illness, such as stroke or MI.

The treatment of DKA in the field depends on making the correct diagnosis. If the patient's history and physical examination are consistent with DKA and your field measurement of the patient's glucose level reveals that it is markedly elevated (more than 300 mg/dL), the physician will probably order treatment for DKA. The goals of prehospital treatment are to begin rehydration and to correct the patient's electrolyte and acid–base abnormalities. In most instances, specific treatment with insulin should await the patient's arrival at the hospital, where therapy can be closely monitored with laboratory determinations of blood sugar, ketones, etc.

Follow the procedure for any comatose patient with regard to airway maintenance and oxygen. Be particularly alert for *vomiting,* and have suction ready.

Start an IV and infuse up to 1 L of NS over the first half hour or at the rate suggested by protocol or online medical control. Remember, a patient in DKA is severely dehydrated, often to the point of shock, and needs volume, usually at a rate of about 1 L/h for at least the first few hours.

Monitor cardiac rhythm. Changes in serum potassium caused by DKA can lead to marked myocardial instability. Note the contour of the T waves on the rhythm strip; if they are sharply peaked, the patient's potassium level may be dangerously high, and you may need to administer sodium bicarbonate. If ordered to do so, proceed with extreme caution—even a little too much can cause serious problems, including death.

Hyperosmolar Nonketotic Coma

Hyperosmolar nonketotic coma (HONK), also called hyperosmolar hyperglycemic nonketotic coma (HHNC), is a metabolic derangement that occurs principally in patients with type 2 diabetes. This condition is characterized by hyperglycemia, hyperosmolarity, and an absence of significant ketosis.

Oddly enough, coma is present in fewer than 10% of cases. Instead, most patients present with severe dehydration and focal or global neurologic deficits. In addition, acute MI is frequently associated with HONK/HHNC. The clinical features of HONK/HHNC and DKA tend to overlap and are often observed simultaneously.

HONK/HHNC often develops in patients with diabetes who have some secondary illness that leads to reduced fluid intake. Although infection (in particular, pneumonia and urinary tract infection) is the most common cause, many other conditions can cause altered mentation or dehydration. In most cases, the secondary illness is not identified.

Hyperglycemia and hyperosmolarity lead to osmotic diuresis and an osmotic shift of fluid to the intravascular space, resulting in further intracellular dehydration. Unlike patients

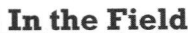

In the Field

Certain medications may contribute to the development of HONK/HHNC by raising serum glucose, inhibiting insulin, or causing dehydration: diuretics, beta blockers, histamine-2 (H_2) blockers, dialysis, total parenteral nutrition, and dextrose-containing fluids.

with DKA, patients with HONK/HHNC do not develop ketoacidosis. Although most patients diagnosed with HONK/HHNC have a known history of diabetes (usually type 2), approximately 30% do not have a prior diagnosis of diabetes. The stress response to any acute illness tends to increase hormones that favor elevated glucose levels; cortisol, catecholamines (epinephrine and norepinephrine), glucagon, and many other hormones have effects that tend to counter those of insulin. Various neurologic changes may be found, including drowsiness and lethargy, delirium and coma, focal or generalized seizures, visual disturbances, hemiparesis, and sensory deficits.

The treatment of HONK/HHNC in the prehospital setting follows the pathway for dehydration and altered mental status. Airway management is the top priority. The comatose patient is

In the Field

Not all patients with increased blood glucose levels have DKA or HONK/HHNC. Many people have glucose intolerance and hyperglycemia with absolutely no symptoms. Look at the patient, not at the number.

often unable to maintain and protect his or her airway. For this reason, endotracheal intubation may be indicated and should be completed as early as possible. Cervical spine immobilization should be used for all unresponsive patients found down, unless witnesses can validate that no fall occurred. Large-bore IV access should be gained as soon as possible, but do not delay transfer while initiating the IV. If necessary, obtain IV access during the transport to the emergency department. Also obtain a blood glucose level as soon as possible.

In the Field

Although oral steroid therapy is the most common cause of exogenous adrenal suppression, inhaled steroids (used for asthma or chronic obstructive pulmonary disease) may also have a similar effect.

Once you have initiated the IV, a bolus of 500 mL 0.9% NS is appropriate for nearly all adults who are clinically dehydrated. In patients with a history of congestive heart failure and/or renal insufficiency, a 250-mL bolus may be a more appropriate starting point. Fluid deficits in HONK/HHNC patients may amount to 10 L or more. These patients may receive 1 to 2 L within the first hour. If the glucose level is less than 60 to 80 mg/dL, then (depending on your local protocols), administer 25 g of D_{50} as soon as possible.

Adrenal Insufficiency

Adrenal insufficiency is characterized by decreased function of the adrenal cortex and consequent underproduction of cortisol

You are the Provider Part 3

You quickly begin to look for an IV site as your partner prepares the equipment and a prefilled syringe of D_{50}. An 18-gauge catheter is successfully inserted into the right antecubital fossa and you administer 25 grams of D_{50}. Within a minute, your patient becomes more alert and is confused and scared about her surroundings.

You explain to the patient what happened while she was in the courtroom. She blushes and becomes embarrassed. She admits to being diabetic and tells you that the trial has been making her stressed and as a result she has not been eating properly and trying to self-regulate her insulin. She denies any other medical history, medications, or allergies.

Reassessment	Recording Time: 11 Minutes
Skin	Pink, warm, and dry
Pulse	85 beats/min, strong and regular
Blood pressure	116/74 mm Hg
Respirations	18 breaths/min, regular
Sao_2	98% on room air
ECG	Sinus rhythm with no ectopy
Pupils	PERLA
Blood glucose	149 mg/dL

5. Which medications besides insulin can be used to control diabetes?

and aldosterone. A decrease in either of these adrenal hormones will result in weakness, dehydration, and the body's inability to maintain adequate blood pressure or to properly respond to stress.

Cortisol affects almost every organ and tissue in the body. Although its primary role is to assist with the body's response to stress, this adrenal hormone also helps maintain blood pressure and cardiovascular function; regulates the metabolism of carbohydrates, proteins, and fats; affects glucose levels in the blood by balancing the effects of insulin; and functions as an anti-inflammatory agent by slowing the inflammatory response.

Aldosterone regulates and maintains the salt and potassium balance in the blood. Secretion of this adrenal hormone is primarily regulated by the renin–angiotensin system, but is also stimulated by increased serum potassium concentrations.

Abnormal adrenal cortical function produces abnormalities in the metabolism of carbohydrates and protein as well as disturbances of salt and water metabolism. This condition is usually well tolerated unless there are coexisting factors (eg, infection, stress). It affects about 4 people per 100,000 in the United States, strikes an equal number of men and women, and is found in patients of all races and ages.

Primary Versus Secondary Adrenal Insufficiency

Adrenal insufficiency is classified as either primary or secondary. Primary adrenal insufficiency (also known as Addison's disease) is caused by atrophy or destruction of both adrenal glands, leading to deficiency of all the steroid hormones produced by these glands. A rare disease (occurring in approximately 1/100,000 persons in the United States), it is most frequently the result of idiopathic atrophy, an autoimmune process in which the immune system creates antibodies that attack the adrenal cortex, which leads to its gradual destruction. This phenomenon accounts for approximately 70% of Addison's disease cases in the United States. Adrenal insufficiency occurs when at least 90% of the adrenal cortex has been destroyed. Less commonly (approximately 30% of cases), the adrenal destruction is caused by tuberculosis; bacterial, viral, or fungal infections; adrenal hemorrhage; or cancer of the adrenal glands. Patients with Addison's disease who receive treatment have a normal life expectancy.

In patients with Addison's disease, the body fails to properly regulate the content of sodium, potassium, and water in body fluids. Blood volume and pressure fall, as does the concentration of sodium in the blood; blood potassium rises. The blood volume may become so reduced that the circulation can

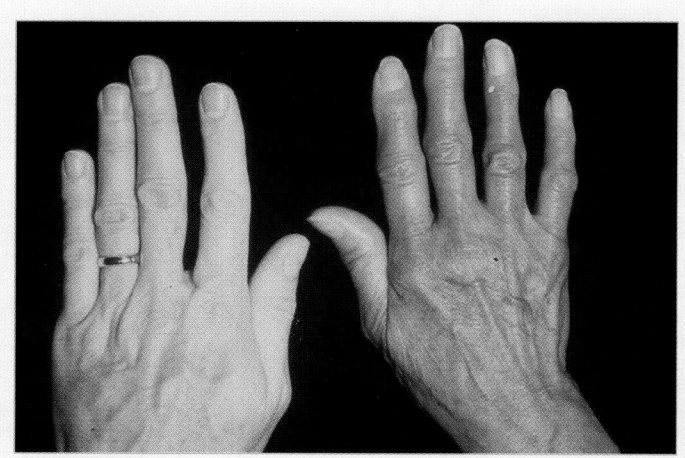

Figure 29-10 The hand of a patient with Addison's disease (right) compared with the hand of a normal subject (left).

no longer be maintained efficiently. Patients with Addison's disease also frequently exhibit increased pigmentation of the skin, which is caused by the increased secretion of hormones Figure 29-10 ▲ .

Secondary adrenal insufficiency (a relatively common condition) is defined as a lack of ACTH secretion from the pituitary gland. ACTH, a pituitary messenger, stimulates the adrenal cortex to manufacture and secrete cortisol. If ACTH secretion is insufficient, cortisol production is not stimulated. Patients who abruptly stop taking corticosteroids (eg, prednisone) may also experience secondary adrenal insufficiency. Corticosteroid treatments suppress natural cortical production; however, aldosterone production is usually not affected with this form of adrenal insufficiency.

Addisonian Crisis

Signs and symptoms of acute adrenal insufficiency may appear suddenly and are referred to as an Addisonian crisis. They may result from an acute exacerbation of chronic insufficiency, usually brought on by a period of stress, trauma, surgery, or severe infection. Steroid withdrawal is the most common cause.

Although most patients with adrenal insufficiency experience symptoms that are severe enough to seek medical treatment prior to a crisis, approximately 25% of patients will develop their first symptoms during an Addisonian crisis. The primary clinical manifestation of adrenal crisis is shock. Patients may also manifest nonspecific symptoms, including weakness; lethargy; confusion or loss of consciousness; low blood pressure (vascular collapse); elevated temperature; severe pain in the lower back, legs, or abdomen; and severe vomiting and diarrhea that leads to dehydration.

Treatment of Adrenal Insufficiency

Adrenal insufficiency is a potentially fatal disease if unrecognized and untreated. Death usually results from hypotension or cardiac dysrhythmias due to hyperkalemia. The treatment for adrenal insufficiency is based on the clinical presentation and

In the Field

Signs of chronic adrenal insufficiency include unexplained weight loss, fatigue, vomiting, diarrhea, anorexia, salt craving, muscle and joint pain, abdominal pain, postural dizziness, and increased pigmentation in the extensor surfaces, palm creases, and oral mucosa.

findings, and is geared toward maintaining the airway, breathing, and circulation until arrival at the emergency department. Other goals of prehospital treatment are to begin rehydration of the patient and to correct the electrolyte and acid–base abnormalities.

Follow the procedure for a patient with altered mental status or comatose patient with regard to airway maintenance and supplemental oxygen. Be alert for *vomiting,* and have suction ready.

Start an IV and infuse up to 1 L of 0.9% NS. If the patient is hypotensive, administer an NS bolus at 20 mL/kg. Remember, a patient in adrenal insufficiency may be severely dehydrated, often to the point of shock, and needs volume.

Check the patient's glucose level. Administer 25 to 50 g of D_{50} to correct the hypoglycemia. D_5NS is the preferred IV fluid, but a second IV, administering D_5W, can be used to maintain the patient's blood glucose level. Monitor cardiac rhythm, as changes in serum electrolytes can lead to marked myocardial instability.

Cushing's Syndrome

Cushing's syndrome is caused by an excess of cortisol production by the adrenal glands or by excessive use of cortisol or other similar steroid (glucocorticoid) hormones. Tumors of the pituitary gland or adrenal cortex can stimulate the production of excess hormone, for example, and lead to Cushing's syndrome. Administration of large amounts of cortisol or other glucocorticoid hormones (eg, hydrocortisone, prednisone, methylprednisolone, or dexamethasone) for the treatment of life-threatening illnesses, such as asthma, rheumatoid arthritis, systemic lupus, inflammatory bowel disease, and some allergies, can also cause this syndrome.

Regardless of the cause, excess cortisol causes characteristic changes in many body systems. Metabolism of carbohydrate, protein, and fat is disturbed, such that the blood glucose level rises. Protein synthesis is impaired so that body proteins are broken down, which leads to loss of muscle fibers and muscle weakness. Bones become weaker and more susceptible to fracture. Other common signs and symptoms related to excess cortisol include the following:

- Weakness and fatigue
- Depression and mood swings
- Increased thirst and urination
- Low blood glucose level
- Weight gain, especially on the abdomen, face ("moon face"), neck, and upper back ("buffalo hump")
- Thinning of the skin, with easy bruising and pink or purple stretch marks (striae) on the abdomen, thighs, breasts, and shoulders
- Increased acne, facial hair growth, and scalp hair loss in women, and cessation of menstrual periods
- Darkening of skin (acanthosis) on the neck
- Obesity and poor growth in height in children

The incidence of Cushing's syndrome is about 5 to 25 cases per 1 million people per year. It generally affects people between the ages of 25 and 45.

Prehospital treatment is generally supportive. Obtain a glucose level, monitor the patient's blood pressure, and treat abnormalities as they present.

Hypothyroidism and Hyperthyroidism

Thyroid hormone is secreted in response to the stimulation of the thyroid gland by the anterior pituitary gland. The anterior pituitary gland secretes thyroid-stimulating hormone (TSH) in response to the hypothalamus's secretion of thyrotropin-releasing hormone (TRH). **Table 29-5 ▶** summarizes the major effects of hypothyroidism and hyperthyroidism. Approximately 20 million Americans suffer some kind thyroid disorder, and many of them will be unaware of their condition.

You are the Provider Part 4

Concerned about the attention she has brought to herself, your patient requests not to be transported to the hospital. She does not want to cause any further delays in the court proceedings or be removed from the jury. You explain to her that although her blood sugar level has returned to normal, it's still very important for her to be transported to the hospital to ensure that it will remain stable. Still hesitant about going to the hospital, the patient asks if she could contact her physician to get his opinion. You agree and help her place the call. After much convincing from her physician, she agrees to be transported to the hospital for observation.

Reassessment	Recording Time: 20 Minutes
Skin	Pink, warm, and dry
Pulse	84 beats/min, strong and irregular
Blood pressure	118/74 mm Hg
Respirations	18 breaths/min, regular
Sao$_2$	98% on room air
ECG	Sinus rhythm with no ectopy

6. Does diabetes affect other organ systems?

Table 29-5	Comparison of Major Effects of Hypothyroidism and Hyperthyroidism	
	Hypothyroidism	**Hyperthyroidism**
Cardiovascular effects	Slow pulse, reduced cardiac output	Rapid pulse, increased cardiac output
Metabolic effects	Decreased metabolism, cold skin, weight gain	Increased metabolism, skin hot and flushed, weight loss
Neuromuscular effects	Weakness, sluggish reflexes	Tremor, hyperactive reflexes
Mental, emotional effects	Mental processes sluggish, personality placid	Restlessness, irritability, emotional lability
Gastrointestinal effects	Constipated	Diarrhea
General somatic effects	Cold, dry skin	Warm, moist skin

In the Field

Both hyperthyroidism and hypothyroidism patients are likely to require supplemental oxygen. Hyperthyroid metabolic activity increases oxygen demand. Hypothyroid conditions may lead to diminished respiratory effort that may require positive-pressure ventilation.

Myxedema Coma

Thyroid hormones are critical for cell metabolism and organ function. If their supply becomes inadequate, organ tissues don't grow or mature (due to the decreased metabolic rate), energy production declines (a cause of the decreased metabolic rate), and the actions of other hormones are affected.

Adult hypothyroidism is sometimes called *myxedema*. The condition is manifested by a general slowing of the body's metabolic processes due to the reduction or absence of thyroid hormone. All organ systems may exhibit symptoms in such a case, with the severity of the symptoms reflecting the degree of hormone deficiency. Frequently, there are localized accumulations of mucinous material in the skin, which gives the disease its name (*myx* = mucin; *edema* = swelling) **Figure 29-11 ◄**.

Symptoms of hypothyroidism include fatigue, feeling cold, weight gain, dry skin, and sleepiness. Because these symptoms are often subtle and can be mistaken for other conditions, the disease may go undiagnosed. Continued decrease of the hormone levels may lead to

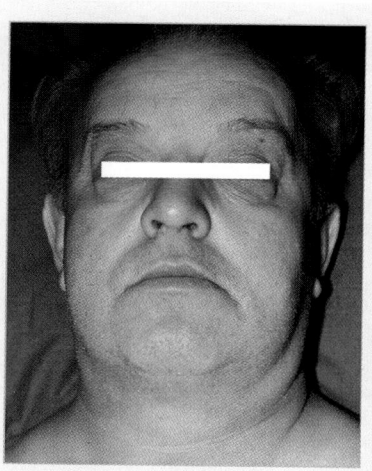

Figure 29-11 Localized accumulations of mucinous material in the neck of a hypothyroid patient.

myxedema coma, an extreme manifestation of untreated hypothyroidism that is accompanied by physiologic decompensation. When hypothyroidism is long standing, physiologic adaptations occur, such as reduced metabolic rate and decreased oxygen consumption, which in turn lead to peripheral vasoconstriction. Triggers such as infection (especially lung and urine infections), exposure to cold, trauma, surgery, and certain medications are often precipitating factors in the progression to myxedema coma.

The hallmark of myxedema coma is deterioration of the patient's mental status. Although family members may not be overly concerned about more subtle changes, such as apathy or decreased intellectual function, more obvious changes, such as confusion, psychosis, and coma, will most certainly elicit a call for emergency assistance.

Most cases of myxedema coma occur during the winter in women older than age 60. The condition is 4 to 8 times more common in women than in men. Just as the incidence of hypothyroidism increases with age, myxedema coma occurs primarily in elderly patients. One consistent finding is hypothermia, and you may need to use a thermometer that records temperatures of less than 90° F in cases of myxedema coma. Thus absence of fever in the presence of infection is a common finding.

Hypothyroidism decreases intestinal motility, and the decreased metabolic rate associated with this condition can lead to drug toxicity, especially in the elderly. A slower metabolic rate causes the levels of medications, especially those that affect the central nervous system, to rise to toxic levels in the blood. This accidental overdose in the hypothyroid patient can actually precipitate myxedema coma.

Myxedema coma is a metabolic and cardiovascular emergency. If not diagnosed and treated immediately, the mortality rates are approximately 50%. Thus the patient's condition must be stabilized as soon as possible.

Administer supplemental oxygen therapy to correct hypoxia. Intubation and ventilation are indicated for patients with diminished respiratory drive or those who are unable to protect their airway; these measures will help prevent respiratory failure.

Monitor the patient's cardiac status. Hypotension may respond to crystalloid therapy, and vasopressive agents may be

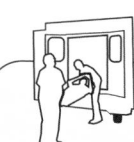

In the Field

Protrusion of the eyeballs (exophthalmos) is common in chronic hyperthyroidism.

necessary (dopamine). Administer 25 to 50 g of D$_{50}$ if glucose levels are less than 60 mg/dL.

Treat hypothermia with passive rewarming methods, as aggressive rewarming may lead to vasodilation and hypotension. Hemodynamically unstable patients with profound hypothermia, however, will require active rewarming. Avoid sedatives, narcotics, and anesthetics because of the delayed metabolism.

Thyrotoxicosis

Thyrotoxicosis is a toxic condition caused by excessive levels of circulating thyroid hormone. Although hyperthyroidism can cause thyrotoxicosis in some patients, the two conditions are not identical. Thyrotoxicosis may also be caused by goiters, autoimmune disease (Grave's disease—the most common cause of hyperthyroidism), and thyroid cancer. Grave's disease, which has an incidence of 1.4 cases per 1,000 persons, has a chronic course with remissions and relapses. If left untreated, it may be fatal.

In the Field

Both hyperthyroidism and hypothyroidism can adversely affect the electrical status of the myocardium. Application of the cardiac monitor may reveal tachyarrhythmias in hyperthyroidism or bradyarrhythmias in hypothyroidism. Treat all arrhythmias according to your local protocols, while keeping in mind that these arrhythmias may be difficult to correct without first fixing the underlying disorder.

A thyroid storm is a rare, life-threatening condition that may occur in patients with thyrotoxicosis. The condition is usually triggered by a stressful event or increased volume of thyroid hormones in the circulation. In addition to the normal signs and symptoms of hyperthyroidism, patients may present with fever, severe tachycardia, nausea, vomiting, altered mental status, and possibly heart failure.

General Assessment

The difficult part of assessing patients with endocrine emergencies is that their problems tend to affect many organ systems and the seriousness of their presentations varies greatly. Many of the patients will have had their conditions for some time and may already be receiving treatment. These patients or their family members will likely share with you that there is a history of an endocrine problem; this information, in addition to the common signs and symptoms associated with each endocrine emergency, should help you determine the cause of the current problem. In any event, don't take these calls lightly, as poor outcomes can result very quickly.

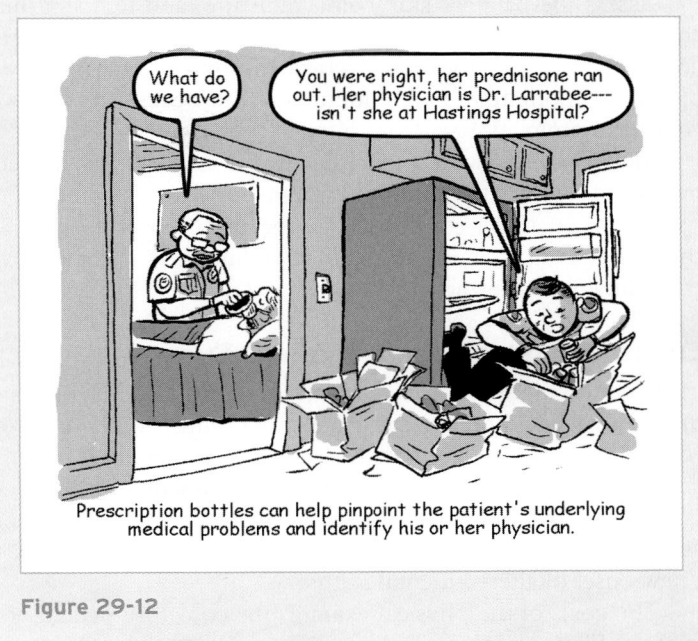

Prescription bottles can help pinpoint the patient's underlying medical problems and identify his or her physician.

Figure 29-12

Scene Size-up

Your initial scene size-up will vary depending on the rate of the progression of deterioration and the patient's symptoms when you arrive. Regardless of the patient's condition or the cause, airway, breathing, and circulation must always be assessed first.

Your observations of the scene in which the patient is found can also furnish valuable information regarding what might have happened. Check bureau tops, bedside tables, and medicine cabinets for medications that might give a clue as to the patient's underlying illness. Check the refrigerator for insulin **Figure 29-12 ▲**. Bring any medication bottles along with the patient to the hospital. They can help pinpoint the patient's underlying medical problems and identify his or her physician, who should be able to provide more information.

Initial Assessment

The initial assessment begins with the basics: airway, breathing, and circulation. Patients in the middle of any endocrine emergency may be in serious distress, so be prepared to assist them if your initial assessment reveals any of these basics to be abnormal.

When patients present with an altered level of consciousness, they may be unable to protect the airway. Many will be very ill and have chronic episodes of vomiting. Maintain the airway as needed through patient positioning, suctioning, or basic airways.

Patients with endocrine emergencies may present with a variety of breathing levels. Supplemental oxygen is recommended in all cases of suspected respiratory involvement. Although pulse oximetry is commonly used, don't let a reading at a normal or above-normal level persuade you to withhold oxygen.

Assess the patient's skin color, moisture, and temperature, and take his or her blood pressure. Because endocrine emergencies may affect the body's compensating systems, IVs or blood component replenishment may be necessary. Follow your local protocols.

Many patients with endocrine disorders are being treated by specialists, and they should be transported to a facility that specializes in these conditions. If the patient is unstable or shows signs of becoming unstable, take him or her to the closest facility for stabilization first.

Focused History and Physical Exam

In diabetic emergencies in particular, the family history can provide very important information. Because diabetes is a genetic disease (passed down through family members), learning that a parent or grandparent has a diabetic history is a major clue, and may prove to be invaluable in your treatment decision. This is especially true if the patient is a child and has a new onset of altered mental status.

The goals of the physical exam in the comatose patient are twofold. First, you want to determine the patient's level of consciousness with precision, so that other examiners who assess him or her later can readily determine whether the patient's condition is improving or deteriorating. Second, you should look for signs that might provide clues to the source of coma.

Begin the physical assessment by observing the patient's general appearance and the position in which he or she is found. Patients found in awkward positions often have brain stem damage; conversely, a natural posture tends to be a good sign. Decorticate or decerebrate posturing should also be noted, if present; both are *bad* signs.

Your physical examination should be geared toward identifying as many atypical findings as possible. Using this information, you can make a more educated decision about treatment. Unless the patient had an endocrine emergency that caused some form of trauma, a rapid trauma assessment is usually not necessary.

Detailed Physical Exam

The detailed physical exam will reveal the finer abnormalities that will provide you with the final determining factors for your treatment.

The condition of the skin may be very informative. Cold, clammy skin is classically a sign of shock but may also signal severe hypoglycemia, as from an insulin reaction. Cold, dry skin may indicate overdose of sedative drugs or alcohol. Hot, dry skin suggests fever or, if the circumstances are appropriate, heat stroke.

In checking the vital signs, look for the combination of hypertension and bradycardia, which suggest increased intracranial pressure. Be alert for abnormal respiratory patterns. Cheyne-Stokes breathing usually points to a nonneurologic source of the coma. More worrisome are other abnormal breathing patterns, such as central neurogenic ventilation or

huffing and puffing that doesn't seem to move much air. Look for "pararespiratory" motions, such as sneezing and yawning. An intact brain stem is required to produce a sneeze or a yawn, so both of those actions have positive prognostic significance. Hiccupping and coughing, by contrast, may indicate brain stem damage.

Ongoing Assessment

Once you've initiated your treatment plan, continually reassess the patient to check for obvious, and subtle, changes. For every action you take, there should be a response. No response *is a* response. Document your findings along the way.

General Management

Management of the ABCs should have been carried out during the initial assessment. Remember that a patient whose gag reflex is absent can't protect his or her own airway from aspiration and should be intubated at the earliest opportunity. If breathing is abnormally slow or shallow, assist breathing with bag-mask ventilation. Give supplemental oxygen whether the patient is breathing spontaneously or being ventilated.

If the patient has altered mental status, establish an IV with 0.9% NS or a saline lock. Make an immediate determination of the blood glucose level and initiate treatment if the reading is less than 60 mg/dL. Give 25 g of D_{50}; this dose will reverse most cases of hypoglycemia. If the patient doesn't come around after a dose of D_{50} or if you have any other reason to suspect narcotics overdosage (pinpoint pupils, needle tracks on the arms, depressed respirations), then consider administration of Narcan.

Monitor the cardiac rhythm of every comatose patient. For the neurologic assessment, the most important consideration is not a single measurement at a single point in time but rather the *trend* shown by several measurements. Recheck vital signs, pupils, and level of consciousness (every 5 minutes in unstable patients and every 10 minutes in stable patients) and *record your findings* immediately.

Transport the comatose patient *supine* if he or she is intubated; otherwise, you may transport the patient in the stable side position (unless injuries preclude that position). If the patient must be supine (eg, because of suspected spine injury) and can't be intubated, keep the mouth and pharynx suctioned free of secretions, vomitus, and blood.

In the Field

Obtaining blood specimens early is particularly important in the diabetic patient because any administration of prehospital dextrose or other medications will significantly change the chemical makeup of subsequent blood samples.

You are the Provider Summary

1. What are some potential differential diagnoses?

On the basis of the signs and symptoms, your patient's potential differential diagnoses can include hypotension, drug overdose, arrhythmias, and hypoglycemia.

2. When do symptoms of hypoglycemia occur?

Signs and symptoms of hypoglycemia usually occur once the blood glucose level falls below 60 mg/dL. However, if the drop in glucose levels is rapid, they can be seen at higher levels.

3. What are some of the causes of hypoglycemia?

The causes of hypoglycemia are very diverse. The more common causes of hypoglycemia in patients with diabetes are taking too much insulin or oral hypoglycemic medications, not eating enough, and unusual or extreme exercise without adequate food intake. Hypoglycemia may also be found in patients who are chronic alcoholics, suffer from malnutrition, or have pancreatic disorders, liver disease, hypothermia, cancer, or sepsis. Be on the lookout for intentional overdoses on insulin and oral hypoglycemic medications. People with a history of eating disorders may take insulin to burn off the "extra calories" of desserts or other foods that may be considered high calorie.

4. How may a patient with hypoglycemia present?

Why, you may actually be exhibiting signs and symptoms of hypoglycemia as you are studying this section! Are you hungry, irritable, shaky, or have a headache? Are you having sugar cravings? These are all signs and symptoms of hypoglycemia. Others include changes in mental status, appearance of intoxication, seizures, and coma. Vital sign changes will include a weak, rapid pulse and pale, cool, diaphoretic skin.

5. Which medications besides insulin can be used to control diabetes?

Patients with type 2 diabetes may be prescribed oral hypoglycemic agents to help regulate their glucose levels. Type 2 diabetics are able to use these medications because they work with the body's own insulin (they have working beta cells). Examples of commonly prescribed oral hypoglycemic agents include chlorpropamide, tolazide, tolbutamide, glipizide, and glyburide. Two newer medications include pioglitizone and metformin.

6. Does diabetes affect other organ systems?

Unfortunately, the answer to this question is yes. Diabetic patients are at risk for developing blindness, kidney disease, peripheral neuropathy, hypertension, atherosclerosis, heart disease, and peripheral vascular disease.

Prep Kit

Ready for Review

- The endocrine system directly or indirectly influences almost every cell, organ, and function of the body.
- Patients with an endocrine disorder often present with a multitude of signs and symptoms that require a thorough assessment and immediate treatment to interrupt life-threatening emergencies.
- The endocrine system comprises a network of glands that produce and secrete hormones. The main function of the endocrine system and its hormone messengers is to maintain homeostasis and promote permanent structural changes.
- Hormones travel in the bloodstream to target tissues.
- The major components of the endocrine system are the hypothalamus, pituitary, thyroid, parathyroid, adrenals, and reproductive organs (gonads). The pancreas is also part of this system; it has a role in hormone production as well as in digestion.
- The pituitary gland is often referred to as the "master gland" because its secretions control, or regulate, the secretions of other endocrine glands.
- The thyroid secretes thyroxine when the body's metabolic rate decreases. Thyroxine, the body's major metabolic hormone, stimulates energy production in cells, which increases the rate at which cells consume oxygen and use carbohydrates, fats, and proteins. The thyroid gland also secretes calcitonin, which helps maintain normal calcium levels in the blood.
- The adrenal glands produce hormones that regulate the body's metabolism, its balance of salt and water, the immune system, and sexual function. Adrenal hormones also help the body cope with physical and emotional stress by increasing the pulse and respiratory rates and the blood pressure.
- The pancreas secretes digestive enzymes as well as the hormones glucagon and insulin, which are responsible for the regulation of blood glucose levels.
- The gonads are the main source of sex hormones (Table 29-3). In men, the gonads, or testes, are located in the scrotum and produce hormones called androgens. The most important androgen in men is testosterone. Androgens regulate body changes associated with sexual development (puberty), including growth spurts, deepening of the voice, growth of facial and pubic hair, and muscle growth and strength.
- In women, the gonads are the ovaries, which release the eggs and secrete the hormones estrogen and progesterone.
- Diabetes is a metabolic disorder in which the body's ability to metabolize glucose is impaired. It is characterized by the passage of large quantities of urine containing glucose, significant thirst, and deterioration of body function.
- In type 1 diabetes, most patients do not produce insulin at all. They require daily injections of supplemental synthetic insulin throughout their lives to control blood glucose levels.
- The most common form of diabetes is type 2 diabetes (sometimes called adult-onset diabetes), in which blood glucose levels are elevated.
- Hypoglycemia in the insulin-dependent diabetic is often the result of having taken too much insulin, too little food, or both. The patient will experience trembling, a rapid pulse rate, sweating, and a feeling of hunger—a result of the actions of epinephrine.
- Hyperglycemia (high blood glucose level) is one of the classic symptoms of diabetes mellitus. Common early signs include frequent and excessive thirst, accompanied by frequent and excessive urination.
- If left untreated, hyperglycemia progresses to the life-threatening condition known as diabetic ketoacidosis (DKA). DKA occurs when certain acids accumulate in the body because insulin is not available.
- Hyperosmolar nonketotic coma (HONK), also called hyperosmolar hyperglycemic nonketotic coma (HHNC), is a metabolic derangement that occurs principally in patients with type 2 diabetes. This condition is characterized by hyperglycemia, hyperosmolarity, and an absence of significant ketosis.
- Adrenal insufficiency is characterized by underproduction of cortisol and aldosterone, which leads to weakness, dehydration, and the body's inability to maintain adequate blood pressure or to properly respond to stress. Primary adrenal insufficiency (also known as Addison's disease) is caused by atrophy or destruction of both adrenal glands, leading to deficiency of all the steroid hormones produced by these glands. Secondary adrenal insufficiency is defined as a lack of ACTH secretion from the pituitary gland.
- Acute adrenal insufficiency is referred to as an Addisonian crisis, which may result from an acute exacerbation of chronic insufficiency, usually brought on by a period of stress, trauma, surgery, or severe infection.
- Cushing's syndrome is caused by an excess of cortisol production by the adrenal glands or by excessive use of cortisol or other similar steroid (glucocorticoid) hormones.
- Thyroid hormones are critical for cell metabolism and organ function. If their supply becomes inadequate, organ tissues don't grow or mature (due to the decreased metabolic rate), energy production declines (a cause of the decreased metabolic rate), and the actions of other hormones are affected.
- Symptoms of hypothyroidism include fatigue, feeling cold, weight gain, dry skin, and sleepiness. Continued decrease of the hormone levels may lead to myxedema coma.
- Thyrotoxicosis is a toxic condition caused by excessive levels of circulating thyroid hormone. A thyroid storm is a rare, life-threatening condition that may occur in patients with thyrotoxicosis.
- Assessing patients with endocrine emergencies can be difficult because their conditions tend to affect many organ systems and the seriousness of their presentations varies greatly. Don't take these calls lightly, as poor outcomes can result very quickly.

Vital Vocabulary

adrenal cortex The outer part of the adrenal glands that produces corticosteroids.

adrenal glands Paired glands located above the kidneys; each adrenal gland consists of an inner adrenal medulla and an adrenal cortex.

adrenal medulla The inner part of the adrenal glands that produces catecholamines (epinephrine and norepinephrine).

adrenocorticotropic hormone (ACTH) Hormone that targets the adrenal cortex to secrete cortisol (a glucocorticoid).

agonists Molecules that bind to a cell's receptor and trigger a response by that cell. Agonists produce some kind of action or biologic effect.

aldosterone Hormone that stimulates the kidneys to reabsorb sodium from the urine and excrete potassium by altering the osmotic gradient in the blood.

androgens Male sex hormones that regulate body changes associated with sexual development (puberty), including growth spurts, deepening of the voice, growth of facial and pubic hair, and muscle growth and strength.

antagonist Molecules that bind to a cell's receptor and block the action of agonists. Hormone antagonists are widely used as drugs.

antidiuretic hormone (ADH) A hormone secreted by the posterior pituitary lobe of the pituitary gland, ADH constricts blood vessels and raises the blood pressure; also called vasopressin.

calcitonin The hormone secreted by the thyroid gland that helps maintain normal calcium levels in the blood.

catecholamines Hormones produced by the adrenal medulla (epinephrine and norepinephrine) that assist the body in coping with physical and emotional stress by increasing the heart and respiratory rates and the blood pressure.

corticosteroids Hormones that regulate the body's metabolism, the balance of salt and water in the body, the immune system, and sexual function.

cortisol Hormone that stimulates most body cells to increase their energy production.

Cushing's syndrome A condition caused by an excess of cortisol production by the adrenal glands or by excessive use of cortisol or other similar steroid (glucocorticoid) hormones.

diabetes mellitus Disease characterized by the body's inability to sufficiently metabolize glucose. The condition occurs either because the pancreas doesn't produce enough insulin or the cells don't respond to the effects of the insulin that's produced.

diabetic ketoacidosis (DKA) A form of acidosis in uncontrolled diabetes in which certain acids accumulate when insulin is not available.

endocrine glands Glands that secrete or release chemicals that are used inside the body. Endocrine glands lack ducts and release hormones directly into the surrounding tissue and blood.

epinephrine Hormone produced by the adrenal medulla that plays a vital role in the function of the sympathetic nervous system.

estrogen One of the three major female hormones. At puberty, estrogen brings about the secondary sex characteristics.

exocrine glands Glands that excrete chemicals for elimination.

glands Cells or organs that selectively remove, concentrate, or alter materials in the blood and then secrete them back into the body.

glucagon Hormone produced by the pancreas that is vital to the control of the body's metabolism and blood sugar level. Glucagon stimulates the breakdown of glycogen to glucose.

gonads The reproductive glands; the main source of sex hormones.

hormones Chemicals secreted by the body that regulate many body functions, such as growth, reproduction, temperature, metabolism, and blood pressure.

hyperglycemia Abnormally high blood glucose level.

hyperosmolar hyperglycemic nonketotic coma (HHNC), also known as hyperosmolar nonketotic coma (HONK), is a metabolic derangement that occurs principally in patients with type 2 diabetes. The condition is characterized by hyperglycemia, hyperosmolarity, and an absence of significant ketosis.

hyperosmolar nonketotic coma (HONK), also known as hyperosmolar hyperglycemic nonketotic coma (HHNC), is a metabolic derangement that occurs principally in patients with type 2 diabetes. The condition is characterized by hyperglycemia, hyperosmolarity, and an absence of significant ketosis.

hypoglycemia Abnormally low blood glucose level.

hypothalamus A small region of the brain that contains several control centers for the body functions and emotions. It is the primary link between the endocrine system and the nervous system.

insulin Hormone produced by the pancreas that's vital to the control of the body's metabolism and blood sugar level. Insulin causes sugar, fatty acids, and amino acids to be taken up and metabolized by cells.

insulin resistance Condition in which the pancreas produces enough insulin but the body can't effectively utilize it.

iodine An essential element in the diet and an important component of thyroxine. Without the proper level of iodine intake, thyroxine can't be produced, and physical and mental growth are diminished.

islets of Langerhans A specialized group of cells in the pancreas where insulin and glucagon are produced.

luteinizing hormone (LH) Hormone that regulates the production of both eggs and sperm, as well as production of reproductive hormones.

myxedema coma A rare condition that can occur in patients who have severe, untreated hypothyroidism.

norepinephrine Hormone produced by the adrenal glands that is vital in the function of the sympathetic nervous system.

ovaries Female gonads; ovaries release eggs and secrete the female hormones.

pancreas The digestive gland that secretes digestive enzymes into the duodenum through the pancreatic duct. The pancreas is considered both an endocrine gland and an exocrine gland.

parathyroid hormone (PTH) A hormone secreted by the parathyroids that acts as an antagonist to calcitonin. PTH is secreted when calcium blood levels are low.

pituitary gland Gland whose secretions control, or regulate, the secretions of other endocrine glands. Often called the "master gland."

primary adrenal insufficiency Also known as Addison's disease. A rare condition in which the adrenal glands produce an insufficient amount of adrenal hormones.

progesterone One of the three major female hormones.

target tissues Tissues to which hormones are directed to act on.

testes Male gonads located in the scrotum that produce hormones called androgens.

testosterone The most important androgen in men.

thyroid Large gland located at the base of the neck that produces and excretes hormones that influence growth, development, and metabolism.

thyroid-stimulating hormone (TSH) Hormone that controls the release of thyroid hormone from the thyroid gland.

thyroid storm A rare, life-threatening condition that may occur in patients with thyrotoxicosis. The condition is usually triggered by a stressful event or increased volume of thyroid hormones in the circulation.

thyrotoxicosis A toxic condition caused by excessive levels of circulating thyroid hormone.

thyroxine The body's major metabolic hormone. Thyroxine stimulates energy production in cells, which increases the rate at which the cells consume oxygen and use carbohydrates, fats, and proteins.

type 1 diabetes The type of diabetic disease that usually starts in childhood and requires daily injections of supplemental synthetic insulin to control blood glucose. Sometimes called juvenile or juvenile-onset diabetes.

type 2 diabetes The type of diabetic disease that usually starts in later life and often can be controlled through diet and oral medications. Sometimes called adult-onset diabetes.

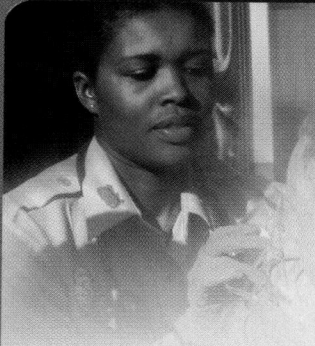

Assessment in Action

You are dispatched to a warehouse for an unconscious man. You arrive on scene and are greeted by the plant manager. He walks you through the plant and advises you that the patient is an insulin-dependent diabetic who got caught up working and was unable to eat lunch on time. When you arrive to the patient's side, you find the patient unresponsive to verbal stimuli; however, he does withdraw purposefully when you attempt to perform your physical assessment. You obtain a baseline set of vitals, which are within normal limits. You initiate an IV of normal saline and you perform a glucose test, which gives a reading of 28 mg/dL. Under the standing orders for your department, you give the patient 25 g of 50% dextrose. The patient slowly responds to the sugar and initially appears lethargic. As the sugar metabolizes through his body, the patient becomes conscious, alert, and oriented and refuses transport to the hospital. After you advise the patient that he should go to the hospital and he still refuses, you advise him that he needs to eat a meal with carbohydrates and explain to him that the dextrose you gave him is short acting.

1. **Glucagon is a hormone that:**
   A. is produced in the pancreatic alpha cells and facilitates the process of glycogenolysis.
   B. is released by the beta cells of the pancreas and facilitates the cellular uptake of glucose.
   C. causes a decrease in circulating blood glucose levels by blocking the conversion of glycogen to glucose.
   D. is typically administered by the paramedic in a dose of 25 g via rapid IV or IO push.

2. **The term diabetes mellitus refers to:**
   A. a metabolic disorder in which the body's ability to metabolize simple glucose is normal.
   B. a metabolic disorder in which the body lacks the ability to produce hormones that stimulate the sympathetic nervous system.
   C. glands that secrete or release chemicals that are utilized inside the body.
   D. a disease that is characterized by an inability to sufficiently metabolize glucose.

3. **The _____ is a digestive gland that is considered both an endocrine gland and an exocrine gland.**
   A. gonad
   B. liver
   C. kidney
   D. pancreas

4. **What is insulin responsible for?**
   A. The removal of glucose from the blood for storage as glycogen, fats, and protein
   B. The maintenance of glucose levels in the blood for storage as glycogen, fats, and protein
   C. The main source of sex hormones
   D. The hormones that regulate the body's metabolism

5. **What causes diabetes mellitus?**
   A. The liver does not produce enough insulin.
   B. There is not enough glucose in the bloodstream.
   C. The pancreas does not produce enough insulin or the cells do not respond to the effects of the insulin produced.
   D. The pancreas produces too much insulin and the cells respond appropriately to the effects of the insulin produced.

6. **What is type 1 diabetes mellitus?**
   A. The type of diabetic disease that usually starts in childhood and requires daily injections of supplemental, synthetic insulin to control blood glucose
   B. The type of diabetic disease that usually starts in later life and often requires daily injections of supplemental, synthetic insulin to control blood glucose
   C. The type of diabetic disease that usually starts later in life and often can be controlled through diet and oral medications
   D. The type of diabetic disease that usually starts in childhood and can often be controlled through diet and oral medications

7. **What is type 2 diabetes mellitus?**
   A. The type of diabetic disease that usually starts in childhood and requires daily injections of supplemental, synthetic insulin to control blood glucose
   B. The type of diabetic disease that usually starts in later life and often requires daily injections of supplemental, synthetic insulin to control blood glucose
   C. The type of diabetic disease that usually starts in later life and often can be controlled through diet and oral medications
   D. The type of diabetic disease that usually starts in childhood and can often be controlled through diet and oral medications

8. _____ in the insulin-dependent diabetic is often the result of having taken too much insulin, too little food, or both and often presents with an altered mental status.
   A. Hyperglycemia
   B. Increase in blood sugar
   C. Hypoglycemia
   D. Hypotension

9. A normal blood glucose level is approximately:
   A. 30 to 120 mg/dL.
   B. 70 to 120 mg/dL.
   C. 70 to 200 mg/dL.
   D. 160 to 500 mg/dL.

Challenging Question

You are dispatched to a private home for a person with weakness. When you arrive, the patient tells you that she has been feeling weak and fatigued for approximately 1 week. She called today because she "can't take it anymore." She states that she has been depressed lately and does not understand why. Her vital signs are within normal limits. Her medical history includes hypertension, cardiac problems (unable to specify), and lupus. Her medications include metoprolol and hydrocortisone. You question her as to whether she has had any increased thirst or urination, and she states yes.

10. What differential diagnosis can you make?

■ Points to Ponder

You are dispatched to a private residence for a patient with an altered level of consciousness. When you arrive, you are greeted by the patient's husband, who tells you that his wife is "not acting right." When you begin to assess her, she does not answer questions appropriately, and she has erratic respirations. She is hot to the touch, dry, and appears pink. Her pulse rate is 132 beats/min, with sinus tachycardia on the monitor; her blood pressure is 140/70 mm Hg. After you initiate an IV of normal saline, you perform a glucose test that reads "high" on your monitor. In your head you understand that this means her sugar is greater than 500 mg/dL. Her husband states that she has not been feeling well for the last 2 days, and they believed she was coming down with the flu. He called today because she appeared confused to him.

What are your priorities in this situation? What do you need to do for this patient?

Issues: Understanding the Importance of the Endocrine System, Understanding the General Assessment Findings Associated With an Endocrine Emergency.

30

Allergic Reactions

Objectives

Cognitive

5-5.1   Define allergic reaction. (p 30.3)

5-5.2   Define anaphylaxis. (p 30.4)

5-5.3   Describe the incidence, morbidity and mortality of anaphylaxis. (p 30.4)

5-5.4   Identify the risk factors most predisposing to anaphylaxis. (p 30.4)

5-5.5   Discuss the anatomy and physiology of the organs and structures related to anaphylaxis. (p 30.5, 30.6)

5-5.6   Describe the prevention of anaphylaxis and appropriate patient education. (p 30.14)

5-5.7   Discuss the pathophysiology of allergy and anaphylaxis. (p 30.7)

5-5.8   Describe the common methods of entry of substances into the body. (p 30.5)

5-5.9   Define natural and acquired immunity. (p 30.7)

5-5.10   Define antigens and antibodies. (p 30.3)

5-5.11   List common antigens most frequently associated with anaphylaxis. (p 30.4)

5-5.12   Discuss the formation of antibodies in the body. (p 30.7)

5-5.13   Describe physical manifestations in anaphylaxis. (p 30.9)

5-5.14   Differentiate manifestations of an allergic reaction from anaphylaxis. (p 30.3)

5-5.15   Recognize the signs and symptoms related to anaphylaxis. (p 30.10)

5-5.16   Differentiate among the various treatment and pharmacological interventions used in the management of anaphylaxis. (p 30.12)

5-5.17   Integrate the pathophysiological principles of the patient with anaphylaxis. (p 30.8)

5-5.18   Correlate abnormal findings in assessment with the clinical significance in the patient with anaphylaxis. (p 30.10)

5-5.19   Develop a treatment plan based on field impression in the patient with allergic reaction and anaphylaxis. (p 30.12)

Affective

None

Psychomotor

None

Introduction

Allergic reactions and anaphylaxis have been documented for many years. One of the earliest accounts may have been noted by the late 17th century clergyman Increase Mather:

> Some men also have strange antipathies in their natures against that sort of food which others love and live upon. I have read of one that could not endure to eat either bread or flesh; of another that fell into a swooning fit at the smell of a rose . . . There are some who, if a cat accidentally comes into the room, though they neither see it, nor are told of it, will presently be in a sweat, and ready to die away.

Although these cases cannot be proven to be anaphylaxis, the descriptions suggest some type of reaction was present—possibly an allergic or anaphylactic reaction given the severity and fatality of the descriptions. This chapter explores these types of reactions, including their typical signs and symptoms, and the steps you should take to manage such patients. In addition, it discusses the common causes of "swooning fit" so we can be better prepared to care for affected patients.

The first task is to clarify the many terms associated with allergic and anaphylactic reactions. An <u>allergen</u> is a substance that produces allergic symptoms in a patient. Most allergens are usually harmless substances that do not pose a threat to other people—for example, milk, eggs, chocolate, and strawberries. An <u>antibody</u> is a protein the body produces in response to an <u>antigen</u>. This protein (globulin) is found in the plasma—hence, its other name *immunoglobulin* (Ig). **Table 30-1 ▾** lists the common antibodies, their actions, and locations.

An <u>allergic reaction</u> is an abnormal immune response the body develops when the person is reexposed to a substance or allergen. In most people, exposure to this substance would not be a problem; in a person with an allergic reaction, however, a local or systemic reaction may occur. In a <u>local reaction</u>, the body limits its response to a specific area after being exposed to a foreign substance; the swelling around an insect bite would be an example. A <u>systemic reaction</u> occurs throughout the body, possibly affecting multiple body systems. It is seen when a person who is allergic to strawberries, for example, has swelling and hives all over his body after eating strawberry

Table 30-1	Antibodies or Immunoglobulins	
Antibody	**Action**	**Location**
IgA	Provides localized protection to mucous membranes. Stress can lower the IgA level, making the body more susceptible to infection.	Tears, saliva, mucus, breast milk, gastrointestinal secretions, blood, and lymph
IgD	Thought to stimulate antibody-producing cells to make antibodies	Blood, lymph, and the surfaces of B cells
IgE*	Responds in allergic reactions	Located on mast and basophil cells
IgG	Provides protection against bacteria and viruses; enhances phagocytosis, neutralizes toxins, triggers the complement system	Blood, lymph, intestines
IgM	One of the first to appear; causes agglutination and lysis of microbes. ABO agglutinins are IgM antibodies.	Blood, lymph, and surface of B cells

*The primary antibody you need to be concerned with during allergic and anaphylactic reactions is the IgE antibody.

You are the Provider Part 1

You are dispatched to a private residence for a 26-year-old man with "trouble breathing." On arrival, you find a young man, Matthew Weil, in the living room of his home, holding his throat and working hard to breathe. You hear wheezes without the use of a stethoscope and notice that he is leaning far forward on the edge of the couch.

His wife tells you that the patient has been sick with "walking pneumonia." She just picked up a new prescription for him, azithromycin, which he took just a few minutes ago. She said her husband is normally very healthy, has no other medical history, and is not taking any other medications.

Initial Assessment	Recording Time: 0 Minutes
Appearance	Sitting on the edge of the couch, appears very anxious
Level of consciousness	A (Alert to person, place, and day)
Airway	Coughing, hoarse voice, and audible wheezing
Breathing	Rapid and labored
Circulation	Weak, fast radial pulse

1. How would you categorize this patient and why?
2. What must you do to correct life-threatening conditions?

Notes from Nancy

The term *anaphylaxis* is not, therefore, really accurate; for in fact the fundamental problem in an anaphylactic reaction is not lack of "protection" but overprotection. That is, anaphylaxis is a form of allergy—a very extreme and devastating form—and allergy represents the body's protective immune system gone overboard.

shortcake. Hypersensitivity occurs when a patient reacts with exaggerated or inappropriate allergic symptoms after coming into contact with a substance perceived by the body to be harmful. Anaphylaxis is an extreme systemic form of an allergic reaction involving two or more body systems. This term was first used in 1902, when Portier and Richet were vaccinating dogs with sea anemone toxin. After the second dose of the toxin, one of the dogs died. Because this response was the opposite of protection, it was referred to as anaphylaxis (meaning "without protection").

Anaphylaxis causes the death of 500 to 1,000 people in the United States each year. It is estimated that more than 40 million Americans are at risk for this life-threatening event. Unfortunately, no exact cause for anaphylaxis can be determined in up to two thirds of patients. To anticipate anaphylaxis, of course, it would be useful to be able to identify people at greatest risk. Neither race nor sex seems to affect the incidence of anaphylaxis. The incidence of insect sting anaphylaxis tends to be higher in men. Women have a greater incidence of anaphylactic reactions to latex, aspirin, and intravenous (IV) muscle relaxants. Anaphylactic reactions have been documented in children as young as 6 months and adults as old as 89 years. Children are more likely to have severe food allergies, whereas adults tend to have anaphylactic reactions to insect stings, anesthetics, and radiocontrast media. **Table 30-2** ▼ lists the common substances associated with anaphylaxis.

Table 30-2	Common Causes of Anaphylactic Reactions	
General Type of Antigen	**Specific Antigen**	**Examples/Comments**
Drugs	Penicillin (antibiotic)	Causes most IgE-mediated drug interactions in the United States
	Beta-lactam antibiotics (cephalosporins)	Possibly a cross-reaction in patients allergic to penicillin
	Other antibiotics	Ampicillin
	Sulfa drugs (antibiotic)	Sulfanomide, sulfisoxazole
	Muscle relaxants, hypnotics, opioids	Acetaminophen with codeine, morphine, meperidine
	Salicylates	Aspirin
	Colloids	
	Local anesthetics	Procaine
	Enzymes	Chymotrypsin, penicillinase
	Mismatched blood transfusion	
	Iodinated radiocontrast dyes used in taking radiographs	Intravenous pyelogram
	Biologic extracts and hormones	Insulin, heparin
	Vaccines	
Insect stings	Bees, yellow jackets, hornets, wasps, fire ants	0.5%–3% of the population will have a systemic reaction after being stung.
Foods (problem worldwide—most common cause of anaphylaxis)	Peanuts	As little as 100 µg of peanut protein can cause a reaction.
	Tree nuts, fish, and shellfish	Most common to all age groups
	Some fruits	Mango, strawberries
	Egg, soy, and milk	Most common in children
Latex (may be seen in myelodysplasia, genitourinary anomalies, patients with frequent exposure to latex, and sensitized health care workers)	Gloves and other materials made from latex	The incidence rate is decreasing owing to awareness and better manufacturing practices. People with allergies to bananas, kiwi, and strawberries may have a cross-reaction to latex.
Immunotherapy	Allergen immunotherapy, skin testing (Note: Patients with atopic diseases are at greater risk for anaphylaxis.)	Rare, associated with asthma, errors in administration, overdose, and beta-blocker use during immunotherapy
Animals	Dander	Long-haired animals
	Animal serum products	Horse serum, gamma globulins

Adapted from Dreskin et al, Anaphylaxis, eMedicine, *www.emedicine.com/med/topic128.htm*. Accessed 5/26/06.

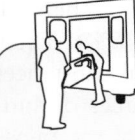

In the Field

It is important to be prepared for latex allergies in the field and to consider a latex-free or latex-safe environment.

Diseases related to allergies, such as allergic rhinitis, asthma, and atopic dermatitis increase the potential for anaphylactic reactions. One third to one half of patients with anaphylaxis have a history of atopic diseases.

The other major factors associated with anaphylaxis are the route of exposure to the allergen and time between exposures. When a substance is ingested (taken by mouth), it is less likely to cause an anaphylactic reaction, and, if a reaction occurs, it usually is not fatal. By contrast, if a substance is injected, the reaction is more likely to be severe. Also, the longer the time between exposures to a substance, the less likely a severe anaphylactic reaction will occur. This is thought to be due to the decreased production of the specific Ig (antibody) cells in the body over time.

Anatomy and Physiology

The Normal Immune Response

The immune system protects the human body from substances and organisms that are considered foreign to the body. Without our immune system for protection, life as we know it would not exist. We would be under constant attack from any bacterium, virus, or other type of invader that wanted to make our bodies their home. Luckily, for the majority of the population, the body is equipped with an amazing immune system that is on patrol 24 hours a day, 7 days a week, to detect unauthorized visits or invading attacks by foreign substances.

The body protects itself via two types of systems: cellular immunity and humoral (that is, related to the body's fluids) immunity. In cellular immunity, the body produces special white blood cells called T cells that attack and destroy invaders. In humoral immunity, the body uses the antibodies dissolved in the plasma and lymph to wage war on invading organisms. The cells producing immunity are located throughout the body in the lymph nodes, spleen, and gastrointestinal tract. Their goal is to intercept foreign forces as they enter the body, thereby limiting the invaders' spread and damage.

Routes of Entry for Allergens

Substances can invade the body through the skin, the respiratory tract, or the gastrointestinal tract. Invasion through the skin may come in the form of injection or absorption. In injection, the invading substance pierces the skin and deposits foreign material into the skin. Bees and hornets prefer this method of invasion. Absorption occurs when foreign material is deposited on the skin and slowly absorbed through the skin. Absorption invaders may take the form of lotions or therapeutic or medicinal creams to trick unsuspecting people into applying them to the skin. Invaders do not stop at the skin, but may also enter the respiratory tract as the patient quietly breathes; this type of raid is referred to as an inhalation exposure. The foreigners advance through the respiratory system and launch their attack from the lungs. Cats, peanuts, and many plants attack in this way. The final way invading armies attack the body is through the gastrointestinal tract via ingestion. That is, invaders may camouflage themselves as some tempting delicacy such as strawberry shortcake, a mushroom-and-cheese omelet, or a peanut butter pie Figure 30-1 ▶ .

You are the Provider Part 2

You take Mr. Weil's vital signs, and your partner immediately applies high-flow oxygen via nonrebreathing mask and obtains a blood pressure while you gain IV access. As you begin your series of interventions, you explain to the patient what is happening to him and what you need to do to correct it. You then administer epinephrine and diphenhydramine via IV per local protocols. You are mentally prepared to aggressively manage this patient's airway but hope that your treatments will result in quick, significant patient improvement. You administer IV normal saline at a wide-open rate using a 16-gauge catheter and 0.3 mg of epinephrine 1:10,000 and 25 mg of diphenhydramine.

Vital Signs	Recording Time: 5 Minutes
Level of consciousness	Alert, with a Glasgow Coma Scale score of 14
Skin	Flushed, hives
Pulse	130 beats/min, weak and slightly irregular
Blood pressure	88/40 mm Hg
Respirations	50 breaths/min
Sao$_2$	90% with oxygen at 15 L/min via nonrebreathing mask

3. Why does the order of the medications matter?
4. Why is knowing all of the medication administration routes important?
5. Would your care change if this patient were geriatric?

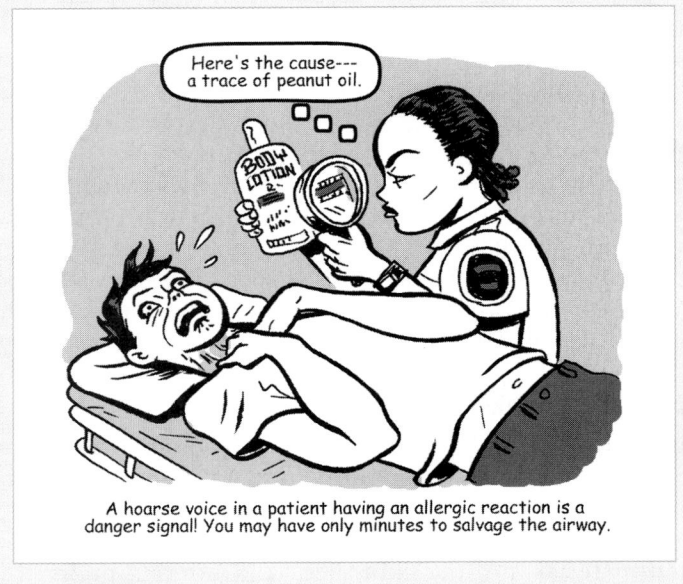

A hoarse voice in a patient having an allergic reaction is a danger signal! You may have only minutes to salvage the airway.

Figure 30-1

The basophils and mast cells produce the body's "chemical weapons"—that is, chemical mediators **Table 30-3 ▶**. These cells contain granules filled with a host of powerful substances that are ready to be released to fight invading forces of antigens. As long as the body is not invaded by one of the previously identified foreign substances, the granules are kept encapsulated in their protective walls and remain inactive. If an antigen invades the body and combines with one of the antibodies, however, the granules are ejected from the mast cells and detonated. The chemical mediators are then released into the surrounding tissue and the bloodstream **Figure 30-2 ▾**.

The chemical mediators launch and maintain the immune response. They summon more white blood cells to the area to battle the invading force. They also increase blood flow to the area under attack by dilating the blood vessels and increasing the capillary permeability. These actions are useful when a small invasion occurs to a limited area but can be extremely dangerous when they spread throughout the body. When they have systemic effects, the chemical mediators cause the signs and symptoms of the allergic and anaphylactic reactions seen in the body.

Physiology

Once a foreign substance invades the body, the body goes on alert and initiates a series of responses. The first encounter with the foreign substance begins the primary response. Cells (macrophages) immediately greet, confront, and engulf the invaders to check their papers or passports to see if they can legally be present in the body. If the body is unable to identify the substance or determines the papers are not in order, it starts a file on the outsider. It fingerprints the invader or takes a "mug shot" of the suspect for later identification by using immune cells to record the salient features of the outside substance. These cells record one or two of the proteins on the surface of the invading substance and then design specific proteins to match each substance. These proteins—called antibodies—are intended to match up with the invader—the antigen—and inactivate it.

Through the primary response, the body develops sensitivity—that is, the ability to recognize the foreigner the next time it is encountered. To determine whether the substance is "one of us," the body records enough details to assist in future identification of the substance and production of antibodies to perfectly fit the invading antigen. The body then sends out these details to the rest of the body, much like sending out "Wanted" posters to "post offices" throughout the body. The Wanted posters are distributed by placing the specific antibodies on two types of cells: basophils and mast cells. Basophils are stationed like guards in specific sites within the tissues. Mast cells are on patrol like police cruisers or bounty hunters through the connective tissues, bronchi, gastrointestinal mucosa, and other vulnerable border areas that act as barriers to foreign invaders.

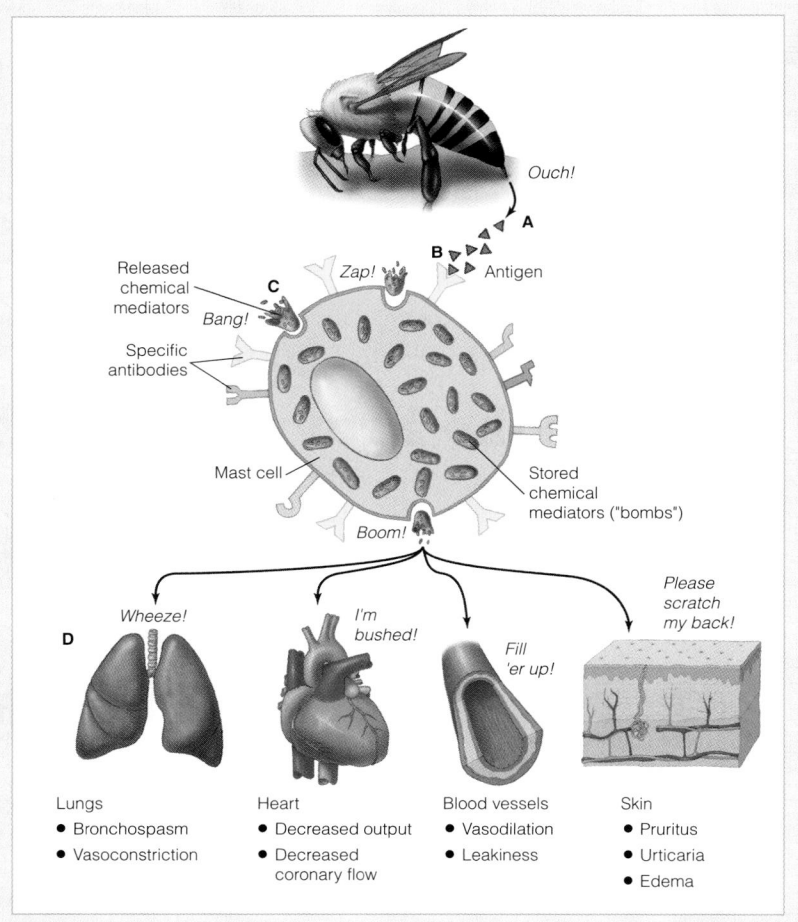

Figure 30-2 The sequence of events in anaphylaxis. **A.** The antigen is introduced into the body. **B.** The antigen-antibody reaction at the surface of a mast cell. **C.** Release of mast cell chemical mediators. **D.** Chemical mediators exert their effects on end organs.

Table 30-3	Chemical Mediators
Mediator	**Physiological Effects**
Histamine	• Systemic vasodilation • Increased permeability of blood vessels • Decreased cardiac contractility • Decreased coronary blood flow • Dysrhythmias • Bronchoconstriction • Pulmonary vasoconstriction
Eosinophil chemotactic factor	• Attracts eosinophils and neutrophils
Arachidonic acid (precursor of the following):	These factors act to produce other inflammatory mediators:
Prostaglandin	• Smooth muscle contraction

Leukotrienes (slow reaction substance of anaphylaxis [SRS-A])	• Vascular permeability
	• Bronchoconstriction
	• Decreased force of cardiac contraction
	• Decreased coronary blood flow
	• Dysrhythmias
	  – More potent than histamine (thousands of times)
	  – React more slowly than histamine

Platelet-activating factor	• Platelet aggregation • Causes histamine release
Serotonin	• Pulmonary vasoconstriction • Bronchoconstriction

Proteoglycans:
  Heparin
  Chondroitin sulfate
  Chemokines
  Cytokines
	• Control the release of histamine. These mediators as a whole work to activate the kinin system and are thought to contribute to prolonged and biphasic reactions.
	• These mediators trigger inflammatory pathways and increase the recruitment of inflammatory cells.

Kinins	• Bradykinin is one of the stronger kinins and is responsible for increased vascular permeability.

As health care providers, we exploit the body's ability to protect itself. For example, we administer vaccines to produce immunity against a disease. The body develops antibodies in response to the vaccine so it can produce an immune response to neutralize the invading disease before it can establish itself and damage the body. Thus, the body develops antibodies in a controlled way. When the hepatitis B vaccine is administered, for example, a small amount of the hepatitis B virus (HBV) enters the body. The body identifies this virus and produces antibodies to it; these antibodies are then distributed throughout the body. Should an immunized person later be exposed to HBV, the virus will invade the body. Once in the body, the virus begins to set up residency and reproduce. At this point, the officer on patrol (the wandering immune cell) identifies the HBV as something that does not belong in the area. It remembers seeing the HBV Wanted poster and radios for backup (activates the immune system). The alarm is sounded, and the body begins aggressive production of the "antihepatitis" antibodies, sending in platoons of immune system soldiers to kill the HBV and clean up residual traces of the invasion. This intense response to the invading virus is called the secondary response. Meanwhile, the "contaminated," immunized person remains blissfully unaware of the battle raging inside his or her body.

This battle is termed acquired immunity. In this type of immunity, the administration of a vaccine allows the body to produce antibodies without having to experience the disease. Vaccinations against measles, mumps, and polio are examples of acquired immunity. In natural immunity, by contrast, the body encounters the antigen and experiences a full immune response with all the pathology of the disease. Having the measles, for example, causes the body to produce antibodies to this pathogen, but the drawback is that the person has the itching, rash, and high fever associated with the disease.

Use of the polio vaccine has resulted in herd immunity, which occurs when a group of individuals are immunized against a substance. This immunization protects vulnerable people in the group and the entire group by decreasing the number of people able to contract the disease, thus protecting the group.

Pathophysiology

Abnormal Immune Reactions

An ever-watchful and responsive immune system is essential to life and health. Unfortunately, sometimes the immune system becomes overzealous in defending the body. The resulting

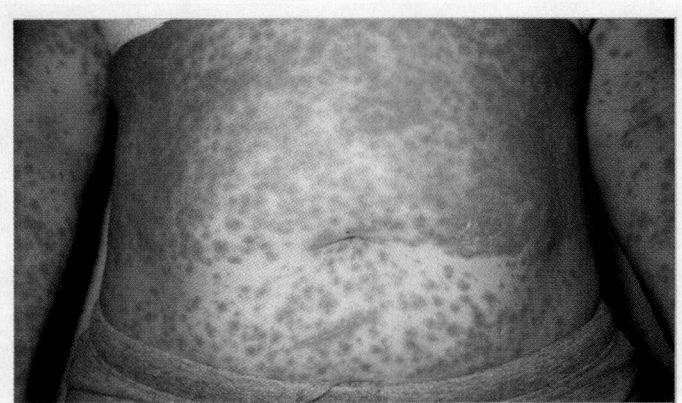

Figure 30-3 A severe allergic reaction to medication. This patient was allergic to penicillin and most other antibiotics.

problems may range in severity from hay fever to anaphylaxis and exist along the spectrum from a simple annoyance to a life-threatening crisis. During these abnormal reactions, the immune system becomes hypersensitive to one or more substances. The body often has these reactions to substances that should not be identified as harmful by the immune system—substances such as ragweed, strawberries, and penicillin Figure 30-3 ▲ . The immune cells of the allergic person are more sensitive and jumpier than the immune cells of a person without allergies. Although these cells are able to recognize and react to dangerous invaders such as bacteria and viruses, they also identify harmless substances as posing a threat. They behave like border guards gone berserk, shooting the smugglers and the tourists!

Not only do the border guards go berserk, but they also call in the special forces. When the invading substance enters the body, the mast cells recognize it as potentially harmful and begin releasing chemical mediators. Histamine, one of the primary chemical weapons, causes the blood vessels in the local area to dilate and the capillaries to leak. Leukotrienes, which are even more powerful, are released and cause additional dilation and leaking. White blood cells are called to the area to help engulf and destroy the enemy, and platelets begin to collect and clump together. In most cases, this overreaction to harmless invaders is usually restricted to the local area being invaded. The runny, itchy nose and swollen eyes associated with hay fever are examples of a local allergic reaction.

In the case of anaphylaxis, the person is not so lucky. The body not only has out-of-control border guards, but also has out-of-control special forces units that do not restrict their activities to the local area. They take their chemical weapons to the remainder of the body and detonate them, causing widespread havoc. Although the same chemical mediators are released, the effect involves more than one system throughout the body. An initial effect may be seen from the histamine release, with secondary effects following a few hours later when the remainder of the chemicals are released.

Histamine release causes immediate vasodilation, which often presents as flushed skin and hypotension. It also increases vascular permeability, which results in tissue swelling and fluid secretion. The tissue swelling can present as hives Figure 30-4 ▶ , narrowing of the airway, and increased fluids in the airway. Histamine likewise causes smooth muscle contraction, especially in the respiratory system and gastrointestinal system. This results in laryngospasm or bronchospasm and abdominal cramping. Finally, histamine decreases the contractility of the heart. When this effect is coupled with vasodilation, the person may experience profound hypotension. Dysrhythmias due to hypoperfusion and hypoxia are also common.

Later responses from the much more powerful leukotrienes compound the effects of histamine. The person's respiratory status will become even more dire as these highly potent

You are the Provider Part 3

Mr. Weil's condition is improving rapidly. He is able to communicate with you and seems fully alert. He still has some shortness of breath, which you treat with a beta-2 agonist. You begin transport, apply the cardiac monitor, and administer epinephrine subcutaneously.

Your quick action and proficient skills saved this patient's life. He is later released, with no permanent deficits. He now wears a medical ID bracelet that identifies his severe allergy to azithromycin.

Reassessment	Recording Time: 15 Minutes
Level of consciousness	Alert, with a Glasgow Coma Scale score of 15
Skin	Warm, pink, and slightly diaphoretic
Pulse	110 beats/min, weak and slightly irregular
Blood pressure	106/70 mm Hg
Respirations	36 breaths/min
Sao_2	95% with oxygen at 15 L/min via nonrebreathing mask

6. If the initial dose of epinephrine was successful, why administer another dose subcutaneously?

7. What other options are available should your patient begin to have the same signs and symptoms you noted initially?

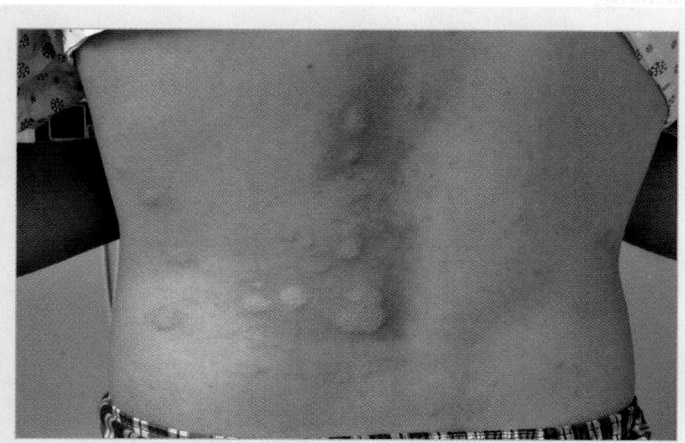

Figure 30-4 Urticaria, or hives, may appear following a sting and are characterized by multiple, small, raised areas on the skin.

bronchoconstrictors are released. In addition, leukotriene release causes coronary vasoconstriction, which contributes to a worsening cardiac condition and myocardial irritability. Leukotrienes are also associated with increased vascular permeability, contributing to a further state of hypoperfusion.

The remaining chemical mediators continue to worsen the situation as they undertake what they see as steps to protect the body from this foreign invader. As a result of these activities, when the body undergoes an anaphylactic reaction, it may not survive without immediate intervention.

Clinical Symptoms of Anaphylaxis

The skin is the body's first line of defense against would-be invaders, so skin symptoms are often the first indications of anaphylaxis. Initially, the person may be aware of feeling warm and flushed. Pruritis (itching) is another early sign, which is due to vasodilation and capillary leaking. The area around the eyes is often susceptible to this effect, which causes swollen, red eyes. Swelling of the face and tongue may contribute to airway compromise. You may also note swelling of the hands and feet. Histamine is responsible for the urticaria (hives) experienced by the anaphylactic patient.

The most common complaints are usually respiratory symptoms, which often present as shortness of breath or dyspnea and tightness in the throat and chest. You may also note stridor and/or hoarseness. These signs and symptoms are often due to upper airway swelling in the laryngeal and epiglottic areas. Affected patients may complain of a lump in the throat. The lower airway is often involved as well. Bronchoconstriction and increased secretions may result in wheezes and crackles. It is not uncommon for the patient to cough or sneeze as the body tries to clear the airway. These symptoms may progress slowly or alarmingly fast. You may have only 1 or 3 minutes to halt this rapid, life-threatening process.

Cardiovascular symptoms are serious complications of anaphylaxis. As noted earlier, histamine and leukotrienes work directly on the heart to decrease its contractility. The resulting decrease in cardiac output is complicated by vasodilation and increased capillary permeability, which further decrease the amount of fluid returned to the heart. As cardiac output declines, perfusion decreases, leading to ischemia and bringing the potential for cardiac dysrhythmias. As the fluid leaks out of the capillaries, the intravascular system is left short on fluid. (As much as 50% of the vascular volume can be shifted to the extravascular space within 10 minutes of exposure to an antigen.) Instead of responding normally to the fluid loss and constricting, the blood vessels do just the opposite: They dilate. The already low vascular volume becomes totally inadequate, and hypotension reigns. In

> **Notes from Nancy**
> Flushing (from vasodilation) and tachycardia are so characteristic of anaphylactic shock that it is very questionable to make the diagnosis without these two signs being present.

response to the low blood pressure, the heart rate increases, putting stress on an already compromised heart. In this situation, tachycardia, flushed skin, and hypotension are synonymous with anaphylactic shock.

Gastrointestinal symptoms may also be part of an anaphylactic response, particularly if the offending antigen has been ingested. Abdominal cramping is a common presentation, but nausea, bloating, vomiting, abdominal distention, and profuse, watery diarrhea may also be present.

Patients may present with central nervous system symptoms in response to decreased cerebral perfusion and hypoxia. These symptoms include headache, dizziness, confusion, and anxiety. A sense of "impending doom" aptly represents the patient's sense of being near death. This observation may be more fact than fiction.

Table 30-4 ▶ summarizes the signs and symptoms of anaphylaxis. Anaphylaxis may present as affecting any two or more of these body systems, so the picture can be confusing at times. Think of a patient with anaphylaxis as experiencing three types of shock: (1) cardiogenic shock due to decreased cardiac output, (2) hypovolemic shock due to fluids leaking into the tissues, and (3) neurogenic shock due to inability of the blood vessels to constrict. You will need to use your assessment skills to identify the potential for anaphylaxis and take aggressive action to manage the patient and stop the anaphylactic process as rapidly as possible.

Assessment of a Patient With Anaphylaxis

Assessment of a patient with an anaphylactic reaction can be highly challenging. You may have to simultaneously assess the patient, identify the problem, and intervene within seconds of arriving on the scene to save the patient's life. Index of suspicion for anaphylaxis must be high on your list if any of the symptoms discussed previously are present. You may not have

Table 30-4	Signs and Symptoms of Anaphylaxis*
System	**Signs and Symptoms**
Skin	• Warm • Flushed • Itching (pruritis) • Swollen, red eyes • Swelling of the face and tongue • Swelling of the hands and feet • Hives (urticaria)
Respiratory	• **Dyspnea** • Tightness in the throat and chest • Stridor • Hoarseness • Lump in throat • Wheezes • Crackles • Coughing • Sneezing
Cardiovascular	• Dysrhythmias • **Hypotension** • **Tachycardia**
Gastrointestinal	• Abdominal cramping • Nausea • Bloating • Vomiting • Abdominal distention • Profuse, watery diarrhea
Central nervous	• Headache • Dizziness • Confusion • Anxiety and restlessness • Sense of impending doom • Altered mental status

*Key indicators are represented by bold type.

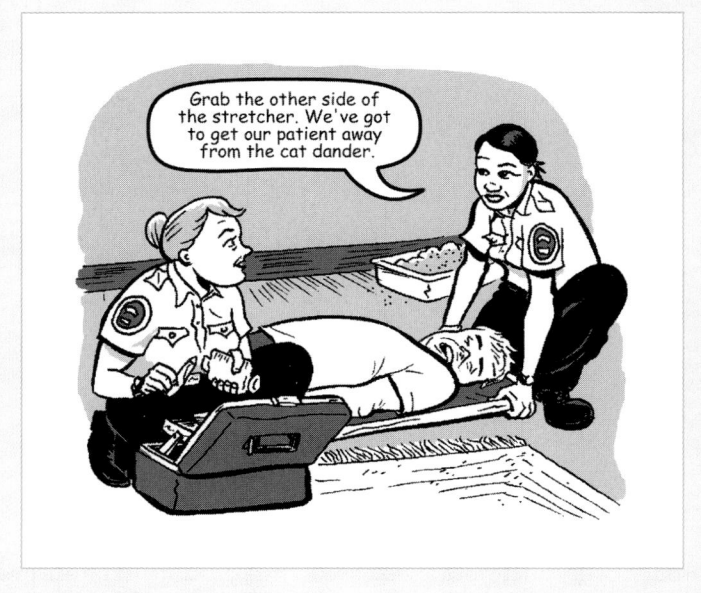

Figure 30-5

a second opportunity because the patient's condition may deteriorate before your eyes.

Scene Size-up

When you arrive on scene, you should observe it for any potential exposure problems. For example, if the patient was out gardening, a bee sting might be a cause of the problem. Dinner at a seafood restaurant might make you suspicious of the shellfish menu items. Because anaphylaxis is a life-threatening event, taking the time to survey the scene for potential anaphylactic hazards is important (Figure 30-5 ▸).

Initial Assessment

Level of Consciousness

The status of the brain is a direct reflection of the patient's oxygenation status. A restless, confused, anxious, or combative patient is most likely hypoxic. As the patient's condition deteriorates and the oxygen level decreases or the carbon dioxide level increases, you are likely to find a patient with a decreased level of consciousness or completely unresponsive. If the

patient is unable to speak, assess the airway for patency before assuming a neurologic problem. Any change in mental status in an anaphylactic patient should direct you to immediate airway evaluation and management.

Upper Airway

A noisy upper airway is a concern in any patient, but even more so in an anaphylactic patient because it may be an early sign of impending airway occlusion due to swelling. You should listen for stridor and hoarseness. In addition, the patient may complain of a tight feeling or a "lump in the throat."

Lower Airway

Observe the patient for tachypnea, labored breathing, accessory muscle use, abnormal retractions, and prolonged expiration. The severity of these findings predicts the stability of the patient's condition. Lung sounds are also a predictor of severity. Initially, you will hear wheezing. As the patient's condition deteriorates and the lungs become tighter and less ventilated (hypoventilation), the diminished lung sounds will be present and the chest may become silent. A silent chest is an ominous finding.

Circulation

Evaluate the skin for redness, rashes, edema, moisture, itching, and urticaria—these symptoms are more commonly associated with an anaphylactic reaction due to histamine release. Pallor and cyanosis may be present as well.

Focused History and Physical Exam

History

Does the patient have any allergies? Has the patient ever had an allergic or anaphylactic reaction? If so, how severe was the incident and how rapidly did it progress? You may want to interview the patient to determine whether he or she had a previous exposure to the antigen. A severe reaction may occur at the second exposure to an antigen, so the patient might not know about the allergy. In some cases, you may not be able to identify the offending antigen. When in doubt, in the presence of a severe reaction, intervention takes precedence over identifying the antigen. To identify where you are in the process, ask when the symptoms began. Because the airway is a major concern, ask about feelings of dyspnea.

You should also determine whether the patient or first responders have administered any treatment before your arrival. This may include using an EpiPen, taking diphenhydramine (Benadryl), or using an inhaler with a beta agonist (such as albuterol or metaproterenol) or aerosolized epinephrine (such as Primatene Mist or racemic epinephrine) ▶ Figure 30-6 ▶ .

Vital Signs

A patient with an allergic reaction will often present with tachypnea, tachycardia, and hypotension. When these signs are noted in conjunction with flushed skin and hives, anaphylaxis should be one of the major considerations. Obviously, the more abnormal the vital signs, the more aggressively you should treat the patient.

Physical Exam

The classic presentation of anaphylaxis includes respiratory symptoms and hypotension. Gastrointestinal symptoms such as abnormal cramping, nausea, vomiting, and diarrhea may be present.

You should use tools such as a cardiac monitor in your assessment because dysrhythmias may be associated with anaphylaxis. A 12-lead electrocardiogram should be considered during the assessment to monitor for cardiac ischemia.

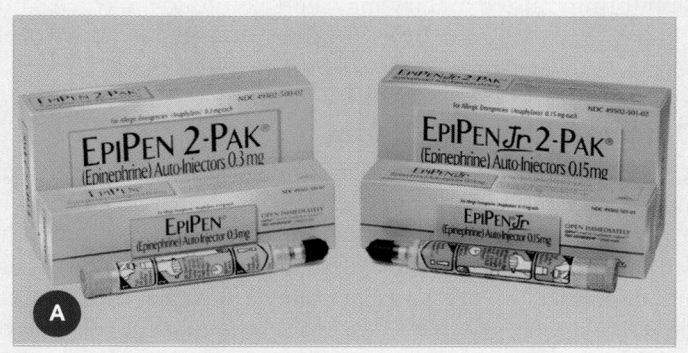

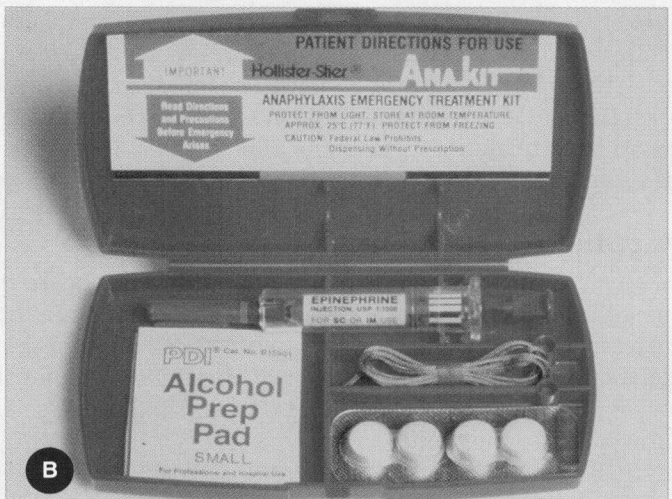

Figure 30-6 Patients who experience severe allergic reactions often carry their own epinephrine, which comes predosed in an auto-injector or a standard syringe. **A.** EpiPen auto-injectors (adult and pediatric sizes). **B.** AnaKit with epinephrine syringe.

You are the Provider Part 4

Mr. Weil's condition remains stable throughout transport. You note ectopy on the electrocardiogram, but this subsides and your patient tells you that he can breathe much more easily. You decide to place a second IV line in case his condition deteriorates, and you administer 2.5 mg of albuterol. You release the patient to emergency department staff who keep close watch on his condition.

Reassessment	Recording Time: 20 Minutes
Level of consciousness	Alert, with a Glasgow Coma Scale score of 15
Skin	Warm, pink, and dry with some hives still noted
Pulse	110 beats/min, weak and regular
Blood pressure	106/70 mm Hg
Respirations	36 breaths/min
Sao2	95% with oxygen at 15 L/min via nonrebreathing mask

8. If your patient had not responded to initial treatment, what would you have anticipated in terms of interventions related to airway management?

9. If you had been unable to obtain IV access, how would this have affected the call?

Monitoring pulse oximetry may alert you to low oxygen saturation. End-tidal carbon dioxide should be monitored because the level may be elevated in anaphylaxis.

Detailed Physical Exam

A patient with a minor allergic reaction will most likely require further examination by paramedics to confirm that no other problems are contributing to his or her condition. Typically, the detailed physical exam is done on trauma patients who have a significant mechanism of injury. For example, a patient with an allergic reaction who may have developed symptoms of anaphylaxis and who has sustained significant trauma will need a detailed physical exam en route to the hospital. The detailed physical exam involves examination of the head, face, eyes, nose, ears, mouth, neck, chest, abdomen, pelvis, all four extremities, back, and buttocks. Do not delay transport of patients with suspected anaphylaxis to perform a detailed physical exam on scene. If the patient has a second EpiPen bring it with you as it may be needed.

Ongoing Assessment

The ongoing assessment is conducted typically en route to the emergency department. In case of anaphylaxis, it involves reassessment of the patient, serial vital signs, and checking interventions (such as the need for another dose of epinephrine, oxygen therapy, Trendelenburg position, and reassessment of the patient's lung sounds).

▌Management of Anaphylactic Reactions

An anaphylactic reaction is a life-threatening emergency and must be treated as such. It takes rapid recognition and rapid intervention to reverse the anaphylactic process and save the patient's life. Although the actions to reverse anaphylaxis will be reviewed here in an orderly manner, in reality, these interventions may be performed simultaneously, especially if multiple providers are available.

Remove the offending agent. When possible, remove the patient from the situation involving the antigen or the antigen from the patient. For example, if the patient is allergic to peanuts and is being exposed to peanuts through inspiration, you may need to remove the patient from the room because you may not be able to eliminate the peanut allergen from the air. If the patient has a stinger from a bee sting still in place, you may need to remove the stinger. Remember to scrape the stinger off because you can inject more venom into the patient if you pinch or squeeze the stinger ◖Figure 30-7 ▶◗.

Maintain the airway—the airway is always a priority regardless of the situation. You will need to be prepared to intubate. If the airway is already swollen shut, you may need to perform a cricothyrotomy to ventilate the patient. Assessing for the presence of stridor and hoarseness should indicate the severity of the airway compromise. If the patient is still awake, allow him or her to

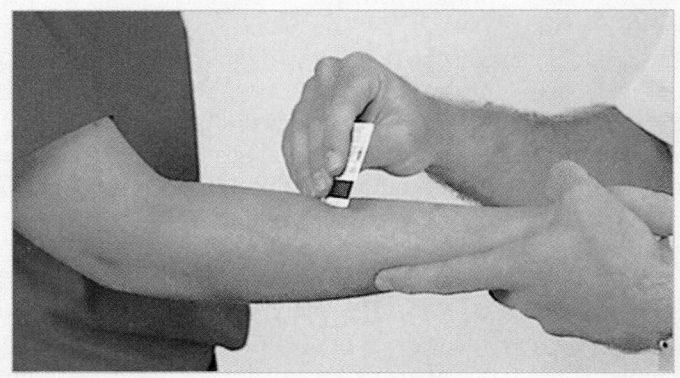

Figure 30-7 To remove the stinger of a honeybee, gently scrape the skin with the edge of a sharp, stiff object such as a credit card.

In the Field

In the absence of an IV site, intramuscular (IM) administration of epinephrine is preferred because it provides more rapid absorption. Subcutaneous (SQ) administration of epinephrine is unpredictable and may have delayed effects in the presence of shock.

assume a position that does not compromise breathing. Use an appropriate oxygen device for supplemental oxygen administration, and consider early transport. Be prepared to assist breathing as needed. *Early administration of epinephrine should be a priority.*

Because epinephrine has immediate action, it can rapidly reverse the effects of anaphylaxis. Administer epinephrine by the IM, SQ, or IV route as soon as possible if airway or respiratory compromise and/or hypotension are present. Epinephrine is the drug of choice for anaphylactic reactions, because it stops the process of mast cell degranulation. In addition, epinephrine reverses the effects of the chemical mediators released via this degranulation. The alpha-adrenergic properties cause the blood vessels to constrict, which reverses vasodilation and hypotension. This, in turn, elevates the diastolic pressure and improves coronary blood flow. The beta-1 adrenergic effects increase cardiac contractility, reversing the depressing effects on the heart and improving the strength of cardiac contractions. The beta-2 adrenergic effects cause bronchodilation, relieving bronchospasm in the lungs. Many patients and EMT-B crews carry epinephrine in the form of an EpiPen and may have administered it before your arrival. The patient may have taken other medications as well, so it important to obtain a medication history.

Maintain circulation by inserting at least one large-bore IV catheter to give an isotonic solution (lactated Ringer's or normal saline) at a wide-open rate. Ideally, you should place two IV lines en route to the ED. This step is crucial, especially if the patient is hypotensive and does not respond to the epinephrine.

Special Considerations

Because epinephrine can stress the heart, it is important to use this drug only as needed in older patients and patients with a cardiovascular disease history. Monitor patients closely for cardiac problems or hypertension.

In the Field

"Mu" (μ) is the Greek letter used as the symbol for "micro." The abbreviation for micrograms is "μg," sometimes written as "mcg." Do not make the mistake of writing "mg" (which stands for "milligrams") when you mean micrograms.

Initially, 1 to 2 L should be administered. If there is no response, you may need to administer up to 4 L. If the patient does not respond after 4 L of fluid, consider a vasopressor in conjunction with fluid administration.

Initiate pharmacologic therapy: oxygen, epinephrine, antihistamines, anti-inflammatory and immunosuppressant agents, and a vasopressor. Administer high-flow oxygen, and be prepared to assist ventilation. Patients who receive epinephrine must be monitored closely for adverse effects. You can do so by using a cardiac monitor to watch for dysrhythmias and reassessing vital signs frequently.

Allergic reactions that are *not* accompanied by signs of cardiovascular collapse (that is, hypotension) or airway compromise can be adequately treated with epinephrine 1:1,000 via the SQ route. For adults, give 0.3 to 0.5 mg of epinephrine; for children, give 0.01 mg/kg.

The adult EpiPen **Figure 30-8 ▾** delivers the medication intramuscularly in a dose of 0.3 mg of a 1:1,000 solution. The EpiPen Jr, which is used for children who weigh less than 33 lb (15 kg), is also administered intramuscularly, but the concentration is 1:2,000 and the dose is 0.15 mg.

Epinephrine should be administered intravenously as soon as possible if hypotension or a reaction involving the airway or respiratory system is suspected or occurring. With IV epinephrine, give adults 0.1 to 0.5 mg of a 1:10,000 solution (during 5 minutes); give children 0.01 mg/kg of the same (1:10,000)

solution. An IV infusion of epinephrine should be administered at 1 to 4 μg/min (that is, 1 mg in 250 mL of saline = 4 μg/mL concentration). The advantage of an IV infusion is that the dose can be more easily controlled if the patient reacts negatively to the epinephrine (such as a geriatric patient or a patient with coronary artery disease). This approach may eliminate the need for repeated doses.

Antihistamine administration should be considered only after epinephrine has been administered. Antihistamines block the histamine 1 (H_1) and 2 (H_2) receptor sites. The antihistamine diphenhydramine (Benadryl) is commonly used in the prehospital setting following the administration of epinephrine. This medication does not prevent histamine release, but rather blocks histamine effects at the H_1 receptor sites. The typical dose of Benadryl is 25 to 50 mg administered slowly via the IM or IV route. H_2 blockers such as cimetidine (Tagamet) and ranitidine (Zantac) are also indicated but are more commonly used in the in-hospital setting. It is recommended that H_1 and H_2 blockers be administered until the anaphylactic symptoms resolve.

Corticosteroids do not have an immediate effect but are useful in preventing late-phase anaphylactic reactions and should be administered early in the treatment process. Common corticosteroids include methylprednisolone (Solu-Medrol), hydrocortisone (Solu-Cortef), and dexamethasone (Decadron).

Glucagon may also be indicated for an anaphylactic patient, especially if the patient does not respond to epinephrine or is taking a beta blocker. The usual dose is 1 to 2 mg IM or IV every 5 minutes. Glucagon increases cardiac contractility.

Vasopressors such as dopamine or levophed should be considered if the patient does not respond to fluid administration to treat the hypotension.

Inhaled beta-adrenergic agents such as albuterol may also be included as part of the care regimen if bronchospasm is present.

Psychological support is a crucial component of management. Anaphylaxis can progress rapidly and has the potential to be a life-threatening event. Patients and their families will

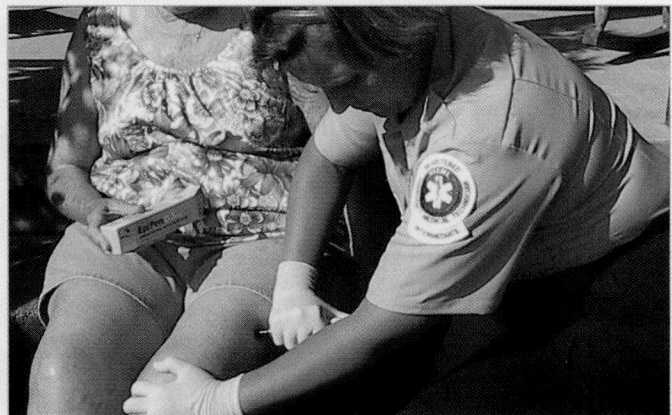

Figure 30-8 Administration of epinephrine with an auto-injector involves stabilizing the leg, pushing the auto-injector firmly against the thigh, and holding it in place until all of the medication is injected.

Special Considerations

Patients taking beta blockers have been reported to have more severe and frequent anaphylactic reactions and can develop a paradoxical reaction to epinephrine. Glucagon and ipratropium should be considered for these patients.

In the Field

Steroids include both corticosteroids such as prednisone or its derivative and anabolic steroids, which are substances used to promote muscle growth and development and have little legitimate medical use.

need reassurance as you perform the necessary interventions. Many of the patients have experienced similar events and may recognize how serious their condition has become. For others, this may be a first-time event. You need to be professional and reassuring and focus on early intervention and transport.

Consider early transport if the patient needs resources beyond your capabilities. Even if you are able to stop the reaction and the patient begins to recover, it is recommended that patients be observed in a medical facility. As many as 20% of patients will have a recurrence of the symptoms within the next 8 hours, even if they have been symptom-free for a time. Once the patient has been symptom-free for 4 hours, he or she can be released from the facility but should be instructed to return or call an ambulance if the symptoms recur.

Management of Allergic Reactions

People having allergic reactions are separated into two groups for management purposes. The first group includes patients who have signs of an allergic reaction—for example, hives—but no respiratory distress or dyspnea. The drug of choice is diphenhydramine. Continue to monitor for changes in condition, but most in this group will recover with no further problems.

The second group includes patients with signs of an allergic reaction and dyspnea. Patients require oxygen, epinephrine, and antihistamines (usually diphenhydramine). Whenever dyspnea is present with signs of an allergic reaction, you should administer epinephrine and monitor the patient for the development of anaphylaxis.

Patient Education

The best management of anaphylaxis and allergic reactions is to educate patients about prevention and self-preservation. At a minimum, discuss the following topics:

- **How to avoid the antigen.** Review information on the offending item. For example, if the patient is allergic to penicillin, he or she should be provided with a list of drugs that include penicillin and the alternative names for penicillin. Drugs that may produce a cross-reaction should also be discussed.
- **Notify all health personnel of the allergy.** Review the need to alert health personnel to the allergy. This is important because people often think only the doctor would need this information, not the EMS provider.
- **Wear identification tags or bracelets.** These items notify providers of allergies in case the patient is unable to do so.
- **Carry an anaphylaxis kit.** A reaction may happen rapidly or worsen before help can arrive. Make sure the patient and his or her family know how to use the kit.
- **Report symptoms early.** Ideally, intervention should begin before the situation becomes life threatening. The patient should recognize that reactions can occur more rapidly and with greater severity with repeated exposures.

You are the Provider Summary

1. How would you categorize this patient and why?

Without always realizing it, you formulate your initial impression in a matter of moments. Factors such as facial expression, body position, and skin signs are noted immediately and provide valuable information about your patient's condition. Owing to this patient's anxious expression, tripod position, flushed skin, and audible wheezing, you know in 10 seconds or less that he is experiencing a life-threatening emergency.

2. What must you do to correct life-threatening conditions?

Given his tachypnea, tachycardia, hypotension, and recent history, you recognize this case as anaphylactic shock. You must apply high-flow oxygen and definitive care by administering epinephrine and diphenhydramine. These drugs will stop the production and absorption of histamine.

3. Why does the order of the medications matter?

Epinephrine should be administered first, because it will stop the production of histamine and correct the hypotension and continued edema, which could affect the airway. Diphenhydramine (Benadryl) should follow immediately. It binds the histamine receptor sites, minimizing the effects from histamine already present in the bloodstream.

4. Why is knowing all of the medication administration routes important?

If you cannot use your first choice of access for drug administration, you must be aware of alternatives. If you are unaware of these choices, you will cause unnecessary delays in patient care.

5. Would your care change if this patient were geriatric?

Because epinephrine has positive beta-1 and alpha-1 properties, its administration increases myocardial oxygen demand. With the current patient, his heart will be able to compensate for this increase without much difficulty. For a patient with a diseased heart, you must provide these interventions judiciously and be prepared for adverse reactions.

6. If the initial dose of epinephrine was successful, why administer another dose subcutaneously?

Like all drugs, epinephrine has a half-life. Providing another dose of epinephrine subcutaneously will maintain the therapeutic level in your patient.

7. What other options are available per medical control should your patient begin to have the same signs and symptoms you noted initially?

Initiating an epinephrine drip via IV piggyback is a choice you should anticipate. This will also provide a continual supply of epinephrine that may be required to counteract the histamine response, particularly because this patient took an oral medication that will likely continue to be released in the body for minutes to hours.

8. If your patient had not responded to initial treatment, what would you have anticipated in terms of interventions related to airway management?

Patients experiencing airway edema can be a particular challenge for paramedics. Endotracheal intubation can become impossible if laryngeal edema is too severe. Anticipate a narrowed glottis, which may require the choice of a smaller tube than would be normally used. If you cannot use bag-mask ventilation and intubation is unsuccessful, you must consider implementing a surgical airway in accordance with your local protocols.

9. If you had been unable to obtain IV access, how would this have affected the call?

All of the medications used in this case could have been administered intramuscularly or subcutaneously. Doing so would have been less effective, however. Certain calls demand skill proficiency; they are literally a matter of life and death. As a paramedic, you must keep your skills sharp. If your call volume is high, you will not struggle as much with this issue. If you work in a location that does not run many calls, you must make up for this infrequency with constant practice and training.

Prep Kit

Ready for Review

- An antigen is a substance the body recognizes as foreign. This recognition causes the body to produce antibodies to destroy the foreign substance.
- The immune system is responsible for the antigen–antibody response.
- An allergic response occurs when the body produces the antigen–antibody response when exposed to a substance that is usually harmless. An allergic response is usually limited to one body system or a local area.
- Anaphylaxis is an extreme form of systemic allergic response involving two or more body systems.
- A person must be sensitized to an antigen before an allergic or anaphylactic reaction can occur.
- The routes of exposure to an antigen include injection, absorption, inhalation, and ingestion.
- Mast cells release chemical mediators to stimulate the allergic reaction.
- Chemical mediators produce signs and symptoms through their effects on the skin, cardiovascular, respiratory, neurologic, and gastrointestinal systems.
- Skin effects include flushing, hives, and itching. Cyanosis and pallor may also be present.
- Cardiovascular effects include vasodilation, hypotension, decreased cardiac output, cardiac ischemia, and dysrhythmias.
- Respiratory effects include upper airway edema and stridor, hoarseness, bronchoconstriction, increased bronchial secretions, wheezes, hypoxia, and hypercapnea.
- Neurologic symptoms include altered level of consciousness, anxiety, restlessness, combativeness, and unconsciousness.
- Gastrointestinal symptoms include nausea, vomiting, diarrhea, and cramping.
- As part of your assessment, you should evaluate the scene, patient history, level of consciousness, upper airway, lower airway, skin, and vital signs. Assessment tools such as a pulse oximeter, cardiac monitor, and capnography are useful.
- Treatment of anaphylaxis includes removing the offending agent; maintaining the airway; administering medications such as epinephrine, antihistamines (diphenhydramine, cimetidine, ranitidine), corticosteroids, inhaled beta-adrenergic agents, and vasopressors; resuscitating with IV fluids; and initiating rapid transport.
- Epinephrine is first-line drug therapy for anaphylaxis.
- Patient education to prevent reexposure, to understand symptoms, and to understand the need to use an anaphylaxis kit is essential.

Vital Vocabulary

absorption In allergic reactions, when foreign material is deposited on and moves into the skin.

acquired immunity The immunity the body develops as part of exposure to an antigen.

allergen A substance that produces allergic symptoms in a patient.

allergic reaction An abnormal immune response the body develops when reexposed to a substance or allergen.

anaphylaxis An extreme systemic form of an allergic reaction involving two or more body systems.

antibody A protein the body produces in response to an antigen; an immunoglobulin.

antigen An agent that, when taken into the body, stimulates the formation of specific protective proteins called antibodies.

basophils White blood cells that work to produce chemical mediators during an immune response.

cellular immunity The immunity provided by special white blood cells called T cells that attack and destroy invaders.

chemical mediators Chemicals that work to cause the immune or allergic response, for example, histamine.

histamine A chemical found in mast cells that, when released, causes vasodilation, capillary leaking, and bronchiole constriction.

humoral immunity The use of antibodies dissolved in the plasma and lymph to destroy foreign substances.

hypersensitivity Occurs when a patient reacts with exaggerated or inappropriate allergic symptoms after coming into contact with a substance the body perceives as harmful.

immune system The system that protects the body from foreign substances.

immunity The body's ability to protect itself from acquiring a disease.

ingestion Eating or drinking materials for absorption through the gastrointestinal tract.

inhalation In allergic reactions, foreign substances are breathed in through the respiratory system.

injection In allergic reactions, when the skin is pierced, and foreign material is deposited into the skin.

local reaction When the body limits a response to a specific area after being exposed to a foreign substance.

mast cells Basophils that are located in the tissues.

natural immunity The immunity the body develops as part of being exposed to an antigen and developing antibodies, for example, exposure to measles, having the measles, and developing immunity to the measles.

primary response The first encounter with the foreign substance to begin the immune response.

pruritis Itching.

secondary response The body's reaction when it is exposed to an antigen for which it already has antibodies, in which it responds by killing the invading substance.

sensitivity The ability to recognize a foreign substance the next time it is encountered.

systemic reaction A reaction that occurs throughout the body, possibly affecting multiple body systems.

urticaria Hives or reddened elevated patches on the skin.

Assessment in Action

You are dispatched to the home of a 30-year-old woman who called because of an allergic reaction. When you enter the home, you see that the patient has bright red hives on her arms and upper part of the chest. She is in obvious respiratory distress. Her friend says that she is being treated for a recent strep infection. Her doctor gave her an antibiotic, and the patient has been taking it for approximately 4 days. When you ask her about allergies, she says that she was allergic to penicillin when she a teenager. She noticed her face and arms were turning red approximately 2 days ago; last night, her eyes began to swell. She called today because she felt as if her throat were closing up and she began having trouble breathing. She also complains of chest tightness. Her vital signs are a heart rate of 104 beats/min, sinus tachycardia on the monitor, pulse oximetry of 93% while breathing room air, blood pressure of 80/64 mm Hg, and a respiratory rate of 28 breaths/min.

1. An _____ is an overreaction by the body's immune response to normally harmless foreign substances, which cause damage to body tissues.
   A. antigen
   B. antibody
   C. allergic reaction
   D. allergy

2. In the preceding scenario, what type of reaction is the patient experiencing?
   A. Local reaction
   B. Systemic reaction
   C. Hypersensitive reaction
   D. Allergen reaction

3. The most common causes of anaphylaxis include all of the following, EXCEPT:
   A. drugs.
   B. insect stings.
   C. blood products.
   D. IV fluids.

4. What are the routes of entry by which substances can invade?
   A. Skin, respiratory tract, and gastrointestinal tract
   B. Skin, respiratory tract, and cardiovascular system
   C. Skin, cardiovascular system, and gastrointestinal tract
   D. Skin, respiratory tract, and urinary tract

5. White blood cells that work to produce chemical mediators during an immune response are:
   A. mast cells.
   B. antibodies.
   C. basophils.
   D. histamines.

6. When an antigen enters the body, it binds to the IgE antibodies on the mast cells. This stimulates the mast cells to release:
   A. chemical mediators.
   B. granules.
   C. antihistamines.
   D. cellular immunity.

7. Itching or pruritis is an early sign of an allergic reaction. What is it caused by?
   A. Vasoconstriction
   B. Vasodilation
   C. Antigens
   D. Bronchodilation

8. What is the preferred route for administering epinephrine to a patient in anaphylactic shock?
   A. IV
   B. IM
   C. SQ
   D. SL

9. What is the IM adult dose of epinephrine?
   A. 1:1,000, 0.3–0.5 mg
   B. 1:10,000, 0.3–0.5 mg
   C. 1:1,000, 1 mg
   D. 1:10,000, 1 mg

Challenging Question

You are dispatched to the local high school to treat an allergic reaction. When you arrive on scene, you find a 17-year-old girl complaining of itchiness and hives. There is no respiratory distress. Her vital signs are all within normal ranges.

10. Is this patient having an allergic reaction or an anaphylactic reaction?

▇ Points to Ponder

You are treating a 46-year-old man for chest pain. You administer nitroglycerin and 324 mg of "baby" aspirin. En route to the hospital, you notice that the patient's skin is beginning to turn red and urticaria is developing. His lips are beginning to swell. You ask the patient about these signs, and he says that he forgot to tell you he is allergic to aspirin. His blood pressure has dropped significantly, his respiratory rate has increased, and his heart rate is increasing.

How urgent is this patient's emergency, and how will you care for it?

Issues: Understanding the Pathophysiology of an Allergic or Anaphylactic Reaction, Knowing Your Treatment Protocols for an Allergic Reaction and Anaphylactic Shock.

31 Gastrointestinal Emergencies

Objectives

Cognitive

5-6.1   Describe the incidence, morbidity and mortality of gastrointestinal emergencies. (p 31.4)

5-6.2   Identify the risk factors most predisposing to gastrointestinal emergencies. (p 31.4)

5-6.3   Discuss the anatomy and physiology of the organs and structures related to gastrointestinal diseases. (p 31.5)

5-6.4   Discuss the pathophysiology of inflammation and its relationship to acute abdominal pain. (p 31.9)

5-6.5   Define somatic pain as it relates to gastroenterology. (p 31.17)

5-6.6   Define visceral pain as it relates to gastroenterology. (p 31.17)

5-6.7   Define referred pain as it relates to gastroenterology. (p 31.17)

5-6.8   Differentiate between hemorrhagic and non-hemorrhagic abdominal pain. (p 31.17)

5-6.9   Discuss the signs and symptoms of local inflammation relative to acute abdominal pain. (p 31.10)

5-6.10 Discuss the signs and symptoms of peritoneal inflammation relative to acute abdominal pain. (p 31.10)

5-6.11 List the signs and symptoms of general inflammation relative to acute abdominal pain. (p 31.10)

5-6.12 Based on assessment findings, differentiate between local, peritoneal and general inflammation as they relate to acute abdominal pain. (p 31.18)

5-6.13 Describe the questioning technique and specific questions the paramedic should ask when gathering a focused history in a patient with abdominal pain. (p 31.15)

5-6.14 Describe the technique for performing a comprehensive physical examination on a patient complaining of abdominal pain. (p 31.16)

5-6.15 Define upper gastrointestinal bleeding. (p 31.10)

5-6.16 Discuss the pathophysiology of upper gastrointestinal bleeding. (p 31.10)

5-6.17 Recognize the signs and symptoms related to upper gastrointestinal bleeding. (p 31.19)

5-6.18 Describe the management for upper gastrointestinal bleeding. (p 31.33)

5-6.19 Integrate pathophysiological principles and assessment findings to formulate a field impression and implement a treatment plan for the patient with upper GI bleeding. (p 31.19)

5-6.20 Define lower gastrointestinal bleeding. (p 31.10)

5-6.21 Discuss the pathophysiology of lower gastrointestinal bleeding. (p 31.10)

5-6.22 Recognize the signs and symptoms related to lower gastrointestinal bleeding. (p 31.19)

5-6.23 Describe the management for lower gastrointestinal bleeding. (p 31.33)

5-6.24 Integrate pathophysiological principles and assessment findings to formulate a field impression and implement a treatment plan for the patient with lower GI bleeding. (p 31.19)

5-6.25 Define acute gastroenteritis. (p 31.13)

5-6.26 Discuss the pathophysiology of acute gastroenteritis. (p 31.13)

5-6.27 Recognize the signs and symptoms related to acute gastroenteritis. (p 31.21)

5-6.28 Describe the management for acute gastroenteritis. (p 31.24)

5-6.29 Integrate pathophysiological principles and assessment findings to formulate a field impression and implement a treatment plan for the patient with acute gastroenteritis. (p 31.24)

5-6.30 Define colitis. (p 31.13)

5-6.31 Discuss the pathophysiology of colitis. (p 31.13)

5-6.32 Recognize the signs and symptoms related to colitis. (p 31.21)

5-6.33 Describe the management for colitis. (p 31.24)

5-6.34 Integrate pathophysiological principles and assessment findings to formulate a field impression and implement a treatment plan for the patient with colitis. (p 31.24)

5-6.35 Define gastroenteritis. (p 31.13)

5-6.36 Discuss the pathophysiology of gastroenteritis. (p 31.13)

5-6.37 Recognize the signs and symptoms related to gastroenteritis. (p 31.21)

5-6.38 Describe the management for gastroenteritis. (p 31.24)

5-6.39 Integrate pathophysiological principles and assessment findings to formulate a field impression and implement a treatment plan for the patient with gastroenteritis. (p 31.24)

5-6.40 Define diverticulitis. (p 31.12)

5-6.41 Discuss the pathophysiology of diverticulitis. (p 31.12)

5-6.42 Recognize the signs and symptoms related to diverticulitis. (p 31.12)

5-6.43 Describe the management for diverticulitis. (p 31.21)

5-6.44 Integrate pathophysiological principles and assessment findings to formulate a field impression and implement a treatment plan for the patient with diverticulitis. (p 31.24)

5-6.45 Define appendicitis. (p 31.12)

5-6.46 Discuss the pathophysiology of appendicitis. (p 31.12)

5-6.47 Recognize the signs and symptoms related to appendicitis. (p 31.20)

5-6.48 Describe the management for appendicitis. (p 31.24)

5-6.49 Integrate pathophysiological principles and assessment findings to formulate a field impression and implement a treatment plan for the patient with appendicitis. (p 31.24)

5-6.50 Define peptic ulcer disease. (p 31.11)

5-6.51 Discuss the pathophysiology of peptic ulcer disease. (p 31.11)

5-6.52 Recognize the signs and symptoms related to peptic ulcer disease. (p 31.20)

5-6.53 Describe the management for peptic ulcer disease. (p 31.24)

5-6.54 Integrate pathophysiological principles and assessment findings to formulate a field impression and implement a treatment plan for the patient with peptic ulcer disease. (p 31.24)

5-6.55 Define bowel obstruction. (p 31.13)

5-6.56 Discuss the pathophysiology of bowel obstruction. (p 31.13)

5-6.57 Recognize the signs and symptoms related to bowel obstruction. (p 31.21)

5-6.58 Describe the management for bowel obstruction. (p 31.25)

5-6.59 Integrate pathophysiological principles and assessment findings to formulate a field impression and implement a treatment plan for the patient with bowel obstruction. (p 31.25)

5-6.60 Define Crohn's disease. (p 31.13)

5-6.61 Discuss the pathophysiology of Crohn's disease. (p 31.13)

5-6.62 Recognize the signs and symptoms related to Crohn's disease. (p 31.21)

5-6.63 Describe the management for Crohn's disease. (p 31.24)

5-6.64 Integrate pathophysiological principles and assessment findings to formulate a field impression and implement a treatment plan for the patient with Crohn's disease. (p 31.24)

5-6.65 Define pancreatitis. (p 31.12)

5-6.66 Discuss the pathophysiology of pancreatitis. (p 31.12)

5-6.67 Recognize the signs and symptoms related to pancreatitis. (p 31.21)

5-6.68 Describe the management for pancreatitis. (p 31.24)

5-6.69 Integrate pathophysiological principles and assessment findings to formulate a field impression and implement a treatment plan for the patient with pancreatitis. (p 31.24)

5-6.70 Define esophageal varices. (p 31.10)

5-6.71 Discuss the pathophysiology of esophageal varices. (p 31.10)

5-6.72 Recognize the signs and symptoms related to esophageal varices. (p 31.20)

5-6.73 Describe the management for esophageal varices. (p 31.23)

5-6.74 Integrate pathophysiological principles and assessment findings to formulate a field impression and implement a treatment plan for the patient with esophageal varices. (p 31.23)

5-6.75 Define hemorrhoids. (p 31.11)

5-6.76 Discuss the pathophysiology of hemorrhoids. (p 31.11)

5-6.77 Recognize the signs and symptoms related to hemorrhoids. (p 31.20)

5-6.78 Describe the management for hemorrhoids. (p 31.23)

5-6.79 Integrate pathophysiological principles and assessment findings to formulate a field impression and implement a treatment plan for the patient with hemorrhoids. (p 31.23)

5-6.80 Define cholecystitis. (p 31.11)

5-6.81 Discuss the pathophysiology of cholecystitis. (p 31.11)

5-6.82 Recognize the signs and symptoms related to cholecystitis. (p 31.20)

5-6.83 Describe the management for cholecystitis. (p 31.24)

5-6.84 Integrate pathophysiological principles and assessment findings to formulate a field impression and implement a treatment plan for the patient with cholecystitis. (p 31.24)

5-6.85 Define acute hepatitis. (p 31.13)

5-6.86 Discuss the pathophysiology of acute hepatitis. (p 31.13)

5-6.87 Recognize the signs and symptoms related to acute hepatitis. (p 31.21)

5-6.88 Describe the management for acute hepatitis. (p 31.25)

5-6.89 Integrate pathophysiological principles and assessment findings to formulate a field impression and implement a treatment plan for the patient with acute hepatitis. (p 31.25)

5-6.90 Integrate pathophysiological principles of the patient with a gastrointestinal emergency. (p 31.15)

5-6.91 Differentiate between gastrointestinal emergencies based on assessment findings. (p 31.17)

5-6.92 Correlate abnormal findings in the assessment with the clinical significance in the patient with abdominal pain. (p 31.17)

5-6.93 Develop a patient management plan based on field impression in the patient with abdominal pain. (p 31.21)

Affective

None

Psychomotor

None

Introduction

Gastrointestinal (GI) problems, in and of themselves, are rarely life-threatening. This fact does not minimize the systemic problems that can erupt from untreated or undertreated disease of the GI system. The appendix—a small, inconsequential portion of the intestine—has no known function, and its removal places the patient at no great health risk. Yet, infect this little dangling outcropping, and the consequences can be deadly.

Almost everyone has suffered from abdominal pain at some point. Diarrhea, nausea, and vomiting are also common occurrences that bring both discomfort and unpleasantness, although they are merely signs and symptoms of an underlying condition. A wide range of conditions are actually responsible for these effects, as suggested by the data in ⬤ Table 31-1 ▶ . For example, some 60 million people in the United States suffer from gastroesophageal reflux disease (GERD), or one in every five US residents.

Certain behaviors or characteristics may predispose patients to GI disorders. For example, alcohol consumption and smoking increase a person's risk for developing stomach disorders. Both alcohol and nicotine increase the release of gastric acids within the stomach. As a result, many people will appreciate a *small* amount of wine or a beer before a meal—it primes the stomach for the food about to enter. Chronic alcohol consumption or smoking, by contrast, increases the acidity within the stomach beyond the limits of the protective mucosal layer, putting the individual at risk for ulcers within the upper GI tract. ⬤ Table 31-2 ▶ lists other activities that place patients at increased risk. Note that some supposed causes of GI disorders are myths. For example, many people incorrectly believe that eating spicy foods can cause esophagus and stomach problems.

Table 31-1	Incidence and Prevalence of Gastrointestinal Disorders
Disorder	**Incidence/Prevalence**
All GI disorders	60–70 million (234,000 deaths per year)
Constipation	3.1 million
Crohn disease	162 new cases/100,000 population
Diverticular disease (diverticulosis, diverticulitis)	2.5 million
Gallstones	20.5 million
Gastritis	3.7 million
GERD	20% of the US population
Hemorrhoids	8.5 million
Hepatitis A	31% of the US population
Hepatitis B	5% of the US population
Hepatitis C	1.8% of the US population
Hepatitis D	15 million people worldwide; occurs in 5% of hepatitis B patients
Hepatitis E	Cases within the US occur in people who have traveled to Central Asia, Southeast Asia, Africa, and Mexico
Infectious diarrhea	16 million new cases
Irritable bowel syndrome	2.1 million
Pancreatitis	17 new cases/100,000 population
Peptic ulcer disease	14.5 million
Ulcerative colitis	246 new cases/100,000 population

You are the Provider Part 1

It's 1:00 AM on a busy Friday the 13th, and you and your partner are finally returning to the station for the first time since lunch. You barely get your boots off and rub your feet when the tones play that familiar song. Dispatch is sending you to a popular bar for a patient with uncontrolled bleeding. No other information is available at this time.

You walk into a dimly lit bar that's enveloped in a haze of cigarette smoke. The bartender signals you over and shouts that the patient is in the men's bathroom. You push your way through the crowd and slowly open the door. Your partner points to an open stall in the corner where a man is slumped over the toilet bowl with bright red blood trickling from the corner of his mouth. He responds appropriately but slowly when you speak to him.

Initial Assessment	Recording Time: 0 Minutes
Appearance	Ill-appearing middle-aged man
Level of consciousness	V (Responsive to verbal stimuli)
Airway	Open and clear
Breathing	Adequate chest rise and volume
Circulation	Weak, rapid radial pulse

1. What is your first priority in this situation?
2. What are some of the potential differential diagnoses?

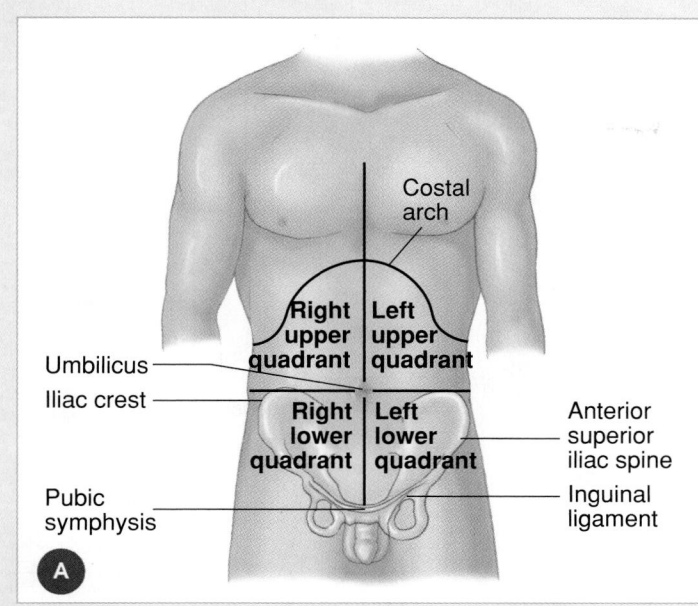

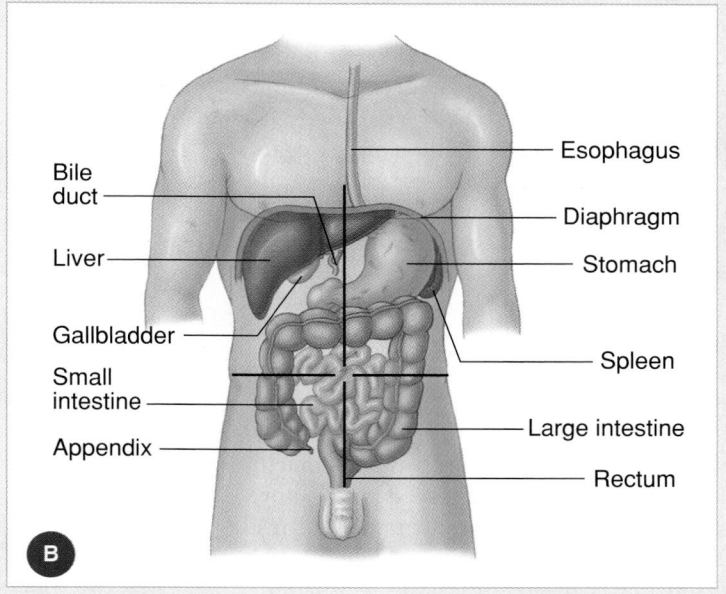

Figure 31-1 The anatomy of the abdomen. **A.** The four quadrants of the abdomen. **B.** Abdominal organs can lie in more than one quadrant.

Table 31-2	Behaviors and Corresponding Risk Factors for GI Disease
Behavior	**Risk factor**
Smoking	Stomach/esophageal disease
Ingestion of caustic agents	Stomach/esophageal disease
Low-fiber diet	Colon disease/constipation
Alcohol	Stomach/esophageal/liver disease
Ingestion of certain medications: acetylsalicylic acid, nonsteroidal anti-inflammatory drugs (NSAIDs), anticoagulants	Stomach/esophageal disease
Stress	Disease throughout the GI tract

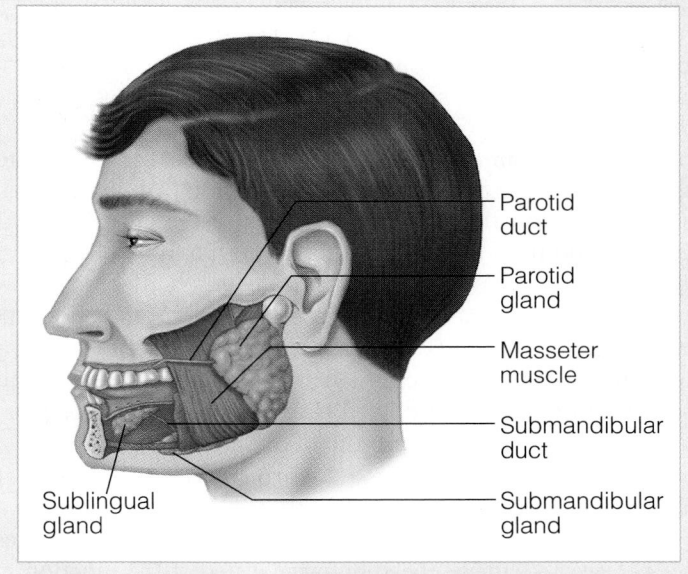

Figure 31-2 Mastication—the first step in the journey of the garden salad.

Anatomy and Physiology

It's dinner time, and Miranda is enjoying one of her favorite meals—a garden salad with lettuce, tomatoes, cucumbers, raisins, peanuts, croutons, carrots, and shrimp with ranch dressing. Examining the journey from food intake to elimination will illuminate the normal anatomy and physiology related to the GI system   Figure 31-1 ▲ .

Miranda takes a bite of her salad. The lettuce, carrots, and cucumbers feel cool and crisp in her mouth, and this pleasant sensation encourages her to chew—a process referred to as mastication   Figure 31-2 ▶ . Miranda's front teeth are mainly

used to tear or cut the food. At the back of her mouth, her molars pound and grind the food into a more easily swallowed consistency. This mechanical activity prepares food to travel down the esophagus more easily and prevents aspiration.

Saliva is secreted into the mouth to help lubricate food. Shrimp, already rather slippery, would have little problem making the transit down the esophagus. The dry and hard croutons, by contrast, would certainly get stuck without the assistance of saliva. The combination of pulverizing and lubrication creates a substance that can be easily moved.

Saliva also contains enzymes that begin the chemical breakdown of foods—in particular, starches. These complex carbohydrates can be disassembled into simple sugars that are more easily absorbed. As Miranda eats the raisins, the simple sugars are released and rapidly absorbed by capillaries within her tongue and mouth. In addition, some initial breakdown of triglycerides occurs.

Now Miranda prepares to swallow. The esophagus is located at the posterior portion of the hypopharynx. This muscular tube is typically collapsed (ie, closed in on itself), which allows for air to easily flow into the lungs but not into the stomach. This collapsed tube idea also explains how gastric dilation and impairment of lung expansion can occur during ventilation. If a person needs positive-pressure ventilation, bag-mask ventilation can push air into the lungs. If the pressure of the breath is too high, then the esophagus dilates; air then follows the path of least resistance. Given the choice between moving through a large tube into a large open space (the stomach) or moving down a series of progressively smaller tubes (the trachea into the right or left mainstem bronchus), air will flow into the stomach.

Intertwined around the esophagus are veins that drain into an even more complex series of veins, which ultimately join together to form the portal vein. The portal vein transports venous blood from the GI tract directly to the liver for processing of the nutrients that have been absorbed. If blood flow through the liver slows for any reason, the blood may back up throughout the entire GI system, because this series of veins lacks any valves. The veins surrounding the stomach and esophagus then become dilated. Even a low amount of pressure may cause leaking or rupture of these vessels.

The esophagus does not absorb nutrients but rather pushes the food along using rhythmic contractions called peristalsis. The food travels through the diaphragm and comes to a doorway—namely, the sphincter located at the junction of the esophagus and the stomach. The cardiac sphincter (which earns its name because people who have regurgitation of acid out of their stomach into their esophagus often feel they are having a heart attack) controls the amount of food that moves back up the esophagus.

When empty, the stomach is rather small, but it is capable of stretching many times beyond its normal size to accommodate meals (**Figure 31-3** ▶). As the food enters this muscular organ, the stomach begins to secrete hydrochloric acid, which helps to break down the food. To mix the acid with the food more evenly, the stomach also contracts, churning the acid and food mixture together until a relatively smooth consistency is achieved. The material that exits the pyloric sphincter, the

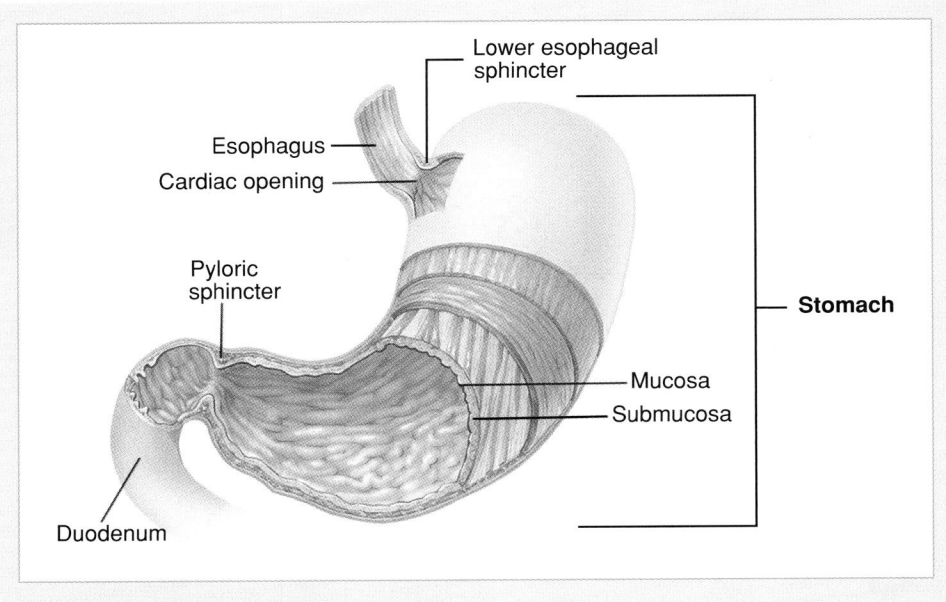

Figure 31-3 The stomach.

doorway at the inferior portion of the stomach, is called chyme.

Because Miranda enjoys her salad, she eats a large helping. This is far too much food for the duodenum, the portion of the small intestine that will begin the very active stage of absorption. The stomach is designed to release only small amounts of the food into the duodenum, thereby enabling the small intestine to better manage digestion.

The stomach absorbs some materials, such as water and fat-soluble substances (eg, alcohol). If Miranda decided to have a glass of wine with her meal, the absorption of the alcohol would begin, slowly, within the stomach. Alcohol is rapidly absorbed within the duodenum. The longer the alcohol remains within the stomach, the slower the rate of its absorption into the bloodstream. Drinking alcohol with a fatty meal will delay gastric emptying, as the stomach works to digest the difficult fats. Miranda's meal is relatively low in fats, however, so she will feel the effects relatively quickly.

The real purpose of the digestive system is revealed in the next portion of the GI system. Why is Miranda eating in the first place? As the levels of nutrients available to her cells begin to drop, she feels hungry. She eats to replenish her resources, keeping her cells supplied with proteins, sugars, fats, electrolytes, and vitamins. The main function of the GI system is to absorb these resources for use by other cells in the body.

The duodenum is the first part of the small intestine. It is where the pancreas, liver, and gallbladder connect to the digestive system. The exocrine portion of the pancreas secretes several enzymes into the duodenum that assist with digestion of fats, proteins, and carbohydrates. In addition, pancreatic juice helps to neutralize gastric acids.

The liver creates bile, which is then stored in the gallbladder. Bile is an enzyme used by the body to help break down

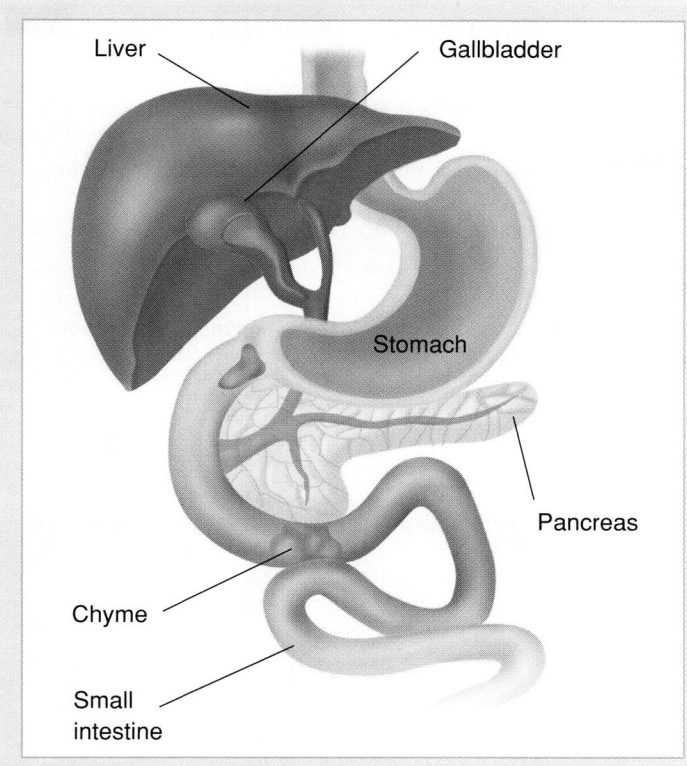

Figure 31-4 The garden salad is broken down into nutrients that the body can use.

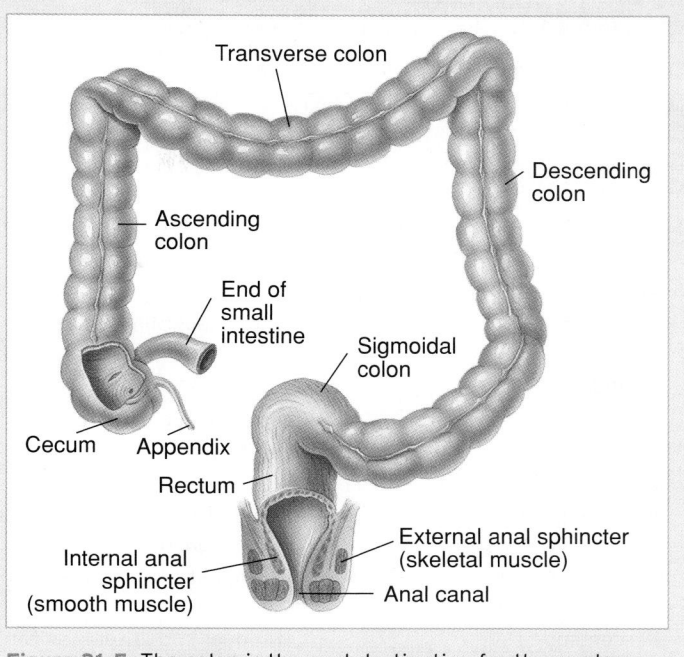

Figure 31-5 The colon is the next destination for the garden salad.

fats. Miranda's salad included shrimp and ranch dressing, both of which contain fat that must be broken down before it can be absorbed into the bloodstream. Bile is released into the duodenum, where it helps to emulsify (ie, dissolve into solution) the fats.

The liver also affects the GI system indirectly, through carbohydrate metabolism. The brain cells can burn only one fuel source—glucose. If blood sugar falls, the liver can convert glycogen into glucose. Dramatic drops in sugar stores will cause the liver to convert fats and proteins into sugar. As blood flows through the liver, fat and protein metabolism continues. Without a functioning liver, Miranda would soon die, because she would not be able to use any of the proteins that were absorbed from the GI system. In addition, the liver detoxifies drugs, completes the breakdown of dead red and white blood cells, and stores vitamins and minerals.

The real workhorse of the digestive system is the small intestine; 90% of all absorption occurs there. This 22′-long structure is divided into three sections: the duodenum (the last section of the upper GI system), the jejunum (the first part of the lower GI system), and the ileum. The small intestine produces enzymes that work with the pancreatic enzymes to turn chyme into substances that can be directly absorbed by the capillaries of the small intestine and thereby move into the bloodstream **Figure 31-4 ▲** .

Blood filled with these nutrients exits the intestinal circulation and heads to the liver, where additional metabolism of fats and proteins takes place. The blood then leaves the liver and enters the subclavian vessels. The water-soluble vitamins from the tomatoes and cucumbers in Miranda's salad are absorbed into the bloodstream for use by cells.

The large intestine, or colon, is the next destination for the remnants of the salad **Figure 31-5 ▲** . The substance that arrives in this 5′-long structure is no longer called chyme, but rather feces. The valve between the ileum and the first portion of the large intestine is called the cecum. Located directly posterior to the ileocecal valve is the appendix. This blind pouch is able to hold small amounts of material. If the feces contains too much bacteria, indigestible foreign bodies are present, or the appendix becomes compressed or twisted, it can become inflamed, resulting in appendicitis.

Rising up from the cecum is the ascending colon. It attaches to the transverse colon, which runs from right to left. After a 90° turn, the descending colon begins. The end of the colon is therefore found near the left lower quadrant. The sigmoid colon then takes an "S" turn, which aligns its most inferior portion in the center of the abdomen. Attached to the sigmoid colon is the rectum, the last portion of the colon. The colon terminates at a sphincter called the anus, where the feces are expelled from the body.

The primary role of the large intestine is to complete the reabsorption of water. Although the majority of water is reabsorbed in the small intestine, the osmotic function within the colon helps to solidify the digested material into a formed

Table 31-3	Abdominal Organs, Location, and Functions	
Organ/Structure	**Location**	**Function**
Mouth	Head	Mechanical breakdown of food. Begins chemical breakdown with saliva.
Esophagus	Substernal, epigastric	Tube that moves food from the mouth to the stomach. Muscular and vascular structure.
Stomach	Left upper quadrant, epigastric	Performs mechanical and chemical breakdown of food. Food in, chyme out.
Small intestine		
Duodenum	Central, upper umbilical	Major site for chemical breakdown of food and major absorption of water, fats, proteins, carbohydrates, and vitamins.
Jejunum	Central, umbilical	
Ileum	Central, hypogastric to lower right abdomen	
Large intestine		
Ascending colon	Right lower quadrant, hypogastric into epigastric	Water reabsorption, formation of feces, bacterial digestion of food.
Transverse colon	Right to left upper quadrant, epigastric	
Descending colon	Left upper and lower quadrant, epigastric to umbilical	
Sigmoid colon	Left lower quadrant, hypogastric	
Rectum	Superpubic, hypogastric	
Anus	Most inferior portion of the large intestine	Sphincter to control release of feces.
Liver	Upper abdomen; mainly right with central upper abdomen	Production of bile; assists with carbohydrate, protein, and fat metabolism of nutrients within the bloodstream; vitamin storage and manufacture; detoxification of blood; elimination of waste.
Pancreas	Posterior to the stomach	Exocrine: enzymes for protein, carbohydrate, and fat breakdown within duodenum. Endocrine: insulin, somatostatin, glucagons.
Gallbladder	Inferior surface of the liver	Storage of bile.
Spleen	Left upper abdomen	Filtering of blood, recycling of dead red blood cells.
Aorta	Central upper abdomen	Main artery to lower body.
Bladder	Suprapubic area	Storage of urine.
Uterus	Suprapubic area	Reproduction.
Iliac arteries	Central abdomen and lower right/left quadrants	Blood supply to legs and pelvis.

stool. Failure of this portion of the bowel can lead to a soft stool, termed diarrhea.

The colon is also the site of bacterial digestion. Bacteria normally found within the colon help to finish the breakdown of the chyme. This breakdown produces gas as a by-product. Flatulence may be considered impolite, but it is certainly normal.

The entire digestion process takes 8 to 72 hours (Table 31-3 ▲ summarizes the organs involved). At this pace, bowel movements normally range between three movements per day and one movement every 3 days. Of course, this number varies based on the types of food you eat, the amount of water consumed, your exercise level, and your stress level.

General Pathology

Three major pathologic conditions are responsible for diseases of the GI tract: hypovolemia, infection, and inflammation.

Hypovolemia

Hypovolemia is caused by either dehydration or hemorrhage. Dehydration occurs from vomiting and/or diarrhea. As the patient loses fluid, the body continues to shift water from inside the cells to the interstitial space and finally into the vascular space in an attempt to maintain adequate fluid volume within the blood vessels. If a person becomes hypotensive

Table 31-4	Electrolyte Imbalances due to Diarrhea	
Condition	Effects	Signs and Symptoms
Hyponatremia: low sodium	Swelling of cells	Muscle weakness, cramping, coma, convulsions
Hypernatremia: high sodium	Shrinking of cells due to excessive water loss	Coma, convulsions
Hypokalemia: low potassium	More stimulation needed to fire nerve/muscle cells	Muscle cramps, weakness, paralysis, heart failure, dysrhythmia
Hyperkalemia: high potassium	Less stimulation needed to fire nerve/muscle cells	Muscle weakness and cramps, bradycardia, asystole

during a dehydration episode, it means that he or she is no longer capable of effectively pulling fluid from the interstitial space and the cellular area.

Electrolytes are also involved in this fluid shift. Although persistent vomiting certainly decreases the amount of food ingestion, diarrhea can alter electrolyte levels even more rapidly, especially sodium and potassium concentrations. Interestingly, diarrhea can cause both excessively high and excessively low electrolyte levels. Electrolytes are naturally lost with the water in the diarrhea. As the diarrhea becomes clearer, meaning that it contains less fecal material and more water, smaller amounts of electrolytes are lost compared to the amount of water lost. Conversely, the less water lost, the thicker the diarrhea, and the less dramatic the change in electrolyte levels. Table 31-4 ▲ summarizes the effects of electrolyte imbalances.

Hypovolemia may also be a consequence of hemorrhage. Bleeding within the GI system typically derives from either the rupture or the destruction of a structure. The GI system's close proximity to the blood supply—while essential to ensure that nutrients are transported to cells—makes damage to this system more likely to cause severe hemorrhage.

Trauma is an obvious mechanism for bleeding from within the GI system. Other potentially damaging events include erosion of the protective mucosal layers, chemical destruction of tissue, or dilation of blood vessels. GI bleeding can occur slowly over several days to weeks, or it can be very sudden with large amounts of blood loss. In either case, fatal hemorrhage from a GI bleed is possible.

With either diarrhea or hemorrhage, the patient will suffer an absolute loss of fluid volume. Consequently, classic signs and symptoms of shock should be present. As discussed in Chapter 18, the body compensates for shock by releasing catecholamines. In an effort to maintain blood pressure, these neurotransmitters increase the heart rate, force contractions of the heart, and increase vasoconstriction. Although the early effects of shock may include patient anxiety and restlessness, the brain fares well initially in the compensated phase of shock, and blood pressure remains near normal. The earliest "sign" will involve tachycardia and pale, cool, clammy skin as the body shunts blood away from the skin and muscles. The pulse pressure narrows as epinephrine causes vasoconstriction, and

respirations increase. If the patient's blood pressure has dropped, then significant volume has been lost and efforts to compensate have failed. Such a patient is critical.

Infection

The food we eat is alive. Bacteria, viruses, and fungi are present throughout our food stream. Infections within the GI system typically occur by either ingestion of severely infectious food or a rupture of the system.

The majority of people who become ill from consumption of contaminated foods have stomach aches, vomiting, or diarrhea. In the United States, an estimated 76 million people get a food-borne illness every year, but only 5,000 die of this cause—a mere 0.007% of those who become ill. People who are immunocompromised (eg, patients who have acquired immunodeficiency syndrome [AIDS] or certain types of cancers, patients who are undergoing chemotherapy, and transplant recipients), the very old, and the very young generally have a harder time fighting off an infection of any type and are more likely to have a poor outcome from food-borne illness. Traveling to other countries can also place a person at greater risk for food intolerances or food-borne infections. "Traveler's diarrhea" affects as many as 33% of all people who travel to countries where food cleanliness is less than adequate, such as in parts of South America, Asia, and Africa.

Infection can also occur when the GI system suffers damage. A breach in the container allows GI contents—which are filled with a variety of organisms—to move into the surrounding tissues. In appendicitis, for example, feces moving through the intestines become trapped in the appendix and prevent the normal flushing of this structure. Bacteria found within the feces then multiply, producing pus and gas as by-products, and possibly exerting pressure on this small structure. If the pressure is too high, the structure will fail, spilling material laden with pus and feces into the peritoneum. This can cause peritonitis, or inflammation of the protective lining of the abdominal cavity.

Regardless of the cause, the body will begin to defend itself against the infection. Fever represents an attempt to slow down the organisms' reproduction. White blood cells are directed to the site of infection to attack the invaders. The patient begins to feel malaise, weakness, chills, and a decreased ability to concentrate as the available energy is mobilized to manage the infection. This response is the body's way of telling a person to sit down, take the day off, and let it fight the infection.

Inflammation

Inflammation is a natural response to injury. If the body is attacked by infectious agents, then vasodilation, mobilization of white blood cells, and changes within cellular metabolic processes occur. All of these effects allow cells to move from a normal operating mode into a state of being under siege. Inflammation assists the white blood cells in either destroying the invading agents or, at the least, walling them off so they cannot spread.

The redness, swelling, and tenderness you feel in your finger when you have an infection are the results of inflammation, for example. The change in capillary permeability and vasodilation enable white blood cells to more effectively get into the area of damage. Swelling can increase the pressure within the finger, which leads to pain.

Localized inflammation within the GI system causes localized signs and symptoms. In hepatitis, for example, the liver becomes inflamed. Patients with hepatitis may initially experience pain in the right upper quadrant of the abdomen due to mild swelling of the liver. In peritonitis, inflammation occurs throughout the abdomen; thus the patient may experience generalized pain that is rebound in nature. In this type of inflammation, the peritoneum becomes irritated. If the inflammation is caused by an infectious agent, then peritonitis can be a sign of movement of bacteria into the abdomen and eventually into the bloodstream; the latter condition is called sepsis.

The body responds to sepsis with a more generalized inflammatory response. One particularly severe consequence of sepsis is the depletion of resources needed to manage the infection. In sepsis, infection is nearly everywhere. The body tries to fight many battles but does not have adequate white blood cells, histamine, blood, or energy to win the war. If the balance between resource demand and supply cannot soon be restored, death will occur.

Sometimes the body attacks and kills its own cells for no particular reason, a situation referred to as an autoimmune condition. A variety of reasons have been postulated to explain this misdirected attack, but no conclusive cause-and-effect relationship has been found. One theory is that the patient ingests food that contains a little-known antigen; this protein substance is identified as foreign, and the body creates antibodies to it. It has also been speculated that the patient comes in contact with a virus that triggers an immune response.

Whatever the cause of the autoimmune disease, the end result is that white blood cells begin to destroy a portion of the GI system, causing damage. Even as the white cells continue to attack, however, the body attempts to repair the damaged area. In colitis, for example, one portion of the body believes that the lining of the colon is a foreign protein. The white blood cells begin to attack and kill the normal cells within this lining. At the same time, the body begins to re-build the damaged colonic wall. As a result, scarred portions of the GI tract appear next to perfectly normal portions.

Notes from Nancy
Not all abdominal pain is from abdominal causes.

Special Considerations

The geriatric population presents paramedics with a number of complicating factors. For example, older people tend to have more than one disease, they may take several medications, and the efficiency of their organ systems is often on the decline. In addition, the nervous system of an older patient with diabetes may be affected by diabetic neuropathy, preventing the patient from feeling pain in a typical manner.

In younger individuals, the pain of appendicitis is periumbilical and then moves to the right lower quadrant. In elderly patients, appendicitis pain is often vague, diffuse, and not well localized. The immune system decreases its intensity of response as we age, so fever may or may not be present. To the paramedic, this older person might appear to be having gastroenteritis caused by one of the many medications he or she is taking.

The prudent paramedic will perform a detailed assessment of the conscious geriatric patient to detect even subtle changes related to bowel habits, eating habits, new foods, travel, new medications, low-grade fevers, or other factors. Don't pummel the patient with nonstop questions as part of this information-gathering expedition, but rather weave the inquiries into the flow of your conversation. With the geriatric population, gathering information may be more difficult, but your efforts will convey your sense of compassion and caring to a population that is all too often ignored or dismissed.

Specific Conditions

Table 31-5 lists the major diseases of the GI system.

Gastrointestinal Bleeding

Bleeding within the GI tract is a symptom of another disease, not a disease itself. **Table 31-6** describes the causes of GI bleeds. The differences between upper and lower GI bleeds are predominately related to the consistency and characteristics of the vomit and stool that may be present. Upper GI bleeds are far more common than lower GI bleeds.

Esophageal Varices

Esophageal varices occur when the amount of pressure within the blood vessels surrounding the esophagus increases. The esophageal blood vessels eventually deposit their blood into the portal system. If the liver becomes damaged and blood cannot flow through it easily, blood begins to back up into these portal vessels, dilating the vessels and causing the capillary network of the esophagus to begin leaking. If pressure continues to build, the vessel walls may fail, causing bleeding.

In industrialized countries, alcohol is the main cause of portal hypertension. Chronic alcohol consumption damages

Disease	Type of Condition	Common Presenting Problems
Table 31-5	**Gastrointestinal Diseases by Type of Condition and Presenting Problem**	
Acute gastroenteritis	Infectious	Pain, diarrhea, dehydration
Acute hepatitis	Infectious	Pain, liver failure
Appendicitis	Acute inflammation	Pain, sepsis
Bowel obstruction	Decreased motility	Pain, sepsis
Cholecystitis	Acute inflammation	Pain
Colitis	Chronic inflammation	Pain, diarrhea, dehydration
Crohn disease	Chronic inflammation	Pain, diarrhea, dehydration
Diverticulitis	Acute inflammation	Pain, sepsis
Esophageal varices	Hemorrhagic	Pain, hemorrhage
Gastroenteritis	Erosive	Pain, diarrhea, dehydration
Hemorrhoids	Hemorrhagic	Pain, hemorrhage
Pancreatitis	Acute inflammation	Pain, hemorrhage
Peptic ulcer disease	Erosive/infectious	Pain, hemorrhage

Table 31-6 Gastrointestinal Bleeding by Organ and Cause

Organ	Causes	Location	Substances
Esophagus	Inflammation (esophagitis) / Varices (varicose veins) / Tear (Mallory Weiss syndrome) / Cancer / Dilated veins (cirrhosis, liver disease)	Upper GI	Melena, hematemesis, vomit with gross blood
Stomach	Ulcers / Cancer / Inflammation (gastritis)	Upper GI	Melena, hematemesis, vomit with gross blood
Small intestine	Ulcer (duodenal)	Upper GI	Melena, hematemesis, vomit with gross blood
	Cancer / Inflammation (irritable bowel disease)	Upper or lower GI	Melena, hematemesis, vomit with gross blood
Large intestine	Infections / Inflammation (ulcerative colitis) / Colorectal polyps / Colorectal cancer / Diverticular disease	Lower GI	Hematochezia
Rectum	Hemorrhoids	Lower GI	Hematochezia, gross bleeding

the interior of the liver (cirrhosis), leading to slower blood flow. In developing countries, viral hepatitis is the main culprit causing liver damage.

Mallory Weiss Syndrome

Mallory Weiss syndrome may lead to severe hemorrhage. In this condition, the junction between the esophagus and the stomach tears, causing severe bleeding and potentially death. During the act of vomiting, pressure within the stomach can increase so greatly as to cause a failure of the structure of the esophagus. Mallory Weiss syndrome affects both men and women equally, but is more prevalent in older adults and older children.

Hemorrhoids

Hemorrhoids are created by swelling and inflammation of the blood vessels surrounding the rectum. They are a common problem, with almost half the population having at least one hemorrhoid by age 50. Hemorrhoids may result from conditions that increase pressure on the rectum or irritation of the rectum. Pregnancy, straining at stool, and chronic constipation cause increased pressure. Anal intercourse and diarrhea cause irritation.

Peptic Ulcer Disease

The stomach and duodenum are subjected to high levels of acidity. To prevent damage to these organs, protective layers of mucus line both organs. In peptic ulcer disease (PUD), the protective layer is eroded, allowing the acid to eat into the organ itself over the course of weeks, months, or even years.

In the past, PUD was thought to be related to the types of food that people were eating. Today, it is known to have a variety of etiologies. The majority of peptic ulcers are the result of infection of the stomach with *Helicobacter pylori*. Another major cause is chronic use of nonsteroidal anti-inflammatory drugs (NSAIDs). Alcohol and smoking can also affect the severity of PUD by increasing gastric acidity.

PUD affects both men and women equally, but tends to occur more often in the older population. As people age, the immune system's ability to fight infection decreases, making *H pylori* infection more likely. The geriatric population, in general, also uses NSAIDs frequently for arthritis and other musculoskeletal complaints.

Cholecystitis

Cholecystitis is caused by obstruction of the cystic duct leading from the gallbladder to the duodenum, usually by gallstones. Gallstones are believed to form due to either increased production of bile or decreased emptying of the gallbladder.

The gallbladder stores bile, an enzyme used to break down fat; when it contracts, it releases this bile. When fatty foods are present within the duodenum, the contraction will occur, but if a blockage is present, the patient may experience severe extreme right upper quadrant pain, radiating to the right shoulder. In addition to the pain, the patient may demonstrate a positive Murphy's sign. Nausea, vomiting, fever, jaundice, and tachycardia are also present with cholecystitis.

Females suffer from cholecystitis two to three times more often than do males. Older people are also more prone to this condition than their younger counterparts. Caucasians have a higher prevalence than African Americans. People who are overweight or have a recent extreme weight loss are also at greater risk. Thus the profile of the "classic" cholecystitis patient is: fair, fat, female, and fifty.

Appendicitis

Appendicitis begins with the accumulation of material, usually feces, within the appendix. Once the normal flushing of this organ is obstructed, pressure may build within the appendix. This pressure decreases the flow of blood and lymph fluid, which in turn hinders the body's ability to fight infection. The combination of the bacteria within the feces and the body's decreased ability to fight any local infection provides an environment ripe for the bacteria's uncontrolled reproduction. If left unchecked, overpressurization of the appendix may eventually result in rupture, peritonitis, sepsis, and death.

Adolescents have the highest incidence of appendicitis, with the number of cases dropping as age increases. Although elderly individuals suffer from appendicitis less often, they have a higher mortality with this condition compared to their younger counterparts. Males are slightly more prone to developing appendicitis than females.

Diverticulitis

Diverticulitis was first recognized around 1900, when the types of foods people ate began to change dramatically. In particular, the amount of fiber within the US diet plummeted as the amount of processed foods eaten increased.

As the amount of fiber consumed as part of the diet decreases, the consistency of the normal stool becomes more solid. This hard stool takes more contractions and subsequently increases pressure within the colon to move. In this environment, small defects within the colonic wall that would otherwise never pose a problem now fail, resulting in bulges in the wall. These small outcroppings eventually turn into pouches, called diverticula.

As feces travel through the colon, some may become trapped within these pouches. When bacteria grow there, they cause localized inflammation and infection. As the body attempts to manage this infection, scarring can occur, along with adhesions and fistulas. A fistula is an abnormal connection between two cavities. In the case of diverticulitis, fistulas are typically between the colon and the bladder, increasing their vulnerability to infection.

The typical patient with diverticulitis is more than 40 years old. More important than sex or race is the amount of fiber within the patient's diet. Decreased fiber increases the patient's risk for this disease. Interestingly, people in the Western world tend to get diverticulitis, whereas people from Africa and Asia are less vulnerable to this condition.

Pancreatitis

The pancreas produces several enzymes that help break down the food we eat into substances that can be absorbed by the intestines. If the tube carrying these enzymes becomes blocked,

You are the Provider Part 2

You begin your assessment while your partner takes a set of vital signs. You are able to find out that the patient's name is Rob, and that he is 47 years old. When asked what happened this evening, all he is able to tell you is that he was drinking at the bar minding his own business when he felt a horrible pain in his stomach. He felt like he needed to throw up so he went to the bathroom. That was the last thing that he remembered. You observe a significant amount of bright red blood (approximately 1 L) on the floor around the toilet.

The patient says that he is still very nauseous and is in extreme pain. He rates his pain as 10 out of 10 on the pain scale. His pain is located in the epigastric area and does not radiate. He describes the pain as knife-like. He denies having any past medical condition or allergies. When questioned about his alcohol intake for the night, he says that he lost count at five Jack Daniels on the rocks and about 10 beers since 8:00 PM.

Vital Signs	Recording Time: 5 Minutes
Level of consciousness	Verbal; confused about day of week
Pulse	118 beats/min, weak and regular
Blood pressure	88/64 mm Hg
Respirations	26 breaths/min, regular
Skin	Jaundiced, warm, slightly diaphoretic
Sao_2	97% on room air

3. What are the signs and symptoms of ruptured esophageal varices?
4. What is the most common cause of esophageal varices?

the enzymes become activated and begin to do their job right where they are. They break down the protein and fat of the pancreas itself, a process referred to as autodigestion of the pancreas. Factors contributing to the development of pancreatitis include increased alcohol consumption and gallstones. Other causes include medication reactions, trauma, cancer, and very high triglyceride levels.

Pancreatitis can occur suddenly, or it may persist over many months. Patients can have singular attacks or episodes of attacks that can retreat for a long time. Men tend to have this condition more than women. It also occurs more often in African Americans aged 35 to 64 years.

Ulcerative Colitis

Ulcerative colitis is caused by generalized inflammation of the colon. It is unclear what causes this chronic inflammation, but genetics, stress, and autoimmunity have been speculated to contribute to its etiology. In ulcerative colitis, the inflammation causes a thinning of the wall of the intestine, resulting in a weakened, dilated colon. The damaged lining of the colon is then prone to infections by bacteria and bleeding.

Ulcerative colitis is a disease of the young; most patients are between 15 and 30 years of age. It occurs with equal incidence in men and women. There is a strong hereditary component to this disease; 20% of patients have a family member with this disease. Ulcerative colitis is also more prevalent in Caucasians and people of Jewish descent.

Crohn Disease

Crohn disease is similar to ulcerative colitis, but may affect the entire GI tract. In this condition, the immune system attacks the GI tract, and the activity of the white blood cells damages all layers of the portion of GI tract involved. The most likely site of inflammation is the ileum, the last portion of the small intestine before this organ joins the large intestine. The result is a scarred, narrowed, stiff, and weakened portion of the small intestine; this damaged patch is found among areas of intestine that are perfectly normal.

To date, no definitive cause for Crohn disease has been identified. However, the presence of signs and symptoms outside the GI system supports the hypothesis that some autoimmune component is operating within this disease. Perhaps the presence of antigens within the GI tract triggers an immune response, or perhaps the immune system itself is not working correctly. Another hypothesis is that the immune system creates antibodies for an antigen that does not exist, initiating a cascade of reactions to a ghost invader.

Most patients with Crohn disease are between the ages of 20 and 30 years. Men are diagnosed as often as women. African Americans tend not to suffer from this condition, whereas people of Jewish descent have an increased incidence. Many of the people with this condition have a blood relative with some type of inflammatory bowel disease, suggesting that these conditions have a familial/genetic component.

Acute Gastroenteritis

Acute gastroenteritis comprises a family of conditions revolving around a central theme of infection combined with diarrhea, nausea, and vomiting. Bacterial and viral organisms that can cause this condition include *Escherichia coli, Salmonella, Shigella, Giardia,* the Norwalk virus, *Clostridium difficile,* and rotavirus. These agents typically enter the body through contaminated food or water. Patients may begin to experience upset stomach and diarrhea as soon as several hours or several days after contact with the matter. The disease can then either run its course in 2 to 3 days or continue for several weeks.

Cholera, a type of acute gastroenteritis that is relatively unknown in the United States, is frequently encountered in the developing world. The Norwalk virus is responsible for the majority of acute viral gastroenteritis in adults, whereas rotavirus causes the same condition in children.

Gastroenteritis

Gastroenteritis is not an infectious disease but has all of the hallmarks of its acute (infectious) cousin. Patients with this condition suffer from nausea, vomiting, and diarrhea from a noninfectious cause, such as medications, toxins from shellfish, or chemotherapy.

Acute Hepatitis

Acute hepatitis is the result of damage to the liver caused by one of several viruses. Hepatitis viruses A, B, C, D, and E are clearly capable of damaging the liver. In the United States, the A, B, and C strains are the predominant organisms that cause this disease. Two other strains, F and G, are also being investigated for their role in causing liver damage. Other causes of acute hepatitis include the Epstein-Barr virus, cytomegalovirus, certain bacterial infections, and liver cancer. The time from the initial infection to the emergence of clinical signs and symptoms can range from 14 to 180 days with acute hepatitis.

Hepatitis viruses are transmitted in a variety of ways. Types A and E move from patient to patient by the fecal–oral route (ie, feces from an infected person is released into the environment and then contaminates either the food or water consumed by another individual). Types B, C, and D are transmitted by person-to-person contact, typically either by sexual intercourse or parenterally (ie, blood-to-blood contact, usually by blood transfusion, accidental needle sticks, or sharing of dirty needles). IV drug users and prostitutes are at higher risk for acquiring hepatitis B, C, and D, whereas people traveling to countries where food and water safety are not adequate are at risk for developing hepatitis A and E.

Bowel Obstruction

With bowel obstruction, the underlying etiology is decreased intestinal motility (ie, abnormally slow movement of material through the intestines). Two major reasons for this problem are paralysis of the intestines or a change in the diameter of their lumen.

Paralysis can be caused by infection, kidney disease, impaired blood flow to the intestines, or medications. In particular, narcotics and anesthetics can paralyze the intestinal muscles. For this reason, patients who undergo major surgery often will not be released from the hospital until they have had at least one bowel movement.

Intestinal lumen diameter compromise can be caused by neoplasms (ie, tumors of the intestines), objects that the patient has swallowed, or strictures (narrowing of the lumen due to damage in the intestinal wall). Other causes include hernia, in which the intestine becomes trapped and compressed; intussusceptions, telescoping of the intestines into themselves; or twisting of the intestines (volvus). The end result is that the diameter of the intestines is narrowed or blocked.

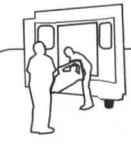

In the Field

All providers should have a clear understanding of the medical terms used to describe findings from a GI patient. This knowledge will avoid confusion.

Assessment

Scene Size-up

Scene safety is the paramount concern for all types of calls. While there are no specific concerns related to patients with GI emergencies, you need to exercise caution to ensure that all personnel remain safe. In terms of additional resources, often these patients need some type of assistance with hygiene, as GI complaints routinely involve body substances. Examples of additional resources for the GI patient include extra gloves, mask, gowns, change of uniform, suction equipment, extra linens, blankets, wash cloths, towels, and adult and child diapers.

The mechanism of injury or nature of illness, as with most medical complaints, will contribute to your initial impression. Early in the call, the only information available may have come from the dispatch center. Use this information to help choose the amount of equipment you will take into the scene. Note that most calls for GI problems will not involve multiple patients. However, a call for assistance at an office building where several people are complaining about GI symptoms should lead you to suspect release of an agent. Biological or chemical agents, for example, can cause people to have abdominal pain, nausea, vomiting, diarrhea, and other GI signs and symptoms.

The last component of the scene size-up is body substance isolation (BSI) precautions. This consideration is particularly important for GI patients. Gloves are needed, as with most calls. Given that you may need to manage vomit, diarrhea, and soiled patient clothing in these calls, additional BSI resources may be called upon. Gowns can be helpful when dealing with

In the Field

Patients tend to assume the most comfortable position. Flexion of the hips reduces movement of the psoas muscle and decreases pain. Ask the patient whether movement, walking, or deep breathing relieves or intensifies the pain. Peritoneal pain, inflammatory in nature, intensifies with movement. Patients with colicky pain (renal, biliary, bowel) often present with restlessness.

patients who have become incontinent. Masks can help with noxious odors.

Initial Assessment

In forming your general impression, closely examine the location where the patient is found, as it can provide hints about what happened. Was the patient walking to the bathroom when he or she passed out? Has the patient been sick for several days and camped out on the couch? Was the patient at work when a sudden bout of pain doubled him or her over Figure 31-6 ?

Notes from Nancy

Any severe abdominal pain that comes on suddenly and lasts more than 6 hours must be considered serious and may require surgery.

In the Field

Remain alert to the four causes of acute abdominal pain that are immediate life threats: acute myocardial infarction (AMI), ruptured abdominal aortic aneurysm, ruptured ectopic pregnancy, and a ruptured viscus (any hollow organ).

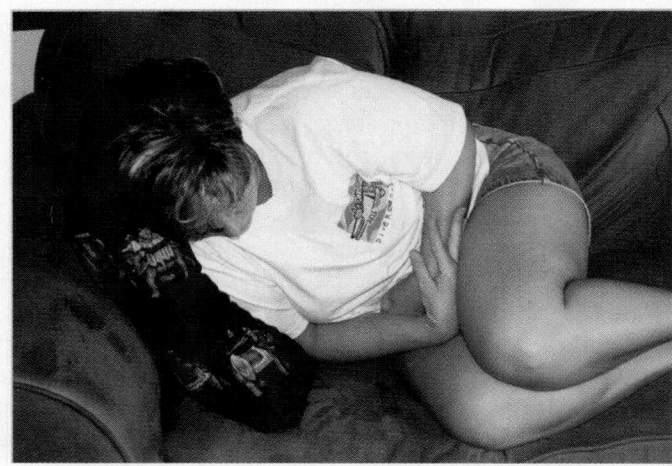

Figure 31-6 A patient experiencing abdominal pain will often curl up into a fetal position to relieve the pressure on the abdomen.

One aspect of the general impression that is different for the GI patient is odor. What is the smell of the room or location of the patient? There are few EMS calls that rise to the level of noxious odor as those that involve upper GI bleeding. The foul-smelling stool that accompanies these calls can make even experienced paramedics nauseous. When dealing with these strong odors, the key is to hold your ground. The sense of smell is the most acute for about 1 minute, but then more than 50% of the intensity of an odor is lost due to the olfactory nerve becoming tired of sending the same signal. If you are faced with a strong odor on a call, stay in the environment. After 2 to 5 minutes, the smell may be hardly noticeable.

Airway patency becomes a more pertinent concern with the GI patient. A patient who is vomiting has a greater chance to aspirate. Open the airway using the appropriate maneuvers, and closely inspect it for foreign bodies. Remove or suction any obstructions that are found. While evaluating the airway, notice any unusual odors emanating from the mouth. Patients who have extremely advanced bowel obstructions can have feculent breath, smelling of stool.

In the Field

Ask your patient about his or her recent food intake. Fatty foods cause the gallbladder to contract, releasing bile. In the patient with gallbladder disease, this leads to distention and pain. Spicy foods act as a direct irritant on the GI tract; when eaten in large amounts, they will cause pain in most individuals. Milk products contain sugar lactose. Lactose intolerance is very common, and patients affected by it will experience bloating, pain, and often violent diarrhea within minutes of ingestion of dairy products.

GI problems rarely affect breathing directly. If a breathing problem is encountered, it typically stems from a severe complication. Ensure that the airway is clear. In particular, if the patient has aspirated, it can affect his or her ability to oxygenate and ventilate.

The assessment of the circulatory system is essential in understanding how the GI disease is affecting the body. As with all patients, assess skin color, temperature, and condition (ie, moisture content). Note findings consistent with shock. Determine the heart rate. Evaluate the peripheral pulses and compare them to the central pulses.

Many GI diseases involve pain and/or hemorrhage. As blood volume begins to drop, the body tries to compensate for this change by releasing catecholamines in the form of epinephrine and norepinephrine. These agents attempt to stabilize blood pressure through vasoconstriction, increased heart rate, and increased force of left ventricular contraction. Pain stimulates similar body responses. Either problem can leave the patient with tachycardia, diminished peripheral pulses, diaphoresis, and pale, cool, clammy skin.

In the Field

Orthostatic changes usually occur when there has been a 15% to 20% loss in circulating volume. Decompensated shock is almost always present when the patient loses more than 30% of the blood volume.

Check the patient's blood pressure. To ensure this measurement's accuracy, obtain a manual pressure before you use one of the automated blood pressure machines. Orthostatic vital signs will help you determine the extent of bleeding that has occurred. First, have the patient assume a position of comfort, usually either seated or lying down. Take an accurate blood pressure and heart rate. Next, have the patient change positions (eg, have the patient stand or sit up). Use caution, because the patient may potentially lose consciousness with a positional change. Wait a minute or two, and then repeat the blood pressure and heart rate measurements. Normally, there should be little change in the blood pressure or heart rate with such a positional change. When a patient has a significant loss of fluid within the vascular space, however, there may be a 10-beat increase in the heart rate and/or a 10-mm Hg drop in blood pressure.

When you examine the GI patient for gross bleeding, it is not unusual to find large amounts of blood. Take note of the amount of blood lost, focusing on being accurate. Many people grossly exaggerate the volume lost due to the emotional effects of seeing large amounts of blood. The amount of blood in a toilet is particularly difficult to estimate due to dilution. To practice volume estimation, measure the amount of water in a glass and then spill it on a carpet; note the size of the puddle. Spill another volume of water on a hard surface such as a tile floor; again note the size of the puddle.

When making your transport decision, integrate the information gathered from the initial assessment. If the patient has a positive tilt test (ie, serial vital signs change with a change in position), then thoughtfully consider how the patient will be moved. Can the patient sit up in a stair chair, or will he or she pass out? Is the patient critical, so that he or she needs to be moved urgently?

In the Field

In females, consider possible sources such as ectopic pregnancy, spontaneous or threatened abortion, ovarian cyst, or pelvic inflammatory disease. Your history should include addressing the gynecologic system and risk factors for these patients.

In pediatrics, consider common causes such as gastroenteritis, appendicitis, and intussusception of the small bowel. Always maintain an index of suspicion for child abuse.

The elderly can be poor historians, have muted symptoms, atypical pain, and low or absence of fever.

Focused History and Physical Exam

For the unstable patient, the head-to-toe examination will provide you with ample opportunities to discover clues as to the underlying problem. Beginning at the head, perform the standard DCAP-BTLS exam. With a GI problem, examination of the head, neck, and chest should not reveal any major changes. Instead, the major effects from GI disease typically relate to the nervous, cardiovascular, and respiratory systems and result from pain, hypovolemia, and infection.

Examining the abdomen can be rather embarrassing for both the patient and the paramedic. Be professional and talk calmly. As you prepare for the abdominal exam, if the patient is stable, place a pillow under his or her knees. Have the patient relax the arms at his or her side. Maintaining straight legs and arms over the head will result in flexed abdominal muscles, which can distort your examination 〔Figure 31-7 ▾〕. Make sure your hands are warm before you touch the abdomen. If the patient is uncomfortable with this examination, try to distract him or her by having a casual conversation. If the patient is unstable, then proceed with the examination in a quick and compassionate manner.

Examine the skin for irregularities. Do you see scars indicating trauma or past surgery? If so, ask the patient about the scarring. Do you notice stretch marks (striae)? These indicate a change in the size of the abdomen over a short period of time. Recent increases or decreases in weight, pregnancy, and severe abdominal edema can all cause striae 〔Figure 31-8 ▸〕.

Is the abdomen symmetric? Looking down at a supine patient, the abdomen should lie flat and gently slope off of the ribs with a gentle upward slope as you approach the pelvis. Tumors, hernia, enlarged or distended organs, pregnancy, and other masses can cause asymmetry.

What is the shape of the abdomen? Is it flat, round, protuberant, or scaphoid? As people gain weight, the weight can be localized to the abdomen, producing a round abdomen. If weight becomes extreme, the abdomen may protrude (ie, become protuberant). Other causes of protuberance include fluid buildup in the abdomen (ascites), pregnancy, and organ enlargement. A scaphoid (concave) abdomen may result from decreased abdominal volume, such as would happen with an abdominal evisceration.

Listen to the abdomen before you touch it, because palpation of the abdomen can alter the bowel sound patterns. Bowel sounds are transmitted easily through the abdominal cavity. Place your stethoscope lightly on the abdominal wall and listen. Listening to one location, such as the right lower quadrant, is usually all that is needed.

Normal bowel sounds sound like gurgles and clicks and occur 5 to 30 times per minute 〔Table 31-7 ▸〕. In your exam, you are merely listening for the presence or absence of these sounds. Sometimes you may hear loud prolonged sounds. This "stomach growling" (borborygmi) indicates strong contractions of the intestines; it can be normal or it may present with diarrhea. Interestingly, hyperperistalsis can also be heard in patients with early bowel obstruction, as the bowel contracts forcefully in an effort to overcome the obstruction.

Decreased bowel sounds—that is, listening over the right lower quadrant and not hearing anything for 15 to 20 seconds—can indicate decreased peristalsis of the intestines. This lack of movement can lead to bowel obstruction. True absent bowel sounds, which are characterized by no sounds heard for 2 minutes, are typically not practical to discover in the prehospital setting. The absence of bowel sounds means that the intestines are not contracting, so any material within them is not in motion.

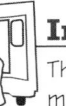

In the Field

The extraneous noise in the prehospital environment makes assessing for bowel sounds difficult.

Many recommend listening for bowel sounds for anywhere from 1 to 5 minutes in each quadrant. In practice, this is rarely done. Follow your local protocols. Most importantly, note whether bowel sounds are present or absent—their absence is more clinically significant than the variations in sounds that are present.

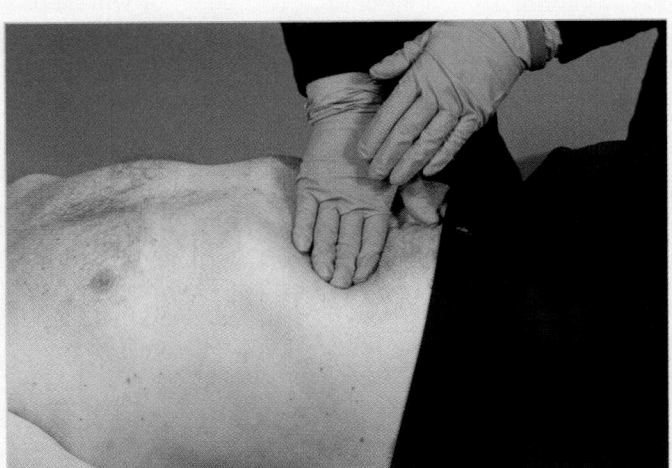

Figure 31-7 Examining a patient's abdomen.

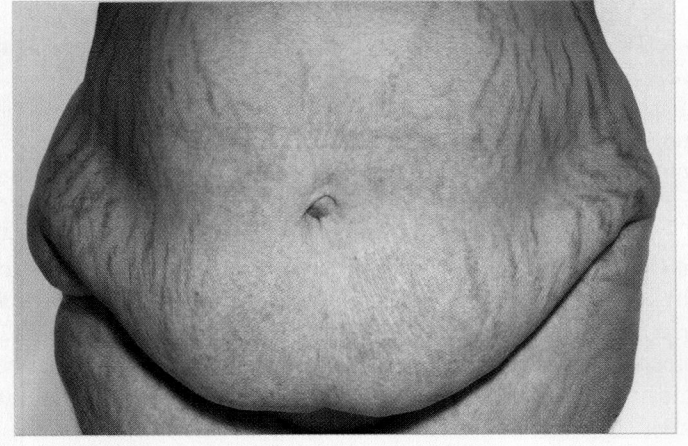

Figure 31-8 Striae.

To palpate the abdomen, place your hand flat on the wall of the abdomen with your fingers together. Choose the quadrant farthest away from where the patient is having the complaint to start your assessment, and then make your way to the quadrant where the complaint is located. Such a cautious approach to an abdominal assessment will decrease the patient's anxiety, help to reveal more accurate information, and allow the patient to focus his or her attention on other portions of the abdomen that he or she may not have considered because of the current discomfort.

With your hand sitting on the wall of the abdomen, raise your wrist so that you indent the abdominal wall with your fingers about 2″ to 4″. As you are palpating, assess the abdomen for the presence of rigidity, discomfort, or masses. Sometimes patients may feel ticklish or otherwise guard the abdomen with flexed muscles, which can make it difficult to determine if the abdomen is rigid or just muscularly guarded. A rigid abdomen may indicate hemorrhage or infection.

Have the patient breathe with an open mouth. It is more difficult to hold the stomach contracted during mouth breathing, so this technique can help to relax the abdomen and allow for a more accurate assessment. You can also hold your fingers slightly depressed into the abdomen during the respiratory cycle.

When the patient exhales, the abdomen typically relaxes. You can also try to coach the patient to relax the abdomen. It

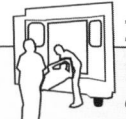
In the Field
Don't forget that cardiac pain may radiate or even originate in the abdomen. Patients typically describe the pain as aching, sharp, "gassy," or indigestion-like.

isn't always possible to get the patient to relax the abdomen, however. Nevertheless, if you're going to report a rigid abdomen, you should take reasonable steps to ensure that your assessment finding is accurate.

Pain is often a finding of importance with GI patients, because it can indicate trauma, hemorrhage, infection, or obstruction. As with the initial assessment, utilize OPQRST to elaborate on the chief complaint. Table 31-8 describes the types of pain that may be experienced with an abdominal problem.

As with all pain evaluations, you also need to determine *when* the patient has pain. Does he or she have pain when the abdomen is not being touched? Does the palpation of the abdomen increase the pain? What is the character of the pain? Does the pain change in character or location during your palpation?

Rebound tenderness (parietal pain) may sometimes accompany abdominal pain and is a finding suggestive of a serious and potentially life-threatening pathology. It occurs when the peritoneum is irritated due to either hemorrhage or infection. The peritoneum is a thin layer within the abdominal cavity that contains most of the abdominal organs. This "bag" normally contains a small amount of fluid.

Your exam goal is to have the peritoneum vibrate. If the peritoneum is irritated, this vibration will cause a sudden increase in pain. There can also be a sudden relocation of pain to another region of the abdomen. Once

Table 31-7	Bowel Sounds	
Sound Name	Description	Possible Causes
Normal	Soft gurgles or clicks occurring at 5 to 30/min	Normal movement of material through the intestines.
Borborygmi	Loud gurgles, often heard without a stethoscope and occurring at greater than 30/min	Hyperperistalsis. Can be normal. If prolonged, can indicate increased intestinal contractions as with diarrhea of any cause.
Decreased	Quiet sounds occurring at less than 1 sound/15 to 20 sec	Hypoperistalsis. Can indicate impending obstruction of the intestines.
Absent	No sounds after 2 min of continuous listening	Bowel obstruction/intestinal paralysis.

Table 31-8	Types of Abdominal Pain		
Abdominal Pain Type	Origin	Description	Cause
Visceral pain	Hollow organs	Difficult to localize; described as burning, cramping, gnawing or aching; usually felt superficially	Organ contracts too forcefully or is distended (stretched)
Parietal pain/ rebound pain	Peritoneum	Steady, achy pain; more easy to localize than visceral. Pain increases with movement.	Inflammation of the peritoneum (blood and/or infection)
Somatic pain	Peripheral nerve tracts	Well localized pain, usually felt deeply	Irritation or injury to tissue, causing activation of peripheral nerve tracts
Referred pain	Peripheral nerve tracts	Pain originating in the abdomen and causing "pain" in distant locations; due to similar paths for the peripheral nerves of the abdomen and the distant location	Usually occurs after an initial visceral, parietal, or somatic pain

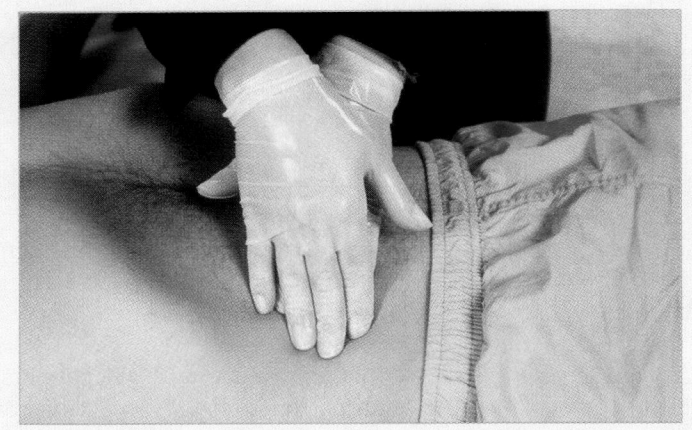

Figure 31-9 Check tenderness by gently palpating each of the four quadrants.

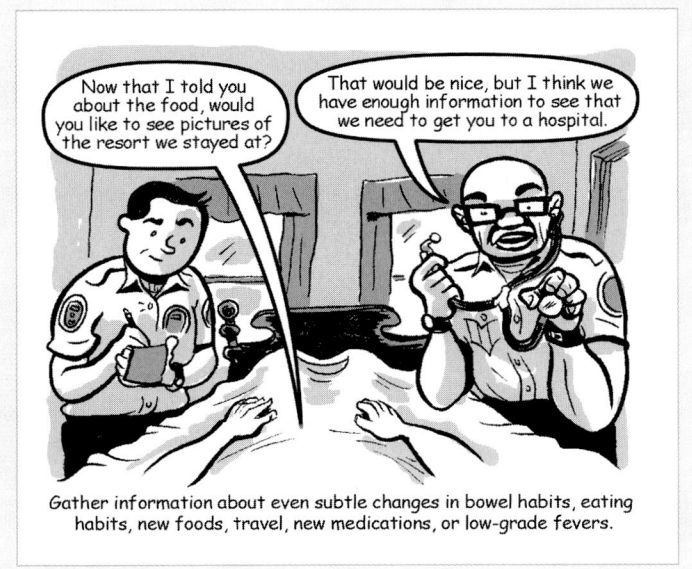

"Now that I told you about the food, would you like to see pictures of the resort we stayed at?"

"That would be nice, but I think we have enough information to see that we need to get you to a hospital."

Gather information about even subtle changes in bowel habits, eating habits, new foods, travel, new medications, or low-grade fevers.

Figure 31-10

you discover an area of the abdomen that is tender to the patient, depress the skin with your fingertips about 2″ to 4″ and then quickly pull your fingers off the abdominal wall. Speed is essential—if you pull the fingers off too slowly, you won't be able to get the desired movement of the peritoneum.

The abdomen should be rather smooth when subjected to light palpation **Figure 31-9 ▲**. While deep palpation can determine some of the organs and structures within the cavity, this requires a level of technique rarely employed within the prehospital setting. As you palpate the abdomen, note the presence of any masses. These will feel like areas of increased density compared to the soft surrounding tissue. Masses may signal the presence of an engorged liver, bowel distention, aortic aneurysm, or cancerous tumors.

In the Field

Be aware of common pain referral patterns:
- Biliary pain commonly radiates around to the right side of the back and angle of the scapula.
- Pancreatic pain goes straight through to the back in the midline of the lower thoracic area.
- Blood/pus under the diaphragm presents as aching pain in the top of the shoulder.
- A leaking or ruptured aneurysm causes pain in the lumbosacral area and usually in the upper thighs.
- Renal colic (kidney stones) pain radiates to the groin and external genitalia.
- Uterine and rectal pain will often be felt in the lower back.

A positive Murphy's sign suggests the presence of cholecystitis. If the patient is experiencing right upper quadrant pain, have the patient breathe out. With the tips of your fingers, palpate deeply along the intercostal margin of the right upper quadrant. You are now applying pressure to the liver and subsequently the gallbladder. Next, have the patient take a deep breath in. As inspiration continues, the diaphragm will drop

and eventually come in contact with the gallbladder. If the patient has cholecystitis, he or she may suddenly stop inspiring due to a sharp increase in pain; this result is reported as a positive Murphy's sign.

Notes from Nancy

Don't spend a lot of time poking at the belly of a patient with abdominal pain.

The SAMPLE history will help the paramedic elicit the relevant current and past medical history **Figure 31-10 ▲**. When asking patients about their complaints, oftentimes you need to discuss subjects that are not commonly described with everyday language. It is important that you and your patient have a common frame of reference. For example, one person's "diarrhea" may be another person's "soft stool." **Table 31-9 ▶** suggests ways to standardize language so that the health care providers taking over care from you will have the same understanding of the patient's condition as you do.

Ongoing Assessment

The goal of the ongoing assessment is to monitor your patient for changes en route to the hospital. Routine monitoring should include heart rate, ECG, blood pressure, respiratory

In the Field

When recording information about the patient's body substances, be as accurate as possible. Describe the substances in detail. Saying the patient had feces covering the legs is adequate if melena is not present. If you see the diarrhea, describe how liquid it is. This information can help to determine the patient's degree of dehydration.

Table 31-9	Body Substances From the GI Tract		
Substance	**Description**		**Possible Cause**
Vomit	Food and partially digested food. Strong acid odor mixed with odor of food eaten.		Influenza, food intolerance
Hematemesis or coffee-ground emesis	Dark, granular material that is the color black or very dark red. This slurry of material may have food within it. The food and blood are indistinguishable.		Blood from the mouth, esophagus, or stomach that has been digested by stomach acids and then vomited
Vomit with gross blood	Vomit with obvious red blood. In this setting there is distinct food and blood that are not incorporated into each other.		Bleeding from the mouth or esophagus that has not been exposed to stomach acids
Diarrhea	Liquid stool that is the consistency of water. It can range in color from clear to dark brown.		Intestinal infections, bowel obstructions; usually associated with small intestinal problems; is always considered abnormal
Acholic stools	Tan-colored, formed stools. May be softer than typical.		Liver problem; bile is released by the liver into the small intestine; bile gives stool its dark color
Steatorrhea	Foamy, foul-smelling, mushy, yellow to gray stools. These oily stools will usually float within water.		Liver or pancreatic disease causing excessive excretion of fat within the stool
Soft stools	Bowel movement that is the consistency of soft-serve ice cream. Can range in color from tan to dark brown.		Normal variant for some people; caused by new foods or rapid change in diet
Hematochezia	Stool and blood that incorporated together into the same substance yet are easily distinguished from each other.		Bleeding from the lower GI tract
Melena	Stool and blood that are blended together into one substance. You are unable to distinguish blood from stool. These are black, tarry, sticky, and very odorous.		Bleeding from the upper GI tract

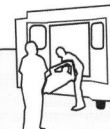

In the Field

Factors that may complicate the abdominal assessment:

- **Young age.** Poor historians; fear
- **Old age.** Poor historians, muted symptoms, atypical presentations
- **Obesity/pregnancy.** A large abdomen can displace or hide abdominal organs
- **Compromised immune systems.** Don't mount a telltale response to infection or inflammatory disease.

rate, and pulse oximetry. If the patient is suffering from a GI bleed, continue to assess him or her for signs of shock. Equally important, you should determine what effect your treatment is having. Before giving additional fluid boluses, listen to the patient's lung sounds to determine whether he or she is developing acute pulmonary edema.

Also monitor the patient's pain level. Many patients with abdominal pain may be receiving pain medication. How effective was your treatment? Does the patient need more medication? What are the blood pressure and respiratory rate?

If the patient's condition undergoes a sudden dramatic change, repeat the rapid and detailed assessments as if this case were a new patient. This will give you the best chance of modifying your care to adequately manage this new development.

Notes from Nancy

It is not necessary to diagnose the specific cause of a patient's abdominal pain in order to appreciate that the patient is in a serious condition.

Assessment of Specific Conditions

Gastrointestinal Bleeding

Presentation of GI bleeding is variable, as it can reflect the presence of a number of diseases. Each of these conditions has its own pattern of disease progression. For example, diverticular disease has a rather gradual onset and tends to strike people in their 50s, 60s, or later decades. Mallory Weiss syndrome has a very sudden onset and affects people of all ages. Gathering the information about how the patient progressed from being healthy to needing an ambulance is critical in forming your field impression.

The patient's medical history and other possible events of abdominal pain or bleeding from the GI tract may also provide important information. Find out which medications the patient is taking; many drugs can irritate the GI tract, precipitating bleeding. Determine how long the patient has had the problem.

The most important component of the physical exam is to determine how much bleeding has occurred. Do you see evidence of bleeding in the environment? If so, estimate the amount of liquid present. Focus your assessment on evaluation for shock. Determine whether the patient is compensating for the fluid loss. Orthostatic vital signs are the key to gauging the degree of fluid loss in the prehospital setting.

Esophageal Varices

Presentation of esophageal varices takes two forms. Initially, the patient shows signs of liver disease—that is, fatigue, weight loss, jaundice, anorexia, edema in the abdomen, pruritus, abdominal pain, nausea, and vomiting. This very gradual disease process takes months to years before the patient reaches a state of extreme discomfort.

By contrast, the rupture of the varices is far more sudden. The patient will complain of sudden-onset discomfort in the throat. He or she may have severe dysphagia, vomiting of bright red blood, hypotension, and signs of shock. If the bleeding is less dramatic, then hematemesis and melena are likely. Regardless of the speed of bleeding, damage to these vessels can be life-threatening.

Mallory Weiss Syndrome

The presentation of Mallory Weiss syndrome is linked to vomiting. In women, this syndrome may be associated with hyperemesis gravidarum (ie, severe vomiting related to pregnancy). The extent of the bleeding can range from very minor, resulting in very little blood loss, to severe bleeding and extreme hypovolemia. In extreme cases, patients may suffer from signs and symptoms of shock, epigastric abdominal pain, hematemesis, and melena.

Hemorrhoids

Hemorrhoids present as bright red blood during defecation. This hematochezia (gross bleeding) tends to be minimal and is easily controlled. Additionally, patients may experience itching and a small mass on the rectum. Typically, this mass is a clot formed in response to the mild bleeding.

Peptic Ulcer Disease

Patients with peptic ulcers experience a classic sequence of burning or gnawing pain in the stomach that subsides or diminishes immediately after eating and then reemerges 2 to 3 hours later. Nausea, vomiting, belching, and heartburn are common as well. If the erosion is severe, gastric bleeding can occur, resulting in hematemesis and melena.

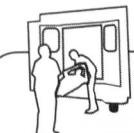

In the Field

Many patients who bleed from a peptic ulcer have had no prior symptoms or history of ulcer disease. When obtaining a history, ask about recent ingestion of alcohol, ibuprofen, or salicylates.

Cholecystitis

In the classic pattern of cholecystitis, the patient originally has no pain. He or she then eats a fatty meal and 2 to 3 hours later develops severe upper right quadrant abdominal pain. This pattern is not absolute, but may vary depending on the consistency of the food being eaten. A fatty steak will remain in the stomach longer than a cheesy casserole, for example. The faster the food is emptied from the stomach, the sooner the complaints will begin after the meal.

Appendicitis

Patients with appendicitis classically present with periumbilical (around the navel) pain that migrates to the right lower quadrant. The duration of the pain is usually less than 48 hours. As the condition progresses, the pain will change characteristics.

You are the Provider Part 3

Your physical exam is significant for jaundice of the skin and eyes, jugular venous distention while sitting, and a swollen abdomen with a palpable liver. You are able to smell an alcohol-like odor on the patient's breath. While completing your exam, the patient leans forward and vomits an additional 250 mL of bright red blood on the floor. You and your partner decide to load the patient on the stretcher and initiate treatment in the back of the ambulance. While you insert two 18-gauge needles in the left and right antecubital region and hang 1,000-mL bags of normal saline running wide open, your partner applies 100% supplemental oxygen via a nonrebreathing mask and attaches the cardiac monitor. A nasogastric tube is inserted in his right nare and returns an additional 100 mL of blood into the suction canister.

Reassessment	Recording Time: 13 Minutes
Skin	Jaundiced, cool, and diaphoretic
Pulse	130 beats/min; weak and regular
Blood pressure	80/56 mm Hg
Respirations	26 breaths/min, regular
Sao$_2$	98% on nonrebreathing mask at 12 to 15 L/min of oxygen
ECG	Sinus tachycardia with no ectopy
Pupils	Pupils equal and reactive to light and accommodation

5. What does this patient need to be monitored for?

6. Is it possible that your patient has aspirated blood? Why or why not?

Rebound tenderness is a sign of perforation of the appendix with resultant peritonitis. Additionally, these patients often develop anorexia, nausea, and fever.

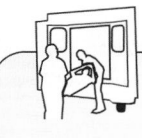

In the Field

Missed appendicitis is more common in the young, the elderly, and in pregnant patients because the symptoms are often atypical.

Diverticulitis

The presentation of diverticulitis is abdominal pain, which tends to be localized to the left side of the lower abdomen. Classic signs of infection include fever, malaise, body aches, chills, nausea, and vomiting. Bleeding is rare with this condition. Due to the local infections of these pouches, adhesions may develop, narrowing the diameter of the colon and resulting in constipation and bowel obstruction.

Pancreatitis

The pain of pancreatitis tends to be localized to the epigastric area or right upper abdomen. It can be sharp and may be quite severe. Radiation of the pain to the back is not uncommon. Patients may also experience nausea, vomiting, fever, tachycardia, hypotension, and muscle spasms in the extremities as a result of hypocalcemia (low blood calcium).

The greatest cause for alarm with pancreatitis is internal hemorrhage. If autodigestion is advanced, blood vessels in and near the pancreas can be compromised. Severe and uncontrolled hemorrhage may then ensue. In these patients, hemodynamic instability can be present. Grey Turner's sign (bruising in the flanks) and Cullen's sign (bruising around the umbilicus) indicate that retroperitoneal bleeding may be present.

Ulcerative Colitis

The presentation of ulcerative colitis entails the gradual onset of bloody diarrhea (hematochezia) and abdominal pain, which can range from mild to severe. Other signs and symptoms may include joint pain and skin lesions, which lends credence to the idea that this disease has an autoimmune component. Finally, patients may experience fever, fatigue, and loss of appetite as a consequence of the infections occurring within the colon.

Crohn Disease

Crohn disease presents with a chronic complaint of abdominal pain, often in the lower right area. This pain corresponds to the location of the ileum. Rectal bleeding, weight loss, diarrhea, arthritis, skin problems, and fever may also be present. The bleeding tends to be small amounts over a long period of time. Acute severe hemorrhage is rare, but chronic bleeding resulting in anemia and hypotension does occur. Patients may experience repeated episodes of mild to severe signs and symptoms.

Acute and Nonacute Gastroenteritis

The presentation of acute gastroenteritis and nonacute gastroenteritis involves diarrhea of various types. Patients may experience large dumping-type diarrhea or frequent small liquid stools. The diarrhea may contain blood and/or pus, and it may have a foul odor or be odorless. Abdominal cramping is frequent as hyperperistalsis continues. Nausea, vomiting, fever, and anorexia are also present.

If the diarrhea continues, dehydration and hemodynamic instability will result. As the volume of fluid loss increases, the likelihood of potassium and sodium imbalance increases. Watch for changes in level of consciousness and other profound signs of shock, as they indicate a critical volume loss.

Acute Hepatitis

All types of acute hepatitis, regardless of their etiology, are associated with the same signs and symptoms. Clinically, the disease occurs in two phases. In the first phase, patients experience joint aches, weakness, fatigue, nausea, vomiting, anorexia, urticaria, and pruritus (itching). At this point in the course of the disease, the patient may be misdiagnosed as having influenza or gastroenteritis.

The second clinical phase of acute hepatitis involves damage to the liver that results in liver failure. It is characterized by acholic stools, darkening of the urine, jaundice, and icteric sclera (yellow sclera). Abdominal pain in the right upper quadrant and an enlarged liver also become apparent at this time. Depending on the disease progression, total liver failure may be only days away.

Bowel Obstruction

The presentation of bowel obstruction varies according to the underlying cause. If this condition is caused by the swallowing of some object, then obstruction can occur within hours. If it is caused by cancer, then the narrowing may take months to become apparent.

Signs of this problem include abdominal pain and fullness. Initially, diarrhea will occur. The slowdown of stool is interpreted as a decrease in water content, so water absorption slows and peristalsis increases as the body tries to overcome the obstruction. If this effort is unsuccessful, constipation results, with decreased bowel sounds. Nausea and vomiting are common in the later stages, with both the emesis and the patient's breath having a feculent odor. Eventually, infection may occur, leading to sepsis.

Management

General Management Guidelines

Often there is little the paramedic can do about the GI disease itself, but you can care for the effects of the disease. Patients may be in extreme amount of pain; they may be suffering from severe dehydration, hypotension, or extreme nausea. Your main goals are to maintain BSI, manage the ABCs, and manage the patient's pain and nausea.

With GI patients, BSI is essential due to the high likelihood of coming in contact with infectious agents. Be prepared to deal with large amounts of vomit, feces, and blood. The following equipment will be helpful to ensure your safety:

- Gloves/gowns/eye protection/surgical mask
- Towels and wash cloths
- Extra linen
- Absorbent pads (Chux)
- Emesis basin
- Disposable basin
- Biohazard bags
- Sterile water for irrigation

Using this equipment to clean the patient also helps to return some degree of dignity to a person who is often quietly humiliated by the circumstances of his or her disease.

The only real airway concern for the GI patient is the potential for aspiration or obstruction of the airway due to vomit or blood. Although these complications are rare, they pose real concerns for the paramedic. Effective positioning of the patient will ensure adequate drainage of material out of the mouth. If the patient has suffered trauma, be prepared to tilt the long backboard. In such a case, the patient needs to be packaged and padded well so that spinal movement is minimized during the board movement. Portable suction should be part of every department's first-in equipment.

If breathing problems are present in association with GI problems, they are often associated with decreased hemoglobin due to bleeding. Be liberal in delivering oxygen to patients with GI bleeds. Don't rely on oxygen saturation readings as evidence that oxygen is not needed. A patient who has been bleeding internally may have a severely decreased hemoglobin level. Although the oxygen saturation may read 96%, if the hemoglobin is low, the patient still needs supplemental oxygen.

Oxygen masks can cause some patients to experience a sense of confinement, especially if they're experiencing nausea. Monitor patients with whom you use a mask to ensure they can get the mask off quickly if they need to vomit.

Listen to lung sounds. This baseline and continuing information is paramount to the safe administration of fluids. In patients who are suffering from dehydration, the overall goal of treatment is to refill the cellular space. The degree of hemodynamic stability will dictate whether you should give the patient a hypotonic or isotonic solution.

A very stable patient should receive a hypotonic solution. Giving one half of the normal saline solution will effectively move fluids from the vascular space into the interstitial space and finally into the intracellular space. In these patients, an infusion rate of 125 mL/h should be sufficient to slowly rehydrate cells without causing dramatic swings in either fluid volume or electrolyte balance.

If the patient is more profoundly dehydrated, then isotonic fluid would be needed to re-expand the vascular space first. Although the cells in this setting are dehydrated, the resultant decrease in blood volume can be life-threatening, so refilling the vascular space takes priority over rehydrating the cells.

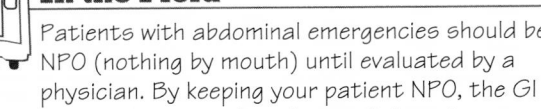

In the Field

Patients with abdominal emergencies should be NPO (nothing by mouth) until evaluated by a physician. By keeping your patient NPO, the GI tract can rest. Food causes the release of digestive enzymes that often worsen most abdominal conditions. Also, it's helpful to minimize stomach contents in the event that surgery is required.

This step is essential to ensure adequate perfusion to the vital organs of the body.

Care for the patient with hemorrhage is directed at maintaining perfusion of vital organs. Internal hemorrhage cannot be controlled in the prehospital setting. Although volume replacement is critical to ensure adequate circulation to the vital organs, very aggressive volume replacement can result in dramatic hemodilution (ie, dilution of the blood) and potentially death. The goal of management is to provide enough volume to keep vital organs from becoming hypoxic but not so much volume as to increase the bleeding. Maintaining peripheral perfusion at the radial artery should be adequate to allow for adequate perfusion to the brain, kidneys, and other vital organs. Once the patient arrives within the hospital, blood administration will be critical to stabilization.

Establish secure IV lines with 1,000 mL of normal saline solution or lactated Ringer's solution with large-bore catheters. If the patient is hypotensive, consider a rapid bolus of 10 to 20 mL/kg and then reassess the patient's status. In the average individual, 20 mL/kg equals approximately one third of the patient's blood volume. Listen to lung sounds before administering any fluid bolus to prevent or limit congestive heart failure, and then administer enough fluid to ensure a peripheral pulse. If the patient is suffering from dehydration, continue the fluid bolus and lung sound assessments until the systolic blood pressure is above 100 mm Hg.

Pain management of the GI patient is a controversial subject. Your system protocols should provide guidance as to which medications, if any, are to be used in this setting. In any event, controlling pain should be a priority with GI patients. The only true contraindication to pain management in the prehospital setting for the GI patient is hypotension. When providing pain management for the GI patient, the goal is to make the patient more comfortable, not to eliminate the pain entirely. Giving enough medication to completely remove the pain may result in severe hemodynamic compromise.

The following five medications provide the paramedic with tools to manage abdominal pain:

- Meperidine hydrochloride (Demerol), 50 to 150 mg IV/IO/IM. This synthetic narcotic can cause hypotension and respiratory depression. It is often given with hydroxyzine to decrease the accompanying nausea.
- Morphine, 4 to 8 mg IV/IO/IM. This narcotic can cause hypotension and respiratory depression.

- Ketorolac (Toradol), 15 to 60 mg IV/IO/IM (IV dose not in excess of 30 mg). This medication is nonnarcotic, so it doesn't cause hypotension or respiratory depression.
- Nalbuphine (Nubain), 10 mg IV/IO/IM. This synthetic narcotic can cause hypotension and respiratory depression.
- Fentanyl (Sublimaze) 1 mcg/kg is a popular opioid agonist because it's rapid-acting, very potent, and has a relatively short duration of action.

The following medications may be administered for management of nausea:

- Diphenhydramine (Benadryl), 10 to 50 mg IV/IO/IM. This medication is typically used for allergic reactions but also has antiemetic properties. It can cause drowsiness and a decline in blood pressure.
- Hydroxyzine (Vistaril), 25 to 100 mg IM. Be cautious when administering this medication to patients who have taken any medication that has central nervous system (CNS) depressive effects, as it acts synergistically to increase the CNS depression.
- Promethazine (Phenergan), 12.5 to 25 mg IV/IO/IM (6.25 mg for elderly patients). Be cautious when administering this medication to patients who have taken any medication that has CNS depressive effects, as it acts synergistically to increase the CNS depression. Because this medication is formulated with phenol, promethazine has a pH between 4 and 5.5, so it produces a marked burning sensation during injection. Administer it very slowly (over 10 to 15 minutes), and dilute the drug in 10 to 20 mL of normal saline if it will be administered by the IV route.

Proper cleaning and maintenance of equipment and uniforms that become soiled during a call is essential to protecting the health of both the EMS crew and its next patient. Hepatitis B, for example, can remain infectious even in dried blood for more than a week.

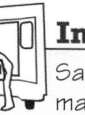

In the Field

Certain medications vary in their effectiveness on specific conditions. Renal colic responds well to Toradol, and gallbladder pain responds better to Demerol. Morphine should be avoided in allergic patients or those with biliary pain because it can cause spasms of the common bile duct, worsening the situation.

Gastrointestinal Bleeding

Treatment for patients with GI bleeding consists of following the general management guidelines. Fluid resuscitation is commonly needed. In most patients—even those with stable vital signs—it is prudent to establish an IV with 1,000 mL of normal saline or lactated Ringer's solution using macrodrip tubing. This type of IV will allow you to provide fluid resuscitation quickly if the patient's condition changes.

In the Field

Saving samples of vomitus, unpleasant as it is, may provide significant diagnostic clues, especially in cases of unknown ingestions, GI bleeding, or an abdominal disease of unknown origins. Follow your local protocols.

Esophageal Varices

Treatment for patients with esophageal varices in the prehospital setting should follow the general management guidelines. As with any GI bleeding disorder, accurate assessment of the extent of blood loss is critical. Be prepared for a very hemodynamically unstable patient who needs volume resuscitation and aggressive suctioning of the airway. If the patient's level of consciousness begins to deteriorate, consider inserting an advanced airway to minimize the potential for aspiration.

In-hospital treatment involves aggressive fluid resuscitation. The bleeding needs to be stopped, so an endoscope is advanced into the esophagus. The physician then attempts to control the bleeding either by using chemicals to cauterize the bleeding veins or placing a type of rubber band to constrict them.

Mallory Weiss Syndrome

Management of Mallory Weiss syndrome is the same as for esophageal varices and is directed at determining the extent of blood loss. The patient may be dehydrated from repeated vomiting, so blood loss can be exaggerated in its effects. In-hospital management includes volume resuscitation as needed, endoscopy to visualize the extent of the damage, and possibly an attempt to repair the damage. In most cases, Mallory Weiss syndrome resolves spontaneously.

Hemorrhoids

Prehospital management of hemorrhoids is largely supportive. In isolation, hemorrhoids are more of an inconvenience than they are a life-threatening condition. Some patients may be at greater risk for serious consequences, however. Cautiously assess the patient who has any bleeding disorder or is taking anticoagulants. In this setting, even a minor bleeding problem can become life-threatening. To ensure that the patient is hemodynamically stable, take the patient's orthostatic vital signs.

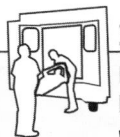

In the Field

Nasogastric (NG) tube placement, if permitted by local protocols, may be beneficial in patients with GI bleeding. The role of iced saline lavage to control ongoing bleeding via vasoconstriction is controversial, and can lead to significant hypothermia and worsen shock states. Follow your local protocols.

The majority of hemorrhoids resolve without treatment in 2 to 3 days. In-hospital management may include creams to help shrink the inflamed tissues. If the condition becomes chronic, surgical removal is a possibility. The best management for hemorrhoids is to prevent them by eating a high-fiber diet.

Peptic Ulcer Disease

The major focus for the prehospital management of patients with peptic ulcers is to accurately assess the extent of blood loss and prepare to manage any hypotension that is present. Orthostatic vital signs are critical in determining fluid needs and transportation/packaging issues.

In-hospital management includes acid neutralization and reduction therapies. Antibiotic therapy is often effective at stopping any new erosion. Management for erosion of the GI tract will be tailored based on the degree of damage to the GI tract. Patients will often need an endoscopic examination, in which a fiber-optic tube is advanced down the esophagus. The stomach wall can then be directly assessed for damage. Surgical repair of the damaged stomach lining in concert with medication therapy is often effective in treating peptic ulcer disease.

Cholecystitis

Prehospital treatment for cholecystitis is directed at making the patient comfortable. This condition is rarely life-threatening, but the extreme pain associated with this condition can make the patient suffer from vasovagal stimulation. Be cautious when transporting any patient in severe pain as syncope, simply from increased pain, is a real possibility.

Medications given to control pain include morphine and meperidine. Morphine is believed to cause a contraction of the sphincter of Oddi, the valve controlling bile movement out of the gallbladder; this contraction can increase the pain linked to cholecystitis. To be cautious, meperidine is an acceptable alternative. To control nausea, use one of the medications mentioned in the standard management guidelines. IV fluids are also indicated, as these patients are often vomiting. In-hospital treatment may include antibiotics, pain medication, ultrasound, and surgical removal of the gallbladder.

Appendicitis

Prehospital management for appendicitis includes keeping a wary eye out for septicemia. If this blood infection is present, septic shock can occur. Volume resuscitation may not be adequate to restore blood pressure. Be prepared to use dopamine if crystalloids are not effective. Administration of pain and antinausea medications is clearly indicated with these patients. At the hospital, these patients will receive antibiotics and typically undergo surgical removal of the appendix.

Diverticulitis

Management of diverticulitis is directed at making the patient comfortable. Examine the patient closely to ensure that severe infection is not present, as sepsis can occur easily in conjunc-

tion with fistulas to the urinary bladder. Patients with diverticulitis may also need large amounts of fluids and/or dopamine to maintain blood pressure. In-hospital treatment includes antibiotics, allowing the GI tract to rest by giving the patient a liquid diet, and possibly surgery to remove the pouches and repair any fistulas.

Pancreatitis

Management for the prehospital patient with pancreatitis should follow the general management guidelines. Pay special attention to assessing the patient for signs of severe hemorrhage. If they are present, begin fluid resuscitation. Given that some of these patients also have gallstones, the most conservative choice for management of abdominal pain is meperidine. Morphine may cause spasms of the gallbladder, increasing the patient's pain.

In-hospital management includes GI rest and fluid resuscitation. In some cases, antibiotics and surgery can be helpful. Although the pancreas cannot be removed unless it is immediately replaced, surgery can be performed to control any bleeding or manage the gallstones and subsequent blockage of bile from the liver.

Ulcerative Colitis

Management of ulcerative colitis consists of determining the degree of hemodynamic instability. Look for signs of shock. If the diarrhea and bleeding have caused sufficient volume loss to make the patient unstable, administer fluids to return the patient to a near-normal volume balance. Otherwise, provide supportive care and follow the general management guidelines.

In-hospital care for these patients will include anti-inflammatory medications, antibiotics, antidiarrheals, and potentially surgical removal of the diseased sections of the colon. Many patients with ulcerative disease suffer for years with periods of diarrhea and abdominal pain, and nearly one third will eventually have part of their colon removed.

Crohn Disease

Management of Crohn disease in the prehospital setting should follow the general management guidelines. Volume resuscitation may be needed because of diarrhea and chronic hemorrhage. Measures to control nausea and pain are commonly needed.

In-hospital care focuses on stopping the inflammation, correcting any fluid imbalances, managing infections, and creating an environment where the GI tract can heal itself. The damage to the intestines can sometimes be so severe that surgical removal of portions is needed.

Acute and Nonacute Gastroenteritis

Prehospital management of both acute and nonacute gastroenteritis follows the general management guidelines. Pay special attention to the problem of determining the degree of fluid deficit. For stable patients, one-half normal saline may be indicated to begin rehydration. Indeed, patients often feel

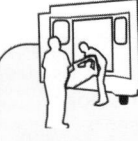

In the Field

Remember to follow strict BSI procedures with these patients. Some of the causative organisms for gastroenteritis are highly contagious.

markedly better after rehydration. Take the orthostatic vital signs to determine the need for isotonic fluid resuscitation. Analgesic and antiemetic medications are also indicated for these patients.

In the emergency department, care is directed to rehydration, control of vomiting and diarrhea, identification of the organism involved, antibiotic therapy, and stabilization of electrolyte imbalances. The patient will have blood evaluation of electrolytes before electrolyte replacement or stabilization therapies are initiated. Once hemodynamically stable, the patient may receive an oral rehydration solution containing water, sodium, potassium, and sugar.

One of the most critical issues when managing acute gastroenteritis is education. It is a food- and water-borne illness, so patients need to be instructed on safe food and water use to prevent future infections.

Acute Hepatitis

Prehospital management for acute hepatitis is supportive and follows the general management guidelines for GI patients. Two important areas on which to focus during patient care are infection control and medication administration.

Patients with acute hepatitis are infectious, so you should take adequate precautions to limit contact with body fluids. Use good handwashing and equipment cleaning techniques, remembering that hepatitis B can remain infectious in dried blood for at least a week. A vaccine for hepatitis A and B is also available.

One of the liver's functions is to detoxify medications. When patients have hepatitis, any drug that is given may remain active within the body for longer than anticipated. As a consequence, when administering medications to patients with signs of liver failure, use the lower ends of the normal dose range. Give medications at longer intervals and watch for signs of cumulative effects.

In-hospital management of hepatitis aims to support liver function. Without a functioning liver, the patient will die within a few days. Antiviral medications may slow the effects of the virus. In extreme cases, a liver transplant is the only effective treatment.

Bowel Obstruction

Management of bowel obstruction follows the general management guidelines. This disease is rarely life-threatening in the prehospital setting. In-hospital management focuses on decompressing the intestines, determining the cause of the obstruction, and treating any side effects such as infection or intestinal perforation.

You are the Provider Part 4

Just as your partner pulls into traffic leaving the parking lot, your patient loses consciousness. A quick reassessment reveals shallow breathing at a rate of 10 breaths/min and an absent radial pulse. You are relieved to discover that a strong carotid pulse is present. Work of breathing is taken over using bag-mask ventilation with 100% supplemental oxygen. Both IV lines are patent. The emergency department is contacted and notified of your impending arrival in approximately 8 minutes.

The emergency room staff is awaiting your arrival in the resuscitation room. The patient is intubated, has a central line inserted for fluid resuscitation, receives 2 units of whole blood, and is taken to the endoscopy suite for diagnosis and treatment. He is diagnosed with bleeding esophageal varices, which were managed medically with vasopressin injected at the site of the bleed. He is admitted to the medical intensive care for 3 days and is discharged from the hospital after the 7th day on propranolol (Inderal).

Reassessment	Recording Time: 20 Minutes
Skin	Jaundiced, cool, and diaphoretic
Pulse	134 beats/min (carotid)
Blood pressure	76/50 mm Hg
Respirations	12 manual ventilations/min via bag-mask
Sao_2	99% on 100% supplemental oxygen
ECG	Sinus rhythm without ectopy

7. Why was the patient discharged on Inderal?

You are the Provider Summary

1. What is your first priority in this situation?

This is an easy one! Scene safety should always be your first priority. In this situation, you're entering a dimly lit bar late at night; many of the customers are more than likely happy to "assist" you in a variety of ways. You're also working in a confined space inside of this establishment, which increases the possibility of something going wrong. It wouldn't be a bad idea to have additional personnel or even law enforcement on scene with you.

2. What are some of the possible differential diagnoses?

The differential diagnoses for upper GI bleeding include peptic ulcer disease, esophageal varices, Mallory Weiss syndrome, and tumors.

3. What are the signs and symptoms of ruptured esophageal varices?

Patients with esophageal varices may present with bright red hematemesis, melena, and signs of shock.

4. What is the most common cause of esophageal varices?

In the adult patient, the most common cause of esophageal varices is cirrhosis of the liver, which is most often caused by alcohol abuse.

5. What does this patient need to be monitored for?

The patient is definitely exhibiting the classic signs and symptoms of decompensated shock: altered mental status, increased heart rate, and decreased blood pressure. We know that he no longer has a radial pulse. He does, however, have a strong carotid pulse. It is vital to frequently reassess the presence of the carotid pulse to ensure that the patient has not developed pulseless electrical activity. His airway is currently being managed by manual ventilations with bag-mask ventilation. Protection of the airway is paramount! Perhaps you thought of other ways that the airway should have been managed, but at the end of the day you need to make sure that the airway remains secure, no matter how it's done.

6. Is it possible that the patient has aspirated blood? Why or why not?

Absolutely! When you arrived on scene, the patient was already experiencing an altered mental status. There is no guarantee that he didn't aspirate blood prior to your arrival. Always assume the worst and be pleasantly surprised with the best!

7. Why was the patient discharged on Inderal?

You might still be scratching your head on this one! Inderal is a beta blocker, right? A review of the properties of beta blockers should have reminded you that they reduce blood pressure. Therefore, a lower pressure should help prevent a recurrence of bleeding by lowering the pressure within the esophageal veins.

Prep Kit

Ready for Review

- Gastrointestinal problems, in and of themselves, are rarely life-threatening. This fact does not minimize the systemic problems that can erupt from untreated or undertreated disease of the GI system.
- Three major pathologies are responsible for diseases of the GI tract:
  - Hypovolemia
  - Infection
  - Inflammation
- Bleeding within the GI tract is a symptom of another disease, not a disease itself.
- Presentation of GI bleeding is variable, as it can reflect the presence of a number of diseases. Each of these conditions has its own pattern of disease progression.
- Often there is little the paramedic can do about the GI disease itself, but you can care for the effects of the disease.
  - Patients may be in extreme amount of pain; they may be suffering from severe dehydration, hypotension, or extreme nausea.
  - Your main goals are to maintain BSI, manage the ABCs, and manage the patient's pain and nausea.

Vital Vocabulary

acholic stools Light, clay-colored stools caused by liver failure.

ascites Abdominal edema typically caused by liver failure.

borborygmi A bowel sound characterized by increased activity within the bowel.

chyme The partially digested food that exits the stomach, entering the duodenum.

diarrhea Liquid stool.

endoscopy The insertion of a flexible tube into the esophagus with the intent of visualizing and repairing damage or disease.

epigastric The right upper region of the abdomen directly inferior to the xyphoid process and superior to the umbilicus.

feculent Smelling of feces.

hematemesis Vomit with blood. Can either be like coffee grounds in appearance, indicating partially digested blood, or bright red blood indicating current active bleeding.

hematochezia Blood with the stool that is separate. Caused by lower GI bleeds.

hyperperistalsis Increased movement within the bowel.

hypoperistalsis Decreased bowel movement.

melena Dark, tarry, very odorous stools caused by upper GI bleeds.

Murphy's sign Pain when pressure is applied to the right upper quadrant of the abdomen in a specific manner; helps detect gallbladder problems.

orthostatic vital signs Assessing vital signs in two different patient positions to determine the degree of hypovolemia.

peptic ulcer disease (PUD) Abrasion of the stomach or small intestine.

peristalsis The rhythmic contractions of the intestines and esophagus that allow material to move.

periumbilical Located around the navel.

portal vein A large vessel created by the intersection of blood vessels from the GI system. The portal vein empties into the liver.

protuberant A convex or distended shape of the abdomen. This can be caused by edema.

pruritus A condition of itching.

scaphoid A concave shape of the abdomen. This can be caused by evisceration.

steatorrhea Foamy, fatty stools caused by liver failure or gallbladder problems.

striae Stretch marks on the abdomen caused by size changes.

suprapubic The region of the abdomen superior to the pubic bone and inferior to the umbilicus.

umbilical The region of the abdomen surrounding the umbilicus.

urticaria An itching rash.

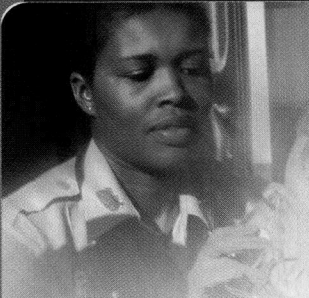

Assessment in Action

You are dispatched to the assisted-living facility for someone who is "bleeding." When you arrive on scene you find the patient supine on the floor. The smell to you indicates lower GI bleeding and you immediately walk into the bathroom to check out the toilet bowl, where you see approximately 200 mL of a substance that resembles coffee grounds. The patient's vital signs are as follows: pulse rate, 120 beats/min; sinus tachycardia on the cardiac monitor; blood pressure, 70 mm Hg by palpation; respiratory rate, 26 breaths/min; and pulse oximetry, 97% on room air.

1. **What are the three main conditions responsible for diseases of the GI tract?**
   A. Hypovolemia, infection, inflammation
   B. Hypertension, hypovolemia, tachycardia
   C. Hypovolemia, infection, hypertension
   D. Hypovolemia, inflammation, gallstones

2. **From what organs does an upper GI bleed originate?**
   A. Small intestine, large intestine, rectum, stomach
   B. Esophagus, stomach, rectum
   C. Rectum, stomach, large intestine
   D. Esophagus, stomach, small intestine

3. **An aspect of the general impression that is often different for the patient with GI bleeding is:**
   A. patient color.
   B. patient vital signs.
   C. odor.
   D. restlessness.

4. **_____ becomes more pertinent with the GI patient.**
   A. Airway patency
   B. Breathing
   C. Circulation
   D. Bleeding

5. **As blood volume begins to drop, the body begins to compensate by releasing:**
   A. antihistamines.
   B. ketoacidosis.
   C. catecholamines.
   D. insulin.

6. **What is the dark red or black granular material called?**
   A. Hematemesis, or coffee ground emesis
   B. Vomit
   C. Diarrhea
   D. Steatorrhea

7. **What is the most important component of the physical exam?**
   A. The length of time the patient has been having complaints
   B. How much bleeding has occurred
   C. Where the abdominal pain, if any, is located
   D. Noting when the last bowel movement occurred

8. **_____ are the key to gauging the degree of fluid loss in the prehospital setting.**
   A. Normal vital signs
   B. Orthostatic vital signs
   C. Abnormal vital signs
   D. No vital signs

Challenging Question

You are dispatched to a private residence for a person with abdominal pain. When you arrive on scene, the patient is doubled over in pain and complains of point tenderness to the upper right quadrant. The patient's vital signs are as follows: pulse rate, 108 beats/min with sinus tachycardia; blood pressure, 110/70 mm Hg; respiratory rate, 24 breaths/min; and pulse oximetry, 100% on room air.

9. **What management is required for this patient with an acute abdomen?**

■ Points to Ponder

You are dispatched to the home of a 37-year-old woman. When you arrive, you find her doubled over in pain, complaining of left upper quadrant pain that radiates to the right upper quadrant. You take the following set of vital signs: pulse rate, 118 beats/min; sinus tachycardia on the cardiac monitor; blood pressure, 140/82 mm Hg; respiratory rate, 24 breaths/min; and pulse oximetry, 99% on room air. Your patient tells you that her last menstrual cycle ended 4 days ago. She also tells you that the pain has been intermittent for approximately 2 weeks. The pain is sharp, like a knife cutting away her abdomen. You initiate IV therapy and administer 15 L of oxygen by nonrebreathing mask. You transport her to the hospital in a position of comfort and give your patient care report to the emergency department staff. Towards the end of your shift, you call the hospital and find out she was admitted with acute pancreatitis.

What are some common causes of abdominal pain? How can pancreatitis affect other body systems?

Issues: Understanding the Importance of a Complete Abdominal Assessment, Appropriate Medical Response to Gastrointestinal Emergencies.

www.Paramedic.EMSzone.com

32 Renal and Urologic Emergencies

Objectives

Cognitive

5-7.1   Describe the incidence, morbidity, mortality, and risk factors predisposing to urological emergencies. (p 32.3)

5-7.2   Discuss the anatomy and physiology of the organs and structures related to urogenital diseases. (p 32.3)

5-7.3   Define referred pain and visceral pain as it relates to urology. (p 32.7)

5-7.4   Describe the questioning technique and specific questions the paramedic should utilize when gathering a focused history in a patient with abdominal pain. (p 32.15)

5-7.5   Describe the technique for performing a comprehensive physical examination of a patient complaining of abdominal pain. (p 32.15)

5-7.6   Define acute renal failure. (p 32.8)

5-7.7   Discuss the pathophysiology of acute renal failure. (p 32.8)

5-7.8   Recognize the signs and symptoms related to acute renal failure. (p 32.8)

5-7.9   Describe the management for acute renal failure. (p 32.18)

5-7.10   Integrate pathophysiological principles and assessment findings to formulate a field impression and implement a treatment plan for the patient with acute renal failure. (p 32.18)

5-7.11   Define chronic renal failure. (p 32.18)

5-7.12   Discuss the pathophysiology of chronic renal failure. (p 32.8)

5-7.13   Recognize the signs and symptoms related to chronic renal failure. (p 32.8)

5-7.14   Describe the management for chronic renal failure. (p 32.18)

5-7.15   Integrate pathophysiological principles and assessment findings to formulate a field impression and implement a treatment plan for the patient with chronic renal failure. (p 32.18)

5-7.16   Define renal dialysis. (p 32.9)

5-7.17   Discuss the common complications of renal dialysis. (p 32.10)

5-7.18   Define renal calculi. (p 32.7)

5-7.19   Discuss the pathophysiology of renal calculi. (p 32.7)

5-7.20   Recognize the signs and symptoms related to renal calculi. (p 32.7)

5-7.21   Describe the management for renal calculi. (p 32.17)

5-7.22   Integrate pathophysiological principles and assessment findings to formulate a field impression and implement a treatment plan for the patient with renal calculi. (p 32.17)

5-7.23   Define urinary tract infection. (p 32.7)

5-7.24   Discuss the pathophysiology of urinary tract infection. (p 32.7)

5-7.25   Recognize the signs and symptoms related to urinary tract infection. (p 32.7)

5-7.26   Describe the management for a urinary tract infection. (p 32.17)

5-7.27   Integrate pathophysiological principles and assessment findings to formulate a field impression and implement a treatment plan for the patient with a urinary tract infection. (p 32.17)

5-7.28   Apply the epidemiology to develop prevention strategies for urological emergencies. (p 32.3)

5-7.29   Integrate pathophysiological principles to the assessment of a patient with abdominal pain. (p 32.15)

5-7.30   Synthesize assessment findings and patient history information to accurately differentiate between pain of a urogenital emergency and that of other origins. (p 32.15)

5-7.31   Develop, execute, and evaluate a treatment plan based on the field impression made in the assessment. (p 32.16)

Affective

None

Psychomotor

None

Introduction

The urinary system performs two main functions for the body. It acts as the body's accounting firm, keeping track of the electrolytes, water content, and acids of the blood; and it acts as the blood's sewage treatment plant, removing metabolic wastes, drug metabolites, and excess fluids. The kidneys perform these functions continuously, filtering 200 L of blood each day.

The most common renal disorder is kidney disease, which affects more than 20 million Americans. Approximately 50,000 Americans die of kidney disease each year, and more than 30,000 require dialysis. The most common acute renal disease is renal calculi (kidney stones), with 2 million cases diagnosed each year. Other common types of renal disease include urinary tract infections, which occur in more than 50% of all women, and noncancerous enlargement of the prostate, which 60% of men will develop by age 50. Many of these conditions can be prevented by diet and hygiene, including proper hydration.

Anatomy and Physiology

The urinary system consists of the kidneys, which filter the blood and produce urine; the urinary bladder, which stores the urine until it is released from the body; the ureters, which transport

the urine from the kidneys to the bladder; and the urethra, which transports the urine from the bladder out of the body. The bean-shaped kidneys are found in the retroperitoneal space (behind the peritoneum), which extends from the twelfth thoracic vertebra to the third lumbar vertebra. The right kidney is slightly lower than the left due to the position of the liver. The medial side of the kidney is concave, forming a cleft called the hilus, where the ureters, renal blood vessels, lymphatic vessels, and nerves enter and leave the kidney   Figure 32-1 ▾ .

A fibrous capsule covers the kidney and protects it against infection. Surrounding this capsule is a fatty mass of adipose tissue, which cushions the kidney and holds it in place in the abdomen. A layer of dense fibrous connective tissue called the renal fascia anchors the kidney to the abdominal wall.

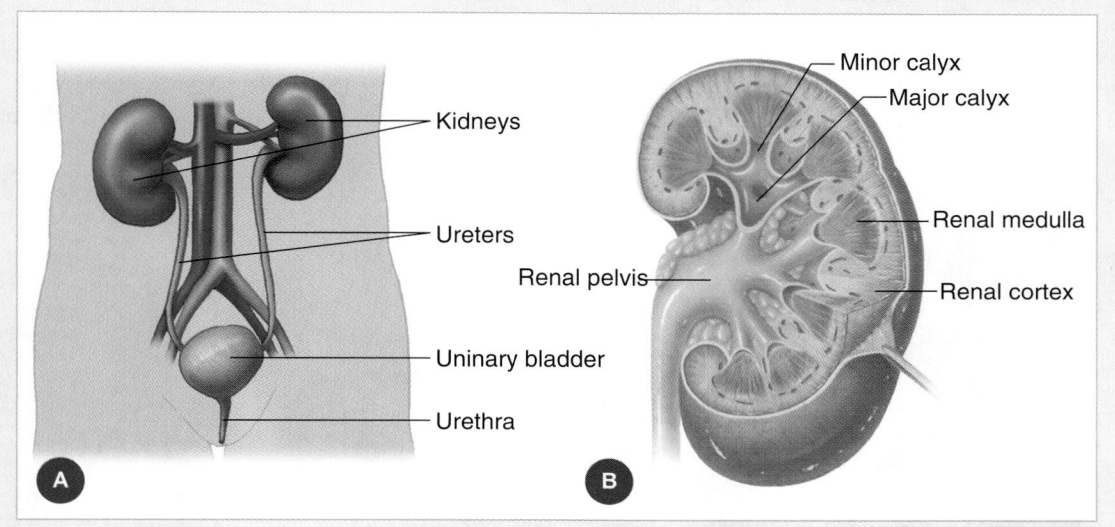

Figure 32-1 The urinary system. **A.** Anterior view showing the relationship of the kidneys, ureters, urinary bladder, and urethra. **B.** Cross-section of the human kidney showing the renal cortex, renal medulla, and renal pelvis.

You are the Provider Part 1

You arrive at a residence of a 71-year-old woman with severe weakness. As you enter the residence, you find the patient seated in a chair in her living room. She is conscious, but somewhat confused, and she clearly appears ill. She tells you that she has missed her last few dialysis treatments because her friend—who usually takes her to and from her treatments—is out of town. Your initial assessment findings are as follows:

Initial Assessment	Recording Time: 0 Minutes
Appearance	Looks ill; skin is slightly jaundiced; hands and feet are edematous
Level of consciousness	V (Responsive to verbal stimuli), somewhat confused
Airway	Patent
Breathing	Tachypneic; adequate tidal volume
Circulation	Radial pulses are rapid and irregular

1. What is the purpose of dialysis?
2. What are the two types of dialysis?

The internal anatomy of the kidney can be divided into three distinct regions: the cortex, the medulla, and the pelvis. The cortex is the lighter-colored outer region closest to the capsule. The medulla (middle layer) includes the cone-shaped renal pyramids (parallel bundles of urine-collecting tubules), and inward extensions of cortical tissue that surround the pyramids, called the renal columns. The renal pelvis is a flat, funnel-shaped tube that fills the sinus at the level of the hilus. The major and minor calyces branch off the pelvis and connect with the renal pyramids to receive the urine draining from the collecting tubules. This arrangement has been described as several strands of uncooked spaghetti (the collecting tubules) sitting in a thimble (the papilla, or tip, of the pelvis). The collected urine flows through the pelvis and into the ureter on its way to the bladder.

Approximately one fourth of the body's systemic cardiac output of blood flows through the kidney each minute. The blood flows from the abdominal aorta into the kidney by way of the renal artery. Once it enters the kidney at the hilus, the artery branches several times to become the afferent arteriole.

The afferent arteriole quickly branches into a tuft of capillaries called a glomerulus, which is the main filter for the blood in the kidney. From the glomerulus, the blood enters the efferent arteriole, which branches into the peritubular capillaries, where tubular resorption occurs. This secondary set of capillaries is unique to the kidney; no other organ in the body has two distinct capillary beds. The capillaries then merge, forming venules and veins, until the renal vein leaves the hilus, carrying the cleansed blood to the inferior vena cava.

Nephrons, found in the cortex, are the structural and functional units of the kidney that form urine. Each nephron is composed of the glomerulus; the glomerular (Bowman's) capsule, which surrounds the glomerulus; the proximal convoluted tubule (PCT); the loop of Henle; and the distal convoluted tubule (DCT), which connects with the kidney's collecting tubules). Each kidney contains approximately 1.25 million nephrons **Figure 32-2**.

The glomerular capsule is a double-layered cup in which the inner layer infiltrates and surrounds the capillaries of the glomerulus. Special cells in the inner membrane called

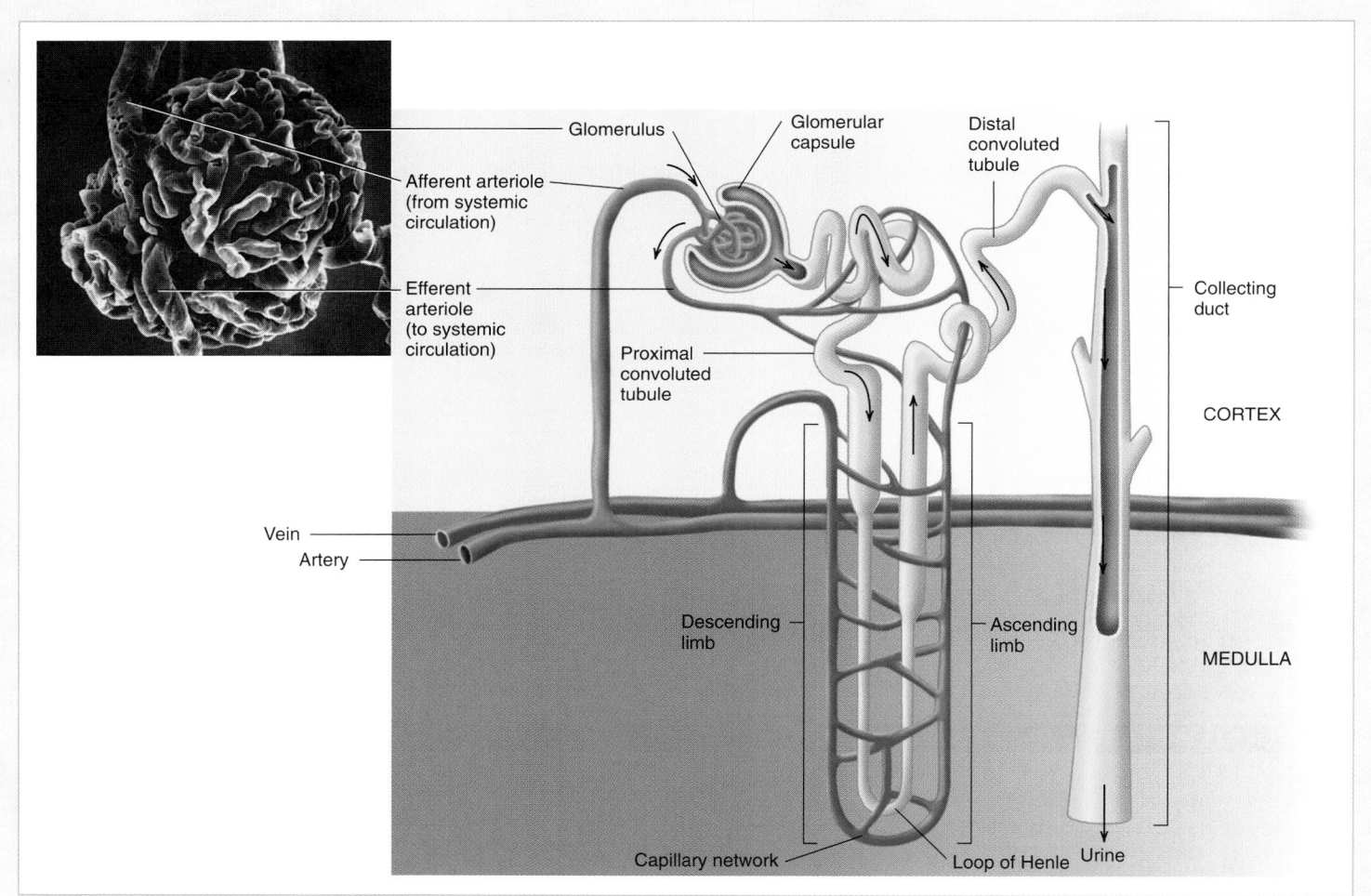

Figure 32-2 The nephrons of the kidney. Part of the nephron is located in the cortex, and part is located in the medulla. Inset at left, Electron micrograph of a glomerulus from a human nephron.

podocytes wrap around the capillaries in the glomerulus, forming filtration slits. The filtrate passes through these slits, across the filtration membrane, and into the capsule. In this manner, the filtration membrane prevents large molecules, such as proteins, from entering the capsule.

Imagine watering your garden with an open-ended hose. If you place your finger over half of the hose's opening, the same amount of water must now pass through half the space. As a consequence, the pressure increases and you can spray the water farther. The same thing happens at the glomerulus. As the blood moves from the relatively large afferent arteriole into the smaller capillaries of the glomerulus, the pressure increases. This effect, along with the smaller diameter of the efferent arteriole, causes the pressure in the glomerulus to become high enough to force the filtrate from the blood into the glomerular capsule **Figure 32-3 ▾** .

The amount of filtrate produced, called the glomerular filtration rate (GFR), is maintained at a relatively constant rate of 125 mL/min in healthy adults. Changes in the GFR cause many of the renal emergencies encountered in the prehospital setting.

Initially, the filtrate contains everything that can pass through the filtration membrane: salts, minerals, glucose, water, and metabolic wastes. As the filtrate passes through the rest of the nephron, tubular resorption and tubular secretion convert the filtrate into urine. As the fluid passes through the PCT, the cells lining the PCT remove all organic nutrients and plasma proteins, as well as some ions from the filtrate. These compounds are deposited in the interstitial fluid surrounding the PCT. As these solutes accumulate, the concentration of the surrounding fluid becomes higher than that of the filtrate. Water will then move from the filtrate by osmosis. The fluid and nutrients in the interstitial fluid, in turn, move into the peritubular capillaries around the PCT. This process re-establishes the homeostatic balance in the blood and reduces the volume of the tubular filtrate.

Additional resorption of water and electrolytes occurs in the loop of Henle. The loop of Henle has two sections—the descending limb, extending toward the medulla, and the ascending limb, moving toward the cortex. The cells in the descending limb are permeable to water, but impermeable to sodium and chloride ions; the cells in the ascending limb are permeable to sodium and chloride ions, but impermeable to water. As a consequence, when the sodium and chloride ions move out of the ascending limb, they increase the solute concentration of the fluid surrounding the descending limb. Water moves by osmosis from the descending limb into the surrounding tissue and eventually into the vasa recta, a series of peritubular capillaries that surround the loop of Henle. This countercurrent multiplier process allows the body to produce either concentrated or diluted urine, depending on the body's needs.

After leaving the loop of Henle, the fluid enters the DCT. At this point, approximately 80% of the water and 85% of the solutes originally forced out of the glomerulus have been reabsorbed. As the urine passes through the DCT and the collecting ducts to which it is attached (both of which are impermeable to solutes), its composition undergoes its final adjustments. Ions are actively secreted or reabsorbed, and the body alters the permeability of the DCT and collecting ducts to water as necessary, depending on the body's homeostatic needs. These adjustments to the final composition of the urine facilitate the removal of metabolic wastes while maintaining the body's fluid-electrolyte balance.

At the site where the efferent arteriole comes in contact with the DCT, a structure called the juxtaglomerular apparatus is formed. The cells in the efferent arteriole (called juxtaglomerular cells) are pressure-sensitive, and monitor the blood pressure. The cells in the DCT (called macula densa cells) are sensitive to chemical changes and monitor the concentration of the filtrate in the DCT. When triggered by changes in the blood pressure of filtrate content, the juxtaglomerular cells release renin. This enzyme initiates a cascade of reactions in the body by converting the plasma protein angiotensinogen into angiotensin I. Other enzymes present in the blood then convert angiotensin I into angiotensin II. A potent vasoconstrictor, angiotensin II promotes smooth muscle contraction in the arterioles throughout the body. This constriction raises the blood pressure by increasing peripheral resistance. Angiotensin II also increases the resorption of sodium from the PCT. Given that water tends to follow sodium, by increasing sodium resorption, the kidney increases water resorption and, in turn, blood pressure.

The final adjustments to the composition of the urine at the DCT and collecting duct are controlled primarily by two

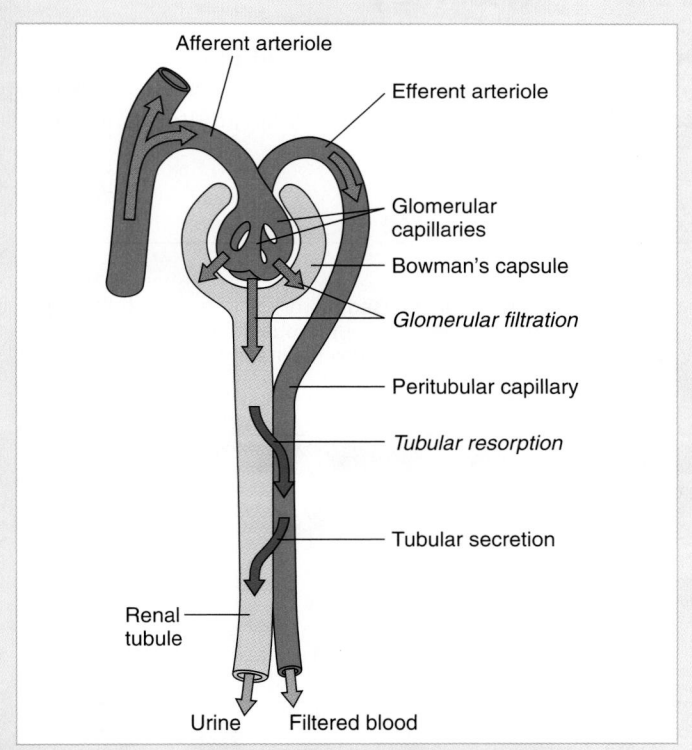

Figure 32-3 The glomerulus of the kidneys. The nephron carries out three blood-filtering processes: glomerular filtration, tubular resorption, and tubular secretion.

hormones: antidiuretic hormone (ADH) and aldosterone. ADH is produced by the hypothalamus and stored in the posterior lobe of the pituitary; aldosterone is produced in the adrenal glands.

Neurons in the hypothalamus monitor the solute concentration of the blood. When the solute concentration of the blood increases (eg, due to sweating or decreased fluid intake), ADH is released into the bloodstream. This hormone travels to the DCT and collecting ducts, increasing these structures' permeability to water. Water therefore leaves the DCT and collecting ducts, and reenters the bloodstream. As the solute concentration returns to normal, secretion of ADH will stop.

Aldosterone increases the rate of active resorption of sodium and chloride ions into the blood; a corresponding increase occurs in water resorption. This hormone also decreases the resorption of potassium ion, resulting in excess potassium being secreted in the urine.

Diuretics, chemicals that increase urinary output, work in a variety of ways. A substance that is not reabsorbed from the filtrate, for example, will increase the amount of water retained in the urine. An example of such an osmotic diuretic is glucose in a patient with diabetes mellitus. Alcohol encourages diuresis by inhibiting the production of ADH. Other diuretics, including caffeine and the diuretics commonly prescribed for hypertension and congestive heart failure (Lasix, Diuril), inhibit the sodium importers in the DCT and collecting ducts.

Once the urine enters the collecting ducts (the renal pyramids of the medulla), it passes through the minor calyx, into the major calyx, and then into the renal pelvis. From there, the urine moves through the ureter (one ureter from each kidney) and is stored in the urinary bladder. Most of the bladder sits in the anterior abdominal cavity, but the dome of the bladder sits in the posterior abdominal cavity, or retroperitoneum, where the ureters and kidneys reside. When empty, the bladder collapses, and the muscular walls fold over onto themselves. In contrast, as urine accumulates, the bladder expands and becomes pear-shaped. The stretching of the bladder walls ultimately stimulates nerve impulses to produce the micturition reflex. This spinal reflex causes contraction of the bladder's smooth muscles, which in turn produces the urge to void as pressure is exerted on the internal urinary sphincter. Normally, the brain exerts control over this urge, keeping the external urinary sphincter contracted until conditions are favorable for urination. At this point, the inhibition of the external urinary sphincter is reduced and the urine passes from the urinary bladder into the urethra.

The beginning of the urethra, through which urine is expelled, sits at the inferior aspect of the bladder. In females, the urethra exits at the site of the external genitalia. The female urethra is shorter than the male urethra (4 cm versus 20 cm) **Figure 32-4 ▶** . The male urethra can be divided into three regions:

- The *prostatic urethra* begins at the bladder and extends through the prostate gland.
- The *membranous urethra* extends from the prostate gland through the abdominal wall and into the penis.
- The *spongy, or penile, urethra* passes through the penis to the external urethral opening.

▌Pathophysiology

Diseases and problems of the renal and urologic system range from mild (urinary tract infections) to true emergencies (acute renal failure). Although the prehospital care for many urologic

You are the Provider Part 2

You have placed the patient on oxygen via a nonrebreathing mask set at 12 L/min. During your focused history, the patient tells you that she has been taking dialysis treatments for over a year for "kidney failure." Additionally, she takes numerous medications and has a history of high blood pressure. Your physical exam reveals scattered crackles in her lungs and edema to her hands and feet. As you apply a cardiac monitor, your partner obtains baseline vital signs.

Vital Signs	Recording Time: 5 Minutes
Level of consciousness	V (Responsive to verbal stimuli), somewhat confused
Skin	Slight jaundice; cool and dry
Pulse	110 beats/min and irregular
Blood pressure	104/58 mm Hg
Respirations	24 breaths/min; adequate tidal volume
Sao_2	97% (on supplemental oxygen)
Blood glucose	104 mg/dL

The 3-lead ECG reveals sinus tachycardia at 110 beats/min with premature ventricular complexes (PVCs) and tall peaked T-waves. The patient denies having any heart problems or diabetes.

3. What condition do you suspect this patient is experiencing?
4. What special concerns should you have regarding the patient's condition?

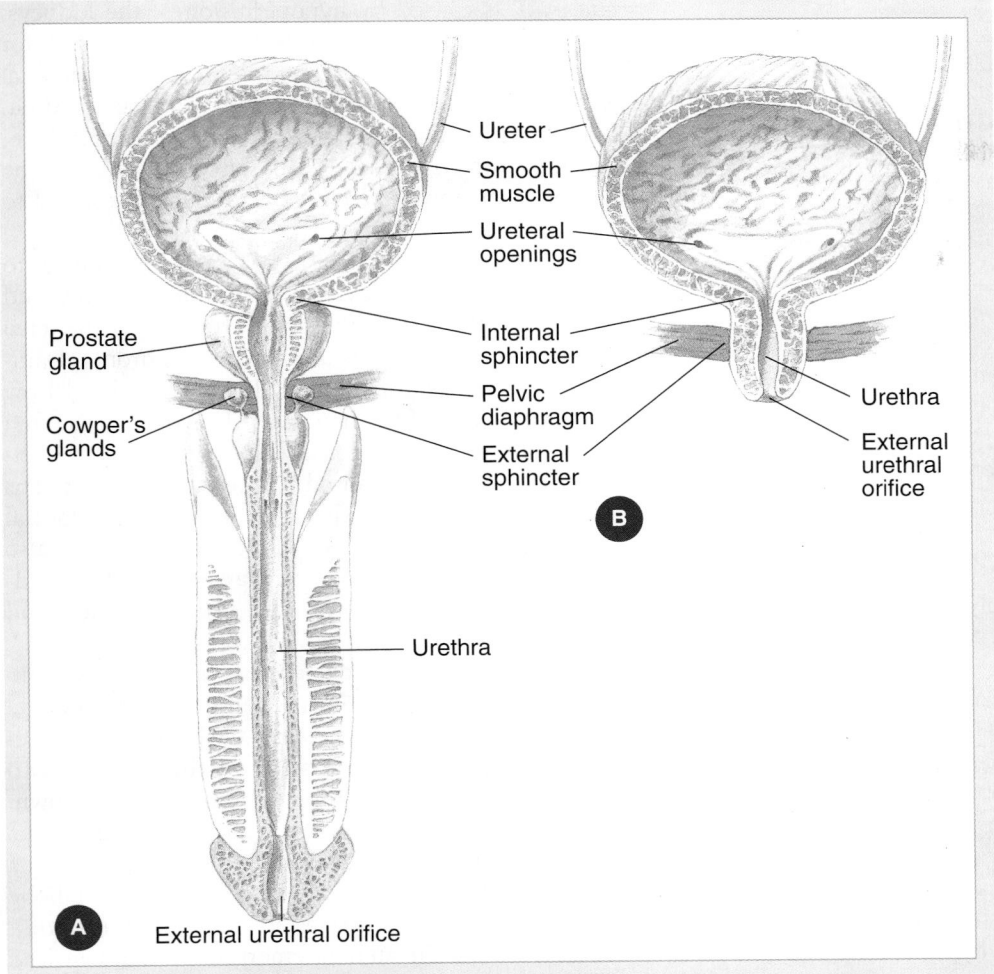

Figure 32-4 The differences in the urethras of (**A**) men and (**B**) women.

Labels in figure:
- Ureter
- Smooth muscle
- Ureteral openings
- Internal sphincter
- Pelvic diaphragm
- External sphincter
- Prostate gland
- Cowper's glands
- Urethra
- External urethral orifice
- Urethra
- External urethral orifice
- B
- A

often perceived as bladder pain in women and as prostate pain in men. Sometimes the pain may be referred to the shoulder or neck. In addition, the urine will have a foul odor and may appear cloudy.

Renal Calculi (Kidney Stones)

Kidney stones originate in the renal pelvis and result when an excess of insoluble salts or uric acid crystallizes in the urine Figure 32-5 ▾ . This excess of salts is typically due to water intake that is insufficient to dissolve the salts. The stones consist of different types of chemicals, depending on the precise imbalance in the urine.

The most common stones—calcium stones—occur more frequently in men than in women and may have a hereditary component. These stones also occur in patients with metabolic disorders such as gout or with hormonal disorders. Struvite stones are more common in women, and may be associated with chronic UTI or frequent catheterization. Uric acid and cystine stones are the least common. Uric acid stones tend to run in families, especially those with a history of gout. Cystine stones are associated with a condition that causes large amounts of amino acids and proteins to accumulate in the urine.

Patients who have kidney stones will almost always be in pain (many rate kidney stone pain as 11 on a scale of 1 to 10). The pain usually starts as a vague discomfort in the flank, but becomes very intense within 30 to 60 minutes. It may migrate forward and toward the groin as the stone passes through the system.

Some patients will be agitated and restless as they walk and move in an attempt to relieve the pain. Others will attempt to remain motionless and

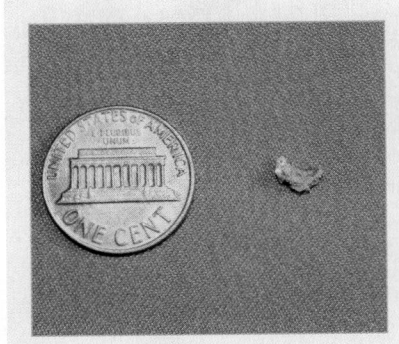

Figure 32-5 A kidney stone.

guard the abdomen. Either behavior makes palpation of the abdomen difficult. Vital signs will vary, depending on the severity of pain. The greater the pain, the higher will be the blood pressure and pulse.

diseases is supportive, your ability to recognize the signs and symptoms of the true emergencies is critical to provide your patients with the best chance of a positive outcome.

Urinary Tract Infections

Urinary tract infections (UTIs) usually develop in the lower urinary tract (urethra and bladder) when normal flora bacteria, which exist naturally on the skin, enter the urethra and grow. These infections are more common in women due to the relatively short urethra and the close proximity of the urethra to the vagina and rectum. UTIs in the upper urinary tract (ureters and kidneys) occur most often when lower UTIs go untreated. Upper UTIs can lead to pyelonephritis (inflammation of the kidney linings) and abscesses, which eventually reduce kidney function. In severe cases, untreated UTIs can lead to sepsis.

Common symptoms in patients with a lower UTI include painful urination, frequent urges to urinate, and difficulty in urination. The pain usually begins as a visceral discomfort, but then converts to an extreme burning pain, especially during urination. The pain, which remains localized in the pelvis, is

If a stone has become lodged in the lower ureter, signs and symptoms of a UTI (frequency and urgency of urination, painful urination, and/or hematuria) may be present, but the patient will not have a fever. If a kidney stone is suspected, be sure to obtain both a patient history and a family history; both can supply important information.

Acute Renal Failure

Acute renal failure (ARF) is a sudden (possibly over a period of days) decrease in filtration through the glomeruli. It is accompanied by an increase of toxins in the blood. ARF accounts for 30% of all ICU patients in the United States, and 5% of all hospitalizations. Patients with ARF have an overall mortality rate of 50%, but the disease is reversible if diagnosed and treated early.

If the urine output drops to less than 500 mL/day, the condition is called oliguria. If urine production stops completely, the condition is called anuria. Whenever ARF occurs, the patient may experience generalized edema, acid buildup, and high levels of nitrogenous and metabolic wastes in the blood. If left untreated, ARF can lead to heart failure, hypertension, and metabolic acidosis.

ARF is classified into three types, based on the area where the failure occurs: prerenal, intrarenal, and postrenal. The signs and symptoms of each type are summarized in   Table 32-1 ▼ .

Table 32-1	Signs and Symptoms of Acute Renal Failure
Prerenal acute renal failure	Hypotension Tachycardia Dizziness Thirst
Intrarenal acute renal failure	Flank pain Joint pain Oliguria Hypertension Headache Confusion Seizure
Postrenal acute renal failure	Pain in lower flank, abdomen, groin, and genitalia Oliguria Distended bladder Hematuria Peripheral edema

Prerenal ARF is caused by hypoperfusion of the kidneys. In other words, not enough blood passes into the glomeruli for them to produce filtrate. The most common causes of prerenal ARF are hypovolemia (hemorrhage, dehydration), trauma, shock, sepsis, and heart failure (congestive heart failure, myocardial infarction). Prerenal ARF is often reversible if the underlying condition can be treated and perfusion restored to the kidney.

Intrarenal acute renal failure (IARF) involves damage to one of three areas in the kidney: the glomeruli capillaries and small blood vessels, the cells of the kidney tubules, or the renal parenchyma (the interstitial cells around the nephrons). Damage to the small vessels and glomeruli hinders blood flow through these vital parts of the nephrons. This damage is often caused by immune-mediated diseases (eg, type 1 diabetes mellitus). Tubule damage can be caused by prerenal ARF or toxins (eg, heavy metals). Chronic inflammation of the interstitial cells surrounding the nephrons (interstitial nephritis) can also produce IARF. This type of renal failure may be caused by medications such as antibiotics, anticancer drugs, alcohol, and drugs of abuse (eg, cocaine).

Postrenal ARF is caused by obstruction of urine flow from the kidneys. The source of this obstruction is often a blockage of the urethra by prostate enlargement, renal calculi, or strictures. This blockage causes pressure on the nephrons to increase, which eventually causes the nephrons to shut down. At this point, the kidneys can no longer carry out their cleansing functions, resulting in the development of hyperkalemia (an increase in the blood potassium levels) and/or metabolic acidosis (an increase in the hydrogen ion content of the blood). Both conditions are life-threatening emergencies that can lead to fatal dysrhythmias of the heart.

Chronic Renal Failure

Chronic renal failure (CRF) is progressive and irreversible inadequate kidney function due to permanent loss of nephrons. This disease develops over months or years. More than half of all cases are caused by systemic diseases, such as diabetes or hypertension. CRF can also be caused by congenital disorders or prolonged pyelonephritis.

As the nephrons become damaged and cease to function, scarring occurs in the kidneys. The tissue begins to shrink and waste away as the scarring progresses, leading to a loss of nephrons and renal mass. As kidney function diminishes, waste products and fluid build up in the blood. Uremia (increased urea and other waste products in the blood) and azotemia (increased nitrogenous wastes in the blood) develop, leading to systemic complications such as hypertension, congestive heart failure, anemia, and electrolyte imbalances.

Patients with CRF exhibit several signs and symptoms, beginning with an altered level of consciousness due to the electrolyte imbalance and the resulting effects on nerve transmission in the brain. In the late stages, seizures and coma are possible. The patients may also present with lethargy, nausea, headaches, cramps, and signs of anemia.

In a case of CRF, the patient's skin will be pale, cool, and moist, and the individual may appear jaundiced due to the buildup of nitrogenous wastes. A powdery accumulation of uric acid called <u>uremic frost</u> may also be present, especially around the face. The skin may appear bruised, and muscle twitching may be present.

Patients with CRF exhibit edema in the extremities and face due to fluid imbalances; they will also be hypotensive and have tachycardia. As hyperkalemia develops, the heart's electrical conduction will decrease. The ECG monitor will show increasing PR and QT intervals. As the hyperkalemia progresses, these dysrhythmias may evolve into an idioventricular rhythm. Pericarditis and pulmonary edema are also common and should be evaluated during auscultation of the chest.

Notes from Nancy

Don't give medications to patients with chronic renal failure unless specifically instructed to do so by medical command.

Renal Dialysis

Although not truly a urologic disorder, <u>renal dialysis</u> and problems associated with it may require prehospital interventions. Renal dialysis is a technique for "filtering" toxic wastes from the blood, removing excess fluid, and restoring the normal balance of electrolytes **Figure 32-6**.

There are two types of dialysis—peritoneal dialysis and hemodialysis. In peritoneal dialysis, large amounts of specially formulated dialysis fluid are infused into (and back out of) the abdominal cavity. This fluid stays in the cavity for 1 to 2 h, allowing equilibrium to occur. Peritoneal dialysis is very effective but carries a high risk of peritonitis; consequently, aseptic technique is essential. With proper training, however, peritoneal dialysis can be performed in the home.

In hemodialysis, the patient's blood circulates through a dialysis machine that functions in much the same way (albeit not as elegantly) as the normal kidneys. Most patients undergoing chronic hemodialysis have some sort of shunt, ie, a surgically created connection between a vein and an artery. The patient is connected to the dialysis machine through this shunt, which allows blood to flow from the body into the dialysis machine and back to the body. A Scribner shunt, for example, consists of two plastic tubes: one fastened in the radial artery, the other in the cephalic vein. These two tubes are joined together near the wrist with a Teflon connector. A Thomas shunt is similar, but this device is usually placed in the groin. Other patients will have a small, button-shaped device, a Hemasite, with a rubber septum that can be punctured with dialysis needles during treatment. Hemasites are usually placed in the upper arm or proximal anterior thigh. Finally, some patients have an <u>internal shunt</u> (an arteriovenous [AV] fistula), which is an artificial connection between a vein and an artery that is usually located in the forearm or upper arm **Figure 32-7**.

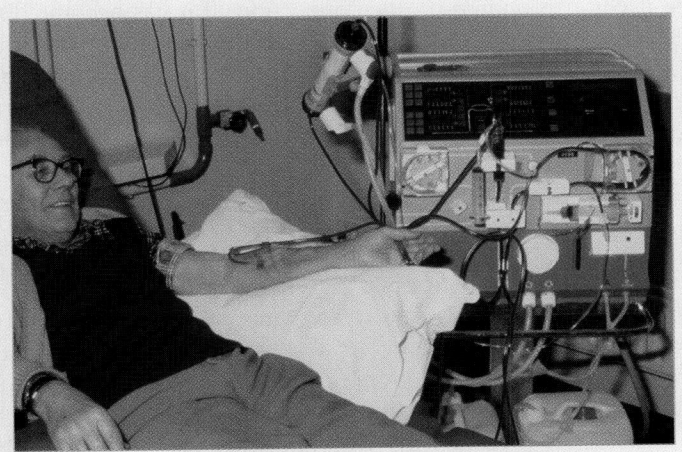

Figure 32-6 A patient undergoing dialysis.

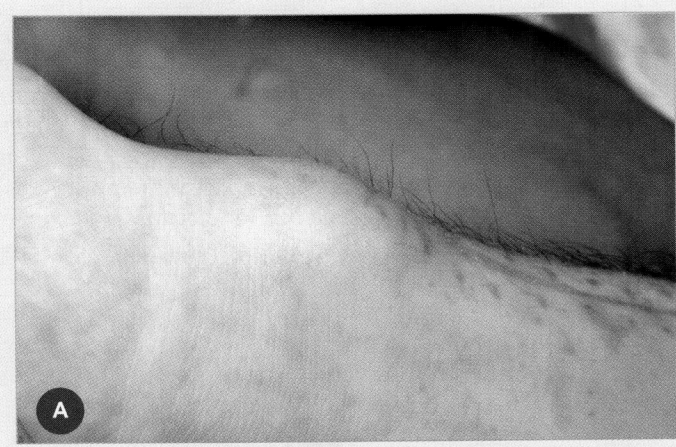

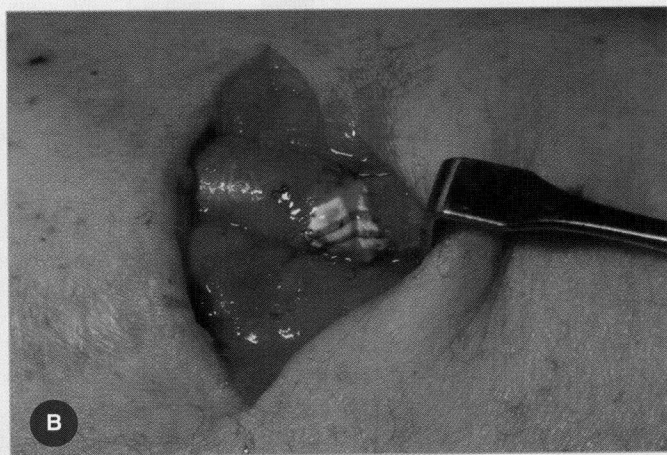

Figure 32-7 **A.** With an AV fistula, a bulge is created by arterial pressure. **B.** An AV graft creates a raised area that looks like a large vessel.

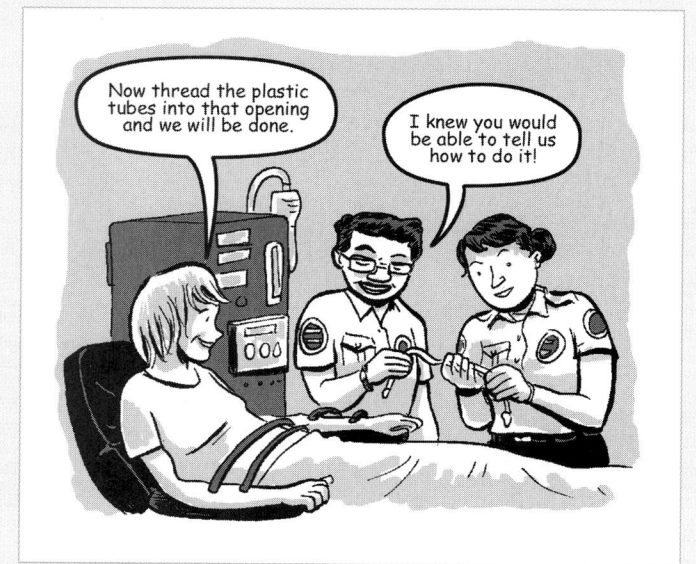

Figure 32-8

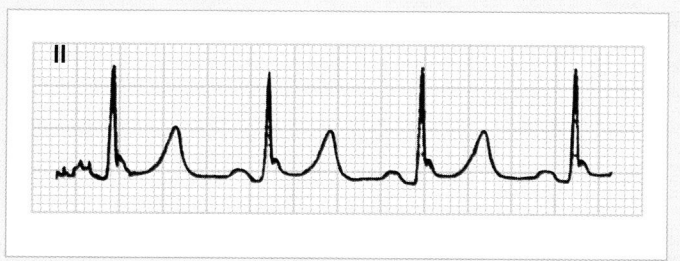

Figure 32-9 Peaked T waves, as shown in this rhythm strip, are a classic sign of hyperkalemia.

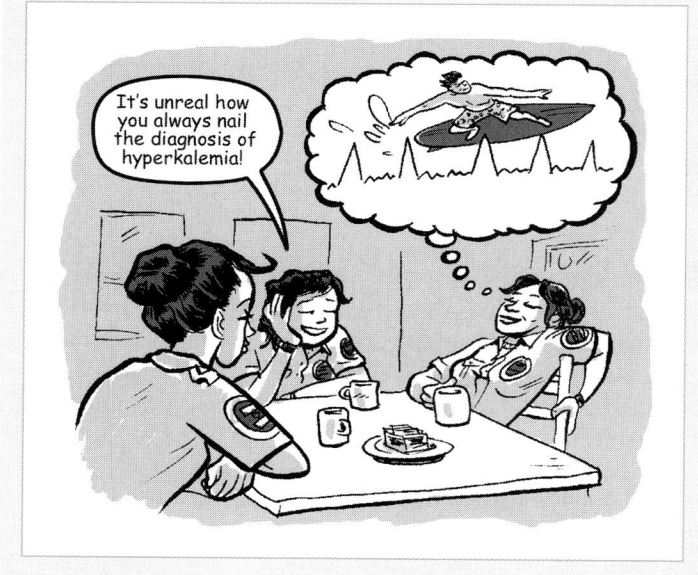

Figure 32-10

Patients requiring chronic dialysis usually go "on the machine" every 2 or 3 days for a period of 3 to 5 hours. Many receive dialysis in the hospital or in community dialysis facilities, but a significant number have home dialysis units. Patients undergoing dialysis at home usually have extensive training in the procedures, and often someone else in the home has also been trained. If a problem with the machine occurs, the patient may know a lot more about it than you do, so always ask what the patient has done prior to your arrival **Figure 32-8 ▲** !

Patients undergoing chronic dialysis can suffer the same spectrum of illnesses and injuries as any other patients. Dialysis patients, however, are particularly vulnerable to certain problems, either because of the dialysis itself or because of the underlying renal failure. Problems associated with dialysis may result from accidental disconnection from the machine, malfunction of the machine, or rapid shifts in fluids and electrolytes that produce hypotension, potassium imbalances, and disequilibrium syndrome.

Notes from Nancy

When you measure the blood pressure in a dialysis patient, use the arm that doesn't have the shunt!

Hypotension and Shock

A sudden drop in blood pressure is not uncommon during or immediately after dialysis, but it can lead to cardiac arrest if not promptly detected and treated. The patient may feel light-headed or become confused, and often he or she yawns more than usual. Because dialysis alters the blood's chemistry, the patient may develop an electrolyte imbalance. For this reason, you should always monitor dialysis patients for cardiac dys-

rhythmias. Shock secondary to bleeding is also possible from any number of causes. Patients with CRF, for example, are very prone to duodenal ulcers; bleeding from those ulcers is not unusual. Bleeding may also occur from the dialysis cannula.

When you find a shunt leaking during the dialysis cycle, see if you can tighten up the connection. If it has become disconnected at the vein, clamp the cannula and disconnect the patient from the machine. In a suicide attempt, the patient may open up the cannula and allow himself or herself to exsanguinate. Keep in mind that these patients have often endured numerous medical interventions to simply survive. If you encounter this situation, immediately *clamp off the cannula* and apply direct pressure.

Potassium Imbalance

One consequence of renal impairment is the inability to excrete ingested potassium. As a consequence, CRF patients are prone to developing hyperkalemia, especially in circumstances of increased potassium intake or catabolic stress. Such a patient may present with profound muscular weakness. On the ECG, the classic signs of hyperkalemia are peaked T waves (**Figure 32-9 ▲** and **Figure 32-10 ▲**), a prolonged QRS

calyces (singular: calyx) Large urinary tubes that branch off the renal pelvis and connect with the renal pyramids to collect the urine draining from the collecting tubules.

chronic renal failure (CRF) Progressive and irreversible inadequate kidney function due to permanent loss of nephrons.

cortex Part of the internal anatomy of the kidney; the lighter-colored outer region closest to the capsule.

countercurrent multiplier The process in which the body produces either concentrated or diluted urine, depending on the body's needs.

distal convoluted tubule (DCT) Connects with the kidney's collecting tubules.

diuretics Chemicals that increase urinary output.

efferent arteriole The structure in the kidney where blood drains from the glomerulus.

glomerular (Bowman's) capsule A double-layered cup with the inner layer infiltrating and surrounding the capillaries of the glomerulus.

glomerular filtration rate (GFR) The rate at which blood is filtered through the glomerula.

glomerulus A tuft of capillaries located in the kidney that serve as the main filter for the blood in the kidney.

hematuria The presence of blood in the urine.

hilus A cleft where the ureters, renal blood vessels, lymphatic vessels, and nerves enter and leave the kidney.

internal shunt Also called an arteriovenous (AV) fistula, this device is an artificial connection between a vein and an artery, usually in the forearm or upper arm.

interstitial nephritis A chronic inflammation of the interstitial cells surrounding the nephrons.

intrarenal acute renal failure (IARF) A type of acute renal failure due to damage in the kidney itself, often caused by immune-mediated diseases, prerenal ARF, toxins, heavy metals, some medications, or some organic compounds.

juxtaglomerular apparatus A structure formed at the site where the efferent arteriole and distal convoluted tubule meet.

kidneys Solid, bean-shaped organs located in the retroperitoneal space that filter blood and excrete body wastes in the form of urine.

kidney stones Solid crystalline masses formed in the kidney, resulting from an excess of insoluble salts or uric acid crystallizing in the urine; may become trapped anywhere along the urinary tract.

loop of Henle The U-shaped portion of the renal tubule that extends from the proximal to the distal convoluted tubule; concentrates the filtrate and converts it to urine.

medulla Part of the internal anatomy of the kidney; the middle layer.

micturition reflex A spinal reflex that causes contraction of the bladder's smooth muscles, producing the urge to void as pressure is exerted on the internal urinary sphincter.

nephrons The structural and functional units of the kidney that form urine; composed of the glomerulus, the glomerular (Bowman's) capsule, the proximal convoluted tubule (PCT), loop of Henle, and the distal convoluted tubule (DCT).

oliguria A decrease in urine output to the extent that total urine output drops below 500 mL/day.

peritubular capillaries A set of capillaries unique to the kidney that branch off from the efferent arteriole; the site of tubular resorption.

podocytes Special cells in the inner membrane of the glomerulus that wrap around the capillaries in the glomerulus, forming filtration slits.

postrenal ARF A type of acute renal failure caused by obstruction of urine flow from the kidneys, commonly caused by a blockage of the urethra by prostate enlargement, renal calculi, or strictures.

prerenal ARF A type of acute renal failure that is caused by hypoperfusion of the kidneys, resulting from hypovolemia (hemorrhage, dehydration), trauma, shock, sepsis, and heart failure (congestive heart failure, myocardial infarction); often reversible if the underlying condition can be found and perfusion restored to the kidney.

priapism A sustained, painful erection of the penis.

proximal convoluted tubule (PCT) One of two complex sections of the nephron, the PCT includes an enlargement at the end called the glomerular capsule.

pyelonephritis Inflammation of the kidney linings.

referred pain Pain that originates in one area of the body but is interpreted as coming from a different area of the body.

renal columns Inward extensions of cortical tissue that surround the renal pyramids.

renal dialysis A technique for "filtering" the blood of its toxic wastes, removing excess fluids, and restoring the normal balance of electrolytes.

renal fascia Dense, fibrous connective tissue that anchors the kidney to the abdominal wall.

renal pelvis Part of the internal anatomy of the kidney; a flat, funnel-shaped tube filling the sinus at the level of the hilus.

renal pyramids Parallel cone-shaped bundles of urine-collecting tubules that are located in the medulla of the kidneys.

renin A hormone produced by cells in the juxtaglomerular apparatus when the blood pressure is low.

uremia The presence of excessive amounts of urea and other waste products in the blood.

uremic frost A powdery buildup of uric acid, especially around the face.

ureters A pair of thick-walled, hollow tubes that transport urine from the kidneys to the bladder.

urethra A hollow, tubular structure that drains urine from the bladder, passing it outside of the body.

urinary bladder A hollow, muscular sac in the midline of the lower abdominal area that stores urine until it is released from the body.

urinary tract infections (UTIs) Infections, usually of the lower urinary tract (urethra and bladder), which occur when normal flora bacteria enter the urethra and grow.

urine Liquid waste products filtered out of the body by the urinary system.

vasa recta A series of peritubular capillaries that surround the loop of Henle, into which water moves after passing through the descending and ascending limbs of the loop of Henle.

visceral pain Crampy, aching pain deep within the body, the source of which is usually hard to pinpoint; common with urologic problems.

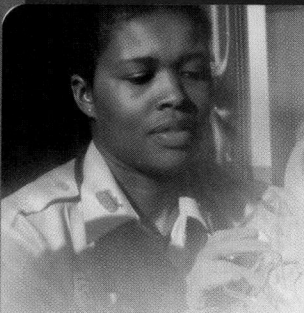

Assessment in Action

You are dispatched to the home of a 54-year-old man complaining of abdominal pain. When you arrive, you find the patient doubled over in pain and he states that this began approximately 2 hours ago. It is the worst pain he has ever had and he tells you that it "burns" when he urinates. His blood pressure is 140/90 mm Hg; pulse rate, 110 beats/min; and respiratory rate, 24 breaths/min. His rhythm on the monitor indicates sinus tachycardia. His pulse oximetry reading on room air is 100%. He has no medical problems and has no allergies.

1. **Which of the following conditions originates in the renal pelvis and is the result of an excess of insoluble salts or uric acid crystallizing in the urine?**
   A. Gall stones
   B. Urinary tract infections
   C. Kidney stones
   D. Pyleonephritis

2. **What is the most common type of stone?**
   A. Struvite
   B. Calcium
   C. Uric
   D. Cystine

3. **If a stone becomes lodged in the lower ureter, signs and symptoms of a _____ may be present.**
   A. UTI
   B. uric event
   C. URI
   D. MRSA

4. **Patients who are experiencing renal problems may exhibit many of the same symptoms as a patient with other abdominal problems. These symptoms include nausea and vomiting, constipation or diarrhea, weight loss, abdominal pain, and:**
   A. chest pain.
   B. headache.
   C. dizziness.
   D. back pain.

5. **What is the most common type of pain associated with urologic problems?**
   A. Referred pain
   B. Pain in the urethra
   C. Visceral pain
   D. Pain that can be pinpointed to a specific location

6. **Pain that may be interpreted by the brain as coming from another area of the body is called:**
   A. visceral pain.
   B. urethra pain.
   C. pleurisy.
   D. referred pain.

Challenging Questions

You are dispatched to the high school for a football player who was injured. When you arrive on scene, you find the patient complaining of right flank pain. You find out that the patient was running with the football and was tackled from the side. He was jolted and immediately felt a sharp pain in his side. He thought the pain would subside, but it hasn't. You observe his abdominal area and see a contusion in the right flank region and some bruising near his spine. You provide spinal precautions and begin transport to the hospital. His vital signs appear to be within normal limits; however, he is in a great deal of pain.

7. **What do you suspect is wrong with the patient?**

8. **How would you begin treatment of this patient?**

Points to Ponder

You and your partner are dispatched to the dialysis center in your town for an unconscious patient. When you arrive on scene, you find a patient sitting in the chair in the dialysis center and the staff tells you that after the patient received dialysis, he had an episode of syncope. The patient's blood pressure is 80/40 mm Hg; pulse rate, 64 beats/min; respiratory rate, 18 breaths/min; and pulse oximetry reading on room air, 97%.

Why might a patient who had received dialysis experience syncope?

Issues: Understanding the Role of the Kidneys, Treating Patients Who Received Dialysis, Understanding Renal Dialysis.

33 Toxicology: Substance Abuse and Poisoning

Objectives

Cognitive

5-8.1 Describe the incidence, morbidity and mortality of toxic emergencies. (p 33.4)

5-8.2 Identify the risk factors most predisposing to toxic emergencies. (p 33.4)

5-8.3 Discuss the anatomy and physiology of the organs and structures related to toxic emergencies. (p 33.5–33.7)

5-8.4 Describe the routes of entry of toxic substances into the body. (p 33.5)

5-8.5 Discuss the role of the Poison Control Center in the United States. (p 33.5)

5-8.6 List the toxic substances that are specific to your region. (p 33.5)

5-8.7 Discuss the pathophysiology of the entry of toxic substances into the body. (p 33.5)

5-8.8 Discuss the assessment findings associated with various toxidromes. (p 33.11)

5-8.9 Identify the need for rapid intervention and transport of the patient with a toxic substance emergency. (p 33.13)

5-8.10 Discuss the management of toxic substances. (p 33.11)

5-8.11 Define poisoning by ingestion. (p 33.5)

5-8.12 List the most common poisonings by ingestion. (p 33.6)

5-8.13 Describe the pathophysiology of poisoning by ingestion. (p 33.6)

5-8.14 Recognize the signs and symptoms related to the most common poisonings by ingestion. (p 33.8)

5-8.15 Correlate the abnormal findings in assessment with the clinical significance in the patient with the most common poisonings by ingestion. (p 33.11)

5-8.16 Differentiate among the various treatments and pharmacological interventions in the management of the most common poisonings by ingestion. (p 33.11)

5-8.17 Discuss the factors affecting the decision to induce vomiting in a patient with ingested poison. (p 33.11)

5-8.18 Integrate pathophysiological principles and the assessment findings to formulate a field impression and implement a treatment plan for the patient with the most common poisonings by ingestion. (p 33.11)

5-8.19 Define poisoning by inhalation. (p 33.6)

5-8.20 List the most common poisonings by inhalation. (p 33.6)

5-8.21 Describe the pathophysiology of poisoning by inhalation. (p 33.6)

5-8.22 Recognize the signs and symptoms related to the most common poisonings by inhalation. (p 33.8)

5-8.23 Correlate the abnormal findings in assessment with the clinical significance in patients with the most common poisonings by inhalation. (p 33.11)

5-8.24 Differentiate among the various treatments and pharmacological interventions in the management of the most common poisonings by inhalation. (p 33.11)

5-8.25 Integrate pathophysiological principles and the assessment findings to formulate a field impression and implement a treatment plan for the patient with the most common poisonings by inhalation. (p 33.11)

5-8.26 Define poisoning by injection. (p 33.6)

5-8.27 List the most common poisonings by injection. (p 33.6)

5-8.28 Describe the pathophysiology of poisoning by injection. (p 33.7)

5-8.29 Recognize the signs and symptoms related to the most common poisonings by injection. (p 33.8)

5-8.30 Correlate the abnormal findings in assessment with the clinical significance in the patient with the most common poisonings by injection. (p 33.11)

5-8.31 Differentiate among the various treatments and pharmacological interventions in the management of the most common poisonings by injection. (p 33.11)

5-8.32 Integrate pathophysiological principles and the assessment findings to formulate a field impression and implement a treatment plan for the patient with the most common poisonings by injection. (p 33.11)

5-8.33 Define poisoning by surface absorption. (p 33.7)

5-8.34 List the most common poisonings by surface absorption. (p 33.7)

5-8.35 Describe the pathophysiology of poisoning by surface absorption. (p 33.7)

5-8.36 Recognize the signs and symptoms related to the most common poisonings by surface absorption. (p 33.8)

5-8.37 Correlate the abnormal findings in assessment with the clinical significance in patients with the most common poisonings by surface absorption. (p 33.11)

5-8.38 Differentiate among the various treatments and pharmacological interventions in the management of the most common poisonings by surface absorption. (p 33.11)

5-8.39 Integrate pathophysiological principles and the assessment findings to formulate a field impression and implement a treatment plan for patients with the most common poisonings by surface absorption. (p 33.11)

5-8.40 Define poisoning by overdose. (p 33.13)

5-8.41 List the most common poisonings by overdose. (p 33.13)

5-8.42 Describe the pathophysiology of poisoning by overdose. (p 33.5)

5-8.43 Recognize the signs and symptoms related to the most common poisonings by overdose. (p 33.8)

5-8.44 Correlate the abnormal findings in assessment with the clinical significance in patients with the most common poisonings by overdose. (p 33.11)

5-8.45 Differentiate among the various treatments and pharmacological interventions in the management of the most common poisonings by overdose. (p 33.13)

5-8.46 Integrate pathophysiological principles and the assessment findings to formulate a field impression and implement a treatment plan for patients with the most common poisonings by overdose. (p 33.12)

5-8.47   Define drug abuse. (p 33.9)

5-8.48   Discuss the incidence of drug abuse in the United States. (p 33.9)

5-8.49   Define the following terms:
a. Substance or drug abuse
b. Substance or drug dependence
c. Tolerance
d. Withdrawal
e. Addiction (p 33.9)

5-8.50   List the most commonly abused drugs (both by chemical name and street names). (p 33.13–33.20)

5-8.51   Describe the pathophysiology of commonly used drugs. (p 33.13–33.20)

5-8.52   Recognize the signs and symptoms related to the most commonly abused drugs. (p 33.13–33.20)

5-8.53   Correlate the abnormal findings in assessment with the clinical significance in patients using the most commonly abused drugs. (p 33.13–33.20)

5-8.54   Differentiate among the various treatments and pharmacological interventions in the management of the most commonly abused drugs. (p 33.13–33.20)

5-8.55   Integrate pathophysiological principles and the assessment findings to formulate a field impression and implement a treatment plan for patients using the most commonly abused drugs. (p 33.13–33.20)

5-8.56   List the clinical uses, street names, pharmacology, assessment finding and management for patients who have taken the following drugs or been exposed to the following substances:
1. Cocaine
2. Marijuana and cannabis compounds
3. Amphetamines and amphetamine-like drugs
4. Barbiturates
5. Sedative-hypnotics
6. Cyanide
7. Narcotics/opiates
8. Cardiac medications
9. Caustics
10. Common household substances
11. Drugs abused for sexual purposes/sexual gratification
12. Carbon monoxide
13. Alcohols
14. Hydrocarbons
15. Psychiatric medications
16. Newer anti-depressants and serotonin syndromes
17. Lithium
18. MAO inhibitors
19. Non-prescription pain medications
  (1) Nonsteroidal anti-inflammatory agents
  (2) Salicylates
  (3) Acetaminophen
20. Theophylline
21. Metals
22. Plants and mushrooms (p 33.13–33.15, 33.17, 33.20–33.26, 33.28–33.33)

5-8.57   Discuss common causative agents, pharmacology, assessment findings and management for a patient with food poisoning. (p 33.35)

5-8.58   Discuss common offending organisms, pharmacology, assessment findings and management for a patient with a bite or sting. (p 33.36)

5-8.59   Integrate pathophysiological principles of the patient with a toxic substance exposure. (p 33.11)

5-8.60   Differentiate between toxic substance emergencies based on assessment findings. (p 33.11)

5-8.61   Correlate abnormal findings in the assessment with the clinical significance in the patient exposed to a toxic substance. (p 33.12)

5-8.62   Develop a patient management plan based on field impression in the patient exposed to a toxic substance. (p 33.12)

Affective

None

Psychomotor

None

Introduction

Paramedics treat patients who have taken drugs of abuse (including alcohol) on an almost daily basis. Given the nature of drug use and abuse, it is impossible to accurately identify how many "users" of such substances exist. Sometimes the abused substance is legal (licit), as in the case of alcohol and oxycodone by prescription **Figure 33-1 ▾** . At other times, the substance is illegal (illicit), as in the case of heroin and ecstasy. Although research indicates that the use of street drugs has stabilized in smaller communities in recent years, larger cities have seen increases in heroin and cocaine use.

Before we actually dig into this very challenging area of paramedic practice, it is important to define some key terms. A poison is a substance that is toxic by nature, no matter how it gets into the body or in what quantities it is taken. At a minimum, a poison will make people ill; in the worst-case scenario,

it will kill them. By contrast, a drug is a substance that has some therapeutic effect (such as reducing inflammation, fighting bacteria, or producing euphoria) when given in the appropriate circumstances and in the appropriate dose. When a drug (licit or illicit) is taken in excess, the person is said to have "overdosed," which is a toxicologic emergency, because the person has been "poisoned." In a nutshell, a poison is always a poison, whereas a licit or illicit substance can poison a person if it is taken to excess.

Types of Toxicologic Emergencies

Toxicologic emergencies usually fall under one of two general headings: intentional and unintentional. Poisoning in adults is commonly intentional. In particular, suicide is often accomplished with the use of drugs.

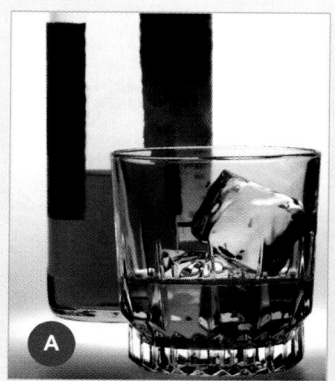 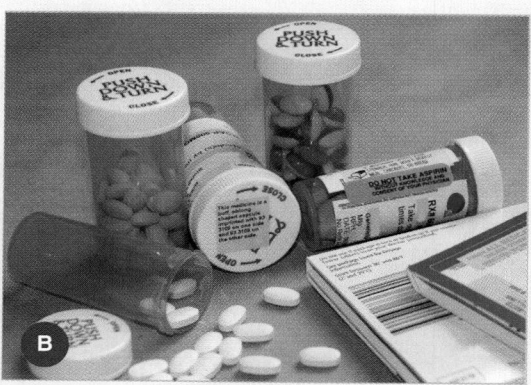 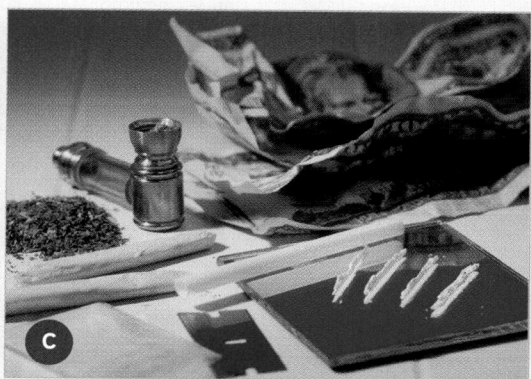

Figure 33-1 A. Alcohol is a legal substance that is a drug. **B.** Medications are legal substances that can be abused. **C.** Illegal drugs can also be abused.

You are the Provider Part 1

You and your partner respond to the local high school for an unknown medical emergency. You are met at the school entrance by the girls' physical education coach, who escorts you to the gymnasium. There, your attention is drawn to a group of young girls surrounding one of their peers, who is lying motionless on the floor.

Your partner makes room for the two of you to reach the patient. You find a 14-year-old girl lying supine on the floor and unresponsive to verbal stimuli. When you apply a sternal rub, she mumbles incoherently. A student steps forward and introduces herself as the patient's best friend. She says that Julie has been sleepy all morning, becoming drowsy during lunch and passing out while getting ready to play volleyball.

Initial Assessment	Recording Time: 0 Minutes
Appearance	Unconscious, no apparent distress
Level of consciousness	P (Responsive to painful stimuli), mumbles incoherently
Airway	Open
Breathing	Adequate rate and volume
Circulation	Radial pulse present

1. What are your priorities at this point?
2. What information do you need to obtain?

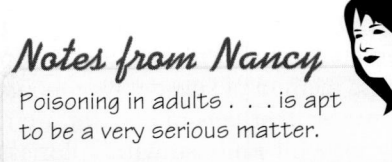

An unintentional toxicologic emergency can occur in many ways. For example, medication dosing errors are common problems in clinical practice. In some cases the event may be idiosyncratic: 2 mg of midazolam (Versed) may simply relax one patient but cause respiratory arrest in another.

Childhood poisonings are quite common, especially in younger children who may put anything into their mouths Figure 33-2 ▼ , such as colorful berries on a house or garden plant that draw a child's attention. A parent's prescription medication may be mistaken for candy.

Even nature is fraught with toxicologic perils, as ask any hiker who has inadvertently wandered through a batch of poison ivy would attest. Wild mushrooms, once in the body, can produce a wide spectrum of results—from being a tasty treat, to being nauseating, to being deadly.

The workplace also harbors its share of toxic hazards. Unfortunately, some of these hazards aren't identified until after the exposure has occurred. For example, countless workers in the electric energy field worked with polychlorinated biphenyls, or PCBs, on a daily basis and developed cancer later in life. Similarly, asbestosis developed in thousands of people after continued exposure to asbestos in the workplace.

Unintentional toxicologic emergencies can also occur from simple neglect or oversight. Consider a geriatric person with diabetes, possibly combined with early-onset dementia or Alzheimer's disease, who takes his or her insulin in the morning, later cannot remember whether the dose was taken, and takes another dose. The result: a call to 9-1-1 for an "unconscious, unresponsive" person in need of assistance.

Biological warfare has drawn increasing attention in recent years owing to the heightened awareness of bioterrorism, but intentional poisoning or overdose may also commonly occur during more intimate crimes. In recent years, "date rape" drugs such as Rohypnol have been used to facilitate sexual assault. Chloral hydrate ("knockout drops") has been used to commit assault for decades, and pharmacologic agents are used in homicide as well.

Poison Centers

Given the variety of illicit drugs coupled with the continued growth of licit drugs, even the most well-read veteran paramedic may find it difficult to keep current with the myriad drugs sold in the streets today. For this reason, Poison Centers (1-800-222-1222) may be an indispensable aid.

Suppose you are called to a home where a frantic mother is hovering over a toddler who sits beside the remains of a potted philodendron, most of which he apparently just ate. Is the plant poisonous? How poisonous? Should you make the child vomit? Is an antidote available? In such a scenario, you can call the Poison Center and get a fast rundown on the ingestion, its toxic potential, and steps to negate its effects, thereby providing proper patient care.

Poison Centers are a virtual gold mine of information that you should add to your toolbox. Never hesitate to tap these resources when confronted with *any toxin* for which you have limited or no familiarity. At the same time, your call helps the center collect data on poisonings in your region. These data may be analyzed to help

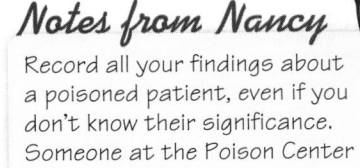

detect trends, spot developing public health problems, and evaluate current treatment protocols for different poisonings.

Routes of Absorption

As nasty as they are, toxins can't exert their effects until they enter the human body. The four primary methods of entry are ingestion, inhalation, injection, and absorption. Just as each of these methods of entry is unique, so is the rate at which a given toxin is absorbed into the body. Once a toxin is in the body, the combination of the amount of toxin and the relative speed at which it is metabolized affect the bioavailability of the toxin and the excretion rate.

Poisoning by Ingestion

Ingested poisons may produce immediate damage to tissues, or their toxic effects may be delayed for several hours. Ingestions of a caustic substance (that is, a strong acid or alkali) occurs immediately. By contrast, some poisons must be absorbed into

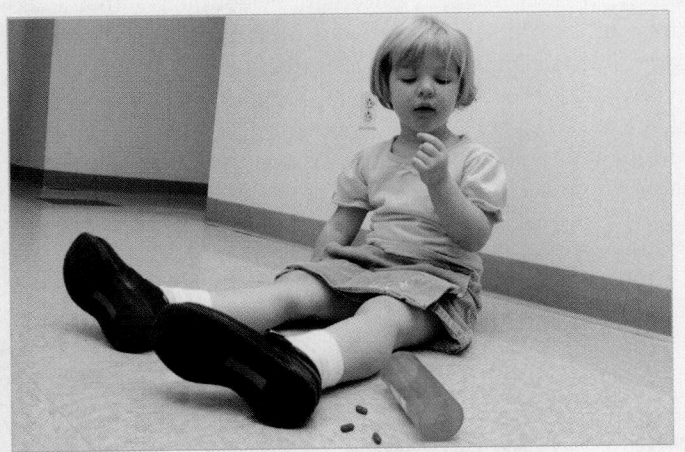

Figure 33-2 Toddlers will put anything into their mouths, including dangerous medications.

the bloodstream before they can produce their toxic effects. Medications around the home and household chemicals (such as cleaning agents) are the most common sources of poisoning by ingestion.

Poisoning by ingestion is marked by a wide range of possibilities regarding *what* is actually ingested and *why* it was ingested. Consider, for example, a curious child who eats the

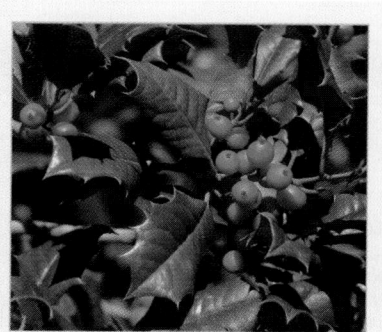

bright red berries of a holly plant or the flowers of a purple foxglove 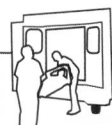 Figure 33-3 ◂ . By contrast, a person who is taking acetaminophen for pain relief may inadvertently increase his or her intake to a toxic level, possibly to the point of destroying the liver and leading to death. Although both of these scenarios would be considered accidental, intentional poisoning by ingestion is also possible—as when someone takes a lethal quantity or combination of drugs in a suicide attempt.

Figure 33-3 Certain berries and flowers are poisonous, such as those of the holly plant and the purple foxglove.

Assessment clues pointing toward ingestion can be as obvious as a plant with partially chewed leaves or a section of plant with berries missing. Stained fingers, lips, or tongue are also worth noting. Any patient complaining of a sudden onset of stomach cramps with or without nausea, vomiting, or diarrhea may have an ingestion-related problem. Empty pill bottles are another obvious clue, as is the date on which the prescription was filled. The bottle for a prescription filled 6 months ago likely wasn't full today; an empty bottle for a prescription filled yesterday is far more ominous.

A toxin that enters the body by the oral route generally provides a more forgiving timeframe for treatment. Little absorption occurs in the stomach; indeed, the ingested substance may stay there for a variable period, with the vast majority of absorption actually taking place in the small intestine. As a consequence, much of the management of poisoning by ingestion aims to remove or neutralize the poison before it gains access to the intestines.

Poisoning by Inhalation

A person can be poisoned by inhalation only if the poison is present in the surrounding atmosphere. That fact, obvious as it seems, has important implications. First, so long as the patient remains in the toxic environment, he or she will keep inhaling the poison—and so will you, if you enter that environment without the appropriate protective breathing apparatus. Second, when poisoning occurs because of a toxic environment, you are likely to encounter more than one patient at the emergency scene. Home medications and household chemical products (such as bleach and cleaning agents) are responsible for the most common types of inhalation emergencies.

Poisoning by inhalation may be accidental or intentional. Consider carbon monoxide (CO) poisoning. Leaving the garage door shut while seated in an automobile with the engine running provides a quick, painless method of suicide. By contrast, an automatic damper on a furnace that fails to open or a bird nest that blocks a chimney may fill a house with colorless, odorless CO, quietly and efficiently poisoning those inside.

From the anatomic and physiologic perspective, inhaled toxins quickly reach the alveoli, providing almost instant access to the circulation. CO, for example, binds to hemoglobin on the red blood cells (RBCs) about 250 times more readily than do oxygen molecules. As a result, rapid systemic distribution can occur with an equally rapid onset of signs and symptoms. For this reason, the window of opportunity for treatment is limited.

When dealing with an inhalation emergency, the first general management consideration is that of scene safety. After donning the appropriate breathing apparatus, remove the patient(s) to a safe environment before beginning any treatment.

In the Field

Scene safety is your primary concern when you are called to an inhalation incident. Whenever you encounter more than one patient but find no evidence of the mechanism of injury (MOI), be suspicious. Toxic fumes may be odorless and colorless, and they do not discriminate between rescuers and victims. Be suspicious of toxic fumes when encountering patients with changes in level of consciousness (LOC), especially at an industrial site or enclosed space.

Inhaled toxins produce a wide range of signs and symptoms, many of which are unique to the toxin involved. A patient with CO poisoning does not exhibit the same signs and symptoms as a person who has sniffed glue, who in turn looks nothing like a patient poisoned by a furniture stripper containing methylene chloride. Frequently, the emergency scene itself contains the clues to the identification of the toxin that is making the patient ill. That information, coupled with the assistance of the Poison Center and direction from the medical control physician, will drive your treatment plan. Correction of hypoxia is a must, so administer a high concentration of supplemental oxygen. Establish vascular access, apply an electrocardiographic (ECG) monitor, and perform pulse oximetry and capnography.

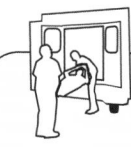

In the Field

Always treat the patient and not the diagnostic tool. Pulse oximeters may give false readings when patients have been exposed to CO.

Poisoning by Injection

Injected poisons usually gain access to the body as the result of stings or bites from a variety of unpleasant creatures. Abuse of intravenously administered drugs such as heroin, cocaine,

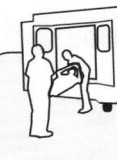

In the Field

Treat all tools used to inject substances as bio-hazards. These needles or devices may have been shared with other drug users and may carry the human immunodeficiency virus or other pathogens.

In the Field

Absorption of toxic substances through the skin is a common problem in agriculture and manufacturing. Most solvents and "cides"—insecticides, herbicides, and pesticides—are toxic and can be readily absorbed through the skin.

amphetamines, and "speedball" (heroin and cocaine together) is also common in the prehospital setting.

Depending on the geographic location, multiple possibilities for poisoning by injection may exist in the environment. Whereas snake bites and scorpion stings are more prevalent in the southwestern United States, paramedics in coastal areas are more likely to encounter patients stung by jellyfish, Portuguese men-of-war, sea urchins, or anemones. Wasps, yellow jackets, and hornets have a wider geographic distribution, and stings from these insects are common occurrences throughout most of the United States.

Some of these injected poisons are neurotoxic, whereas others produce localized or systemic reactions. When a bite or sting hits a vein or artery and results in a toxin immediately entering the bloodstream, the outcome is much more dangerous than when the same toxin enters a muscle mass such as the calf, which has a much slower rate of absorption and distribution.

When assessing bites and stings, physical findings will usually provide the most clues, especially local reactions such as pain at the wound site. Depending on the specific toxin, signs and symptoms can vary greatly. Frequently, the patient may be able to identify the culprit, greatly simplifying the assessment process.

Poisoning by Absorption

Some poisons gain access to the body by being absorbed through the skin. Of the poisonings that occur by absorption,

those caused by pesticides such as organophosphates and similar substances are often the most serious.

Understanding and Using Toxidromes

Although the sheer number of substances of abuse may seem daunting, the good news is that many drugs, on entering the body, result in similar signs and symptoms. Consider narcotics. Irrespective of whether it is a natural product derived from opium (that is, an opiate) or a synthetic, non–opium-derived narcotic (that is, an opioid), all drugs in this group work in a similar manner, so they produce similar signs and symptoms. The syndrome-like symptoms of a poisonous agent are termed a toxic syndrome or <u>toxidrome</u>. Toxidromes are useful for remembering the assessment and management of different substances that fall under the same clinical umbrella. The major toxidromes are produced by stimulants, narcotics, cholinergics, anticholinergics, sympathomimetics, and sedative and hypnotics **Table 33-1 ▸** .

Table 33-2 ▸ lists common signs and symptoms of poisoning. If you look at your history and physical examination findings in conjunction with the vital signs, more often than not you can develop a working diagnosis that will allow you to provide appropriate care until you can deliver the patient to the receiving facility.

You are the Provider Part 2

You conduct your initial assessment of the patient. A rapid trauma assessment reveals no life-threatening conditions. As you prepare to perform a detailed physical exam, you ask the coach to find out if the patient has any relevant medical history and to get a contact number for her mother. You also ask the patient's friend if she knows of any information that might be helpful. She says that Julie has been depressed lately over problems with her boyfriend and thinks that she might be taking some medication to help her cope. The friend seems to remember something and suddenly runs off.

Vital Signs	Recording Time: 5 Minutes
Skin	Flushed, warm, and dry
Pulse	140 beats/min, regular, and weak
Blood pressure	88/58 mm Hg
Respirations	10 breaths/min
Sao$_2$	93% on nonrebreathing mask at 12 L/min of supplemental oxygen

3. What are some potential differential diagnoses?

4. Which interventions should you consider at this point, if any?

Table 33-1 Major Toxidromes

Toxidrome	Drug Examples	Signs and Symptoms
Stimulant	Amphetamine, methamphetamine, cocaine, diet aids, nasal decongestants	Restlessness, agitation, incessant talking; insomnia, anorexia; dilated pupils, tachycardia; tachypnea, hypertension or hypotension; paranoia, seizures, cardiac arrest
Narcotic (opiate and opioid)	Heroin, opium, morphine, hydromorphone (Dilaudid), fentanyl, oxycodone-aspirin combination (Percodan)	Constricted (pin-point) pupils, marked respiratory depression; needle tracks (IV abusers); drowsiness, stupor, coma
Sympathomimetic	Pseudoephedrine, phenylephrine, phenylpropanolamine, amphetamine, and methamphetamine	Hypertension, tachycardia, dilated pupils (mydriasis), agitation and seizures, hyperthermia
Sedative and hypnotic	Phenobarbital, diazepam (Valium), thiopental	Drowsiness, disinhibition, ataxia, slurred speech, mental confusion, respiratory depression, progressive central nervous system depression, hypotension
Cholinergic	Diazinon, orthene, parathion, sarin, tabun, VX	Increased salivation, lacrimation, gastrointestinal distress, diarrhea, respiratory depression, apnea, seizures, coma
Anticholinergic	Atropine, scopolamine, antihistamines, antipsychotics	Dry, flushed skin, hyperthermia, dilated pupils, blurred vision, tachycardia; mild hallucinations, dramatic delirium

Table 33-2 Common Signs and Symptoms of Poisoning

Sign or Symptom	Type	Possible Causative Agents
Odor	Bitter almonds	Cyanide
	Garlic	Arsenic, organophosphates, phosphorus
	Acetone	Methyl alcohol, isopropyl alcohol, aspirin, acetone
	Wintergreen	Methyl salicylate
	Pears	Chloral hydrate
	Violets	Turpentine
	Camphor	Camphor
	Alcohol	Alcohol
Pupils	Constricted	Narcotics, organophosphates, Jimson weed, nutmeg, propoxyphene (Darvon)
	Dilated	Barbiturates, atropine, amphetamine, glutethimide (Doriden), lysergic acid diethylamide (LSD), cyanide, CO
Mouth	Salivation	Organophosphates, arsenic, strychnine, mercury, salicylates
	Dry mouth	Atropine (belladonna), amphetamines, diphenhydramine (Benadryl), narcotics
	Burns in mouth	Formaldehyde, iodine, lye, toxic plants, phenols, phosphorous, pine oil, silver nitrate, acids
Skin	Pruritis	Jimson weed, belladonna, boric acid
	Dry, hot skin	Atropine (in belladonna), botulism, nutmeg
	Sweating	Organophosphates, arsenic, aspirin, amphetamines, barbiturates, mushrooms, naphthalene
Respiratory	Depressed respirations	Narcotics, alcohol, propoxyphene, CO, barbiturates
	Increased respirations	Aspirin, amphetamines, boric acid, cyanide, kerosene, methyl alcohol, nicotine
	Pulmonary edema	Organophosphates, petroleum products, narcotics, CO
Cardiovascular	Tachycardia	Alcohol, amphetamines, arsenic, atropine, aspirin, cocaine, some antiasthma drugs
	Bradycardia	Digitalis, gasoline, nicotine, mushrooms, narcotics, cyanide, mistletoe, rhododendron
	Hypertension	Amphetamines, lead, nicotine, antiasthma drugs
	Hypotension	Barbiturates, narcotics, tranquilizers, house plants, mistletoe, nitroglycerin, antifreeze
Central nervous system	Seizures	Amphetamines, camphor, cocaine, strychnine, arsenic, CO, petroleum products, scorpion sting
	Coma	All depressant drugs (such as narcotics, barbiturates, tranquilizers, alcohol), CO, cyanide
	Hallucinations	Atropine, LSD, mushrooms, organic solvents, phencyclidine (PCP), nutmeg
	Headache	CO, alcohol, disulfiram (Antabuse)
	Tremors	Organophosphates, CO, amphetamine, tranquilizers, poisonous marine animals
	Weakness or paralysis	Organophosphates, botulism, eel, hemlock, puffer fish, pine oil, rhododendron
Gastrointestinal	Cramps, nausea, vomiting, and/or diarrhea	Many, if not most, ingested poisons

Overview of Substance Abuse

Human beings have a long history of abusing drugs and alcohol. With the passing of time, the physiologic and societal effects of alcohol abuse have become well known and thoroughly documented. Unfortunately, the area of medicine dealing with drugs of abuse is highly challenging because of uncertainty about the prevalence of the problem and the continual evolution of the substances themselves. In the 1980s, creative chemists took existing pharmacologic agents and structurally manipulated them to create new or different drugs ("designer drugs") that were often far more potent than the original drugs. For example, cocaine was made into crack, a far more addictive form of the drug.

Substance abuse can be broadly defined as the self-administration of licit or illicit substances in a manner not in accord with approved medical or social practice. Part of that definition is cultural—and there is great variation in what is considered substance abuse. In our society, for example, it is acceptable to administer narcotics under medical supervision for the relief of pain; conversely, self-administration of the same drugs for the purpose of inducing euphoria is regarded as drug abuse.

Any given society's definition of abuse may have little relation to the potential harm from the abused substance. For example, our culture places no restrictions on the long-term and compulsive use of tobacco, even though it is a major contributor to cardiovascular and respiratory disease 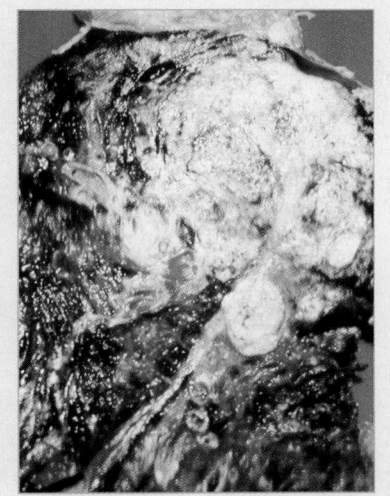 Figure 33-4 . By comparison, use of marijuana, which has less damaging effects, may be punishable by fines or imprisonment.

Figure 33-4 A diseased lung as a result of tobacco use.

Let's formally define some basic terms and concepts related to substance abuse:

- **Drug abuse.** Any use of drugs that causes physical, psychological, economic, legal, or social harm to the user or to others affected by the drug user's behavior.
- **Habituation.** Psychological dependence on a drug or drugs.
- **Physical dependence.** A physiologic state of adaptation to a drug, usually characterized by tolerance to the drug's effects and a withdrawal syndrome if the drug is stopped, especially if it is stopped abruptly.
- **Psychological dependence.** The emotional state of craving a drug to maintain a feeling of well-being.

- **Tolerance.** Physiologic adaptation to the effects of a drug such that increasingly larger doses of the drug are required to achieve the same effect.
- **Withdrawal syndrome.** A predictable set of signs and symptoms, usually involving altered central nervous system (CNS) activity, that occurs after the abrupt cessation of a drug or after rapidly decreasing the usual dosage of a drug.
- **Drug addiction.** A chronic disorder characterized by the compulsive use of a substance resulting in physical, psychological, or social harm to the user, who continues to use the substance despite the harm.
- **Antagonist.** Something that counteracts the action of something else. In relation to drugs, a drug that is an antagonist has an affinity for a cell receptor; by binding to the receptor, the antagonist prevents the cell from responding.
- **Potentiation.** Enhancement of the effect of one drug by another drug.
- **Synergism.** The action of two substances, such as drugs, in which the total effects are greater than the sum of the independent effects of the two substances (that is, 2 + 2 = 5).

Drug abuse is not limited to members of the younger generation or to any particular stratum of society. It occurs in all age groups and at all social levels.

Alcoholism

Alcohol is the most widely abused drug in the United States. More than 100 million Americans regularly consume alcohol, of which slightly more than 10% have alcoholism. Alcoholism remains one of the top five causes of death in the United States. Furthermore, because of its harmful effects on organs, including the liver, stomach, heart, pancreas, brain, and CNS, alcoholism decreases a person's life span by 10 to 20 years. In addition, people with alcoholism tend to have chronic malnutrition and fall frequently, increasing the likelihood of head injury or other trauma.

Alcoholism usually consists of two distinct phases. The first phase is problem drinking, during which alcohol is used increasingly more often to relieve tensions or other emotional difficulties. Because of the disinhibition, relaxation, and sense of well-being mediated by alcohol, some degree of psychological dependence often develops with its use. Unfortunately, many people become so dependent on the psychological influences of alcohol that they become compulsive consumers. As a person becomes more dependent on drinking, his or her performance at work and relationships with friends, family, and coworkers may deteriorate. Increased absence from work, emotional disturbances, and automobile crashes become more frequent.

Physical dependence also results from the regular consumption of large quantities of alcohol. This becomes apparent when a person abruptly stops consuming alcohol and withdrawal symptoms result. The severity of the withdrawal can

Notes from Nancy

The patient found stuporous with alcohol on his or her breath must not be assumed to be intoxicated.

vary according to the length and intensity of the alcoholic habit. Minor withdrawal is characterized by restlessness, anxiousness, sleeping problems, agitation, and tremors.

In the second phase of alcoholism, true addiction, abstinence causes major withdrawal symptoms—for example, increased blood pressure, vomiting, and hallucinations. Delirium tremens, or alcohol withdrawal delirium, results in fever, disorientation, confusion, seizures, and possibly death.

Alcoholism occurs in all social strata, and only a small minority of people with alcoholism fit the "skid row" stereotype. Red flags pointing to alcoholism include the following:

- Drinking early in the day
- Drinking alone or in "secret"
- Periodic binges
- Loss of memory or "blackouts"
- Tremulousness and anxiety
- Cigarette burns on clothing from falling asleep with a lit cigarette
- "Green tongue syndrome," caused by the use of chlorophyll-containing compounds to disguise the smell of alcohol on the breath
- Chronically flushed face and palms

Medical Consequences of Alcohol Abuse

Because of the toxic effects of alcohol, a person with alcoholism is considerably more prone than sober counterparts to a number of serious illnesses and injuries Table 33-3 ▶ . Chronic damage to the CNS, for example, leads to deterioration in higher mental functions, such as memory and logical thinking. Damage to the cerebellum results in problems of balance, which in turn contribute to the frequent falls experienced by people with alcoholism. Damage to the peripheral nerves leads to decreased sensation in the extremities, making the person prone to burns and similar injuries that an intact pain sense would ordinarily prevent.

As alcohol travels through the digestive system, it irritates tissue and can damage the lining of the stomach by causing acid imbalances, inflammation, and acute gastric distress. Often, the result is gastritis (an inflamed stomach) and heartburn. The more frequently consumption takes place, the greater the irritation. One of every three heavy drinkers has chronic gastritis. Heavy drinkers also have double the risk of cancer of the mouth and esophagus. Prolonged heavy use of alcohol may cause ulcers, hiatal hernias, and cancers throughout the digestive tract.

The toxic effects of alcohol on the liver produce a variety of complications, such as coagulopathies (easy bleeding and poor clotting ability), hypoglycemia, and gastrointestinal (GI) bleeding. In addition, people with alcoholism are at high risk of acute pancreatitis, pneumonia, and cardiomyopathy.

Table 33-3	Medical Problems to Which People With Alcoholism Are Particularly Susceptible	
Condition	**Contributing Factors**
Subdural hematoma	Frequent falls; impaired clotting mechanisms
GI bleeding	Irritant effect of alcohol on the stomach lining (leading to gastritis); impaired clotting mechanisms; cirrhosis of the liver, leading to engorgement of esophageal veins (esophageal varices)
Pancreatitis	Indirect effect on alcohol of the pancreas
Hypoglycemia	Damage to the liver, which normally mobilizes sugar into the blood
Pneumonia	Aspiration of vomitus occurring during intoxication and coma; suppression of immune system by alcohol
Burns	Relative insensitivity to pain occurring during intoxication; falling asleep with a lit cigarette while intoxicated
Hypothermia	Insensitivity to extremes of temperatures while intoxicated; falling asleep outside in the cold
Seizures	Effect of withdrawal from alcohol
Arrhythmias	Toxic effects of alcohol on the heart
Cancer	Mechanism not known (perhaps related to suppression of the immune system), but people with alcoholism are 10 times more likely than the general population to have cancer
Esophageal varices (abnormally enlarged veins in the lower part of the esophagus)	Develop when normal blood flow to the liver is blocked and blood backs up into smaller, more fragile blood vessels in the esophagus; do not produce symptoms unless they rupture and bleed (a life-threatening condition that requires immediate medical care; can be fatal when not controlled)

Alcohol Emergencies

Any of the conditions previously mentioned may contribute to an emergency. In addition, acute consumption of and acute abstinence from alcohol may produce serious problems, including withdrawal seizures.

Acute Alcohol Intoxication

Severe alcohol intoxication is a form of poisoning and carries the same lethal potential as poisoning with any other CNS depressant. Death from alcohol intoxication has been reported with blood alcohol levels of 400 mg/dL, which can be attained by the relatively rapid consumption of as little as a half-pint of whiskey. The most immediate danger to an acutely intoxicated person is death of respiratory depression and/or aspiration of vomitus or stomach contents secondary to a suppressed gag reflex.

If an intoxicated patient is unconscious, treat him or her as you would any unconscious patient. As always, first establish and maintain the airway. With an intact gag reflex, place the patient in left lateral recumbent position with suction ready. If there is no gag reflex, intubate the patient. In addition, give high-concentration supplemental oxygen, and assist ventilation as needed. Establish vascular access. Monitor the ECG rhythm. Assess the patient's blood glucose level, treating hypoglycemia if it is found. If directed to do so by medical control, administer thiamine 100 mg via slow intravenous (IV) push. Finally, transport the patient to an appropriate facility.

Withdrawal Seizures

A person who has been drinking heavily for an extended period and suddenly stops drinking may have a variety of withdrawal phenomena. Seizures usually occur within about 12 to 48 hours of the last drink. Use the same care plan described for alcohol intoxication, and consult with medical control about giving benzodiazepines for seizure control.

Delirium Tremens

One of the most serious and lethal complications of alcohol withdrawal is delirium tremens (DTs). Symptoms usually start 48 to 72 hours after the last alcohol intake, although a week to 10 days may pass before the onset of symptoms in some cases. Delirium tremens is a serious and potentially fatal syndrome with mortality reported as high as 15%. Signs and symptoms include confusion, tremors and restlessness, fever and diaphoresis, hallucinations (extremely frightening—such as snakes, spiders, and rats), and hypotension, often secondary to dehydration.

The treatment for a patient in DTs is aimed at protecting him or her from injury and supporting the cardiovascular system. The often-terrifying hallucinations associated with DTs typically make for an agitated, often combative patient. Try to keep the patient calm. In addition, you should administer supplemental oxygen by nasal cannula and establish vascular access. Manage hypotension with an infusion of normal saline, and, during the ongoing assessment, reassess breath sounds. Maintain an ongoing dialogue with the patient throughout transport to help orient and reassure the patient.

General Principles of Assessment and Management for Toxicologic Emergencies

Generally, patients with toxicologic emergencies are considered medical patients, although toxicologic emergencies may lead to

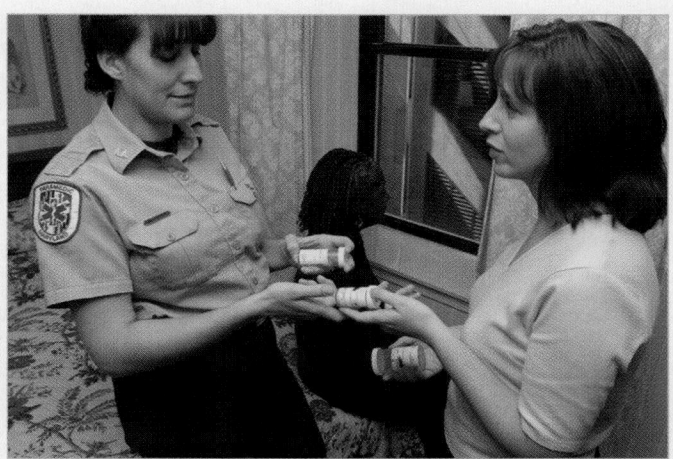

Figure 33-5 Take any bottles, containers, and their remaining contents to the ED.

trauma, too. The general assessment approach is the same for all patients: scene size-up, initial assessment, and then focused history and physical exam. If the mental status is altered, monitor the patient's airway and breathing diligently to ensure that he or she does not aspirate and is adequately filling the chest with air. If the patient is responsive, use the OPQRST mnemonic to elaborate on the chief complaint, take the patient's vital signs, take a SAMPLE history, and perform a focused physical examination. If the patient is not responsive, obtain vital signs and complete a rapid medical assessment; obtain the OPQRST and SAMPLE history from bystanders and family members, if possible.

To choose the appropriate course of action in a toxicologic emergency, obtain at least the following specific information:

- *What is the agent?* If the patient has overdosed on a prescription drug, take the pill bottle and the remaining pills in with the patient **Figure 33-5 ▲**. If the substance was a commercial product, take the container and its remaining contents to the emergency department (ED). If the patient ingested a plant, find out what part (roots, leaves, stem, flower, or fruit) and take a sample of the plant to the ED for identification. If the patient vomits, save a sample of the vomitus in a clean, closed container, and take it with you to the emergency department **Figure 33-6 ▶**.
- *When was the poison ingested, injected, absorbed, or inhaled?* The decision to induce vomiting (infrequently done—check local protocols) or to flush out (lavage) the stomach is strongly influenced by the amount of time that has elapsed since the exposure. The likelihood of retrieving significant quantities of the poison from the stomach decreases rapidly after the first 30 to 60 minutes. Also, acute-onset events often indicate a more serious patient scenario—for example, if the patient smoked crack cocaine 15 minutes ago and immediately began to have crushing chest pain.
- *How much was taken, injected, absorbed, or inhaled?* Street drugs are commonly sold in single-dose "hits" or "tabs" (tablets). If the patient says he has taken "three hits of

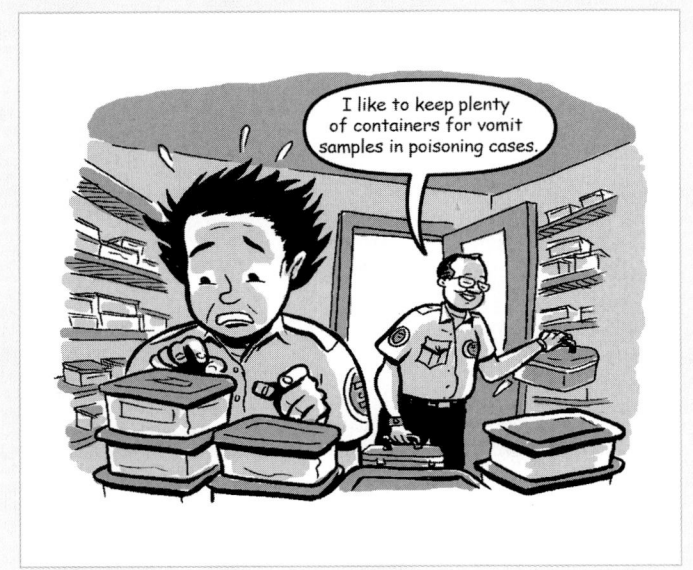

Figure 33-6

Documentation and Communication

While at the scene, make thorough (and legible) notes about the nature of the poisoning. You can then quickly state the type and amount of substance and the time and route of exposure in your radio, verbal, and written reports. Clear notes that can be handed over on arrival will be appreciated by busy hospital staff.

acid," you know he has taken three times the "normal dose" of LSD. If the patient says that she took 4 tabs of ecstasy, that's four times a single dose. There is almost always a distinct correlation between dose and toxic effects.

- *What else was taken?* A majority of intentional self-poisonings (suicide attempts) or illicit drug overdoses involve polydrug ingestions, often with alcohol as one of the drugs. The patient may also have tried to take something as an antidote (that is, something to counteract the effect of the poison). This information can be invaluable to ED staff when deciding which tests to order.
- *Has the patient vomited or aspirated?* If so, how soon after the ingestion or exposure? How much?
- *Why was the substance taken?* Although you may not get a reliable answer from someone abusing illicit drugs, this is still a question worth asking. Don't assume that every patient is trying to get high. Drug use could be a coping mechanism for a person who is being abused, or it could be a suicide attempt. Put the reason in "quotation marks" on your patient care report.

Scene Size-up

Patients who have taken an overdose may be extremely dangerous, so make sure you do a scene size-up in every case. If necessary, call for law enforcement backup or a crisis unit to minimize potential for injury to EMS providers.

Initial Assessment

The initial assessment of a drug-overdosed or poisoned patient begins with your general impression. It can be as simple as "a young adult man snoring in a public bathroom stall." The initial assessment seeks to rapidly identify concerns with mental status, airway, breathing, and circulation. Threats to life need to be quickly managed by measures such as a head tilt–chin lift, suctioning, or ventilation assistance with a bag-mask device. The initial assessment may identify the MOI or nature of illness and the need for additional units and set the priority and "tone" of the call.

Focused History and Physical Exam

After completing the initial assessment, begin the focused history and physical exam. With a trauma case, you will need to classify the patient as having a significant or nonsignificant MOI. With a significant MOI, you must quickly perform a rapid trauma assessment of the major body regions—head, neck, chest, abdomen, pelvis, back, buttocks, and four extremities. Obtain a set of baseline vital signs and a SAMPLE history. This patient should also receive a detailed physical exam en route to the hospital. If the patient does not have a significant MOI, perform a focused exam of the injured body part—that is, evaluate distal pulse, motor, and sensory functions, and range of motion.

Special Considerations

In an accidental overdose or poisoning, a geriatric patient may have become confused about his or her drug regimen. The person may have forgotten that the medication had been taken and repeat the dose one or more times. The patient could also have forgotten the doctor's instructions to discard leftover medication and might have taken the current and the older drug, resulting in increased effects or unwanted drug interactions. A geriatric patient may also intentionally overdose in a suicide attempt.

Most poisoning and overdose cases involve patients with medical conditions, so you will need to elaborate on their chief complaint using the OPQRST questions. If the patient is not responsive, perform a rapid medical assessment (basically the same as the rapid trauma assessment), obtain baseline vital signs, and ask the SAMPLE history questions of the family or bystanders, if possible. If the patient is responsive, complete the SAMPLE history, obtain the baseline vital signs, and conduct a focused exam targeting the body system most relevant to the complaint (for example, cardiovascular, pulmonary, neurologic, trauma).

Detailed Physical Exam

The detailed physical exam should be conducted en route to the ED, unless you are delayed on the scene and have the time to complete it there. Such an exam is usually conducted on a patient who has trauma with a significant MOI—as may occur in an overdosed or a poisoned patient who fell, was assaulted, or decided he or she could "fly." The detailed physical exam is similar to the rapid trauma assessment except that it is slower, is more involved, and looks more closely at the head. After completing the detailed physical exam, prioritize the injuries, manage them appropriately, and document your findings on the patient care report.

Ongoing Assessment

The ongoing assessment includes reassessment, reprioritizing, and checking the effectiveness of interventions provided. It is done en route to the ED. Continually monitor all patients who have ingested, injected, absorbed, or inhaled a poisonous substance, and be aware that they may vomit at any point.

▌Assessment and Management of Overdose With Specific Substances

From a management perspective, ALS care builds on the basics:

- Ensure the scene is safe for access and egress.
- Maintain the airway.
- Ensure that breathing is adequate.
- Ensure that circulation isn't compromised (that is, by hypoperfusion or arrhythmia).
- Administer high-concentration supplemental oxygen.
- Establish vascular access.

- Be prepared to manage shock, coma, seizures, and arrhythmias.
- Transport the patient as soon as possible. Place the patient in the left lateral recumbent position if there is any risk of vomiting to reduce the risk of aspiration.

Stimulants

Few drugs compare with stimulants in potential for abuse—particularly cocaine, amphetamines, and methamphetamine. A first-time user may become an addict to one of these substances within just a few days. If the person decides to quit using the stimulant, the likelihood that he or she will succeed over the long haul is virtually nil. Sadly, the only way out of methamphetamine or cocaine addiction is often an early death.

Depending on the formulation, stimulant drugs may be taken orally, smoked, or injected intravenously. The clinical presentation of the stimulant abuser includes excitement, delirium, tachycardia, hypertension with a fast pulse rate or hypotension with a fast pulse rate, and dilated pupils. As toxic levels are reached, the patient may develop outright psychosis, hyperpyrexia, tremors, seizures, and cardiac arrest.

The chronic "speed freak" or "tweaker" is easily recognized by a wild-eyed but thin-as-a-rail appearance, nervous or jittery movements, and often picked-raw skin. For a serious abuser, week-long runs without sleeping are not unusual, and the person often goes days without eating during such a period. As the days pass, increasing paranoia makes encounters risky. Patients are usually "amped up" when you encounter them, and it often takes very little to set off a violent tirade.

Cocaine

Cocaine is a naturally occurring alkaloid that is extracted from the *Erythroxylon coca* plant leaves found in South America. In the sixth century, the chewing of coca leaves was a daily event for people living in the coca-growing region of South America. With a relative purity of only about 2%, the leaves served as a mild stimulant, with no real potential for overdose. Chewing coca leaves also produced anorexia, euphoria, and improved energy. Once processed into cocaine hydrochloride, however, the active ingredient in the leaves goes from 2% to 100% pure, drastically increasing its toxic potential.

During the 1800s, cocaine and opium were commonly found in the elixirs, potions, and syrups sold by traveling medicine shows in the United States. Although neither substance cures anything, the people who used these products did not complain, given the drugs' euphoria-producing capabilities.

In more recent times, use of cocaine has had devastating effects on the US population. Since 1988, ED visits by cocaine abusers have tripled, and more than 50 tons of cocaine makes its way into the United States every year. Cocaine is sold under many street names (blow, flake, lady, nose candy, snow, toot). When the National Household Survey on Drug Abuse was conducted in 2000, approximately 1.2 million Americans were current cocaine users. Once addicted to the drug, people will spend their last penny trying to replicate the intensity and unique euphoria from their first cocaine experience. Cocaine addicts will sell everything they own and anything they can steal to support their addiction. Along the way, they inevitably lose their jobs, their homes, and their family and friends.

Cocaine is a local anesthetic and a CNS stimulant. It also has the ability to create a euphoria that features enhanced alertness and a tremendous sense of well-being. Collectively, this constellation of effects makes cocaine one of—if not the most—psychologically addictive drug available.

Today, cocaine has limited use in clinical medicine, mostly in ear, nose, throat, and eye surgery. This water-soluble hydrochloride salt is quickly absorbed across all mucosal membranes, allowing it to be applied topically, swallowed, or injected intravenously. In higher societal strata, cocaine is usually insufflated (snorted) and occasionally injected. In the lower societal strata, crack cocaine and IV drug abuse are more prevalent. Crack cocaine is simply cocaine mixed with two inexpensive ingredients, baking soda and water. Once mixed together into a pastelike slurry and cooked or baked, the end result is smokable cocaine (crack).

When cocaine is snorted nasally, effects are felt within 1 to 2 minutes, and peak effects occur in 20 to 30 minutes. After the intense, initial high, only 15 to 30 minutes passes before the user wants to redose. When cocaine is smoked and the alveoli are literally bathed in cocaine-laden smoke, the onset of effects is much more rapid (in the 8- to 10-second range) and the high is even more intense than when cocaine is snorted.

When the effects of cocaine wear off, a predictable cycle of events occurs. The user experiences a "crash," which is characterized by depression, irritability, sleeplessness, and exhaustion. To avoid this crash, the user will often seek more cocaine. Men commonly turn to theft to support their habit, whereas women often turn to prostitution.

Adding to the problem, a cocaine addict who is trying to escape the unpleasant effects of a crash often takes a sedative (such as diazepam [Valium], alcohol, or heroin). Thus, a chronic cocaine user probably practices polypharmacy and may be dependent on more than cocaine, increasing the likelihood that he or she will need EMS care, possibly overdosed on uppers, downers, or both.

A person who has overdosed on cocaine may exhibit any of the signs and symptoms for stimulants in general (discussed earlier). Furthermore, cocaine has been reported to cause a variety of serious—sometimes fatal—complications: lethal ECG arrhythmias, acute myocardial infarction, seizures, stroke, apnea, and hyperthermia. In addition, a crack smoker risks pneumothorax and pneumomediastinum.

Give particular attention to the ECG rhythm in case of suspected cocaine overdose. Cocaine has quinidinelike effects on cardiac conduction, causing widening of the QRS and QT prolongation. With increased dosing levels, cocaine exerts potentially deadly, toxic effects on the myocardium, which may present as wide-complex arrhythmias, negative inotropic effects with decreased cardiac output, hypotension, or tachycardia initially, followed by bradycardia.

Speedballing refers to the combined use of heroin and cocaine. Heroin addicts may use cocaine to withdraw or detoxify themselves from heroin by gradually decreasing the amounts of heroin taken while increasing the amounts of cocaine used. Addicts claim that cocaine provides relief from the unpleasant withdrawal effects that accompany heroin abstinence in a dependent user.

Amphetamine, Methamphetamine, and Amphetamine-like Drugs

Amphetamines are structurally similar to the derivatives of phenylethylamine and include methamphetamine (crank or ice), methylenedioxyamphetamine (MDA, Adam), and methylenedioxymethamphetamine (MDMA, Eve, ecstasy). Amphetamine and amphetamine-like drugs have a number of legitimate clinical applications. Most nasal decongestants and diet pills are members of this family, as are the drugs used to treat narcolepsy, attention-deficit disorder, and attention-deficit/hyperactivity disorder **Figure 33-7 ▾**.

Methamphetamine is problematic because it is a low-cost, long-acting (up to 12 hours) stimulant that is extremely addictive. Little of the United States has escaped the scourge of this drug. Because the ingredients to cook methamphetamine are available locally within the United States and the drug is easily and quickly made, its manufacture avoids the hassle, risk, and high cost associated with importing cocaine. "Meth labs" are dangerous and should be treated as a hazardous materials incident (see Chapter 50).

The clinical presentation of the patient abusing amphetamine or methamphetamine is almost identical to that of a person abusing cocaine, with the primary exception that the effects of the former drugs last many hours longer than those of cocaine. Patient management remains the same as well. In the majority of cases, prehospital management is primarily supportive. Never forget about the potential emotional and psychological instability, particularly in patients who have been on a "run." With each passing day of no sleep and little or no

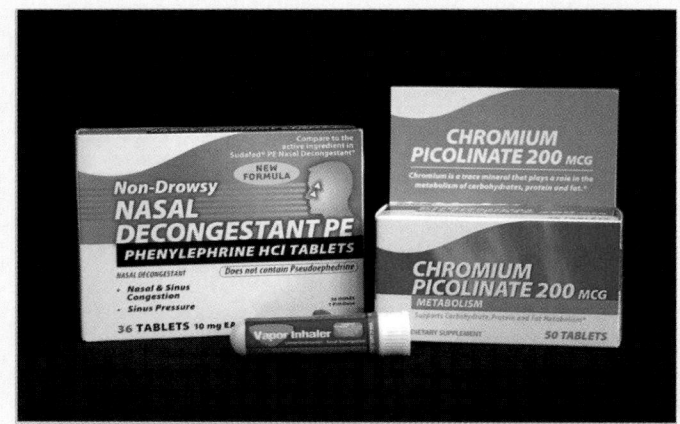

Figure 33-7 Drugs such as nasal decongestants and diet pills stimulate the sympathetic nervous system and can be detrimental to patients with an underlying cardiovascular disease.

food, they become increasingly paranoid and even psychotic. In the blink of an eye, their behavior can become violent, so consider the situation a potential hazard. At the first hint of trouble, contact law enforcement for support. (Chapter 37 deals with the issue of restraint in detail.)

Management of Stimulant Abuse

The treatment for patients abusing cocaine, amphetamine, or methamphetamine is fundamentally the same: maintain maximum oxygen saturation levels, prevent seizures with adequate sedation, and monitor serial vital signs.

- Establish and maintain the airway. Consider an advanced airway as needed.
- Give high-concentration supplemental oxygen.
- Establish vascular access.
- Apply the ECG monitor, pulse oximeter, and capnometer.
- To control anxiety and seizures, administer benzodiazepines per local protocol.
- Manage hypotension with a fluid infusion of normal saline.
- For uncontrolled hypertension, contact medical control regarding administration of nitroprusside.
- For violent behavior, contact medical control for consideration of intramuscular (IM) haloperidol (Haldol; chemical restraint).
- Transport to the appropriate facility.
- The administration of beta-adrenergic antagonist agents is *absolutely contraindicated* for patients abusing stimulants.

In severe cases of stimulant overdose, the patient may present with hyperthermia, which can be lethal. Application of ice packs or misting the patient's skin may reduce his or her temperature.

Throughout the resuscitation process, it is essential to maintain urine output with aggressive fluid therapy. Regular assessment of breath sounds to avoid inadvertent overhydration is a must.

If the patient has a seizure, benzodiazepines constitute first-line therapy. Should the situation worsen into status epilepticus, phenobarbital may be administered. In addition, neuromuscular blockade may be needed to control motor activity to avoid hyperthermia, acidosis, and, potentially, rhabdomyolysis.

Marijuana and Cannabis Compounds

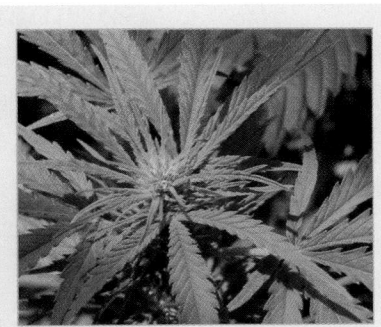

Figure 33-8 A marijuana plant.

When the leaves and flower buds of the *Cannabis sativa* plant are harvested and dried, the end product is referred to as marijuana (also known as weed, pot, dope, and smoke; Figure 33-8 ◄). The resin produced by the maturing flower tops can also be harvested and used to produce hashish (also known as hash). Clinical uses of marijuana are limited but include the treatment of glaucoma and relief of nausea and appetite loss for patients undergoing chemotherapy.

The primary psychoactive ingredient in marijuana and hashish is delta 9-tetrahydrocannabinol. Marijuana is usually smoked but can be ingested (such as when baked in cookies or brownies). The onset of effects from smoking marijuana is a matter of minutes; oral ingestion slows the onset time to several hours. When smoked, the effects generally last 2 to 4 hours. When ingested, the effects can last twice as long.

Although classified as a hallucinogen, marijuana does not produce true hallucinations (unlike PCP, LSD, and mescaline), but users may have a distorted sense of time and space and, occasionally, a feeling of unreality. Smoking marijuana results in bronchodilation and slight tachycardia. Other signs and symptoms of marijuana use include euphoria, drowsiness, decreased short-term memory, diminished motor coordination, increased appetite, and bloodshot eyes.

Management focuses on supportive care because the likelihood of serious medical complication is small. A novice user may exhibit some behavioral symptoms such as paranoia and (rarely) psychosis. Psychological first aid and reassurance generally suffices to address either issue. If the patient remains anxious, low-dose benzodiazepines may be administered. Transport for continued evaluation is rarely warranted, but providing information for support and counseling services can be helpful.

Hallucinogens

A hallucinogen is a substance that causes some distortion of sense perception—seeing, hearing, or feeling things that are not actually present. These outcomes are termed psychedelic effects. Experiences involving hallucinogens can vary markedly, with people taking the same dose of the same drug from the same batch experiencing totally different effects. The overall drug experience is affected by the user's previous drug experience, the dose taken, the user's expectations, and the social setting.

A wide variety of substances have been used over the centuries for their hallucinogenic properties, and these substances can be classified into two categories: synthetic and naturally occurring. The synthetic class includes LSD, PCP, and ketamine. The naturally occurring hallucinogens include mescaline, psilocybin mushroom, and the seeds of the Jimson weed plant.

LSD

In 1947, Dr Albert Hoffman discovered what would be the prototype for synthetic hallucinogens, LSD. Use of this drug peaked in the 1960s and then faded, but LSD resurfaced with a vengeance in the 1990s. LSD is considered a non–habit-forming drug, although tolerance can occur if it is taken for several days in a row.

LSD primarily affects the senses rather than changing physiologic functions. Synthesthesias (crossing of the senses) often prompt a user to respond to the question "What were you doing?" with a reply such as "I was watching the music play" or "I was listening to that painting." Users often experiment with LSD for self-exploration, for religious reasons, or to experience its often stunning visual and auditory effects.

Because of LSD's high potency, as little as 25 µg can produce CNS effects. A single dose or "hit" is 25 to 100 µg, although many users take three or more hits. As dosing increases to about 1,000 µg, there is a proportional increase in the drug's effects, which may last as long as 12 hours, although 3 to 4 hours is more typical.

From a physiologic perspective, the effects of LSD are mostly sympathomimetic, often consisting of tachycardia, mild hypertension, and dilated pupils. In a "bad trip," the user has a frightening experience, resulting in an acute anxiety attack and the physical effects secondary to increased anxiety.

The treatment for a patient using LSD is primarily supportive, focusing on the psychological aspects of the drug experience. For a person having a bad trip, think of it as being in a living nightmare or a dream that is as real as reality; this dream doesn't end until the drug wears off, however. Try to limit sensory stimulation as much as possible—for example, by avoiding the use of emergency lights and sirens. Routine transport to the appropriate facility plus psychological support are usually all that is required in the prehospital setting.

Phencyclidine

PCP, also called angel dust or dust, was developed in the late 1950s. In clinical trial, problems with the drug—namely, delirium and psychoticlike symptoms—led to PCP to be relegated to use as an animal tranquilizer (Syrnalan). PCP abuse was first noted in the 1970s. The majority of PCP available on the streets today is manufactured in clandestine laboratories, so variations in potency and purity are common. PCP is also a contaminant in many other street drugs.

Although PCP is grouped with the hallucinogens here, it is actually classified as a dissociative anesthetic. It is typically smoked or snorted, although it can be injected. Small doses (25–50 mg) can produce signs and symptoms of intoxication in an adult, with the high from a single dose typically lasting 4 to 6 hours. Slurred speech, staggering gait, tachycardia, hypertension, staring blankly for extended periods, and horizontal nystagmus (involuntary, rhythmic movement of the eyes) are common with PCP use. Muscle rigidity and especially grinding of the teeth prompt many users to resort to pacifiers in an effort to avoid pronounced jaw aches.

More problematic are the mind-body separation, related hallucinations, and violent outbreaks that are hallmarks of PCP use. Users may make bizarre comments such as "I can fly" and then jump off a balcony to prove it. Users have an almost unfathomable ability to take pain with no reaction and exhibit almost superhuman strength. In one case, it took four very large fire fighters to subdue and contain a young female weighing approximately 100 pounds who was intoxicated on PCP. Police who use taser-type devices often tell stories of PCP victims not even being bothered by its effects.

PCP can cause some of the most violent and difficult behavior you will encounter in the field, so care focuses on protecting the patient and the EMS team from attacks involving poor judgment and impaired behavior. Given that no PCP antagonist exists, there is little reason to insert an IV line—especially because even the slightest event can send a PCP abuser into a violent tirade. If you can safely establish vascular access, you will have a route to administer benzodiazepines if the patient starts to act inappropriately. Haloperidol can be given by the IM route in an emergency situation. Give high-flow oxygen, monitor vital signs, and provide safe transport to an appropriate facility.

Ketamine

Ketamine (special K, vitamin K; also discussed in Chapter 38) is an analog of PCP and another dissociative anesthetic. Most ketamine available on the street is stolen from veterinary clinics, although this drug is used in clinical medicine, primarily for pediatrics. Ketamine, which is colorless and odorless, is commonly found in powdered form. It is often mixed in a drink, although it can be snorted. It is physically and psychologically addicting.

Typical oral dosing is 75 to 300 mg. When snorted, the dose is reduced slightly, to 15 to 200 mg. At low doses, a user presents with mild inebriation, dreamy or erotic thoughts, and increased sociability. At higher doses, a patient may have pronounced nausea, difficulty moving, and a complaint of "entering another reality." In extreme cases, users will enter the "K hole," which involves out-of-body experiences.

Although violent outbreaks are much less likely with ketamine than with PCP, the principles of management are the same for the two drugs. Secure the patient well, assess and manage the ABCs, provide oxygen therapy, and establish vascular access if time and the situation allow as you provide safe transport to the appropriate facility. Keep a close eye on the patient because violent behavior can occur in the blink of an eye.

Peyote and Mescaline

Native tribes in the southwestern United States and Mexico have been using hallucinogens for thousands of years, primarily for religious purposes, with their primary drug of choice being mescaline. Ingesting between 3 and 12 of the dried flower "buttons" of the peyote cactus delivers a dose of 200 to 500 mg of mescaline **Figure 33-9 ▶**. The buttons have a bitter taste and act as a gastric irritant, with profound vomiting occurring shortly after their ingestion. The psychedelic experience then typically begins with feelings of increased sensitivity to sensory stimulation. Flashes of color, commonly in geometric

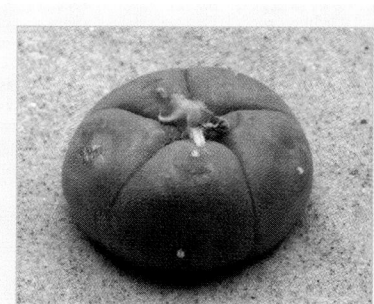

Figure 33-9 A peyote cactus. Dried flower buttons of the peyote cactus contain mescaline and produce a hallucinogenic effect if ingested.

patterns, are noted, although images of animals and people may also arise. Users experience a distortion of time and space, and out-of-body experiences are commonly reported.

The chemical structure of mescaline does not resemble that of LSD, although the two drugs produce similar psychedelic effects. Structurally, mescaline looks more like amphetamine, which accounts for its physical effects: dilated pupils, increased heart rate, mild hypertension, and increased body temperature.

Care in the field setting is primarily supportive. Pay attention to the ABCs, give supplemental oxygen therapy, monitor vital signs, provide positive psychological support, and arrange safe transport to the receiving facility.

Psilocybin Mushrooms

After LSD, psilocybin mushrooms **Figure 33-10 ▾** are probably the most frequently used hallucinogens in the United States. Use of hallucinogenic mushrooms dates from at least 100 to 1400 AD in Mexico and Central America. In Guatemala, mushroom artifacts that suggest use of psilocybin tea as an after-dinner drink have been traced back as far as 500 BC.

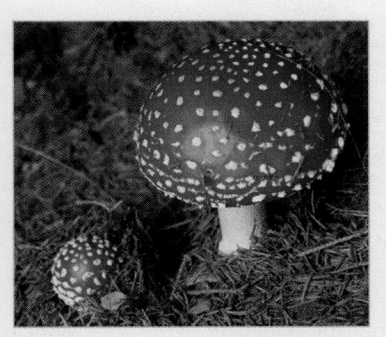

Figure 33-10 Certain mushrooms are hallucinogenic if ingested.

Hallucinogenic mushrooms come from several different genera, including *Psilocybe*. In the United States, the most commonly abused are the *Psilocybe mexicana* and *Psilocybe cyaescens* varieties. The typical dose is estimated to be 4 to 10 mg (approximately 2–4 mushrooms). Consumption of 100 mushrooms or more as a single dose has been reported.

The onset of symptoms and hallucinogenic effects (similar to LSD but less intense) is within 30 minutes of ingestion, and effects usually last 4 to 6 hours. Signs and symptoms include nausea and vomiting, mydriasis, mild tachycardia, and mild hypertension. The likelihood of any serious medical side effects is low, although the literature describes seizures and hyperthermia in some cases.

Treat the patient with supportive care. Attention to the ABCs and monitoring vital signs are usually all that is required, along with safe transport to the appropriate facility. If time and circumstances allow, establish vascular access to facilitate seizure control with benzodiazepines, if necessary.

Sedatives and Hypnotics

The drugs in the sedative-hypnotic category have a wide range of applications. Drugs with sedative qualities are used to reduce anxiety and to calm agitated patients. Drugs with hypnotic qualities are used as sleep aids, helping produce drowsiness and sleep. In either case, sedative-hypnotic drugs function primarily as CNS depressants.

Barbiturates

The barbiturates have a long history of use as sleep aids, antianxiety drugs, and seizure control medications. Barbiturate use and abuse reached its peak in the late 1970s, when these drugs were often tagged with street names that coincided with the color of the pill or capsule: reds (secobarbital), yellows or yellow jackets (pentobarbital), blues or blue heavens (amobarbital), and rainbows (amobarbital plus secobarbital).

The frequent combination of alcohol and barbiturates as a suicide mechanism, coupled with the high incidence of accidental overdoses, pushed researchers to develop sedative-hypnotic drugs that had fewer depressive effects on the respiratory system and were less lethal. Today, the likelihood of death after the ingestion of a single-entity sedative-hypnotic such as diazepam is small.

Barbiturates come in four basic configurations: long-acting, intermediate-acting, short-acting, and ultra–short-acting. The long-acting barbiturates tend to be less lipid soluble, which results in a delayed onset and long duration of action. By comparison, the short- and ultra–short-acting barbiturates are highly lipid soluble, so they can quickly move across the blood-brain barrier and exert their effects in a matter of minutes. Phenobarbital, for example, is a long-acting barbiturate, which makes it ideal for use in seizure control. If the patient delays taking this medication for a few hours, there is no real impact. Conversely, delaying a dose of an ultra–short-acting barbiturate might lead to a seizure. The liver metabolizes most barbiturates into inactive waste products, although drugs that bind less tightly to proteins tend to be excreted unchanged in the urine.

Your assessment findings will reflect the dosing and the configuration of the barbiturate. With mild to moderate barbiturate intoxication, patients present much like alcohol intoxication; their symptoms include drowsiness, decreased inhibitions, ataxia, mental confusion, and staggering gait. As the dose increases, the patient moves farther down the scale of CNS depression, becoming increasingly lethargic and demonstrating an increasingly lower level of responsiveness until he or she is comatose (that is, no neurologic response and a Glasgow Coma Scale score of 3).

Care for a patient who has overdosed on barbiturates follows a logical and predictable path. Because of the CNS depressant effects of these drugs, airway control is the first management priority, often requiring intubation to secure the airway and prevent aspiration should the patient vomit. Next, you should administer high-concentration supplemental oxygen, monitor the ECG rhythm, and establish venous access. It is prudent to use pulse oximetry and capnography to monitor hemoglobin saturation and the effectiveness of respiration and ventilation.

If shock develops, rapid infusion of 1 to 2 L of crystalloids may be needed—specifically, as sequential boluses of normal saline. Assess breath sounds before and after each bolus, rather than simply infusing an entire liter and then assessing breath sounds. The bolus approach is particularly indicated for older patients and for patients with renal disease or decreased cardiac function. If hypotension persists, administer a vasopressor such as dopamine.

For the long-acting barbiturates such as phenobarbital, administering a dose of 1 to 2 mEq of sodium bicarbonate helps alkalinize the urine and traps the drug in its ionized form, promoting effective excretion in the urine. This therapy is not effective for shorter-acting barbiturates, however. Use of fluid loading coupled with forced diuresis can further supplement urine alkalinization efforts, but again is limited to the long-acting barbiturates. Administration of IV furosemide will accomplish the task but is contraindicated for patients who are hypotensive or in shock.

Gastric emptying is not recommended unless you have good reason to believe that the patient ingested a life-threatening dose of barbiturates *and* the procedure can be implemented within 60 minutes of ingestion. In such a case, perform intubation to protect the airway before instituting gastric lavage. For patients outside the 1-hour window, use of activated charcoal is an option. Studies have shown that activated charcoal is at least as effective as gastric lavage and may be a better option because it almost immediately reduces serum barbiturate levels.

In the Field

While one provider explains the use of charcoal to the patient, the other can prepare a large plastic garbage bag to hang on the patient as a bib. This will help contain the charcoal solution if the patient vomits.

Barbiturate abusers quickly develop tolerance and require ever-larger doses to produce the desired effects. Long-term use results in physical addiction. Abrupt cessation in a long-term barbiturate abuser will produce typical signs and symptoms of withdrawal syndrome in approximately 24 hours, with potentially life-threatening signs and symptoms arising during a period of several days to a week. In the case of minor withdrawal, the patient may present with symptoms similar to those observed in a patient with alcohol withdrawal: restlessness and anxiety, depression, insomnia, diaphoresis, abdominal cramping, and nausea and vomiting. With severe cases of withdrawal, expect delirium, hallucinations, psychosis, seizures, hyperthermia, and cardiovascular collapse.

Notes from Nancy

Consider the possibility of a drug-related problem in any patient presenting with unexplained behavioral changes, stupor, coma, or seizures.

If you encounter barbiturate abstinence syndrome in the prehospital setting, focus your treatment efforts on preventing seizures (IV benzodiazepines are a common choice) and cardiovascular collapse. Rapid transport to an ED, with subsequent intensive care, will be required to best manage the patient over the long-term.

Benzodiazepines

Benzodiazepines are also members of the sedative-hypnotic family. They are most commonly used to treat anxiety, seizures,

You are the Provider Part 3

Upon completing your detailed physical exam, you determine that the cause of Julie's altered mental status is a possible overdose. As you insert an 18-gauge IV catheter in her right arm, your partner begins to prepare the equipment for intubation. You secure the IV line, begin to run a fluid challenge with normal saline, and turn your attention to securing an airway. Under direct visualization of the vocal cords, you insert a 6.5 endotracheal tube. Correct placement of the endotracheal tube is confirmed with auscultation of bilateral breath sounds, bilateral chest rise, and a positive color change on the end-tidal carbon dioxide detector. You secure the tube at the 23-cm mark at the teeth and ask your partner to ventilate via a bag-mask device at a rate of 12 breaths/min. You administer 0.4 mg of naloxone (Narcan) in case Julie ingested narcotics, but you do not get a response.

As you begin to package Julie for transport, her friend returns with an empty pill bottle that she found next to Julie's backpack in the locker room. The label reveals a prescription for amitriptyline (Elavil) filled the day before; the prescription was for 60 pills.

Reassessment	Recording Time: 10 Minutes
Skin	Flushed, warm, and dry
Pulse	160 beats/min; regular and weak
ECG	Possible wide complex tachycardia
Blood pressure	80/50 mm Hg
Respirations	12 breaths/min via bag-mask device
Sao_2	97% on 100% supplemental oxygen via bag-mask device
Pupils	Dilated
Blood glucose	76 g/dL

5. Given the current situation, should you consider treating the patient on the scene or continuing treatment on the way to the hospital?

6. How should your patient management progress?

and alcohol withdrawal. In recent years, the use of fast-acting benzodiazepines such as zolpidem tartrate for treatment of insomnia has grown rapidly. Drugs such as zolpidem tartrate can be easily obtained from Internet sources, increasing the likelihood of abuse.

Benzodiazepines exert their effects by stimulating the gamma-aminobutyric acid pathways, resulting in sedation, reduced anxiety, and relaxation of striated muscle. When taken orally, these medications are readily absorbed from the GI tract. IV administration allows for more rapid onset of action and more controlled dosing. Because IM injections of benzodiazepines other than lorazepam and midazolam often result in variable rates of absorption, the IV route is more desirable when administering benzodiazepines in the prehospital setting. These drugs are metabolized primarily by the liver.

Assessment of a patient who is abusing benzodiazepines can be complicated because the person is also likely to use other drugs and alcohol. In a single-entity overdose, benzodiazepines have a relatively low rate of morbidity and mortality. The most common clinical effects of benzodiazepine overdose include altered mentation, drowsiness, confusion, slurred speech, ataxia, and general incoordination. For a suspected overdose in which the patient presents with severe respiratory depression, hypotension, or coma, you need to think beyond a simple benzodiazepine event to other CNS depressants and alcohol. On occasion, extrapyramidal reactions may occur in tandem with hepatotoxic or hematologic reactions.

Treatment of benzodiazepine overdose is relatively straightforward:

- Assess and manage the airway, inserting an advanced airway as needed.
- Give high-concentration supplemental oxygen.
- Establish vascular access.
- Apply the ECG monitor, pulse oximeter, and capnometer.
- Consider administering flumazenil (a benzodiazepine antagonist) via slow IV push (0.2 mg IV/min) up to a total of 3 mg. Flumazenil is contraindicated for patients with head injuries and elevated intracranial pressure, and for patients who are dependent on benzodiazepines because it will precipitate seizures.
- Transport to the appropriate facility.

Narcotics, Opiates, and Opioids

A narcotic is a drug that produces sleep or altered mental status. Historically, narcotics have been classified into two major divisions: opiates and opioids. The term opiate is used to describe natural drugs derived from opium (that is, from poppy juice); the term opioid refers to non–opium-derived synthetics. We use the term *opioids* to describe licit therapeutic agents and illicit substances in this group.

Narcotics have a long history of use and abuse, with writings as far back as the third century BC mentioning the use of poppy juice. Today, abuse of narcotics remains one of the most common causes of overdose deaths reported to Poison Centers.

Narcotic agents include morphine, codeine, heroin, fentanyl, oxycodone, meperidine, propoxyphene, and dextromethorphan.

Although these drugs share certain commonalities, they exhibit highly diverse effects and vary widely in their potency. Opioids are used primarily in clinical medicine for analgesia, whereas the illicit drug heroin is abused for the unique euphoria it produces. In terms of potency, 80 to 100 mg of meperidine (Demerol) produces analgesia for 2 to 4 hours; 10 mg of morphine produces a similar effect for 4 to 5 hours; and just 2 mg of hydromorphone (Dilaudid) has an analgesic effect, which also lasts for 4 to 5 hours.

Opioids produce their major effects on the CNS by binding with receptor sites in the brain and other tissues. The highest concentrations of receptor sites are found in the limbic system, frontal and temporal cortices, thalamus, hypothalamus, midbrain, and spinal cord.

Opioids are readily absorbed from the GI tract but can also be absorbed from the nasal mucosa (when snorted) or from the lungs (opium smoking). When taken orally, the effects of these drugs are lessened owing to their significant first-pass metabolism through the liver compared with their effects when given parenterally. When heroin passes through the liver, it is metabolized into acetyl-morphine, which continues to exert narcotic effects that may outlast the effects of naloxone. A paramedic who does not understand this concept can be fooled into thinking that a dose of naloxone has permanently reversed the effects of the heroin, only to have the patient lapse into unconsciousness 15 or 20 minutes later.

Morphine is a commonly used analgesic in the prehospital setting and is a potent vasodilator. When given to young adults, its half-life is roughly 2 to 3 hours, but it typically takes longer to metabolize in older adults.

Assessment

The classic presentation of opioid use features euphoria, hypotension, respiratory depression, and pinpoint pupils. Depending on the particular agent, nausea, vomiting, and constipation may occur as well. Allergic phenomena may also occur with opioid use, albeit rarely. With increased doses, coma, seizures (usually secondary to hypoxia), and cardiac arrest (usually secondary to respiratory arrest) are common.

Morphine (named after Morpheus, the god of dreams) and heroin produce an impressive dreamlike state. Shortly after injecting heroin, a user will appear to pass out (in street terms, "going on the nod"). However, the user is typically quite lucid and remains aware of what is being done or said.

Management

Because of the CNS depressant effects, patient management initially focuses on establishing and maintaining a patent airway and providing adequate ventilation. A patient who has overdosed on opioids is almost always hypoventilating, sometimes breathing as few as 4 or 5 breaths/min, and is consequently hypoxic and hypercarbic. Rather than moving immediately to intubation, place an oropharyngeal airway and provide bag-mask ventilation with 15 L/min of supplemental oxygen.

Next, establish vascular access and administer 0.4 to 2 mg of naloxone. For street heroin, which can range in purity from 5% to 30%, as little as 0.4 mg of naloxone may bring a patient back to consciousness before you can remove the needle from the injection port. This abrupt reversal can have clinical and safety implications—the fact that you've just reversed a $40 buzz with a few pennies' worth of naloxone will not make you popular. The best approach is to draw up 2 mg of naloxone in a 10-mL syringe and fill the rest of the syringe with normal saline. Administer the naloxone just to the point that the patient's respirations improve, rather than waking the patient up completely.

Sometimes the patient may not respond to naloxone. Perhaps the patient has taken a potent synthetic drug such as fentanyl, which may require a much higher dose of naloxone to reverse its effects. In one case, a patient presented with the classic signs and symptoms of opioid overdose. When he showed no response to 2.0 mg of naloxone, medical control ordered 10 mg of naloxone, which aroused the patient for only approximately 30 seconds, after which he became unconscious again. Ultimately, it took 40 mg of naloxone at the hospital to bring the patient back to consciousness. It was determined that the patient had taken a dose of a fentanyl analog that was several thousand times more potent than a typical dose of heroin.

A second possibility if the patient doesn't respond to naloxone is that the person has a "mixed-bag overdose"—that is, the patient may have taken multiple drugs, some of which aren't opioids and won't respond to naloxone. Alternatively, the coma may be from another source altogether, such as a head injury. In such a scenario, insert an advanced airway (endotracheal tube, Combitube, or laryngeal mask airway), provide other care as needed, and transport the patient to an appropriate facility.

Cardiac Medications

The medications used to treat patients with cardiac and cardiac-related problems continue to increase in number and sophistication. The major classes of drugs used as part of these treatment regimens include antiarrhythmics, beta blockers, calcium channel blockers, cardiac glycosides, and angiotensin-converting enzyme inhibitors. Many patients take a combination of drugs, sometimes three or more, in attempts to control hypertension, ECG rhythm disturbances, or other problems. Overdoses with these drugs are usually accidental—a result of the multidrug approach to cardiac care—because these types of drugs do not produce effects desirable to recreational drug abusers.

Signs and symptoms of overdose with cardiac drugs vary but may include hypotension, weakness or confusion, nausea and vomiting, rhythm disturbances (most commonly bradycardia or heart block), headache, and difficulty breathing. As with all emergencies, ensure a patent airway, provide adequate ventilation, and administer high-flow supplemental oxygen.

Establish vascular access in case of overdose with these agents because several therapeutic interventions and antidotes are available if the specific agent is identified. For a beta blocker overdose, glucagon is the drug of choice. For a calcium channel blocker overdose, calcium gluconate and calcium

chloride are options. Among the most problematic cardiac medications in propensity to reach toxic levels are the cardiac glycosides (such as digoxin), which typically have very small therapeutic windows. For an overdose with these agents, digoxin immune Fab (Digibind) is the antidote of choice. In case of hypotension, sequential fluid boluses of normal saline will often bring the blood pressure into an acceptable range.

Because of the sophistication of cardiac drugs and the likelihood that the patient maybe taking multiple cardiac and other medications, making contact with medical control to consult with a physician is prudent.

Organophosphates

Organophosphates are a major component in many insecticides used in agriculture and in the home; they include orthene, Diazinon, and Malathion. Similar-performing compounds are used in chemical warfare. Although carbamates were introduced as replacements for organophosphates, carbamates continue to cause thousands of cases of poisoning each year, with about 10% of victims requiring hospitalization. The death rate is around 10% for adults and nearly 50% for children.

Suicide attempts account for a considerable share of organophosphate poisonings. When suicide is the goal, the poison is usually taken by mouth. Accidental agricultural exposure is another common source, and persons involved in the manufacture of organophosphates and similar compounds are at risk. In one case, a farmer decided to burn the empty chemical bags after applying the pesticide and then did some work downwind of the fire. The smoke contained enough organophosphate residue to result in a 9-1-1 call and a trip to the ED.

US soldiers serving in the Persian Gulf, along with civilian populations within range of Iraqi missiles, were put at risk of mass organophosphate poisoning during the Gulf War. The nerve gases used in chemical weapons are members of the same family as agricultural pesticides, with nerve gases used in the military setting differing chiefly by increased potency.

Organophosphates exert their toxic effects at junctions (synapses) of the nerve cells of the autonomic nervous system. The conduction of an impulse from one nerve to another occurs through the release of acetylcholine at the synapse. Acetylcholine works as a chemical messenger, crossing the synapse to depolarize the nerve on the other side of the junction. Once it has delivered its message, the acetylcholine molecule must be inactivated or it would continue to stimulate the target nerve cell indefinitely, leaving the nerve cell unable to receive another message from the brain.

The symptoms of organophosphate poisoning are fundamentally the same regardless of entry by ingestion, inhalation, or absorption: anxiety and restlessness; headache, dizziness, and confusion; tremors or seizures; dyspnea, diffuse wheezing, and respiratory depression; and loss of consciousness. A patient poisoned with organophosphates will usually present with signs and symptoms within the first 8 hours. In addition, the CNS signs and symptoms associated with cholinergic excess are often expressed; the SLUDGE mnemonic, Salivation,

Lacrimation, Urination, Defecation, Gastric upset, and Emesis, is helpful in assessment.

Assessment and management of a patient with organophosphate poisoning start with decontamination and removal of all contaminated clothing *before* initiating care or loading the patient into the ambulance. Contaminated clothing should be placed in plastic bags and disposed of as hazardous materials. Ideally, the patient should be scrubbed with soap and water. After that, patient care includes the following measures:

- Establish and maintain the airway. Consider an advanced airway as needed.
- Suction as needed.
- Give high-flow supplemental oxygen.
- Establish vascular access.
- Administer 1.0 mg atropine IV push, and repeat the dose every 3 to 5 minutes until symptom reversal (that is, atropinization) occurs.
- Administer 1 to 2 g of pralidoxime (2-PAM) infused with normal saline during 5 to 10 minutes.
- Apply the ECG monitor, pulse oximeter, and capnometer.
- Immediately transport to the appropriate facility.

Carbon Monoxide

CO causes more poisoning deaths than any other toxic substance. CO is produced during the incomplete combustion of organic fuels, such as in an automobile engine or a home-heating device. CO poisoning is often a winter phenomenon, occurring when a flue or ventilating system becomes blocked. However, approximately half of successful adult suicides are caused by CO: An automobile running in a closed garage can generate a lethal concentration of CO in as little as 30 minutes. CO is also a major contributor to death in house fires.

CO is a colorless, odorless, tasteless gas, so people exposed to CO have no idea that they are inhaling a toxic substance until it is too late. The toxicity arises primarily from CO's affinity for hemoglobin in RBCs; CO displaces oxygen, thereby preventing the RBCs from carrying oxygen to the tissues and leading to suffocation at the cellular level. Hemoglobin's affinity for CO is more than 250 times its affinity for oxygen, so the atmospheric level of CO does not need to be very high for poisoning to occur. Even relatively small concentrations of CO in the atmosphere can convert a significant proportion of hemoglobin into carboxyhemoglobin (hemoglobin combined with carbon dioxide), making it ineffective as an oxygen carrier.

Because the overall ability of the blood to transport oxygen is so drastically reduced when CO reaches toxic levels, anything that increases the body's oxygen requirements, such as physical exertion or a fever, will increase the severity of the poisoning. Children, whose metabolic rate is intrinsically higher than that of adults, tend to have more severe symptoms at any given level of exposure.

CO poisoning can be difficult to diagnose in the field unless it is the direct result of an easily identifiable cause such as a fire or intentional exposure to exhaust fumes from an automobile. Its signs and symptoms are highly variable and quite vague,

In the Field

CO is a hazard for rescuers as well as for patients. Multiple patients with medical complaints—at the same time and inside the same building—equals poisoning until proven otherwise!

often resembling early onset of the flu—for example, headache, nausea, and vomiting. With acute CO poisoning, the patient may be confused and unable to think clearly. Complaints of a sensation of pressure in the head or roaring in the ears are common. Physical examination often reveals bounding pulses, dilated pupils, and pallor or cyanosis. Consider the possibility of CO poisoning whenever you are confronted with several (possibly many) people who have shared the same accommodations for any period, especially if they have been quartered together in a closed area, such as one house in the winter.

The cherry red color of the skin that is mentioned in many textbooks is a very late sign of CO poisoning. Put bluntly, cherry red usually means really dead.

Recent developments in technology have given paramedics the ability to perform noninvasive identification of CO poisoning (% SpCO) in the field, which helps address the problem of delayed diagnosis. Note that pulse oximetry *will not* provide a true assessment of arterial oxygenation because the device cannot determine whether CO or oxygen is bound to the hemoglobin. A reading of 99% on the pulse oximeter would be excellent in a normal environmental setting but would be a grave error in the presence of carboxyhemoglobin because the hemoglobin is saturated with the wrong chemical! Application of the ECG monitor to assess for cardiac ischemia can further support diagnostic and treatment efforts when CO is the suspected culprit.

Treatment of CO poisoning in the field is aimed at providing the highest concentration of oxygen possible to attempt to displace CO molecules from the hemoglobin. For patients with only mild symptoms, such as headache, nausea, and flulike symptoms, the elimination half-time of carboxyhemoglobin is roughly 4 hours. By comparison, if the patient is breathing 100% oxygen, the half-time can be reduced to about 1.5 hours. Hyperbaric oxygen therapy at 2.5 atmospheres of pressure can further reduce the elimination time to 15 to 20 minutes.

If you suspect CO poisoning:
- Remove the patient from the exposure environment.
- Establish and maintain the airway, inserting an advanced airway as needed.
- Give high-flow supplemental oxygen by tight-fitting nonrebreathing mask.
- Establish vascular access.
- Keep the patient quiet and at rest to minimize oxygen demand.
- Monitor the ECG rhythm and LOC.
- Transport to the appropriate facility. If the patient is unresponsive or has signs of serious CO poisoning, direct

transport to a facility capable of providing hyperbaric medicine is preferred.

- For patients with injuries or illness from a structural or vehicular fire, consider the possibility of combined CO/cyanide poisoning, especially if the patient has signs of shock. Contact medical control for an order to administer amyl nitrite or sodium thiosulfate, if available.

CO poisoning can be reversed if it is diagnosed and treated in time. Even if the patient recovers, however, acute CO poisoning may result in permanent damage to vital organs and lead to mild to severe neurologic deficits.

Chlorine Gas

Incidents involving chlorine gas are relatively common because of the widespread use of chlorine compounds in the home and occupational settings. Household exposures usually occur when someone mixes a cleaning agent containing sodium hypochlorite (such as bleach) with a strong acid in an overzealous attempt to "really clean" a toilet bowl Figure 33-11 . The resulting chemical reaction releases chlorine gas, often in high concentrations. Most cases of chlorine gas exposure occur outside the home, however. The chlorination of large swimming pools, which tends to rely on gaseous rather than liquid or solid forms of chlorine, has led to mass exposures at hotels and community recreation centers. Leakage of chlorine gas from an industrial storage tank, truck, or rail car can also result in a mass-casualty incident.

The signs and symptoms of chlorine gas exposure depend on the concentration of the inhaled gas and the duration of exposure. Chlorine gas is extremely irritating to all mucous membranes. When it comes in contact with the moisture on those surfaces, it can form hydrochloric and other acids that are damaging to human tissue. With a minor exposure, the patient

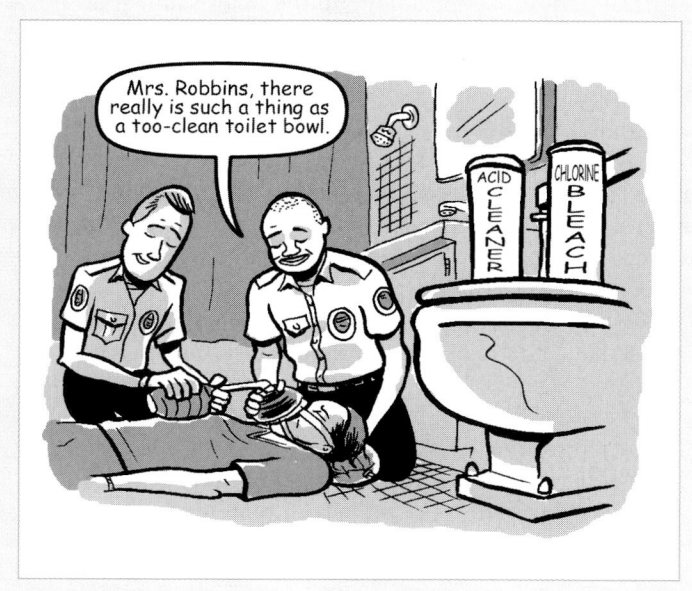

Figure 33-11

will experience burning sensations in the eyes, nose, and throat along with a slight cough. More intense exposure to chlorine gas causes chest tightness, choking, paroxysmal cough, headache, nausea and vomiting, and diffuse wheezing. Patients with more severe exposures may also develop cyanosis, crackles in the chest, shock, seizures, and loss of consciousness.

When treating patients who have been exposed to chlorine gas, your first priority is to remove them from the area of exposure. If the incident involves a serious gas spill, an upwind location for parking the ambulance is a must. Also make sure that all rescuers wear protective breathing apparatus.

Once in a safe environment, quickly triage the patients. People with dyspnea, wheezing, severe cough, or other signs of respiratory distress are priority patients and should ideally receive high-concentration, humidified oxygen by mask. Intubation and rapid-sequence intubation (RSI) are considerations as well. Irrigate burning or itching eyes with water, as well as any areas of the skin that have come in contact with the chlorine.

Cyanide

Cyanide is used in industry for electroplating, ore extraction, and fumigation of structures. In addition to industrial exposures, poisoning can occur after ingestion of cyanide contained in commercial products such as silver polish or from the seeds of cherries, apples, pears, and apricots. More commonly, cyanide poisoning occurs when a household fire results in the combustion of nitrogen-containing materials (such as plastic items or furnishings, wool carpeting, polyurethane silk).

Cyanide is one of the most rapid-acting and deadly poisons. This toxin does its damage by combining with a crucial cellular enzyme, cytochrome oxidase, which in turn blocks the utilization of oxygen at the cellular level. The results are cellular suffocation and death of the patient within seconds if the cyanide was inhaled or within minutes to possibly an hour or two if it was ingested.

Physical examination of a patient who has been poisoned with cyanide may reveal an altered mental state. If awake enough to answer questions, the patient may complain of headache, palpitations, or dyspnea. The classic odor of bitter almonds on the patient's breath is highly suggestive of cyanide poisoning but is not diagnostic. Respirations are usually rapid and labored early on; as the poisoning progresses, they become slow and gasping. The pulse is usually rapid and thready. Vomiting, seizures, and coma are common. The patient's venous blood and sometimes the patient's body may be bright red—even though oxygen is available in the bloodstream, it is not being taken up by the tissues. Thus, a patient who is cyanotic has either not been poisoned with cyanide or is very close to death.

Cyanide poisoning is a dire emergency that requires prompt treatment. The aim of treatment is to displace the cyanide from the cytochrome oxidase by introducing another chemical that will "attract" the cyanide. This involves administering three drugs—amyl nitrite, sodium nitrite, and sodium thiosulfate—which are contained in a commercially available cyanide antidote kit. If given in time, the treatment is usually effective.

If the cyanide poisoning occurred as the result of a toxic inhalation, have the patient *safely* removed from the source of the cyanide (the toxic environment). Establish a patent airway, administer 100% oxygen, and assist ventilation as necessary.

If a commercially available cyanide antidote kit is available, follow the instructions supplied with the kit. Break a vial of amyl nitrite into a gauze pad and hold it over the patient's nose for 20 seconds, and then remove it to allow the patient to breathe 100% oxygen for 40 seconds. Thus, in each minute, the patient should inhale amyl nitrite one third of the time and breathe 100% oxygen two thirds of the time. Alternate the amyl nitrite and oxygen until vascular access is available. Once vascular access is available, discontinue the amyl nitrite (continue the 100% oxygen) and administer 300 mg (10 mL) of sodium nitrite via slow (over 2 to 4 minutes) IV push, followed by 12.5 g (50 mL) of sodium thiosulfate via IV push.

Notes from Nancy

The most important aspect of treatment in toxic inhalations is to remove the patient from the toxic environment, but do not enter a known toxic environment without protective breathing apparatus.

Anticipate hypotension as a consequence of nitrite therapy. If the patient becomes hypotensive, stop the nitrite, elevate the patient's legs and treat for shock, and contact medical control about whether to administer an IV vasopressor. Monitor the patient's cardiac rhythm and vital signs closely, transport to an appropriate facility, and notify the receiving staff as early as possible.

Caustics

Caustics include strong acids (pH < 2.0) and strong alkalis (pH > 12.0). Both types of chemicals are commonly used in industry, agriculture (anhydrous ammonia), and the home **Table 33-4** and **Figure 33-12**. According to the American Association of Poison Control Centers (AAPCC), approximately 100,000 caustic exposures occur each year in the United States. Most cases involve accidental dermal or ocular exposure, although occasionally you may encounter oral ingestions. If the patient is an adult, oral ingestion of caustics is usually an intentional suicide attempt. Although many serious burns occur from caustics, including results such as cataracts and blindness, only about 20 people die each year of caustic exposure.

Caustic substances cause direct chemical injury to the tissues they contact. Signs and symptoms of a caustic exposure include severe pain, burns, difficulty talking or swallowing (with oral ingestions), and hypoperfusion or shock (rarely, usually secondary to internal bleeding).

The widespread practice of storing such substances in beverage containers (such as soft drink or milk bottles), usually

Table 33-4	**Common Caustic Substances**	
Substance	Example	Source
Acids	Hydrochloric acid	Toilet bowl cleaners, swimming pool cleaners
	Sulfuric acid	Battery acid, toilet bowl cleaners (as bisulfate)
	Others	Bleach disinfectants, slate cleaners
Alkalis	Lye (sodium or potassium hydroxide)	Paint removers, washing powders, drain cleaners (such as Drano, Liquid Plumr, Plunge), button-shaped batteries, Clinitest tablets
	Sodium hypochlorite	Bleach (Clorox)
	Sodium carbonate	Bleach (Purex), nonphosphate detergents
	Ammonia	Hair dyes, jewelry cleaners, metal cleaners or polishes, antirust agents
	Potassium permanganate	Electric dishwasher detergents

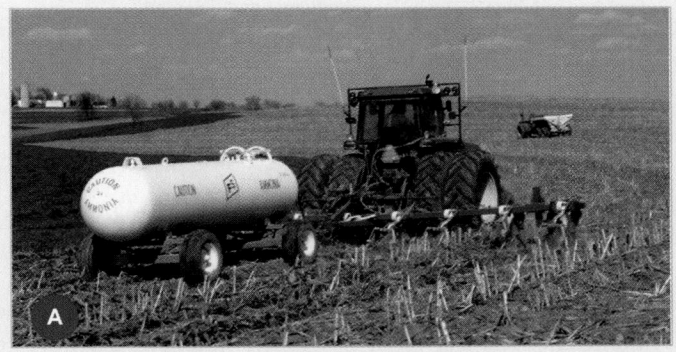

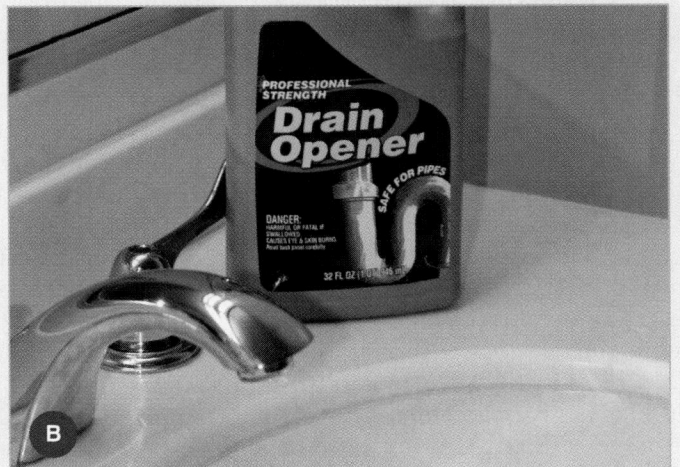

Figure 33-12 Caustic chemicals are commonly used in industry. **A.** Anhydrous ammonia tank used in agriculture. **B.** Plumbing agents used in the home.

because the original container has started to leak, increases the likelihood that a child will regard the substance as a tasty drink. As the liquid enters the mouth and begins to burn, the child may simultaneously remove the bottle and turn the head, resulting in burns to the mouth, tongue, and face.

Most patients who have swallowed caustic substances present with severe pain in the mouth, throat, or chest. Usually the airway is not a problem, nor is the patient in shock. Respiratory distress, if present, is most probably due to soft-tissue swelling in the larynx, epiglottis, or vocal cords, which means that the patient is in immediate danger of complete airway obstruction. For a caustic ingestion in an alert patient, giving milk—at least 6 to 8 ounces for a child and 8 to 12 ounces for an adult—may help if the Poison Center or medical control agrees. Establish vascular access, usually en route, because immediate transport to the ED is indicated.

Notes from Nancy

If a patient who swallowed a caustic agent is in respiratory distress, get moving without further delay to the hospital. Have your cricothyrotomy kit ready.

In the Field

Some chemicals react with water. Although small amounts can usually be flushed safely with large quantities of water, larger amounts of such chemicals can give off toxic fumes or explode when wet. Be sure to check the relevant warnings or placards.

With dermal exposure to a strong acid, the result is immediate and excruciating pain. For a strong alkali, the onset of pain is somewhat delayed, allowing more time before the patient reacts and increasing the severity of the burn. In such an injury, diluting and flushing away the caustic substance is the main goal of field treatment. Acids tend to be more water-soluble than alkalis, so they are often diluted relatively quickly. With alkalis, it is more important to keep water continually flowing because it usually takes much longer to rinse an alkali away (compared with an acid).

For an eye exposure, cut the prong section off a nasal cannula, place it on the bridge of the patient's nose, and plug in a macro IV administration set and run it wide open to provide continuous irrigation. This also frees you up to perform other tasks. A Morgan lens may also be used after the initial gross flushing has been accomplished.

One of the most common caustic exposures in the agricultural setting involves anhydrous ammonia. The exposure usually occurs during the hook-up or disconnection of a nurse tank. Farmers often keep a small water bottle in the shirt pocket, allowing them to immediately rinse their eyes should

an exposure occur. Without treatment, eye exposure to anhydrous ammonia can cause devastating damage in less than a minute, resulting in cataracts or blindness.

There are a number of significant "don'ts" for caustic ingestions:

- *Don't* give any "neutralizing substances." Some product laboratories incorrectly advise neutralizing the caustic agent—for example, by giving lemon juice or dilute vinegar (both weak acids) to a patient who has swallowed an alkali. Mixing an acid and an alkali produces *heat,* adding a thermal injury to the chemical injury.
- *Don't* induce vomiting—what burned on the way down will burn on the way up.
- *Don't* perform gastric lavage.
- *Don't* give activated charcoal. It is not effective in acid or alkali ingestion, and it may interfere with the patient's subsequent care by blackening the field of vision for an endoscopist who tries to inspect the esophagus and stomach for damage.

Common Household Items

From a toxicologic perspective, the average home is a nightmare. Many house plants have poisonous leaves or berries. All pesticides and herbicides used in lawn and garden care are potentially poisonous. All hydrocarbon products (such as paint thinners, solvents, gas) can cause permanent neurologic damage or death if inhaled in the right amount; the same is true of glue fumes (often called "huffing"). Many household cleaning agents are also toxic if ingested.

It is not possible within the scope of this chapter to discuss all of the possibilities when it comes to household poisonings. Some of the more likely culprits are covered in several of the other sections to assist in preparing you to handle the myriad possibilities. As always, keep in mind that the Poison Center is an invaluable resource.

Drugs Abused for Sexual Purposes

Drugs that are abused for sexual purposes include those that increase sexual gratification and those that are used to facilitate sexual assault.

Drugs That Increase Sexual Gratification

Drugs that increase sexual gratification constitute a long and varied list. Clearly, the most dangerous include erectile dysfunction medications such as sildenafil (Viagra), which are contraindicated for patients who take nitrates for cardiac problems. Their use by people taking nitrates may result in severe hypotension or total cardiovascular collapse, ultimately leading to death. For hypotension, repeated boluses of normal saline can bring the blood pressure up to an acceptable level. If cardiac arrest occurs, follow your protocols.

For some people, the relaxed dreamy high of marijuana is very desirable for sexual gratification. There is no overdose potential for marijuana. Supportive care is all that is required.

Cocaine and other stimulant drugs (such as amphetamines and methamphetamine) are popular choices for people seeking a more intense sexual experience. Should the patient have sustained tachycardia in such a case, hypotension can occur as a result of inadequate preload. Be alert for this possibility when the heart rate is in the range of 170 to 180 beats/min or higher, although a rate in the 160s could cause problems for a patient with an extensive cardiac history. Serial boluses of normal saline will usually stabilize the blood pressure. If fluid boluses are not effective, a vasopressor (such as dopamine or dobutamine) may be required.

Another drug that increases sexual gratification is amyl nitrite (poppers, rush, happy snaps). This organic nitrate drug can be crushed and inhaled, again producing an intense sexual experience. As with any nitrate, hypotension may result from blood pooling in the periphery owing to the drug's vasodilatory effects.

One of the most unique drugs in this group is ecstasy (the love drug, hug drug). Although this so-called club drug is an analog of methamphetamine, the effects of ecstasy hardly resemble the action of methamphetamine. Ecstasy would be more correctly termed an "euphorogenic"—it creates an incredible sense of well-being.

Dextromethorphan (DXM), which is found in almost 150 over-the-counter (OTC) cough suppressants, can produce a euphoric floating sensation or out-of-body experience. At a plateau level of approximately 6 tablets (180-mg dose), DXM produces a mild stimulant effect that may enhance a sexual experience. DXM or "Robo" (Robitussin) abusers are often called "Roboheads"; this kind of abuse is common among teenagers because this drug is readily available in pharmacies and online. Consuming large quantities of DXM can lead to hallucinations, psychedelic visions, loss of motor control, confusion, blurred vision, dreamlike euphoria, and out-of-body sensations.

Drugs Used to Facilitate Sexual Assault

Drugs used to facilitate sexual assault are often administered unknowingly to a woman, frequently in an alcoholic drink. These substances are used by sexual predators, which explains why they are called "date rape" drugs. They are discussed further in Chapter 38.

Gamma-hydroxybutyrate (GHB) is an endogenous metabolite of gamma-aminobutyric acid, a neuromodulator involved with sleep cycles, memory retention, and emotional control. GHB was used as anesthetic in Europe for about 40 years before it appeared in the United States, where it was originally sold in health food stores for body building purposes (it supposedly "burned fat" while the person was sleeping). By the late 1980s, GHB had gained popularity with young people as a club drug, earning the name "liquid ecstasy" from its euphoric effects at raves (all-night dance parties). In the mid 1990s, GHB became increasingly associated with sexual assaults. In 1990, the US Food and Drug Administration banned this drug from OTC sales. In 1996, the federal government enacted the Drug-Induced Rape Prevention and Punishment Law. This law allows

prison terms of up to 20 years for anyone who commits a violent crime, including sexual assault, with any controlled substance.

Although GHB is available as an odorless and colorless liquid, it has a salty taste. Reportedly, it cannot be tasted when placed in a drink such as a margarita in a salt-ringed glass. Once ingested, GHB quickly crosses the blood-brain barrier, exerting its effects within 30 to 60 minutes. As little as 0.5 mg of GHB can produce a pronounced hypnotic effect along with disinhibition, severe passivity (that is, a lack of the will to resist), and antegrade amnesia. When taken with alcohol, GHB increases the risk of devastating CNS depression (culminating in coma or death); when taken with methamphetamine and similar drugs, it increases the risk of seizures.

Treatment for GHB intoxication focuses on the CNS depression and the risks of the patient being unable to protect the airway. First, establish and maintain the airway, inserting an advanced airway as needed. Carefully monitor the patient's LOC. Assist breathing as necessary, and give high-flow supplemental oxygen. Establish vascular access. Apply the ECG monitor, pulse oximeter, and capnometer. Finally, provide rapid transport to the ED.

Poisonous Alcohols

The form of alcohol consumed by humans in alcoholic beverages is ethyl alcohol (or ethanol). It is not conventionally recognized as a poison, even though it has many properties of a poison when ingested in sufficient quantities. Instead, "poisonous alcohols" are generally considered alcohols manufactured for industrial or nongastronomic purposes, such as methyl alcohol and ethylene glycol.

Methyl Alcohol

Methyl alcohol (also known as wood alcohol or methanol) is present in paints, paint remover, windshield washer fluids, varnishes, antifreeze, and canned fuels such as Sterno Figure 33-13 ▶ . Methanol poisoning can occur after inadvertently drinking contaminated whiskey or moonshine or from intentional ingestion in a suicide attempt. Methanol is a popular substitute for ethanol among desperate people with alcoholism when they don't have the means to obtain ethanol. This colorless liquid has a unique odor.

Methanol itself is not harmful. Rather, its metabolic breakdown products, formaldehyde and formic acid, are responsible for the characteristic signs and symptoms of methanol poisoning. A dose of as little as 30 mL (2 tablespoons) can produce toxicity and even death. Once ingested, methanol is quickly absorbed from the GI tract, with peak blood levels attained within 30 to 90 minutes. In mild toxicity, the half-life of methanol is 14 to 20 hours. As toxicity increases, the half-life increases to 24 to 30 hours. The liver eliminates 90% to 95% of the methanol.

The symptoms of methanol poisoning do not usually appear immediately but begin from 12 to 18 hours, occasionally up to 72 hours, after ingestion. As a consequence, the patient may or may not connect the symptoms to what he or she drank

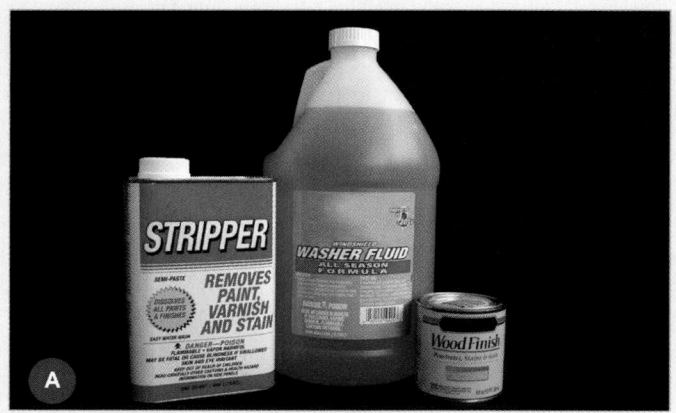

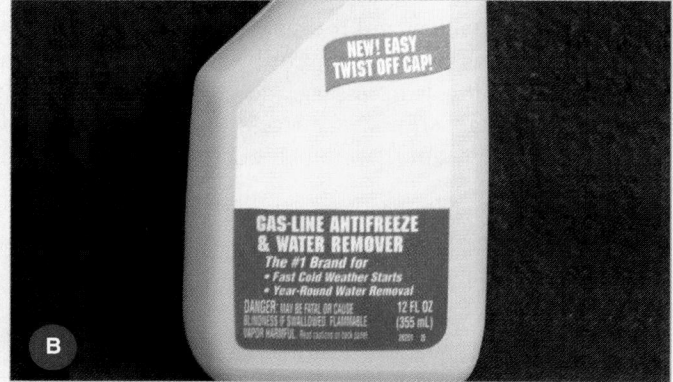

Figure 33-13 Methyl alcohol is present in paints, paint remover, windshield washer fluids, and varnishes (**A**) and in antifreeze and canned fuels (**B**).

yesterday or several days ago. Patient complaints include nausea and vomiting (in almost 50% of cases), headache or vertigo, abdominal pain (often from pancreatitis), and blurred vision ("looks like a snowstorm") or, possibly, blindness. Findings on the physical exam may include an odor of alcohol on the breath, altered mental status ranging from drunken behavior to seizures or coma, dilated pupils with sluggish or no reaction, hyperpnea and tachypnea from metabolic acidosis, and bradycardia and hypotension (very late signs).

Field care for methanol poisoning is primarily supportive. Establish and manage the airway, considering advanced airway placement as needed. Establish vascular access. Assess the blood glucose level, and administer glucose if the patient has hypoglycemia. In addition, administer thiamine per local protocol. Consult medical control for consideration of sodium bicarbonate. Provide immediate transport to an appropriate facility.

If the patient is alert, the ingestion took place within the last 30 minutes, and if local protocol allows it, insert a nasogastric tube and provide gastric aspiration. You should also assess the patient for other drug involvement. Administration of activated charcoal is contraindicated unless other drugs have been ingested that are adsorbable, in which case you should follow your local protocol.

Ethylene Glycol

Ethylene glycol is a colorless, odorless liquid found in a variety of commercial products, including antifreeze, coolant, deicers, polishes, and paints. Its relatively pleasant taste has made it a favorite substitute among people with alcoholism when the beverage of choice is unavailable. The lethal dose of ethylene glycol is estimated at 2 mL/kg, or as little as 150 mL in the average-size adult.

Ethylene glycol is very water-soluble. With oral intake, it is absorbed rapidly, with peak blood levels attained within 1 to 4 hours after ingestion. The liver and kidneys metabolize ethylene glycol into a number of toxic metabolites, including aldehydes, lactate, oxalate, and glycolate. In turn, these metabolites produce metabolic acidosis.

Toxicity from ethylene glycol occurs in three stages, so the signs and symptoms vary depending on when you encounter the patient relative to the time of ingestion:

- **Stage 1.** 20 minutes to 12 hours after ingestion. The patient presents with CNS depression and may appear intoxicated, as evidenced by slurred speech and ataxia, although the odor of ethanol on the breath is notably absent. The patient may also experience nausea, vomiting, seizures, or coma.
- **Stage 2.** 12–24 hours after ingestion. Pulmonary edema produces tachypnea, tachycardia, mild hypertension, and rales (or crackles). In severe cases, acute respiratory distress syndrome, congestive heart failure, and cardiovascular collapse may be apparent.
- **Stage 3.** 24–72 hours after ingestion. The renal damage produced by the ethylene glycol becomes evident with patient complaints of flank pain and anuria (absence of urine formation).

The care plan for a patient with suspected ethylene glycol poisoning is the same as for methanol poisoning, with the exception of possibly getting an order from medical control to administer 10 mL of 10% calcium gluconate via slow IV push to treat the hypocalcemia that accompanies ethylene glycol toxicity. This medication is usually ordered only after good urine flow is established and after the IV line is flushed clear of sodium bicarbonate. Once at the hospital, care focuses on correction of acidosis, administration of fomepizole or ethanol (to reduce the conversion of the methanol to its toxic metabolites), and, potentially, renal dialysis.

Hydrocarbons

Hydrocarbons are compounds made up principally of hydrogen and carbon atoms, with most, but not all, obtained from the distillation of petroleum. Hydrocarbons are found in a variety of products around the home, including cleaning and polishing agents, glues, spot removers, lighter fluids, paints, paint thinners and paint removers, other fuels, and pesticides.

Hydrocarbon Inhalation

The vast majority of intentional hydrocarbon inhalations are "recreational." Frequently, people who "bag" or huff are young—middle-school age and, occasionally, younger children. The profile adds up with deadly simplicity: Young children who see their siblings and parents abuse alcohol or drugs may seek to emulate that behavior but may not have the cash to make that wish a reality, so they turn to a variety of everyday products: paint thinner, solvents, paint strippers, gasoline, nonstick cooking spray (such as Pam), and glues. The rich alveolar capillary network makes the lungs a highly efficient mechanism for providing a quick and inexpensive drug high. Unfortunately, long-term inhalant abuse can lead to permanent loss of mental function as evidenced by a variety of neuropathies, such as loss of hearing, loss of fine motor function, balance and equilibrium disorders, and occasionally death.

The modern epidemic of inhalation began in the early 1960s, when the first reports of glue sniffing and its consequences appeared. Within a short time, the number of agents being inhaled to get high had increased exponentially, as had the techniques for inhalation. Simple sniffing over the opening of a glue bottle did not provide an intense enough exposure for serious abusers. Pouring the volatile material onto a rag, placing it in a trash bag, and holding the bag over one's face to breathe in the fumes proved far more efficient, producing a more intense high more quickly. Breathing fumes directly off a soaked rag or towel is termed huffing, whereas the use of a trash bag is termed bagging. Table 33-5 ▼ lists commonly abused inhaled compounds.

The primary goals when dealing with a patient who has inhaled hydrocarbons focus on removal from the noxious environment, giving high-concentration supplemental oxygen, and prompt transport to the appropriate facility.

Hydrocarbon Ingestion

Given the ready accessibility of hydrocarbons and the high likelihood that they might be mistaken for potable beverages, it is not surprising that hydrocarbon poisonings are common among children younger than 5 years. The potential hazards of swallowing a given hydrocarbon are directly related to the viscosity of the agent: The lower the viscosity, the higher the risk of aspiration and other complications. The vast majority of hydrocarbon ingestions do *not* produce lasting damage. Patients who develop symptoms within a few minutes of ingestion are likely to have aspirated and need immediate attention.

Low-viscosity hydrocarbons (such as kerosene, naphtha, and toluene) can easily enter the lungs during swallowing. If the patient reports coughing, choking, or vomiting immediately after swallowing the substance, assume that aspiration occurred. Similarly, any signs of respiratory distress—air hunger, intercostal retractions, tachypnea, cyanosis—must be considered danger signals.

Low viscosity also facilitates the uptake of a hydrocarbon by tissues of the CNS and, therefore, its anesthetic effects. At first, the patient may experience excitement and euphoria, followed

Table 33-5	Compounds Commonly Abused by Sniffing and Bagging	
Example	**Sources**	**Signs and Symptoms of Toxicity**
Halogenated hydrocarbons		
1,1,1-Trichloroethane (methylchloroform)	Cleaning solvents, typewriter correction fluid, aerosol propellant	Eye irritation, light-headedness, incoordination, CNS depression, respiratory failure, cardiac arrhythmias, sudden death
Trichloroethylene	Degreasing solvent, aerosol propellant, rubber cement, plastic cement	Euphoria, anesthesia, weakness, vomiting, abdominal cramps, loss of coordination, neuropathy, blindness, cardiac arrhythmias, "degreaser's flush" (flushed face, neck, and shoulders when taken along with alcohol)
Tetrachloroethylene (perchloroethylene)	Solvent, dry cleaning agent	Drunken behavior, dizziness, lightheadedness, difficulty walking, numbness, sleepiness, visual disturbances, memory impairment, eye irritation, cutaneous flushing, sudden death
Methylene chloride (dichloromethane)	Refrigerant, paint remover, aerosol propellant	Fatigue, weakness, chills, sleepiness, nausea, dizziness, incoordination, pulmonary edema
Carbon tetrachloride	Cleaning fluid	Narcosis, sudden death
Petroleum hydrocarbons		
Benzene	Cable cleaner, industrial solvents, rubber cement	Delirium, agitation, seizures, sudden death
Toluene	Spray paint, model and plastic cements, lacquer thinner	Narcosis, hallucinations, mania; impulsive, destructive, accident-prone behavior; sudden death
Gasoline	Gas tank	Sudden death

by weakness, incoordination, drowsiness, confusion, and coma. Some petroleum products—notably gasoline—can produce hypoglycemia and cardiac arrhythmias, so you should always monitor the patient's ECG rhythm.

Many hydrocarbon products cause gastric irritation, which results in severe abdominal pain, diarrhea, and belching, sometimes lasting for hours after the incident. At the other end of the spectrum, just a single hydrocarbon substance exposure may cause life-threatening toxicity and, on occasion, sudden death.

If a patient who has swallowed a hydrocarbon product is asymptomatic when you arrive and remains so while you are on scene, he or she is highly unlikely to experience significant complications. In such a scenario, and after discussion with medical control, some patients may not warrant transport because they can be safely observed at home. In one study involving 211 patients suspected of hydrocarbon ingestion, fewer than 1% required physician intervention.

By contrast, all symptomatic patients suspected of ingesting a hydrocarbon product—especially patients with respiratory symptoms—should be transported immediately to the ED for further evaluation and care. Management should include the following measures:

- Remove contaminated clothing and decontaminate the patient, ideally before placing the patient in the ambulance.
- Establish and maintain the airway, and ensure adequate ventilation.
- Give high-flow supplemental oxygen.
- Establish vascular access.
- Continuously monitor the ECG rhythm; consider running a 12-lead.
- Administer sequential bolus infusions of normal saline to treat hypotension.
- Transport the patient to the most appropriate facility.

Psychiatric Medications

One only needs to consider what is trying to be accomplished with psychiatric medications—altering dysfunctions of mood and affect (most commonly depression) and of thought, orientation, or perception—to appreciate the sophistication of these pharmacologic agents. When patients taking psychiatric medications have toxicologic emergencies, you should expect to be challenged with matters of patient care and scene management.

Tricyclic Antidepressants

In their heyday, the tricyclic antidepressants (TCAs) were the drugs of choice to treat depression. Unfortunately, TCAs require close attention to compliance with dosing regimens—and patients who need them have difficulty following the regimen. Patients are depressed, and many also have problems with alcohol (a CNS depressant). Consequently, they are at high risk of intentional overdose.

Making matters worse, TCAs have a small therapeutic window—that is, the difference between "minimum dosing" (the least amount of drug needed for the desired effect) and "maximum dosing" (the amount at which the drug becomes toxic). With some drugs, the therapeutic window spans several thousand milligrams. With TCAs, even minimal dosing errors may produce toxic effects.

According to a 2001 report from the AAPCC, TCAs were involved in more deaths than any other class of medication. Of the eight TCAs currently available in the United States, the five most likely to be involved in drug-related events are amitriptyline (40%), imipramine (Tofranil; 17%), doxepin (Sinequan, Zonalon; 14%), nortriptyline (Aventyl, Pamelor; 12%), and desipramine (Norpramin, Pertofrane; 6%). Although they are no longer first-line therapy for depression, TCAs still have other applications, such as pain management.

You are the Provider Part 4

Now that you have identified the substance that Julie might have taken, you contact the hospital for medical guidance once you are situated in the back of the unit. Once you establish contact with the ED physician, you explain what you found on arrival, your physical assessment findings (including your suspicion of amitriptyline overdose), the interventions undertaken, and the current reassessment findings. The physician agrees with your assessment and orders the IV administration of 50 mEq of sodium bicarbonate.

Reassessment	Recording Time: 18 Minutes
Skin	Flushed, warm, and dry
Pulse	165 beats/min; regular and weak
ECG	Possible wide complex tachycardia
Blood pressure	88/56 mm Hg
Respirations	12 breaths/min via bag-mask device
Sao$_2$	99% via bag-mask device on 100% supplemental oxygen
Pupils	Dilated

7. Can the information you provide to hospital staff during your radio report contribute to a negative patient outcome?

8. Are there any potential complications that can arise during transport relative to the patient's condition?

The signs and symptoms of TCA overdose may vary dramatically among patients. One patient may present with only a mild antimuscarinic symptom such as a dry mouth, whereas another may have cardiotoxic effects, such as life-threatening or fatal arrhythmias. The most common signs and symptoms of a TCA overdose are altered mental status (drowsy, confused, slurred speech), arrhythmias (usually sinus tachycardia or supraventricular tachycardia), dry mouth, blurred vision or dilated pupils, urinary retention, constipation, and pulmonary edema. With a more serious toxic exposure, be alert for ventricular tachycardia, hypotension, respiratory depression, QT prolongation on the ECG, and seizures.

When TCAs exert their toxic effects, the most common cause of death is cardiac arrhythmia. A significant number of the drug overdoses involving TCAs also involve other drugs and frequently alcohol, which contributes to increased morbidity and mortality. A patient who presents with serious signs and symptoms within 6 hours of the ingestion should be considered in critical condition.

Management of patients with a TCA overdose includes the following measures:

- Maintain the airway. If the patient's mental status suddenly deteriorates, as is often the case, insert an advanced airway.
- Give high-flow supplemental oxygen.
- Establish vascular access.
- Provide continuous ECG monitoring (watch for widening of the QRS).
- Administer activated charcoal per medical control orders.
- Consult with medical control to consider sodium bicarbonate administration (if the QRS is widened).
- Manage hypotension with sequential boluses of normal saline. Be alert to the possibility of pulmonary edema; it occurs frequently in cases of TCA overdose.
- Assess blood glucose levels. Give D_{50} if the patient is hypoglycemic.
- Rule out head trauma as a possible cause of decreased mental status.
- Be alert for agitation or violence. Manage this problem with reassurance and benzodiazepines.
- *Do not give* flumazenil (Romazicon; may cause seizures) or physostigmine (Eserine, Antilirium).
- For seizures, consider RSI and intubation.
- Provide rapid transport to the appropriate facility.

Monoamine Oxidase Inhibitors

Monoamine oxidase inhibitors (MAOIs) are used primarily to treat atypical depression. They work by increasing norepinephrine and serotonin levels within the CNS. Unfortunately, the potential for drug interactions is a major issue for patients receiving MAOI therapy. A very tight therapeutic window also contributes to the limited popularity of MAOIs—as little as 2 mg/kg may produce a life-threatening event. In addition, MAOIs can precipitate a hypertensive crisis if taken in conjunction with tyramine-containing foods (such as beer, wine, aged cheese, chopped liver, pickled herring, sour cream, yogurt, fava beans).

When taken in toxic levels, MAOIs can be lethal because they can produce hyperkalemia, metabolic acidosis, and rhabdomyolysis. Symptoms of MAOI toxicity are often delayed, occurring 6 to 12 hours after ingestion and, in some cases, as long as 24 hours later. Once signs and symptoms begin to appear, you should prepare to manage a life-threatening event. When death occurs from an MAOI overdose, it is usually secondary to multiple-system organ failure.

Early signs and symptoms of MAOI overdose include hyperactivity, arrhythmias (usually sinus tachycardia), hyperventilation, and nystagmus. With increased levels of toxicity, be alert for chest pain, palpitations, hypertension, diaphoresis, agitated or combative behavior, marked hyperthermia, and hallucinations. With a severe MAOI overdose, expect bradycardia, hypotension, seizures, worsening hyperthermia, pulmonary edema, coma, or cardiac arrest.

Unfortunately, there is no antidote available for an MAOI overdose. With any suspected MAOI overdose, you should establish and maintain the airway, inserting an advanced airway as needed. In addition, give high-flow supplemental oxygen. Establish large-bore vascular access. Monitor the ECG rhythm, staying alert for changes indicative of hyperkalemia. After consultation with medical control, you may administer a single dose of activated charcoal. However, you should *not* give syrup of ipecac.

With a patient in deteriorating condition, treat hypotension with sequential fluid boluses of normal saline. If seizures occur, treat them with benzodiazepines per local protocol because persistent seizures may contribute to the combined problems of metabolic acidosis, hyperkalemia, and rhabdomyolysis. If the patient is hypertensive, contact medical control to consider administration of phentolamine (Regitine) boluses every 10 to 15 minutes until normotension is obtained. If RSI is required, the use of a nondepolarizing paralytic such as vecuronium (Norcuron) is recommended because MAOIs may enhance the actions of succinylcholine.

Selective Serotonin Reuptake Inhibitors

A larger therapeutic window, which increases their safety margin, has helped make selective serotonin reuptake inhibitors (SSRIs) a top choice for managing depression. In addition, SSRIs have far fewer anticholinergic and cardiac effects than the TCAs. Popular SSRIs include fluoxetine (Prozac), paroxetine (Paxil), and sertraline (Zoloft).

As many as 50% of adult patients may be asymptomatic with an SSRI overdose. When symptoms are present, the most commonly seen include nausea, vomiting, arrhythmias (usually sinus tachycardia), sedation, and tremors. Other symptoms that occur much less often include dilated pupils, agitation, blood pressure changes (hypotension or hypertension), seizures, and hallucinations, When SSRIs are taken in conjunction with alcohol, look for tachycardia, mild hypotension, and generally lethargy as the most common signs and symptoms.

A pure SSRI overdose with no other drugs or alcohol involved usually produces limited toxic effects, with the exception of seizures or serotonin syndrome (discussed later in this section). As such, management of an SSRI overdose follows the general approach for poisoned patients:

- Establish and maintain the airway.
- Administer high-flow supplemental oxygen.
- Establish vascular access.
- Provide continuous ECG monitoring.
- Consider a single dose of activated charcoal per medical control.
- Treat seizure activity with benzodiazepines per local protocol.
- Should widening of the QRS occur, consult with medical control for consideration of sodium bicarbonate administration.
- Transport to the appropriate facility.

Serotonin syndrome is an idiosyncratic complication that occasionally occurs with antidepressant therapy. This condition is not limited to patients taking SSRIs, but also can occur when patients take any combination of drugs that increase central serotonin neurotransmission. Because no laboratory test can pinpoint serotonin syndrome and the symptomatology is vague at best, it is a difficult diagnosis based on clinical suspicion after other psychiatric or medical causes have been ruled out. Lower extremity muscle rigidity is one of the few classic signs, with approximately half of patients presenting with confusion or disorientation and one third with agitation.

Although serotonin syndrome is rare, it is potentially lethal: 1 of every 10 patients dies. The primary treatment is to discontinue drug therapy, which is clearly not a field intervention. In the field, management is primarily supportive. Pay close attention to the patient's ability to protect the airway because 25% of patients with serotonin syndrome eventually require intubation.

Lithium

Despite the major advances made in many areas of psychiatric medicine, lithium remains the cornerstone drug for the treatment of bipolar disorder. In 1949, lithium salts made their debut for the treatment of mania. Eventually, they were found to be much more efficacious for the treatment of bipolar disorder, and they retain their position as first-line treatment for this condition.

Lithium is almost completely absorbed in the GI tract roughly 8 hours after ingestion. Bioelimination occurs relatively slowly, with approximately 95% of the lithium eliminated in the urine; although two thirds of the lithium dose is excreted within 12 hours after ingestion, the remainder is excreted during the next 2 weeks. Given its small therapeutic window and slow excretion process, the threat of toxic levels and overdosing is ever present.

Early signs and symptoms of lithium overdose include nausea, vomiting, hand tremors, excessive thirst, and slurred speech. With increased toxicity come increased neurologic symptoms: ataxia, muscle weakness and incoordination, blurred vision, and hyperreflexia (twitching). Eventually, the patient may have seizures and become comatose.

Management of a patient suspected of a lithium overdose is mostly supportive. Establish and maintain the airway, inserting an advanced airway as needed. Give high-flow supplemental oxygen, and ensure vascular access. If the patient experiences hypotension, administer serial boluses of normal saline. Maintain continuous ECG monitoring, being alert for AV blocks and ventricular arrhythmias. Finally, transport the patient to an appropriate facility.

Nonprescription Pain Medications

Medications used for pain management make up a huge part of the OTC drug market. In the OTC and prescription drug markets, nonsteroidal anti-inflammatory drugs (NSAIDs) are some of the most popular options for pain relief, fever control, and anti-inflammatory action. Their convenient dosing schemes and large therapeutic windows, coupled with their safe track records relative to acute ingestion and overdose, enhance their popularity.

NSAIDs are rapidly absorbed from the GI tract before being eliminated from the body in urine and feces. The half-lives of these agents vary widely, ranging from 2 to 4 hours for ibuprofen, to approximately 15 hours for selective cyclooxygenase-2 inhibitors, to 50 hours for some long-acting agents. Patients who take lithium and NSAIDs have slowed renal clearance of the lithium, increasing the likelihood that they will inadvertently reach a toxic lithium level.

Most of the problems associated with NSAID use involve long-term use; patients may experience GI bleeding and kidney dysfunction. Acute ingestion and overdoses are rare, with ibuprofen being the NSAID most commonly encountered in the acute setting. At toxic levels, the signs and symptoms of NSAID overdose may include headache, altered mentation (cognitive difficulties, behavioral changes), seizures, bradyarrhythmia, hypotension, abdominal pain, nausea, and vomiting. Many patients who experience NSAID overdose remain asymptomatic, however.

For symptomatic patients, care in the prehospital setting is usually supportive. Establish and maintain the airway, inserting an advanced airway as needed. Give high-flow supplemental oxygen, and establish vascular access. If hypotension develops, administer fluid boluses of normal saline. If hypotension persists after sequential fluid boluses, consider giving a vasopressor. Treat seizures with benzodiazepines per local protocol. Finally, transport the patient to an appropriate facility.

A unique side effect of NSAID use is aseptic meningitis, in which a patient presents with complaints of a stiff neck, headache, and fever within several hours after taking an NSAID. Discontinuing the NSAID therapy generally resolves the problem, but patients must be evaluated at the hospital to rule out other causes.

Salicylates

Although aspirin (acetylsalicylic acid, or ASA) can be involved in a toxic event, more typically OTC products containing salicylates cause toxicity. For example, a single 30-mL dose of

Pepto-Bismol (bismuth subsalicylate) contains 261 mg of salicylate (two thirds the total dose of one aspirin). Similarly, many of the liniments used with hot-air vaporizers contain high levels of methyl salicylate. With continued use of these products for a period of days, infants or young toddlers may ingest toxic levels of the salicylate.

The clinical presentation of salicylate overdose can change based on three primary variables: the patient's age, the dose ingested, and the duration of the exposure. Ingestion of 150 mg/kg or less will usually make a person "mildly toxic." At this level, chief complaints are usually nausea, vomiting, and abdominal pain. With a dosing range of 150 to 300 mg/kg, moderate toxicity results, with signs and symptoms including vomiting, diaphoresis, hyperpnea, ringing in the ears, pulmonary edema, and acid-base disturbances. At levels of 300 mg/kg, severe toxicity may produce metabolic acidosis or combined respiratory alkalosis–metabolic acidosis.

When pediatric patients have an acute salicylate episode, the ingestion is usually accidental, the symptoms are mild, and they recover swiftly. A chronic event (possibly from several days of vaporizer use) is usually much more serious in pediatric patients.

By comparison, an acute salicylate event with an adult usually involves an intentional overdose, with the most common patient profile being young women with a history of drug abuse or psychiatric problems. A fatal event is possible if an adult with suspected salicylate overdose is unconscious during initial assessment and presents with a high fever, seizures, or cardiac arrhythmias.

No salicylate antidote or antagonist is available, so field management is primarily supportive. Establish and maintain the airway, inserting an advanced airway as needed. Give high-flow supplemental oxygen, and establish vascular access. If hypotension develops (from volume depletion), administer serial boluses of normal saline. Monitor carbon dioxide levels with capnometry. Following consultation with medical control, administer one dose of activated charcoal. In addition, consult with medical control regarding urine alkalinization with sodium bicarbonate. Finally, transport the patient to an appropriate facility.

Acetaminophen

Acetaminophen is a well-tolerated drug with few side effects that is available on an OTC basis. These characteristics have made this drug one of the best-selling analgesics in the United States—and one of the most common culprits in toxic exposures. In 2000, the Toxic Drug Exposure System revealed that acetaminophen was involved in 5% of all toxic exposures and produced 23% of all deaths from this cause. Its lethality is believed to stem from two sources: a widely held belief that acetaminophen is not a dangerous drug and a general lack of awareness that acetaminophen is an ingredient in many other preparations.

Once ingested, acetaminophen is rapidly absorbed from the GI tract, producing peak serum levels in 30 to 120 min-

Table 33-6	Signs and Symptoms of Acetaminophen Toxicity	
Stage	**Timeframe**	**Signs and Symptoms**
I	< 24 h	Nausea, vomiting, loss of appetite, pallor, malaise
II	24–72 h	Right upper quadrant abdominal pain; abdomen tender to palpation
III	72–96 h	Metabolic acidosis, renal failure, coagulopathies, recurring GI symptoms
IV	4–14 d (or longer)	Recovery slowly begins, or liver failure progresses and the patient dies

utes. Absorption slows when the drug is combined with diphenhydramine (Tylenol PM) or with propoxyphene (Darvocet). One unique aspect of acetaminophen toxicity is that the signs and symptoms appear in four distinct stages **Table 33-6 ▲** .

It is important to try to accurately estimate the time of ingestion because this information drives the decision-making process for patient care in the field and the hospital. Although an antidote for acetaminophen toxicity exists—namely, acetylcysteine (Acetadote)—ideally this drug should be given less than 8 hours after the ingestion. Typically, however, it is administered based on the patient's laboratory results; as such, it is not a field intervention.

Management of the patient in the field first focuses on establishing and maintaining the airway, with an advanced airway being inserted as needed. Give high-flow supplemental oxygen, and establish vascular access. For recent ingestions, administer activated charcoal after consulting with medical control. Finally, transport the patient to an appropriate facility.

Theophylline

Theophylline, caffeine, and theobromine are naturally occurring alkaloids found in a variety of plants around the world; they belong to the family of drugs called methylated xanthines. It is estimated that half the world's population drinks tea, which contains caffeine and theophylline. Cocoa and chocolate contain caffeine and theobromine as well.

For many years, theophylline was used to treat patients with chronic obstructive pulmonary disease and asthma, primarily because of its bronchodilatory effects. In addition, theophylline is a potent CNS stimulant. Even when taken in normal therapeutic doses, it can cause a variety of ECG rhythm disturbances, including sinus or atrial tachycardia, frequent premature atrial contractions, atrial fibrillation, and atrial flutter. Even more problematic is the occurrence of premature ventricular contractions and ventricular arrhythmias, including ventricular tachycardia. Theophylline has a very small therapeutic window. This narrow safety range, coupled with the prevalence of CNS and cardiovascular side effects and the continued development of beta-2 agonists for chronic obstructive pulmonary disease and asthma treatment, has led to decreased use of theophylline.

Peak levels of theophylline are reached within 90 to 120 minutes after ingestion, except in the case of sustained-release preparations, which may take as long as 8 hours to produce peak serum levels. Absorption rates increase if the drug is taken on an empty stomach or with large amounts of fluids, but also can decrease when theophylline is taken with certain foods. Approximately 85% to 90% of the drug is metabolized by the liver, with the remainder excreted in the urine.

Most toxic exposures of theophylline in adults involve unintentional overdoses, usually resulting from the drug's variable absorption rate and small therapeutic window. The toxic effects may range from mild GI distress (nausea and vomiting) to life-threatening or fatal cardiac arrhythmias. Indeed, a patient taking theophylline can quickly go from being asymptomatic to a life-threatening state with little to no warning. Complaints of restlessness, insomnia, tremors, agitation, and other signs and symptoms of CNS overstimulation are common, as are cardiac arrhythmias.

Because of the rapidity with which a patient's condition may deteriorate, prompt intervention is essential, especially in regard to the use of activated charcoal, which can greatly reduce the half-life of theophylline. First, establish and maintain the airway, inserting an advanced airway as needed. Give high-flow supplemental oxygen, and establish vascular access. Continuously monitor the ECG rhythm. After consulting with medical control, administer activated charcoal, repeating the dosing as necessary. If hypotension develops, administer fluid boluses; if they fail to relieve the problem, administer a vasopressor. You may also consider low-dose beta blockers, per your local protocol. For symptomatic reentry supraventricular tachycardia, you may give adenosine, but stay alert for bronchospasm (a potential side effect of adenosine). Finally, treat arrhythmias per ACLS (see Chapter 27).

Metals and Metalloids

Although acute metal and metalloid toxic exposures are relatively rare, when they occur, they can produce devastating results, usually because of delayed diagnosis or misdiagnosis. The difficulty reaching the correct diagnosis may contribute to increased mortality or morbidity because of delayed or inadequate treatment. Toxic exposures involving metals or metalloids usually manifest by affecting four body systems: neurologic, hematologic, renal, and GI.

Lead

Despite the bans on lead in gasoline, paint, canning processes, and plumbing, lead poisoning remains the leading cause of chronic metal poisoning. It has long been known that elevated lead levels may significantly hamper intellectual development in children.

With inorganic lead, absorption usually occurs via the respiratory or GI tract. Once in the body, approximately 90% of

Table 33-7	Systems Affected by Lead Poisoning
System	**Signs and Symptoms**
CNS	Altered mentation, including irritability, mood changes, memory deficit, sleep disturbances; headache; seizures; ataxia
GI	Abdominal pain (usually occurs with acute poisoning); constipation; diarrhea
Renal	Renal insufficiency; hypertension; gout
Hematologic	Anemia

the lead is stored in bone. From this site, it eventually makes its way into the bloodstream. Inorganic lead can also cross the placental barrier and negatively affective fetal development. Its excretion from the body is incredibly slow, with the half-life of lead in bone estimated at 30 years.

Most organic lead (tetraethyl lead) exposures occur in the occupational setting, although they can also occur from gas sniffing where leaded gasoline is available. Once in the body, tetraethyl lead is metabolized to inorganic lead and triethyl lead, with triethyl lead the primary cause of CNS toxicity.

Lead poisoning is associated with a long list of signs and symptoms **Table 33-7 ▲** . In particular, encephalopathy is a major cause of mortality and morbidity from lead poisoning.

In the field, you have few treatment options for lead poisoning. Your most helpful move may be identification of the source of the lead, which can assist the appropriate government agency to prevent more occurrences by removing the toxin. When managing the patient, first establish and maintain the airway, inserting an advanced airway as needed. Give high-flow supplemental oxygen. Establish vascular access with a saline or heparin lock. Unless hypotension is present, don't provide fluid therapy—it may worsen cerebral edema. Transport the patient to an appropriate facility.

Iron

The AAPCC's 2000 annual report identified 30,000 calls specific to iron supplement ingestion. Although only a small amount of iron is required as part of a healthy diet, many adult and pediatric multivitamins contain iron. Children younger than 6 years have frequent iron exposures, usually secondary to ingesting chewable vitamins. By comparison, most toxic exposures in adults are intentional.

In the average 70-kg adult, the body's entire iron supply consists of only about 4 g. Of that total, roughly 65% is found in hemoglobin, with the remainder sequestered elsewhere. Because of its toxic potential, iron is stored in the body by several mechanisms, which permit access to the supply as needed. The body of a healthy person does not contain "free" (unbound) iron.

From a practical perspective, the toxic effects of an iron exposure reflect the amount of elemental iron ingested. With ingestion of 20 to 60 mg/kg, mild to moderate toxicity should be expected. With dosing of more than 60 mg/kg, severe and potentially lethal toxicity is a possibility.

Two broad categories of iron poisoning can be distinguished: GI and systemic. With GI toxicity, the symptoms consist of abdominal pain, vomiting (the most common sign), and diarrhea. With systemic toxicity, patients may be hypotensive or in frank shock from coagulopathy and vomiting blood. They are commonly in metabolic acidosis and become tachypneic as the body attempts to adjust pH by increasing the elimination of carbon dioxide.

Children typically remain asymptomatic when they have a low-level iron exposure. However, children who ingest a large dose of iron are at risk of dying unless aggressive and timely interventions take place. Unfortunately, little can be done in the field for iron poisoning, other than providing basic attention to the ABCs and transporting to the hospital for further evaluation and laboratory studies.

Mercury

Mercury exists in a variety of organic and inorganic forms. In the human body, all forms produce toxic effects. Although accidental exposures to mercury often occur in the occupational setting, mercury can be found in the home in thermometers and in some switches used in heating and air conditioning.

Organic mercury is very lipid-soluble and quickly accumulates in the liver, CNS, and kidneys. It can also cross the placental membrane into the fetus.

Mercury poisoning can present differently depending on the type of mercury and its route of entry into the body. Most signs and symptoms involve the CNS and GI and renal systems. CNS alterations may include anxiety, depression, irritability, sleep disturbances, and memory loss. In addition, tremors, ataxia, paresthesias, muscle weakness or rigidity, and excessive drooling may develop.

In the occupational setting, safe removal from the exposure source is the primary intervention. In all cases of suspected mercury poisoning, EMS management is supportive and includes basic attention to the ABCs and transport to the hospital. In the hospital setting, the patient may undergo aggressive GI decontamination and receive dimercaprol (BAL), succimer (DMSA), or other chelating agents.

Arsenic

The most common cause of acute metal poisoning and the second leading cause of chronic metal poisoning is arsenic. This metal is used in a variety of industries and appears in a variety of compounds, so it is often the source of unintentional exposures. Intentional exposures include the use of arsenic in homicide and suicide.

Arsenic can enter the body by ingestion, inhalation, and absorption and dermally through a wound. It is eliminated from the body through the kidneys.

The clinical presentation of arsenic poisoning depends on the type, amount, and concentration of arsenic that enters the body and the rate of absorption and elimination. In general, symptoms appear within 30 minutes to several hours of arsenic ingestion. Arsenic poisoning should be suspected with patients who present with hypotension of unknown cause following a bout of severe gastroenteritis.

Signs and symptoms of arsenic poisoning include severe abdominal pain, nausea, explosive diarrhea, "metal taste" in the mouth, skin rash, general malaise, weakness, hypotension secondary to fluid loss, pulmonary edema, rhabdomyolysis, and renal failure. ECG changes and arrhythmias (usually sinus tachycardia) may be apparent, but nonspecific ST-segment and T-wave changes are also possible, as is QT prolongation. Ventricular tachycardia and torsade de pointes can occur.

A patient with acute arsenic toxicity is in critical condition and requires aggressive interventions. Establish and maintain the airway, inserting an advanced airway as needed. Give high-flow supplemental oxygen, and establish vascular access. For hypotension, administer sequential boluses of normal saline. If the hypotension proves refractory to fluid therapy, administer a vasopressor (dopamine or dobutamine). Continuously monitor the ECG, and follow ACLS algorithms for arrhythmias—uncorrected hypotension arrhythmias may lead to death. For torsade de pointes, consider administration of magnesium after consulting with medical control. Finally, provide rapid transport to an appropriate facility.

Poisonous Plants

Of the thousands of plant varieties, only a few are poisonous **Figure 33-14**. Oddly enough, poisonous plants represent some of the most common ornamental garden shrubs and houseplants. Perhaps for that reason, 70% to 80% of plant-related exposures involve children younger than 6 years. In the AAPCC's 2001 report, plant ingestions ranked fourth on the list of most common reasons to contact a Poison Center. Thankfully, deaths from plant ingestions are rare (< 0.001% of all cases). **Table 33-8** lists plants that can cause toxic results and, in some cases, death.

The ubiquitous dieffenbachia is a lovely green plant with broad, variegated leaves. It is nicknamed "dumb cane," because eating dieffenbachia can result in a person being unable to speak. All parts of the dieffenbachia plant—leaves, stems, roots—contain sharp caladium oxalate crystals. When ingested, the crystals cause burns of the mouth and tongue and, sometimes, paralysis of the vocal cords. In severe cases, edema of the tongue and larynx may lead to airway compromise.

Caladium, with its stunning multicolored leaves, is another hazard lurking in the flowerpot. Like dieffenbachia, it contains caladium oxalate crystals and produces the same results when ingested. Nausea, vomiting, and diarrhea commonly occur after ingestion of either plant.

Lantana (also known as red sage or wild sage) is a perennial flowering shrub with clusters of little red berries. These berries—particularly when ripe—can lead to serious poisoning. Even when still green, the berries contain lantadene A, a poison that causes stomach upsets, muscle weakness, shock, and sometimes death.

Then there's the real killer in the flowerpot: castor bean. The seeds of this attractive shrub are highly poisonous—chewing on

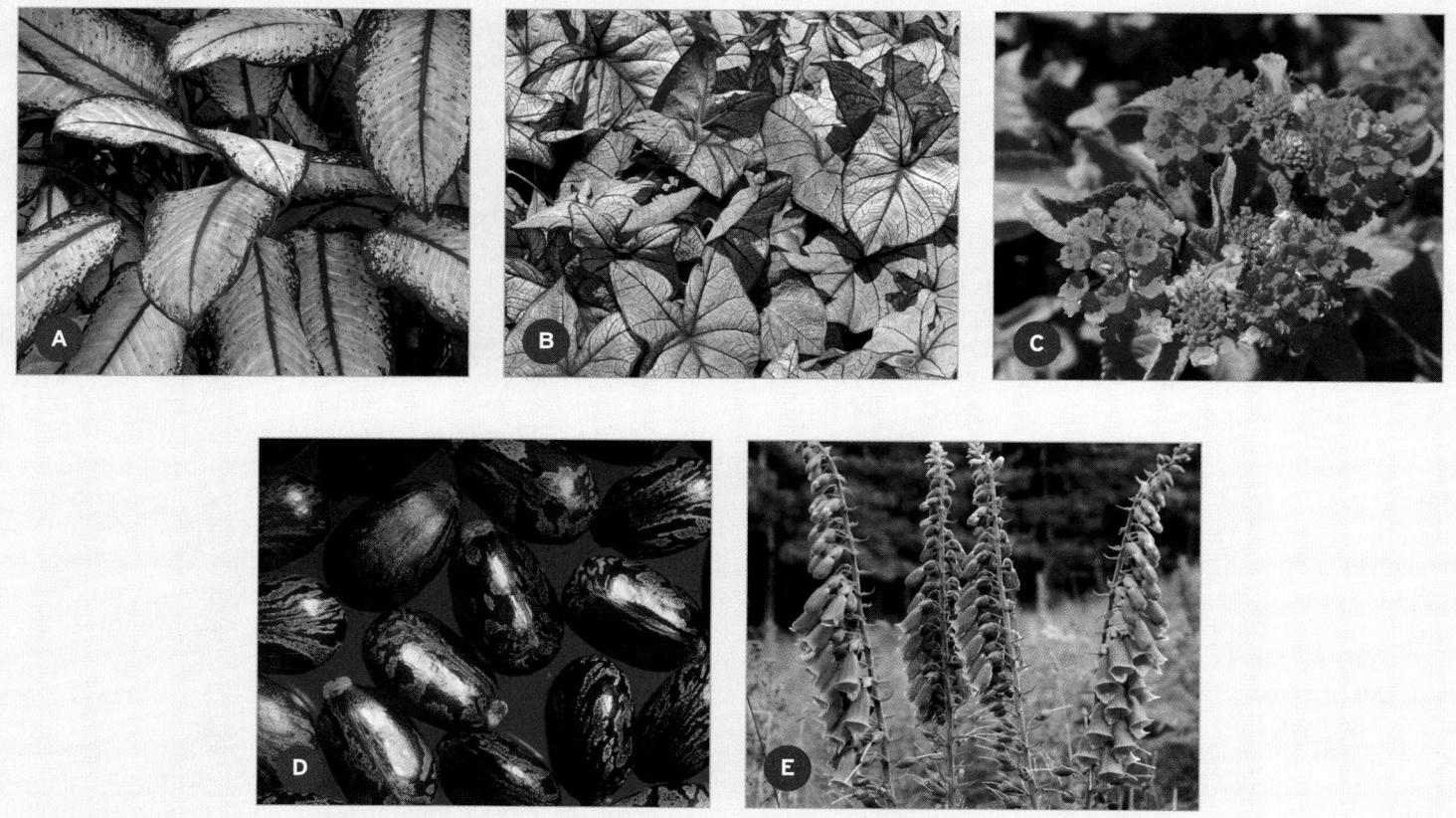

Figure 33-14 Poisonous plants. **A.** Dieffenbachia. **B.** Caladium. **C.** Lantana. **D.** Castor beans. **E.** Foxglove.

just a few seeds (and, in some cases, just one) can kill a child. Ricin, the poison in castor beans, causes a variety of toxic effects: burning of the mouth and throat; nausea, vomiting, diarrhea, and severe stomach pains; prostration; failing vision; and kidney failure (the usual cause of death).

Foxglove, which has beautiful trumpetlike flowers, contains cardiac glycosides and is used in making the drug digitalis. Along with nausea, vomiting, diarrhea, and abdominal cramps, ingestion of foxglove can produce hyperkalemia and cardiac arrhythmias.

When you encounter a case of plant poisoning, get all the information you can from the parent, and then consult your regional Poison Center for advice:

- *When was the plant ingested?* If it was more than 12 hours ago and the patient is still asymptomatic, chances are good that the patient will emerge unscathed. Most plant poisonings produce signs and symptoms of toxicity, if they are going to do so, within 4 hours of ingestion. One notable exception is castor bean, for which symptoms may not appear until 1 to 3 days after ingestion.
- *What, exactly, did the child eat?* Try to find out not just what type of plant, but also what parts of the plant (leaves, root, stem, flower, or fruit) were eaten. If possible, estimate how much was ingested (such as a bite or two from a leaf, three

or four leaves). If you transport the child to the hospital, take the offending plant—or whatever is left of it.

- *What signs or symptoms, if any, does the child have?*

The vast majority of plant-related exposures require no treatment, a decision that can be made after consulting with the Poison Center and medical control per local protocol. If there is a responsible adult who can keep a close eye on the child for at least 4 to 6 hours after the ingestion, there is no need to transport the child to the hospital. Conversely, a child with any signs and symptoms should be evaluated in the ED.

Poisonous Mushrooms

Four groups of people are most likely to be the victims of poisoning related to mushroom ingestion: wild mushroom pickers, people looking for hallucinogenic mushrooms to get high, people attempting suicide or homicide, and young children who eat them by accident. Even among educated people who like to gather their own mushrooms in the wild, mistakes can happen. In 2001, Poison Centers received 8,400 calls related to mushroom ingestions, with 70% occurring in children younger than 6 years. Thankfully, the majority of these events result in limited or no toxic effects.

A variety of factors determine whether a mushroom ingestion will produce toxic results: the age of the mushroom, the season in which it was gathered, the amount ingested, and the

Table 33-8	Poisons in Some Common Plants		
Plant	**Poisonous Part**	**Poison**	**Signs and Symptoms of Poisoning**
Apricot	Seeds	Cyanide	Headache, dizziness, weakness, nausea, vomiting, coma, seizures
Autumn crocus	Entire plant	Colchicine	Cramps, nausea, hematuria, diarrhea, coma, shock
Bird of paradise	Pod	Multiple	Vomiting, diarrhea
Bloodroot	Root	Sanguinarine	Cramps, diarrhea, dizziness, paralysis, coma
Buttercup	Entire plant	Protoanemonin	Gastroenteritis, seizures
Caladium	Leaves and roots	Calcium oxalate	Burning of mucous membranes, swelling of the tongue and throat, salivation, gastroenteritis
Cherry	Bark, leaves, seed	Amygdalin	Stupor, vocal cord paralysis, seizures, coma
Daffodil	Bulb	Multiple	Gastroenteritis
Deadly nightshade	Berry, leaf, root	Atropine	Fever; tachycardia; dilated pupils; hot, red, dry skin
Dieffenbachia	Leaves and roots	Calcium oxalate	Same as for caladium
Elderberry	Leaf, shoot, bark	Sambunigran	Gastroenteritis
Holly	Berries	Ilicin	Gastroenteritis, coma
Hyacinth	Bulb	Multiple	Severe gastroenteritis
Jack-in-the-pulpit	All parts	Calcium oxalate	Severe gastroenteritis
Jimson weed	All parts	Atropine	Dry mouth; hot, red skin; headache; hallucinations; tachycardia; hypertension; delirium; seizures
Laurel	All parts	Andromedotoxin	Salivation, lacrimation, rhinorrhea, vomiting, seizures, bradycardia, hypotension, paralysis
Lily of the valley	Leaf, flowers	Glycosides	Cardiac arrhythmias, nausea
Mistletoe	All parts	Tyramine	Bradycardia, gastroenteritis, hypertension, dyspnea, delirium, sweating, shock
Morning glory	Seeds	LSD	Hallucinations
Narcissus	Bulb	Multiple	Gastroenteritis
Oleander	Entire plant	Oleanin	Cramps, bradycardia, dilated pupils, bloody diarrhea, coma, apnea (one leaf is lethal)
Philodendron	Entire plant	Calcium oxalate	Edema of tongue, throat
Poinsettia	Leaves, stem, sap	Multiple	Contact dermatitis, gastroenteritis
Potato	Green tubers, new sprouts	Solanine	Severe gastroenteritis, headache, apnea, shock
Rhododendron	Entire plant	Andromedotoxin	Salivation
Rhubarb	Leaves only	Oxalic acid	Cramps, nausea, vomiting, anuria
Wisteria	Pods	Glycoside	Severe gastroenteritis, shock

preparation method. Toxic effects vary from mild GI signs and symptoms to severe cytotoxic—even lethal—effects. In the United States, almost all deaths due to mushroom ingestion involve the *Amanita* species (*Amanita phalloides, Amanita virosa,* and *Amanita verna*) Figure 33-15 ▸ .

Time of symptom onset can serve as a predictor of potential severity. If the patient presents with symptoms within approximately 2 hours of ingestion, the event is most likely to be non–life-threatening. By comparison, if symptom onset occurs 6 hours or later, there is a much greater likelihood the event will be serious and potentially fatal. The most common patient complaints involve GI signs or symptoms, including abdominal cramping and watery or bloody diarrhea. Patients may also experience chills or headaches.

Management for a symptomatic patient with a toxic mushroom ingestion includes the usual measures. Establish and main-

tain the airway, and establish vascular access. For hypotension secondary to vomiting and diarrhea, administer fluid boluses of normal saline. Contact the Poison Center and medical control per local protocol, and administer activated charcoal if directed to do so. Finally, transport the patient to an appropriate facility.

Food Poisoning

Whenever you encounter two or more people sick at the same time and at the same scene, think food poisoning or CO poisoning—your hunch will likely be correct. In the United States, an estimated 76 million food-related illnesses occur each year, requiring 325,000 hospitalizations and producing 5,000 deaths. Almost half of these food poisonings take place in restaurants, cafeterias, and delicatessens.

Three toxins—*Salmonella, Listeria,* and *Toxoplasma*—produce roughly 35% of all food-related deaths. Poisoning

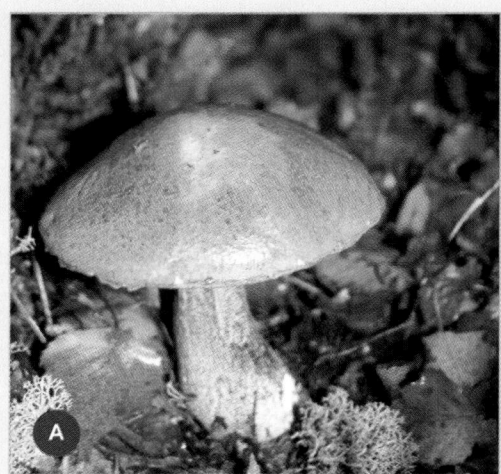 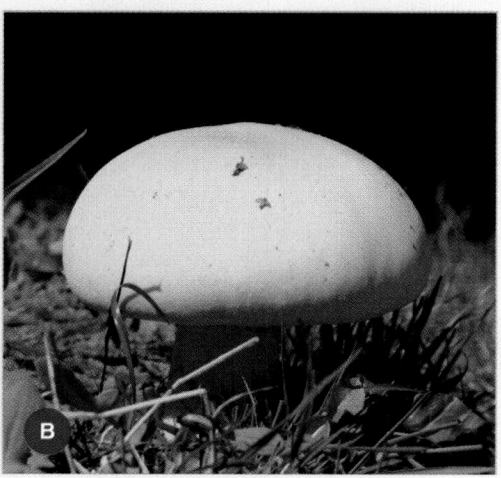

Figure 33-15 **A.** The deadly *Amanita* mushroom. **B.** A nonpoisonous, edible mushroom.

with *Clostridium botulinum,* an extremely deadly toxin, is usually the result of improper food storage or canning. In addition, the toxins produced by dinoflagellates in "red tides" may contaminate bivalve shellfish such as oysters, clams, and mussels and produce life-threatening or fatal paralytic shellfish poisoning. Cooking does not kill these toxins.

Depending on the toxin, onset of signs and symptoms can range from several hours after ingestion to days or weeks. The longer the time until symptom onset, the more difficult it will be to link the patient's problem to the event at which the toxin was ingested. Gastrointestinal complaints are the most common and include abdominal pain and cramping, nausea, vomiting, and diarrhea. With prolonged episodes of vomiting or diarrhea, hypotension secondary to fluid loss and electrolyte imbalance becomes likely. Respiratory distress or arrest can occur with toxins such as *C botulinum* or those found in paralytic shellfish poisoning.

Management for patients with food poisoning is usually supportive because the vast majority of cases you encounter will not be life threatening, and the signs and symptoms of acute gastroenteritis are typically self-limiting. Establish and maintain the airway, inserting an advanced airway as needed. Give high-flow supplemental oxygen, and establish vascular access. For hypotension secondary to fluid loss, administer fluid boluses of normal saline. Consider administration of antiemetics, per local protocol. For patients with facial flushing (most likely secondary to histamine release), consider administration of diphenhydramine per local protocol. Finally, transport the patient to an appropriate facility.

Bites, Stings, and Injected Poisons

Injected poisons usually gain access to the body as the result of stings or bites from a variety of creatures. This section considers the ill effects that may result from unfriendly encounters with creatures from the land, air, and sea.

Arthropod Bites and Stings

If sheer numbers were the sole criterion determining such things, arthropods would rule the world. The phylum Arthropoda includes at least 1.5 million species of "joint-footed" animals, ranging from the lobster to the mite. The classes of arthropods of most medical importance, because of their ability to inject venom, are the arachnids (including spiders, scorpions, and ticks), Chilopoda (centipedes), and insects (including the Hymenoptera).

Hymenoptera Stings

The Hymenoptera family of insects includes bees, wasps, hornets, yellow jackets, and ants **Figure 33-16 ▾**. Collectively, they kill more people each year than any other venomous animals, including snakes. Death from a Hymenoptera stings usually occurs from anaphylaxis, which is covered in detail in Chapter 30.

The diagnosis of a bee sting is usually not difficult—indeed, in most cases, the patient will have already made the diagnosis. There is almost always an immediate local reaction consisting of pain (sometimes extreme), redness and swelling, and sometimes itching at the site of the sting. Honeybees sting once, usually leaving the barbed stinger and the venom sac attached to the patient's skin. By comparison, wasps, hornets, yellow jackets, and fire ants can sting repeatedly until they are chased away or the patient is removed.

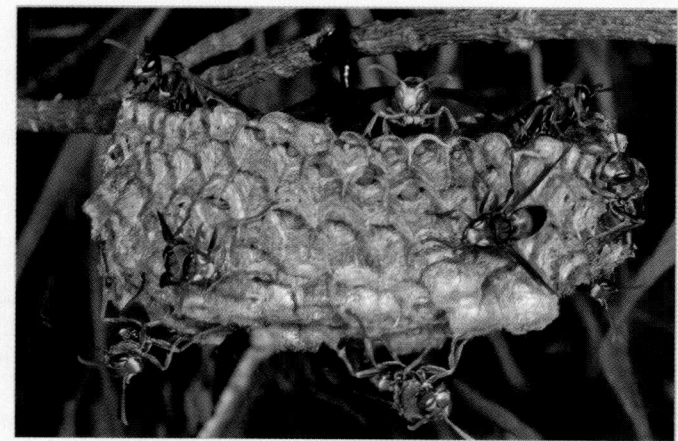

Figure 33-16 Hymenoptera stings include those from bees, wasps, hornets, yellow jackets, and ants.

If the patient has no history of allergy to bee stings and does not have a systemic reaction, transport to the hospital is usually unnecessary. When this decision is made, advise the patient of the warning signs of anaphylaxis and the urgency of calling 9-1-1 in such an event. Instruct the patient to have the wound checked by a doctor if it does not improve markedly within 24 hours. Bee stings, especially those to the extremities, often become infected and require antibiotic treatment. Infection is particularly likely after the stings of fire ants, which roam the southeastern United States throughout the late spring and early summer. Fire ant stings typically produce small pustules at the sting site about 6 hours after the sting. When the pustules are broken open—as they invariably are when the patient starts to scratch—the affected area is vulnerable to secondary infection.

Treatment of a Hymenoptera sting focuses primarily on pain relief and minimization of the risk of infection. First, determine whether the stinger and venom sac are still attached to the skin. If so, use a scalpel blade to gently scrape the stinger and venom sac from the wound. Do not try to pluck the stinger out with tweezers or forceps. If you squeeze the stinger or the venom sac, you will pump more venom into the wound!

After removing the stinger, clean the wound thoroughly with soap and water or an antiseptic solution such as povidone-iodine. Apply cold packs to the site for pain relief.

Tick Bites

Ticks are blood-sucking arthropods found around the world, often in rural, wooded areas Figure 33-17. Ordinarily, tick bites are not a medical emergency, but they are of concern because ticks serve as disease vectors. Bacteria, viruses, and protozoa can be transmitted via a tick bite, and they are linked to a variety of serious illnesses, including Lyme disease, Rocky Mountain spotted fever, and tularemia.

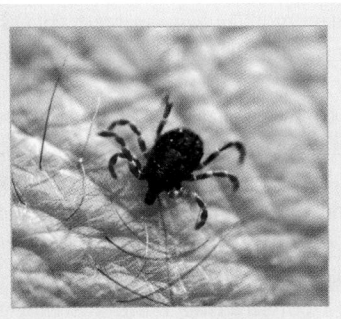

Figure 33-17 Ticks typically attach themselves directly to the skin.

In rare cases, a tick bite on the back of the head, neck, or spine may produce potentially life-threatening paralysis, which cannot be reversed unless the tick is removed. The clinical presentation mirrors that of Guillain-Barré syndrome. Although this is a rare occurrence, consider this possibility in unexplained weakness or paralysis after a person (especially a child) has recently been out in the woods.

The principal treatment of a tick bite is careful removal of the tick. Ticks attach themselves tenaciously to their victims using their mouth parts and a cementlike adhesive. If you try to pull the tick away from the skin, the mouth parts may remain embedded. To remove the tick, after putting on gloves, use a curved forceps to grasp the tick by the head, as close to the skin as possible, and pull straight upward using steady gentle traction. Use even pressure as you pull, and avoid twisting or jerking the tick. Do not squeeze or crush the tick's body. Dispose of the tick in a container of alcohol.

Once you have removed the tick, wash the area around the bite with soap and water. There is no reason to transport the patient if he or she remains asymptomatic. In case of tick paralysis, transport the patient with spinal motion restriction to an appropriate facility.

Spider Bites

There are an estimated 34,000 species of spiders worldwide. All of these carnivores can bite; they normally use their venom to subdue their prey. Two types of spiders are of medical concern in the United States: the black widow and the brown recluse.

Black Widow Spider

Only the female black widow spider poses a danger to humans. Her name derives from her rather disagreeable practice of devouring her mate. This spider is glossy black with a half-inch oval body, a leg span of about 1.5″, and a characteristic orange or reddish hourglass mark on the abdomen Figure 33-18.

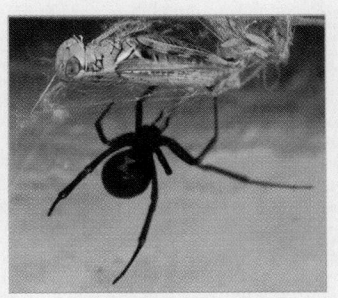

Figure 33-18 Black widow spiders are distinguished by their glossy black body and bright red-orange hourglass marking on the abdomen.

The black widow spider is found throughout the United States, but especially in the southeast. Most of the 500 or 1,000 or so black widow spider bites that occur each year in the United States happen between the months of April and October. This spider makes its home in sheds, basements, garages, woodpiles, and similar areas. Because it likes to hang out in outhouses, bites may occur in some rather unusual—and highly sensitive areas—of the anatomy. Nevertheless, most wounds involve the hands or forearms.

A history of a spider bite is not often confirmed. Instead, the patient may report a sudden, sharp prick followed by a cramping or numbing pain that begins at the bite area and gradually spreads. Extreme restlessness is the classic sign of the reaction to a black widow spider bite.

A careful search on the physical examination often reveals slight swelling in the area of the bite and tiny red bite marks. Because the bite itself is not obvious, many patients with black widow spider bites are often misdiagnosed with an acute abdomen. Notably, the abdomen is not tender to palpation, even though it may be rigid from muscle spasms. Other signs and symptoms may include excruciating pain; muscular rigidity, especially in the abdomen; severe respiratory distress and dyspnea; nausea and vomiting; hypertension; hypersalivation; and paresthesias (pins and needles sensations).

Despite the fact that black widow spider bites have a mortality rate of about 5%, treatment in the prehospital setting is largely supportive. Establish and maintain the airway, inserting an advanced airway as needed. Give high-flow supplemental oxygen, and establish vascular access. Manage pain by giving opioids or benzodiazepines per local protocol. For severe muscle spasms, contact medical control for consideration of calcium gluconate administration, although this therapy remains controversial.

Brown Recluse Spider

The brown recluse spider is not large—only ½″ long and ¼″ wide—but it can deliver a nasty bite. As its name implies, this

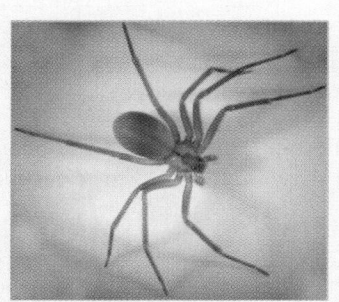

spider is usually brown or tan and has a violin-shaped band of a darker color that extends backward from its eyes; this feature is responsible for its alternative name, "fiddleback" spider Figure 33-19 . Brown recluse spiders are found most commonly in the southern and midwestern United States but can be found in a much larger geographic area. Abandoned buildings, sheds, and workshops are favorite haunts for these creatures.

Figure 33-19 Brown recluse spiders are dull brown and have a dark, violin-shaped mark on the back.

The bite of a brown recluse spider may not result in immediate symptoms Figure 33-20 . Indeed, several hours may pass before the local reaction is noticed. That reaction consists of a painful, reddened area with overlying blister formation and a white surrounding area of ischemia. During the next few days (or longer), the area turns dark and becomes deeply ulcerated. It is usually at this point that the patient seeks care. Systemic reactions may accompany the local reaction and can be quite severe; they may include weakness, nausea, vomiting, rash, and anxiety.

Prehospital treatment for a patient with a brown recluse spider bite consists of providing the general care given to any other ill patient.

Scorpion Stings

Arguably some of the scarier-looking creatures in nature, scorpions live in warm climates around the world, including Mexico, India, Africa, South America, and the Caribbean. In the United States, they are found principally in the southwest—namely, Arizona, New Mexico, and southern California. Of the many species of scorpions, all of which can deliver a painful sting, only the bark scorpion is commonly associated with deaths in the United States Figure 33-21 .

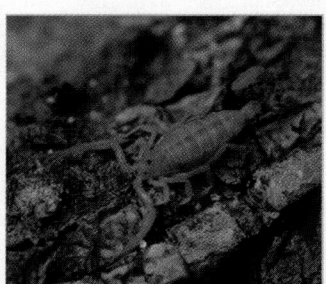

Figure 33-21 The bark scorpion.

Scorpions tend to be nocturnal creatures, living under decks, in the bark or rotted trunk of trees, or in brush piles. They may occasionally stray into a house. If touched or stepped on, the scorpion releases its venom from the stinger on its whiplike tail. A scorpion sting causes immediate pain at the wound site, followed by numbness or tingling. The pain is usually exacerbated by pressure to the wound site. Eventually, the peripheral area around the wound becomes hypersensitive to touch and temperature changes.

The sting of the bark scorpion, especially with severe envenomation, can cause dramatic neuromuscular signs and symptoms: uncontrolled roving movements of the eyes, blurred vision, drooling, difficulty swallowing, slurred speech, severe agitation, nausea, vomiting, muscle twitching or spasms, and, possibly, seizures.

The initial field treatment for a scorpion bite focuses on pain relief with analgesics and transport to the appropriate facility. For a bark scorpion sting in which the patient shows signs of severe toxicity, a goat-derived antivenin may be used. This antivenin has been associated with immediate and delayed allergic reactions and serum sickness.

In the field, application of a constricting band just above the wound site (but not tight enough to occlude the pulse) may reduce lymph flow and the subsequent spread of venom; follow your local protocol. In the unlikely event of seizures, treat with benzodiazepines per local protocol and transport the patient to an appropriate facility.

Snakebites

Venomous snakes cause an estimated 3 million bites and 150,000 deaths worldwide each year. Approximately 120 species of snakes are indigenous to the United States, but fewer than 20% are venomous. Most venomous snakebites in the United

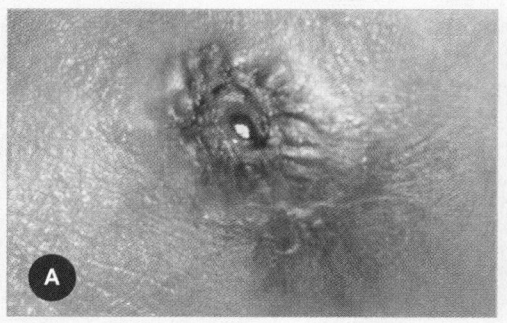
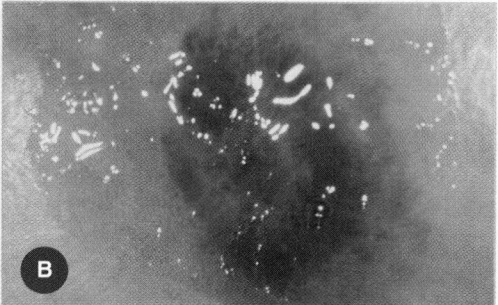

Figure 33-20 Brown recluse spider bite in early stage (**A**) and late stage (**B**).

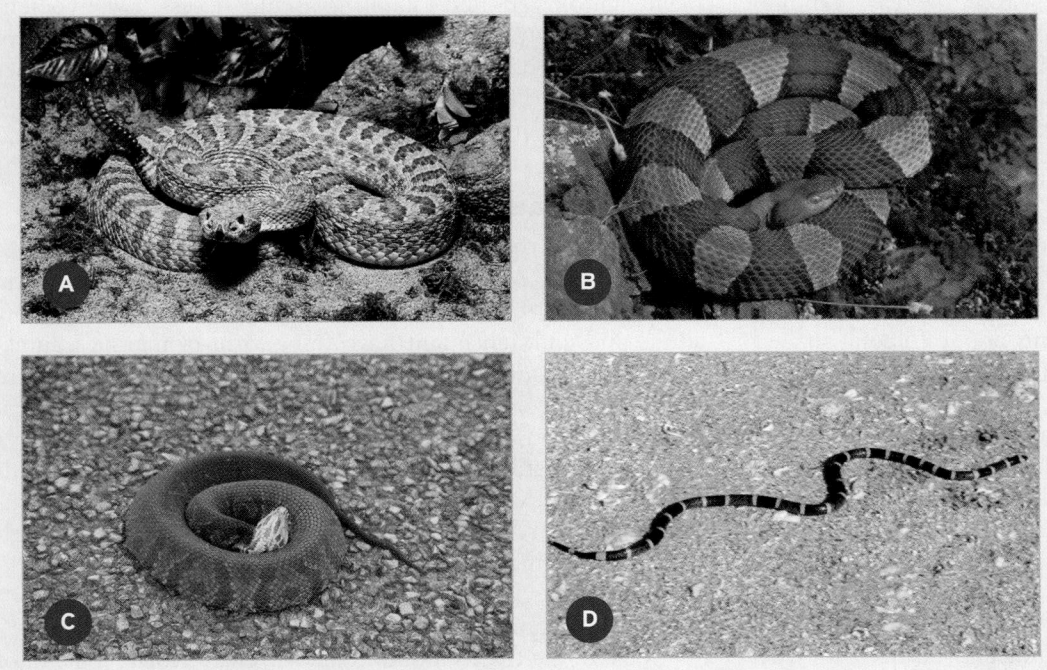

Figure 33-22 **A.** Rattlesnake. **B.** Copperhead. **C.** Cottonmouth. **D.** Coral snake.

This venom is composed of a mix of enzymes that cause local tissue damage, hemolysis, increased permeability of the vasculature, coagulopathy, and neuromuscular dysfunction.

Although one of every four pit viper bites is "dry" (that is, no signs or symptoms of venom release), envenomation, when it occurs, may produce a variety of signs and symptoms. The most common are fang marks, localized pain, and rapidly developing edema around the area of the bite, usually within 15 to 30 minutes. Other signs and symptoms of a pit viper bite include nausea and vomiting, dizziness or weakness, oral numbness or tingling of the mouth and tongue, tachycardia and hypotension, tachypnea, and muscle fasciculations.

First and foremost, make certain that the scene is safe—that is, that the snake is dead, trapped, or gone. In short, make absolutely certain that the snake is *not* a threat to the EMS team or the patient. In addition, you should establish and maintain the airway, give high-flow supplemental oxygen, and establish vascular access. Keep

States involve pit vipers and coral snakes, although other venomous, exotic species may be imported. Of the 6,000 bites reported to the AAPCC each year, only a small number (0.5%) produce death.

Pit Vipers

Pit vipers include rattlesnakes, copperheads, and cottonmouth moccasins, with the rattlesnake the most common Figure 33-22 ▲ . In the United States, one of the most impressive snakes is the diamondback rattlesnake, which can be 8′ long and weigh close to 30 lb—clearly, a creature best left in peace.

The head of a pit viper is triangular, somewhat resembling an arrowhead. Just beneath the eyes on either side is an indentation or pit, which is a heat-sensing organ that helps the snake locate its prey Figure 33-23 ▶ . Pit vipers also have vertical pupils (most other snakes have round pupils). Their long, erectile fangs are used to puncture the skin, leaving a distinctive mark.

Pit vipers are not naturally aggressive, although some (such as cottonmouths) seem to be more easily irritated than others. Pit vipers usually attack people in self-defense or when surprised, such as when a hiker accidentally steps on a snake. A pit viper strikes with lightning speed. Its fangs snap forward from their folded-back position, and they inject a variable amount of venom—ranging from no venom to a potentially lethal dose.

Notes from Nancy

Not every snakebite contains venom.

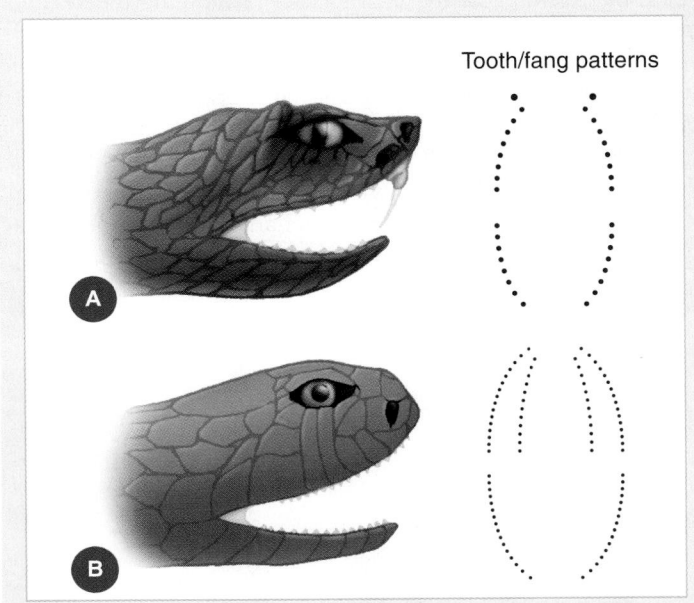

Tooth/fang patterns

Figure 33-23 Characteristics of pit vipers and nonpoisonous snakes. **A.** Pit vipers have vertical pupils, a pit between the eye and the nostril, a single row of teeth, and two erectile fangs. **B.** Nonpoisonous snakes have round pupils and often a double row of upper teeth; they do not leave fang marks.

the patient calm, supine, and motionless to decrease venom spread and absorption. Immobilize the extremity with the bite in a neutral position below the level of the heart. For hypotension, administer fluid boluses of normal saline. Finally, begin immediate transport to a facility where the patient can receive antivenin.

Coral Snakes

Coral snakes are found around the world, most commonly in warm or tropical areas. In the United States, they are primarily found in the southeast, although Arizona and Texas have coral snake species named after the state. Only about 25 coral snake bites occur each year in the United States.

Coral snakes are brightly colored with red, yellow, and black rings (Figure 33-22D). On a coral snake, the red and yellow rings touch; on nonpoisonous snakes, there is a black ring between the red and yellow rings. This difference leads to the helpful saying, "Red on yellow, kill a fellow; red on black, venom they lack."

Because coral snake venom mostly consists of neurotoxins, the patient with a bite will usually present with neurologic signs and symptoms rather than a significant localized injury. Even when a bite results in significant envenomation, the patient may report feeling fine and may remain asymptomatic for 12 hours or longer. Once signs and symptoms begin to appear, you should expect nausea and vomiting; tremors or seizures; drooling; paralysis of the face, mouth, or vocal cords; fixed, dilated pupils; blurred vision; ataxia; muscle weakness (but possibly a stiff neck); dyspnea; respiratory failure (the usual cause of death); hypotension; and loss of consciousness.

Along with the usual assessment and initial attention to the ABCs, management in the field focuses on limiting the systemic spread of the venom by containing it within the lymphatic vessels. Apply a compression bandage starting at the bite site, and then wrap the entire extremity. Use the same pressure with which you would wrap a sprained ankle—not tight enough to occlude pulses, but not loose and hanging off. Place the patient supine, and splint the injured extremity, keeping it at the level of the heart.

In addition, you should establish and maintain the airway, inserting an advanced airway as needed. Give high-flow sup-

plemental oxygen, and establish vascular access. For hypotension, administer serial boluses of normal saline. Control seizures with benzodiazepines or phenytoin (Dilantin), per local protocol. Finally, transport the patient immediately to an appropriate facility.

Marine Trauma and Envenomations

Almost half of the world's population lives within 125 miles of a coastal area. Add to that the huge number of people who enjoy marine recreation activities, and it's easy to see how adults and children might have some form of marine trauma. In one US study, the most common marine injuries were reported to involve jellyfish stings (31%); venomous fish stings, including catfish, rockfish, and lionfish (28%); stingrays (16%); and gastropods (6%). Most marine trauma is the result of accidental exposures, such as swimming into a jellyfish, stepping on a sea urchin, or scraping against coral. Although shark attacks make for great news coverage, fewer than 100 shark attacks occur worldwide each year, and they result in 5 to 15 deaths annually on average.

Most of the toxins found in marine creatures are a blend of protein and peptide toxins that have an impressive ability to produce excruciating pain from even a tiny injury. These toxins tend to be unstable and, in most cases, can be deactivated by applying a hot compress. In addition to the toxins, microorganisms and contaminants found in saltwater and fresh water greatly increase the likelihood of a secondary infection in marine trauma.

Signs and symptoms vary greatly, depending on the creature involved, but may include nausea and vomiting, extreme pain, localized swelling, tachycardia, and dyspnea. Most marine trauma is not life threatening, so treatment focuses primarily on wound irrigation, removal of foreign bodies (spines, teeth), pain relief, and transport. In addition, establish and maintain the airway. Apply hot compresses or hot water to the wound (about 110°F—just slightly hotter than hot tub water). Carefully remove nematocysts or stingers. Treat pain with opioids per local protocol, and transport the patient to an appropriate facility.

You are the Provider Summary

1. What are your priorities at this point?

Safety is the main priority at all times. In this scenario, crowd control might be a factor. Once you are confident of scene safety, turn your attention to addressing the patient's ABCs. Additional priorities include obtaining as much pertinent information as possible and appointing someone to contact the patient's parents or caregivers.

2. What information do you need to obtain?

This scenario emphasizes the need to obtain as much information related to SAMPLE as possible. Because the patient cannot provide information, your sources will be her friends and the coach. Patients with altered mental status can have a wide variety of problems, and SAMPLE will be one of the keys to providing successful treatment.

3. What are some potential differential diagnoses?

Although your rapid trauma survey did not reveal life-threatening injuries, you cannot rule out a head injury as the cause of Julie's altered mental status. Based on the information you have at this point, other differential diagnoses include overdose, hypoglycemia, and infection.

4. Which interventions should you consider at this point, if any?

By now, you should have delegated the role of cervical-spine immobilization. The patient is already receiving supplemental oxygen. While you perform a detailed physical assessment, you can ask your partner to obtain a glucose level and apply the cardiac monitor. Until you obtain more information, no further interventions are needed.

5. Given the current situation, should you consider the patient treating on the scene, or continuing treatment on the way to the hospital?

In this case, it is best to package the patient and continue treatment on the way to the hospital. If the patient's condition continues to deteriorate, the optimal place for treatment to be given would be the ED.

6. How should your patient management progress?

Maintenance of the ABCs should take priority. Now that you have ruled out trauma as a potential MOI, the patient no longer requires cervical-spine immobilization. Field management for a tricyclic antidepressant overdose such as Elavil is administration of sodium bicarbonate. Depending on your department's protocol, you might have to contact the receiving hospital for orders. Remember to bring the medication bottle to the hospital. Also, keep a watchful eye on the cardiac monitor for the development of ventricular rhythms associated with the drug's toxicity.

7. Can the information you provide to the hospital staff during your radio report contribute to a negative patient outcome?

Absolutely! Not providing the proper information to the hospital staff can lead to mistreatment of your patient. In this case, not making the ED staff aware of the ingestion of amitriptyline, including the dose and number of pills taken, might delay lifesaving treatment or lead to the administration of incorrect treatment that produces unwanted complications, including death. You are the eyes and ears of the ED physician—it is your responsibility to paint an accurate picture that enables the physician to make proper treatment decisions.

8. Are there any potential complications that can arise during transport relative to the patient's condition?

Tricyclic antidepressants are extremely toxic medications. Life-threatening events potentially include the development of ventricular arrhythmias, seizures, and pulmonary edema. Sound knowledge of the effects of tricyclic antidepressants and good assessment skills are paramount to the delivery of effective patient care.

Prep Kit

■ Ready for Review

- Toxicologic emergencies usually fall under one of two general headings: intentional and unintentional.
- Given the variety of illicit drugs coupled with the continued growth of licit drugs, even the most well-read veteran paramedic may find it difficult to stay current with the myriad drugs sold in the streets today. For this reason, Poison Centers may be an indispensable aid.
- The four primary methods whereby a toxin commonly enters the body are ingestion, inhalation, injection, and absorption.
- Although the sheer number of substances of abuse may seem daunting, the good news is that many drugs, on entering the body, produce similar signs and symptoms.
- Human beings have a long history of abusing drugs and alcohol. With the passing of time, the physiologic and societal effects of alcohol abuse have become well known and thoroughly documented. Unfortunately, the area of medicine dealing with drugs of abuse is challenging because of uncertainty about the prevalence of the problem and the continual evolution of the substances themselves.
- Alcohol is the most widely abused drug in the United States.
- Generally, patients with toxicologic emergencies are considered medical patients, although toxicologic emergencies may lead to trauma, too.
- From a management perspective, ALS care builds on the basics:
  - Ensure the scene is safe for access and egress.
  - Maintain the airway.
  - Ensure that breathing is adequate.
  - Ensure that circulation isn't compromised (by hypoperfusion or arrhythmia).
  - Administer high-concentration supplemental oxygen.
  - Establish vascular access.
  - Be prepared to manage shock, coma, seizures, and arrhythmias.
  - Transport the patient as soon as possible. Place the patient in the left lateral recumbent position if there is any risk of vomiting to reduce the risk of aspiration.

■ Vital Vocabulary

alcoholism A state of physical and psychological addiction to ethanol.

amphetamines A class of drugs that increase alertness and excitation (that is, stimulants); includes methamphetamine (crank or ice), methylenedioxyamphetamine (MDA, Adam), and methylenedioxymethamphetamine (MDMA, Eve, ecstasy).

antagonist Something that counteracts the action of something else; in relation to drugs, a drug that is an antagonist has an affinity for a cell receptor and, by binding to it, the cell is prevented from responding.

barbiturates Potent sedative-hypnotics historically used as sleep aids, antianxiety drugs, and as part of the regimen for seizure control.

benzodiazepines The family of sedative-hypnotics most commonly used to treat anxiety, seizures, and alcohol withdrawal.

caladium A common houseplant that contains caladium oxalate crystals; ingestion leads to nausea, vomiting, and diarrhea.

castor bean A seed that contains the poison ricin; causes a variety of toxic effects: burning of the mouth and throat; nausea, vomiting, diarrhea, and severe stomach pains; prostration; failing vision and kidney failure, which is the usual cause of death.

caustics Chemicals that are acids or alkalis; cause direct chemical injury to the tissues they contact.

delirium tremens (DTs) A severe withdrawal syndrome seen in people with alcoholism who are deprived of ethyl alcohol; characterized by restlessness, fever, sweating, disorientation, agitation, and seizures; can be fatal if untreated.

dieffenbachia A common houseplant that resembles "elephant ears"; ingestion leads to burns of the mouth and tongue and, possibly, paralysis of the vocal cords and nausea and vomiting; in severe cases, may be edema of the tongue and larynx, leading to airway compromise.

drug Substance that has some therapeutic effect (such as reducing inflammation, fighting bacteria, or producing euphoria) when given in the appropriate circumstances and in the appropriate dose.

drug abuse Any use of drugs that causes physical, psychological, economic, legal, or social harm to the user or others affected by the user's behavior.

drug addiction A chronic disorder characterized by the compulsive use of a substance that results in physical, psychological, or social harm to the user who continues to use the substance despite the harm.

foxglove A plant that contains cardiac glycosides used in making digitalis; ingestion of leaves causes nausea, vomiting, diarrhea, abdominal cramps, hyperkalemia, and a variety of arrhythmias.

habituation The situation in which there is a physical tolerance and psychological dependence on a drug or drugs.

hallucinogen An agent that produces false perceptions in any one of the five senses.

hydrocarbons Compounds made up principally of hydrogen and carbon atom mostly obtained from the distillation of petroleum.

illicit In relation to drugs, illegal drugs such as marijuana, cocaine, and LSD.

lantana A perennial flowering shrub with clusters of red berries that can lead to serious and even fatal poisoning; Also known as red sage or wild sage; ingestion causes stomach upsets, muscle weakness, shock, and, sometimes, death.

licit In relation to drugs, legalized drugs such as coffee, alcohol, and tobacco.

lithium The cornerstone drug for the treatment of bipolar disorder.

marijuana The dried leaves and flower buds of the *Cannabis sativa* plant that are smoked to achieve a high.

methamphetamine A highly addictive drug in the amphetamine family.

monoamine oxidase inhibitors (MAOIs) Psychiatric medication used primarily to treat atypical depression by increasing norepinephrine and serotonin levels in the central nervous system.

narcotic The generic term for opiates and opioids, drugs that act as a CNS depressant and produce insensibility or stupor.

opiate Various alkaloids derived from the opium or poppy plant.

opioid A synthetic narcotic not derived from opium.

organophosphates A class of chemical found in many insecticides used in agriculture and in the home.

physical dependence A physiologic state of adaptation to a drug, usually characterized by tolerance to the drug's effects and a withdrawal syndrome if use of the drug is stopped, especially abruptly.

poison A substance whose chemical action could damage structures or impair function when introduced into the body.

potentiation Enhancement of the effect of one drug by another drug.

psychological dependence The emotional state of craving a drug to maintain a feeling of well-being.

salicylates Aspirinlike drugs.

sedative-hypnotic A drug used to reduce anxiety, calm agitated patients, and help produce drowsiness and sleep (CNS depressants).

selective serotonin reuptake inhibitors (SSRIs) A class of antidepressants that inhibit the reuptake of serotonin.

serotonin syndrome An idiosyncratic complication that occurs with antidepressant therapy in which patients have lower extremity muscle rigidity, confusion or disorientation, and/or agitation.

synergism The action of two substances such as drugs, in which the *total effects are greater than the sum of the independent effects* of the two substances.

theophylline A naturally occurring alkaloid found in a variety of plants (such as tea leaves).

tolerance Physiologic adaptation to the effects of a drug such that increasingly larger doses of the drug are required to achieve the same effect.

toxicologic emergencies Medical emergencies caused by toxic agents such as poison.

toxidrome The syndrome-like symptoms of a poisonous agent.

tricyclic antidepressants (TCAs) A group of drugs used to treat severe depression and manage pain; minimal dosing errors can cause toxic results.

withdrawal syndrome A predictable set of signs and symptoms, usually involving altered central nervous system activity, that occurs after the abrupt cessation of a drug or after rapidly decreasing the usual dosage of a drug.

Points to Ponder

You and your partner are called to a single-family residence near a college campus. When you arrive in front of the residence, you notice a large number of college-age people gathered around someone lying supine on the front lawn. A law enforcement officer arrives on the scene at the same time you do. You approach the patient and find a female who looks to be in her late teens or early 20s. You hear snoring respirations and notice that the patient is covered in emesis. As your partner is rolling the patient to her side and clearing her airway, you ask some of the bystanders what happened. They back away, saying, "We were just having a party, and she wasn't feeling good so we brought her outside." Your partner reports that the patient is breathing and responds to deep painful stimuli but does not have a gag reflex.

What is your first treatment priority? Can you immediately assume that the signs and symptoms you are seeing are caused by alcohol ingestion? What other assessment points should you consider?

Issues: Assessing a Potential Alcohol Overdose, Obtaining Information From Bystanders.

Assessment in Action

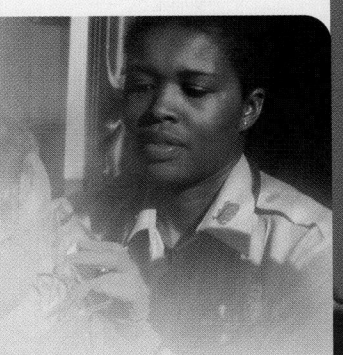

You and your partner have arrived on the scene of a reported diabetic emergency. When you arrive at the patient's side, you see a 50-year-old man who seems to be unconscious on the floor. The patient's wife states that her husband had been at work all day. When he arrived at home, he stated he had a very bad headache and then collapsed to the floor. The wife confirms that the patient has type 1 diabetes.

As you and your partner begin your assessment, you notice that he is drooling severely, is diaphoretic, and has been incontinent. You direct your partner to obtain a blood glucose level, which comes back as 180 mg/dL. You were assuming that this call was for a diabetic emergency, but now that does not seem to be the case. As you return to your assessment, the patient vomits a large amount, which has a distinct chemical smell. You suction the patient aggressively and complete airway management measures. When you ask the wife what the patient may have been around at work, she says that her husband works at a landscaping business.

1. **What are the two types of toxicologic emergencies?**
   A. Licit and illicit
   B. Prescribed and OTC
   C. Intentional and unintentional
   D. Drug or poison

2. **The patient in this scenario may be experiencing signs and symptoms of which toxidrome?**
   A. Stimulant
   B. Narcotic
   C. Sedative-hypnotic
   D. Cholinergic

3. **You determine through further questioning that the patient was using some kind of chemical at work, but the wife does not know what it was. What is your primary concern at this point in your assessment?**
   A. Determine what your crew and bystanders have potentially been exposed to.
   B. Move the patient quickly to your ambulance and transport immediately.
   C. Obtain IV access and administer naloxone per protocol.
   D. Determine the potential for the patient to become violent.

4. **A patient with signs and symptoms of SLUDGE may have been exposed to:**
   A. carbon monoxide.
   B. organophosphates.
   C. barbiturates.
   D. chlorine.

5. **Organophosphates exert their toxic effects on which body system?**
   A. Integumentary
   B. Cardiac
   C. Nervous
   D. Endocrine

6. **The approach to a patient with organophosphate poisoning should start with:**
   A. decontamination and removal of contaminated items.
   B. administering atropine 1.0 mg IV push immediately.
   C. contacting law enforcement personnel to prevent violence.
   D. obtaining an oxygen saturation level on your patient.

Challenging Question

7. **Given that your crew and the patient's wife have potentially been contaminated through contact with the patient's clothing and emesis, which component becomes the most important part of decontamination—the patient or everyone else in the room?**

Hematologic Emergencies

Objectives

Cognitive

5-9.1   Identify the anatomy of the hematopoietic system. (p 34.4)

5-9.2   Describe volume and volume-control related to the hematopoietic system. (p 34.4)

5-9.3   Identify and describe the blood-forming organs. (p 34.5)

5-9.4   Describe normal red blood cell (RBC) production, function and destruction. (p 34.5)

5-9.5   Explain the significance of the hematocrit with respect to red cell size and number. (p 34.4)

5-9.6   Explain the correlation of the RBC count, hematocrit and hemoglobin values. (p 34.4)

5-9.7   Define anemia. (p 34.6)

5-9.8   Describe normal white blood cell (WBC) production, function and destruction. (p 34.5)

5-9.9   Identify the characteristics of the inflammatory process. (p 34.5)

5-9.10   Identify the difference between cellular and humoral immunity. (p 34.5)

5-9.11   Identify alterations in immunologic response. (p 34.5)

5-9.12   Describe the number, normal function, types and life span of leukocytes. (p 34.3)

5-9.13   List the leukocyte disorders. (p 34.7)

5-9.14   Describe platelets with respect to normal function, life span and numbers. (p 34.4)

5-9.15   Describe the components of the hemostatic mechanism. (p 34.4)

5-9.16   Describe the function of coagulation factors, platelets and blood vessels necessary for normal coagulation. (p 34.4)

5-9.17   Describe the intrinsic and extrinsic clotting systems with respect to identification of factor deficiencies in each stage. (p 6.39, 6.40)

5-9.18   Identify blood groups. (p 34.5)

5-9.19   Describe how acquired factor deficiencies may occur. (p 34.8)

5-9.20   Define fibrinolysis. (p 34.8)

5-9.21   Identify the components of physical assessment as they relate to the hematologic system. (p 34.10)

5-9.22   Describe the pathology and clinical manifestations and prognosis associated with:
  1. Anemia
  2. Leukemia
  3. Lymphomas
  4. Polycythemia
  5. Disseminated intravascular coagulopathy
  6. Hemophilia
  7. Sickle cell disease
  8. Multiple myeloma (p 34.6–34.9)

5-9.23   Integrate pathophysiological principles into the assessment of a patient with hematologic disease. (p 34.9)

Affective

5-9.24   Value the sense of urgency for initial assessment and interventions for patients with hematologic crises. (p 34.9)

Psychomotor

5-9.25   Perform an assessment of the patient with hematologic disorder. (p 34.9)

Introduction

Most EMS systems rarely respond to hematologic emergencies. Hematologic disorders can be complex, difficult to assess, and challenging to treat in the out-of-hospital setting. Although you may be able to provide only limited interventions, your actions may not only offer support, but actually save the patient's life. As a paramedic, you should have a basic understanding of the hematopoietic system (the blood components and the organs involved in their development and production) and hematologic disorders, and you should know how to respond to these kinds of emergencies appropriately.

Anatomy and Physiology

Blood and Plasma

Blood is "the fluid of life": Without it, we would not be able to live. Blood performs the following functions:

- **Respiratory function.** Transports oxygen from the lungs to the tissues and carbon dioxide from the tissues to the lungs
- **Nutritional function.** Carries nutrients (glucose, proteins, and fats) from the digestive tract to cells throughout the body
- **Excretory function.** Ferries the waste products of metabolism from the cells where they are produced to the excretory organs
- **Regulatory function.** Transports hormones to their target organs and transmits excess internal heat to the surface of the body to be dissipated
- **Defensive function.** Carries defensive cells and antibodies, which protect the body against foreign organisms

Blood is made up of two main components: plasma and formed elements (cells). Plasma is essentially 92% water and 6% to 7% proteins; the remainder consists of a variety of other elements (including electrolytes, clotting factors, glucose). Plasma accounts for 55% of the total blood volume. It has a specific gravity of around 1.03. Specific gravity is a substance's weight compared with that of water. Water has a specific gravity of 1.0, so anything with a specific gravity greater than 1.0 is "heavier" than water and anything with a specific gravity less than 1.0 is "lighter."

The formed elements account for 45% of the total blood volume. These elements include red blood cells (RBCs) or erythrocytes, white blood cells (WBCs) or leukocytes, and platelets or thrombocytes Figure 34-1 . Most of these elements (99%) are RBCs.

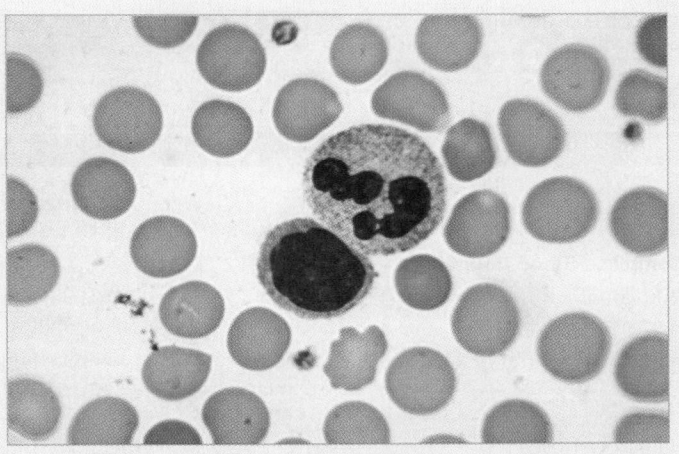

Figure 34-1 The components of blood include RBCs, WBCs, platelets, and plasma.

You are the Provider Part 1

It is early evening, and you have just been dispatched to 1355 Northwest Lane for a 30-year-old man complaining of shortness of breath and severe abdominal pain. Per department standard operating procedures, the engine crew, consisting of a paramedic lieutenant, two fire fighters (EMT-Bs), and engineer (EMT-B), respond along with you to provide additional assistance.

When you arrive, you are greeted at the front door by a concerned family member. The woman points to the bedroom and says, "He's in there! He's having another attack!" When you enter the bedroom, you see an African-American man sitting on the edge of the bed holding his stomach.

Initial Assessment	Recording Time: 0 Minutes
Appearance	Eyes open with pained expression
Level of consciousness	A (Alert to person, place, and day)
Airway	Patent
Breathing	Fast, labored, and shallow
Circulation	Weak, fast radial pulse; diaphoretic skin

1. What, if anything, about his appearance gives you cause for concern?
2. What information do you already have at your disposal?

RBC production occurs within stem cells; this production is stimulated by a protein secreted by the kidneys in response to circulatory need. RBCs may take as long as 5 days to mature and have an average life of about 4 months. Their specific gravity is approximately 1.09. Within the RBCs, iron-rich hemoglobin is responsible for carrying oxygen to the tissues. Oxygen attached to hemoglobin gives blood its characteristic red color, although many other factors can change the color of blood (such as carbon monoxide poisoning).

Three laboratory tests are commonly performed on blood: RBC count, hemoglobin level, and hematocrit. The RBC count measures the number of RBCs in a sample of blood. The hemoglobin level identifies the percentage of hemoglobin found within the RBCs. The hematocrit gives the overall percentage of RBCs in the blood. The patient's blood is considered balanced (even if the numbers are too high or low) if the hemoglobin level is one third of the hematocrit and the RBC count is one third of the hemoglobin level. **Table 34-1 ▾** describes these tests in more detail.

WBCs, which are larger than RBCs, provide the body with immunity against "foreign invaders." They are derived from the stem cells, or cells that develop into other types of cells in the body. Several types of WBCs exist, each of which performs a specific task in relation to maintaining the immune system.

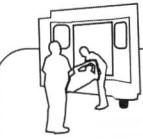

In the Field

Platelets form the initial plug following vascular injury. The clotting proteins then toughen and complete the blood clot.

Platelets are the smallest of the formed elements and are responsible for the clotting of the blood. (The coagulation process or hemostasis is described in more detail in Chapter 6.) Approximately two thirds of the platelets circulate throughout the blood; the rest are stored in the spleen. Platelets are also derived from stem cells. They have an average life span of up to 11 days.

Table 34-1	RBC and WBC Tests		
Name	**Normal Values**	**Conditions Associated With Low Readings**	**Conditions Associated With High Readings**
Complete Blood Count Test			
RBC count	4.5–6.0 adult 3.3–5.5 child	Anemia, hemorrhage, certain leukemias, overyhydration, chronic infections	Polycythemia, cardiovascular disease, hemoconcentration, dehydration
Hemoglobin (Hgb)	12.0–16.0 female 14.0–18.0 male 10.7–17.1 child	Anemia, hyperthyroidism, liver disease, hemorrhage, hemolytic reactions	COPD, CHF, polycythemia, high altitude sickness
Hematocrit (HCT)	35%–45% female 40%–50% male 32%–55% child	As above, including leukemia, lupus, endocarditis, rheumatic fever, nutritional disorders	Polycythemia and usually anything that produces severe dehydration
WBC Count and Differential			
WBC count	5,000–10,000 adult 4,500–15,500 child 9,400–34,000 infant	Viral infections, bone marrow diseases or disorders, leukemia, radiation, late-stage AIDS	Viral and bacterial infections, hemorrhage, traumatic tissue injuries, leukemia, cigarette smoking
Neutrophils (segmented and unsegmented)	50%–60%* 2,500–8,000/mm^3	Leukemia, infections, rheumatoid arthritis, vitamin B12 deficiency, enlarged spleen	Bacterial infections, tissue breakdown, hemolytic reactions, tumors, MI, surgical stress, and cancer
Basophils (also known as mast cells)	0.5%–1%* 25–100/mm^3	Allergic reactions, hyperthyroidism, MI, bleeding ulcers, stress	Certain leukemias, inflammations, allergy, polycythemia, hemolytic anemia
Eosinophils	1%–4%* 50–500/mm^3	Mononucleosis, CHF, Cushing disease	Addison disease, tumors, skin infections, allergies
Lymphocytes	20%–40%* 1,000–4,000/mm^3	Hodgkin disease, burns, trauma, lupus, Cushing disease, immunodeficiency states	Numerous bacterial and viral infections, hepatitis, leukemia, toxoplasmosis, Graves' disease
Monocytes	2%–6%* 100–700/mm^3	Steroid use, infections, rheumatoid arthritis, HIV	Numerous bacterial and parasitic infections, recovery of acute infections, TB, hematologic disorders
Thrombocytes (platelets)	150,000–400,000 μL	Thrombocytopenia, certain cancers, certain leukemias, sickle cell disease, systemic lupus erythematosus	Pulmonary embolism, polycythemia, acute hemorrhage, metastatic cancer, surgical stress

COPD indicates chronic obstructive pulmonary disease; CHF, congestive heart failure; MI, myocardial infarction; and TB, tuberculosis.
*Percentage of the total WBC count.
Example: If the WBC is 5,000, neutrophils should account for 2,500 to 3,000 of this count.

Challenging Questions

You are dispatched to the local mall for a fall victim. On arrival, you find a 42-year-old man sitting at the base of the steps. According to witnesses, he tripped up the steps, lost his balance, and then fell down four steps. He is alert to his name but is confused about what happened. The patient complains of pain to his left axillary area and his left knee. During your assessment, you find him to be tachycardic, tachypneic, and grossly diaphoretic. His blood pressure is 70/30 mm Hg, pulse rate is 118 beats/min, and respiratory rate is 30 breaths/min. While you and your partner are providing the patient with full cervical-spine precautions, you note a bruise on his left flank area. You provide the patient with 100% supplemental oxygen via a nonrebreathing mask and take him to the ambulance for transport to the emergency department.

During your focused exam, you note a medical ID tag that reads "Hemophilia A." You initiate IV therapy and provide a fluid bolus. The patient is transported to the hospital without any further incident. You give report to the emergency department nurse and physician. You overhear the physician order "factor VIII" from the pharmacy.

14. **What is your primary care in the field for a patient with hemophilia?**

15. **What would your primary care be for any patient with a hematopoietic problem?**

▒ Points to Ponder

You respond to a private residence, where you find a 28-year-old African-American woman lying in bed. She complains of pain in her chest with associated shortness of breath. You note swelling of her hands and feet. The patient says that she has had the flu for the past 2 days and has vomited at least four times. She has also had a low-grade fever and generalized body aches. Your physical exam reveals nothing truly remarkable. The patient has a history of high blood pressure and sickle cell disease.

What is happening with this patient physiologically? What, if any, treatment should you administer?

Issues: Understand the Urgency for Assessment and Intervention in Patients With Hematologic Crises.

35

Environmental Emergencies

Objectives

Cognitive

Affective

None

Psychomotor

None

Introduction

According to the Centers for Disease Control and Prevention, 4,607 people died of hypothermia-related causes from 1999 to 2002. During 1979 to 2002, 4,780 deaths were classified as heat-related. Environmental emergencies are medical conditions caused or worsened by the weather, terrain, or unique atmospheric conditions such as high altitude or underwater. Most EMS providers would recognize the obvious problem of a child who has fallen into an icy lake. The challenge lies in recognizing patients with environmental emergencies in the unusual settings of endurance sports events or at mass gatherings, and even acutely confused older patients Figure 35-1 ▾ .

Unique to environmental emergencies are the conditions that directly cause harm or complicate treatment and transport considerations. Wind, rain, snow, temperature extremes, and humidity may all affect the body's ability to adapt to its environment. Unprepared hikers can experience cold illnesses during summer rainstorms as easily as overdressed snow sports enthusiasts can die of heat illnesses during strenuous outings. The locations of these outings can also have a huge impact on the ability to know about, respond to, and rescue people in remote settings Figure 35-2 ▾ .

Certain generic risk factors predispose people to environmental emergencies. In addition, very young and old people have unique disadvantages when it comes to thermoregulation. Conditions such as diabetes, cardiac disease (for example, coronary artery disease, congestive heart failure), restrictive lung disease, thyroid disease, and psychiatric illnesses can alter the body's ability to compensate for environmental extremes.

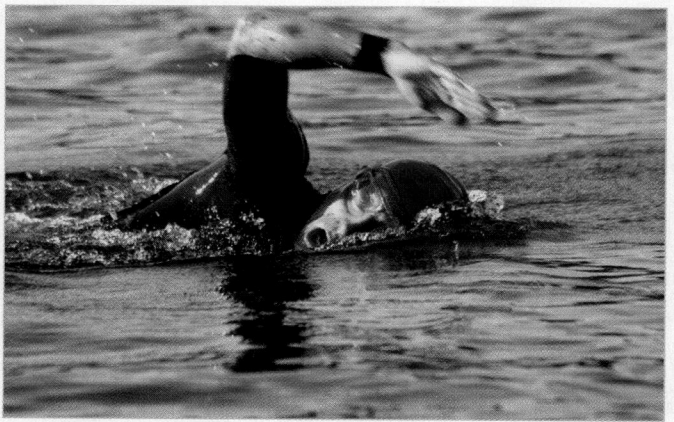

Figure 35-1 Environmental emergencies can occur in a variety of settings, including endurance sports events.

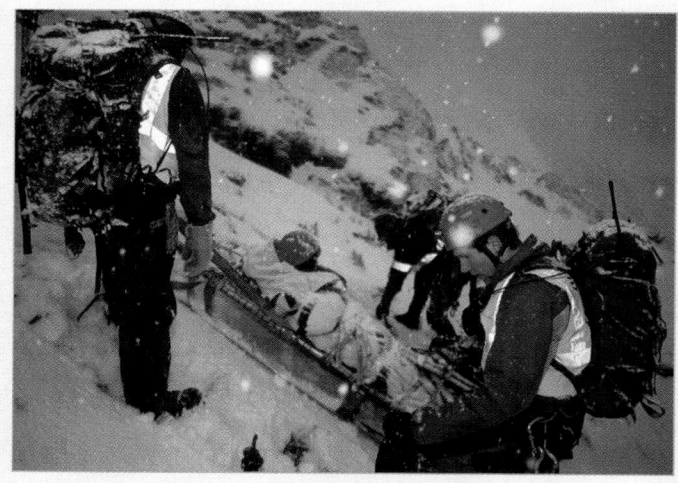

Figure 35-2 Medical attention may be needed in some extreme environments.

You are the Provider Part 1

You and your partner are called to the public library because of a man "acting strangely." You notice that the spring day has turned cooler as you respond and begin to consider why someone would be acting strangely at the library.

When you arrive, you run through the downpour and wind to the entrance. You recognize one of the police officers. She tells you, "I think he's just drunk," and notes that she arrested the man a month ago after a bar disturbance. After you confirm that the police officer has checked the man for weapons, you ask the bystander who has given up his coat to the patient what is going on. He reports that the patient was standing outside trying to remove his shirt and pants. The patient told him that he was "too hot."

Initial Assessment	Recording Time: 0 Minutes
Appearance	Eyes open, no obvious distress
Level of consciousness	V (Responsive to verbal stimuli); slurs words
Airway	Open; odor of alcohol on breath
Breathing	Adequate rate and tidal volume
Circulation	Radial pulse present; cold hands

1. What are three things that could medically harm this man in the next hour?
2. Do you believe the scene to be adequately secured?
3. Where do you believe is the best place to properly assess the patient?

Finally, the patient's overall health and fitness status and ability to acclimatize (that is, adjust to the new environment) can mean the difference between life and death.

This chapter first describes the techniques that the healthy body uses to respond to changes in temperature. It then assesses factors that can interfere with the body's ability to shed or gain heat, thereby increasing a person's risk of experiencing an environmental emergency. Next, it examines the pathophysiology, recognition, and treatment of environmental illnesses. Finally, the chapter considers preventive measures for environmental illnesses.

Homeostasis and Body Temperature

Homeostasis refers to body processes that balance the supply and demand of the body's needs. Ensuring the balance between heat production and heat excretion (thermoregulation) is the job of thermosensitive neurons in the anterior hypothalamus. Like a car thermostat, the hypothalamus—the "master thermostat" in the brain—operates according to the principle of negative feedback control: A rise in core body temperature elicits responses that increase heat loss and shut off normal heat production pathways (thermogenesis); a fall in core body temperature prompts heat production and conservation and turns off normal heat-liberating pathways (thermolysis) **Figure 35-3**.

The human body stubbornly defends a constant core temperature of approximately 98.6°F (37°C) that represents a bal-

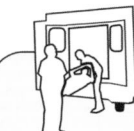

In the Field

Do not become a victim yourself. Dress for the weather.

ance between the heat produced or absorbed by the body and the heat eliminated to the outside. At this temperature, the metabolic reactions of the body proceed at their optimal level. Temperatures in the core (the brain and thoracoabdominal organs) remain relatively constant. The temperature of the periphery (the skin) can fluctuate a great deal, so this part of the body has a major role in thermoregulation. The lowest body temperature at which human survival of accidental hypothermia has been reported is 56.7°F (13.7°C). More generally, hypothermia is defined as a body temperature starting at 95°F (35°C) and heat stroke at 104°F (40°C).

In the field, the oral temperature is commonly used and is a suitable measurement for general medical conditions such as suspected pneumonia. It can vary dramatically from the core temperature if the patient has been mouth breathing or drinking hot or cold liquids. The axillary temperature, taken in the armpit, is typically 1°F cooler than the oral temperature. Tactile temperatures taken by parents are remarkably accurate but only in terms of knowing whether a child has a fever, not in determining the actual temperature. In environmental situations, the most accurate means of determining core temperatures is to use a rectal thermometer capable of measuring extremes of temperatures **Figure 35-4**. Tympanic temperatures, which are taken with a device that measures the heat reflected off the eardrum, also provide accurate core measurements.

Thermoregulatory Mechanisms

The body's main thermoregulatory center is located in specialized tissue found in the hypothalamus. The thermogenic (heat-generating) tissues in the hypothalamus are mediated by the sympathetic nervous system; the thermolytic (heat-liberating) tissues are mediated by the parasympathetic nervous system. The hypothalamus receives signals from peripheral receptors (located primarily in the skin and muscles) and central receptors (triggered by changes in blood temperature; located in the core).

At rest, the body produces heat chiefly by the metabolism of nutrients (carbohydrates, fats, and rarely proteins), with the subsequent liberation of primarily water and carbon dioxide. Liver and skeletal muscles are the major contributors to the basal metabolic rate (BMR), the heat energy produced at rest from normal body metabolic reactions. The BMR can be thought of as the minimal caloric energy requirement to sit on

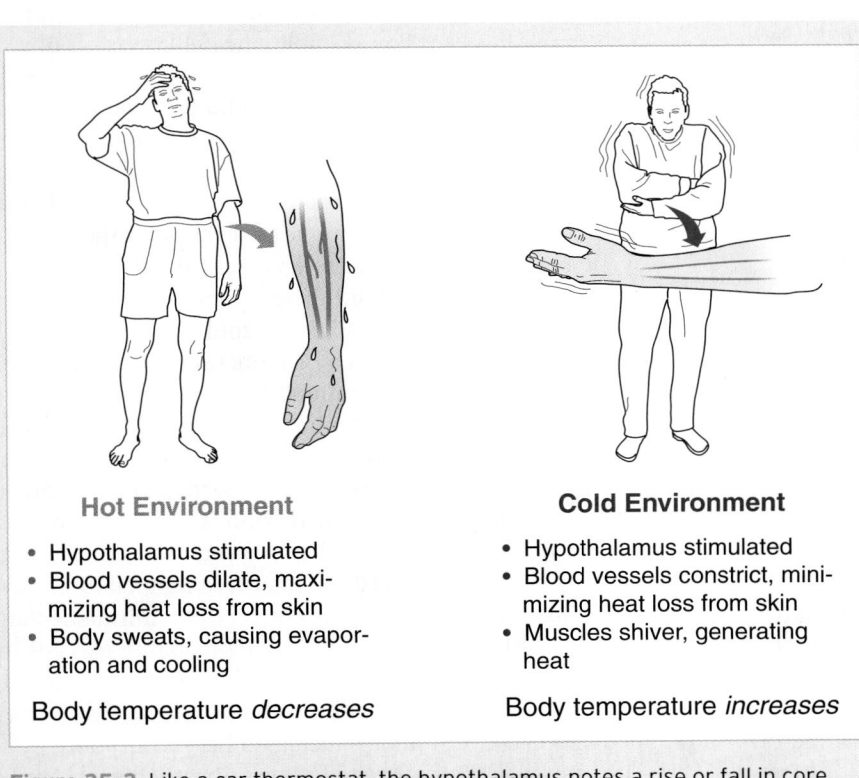

Hot Environment
- Hypothalamus stimulated
- Blood vessels dilate, maximizing heat loss from skin
- Body sweats, causing evaporation and cooling

Body temperature *decreases*

Cold Environment
- Hypothalamus stimulated
- Blood vessels constrict, minimizing heat loss from skin
- Muscles shiver, generating heat

Body temperature *increases*

Figure 35-3 Like a car thermostat, the hypothalamus notes a rise or fall in core body temperature and elicits responses to regulate it.

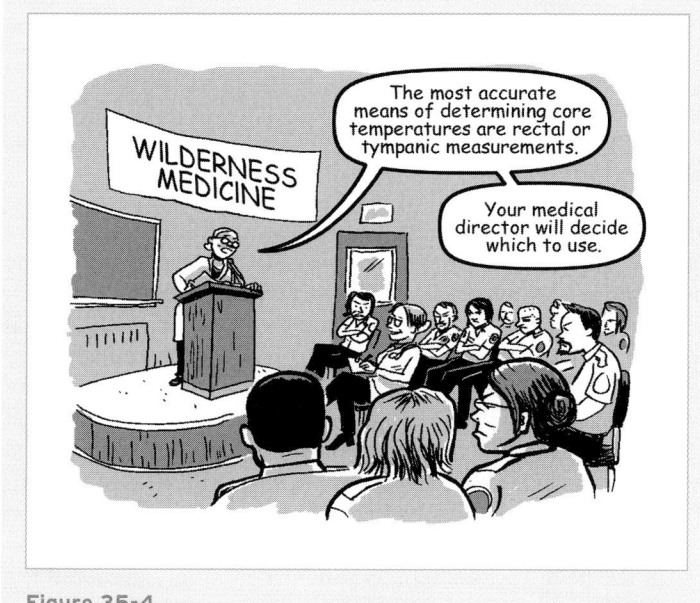

Figure 35-4

the couch all day! The BMR of the average 70-kg adult is in the range of 60 to 70 kilocalories per hour. Many factors affect this rate, including age, sex, stress, and hormones. The most important factor, however, is body surface area. As the ratio of body surface area to body volume increases, heat loss to the environment increases. Thus, when two people have the same weight, the shorter person will have a higher BMR.

Exertion also affects the metabolic rate. A brisk walk can produce heat totaling 300 kcal/h, for example. The recommended daily caloric intake is 2,000 to 2,500 kcal (a food "calorie" is actually a kilocalorie).

Some of the heat generated by metabolism and glycogen breakdown for muscular work is used to warm the body; the excess is excreted, ordinarily by taking advantage of the temperature gradient between the body and the outside environment. If the environmental temperature is higher than the body temperature, there is a third potential source of body heat: absorption of heat from the outside. Standing in bright sunshine on a hot, breezeless day, for example, can add up to 150 kcal/h to the internal heat load.

Physiologic Responses to Heat and Cold
Thermolysis
The body reacts to its daily production of heat energy and to hot environmental conditions in much the same way—thermolysis, the release of stored heat and energy from the body. An increase in core temperature causes the hypothalamus to send signals via efferent pathways in the parasympathetic nervous system, causing vasodilatation and sweating.

Because of cutaneous vasodilation, the effective volume of the vascular system is increased (when the diameter of a tube, such as an artery, is increased, its volume increases); the heart must increase its output to compensate for this effect. Heart

rate and stroke volume increase, but the work of the heart is markedly increased. If vasodilation increases dramatically, the person may have a complete loss of vasomotor control (that is, the ability of the arteries to constrict in response to sympathetic stimulation). In that case, blood pools in the periphery, and the patient could experience neurogenic shock.

When warmed blood from the core and overheated muscles heads for the peripherally dilated cutaneous vessels, it may be cooled in four major ways (in addition to behavioral changes, such as slowing down or seeking shade):

- **Radiation**, the transfer of heat via electromagnetic waves, accounts for more than 65% of heat loss in a cooler setting. Heat loss through the head is especially notable. If the ambient temperature is high (68°F or greater), body heat will be gained.
- **Conduction** is the transfer of heat from a hotter object to a cooler object by direct physical contact. Air is a poor conductor of heat (only 2% of body heat is lost to it), whereas the ground is a good conductor. Water is the best conductor. A person who falls into a cold lake will lose heat 25 times faster than a dry person exposed to air of the same temperature. Clothing soaked with rain, snow, or perspiration can be just as dangerous.
- **Convection** refers to the loss of heat that takes place when moving air picks up heat and carries it away. A person instinctively uses this principle when blowing on hot food to cool it. Likewise, air moving across the body surface can pick up heat and carry it away. The faster the air is moving, the faster it can remove heat from the body. The windchill factor measures the chilling effect of a given temperature at a given wind speed. For example, the chilling effect of a 30°F temperature with a 35 mph wind is −4°F.
- **Evaporation**, the conversion of a liquid to a gas, liberates 1 kcal per 1.7 mL of sweat. Sweating and heat dissipation by evaporation normally account for about 30% of cooling. Evaporation is the main mode of cooling in higher temperatures until a high humidity level slows the rate of evaporation. It has a minor role via respiration. This phenomenon is also behind the evaporative method of cooling for heat stroke patients. In cold conditions, wet clothes can cause heat loss by conduction and, as they dry, further heat loss by evaporation.

These four mechanisms require a thermal gradient between the body and its surroundings; that is, the mechanisms work only as long as the temperature of the skin surface is higher than that of the outside environment (and metabolism does not produce an overwhelming heat load). When the outside temperature approaches or exceeds skin surface temperature, however, heat loss by radiation and convection diminishes and finally ceases. When the environmental temperature exceeds the skin temperature, the body absorbs heat. In those circumstances, the increase in blood flow to the skin becomes counterproductive because it promotes increased heat absorption.

The only way the body can dissipate heat when the ambient temperature approaches body temperature is by the evaporation of sweat, up to a point. A healthy adult can sweat a maximum of about 1 L/h but cannot maintain that rate for more than a few hours at a time. Furthermore, for effective evaporation of sweat, the ambient air must be relatively unsaturated with water. As the relative humidity increases, the rate of evaporation decreases; effective sweat evaporation ceases when the relative humidity reaches about 75%.

Thermogenesis

In a cold environment, the skin serves as the body's thermostat. If your skin is cold, your body will shiver even if your core body temperature is not lowered. Thermogenesis, the production of heat and energy for the body, is the main method of dealing with cold stressors. In addition to normal heat production from the BMR and physical exertion, the sympathetic nervous system can increase muscle tone and initiate shivering in the short-term and increase thyroid levels in the long-term. The hypothalamus also stimulates peripheral vasoconstriction, thereby shunting blood to the core. Sweating decreases. The thicker the outer shell, the better the insulation. All other factors being equal, heavier people are more effectively insulated from the cold. This conservation of heat for the sake of the core continues until the body's ability to generate heat becomes overwhelmed, resulting in hypothermia.

Heat Illness

Heat illness is an increase in core body temperature (CBT) due to inadequate thermolysis. The fundamental problem is the inability to get rid of the heat buildup in the body, often because of hot and humid conditions. A person's general state of health, clothing, mobility, age, preexisting illnesses, and certain medications (Table 35-1 ▶) can add to the problem. When the thermoregulatory system is taxed beyond its limits or fails for any reason, the core body temperature soars, sometimes rising from normal to about 106°F (41°C) in less than 15 minutes. That is the situation in heat stroke, for example.

Risk Factors for Heat Illness

Certain factors increase a person's risk for ill effects from any given heat stress; the factors are summarized in (Table 35-2 ▾). Older people are at particular risk because they do not adjust as well to the heat: They perspire less; they acclimatize more slowly; they feel thirst less readily in response to dehydration; and decreased mobility may make getting a glass of water difficult. Older people are also more likely to have chronic conditions, such as diabetes and cardiovascular disease, that interfere with normal heat excretion. In addition, they are more apt to be taking medications that disrupt the body's mechanisms for dissipating heat. For example, diuretics taken for hypertension may result in an older person being dangerously close to dehydration and electrolyte disturbances and interfere with the peripheral vasodilation necessary for heat transfer. Beta blockers can lessen a tachycardic response to heat stress, as can normal age-related decreased

Table 35-1	Medications Contributing to Heat Illness
■ Alcohol ■ Alpha agonists ■ Amphetamines ■ Anticholinergic medications (atropine sulfate, scopolamine, benztropine mesylate, belladonna, and synthetic alkaloids) ■ Antihistamines ■ Antiparkinsonian agents ■ Antipsychotics (such as haloperidol) ■ Beta blockers ■ Calcium channel blockers ■ Cocaine ■ Diuretics (furosemide, hydrochlorothiazide, bumetanide) ■ Heroin	■ Laxatives ■ Lithium ■ Lysergic acid diethylamide (LSD) ■ Monoamine oxidase inhibitors ■ Phencyclidine hydrochloride ■ Phenothiazines (prochlorperazine, chlorpromazine, promethazine) ■ Sympathomimetic medicines (amphetamines, epinephrine, ephedrine, cocaine, norepinephrine) ■ Thyroid agonists (levothyroxine) ■ Tricyclic antidepressants (amitriptyline, imipramine, nortriptyline, protriptyline)

Table 35-2	Factors That Predispose to Heat Illness	
Factors That Increase Internal Heat Production	**Factors That Interfere With Heat Dissipation**
■ Physical exertion ■ Response to infection (fever) ■ Hyperthyroidism ■ Agitated and tremulous states (Parkinson, psychosis, mania, drug withdrawal—opiate and alcohol) ■ Drug overdoses (such as sympathomimetics, cocaine, caffeine, lysergic acid diethylamide, phencyclidine hydrochloride, methamphetamine, ecstasy)	■ High ambient temperature ■ High humidity ■ Obesity (insulation effect, less efficient dissipation) ■ Impaired vasodilatation ■ Diabetes ■ Alcoholism ■ Drugs: diuretics, tranquilizers, beta blockers, antihistamines, phenothiazines ■ Impaired ability to sweat (cystic fibrosis, skin diseases, healed burns) ■ Heavy or tight clothing
Factors That Increase Heat Absorption	**Factors That Impair the Body's Response to Heat Stress**
■ Confined, unventilated, hot living quarters ■ Working in hot conditions (bakeries, steel mills, construction sites) ■ Being in parked automobiles in summer	■ Dehydration ■ Prior heat stroke ■ Hypokalemia ■ Cardiovascular disease ■ Previous stroke or other central nervous system lesion

Table 35-3	Comparing Conditions Resulting From Heat Stress		
Variable	Heat Cramps	Heat Exhaustion	Heat Stroke
Pathophysiology	Sodium and water loss	Sodium and water loss, hypovolemia	Failure of heat-regulating mechanisms
Mental status	Normal	Normal or mild confusion	Altered, delirium, seizures
Temperature	May be mildly elevated	Usually mildly elevated	>105°F (40.5°C)
Skin	Cool, moist	Pale, cool, moist	Dry, hot, but sweating may persist, especially with exertional heat stroke
Muscle cramping	Severe	May or may not be present	Absent

maximum heart rates. Acclimatazation can decrease the likelihood of heat illness, but it takes days of progressive exertion in a hot environment to be effective.

Among the young and healthy, people most vulnerable to heat stress include infants and young children exposed to a hot environment. Children, compared with adults, have proportionately higher metabolic heat production, have a CBT that rises faster during dehydration, and do not dissipate heat as well owing to their smaller organ and vascular systems. Athletes and military recruits engaging in heavy exertion in hot conditions are also at increased risk.

The following subsections discuss the major types of heat illness Table 35-3 ▲ .

Heat Cramps

Heat cramps are acute and involuntary muscle pains, usually in the lower extremities, the abdomen, or both, that occur because of profuse sweating and subsequent sodium losses in sweat. Three factors contribute to heat cramps: salt depletion, dehydration, and muscle fatigue. Heat cramps most often afflict people in good physical condition—for example, athletes, military personnel, and physical laborers. In fact, British coal miners would add salt to their beer to prevent cramps. A recent study of US college football players showed a twofold increase in sweat sodium losses in athletes prone to heat cramps. Usually a person exerting himself or herself in a hot environment will become thirsty and increase the intake of fluids. But if the person is sweating heavily, he or she is losing fluids and salt through the skin. If the person drinks plain water, he or she will not replace sweat sodium losses Figure 35-5 ▸ . Hence, the rehabilitation sector at a fire should have watered-down sports drinks available instead of just water.

Heat cramps usually start suddenly during strenuous and/or prolonged physical activity. They may be mild, characterized by only slight abdominal cramping and tingling in the extremities. More often, however, they present with severe, incapacitating pain in the extremities and abdomen. The patient may become hypotensive and nauseated but remains alert. The pulse is generally rapid, the skin pale and moist, and the temperature normal.

Treatment of heat cramps aims to eliminate the exposure and restore lost salt and water to the body:

- Move the patient to a cool environment. Have the patient lie down if he or she feels faint.

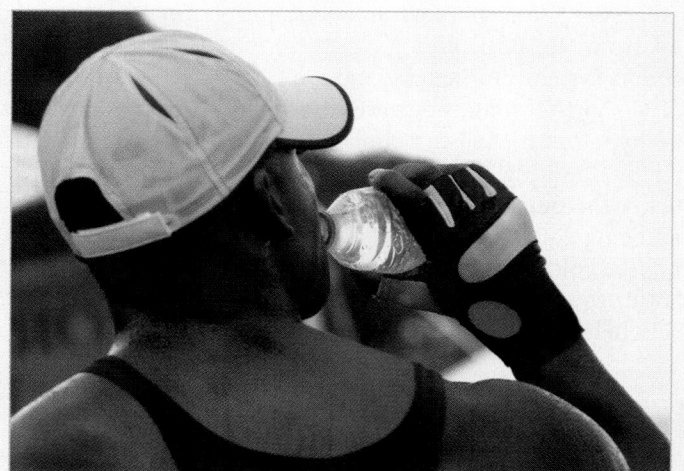

Figure 35-5 If you drink plain water, you will not replace the sweat salt losses.

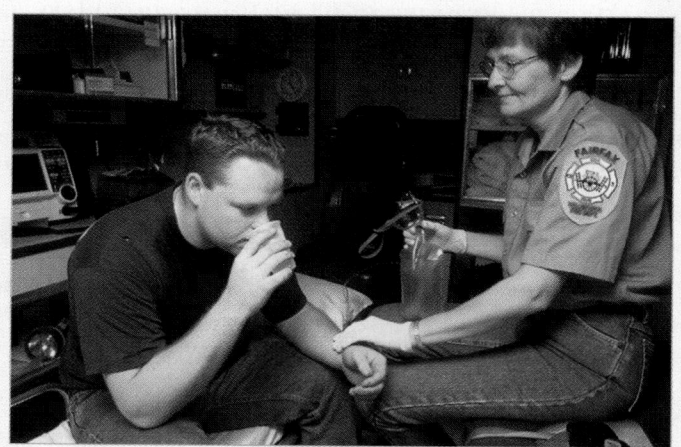

Figure 35-6 Give the patient with heat cramps one or two glasses of a salt-containing solution if he or she is not nauseated.

- If the patient is not nauseated, give one or two glasses of a salt-containing solution (such as lemonade with ½ teaspoon of salt added or a commercial sports drink) Figure 35-6 ▲ . Instruct the patient to drink the solution slowly. Have the patient munch on salty chips or pretzels. Salt tablets can irritate the stomach lining and may precipitate or worsen nausea.

■ If the patient is too nauseated to take liquids by mouth, insert an intravenous (IV) catheter and infuse normal saline rapidly. (Consult medical control for the IV rate.)

■ Do not massage the cramping muscles. That tactic may actually aggravate the pain.

■ As the patient's salt balance is restored, the symptoms will abate and the patient may want to resume activity. In the prehospital setting, this decision is best made with medical control.

Heat Syncope

Heat syncope is an orthostatic syncopal, or near-syncopal, episode that typically occurs in nonacclimated people who may be under heat stress. It can occur with prolonged standing, as in mass outdoor gatherings, or when standing suddenly from a sitting or lying position. Peripheral vasodilatation, possibly exacerbated by some degree of dehydration, is thought to be the cause. Treatment involves placing the patient in a supine position and replacing fluid deficits. If the patient does not recover quickly in the supine position, suspect heat exhaustion or heat stroke.

Heat Exhaustion

Heat exhaustion is a clinical syndrome thought to represent a milder form of heat illness on a continuum leading to heat stroke. Its hallmarks are volume depletion and heat stress. Classically, two forms are described: water-depleted and sodium-depleted. Water-depleted heat exhaustion occurs primarily in geriatric patients owing to immobility, medications that contribute to dehydration, and decreased thirst sensitivity and in active younger workers or athletes who do not adequately replace fluids in a hot environment. Sodium-depleted heat exhaustion may take hours or days to develop and results from huge sodium losses from sweating but replacing only free water, not sodium.

A concept closely related to sodium-depleted heat exhaustion is exertional hyponatremia. Studies from the Boston Marathon, the Grand Canyon National Park, and the military point to a common thread: prolonged exertion in a hot environment coupled with excessive hypotonic fluid intake. This phenomenon leads to nausea, vomiting, weight gain, and, in severe cases, mental status changes, cerebral edema, and seizures. The practical field concern is older, debilitated patients and patients who participate in extreme endurance sports events such as marathons and Ironman competitions.

Symptoms of heat exhaustion may include headache, fatigue, dizziness, nausea, vomiting, and, sometimes, abdominal cramping. The patient is usually sweating profusely, and the skin is pale and clammy. He or she may be slightly disoriented. The temperature may be normal or slightly elevated (< 104°F or 40°C). Tachycardia is present, although this response may be blunted if the patient is taking a beta blocker. Respirations are fast and shallow. Tachypnea may produce

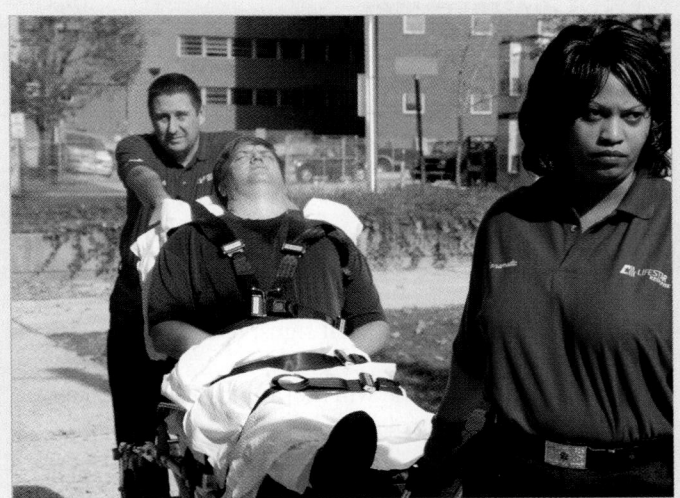

Figure 35-7 Remove the patient from the heat.

symptoms of hyperventilation: carpopedal spasm, perioral numbness, and a low end-tidal carbon dioxide level. Blood pressure may be decreased due to peripheral pooling of blood or volume depletion; if not decreased at rest, blood pressure will almost certainly drop when the patient tries to sit or stand from a recumbent position (orthostatic hypotension). If the patient reports brown urine, suspect rhabdomyolysis (the destruction of muscle tissue leading to a release of potassium and myoglobin).

Heat exhaustion is sometimes mistaken for "summer flu," and the condition may be misdiagnosed. If untreated, heat exhaustion may progress to heat stroke. The treatment of heat exhaustion is aimed at removing the patient from exposure to heat and repairing the derangement in fluid and electrolyte balance:

■ Move the patient to a cool environment (Figure 35-7 ▲); remove excess clothing, and place supine with legs elevated.

■ If the patient's temperature is elevated, sponge, spray, or drip the patient with tepid water and fan gently to make him or her more comfortable—but don't overdo it. Heroic measures to lower body temperature rapidly are unnecessary, and chilling the patient can cause shivering and thermogenesis.

■ Consider specially designed cooling chairs for hand and forearm immersion in cold water for rehabilitation at fire scenes, mass gatherings, and endurance sports.

■ Oral hydration with sports drinks may be appropriate. If nausea and vomiting are present, start a normal saline IV and draw blood for electrolyte determinations. Use the heart rate and blood pressure to guide the fluid amounts administered.

■ If exertional hyponatremia is suspected, do not give fluids by mouth. Instead, draw blood for checking the blood sodium level and administer IV normal saline.

Controversies

Care of endurance sports athletes is controversial. We no longer automatically give them fluids via large-bore IV and lots of oral fluid without first ruling out hypoglycemia and letting them lie down for a few minutes because they may actually be hyponatremic. In that case, the IV fluid would cause iatrogenic hyponatremia, irritable heart, and dysrhythmias.

- Monitor cardiac rhythm, vital signs, temperature, and end-tidal carbon dioxide.
- If you cannot determine whether the patient has heat exhaustion or heat stroke, treat for heat stroke.

Heat Stroke

Of all heat illnesses, heat stroke is the least common but the most deadly. It is caused by a severe disturbance in the body's thermoregulation and is a profound emergency, with mortality rates as high as 10% in treated patients and 30% to 80% in untreated patients. Experts typically rely on two findings to make this diagnosis: core temperature more than 104°F (40°C) and altered mental status.

Two heat stroke syndromes are distinguished: classic and exertional **Table 35-4 ▾**. Classic heat stroke (passive heat stroke), which usually occurs during heat waves, is most likely to strike very old, very young, or bedridden people. Patients with chronic illnesses, such as diabetes or heart disease, are particularly susceptible, as are people with alcoholism and patients taking certain medications (diuretics, sedatives, anticholinergics). In this syndrome, high environmental temperatures initially elicit thermolysis, but the CBT eventually soars, and the typical signs and symptoms of heat stroke appear.

Exertional heat stroke is typically an illness of young and fit people exercising in hot and humid conditions. When the ambient temperature approaches body temperature, radiation

and convection are no longer effective means of shedding excess heat. If the relative humidity rises above 75%, evaporative cooling becomes ineffective. A person who continues exercising in such conditions will continue generating heat without any means of excreting that heat. Heat will then build up within the body, causing the CBT to skyrocket.

The Clinical Picture of Heat Stroke

Both types of heat stroke present with similar signs and symptoms, which may or may not be recognized as the consequence of heat exposure. Patients almost certainly won't be able to give a coherent history because they will be confused, delirious, or comatose. Often the very earliest signs of heat stroke are changes in behavior—irritability, combativeness, signs the patient is hallucinating—which may mislead bystanders and EMS workers into thinking the patient is having a behavioral or substance-related emergency. Older patients with heat stroke may present with signs resembling those of a suspected stroke. Other central nervous system disturbances—including tremors, seizures, constricted pupils, and decerebrate or decorticate posturing—may also be prominent features of heat stroke.

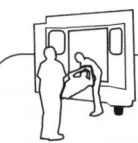

In the Field

Suspect heat stroke and check a core temperature in any person behaving strangely in a hot environment.

The diagnostic vital sign is, of course, a markedly elevated temperature, usually greater than 104°F (40°C). Signs of a hyperdynamic state are usually present: tachycardia, hyperventilation with an end-tidal carbon dioxide of less than 20 mm Hg, and lowered peripheral vascular resistance from efforts of the body to cool itself with vasodilatation. Heat stroke is characterized by some degree of dehydration, which worsens the problem by decreasing the body's ability to get the hotter core blood to the periphery for thermolysis. Blood pressure can be normal or decreased depending on the level of dehydration. The skin can be dry, red, and hot in classic heat stroke or pale and sweaty in exertional heat stroke.

The diagnosis of heat stroke is easy to miss. It may develop rapidly in a patient whose heat exhaustion was mistaken for the flu, or it may present as coma of unknown origin. Unless you keep the possibility of heat stroke constantly in mind during the hot months of the year and routinely take the temperature as part of the vital signs, you may waste precious time searching for some other cause of the patient's symptoms.

Fever and Conditions That Mimic Heat Stroke

New paramedics may face a perplexing challenge: Why is this nursing home patient's temperature elevated? Is it heat stroke, a febrile illness, or sepsis? Neurologic changes can be present in either case. The history, however, may suggest infectious causes. For example, a change in the urine color in a catheter bag, a recent complaint of cough and dyspnea, an obvious skin

Table 35-4	Classic Versus Exertional Heat Stroke	
Characteristic	**Classic Heat Stroke**	**Exertional Heat Stroke**
Age	Older	Younger
General health	Chronic diseases, schizophrenia	Healthy person
Medications	Beta blockers, diuretics, anticholinergics	Often none, consider stimulant abuse
Activity	Very little to bedridden	Strenuous
Sweating	Absent	Present
Skin	Hot, red, dry	Moist, pale
Blood glucose level	Normal	Hypoglycemic
Rhabdomyolysis	Rare	Common
Acute renal failure	Rare	Common

infection, or complaints of a fever, rash, photophobia, and stiff neck may point to meningitis. An intermittent shaking chill also favors infectious causes of increased temperature.

A fever can signal that the body is fighting an infection by inhibiting reproduction of harmful toxins. Pyrogens (proteins secreted by infective organisms and the body's immune system) act on the hypothalamus by increasing the thermal set point, which results in a fever. The body then uses its thermoregulatory tools to maintain the new temperature setting. The patient with a reset temperature may adapt to this change by wearing more clothes, and sometimes the body creates more heat via shivering. Although aspirin and nonsteroidal anti-inflammatory drugs can lower a fever (by blocking prostaglandins), they are dangerous in treating heat illnesses.

Anticholinergic poisoning presents with an elevated temperature; dry, red skin; mental status changes; and tachycardia. Anticholinergic poisonings usually cause dilated pupils, whereas patients with heat stroke usually have constricted pupils.

Two rare syndromes must also be considered. Neuroleptic malignant syndrome (NMS) is caused by antipsychotic and some antiemetic medications and presents with hyperthermia, muscular rigidity, altered mental status, and a hyperdynamic state. Malignant hyperthermia can occur as a result of common anesthesia medications (notably succinylcholine) and presents similarly to NMS. Researchers are exploring a common genetic contributor to malignant hyperthermia and heat stroke.

Treatment of Heat Stroke

If you are unsure about what exactly is causing the elevated temperature, the prudent step is to treat for heat stroke given the deadly consequences of missing it. Online medical control may also help with treatment plans.

Treatment of heat stroke aims at removing the patient from the environment and promoting rapid cooling. Two main methods are used for rapid cooling: ice water body immersion and evaporative cooling by spraying tepid water over the patient accompanied by the use of fans to promote convection. Placing ice packs on the neck, groin, and axillae can augment the evaporative method. Research has shown that ice water immersion is probably the more effective means of rapid cooling but has obvious limitations in the back of an ambulance, including the need for ice. Conscious patients do not tolerate this measure well, and patients with altered mental status can be challenging to manage in an ice bath. You must also monitor CBT to avoid overshoot, resulting in shivering and even hypothermia.

- Evaluate the ABCs, administer supplemental oxygen, and be prepared to intubate.
- Move the patient to a cool environment, and strip the patient to underclothing. Monitor the rectal temperature every 10 minutes. Cooling efforts should continue until the rectal temperature has fallen below about 102°F (39°C).
- Cool as rapidly as possible by the most expeditious means available.
  - Spray the patient with tepid water while fanning constantly to promote rapid evaporation. The ambulance should carry a portable fan during the

summer months for this purpose. Apply ice packs to the patient's neck, groin, and axillae to aid in cooling from evaporative techniques.
  - Consider ice water immersion in cases of prolonged transport or delayed evacuation. Cooling with ice water–soaked blankets and fanning is nearly as effective as immersion. Pay close attention to airway status; watch for seizures and CBT to avoid overcooling.
- Start an IV line, give normal saline, and check the blood glucose level. Be careful with fluids—pulmonary edema is a known complication of heat stroke. Remember that cooling promotes peripheral vasoconstriction that can raise the blood pressure.
- Monitor cardiac rhythm, and remember that rhabdomyolysis can occur with resultant hyperkalemia.
- Be prepared to treat seizures with common antiseizure medicines (lorazepam, midazolam, or diazepam).

A few measures are *not* helpful: Covering the patient with wet sheets may impede heat loss by evaporation. Dantrolene, a medication once thought to aid in lowering the temperature, has not been shown to be effective. Last, massaging muscles to combat cutaneous vasoconstriction from cooling too much is not beneficial.

Prevention of Heat Illness

The following measures can help protect you, your colleagues, and the communities you serve from heat illness:
- Paramedics working in hot climates should have appropriate summer uniforms.
- If you are standing by at a post or street location, park the ambulance in the shade and make sure the air conditioning works.
- Increase your daily intake of fluid. Do not rely on thirst to gauge your need. Try to drink something every hour during very hot weather, aiming for urination every 2 hours. Dark urine is concentrated, indicating that the body is dehydrated. Avoid beverages with a high sugar content and those that promote diuresis (such as caffeinated or alcoholic drinks).
- Install or carry a portable fan in the ambulance to improve convection, supplement the air conditioning, and treat patients with heat illness.
- Carry a portable cooler or—if you are lucky enough—an onboard refrigerator for hot weather. Fill the cooler about half full with crushed ice, and stock it with sports drinks or other salt-containing drinks for patients and the ambulance crew.
- Review **Figure 35-8 ▶** outlining the relationship of heat and humidity to heat stress.
- Conduct community-based programs aimed at high-risk populations—for example, nursing home risk assessments.

Be alert for early symptoms of heat illness, such as headache, nausea, cramps, and dizziness. If you experience any of those symptoms, get out of the hot environment immediately and get medical attention.

Heat Index

Temperature (°F)

Relative Humidity (%)	80	82	84	86	88	90	92	94	96	98	100	102	104	106	108	110
40	80	81	83	85	88	91	94	97	101	105	109	114	119	124	130	136
45	80	82	84	87	89	93	96	100	104	109	114	119	124	130	137	
50	81	83	85	88	91	95	99	103	108	113	118	124	131	137		
55	81	84	86	89	93	97	101	106	112	117	124	130	137			
60	82	84	88	91	95	100	105	110	116	123	129	137				
65	82	85	89	93	98	103	108	114	121	128	136					
70	83	86	90	95	100	105	112	119	126	134						
75	84	88	92	97	103	109	116	124	132							
80	84	89	94	100	106	113	121	129								
85	85	90	96	102	110	117	126	135								
90	86	91	98	105	113	122	131									
95	86	93	100	108	117	127										
100	87	95	103	112	121	132										

Likelihood of heat disorders with prolonged exposure or strenuous activity:

☐ Caution   ☐ Extreme caution   ☐ Danger   ☐ Extreme danger

Figure 35-8 Likelihood of heat disorders.
Reprinted from: US National Weather Service. Available at: http://www.nws.noaa.gov/om/heat/index.shtml. Accessed May 2006.

■ Local Cold Injury

Most injuries from the cold are localized to the extremities or exposed parts of the body, such as the tips of the ears, nose, upper cheek, and tips of the fingers or toes (Figure 35-9 ▶). Local freezing injuries fall under the general heading of frost-bite. Frostbite is an ischemic injury that is classified as superficial or deep depending on whether tissue loss occurs.

A very mild form of frostbite, sometimes called frostnip, comes on slowly and generally is not painful, so the victim tends to be unaware of its occurrence. This problem is easily treated by placing a warm hand firmly over the chilled nose or ear or, when the fingers are frost-nipped, by placing the fingers into the armpit. The return of warmth to a frost-nipped area is usually signaled by some redness and tingling. Windmilling involves rapidly making a large circle with your hand, starting with your hand next to your side, raising it backward and up until you are reaching straight up, and moving it rapidly down frontward. This technique forces blood into the cold hand.

Deeper degrees of frostbite involve freezing of tissues and can occur only in ambient temperatures well below the freezing point. Cells are composed chiefly of water, so when they are subjected to low enough temperatures, the water within them turns into ice crystals, which can damage or destroy the cells. This problem is further complicated by increased viscosity accompanied by "sludging," poor flow, capillary leakage, and resultant thrombus and ischemic injury.

Risk Factors for Frostbite

Several factors predispose a person to frostbite:

- Going out on a cold, windy day without earmuffs, mittens, a scarf, or a hat.

You are the Provider Part 2

You ask the patient what is going on as you assist him to the ambulance. His gait is unsteady. Your partner obtains an initial set of vital signs. The patient takes a moment and tells you that he had been drinking earlier and got caught in the rain. You notice that the coat he is wearing is dry. When you ask him if it is his coat, the patient says "no." Your EMT-B partner informs you that the coat belongs to the bystander who initially helped him and that his identification says he is 44 years old.

As you begin to undress the patient, you notice that his clothes are wet and his appearance is unkempt. The patient states that his head hurts. He says "no" when asked about dizziness, visual disturbances, chest pain, and trouble breathing. He says that his stomach "always hurts," and that he has trouble with his pancreas but can offer no more clarification on his pain or history. There is no nausea, vomiting, diarrhea, or unusually colored stools. The patient states he has been drinking most of the afternoon but does not know where he is or what day it is. He denies any psychiatric history.

Vital Signs	Recording Time: 5 Minutes
Skin	Pink, cool, and dry
Pulse	112 beats/min; irregular and weak
Blood pressure	108/60 mm Hg
Respirations	24 breaths/min
Sao$_2$	Not reading

4. Does the additional information narrow the diagnostic possibilities?
5. What interventions might benefit the patient?
6. Why is the pulse oximetry not working?

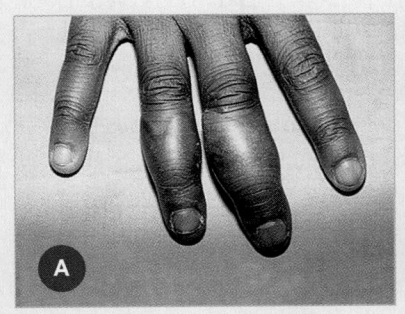 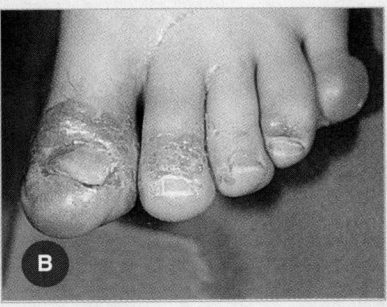 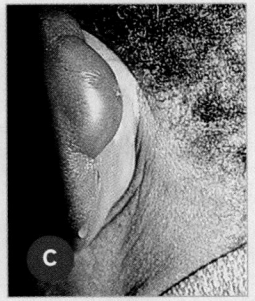

Figure 35-9 The extremities (**A** and **B**) and the ears (**C**) are particularly susceptible to frostbite.

■ Impeding the circulation to the extremities:
  - Wearing tight gloves and shoes and too many socks.
  - Lacing boots very tightly and remaining in a cramped position for a while.
  - Wearing plastic boots that won't expand. Preferably, boots should be lined with felt, which will expand when wet.
  - Smoking, which constricts arteries.
  - Drinking, which helps peripherally dilate blood vessels, helping the person to get colder.
■ Going out in the cold when tired, dehydrated, or hungry.
■ Coming in direct contact with cold objects.
■ Not staying hydrated, which would otherwise promote increased blood flow.
■ Allowing oneself to become thoroughly chilled. Generalized hypothermia is the most effective way to sustain local cold injury.

To avoid getting frostbite, avoid all of the preceding behaviors! Note the windchill, and always cover your face when you are outside for a long time (such as when skiing). Keep your feet dry and warm, and come in often to warm up. This precaution is especially important for children.

Superficial Frostbite

The most common symptom of frostbite is an altered sensation: numbness, tingling, or burning. The skin typically appears white and waxy and has been compared with frozen halibut Figure 35-10 ▸. Because it is frozen, the skin is firm to palpation, but the underlying tissues remain soft. Once thawing occurs, the injured area turns cyanotic, and the patient experiences a hot, stinging sensation. Capillary leakage produces edema in the frostbitten area, and blebs develop within a few hours after thawing. Dull or throbbing pain may persist for days or weeks after the injury.

The prehospital treatment of superficial frostbite differs significantly from that of deep frostbite, so it is very important to distinguish between the two. Usually it is difficult to determine the depth of the injury when you first see it—even a shallow frostbite injury can appear to be frozen solid. If the tissues beneath the skin are soft when you press down on the skin surface, the frostbite is probably superficial. If not, or if there is

any doubt, treat the injury as deep frostbite.

Mild cold injuries are generally managed by a combination of dressing, rest, food, and limiting exposure to the cold. Once you have determined that the patient has superficial frostbite only, proceed as follows:

■ *Get the patient out of the cold.* Take the patient indoors or into a heated ambulance so the body can stop hoarding its warm blood in the core and instead send some warm blood to the periphery, where it is urgently needed.
■ *Rewarm the injured part with body heat.* If an ear, nose, or foot is frostbitten, apply firm, steady pressure against the area with a warm hand. If a hand is frostbitten, have the patient insert the hand into the armpit and hold it there without moving. Do not try to rewarm a frostbitten part with radiant or dry heat.
■ *Do not rub or massage the frostbitten area;* massage will cause further damage to injured tissues.
■ *Cover blisters with a dry, sterile dressing,* and protect the area from further injury.
■ *Transport the patient to the hospital* with the injured area elevated and protected from the cold.

Deep Frostbite

Deep frostbite usually involves the hands or the feet. A frozen extremity looks white, yellow-white, or mottled blue-white, and it is hard, cold, and without sensation. The major tissue damage occurs not from the freezing of the tissues, but rather when the tissues thaw out, particularly if thawing occurs gradually. When tissues thaw slowly, partial refreezing of melted water may

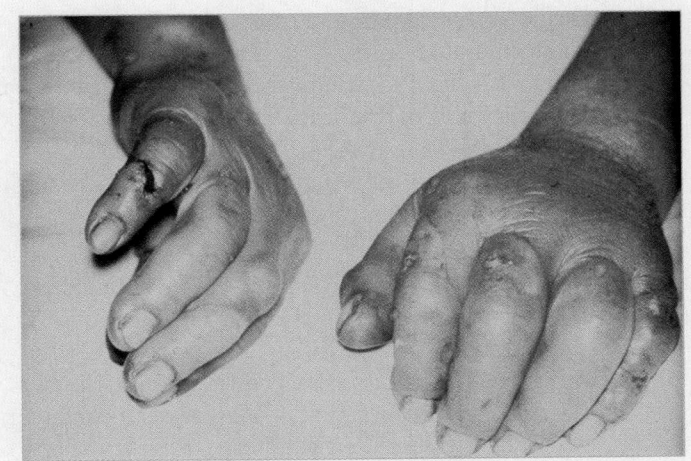

Figure 35-10 Frostbitten parts are hard and usually waxy to the touch.

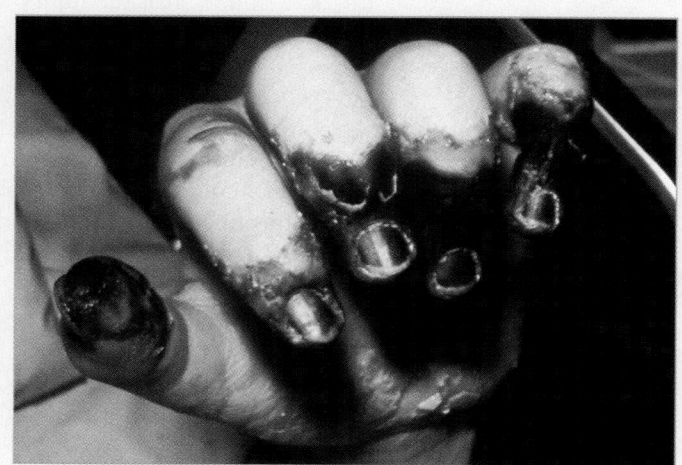

Figure 35-11 Gangrene can occur when tissue is frozen and chemical changes occur in the cells.

occur. Because these new ice crystals tend to be much larger than those formed during the original freeze, they cause even greater tissue damage. As thawing occurs, the injured area turns purple and becomes excruciatingly painful. Gangrene (permanent cell death) may set in within a few days, requiring amputation of all or part of the injured limb Figure 35-11 .

The prehospital treatment of deep frostbite depends on two factors: (1) whether the injured extremity has been partially or completely thawed before you arrive and (2) how far the patient is from the hospital.

- If the extremity is still frozen when you find the patient, leave it frozen until the patient reaches the hospital; rapid rewarming is extremely difficult to carry out properly in the field. If you are within about an hour's drive of a medical facility:
  1. Leave the frozen extremity frozen. As long as the limb is not thawed, the patient may even walk on it if necessary.
  2. Once you get the patient into the ambulance, pad the injured extremity to protect the tissues from further trauma, and keep the extremity away from the heater or any other sources of dry heat.
  3. Do not massage the extremity. The cells are full of ice crystals, and massaging the extremity will cause the ice crystals to lacerate delicate tissues.
  4. Transport without delay.
- If the extremity is already partially thawed or if the evacuation or transport will be delayed, contact medical control to discuss field rewarming.
  1. Rewarm the injured extremity before transport. To do so, you will need a water bath—a large, clean container in which the extremity can be immersed without touching the container's side or bottom. Water should be heated in a second container and then stirred into the water bath until the temperature of the bath is

between 95°F and 104°F (35°C and 40°C). While you are heating the water, administer intravenous analgesia such as fentanyl or morphine. The patient will experience very severe pain as the limb thaws out, and you want to mitigate that pain as much as possible.
  2. When the water bath has reached the appropriate temperature, gently immerse the injured extremity. Keep a thermometer in the water. When the water temperature falls below 38°C, temporarily remove the injured extremity from the bath while you add more hot water to the container. Stir the water around and keep adding more hot water until the bath is again in the appropriate temperature range; then reimmerse the injured extremity.

The rewarming procedure typically takes 10 to 30 minutes. It is complete when the frozen area is warm to the touch and is deep red or bluish (and remains red when you remove the limb from the water bath). While rewarming is in progress, the patient should be kept warm, preferably indoors, with insulated clothing and blankets. Do not permit the patient to smoke, because nicotine causes vasoconstriction and, therefore, interferes with blood flow to the injured area.
  3. Once rewarming is complete, dry the extremity and apply sterile dressings very gently. Use sterile gauze to separate frostbitten fingers and toes.

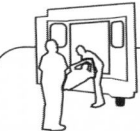

In the Field

Do not attempt rewarming in the field if there is any possibility of refreezing or if the patient must walk on the frostbitten foot.

Trench Foot

Trench foot involves a process similar to frostbite but can occur at temperatures as high as 60°F. It is caused by prolonged exposure to cool, wet conditions. The mechanism of injury can be explained by conduction: Wet feet lose heat 25 times faster than dry feet. Vasoconstriction and an ischemic cascade similar to that seen with frostbite then set in. Prevention—keeping the feet dry and warm—is the best treatment.

Hypothermia

Hypothermia is defined as a decrease in CBT generally starting at 95°F (35°C) owing to inadequate thermogenesis and/or excess environmental cold stress. Any temperature below the body's temperature can result in hypothermia. For example, a geriatric patient with alcoholism who has had a stroke and is now living alone can become hypothermic in a 60°F home. An unprepared hiker caught in a summer wind and rainstorm is another classic example, as is a person who becomes submerged in icy water Figure 35-12 .

The body regulates cold stress by increasing thermogenesis, decreasing thermolysis, and pursuing adaptive behavioral changes. Table 35-5 ▾ summarizes the factors contributing to thermoregulation and hypothermia.

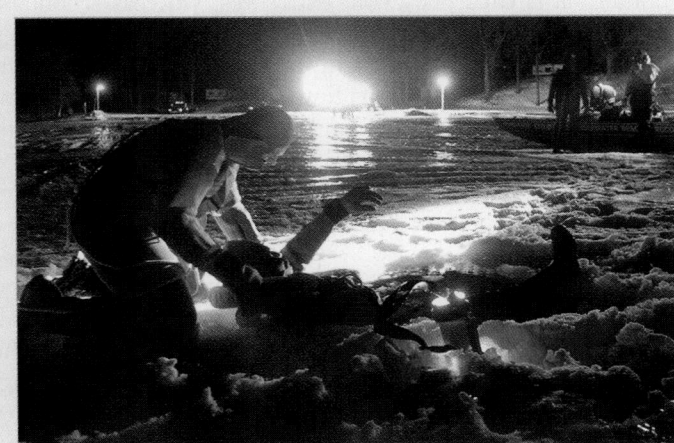
Figure 35-12 Patients who have been submerged in cold water are at high risk for hypothermia.

Table 35-5	Factors Contributing to Thermoregulation and Hypothermia	
If thermogenic factors plus heat retention factors are less than cold factors, then hypothermia results.		
Thermogenic Factors	Heat Retention Factors	Cold Factors
Muscular exertion	Vasoconstriction	Radiation • Temperature • Surface areas
Shivering (↑ BMR 2–5 times)	Body surface area	Convection • Windchill
Energy stores	Adipose tissue	Conduction • Wetness

Risk Factors for Hypothermia

People at risk for hypothermia have increased thermolysis, decreased thermogenesis, impaired thermoregulation, or other contributing factors. Many issues can lead to the development of a hypothermic condition, including cold temperatures, fatigue, improper gear for adverse conditions, wetness, dehydration, malnutrition, and the length of exposure and intensity of weather conditions Table 35-6 ▾ .

Work in the 1980s in New York City and other major urban areas showed that alcohol is by far the most common cause of heat loss in urban settings. It predisposes the patient to hypothermia by impairing shivering thermogenesis (decreased thermogenesis) and by promoting cutaneous vasodilatation (increased thermolysis), which hinders the body's attempts to create an insulating shell around its warm core. Liver disease, which leads to inadequate glycogen stores, and the subnormal nutritional status of most people with alcoholism further impair metabolic heat generation. Finally, alcohol impairs judgment, which often leads to inappropriate behavior in cold conditions. Impaired thermoregulation can also occur with therapeutic or overdoses of sedative medications, tricyclic antidepressants, and phenothiazines, primarily by interfering with central nervous system (CNS)-mediated vasoconstriction.

Older people often cannot generate heat effectively because of reduced muscle mass and a diminished shivering response. Atrophy of subcutaneous fat also reduces elderly patients' insulation against heat loss. Medications commonly prescribed to older people may interfere with vasoconstriction as well. Hypothyroidism and malnutrition may further contribute to an older person's vulnerability (decreased thermogenesis).

Special Considerations
Older people on fixed budgets should be checked on during cold spells. Infants and toddlers, who have a large head-to-body surface area, should always have their heads covered during the winter.

Table 35-6	Factors That Predispose to Cold Illness		
Factors That Increase Heat Loss	Factors That Impair Thermoregulatory Mechanisms	Factors That Decrease Heat Production	Miscellaneous Causes
■ Cold water drowning ■ Wet clothes ■ Windchill ■ Impaired judgment from drugs or alcohol ■ Vasodilatation from: 　– Alcohol 　– Acute spinal cord injury ■ Diabetic peripheral neuropathies	■ Dehydration ■ Parkinson's disease or dementias ■ Multiple sclerosis ■ Anorexia nervosa ■ Central nervous system bleeding or ischemic cerebrovascular accident ■ Multisystem trauma ■ Drugs interfering with vasoconstriction: 　– Alcohol 　– Benzodiazepines 　– Phenothiazines 　– Tricyclic antidepressants	■ Hypothyroidism ■ Age extremes ■ Hypoglycemia ■ Malnutrition ■ Inability to shiver and immobility	■ Sepsis ■ Meningitis ■ Overzealous heat stroke treatment

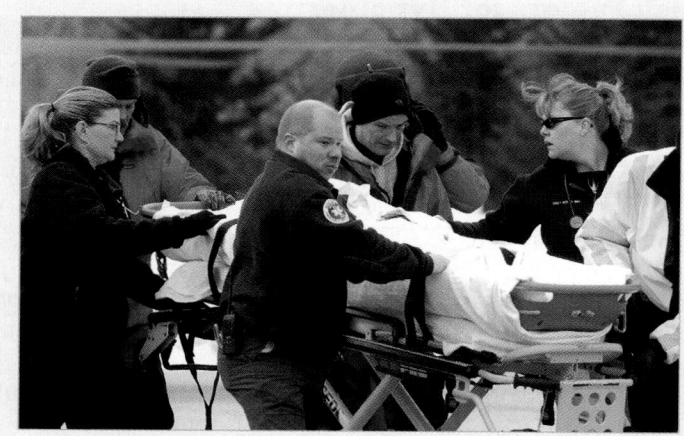

Figure 35-13 Trauma patients need to be moved to the backboard or stretcher with a blanket on it as soon as is safe and medically appropriate.

In the Field

Simply covering a patient hit by a car and lying in the street is not good enough; body heat continues to be conducted away into the cold pavement. Remove the patient from the street onto a blanket or backboard quickly.

The most important of the other factors contributing to hypothermia is trauma. Hypotension and hypovolemia can interfere with normal thermoregulation. Patients with CNS trauma or shock will not be able to mount a shivering response owing to the nature of their injuries. Last, hypothermia in trauma patients can lead to serious coagulation problems. If you are wearing protective gear in the cold, make sure your ambulance is toasty, ask the patient if he or she is cold, and do what you can to conserve the patient's body heat **Figure 35-13 ▲** .

The Clinical Picture of Hypothermia

The National Institutes of Health has initiated a public awareness campaign informing the public to watch for "umbles"—stumbles, mumbles, fumbles, and grumbles. These behaviors are good indicators of how the cold affects the cerebral and cognitive functioning of patients in the early stages of hypothermia.

The clinical definition of mild hypothermia is a CBT greater than 90°F (32.2°C). Below this CBT, the condition is considered severe hypothermia. In the early stage of hypothermia, the CBT is more than 95°F, but the patient shows obvious signs and symptoms of hypothermia. Luckily, the body may compensate for this condition through thermogenesis until the patient finds a way to increase heat production or the glycogen energy stored in muscles and liver is exhausted.

Hypothermia may also be classified according to the time to onset. Acute occurs rapidly (as in cold water drownings), subacute during a short time (as in exposure to cold conditions during a short time), and chronic that may occur over days (for example, an urban homeless person or a poorly heated home with an elderly resident). In yet another classification, primary hypothermia is caused by cold exposures, whereas secondary hypothermia is due to problems such as severe sepsis.

In mild hypothermia, the shivering is in full force and the umbles are noticeable. Often, however, the initial symptoms are vague. Older people may simply have a more flat affect, be slightly more confused, or develop symptoms suggestive of a possible stroke, including dysarthria and ataxia. No strong correlation has been observed between signs or symptoms and a specific CBT.

The net effect of hypothermia is to slow things down, but different body systems react in different ways. The overall slowdown of function is most dramatically apparent in the CNS, where just about everything slows—thinking, feeling, speaking. A hypothermic patient is typically apathetic and often shows impaired reasoning ability. Speech is slow and may be slurred; coordination is impaired; the gait is ataxic. This picture may closely resemble that associated with stroke, head injury, or alcohol intoxication, which probably explains why so many cases of hypothermia are initially misdiagnosed.

In the cardiovascular system, hypothermia induces several changes. Initially, as peripheral vasoconstriction shunts blood to the body core, the body's volume receptors interpret the increased flow as an increase in volume. They therefore stimulate the kidneys to start producing more urine (cold diuresis). At the same time, cooling of the tissues induces a flow of water from the intravascular to the extravascular spaces. The net effects are to increase the viscosity of the blood, thereby impairing circulation, and to produce a state of hypovolemia. Meanwhile, the heart is suffering from the drop in body temperature. Cold initially speeds up the heart, then slows the rate and disrupts the electric conduction system. At a CBT of approximately 90°F (32.2°C), the body experiences cardiac dysrhythmias, including atrial fibrillation. A unique Osborn wave may be observed if shivering does not obscure the tracing **Figure 35-14 ▼** . Of special concern is ventricular fibrillation (V-fib), to which a hypothermic heart becomes susceptible at a CBT around 82.4°F (28°C). Once the heart fibrillates, repeated defibrillation is not recommended until the CBT is greater than 86°F (30°C).

Initially, the respiratory rate speeds up, but later it slows, leading to a decrease in minute volume. Tracheobronchial secretions increase, and

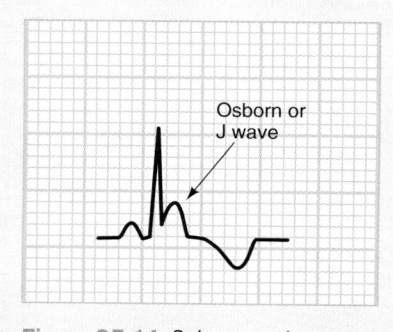

Figure 35-14 Osborn or J wave.

bronchospasm may occur. At 90°F (32.2°C), hypoventilation is profound, protective airway reflexes decline, and oxygen consumption decreases by about half.

The muscular system also slows down in response to cold. Although the initial muscular reaction to cold is shivering, that reaction is a mixed blessing. It generates heat, but it also makes skilled movements more difficult. Shivering, in any case, ceases when the CBT falls below 91°F (32.7°C). Thereafter, cold muscles become progressively weaker and stiffer, impairing the exposed person's ability to save himself or herself.

Finally, cold affects the body's metabolism. Shivering can deplete the body of glucose, leading to hypoglycemia. Meanwhile, insulin levels fall, making further glucose metabolism impossible, so the body switches to the metabolism of fat. The liver's metabolism of drugs is also affected by the cold. Because medications are metabolized more slowly than normal, the effects of those drugs last much longer.

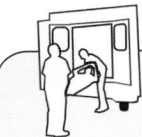

In the Field

If a patient in a car crash is shivering, this is not a good sign. If you need heavy clothing, remember that the patient will also be cold.

Treatment of Hypothermia

This section first discusses general care and then explains how to manage cardiac arrest in a hypothermic patient. General care is aimed at preserving further heat loss and rewarming. The victim should be stripped of wet clothes and insulated from further heat loss. The 2005 Advanced Cardiac Life Support (ACLS) guidelines divide hypothermia into three classes and base treatment on the CBT and the presence (or absence) of a perfusing rhythm. **Figure 35-15** summarizes and adapts these recommendations for prehospital care.

Breathing Patients With a Pulse
Mild Hypothermia Cases: 93.2°F (34°C)
The treatment is passive rewarming, which involves removing wet clothing, drying the patient's skin, moving the patient into a warmed ambulance, and using warm blankets or "space" blankets to prevent further conductive heat loss. Depending on the patient's location and the relative ease of transport, you may have to promote heat generation by feeding the patient, giving warm fluids (not caffeine or alcohol), and getting the person to move about.

Moderate Hypothermia Cases: 86°F to 93.2°F (30°C to 34°C)
The treatment is passive rewarming and active external rewarming of the truncal areas. This approach involves the use of several means to directly warm the patient's skin, including heating blankets or radiant heat from hot packs in the groin, neck, and axillae; forced hot air; and warmed IV fluids. Fluids at temperatures from 102°F to 105°F may be infused. It is prudent to administer a 500-mL bolus (unless

otherwise contraindicated) to counter the hypovolemia commonly encountered in hypothermia. Commercial warming devices that use special blankets and a heated fan unit can warm patients at a rate of up to 4.3°F per hour, which is much faster than warm blankets (2.2°F). Carefully monitor the patient for hemodynamic changes and direct thermal tissue injury because active external rewarming measures can cause "afterdrop." Afterdrop, the continued lowering of CBT even after the patient is removed from the cold, is more common in chronic hypothermia and hypothermia complicated by frostbitten extremities. Nevertheless, the 2005 American Heart Association guidelines point out that forced air rewarming can be effective for some patients, even patients with severe hypothermia.

Paramedics working in regions where winter wilderness rescue operations are routine should carry specialized gear for prehospital management of hypothermia. The hydraulic sarong, for example, is a thin, double-layered blanket with a network of plastic tubing running between the two layers **Figure 35-16**. This blanket is wrapped around the hypothermia victim, and water heated over a camp stove is pumped through the tubing. Other devices have been developed to help deliver heated, humidified supplemental oxygen to aid in core rewarming. Note that the oxygen must be heated *and* humidified to be effective, which generally requires the use of commercial devices.

Severe Hypothermia Cases: Less Than 86°F (30°C)
The active internal rewarming sequence used to treat severe hypothermia is accomplished in-hospital using the following modalities: warm IV fluids; warm, humid oxygen; peritoneal lavage (potassium chloride–free fluid); extracorporeal rewarming; and esophageal rewarming tubes. Rewarming should continue until the CBT is greater than 95°F (35°C), spontaneous circulation returns, or resuscitative efforts cease.

Patients With No Pulse or Not Breathing
You may need to "look, listen, and feel" for a good 60 seconds to determine whether breathing and a pulse are present and, perhaps, use a portable Doppler device. Patients in cardiac arrest require high-quality CPR (push hard and fast, and allow full chest recoil) and a single shock if in V-fib/V-tach. Resume CPR immediately. Establish IV access. Infuse warm normal saline. Attempt to insert an advanced airway, and ventilate with warm, humid oxygen.

Cases of Hypothermia Less Than 86°F (30°C)
Continue CPR, attempt a single defibrillation for V-fib/V-tach, establish IV access, withhold IV medications, and transport to the hospital.

Cases of Hypothermia Greater Than 86°F (30°C)
Continue CPR, and administer IV medications as indicated by the electrocardiographic rhythm, but space them at longer than standard intervals. Repeat defibrillation for V-fib/V-tach as the core temperature rises. Transport the patient to the hospital to provide active internal rewarming.

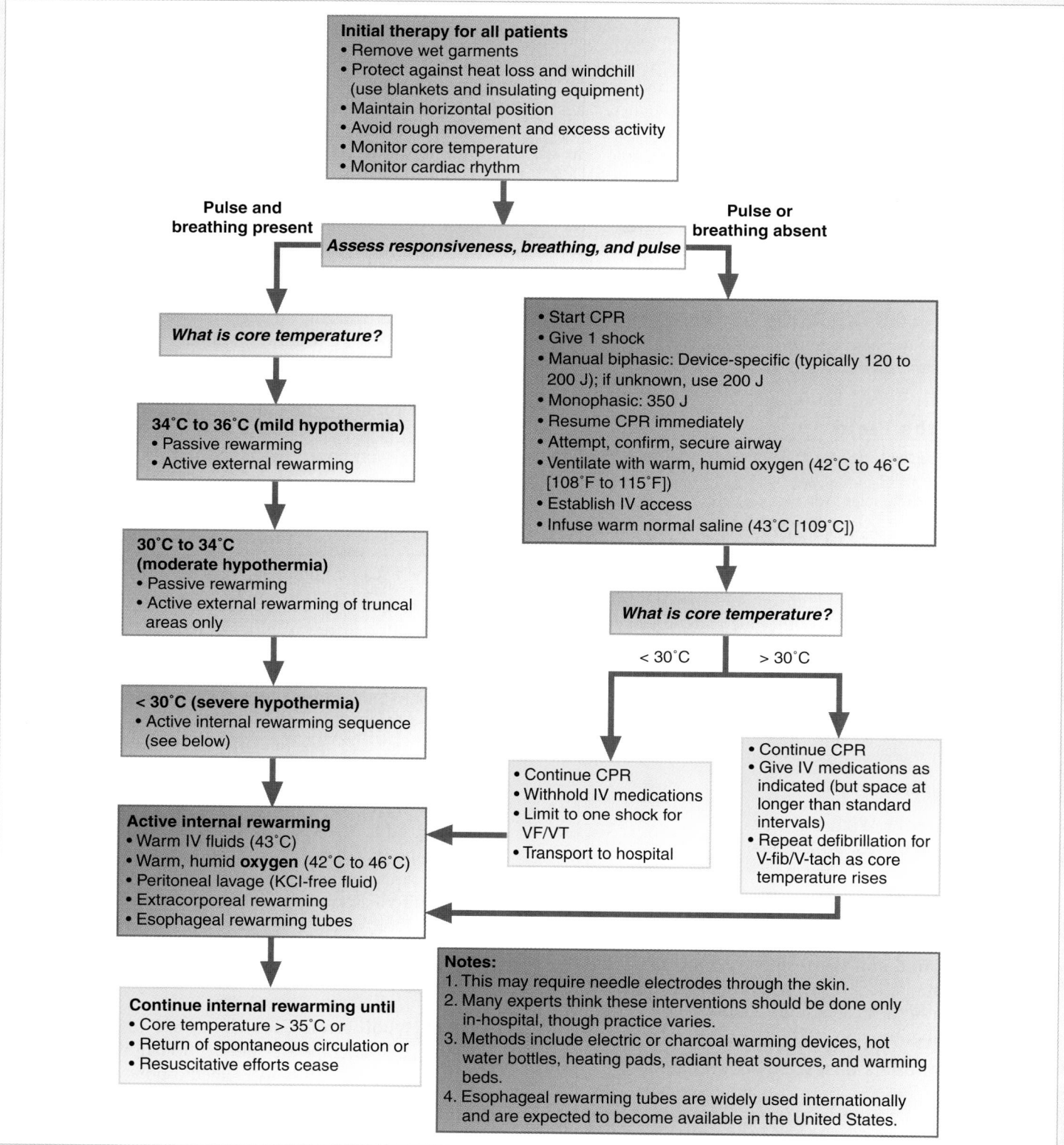

Figure 35-15 Prehospital hypothermia treatment algorithm.

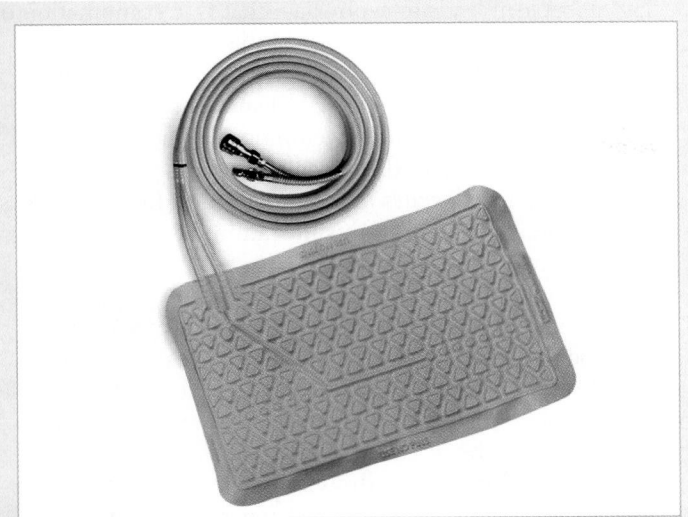

Figure 35-16 The hydraulic sarong can be wrapped around a patient with hypothermia and warms the patient via warm water fed through tubes.

Withholding and Cessation of Resuscitative Efforts

In the field, patients with obvious lethal traumatic injuries or those so frozen as to block the airway or chest compression efforts generally are dead. If submersion preceded the arrest, successful resuscitation is unlikely, with the possible exception of immersion in icy waters. Trauma and alcohol and drug overdoses could have led to hypothermia in the first place and can hamper resuscitation efforts. Try to factor these conditions into your treatment decisions. For example, a heroin user who was

Controversies

There is a widespread belief that rough handling of a hypothermic heart may cause V-fib. Although people in severe hypothermia are prone to a V-fib arrest, it has not been clearly demonstrated that intubation or roughly handling the patient causes V-fib. In fact, Danzl's multicenter hypothermia survey showed no case of V-fib in 117 hypothermic patients who were intubated. Do not let your concern for possible V-fib prevent you from inserting an advanced airway or moving the patient.

found outdoors and quickly recovers after naloxone administration should have a temperature check and should not be left at the scene.

Some believe that patients who appear dead after prolonged exposure to cold temperatures are not dead until "warm and dead." The effects of hypothermia may essentially protect the brain and organs if hypothermia develops quickly, a fact that is being used to successfully treat some cardiac arrest patients. Sometimes it may be impossible to know which came first—a cardiac arrest and then hypothermia or vice versa. In those situations, it is prudent to attempt resuscitation.

Drowning or Submersion

According to the Centers for Disease Control and Prevention, 3,482 unintentional drownings occurred in the United States in 2000, for an average of nine people per day. In the United States, drowning is the second leading cause of injury-related death among children younger than 15 years. The good news

You are the Provider Part 3

After getting the patient out of his wet clothes, you begin your exam. He is barely shivering. He has trouble following your commands but does not seem to have any focal weakness. His pupils are equal, round, and reactive to light. His voice is slurred, but his facial muscles are symmetric and intact. The spine is nontender; the lungs are clear; and there is moderate epigastric tenderness to palpation. You find no evidence of trauma.

You insert an 18-gauge IV catheter, draw a blood sample, and check the patient's glucose level. It is 162. Your partner has hung a bag of warm normal saline. The rectal temperature is 91.4°F (33°C). You begin to remove the patient's clothes and place hot packs in the groin, axillae, and neck. You wrap the IV fluid warmer around the bag of the nonrebreathing mask and wrap the oxygen tubing in a hot pack.

Reassessment	Recording Time: 15 Minutes
Skin	Getting pinker, cold, dry
Pulse	108 beats/min; regular and strong
Blood pressure	110/64 mm Hg
Respirations	24 breaths/min
Sao2	100% on nonrebreathing mask at 10 L/min supplemental oxygen; good waveform

7. What information is important to convey to the emergency department staff when you call?
8. What effect does alcohol have on hypothermia?
9. Why did the patient remove his clothing if he was hypothermic?

Table 35-7	Risk Factors for Drowning and Submersion

- Male sex
- Younger than 20 years (even higher for < 5 years)
- Preexisting conditions, such as seizure disorder
- Alcohol use
- Ineffective safety barriers (gates, locks, or use of a solar panel on a pool)
- Hyperventilation (may lead to shallow water blackout syndrome)

is that these numbers are declining as more groups tout the virtues of prevention.

The first task in understanding drowning is to define this condition. At one point, 33 different definitions existed. In 2002, the first World Congress on Drowning developed the definition now in use: Drowning is the process of experiencing respiratory impairment from submersion/immersion in liquid. The "Utstein style" guidelines were then modified for drowning, and the term "near-drowning" was abandoned.

People may live or die based on what happens when a liquid-air interface occurs at the airway's entrance. Consequently, the drowning continuum progresses from breath holding, to laryngospasm, to the accumulation of carbon dioxide and the inability to oxygenate the lungs, to subsequent respiratory and cardiac arrest from multiple-organ failure due to tissue hypoxia. The victim can be resuscitated at any point along this continuum.

Table 35-7 lists the risk factors for drowning. Note that toddlers typically drown in bathtubs, school-age children in pools, and teens in lakes or rivers.

Pathophysiology of Drowning and Submersion

Drowning generally follows a predictable sequence starting when the victim cannot keep his or her face out of the liquid medium:

- The length of breath holding depends on the victim's state of health and fitness, his or her level of panic, and the water temperature.
- As the victim goes under and water enters the mouth and nose, coughing and gasping ensue, and the victim swallows considerable amounts of water. Note that while some theoretical differences distinguish saltwater and freshwater drownings, this information is neither clinically significant nor useful in resuscitating a patient. In fact, 11 mL of water per kilogram of body weight is required to produce significant blood problems, and 22 mL/kg is needed to create electrolyte problems. Both types of water can lead to pulmonary injuries.
- A very small amount of water is aspirated into the posterior pharynx and perhaps the trachea, setting off spasms of the laryngeal muscles (laryngospasm) that effectively seal off and protect the airway—at least temporarily—from further aspiration.

- Laryngospasm leads to asphyxia—that is, a combination of hypoxemia and hypercarbia—and the patient may lose consciousness. Hypoxemia stimulates the body to shift from aerobic to anaerobic metabolism, with the ensuing production of lactate and development of metabolic acidosis. If the patient dies during this phase of laryngospasm, as occurs in 10% to 15% of drowning cases, it is essentially a death from suffocation, because the lungs are still dry ("dry drowning").
- At a certain point, which varies from person to person, water begins to enter the lungs. That event may occur because the hypercarbic and hypoxic drives stimulate inhalation or, if the patient has lost consciousness, because progressive asphyxia causes the laryngeal muscles to relax. In either case, the net effect is to permit water to gain access to the lungs ("wet drowning"). Its entry triggers an increase in peripheral airway resistance along with constriction of pulmonary vessels, all of which decrease the compliance of the lungs. In other words, the lungs become stiff.
- The decompensation stage of drowning occurs next. The victim gasps for air, inhaling yet more water, which mixes with air and chemicals in the lungs to form froth. Apnea recurs, and the patient loses consciousness (if he or she has not already done so). The process of hypoxic brain damage begins, and cardiac arrest occurs.

Response to Drowning and Submersion Incidents

In general terms, the resuscitation of a victim of a submersion is the same as that for any other patient in respiratory or cardiac arrest, albeit with a few new logistic problems.

First, of course, you must reach the victim. People who have specialized training and experience in water rescue are best able to accomplish this task Figure 35-17 . Many fire departments and law enforcement agencies have water rescue teams, as does the US Coast Guard.

When you reach the victim, the steps of treatment follow the usual sequence of ABCs. The first priority is establishing the airway. Cervical spine precautions should then be taken if necessary. The American Heart Association, as part of its 2005 ACLS revisions, suggests that routine cervical spine stabilization is not needed in cases involving drowning or submersion. The exceptions are patients who have a history of diving or using a water slide before the drowning or who have obvious traumatic injury signs and when witnesses claim alcohol was involved.

Assist ventilation as soon as possible, even before the patient is removed from the water. Do not perform manual thrusts (Heimlich maneuver) to remove water from the lungs because they may displace water from the stomach into the lungs.

Start supplementary oxygen at the same time that you quickly determine whether a pulse is present. If there is no pulse, begin high-quality CPR. You may need to suction. One Australian study of drowning victims noted that 66% of

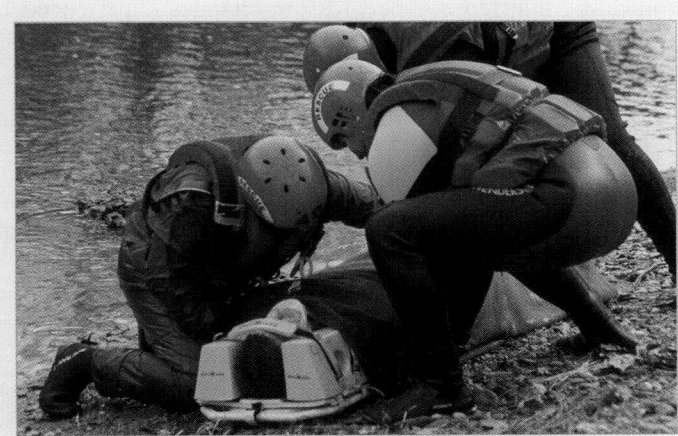

Figure 35-17 Rescuers must wear proper personal protective equipment, including a personal flotation device, when performing a water rescue.

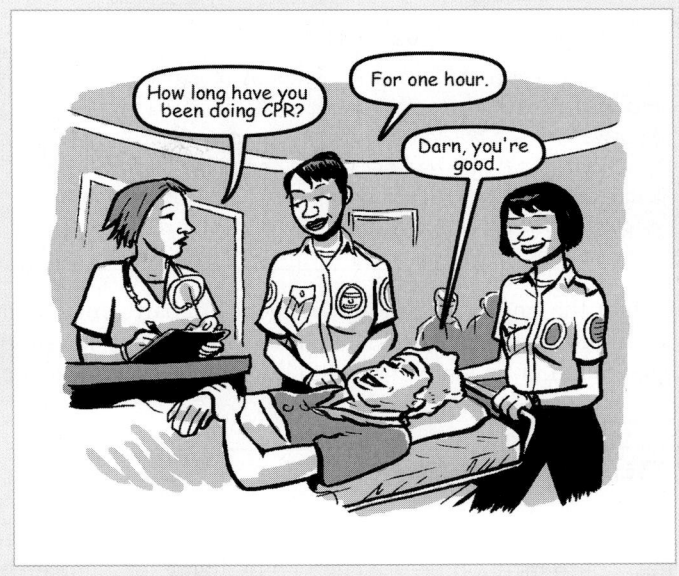

Figure 35-18

patients receiving rescue breathing and 86% getting compressions vomited; one of your primary goals will be to prevent vomiting. In any event, protect the airway from aspiration during vomiting. Advanced airway placement may be appropriate if BLS airway interventions fail.

During normal, spontaneous breathing, the pressure in the airways at the end of exhalation is effectively zero. As a result, some alveoli normally collapse during the expiratory phase of the respiratory cycle. When there is widespread atelectasis and shunt—as in drowning—it is desirable to maintain some positive pressure at the end of exhalation to keep alveoli open and to drive any fluid that may have accumulated in the alveoli back into the interstitium or capillaries. The technique called positive end-expiratory pressure (PEEP) focuses on maintaining some degree of positive pressure at the end of the expiratory phase of respiration. In the field, PEEP is indicated for intubated patients who must be transported over long distances to the hospital after submersion or who have other conditions that produce significant shunt. Several commercial devices are designed to allow PEEP via an endotracheal tube. In addition, portable ventilators usually have a PEEP setting.

If an endotracheal tube has been inserted (not before insertion!), insert a nasogastric tube to decompress the stomach (discussed in Chapter 11). If a pulse is absent, implement advanced life support measures similar to those used in any other case of cardiopulmonary arrest: establish IV access, administer epinephrine, perform cardiac monitoring, and ensure electric conversion of V-fib.

Patients rescued from submersion are prone to bronchospasm from the irritation to their airways. If you hear wheezes, administer a beta-2 adrenergic drug, such as albuterol by nebulizer, as you would for a patient having an acute asthmatic attack.

Do not give up on the victim of submersion, especially if the patient is a child and the incident occurred in icy water Figure 35-18 ▸ . Successful resuscitations with complete

Table 35-8	Management of Drowning and Submersion

- Rescuers trained and practiced in doing so should perform the water rescue.
- Ensure basic life support measures are being carried out with an emphasis on airway and oxygenation.
- Anticipate vomiting.
- Administer supplemental oxygen and intubate if needed.
- Establish IV access.
- Measure core temperature, and prevent or treat hypothermia.
- Give a beta-2 adrenergic by metered-dose inhaler or nebulizer for wheezing.
- Monitor end-tidal carbon dioxide and pulse oximetry.
- Insert a nasogastric tube in intubated patients.
- Transport every submersion patient to the hospital, including patients who seem to recover at the scene.

neurologic recovery have been reported even in cases in which the victim had been submerged for more than an hour in icy water. Remember to consider the effects of hypothermia on a drowning patient, including measuring a core temperature and using the hypothermia algorithm. Studies indicate that the length of submersion and the response to field resuscitation are major predictors of outcome. In other words, if patients are awake on hospital arrival, they will do better.

Table 35-8 ▴ summarizes the management of drowning and submersion.

Postresuscitation Complications

Adult respiratory distress syndrome, chemical or bacterial pneumonitis, and renal failure are common complications that can occur hours to days after a submersion. These factors highlight the importance of an emergency department evaluation of submersion victims. Their symptoms may be subtle (slight cough, mild tachypnea), or they may be asymptomatic.

Diving Injuries

There are 5 million recreational scuba divers in the United States, not to mention people engaged in diving for commercial and military purposes, and about 200,000 Americans receive scuba instruction every year. Paramedics who work in coastal or lakefront areas are likely to encounter a diving casualty. Paramedics who operate in areas where diving is popular should become at least as conversant with diving medicine as enthusiasts of the sport are.

Four modes of diving are distinguished:

- **Scuba diving.** The most popular form of diving, scuba diving is named for the self-contained underwater breathing apparatus that the diver carries on his or her back.
- **Breath-hold diving.** Also called free diving, it does not require any equipment, except sometimes a snorkel.
- **Surface-tended diving.** Air is piped to the diver through a tube from the surface.
- **Saturation diving.** The diver remains at depth for prolonged periods.

All divers, irrespective of the type of diving they do, are subject to the increased ambient pressures that occur under water.

Pressure Effects: Physical Principles

Pressure, which is defined as force per unit area, may be expressed in a number of ways. The weight of air at sea level, for example, can be expressed as 14.7 pounds per square inch (psi), as 760 mm Hg, or as 1 atmosphere absolute (ATA). The latter system—measurement in atmospheres absolute—is used most commonly in diving medicine. Because water is much denser than air, relatively small changes in depth produce large changes in pressure. For every 33 feet of seawater (fsw), the pressure increases 1 ATA. The depth of the dive can be used to estimate the pressure to which the diver was exposed: At a depth of 33 fsw, the pressure is 2 ATA; at 66 fsw, it is 3 ATA; and so forth. The majority of scuba diving is done at depths between 60 and 120 fsw.

The body and its tissues, because they are composed primarily of water, are not compressible and, therefore, are not significantly affected by the pressure changes experienced in descent or ascent through water. Gas-filled organs are another matter, however, because they *are* compressible:

- Nitrogen, an inert gas, is fat-soluble (it prefers to dissolve in fatty or lipid-rich tissues), exists safely as gas nuclei in body tissues, and is found in 79% of the air we breathe. It produces nitrogen narcosis in humans at a depth of 100 fsw. Nitrogen can cause decompression sickness (decompression illness) on ascent because of the bubbles that form on reduction of pressure. For this reason, commercial divers use a decompression schedule. Recreational divers usually adhere to a "no-decompression" limit (a table outlining safe times at various depths) so they do not have to decompress on surfacing.
- Boyle's law states that at a constant temperature, the volume of a gas is inversely proportional to its pressure (if you double the pressure on a gas, you halve its volume): $PV = K$, where P = pressure, V = volume, and K = a constant. This equation tells us that as a diver descends (and the pressure goes up), gas volume is reduced; as the diver ascends (pressure goes down), gas volume increases **Figure 35-19 ▸**. This law explains the problems that can occur in gas-filled spaces in the body (eg, lungs, gastrointestinal tract, sinuses, and parts of the ear).
- Dalton's law deals with the pressures exerted by mixtures of different gases. Dalton's law states that each gas in mixture exerts the same partial pressure that it would exert if it were alone in the same volume and that the total pressure of a mixture of gases is the sum of the partial pressures of all gases in the mixture. Thus, for fresh air:

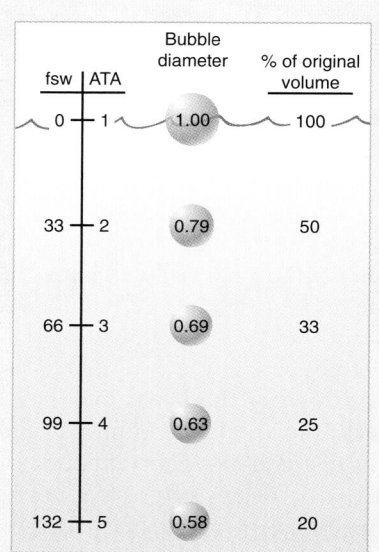

fsw	ATA	Bubble diameter	% of original volume
0	1	1.00	100
33	2	0.79	50
66	3	0.69	33
99	4	0.63	25
132	5	0.58	20

Figure 35-19 Boyle's law: As a bubble descends through water, its volume changes in inverse proportion to the ambient temperature.

$$P_{total} = P_{O_2} + P_{CO_2} + P_{N_2}$$

This law helps explain nitrogen narcosis, oxygen toxicity, and the dangers of contamination in pressurized breathing systems. It also explains why pulse oximetry readings in divers with nitrogen narcosis remain unaffected.

- **Henry's law** states that the amount of gas dissolved in a liquid is directly proportional to the partial pressure of the gas above the liquid. A classic example of this law is when a sealed bottle that has dissolved carbon dioxide is opened: The lowering of the pressure of the gas in solution (in this case, a mixture of a liquid and a gas) allows its volume to increase and the gas to escape as bubbles.

Diving History

It is very important to obtain as many details as you can about the dive and the onset of the patient's symptoms. It is helpful to use a special form for taking the diving history that records the following information:

- Onset of symptoms (during ascent or descent). Decompression sickness will usually manifest within the first hour of surfacing and certainly within 6 hours. Symptoms occurring within 10 minutes suggest air embolism, especially when they are accompanied by a loss of consciousness.
- Type of diving and the type of equipment used
- Type of tank used (compressed air or a Nitrox system with distinctive yellow and green stripes on the tank)
- Site of diving and water temperature
- Number of dives made during the past 72 hours, along with the depth, bottom time, and surface interval for each. Was a dive computer used?
- Were safety stops used?
- Were there any attempts at in-water decompression (a no-no!)?
- Dive complications, if any
- Predive and postdive activities

Injuries During Descent

The major problem encountered during descent is barotrauma ("squeeze"). This injury results from a pressure imbalance between gas-filled spaces inside the body and the external atmosphere. Barotrauma can result from two different mechanisms: compression of gases within body spaces during descent or expansion of gases within those spaces during ascent (discussed later). Barotrauma can affect any gas-filled space in the body, including the sinuses, the inner and middle ears, and even teeth. **Table 35-9** summarizes the types of barotrauma.

A person who is scuba diving is theoretically protected from barotrauma by breathing compressed air, which will match the pressure of the surrounding environment. Thus, as long as the air-filled cavities of the body can equilibrate freely, they will not implode, unless there is an obstruction.

If there is blockage in the eustachian tube, which connects the middle ear with the nasopharynx, or if the diver cannot equalize ear pressures with a Valsalva maneuver, the pressure in the middle ear cannot be equalized with that of the outside water. A characteristic "middle ear squeeze" syndrome then develops with severe ear pain. If the tympanic membrane ruptures, nausea, vomiting, and vertigo may occur. This effect is especially likely in colder waters. At

depths, this reaction may cause panic, rapid ascent, and the problems associated with such an ascent. Treatment involves a loose dressing for ear bleeding; some patients may require IV antiemetics or sedatives.

Injuries at Depth

Nitrogen narcosis ("rapture of the deep," "narc'ed") is a state of altered mental status caused by breathing compressed air (including nitrogen) at depth. The human body does not use nitrogen for metabolism; thus, in a breathing gas mixture, nitrogen dilutes the concentration of oxygen. A problem may occur when a diver descends to a depth of 99 ft (30 m), for example, where the ambient pressure is 4 ATA. For the person to be able to breathe, the inspired air pressure must be the same as the ambient pressure. Thus, the inspired partial pressure of nitrogen is 80% times 4 ATA, or 3.2 ATA (per Dalton's law).

Nitrogen narcosis typically occurs around 100 ft, becomes more pronounced at 150 fsw, and is why sport divers should not use compressed air only for dives greater than 120 ft. Signs and symptoms include a euphoric feeling; inappropriate behavior at depth, including lack of concern for safety, apparent stupidity or inappropriate laughter; and tingling of lips, gums, and legs. Divers report tolerance over their diving lifetime. A diver may suddenly become panicked and spit out the regulator or surface too quickly. The only effective way to counteract the narcotic effect of nitrogen is to lower the nitrogen partial pressure through controlled ascent or by using a Nitrox system.

Injuries During Ascent
Barotrauma

As the diver ascends and the ambient pressure around him or her decreases, the gases within the body's air-filled spaces will expand. For example, the lung volume of a scuba diver who has inhaled to his total lung capacity at a depth of 33 fsw would double by the time the diver reached the surface if he were to hold his breath during ascent. For that reason, all diving students are trained to exhale constantly as they are ascending so as to vent air from their lungs. A common scenario in which barotrauma occurs involves a diver who has used decongestants before a dive. If the medication begins to wear off before ascent, air may become trapped in the sinuses and ears, creating a "reverse squeeze" in which the increasing pressure cannot equalize during ascent. Symptoms are identical to those observed during descent.

A more dangerous situation can occur in an emergency ascent—for example, when the diver experiences difficulty with his or her equipment and panics—and gives in to the instinctive impulse to hold his or her breath under water. The result is one of the worst forms of barotrauma of ascent—pulmonary overpressurization syndrome (POPS), also known as "burst lung." It can cause pneumothorax, mediastinal and subcutaneous emphysema, alveolar hemorrhage, and a lethal arterial gas embolism (AGE). Because the relative pressure and volume changes are greatest near the surface of the water,

Table 35-9	Diving Injuries

Mechanisms and Pathophysiology	Body Region	Condition	Clinical Features	Treatment
Barotrauma				
During *descent*: compression of gas in closed spaces	Ear	External ear squeeze (*barotitis externa*)	Otalgia, bloody otorrhea	Keep ear canal dry; no swimming or diving until healed
		Middle ear squeeze (*barotitis media*)	Severe ear pain, tympanic membrane can rupture; emesis, vertigo, nystagmus	Decongestants; no diving until healed, may need IV antinausea medications
		Inner ear squeeze	Tinnitus, vertigo, hearing loss; emesis, pallor, diaphoresis	May need IV antinausea medications, surgical repair
	Paranasal sinuses	Sinus squeeze	Severe pain over affected sinuses and upper teeth, epistaxis	Topical and oral decongestants; antibiotics
	Face	Face mask squeeze	Ecchymoses and petechiae of skin beneath face mask; scleral/conjunctival hemorrhage	Cold compresses, prevent by forced exhalation through nose
During *ascent*: expansion of gas in closed spaces	Gastrointestinal tract	"Gas in gut" (*aerogastralgia*)	Colicky belly pain, belching, flatulence	Rare reports of rupture; usually, no care needed
	Lungs	Pulmonary barotrauma "burst lung," pulmonary overpressurization syndrome (POPS)	Dyspnea, dysphagia, hoarseness, substernal pain; subcutaneous emphysema around neck; pneumothorax, syncope	100% oxygen; decompress pneumothorax
		Arterial gas embolism (AGE)—complication of POPS	Altered mental status, vertigo, dizziness, seizures, dyspnea, pleuritic chest pain, sudden loss of consciousness on surfacing; sudden death	100% oxygen; transport supine; hyperbaric therapy; steroids
Decompression sickness	Skin		Pruritus, subcutaneous emphysema, swelling, rashes	Symptomatic; observe for complications
	Joints and muscles	Bends ("pain-only bends")	Arthralgias, especially in elbows and shoulders, relieved by pressure	Analgesia; observe
	Cerebrum		Multiple sensory and motor disturbances	Hyperbaric therapy; IV fluids
	Cerebellum	The "staggers"	Unsteadiness, incoordination, vertigo	Corticosteroids for all patients with anything more than skin and musculoskeletal involvement
	Spinal cord		Paraplegia, paraparesis, bladder dysfunction (inability to void), back pain	See above
	Lungs	Venous air embolism (the "chokes")	Chest pain, cough, dyspnea, signs of pulmonary embolism	See above
Dissolved nitrogen	Central nervous system	Nitrogen narcosis ("rapture of the deep")	Symptoms like those of alcohol intoxication	Ascent to shallower water
Hyperventilation before dive	Central nervous system	Shallow water blackout (in breath-hold dives)	Loss of consciousness just before reaching surface	100% oxygen; assisted breathing

- Treatment of barotrauma depends on whether an air embolism is present. A pneumothorax may require needle decompression. With an air embolism, the patient must receive treatment in a hyperbaric chamber.
- Decompression sickness encompasses a broad range of signs and symptoms caused by nitrogen bubbles in blood and tissues coming out of solution on dive ascent. Symptoms include itchy skin, subcutaneous emphysema, swelling, rashes, joint and muscle pain, sensory and motor disturbances, incoordination, paralysis, chest pain, and dyspnea. Treatment is 100% oxygen, IV normal saline, and transport to a hyperbaric facility.
- Shallow water blackout occurs when a person hyperventilates just before diving underwater and passes out before resurfacing. Treatment is the same as for any other submersion.
- The Divers Alert Network is a valuable resource for diving-related injuries. Callers are immediately connected to a physician experienced in diving medicine who can provide advice regarding specific management.
- Altitude illness occurs when unacclimatized people ascend to altitude. Types of altitude illness include acute mountain sickness (AMS), high-altitude cerebral edema (HACE), and high-altitude pulmonary edema (HAPE).
- Symptoms of AMS include headache plus fatigue, weakness, gastrointestinal symptoms, dizziness, lightheadedness, and difficulty sleeping.
- Symptoms of HACE include a change in mental status and/or ataxia in a person with AMS or the presence of both in a person without AMS.
- Symptoms of HAPE include at least two of the following: dyspnea at rest, cough, weakness, or chest tightness or congestion and at least two of the following: central cyanosis, audible rales, wheezing, tachypnea, or tachycardia.
- Treatment of altitude illnesses includes descending or using a portable hyperbaric chamber, providing oxygen, and giving certain IV medications.

■ Vital Vocabulary

acute mountain sickness (AMS) An altitude illness characterized by headache plus at least one of the following: fatigue or weakness, gastrointestinal symptoms (nausea, vomiting or anorexia), dizziness or lightheadedness, or difficulty sleeping.

afterdrop Continued fall in core temperature after a victim of hypothermia has been removed from a cold environment, due at least in part to the return of cold blood from the body surface to the body core.

altitude illnesses Conditions caused by the effects from hypobaric (low atmospheric pressure) hypoxia on the CNS and pulmonary systems as result of unacclimatized people ascending to altitude; range from acute mountain sickness to high altitude cerebral edema (HACE) and high altitude pulmonary edema (HAPE).

arterial gas embolism (AGE) The resultant gaseous emboli from the forcing of gas into the pulmonary vasculature from barotrauma.

ataxia Inability to coordinate the muscles properly; often used to describe a staggering gait.

atmosphere absolute (ATA) A measurement of ambient pressure; the weight of air at sea level.

barotrauma Injury resulting from pressure disequilibrium across body surfaces.

basal metabolic rate (BMR) The heat energy produced at rest from normal body metabolic reactions, determined mostly by the liver and skeletal muscles.

Boyle's law At a constant temperature, the volume of a gas is inversely proportional to its pressure (if you double the pressure on a gas, you halve its volume); written as $PV = K$, where P = pressure, V = volume, and K = a constant.

breath-hold diving Also called free diving, this type of diving does not require any equipment, except sometimes a snorkel.

classic heat stroke Also called passive heat stroke, this is a serious heat illness that usually occurs during heat waves and is most likely to strike very old, very young, or bedridden people.

cold diuresis Secretion of large amounts of urine in response to cold exposure and the consequent shunting of blood volume to the body core.

conduction Transfer of heat to a solid object or a liquid by direct contact.

convection Mechanism by which body heat is picked up and carried away by moving air currents.

core body temperature (CBT) The temperature in the part of the body comprising the heart, lungs, brain, and abdominal viscera.

Dalton's law Each gas in mixture exerts the same partial pressure that it would exert if it were alone in the same volume, and the total pressure of a mixture of gases is the sum of the partial pressures of all the gases in the mixture.

decompression sickness (DCS) A broad range of signs and symptoms caused by nitrogen bubbles in blood and tissues coming out of solution on ascent.

deep frostbite A type of frostbite in which the affected part looks white, yellow-white, or mottled blue-white and is hard, cold, and without sensation.

drowning The process of experiencing respiratory impairment from submersion or immersion in liquid.

dysphagia Difficulty in swallowing.

environmental emergencies Medical conditions caused or exacerbated by the weather, terrain, or unique atmospheric conditions such as high altitude or underwater.

evaporation The conversion of a liquid to a gas.

exertional heat stroke A serious type of heat stroke usually affecting young and fit people exercising in hot and humid conditions.

exertional hyponatremia A condition due to prolonged exertion in hot environments coupled with excessive hypotonic fluid intake that leads to nausea, vomiting, and, in severe cases, mental status changes and seizures.

frostbite Localized damage to tissues resulting from prolonged exposure to extreme cold.

frostnip Early frostbite, characterized by numbness and pallor without significant tissue damage.

fsw Abbreviation for feet of seawater, an indirect measure of pressure under water.

gangrene Permanent cell death.

heat cramps Acute and involuntary muscle pains, usually in the lower extremities, the abdomen, or both, that occur because of profuse sweating and subsequent sodium losses in sweat.

heat exhaustion A clinical syndrome characterized by volume depletion and heat stress that is thought to be a milder form of heat illness and on a continuum leading to heat stroke.

heat illness The increase in core body temperature due to inadequate thermolysis.

heat stroke The least common and most deadly heat illness, caused by a severe disturbance in thermoregulation, usually characterized by a core temperature of more than 104°F (40°C) and altered mental status.

heat syncope An orthostatic or near-syncopal episode that typically occurs in nonacclimated individuals who may be under heat stress.

Henry's law The amount of gas dissolved in a liquid is directly proportional to the partial pressure of the gas above the liquid.

high-altitude cerebral edema (HACE) An altitude illness in which there is a change in mental status and/or ataxia in a person with AMS or the presence of mental status changes and ataxia in a person without AMS.

high-altitude pulmonary edema (HAPE) An altitude illness characterized by dyspnea at rest, cough, severe weakness, and drowsiness that may eventually lead to central cyanosis, audible rales or wheezing, tachypnea, and tachycardia.

homeostasis Body processes that balance the supply and demand of the body's needs.

hyperthermia Unusually elevated body temperature.

hypothalamus Portion of the brain that regulates a multitude of body functions, including core temperature.

hypothermia Condition in which the core body temperature is significantly below normal.

laryngospasm Severe constriction of the larynx in response to allergy, noxious stimuli, or illness.

lassitude Condition of listlessness and fatigue.

malignant hyperthermia A condition that can result from common anesthesia medications (notably succinylcholine) and present with hyperthermia, muscular rigidity, altered mental status, and a hyperdynamic state.

neuroleptic malignant syndrome (NMS) A condition caused by antipsychotic and even common antiemetic medications that presents with hyperthermia, muscular rigidity, altered mental status, and a hyperdynamic state.

nitrogen narcosis A state resembling alcohol intoxication produced by nitrogen gas dissolved in the blood at high ambient pressure; also called rapture of the deep.

orthostatic hypotension A fall in blood pressure that occurs when moving from a recumbent to a sitting or standing position.

partial pressure The amount of the total pressure contributed by various gases in solution.

pulmonary overpressurization syndrome Also called "POPS" or "burst lung," this diving emergency can occur during ascent and can cause pneumothorax, mediastinal and subcutaneous emphysema, alveolar hemorrhage, and the lethal arterial gas embolism (AGE).

radiation Emission of heat from an object into surrounding, colder air.

saturation diving A type of diving in which the diver remains at depth for prolonged periods.

self-contained underwater breathing apparatus The expansion of the acronym (SCUBA) for specialized underwater breathing equipment.

shallow water blackout A diving emergency that occurs when a person hyperventilates just before submerging underwater and loses consciousness before resurfacing due to hypoxemia and cerebral vasoconstriction.

superficial frostbite A type of frostbite characterized by altered sensation (numbness, tingling, or burning) and white, waxy skin that is firm to palpation, but the underlying tissues remain soft.

surface-tended diving A type of diving in which air is piped to the diver through a tube from the surface.

thermogenesis The production of heat in the body.

thermolysis The liberation of heat from the body.

thermoregulation The process by which the body compensates for environmental extremes, for example, balancing between heat production and heat excretion.

trench foot A process similar to frostbite but caused by prolonged exposure to cool, wet conditions.

windchill factor The factor that takes into account the temperature and wind velocity in calculating the effect of a given ambient temperature on living organisms.

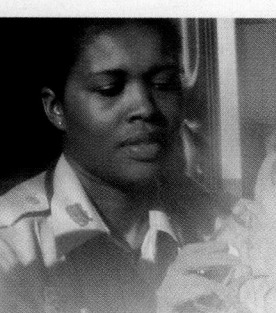

Assessment in Action

You are dispatched to the senior citizen complex for an unconscious person. When you arrive on scene and enter the apartment, you find the patient lying on floor. This is the fourth day of a heat wave and the patient did not have her air conditioning unit on. The patient's heart rate is 120 beats/min; the respiratory rate is 36 breaths/min.

1. **What do you suspect is wrong with this patient?**
   A. Heat exhaustion
   B. Heat cramps
   C. Heat stroke
   D. Frostbite

2. **What are the two types of heat stroke?**
   A. Classic heat stroke and exertional heat stroke
   B. Thermolysis and thermoregulation
   C. Orthostatic hypotension and classic hypotension
   D. Classic heat stroke and orthostatic hypotension

3. **A clinical syndrome thought to represent a milder form of heat illness and on a continuum leading to heat stroke is:**
   A. heat cramps.
   B. classic heat stroke.
   C. hyponatremia.
   D. heat exhaustion.

4. **A condition closely related to sodium-depleted heat exhaustion is:**
   A. classic heat stroke.
   B. exertional heat stroke.
   C. exertional hyponatremia.
   D. heat exhaustion.

5. **Medical conditions caused or worsened by the weather, terrain, or unique atmospheric conditions such as high altitude or underwater are called:**
   A. hypothermia.
   B. hyperthermia.
   C. weather-related emergencies.
   D. environmental emergencies.

6. **Which of the following terms refers to the body processes that balance the supply and demand of the body's needs?**
   A. Homeostasis
   B. Thermoregulation
   C. Hypothalamus
   D. Body temperature

7. **The body's reaction to its daily production of heat energy and to hot environmental conditions is:**
   A. thermogenesis.
   B. thermolysis.
   C. hypothermia.
   D. hyperthermia.

8. **When warmed blood from the core and overheated muscles heads for the peripherally dilated cutaneous vessels, the four major means of cooling it are:**
   A. thermogenesis, thermolysis, hypothermia, and hyperthermia.
   B. radiation, conduction, convection, and evaporation.
   C. hypothermia, radiation, conduction, and hyperthermia.
   D. conduction, convection, evaporation, and thermogenesis.

Challenging Questions

You are treating a severely hypothermic middle-aged male who is in cardiac arrest. The man was found in a wilderness area after being lost for 12 hours. The ambient temperature is 28°F. CPR is in progress and the patient has been successfully intubated. Medical control orders you to attempt defibrillation one time if indicated, withhold all cardiac medications, and rapidly transport the patient to the closest appropriate facility.

9. **What affect would repeated defibrillation attempts have on this patient?**

10. **Why should medication therapy be withheld in cardiac arrest patients with severe hypothermia?**

◼ Points to Ponder

You are dispatched for a man down outdoors. When you arrive, you find a man lying on the ground responsive to painful stimuli only. It is the middle of winter and is very cold. The patient is wearing only a light jacket and regular clothes. You immediately put the patient in the ambulance and begin assessing the patient. You turn the heat up in the back of the ambulance. The patient is extremely cold to the touch. His heart rate is 50 beats/min; blood pressure is 100/60 mm Hg; and the respiratory rate is 12 breaths/min. You are unable to obtain a pulse oximetry reading.

What are your main concerns for this patient?

Issues: Understanding the Pathophysiology of Environmental Emergencies. Understanding the Treatment Modalities for Hypothermia. Understanding How Young and Old People Are at Risk for Hypothermia.

36

Infectious and Communicable Diseases

Objectives

Cognitive

5-11.1   Review the specific anatomy and physiology pertinent to infectious and communicable diseases. (p 36.4)

5-11.2   Define specific terminology identified with infectious/communicable diseases. (p 36.5)

5-11.3   Discuss public health principles relevant to infectious/communicable disease. (p 36.7)

5-11.4   Identify public health agencies involved in the prevention and management of disease outbreaks. (p 36.4)

5-11.5   List and describe the steps of an infectious process. (p 36.5)

5-11.6   Discuss the risks associated with infection. (p 36.5)

5-11.7   List and describe the stages of infectious diseases. (p 36.6)

5-11.8   List and describe infectious agents, including bacteria, viruses, fungi, protozoans, and helminths (worms). (p36.6)

5-11.9   Describe host defense mechanisms against infection. (p 36.6)

5-11.10   Describe characteristics of the immune system, including the categories of white blood cells, the reticuloendothelial system (RES), and the complement system. (p 36.4)

5-11.11   Describe the processes of the immune system defenses, to include humoral and cell-mediated immunity. (p 36.4)

5-11.12   In specific diseases, identify and discuss the issues of personal isolation. (p 36.8)

5-11.13   Describe and discuss the rationale for the various types of PPE. (p 36.8)

5-11.14   Discuss what constitutes a significant exposure to an infectious agent. (p 36.7)

5-11.15   Describe the assessment of a patient suspected of, or identified as having, an infectious/communicable disease. (p 36.12)

5-11.16   Discuss the proper disposal of contaminated supplies (sharps, gauze sponges, tourniquets, etc.). (p 36.10)

5-11.17   Discuss disinfection of patient care equipment, and areas in which care of the patient occurred. (p 36.26)

5-11.18   Discuss the following relative to HIV—causative agent, body systems affected and potential secondary complications, modes of transmission, the seroconversion rate after direct significant exposure, susceptibility and resistance, signs and symptoms, specific patient management and personal protective measures, and immunization. (p 36.20)

5-11.19   Discuss hepatitis A (infectious hepatitis), including the causative agent, body systems affected and potential secondary complications, routes of transmission, susceptibility and resistance, signs and symptoms, patient management and protective measures, and immunization. (p 36.22)

5-11.20   Discuss hepatitis B (serum hepatitis), including the causative agent, the organ affected and potential secondary complications, routes of transmission, signs and symptoms, patient management and protective measures, and immunization. (p 36.19)

5-11.21   Discuss the susceptibility and resistance to hepatitis B. (p 36.19)

5-11.22   Discuss hepatitis C, including the causative agent, the organ affected, routes of transmission, susceptibility and resistance, signs and symptoms, patient management and protective measures, and immunization and control measures. (p 36.20)

5-11.23   Discuss hepatitis D (hepatitis delta virus), including the causative agent, the organ affected, routes of transmission, susceptibility and resistance, signs and symptoms, patient management and protective measures, and immunization and control measures. (p 36.20)

5-11.24   Discuss hepatitis E, including the causative agent, the organ affected, routes of transmission, susceptibility and resistance, signs and symptoms, patient management and protective measures, and immunization and control measures. (p 36.22)

5-11.25   Discuss tuberculosis, including the causative agent, body systems affected and secondary complications, routes of transmission, susceptibility and resistance, signs and symptoms, patient management and protective measures, and immunization and control measures. (p 36.14)

5-11.26   Discuss meningococcal meningitis (spinal meningitis), including causative organisms, tissues affected, modes of transmission, susceptibility and resistance, signs and symptoms, patient management and protective measures, and immunization and control measures. (p 36.14)

5-11.27   Discuss other infectious agents known to cause meningitis including streptococcus pneumonia, hemophilus influenza type b, and other varieties of viruses. (p 36.14)

5-11.28   Discuss pneumonia, including causative organisms, body systems affected, routes of transmission, susceptibility and resistance, signs and symptoms, patient management and protective measures, and immunization. (p 36.15)

5-11.29   Discuss tetanus, including the causative organism, the body system affected, modes of transmission, susceptibility and resistance, signs and symptoms, patient management and protective measures, and immunization. (p 36.23)

5-11.30   Discuss rabies and hantavirus as they apply to regional environmental exposures, including the causative organisms, the body systems affected, routes of transmission, susceptibility and resistance, signs and symptoms, patient management and protective measures, and immunization and control measures. (p 36.23)

5-11.31   Identify pediatric viral diseases. (p 36.12)

5-11.32   Discuss chickenpox, including the causative organism, the body system affected, mode of transmission, susceptibility and resistance, signs and symptoms, patient management and protective measures, and immunization and control measures. (p 36.13)

5-11.33   Discuss mumps, including the causative organism, the body organs and systems affected, mode of transmission, susceptibility and resistance, signs and symptoms, patient management and protective measures, and immunization. (p 36.13)

5-11.34 Discuss rubella (German measles), including the causative agent, the body tissues and systems affected, modes of transmission, susceptibility and resistance, signs and symptoms, patient management and protective measures, and immunization. (p 36.12)

5-11.35 Discuss measles (rubeola, hard measles), including the causative organism, the body tissues, organs, and systems affected, mode of transmission, susceptibility and resistance, signs and symptoms, patient management and protective measures, and immunization. (p 36.12)

5-11.36 Discuss the importance of immunization, and those diseases, especially in the pediatric population, which warrant widespread immunization (MMR). (p 36.12)

5-11.37 Discuss pertussis (whooping cough), including the causative organism, the body organs affected, mode of transmission, susceptibility and resistance, signs and symptoms, patient management and protective measures, and immunization. (p 36.14)

5-11.38 Discuss influenza, including causative organisms, the body system affected, mode of transmission, susceptibility and resistance, signs and symptoms, patient management and protective measures, and immunization. (p 36.16)

5-11.39 Discuss mononucleosis, including the causative organisms, the body regions, organs, and systems affected, modes of transmission, susceptibility and resistance, signs and symptoms, patient management and protective measures, and immunization. (p 36.16)

5-11.40 Discuss herpes simplex type 1, including the causative organism, the body regions and system affected, modes of transmission, susceptibility and resistance, signs and symptoms, patient management and protective measures, and immunization. (p 36.17)

5-11.41 Discuss the characteristics of, and organisms associated with, febrile and afebrile respiratory disease, to include bronchiolitis, bronchitis, laryngitis, croup, epiglottitis, and the common cold. (p 36.15)

5-11.42 Discuss syphilis, including the causative organism, the body regions, organs, and systems affected, modes of transmission, susceptibility and resistance, stages of signs and symptoms, patient management and protective measures, and immunization. (p 36.17)

5-11.43 Discuss gonorrhea, including the causative organism, the body organs and associated structures affected, mode of transmission, susceptibility and resistance, signs and symptoms, patient management and protective measures, and immunization. (p 36.16)

5-11.44 Discuss chlamydia, including the causative organism, the body regions, organs, and systems affected, modes of transmission, susceptibility and resistance, signs and symptoms, patient management and protective measures, and immunization. (p 36.17)

5-11.45 Discuss herpes simplex 2 (genital herpes), including the causative organism, the body regions, tissues, and structures affected, mode of transmission, susceptibility and resistance, signs and symptoms, patient management and protective measures, and immunization. (p 36.17)

5-11.46 Discuss scabies, including the etiologic agent, the body organs affected, modes of transmission, susceptibility and resistance, signs and symptoms, patient management and protective measures, and immunization. (p 36.18)

5-11.47 Discuss lice, including the infesting agents, the body regions affected, modes of transmission and host factors, susceptibility and resistance, signs and symptoms, patient management and protective measures, and prevention. (p 36.18)

5-11.48 Describe Lyme disease, including the causative organism, the body organs and systems affected, mode of transmission, susceptibility and resistance, phases of signs and symptoms, patient management and control measures, and immunization. (p 36.22)

5-11.49 Discuss gastroenteritis, including the causative organisms, the body system affected, modes of transmission, susceptibility and resistance, signs and symptoms, patient management and protective measures, and immunization. (p 36.22)

5-11.50 Discuss the local protocol for reporting and documenting an infectious/communicable disease exposure. (p 36.7)

5-11.51 Articulate the pathophysiological principles of an infectious process given a case study of a patient with an infectious/communicable disease. (p 36.5)

5-11.52 Articulate the field assessment and management, to include safety considerations, of a patient presenting with signs and symptoms suggestive of an infectious/communicable disease. (p 36.12)

Affective

5-11.53 Advocate compliance with standards and guidelines by role modeling adherence to universal/standard precautions and BSI. (p 36.8)

5-11.54 Value the importance of immunization, especially in children and populations at risk. (p 36.8)

5-11.55 Value the safe management of a patient with an infectious/communicable disease. (p 36.12)

5-11.56 Advocate respect for the feelings of patients, family, and others at the scene of an infectious/communicable disease. (p 36.2)

5-11.57 Advocate empathy for a patient with an infectious/communicable disease. (p 36.12)

5-11.58 Value the importance of infectious/communicable disease control. (p 36.7)

5-11.59 Consistently demonstrate the use of body substance isolation. (p 36.8)

Psychomotor

5-11.60 Demonstrate the ability to comply with body substance isolation guidelines. (p 36.8)

5-11.61 Perform an assessment of a patient with an infectious/communicable disease. (p 36.12)

5-11.62 Effectively and safely manage a patient with an infectious/communicable disease, including airway and ventilation care, support of circulation, pharmacological intervention, transport considerations, psychological support/communication strategies, and other considerations as mandated by local protocol. (p 36.12)

Introduction

In 1913, Randolph Borne said "We can become as much slaves to precaution as we can to fear." This statement is particularly relevant to EMS care in the streets today, because many care providers are fearful when caring for patients who have or are suspected to have a communicable disease. A paramedic who does not understand how communicable diseases are transmitted and how to take sensible precautions will be hesitant in caring for some patients, no matter what the cause of their illness. This chapter examines the ways in which communicable diseases are transmitted from one person to another. The communicable diseases that paramedics are most likely to encounter in the course of their work are examined, as well as those illnesses that create the greatest anxiety among EMS personnel and the public at large. Finally, the chapter reviews the measures that a paramedic can take to protect against communicable disease.

Agencies Responsible for Protecting the Public Health

A number of government agencies are responsible for protecting the health of the general public. Agencies at the national level include the Occupational Health and Safety Administration (OSHA), which has promulgated rules and regulations designed to protect the employees of public and private organizations. This chapter refers to several OSHA regulations, for example, CFR 1910.1030, commonly known as the Bloodborne Pathogen Standard. Data on the numbers of patients infected as well as research and guidance for health care providers and the general public are available from the Centers for Disease Control and Prevention (CDC).

On the state and local levels, both state and county public health departments bear the responsibility for protection of the public health from disease, prevention of epidemics, and management of outbreaks. Although paramedics may not feel that supervision of water quality, cleanliness of restaurants, and routine inoculation programs relate directly to emergency care, clearly it's beneficial for EMS agencies to know their local public health officials and work with them. When potential threats to a community's health exist—such as the anthrax and smallpox scares from September 11 and Hurricane Katrina, and bird flu—a close working relationship between EMS providers and public health agencies is essential. If you don't know the public health professionals and officials in your county or parish, reach out to them and learn who they are.

Host Defense Mechanisms

The human body provides "built-in protection" from pathogenic organisms with several defenses that protect you against infection.

Skin, which covers the entire exterior of the body, offers a primary protective barrier blocking pathogens' ability to enter through the intact surface. The normal secretions of the skin also provide an antibacterial property that protects against pathogen entry. This is why antibacterial handwashing solutions should not be used; these solutions kill off all bacteria and viruses on the skin, including normal flora.

Mucous membranes offer another protective barrier. For example, the eyes produce tears that dilute and remove foreign substances. The mucous membranes that line the urinary, respiratory, and gastrointestinal (GI) tract also trap and remove organisms. Cells that line the respiratory tract secrete lysozymes that destroy bacteria, while macrophages trap and

You are the Provider Part 1

You are dispatched to a private residence for an older woman who is "not feeling well." You are greeted by a family member who identifies herself as the 9-1-1 caller. She tells you that she found her 70-year-old grandmother, Laverne, lying on the bathroom floor complaining of "feeling sick and hurting all over." She thinks that her grandmother has been on the floor since sometime yesterday.

You are unable to bring all of your bags and equipment into the bathroom because of the cramped space, and your patient is wedged behind the bathroom door. Before entering, you peek around the door to perform a quick initial assessment. After you squeeze through the doorway, you must close the door to gain complete access to the patient's face and head.

Initial Assessment	Recording Time: 0 Minutes
Appearance	Fetal position, appears tired
Level of consciousness	A (Alert to person, place and day)
Airway	Patent, occasional cough
Breathing	Rapid and shallow
Circulation	Flushed face, sweaty skin, rapid pulse

1. Given your initial findings, what do you know about the patient's overall condition?
2. What are your immediate concerns?

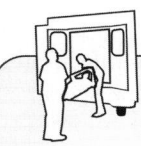

In the Field

Your body (intact skin) offers the first line of defense against infection.

destroy bacteria; thus these mucous membranes serve as the first line of defense against airborne and droplet-transmitted diseases. Goblet cells lining the GI tract produce highly acidic and alkaline secretions, which form barriers that prevent penetration by bacteria and some viruses.

The immune system contains proteins that kill viruses. Immune response ignites the production of antibodies that are directed against a specific invading organism. Both B cells and T cells work together to fight infection.

The Cycle of Infection

Infection involves a chain of events through which the communicable disease spreads. In some cases, solving the puzzle of why a particular individual or group of individuals developed a specific disease may be as simple as retracing steps to find the source of exposure. In other cases, the puzzle is more difficult to solve, with infectious disease experts taking years to find a pattern in the spread of a disease and then plan a strategy to break the chain of the infection. The study of infectious diseases takes into consideration population demographics that can affect the spread of a disease, such as age distributions; genetic factors; income levels; ethnic groups; workplaces and schools; geographic boundaries; and the expansion, decline, or movement of the disease.

Here's a classic tale that illustrates how easily disease may spread. In a local hospital pediatric unit, a visitor brought a box of candy for a child. Because of the "no food" rule, his attentive nurse placed the candy at the nurses' station. Another nurse had emptied a bedpan of stool from a child admitted for hepatitis A infection, but was in such a rush that she forgot to wash her hands. She then noticed the box of candy, poked a few selections, and finally found one she wanted to eat. The candy, being out in a public place, was consumed throughout the morning. Subsequently, another nurse came down with hepatitis A, a disease that is typically spread by the oral–fecal route. Obviously, the chain of infection in this scenario could have been broken by handwashing and following a few simple rules 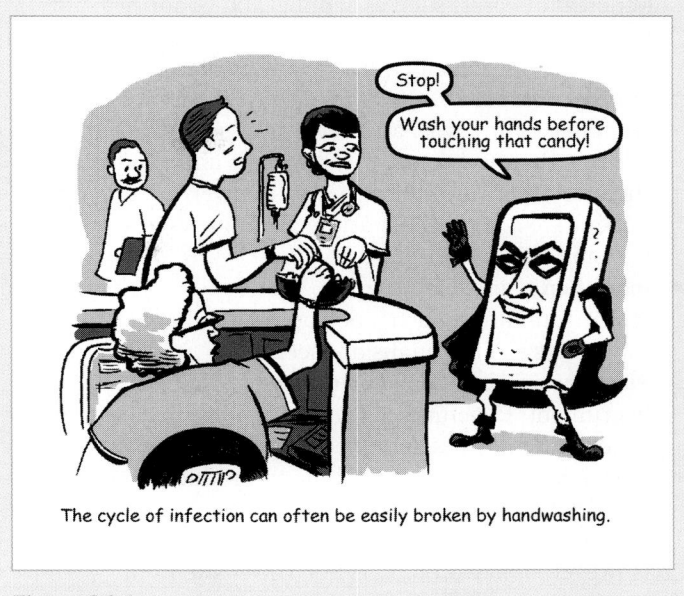 **Figure 36-1 ▸**.

Transmission of Communicable Diseases

By the very nature of their work, health care providers come in contact with sick people; a certain proportion of those sick people have contagious diseases. Communicable diseases can

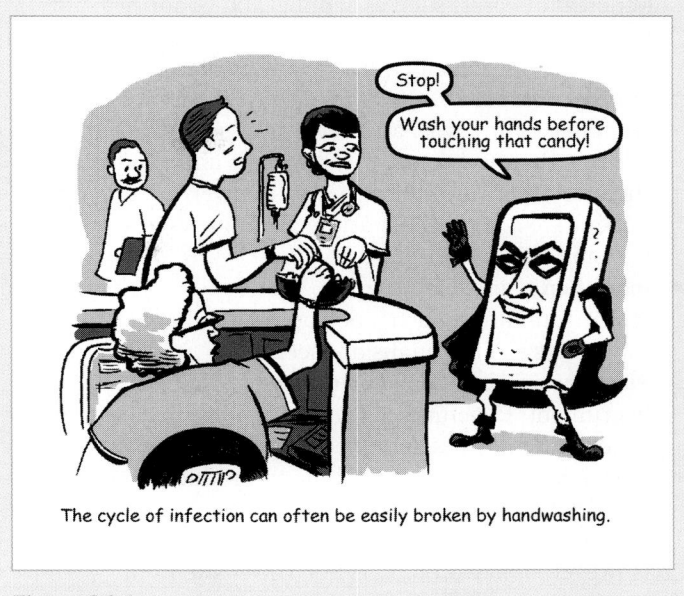

The cycle of infection can often be easily broken by handwashing.

Figure 36-1

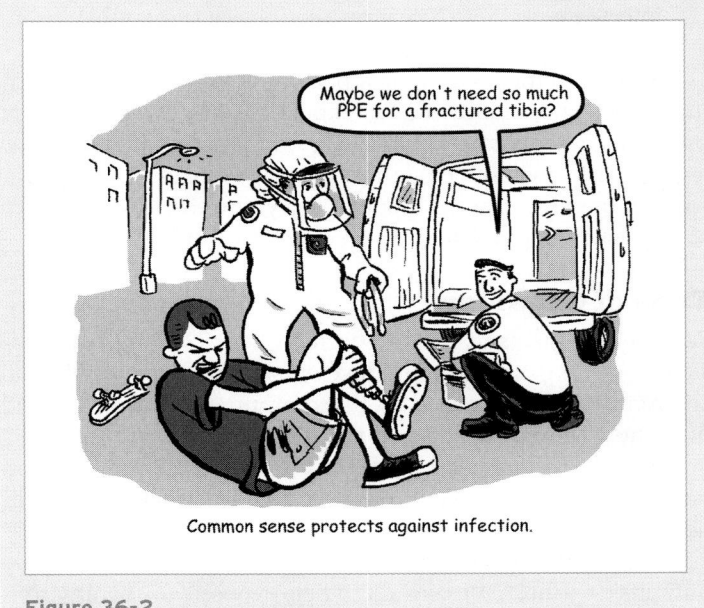

Common sense protects against infection.

Figure 36-2

be transmitted from one person to another under certain conditions **Figure 36-2 ▴**.

To understand the principles of prevention, you must first understand how diseases are spread. Communicable diseases are caused by microorganisms—usually bacteria or viruses, but sometimes fungi and parasites. They spread from person to person by several specific mechanisms:

- **Direct contact** with the infected person—that is, by touching. Direct contact may be as brief as touching one patient after caring for another patient or as intimate as sexual intercourse. Most cases of the common cold are thought to be transmitted through casual direct contact.

Venereal diseases, such as syphilis and gonorrhea, are transmitted principally by sexual contact, and are therefore referred to as sexually transmitted diseases (STDs).

- **Indirect contact**—for example, touching a bloody stretcher railing with an open cut or sore on your hand. Objects that harbor micro-organisms and can transmit them to others are called <u>fomites</u>. Towels used by a patient are a good illustration of fomites that could transmit the infection.
- **Inhalation** of infected droplets, such as those released into the surroundings when a person with pulmonary tuberculosis (TB) coughs or sneezes.
- **Puncture by a contaminated needle** or other sharp instrument. Punctures may occur if a health care provider is not using needlesafe or needleless devices.
- **Transfusion** of contaminated blood products. Screening tests for bloodborne disease have vastly reduced the risks of contracting illnesses from contaminated blood. However, donated blood is not 100% safe from <u>bloodborne pathogens</u>.
- **Vectorborne.** A vector is a vehicle that transmits infection from a reservoir to a host. For example, a mosquito infected with West Nile virus that bites a susceptible person may transmit the disease.

Several factors determine a person's actual risk of contracting an infection following an exposure. An organism's mere presence presents a risk. However, other factors influence the level of risk, including the dosage of the organism, the virulence of the organism, its mode of entry, and the host resistance of the health care provider.

Type of Organism

Pathogenic organisms may be bacteria, viruses, fungi, or parasites. <u>Bacteria</u> grow and reproduce outside the human cell in an environment characterized by the appropriate temperature and nutrients. They cause disease when they invade and multiply in the host. Salmonella bacteria, for example, can multiply in potato salad that has been unrefrigerated, leading to human illness when the food is eaten.

<u>Viruses</u> are much smaller than bacteria and can multiply only inside a host. Viruses die when exposed to the environment. For example, the human immunodeficiency virus (HIV) does not multiply or maintain its infectiousness outside a living host.

<u>Fungi</u> are similar to bacteria in that they can grow rapidly in the presence of nutrients and organic material. Most fungal infections are acquired from contact with decaying organic matter or from airborne spores in the environment (eg, molds).

<u>Parasites</u> live in or on another living creature. They take advantage of their host by feeding off its cells and tissues. Scabies and lice are examples. Parasites include both <u>protozoans</u>—single-celled, usually microscopic, eukaryotic organisms (eg, amoebas, ciliates, flagellates, and sporozoans)—and <u>helminths</u> (commonly called worms), which are invertebrates with long, flexible, rounded or flattened bodies.

Dosage of the Organism

A certain number of organisms must be present for infection to occur. For example, the laboratory report on a urine specimen sent for culture may note "greater than 100,000 colonies of bacteria per milliliter" of urine or infection is not present.

Virulence of the Organism

<u>Virulence</u> is the ability of an organism to invade and create disease in a host. It also encompasses the organism's ability to survive outside the living host. For example, HIV does not pose a risk outside the human body because it dies upon exposure to light and air.

Mode of Entry

If the organism does not enter the body by the correct route, infection cannot occur. Thus if you suspect a patient has a respiratory communicable disease and you mask the patient, you can't inhale the droplets.

Host Resistance

The healthier you are, the less susceptible you are to infection. Your ability to fight off infection is called <u>host resistance</u>. Your immune system will protect you from acquiring disease even though all of the other risk factors may be present. Wellness programs and vaccine/immunization programs serve to boost host resistance.

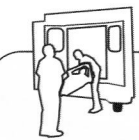

In the Field

Exposure does not mean infection.

Once a susceptible person has been exposed to an organism, it takes time for the organism to multiply within the body and produce symptoms. That time period—between exposure to the organism and the first symptoms of illness—is called the <u>incubation period</u>. For example, it usually takes 12 to 26 days from a susceptible person's exposure to the mumps virus until the patient begins to feel feverish and unwell. The incubation period for the influenza virus is much shorter—usually 24 to 72 hours.

Most communicable diseases are contagious only during a portion of the illness. A person may be sick with chickenpox for 2 to 3 weeks, but is capable of transmitting the virus to another individual for only about 1 week—from 1 day before the <u>vesicles</u> appear on the skin to about 6 days after. The period during which a person can transmit the illness to someone else is called the <u>communicable period</u>.

Just as exposure and infection are different concepts, we also need to distinguish between contamination and infection. An object that has organisms on or in it is <u>contaminated</u>. This term applies to water, food, dressing materials, linens, sharps, equipment, and even the ambulance. A person is not infected, however, unless the organisms actually produce an illness. With some diseases, such as hepatitis B or C viral infection, a person may have the disease and not be aware of it; there are no signs or symptoms, and the person is not ill. However, such carriers can pass the disease on to others through their blood or through sexual contact.

In the context of communicable disease, a reservoir is a place where organisms may live and multiply. In institutional settings, for example, air-conditioning systems and shower-heads have been identified as reservoirs for the bacterium that causes Legionnaires' disease. In ambulances, the oxygen humidifier is commonly implicated as a reservoir for infection. Obviously, health care personnel have a responsibility not only to protect themselves from contracting communicable diseases, but also to ensure that they and their equipment do not transmit illness to others.

▌ Precautions for the Health Care Provider

Although the risk of contracting a communicable disease is real, it should not be exaggerated and certainly should not be a source of fear and stress. Fear comes from lack of proper education and training, and there is no reason a paramedic should not be properly educated about disease issues.

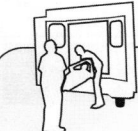

In the Field
Infection control works for the patient and the health care provider.

Designated Infection Control Officer

The federal Ryan White Law, Subpart II, requires that every emergency response agency have a designated infection control officer (DICO). This individual is charged with ensuring that proper postexposure medical treatment and counseling is provided to the exposed employee/volunteer. Postexposure medical treatment is offered to prevent the exposed health care provider from contracting the disease to which he or she was exposed. Treatment should be offered within 24 to 48 hours following an exposure, with the actual time frame being based on the diagnosis; exposure to bacterial meningitis, for example, would require treatment within 24 hours. The DICO tracks and follows the correct time frames, serves as a liaison between the exposed employee and the medical facility, ensures that confidentiality is maintained, and makes sure that documentation adheres to guidelines. This is important for workers' compensation issues and, in some states, presumption issues.

The communication network for exposure reporting involves three individuals: the exposed paramedic, the DICO, and the treating physician. If you feel you sustained an exposure, call your DICO directly. It is the DICO's job to make the initial determination as to whether an actual exposure occurred. Each department must have a reporting system that complies with the Ryan White Law and the OSHA-required Exposure Control Plan.

Public Health Department

State and local health departments are responsible for many activities related to infectious diseases, including collecting data on the incidence of diseases, performing contact follow-up, and running TB and immunization clinics. Public health departments (PHDs) also play a major role in outbreak investigations. The PHD acts as a backup for exposure notification and determination of the need for medical follow-up treatment. Under the Ryan White Law, the local PHD must know who the DICO is for each department. The PHD director

You are the Provider Part 2

Because of the problem with access, you decide to carry the patient to the stretcher in the next room using the front cradle method (patient's arms around your neck, your arms under her torso and legs). During your carry, you notice that your patient is quite warm and coughs occasionally. When you ask about her flu-like symptoms, she says that she has had chills and a dry cough for a few days.

Vital Signs	Recording Time: 7 Minutes
Level of consciousness	A (Alert to person, place, and day)
Skin	Flushed, warm, and sweaty
Pulse	110 beats/min, weak radial pulse
Blood pressure	118/72 mm Hg
Respirations	36 breaths/min, shallow
Sa_{O_2}	90% on room air

3. Think of a few potential illnesses that could cause these signs and symptoms.

4. Of those, which are the most serious and why?

serves as a liaison for problems that may arise regarding exposure notification by the medical facility and the sharing of source-patient testing results. The PHD collects all disease statistics for each locality and shares the information with the state PHD, which then sends the state totals to the CDC.

Standard Precautions

The term standard precautions is used to describe infection control practices that reduce the opportunity for an exposure to occur in the daily care of patients. It replaces the older terms "universal precautions" and "body substance isolation (BSI)." BSI precautions have commonly been taught to EMS providers for the past decade; this approach assumes that all blood and body fluids are infectious. Standard precautions add another element— protection from moist body substances that may transmit other bacterial or viral infections. For example, if a patient has oral herpes lesions and you are suctioning without a glove and have an open cut or sore, your finger could become infected with herpes. These precautions apply to all body substances except sweat.

CDC-Recommended Immunizations and Vaccinations

Keeping current with recommended vaccines and immunizations boosts host resistance and the immune response. In 1997, the CDC published guidelines for the recommended vaccinations and immunizations that should be offered to health care providers. **Table 36-1 ▸** lists the CDC recommendations for health care providers. OSHA began enforcing these guidelines in 1999.

Each employer must offer the CDC-recommended vaccinations and immunizations to staff and pay for them. You have the right to decline them, but will be required to sign a waiver if you do not wish to participate.

Personal Protective Equipment

Personal protective equipment (PPE) serves as a secondary protective barrier beyond what your body provides. The selection and use of PPE depends on the task and procedure at hand. Your department's Exposure Control Plan should contain a listing of its risk procedures and the recommended use of PPE. The CDC has also developed guidelines for PPE **Table 36-2 ▾** .

Handwashing is your major protective measure. The current standard for handwashing is the use of antimicrobial,

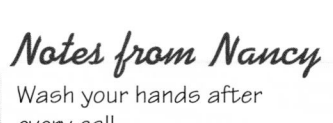 *Notes from Nancy*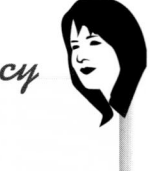
Wash your hands after every call.

Table 36-1	Recommended Immunizations/ Vaccinations for Health Care Providers
■ Hepatitis B vaccine ■ Measles, mumps, rubella (MMR) ■ Chickenpox vaccine ■ Tuberculosis (TB) testing ■ Tetanus (every 10 years) ■ Flu vaccine (annually)	

Adapted from: Centers for Disease Control and Prevention, 1997.

Table 36-2	Recommended Personal Protective Equipment for Prevention of Transmission of HIV and Hepatitis B Virus in the Prehospital Setting			
Task or Activity	**Disposable Gloves**	**Gown**	**Mask**	**Protective Eyewear**
Bleeding control with spurting blood	Yes	Yes	Yes	Yes
Bleeding control with minimal bleeding	Yes	No	No	No
Emergency childbirth	Yes	Yes	Yes, if splashing is likely	Yes, if splashing is likely
Blood drawing	Not required by CDC, but recommended for EMS	No	No	No
Starting an intravenous line	Yes	No	No	No
Endotracheal intubation, laryngeal mask airway, Combitube use	Yes	No	No, unless splashing is likely*	No, unless splashing is likely*
Oral/nasal suctioning, manually cleaning airway	Yes	No	No, unless splashing is likely*	No, unless splashing is likely*
Handling and cleaning instruments with microbial contamination	Yes	No, unless soiling is likely	No	No
Measuring blood pressure	No	No	No	No
Measuring temperature	No	No	No	No
Giving an injection	Not required by CDC, but recommended for EMS	No	No	No

*Splashing is often likely, so use PPE accordingly.
Adapted from: Centers for Disease Control and Prevention.

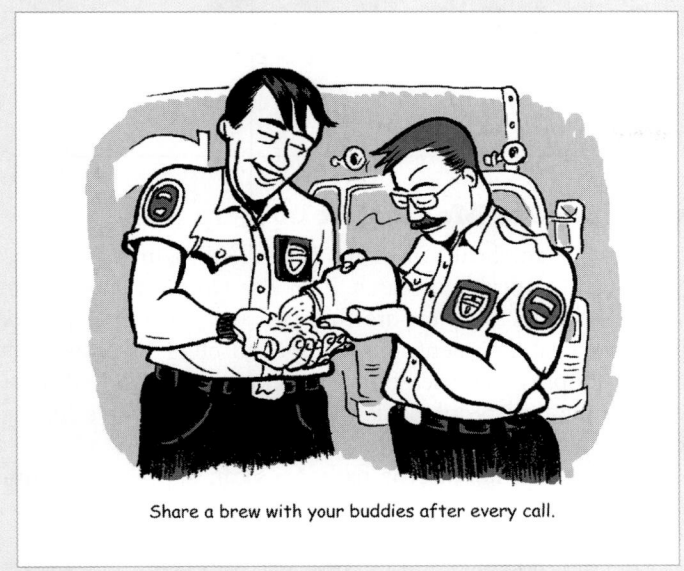

Share a brew with your buddies after every call.

Figure 36-3

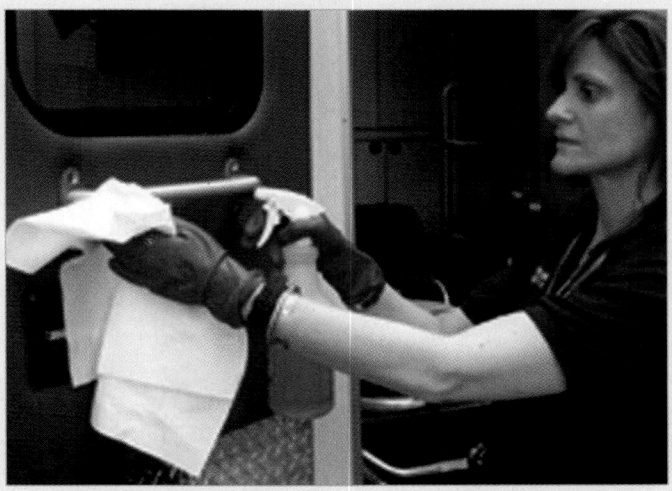

Figure 36-5 Utility-style gloves are washable and reusable as long as they are free of tears or holes.

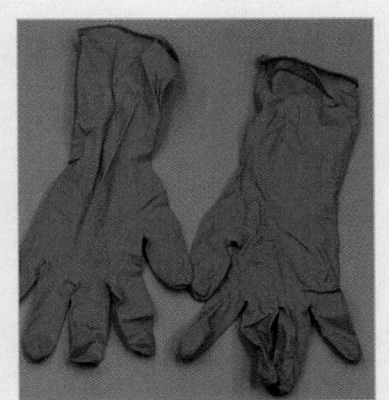

Figure 36-4 Gloves should be nonlatex, vinyl, nitrile, or rubber to reduce the risk for developing latex allergy/sensitivity.

alcohol-based foams or gels Figure 36-3 ▲. Use of antibacterial products is not recommended. The friction used to get alcohol-based foams and gels to evaporate removes surface organisms and kills viruses, but leaves the normal flora intact.

According to the CDC and OSHA, health care providers who have open cuts or sores on their hands should cover the area with a dressing. If the area is too large to cover, the provider should not perform high-risk tasks and procedures. Health care providers caring for high-risk patients are not permitted to wear artificial nails.

PPE should consist of, but not be limited to, disposable gloves, protective eyewear, cover gowns, surgical masks, N95 respirators (in some cases), waterless handwashing alcohol-based foam or gel, needlesafe or needleless devices, biohazard bags, and resuscitative equipment.

Gloves should be nonlatex, vinyl, nitrile, or rubber, to help reduce the risk for developing latex allergy/sensitivity Figure 36-4 ▲. (All PPE and patient care equipment should be latex-free.) Gloves are not needed for intramuscular or subcutaneous injections or contact with sweat. However, they are recommended for IV starts, suctioning, intubation,

In the Field

Other potentially infectious materials (OPIM) include cerebrospinal fluid (CSF), pericardial fluid, amniotic fluid, synovial fluid, peritoneal fluid, and any fluid containing visible blood.

contact with blood or other potentially infectious materials (OPIM), and contact with patient mucous membranes or nonintact skin. For cleaning activities, OSHA requires the use of utility-style gloves (dishwashing gloves). These are washable and reusable as long as they are free of tears or holes Figure 36-5 ▲. Hands should be washed after glove removal, because gloves are not a primary protection. Many gloves contain holes and absorb viruses and bacteria.

Surgical masks protect against splatter into the mouth or up the nose. They are also placed on patients deemed to have a respiratory or droplet-transmitted disease, because they filter what goes out through the mask.

N95 or P100 respirators are indicated for smallpox. Interim CDC guidelines also indicated N95 or P100 respirators for severe acute respiratory syndrome (SARS). A full respiratory protection program that complies with OSHA's respiratory protection program 1910.134 must be in place if these devices are on EMS vehicles. A respirator filters what comes in through the mask. Never place a respirator on a patient!

Protective eyewear blocks splatter into the eye. Prescription glasses may be worn with disposable or reusable side shields. Goggles should not be worn over prescription glasses because vision may be distorted Figure 36-6 ▶.

Cover garments are recommended for large-splash situations. These could be washable or disposable jackets or gowns. Uniforms may also serve as PPE if the employer purchases them, maintains them, and launders them.

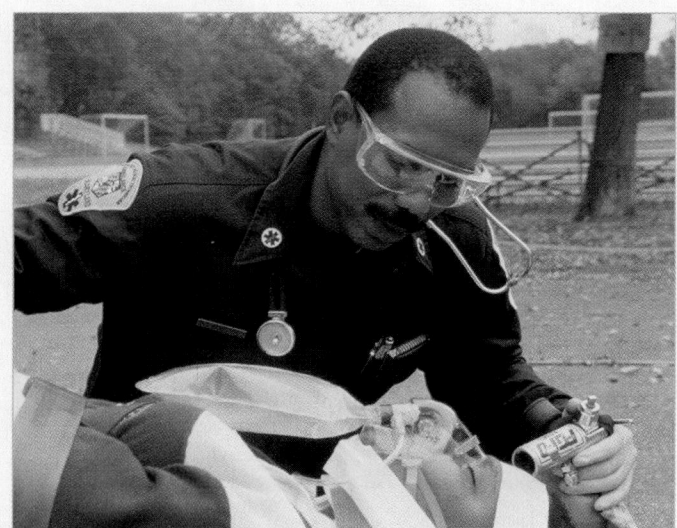

Figure 36-6 Wear eye protection to prevent blood and oral secretions from splattering into your eyes.

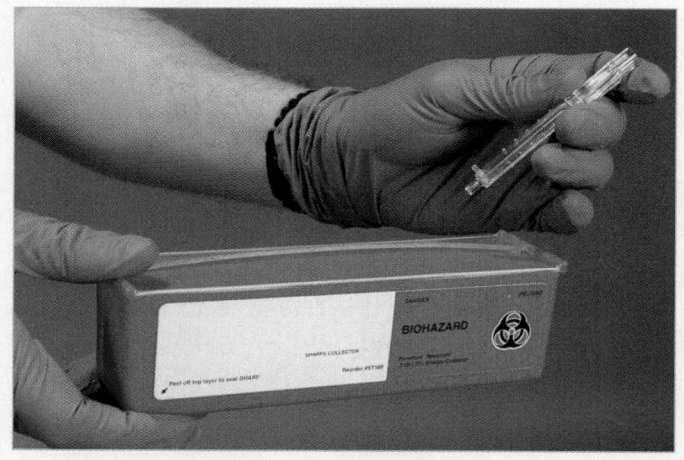

Figure 36-7 All sharps must be placed into containers that are puncture-resistant, closable, leakproof, and contain the biohazard symbol.

Booties and hair covers are not needed in the prehospital setting. Pocket masks and/or respiratory assistive devices (eg, bag masks) must be readily available.

More than 80% of exposures of health care providers to infectious agents come through sharps injuries. In 2000, Congress passed the Needlestick Safety and Prevention Act, which required that all sharps be either needlesafe or needle-less systems. The systems that have adopted needlesafe and needleless devices have reported no sharps injuries. All sharps must be placed into sharps containers that are puncture-resistant, closable, leakproof, and contain the biohazard symbol (**Figure 36-7** ▲).

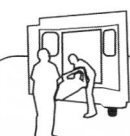
In the Field
PPE is your second line of protection!

Postexposure Medical Follow-up

Postexposure medical follow-up is your third line of defense against communicable diseases. If all else fails and an exposure occurs, the DICO will ensure that you receive proper postexposure medical treatment, including counseling, to protect you from developing the disease to which you were exposed. Postexposure medical prophylaxis (prevention) is available for diseases except hepatitis C.

Exposure to bloodborne pathogens can happen in a number of different ways:

- A contaminated needlestick injury
- Blood/OPIM splattered into the eye, up the nose, or in the mouth
- Blood/OPIM in contact with an open area of the skin (fresh cut/abrasion/dermatitis)
- Cuts with a sharp object covered with blood/OPIM
- Human bites involving blood exposure (The source is the person who is bleeding, not the biter.)

If one of these events occurs, you should immediately contact your DICO.

For airborne transmissible diseases, the DICO will review the following criteria: the organism involved, the amount of time spent with the patient, the provider's distance from the patient, the procedure or task being performed, and the ventilation present.

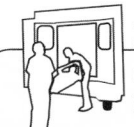
In the Field
Contaminated laundry has been soiled with blood or OPIM or may contain sharps. A contaminated sharp is any contaminated object that can penetrate the skin.

Postexposure medical management begins with the source individual, not the exposed employee. OSHA clarified this point in 1999. Employers must pay for all costs related to exposure events, including testing the source individual.

Blood work for the source patient should include rapid HIV testing, hepatitis B virus (HBV) antigen, rapid hepatitis C virus (HCV) antibody, and, if the HIV or HCV test is positive, syphilis testing. The HIV and hepatitis C results should be available in less than one hour, and HBV usually by the following day. HIV testing requires patient consent in roughly half the states in the United States, but state law often makes exceptions for occupational exposure of health care providers. In the other states, there is "deemed consent"—that is, the state assumes consent to be tested.

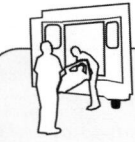
In the Field

Postexposure medical follow-up is your third protective level.

Under the Ryan White Law, the medical facility must release the source patient's tests results to the DICO; this release is not considered a HIPAA (privacy) violation. This information is then shared with the exposed employee, and proper care and counseling begin. The blood work drawn as a baseline on the exposed paramedic does not yield information on the exposure that just occurred; rather, it documents whether the provider already has one of these diseases. Postexposure medical counseling and treatment should begin within 24 to 48 hours, unless testing of the source patient yields information that necessitates more rapid follow-up.

Department Responsibilities

Under OSHA's mandate to protect staff from exposure to bloodborne pathogens, each EMS department is required to have a comprehensive Exposure Control Plan. This document lays out the specifics of how the department plans to reduce the risk of exposure to infectious agents and provide postexposure medical follow-up if needed. Key elements of the Exposure Control Plan include proper education and training related to bloodborne pathogens and TB and establishment of postexposure medical follow-up procedures **Table 36-3 ▶**.

Another key component of the plan is compliance monitoring. Management must make spot checks to ensure that staff members are following the Exposure Control Plan and that the plan is working effectively. Although management is responsible for developing and implementing the plan, OSHA has made it clear that the employees are required to follow the plan.

A part of the Exposure Control Plan that will benefit both department personnel and patients is the work restriction guidelines. These guidelines, which were published by the CDC and are enforced by OSHA, indicate when employees with various illnesses may or may not be at work and when they may not care for high-risk patients. Work restriction guidelines require employees to use sick time unless the illness is the result of an occupational exposure; in which case it is covered under workers' compensation.

Table 36-3 | Exposure Control Plan Components

- Exposure determination
- Education and training
- Hepatitis B vaccine program
- TB testing program
- Personal protective equipment (PPE)
- Engineering controls/work practices
- Postexposure management
- Medical waste management
- Compliance monitoring
- Recordkeeping

You are the Provider Part 3

To gather more information about the patient, you request that her granddaughter ride with you in the ambulance on the way to the hospital. She reveals that her grandmother has recently returned home from a nursing care facility. After a fall, the patient had required several weeks of full-time nursing care that her family was unable to provide. She has been in her own home for about 7 days, and the first flu-like symptoms occurred a few days ago. The patient now complains of headache, weakness, and some difficulty breathing. As you consider her signs, symptoms, and history, you begin to hone your differential diagnosis, and immediately don additional PPE. You administer oxygen at 12 L/min via a nonrebreathing mask and establish a 20-gauge IV of normal saline in her right hand, giving a 150-mL bolus.

Reassessment	Recording Time: 17 Minutes
Skin	Flushed, warm, and sweaty
Pulse	110 beats/min, weak radial pulse
Blood pressure	118/68 mm Hg
Respirations	36 breaths/min, shallow
Sao$_2$	94%
Temperature	38°C
Lung sounds	Inspiratory crackles (bilateral lower lobes)
Blood glucose	80 mg/dL
ECG	Sinus tachycardia (no ectopy)

5. Why is it important to periodically reconsider your differential diagnosis throughout the call?
6. Given your updated differential, what would be considered "high-risk" procedures for this patient?

General Assessment Principles

The assessment of a patient suspected to have an infectious disease should be approached much like any other medical patient. First the scene must be sized up and standard precautions taken. Once you can be assured that the scene is safe, proceed with the initial assessment by following the MS-ABC plan—assess the patient's mental status, airway, breathing, and circulation and prioritize treatment of the patient. With most patients who have a potentially infectious disease and are being seen in the prehospital setting, the next step will be a focused history and physical exam, using the OPQRST to elaborate on their chief complaint. Typical chief complaints include fever, nausea, rash, pleuritic chest pain, and difficulty breathing. Be sure to take a SAMPLE history and obtain a set of baseline vital signs, paying particular attention to medications the patient is currently taking, and the events leading up to today's problem and also whether the patient has recently traveled. Always show respect for the feelings of patients, family, and others at the scene.

General Management Principles

The general management of the patient with a suspected infectious disease first focuses on any life-threatening conditions that were identified in the initial assessment (airway maintenance, oxygen and ventilatory assistance, bleeding control, and circulatory support). Remember to be empathetic. Because most of these patients will have a fever of an unexplained origin or mild breathing problems, place the patient in the position of comfort on the stretcher and keep him or her warm. If the patient has early signs of dehydration, a preliminary IV and a fluid infusion of normal saline or lactated Ringer's solution may be appropriate. Remember to use standard precautions for your own safety and to properly dispose of sharp, even needlesafe devices. Always follow your agency's exposure control plan in cleaning the suction unit and any reusable equipment and properly discard any disposable supplies as well as linens.

Airborne Transmitted Diseases

Common Communicable Diseases of Childhood

The most striking aspect of "common" communicable diseases of childhood is that they are no longer so common, at least not in developed countries. Thirty years ago, few children reached their teens without having had measles, chickenpox, and usually mumps. Since the US government initiated Goals 2000, almost all children in this country are being inoculated against all vaccine-preventable diseases. Nonetheless, there are still sporadic cases and even occasional epidemic outbreaks of those diseases, including some related to religious waivers from vaccination.

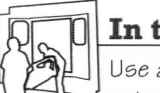

In the Field

Use a surgical mask on any patient who presents with fever and a rash. Most droplet and airborne disease exposure can be prevented by following this simple rule.

Measles

Measles—also known as rubeola, hard measles, or red measles—is a highly communicable viral disease characterized by fever, conjunctivitis, coughing, a blotchy red rash, and whitish gray spots on the buccal (mouth) mucosa **Figure 36-8 ▾**. Transmission occurs by airborne aerosolized droplets or direct contact with the nasal or pharyngeal secretions of an infected person. Less commonly, measles can be spread by contact with articles recently soiled by the patient's nasal or throat sections (tissues). The incubation period is about 10 days. The onset of fever is generally between days 7 to 18 (after exposure) and the rash appears about day 14 after exposure. The communicable period begins when the first symptoms appear (about 4 days before the rash) and then diminishes rapidly to end about 2 days after the rash appears.

Although placing a mask on the patient may prevent droplet transmission, the only certain protection against measles is immunity. Anyone who has had measles or received live virus measles vaccine after 1968 can be assumed to be immune to measles. If you did not receive live virus vaccine, you should be revaccinated. Postexposure treatment includes a vaccine if you are not immune.

No special disinfection measures are required for the ambulance after carrying a patient known to have measles. (Routine disinfection for the ambulance is described later.) Simply washing patient contact areas and laundering any soiled linens is sufficient.

Rubella

Rubella, also known as German measles or three-day measles, is characterized by a low-grade fever, headache, runny nose, swollen lymph glands, and usually a diffuse rash that may look a bit like

Figure 36-8 A blotchy red rash is characteristic of measles.

the rash of measles. When it occurs in children, rubella is ordinarily a mild, uncomplicated illness. When it occurs in women during the first 3 to 4 months of pregnancy, however, rubella may cause severe abnormalities in the developing fetus, including deafness, cataracts, mental retardation, and heart defects.

Rubella occurs most commonly during the winter and spring and is highly communicable to susceptible individuals. Transmission occurs by direct contact with the nasopharyngeal secretions of an infected person—either by droplet spread or by touching the patient or articles freshly contaminated with the patient's secretions. The incubation period is 14 to 23 days. The communicable period starts about a week before the rash appears and continues until 4 days after the rash becomes evident.

As with measles, the only certain protection against rubella is immunity. All paramedics should be immunized against rubella before starting their employment. No special measures are needed to disinfect the ambulance after carrying a patient known to have rubella. Prevention measures include masking the patient with a surgical mask. Postexposure treatment includes a vaccine if you are not immune. Practice standard precautions and routine cleaning after transport of a rubella patient.

Mumps

Mumps is a viral disease that occurs most commonly in winter and spring. Signs and symptoms in children include fever plus swelling and tenderness of one of the salivary glands, usually the parotid. Mumps in males past the age of puberty may have a very painful complication; inflammation of the testicles occurs in up to 25% of cases, but this does not result in sterility. Thus while rubella is a matter of particular concern for female paramedics, mumps should worry any male paramedic who did not have the illness or receive immunization against it as a child. All paramedics should be immunized against mumps before starting employment if they are not already immune.

Transmission of mumps occurs by droplet spread or direct contact with the saliva of an infected person. The incubation period is 12 to 26 days. The communicable period lasts 9 days after the salivary glands swell up. As a precaution, place a surgical mask on the mumps patient. Wear gloves when in contact with drainage, and carry out routine cleaning following patient transport. Postexposure treatment with a vaccine is not recommended. Work restriction will apply.

Chickenpox

Chickenpox, also known as varicella, is a highly contagious viral disease that produces a slight fever, photosensitivity, and a vesicular rash that gradually crusts over, leaving a series of scabs Figure 36-9 ▾ . The rash comes in crops, moving from the covered areas of the body to uncovered areas. The same virus can lead to herpes zoster ("shingles") in adults. Herpes zoster arises when the chickenpox virus takes up residence in the ganglion of a nerve. When the individual later becomes stressed (physically or emotionally), lesions may appear along the affected nerve pathway. Herpes zoster can be extremely painful.

Transmission of varicella virus occurs by direct contact or droplet spread of respiratory secretions from patients with chickenpox. Contact with the vesicular fluid of patients with either chickenpox or herpes zoster, and probably contact with articles recently contaminated by that fluid, can also transmit the virus. The incubation period for chickenpox is 10 to 21 days. The communicable period starts 1 to 2 days before the appearance of the rash and lasts about 5 days after the first vesicles become apparent.

Having chickenpox as a child usually provides lifelong immunity against infection. When transporting a patient suspected to have chickenpox, place a surgical mask on the patient. Wear gloves when in contact with discharges or drainage from lesions. Post-exposure treatment includes a vaccine if not immune. If the exposed person is pregnant or immunocompromised, varicella zoster immune globulin

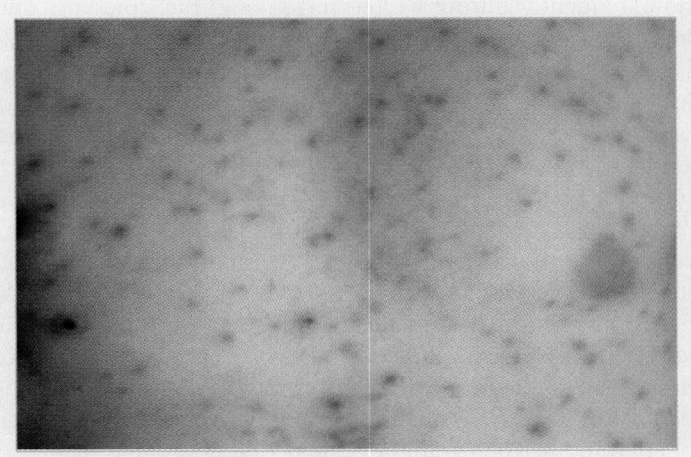

Figure 36-9 The distinctive rash produced by chickenpox.

should be offered. All paramedics not immune to chickenpox should be offered the vaccine when hired.

Pertussis

Pertussis (whooping cough) is a bacterial infection. It has an insidious onset and is characterized by an irritating cough that becomes paroxysmal in about 1 to 2 weeks; this cough may last for 1 to 2 months. In recent years, the incidence of this disease has been increasing in adolescents and young adults. Some cases have occurred in previously vaccinated persons who have diminished immunity.

Transmission takes place through direct contact with discharges from mucous membranes and/or airborne droplets. The incubation period is 7 to 14 days. This disease is highly communicable in its early stages before the cough becomes paroxysmal, and then becomes negligible in about 3 weeks. Prevention includes placing a surgical mask on the patient. If coughing makes this placement difficult, try a nonrebreathing mask. Postexposure care may include antibiotic treatment. Good handwashing and routine cleaning of the vehicle are the only special measures required after transporting a patient with pertussis. All paramedics should be assessed for vaccination with DPT (diphtheria, pertussis, tetanus).

Other Common or Serious Communicable Diseases

Meningitis

Meningitis is an inflammation of the membranes that cover the brain and spinal cord, called the meninges. Two types of meningitis are distinguished: bacterial and viral. The bacterial form is communicable, and the viral form is not. Meningitis is not transmitted through the air, but rather is a droplet-transmitted disease. The most common bacterial organisms implicated in meningitis are *Neisseria meningitidis, Streptococcus pneumoniae, Haemophilus influenzae,* group B *Streptococcus,* and *Listeria monocytogenes.*

The type of meningitis most often involved in epidemic outbreaks is meningococcal meningitis, which is caused by *N meningitidis.* Sporadic cases of meningococcal meningitis occur most frequently during winter and spring, but epidemic outbreaks can occur at any time, especially where young people live together under crowded conditions, such as in college dorms or military barracks. The classic signs and symptoms of meningitis are the same for both the viral and bacterial forms: sudden-onset fever, severe headache, stiff neck, photosensitivity, and a pink rash that becomes purple in color. The patient almost always experiences changes in mental status, ranging from apathy to delirium. Projectile vomiting is common. Diagnosis is made by Gram's stain.

Transmission occurs following direct contact with the nasopharyngeal secretions of an infected person (mouth-to-mouth, suctioning/intubation with spraying of secretions). The incubation period for meningococcal meningitis lasts between 2 and 10 days. The communicable period is variable, as it lasts as long as meningococcal bacteria are present in the patient's

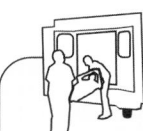

In the Field

Meningitis is *not* transmitted via airborne means. Viral meningitis is not communicable.

nasal and oral secretions. The microorganisms generally disappear from the patient's upper respiratory tract within 24 hours after antibiotic treatment begins.

When treating a patient with meningitis, place a surgical mask or nonrebreathing mask on the patient. If this is not possible, mask yourself. Transmission from patient to health care provider is rare. Postexposure treatment typically includes ciprofloxacin (one dose given orally) or rifampin for 2 days. This treatment is not appropriate if the person is taking birth control pills, and it should not be offered to pregnant personnel. Meningitis vaccine is not recommended for any health care provider group; it is recommended for college students entering dormitory living for the first time, military recruits, and middle school and high school students.

Tuberculosis

Tuberculosis (TB) was once widespread in the United States, but no longer. This disease remains an important cause of disability and death in much of the developing world, however. In 2004, the lowest incidence of TB in US history was documented. About 75% of all cases reported in this country occur in California, New York, New Jersey, Florida, Illinois, Texas, and Georgia.

TB is *not* a highly communicable disease. Three types of TB exist: typical, which is communicable, and atypical and extrapulmonary (TB of the bone, kidney, lymph glands, and so on), which are not communicable.

TB infection means that the individual has tested positive for exposure to TB but does not have, and may never develop, active disease. People with TB infection do not pose a risk to others. *TB disease* means that the individual has active TB disease verified by laboratory testing and a positive chest radiograph.

The first case of multidrug-resistant TB was identified in Boston in 1985. Although it was initially an untreatable disease, therapies for it are now available. Multidrug-resistant TB occurs in immunocompromised people who have not complied with their full course of treatment, but its incidence is quite low. In 2003, ninety cases were reported in the United States (out of a total population of almost 300 million people).

Signs and symptoms of TB include a persistent cough for more than 3 weeks plus one of more of the following: night sweats, headache, weight loss, hemoptysis, or chest pain. Transmission occurs by airborne droplets from a person with active untreated disease. In general, that type of spread occurs among people who have continued, intimate exposure to the infected individual (primarily those living in the same household). For the paramedic, such intense exposure is likely to occur only when mouth-to-mouth ventilation is

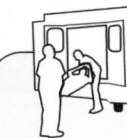

In the Field

Notify your DICO if you believe you may have been exposed to TB. The medical facility is required to notify the DICO if a patient you have transported may have TB.

given to a patient with active untreated TB. Thanks to new medications, 10% of people are no longer communicable after 2 days of treatment.

The incubation period for TB is 4 to 12 weeks. The disease is communicable only when an active lesion develops in the lungs and droplets are expelled into the air by coughing. Ten percent of patients are no longer communicable after 2 days of treatment. After 14 days of treatment virtually all patients are no longer communicable.

Early infection with TB can be detected either by a tuberculin skin test or by the QFT-TB Gold blood test. All health care providers, including paramedics, should have a tuberculin test at the beginning of employment and periodically based on the TB risk assessment for the department. If a known positive history is present on hire, then a questionnaire must be completed. A chest radiograph is indicated only for a first positive test.

As a preventive measure, place a surgical mask on the suspected TB patient. If prevention was not taken, report the incident to your DICO. Given that the incubation period for TB is

Notes from Nancy

TB is *not* a highly communicable disease.

4 to 12 weeks, the paramedic who suspects he or she has been exposed to TB should assess the need for baseline testing and then be retested in 8 to 10 weeks. If the test has become positive at that time, the individual will have a chest radiograph to rule out infection and usually will be offered a 6- to 9-month course of antibiotic therapy. Because these drugs are toxic to the liver, the individual should not consume alcohol while on the drugs and liver function tests should be done monthly.

No special measures are required after transporting a patient suspected of having active TB. The vehicle should be cleaned as usual.

Pneumonia

Each year more than 60,000 people in the United States die from pneumonia, which is an inflammation of the lungs. The cause of pneumonia may be bacteria, viruses, fungi, or other organisms. More than 50 types of pneumonia have been identified, ranging from mild to life-threatening. Individuals who are most susceptible to pneumonia are older adults, heavy smokers or alcoholics, individuals with chronic illnesses, and immunocompromised individuals. Worldwide, pneumonia is a leading cause of death in pediatric patients, particularly infants. Although antibiotics have been very successful in treating the

most common forms of bacterial pneumonia, some antibiotic-resistant strains pose a very serious therapeutic challenge.

Other Respiratory Conditions

A number of "other respiratory conditions" may (or may not) be associated with a fever and may (or may not) be infectious. These conditions run the gamut from basic annoyance to potentially life-threatening conditions.

Bronchiolitis is an infection of the lungs and airways that usually occurs in children 3 to 6 months of age. The child starts with a runny nose and slight fever. After 2 to 3 days, the child is wheezing and coughing with tachypnea and tachycardia. The cause is usually viral (eg, respiratory syncytial virus, parainfluenza, influenza). Transmission of bronchiolitis generally occurs by inhaling droplets of infected mucus or respiratory secretions.

Bronchitis arises when the inner walls of the bronchioles become infected and inflamed. Symptoms include soreness in the chest and throat, congestion, wheezing, dyspnea, and a slight fever. This condition is caused by the same virus that produces the common cold and gastric reflux disease, as well as by common pollutants and smoking or secondhand smoke. "Chronic" bronchitis patients cough most days for spans of 3 months or more a year, for two or more consecutive years. Chronic bronchitis is discussed further in Chapter 26.

Laryngitis is an inflammation of the voice box due to overuse, irritation, or infection. Its cause is usually viral but can be bacterial. Symptoms include hoarseness, weak voice, sore throat, dry throat, and cough.

Croup is the inflammation of the larynx and airway just below it. It primarily affects children 5 years old or younger. Croup comes on strongest in the nighttime and may last 3 to 7 days. Symptoms include a loud, harsh, barking cough; fever; noisy inhalations; hoarse voice; and mild to moderate dyspnea. This infection is caused by a virus, similar to the common cold, as well as by other viruses (eg, parainfluenza, respiratory syncytial virus, measles, adenovirus). It is spread by respiratory secretions or droplets from coughing, sneezing, and breathing.

Epiglottitis is a life-threatening condition that causes the epiglottis and supraglottic tissue to swell. The pus-filled flap of tissue then partially or completely occludes the glottic opening. Although this disease can affect any age group, it is most prevalent in 2- to 7-year-olds. Its incidence has fallen sharply since 1985, when administration of the Hib vaccine to 2-month-old infants became routine. Symptoms include difficulty breathing and swallowing with stridor and drooling. Patients are very anxious, are cyanotic, and have a muffled voice and fever. Epiglottitis is caused by the *Haemophilus influenzae* type b (Hib) bacteria and is contagious by the droplet route via coughing and sneezing.

The common cold is an infection of the upper respiratory system characterized by a runny nose, sore throat, cough, congestion, and watery eyes. Any one of 200 viruses can cause the cold, so symptoms may vary. Patients do not have a fever. Colds are very common in preschoolers but can occur in patients of all ages. Colds usually last about a week and are spread by droplets, coughing, hand-to-hand contact, and shared utensils.

Respiratory Syncytial Virus

Respiratory syncytial virus (RSV) is the leading cause of lower respiratory tract infections in infants, older people, and immunocompromised individuals. This virus spreads in the hospital environment as well as in the community. In the community setting, outbreaks generally occur in late fall, winter, and early spring.

Signs and symptoms include those of upper respiratory infection—sneezing, runny nose, nasal congestion, cough, and fever. The disease progression moves to the lower respiratory tract, leading to pneumonia, bronchiolitis, and tracheobronchitis. Hypoxemia and apnea are often seen in infants and are usually the leading cause for the child's hospitalization.

Transmission may occur in two ways: (1) by direct contact with large droplets that do not extend more than 3′, or (2) by indirect contact with contaminated hands or contaminated items. Research has shown that RSV can survive on hands for less than 1 hour; however, the virus has been shown to survive on other surfaces for as long as 30 hours. The infection's incubation period ranges from 2 to 8 days.

Prevention of RSV transmission relies on proper use of PPE. Gloves should be worn when caring for the RSV-infected patient, and their removal must be followed by good handwashing. The use of alcohol-based foams or gels is acceptable. Post-transport cleaning of the vehicle is important, but special cleaning solutions are not required.

Postexposure treatment consists of supportive care. If you have been exposed, your DICO will follow your health status. Health care providers who develop RSV infection should be placed on work restrictions—in particular, they should not care for immunocompromised patients.

Mononucleosis

Mononucleosis is caused by the Epstein-Barr virus, a herpesvirus. This virus is also suspected of causing a related disease, chronic fatigue syndrome. The virus grows in the epithelium of the oropharynx and sheds into saliva—hence the name "kissing disease" for mononucleosis.

Transmission occurs via direct contact with the saliva of an infected person. Some cases have also been linked to contaminated blood transfusions. The incubation period is 4 to 6 weeks following exposure, with a prolonged communicable period. Pharyngeal excretions may persist for a year or more after infection. Signs and symptoms include sore throat, fever, secretions from the pharynx, and swollen lymph glands, with or without malaise, anorexia, headache, muscle pain, and an enlarged liver and spleen.

Prevention involves the use of gloves and good handwashing techniques when in direct contact with patient oral secretions. No special cleaning solutions are required following patient transport.

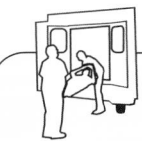

In the Field

A paramedic with a cold or flu can be extremely hazardous to a patient who is immunocompromised.

Influenza

Influenza (flu) viruses cause acute respiratory illnesses generally presenting as winter epidemics. In the United States, the flu causes approximately 36,000 deaths each year. Infection rates are high in children, but the most deaths occur in the over-65 age group, especially in patients with medical conditions such as chronic pulmonary or heart disease.

For this droplet-transmitted disease, transmission occurs from person to person by coughing and sneezing. The incubation period is about 1 to 4 days following exposure. The communicable period in adults lasts from the day before symptoms begin until about 5 days after the onset of the illness. Signs and symptoms include systemic fever, shaking chills, headache, muscle pain, malaise, and loss of appetite. Respiratory symptoms include dry cough, hoarseness, and nasal discharge. The duration of illness is about 3 to 4 days, and complications may include viral or bacterial pneumonia.

Prevention involves placing a surgical mask or nonrebreathing mask on the patient. The key preventive measure, however, is an annual flu shot. Each year, a new vaccine is developed based on the anticipated strains for that year. The injectable form of the vaccine does not contain live virus, so you cannot get the disease from the flu shot. An alternative to the injectable form is the nasal spray, which contains live attenuated virus. This is an option for people younger than age 49. If you do not receive a vaccine and have an exposure, antiviral drugs may be offered within 48 hours to reduce the severity of the flu should you contract it.

■ Sexually Transmitted Diseases

As the name implies, sexually transmitted diseases (STDs) are usually acquired by sexual contact. While the term STD ordinarily conjures up diagnoses such as gonorrhea or syphilis, in fact the range of diseases that are transmitted sexually is very wide and includes such conditions as herpes, hepatitis, and HIV infection. Hepatitis and HIV/AIDS are considered separately in this chapter. This section reviews the features of gonorrhea, syphilis, scabies, and genital herpes infections.

Gonorrhea

Gonorrhea is an infection caused by the gonococcal bacteria, *Neisseria gonorrhoeae*. In 2005, more than 300,000 cases of gonorrhea were reported to the CDC. Transmission occurs sexually, by contact with the pus-containing fluid from mucous membranes of infected persons. The incubation period is usually 2 to 7 days but may be longer. This infection is communicable for months if not treated. If treated, the individual is noncommunicable within hours.

Signs and symptoms of gonorrhea differ between males and females. Males usually see a pus-containing discharge from the urethra and often experience pain on urination (dysuria) starting a few days after the exposure. In females, the initial inflammation of the urethra or cervix may be so mild that it passes unnoticed, and the illness may progress until it presents as pelvic inflammatory disease, with signs and symptoms of an acute abdomen. Depending on the patient's sexual practices, gonorrheal infection may also involve the anus and throat.

The risk of acquiring any STD through a route other than sexual contact is remote. Prevention includes glove use if touching drainage from the genital area and thorough handwashing.

Syphilis

Syphilis is an acute and chronic disease caused by the spiral-shaped bacteria *Treponema pallidum*. Its incidence has been increasing in the United States for the past 5 years. The groups with the highest incidence rates are young people aged 20 to 35 years. High numbers of cases are also reported in urban areas.

Transmission occurs by direct contact with the infectious fluids of the primary lesion(s). The bacteria can be transmitted across the placenta from an infected mother to her fetus and by sexual contact. In some cases, transmission has occurred via blood transfusion. The incubation period is 10 days to 3 months; the communicable period has a variable length. If treated with penicillin, the individual is considered noncommunicable within 24 to 48 hours.

The initial infection with syphilis produces an ulcerative lesion, called a chancre, of the skin or mucous membrane at the site of infection   Figure 36-10 ▶ . Chancres are most commonly located in the genital region. "Secondary infection" is the term used to describe the presence of skin rash, patchy hair loss, and swollen lymph glands. Complications of syphilis can include cardiac, ophthalmic, auditory, and central nervous system complications, as well as lesions of the tissues and bone.

Prevention measures include use of gloves and good handwashing techniques. No special cleaning precautions are required.

Genital Herpes

Genital herpes is a chronic, recurrent illness produced by infection with the herpes simplex virus. The herpes simplex virus is further classified into two types: type 1 is generally transmitted via contact with oral secretions, and type 2 is spread through sexual contact. Genital herpes is characterized by vesicular lesions   Figure 36-11 ▶ . In women, the vesicles occur initially on the cervix; during recurrent infections, vesicles may also appear around the vulva, legs, and buttocks. In men, lesions commonly occur on the penis, as well as around the anus,

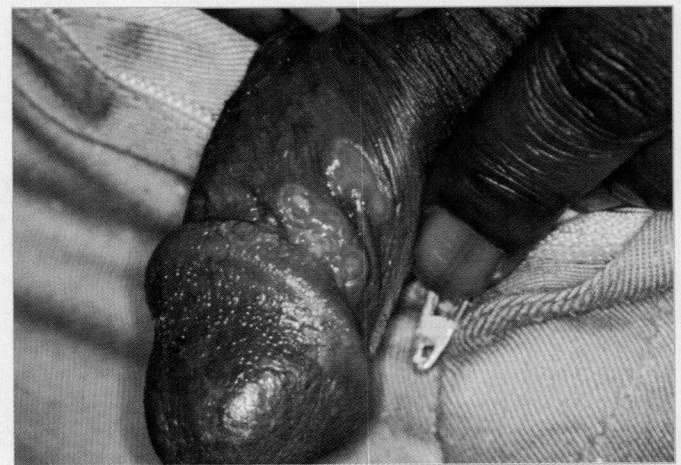

Figure 36-10 A chancre is a sign of syphilis.

depending on sexual practices. Lesions may also be present on the mouth as the result of oral sex.

Transmission usually occurs through sexual contact, but infants may become infected if delivered through the birth canal of a woman with active disease. The incubation period is 2 to 12 days. Secretion of the virus in saliva has been noted to persist for up to 7 weeks following the appearance of a lesion. Genital lesions are infectious for 4 to 7 days.

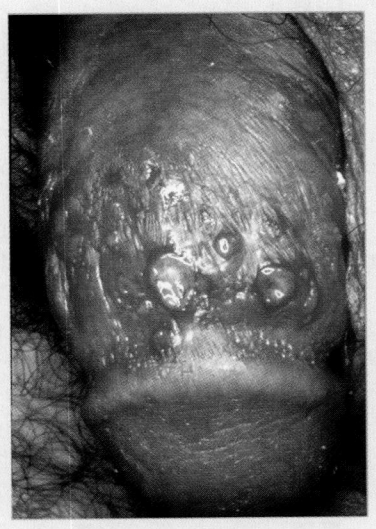

Figure 36-11 Genital herpes.

This disease is elusive; it can suddenly become reactivated, often repeatedly, over many years. Outbreaks are often stress-related. This disease can be treated with acyclovir, valacyclovir, or famciclovir for 7 to 10 days to reduce outbreaks. There is no cure, however. Preventive measures include the use of gloves when touching drainage from lesions and good handwashing techniques. No special cleaning precautions are necessary.

Chlamydia

Chlamydia infections have the highest incidence of all STDs. In 2005, more than 900,000 cases were reported to the CDC; the growth in this number is believed to be due to the availability of more sensitive screening tests and the trend toward routine screening. In most women, this infection initially remains asymptomatic. However, many women who are infected with *Chlamydia trachomatis* go on to develop pelvic inflammatory disease. In men, infection may lead to epididymitis, prostatitis, proctitis, and proctocolitis.

Transmission occurs through sexual contact. Perinatal infections may result in premature rupture of membranes, premature birth, or stillbirth. The incubation period is believed to be 7 to 14 days or longer. The communicable period is unknown. Signs and symptoms include inflammation of the urethra, epididymis, cervix, and fallopian tubes when the infection is acquired through sexual transmission. Urethral discharge may appear gray or white in color. The amount of discharge is variable.

Chlamydia infection is treated with antibiotics. Preventive measures include wearing gloves when in contact with discharge from the genital area and using good handwashing techniques. There are no special cleaning requirements for the EMS vehicle or linens.

Scabies

Scabies is caused by infection with *Sarcoptes scabiei,* a parasite. Incidence of this disease has been increasing over the past few years in both the United States and Europe. This infection commonly affects families, children, sexual partners, chronically ill patients, and persons in communal living.

Transmission occurs via direct skin-to-skin contact, such as through wrestling, sexual contact, undergarments, towels, and linens. The incubation period is 2 to 6 weeks for persons with no prior exposure to the pathogen. The communicable period lasts until the mites and eggs are destroyed by treatment. Signs and symptoms include nocturnal itching and the presence of a rash involving the hands, flexor aspects of the wrists, axillary folds, ankles, toes, genital area, buttocks, and abdomen **Figure 36-12 ▶** .

Prevention consists of wearing gloves and practicing good handwashing techniques. Vehicle linens require only routine washing in hot water, with routine cleaning of the vehicle after patient transport. Lindane is a topical treatment for scabies, but no treatment cream or lotion should be applied on a routine basis because of reports of lindane toxicity. In case of documented exposure, treatment will be undertaken and work restrictions from patient care may be ordered.

Lice

Lice are small insects that live in hair and feed on blood through the skin. There are three types of lice: head lice, body lice, and pubic lice. All types of lice are acquired through direct contact with an infested person. Head and body lice can also be acquired from objects such as hats, combs, or clothes

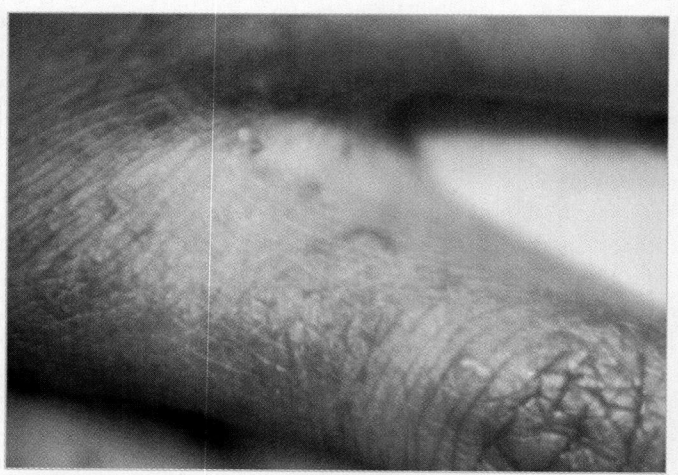

Figure 36-12 Rash produced by scabies.

You are the Provider Part 4

When you arrive at the emergency department, you are met by the staff as you open your ambulance doors. They are wearing full PPE, including gloves, gowns, goggles, and N95 masks. With the information you provided in your radio report, the hospital staff confirmed your suspicions (due to other recent admissions from this same nursing care facility) that your patient likely has SARS and will have to be placed in isolation.

Reassessment	Recording Time: 25 Minutes
Skin	Flushed, warm, and sweaty
Pulse	108 beats/min, weak radial pulse
Blood pressure	116/56 mm Hg
Respirations	36 breaths/min, shallow
Sao$_2$	94%
ECG	Sinus tachycardia (no ectopy)

7. After the transfer of care, what steps must be taken with regard to exposure?

8. Will this alter your immediate lifestyle or work habits? If so, how?

9. What are some other considerations with respect to this patient's family?

infested with lice. Lice eggs look like small white or tan dots on the skin. The eggs hatch after about one week, and then the new lice mature in one to two weeks. Head lice can be found in the hair, as well as in other hairy areas of the head such as eyebrows, eyelashes, mustaches, and beards. Body lice is usually found in the seams of clothing, and can transfer certain diseases. Signs and symptoms of lice include itching and irritation, and possibly sores.

When discussing lice as an STD, the focus is on pubic or crab lice. *Phthirus pubis* is a parasite that is usually grayish in color. Lice are common in individuals with poor hygiene, communal lifestyles, and multiple sexual partners.

Transmission of pubic lice occurs through intimate physical or sexual contact. The incubation period lasts approximately 8 to 10 days after the eggs hatch. The communicable period ends when all lice and eggs are destroyed by treatment. Signs and symptoms include slight to severe itching and visual nits clinging to the pubic, perianal, or perineal hair. Pubic lice can also infest eyelashes, eyebrows, axilla, scalp, and other body hairs.

Preventive measures include wearing gloves and practicing good handwashing techniques. Routine cleaning of the vehicle after transport is sufficient. In case of documented exposure, permethrin cream treatment may be prescribed and restrictions from patient care may be indicated until the paramedic is free of lice.

Bloodborne Diseases

Viral Hepatitis

Viral hepatitis is an inflammation of the liver produced by a virus. Five distinct forms of viral hepatitis exist (A, B, C, D, and E) that are produced by different viruses and vary somewhat in their means of transmission. All five types present with the same signs and symptoms, so the type causing illness is ultimately determined by blood testing. Hepatitis A and hepatitis E will be discussed as enteric (intestinal) diseases in this chapter, because they are not bloodborne infections.

Hepatitis B Virus Infection

Hepatitis type B virus (HBV), also known as serum hepatitis, cases have greatly diminished in the US population due to vaccine programs geared toward health care providers and all children and young adults. By 2004, the CDC had noted an 89% decrease in cases in the US population. Transmission is through sexual contact, blood transfusion, or puncture of the skin with contaminated needles. Occasionally other objects, such as shared razors, tattoo needles, or acupuncture needles, have been implicated in transmission. Type B hepatitis is particularly common in intravenous drug users who share needles. Health care providers, especially those involved in surgery, dentistry, and emergency medicine, were deemed to carry a particularly high risk of contracting hepatitis through accidental needlestick injuries until vaccination programs began in 1982. Since then, the incidence rate for occupationally acquired HBV infection has fallen by 95%.

Limited data suggest that this virus can survive outside the body in the presence of dried blood for as long as 7 days. The incubation period for HBV varies widely—from 45 to 200 days. The communicable period starts weeks before the first symptoms appear and may persist for years in chronic carriers. It is estimated that 2% to 10% of all HBV-infected individuals will become chronic carriers. Approximately 3% to 5% of infected persons will eventually develop cirrhosis of the liver or liver cancer.

Signs and symptoms of HBV infection include loss of appetite, nausea, vomiting, general fatigue and malaise, low-grade fever, vague abdominal discomfort, and sometimes aching in the joints. The very smell of food may provoke nausea, and smokers often notice a sudden distaste for cigarettes. Signs and symptoms may subside at this point for 50% to 60% of infected persons, which explains why many infected individuals never know that they have acquired the disease. For those who progress into the second phase of the disease, the urine begins to turn dark, and then a day or two later, the patient develops jaundice, a yellowing of the skin, and scleral icterus, a yellowing of the eyes **Figure 36-13 ▼**. Type B hepatitis usually lasts several weeks, although complete recovery may take 3 to 4 months.

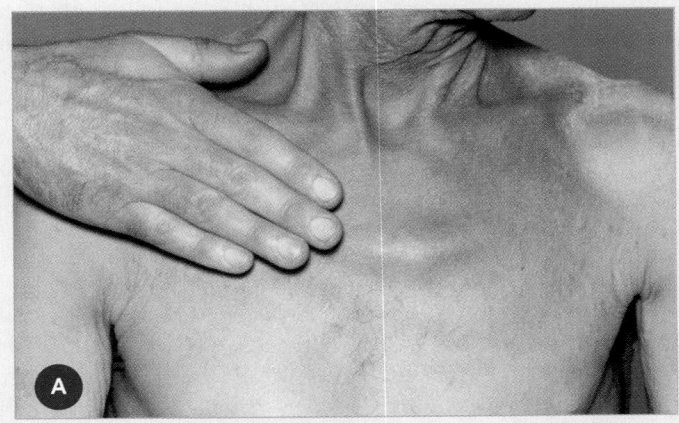

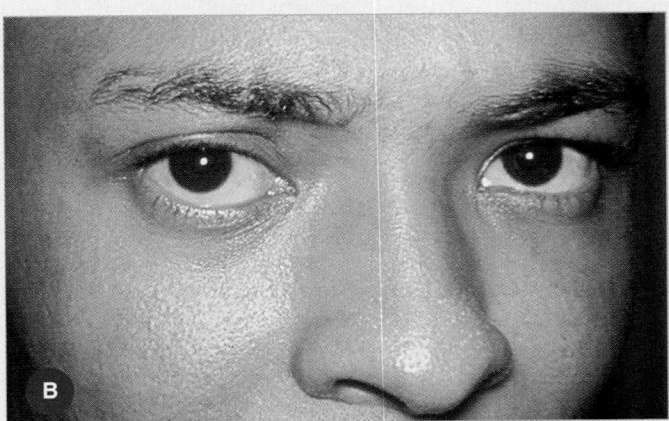

Figure 36-13 Signs of HBV infection. **A.** Jaundice. **B.** Scleral icterus.

Table 36-4	Vaccine Series for Hepatitis B

- Initial dose
- Second dose: 4 weeks from first dose
- Third dose: 6 months from first dose
- Titer: 1 to 2 months after completion of the three-dose series

Prevention of HBV transmission focuses on using gloves when handling blood, OPIM, or materials containing "gross visible" blood. Good handwashing technique is essential. Paramedics should be immunized against HBV when hired. Vaccination, which is both safe and effective, protects only against HBV but offers that protection for life; it indirectly protects against hepatitis D infection because one must be infected with type B to acquire type D. OSHA requires that employers offer the HBV vaccine at no cost to at-risk staff members. If you are allergic to yeast or mercury (Thimerisol), notify the vaccine administrator and arrangements will be made to obtain the proper vaccine to meet your needs. Vaccine is administered in a three-dose series Table 36-4 ▲ . After the series is completed, you should have a blood test (titer) performed 1 to 2 months later to ensure that you responded to the vaccine.

Practice routine standard precautions. If you are exposed, notify your DICO. The DICO will verify the source patient's test results. If you have a positive titer on file, no follow-up treatment is needed. If you do not have a titer report on file and the patient is positive for HBV infection, a titer will be ordered on you. Treatment will depend on the results of that titer report. If you have not been vaccinated and the patient is positive for HBV, you will be offered hepatitis B immune globulin and the vaccine series. The risk of infection is 6% to 30% only if you were not vaccinated and did not report the exposure event.

Hepatitis C Virus Infection

The hepatitis C virus (HCV) is the most common chronic bloodborne infection and the leading cause of liver transplant in the United States. An estimated 1% to 4% of health care providers are antibody-positive for HCV. However, this disease is not efficiently transmitted through occupational exposure, and no health care provider group is at increased risk for occupationally acquired HCV infection. Instead, occupational risk is related to a contaminated deep needlestick with visible blood on the sharp, a sharp that has been in the patient's vein or artery, a hollow-bore needle, and a source patient with a high viral load.

Transmission may occur by blood-to-blood contact with an open area of the skin, sexual contact, blood transfusion, organ donation, unsafe medical practices, and from an infected mother to her infant. Transmission through mucous membrane or nonintact skin exposure is rare. The virus cannot survive in the environment long enough to pose a risk for any means of transmission except via bloodborne contact.

Approximately 75% to 80% of HCV-infected individuals progress to long-term chronic infection. The incubation period ranges from 2 to 24 weeks (average is 6 to 7 weeks). Signs and symptoms are the same as those for hepatitis B, and diagnosis is established by testing for HCV antibody. Some 75% of infected persons remain unaware that they acquired the infection because they do not develop phase 2 signs and symptoms.

To prevent HCV transmission, use gloves when in direct contact with blood or OPIM, and use needlesafe or needleless devices. No special cleaning requirements apply—just perform routine cleaning of the vehicle and equipment.

If you have sustained an exposure, testing will begin with the source patient in accordance with your state's testing law. If the source is HCV-positive, you will have a baseline HCV antibody test and liver function test. You should have an HCV-RNA test 4 to 6 weeks following the exposure event. If it is negative, you did not acquire HCV from the exposure. If it is positive, you will begin treatment. There is no vaccine to protect against HCV infection, nor can any medication offer postexposure prevention against infection, however, treatment is available, which is highly successful in preventing chronic infection.

Hepatitis D Virus Infection

Hepatitis type D, also called delta hepatitis, requires that the host be infected with hepatitis B for hepatitis D virus (HDV) infection to occur. For this reason, HDV is considered a parasite for HBV. Approximately 5,000 to 7,000 HDV cases occur each year in the United States, with the highest incidence noted in IV drug users. Transmission is generally by percutaneous exposure, as HDV is not effectively transmitted through sexual contact. Perinatal transmission is rare.

The incubation period for HDV infection ranges from 30 to 180 days. Blood is considered to be infectious during all phases of the illness. Signs and symptoms are the same as those associated with hepatitis B.

To protect against HDV transmission, use gloves when in contact with blood or OPIM, use needlesafe or needleless devices, and perform routine cleaning of the vehicle following patient transport. Remember that you should not go through the pockets of known IV drug users who are found unconscious, as you may get cut with a contaminated sharp. If a documented exposure occurs, testing begins with the source patient in accordance with state testing laws. If the source is positive for HDV and you are protected against HBV, no further treatment is indicated.

Notes from Nancy

Assume that every patient you treat is HIV-positive, even your grandmother.

Human Immunodeficiency Virus Infection

Human immunodeficiency virus (HIV) type 1 was first identified in the late 1970s. Today, an estimated 60 million people worldwide are infected with this virus. In the United States, HIV infection is not a reportable disease in all states.

Although HIV is primarily a sexually transmitted disease, it is also bloodborne and can be transmitted from mother to infant in the birthing process. In the United States, the rate of infection from mother to child is only 1% to 3% because infected mothers are treated with antiretroviral drugs beginning in the second trimester. HIV is also transmitted through blood transfusions, albeit at a very low rate since the initiation of testing for the presence of P24 (a protein present from the beginning of the HIV life cycle) in donated blood. With P24 testing, the virus can now be detected 1 to 6 days after infection.

HIV is not transmitted through casual or even household contact. Even among individuals who routinely share eating utensils, toothbrushes, and razors with HIV-infected patients, there is no evidence of an increased rate of HIV infection. This disease is not airborne or droplet transmitted.

The HIV pathogen envelops infected cells and attacks the immune system and other body organs. The immune system is then unable to assist in protecting the infected individual from other diseases. It takes about 7 days for the virus to envelop a cell, and this process may occur 4 to 6 weeks after the exposure event. The communicable period is unknown, but is believed to span from the onset of infection possibly throughout life.

Signs and symptoms may include acute febrile illness, malaise, swollen lymph glands, headache, and possibly rash. Following initial infection, most individuals present with enlargement of the lymph nodes and appear healthy. However, the number of T-helper lymphocytes (CD4 cells) gradually declines. T-helper cells are essential components of the immune system that mediate both cellular and humoral immunity. Seroconversion occurs, meaning that antibodies can be detected in the blood; this usually occurs within the first three months. Persons who are seropositive for HIV are placed on antiretroviral drug treatment.

Prevention focuses on the use of gloves when in direct contact with patient blood or OPIM, the use of needlesafe or needleless devices, good handwashing technique, and routine cleaning of the vehicle after transport. Postexposure medical follow-up is covered in the AIDS section that follows.

The risk for acquiring HIV infection is sharps-related. As of November 2005, 58 health care providers had developed documented occupationally acquired HIV infection; none were fire/EMS personnel. Of these 58 occupational infections, 48 were the result of a high-risk exposure. A high-risk exposure to HIV includes *all* of the following: a deep stick with a large-gauge hollow-bore needle, the device has visible blood on it, the patient is HIV-positive with a high viral load, and the device had been in the patient's vein or artery. Following this type of exposure, the risk of transmission is 0.3% for mucous membrane exposure to the eye and 0.09% for nonintact skin.

Acquired Immunodeficiency Syndrome

Acquired immunodeficiency syndrome (AIDS) is the end-stage disease process caused by HIV. The patient with AIDS is extremely vulnerable to numerous bacterial, viral, and fungal infections that would not affect a person with an intact immune system. These *opportunistic infections* include pneumonia in infants or people with compromised immune systems,

loss of vision due to cytomegalovirus, reddish/purple skin lesions, atypical TB, and cryptococcal meningitis.

Notes from Nancy
AIDS is not a highly communicable disease.

The incubation period of AIDS spans the time between documented infection (ie, becoming HIV-positive) and development of the end-stage disease; it is determined by the CD4 cell count and the presence of opportunistic infections. The communicable period is presumed to last as long as the patient is seropositive, *even before clinically apparent AIDS develops.* Surveys of patients presenting to emergency departments have shown that around 6% of seriously ill or injured patients are HIV-positive.

Prevention involves following standard precautions. Use gloves when in contact with blood or OPIM, use needlesafe or needleless devices, and perform routine cleaning of the vehicle and equipment. There is no need to restrict pregnant care providers from contact with known HIV/AIDS patients.

If an actual exposure occurs, the source patient will be tested in accordance with state law, ideally using the rapid HIV testing method. Its results are accurate and are available in less than 1 hour. If the test is negative, then no further testing is indicated for the paramedic. If the source is positive, then blood is sent for assessment of viral load and the paramedic may be offered antiretroviral drugs for a period of 4 weeks; the criteria for use of these drugs are published by the CDC. The CDC guidelines for post-exposure prophylaxis are enforced by OSHA under the bloodborne pathogens regulation (CFR 1910.1030).

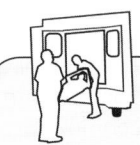
In the Field
Body fluids that do *not* transmit bloodborne disease: tears, sweat, urine, stool, vomitus, nasal secretions, and sputum.

Antiretroviral drugs are toxic, so careful and complete counseling should be provided to the exposed health care provider. The CDC recommends that a physician knowledgeable in the use of these drugs be consulted. If one is not available, then the physician should contact the 24-hour Post-Exposure Prophylaxis (PEP) Hotline at 1-888-448-4911 before prescribing these drugs. Before initiating antiretroviral therapy, baseline laboratory testing should be done—CBC, liver function, and kidney function. For a female of childbearing age, pregnancy testing is appropriate. These tests should be repeated every 2 weeks while on the drugs.

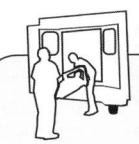
In the Field
Bloodborne pathogens are considered "protected handicaps" under the Americans With Disabilities Act.

■ Enteric (Intestinal) Diseases

Gastroenteritis

Gastroenteritis, also known as the stomach flu, comprises many types of infections and irritations of the gastrointestinal tract. Patients experience symptoms such as nausea and vomiting, fever, abdominal cramps, and diarrhea. In healthy individuals, gastroenteritis is usually not serious. In children, elderly persons, and patients with chronic illness, severe complications such as dehydration may develop.

Hepatitis A Virus Infection

Hepatitis type A, or infectious hepatitis, is the most common type of hepatitis in the United States. In the past, outbreaks of this disease have been reported in several states. Transmission is by the fecal–oral route—that is, by ingestion of food or water that has been contaminated by infected feces. Epidemic outbreaks are most often traced to contaminated drinking water, milk, sliced meats, and undercooked shellfish. Hepatitis A is often described as a "benign" disease because once you acquire the disease you have lifelong immunity to it. Since 2000, all US children have received a vaccine to protect them from acquiring this disease.

The incubation period is usually about 2 to 4 weeks, although it can range from 15 to 50 days after ingestion of the virus. The communicable period probably starts toward the end of the incubation period and continues for a few days after the patient becomes jaundiced. Signs and symptoms in phase 1 include fatigue, loss of appetite, fever, nausea, and abdominal pain; smokers will lose their interest in smoking. In phase 2, patients have jaundice, dark-colored urine, and whitish stools.

Prevention includes use of gloves and good handwashing technique if in contact with patient stool. No special cleaning of the vehicle is needed. Hepatitis A vaccine is recommended for Federal Emergency Management Agency response team members who may work outside the United States, but not for any other health care provider groups.

Hepatitis E Virus Infection

Hepatitis E virus (HEV) infection is also referred to as enterically transmitted non-A, non-B hepatitis (ET-NANB). It accounts for an estimated 50% of hepatitis cases in developing countries. Transmission occurs via the fecal–oral route by ingestion of contaminated water. In developing countries, there is a strong association between HEV and floods, poor sanitation, and primitive hygiene. Rare cases of transmission via transfusion have been documented, and sexual transmission is on record.

This disease is not chronic. Its incubation period is about 15 to 64 days. The communicable period is believed to be the same as for hepatitis A. Signs and symptoms are the same as for other forms of hepatitis. Prevention includes the use of gloves when in contact with stool, good handwashing technique, and cleaning contaminated equipment.

■ Vectorborne Diseases

West Nile Virus

West Nile virus (WNV) is a relatively new disease in the United States. The virus was first discovered in Uganda in the 1930s; its first identified appearance in the Western Hemisphere was in New York City in 1999.

Transmission is via bite from a mosquito carrying the virus (only about 1% of mosquitoes carry WNV). This infection is not transmitted from person to person, so there is no period of communicability. WNV has been transmitted via donated blood and organs, as well as during hemodialysis; two cases have involved needlestick injuries in laboratory workers working with this virus. The incubation period is from 3 to 14 days following the bite.

In the majority of cases, this disease is mild and uneventful. Indeed, 80% of persons who acquire WNV infection remain unaware that they have it. The 20% of persons who are symptomatic exhibit fever, headache, body rash, and swollen lymph glands. Mild symptoms appear in older people and immunocompromised persons. In healthy individuals, the immune system fights off the disease. About 1 in 150 symptomatic individuals will go on to develop severe signs and symptoms, which include encephalitis, meningitis that can lead to neurologic complications, and death.

Use needlesafe devices systems to avoid a contaminated sharps injury when WNV infection is suspected. If you sustain a contaminated sharps injury involving a patient with WNV, notify your DICO. There is no recommended medical follow-up treatment. No special cleaning of the vehicle is needed or recommended.

Lyme Disease

Lyme disease is the most common tick-borne disease in the United States. In 1982, a national reporting system was established for this infection. The highest prevalence of this disease is found along the Atlantic coast, the upper Midwest, and the Pacific coast. Peak season is between June and August; incidence rates decrease in the early fall.

Lyme disease primarily affects the skin, heart, joints, and nervous system. Some patients remain asymptomatic. This disease occurs more often in children younger than age 10 years and in middle-aged adults. Lyme disease is not transmitted from person to person. Its incubation period ranges from 3 to 32 days.

Lyme disease is usually divided into three stages: early localized, early disseminated, and late manifestations. The early stage is characterized by a round, red skin lesion. This bull's-eye rash (so called because it extends outward with a ring in the center) is most common in the area of the groin, thigh, or axilla **Figure 36-14 ▶**. If present, it is warm to the touch, and may blister or scab. In the early disseminated stage, secondary lesions may develop within days and the patient may complain of flu-like symptoms—fever, chills, headache,

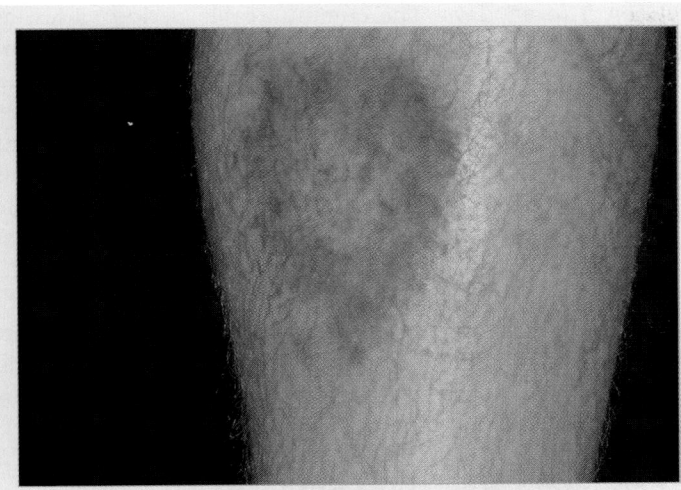

Figure 36-14 The bull's-eye rash of Lyme disease is most common in the area of the groin, thigh, or axilla.

malaise, and muscle pain. Nonproductive cough, testicular swelling, sore throat, enlarged spleen, and enlarged lymph nodes may be present. Neurologic involvement may occur in 15% to 20% of untreated patients within 2 to 8 weeks; cardiac involvement may occur in 10% of untreated patients. In the third phase of the illness, arthritis occurs in about 60% of untreated patients, beginning days to years after the initial infection. Intermittent joint pain affects about 50% of patients, and lasts from days to months. Chronic neurologic symptoms are uncommon. In the United States, memory impairment, depressed mood, and severe fatigue are the most common symptoms of Lyme disease.

Prevention includes wearing long sleeves and pants when in tick-infested areas, plus use of insecticides that contain carbaril, diazinon, chlorpyrifos, or cyfluthrin. If you sustain a tick bite, use proper technique for removing ticks. Postexposure treatment with antibiotics is not warranted or recommended.

Zoonotic (Animal-borne) Diseases

Hantavirus

Hantavirus, also known as hemorrhagic fever with renal syndrome, is associated with the deer mouse, white-footed mouse, and cotton rat. It has also been found in rats in urban areas. This disease was first identified in Korea in the early 1950s and in the Southwestern United States in 1993. By 2000, about 330 cases had been reported in the United States.

Hantavirus is found in the urine, feces, and saliva of chronically infected rodents. Transmission occurs via direct contact with rodent waste matter, often through aerosol inhalation. The incubation period usually lasts 12 to 16 days following exposure but has been noted to range from 5 to 42 days. This disease is not transmitted from person to person, so there is no period of communicability. Signs and symptoms begin with the sudden onset of fever, which lasts 3 to 8 days. It is accompanied by headache, abdominal pain, loss of appetite, and vomiting.

Prevention focuses on standard precautions. Routine cleaning of the vehicle is all that is indicated.

Rabies

Rabies (hydrophobia) is found worldwide and accounts for about 300,000 deaths each year in developing countries. In the United States, cases have been declining since rabies control programs began in the 1940s. The vaccination of domestic animals and the development of vaccine and rabies immunoglobulin have greatly reduced the number of deaths in humans who contract rabies. However, as many as 39,000 people still receive postexposure prophylaxis annually worldwide.

Transmission is primarily related to the direct bite of an infected animal. The virus is shed in the saliva of the infected animal from the time it becomes infected. Other routes of transmission include contamination of mucous membranes (eyes, mouth) and one case suspected to be related to a cornea organ transplant. In general, however, nonbite exposures to rabies—scratches, abrasions, open wounds, or mucous membranes contaminated with saliva or other potentially infectious material from a rabid animal—are rare. There are no documented cases of human-to-human transmission of rabies.

The incubation period is usually 2 to 8 weeks, but varies depending on the severity of the bite and the location of the wound. Signs and symptoms in human infection are generally nonspecific: fever, chills, sore throat, malaise, headache, and weakness. Paresthesia (skin sensation with no apparent cause) may develop at or near the site of exposure. Following these initial signs, the neurologic phase of the disease begins—hyperactivity, seizures, bizarre behavior, and hydrophobia. Patients also have fear of the sight of water or while drinking it as a result of severe spasms of the throat and masseter (chewing) muscles. As the disease progresses, patients may develop paralysis and deterioration of mental status leading to coma. Although rabies is generally viewed as a fatal disease, several cases of survival have been reported recently.

For prevention, follow standard precautions for patient care and cleaning of the vehicle. If you are bitten by a suspect animal, you will be offered human rabies vaccine if deemed appropriate.

Tetanus

In the United States, 50 to 90 cases of tetanus (lockjaw) occur annually, with a death rate of 20 to 30. About 60% of cases occur in persons older than 60 years of age. Tetanus is more common in agricultural areas and in underdeveloped areas, where contact with animal waste is common and immunization is inadequate. The tetanus bacillus is found in the intestines of horses and other animals, but some cases have been linked to use of IV drugs.

Transmission occurs when tetanus spores enter the body by either of two means: (1) a puncture wound contaminated with animal feces, street dust, or soil, or (2) contaminated street drugs. Tetanus is not transmitted from person to person. Occasionally, cases have occurred postoperatively or following seemingly minor injuries.

The incubation period is usually about 14 days from the exposure but has been documented to be as short as 3 days. The cases that have short incubation periods tend to feature a higher level of contamination. Signs and symptoms begin at the site of the wound, followed by painful muscle contractions in the neck and trunk muscles. The key sign that suggests tetanus is abdominal rigidity, although this rigidity may be confined to the location of the injury.

Prevention involves the use of gloves when handling any patient wounds and drainage. Paramedics should be offered tetanus booster doses every 10 years. No special cleaning routines are necessary after transport of a patient with tetanus.

Antibiotic-Resistant Organisms

The overuse and misuse of antibiotics has led some pathogens to develop resistance to the antibiotic drugs commonly prescribed to eradicate them. As a consequence, both medical facility pharmacies and the CDC now restrict the use of many antibiotics. There has also been an attempt to educate the population regarding the risks associated with the overuse of antibiotics.

Methicillin-Resistant *Staphylococcus aureus*

Staphylococcus aureus became resistant to penicillin in the late 1950s. Today almost 90% of community (CA-MRSA) and hospital isolates are resistant to penicillin. The drug methicillin was made available in the early 1960s to treat infections with this pathogen. By the mid-1970s, methicillin-resistant *S aureus* (MRSA) was present in US hospitals; it has since moved into the larger community. MRSA strains are also resistant to some other antibiotics, including cephalosporins, erythromycins, clindamycin, tetracyclines, and aminoglycosides. Although vancomycin has been shown to effectively treat MRSA, some mild strains are showing resistance to this drug as well. Other drugs used to treat MRSA include Synercid, linezolid, and daptomycin.

In health care settings, MRSA is believed to be transmitted from patient to patient via unwashed hands of health care providers. Studies have shown that 50% to 90% of health care providers carry MRSA in their nares; the pathogen can subsequently be transferred to skin and other areas of the body through a break in the skin. Surfaces contaminated with MRSA do not seem to be important in transmission. Factors that increase the risk for developing MRSA include antibiotic therapy, prolonged hospital stays, a stay in intensive care or a burn unit, and exposure to an infected patient. Many patients who contract MRSA live in long-term care facilities.

Patients with MSRA may be either colonized with this organism or infected. The incubation period appears to be

between 5 to 45 days. The communicable period varies, as patients who have active infection may carry MRSA for months. MRSA results in soft-tissue infections. Its signs and symptoms may involve localized skin abscesses and cellulites, empyemas, and endocarditis. Sepsis is found in older patients with *S aureus* infections. After bloodstream infection with this organism, secondary infections such as osteomyelitis and septic arthritis may develop at other body sites.

To prevent MRSA transmission, use standard precautions (gloves and good handwashing technique) when in contact with patient wounds and nonintact skin. If you are in direct contact with wound drainage but your skin is intact, no exposure will occur. If you have a true exposure, no postexposure treatment is recommended. The incident must still be documented, however.

Vancomycin-Resistant Enterococci

Enterococcus is a common, normal organism of the GI tract, urinary tract, and genitourinary tract. More than 450 species of enterococci exist, many of which are resistant to antimicrobial agents. These organisms grow under both reduced and oxygenated conditions. When they become resistant to the main drug used for treating enterococcal infection, vancomycin, the patient is said to have vancomycin-resistant enterococci (VRE). VRE is primarily a hospital-acquired (nosocomial) infection. Patients identified with VRE outside the hospital setting typically reside in nursing homes or visit hemodialysis centers.

VRE may be found in urinary tract infections and bloodstream infections; it has also been identified in livestock stool, uncooked chicken, and persons who work at farms or processing plants. The infectious organisms can live on surfaces for long periods of time, so transmission may occur by direct contact with contaminated surfaces or equipment. A person can be either colonized or infected with VRE, but only infected patients can transmit this organism. Thus transmission may occur when you have direct contact with wound drainage and an open cut or sore allows entry of the organism. This illness can be treated with a new synthetic antibiotic, linezolid.

Prevention relies on the use of standard precautions, gloves, and good handwashing technique when in contact with wound drainage. A cover gown is necessary only if your uniform may come in contact with wound drainage. Post-transport cleaning of all areas that came in contact with the patient is important, but no special cleaning solution is required. If you sustain direct contact with an open wound and VRE body fluids, notify your DICO and complete an exposure report. No postexposure medical treatment is indicated.

Patients with VRE (or MRSA) may be protected by the Americans With Disabilities Act. It is important not to "overdo" the use of PPE, as this may be considered discrimination.

New and Emerging Diseases

In the past, a disease would jump from animals to humans every 20 to 30 years. Today, this transmission is occurring much more frequently. Recent examples include HIV infection, monkeypox, SARS, and avian flu. The latter two are discussed here.

Severe Acute Respiratory Syndrome

Severe acute respiratory syndrome (SARS) is a new disease that arose from the merger of two viruses, one from mammals and one from birds. The source of this virus has been identified as bats found in Hong Kong. SARS was first reported in Asia in February 2003. Within a few months, the disease had spread from Asia to Canada, South America, and Europe. By early 2003, the World Health Organization (WHO) reported a total of 8,098 cases worldwide and 774 deaths. In the United States, there were eight confirmed cases (all mild) and no deaths; all of the US cases involved people who had traveled to areas where SARS cases had previously been reported. The latest cases of SARS were reported in April 2004 in China and resulted from a laboratory accident. In the United States, no health care providers have contracted SARS.

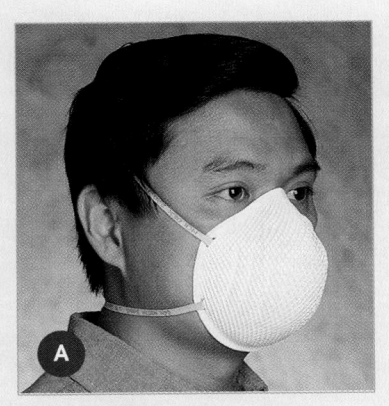

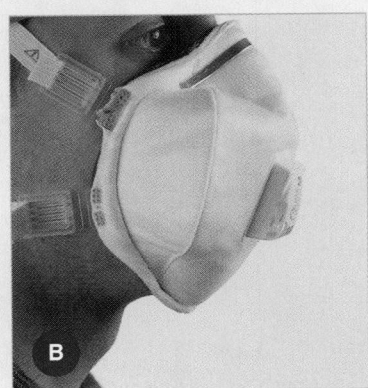

Figure 36-15 Wear an N95 respirator (**A**) or P100 respirator (**B**) that has been properly fit-tested to protect yourself from SARS.

Transmission is by close personal contact—that is, living with and caring for a person with the disease or having direct contact with respiratory secretions or body fluids of an infected person (eg, kissing or hugging, talking within 3´, sharing eating utensils). The incubation period is about 10 days from the date of exposure; the communicable period has not been well defined. Signs and symptoms include a fever of greater than 100.4°F, headache, overall feeling of discomfort, and body aches. SARS resembles any general flu-like illness; however, after 2 to 7 days a dry cough appears, and patients with severe illness progress to pneumonia and may need respiratory support.

Care for a person suspected of having SARS begins with an assessment and taking of a travel history. Place a surgical mask on a patients who presents with signs and symptoms of SARS in order to contain secretions. Interim CDC guidelines indicate that the paramedic should wear an N95 or P100 respirator that has been properly fit-tested 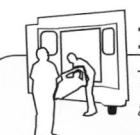 Figure 36-15 ▲. Under the cur-

rent reporting system, medical facilities are required to notify the DICO if a patient transported is later diagnosed with SARS. If an unprotected exposure occurs, notify the DICO and complete an exposure report form. If a true exposure occurred, a 10-day quarantine may be recommended. This time off will be covered by workers' compensation. The exposed paramedic will be asked to take a temperature check at least daily.

Avian Flu

Avian (bird) flu is caused by a virus that occurs naturally in the bird population. This virus is carried in the intestinal tract of wild birds and does not usually cause illness. However, in domestic bird populations (eg, chickens, ducks, and turkeys), it is very contagious. Birds acquire the illness from contact with contaminated excretions or surfaces that are contaminated with excretions. If an infected bird is used for food and is cooked, it does not pose a risk to those who eat it.

The first cases of avian flu in humans were reported in Hong Kong in 1997; 18 people became infected and 6 died in this outbreak. In the cases that have occurred since then, the death rate is approximately 25%. No rapid human-to-human cases of this disease has been reported. Instead, the cases occurring in humans have involved close contact with infected birds. The transmission risk for humans is quite low.

Signs and symptoms of avian flu include fever, sore throat, cough, and muscle aches; some eye infections have also been noted. Illness may eventually progress to pneumonia and severe respiratory distress.

In the Field

Travel history should be a routine part of patient assessment.

Preventive measures include placing a surgical mask on the patient to contain secretions. If the patient's condition does not permit this action, the paramedic can wear a surgical mask for protection. Follow current CDC guidelines regarding protection for health care providers. Under the current information-sharing system, the medical facility is required to notify the DICO if a patient transported is later

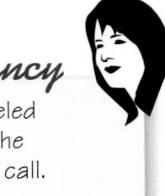

Notes from Nancy

Don't drive a four-wheeled fomite. Clean and air the ambulance after every call.

diagnosed with avian flu. If an exposure is documented, then an antiviral drug may be offered within 48 hours of exposure. Antiviral drugs do not prevent the flu, but rather reduce the severity of the illness. It is also important to get an annual flu shot to ensure protection from type A viruses. Some concern exists that someone infected with a regular type A flu virus may become co-infected with avian flu, allowing the two to merge and form a new virus.

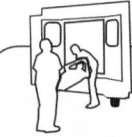

In the Field

The lead agency for responding to potential pandemic diseases is the Department of Health and Human Services. The CDC is part of this agency.

Ambulance Cleaning and Disinfection

The paramedic has an obligation to protect patients from nosocomial infections (infections acquired from a health care setting—in this instance, an ambulance). One way to protect patients is by complying with work restriction guidelines: Reporting for work when you have a sore throat or the flu is *not* in the best interests of your patients or your coworkers.

Another way to protect patients from nosocomial infections is to keep the ambulance interior and its equipment clean and disinfected. When cleaning equipment, select cleaning solutions to fit the equipment category:

- **Critical equipment:** items that come in contact with mucous membranes; laryngoscope blades, endotracheal tubes, Combitubes. High-level disinfection—that is, use of EPA-registered chemical "sterilants"—is the minimum level for this equipment.
- **Semicritical equipment:** items that come in direct contact with intact skin; stethoscopes, blood pressure cuffs, splints, pneumatic antishock garments. Clean with solutions that have a label claiming to kill HBV. Bleach and water at 1:100 dilution fits this requirement.
- **Noncritical equipment:** cleaning surfaces, floors, ambulance seats, work surfaces. EPA-registered hospital-grade cleaner or bleach and water mixture is effective for this equipment.

General cleaning routines need to be listed in the department's Exposure Control Plan. A basic rule of thumb is to do the following after *every* call:

1. Strip used linens from the stretcher immediately after use, and place them in a plastic bag or in the designated receptacle in the emergency department.
2. In an appropriate receptacle, discard all disposable equipment used for care of the patient that meets your state's definition of medical waste. Most items will be considered general trash.
3. Wash contaminated areas with soap and water. For disinfection to be effective, cleaning must be done first.
4. Disinfect all nondisposable equipment used in the care of the patient. For example, disassemble the bag-mask device and place the components in a liquid sterilization solution as recommended by the manufacturer.
5. Clean the stretcher with an EPA-registered germicidal/virucidal solution or bleach and water at 1:100 dilution.
6. If any spillage or other contamination occurred in the ambulance, clean it up with the same germicidal/virucidal or bleach/water solution.
7. Create a schedule for routine full cleaning for the vehicle, as required by the Exposure Control Plan. Name the brands of solution to be used.
8. Have a written policy/procedure for cleaning each piece of equipment. Refer to the manufacturer's recommendations as a guide.

You are the Provider Summary

1. Given your initial findings, what do you know about the patient's overall condition?

Her flushed, sweaty skin points to the possibility of fever and infection. Depending on her health history, she may or may not be able to compensate for the vasodilation and the resultant increased myocardial workload and oxygen consumption.

2. What are your immediate concerns?

Before moving this patient, you must determine that no trauma has occurred. Also note the length of time that this patient has been on the floor and whether any loss of consciousness occurred.

3. Think of a few potential illnesses that could cause these signs and symptoms.

Viral, bacterial, fungi, and other parasitic infections can result in pneumonia, bronchitis, and influenza, to name just a few.

4. Of those, which are the most serious and why?

Communicable, contagious, or infectious diseases not only place your patient at risk but all those individuals around the patient, including friends, family, health care providers, and the general public.

5. Why is it important to periodically reconsider your differential diagnosis throughout the call?

You must remain mentally flexible and periodically rethink your list of possible causes related to the patient's signs and symptoms. Failure to do so can result in a pigeon-holing of your differentials and can cause you to make errors in patient care. Critical thinking skills are the key to delivering good medicine.

6. Given your updated differential, what would be considered "high-risk" procedures for this patient?

Any airway maneuvers, procedures, or treatment that could potentially spread the disease and/or place the health care provider at elevated risk for exposure would be considered "high risk." Examples include endotracheal intubation, laryngeal mask airway, Combitube, CPAP, BiPAP, bag-mask ventilations (without appropriate filtration), and use of nebulizer treatments.

7. After the transfer of care, what steps must be taken with regard to exposure?

Immediately notify your department's DICO and complete an exposure report form. During this call, which included close patient contact in an enclosed space as well as carrying the patient to the gurney, you have received a true exposure. Your DICO and medical director will likely remove you from duty and place you on a 10-day quarantine. Because your partner did not receive the same level of exposure, he or she may or may not be removed from active duty.

8. Will this alter your immediate lifestyle or work habits? If so, how?

Yes—a 10-day quarantine means that you will not be going to work on an EMS unit and potentially coming in contact with sick patients (for your sake and theirs).

9. What are some other considerations with respect to this patient's family?

The granddaughter and any other family members will need to be notified and watched for signs and symptoms of SARS. Due to family stressors and mortality rates associated with SARS in older people, they may also need some form of mental health counseling.

Prep Kit

Ready for Review

- Government agencies such as OSHA, the CDC, and state and county public health departments bear the responsibility for protection of the public health, prevention of epidemics, and management of outbreaks.
- The human body offers several defenses to protect against infection, such as skin, the mucous membranes, and the immune system.
- Infection involves a typical chain of events through which the communicable disease spreads.
- Communicable diseases can be transmitted from one person to another under certain conditions.
- Precautions against communicable diseases include the designated infection control officer, the public health department, standard precautions, immunizations and vaccinations, personal protective equipment, postexposure medical follow-up, and an exposure control plan.
- The overuse and misuse of antibiotics has led some pathogens to develop resistance to the antibiotic drugs commonly prescribed to eradicate them.
- New and emerging diseases of concern include SARS and the avian flu.
- Clean and disinfect the ambulance and your equipment to protect patients from infection.

Vital Vocabulary

acquired immunodeficiency syndrome (AIDS) The end-stage disease process caused by the human immunodeficiency virus (HIV). A person with this is extremely vulnerable to numerous bacterial, viral, and fungal infections that would not affect a person with an intact immune system.

avian (bird) flu A disease caused by a virus that occurs naturally in the bird population. Signs and symptoms include fever, sore throat, cough, and muscle aches.

bacteria Small organisms that can grow and reproduce outside the human cell in the presence of the temperature and nutrients, and cause disease by invading and multiplying in the tissues of the host.

bloodborne pathogens Pathogenic microorganisms that are present in human blood and can cause disease in humans. These pathogens include, but are not limited to, hepatitis B virus (HBV) and human immunodeficiency virus (HIV).

carrier An individual who harbors an infectious agent and, although not personally ill, can transmit the infection to another person.

chancre The primary hard lesion or ulcer of syphilis that occurs at the entry site of the infection.

chickenpox A very contagious disease caused by varicella zoster virus, which is part of the herpes virus family, occurring most often in the winter and early spring.

Chlamydia A sexually transmitted disease that has the highest incidence. Signs and symptoms include inflammation of the urethra, epididymis, cervix, fallopian tubes, and discharge from the urethra.

communicable disease A disease that can be transmitted from one person to another under certain conditions.

communicable period The period during which an infected person is capable of transmitting illness to someone else.

contaminated The presence or the reasonably anticipated presence of blood or other potentially infectious materials on an item or surface.

designated infection control officer (DICO) An individual trained to ensuring that proper post-exposure medical treatment and counseling is provided to an exposed employee or volunteer.

enterococcus A common, normal organism of the GI tract, urinary tract, and genitourinary tract, and which may become resistant to vancomycin.

fomite An inanimate object contaminated with microorganisms that serves as a means of transmitting an illness.

fungus (plural: fungi) A small organism that can grow rapidly in the presence of nutrients and organic material, and can cause infection related to contact with decaying organic matter or from airborne spores in the environment such as molds.

gastroenteritis A term that comprises many types of infections and irritations of the gastrointestinal tract; symptoms include nausea and vomiting, fever, abdominal cramps, and diarrhea.

gonorrhea An sexually transmitted disease which results in infection caused by the gonococcal bacteria, *Neisseria gonorrhea*. Signs and symptoms include pus-containing discharge from the urethra and painful urination in males, and signs and symptoms of an acute abdomen in females.

hantavirus Also known as hemorrhagic fever with renal syndrome, this is a type of virus found in wild rodents, which can also cause disease in humans, characterized by fever, headache, abdominal pain, loss of appetite, and vomiting.

helminths Invertebrates with long, flexible, rounded, or flattened bodies, commonly called worms; a type of parasite.

host resistance One's ability to fight off infection.

human immunodeficiency virus (HIV) AIDS (acquired immunodeficiency syndrome) is caused by HIV, which kills or damages the cells in the body's immune system so that the body is unable to fight infections and certain cancers.

icterus Jaundice; the yellow appearance of the skin and other tissues caused by an accumulation of bile pigments.

incubation period The time period between exposure to an organism and the first symptoms of illness, during which the organism multiplies within the body and starts to produce symptoms.

infection The abnormal invasion of a host or host tissue by organisms such as bacteria, viruses, or parasites, with or without signs or symptoms of disease.

infectious hepatitis Another name for hepatitis A, an Inflammation from a virus that causes mild fatigue, loss of appetite, fever, nausea, abdominal pain, and eventually, jaundice, dark-colored urine, and whitish stools.

influenza The flu, a respiratory infection caused by a variety of viruses. It differs from the common cold in that the flu involves a fever, headache, and extreme exhaustion.

jaundice The presence of excessive bile pigments in the bloodstream that give the skin, mucous membranes, and eyes a distinct yellow color; jaundice is often associated with liver disease.

lice Tiny, wingless, parasitic insects that feed on the patient's blood. This infestation is easily spread through close personal contact. Several types exist: head, body, and pubic lice.

Lyme disease A tick-borne disease which primarily affects the skin, heart, joints, and nervous system, and characterized by a round, red lesion or bull's-eye rash.

measles An infectious viral disease that occurs most often in late winter and spring. It begins with a fever followed by a cough, running nose, and pink eye. Then a rash spreads from the face and neck down the back and trunk.

meningitis An inflammation of the meningeal coverings of the brain and spinal cord; it is usually caused by a virus or bacterium.

meningococcal meningitis An infection of the fluid of a person's spinal cord and the fluid that surrounds the brain. Sometimes referred to as spinal meningitis, it is caused by bacteria or virus. The viral type is less severe than the bacterial; the bacterial type can result in brain damage, hearing loss, learning disability, or death.

mononucleosis Infectious mononucleosis or mono (glandular fever), caused by the Epstein-Barr virus, is often called the kissing disease. It is also spread by coughing or sneezing.

mumps A viral infection that primarily affects the parotid glands, which are one of the three pairs of salivary glands, causing swelling in front of the ears.

needleless systems A device that does not use needles for: (1) collection of body fluids or withdrawal of body fluids after initial venous or arterial access is established; (2) administration of medication or fluids; or (3) any other procedure involving the potential for occupational exposure to bloodborne pathogens due to percutaneous injuries from contaminated sharps.

nosocomial infection An infection acquired from a health care setting.

OPIM An acronym that stands for other potentially infectious materials. These include CSF, pericardial fluid, synovial fluid, pleural fluid, amniotic fluid, peritoneal fluid, and any fluid containing gross visible blood.

parasite Any living organism in or on any other living creature; takes advantage of the host by feeding off cells and tissues.

pertussis An acute infectious disease characterized by a catarrhal stage, followed by a paroxysmal cough that ends in a whooping inspiration. Also called whooping cough.

pneumonia An inflammation of the lungs caused by bacteria, viruses, fungi, or other organisms.

protozoans Single-celled, usually microscopic, eukaryotic organisms such as amoebas, ciliates, flagellates, and sporozoans; a type of parasite.

rabies A fatal infection of the central nervous system caused by a bite from an animal that has been infected with the rabies virus.

reservoir In the context of communicable disease, a place where organisms may live and multiply.

respiratory syncytial virus (RSV) A labile paramyxovirus that produces its characteristic fusion of human cells in a tissue culture known as the syncytial effect. Two subtypes, A and B, have been identified. RSV can affect both the upper and lower respiratory tracts but is more prevalent with the lower, causing pneumonias and bronchiolitis.

rubella A viral disease similar to measles, best known by the distinctive red rash on the skin. It is not nearly as infectious or severe as measles.

scabies An infestation of the skin with the mite Sarcoptes scabei. It spreads rapidly when there is skin-to-skin contact.

seropositive Having a positive blood test for an infectious agent, such as HIV or hepatitis B or C virus.

serum hepatitis The hepatitis type B virus (HBV), which is transmitted through sexual contact, blood transfusion, or puncture of the skin with contaminated needles, and whose signs and symptoms include loss of appetite, nausea, vomiting, general fatigue and malaise, low-grade fever, vague abdominal discomfort, and sometimes aching in the joints. Eventually, jaundice will occur.

severe acute respiratory syndrome (SARS) Potentially life-threatening viral infection that usually starts with flu-like symptoms.

sexually transmitted diseases (STDs) A group of diseases usually acquired by sexual contact, and which include gonorrhea, syphilis, chlamydia, scabies, pubic lice, herpes, hepatitis, and HIV infection.

source individual Any individual, living or dead, whose blood or other potentially infectious materials may be a source of occupational exposure to the member/volunteer. Examples include, but are not limited to, hospital and clinic patients; clients in institutions for the developmentally disabled; trauma victims; clients of drug and alcohol treatment facilities; residents of hospices and nursing homes; human remains; and individuals who donate or sell blood or blood components.

standard precautions The new term used to describe the infection control practices that will reduce the opportunity for exposure of providers in the daily care of patients.

Staphylococcus aureus A strain of bacteria that became resistant to the drug methicillin, creating a new strain called methicillin-resistant staphylococcus aureus; symptoms include infection and possibly localized skin abscesses and cellulites, empyemas, and endocarditis.

syphilis A sexually transmitted disease caused by the spiral-shaped bacteria Treponema pallidum and whose signs and symptoms include an ulcerative lesion or chancre of the skin or mucous membrane at the site of infection, commonly in the genital region.

tetanus A disease caused by spores that enter the body through a puncture wound contaminated with animal feces, street dust, or soil, or which can enter through contaminated street drugs, and whose signs and symptoms include pain at the wound site and painful muscle contractions in the neck and trunk muscles.

tuberculin skin test A test to determine if a person has ever been infected with tuberculosis.

tuberculosis (TB) An infection which can progress to a disease characterized by a persistent cough for 2 to 3 weeks plus night sweats, headache, weight loss, hemoptysis, or chest pain.

vesicle A tiny fluid-filled sac; a small blister.

viral hepatitis An inflammation of the liver produced by one of five distinct forms a virus—A, B, C, D, and E. The five types differ in transmission but present with the same signs and symptoms.

virulence The ability of an organism to invade and create disease in a host. Also refers to the ability of an organism to survive outside the living host.

virus A small organism that can only multiply inside a host, such as a human, and cause disease.

West Nile virus (WNV) A type of virus that is transmitted by mosquitos, and which usually only causes mild disease in humans, but can cause encephalitis, meningitis, or death. Symptoms, if exhibited, include fever, headache, body rash, and swollen lymph glands.

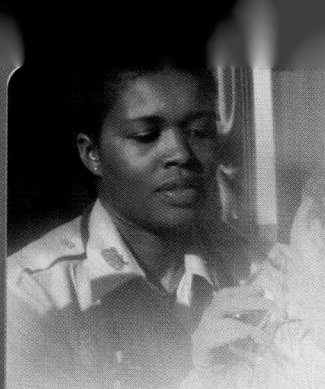

Assessment in Action

A call goes out for a patient complaining of fever, rash, and weakness. The location given is the local university. When the paramedics arrive, they are taken to a dorm room where a student is lying on the sofa. Patient assessment reveals a pinkish-colored rash, rapid onset of a headache, and stiff neck; also, the patient does not want to be in bright light.

During transport to the local hospital, the patient vomits. The next day, a rumor circulates that the student was diagnosed with bacterial meningitis. The medical facility contacts the DICO, who then contacts the crew members who were on the call.

1. **What is meningitis?**
   A. Inflammation of the lining of the myocardium
   B. Inflammation of the meninges, the membranes that cover the brain and spinal cord
   C. Inflammation of the pleura
   D. Inflammation of the endocrine system

2. **What is the transmission mode for meningitis?**
   A. Vectorborne
   B. Direct contact with the nasopharyngeal secretions of an infected person
   C. Indirect contact
   D. Inhalation of infected droplets

3. **How is the diagnosis of meningitis made?**
   A. Gram's stain
   B. Standard blood work
   C. Chest radiographs
   D. Arterial blood gas analysis

4. **What is the incubation period of meningitis?**
   A. 12 to 24 hours
   B. 8 to 36 hours
   C. 2 to 10 days
   D. 10 to 21 days

5. **Which type of meningitis is communicable?**
   A. Viral
   B. Bacterial

6. **Communicable diseases are caused by microorganisms. How many means of transmission are there?**
   A. 3
   B. 6
   C. 8
   D. 4

7. **What are bacteria?**
   A. Small organisms that can grow and reproduce outside the human cell in the presence of the right temperature and nutrients
   B. Small organisms that multiply inside a host; they die when exposed to the environment
   C. Organisms that grow rapidly in the presence of nutrients and organic material
   D. Small living organisms in or on any living creature

8. **Who does the postexposure medical management begin with?**
   A. Employee
   B. Source individual
   C. Family members
   D. DICO

9. **The liaison who handles notification between the hospital and an exposed responder is the:**
   A. medical director.
   B. DICO.
   C. chief supervisor.
   D. dispatcher

10. **In an approach to infection control, which of the following is based on the assumption that all blood and body fluids are potentially infectious?**
    A. PPE
    B. Handwashing
    C. Biohazard labeling
    D. Standard precautions

Challenging Question

It's 2:00 AM and you are dispatched to a private residence for a man who doesn't feel well. When you arrive on the scene, the patient tells you he has been coughing for approximately 2 weeks. During that time he has had a headache, unexplained weight loss, and night sweats. On the way to the hospital, the patient begins to cough uncontrollably, including in your face.

11. **What are some communicable diseases this patient may possibly have, and how can you prevent becoming exposed to them?**

■ Points to Ponder

You are dispatched to a private residence for a 42-year-old man complaining of right-sided chest pain. During your assessment you find the patient to be in supraventricular tachycardia at a rate of 220 beats/min, with blood pressure of 100/70 mm Hg and a respiratory rate of 22 breaths/min. He is pale in color and slightly diaphoretic. Before starting an IV, your partner practices the appropriate standard precautions. You are helping your partner clean up when you suddenly feel a sharp prick in the palm of your hand. You have just received a needlestick from the used catheter. Your palm has small specks of blood coming from it. When you arrive at the hospital, the patient informs you that he has hepatitis C virus and is currently under treatment for this disease.

What should you do now? Could you have prevented this exposure?

Issues: Safe Management of a Patient With an Infectious and Communicable Disease, Compliance With Standard Precautions and BSI, Managing an Exposure.

37 Behavioral Emergencies

Objectives

Cognitive

5-12.1   Define behavior and distinguish between normal and abnormal behavior. (p 37.1)

5-12.2   Define behavioral emergency. (p 37.1)

5-12.3   Discuss the prevalence of behavior and psychiatric disorders. (p 37.16)

5-12.4   Discuss the factors that may alter the behavior or emotional status of an ill or injured individual. (p 37.4)

5-12.5   Describe the medical-legal considerations for management of emotionally disturbed patients. (p 37.8)

5-12.6   Discuss the pathophysiology of behavioral and psychiatric disorders. (p 37.4)

5-12.7   Describe the overt behaviors associated with behavioral and psychiatric disorders. (p 37.5)

5-12.8   Define the following terms:
  a. Affect (p 37.6)
  b. Anger (p 37.2–37.3)
  c. Anxiety (p 37.13)
  d. Confusion (p 37.5)
  e. Depression (p 37.15)
  f. Fear (p 37.13)
  g. Mental status (p 37.10)
  h. Open-ended question (p 37.9)
  i. Posture (p 37.24)

5-12.9   Describe the verbal techniques useful in managing the emotionally disturbed patient. (p 37.9)

5-12.10   List the reasons for taking appropriate measures to ensure the safety of the patient, paramedic and others. (p 37.25)

5-12.11   Describe the circumstances when relatives, bystanders and others should be removed from the scene. (p 37.11)

5-12.12   Describe the techniques that facilitate the systematic gathering of information from the disturbed patient. (p 37.9)

5-12.13   List situations in which the EMT-P is expected to transport a patient forcibly and against his will. (p 37.25)

5-12.14   Identify techniques for physical assessment in a patient with behavioral problems. (p 37.9)

5-12.15   Describe methods of restraint that may be necessary in managing the emotionally disturbed patient. (p 37.25)

5-12.16   List the risk factors for suicide. (p 37.16)

5-12.17   List the behaviors that may be seen indicating that patient may be at risk for suicide. (p 37.17)

5-12.18   Integrate the pathophysiological principles with the assessment of the patient with behavioral and psychiatric disorders. (p 37.10)

5-12.19   Differentiate between the various behavioral and psychiatric disorders based on the assessment and history. (p 37.10)

5-12.20   Formulate a field impression based on the assessment findings. (p 37.8)

5-12.21   Develop a patient management plan based on the field impressions. (p 37.13)

Affective

5-12.22   Advocate for empathetic and respectful treatment for individuals experiencing behavioral emergencies. (p 37.8)

Psychomotor

5-12.23   Demonstrate safe techniques for managing and restraining a violent patient. (p 37.25)

Introduction

Problems related to abnormal behavior are commonly the result of "mental problems," implying that they originate in some ephemeral place called the mind, as opposed to "real" medical problems, which originate in the solid, tangible structures of the body. In reality, the mind and the body are not separate entities; they are inseparable parts of a whole human being. When a person becomes ill with any disease, that illness will inevitably affect the individual's behavior—often making him or her anxious or depressed. Similarly, changes in mental state influence the body's physical health. A depressed person, for example, may lose appetite or become more susceptible to bodily disease. Thus, whenever we examine a patient, it is important to view the patient as a whole person and try to understand both the physical and the mental factors that contribute to the patient's distress Figure 37-1 ▸ .

Notes from Nancy

Abnormal behavior may be due to many conditions other than mental illness.

What Is a Behavioral Emergency?

The concept of behavior has been widely debated over the years. Most experts define it as the way people act or perform—for example, how they react to a situation. Behavior includes all the things people do and the reasons why they do those things. Who defines when the behavior becomes abnormal is also a source of debate, as is who defines what is normal—society in general, a particular community or social group, a parent, a boss, a friend, or even a stranger. Abnormal behavior in and of itself may not be a medical problem and is hardly cause for alarm. The real questions are "When does abnormal behavior require medical intervention?" and "When does it require EMS?" Almost all disordered behavior represents the individual's effort to adapt to some stress, whether internal or external. In most cases the disruptive behavior is a temporary action, abating when the individual has managed to mobilize his or her psychological defense mechanisms.

Behavioral emergencies are situations in which the patient's presenting problem is some disorder of mood, thought, or behavior that interferes with his or her activities of daily living (ADLs); ADLs are normal, everyday activities such as getting dressed and taking out the garbage. When a person becomes so depressed that he or she cannot get up in the morning,

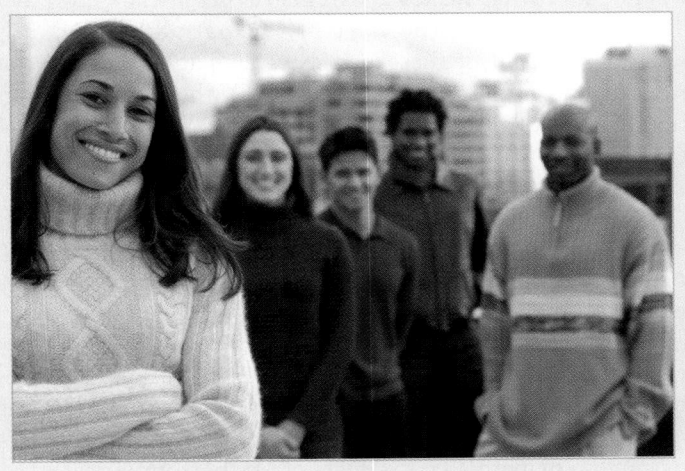

Figure 37-1 Which of these people is battling mental illness?

You are the Provider Part 1

You are dispatched to 1022 Pierce Lane for a 39-year-old man who is "acting crazy." Per dispatch protocols, law enforcement officers have been sent as well. You stage two blocks from the scene and wait for an update from law enforcement. A few minutes later, a police officer notifies you that the scene is safe and one man is in custody.

You arrive to find a man in his 30s lying on the ground with his hands cuffed behind his back. He is yelling about seeing flashing green and yellow lights from the sky. After you introduce yourself, he tells you that his name is Eugene.

Initial Assessment	Recording Time: 0 Minutes
Appearance	Sweaty, anxious
Level of consciousness	A (Alert to person, place, and day)
Airway	Patent
Breathing	Fast and deep
Circulation	Fast, slightly irregular pulse

1. What are some medical conditions that can give the appearance of "acting crazy?"
2. What are some considerations to discuss with your partner while you stage the scene?

shower, and make breakfast, or when someone has delusions or hallucinations that prohibit holding a job, a behavioral emergency exists.

A psychiatric emergency exists when the abnormal behavior threatens an individual's health and safety or the health and safety of another. The most extreme examples are situations in which a person becomes suicidal, homicidal, or has a psychotic episode. In a psychotic episode, a person often experiences delusions (false beliefs) or hallucinations (false perceptions) that result in loss of contact with reality. For example, a patient who has taken illicit drugs may experience an alteration of reality—a "bad trip." Psychotic episodes can have very dangerous consequences because the individual's behavior becomes violent, usually from exaggerated fear or paranoia.

No matter what definition of a psychiatric emergency a textbook may furnish, the *operative* definition of a behavioral or psychiatric emergency is provided by the person who dials 9-1-1. Often what makes a psychiatric emergency an "emergency" is panic on the part of the patient, the family, bystanders, or all of these parties. That panic, in turn, may translate into a demand for action, and the paramedic may therefore face intense pressure to do something (such as transport the patient to an emergency department with a crisis unit).

Paradoxically, it is precisely in this situation—when the patient is behaving strangely and bystanders are clamoring for action—that the paramedic usually feels least *able* to do something. Most paramedics would much prefer to deal with a train wreck than with the tangle of confused and frayed feelings presented by a psychiatric emergency. Most people prefer to operate in areas in which they feel competent. For paramedics, that means dealing with problems like broken legs, cardiac dysrhythmias, or narcotic overdoses. EMS personnel feel much less confident of their ability to deal with emotional disturbances—especially since most paramedic training programs don't delve into such matters. Furthermore, paramedics tend to be action-oriented people. They like to see tangible results of what they do—a hypoglycemic patient coming around after a bolus of glucose, a clinically dead patient restored to life by CPR and defibrillation. What tangible rewards can there be in escorting a confused, hallucinating patient to the hospital, let alone in dealing with a belligerent and violent patient who's screaming obscenities?

In fact, prehospital intervention *is* possible and often critical in behavioral emergencies. Paramedics can make a huge difference in the life of a disturbed patient, and the skills for doing so can be learned just like any other skill. Indeed, the skills for dealing with abnormal behavior may ultimately be much more important to the paramedic's work than skills such as endotracheal intubation. After all, how many calls require placing an advanced airway? Many more calls require the paramedic to deal with people who are angry, depressed, agitated, panicky, or out of control. Clearly, it's worthwhile learning an organized and systematic approach to emergencies that involve abnormal behavior.

Causes of Abnormal Behavior

Anyone who has seen a paranoid, belligerent diabetic transformed into a paragon of courtesy and charm by the mere addition of 25 g of glucose to the bloodstream knows that not everyone who acts crazy *is* crazy. Similarly, no one would diagnose mental illness in a person who was stunned and mute after the unanticipated death of a husband or wife. Abnormal behavior typically results from a complex interaction of biological or organic causes, developmental factors, psychological stressors, emotional stimuli, and sociocultural influences. Those causes can be classified into three broad categories: (1) biological or organic causes, (2) psychosocial causes, and (3) sociocultural causes.

Biological or Organic Causes of Abnormal Behavior

Many patients presenting with psychiatric symptoms are actually suffering from a physical illness or are under the influence of a substance that interferes with normal cerebral function. Such patients are generally classified as having organic brain syndrome. Diabetes, seizure disorders, severe infections, metabolic disorders, head injury, stroke, alcohol, tumors in the brain, and drugs may all cause derangements in behavior. When faced with abnormal behavior, always look for situational and organic causes, as they're the ones you'll be best able to treat in an acute emergency.

The conditions and substances that can produce psychiatric symptoms are summarized in **Table 37-1 ▸**. Probably the most common offenders are alcohol and drugs. Besides intoxication with alcohol or drugs, other common forms of organic brain syndrome include delirium and dementia. Delirium is characterized by a global impairment of cognitive function that comes on quite rapidly and may fluctuate in severity over the course of a day. Delirium is almost always a disturbance in mental status. Dementia is a more chronic process that produces severe deficits in memory, abstract thinking, and judgment.

Psychosocial Causes of Abnormal Behavior

Normal individuals may develop abnormal reactions to stressful psychosocial events (eg, childhood trauma) or developmental influences (eg, parents who deprived them of love, caring, support, and encouragement). When a person's basic needs are threatened, that individual faces a crisis. A person in crisis has two alternatives for dealing with this threat: (1) cope with it, finding ways to alter the situation or his or her perception of it so that it is no longer so stressful, or (2) attempt to alleviate the discomfort by escaping from the stress. Escape may take many forms, including alcohol, drugs, psychiatric symptoms, and even suicide.

Sociocultural Causes of Abnormal Behavior

Chapter 2 considered the responses of patients, their families, bystanders, and rescue personnel to the stresses of emergencies

Table 37-1	Selected Disease States That May Produce Psychotic Symptoms
Disease State	**Psychotic Symptoms**
Toxic and deficiency states	Drug-induced psychoses, especially from: • Digitalis • Steroids • Disulfiram • Amphetamines • LSD, PCP, and other psychedelics Nutrition disorders: • Alcohol abuse • Vitamin deficiencies Poisoning with bromide or other heavy metals Kidney failure Liver failure
Infections	Syphilis Parasites Viral encephalitis (eg, after measles) Brain abscess
Neurologic disease	Seizure disorders (especially temporal lobe seizures) Primary and metastatic tumors of the brain Dementia Cerebrovascular accident Closed-head injury
Cardiovascular disorders	Low cardiac output (eg, in heart failure)
Endocrine disorders	Thyroid hyperfunction (thyrotoxicosis) Adrenal hyperfunction (Cushing's syndrome)
Metabolic disorders	Electrolyte imbalances (eg, after severe diarrhea) Hypoglycemia Diabetic ketoacidosis

and the various ways that people react to death and dying. Humans are social animals; we prefer to live in groups. Not surprisingly, then, social and cultural factors directly affect biology, behavior, and responses to the stress of emergencies. For example, the effects of assault, rape, and racial attacks or the death of a loved one may produce significant changes in an individual's behavior.

Psychopathology

Many factors contribute to disturbances of behavior. Some of these influences are easily identified and treated, while others may never be clearly understood. The causes, signs, symptoms, and management of abnormal behavior can be grouped into several common areas of psychopathology:

- Anxiety disorders
- Mood disorders and suicide
- Personality disorders

- Somatoform (a disorder involving excessive concern with one's physical health and appearance) and dissociative disorders
- Eating, impulse control, and substance-related disorders
- Schizophrenia and other psychotic disorders
- Hostile and violent patients

The remainder of this chapter focuses on these areas of psychopathology. Before considering those categories in detail, however, you need to learn about assessing a patient with a behavioral emergency.

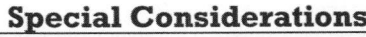

Special Considerations

The American Psychiatric Association (APA) is a scientific and professional organization whose goals are to promote quality care, education, and research in mental health.

The APA publishes the *Diagnostic and Statistical Manual of Mental Disorders, Fourth Edition, Text Revision (DSM IV TR)*, a comprehensive reference manual focusing on mental health disorders, including symptomatic and diagnostic information.

Psychiatric Signs and Symptoms

When an organ begins functioning abnormally, the human body mobilizes various defenses to correct the abnormality. The patient experiences those corrective measures as symptoms, and the paramedic observes their effects as signs. Physical symptoms and signs reflect the body's attempts to maintain its balance in the face of physical stress.

Psychiatric signs and symptoms serve the same function for the mind: They reveal the personality trying to maintain the optimal internal balance in the face of a stressor. Like the symptoms and signs of physical illness, psychiatric symptoms and signs can be grouped according to the "systems" they affect. Here, however, the focus is on systems of psychological (rather than physiologic) functioning. The psychological functions involved are consciousness, motor activity, speech, thought, affect, memory, orientation, and perception. Psychiatric signs and symptoms are categorized by disorder in **Table 37-2 ▸**.

Disorders of Consciousness

Consciousness refers to the degree to which a person is aware of and attentive to the external world. Disorders of consciousness such as delirium, stupor, and coma usually indicate an organic basis for the patient's disorder. Other disorders of consciousness, however, are seen in psychiatric patients. Inattention in patients means that it is difficult to gain their attention; with distractibility, their attention is easily diverted; and confusion refers to impaired understanding of their surroundings.

Table 37-2	Classification of Psychiatric Signs and Symptoms
Disorder	**Psychiatric Signs and Symptoms**
Disorders of consciousness	Distractibility and inattention Confusion Delirium Stupor and coma
Disorders of motor activity	Restlessness Stereotyped movements Compulsions Retarded movements
Disorders of speech	Retarded speech Acceleration or pressure of speech Neologisms (words the patient invents) Echolalia (the patient echoes words he or she hears) Mutism
Disorders of thinking	Disordered thought progression: • Flight of ideas • Retardation of thought • Perseveration • Circumstantial thinking Disordered thought content: • Delusions • Obsessions • Phobias
Disorders of mood and affect	Anxiety Euphoria Depression Inappropriate affect Flat affect
Disorders of memory	Amnesia Confabulation
Disorders of orientation	Disoriented to person, place, and time
Disorders of perception	Illusions Hallucinations
Disorders of intelligence	Mental retardation

Disorders of Motor Activity

Motor activity in a disturbed patient may be increased, decreased, or bizarre in some way. Restlessness refers to the situation in which a patient cannot sit still; when restlessness occurs in association with extreme anxiety, it's called agitation. At the other end of the spectrum, a very depressed or psychotic patient may exhibit exceptionally slow or retarded movements. In some cases, the patient appears to have little or no control over motor activity. Stereotyped activity involves a repetition of movements that don't seem to serve any useful purpose—for instance, a patient's repetitive touching of the elbow, nose, and forehead in succession. Compulsions are repetitive actions that are carried out to relieve the anxiety of obsessive thoughts.

Disorders of Speech

Like motor activity, speech may be abnormally fast or abnormally slow. Retardation of speech is seen in severely depressed patients, whereas manic patients often show accelerated speech and pressure of speech (ie, words pour out like water escaping under pressure). The words the patient uses may themselves be strange or unusual. Neologisms are words that the patient invents. In echolalia, the patient echoes the words of the examiner. When the patient doesn't speak at all, the condition is called mutism.

Disorders of Thinking

Thinking is the highest of the mental functions, requiring integration of knowledge, perception, and memory. Thinking may be disordered in its progression or in its content.

The *progression* of thought, like motor activity and speech, may be speeded up or slowed down. Flight of ideas, which occurs in some manic conditions, refers to accelerated thinking in which the mind skips so rapidly from one idea to another that the listener finds it difficult to grasp the connection between them. At the other end of the spectrum, depressed patients may experience retardation of thought, in which it seems to take a very long time to get from one thought to the next. In circumstantial thinking, the patient includes many irrelevant details in his or her account of things. Perseveration refers to repetition of the same idea over and over again.

The *content* of thought may also be abnormal in a patient with psychiatric problems. The patient may, for example, express delusions—fixed beliefs that are not shared by others of the same culture or background and that the patient is not willing to change by reasonable explanation. With delusions of persecution, the individual believes that others are plotting against him or her. With delusions of grandeur, the patient believes he or she is someone of great importance. Other delusions that suggest psychoses include thought broadcasting (the belief that others can hear one's thoughts) and thought control (the belief that outside forces are controlling one's thoughts).

Obsessions are thoughts that will not go away, despite attempts to forget them. Usually the person with an obsession knows that the idea is unreasonable, but can't stop thinking about it. Patients may, for example, have an obsessional belief that the gas stove hasn't been turned off, so they'll return again and again to the kitchen to make sure. Each time they do so, their anxiety will be relieved for a short time, but then they must go back and check yet again. Phobias are obsessive, irrational fears of specific things or situations, such as fear of heights, fear of open places, fear of confined places, or fear of certain animals Figure 37-2 ▸.

Disorders of Mood and Affect

Mood refers to a person's sustained and pervasive emotional state; affect is the outward expression of a person's mood. A person's mood may be described as *depressed, euphoric,* or *anxious.* Affect is described as *appropriate* or *inappropriate.* A

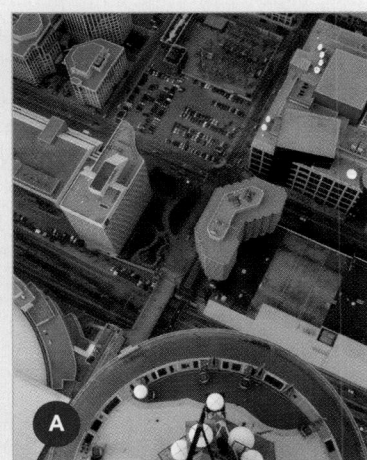

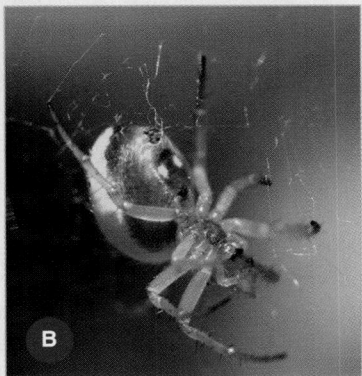

Figure 37-2 Phobias are irrational fears of specific things, such as fear of heights (**A**) or fear of certain animals (**B**).

patient who puts on a waxy smile as he tells you of a parent's death would be considered to be showing inappropriate affect—that is, the emotion expressed is out of synch with the situation. Affect is characterized as labile when it shifts rapidly, as in the patient who is laughing one moment and crying the next. With a flat affect, the patient does not seem to feel much of anything at all.

Disorders of Memory

The most profound disorder of memory is amnesia, the loss of memory. Memory is a complex process consisting of four separate functions: registration, the ability to add new items to the cerebral data bank; retention, the ability to store those items in an accessible place in the mind;

recall, the ability to retrieve a specific piece of stored information on demand; and recognition, the ability to identify information that one has encountered before. Amnesia may reflect the disruption of one or several of those functions. In delirium, for example, a person may be unable to register events properly and thus can't recall what happened while he or she was delirious. When painful memories are repressed, recall is impaired.

Sometimes patients with severe memory deficits from organic brain disease will invent experiences to "paper over" the gaps in memory; this behavior is called confabulation.

Disorders of Orientation

Orientation refers to a person's sense of who one is (person), where one is (place), and at what day of the week one finds himself or herself (day). A person who is confused about those particulars is said to be disoriented. Disorientation is most common in organic brain syndromes.

Disorders of Perception

Perception refers to the way a person processes the data supplied by the five senses. Two disorders of perception are illusions and hallucinations. An illusion is a misinterpretation of sensory stimuli—for example, mistaking a piece of rope for a snake or a cat's meowing for a human voice. A hallucination is a perception that has no basis in reality and occurs without any external stimuli. Hallucinations may involve any of the five senses—a person may hear, see, feel, taste, or smell something that isn't there. Auditory hallucinations (eg, hearing voices) are the most common. Hallucinations involving other senses (eg, the frightening visual hallucinations in delirium tremens) suggest an organic cause.

You are the Provider Part 2

After a few minutes, you are able to calm the patient. When you ask why he's upset, he tells you that he came home from work to find the neighbor's dog barking. He tells you that the barking changed into understandable words. The dog said that it would tell his boss that he was stealing at work. Your patient also tells you that things have been stressful at work with many cutbacks and layoffs, and he's afraid he might lose his job if his boss thought he was stealing. After you display concern for his well-being, the patient agrees to let you "check him out."

Vital Signs	Recording Time: 5 Minutes
Skin	Sweaty, flushed, and warm
Pulse	100 to 120 beats/min (dependent upon emotional state)
Blood pressure	146/90 mm Hg
Respirations	24 to 42 breaths/min (dependent upon emotional state)
Sao₂	99% ambient air

3. What are the medical implications when police control the scene of a violent patient?

4. Is it wise to agree with or validate a patient's hallucinations?

Disorders of Intelligence

Intelligence refers to a person's intellectual ability. A person's intelligence is not necessarily a function of his or her education. For example, a person with a disorder of intelligence may have been born with mental retardation or may have suffered from a disease that makes it more difficult to process, remember, and communicate information.

In the Field

Many people have mental disorders, and many individuals who don't currently have such a disorder may develop one at some point in their lives. It's no cause for shame. With so many stressors in today's society, it's quite understandable.

■ Assessment of the Patient With a Behavioral Emergency

Assessment of the patient with a behavioral emergency differs in at least two ways from the methods of patient assessment studied so far. In assessing the patient with trauma or acute illness, you use a variety of diagnostic instruments to measure vital functions and detect abnormalities—a stethoscope to evaluate breath sounds, a sphygmomanometer to measure the blood pressure, and so forth. In assessing the disturbed patient, *you* are the diagnostic instrument. You must use your thinking processes to evaluate someone else's thinking processes, your perceptions to test the validity of someone else's perceptions, your feelings to measure someone else's feelings. That takes practice, because most EMS providers are not accustomed to using their feelings in this way. For example, if someone makes you feel very angry, your reaction is apt to be "That guy infuriates me. I'd like to knock his teeth in." In conducting the psychiatric examination, however, a more useful paradigm is "That guy infuriates me, so it is quite likely he's paranoid, because paranoid patients often elicit anger in others."

A second way in which the assessment of a patient with a behavioral emergency differs from that of a patient with a non-mental medical problem is that the assessment is part of the treatment. As soon as you speak to the patient, your voice and manner will influence his or her condition, for better or worse. The very process of listening to the patient describe the issue at hand can also mitigate the problem.

Scene Size-up

The patient's overall condition and the nature of his or her psychiatric problem will determine how much of the assessment you are able to perform. A disturbed patient may prefer not to be touched, and you must respect that wish unless there's a compelling medical reason for doing otherwise (eg, profuse bleeding from slashed wrists or a decreased level of consciousness from an overdose). At the very least, you should be able to assess the patient's general appearance—for example, the patient's dress, cleanliness, and grooming, all of which provide clues to the way the patient perceives himself or herself. Pay attention to the patient's posture. Does the patient appear frustrated, angry, sobbing, or catatonic (lacking expression or movement, or appearing rigid)? Observe the scene carefully for weapons, remembering that almost anything—a chair, a lamp, or a book—can be used as a weapon. If you have any questions about your ability to manage the situation safely, call for assistance.

Initial Assessment

Identify yourself clearly. Tell the patient who you are and what you are trying to do. If the patient is confused or delusional, you may have to explain who you are at frequent intervals. Do so without arguing, in an emotionally neutral tone of voice. ("No, Mr. Jones, I'm not from the CIA. I'm a paramedic with the city ambulance service, and I'm here to help you.")

Attend first to priority problems—airway, breathing, or circulatory concerns. In most patients with behavioral emergencies, the problem will be more psychiatric than physiologic in presentation. However, your assessment must look for signs and symptoms of abnormal functioning as well as abnormal behavior.

Be prepared to spend time with the disturbed patient. Don't be in a hurry; rather, convey the message that you have the time and concern to learn what's bothering the patient. Assess the patient wherever the emergency occurs. Don't rush off immediately to the hospital, because the hospital is likely to be a strange, intimidating place for the patient; your haste to get there may reinforce the patient's belief that something is terribly wrong. Let the patient recover his or her bearings in familiar surroundings when medically possible.

Patients who are seriously disturbed should be seen by a physician and evaluated for possible hospitalization. Many of these patients will agree to their transport to the hospital. Others may not want your help and try to prevent you from taking them to a hospital. Because this kind of transport deprives the patient of his or her civil liberties, it must never be undertaken lightly. Even an experienced psychiatrist may find it difficult to define what kind of behavior justifies removing a person from society or what constitutes "dangerous behavior." Furthermore, laws vary from one region to another, so it's important to be familiar with the legal requirements in your community.

As a general rule, a conscious adult must consent to be taken to the hospital. If the patient withholds this consent, he or she may be taken against his or her will only at the express request of the police or the county mental health physician (in many jurisdictions). The same policy applies to the use of forcible restraint. Where such measures are deemed necessary, law enforcement officers should be summoned. In addition, every ambulance service should have clearly defined protocols, drawn up with legal advice, for dealing with patients who require involuntary commitment. Follow those protocols to the letter and consult medical command as necessary.

Focused History and Physical Exam

Begin your focused history and physical exam for individuals who are behaving abnormally by obtaining both their past medical history and their history of present illness. To gather the needed information, talk with the patient and use your interviewing skills. Set some ground rules for your interview. Let the patient know what you expect, and what he or she may expect of you. ("It's okay to cry or even scream, but we aren't going to let you hurt yourself or anyone else.") Allow the patient tell the story in his or her own way. Don't attempt to direct the conversation, but allow the patient to vent his or her feelings.

Interviewing Techniques

When evaluating a trauma patient, you can generally obtain enough information to provide appropriate initial treatment just from the physical examination, even if the patient is unconscious and can't give a history. When evaluating a patient with a behavioral emergency, by contrast, virtually all of the diagnostic information (and much of the therapeutic benefit) must come from talking with the patient. Skill in interviewing a disturbed person, therefore, is central to dealing with psychiatric emergencies. Here are some guidelines:

- *Begin the interview with an open-ended question*. An open-ended question doesn't provide possible answers for the patient, but rather allows the patient to select the answer. For example, say "It's clear you've been feeling bad. Tell me something about the kind of troubles you've been having." (The only circumstance in which you should begin with more direct questioning is when it is essential to obtain specific information in a hurry, such as "What kind of pills did you take? How many?")
- *Let the patient talk* and tell the story in his or her own way, even if it takes a little more time. Letting patients talk allows them to gain some control over themselves and their situation. At the same time, it enables *you* to assess the patient's speech, affect, and thought processes.
- *Listen, and show that you're listening*. Your facial expression, posture, eye contact, an occasional nod—all of these things can convey to the patient that you're paying close attention to what he or she is saying **Figure 37-3 ▸**.
- *Don't be afraid of silences*, even though they may seem intolerably long. Maintain an attentive and relaxed attitude until the patient takes up the story again. It's especially important to be silent when the patient stops speaking because of overwhelming emotion. Avoid the temptation to jump into the silence with a hasty "There, there," to forestall the patient's expressions of emotion, such as crying. The expression of feelings is often therapeutic in itself—that's why people speak of having "a good cry"—and the patient will likely be better able to express himself after intense emotion has been released. Furthermore, your

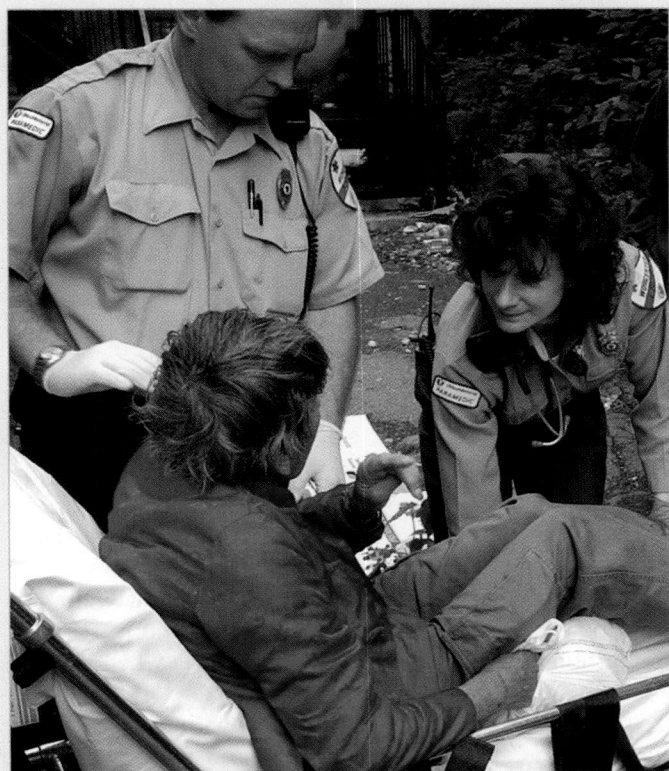

Figure 37-3 Making eye contact with a patient can provide useful clues about his or her emotional state—but don't stare at the patient.

silence gives patients a chance to get control of themselves in their own way.

- *Acknowledge and label the patient's feelings*. The disturbed patient may feel overwhelmed by intense and chaotic feelings. Identifying those feelings and giving them a name (eg, "You seem very angry") can help the patient gain control over them.
- *Don't argue*. If the patient misperceives reality, make note of the misperceptions, but don't try to talk the patient out of them. When a misperception is very frightening or distressing to the patient, you might try just once to provide a simple and factual statement, in a neutral tone of voice ("Yes, that does look a lot like a snake, but actually it's just a shadow."). But don't get into a dispute on the nature of reality.
- Facilitation is a technique of encouraging the patient to communicate by using gestures or noncommittal words, such as a nod of the head or a phrase like "Go on," "I see," or "What happened after that?" You can also use facilitation to return the patient to a topic on which you'd like some elaboration. For example, a patient may have made a passing reference to suicidal thoughts and then moved on to another subject. When the patient

finishes, you might comment, "You say you've had thoughts of suicide?" This remark tells the patient that you've been paying attention to the story and would like to learn more.

■ Confrontation refers to pointing out something of interest in the patient's conversation or behavior, thereby directing the patient's attention to something he or she may have been unaware of. Confrontations describe how the patient appears to the interviewer based on observations, *not* judgments. For example, the interviewer might remark, "You seem worried" or "You look very sad." Such comments often elicit a freer expression of feelings from the patient. Confrontations must be carefully phrased, so they won't sound nagging or condescending.

■ When the patient finishes giving the initial account of the problem, you will have to *ask questions*. Keep the questions as nondirective as possible. Avoid asking questions that can be answered with a yes or no ("Are you very angry?") or asking leading questions ("Do you think that your husband is a part of the problem?"). *How* and *what* questions are preferred ("How did you feel when that happened?").

Some patients find it difficult to deal with the unstructured situation of nondirective questioning and may become very anxious during silences. That response is particularly likely among adolescents, severely depressed patients, and confused or disorganized patients. When your open-ended questions meet with uncomprehending silence, try another approach and perform a more structured interview.

The Mental Status Examination

The mental status examination (MSE) is a key part of your focused physical exam of a patient who is experiencing an acute psychiatric problem. To conduct the MSE, you must check each of the "systems" of mental function in an orderly way. A useful mnemonic for the elements of the MSE is COASTMAP, also discussed in Chapter 14 **Figure 37-4 ▸** :

■ **Consciousness.** Determine the patient's level of consciousness (alert, confused, responds to pain, unresponsive). Note the patient's ability to *pay attention* to a discussion and *concentrate*. Is the patient easily distracted, or can he or she focus on the events at hand?

■ **Orientation.** Ask what the year or month is. Ask the patient to state where he or she is at the moment—the country, state, town, or specific location. If the patient is not sure, have the patient make a best guess.

■ **Activity.** Examine the patient's behavior. Is the patient restless and agitated, pacing up and down? Experiencing tremors? Sitting very still, scarcely moving at all? Making any strange or repetitive movements (scanning of the environment, odd or repetitive gestures)?

■ **Speech.** Identify the form, rather than the content of the patient's speech. Note the rate, volume, flow, articulation, and intonation of speech. Is it too fast or too slow? Too

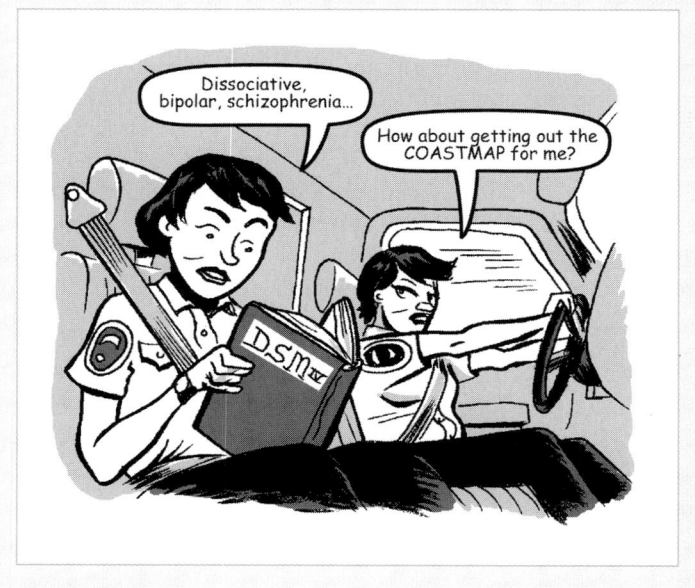

Figure 37-4

loud or too soft? Is the speech garbled or slurred (dysarthria)? Is the patient stuttering or mumbling? Using any strange words?

■ **Thought.** Listen to the patient's story. What's on his or her mind? Is the patient making sense? Is there anything unusual about his or her reasoning? Is the patient expressing apparently false ideas (delusions), such as a belief that the CIA is after him/her? Is the patient experiencing any false sensory impressions (hallucinations), such as hearing voices? Is he/she experiencing a flight of ideas?

■ **Memory.** Form an impression of the patient's memory—recent, remote, and immediate. If memory loss is present, determine whether it is constant or variable. Some patients may create memories to take the place of things they can't recall (confabulation).

■ **Affect and mood.** The patient's mood may be objectively noted via body language. Is the mood euphoric or sad? Is it labile? Does the affect—the expression of inner feelings—seem appropriate to the situation or is it animated, angry, flat, or withdrawn?

■ **Perception.** Detecting disorders of perception may be difficult, because patients often hesitate to answer direct questions about hallucinations or illusions. Sometimes it is helpful to ask the patient, "Do you ever hear things that other people can't hear?"

You can conduct nearly all of the MSE just by watching and listening (and knowing what to watch and listen *for!*). Only the assessment of memory, orientation, and perhaps perception requires you to ask some direct questions. Practice being an observer. As you sit in a diner drinking your coffee, eavesdrop on the waitress talking to other customers and

Table 37-4	Medications for Anxiety	
Class	Generic Name	Trade Name
Antidepressants		
Selective serotonin reuptake inhibitors	Citalopram	Celexa
	Escitalopram	Lexapro
	Fluoxatine	Prozac
	Fluvoxamine	Luvox
	Paroxetine	Paxil
	Sertraline	Zoloft
Monoamine oxidase inhibitors	Phenelzine	Nardil
Serotonin-norepinephrine reuptake inhibitors	Venlafaxine	Effexor
Anxiolytics		
Benzodiazepines	Alprazolam	Xanax
	Chlordiazepoxide	Librium
	Clonazepam	Klonopin
	Clorazepate	Tranxene
	Diazepam	Valium
	Lorazepam	Ativan
Nonbenzodiazepines	Buspirone	BuSpar
Other Classes		
Antihistamines	Hydroxyzine	Atarax / Vistaril
Beta blockers	Propanolol	Inderol
Anticonvulsants	Carbamazepine	Tegretol
	Gabapentin	Neurontin
	Valproic acid	Depakote

One symptom commonly associated with PTSD is flashbacks—sudden memories in which the victim relives the event. Sleep disturbances, including nightmares, and depression or survivor guilt are other signs and symptoms of PTSD. Treatment in the prehospital setting is intended to protect the patient, support the individual in a positive way, and transfer the individual to a medical facility for a more thorough evaluation.

Medications for Anxiety

Several classes of medications are effective in the treatment of anxiety disorders, including many antidepressants Table 37-4. In the past, drugs that exert a tranquilizing or sedative effect, thereby reducing anxiety, were the most commonly prescribed (and overprescribed) psychotropic agents. Today, much safer drugs such as the selective serotonin reuptake inhibitors are more frequently prescribed.

Benzodiazepines serve such functions—as antianxiety agents, muscle relaxants, anticonvulsants, and sedatives. Unfortunately, they are often the source of overdoses. In addition to use of these drugs for chemical restraint, paramedics can administer benzodiazepines to treat status epilepticus, for pain for external pacing or synchronized cardioversion, or to assist with rapid sequence intubation. Beware of the signs and symptoms of potential overdose: severe hypotension, bradycar-

dia, slurred speech, altered mental status, and impaired coordination. Management of a benzodiazepine overdose includes airway management, IV fluids for hypotension, and the potential medical control option of flumazenil to reverse the effects of the benzodiazepine.

Mood Disorders

Mood disorders, formally known as affective disorders, are among the most prevalent psychiatric disorders. As much as 10% of the US population will experience a mood disorder, such as a major depression or a manic-depressive illness, at some point in their lives. Although feelings such as depression and joy are universal, mood disorders differ from normal bouts of sadness or happiness. In mood disorders, the changes in affect are accompanied by other symptoms, and the net effect is to cause a major disturbance in the person's ability to function. Patients who experience either depression or mania suffer from a unipolar mood disorder; that is, their mood remains at only one pole of the depression-mania continuum. Patients who alternate between mania and depression (both poles of the continuum) have bipolar mood disorder. The majority of patients with a unipolar mood disorder are depressed. Unipolar mania is relatively rare.

Depression and Suicidal Behavior

Depression is the leading cause of disability in people between 15 and 44 years of age. It affects women more frequently than men and may occur at any age (the mean age of onset is 32 years). The depressed patient is often readily identified by a sad expression, bouts of crying, and listless or apathetic behavior. He or she expresses feelings of worthlessness, guilt, and pessimism. These patients may want to be left alone, asserting that no one understands or cares and that their problems are hopeless.

Depression may occur in episodes with a sudden onset and limited duration; this is common in major depressive disorder, in which the patient feels substantial suffering and pain that interfere with social or occupational functioning. In other cases, the onset of depression may be insidious and chronic in nature. When a person experiences signs and symptoms of depression for more days than not for a period of at least two years, he or she may be suffering from a chronic form of depression known as dysthymic disorder. The signs and symptoms of dysthymic disorder cause social and occupational distress but rarely require hospitalization unless the individual becomes suicidal.

The diagnostic features of depression are most easily remembered by the mnemonic GAS PIPES:

- **Guilt** and self-reproach are characteristic features of depression. One way to try to get at the patient's guilt feelings is to ask a question such as "Are you down on yourself?" or "Do you ever feel as if you're worthless?"
- **Appetite** is abnormal in depression. Usually it is *decreased,* but a minority of depressed patients may report increased appetite.

- **Sleep disturbance** usually takes the form of insomnia. The typical depressed patient will report that he or she awakens at 3:00 or 4:00 AM and can't get back to sleep again.
- **Paying attention.** The depressed patient has difficulty paying attention; that is, the ability to concentrate is impaired, sometimes severely. Ask the patient, "When you're reading a book or a newspaper, can you get all the way through what you're reading, or does your mind start to wander after a couple of minutes?"
- **Interest.** The depressed patient loses interest in things that were once important. He or she can no longer summon enthusiasm for work or hobbies. You might ask the patient, "Are you a [local team name] fan?" If the answer is yes, ask, "How are they doing this season?" The depressed patient will tell you, "Well, I haven't really been following them lately."
- **Psychomotor abnormalities** in the depressed patient can take the form of either retardation or agitation. Although many depressed patients seem to do everything in slow motion, a significant percentage show agitated behavior, such as pacing, wringing their hands, or picking at themselves.
- **Energy.** Depressed people have no energy. They are tired all the time and don't feel like doing anything.
- **Suicide.** Most worrisome, depressed people tend to have pervasive and recurrent thoughts of suicide.

Medications for Depression

Antidepressants are prescribed to combat the symptoms of depressive illness **Table 37-5**. They are classified into three categories:

- *Tricyclic antidepressants (TCAs) and related drugs,* like the neuroleptics, produce atropine-like side effects and may cause orthostatic hypotension.
- *Monoamine oxidase (MAO) inhibitors* are usually prescribed when TCAs are not effective. Their most notable side effect is *hypertensive crisis,* which may occur in patients taking MAO inhibitors if they receive certain other drugs (eg, sympathomimetics, narcotics) or if they eat certain foods (eg, cheese, yogurt, sour cream, beer, wine, chopped liver).
- *Other agents* include the very widely prescribed fluoxetine (Prozac).

Suicidal Ideation

Suicide is any willful act designed to end one's own life. It is the third leading cause of death among 15- to 25-year-olds and the fourth leading cause of death in the 25- to 44-year age group. For people aged 45 to 64 years, suicide rates are the eighth leading cause of death. Suicide is more common among men, especially those who are Caucasian and single, widowed, or divorced. The risk

Notes from Nancy
Evaluate the suicide risk in every depressed patient.

of suicide is also high among depressed patients, one sixth of whom will succeed in taking their own lives. Alcoholism is another important risk factor. Notably, more than half of all successful suicides have made a previous attempt, and three fourths have given a clear warning of their intent to kill themselves. The risk factors for suicide are summarized in **Table 37-6**.

Suicide attempts typically occur when a person feels that close emotional attachments are endangered or when the person has lost someone or something important in his or her life. The suicidal person may also have feelings characteristic of depression—feelings of worthlessness, lack of self-esteem, and a sense of being unable to manage his or her life.

Table 37-5	Medications for Depression		
Class		**Generic Name**	**Trade Name**
Tricyclic antidepressants and related drugs		Amitriptyline	Amitril, Endep, Elavil
		Amoxapine	Asendin
		Desipramine	Norpramin, Pertofrane
		Doxepin	Adapin, Sinequan
		Imipramine	Imavate, Janimine, Pramine, Presamine, Tofranil
		Maprotiline	Ludiomil
		Nortriptyline	Aventyl, Pamelor
		Protriptyline	Vivactil
		Trimipramine	Surmontil
MAO inhibitors		Isocarboxazid	Marplan
		Phenelzine	Nardil
		Tranylcypromine	Parnate
Serotonin reuptake inhibitors		Bupropion Fluoxetine	Wellbutrin Prozac
Others		Trazodone	Desyrel

Table 37-6	Risk Factors for Suicide
■ Depression, or sudden improvement in depression ■ Male sex, age > 55 ■ Single, widowed, or divorced ■ Alcohol or other drug abuse ■ Recent loss of spouse or significant relationship ■ Chronic, debilitating illness ■ Schizophrenia	■ Expresses suicidal thoughts and concrete plans for carrying them out ■ Caucasian ■ Social isolation ■ Previous suicide attempt(s) ■ Financial setback or job loss ■ Family history of suicide

In the Field

Patients with suicidal thoughts, especially those who have made a threat or unsuccessful attempt, may not be thinking clearly and may behave in very unpredictable ways. Some recognize that if they get into the ambulance or enter the hospital, they won't have the opportunity to complete their threat or gesture. They may therefore make a last effort to kill themselves. Suicidal and/or homicidal patients won't hesitate to hurt you or your partner. Be very careful how you assess the situation, making certain that you, your team, and the patient are safe.

Evaluation of Suicide Risk

The assessment of *every* depressed patient must include an evaluation of the suicide risk. Many paramedics are reluctant to ask a patient directly about suicidal thoughts, because they fear that they might "put ideas into the patient's head" **Figure 37-8**. The paramedic should realize, however, that suicide is not such an original idea that a depressed patient will not have thought of it. Most depressed patients, in fact, are relieved when the topic is brought up, as this discussion gives them "permission" to talk about their suicidal ideas. Often it is easier for both the paramedic and the patient to broach the subject in a stepwise fashion. You might start by asking, "Have you ever thought that life wasn't worth living?" From there, you may proceed by degrees: "Did you ever feel that you would be better off dead? Have you ever thought of harming yourself? Do you feel that way now? Do you have a plan of how you would go about it?

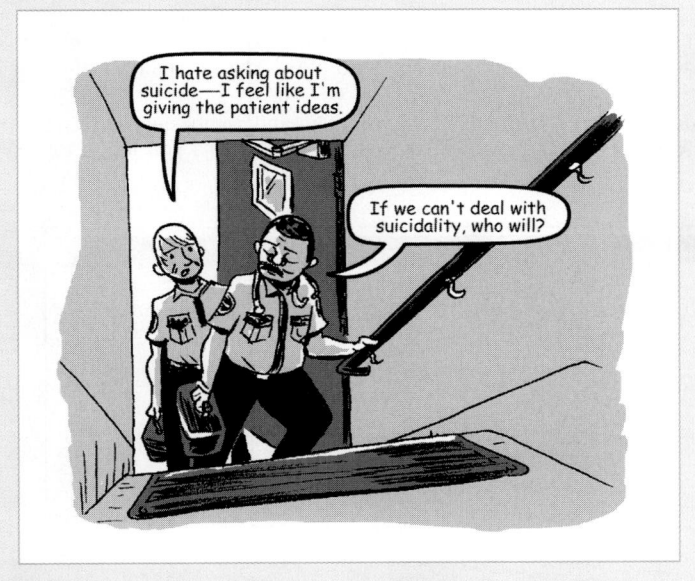

Figure 37-8

Do you have the things you need to carry out the plan? Has anyone in your family ever committed suicide? Have you ever tried to kill yourself before?" Patients who have made previous attempts; who have fashioned detailed, concrete plans for suicide; or who have a history of suicide among close relatives are at higher risk and must be evaluated at the hospital.

Many patients make last-minute efforts to communicate their suicidal intentions. When an individual phones to threaten suicide, someone should stay on the line until the rescue squad has reached the scene. On arrival, quickly survey the area for

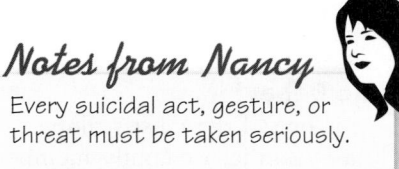

Notes from Nancy

Every suicidal act, gesture, or threat must be taken seriously.

any implements that the patient might use to injure himself or herself and discreetly remove those items. Make certain that you account for your own safety. Talk with the patient, and encourage him or her to discuss feelings. Ask the same questions mentioned earlier regarding the patient's suicidal ideas and plans.

Management of the Patient at Risk of Suicide

Whenever you find a patient to be severely depressed or you have another reason to suspect that a patient is at risk of suicide, follow these guidelines:

- Don't leave the patient alone. The patient's well-being is your responsibility until transferred to the care of another medical professional.
- Bring any implements of potential self-destruction you may have found at the scene (pill bottles, weapons) to the hospital.
- Acknowledge the patient's feelings. Don't argue with the wish to die, but provide honest reassurance. ("It's not unusual for a person to feel like you do after losing someone close to them. Sometimes it helps to talk about it.")
- If the patient refuses transport, try to involve persons close to him or her in eliciting cooperation. If resistance persists, it may be necessary to obtain police assistance.

When a person has *attempted* suicide, medical treatment has priority. The patient who has taken an overdose of sedative or depressant drugs must be managed for possible respiratory depression or circulatory collapse; the patient who has slashed his or her wrists must be treated to control bleeding and restore circulating volume. Nonetheless, if the patient is conscious, try to establish communication and ask the patient to talk about the situation.

A person who attempts suicide is in enormous distress. Among the most important skills that any health care provider can acquire is the ability to see beyond another person's behavior to the underlying distress. When called to treat a person who has attempted suicide, it's worthwhile to say to the person, and to remind yourself, "You must have been very unhappy to do something like this. It's time to get some help."

Table 37-7	Medications for Mania
Generic Name	**Trade Name**
Lithium carbonate	Eskalith, Lithane, Lithobid, Lithonate, Lithotabs
Lithium citrate	Cibalith
Carbamazepine	Tegretol
Valproic acid	Depakote

Manic Behavior

Mania is one of the most striking psychiatric conditions. Typically a bystander or family member calls for an ambulance, because the patient is unlikely to believe there's anything wrong. To the contrary, the manic patient is more apt to report being "on top of the world—never felt better in my life." Individuals experiencing mania typically have abnormally exaggerated happiness, joy, or euphoria with hyperactivity and insomnia.

Medications for Mania

Drug therapy for bipolar (manic-depressive) disorder usually requires multiple medications **Table 37-7 ▲**. Antianxiety drugs may help reduce agitation or anxiety, while antipsychotic drugs may help reduce psychomotor activity and delusions or hallucinations. Antidepressants may help reduce depression. While these agents may be used for a limited period of time, mood stabilizers are considered lifetime therapy for bipolar patients. Lithium carbonate and valproic acid (Depakote) are most often used as first-line therapy. Unfortunately, some patients taking lithium preparations develop symptoms of toxicity, including nausea and vomiting, dysarthria, tremors, and lethargy. Lithium toxicity may lead to brain damage if not treated, so patients showing signs of toxicity require medical attention. Antiepileptic medications such as valproic acid (Depakote) or carbamazepine (Tegretol) are frequently used for lithium nonresponders, who account for 20% to 40% of bipolar patients.

The Mental Status Examination in the Manic Patient

In manic patients, the MSE is likely to reveal the following findings:

- **Consciousness**—awake and alert, but easily distracted. The patient may complain of an inability to concentrate.
- **Orientation to time and place**—commonly disturbed in manic patients.
- **Activity**—markedly hyperactive. Almost all manic patients report a significantly decreased need for sleep, and they may go for days without sleeping.
- **Speech**—pressured and rapid. The patient is also very talkative.
- **Thought**—flight of ideas and delusions of grandeur. Patients may report that their thoughts are racing; their monologues may skip rapidly from one topic to another (tangential thinking). Their ideas are often grandiose, such as unrealistic plans to embark on a large business venture or to run for high public office. Patients may also believe that they have special powers or they are famous and wealthy.
- **Memory**—usually intact in manics, but may be distorted by underlying delusions.

You are the Provider Part 4

You establish a 20-gauge IV of normal saline in the patient's right hand to keep the vein open. You contact the hospital via cell phone and notify them of your patient's status. Hospital personnel in turn contact the crisis response team and other mental health professionals who will evaluate the patient in the emergency department.

Upon arrival at the emergency department, you are met by a nurse and a security guard. They are very calm and compassionate, and the patient readily trusts both of them. He remains calm throughout your stay there, even falling asleep just before you leave for another call.

Reassessment	Recording Time: 20 Minutes
Skin	Warm, pink and slightly moist
Pulse	90 beats/min, regular
Blood pressure	138/68 mm Hg
Respirations	20 breaths/min
Sao₂	100% ambient air
Temperature	37°C
Pupils	4 mm/PEARRL
Blood glucose	90 mg/dL
ECG	Sinus rhythm

8. How can your professionalism and general demeanor affect patient care in scenarios such as these?

9. What would you tell the hospital in your radio report to help personnel there prepare for the patient?

- **Affect**—an apparently elated affect (the hallmark of mania). The patient seems to be on a "high," and is unusually and infectiously cheerful. The good cheer may be quite brittle, however, and the person may quickly become irritable, sarcastic, and hostile with very little provocation.
- **Perception**—may be disturbed. A person having an acute manic episode may show psychotic symptoms such as hallucinations.

Management of the Manic Patient

Individuals experiencing acute manic episodes have a high probability of getting themselves into trouble of one sort or another—for example, going on wild spending sprees, making foolish business investments, driving recklessly, committing sexual indiscretions, or picking fights. Generally it is when the person has gotten into some sort of trouble, or when his or her behavior has become intolerably disruptive, that an ambulance is summoned.

Because manic patients are unlikely to consider themselves ill, they may not agree that they need treatment. In dealing with the manic patient, be calm, firm, and patient; don't argue or get into a power struggle. Minimize external stimulation. Talk to the patient in a quiet place, away from other people. (Meanwhile, have your partner obtain the history separately from relatives or bystanders.) When it's time to transport, don't use sirens.

If the patient refuses transport, consult medical control. Obtain police assistance for transport if your medical director indicates that hospital evaluation is necessary.

Personality Disorders

According to the American Psychiatric Association, personality disorders are "enduring patterns of perceiving, relating to and thinking about the environment and one's self that are exhibited in a wide range of social and personal contexts" and are "inflexible and maladaptive, and cause significant functional impairment or subjective distress." Common definitions of "personality" include the ways a person behaves or thinks. How people think or behave in the world and with others may be suspicious, outgoing, fearful, or overly dramatic. When these ways of relating to others become dysfunctional or cause distress to other people, that person is considered to have a personality disorder. Many times the person with the personality disorder doesn't feel any subjective distress but such distress may be acutely felt by others. The *Diagnostic and Statistical Manual of Mental Disorders, Fourth Edition, Text Revision (DSM IV TR),* classifies personality disorders into three categories: odd or eccentric disorders; dramatic, emotional or erratic disorders; and anxious or fearful disorders.

True personality disorders are rare in the general population. When a person does have a personality disorder, another psychiatric illness is likely to be present at the same time. Such patients tend to do poorly during treatment. For example, individuals who are depressed in addition to having a personality disorder usually have more difficulty managing the depression.

EMS providers will have difficulty influencing personality disorders over the long term because of their limited interaction with patients. Nevertheless, they need to understand these abnormal behaviors to be aware of how they should react in the current situation. A patient with an antisocial personality will not think twice about hurting you if agitated. One with a histrionic personality may be demanding and dictate the level of care. Be calm and professional in your interactions with patients exhibiting these traits.

Somatoform Disorders

People who are overly concerned with their physical health and appearance may have a somatoform disorder if their preoccupation dominates their life. A hypochondriac provides the classic example of a somatoform disorder. In hypochondriasis, patients have a great deal of anxiety or fear that they may have a serious disease. They are so convinced that they're ill that even a physician can't convince them otherwise. Although the problem in hypochondriasis is anxiety, the individual is preoccupied with other supposed symptoms. With somatization disorder, individuals also have multiple complaints, but are more concerned with the symptoms than with their meaning. In conversion disorders, a physical problem (eg, paralysis, blindness, or seizures) has no identifiable pathophysiology, but results from malingering or faking a physical disorder.

Similar to conversion disorder and malingering are factitious disorders, in which the symptoms the patient is experiencing are under voluntary control but there is no obvious reason for producing the symptoms except to assume the "sick role" and receive extra attention. This type of behavior has also been referred to as Munchausen syndrome. When a parent (typically a mother) intentionally makes a child sick to garner attention and pity, it is referred to as factitious disorder by proxy or Munchausen syndrome by proxy. This is an atypical form of child abuse.

Dissociative Disorders

People who have mild feelings of being detached from themselves, as if they were dreaming, are said to be having a dissociative experience. When this dissociation becomes so intense that they lose their identity and assume new ones or are unable to function because they have lost their memory or sense of reality, a dissociative disorder may be present. Somatoform and dissociative disorders have been linked historically and share many common traits. Management of these patients centers on careful observation to prevent injury and management of symptomatic signs and symptoms based on local protocols. Because treatment to correct the disorder is difficult and often unsuccessful, it should be carried out in the safety and security of a hospital. Talk with the patient about what is happening so you have detailed information to report to the hospital staff.

A stressful event, exhaustion, or physical or mental pressures—usually extreme in nature—may cause a feeling of dreaming or slow motion. These alterations in perceptions of reality are often referred to as dissociative experiences; they can be either mild and readily explained or extraordinarily frightening. Two types of experiences are distinguished—depersonalization and derealization. As a paramedic, you may have responded to a horrible automobile crash where a patient described the event as "dreamlike" or "as if time had stopped." In such a case of depersonalization, the patient loses his or her own sense of reality. In derealization, objects seem to change size or shape; people may seem dead or behave like robots. In their most severe forms, dissociative disorders result in abnormal functioning, amnesia, a trance, or even a new identity (formerly known as multiple personality disorder).

Eating, Impulse Control, and Substance-Related Disorders

Disorders of personal control, motivation, and substance use generally evolve over a relatively long period of time. Because of the chronic nature of these problems, EMS will typically be called when an acute exacerbation of the underlying problem occurs—for example, when a bulimic patient experiences electrolyte imbalances that produce a sudden onset of weakness, dizziness, cardiac or respiratory complaints, or seizures, or when an alcoholic suffers respiratory depression from binge drinking. Emergency management of these patients typically focuses on treating symptomatic complaints and the presenting signs and symptoms.

Eating Disorders

Eating disorders have been around for many decades, although their incidence began to increase rapidly in the 1950s and 1960s. Today, eating disorders are widespread in the developed world and are emerging as a problem in developing countries: Some countries are experiencing a fourfold increase in eating disorders. Individuals most likely to be affected by these disorders are young females of upper-middle-class or upper-class socioeconomic status who live in socially competitive surroundings.

There are two major types of eating disorders: bulimia nervosa and anorexia nervosa. In both forms, individuals may experience severe electrolyte imbalances leading to cardiac problems, seizures, and renal failure as well as less severe erosion of dental enamel and salivary gland enlargement. Anxiety, depression, and substance abuse disorders are noted in as many as two thirds of those diagnosed with eating disorders.

Bulimia nervosa is characterized by consumption of large amounts of food, typically more junk food than fruits and vegetables; many individuals with this disorder describe their eating as "out of control." Most patients compensate for the binge eating by using purging techniques such as vomiting, laxatives, diuretics, or excessive exercise. Individuals with bulimia are humiliated by both their problem and their lack of control.

People with anorexia differ from those with bulimia in one important characteristic—they are successful at losing weight. Unfortunately, they are so effective at losing weight that they jeopardize their health and even their lives. They may even

binge, albeit on smaller quantities of food. These individuals diet by exerting extraordinary control over their eating. The typical anorexic has decreased body weight based on age and height, demonstrates an intense fear of obesity even though the person is underweight, and experiences amenorrhea (the absence of menstruation).

Impulse Control Disorders

Individuals who have impulse control disorders lack the ability to resist a temptation or can't avoid acting on a drive. Examples of impulse control disorders include intermittent explosive disorder (acting on aggressive impulses involving the destruction of property), kleptomania (acting on the urge to steal things), pyromania (acting on the urge to set fires), and pathological gambling.

Of course, not every arsonist is a pyromaniac, nor is everyone who steals a kleptomaniac. Impulse control disorders are typically associated with other disorders, such as depression, antisocial or borderline personality disorders, and Alzheimer's disease. Treatment relies on cognitive and behavioral interventions to identify underlying triggers and influences. This group of disorders is rare; only 4% of arsonists are diagnosed with pyromania, for example.

Substance-Related Disorders

Substance-related disorders include psychological disorders associated with the use of alcohol, cigarettes, illicit drugs, and other substances that change the way a person feels, behaves, or thinks. These disorders have been known for thousands of years and now cost thousands of lives and billions of dollars annually. It was not until 1980 that substance-related disorders were recognized as a complex biological and psychological problem rather than a sign of moral weakness, however. An estimated 8% of the US population used illegal drugs in 2003.

Substance-related disorders are regarded on four levels. In substance use, a person may use moderate amounts of a substance without seriously affecting ADLs (eg, a social drinker). Substance intoxication describes use that results in impaired thinking and motor function (eg, a drunk driver). Substance abuse occurs when the use of a substance disrupts ADLs (eg, a person has difficulty with work, school, or relationships). Substance dependence describes an addiction to a substance. The person is physiologically dependent and requires increasingly larger amounts to produce the same effect. An addict may display "drug-seeking behaviors" such as the repeated use of the substance or taking desperate measures to ingest more of the substance (stealing money, standing out in the cold for a smoke).

Determining the most effective treatment for substance-related disorders requires an integrative approach of examining the social, biological, cultural, cognitive, and psychological dimensions of the problem. As a paramedic, it will be difficult to explore these areas during a short transport to the hospital, particularly given that much of your time will be devoted to ensuring the safety of your crew and the patient's ABCs. Understanding the complex nature of substance-related disorders is the first step in providing professional, competent, and compassionate care to the homeless drug addict as well as the substance-dependent businessperson.

Psychosis

Psychosis is a state of delusion in which the individual is out of touch with reality. Affected people are tuned into their own internal reality of ideas and feelings, which they mistake for the reality of the external world. To the person experiencing a psychotic episode, the line differentiating reality from fantasy is blurred—not distinct, as it is in those without psychoses. That internal reality may make patients belligerent and angry toward others. Alternatively, they may become mute and withdrawn as they give all their attention to the voices and feelings within. Psychoses or psychotic episodes occur for many reasons; the use of mind-altering substances is one of the most common causes, and that experience may be limited to the duration of the substance within the body. Other causes include intense stress, delusional disorders, and, more commonly, schizophrenia. Some psychotic episodes last for brief periods; others last a lifetime.

Schizophrenia

Schizophrenia is a complex disorder that is neither easily defined nor readily treated, yet has a dramatic effect on society. One in 100 people will be affected by schizophrenia in their lifetimes. An estimated 0.2% to 1.5% of the world's population has schizophrenia. The typical onset occurs during early adulthood, with dysfunctional symptoms becoming more prominent over time. Some individuals diagnosed with schizophrenia display signs during early childhood; their disease may be associated with brain damage suffered early in life. Other influences thought to contribute to this disorder include genetics, neurobiological influences, and psychological and social influences.

Persons with schizophrenia may experience positive, negative, or disorganized symptoms. Positive symptoms include delusions and hallucinations. Negative symptoms (a lack of normal behavior) include apathy, mutism, a flat affect, and a lack of interest in pleasure. Disorganized symptoms include erratic speech, emotional responses, and motor behavior.

Schizophrenia can be divided into several subclasses. The paranoid type is characterized by delusions or hallucinations usually centered on a specific theme, while cognitive functions remain intact. Individuals with the disorganized type of schizophrenia usually display the wrong emotion for a particular situation and are often self-absorbed. Patients with the catatonic type display odd motor activity, such as strange expressions in their face or remaining rigid, while the undifferentiated type features behaviors that don't fit neatly into another category.

Medications for Psychosis

Antipsychotic drugs are separated into two groups: atypical antipsychotic (AAP) agents and typical (traditional) antipsychotic agents (also known as neuroleptics). Both classes are prescribed to control psychotic symptoms, no matter what their cause. Antipsychotic medications are listed in **Table 37-8 ▶**.

Table 37-8	Antipsychotic Medications	
Type	**Generic Name**	**Trade Name**
Atypical antipsychotic (AAP) agents	Clozapine	Clozaril
	Olanzapine	Zyprexa
	Quetiapine	Seroquel
	Risperidone	Risperidal
	Ziprasidone	Geodon
	Aripiprazole	Abilify
Traditional antipsychotics	Chlorpromazine	Thorazine
	Chlorprothixene	Taractan
	Fluphenazine	Prolixin, Permitil
	Haloperidol	Haldol
	Loxapine	Loxitane, Daxolin
	Mesoridazine	Serentil
	Molindone	Moban
	Perphenazine	Trilafon
	Thioridazine	Mellaril
	Thiothixene	Navane
	Trifluoperazine	Stelazine

Patients taking typical antipsychotic agents may occasionally experience an acute dystonic reaction, in which the individual develops muscle spasms of the neck, face, and back within a few days of starting treatment with the drug. An acute dystonic reaction can be rapidly corrected by giving diphenhydramine (Benadryl), 25 to 50 mg IV, but the muscle spasms are apt to recur after the diphenhydramine wears off. Neuroleptics also have atropine-like effects (anticholinergic effects), so patients taking antipsychotic medications may suffer the side effects associated with atropine use, such as dry mouth, blurred vision, urinary retention, and cardiac dysrhythmias.

The AAP agents are often used as first-line therapy because they not only relieve symptoms such as delusions and hallucinations but also enhance the quality of life for schizophrenics by improving the affective symptoms of anxiety and depression and decreasing suicidal tendencies. However, the AAP medications may cause metabolic side effects such as glucose deregulation, hypercholesterolemia, and hypertension.

The Mental Status Examination of the Psychotic Patient

The most characteristic feature of psychosis is a profound thought disorder, often accompanied by disturbances in mood and perception. The following list outlines disturbances of mood and perception.

- **Consciousness.** The psychotic is awake and alert, but may be easily distracted, especially if paying attention to hallucinations. If the level of consciousness is fluctuating, suspect an organic brain syndrome.

- **Orientation.** Disturbances in orientation are more common in organic disorders than in psychoses, but the severely psychotic patient may be disoriented as to time and place.
- **Activity.** Activity is most commonly accelerated, with agitation and hyperactivity, but can be retarded. Bizarre, stereotyped movements are common.
- **Speech.** Speech may be pressured or sound strange because of unusual words that the patient has invented (neologisms).
- **Thought.** Thought is disturbed in progression and content and may show any of the following disorders:
  - Flight of ideas, the headlong plunge from one thought to another.
  - Loosening of associations, in which the logical connection between one idea and the next becomes obscure, at least to the listener. In extreme cases, the patient's speech may be entirely incomprehensible.
  - Delusions, especially of persecution.
  - Thought broadcasting (the belief that thoughts are broadcast aloud and can be heard by others.)
  - Thought insertion (the belief that thoughts are being thrust into his or her mind by another person) and thought withdrawal (the belief that thoughts are being removed).
- **Memory.** Memory can be relatively or entirely intact in psychosis. It may be difficult to obtain the cooperation of the patient for formal memory testing.
- **Affect and mood.** Mood is likely to be disturbed in psychosis. The disturbance may take the form of euphoria, sadness, or wide swings in mood; affect may reflect those inner states or be flat.
- **Perception.** Auditory hallucinations are common in psychosis. Patients hear voices commenting on their behavior or telling them what to do. Suspect that patients are hearing such voices when they seem to be attending a conversation other than yours or talking to themselves.

Management of the Patient With Psychotic Symptoms

Dealing with a psychotic patient is difficult. The usual methods of reasoning with a patient are unlikely to be effective, because the psychotic person has his or her own rules of logic that may be quite different from those that govern nonpsychotic thinking. Furthermore, the paramedic is likely to feel uncomfortable in the presence of a psychotic person. Those uncomfortable feelings are one of your built-in diagnostic instruments. They are elicited by the fear, suspicion, and hostility that the patient is

Notes from Nancy

Warning! The patient who hears voices commanding him to hurt himself or others must be considered dangerous.

broadcasting through body language. Use your uncomfortable feelings to help make a tentative diagnosis of a psychotic problem. Then proceed as follows:

- *Assess the situation for danger* to yourself or others.
- *Identify yourself clearly*, and explain your mission. ("I'm Gloria Goodheart. I'm a paramedic with the ambulance service, and this is my partner, Stan Steadfast. We've come to see if we can help. Can you tell us about your problem?")
- *Be calm, direct, and straightforward*. Your calmness and confidence can do a great deal toward calming the patient.
- *Maintain an emotional distance*. Don't touch the patient, and don't be overly friendly or effusively reassuring. Convey an attitude of emotional neutrality.
- *Don't argue*. Don't challenge patients regarding the reality of their beliefs or the validity of their perceptions. Don't go along with their delusions simply to humor them, but don't make an issue of the delusions either. Talk about real things.
- *Explain your expectations of the patient*. ("We're not going to let you hurt anyone with that baseball bat. . . .")
- *Explain each step of management*. ("Let's walk downstairs to the ambulance.")
- *Involve people the patient trusts*, such as family or friends, in managing the patient and gaining cooperation.

Special Considerations

Pediatric Behavioral Problems

Behavioral disorders are estimated to affect as many as one in five children and adolescents, with two thirds of those having a mental health problem not receiving proper treatment. When not treated properly, such a problem will most likely persist into adulthood. Given that suicide is the third leading cause of death in adolescents and the seventh leading cause of death in school-aged children, more attention has been given to mood disorders, anxiety, and other behavioral problems in this population. Children are also more likely to have coexisting problems (eg, attention deficit hyperactivity disorder, conduct disorder, and oppositional defiant disorder) along with the more traditional mental health disorders.

Mental health problems in children are difficult to diagnose because the lines between normal and abnormal behavior are less clear in this population. Diagnosis and treatment may be difficult when trying to distinguish between organic, genetic, and environmental causes. Cultural and ethnic factors also blur the line between normal and abnormal coping mechanisms. The mental status assessment of the child is similar to that of an adult, but takes the child's developmental level into consideration. Abnormal findings in the developmental and MSE are often related to adjustment disorders and stress rather than the more serious disorders. Your assessment must

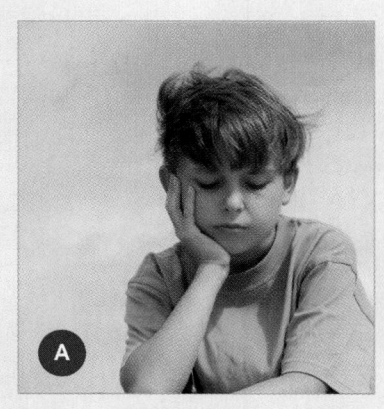

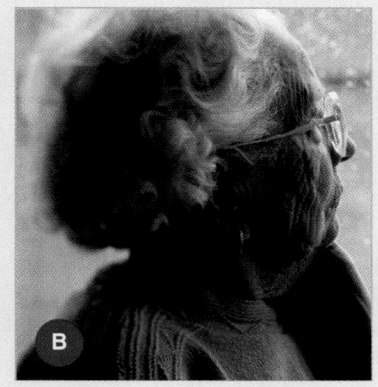

Figure 37-9 Children as well as older adults are affected by behavioral problems.

include an assessment of suicide risk in any child 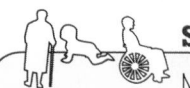.

Geriatric Behavioral Problems

As people age, they are exposed to new experiences and alterations to routines that may have become well established over the course of many years. Some of these experiences may result in physical and psychological changes in the older adult. For example, dementia, a gradual loss of mental capabilities, may result from Alzheimer's disease, chronic alcohol abuse, aftereffects of multiple strokes, or nutritional deficiencies. The loss of loved ones or family moving away may cause loneliness. Financial worries, dissatisfaction with living arrangements, or doubts about the significance of one's life accomplishments may become a significant concern as well. These issues often produce psychological distress and physical pain, which may manifest as abnormal behavior. Anxiety disorders, substance abuse disorders (particularly alcohol abuse), and mood disorders such as depression and even suicide are common among older people.

An elderly person is less likely to be accurately diagnosed with a mental illness than a similarly affected younger person. All too often, anxiety and depression are incorrectly considered a normal part of aging. Agism is discrimination against older people because of their age. To avoid engaging in agism and to provide proper care for the geriatric population, particularly those with mental health issues, you must first take stock of your own attitudes toward older people and the mentally ill. With this awareness, you will be able to perform a complete physical and psychosocial assessment without bias, and will understand the complex issues surrounding the care of older people.

▌Hostile and Violent Patients

Few situations are as difficult for the paramedic as dealing with a hostile, angry patient. It takes a great deal of maturity and a lot of experience to understand that anger may be a response to illness and aggressive behavior may be the patient's way of dealing with feelings of helplessness. Sometimes the patient seems to be implying, "There's something very wrong with me, and you're not doing everything possible to help." The temptation is to respond with anger, but doing so rarely serves any useful purpose. Most angry patients can be calmed by a trained person who conveys an impression of confidence that the patient will behave well. It may be helpful to ask the patient directly about his or her anger: "Can you explain why you're so angry with me?" Giving the patient a chance to talk about these feelings often enables the patient to gain mastery over those feelings.

A patient who is violent or threatening violence poses one of the most difficult management problems for EMS personnel. Most EMTs and paramedics see themselves as caregivers, not as "heavies," and often find themselves unprepared—both psychologically and tactically—to deal with hostile or violent behavior. Furthermore, the encounter with a violent patient carries the constant risk that someone may get hurt—the patient, a bystander, the paramedics, or all of them. The best way to ensure that no one is harmed is to take preventive action—that is, to assess the potential for violence in *every* call and to take steps to prevent violence from happening.

Assessing the potential for violence is not merely an academic exercise. A 1993 survey of EMS agencies in 25 US cities reported high rates of violence against on-duty EMS personnel. In Chicago, for example, 92% of the fire department paramedics reported that they had been assaulted at least once

Special Considerations

Many law enforcement agencies use TASER® devices Figure 37-10 ▶ to immobilize people who are behaving in a violent or aggressive manner. TASER® devices were designed as an alternative to more violent immobilization methods. There is some controversy in the use of these weapons in the in-custody death phenomenon. There is data supporting the assertion that these weapons are temporally, but not causally, related to these deaths in custody. More studies are being done. EMS personnel need to be aware that many of the patients subjected to a TASER® exposure are at high risk for medical problems due to the underlying condition which is affecting their behavior. It is important for EMS personnel to identify these underlying conditions and to ensure appropriate medical care. Conditions to be vigilant for include: drug overdose syndromes, excited delirium, acute psychiatric decompensation, hypoglycemia, heat stroke, hepatic encephalopathy, seizure disorders, dementia, and encephalitis. Police officers are not routinely trained to recognize these conditions, and will rely on EMS personnel to make appropriate disposition decisions at the scene.

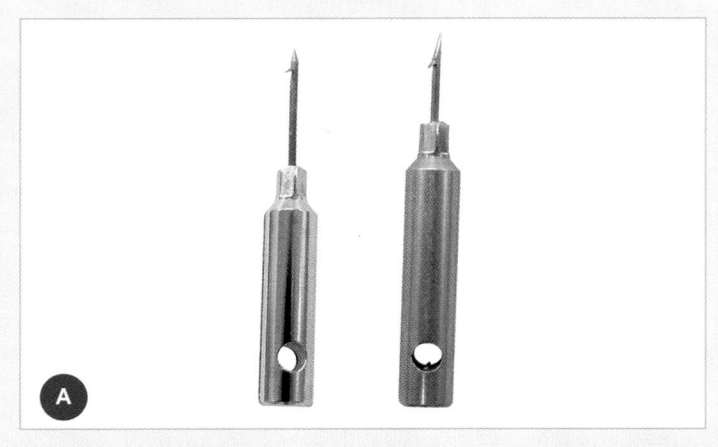
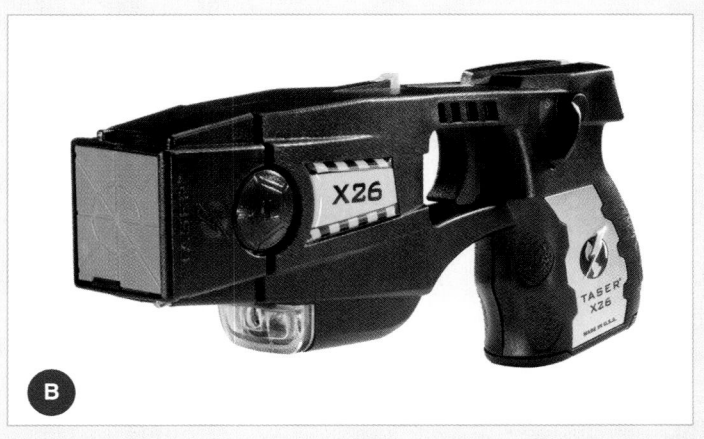

Figure 37-10 A. TASER® probes. **B.** TASER® Electronic Control Device.

while on duty (68% sustained blunt trauma, 33% were cut or stabbed, and 64% were shot at). The paramedic who does *not* look out for a possible violent encounter may become a statistic like those just cited.

Identifying Situations With the Potential for Violence

Preventive action starts with being psychologically prepared for a possible violent encounter and keeping that possibility somewhere in the back of your mind in your response to *every* call. Don't rely too heavily on the information you get from your dispatcher—the "old woman with a possible stroke" may have a disgruntled son with an M-16 rifle! Being psychologically prepared for violence does *not* mean becoming paranoid or treating every patient with distrust. It *does* mean developing a "nose for danger," also known as "survival awareness."

Risk Factors for Violence

Scenarios in which violence is more likely to occur include any situation where alcohol or illicit drugs are being consumed (eg, tavern, party), crowd incidents, and incidents in which violence has already occurred (eg, shooting, stabbing, domestic disturbances). People who are more likely to be violent include those who are intoxicated with alcohol or drugs (especially PCP, LSD, amphetamines, and cocaine), experiencing withdrawal from alcohol or drugs, psychotic (especially manic and paranoid types), or delirious from any cause (eg, hypoglycemia, sepsis).

The most important clues to the patient's potential for violence are found in the individual's behavior and body language. Look for these warning signals:

- **Posture**—the patient who sits tensely at the edge of the chair or grips at the armrest.
- **Speech**—loud, critical, threatening, full of profanity.

- **Motor activity**—unable to sit still; pacing back and forth or in circles; easily startled.
- **Other body language**—clenched fists, avoidance of eye contact, turning away when spoken to.
- **Your own feelings**—your own "gut" response to the patient. If your instinct tells you that you're in danger, pay attention!

Management of the Violent Patient

Once you have concluded, for *any* reason, that there is a potential for violence in a situation, take the following steps.

Assess the whole situation. Are factors in the surroundings contributing to the escalation of violence (eg, friends who are egging the patient on)? Can those factors be removed? Does evidence suggest drug use, alcohol use, head injury, or diabetes? Can anyone present give you some background information? (Did the patient's behavior come on gradually or suddenly? Does he or she have a history of violent behavior? Are there any known medical problems, such as diabetes?)

Observe your surroundings. Make sure you have an escape route. Place yourself between the patient and the door, but don't move behind an agitated patient. Don't turn your back on the patient—not even for a moment. Note any furniture or other potential barriers. Scan the area for anything that could be used as a weapon (eg, heavy or sharp objects) if the level of violence escalates. If a violent patient is armed with a weapon, don't try to deal with the situation yourself; back off and notify law enforcement authorities. Make sure that others at the scene are not endangered while you await the arrival of the police.

Maintain a safe distance. Moving too close to a potentially violent patient is likely to increase his or her anxiety level. Maintain a safety zone of two arm lengths; if the patient is backing away from you, it's a sign that you're too close. Let the patient find a comfortable distance. Don't position yourself

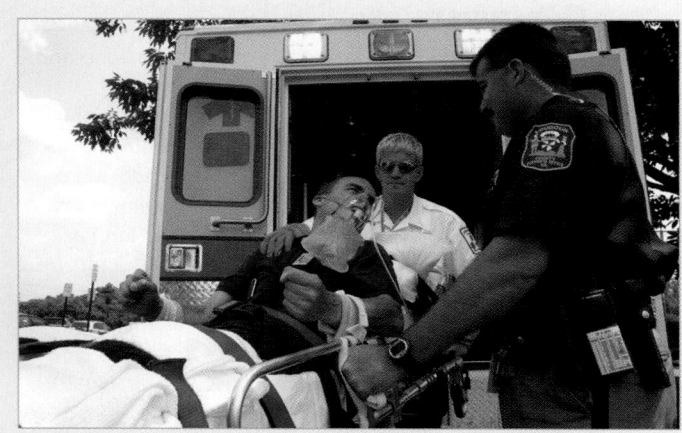

Figure 37-11 You may use physical restraints only to protect yourself or others or to prevent a patient from causing injury to himself or herself.

directly face-to-face with the patient but rather slightly to the side at a 45° angle, with your escape route unobstructed.

Try verbal restraints first. Anger and aggressive behavior are often responses to illness or to feelings of helplessness. Just talking to the angry person in a calm, sympathetic way may defuse some of the anger.

- Take a moment to concentrate your own thoughts so that you can convey an impression of calmness and self-control to the patient.
- Identify yourselves as medical personnel who are there to try to help. Keep your voice low—that forces the patient to stop what he or she is doing to focus on what you are saying.
- Acknowledge the patient's behavior, and restate your willingness to help. ("You look very upset. How can we help you?").
- Encourage the patient to talk about what is bothering him or her. *Listen* to what is said, and *show* that you are listening by paraphrasing the words back to the patient. ("I think I understand. Are you saying that . . .?")
- Ask the patient specifically if he or she might lose control or is carrying any sort of weapon.
- Define your expectations of the patient's behavior. Acknowledge his or her potential to do harm ("You could really hurt someone with that crowbar . . ."), but assure the patient that losing control won't be permitted.
- If "verbal de-escalation" isn't working, back off and get help. ("Look, I've been trying to talk to you for the past 15 minutes and we're just going in circles. I'm going to leave you alone for a few minutes and see if you can get hold of yourself. When I come back, we'll try talking again, but if that still doesn't work, I'm going to have some people with me to keep you from hurting anyone.")

When verbal restraint fails, use physical restraint Figure 37-11 ▲ . Some restraint devices may be improvised

from materials on the ambulance; others are commercially made from leather or nylon that is padded for comfort and safety. Most commercial restraints are applied to the wrists and ankles to prevent movement of the arms and legs. Some are placed around the waist to restrict movement of the torso. Vest-type restraints are applied from the front of the patient and may include sleeves to restrain the arms from moving. Make sure you are familiar with the restraints used by your agency before you enter a situation requiring their application.

Make sure you have sufficient personnel before you attempt to overpower the patient. You will need police assistance. In most jurisdictions, paramedics (or anyone else) are not allowed to restrain or transport persons against their will except possibly at the express order of a county mental health physician. You must have overwhelming force to apply a physical restraint, which means a *minimum* of five trained, able-bodied people— one for each limb (assign a specific limb in advance to each responder) and one for the head. Appoint one leader, who will direct the team and maintain verbal contact with the patient.

Sometimes the show of force may be enough to calm the patient. The mere sight of five 6′ police officers, for example, has been known to have a remarkably tranquilizing effect on even the most belligerent patient. Don't move toward the patient immediately; give him or her a chance to make a graceful retreat to a nonviolent alternative behavior.

If the show of force doesn't calm the patient down (eg, someone under the influence of drugs such as PCP), you must move quickly to restrain the patient. First, remove any equipment or jewelry from your own person that could be used as a weapon (eg, name badge, scissors worn on the belt, key chain, earrings). Make sure you have adequate restraining devices— preferably padded leather or nylon restraints—immediately available. Then, at a signal from the leader, move in *fast* from the patient's sides. Grasp the patient at the elbows, knees, and head, and apply restraints to all four extremities. Probably the best position in which to secure the patient to the stretcher is supine, with legs spread-eagled and both arms secured to one side of the stretcher. This position will turn the patient's head to the side, so that he or she won't aspirate in case of vomiting. Never "hog tie" a patient (tying the ankles and wrists together as one); this type of restraint has been known to result in death. Never "hobble tie" a patient (tying just the feet together). Placing a patient face down in a Reeves stretcher can also be dangerous and lead to positional asphyxia or aspiration.

Throughout the entire restraint procedure and transport, the leader should maintain verbal contact with the patient, even if the patient does not appear to be paying attention to what you're saying. When only the leader speaks, the patient can focus on what the leader is saying. This will decrease the amount of stimuli experienced by the patient. Avoid being bitten by the patient during the restraining procedure. Once the restraints are in place, don't remove them. Don't negotiate or make deals. If the patient is spitting, you can place an oxygen mask over the face with a normal flow rate.

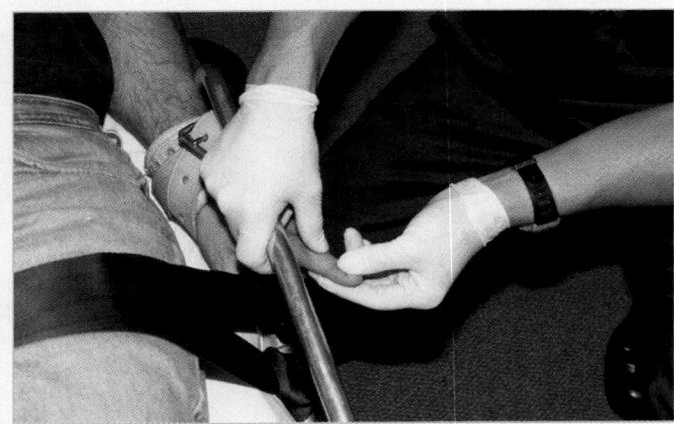

Figure 37-12 Assess circulation frequently while a patient is restrained.

Check the patient's peripheral circulation every few minutes to make sure the restraints aren't too tight Figure 37-12 ▲. Check the radial pulses in the arms and the dorsalis pedis pulses in the feet.

Document everything in the patient's chart—the reasons for using restraints (be specific, giving examples of the patient's behavior and the indications of the violence potential); the number of people used to subdue the patient; the restraining devices used; and the status of the peripheral circulation after restraints were applied.

Proper restraint is summarized in the following steps, shown in Skill Drill 37-1 ▶:

1. Assemble four or five rescuers and have the stretcher or carrying device and soft restraints (wide cloth or commercial leather restraints) nearby Step 1.
2. Designate a leader who will communicate with both the team and the patient.

Controversies

Physical restraint is not without complications and hazards. One alternative is to use chemical restraints, although this option should be used only with medical control approval following local protocols. Until recently, benzodiazepines, droperidol, and haloperidol were the only medications available for chemical restraint in the prehospital arena. The Food and Drug Administration has issued a black box warning for droperidol due to its association with prolonged QT syndromes. Benzodiazepines and haloperidol carry their own risks. Newer atypical antipsychotic (AAP) agents, such as the injectable ziprasidone (Geodon), hold promise for preventing injuries to patients and providers.

3. Assign positions to each team member: four extremities and the head Step 2.
4. If possible, corner the patient in a safe area with the least obstruction and no glass Step 3.
5. On the direction of the team leader, who will be talking to the patient calmly, move together toward the patient Step 4.
6. Each team member should grasp the assigned body part and carefully, with the least amount of force, bring the patient to the ground Step 5.
7. Carefully place the patient on the stretcher or carrying device in a face-up position Step 6.
8. Tie the patient with soft restraints at each wrist and ankle as well as over the chest and pelvis with sheets Step 7. If the patient is spitting, place an oxygen mask or surgical mask on his or her face.

Skill Drill 37-1: Restraining a Patient

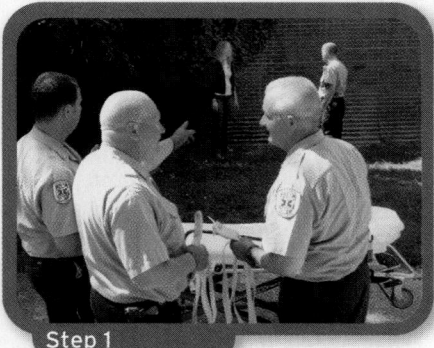

Step 1

Assemble 4 or 5 rescuers and have the stretcher or carrying device and soft restraints nearby. Designate a leader.

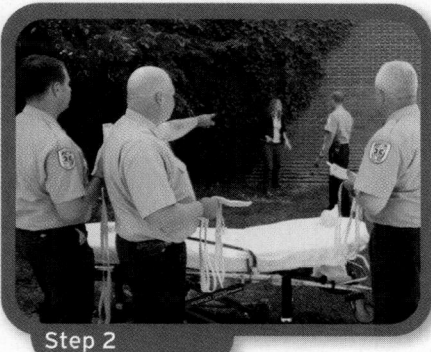

Step 2

Assign positions to each team member: four extremities and the head.

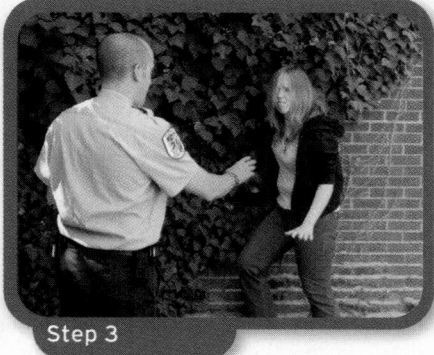

Step 3

If possible, corner the patient in a safe area.

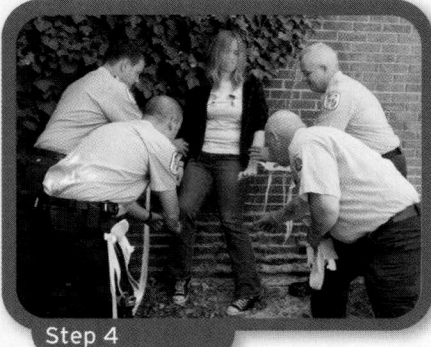

Step 4

On the direction of the team leader, move together toward the patient.

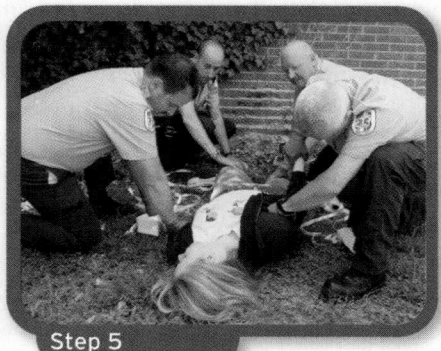

Step 5

Each team member should grasp the assigned body part and carefully, with the least amount of force, bring the patient to the ground.

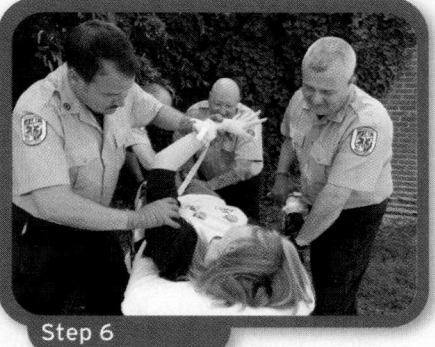

Step 6

Carefully place the patient on the stretcher or carrying device in a face-up position.

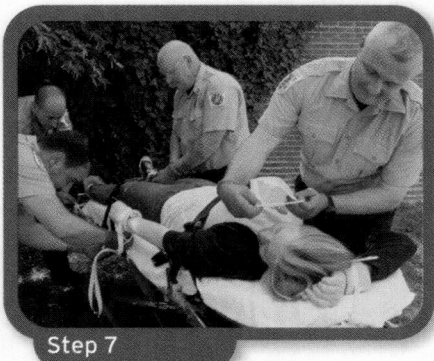

Step 7

Tie the patient with soft restraints at each wrist and ankle as well as the chest and pelvis with sheets. If the patient is spitting, place an oxygen mask or surgical mask on his or her face.

You are the Provider Summary

1. What are some medical conditions that can give the appearance of "acting crazy"?

Abnormal behavior may have many medical causes. It is very important to look at all of the possible reasons that could result in combative and aggressive behavior. Hypoxia and hypoglycemia are two of the most common underlying medical conditions that can manifest themselves in ways similar to this patient's behavior.

2. What are some considerations to discuss with your partner while you stage the scene?

Every situation has a potential for danger. Situations you have been asked to stage in which the police are on scene are even more likely to have problems. Good mental preparation and careful observation of the scene are your best defenses against harm. Follow the lead of the police, but realize that even they are caught off guard at times.

3. What are the medical implications when police control the scene of a violent patient?

When the police are present, they control the scene. Medical responders should follow their direction on when and how to approach. Police officers are not responsible for medical care unless protocol dictates that they are and they are appropriately trained. The most important rule is for everyone to work together to ensure the safety of the responders and safeguard the best interest of the patient.

4. Is it wise to agree with or validate a patient's hallucinations?

If the patient asks you what a dog is saying, truthfully and neutrally answer that you don't hear it. This response does not deny the patient's own experience, but does inform the patient that others are not having the same experience.

5. How important is police involvement if the patient apparently becomes agreeable?

A patient's attitude and general demeanor can change in a flash. You must always consider this potential for change, especially if you will be providing patient care while alone in the back of the ambulance. Ask for escorts, including an officer in the back if you feel it's appropriate. When the patient is restrained, check the extremities every five minutes to ensure that circulation and neurologic function are not compromised.

6. What are the risk factors for suicide, and do they apply in this situation?

This man is in danger of losing his job, he has an altered perception of reality, he is recently divorced, and he is under the influence of drugs. He has several risk factors for suicide even if he doesn't express the intent.

7. Would you talk with Eugene about his comment or wait and let the hospital explore these issues?

Every statement regarding suicide must be taken seriously, even if it's made impulsively or casually. You must determine the patient's seriousness by asking whether he or she has plans or has made preparations. The patient's responses may affect your immediate safety.

8. How can your professionalism and general demeanor affect patient care in scenarios such as these?

Talking with the patient is therapeutic. Take the time to build trust and rapport. Let the patient tell the story in his or her own way. Listen. Don't argue or dispute the nature of reality.

9. What would you tell the hospital in your radio report to help personnel there prepare for the patient?

Hospital personnel need to know the basics of the patient's thinking and state of mind. They also need to know if and why the patient is restrained. If a patient is out of control, the hospital may want additional security or chemical restraints immediately available. Don't bring behavioral emergency patients into the emergency department unannounced.

Prep Kit

■ Ready for Review

- Behavior includes the things we do—how we act or react to situations.
- Behavior may be abnormal as defined by society, your boss, a parent, or friend. Abnormal behavior by itself may not be an emergency.
- In a behavioral emergency, the individual's presenting problem is a disorder of thought, mood, or behavior that interferes with the activities of daily living.
- The behavioral emergency becomes a psychiatric emergency when the patient becomes suicidal, homicidal, or acutely psychotic.
- Abnormal behavior can stem from a situational crisis, organic problems, or psychiatric causes.
- When assessing psychiatric problems, you collect information about the person's state of mind and thinking. Your actions and attitude often provide some of the therapy sought by the patient. Be prepared to spend some time with the patient as you assess his or her thinking.
- Dissociative disorders are characterized by depersonalization (stepping out of one's current experience) and derealization (an altered perception of objects or people in an experience). In the most severe form of dissociative disorders, multiple personalities may emerge.
- The mind generates specific signs and symptoms when it is not functioning well. Paramedics must sharpen their assessment skills to properly identify how the patient is functioning mentally. The COASTMAP mnemonic can be used to remember various disorders of behavior.
- In anxiety disorders, the dominant mood is fear and apprehension. Fear can turn into a phobia when it becomes unreasonable. Anxiety, when sudden and overwhelming, may become a panic disorder. Anxiety, phobias, and panic disorder may complicate your efforts to treat a person.
- Mood disorders are the most common psychiatric disorders. In mania, the patient often feels great to the point of exaggeration, with hyperactivity, insomnia, and grandiose ideas. Feelings of depression can be accompanied by guilt, apathy, and sleep disturbances. Depression may become so severe that the person may attempt suicide.
- Suicide and attempted suicide are problems affecting all age groups and people of all socioeconomic status. Men are often more successful at suicide because they use more lethal means, although women make more attempts. Every suicidal gesture must be assessed and taken very seriously. Don't be afraid to talk with patients about their suicidal thoughts.
- Personality disorders are exaggerations in how people think about or perceive their environment and surroundings. They are classified into three categories: odd or eccentric behaviors; dramatic, emotional, or erratic behaviors; and anxious or fearful behaviors.
- In somatoform disorders, such as factitious disorders and hypochondriasis, patients are overly concerned with their physical health or appearance to the point that this concern dominates their lives.
- Eating disorders, such as anorexia nervosa and bulimia nervosa, are disorders of personal control related to eating. They can result in acute and chronic problems.
- Impulse control disorders include impulsive gambling, kleptomania, and pyromania. They reflect the inability to resist temptation.

- Substance-related disorders are associated with the use of alcohol and drugs. A variety of social, biological, cultural, and physiologic dimensions define substance-related disorders.
- Psychosis is a state of delusion in which individuals are out of touch with reality. Causes include psychiatric problems (eg, schizophrenia), drug-induced psychotic states, and intense stress.
- Individuals with schizophrenia may display positive symptoms (hallucinations and delusions), negative symptoms (apathy and a flat affect), or disorganized symptoms (erratic speech or motor function). Dealing with psychotic patients is difficult because their behavior may be dangerous.
- Disorganization and disorientation describe how conditions may present themselves. Disorganized patients have uncontrolled and disconnected thoughts. They need structure, explanations, and directions. Disoriented patients may not know where they are, what day it is, or even who they are. These patients need continuous orienting.
- Dealing with hostile, combative, and violent patients can be emotionally and physically demanding for emergency responders. Be cautious when approaching these individuals and evaluating situations where violent or potentially violent patients may be. Know the specific risk factors and signs of hostile situations.
- Combative patients may need to be restrained. In such cases, make sure you have enough experienced people and work quickly. Follow the legal guidelines for restraining patients.

■ Vital Vocabulary

activities of daily living (ADLs) Normal everyday activities such as getting dressed, brushing teeth, taking out the garbage, etc.

acute dystonic reaction A syndrome that may occur in patients taking typical antipsychotic agents. The patient develops muscle spasms of the neck, face, and back within a few days of starting treatment with the drug.

affect The outward expression of a person's mood.

agitation Extreme restlessness and anxiety.

agoraphobia Literally, "fear of the marketplace"; fear of entering a public place from which escape may be impeded.

amnesia Loss of memory.

anger A strong, negative emotion that may be a response to illness, and which could result in aggressive behavior on the part of the patient.

anorexia nervosa An eating disorder in which a person diets by exerting extraordinary control over his or her eating, and losses weight to the point of jeopardizing his or her health and life.

antipsychotic drugs Medications used to control psychosis.

anxiety disorder A mental disorder in which the dominant mood is fear and apprehension.

atropine-like effects Results of some antipsychotic medications that include side effects similar to atropine, resulting in dry mouth, blurred vision, urinary retention, and cardiac dysrhythmias.

behavior The way people act or perform, for example how they react/respond to a situation.

behavioral emergencies An emergency in which the patient's presenting problem is some disorder of mood, thought, or behavior that interferes with their activities of daily living (ADLs).

bipolar mood disorder A disorder in which a person alternates between mania and depression.

borderline personality disorder A disorder characterized by disordered images of self, impulsive and unpredictable behavior, marked shifts in mood, and instability in relationships with others.

bulimia nervosa An eating disorder characterized by consumption of large amounts of food, and for which the patient then sometimes compensates by using purging techniques.

catatonic Lacking expression or movement, or appearing rigid.

catatonic type A type of schizophrenia in which the person displays odd motor activity, such as strange facial expression or rigidity.

circumstantial thinking Situation in which a patient includes many irrelevant details in his or her account of things.

compulsion A repetitive action carried out to relieve the anxiety of obsessive thoughts.

confabulation The invention of experiences to cover gaps in memory, seen in patients with certain organic brain syndromes.

confrontation Interviewing technique in which the interviewer points out to the patient something of interest in his/her conversation or behavior.

confusion An impaired understanding of one's surroundings.

delirium An acute confessional state characterized by global impairment of thinking, perception, judgment, and memory.

delusion A fixed belief that is not shared by others of a person's culture or background and that can't be changed by reasonable argument; a false belief.

delusions of grandeur A state in which a person believes oneself to be someone of great importance.

delusions of persecution A state in which a person believes that others are plotting against him or her.

dementia Chronic deterioration of mental function.

depersonalization A type of dissociative disorder in which a person loses his or her sense of reality, and may experience events as being "dream-like."

depression A persistent mood of sadness, despair, and discouragement; may be a symptom of many different mental and physical disorders, or it may be a disorder on its own.

derealization A symptom of a dissociative disorder in which objects seem to change size or shape; people may seem dead or behave like robots when viewed during a moment of acute stress.

disorganization A condition in which a person is characterized by uncontrolled and disconnected thought, is usually incoherent or rambling in speech, and may or may not be oriented to person and place.

disorganized symptoms Refers to erratic speech, emotional responses, and motor behavior.

disorganized type A type of schizophrenia in which the person usually displays the wrong emotion for a particular situation, often self-absorbed.

disorientation Confusion regarding a person's sense of who one is (person), where one is (place), and at what point in time one finds oneself (time).

dissociation Feelings of being detached from yourself, as if you were dreaming.

distractibility The patient's attention is easily diverted.

echolalia Meaningless echoing of the interviewer's words by the patient.

facilitation An interviewing technique in which the interviewer uses noncommittal words and gestures to encourage the patient to proceed.

fear Also sometimes referred to as a phobia, this is an anxious feeling, usually about specific things or situations.

flat Used to describe behavior in which the patient doesn't seem to feel much of anything at all.

flight of ideas Accelerated thinking in which the mind skips very rapidly from one thought to the next.

generalized anxiety disorder (GAD) A disorder in which a person worries about everything for no particular reason, or their worrying is unproductive and they can't decide what to do about an upcoming situation.

hallucination A sense perception not founded on objective reality; a false perception.

illusion A misinterpretation of sensory stimuli.

impulse control disorders A condition in which an individual lacks the ability to resist a temptation or can't stop acting on a drive.

inattention Used to describe patients with whom it is difficult to gain their attention or focus.

labile Used to describe a rapid shift in mood.

loosening of associations A situation in which the logical connection between one idea and the next becomes obscure, at least to the listener.

mania A mental disorder characterized by abnormally exaggerated happiness, joy, or euphoria with hyperactivity, insomnia, and grandiose ideas.

manic-depressive illness A bipolar disorder in which mood fluctuates between depression and mania. The alterations in mood are usually episodic and recurrent.

mental status examination (MSE) A way of measuring the "mental vital signs" in a disturbed patient. The mnemonic COASTMAP can be used to conduct this exam, assessing consciousness, orientation, activity, speech, thought, memory, affect and mood, and perception.

mood A person's sustained and pervasive emotional state.

mood disorder A group of disorders in which the disturbance of mood is accompanied by full or partial manic or depressive syndrome.

mutism The absence of speech.

negative symptoms Evidence of a disease or condition, noted by lack of normal circumstances, rather than the presence of new physical evidence or a physical change; with regard to schizophrenia, refers to a lack of normal behavior, and apathy, mutism, a flat affect, and a lack of interest in pleasure.

neologism An invented word that has meaning only to its inventor.

obsession A persistent idea that a person cannot dismiss from his or her thoughts.

organic brain syndrome Temporary or permanent dysfunction of the brain, caused by a disturbance in the physical or physiologic functioning of brain tissue.

orientation A person's sense of who one is (person), where one is (place), and at what day of the week one finds oneself (day).

paranoid type A type of schizophrenia in which the person experiences delusions or hallucinations usually centered around a specific theme, where their cognitive functions remain intact.

perception The way a person processes the data supplied by the five senses.

perseveration Repeating the same idea over and over again.

personality disorder The term used to describe a condition a person has when he or she behaves or thinks in a way that is dysfunctional or causes distress to other people.

phobia An abnormal and persistent dread of a specific object or situation.

positive symptoms Evidence of or physical change due to a disease or condition, which can be physically noted by the patient or health care provider; with regard to schizophrenia, refers to delusions and hallucinations.

posttraumatic stress disorder (PTSD) A severe form of anxiety that stems from a traumatic experience. PTSD is characterized by the reliving of the stress and nightmares of the original situation.

posture The position of one's body.

pressure of speech Speech in which words seem to tumble out under immense emotional pressure.

psychiatric emergency An emergency in which abnormal behavior threatens an individual's health and safety or the health and safety of another person, for example when a person becomes suicidal, homicidal, or has a psychotic episode.

psychosis A mental disorder characterized by loss of contact with reality.

psychotropic drugs Drugs that affect mood, thought, or behavior.

recall The ability to retrieve a specific piece of stored information on demand.

recognition The ability to identify information that one has encountered before.

registration The ability to add new items to the cerebral data bank.

restlessness A situation in which the patient can't sit still.

retardation of thought The patient seems to take a very long time to get from one thought to the next.

retention The ability to store items in an accessible place in the mind.

simple phobia A fear that is focused on one class of objects (eg, mice, spiders, dogs) or situations (eg, high places, darkness, flying).

somatoform disorder A condition in which a person is overly concerned with physical health and appearance to the point that it dominates his or her life; an example is hypochondria.

stereotyped activity Repetitive movements that don't appear to serve any purpose.

substance abuse Use of a substance that disrupts activities of daily living.

substance dependence Use of a substance that results in addiction and physiologic dependence on the substance.

substance intoxication Use of a substance that results in impaired thinking and motor function.

substance use Use of moderate amounts of a substance without seriously affecting activities of daily living.

suicide Any willful act designed to bring an end to one's own life.

tangential thinking Leaving the current topic midconversation to talk about something else, inhibiting interpersonal communication.

thought broadcasting The belief that others can hear one's thoughts.

thought control The belief that outside forces are controlling one's thoughts.

thought insertion The belief that thoughts are being thrust into one's mind by another person.

thought withdrawal The belief that thoughts are being removed from one's mind.

undifferentiated type Schizophrenia that does not fit neatly into another category.

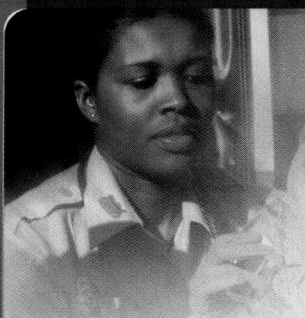

Assessment in Action

Dispatch requests that you respond with the police department to "check the welfare" of an older woman. Dispatch received a call from the woman's niece, who lives out of state. She said her aunt called and told her that her house was being robbed by an "invisible man." This behavior is not normal for her.

On your arrival, the police department has to use force to gain access to the apartment. You find the patient squatting in the corner. She is belligerent and screaming obscenities to the "invisible robber." You spend some time trying to speak with her, but she isn't cooperative. It is time to transport the patient to hospital, but she refuses to go.

1. **This patient is more than likely having a(n) _____ type of behavioral emergency.**
   A. organic
   B. situational
   C. psychiatric
   D. depressive

2. **What type of psychiatric disorder could this be considered?**
   A. Mood disorder
   B. Eating disorder
   C. Somatoform disorder
   D. Schizophrenic/psychotic disorder

3. **Which of the following statements regarding open-ended questions is not true?**
   A. They can lead patients to give a specific answer.
   B. They give patients an opportunity to express themselves.
   C. They encourage better patient responses.
   D. They are less likely to provoke unwanted answers.

4. **Classifications of psychiatric signs and symptoms include:**
   A. disorders of consciousness.
   B. disorders of motor activity.
   C. disorders of speech.
   D. all of the above.

5. **Delusions of persecution fall under which classification?**
   A. Disorders of thinking
   B. Disorders of orientation
   C. Disorders of perception
   D. Disorders of memory

6. **Disorder of perception refers to a:**
   A. person's sense of who one is, where one is, and what time it is.
   B. person's ability to process the data supplied by the five senses.
   C. person's intellectual ability.
   D. person's sustained and pervasive emotional state.

7. **The patient in the above scenario is having which of the following?**
   A. A hallucination
   B. An illusion
   C. Acute depression
   D. Organic symptoms

8. **When examining a patient's mental status, use the mnemonic:**
   A. SAMPLE.
   B. AMPLE.
   C. MSE.
   D. COASTMAP.

9. **Psychosis is defined as a(n):**
   A. state of delusion and describes individuals who are out of touch with reality.
   B. complex disorder that is neither easily defined nor easily treated, and that dramatically affects today's society.
   C. inability to resist a temptation.
   D. eating disorder.

10. **The best way to deal with a patient having hallucinations is to:**
   A. use physical restraints.
   B. use the talk-down method.
   C. administer antipsychotic medications.
   D. scream at the patient.

Challenging Question

You are dispatched to a private residence for a 96-year-old woman. The patient's daughter found her sitting in a chair, not responding as she would normally. Her daughter initially thought she might have awakened her mother, and her mother was just "a little slow." After approximately 30 minutes, she called 9-1-1. Upon your arrival, you find the patient to be resting comfortably in her chair. She is alert and responsive to her name and address only. She doesn't remember her daughter's name, nor does she know what month or year it is. Her daughter states that she has had a stroke in the past and has a history of high blood pressure. The patient denies any complaints, has no chest pain, and no shortness of breath. During your assessment you find no neurologic deficits, and the patient has equal hand grips, negative facial droop, and negative slurred speech. Her blood glucose level is 112 mg/dL. She doesn't remember getting out of bed this morning and doesn't remember going to her chair. She continuously asks you who you are and why you're there.

11. **As the paramedic, what field differential diagnosis could you make?**

■ Points to Ponder

Toward the end of your shift, you are dispatched to a private residence for a 24-year-old man having chest pain. When you arrive on scene, you find the young man lying on the ground, complaining of reproducible chest pain and trembling. He appears to be hyperventilating. He does not answer questions, but does follow commands. His vital signs are all within normal limits, except he's breathing approximately 30 times per minute. As you attempt to speak to the patient, his father keeps interrupting, wanting to know whether his son is having a heart attack. The father is upset that you're not transporting right away. While you're attempting to take control of the scene, his sister tells you that the patient was on the phone with his girlfriend and she was breaking up with him. He became very agitated, and then began to breathe "very fast." She called 9-1-1. The patient has a history of anxiety/panic attacks, but this episode was different than in the past.

What are some possibilities for what could be happening with this patient? How can you calm this patient down?

Issues: Empathy for Patients With Behavioral Emergencies, Respectful Approach to Patients and Family Members.

38

Gynecologic Emergencies

Objectives

Cognitive

5-13.1 Review the anatomic structures and physiology of the female reproductive system. (p 38.3)

5-13.2 Identify the normal events of the menstrual cycle. (p 38.4)

5-13.3 Describe how to assess a patient with a gynecological complaint. (p 38.12)

5-13.4 Explain how to recognize a gynecological emergency. (p 38.15)

5-13.5 Describe the general care of any patient experiencing a gynecological emergency. (p 38.17)

5-13.6 Describe the pathophysiology, assessment, and management of specific gynecological emergencies. (p 38.18)

Affective

5-13.7 Value the importance of maintaining a patient's modesty and privacy while still being able to obtain necessary information. (p 38.13)

5-13.8 Defend the need to provide care for a patient of sexual assault, while still preventing destruction of crime scene information. (p 38.20)

5-13.9 Serve as a role model for other EMS providers when discussing or caring for patients with gynecological emergencies. (p 38.13)

Psychomotor

5-13.10 Demonstrate how to assess a patient with a gynecological complaint. (p 38.13)

5-13.11 Demonstrate how to provide care for a patient with:
a. Excessive vaginal bleeding
b. Abdominal pain
c. Sexual assault (p 38.16, 38.17, 38.20)

Introduction

The *Merriam-Webster Dictionary* defines gynecology as "a branch of medicine that deals with the diseases and routine physical care of the reproductive system of women" and obstetrics as "a branch of medical science that deals with birth and with its antecedents and sequels." Although the medical specialties of obstetrics and gynecology are separate fields of study, the two are so inextricably entwined—as these definitions make clear—that it is virtually impossible to write about one without referencing the other.

Before the 20th century, both fields of study were relegated to the realm of "subjects not discussed in polite society." Despite the work of pioneering doctors dating back as far as 98 AD, most of the knowledge of these two sciences was held by midwives, who jealously guarded the "secrets" of womankind with religious fervor.

One of the earliest medical texts covering obstetrics and gynecology was written by Soranus (98 AD), a Greco-Roman physician. His obstetric textbook, which was used until the 1600s, described podalic version (delivery of the infant feet first), the obstetric chair, and instructions for the newborn: "boiled water and honey for the child for the first two days, then on to the mother's breast." Unfortunately for women, the enlightened science of the Romans did not survive their empire. In 1522, a German physician named Wert masqueraded as a woman to sneak a peek at the mysteries of the birthing room. He was unmasked and burned at the stake for his intellectual curiosity.

Three other physicians of the 1500s fared better than the hapless Dr Wert. Ambrose Pare was a surgeon-barber who apprenticed at the famous Paris Hotel Dieu, the first midwife school in Paris, and was one of the first physicians to record dilating the cervix to induce labor. Thomas Raynalde penned *The Birth of Mankynde* in 1544, which described cesarean sec-

tion. In 1554, Jacob Rueff published *De Conceptu Generationis Hominis,* which described the whole process of pregnancy.

Despite the advances of these forward-thinking minds, childbirth and female medical conditions remained in the realm of superstition and folk medicine until well into the 1900s. The women's suffrage movement (1848–1920) and the women's liberation movement of the 1960s not only catalyzed progress in equal rights, but also made strides in the scientific study of women's unique medical problems.

It has often been said that human males and females are actually two separate species, which just happen to be able to reproduce. The physiologic, emotional, and mental processes experienced by the two sexes are widely disparate, despite sharing many similarities. The physiologic, chemical, hormonal, and even mental differences between men and women are beyond the scope of this book. The most obvious difference between the two sexes, however, is that women are uniquely designed to conceive and give birth. This difference makes women susceptible to a variety of problems that do not occur in men.

This chapter examines a few of those problems. It first discusses the female anatomy, then outlines issues that are unique to female patients, including problems that may be encountered in the emergency setting. We next consider the gynecologic causes of abdominal pain in women and look in detail at life-threatening conditions. We also briefly examine vaginal bleeding, both traumatic and organic, and discuss how it should be managed in the field. Finally, we consider the principles of managing a woman who has been the victim of sexual assault.

Female Anatomy

The female external genitalia, collectively called the pudendum or vulva, are the structures seen from the outside of the body Figure 38-1 ▸ . The mons veneris (mons pubis) is a rounded

You are the Provider Part 1

You are dispatched to a private residence for a 40-year-old woman with abdominal pain and vaginal bleeding. You arrive to find an apparently healthy middle-aged woman, Maria Medina, lying on her side on the couch with her knees drawn up.

The patient tells you that she has been experiencing spotting for 10 to 15 minutes and is now having abdominal pain and cramping. She is 6 weeks' pregnant, and this is her first pregnancy. She immediately phoned her doctor when the spotting started and was headed out the door to his office when the pain began.

Initial Assessment	Recording Time: 0 Minutes
Appearance	Anxious and tearful
Level of consciousness	A (Alert to person, place, and day)
Airway	Patent; patient is talking
Breathing	Rapid with adequate tidal volume
Circulation	Strong, slightly fast radial pulse

1. Based on your general impression and initial assessment, how would you categorize this patient?
2. What interventions would you choose to initiate at this point?

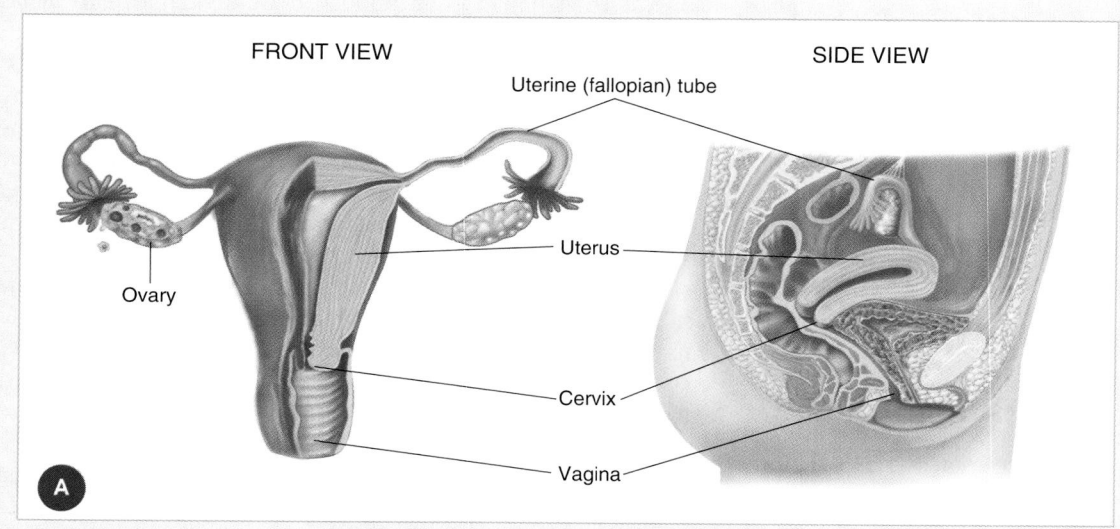

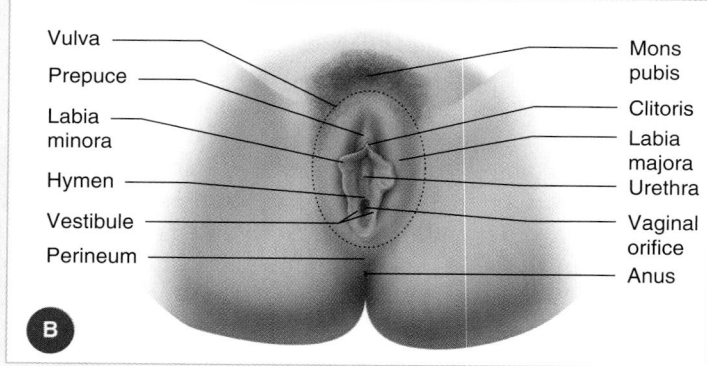

Figure 38-1 The anatomy of the female reproductive system. **A.** Front and side views. **B.** External genitalia.

This short length is one reason why women are more prone than men to urinary tract infections and bladder infections.

The vagina, or lower portion of the birth canal, serves as a passage for menstrual flow and as the receptacle of the penis during sexual intercourse. Just inside the lower vagina are two tiny openings that lead to the Bartholin glands. These glands secrete mucus that acts as a lubricant during intercourse. Bacterial infection, particularly gonorrhea, may cause these openings to become abscessed and cystic.

Before first intercourse, the vaginal orifice is protected by the hymen. This membrane forms a border around the vaginal orifice, partially enclosing it. The hymen may be ruptured before first intercourse by trauma or by such mundane events as horseback riding, gymnastics, or other sports. Pain and vaginal bleeding

pad of fatty (adipose) tissue that overlies the symphysis pubis, located anterior to the urethral and vaginal openings. The mons veneris is not an organ, but rather a "landmark." Coarse, dark hair normally appears over the mons in early puberty, becoming sparser later in life with the advent of menopause. The labia majora and labia minora, described as "lips," surround and protect the vaginal opening together with the more anterior opening of the urethra. The labia majora are covered with pubic hair, but the labia minora are devoid of it. The area between the vaginal opening and the anus is called the perineum. The clitoris is located at the anterior junction of the labia minora, just below a layer of skin called the prepuce. The clitoris is a small, cylindrical mass of erectile tissue and nerves that is homologous to the glans penis of the male. Like the male penis, the clitoris becomes enlarged with blood flow on tactile stimulation, and it has an important role in the sexual excitement of the female.

Between the labia minora is a cleft referred to as the vestibule. Located within the vestibule is the urethral opening (orifice), the vaginal opening (orifice), and the hymen. The urethra, which leads to the bladder, allows for passage of urine. The length of the urethra in females averages approximately 3.8 cm.

will generally be present in such an event; because this usually occurs in young women, it may be of concern to the patient and her parents. In some cases, the hymen may completely cover the vaginal orifice, a condition called imperforate hymen. If it remains undetected until puberty, this condition will block the flow of first menses, resulting in relatively acute pain, with severe constipation and low back pain among the presenting symptoms. Such a condition may lead to endometriosis or cause other secondary painful effects as well. Imperforate hymen can also be caused by childhood sexual abuse, in which the imperforation results from scarring from digital or penile penetration.

About an inch below the vaginal opening is the anal opening, which allows for the passage of feces and bowel gases. The area of skin between the vagina and the anus is called the clinical perineum.

Menstruation

Of the many emergencies that paramedics are called on to treat, one of the most common calls is bleeding. For gynecologic emergencies, that would translate into "vaginal bleeds." However,

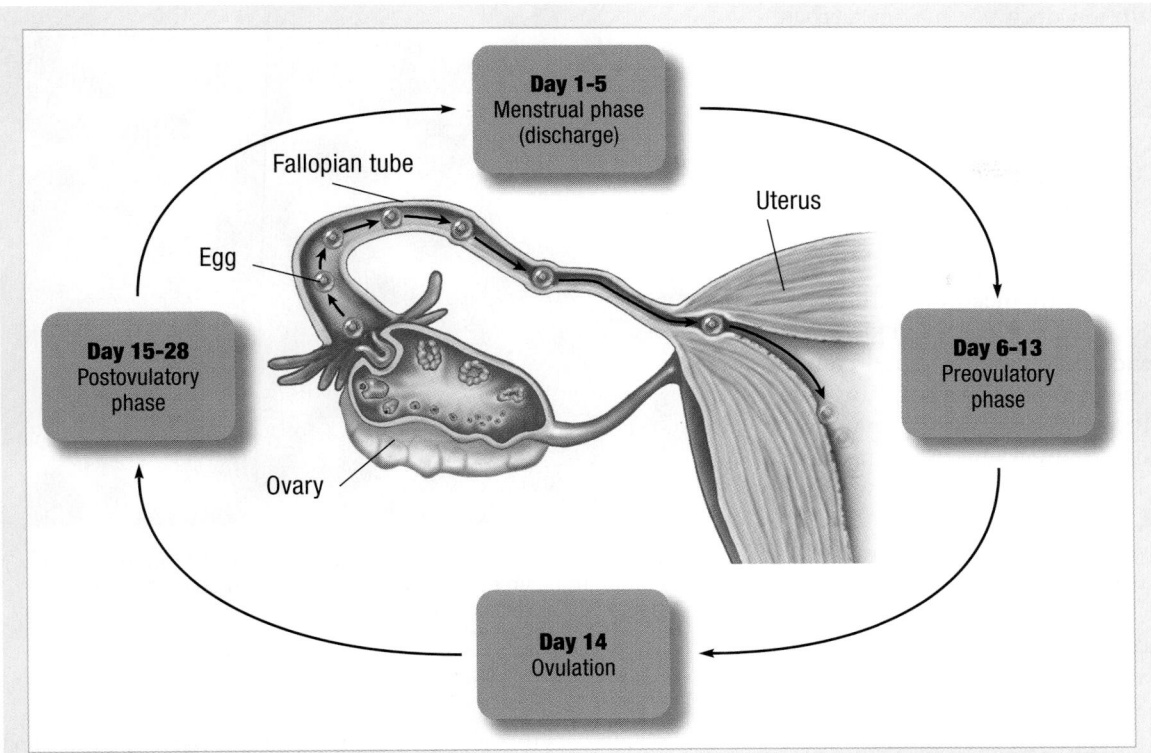

Figure 38-2 The menstrual cycle, based on an average 28-day cycle. The length of the cycle and number of days in each phase vary from woman to woman, but generally fall within a range of 24 to 35 days.

The onset of first menses, when a female reaches childbearing age, is called menarche. Depending on genetics, socioeconomic factors, and individual health, this event may take place anywhere between the ages of 11 and 14 years. The last menses, when a woman has reached the end of childbearing age, is called menopause. The advent of menopause typically begins between the ages of 40 and 50, with menstrual cycles becoming less frequent. This last phase of a woman's entire birth cycle, including the period of life that follows it, is called the climacteric.

Owing to gradually decreasing production of estrogen and other hormones during the climacteric, a woman may experience a range of symptoms due to hormonal imbalance. These symptoms may be as benign as copious diaphoresis, hair loss, and hot flashes (sometimes accompanied by tachycardia) or as ominous as the symptoms seen often in the emergency setting such as severe muscle aches and pains, headache, dyspnea, vertigo, digestive problems, and emotional instability. Postmenopausal women no longer have to deal with the discomfort and irritation of monthly menses, but the decreased hormone production makes them more susceptible to atherosclerosis, osteoporosis, and coronary heart disease. Diminished estrogen may also result in atrophy of genitourinary organs, resulting in vaginal dryness and discomfort. Atrophy of the bladder and urethral mucosa can result in urinary frequency, nocturia, and incontinence.

Menstruation is predominantly related to the discussion of obstetrics, but is also a necessary component of the gynecologic examination. Disorders of the menstrual cycle may be seen in the prehospital setting, actually putting the call for emergency service in motion. Some of these disorders are classified in the following paragraphs.

Premenstrual syndrome (PMS) (also called premenstrual tension) is a cluster of all or some of the troubling symptoms mentioned in the discussion of the menstrual cycle. It normally occurs 7 to 14 days before the onset of the menstrual flow, then generally subsides once the flow begins. Premenstrual syndrome affects about one third of all premenopausal women, particularly in the 30- to 40-year-old group, and may be significantly debilitating. Stress, diet, alcohol consumption,

before we embark on the emergency treatment of vaginal bleeding, we must first broach what is "normal" vaginal bleeding.

One way in which women are uniquely different from men is the physiologic phenomenon of menstruation. Also called the menses, period, or menstrual cycle, menstruation is the cyclic and periodic vaginal discharge of 25 to 65 mL of blood, epithelial cells, mucus, and tissue. The duration of the cycle differs from woman to woman, ranging from an average of 24 days to 35 days. Unless told otherwise by the patient, assume the average cycle to be 28 days. Three phases make up the entire menstrual cycle: the menstrual phase (the first phase), the preovulatory phase, and the postovulatory phase. Based on a 28-day cycle, the menstrual (discharge) phase lasts about 5 days. The preovulatory phase lasts from about day 6 to 13, and the postovulatory phase lasts from day 15 to 28 **Figure 38-2** .

During the menstrual cycle, a woman experiences several systemic changes as her hormonal levels ebb and flow. She may experience a weight gain of several pounds due to extracellular edema (fluid retention) that tends to localize in the abdomen, fingers, and ankles; muscle sensitivity due to the extracellular edema (hypertonicity); vascular alterations that increase her susceptibility to bruising; breast pain and tenderness resulting from swelling; mild to severe headache, including "menstrual migraine" (a vascular headache resulting from the hormonal "dump"); severe cramping; and emotional changes, such as agitation, irritability, depression, anger, and moodiness.

and prescription or nonprescription drug use may exacerbate symptoms. In addition, some women may experience reactive hypoglycemia, resulting in increased fatigue. This may be a strong clue as to what is troubling the patient, especially if the history elicits a recent intense craving for sweets or decreased alcohol tolerance. Prehospital treatment is predominantly supportive; the root cause of the symptomology must be defined by differential medical diagnosis. Supportive field treatment may include administration of oral or intravenous (IV) glucose, if blood glucose levels support the need, or administration of a small dose of analgesics to reduce patient anxiety.

Some women may experience abdominal pain and cramping in the 2 weeks before the beginning of menses. This pain and its accompanying symptoms result from the ovulatory process and are collectively called mittelschmerz (pronounced "MITT-ul-shmurz"; German for "middle pain"). Mittelschmerz, which may start at any time during ovulation (midcycle), affects approximately 20% of women. In most cases, the pain is not severe; it may last only a few minutes or as long as 48 hours (average, 6 to 8 hours). Signs and symptoms include sharp, cramping pain in the lower abdomen, localized to one side, beginning midcycle, with a history of similar pain episodes during previous periods. The pain may also be reported as "switching sides" from month to month. Some women also report feeling nauseated or experiencing minor blood spotting. The condition itself is not serious, and the pain can often be relieved by over-the-counter analgesics. Any persistent pain or any abnormal symptoms are cause for concern and should be evaluated by a physician.

Dysmenorrhea is painful menses. It is classified into two categories: primary and secondary. Primary dysmenorrhea occurs with the advent of the menstrual flow and normally lasts for the first 1 to 2 days with gradual relief. Severe cramping may precede the period, with pain originating in the area of the symphysis pubis and radiating downward to the vulva and outward to the thighs. Nausea, vomiting, and diarrhea may accompany the pain. Primary dysmenorrhea accounts for about 80% of patients presenting with painful menses and accompanies a "regular" period. Secondary dysmenorrhea is pain that is present before, during, and after the menstrual flow. It is generally organic in nature (not hormonal) and may signal an underlying illness or dysfunction. As with premenstrual syndrome, prehospital treatment is largely supportive.

At this point, you may be asking why this information is important and whether anyone would actually call EMS for "menstrual" problems. In fact, people call EMS for virtually anything. If the situation is an emergency to the patient, professionally, it should be an emergency to you as well. Generally, for menstrual-related conditions, EMS is called because (1) the symptoms are new for the patient, (2) the symptoms are worse than in the past, or (3) the patient innately "feels" that something is wrong **Figure 38-3 ▶** . You are in the unique position of being one of the few remaining medical specialties that make "house calls." As a consequence, you are able to examine the patient's living conditions, estimate familial tensions (if evident),

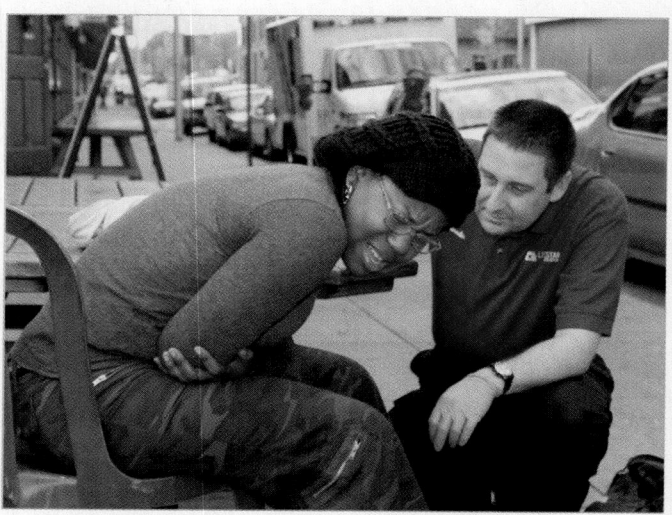

Figure 38-3 A patient may call EMS because she perceives her condition to be an emergency. Make sure you take each call seriously.

and obtain data that a patient might not otherwise bring to a clinician's office (for example, a menstrual chart). Your history taking and inferences can provide important information for the treating physician and contribute to the overall well-being and recovery of the patient. Of course, for you to ascertain what is "abnormal," you must know what is "normal."

Amenorrhea is the absence or cessation of menses. This condition may be caused by a number of factors, but *the most common cause is pregnancy.* Exercise-induced amenorrhea is common in female athletes, particularly those who participate in physically intense sports. Amenorrhea can also be caused by emotional problems or extreme stress. In an adolescent or young adult, the condition may have its origination in anorexia nervosa; in this case, it is a symptom of the patient's malnutrition and emotional state.

> **Notes from Nancy**
> The most common cause of amenorrhea is pregnancy.

Vaginal bleeding is one of the most frequent reasons that women consult a gynecologist. The assessment and management of a patient with this chief complaint depend largely on whether there is a mechanism of injury. Vaginal bleeding, when not in the course of regular menstruation, is always an abnormal finding. The cause may be as benign as emotional stress or as serious as pelvic, cervical, or uterine cancer. Likewise, a disturbance in the normal menstrual cycle is cause for concern. If the flow of blood lasts several days longer than normal or is excessive, the condition is called hypermenorrhea. If the blood flow occurs more often than a 24-day interval, it is termed polymenorrhea (usually caused by physical or emotional stress). Blood flow or intermittent spotting of blood occurring irregularly but frequently is termed metrorrhagia. Metrorrhagia is of greatest concern to paramedics because its causes range from hormonal imbalance to malignancies to spontaneous abortion (miscarriage). Endometritis, inflammation of the endometrium, often associated with a bacterial infection, may be another cause of vaginal bleeding, with postabortal issues or tuberculosis as the underlying factor.

Pathophysiology

Causes of gynecologic emergencies range from disease to ectopic pregnancy to trauma.

Endometritis

Endometritis is an inflammation or irritation of the endometrium (uterine lining), most commonly caused by infection. Sexually transmitted diseases are a frequent culprit (gonorrhea and chlamydia, predominantly), but endometritis may also occur after gynecologic surgery, abortion (elective, miscarriage, or therapeutic), or use of an intrauterine device (IUD). Symptoms may include malaise, fever (high- or low-grade), constipation or uncomfortable bowel movements, vagi-

nal bleeding or discharge (or both), abdominal distention, and lower abdominal or pelvic pain. Abdominal auscultation may reveal decreased bowel sounds, and pain may be elicited by palpation of the abdomen. Left untreated, endometritis may lead to septic shock or cause spontaneous abortion in a pregnant patient.

Endometriosis

Endometriosis affects an estimated 5.5 million women in the United States. This condition can be extremely painful, or there may be no symptoms. It results when endometrial tissue grows outside the uterus, generally on the surface of abdominal and pelvic organs. Organs of the pelvic cavity are the most common locations for the ectopic growths, but endometrial tissue can occasionally be found in the lungs or other parts of the body. This condition is one of the leading causes of infertility in women, with 30% to 40% of affected women unable to conceive. Many women do not even realize they have endometriosis until they encounter difficulties trying to get pregnant.

In women who experience symptoms, the most common complaint is pain, generally localized in the lower back, pelvic, and abdominal regions, that may be chronic. Other symptoms include painful coitus (during and after), gastrointestinal pain, dysuria and painful bowel movements during the menstrual cycle, fatigue (perhaps leading to misdiagnosis as chronic fatigue syndrome), extremely painful and escalating menstrual cramping, and very heavy menstrual periods. Patients may also experience bleeding between periods or report premenstrual spotting.

Pelvic Inflammatory Disease

Approximately one of every seven women in the United States will contract pelvic inflammatory disease (PID) at some point,

You are the Provider Part 2

You administer oxygen to the patient, obtain vital signs, insert an IV line, and apply the cardiac monitor and note sinus rhythm. As you continue your assessment, she says, "Please just take me to the hospital. Please." You can tell that she is very frightened. You assist her to the gurney, where she finds her original position of comfort.

Vital Signs	Recording Time: 5 Minutes
Level of consciousness	Alert, with a Glasgow Coma Scale score of 15
Skin	Warm, pink, and dry
Pulse	90 beats/min and regular
Blood pressure	110/68 mm Hg
Respirations	30 breaths/min
Sa_{O_2}	100% with oxygen at 4 L/min via nasal cannula

3. What other information would you like to know?

4. What issues do you foresee that will likely impact patient care?

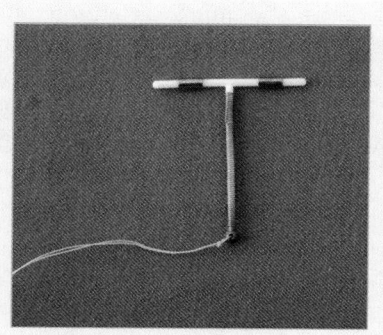

Figure 38-4 The IUD contraceptive device can increase a woman's risk of developing PID and ectopic pregnancy and may cause pain and bleeding.

or more than 1 million women per year. One fourth of the women will require hospitalization. PID is one of the most common causes of women presenting to an emergency service with a chief complaint of abdominal pain. One of every four women who contract PID will have severe abdominal pain or experience sterility or childbirth complications. Many women may have PID for years but do not realize it until they learn they are infertile.

PID is an infection of the female upper organs of reproduction—specifically, the uterus, ovaries, and fallopian tubes—that occurs almost exclusively in sexually active women. Disease-causing organisms enter the vagina, generally by the process of sexual activity, and migrate through the opening of the cervix and into the uterine cavity, where they invade the mucosa. The infection may then expand to the fallopian tubes (producing scarring that can lead to life-threatening ectopic pregnancy or sterility), eventually involving the ovaries (leading to the development of a life-threatening tubo-ovarian abscess) and the peritoneal cavity. Although PID itself is seldom a threat to life, its ultimate consequences can be lethal.

Risk factors for PID include the use of an IUD as a contraceptive device Figure 38-4 ▲ , frequent sexual activity with multiple partners, and a history of previous PID. The disease is most prevalent in the collegiate age group (20 to 24 years) and statistically decreases after age 30 years (the typical monogamy and marriage years).

Gardnerella Vaginitis

The *Gardnerella* bacterium normally resides in the genital area in women. It can cause an infection called Gardnerella vaginitis if the bacteria become too numerous. Young, sexually active women are the most likely to be affected, but it can develop in any female—adult or child. This infection can also occur in the urethra of males. It can be associated with PID, and recent use of antibiotics can increase the risk of contracting the infection. Gardnerella vaginitis can cause complications in pregnant women.

Gardnerella vaginitis is often confused with a yeast infection. Signs and symptoms include a "fishy" vaginal odor, itching, irritation, and a smooth, thin, sticky, white or gray discharge. Patients often describe their symptoms as being worse after intercourse or menstruation. Patients, although they are not in acute distress, should be seen by a physician, who will most likely treat the condition with antibiotics.

Interstitial Cystitis

An estimated 850,000 people in the United States have been diagnosed with interstitial cystitis/painful bladder syndrome (IC/PBS). Although this condition affects men and women, 94% of diagnosed cases have been women. IC/PBS is a chronic bladder condition with an unknown cause; it results in an inflamed or irritated bladder wall. In severe cases, the irritation can lead to the formation of ulcers in the bladder and bleeding into the bladder lining. The bladder may become internally scarred and stiff, resulting in markedly reduced bladder capacity. Symptoms vary but may mimic the symptoms associated with urinary tract infections and sexually transmitted diseases: pressure or tenderness in the bladder and surrounding pelvic region, pain that ranges from mild discomfort to severe, and urinary frequency or urgency. Some patients report urinating as many as 60 times per day. Painful coitus is not uncommon, and many women report that their symptoms become worse during their menstrual cycle.

There is currently no cure for IC/PBS (antibiotics are ineffective), so patients are generally treated so as to provide symptomatic relief. Some physicians may prescribe antihistamines or antidepressants, whereas others give ibuprofen, aspirin, or even narcotics for severe cases. The only US Food and Drug Administration–approved oral medication for treatment of IC/PBS is pentosan polysulfate sodium (Elmiron).

Ectopic Pregnancy

The word *ectopic* means "located away from a normal position." In ectopic pregnancy, a fertilized egg is implanted somewhere besides the uterus Figure 38-5 ▶ . In 97% of cases, the egg is fertilized inside one of the fallopian tubes and has been blocked from passing into the uterus, generally by an obstruction, such as PID-related tubal scarring or as a result of tubal surgery (ligation or reverse ligation). The other 3% of ectopic pregnancies occur in the abdomen, within the cervix, or on an ovary. Ectopic pregnancy is the leading cause of maternal death in the first trimester. Nearly 1 in 66 women will experience an ectopic pregnancy. More than 100,000 cases occur in the United States each year. Although PID is the most common cause of ectopic pregnancy, other causes include pelvic surgery, smoking, IUD use (IUDs do not cause ectopic pregnancy but, by blocking uterine pregnancy, may cause fertilization to occur higher up), fibroids, tumors or cysts in the tubes, fallopian endometriosis, hormonal imbalance, and fertility treatments.

With a tubal pregnancy, the fertilized egg implants in the fallopian tube, then begins to grow and produce hormones in the same way a normally implanted egg does, taking nourishment from the maternal blood supply. Owing to the production of hormones, the woman begins to experience the early physiologic changes of pregnancy. Her period stops, her breasts become enlarged and tender, and the uterine environment changes just as it would with a normal pregnancy. The fallopian tube, lacking the expansive muscle capacity of the uterus, has little stretching ability, so the developing embryo will soon run out of growing room. When this occurs, the

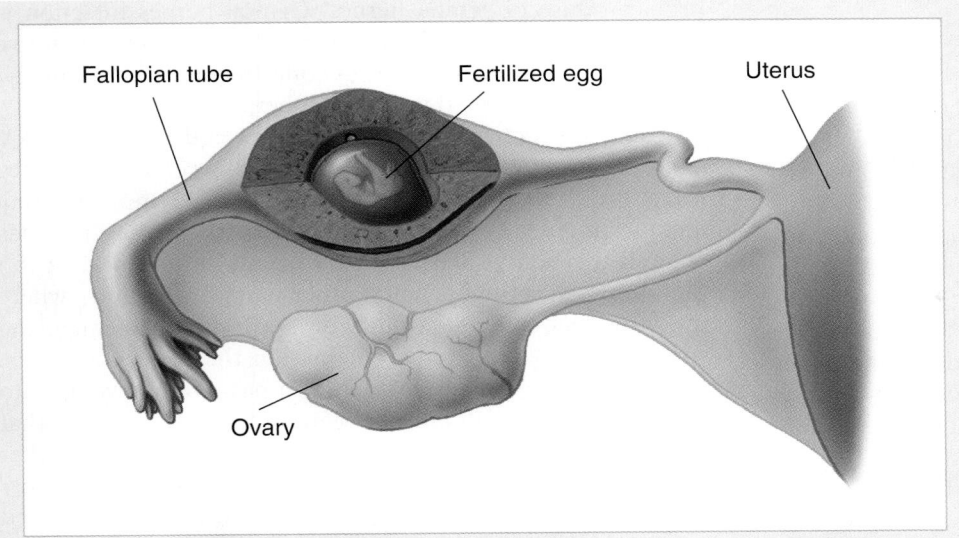

Figure 38-5 In an ectopic pregnancy, a fertilized egg implants somewhere other than the uterus. Here it is implanted in one of the fallopian tubes.

tube is likely to rupture, causing massive intra-abdominal hemorrhage and shock.

Ruptured Ovarian Cyst and Tubo-ovarian Abscess

Ruptured ovarian cysts and tubo-ovarian abscesses present with similar findings to ectopic pregnancy, so their field management is identical to that for ectopic pregnancy.

An ovarian cyst is essentially a fluid-filled sac that forms on or within an ovary. Of the many types of cysts, the most common is the *functional cyst,* which generally develops during the menstrual cycle. During the cycle, the ovaries form tiny sacs (cysts) to hold the eggs. Once an egg matures, the sac breaks open and releases the egg, which then begins its journey through the fallopian tube for fertilization; the sac itself dissolves. If the sac fails to break open, however, the egg may continue to mature and form a *follicular cyst.* Under normal circumstances, this type of cyst spontaneously disappears within a 1- to 3-month period. A *corpus luteum cyst* develops if the sac seals itself after release of the egg. Fluid then accumulates inside the cyst, and the cyst continues to grow. These cysts usually resolve spontaneously but may grow up to 4 inches. At this size, they can twist the ovary, causing bleeding and pain. Fertility drugs can increase the chances of corpus luteum cysts developing.

If the cycle of forming sacs is repeated excessively and the eggs do not release, *polycystic ovaries* may develop. This hormonal reproductive disorder is characterized by lack of progesterone and high levels of androgens (male hormone). It can have a negative impact on normal insulin production, leading to diabetes (especially gestational). It can also initiate heart and blood vessel problems, such as hypertension, and produce pelvic pain and irregular menstrual cycles.

Dermoid cysts lead to growths of formational tissue, such as teeth and hair, and may become very large and painful. Endometriomas form in women who have endometriosis, when uterine tissue attaches to the ovaries and begins to grow. Pain from this type of cyst usually manifests during menstruation or sexual intercourse. Cystadenomas are formed from cells on the outer surface of the ovary. These cysts are usually filled with a sticky gel substance or other fluid. They can become large and cause pain. A hemorrhagic cyst forms when a blood vessel bursts in the cyst wall and the blood fills the sac. Occasionally, these cysts will rupture and spill blood into the abdominal cavity, resulting in great pain.

Tubo-ovarian abscess is encountered secondary to a primary infectious agent—typically, the ones that cause PID. The most common underlying cause is gonorrhea. Diverticulitis and appendicitis have also been found to be causative agents. In this condition, the fallopian tubes or ovaries become blocked by an infectious mass, which grows and forms an abscess.

Toxic Shock Syndrome

Toxic shock syndrome (TSS) is a form of septic shock. The disease made headlines in the 1980s, when it was identified as a syndrome affecting women who used tampons. A connection was made between the use of super-absorbancy tampons and a risk of contracting the disease, but the panic that ensued was out of proportion to the actual threat. The disease has been identified as having *Streptococcus pyogenes* (group A strep) or *Staphylococcus aureus* as the causative agent. TSS affects men and women, and it can involve several of the body's systems, including the hepatic, cardiovascular, central nervous, and renal systems. It can result when minor infections of the lungs, sinuses, skin lesions, or the vagina progress to actual TSS, which can be lethal. Menstruating women appear particularly prone to developing TSS—hence, the original association between the syndrome and tampon use. Initial symptoms include syncope, myalgia, diarrhea, vomiting, headache, fever, and sore throat. Other symptoms may include diverse petechiae, light rash, and scleral injection (bloodshot eyes). As the disease progresses, signs of systemic shock will begin to appear. Disseminated intravascular coagulation, severe hypotension, adult respiratory distress syndrome, and dysrhythmias may develop, and the patient may show signs of kidney and liver failure.

Rapid transport is indicated in cases of TSS. Provide high-flow supplemental oxygen, IV therapy, and cardiac monitoring. Little more can be done for a patient with TSS in the field because aggressive antibiotic therapy and possible surgical intervention are required.

Sexually Transmitted Diseases

As mentioned earlier, PID results from infective organisms crossing the cervix. It is typically a secondary infection, with the primary infection being a sexually transmitted disease (STD)—often chlamydia or gonorrhea. STDs are reviewed briefly here, with the exception of the human immunodeficiency virus (HIV), which is discussed in Chapter 36.

Bacterial vaginosis is one of the most common conditions to afflict women. In this infection, normal bacteria in the vagina are replaced by an overgrowth of other bacterial forms. Symptoms may include itching, burning, or pain and may be accompanied by a "fishy," foul-smelling discharge. Left untreated, bacterial vaginosis can lead to premature birth or low birthweight in case of pregnancy, make the patient more susceptible to more serious infections, and result in PID. It is treated with metronidazole, an antibiotic. If the patient consumes alcohol while taking this therapy, severe nausea and vomiting may develop.

Chancroid is caused by infection with the bacterium *Haemophilus ducreyi*. This highly contagious yet curable disease causes painful sores (ulcers), usually of the genitals. Swollen, painful lymph glands or inguinal buboes in the groin area may be present as well. Women may be asymptomatic and, thus, unaware they have the disease. Chancroid is known to facilitate the transmission of HIV.

Chlamydia is caused by the bacterium *Chlamydia trachomatis*. A very common STD, it affects an estimated 2.8 million Americans each year. Although symptoms of chlamydia are usually mild or absent, some women may have symptoms including lower abdominal pain, low back pain, nausea, fever, pain during intercourse, to bleeding between menstrual periods. Chlamydial infection of the cervix can spread to the rectum, leading to rectal pain, discharge, or bleeding. Left untreated, the disease can progress to PID. In rare cases, chlamydia causes arthritis that may be accompanied by skin lesions and inflammation of the eye and urethra (Reiter syndrome).

Cytomegalovirus (CMV) is a member of the herpesvirus family. This very common viral infection has no known cure, and the virus can remain dormant in the body for years. An estimated 80% of the US population has been exposed to CMV. In its active stages, CMV may produce symptoms including prolonged high fever, chills, headache, malaise, extreme fatigue, and an enlarged spleen. People with an increased risk for developing active infection and more serious complications (such as fever, pneumonia, liver infection, and anemia) include people with immune disorders, people receiving chemotherapy, and pregnant women. Newborns who acquire CMV are susceptible to lung problems, blood problems, liver problems, swollen glands, rash, and poor weight gain.

Genital herpes is an infection of the genitals, buttocks, or anal area caused by herpes simplex virus, type I or type II. Type I, which is the most common form, infects the mouth and lips, causing cold sores or "fever" blisters; it may also produce sores on the genitals. Type II, the more serious infection, can affect the mouth as well, but is more commonly known as the primary cause of genital herpes. Genital herpes infection is more prevalent in women than in men. While over one in five Americans have genital herpes, one in four women in the United States is infected with type II herpes.

In an active herpes infection (called an outbreak), symptoms generally appear within 2 weeks of primary infection and can last for several weeks. Symptoms may include tingling or sores near the area where the virus has entered the body, such as on the genital or rectal area, on the buttocks or thighs, or on other parts of the body where the virus has entered through broken skin. In women, the sores may occur inside the vagina, on the cervix, or in the urinary passage. Small red bumps appear first, develop into small blisters, and finally become itchy, painful sores that might develop a crust and heal without leaving a scar. Other symptoms that may accompany the first outbreak, and possibly subsequent outbreaks, include fever, muscle aches and pains, headache, dysuria, vaginal discharge, and swollen glands in the groin area.

Gonorrhea is caused by *Neisseria gonorrhoeae,* a bacterium that can grow and multiply rapidly in the warm, moist areas of the reproductive tract, including the cervix, uterus, and fallopian tubes in women and in the urethra in women and men. The bacterium can also grow in the mouth, throat, eyes, and anus. Symptoms, which are generally more severe in men than in women, appear approximately 2 to 10 days after exposure. Women may be infected with gonorrhea for months but experience virtually no symptoms until the infection has spread to other parts of the reproductive system. When symptoms do appear in women, they generally manifest as dysuria (painful urination), with associated burning or itching, a yellowish or bloody vaginal discharge, usually with a foul odor, and occult blood associated with vaginal intercourse. More severe infections may present with cramping and abdominal pain, nausea and vomiting, and bleeding between periods; these symptoms indicate that the infection has progressed to PID. Rectal infections generally present with anal discharge and itching, plus occasional painful bowel movements with fecal blood spotting. Infection of the throat (for which oral sex is the introducing factor) is called gonococcal pharyngitis. Its symptoms are usually mild, consisting of painful or difficult swallowing, sore throat, swollen lymph glands, and fever. Headache and nasal congestion may also be present. If the infection is not treated, the bacterium may enter the bloodstream and spread to other parts of the body, including the brain—a condition known as disseminated gonococcemia.

Genital warts (also called condylomata acuminata and venereal warts) are caused by the human papillomavirus (HPV). Of the more than 100 types of HPV that have been identified (most are harmless), about 30 types are spread through sexual contact. HPV is the most common STD, with almost 6 million new cases being reported every year and more than 20 million open cases being treated. Some infected people have no symptoms. In others, multiple growths develop in the genital areas—that is, the vagina, vulva, cervix, or rectum, or the penis and scrotum in men. HPV has been identified as a causative agent in cervical, vulvar, and anal cancers. In pregnant women, warts may develop that become large enough to impede urination or obstruct the birth canal. If the virus is passed to the fetus, the child may develop *laryngeal papillomatosis* (throat warts that block the airway), a potentially life-threatening condition.

Syphilis is caused by the bacterium *Treponema pallidum*. Because many of its signs and symptoms mimic other diseases, syphilis is sometimes called the "great imitator" by clinicians. The disease manifests in three stages: primary, secondary, and late. Approximately 20,000 to 30,000 cases of syphilis are reported each year in the United States, mostly in the 20- to 40-year-old group; the highest incidence is found in women aged 20 to 24 years. Transmission occurs through direct contact with open sores, which may arise anywhere on the body, but tend to appear on the genitals, anus, rectum, lips, or mouth. A person with syphilis may remain asymptomatic for years, not realizing that his or her sores are manifestations of a disease.

The primary stage of syphilis is usually marked by the appearance of a single sore (a chancre), although in some people, multiple sores develop. The chancre is usually painless and is small, firm, and round. It usually goes away after 3 to 6 weeks, at which point the disease has progressed to the second stage.

The secondary stage of syphilis is characterized by the development of mucous membrane lesions and a skin rash. The characteristic rash may manifest on the palms of the hands and the bottoms of the feet as rough, red or reddish brown spots. Alternatively, it may be barely discernible or resemble rashes from other diseases. The rash generally does not itch. Symptoms of secondary syphilis may include fever, swollen lymph glands, sore throat, patchy hair loss, headaches, weight loss, muscle aches, and fatigue. Like the chancre of the primary stage, these symptoms will resolve without treatment. Left untreated, the secondary stage invariably leads to late-stage syphilis.

In the late stage, syphilis has no signs or symptoms, but internal damage is accumulating. Syphilis attacks the brain, nerves, eyes, heart, blood vessels, liver, bones, and joints, although the damage may not become evident for years. Paralysis, numbness, dementia, gradual blindness, and difficulty coordinating muscle movements are possible physical manifestations and may be serious enough to cause death. Pregnant women with syphilis may have stillborn babies, babies who are born blind, developmentally delayed babies, or babies who die shortly after birth.

Trichomoniasis is caused by a single-celled protozoan parasite, *Trichomonas vaginalis*. This parasite is transmitted through sexual contact, with the vagina being the most common site of infection. The infected person may be asymptomatic or may experience signs and symptoms including a frothy, yellow-green vaginal discharge with a strong odor. The infection may also cause irritation and itching of the female genital area, discomfort during intercourse, dysuria, and lower abdominal pain. When present, symptoms usually appear in women within 5 to 28 days of exposure to *T vaginalis*. Left untreated, the infection can lead to low birthweight or premature birth in pregnant women and to increased susceptibility to HIV infection. Approximately 7 million cases of trichomoniasis are reported in the United States each year.

Vaginal yeast infections are typically caused by the *Candida albicans* fungus. Yeasts are tiny organisms that normally live in small numbers inside the vagina and on the skin. The normal acidic environment of the vagina helps keep yeast from growing. If the vagina becomes less acidic, however, the yeast population may increase dramatically and result in infection. Conditions that may alter the acidic balance of the vagina include the use of oral contraceptives, menstruation, pregnancy, diabetes, and some antibiotics. Moisture and irritation of the vagina also seem to encourage yeast growth. Stress from lack of sleep, illness, or poor diet are other contributing factors. Women with immunosuppressive diseases such as HIV infection or diabetes are also at increased risk. Approximately 75% of all women will likely experience at least one infection during their lifetime. Symptoms include itching, burning, soreness in the vagina and around the vulva, and vulvar swelling. Some women may report a thick, white vaginal discharge ("cottage cheese" appearance), pain during sexual intercourse, and burning on urination.

Patient Assessment

Obtaining an accurate and detailed patient assessment is of utmost importance when dealing with gynecologic issues. You may not be able to make a specific diagnosis in the field, but a thorough detailed examination and patient history will help determine just how sick the patient is and whether lifesaving measures should be initiated. This is especially true when dealing with abdominal pain.

Women have many of the same conditions that cause abdominal pain in men—for example, renal colic, ulcers, gastroenteritis, cholecystitis, diverticulitis, pancreatitis, appendicitis, mesenteric ischemia, and dissecting aneurysm. In addition, there are numerous gynecologic causes of abdominal pain. An old medical axiom states, "Anyone who neglects to consider a gynecologic cause in a woman of childbearing age who complains of abdominal pain will miss the diagnosis at least 50% of the time." Missing the diagnosis may be fatal for the patient.

Scene Size-up

Every emergency call—including calls involving gynecologic emergencies—begins with a thorough scene size-up. Is the scene safe? Will you need assistance? Is it a medical call, a trauma call, or both? How many patients do you have? What is the mechanism of injury or nature of illness? Have you taken proper body substance isolation precautions? Gynecologic emergencies can be very messy, sometimes involving large amounts of blood and body fluids contaminated with communicable diseases.

Where is the patient found? If she is at home, what is the condition of the residence? Is it clean, filthy, or wrecked? Do you see evidence of a fight? Are alcohol, tobacco products, or drug paraphernalia present? Are there pictures of loved ones or, conversely, a noticeable absence of pictures? Does the patient live alone or with other people? All information you obtain will contribute to your assessment of the patient's overall health and the safety of the scene. In case of a crime scene, you may also be required to testify in court regarding the conditions on your arrival.

Initial Assessment

What is the overall presentation of the patient? Are there any obvious life threats? Is she conscious? Does she have obvious breathing difficulty or evidence of injury? Does she appear pale, cyanotic, red, or gray? Is she alert and oriented or confused? Is she calm or not? What is her emotional state? What is her physical appearance—well kept or dirty? Do you find the patient sitting up, lying down, prone, supine, in the fetal position, in the tripod position, in the bathtub, or on all fours? (The last position is common for patients in severe pain from renal colic.)

Once you have answered these basic questions and treated any immediate threats to airway, breathing, or circulation, you can proceed with the focused physical exam, rapid medical assessment, or rapid trauma assessment as the situation dictates. Conduct rapid medical or trauma assessment if the patient is not responsive or has a significant mechanism of injury but life threats are not immediately obvious. In the focused history and physical exam, pay special attention to gynecologic and reproductive history in addition to the usual criteria.

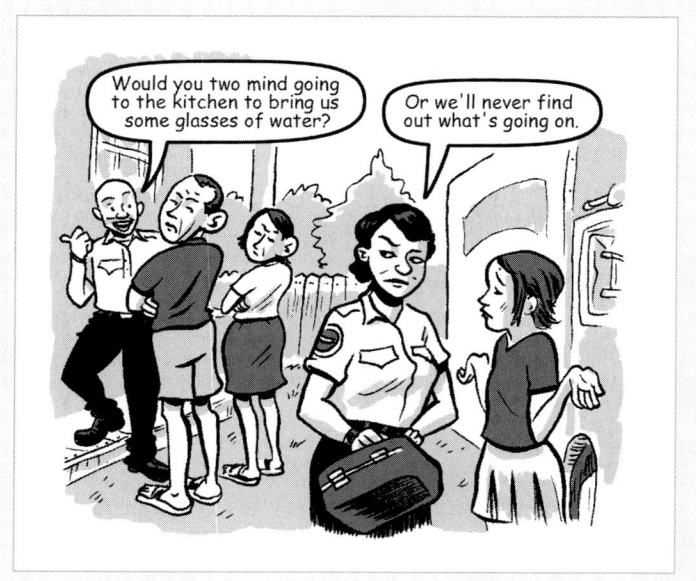

Figure 38-6

Try to protect the patient's modesty at all times during your history and physical examination. Gynecologic emergencies can be highly embarrassing for the patient, and many women may be extremely uncomfortable about discussing their sexual history in front of strangers or even close family members **Figure 38-6 ▲** . A teenage or adolescent girl may want to keep her sexual history from her parents, and few women are comfortable with having their genitals exposed to a crowd of family, neighbors, paramedics, police officers, or fire fighters. Limit the crowd to

You are the Provider Part 3

You continue to ask questions about Mrs. Medina's pain and pregnancy using the LORDS TRACHEA mnemonics (see the "Focused Physical Exam" section of this chapter). You obtain her orthostatic vital signs and perform a focused physical exam. No changes in positional vital signs are noted, and you find no signs of shock or trauma. You believe that Mrs. Medina is in stable condition but requires immediate physician evaluation. En route to the receiving facility, you advise emergency department personnel of the patient's signs, symptoms, and other pertinent information regarding your assessment and interventions.

Vital Signs	Recording Time: 15 Minutes
Level of consciousness	Alert, with a Glasgow Coma Scale score of 15
Skin	Warm, pink, and dry
Pulse	86 beats/min and regular
Blood pressure	110/66 mm Hg
Respirations	24 breaths/min
Sao_2	100% with supplemental oxygen at 4 L/min via nasal cannula

5. Given the information you have so far, will this patient require aggressive prehospital care?

6. What are the three true life-threatening gynecologic emergencies?

7. Does your differential diagnosis include any of these conditions?

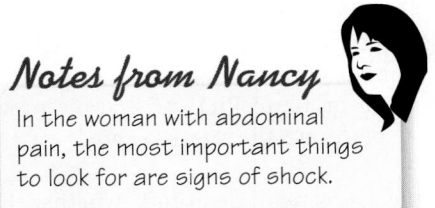

Notes from Nancy

In the woman with abdominal pain, the most important things to look for are signs of shock.

personnel required to perform the necessary tasks, and show the patient you respect her by being the advocate for her modesty. You also serve as a role model for other EMS providers when you act this way.

Documentation and Communication

By properly documenting your general impression, level of consciousness, chief complaint, life threats, and ABCs (the initial assessment), you provide vital information that is necessary for good, ongoing patient care.

Focused History and Physical Exam
Obtaining the History

What is the patient's chief complaint? If it is excessive bleeding, you can move on to getting the gynecologic history. If the chief complaint is abdominal pain, you need to find out more about the pain itself. Although the OPQRST (Onset; Provoking factors; Quality of pain; Region of pain and whether it radiates or refers; Severity; and Time [duration]) method discussed in previous chapters works well, a more specific approach is the LORDS TRACHEA mnemonic.

L What is the *Location* of the pain? Can the patient point to where the pain originates? Are multiple areas producing pain? Pain located in the midline may indicate spontaneous abortion (miscarriage). An achy pain that is diffused throughout the lower abdomen may be PID. Pain localized to one side of the abdomen may be an ectopic pregnancy.

O What was the *Onset* of the pain? When did the pain start? What activity was the patient performing when the pain started? A patient who reports the pain began during exercise may have a ruptured ovarian cyst.

R Does the pain *Radiate*? That is, does the pain stay centralized or does it travel? Pain that radiates to the shoulder may indicate large amounts of blood in the abdomen.

D What is the *Duration* of the pain? Is it constant or intermittent? If intermittent, how long does the pain last?

S What is the *Severity* of the pain, on a scale of 1 to 10? Is the pain excruciating or tolerable? Excruciating pain usually points to a nongynecologic cause, such as renal colic or aortic dissection.

T What is the *Timing* of the pain? Did it start after the patient took an oral contraceptive? Is there a temporal relationship between the onset of the pain and the last menstrual period? Pain that originates with PID generally starts after

the last menstrual flow. Which symptoms presented first? In cases of spontaneous abortion, pain generally *follows* bleeding. With ectopic pregnancy, the pain usually develops *before* bleeding.

R Does anything *Relieve* the pain? Does holding still, posturing a particular way, or lying down diminish the pain? Has the patient taken any medication for the pain? If so, what? Did the medication help?

A What *Aggravates* the pain? Does physical activity such as walking, sitting, or turning make the pain worse? Is the pain aggravated by physiologic activities, such as urinating, defecating, breathing, or swallowing? A patient with PID may (or may not) volunteer that the pain is made worse by sexual intercourse.

C What is the *Character* of the pain? Is it crampy? Aching? Sharp? Dull? Squeezing? Shooting? Stabbing? A patient experiencing a spontaneous abortion generally presents with "cramping" pain. The pain of PID will most likely be dull and steady.

H Is there a *Historic* precedent? Has the patient ever had this pain before? If yes, what was the cause? Is the pain now the same as or different from the earlier pain? What is the difference?

E Has the patient *Eaten* anything? If so, what? How much? How long ago? Did the symptoms appear after eating? If not, did eating alleviate any of the symptoms? Fluctuating hormonal levels frequently give rise to digestive problems, so it is just as important to rule out the obvious (indigestion) as it is to pinpoint the obscure.

A Are there *Associated* symptoms? Ask specifically about bleeding and symptoms of significant blood loss. Has the patient experienced any nausea, vomiting, or vertigo?

Once you have ascertained all that you can about the chief complaint and have developed a feeling for the patient's pain, you can proceed to obtain the gynecologic history. Probably the single most important question to ask is, "When did you have your last menstrual period (LMP)?" If the patient knows for certain, record the beginning and ending dates of the LMP. If she is unsure, record the approximate dates. Ask the patient whether she noticed anything unusual about the LMP. Was it longer or shorter than usual? Was the flow heavier or lighter than usual? Was there more or less cramping involved? Was the period late or on time? Did she have any spotting or bleeding between periods? Was any unusual pain involved?

Does the patient suspect that she might be pregnant, or is there any possibility of pregnancy? Many patients may find this question highly personal and may be uncomfortable answering it. They do not want you making a character judgment of their sexual history. Be patient, reassuring, professional, and non-judgmental in your questioning. If the answer is a strong "No way," find out why. Younger, sexually active women may incorrectly presume that birth control methods are 100% effective against pregnancy; in truth, most current methods are only 98% effective at best, and only if used correctly. If not using any contraceptive, 25% of women will become pregnant within

In the Field

Use the mnemonic ACHES-S to help isolate the "symptom cluster" associated with oral contraceptives: Abdominal pain, Chest pain, Headache (severe), Eyes (blurred vision), Spotting, and Sharp leg pain.

1 month and 85% within 1 year. If the patient insists she cannot be pregnant, ask about other symptoms such as breast enlargement and tenderness, morning sickness (nausea and vomiting on waking), weight gain, and urinary frequency.

Does the patient use contraception and, if so, what kind? Does the patient use birth control pills and, if so, what kind? (**Table 38-1 ▾** shows several currently used birth control methods.) Are they uniquely prescribed for her or does she borrow them from a friend? Did the patient just start using birth control pills? (Vaginal spotting is sometimes a side effect of a new prescription.) Does she use spermicides, condoms, or a diaphragm? Does she use an implanted device (such as, Norplant) or an IUD? Woman who use an IUD (also called the "loop" or "coil") are more prone to PID and ectopic pregnancy. The IUD may also perforate the uterus, causing pain and bleeding.

Continuing on with the assessment, determine whether the patient has experienced vaginal bleeding. If yes, try to quantify the amount of blood. Try to obtain an accurate description of the bleeding. Is the blood bright red, dark, or a combination? Are there clots? When did the bleeding start? Is it intermittent or continuous? Is the bleeding excessive? Are signs of shock present? If so, initiate standard fluid therapy with a large-bore IV catheter but run to keep the vein open unless otherwise ordered by medical direction. The systolic blood pressure should be maintained at approximately 70 to 84 mm Hg. Anything higher may worsen the bleeding, and a wide-open infusion can destroy clotting factors and significantly reduce

Table 38-1	Birth Control Methods
Type of Contraceptive	**Description**
Male condom latex/polyurethane	A sheath placed over the erect penis blocking the passage of sperm; the only method that provides good protection against STDs
Female condom	A lubricated polyurethane sheath shaped similarly to the male condom; closed end has a flexible ring that is inserted into the vagina; may give some STD protection
Diaphragm	A dome-shaped rubber disk with a flexible rim that covers the cervix so that sperm cannot reach the uterus; spermicide is applied to the diaphragm before insertion
Lea's shield	A dome-shaped rubber disk with valve and a loop that is held in place by the vaginal wall; covers the upper vagina and cervix so that sperm cannot reach the uterus; spermicide is applied before insertion
Cervical cap	A soft rubber cup with a round rim, which fits snugly around the cervix
Sponge	A disk-shaped polyurethane device containing the spermicide nonoxynol-9
Spermicide	A foam, cream, jelly, film, suppository, or tablet that contains nonoxynol-9, a sperm-killing chemical
Oral contraceptives	Pills that suppress ovulation by the combined actions of the hormones estrogen and progestin; chewable form approved in November 2003 • The progestin-only version reduces and thickens cervical mucus to prevent sperm from reaching the egg. • The 91-day regimen, which contains estrogen and progestin, is taken in 3-month cycles of 12 weeks of active pills followed by 1 week of inactive pills.
Patch	A skin patch worn on the lower abdomen, buttocks, or upper body that releases progestin and estrogen into the bloodstream
Vaginal contraceptive ring	A flexible ring about 2 inches in diameter that is inserted into the vagina and releases progestin and estrogen
Postcoital contraceptives	Pills containing progestin alone or progestin plus estrogen
Injection	An injectable progestin or a combination of progestin and estrogen that inhibits ovulation, prevents sperm from reaching the egg, and/or prevents the fertilized egg from implanting in the uterus
Implant	Six matchstick-size rubber rods that are surgically implanted under the skin of the upper arm, where they steadily release the contraceptive steroid levonorgestrel
IUD	A T-shaped device inserted into the uterus by a health care professional
Periodic abstinence	Deliberately refraining from having sexual intercourse during times when pregnancy is more likely
Transabdominal surgical sterilization—female	Blocking of the woman's fallopian tubes so the egg and sperm cannot meet in the fallopian tube, preventing conception
Sterilization implant—female	Small metallic implant placed into the fallopian tubes; causes scar tissue formation, blocking the fallopian tubes and preventing conception
Surgical sterilization—male	Sealing, tying, or cutting a man's vas deferens so that the sperm cannot travel from the testicles to the penis

Source: Adapted from the Food and Drug Administration. Available at: www.fda.gov/fdac/features/1997/babytabl.html. Accessed May 11, 2006.

Notes from Nancy

Abnormal vaginal bleeding is a complication of pregnancy until proved otherwise.

the blood's oxygen-transporting capacity. An initial fluid bolus of 100 to 200 mL can be administered (as long as you have ruled out pulmonary edema) to improve the patient's perfusion status.

In the Field

Vaginal bleeding is a sign of internal bleeding and should not be taken lightly. Apply a pad over the vaginal area, and transport all used pads with the patient to the hospital for analysis.

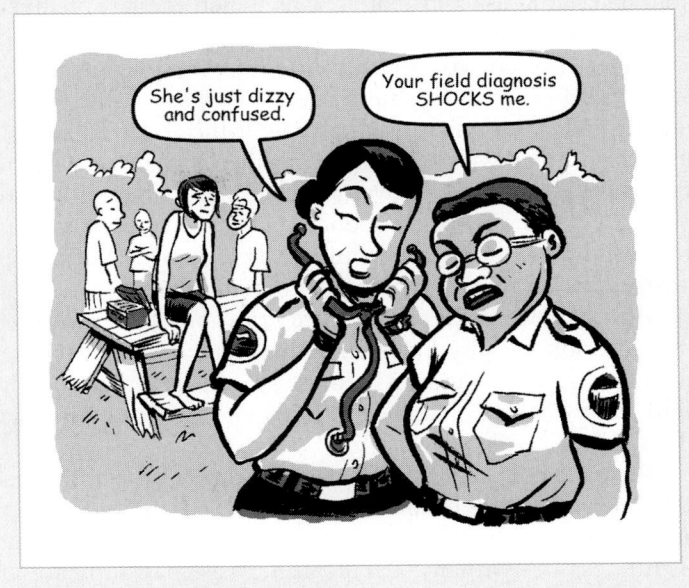

Figure 38-7

Has the patient experienced any vaginal discharge? If so, what was its nature? Did the discharge have an odor? What color was it? Was it clear fluid or mucus? Was it frothy, lumpy, or stringy? Was any blood observed with the fluid? Has the patient or her partner ever had an STD? If yes, which one? Has she ever been treated for an STD?

What is the woman's obstetric history? Has she ever been pregnant? How many times? Has she ever had a live birth? How many? (The medical term for any pregnancy is gravid or gravidity; the term for delivery of an infant is parity. Thus a woman who has been pregnant three times, with one live birth, one miscarriage, and one abortion would be documented as gravida 3, parity [or para] 1.) Have any of the deliveries been complicated? How? Were any of the pregnancies complicated? How? What kind of deliveries did she experience—vaginal or cesarean? How much time passed between pregnancies? Has she had any miscarriages and, if so, how many? Has she had any abortions? Were they spontaneous or elective? If elective, what form of abortion was used—medical or surgical? Elective abortion statistically increases the risks of future miscarriage, ectopic pregnancy, and development of certain cancers. A recent elective abortion may also be the underlying cause of the current emergency.

Does the patient have a history of gynecologic problems? Any known issues such as bleeding or infections? Any ectopic pregnancies?

Does the patient have any known medical conditions? Any personal or familial history of diabetes, cancer, hypertension, or cardiovascular disease? Is the familial history maternal or paternal? Is the patient being treated for a known medical condition? Does she take antihypertensives, anticoagulants, or diuretics? Make sure all of the components of the SAMPLE history are completed at this point.

The Physical Examination

When you are conducting an examination of a woman with abdominal pain, essentially one fundamental question needs to

be answered in the prehospital setting: Is the pain a symptom of a life-threatening condition? Only three life-threatening gynecologic conditions present with pain (ectopic pregnancy, ruptured ovarian cyst, and tubo-ovarian abscess), all of which typically present with similar findings. Other gynecologic causes of pain are not immediately (if at all) life-threatening, but any manifestation of pain will naturally be worrisome to the patient.

Your chief concern is to identify any signs of shock **Figure 38-7 ▲**. Thus, the points of emphasis in the focused history and physical exam are as follows:

- What is the patient's general presentation? Does she appear anxious? Is she restless or apprehensive? Is she fatigued? Is she thirsty?
- What is the condition of the skin and mucous membranes? Is the skin warm and dry? Feverish? Diaphoretic? Cold and clammy? Is there pallor or cyanosis? Does the patient appear dehydrated? Are the mucous membranes pale?
- What are the patient's vital signs? Are there any variations in the pulse? Is it fast, slow, or irregular? Strong or weak and thready? Is the blood pressure normal, low, or elevated? What is normal for the patient? Check the pressure in sitting and standing positions. Are there significant orthostatic changes? If yes, the patient must be presumed to be in shock.

Next, examine the patient's abdomen. Examination of the abdomen is a process of inspection, auscultation, percussion, and palpation.

Inspect the abdomen for signs of abuse, such as bruising. The abdomen is a favorite target of abusers, especially if a woman is pregnant. Note whether there are several bruises in various stages of healing. Do you see any surgical scarring from abdominal surgery or previous cesarean section or stretch marks from previous pregnancies? Is evidence of needle tracks from illicit drug use apparent? The abdomen is a favorite injection spot for chronic drug abusers because clothing hides the evidence. Also look for a positive Cullen's sign (ecchymosis at the umbilicus) or Grey Turner's sign (ecchymosis at the flanks); either is indicative of internal bleeding. Is the abdomen swollen and distended (possibly indicative of pregnancy, internal bleeding, bowel obstruction, or liver problems)? Is it flat and flaccid? Is there any guarding of the abdomen? Are any rashes or lesions present? Is the abdomen symmetrical? Is the liver or spleen enlarged and protruding from under the rib cage?

Auscultate the abdomen before you undertake palpation or percussion because the latter activities tend to alter the frequency of bowel sounds. The most significant finding in the field is *lack of bowel sounds*, which may indicate internal bleeding.

Percussion is a skill not widely practiced by paramedics, but it may yield useful information and guide palpation. Percuss all four quadrants of the abdomen (lightly) to elicit areas of dullness or tympany. Large, dull areas may indicate an underlying mass or enlarged organ. Tympanic areas indicate areas of gas. If the abdomen is distended and tympanic throughout, it generally indicates an intestinal obstruction.

Palpate the abdomen. Examine all quadrants, starting at the quadrant farthest from the pain and working toward the quadrant where the pain is located. Examine this quadrant last. Is the abdomen rigid (possibly indicative of internal bleeding)? Is there point tenderness? Does the palpation elicit more pain? Is rebound tenderness present (indicative of infection, such as may be associated with appendicitis)? Are there masses present? If yes, are they pulsating (abdominal aortic aneurysm)?

Pain Presentations

There are essentially three categories of abdominal pain: visceral pain, parietal pain, and referred pain.

Visceral pain is caused by some dysfunction of the hollow abdominal organs. It is generally poorly localized and diffuse but is typically felt near the midline. Right upper quadrant pain that mediates to the midline may have its origin in the liver or biliary tree. Epigastric pain that mediates to the midline is generally pain from the stomach, pancreas, or duodenum. Midline periumbilical pain typically has its origin in the proximal colon, small intestine, or appendix. Most hypogastric pain is from the colon, bladder, or uterus. Suprapubic pain generally indicates disorders in the rectum.

Parietal pain is caused by inflammation of the parietal peritoneum. It is generally described as a steady, aching pain that is aggravated by movement (such as coughing). The patient will usually try to lie as still as possible to avoid triggering the pain.

Referred pain develops as pain levels become more intense, and the pain seems to radiate or travel. Gallbladder pain tends to radiate and localize to the right shoulder or posterior part of the chest. Pancreatic or duodenal pain may be referred to the patient's back. Pleuritic pain from lungs or ischemic pain from acute coronary syndrome may be referred to the upper abdominal area; the same is true for pain from the pelvis, chest, and spine.

General management of abdominal pain is mostly psychologically supportive. Local protocols may allow for administration of morphine or meperidine (Demerol) for pain management, but you should always check with the receiving facility first. Many physicians are wary of masking abdominal pain until a definitive diagnosis is reached and will likely tell you to withhold administration of an analgesic. If you have obtained a complete history, however, the attending physician may feel comfortable enough to allow administration. Pain-free or reduced pain transport will greatly reduce your patient's anxiety. Just remember to ask the physician first.

Detailed Physical Exam

The overall detailed physical exam is intended to get a complete picture of your patient's health and needs. When you are conducting this exam, pay special attention to the details that are specific to women.

You are the Provider Part 4

The patient's husband greets her as she is brought into the emergency department. She is taken immediately to the obstetric wing, where her physician awaits her. As you transfer care, the husband thanks you for getting her to the hospital so quickly. He said he felt much better knowing she was not alone.

Vital Signs	Recording Time: 20 Minutes
Level of consciousness	Alert, with a Glasgow Coma Scale score of 15
Skin	Pink, warm, and dry
Pulse	82 beats/min and regular
Blood pressure	110/60 mm Hg
Respirations	24 breaths/min
Sao$_2$	100% with oxygen at 4 L/min via nasal cannula

8. What do you believe is the source of her bleeding, cramping, and pain?

Starting at the head, examine the condition of the patient's hair. Is it clean, dirty, oily, or dry and brittle? Most women take great care in their physical appearance; failure to do so may indicate depression. Dry and brittle hair may indicate vitamin deficiencies or chronic methamphetamine use. Examine the way the hair is styled. Does it cover one side of the face more than the other, as if the patient is trying to hide signs of physical abuse. Examine the teeth. Rotting teeth may also be a sign of methamphetamine use. Are there any sores on the patient's face? If yes, they may indicate an underlying condition or may signify illicit drug use.

How is the patient dressed? Long sleeves in hot weather may be an attempt to hide signs of abuse. Is the patient dressed too warmly for the season? This may indicate an illness affecting the body's thermoregulation ability. Do you see signs of bruising on the patient's upper torso or linear or odd-shaped bruises in various stages of healing? Again, these are potential signs of abuse. Do not palpate or examine the breasts unless there is a specific and documentable necessity to do so.

Is small scarring present on the abdomen? It may indicate diabetes and daily insulin shots, or it may signal illicit drug use. Examine the abdomen for the presence of bruising as well, then perform the same examination for the hips and legs. If drug use is suspected, inspect the webs between the toes and fingers because these spots may be used as injection sites in an attempt to hide the signs of use.

Last, check distal pulses and motor and sensory function, and note any deficits or remarkable findings.

Ongoing Assessment

En route to the hospital, recheck your interventions and note any improvement (or decline) in the patient's condition. Remember to obtain serial vital signs. Pay specific attention to the needs of your patient, and accommodate her desire for conversation or silence. Do not focus on your paperwork. You are caring for a human being—the paperwork can wait until the patient has been delivered to the receiving facility.

General Management

The general management of a gynecologic patient is actually simple because there are few interventions you can initiate in the field. Primary management will be directed at mitigating life threats, being supportive and compassionate, and protecting the patient's modesty. In most gynecologic emergencies, your role will be primarily investigatory. The more accurate and detailed the history and examination are, the better you will be at differentiating gynecologic and nongynecologic pathology. For all patients, assess and supply the appropriate oxygen needs. Obtain baseline vital signs, and continue to monitor vital signs throughout patient care for trends. Obtain a baseline electrocardiogram (ECG), preferably a 12-lead ECG. Initiate fluid therapy, providing for pharmacologic interven-

tions (pain management) or volume replacement as necessary. Provide transport. Protect the patient's modesty, and provide psychological care with a supportive attitude.

Management of Gynecologic Trauma

The female genital area is highly vascularized and very susceptible to trauma. Trauma sustained from motor vehicle collisions, sporting events, assault, and even consensual sex are common mechanisms of injury. Bleeding from genital trauma may be profuse (and very painful), and, if the patient is currently having her period, trying to differentiate between menstrual blood and trauma-related blood can be difficult.

Applying simple external pressure over the area of the laceration is usually sufficient to control bleeding. Bleeding from the *internal* genitalia, by contrast, can be massive and very difficult to control. Blindly packing the vagina is dangerous and is *not* recommended or even useful. A woman with exsanguinating vaginal hemorrhage must be treated as any other injured patient with exsanguinating hemorrhage—that is, she must be treated for shock and rapidly transported to the hospital.

Assessment of a patient with gynecologic trauma will focus on the following questions: What are her symptoms? Is there a mechanism of injury? Is the patient pale, cool, and diaphoretic? Does she appear fatigued? Anxious? Irritable? Is the patient using sanitary pads or tampons? Can she tell you how many pads have been soaked? An average pad holds about 30 mL of blood and a tampon about 20 mL. Is the blood a normal color? Is it brighter or darker than normal? Do any clots appear in the flow? Is the abdomen tender or distended? Affirmative answers may indicate that the patient is in the early stages of shock. Keep the patient recumbent. Ensure an adequate airway, administer oxygen, insert a large-bore IV catheter and give normal saline or lactated Ringer's solution, and monitor the ECG Figure 38-8 . Assess vital signs frequently.

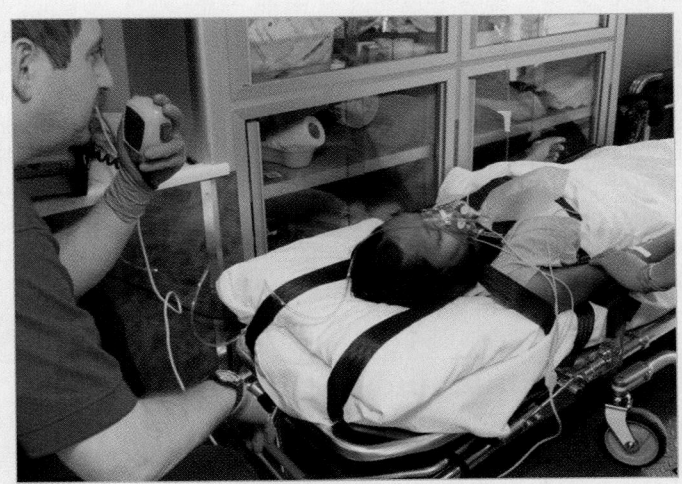

Figure 38-8 A patient with gynecologic trauma should be kept lying down. Manage the airway, administer supplemental oxygen and IV fluids, and monitor the ECG.

Table 38-2	Estimating Blood Volume Loss			
Grade of Hemorrhage/ Blood Loss	Heart Rate	Respiratory Rate	Blood Pressure	Central Nervous System
First/< 15%	Minor tachycardia	No change	No change	No change
Second/15%–30%	Tachycardia	Tachypnea	Decreased pulse pressure	Anxiety or combativeness
Third/30%–40%	Marked tachycardia	Marked tachypnea	Systolic hypotension	Altered mental status
Fourth/> 40%	Marked tachycardia	Marked tachypnea	Severe systolic hypotension	Comatose/unresponsive

Source: Adapted from United States Department of Defense. *Emergency War Surgery Nato Handbook.* 2004:Table 7-1. Available at: http://www.bordeninstitute .army.mil/emrgncywarsurg/Chp7Shock&Resuscitation.pdf. Accessed May 18, 2006.

Consider transport in the Trendelenburg position. Do *not* perform an interior vaginal exam. Examination of the external genitalia is warranted in the presence of genital trauma only.

Estimating Blood Loss

Estimating blood volume loss in the field is a tricky business and cannot be done accurately, especially in female patients, in whom trauma and the menses may be found together. Nevertheless, some physicians may want you to make a field estimate before arrival at the hospital. Myriad techniques are used for estimating blood loss in the field—the soaked tampon method, the soaked chux pad used in nursing, and the "palmar" method used by "old-timer" street medics. These methods provide a very rough guess of total blood loss and fail to take into consideration blood that may be leaking into an internal cavity. The most reliable field method is based on symptomology. **Table 38-2 ▲** shows estimated blood loss based on the patient's symptoms.

One rule of thumb is that for the average patient, 7% to 8% of body weight is the available circulating blood volume (70 mL/kg body weight). For example, a 70-kg patient has approximately 4,900 mL of available circulating blood. Thus, if the patient has the symptoms listed in Table 38-2 for 30% to 40% blood loss, you would estimate 1,470 to 1,960 mL of blood lost. Even the pulse changes listed in Table 38-2 are not highly reliable indicators—recent military studies have shown that that the heart rate can remain fairly stable even in severe cases of shock. Instead, consider the overall presentation of the patient. What are her symptoms? Is she pale, cool, or diaphoretic? Is she thirsty? Do the symptoms include restlessness or nausea? This information paints a fuller picture regarding how much blood the patient has lost.

Assessment and Management of Specific Conditions

Of the several diverse gynecologic conditions that you may be called on to treat, only three are truly life-threatening emergencies: ectopic pregnancy, ruptured ovarian cyst, and tubo-ovarian abscess. Each of these manifests with similar symptoms, so they

are virtually impossible to definitively diagnose in the field. You may also be called on to treat conditions related to PID.

Pelvic Inflammatory Disease

A patient with PID will present with abdominal pain in virtually every scenario encountered by paramedics. The pain generally starts during or after normal menstruation, so eliciting the LMP is an important component of the history. The pain is typically diffuse and is spread over both quadrants of the lower abdomen. It may be described as "achy," and the patient may volunteer that the pain is made worse by walking or by sexual intercourse. The latter revelation usually indicates cervical involvement in the infective process. Pain localized to the right upper quadrant is indicative of infection that has spread to the abdominal cavity. Associated symptoms may include vaginal discharge, fever and chills, and pain or burning on urination (dysuria).

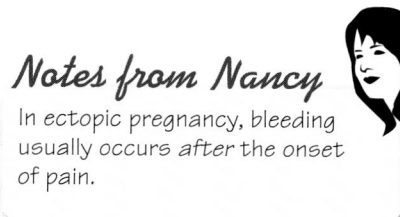

Notes from Nancy

In ectopic pregnancy, bleeding usually occurs *after* the onset of pain.

Any woman with PID who feels sick enough to call for an ambulance probably has a severe infection and is likely to present as febrile and look ill. Physical examination findings may be sparse or may include the entire textbook profile. Be alert for signs of peritoneal irritation (that is, the patient winces on palpation of the abdomen or every time the ambulance hits a bump). Be very gentle should you decide to palpate this patient's abdomen as part of the examination.

PID cannot be treated in the field because it generally requires administration of an appropriate antibiotic for 10 to

In the Field

The ambulance does not carry the appropriate supplies and equipment for a definitive diagnosis in the field. Look for life threats, treat for shock, and transport in a position of comfort.

14 days. The best you can do is obtain a thorough history, make the patient as comfortable as possible, and transport with as gentle a ride as can be managed.

Ectopic Pregnancy

Nearly all women with ectopic pregnancy will present with a chief complaint of abdominal pain. This pain will generally be localized to one side of the abdomen and, in the early stages, will be described as crampy and intermittent. As the pregnancy progresses, the embryo will abort or the tube will rupture. Either event will produce severe abdominal pain, localized to one side. By the time EMS is involved, the patient is likely to be in constant pain, which will be diffused throughout the abdomen. Diffuse pain is especially likely if there is significant hemoperitoneum (blood in the abdominal cavity). Referred pain to the shoulder is ominous because it indicates massive hemoperitoneum. Vaginal bleeding is another sign of ectopic pregnancy, occurring in approximately 65% of women. This bleeding will usually occur *after* onset of pain in ectopic pregnancy, in contrast with spontaneous abortion, in which bleeding usually *precedes* pain.

In the history, you need to establish the intervals between the manifestations of the various symptoms. Part of the blood volume in ectopic pregnancy originates in the shedding of the uterine lining as the embryo is displaced from its site of implantation and the production of hormones ceases. Vaginal bleeding may itself be light, so it is not a good indicator of internal blood loss. Look for a positive Cullen's sign or Grey Turner's sign and for signs of shock and abdominal distention and tenderness to help gauge internal bleeding. Signs of shock will generally be a pulse greater than 100 beats/min; systolic blood pressure less than 90 mm Hg, cold, moist skin; fatigue; and restlessness and anxiety.

The classic triad for diagnosing ectopic pregnancy is amenorrhea (75% of patients), vaginal bleeding, and abdominal pain. A history of ectopic pregnancy, IUD use, and a history of PID also significantly raise the index of suspicion. *Always treat for shock in any woman presenting with abdominal pain and vaginal bleeding, regardless of whether shock symptoms are actually present* **Figure 38-9 ▶**. Follow these steps in the management of a patient with a suspected ectopic pregnancy:

- Ensure an adequate airway, and administer high-concentration supplemental oxygen.
- Keep the patient left laterally recumbent, even if unconscious and intubated.
- Insert at least one large-bore IV catheter and administer lactated Ringer's solution or normal saline; be prepared to run it wide open if signs of shock develop.
- Give nothing by mouth, including water.
- If local protocols allow, consider urethral catheterization, filling the bulb with normal saline. This can help tamponade the bleeding and will drain the bladder. A full bladder can exacerbate bleeding from uterine relaxation.
- Anticipate vomiting. Have an emesis bag and suction close at hand.

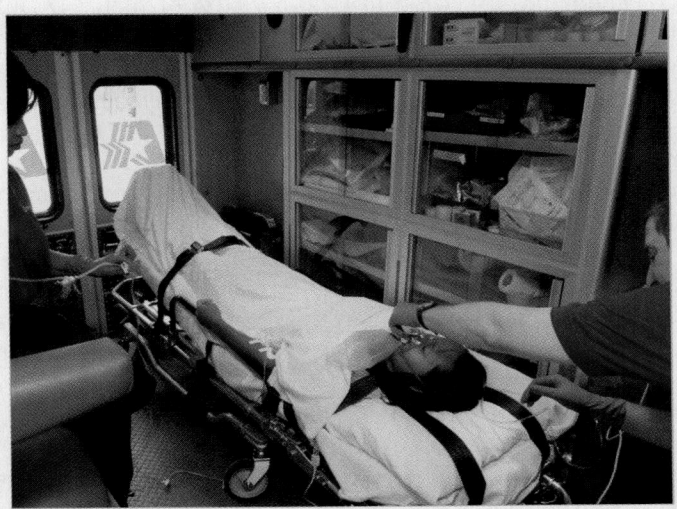

Figure 38-9 Always treat for shock in any woman with abdominal pain and vaginal bleeding.

- Keep the patient warm.
- Monitor the patient's ECG.
- Transport.
- Notify the receiving hospital of the patient's suspected diagnosis, her condition, and your estimated time of arrival.
- Do not give pain management drugs because they may hinder accurate diagnosis in the ED.
- Recheck vital signs frequently during transport.

Ruptured Ovarian Cyst and Tubo-ovarian Abscess

A patient with an ovarian cyst may complain of dull, achy pain in the lower back and thighs, abdominal pain or pressure, nausea and vomiting, breast tenderness, abnormal bleeding and painful menstruation, and painful intercourse. A patient with a tubo-ovarian abscess may present with severe abdominal pain, guarding and rebound tenderness, nausea and vomiting, abdominal distention, and fever. If the abscess ruptures, infectious matter can spread throughout the entire body. The prehospital management of ruptured ovarian cyst and tubo-ovarian abscess are the same as for ectopic pregnancy.

▌Sexual Assault

Sexual assault is a crime that is as old as humankind. It can take many forms, but the most common is rape. Among the crimes that humans perpetrate against their fellow humans, rape ranks as one of the most perverse and devastating. In the United States, one of every three women will be raped in her lifetime, and one of every four will be sexually molested, often before the age of 12 years.

Paramedics called on to treat a victim of sexual assault, molestation, or actual or alleged rape face many complex issues, ranging from obvious medical ones to serious psychological and legal issues. In particular, you may be the first person the victim has contact with after the encounter, and how the situation is managed from first contact throughout treatment and transport may have lasting effects for the patient and you. Professionalism, tact, kindness, and sensitivity are of paramount importance.

Because rape is a *crime,* you can generally expect police involvement early in the situation. In many cases, EMS may be called by the police. Police officers generally have rudimentary medical training, with many states requiring at least basic training at the first responder level. Nevertheless, primary training for police officers focuses on *investigation,* not patient care.

A rape victim has just experienced a purposeful "major vehicle crash" of her mind and body. The act was most likely perpetrated by someone she knew and trusted. The last thing she wants to do is give a concise, detailed report of what she has just experienced, and attempting to elicit information in this manner most likely will cause the victim to "shut down." Whenever possible, a female rape victim should be given the option of being treated by a female paramedic because the patient may be experiencing ambivalent feelings toward men in general; these feelings will hinder assessment and the patient's well-being.

The job of the police is to solve the crime, arrest the perpetrator, and see justice served. The job of paramedics is to deal with the medical aspects of the case and to act as the patient advocate. In this capacity, it is important for you to focus on several key issues.

The first issue is the medical treatment of the patient. Is she physically injured? Are any life-threatening injuries present? Does the patient complain of any pain?

The second issue is your psychological care of the patient. Do not cross-examine her or attempt to elicit information for the benefit of the police. These issues will be handled later in the ED setting. Do not pass judgment on the patient, and protect her from the judgment of others on the scene. It does not matter how the patient is dressed, what her local reputation is, where she was, or what she was doing when the assault occurred. The concept of a woman "deserving" to be raped is just as ludicrous as you "deserving" to be assaulted for wearing the colors of a rival sports team. A crime has been committed, and you need to remain cognizant of that fact. Many women report feeling "reraped" when subjected to interrogation, criticism, or incredulity.

Last, remember that you are at a crime scene. Although your job is to treat the *medical* aspects of the incident and not collect evidence, you still have a responsibility to *preserve* evidence. Do not cut through any clothing or throw away anything from the scene. Place bloodstained articles in separate paper (not plastic) bags. Obtain evidentiary bags from the police if necessary. Paper bags allow wet items to dry naturally, whereas plastic allows mold to grow and may destroy biologic evidence.

It may also be necessary to gently persuade the patient to *not* clean herself up. This will be a natural desire on the part of the patient, stemming from the desire to "wash away" the humiliation and embarrassment of the assault. Valuable evidence can be destroyed in this process. The patient also needs to be discouraged from urinating, changing clothes, moving her bowels, or rinsing out her mouth. She will need to be photographed by law enforcement personnel as well, and the photographic record needs to be as accurate as possible. If the patient cannot be dissuaded from taking these actions, respect her feelings. Some patients may refuse transport altogether, and they have the right to do so. Do not simply accept this refusal and leave. Instead, try to persuade the patient to allow you to call a friend or relative who can stay with her or, better yet, with whom the victim can stay. Getting the patient away from the scene keeps her from having to constantly relive the experience by being subjected to the environment where the assault occurred. Many churches offer pastoral care to rape victims, and the patient may benefit from this resource if she has religious inclinations. Many communities also have rape crisis centers, with victim advocates on-call. Getting a professional advocate to the scene may help the patient deal with the trauma, and the advocate can better explain the necessities of evidence preservation in more compassionate detail. Many victim advocates are rape-trauma survivors themselves.

Notes from Nancy

Find out if the woman has been injured. Do not ask questions about the incident itself.

Documentation and Communication

Just as you might be uncomfortable talking about your last sexual encounter to a total stranger, so your patient might feel a mix of emotions, including shame and frustration after being assaulted. A calm, nonjudgmental approach from a same-sex paramedic will be helpful.

Limit any physical examination to a brief survey for life-threatening injuries. Expose and examine the vaginal area only if there is evidence of bleeding that needs to be treated. Do everything possible to protect the patient's privacy. Examine and interview the patient with a minimum of people present, moving her to the ambulance if necessary.

The patient report is a legal document and, should the case result in an arrest and subsequent trial, may be subpoenaed. Keep the report concise, and record only what the patient stated in her own words. Use quotation marks to indicate that you are reporting the patient's version of events. Do not insert your own "opinion" as to whether the patient was raped or offer any conclusions that would validate or invalidate the patient's account of the event. Focus on the facts. Record all of your observations during the physical exam—the patient's emotional state, the condition of her clothing, obvious injuries, and so forth. Bear in mind that rape is a *legal* diagnosis, not a medical diagnosis. The medical team can establish only whether sexual intercourse occurred; a court must decide whether intercourse was inflicted forcibly on the victim, against her will.

Sexual Practices and Medical Emergencies

The human race is fascinated by sex. Indeed, the various ways humankind can engage in sexual acts has been a source of intense study and curiosity since the beginnings of recorded history. The Bible records the first sexual act between human beings in the book of Genesis. Other works that record the sexual interactions of men and women range from the *Kama Sutra* of ancient India to the modern lab reports of Masters and Johnson. Of particular interest to paramedics, however, is when private sexual practices go bad, resulting in an embarrassing call to 9-1-1.

The most common sexual gynecologic emergency you may encounter is simply a foreign object (for example, a soda pop or beer bottle or a sex toy) that has become stuck in the vagina or anus. For example, a bottle may develop a vacuum inside of the body and stick to an interior structure. Attempts at removal by the patient may result in intense pain or even vaginal bleeding as internal structures tear. Bleeding and pain cause the patient to panic. With this type of call, keep the patient calm, protect his or her dignity as much as possible, and transport. Overpenetration of any item may lead to internal injury, and should be managed as such.

Some cases of bottle insertion may be associated with rape, so bear in mind that the patient may be an assault victim. Some gangs have been known to insert beer bottles in a woman's vagina after rape, then take turns punching the woman in the lower abdomen until the bottle breaks. If this is the case, use extreme care and do not move the patient more than necessary to prevent even more internal damage.

Among some of the more bizarre practices you may encounter include a technique known as "fisting" and the insertion of live animals into the vagina, including fish, eels, snakes, worms, and hamsters. The patient becomes alarmed when the animal goes in but does not come out. Treat such a case as you would with any other foreign object, remain nonjudgmental, and transport. Do not attempt to retrieve the animal from inside the vagina. Transport the patient in a knees-flexed, legs-together position. Having a live snake make a sudden reappearance in the back of a moving ambulance is a recipe for disaster.

Documentation and Communication

"Fisting" involves placing the closed fist and wrist into a body orifice (vagina or rectum) for sexual stimulation. Whether the patient is male or female, organ rupture (rectum, vagina) is likely. Life-threatening peritonitis may result. As with other sexually related injuries, patients are often reluctant to divulge correct historical information.

Drugs Used to Facilitate Rape

Although rape may be second only to murder as the oldest crime, the use of drugs to facilitate rape is just about as old. Alcohol was probably the first drug used to facilitate rape and, even in this modern age, remains the most common element to rape scenes. The rapist and the victim may be intoxicated; as the central nervous system becomes depressed, the rapist becomes more aggressive and the victim more vulnerable. Some of the earliest reports in the United States of a drug other than alcohol used in crimes date back to the late 1800s, when legend has it that a Chicago bar owner named Mickey Finn would slip patrons drops of chloral hydrate in their drinks, for the purpose of knocking them out for robbery. Today, the drugs of choice for commission of the crime of rape are "club drugs" such as gamma-hydroxybutyric acid (GHB), ketamine, ecstasy, and Rohypnol.

Gamma-Hydroxybutyric Acid

Gamma-hydroxybutyric acid (GHB) is the best known of the date-rape drugs. During the 1980s, it was available over-the-counter in nutrition stores as a body-building aid, sexual aid, and sleep aid. Today, its only legal use in the United States is by prescription for treatment of a rare form of narcolepsy. Illegally produced GHB is very common in the "rave" and "club" crowds. This colorless liquid generally has a salty taste that is disguised when mixed in with a drink. Street names for GHB include Georgia home boy, grievous bodily harm, easy lay, G, scoop, liquid X, soap, and salty water.

GHB is a depressant and has amnestic properties. Symptoms of GHB intoxication range from sleepiness, loss of muscle tone, and forgetfulness to seizurelike activity. Respirations and heartbeat are depressed, progressing to a comalike state that generally last about 2 hours. Emergency care is supportive, making sure that adequate ventilatory support is initiated for patients in respiratory depression. There is no current antidote for GHB ingestion, and naloxone (Narcan) and flumazenil (Romazicon, a benzodiazepine agonist) are of no benefit.

Ketamine Hydrochloride

Ketamine hydrochloride (Ketalar, Ketaset) is predominantly marketed in the United States as a veterinary anesthetic. It works well in this capacity owing to its ability to block pain pathways without affecting respiratory or circulatory function. Ketamine also has some use in human medicine owing to its dissociative effects, and it can be effective in cases of major trauma, such as burn injuries. It creates an "out of body" sensation that removes the patient from the pain stimulus. In some people, it may produce frightening hallucinations. The hallucinatory effects make this drug popular with the club crowd, and the anesthetic and dissociative effects make it a popular date-rape drug. Street names for this agent include special K, vitamin K, cat Valium, and Fort Dodge.

A phencyclidine hydrochloride (PCP) derivative, ketamine has physical effects similar to those of PCP, plus psychedelic effects resembling those associated with LSD (lysergic acid diethylamide). It is available in liquid and powder form and can be inhaled, injected, or mixed into a drink. Symptoms of ketamine use include loss of coordination, muscle rigidity, slurred speech, and a catatonic or "blank" stare. The anesthetic properties may also produce a general sense of "numbness." Like PCP, ketamine can lead to aggressive and violent behavior and an exaggerated sense of strength. Physiologic symptoms of overdose include nausea and vomiting, hypertension, and respiratory impairment leading to oxygen deprivation of the brain. There is no field antidote for ketamine.

Ecstasy

Methylenedioxymethamphetamine (MDMA), also known as ecstasy, is a methamphetamine derivative with hallucinogenic properties. It is generally sold in capsule or tablet form but can also be found as a powder. It can be injected, snorted, ingested, or smoked. The tablets come in many colors and may be imprinted with the Superman, Batman, Nike, Mercedes, Rolls Royce, or any of many other logos. Street names for ecstasy include XTC, Adam, X, lover's speed, and clarity. Although law enforcement reports cite it as a date-rape drug, ecstasy is actually a stimulant. Mental confusion is a side effect of its ingestion, and overdose can result in unconsciousness and death. Ecstasy affects serotonin levels in the brain, which probably explains the reports of heightened sexual experiences and feelings of tranquility the drug allegedly produces. These effects also explain why it is included in the date-rape category—the powder can be mixed in an alcoholic drink to get the victim "in the mood."

The signs and symptoms of ecstasy use are similar to those of cocaine and speed. The most serious are a rapid heart rate and rapid increase of body temperature, often to deadly levels. Other symptoms include anxiety, hypertension, blurred vision, mental confusion, nausea, and excessive sweating, leading to dangerous levels of dehydration. Rapid eye movement and tremors have also been reported. Bruxism (teeth clenching) is another common side effect, and regular users may use paraphernalia such as rubber or candy pacifiers to ease the effects. A surgical mask smeared with Vicks VapoRub is also a clue of ecstasy use because the vapors reportedly increase the effect of the "rush."

Rohypnol

Rohypnol is one of the latest drugs to hit the club scene and be used as a date-rape drug. Rohypnol is illegal in the United States but is legally marketed outside the United States by Roche Pharmaceutical as a sedative and preoperative anesthetic. This benzodiazepine has sedative-hypnotic, amnestic, and anesthetic properties. Street names for Rohypnol include roofies, roof, roachies, rocha, and Mexican Valium.

Rohypnol is sold as a white, scored tablet, with the word "Roche" appearing on one side. The tablet can be dissolved in a drink, where it is undetectable. Roche Pharmaceuticals has recently added a color base of royal blue to the tablet; if the drug is mixed with a drink, the color will appear.

When ingested, Rohypnol impairs judgment and motor skills, creating a condition in which the victim is unable to resist a sexual attack. Its sedative-hypnotic effects also make victims highly prone to suggestion. Losing social inhibitions (disinhibition) is a reported side effect of Rohypnol when taken alone or in combination with alcohol. The potentiated effect of alcohol on Rohypnol creates a significant danger.

Effects generally begin within 30 minutes after Rohypnol is consumed and last for about 8 hours, with peak effects occurring about 2 hours after ingestion. Symptoms include decreased blood pressure, drowsiness, dizziness, confusion, and memory loss. This last effect makes Rohypnol a particularly popular date-rape drug because the victim has no memory of the last 15 to 20 minutes or longer before blacking out. Overdose can lead to death due to central nervous system depression. Treatment in the field is ALS supportive, with possible administration of flumazenil. Naloxone (Narcan) has no effect on Rohypnol, but its administration may be considered because Rohypnol is sometimes used in conjunction with other drugs.

Documentation and Communication
In some states, you will be required to report assaults.

You are the Provider Summary

1. Based on your general impression and initial assessment, how would you categorize this patient?

Based on her mentation, skin signs, and vital signs, Mrs. Medina appears to be in no immediate danger. At this point, she is in stable condition, which allows for more thorough history taking and assessment. Be aware that her condition could change, though.

2. What interventions would you choose to initiate at this point?

Although she appears to be well ventilated and oxygenated and shows no signs of shock, your patient will benefit from supplemental oxygen and IV access. Keeping her on her side and covering her to preserve body temperature are other important aspects of care.

3. What other information would you like to know?

Obtaining a SAMPLE history is very important, as is conducting a thorough physical exam, including inspection, auscultation, and palpation of the abdomen. You also need to estimate blood loss, which can be done by asking your patient about the number and type of pads she has used since the spotting began.

4. What issues do you foresee that will likely impact patient care?

The patient is understandably very frightened. Your management of her will require gentle care, compassion, and utmost respect for preserving her modesty. When you perform your assessment, explain everything that you are doing and why you are doing it. Establishing and maintaining trust with your patient will go a long way for both of you.

5. Given the information you have so far, will this patient require aggressive prehospital care?

Sometimes your job is to "hover." Because most paramedics have an inherent drive to "take action," sometimes watching and anticipating problems can be quite a challenge.

6. What are the three truly life-threatening gynecologic emergencies?

The three truly life-threatening emergencies discussed in this chapter are ectopic pregnancy, ruptured ovarian cysts, and tubo-ovarian abscesses. None of your findings correspond to those found in any of these conditions. In particular, this patient does not present with signs of shock.

7. Does your differential diagnosis include any of these conditions?

Based on this information, your differential diagnosis would not include ectopic pregnancy, ruptured ovarian cyst, and tubo-ovarian abscess. The patient could be experiencing the onset of a spontaneous abortion, hormonal imbalances, or stress.

8. What do you believe is the source of her bleeding, cramping, and pain?

Sometimes we find ourselves scratching our heads as to the underlying condition that causes a specific patient presentation. Sometimes we are never certain. Focus on recognizing and treating life-threatening emergencies and keep a suspicious eye out for the worst-case scenarios.

Prep Kit

■ Ready for Review

- Gynecology is the study of and care for diseases of the female reproductive system.
- The external anatomy of the female genitalia, sometimes referred to as the pudendum, includes the mons veneris, labia majora, labia minora, perineum, clitoris, prepuce, and vestibule.
- The internal anatomy of the female genitalia includes the vagina, Bartholin glands, and the hymen (before rupture).
- Menstruation (menses or period) is the vaginal discharge of primarily blood that generally occurs every 25 to 34 days in premenopausal women.
- A woman can experience physical changes during the menstrual cycle that result in fluid retention, breast pain and tenderness, headache, cramping, and more intense emotional states. This premenstrual syndrome can be debilitating.
- The last menses is called menopause; it generally occurs between the ages of 40 and 50 years. Women may experience physical symptoms of menopause, including diaphoresis, hair loss, hot flashes, muscle aches and pains, headache, dyspnea, vertigo, digestive problems, and emotional instability.
- Mittelschmerz is abdominal pain and cramping that occur about 2 weeks before menstruation. Dysmenorrhea is painful menstruation. Prehospital treatment is supportive.
- Amenorrhea is the absence or cessation of menses. The most common cause is pregnancy. Amenorrhea can also occur in athletes and in people with anorexia nervosa or emotional problems.
- Endometritis is inflammation or irritation of the endometrium. Symptoms include malaise, fever, bowel problems, vaginal bleeding, abdominal distention, and lower abdominal or pelvic pain.
- Endometriosis is the growth of endometrial tissue outside of the uterus. It can cause infertility. Symptoms include low back, pelvic, or abdominal pain; painful coitus; elimination problems during menstruation; menstrual cramping; and heavy menstruation.
- Pelvic inflammatory disease (PID) is an infection of the female upper reproductive organs. One of the most common causes of abdominal pain in women, it can cause infertility.
- Interstitial cystitis is a chronically inflamed or irritated bladder wall. Symptoms may mimic those of gynecologic origin.
- In ectopic pregnancy, a fertilized egg implants somewhere other than the uterus, usually in a fallopian tube, which can lead to rupture of the fallopian tube.
- Ruptured ovarian cyst and tubo-ovarian abscess are other gynecologic conditions that can become an emergency.
- Toxic shock syndrome is a form of septic shock that can result from an infection in the body. Symptoms include syncope, mylagia, diarrhea, vomiting, headache, fever, sore throat, petechiae, rash, and bloodshot eyes. Transport patients rapidly.
- Sexually transmitted diseases (STDs) can cause PID. STDs include bacterial vaginosis, chancroid, chlamydia, cytomegalovirus, genital herpes, gonorrhea, syphilis, and trichomoniasis.
- Symptoms of STDs can include itching, burning, pain, fishy smelling discharge, sores around the genitals, swollen or painful lymph glands, lower abdominal or back pain, nausea, fever, painful intercourse, bleeding between menstrual periods, fatigue, headache, and painful urination.
- When assessing a patient with a gynecologic emergency, begin by focusing on the ABCs.
- Protect the patient's modesty at all times. Gynecologic emergencies can be very embarrassing for the patient.
- If the chief complaint is abdominal pain, investigate the pain by following the mnemonic LORDS TRACHEA: Location, Onset, Radiation, Duration, Severity, Timing, Relief, Aggravation, Character, History, Eating, and Associated symptoms.

- Determine when the patient had her last menstrual period, if it is unusual in any way, whether she could be pregnant, and whether she uses contraception.
- Vaginal bleeding that does not occur during the course of regular menstruation is cause for concern. Consider whether there is a mechanism of injury. Try to obtain an accurate description of the bleeding.
- During the patient history, obtain the patient's obstetric history, including any previous pregnancies, miscarriages, or abortions. If the patient has a vaginal discharge, obtain a description of it.
- During the physical exam, determine whether there is a life-threatening condition. Inspect the abdomen for signs of abuse. Palpate the painful quadrant last.
- Abdominal pain can be visceral, parietal, or referred. Management should be psychologically supportive.
- General management for gynecologic emergencies is simple, including addressing life threats, being supportive, and protecting the patient's modesty.
- Gynecologic trauma may cause profuse bleeding. Control external bleeding using pressure over the area, but never pack the vagina. Attempt to estimate the patient's blood loss.
- Patients with PID will present with abdominal pain starting during or after menstruation. Take a thorough history and transport gently.
- The three life-threatening gynecologic emergencies are ectopic pregnancy, ruptured ovarian cyst, and tubo-ovarian abscess. Patients will present with abdominal pain and possibly vaginal bleeding, nausea, vomiting, or fever. Identify when each symptom began. Management includes airway maintenance, supplemental oxygen, positioning the patient on the left side, IV fluids, keeping the patient warm, monitoring the ECG, and transporting.
- Sexual assault is a category of crime that includes molestation and rape. Your compassion and professionalism in these situations are of the utmost importance.
- It may be difficult to obtain a history from a victim of rape. Have a female paramedic treat the patient when possible.
- Remember that your job is to medically treat the patient. Ask only medical questions, and do not judge the patient. Limit the physical exam to addressing life-threatening injuries.
- Preserve evidence when possible. Try to persuade the rape victim not to clean herself.
- If a rape victim refuses transport, try to call a friend or relative with whom she can stay.
- Document cases of sexual assault properly and professionally. Report the patient's words in quotation marks. Record facts obtained from the physical examination.
- Sexual emergencies may involve foreign objects stuck in the vagina or anus, which may potentially lead to internal injury. Do not remove the object. Remain professional, and transport the patient.
- Drugs used to facilitate rape include gamma-hydroxybutyric acid, ketamine hydrochloride, ecstasy, and Rohypnol. These drugs can cause sleepiness, forgetfulness, numbness, loss of inhibitions, or rapid heart rate and increase in body temperature, depending on the drug.

■ Vital Vocabulary

amenorrhea Absence of menstruation.

bacterial vaginosis An overgrowth of bacteria in the vagina, characterized by itching, burning, or pain, and possibly a "fishy" smelling discharge.

Bartholin glands The glands that secrete mucus for sexual lubrication.

chancroid A highly contagious sexually transmitted disease caused by the bacteria *Haemophilus ducreyi*, which causes painful sores (ulcers), usually of the genitals.

chlamydia A sexually transmitted disease caused by the bacterium *Chlamydia trachomatis*.

climacteric End phase of a woman's life menstrual cycle.

clitoris A small, cylindrical mass of erectile tissue and nerves located at the anterior junction of the labia minora, homologous to the glans penis of the male.

contraceptive device A device used to prevent pregnancy.

cystadenomas Fluid-filled cysts that form on the outer ovarian surface.

cytomegalovirus (CMV) A herpesvirus that can produce the symptoms of prolonged high fever, chills, headache, malaise, extreme fatigue, and an enlarged spleen.

dermoid cysts Ovarian cysts containing formational tissue, such as hair and teeth.

dysmenorrhea Painful menstruation.

ecstasy A drug officially named methylenedioxymethamphetamine (MDMA) that is sometimes used to facilitate date rape; a methamphetamine derivative with hallucinogenic properties; street names include XTC, Adam, X, lover's speed, and clarity.

ectopic pregnancy A pregnancy in which the ovum implants somewhere other than the uterine endometrium.

endometriomas Ovarian cysts formed from endometrial tissue.

endometriosis A condition in which endometrial tissue grows outside the uterus.

endometritis An inflammation of the endometrium that often is associated with a bacterial infection.

endometrium The inner mucous membrane of the uterus.

gamma-hydroxybutyric acid (GHB) A drug used to facilitate date rape; is colorless with a salty taste disguised when mixed with a drink; street names include Georgia home boy, grievous bodily harm, easy lay, G, scoop, liquid X, soap, and salty water.

Gardnerella vaginitis An infection caused by a bacterium that normally resides in the genital area in women but that can cause infection if the bacteria become too numerous; signs and symptoms include a vaginal odor that may be fishy, itching, irritation, and, possibly, a smooth, thin, sticky, white or gray discharge.

genital herpes An infection of the genitals, buttocks, or anal area caused by herpes simplex virus (HSV), which may cause sores of the genitals, mouth, or lips.

genital warts Warts caused by the human papillomavirus (HPV), a sexually transmitted disease; also called condylomata acuminata or venereal warts.

gonorrhea A sexually transmitted disease caused by *Neisseria gonorrhoeae*.

gravid Pregnant; the number of times a woman has been pregnant is indicated by gravida, for example, gravida 3 indicates three pregnancies.

hemoperitoneum Blood in the peritoneal cavity.

hemorrhagic cyst A blood-filled sac that forms when a blood vessel bursts in a cyst wall and the blood fills the sac.

hymen A membrane that protects the vaginal orifice before first intercourse.

hypermenorrhea Menstrual blood flow that lasts several days longer than it should or flow that is abnormally excessive.

imperforate hymen A situation in which the hymen completely covers the vaginal orifice.

ketamine hydrochloride A drug used to facilitate date rape but that is predominantly marketed in the United States as a veterinary anesthetic and is a phencyclidine hydrochloride derivative; street names include special K, vitamin K, cat Valium, and Fort Dodge.

labia majora Outer fleshy "lips" covered with pubic hair that protect the vagina.

labia minora Inner fleshy "lips" devoid of pubic hair that protect the vagina.

menarche The beginning phase of a woman's life cycle of menstruation.

menopause The ending phase of a woman's life cycle of menstruation.

menstrual cycle The entire monthly cycle of menstruation from start to finish.

menstruation Monthly flow of blood.

metrorrhagia Irregular but frequent vaginal bleeding.

mons veneris Also called the mons pubis, this is a rounded pad of fatty tissue that overlies the symphysis pubis and is anterior to the urethral and vaginal openings.

parietal pain Pain caused by inflammation of the parietal peritoneum that is generally described as steady, aching, and aggravated by movement.

parity The number of times a woman has delivered an infant or infants.

perineum The area between the vaginal opening and the anus.

pelvic inflammatory disease (PID) An infection of the female upper organs of reproduction, specifically the uterus, ovaries, and fallopian tubes.

polymenorrhea Menstrual blood flow that occurs more often than a 24-day interval.

premenstrual syndrome (PMS) A cluster of all or some of the troubling symptoms that occur during a woman's menstrual phase that can include fluid retention, breast pain and tenderness, headache, severe cramping, and emotional changes, including agitation, irritability, depression, and anger.

prepuce In the anatomy of the female genitalia, a layer of skin directly above the clitoris.

pudendum The female external genitalia.

rape Sexual intercourse inflicted forcibly on another person, against that person's will.

referred pain Pain that seems to radiate or travel as it becomes more intense.

Rohypnol A benzodiazepine used to facilitate date rape and that can create memory loss; street names include roofies, roof, roachies, rocha, and Mexican Valium.

ruptured ovarian cyst A fluid-filled sac within the ovary that bursts from internal pressure.

sexual assault An attack against a person that is sexual in nature, the most of common of which is rape.

syphilis A sexually transmitted disease caused by the bacterium *Treponema pallidum*, which manifests in three stages—primary, secondary, and late—and is transmitted through direct contact with open sores.

toxic shock syndrome (TSS) A form of septic shock caused by *Streptococcus pyogenes* (group A strep) or *Staphylococcus aureus*; initial symptoms include syncope, myalgia, diarrhea, vomiting, headache, fever, and sore throat.

trichomoniasis A parasitic infection.

tubo-ovarian abscess An infectious mass growing within the ovaries and fallopian tubes.

vagina The lower portion of the birth canal, which also serves as a passage for menstrual flow and as the receptacle of the penis during sexual intercourse.

vaginal bleeding Bleeding from the vagina.

vaginal yeast infection An infection caused by the fungus, *Candida albicans*, in which fungi overpopulate the vagina.

vestibule A cleft between the labia minora, where the urethral opening (orifice), the vaginal opening (orifice), and the hymen are located.

visceral pain Pain caused by some dysfunction of the hollow abdominal organs and is generally poorly localized and diffuse.

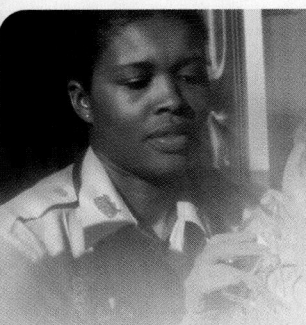

Assessment in Action

You are dispatched to a call for abdominal pain in an office building. When you arrive on scene, you are led to the cubicle of a 21-year-old woman who is bent over at the waist complaining of severe pain in her pelvic region. She states her pain began last night while she was watching TV and states that it's becoming unbearable. Her vital signs are a respiratory rate of 24 breaths/min, blood pressure of 130/74 mm Hg, a heart rate of 120 beats/min, sinus tachycardia on the ECG monitor, and a pulse oximetry reading of 100% while breathing room air. She tells you that she is currently menstruating so there is no chance she is pregnant. Her bleeding is normal. She takes birth control pills.

1. **How long does the normal menstrual cycle last?**
   A. Generally 14 days and occurs at regular intervals from puberty to menopause
   B. Generally 21 days and occurs at regular intervals from puberty to menopause
   C. Generally 28 days and occurs at regular intervals from puberty to menopause
   D. Generally 35 days and occurs at regular intervals from puberty to menopause

2. **When should you ask about sexual activity?**
   A. Whenever you have a patient who might be pregnant
   B. In all patients with abdominal pain
   C. In all adult women but not children
   D. In all women except older women

3. **Some potential causes of this patient's pain include all the following, EXCEPT:**
   A. ectopic pregnancy.
   B. pelvic inflammatory disease.
   C. ruptured ovarian cyst.
   D. none of the above.

4. **An infection in the female reproductive system and surrounding organs that can lead to sepsis and infertility is called:**
   A. ruptured ovarian cyst.
   B. endometriosis.
   C. pelvic inflammatory disease.
   D. spontaneous abortion.

5. **The inflammation of PID frequently follows the onset of menstrual bleeding by:**
   A. 1 to 3 days.
   B. 4 to 6 days.
   C. 7 to 10 days.
   D. 14 to 21 days.

6. **A ruptured ovarian cyst may mimic all of the following, EXCEPT:**
   A. appendicitis.
   B. cholecystitis.
   C. ectopic pregnancy.
   D. salpingitis.

7. **Ectopic pregnancy usually presents with:**
   A. missed periods, watery periods, nausea, vomiting, or frequent urination.
   B. the Kehr sign, breast tenderness, nausea, vomiting, and shortness of breath.
   C. chest pain, low blood glucose level, and frequent urination.
   D. elevated white blood cell count, low Sao_2, and hyperglycemia.

8. **Gynecologic emergencies are classified into which of the following three groups?**
   A. Nontraumatic, traumatic, and sexual assault
   B. Normal, traumatic, and sexual assault
   C. Self-inflicted, nontraumatic, and sexual assault
   D. Sexual assault, nontraumatic, and hereditary

9. **What is mittelschmerz?**
   A. Lower abdominal pain experienced by some women at the time of ovulation
   B. Upper abdominal pain experienced by some women at the time of ovulation
   C. The absence of pain during menstruation
   D. Painful menses but also may be associated with headache, syncope, backache, and leg pain

10. **Endometritis is inflammation of the:**
    A. uterine lining.
    B. ovaries.
    C. fallopian tubes.
    D. endometrial wall.

11. **What are the complications of vaginal bleeding?**
    A. Uncontrolled vaginal bleeding can lead to hypovolemia, shock, and death.
    B. Uncontrolled vaginal bleeding can lead to hypertension.
    C. Uncontrolled vaginal bleeding can lead to endometriosis.
    D. Uncontrolled vaginal bleeding can lead to cystitis.

Challenging Questions

12. **What is the treatment for a ruptured ectopic pregnancy?**

9. **Pregnant patients are described by their gravid and parous states. What is the correct terminology?**
   A. Gravida and parachute
   B. Gravida and para
   C. Live and aborted
   D. Para and gravitation

10. **Uterine rupture refers to:**
    A. painless, bright red bleeding without uterine contraction.
    B. localized uterine tenderness.
    C. absent fetal heart tones.
    D. spontaneous or traumatic rupture of the uterine wall.

Challenging Question

11. **What special considerations will you need to take into account for this trauma patient?**

▄▄ Points to Ponder

You respond to an obstetric emergency. On arrival you find a 23-year-old woman in the final trimester of pregnancy. She is seated in the living room on a chair. She is sobbing uncontrollably. You notice that she is sitting on a towel that has blood on it. Her chief complaint is a sudden onset of vaginal bleeding that has been occurring for 20 minutes. You ask if she is in pain, and she replies "a little." You ask if she has ever been pregnant, and she replies "once before, and I began hemorrhaging 2 weeks before delivery. I delivered a stillborn baby." She sobs.

How will you address this patient's emotions?

Issues: Dealing With Personal Tragedy, Determining a Pregnant Woman's History, Empathetic Response, Implementing a Treatment Plan.

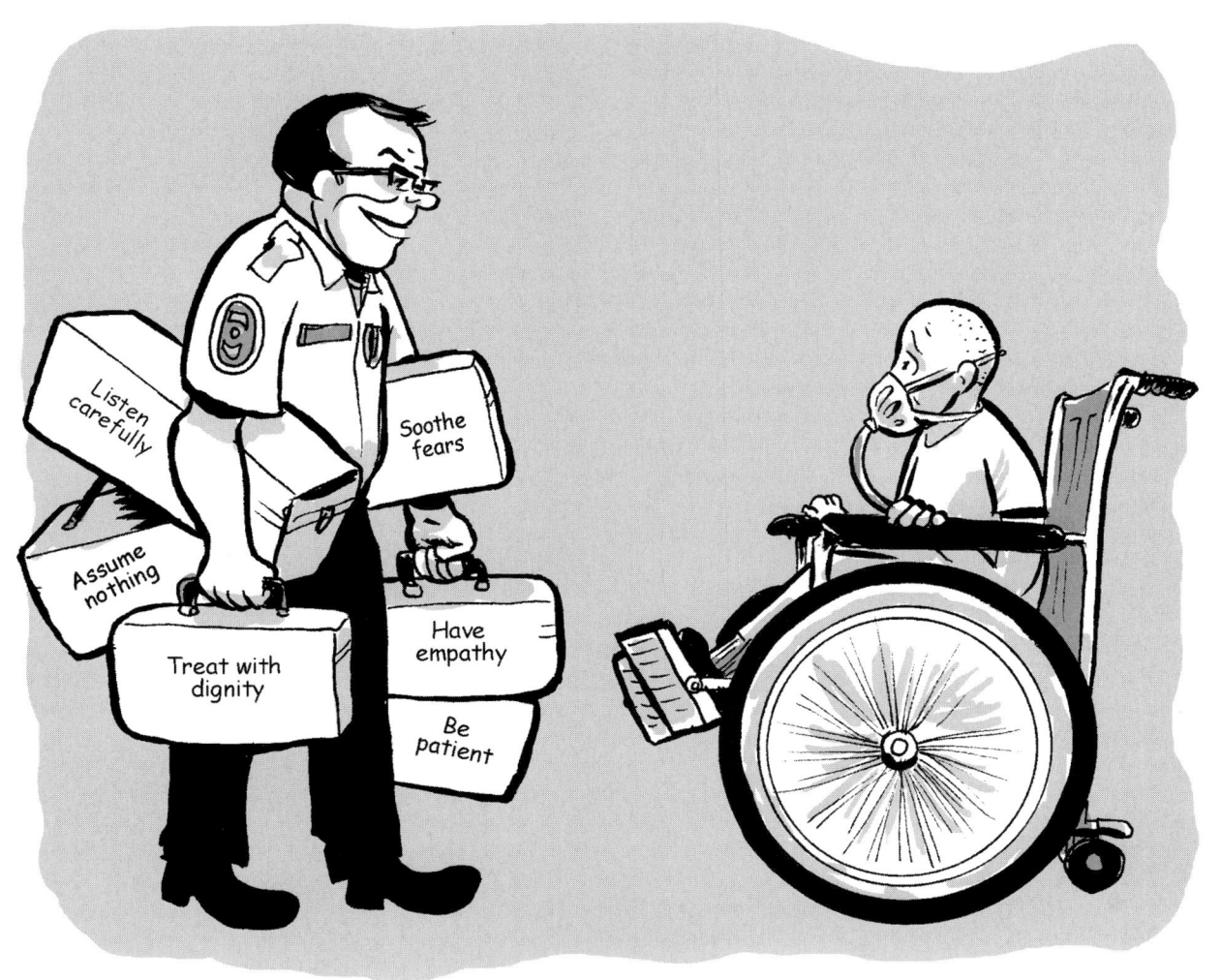

Special problems . . . require special approaches."

—Nancy L. Caroline, MD

Special Considerations

40 Neonatology

Objectives

Cognitive

6-1.2   Define the term newborn. (p 40.6)

6-1.3   Define the term neonate. (p 40.6)

6-1.4   Identify important antepartum factors that can affect childbirth. (p 40.6)

6-1.5   Identify important intrapartum factors that can term the newborn high risk. (p 40.6)

6-1.6   Identify the factors that lead to premature birth and low birth weight newborns. (p 40.20)

6-1.7   Distinguish between primary and secondary apnea. (p 40.20)

6-1.8   Discuss pulmonary perfusion and asphyxia. (p 40.10)

6-1.9   Identify the primary signs utilized for evaluating a newborn during resuscitation. (p 40.10)

6-1.10   Formulate an appropriate treatment plan for providing initial care to a newborn. (p 40.8)

6-1.11   Identify the appropriate use of the APGAR score in caring for a newborn. (p 40.9)

6-1.12   Calculate the APGAR score given various newborn situations. (p 40.9)

6-1.13   Determine when ventilatory assistance is appropriate for a newborn. (p 40.10)

6-1.14   Prepare appropriate ventilation equipment, adjuncts and technique for a newborn. (p 40.10)

6-1.15   Determine when chest compressions are appropriate for a newborn. (p 40.15)

6-1.16   Discuss appropriate chest compression techniques for a newborn. (p 40.15)

6-1.17   Assess patient improvement due to chest compressions and ventilations. (p 40.15)

6-1.18   Determine when endotracheal intubation is appropriate for a newborn. (p 40.13)

6-1.19   Discuss appropriate endotracheal intubation techniques for a newborn. (p 40.13)

6-1.20   Assess patient improvement due to endotracheal intubation. (p 40.13)

6-1.21   Identify complications related to endotracheal intubation for a newborn. (p 40.14)

6-1.22   Determine when vascular access is indicated for a newborn. (p 40.16)

6-1.23   Discuss the routes of medication administration for a newborn. (p 40.16)

6-1.24   Determine when blow-by oxygen delivery is appropriate for a newborn. (p 40.10)

6-1.25   Discuss appropriate blow-by oxygen delivery devices and technique for a newborn. (p 40.10)

6-1.26   Assess patient improvement due to assisted ventilations. (p 40.10)

6-1.27   Determine when an orogastric tube should be inserted during positive-pressure ventilation. (p 40.14)

6-1.28   Discuss the signs of hypovolemia in a newborn. (p 40.18)

6-1.29   Discuss the initial steps in resuscitation of a newborn. (p 40.10)

6-1.30   Assess patient improvement due to blow-by oxygen delivery. (p 40.10)

6-1.31   Discuss the effects maternal narcotic usage has on the newborn. (p 40.18)

6-1.32   Determine the appropriate treatment for the newborn with narcotic depression. (p 40.18)

6-1.33   Discuss appropriate transport guidelines for a newborn. (p 40.27)

6-1.34   Determine appropriate receiving facilities for low and high risk newborns. (p 40.27)

6-1.35   Describe the epidemiology, including the incidence, morbidity/mortality, risk factors and prevention strategies for meconium aspiration. (p 40.19)

6-1.36   Discuss the pathophysiology of meconium aspiration. (p 40.19)

6-1.37   Discuss the assessment findings associated with meconium aspiration. (p 40.19)

6-1.38   Discuss the management/treatment plan for meconium aspiration. (p 40.19)

6-1.39   Describe the epidemiology, including the incidence, morbidity/mortality, risk factors and prevention strategies for apnea in the neonate. (p 40.19)

6-1.40   Discuss the pathophysiology of apnea in the neonate. (p 40.20)

6-1.41   Discuss the assessment findings associated with apnea in the neonate. (p 40.20)

6-1.42   Discuss the management/treatment plan for apnea in the neonate. (p 40.20)

6-1.43   Describe the epidemiology, pathophysiology, assessment findings, management/treatment plan for diaphragmatic hernia. (p 40.19)

6-1.44   Describe the epidemiology, including the incidence, morbidity/mortality and risk factors for bradycardia in the neonate. (p 40.10)

6-1.45   Discuss the pathophysiology of bradycardia in the neonate. (p 40.10)

6-1.46   Discuss the assessment findings associated with bradycardia in the neonate. (p 40.10)

6-1.47   Discuss the management/treatment plan for bradycardia in the neonate. (p 40.17)

6-1.48   Describe the epidemiology, including the incidence, morbidity/mortality and risk factors for premature infants. (p 40.20)

6-1.49   Discuss the pathophysiology of premature infants. (p 40.20)

6-1.50   Discuss the assessment findings associated with premature infants. (p 40.20)

6-1.51   Discuss the management/treatment plan for premature infants. (p 40.20)

6-1.52   Describe the epidemiology, including the incidence, morbidity/mortality and risk factors for respiratory distress/cyanosis in the neonate. (p 40.10)

6-1.53   Discuss the pathophysiology of respiratory distress/cyanosis in the neonate. (p 40.10)

6-1.54   Discuss the assessment findings associated with respiratory distress/cyanosis in the neonate. (p 40.10)

6-1.55   Discuss the management/treatment plan for respiratory distress/cyanosis in the neonate. (p 40.10)

6-1.56   Describe the epidemiology, including the incidence, morbidity/mortality and risk factors for seizures in the neonate. (p 40.21)

6-1.57   Discuss the pathophysiology of seizures in the neonate. (p 40.21)

6-1.58   Discuss the assessment findings associated with seizures in the neonate. (p 40.22)

6-1.59   Discuss the management/treatment plan for seizures in the neonate. (p 40.22)

6-1.60   Describe the epidemiology, including the incidence, morbidity/ mortality and risk factors for fever in the neonate. (p 40.22)

6-1.61   Discuss the pathophysiology of fever in the neonate. (p 40.22)

6-1.62   Discuss the assessment findings associated with fever in the neonate. (p 40.23)

6-1.63   Discuss the management/treatment plan for fever in the neonate. (p 40.23)

6-1.64   Describe the epidemiology, including the incidence, morbidity/mortality and risk factors for hypothermia in the neonate. (p 40.23)

6-1.65   Discuss the pathophysiology of hypothermia in the neonate. (p 40.23)

6-1.66   Discuss the assessment findings associated with hypothermia in the neonate. (p 40.23)

6-1.67   Discuss the management/treatment plan for hypothermia in the neonate. (p 40.23)

6-1.68   Describe the epidemiology, including the incidence, morbidity/mortality and risk factors for hypoglycemia in the neonate. (p 40.24)

6-1.69   Discuss the pathophysiology of hypoglycemia in the neonate. (p 40.24)

6-1.70   Discuss the assessment findings associated with hypoglycemia in the neonate. (p 40.24)

6-1.71   Discuss the management/treatment plan for hypoglycemia in the neonate. (p 40.24)

6-1.72   Describe the epidemiology, including the incidence, morbidity/mortality and risk factors for vomiting in the neonate (p 40.24)

6-1.73   Discuss the pathophysiology of vomiting in the neonate. (p 40.24)

6-1.74   Discuss the assessment findings associated with vomiting in the neonate. (p 40.25)

6-1.75   Discuss the management/treatment plan for vomiting in the neonate. (p 40.25)

6-1.76   Describe the epidemiology, including the incidence, morbidity/mortality and risk factors for diarrhea in the neonate. (p 40.26)

6-1.77   Discuss the pathophysiology of diarrhea in the neonate. (p 40.26)

6-1.78   Discuss the assessment findings associated with diarrhea in the neonate. (p 40.26)

6-1.79   Discuss the management/ treatment plan for diarrhea in the neonate. (p 40.26)

6-1.80   Describe the epidemiology, including the incidence, morbidity/mortality and risk factors for common birth injuries in the neonate. (p 40.26)

6-1.81   Discuss the pathophysiology of common birth injuries in the neonate. (p 40.26)

6-1.82   Discuss the assessment findings associated with common birth injuries in the neonate. (p 40.26)

6-1.83   Discuss the management/treatment plan for common birth injuries in the neonate. (p 40.27)

6-1.84   Describe the epidemiology, including the incidence, morbidity/mortality and risk factors for cardiac arrest in the neonate. (p 40.10)

6-1.85   Discuss the pathophysiology of cardiac arrest in the neonate. (p 40.10)

6-1.86   Discuss the assessment findings associated with cardiac arrest in the neonate. (p 40.10)

6-1.87   Discuss the management/treatment plan for cardiac arrest in the neonate. (p 40.15)

6-1.88   Discuss the pathophysiology of post arrest management of the neonate. (p 40.27)

6-1.89   Discuss the assessment findings associated with post arrest situations in the neonate. (p 40.27)

6-1.90   Discuss the management/treatment plan to stabilize the post arrest neonate. (p 40.27)

Affective

6-1.91   Demonstrate and advocate appropriate interaction with a newborn/neonate that conveys respect for their position in life. (p 40.6)

6-1.92   Recognize the emotional impact of newborn/neonate injuries/illnesses on parents/guardians. (p 40.6)

6-1.93   Recognize and appreciate the physical and emotional difficulties associated with separation of the parent/guardian and a newborn/neonate. (p 40.6)

6-1.94   Listen to the concerns expressed by parents/guardians. (p 40.6)

6-1.95   Attend to the need for reassurance, empathy and compassion for the parent/guardian. (p 40.6)

Psychomotor

6-1.96   Demonstrate preparation of a newborn resuscitation area. (p 40.8)

6-1.97   Demonstrate appropriate assessment technique for examining a newborn. (p 40.8)

6-1.98   Demonstrate appropriate assisted ventilations for a newborn. (p 40.10)

6-1.99   Demonstrate appropriate endotracheal intubation technique for a newborn. (p 40.13)

6-1.100   Demonstrate appropriate meconium aspiration suctioning technique for a newborn. (p 40.19)

6-1.101   Demonstrate appropriate insertion of an orogastric tube. (p 40.15)

6-1.102   Demonstrate needle chest decompression for a newborn or neonate. (p 40.18)

6-1.103   Demonstrate appropriate chest compression and ventilation technique for a newborn. (p 40.15)

6-1.104   Demonstrate appropriate techniques to improve or eliminate endotracheal intubation complications. (p 40.14)

6-1.105   Demonstrate vascular access cannulation techniques for a newborn. (p 40.16)

6-1.106   Demonstrate the initial steps in resuscitation of a newborn. (p 40.10)

6-1.107   Demonstrate blow-by oxygen delivery for a newborn. (p 40.10)

Introduction

The care of a newborn or neonate must be tailored to meet the unique needs of this population. A newborn refers to an infant within the first few hours after birth; a neonate refers to an infant within the first month after birth. A healthy neonate is completely dependent on others for nourishment, warmth, and protection from the environment. Most parents recognize this need and instinctively wish to fulfill the role of nurturer and caregiver. When a newborn needs special support that necessitates intervention by trained caregivers, the parents may feel isolated and inadequate. It is important for you to support the needs of both the newborn and the parents or other caregivers by allowing them to be physically close as much as possible, explaining what is being done, and providing details of the plan for transport to the next level of care.

This chapter reviews the physiologic changes that occur in a newborn during birth, the care that should be provided during and immediately after birth, and the special needs of premature births or births complicated by other factors. It also reviews the steps involved in neonatal resuscitation and outlines the process of transporting an infant to a hospital or between hospitals.

General Pathophysiology and Assessment

Additional skilled care intervention is needed for approximately 6% of newborn deliveries, with the rate of complications increasing as the newborn's birth weight and gestational age decrease. In the United States, approximately 80% of the 30,000 babies born each year weighing less than 3 lb (1,500 g)

require resuscitation. Table 40-1 ▲ and Table 40-2 ▲ outline risk factors for complications before and during birth. Because both short- and long-term outcomes in newborns have been linked to initial stabilization efforts, it is imperative that you anticipate problems with newborns, are knowledgeable about how to deal with them, have the appropriate resuscitation equipment readily available, and carefully consider the newborn's ultimate transport destination.

Table 40-1	Antepartum (Before Birth) Risk Factors
■ Multiple gestation ■ Pregnant woman's age < 16 y or > 35 y ■ Post-term (> 42 weeks') gestation ■ Toxemia, hypertension, diabetes ■ Polyhydramnios (excessive amount of amniotic fluid) ■ Premature rupture of the membrane and fetal malformation	■ Inadequate prenatal care ■ History of perinatal morbidity or mortality ■ Use of drugs/medications ■ Fetal anemia ■ Oligohydramnios (decreased volume of amniotic fluid during a pregnancy)

Table 40-2	Intrapartum (During Birth) Risk Factors
■ Premature labor ■ Rupture of membranes > 24 hours before delivery ■ Abnormal presentation ■ Prolapsed cord ■ Chorioamnionitis	■ Meconium-stained amniotic fluid ■ Use of narcotics within 4 hours of delivery ■ Prolonged labor or precipitous delivery ■ Bleeding ■ Placenta previa

You are the Provider Part 1

You are called to the home of a 24-year-old woman who is 39 weeks' pregnant. She was alone when her amniotic sac ruptured. She is experiencing regular contractions that are 3 minutes apart and was afraid to drive to the hospital, so she called 9-1-1. When you and your partner arrive, you find your patient sitting on the couch. After you introduce yourselves, the patient tells you that she has already called her husband, who said he will meet her at the hospital. According to the patient, her water broke and the fluid was clear.

Initial Assessment	Recording Time: 0 Minutes
Appearance	Obviously pregnant; very nervous and in pain
Level of consciousness	A (Alert to person, place, and day)
Airway	Patent
Breathing	Respirations, increased; adequate tidal volume
Circulation	Radial pulses, increased rate and regular; no gross bleeding

1. Why is it important to determine the color of the amniotic fluid?
2. What are some reliable indicators of imminent delivery?
3. What specific questions should you ask that will allow you to anticipate the need for resuscitation of the newborn?

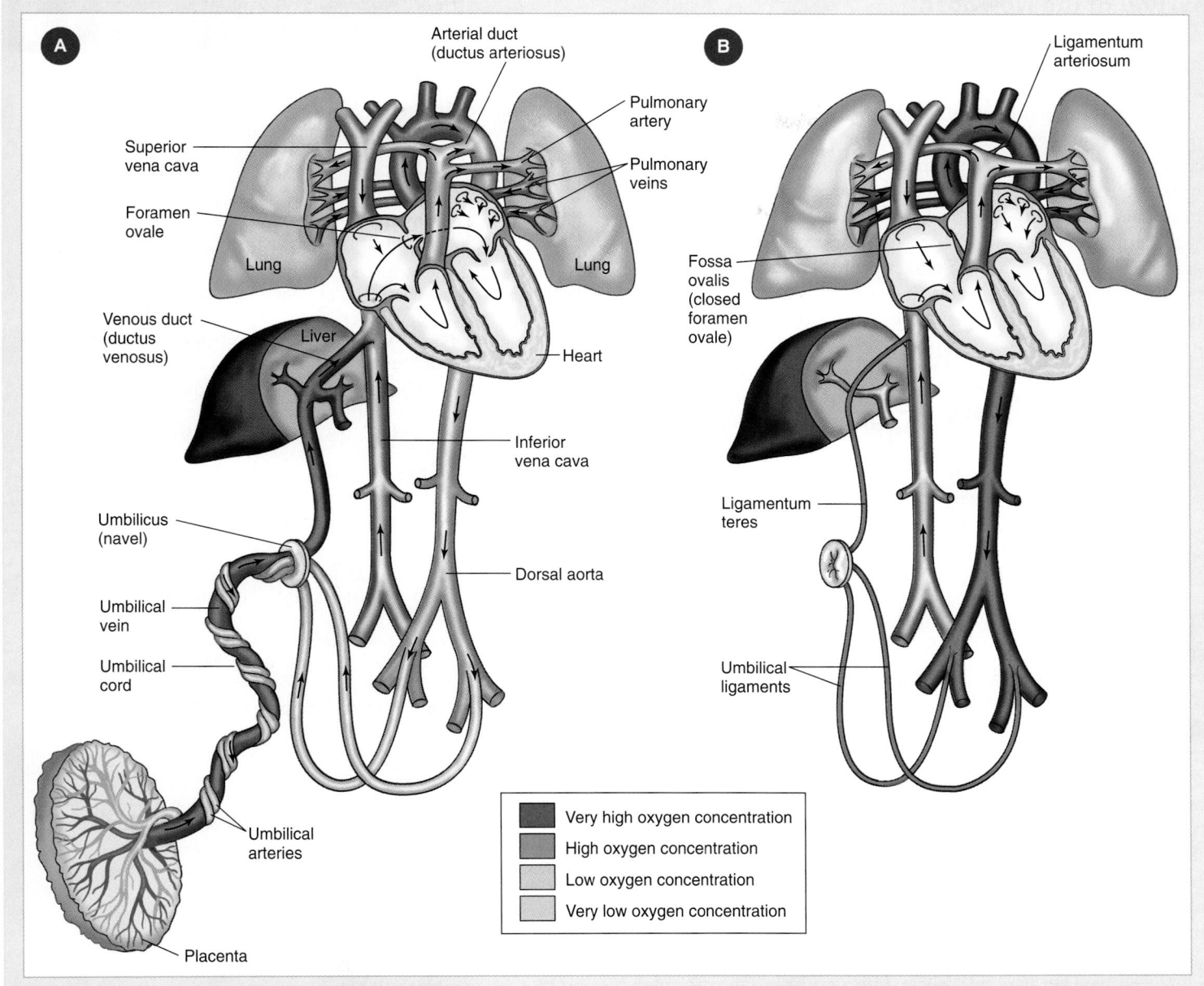

Figure 40-1 Fetal circulation. **A.** Oxygenated blood from the placenta reaches the fetus through the umbilical vein. Blood returns to the placenta via two umbilical arteries. Right-to-left shunts occur at the foramen ovale and the ductus arteriosus. **B.** Fetal circulation following transition.

Transition From Fetus to Newborn

In utero (ie, in the pregnant woman's womb), a fetus receives its oxygen from the placenta **Figure 40-1 ▲** . The fetal lung is collapsed and filled with fluid, and most of the fetal blood flow is diverted away from the lungs. As the baby is delivered, a rapid series of events needs to occur to enable the baby to breathe; this process is called fetal transition. During fetal transition, the newborn's lungs need to expand with air within seconds. As the baby's lungs become filled with air, the pulmonary pressure drops and blood begins to flow to the lungs, picking up oxygen. Anything that delays this decline in pulmonary pressure can lead to delayed transition, hypoxia, brain damage, and, ultimately, death **Table 40-3 ▶** .

Table 40-3	Causes of Delayed Transition in Newborns
■ Hypoxia	■ Hypothermia
■ Meconium or blood aspiration	■ Pneumonia
■ Acidosis	■ Hypotension

An infant delivered at less than 37 completed weeks of gestation is considered preterm; an infant born at 38 to 42 weeks of gestation is described as term; and an infant born at more than 42 weeks of gestation is described as post-term (or post-dates). These gestational lengths change if there is more than one fetus in the uterus.

Arrival of the Newborn

Use any time available before the infant arrives to take a patient history and prepare the environment and equipment that may be necessary. Key questions you need to ask when you are at a scene involving a pregnant woman or a recent home birth include the mother's age; length of the pregnancy (preferably expressed in weeks); the presence and frequency of contractions; the presence or absence of fetal movement; whether there have been any pregnancy complications (eg, diabetes, hypertension, fever); whether membranes have ruptured, including its timing and the makeup of the fluid (clear, meconium stained, or bloody); and the medications being taken. In the excitement of the moment these questions may seem trivial, but they help determine what resuscitation and equipment may be needed.

Even if a piece of equipment is in a sealed sterile wrap, having it near at hand will expedite its use once the infant is delivered. At a minimum, you will need warm, dry blankets, a bulb syringe, two small clamps or ties, and a pair of clean scissors to cut the umbilical cord. Table 40-4 ▶ lists additional equipment that may be needed if more extensive resuscitation becomes necessary.

If the infant is delivered in the ambulance, the foot of the mother's bed, covered with clean, warm blankets, can be used for the initial stabilization steps. The newborn can then be placed on mother's chest after you confirm adequate patency of the airway, breathing, and pulse rate. If more extensive resuscitation is needed, this area can be used as needed initially, optimally transitioning to a second ambulance equipped with a neonatal transport incubator to allow maintenance of a thermoneutral environment and observation of the newborn's color and tone.

If the umbilical cord comes out ahead of the baby (which is more common with polyhydramnios, a condition characterized by extra amniotic fluid), the blood supply through the umbilical cord may be cut off. In this case, relieving pressure on the cord (by gently moving the presenting part of the body off the cord and pushing the cord back) can be lifesaving.

When the baby's head is delivered, suction the mouth and nose with a bulb syringe. After the infant is delivered, keep the

Notes from Nancy

Steps to Improve Fetal Circulation

- Roll the mother onto her side, to take the weight of her uterus off the great vessels.
- Administer 100% oxygen by mask to the mother.

Special Considerations

A delay in clamping the umbilical cord and keeping the infant below the placenta may allow blood to flow into the infant, which can in turn lead to polycythemia (an abnormally high red blood cell count).

Table 40-4	Preparation of Area for Newborn Resuscitation*

Resuscitation Equipment and Supplies
- Suction equipment
- Bulb syringe, mechanical suction and tubing, suction catheters, 5F or 6F
- 8F feeding tube and 20-mL syringe
- Meconium aspirator

Bag-Mask Equipment
- Device for delivering positive-pressure ventilation, capable of delivering 90% to 100% oxygen
- Face masks, newborn and premature infant size (cushioned-rim masks preferred)
- Oxygen source with flow meter (flow rate up to 10 L/min)

Intubation Equipment
- Laryngoscope with straight blades, size 0 (preterm) and 1 (term)
- Extra bulb, batteries for laryngoscope
- Endotracheal tubes size 2.5, 3.0, 3.5, and 4.0
- Stylet (optional)
- Scissors and tape for securing endotracheal tube
- CO_2 detectors
- Laryngeal mask airway (optional)

Medications
- Epinephrine 1:10,000 (0.1 mg/mL), 3- or 10-mL ampules
- Isotonic crystalloid (normal saline or lactated Ringer's solution), 100- or 250-mL bag
- Sodium bicarbonate, 4.2% (5 mEq/10 mL)
- Naloxone hydrochloride, 0.4- or 1.0-mg/mL ampule
- Dextrose, 10%, 250 mL

Umbilical Catheterization Equipment
- Sterile gloves
- Scalpel or scissors
- Antiseptic solution
- Umbilical tape
- Umbilical catheters, 3.5F, 5F (a sterile 3.5F feeding tube can be used in an emergency)
- Three-way stopcock
- Syringes, 1, 3, 5, 10, 20, and 50 mL
- Needles, 25, 21, and 18 gauge

Miscellaneous
- Gloves and appropriate BSI protection
- Radiant warmer or other heat source
- Firm, padded resuscitation surface
- Clock with second hand, timer optional
- Towels, linen
- Stethoscope, neonatal or pediatric preferred
- Cardiac monitor or saturation monitor (optional at delivery)
- Oropharyngeal airways (0, 00, and 000 sizes or 30-, 40-, and 50-mm long)

*adapted from the American Academy of Pediatrics Neonatal Resuscitation Program

baby at the level of the mother, with the head slightly lower than the body, while you clamp the umbilical cord in two places and then cut between the clamps Figure 40-2 ▶ .

Your initial rapid assessment of the newborn may be done simultaneously with any treatment interventions. Note the time of delivery, and monitor the ABCs. In particular, assess respiratory rate, respiratory effort, pulse rate, color, and capillary refill.

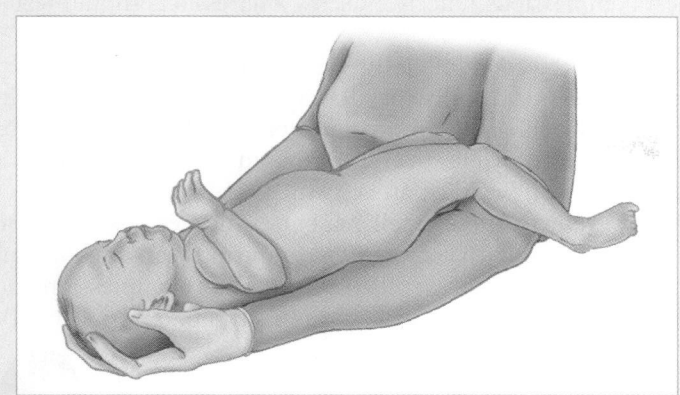

Figure 40-2 Positioning. Immediately after delivery, hold the baby with the head slightly lower than the body to facilitate drainage of secretions.

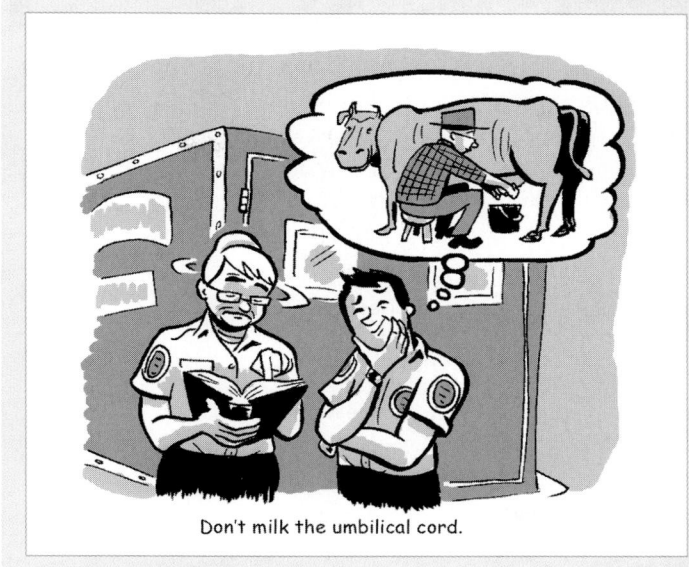

Don't milk the umbilical cord.

Figure 40-3

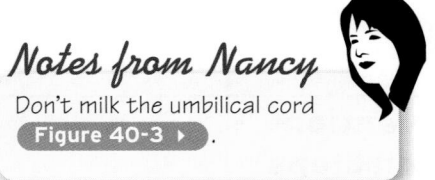

Notes from Nancy

Don't milk the umbilical cord Figure 40-3 ▶ .

Nearly 90% of newborns are vigorous term babies. To ensure thermoregulation in a healthy newborn, put the baby directly on the mother's chest after birth, drying, and then covering with a dry towel. Position the baby to ensure a patent airway, clear the airway of secretions as needed, and assess the baby's color. All newborns are cyanotic immediately after birth. If the newborn remains vigorous and quickly becomes pink, ongoing observation and continued thermoregulation with direct skin-to-skin contact with the mother should be maintained while on the way to a local hospital. Bonding with the mother should be encouraged in a well-appearing newborn.

The Apgar Score

The Apgar score, named after Dr. Virginia Apgar, who developed this measure in 1953, helps determine the need for and the effectiveness of resuscitation. The Apgar score is determined on the basis of the newborn's condition at 1 and 5 minutes after birth   Table 40-5 ▶ . If the 5-minute Apgar score is less than 7, the newborn's condition should be reassessed and a new score assigned every 5 minutes until 20 minutes after birth. If resuscitation is necessary, the Apgar score is completed by determining the result of the resuscitation.

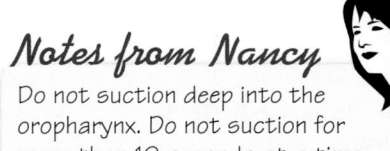

Notes from Nancy

Do not suction deep into the oropharynx. Do not suction for more than 10 seconds at a time.

You are the Provider Part 2

Your patient tells you that this is her third pregnancy and that her first two pregnancies resulted in normal deliveries. At her last doctor's appointment, her obstetrician told her that he did not anticipate any problems and that the baby was in a head-down position in the uterus (fully engaged).

Your partner obtains baseline vital signs as you perform a visual exam of the patient's vaginal area and put on appropriate BSI attire. Your exam reveals crowning of the baby's head. You immediately position the patient appropriately and open the OB kit.

Vital Signs	Recording Time: 3 Minutes
Skin	Pink, warm, and moist
Pulse	110 beats/min, strong and regular
Blood pressure	106/60 mm Hg
Respirations	24 breaths/min; adequate tidal volume
SaO_2	98% on room air

4. What equipment and supplies should be available in case the infant requires resuscitation?

Table 40-5	The Apgar Score	
Condition	Description	Score
Appearance—skin color	Completely pink	2
	Body pink, extremities blue	1
	Centrally blue, pale	0
Pulse rate	> 100	2
	< 100, > 0	1
	Absent	0
Grimace—irritability	Cries	2
	Grimaces	1
	No response	0
Activity—muscle tone	Active motion	2
	Some flexion of extremities	1
	Limp	0
Respiratory—effort	Strong cry	2
	Slow and irregular	1
	Absent	0

Need for Resuscitation

Not all deliveries go so smoothly. Approximately 10% of newborns need additional assistance and 1% need major resuscitation to survive. If a problem arises, it is important to follow the clearly defined algorithm developed by the American Academy of Pediatrics and the American Heart Association to optimize the outcome **Figure 40-4**. In this algorithm, interventions, assessment, and determination of need to progress to the next level of resuscitation are delineated in 30-second intervals.

After the initial steps following delivery (bulb suctioning mouth and nose, drying, stimulating) are followed for 30 seconds, if the newborn has not responded, further intervention is indicated. Assess the newborn's respiratory rate, respiratory effort, pulse rate, and color. Count the respiratory rate and pulse rate for 6 seconds and then multiply by 10 to quickly determine the rate per minute. The pulse rate can be determined either by auscultation or by feeling the base of the umbilical cord at the baby's abdomen, as the umbilical artery should still have pulsatile flow **Figure 40-5**. Many newborns become centrally pink but have blue hands and feet (acrocyanosis). If the baby maintains central cyanosis of the trunk or mucous membranes, however, provide supplemental free-flow oxygen as stimulation. Keep the baby on the mother's chest and continue to manage the airway.

If the baby is apneic (ie, has a 20-second or longer respiratory pause) or has a pulse rate less than 100 beats/min after 30 seconds of drying and stimulation and supplemental free-flow (blow-by) oxygen, begin positive-pressure ventilation (PPV) by bag-mask device, being sure to use a newborn sized bag-mask. You should use caution when squeezing the bag in order to avoid inadvertently delivering too much volume, potentially resulting in a pneumothorax. After 30 seconds of adequate ventilation by PPV with 100% oxygen via a bag-mask device, if the infant's pulse rate is less than 60 beats/min, begin

chest compressions. Effective chest compressions should result in palpable pulses.

Fewer than 1% of deliveries involve bradycardia that requires treatment with chest compressions. The most common etiology for bradycardia in a neonate is hypoxia, which is readily reversed by effective PPV. Profound hypoxia or shock is also the cause of cardiac arrest, which is almost always a secondary event in these small patients. Another less common etiology—but one that requires prompt intervention—is tension pneumothorax. If ventilation and chest compressions do not improve the bradycardia, administer epinephrine via IV line or endotracheal (ET) intubation. Even infants who have been resuscitated for 20 minutes can have positive long-term outcomes. Newborns are very resilient, and most respond readily to interventions.

Notes from Nancy

Do not wait until you have measured the 1-minute Apgar score before you start resuscitation.

Specific Intervention and Resuscitation Steps

Drying and Stimulation

After ensuring the patency of the airway by bulb suctioning of the newborn's mouth and nose, dry and stimulate the infant (in the absence of meconium-stained fluid). Flick the soles of the baby's feet and gently rub the baby's back. Avoid rubbing too roughly or slapping the baby, since these actions may lead to traumatic injury.

Free-Flow Oxygen

If an infant is cyanotic or pale, provide supplemental oxygen. Given that 5 g/dL of deoxygenated hemoglobin is needed before clinical cyanosis becomes apparent, a severely anemic hypoxic infant will be pale, but not cyanotic. Warm and humidify the oxygen if it will be provided for more than a few minutes. If PPV is not indicated (ie, the pulse rate is greater than 100 beats/min and the infant has adequate respiratory effort), oxygen can initially be delivered through an oxygen mask or via oxygen tubing within a hand that is cupped and held close to the infant's nose and mouth **Figure 40-6**. The oxygen flow rate should be set at 5 L/min. Do not blow oxygen directly into the newborn's eyes.

Oral Airways

Oral airways are rarely used for neonates, but they can be life-saving if airway obstruction leads to respiratory failure. Bilateral choanal atresia (bony or membranous obstruction of the back of the nose preventing air flow) can be rapidly fatal, but usually responds to placement of an oral airway (or a gloved finger until an adequate oral airway is located). The Pierre

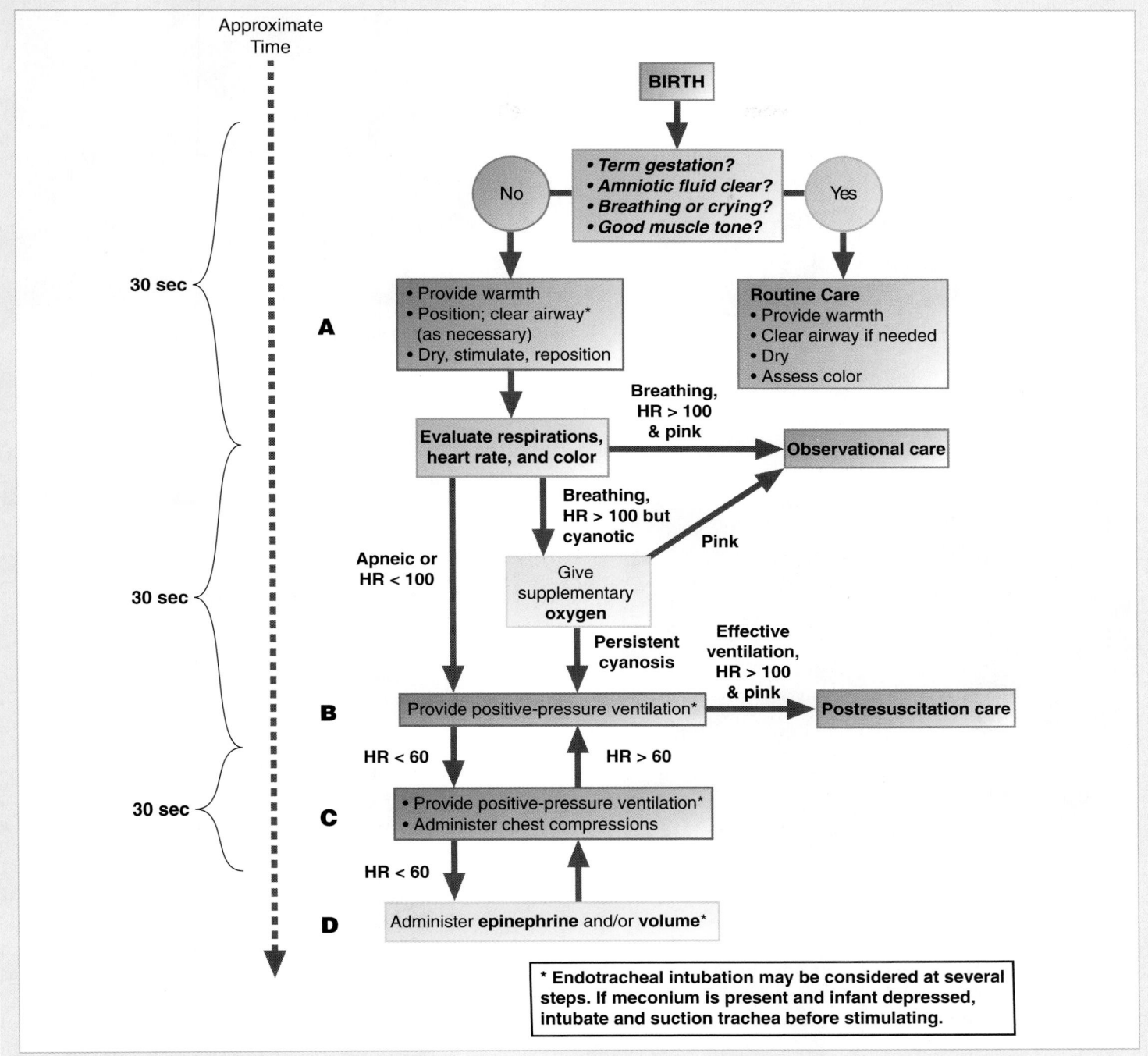

Approximate
Time

BIRTH

• *Term gestation?*
• *Amniotic fluid clear?*
• *Breathing or crying?*
• *Good muscle tone?*

No   Yes

30 sec

A
• Provide warmth
• Position; clear airway*
  (as necessary)
• Dry, stimulate, reposition

Routine Care
• Provide warmth
• Clear airway if needed
• Dry
• Assess color

**Evaluate respirations,
heart rate, and color**

Breathing,
HR > 100
& pink
→ **Observational care**

Breathing,
HR > 100 but
cyanotic

Apneic or
HR < 100

Give
supplementary
oxygen

Pink

30 sec

Persistent
cyanosis

Effective
ventilation,
HR > 100
& pink

B   Provide positive-pressure ventilation*   → **Postresuscitation care**

HR < 60   HR > 60

30 sec

C
• Provide positive-pressure ventilation*
• Administer chest compressions

HR < 60

D   Administer **epinephrine** and/or **volume***

* Endotracheal intubation may be considered at several
steps. If meconium is present and infant depressed,
intubate and suction trachea before stimulating.

Figure 40-4 Neonatal Resuscitation Algorithm.

Reproduced with permission, *2005 American Heart Association Guidelines for Cardiopulmonary Resuscitation and Emergency Cardiovascular Care.* © 2005, American
Heart Association.

Robin sequence is a series of developmental anomalies including a small chin and posteriorly positioned tongue that frequently lead to airway obstruction. Positioning the patient
prone (chest down) may relieve the obstruction. If not, insert
an oral airway. As with infants and small children, use a tongue
blade to depress the tongue and insert the oral airway without
rotating it.

Bag-Mask Ventilation

Bag-mask ventilation is indicated when an infant is apneic, has
inadequate respiratory effort, or has a pulse rate less than
100 beats/min (bradycardia) after you clear the airway of secretions, relieve obstruction from the tongue, and dry and stimulate the infant. Signs of respiratory distress that suggest a need

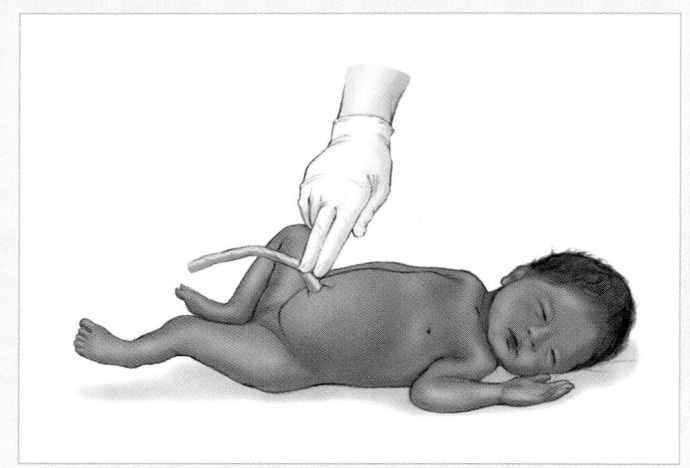

Figure 40-5 Feel for a pulse at the base of the umbilical cord.

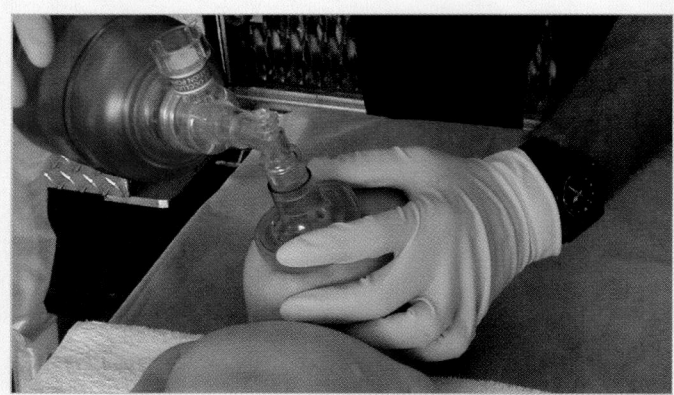

Figure 40-7 Bag-mask ventilation of the newborn. Hold the mask securely to the face with your thumb and index finger. Apply countertraction under the bony part of the chin with your middle finger.

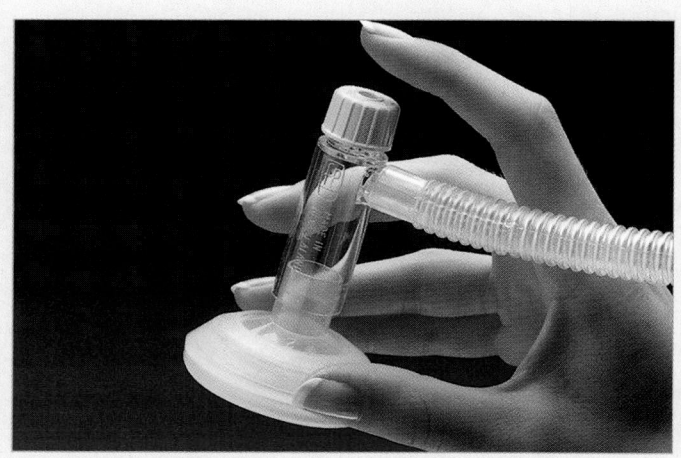

Figure 40-6 Free-flow oxygen device.

Table 40-6	Common Causes of Respiratory Distress
■ Lung or heart disease	■ Persistent pulmonary hypertension
■ Central nervous system disorders	■ Mucous obstruction of nasal passages
■ Pneumothorax	■ Choanal atresia
■ Meconium aspiration	■ Amniotic fluid aspiration
■ Lung immaturity	■ Pneumonia
■ Shock and sepsis	■ Metabolic acidosis
■ Diaphragmatic hernia	

for bag-mask ventilation include periodic breathing, intercostal retractions (sucking in between the ribs), nasal flaring, and grunting on expiration. Respiratory distress occurs in approximately 8 of every 1,000 live births and accounts for approximately 15% of neonatal deaths. **Table 40-6 ▶** summarizes the most common conditions leading to respiratory distress.

Three devices may be used to deliver bag-mask ventilation to a neonate. First, you may use a self-inflating bag with an oxygen reservoir (an oxygen source is not necessary to provide PPV but is necessary to provide supplementary oxygen). Second, you may use a flow-inflating bag, though it needs a gas source to provide PPV; this technique is therefore more common in the operating room. Third, you may apply a T-piece resuscitator (mostly found in neonatal intensive care units).

In the field, you will most likely use a self-inflating bag for bag-mask ventilation. If available, always use the infant size (240 mL). Given that the breath size (tidal volume) of a neonate is only 5 to 8 mL/kg, only one tenth of the bag's volume will be used for each breath—which explains why a larger bag can easily create problems. If a neonatal bag is not available and the infant is in severe respiratory distress, has apnea, or has bradycardia, you can use a bag designed for adults or older children (750 mL or greater volume) as long as you keep the delivered breath size appropriately small and monitor chest rise to avoid excessive volumes of delivered breaths.

When you are administering bag-mask ventilation with 100% oxygen, the face mask needs to provide an airtight seal, fitting over the newborn's mouth and nose, and extending down to the chin but not over the eyes **Figure 40-7 ▲** . The newborn needs to have a patent airway, cleared of secretions, with his or her neck slightly extended in the sniffing position **Figure 40-8 ▶** . The first few breaths after birth will frequently require higher pressures (perhaps 30 mm Hg or even higher) because the lungs are not yet expanded and are still full of fluid. To deliver these initial breaths, you may need to manually (cover with your finger) disable the spring-loaded pop-off valve (it is usually set by the manufacturer at 30 to 40 cm Hg).

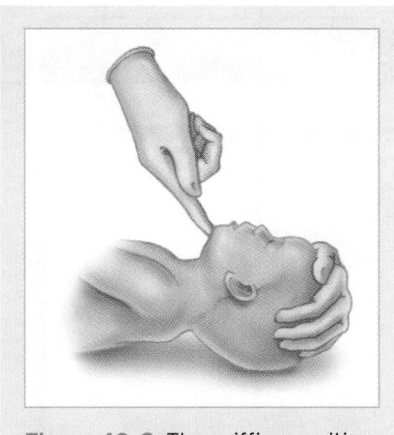

Figure 40-8 The sniffing position.

Subsequent breaths should be delivered with sufficient pressure to result in visible but not excessive chest rise.

In a newborn, the correct timing for ventilation is 40 to 60 breaths/min. In the excitement of the moment, with your adrenaline surging, it is easy to inadvertently deliver breaths at a much higher rate, which can lead to hypocapnia, air trapping, or pneumothorax. To help with the timing, count "breath–two–three, breath–two–three" as you ventilate: Give a breath on "breath," and release on "two–three." Continue PPV as long as the pulse rate remains less than 100 beats/min or respiratory effort is ineffective. If prolonged PPV is needed, hook the system to a pressure manometer to aid in monitoring and minimizing excessive pressures (target peak inspiratory pressure less than 25 mm Hg in full-term newborns, less in preterm infants).

The most common reasons for ineffective bag-mask ventilation are inadequate seal of the mask on the face and incorrect head position. Other causes such as mucous plug, pneumothorax, or equipment malfunction need to be considered as well.

Intubation

Bag-mask ventilation provides successful resuscitation of most newborns. Intubation, however, may be necessary if the newborn requires resuscitation beyond simple interventions (Figure 40-9 ▶). Intubation is indicated in the following situations:

- Meconium-stained fluid is present and the infant is not vigorous (ie, poor muscle tone, bradycardia, inadequate

> ### Notes from Nancy
> **Indications for Artificial Ventilation of the Newborn**
> - Apnea
> - Pulse rate less than 100 beats/min
> - Persisting central cyanosis despite breathing 100% oxygen

> ### Controversies
> While resuscitation with 100% oxygen is the norm in the United States and is currently recommended by the American Academy of Pediatrics, a growing body of evidence suggests that resuscitation with room air is a safe alternative. Bag-mask ventilation can be initiated with room air while an oxygen source is being secured.

ventilation), a condition for which tracheal suctioning is indicated.

- Congenital diaphragmatic hernia (a congenital defect in which abdominal organs herniate through an opening in the diaphragm into the chest cavity) is suspected and respiratory support is indicated.
- The infant does not respond to bag-mask ventilation and chest compressions, necessitating endotracheal administration of epinephrine (ie, no intraosseous site has been established).
- Prolonged positive-pressure ventilation is needed.

Before you begin ventilation, make sure that you have the following equipment available:

- Suction equipment (10F tubing, with 5F to 8F being available, suction set to 100 mm Hg)
- Laryngoscope (check the light to ensure that the bulb is bright and screwed in tightly)
- Blades—straight: No. 1 for full-term infants, No. 0 for preterm infants
- Shoulder roll
- Adhesive tape, to tape the endotracheal tube
- Endotracheal tube: 2.5 to 4.0 mm (2.5 mm if the newborn is delivered before 28 weeks of gestation, 3.0 mm if delivered before 28 to 34 weeks of gestation, 3.5 mm if delivered before 34 to 38 weeks of gestation, and 4.0 mm if delivered after 38 weeks of gestation)

Some paramedics use a stylet to provide rigidity to the ET tube. In such a case, you must secure the stylet (bending it over at the top of the ET tube so it can't advance) and make sure that it does not extend beyond the ET tube, or tracheal perforation may occur.

Intubation of the neonate is discussed in the following steps and shown in Skill Drill 40-1 ▶ :

1. Be sure the newborn is preoxygenated by bag-mask ventilation with 100% supplemental oxygen prior to making an intubation attempt Step 1 .

2. Suction the oropharynx to remove any secretions Step 2 . This is a vagal stimulus, so pay close attention to pulse rate. Bag-mask ventilation may be needed if the newborn develops bradycardia at this point.

3. Place the laryngoscope blade in the oropharynx and then visualize the vocal cords Step 3 . Avoid applying torque to the blade, as it increases the risk of trauma. Place the ET tube between the vocal cords until the black line on the tube is at the level of the cords. For full-term babies, the ET tube is usually advanced until it is at 9 cm at the lip. A premature baby may need to have the ET tube advanced to only 6½ to 7 cm at the lip. Limit the intubation attempt to 20 seconds, and initiate bag-mask ventilation if it is unsuccessful or if significant bradycardia develops.

4. Confirm placement Step 4 by observing chest rise when applying positive pressure through the ET tube, auscultating laterally and high on the chest, noting the absence of significant air sounds over the stomach, noting mist in the ET tube (seen when the patient exhales

Skill Drill 40-1: Intubation of a Neonate

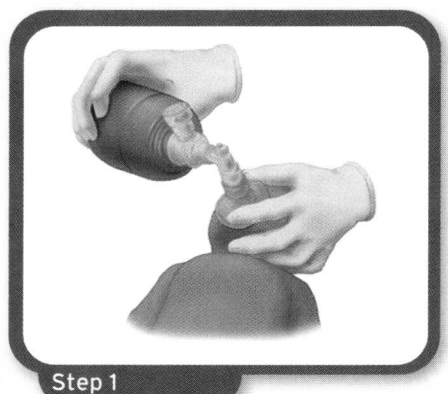

Step 1

Preoxygenate the infant by bag-mask ventilation with 100% supplemental oxygen.

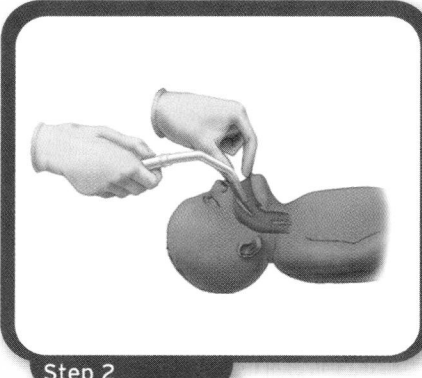

Step 2

Suction the oropharynx. Provide bag-mask ventilation if bradycardia results.

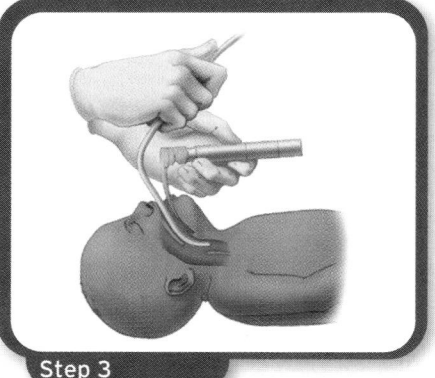

Step 3

Place the laryngoscope blade in the oropharynx. Visualize the vocal cords. Place the ET tube between the vocal cords until the black line on the ET tube is at the level of the cords.

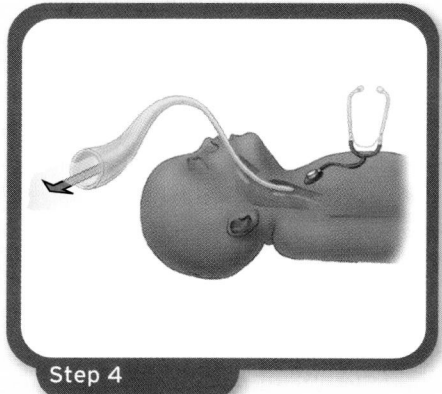

Step 4

Confirm placement. Observe chest rise, auscultate laterally and high on the chest, note the absence of significant air sounds over the stomach, and note mist in the ET tube.

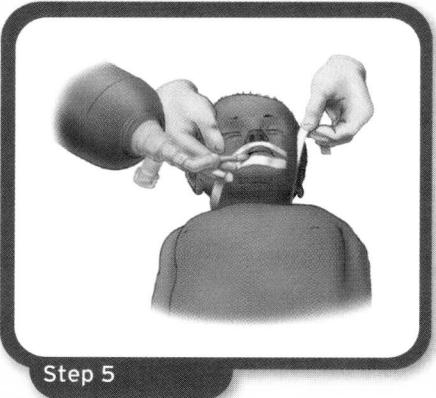

Step 5

Tape the ET tube in place. Monitor the newborn closely for complications.

through the tube from condensation of humidified air leaving the lungs), and observing for clinical improvement.

5. Tape the ET tube in place on the face to minimize the risk of the tube dislodging (**Step 5**). Monitor the infant closely for complications such as tube dislodgement, tube occlusion by mucous plug or meconium, or pneumothorax.

Notes from Nancy

Indications for Endotracheal Intubation of the Newborn

- Inability to ventilate effectively by bag-mask device
- Necessity to perform tracheal suctioning, especially if meconium is present and infant depressed at birth
- When prolonged ventilation will be necessary

Complications of ET tube placement include oropharyngeal or tracheal perforation, esophageal intubation with subsequent persistent hypoxia, and right mainstem intubation that can lead to atelectasis, persistent hypoxia, and pneumothorax. You can minimize these risks by ensuring optimal placement of the laryngoscope blade and carefully noting how far the ET tube is advanced.

Gastric Decompression

Gastric decompression using an orogastric tube is indicated for prolonged bag-mask ventilation (more than 5 to 10 minutes), if abdominal distention is impeding ventilation, or in the presence of diaphragmatic hernia. Many diaphragmatic hernias are diagnosed prenatally by routine ultrasound; they are suspected clinically if there are decreased breath sounds

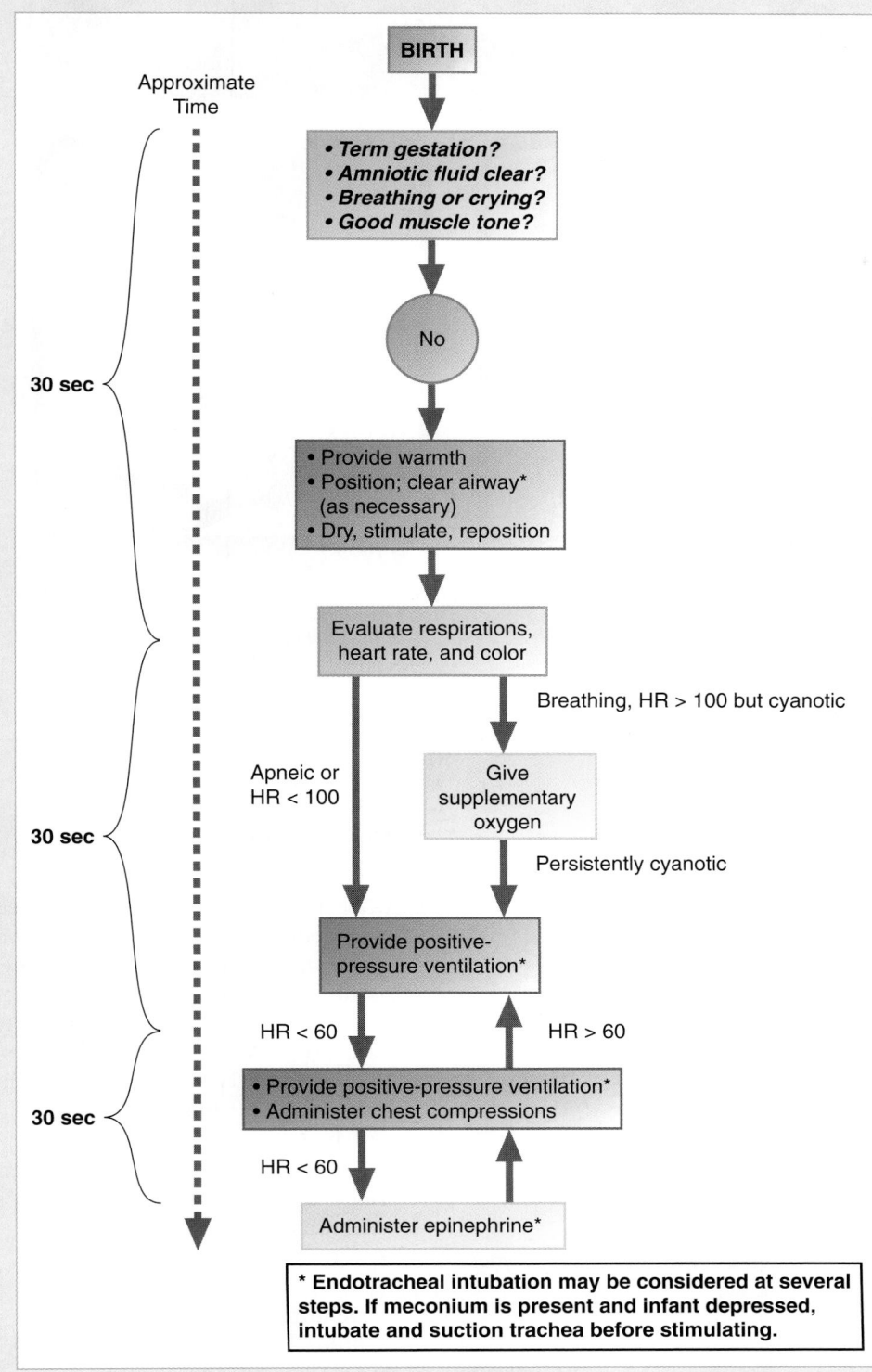

Figure 40-9 Resuscitation algorithm for the distressed newborn.

Within the figure:

BIRTH

- *Term gestation?*
- *Amniotic fluid clear?*
- *Breathing or crying?*
- *Good muscle tone?*

No

- Provide warmth
- Position; clear airway* (as necessary)
- Dry, stimulate, reposition

Evaluate respirations, heart rate, and color

Breathing, HR > 100 but cyanotic

Apneic or HR < 100

Give supplementary oxygen

Persistently cyanotic

Provide positive-pressure ventilation*

HR < 60 / HR > 60

- Provide positive-pressure ventilation*
- Administer chest compressions

HR < 60

Administer epinephrine*

* Endotracheal intubation may be considered at several steps. If meconium is present and infant depressed, intubate and suction trachea before stimulating.

Approximate Time: 30 sec / 30 sec / 30 sec

(90% of diaphragmatic hernias are on the left), a scaphoid or concave abdomen (many of the abdominal contents are in the chest), and increased work of breathing. **Skill Drill 40-2 ▶** shows gastric decompression in a neonate.

1. To determine the length of tube to insert, use an 8F feeding tube and measure the length from the bottom of the earlobe to the tip of the nose to halfway between the xiphoid process (lower tip of sternum) and the umbilicus **Step 1.**
2. Insert the tube through the mouth **Step 2**.
3. Attach a 20-gauge syringe and suction the stomach contents **Step 3**. Tape the tube to the baby's cheek. Remove the syringe from the feeding tube to allow venting of air from the stomach, and intermittently suction the feeding tube.

Chest Compressions

Chest compressions are indicated if the pulse rate remains less than 60 beats/min despite positioning, clearing the airway, drying and stimulation, and 30 seconds of effective PPV. Two techniques are used, depending on the number of rescuers available **Figure 40-10 ▶**. With the thumb (two-rescuer) technique, two thumbs are placed side by side over the sternum between the nipples, and the hands encircle the torso. With the two-finger (one-rescuer) technique, the tips of the index and middle fingers are placed over the sternum between the nipples and the sternum is compressed between the fingers and a hand behind the baby's back.

The depth of compression is one third of the anteroposterior diameter of the chest. Your fingers should remain in contact with the chest at all times. In neonates, the chest compressions occur in synchrony with artificial ventilation, which you continue during chest compressions. The person delivering the chest compression counts out loud, "One and two and three and breath and. . . ." Downward strokes of chest compressions should be delivered while saying, "One and two and three." Release of the strokes should occur while saying "and." The

Skill Drill 40-2: Inserting an Orogastric Tube in the Newborn

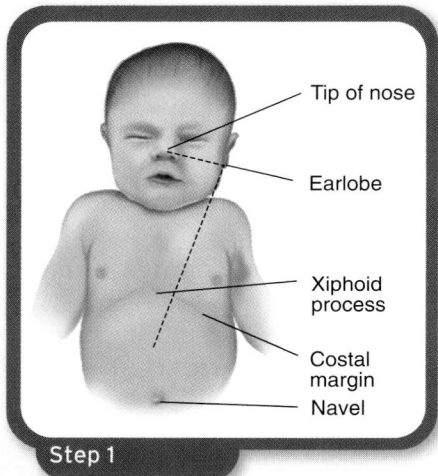

Step 1

Measure for correct depth—from the bottom of the earlobe to the tip of the nose to halfway between the xiphoid process (lower tip of sternum) and the umbilicus.

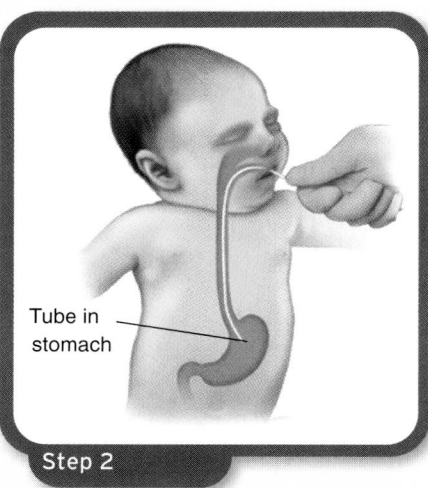

Step 2

Insert the tube to the appropriate depth. Leave the nose open to allow for ventilations.

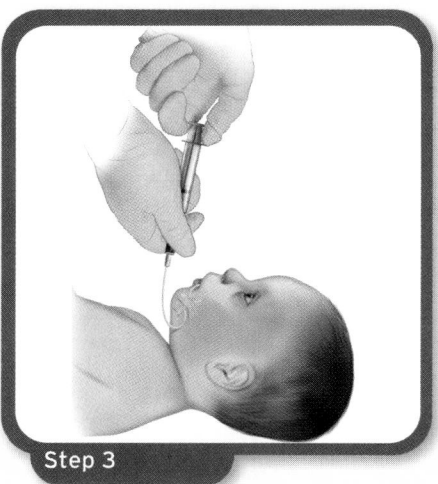

Step 3

Remove the gastric contents with a 20-mL syringe. Remove the syringe and leave the tip of the tube open to allow air to vent from the stomach. Tape the tube to the newborn's cheek.

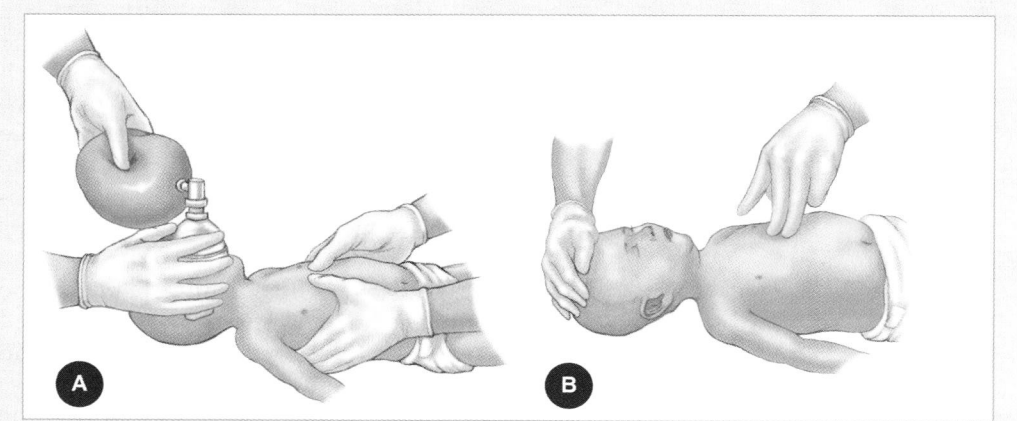

Figure 40-10 Chest compressions in the newborn. **A.** When there are two rescuers, use your thumbs side by side, placed just below an imaginary line drawn between the two nipples. **B.** When working alone, or when the baby is large, use two fingers to depress the sternum.

person ventilating delivers a breath during the sequence "breath and." This results in 90 compressions and 30 breaths/min. Pulse rate is assessed at 30-second intervals, and chest compressions stop when the pulse rate is greater than 60 beats/min. Liver laceration and rib fractures are possible risks of delivering chest compressions. Refer to Appendix A for coverage of infant CPR.

Venous Access

Emergent access becomes necessary when fluid administration is needed to support circulation, when resuscitation medications (eg, epinephrine, sodium bicarbonate) must be administered IV, and when therapeutic drugs (eg, IV dextrose, antibiotics) must be given IV. Establishing peripheral access in an infant can prove difficult, however.

The umbilical vein can be catheterized using an umbilical vein line in a newborn using the following steps:

1. Clean the cord with alcohol or another antiseptic. Place a sterile tie firmly, but not too tightly, around the base of the cord to control bleeding. Place a sterile drape over the site. Although the line must be placed quickly in a code situation, maintain sterile technique as much as possible.
2. Prefill a sterile 3.5F to 5F umbilical vein line catheter (a comparable-size sterile feeding tube can be used in an emergency) with normal saline using a 3-mL syringe.
3. Cut the cord with a scalpel below the clamp placed on the cord at birth about 1 to 2 cm from the skin (between the clamp and the cord tie).

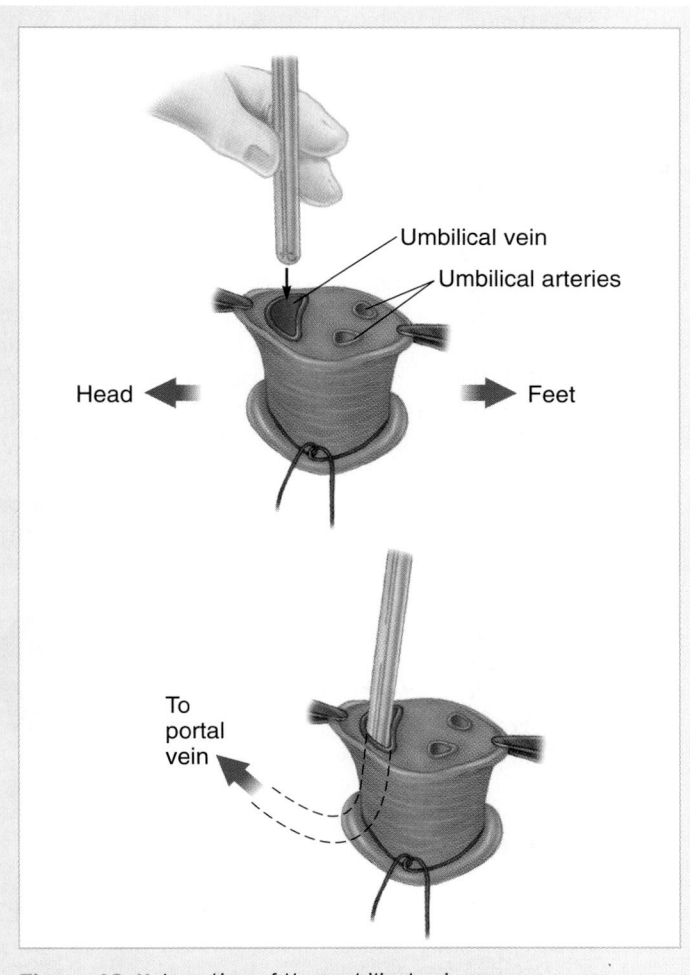

Figure 40-11 Location of the umbilical vein.

4. The umbilical vein is a large, thin-walled vessel usually found at the 12 o'clock position, as compared to the two thick-walled umbilical arteries usually found at 4 and 8 o'clock (Figure 40-11 ◄). Insert the catheter into this vein for a distance of 2 to 4 cm (less in preterm infants) until blood can be aspirated. If the catheter is advanced into the liver, the infusion of hypertonic solutions may lead to irreversible damage (Figure 40-12 ▼). If the catheter is advanced into the heart, arrhythmias may develop.

5. Flush the catheter with 0.5 mL of normal saline and tape it in place.

Pharmacologic Interventions

Medications are rarely needed in neonatal resuscitation, as most infants can be resuscitated with ventilatory support. Medications in neonates are based on weight, so you may need to estimate the infant's weight for dosing. A full-term infant usually weighs 6½ to 9 lb (3 to 4 kg); an infant born at 28 weeks of gestation, on average, weighs 2½ lb (1 kg) and is approximately 14¾″ (37.5 cm) long.

Epinephrine

Administration of epinephrine is indicated when the infant has a pulse rate of less than 60 beats/min after 30 seconds of effective ventilation and 30 seconds of chest compressions. The recommended concentration for newborns is 1:10,000. The recommended dose is 0.1 to 0.3 mL/kg of 1:10,000 epinephrine IV, equal to 0.01 to 0.03 mg/kg, administered rapidly, followed by a 0.5- to 1-mL normal saline flush to clear the line. If IV access is not yet established, consider starting with the higher dose of 0.3 up to 1 mL/kg of 1:10,000 epinephrine given via the ET tube. Dosing may be repeated every 3 to 5 minutes in case of persistent bradycardia.

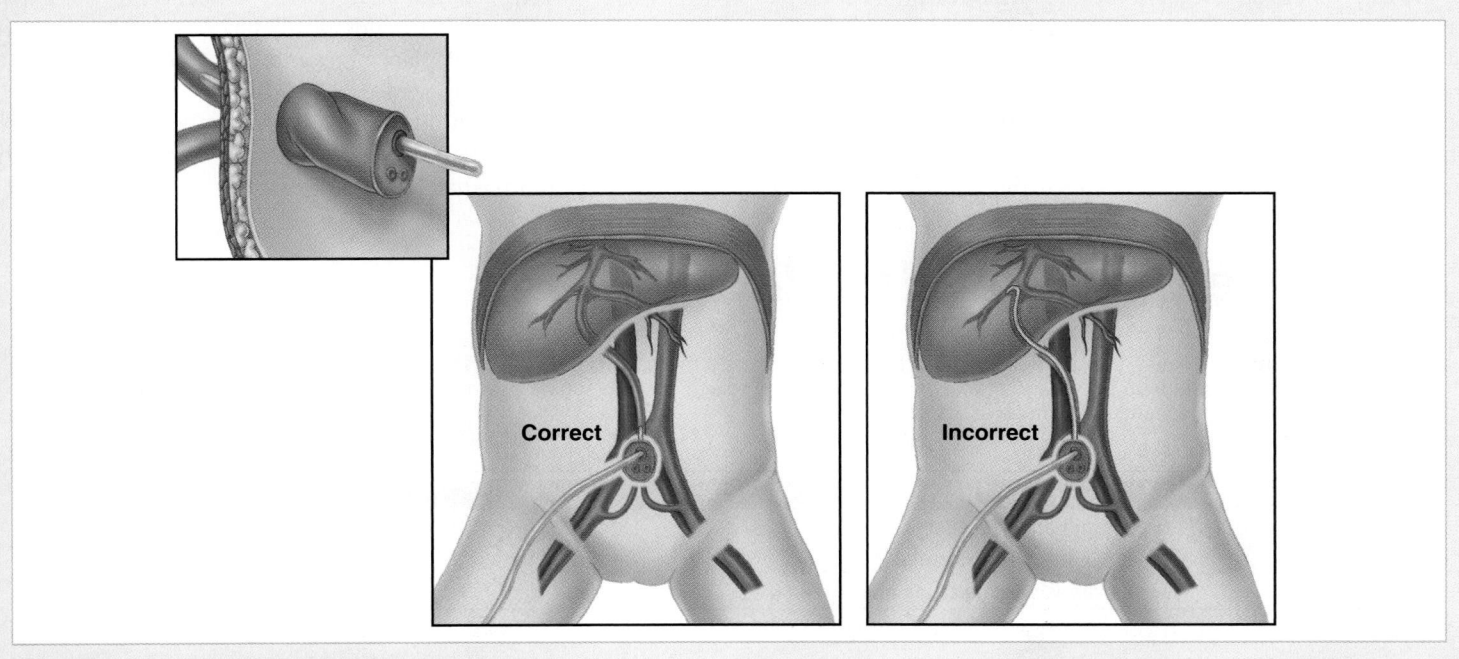

Figure 40-12 Umbilical vein catheterization.

Volume Replacement

If the infant has significant intravascular volume depletion owing to conditions such as placental abruption (separation of the placenta from the uterus, which leads to excessive bleeding) or septic shock, fluid resuscitation may be needed. In a newborn, place a low umbilical vein line as outlined earlier. In a newborn more than a few days old, place a peripheral IV or intraosseus (IO) line. Placement of an intraosseus line is discussed in Chapter 8. While the technique for placing an IO line is similar to that used with older children or adults, a smaller needle should be used in neonates to avoid exiting the far side of the bone. A fluid bolus in an infant consists of 10 mL/kg of normal saline IV given over 5 to 10 minutes. Multiple boluses may be administered if the patient remains clinically hypovolemic. Signs of hypovolemia include pallor, delayed capillary refill, and weak pulses despite a good pulse rate or high-quality chest compressions.

Specific Conditions

Acidosis

If bradycardia persists after adequate ventilation, chest compressions, and volume expansion, and you suspect metabolic acidosis, sodium bicarbonate may be indicated. Medical control may suggest an initial dose of 2 mEq/kg of 4.2% solution (0.5 mg/mL) IV to be administered over 5 to 10 minutes. Avoid rapid administration, especially in premature infants—a rapid change in pH may increase the risk of bleeding into the brain.

Respiratory Suppression Secondary to Narcotics

In the case of a drug-addicted mother, administration of naloxone to the newborn to reverse the narcotic effect may precipitate seizures that can potentially cause death, so this intervention is no longer recommended as a first line drug in resuscitation. In the case of respiratory suppression from chronic narcotics in the field, provide ventilatory support and transport immediately. If respiratory depression is from the mother being treated acutely with narcotics, and there is no chronic narcotic exposure, naloxone, 0.1 mg/kg, may be administered to the newborn via the IV (preferred) or IM route to reverse the narcotic effect.

Pneumothorax Evacuation

If an infant has signs of a significant pneumothorax—severe respiratory distress unresponsive to PPV with unilateral decreased breath sounds and (if the pneumothorax is on the right) shift of heart sounds—a needle evacuation of the pneumothorax may be necessary. On the side of the suspected pneumothorax, clean the area around the second intercostal space, midclavicular line (usually just above the nipple), with alcohol. Prepare the equipment needed: a 22-g butterfly needle attached to extension tubing, a three-way stopcock, and a 20-mL syringe. Insert the needle above the second rib as a second provider pulls back on the syringe (which is open to the patient). The nerves and blood vessels run below the ribs, so avoid piercing this area. Continue to slowly advance the needle until air is recovered. The butterfly needle is rigid, so be gentle so as to avoid further tearing the lung. If the 20-mL syringe becomes filled with air, turn the stopcock off to the newborn, push out the air from the syringe, open the stopcock to the newborn, and continue withdrawing air. Once no more air can be withdrawn, remove the needle.

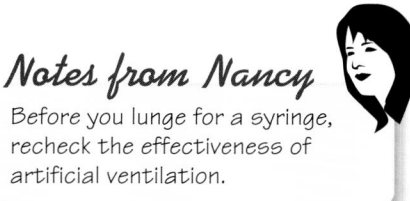

Notes from Nancy

Before you lunge for a syringe, recheck the effectiveness of artificial ventilation.

If there is a symptomatic ongoing air leak, a 22-g angiocatheter can be inserted in a similar location, the introducer needle removed, and the angiocatheter attached to the extension tubing. Note that the angiocatheter may further tear the lung during its initial placement and that it is more likely to kink than the butterfly needle.

Remove as much air as possible with the syringe. At this point, the tubing may be briefly occluded while you place the end of the tubing that had been attached to the syringe in a

You are the Provider Part 3

As the baby's head delivers, you suction the mouth and nose. Shortly thereafter, the rest of the baby delivers. It is a little girl. There is no evidence of meconium on the infant's face. You dry the infant, place her in a supine position with her head slightly extended, resuction her mouth and nose, and perform an assessment.

Newborn Assessment	Recording Time: 9 Minutes
Respiratory effort	Rapid and irregular; strong cry
Pulse rate	130 beats/min, regular
Color	Cyanosis to the trunk and extremities

5. What treatment is indicated for this infant?

6. When is positive-pressure ventilation indicated for the newborn?

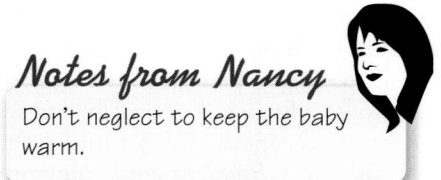
Notes from Nancy
Don't neglect to keep the baby warm.

small bottle of sterile water and release the tubing occlusion. This can relieve the pressure buildup from the pneumothorax until the patient can be transferred to a facility for placement of a chest tube. During transport, monitor the infant very closely for signs of a reaccumulation of the pneumothorax.

While performing the pneumothorax evacuation, continue your ongoing patient assessment—use proper positioning to maintain the airway and avoid aspiration, take steps to maintain thermoregulation, and ensure adequate communication with the family and with the medical team receiving the newborn. If the newborn is distressed, transport rapidly.

In the Field

While positive-pressure ventilation and chest compressions can be performed in a moving emergency vehicle, you should pull the vehicle over to the side of the road while placing and securing an advanced airway.

Meconium-Stained Amniotic Fluid

Meconium-stained amniotic fluid, which is present in 10% to 15% of deliveries, carries a high risk of morbidity. Passage of meconium may occur either before or during delivery. It is more common in post-term infants and in those who are small for their gestational age (weigh less than the 10th percentile for their age). Infants do not normally pass stool before birth, but if they do and then inhale the meconium-stained amniotic fluid either in utero or at delivery, their airways may become plugged and hypoxia may ensue. This, in turn, can lead to atelectasis, persistent pulmonary hypertension (delayed transition from fetal to neonatal circulation), pneumonitis, or pneumothorax, which may require needle aspiration.

When a newborn is delivered through meconium-stained amniotic fluid, determine whether the fluid is thin and green stained versus thick and particulate. Assess the newborn's activity level. If the baby is crying and vigorous, employ standard interventions. If the baby is depressed, do not dry or stimulate him or her. Intubate the trachea, attach a meconium aspirator and suction catheter to the end of the ET tube, and suction the ET tube while withdrawing the tube from the trachea. Be sure to cover the hole of the meconium aspirator with your finger while you are suctioning 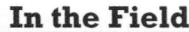 **Figure 40-13 ▶**.

After tracheal suctioning, drying and stimulation are often enough to establish adequate breathing and pulse rate; in many cases, however, oxygen and PPV are needed. If intubation for direct tracheal suctioning is unsuccessful and the newborn has significant bradycardia, continue with standard resuscitation per NRP guidelines, recognizing that the newborn will be at

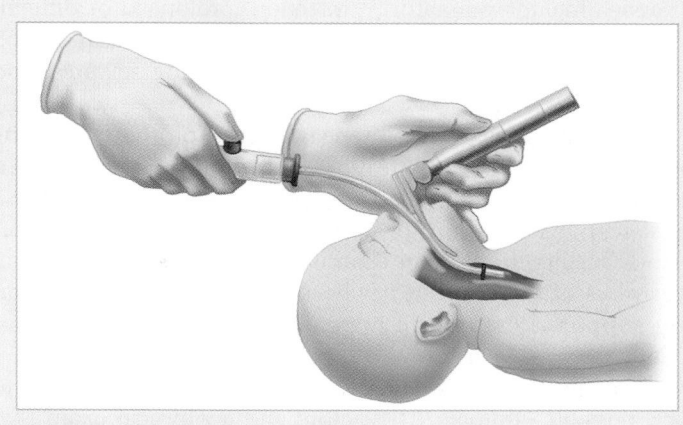
Figure 40-13 Meconium aspiration.

very high risk of meconium aspiration. If the newborn has prolonged hypoxia after significantly delayed resuscitation, the outcome will likely be poor. When transporting such an infant with respiratory symptoms, stay in communication with a facility skilled at managing high-risk newborns to help with management and identification of an appropriate transport destination. To help support the family, explain what is being done for the newborn but do not discuss "chance of survival."

Diaphragmatic Hernia

Diaphragmatic hernia—that is, an abnormal opening in the diaphragm, most commonly on the left side—has an incidence of 1 in 2,200 live births. This diagnosis is often made on prenatal ultrasound before the baby's birth. The diagnosis is suspected clinically in a newborn with respiratory distress, heart sounds shifted to the right, decreased breath sounds on the left (which can also be signs of a pneumothorax), and scaphoid abdomen (ie, the abdomen, rather than being round, is sunken due to the abdominal contents being in the chest cavity). Mortality may be as high as 50% for this condition.

If a newborn has a diaphragmatic hernia, bag-mask ventilation will introduce air that distends the intestines in the chest cavity, further compromising the newborn's ability to ventilate. If PPV is needed in such a newborn, place an ET tube and deliver a peak ventilatory pressure of 25 mm Hg or less to minimize barotrauma—these babies have poorly developed lungs. Put an OG tube in place and intermittently suction the newborn to minimize intestinal distention. Ultimately, a newborn with a diaphragmatic hernia will require surgical correction, so transport him or her to a facility with a neonatal intensive care unit and a pediatric surgical team.

Apnea

Apnea is common in infants delivered before 32 weeks of gestation, but is rarely seen in the first 24 hours after delivery, even in premature infants. If prolonged (more than 20 seconds), it can lead to hypoxemia and bradycardia. Risk factors for apnea include prematurity, infection, prolonged or difficult labor and delivery, drug exposure, gastroesophageal reflux, central nervous system abnormalities including seizures, and metabolic disorders.

The pathophysiology of apnea depends on the underlying etiology. Apnea of prematurity is due to an underdeveloped central nervous system. Gastroesophageal reflux can trigger a vagal response, leading to apnea. Drug-induced apnea frequently results from direct central nervous system depression. Regardless of the cause, a newborn with apnea needs respiratory support to minimize hypoxic brain damage and other organ damage.

Assessment of an apneic infant includes a careful history to elicit possible etiologic risk factors and a physical exam that focuses on neurologic signs and symptoms or signs of infection. At birth it is important to differentiate between primary apnea and secondary apnea. If the newborn has experienced a relatively short period of hypoxia, he or she will have a period of rapid breathing, followed by apnea and bradycardia. At this point, drying and stimulation may suffice to cause a resumption of breathing and improvement in pulse rate. If hypoxia continues during primary apnea, the infant will gasp and enter secondary apnea. At this point, stimulation alone will not restart the baby's breathing. Instead, PPV by bag-mask device is required.

Additional Conditions

Additional conditions that you may encounter and your treatment response include the following:

- **Choanal atresia.** Place an oral airway.
- **Pierre Robin sequence.** Position the infant prone to maintain the airway. Use an oral airway if needed.
- **Cleft lip and/or palate.** Airway resuscitation is not needed, but you may need to apply some cricoid pressure if intubation becomes necessary. Consider delivering PPV via bag-mask device. You may need to use a little extra positive pressure in the case of a cleft palate. Owing to the risk of aspiration and regurgitation, do not feed the newborn with a cleft lip and palate in the field.
- **Exposed abdominal contents.** A developmental defect may lead to intestines appearing outside the abdomen. In this situation, while providing standard resuscitation, place the newborn from the waist down into a sterile, clear plastic bag to keep the bowel clean and minimize heat/fluid loss. Monitor the color of the intestines (pink is good, blue/black is bad) and, if necessary, reposition the newborn, and if necessary the intestines, so that the intestines remain pink and he or she cannot turn and cut off the blood supply.

Premature and Low Birth Weight Infants

Infants delivered before 37 completed weeks of gestation are considered premature **Figure 40-14** . Infants born weigh-

ing less than 5½ lb (2,500 g) are considered low birth weight. The most common etiology for low birth weight is prematurity. A number of factors can predispose a woman to deliver prematurely, including genetic factors, infection, cervical incompetence (early opening of cervix), abruption (blood under the placenta), multiple gestations (eg, twins, triplets), previous delivery of a premature infant, drug use, and trauma. Other factors that may contribute to low birth weight include chronic maternal hypertension, smoking, placental anomalies, and chromosomal abnormalities. If an infant is delivered prior to 24 weeks of gestation or weighs less than 1 lb (500 g) and is born outside of a center that is equipped to manage such deliveries, the baby is unlikely to survive. The degree of immaturity can be estimated by physical characteristics such as skin appearance (more thin and translucent in more premature infants). If you observe signs of life, it is advisable to attempt resuscitation until the newborn can be transported to an appropriate facility.

Approximately 12% of births in the United States are preterm (< 37 weeks of gestation). Morbidity and mortality in this population are, in large part, related to the degree of prematurity. Most infants delivered after 28 weeks of gestation who receive needed cardiovascular support after birth survive and do well over the long term. Infants delivered at 24 weeks of gestation have a high morbidity and mortality. Approximately one third die and one third experience significant long-term problems—typically respiratory issues, related to the need for long-term ventilation and oxygen treatment, and neurologic issues, related to bleeding into the brain.

If an infant is delivered prematurely in the field, providing cardiorespiratory support and a thermoneutral environment will optimize his or her survival and long-term outcome.

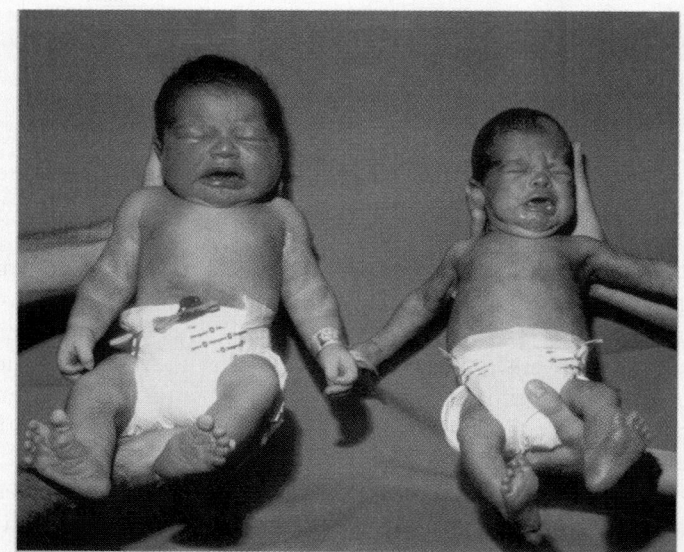

Figure 40-14 Premature infants (right) are smaller and thinner than full-term infants (left).

Premature infants are at higher risk for respiratory distress owing to surfactant deficiency. Their thermoregulation can be improved with careful environmental control (eg, warm blankets, plastic wrap, plastic bag up to head). The lungs of a premature infant are weak, so use only the minimum pressure necessary to move the chest when you are providing PPV. Brain injury can result from hypoxemia, rapid changes in blood pressure, or hyperosmolarity leading to intraventricular hemorrhage. Premature infants are also at risk of retinopathy of prematurity (abnormal vascular development of the retina), which may be worsened by long-term oxygen exposure. Because hypoxia causes irreparable brain damage, however, do not withhold oxygen from a cyanotic premature infant.

Seizures in the Neonate

Seizures are the most distinctive sign of neurologic disease in the newborn. A seizure is defined clinically as a paroxysmal alteration in neurologic function (ie, behavioral and/or autonomic function). Seizures are more common in premature infants. The incidence in this population can be as high as 57.5 per 1,000 infants who weigh less than 3 lb (1,500 g) at birth, compared with 2.8 per 1,000 infants who weigh between 5½ lb and 9 lb (2,500 g and 3,999 g) at birth. In the field, seizures are identified by direct observation; in the hospital, an electroencephalogram is used to confirm the diagnosis of seizures.

Newborns may exhibit normal motor activity that can sometimes be mistaken for seizures. These myoclonic, dysconjugate eye movements or sucking movements are often seen when the newborn is drowsy or asleep. In addition, jitteriness is often confused with a seizure Table 40-7. Jitteriness is characteristically a disorder of the newborn and is rarely seen at a later age. Jitteriness is most commonly seen with hypoxic-ischemic encephalopathy, hypocalcemia, hypoglycemia, and drug withdrawal.

Seizures, by contrast, represent a relative medical emergency. They are usually related to a significant underlying abnormality—one that often requires specific therapy. Seizures may also interfere with cardiopulmonary function, feeding, and metabolic function. Finally, prolonged seizures may even cause brain injury.

Types of Seizures
Four major types of seizures are distinguished as follows:
- **Subtle seizure.** A seizure characterized by eye deviation, blinking, sucking, and pedaling movements of the legs and apnea.
- **Tonic seizure.** A seizure characterized by tonic extension of the limbs. Less commonly, flexion of the arms and extension of the legs may also occur. This type of seizure is more common in premature infants, especially in those with intraventricular hemorrhage.
- **Focal clonic seizure.** A seizure characterized by clonic localized jerking. This type of seizure can occur in both full-term and premature infants.
- **Myoclonic seizure.** A seizure characterized by flexion jerks of the upper or lower extremities. This type of seizure may occur singly or in a series of repetitive jerks.

When describing seizures, *multifocal* refers to clinical activity that involves more than one site, is asynchronous, and is usually migratory. *Generalized* refers to activity that is bilateral, synchronous, and nonmigratory.

Causes of Seizures
Table 40-8 lists the most common (and important) causes of neonatal seizures. The time of onset for hypoxic ischemic encephalopathy, hypoglycemia, and other metabolic disturbances is up to 3 days after delivery. With all other causes listed in Table 40-8, seizures may begin 3 days or longer after birth.

Hypoxic ischemic encephalopathy, usually secondary to perinatal asphyxia (lack of oxygen to tissues) is the single most common cause of seizures in both term and preterm infants. Seizures characteristically occur in the first 24 hours and usually become severe. Metabolic abnormalities include disturbances in the levels of glucose, calcium, magnesium, or electrolytes. Other metabolic disturbances include abnormalities of amino acids, organic acids, blood ammonia, and certain toxins.

Hypoglycemia is most frequently seen in infants who are small for their gestational age, those who are large for their gestational age, and those whose mothers were diabetic during

Table 40-7	Jitteriness Versus Seizures in the Newborn	
Characteristic	Jitteriness	Seizures
Ocular phenomenon (deviation or fixation of the eyes)	Not seen	Commonly associated
Stimulus sensitive (may be triggered by a stimulus)	Yes	No
Dominant movement	Tremor	Clonic jerking
Application of gentle pressure to limb	Stops jitteriness	Does not stop seizures
Autonomic phenomenon	Not associated	Common association

Table 40-8	Causes of Neonatal Seizures	
Hypoxic ischemic encephalopathy		Intracranial hemorrhage
Intracranial infections (meningitis)		Development defects
Hypoglycemia		Hypocalcemia
Other metabolic disturbances		
Epileptic syndromes		

pregnancy. Neurologic symptoms consist of jitteriness, stupor, hypotonia (floppy), apnea, poor feeding, and seizures.

Hypocalcemia has two major peaks of incidence. The first peak occurs at 2 to 3 days after delivery and is most commonly seen in low birth weight infants and in infants of diabetic mothers. Late-onset hypocalcemia is rare in the United States but may be seen in infants who consume cow's milk or synthetic formulas high in phosphorus.

Other metabolic disturbances are uncommon in neonates, although hyponatremia, hyperammonemia, other amino acid and organic acid abnormalities, or seizures from drug withdrawal (eg, narcotic analgesics, sedative hypnotics, tricyclic antidepressants, cocaine, or alcohol) may be seen.

Assessment and Management of Seizures

Evaluation of a newborn with seizures must include a quick evaluation of prenatal and birth history and a careful physical exam. You may observe a quiet, often hypotonic infant. The newborn may be lethargic or apneic. Hypoglycemia must be recognized quickly and treated promptly. In these cases, blood glucose measurement and administration of dextrose may be lifesaving in the field. Obtain the newborn's baseline vital signs and oxygen saturation readings and provide additional oxygen, assisted ventilation, blood pressure evaluation, and IV access as necessary. A 10% dextrose solution may be given as an IV bolus (2 mL/kg) if the newborn's blood glucose level is less than 40 mg/dL, with a recheck of the blood glucose level in about 30 minutes. IV administration of dextrose often needs to be followed by a 10% dextrose infusion.

Consult with medical control if you are considering giving the newborn anticonvulsant medication. Phenobarbitol (Luminal) and phenytoin (Dilantin)—the drugs most commonly used in such cases—require care in administration and may interfere with respiratory and cardiac function. Lorazepam (Ativan) is a benzodiazepine that may be administered IV or rectally.

Monitor the newborn's respiratory status and saturations carefully. Maintain the newborn's normal body temperature and keep the family informed about what you are doing for their infant as transport gets under way.

▊ Thermoregulation

Thermoregulation is the body's ability to balance heat production and heat loss so as to maintain normal body temperature. This ability is very limited in the newborn. The average normal temperature of a newborn is 37.5°C (99.5°F). For the neonate, the thermoneutral temperature range is 36.6 to 37.2°C.

Nonshivering thermogenesis, the production of heat by metabolism, is the primary source of heat production in the neonate. Brown fat (deposited in the fetus after 28 weeks of gestation, and principally stored around the scapula, kidneys, adrenal glands, neck, and axilla) is a thermogenic tissue unique to the newborn.

Heat loss occurs when heat is lost to the environment, through any of the following four mechanisms. In evaporation, heat is lost when water evaporates from the skin and respiratory tract. In convection, heat is lost to cooler surrounding air; the extent of heat loss depends on the air temperature and air movement. In conduction, heat is lost to cooler solid objects in direct contact with the body. In radiation, heat is lost to cooler surrounding objects not in direct contact with the body.

Fever

Fever is defined as a rectal temperature greater than 38°C (100.4°F). Oral and axillary temperatures are, respectively, 0.6°C (1°F) and 1.1°C (2°F) lower than the rectal temperature on average.

A newborn's temperature regulation system is relatively immature, so fever may not always be a presenting feature with infection or illness. In fact, neonates may become hypothermic with infection. No matter what the presenting symptoms are, it is important to identify newborns with serious bacterial infection (eg, bacteremia, urinary tract infection, meningitis, bacterial gastroenteritis, and pneumonia) or serious viral infection (eg, herpes simplex) for which treatment is available. Approximately 13% of infants younger than 28 days with a temperature of more than 38.1°C will have a serious bacterial infection.

Fever may also be caused by overheating. Babies can easily become too hot when dressed in many layers of clothing, overbundled in a heated car, or placed in direct sunlight, even through a window, or near heating vents at home. Fever related to dehydration is an important consideration in breastfeeding babies, especially in the first week after birth. These infants have often lost more than 10% of their weight and may have a history of difficulty in initiating breastfeeding.

Newborns have limited ability to control their temperature. They do not sweat when they are hot to allow cooling, and they do not shiver to raise their temperature when they are cold. Term infants may produce sweat over their brow but not the rest of their body. Premature infants do not produce sweat.

You are the Provider Part 4

After delivery of blow-by oxygen, the baby's trunk is now pink; her hands and feet, however, remain cyanotic. You take appropriate actions to keep her warm. Further assessment reveals that her respirations are rapid and her pulse rate is 120 beats/min. She resists your attempts to straighten her hips and knees and moves her foot away when you snap your finger against it.

7. What is the infant's Apgar score?

8. Is it safe to clamp and cut the umbilical cord?

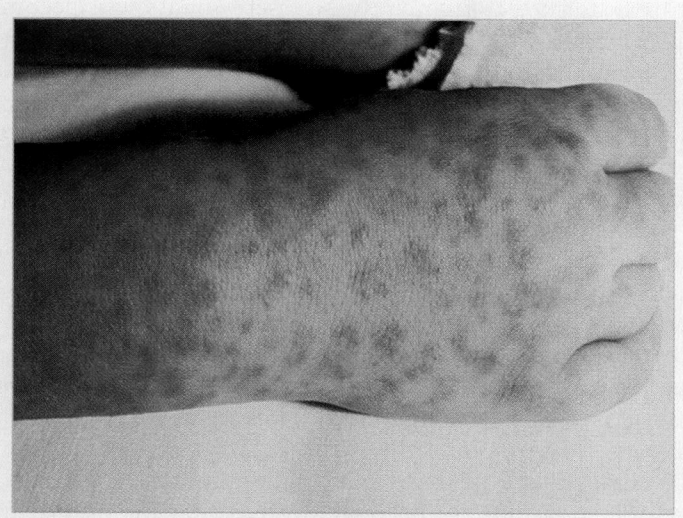

Figure 40-15 A newborn with a fever may also have petechiae or pinpoint pink or red skin lesions.

Table 40-9	Risk Factors for Hypothermia

- All neonates in the first 8 to 12 hours after birth
- Home delivery
- Prolonged resuscitation
- Small for gestational age infant
- Infant with central nervous system problems
- Prematurity
- Sepsis
- Inadequate measures to keep the infant warm during transport

Moreover, many newborns with serious life-threatening infections may actually see their core temperature drop; these infants are at a higher risk for hypoglycemia and metabolic acidosis. A careful examination will reveal irritability, somnolence, and decreased feeding. The infant may feel warm to touch. Some infants with fever, however, may be initially asymptomatic.

When fever is suspected, observe the newborn for the presence of rashes, especially petechiae or pinpoint pink or red skin lesions Figure 40-15 . Obtain a careful history regarding general activity, feeding, voiding, and stooling. Obtain the newborn's vital signs and ensure adequate oxygenation and ventilation, providing free-flow supplemental oxygen if necessary. Perform chest compressions, if indicated. Administration of antipyretic agents such as acetaminophen or ibuprofen is controversial in the prehospital setting; do not give ibuprofen to an infant. To cool the newborn, remove additional layers of clothing and improve ventilation in the environment.

Hypothermia

Hypothermia is a drop in body temperature to less than 35°C (95°F). Hypothermia in the newborn occurs in all climates, but is more common during the winter months. It has been linked to impaired growth and may make the newborn vulnerable to infections. Moderate hypothermia is associated with an increased risk of death in low birth weight infants. Sick or low birth weight infants admitted to hospital with hypothermia are more likely to die than those admitted with normal temperature. Infants may die of cold exposure at temperatures adults find comfortable. Table 40-9 lists risk factors for hypothermia.

Newborn infants have increased surface area-to-volume ratio, making the newborn extremely sensitive to environmental conditions, especially when wet after delivery. An increase in metabolic function in an attempt to overcome the heat loss can cause hypoglycemia, metabolic acidosis, pulmonary hypertension, and hypoxemia. Every hypothermic newborn should also be investigated for infection.

Hypothermic neonates are cool to the touch, initially in the extremities; as their temperature drops, however, the skin becomes cool all over. The infant may also be pale and have acrocyanosis. The hypothermic newborn may present with apnea, bradycardia, cyanosis, irritability, and a weak cry. As a newborn's temperature drops, he or she may become lethargic and obtunded. In severely hypothermic babies, the face and extremities may appear bright red. Sclerema—hardening of the skin associated with reddening and edema—may be seen on the back, limbs, or all over the body. Thermal shock, disseminated intravascular coagulopathy, and death may occur in more serious cases.

Preventive measures include warming your hands before touching the baby. Dry the newborn thoroughly after birth and remove any wet blankets. Place a cap on the newborn's head, as the head is the largest source of heat loss. Place the infant "skin to skin" with the mother, if possible. This serves two purposes: The mother keeps the baby warm, and mother and baby can more readily bond. Ensure adequate oxygenation and ventilation, and perform chest compressions if necessary. If the infant is hypoglycemic, you may administer $D_{10}W$. Warm IV fluids can assist in rewarming the newborn. The critically ill newborn, once stabilized, should be placed in a prewarmed incubator or, if none is available, covered with warm blankets and kept on mother's chest.

At home, skin-to-skin contact is the best method to rewarm a baby with mild hypothermia. Ideally, the room should be warm (24°C to 26.5°C), and the baby should be covered with a warm blanket and wear a prewarmed cap. Continue the rewarming process until the baby's temperature reaches the normal range or his or her feet are no longer cold. Do not use hot water bottles—they may cause burns because blood circulation is poor in the cold skin of babies.

Recent studies in neonates with hypoxic-ischemic injury indicate improved outcomes when the infant is provided mild therapeutic hypothermia within 6 hours of birth. This approach is not recommended in the field, although it is prudent to prevent hyperthermia. Maintain the infant at the lower margin of normal temperature (axillary temperature no higher than 36.5°F).

Hypoglycemia

In full-term or preterm infants, hypoglycemia is a blood glucose level of less than 40 mg/dL. This condition represents an imbalance between glucose supply and utilization. Glucose levels may be low due to inadequate intake or storage or increased utilization of glucose. Most infants remain asymptomatic until the glucose falls below 20 mg/dL for a significant period of time. Because the brain relies on glucose as its primary fuel, hypoglycemia may result in seizures and severe, permanent brain damage. **Table 40-10** lists risk factors for hypoglycemia in the newborn.

The fetus receives glucose from the mother and deposits glycogen in the liver, lung, heart, and skeletal muscle in utero. The infant then begins to utilize those glycogen stores to meet glucose needs after birth; most full-term infants will have sufficient glycogen stores to meet their glucose needs for 8 to 12 hours. Disorders related to decreased glycogen stores (small for gestational age, prematurity, postmaturity) or to increased utilization of glucose (infant of a diabetic mother, large for gestational age, hypoxia, hypothermia, sepsis) place the infant at increased risk for hypoglycemia. Metabolic adaptations to maintain normal glucose levels are regulated by counterregulatory hormones such as glucagon, epinephrine, cortisol, and

Table 40-10	Risk Factors for Hypoglycemia in the Newborn
Risk Factor	**Specific Indicators**
Disorders of fetal growth and maturity	Small for gestational age
	Smaller of discordant twins (weight difference > 25%)
	Large for gestational age
	Low birth weight infant (birth weight < 2,500 g)
Prematurity	Less than 37 weeks of gestation or less than 5.5 pounds (2.5 kg)
Disorders of maternal glucose regulation	Insulin-dependent diabetic mother
	Gestational diabetic mother
	Morbid obesity in mother
Neonatal conditions with disturbed oxidative metabolism	Perinatal distress (eg, 5-minute Apgar score < 5)
	Hypoxemia due to cardiac or lung disease
	Shock, hypoperfusion, sepsis, cold stress
Severe anemia	Pallor (in the absence of hypovolemia)
Congenital anomalies and genetic disorders	Visible anatomic deformities/abnormalities

growth hormone. Frequently, stressed infants will become hypoglycemic.

Symptoms of hypoglycemia may include cyanosis, apnea, irritability, poor sucking or feeding, and hypothermia. These symptoms may also be associated with lethargy, tremors, twitching or seizures, and coma. They may also have tachycardia, tachypnea, or vomiting.

Check the blood glucose level in all sick newborns (by heel stick) and evaluate the newborn's vital signs. After you establish good oxygenation, ventilation, and circulation (ABCs), manage the hypoglycemia. Medical control personnel may order the administration of a 10% dextrose solution as a bolus at 2 mL/kg via IV access if the newborn's blood glucose level is less than 40 mg/dL. This intervention may be followed by an IV infusion of 10% dextrose based on the infant's gestational age (60 mL/kg/d for a full-term infant; adjust upward based on the recommendations of the referring hospital for premature infants). As always, maintain normal body temperature—hypothermia places additional stress on glucose demand.

Vomiting

Vomiting is very common in newborns. Approximately 85% of infants vomit during the first week of life, and another 10% have vomited by 6 weeks of age. Vomiting ranges from "spitting up" to severe, bloody or bilious, projectile vomiting. Most episodes of vomiting are benign and do not result in weight loss, dehydration, or other ill effects. Bilious and/or bloody emesis (vomiting) indicates a pathologic condition that needs medical attention. Persistent vomiting is a warning sign and can cause excessive loss of fluid, dehydration, and changes in electrolyte levels (ie, sodium, potassium, and glucose).

Vomiting mucus, occasionally blood streaked, in the first few hours of life is not uncommon. Persistent vomiting in the first 24 hours of life suggests obstruction in the upper digestive tract or increased intracranial pressure. Vomitus containing dark blood is often a sign of a life-threatening illness; it indicates bleeding in the gut. Sometimes, vomitus may be accompanied by bloody or tarry stool, another worrisome sign. Aspiration of vomitus can cause respiratory insufficiencies or obstruction of the airway.

Causes of Vomiting

A newborn's presenting symptoms may give a clue to the site of obstruction or other problem that is causing the vomiting. One possible cause is esophageal atresia (narrowing) with or without tracheoesophageal fistula. Its incidence is 1 case per 3,000 to 4,500 births. Infants are seen with excessive frothing soon after birth and may choke when attempting to feed, because the swallowed milk is returned promptly. This condition can also lead to an acute gastric perforation when the infant cries or strains and the air from the fistula enters the stomach; this problem is often lethal.

Another possible cause of vomiting, pathogenic gastro-esophageal reflux (GER), is common in infants, with a reported prevalence of 2% to 10%. GER is most commonly seen in infancy, with its incidence peaking in the 1- to 4-month age group. The infant may vomit either immediately or a few hours after a feeding. The vomiting may not be forceful. In uncomplicated GER, the vomitus is not bile stained or bloody. GER in infants and young children can present as typical or atypical crying and/or irritability, apnea and/or bradycardia, poor appetite, apparent life-threatening event, vomiting, wheezing, stridor, weight loss or poor growth (failure to thrive), hoarseness, and/or laryngitis.

In infantile hypertrophic pyloric stenosis (IHPS), marked hypertrophy and hyperplasia of the two (circular and longitudinal) muscular layers of the pylorus occur. As a consequence, the pylorus becomes thickened and obstructs the end of the stomach. The incidence of IHPS is 2 to 4 cases per 1,000 live births, with a male-to-female predominance of 4:1; 30% of patients with IHPS are first-born males. The usual age of presentation is approximately 3 weeks of life (range, 1 to 18 weeks). In IHPS, the stomach muscles contract forcibly to overcome the obstruction. Affected infants usually present with projectile vomiting, dehydration, malnutrition, and electrolyte changes. The vomitus in this case is not bile stained, but it can be brown or coffee colored due to blood, resulting from gastritis or to a Mallory Weiss tear at the gastroesophageal junction.

Malrotation is a congenital anomaly of rotation of the midgut. In this condition, the small bowel is found predominantly on the right side of the abdomen; the cecum is found in the epigastrium–right hypochondrium. In cases of malrotation, the vomitus is bile stained and may be feculent (like feces/stool) if the obstruction is distal in the intestines. Malrotation is estimated to occur in 1 of every 500 live births. Approximately 40% of patients are diagnosed within the first week of life; 75% are diagnosed by 1 year of age; and the remaining 25% are diagnosed later in life. With symptomatic malrotation, 75% to 90% of cases occur in infants younger than 1 year, 50% to 64% of cases occur in infants younger than 1 month, and 25% to 40% of cases occur in the first week of life. During the first week of life, the ratio of male-to-female presentation is 2:1. Since the advent of corrective surgical procedures, the morbidity and mortality have decreased significantly. Early mortality rate ranged from 23% to 33%, with most deaths resulting from bowel dysfunction and malnutrition.

Another cause of vomiting, meconium plug, is seen in Hirschsprung disease, wherein the last segment of colon fails to relax and causes mechanical obstruction. The infant usually has a history of not passing meconium in the first 24 hours of life.

Vomiting may also happen in conjunction with asphyxia, meningitis (infection of the layers covering the brain and spine), and hydrocephalus (large head size is a clue). It is often sudden, unexpected, and forceful in such cases, and it may be accompanied by persistent irritability. Meningitis and hydrocephalus may also be associated with increased intracranial pressure (ICP).

Use of drugs during pregnancy can lead to several withdrawal symptoms in infants, including vomiting. The drugs that most commonly cause vomiting in newborns are barbiturates.

Assessment and Management of Vomiting

On physical exam, you may note a distended stomach that has been caused by vomiting. Suspect an infection if the newborn has a fever or a history of contact with sick people.

Initial management steps for a newborn with vomiting start with the ABCs. Maintain a patent airway, while staying aware that a vomiting infant can aspirate the vomitus and compromise the airway. Keep the infant's face turned to one side to prevent further aspiration. Suction or clear the vomitus from the airway with the help of a suction catheter or suction bulb. Ensure adequate oxygenation, providing either free-flow supplemental oxygen or bag-mask ventilation as necessary. Bradycardia may be caused by vagal stimulus and is usually transient; it may resolve with stimulation and free-flow oxygen.

Antiemetics should not be administered in the field. The infant may be dehydrated, however, and need fluid resuscitation. Dry mucous membranes, tachycardia, or a sunken fontanelle are clues that the patient needs hydration. Normal saline (10 mL/kg per bolus) may be required in that case.

On transport, place the newborn on his or her side, identify a facility capable of managing a high-risk infant, and explain what is being done for the infant to the family.

Diarrhea

A normal number of stools per day for an infant is five to six, especially if the infant is breastfeeding, when infants often stool after every feeding. Diarrhea is an excessive loss of electrolytes and fluid in the stool. In the United States, infants younger than 3 years have 1.3 to 2.3 episodes of diarrhea each year. The prevalence is higher in infants attending daycare centers. Nine percent of all hospitalizations of children younger than 5 years of age are for diarrhea.

The most common cause of acute diarrhea in children is viral infection (especially rotavirus infection during the winter months). Less frequently encountered causes include poisoning due to insecticides, organophosphates, and carbamates. Diarrhea related to these agents is accompanied by profuse sweating, lacrimation, hypersalivation, and abdominal cramps, or more serious conditions such as intussusception, malrotation, increased ICP, and metabolic acidosis. Other causes of diarrhea include gastroenteritis, lactose intolerance, neonatal abstinence syndrome, thyrotoxicosis, and cystic fibrosis.

Severe cases of diarrhea can cause dehydration and subsequent electrolyte imbalance. Combinations of physical signs—such as ill general appearance, poor vital signs, capillary refill of greater than 2 seconds, dry mucous membranes, absent tears, weight loss, and low urine output—are good objective predictors of the degree of dehydration.

Assessment and Management of Diarrhea

Assessment includes estimating the number and volume of loose stools, decreased urinary output, and degree of dehydration based on skin turgor, mucous membranes, presence of sunken eyes, and other signs. Patient management, as always, begins with the ABCs. The newborn's airway and ventilation may be compromised if he or she is severely dehydrated and is obtunded, so ensure adequate oxygenation and ventilation. Perform chest compressions in addition to PPV in a newborn if the pulse rate is less than 60 beats/min.

Fluid therapy may be indicated when a newborn has diarrhea. Normal saline (10-mL/kg boluses) may be needed immediately to fluid resuscitate the infant.

Common Birth Injuries in the Newborn

Birth trauma includes both avoidable and unavoidable injuries to the infant resulting from mechanical forces (ie, compression, traction) during the delivery process. Such trauma is estimated to occur in 2 to 7 of every 1,000 live births. Most birth injuries are self-limiting and have a favorable outcome. Nearly half are potentially avoidable with recognition and anticipation of obstetric risk factors.

Birth injuries account for 2% to 3% of all infant deaths, with 5 to 8 of every 100,000 newborns dying of birth trauma and 25 of every 100,000 newborns dying of anoxic injury. Separating the effects of a hypoxic ischemic insult from the effects of a traumatic birth injury may prove difficult.

A difficult birth or injury to the baby can occur because of the infant's size or position during labor and delivery. Conditions associated with a difficult birth include primigravida (first pregnancy), prolonged labor, cephalopelvic disproportion (the size and shape of the maternal pelvis are not adequate for the vaginal delivery of the infant), prolonged or rapid labor, abnormal presentation (eg, breech), large size (birth weight exceeding 9 lb, or 4,000 g), prematurity, or low birth weight.

Birth trauma includes a variety of injuries. For example, abrasions, lacerations, bruises, and subcutaneous fat necrosis can occur with deliveries that involve instruments (eg, a vacuum or forceps). Molding of the head and overriding parietal bones are part of the normal process of labor, but occasionally excessive molding may be seen.

Caput succedaneum is swelling of the soft tissue of the baby's scalp as it presses against the dilating cervix. This type of cranial injury is very common. The swelling usually disappears in the first day or two after birth.

A cephalhematoma is an area of bleeding between the parietal bone and its covering periosteum. It often appears several hours after birth as a raised lump on the newborn's head, is limited by the boundaries of the bone, and may take 2 weeks to 3 months to resolve. If the bleeding is severe, jaundice may be seen as the red blood cells break down. Babies born by instrumental vaginal delivery are more likely to have a cephalhematoma. Do not try to drain a rapidly expanding scalp hematoma, as this may worsen or prolong the bleeding.

Linear fractures are occasionally seen with difficult births (spontaneous vaginal deliveries or deliveries using instruments).

Brachial plexus injuries typically occur in large babies and have an incidence of 0.5 to 2.0 cases per 1,000 live births. The most common brachial plexus injury is Erb palsy (involvement of C5, C6). Klumpke paralysis (C7–C8, T1) is rare and results in the weakness of the intrinsic muscles of the hand.

Although branches of the facial nerve may be injured in forceps delivery, most facial nerve palsy is unrelated to trauma. Physical findings include asymmetric facies with crying (lack of

You are the Provider Part 5

You prepare both the infant and mother for transport, load them into the ambulance, and begin transport to a hospital located 20 miles away. En route, the mother experiences mild vaginal bleeding, which you control with fundal massage. As the infant is nursing, you establish an IV of normal saline on the mother and administer supplemental oxygen at 4 L/min via nasal cannula. After delivery of the placenta, you reassess the mother.

Reassessment	Recording Time: 19 Minutes
Skin	Pink, warm, and moist
Pulse	84 beats/min, strong and regular
Blood pressure	104/58 mm Hg
Respirations	20 breaths/min; adequate tidal volume
Sao₂	99% on oxygen via nasal cannula

When you arrive at the emergency department, you are met by a neonatologist and an emergency physician. Both the mother and baby are hemodynamically stable and are admitted to the hospital.

9. When are chest compressions indicated for the newborn?
10. When is epinephrine indicated during newborn resuscitation?

movement on the affected side makes the face appear to be "pulled" to the opposite side). Full resolution of cranial nerve injuries may take several weeks.

Diaphragmatic paralysis may occur as an isolated finding when the cervical roots supplying the phrenic nerve are injured or in association with brachial plexus injury. The newborn may experience respiratory distress with hypoxemia, hypercapnea, and acidosis. Approximately 80% of the lesions are on the right side, and 10% are bilateral.

Laryngeal nerve injury appears to result from an intrauterine posture in which the head is rotated and flexed laterally. The infant presents with stridor or a hoarse cry. Bilateral injury may be associated with severe respiratory distress needing respiratory support. The paralysis often resolves in 4 to 6 weeks, but may occasionally take as long as 6 to 12 months to clear up.

Spinal cord injury may result from excessive traction (in a breech delivery) or rotation and torsion (in a vertex delivery). The clinical presentation is stillbirth or rapid neonatal death with failure to establish an adequate airway.

The clavicle is the most frequently fractured bone in the newborn; such a bone injury is most often an unpredictable, unavoidable complication of normal birth. Risk factors may include large size, mid-forceps delivery, and shoulder dystocia (ie, the baby's shoulders get stuck in the birth canal). The infant may present with pseudoparalysis as he or she tries not to move the affected extremity to minimize pain. Examination will show crepitus and palpable bony irregularity.

Loss of spontaneous arm or leg movement is an early sign of long bone fracture. The femur and humerus are the most commonly affected long bones. The fractures are treated by splinting. Look for signs of radial nerve injury with a humerus fracture. Intra-abdominal injury is uncommon and may be overlooked as a cause of death in a newborn. Hemorrhage is the most serious complication, and the liver is the organ most commonly injured. The bleeding may be catastrophic or insidious, and the patient presents with circulatory collapse. Consider intra-abdominal bleeding in every infant presenting with shock, or unexplained pallor, plus abdominal distention.

Family and Transport Considerations

Once the infant is stabilized as much as possible in the field, transport the patient to the nearest facility that can provide the next level of care. This facility will not necessarily be a tertiary hospital. A nearby community hospital, if it is located much closer, may be able to perform additional stabilization procedures for a very ill baby, such as placement of a chest tube for a clinically significant pneumothorax. Ideally, someone will contact this facility to discuss the situation and obtain advice regarding care and disposition. Throughout the process, ongoing communication with the family regarding what is being done for the infant and what care is planned will help allay fears. Do not be specific about survival statistics. Many factors play into mortality and morbidity, and you don't want to be misleading. If family members have questions you can't answer, be straightforward. Tell them that you don't have a definite answer, but you will help put them in touch with the people who do (ie, the center to which the infant is being transferred) **Figure 40-16 ▾**.

During transport, ongoing observation and frequent reassessment will ensure timely intervention should the newborn's status change. Attention to thermoregulation, respiratory effort, patency of airway, skin color, and pulse rate is vital. If the infant is being transferred between facilities after the initial stabilization, continue to provide close observation and assessment of these factors to facilitate initiation of interventions should the infant's condition change.

The development of new and more sophisticated techniques for the care of newborn infants, especially premature infants, together with round-the-clock care by expert medical personnel, has significantly reduced the mortality among high-risk newborns in hospitals where such capabilities are available. Because the average community hospital cannot provide the specially trained doctors and nurses or the expensive equipment needed for such care, it sometimes becomes necessary to transfer the critically ill infant to a regional center, where the infant may benefit from highly skilled personnel and sophisticated equipment. In the well-organized regional referral system, transport of a high-risk newborn proceeds through the following several steps:

1. A physician at the referring hospital initiates a request for transport. A physician in the regional control center decides which intensive care nursery can accommodate the patient and gives the referring physician advice on management of the infant until the transport team arrives.

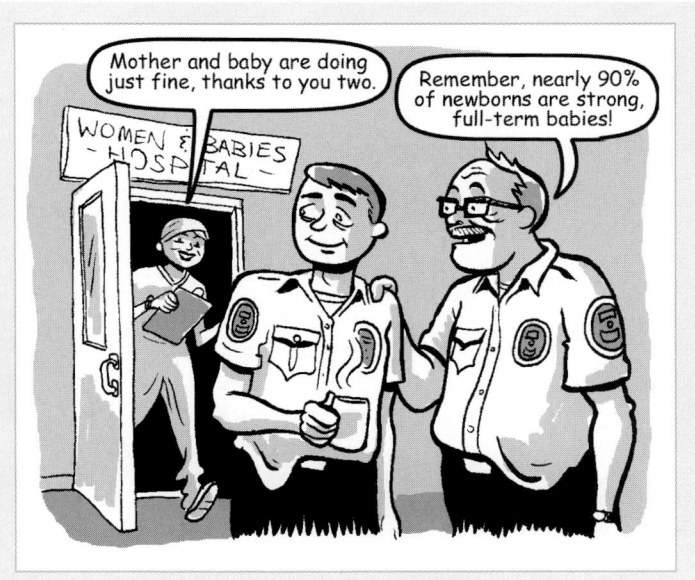

Figure 40-16

2. A mode of transportation is chosen—ground transportation, helicopter, or fixed-wing aircraft, depending on the distance, availability of services, and weather conditions.

3. The transport team is mobilized, and equipment is assembled. The ideal team consists of a nurse with special training in neonatal intensive care, a respiratory therapist with similar special training, and a paramedic who has spent a period of apprenticeship in a neonatal intensive care unit. For particularly critical patients, a physician may also attend. The equipment is highly specialized, requiring appropriately designed ventilation and oxygenation units and an incubator meeting stringent criteria.

4. On arriving at the referring hospital, the transport team continues to stabilize the infant before embarking on transport. Conditions such as hypoxemia, acidosis, hypoglycemia, and hypovolemia must be treated before leaving the referring hospital.

5. While stabilizing the infant, the team collects information and materials including a copy of the mother's and infant's charts and any x-rays taken of the infant.

You are the Provider Summary

1. Why is it important to determine the color of the amniotic fluid?

A crucial part of your predelivery evaluation is to determine the color of the amniotic fluid. Normally, it should be clear. Amniotic fluid that is brown or contains thick, particulate meconium—the baby's first bowel movement—indicates that the newborn may have aspirated the meconium. In such a case, the newborn may be severely hypoxic and may require aggressive resuscitation.

2. What are some reliable indicators of imminent delivery?

When determining whether you have time to transport the mother to the hospital or must prepare for imminent delivery, there are some key questions to ask and some key observations to make. Regular contractions that are less than 5 minutes apart—even if the amniotic sac has not ruptured—should be considered a sign of impending delivery. If the woman says that she feels the urge to move her bowels, the baby is pressing on her rectum and is in the birth canal. Clearly, crowning of the baby's head indicates that delivery is in progress. Perhaps one of the most reliable indicators of impending delivery is when the mother states that she is going to have her baby "now!" If she tells you this, believe her—even if it is her first baby.

3. What specific questions should you ask that will allow you to anticipate the need for resuscitation of the newborn?

Although it's impossible to predict all of the complications that might potentially occur following delivery, a thorough maternal assessment—if time permits—will enable you to identify risk factors that should increase your suspicion for a distressed newborn who will require resuscitation. Establishing how far along a woman is into her pregnancy is a key consideration. If a fetus is less than 37 weeks of gestation—in which case the woman would be in premature labor—the risk for a distressed newborn increases. You should also ask if the patient is carrying more than one baby. Of course, if she has had regular prenatal care—which typically includes an ultrasound—she will know the answer. Inquire about the use of drugs (legal and illicit), alcohol, or cigarettes during the mother's pregnancy; these factors clearly increase the risk of newborn distress. Finally, ask about her medical history, focusing specifically on conditions that can complicate pregnancy (ie, pregnancy-induced hypertension [preeclampsia] or gestational diabetes).

4. What equipment and supplies should be available in case the infant requires resuscitation?

Although approximately 90% of babies are born normal and require little more than drying, warming, and suctioning, you should be adequately prepared in the event that the infant requires more aggressive resuscitative measures. In addition to the sterile OB kit, you should have a neonatal-size bag-mask device, equipment and supplies required to perform tracheal suctioning of meconium (ie, newborn-size ET tubes, meconium aspirator, suction, laryngoscope and blades), and epinephrine (1:10,000 only) for refractory cardiopulmonary depression. Consider carrying this equipment and supplies in a special newborn resuscitation kit, which should be checked daily, along with the other equipment and supplies on the ambulance.

5. What treatment is indicated for this infant?

Although the infant is breathing adequately and has a pulse rate greater than 100 beats/min, the presence of central cyanosis indicates the need for free-flow supplemental oxygen. It can be delivered using an oxygen mask or oxygen tubing held near the baby's nose and mouth. Set the oxygen flow rate at 5 L/min and observe the infant for improving color. Avoid blowing oxygen directly into the baby's eyes, as it may dry out the mucosa.

6. When is positive-pressure ventilation indicated for the newborn?

PPV is indicated in the newborn if the infant is apneic or has gasping respirations, if the infant's pulse rate is less than 100 beats/min, or if central cyanosis persists despite the delivery of free-flow supplemental oxygen. The proper ventilation rate for the newborn is 40 to 60 breaths/min.

7. What is the infant's Apgar score?

On the basis of your evaluation of the infant, her Apgar score is 9:

1. Appearance: pink body; cyanotic hands and feet (1)
2. Pulse: greater than 100 beats/min (2)
3. Grimace/irritability: infant moves her foot away when you snap your finger against her (2)
4. Activity/muscle tone: infant resists attempts to straighten hips and knees (2)
5. Respirations: rapid (2)

8. Is it safe to clamp and cut the umbilical cord?

The umbilical cord should not be clamped and cut until the baby is breathing adequately on its own and the cord has stopped pulsating. If neither of these has occurred, do not clamp and cut the cord. Instead, keep the baby at the level of the perineum, wrap the cord with sterile, moist dressings, and transport immediately with continued resuscitation en route to the hospital. The infant in this case has adequate breathing and a pulse rate greater than 100 beats/min; therefore, it is hemodynamically stable, and it is safe to clamp and cut the umbilical cord.

9. When are chest compressions indicated for the newborn?

Chest compressions are rarely needed during newborn resuscitation. However, if there is no pulse or if the pulse rate falls below 60 beats/min despite *adequate* oxygenation and ventilation, begin chest compressions immediately. In the newborn, chest compressions are delivered using the two-finger technique (one rescuer) or the two-thumb encircling-hands technique (two rescuers). Compress the chest one-third to one-half the anteroposterior depth of the chest at a rate of 120 compressions/min. After 30 seconds of chest compressions, reassess the infant.

10. When is epinephrine indicated during newborn resuscitation?

As with chest compressions, medication therapy is rarely needed during newborn resuscitation. However, if the pulse is absent *or* less than 60 beats/min despite 30 seconds of *adequate* oxygenation and ventilation *plus* an additional 30 seconds of chest compressions (1 minute total), you should administer epinephrine. The proper newborn dose for epinephrine is 0.1 to 0.3 mL/kg of a 1:10,000 solution via rapid administration. *Never use epinephrine 1:1,000 during newborn resuscitation; it is too concentrated and may result in a spontaneous intracranial hemorrhage!* Epinephrine can be administered via a peripheral IV line or through the umbilical vein (if you are able to cannulate the umbilical vein). If epinephrine is administered via the ET tube, consider giving a higher dose—0.3 to 1 mL/kg.

Prep Kit

■ Ready for Review

- The care of a newborn or neonate must be tailored to meet the unique needs of this population.
- Additional skilled care intervention is needed for approximately 6% of newborn deliveries, with the rate of complications increasing as birth weight and gestational age decrease.
- In the United States, approximately 80% of the 30,000 babies born each year weighing less than 1,500 g require resuscitation.
- Both short- and long-term outcomes have been linked to initial stabilization efforts.
- Your initial rapid assessment of the infant may be done simultaneously with any treatment interventions.
- Nearly 90% of newborns are vigorous full-term babies.
- Not all deliveries go so smoothly. Approximately 10% of newborns need additional assistance and 1% need major resuscitation to survive.
- Infants born before 37 weeks of gestation are considered premature.
- Seizures are the most distinctive sign of neurologic disease in the newborn.
- Thermoregulation is very limited in the newborn, so the paramedic must take an active role in keeping the newborn's body temperature in the normal range.
- In full-term or preterm neonates, hypoglycemia is a blood glucose level of less than 40 mg/dL.
- Vomiting is common in infants.
- For an infant who is breastfeeding, five to six stools per day is normal.
- Birth trauma includes both avoidable and unavoidable injuries to the infant resulting from mechanical forces during the delivery process. A difficult birth or injury to the baby can occur because of the infant's size or position during labor or delivery.
- Once the infant is stabilized as much as possible in the field, he or she needs to be transported to the nearest facility that can provide the next level of care.

■ Vital Vocabulary

acrocyanosis A decrease in the amount of oxygen delivered to the extremities. The hands and feet turn blue because of narrowing (constriction) of small arterioles (tiny arteries) toward the end of the arms and legs.

amniotic fluid A clear, slightly yellowish liquid that surrounds the unborn baby (fetus) during pregnancy; contained in the amniotic sac.

Apgar score Scale used to assess newborn infant status (range, 0 to 10).

apnea Respiratory pause greater than or equal to 20 seconds.

asphyxia Condition of severely deficient supply of oxygen to the body leading to end organ damage.

bradycardia A pulse rate of less than 100 beats/min in the newborn.

central cyanosis Bluish coloration of the skin due to the presence of deoxygenated hemoglobin in blood vessels near the skin surface.

choanal atresia A narrowing or blockage of the nasal airway by membranous or bony tissue; a congenital condition, meaning it is present at birth.

cleft lip An abnormal defect or fissure in the upper lip that failed to close during development. It is often associated with cleft palate.

cleft palate A fissure or hole in the palate (roof of the mouth) that forms a communicating pathway between the mouth and nasal cavities.

diaphragmatic hernia Passage of loops of bowel with or without other abdominal organs, through the diaphragm muscle; occurs as the bowel from the abdomen "herniates" upward through the diaphragm into the chest (thoracic) cavity.

Erb palsy Lack of movement at the shoulder due to nerve injury resulting from the stretching of the cervical nerve roots (C5 and C6 most commonly) during delivery of the baby's head during birth. The effect is usually transient, but can be permanent

free-flow oxygen Oxygen administered via oxygen tube and a cupped hand on patient's face.

gestation Period of time from conception to birth. For humans, the full period is normally 9 months (or 40 weeks).

grunting Noises heard when a baby is having difficulty breathing; short inarticulate guttural sounds as effort is expended.

hypoglycemia A deficiency of glucose in the blood caused by too much insulin or too little glucose; in the newborn it is a level less than 40 mg/dL, and in older neonates it is a level less than 60 mg/dL.

hypotonia Low or poor muscle tone (floppy).

hypovolemia An abnormal decrease in blood volume or, strictly speaking, an abnormal decrease in the volume of blood plasma.

hypoxic ischemic encephalopathy Damage to cells in the central nervous system (the brain and spinal cord) from inadequate oxygen.

intercostal retractions Skin sucking in between the ribs, seen when a patient creates increased negative intrathoracic pressure to breathe.

intussusception An event where one part of the intestine folds into another part of the intestines lead to a blockage.

Klumpke paralysis An injury of childbirth affecting the spinal nerves C7, C8, and T1 of the brachial plexus. It can be contrasted to Erb palsy, which affects C5 and C6.

malrotation A congenital anomaly of rotation of the midgut, the small bowel is found predominantly on the right side of the abdomen.

meconium A dark green fecal material that accumulates in the fetal intestines and is discharged around the time of birth.

nasal flaring Intermittent outward movements of the nostrils with each inspiration; indicates an increase in the work needed to breathe.

neonate Infant during the first month after birth.

newborn Infant within the first few hours after birth.

oligohydramnios Decreased volume of amniotic fluid during a pregnancy; a risk factor associated with abnormalities of the urinary tract, postmaturity (birth after a prolonged pregnancy), and intrauterine growth retardation.

persistent pulmonary hypertension Delayed transition from fetal to neonatal circulation.

Pierre Robin sequence A condition present at birth marked by a very small lower jaw (micrognathia). The tongue tends to fall back and downward (glossoptosis), and there is a cleft soft palate.

placenta previa Abnormal location of the placenta in the lower part of the uterus, near or over the cervix.

polycythemia Abnormally high red blood cell count.

polyhydramnios An excessive amount of amniotic fluid. May cause preterm labor.

positive-pressure ventilation (PPV) Method for assisting ventilation (bag-mask or intubated) with high-flow air or supplemental oxygen.

post-term Any pregnancy that lasts more than 42 weeks.

premature Underdeveloped; the condition of an infant born too soon. Refers to infants delivered before 37 weeks from the first day of the last menstrual period.

preterm Used to describe an infant delivered at less than 37 completed weeks.

primary apnea Apnea caused by oxygen deprivation; usually corrected with stimulation, such as drying or slapping the newborn's feet. Primary apnea is typically preceded by an initial period of rapid breathing.

primigravida First pregnancy.

prolapsed cord When the umbilical cord presents itself outside of the uterus while the fetus is still inside; an obstetric emergency during pregnancy or labor that acutely endangers the life of the baby; can happen when the water breaks and with the gush of water the cord comes along.

pulmonary hypertension Elevated blood pressure in the pulmonary arteries from constriction; causes problems with the blood flow in the lungs, and makes the heart work harder.

retinopathy of prematurity A disease of the eye that affects prematurely born babies, thought to be caused by disorganized growth of retinal blood vessels resulting in scarring and retinal detachment; can lead to blindness in serious cases.

secondary apnea When asphyxia continues after primary apnea, infant responds with a period of gasping respirations, falling pulse rate and falling blood pressure.

seizure A paroxysmal alteration in neurologic function, ie, behavioral and/or autonomic function.

small for gestational age An infant whose size and weight are considerably less than the average for babies of the same age.

surfactant A substance formed in the lungs that helps keep the small air sacs or alveoli from collapsing and sticking together; a low level in a premature baby contributes to respiratory distress syndrome.

term Used to describe an infant delivered at 38 to 42 weeks of gestation.

umbilical vein Blood vessel in umbilical cord used to administer emergency medications.

Assessment in Action

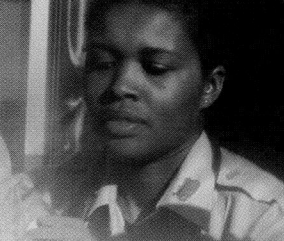

A 21-year-old woman who is 41 weeks' pregnant felt a few contractions and had the urge to go the bathroom. Her membranes ruptured (her "water broke") during this process, and she noticed it looked like "pea soup." She remembered from her prenatal visits that this wasn't a good sign and called 9-1-1. You arrive at the scene and find the infant's head presenting at the perineum.

1. **What does the "pea soup" appearance of the amniotic fluid indicate?**
   - **A.** Dehydration of the newborn
   - **B.** Meconium staining
   - **C.** Cardiac arrest of the newborn
   - **D.** Normal delivery

2. **How are delivery and resuscitation of a meconium-stained infant different from other full-term deliveries?**
   - **A.** Higher rate of morbidity
   - **B.** Lower rate of morbidity
   - **C.** Higher rate of breech presentation
   - **D.** Lower rate of breech presentation

3. **What is the most essential piece of equipment you need to prepare for this delivery?**
   - **A.** Items to warm and dry the newborn
   - **B.** Bulb syringe
   - **C.** Cardiac monitor
   - **D.** ET tube and meconium aspirator

4. **What is the primary use of the ET tube once you have it placed in the meconium-stained newborn?**
   - **A.** It supplies positive-pressure ventilation.
   - **B.** It serves as a suction device.
   - **C.** It holds the airway open.
   - **D.** It provides standard ventilation.

5. **What scale will you use to assess the newborn?**
   - **A.** AVPU
   - **B.** GCS
   - **C.** Apgar
   - **D.** SAMPLE

Challenging Question

6. **What measures will you take to care for the mother of this child?**

■ Points to Ponder

For the infant born through meconium-stained amniotic fluid discussed previously, the infant is depressed and you intubated and suctioned the trachea using a meconium aspirator while providing free-flow oxygen. You've dried and stimulated the newborn without causing injury. It is almost 2 minutes past delivery. The infant's pulse rate is 85 beats/min.

What is the next step in managing the airway—PPV or intubation?

Issues: Infant Airway Intubation, Neonatal Resuscitation.

41 Pediatrics

Objectives

Cognitive

6-2.2   Discuss the paramedic's role in the reduction of infant and childhood morbidity and mortality from acute illness and injury. (p 41.5)

6-2.3   Identify methods/mechanisms that prevent injuries to infants and children. (p 41.59)

6-2.4   Describe Emergency Medical Services for Children (EMSC). (p 41.58)

6-2.5   Discuss how an integrated EMSC system can affect patient outcome. (p 41.58)

6-2.6   Identify key growth and developmental characteristics of infants and children and their implications. (p 41.6)

6-2.7   Identify key anatomical and physiological characteristics of infants and their implications. (p 41.6)

6-2.8   Describe techniques for successful assessment of infants and children. (p 41.6–41.8)

6-2.9   Describe techniques for successful treatment of infants and children. (p 41.5)

6-2.10 Identify the common responses of families to acute illness and injury of an infant or child. (p 41.8)

6-2.11 Describe techniques for successful interaction with families of acutely ill or injured infants and children. (p 41.8)

6-2.12 Outline differences in adult and childhood anatomy and physiology. (p 41.6)

6-2.13 Identify "normal" age group related vital signs. (p 41.12)

6-2.14 Discuss the appropriate equipment utilized to obtain pediatric vital signs. (p 41.11, 41.12)

6-2.15 Determine appropriate airway adjuncts for infants and children. (p 41.21)

6-2.16 Discuss complications of improper utilization of airway adjuncts with infants and children. (p 41.22, 41.23)

6-2.17 Discuss appropriate ventilation devices for infants and children. (p 41.24)

6-2.18 Discuss complications of improper utilization of ventilation devices with infants and children. (p 41.25)

6-2.19 Discuss appropriate endotracheal intubation equipment for infants and children. (p 41.26)

6-2.20 Identify complications of improper endotracheal intubation procedures for infants and children. (p 41.28)

6-2.21 List the indications and methods for gastric decompression for infants and children. (p 41.29)

6-2.22 Define respiratory distress. (p 41.15)

6-2.23 Define respiratory failure. (p 41.15)

6-2.24 Define respiratory arrest. (p 41.16)

6-2.25 Differentiate between upper airway obstruction and lower airway disease. (p 41.17–41.20)

6-2.26 Describe the general approach to the treatment of children with respiratory distress, failure, or arrest from upper airway obstruction or lower airway disease. (p 41.16)

6-2.27 Discuss the common causes of hypoperfusion in infants and children. (p 41.31)

6-2.28 Evaluate the severity of hypoperfusion in infants and children. (p 41.31)

6-2.29 Identify the major classifications of pediatric cardiac rhythms. (p 41.36)

6-2.30 Discuss the primary etiologies of cardiopulmonary arrest in infants and children. (p 41.39)

6-2.31 Discuss age appropriate vascular access sites for infants and children. (p 41.32)

6-2.32 Discuss the appropriate equipment for vascular access in infants and children. (p 41.32, 41.33)

6-2.33 Identify complications of vascular access for infants and children. (p 41.33)

6-2.34 Describe the primary etiologies of altered level of consciousness in infants and children. (p 41.42)

6-2.35 Identify common lethal mechanisms of injury in infants and children. (p 41.50)

6-2.36 Discuss anatomical features of children that predispose or protect them from certain injuries. (p 41.49)

6-2.37 Describe aspects of infant and children airway management that are affected by potential cervical spine injury. (p 41.21, 41.22, 41.50)

6-2.38 Identify infant and child trauma patients who require spinal immobilization. (p 41.52)

6-2.39 Discuss fluid management and shock treatment for infant and child trauma patients. (p 41.32–41.35)

6-2.40 Determine when pain management and sedation are appropriate for infants and children. (p 41.53)

6-2.41 Define child abuse. (p 41.47)

6-2.42 Define child neglect. (p 41.47)

6-2.43 Define sudden infant death syndrome. (p 41.46)

6-2.44 Discuss the parent/caregiver responses to the death of an infant or child. (p 41.46)

6-2.45 Define children with special health care needs. (p 41.55)

6-2.46 Define technology assisted children. (p 41.55)

6-2.47 Discuss basic cardiac life support (CPR) guidelines for infants and children. (p 41.36, 41.37)

6-2.48 Identify appropriate parameters for performing infant and child CPR. (p 41.36, 41.37)

6-2.49 Integrate advanced life support skills with basic cardiac life support for infants and children. (p 41.31)

6-2.50 Discuss the indications, dosage, route of administration and special considerations for medication administration in infants and children. (p 41.33, 41.34, 41.39, 41.43)

6-2.51 Discuss appropriate transport guidelines for infants and children. (p 41.52)

6-2.52 Discuss appropriate receiving facilities for low and high risk infants and children. (p 41.57)

6-2.53 Describe the epidemiology, including the incidence, morbidity/mortality, risk factors and prevention strategies for respiratory distress/failure in infants and children. (p 41.15)

6-2.54 Discuss the pathophysiology of respiratory distress/failure in infants and children. (p 41.15)

6-2.55 Discuss the assessment findings associated with respiratory distress/failure in infants and children. (p 41.15, 41.16)

6-2.56 Discuss the management/treatment plan for respiratory distress/failure in infants and children. (p 41.15, 41.16)

6-2.57 Describe the epidemiology, including the incidence, morbidity/mortality, risk factors and prevention strategies for hypoperfusion in infants and children. (p 41.31)

6-2.58 Discuss the pathophysiology of hypoperfusion in infants and children. (p 41.31)

6-2.59 Discuss the assessment findings associated with hypoperfusion in infants and children. (p 41.31)

6-2.60 Discuss the management/treatment plan for hypoperfusion in infants and children. (p 41.32–41.35)

6-2.61 Describe the epidemiology, including the incidence, morbidity/mortality, risk factors and prevention strategies for cardiac dysrhythmias in infants and children. (p 41.36)

6-2.62 Discuss the pathophysiology of cardiac dysrhythmias in infants and children. (p 41.36)

6-2.63 Discuss the assessment findings associated with cardiac dysrhythmias in infants and children. (p 41.36)

6-2.64 Discuss the management/treatment plan for cardiac dysrhythmias in infants and children. (p 41.36–41.40)

6-2.65 Describe the epidemiology, including the incidence, morbidity/mortality, risk factors and prevention strategies for neurological emergencies in infants and children. (p 41.42)

6-2.66 Discuss the pathophysiology of neurological emergencies in infants and children. (p 41.42)

6-2.67 Discuss the assessment findings associated with neurological emergencies in infants and children. (p 41.42)

6-2.68 Discuss the management/treatment plan for neurological emergencies in infants and children. (p 41.42)

6-2.69 Describe the epidemiology, including the incidence, morbidity/mortality, risk factors and prevention strategies for trauma in infants and children. (p 41.49)

6-2.70 Discuss the pathophysiology of trauma in infants and children. (p 41.49)

6-2.71 Discuss the assessment findings associated with trauma in infants and children. (p 41.50)

6-2.72 Discuss the management/treatment plan for trauma in infants and children. (p 41.50)

6-2.73 Describe the epidemiology, including the incidence, morbidity/mortality, risk factors and prevention strategies for abuse and neglect in infants and children. (p 41.47)

6-2.74 Discuss the pathophysiology of abuse and neglect in infants and children. (p 41.47)

6-2.75 Discuss the assessment findings associated with abuse and neglect in infants and children. (p 41.47, 41.48)

6-2.76 Discuss the management/treatment plan for abuse and neglect in infants and children. (p 41.47, 41.48)

6-2.77 Describe the epidemiology, including the incidence, morbidity/mortality, risk factors and prevention strategies for SIDS in infants and children. (p 41.46)

6-2.78 Describe the epidemiology, including the incidence, morbidity/mortality, risk factors and prevention strategies for children with special health care needs including technology assisted children. (p 41.55)

6-2.79 Discuss the pathophysiology of children with special health care needs including technology assisted children. (p 41.55)

6-2.80 Discuss the assessment findings of children with special health care needs including technology assisted children. (p 41.57)

6-2.81 Discuss the management/treatment plan for children with special health care needs including technology assisted children. (p 41.57)

6-2.82 Describe the epidemiology, including the incidence, morbidity/mortality, risk factors and prevention strategies for SIDS in infants and children. (p 41.46)

6-2.83 Discuss the pathophysiology of SIDS in infants and children. (p 41.46)

6-2.84 Discuss the assessment findings associated with SIDS in infants and children. (p 41.46)

6-2.85 Discuss the management/treatment plan for SIDS in infants and children. (p 41.46)

Affective

6-2.86 Demonstrate and advocate appropriate interactions with the infant/child that conveys an understanding of their developmental stage. (p 41.6)

6-2.87 Recognize the emotional dependence of the infant/child to their parent/guardian. (p 41.6–41.8)

6-2.88 Recognize the emotional impact of the infant/child injuries and illnesses on the parent/guardian. (p 41.8)

6-2.89 Recognize and appreciate the physical and emotional difficulties associated with separation of the parent/guardian of a special needs child. (p 41.8)

6-2.90 Demonstrate the ability to provide reassurance, empathy and compassion for the parent/guardian. (p 41.8)

Psychomotor

6-2.91 Demonstrate the appropriate approach for treating infants and children. (p 41.6, 41.7)

6-2.92 Demonstrate appropriate intervention techniques with families of acutely ill or injured infants and children. (p 41.8)

6-2.93 Demonstrate the appropriate assessment for different developmental age groups. (p 41.6, 41.7)

6-2.94 Demonstrate an appropriate technique for measuring pediatric vital signs. (p 41.11, 41.12)

6-2.95 Demonstrate the use of a length-based resuscitation device for determining equipment sizes, drug doses or other pertinent information for a pediatric patient. (p 41.11)

6-2.96 Demonstrate the appropriate approach for treating infants and children with respiratory distress, failure, and arrest. (p 41.15, 41.16)

6-2.97 Demonstrate proper technique for administering blow-by oxygen to infants and children. (p 41.24)

6-2.98 Demonstrate the proper utilization of a pediatric non-rebreather oxygen mask. (p 41.24)

6-2.99 Demonstrate proper technique for suctioning of infants and children. (p 41.11)

6-2.100 Demonstrate appropriate use of airway adjuncts with infants and children. (p 41.21–41.23)

6-2.101 Demonstrate appropriate use of ventilation devices for infants and children. (p 41.24)

6-2.102 Demonstrate endotracheal intubation procedures in infants and children. (p 41.26)

6-2.103 Demonstrate appropriate treatment/management of intubation complications of infants and children. (p 41.28)

6-2.104 Demonstrate appropriate needle cricothyroidotomy in infants and children. (p 41.50)

6-2.105 Demonstrate proper placement of a gastric tube in infants and children. (p 41.30)

6-2.106 Demonstrate an appropriate technique for insertion of peripheral intravenous catheters for infants and children. (p 41.33)

6-2.107 Demonstrate an appropriate technique for administration of intramuscular, inhalation, subcutaneous, rectal, endotracheal and oral medication for infants and children. (p 41.32–41.34, 41.39)

6-2.108 Demonstrate an appropriate technique for insertion of an intraosseous line for infants and children. (p 41.33)

Introduction

Children differ anatomically, physiologically, and emotionally from adults. In addition, the types of illnesses and injuries they sustain and their responses to them vary across the pediatric age span. For these reasons, you must tailor your approach to accommodate the developmental and social issues unique to pediatrics. Some children may be afraid of the EMS crew. Depending on the age of the child, he or she may not be able to tell you what is wrong. Also, each pediatric call involves one or more caregivers who may be stressed or frightened themselves.

This chapter addresses some of the special considerations that will enhance your effectiveness in caring for an ill or injured child. It begins by discussing the approach to pediatric patients, with an eye toward their developmental level and the anatomic or physiologic differences unique to the age group. This information is used to outline an approach to pediatric assessment, review specific pediatric emergencies, and address their prehospital management. Finally, the chapter details the skills needed to care efficiently and effectively for pediatric patients, regardless of the diagnosis.

Approach to Pediatric Patients

Sick or injured children present unique challenges in evaluation and management. Their perceptions of their illness or injury, their world, and you differ from the perceptions of adults. Depending on their age, they may not be able to report what is bothering them. Fear or pain may make children difficult to assess as well. In addition, you will have to work with

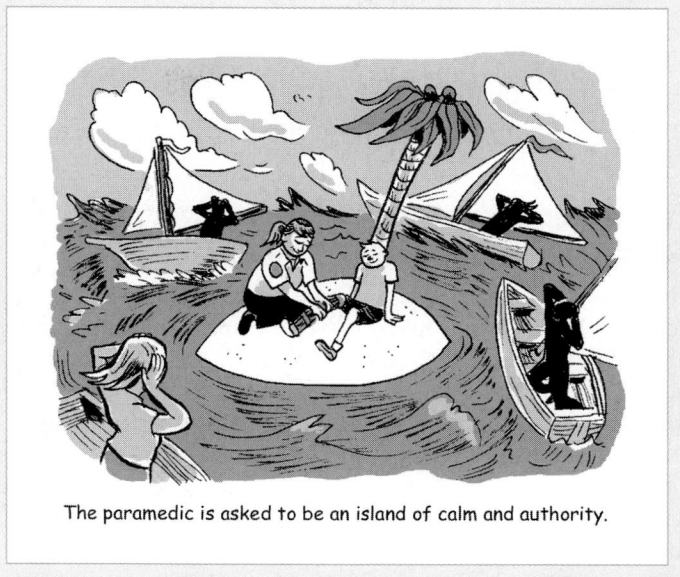

The paramedic is asked to be an island of calm and authority.

Figure 41-1

concerned parents and caregivers who may themselves be acting irrationally. In the midst of this chaos, you are expected to be an island of calm and authority, carrying out your job systematically, carefully, and confidently **Figure 41-1 ▲**.

The manner in which you approach a sick or injured child will depend on the child's age and developmental level. Childhood extends from the neonatal period, just after birth, until age 18 years. An enormous amount of physical and psychological development occurs in these 18 years. A child's anatomy, physiology, and psychosocial development will all influence your assessment and treatment.

You are the Provider Part 1

You and your partner are completing morning chores at the station when you are dispatched to treat a child who fell from a third-story balcony. When you arrive in the quiet subdivision, you are flagged down by a frantic mother who points toward her 2-year-old son. You then see a toddler lying face up on the driveway approximately 3' from the house. The mother tells you that she turned her son over but did not move him any further.

The toddler is lying motionless. His eyes are open, but he does not focus on you or his mother as she stands crying beside him. You observe an adequate respiratory rate with good bilateral chest expansion. The boy appears pale and has cool, dry skin.

Initial Assessment	Recording Time: 0 Minutes
Appearance	Pale toddler, lying motionless, making no eye contact
Level of consciousness	V (Responsive to verbal stimuli)
Airway	Open
Breathing	Adequate rate and volume; no retractions or audible sounds
Circulation	Weak radial pulses with pale, cool, dry skin

1. What assessment tool will you use to form your general impression of your patient?
2. What can you do to assist the panicked mother?

Special Considerations

Children have more head injuries than adults because of their large heads.

Pediatric Anatomy and Physiology

Head

You may have seen an infant or young child and noted the size of the child's head: Little children have very big heads. In fact, an infant's head is already two thirds the size it will be in adulthood. The large head means more surface area for heat loss. It also means more mass relative to the rest of the body—an important factor in the incidence of head injuries in young patients, who tend to lead with the head in a fall. During the school-age years, the head and body become more proportional.

Neck and Airway

Children have short, stubby necks, which can make it difficult to feel a carotid pulse or see jugular veins. Not surprisingly, the airway of a young child is also much smaller than an adult airway. That smaller diameter makes the airway more prone to obstruction, either by foreign body inhalation, inflammation with infection, or the child's disproportionately large tongue. During the first few months of life, infants are obligate nose breathers, and nasal obstruction with mucus can result in significant respiratory distress. Their epiglottis is quite floppy and U-shaped, which can make it difficult to visualize the cords during intubation. Finally, the narrowest part of a young child's airway occurs at the level of the cricoid cartilage, rather than at the vocal cords as in adults; this issue should influence your choice of endotracheal (ET) tubes.

Chest and Lungs

A child's chest wall is quite thin, with less musculature and less subcutaneous fat than in an adult. The thin chest wall makes it easy to hear heart and lungs sounds but also means that sounds are readily transmitted throughout the chest. Sounds originating from the nose or throat can be heard quite clearly on auscultation, for example. The rib cage is more compliant, making retractions easy to see. Use of the diaphragm as a muscle of respiration is pronounced in infants, leading to belly breathing at baseline.

Heart

Circulation in the fetus is much different from that in the newborn, and large right-sided forces on the electrocardiogram (ECG) are normal in young infants. During the first year of life, the ECG axis and voltages shift to reflect left ventricular dominance. Cardiac output is rate-dependent in infants and young children. They have relatively poor ability to increase stroke volume, which is reflected in their normal heart rates (higher in newborns than in older children and adults) and in rate response to physiologic stress and hypovolemia.

Abdomen

The appearance of abdominal distention in a healthy infant is due to two factors: the weak abdominal wall muscles and the size of the solid organs. The liver extends below the ribcage in infants, making it more vulnerable to injury. As the child grows, the liver becomes more proportionate and is better protected by the bony ribcage.

Special Considerations

Because of children's shorter ribcages and less well-developed abdominal musculature, expect more intra-abdominal injuries in pediatric patients than in adults.

Musculoskeletal System

Reaching adult height requires active bone growth. The growth plates (ossification centers) of a child's bones are made of cartilage, are relatively weak, and are easily fractured. As a consequence, the bones of growing children are weaker than their ligaments, making fractures more common than sprains. Bones finish growing at differing times, but most growth plates will be closed by late adolescence.

Brain and Nervous System

The brain and nervous system continue to develop once the baby is born. As the brain matures, the infant's responses to the environment, outside stimuli, and even pain become more organized and purposeful. The rapidity of brain development can be appreciated by comparing the abilities and interactions of a 4-day-old baby, whose repertoire is limited to eating, sleeping, and defecating, with those of a 4-month-old, who smiles socially, rolls over, and plays with a rattle, and with those of a 12-month-old, who walks, is beginning to talk, and expresses preferences for individuals and activities.

Developmental Stages

Neonate and Infant

The first month of life is called the neonatal period, whereas infancy refers to the first 12 months of life. A lot of development occurs in this interval. Neonates don't do very much, other than eat, sleep, and cry. During the first months of life, a baby will have longer awake periods and interact more with the environment. Infants between 2 and 6 months of age are more active and social and can recognize their caregivers. By 4 months of age, infants are able to hold their heads up. Infants between 6 and 12 months of age babble, can sit unsupported, reach for objects, and are becoming more mobile—crawling and even walking. At 9 months of age, most infants develop stranger anxiety, with a strong preference for known caregivers.

Because infants cannot communicate their feelings or needs verbally, it is especially important to respect a caregiver's perception that "something is wrong." Nonspecific concerns about a young infant's behavior, feeding, or sleep pattern may be tip-offs to a serious underlying illness or injury.

Consider the best location for performing your initial assessment. Although separating a 2-week-old from a parent will not cause distress, an older infant in stable condition will be calmest in a parent's arms. Make sure that your hands and stethoscope are warm—a startled, crying infant will be difficult to examine. Be opportunistic with your exam. If the child is quiet, listen to the heart and lungs first, perhaps listening over the clothes before you expose the chest and disturb the infant. If a young infant starts crying, letting the baby suck on a pacifier or gloved finger may quiet the child enough to allow you to complete your assessment. Jingling keys or shining a penlight may distract an older infant for long enough for you to finish an exam.

Toddler

The toddler period includes the ages from 1 to 3 years. It includes the "terrible twos," a behavioral manifestation of the child's struggle between continued dependence on caregivers for food, shelter, and love and his or her emerging drive for independence. Children in this age group are not capable of reasoning, and they have a poorly developed sense of cause and effect. Language development is occurring rapidly, as is the ability to explore the world by crawling, walking, running, and climbing. Many toddlers will begin to have associations—possibly negative—with health care providers.

Your assessment of a toddler begins with observation of the child's interactions with the caregiver, vocalizations, and mobility, measured through the Pediatric Assessment Triangle (PAT), which is described in detail later. Examine a toddler in stable condition on the parent's lap. Get down to the child's level, sitting or squatting for the exam. You may need to be creative to get a good exam on a toddler with stranger anxiety: Use a parent to lift the shirt so that you can count respiratory rate, or have the parent press on the abdomen to see if that appears painful. Use play and distraction techniques whenever possible—listening to the doll's chest first may buy you a few minutes of cooperation. Offer toddlers limited choices when possible because they like to be in control. If you ask yes or no questions, the answer is likely to be "No!" Consider doing the more upsetting parts of the exam, such as palpating a tender abdomen or examining an injured extremity, for last. Be flexible in your approach—some toddlers will not let you complete an orderly head-to-toe exam.

Preschool-Age Child

During the preschool years (3 to 6 years), the child is becoming much more verbal and interactive. He or she can understand directions and be engaged with an activity or set of goals.

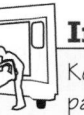

In the Field

Keep infants and young children close to their parents during your assessment to help them feel safe and to improve your ability to perform the assessment.

Generally, a preschooler will be able to tell you what hurts and may have a story to share about the illness or injury. Preschoolers will understand as you explain what you are going to do, but choose your words carefully because preschoolers are very literal. Saying "I'm going take your pulse" may lead preschoolers to believe that you are taking something from them and wonder if you plan to give it back! Speak to them in very plain language about what you are going to do and provide lots of reassurance—this is the stage of monsters under the bed and many other fears.

As you perform your assessment, take advantage of the child's curiosity and desire to cooperate. If the patient is in medically stable condition, offer to take turns with the child in listening to the heart and lungs. Let the preschooler play with or hold equipment that is safe. To help give the child some sense of control, offer simple choices. Avoid yes or no questions. Set limits on behavior if the child acts out. For the most part, you should be able to talk a preschooler through an orderly head-to-toe exam.

School-Age Child

As a child enters the school-age period (6 to 12 years), he or she becomes much more analytic and capable of abstract thought. At this age, the child can understand cause and effect. School-age children will have their own stories to tell about the illness or injury and may have their own ideas about the care to be given. By 8 years, the child's anatomy and physiology are similar to those of adults.

Ask the child about the history leading to calling 9-1-1 and let the child describe the symptoms, rather than focusing on the caregiver. Explain what you plan to do in simple language, and answer the child's questions. Give the child appropriate choices and control whenever possible, and provide ongoing reassurance and encouragement.

Adolescent

The adolescent years, from 13 to 18 years, can be difficult. Adolescents are struggling with issues of independence, body image, sexuality, and peer pressure. Friends are key support figures, and this is a time of experimentation and risk-taking behaviors.

With respect to CPR and foreign body airway obstruction procedures, once secondary sexual characteristics have developed (breasts or facial/axillary hair), the child should be treated as an adult. During the assessment, you must address the patient. Failure to do so can result in the adolescent feeling left out of his or her own care, which can alienate the patient, making it difficult to get an accurate assessment or give appropriate treatment. Encourage the patient's questions and involvement. Also, provide accurate information—a teen may become alienated and uncooperative if you are suspected of being misleading. When you perform the physical exam, respect the patient's privacy. If possible, address the adolescent without a caregiver present, especially about sensitive topics such as sexuality or drug use. If the adolescent's friends are on scene, he or she may want them to remain during the assessment. Let the patient have as much control over the situation as appropriate. Of course, do not let down your guard regarding scene safety: In a gang situation, members may have weapons and a reputation to earn.

Parents of Ill or Injured Children

The majority of children you will treat will come with at least one parent or caregiver. Thus, in many pediatric calls, you will be dealing with more than one patient—even if only the child is ill or injured. Serious illness or injury to a child is one of the most stressful situations caregivers can face. Some may react to this stress by becoming angry—at the fact that their child is sick, at the person or situation that caused the injury, or at you simply because they need someone to blame! Other parents will be frightened or guilty about the circumstances that led to the illness or injury. Establishing rapport with caregivers is vital, however, because they will be a source of important information and assistance. Children look to their parents when they are frightened and often mimic their response, so helping calm a parent may also help the patient cope.

Approach stressed caregivers in a calm, quiet, and professional manner. Enlist their help in caring for the child. Along the way, explain what you are doing and provide honest reassurance and support. Above all, don't blame the parent for what has happened. Finally, transport at least one caregiver with the child.

If the parent is extremely emotional, provide support, but remember that your first priority is the child. Don't let a distraught or aggressive parent interfere with your care. If necessary, enlist the help of other family members or law enforcement personnel.

Pediatric Assessment

Just as your general approach to a pediatric patient differs somewhat from your approach to an adult patient, so, too, will your assessment. In particular, you may need to adapt your assessment skills.

General Impression Using the Pediatric Assessment Triangle

After ensuring scene safety, the first step in an initial assessment of any patient begins with your general assessment of how the patient looks (the "sick–not sick" classification). An assessment tool called the Pediatric Assessment Triangle (PAT) **Figure 41-2 ▶** has been developed to help EMS providers form a "from-the-doorway" general impression of pediatric patients. Providers with experience in treating ill and injured children intuitively use some version of the PAT to make the important distinction between sick and not-sick patients. The PAT standardizes this approach by including three elements— the child's appearance, work of breathing, and circulation—

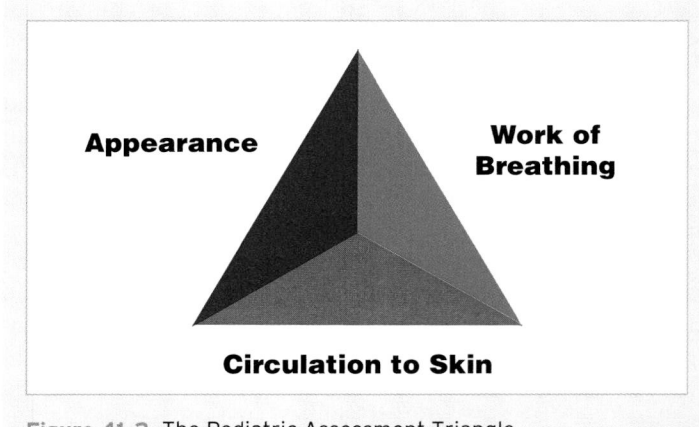

Figure 41-2 The Pediatric Assessment Triangle.

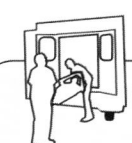

In the Field

Use the PAT to help with your hands-off, from-the-doorway general impression of pediatric patients.

that collectively paint an accurate clinical picture of the patient's cardiopulmonary status and level of consciousness. It applies a rapid, hands-off systematic approach to observing an ill or injured child and helps answer three questions:

- Is this patient sick or not sick?
- What is the most likely physiologic abnormality?
- Does this child require emergency treatment?

Appearance

The first element of the PAT is the child's appearance. In many cases, this is the most important factor in determining the severity of illness, the need for treatment, and the response to therapy. Appearance reflects the adequacy of ventilation, oxygenation, brain perfusion, body homeostasis, and central nervous system (CNS) function. The TICLS (tickles) mnemonic highlights the most important features of a child's appearance: Tone, Interactiveness, Consolability, Look or gaze, and Speech or cry **Table 41-1 ▶**.

To assess appearance, observe the child from a distance, allowing the child to interact with the caregiver as he or she chooses. Walk through the characteristics of the TICLS mnemonic while observing the child from the doorway. Delay touching the patient until you have developed your general impression because the child may become agitated by your touch. Unless a child is unconscious or critically ill, take your time in assessing his or her general appearance by observation before you begin the hands-on assessment and take vital signs. **Figure 41-3 ▶** and **Figure 41-4 ▶** demonstrate examples of an infant with a normal appearance and one with a worrisome appearance.

Table 41-1	Characteristics of Appearance: The TICLS Mnemonic
Characteristic	**Features to Look For**
Tone	Is the child moving or resisting examination vigorously? Does the child have good muscle tone? Or is the child limp, listless, or flaccid?
Interactiveness	How alert is the child? How readily does a person, object, or sound distract the child or draw the child's attention? Will the child reach for, grasp, and play with a toy or exam instrument, like a penlight or tongue blade? Or is the child uninterested in playing or interacting with the caregiver or prehospital professional?
Consolability	Can the child be consoled or comforted by the caregiver or by the prehospital professional? Or is the child's crying or agitation unrelieved by gentle reassurance?
Look or gaze	Does the child fix his or her gaze on a face, or is there a "nobody home," glassy-eyed stare?
Speech or cry	Is the child's cry strong and spontaneous or weak or high-pitched? Is the content of speech age-appropriate or confused or garbled?

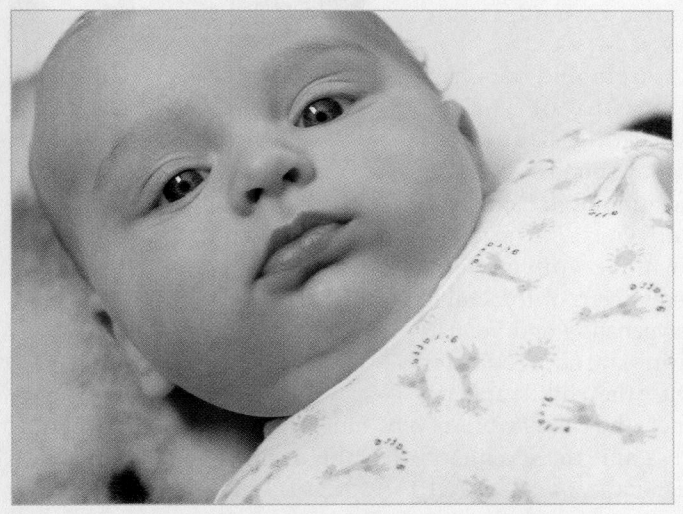

Figure 41-3 A child with a normal appearance. An infant or child who is not very sick will make good eye contact.

An abnormal appearance may result from numerous underlying physiologic abnormalities. A child may show evidence of inadequate oxygenation or ventilation, as in respiratory emergencies; inadequate brain perfusion, as from cardiovascular emergencies; systemic abnormalities or metabolic derangements, such as with poisoning, infection, or hypoglycemia; or

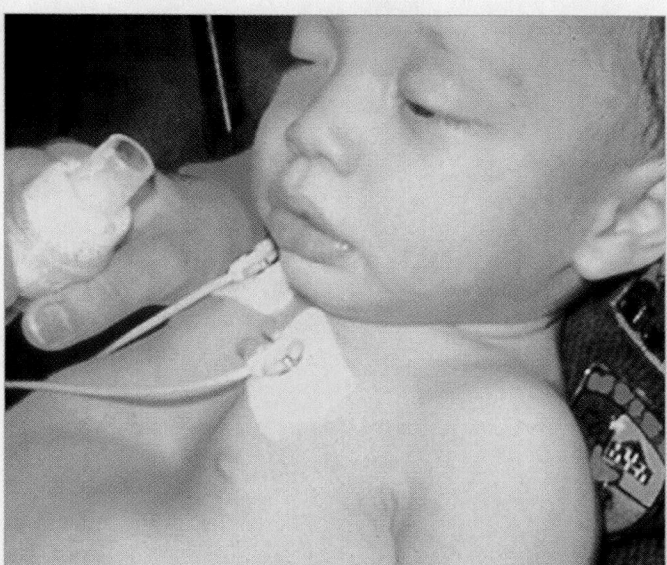

Figure 41-4 A child with an abnormal appearance. A limp child unable to maintain eye contact may be critically ill or injured.

acute or chronic brain injury. In any event, a child with a grossly abnormal appearance is seriously ill and requires immediate life-support interventions and transportation. The remainder of the PAT—work of breathing and circulation—plus the initial assessment may help identify the cause of the abnormal appearance and determine the severity of a child's illness and the need for treatment and transportation.

Work of Breathing

A child's work of breathing is often a better assessment of his or her oxygenation and ventilation status than the auscultation or respiratory rate. The work of breathing reflects the child's attempt to compensate for abnormalities in oxygenation and ventilation and, therefore, it is a proxy for effectiveness of gas exchange. The hands-off assessment of work of breathing includes listening for abnormal airway sounds and looking for signs of increased breathing effort Table 41-2 ▶ .

Some abnormal airway sounds can be heard without a stethoscope and can indicate the likely physiology and anatomic location of the breathing problem. For example, snoring, muffled or hoarse voice, or stridor can indicate obstruction at the level of the oropharynx, glottis or supraglottic structures, or glottis or subglottic structures, respectively. Such an upper airway obstruction may result from croup, bacterial upper airway infections, or bleeding or edema.

Lower airway obstruction is suggested by abnormal grunting or wheezing. Grunting is a form of auto-PEEP (positive end-expiratory pressure), a way to distend the lower respiratory air sacs or alveoli to promote maximum gas exchange. Grunting involves exhaling against a partially closed glottis. This short, low-pitched sound is best heard at the end of exhalation and is often mistaken for whimpering. Grunting suggests moderate to severe hypoxia and is seen with lower airway conditions such as

Table 41-2	Characteristics of Work of Breathing
Characteristic	**Features to Look For**
Abnormal airway sounds	Snoring, muffled or hoarse speech, stridor, grunting or wheezing
Abnormal posturing	Sniffing position, tripod position, refusing to lie down
Retractions	Supraclavicular, intercostal, or substernal retractions of the chest wall; head bobbing in infants
Flaring	Flaring of the nares on inspiration

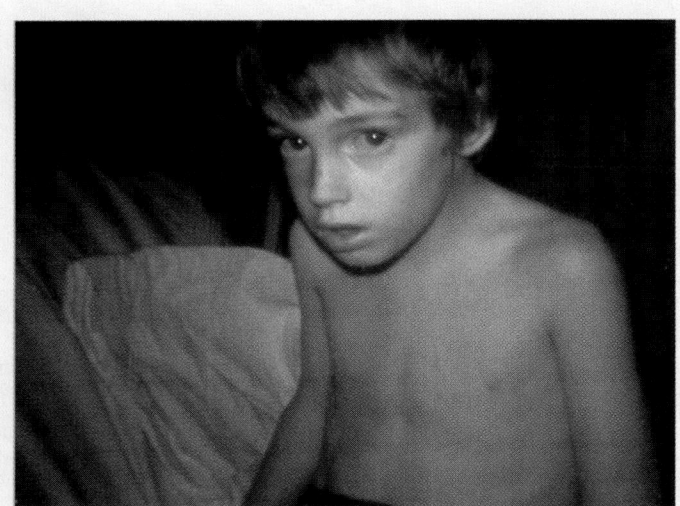

Figure 41-5 A child in a sniffing position is trying to align the airway to increase patency and improve airflow.

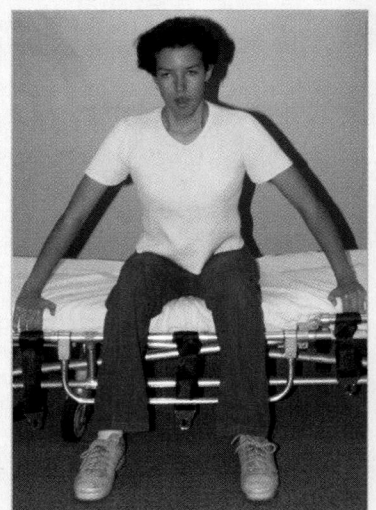

Figure 41-6 A child in a tripod position is maximizing his or her accessory muscles of respiration.

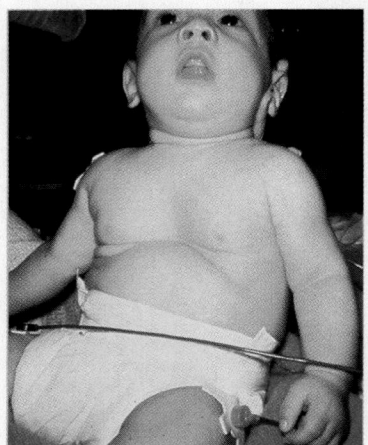

Figure 41-7 Retractions can occur in the suprasternal, intercostal, and substernal areas and indicate increased work of breathing.

adults because a child's chest wall is less muscular, so the inward excursion of skin and soft tissue between the ribs is more apparent. Retractions may be evident in the supraclavicular area (above the clavicle), the intercostal area (between the ribs), or the substernal area (under the sternum) **Figure 41-7**. Another form of retractions that is seen only in infants is head bobbing, the use of neck muscles to help breathing during severe hypoxia. The infant extends the neck as he or she inhales, then allows the head to fall forward during exhalation. Nasal flaring is the exaggerated opening of the nostrils during labored inspiration and indicates moderate to severe hypoxia.

Combine the characteristics of work of breathing—abnormal airway sounds, abnormal positioning, retractions, and nasal flaring—to make your general assessment of the child's oxygenation and ventilation status. Together with the child's appearance, the child's work of breathing suggests the severity of the illness and the likelihood that the cause is in the airway or is respiratory.

pneumonia and pulmonary edema. It reflects poor gas exchange because of fluid in the lower airways and air sacs. Wheezing is a musical tone caused by air being forced through constricted or partially blocked small airways. It often occurs during exhalation only but can occur during inspiration and expiration during severe asthma attacks. Although this sound is often heard only by auscultation, severe obstruction may result in wheezing that is audible even without a stethoscope.

Abnormal positioning and retractions are physical signs of increased work of breathing that can easily be assessed without touching the patient. A child who is in the sniffing position is trying to align the axes of the airways to improve patency and increase air flow **Figure 41-5**; such a position often reflects a severe upper airway obstruction. The child who refuses to lie down or who leans forward on outstretched arms (tripoding) is creating the optimal mechanical advantage to use accessory muscles of respiration **Figure 41-6**.

Retractions represent the recruitment of accessory muscles of respiration to provide more "muscle power" to move air into the lungs in the face of airway or lung disease or injury. To optimally observe retractions, expose the child's chest. Retractions are a more useful measure of work of breathing in children than in

Circulation

The goal of rapid circulatory assessment is to determine the adequacy of cardiac output and core perfusion. When cardiac output diminishes, the body responds by shunting circulation from nonessential areas (eg, skin) toward vital organs. Therefore, circulation to the skin reflects the overall status of core circulation. The three characteristics considered when assessing the circulation are pallor, mottling, and cyanosis **Table 41-3**.

Pallor may be the initial sign of poor circulation or even the only visual sign in a child with compensated shock. It indicates

Table 41-3	Characteristics of Circulation to Skin
Characteristic	**Features to Look For**
Pallor	White or pale skin or mucous membranes from inadequate blood flow
Mottling	Patchy skin discoloration due to vasoconstriction or vasodilation
Cyanosis	Bluish discoloration of skin and mucous membranes

In the Field

Note the line of demarcation of any mottling or pallor on the child's limbs during your initial assessment. An increase in mottling or pallor with movement toward the core of the body indicates a worsening "shell to core" shunt from peripheral vasoconstriction.

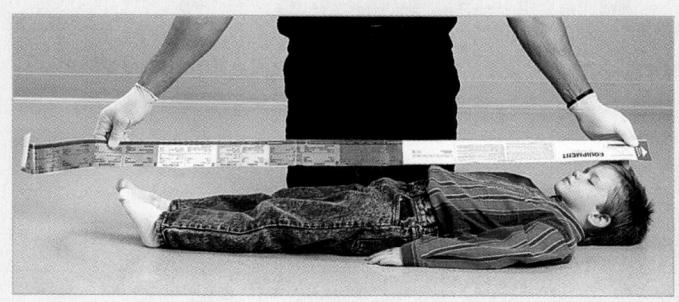

Figure 41-8 Use of a length-based resuscitation tape is one way to estimate a child's weight and identify the correct size for pediatric equipment and medication doses.

reflex peripheral vasoconstriction that is shunting blood toward the core. Pallor may also indicate anemia or hypoxia.

Mottling reflects vasomotor instability in the capillary beds demonstrated by patchy areas of vasoconstriction and vasodilation. It may also be a child's physiologic response to a cold environment.

Cyanosis, a bluish discoloration of the skin and mucous membranes, is the most extreme visual indicator of poor perfusion or poor oxygenation. Acrocyanosis, blue hands or feet in an infant younger than 2 months, is distinct from cyanosis; it is a normal finding when a young infant is cold. True cyanosis is seen in the skin and mucous membranes and is a late finding of respiratory failure or shock.

After assessing the child's appearance and work of breathing, visually scan the child's skin and mucous membranes looking for pallor, mottling, and cyanosis. You can then combine the three pieces of the PAT to estimate the severity of illness and the likely underlying pathologic cause. For example, a child with an abnormal appearance with poor circulation may be in shock from a cardiovascular cause.

Initial Assessment

After using the PAT to form a general impression of the patient, you will need to complete the rest of the initial assessment—that is, you must assess the child's mental status and ABCs and prioritize the care and need for transport. Threats to the ABCs are managed as they are found, providing a prioritized sequence of life-support interventions to reverse critical physiologic abnormalities. The steps are the same as with adults, albeit with differences related to the child's anatomy, physiology, and signs of distress.

Early in your assessment of a young child, you will need to estimate the child's weight, because much of your care will depend on the child's size. Ask a caregiver how much the child

weighs or make your own estimate, using a tool such as a length-based resuscitation tape Figure 41-8 ▲.
1. Measure the child's length, from head to heel, with the tape (with the red portion at the head).
2. Note the weight in kilograms that corresponds to the child's measured length at the heel.
3. If the child is longer than the tape, use adult equipment and medication doses.
4. From the tape, identify appropriate equipment sizes.
5. From the tape, identify appropriate medication doses

Airway
The PAT may suggest the presence of an airway obstruction based on abnormal airway sounds and increased work of breathing. As with adults, determine if the airway is open and the patient has adequate chest rise with breathing. Check for mucus, blood, or a foreign body in the mouth or airway. If there is potential obstruction from the tongue or soft tissues, position the airway and suction as necessary. Determine whether the airway is open and patent, partially obstructed, or totally obstructed. Do not keep the suction tip or catheter in the back of a child's throat too long because young patients are extremely sensitive to vagal stimuli and the heart rate may plummet.

Breathing
The breathing component of the initial assessment involves calculating the respiratory rate, auscultating breath sounds, and checking pulse oximetry for oxygen saturation. Verify the respiratory rate per minute by counting the number of chest rises in 30 seconds and then doubling that number. Healthy infants may show periodic breathing, or variable respiratory rates with short periods of apnea (< 20 s). As a consequence, counting for only 10 to 15 seconds may give a falsely low respiratory rate. Interpreting the respiratory rate requires knowing the normal values for the child's age Table 41-4 ▶ and putting the respiratory rate in context with the rest of the PAT and initial assessment. Rapid respiratory rates may simply reflect high fever, anxiety, pain, or excitement. Normal rates, by contrast, may occur in a child who has been breathing rapidly with increased work of breathing and is becoming fatigued. Serial

Table 41-4	Normal Respiratory Rate by Age
Age	**Respiratory Rate (breaths/min)**
Infant	25–50
Toddler	20–30
Preschool-age child	20–25
School-age child	15–20
Adolescent	12–16

Table 41-5	Normal Pulse Rates for Age
Age	**Pulse Rate (beats/min)**
Infant	100–160
Toddler	90–150
Preschool-age child	80–140
School-age child	70–120
Adolescent	60–100

In the Field

Consider pulse oximetry readings in terms of the environmental context and the physiologic status of the child. Peripheral vasoconstriction from hypothermia or poor perfusion may alter these readings. Always correlate the pulse oximetry waveform with the patient's pulse rate and ECG reading.

assessment of respiratory rates may be especially useful because the trend may be more accurate than any single value.

Auscultate the breath sounds with a stethoscope over the midaxillary line to hear abnormal lung sounds during inhalation and exhalation. Listen for extra breath sounds such as inspiratory crackles, wheezes, or rhonchi; rhonchi often indicate harsh breath sounds or sounds that may be transmitted from the upper airways. If you cannot determine whether the sounds are being generated in the lungs or the upper airway, hold the stethoscope over the nose or trachea and listen. Also, listen to the breath sounds for adequacy of air movement. Diminished breath sounds may signal severe respiratory distress. Auscultation over the trachea may also help distinguish stridor from other sounds.

Check the pulse oximetry reading to determine the oxygen saturation while the child breathes ambient air. You can place the pulse oximetry probe on a young child's finger just as you would with an adult. In infants or young children who try to remove the probe, it may be helpful to place the probe on a toe, possibly with a sock covering it. A pulse oximetry reading of greater than 94% saturation while breathing room air indicates good oxygenation.

As with the respiratory rate, evaluate the pulse oximetry reading in the context of the PAT and remainder of the initial assessment. A child with a normal pulse oximetry reading, for example, may be expending increasing amounts of energy and increasing the work of breathing to maintain his or her oxygen saturation. The PAT and initial assessment would identify the respiratory distress and point to the need for immediate intervention despite the normal oxygen saturation.

Circulation

The information obtained from the PAT about circulation to the skin directs the next step of the initial assessment. Integrate this assessment of circulation with the pulse rate and quality, skin CTC (color, temperature, and condition plus capillary refill time), and blood pressure to obtain an overall assessment of the child's circulatory status.

Obtain the child's pulse rate by listening to the heart or feeling the pulse for 30 seconds and doubling the number. As with respiratory rates in pediatric patients, it is important to know normal pulse rates based on age (Table 41-5 ▲). Interpret the pulse rate within the context of the overall history, PAT, and initial assessment. Tachycardia may indicate early hypoxia or shock or a less serious condition such as fever, anxiety, pain, or excitement.

Feel for the pulse to ascertain the rate and quality of pulsations. If you cannot find a peripheral (distal) pulse (that is, radial or brachial), feel for a central pulse (that is, femoral or carotid). Check the femoral pulse in infants and young children and the carotid pulse in older children and adolescents. As with adults, if there is no pulse, start CPR.

After checking the pulse rate, do a hands-on evaluation of skin CTC. Check whether the hands and feet are warm or cool to the touch. Check capillary refill time in the fingertip, toe, heel, or pads of the fingertips; a normal refill time is less than 2 seconds. These two pieces of information need to be placed in context with the PAT and remainder of initial assessment because cool extremities and delayed capillary refill are commonly seen in a child in a cool environment.

The last step in the circulation assessment is to measure the blood pressure. It may be difficult to obtain an accurate measurement in a young child or infant because of a lack of cooperation and need for proper cuff size. Nevertheless, you should attempt to measure the blood pressure on the upper arm or thigh, making sure the cuff has a width two thirds the length of the upper arm or thigh. One formula for determining the lower limit of acceptable blood pressure in children ages 1 to 10 years is this: minimum systolic blood pressure = 70 + (2 × age in years).

In the Field

Blood pressure is just one component of the overall assessment of pediatric patients. Determination of physiologic stability should be based on all data collected from the PAT, physical exam, and initial vital signs. Remember that compensated shock can exist in the face of adequate blood pressure.

Table 41-6	Normal Blood Pressure for Age
Age	Minimum Systolic Blood Pressure (mm Hg)
Infant	> 60
Toddler	> 70
Preschool-age child	> 75
School-age child	> 80
Adolescent	> 90

Table 41-7	AVPU Scale		
Category	Stimulus	Response Type	Reaction
Alert	Normal environment	Appropriate	Normal interactiveness for age
Verbal	Simple command or sound stimulus	Appropriate	Responds to name
		Inappropriate	Nonspecific or confused
Painful	Pain	Appropriate	Withdraws from pain
		Inappropriate	Makes sound or moves without purpose or localization of pain
		Pathologic	Posturing
Unresponsive			No perceptible response to any stimulus

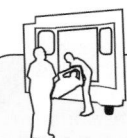

In the Field

For children 1 to 10 years, calculate the lower limit of acceptable blood pressure for age with the following formula:

Minimum systolic blood pressure = 70 + (2 × age in years)

For example, a 2-year-old toddler should have a minimum systolic blood pressure of 74; a lower reading indicates decompensated shock. (Table 41-6 ▲ shows normal minimal systolic blood pressure values for different ages.) Given the technical difficulty of trying to measure a blood pressure, make one attempt in the field; if unsuccessful, move on to the rest of the assessment.

Mental Status

Your general impression of the patient should provide the first clues about the child's neurologic status. As you begin the initial assessment, use the AVPU scale (Table 41-7 ▲ to evaluate the cerebral cortex. The AVPU scale is a conventional way of assessing any patient's level of consciousness (LOC) or mental status. It categorizes motor response based on simple response to stimuli, classifying the patient as alert, responsive to verbal stimuli, responsive to painful stimuli, or unresponsive.

After evaluating the patient's response with the AVPU scale, assess the pupillary response to a beam of light to assess brain stem response. Next, evaluate motor activity, looking for symmetric movement of the extremities, seizures, posturing, or flaccidity. Combine this information with the PAT results to determine the child's neurologic status.

Exposure Considerations

Proper exposure of the child is necessary to complete the initial assessment. During the PAT, the child will have been at least partially undressed to assess the work of breathing and circulation. It is also important to evaluate the child from head to toe and to look at the child's back during the initial assessment. Be careful to avoid heat loss, especially in infants, by covering the child up as soon as possible. Keep the temperature in the ambulance high, and use blankets when necessary.

Assessment of Pain

Numerous studies have found that children are much less likely than adults to receive effective pain medications. Inadequate treatment of pain has many adverse effects on the child and family. Pain causes morbidity and misery for the child and caregivers, and it interferes with your ability to accurately assess physiologic abnormalities. Children who do not receive appropriate analgesia may be more likely to have exaggerated pain responses to subsequent painful procedures. Also, posttraumatic stress may be more common among children who experience pain during an illness or injury.

Assessment of pain must consider developmental age. The ability to identify pain improves with the age of the child. In infants and preverbal children, it may be difficult to distinguish crying and agitation due to hypoxia, hunger, or pain. Further assessment and discussion with caregivers about their perceptions of the child's pain are essential to identify pain in this age group. For verbal children, pain scales using pictures of facial expressions, such as the Wong-Baker FACES scale, may prove helpful Figure 41-9 ▶ .

Remaining calm and providing quiet, professional reassurance to parents and child is critical for managing pediatric pain and anxiety. A calm parent will help keep the child calm and more at ease. Distraction techniques with toys or stories may prove helpful in reducing pain, as may visual imagery techniques and music. Sucrose pacifiers may reduce pain in neonates. Pharmacologic methods for reducing pain—such as acetaminophen, opiates, benzodiazepines, and nitrous oxide—are available to paramedics in a number of EMS systems. The benefit of such analgesic or anxiolytic medication must be weighed against the risks of its administration (respiratory depression, bradycardia, hypoxemia, and hypotension are potential side effects of sedatives), including the potential route of administration. Medications that are given intravenously are often most effective at reducing pain, but they

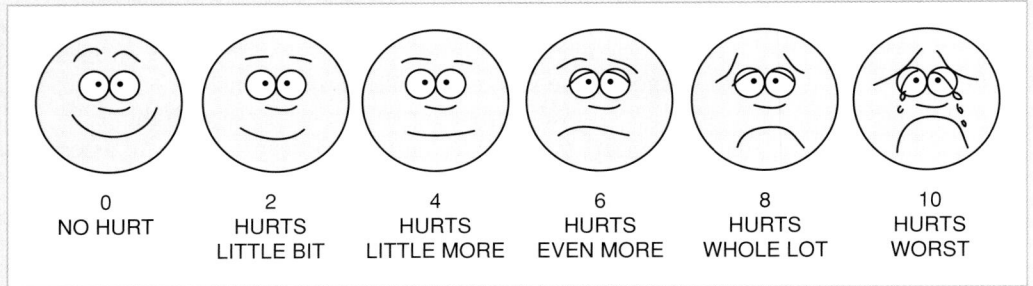

Figure 41-9 Pictures such as the Wong-Baker FACES Pain Rating Scale allow for self-assessment of pain in young children.

From Hockenberry MJ, Wilson D, Wikelstein ML: *Wong's Essentials of Pediatric Nursing*, ed. 7, St. Louis, 2005, p. 1259. Used with permission. Copyright, Mosby.

Special Considerations

Consider pain to be a vital sign in pediatric patients. Assess and reassess pain along with the other vital signs. Treat pain accordingly.

require establishing intravenous (IV) access, which itself is a painful procedure.

Today, assessment of pain is recognized as part of vital sign assessment, and management of pediatric pain and anxiety should be a routine part of field care. This effort requires a thorough understanding of nonpharmacologic techniques, drugs, potential drug contraindications and complications, and management of the complications.

Transport Decision

After completing the initial assessment and beginning resuscitation when necessary, you must make a crucial decision: whether to immediately transport the child to the emergency department (ED) or continue the additional assessment and treatment on scene. Immediate transport is imperative if the emergency call is for trauma and the child has a serious mechanism of injury (MOI), a physiologic abnormality, or a potentially significant anatomic abnormality or if the scene is unsafe. In these cases, stabilize the spine, manage the airway and breathing, stop external bleeding, and begin transport. Attempt vascular access on the way to the ED. If the emergency call is for an illness, the decision to stay or go is less clear-cut and depends on the following factors: expected benefits of treatment, EMS system regulations, comfort level, and transport time.

Additional Assessment
Focused History and Physical Exam

The focused history and physical exam, which is performed on medical and trauma patients, has four objectives:

- To obtain a complete description of the chief complaint (for example, OPQRST and SAMPLE)
- To determine the MOI or nature of an illness

You are the Provider Part 2

You use the PAT to form a general impression of the patient. Based on his abnormal appearance and circulation, you determine that the child is sick and requires rapid treatment. The combination of your knowledge that children are more prone to head injuries than adults because of the larger size and weight of their heads compared with rest of their bodies, the MOI, and your general impression of the patient leads you to suspect that the child may have a closed head injury.

You immediately assign one of the fire fighters the task of maintaining manual cervical spine immobilization. You ask your partner to apply 100% supplemental oxygen via nonrebreathing mask as you expose the child to complete a rapid trauma assessment. This examination reveals a mildly distended abdomen and an obviously deformed right thigh. You ask the lieutenant to issue a trauma alert, citing the combination of your physical assessment findings and the MOI.

Vital Signs	Recording Time: 5 Minutes
Skin	Pale, cool, and dry
Pulse	170 beats/min, regular; weak distally but strong centrally
Blood pressure	86/48 mm Hg
Respirations	40 breaths/min; unlabored, clear breath sounds
Sao$_2$	99% on nonrebreathing mask at 12 L/min of oxygen
Capillary refill	2–3 seconds

3. What do you need to carefully monitor the patient for?

4. Which interventions should you consider at this point, if any?

Table 41-8	Pediatric SAMPLE Components
Component	**Explanation**
Signs and symptoms	Onset and nature of symptoms of pain or fever Age-appropriate signs of distress
Allergies	Known drug reactions or other allergies
Medications	Exact names and doses of ongoing drugs (including over-the-counter, prescribed, herbal, and recreational drugs) Timing and amount of last dose Time and dose of analgesics or antipyretics
Past medical history	Previous illnesses or injuries Immunizations History of pregnancy, labor, delivery (infants and toddlers)
Last oral intake	Timing of the child's last food or drink, including bottle or breastfeeding
Events leading to illness or injury	Key events leading to the current incident Fever history

- To perform a rapid trauma or medical assessment or a focused or vectored physical exam of a specific body part or body system
- To obtain baseline vital signs

If the child seems to be in physiologically unstable condition based on the initial assessment, you may decide to begin transport immediately and conduct the focused history and physical exam in the ambulance. If the child is in stable condition and the scene is safe, perform the focused history and physical exam on the scene, before transport. The detailed physical exam is conducted en route to the hospital for trauma patients with a significant MOI. It can be done on the scene if you are waiting for the ambulance to arrive or if patient removal is delayed because of entrapment. As opposed to the initial assessment, which addresses immediately life-threatening pathologic problems, the focused history and physical exam narrows the focus to assessing the body part or body system specifically involved, obtaining a complete set of baseline vital signs, elaborating on the chief complaint (ie, OPQRST), and obtaining a patient history (ie, SAMPLE).

To obtain the focused history, use the SAMPLE mnemonic **Table 41-8 ▲**. Tailor the physical exam to the child's age and developmental stage. In trauma patients, after the detailed physical exam is complete, reconsider the need for immediate transport.

Ongoing Assessment

The elements in the ongoing assessment include the PAT, reassessment of patient priority, vital signs (every 5 minutes if unstable condition and every 15 minutes if stable), assessment of the effectiveness of interventions (eg, medications adminis-

Documentation and Communication

Perform frequent reassessment of serial vital signs, and record them on your documentation form. By recording each set of vital signs, you can visualize trends and transfer important information to the accepting physicians.

tered, splints applied, bleeding controlled), and reassessment of the focused exam areas. Perform this kind of ongoing assessment on all patients to observe their response to treatment, to guide ongoing treatments, and to track the progression of identified pathologic and anatomic problems. New problems may also be identified on reassessment. The elements in the ongoing assessment also guide the choice of an appropriate transport destination and your radio or telephone communications with medical oversight or ED staff.

Respiratory Emergencies

Respiratory problems are among the medical emergencies that you will most frequently encounter in children. Pediatric patients with a respiratory chief complaint will span the spectrum from mildly ill to near death. In pediatrics, respiratory failure and arrest precede the majority of cardiopulmonary arrests; by contrast, a primary cardiac event is the usual cause of sudden death in adults. Early identification and intervention can stop the progression from respiratory distress to cardiopulmonary failure and help to avert much pediatric morbidity and mortality.

General Assessment and Management

When faced with a respiratory emergency, the first step is to determine the severity of the disease: Is the patient in respiratory distress, respiratory failure, or respiratory arrest?

Respiratory distress entails increased work of breathing to maintain oxygenation and/or ventilation; that is, it is a compensated state in which increased work of breathing results in adequate pulmonary gas exchange. The hallmarks of respiratory distress—which is classified as mild, moderate, or severe—are retractions (suprasternal, intercostal, subcostal), abdominal breathing, nasal flaring, and grunting.

A patient in respiratory failure can no longer compensate for the underlying pathologic or anatomic problem by increased work of breathing, so hypoxia and/or carbon dioxide retention occur. Signs of respiratory failure may include decreased or absent retractions owing to fatigue of the chest wall muscles, altered mental status owing to inadequate oxygenation and ventilation of the brain, and an abnormally low respiratory rate **Table 41-9 ▶**. Respiratory failure is a decompensated state, requiring urgent intervention to ensure adequate oxygenation and ventilation and prevent respiratory arrest. Do not be afraid to assist ventilations at this point if you judge the tidal volume or respiratory effort to be inadequate.

Table 41-9	Signs of Impending Respiratory Failure
Assess	**Sign**
Mental status	Agitation, restlessness, confusion, lethargy (VPU of AVPU)
Skin color	Cyanosis, pallor
Respiratory rate	Tachypnea → bradypnea → apnea
Respiratory effort	Severe retractions, nasal flaring, grunting, paradoxical abdominal motion, tripod positioning
Auscultation	Stridor, wheezing, rales, or diminished air movement
Blood oxygen saturation	< 90% with supplemental oxygen
Pulse rate	Tachycardia, bradycardia, or cardiac arrest

Table 41-10	Key Questions in Respiratory Emergencies
Component	**Key Questions**
Signs and symptoms	Shortness of breath? Hoarseness? Stridor? Wheezing? Cough? Chest pain? Choking? Rash/Hives? Cyanosis?
Allergies	Known drug or food allergies; smoke exposure
Medications	Names and doses of ongoing medications; recent use of corticosteroids
Past medical history	History of asthma, chronic lung disease, heart problems, prematurity; prior hospitalizations and intubation for breathing problems; history of choking or anaphylaxis; immunizations
Last oral intake	Timing of last food, including bottle or breastfeeding
Events leading to illness or injury	Fever history or recent illness; history of injury to chest; history of choking on food or object

In the Field

Initiate aggressive airway management and ventilatory support with a bag-mask device and supplemental oxygen as soon as possible for a child with respiratory failure.

Respiratory arrest implies that the patient is not breathing spontaneously. Administer immediate bag-mask ventilation with supplemental oxygen to prevent progression to cardiopulmonary arrest. Resuscitation of a child from respiratory arrest is often successful, whereas resuscitation of a child in cardiopulmonary arrest usually fails.

By combining the three components of the PAT, you can determine the severity of disease before you even touch the patient. The child's appearance will give you clues about the adequacy of CNS oxygenation and ventilation. If a child with trouble breathing is sleepy, assume the child is hypoxic. Assess the work of breathing by noting the patient's position of comfort, presence or absence of retractions, and grunting or flaring. A patient who prefers to sit upright, in the sniffing position, or to use his or her arms for support is trying to optimize breathing mechanics. Deep retractions herald the use of accessory muscles of respiration to move air. Assessment of circulation for the presence of pallor or cyanosis will give further information on the adequacy of oxygenation.

After forming a general impression using the PAT, move on to the hands-on initial assessment. For respiratory emergencies, focus on the child's airway and breathing. Assess the airway by listening for stridor in awake patients or checking for obstruction in obtunded patients. Assess breathing by determining the child's respiratory rate, listening to the lungs for adequacy of air entry and abnormal breath sounds, and checking pulse oximetry readings. A rate that is too low may be more worrisome than a rate that is too high for the child's age. The presence of abnormal breath sounds may identify the anatomic or pathologic abnormality and suggest a likely diagnosis. For example, symmetric, diffuse wheezing implies bronchospasm and possibly asthma, whereas diffuse rhonchi, rales, and wheezing in an infant or toddler are typical signs of lower airway inflammation associated with bronchiolitis. The presence of stridor in the context of clear lung fields is consistent with upper airway obstruction, often due to croup. Poor air entry with decreased breath sounds is an ominous sign that must be addressed immediately. Determine oxygen saturation by assessing pulse oximetry via a finger or toe or, in a small infant, around the foot.

Your determination of whether the patient is in respiratory distress, respiratory failure, or respiratory arrest will drive your next steps, by indicating the urgency for treatment and transport. You can obtain the SAMPLE history at the scene or during transport, depending on the patient's stability. **Table 41-10 ▲** lists key questions to ask during a respiratory emergency.

Most pediatric patients with a primary respiratory complaint will have respiratory distress and require only generic treatment. Allow the child to assume a position of comfort, and provide supplemental oxygen. The choice of oxygen delivery method will depend on the severity of illness and the child's developmental level. Young children may become agitated by a nasal cannula or face mask. Because crying and thrashing increase metabolic demands and oxygen consumption, you must weigh the benefits of this therapy against the potential cost. Allowing a caregiver to deliver blow-by oxygen to a calm toddler may be your best choice, if the child does not show signs of respiratory failure.

As a child becomes fatigued, respiratory distress may progress to respiratory failure. As part of your ongoing assessment, electronically monitor the patient's pulse rate, respiratory rate, and oxygen saturation. A significant change or trend in any of these variables requires prompt patient reassessment. You should also perform frequent reassessment to evaluate the effects of your treatment.

Upper Airway Emergencies
Foreign Body Aspiration or Obstruction

Infants and toddlers explore their environment by putting everything and anything into their mouths, resulting in a high risk of foreign body aspiration. Any small object or food item has the potential to obstruct a young child's narrow trachea. Peanuts, hot dogs, grapes, balloons, and small toys or pieces of toys are frequent offenders. Swallowed foreign bodies can also cause respiratory distress in infants and young children because a rigid esophageal foreign body can compress the relative pliable trachea. In addition, the tongue, owing to its large size relative to the upper airway, frequently causes mild upper airway obstruction in a child with a decreased LOC and diminished muscle tone.

Suspect foreign body aspiration when you encounter signs of mild or severe airway obstruction on the PAT or initial assessment. An awake patient with stridor, increased work of breathing, and good color on the PAT has mild upper airway obstruction. Auscultation may reveal fair to good air entry, and the presence of unilateral wheezing may tip you off to a foreign body lodged in a mainstem bronchus. In contrast, a patient with severe airway obstruction is likely to be cyanotic and unconscious when you arrive, owing to profound hypoxia. If the child has spontaneous respiratory effort, you will hear poor air entry, but you may *not* hear stridor owing to minimal air flow through the trachea. A typical SAMPLE history for foreign body aspiration reveals a previously healthy child with sudden onset of coughing, choking, or gagging while eating or playing.

Initial management of mild airway obstruction involves allowing the patient to assume a position of comfort, providing supplemental oxygen as tolerated, and transporting the child to an appropriate treating facility. Avoid agitating the child because this stimulus could worsen the situation. Continuous monitoring and frequent reassessments are needed to ensure that the problem does not progress to severe airway obstruction.

In severe airway obstruction, the initial management steps follow BLS guidelines for attempted removal. For a conscious infant, deliver five back slaps and five chest thrusts
Figure 41-10 ▶ :

1. Hold the infant face down, with the body resting on your forearm. Support the infant's head and face with your hand, and keep the head lower than the rest of the body.

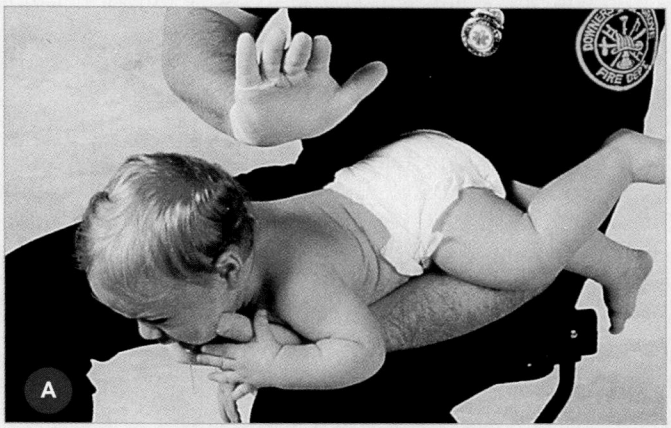
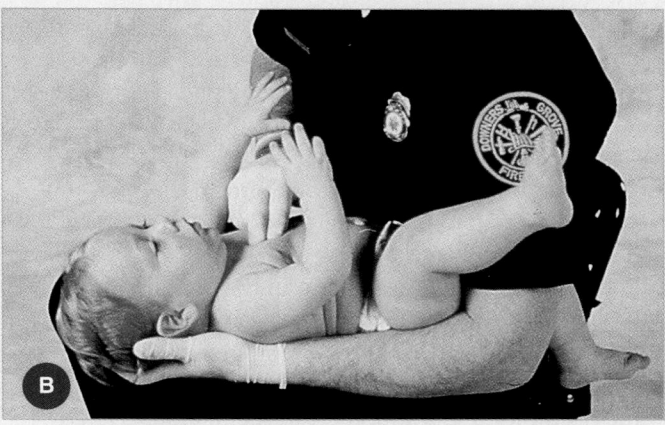

Figure 41-10 Perform back slaps and chest thrusts to clear a foreign body airway obstruction in an infant. **A.** Hold the infant face down with the body resting on your forearm. Support the jaw and face with your hand, and keep the head lower than the rest of the body. Give the infant five back slaps between the shoulder blades, using the heel of your hand. **B.** Give the infant five quick chest thrusts, using two fingers placed on the lower half of the sternum.

2. Deliver five back slaps between the shoulder blades using the heel of your hand.
3. Place your free hand behind the infant's head and back, and bring the infant upright on your thigh, sandwiching the infant's body between your two hands and arms. The infant's head should remain below the level of the body.
4. Give five quick chest thrusts in the same location and manner as for chest compressions, using two fingers placed on the lower half of the sternum. For larger infants, or if you have small hands, you can place the infant in your lap and turn the infant's whole body as a unit between back slaps and chest thrusts.
5. Repeat the sequence of back slaps and chest thrusts until the object is expelled or the infant becomes unresponsive.
6. If the infant with a severe airway obstruction becomes unresponsive, begin CPR.

If the infant regains consciousness, place him or her in the recovery position, administer 100% supplemental oxygen, and transport immediately. If you are unable to relieve the obstruction after several attempts, begin immediate transport.

If you have reason to believe that an unresponsive child has a foreign body obstruction, check the upper airway to see whether an object is visible. If so, try to remove it using a finger sweep motion. Never perform blind finger sweeps; doing so may push the object farther into the airway.

Abdominal thrusts (Heimlich maneuver) are recommended to relieve a severe airway obstruction in a conscious child. They increase the pressure in the chest, creating an artificial cough that may force a foreign body from the airway. Follow these steps to remove a foreign body obstruction from a conscious child who is in a standing position (Figure 41-11 ▾):

1. Kneel on one knee behind the child, and circle his or her body by placing both arms around the child's chest. Prepare to give abdominal thrusts by placing your fist just above the patient's umbilicus and well below the xiphoid process. Place your other hand over that fist.
2. Give the child rapid, distinct abdominal thrusts in an upward direction. Be careful to avoid applying force to the lower ribcage or sternum.
3. Repeat this standing technique until the child expels the foreign body or becomes unresponsive.
4. If the child becomes unresponsive, place him or her supine on a firm, flat surface and inspect the airway using the head tilt–chin lift. If you can see the foreign body, try to remove it. Do not perform blind finger sweeps.
5. Attempt rescue breathing. If the first attempt fails, reposition the head and try again.
6. If the airway remains obstructed, begin CPR with chest compressions at the 30:2 compression/ventilation ratio and prepare for immediate transport.

If you manage to clear the airway obstruction in an unresponsive child (older than 1 year), but he or she remains apneic and pulseless, begin CPR and attach the automated external defibrillator (AED) as soon as possible, using appropriately sized AED pads. If you are unable to relieve the obstruction after several attempts, transport immediately.

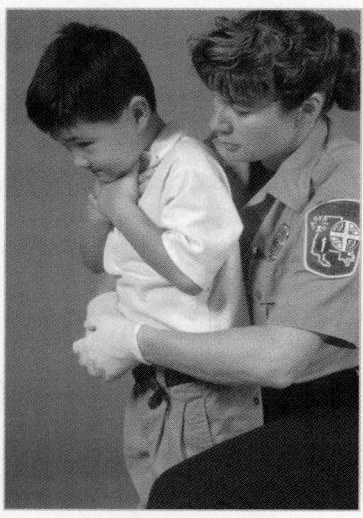

Figure 41-11 To relieve a foreign body obstruction in a responsive child who is standing, kneel behind the child, wrap your arms around his or her body, and place your fist just above the umbilicus and well below the xiphoid process.

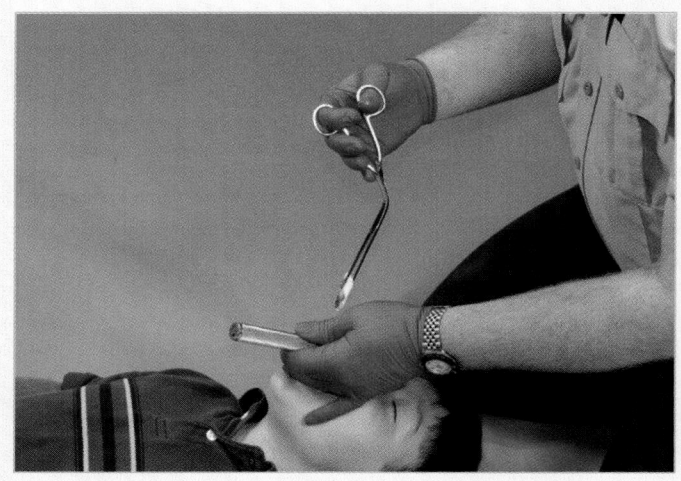

Figure 41-12 Using Magill forceps and direct laryngoscopy to remove foreign body airway obstruction.

If the BLS procedures do not dislodge the obstruction and severe airway obstruction remains, advanced airway procedures may be required. If the obstruction is more proximal, direct laryngoscopy with removal of the foreign body with Magill forceps may be successful (Figure 41-12 ▴):

1. Hold the laryngoscope handle with your left hand.
2. Open the mouth by exerting thumb pressure on the chin.
3. Insert a pediatric straight blade into the mouth, and lift the tongue with the blade.
4. Exert gentle traction upward along the axis of the laryngoscope handle at a 45° angle, and advance the blade. Do not use the teeth or gums for leverage.
5. Watch the tip until the foreign body is visible. Do not go past the vocal cords.
6. Use suction to improve visibility if secretions are present.
7. Insert the Magill forceps into the mouth with the tips closed.
8. Grasp the foreign object and remove while looking directly at it.
9. Look at the airway to ensure that it is clear of debris. Remove the laryngoscope blade.

If you manage to remove the object, recheck the patient's breathing and circulation. Begin rescue breathing and CPR as needed and arrange for immediate transport. If direct laryngoscopy does not reveal the foreign body, use bag-mask ventilation. If bag-mask ventilation does not provide adequate ventilatory support, attempt to insert an advanced airway (such as ET tube, laryngeal mask airway, or Combitube). Immediate transportation to an appropriate facility is required.

Anaphylaxis

Anaphylaxis is a potentially life-threatening allergic reaction, triggered by exposure to an antigen (foreign protein). Food—especially nuts, shellfish, eggs, and milk—and bee stings are among the most common causes, although anaphylaxis to antibiotics and other medications can occur as well. Exposure to the antigen stimulates the release of histamine and other vasoactive chemical mediators from white blood cells, leading to multiple organ system involvement. Onset of symptoms generally occurs immediately after the exposure and may include hives, respiratory distress, circulatory compromise, and gastrointestinal symptoms (vomiting, diarrhea, abdominal pain).

Although a child with mild anaphylaxis may experience only hives and some wheezing, a child with severe anaphylaxis may be in respiratory failure and shock when you arrive. The PAT may reveal an anxious child (many adults describe a sense of impending doom at the onset of anaphylaxis). With severe anaphylaxis, the child may be unresponsive due to respiratory failure and shock. He or she may have increased work of breathing due to upper airway edema or bronchospasm and poor circulation. The initial assessment will usually reveal hives, with other findings potentially including swelling of the lips and oral mucosa, stridor and/or wheezing, and diminished pulses. If the child has a known allergy, the SAMPLE history may reveal recent contact with or ingestion of the potentially offending agent (including consumption of prepared foods containing traces of eggs, nuts, and milk at daycare or school).

The "gold standard" treatment for anaphylaxis is epinephrine. Epinephrine's alpha-agonist effect decreases airway edema by vasoconstriction and improves circulation by increasing peripheral vascular resistance. Its beta-agonist effect causes bronchodilation, resulting in improved oxygenation and ventilation. Epinephrine should be given by the subcutaneous (SQ) or intramuscular (IM) route at a dose of 0.01 mg/kg of the 1:1,000 solution, to a maximum dose of 0.3 mg. This dose may be repeated as necessary every 5 minutes. If several doses are needed, the child may require a continuous IV epinephrine drip. In addition to epinephrine, treatment of anaphylaxis should include supplemental oxygen, fluid resuscitation for shock, diphenhydramine for its antihistamine effect (dose: 1 to 2 mg/kg IV to a maximum of 50 mg), and bronchodilators for wheezing.

Many children with a history of anaphylaxis will have been treated with IM epinephrine by a caregiver before EMS activation. Given the short half-life of this drug, the child should be transported, even if asymptomatic on your arrival.

Croup

Croup (laryngotracheobronchitis) is a viral infection of the upper airway and the most common cause of upper airway emergencies in young children. The parainfluenza virus is the pathogen most commonly responsible for croup, but respiratory syncytial virus (RSV), influenza, and adenovirus have also been implicated. The virus is transmitted by respiratory secretions. Croup most commonly affects children 6 months to 6 years, with most cases occurring in the fall and winter months. The virus has an affinity for the subglottic space—the narrowest part of the pediatric airway—and causes edema and progressive airway obstruction. Turbulent air flow through the narrowed subglottic airway causes the hallmark sign of croup—stridor.

Most cases of croup are mild. EMS may be called when the symptoms come on abruptly or cause moderate to severe respiratory distress. The PAT for a child with croup will typically reveal an alert infant or toddler who has audible stridor with activity or agitation, a barky cough, some increased work of breathing, and normal skin color. If a child with a history compatible with croup is sleepy or obtunded or has significant respiratory distress or cyanosis, be concerned about critical airway obstruction. On your initial assessment, breath sounds will likely be clear over the lung fields, although you may hear stridor (originating at the level of the subglottic space). Because the pathophysiology of croup largely involves the upper airway, hypoxia is uncommon, and its presence should alert you to critical obstruction and the need for immediate treatment. The SAMPLE history usually reveals several days of cold symptoms and low-grade fever, followed by onset of a barky cough, stridor, and trouble breathing. The cough and respiratory distress are often worse at night.

The initial management of croup is the same as for most respiratory emergencies. Allow the child to assume a position of comfort, and avoid agitating him or her. The use of cool mist or nebulized saline is controversial. For patients with stridor at rest, moderate to severe respiratory distress, poor air exchange, hypoxia, or altered appearance, nebulized epinephrine is the treatment of choice. It works by causing vasoconstriction and decreasing upper airway edema. Nebulized epinephrine is available in two formulations: racemic epinephrine and L-epinephrine. The dose for racemic epinephrine (2.25%) is 0.5 mL mixed in 3 mL of normal saline. The dose for L-epinephrine is 0.25 to 0.5 mg/kg of the 1:1,000 solution (maximum, 5 mg per dose); this form can be diluted with normal saline to bring the volume to 3 mL. Although only a small amount of epinephrine is absorbed via the nebulized route, side effects may include tachycardia, agitation, tremor, and vomiting.

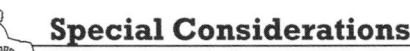

Special Considerations

The presence of hypoxia in a child with croup is a potentially ominous finding, indicating significant subglottic edema. Assess and transport quickly.

In the case of croup and respiratory failure, nebulized epinephrine alone may not be adequate and assisted ventilation may be necessary. Assisted ventilation with bag-mask ventilation will often succeed in overcoming the upper airway obstruction. Advanced airway placement is rarely needed in croup. If performed, choose an ET tube one-half to one size smaller than normal for age or size to accommodate the subglottic edema. Children requiring nebulized epinephrine or assisted ventilation need to be transported immediately to an appropriate treatment facility.

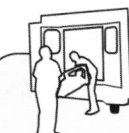

In the Field

Bag-mask ventilation is the mainstay of treatment for most upper airway emergencies.

Epiglottitis and Bacterial Infections

Epiglottitis, a once-dreaded inflammation of the supraglottic structures, usually due to bacterial infection, is now rare in children. Since the introduction of a childhood vaccine against *Haemophilus influenzae,* type B, the incidence of this life-threatening condition has decreased dramatically. Nevertheless, sporadic cases have been reported among adolescents, adults, and unimmunized children.

The classic presentation of epiglottitis is easily distinguishable using the PAT and the initial assessment. A child with epiglottitis looks sick and will be anxious, will sit upright in the sniffing position with the chin thrust forward to allow for maximal air entry, and may be drooling because of an inability to swallow secretions. The work of breathing is increased, and pallor or cyanosis may be evident. The initial assessment may reveal stridor on auscultation over the neck, a muffled voice, decreased or absent breath sounds, and hypoxia—all signs of a significant airway obstruction. The SAMPLE history will reveal a sudden onset of high fever and sore throat in preschool- or school-age children. Because symptoms progress rapidly, children with epiglottitis are generally sick for only a few hours before they come to medical attention. Remember to ask about immunizations as part of the pertinent medical history for patients suspected of having epiglottitis.

Your goal is to get the child with epiglottitis to an appropriate hospital with a maintainable airway. Because rapidly progressive disease carries a risk for acute airway obstruction and respiratory arrest, you should minimize your scene time and not attempt procedures that might agitate the child. Allow the patient to assume a position of comfort, and give supplemental oxygen only if tolerated by the patient. Do not attempt to look in the mouth because this can precipitate complete airway obstruction, and do not insert an IV line. Be prepared with a bag-mask device and an ET tube one to two sizes smaller than anticipated for the child's age and length in case of complete obstruction during transport and the need for assisted ventilation. Endotracheal intubation of a child with epiglottitis is notoriously difficult owing to the extreme distortion of the airway anatomy. Alert personnel at the receiving facility to the suspected diagnosis and patient's condition because they will need to mobilize a team for the management of this difficult airway.

Some uncommon conditions can also cause upper airway obstruction, including retropharyngeal abscess, peritonsillar abscess, tracheitis, and diphtheria. Presentation may include fever, stridor, difficulty handling secretions, and respiratory distress. Regardless of the underlying diagnosis, initial assessment and management will be the same as for croup.

Lower Airway Emergencies

The underlying pathophysiology in upper airway emergencies involves restriction of air flow *into* the lungs (inhalation). By contrast, the pathophysiology of lower airway respiratory emergencies involves restriction of air flow *out* of the lungs (exhalation).

Asthma

Asthma is the most common chronic illness of childhood and the most common respiratory complaint encountered by prehospital providers. An estimated 5% to 10% of children are affected by asthma, many of whom will be treated in the ED. Recent studies indicate that the incidence and mortality of this disease are increasing.

In this disease of the small airways, three main components lead to obstruction and poor gas exchange: bronchospasm, mucus production, and airway inflammation. Lower airway inflammation in asthma results in hypoxia because of ventilation-perfusion mismatch, a situation in which blood flowing to parts of the lung is poorly oxygenated. Triggers for asthma attacks include upper respiratory infections, environmental allergies, exposure to cold, changes in the weather, and secondhand smoke. Clinical signs include frequent cough, wheezing, and more general signs of respiratory distress.

The initial assessment of a child with an acute exacerbation of asthma will vary based on the degree of obstruction and the presence or absence of respiratory fatigue. A child with mild to moderate respiratory distress will be awake and alert, sometimes preferring a seated posture. Although increased work of breathing may be evident by retractions and nasal flaring, circulation will seem normal. Decreasing alertness, assumption of the tripod position, deep retractions, and cyanosis are signs of severe respiratory distress and impending respiratory failure. The initial assessment will reveal shortness of breath as evidenced by inability to speak in full sentences, increased respiratory rate, prolonged expiration phase, and wheezes noted on auscultation. Expiratory wheezing alone may be heard in patients with mild to moderate asthma attacks, but wheezing may be heard on inspiration and expiration in patients with moderate to severe disease. Decreased air movement and the absence of wheezes in a person with asthma who has activated the EMS system suggest severe lower airway obstruction and respiratory fatigue and signal the need for immediate treatment to prevent respiratory arrest.

The SAMPLE history for a patient suspected of having asthma should reveal the frequency and severity of previous asthma attacks, as reflected by ED visits and hospitalizations. A patient who has previously been admitted to an intensive care unit or intubated for asthma is at increased risk for severe—even possibly fatal—attacks. The medication history should identify any preventive treatment (controller medications) and any rescue medications administered by the caregiver before your arrival. Inhaled steroids are the most common controller medications used in pediatrics, whereas inhaled albuterol is the most common beta-2 agonist drug used as a rescue medication.

The initial management of an asthma exacerbation remains basic respiratory care: Allow the patient to remain in a position of comfort, and start supplemental oxygen. The gold standard treatment consists of bronchodilators, beta-agonists that act to relax smooth muscles in the bronchioles, thereby decreasing bronchospasm and improving air movement and oxygenation.

Bronchodilators may be delivered by nebulizer or metered-dose inhaler (MDI) with a spacer-mask device. Unit doses of 2.5 mg of albuterol premixed with 3 mL of normal saline are often used for nebulization and represent an acceptable starting dose for most young children. For a larger child or a child of any age who is in severe distress, consider administering 5 mg of albuterol as the initial dose. If nebulized albuterol is used, four puffs is equivalent to 2.5 mg administered by nebulizer. Children with moderate to severe respiratory distress can be given treatments every 20 minutes during transport, including back-to-back nebulizer treatments.

Although albuterol is a relatively safe medication, its potential side effects include tachycardia, tremor, and mild hyperactivity. An isomer of albuterol, levalbuterol, reportedly has fewer side effects. It has not been studied in the prehospital setting but is likely an acceptable alternative to albuterol.

Children with moderate to severe respiratory distress may also benefit from treatment with inhaled ipratropium, an anticholinergic bronchodilator. Studies have shown that the combination of albuterol and ipratropium (which may be mixed and delivered together by nebulizer) is more effective than albuterol given alone. The dose of ipratropium given is based on the patient's weight: a 0.25-mg unit dose nebulized or one puff by MDI for children weighing less than 10 kg; a 0.5-mg unit dose nebulized or two puffs by MDI for children weighing more than 10 kg.

If a child is in severe respiratory distress, is obtunded, or has markedly diminished air movement on auscultation, a dose of SQ or IM epinephrine may be required. Epinephrine will cause immediate relaxation of bronchial smooth muscles, opening the airways to allow bronchodilators to work. The dose is 0.01 mg/kg of 1:1,000 epinephrine injected SQ or IM; single doses should not exceed 0.3 mg. Initiate bronchodilator therapy immediately after administering the epinephrine.

Assisted ventilation is problematic for patients with an asthma exacerbation. High inspiratory pressures force air into the lungs, but exhalation is compromised by bronchospasm, mucus production, and inflammation, leading to air trapping and a high risk of pneumothorax and pneumomediastinum. Assisted ventilation should be undertaken only if the patient has respiratory failure and has failed to respond to SQ or IM epinephrine and high-dose bronchodilators. If this therapy is performed, use very slow rates to allow time for adequate exhalation: Your goal is adequate oxygenation.

Bronchiolitis

Bronchiolitis is an inflammation of the small airways (bronchioles) in the lower respiratory tract due to viral infection. The most common source of this disease is respiratory syncytial virus (RSV), although a new virus, Metapneumovirus, has also been found to cause this illness. These viruses occur with highest frequency during the late fall and winter months, and they primarily affect infants and children younger than 2 years. Severity ranges from mild to moderate respiratory distress with hypoxia and respiratory failure. Younger infants are at particularly high risk for episodes of apnea associated with RSV infection, which may not be associated with severe respiratory distress.

The signs and symptoms of bronchiolitis can be difficult to distinguish from those of asthma. One clue is the child's age: Asthma is rare in children younger than 1 year. An infant with a first-time wheezing episode occurring in late fall or winter likely has bronchiolitis. Mild to moderate retractions, tachypnea, diffuse wheezing, diffuse crackles, and mild hypoxia are characteristic findings on the PAT and initial assessment. As with asthma, a sleepy or obtunded patient or one with severe retractions, diminished breath sounds, or moderate to severe hypoxia (oxygen saturation < 90%) is in danger of respiratory failure and requires immediate transport. Infants in the first months of life or who have a history of prematurity, underlying lung disease, congenital heart disease, or immunodeficiency are at greatest risk for respiratory failure and arrest.

The management of infants and young children with bronchiolitis is entirely supportive. Leave the patient in a position of comfort (eg, in the caregiver's arms, if the child does not seem to be in respiratory failure), and provide supplemental oxygen. Although bronchodilator therapy has not proved effective in the majority of cases, inhaled albuterol or nebulized racemic epinephrine (0.5 mL of a 2.25% solution for inhalation) may be given as a therapeutic trial in children with moderate to severe respiratory distress. Be prepared to assist ventilation with bag-mask ventilation or endotracheal intubation if needed.

Management of Respiratory Emergencies

Infants and young children with severe tachypnea and retractions, in association with hypoxia, bradycardia, or altered mental status, are in respiratory failure and need immediate intervention to prevent respiratory arrest. A respiratory rate too slow for age in a child with a history of respiratory distress should also raise concerns for respiratory fatigue and failure.

Airway Management

The first step in managing any respiratory emergency is to start with the airway. Check for obstruction, and position the airway using the head tilt–chin lift or jaw-thrust maneuver **Figure 41-13 ▶** . In a young infant, place a small roll under the shoulders to align the airway **Figure 41-14 ▶** .

An airway adjunct may be helpful if the patient is unresponsive and cannot maintain a patent airway. The use of a nasal or oral airway will help to maintain an open airway, improve bag-mask ventilation, and may avert the need for an advanced airway (such as an ET tube, laryngeal mask airway, or Combitube). When placing the adjunct, make sure to start by choosing the appropriately sized equipment.

Oropharyngeal Airway

An oropharyngeal (oral) airway is designed to keep the tongue from blocking the airway, and it makes suctioning the airway easier. This kind of airway should be used for pediatric patients who are unresponsive and cannot maintain their own airway

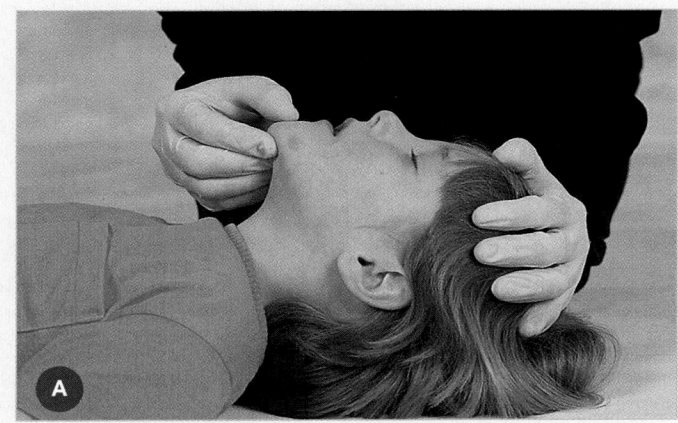

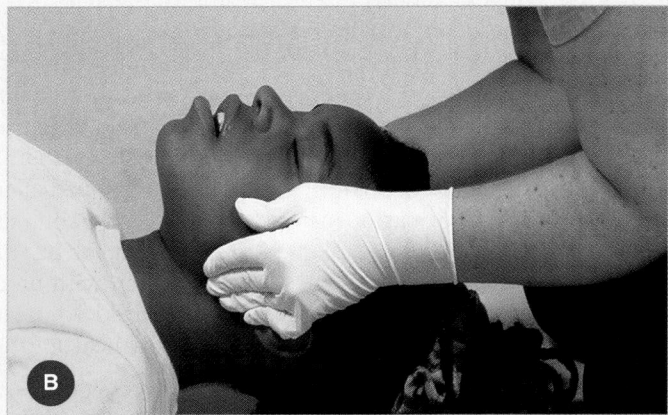

Figure 41-13 A. Use the head tilt–chin lift maneuver to open the airway of a child without trauma. **B.** For a child with suspected spinal injury, use the jaw-thrust maneuver to open the airway.

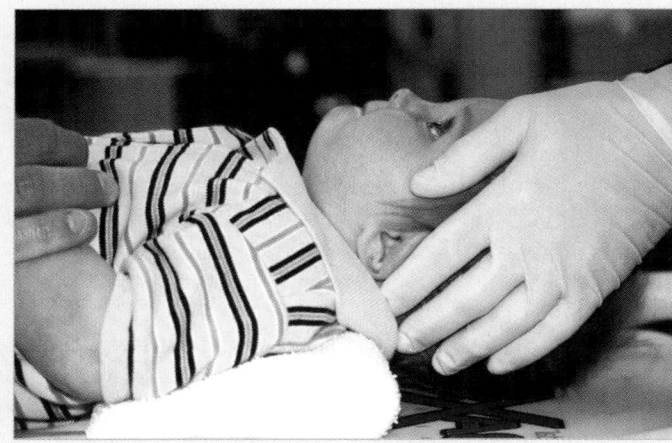

Figure 41-14 Use a shoulder roll in an infant without trauma to position the airway in a neutral position.

spontaneously. It should *not* be used for conscious patients or patients with a gag reflex—an oropharyngeal airway may stimulate vomiting, thereby increasing the risk of aspiration. In addition, this adjunct should *not* be used for children who have ingested a caustic (corrosive) or petroleum-based product.

Skill Drill 41-1 ▸ shows the preferred technique for inserting an oropharyngeal airway in a child.

1. Determine the appropriately sized airway by measuring from the corner of the mouth to the earlobe or by using the length-based resuscitation tape to measure the patient.
2. Place the airway next to the face, with the flange at the level of the central incisors and the bite block segment parallel to the hard palate. The tip of the airway should reach the angle of the jaw (Step 1).
3. Position the patient's airway. For medical patients, use the head tilt–chin lift maneuver, avoiding hyperextension; you may place a towel under the patient's shoulders. If the patient has a traumatic injury, use the jaw-thrust maneuver and provide in-line spinal stabilization (Step 2).
4. Open the mouth by applying pressure on the chin with your thumb.
5. Insert the airway by depressing the tongue with a tongue blade on the base of the tongue and inserting the airway directly over the tongue blade. If a tongue blade is not available, point the airway tip toward the roof of the mouth to depress the tongue. Gently rotate the airway into position as it passes through the mouth toward the curve of the tongue. Insert the airway until the flange rests against the lips.
6. Reassess the airway after insertion (Step 3).

Take care to avoid injuring the hard palate as you insert the airway. Rough insertion can cause bleeding, which may aggravate airway problems and cause vomiting. If the oropharyngeal airway is too small, the tongue may be pushed back into the pharynx, obstructing the airway. If it is too large, it may obstruct the larynx.

Nasopharyngeal Airway

A nasopharyngeal (nasal) airway is usually well tolerated and is not as likely as the oropharyngeal airway to cause vomiting. The nasopharyngeal airway is used for conscious patients and patients with altered levels of consciousness. In pediatric patients, it is typically used in association with respiratory failure. It is also a good choice for patients having a seizure or in a postictal state as a way of maintaining an airway. This type of airway is rarely used for children younger than 1 year because of the small diameter of their nares, which tend to become easily obstructed by secretions.

Follow the steps in **Skill Drill 41-2 ▸** to insert a nasopharyngeal airway in a child.

1. Determine the appropriately sized airway. The external diameter of the airway should not be larger than the diameter of one of the external openings of the nose (nares), and there should be no blanching (turning white) of the nare after insertion.
2. Place the airway next to the patient's face to make sure the length is correct. The airway should extend from the tip of the nose to the tragus of the ear (that is, the small cartilaginous projection in front of the opening of the ear).
3. Position the patient's airway, using the techniques described for the oropharyngeal airway (Step 1).

Table 41-11 DOPE: Troubleshooting the ET Tube

Problem	Assessment	Intervention
Dislodgment		
Esophageal intubation	No ETCO$_2$ reading or color change Oxygen saturation < 90% Bradycardia Lack of chest rise with ventilation Auscultation of bubbling over stomach	Extubate Bag-mask ventilation Reintubate
Mainstem bronchus intubation	Asymmetric chest rise Asymmetric breath sounds	Pull tube back until breath sounds and chest rise are symmetric
Accidental extubation	Same as esophageal intubation Poor or absent air movement on auscultation	Bag-mask ventilation Reintubate
Obstruction		
Tube blocked with blood, secretions, or kink	Decreased chest rise Decreased breath sounds bilaterally Oxygen saturation < 90% Increased resistance to bagging	Suction Extubate Bag-mask ventilation Reintubate
Pneumothorax		
Tension pneumothorax, spontaneous or induced	Asymmetric chest rise Asymmetric breath sounds Shock Oxygen saturation < 90% Jugular venous distention* Tracheal deviation*	Needle thoracostomy
Equipment		
Big air leak around tube Activated pop-off valve on resuscitator Oxygen tubing disconnected Oxygen tank empty		Check equipment "patient to tank"

*Not easily accessed or frequently seen in young children.

- Presence of epigastric gurgling sounds or vomitus in the ET tube
- Failure to confirm proper tube position with detection devices

In a patient with spontaneous circulation, lack of a color on a colorimetric device indicates esophageal intubation. In such a case, the ET tube should be removed, bag-mask ventilation resumed for 2 minutes, and endotracheal intubation reattempted.

If an intubated patient experiences a sudden decline in respiratory status, use the DOPE mnemonic (Dislodgment, Obstruction, Pneumothorax, Equipment) to identify the potential problem, and institute an appropriate intervention **Table 41-11 ▲**.

In the Field

Calculate the endotracheal tube size for a child older than 1 year as follows:

$$\frac{(Age + 16)}{4} = \text{Size of ET tube (in mm)}$$

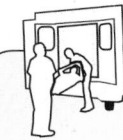

Documentation and Communication

Vital signs, especially pulse rate and oxygen saturation, should be recorded before and after each intubation attempt. Record the size of the ET tube and the depth of insertion as measured at the patient's lip.

Orogastric and Nasogastric Tube Insertion

During positive-pressure ventilation, it is common to inflate the stomach, as well as the lungs, with air. Gastric distention slows downward movement of the diaphragm and decreases tidal volume, making ventilation more difficult and necessitating higher inspiratory pressures. It also increases the risk that the patient will vomit and aspirate stomach contents into the lungs. Placement of a nasogastric (NG) tube or an orogastric (OG) tube decompresses the stomach and makes assisted ventilation easier.

Gastric decompression with an NG or OG tube is contraindicated in unresponsive children with a poor or absent gag reflex and an unsecured airway. Instead, you should perform

Special Considerations

A single intubation attempt should be limited to 20 seconds. If the attempt is not successful after 20 seconds, resume bag-mask ventilation and preoxygenate the child for the next attempt.

endotracheal intubation first to decrease the risk of vomiting and aspiration.

Preparation of Equipment

To perform NG or OG tube insertion, you will need an appropriately sized NG or OG tube; a 30- to 60-mL syringe with a funnel-tipped adapter for manual removal of stomach contents through the tube; mechanical suction; adhesive tape; and a water-soluble lubricant. To prepare the patient and the equipment for NG or OG tube placement:

1. Select the proper size of tube. Use a length-based resuscitation tape to determine the proper size, or use a tube size twice the ET tube size that the child would need. For example, a child who needs a 5.0-mm ET tube requires a 10F OG or NG tube.
2. Measure the tube on the patient. The length of the tube should be the same as the distance from the lips or tip of the nose (depending on whether the OG or NG route is used) to the earlobe *plus* the distance from the earlobe to the xiphoid process **Figure 41-19 ▶**.
3. Mark this length on the tube with a piece of tape. When the tip of the tube is in the stomach, the tape should be at the lips or nostril.

4. Place the patient in a supine position.
5. Assess the gag reflex. If the patient is unresponsive and has a poor or absent gag reflex, perform endotracheal intubation before gastric tube placement.
6. In a trauma patient, maintain in-line stabilization of the cervical spine if a neck injury is possible. Choose the OG route of insertion if the patient has a severe head or midfacial injury.
7. Lubricate the end of the tube.

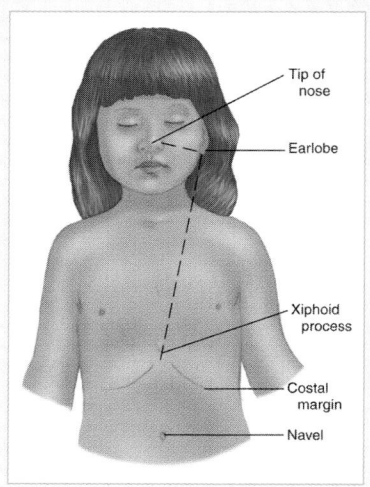

Figure 41-19 Technique for measuring the distance to insert an NG or OG tube.

OG Tube Insertion

Follow these steps to insert an OG tube in an infant or child:

1. Insert the tube over the tongue, using a tongue blade if necessary to facilitate insertion.
2. Advance the tube into the hypopharynx, then insert it rapidly into the stomach.

You are the Provider Part 3

As you prepare to immobilize the patient for transport, he begins to vomit. You, your partner, and the fire fighter maintaining manual cervical spine stabilization log roll the child using a coordinated movement directed by the fire fighter. You suction what appear to be chunks of French toast from the child's mouth and back of his throat. After suctioning, the child's oxygen saturation falls to 90%, his respiratory rate decreases to 16 breaths/min, and work of breathing increases. Your partner immediately begins bag-mask ventilation using 100% oxygen, while you quickly measure the child using a length-based resuscitation tape and gather the appropriate intubation equipment.

The child is successfully intubated with a 4.5 uncuffed ET tube using in-line cervical spine stabilization for potential cervical spine injury. You confirm ET tube placement by direct visualization of the vocal cords, bilateral breath sounds, and a positive color change on the colorimetric ETCO$_2$ detector. You then secure the ET tube at the 14-cm mark at the child's lip. Your partner continues to provide bag-mask ventilation at a rate of 20 breaths/min with 100% supplemental oxygen while you reassess the patient.

Reassessment	Recording Time: 10 Minutes
Skin	Pale, cool, and dry
Pulse	190 beats/min, regular; weak distally but strong centrally
ECG	Narrow complex tachycardia
Blood pressure	78/46 mm Hg
Respirations	20 breaths/min via bag-mask ventilation
Sao$_2$	97% on bag-mask ventilation at 100% oxygen
Pupils	Equal and reactive to light
Capillary refill	4 seconds

5. Is this child in shock? If so, is it compensated or decompensated?
6. How should your patient management progress?

3. If the child begins coughing or choking or has a change in voice, immediately remove the tube; it may be in the trachea.

NG Tube Insertion

Follow these steps to insert an NG tube in an infant or child:

1. Insert the tube gently through the nostril, directing the tube straight back. Do not angle the tube superiorly.
2. If the tube does not pass easily, try the opposite nostril or a smaller tube. Never force the tube.
3. If NG passage is unsuccessful, use the OG approach.

Assessing Placement of OG and NG Tubes

Follow these steps to confirm successful placement of an NG or OG tube:

1. Check tube placement by aspirating stomach contents. Use a syringe with an appropriate adapter to quickly instill 10 to 20 mL of air through the tube while auscultating over the left upper quadrant. If you hear a rush of air (or gurgling) over the stomach, the placement is correct.
2. If correct placement cannot be confirmed, remove the tube.
3. Secure the tube to the bridge of the nose or to the cheek, using adhesive tape.
4. Aspirate air from the stomach, using a 30- to 60-mL catheter-tipped syringe, or connect the tube to mechanical suction at a low, continuous suction of 20 to 40 mm Hg or to the intermittent setting.

Complications of OG or NG Tube Insertion

As with endotracheal intubation, you must be aware of the potential complications associated with the placement of an NG or OG tube—namely, placement of the tube into the trachea, resulting in hypoxia; vomiting and aspiration of stomach contents; airway bleeding or obstruction; and passage of the tube into the cranium. The last complication can occur if you insert an NG tube into a patient with severe head or midfacial trauma because the tube may be passed through the fracture and into the brain.

Cardiovascular Emergencies

Cardiovascular emergencies are relatively rare in children. When such problems arise, they are often related to volume or infection rather than a primary cardiac cause, unless the child has congenital heart disease. Through the PAT and initial assessment, you can quickly identify a cardiovascular emergency, understand the likely cause, and institute potentially lifesaving treatment.

General Assessment and Management

As with all pediatric emergencies, when called to a scene for a suspected cardiac complaint, begin the hands-off assessment by using the PAT and then move on to the initial assessment using the ABCs. The child's appearance gives an overview of perfusion, oxygenation, ventilation, and neurologic status. For a suspected cardiovascular problem, an abnormal appearance may indicate inadequate brain perfusion and the need for rapid intervention. Tachypnea, without retractions or abnormal airway sounds, is common in an infant or child with a primary cardiac problem; it is a mechanism for blowing off carbon dioxide to compensate for metabolic acidosis related to poor perfusion. In contrast, when cardiac compromise progresses to congestive heart failure, pulmonary edema leads to increased work of breathing and a fast respiratory rate. The presence of pallor, cyanosis, or mottling may tip you off to this problem.

For suspected cardiovascular compromise, start with airway and breathing, and provide supportive care as needed. Ensure adequate oxygenation and ventilation, and then assess the circulation by checking heart rate, pulse quality, skin CTC, and blood pressure when possible. Combine information from the PAT and initial assessment to make an initial decision about the likely underlying cause, the patient's priority, and the need for immediate treatment or transport.

If you determine that the patient's condition is stable enough for you to continue the assessment on site, continue with the SAMPLE history and the focused physical exam. (Table 41-12 ▸ reviews key elements of a cardiovascular SAMPLE history.) Repeat the PAT and ABCs after each intervention, and monitor trends over time.

Shock

Shock is defined as inadequate delivery of oxygen and nutrients to tissues to meet metabolic demand. The types of shock that you may encounter are the same in adults and children: hypovolemic, distributive, and cardiogenic.

Besides determining the cause of shock, you must quickly determine whether the child is in a compensated or decompensated state. In compensated shock, although the child has critical abnormalities of perfusion, his or her body is (for the moment) able to mount a physiologic response to maintain adequate perfusion to vital organs by shunting blood from the periphery, increasing the heart rate, and increasing the vascular tone. A child in compensated shock will have a normal appearance, tachycardia, and signs of decreased peripheral perfusion, such as cool extremities with prolonged capillary refill. Timely intervention is needed to prevent a child in compensated shock from decompensating.

Decompensated shock is a state of inadequate perfusion in which the body's own mechanisms to improve perfusion are no longer sufficient to maintain a normal blood pressure. By definition, a child in decompensated shock will be hypotensive for age Table 41-13 ▸ . In addition to being profoundly tachycardic and showing signs of poor peripheral perfusion, a child in decompensated shock may have an altered appearance, reflecting inadequate perfusion of the brain. Because children typically have strong cardiovascular systems, they are able to compensate for inadequate perfusion by increasing heart rate and peripheral vascular resistance more efficiently than adults. Hypotension is, therefore, a late and ominous sign in an infant

Table 41-12	SAMPLE Components for a Child With Cardiovascular Problems
Components	**Features**
Signs and symptoms	Presence of vomiting or diarrhea Number of episodes of vomiting or diarrhea Vomiting blood or bile; blood in stool External hemorrhage Presence or absence of fever Rash Respiratory distress or shortness of breath
Allergies	Known allergies History of anaphylaxis
Medications	Exact names and dosages of ongoing medications Use of laxative or antidiarrheal medications Long-term diuretic therapy Potential exposure to other medications or drugs Timing and dosages of analgesics or antipyretics
Past medical problems	History of heart problems History of prematurity Prior hospitalizations for cardiovascular problems
Last oral intake	Timing of the child's last food or drink, including bottle or breastfeeding
Events leading to injury or illness	Travel Trauma Fever history Symptoms in family members Potential toxic exposure

Table 41-13	Lower Limits of Normal Systolic Blood Pressure by Age
Age	**Minimum Systolic Blood Pressure**
Infant (1 month to 1 year)	> 70 mm Hg
1-year-old child	> 80 mm Hg
Child (1–10 years)	70 + (2 × age in years)
Child or adolescent > 10 years	> 90 mm Hg

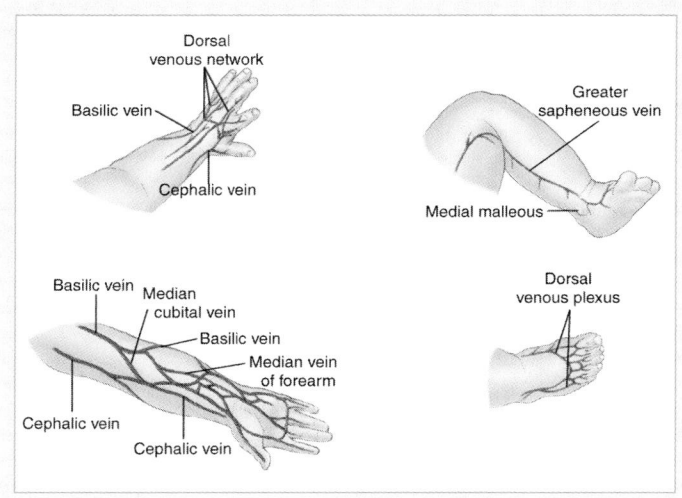

Figure 41-20 Sites for IV access in infants and children include the hands, antecubital fossa, saphenous veins at the ankle, and feet.

Hypovolemic Shock

Hypovolemia is the most common cause of shock in infants and young children, with loss of volume occurring due to illness or trauma. Because of their small blood volume (80 mL/kg body weight), a combination of excessive fluid losses and poor intake in an infant or a young child with gastroenteritis ("stomach flu") can result in shock relatively quickly. The same vulnerability exists with hemorrhage from trauma.

A patient with hypovolemic shock will often appear listless or lethargic and may have compensatory tachypnea. The child may appear pale, mottled, or cyanotic. In medical shock, further assessment may identify signs of dehydration such as sunken eyes, dry mucous membranes, poor skin turgor, or delayed capillary refill with cool extremities. In an injured child, the site of bleeding may be identified on the initial assessment or detailed physical exam.

Allow the child to remain in a position of comfort, administer supplemental oxygen, and keep the child warm. Apply direct pressure to stop any external bleeding. Volume replacement is the mainstay of treatment for hypovolemic shock, whether medical or traumatic in origin.

If the child is in compensated shock, you can attempt to establish IV or intraosseous (IO) access en route to the hospital. As with all procedures, gather all the equipment necessary before beginning this step. Catheters—preferably an over-the-needle catheter—are available in pediatric sizes of 20, 22, and 24 gauge. A butterfly needle is a temporary alternative if an over-the-needle catheter is unavailable; this stainless steel needle stays in the vein, predisposing it to infiltration.

Many of the sites used for IV access in adults are the same for children. The most commonly used sites are the dorsum of the hand and the antecubital fossa. In children, veins in the foot may also be used **Figure 41-20 ▲**. Scalp veins and the external jugular veins are used less commonly.

or a young child, and urgent intervention is needed to prevent cardiac arrest.

Initial management involves allowing the child to assume a position of comfort and starting supplemental oxygen. After completing the initial assessment, make a transport decision based on the severity of the problem. Start resuscitation on scene for any child who shows signs of decompensated shock. While rapid transport is imperative, the risk of deterioration to cardiac arrest is too high to permit a "load-and-go" approach.

The procedure for establishing IV access is as follows:

1. Select the vein that you will use.
2. Secure the appropriate limb to minimize movement during the procedure.
3. Apply a tourniquet proximal to the selected site.
4. Clean the site with alcohol.
5. Insert the catheter through the skin with the bevel facing upward. Be sure to enter the skin at a shallow angle parallel to the vein.
6. Advance the catheter until you see blood return into the hub.
7. Continue to gently advance the catheter over the needle into the vein until the hub of the catheter is flush with the skin.
8. Completely remove the needle and attach IV tubing.
9. Flush the catheter with saline. Note if the line is easily flushed or if there is resistance. Resistance may mean that the catheter has infiltrated the vein. Carefully look at the surrounding skin for infiltration of fluids. If the line is infiltrated, remove it.
10. Secure the catheter with tape or a clear plastic dressing. Wrap the IV tubing with extra gauze to prevent the child from pulling out the IV catheter.

Once IV access is established, fluid resuscitation should begin with isotonic fluids *only,* such as normal saline or lactated Ringer's. Begin with 20 mL/kg of isotonic fluid, and then reassess the patient's status. The use of warm IV fluids (when possible) can counteract the effects of systemic hypothermia from environmental exposure, blood loss, or open wounds. Multiple fluid boluses may be necessary during transport.

Volume resuscitation should be addressed separately from treatment of hypoglycemia. In a child with shock due to medical illness, perform a bedside glucose check; treat with dextrose-containing fluid only for a documented low blood glucose level. Hypoglycemia is unlikely in shock due to acute injury.

If a child is in decompensated shock with hypotension, begin initial fluid resuscitation at the scene. Make one attempt at IV access. If it is unsuccessful, begin IO infusion. When an IO needle is placed correctly, it will rest in the medullary canal, the space within the bone that contains bone marrow. An IO infusion is contraindicated if a secure IV line is available or if a fracture (or possible fracture) exists in the same bone in which you plan to insert the IO needle. Anything that can be administered IV can be administered through an IO line (such as isotonic fluids, medications).

The IO needles are usually double needles, consisting of a solid-bore needle inside a sharpened hollow needle **Figure 41-21 ▶**. This double needle is pushed into the bone (usually the proximal tibia) with a screwing, twisting action. Once the needle pops through the bone, the solid

Notes from Nancy

Be alert for signs of shock or respiratory insufficiency in any child who has sustained blunt chest trauma.

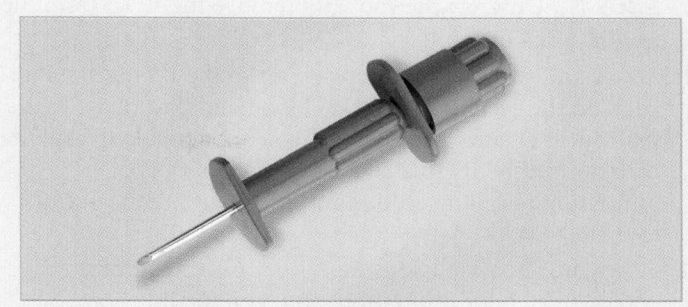

Figure 41-21 Standard pediatric IO needle.

needle is removed, leaving the hollow steel needle in place. Standard IV tubing is attached to this catheter.

The IO lines require full and careful immobilization because they rest at a 90° angle to the bone and are easily dislodged. Stabilize the IO needle, thereby ensuring adequate flow, in the same manner that you would any impaled object. As with any invasive procedure, several complications may be associated with IO infusion: compartment syndrome, failed infusion, growth plate injury, bone inflammation caused by infection (osteomyelitis), skin infection, and bony fracture. Proper technique will help to minimize these complications.

Follow the steps in **Skill Drill 41-5 ▶** to establish an IO infusion in pediatric patients:

1. Check the IV fluid for proper fluid, clarity, and expiration date. Look for any discoloration or particles floating in the fluid. If any are found, discard and choose another bag of fluid.
2. Select the appropriate equipment, including an IO needle, syringe, saline, and extension set **Step 1**. A three-way stopcock may also be used to facilitate easier fluid administration.
3. Select the proper administration set. Connect the administration set to the bag. Prepare the administration set. Fill the drip chamber, and flush the tubing. Make sure no air bubbles remain in the tubing.
4. Prepare the syringe and extension tubing **Step 2**.
5. Cut or tear the tape. This can be done at any time before the IO puncture.
6. Take BSI isolation precautions. This must be done before the IO puncture.
7. Identify the proper anatomic site for IO puncture **Step 3**. To miss the epiphyseal (growth) plate, you should measure two fingerbreadths below the knee on the medial side of the leg.
8. Cleanse the site using aseptic technique (that is, in a circular manner from the inside out).
9. Stabilize the tibia. Place a folded towel under the knee, and hold it so that you keep your fingers away from the puncture site.
10. Insert the needle at a 90° angle to the leg. Advance the needle with a twisting motion until you feel a "pop"

Step 4 . Unscrew the cap, and remove the stylet from the needle Step 5 .

11. Attach the syringe and extension set to the IO needle. Pull back on the syringe to aspirate blood and particles of bone marrow to ensure placement. If you are not able to aspirate marrow but the IO flushes easily with no signs of infiltration (swelling around insertion site), then continue to flush.

12. Slowly inject saline to ensure proper placement of the needle. Watch for infiltration, and stop the infusion immediately if any is noted.

13. It is possible to fracture the bone during insertion of the IO. If this happens, you should remove the IO needle and switch to the other leg.

14. Connect the administration set, and adjust the flow rate. Fluid does not flow well through an IO needle, and boluses are given by administering the fluid using the syringe and a three-way stopcock Step 6 .

15. Secure the needle with tape, and support it with a bulky dressing. Be careful not to tape around the entire circumference of the leg, which could impair circulation and create compartment syndrome.

16. Dispose of the needle in the proper container Step 7 .

As with IV administration, give 20-mL/kg boluses of isotonic fluid via IO infusion to treat hypovolemia, reassessing after each bolus and repeating as needed based on physiologic response. As much as 60 mL/kg may be needed during transport to improve the child's blood pressure, pulse rate, mental status, and peripheral perfusion. Rapidly transport the patient to an appropriate treatment facility.

Distributive Shock

In distributive shock, decreased vascular tone develops, resulting in vasodilation and third spacing of fluids due to increased vascular permeability (leakage of plasma out of the blood vessels and into the surrounding tissues). This results in a drop in effective blood volume and functional hypovolemia. Distributive shock may be due to sepsis, anaphylaxis, and spinal cord injury; sepsis accounts for the bulk of pediatric cases.

Early in distributive shock, the child may have warm, flushed skin and bounding pulses as a result of peripheral vasodilation. In contrast, the symptoms and signs of *late* distributive shock will look much like hypovolemic shock on initial assessment. Fever is a key finding in septic shock, whereas urticarial rash and wheezing may be noted in anaphylaxis, and neurologic deficits are apparent in shock due to spinal cord injury.

Front-line treatment of distributive shock is volume resuscitation because the child is in a state of relative hypovolemia. In a child with apparent sepsis who remains persistently hypotensive despite a total of 60 mL/kg of isotonic fluid, vasopressor support to improve vascular tone may be considered.

Anaphylactic shock should be treated immediately with SQ or IM epinephrine, 0.01 mg/kg of 1:1,000 solution (maximum dose, 0.3 mg). This dose should be repeated as necessary every 5 minutes. If several doses are needed, the child may require a low-dose, continuous epinephrine IV drip. The decision about timing of IV access and transport for distributive shock considers the same factors as for hypovolemic shock.

Cardiogenic Shock

Cardiogenic shock is the result of pump failure: Intravascular volume is normal, but myocardial function is poor. This type of shock is uncommon in the pediatric population but may be present in children with underlying congenital heart disease, myocarditis, or rhythm disturbances. It is important to recognize cardiogenic shock by the child's history or from the initial assessment because the treatment for this type of shock is very different from that for hypovolemic or distributive shock.

A child in cardiogenic shock will appear listless or lethargic (like children in hypovolemic or distributive shock) but is likely to show signs of increased work of breathing owing to congestive heart failure and pulmonary edema. Circulation will be impaired, and skin will look pale, mottled, or cyanotic. Your initial assessment may reveal an abnormal heart rate or rhythm or a murmur or gallop. The child's skin may feel clammy, and you may feel an enlarged liver. The caregiver may describe the infant sweating with feeding and, in many cases, will recount a history of congenital heart disease.

Special Considerations
Shock in children is most likely due to hypovolemia. Fluid resuscitation with isotonic fluid is the mainstay of treatment.

If you suspect cardiogenic shock, allow the child to remain in a position of comfort (often sitting upright), administer supplemental oxygen, and transport. The transport destination is a critical decision because the ultimate management requires pediatric critical care capability. Supplemental oxygen may not increase the SaO$_2$ in children with particular types of congenital heart disease, and parents will often alert you to this fact. Consider establishing IV access en route to the receiving facility. Unless you are sure of the diagnosis of cardiogenic shock (the child has a history of congenital heart disease, is afebrile, and has no history of volume loss), err on the side of fluid resuscitation. If you suspect cardiac dysfunction, administer a single isotonic fluid bolus slowly, and monitor carefully to assess its effect. Increased work of breathing, a drop in oxygen saturation, or worsening perfusion after a fluid bolus will confirm your suspicion of cardiogenic shock. Although inotropic agents may be needed to improve cardiac contractility and improve perfusion, they are rarely administered in the field.

In the Field
A child with decompensated shock from hypovolemia needs fluid resuscitation. Do not waste time with multiple IV insertion attempts. Insert an IO needle, and begin fluid therapy.

Skill Drill 41-5: Pediatric IO Infusion

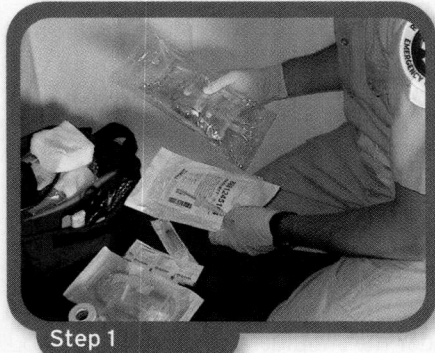

Step 1

Check selected IV fluid for proper fluid, clarity, and expiration date.
Select the appropriate equipment, including an IO needle, syringe, saline, and extension.

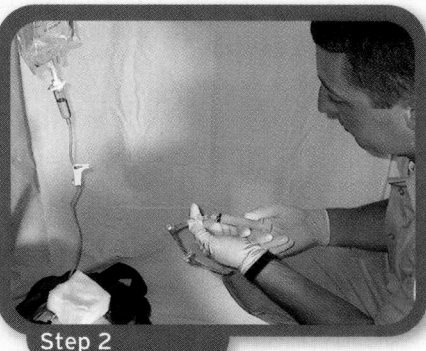

Step 2

Select the proper administration set. Connect the administration set to the bag. Prepare the administration set. Prepare the syringe and extension tubing.

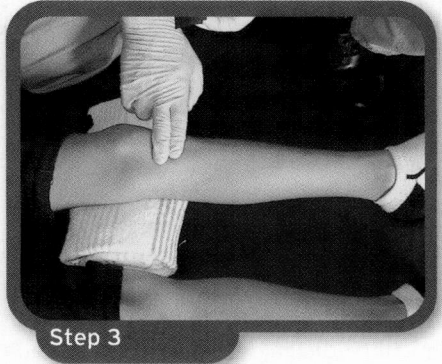

Step 3

Cut or tear the tape. Take BSI precautions.
Identify the proper anatomic site for IO puncture.

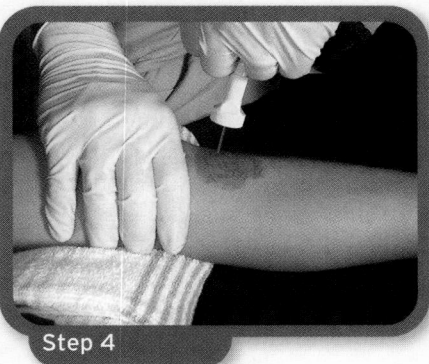

Step 4

Cleanse the site appropriately.
Stabilize the tibia.
Insert the needle at the proper angle.
Advance the needle with a twisting motion until a "pop" is felt.

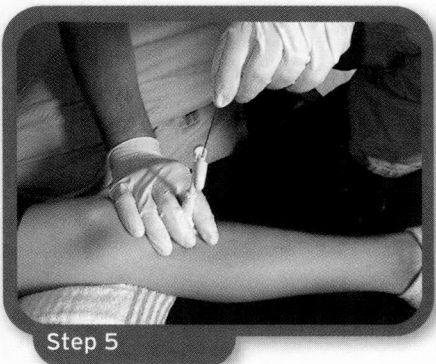

Step 5

Unscrew the cap, and remove the stylet from the needle.

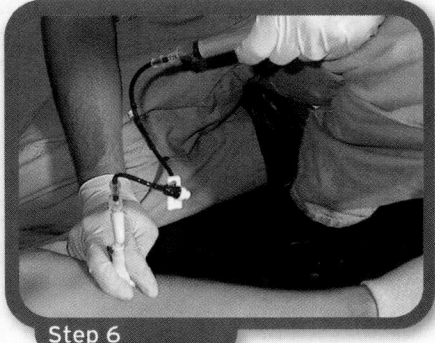

Step 6

Attach the syringe and extension set to the IO needle.
Pull back on the syringe to aspirate blood and particles of bone marrow to ensure placement.
Slowly inject saline to assure proper placement of the needle.
Watch for infiltration, and stop the infusion immediately if noted.
Connect the administration set, and adjust the flow rate as appropriate.

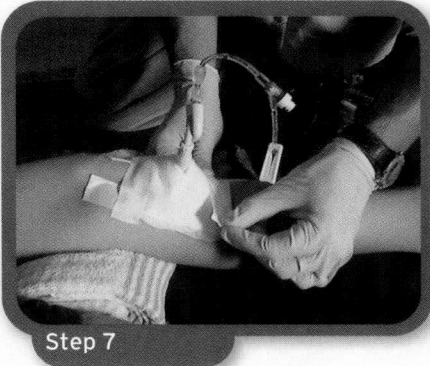

Step 7

Secure the needle with tape, and support it with a bulky dressing.
Dispose of the needle in the proper container.

Arrhythmias

Rhythm disturbances can be classified based on whether the heart beat is too slow (bradyarrhythmias), too fast (tachyarrhythmias), or absent (pulseless). The signs and symptoms associated with a rhythm disturbance are often nonspecific—for example, the patient or caregiver may report fatigue, irritability, vomiting, chest or abdominal pain, palpitations, and shortness of breath. If you suspect a rhythm disturbance, quickly move through the PAT and initial assessment, supporting the airway and breathing as necessary. An ECG or rhythm strip will help to identify the underlying rhythm and suggest which specific management steps should be initiated. Address reversible causes of arrhythmias such as hypoxemia. The decision to stay on scene to obtain additional history and perform a focused physical exam will be dictated by the child's overall physiologic status.

Bradyarrhythmias

Bradyarrhythmias in children most often occur secondary to hypoxia, rather than as a result of a primary cardiac problem (such as heart block). Airway management, supplemental oxygen, and assisted ventilation as needed are always first-line treatment. Also, treat any underlying respiratory problem. Less common causes of bradycardia include congenital or acquired heart block and toxic ingestion of beta blockers, calcium channel blockers, or digoxin. Elevated ICP can also cause bradycardia and should be considered in children with ventricular shunts, a history of head injury, or suspected child abuse without a consistent injury history.

Initiate electronic cardiac monitoring as part of your initial assessment. If the child is asymptomatic, no further treatment is indicated in the field. Healthy, athletic adolescents may have bradycardia as an incidental finding and should be transported to a hospital for further evaluation.

If the child's pulse rate is lower than normal for age despite oxygenation and ventilation and perfusion is poor, begin chest compressions and attempt IV or IO access. For chest compressions to be effective, the patient should be placed on a firm, flat surface with the head at the same level as the body. If you need to carry an infant while providing CPR, your forearm and hand can serve as the flat surface.

Follow the steps in **Skill Drill 41-6** ▾ to perform infant chest compressions:

1. Place the infant on a firm surface, using one hand to keep the head in an open airway position. You can also use a pad or wedge under the shoulders and upper body to keep the head from tilting forward.

2. Imagine a line drawn between the nipples. Place two fingers in the middle of the sternum, one fingerbreadth below the imaginary intermammary line (**Step 1**).

3. Using two fingers, compress the sternum about one third to one half the depth of the chest. Push hard and fast (100 compressions/min), and allow full chest recoil. Minimize interruptions in chest compressions.

4. After each compression, allow the sternum to return briefly to its normal position. Allow equal time for compression and relaxation of the chest. Avoid jerky movements of your compressing fingers (**Step 2**).

5. Coordinate rapid compression and ventilation in a 30:2 ratio, making sure the infant's chest rises with each ventilation. You will find this easier to do if you use your

Skill Drill 41-6: Performing Infant Chest Compressions

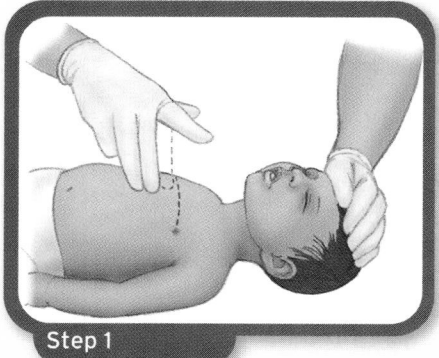

Step 1

Position the infant on a firm surface while maintaining the airway. Place two fingers in the middle of the sternum, one fingerbreadth below the imaginary intermammary line.

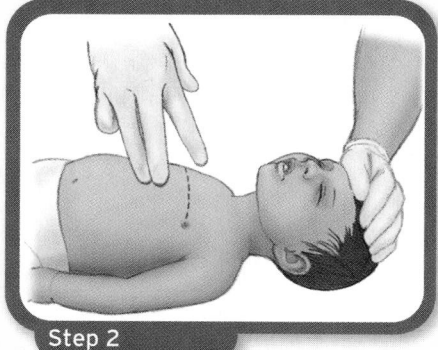

Step 2

Using two fingers, compress the sternum about one third to one half the depth of the chest. Push hard and fast, at a rate of 100 compressions/min. Allow the sternum to return briefly to its normal position between compressions.

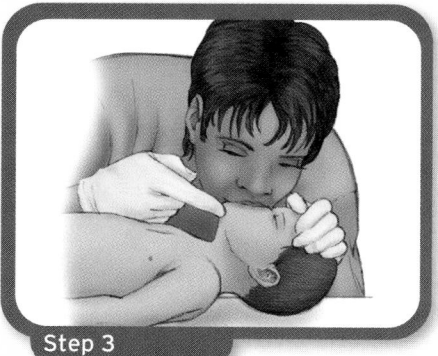

Step 3

Coordinate rapid compression and ventilation in a 30:2 ratio. Check for return of breathing and pulse after 2-minute intervals.

free hand to keep the head in the open airway position. If the chest does not rise or rises only a little, use a chin lift to open the airway. The compression/ventilation ratio can be 15:2 if there are two rescuers doing CPR.

6. Reassess the infant for signs of spontaneous breathing or pulses after 2 minutes (5 cycles) and again at each 2-minute interval (**Step 3**).

Skill Drill 41-7 ▶ shows the steps for performing chest compressions in children between 1 year and puberty (approximately 12 years):

1. Place the child on a firm surface, and use one hand to maintain the head tilt–chin lift (**Step 1**).
2. Place the heel of your hand over the middle of the sternum (between the nipples). Avoid compression over the lower tip of the sternum, which is called the xiphoid process (**Step 2**).
3. Compress the chest about one third to one half its total depth. Push hard and fast (100 compressions/min), and allow full chest recoil. Minimize interruptions in chest compressions. Compression and relaxation should be about the same duration. Use smooth movements, and hold your fingers off the child's ribs.
4. Coordinate rapid compression and ventilation in a 30:2 ratio, making sure that you see a visible chest rise with each ventilation (**Step 3**).
5. Reassess the child for signs of spontaneous breathing and pulses after 2 minutes (5 cycles of 30:2) and at 2-minute intervals.
6. If the child resumes effective breathing, place him or her in the recovery position (**Step 4**).

Quickly transport the patient to an appropriate receiving facility, while performing ongoing reassessments. If the child still has symptomatic bradycardia, medications are indicated. Epinephrine is the initial medication of choice; the dose should be repeated every 3 to 5 minutes as needed for symptomatic bradycardia. If you identify heart block, give atropine as the second medication. If the child continues to have symptomatic bradycardia, cardiac pacing may be indicated.

If the child's rhythm deteriorates, switch to the appropriate treatment algorithm.

Tachyarrhythmias

Sinus tachycardia, a pulse rate higher than normal for age, is common in children. Although it may be a sign of serious underlying illness or injury, it may also be due to fever, pain, or anxiety. Interpret the presence of tachycardia in the context of the remainder of the PAT and initial assessment. For example,

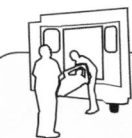

In the Field

The preferred agent for pediatric bradycardia is epinephrine unless the bradycardia is suspected to be from increased vagal tone.

Skill Drill 41-7: Performing Chest Compressions on a Child

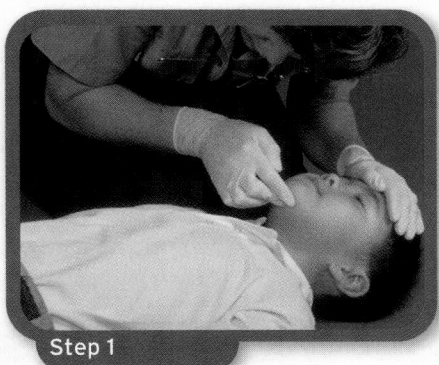

Step 1

Place the child on a firm surface, and use one hand to maintain the head tilt-chin lift.

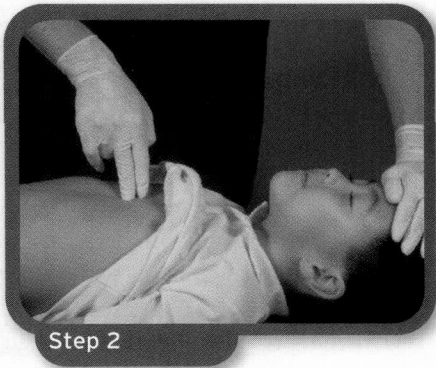

Step 2

Place the heel of your hand over the middle of the sternum (between the nipples); avoid compression of the xiphoid process.

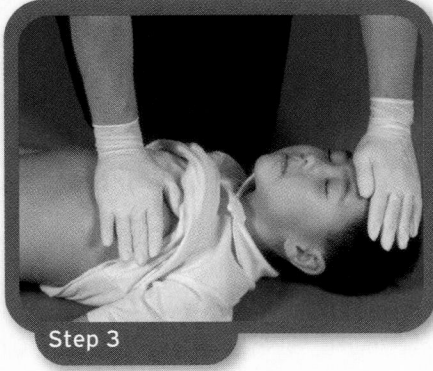

Step 3

Coordinate compression with ventilation in a 30:2 ratio, pausing for ventilation.

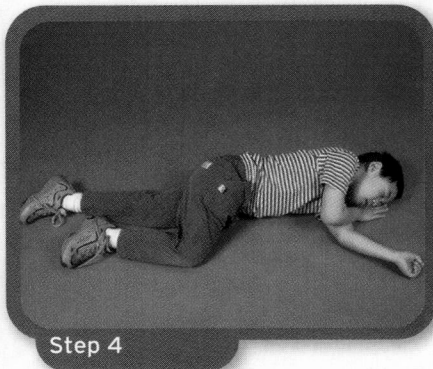

Step 4

Reassess breathing and pulse after 2 minutes and at 2-minute intervals thereafter. If the child resumes effective breathing, place him or her in the recovery position.

if a child appears well but has a fever, sinus tachycardia is likely and treatment with antipyretics is all that is necessary. If a tachycardic child has a history of copious vomiting or diarrhea, fluid resuscitation is the appropriate treatment.

If a tachycardic child appears ill and has poor perfusion with no history of fever, trauma, or excessive volume loss, continue your assessment for a primary cardiac cause while initiating resuscitation. Your assessment should include determination of pulse rate along with interpretation of an ECG or rhythm strip.

Tachyarrhythmias are subdivided into two types based on the width of the QRS complex. A narrow complex tachycardia exists when the QRS complex is 0.08 second or less (less than two standard boxes on the rhythm strip); a wide complex tachycardia exists when the QRS complex is greater than 0.08 second (more than two standard boxes on the rhythm strip).

Narrow Complex Tachycardia

Although sinus tachycardia is the most common arrhythmia in children, supraventricular tachycardia (SVT) is the most frequent tachyarrhythmia requiring antiarrhythmic treatment. Table 41-14 compares sinus tachycardia, reentry SVT, and ventricular tachycardia (V-tach). You may identify sinus tachycardia based on the presence or absence of P waves, pulse rate, and history of preceding illness or injury. Its treatment is geared toward the underlying cause and may include oxygen, fluids, splinting, and analgesia.

SVT, which involves abnormal conduction pathways, can be identified by a narrow QRS complex, absence of P waves, and an unvarying pulse rate of more than 220 beats/min in an infant or more than 180 beats/min in a child. The child may have a history of SVT or exhibit nonspecific signs and symptoms, including irritability, vomiting, and chest or abdominal pain. Parents of young infants may report poor feeding for sev-

eral days. The treatment of SVT depends on the patient's perfusion and overall stability. If the child is in stable condition, consider attempting vagal maneuvers while obtaining IV access: Have an older child hold his or her breath, blow into a straw with the end crimped over, or bear down as if having a bowel movement; in a younger child, place an exam glove filled with ice firmly over the midface, being careful not to obstruct the nose and mouth. Attempt these techniques only once, while continually monitoring the child's rhythm.

If the child has adequate perfusion and vagal maneuvers do not succeed in converting SVT to a sinus rhythm, consider administering adenosine. Adenosine has a short half-life and must be injected quickly into a vein near the heart, usually an antecubital vein. Its administration will be followed by a brief run of bradycardia, ventricular tachycardia, ventricular fibrillation, or asystole, which will convert spontaneously to sinus rhythm. Persistence of any of these rhythms is rare, but be prepared to switch arrhythmia algorithms if necessary.

For a child with SVT who has poor perfusion, synchronized cardioversion is recommended. Synchronized cardioversion is the timed administration of electrical energy to the heart to correct an arrhythmia. If the child is generating a regular but ineffective rhythm, it's important to time the jolt of electricity with the appropriate phase of the electrical activity (corresponds with the R wave on an ECG). A burst of electricity to the myocardium during the relative refractory period (the downward slope of the T wave) can precipitate ventricular fibrillation (V-fib)—a potentially lethal effect. Follow the same steps with synchronized cardioversion as with defibrillation, except that you must press the "sync" button on the defibrillator to alert the machine to time the electrical jolt. The dose of the initial synchronized cardioversion attempt is 0.5 to 1.0 joules per kilogram of body weight (J/kg). If the first dose is unsuccessful, a

Table 41-14 | **Features of Sinus Tachycardia, SVT, and V-tach**

	History	Pulse Rate	Respiratory Rate	QRS Interval	Assessment	Treatment
Sinus tachycardia	Fever, Volume loss, Hypoxia, Pain, Increased activity or exercise	< 220 beats/min (infant), < 180 beats/min (child)	Variable	Narrow: < 0.08 s	Hypovolemia, Hypoxia, Painful injury	Fluids, Oxygen, Splinting, Analgesia or sedation
Supraventricular tachycardia	Congenital heart disease, Known SVT, Nonspecific symptoms (such as poor feeding, fussiness)	> 220 beats/min (infants), > 180 beats/min (child)	Constant	Narrow: < 0.08 s	CHF* may be present	Vagal maneuvers (ice to face), Adenosine, Synchronized electrical cardioversion
Ventricular tachycardia	Serious systemic illness	> 150 beats/min	Variable	Wide: > 0.08 s	CHF may be present	Synchronized electrical cardioversion, Amiodarone, Procainamide

*CHF indicates congestive heart failure.

repeated dose of 2 J/kg can be given. In the hospital setting, sedation is provided before cardioversion, but its administration must not delay the procedure in a child in unstable condition.

An alternative approach to treating the child in SVT with poor perfusion is to give a dose of IV adenosine if vascular access is readily available. Do not delay synchronized cardioversion if vascular access is not already established, however. If the child remains in SVT and is in unstable condition or shock or is unconscious, you may give additional antiarrhythmic medications in conjunction with cardiology consultation.

Wide Complex Tachycardia

A child with a wide QRS complex tachycardia with a palpable pulse is likely in V-tach, a rare, but potentially life-threatening rhythm in children. Its presence may reflect underlying cardiac pathology. SVT may sometimes manifest as a wide complex rhythm, and distinguishing between the two can be challenging.

If a child with suspected V-tach is in hemodynamically stable condition and IV access is available, consider giving antiarrhythmic medication. Amiodarone is the drug of choice for V-tach with a pulse, although procainamide is an acceptable alternative. Do not give amiodarone *and* procainamide because both prolong the QT interval. If a child with V-tach is in unstable condition or shock or is unconscious, the treatment is synchronized cardioversion. Prior sedation is ideal, but do not delay cardioversion for this reason. The same dose of synchronized cardioversion is used for SVT and V-tach.

Special Considerations

The most common cause of tachycardia in an infant or a young child is sinus tachycardia from fever, dehydration, or pain.

If a child with a tachyarrhythmia is or becomes pulseless, begin CPR and follow the pulseless arrest treatment guidelines. Prepare to immediately transport any child with an arrhythmia to an appropriate receiving facility. Copies of rhythm strips or ECG tracings will be helpful to hospital personnel for diagnostic and therapeutic purposes.

Pulseless Arrest

Cardiopulmonary arrest exists when the child is unresponsive, apneic, and pulseless. In children, this type of arrhythmia is usually a secondary event—that is, the end result of profound hypoxemia and acidosis owing to respiratory failure. Asystole is the most common arrest rhythm. Pulseless electrical activity (PEA), V-tach, and V-fib are seen with lower frequency in children than in adults. The survival rate for children with asystolic arrest in the prehospital setting is poor, and few survivors have good neurologic outcomes. The survival rate for children with V-fib arrest is slightly better and, as in adults, depends on early defibrillation.

When confronted with a pediatric patient in cardiopulmonary arrest, the most important consideration is to provide high-quality BLS skills. Support the airway and breathing, and

Table 41-15	Pediatric Defibrillation Paddle Size	
Age/Weight	**Paddle Size**
Older than 12 mo or > 10 kg	8-cm (adult) paddles
Up to 12 mo or < 10 kg	4.5-cm (pediatric) paddles

begin chest compressions. Attempt IV or IO access. Attach a monitor or defibrillator to determine the underlying cardiac rhythm. If it is asystole or PEA, defibrillation is not indicated, and additional treatment is limited to epinephrine. After administering the medication, perform five cycles of CPR (approximately 2 minutes) before rechecking the rhythm and assessing for the presence of a pulse. If asystole or PEA persists, continue with CPR and epinephrine. High-dose epinephrine is not routinely recommended, however. Consider the "Hs" as the potential causes—for example, Hypoxia, Hypothermia, or Hypovolemia.

Defibrillation is performed before administration of medication in the treatment of V-fib or pulseless V-tach. Follow these steps to perform manual defibrillation in an infant or a child:

1. Confirm unresponsiveness, pulselessness, and apnea.
2. Begin CPR if a defibrillator is not immediately available.
3. Select the proper paddle size Table 41-15 ▲ .
4. Apply conductive gel to the paddles. Place one paddle on the anterior chest wall to the right of the sternum, inferior to the clavicle; place the other paddle on the left midclavicular line at the level of the xiphoid process Figure 41-22 ▶ . Apply firm pressure to the paddles. For children who are younger than 12 months or who weigh less than 10 kg, you may use anterior-posterior paddle placement Figure 41-23 ▶ .
5. Assess the cardiac rhythm to confirm the presence of V-fib or pulseless V-tach.
6. Select the appropriate energy setting, and charge the defibrillator.
7. Verbally and visually ensure that no one is in contact with the patient; stop CPR if it is in progress.
8. Deliver the shock at the appropriate energy setting.
9. Give 5 cycles of CPR (approximately 2 minutes).
10. Reassess the rhythm.

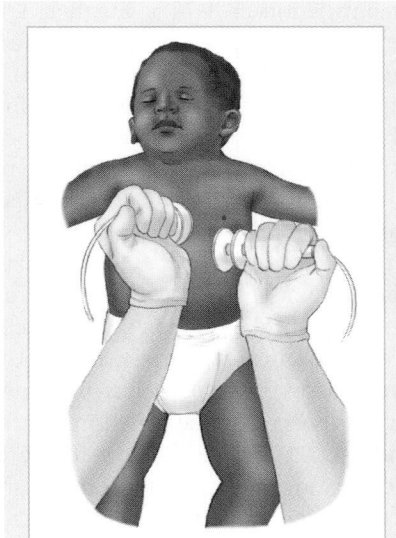

Figure 41-22 Site for defibrillation paddles on anterior chest wall in small infants.

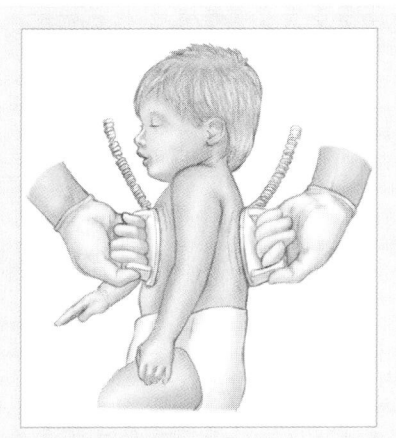

Figure 41-23 Site for defibrillation paddles placed in anterior-posterior position for larger infants and children.

11. If a shockable rhythm persists, give an additional shock at an increased or the same energy, and immediately resume CPR.

12. Insert an advanced airway, establish IV access, and begin medication therapy if indicated. Repeat the defibrillation after 5 cycles of CPR (approximately 2 minutes) if refractory V-fib or pulseless V-tach persists.

Many EMS systems use pregelled defibrillator pads instead of paddles. If your system uses defibrillator pads, place them in the same location as you would when using an AED. When applying the pads, ensure that there are no air pockets in the pad-skin interface because they may result in skin burns and decreased defibrillation effectiveness.

The initial energy setting for defibrillation of pediatric patients is 2 J/kg. If this level does not succeed, repeat the defibrillation at 4 J/kg. Further defibrillation should occur at 4 J/kg after cycles of CPR, as needed. With ongoing CPR, remember to search for and treat any underlying reversible causes. Give epinephrine only after you have delivered two shocks, doubling the dose for the second attempt.

As soon as possible, transport patients in cardiopulmonary arrest to an appropriate receiving facility. Early return of spontaneous circulation (< 5 min) and V-fib or V-tach as a presenting rhythm are associated with improved neurologic outcome for survivors of pediatric cardiopulmonary arrest.

Many EMS systems permit declaration of death in the field if a child in cardiac arrest does not respond to resuscitation. In some cases, you may elect to transport the patient to an ED, even when resuscitation efforts are not successful, so as to provide social service support to the family. A child's death is a devastating event for the family and the EMS crew, and this may be one of your most difficult calls.

Medical Emergencies

Approximately half of all prehospital calls for pediatric patients are trauma-related; the other half are medical. Medical calls

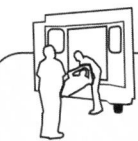

In the Field

Keep a laminated copy of the pediatric algorithms with you at all times for your reference during a cardiovascular emergency.

may include respiratory complaints (as previously discussed in this chapter), fever, seizures, and altered LOC.

Fever

Fever is a common pediatric complaint but often not a true medical emergency. A symptom of an underlying infectious or inflammatory process, fever can have multiple causes. Most pediatric fevers are caused by viral infections, which are often mild and self-limiting. In other cases, fever is a symptom of a more serious bacterial infection.

Your general impression and initial assessment will help you determine the severity of illness. Remember that young children with a fever can look quite ill—even if they only have a "bug"—because increased body temperature causes increased metabolism, tachycardia, and tachypnea. Record temperature as part of the vital signs, but recognize that the height of the fever does not reflect the severity of the illness. If the patient is a young infant, a rectal temperature is most accurate, but recognition that fever is present is more important than the exact temperature. As you move through the initial assessment, look for signs of respiratory distress, shock, seizures, stiff neck, petechial or purpuric rash, or a bulging fontanelle in an infant. These signs may tip you off to the presence of pneumonia, sepsis, or meningitis, all of which can be life threatening and require prompt transport to an appropriate facility.

Very young infants (younger than 2 months) should always be considered at risk for serious infection. Young infants have few ways of interacting with the world, and a fever (defined as body temperature >100.4°F [>38°C]) may be the only sign of a potentially life-threatening illness. Regardless of how well a child in this age group looks, he or she should be assessed and transported quickly to a hospital for a full sepsis workup, including blood, urine, and cerebrospinal fluid (CSF) analysis.

The focused history and physical exam will help to determine the underlying cause of the fever and the severity of illness. Perform this assessment on scene if the child is in stable condition or en route to the hospital if the child appears seriously ill. Ask about the presence of vomiting, diarrhea, poor feeding, headache, neck pain or stiffness, and rash. A history of infectious exposure may provide clues to the likely cause of the child's current illness. The focused medical history may also identify a child at high risk for serious bacterial illness. For example, sickle cell disease, human immunodeficiency virus infection, and childhood cancers may all lead to an immunocompromised state.

A child with a fever may require little intervention in the field. Simply support the ABCs as needed. Although fever by itself is not dangerous, temperature control will make the child with a minor acute illness look and feel better. Consider treating with acetaminophen or ibuprofen, but avoid aspirin in children. Use of aspirin in

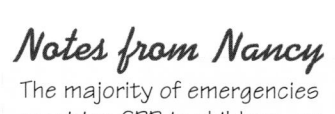

Notes from Nancy

The majority of emergencies requiring CPR in children are preventable.

children has been linked with a rare illness called Reye syndrome, which can result in cerebral edema and liver failure. Other cooling measures should be limited to undressing the child. Transport the patient to an appropriate medical facility with ongoing reassessment for clinical deterioration.

Meningitis

Meningitis entails inflammation or infection of the meninges, the covering of the brain and spinal cord. It is most often caused by a viral or bacterial infection. Although children may look and feel quite ill, viral meningitis is rarely a life-threatening infection. By contrast, bacterial meningitis is potentially fatal. Children with bacterial meningitis can progress rapidly from mildly ill-appearing to coma and even death. In the early stages of illness, it is difficult to tell which type of infection is present, so take the safe route: Always proceed as if the child may have bacterial meningitis.

The symptoms of meningitis vary depending on the age of the child and the agent causing the infection. In general, the younger the child, the more vague the symptoms. A newborn with early bacterial meningitis may have fever as the only symptom. Young infants will often have fever and perhaps localizing signs such as lethargy, irritability, poor feeding, and a bulging fontanelle. Young children rarely show typical "meningeal signs" such as nuchal rigidity (neck stiffness with movement of the neck) until they are a bit older. Verbal children will often complain of headaches and neck pain. An altered LOC and seizures are ominous symptoms at any age.

Neonates most often contract meningitis-causing bacteria during the birthing process: The bacteria that are a normal part of the mother's vaginal tract—*Escherichia coli,* group B *Streptococcus,* and *Listeria monocytogenes*—can produce serious infections in newborns. Older infants and young children are at risk for contracting viral meningitis from enteroviruses, which are widespread during the summer and fall. Bacterial meningitis in this age group most often involves *Streptococcus pneumoniae* (also known as pneumococcus) and *Neisseria meningitidis* (also known as meningococcus), although pneumococcus infection is becoming less frequent as more young children are vaccinated against this bacterium. Meningitis from *H influenzae* is rare because a vaccine against this pathogen was introduced several years ago.

Neisseria meningitidis may also cause sepsis (an overwhelming bacterial infection in the bloodstream). Meningococcal meningitis with sepsis is typically characterized by a petechial (small, pinpoint red spots) or purpuric (larger purple or black spots) rash in addition to the other symptoms of meningitis Figure 41-24 ▶ .

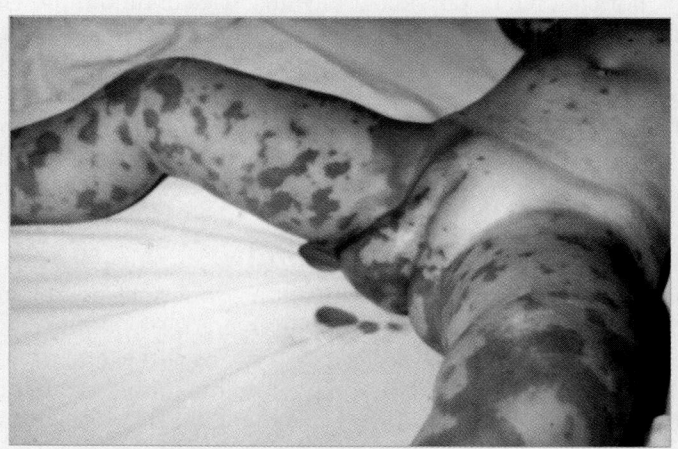

Figure 41-24 Purpura in a child with meningococcal sepsis.

Table 41-16	Pediatric SAMPLE History for Suspected Meningitis	
Component	**Explanation**	
Signs and symptoms	Onset and duration of illness, including "cold symptoms"–runny nose, cough Onset and duration of fever Rash? Headache? Neck pain? Photophobia? Irritability?	
Allergies	Known drug reactions or other allergies	
Medications	Exact names and doses of ongoing drugs Timing and amount of last dose Time and dose of analgesics and antipyretics	
Past medical history	Previous illnesses or injuries Immunizations Perinatal history for young infants	
Last oral intake	Timing of the child's last food or drink, including bottle or breastfeeding	
Events leading to illness or injury	Any known exposures to children with illnesses and what kind of illnesses	

Infection control is an important part of managing a child who may have meningitis. Meningococcus, in particular, is quite contagious. Protect yourself and others from contracting this illness by being vigilant about using standard and respiratory precautions. Wear a gown, gloves, and a mask if meningitis is a possibility.

Children with meningococcal sepsis and meningitis get very sick, very fast, so move quickly through your assessment. Form your general impression, and perform the initial assessment as usual, while recognizing that the initial presentation of a child with meningitis can be highly variable. Look for fever, altered mental status, bulging fontanelle, photophobia, nuchal rigidity, irritability, petechiae, purpura, and signs of shock. Perform a bedside glucose check because hypoglycemia may result from the hypermetabolic state. Helpful components of a SAMPLE history are shown in Table 41-16 ▲ .

For children in physiologically unstable condition, provide lifesaving interventions as needed and transport them quickly, ideally to a facility with a pediatric intensive care unit. En route, perform frequent reassessments—one of the hallmarks of this disease is rapid deterioration. Monitor vital signs and changes in physical exam findings closely to anticipate a child's needs and intervene early.

Altered LOC and Mental Status

An altered LOC or mental status is an abnormal neurologic state in which a child is less alert and interactive with the environment than normal. **Table 41-17 ▼** uses the mnemonic AEIOU-TIPPS to highlight some common causes of altered LOC. Without a good history, it may be difficult to determine the underlying cause, and you may find yourself simply identifying and treating concerning symptoms.

Run through the PAT and ABCs quickly to determine possible points of intervention. Pay special attention to possible disability and dextrose issues. Use the AVPU scale (Alert, responsive to Voice, responsive to Pain, Unresponsive) to identify the level of disability. In addition, check the patient's glucose level because hypoglycemia (defined as a serum glucose concentration < 40 mg/dL in a newborn and < 60 mg/dL in all other infants and children) is easily treatable.

The focused history and physical exam, whether performed at the scene or en route to the hospital, may also pro-vide clues about the underlying cause. For example, a child with a history of epilepsy may be in a postictal state after an unwitnessed seizure; a child with diabetes may be hypoglycemic or in diabetic ketoacidosis. A history of toxic ingestion, recent illness, or injury may also reveal the cause of the altered mental status.

Regardless of the cause, the initial management of altered mental status is the same. Support the ABCs by carefully assessing the patient's airway and breathing. Provide assisted ventilation or airway support as needed. If the child is hypoglycemic, give glucose at a targeted dose of 0.5 g/kg. Depending on which glucose solution is available, this dose can be given as 5 mL/kg of D_{10} solution, 2 mL/kg of D_{25} solution, or 1 mL/kg of D_{50} solution. Always recheck the blood glucose level after giving IV glucose. The goal is to maintain a *normal* glucose level: Hyperglycemia is associated with worse neurologic outcomes in patients with cerebral ischemia. For children with altered mental status and signs or symptoms suggestive of an opiate toxidrome **Table 41-18 ▼**, consider giving naloxone. All patients with altered mental status should be transported expeditiously to an appropriate medical facility.

Seizures

Seizures result from abnormal electrical discharges in the brain. Although many types of seizures exist, generalized seizures manifest as abnormal motor activity and an altered LOC. Some children are predisposed to seizures because of underlying brain abnormalities, whereas others experience seizures as a result of trauma, metabolic disturbances, ingestion, or infection. Seizures associated with fever (febrile seizures) are unique to young children.

The physical manifestation of a seizure will depend on the area of the brain firing the electrical discharges and the age of the child. Infants have immature brains, so seizures in this age group may be subtle. Repetitive movements such as lip smacking,

Table 41-17	AEIOU-TIPPS: Possible Causes of Altered LOC and Mental Status
A	Alcohol
E	Epilepsy, endocrine, electrolytes
I	Insulin
O	Opiates and other drugs
U	Uremia
T	Trauma, temperature
I	Infection
P	Psychogenic
P	Poison
S	Shock, stroke, space-occupying lesion, subarachnoid hemorrhage

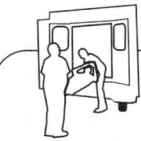

In the Field

Always check the glucose level for a patient with altered mental status.

Table 41-18	Common Toxidromes	
Toxidrome	**Agent**	**Signs and Symptoms**
Anticholinergic	Antihistamines, cyclic antidepressants	"Hot as a hare, red as a beet (hot, dry skin; hyperthermia), blind as a bat (dilated pupils), mad as a hatter (delirium, hallucinations)"
Cholinergic	Organophosphates	DUMBELS: Diarrhea/diaphoresis, Urination, Miosis, Bradycardia/bronchoconstriction, Emesis, Lacrimation, Salivation
Narcotic	Morphine, methadone	Bradycardia, hypoventilation, miosis, hypotension
Sympathomimetic	Cocaine, amphetamines	Tachycardia, hypertension, hyperthermia, mydriasis (dilated pupils), diaphoresis (sweating)

chewing, and "bicycling" suggest seizure activity. Apnea and cyanosis can also be signs of underlying seizure activity.

The prognosis following a seizure is closely linked to the underlying cause. For example, a child with a febrile seizure will not have brain damage as a consequence of the event, whereas a child who has a seizure as a complication of a head injury or meningitis may have long-term neurologic abnormalities. All types of seizures (but especially first-time seizures) are frightening to caregivers, and they often result in 9-1-1 calls.

Types of Seizures

The classification system for seizures is the same for children and adults (see Chapter 28 for an in-depth discussion of seizures). Briefly, seizures that involve the entire brain are considered generalized seizures, whereas those that involve only one part of the brain are called partial seizures. The most common type of seizures are generalized tonic-clonic seizures (grand mal), which involve jerking of both arms and/or legs. Absence seizures (petit mal) are generalized seizures that involve brief loss of attention without abnormal body movements. Partial seizures can be further subclassified into simple partial seizures, which involve focal motor jerking without loss of consciousness, and complex partial seizures, which feature focal motor jerking with loss of consciousness.

Febrile Seizures

Febrile seizures occur in about 25% of young children. To make this diagnosis, the child must be between 6 months and 6 years old, have a fever, and have no identifiable precipitating cause (such as head injury, ingestion, or meningitis). Most febrile seizures occur in children between the ages of 6 months and 3 years. The strongest predictor for having a febrile seizure is a history of this diagnosis in a first-degree relative.

Simple febrile seizures are brief, generalized tonic-clonic seizures (lasting < 15 minutes) that occur in a child without underlying neurologic abnormalities. Complex febrile seizures are longer (lasting > 15 minutes), are focal, or occur in a child with baseline developmental or neurologic abnormality. They may also be associated with serious illness.

The majority of your calls for fever and seizures will involve simple febrile seizures. The postictal phase after a brief seizure tends to be short, so the child will often be waking up or back to baseline by the time you arrive at the scene. Depending on your agency's policy, a well-appearing child who has a history consistent with a simple febrile seizure may be transported by EMS or by parents but always needs urgent physician evaluation.

The prognosis for children with simple febrile seizures is excellent. Although one third of children who have one simple

Special Considerations

Febrile seizures are unique to children. Reassure the parents of a child with a simple febrile seizure that the child has an excellent prognosis.

febrile seizure will have another such seizure, their prognosis does not change. There is no relationship between simple febrile seizures and brain damage or future developmental or learning disabilities, and children with this diagnosis have only a slightly increased risk for subsequent development of epilepsy.

Assessment of Seizures

The general impression and initial assessment of a child with a history of seizures should give special attention to compromised oxygenation and ventilation and signs of ongoing seizure activity. Seizures place a child at risk for respiratory distress or failure because of airway obstruction (often from the tongue), aspiration, or depressed respiratory drive. Given the typical EMS response time, any child who is still having a seizure when you arrive has likely been having seizure activity for at least 10 minutes and should be considered to be in status epilepticus; initiate treatment to stop the seizure in such cases. Status epilepticus has historically been defined as any seizure lasting more than 20 minutes or two or more seizures without return to neurologic baseline between seizures. In recent years, however, neurologists have begun urging treatment for any seizure lasting more than 5 minutes. As part of your SAMPLE history, ask about prior seizures; anticonvulsant medications; recent illness, injury, or suspected ingestion; duration of the seizure activity; and the character of the seizure.

Treatment of Seizures

Treatment at the scene will be limited to supportive care if the seizure has stopped by your arrival, but status epilepticus requires more extensive intervention. For a child with ongoing seizure activity, open the airway using the chin-lift or jaw-thrust maneuver. Very proximal airway obstruction is common during a seizure or postictal state because the tongue and jaw fall backward owing to the decreased muscle tone associated with altered mental status. If the airway is not maintainable with positioning, consider inserting a nasopharyngeal airway. Suction for secretions or vomitus, and consider the lateral decubitus position in case of ongoing vomiting. Do not attempt to intubate during an active seizure because endotracheal intubation in this setting is associated with serious complications and is rarely successful. You are better off using BLS airway management, stopping the seizure, and then considering the child's need for ALS airway support.

Provide 100% supplemental oxygen to the patient, and start bag-mask ventilation as indicated for hypoventilation. Consider placing an NG tube to decompress the stomach if the patient requires assisted ventilation.

Assess the child for IV sites. Measure the serum glucose level, and treat any documented hypoglycemia.

Consider your options for anticonvulsant administration. Insertion of an IV line can be difficult in a child having a seizure, and alternative routes for medication delivery may be needed. The goal of medical therapy is to stop the seizure while minimizing anticonvulsant side effects.

First-line anticonvulsant treatment consists of a benzodiazepine—lorazepam, diazepam, or midazolam. All benzodiazepines can cause respiratory depression, so monitor oxygenation and ventilation carefully, especially when you give repeated doses or combinations of anticonvulsants. Lorazepam is an excellent choice for seizure management because of its rapid onset, lower risk of respiratory depression, and relatively long half-life. Its usefulness in the field is limited because it must be refrigerated. Diazepam is frequently used in the prehospital setting, given by the IV or rectal route. The advantages of rectal administration include ease of access and a lower rate of respiratory depression, although onset of action is longer (approximately 5 minutes). The half-life of diazepam is relatively short, however, and breakthrough seizures may occur with longer transport times. Midazolam may be administered by the IV, IM, and intranasal (using an atomizer) routes. Although it has excellent anticonvulsant effects, it has the shortest duration of action of the three benzodiazepines mentioned. Be prepared to repeat dosing for recurrent seizures.

If the seizures do not stop after two or three doses of a benzodiazepine, a second-line agent is necessary. Phenobarbital is the second-line agent of choice for neonates. Phenobarbital, phenytoin, and fosphenytoin are acceptable second-line agents for infants and children outside of the neonatal age group. Phenobarbital has sedative effects and causes respiratory depression, so be vigilant if you give it after a benzodiazepine. Although phenytoin has the advantage of not compromising the respiratory system or causing sedation, it is difficult to administer and can cause hypotension and bradycardia. Fosphenytoin, a drug that is metabolized to phenytoin, allows for more rapid infusion with fewer side effects; it may be administered by the IV or IM route.

Any child with a history suggestive of seizures requires physician evaluation to look for the cause. Although treatment at the scene is appropriate for a child in status epilepticus, detailed assessment should be performed during transport. Monitor cardiorespiratory status in any postictal child, and reassess frequently for recurrent seizure activity.

■ Toxicology Emergencies

Toxic exposures account for a significant number of pediatric emergencies. In 2004, almost 2.5 million poisoning cases were reported to poison centers. More than half of these poisonings occurred in children younger than 6 years, and 65% (> 1.5 million cases) occurred in patients younger than 20 years.

Toxic exposures can take the form of ingestion, inhalation, injection, or application of a substance (see Chapter 33 for more on specific exposures). A toddler or preschool-age child is most likely to have an unintentional exposure, the result of developmentally normal exploration. In this age group, ingestion tends to involve small quantities of a single cleaning product, cosmetic, or plant or a few pills. In contrast, toxic exposures in adolescents are typically the result of recreational drug use or suicide attempts and often involve multiple agents. Although intentional exposures among adolescents lead to greater morbidity and mortality, in small children, the toxic effects of some medications are such that "one pill can kill" **Table 41-19 ▸** .

Assessment

The evaluation of a child who has experienced a potentially toxic exposure follows the standard assessment sequence. Take a focused history to identify the agents to which the child was

You are the Provider Part 4

Based on the patient's vital signs and condition, you determine that he is in compensated shock. You insert a 20-gauge peripheral IV catheter in both antecubital fossae, and initiate a normal saline bolus. When you used the length-based resuscitation tape earlier, you estimated the child's weight to be approximately 12 kg, so you plan to administer a total of 240 mL (20 mL/kg). While the fluid is being delivered, you and your crew apply a cervical collar, secure the child to a pediatric spine board, and pad the voids with a blanket. You then load the patient in the ambulance, making sure to keep him warm, and contact the receiving facility. The physician agrees with your assessment and treatment and advises no further orders at this time.

Reassessment	Recording Time: 18 Minutes
Skin	Pale, cool, and dry
Pulse	165 beats/min, regular; weak distal pulses but strong central pulses
ECG	Narrow complex tachycardia
Blood pressure	84/56 mm Hg
Respirations	20 breaths/min via bag-mask ventilation
Sao₂	98% on bag-mask ventilation with 100% supplemental oxygen
Pupils	Equal and reactive to light

7. What do you think is the cause for shock in this patient?

8. What criteria were used to determine that this patient was a "trauma alert"?

Table 41-19	One Pill Can Kill: Potentially Lethal Toddler Ingestion
Medicine	**Lethal Dose**
Camphor	One teaspoon of oil
Chloroquine	One 500-mg tablet
Clonidine	One 0.3-mg tablet
Glyburide	Two 5-mg tablets
Imipramine	One 150-mg tablet
Lindane	Two teaspoons of 1% lotion
Diphenoxylate/atropine	Two 2.5-mg tablets
Propranolol	One or two 160-mg tablets
Theophylline	One 500-mg tablet
Verapamil	One or two 240-mg tablets

Table 41-20	The Pediatric SAMPLE for Toxic Exposures	
Components	**Features**	
Signs and symptoms	Time of suspected exposure Behavior changes in child Emesis and content of vomit	
Allergies	Known drug reactions or other allergies	
Medications	Identity of suspected toxin Amount of toxin exposure (count pills or measure volume) Pill or chemical containers on scene Exact names and doses of prescribed medications	
Past medical problems	Previous illnesses or injuries	
Last oral intake	Timing of the child's last food or drink Type and time of home treatment (such as ipecac)	
Events leading to injury or illness	Key events leading to the exposure Type of exposure (inhaled, injected, ingested, or absorbed through the skin) Poison Center contact	

exposed, the quantity, and the route and time of exposure. Findings of physical assessment will vary widely based on these factors. Make special note of vital signs, pupillary changes, skin temperature and moisture, and any unusual odors. Putting together these pieces of the puzzle may allow you to identify a toxidrome—a pattern of symptoms and signs typical of a particular poisoning.

When performing the initial assessment, attend to airway, breathing, and circulatory support as indicated. A dextrose (glucose) check is an important test because ingestion of some common substances can lead to hypoglycemia—namely, ethanol and other alcohols, insulin, oral hypoglycemic agents, and beta blockers. Treat documented hypoglycemia as part of your resuscitation.

If the child is in stable condition without physiologic abnormalities and without a serious toxic exposure, stay on scene to obtain additional history and perform an expanded physical exam. See **Table 41-20** for the SAMPLE history for a pediatric patient with a potential toxic exposure. During the expanded physical exam, look for toxidromes by assessing the patient's mental status, pupillary changes, skin CTC, gastrointestinal activity (bowel sounds, emesis, or diarrhea), and abnormal odors. Perform frequent reassessments because the child's condition may change.

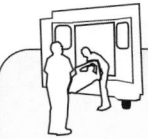
In the Field

Have the national Poison Center number (1-800-222-1222) handy for suspected poisonings.

Children with potentially life-threatening toxic exposures may be asymptomatic on your arrival, and the dose of drug in an accidental toddler ingestion may be high. Always attempt to collect any pill containers or bottles and transport them with the patient to the hospital to assist the ED staff in making treatment decisions.

Management

The management of any potential toxic exposure begins with supportive care and attention to the ABCs. Other management options include reducing the absorption of the substance by decontamination, enhancing elimination of the substance, and/or providing an antidote. Give special attention to the risks of environmental exposures for the EMS crew, who may also require decontamination measures.

Decontamination

If the substance has been applied to the skin, reducing absorption involves removal of all clothing and a thorough washing of the skin. With ocular exposure, immediately wash out the eyes. For ingested toxins, options to reduce gastric absorption include dilution, gastric lavage, and activated charcoal.

Depending on the substance ingested, it may be useful to dilute the substance by having the child drink a glass of milk or water. This decision should be made in conjunction with a Poison Center consultant or your medical control physician or nurse. If the child has any airway or breathing concerns, do not to allow the child to drink.

Although parents were once encouraged to keep syrup of ipecac available to induce vomiting in young children, this treatment is no longer recommended by the American Academy of Pediatrics. Ipecac does not remove significant amounts of ingested toxins and can cause prolonged emesis, and it should not be used in the prehospital management of pediatric toxic ingestion.

The most common method currently used for gastrointestinal decontamination in the ED setting is the administration of

Table 41-21 Common Antidotes

Poison	Antidote
Carbon monoxide	Oxygen
Organophosphate	Atropine/pralidoxime
Tricyclic antidepressants	Bicarbonate
Opiates	Naloxone
Beta blockers	Glucagon
Calcium channel blockers	Calcium
Benzodiazepine	Flumazenil

activated charcoal. Activated charcoal absorbs many ingested toxins in the gut, making less drug available for systemic absorption. If it is administered within the first hour after exposure, however, some common toxins do not bind to charcoal—for example, heavy metals, alcohols, hydrocarbons, acids, and alkalis. Activated charcoal is messy to administer and is rarely readily accepted by pediatric patients. For these reasons, as well as the risk of severe chemical pneumonia if a child with altered mental status or vomiting aspirates the charcoal, this treatment may be best given in the hospital setting. If activated charcoal is given in the field, the ideal dose is 10 times the mass of the ingested substance. The amount of drug ingested is often not known, so the typical dose is 1 to 2 g/kg.

Enhanced Elimination

Cathartics such as sorbitol are sometimes combined with activated charcoal. They work by speeding up elimination. In general, cathartics are not recommended for young children because they have been known to cause significant diarrhea with serious—sometimes life-threatening—electrolyte abnormalities. Hospital providers have additional options for enhancing elimination, such as whole bowel irrigation, urinary alkalinization for salicylate overdoses, dialysis, and hemoperfusion.

Antidotes

Antidotes can be lifesaving but are available for only a few poisonings. They work by reversing or blocking the effects of the ingested toxin. **Table 41-21** lists some of the more commonly available antidotes; indications for their use are the same for young children as for adults. The dose depends on the weight of the child.

Notes from Nancy
Any child with unexplained hyperpnea should be suspected to have salicylate poisoning.

Sudden Infant Death Syndrome

Sudden infant death syndrome (SIDS), formerly known as crib death, is the sudden and unexpected death of an infant younger than 1 year for whom a thorough postmortem examination (autopsy) fails to demonstrate an adequate cause of death. Whatever the cause, the sudden death of an apparently healthy baby is devastating to families and to the EMS crew that responds to the call. Risk factors associated with SIDS include male sex; prematurity; low birth weight; young maternal age; sleeping in the prone position; sleeping with soft, bulky blankets or soft objects; sleeping on soft surfaces; and exposure to tobacco smoke.

SIDS is the leading cause of death in infants aged 1 month to 1 year, with a peak incidence between 2 and 4 months. Approximately 250,000 SIDS deaths occur each year in the United States.

Assessment and Management

The typical scenario for a SIDS call is that of a healthy infant who was put down for a nap and later found dead in bed. On arrival of EMS, the baby will be lifeless and, depending on discovery time, may have rigor mortis and dependent lividity (pooling of blood on the underside of the body). The presence of frothy or blood-tinged fluid in the mouth or nose or on the bedding is typical of SIDS. Be alert for clues to other potential causes of death, such as trauma, suffocation, or maltreatment.

Your decision to start resuscitative efforts, or to stop CPR that was started by first responders or family members, can be difficult in cases of suspected SIDS. Your actions will be guided by local protocols on declaring death in the field and by your assessment of the patient and the needs of the family. Although a victim of SIDS cannot be resuscitated, failure to initiate care may not be acceptable to the shocked family. Likewise, ED care will not change the outcome for the infant, but hospital-based social services for the family may be an important resource. In cases that meet the criteria for declaring death at the scene and nontransport, notify the coroner, medical examiner, or law enforcement personnel, as dictated by local protocol, so that appropriate scene investigation can be undertaken. You also have an important role in mobilizing support for the survivors—for example, a chaplain or minister, SIDS team, social worker, or other family members.

Despite the emotionally charged atmosphere, doing a thorough scene size-up and obtaining the pertinent history is important. A history of recent illnesses, chronic conditions, medications, or trauma may decrease the likelihood of SIDS as the cause of death. The presence of pillows, stuffed toys, window blind cords, or sheepskin in the baby's crib may make suffocation a possibility.

Death of a Child

Whatever you suspect as the cause of death, be compassionate and nonjudgmental in dealing with caregivers. Find out the infant's name, and use it. Don't hesitate to tell the family how sorry you are. Families in this situation will often look to you for answers. Even when there is nothing to do medically, you can make a big impact by providing emotional support and care to the surviving family members.

Apparent Life-Threatening Event

An apparent life-threatening event (ALTE) is an episode during which an infant becomes pale or cyanotic; chokes, gags, or has an apneic spell; or loses muscle tone. These changes are sufficiently dramatic that the caregiver becomes frightened and may think that the baby is dying. ALTEs frequently prompt 9-1-1 calls. Their causes may include benign diagnoses, such as a brief episode of laryngospasm during feedings or gastroesophageal reflux, and serious diagnoses, such as sepsis, congenital heart disease, and seizures.

ALTEs were once thought of as existing along a spectrum with SIDS; hence they were called near-miss or aborted SIDS. More recent evidence demonstrates that although both events occur in early infancy, the two are not related.

It is common to find a distraught caregiver and a well-appearing baby on arrival at the scene of an ALTE call. Provide life support if the infant shows signs of cardiorespiratory compromise or altered mental status, and transport all infants with a history of an ALTE to an appropriate medical facility for evaluation. This is a challenging age group to assess, and overtriage is the safest path.

Child Abuse and Neglect

Sadly, child abuse is prevalent in our society. In 2002, national child protective services reported more than 900,000 confirmed cases of child abuse in the United States. Approximately 1,500 of these patients died as a result of maltreatment.

Child abuse or maltreatment comes in many forms: physical abuse, sexual abuse, emotional abuse, and child neglect. Physical abuse involves the infliction of injury to a child. Sexual abuse occurs when an adult engages in sexual activity with a child; it can range from inappropriate touching to intercourse. Emotional abuse and child neglect are often difficult to identify and may go unreported.

Keep the possibility of child abuse and neglect in mind when you are called to assist with an injured child. The information you gather from the initial scene size-up and interviews may prove invaluable. If you suspect child abuse, you should act on your suspicions because child abuse involves a pattern of behavior. A child who is abused once is likely to be abused again—and next time, it may be more serious or even fatal.

Risk Factors for Abuse

No child asks to be abused, but certain risk factors make abuse more likely. Younger children are more often abused than older children, perhaps a function of their helplessness and limited ability to communicate their needs. Children who require a lot of extra attention, such as children with handicaps, chronic illnesses, or other developmental problems, are also more likely to be abused.

Table 41-22	CHILD ABUSE Mnemonic for Suspicion of Child Abuse
C	Consistency of the injury with the child's developmental age
H	History inconsistent with injury
I	Inappropriate parental concerns
L	Lack of supervision
D	Delay in seeking care
A	Affect (of the parent or caregiver and the child in relation to the caregiver)
B	Bruises of varying ages
U	Unusual injury patterns
S	Suspicious circumstances
E	Environmental clues

Child abuse occurs across all socioeconomic levels, although it is more prevalent in lower-socioeconomic families. Divorce, financial problems, and illness can contribute to the overall stress level of parents, placing them at higher risk to abuse their children. Drug and alcohol abuse can also interfere with a caregiver's ability to parent, and both are associated with higher rates of abusive behavior. Domestic violence in the home places a child at a much higher risk for child abuse.

Suspecting Abuse

When you are called to the home of an injured child and suspect abuse or neglect, trust your instincts. Use your scene size-up, focused history, and physical exam to gather additional information. Look for "red flags" that could suggest child maltreatment (summarized in the mnemonic CHILD ABUSE; **Table 41-22 ▲**):

- A history inconsistent with the type of injury sustained—for example, a child who fell from a tree but whose bruises are only on the buttocks
- An account of the injury that is inconsistent with the developmental abilities of the child—for example, a 2-month-old child rolling off a bed
- An old injury that went unreported
- Inappropriate actions or language from the caregiver

Assessment and Management
Scene Size-up

To recognize abuse, you first have to suspect it. Once you begin to question whether abuse or neglect is involved, it becomes important to carefully document what you see. Although it may be difficult to remain impartial when child abuse or neglect is suspected, it is an important part of professionalism. Record what you see and hear, but do not editorialize. Be detailed in your incident report about the child's environment, noting the condition of the home and the interactions among the caregivers, the child, and the EMS crew. Record concerning comments verbatim.

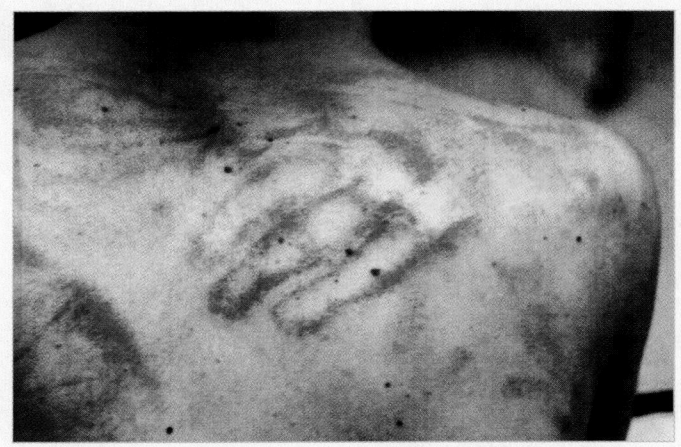

Figure 41-25 Bruises from child abuse. Look for bruises that look like finger or hand marks.

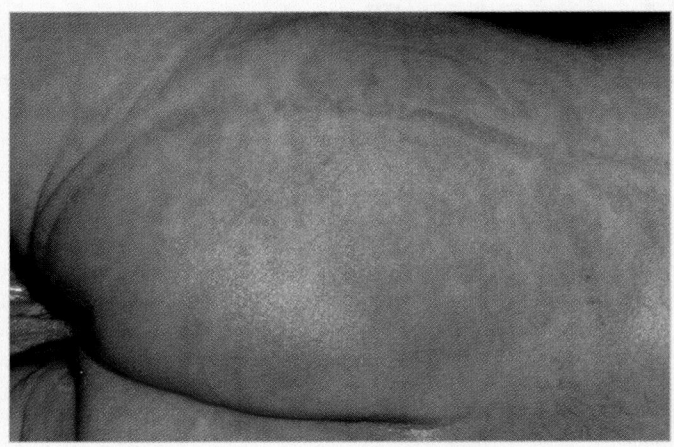

Figure 41-27 A Mongolian spot is a birthmark that can mimic a bruise. It may be on the back, buttocks, or extremities.

Documentation and Communication

If you suspect child abuse, take extra care with your documentation. Record conversations verbatim (in quotes) and document on your patient care report what you see and hear.

Do not approach the caregiver with your concerns, but make sure that you pass them on to staff at the receiving hospital. In many states, EMS providers are mandatory reporters of suspected child abuse. Be aware of local regulations; you may have a legal—and an ethical—obligation to ensure that a report is made to the local child protection services.

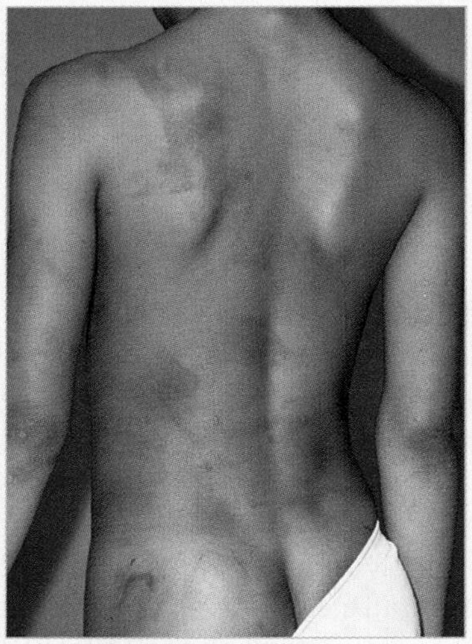

General and Initial Assessments

Although child abuse can generate a big emotional response from the EMS crew, remember that your primary focus should be on trauma assessment and management and on ensuring the safety of the child. Base your general impression on the PAT, which may range from normal in a child with minor inflicted injuries to grossly abnormal in a child with severe internal or CNS injuries. In shaken baby syndrome you may encounter a child with a very abnormal appearance but no external signs of injury. In such a case, the child receives a severe brain injury when a caregiver violently shakes the infant, often when the child is crying inconsolably. Given that few caregivers will admit to having hurt the child, be alert for a history that is inconsistent with the clinical picture.

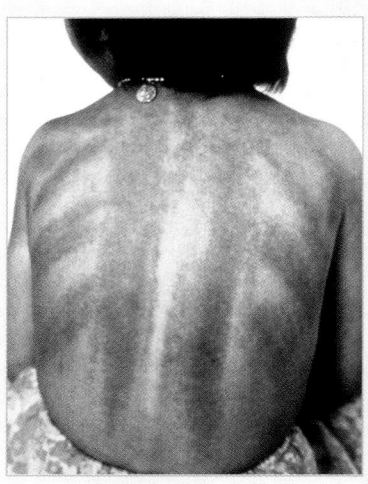

Figure 41-28 Coining, the practice of rubbing hot coins on the back as a treatment of medical illnesses, can leave impressive markings that can mimic child abuse.

Give special attention to the child's skin while looking for bruises, especially of different ages or in concerning locations. Active toddlers often have bruises on their shins from falls and active playing but rarely on their backs or buttocks. Bruises in identifiable patterns such as belt buckles, looped cords, or straight lines are rarely incurred accidentally. **Figure 41-25 ◄** and **Figure 41-26 ◄** are examples of bruises that are suggestive of abuse.

Use the CHILD ABUSE mnemonic when you obtain additional history. Ask yourself, "Does the caregiver's explanation make sense? Could this child produce this bruise or injury through his or her normal activities?"

Figure 41-26 Bruises from child abuse. Multiple bruises or injuries that are in different stages of healing are concerns for abuse.

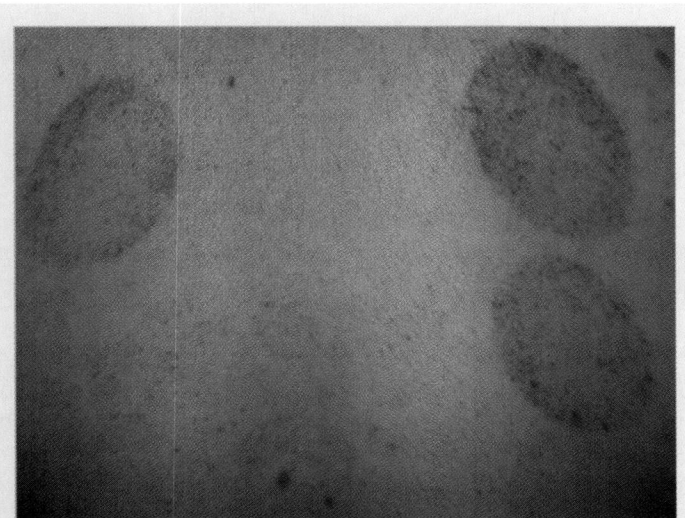

Figure 41-29 Round, flat, red circles on a child's back may be from the practice of cupping—placing warm cups on the skin to draw out illness from the body.

Mimics of Abuse

It can be difficult to distinguish some normal skin findings from inflicted injuries. For example, <u>Mongolian spots</u> Figure 41-27 ◄ can mimic bruises. These birthmarks are generally found on the lower back and buttocks of children of Asian or African-American descent; they may be mistaken for bruises because of their unique bluish coloring.

Certain cultural customs also produce skin markings that can mimic child abuse. Coining and cupping Figure 41-28 ◄ and Figure 41-29 ▲ are traditional Asian healing practices, often used in the treatment of fever. Although the skin markings can be impressive, the practice is not harmful and does not represent abuse.

Trauma

Pediatric trauma is the leading cause of death among children older than 1 year. Motor vehicle collisions cause the most deaths in this age group, followed by falls and submersions. Among adolescents, homicide and suicide are major causes of death.

Children's age-related anatomy and physiology make their injury patterns and responses to trauma different from those seen in adults. In addition, a child's developmental stage will affect his or her response to injury. For a young child, being strapped to a backboard may be as traumatic as the injury leading to the EMS call!

Anatomic and Physiologic Differences

Head

Recall that infants and young children have heads that are large relative to the rest of their bodies. The head also has a larger mass compared with adults. The head's larger size and weight make it more prone to injury. A young child falling from a height, for example, is more likely to fall on his or her head. Traumatic brain injury is the leading cause of death and significant disability in pediatric trauma patients.

Spinal Column

The vertebral column continues to develop along with the child. When the child is younger, the cervical spine fulcrum (or bending point) is higher because the head is heavier. As the child grows, the fulcrum descends to "adult level," around C5 through C7. An infant who sustains blunt head trauma involving acceleration-deceleration forces is at high risk for a fatal, high cervical spinal injury. By comparison, a school-age child who experiences the same injury will likely sustain a lower cervical spinal injury and be paralyzed.

Fortunately, vertebral fractures and spinal cord injuries in young children are uncommon. Spinal ligaments are more lax in children than in adults, leading to increased mobility and the phenomenon of cord injury in the absence of identifiable vertebral bony fracture or dislocation.

Thoracic and lumbar spinal injuries are also encountered relatively infrequently until a child is pursuing adult activities, such as driving and diving. Nevertheless, these injuries are seen in children in association with specific mechanisms—for example, seatbelt-associated lumbar spine injuries (often associated with abdominal injury) and compression fracture due to axial loading in a fall. When confronted with a significant MOI, the safest course is to assume that the child has a bony injury and transport with spinal immobilization precautions.

Chest

Chest trauma is the third leading cause of serious injury in pediatric trauma. A child's chest wall is more pliable and flexible than that of an adult. As a result, children have fewer rib fractures and flail chest events, but injuries to the thoracic organs may be more severe because the pliable ribcage is more easily compressed during blunt trauma. As a consequence, children are more vulnerable than adults to pulmonary contusions, pericardial tamponade, and diaphragmatic rupture. Be sure to look for signs of these injuries in a child with suspected chest trauma, but note that the signs of pneumothorax or hemothorax in children are often subtle. You may not see signs such as neck vein distention, and it may be difficult to determine tracheal deviation.

Abdomen and Pelvis

Abdominal injuries are the second leading cause of serious trauma in children (after head injuries). In pediatric patients, the intra-abdominal organs are relatively large, making them vulnerable to blunt trauma. For example, the abdomen in an infant or toddler often seems protuberant because of the large liver. The liver and the spleen extend below the ribcage in young children and, therefore, do not have as much bony protection as they do in an adult. These organs have a rich blood supply, so injuries to them can result in large blood losses. The kidneys are also more vulnerable to injury in children because they are more mobile and less well supported than in adults. Finally, the duodenum and pancreas are likely to be damaged in handlebar injuries.

Pelvic fractures are relatively rare in young children and are generally seen only with high-energy MOIs. The risk for pelvic fracture increases in adolescence, when the skeleton and MOIs become more like those of adults.

Extremities

The bones of young children continue growing until well into adolescence, resulting in a higher rate of fractures than in adults. This susceptibility to fractures is a function of bone density and the presence of cartilaginous growth plates. Growth plate fractures can be seen with low-energy MOIs, and they may not evidence the degree of tenderness, swelling, and bruising usually associated with a broken bone. Because a young child's ligaments are sturdier than the long bones, sprains are relatively uncommon, and joint dislocations without associated fractures are not often encountered.

Injury Patterns

Blunt trauma is the MOI in more than 90% of pediatric injury cases. Because they have less muscle and fat mass than adults, children have less protection against the forces transmitted in blunt trauma.

Falls are common in pediatric patients, and the injuries sustained will reflect the anatomy of the child and the height of the fall. For example, a 6-year-old playing on the monkey bars is most likely to sustain an upper extremity fracture when falling onto an outstretched arm. Internal or head injuries would be uncommon with this mechanism. Conversely, an infant, with a big head and no protective reflexes, who pitches out of a backpack or shopping cart will commonly have a skull fracture and could have an intracranial hemorrhage. Falls from a standing position usually result in isolated long bone injuries, whereas high-energy falls (such as from a window, ejection from a motor vehicle, car-versus-pedestrian collision) may result in multiple trauma.

Injuries from bicycle handlebars typically produce compression injuries to the intra-abdominal organs. Duodenal hematomas and/or pancreatic injuries are common with this MOI, as are upper extremity injuries. You must also consider a head injury if the patient went over the handlebars, especially if not wearing a helmet.

Motor vehicle collisions can result in a variety of injury patterns depending on whether the child was properly restrained and where the child was seated in the car. For unrestrained passengers, assume multiple trauma. Restrained passengers may sustain chest and abdominal injuries associated with seatbelt use. If you see chest or abdominal bruising in a seatbelt pattern, have a high suspicion for spinal fractures. Air bags pose a particular threat for head and neck injuries in young children.

A child who is the victim of a car-versus-pedestrian collision is likely to sustain multisystem trauma. Depending on the child's height and the height of the vehicle's bumper, a child

Special Considerations

Always consider multiple trauma in pediatric patients. Consider head or abdominal injuries, even if they are not readily apparent.

may receive chest, abdominal, and lower extremity injuries at impact. Head and neck injuries may result from the fall when the child is thrown.

Assessment and Management

The first steps in managing pediatric trauma are the same as for medical emergencies. Use your hands-off assessment to establish a general impression. If the PAT findings are grossly abnormal, quickly move to initial assessment and management to prevent death or disability. Abnormal appearance should make you think immediately of a head injury. With an isolated closed head injury, the child's breathing and circulation may be normal. Of course, abnormal appearance may also reflect inadequate oxygenation of the brain owing to shock or respiratory failure. Abnormalities in work of breathing will tip you off to chest or airway injury and abnormal circulation to a hemorrhage problem. If multisystem injuries are present, all three sides of the PAT may be abnormal.

Begin the initial assessment, initiating life support interventions as you identify problems. Assess the airway for obstruction with teeth, blood, vomit, or edema. Suction as needed. For cervical spinal injury, open the airway using the jaw-thrust maneuver. If the child cannot maintain the airway, consider placement of a nasopharyngeal or oropharyngeal airway. If you attempt endotracheal intubation, maintain cervical spinal precautions. Establishment of an emergency surgical airway in a child is fraught with complications, and the failure rate is high; for these reasons, tracheotomy should be reserved for the most expert surgeons in a controlled setting. The chances of needing to perform a needle cricothyrotomy in a child are remote. In younger children, identification of the cricothyroid membrane is difficult. Appropriate needle cricothyrotomy is described in Chapter 11.

Breathing assessment includes evaluation for symmetric chest rise and equal breath sounds. Provide 100% supplemental oxygen, give bag-mask ventilation as needed, and place an NG or OG tube for stomach decompression.

Pneumothorax is not common in pediatric blunt chest injury, but it may be present with penetrating trauma of the chest or upper abdomen. Remember that you are less likely to see jugular venous distention and tracheal deviation in a child. If the mechanism suggests a possible tension pneumothorax and the patient is in significant respiratory distress, perform needle decompression **Skill Drill 41-8 ▶**:

1. Assess the patient to ensure that the presentation is due to a tension pneumothorax.
2. Prepare and assemble the necessary equipment: large-bore IV catheter, preferably 14 to 16 gauge, alcohol or povidone iodine preps, and adhesive tape.

3. Locate the appropriate site. Find the second or third intercostal space in the midclavicular line on the affected side.

4. Cleanse the appropriate area using aseptic technique.

5. Insert the needle at a 90° angle, just superior to the third rib (nerves, arteries, and veins run along the inferior borders of each rib), and listen for the release of air Step 1 .

6. Advance the catheter over the needle, and place the needle in the sharps container.

7. Secure the catheter in place the same way you would secure an impaled object.

8. Monitor the patient closely for recurrence of the tension pneumothorax.

Any trauma patient should be considered to be at risk for developing shock from visible external bleeding or internal bleeding. Assess the child's circulation by checking the heart rate and quality, capillary refill, skin temperature, and blood pressure. In pediatric patients, the only sign of compensated shock might be an elevated heart rate—children have a remarkable capacity for peripheral vasoconstriction and can maintain their blood pressure despite significant blood loss. If the MOI is concerning and the child is tachycardic, assume the presence of compensated shock and initiate volume resuscitation with 20 mL/kg of isotonic fluid (normal saline or lactated Ringer's). Ideally, you will insert two peripheral IV lines, but an

IO line may be best in a child with hemorrhagic shock. Control external bleeding as you would in any trauma patient. Once the ABCs are stabilized, continue your assessment of disability with the AVPU scale. Your assessment of appearance in the PAT will already have identified an altered LOC. Check the child's pupils and motor function. Place a cervical collar, and immobilize the child on a long backboard as indicated.

If increased ICP is a concern, keep the head midline to facilitate jugular venous return to the heart. If the patient is not in shock, elevate the backboard or head of the stretcher to 30°. Perform shock resuscitation with IV fluids—brain hypoperfusion will make matters worse. If the child has acute signs of herniation such as a "blown" pupil or the Cushing's triad (elevated blood pressure, bradycardia, abnormal respiratory pattern), consider mild hyperventilation guided to an $ETCO_2$ of 32 to 35 mm Hg and giving mannitol.

The last piece of the initial assessment will be "exposure"—that is, a head-to-toe exam to identify all injuries. Log roll the child, and examine the back and buttocks. Once you have completed this exam, cover the child in blankets. Don't forget to cover the head, especially in infants and young children, and avoid drafts from heating or air-conditioning units. Children have a relatively large skin surface area–body mass ratio, increasing their risk for heat loss and hypothermia. Consider the use of warm IV fluids, warm oxygen, and a warm patient transport environment and keeping the patient covered. Also be sure to remove any wet clothing that could conduct heat away from the patient.

Skill Drill 41-8: Decompression of a Tension Pneumothorax

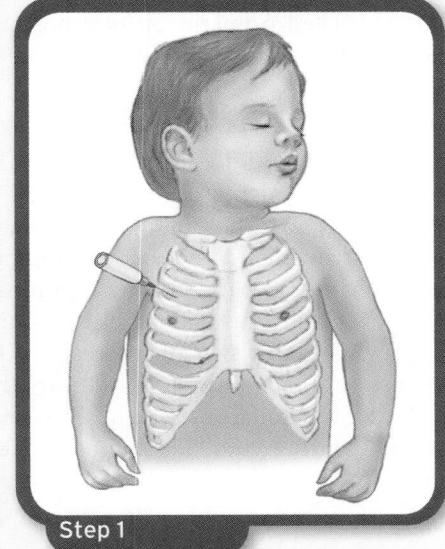

Step 1

Locate the appropriate site. Find the second or third intercostal space in the midclavicular line on the affected side.

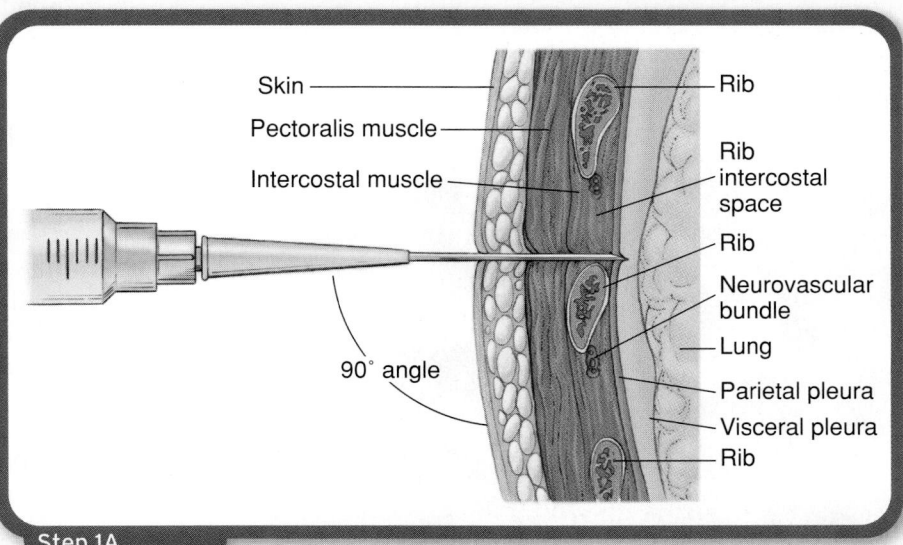

Step 1A

Cleanse the appropriate area using aseptic technique. Insert the needle at a 90° angle and listen for the release of air.

Treat any fractures—open or closed—as you would in an adult. Check out your equipment ahead of time to ensure that you have splints appropriate for smaller children.

Transport Considerations

After initial assessment and stabilization, you are faced with the transport decision. Some traumas are load-and-go situations because of the severity of injuries and the patient's unstable condition. Examples include trauma involving an ominous MOI regardless of how the patient looks on scene, a child with an unstable or compromised airway, a child in shock, a child with difficulty breathing, and a child with a severe neurologic disability. For these patients, perform lifesaving procedures on scene or en route, and quickly transfer them to an appropriate trauma center according to local trauma triage protocols.

All trauma victims for whom spinal injury is suspected require appropriate spinal stabilization. The indications are the same for children and adults. You may have difficulty finding an appropriately sized cervical collar for infants or very young children. Do not attempt to place a collar that is too big on a small child—use towel rolls and tape to immobilize the head. Apply the tape across the temples and forehead, but avoid tape over the chin or throat because it may impair ventilation. Choose a pediatric immobilizer with a recess for the child's large occiput, or place a towel or small blanket under the shoulders and back to prevent neck flexion in infants and toddlers **Figure 41-30 ▼**.

Immobilize a child with the following steps **Skill Drill 41-9 ▶**:

1. Maintain a small child's head in a neutral position by placing a towel under the a small child's shoulders **Step 1**.
2. Place an appropriately sized cervical collar on the patient **Step 2**.
3. Carefully log roll the child onto the immobilization device **Step 3**.

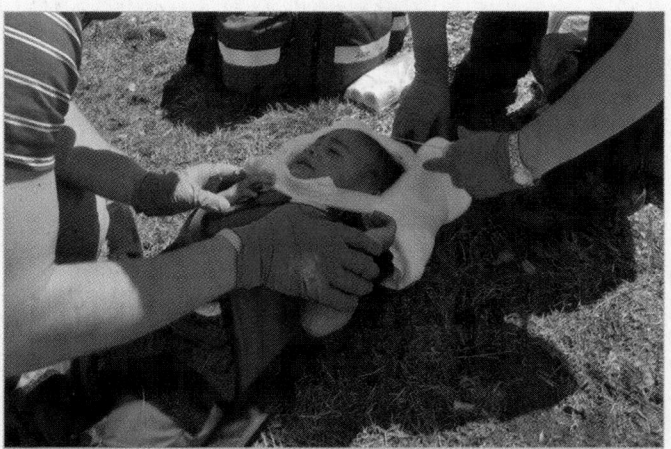

Figure 41-30 Cervical spinal stabilization with towels and tape for a young infant.

4. Secure the patient's torso to the immobilization device first **Step 4**.
5. Secure the child's head to the immobilization device **Step 5**.
6. Complete immobilization by ensuring that the child is strapped in properly **Step 6**.

Secure the child firmly onto the backboard but leave room for adequate chest expansion. Being immobilized is a frightening experience, especially for a young child who cannot understand your intent. Use developmentally appropriate language to explain what you are doing and why, and keep a parent close by when possible.

Follow the steps in **Skill Drill 41-10 ▶** to immobilize an infant:

1. Carefully stabilize the infant's head in a neutral position and lay the seat down into a reclined position on a hard surface **Step 1**.
2. Position a pediatric board or other similar device between the patient and the surface on which the infant is resting **Step 2**.
3. Carefully slide the infant into position on the board **Step 3**.
4. Make sure the infant's head is in a neutral position by placing a towel under the infant's shoulders **Step 4**.
5. Secure the torso first, and place padding to fill any voids **Step 5**.
6. Secure the infant's head to the backboard **Step 6**.

The identification of the nearest appropriate facility depends on local protocols and the capabilities of local hospitals. In some areas of the country, you may be directed to take the patient directly to a pediatric trauma center or to arrange for air transport to a pediatric trauma center. In other areas of the country, children are evaluated primarily at local hospitals and then transferred to a pediatric trauma center.

Expanded History and Exam

If the patient is in stable condition and does not meet the load-and-go criteria, obtain additional history as outlined in **Table 41-23 ▶** and perform a more thorough physical exam. A head-to-toe, back-to-front detailed physical examination should be performed on all trauma patients with significant MOI en route to the ED. For infants, this will include checking the anterior fontanelle for bulging (a sign of increased ICP). Look for bruises, abrasions, or other subtle signs of injury that may have been missed during the initial assessment. Be sure to revisit the initial assessment during your ongoing assessment on the way to the hospital because the patient's condition can change quickly.

Pain Management

Pain is often undertreated in young children. Whether a child can communicate with you verbally, do not overlook signs of pain in pediatric trauma patients. Consider pain assessment as

Skill Drill 41-9: Immobilizing a Child

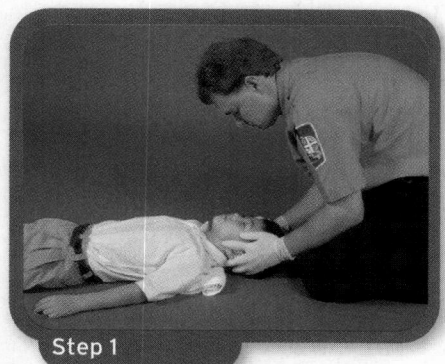

Step 1

Use a towel under the shoulders of a small child to maintain the head in a neutral position.

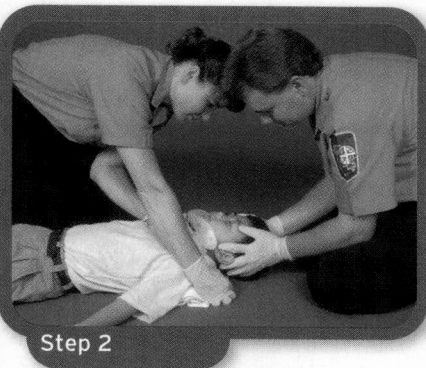

Step 2

Apply an appropriately sized cervical collar.

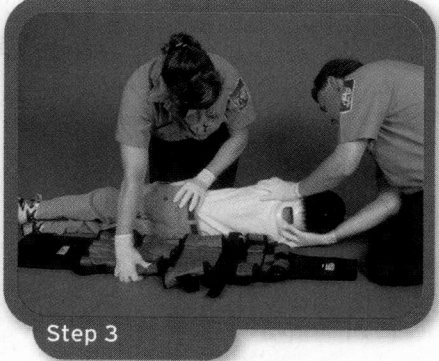

Step 3

Log roll the child onto the immobilization device.

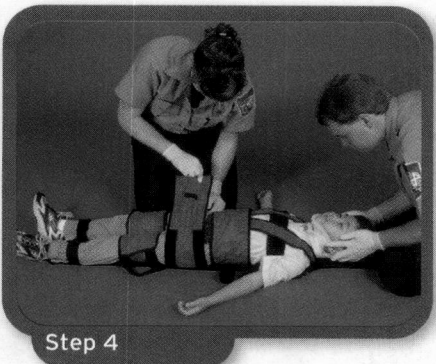

Step 4

Secure the torso first.

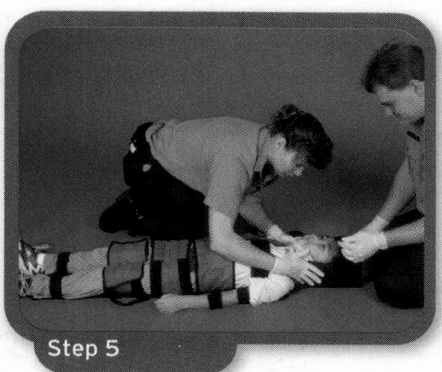

Step 5

Secure the head next.

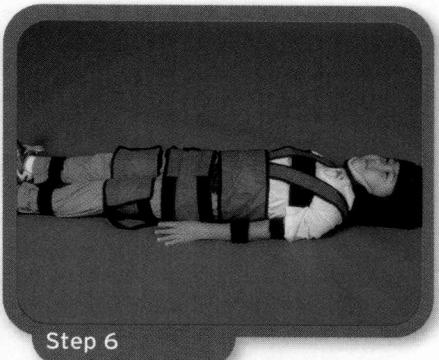

Step 6

Ensure that the child is strapped in properly.

Table 41-23	SAMPLE History in Pediatric Trauma
Component	**Explanation**
Signs and symptoms	Time of event Nature of symptoms or pain Age-appropriate signs of distress
Allergies	Known drug reactions or other allergies
Medications	Timing and last dose of long-term medications Timing and dose of analgesics or antipyretics
Past medical history	Prior surgeries Immunizations, especially last tetanus
Last oral intake	Time of child's last food and drink, including bottle or breastfeeding
Events leading to the injury	Key events leading to the current incident MOI Hazards at the scene

important as the vital signs, and use one of the many tools available to elicit the child's self-report of pain level. Tachycardia and inconsolability may be the only way a child has to express pain, and findings may be similar to those of early shock or plain old fear.

Pain treatment includes use of a calm, reassuring voice, distraction techniques, and, when appropriate, medications. Commonly used pain medications include morphine and fentanyl. Patients who are intubated should receive pain medication and sedation (such as diazepam and midazolam) if they are in hemodynamically stable condition. These medications, which may need to be redosed depending on transport time, can also be used in conjunction with narcotics for patients in stable condition. Side effects of narcotics and benzodiazepines include respiratory depression, hypoxemia, bradycardia, and hypotension.

You must weigh the risks and benefits when deciding to administer these medications. Children who are in shock and hemodynamically unstable condition are not good candidates

Skill Drill 41-10: Immobilizing an Infant

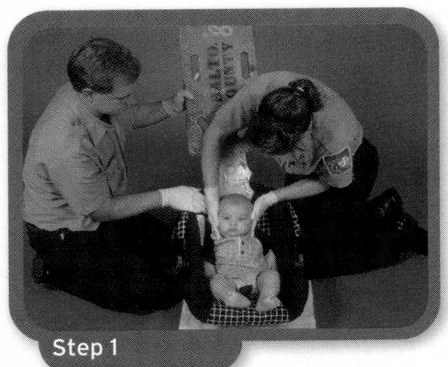

Step 1

Stabilize the head in a neutral position.

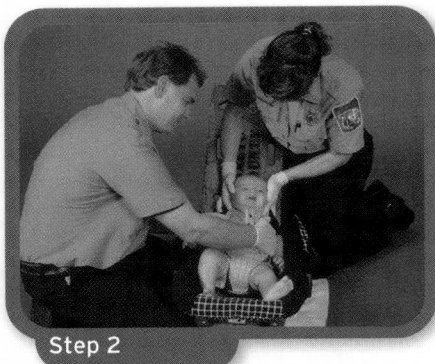

Step 2

Place an immobilization device between the infant and the surface on which he or she is resting.

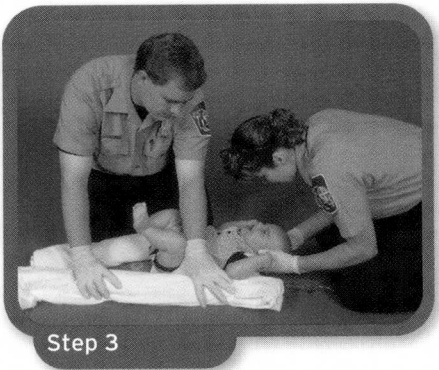

Step 3

Slide the infant onto the board.

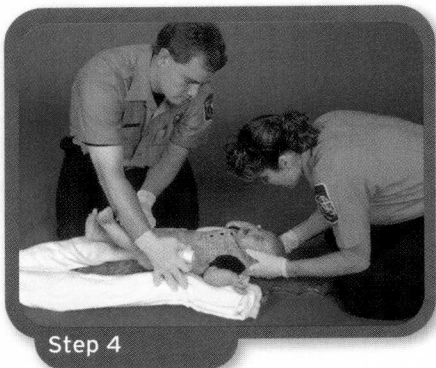

Step 4

Place a towel under the shoulders to ensure neutral head position.

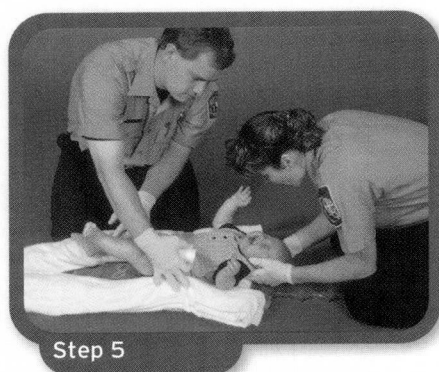

Step 5

Secure the torso first; pad any voids.

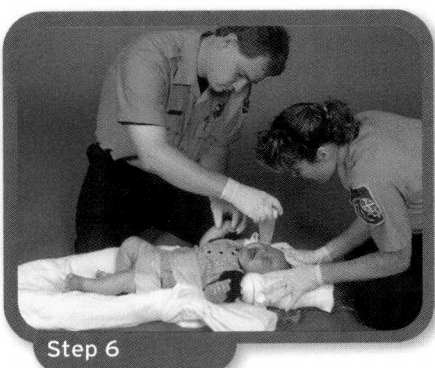

Step 6

Secure the head.

for narcotics or sedatives; these medications may worsen their already precarious status. All children receiving such medications should be carefully monitored in terms of their pulse rate, respiratory rate, pulse oximetry, and blood pressure.

Burns

The initial assessment and management of pediatric burn victims is similar to that of adults, with a few key differences. The larger skin surface–body mass ratio of children makes them more susceptible to heat and fluid loss. Worrisome patterns of injury or suspicious circumstances should also raise concerns of child abuse.

Assessment

The assessment of scene safety is an important element in a burn call. Check for ongoing dangers such as fire, chemicals, or other hazardous materials. Your from-the-doorway assessment may identify signs of smoke inhalation, such as abnormal airway sounds and respiratory distress, or soot around the nose. Quickly move the patient and crew to a well-ventilated area.

An estimation of the percentage of body surface area burned may affect your decision to start fluid resuscitation in the field and influence the transport destination. For adolescents, use the same rule of nines that you use for adult burn victims. For younger children, this rule of nines is modified to account for a child's disproportionately larger head size. For infants, the head and trunk each account for 18% of body surface area, the arms each count as 9%, and the legs each count as 14%. The size of a child's palm (not including fingers) represents about 1% total body surface area. You can also use this rule of palm to assess the extent of the burn **Figure 41-31 ▶** .

Burns suggestive of abuse include those in which the mechanism or pattern observed does not match the history or the child's developmental capabilities. For example, a child who cannot stand independently is unlikely to pull a hot cup

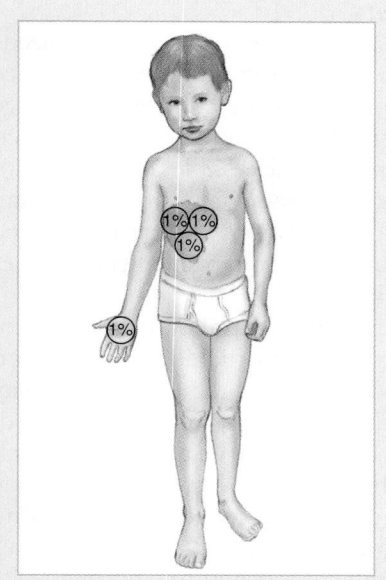

Figure 41-31 Using the child's palm to estimate burned body surface area.

of coffee off a table. Splash burns—as from tipping over a pot of boiling water—should have an irregular configuration because the hot liquid runs down the child's body. Be suspicious if a burn has clear demarcation lines or is on the buttocks.

Management

Initial management begins with removal of burning clothing and support of the ABCs. If you observe signs of smoke inhalation, consider early intubation. Make sure that you have a range of tubes available because airway edema and sloughing may mandate use of a smaller tube than originally estimated.

All burn victims should be provided 100% supplemental oxygen, regardless of the presence or absence of signs of respiratory distress. Smoke inhalation may cause bronchospasm resulting in wheezing and mild respiratory distress. Consider using a bronchodilator such as albuterol or epinephrine (SQ or IM).

If possible, insert an IV line and initiate fluid resuscitation in transport for patients with more than 5% of burned body surface area. Start with 20 mL/kg of isotonic fluid, and reassess the need for additional boluses—as large burns can lead to huge fluid shifts.

Clean burned areas minimally to avoid hypothermia, and cover them with clean, dry cloth. Avoid putting lotions or ointments on burned skin because they can trap heat and bacteria. Avoid heat loss by covering the burn and the patient as needed.

Analgesia is a critical part of the early management of burns; these injuries can be incredibly painful. Assess and treat pain and anxiety as discussed previously. Carefully monitor any child given narcotics or benzodiazepines for signs of respiratory or hemodynamic compromise.

Once the patient's condition is stabilized, begin transport to an appropriate medical facility. Larger burns, full-thickness burns, and burns involving the face and neck are best treated at a regional burn center.

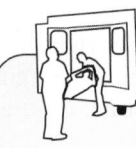

In the Field

Use the rule of palm to estimate the percentage of body surface area burned in a young child or infant: A child's palm is equal to 1% of body surface area.

Children With Special Health Care Needs

Children with special health care needs include those with physical, developmental, and learning disabilities. The disabilities have a broad range of causes, including premature birth, traumatic brain injury, congenital anatomic anomalies, and acquired illnesses. Advances in technology and drugs have enabled an increasing number of children with disabilities to receive care in the community, leading to a corresponding increase in the number of EMS calls for this medically complex population.

Technology-Assisted Children

Technology-assisted children constitute a subset of children with special health care needs that may require your assistance. It is important to familiarize yourself with the various types of medical technology that you may encounter and have to troubleshoot.

Tracheostomy Tubes and Artificial Ventilators

Tracheostomy is surgical procedure, involving creation of a stoma—in this case, a permanent connection between the skin of the throat and trachea—through which a tracheostomy tube can be placed for long-term ventilatory needs

Figure 41-32 ▶ . A child might need a tracheostomy for a variety of reasons, including long-term ventilator support for chronic lung disease, inability to protect the airway because of neurologic impairment, and a congenital airway anomaly leading to airway obstruction. Caregivers have been trained in the use and care of their child's tracheostomy and are a source of valuable information. In general, they will have a spare tracheostomy tube available.

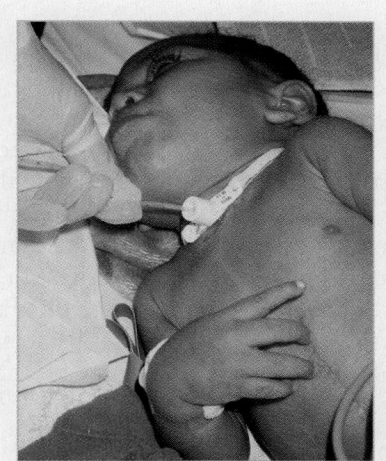

Figure 41-32 A tracheostomy is a surgical opening in the neck into the trachea, creating an artificial airway.

A child with a tracheostomy tube may breathe spontaneously with room air, if the function of the tube is simply to bypass mechanical upper airway obstruction. Alternatively, the child may be dependent on a home ventilator and supplemental oxygen if he or she has severe lung disease or problems with respiratory drive.

Although a tracheostomy tube is intended to provide a secure, permanent airway, problems can arise, as with any mechanical device. The most common problem is obstruction

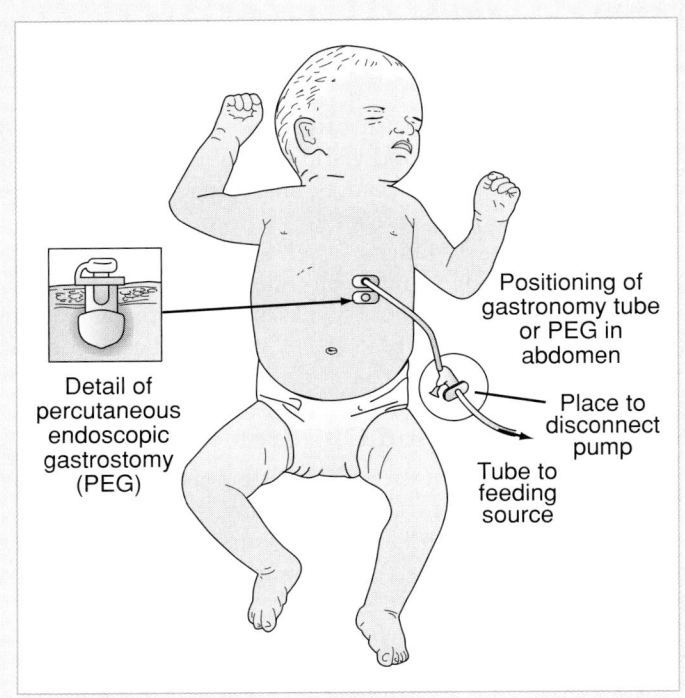

Figure 41-33 A G-tube is an opening through the skin directly into the stomach.

of the tracheostomy tube with secretions, resulting in respiratory distress or respiratory failure. Displacement of the tube is another potential problem. If you are faced with a child with a tracheostomy tube and respiratory distress, start by assessing tube position and suctioning the tube. If the child is using a home ventilator, disconnect the circuit and provide bag-mask ventilation. If these measures fail to lead to improvement or if the child is cyanotic or in severe distress, you may need to remove and replace the tracheostomy tube, preferably using a tube of the same diameter and length. Confirmation of tube position is done in the same manner as for an ET tube.

Gastrostomy Tubes

Gastrostomy tubes (G-tubes) are surgically placed directly into the patient's stomach through the skin Figure 41-33 ▲ . They provide nutrition or medications directly into the stomach, bypassing the oropharynx and esophagus. Some children are unable to take food or medication by mouth and depend on a G-tube for all of their nutrition; for other patients, the tube is used to supplement intake and ensure adequate nutrition.

Problems such as obstruction, dislodgment, or leakage of a G-tube are not uncommon but rarely represent an emergency. Most such calls can be managed by supportive care and transport. Urgent physician evaluation is needed if a G-tube has been pulled out because the opening on the abdominal wall tends to constrict quickly, making replacement difficult.

Central Venous Catheters

A central venous catheter may be inserted when a child needs long-term IV access for medications or nutrition. Such a device is placed surgically or by interventional radiologists into large central veins, such as the subclavian. Completely implanted central lines, with a port or reservoir accessible under the skin, may be left in place for months to years. For example, they are commonly placed in children with cancer who are undergoing long courses of chemotherapy. Partially implanted central lines have tubing external to the skin.

Complications associated with central venous catheters include infections, obstruction, and dislodged or broken catheters. Children with an infection of the central line may have redness, swelling, tenderness, or pus at the skin site of insertion; they may also have systemic signs of infection (such as fever) or signs of septic shock. Central line obstruction may be a medical emergency, depending on what is infusing through the line. If the child is not in urgent need of the infusion, simply assess the patient and transport to a hospital. Dislodged or broken catheters may result in leakage of fluid or blood. In such a case, use sterile technique to clamp off the broken line to minimize risk of infection or air embolus.

On rare occasions, you will be confronted with a child who has a functioning central line but requires emergency IV access for field treatment. Because these permanent lines carry a high risk for infection, look for peripheral access and avoid using the central line whenever possible.

CSF Shunts

Hydrocephalus is a condition resulting from impaired circulation and absorption of CSF, leading to increased size of the ventricles (fluid-filled spaces in the brain) and increased ICP. Hydrocephalus may be congenital or acquired; it is most commonly seen in children born with brain malformations as a complication of prematurity or following surgery for a brain tumor. Cerebrospinal fluid shunts are inserted to drain excessive fluid from the brain, thereby normalizing ICP Figure 41-34 ▶ . A neurosurgeon places the tube and connects it to a one-way, pressure-sensitive valve that runs from the enlarged ventricle subcutaneously into the abdominal peritoneal space. When pressure builds up in the ventricle, the one-way valve opens, and CSF drains into the peritoneum, where it is reabsorbed.

A CSF shunt obstruction occurs when the drainage of fluid from the brain through the shunt tubing becomes blocked—perhaps due to a break in the tubing, problems with the valve, or buildup of debris in the tubing. Without adequate fluid drainage, the CSF fluid continues to accumulate, resulting in hydrocephalus. A child with a shunt obstruction will show signs of increased ICP, which may range from subtle changes in behavior to impending brain herniation. Typical symptoms include headache, fatigue, vomiting, and even coma. Late signs include the Cushing's triad (hypertension, bradycardia, respiratory compromise).

A CSF shunt infection results from bacterial contamination during the surgery to place the shunt or from bacteria in the

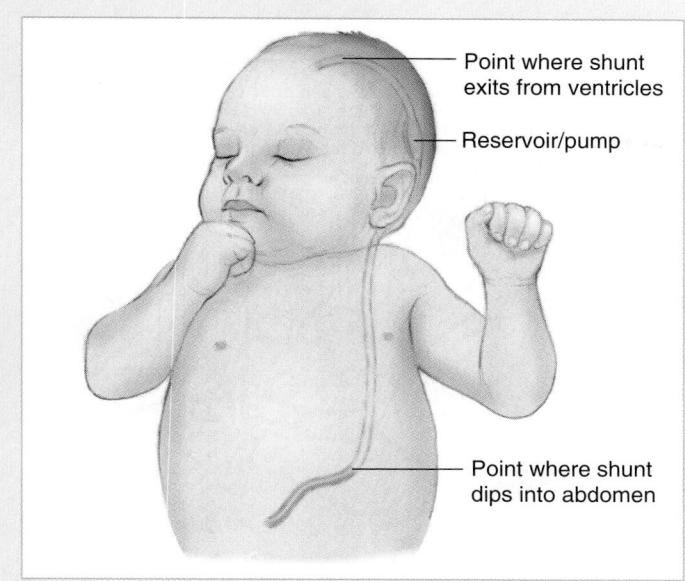

- Point where shunt exits from ventricles
- Reservoir/pump
- Point where shunt dips into abdomen

Figure 41-34 A CSF shunt directs CSF away from the ventricles in the brain to the abdomen to relieve pressure.

blood adhering to and infecting the hardware. Infections are encountered most frequently within months of shunt surgery. Children with shunt infections are generally very sick and have fever and signs of shunt obstruction.

Shunt obstructions and shunt infections are true medical emergencies. The patient should be transported to appropriate treatment facilities where neurosurgical evaluation is available. The child's condition can deteriorate rapidly, so maintain continuous cardiopulmonary monitoring during transport.

Assessment and Management

Follow the standard pediatric assessment sequence when approaching children with special health care needs. Ask questions of the parent or caregiver to establish the child's baseline level of neurologic function and baseline physiologic status. Meet every child at his or her unique developmental level. An otherwise healthy 10-year-old with a perinatal brain injury may have the developmental skills of a toddler. Conversely, a 6-year-old with severe cardiopulmonary compromise may be ventilator-dependent and have oxygen saturation in the 80s but be cognitively intact.

Your treatment goal is to restore a child to his or her own physiologic baseline, which will require collaboration with caregivers to determine what is normal for the child and management strategies that have been successful in the past.

Special Considerations

Caregivers will be key resources when managing a child with special health care needs. Draw on their expertise to assist you in assessing and managing the child.

Transport

Most children with special health care needs will have a medical home—that is, a hospital, clinic, or private practice where they receive their care. Transporting to a facility where the clinical team is familiar with the patient's history and needs will streamline their care. If this is not possible, take along any medical records available to assist the team at the receiving facility to sort out the potentially complex issues faced by the patient. Take any assistive devices as well, including home ventilators and feeding pumps. Most important, take the parent or caregiver of the child! Children with special health care needs rely on their caregivers for much—if not all—of their care-taking needs, so it can be emotionally difficult for the child to be separated from the caretaker.

■ Pediatric Mental Health

During your time as a paramedic, you will undoubtedly encounter children with behavioral and psychiatric problems. The call may be for out-of-control behavior or for a suicide attempt. Unfortunately, EMS calls for behavioral emergencies are increasing, reflecting in part the limited community resources available for children with mental health problems. A recent study of one pediatric ED found that 5% of all pediatric ED visits were for mental health concerns.

Safety

When you are called to a home for a behavioral or psychiatric emergency, safety should be your first priority. Assess the scene for your own safety and for the safety of your patient. If weapons are involved or you cannot determine the degree of risk, call for law enforcement backup.

Approach the child calmly, letting him or her know you are there to help. Address the patient directly when obtaining the history, and explain clearly what you are doing and why. Some children are flight risks, so determine how best to deploy your squad so that they do not leave the scene. As always, answer questions as honestly as possible.

A small percentage of children cannot be safely talked down for transport and must be mechanically restrained for their own protection and the protection of the EMS crew. Applying these restraints may be a task for EMS or for law enforcement personnel. If you decide to apply restraints, carefully document the reason and keep the restraints in place until arrival at the ED. An out-of-control, 60-lb 8-year-old can make a transport dangerous! Try to avoid using chemical restraint (that is, tranquilizing drugs) in the prehospital setting.

Assessment and Management

The PAT will give you a general impression of the child's mental status and cardiovascular stability. A child who has attempted suicide by ingestion may have life-threatening medical complications that trump his or her psychiatric concerns.

Table 41-24	SAMPLE History for Behavioral Problems in Children
Component	**Features**
Signs and symptoms	Out-of-control behavior? Suicidal or homicidal thoughts or actions? Harm to self, others, or pets? Recent change in behavior? Recent change in medication? Auditory or visual hallucinations?
Allergies	Known food or drug allergies and their reactions
Medications	List of all patient's medications and vitamins, prescribed and over-the-counter
Past medical history	History of any behavior or psychiatric problems? Therapist, counselor, or psychiatrist contact information? Prior psychiatric or behavioral hospitalizations? Any medical illnesses?
Last oral intake	Timing and identification of last food and drink
Events leading to behavioral problems	Ongoing or new stressors? Argument or fight with boyfriend, girlfriend, or family members?

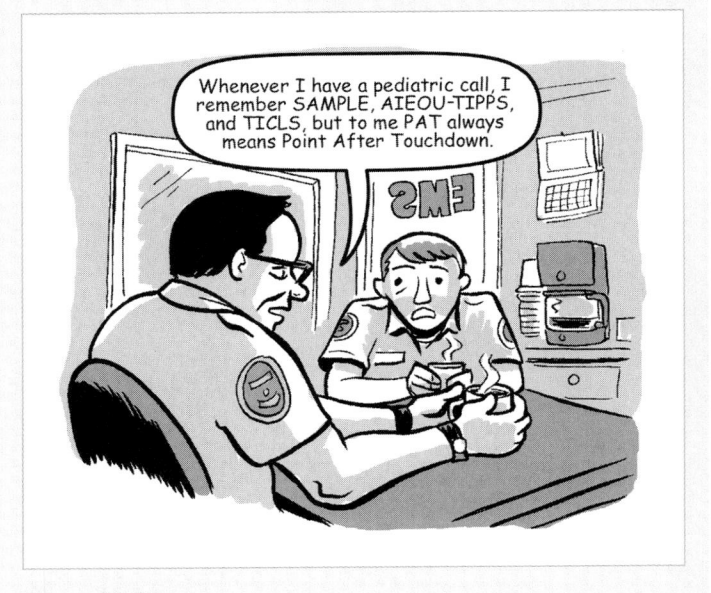

Figure 41-35

In the absence of acute medical issues, the bulk of your assessment will be based on observation and history. In cases involving a very agitated child, your hands-on exam may be limited. **Table 41-24 ▲** lists specific SAMPLE questions for behavioral emergencies. As always, treat any existing medical problems or injuries by using standard protocols.

■ An Ounce of Prevention

Emergency care for children involves a team approach by health care professionals in the community and in the hospital. Paramedics are a critical part of the community responsible for caring for sick and injured children, but their role in prevention is not always highlighted, even though this is an area where they can have a greater public health impact than possible by running a code or controlling an airway **Figure 41-35 ▲**. To be an effective child safety advocate, you must be knowledgeable about local and national prevention programs, such as those conducted through the Emergency Medical Services for Children (EMSC) initiative.

Emergency Medical Services for Children

EMSC is a federally funded program that was created more than 20 years ago in an effort to reduce child disability and death due to severe illness and injury. EMSC works with local communities and hospitals to improve care for children in and out of the hospital. It also works with existing EMS systems to improve the quality of children's emergency care, such as by creating pediatric-specific protocols and procedures. For example, EMSC has helped provide ambulances and EDs with child-appropriate equipment. The program also supports training EMTs, paramedics, and other emergency care providers in pediatric-specific emergency care.

Prevention of Injuries

Most injuries are not accidents, but rather are predictable and preventable events. Knowledge of injury patterns helps target potential areas for intervention and prevention. For example, childhood poisonings can be prevented by effective storage of medications and chemicals. Toddler drowning and submersion can be virtually eliminated by installation of four-sided pool fencing. The risk of serious injury from a bike crash is lessened by use of a helmet. The morbidity and mortality from motor vehicle crashes is dramatically decreased by the appropriate use of child restraint devices.

Notes from Nancy

In the seriously injured child, all organ systems must be assumed to be injured until proved otherwise.

As you care for children, you may be frustrated by the illnesses and injuries that you encounter, especially when they are preventable. Take this frustration as a call to action. Get involved in your community. Participate in existing prevention programs or start your own program. Numerous types of pediatric injury can be targeted (Table 41-25 ▶); choose something that interests you, and take a leadership role.

Table 41-25	Examples of Common Injuries and Possible Prevention Strategies	
Injury	**Preventive Measures**
Vehicle trauma	Infant and child restraint seats Seatbelts and air bags Pedestrian safety programs Motorcycle helmets
Cycling	Bicycle helmets Bicycle paths separate from vehicle traffic

Recreation	Appropriate safety padding and apparel
	Cyclist, skateboard, and skater safety
	  programs
	Soft, energy-absorbent playground
	  surfaces

Drowning and submersion	Four-sided locked pool enclosures Pool alarms Immediate adult supervision Caretaker CPR training Swimming lessons Pool and beach safety instruction Personal flotation devices

Poisoning and
  household injuries
	Proper storage of chemicals
	  and medications
	Child safety packaging

Burns	Proper maintenance and monitoring
	  of electrical appliances and cords
	Fire and smoke detectors
	Proper placement of cookware on
	  stove top

Other	Discouragement of infant walker use Gated stairways Babysitter first-aid training Child care worker first-aid training

You are the Provider Summary

1. What assessment tool will you use to form your general impression of your patient?

The PAT provides emergency care providers with a quick hands-off approach to patient assessment. It can provide you with information about your patient in less than 30 seconds and without touching the patient. The three legs of the PAT—appearance, breathing, and circulation—will aid you in determining whether the child is sick or not sick. The PAT will also assist you in figuring out the physiologic status of your patient: Is he or she in respiratory distress or failure; in shock; or experiencing a neurologic problem?

2. What can you do to assist the panicked mother?

If you are a parent, you can probably relate to the fear and panic the mother is experiencing. Your best approach is to let the mother know everything that you are doing as you are doing it. Reassure her that you are doing everything possible to take care of her child, but be careful not to offer false hope by saying "Everything will be okay." Above all, remain calm and in charge of the scene. The mother needs to see that you are confident and secure with what you are doing. If possible, ask the mother to help care for the child and allow her to accompany her child to the hospital.

3. What do you need to carefully monitor your patient for?

Although the patient seems to be in stable condition at this time, he can begin to decompensate at any time without warning. The physical exam revealed a potential head injury, abdominal injury with bleeding, and a fractured femur. Any of these injuries can cause rapid deterioration of the patient's condition. Be alert for further changes in mental status, decline in respiratory status, and signs of shock.

4. Which interventions should you consider at this point, if any?

You have delegated the role of cervical spine immobilization, and the patient is receiving supplemental oxygen. At this time, you can consider establishing IV access, applying a cardiac monitor, applying a cervical collar, and immobilizing the child on a backboard.

5. Is this child in shock? If so, is it compensated or decompensated?

Yes, the child is in shock. Your patient assessment reveals an increased pulse rate, decreased respiratory status, decreased blood pressure, and increased capillary refill. Currently, he is in compensated shock based on the blood pressure, which remains higher than the minimal acceptable blood pressure. The formula for calculating minimal acceptable blood pressure for children younger than 10 years is $80 + (2 \times \text{age in years})$; this patient is 2 years old, so the minimal acceptable blood pressure would be 84 mm Hg.

6. How should your patient management progress?

Once the airway has been secured, you should focus on correcting the problems with circulation. Establish vascular access so you can administer fluids. Time is of the essence, meaning you should not spend a great deal of time trying to secure peripheral IV access. If you experience difficulty trying to find a vein, obtain vascular access using an IO needle. After securing vascular access, administer a fluid bolus at 20 mL/kg.

7. What do you think is the cause for shock in this patient?

This child has two potential causes for shock: abdominal injury with bleeding and a fractured femur. Both injuries could lead to a significant blood loss. Head injury will cause the blood pressure to increase as the pressure within the skull rises.

8. What criteria were used to determine that this patient was a "trauma alert"?

A trauma alert was called for this patient owing to the MOI, potential for a closed head injury, possible abdominal bleeding, and a femoral fracture.

Prep Kit

Ready for Review

- Children differ anatomically, physiologically, and emotionally from adults.
- Sick or injured children present unique challenges in evaluation and management. Their perceptions of their illness or injury, their world, and of paramedics differ from the perceptions of adults.
- The majority of children you treat will come with at least one parent or caregiver. Thus, in many pediatric calls, you will be dealing with more than one patient—even if only the child is ill or injured.
- Serious illness or injury to a child is one of the most stressful situations caregivers can face.
- An assessment tool called the Pediatric Assessment Triangle (PAT) has been developed to help EMS providers form a from-the-doorway general impression of pediatric patients.
- Respiratory problems are among the medical emergencies that you will most frequently encounter in children. Pediatric patients with a respiratory chief complaint will span the spectrum from mildly ill to near death.
- In pediatrics, respiratory failure and arrest precede the majority of cardiopulmonary arrests; by contrast, a primary cardiac event is the usual cause of sudden death in adults.
- Cardiovascular emergencies are relatively rare in children. When such problems arise, they are often related to volume or infection rather than to a primary cardiac cause, unless the child has congenital heart disease.
- Through the PAT and initial assessment, you can quickly identify a cardiovascular emergency, understand the likely pathologic cause, and institute potentially lifesaving treatment.
- Pediatric medical calls may include respiratory complaints, fever, seizures, and altered LOC.
- Toxic exposures account for a significant number of pediatric emergencies.
- The sudden death of an apparently healthy baby is devastating to families and the EMS crew that responds to the call.
- An apparent life-threatening event (ALTE) is an episode during which an infant becomes pale or cyanotic; chokes, gags, or has an apneic spell; or loses muscle tone.
- Child abuse or maltreatment comes in many forms: physical abuse, sexual abuse, emotional abuse, child neglect.
- Pediatric trauma is the leading cause of death among children older than 1 year.
  - Motor vehicle collisions cause the most deaths in this age group, followed by falls and submersions.
  - Among adolescents, homicide and suicide are major causes of death.
- The initial assessment and management of pediatric burn victims is similar to that of adults, with a few key differences.
  - The larger skin surface–body mass ratio of children makes them more susceptible to heat and fluid loss.
  - Worrisome patterns of injury or suspicious circumstances should raise concerns of child abuse.
- Children with special health care needs include children with physical, developmental, and learning disabilities.
  - These disabilities have a broad range of causes, including premature birth, traumatic brain injury, congenital anatomic anomalies, and acquired illnesses.
  - Advances in technology and drugs have enabled an increasing number of children with disabilities to receive care in the community, leading to a corresponding increase in the number of EMS calls for this medically complex population.
- During your time as a paramedic, you will undoubtedly encounter children with behavioral and psychiatric problems.
  - The call may be for out-of-control behavior or for a suicide attempt.
  - EMS calls for behavioral emergencies are increasing, reflecting in part the limited community resources available for children with mental health problems.

Vital Vocabulary

absence seizures The type of seizures characterized by a brief lapse of attention in which the patient may stare and not respond; formerly known as petit mal seizures.

acrocyanosis Cyanosis of the extremities.

apparent life-threatening event (ALTE) An unexpected sudden episode of color change, tone change, or apnea that required mouth-to-mouth resuscitation or vigorous stimulation.

blow-by technique A method of delivering oxygen by holding a face mask or similar device near an infant's or a child's face; used when a nonrebreathing mask is not tolerated.

bronchiolitis A condition seen in children younger than 2 years, characterized by dyspnea and wheezing.

central venous catheter A catheter inserted into the vena cava to permit intermittent or continuous monitoring of central venous pressure and to facilitate obtaining blood samples for chemical analysis.

cerebrospinal fluid shunts Tubes that drain fluid manufactured in the ventricles of the brain from the subarachnoid space to another part of the body outside of the brain, such as the peritoneum; lowers pressure in the brain.

complex febrile seizures An unusual form of seizures that occurs in association with a rapid increase in body temperature.

complex partial seizures Seizures characterized by alteration of consciousness with or without complex focal motor activity.

cricoid pressure The application of posterior pressure to the cricoid cartilage; minimizes gastric distention and the risk of vomiting and aspiration during ventilation; also referred to as the Sellick maneuver.

croup A childhood viral disease characterized by edema of the upper airways with barking cough, difficult breathing, and stridor.

cyanosis Slightly bluish, grayish, slatelike, or dark purple discoloration of the skin due to hypoxia.

epiglottitis Inflammation of the epiglottis.

generalized seizures The seizures characterized by manifestations that indicate involvement of both cerebral hemispheres.

grunting A short, low-pitched sound at the end of exhalation, present in children with moderate to severe hypoxia; reflects poor gas exchange because of fluid in the lower airways and air sacs.

head bobbing A sign of increased work of breathing in which the head lifts and tilts back during inspiration, then moves forward during expiration.

hydrocephalus The increased accumulation of cerebrospinal fluid within the ventricles of the brain.

meningitis Inflammation of the membranes of the spinal cord or brain.

Mongolian spots Blue-gray areas of discoloration of the skin caused by abnormal pigment, not by trauma or bruising.

mottling A condition of abnormal skin circulation, caused by vasoconstriction or inadequate circulation.

nasal flaring The flaring out of the nostrils, indicating increased work of breathing and hypoxia.

neonatal period The first month of life.

nuchal rigidity A stiff or painful neck; commonly associated with meningitis.

obtunded A condition when the patient is dulled to pain and sensation.

ossification centers Areas where cartilage is transformed through calcification into a new area of bone.

osteomyelitis Inflammation of the bone due to infection; a potential complication of intraosseous infusion.

pallor Lack of color; paleness.

Pediatric Assessment Triangle (PAT) An assessment tool that allows rapid formation of a general impression of the type and level of illness or injury in an infant or child without touching him or her; consists of assessing appearance, work of breathing, and circulation to the skin.

petechial Characterized by small purplish, nonblanching spots on the skin.

purpuric Pertaining to bruising of the skin.

respiratory arrest The absence of respirations with detectable cardiac activity.

respiratory distress A clinical state characterized by increased respiratory rate, effort, and work of breathing.

respiratory failure A clinical state of inadequate oxygenation, ventilation, or both.

respiratory syncytial virus (RSV) A virus that commonly causes bronchiolitis; usually results in lifelong immunity following exposure.

retractions Physical drawing in of the chest wall between the ribs that occurs with increased work of breathing.

rhonchi Rattling respiratory sounds; also called crackles.

sepsis A pathologic state, usually in a febrile patient, resulting from the presence of invading microorganisms or their poisonous products in the bloodstream.

shaken baby syndrome A syndrome seen in abused infants and children; the patient has been subjected to violent, whiplash-type shaking injuries inflicted by the abusing individual that may cause coma, seizures, and increased intracranial pressure due to tearing of the cerebral veins with consequent bleeding into the brain.

simple febrile seizures A brief, self-limited, generalized seizure in a previously healthy child between the ages of 6 months and 6 years that is associated with the onset of or sudden increase in fever.

simple partial seizures Focal seizures that involve a motor or sensory abnormality in a patient who remains conscious.

sinus tachycardia Rapid heart rate in a child with normal conduction.

sniffing position An upright position in which the patient's head and chin are thrust slightly forward to keep the airway open; appears to be sniffing.

status epilepticus A state of continuous seizures or multiple seizures without a return to consciousness for 20 minutes.

stoma A small opening, especially an artificially created opening, such as that made by tracheostomy.

stridor A harsh sound during inspiration, high-pitched due to partial upper airway obstruction.

subglottic space The narrowest part of the pediatric airway.

sudden infant death syndrome (SIDS) The abrupt and unexplained death of an apparently healthy child younger than 1 year.

supraventricular tachycardia (SVT) An abnormal heart rhythm with a rapid, narrow QRS complex.

synchronized cardioversion The timed delivery of energy into the myocardium to correct rapid, regular cardiac rhythms in patients who are in unstable condition.

tonic-clonic seizures Seizures that feature rhythmic back-and-forth motion of an extremity and body stiffness.

tripoding An abnormal position to keep the airway open; involves leaning forward onto two arms stretched forward.

vasoconstriction A decrease in the caliber of blood vessels.

ventilation-perfusion mismatch A pathologic state in which the oxygen entering the lungs is not mixing properly with the blood circulating through the lungs.

wheezing The production of whistling sounds during expiration such as occurs in asthma and bronchiolitis.

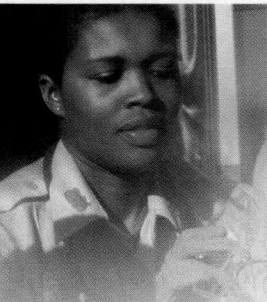

Assessment in Action

You arrive on the scene of a 6-year-old girl having difficulty breathing. Your assessment reveals that she is breathing about 40 times per minute. Her chest muscles seem to be tight and sunken between her ribs. She appears to be working very hard to breathe, and you hear grunting sounds, but the patient's skin color and mentation seem within normal limits.

1. **Which phase of physiologic response is this patient in?**
   A. Respiratory distress
   B. Respiratory failure
   C. Respiratory arrest
   D. Cardiac arrest

2. **A child who appears to be sleepy or drowsy in addition to having difficulty breathing is called:**
   A. obtuse.
   B. obstructed.
   C. obtunded.
   D. objective.

3. **A child who uses chest muscles to help breathe is said to be using:**
   A. excessive muscles.
   B. accessory muscles.
   C. retractive muscles.
   D. tripod muscles.

4. **When counting the respiratory rate in a pediatric patient, count chest rise for:**
   A. 10 seconds and multiply by 6.
   B. 15 seconds and multiply by 4.
   C. 30 seconds and multiply by 2.
   D. a full 60 seconds.

5. **Which phase of physiologic response represents the point at which the patient will decompensate?**
   A. Respiratory distress
   B. Respiratory failure
   C. Respiratory arrest
   D. Cardiac arrest

6. **What is the best way to manage a pediatric patient in respiratory arrest?**
   A. Face mask with oxygen at 15 L/min
   B. Bag-mask ventilation with oxygen at 15 L/min
   C. ET tube with bag-mask ventilation
   D. Chest compressions, ET tube with bag-mask ventilation

Challenging Question

7. **Why are pediatric patients more likely to have respiratory arrest before cardiac arrest?**

▆▆ Points to Ponder

You have been dispatched to care for a pediatric patient who has a low oxygen saturation level. During your response, you wonder how this call came in for a specific problem like "low oxygen saturation level," so you ask your dispatcher to find out more about the call. The dispatcher reports that the call came from the child's mother. When you arrive at the scene, you find a child lying on a bed. The patient is connected to a number of tubes, and you notice a tracheostomy tube in place. The mother states that his saturation level is lower than nor-mal and she is concerned that one of the drains is not working. When you look around the room, you realize that you are not familiar with any of the equipment present.

What is the best way to proceed with your assessment and treatment of this child?

Issues: Technology-Assisted Children, Work of Breathing, Airway Obstruction.

Objectives

Cognitive

6-3.1   Discuss population demographics demonstrating the rise in elderly population in the U.S. (p 42.5)

6-3.2   Discuss society's view of aging and the social, financial, and ethical issues facing the elderly. (p 42.5)

6-3.3   Assess the various living environments of elderly patients. (p 42.5)

6-3.4   Describe the local resources available to assist the elderly and create strategies to refer at risk patients to appropriate community services. (p 42.5)

6-3.5   Discuss issues facing society concerning the elderly. (p 42.5)

6-3.6   Discuss common emotional and psychological reactions to aging to include causes and manifestations. (p 42.5)

6-3.7   Apply the pathophysiology of multi-system failure to the assessment and management of medical conditions in the elderly patient. (p 42.17)

6-3.8   Discuss the problems with mobility in the elderly and develop strategies to prevent falls. (p 42.15)

6-3.9   Discuss the implications of problems with sensation to communication and patient assessment. (p 42.19)

6-3.10   Discuss the problems with continence and elimination and develop communication strategies to provide psychological support. (p 42.24)

6-3.11   Discuss factors that may complicate the assessment of the elderly patient. (p 42.19)

6-3.12   Describe principles that should be employed when assessing and communicating with the elderly. (p 42.19)

6-3.13   Compare the assessment of a young patient with that of an elderly patient. (p 42.19)

6-3.14   Discuss common complaints of elderly patients. (p 42.19)

6-3.15   Compare the pharmacokinetics of an elderly patient to that of a young adult. (p 42.14)

6-3.16   Discuss the impact of polypharmacy and medication non-compliance on patient assessment and management. (p 42.14)

6-3.17   Discuss drug distribution, metabolism, and excretion in the elderly patient. (p 42.14)

6-3.18   Discuss medication issues of the elderly including polypharmacy, dosing errors and increased drug sensitivity. (p 42.24)

6-3.19   Discuss the use and effects of commonly prescribed drugs for the elderly patient. (p 42.25)

6-3.20   Discuss the normal and abnormal changes with age of the pulmonary system. (p 42.7)

6-3.21   Describe the epidemiology of pulmonary diseases in the elderly, including incidence, morbidity/mortality, risk factors, and prevention strategies for patients with pneumonia, chronic obstructive pulmonary diseases and pulmonary embolism. (p 42.11)

6-3.22   Compare and contrast the pathophysiology of pulmonary diseases in the elderly with that of a younger adult, including pneumonia, chronic obstructive pulmonary diseases, and pulmonary embolism. (p 42.11)

6-3.23   Discuss the assessment of the elderly patient with pulmonary complaints, including pneumonia, chronic obstructive pulmonary diseases, and pulmonary embolism. (p 42.22)

6-3.24   Identify the need for intervention and transport of the elderly patient with pulmonary complaints. (p 42.22)

6-3.25   Develop a treatment and management plan of the elderly patient with pulmonary complaints, including pneumonia, chronic obstructive pulmonary diseases, and pulmonary embolism. (p 42.22)

6-3.26   Discuss the normal and abnormal cardiovascular system changes with age. (p 42.6)

6-3.27   Describe the epidemiology for cardiovascular diseases in the elderly, including incidence, morbidity/mortality, risk factors, and prevention strategies for patients with myocardial infarction, heart failure, dysrhythmias, aneurism, and hypertension. (p 42.10)

6-3.28   Compare and contrast the pathophysiology of cardiovascular diseases in the elderly with that of a younger adult, including myocardial infarction, heart failure, dysrhythmias, aneurism, and hypertension. (p 42.10)

6-3.29   Discuss the assessment of the elderly patient with complaints related to the cardiovascular system, including myocardial infarction, heart failure, dysrhythmias, aneurism, and hypertension. (p 42.21)

6-3.30   Identify the need for intervention and transportation of the elderly patient with cardiovascular complaints. (p 42.21)

6-3.31   Develop a treatment and management plan of the elderly patient with cardiovascular complaints, including myocardial infarction, heart failure, dysrhythmias, aneurism and hypertension. (p 42.21)

6-3.32   Discuss the normal and abnormal changes with age of the nervous system. (p 42.9)

6-3.33   Describe the epidemiology for nervous system diseases in the elderly, including incidence, morbidity/mortality, risk factors, and prevention strategies for patients with cerebral vascular disease, delirium, dementia, Alzheimer's disease and Parkinson's disease. (p 42.13)

6-3.34   Compare and contrast the pathophysiology of nervous system diseases in the elderly with that of a younger adult, including cerebral vascular disease, delirium, dementia, Alzheimer's disease and Parkinson's disease. (p 42.13)

6-3.35   Discuss the assessment of the elderly patient with complaints related to the nervous system, including cerebral vascular disease, delirium, dementia, Alzheimer's disease and Parkinson's disease. (p 42.23)

6-3.36   Identify the need for intervention and transportation of the patient with complaints related to the nervous system. (p 42.23)

6-3.37   Develop a treatment and management plan of the elderly patient with complaints related to the nervous system, including cerebral vascular disease, delirium, dementia, Alzheimer's disease and Parkinson's disease. (p 42.24)

6-3.38   Discuss the normal and abnormal changes of the endocrine system with age. (p 42.12)

6-3.39 Describe the epidemiology for endocrine diseases in the elderly, including incidence, morbidity/mortality, risk factors, and prevention strategies for patients with diabetes and thyroid diseases. (p 42.12)

6-3.40 Compare and contrast the pathophysiology of diabetes and thyroid diseases in the elderly with that of a younger adult. (p 42.12)

6-3.41 Discuss the assessment of the elderly patient with complaints related to the endocrine system, including diabetes and thyroid diseases. (p 42.24)

6-3.42 Identify the need for intervention and transportation of the patient with endocrine problems. (p 42.24)

6-3.43 Develop a treatment and management plan of the elderly patient with endocrine problems, including diabetes and thyroid diseases. (p 42.24)

6-3.44 Discuss the normal and abnormal changes of the gastrointestinal system with age. (p 42.8)

6-3.45 Discuss the assessment of the elderly patient with complaints related to the gastrointestinal system. (p 42.22)

6-3.46 Identify the need for intervention and transportation of the patient with gastrointestinal complaints. (p 42.22)

6-3.47 Develop and execute a treatment and management plan of the elderly patient with gastrointestinal problems. (p 42.22)

6-3.48 Discuss the assessment and management of an elderly patient with GI hemorrhage and bowel obstruction. (p 42.22)

6-3.49 Compare and contrast the pathophysiology of GI hemorrhage and bowel obstruction in the elderly with that of a young adult. (p 42.12)

6-3.50 Discuss the normal and abnormal changes with age related to toxicology. (p42.14)

6-3.51 Discuss the assessment of the elderly patient with complaints related to toxicology. (p 42.24)

6-3.52 Identify the need for intervention and transportation of the patient with toxicological problems. (p 42.24)

6-3.53 Develop and execute a treatment and management plan of the elderly patient with toxicological problems. (p 42.24)

6-3.54 Describe the epidemiology in the elderly, including the incidence, morbidity/mortality, risk factors, and prevention strategies, for patients with drug toxicity. (p 42.14)

6-3.55 Compare and contrast the pathophysiology of drug toxicity in the elderly with that of a younger adult. (p 42.14)

6-3.56 Discuss the assessment findings common in elderly patients with drug toxicity. (p 42.24)

6-3.57 Discuss the management/considerations when treating an elderly patient with drug toxicity. (p 42.24)

6-3.58 Describe the epidemiology for drug and alcohol abuse in the elderly, including incidence, morbidity/mortality, risk factors, and prevention strategies. (p 42.14)

6-3.59 Compare and contrast the pathophysiology of drug and alcohol abuse in the elderly with that of a younger adult. (p 42.14)

6-3.60 Discuss the assessment findings common in elderly patients with drug and alcohol abuse. (p 42.15)

6-3.61 Discuss the management/considerations when treating an elderly patient with drug and alcohol abuse. (p 42.15)

6-3.62 Discuss the normal and abnormal changes of thermoregulation with age. (p 42.15)

6-3.63 Discuss the assessment of the elderly patient with complaints related to thermoregulation. (p 42.15)

6-3.64 Identify the need for intervention and transportation of the patient with environmental considerations. (p 42.15)

6-3.65 Develop and execute a treatment and management plan of the elderly patient with environmental considerations. (p 42.15)

6-3.66 Compare and contrast the pathophysiology of hypothermia and hyperthermia in the elderly with that of a younger adult. (p 42.15)

6-3.67 Discuss the assessment findings and management plan for elderly patients with hypothermia and hyperthermia. (p 42.15)

6-3.68 Discuss the normal and abnormal psychiatric changes of age. (p 42.15)

6-3.69 Describe the epidemiology of depression and suicide in the elderly, including incidence, morbidity/mortality, risk factors, and prevention strategies. (p 42.15)

6-3.70 Compare and contrast the psychiatry of depression and suicide in the elderly with that of a younger adult. (p 42.15)

6-3.71 Discuss the assessment of the elderly patient with psychiatric complaints, including depression and suicide. (p 42.25)

6-3.72 Identify the need for intervention and transport of the elderly psychiatric patient. (p 42.25)

6-3.73 Develop a treatment and management plan of the elderly psychiatric patient, including depression and suicide. (p 42.25)

6-3.74 Discuss the normal and abnormal changes of the integumentary system with age. (p 42.9)

6-3.75 Describe the epidemiology for pressure ulcers in the elderly, including incidence, morbidity/mortality, risk factors, and prevention strategies. (p 42.9)

6-3.76 Compare and contrast the pathophysiology of pressure ulcers in the elderly with that of a younger adult. (p 42.9)

6-3.77 Discuss the assessment of the elderly patient with complaints related to the integumentary system, including pressure ulcers. (p 42.25)

6-3.78 Identify the need for intervention and transportation of the patient with complaints related to the integumentary system. (p 42.25)

6-3.79 Develop a treatment and management plan of the elderly patient with complaints related to the integumentary system, including pressure ulcers. (p 42.25)

6-3.80 Discuss the normal and abnormal changes of the musculoskeletal system with age. (p 42.8)

6-3.81 Describe the epidemiology for osteoarthritis and osteoporosis, including incidence, morbidity/mortality, risk factors, and prevention strategies. (p 42.13)

6-3.82 Compare and contrast the pathophysiology of osteoarthritis and osteoporosis with that of a younger adult. (p 42.13)

6-3.83 Discuss the assessment of the elderly patient with complaints related to the musculoskeletal system, including osteoarthritis and osteoporosis. (p 42.13)

6-3.84 Identify the need for intervention and transportation of the patient with musculoskeletal complaints. (p 42.13)

6-3.85 Develop a treatment and management plan of the elderly patient with musculoskeletal complaints, including osteoarthritis and osteoporosis. (p 42.13)

6-3.86 Describe the epidemiology for trauma in the elderly, including incidence, morbidity/mortality, risk factors, and prevention strategies for patients with orthopedic injuries, burns and head injuries. (p 42.15)

6-3.87 Compare and contrast the pathophysiology of trauma in the elderly with that of a younger adult, including orthopedic injuries, burns and head injuries. (p 42.15)

6-3.88   Discuss the assessment findings common in elderly patients with traumatic injuries, including orthopedic injuries, burns and head injuries. (p 42.26)

6-3.89   Discuss the management/considerations when treating an elderly patient with traumatic injuries, including orthopedic injuries, burns and head injuries. (p 42.26)

6-3.90   Identify the need for intervention and transport of the elderly patient with trauma. (p 42.26)

Affective

6-3.91   Demonstrate and advocate appropriate interactions with the elderly that conveys respect for their position in life. (p 42.19)

6-3.92   Recognize the emotional need for independence in the elderly while simultaneously attending to their apparent acute dependence. (p 42.19)

6-3.93   Recognize and appreciate the many impediments to physical and emotional well being in the elderly. (p 42.19)

6-3.94   Recognize and appreciate the physical and emotional difficulties associated with being a caretaker of an impaired elderly person, particularly the patient with Alzheimer's disease. (p 42.5)

Psychomotor

6-3.95   Demonstrate the ability to assess a geriatric patient. (p 42.18)

6-3.96   Demonstrate the ability to adjust their assessment to a geriatric patient. (p 42.19)

Introduction

Geriatrics is the assessment and treatment of disease in someone 65 years or older. In 2003, elderly Americans accounted for 12% of the US population; by 2030, this percentage is expected to grow to 20%, largely driven by aging of the "baby boomers" (born in the period 1946–1964). Furthermore, the elderly population is itself growing older; indeed, the most rapidly growing segment of the US population is people 85 years and older.

Elderly people constitute an ever-increasing proportion of patients in the health care system, particularly the emergency care sector. Individuals 65 years of age and older account for 36% of all hospital stays in the United States. People are receiving more of their care out of hospital, and with insurance issues, this trend will continue in the future. This population also has more contacts with doctors than those under 65 years of age.

The old-age dependency ratio depicts the dependency individuals place upon society as they age. It is defined as the number of older people for every 100 adults (potential caregivers) between the ages of 18 and 64. In 1990, there were 20 older people for every 100 "caregivers." By 2025, it is projected that there will be 32 older people for every 100 "caregivers." The supply of caregivers is not keeping pace with the growth of the older population. The need for caregivers is going to increase, and society is going to have difficulty keeping up with the demand for services as the population continues to age. As the older population grows, EMS providers will be required to offer services that are cost effective and efficient. Insurance regulations, costs associated with providing care, and facility issues will make cost a continuing concern.

Most of your geriatric patients will not reside in nursing homes. Although nursing home admissions are increasing owing to the larger number of older persons in the United States, a countertrend is for elderly people to maintain independent lives. Many older adults continue to live at home with support from a spouse or family member and a visiting nurse; others live in a more dependent care environment such as a senior center facility. Still others may seek an assisted-living facility or a total care nursing home.

Determining how and where older adults will spend their retirement years is a difficult and complex process involving numerous social and economic issues such as the person's marital status, financial resources, religious beliefs, ethnicity, sex, and general health. Because such decisions may place a burden on family members, their wishes must be considered by health care providers. When making these decisions, older adults and their families can seek advice from medical social workers, professional care managers, discharge planners at health care facilities, and a large number of private and public resources. The range of services available includes delivered meals, personal care, housekeeping, adult day care, transportation, caregiver support, respite care, and emergency response systems, including EMS services and lifelines ◀ Figure 42-1 ▶ .

Psychosocial factors may influence successful aging. For example, at retirement, a person may no longer feel useful or productive in society and may experience diminished self-esteem. Age also brings bereavement—sadness over the loss of friends and loved ones. Notably, the likelihood of death increases during the year following the death of one's spouse. As friends and family die, elderly persons tend to experience increasing loneliness and isolation—factors shown to have negative effects on health.

Finally, the health problems of older people are quantitatively and qualitatively different from the problems of younger people. One cannot simply transfer the principles of caring for

You are the Provider Part 1

You have been assigned to orient a newly hired paramedic, Mike, who graduated paramedic school 7 months ago. Your focus for the day has been on geriatric emergencies because your territory provides service to six nursing homes and assisted-living facilities. As luck would have it, your unit is dispatched to one of the smaller community nursing homes for a sick person.

Upon arrival you are escorted to the day room where the residents spend most of their time. A nurse sitting next to a patient seated in a wheelchair by the window waves you over. She introduces you to Mrs. Howard, a frail-appearing 86-year-old widow. The nurse explains that Mrs. Howard has been running a low-grade fever since last evening and is "not acting like her normal self." The physician has requested that she be transferred to the hospital to be evaluated. When asked how she is feeling, Mrs. Howard slowly turns her head way from the window toward you and replies "not well."

Initial Assessment	Recording Time: 0 Minutes
Appearance	Frail, weak, elderly woman
Level of consciousness	A (Alert to person, place, and day)
Airway	Open and clear
Breathing	Adequate chest rise and volume
Circulation	Strong, rapid radial pulse, slightly irregular

1. Why is it important to review common medical problems of elderly people?
2. Which organ systems are greatly affected by age-related changes?

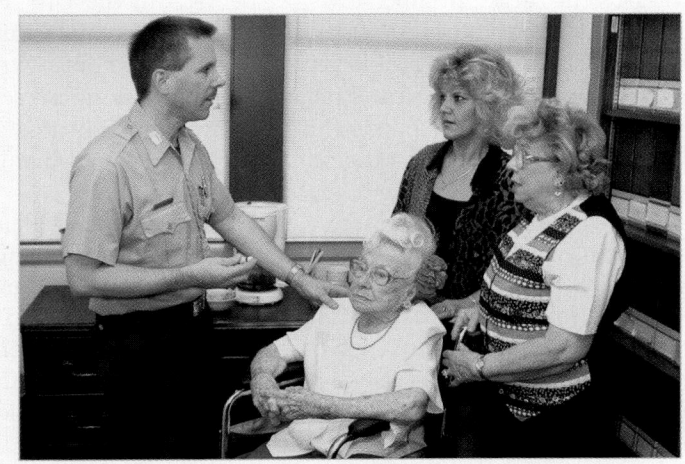

Figure 42-1 EMS professionals should be familiar with available resources.

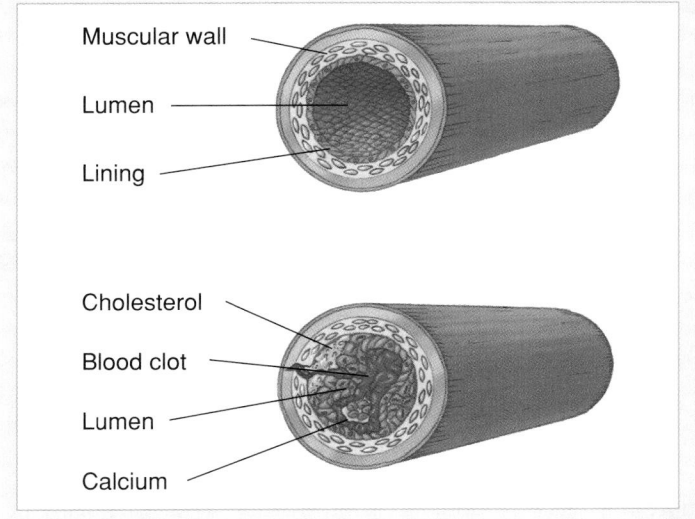

Figure 42-3 Atherosclerosis, the buildup of fatty plaque on arterial walls.

the younger population without modification. The special problems of older people require special approaches.

Anatomy and Physiology

Human growth and development peaks in the late 20s and early 30s, at which point the aging process sets in. Aging is a *linear* process; that is, the rate at which we lose functions does not increase with age. A 35-year-old is aging just as fast as an 85-year-old, but the older person exhibits the cumulative results of a longer process. Of course, the aging process can vary dramatically from one person to another. Most of us can report having seen 60-year-olds who look frail and elderly and 80-year-olds who run marathons 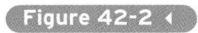 Figure 42-2 ◄ .

The aging process is inevitably accompanied by changes in physiologic function, such as a decline in the function of the liver and kidneys. All tissues in the body undergo aging, albeit not at the same rate. The decrease in the functional capacity of various organ systems is normal but can affect the way in which a patient responds to illness.

It can also affect the way health professionals respond to a patient's illness. For example, a health care provider

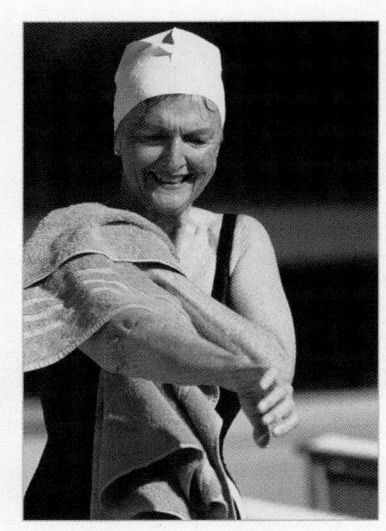

Figure 42-2 Many older people, especially those who have hobbies and activities, are healthy and vital.

who is unaware of the normal changes of aging may mistake the changes for signs of illness and be tempted to give treatment when none is necessary. At the other end of the spectrum, there is a widespread—and unfortunate—tendency to attribute genuine disease symptoms to "just getting old" and to neglect their treatment.

Changes in the Cardiovascular System

A variety of changes occur in the cardiovascular system as a person grows older, with their net effect being to decrease the efficiency of this system. Specifically, the heart hypertrophies (enlarges) with age, probably in response to the chronically increased afterload imposed by stiffened blood vessels. Bigger is not better, however. Over time, cardiac output declines, mostly as a result of a decreasing stroke volume. Arteriosclerosis—the stiffening of vessel walls—contributes to systolic hypertension in many older patients, which places an extra burden on the heart. This phenomenon may be a consequence of disease states such as diabetes, atherosclerosis Figure 42-3 ▲ , and renal compromise, and it is associated with an increased risk of cardiovascular disease, dementia, and death. Compliance of vascular walls depends on the production of collagen and elastin, proteins that are the primary components of muscle and connective tissue. An increase in pressure (normal hypertension seen in aging) leads to overproduction of abnormal collagen and decreased quantities of elastin, both of which contribute to vascular stiffening. The result is a widening pulse pressure, decreased coronary artery perfusion, and changes in cardiac ejection efficiency.

At the same time, the electric conduction system of the heart deteriorates over time. For example, the number of pacemaker cells in the sinoatrial node decreases dramatically as a person ages. In many cases, the changes in the conduction system lead to bradycardia, which can in turn contribute to the decline in cardiac output.

Some changes in cardiovascular performance are probably not a direct consequence of aging, but rather reflect the deconditioning effect of a sedentary lifestyle. Whether because of other disabilities (such as arthritis) or for psychological reasons, many people tend to limit physical activity as they grow older. The bodybuilder's slogan, "Use it or lose it," applies just as much to the cardiac muscle as to the biceps.

Changes in the Respiratory System

A person's respiratory capacity also undergoes significant reductions with age, largely due to decreases in the elasticity of the lungs and in the size and strength of the respiratory muscles. In addition, calcification of costochondral cartilage tends to make the chest wall stiffer. As a result of these changes, the vital capacity (the amount of air that can be exhaled following a maximal inhalation) decreases, and the residual volume (the amount of air left in the lungs at the end of a maximal exhalation) increases. Thus, although the total amount of air in the lungs does not change with age, the proportion of that air usefully used in gas exchange progressively declines. Air flow, which depends largely on airway size and resistance, also deteriorates somewhat with age.

Meanwhile, changes in the distribution of blood flow within the lungs result in declining Pa_{O_2}. At age 30, the Pa_{O_2} of a healthy person breathing ambient air is usually around 90 mm Hg; at 80 years, the Pa_{O_2} under the same conditions is around 75 mm Hg ($Pa_{O_2} = 100 - age/3$). Furthermore, the respiratory drive becomes dulled as a person ages because of decreased sensitivity to changes in arterial blood gases or decreased central nervous system (CNS) response to such changes. As a consequence, elderly people have a slower reaction to hypoxemia and hypercarbia.

Musculoskeletal changes, such as kyphosis (outward curvature of the thoracic spine; also called hunchback), may also affect pulmonary function by limiting lung volume and maximal inspiratory pressure. In addition, the lung's defense mechanisms become less effective as a natural consequence of aging. The cough and gag reflexes decrease with age, increasing the risk of aspiration. Furthermore, the ciliary mechanisms that normally help remove bronchial secretions are markedly slowed.

Changes in the Renal System

Age brings changes in the kidneys as well. The kidneys are responsible for maintaining the body's fluid and electrolyte balance and have important roles in maintaining the body's long-term acid-base balance and eliminating drugs from the body. In a young adult, the kidneys weigh 250 to 270 g; in a healthy 70-year-old, they weigh 180 to 200 g. This decline in weight results from a loss of functioning nephron units, which translates into a smaller effective filtering surface. At the same time, renal blood flow decreases by as much as 50% as a person ages.

Although the kidneys of an elderly person may be capable of dealing with day-to-day demands, they may not be able to meet unusual challenges, such as those imposed by illness. For that reason, acute illness in elderly patients is often accompanied by derangements in fluid and electrolyte balance. Aging kidneys, for example, respond sluggishly to sodium deficiency. An elderly patient may lose a great deal of sodium before the

You are the Provider Part 2

Recognizing an opportunity to complement your earlier review of elderly emergencies with hands-on experience, you ask Mike to begin a physical exam while your partner obtains a set of vital signs. The nurse caring for your patient is new to the facility and is not very familiar with her. She is able to tell you that your patient has a history of atrial fibrillation, congestive heart failure, diabetes, and hypertension. She is currently prescribed digoxin, pioglitazone (Actos), enalapril (Vasotec), and simvastatin (Vytorin).

While you are speaking with the nurse, another patient approaches you and sets her hand on your patient's shoulder. She introduces herself as Mrs. Jessup, a good friend of Mrs. Howard. She tells you that it is normal for them to go for a walk every night after dinner; however, they have not walked for the past couple of evenings because Mrs. Howard has been feeling weak. She also volunteers that Mrs. Howard has not been eating much the past few days. Mrs. Howard brushes off her friend's concerns. You are able to ascertain from Mrs. Howard that the last meal she had was a bowl of soup yesterday at lunch.

Vital Signs	Recording Time: 5 Minutes
Level of consciousness	Alert
Pulse	110 beats/min, strong and irregular
Blood pressure	168/94 mm Hg
Respirations	22 breaths/min, regular
Skin	Hot, pink, and dry
Sa_{O_2}	93% on room air

3. Why might obtaining an accurate medical history and history of the present illness be challenging when interviewing an elderly patient?

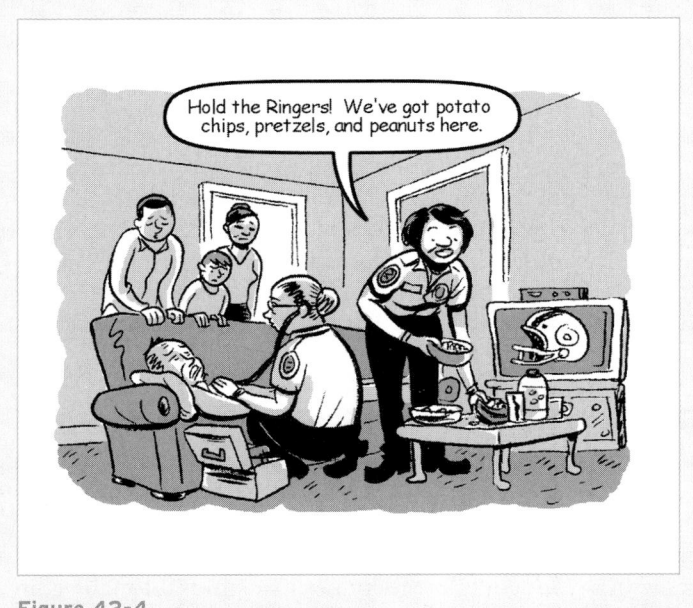

Hold the Ringers! We've got potato chips, pretzels, and peanuts here.

Figure 42-4

kidneys halt urinary sodium excretion, a problem that is exacerbated by the markedly decreased thirst mechanism in elderly people. The net result may be a rapid development of severe dehydration.

Conversely, elderly patients are at considerable risk of overhydration if they are exposed to large sodium loads (such as from intravenous [IV] saline solutions or heavily salted foods) **Figure 42-4 ▲**. Because of its lower glomerular filtration rate, the aging kidney is less able than its younger counterpart to excrete a large sodium load, making the patient vulnerable to acute volume overload.

The same factors that reduce an older person's ability to handle sodium also affect the body's ability to handle potassium. Thus, elderly patients are prone to hyperkalemia, which can reach serious—even lethal—levels if the patient becomes acidotic or if the potassium load is increased from any source.

Bowel and bladder continence require anatomically correct gastrointestinal (GI) and genitourinary tracts, functioning and intact sphincters, and properly working cognitive and physical functions. Urinary incontinence (involuntary loss of urine) can have significant social and emotional impact, but relatively few people admit to the problem and even fewer seek treatment. Incontinence is not a normal part of aging and can lead to skin irritation, skin breakdown, and urinary tract infections. As people age, the capacity of the bladder decreases. As a consequence, an older person may find it difficult to postpone voiding or may have involuntary bladder contractions. Two major types of incontinence are distinguished: stress and urge. Stress incontinence occurs during activities such as coughing, laughing, sneezing, lifting, and exercise. Urge incontinence is triggered by hot or cold fluids, running water, and even thinking about going to the bathroom. Treatment of incontinence consists of medications, physical therapy, and, possibly, surgery.

The opposite of incontinence is urinary retention or difficulty urinating. Patients may have difficulty voiding or absence of voiding as a result of many medical causes. In men, enlargement of the prostate can place pressure on the urethra, making voiding difficult. Bladder and urinary tract infections can also cause inflammation. In severe cases of urinary retention, patients may have acute or chronic renal failure.

Changes in the Digestive System

The process of digestion begins in the mouth, which is also where aging-related changes in the digestive system may first be noted. A decrease in the number of taste buds and changes in olfactory receptors may diminish an older person's senses of taste and smell, which may in turn interfere with the enjoyment of food. The consequent decrease in appetite may lead to malnutrition. Other changes in the mouth include a reduction in the volume of saliva, with a resulting dryness of the mouth. Dental loss is *not* a normal result of the aging process, but rather the result of disease of the teeth and gums; nevertheless, dental loss is widespread in the elderly population and contributes to nutritional and digestive problems.

Like oral secretions, gastric secretions are reduced as a person ages—although enough acid is still present to produce ulcers under certain conditions. Changes in gastric motility also occur, which may lead to slower gastric emptying—a factor of some importance when assessing the risk of aspiration.

Function of the small and large bowel changes little as a consequence of aging, although the incidence of certain diseases involving the bowel (such as diverticulosis) increases as a person grows older.

In the liver, there are changes in hepatic enzyme systems, with some systems declining in activity and others increasing. Notably, the activity of the enzyme systems concerned with the detoxification of drugs *declines* as a person ages.

Changes in the Musculoskeletal System

Aging brings a widespread decrease in bone mass in men and women, but especially among postmenopausal women. Bones become more brittle and tend to break more easily. Narrowing of the intervertebral disks and compression fractures of the vertebrae contribute to a decrease in height as a person ages, along with changes in posture. Joints lose their flexibility and may be further immobilized by arthritic changes. In fact, more than half of all elderly people have some form of arthritis. Muscle mass decreases throughout the body, with an accompanying decrease in muscle strength. From your perspective, the

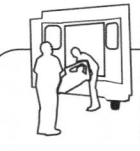

In the Field

Growing old does not naturally or normally include confusion, dementia, delirium, depression, falls, weakness, syncope, and other conditions related to disease processes.

changes in the musculoskeletal system most often translate into fractures incurred as the result of falls.

Changes in the Nervous System

Aging produces changes in the nervous system that are reflected in the neurologic examination. Changes in thinking (cognitive) speed, memory, and postural stability are the most common normal findings in older people. Studies have documented age-associated declines in mental function, especially slower central processing of sensory stimuli and language, and longer retrieval times for short- and long-term memory. Collectively, these changes affect performance on the mental status portion of the neurologic examination, with common findings including slow responses to questioning or requests to repeat a question.

The brain decreases in terms of weight (5% to 10%) and volume as a person ages. The functional significance of these changes is not clear, however. The human brain has an enormous reserve capacity, and having a smaller and lighter brain does not interfere with the mental capabilities of productive elderly people.

Undeniably, though, the performance of most of the sense organs suffers with increasing age. The senses of taste and smell become diminished as a person ages.

Visual changes may begin as early as 40 years, such that as many as 50% of patients older than 65 years have vision problems. Causes of visual impairment in elderly people may include diabetic retinopathy and age-related macular degeneration.

The two most common causes of visual disturbances in elderly people, however, are cataracts and glaucoma. Cataracts are a result of hardening of the lenses over time. The lenses eventually become opaque, which prevents light and images from being transmitted to the rear of the eye. Patients with cataracts may complain of blurred vision, double vision, spots, and/or ghost images. Surgical repair may be required to gain vision. By contrast, glaucoma is caused by an increase in intraocular pressure severe enough to damage the optic nerve, potentially resulting in permanent loss of peripheral and central vision. Treatment of glaucoma consists of oral medications and eye drops.

Decreases in visual acuity are common in older people, even without disease processes such as cataracts. Night vision becomes impaired, as does the ability to adjust to rapid changes in lighting conditions, depth perception, and perception of color. Changes in a patient's vision can affect independence, ability to read, and ability to drive a vehicle.

The possibility of hearing loss increases with age. A common cause of hearing impairment in geriatric patients is presbycusis, a progressive hearing loss, particularly in the high frequencies, along with lessened ability to discriminate between a particular sound and background noise. Patients who lose the ability to interpret most speech experience a decreased ability to communicate, which may lead to isolation and depression.

Another hearing-related impairment noted in the elderly population is Meniere disease (prevalence, 2 people per 1,000 population). Onset of symptoms usually occurs in early

middle age, with symptoms presenting in cycles that last several months at a time. The typical symptoms include vertigo (a sudden loss of normal balance or equilibrium), hearing loss, tinnitus, and pressure in the ear.

For many older people, physiologic changes make it difficult to produce speech that is loud enough, clear, and well spaced. Weakness, paralysis, poor hearing, or brain damage can damage the delicate functions that make these abilities possible.

Sense of body position (proprioception) also becomes impaired with age. Proprioception enables us to maintain postural stability by using a variety of receptors in the joints and information provided by the eyes. As these mechanisms fail with age, people become less steady on their feet, and the tendency to fall increases markedly.

Changes in the Integumentary System

Wrinkling and loss of resiliency of the skin are the most visible signs of aging. Wrinkling occurs because the skin becomes thinner, drier, less elastic, and more fragile. Subcutaneous fat becomes thinner, making for a loosened outer cover for the body. Elastin (the substance that makes the skin pliable) and collagen (the substance that makes the skin strong) decrease with age. Thinner skin tears much more easily, and the loss of elasticity allows for more bleeding before tamponade occurs.

As a person ages, the sebaceous glands produce less oil, making dryer skin. Sweat gland activity also decreases, hindering the ability to sweat and to regulate heat. Hair follicles produce thinner hair or may stop producing hair. Follicles produce less melanin (the pigment that gives hair color), making the hair color revert to gray or white.

The blood vessels that supply the skin also are affected by atherosclerosis and provide less oxygenated blood at the cellular level. As a consequence of the skin's lower metabolism, epidermal cells develop more slowly and do not replace outgoing cells as quickly as with younger skin. Elderly patients, therefore, are at higher risk for secondary infection after the skin breaks, for skin tumors, and for fungal or viral infections of the skin.

Homeostatic and Other Changes

Homeostasis is the process by which the body maintains a constant internal environment. Many homeostatic mechanisms work on a feedback principle, much like the thermostat in a house—that is, a change in the internal environment feeds back to the control system to induce a corrective response. For example, when the body temperature starts to rise, temperature sensors are activated, which in turn activate compensatory responses: Cutaneous blood vessels dilate, and excess heat is transferred from the body to the environment. Similarly, when the concentration of glucose in the blood rises, the pancreas is stimulated to secrete insulin, which leads to uptake of glucose by cells and reduction of the blood glucose level back toward normal.

Across the board, aging is accompanied by a progressive loss of these homeostatic capabilities. For that reason, a specific illness or injury in elderly people is more likely to result in generalized deterioration. For example, the thirst mechanism, which ordinarily protects a person from dehydration, becomes depressed in elderly patients. Likewise, temperature-regulating mechanisms tend to become disordered, which makes elderly patients much more vulnerable to environmental stresses such as heat exhaustion and accidental hypothermia after relatively minor exposures. A defect in temperature regulation also may account for the absence of a febrile response to illness in many elderly people. Infections that would ordinarily produce high fever, such as pneumococcal pneumonia, may produce only a low-grade or no fever in elderly people.

Notes from Nancy

A specific illness or injury in the elderly is more likely to result in generalized deterioration.

The regulatory system that manages the blood glucose level similarly becomes impaired with increasing age, such that an elevated blood glucose level occurs quite commonly in older patients. Ordinarily, moderate hyperglycemia does no harm, but overly aggressive treatment of this problem may produce damaging hypoglycemia.

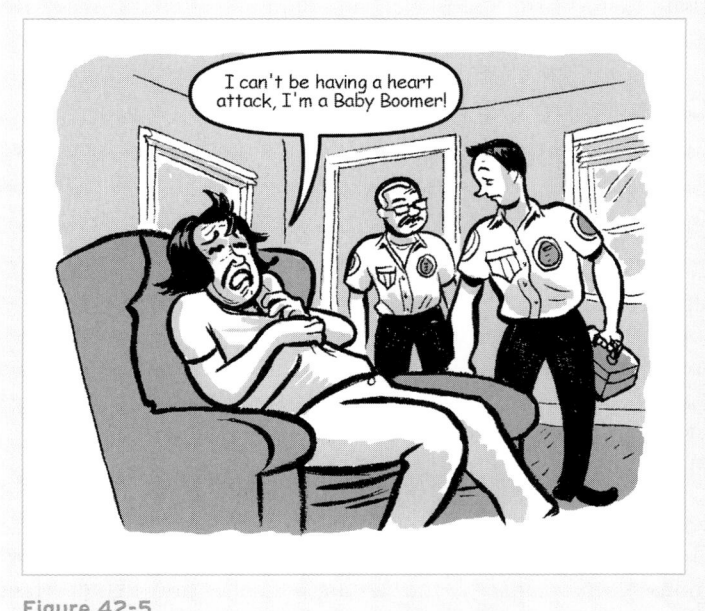

Figure 42-5

Pathophysiology

Cardiovascular System

Diseases of the heart remain the leading cause of death among older adults in the United States, and coronary artery disease (CAD) is the number one culprit. Heart attack is the major cause of morbidity and mortality in people older than 65 years, and its potential for mortality increases significantly after a person reaches 70 years **Figure 42-5 ▶**.

Myocardial infarction (MI) is the death of part of the heart muscle due to the blockage of one of the coronary arteries. Although chest pain is a common presentation for acute myocardial infarction in older patients, it may be decreased in intensity or atypical. In fact, it may even be absent, with the patient complaining primarily of dyspnea or fatigue. Major risk factors for MI include tobacco use, hypertension, diabetes, obesity, psychosocial factors, physical activity, and alcohol consumption. Preventive strategies include measures to prevent the first MI, avoidance of recurring MIs, and lifestyle interventions. Lifestyle changes include the cessation of tobacco use, eating a healthy diet, good control of blood glucose (in diabet-

ics), exercise, weight control, and control of hypertension. A physician may also order aspirin to help reduce the risk of heart attack.

People 65 years and older are a high-risk group for heart failure. In fact, this problem is the most common reason for hospitalization in the geriatric population. Heart failure is on the rise in this cohort for two paradoxical reasons: better care of the diseases that might otherwise result in failure (such as CAD and hypertension), which enables patients to live long enough to develop heart failure, and more effective management of heart failure once it develops. Risk factors include sex, ethnicity, family history and genetics, long-term alcohol abuse, and multiple medical conditions—CAD, emphysema, hyperthyroidism, thiamine (vitamin B) deficiency, and human immunodeficiency virus infection, among others. As with MI, prevention is aimed at lifestyle changes: cessation of tobacco use, eating a healthy diet, good control of blood glucose (in diabetics), exercise, weight control, and control of hypertension.

Rhythm disturbances (arrhythmias) of the heart occur when the electrical system controlling the heartbeat experiences an interruption or malfunction. These irregularities cause heartbeats that are too fast, too slow, irregular, or absent. Many people experience an occasional or harmless arrhythmia, which they may describe as a skipping, fluttering, or fast heartbeat. Arrhythmias in older people are generally a result of age-related changes in the heart, existing cardiac disease, adverse drug effects, or a combination of these factors.

Cardiac arrhythmias are classified by the part of the heart from which they originate. Unlike tachyarrhythmias or bradyarrhythmias, which speed up or slow down the heart, premature beats signify no change in speed but rather alter the regularity of the heartbeat. In contrast, atrial fibrillation (coming from the atria), which is the most common arrhythmia among elderly people, increases the risk of stroke and heart failure. The fibrillating atria allow stasis of the blood, thereby encouraging clot formation and increasing the chances that a clot fragment might travel to the brain and cause a stroke. Most of the blood in the atria enters the ventricles when the valves open, with about 20% being kicked in by contraction of the atria. The aging heart may function adequately when preload provided by the atria ends up in the ventricles; however, when that 20% remains in the atria, new signs or symptoms of heart failure may develop or stable heart failure may decompensate.

Bradycardias are also more common in elderly people. The aging conduction system may produce sinus abnormalities such as sick sinus syndrome. CAD may produce high-degree blocks, whereas medications such as beta blockers or calcium channel blockers can slow the heart too much.

The human heart beats 2.5 billion times and moves 200 million liters of blood in an average lifetime. Not surprisingly, this workload affects the cardiovascular system throughout the entire body over the lifespan. For example, the incidence of aneurysm increases with age. An aneurysm is a weakness in any artery that produces a balloon defect, weakening the arterial wall. This weakness may be congenital (present at birth) or acquired. In the latter case, hypertension, atherosclerotic disease, and obesity are contributing factors to development of such a defect. For example, blood pressure greater than 160/95 mm Hg doubles the mortality risk in men and can lead to kidney loss and blindness by damaging the blood vessels that supply the kidney and eyes. Life-threatening aneurysms can develop in the brain, chest, or abdomen. A new headache or a change in chronic headache patterns, for example, may signal early cerebral bleeding from an aneurysm; all too often, the first manifestation is a sudden and devastating stroke. Preventive measures—proper diet, exercise, smoking cessation, and cholesterol control—aim to control the risk factors associated with hypertension and atherosclerotic diseases.

Aortic dissection occurs when the inside wall of the artery becomes torn and allows blood to collect between the arterial wall layers. It may occur with trauma or sustained hypertension. Dissection weakens the arterial wall, making it prone to rupture. A thoracic dissection, for example, can produce chest pain that is difficult to differentiate from cardiac ischemia. Therefore, it is helpful to take blood pressure readings in both arms in all patients with chest pain. A systolic blood pressure difference of 15 mm Hg or higher suggests a thoracic dissection.

More than half of all older persons are hypertensive. The majority have isolated systolic hypertension resulting from a loss of arterial elasticity. Controlling systolic and/or diastolic hypertension in elderly people helps prevent strokes and MIs. Geriatric hypertensive emergencies require a controlled decline in blood pressure that often cannot be achieved in the field.

Stroke is a significant cause of death and disability in elderly people. More than 80% of all stroke deaths occur in persons older than 65 years, and stroke is the leading cause of long-term disability at any age. Strokes, which are mainly caused by atherosclerosis, are responsible for 1 of every 15 deaths in the United States. The risk of stroke doubles each decade after 35 years, mirroring the increase in risk factors such as hypertension and atrial fibrillation. Hypertension is the primary risk for stroke, but age, family history, smoking, diabetes, high cholesterol, and heart disease also contribute. Prevention is aimed at reduction of risk factors, improving diet and exercise, and lowering cholesterol.

Transient ischemic attacks (also called TIAs and mini-strokes) entail a temporary disturbance of blood supply to the brain that results in a sudden, temporary decrease in brain function. The symptoms are the same as those for a stroke but generally last less than 24 hours; they are warning signs of a future stroke.

Respiratory System

Although tobacco abuse seems to be decreasing among elderly people, chronic lower respiratory disease, influenza, and pneumonia remain in the top five causes of geriatric deaths. In fact, one of the most common causes of death in older patients is infection with *Pneumococcus* bacteria.

Pneumonia involves an inflammation of the lung, secondary to infection by bacteria, viruses, or other organisms. Although it can affect people at any age, this disease has its biggest impact on very young and elderly people, typically during the colder seasons (winter and early spring). People considered at risk include elderly people; people with underlying health problems such as chronic obstructive pulmonary disease (COPD), diabetes mellitus, and vascular diseases; and any person with a depressed immune system because of acquired immunodeficiency syndrome, cancer therapy, or organ transplantation. Treatment is primarily supportive, consisting of bed rest, fluids, oxygen therapy via nasal cannula or mask to relieve dyspnea, analgesics to reduce fever, and antibiotics. Preventive measures include a vaccine given once and boosters after 3 to 5 years.

COPD includes chronic asthma, chronic bronchitis, and emphysema, all of which are characterized by the presence of bronchial obstruction and airway inflammation. Distinguishing these diseases can be difficult, so the problem may not be diagnosed or treated correctly. COPD affects approximately 10% of the older population, mostly owing to tobacco use. Its effects reflect the age-related loss of elastic tissue in the lungs (*senile emphysema*) and a decreased ability to defend against infection. These factors may increase the baseline disability of COPD and set up older patients for an increased risk of acute exacerbation, often caused by infection.

Preventive measures for COPD-related complications include immunization for influenza and pneumococcal pneumonia. Long-term oxygen therapy has proven helpful in hypoxemic patients. In addition, pulmonary rehabilitation may improve functional status and the quality of life for some patients.

Approximately 1 in 20 elderly people has a history of asthma or is affected by it. Onset can occur in old age with presenting symptoms of shortness of breath (especially with effort), chronic or nocturnal cough, and wheezing.

A pulmonary embolus arises when a blood vessel supplying the lung becomes blocked by a clot. Any obstruction in blood flow to the lung can result in irreversible damage or infarction. An embolus is often released from a vein in a lower extremity, the pelvis, or the abdomen but could also result from a damaged heart. The risk of pulmonary embolus increases with age because of increasing immobility. Older patients may also be bedridden after recent surgery (such as abdominal procedures). Finally, elderly patients have an increased incidence of diseases associated with a higher risk of pulmonary embolus, such as cancer, heart attack, cardiac arrhythmias, and clotting disorders.

Prevention of thromboembolism is based on the patient's risk level—high, moderate, or low. Surgical patients are in the highest-risk category for potential emboli, and prophylaxis is recommended, including warfarin (Coumadin) and/or heparin and compression stockings.

Endocrine System

Diabetes arises when the body cannot oxidize complex carbohydrates (sugars) due to impaired pancreatic activity—namely, production of insulin. Insulin moves carbohydrates out of the bloodstream, through the cellular walls, and into the cells to be metabolized. With diabetes, more glucose is present in the blood than the body can handle. Geriatric patients with diabetes are at increased risk for hypoglycemia for several reasons: medications, inadequate or irregular dietary intake, inability to recognize the warning signs due to cognitive problems, and/or blunted warning signs. Delirium may be the only indication of hypoglycemia in an elderly patient.

After 65 years, one of every five people in the United States has diabetes—primarily type 2 diabetes (adult-onset, or non–insulin-dependent diabetes). The most common risk factor for this disease is having more than one chronic disease, and many elderly people with diabetes also have hypertension, heart disease, and stroke. Other risk factors for diabetes include a family history of diabetes, genetics, age, diet, obesity, and a sedentary lifestyle. Symptoms of an elevated blood glucose level (that is, hyperglycemia) include fatigue, poor wound healing, blurred vision, and frequent infections. Other symptoms of diabetes include the three Ps: Polyuria, Polydipsia, and Polyphagia. Prevention of type 2 diabetes is aimed at changes in lifestyle that include dietary restrictions, exercise, and controlling obesity.

Older diabetics whose blood glucose levels tend to be high are more prone to hyperosmolar hyperglycemic nonketotic (HHNK) coma than diabetic ketoacidosis. The most frequent cause for HHNK coma is infection. Presentation is likely to be acute confusion with dehydration, although signs of dehydration may be altered in elderly patients **Table 42-1**. Prehospital treatment remains the same as for younger patients, albeit with a cautious approach to fluid resuscitation.

Thyroid abnormalities also increase with aging. Many older patients remain asymptomatic, and the disease is diagnosed only when a routine blood test reveals a thyroid prob-

Table 42-1	Signs of Dehydration in Elderly People

- Dry tongue
- Longitudinal furrows in the tongue
- Dry mucous membranes
- Weak upper body musculature
- Confusion
- Difficulty in speech
- Sunken eyes

lem. With hypothyroidism, for example, the signs and symptoms may match those seen with normal aging: cold intolerance, constipation, dry skin, weakness, and so on. For acute-onset hyperthyroidism (thyrotoxicosis), the presentation can be blunted; although tachycardia is generally present, older patients may experience less tremor, anxiety, or hyperactive reflexes than their younger counterparts. Atrial fibrillation is more likely to be induced by an overactive thyroid gland in a geriatric patient. A smaller percentage of elderly hyperthyroid patients present with symptoms opposite those expected: weakness, lethargy, and depression. Field care is supportive.

Gastrointestinal System

Constipation is a frequent and significant problem in elderly people. Although it can cause acute abdominal pain, it should not be the initial suspect when a patient experiences such discomfort. Instead, causes with high mortality, such as bleeding from an acute abdominal aneurysm or dead bowel from mesenteric ischemia, should be investigated first. Many elderly people have diverticulosis (small outward pouches in the colon wall) and are at risk for diverticulitis and/or perforation. Appendicitis can be difficult to diagnose in older people, which probably accounts for the high perforation rate (50%) seen with this condition. The incidence of peptic ulcer disease is also increased among the older population, likely because of their relatively high use of nonsteroidal anti-inflammatory drugs (NSAIDs) for pain management.

Large bowel obstructions in elderly people are likely to be caused by cancer, impacted stool, or sigmoid volvulus. In addition, small bowel obstruction secondary to gallstones increases significantly with age. One third to one half of all elderly people have cholelithiasis (gallstones), although most remain asymptomatic for life. With one or more episodes of cholecystitis (inflammation of the gallbladder), the gallbladder adheres to the small bowel and, over time, creates an opening or fistula. The stone(s) drop into the bowel and produce the obstruction. Such a gallstone ileus may account for as many as 25% of geriatric small bowel obstructions. The large and small intestines are at risk for obstruction from adhesions due to previous surgery or infection or when a segment of bowel is forced into a fascial defect (hernia) in the abdominal wall.

Older patients are more likely than younger ones to have stomach or duodenal ulcers (peptic ulcer disease). The main risk factors for peptic ulcers are regular use of NSAIDs and infection with *Helicobacter pylori* (an ulcer-associated bacteria of the stomach), both of which are more common in older patients. Other medications have also been implicated in ulcer formation. The main symptom of peptic ulcer disease is dyspepsia (gnawing, burning pain in the upper abdomen), which usually improves immediately after eating but returns several hours later. Other causes of dyspepsia include acid reflux, gastritis, and gastric cancer.

Musculoskeletal System

Changes in physical abilities can affect older adults' confidence in their mobility. The muscle system atrophies and weakens with age. Muscle fibers become smaller and fewer, motor neurons decline in number, and strength declines. The ligaments and cartilage of the joints lose their elasticity. Cartilage also goes through degenerative changes with aging, contributing to arthritis.

The stooped posture of older people comes from atrophy of the supporting structures of the body. Two of every three older patients will show some degree of kyphosis (also called humpback, hunchback, and Pott curvature). Lost height in older adults generally results from compression in the spinal column, first in the disks and then from the process of osteoporosis in the vertebral bodies.

Osteoporosis, a condition that affects men and women, is characterized by a decrease in bone mass leading to reduction in bone strength and greater susceptibility to fracture. The extent of bone loss that a person undergoes is influenced by numerous factors, including genetics, smoking, level of activity, diet, alcohol consumption, hormonal factors, and body weight. The most rapid loss of bone occurs in women during the years following menopause, and many postmenopausal women use hormone replacement therapy as a means to reduce the loss of bone. Calcium and vitamin D supplementation is another treatment for the condition, and many other medications are available to improve bone strength. Older people should remain active and perform low-impact exercises to maintain bone and muscle strength.

Osteoarthritis is a progressive disease of the joints that destroys cartilage, promotes the formation of bone spurs in joints, and leads to joint stiffness. This type of arthritis is thought to result from "wear and tear" and, in some cases, from repetitive trauma to the joints. It affects 35% to 45% of the population older than 65 years. Typically, osteoarthritis affects several joints of the body, most commonly those in the hands, knees, hips, and spine. Patients complain of pain and stiffness that gets worse with exertion. The end result is often substantial disability and disfigurement. Patients are typically treated with anti-inflammatory medications and physical therapy to improve the range of motion.

Nervous System

Normal age-related cognitive changes have two major features: (1) They are relatively isolated (that is, they are not associated with multiple abnormal neurologic findings that suggest specific disease states), and (2) the onset and progression of these findings are "in time" with the person's aging process (that is, the findings are not sudden or extreme, and they do not extend to other abnormalities).

Delirium (also known as acute brain syndrome or acute confusional state) is a symptom, not a disease. A reflection of an underlying disturbance to a person's well-being (usually a treatable physical or mental illness), this temporary, usually reversible condition results in rapid changes in brain function. In elderly people, delirium often replaces or confounds the typical presentation caused by a medical problem, an adverse medication effect, or drug withdrawal. Disorders that cause delirium may also include poisons, electrolyte imbalances, nutritional deficiencies, and infections such as urinary tract infections and pneumonia. Onset of confusion or disorientation is abrupt (occurring during hours to days) but generally resolves with treatment of the underlying problem. The confusion and disorientation fluctuate with time, and hallucinations may occur. The patient experiences a rapid alteration between mental states, such as lethargy and agitation, serious attention disruption, disorganized thinking, and changes in perception and sensation.

Unlike delirium, dementia is a disease that produces irreversible brain failure. Disorders that cause dementia include conditions that impair vascular and neurologic structures within the brain, such as infections, strokes, head injuries, poor nutrition, and medications. The two most common degenerative types of dementia in older people are Alzheimer's disease (one of the fastest-growing health care problems in the United States) and multi-infarct or vascular dementia, both of which cause structural damage to the brain. An estimated 6% to 10% of elderly people will eventually have dementia, although this percentage increases with advancing age. Dementia may be diagnosed when two or more brain functions are impaired. These cognitive and psychomotor functions consist of language, memory, visual perception, emotional behavior and/or personality, and cognitive skills. Other risk factors that may predispose a patient to dementia include lower level of education, female sex, and African-American ethnicity. Although most cases of dementia cannot be prevented, some experts suggest that low-fat diets and exercise may help ward off vascular dementia.

Experts have not identified a single cause for Alzheimer's disease, but most believe it is not a normal part of the aging process. Although age is a significant risk factor for this disease (Alzheimer's disease typically affects patients older than 60 years), but age alone is not the cause. This progressive disease cannot be cured or reversed by any known treatment or intervention. Symptoms are subtle at onset. Over time, patients lose their ability to think, reason clearly, solve problems, and concentrate; they may present with altered behavior that includes paranoia, delusions, and social inappropriateness. In the later stages of Alzheimer's disease, patients cannot take care of themselves and may lose the ability to speak. People with severe Alzheimer's disease become completely debilitated and totally dependent on others.

Patients with Parkinson's disease—another age-related neurologic disorder—have two or more of the following symptoms: resting tremor of an extremity, slowness of movement (bradykinesia), rigidity or stiffness of the extremities or trunk, and poor balance. Parkinson's disease is caused by degeneration of the substantia nigra, an area of the brain that controls voluntary movement by producing the neurotransmitter dopamine. Cells use dopamine to transmit impulses, so a loss of dopamine results in the loss of muscle function. Parkinson's disease can affect one or both sides of the body and produces a wide range of functional loss.

The incidence of seizures (including status epilepticus) is also increased in elderly people, partly because of the increase in risk factors such as stroke, dementia, primary or metastatic brain tumors, and acute metabolic disorders (such as hyperglycemia, hyponatremia, alcohol withdrawal). Prehospital treatment for seizures is the same for younger and older patients.

Toxicology

As the number of uses for medications increases, there is a proportional increase in the likelihood of adverse drug reactions and interactions. Elderly people are particularly prone to adverse reactions, even when they take drugs at doses that would be safe in younger people. This increased incidence of adverse drug reactions among elderly people seems to reflect changes in drug metabolism because of diminished hepatic function; in drug elimination because of diminished renal function; in body composition, including increased body fat and decreased body water, altering the distribution of drugs through the various body compartments; and in the responsiveness to drugs that affect the CNS. A change in any one of these processes can lead to toxic effects in elderly people.

Other body changes may affect medication use by geriatric patients in a more general way. As vision declines with age, reading small print becomes more difficult. Night vision becomes less acute, so reading labels in dim light can lead to errors. Short-term memory loss may lead to forgetfulness about whether medications have been taken. An inability to distinguish flavors may cause patients to take multiple doses of medications before they detect problems.

Elderly people consume more than 25% of all prescribed and over-the-counter drugs sold in the United States. Community-dwelling older persons take an average of three to five medications per day. Nursing home patients take an average of six to seven routinely scheduled medications daily (polymedicine) and two to three additional medications on an as-needed basis. This kind of polypharmacy may be therapeutic when multiple drugs are needed to manage different medical problems, but it may prove harmful when these medications interact. Elderly patients are particularly prone to having multiple chronic diseases, which may lead to a vicious circle: The presence of multiple disease states leads to the use of multiple medications, which increases the likelihood of adverse reactions, which in turn leads to treatment with more medications. In turn, a person's chance of ending up in the hospital because of an adverse reaction to a medication increases with the number of drugs taken. Ultimately, the best dosage of a drug for an elderly patient is the lowest dosage that will achieve a therapeutic effect.

Medication noncompliance in older patients is also associated with negative effects on health. Many patients—not just older patients—do not follow instructions or advice on the use of their medications. Because elderly people use more medications than the rest of the population, noncompliance issues are more likely. Noncompliance issues include failure to fill a prescription (for example, the patient doesn't have the money to pay for the drug or doesn't see the benefits of it), improper administration of medication (for example, the patient decreases the dosage to make the prescription last longer), discontinuation of medication (for example, the patient feels better and decides not to take the medication), and taking inappropriate medications (for example, the patient had medication left over from a previous prescription or shares the medicine with family or friends).

Geriatric patients are predisposed to medicine-related reactions owing to the previously mentioned age-related physiologic changes that occur in body systems and body composition. For example, an increase in the proportion of adipose tissue can prolong the half-life of a drug. In particular, medications that affect the CNS are the most common source of adverse or unexpected reactions, and barbiturates and benzodiazepines are the drugs most often associated with toxic effects. A reduction in the nervous system response—especially the decrease in parasympathetic activity typically seen with the aging process—increases the risk that adverse anticholinergic effects will occur. Reduced beta-adrenergic receptor sensitivity (which is responsible for bronchodilation) makes most bronchodilator medications less effective. The use of diuretics and antihypertensive

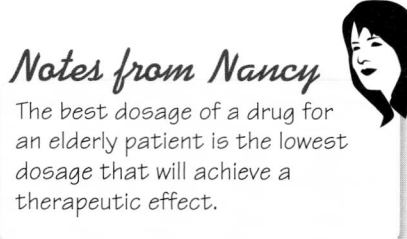

Notes from Nancy

The best dosage of a drug for an elderly patient is the lowest dosage that will achieve a therapeutic effect.

medications by geriatric patients can cause hypotension and orthostatic changes due to reduced cardiac output and a decrease in total body water. Finally, decreased glucose tolerance may cause medications such as diuretics and corticosteroids to have hyperglycemic effects.

Drug and Alcohol Abuse

Alcohol is the preferred substance of abuse among older persons, in whom its use is on the rise. A much smaller but increasing segment of the geriatric population uses illicit drugs. Most users are men, and more than half carry their addiction into old age. About one third develop an abuse problem after reaching 65 years, often in response to a life-changing event such as the loss of a spouse, declining health, or low self-esteem.

The prevalence of alcohol and drug misuse among older people is also attributable to the multiplicity of medications that are prescribed for them and their heightened vulnerability to abuse owing to the effects of aging. Decreased body mass and total body water means higher concentrations of blood alcohol; at the same time, the combination of digestive, renal, and hepatic system changes means slower elimination of alcohol from the body.

As the geriatric population continues to grow and experiences even more chronic disabilities, the likelihood of substance abuse–related problems in this group will increase. Recognizing substance abuse in older people can be difficult. If they have engaged in this behavior for a long time, it may be well hidden from—or even accepted by—family and friends. Because substance abuse can complicate your field assessment and treatment, it is important to ask about this issue.

Psychiatric Conditions

Depression is not part of normal aging, but rather a medical disease that occurs in about 6% of the population older than 65 years. The good news is that it is treatable with medication and therapy. The bad news is that if depression goes unrecognized or untreated, it is associated with a higher suicide rate in the elderly population than in any other age group. Depression in elderly patients can mimic the effects of many other medical problems (such as dementia). Risk factors for depression in older people include a history of depression, chronic disease, and loss (function, independence, or significant others). This condition may be difficult to recognize in older people because many don't want to complain about feeling sad, worthless, or unwanted.

Disturbingly, the majority of elder suicides occur in people who have recently been diagnosed with depression. In addition, the majority of suicide victims have seen their primary care physician within the month before the event. Unlike younger people, geriatric patients typically do not make suicidal gestures or attempt to get help. Instead, the rate of completed suicide is disproportionately high in the geriatric population. Many geriatric patients see no other way out when they have a terminal illness or debilitating cardiac or neurologic condition (such as severe heart disease or stroke). At highest risk are white men 85 years and older who use firearms as their suicide method of choice.

Injury in Elderly People
Environmental Injury

Internal temperature regulation is slowed in elderly people and gets slower with increasing age. The body's ability to recognize fluctuations in temperature becomes delayed owing to a slowed endocrine system. Heat gain or loss in response to environmental changes is delayed by atherosclerotic vessels, slowed circulation, and decreased sweat production in the skin. In addition, thermoregulation can be adversely affected by chronic disease, medications, and alcohol use, all of which are more frequent in elderly people.

Not surprisingly, about half of all deaths of hypothermia occur in elderly people, and most *indoor* hypothermia deaths involve geriatric patients. Although living where harsh winters occur is a risk factor, hypothermia can develop at temperatures above freezing when an older person is exposed for a prolonged period.

The death rates from hyperthermia are more than doubled in elderly people compared with younger persons; people older than 85 years are at highest risk. Arizona has more heat-related deaths than all other states combined, reflecting its very long, hot summers and large geriatric population.

Trauma in Elderly People

Trauma is one of the top 10 causes of death among elderly people. The mortality rate for trauma in patients older than 65 years is 191 per 100,000, versus 50 per 100,000 for all other age groups. Deaths from injury in people older than 65 years account for one fourth of all trauma deaths in the United States, and injury is the seventh leading cause of death in the older population.

Several factors place an elderly person at higher risk of trauma than a younger person—namely, slower reflexes, visual and hearing deficits, equilibrium disorders, and an overall reduction in agility. In particular, changes in the body's homeostatic compensatory mechanisms combined with the effects of aging on body systems and any preexisting conditions usually add up to less-than-favorable outcomes in trauma situations. Compensation in trauma is successful when increased heart rate, increased respiration, and adequate vasoconstriction make up for trauma-related deficits. Reduced cardiac reserve, decreased respiratory function, impaired renal activity, and ineffective vasoconstriction, by contrast, may lead to unsuccessful recovery from traumatic situations. Furthermore, an elderly person is more likely to sustain serious injury in case of trauma because stiffened blood vessels and fragile tissues tear more readily, and brittle, demineralized bone is more vulnerable to fracture.

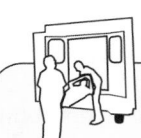 **In the Field**

Compensatory mechanism changes + aging systems + preexisting conditions = bad outcomes.

Most geriatric trauma cases involve falls or motor vehicle crashes. The incidence of falls, for example, increases with increasing age. Although most falls do *not* produce serious injury, elderly people account for 75% of all fall-related deaths. This increased mortality in geriatric patients is directly related to the patient's age, preexisting disease processes, and complications related to the trauma. Falls are associated with a higher incidence of anxiety and depression, a loss of confidence, and postfall syndrome. With this syndrome, geriatric patients develop a lack of confidence and anxiety about potential falls.

Table 42-2	Causes of Falls in the Elderly	
Cause	**Clues to Suggest This Cause**
Extrinsic (accidental)	Obvious environmental hazard at the scene, such as poor lighting, scatter rugs, uneven sidewalk, ice or other slippery surface
Intrinsic drop attacks	Sudden fall; patient found on the ground somewhat confused, often temporarily paralyzed and unable to get up; no premonitory symptoms
Postural hypotension	Fall when getting up from a recumbent or sitting position (Check medications the patient is taking, and ask about occult blood loss, such as presence of black stools. Measure blood pressure in recumbent and sitting positions.)
Dizziness or syncope	Marked bradycardia or tachyarrhythmias
Stroke	Other characteristic signs of stroke, such as hemiparesis, hemiplegia, or aphasia
Fracture	Patient felt something snap before falling.

Ultimately, they may become immobile, risk incontinence, and develop pneumonia or pressure ulcers from lack of movement.

Falls among elderly people are evenly divided between those resulting from extrinsic (external) causes, such as tripping on a loose rug or slipping on ice, and those resulting from intrinsic (internal) causes, such as a dizzy spell or a syncopal attack (Table 42-2 ▲). The risk of falls increases in people with preexisting gait abnormalities (such as from neurologic or musculoskeletal impairment) and cognitive impairment. Older patients with osteoporosis have lower-density bones, so even a sudden, awkward turn may fracture a bone. When treating a patient who has fallen, you need to take a careful history. Although the patient often attributes the fall to an accidental cause ("I must have tripped over the rug"), meticulous questioning often reveals a period of dizziness or palpitations just before the fall, suggesting a different cause. Home safety assessments by EMS—during a routine visit or as part of an outreach program—may reduce fall incidence.

After falls, motor vehicle accidents are the second leading cause of accidental death among elderly people. Of licensed drivers, 10% are elderly people. They account for 10% of all traffic deaths, 11% of all vehicle occupant deaths, and 16% of all pedestrian deaths. Impaired vision, errors in judgment, and underlying medical conditions contribute to the higher risk. Impairments in vision and hearing, along with diminished agility, also contribute to pedestrian deaths involving elderly people.

Types of Injuries Commonly Seen in Elderly People

Changes associated with normal aging and with diseases of aging make elderly people particularly vulnerable to certain types of injuries. In particular, head trauma or injury is a serious problem. The increased fragility of cerebral blood vessels, enlargement of the subdural space, and a decrease in the supportive tissue of the meninges all contribute to make an elderly person more vulnerable than a younger person to intracranial bleeding, particularly subdural hematoma. In many cases, the hematoma develops slowly, during days or weeks. By the time the patient becomes symptomatic, the person or his or her caretakers may not remember the incident, or the family or caretakers may feel guilty about their own negligence in the incident. As a result, it

may be difficult to obtain an accurate history of the initial trauma. The most important early symptom of a subdural hematoma is headache, which may be worse at night. Sometimes the headache occurs on the same side of the head as the blood clot. With increasing intracranial pressure, the state of consciousness becomes depressed, and the patient becomes increasingly drowsy.

Elderly people are also more vulnerable than their younger counterparts to cervical spinal cord injury and cord compression, even after apparently minor trauma. Degenerative changes in the cervical spine (cervical spondylosis) cause arthritic "spurs" and narrowing of the vertebral canal; the nerve roots exiting from the cervical spine gradually become compressed, and pressure on the spinal cord increases. Any injury to the cervical spine, therefore, is much more likely to injure the already compromised spinal cord. Even a sudden movement of the neck may result in spinal cord injury.

Injuries to the chest in elderly people are much more likely to produce rib fracture and flail chest, owing to the brittleness of the ribs and overall stiffening of the chest wall as the costochondral cartilage becomes calcified. Abdominal trauma often produces liver injury, perhaps because the liver is less protected by abdominal musculature.

Orthopedic injuries are a common result of falls in geriatric patients, with hip fractures the most common acute orthopedic injury, followed, in severity and frequency, by fractures of the femur, pelvis, tibia, and upper extremities. Hip fracture may also occur without trauma, simply because of vigorous contracture of the hip musculature. The most important risk factor for hip fracture is osteoporosis: Approximately half of older women and one of eight older men will have an osteoporosis-related fracture (hip or other). An estimated 15 to 20 million people in the United States older than 45 years have osteoporosis, and it leads to nearly 1.3 million fractures annually.

Burns are a significant risk of morbidity and mortality in elderly people because of physiologic and pathophysiologic changes. The risk of mortality is increased when preexisting medical conditions exist, defense mechanisms to protect against infection are weakened, and fluid replacement is complicated by renal compromise. In the assessment of a burn patient, prehospital providers need to monitor the patient's hydration status by assessing current vital signs, mucous membranes, and urine output, which is typically 50 to 60 mL/h or 1 to 2 mL/kg/h.

■ Assessment of Geriatric Patients

Although illness is common among elderly people, it is *not* an inevitable part of aging. Complaints of elderly people cannot be ascribed simply to "getting old." Aging is a continuous process and a normal development sequence that affects people in multiple ways. The normal wear-and-tear concept and genetic makeup are two theories that have been suggested to explain the biologic effects of aging.

Along the same lines, there is a widespread misconception that elderly people tend to be hypochondriacs, with dozens of imaginary or minor complaints. In reality, hypochondria is far less common among elderly than among younger patients. Indeed, older patients tend *not* to complain, even when they have legitimate symptoms. When an elderly person calls for an ambulance, he or she usually has a very real problem.

Knowing what is and what is not part of the aging process constitutes the first challenge in assessing elderly people. A second challenge is that signs and symptoms of disease may be altered from their presentation in younger patients as a consequence of the aging process. An MI may present without chest pain; fever may be minimal in pneumonia; uncontrolled diabetes is more likely to present as HHNK coma

than as ketoacidosis. A variety of acute illnesses—from congestive heart failure to an acute abdomen—may present simply as delirium.

Another challenge relates to the fact that the older the patient, the more likely are multiple problems—medical, psychological, and social. Interestingly, the proportion of older people with a disability has decreased; however, the total number of older people with a chronic disability has increased simply because there are more elderly people. Debilitating health conditions often found in this population include hypertension, arthritic symptoms, heart disease, cancer, diabetes, stroke, and COPD. The incidence of depression also increases with age, with 15% to 20% of people older than 85 years having some form of depression.

The co-occurrence of multiple pathologic conditions has several consequences for patients and health care providers alike. The symptoms of one disease or disability may alter or hide the symptoms of another condition. The patient with severe leg pain from arthritis, for example, may not pay much attention to new pain caused by thrombophlebitis. In addition, when several organ systems are in borderline condition, a disturbance in function in only one of the systems may have repercussions throughout the body, leading to failure of multiple organs in a dominolike manner. The presence of multiple underlying illnesses also makes it much more difficult for health professionals to sort out which problem is causing which symptom. Furthermore, chronic comorbidities may make it much more difficult to treat the patient's acute problem. For example, the medication a patient needs for a cardiac problem may be contraindicated because of a renal or hepatic problem or, at the least, may require major modification in dosage.

Notes from Nancy
Getting old is not a disease, and it does not by itself produce symptoms of disease.

Notes from Nancy
When an elderly person calls for an ambulance, there is usually a very good reason, even if it is not the reason the patient tells you.

You are the Provider Part 3

After gathering the information from the nurse and Mrs. Jessup, you ask Mike what he found during his physical exam. He tells you that he found the patient to have signs of dehydration as demonstrated by tenting of the skin and dry mucous membranes, diminished breath sounds bilaterally with rales at the right base, a slightly elevated irregular heartbeat, and an oral temperature of 102°F. He asks what treatment you would like to him to give.

At this point you ask your partner to establish IV access so that you can administer fluids to help with the dehydration and fever. He is able to successfully insert a 20-gauge needle in the left hand. Supplemental oxygen is administered via nasal cannula at 3 L/min, and the cardiac monitor is applied.

Reassessment	Recording Time: 11 Minutes
Skin	Pink, hot, and dry
Pulse	106 beats/min, weak
Blood pressure	164/92 mm Hg
Respirations	22 breaths/min, regular
Sao$_2$	98% with supplemental oxygen at 3 L/min by nasal cannula
ECG	Atrial fibrillation with no ectopy
Pupils	PERLA
Blood glucose level	178 mg/dL

4. What are some specific respiratory illnesses commonly seen in elderly people?
5. What are the risk factors for pneumonia in elderly people? Are any present here?

The GEMS Diamond

There are many acronyms in the prehospital setting to help you remember steps in your assessment and treatment. The GEMS diamond was created to help providers recall key themes when dealing with geriatric patients (Table 42-3 ▾). It was designed to assist the prehospital professional in the assessment and treatment of elderly patients.

"G" of the GEMS diamond is to recognize that the patient is a *geriatric* patient. The provider's thought process needs to be geared to the possible problems of an aging patient. When responding to an emergency involving an older patient, you should consider that older patients are different from younger patients and may present atypically.

"E" of the GEMS diamond stands for an *environmental* assessment. Assessment of the environment can help give clues to the patient's condition or the cause of the emergency. Is the home too hot or cold? Is the home well kept and secure? Are there hazardous conditions? Preventive care is also very important for a geriatric patient, who may not carefully study the environment or may not realize where risks exist.

"M" of the GEMS diamond stands for *medical* assessment. Older patients tend to have a variety of medical problems and may be taking numerous prescription, over-the-counter, and herbal medications. Obtaining a thorough history is very important in older patients.

"S" stands for *social* assessment. Older people may have less of a social network, because of the death of a spouse, family members, or friends. Older people may also need assistance with activities of daily living, such as dressing and eating. There are numerous social agencies that are readily available to help geriatric patients. Consider obtaining information pamphlets about some of the agencies for older people in your area. If you have these brochures with you and encounter a person in need, you can provide this valuable information. Social agencies that deal with the older population will be more than happy to share a listing of the services they provide.

The GEMS diamond provides a concise way to remember the important issues for older patient. Using this concept will help you make appropriate referrals, and as a result, you will help older patients maintain their quality of life.

Scene Size-up and Initial Assessment

As you move from scene size-up to the initial assessment of a patient, gather information that may prove relevant to the case. Look for potential clues from the patient's social history;

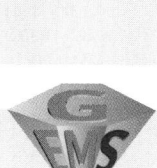

Notes from Nancy

Always assume that an elderly patient's mental status is normal until you have evidence to the contrary.

Table 42-3	The GEMS Diamond

G—Geriatric Patients

- Present atypically.
- Deserve respect.
- Experience normal changes with age.

E—Environmental Assessment

- Check the physical condition of the patient's home: Is the exterior of the home in need of repair? Is the home secure?
- Check for hazardous conditions that may be present (for example, poor wiring, rotted floors, unventilated gas heaters, broken window glass, clutter that prevents adequate egress).
- Are smoke detectors present and working?
- Is the home too hot or too cold?
- Is there an odor of feces or urine in the home? Is bedding soiled or urine-soaked?
- Is food present in the home? Is it adequate and unspoiled?
- Are liquor bottles present? If so, are they lying empty?
- If the patient has a disability, are appropriate assistive devices (for example, a wheelchair or walker) present?
- Does the patient have access to a telephone?
- Are medications out of date or unmarked, or are prescriptions for the same or similar medications from many physicians?
- If living with others, is the patient confined to one part of the home?
- If the patient is residing in a nursing facility, does the care appear to be adequate to meet the patient's needs?

M—Medical Assessment

- Older patients tend to have a variety of medical problems, making assessment more complex. Keep this in mind in all cases—both trauma and medical. A trauma patient may have an underlying medical condition that could have caused or may be exacerbated by the injury.
- Obtaining a medical history is important in older patients, regardless of the chief complaint.
- Initial assessment
- Ongoing assessment

S—Social Assessment

- Assess activities of daily living (eating, dressing, bathing, toileting).
- Are these activities being provided for the patient? If so, by whom?
- Are there delays in obtaining food, medication, or other necessary items? The patient may complain of this, or the environment may suggest this.
- If in an institutional setting, is the patient able to feed himself or herself? If not, is food still sitting on the food tray? Has the patient been lying in his or her own urine or feces for prolonged periods?
- Does the patient have a social network? Does the patient have a mechanism to interact socially with others on a daily basis?

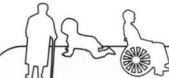
general living conditions; availability of social and family support; activity level; medications; overall appearance with respect to nutrition, general health, cleanliness, personal hygiene; and attitude and mental well-being. Prehospital providers also need to be aware of the numerous factors that affect the assessment process in geriatric patients: sensory alterations, verbal communication skills, mental and physical capabilities, and the ability of health care providers to accommodate and comprehend these conditions.

Patient History

Explain everything you plan to do, especially if the patient seems confused. Is this confused state normal, a new manifestation of a preexisting medical problem, or a patient's lack of understanding? A comprehensive patient history includes many elements—the patient's chief complaint, present illness or injury, pertinent medical history, and current health care status and needs. Pertinent medical history would *not* include information about the removal of a patient's appendix more than 50 years ago but would consider current cardiovascular health (such as palpitations or flutters), exercise tolerance, diet history, medications, smoking and drinking habits, sleep patterns, and other intrinsic and extrinsic factors.

The ability to elicit a good patient history comes from education and experience. The object is to reduce anxiety, not increase it—and if you simply whip out a lot of strange equipment and start, for example, sticking electrodes onto the patient's chest, the patient may well become frightened and wonder what is going to happen.

Communication

The ability to elicit a thorough patient history reflects education and experience. Good communication skills will help you gather the information you need during your assessment. Without good communication skills, you could frighten, alienate, insult, anger, or even harm your patients. Your first words should focus on gaining the patient's trust. Introduce yourself. Use respect when addressing the patient; use his or her name, if you know it; and avoid terms such as "honey," "dear," and "grandma" when addressing an older patient. Speak slowly, distinctly, and respectfully. Attempt to get the patient history from the patient, rather than family and bystanders, whenever possible.

Communication is not just talking; it is also listening. When asking questions of older patients, wait for their answers. Older people may need more time to process your questions, and they may speak slowly when responding. Active listening also involves paying attention to the patient's tone, especially if it conveys fear or confusion.

Nonverbal communication is just as important as verbal communication. Eye contact, hand gestures, body position,

facial expressions, and touch communicate a message. When speaking with patients, get face to face with them and make sure there is plenty of light. Have patients put in hearing aids or wear glasses to facilitate better communication, and be sure to take these aids with the patients to the hospital so other health care providers can communicate as well.

Part of your task in the assessment is to determine whether this confused state is normal, a new manifestation of a preexisting medical problem, or a result of the patient's lack of understanding. Preserve the patient's dignity during exposure and when discussing his or her history around others.

Chief Complaint

Obtaining the chief complaint would seem to be a straightforward procedure, but it may not be simple with some elderly patients. Older patients tend not to report significant symptoms for several reasons. Many share the misconception that illness and assorted aches and pains are simply part of aging. Other older people may not mention even legitimate symptoms to avoid being identified as old and a hypochondriac. Some patients fear that mentioning a symptom will lead to a diagnosis or treatment that will jeopardize their independence. "If I mention those pains in my stomach," the old person may reason, "they'll put me in the hospital, and I may never come out of that place again."

Whereas elderly patients tend to underreport serious symptoms, the symptoms they *do* report are often vague and apparently trivial. Furthermore, elderly patients are likely to have several chief complaints, each of which may have a different source.

When a patient's chief complaint seems trivial, it may be necessary to go through a standard list of screening questions to confirm that you are not missing important pieces of information. In such a review of systems, questions are designed to evaluate the functions of the body's major organ systems. In the field, there is not sufficient time to conduct a complete review of systems, but a few well-chosen questions can provide a great deal of information about the function of the patient's more important systems:

Cardiovascular

- Have you had any pain or discomfort in your chest? When?
- Have you noticed any fluttering in your chest or fast heartbeats?

Respiratory

- Do you ever get short of breath? When?
- Have you had a cough lately?

Neurologic

- Have you had any dizzy spells? Have you fainted?
- Have you had any trouble speaking?
- Have you had headaches recently?
- Have you noticed any unusual weakness or funny sensations in your arms or legs?

Gastrointestinal

- Have there been any changes in your appetite lately?
- Have you gained or lost any weight?
- Have there been any changes in your bowel movements?

Genitourinary

- Do you have any pain or difficulty urinating?
- Have you noticed any change in the color of your urine?

If any of these screening questions yields a positive answer, follow up with further questions. For example, if the patient states that he has been coughing lately, find out whether he is bringing up sputum and, if so, what the sputum looks like (for example, Is there blood in the sputum?).

Once you have elicited what you believe to be the chief complaint, go through the usual process of assembling the history of the present illness. This history may be complicated if other chronic problems are affecting the acute problem. To sort out which symptoms relate to the current chief complaint and which are chronic difficulties, try asking questions such as "How does this problem differ from what it was like last week?" or "What happened today to make you decide to get help?"

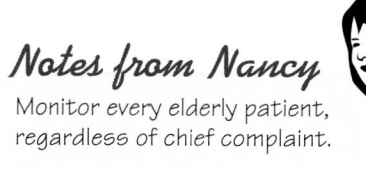

Notes from Nancy

Monitor every elderly patient, regardless of chief complaint.

Obtaining a history from an elderly patient requires patience. You must be prepared to listen, often for an extended period. But your listening will be rewarded—not only by helping you discover the patient's problem, but also by allowing you to provide part of the solution to the problem. Listening is a demonstration of caring, and your caring can mean a great deal to a lonely or frightened older person.

Other Medical History

Just as it is not practical to go through a comprehensive review of systems in the field, it is not usually feasible to obtain a complete medical history in the prehospital setting. Nevertheless, you should inquire about recent hospitalizations and allergies.

Most important, you should obtain the most detailed history possible of the patient's medications, because medications account for a significant percentage of medical problems in elderly people. A medication history should include *all* medications, not just prescription drugs, because many people do not think to mention common over-the-counter preparations such as aspirin, antacid tablets, and herbal medicines. Ask the patient to list the medications by name, and determine the dosing and frequency for each one. Also, inquire about medications that are prescribed but not taken (such as because of cost issues or side effects) and medications that may have been provided by other sources (such as a spouse's medication). Obtain the patient's permission to take medications to the hospital, and then collect them all—prescription and nonprescription drugs. If the patient cannot tell you where the medicines are stored, check the bathroom medicine cabinet, the bedside table, the kitchen table and counters, and the refrigerator.

Physical Exam

The physical examination of an elderly patient may be fraught with difficulties. Poor cooperation and easy fatigability may require that you keep manipulations of the patient to a minimum. You may have to peel many layers of clothing off an elderly patient to perform an adequate exam. Despite these obstacles, an ill or injured geriatric patient deserves as thorough an evaluation as a younger counterpart.

Begin by observing the patient's general appearance, including dress and grooming. In some cases, inattention to appearance may be one of the first signs of depression or a serious medical condition. Evaluate the level of consciousness as you would for any patient. In a critically ill or injured patient, use the AVPU scale. If you have more time, try to perform a more detailed assessment of the patient's cognitive function. Is the patient fully alert? Is he or she oriented to place and time? Does the patient's affect seem appropriate to the situation? Are there obvious disorders in thinking, such as delusions (false beliefs)?

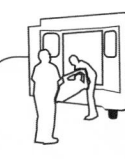

In the Field

Cover the patient with a blanket to protect privacy and keep the patient warm. This action shows respect for the patient and will improve your exam.

Note the patient's position and degree of distress. Check the color, moisture, and temperature of the skin, bearing in mind that the loss of elasticity in the skin of elderly patients may produce apparent signs of dehydration (such as tenting) when hydration is normal.

If you are examining the patient in his or her home, take a good look at the patient's surroundings, as well as at the patient. Try to assess the patient's self-care capability. Is everything neat and well maintained? Or is the home a mess, with dishes piled in the sink and rubbish accumulating? Do you see evidence of alcohol consumption (such as empty bottles)? Are there signs of violence, such as broken glassware, that might provide clues to elder abuse? Are the patient's quarters adequately heated or cooled? Is the patient living alone? Does the patient have pets? (If so, you should make arrangements for someone, such as a neighbor, to assume their care until the patient returns.) Record these observations on the patient care report to enable social service personnel to make appropriate arrangements for follow-up care.

Measure the patient's vital signs carefully. Postural changes in blood pressure vary among elderly people, but changes increase with increasing frailty and heighten the person's risk for falls. Marked postural changes in blood pressure and pulse may indicate hypovolemia or overmedication. As you measure the vital signs, bear in mind that normal blood pressure for a young person may represent significant hypotension in an elderly patient. If possible, determine the patient's baseline blood pressure. When obtaining a patient's blood pressure, be aware of the possibility of significant hypertension and orthostatic changes. Consider taking vital signs in both arms and checking pulses proximally and distally in all extremities. This process will allow you to gather information and observe for signs of dependent edema, dehydration, and the patient's circulatory status without raising his or her anxiety level.

Pay attention to the respiratory rate. Tachypnea can be a very sensitive indicator of acute illness in elderly people—especially pulmonary infection—even when patients show few, if any, other signs. When assessing the patient's respirations, listen to lung sounds in all fields, noting adventitious sounds that might aid in development of a treatment plan. You can also use the stethoscope to listen for carotid bruits; note jugular vein distention.

Notes from Nancy

Consider the possibility of hypovolemia in any elderly person whose systolic blood pressure is less than 120 mm Hg.

Detailed Physical Exam

Conduct the detailed physical exam as you would for any other patient. When examining the mouth, make a note of any upper or lower dentures. In the chest examination, keep in mind that elderly people may have pulmonary crackles without apparent pathology—so don't lunge for the nitroglycerin and furosemide at the first crackle you hear in the chest. Similarly, edema in the legs may be the result of chronic venous insufficiency and not right-sided heart failure.

Assessment and Management of Medical Complaints in Elderly People

Cardiovascular Complaints

Prehospital treatment for chest pain remains essentially unchanged in elderly patients, albeit with extra cautions because of the increased potential for medication side effects.

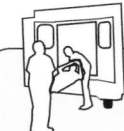

In the Field

If the patient is hypotensive and is wearing a nitroglycerin patch, remove it. The patient's complaint could be caused by too much or too little of this medication.

As in all prehospital emergencies, health care providers must prioritize the patient's airway, breathing, and circulatory status. Nitroglycerin and morphine may produce more hypotension or respiratory compromise than in younger patients or may react adversely with long-term medications. Aspirin may increase bleeding in a patient who is already taking anticoagulants. For patients 75 years or older with ST-segment elevation infarcts, angioplasty offers a better outcome than peripheral fibrinolysis.

The presentation of heart failure in an older person can be confused by symptoms and signs symbolic of old age and shared by a number of chronic diseases—for example, dyspnea on exertion, easy fatigability (especially with left-sided heart failure), confusion, crackles on lung exam, orthopnea, dry cough progressing to productive cough, and dependent peripheral edema in right-sided heart failure. Acute exacerbations of heart failure are often related to poor diet, medication noncompliance, onset of arrhythmias such as atrial fibrillation, or acute myocardial ischemia.

Prehospital treatment is unchanged from that of younger patients, although greater consideration is given to becoming familiar with the patient's medications and their implications for your proposed treatment. For example, the patient taking long-term furosemide (Lasix) may not respond to the usual dose of the same drug that you administer as an acute therapy. Additional treatments by prehospital providers should include close monitoring of fluids and avoidance of excessive fluid overload, use of beta blockers in patients with systolic dysfunction (low ejection fraction), use of digoxin or diltiazem (Cardizem) in patients with atrial fibrillation or atrial flutter, and, possibly, use of anticoagulation therapy in patients with atrial arrhythmias to prevent thromboembolism.

Nonperfusing rhythms receive the same treatment as given to younger adults. Survival depends on the prearrest health of the patient and the usual factors: early recognition, prompt and effective CPR, and early defibrillation.

Thoracic aneurysms generally remain asymptomatic until they become large or rupture. Early symptoms may be related to compression by the aneurysm, such as difficulty swallowing or hoarseness from laryngeal nerve pressure. Abdominal aortic aneurysms present typically with abdominal pain or possibly only with back pain. Asymptomatic thoracic and abdominal aneurysms that do not exceed a certain size and are not expanding are generally treated without surgery but are reassessed on a regular schedule. In an older patient with back pain, examine the chest and abdomen carefully. The treatment of abdominal emergencies is surgical, so early recognition, assessment, stabilization, and rapid transport to an appropriate medical facility are essential.

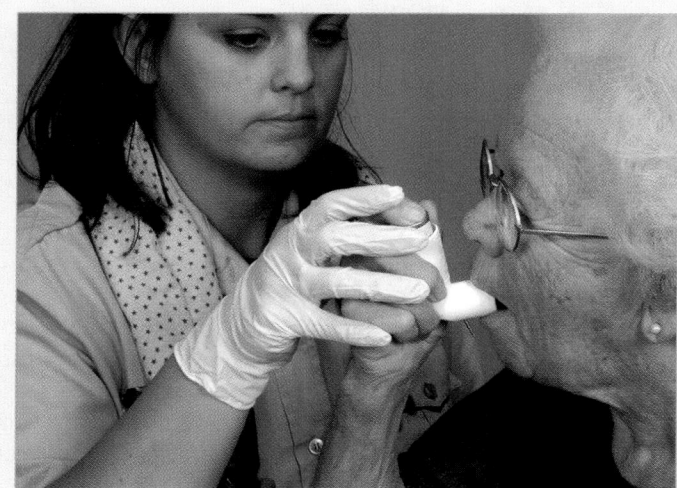

Figure 42-6 A patient having an asthma attack may have a bronchodilator medication in a metered-dose inhaler. Older patients often do not use an inhaler correctly, so you may need to help with its use if your protocols allow it.

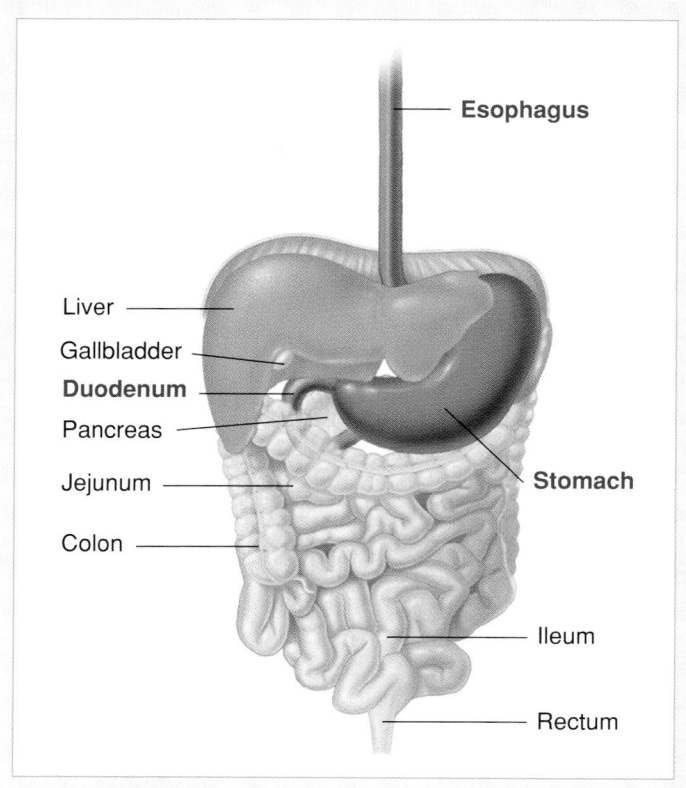

Figure 42-7 Upper GI bleeding occurs in the stomach, esophagus, and duodenum.

The usual treatments for systolic hypertension usually prove safe and effective in geriatric patients. In case of rapid onset of symptomatic systolic hypertension, treatment aims to reduce the systolic pressure with antihypertensive therapy, which can minimize cardiovascular and cerebrovascular morbidity and mortality.

Respiratory Complaints

An older patient with pneumonia often does not have the classic presentation of chills, fever, and productive cough. Instead, these symptoms are often supplanted by acute confusion (delirium), normal temperature, and a minimal to absent cough. Prehospital treatment is supportive and includes oxygen and IV access as indicated. At the receiving facility, providers will determine whether antibiotics or admission is appropriate.

Asthma clinical practice guidelines are the same for younger and older patients **Figure 42-6 ▲**. On rare occasions, epinephrine may be indicated for a life-threatening asthma exacerbation.

In a patient of any age, treatment goals for COPD are to reduce the symptoms and complications. Along with shortness of breath, presenting symptoms may include fatigue and a decreased activity level. Treatment consists of immediate assessment and correction of respiratory difficulties with the application of supplemental oxygen. The patient may also receive bronchodilators to decrease the shortness of breath, inhaled or oral steroids to decrease inflammation, and antibiotics to treat infection.

Many pulmonary emboli are silent or present with tachypnea alone—that is, the classic triad of dyspnea, chest pain, and hemoptysis is often altered or absent. If you suspect a pulmonary embolus, check for swelling, erythema, and warmth or tenderness of the lower leg; all of these are signs of a deep venous thrombosis, which is a common cause of pulmonary embolus. If deep venous thrombosis might be present, handle the leg gently and monitor the patient for respiratory changes. Prehospital treatment is largely supportive after ensuring that airway and ventilation are adequate. Lysing the thrombus and use of anticoagulation therapies may be considered after a risk assessment is performed, with these measures being followed by rapid transport.

GI Complaints

Many causes are possible for gastric complaints. Constipation and its accompanying abdominal pain, for example, are some of the more common complaints of geriatric patients. In your assessment of a gastric emergency, ask the patient about food and fluid intake, history of abdominal complaints, current bowel and bladder habits, and medications and supplements before proceeding with a physical exam. Symptoms are often vague and manifest only as diffuse abdominal pain with no particular point of origin. Abdominal and gastric complaints often require surgical treatment, so early recognition and rapid transport for definitive hospital care are the best practice.

Upper GI hemorrhage occurs when there is bleeding from the esophagus, stomach, or duodenum **Figure 42-7 ▲**. When severe, this condition is a true medical emergency that must be recognized and assessed quickly. Not only are older people more prone to upper GI bleeding, they are also at a greater risk of complications, the need for urgent surgery, and death.

It is not possible to determine the cause of upper GI bleeding without an endoscopic examination (inspection of the inside of a hollow organ or body cavity) of the esophagus, stomach, and duodenum. However, the history can offer clues to the cause. Regular use of NSAIDs or alcohol may result in bleeding from irritation of the lining of the stomach or from ulcers (a hollowing out or disintegration of tissue) in the stomach or duodenum. Forceful vomiting can cause tears in the esophagus that may bleed. Cirrhosis of the liver from long-term alcohol use or chronic infectious hepatitis may cause enlargement of the veins (varices) in the esophagus. These varices can rupture and result in massive bleeding. Stomach cancer or esophageal cancer can also produce upper GI bleeding. Recent weight loss or difficulty swallowing would raise the suspicion of cancer as the source of bleeding.

On arrival at the scene, even more important than knowing the cause of bleeding is being able to assess its severity. Slower bleeding is characterized by emesis with coffee-grounds appearance. With minor bleeding, the heart rate and systolic blood pressure are normal. Brisk bleeding presents with hematemesis (vomiting red blood) or melena (black, tarlike stools). It is important to note that melena, not pain, is the most common presenting symptom of GI bleeding. Prehospital treatment is supportive, including adequate pain control.

Lower GI hemorrhage primarily describes bleeding from the colon and rectum (**Figure 42-8 ▸**) and should never simply be attributed to hemorrhoids. Colon polyps and colon cancer are also possible causes, among others. Minor lower GI bleeding is characterized by small amounts of red blood covering formed brown stools or scant amounts of red blood noticed on the toilet paper. Severe lower GI bleeding is characterized by passing significant amounts of red blood or maroon-colored stools.

Assessment should begin with identifying risk factors such as a history of previous lower GI bleeding, symptoms or signs suggestive of colon cancer, recent constipation or diarrhea, and use of medications such as blood thinners. Treat for shock. Severe lower GI bleeding requires immediate transportation to the nearest emergency department.

Neurologic and Endocrine Complaints

Effective prehospital acute stroke care includes early recognition, discovery of stroke-mimics such as hypoglycemia or hypoxia, and timely transport to the most appropriate facility. Use a stroke assessment tool as appropriate, taking the patient's history into account when assessing the components of the scale. An older person with severe arthritis may not move as well on one side, or damage from a previous stroke may make his or her speech difficult to assess. Always ask family or caregivers for information that may help you identify deviations from the patient's normal pattern of behavior or activity. Assess for new weakness, fatigue, syncope, and near

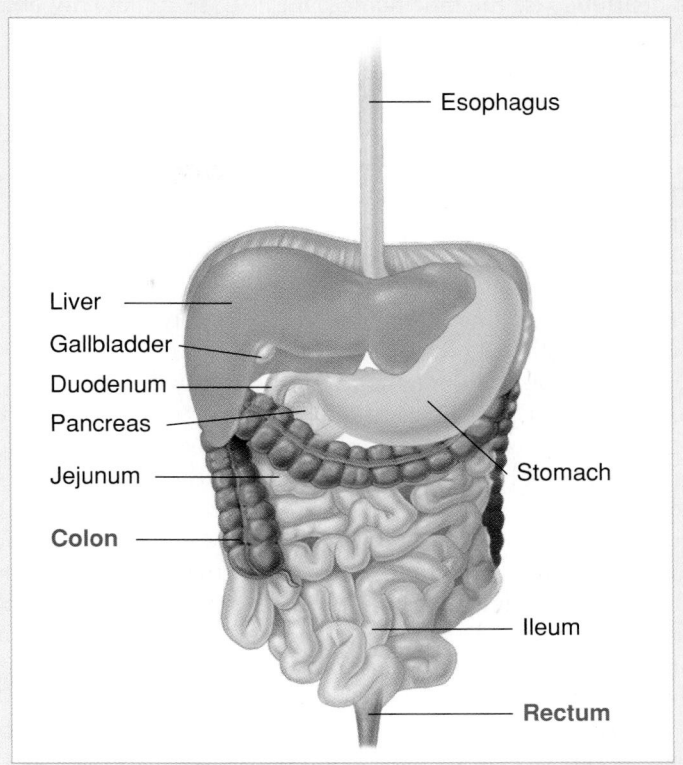

Figure 42-8 Lower GI bleeding takes place primarily in the colon and rectum.

Documentation and Communication

A stroke is a traumatic and emotional event for the patient, and a sensitive and compassionate approach is essential. Even though the patients may not be able to communicate with you, they can often understand. Communicate with them as you would any other patient—in a calm and reassuring manner.

syncope and for changes in these symptoms and in mood and sleep patterns.

Dementia signs and symptoms take months to years to become apparent and may include short-term memory loss or shortened attention span, jargon aphasia (talking nonsense), hallucinations, confusion, disorientation, difficulty in learning and retaining new information, and personality changes such as social withdrawal or inappropriate behavior. Dementia is not synonymous with delirium, however, and a patient with dementia can also have delirium. In delirium, assess for recent changes in the patient's level of consciousness or orientation. Specifically, look for an acute onset of anxiety, an inability to think logically or maintain attention, and an inability to focus. Also assess for changes in vital signs, temperature (indicating infection), glucose level, and medications—all frequent causes of delirium. Use the mnemonic "DELIRIUMS" to identify other causes of delirium:

D Drugs or toxins

E Emotional (psychiatric)

L Low Pao_2 (carbon monoxide poisoning, COPD, congestive heart failure, acute myocardial infarction, pneumonia)

I Infection (pneumonia, urinary tract infection, sepsis)

R Retention of stool or urine

I Ictal (seizures)

U Undernutrition or underhydration

M Metabolism (thyroid or endocrine, electrolytes, kidneys)

S Subdural hematoma

Altered mental status is a symptom, not a disease. As a consequence, the assessment and subsequent management of its numerous causes is complicated. Always consider head injury (medical or traumatic), heart rhythm disturbances, dementia, medications, fluid balance changes (such as blood loss), respiratory disorders (such as hypoxia), endocrine changes (such as blood glucose level fluctuations), hyperthermia or hypothermia, and infection. Most important, prehospital providers need to consider neurologic causes (such as Alzheimer's disease and Parkinson's disease) and endocrine changes (such as diabetes).

In Alzheimer's disease, symptoms may present as confusion (lack of familiarity with surroundings), changes in personality or judgment, and extreme difficulty with daily activities, such as feeding, bathing, and bowel and bladder control. Parkinson's disease may present as dyskinesia (involuntary movements or tremors affecting one or both sides of the body), dementia, depression, autonomic dysfunction (bladder and GI problems), and postural instability (loss of reflexes or inability to "right oneself").

Many endocrine changes may have occurred earlier in life and been diagnosed before intervention by prehospital providers became necessary. Geriatric patients may have diseases such as Grave's disease (hyperthyroidism), Addison's disease (hypoadrenalism), Cushing's syndrome (hyperadrenalism), osteoporosis, or diabetes. In the assessment of geriatric patients with diagnosed diabetes, look for signs of dehydration or hyperglycemia (the three Ps: Polyuria, Polydipsia, and Polyphagia). New-onset diabetes in geriatric patients is often a mild progression that produces no symptoms.

Notes from Nancy

Delirium in the elderly is always a sign of physical illness or drug intoxication and is always an emergency.

Toxicologic Complaints

The most common therapeutic error in cases of reported poison exposure is "inadvertently took/given medication twice" or "double dosing." In essence, medications are poisons with beneficial side effects. This definition emphasizes the need for obtaining a careful history and collecting and transporting all medications with the patient.

As mentioned earlier, many elderly people take a variety of drugs. Patients may be taking medications prescribed by more than one physician, each dispensing prescriptions without knowledge of the others' orders. Patients may also take over-the-counter medications or medications prescribed for a family member or friend.

Another factor contributing to the toxic effects of drugs in elderly people is aging-related alterations in pharmacokinetics (that is, the absorption, distribution, metabolism, and excretion of drugs). Pharmacokinetics may also be influenced by diet, smoking, alcohol consumption, and use of other drugs. Drugs such as digoxin that depend on the liver and kidney for metabolism and excretion are particularly likely to accumulate to toxic levels in older patients. With most drugs, we know little about the optimal dosage for elderly people because nearly all clinical trials to establish the safe dosages of drugs are performed in young populations. For the most part, dosages for elderly people need to be *reduced* compared with those for younger patients ("Start low, go slow").

Although almost any drug can produce toxic effects in an older person, certain drugs and classes of drugs are implicated more often than others; **Table 42-4 ▸** lists the "dirty dozen." Typically toxic effects present with psychiatric symptoms (such as hallucinations, paranoia, delusions, agitation, and psychosis) and cognitive impairment (such as delirium, confusion, disorientation, amnesia, stupor, and coma) **Figure 42-9 ▾**.

Notes from Nancy

Bring all of the patient's medications—prescription and nonprescription—to the hospital.

Sepsis

Infections in older persons can be severe and dangerous. Sepsis is the disease state that results from the presence of microorganisms or their toxic products in the bloodstream. This is a serious

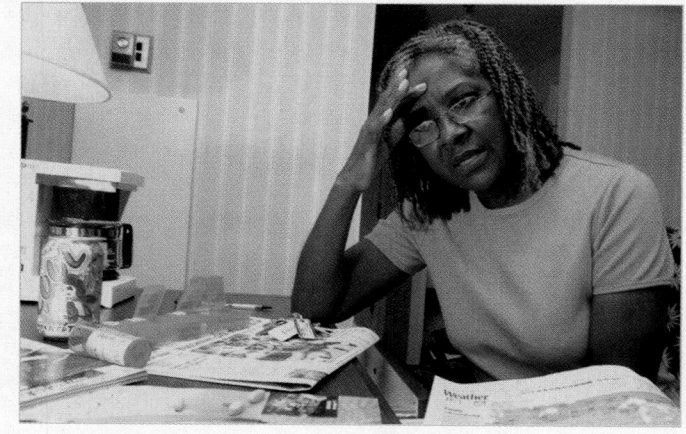

Figure 42-9 The toxic effects of drugs may initially manifest in the form of confusion.

Table 42-4	Drugs Most Commonly Causing Toxic Reactions in Elderly People
Medication	**Symptoms**
Anti-inflammatory agents (NSAIDs, steroids)	Drowsiness, dizziness, confusion, anxiety, bradypnea, tachypnea, GI bleeding
Antibiotics	GI signs, altered mental status, seizures, coma
Anticholinergics and antihistamines	Urination difficulty, constipation, drowsiness, restlessness, irritability, hypertension
Anticoagulants (warfarin)	Ecchymosis, epistaxis, hematuria, abdominal pain, vomiting, fecal blood
Antiarrhythmics (amiodarone, lidocaine)	Restlessness, hypotension, bradycardia, tachycardia, palpitations, angina
Antidepressants (tricyclics, long-acting selective serotonin reuptake inhibitors)	Confusion, delirium, disorientation, memory impairment
Antihypertensives (diuretics, alpha blockers, beta blockers; angiotensin-converting enzyme inhibitors)	Hypotension, palpitations, angina, fluid retention, headache
Antipsychotics (phenothiazines, atypicals)	Drowsiness, tachycardia, dizziness, restlessness
Digoxin	Headache, fatigue, malaise, drowsiness, depression
Insulin and oral antidiabetic medications	Hypoglycemia presenting as confusion
Narcotics	Delirium, respiratory depression, apnea, involuntary muscle movements
Sedative-hypnotics (benzodiazepines, barbiturates)	Incoordination, dizziness, disturbances in cognitive function

problem that every EMS provider should know how to recognize and treat. Think of sepsis whenever you see a hot, flushed patient who is also tachycardic and tachypneic. Other signs of sepsis include an oral temperature greater than 38°C or less than 36°C, a respiratory rate of more than 20 breaths/min or $Paco_2$ less than 32 mm Hg, and pulse rate of greater than 90 beats/min. Sepsis can be caused by bacteria, fungi, and viruses.

Skin Complaints

Herpes zoster (shingles) is caused by the reactivation of varicella virus on nerve roots. This condition is more common in the older population. Most people with herpes zoster are in good health, but people with cancer or immunosuppression are at higher risk. This condition affects any nerve in the body, but the thoracic nerves and the ophthalmic division of the trigeminal nerve are most common. The disease usually starts with pain in the affected area. Subsequently, a cluster of tiny blisters (vesicles) erupts on reddened skin in the same area. The rash is typically unilateral; it rarely crosses the midline.

One of the most common complications of herpes zoster is pain, or postherpetic neuralgia. During the acute phase of the infection, the person may have severe pain and require narcotic pain relievers. Antiviral medications such as acyclovir and famciclovir can be used, preferably within 48 hours of the activation of the disease. These medications decrease healing time, new lesion formation, and pain.

Cellulitis is an acute inflammation in the skin caused by a bacterial infection Figure 42-10 . This condition usually affects the lower extremities. Symptoms include fever, chills,

and general malaise. Cellulitis can cause warmth, swelling, redness, tenderness, and enlarged nodes in the affected area. Blood tests may show elevation of the white blood cell count and the presence of bacteria. Treatments include antibiotic therapy, ensuring adequate fluid intake, and local dressings if there is an open sore.

Psychological Complaints

Depression can be a normal, short-term reaction to a particular event. When sadness, restlessness, fatigue, and hopelessness persist for weeks, however, it becomes a larger concern. Depression in the geriatric population is a major health problem with an incidence growing in tandem with the progressive aging of the population. This trend can be attributed to increases in polypathology, psychosocial stress, and aging-related changes in the brain that collectively lead to greater cognitive impairment, increased medical illness, dependency on health care services, and more suicide attempts Figure 42-11 . Depression may also occur when a patient takes a variety of medications; such polypharmacy is more likely when the person has multiple medical conditions that result in more vulnerability to toxic effects.

When dealing with psychological emergencies with geriatric patients, health care providers need to determine whether the situation is a true behavioral emergency or a behavioral crisis. A behavioral emergency implies a significant risk of serious

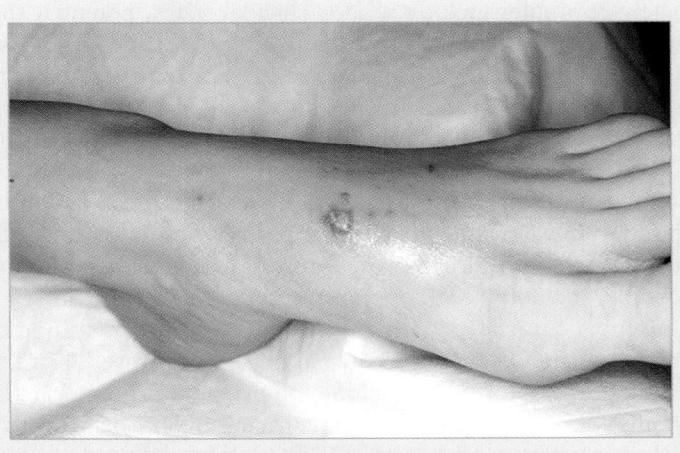

Figure 42-10 Cellulitis is a diffuse, acute inflammation in the skin caused by bacterial infection.

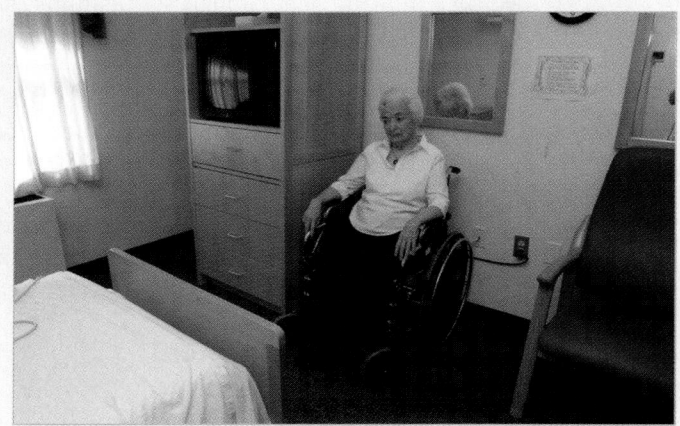

Figure 42-11 Isolation and chronic medical problems are among the factors that contribute to depression in older adults.

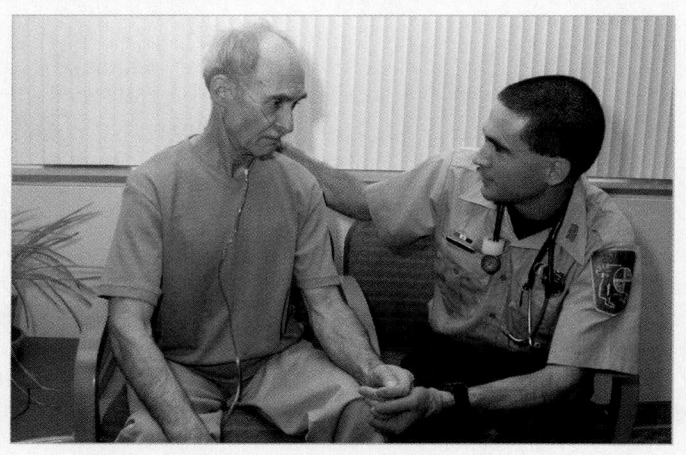

Figure 42-12 A patient in a behavioral crisis may be searching for alternative methods of coping.

harm to self or others unless intervention is undertaken immediately. Examples include serious suicidal states, potential violence, and impaired judgment that could leave a person at risk of injury or death. In a behavioral crisis, the patient's ability to cope is insufficient and becomes overwhelmed, sending the patient in search of alternative methods of coping Figure 42-12 ▲ .

When dealing with a patient's mental illness or psychotic episodes, always remember that a person who is psychotic is out of touch with reality. Many forms of psychotic behavior are possible, including schizophrenic and paranoid behaviors. All symptoms associated with psychotic conditions may not be present when a patient is having an episode, however. Clues to psychotic behavior might include the patient becoming excited or angry for no apparent reason, engaging in antisocial activity or being a loner, and sleeping during the day and staying awake at night. Information about changes in the patient's normal routine may be obtained from family, friends, or caregivers.

Management of Medical Emergencies in Elderly People

The assessment and management of medical emergencies in geriatric patients can be complex. If you are well prepared to deal with these complex situations, you will not feel quite so overwhelmed and helpless.

In every emergency, you should first complete a scene size-up to confirm the scene safety, determine the nature of the call, identify the number of potential patients, and ascertain the need for additional resources. Next, you should perform an initial assessment, which consists of several quick, yet complex observations. First, formulate a general impression based on the patient's mental status and the status of his or her airway, breathing, and circulatory systems. Then, determine transportation priorities.

With the exception of patients who require immediate interventions to maintain a patent airway, adequate and supportive breathing, or circulatory status, most prehospital care is supportive and focuses on pain relief and palliative interventions. Additional steps in the patient treatment plan will depend on the patient's specific medical emergency and chief complaint.

Table 42-5 ▶ reviews common medical complications encountered with geriatric patients and their management strategies.

Assessment and Management of Trauma in Elderly Patients

Begin the assessment by looking at the mechanism of injury. Falls account for the largest number of injuries in elderly people, followed by injuries related to motor vehicles (including passenger and pedestrian trauma) and then burns and other injuries. Always look for signs or symptoms that the patient may have experienced a medical problem before the trauma. A syncopal event while driving, for example, may result in a collision.

The initial management of an injured elderly patient follows the basic ABC pattern of trauma care with some special concerns.

While securing the airway, check for dentures. If they are intact and in place, leave them where they are; if the dentures are broken or loose in the mouth, remove them and place them in a safe container. Aggressive suctioning of blood or secretions is required because of the older patient's lessened airway and gag reflexes Figure 42-13 ▶ .

When assessing breathing, check for rib fracture. If assisted ventilation is required, use a bag-mask gently, exerting just enough pressure to inflate the lungs so as to lessen the chance of creating a pneumothorax. Administer supplemental oxygen early to assist the body in compensating for early states of trauma.

Table 42-5 | Common Medical Complications in Elderly People and Their Management

Medical Complication	Management
Incontinence	Some cases are managed surgically. Other considerations include absorptive devices for fecal and urinary incontinence, placement of catheters, and awareness of the patient's self-esteem and social issues.
COPD	Nebulizer treatment with a bronchial dilator could include metaproterenol (Alupent), racemic epinephrine, isoetharine (Bronkosol), ipratropium (Atrovent), and albuterol (Ventolin) or an IV dose of methylprednisolone (Solu-Medrol).
Pulmonary emboli	Lysing the thrombus and anticoagulation therapies are indicated. Once all risk factors for bleeding have been reviewed, anticoagulants such as heparin or enoxaparin (Lovenox) can be considered.
Heart failure	Heart failure that produces signs and symptoms of pulmonary edema can be managed with sublingual nitroglycerin, IV furosemide (Lasix), and IV morphine. Providers can also consider a vasoactive medication such as dopamine (Intropin) for patients with hemodynamically unstable hypotension.
Arrhythmias	Unless a patient is in unstable condition, arrhythmias are handled with supportive care only. Unstable arrhythmias are treated following current CPR and electrocardiographic guidelines.
Aneurysm	Treatment is handled surgically, and prehospital interventions focus on supportive care.
Hypertension	Hypertensive emergencies require a controlled decline in blood pressure, which is not often feasible in prehospital care. A hypertensive crisis or urgency may be addressed by using labetalol (Normodyne) or sodium nitroprusside (Nipride).
Cerebral vascular disease	Prehospital management targets recognition and support. Definitive treatment is surgery.
Delirium	Recognize and treat the underlying cause, and provide supportive interventions.
Dementia, Alzheimer's disease, Parkinson's disease	Provide supportive care.
Diabetes	In hypoglycemia, treatments address the elevation of the blood glucose level with intramuscular or IV injections when not contraindicated. In hyperglycemia, treatment aims to eliminate additional glucose by using fluid boluses for patients with adequate renal function.
GI problems	Few treatments using medications for GI problems are possible in the prehospital environment, other than antiemetics. For nausea and vomiting, consider promethazine (Phenergan), dimenhydrinate (Dramamine; especially for narcotic-induced nausea and vomiting), or prochlorperazine (Compazine; for severe nausea and vomiting or acute psychosis).
Drug toxic effects	• Lidocaine: CNS depression may occur, so be alert for respiratory changes. No antidote is used in prehospital care to reverse its effects. • Beta blockers: Provide supportive care; give activated charcoal; and consider the use of atropine, epinephrine, and glucagon in symptomatic patients. • Antihypertensives: Provide supportive care. No antidote is used in prehospital care to reverse the drugs' effects. • Diuretics: Provide supportive care. Consider treatments aimed at restoring volume depletion and electrolyte imbalance. No antidote is used in prehospital care to reverse the drugs' effects. • Digitalis: Provide supportive care. Consider fluid replacement, vasoactive medications such as dopamine, and activated charcoal. • Psychotropics: Provide supportive care. Consider aggressive fluid replacement. • Antidepressants: Provide supportive care. Give fluid therapy for hypotension and sodium bicarbonate.
Alcohol abuse	Provide supportive care. Later care includes identification of abuse potential and referral to an appropriate treatment facility.
Behavioral disorders	Use psychological support and communication strategies. Consider haloperidol (Haldol), droperidol (Inapsine), or chlorpromazine (Thorazine).
Depression, suicide	Provide supportive care. Later care includes identification of the potential condition and referral to an appropriate treatment facility.

When evaluating circulation, remember that what is a normal blood pressure in a younger person may mean hypotension in an older person. If possible, try to determine the patient's normal baseline blood pressure and circulatory status.

The initial assessment of disability (neurologic status) should include an evaluation of the pupils and the level of consciousness, according to the AVPU scale. Finally, be sure to expose the entire injured area, even if it means peeling away many layers of clothing.

Once the initial assessment is complete, try to obtain a complete history of the trauma event from the patient and from anyone who may have witnessed the event Figure 42-14 ▶. If the patient fell, from what height? Did the patient have any symptoms beforehand, such as dizziness? If the patient was

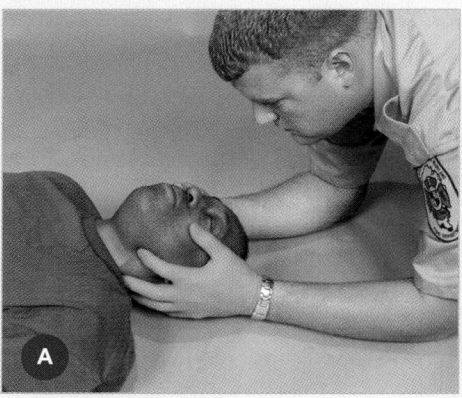 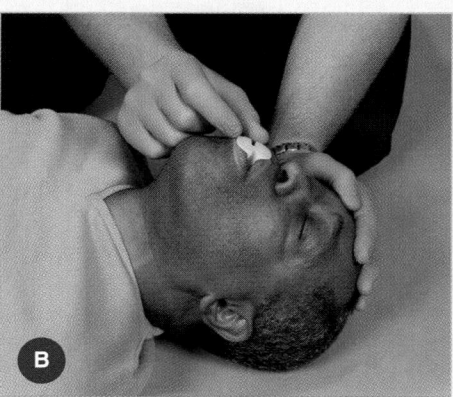 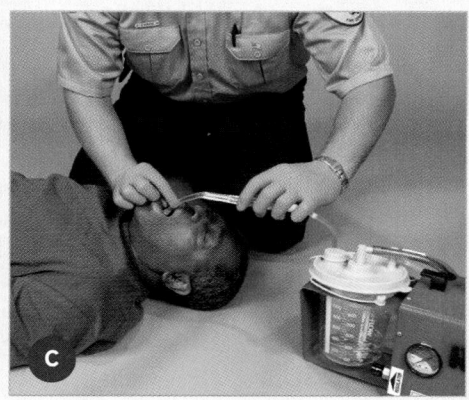

Figure 42-13 The airway should initially be addressed using simple techniques, such as (**A**) the modified jaw-thrust, (**B**) placement of an oropharyngeal or nasopharyngeal airway, and (**C**) suctioning.

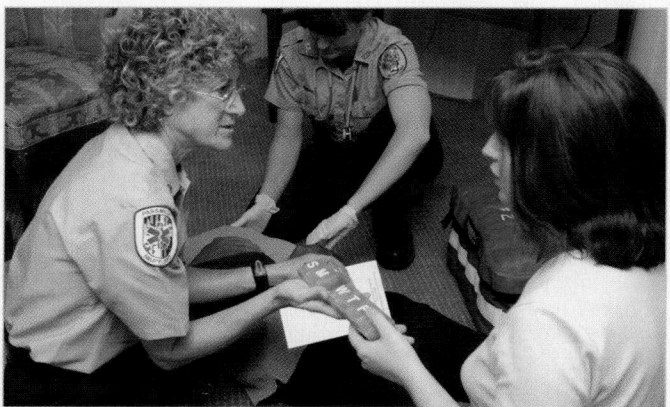

Figure 42-14 History is especially important in older patients who have lost consciousness.

struck by a car, how fast was the car moving? If the patient was the driver of a car involved in an accident, did he or she feel dizzy or black out before the crash? Did the patient have chest pain? Did witnesses notice the car moving erratically before it crashed?

Obtain a complete list of all medications the patient takes regularly. Inquire in particular about beta blockers, antihypertensives, and medications for diabetes because they may affect the patient's response to resuscitation measures and to anesthesia.

Conduct the focused physical exam as usual, staying particularly alert for signs of injuries to the head, cervical spine, ribs, abdomen, and long bones. Pain from fractures or peripheral injury may be difficult to assess if the patient has decreased pain perception.

You are the Provider Part 4

You place your patient on a stretcher in a semi-Fowler's position and move her to the ambulance. While en route to the hospital, she begins to complain of a being "a little winded." A reassessment reveals no changes in her status. Your partner suggests administering a nebulizer treatment with albuterol. You agree, and the patient receives a nebulizer treatment with 0.5 mg of albuterol with 3 mL of normal saline. Report is called en route to the emergency department, and no further orders are given.

As you arrive at the emergency department your patient says that she is breathing easier and thanks you for being so caring. She is observed in the emergency department for a few hours, and right lower lobe pneumonia is diagnosed by chest radiograph. She is admitted to the hospital for treatment with IV antibiotics and is discharged to the nursing home on the fifth day.

Reassessment	Recording Time: 20 Minutes
Skin	Pink, hot, and dry
Pulse	113 beats/min, strong and irregular
Blood pressure	158/96 mm Hg
Respirations	22 breaths/min regular
Sao$_2$	95% with supplemental oxygen at 3 L/min by nasal cannula
ECG	Atrial fibrillation

6. Does pneumonia present the same in elderly people as in younger people?

7. How is pneumonia managed in the prehospital setting?

Additional treatment will depend on the patient's specific injuries, although there are a few general principles to keep in mind:

- Insert an IV catheter and give an isotonic solution, but use caution. It is very easy to overload an elderly person with sodium, and you must balance that with the need to maintain adequate perfusion pressure. Use small boluses, and reassess the patient frequently, especially for signs of pulmonary edema.
- Monitor cardiac rhythm throughout care of the patient, and be alert for changes. Previous or continuing cardiac disease predisposes a person to ECG changes.
- Take steps to preserve temperature in elderly trauma patients. Regulation of temperature is slowed in elderly people, and the blood in cold patients does not clot as well.
- Frail elderly patients may not do very well with a traction splint for a femoral fracture. If possible, place the patient on a well-padded backboard and buttress him or her well with pillows secured firmly in place.
- Immobilize the cervical spine before transporting the patient. Pad the backboard generously, because the skin of an older person may be damaged by the direct trauma of the pressure and the decrease in blood flow. Target areas where the bone is near the surface, from top to bottom: occiput, scapula, spinous processes, elbows, sacrum, and heels. A pressure ulcer can develop in as little as 45 minutes and can complicate the original injury.

Elder Abuse

One category of geriatric trauma that deserves special mention is elder abuse—that is, any form of mistreatment that results in harm or loss to an older person. Five types of abuse are distinguished: physical, sexual, emotional, neglect, and financial. The first four are similar to the forms found in child abuse. Financial abuse involves improper use of an older person's funds, property, or assets. The average victim of elder abuse is 80 years old, is female, and has multiple chronic conditions. These conditions make patients unable to function on their own, leaving them dependent on others for at least part of their care. The abuser is almost always known to the abused and is often a family member (such as adult children or a spouse).

One clue to elder abuse is unexplained injuries that do not fit the stated cause. Assessment of elder abuse must include not only the physical exam, but also the environmental and social clues. Look at the patient's overall hygiene, and review how he or she interacts with caregivers. Take adequate time to listen patiently to any concerns expressed by older patients about their care (or lack of it) **Figure 42-15**. If the patient's condition is stable but the situation is unsafe, see if the patient will

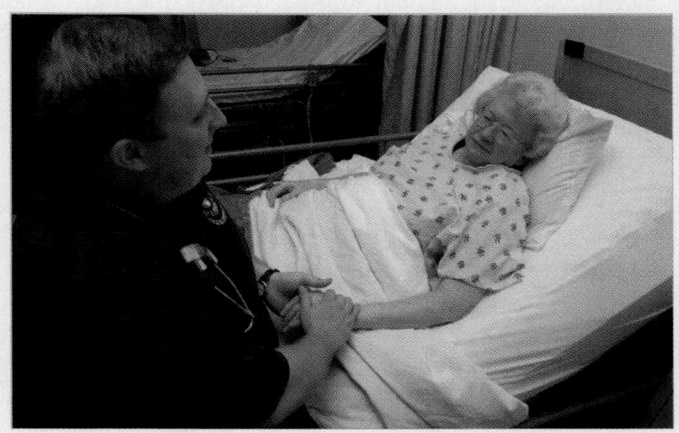

Figure 42-15 Take time to listen patiently to older patients.

accept transportation to the hospital. If the patient refuses transport, see if he or she will accept help from the local adult protective services. If the situation is immediately unsafe, notify law enforcement personnel and remain with the patient only if the scene remains safe to do so.

Many states have elder abuse statutes, and the reporting of suspected abuse is mandatory in some jurisdictions. Nevertheless, only one of five cases of elder abuse is ever reported. The way elder abuse is defined varies considerably from state to state, so it is advisable to become familiar with the legislation that applies to your own area. However, regardless of the legislation, if you have any reason to suspect elder abuse in a given case of geriatric injury—for example, if you found evidence of gross patient neglect in the patient's residence—carefully document your observations and report your findings and suspicions to the receiving facility. For more information on this topic, see Chapter 43.

End-of-Life Care

You will inevitably be involved with end-of-life care for many patients. Of course, "do not resuscitate" (DNR) does *not* mean "do not respond to the needs of a terminal patient." There is much you can do, beginning with demonstrating a caring and concerned attitude and approach. Many of your visits may be "no transport" decisions and may not be perceived as valuable by those who decide on reimbursement, but they prove no less

Controversies

Is a DNR order from a state other than yours valid? It depends on your state's law. About a dozen states recognize out-of-state DNR orders.

valuable to the patient than more aggressive measures. Many communities have a local hospice, an organization that provides terminal care for patients and support for their families. If one exists in your community, consider how you or your service might collaborate on providing quality care for a person at the end of life **Figure 42-16 ▶**.

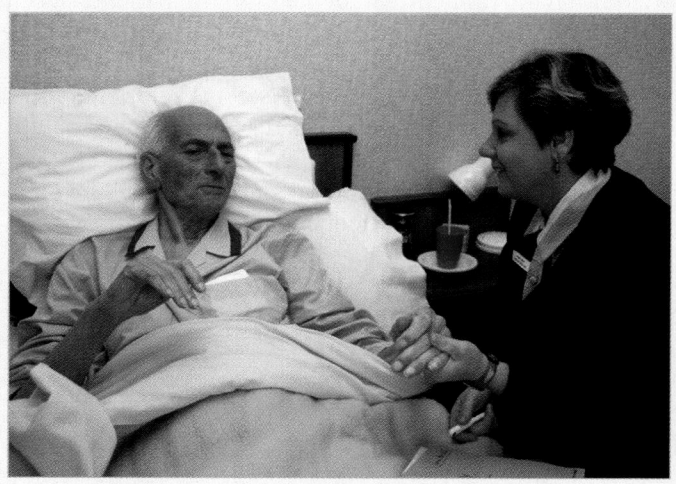

Figure 42-16 Hospice care allows people with terminal illnesses to receive palliative care in their own homes.

You are the Provider Summary

1. Why is it important to review common medical problems of elderly people?

Well, like it or not, we are not getting any younger. As a matter of fact, more than 34 million Americans are older than 65 years; that is 12% of the population! It is predicted that by the year 2050, nearly 25% of Americans will be eligible for Medicare. As we age, our bodies undergo numerous physical changes that affect the way we respond to illness and disease. Keeping up-to-date with medical problems of elderly people is just as important as staying current on other kinds of emergencies.

2. Which organ systems are greatly affected by age-related changes?

Although the aging process affects all body systems, the organ systems most relevant to older patients are the respiratory, cardiovascular, renal, nervous, and musculoskeletal.

3. Why might obtaining an accurate medical history and history of the present illness be challenging when interviewing an elderly patient?

The elderly patient can present with numerous challenges that might make patient assessment tricky. These include having more than one chronic illness, not feeling pain the same way a younger person might, difficulty distinguishing acute from chronic problems, fear of being hospitalized, and fear of losing control over their ability to care for themselves. It is important to be patient and look for subtle clues when assessing an older person.

4. What are some specific respiratory illnesses commonly seen in elderly people?

Respiratory illnesses commonly seen in elderly people include pneumonia, COPD, and pulmonary embolism.

5. What are the risk factors for pneumonia in elderly people? Are any present here?

Residing in an institutional environment, chronic illness, and a compromised immune system are all risk factors for contracting pneumonia. In our case, Mrs. Howard resides in a nursing home and has diabetes, which increases her chances of getting pneumonia.

6. Does pneumonia present the same in elderly people as it does in younger people?

If you are expecting to find a patient presenting with fever, productive cough, chest discomfort, and chest congestion, keep looking! The clinical presentation of pneumonia in elderly people will fool you. Rather than presenting with the "classic clinical picture" described above, an elderly person with pneumonia might present with altered mental status, cough, fever, shortness of breath, tachycardia, and tachypnea.

7. How is pneumonia managed in the prehospital setting?

Prehospital management of pneumonia is aimed at supportive care. Ensuring an adequate airway and oxygenation and a little tender loving care will go a long way for most of your patients. Definitive treatment for pneumonia is the administration of antibiotics.

Ready for Review

- Elderly people constitute an ever-increasing proportion of patients presenting to the health care system, particularly to the emergency care sector.
- The health problems of older people are quantitatively and qualitatively different from those of younger people. The special problems of older people require special approaches.
- The aging process is accompanied by changes in physiologic function. The decrease in the functional capacity of various organ systems can affect the way in which the patient responds to illness.
- A variety of changes occur in the cardiovascular system as a person ages. The heart hypertrophies (enlarges), arteriosclerosis (the stiffening of vessel walls) develops, and the electric conduction system of the heart deteriorates.
- A person's respiratory capacity also undergoes significant reductions with age due to decreases in the elasticity of the lungs and in the size and strength of the respiratory muscles, calcification of costochrondral cartilage in the chest wall, and musculoskeletal changes.
- Geriatric patients may experience renal system changes. Although the kidneys of an elderly person may be capable of dealing with day-to-day demands, they may not be able to meet unusual challenges, such as those imposed by illness. Therefore, acute illness in elderly patients is often accompanied by derangements in fluid and electrolyte balance.
- Changes in the endocrine system may lead to diabetes and thyroid abnormalities in older patients.
- Aging brings a widespread decrease in bone mass in men and women, but especially among postmenopausal women. Bones become more brittle and tend to break more easily.
- Changes in the nervous system lead to a decrease in the performance of sense organs, as evidenced by visual changes (glaucoma and cataracts are common) and hearing loss.
- Diseases of the heart remain the leading cause of death among older adults in the United States. Heart attack is the major cause of morbidity and mortality in people older than 65 years, and its potential for mortality increases significantly after 70 years.
- Stroke is a significant cause of death and disability in elderly people. More than 80% of all stroke deaths occur in persons older than 65 years, and stroke is the leading cause of long-term disability at any age.
- Chronic lower respiratory disease, influenza, and pneumonia remain in the top five causes for geriatric deaths.
- A geriatric patient with diabetes is at increased risk for hypoglycemia for several reasons: medications, inadequate or irregular dietary intake, inability to recognize the warning signs due to cognitive problems, and/or blunted warning signs. Delirium may be the only indication of hypoglycemia in an elderly patient.
- Older diabetics whose blood glucose levels tend to be high are prone to hyperosmolar hyperglycemic nonketotic (HHNK) coma. The most frequent cause for HHNK is infection. Presentation is likely to be acute confusion with dehydration.
- Gastrointestinal problems in elderly people include peptic ulcer disease, small bowel obstruction due to gallstones, and stomach or duodenal ulcers (peptic ulcer disease).
- Osteoporosis is characterized by a decrease in bone mass leading to reduction in bone strength and greater susceptibility to fracture. Osteoarthritis is a progressive disease process of the joints that destroys cartilage, promotes the formation of bone spurs in joints, and leads to joint stiffness.
- In elderly people, delirium often replaces or confounds the typical presentation caused by a medical problem, an adverse medication effect, or drug withdrawal. Disorders that cause delirium may also include poisons, electrolyte imbalances, nutritional deficiencies, and infections such as urinary tract infections and pneumonia.
- Unlike delirium, dementia is a disease that produces irreversible brain failure. Disorders that cause dementia include conditions that impair vascular and neurologic structures within the brain, such as infections, stroke, head injuries, poor nutrition, and medications.
- The two most common degenerative types of dementia in older people are Alzheimer's disease and multi-infarct or vascular dementia, both of which cause structural damage to the brain.
- Elderly people are particularly prone to adverse drug reactions because of changes in the following: drug metabolism because of diminished hepatic function; drug elimination because of diminished renal function; body composition, including increased body fat and decreased body water, altering the distribution of drugs through the various body compartments; and the responsiveness to drugs of the central nervous system.
- Alcohol is the preferred substance of abuse among older persons, in whom its use is on the rise. A much smaller but increasing segment of the geriatric population uses illicit drugs.
- Depression in elderly patients can mimic the effects of many other medical problems (such as dementia). Risk factors for depression in an older person include a history of depression, chronic disease, and loss (function, independence, or significant others).
- Several factors place an elderly person at higher risk of trauma than a younger person: slower reflexes, visual and hearing deficits, equilibrium disorders, and an overall reduction in agility.
- Most geriatric trauma cases involve falls or motor vehicle crashes. Falls among elderly people are evenly divided between those resulting from extrinsic (external) causes, such as tripping on a loose rug or slipping on ice, and those resulting from intrinsic (internal) causes, such as a dizzy spell or a syncopal attack.
- Knowing what is and what is not part of the aging process constitutes the first challenge in assessing elderly patients. A second challenge is that signs and symptoms of disease may be altered from their presentation in younger patients as a consequence of aging.
- When a patient's chief complaint seems trivial, it may be necessary to go through a review of systems to confirm that you are not missing important pieces of information. If any of the screening questions yields a positive answer, follow up with further questions.
- The physical exam of older patients can be difficult. Poor cooperation and easy fatigability may require that you keep manipulations of the patient to a minimum. You may have to peel many layers of clothing off elderly patients to perform an adequate exam.
- Infections in older persons can be severe and dangerous. Consider sepsis whenever you see a hot, flushed patient who is also tachycardic and tachypneic.
- Elder abuse is any form of mistreatment that results in harm or loss to an older person. Five types of abuse are distinguished: physical, sexual, emotional, neglect, and financial.

Vital Vocabulary

bereavement Sadness from loss; grieving.

delirium An acute confusional state characterized by global impairment of thinking, perception, judgment, and memory.

dementia A chronic deterioration of mental functions.

geriatrics The assessment and treatment of disease in someone 65 years or older.

homeostasis A tendency to constancy or stability in the body's internal milieu.

hospice An organization that provides end-of-life care to patients with terminal illnesses and their families.

osteoporosis A decrease in bone mass and density.

polypharmacy The use of multiple medications.

presbycusis Progressive hearing loss, particularly in the high frequencies, along with lessened ability to discriminate between a particular sound and background noise.

proprioception The ability to perceive the position and movement of one's body or limbs.

review of systems A systematic survey of the patient's symptoms according to the major organ systems.

sepsis A disease state that results from the presence of microorganisms or their toxic products in the bloodstream.

spondylosis Immobility and consolidation of a vertebral joint.

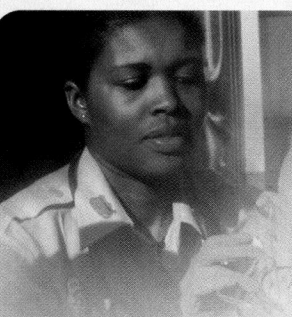

Assessment in Action

You are dispatched to a private residence for a fall. When you arrive on scene, you find an elderly man lying on his back. A large pool of blood is around his head. The patient is conscious, alert, and oriented to person, place, and day. He denies experiencing any loss of consciousness. He states that he was trying to get around the corner and tripped over his feet. His wife tells you that he has neuropathy to both his lower legs, bilateral knee replacements, and a hip replacement. He also has a history of blood clots and hypertension. His medications include lisinopril (Zestril) and warfarin (Coumadin). He has a large laceration to the back of his head. His vital signs are stable.

1. A common change seen in the cardiovascular system of the elderly patient is:
   A. neuropathy.
   B. hypertrophy.
   C. increased inotropy.
   D. increased automaticity.

2. Changes in thinking, speed, memory, and postural stability are effects of the:
   A. cardiovascular system.
   B. nervous system.
   C. pulmonary system.
   D. renal system.

3. What is homeostasis?
   A. Maintaining the constancy of the external environment
   B. An acute confusional state
   C. A decrease in bone mass and density
   D. Maintaining the constancy of the internal environment

4. What is osteoarthritis?
   A. A progressive disease process of the joints resulting in the destruction of cartilage
   B. A condition that affects only women and is characterized by a decrease in bone mass
   C. Atrophy of the supporting structures of the body
   D. A condition in which muscle fibers are smaller and fewer in numbers

5. For what reasons are elderly persons particularly prone to adverse drug reactions?
   A. Changes in drug metabolism because of diminished hepatic function
   B. Changes in drug elimination because of diminished renal function
   C. Changes in body composition, increased body fat, and decreased body water
   D. Changes in responsiveness to drugs that affect the central nervous system
   E. All of the above

6. The underlying causes of falls among the elderly are classified as being:
   A. extrinsic and intrinsic.
   B. medical illness and trauma.
   C. extrinsic and external.
   D. intrinsic and internal.

7. In the elderly, _____ are MOST common after a fall.
   A. epidural hematomas
   B. subdural hematomas
   C. intracerebral aneurysms
   D. ruptured cerebral arteries

Challenging Question

8. Why do many geriatric patients present atypically when they experience and injury or illness that causes shock?

Points to Ponder

It's 7:00 AM and your shift has just begun. You are dispatched to the assisted-living facility across town for an 86-year-old woman with chest pain. You recognize the address and apartment number as one that you have been to on several occasions. When you arrive, the patient's condition appears stable, but she has chest pain on palpation, inspiration, and movement. Her vital signs are as follows: pulse rate, 58 beats/min with sinus bradycardia on the cardiac monitor; blood pressure, 110/72 mm Hg; respiratory rate, 16 breaths/min; and pulse oximetry, 95% on room air. The patient tells you that this pain began after she received a phone call from her daughter, who was supposed to come and visit her and is now unable to do so.

Does this patient need to be transported immediately? How will you manage this patient?

Issues: Being an Advocate for the Elderly, Recognizing the Need for Independence in the Elderly.

43 Abuse, Neglect, and Assault

Objectives

Cognitive

6-4.1   Discuss the incidence of abuse and assault. (p 43.3)

6-4.2   Describe the categories of abuse. (p 43.3)

6-4.3   Discuss examples of spouse abuse. (p 43.9)

6-4.4   Discuss examples of elder abuse. (p 43.6)

6-4.5   Discuss examples of child abuse. (p 43.3)

6-4.6   Discuss examples of sexual assault. (p 43.11)

6-4.7   Describe the characteristics associated with the profile of the typical abuser of a spouse. (p 43.9, 43.10)

6-4.8   Describe the characteristics associated with the profile of the typical abuser of the elder. (p 43.7)

6-4.9   Describe the characteristics associated with the profile of the typical abuser of children. (p 43.4)

6-4.10   Describe the characteristics associated with the profile of the typical assailant of sexual assault. (p 43.10)

6-4.11   Identify the profile of the "at-risk" spouse. (p 43.9)

6-4.12   Identify the profile of the "at-risk" elder. (p 43.7)

6-4.13   Identify the profile of the "at-risk" child. (p 43.4)

6-4.14   Discuss the assessment and management of the abused patient. (p 43.5, 43.10)

6-4.15   Discuss the legal aspects associated with abuse situations. (p 43.6, 43.9–43.11)

6-4.16   Identify community resources that are able to assist victims of abuse and assault. (p 43.6, 43.9, 43.11)

6-4.17   Discuss the documentation associated with abused and assaulted patient. (p 43.10, 43.11)

Affective

6-4.18   Demonstrate sensitivity to the abused patient. (p 43.10)

6-4.19   Value the behavior of the abused patient. (p 43.8, 43.9)

6-4.20   Attend to the emotional state of the abused patient. (p 43.5, 43.8, 43.9)

6-4.21   Recognize the value of non-verbal communication with the abused patient. (p 43.8, 43.9)

6-4.22   Attend to the needs for reassurance, empathy and compassion with the abused patient. (p 43.10)

6-4.23   Listen to the concerns expressed by the abused patient. (p 43.8–43.10)

6-4.24   Listen and value the concerns expressed by the sexually assaulted patient. (p 43.11)

Psychomotor

6-4.25   Demonstrate the ability to assess a spouse, elder or child abused patient. (p 43.5, 43.8, 43.10)

6-4.26   Demonstrate the ability to assess a sexually assaulted patient. (p 43.11)

Introduction

Abuse, neglect, and assault are, unfortunately, all too common in the United States (Table 43-1 ▾). Because these issues are frequently encountered reasons for calls to EMS, it is important for you to recognize the signs and symptoms. You must know not only how to recognize and differentiate among abuse, neglect, and assault, but also how to protect yourself from injury while maintaining optimal care for the patient. Victims who survive abuse or neglect often have permanent disabilities, mental and physical. Although prevention strategies have improved in recent years, paramedics may be on the front lines for getting help to victims of abuse (Figure 43-1 ▸).

Table 43-1	Incidence of Child Abuse	
Type of Abuse	**Percentage**	
Neglect	48	
Physical abuse	15	
Sexual abuse	8	
Psychological abuse	6	
Medical neglect	2	
Other	21	

Source: National Reports of Child Abuse by Type, 1997–2001. Available at: http://www.vcu.edu/vissta/training/va_teachers/images/gif/abuse/type_sm.gif. Accessed July 31, 2006.

Child Abuse

Child abuse includes any improper or excessive action that injures or otherwise harms a child or infant, including physical abuse, sexual abuse, neglect, and emotional abuse. Many survivors are negatively affected by such abuse for the rest of their

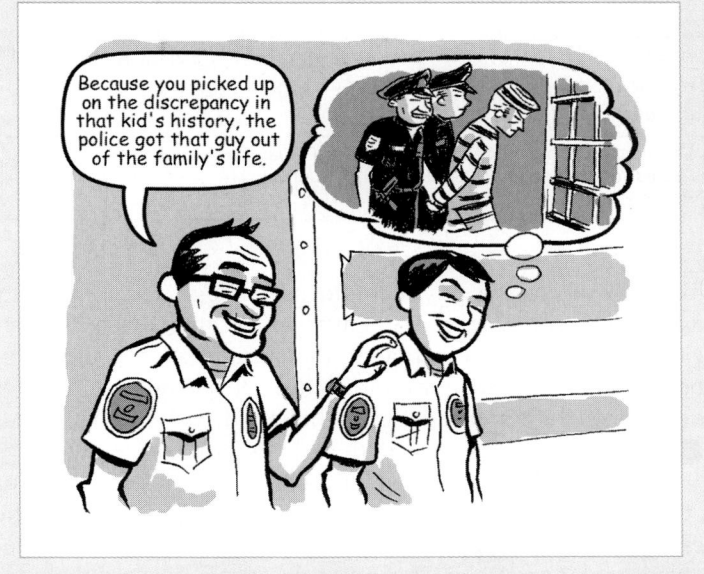

Figure 43-1

You are the Provider Part 1

You respond to a call for a "child who fell." On arrival, you find an unconscious 5-month-old boy. The mother just came home from work; her boyfriend had been watching the baby. The boyfriend states that the baby "fell off the couch" approximately 13″ from the carpeted floor. The child is comatose and has ataxic breathing.

The boyfriend appears nervous. He tries to answer all questions asked of the mother and to control the scene. In the same apartment, you find a 7-year-old girl with wheezing in all fields. The mother states that the child has a puffer, but it is empty and the mother has no insurance to obtain a refill. Five other children are in the cramped apartment, all under 10 years of age. The one-bedroom apartment is clean but very small, and children must sleep on a bare mattress in the living room. The mother sleeps in the bedroom with the baby (in the same bed).

Initial Assessment	Recording Time: 0 Minutes	
	5-month-old patient	**7-year-old patient**
Appearance	Comatose	Agitated, pensive
Level of consciousness	U (Unresponsive)	A (Alert to person, place, and day)
Airway	Mildly obstructed	Mildly obstructed
Breathing	22 breaths/min, irregular	> 40 breaths/min, shallow
Circulation	78 beats/min; irregular	> 140 beats/min; regular
Skin	Acrocyanotic	Flushed

1. What are your first priorities after assessing scene safety?
2. What should raise your index of suspicion?
3. What is the 5-month-old patient's transport and treatment status, in your judgment?

Table 43-2	Potential Complications of Maltreatment	
■ Low self-esteem and underachievement ■ Abnormal growth and development ■ Poor school performance ■ Social withdrawal ■ Substance abuse ■ Criminal behavior beginning in young adulthood ■ Suicidal tendencies ■ Death	■ Psychological disorders or psychiatric symptoms ■ Permanent physical or neurologic damage ■ Teen promiscuity and pregnancy ■ Eating disorders ■ Negative learned behavior ■ Vulnerability to further abuse ■ Increased survivor health care costs to family and society	

Source: American Academy of Pediatrics. *Pediatric Education for Prehospital Professionals*, 2nd ed. Table 12-1, p. 244. Sudbury, MA: Jones and Bartlett Publishers, Inc.

Table 43-3	Risk Factors for Child Abuse
Parent or Caregiver	
■ Parental history of abuse as a child ■ Substance abuse by parents ■ Insufficient or inaccurate parental knowledge about child development	
Family	
■ Disorganized and disruptive family structure ■ Marital or partner discord ■ Financial or outside stressors present ■ Inappropriate or dysfunctional parent–child interaction	
Child	
■ Disability of the child ■ Attention deficits or difficult temperament of child	
Environment	
■ Home life affected by poverty or unemployment ■ Isolation of caregivers; lack of social support ■ Violent, crime-filled community	

Source: Child Welfare Information Gateway. Available at: http://www.childwelfare.gov/pubs/usermanuals/foundation/foundatione.cfm. Accessed July 24, 2006.

lives. Owing to the physical and psychological damage they experience, survivors may themselves become abusive or neglectful caregivers, perpetuating the cycle of abuse. The number of children with long-term effects from neglect has not been well documented but is believed to be substantial. Table 43-2 ▲ lists some of these long-term complications.

Child neglect occurs when a child's physical, mental, or emotional condition is harmed or endangered because the caregiver fails to supply basic necessities or engages in inadequate or dangerous child-rearing practices. Neglect includes failure to provide adequate food, clothing, or shelter; the caregiver's misuse of drugs or alcohol; failure to provide support or affection necessary to the child's psychological and social development; or child abandonment. Children who are neglected are often dirty or too thin or appear developmentally delayed because of a lack of stimulation.

As a paramedic, you will often be called to scenes because of a reported injury to a child. Many abused children have permanent or life-threatening injuries, and some die. If suspected child abuse is not reported, the child is likely to be victimized repeatedly. Therefore, you must be aware of the signs of child abuse and neglect and cognizant of your responsibility to report suspected abuse to law enforcement or child protection agencies. When in doubt as to whether it is an abuse or neglect situation, it is always better to err on the side of caution to protect the victim.

Profile of an At-Risk Child

Child abuse and neglect occurs in all communities and among all socioeconomic strata. Younger children are at higher risk for fatal abuse and neglect than are older children. Approximately 85% of abused or neglected children who die are younger than 6 years; more than 40% are younger than 1 year. Although no geographic, ethnic, or economic setting is free of child abuse or neglect, children from low-income or single-parent families have more *reported* occurrences of abuse and neglect than children from higher-income families. Table 43-3 ▶ lists other factors that put a child at risk of abuse.

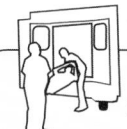

In the Field

It is a good idea to establish a "code" between you and your partner indicating that the provider should discreetly call for police. This signal can be as simple as "Could you go to the ambulance and get the extra set of latex-free gloves?" This way, you will not aggravate or "tip off" the abuser to your request for police, further riling the abuser.

When assessing a potential child abuse case, be attuned to suspicious behavioral traits. A child who does not become agitated when a parent leaves the room or who does not look to a parent for reassurance may be abused. Children who are abused may also cry excessively or not at all, may be wary of physical contact, or may appear apprehensive.

People Who Abuse Children

Child maltreatment can be done by any person who has care, custody, or control of the child, including parents, step-parents, foster parents, babysitters, and relatives. Abusive parents frequently receive little enjoyment from parenting and are more isolated from the community than are nonabusive parents. They have unrealistic expectations of their child and try to control the child through negative and authoritarian means. Abusive parents are often afraid of, or emotionally unable to ask for help from, sources of support in their community. Most were themselves abused or neglected as children. Many view themselves as victims in life generally or in the parent–child relationship in particular. They feel that they have lost control of their children and their own lives. When their children behave in a manner

Table 43-4	"Red Flag" Caregiver Behaviors

- Apathy
- Bizarre or strange conduct
- Little or no concern about the child
- Overreaction to child misbehavior
- Not forthcoming with events surrounding injury
- Intoxication
- Overreaction to child's condition

Source: American Academy of Pediatrics. *Pediatric Education for Prehospital Professionals*, 2nd ed. Table 12-7, p. 250. Sudbury, MA: Jones and Bartlett Publishers, Inc.

that parents perceive as disrespectful, they lash out in an effort to establish control. Abusive caregivers may prefer to discipline using other means but are pushed to violence by stress.

Characteristics shared by caregivers of maltreated children include drug use, poor self-concept, immaturity, lack of parenting knowledge, and lack of interpersonal skills. **Table 43-4 ▲** lists additional "red flag" caregiver behaviors.

Assessment and Management of Child Abuse

One of the most important indicators of possible abuse is repeated calls to the same home or family for a child injury or medical problem. Nevertheless, the best indicator by far is the physical examination of the child, conducted with a keen ear for inconsistencies in the history. The physical exam must take into consideration the mental and emotional age of the child. Examining the child from toe to head may work best on toddlers and preschoolers, whereas an infant may be best examined in a parent's arms. Preadolescents and teenagers have modesty and body awareness concerns, which should be respected.

If possible, do the exam with another colleague. This approach will verify your findings and help prevent false accusations of impropriety. Also, make certain that you are very objective on your documentation. Do not include opinions or draw nonmedical conclusions; list only the objective information, and stick to the facts.

When assessing for possible child abuse, you may find the CHILD ABUSE mnemonic helpful:

- **C** *Consistency* of the injury with the child's developmental age
- **H** *History* inconsistent with injury
- **I** *Inappropriate* parental concerns
- **L** *Lack* of supervision
- **D** *Delay* in seeking care
- **A** *Affect*
- **B** *Bruises* of varying ages
- **U** *Unusual* injury patterns
- **S** *Suspicious* circumstances
- **E** *Environmental* clues

Soft-tissue injuries are the most common findings in the physical exam of an abused child. Multiple bruises in various stages of healing are another red flag **Figure 43-2 ▶**. Be alert for bruises on areas of the body where they would not be expected, such as the buttocks **Figure 43-3 ▶**, back, face, and upper legs. Bites and burns may also be noted. Stocking/glove burns and doughnut burns occur when a child is immersed in hot water **Figure 43-4 ▶**.

Fractures can result from falls, twisting, or jerking injuries. Multiple fractures or fractures in various stages of healing are indicators of abuse, as are "self-healing" fractures. Head injuries are the most deadly for children; even if not fatal, they can easily produce permanent disability. Look for scalp wounds, signs and symptoms of hematoma, and concussion **Figure 43-5 ▶**.

You are the Provider Part 2

You decide to call the police to the scene, owing to the injuries and current history of the 5-month-old patient. The boyfriend becomes visibly agitated when he hears you on the radio. "What do we need cops for? Just take care of the kid," he states. After making sure you have a visible escape route, you continue caring for the child and tell the man, "It's just routine." You then ask the mother for the medical history of the child, hoping to deflect the man's attention. At this time, the 5-month-old boy is having difficulty in breathing, his extremities are becoming cyanotic, and he does not respond to external stimuli. The 7-year-old girl with asthma is in moderate distress as your partner sets up the nebulizer with the pediatric dose of albuterol.

Vital Signs	Recording Time: 5 Minutes	
	5-month-old patient	7-year-old patient
Skin	Cool and dry, cyanotic extremities	Warm, wet
Pulse	62 beats/min	120 beats/min
Blood pressure	Unobtainable	96/50 mm Hg
Respirations	20 breaths/min; irregular	32 breaths/min
Sao$_2$	89 mm Hg on room air	97 mm Hg on room air

4. Do you think you will have to intubate the 5-month-old boy? Why or why not?
5. Do you think you will have to intubate the 7-year-old girl? Why or why not?

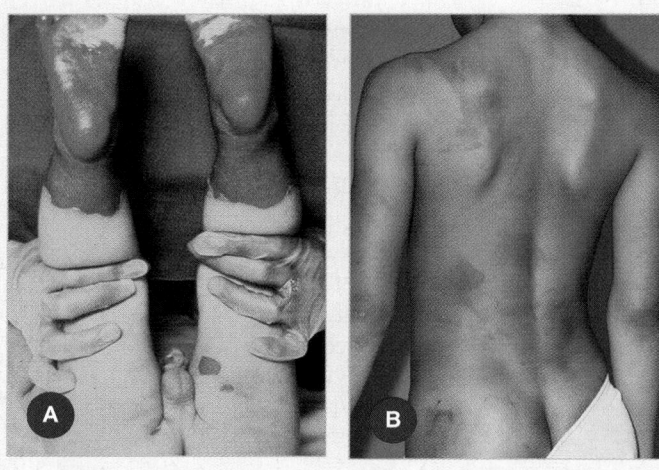

Figure 43-2 Signs of child abuse. **A.** Scald. **B.** Multiple injuries at different stages of healing.

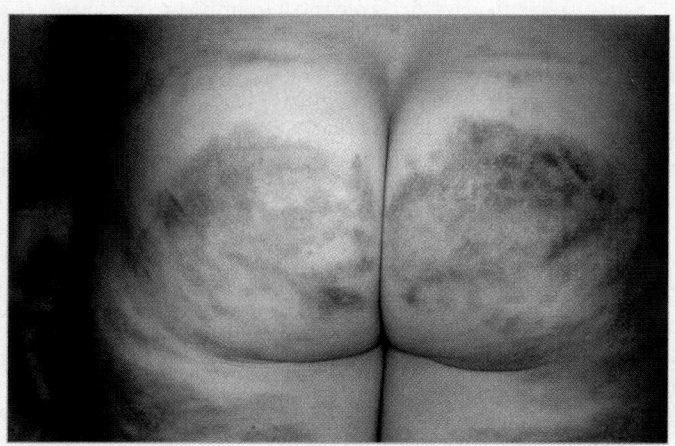

Figure 43-3 Bruises on the buttocks are usually inflicted injuries.

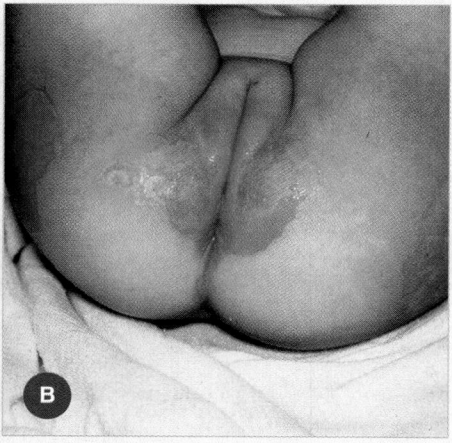

Figure 43-4 **A.** Stocking/glove burns of the feet or hands in an infant or a toddler are almost always inflicted injuries. **B.** A doughnut burn occurs when a child is held in a hot bath and the area in contact with the cooler porcelain is spared.

Although abdominal injuries are rare in child abuse cases, they are usually serious. Remember, small children have thin and underdeveloped abdominal muscles. Note the color and rigidity of the abdomen and tenderness to palpation. Injuries to the abdomen may result in injuries to the intestines or rupture of the liver.

Sometimes, normal physical findings may suggest an inflicted injury. Other benign skin findings can also suggest abuse, although the lesions are actually produced by cultural rituals intended to treat illness. Some medical or folk remedies may be foreign to you or inconsistent with your training. For example, cupping **Figure 43-6** and coin rubbing **Figure 43-7** are alarming to most paramedics, but a reasonable explanation of the practice, which is common in some Asian cultures, should allay your suspicions.

It is important to observe the scene, including the household dynamics, as you care for the patient. In the "You are the Provider" scenario in this chapter, the first responders discovered two patients; be aware that more than one victim may be encountered. It is important to keep the scene as safe and calm as possible while still providing life support for any critical and moderately distressed patients.

In a case involving child abuse or neglect, the patient care reports (PCRs), with objective observations, will be very important to the police and child protective services (CPS). In most states, the paramedic is a mandated reporter in child abuse or neglect cases. Most states have also established toll-free numbers for reporting suspected child abuse or neglect. Don't assume that someone else has already called or that the emergency department will call! It is better to have more than one person call the hotline for the same case than to see the case "fall through the cracks." Most communities also have parenting classes available through county social services.

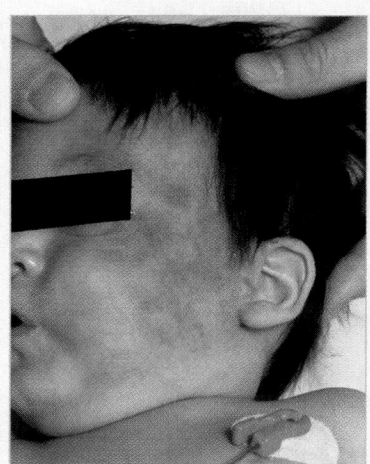

Figure 43-5 The face is a common target for physical abuse.

Elder Abuse

The incidence of older patient abuse and neglect is growing in the United States. The

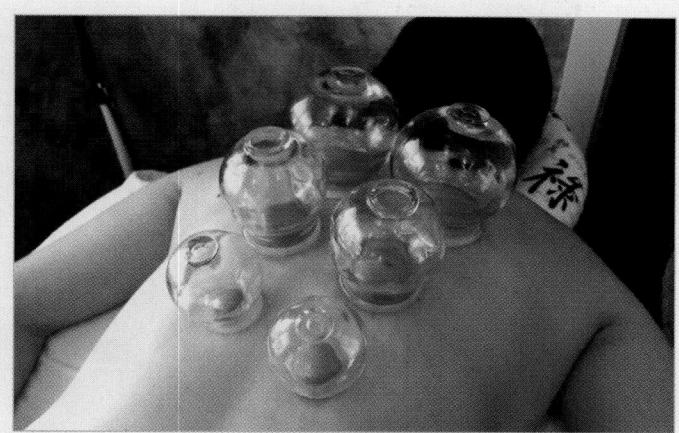

Figure 43-6 Cupping is the cultural practice of placing warm cups on the skin to pull out illness from the body. The red, flat, rounded skin lesions are often more intensely red at the borders.

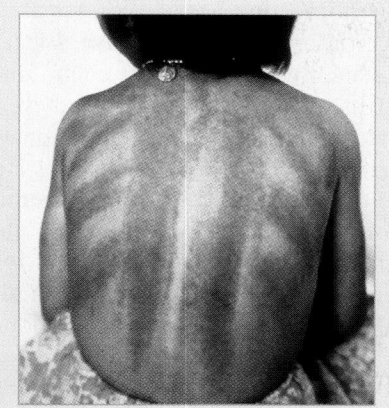

Figure 43-7 Rubbing hot coins, often on the back, produces rounded and oblong red, patchy, flat skin lesions.

aging of the population and the strains placed on caregivers and the nursing home systems contribute to this problem. You must use sound judgment and learn to develop good observational skills. Because geriatric patients present much differently than children and younger adults, you must be especially attuned to the possibility of abuse in this population. Consider the following scenario:

You respond to a call for "man down." On arrival, you find an 86-year-old man lying on his side in the living room, bleeding from the mouth and nose. He appears confused, and you cannot understand what he is trying to say. His 56-year-old daughter states that her father tripped and fell. His vital signs are as follows: pulse, 68 beats/min; respirations, 14 breaths/min; and blood pressure, 100/68 mm Hg. The patient's skin is warm and wet. You see a walker device in the kitchen approximately 25′ away. The daughter states that the patient doesn't really need it, stating, "He just uses it to get sympathy." The daughter is very upset that the police have just pulled up. Your partner tells you that she has been to this home several times before for falls, that the patient has Alzheimer's disease, and that the daughter seems to lose patience with him, sometimes refusing to cooperate with EMS. The daughter then states, "Would you people hurry up and get him out of here? He's getting blood all over the rug."

In this scenario, the elderly patient clearly needs assistance, but his caregiver also seems to be overwhelmed. This situation is not unusual: Because people are living longer than

Table 43-5	Profile of Abused Older Patients

- Women
- Persons older than 75 years
- Persons with one or more chronic physical or mental impairments placing them in a care-dependent position
- Persons who live with their abusers
- Socially isolated people
- Persons who exhibit problematic behavior (such as incontinence or shouting)

Table 43-6	Profile of a Person Who Abuses Elders

- Lives with the victim
- Has drug or alcohol dependency problems
- Is older than 50 years
- Depends on the victim for financial support
- Has poor impulse control
- Is ill prepared or reluctant to provide care
- Has a history of domestic violence

ever before, their children (often baby boomers) must assume responsibility for their care. The stress on these caregivers is real—physical, emotional, and financial burdens can wear them down. Your crews should be familiar with local resources to assist caregivers and patients. This assistance can be as simple as a visiting nurse or a handy-van agency to take the patient to his or her doctor's appointments.

As with child abuse, elder abuse involves a direct action causing harm to the victim. Abuse of older patients includes sexual abuse, psychological or emotional abuse, neglect, and abandonment. Neglect can be active or passive. Active neglect refers to the deliberate withholding of companionship, medicine, food, exercise, or assistance with mobility; passive neglect occurs when an older person is ignored, left alone, isolated, or forgotten. Abandonment is the desertion of an older person by a person who has physical custody of the older person or by a person who has assumed responsibility for providing care. Table 43-5 ▲ lists the characteristics of older abused patients. In domestic abuse cases, the abusers are quite often the children of the abused person Table 43-6 ▲.

Factors Contributing to Elder Abuse

Although EMS providers are concerned with treating and managing the results of abuse and neglect, an understanding of why these problems occur can be beneficial in the field. In some cases, the violence may be a learned response. Children who were abused may ultimately be in a position to abuse their elderly parents. The stress of caring for an older person may push some caregivers into abuse or neglect. Factors such as a diminishing social network, frailty, and medical illness also put older people at risk for maltreatment. Older people are at an increased risk for abuse in nursing facilities that have a history of providing inadequate care, are understaffed, and provide poor training for their employees.

Signs of Elder Abuse

The signs and symptoms of elder abuse and neglect can be subtle and, in the emergency setting, can often be overlooked. Evaluate each situation involving an older person with a critical eye toward potential abuse and neglect.

Be on the lookout for a fearful patient with unexplained bruises or sores that have not been tended to. Of course, the patient may naturally be fearful of the whole emergency situation, and there may well be a reasonable explanation for the marks on the body. Be alert for a situation in which you find an unkempt, dirty patient while the caregiver is clean. Generally speaking, a solicitous caregiver will keep the patient and the patient's surroundings tidy. Watch for a patient who allows the caregiver to answer all of your questions, while appearing mentally competent to do so; this person may look to the caregiver for approval when you ask the patient a direct question. If a patient tells you that items are being taken or money confiscated, such a complaint may be an indication of paranoia or a symptom of dementia—but it could very well be true. Don't investigate these claims; simply document them thoroughly. Be wary if a patient states that he or she is not allowed to socialize with peers and is kept in isolation.

Generally speaking, abused elders do not seek help. This reluctance may be due to fear of being institutionalized, fear of getting the abuser into "trouble," polypharmacy, confusion, or brain disorders such as Alzheimer's disease. In such cases, the physical exam, history, and observation of scene surroundings and patient interaction with caregivers are of paramount concern. The physical exam and history should address the following issues:

- Is the patient capable of answering your questions in an appropriate way?
- Is the patient fearful?
- Does the patient look clean?
- Are the pill bottles marked appropriately and consistent with purchase dates and use?
- Does the patient have bruises or sores?
- Is the patient's current history consistent with the report given by the caregiver?

Objectively record your observations on the PCR, avoiding drawing conclusions and giving opinions. Adult protective services (APS) could use these observations as an indicator of whether assistance is required.

As far as the scene goes, ask these questions **Figure 43-8 ▸**:

- Is the home tidy, and are the surroundings orderly?
- Is there food in the refrigerator?
- What is the heating or cooling situation, and is it appropriate to the weather?
- Does the patient use a walking or wheelchair device?

For patients who reside in nursing homes, signs of abuse include undocumented decubitus ulcers, tied-off catheters, and dangerous use of restraints. Some nursing home residents who are victims of abuse may not have a way to report the abuse, may not know how to report the abuse, may not be physically able to report it, or may fear retaliation for reporting it. Others may be victims of abuse by visiting family members.

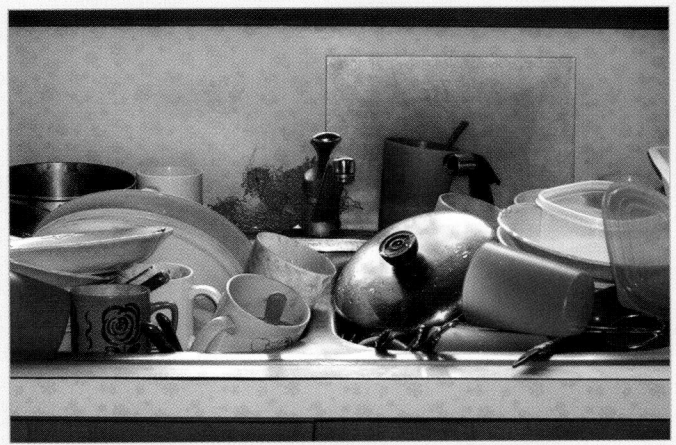

Figure 43-8 The patient's environment can provide clues to abuse or neglect.

Although the aging of the population has placed increased demands on the system, institutional caregivers have a legal obligation to meet accepted standards of care. Most communities have county health departments that provide care and even transportation for elderly citizens. If the patient is institutionalized and abuse or neglect is suspected, you may notify the state or county regulatory commission responsible for overseeing the facility; these organizations are listed in the telephone book. In addition, APS usually maintains a toll-free line for your use. You should thoroughly familiarize yourself with all local assistance and keep an up-to-date directory with 24-hour phone numbers.

▮ Domestic Abuse

Violence within the family has a long history. In ancient Rome, for example, husbands had the legal right to administer physical punishment to their wives within their own homes and in public. Today, EMS providers are frequently called for assault and battery in the home. The statistics on intimate-partner abuse are sobering: Millions of women are abused by an intimate partner each year.

Calls of this nature challenge the skills of EMS professionals. Scene safety is a paramount concern, and preservation of evidence is a necessity. Consider the following scenario:

> You are called for a "woman bleeding." When you arrive, a man opens the door and tells you that his wife fell down the stairs. You find a 42-year-old woman crying and bleeding from her mouth. She has obvious contusions and abrasions on her face. Vital signs are a pulse of 124 beats/min, respirations of 28 breaths/min, and blood pressure of 132/84 mm Hg. The patient is alert and oriented to person, place, and day; her skin is warm and dry. Her husband tries to answer all of the questions you pose to her. The stairwell is carpeted and has only seven risers, but there is no blood on the stairs. Two children, ages 6 and 12, are crying in an

In the Field

If you and your partner can safely get the patient and the person suspected of abuse away from each other, by all means do so. This separation will help make the scene safer; it also gives you a chance to compare current histories.

adjacent bedroom. The father tells them to stay in the bedroom. Police have not been dispatched to this call yet.

Is there significance to the husband dominating the patient interview? Should the crying children raise any red flags? The children's concern and the husband's control of the scene could be perfectly normal behavior. You must look at all the pieces of the puzzle. Document what you have observed, not what you think.

As a paramedic, you must be able to recognize the scope of domestic abuse and understand its various forms:

- **Physical abuse**—hitting, kicking, pushing, shoving, choking, beating
- **Emotional abuse**—making negative comments, calling names, playing mind games
- **Economic abuse**—trying to keep a person from getting a job and gaining his or her own economic independence
- **Sexual abuse**—making a person perform sexual activities against his or her will

Even though the awareness of domestic abuse has been raised in recent years, dealing with these cases in the field presents a challenge to the paramedic. Battered patients may not give accurate details about their injuries, and they may avoid seeking help. Indeed, victims typically report their abuse only as a last resort, for many reasons—for example, embarrassment, financial considerations, and low self-esteem. Many times they believe the behavior will change, as is often promised by the abuser. Sometimes the victim believes that he or she is the reason for the abuse and somehow deserved it (also called the Stockholm syndrome).

Profile of an Abused Spouse

Physical injuries from abuse include broken bones, cuts, head injuries, bruises, burns, scars from old injuries, and internal injuries. An abused spouse may have feelings of anxiety, distress, or hopelessness and may show signs of depression, make suicide attempts, or engage in substance abuse.

Although in the overwhelming majority of cases the victim is a woman, men also are abused. Men who are battered may be too humiliated to report the incident as it happened but still feel the same emotions as their female counterparts: guilt, loss of control, and shame. Because society tends to be less empathetic toward abused men and because fewer resources exist for them, the situation can be all the more difficult.

Same-sex relationships can be as fraught with peril as heterosexual unions. A common misconception is that participants in same-sex relationships are "on an equal playing field," so that the abuse cannot be as serious as that found in heterosexual relationships. In reality, concerns about "coming out" may prevent these victims from seeking help. You must be aware of and sensitive to their concerns.

Battered patients may appear fearful, apprehensive, or non-verbal. They may avoid eye contact, and their answers may be incorrect or inconsistent. Be alert for verbal clues such as "It was my fault—I really shouldn't push him" or "He's a good person—it's just that when he drinks . . ." In many states, if a person shows physical signs of having been abused, the police must make an arrest at the scene **Figure 43-9 ▶**.

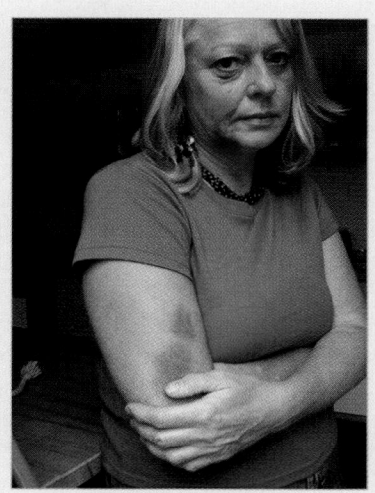

Figure 43-9 Injuries associated with intimate-partner abuse.

People Who Abuse Their Partners

Persons who commit domestic abuse may be paranoid, overly sensitive, obsessive, or threatening. They often abuse alcohol or drugs and have access to weapons. **Table 43-7 ▼** lists other characteristics of abusers.

People who abuse partners or spouses may use intimidation and threats to maintain their control over the person. They may throw objects in a rage or threaten regarding what he or she will do if the spouse leaves or reports the abusive behavior. An abusive spouse may also use isolation as a means to dominate the partner, not allowing the spouse to visit friends or talk openly with others, and may feel that he or she is providing discipline or is justified in these actions. Many times, an abusive person is immediately remorseful and promises never to let the problem happen again. Historically, this is rarely true; the abuse usually continues and becomes even more violent.

Never forget that domestic violence calls can be dangerous. You may be dealing with a potentially violent person, and

Table 43-7	Characteristics of a Person Who Abuses a Partner
<ul><li>Was abused as a child</li><li>Becomes more violent with each ensuing attack</li><li>Usually comes from a family of abusers</li><li>Very low self-esteem</li><li>Remorseful after the attack; promises it will never happen again (but it does)</li><li>May direct violence at children, especially children from a partner's previous relationship(s)</li></ul>	

emotions on the scene will be highly charged. If the person appears to be hostile or violent, remove all unnecessary people (such as family, friends, and bystanders) from the scene. It is imperative that you put your safety and the safety of your partner first. If there is any doubt about scene safety, call for law enforcement assistance (see Chapter 51) **Figure 43-10 ▶** .

Assessment and Management of Domestic Abuse

Identifying a battered patient can be difficult because the victim may be protective of the attacker, frightened, or honestly unable to recall details. Patients may avoid eye contact or be otherwise evasive about their injuries. Listen for verbal clues regarding the incident, such as "We've been having some problems." On approach to the patient, use direct questioning to ascertain whether the domestic problems led to the physical harm. Try to empathize and reassure the patient; this caring attitude alone may instill confidence. Be as objective and nonjudgmental as possible. Listen attentively, and be supportive. Give the patient a sense of control as much as possible. You may be the last or only chance a victim has to escape this situation, so encourage the patient to consider where he or she can go or whom he or she can call for help.

In cases involving domestic abuse, the PCR is more than just documentation of the transfer of care; it is a permanent record of treatment and disposition. More important, from a legal viewpoint, it represents hard evidence for the prosecution and the defense. Your statements and assessments must be objective, nonjudgmental, exact (when quoting a statement from the scene), and as neat as possible. If you make an error and want to change it, draw a line through the error and initial the lined-out statement. Usually, before testifying in court, you are allowed to review your PCR, but remember that your testimony may come many years and many patients later.

Intimate-partner abuse is not simply a "family issue;" it is a crime to beat another person, regardless of the relationship. The presence of law enforcement personnel is always helpful in these cases. If the patient refuses to be transported, consider

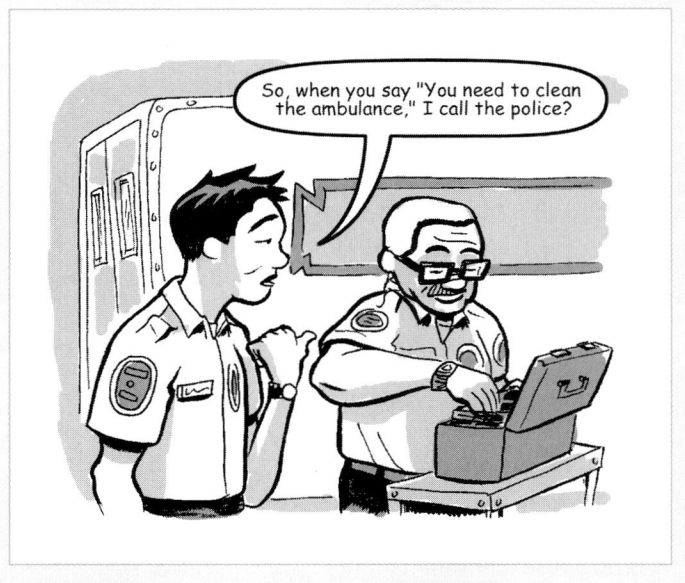

Figure 43-10

leaving information on victim-witness assistance programs, such as domestic abuse shelters, that the patient may reference later. Learn what services are available in your area.

■ Sexual Assault

Sexual assault is another call that EMS receives all too often. Although most victims are women, men and children may also be attacked sexually. There are no typical characteristics of sexual offenders and unfortunately, they are very difficult to detect. Often, you can do little beyond providing compassion and transportation to the emergency department. On some occasions, patients may have multiple-system trauma and need treatment for shock. Your actions will go a long way toward providing relief. From arrival on scene to possible judicial system involvement, your professionalism is the key to proper care.

You are the Provider Part 3

Vital Signs	Recording Time: 10 Minutes	
	5-month-old patient	7-year-old patient
Skin	Good color; cool and dry	Warm, wet
Pulse	98 beats/min	110 beats/min
Blood pressure	60/P	96/50 mm Hg
Respirations	Intubated	Nebulizer treatment; normal breaths/min
Sao₂	98 mm Hg	100 mm Hg

6. What further treatment do you need for the 5-month-old boy? How can you check for level of consciousness at this point?

7. Is the small-volume nebulizer treatment working for the 7-year-old girl? Does this patient need to go to the hospital? Why or why not?

In the Field

It is usually preferable to have a same-gender caregiver assist with the victim of sexual abuse. If you have this capability and there is no unreasonable time lag for that type of response (including rape crisis teams), you should consider this option as a treatment modality.

Consider the following scenario:

You are sent to an "assist police" call. On arrival at the scene, you find a 20-year-old woman covered in a blanket and bleeding from several abrasions on her face. The police officer pulls you aside and states that the patient may have been assaulted in the alleyway on her way home from night class. Vital signs include a pulse of 134 beats/min, respirations of 32 breaths/min and irregular, and blood pressure of 122/80 mm Hg. The patient is alert and oriented to person, place, and day; her skin is warm and wet. She is very quiet, appears confused, and tells you she doesn't remember what happened. She wants to go home and shower.

The victim of sexual assault is often found in a state of denial or disbelief. Likewise, the desire to shower or douche is common. The patient should be encouraged to go to the hospital, where evidence can be collected and where access to professional services is more readily available.

Sexual assault and rape are crimes of power, force, and violence. The legal definitions of these crimes differ from state to state, but essentially *sexual assault* refers to any unwanted sexual contact and *rape* means penile penetration of the genitalia without the victim's consent. When the victim is underage, it is called statutory rape. Rape is a felony offense, and you have a responsibility to preserve the crime scene in addition to treating the patient (see Chapter 51).

Treatment and Documentation

A victim of sexual assault may be hysterical, embarrassed, and/or frightened. You must be vigilant, but above all, you must be professional and compassionate. If you do not observe life-threatening signs and symptoms on arrival, avoid any aggressive treatment behavior. Leave evidence as untouched as possible, and take care to establish a chain of custody as required. The police should be notified as per protocol. Encourage the patient not to bathe, douche, urinate, or defecate, if possible. If oral penetration has occurred, advise the patient not to eat, drink, brush the teeth, or use mouthwash until he or she has been examined.

Treat all other injuries according to appropriate procedures and protocols for your EMS system. Observe BSI precautions. Take the patient's history, perform a limited physical exam, and provide treatment as quickly, quietly, and calmly as possible.

Take care to shield the patient from onlookers. Help the patient regain a sense of control by posing open-ended questions and allowing him or her to make decisions.

The patient may refuse assistance or transport, often because he or she wants to maintain privacy and avoid public exposure. Adult patients have the right to decline care. In these cases, you should follow your system's refusal of treatment policy or procedure for sexual assault victims without being judgmental or condescending to the patient. Your compassion is the best tool to win the patient's confidence to get further help.

Because you may need to appear in court as much as 2 or 3 years later, you should document the patient's history, assessment, treatment, and response to treatment in detail. Record only the objective facts. Subjective statements made by those on the scene or the patient should be in quotes on the PCR. Thoroughly document all patient statements pertaining to the crime, as well as statements, names, addresses, and contact information of any witnesses.

Like a battered partner, a victim of sexual abuse must be treated and protected by the EMS and police. Conscientious caregivers will make a huge difference in the recovery of patients through their professional conduct. Many states offer rape crisis teams to assist patients. Your EMS system should keep an up-to-date directory of all sexual abuse hotlines and assistance available, with 24-hour telephone numbers.

Child Victims

In most cases of child sexual abuse, the person who abused the child is an adult who knows the child and may be living under the same roof. Children of any age and either sex can be victims of sexual abuse. Although most victims of rape are older than 10 years, younger children may also be victims.

Child sexual abuse usually does not occur as a single incident. It does not always involve violence and physical force, and it commonly leaves no visible signs. The power of authority or the parent–child bond may be used to victimize the child instead of force or violence. The child may be manipulated into thinking that the acts are acceptable and normal behavior. The child may also be made to feel deeply ashamed and powerless or even be kept silent by threats. The insidious nature of this abuse makes it difficult to detect unless the child discloses the information to a confidant or a prehospital professional.

Your assessment of a child who has been sexually abused should be limited to determining the type of dressing any injuries require. Sometimes, a sexually abused child is also beaten. In such cases, you should treat bruises and fractures as well. Do not examine the genitalia of a young child unless you see evidence of bleeding or an injury to this region that must be treated. In some cases, the child may present with behavioral or physical problems, such as hostility or restlessness.

You are the Provider Summary

1. What are your first priorities after assessing scene safety?

Your first priority in the scenario should be to open the airway of the 5-month-old boy. Your next priority is to call for a second paramedic unit to help care for the second patient you identified. Additional patient care resources such as a supervisor and engine company may also be helpful, if available in your local area.

2. What should raise your index of suspicion?

Your index of suspicion should be raised by the nervousness of the boyfriend and his attempts to control the scene.

3. What is the 5-month-old patient's transport and treatment status, in your judgment?

The 5-month-old boy should be considered in unstable condition, and treatment and transport should occur as rapidly as possible after airway maneuvering.

4. Do you think that you will have to intubate the 5-month-old boy? Why or why not?

You will have to intubate this patient on the scene because you can control his airway better than the boy can himself.

5. Do you think you will have to intubate the 7-year-old girl? Why or why not?

This patient does not have to be intubated at this point; give the albuterol and/or ipratropium (Atrovent) treatment a chance to work before you take this step.

6. What further treatment do you need for the 5-month-old boy? How can you check for level of consciousness at this point?

This patient needs to be evaluated for brain damage due to the "fall" or to hypoxia. At this point, it is a good idea to check for painful stimuli and watch the boy's reaction, if any. A pinch of the foot may provide a response.

7. Is the nebulizer treatment working for the 7-year-old girl? Does this patient need to go to the hospital? Why or why not?

The nebulizer seems to be working for the 7-year-old girl; however, she should still be transported to the hospital. There the patient can be interviewed by professionals and, at the very least, receive another prescription for her metered-dose inhaler.

Prep Kit

Ready for Review

- Abuse, neglect, and assault occur at all levels of society. Because maltreatment and assault are common reasons for calls to EMS, you must recognize the signs and symptoms of these problems.
- Child abuse includes any improper or excessive action that injures or otherwise harms a child or infant, including physical abuse, sexual abuse, neglect, and emotional abuse. Many survivors are negatively affected for the rest of their lives.
- Reporting of child abuse or neglect is mandatory in most states.
- Watch for the telltale signs of abused children and people who abuse children.
- Abuse and neglect of elderly people are on the rise. Because geriatric patients present much differently than child and adult patients do, you must be especially attuned to the possibility of abuse in the elderly population.
- Elder abuse can be domestic or institutional. Adult children are often the ones who abuse their elderly parents.
- Adult protective services exist for caregivers and victims alike.
- Domestic abuse happens in heterosexual and homosexual relationships.
- Victims of sexual abuse may not be inclined to report the crime.

Vital Vocabulary

abuse Any form of maltreatment that results in harm or loss. Maltreatment may be physical, sexual, psychological, or financial/material.

active neglect The refusal or failure to fulfill a caregiving obligation; a conscious or intentional attempt to inflict physical or emotional stress. Examples include abandonment and denial of food or health-related services.

adult protective services (APS) Organizations that investigate cases involving abuse and neglect and provide case management services in some cases.

assault Unlawfully placing a person in fear of immediate bodily harm.

battery Unlawfully touching a person; this includes providing emergency care without consent.

child protective services (CPS) An agency that is the community legal organization responsible for protection, rehabilitation, and prevention of child maltreatment and neglect; it has the legal authority to temporarily remove from home children who are at risk for injury or neglect and to secure foster placement.

coin rubbing A cultural ritual intended to treat an illness by rubbing hot coins, often on the back, which produces rounded and oblong red, patchy, flat skin lesions.

cupping The cultural practice of placing warm cups on the skin to pull out illness from the body. The red, flat, rounded skin lesions are often more intensely red at the borders.

mandated reporter A category of professional required by some states to report suspicions of child maltreatment. Prehospital professionals may be included.

neglect Refusal or failure on the part of the caregiver to provide life necessities, such as food, water, clothing, shelter, personal hygiene, medicine, comfort, and personal safety.

passive neglect An unintentional refusal or failure to fulfill a caregiving obligation, which results in physical or emotional distress. Examples include forgetting or isolating the person.

polypharmacy Simultaneous use of many medications.

rape Sexual intercourse inflicted forcibly on another person, against that person's will.

sexual assault An attack against a person that is sexual in nature, the most common of which is rape.

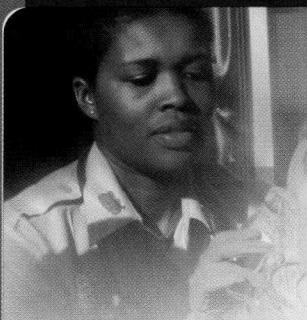

Assessment in Action

You have responded to a report of a female patient in her 40s with a possible fractured arm. As you enter the residence, you notice it is immaculately clean. Your patient is sitting on a sofa holding her left forearm, which is bruised and appears to be very tender. You ask the woman what happened, and she says that she fell on a wet floor that she had just finished mopping. As you begin your assessment, you notice a man has walked into the room. He tells you that his wife is very clumsy and "runs into everything." He states that he is sure it is not as bad as she is making it sound. As the husband is speaking, you notice the patient looks down at the floor and will not make eye contact with you.

1. **What is your primary concern in this situation?**
   A. Gathering more information about the patient
   B. Crew safety
   C. Splinting the patient's arm
   D. Questioning the husband further

2. **When you begin your assessment of the patient, you notice some bruising on her right arm. When you ask the patient how that happened, she states that she must have obtained the bruising when she fell today. How can you tell if bruising is new or old?**
   A. The bruise is larger if it is a new injury.
   B. The bruise is smaller if it is a new injury.
   C. The bruise will be a different color or appearance.
   D. The bruise will be the same color or appearance.

3. **As you ask the patient further about her medical history, she states that she is very clumsy and has broken that arm before. When you ask her when this occurred and what hospital treated her injuries, she states she cannot remember. The husband states that the injury was years ago and it does not matter in this case. What action should you take at this point?**
   A. If it is safe to do so, interview the husband away from the wife.
   B. Immediately remove the patient to the safety of your ambulance.
   C. Ask the patient if there are any children in the home.
   D. You and your partner should leave the scene and call law enforcement.

4. **When you and your partner come back together, you find that the history of events does not match between husband and wife. You choose to splint the patient's arm and transport her to the facility of her choice. When you advise her of your intentions, she states that she does not want to go to the hospital. What is your next course of action?**
   A. Have the patient sign a refusal, and leave the scene.
   B. Have your partner go outside and contact law enforcement.
   C. Have a neighbor come over to take the patient to the hospital.
   D. Contact your supervisor.

5. **After law enforcement personnel arrive, you are able to treat and transport the patient to the hospital of her choice. Once inside your ambulance, what is a recommended way to obtain more information on how the injury occurred?**
   A. Have a law enforcement officer ride in with you and the patient.
   B. Do not ask direct questions because they will upset the patient.
   C. Ask direct questions about the potential that the injury was caused by abuse.
   D. Wait until you arrive at the hospital, and let the physician obtain the information.

Challenging Question

6. **You and your partner begin to write your PCR concerning this call for service. What should you be cognizant of during your documentation?**

◼ Points to Ponder

You and your partner are called to a local kindergarten for an ill child. When you arrive at the school office, you find a 5-year-old Asian child who appears to have a common cold. You notice the child is coughing and is tugging at his ears. The school administrator pulls you aside and says that she suspects child abuse. When you ask why, she directs the child to come into her office and asks him to raise up his shirt. You notice large, red marks extending from the shoulders to the lumbar region of the child's back. You ask the child what happened to make these marks and the child states, "my grandmother is trying to make me better." The school administrator insists that law enforcement personnel be contacted to arrest the grandmother.

What is your opinion?

Issues: Abuse, Cultural Differences, Child Abuse, Physical Abuse.

44 Patients With Special Needs

Objectives

Cognitive

6-5.1   Describe the various etiologies and types of hearing impairments. (p 44.4)

6-5.2   Recognize the patient with a hearing impairment. (p 44.5)

6-5.3   Anticipate accommodations that may be needed in order to properly manage the patient with a hearing impairment. (p 44.5)

6-5.4   Describe the various etiologies of visual impairments. (p 44.7)

6-5.5   Recognize the patient with a visual impairment. (p 44.7)

6-5.6   Anticipate accommodations that may be needed in order to properly manage the patient with a visual impairment. (p 44.7, 44.8)

6-5.7   Describe the various etiologies and types of speech impairments. (p 44.6)

6-5.8   Recognize the patient with speech impairment. (p 44.6)

6-5.9   Anticipate accommodations that may be needed in order to properly manage the patient with speech impairment. (p 44.7)

6-5.10   Describe the various etiologies of obesity. (p 44.8)

6-5.11   Anticipate accommodations that may be needed in order to properly manage the patient with obesity. (p 44.8, 44.9)

6-5.12   Describe paraplegia/quadriplegia. (p 44.8)

6-5.13   Anticipate accommodations that may be needed in order to properly manage the patient with paraplegia/quadriplegia. (p 44.8)

6-5.14   Define mental illness. (p 44.9)

6-5.15   Describe the various etiologies of mental illness. (p 44.10)

6-5.16   Recognize the presenting signs of the various mental illnesses. (p 37.5–37.8)

6-5.17   Anticipate accommodations that may be needed in order to properly manage the patient with a mental illness. (p 37.11–37.12)

6-5.18   Define the term developmentally disabled. (p 44.10)

6-5.19   Recognize the patient with a developmental disability. (p 44.10)

6-5.20   Anticipate accommodations that may be needed in order to properly manage the patient with a developmental disability. (p 44.11)

6-5.21   Describe Down's syndrome. (p 44.10)

6-5.22   Recognize the patient with Down's syndrome. (p 44.10)

6-5.23   Anticipate accommodations that may be needed in order to properly manage the patient with Down's syndrome. (p 44.10)

6-5.24   Describe the various etiologies of emotional impairment. (p 44.11)

6-5.25   Recognize the patient with an emotional impairment. (p 44.11)

6-5.26   Anticipate accommodations that may be needed in order to properly manage the patient with an emotional impairment. (p 44.11, 44.12)

6-5.27   Define emotional/mental impairment (EMI). (p 44.11)

6-5.28   Recognize the patient with an emotional or mental impairment. (p 44.11)

6-5.29   Anticipate accommodations that may be needed in order to properly manage patients with an emotional or mental impairment. (p 44.11, 44.12)

6-5.30   Describe the following diseases/illnesses:
a. Arthritis
b. Cancer
c. Cerebral palsy
d. Cystic fibrosis
e. Multiple sclerosis
f. Muscular dystrophy
g. Myasthenia gravis
h. Poliomyelitis
i. Spina bifida
j. Patients with a previous head injury (p 44.12–44.15)

6-5.31   Identify the possible presenting sign(s) for the following diseases/illnesses:
a. Arthritis
b. Cancer
c. Cerebral palsy
d. Cystic fibrosis
e. Multiple sclerosis
f. Muscular dystrophy
g. Myasthenia gravis
h. Poliomyelitis
i. Spina bifida
j. Patients with a previous head injury (p 44.12–44.15)

6-5.32   Anticipate accommodations that may be needed in order to properly manage the following patients:
a. Arthritis
b. Cancer
c. Cerebral palsy
d. Cystic fibrosis
e. Multiple sclerosis
f. Muscular dystrophy
g. Myasthenia gravis
h. Poliomyelitis
i. Spina bifida
j. Patients with a previous head injury (p 44.12–44.15)

6-5.33   Define cultural diversity. (p 44.17)

6-5.34   Recognize a patient who is culturally diverse. (p 44.17)

6-5.35 Anticipate accommodations that may be needed in order to properly manage a patient who is culturally diverse. (p 44.17)

6-5.36 Identify a patient that is terminally ill. (p 44.15)

6-5.37 Anticipate accommodations that may be needed in order to properly manage a patient who is terminally ill. (p 44.16)

6-5.38 Identify a patient with a communicable disease. (p 44.17)

6-5.39 Recognize the presenting signs of a patient with a communicable disease. (p 44.17)

6-5.40 Anticipate accommodations that may be needed in order to properly manage a patient with a communicable disease. (p 44.17)

6-5.41 Recognize sign(s) of financial impairments. (p 44.18)

6-5.42 Anticipate accommodations that may be needed in order to properly manage the patient with a financial impairment. (p 44.18)

Affective

None

Psychomotor

None

Introduction

Throughout the ages, humans have learned to adapt to the challenges they encounter. In the field, you will encounter patients who face a variety of special challenges. Some conditions or anomalies are congenital; others have developed during the patient's lifetime or occurred as the result of a sudden event (eg, the transection of the spinal cord during a diving accident). Whatever the source of the challenge, these patients will require you to adapt your assessment and management to accommodate their needs.

Although you can still use the standard assessment plan with these patients, sometimes you may find it necessary to adapt so as to best meet a patient's unique needs. Can the patient see you? Can the patient hear you? Can the patient normally move all extremities? You will need to formulate a plan to care for these patients in a short amount of time. Be willing to incorporate "the experts" (ie, the patient, family members, or caregivers) as essential teammates. Learn to solve problems as part of a group, and remember your ultimate goal: to give the patient the best care possible, in the most efficient way, and still accommodate for his or her individual needs. Your confidence and caring attitude will promote trust between you, your patient, and the other members of your team.

Physical Challenges

Humans use all five senses to gather information, but we often take that sensory feedback for granted. Imagine what it would be like to go bowling while blindfolded. You hear the pins dropping—but did you knock down a couple of pins, get a strike, or just leave a 7–10 split? Imagine how frustrating it

might be to see that you need to tie your shoe but to be unable to do so because an injury resulted in the loss of motor function in your hand.

Hearing Impairments

Hearing challenges are generally classified into two types: conductive and sensorineural deafness. Conductive deafness is a usually curable temporary condition caused by an injury to the eardrum, an infection, or simply a buildup of earwax in the external auditory canal. Sensorineural deafness, which is permanent, may be caused by a lesion or damage of the inner ear, or damage to the eighth cranial nerve. This type of hearing impairment may be congenital or secondary to a birth injury, but it may also have occurred over time from disease, medication complications, viral infections, or tumors. People may also lose their hearing due to aging (called *presbycusis*) or from prolonged exposure to loud noise.

Hearing impairment may range from a slight hearing loss to total deafness. Some patients may have difficulty with pitch, volume, and speaking distinctly. Some have learned to speak even though they have never heard speech. Others may have heard speech and learned to talk, but have since lost some or all of their hearing, leading them to speak too loudly. Parkinson's disease or other disease processes may cause the patient to slur words, speak very slowly, or speak in a monotone voice.

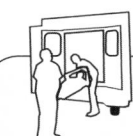

In the Field

Consider sirens and protect your hearing . . . before it's too late.

You are the Provider Part 1

You and your partner are dispatched to a state park for a child in respiratory distress. When you arrive at the entrance you are guided by a park officer to pavilion 4, where you find a group of active 8-year-olds enjoying a class picnic. The scene appears ordinary until you get closer to the pavilion and realize that all the children in this group have Down syndrome.

Seated on one of the picnic benches is a girl in obvious respiratory distress. You observe that she is in a tripod position and is using accessory muscles to breathe. As you get closer, you are able to hear audible expiratory wheezes. Her teacher is next to her trying to provide reassurance.

Initial Assessment	Recording Time: 0 Minutes
Appearance	Anxious; child seated in a tripod position
Level of consciousness	A (Alert to person, place, and day)
Airway	Open
Breathing	Increased work of breathing with accessory muscle use
Circulation	Strong radial pulse, slightly elevated

1. What is Down syndrome?
2. What are the characteristic physical features of Down syndrome?

Interaction With a Hearing-Impaired Patient

Clues that a person could be hearing impaired include the presence of hearing aids, poor pronunciation of words, or failure to respond to your presence or questions. While communicating, face the patient so that he or she can see your mouth; don't exaggerate your lip movements or look away. Position yourself approximately 18″ directly in front of the patient. Most people who are hearing impaired have learned to use body language, such as hand gestures and lipreading. Because hearing-impaired patients typically have more difficulty hearing higher-frequency sounds, if the patient seems to have difficulty hearing you, don't just speak louder—try lowering the pitch of your voice.

Ask the patient, "How would you like to communicate with me?" American Sign Language (ASL) may be his or her preferred method of communication   Figure 44-1 ▾ . An interpreter, family member, or friend may prove to be a valuable teammate. If an interpreter is not readily available, call your receiving facility early on to request one. Ideally, an interpreter will arrive before you begin your assessment. Other patients may prefer written communication or communication of concepts or procedures with gestures or pictures. Simply asking a team member to retrieve the patient's hearing aid or auditory electronic enhancement device may help a great deal.

Here are some helpful hints for working with patients with hearing impairments:

- Speak slowly and distinctly into a less impaired ear, or position yourself on that side.
- Change speakers. Given that 80% of hearing loss is related to inability to hear high-pitched sounds, look for a team

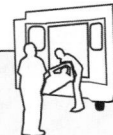

In the Field

Some hearing-impaired patients' ears are overly sensitive to very loud noises close to their ears. Remember to use a normal tone of voice when speaking to them.

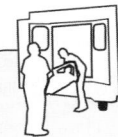

In the Field

When caring for a hearing-impaired patient, one easy solution is to place the ear pieces of your stethoscope into the patient's ears while you speak into the bell of the stethoscope.

member with a low-pitched voice if you think this may be the issue.

- Provide paper and pencil so that you may write your questions and the patient may write his or her responses.
- Only one person should ask interview questions, to avoid confusing the patient.
- Try the "reverse stethoscope" technique: put the earpieces of your stethoscope in the patient's ear and speak softly into the diaphragm of the stethoscope. This will amplify your voice.

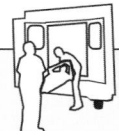

In the Field

Many patients with borderline hearing impairments may not be aware of the extent of their problem. The distracting and noisy EMS environment may worsen the situation. If a patient frequently asks you to repeat things, suspect a hearing impairment.

Hearing Aids

A hearing aid is essentially a device that makes sound louder. Hearing aids cannot restore hearing to normal, but they do improve hearing and listening ability. Several types of hearing aids are available   Figure 44-2 ▸ :

- *In-the-canal* and *completely in-the-canal*. These hearing aids are contained in a tiny case that fits partly or completely into the ear canal.
- *In-the-ear*. All parts are contained in a shell that fits in the outer part of the ear.

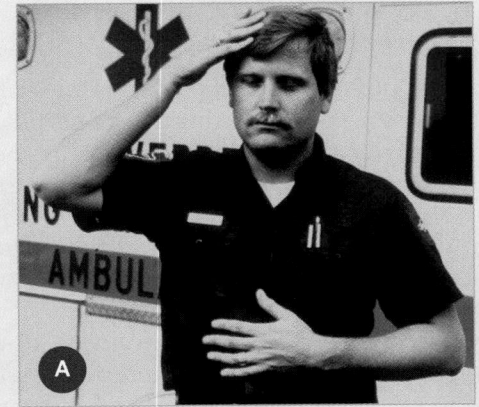
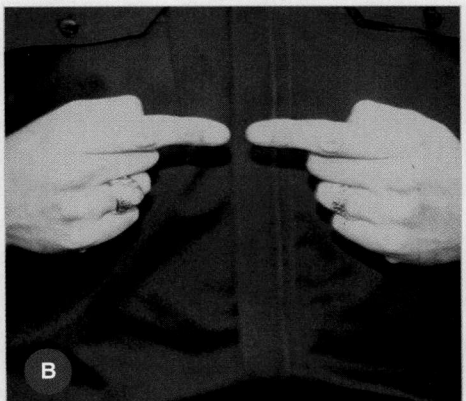
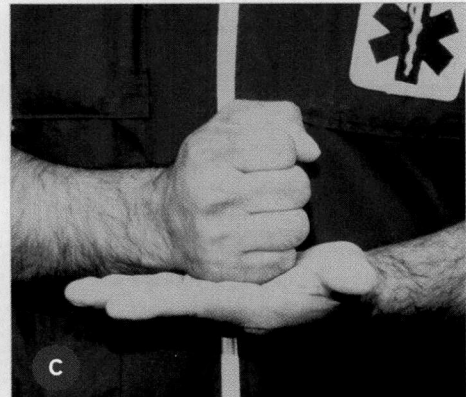

Figure 44-1 Consider learning the ASL signs for common terms related to illness and injury. **A.** Sick. **B.** Hurt. **C.** Help.

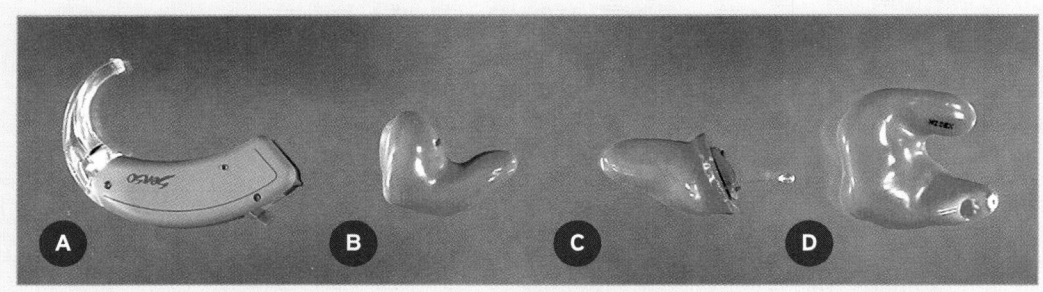

Figure 44-2 Different types of hearing aids. **A.** Behind-the-ear type. **B.** Conventional body type. **C.** In-the-canal type. **D.** In-the-ear type.

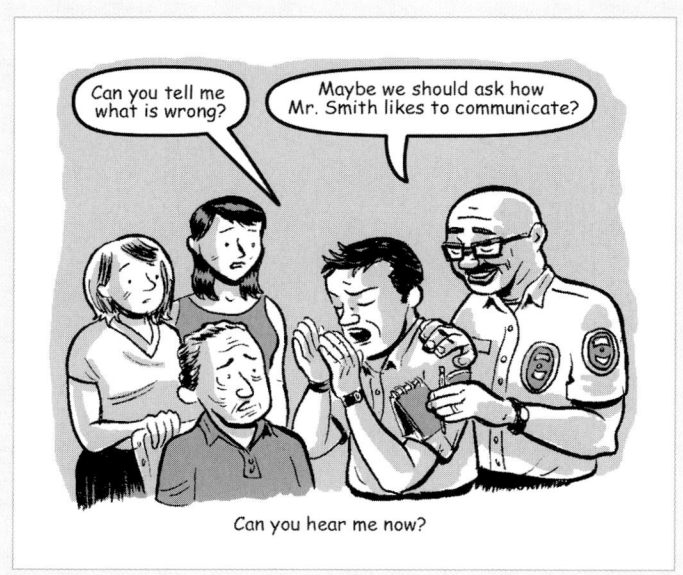

Figure 44-3

- *Behind-the-ear.* All parts are contained in a plastic case that rests behind the ear.
- *Conventional body type.* This older style is generally used by people with profound hearing loss.

Implantable hearing aids are also an option for patients with less profound hearing loss.

To insert a hearing aid, follow the natural shape of the ear. The device needs to fit snugly without forcing. If you hear a whistling sound, the hearing aid may not be in far enough to create a seal, or the volume may be too loud. Try repositioning the hearing aid, or remove it and turn down the volume. If you can't insert the hearing aid after two tries, put it in the box, take it with you, and document the transport and transfer of hearing aids to hospital personnel. Never try to clean hearing aids, and never get them wet.

If a patient's hearing aid is not working, try troubleshooting the problem. First, make sure the hearing aid is turned on **Figure 44-3 ▲** . Try a fresh battery, and check the tubing to make sure it isn't twisted or bent. Check the switch to make sure

it's set on M (microphone), not T (telephone). For a body aid, try a spare cord, as the old one may be broken or shorted. Finally, check the ear mold to make sure it isn't plugged with wax.

Speech Impairments

For most people, the spoken word is the primary mechanism for communicating thoughts and ideas. For some, speech may be delayed by psychological or psychosocial factors. For others, it may be altered by injury, illness, or hearing impairment.

Articulation Disorders

Articulation disorders cause the majority of speech difficulties. Dysarthria—the inability to make speech sounds correctly—results from a lack of muscle control and coordination of the larynx, tongue, mouth, and lips. Speech can be slurred, indistinct, slow, or nasal. Commonly, articulation disorders result from damage to nerve pathways passing from the brain to muscles in the larynx, mouth, or lips; delayed development from hearing problems; or slow maturation of the nervous system due to brain damage or motor disability. Articulation disorders affect both children and adults.

Language Disorders

Stroke, traumatic head/brain injury, brain tumor, delayed development, hearing loss, lack of stimulation, or emotional disturbance may cause damage to the language center of the brain and lead to aphasia. Aphasia is the loss of ability to communicate in speech, writing, or signs. It can range from being very mild to making communication with the patient almost impossible. Aphasia may affect primarily a single aspect of language use, such as the ability to recall the names of objects, to put words into sentences, or to read.

When communicating with an aphasic patient, remember to talk to the patient as an adult, not as a child. Use focused questions rather than open-ended questions, and minimize background noise.

Fluency Disorders

In fluency disorders, the person's speech pattern is broken, interrupted, or repetitious. An example of this type of disorder is stuttering. Stuttering may be noticed only when the person attempts certain words or sounds, and it may become worse when the individual is under stress. Stuttering is normal for young children and will disappear gradually over time. The specific causes of stuttering are unknown.

When dealing with a person who has a fluency disorder, patience is the key. Impatience with or interruption of a patient who stutters may frustrate the patient more and cause the stuttering to get worse, making assessment and history-taking difficult.

Voice Production Disorders

Voice production disorders refer to the way the voice sounds and may be slightly easier to understand than other speech impairments. Signs of these disorders include hoarseness, harshness, inappropriate pitch, or abnormal nasal resonance. Causes include the closure of vocal cords, hormonal or psychiatric disturbance, or severe hearing loss.

Hypernasality may be a complication of a cleft palate, a deformity in which the two sides of the palate fail to fuse in the midline during in utero development Figure 44-4 ◄ , or it may accompany enlarged adenoids.

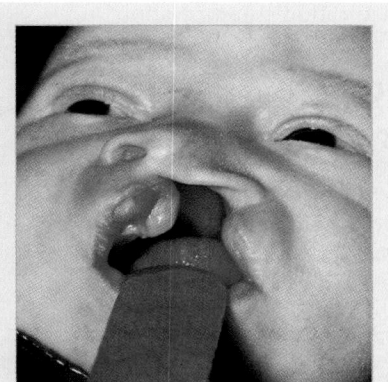

Figure 44-4 Cleft palate.

Inflammation of the larynx may produce laryngitis. Laryngitis is a common occurrence in cases involving overuse of the voice, throat infections, heavy smoking, smoke inhalation, allergic reaction, or exposure to fumes. The cause of the laryngitis may provide clues about the patient's reason for calling for your services and the severity of the situation.

Chronic laryngitis may point to long-term exposure to laryngeal irritants, which may cause polyps to develop in the larynx. Occurring more commonly in men, progressive hoarseness is usually the chief complaint in such cases. Long-term exposure to toxins such as chemicals, smoking, or weakened vocal cords from continuous strain are other risk factors.

The most ominous cause of chronic laryngitis is carcinoma of the larynx. A laryngectomy—either partial or total removal of the larynx—may be performed to battle the cancer. In case of a total laryngectomy, the patient would have *aphonia,* an inability to produce normal speech sounds. The patient would receive a stoma, and might communicate by burping sounds or by using an electronic or mechanical device.

Interaction With a Speech-Impaired Patient

When establishing communication, ask the speech-impaired patient how he or she would be most comfortable communicating with you. Allow an appropriate amount of time for a response, and listen carefully to establish an understanding or enlist someone who knows the patient to interpret. For instance, small children often have speech difficulties that spontaneously resolve, but may be difficult for a stranger to understand. If the patient prefers to speak, your ability to understand the patient will likely be affected.

When working with a patient with a voice production disorder, offer a pencil and paper or listen carefully if the patient prefers to speak. Repeat what the patient said to allow for correction or further clarification. Avoid speaking for the patient or finishing sentences for him or her. And above all, be patient!

Visual Impairments

Visual impairments may result from a multitude of causes—congenital defect, disease, injury, infection (eg, cytomegalovirus), or degeneration of the eyeball, optic nerve, or nerve pathway (eg, with aging). The degree of blindness may range from partial to total. Some patients lose peripheral or central vision; others can distinguish light from dark or discern general shapes.

Visual impairments may be difficult to recognize. During your scene size-up, look for signs that indicate the person is visually impaired, such as the presence of eyeglasses, a white cane, or a service dog. Make yourself known when you enter the room, and introduce yourself and others in the room or have them introduce themselves so that the patient can identify their placement and voice. In addition, retrieve any visual aids to make the interaction more comfortable for your patient Figure 44-5 ▼ .

A visually impaired person may feel vulnerable, especially during the chaos of an accident scene. He or she may have learned to use other senses such as hearing, touch, and smell to compensate for the loss of sight, and the sounds and smells of an accident may be disorienting. Remember to tell the patient what is happening, identify noises, and describe the situation and surroundings, especially if you must move the patient.

In the Field

As with all barriers to communication, remember to document whenever you enlist the help of an interpreter or a person who signs. Also remember that conclusions reached based on the information from interpreters may not be valid.

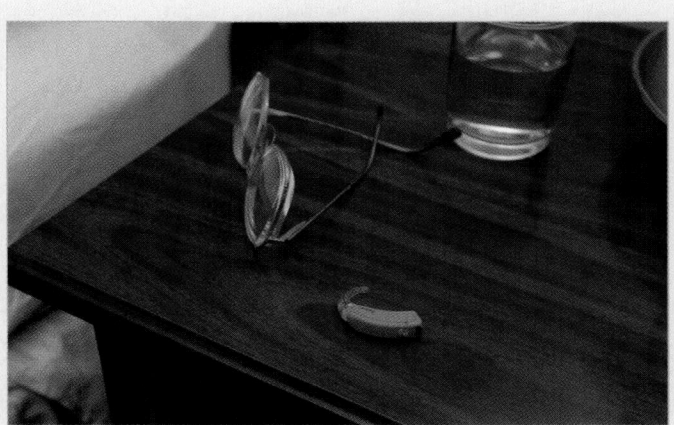

Figure 44-5 Ensuring that a patient with eyeglasses or a hearing aid is using it may reduce the patient's disorientation and stress, and will likely improve your communication with the patient during assessment.

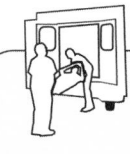

In the Field

Remember that service dogs are "working dogs." Don't allow your crew or bystanders to play with the animal or distract it unless the patient gives permission to do so.

To ambulate safely, the patient may use a cane or walker. Even if the individual will be carried out on your gurney, don't forget to take the patient's cane or walker. Unless the patient is critical, the service dog can remain in the room and will provide reassurance for the patient and prevent delays in transport; however, you may need to make arrangements for the care or accompaniment of the dog. A friend or animal control officer can be helpful in this situation.

An ambulatory patient may be led by a light touch on the arm or elbow. You may also allow the patient to rest his or her hand on your shoulder, as this may enhance the patient's sense of balance and security while moving. You may also ask the patient which method he or she prefers to use while traveling to the ambulance. Patients should be gently guided but never pushed. Obstacles need to be communicated in advance. Statements such as "You're approaching the stairs," and instructions about how many stairs to expect, will allow the patient to anticipate and navigate the obstacles safely. They will also appreciate your consideration and concern.

Paralysis

Paralysis is the inability to voluntarily move one or more body parts. It may be caused by cerebrovascular accidents (CVAs), trauma, or birth defects, among other things. Paralysis does not always entail a loss of sensation, however. In some cases, the patient will have normal sensation or hyperesthesia (increased sensitivity), which may cause the individual to interpret touch as pain in the affected area. Paralysis of one side of the face may cause subsequent communication challenges as well.

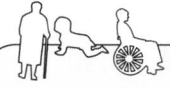

Special Considerations

- Hemiplegia. Paralysis of one side of the body, possibly from CVA or head injury
- Paraplegia. Paralysis of the lower part of the body, possibly from thoracic or lumbar spinal injury or spina bifida
- Quadriplegia. Paralysis of all four extremities and the trunk, possibly from a cervical spine injury

Paralyzed patients may have diaphragmatic involvement requiring the use of a ventilator. They may also rely on specialized equipment such as halo traction, Foley catheters, tracheotomies, colostomies, or feeding tubes. Each spinal cord procedure requires its own equipment and may have its own complications (see Chapter 45).

Dysphagia, caused by a partial paralysis of the esophagus, is the inability to swallow. Patients with dysphagia may choke or aspirate food and drink very easily, leading to the need for emergency airway interventions.

If patients have lost some or all of the sensation in the affected limbs, they cannot tell you when you are hurting them. Always take great care when lifting or moving a paralyzed patient. Because paralyzed limbs lack muscle tone, provide intravenous access and medication administration on the nonaffected side whenever possible. Check intravenous sites frequently for infiltration, especially after medication administration.

Special Considerations

Moving the patient without dislodging or compromising his or her extra equipment takes planning and coordination. You may need to recruit more team members so that you can efficiently move the patient without causing further complication. Strategically placed padding or pillows may also keep the patient more comfortable during transport.

Obesity

Obesity is the result of an imbalance between food eaten and calories used. The solution to the obesity problem may sound relatively simple—reestablish the balance and cure the problem. Unfortunately, obesity can be a much more complex situation. Causes of obesity are not fully understood and, in many cases, are unknown. Oftentimes, this problem may be attributed to low basal metabolic rate or genetic predisposition.

The term obese is used when someone is 20% to 30% over his or her ideal weight. In severe or morbid obesity, the person is 50 to 100 pounds over the ideal weight. Severe obesity afflicts about 9 million adult Americans. These individuals are often ridiculed publicly and sometimes are victims of discrimination. Mobility and the patients' general quality of life are often negatively affected by their oversized status, and the extra weight can cause a myriad of health problems.

Interaction With an Obese Patient

Obese patients may be embarrassed by their condition or fearful of ridicule as a result of past experiences. Some of those negative interactions may have occurred at the hands of an insensitive health care professional. As with any patient, work hard to put these individuals at ease early. Establish the patient's chief complaint and then communicate your plan to help. Many severely obese patients have a complex and extensive past medical history, so mastering the art of conducting a patient interview will serve you well in your interactions with these individuals.

If transport is necessary, plan early for extra help and don't be afraid to call for more help if necessary. In particular, send a member of your team to find the easiest and safest exit. Remember, everyone's safety is at stake! You don't want to risk dropping the patient or injuring a team member by trying to lift too much weight. Moves, no matter how simple they may seem, become far more complex with an oversized patient.

Interaction With a Morbidly Obese Patient

Morbidly obese patients may overcome mobility difficulties by pulling, rocking, or rolling into a position. The constant strain on their body's structures may leave them with chronic joint injuries or osteoarthritis.

Some morbidly obese patients suffer from a condition called obesity hypoventilation syndrome, also known as Pickwickian syndrome. Patients with Pickwickian syndrome are usually *extremely* obese. They experience hypoxemia (deficient oxygenation of the blood), hypercapnia (excess carbon dioxide in the blood), and polycythemia (overabundance or overproduction of red blood cells). Physical findings may include headache, apnea (especially during sleep), sleepiness, red face, muscle twitching, and signs of right-sided heart failure. Some of these symptoms may necessitate emergency intervention in the field.

Weight reduction is the ultimate remedy for Pickwickian syndrome. Some patients may be on a carefully monitored diet; others may benefit from surgical intervention, such as gastric bypass surgery. Surgery carries a high risk of complications, however, and not all patients are suitable candidates.

When you are moving a morbidly obese patient, follow these helpful tips:

- Treat the patient with dignity and respect.
- Ask your patient how best to move him or her before attempting to do so.
- Avoid trying to lift the patient by only one limb, which would risk injury to overtaxed joints.
- Coordinate and communicate all moves to all team members *prior* to starting.
- If the move becomes uncontrolled at any point, stop, reposition, and resume.

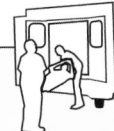

In the Field

When transporting an obese or bariatric patient, be sure to alert the receiving facility in advance if special accommodations, equipment, or other resources may be needed.

- Look for pinch or pressure points from equipment, as they could cause a deep venous thrombosis.
- Very large patients may have difficulty breathing if you lay them flat. Keep this possibility in mind when you position these individuals.
- Many manufacturers now make specialized equipment for morbidly obese patients, and some areas have specially equipped bariatric ambulances for such patients. Become familiar with the resources available in your area.
- Plan egress routes to accommodate for a large patient, equipment, *and* the lifting crew members. Remember: Do no harm!
- Notify the receiving facility early to allow special arrangements to be made prior to your arrival to accommodate the patient's needs.

Mental Challenges

Mental Illness

Mental illness is a generic term for a variety of illnesses that result in emotional, cognitive, or behavioral dysfunction. These

You are the Provider Part 2

You kneel down in front of the young girl, introduce yourself, and ask her name. She tells you that her name is Allison. You note that she has to take a breath after two words. She tells you that she is having a hard time "catching air," points to her bracelet, and starts to cry. You hold her hand and reassure her that you are going to help her feel better very soon. While you are doing this you look at a medical identification bracelet on her right wrist, which reveals that Allison has asthma and is allergic to penicillin. You ask the teacher if she can provide any additional information. She relates that Allison was playing kickball with her classmates when she sat down on the field. One of the aides went over to Allison and found her to be having a hard time breathing. She was brought over to the pavilion and 9-1-1 was called. Allison normally has a rescue inhaler of albuterol (Ventolin), but it was accidentally left at the school. She has no other medical history or drug allergies. She has the emotional and developmental skills of a 4-year-old. A call was placed to her mother who authorized treatment. She will meet you at the hospital.

Vital Signs	Recording Time: 5 Minutes
Level of consciousness	Alert
Pulse	116 beats/min, regular
Blood pressure	106/72 mm Hg
Respirations	28 breaths/min, labored
Skin	Pale, warm, and dry
Sao$_2$	95% on room air

3. What medical conditions are commonly seen in patients with Down syndrome?
4. Why is it important to physically be at the patient's level to speak with her?

conditions include bipolar disorder, depression, schizophrenia, and drug or alcohol abuse. See Chapter 37 for more detail.

Developmental Disabilities

Developmental disability (mental retardation) is insufficient development of the brain resulting in the inability to learn and socially adapt at the usual rate. It may be caused by genetic factors, congenital infections, complications at birth, malnutrition, or environmental factors. Prenatal drug or alcohol use may also cause disability, as in fetal alcohol syndrome. Postnatal causes may include traumatic brain injury or poisoning (eg, with lead or other toxins).

Although IQ testing can identify the extent of the person's ability to learn and reason, just speaking to the patient and family members will give you a good idea of how well the patient can understand you and interact. A person with a slight impairment may appear slow to understand or have a limited vocabulary. Such an individual will often act "immature" in comparison to "normal" peers. Because the individual may also have difficulty adjusting to change or a break in routine, an emergency call that generates a roomful of strangers can be overwhelming. The patient may become more difficult to interact with as his or her anxiety level increases. A severely disabled person may not have the ability to care for himself or herself, communicate, understand, or respond to the surroundings.

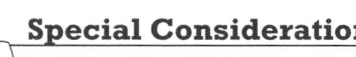

Special Considerations

Mild retardation: IQ = 52–68
Moderate retardation: IQ = 36–51
Severe retardation: IQ = 20–35
Profound retardation: IQ ≤ 19

Treatment of these patients should be based on the complaint unless the illness is related to the mental disability. Patients with developmental disabilities are prone to the same disease processes as any other patients, including diabetes, heart attacks, and respiratory difficulties. Transport should be accomplished without causing any more stress than necessary. In most cases, supportive care is all that is needed.

Down Syndrome

Down syndrome is characterized by a genetic chromosomal defect that can occur during fetal development, resulting in mild to severe mental retardation **Figure 44-6 ▶**. The normal human somatic cell contains 23 chromosomes. Down syndrome, which is also known as trisomy 21, occurs when chromosome 21 fails to separate, so that the ovum contains 24 chromosomes. When the ovum is fertilized by a normal sperm with 23 chromosomes, a triplication ("trisomy") of chromosome 21 occurs.

Increased maternal age (more than 35 years old) and a family history of Down syndrome are known risk factors for this condition. A variety of abnormalities are associated with Down syndrome: a round head with a flat occiput; an enlarged,

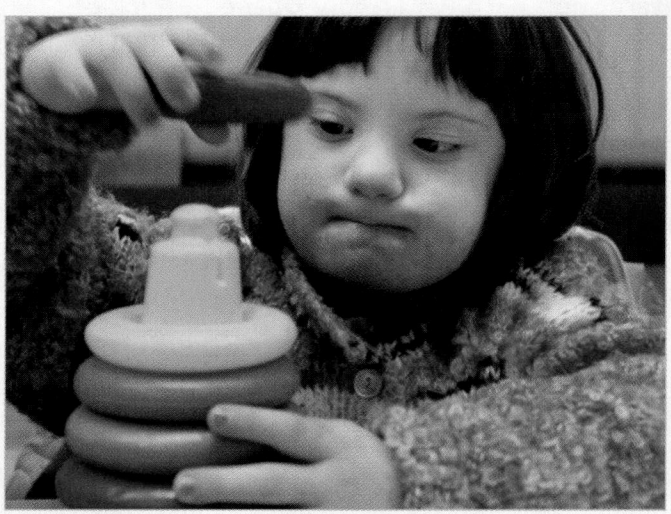

Figure 44-6 A child with Down syndrome.

protruding tongue; slanted, wide-set eyes and folded skin on either side of the nose, covering the inner corners of the eye; short, wide hands; a small face and features; congenital heart defects; thyroid problems; and hearing and vision problems. Patients do not usually have all of these symptoms, but will have a combination of them to such a degree that the diagnosis is rapidly made at birth.

Patients with Down syndrome are at increased risk for medical complications, including those that affect the cardiovascular, sensory, endocrine, orthopaedic, dental, gastrointestinal, neurologic development, and hematologic systems. As many as 40% may suffer from heart conditions and hearing and vision problems. In particular, two thirds of children born with Down syndrome have congenital heart disease (eg, endocardial cushion defects, or ventricular or atrial septal defects). Emergency treatment should therefore include airway management, supplemental oxygen, and IV access. In patients with heart failure, administer diuretics with judicious fluid resuscitation only if necessary.

Because people with Down syndrome often have large tongues and small oral and nasal cavities, intubation of these patients may be difficult. These individuals may also have malocclusions and other dental anomalies (eg, abnormal contact of the upper and lower teeth). The enlarged tongue and dental anomalies can lead to speech abnormalities as well. In an emergency situation, if airway management is necessary, mask ventilation and intubation can be challenging. In the case of airway obstruction, a simple jaw-thrust maneuver may be all that is needed to clear the airway. In an unconscious patient, either the jaw-thrust maneuver or a nasopharyngeal airway may be necessary.

Many people with Down syndrome have epilepsy. Most of the seizures are of the tonic-clonic type. Management is the same as with other patients with seizures.

Interaction With a Mentally Impaired Patient

When caring for a mentally impaired patient, obtain a complete history, treat the presenting illness, and provide supportive care. It is normal to feel somewhat uncomfortable when initiating contact with a mentally impaired patient, especially if you've encountered such situations infrequently. Simply treating the patient as you would anyone else is the best plan.

Approach the mentally impaired patient in a calm and friendly manner, watching him or her for signs of increased anxiety or fear. Remember, you are a "stranger" and are approaching with a group of people. The patient may not understand your uniform or realize that you and your crew are there to help. It may be helpful to have the members of your team hold back slightly until you can establish a rapport with the patient. You can then introduce the team members and explain what they are going to do. This method will slowly bring forward the other providers, instead of "mobbing" the patient all at once.

You might interact with a patient as follows: "Hello Mr. Pemberton. My name is Jerry Booker." (Shake Mr. Pemberton's hand if he will allow it.) "We're here to help you. Your sister called us. She says you're not feeling well today, and we're here to help you feel better. My friend Tim is going to take your blood pressure. Do you remember having that done before?" (Allow Mr. Pemberton to see and touch the blood pressure cuff as Tim moves forward. Move slowly but deliberately, explaining beforehand what you are going to do, just like you would with any other patient. Watch carefully for signs of fear or reluctance from the patient.)

Do your best to soothe the patient's anxiety and/or discomfort as you work through your assessment and treatment. By initially establishing trust and communication, you'll have much better luck successfully executing your treatment plan, even if you eventually need to do something painful such as starting an IV.

Emotional/Mental Impairment

In the Victorian era, an emotional stress condition associated with chronic fatigue, anxiety, depression, sleep disturbances, headache, and sexual dysfunction might be lumped into the category known as *neurasthenia*—in modern terms, a "nervous breakdown." Today, physicians diagnose specific disorders such as anxiety, neurosis, compulsion, or hysteria.

Mental illness can occur in persons with mental or emotional disability just as it can arise in normal people. (The care of mentally ill patients is discussed in depth in Chapter 37.) In the broader sense, a person's mental status can influence his or her physical well-being, and vice versa. Emotionally or mentally impaired individuals may be difficult to assess due to the body's normal stress response, which may alter their respiratory rate, heart rate, or perception of physical illness. Gathering a detailed history will be useful in the assessment and development of a treatment plan for these patients. Calmly ascertain the chief complaint and treat the patient accordingly, with care and understanding.

One of the key components of effective communication—with any type of patient—is to be a good listener. Always "listen" carefully to your patient—not just the words spoken, but also heeding the patient's tone, facial expressions, and body language. Watch for signs of aggression, clenched fists, or aggressive agitated movements or speech; they may be your only warning of an impending dangerous confrontation. Implementing active listening skills by repeating what you heard will reassure the patient that you understand and are there to help.

You are the Provider Part 3

Your partner prepares a nebulizer containing 2.5 mg of albuterol and 3 mL of normal saline and you begin your assessment, taking care to let your patient know everything that you are doing. Your physical exam is significant for diminished air movement bilaterally with faint expiratory wheezes. You ask your partner to prepare an IV and the cardiac monitor. You load the patient onto the stretcher and into the truck to continue your treatment prior to leaving for the hospital.

In the back of the truck you give the patient a teddy bear and tell her how brave she is being. She responds with a weak smile. A 20-gauge IV is started in the left antecubital and an infusion of normal saline is started. As the ambulance departs you refill the nebulizer with 2.5 mg of albuterol and 0.5 mg of ipratropium (Atrovent) inhalation solution.

Reassessment	Recording Time: 12 Minutes
Skin	Pale, warm, and dry
Pulse	120 beats/min, regular
Blood pressure	110/72 mm Hg
Respirations	28 breaths/min, labored
Sao$_2$	98% on nebulizer treatment
ECG	Sinus tachycardia with no ectopy
Pupils	Reactive to light

5. What anatomic features of Down syndrome can make airway management challenging?

Although mentally ill patients may present an assessment challenge, they are still patients and are prone to the same illnesses and disease processes as anyone else. Consequently, treatment and transport of such patients should focus on the chief complaint and supportive care.

When treating patients with emotional/mental impairment, take care in establishing communication with the patient and/or the caregiver. Establish a baseline for the patient's emotional/mental ability so that you will be able to identify any changes. Speak in a calm voice, even if the patient does not have the ability to understand, and explain what you're going to do before doing it.

Pathologic Challenges

Pathologic challenges require special consideration when you formulate your treatment plan. Pathologies you may encounter during your career may include arthritis, cancer, cerebral palsy, cystic fibrosis, multiple sclerosis, muscular dystrophy, poliomyelitis, previous head injury, spina bifida, and myasthenia gravis. Many of these patients will be well versed in the progression, treatment, and unique nuances of their current health status.

Cancer

Simply stated, cancer is the uncontrolled overgrowth of normal tissue cells. If this growth is left unchecked, these cells have the ability to spread, destroy body systems, and kill. More than 200 different kinds of cancer are believed to exist; the type is determined by where the cancer originates. (Cancer is discussed in greater detail in Chapters 6 and 45.)

Numerous types of treatment regimens are available for cancer—surgery, medications, radiation, and chemotherapy, to name a few. Cancer treatment may follow a single pathway, or be orchestrated into a complex combination of therapies and medications. Surgical removal has long been one of the primary methods of controlling or terminating cancer's progression; it is often used in tandem with other therapies.

Arthritis

Arthritis is a joint inflammation that causes pain, swelling, stiffness, and decreased range of motion, all of which leave patients more vulnerable to falls. Many types of arthritis are distinguished, with symptoms ranging from mild to debilitating. For example, osteoarthritis is a degenerative joint disease associated with aging (Figure 44-7 ▶). It initially targets the joints of the lower extremities. The pain of osteoarthritis usually grows throughout the day, with stiffness increasing following prolonged rest. In contrast, rheumatoid arthritis is an autoimmune disorder that causes inflammation and destruction of the joints and connective tissues. Some patients may experience periods of remission while others may have rapid progression of the disease.

Be sure to ask the patient with arthritis about his or her current medications before administering additional ones. Take

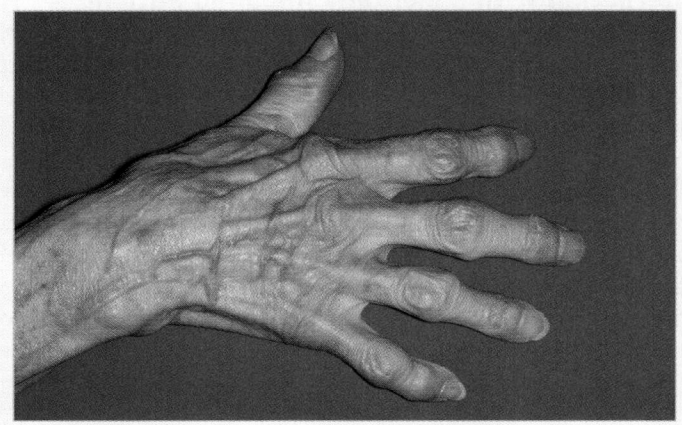

Figure 44-7 Osteoarthritis may cause substantial disfigurement.

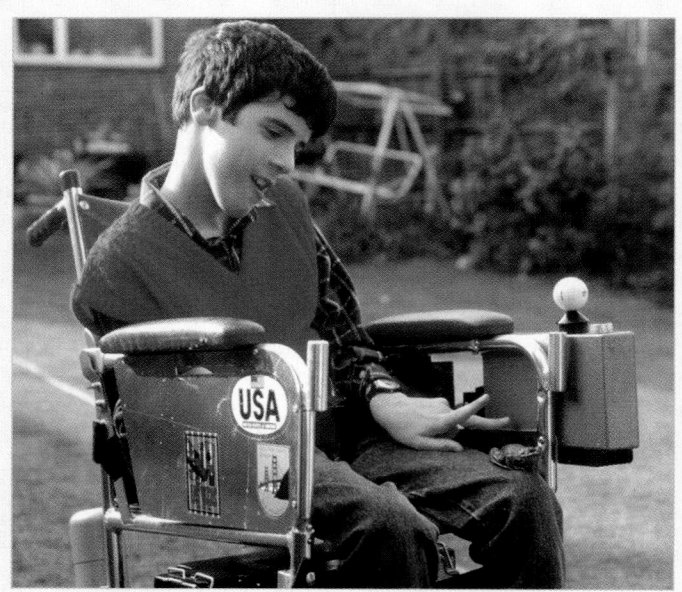

Figure 44-8 A person with cerebral palsy.

special care when moving such a patient so as to incur the least amount of discomfort. Make sure the patient is as comfortable as possible and remember to use equipment that fits the patient properly.

Cerebral Palsy

Cerebral palsy is a nonprogressive, bilateral neuromuscular disorder in which voluntary muscles are poorly controlled. It results from developmental brain defects in utero (eg, cerebral hypoxia, maternal infection, or kernicterus), brain trauma at birth or in early childhood, or postpartum infections (eg, encephalitis or meningitis). Patients often have spastic movements of their limbs and display poor posture (Figure 44-8 ▲), which impairs their ability to move in a controlled manner.

Symptoms of cerebral palsy can range from mild to severe. As children grow, these symptoms may either become exaggerated or stay the same. Related complications include visual impairments, hearing and language difficulties, seizures, and mental retardation.

Some children with severe cases of cerebral palsy are able to learn to walk with assistive devices, whereas others need support even to sit and cannot stand, walk, or speak. If the patient is able to speak, grimacing and uncontrolled movement may make speech difficult and hard to understand. To cope with ordinary tasks, many patients use computerized household controls and speaking aids. Mechanized wheelchairs may be controlled with a joystick or mouth control. Specially shaped chairs and pillows may be custom-built to facilitate the patient's comfort and ease movement. Toys may also be adapted to allow for learning and play. In addition, computers may be specially configured to aid the patient with speech simulation and provide the ability to perform household tasks, such as temperature control and lighting. Thanks to these technologies, many patients with cerebral palsy lead near-normal lives and live independently.

When caring for a patient with cerebral palsy, note the following:

- Do not assume that patients with cerebral palsy are always mentally disabled. Although 75% of patients have some mental retardation, many people with cerebral palsy have a normal IQ or only slight mental impairment.
- Patients' limbs are often underdeveloped and are prone to injury (eg, from a fall from a wheelchair).
- Patients who have the ability to walk may have an ataxic or unsteady gait and are prone to falls.
- If the patient has a specially made pillow or chair (pediatric patients), the patient may prefer to use it during transport. Remember to pad the patient to ensure his or her comfort, and never force a patient's extremities into any position.
- Whenever possible, take walkers or wheelchairs along during transport.
- Approximately 25% of patients with cerebral palsy also have seizures. Be prepared to care for a seizure if one occurs, and keep suctioning available.

Cystic Fibrosis

Cystic fibrosis (mucoviscidosis) is a chronic dysfunction of the endocrine system that targets multiple body systems, but primarily the respiratory and digestive systems. This inherited disease affects approximately 30,000 Americans. Although it is found in all races and ethnic groups, it most commonly occurs in Caucasian individuals of Northern European descent. The disease is usually fatal, with most children not living past their teens; with aggressive management and careful monitoring, however, some patients may live well into their thirties.

Cystic fibrosis is caused by a defective gene, which makes it difficult for chloride to move through cells. This causes unusually high sodium loss (resulting in salty skin) and abnormally thick mucus secretions. The secretions in the lungs cause breathing difficulties and provide an ideal growing medium for bacteria, leaving the patient highly susceptible to infection. Ultimately, the lung damage from the condition leads to lung disease, which is the primary cause of death in affected individuals.

Respiratory difficulties associated with cystic fibrosis include tachypnea, productive cough, shortness of breath, barrel chest, clubbed fingers, and cyanosis. The thick mucus may also collect in the intestines. Malnutrition and poor growth rate are not uncommon symptoms, as are intestinal blockages. Physicians strive to reduce the progression of the disease with physical therapy, exercise, vitamin supplements, and medications. Some patients may also benefit from a lung transplant.

Care of these patients should primarily focus on treating the individual's chief complaint. Keep a keen eye out for respiratory insufficiency, signs of a respiratory infection, intestinal blockage, or cardiac dysrhythmias (as a result of the electrolyte imbalance). Suctioning, high-flow supplemental oxygen, and breathing therapies may also be required during transport.

Multiple Sclerosis

Multiple sclerosis is a chronic disease of the central nervous system characterized by destruction of the myelin and nerve axons within the brain and spinal cord. It has no known cause, but is an autoimmune disorder or in some cases is genetically inherited. This disease strikes women in their 20s to 40s two to three times more often than men. Approximately 400,000 Americans have multiple sclerosis, some with serious handicaps.

Myelin is a fatty covering that shields the axons; axons are responsible for electrical conduction from neurons to muscles, leading to muscle response and communication from the body to the brain. Multiple sclerosis causes areas of myelin in random places to become inflamed, detach from the axon, and ultimately self-destruct. The area of destruction becomes scarred over—hence the name multiple (*many*) sclerosis (*to harden*) **Figure 44-9 ▶** .

Two types of multiple sclerosis are distinguished: relapsing/remitting and progressive. The relapsing/remitting form, which affects 90% of patients, presents with bouts of worsening symptoms. Signs and symptoms of multiple sclerosis can be divided into those associated with the brain and those associated with the spinal cord **Table 44-1 ▶** and include numbness or tingling in parts of the body, unexplained weakness, dizziness, fatigue, double or blurry vision, and vision impairment. Periods of relapse leave the patient feeling marked improvement, with stiffness and weakness lingering for some. The other 10% of patients have the progressive form, in which symptoms get progressively worse with no periods of improvement or relief. Half of all people who have the relapsing/remitting form of the disease will develop the progressive form within 15 years if they remain untreated.

There is no cure for multiple sclerosis, although many treatments can significantly reduce the frequency of attacks and lessen symptoms when they occur. As with other illnesses, your treatment may be limited to supportive care. You may also be called to the patient's side due to tertiary complications

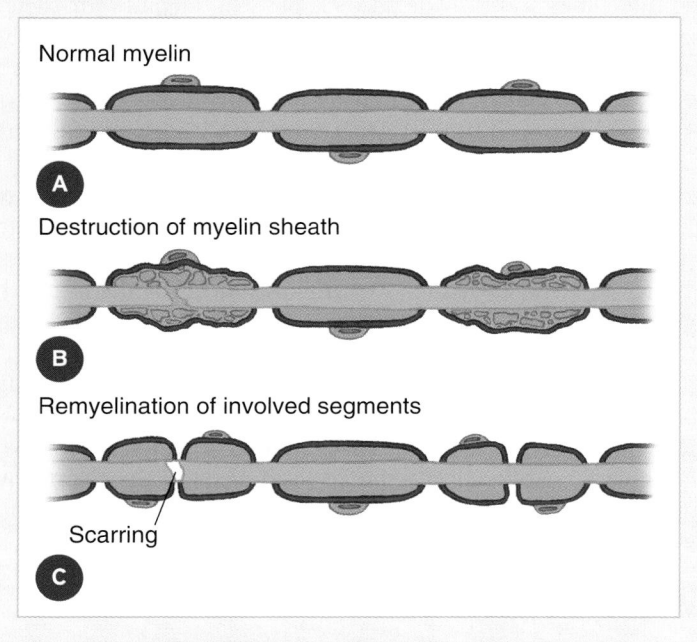

Figure 44-9 Progression of multiple sclerosis. **A.** Normal myelin. **B.** Destruction of myelin sheath. **C.** Scarring.

Normal myelin

A

Destruction of myelin sheath

B

Remyelination of involved segments

Scarring

C

Table 44-1	Signs and Symptoms of Multiple Sclerosis	
Brain-Affected	**Spinal Cord-Affected**	
■ Slurred speech	■ Stiffness	
■ Confusion	■ Muscle spasms	
■ Forgetfulness	■ Bowel and bladder problems	
■ Pain	■ Sexual dysfunction	
■ Depression	■ Paralysis	
	■ Numbness	
	■ Muscle weakness	

of multiple sclerosis, such as a fall. Because of the disease process, the patient may lack feeling, so the physical examination may be difficult. A detailed medical history will help elucidate the diagnosis.

As with paralyzed patients, you must take special care when lifting and moving patients with multiple sclerosis. When these individuals are in crisis, they may not be able to walk even with their assistive devices.

Muscular Dystrophy

Muscular dystrophy is an inherited muscular disease that causes degeneration of the muscle fibers. In many cases, the destroyed fibers are replaced by fat or connective tissue. The result is a gradual weakening of muscles, slowing of motor development, and loss of muscle contractility. More than 30 types of muscular dystrophy have been identified. Some strike in early childhood and progress rapidly. Others don't strike until the late teens into the forties and progress much

more slowly. Duchenne muscular dystrophy, the most common type, chiefly affects boys (1 of every 3,500 male births).

Muscular dystrophy may not be apparent in infancy, but rather appears as the child grows, presenting as muscle weakness during childhood or early adulthood. Parents or physicians may notice a delay in the normal developmental landmarks such as sitting, walking, or climbing stairs. The wasting of skeletal muscles ultimately leads to increasing disability and deformity. Kyphoscoliosis—an outward hump of the upper spine accompanied by curvature of the lower spine—may compromise pulmonary function. Cardiac involvement may also be present in as many as 95% of patients. Unfortunately, only 25% of those affected live to age 21 years, with pulmonary or cardiac complications usually being the cause of death.

Poliomyelitis

Poliomyelitis (commonly known as polio) is a highly contagious viral infection. First identified in 1789, it was once a worldwide plague, with its incidence growing to epidemic proportions from late spring through fall. In the United States, documented cases once ranged from 13,000 to 21,000 cases each year. Following the release of the Salk and Sabin polio vaccines in 1955, the number of cases of polio declined rapidly and the disease is now rare in the United States. Most cases involve vaccine-associated paralytic polio (VAPP), which is caused by contact between an unvaccinated individual and a person who has recently been inoculated with the live vaccine. Although live vaccines have not been used in the United States since 2000, they are still administered in many other parts of the world. Thanks to worldwide vaccination programs, it is anticipated that polio will be completely eradicated within the next decade.

Humans are the only known hosts for the poliomyelitis virus. This pathogen enters the body by direct contact through the mouth, replicating in the pharynx, gastrointestinal system, and local lymphatic system. The virus then enters the bloodstream and spreads to the central nervous system. The spinal cord and brain are affected, which may cause paralysis or death.

In 80% to 90% of cases (usually involving young children), the illness is mild, presenting with malaise, sore throat, headache, vomiting, and slight fever. The initial symptoms are followed by a period of apparent wellness. Symptoms of major illness—fever, severe headache, stiff neck and back, deep muscle pain, or paralysis—then appear after a few days. In nonparalytic forms of polio, recovery is complete. In paralytic forms, muscle function returns gradually and completely. Any weakness or paralysis lasting longer than 12 months after the infection is a sign of permanent damage and disability.

Patients with paralysis will need special attention in order to safely lift, move, and position them. They may also need special equipment such as ventilatory assistance via an endotracheal tube or tracheotomy if they experience respiratory paralysis. They also may have an indwelling catheter in place if the lower extremities are paralyzed.

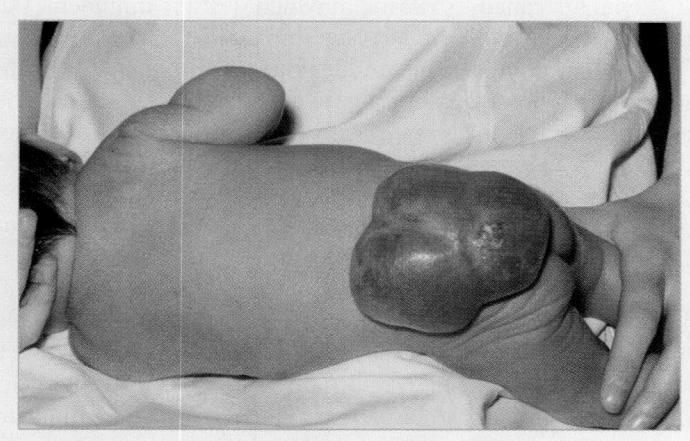

Figure 44-10 Spina bifida is characterized by exposure of part of the spinal cord.

Spina Bifida

Spina bifida is the most common permanently disabling birth defect. It affects approximately 70,000 people in the United States, or 7 of every 10,000 births. In this disorder, during the first month of pregnancy, the fetus's spinal column does not close properly or completely and vertebrae do not develop, leaving a portion of the spinal cord exposed Figure 44-10 ▲. Faithfully taking the B vitamin folic acid prior to becoming pregnant reduces the risk of spinal defects. Other maternal risk factors for spina bifida include previous neural tube defect pregnancy (increases risk by 20%), diabetes, medically diagnosed obesity, some antiseizure medications, exposure to increased temperature in early pregnancy (ie, hot baths or hot tubs, infection resulting in fever), Caucasian or Hispanic ethnicity, and lower socioeconomic status.

Symptoms of spina bifida may include partial or full paralysis (usually of the lower extremities), bladder or bowel control difficulties, learning disabilities, and latex allergy. In addition, as many as 70% to 90% of individuals with the most severe form of spina bifida also have hydrocephalus. In hydrocephalus, an increase in the amount of cerebral spinal fluid results in increased pressure on the brain. A shunt is inserted to relieve this pressure on the brain by draining excess cerebral spinal fluid; the shunt will stay in place throughout the patient's lifetime.

Spina bifida patients will likely benefit from the same considerations that you offer when treating a patient with paralysis or difficulty moving. When you are caring for these patients, ask how best to move them if possible. Remember to rule out a fall or other event that may have caused an injury. Check carefully for injuries, as patients may not be able to feel them—or the pain of an infiltrated IV, for that matter. Also, be aware that these patients may have urinary catheters or other aids in place.

Patients With Previous Head Injuries

Patients who previously experienced head injuries may be difficult to assess and treat. Brain-injured patients may face a complex array of challenges related to their injury. In such cases, gathering a complete medical history from the patient, family, and friends will assist you in the formation of a treatment plan. (Treatment will be primarily supportive care.) Your interaction with the patient will need to be tailored to his or her specific abilities. Take the time to speak with the patient and the family to establish what is normal for the patient—for example, whether the patient has cognitive, sensory, communication, motor, behavioral, or psychological deficits.

When you are caring for a patient with a previous head injury, talk to him or her in a calm and soothing tone, and watch the patient closely for signs of anxiety or aggression. In some cases, the patient may need to be specially positioned or restrained to ensure the safety of both you and the patient. Do not expect such an individual to walk to the ambulance or stretcher. As always, treat the patient with respect, use his or her name, explain procedures, and reassure the patient throughout your care.

Myasthenia Gravis

Myasthenia gravis is an abnormal condition characterized by chronic fatigability and weakness of muscles, especially in the face and throat. It is the result of a defect in the conduction of nerve impulses at the nerve junction, caused by a lack of acetylcholine. In myasthenia gravis, antibodies keep acetylcholine from reaching the muscles by blocking or damaging the receptor sites. This interruption in communication results in sudden bouts of muscle weakness, usually during activity, although the condition improves with rest. Although it affects all ethnic groups and sexes, myasthenia gravis is most commonly found in women younger than age 40 and men older than age 60.

The first symptoms usually present as weakness in eye or eyelid movement. Myasthenia gravis may also affect facial muscle control, changing the person's facial expression. In many cases, the disease is noticed initially as a sudden difficulty swallowing or chewing, or as slurred speech. Other symptoms may include blurry vision, weakness or difficulty moving the neck, shortness of breath, and weakness or difficulty moving limbs. Myasthenia gravis may be difficult to diagnosis because these symptoms can be attributed to many illnesses and disease processes.

A crisis may occur if the patient's respiratory muscles are damaged by infection, stress, or side effects of medications. These muscles could become so weak that the patient suffers an acute onset of respiratory failure. In such a case, you need to intervene immediately with airway management, ventilatory support, and possibly intubation.

▌Terminally Ill Patients

Unfortunately, some illnesses cannot be cured. As health care providers, you and your team will often be called upon to assist a patient who is facing imminent death, or terminal illness

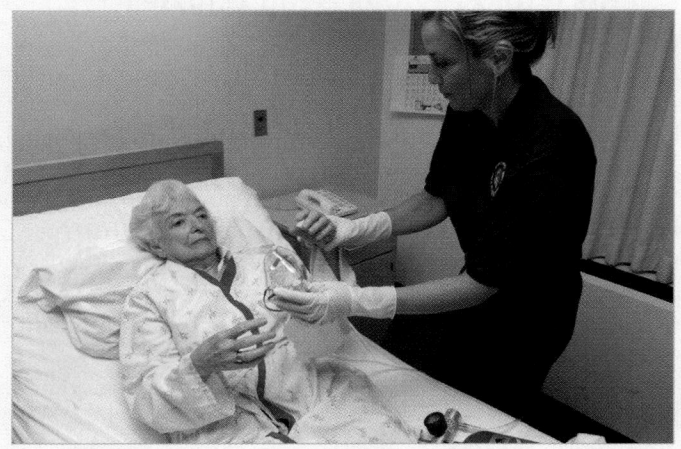

Figure 44-11 You will sometimes encounter patients with a terminal illness.

Figure 44-11 ▲ . Signs of impending death include decreased intake of food and drink, decreased orientation, irregular breathing patterns, and bradycardia or tachycardia. If you recognize these signs, you should help to reassure the family.

Although the goal of end-of-life care is to provide patients with a meaningful, dignified, and comfortable death, there is a surprising lack of data describing what patients and their families believe constitutes a "good death." While some patients with terminal illness choose to have the most aggressive care possible, others have a goal of comfort rather than cure or prolongation of life. In general, seriously ill patients identify pain and symptom management, preparation for death, and achieving a sense of completion as important factors in a good death.

If you are called to a scene in which death is imminent, the actions you take will have a lasting impact on the family. This is a time when compassion, understanding, and sensitivity are most needed. Some scenes may be chaotic. The family may be having a difficult time coping with the situation, and they may act out with anger and hostility. Treat everyone with compassion and understanding. The other members of your team may be able to separate individuals and speak with them individually to diffuse intense emotions and restore order to the situation.

Terminally ill patients usually need only supportive care. Therapy is usually aimed at making the patient as comfortable as possible. The individual may have a displaced urinary catheter, need assistance in returning to bed, or need intervention in a pain crisis. Some patients may also be receiving care from hospice or a home health nurse. You may have been called because of a delay in the arrival of the regular care provider or for transport to take care of an immediate need in a clinical setting. Because terminally ill patients may use a complex array of pain medications, transdermal patches, or self-administered pain management devices, you may need to consult medical direction for guidance in their care.

If the patient has a valid do not resuscitate (DNR) order, CPR is not indicated or appropriate if the patient's heart stops and/or he or she stops breathing. If you have any question regarding the validity of a DNR or the level of interventions the patient wants, you should start resuscitation while contacting medical control for further instructions. When no resuscitative measures are attempted, aggressive comfort measures are required, for example, oxygen administration, albuterol-based breathing treatments, and morphine as needed for pain and respiratory distress per local protocol. Place the patient in a comfortable position. Although the decision for a DNR order had already been made, family members may not understand

You are the Provider Part 4

En route to the hospital you contact the receiving emergency department for orders. You explain your patient's condition and her failure to improve. Your estimated time of arrival is approximately 20 minutes. The emergency department physician asks you to administer another nebulizer treatment of 2.5 mg of albuterol and 3 mL of normal saline, and a 70-mg prednisone (Solumedrol) IV.

Upon your arrival to the emergency department you are met by Allison's mother, who is anxious to be with her daughter. A respiratory therapist is waiting at the patient's bedside to begin a continuous breathing treatment with albuterol and Atrovent. The patient is admitted into pediatric intensive care for observation and possible intubation.

Reassessment	Recording Time: 17 Minutes
Skin	Pale, warm, and dry
Pulse	120 beats/min, strong and regular
Blood pressure	114/70 mm Hg
Respirations	24 breaths/min, labored
Breath sounds	Diminshed bilaterally with faint expiratory wheezes
Sao$_2$	99% on nebulizer treatment
ECG	Sinus tachycardia without ectopy

6. Are patients with Down syndrome capable of taking an active role in their care?

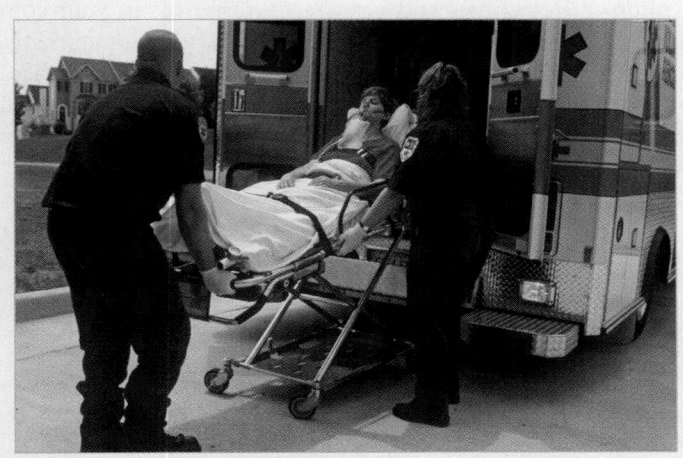

Figure 44-12 Some families may call for transport of a patient with a terminal illness.

what to do, and they may not be ready to face the death of a loved one. In such a case, take a thorough history and compassionately discuss the patient's wishes. Ask to review the DNR and keep it with the patient during transport.

Ascertain the family's wishes about having the patient remain in the home versus transport to the hospital **Figure 44-12 ▲**. During transport, contact medical control and advise the receiving hospital of the situation. If a family member requests to accompany the patient, he or she should

👥 Controversies

On some occasions, the family may disagree with the DNR but the patient is unable to speak for himself or herself. The patient's wishes should be respected with regard to resuscitation when those wishes are clear and no reasonable doubt exists with regard to those specific wishes. If a family wants CPR started, but a DNR order states otherwise, make certain that the family is aware of the existence of the DNR order. Once aware, if they maintain their desire to initiate resuscitative efforts, you should do so.

When the family indicates a desire to start CPR in the face of a DNR order, reasonable doubt about the validity of that order is present. In such a situation, you simply cannot be certain whether the patient or another relative with medical authority for the patient initiated the DNR order or whether an individual with legal authority to make medical decisions for the patient is present. Sorting out those issues is best left for the physicians in the emergency department where more information can be obtained and more thorough discussions with the family about the gravity of the medical condition are possible.

You should thoroughly understand your local or state laws and protocols with regard to DNR orders and carefully consider how you would handle difficult situations with regard to DNR controversies before you face them.

be allowed to do so. If the family wishes the patient to remain at home, this request should be honored provided it is in accordance with your local or state protocol.

Local protocols for handling the death of a patient vary, so you must learn your local or state regulations. Your protocol will identify whether the coroner needs be to called to report the death and, if so, who is responsible for contacting the coroner. Also determine whether a pronouncement of death is required and, if so, who makes it.

▌Patients With Communicable Diseases

Some patients may have communicable diseases, which explains why appropriate BSI procedures need to be followed with every patient, every time **Figure 44-13 ▾**. Gloves and eye protection should be considered basic attire. Gowns, masks, and other protective measures should be deployed if the situation warrants. Safety for yourself, your crew, and your patient is paramount. At the same time, you should treat patients with communicable diseases with the same compassion you would give to any other patient.

Clues that a patient has a communicable disease include rashes, coughing, ill appearance, health history, and medications. Offer

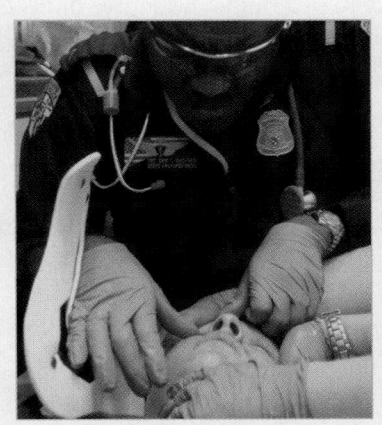

Figure 44-13 Always wear gloves and eye protection as a bare minimum.

AIDS patients or other immunocompromised individuals a mask prior to their arrival at a hospital to safeguard them from further exposure to illness. Masking a patient early during your assessment may be the quickest and easiest method of preventing disease transmission (see Chapters 2 and 36 for more details).

▌Culturally Diverse Patients

As discussed in Chapter 10, acceptance of and awareness of the cultural backgrounds and customs of others will allow you to be a more effective paramedic and a valuable member of your community. Chapter 10 also discusses how to recognize a culturally diverse patient. Cultural diversity requires respect for all cultures, languages, and communities. In many areas, particularly large urban centers, major segments of the population do not speak English. Your job will be much easier if you learn some common words and phrases (especially medical terms) in their language.

As part of the focused history and physical exam, you must obtain a medical history. You cannot skip this step simply because the patient doesn't speak English. Most patients who don't speak English fluently will still know important words or phrases. First, find out how much English the patient can speak. Then, use short, simple questions and simple words whenever possible. Avoid difficult medical terms, and point to specific parts of the body as you ask questions.

Financial Challenges

"I can't go to the hospital. I don't have the money!" These statements are heard from many patients. Many of these individuals do not have health insurance, or are worried about the mounting bills generated by a chronic illness. By engaging in careful, compassionate communication with your patient, you should try to determine the source of his or her anxiety. Share with the patient your concerns about his or her current health Figure 44-14 ▶ .

Fears about payment should not keep any patient from seeking help. Federal laws allow patients to be seen and evaluated regardless of their ability to pay. Indeed, many hospitals have a mechanism for providing free treatment or reduced rates for indigent individuals, and the facility will always be willing to work out a payment plan. You should research the

location of free clinics and health care resources in your community for those patients who may benefit from an alternative in a nonemergency situation. Consult with your medical director to see if your service is allowed to transport to these facilities. Remember—no patient should be refused transport to an emergency care facility based on his or her ability to pay.

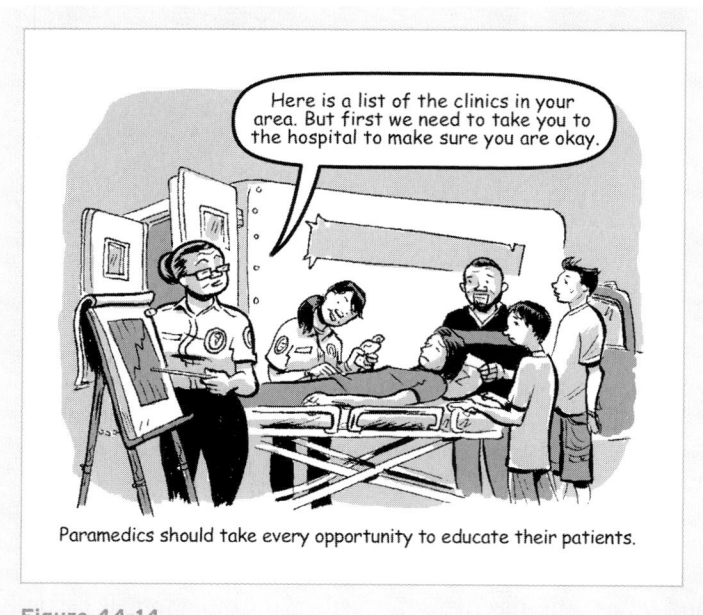

Paramedics should take every opportunity to educate their patients.

Figure 44-14

You are the Provider Summary

1. What is Down syndrome?

Down syndrome, also known as trisomy 21, is a congenital abnormality that occurs from a failure of the number 21 chromosome to divide properly during the first stage of sperm or egg cell development. As a consequence, there are three number 21 chromosomes instead of the normal pair. This extra chromosome is then passed onto the fetus and causes the abnormality.

2. What are the characteristic physical features of Down syndrome?

Classic physical features of Down syndrome include:

- Eyes that slope upward at the outer corners
- Folds of skin on either side of the nose that cover the inside corners of the eyes
- A small face and small facial features
- A large protruding tongue
- Flattening of the back of the head
- Short and broad hands

3. What medical conditions are commonly seen in patients with Down syndrome?

Children with Down syndrome may also have congenital heart defects, intestinal disorders, epilepsy, and hearing defects. They also have an increased risk of having respiratory infections.

4. Why is it important to physically be at the patient's level to speak with her?

How would you feel if you couldn't breathe, were scared, and were approached by a stranger carrying strange machines? Remember with any child it is important to make contact at eye level so you can earn his or her trust.

5. What anatomic features of Down syndrome can make airway management challenging?

Keep in mind that individuals with Down syndrome have smaller faces and facial features, a large protruding tongue, and a flattened back portion of the head. These differences may make the use of airway adjuncts a bit tricky. Be prepared to use smaller size equipment than normal, provide padding under the head, and be patient when airway management is required.

6. Are patients with Down syndrome capable of taking an active role in their care?

Many individuals with Down syndrome are capable of being functional members of society. Others may only need the assistance provided by a group home or assisted-living facility. These people would be able to take an active role in their health care and assist you in the case of an emergency.

Prep Kit

Ready for Review

- In the field, you will encounter patients who face a variety of special challenges.
- Humans use all five senses to gather information, but we often take that sensory feedback for granted.
- Mental illness is a generic term for a variety of illnesses that result in emotional, cognitive, or behavioral dysfunction.
- Developmental disability (mental retardation) is insufficient development of the brain, resulting in the inability to learn and socially adapt at the usual rate.
- Pathologic challenges require special consideration when you formulate your treatment plan. Pathologies you may encounter during your career may include arthritis, cancer, cerebral palsy, cystic fibrosis, multiple sclerosis, muscular dystrophy, poliomyelitis, previous head injury, spina bifida, and myasthenia gravis.
- Unfortunately, some illnesses cannot be cured. As health care providers, you and your team will often be called upon to assist a patient who is facing imminent death from terminal illness.
- Some patients may have communicable diseases, which explains why appropriate BSI procedures need to be followed with every patient, every time.
- Fears about payment for emergency medical services should not keep any patient from seeking help. By engaging in careful, compassionate communication with your patient, you should try to determine the source of his or her anxiety. Share with the patient your concerns about his or her current health.

Vital Vocabulary

aphasia The loss of the ability to communicate in speech, writing, or signs.

arthritis Joint inflammation that causes pain, swelling, stiffness, and decreased range of motion.

cerebral palsy A nonprogressive bilateral neuromuscular disorder in which voluntary muscles are poorly controlled.

conductive deafness A curable temporary condition, caused by an injury to the eardrum.

cystic fibrosis Chronic dysfunction of the endocrine system that affects multiple body systems, primarily the respiratory and digestive systems.

developmental disability Insufficient development of the brain, resulting in some level of dysfunction or impairment.

Down syndrome A genetic chromosomal defect that can occur during fetal development and that results in mental retardation as well as certain physical characteristics, such as a round head with a flat occiput and slanted, wide-set eyes.

emotional/mental impairment Illnesses that cause a person's emotions to become out of control.

hemiplegia Paralysis of one side of the body.

mental illness A generic term for a variety of illnesses that result in emotional, cognitive, or behavioral dysfunction.

multiple sclerosis A chronic disease of the central nervous system in which there is destruction of the myelin and nerve axons within several regions of the brain and spinal cord.

muscular dystrophy An inherited muscular disease causing degeneration of the muscle fibers.

myasthenia gravis An abnormal condition characterized by the chronic fatigability and weakness of muscles, especially in the face and throat. It is the result of a defect in the conduction of nerve impulses at the nerve junction. This deficit is caused by a lack of acetylcholine.

obesity A term generally used when someone is 20% to 30% over their ideal weight.

osteoarthritis A degenerative joint disease associated with aging.

paraplegia Paralysis of the lower part of the body.

poliomyelitis A highly contagious viral infection that can cause paralysis and death, and created a serious epidemic in the past but is now prevented in the US through a vaccine.

quadriplegia Paralysis of all four extremities and the trunk.

sensorineural deafness A permanent lack of hearing caused by a lesion or damage of the inner ear.

spina bifida The most common permanently disabling birth defect in which, during the first month of pregnancy, the spinal column of the fetus does not close properly or completely and vertebrae do not develop, leaving a portion of the spinal cord exposed.

terminal illness A sickness that the patient cannot be cured of; death is imminent.

Assessment in Action

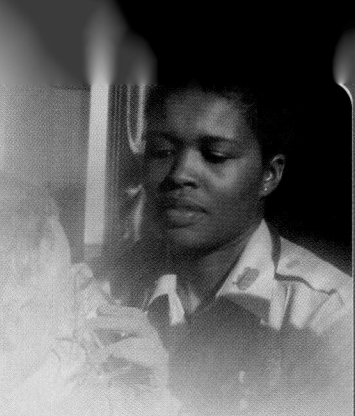

You are dispatched to a private residence for a 32-year-old patient with shortness of breath. When you arrive on scene, you find a male patient supine in his bed. You observed multiple handicapped equipment devices while walking to the patient. You are told by his family that he had a spinal cord injury a year ago and is paralyzed from the neck down. They inform you that the patient is prone to pneumonia and they believe he has it now. His blood pressure is 140/70 mm Hg; pulse rate, 120 beats/min; respiratory rate, 26 breaths/min; pulse oximetry reading on room air, 95%; and the ECG shows sinus tachycardia.

1. _____ is paralysis of all four extremities and the trunk, possibly from a cervical spine injury.
   A. Hemiplegia
   B. Paraplegia
   C. Quadriplegia
   D. Hyperesthesia

2. True or false? Paralyzed patients always have diaphragmatic involvement.
   A. True
   B. False

3. A paralyzed patient may have normal sensation or:
   A. hyperesthesia.
   B. hypoesthesia.
   C. diaphragmatic involvement.
   D. hemiparesis.

4. _____ is paralysis of one side of the body.
   A. Hemiplegia
   B. Hyperesthesia
   C. Hemiparesis
   D. Paraplegia

5. _____ is defined as a nonprogressive bilateral neuromuscular disorder in which voluntary muscles are poorly controlled.
   A. Arthritis
   B. Osteoarthritis
   C. Cerebral palsy
   D. Cystic fibrosis

6. _____ is a chronic dysfunction of the endocrine system that affects multiple body systems.
   A. Arthritis
   B. Cerebral palsy
   C. Pleurisy
   D. Cystic fibrosis

7. _____ is a chronic disease of the central nervous system in which destruction of the myelin and nerve axons occur within several regions of the brain and spinal cord.
   A. Cerebral palsy
   B. Multiple sclerosis
   C. Cystic fibrosis
   D. Arthritis

Challenging Questions

You are dispatched to a private home for an unresponsive patient. When you arrive on scene, you are greeted by the patient's daughter, who tells you she believes her mother is dead, or is dying. After speaking to the daughter, you find out the patient is home with terminal liver cancer. The patient is taking agonal respirations at a rate of 2 to 4 breaths/min. She has weak, slow pulses and an unpalpable blood pressure.

8. What should you do for this patient?

9. What should you do for the family?

■ Points to Ponder

You and your partner are dispatched to a local residential facility for a seizure. You are familiar with this facility, as it is known as the home of severely impaired individuals. When you arrive, you find a female patient who appears postictal. The patient is normally nonverbal, and her body is severely contracted. She has a history of severe mental retardation, seizures, diabetes, and CVA. The patient's vital signs are as follows: blood pressure, 180/90 mm Hg; respiratory rate, 24 breaths/min; pulse rate, 110 beats/min; pulse oximetry reading on room air, 96%; and the ECG shows sinus tachycardia.

How do you assess her mental status?

Issues: Understanding the Challenges of Caring for Patients With Special Needs.

45 Acute Interventions for the Chronic Care Patient

Objectives

Cognitive

6-6.1 Compare and contrast the primary objectives of the ALS professional and the home care professional. (p 45.5)

6-6.2 Identify the importance of home health care medicine as related to the ALS level of care. (p 45.5)

6-6.3 Differentiate between the role of EMS provider and the role of the home care provider. (p 45.5)

6-6.4 Compare and contrast the primary objectives of acute care, home care and hospice care. (p 45.4)

6-6.5 Summarize the types of home health care available in your area and the services provided. (p 45.4)

6-6.6 Discuss the aspects of home care that result in enhanced quality of care for a given patient. (p 45.5)

6-6.7 Discuss the aspects of home care that have a potential to become a detriment to the quality of care for a given patient. (p 45.5)

6-6.8 List complications commonly seen in the home care patients which result in their hospitalization. (p 45.7)

6-6.9 Compare the cost, mortality and quality of care for a given patient in the hospital versus the home care setting. (p 45.5)

6-6.10 Discuss the significance of palliative care programs as related to a patient in a home health care setting. (p 45.5)

6-6.11 Define hospice care, comfort care and DNR/DNAR as they relate to local practice, law and policy. (p 45.26)

6-6.12 List the stages of the grief process and relate them to an individual in hospice care. (p 45.27)

6-6.13 List pathologies and complications typical to home care patients. (p 45.9)

6-6.14 Given a home care scenario, predict complications requiring ALS intervention. (p 45.6)

6-6.15 Given a series of home care scenarios, determine which patients should receive follow-up home care and which should be transported to an emergency care facility. (p 45.6)

6-6.16 Describe airway maintenance devices typically found in the home care environment. (p 45.9)

6-6.17 Describe devices that provide or enhance alveolar ventilation in the home care setting. (p 45.9)

6-6.18 List modes of artificial ventilation and an out-of-hospital situation where each might be employed. (p 45.10)

6-6.19 List vascular access devices found in the home care setting. (p 45.14)

6-6.20 Recognize standard central venous access devices utilized in home health care. (p 45.15)

6-6.21 Describe the basic universal characteristics of central venous catheters. (p 45.14)

6-6.22 Describe the basic universal characteristics of implantable injection devices. (p 45.15)

6-6.23 List devices found in the home care setting that are used to empty, irrigate or deliver nutrition or medication to the GI/GU tract. (p 45.17)

6-6.24 Describe complications of assessing each of the airway, vascular access, and GI/GU devices described above. (p 45.17)

6-6.25 Given a series of scenarios, demonstrate the appropriate ALS interventions. (p 45.6)

6-6.26 Given a series of scenarios, demonstrate interaction and support with the family members/support persons for a patient who has died. (p 2.15–2.18)

6-6.27 Describe common complications with central venous access and implantable drug administration ports in the out-of-hospital setting. (p 45.17)

6-6.28 Describe the indications and contraindications for urinary catheter insertion in an out-of-hospital setting. (p 45.18)

6-6.29 Identify the proper anatomy for placement of urinary catheters in males or females. (p 45.21)

6-6.30 Identify failure of GI/GU devices found in the home care setting. (p 45.21)

6-6.31 Identify failure of ventilatory devices found in the home care setting. (p 45.12)

6-6.32 Identify failure of vascular access devices found in the home care setting. (p 45.15)

6-6.33 Identify failure of drains. (p 45.24)

6-6.34 Differentiate between home care and acute care as preferable situations for a given patient scenario. (p 45.5)

6-6.35 Discuss the relationship between local home care treatment protocols/SOPs and local EMS Protocols/SOPs. (p 45.7)

6-6.36 Discuss differences in individual's ability to accept and cope with their own impending death. (p 45.27)

6-6.37 Discuss the rights of the terminally ill. (p 45.28)

Affective

6-6.38 Value the role of the home-care professional and understand their role in patient care along the life-span continuum. (p 45.5)

6-6.39 Value the patient's desire to remain in the home setting. (p 45.5)

6-6.40 Value the patient's desire to accept or deny hospice care. (p 45.26)

6-6.41   Value the uses of long term venous access in the home health setting, including but not limited to:
a. Chemotherapy
b. Home pain management
c. Nutrition therapy
d. Congestive heart therapy
e. Antibiotic therapy (p 45.14, 45.21, 45.26, 45.27)

Psychomotor

6-6.42   Observe for an infected or otherwise complicated venous access point. (p 45.15)
6-6.43   Demonstrate proper tracheotomy care. (p 45.12)

6-6.44   Demonstrate the insertion of a new inner cannula and/or the use of an endotracheal tube to temporarily maintain an airway in a tracheostomy patient. (p 45.12)
6-6.45   Demonstrate proper technique for drawing blood from a central venous line. (p 45.15)
6-6.46   Demonstrate the method of accessing vascular access devices found in the home health care setting. (p 45.15)

Introduction

Breakthrough technologies, newer drugs, and research have combined to increase the average life expectancy. Thanks to these advances, persons who might have died from injuries or illnesses 50 years ago may now continue to lead satisfying and productive lives. Many of these persons, however, require physical support and care of chronic illnesses—care that may take place in the home setting. As a result of this trend, paramedics are being called upon more frequently to interact with chronic care providers and patients who are receiving home care Table 45-1 ▾ .

Quality patient care is the ultimate goal for providers, but the aims for specific patient populations are often quite different. In the acute care setting (hospital), objectives include stabilization, diagnosis, and treatment. In the prehospital setting, emergency care has historically been associated with these objectives.

In rehabilitation care, the objective is to restore a person with disabilities to his or her maximum potential in several areas: physical, social, spiritual, psychological, and vocational. Formerly, this kind of healing, exercise, and development of skills took place in hospitals. In recent years, however, rehabilitation programs have shifted from the hospital to specialized rehabilitation centers and expanded home health care programs. Rehabilitation centers are designed to promote healing and the gradual return of the patient to the community.

In patients who are unable to return to their homes, the long-term care objectives include maintenance of a safe, stimulating environment for the patient. Although prehospital providers often equate long-term care with nursing homes for the elderly, facilities also exist for children and patients with specific health care needs. Some long-term care facilities offer custodial care; others provide life enhancement. Clearly, long-term care covers a broad range of services.

The philosophy of hospice care began in England in the 1960s. This multidisciplinary approach seeks to improve the quality of a person's life at the end through pain and symptom management. Because many patients feel more comfortable in their own homes, surrounded by familiar people and objects, and living on their own schedule, ensuring this comfort is the primary part of the palliative plan of care.

Originally, patients resided in *hospices* (from the same Latin root as *hospitality*) to receive end-of-life care that included pain management without cure management. Over time, hospice care grew to include home and in-hospital care designed to support the dying patient and his or her family during the terminal illness and afterward through the bereavement process. Patients admitted to hospice care have a life-threatening or terminal illness that is expected to result in death within 6 months.

Home care used to be the norm for terminally ill patients because few patients could afford

Table 45-1	Home Care Patients in the United States, 1992 and 2000				
Year	Number of Persons Receiving Home Care	> 65 Years Old	< 65 Years Old	Female	Male
1992	1,232,200	23.1%	76.9%	66.8%	33.2%
2000	1,355,290	29.5%	70.5%	64.8%	35.2%

Source: www.cdc.gov/nchs/fastats/homehealthcare.htm (retrieved August 1, 2006).

You are the Provider Part 1

You and your partner are dispatched to a private residence for a severe headache. As your partner approaches the address, you both make mention of the wheelchair access ramp leading up to the side entrance. The door is opened by a young woman as you make your way up the walkway. She leads you into the home, explaining that her 36-year-old husband, Michael, has been experiencing a severe headache for the past 2 hours and has not experienced any relief from his normal medication.

You are taken by surprise when you enter the living room and find the patient sitting in a wheelchair. He is awake, alert, and in obvious distress. You observe that he has a tracheostomy tube in place although he is not receiving supplemental oxygen. His wife tells you that he is able to breathe on his own during the day without additional oxygen, but needs a ventilator for support at night. He does not require any other special equipment or treatment.

Initial Assessment	Recording Time: 0 Minutes
Appearance	Seated upright in an electric wheelchair, face wet with sweat, grimacing
Level of consciousness	A (Alert to person, place, and day)
Airway	Open and clear
Breathing	Adequate chest rise and volume
Circulation	Slow, strong radial pulse

1. Does treating a patient with chronic health problems affect the way you deliver emergency care?
2. What types of patients are likely to benefit from home care?

Special Considerations

Chronic conditions necessitating home care occur across all ages. Different conditions are more prevalent in certain age groups. In addition, the age of the person affects his or her response to the chronic condition.

In childhood, chronic conditions may impede the attainment of normal developmental milestones and affect trust and autonomy. In adolescence, body image and peer acceptance become primary concerns, and normal teenage rebellion may interfere with treatment plans. The development of intimate relationships and achievement of vocational goals may be impaired when chronic illness strikes in early adulthood. Chronic illness in middle age may hinder professional or career growth, resulting in early retirement and the need to use retirement income for medical expenses. Spouses of older patients may become the primary caregiver even though they are experiencing a similar decline in health.

expensive hospital care and, therefore, were cared for at home. To assist some families with care of the sick, certain religious groups provided home health care, while public health nurses and visiting nurse societies provided education to home health care providers on cleanliness and prevention of disease in addition to care. Over the years, visiting nursing has evolved into a multidisciplinary specialty. Today, home health care providers are usually referred by a physician and associated with a hospital or agency.

Previously, patients receiving home health care often relied on expensive emergency department visits for management of acute incidents even when the incident could be managed at home. As a paramedic, your role in the care of these patients has expanded as more advanced technology emerges.

Home health care has become an increasingly attractive alternative both to patients, who often want to maintain control over their health care decision making, and to the federal government, which wants to control acute care costs. During the 1990s, however, changes in reimbursement rules severely restricted home health care agencies in terms of who they could serve, which services could be provided, and how many visits could occur each year. Many home health agencies found that they could profitably provide care only to less ill or injured patients, leaving those patients who needed the greatest care to rely on assistance from family members or friends. Unfortunately, these informal caregivers may become overwhelmed by the care requirements and experience stress-related illnesses themselves.

Because the federal government pays for the majority of home services that are reimbursed, it regulates home health care agencies to ensure they meet certain quality standards. Many types of agencies care for patients at home, including those reimbursed by Medicare, Medicaid, the Older Americans Act, state and local funds, private insurance, out-of-pocket, and combinations of payers. In addition, each public program

has its own method of determining reimbursement (ie, through reimbursement guidelines and ceilings).

Costs for similar home care services vary substantially. Nevertheless, studies show that home-based health care costs less than institutional health care, gives more satisfaction to those who receive it because they can remain in familiar surroundings, and often results in fewer and shorter hospital stays.

Measurement of the quality of health care is difficult in any setting but is particularly complex when care is delivered in the home. Consumers of home health care are vulnerable, are frequently too sick to advocate for themselves, and may lack advocates. Paramedics have a unique opportunity to listen to these patients and their families, observe the home care situation, and assist in securing additional resources or reporting to protective agencies. In addition, you can offer guidance for in-home injury prevention as you observe the patient at home.

The Role of the Paramedic in Injury Prevention in the Home Care Setting

The role of the paramedic is ideal for identifying and preventing illness and injury in the home care setting. You may be able to help identify causes of illness or injury, or prevention of either, in the future. For example, you may be called to the home of a patient who has fallen while trying to walk to the bathroom unassisted. As you arrive, you observe that the patient has tripped over a bath rug which caught under her walker leg. Your teachable moment comes in assisting the patient and family to recognize the need to remove scatter rugs and other hazards that might add to the cause of falls. Injuries include unintentional injuries, such as those caused by motor vehicle crashes, drowning, falls, and fires, and intentional injuries, such as suicide and violence.

An injury is defined by the Centers for Disease Control (CDC) as "unintentional or intentional damage to the body resulting from acute exposure to thermal, mechanical, electrical or chemical energy, or from the absence of such essentials as heat or oxygen." Injuries and illness may be preventable by changing the environment or individual behavior. One useful framework for injury prevention is the Haddon Matrix.

The Haddon matrix, developed by Dr. William Haddon, who was the first administrator of what is now the National Highway Traffic Safety Administration, can be a useful tool for identifying injury prevention opportunities. According to the Haddon matrix framework, injuries occur in a certain time sequence: the pre-event phase, the event phase, and the post-event phase. Each event has a host (the person who is involved in the injury) and the equipment that is involved in the injury. There are also different environmental situations in which an injury might occur. Prevention can be focused in any "cell" of the matrix. For example, teaching the patient and family about the hazards of having scatter rugs is an intervention that addresses the host/pre-event cell; removing the rugs may address the pre-event/equipment cell.

Assessment of the Chronic Care Patient

Scene Size-up

Scene safety follows the same guidelines as for any call. Pets that live in homes with chronically ill persons may be agitated because the household has changed from a living quarters to a care facility—full of strange noises, new faces, and smells. Remember, however, that you are entering someone's home, not a health care facility. Families may keep a variety of weapons (or equipment that can function as a weapon) on hand. Caregiver stress, exhaustion, and pressure may cause some family members to react negatively to your presence or rely on you to help relieve stress Figure 45-1 ▼ . The house may have been renovated to accommodate large equipment that may make entrances unsafe (eg, ramps intended to accommodate a wheelchair).

In addition to the usual scene size-up, perform a quick assessment of the supporting equipment. How can it be moved safely? Are backup batteries for the equipment available? Is the equipment compatible with the ambulance electrical system? Will the equipment fit?

When you assess the patient's environment, note whether nutritional support is adequate; basic needs such as a reliable, safe heat source, good ventilation, electricity, and available water are important.

Body Substance Isolation

BSI precautions in the home care scenario are the same as in any setting. Keep contaminated supplies and equipment together and off the floor and furniture. Bring two disposable bags for supplies: Contaminated but disposable supplies can go

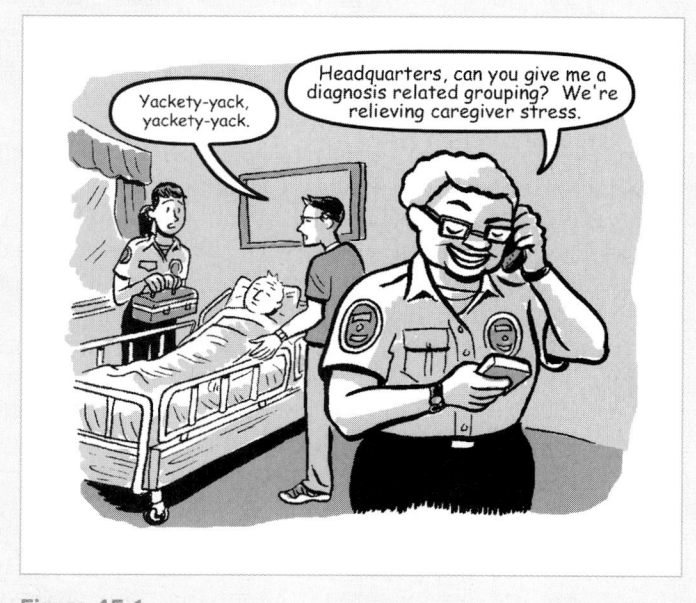

Yackety-yack, yackety-yack.

Headquarters, can you give me a diagnosis related grouping? We're relieving caregiver stress.

Figure 45-1

in one bag, while contaminated but reusable supplies go in the other. Follow your agency's plan for cleaning supplies and returning them to use.

The most effective means of preventing transmission of microorganisms is handwashing. Use a waterless gel with at least 60% alcohol content before applying your gloves and after removing them. Use running water and soap to clean your hands if they are visibly soiled or if your patient has a diagnosed infection or is taking immunosuppression drugs. Use a mask, goggles, and gown if you will be exposed to respiratory secretions or if your patient is immunosuppressed and should be protected from the provider. Most chronically ill patients have had multiple exposures to latex, so avoid wearing latex gloves when caring for these patients. This consideration is especially critical in the pediatric population, particularly for children with spina bifida.

Basic principles of infection control should be applied to the home care setting. The Centers for Disease Control and Prevention suggests a focus on infection control strategies in home care that target reducing infections related to home infusion therapy, urinary tract care, respiratory care, wound care, and enteral therapy. As a paramedic you should adhere to standard and droplet precautions for home care patients to protect your health as well as the health of others you will come in contact with.

Initial Assessment

To conduct the initial assessment of patients with chronic illness, first gather a general impression. Does the patient appear to be on the point of death? If so, do not try to troubleshoot any home care devices. Instead, remove the patient as quickly as possible from the equipment and transfer him or her to your EMS equipment. Apply portable oxygen while you assess the situation, but troubleshoot any malfunctioning devices later if you cannot fix the malfunction or failure.

Assess the patient's airway. Many patients receiving home care have artificial or altered airways such as tracheostomies or laryngectomies. Your evaluation of patients receiving home oxygen or support ventilation are no different than for any other patient. Assess the work of breathing. Look for accessory muscle use, posture, grunting, or pursed lip breathing to keep the alveoli open. Listen to the patient's breath sounds and compare them on a side-to-side basis. Finally, assess pulse oximetry.

Assess the patient's level of consciousness (LOC) or mental status. In the chronic care patient, a common alteration in LOC is dementia. Document the patient's behavior, including accusations, but remain nonjudgmental toward caregivers. Another

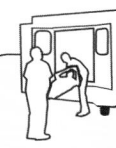

In the Field

Pulse oximetry varies according to patient age and gender. Compare your result to the usual patient results and intervene based on your overall assessment.

possible change in LOC is delirium, an often acute, reversible change in behavior that may be caused by glucose or electrolyte imbalances, nutritional deficiencies, hypothermia, or hyperthermia.

Focused History and Physical Exam

In a trauma patient, stabilize the patient's cervical spine, perform a rapid physical exam, provide comfort, and assess for other injuries. In a medical patient, gather a SAMPLE history, perform an assessment of the chief complaint, and take the patient's vital signs before you develop the plan of care. Once you have obtained the history, you may complete a physical exam. Treatment is based on both history and exam.

Medication Interactions in Home Care

Each patient may react differently to a particular medication. You are expected to treat any possible medication interactions by maintaining the patient's airway, breathing, and circulation.

Untoward reactions to medication interactions may be accidental. Observe the scene for signs of unsafe medication administration practices (eg, Does the patient understand his or her dosing requirements? Could similar-sounding medications cause confusion?), inadequate lighting, or problematic equipment (eg, faulty infusion pumps or failing power systems). Not all medications are meant to be crushed, yet some patients or caregivers may crush tablets before placing them in a gastric tube. Crushed extended-release medications may enter the patient's bloodstream too rapidly, causing an accidental overdose. Be suspicious for potential, accidental, or deliberate overdosing by the patient or caregiver. Report any suspicion of abuse to the proper social service agency.

Using the Home Health History

Home care providers may range from licensed personnel to friends, family, or members of fraternal or church groups. Informal caregiving networks often keep few records about the patient's care. In contrast, when home care is more formal—for example, occurring through hospitals or home care agencies—

providers may be required to keep detailed records similar to those in hospitals or nursing homes. In particular, medical insurance agencies expect detailed records to support a claim for benefits. HIPAA promotes the access of information sharing and permits paramedic access to such records for the treatment and transport of the patient. For more information on HIPAA, see Chapter 4.

Compliance Issues

Calls to patients receiving home care sometimes result from inoperative or damaged equipment such as IVs, tubes, artificial airways, and ventilators. Always consider that a call to a chronically ill patient may result from equipment failure rather than a worsening of the patient's condition. In such a case, care should be directed toward maintaining the patient on EMS equipment while the patient's own equipment is repaired or the patient can be transferred to new equipment. Inability to easily or expeditiously repair or replace the equipment should result in a transfer to the hospital.

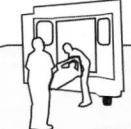

Special Considerations

Culture plays a significant role in determining what the patient and family consider adequate care. Assess the adequacy of care by speaking with the patient and family—not by making assumptions about what would be adequate in your own home. Learn the customs and cultural needs of persons in your area.

Assessing Dementia

When you are assessing a patient with dementia (or any patient, for that matter), ask two critical questions: What is the patient's usual baseline functioning? How does function today vary from baseline? Once you have identified a change from baseline behavior, either from caregivers or from a health record, determine whether a reversible condition needs to be treated—for example, hypoglycemia, hypoxia, or hypothermia.

If no reversible conditions exist, transport the patient to the emergency department for further evaluation. Dementia

Documentation and Communication

Paramedics are often frustrated because they expect a certain level of reporting, including written transfer paperwork from a patient's home care provider. Respectfully ask the home care provider about his or her involvement with the patient. Treat this provider in the same manner as you would a close family member if he or she is unable to answer all of your questions. Whenever possible, explain the rationale for your treatment plan. Remember—you have been called because the home care treatment is not working or the situation has changed. In addition, explain that once you arrive on the scene, the law requires you to assume responsibility of the patient since you are now the primary care provider. You can have the home care provider speak with your medical command only if time permits.

In the Field

Use the mnemonic AEIOU-TIPS to determine possible causes of altered mental status:

A Alcohol or acidosis
E Epilepsy, environment, electricity
I Insulin
O Overdose
U Uremia
T Trauma
I Infection
P Poisoning or psychosis
S Seizure, stroke, or shock

alone does not render a patient incompetent. In many states, patients cannot be transported against their will unless they are a hazard to themselves or others. Call medical control for assistance if the patient is unwilling to be transported. Document all assessments and interventions on your PCR.

Detailed Physical Exam

The detailed physical exam assesses a specific region or body system in the case of trauma with significant MOI. Most calls to the chronic care home will be medical in nature. The chief complaint may clue you into the mechanism or cause of the illness. The level of detail required for a physical exam in the home care setting is similar to any other physical exam encountered in paramedic practice. The need for a comprehensive examination depends on the acuity of the patient and the risk factors for further injury or illness.

Ongoing Assessment

If you are unable to resolve the patient's problem, plan to transport the patient to the appropriate facility per protocol. Streamline the patient's equipment by removing components that will not be used during transport (eg, a humidification device for a home ventilator). Document your care on the PCR or run sheet.

If the patient's own equipment will be used during transport, be sure to have battery backup for electrical devices in case of ambulance mechanical difficulties. Home care equipment is either purchased (usually as an insurance benefit) or rented, and the patient may be financially liable if it is lost or damaged. Be sure that all equipment is clearly labeled with the

patient's name and contact information **Figure 45-2 ▼**. Document which pieces of equipment were transported as well as the name of the person assuming responsibility for the patient and equipment at the receiving facility.

Should the patient's problem resolve before transport, call medical control or follow your protocol for referring the patient to his or her own physician.

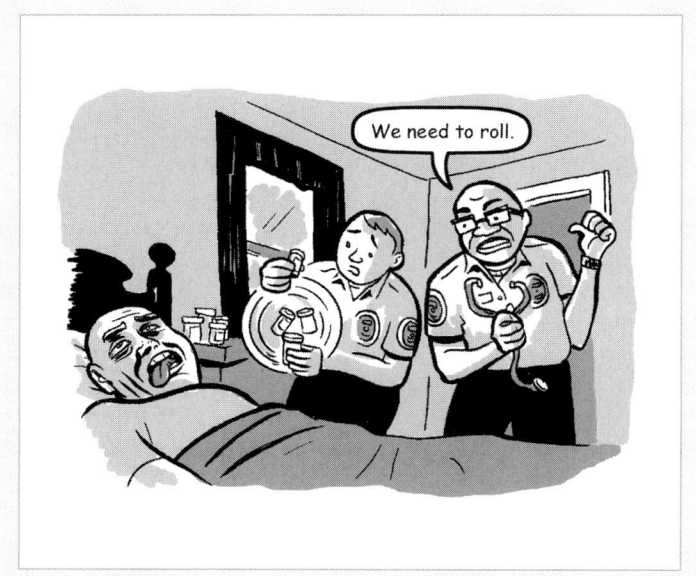

Figure 45-2

You are the Provider Part 2

You begin your assessment while your partner takes a set of vital signs. The patient was involved in a motor vehicle crash 6 months ago, resulting in a ruptured spleen, multiple rib fractures, a fractured left arm, and a C4 fracture of the neck. The spinal fracture and resulting spinal cord injury left your patient a quadriplegic. He is able to move using an electronic wheelchair. His wife was taught to straight catheterize her husband every 6 to 8 hours and assist with a bowel regimen. She is also skilled in providing tracheostomy care and setting up the ventilator at night. A home health nurse visits five times a week to provide additional assistance. He is prescribed 15 mg of baclofen three times a day to help with muscle spasms and cramping and acetaminophen (Tylenol) as needed for pain or fever.

The patient tells you that his headache began approximately 2 hours earlier while watching a football game on television. He had taken the Tylenol as prescribed with no relief. The pain has gradually gotten worse and is now a 10 on a scale of 1 to 10. He describes the pain as a relentless pounding that does not radiate. He does admit to having blurred vision. At this time he denies having experienced nausea, vomiting, chest pain, or shortness of breath.

Vital Signs	Recording Time: 5 Minutes
Level of consciousness	Alert
Pulse	56 beats/min, regular
Blood pressure	194/100 mm Hg
Respirations	16 breaths/min, regular
Skin	Flushed, warm, and diaphoretic about the face; cool, pale, and clammy elsewhere
Sao$_2$	99% on room air

3. What type of equipment might you encounter with patients receiving home health care?

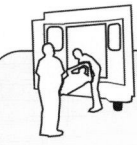

In the Field

Transporting equipment not designed to be used during a transport may increase the risk of injury to patients and EMS professionals.

Types of Patients Who Receive Home Health Care

Chronically ill patients are cared for at home by a wide range of caregivers who may include family members, unlicensed caregivers, licensed nonprofessional caregivers, licensed professionals, or a combination of these. Many family members who care for chronically ill patients are medically knowledgeable and are often the paramedic's best source of information and care guidelines.

In addition to frail or chronically ill elderly patients in the home care setting, you may encounter individuals, for example, who have recently had a hospital stay, surgery, or a high-risk pregnancy, or a newborn with medical complications. Chronic illness or permanent injury may also necessitate home care (Table 45-2 ▾). Many of these patients experience similar physical problems regardless of the initial cause.

Table 45-2	Chronic Illnesses and Injuries Encountered in the Home Care Setting
Type of Disease, Injury, or Abnormality	**General Long-Term Problem**
Neuromuscular disease	Hypoventilation
Guillain-Barré syndrome	Decreased cough mechanism
Muscular dystrophy	Inability to maintain airway
Amyotrophic lateral sclerosis Multiple sclerosis Polio/postpolio syndrome Spinal cord injury Central apnea	Immobility: deep vein thrombosis, pulmonary embolus, pressure ulcers

Musculoskeletal abnormalities:
  Scoliosis or lordosis
  Pectus excavatum
  Pectus carinatum
  Pickwickian syndrome
	Hypoventilation

Pulmonary abnormalities:
  Bronchopulmonary dysplasia
  Chronic obstructive pulmonary disease
  Cystic fibrosis
	Decreased oxygen diffusion, infection

Cardiac abnormalities: Advanced-stage congestive heart failure	Decreased oxygen diffusion

Patients With Abnormal Airway Conditions

Patients with respiratory compromise generally are unable to adequately ventilate themselves. In chronic obstructive pulmonary disease (COPD), loss of alveolar surface area or damage to the bronchial lining reduces the volume of air delivered to the alveoli and increases the work of breathing. Cystic fibrosis increases the amount of mucus present in the airway, limiting air flow and reducing diffusion across the pulmonary capillary membrane. Bronchopulmonary dysplasia results from early oxygen administration to (usually premature) newborns and causes permanent changes in the cells of the respiratory tract. Musculoskeletal changes such as scoliosis and chest wall abnormalities make it difficult to expand the chest adequately. Excess weight over the chest (Pickwickian syndrome) or sleep apnea may leave the patient hypoventilated during sleep. In isolated cases, ventilation would normally be adequate but the patient is experiencing an increased metabolic demand from fever or infection.

Home Oxygen-Delivery Systems

With any type of respiratory abnormality, the home care treatment plan is designed to supplement the patient's respiratory effort. Any stressor such as infection, exposure to an allergen, or psychological upset can increase the severity of signs and symptoms and render the current respiratory support inadequate.

The simplest home oxygen systems involve a nasal cannula and oxygen in various delivery systems, ranging from small portable cylinders to large oxygen-enrichment systems (Figure 45-3 ▸). The patient usually contracts with a respiratory home care company to purchase the cannulas, oxygen tubing, and oxygen. Patients who are anxious breathe faster, use more of the oxygen, and may run out prior to delivery; you may be called when a person's

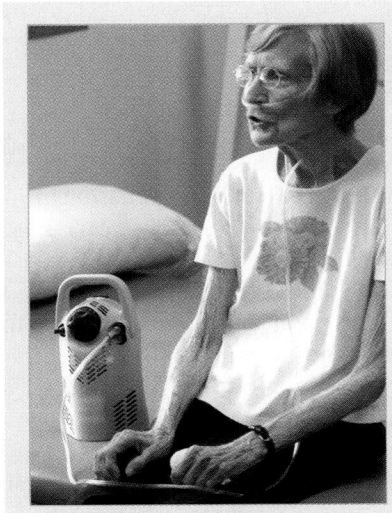

Figure 45-3 Home oxygen systems involve a nasal cannula and oxygen.

oxygen demand exceeds the current supply. If your assessment reveals that the patient needs to have more stored oxygen available, call the home care company. Meanwhile, use your cylinders to keep the patient calm and prevent decompensation. Be sure the cylinders are stored safely and within reach of the patient or caregiver.

Some patients use oxygen concentrators, which are large electrical devices that concentrate the oxygen in ambient air and eliminate other gases. Such a system eliminates frequent delivery of oxygen cylinders, is less expensive, and is easy to maintain. Its large size means that the device is not portable, however, and many concentrators are noisy and give off heat. Patients should have backup oxygen cylinders available in the event of electrical failure.

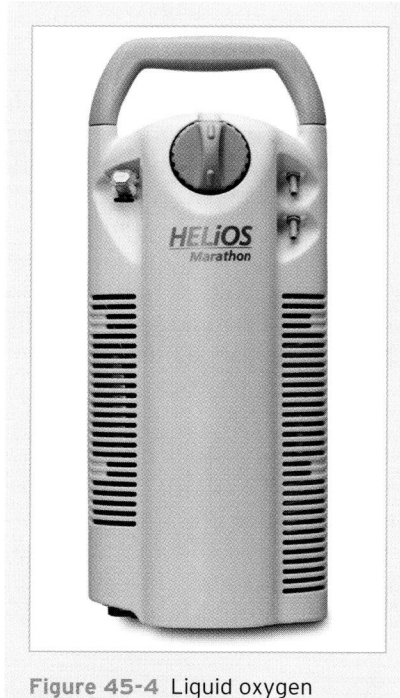

Figure 45-4 Liquid oxygen system.

A liquid oxygen system **Figure 45-4** may also be used. With this system, more gas can be kept in a smaller container, making it an attractive option for active patients. Oxygen cannot be stored as a liquid for long as it will evaporate.

To decrease the work of breathing by keeping the air passages and alveoli open during the expiratory phase, patients may use continuous positive airway pressure (CPAP) **Figure 45-5** . By keeping the airway pressure slightly higher than atmospheric pressure, CPAP keeps alveoli and airway passages stented open and decreases the work of breathing. It also increases the driving (diffusing) force of oxygen and improves overall oxygenation if a supplemental oxygen line is attached. In the home care setting, CPAP is typically used for sleep apnea. The device consists of a tight-fitting mask or nasal prongs with a thick pillow of air to decrease pressure and prevent damage to the nose and upper lip. A continuous pressure measured in centimeters of H_2O assists the patient in taking a breath and makes it difficult to completely exhale.

Bilevel airway pressure (BiPAP) exerts a different level of inspiratory pressure versus expiratory pressure. This type of support is used less often in the home care setting and does not ventilate the patient.

A ventilator, also called a respirator, mechanically delivers air to the lungs. Home ventilators are smaller than most

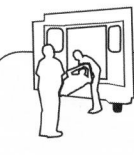

In the Field

Both CPAP and BiPAP can be administered in the home by nasal or face mask without endotracheal intubation. This technique is referred to as "noninvasive ventilation."

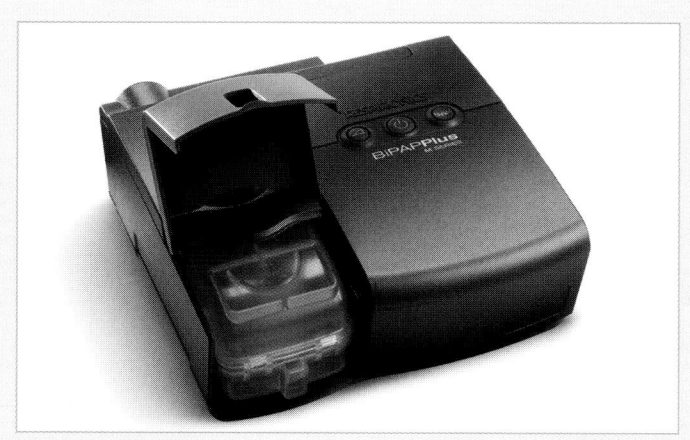

Figure 45-5 Continuous positive airway pressure machine.

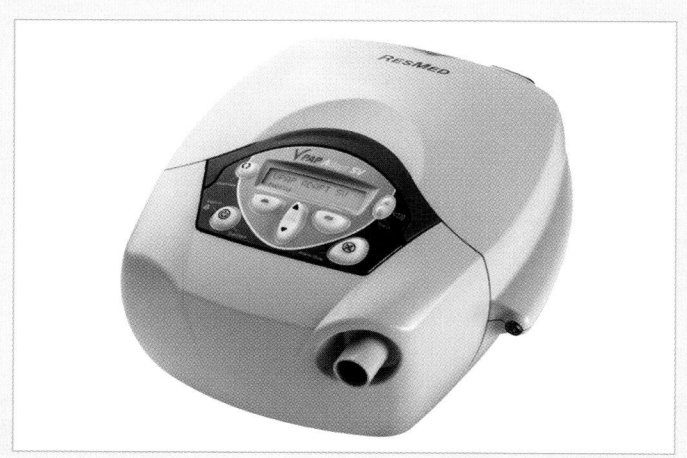

Figure 45-6 Home ventilator.

microwave ovens, use regular household electricity, and may include a battery backup **Figure 45-6** . It is important for you to become familiar with the types of units available to effectively transport your patient or assist with an equipment malfunction.

Ventilators may be set to deliver a certain volume of gas to the lungs. For example, the machine setting may specify the tidal volume (volume of air breathed in and out during a normal breath) to be delivered. This target tidal volume is based on patient-specific factors, such as resistance to flow or lung compliance (elasticity), and physician preference. Other ventilators are designed to deliver a certain pressure. Volume ventilators and pressure ventilators are used most often with an invasive airway, endotracheal intubation, or tracheostomy (discussed later in this section).

Normal breathing relies on increasing the size of the chest so that intrapulmonary and intrapleural pressures fall and air

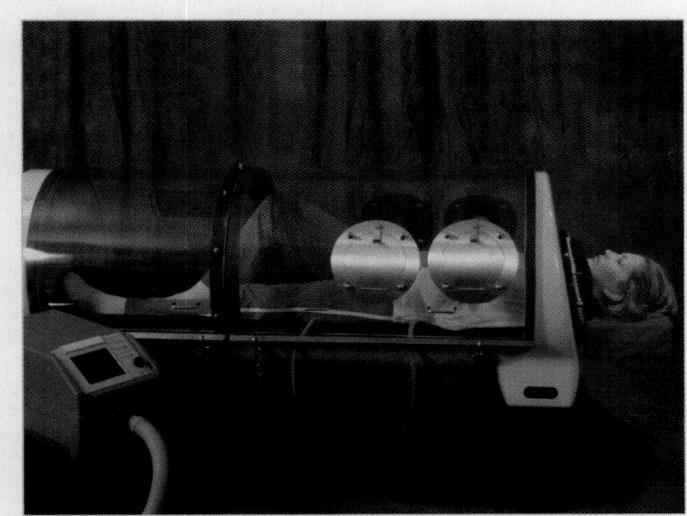

Figure 45-7 Negative-pressure ventilator.

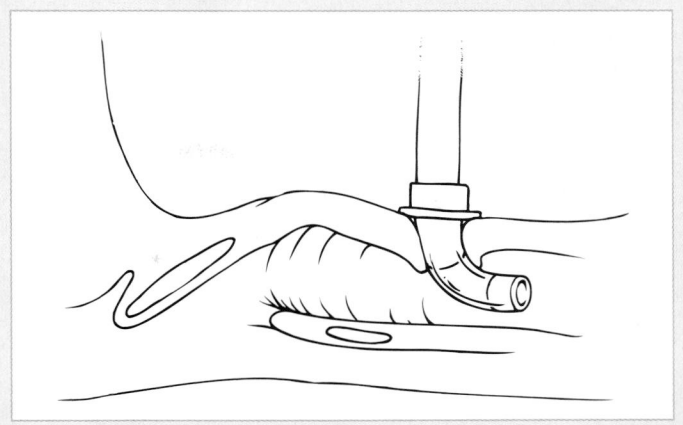

Figure 45-8 A tracheostomy is a planned surgical procedure in which an opening is placed in the trachea below the cricoid ring.

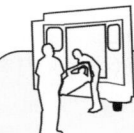

In the Field

Monitor the patient's blood pressure and pulse if you are going to begin positive-pressure ventilation after a period of normal breathing.

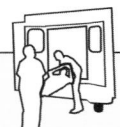

In the Field

If a tracheostomy becomes plugged, the patient may be ventilated by deflating the cuff, covering the nose and mouth with a mask, and using the bag-mask device. If you are unable to ventilate the patient through the tracheostomy, plug the tracheostomy stoma and attempt to ventilate the patient in the traditional manner with a bag-mask device.

rushes in (<u>negative-pressure ventilation</u>). Most mechanical ventilators rely on <u>positive-pressure ventilation</u>—that is, air is pushed into the lungs. (You may be most familiar with positive-pressure ventilation when you are using the bag-mask device.) This type of ventilation alters the hemodynamics of the body by decreasing venous return to the heart; the thoracic pump pulls blood back to the heart when the pressure within the chest is less than atmospheric pressure. During positive-pressure ventilation, the pump is not as effective and cardiac output can drop.

Negative-pressure ventilators mimic the body's normal method of breathing. These devices—which may be called ponchos, turtleshells, or belts **Figure 45-7 ▲**—enlarge the chest, dropping intrapulmonary pressure below the atmospheric pressure and allowing air to rush in. Negative-pressure ventilators do not need an invasive airway and do not alter hemodynamics. They depend on a patent airway.

Invasive Airways

Improvements in artificial ventilation have transformed many homes into satellite intensive care units. As a consequence, paramedics may encounter patients who are ventilated through a <u>tracheostomy</u>, a surgical airway in which an opening is placed in the trachea below the cricoid ring **Figure 45-8 ▶**. A tracheostomy may become necessary when prolonged use of an endotracheal (ET) tube might predispose the patient to tra-

cheal necrosis, tracheoesophageal fistula, ventilator-acquired pneumonia, or oral damage. (ET tubes and intubation are covered in depth in Chapter 11.)

A <u>laryngectomy</u> is a surgical procedure in which the larynx is removed, usually because of cancer. The trachea is then curved anteriorly and sewn to tissues of the neck. The opening that is created in the neck is called a stoma. A patient with a laryngectomy cannot be manually bagged through the nose and mouth, and you must be careful not to introduce liquids into the stoma. Most of these patients use a stoma cover to act as a filter and prevent mucus from being coughed onto others. A patient with a laryngectomy cannot produce normal speech and must learn to swallow and regurgitate air from the stomach or use an assistive device **Figure 45-9 ▶**.

Tracheostomy tube designs vary, so ask the caregiver about the tube prior to beginning care. General types of tracheostomy

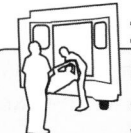

In the Field

If you are transporting a child with a tracheostomy in a standard car seat, avoid using seats with a tray or shield. The tray or shield could come into contact with the tracheostomy and injure the child or block the airway.

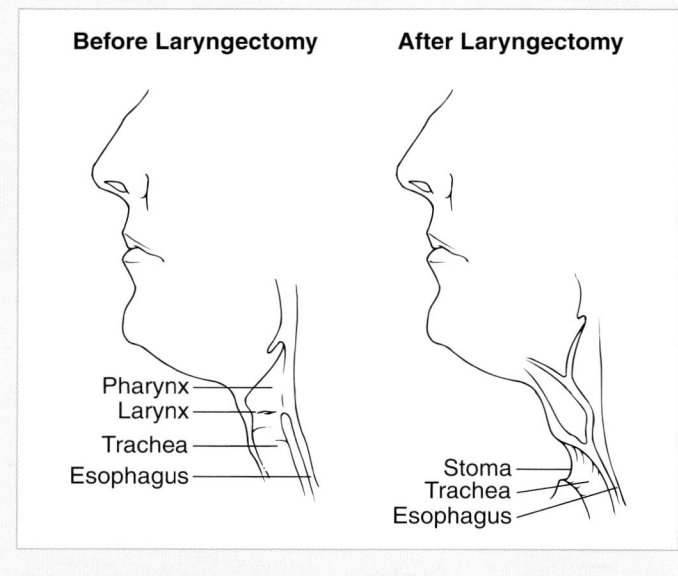

Before Laryngectomy   **After Laryngectomy**

Pharynx
Larynx
Trachea
Esophagus

Stoma
Trachea
Esophagus

Figure 45-9 Laryngectomy.

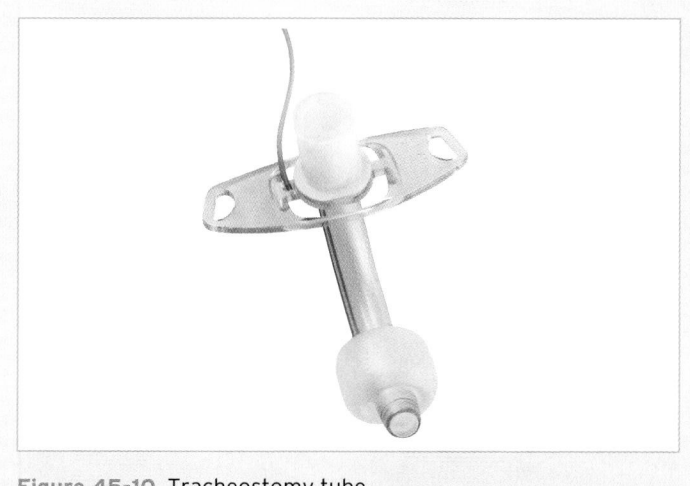

Figure 45-10 Tracheostomy tube.

In the Field

For infants and small children, the tracheostomy tube is usually a single-cannula plastic tube and is generally not cuffed (even if mechanical ventilation is required).

tubes include a one-piece metal tube that can be plugged for speech. Such tubes are usually placed in patients weeks to months after the tracheostomy surgery when the opening has healed well.

Airway Management

It is important to assess for airway patency in all patients, but it is especially important in patients with artificial airways. The basic airway techniques of opening, repositioning, and clearing (especially suctioning) the airway are the most critical steps in improving airway clearance and patency, thereby improving oxygenation and ventilation.

Assess the flow of oxygen and ensure that there is sufficient oxygen in the system. If you are uncertain about the oxygen flow, transfer the patient to the transport oxygen source. If a patient is on a ventilator when you arrive, assess the patient's chest for synchronous movement with the ventilator. If you have any doubt about ventilator function, do not be afraid to remove the patient from the ventilator and use manual positive-pressure ventilation. Avoid adjusting home ventilator settings unless you are specifically credentialed to work with the particular device. Soliciting the help of the patient, family, and caregivers can assist in assessment and troubleshooting of equipment.

Occasionally an artificial airway will need to be exchanged or replaced. Tracheostomy tubes are easily removed Figure 45-10 ▶ . Untie the tracheostomy strings or device used to secure the tube, and gently slide the tube out on exhalation. When replacing this tube, have the patient take a deep breath and gently follow the contour of the tube during inhalation.

One-piece plastic tubes come either with or without cuffs. When you are working with plastic tubes, suction the patient orally with a whistle-tip catheter. Deflate the cuff and remove it

during exhalation. To replace the tracheostomy, insert an obturator (guide) into it, gently guide the tube in on inhalation, remove the obturator, and add air to the cuff.

Two-piece tracheostomies have an outer cannula that is guided into place by the obturator. When the obturator is removed, insert the inner cannula and turn the standard connector until it clicks or locks into place. Add air to the cuff, and apply the holder to secure the device around the neck. Never let go of the tube until it is secured.

On rare occasions, the paramedic will need to replace a tracheostomy with an ET tube. The easiest method is to remove the tracheostomy tube and gently guide a slightly smaller ET tube into place. (The size of the tracheostomy tube appears on its neck piece.) The ET tube will extend out from the neck, so take care to stabilize the tube. Confirm chest rise with ventilation, as it is possible—especially with new tracheostomies—to misplace the tube within the neck but outside of the trachea.

If the tracheostomy has inadvertently closed, you may intubate the patient orally or nasally. Place an occlusive dressing over the tracheostomy site to prevent air loss and observe the patient carefully for adequate chest rise.

To suction and clean a tracheostomy, follow the steps given here and in Skill Drill 45-1 ▶ :

1. Wash your hands and apply a mask, goggles, and clean nonlatex gloves. Suctioning a home care patient is a clean procedure, not a sterile one.

2. Open supplies may be used. For cost reasons, home care patients often reuse their suction catheters. If the catheters

Skill Drill 45-1: Cleaning a Tracheostomy

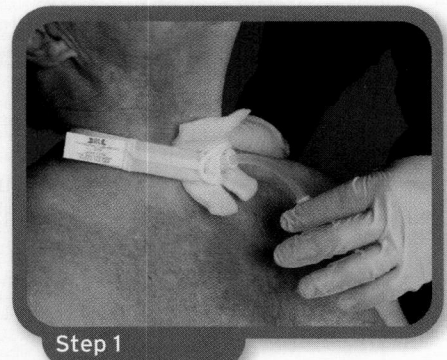

Step 1

Remove the inner cannula and place the device to soak in the proper solution.

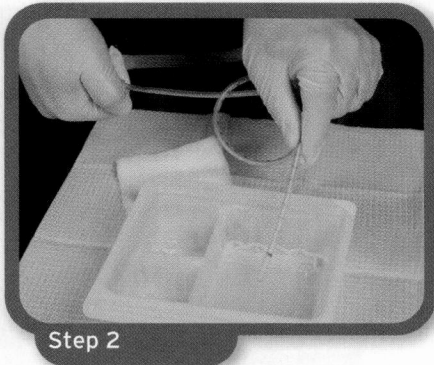

Step 2

Attach the catheter to negative pressure. Check the suction and clear the catheter by drawing up a small amount of saline.

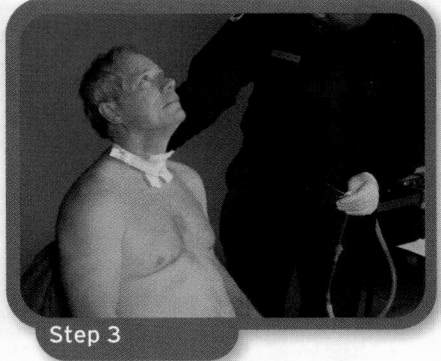

Step 3

Have the patient take a deep breath or pre-oxygenate him or her using the ventilator.

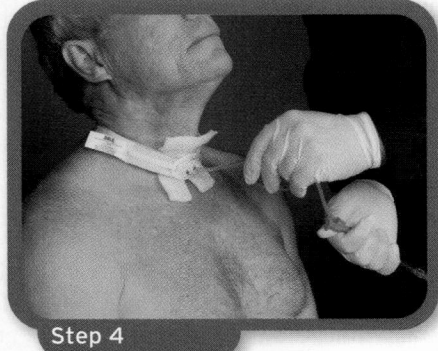

Step 4

Insert the catheter into the trachea without suction. Apply intermittent suction while removing the catheter. Repeat as necessary.

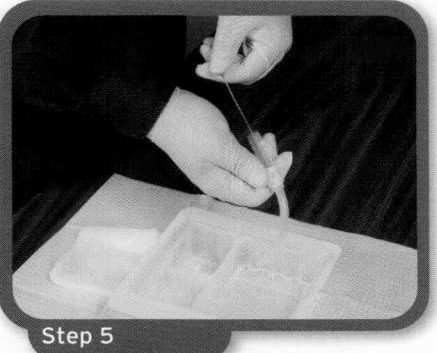

Step 5

Clean the inner cannula with the tracheostomy brush, rinse, and replace and lock into place.

do not have visible contamination and have been stored in a clean manner, they are acceptable for use.

3. Remove the inner cannula. Check with your patient's caregiver, if available, and place the device to soak in the appropriate recommended solution. If the caregiver is not available, use a mixture of hydrogen peroxide and water. Placing the cannula in plain water is acceptable in short-term situations. With one-piece tracheostomy tubes, this step is unnecessary. If the patient is dependent on a ventilator, have a replacement cannula immediately available (Step 1).

4. Attach the catheter to negative pressure. Check the suction and clear the catheter by drawing up a small amount of saline (Step 2).

5. Have the patient take a deep breath or preoxygenate him or her (Step 3).

6. Insert the catheter into the trachea without suction. Apply intermittent suction while removing the catheter. Repeat as

necessary. Keep the patient well oxygenated during the procedure (Step 4).

7. Clean the inner cannula with the tracheostomy brush, rinse, and replace and lock into place. Omit this step for a one-piece tracheostomy (Step 5).

8. Remove your gloves and wash your hands.

9. Document the procedure and assessment on your PCR.

In asthmatic patients, peak flow readings are usually obtained immediately before and after treatment for bronchospasm. A peak flow meter measures the rate of air being expired in liters per minute and gives the provider an indication about the condition of the larger airways. To take a peak flow reading, follow the steps in **Skill Drill 45-2 ▶** :

1. Help the patient into a position of comfort, either sitting upright or standing upright, if safe to do so.

2. Place the indicator at the base of the numbered scale (Step 1).

3. Have the patient take a deep breath through the mouth.

Skill Drill 45-2: Obtaining a Peak Flow Reading

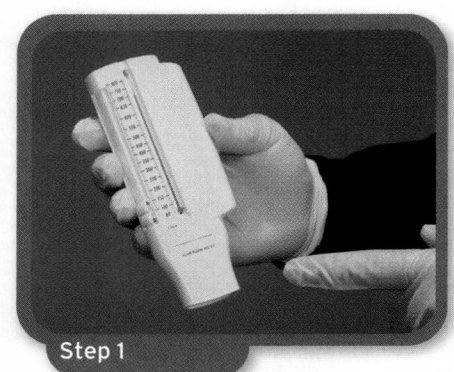

Step 1

Help the patient into a position of comfort. Place the indicator at the base of the numbered scale.

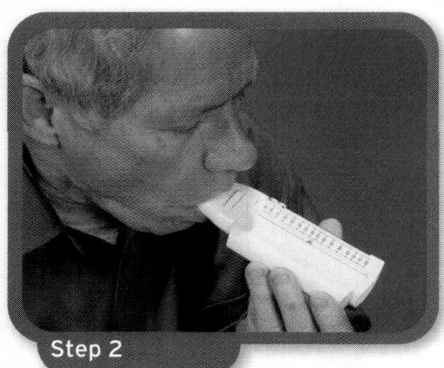

Step 2

Have the patient take a deep breath through the mouth and put the meter in the mouth. Patient blows out as hard as possible through the device for approximately 1 second. If possible, repeat two more times to obtain an average result.

4. Have the patient put the meter in the mouth and close his or her lips around the end.
5. Have the patient blow out as hard as possible through the device for approximately 1 second (**Step 2**).
6. If time and conditions permit, have the patient repeat steps 2 through 5 two more times to obtain an average result. Allow rest periods.
7. Document the results on the patient care record/run record.
8. Assist in cleaning the device and storing it correctly.

Patients With Acute Cardiovascular Disease and Vascular Access

Patients who have chronic cardiovascular disease are often cared for in the home setting. Many patients have cardiac insufficiency or heart failure, an inability of the heart to keep up with the demands placed on it and failure of the heart to pump blood efficiently. The heart is then unable to provide adequate blood flow to other organs. The signs and symptoms of heart failure depend on which side of the heart is failing and include dyspnea, cardiac asthma, pooling of blood (stasis) systemically or in the liver's circulation, edema, cyanosis, and hypertrophy (enlargement) of the heart. There are many causes of congestive heart failure: coronary artery disease, leading to heart attacks and heart muscle weakness; primary heart muscle weakness from viral infections or toxins such as prolonged alcohol exposure; heart valve disease causing heart muscle weakness due to too much leaking of blood; heart muscle stiffness from a blocked valve; and hypertension. Treatment is aimed at improving the pumping function of the heart.

Some patients may have an implantable pacemaker that delivers synchronized electrical stimulation to three chambers of the heart, enabling the heart to pump blood more efficiently throughout the body.

Cardiomyopathy, a condition in which the heart muscle does not work at the optimal level, can be caused by many disease processes. Primary cardiomyopathy cannot be traced to a single cause. Hypertension, coronary artery disease, and viral infections might combine to decrease the ability of the muscle to eject blood. Secondary cardiomyopathy can be traced to a single cause, usually one that affects other body organs at the same time. All types of cardiomyopathy result in inadequate cardiac output, limiting the patient's activity. Many treatments require long-term venous access devices.

The heart never ejects 100% of the blood in the left ventricle during a heartbeat, but an ejection fraction greater than 55% is considered adequate. An ejection fraction less than 55% may limit the patient's activity level and indicates the presence of cardiomyopathy. An ejection fraction less than 20% can significantly alter a patient's lifestyle. In a home care patient, a change in the previous level of activity is a red flag that the heart may be temporarily or permanently deteriorated.

Vascular Access

A central venous catheter—a venous access device with the tip of the catheter in the vena cava—is used for many types of home care patients, including those receiving chemotherapy, long-term antibiotic or pain management, high-concentration glucose solutions, and hemodialysis. In contrast, a midline catheter is located in a large vessel but not the vena cava (**Table 45-3 ▶**).

Because the devices are used intermittently, they must be flushed to keep them open. In the past, low-concentration heparin has been the flush of choice. However, research has shown that low platelet counts develop in some patients following long-term use of heparin even at low concentrations, a condition known as heparin-induced thrombocytopenia. Flushing the device with saline eliminates the possibility of heparin-induced thrombocytopenia but means the patency of the device must be assessed frequently. Patients who are chronically ill or fragile may have devices that allow medications and fluids to be infused or body fluids to be removed and monitored. These devices place the patient at increased risk for cardiovascular complications including anticoagulation, embolus

Table 45-3	Venous Access Devices		
Type	**Use**		**Prehospital Precautions**
Midline catheters	Short-term fluids, analgesia, antibiotics		Moderate-length catheter, not good for rapid fluid resuscitation
Peripherally inserted central catheter	Long-term fluids, analgesia, chemotherapy, antibiotic therapy		Long catheter; not good for fluid resuscitation; may require online medical direction for use
Central lines, tunneled implanted	Long-term fluids, analgesia, chemotherapy, antibiotic therapy, multiple blood draws		Have a noncutting/crush clamp available, as not all have a clamp; may require online medical direction for use
Implanted infusion device	Long-term fluids, analgesia, chemotherapy, antibiotic therapy		Use a noncutting or nonbeveled needle for access; may require online medical direction for use

formation, stasis, air embolus, and obstructed or malfunctioning devices.

Catheter dysfunction occurs frequently in patients receiving home infusions. Catheter-associated thrombosis can be life threatening and limit future vascular sites. Both of these complications can be minimized and treated when the paramedic is aware of preventative measures.

If a device does not seem to be working properly, ensure that it is not used for medications or any other purpose. If the patient has a gastric tube (which places him or her at increased risk for aspiration of stomach contents), position the patient in a semi-Fowler's or upright position if tolerated. Inspect and secure all external devices prior to moving the patient, especially when preparing for transport—it takes relatively little tension to inadvertently displace a tube, line, or device.

There are several things that a paramedic can do to reduce or prevent complications of vascular access devices: check the devices carefully before any treatment; keep device area clean; check that the correct medication and dose or nutrition are being infused into the device; use the device site only for what it was designed for (eg, dialysis catheters should only be used for dialysis treatment); avoid placing a blood pressure cuff on an arm that has an device port; and check pulses carefully in the device area.

Occasionally, it will be necessary to access a device for assessment, to draw blood, or to infuse medications. Proper technique is important. Patients and their caregivers will be your best resource in performing these functions. In addition, check with your local medical control officer regarding accessing a venous access device when there is a need for resuscitation and you are unable to obtain any other vascular access.

Drawing Blood From a Central Venous Catheter

Central venous catheters (CVCs) offer easy access to the venous system but may present resistance to rapid fluid infusion due to their length. Because they enter the central circulation in the chest, negative pressure may draw in air (air embolus) or provide entry to microorganisms. To draw blood from a CVC, follow the steps illustrated in **Skill Drill 45-3 ▶**:

1. Wash your hands and apply a mask, goggles, and nonlatex gloves.
2. Draw the flush solution (usually normal saline but may be a heparin solution) into a syringe (Step 1).

3. Set up the supplies, including the port access kit.
4. Swab the port with an appropriate cleansing solution (eg, Betadine) *or* clamp the catheter and remove the cap (Step 2).
5. Attach an empty syringe or Vacutainer adapter to the hub or port (Step 3).
6. Release the clamp (if clamped), and aspirate 5 mL of blood (Step 4).
7. Reclamp the catheter if necessary and discard the aspirated blood (Step 5).
8. Attach a new syringe or adapter (Step 6).
9. Obtain the blood samples (Step 7).
10. Reclamp the catheter if necessary and attach the syringe with the flush solution (Step 8).
11. Release the clamp and flush the line (Step 9).
12. Reclamp and recap the line (Step 10).
13. Identify the tubes of blood by writing the date and time drawn and the paramedic's name on the side of the tube, and ready them for transport by securing them in a leak-proof protected container. Transport tubes to the patient's physician, hospital personnel, or usual lab. Do not shake blood collection tubes, as this may cause the blood to hemolyze.
14. Document the procedure and assessment on the PCR.
15. Dispose of contaminated equipment.

Accessing an Implantable Venous Access Device

To access an implantable venous access device, follow the steps in **Skill Drill 45-4 ▶**:

1. Wash your hands and apply a mask, goggles, and nonlatex gloves.
2. Open supplies including the port access kit.
3. Palpate the skin over the device (Step 1).
4. Cleanse the skin over the device using a cleansing solution (eg, Betadine) (Step 2).
5. Prime the needle tubing and needle with saline. Use a special access needle called unbeveled or noncutting to avoid slicing the silicone reservoir wall (Step 3).
6. While stabilizing the device, insert the needle at a 90° angle to the skin until the needle tip reaches the back of the device (Step 4).

Skill Drill 45-3: Drawing Blood From a Central Venous Catheter

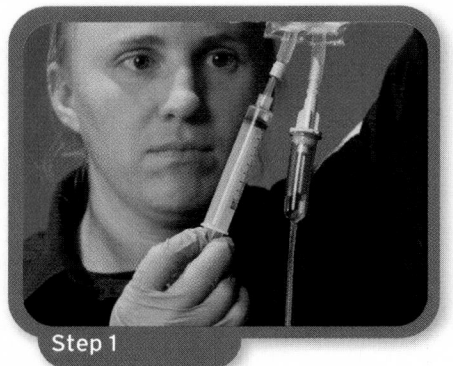

Step 1

Draw the flush solution into a syringe.

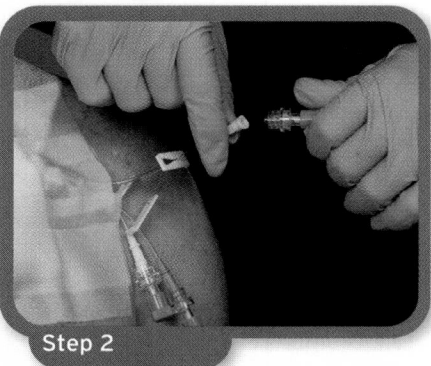

Step 2

Swab the port with an appropriate cleansing solution *or* clamp the catheter and remove the cap.

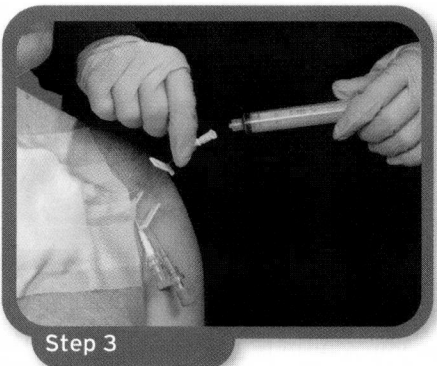

Step 3

Attach an empty syringe or Vacutainer adapter to the hub or port.

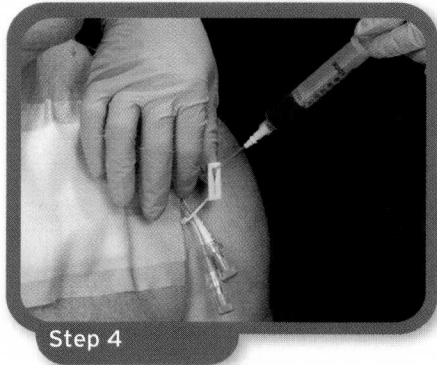

Step 4

Release the clamp (if clamped), and aspirate 5 mL of blood.

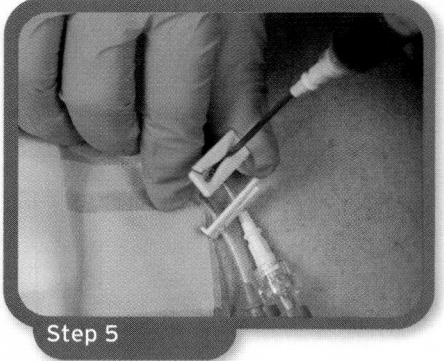

Step 5

Reclamp if necessary and discard the aspirated blood per your exposure control plan.

7. Aspirate 5 mL of blood (Step 5).

8. Discard the aspirate and obtain blood samples if necessary (Step 6).

9. Flush the line with normal saline (Step 7).

10. Administer medications or fluids as directed (Step 8).

11. Flush the device (Step 9).

12. Secure the needle with a sterile dressing *or* remove by pulling straight out of the device (Step 10).

13. Apply a dressing to the skin over the device if the needle was removed.

14. Identify the tubes of blood by writing the date and time drawn and the paramedic's name on the side of the tube, and ready them for transport by securing them in a leak-proof protected container. Transport tubes to the patient's physician, hospital personnel, or usual lab. Do not shake blood collection tubes, as this may cause the blood to hemolyze.

15. Document the procedure and assessment on the PCR.

16. Dispose of contaminated equipment.

Anticoagulant therapy is common in home care patients, so you should consider covert bleeding as a likely cause of hypovolemic shock in such individuals. A sudden onset of chest pain, shortness of breath, and decreased cardiac output during or immediately after opening an implanted or tunneled port may be indicators of an air embolus. Turn the patient on his or her left side to keep the embolus sequestered in the right atrium, so that air can be absorbed a little at a time, and transport the patient in that position.

Management of Vascular Access Devices

Vascular access devices relieve anxiety and the pain of frequent insertion attempts for patients. At the same time, they create potential complications. Common complications resulting from vascular access, assessment findings, and emergency interventions are shown in Table 45-4 ▶. If a device

Skill Drill 45-3: Drawing Blood From a Central Venous Catheter (*continued*)

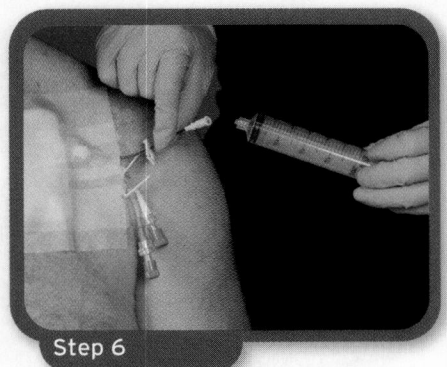

Step 6

Attach a new syringe or adapter.

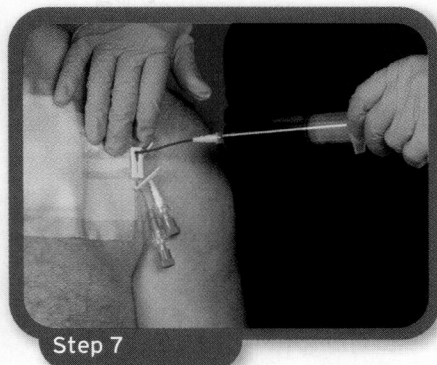

Step 7

Obtain the blood samples.

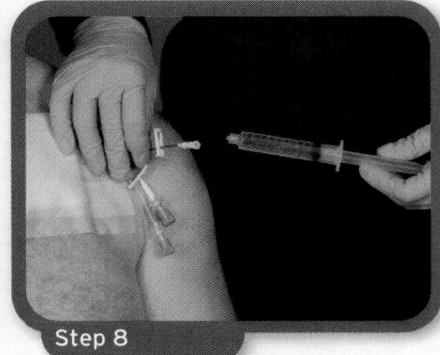

Step 8

Reclamp if necessary and attach the syringe with the flush solution.

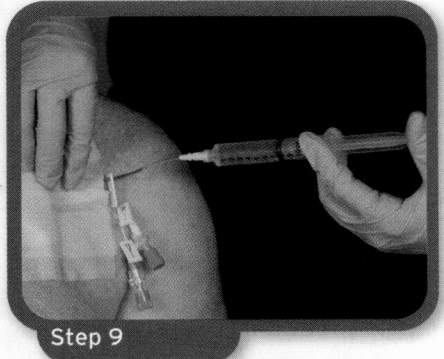

Step 9

Release the clamp and flush the line.

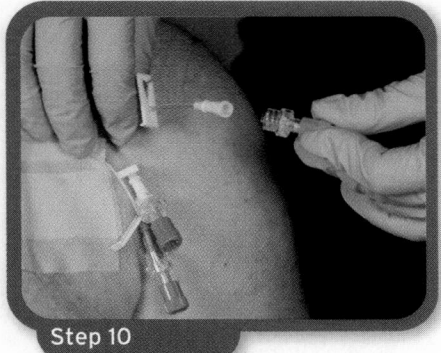

Step 10

Reclamp and recap the line.

Table 45-4	Serious Complications Associated With Vascular Access Devices
Complication	**Assessment Findings**
Occlusion	Cannot aspirate blood; infusion doesn't run
Catheter thrombosis	Swelling of arm, neck, or shoulder; pain
Sepsis	Fever, chills, malaise
Catheter migration	Change in length of exposed catheter
Catheter breakage	Leaking or bleeding from catheter
Embolism (air)	Chest pain, shortness of breath, tachycardia, hypotension, decreased level of consciousness
Embolism (PICC/midline catheter)	Inadvertent removal with distal portion of catheter missing

complication is suspected, the paramedic should not attempt to access the device. A device complication requires additional medical intervention. While not all patients will need to be transported immediately to a hospital, contact should be established and a plan made with the patient's usual health care professional. Serious complications require immediate transport of the patient to an acute care facility for further evaluation and treatment.

Patients With Gastrointestinal/Genitourinary Access

A gastric tube may be placed when the patient cannot ingest fluids, food, or medications by mouth. Tubes may be inserted through the nose or mouth into the stomach (using nasogastric or orogastric tubes). Alternatively, endoscopy procedures may be undertaken to guide the surgical entrance of the tube into the stomach, such as a percutaneous endoscopic gastric tube or placement of a percutaneous endoscopic jejunum tube into the

Skill Drill 45-4: Accessing an Implantable Venous Access Device

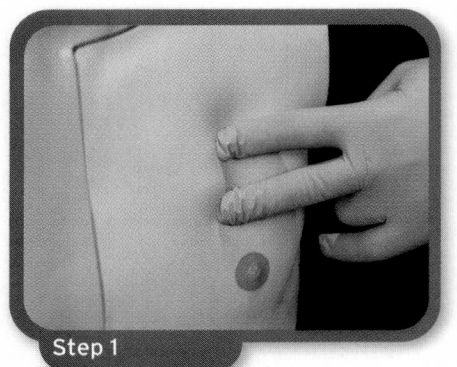

Step 1

Palpate the skin over the device.

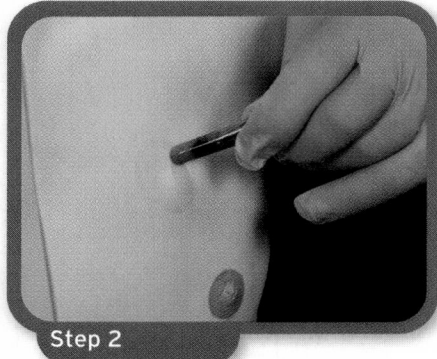

Step 2

Cleanse the skin over the device (Betadine solution).

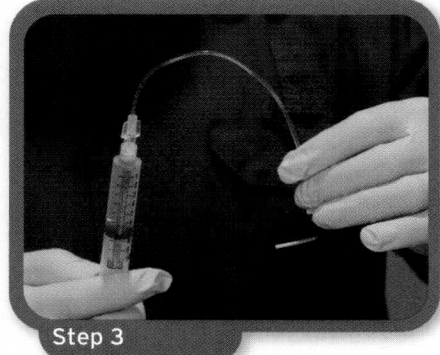

Step 3

Prime the needle tubing and needle with saline.

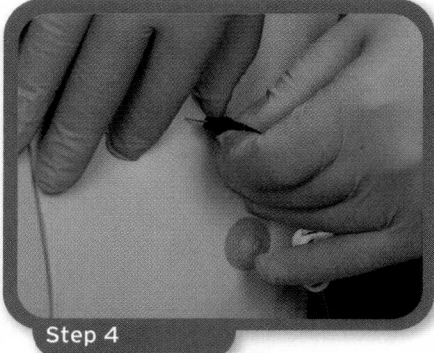

Step 4

While stabilizing the device, insert the needle at a 90° angle to the skin until the needle tip reaches the back of the device.

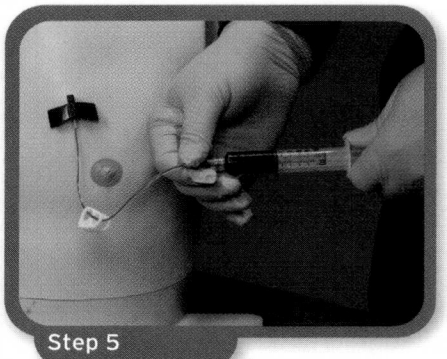

Step 5

Aspirate 5 mL of blood.

---

jejunum. The patient must have adequate stomach function to support use of a gastric tube. If there has been damage to the stomach, the tube may be placed into the jejunum of the small intestine.

Patients who have gastric tubes in place may still be at increased risk for aspiration. To minimize the risk of regurgitation and aspiration, the patient should be upright, at least to 30° when medications or nutrition is being infused. They should ideally be kept upright for 30 to 60 minutes after feeding. To prevent further complications such as cramping, nausea, vomiting, and diarrhea, liquids should be infused slowly. Some home care patients with gastric tubes may have their liquids delivered by an infusion pump. Occasionally a gastric tube may become nonfunctional when noncommercial foods are infused through it. This practice is highly discouraged by nutrition experts. Gastric tubes should be flushed, usually with water, after infusing medications or nutritional fluids.

Any abdominal surgery places the patient at risk for development of adhesions. Adhesions are scar tissue that may connect one loop of bowel to another or encircle a segment of bowel, constricting it and resulting in a bowel obstruction. A large-bowel obstruction (ie, obstruction in the colon) usually results from a growth within the bowel rather than adhesions. A small-bowel obstruction occurs when the small intestine becomes blocked. Improperly dissolved medications, food supplements, or the actions of certain types of medications can all lead to bowel obstruction.

Chronically ill patients who receive care at home are especially vulnerable to difficulties with normal elimination, especially normal urinary function. Such patients may require a long-term indwelling urinary catheter. Conversely, patients with neurologic damage may require intermittent urinary catheterization or placement of an indwelling catheter. The bladder is normally sterile, so introduction of any device can

Skill Drill 45-4: Accessing an Implantable Venous Access Device (*continued*)

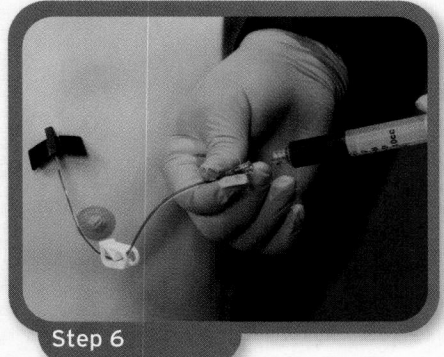
Step 6
Discard the aspirate and obtain blood samples if necessary.

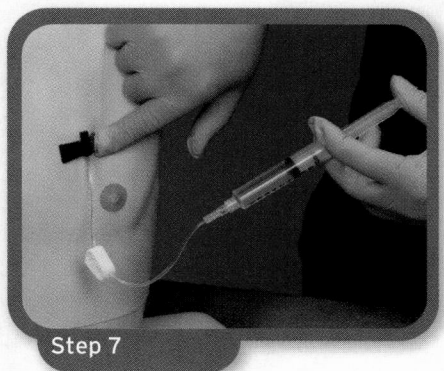
Step 7
Flush the line with normal saline.

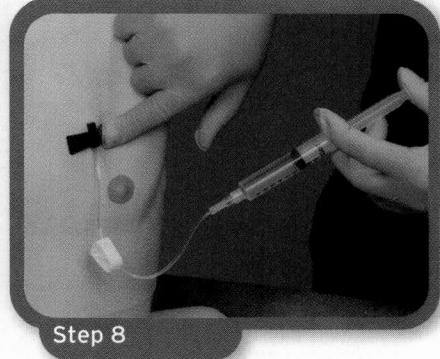
Step 8
Administer medications or fluids as directed.

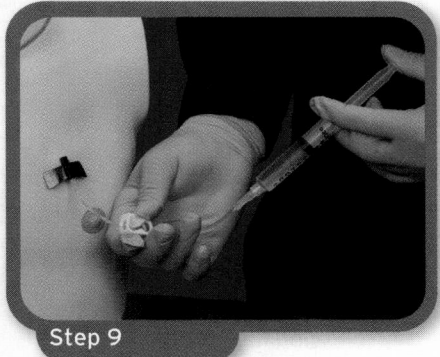
Step 9
Flush the device.

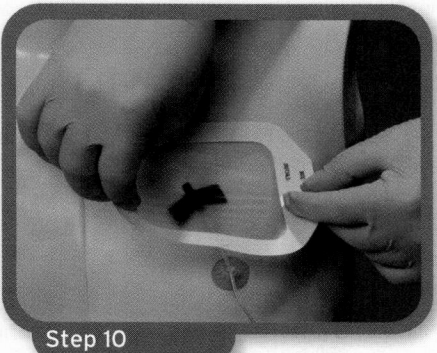
Step 10
Secure the needle with a sterile dressing.

You are the Provider Part 3

You perform a physical examination and find that the patient's abdomen is distended and firm upon palpation. No other significant findings are observed. Unsure of what to make of your clinical findings and the patient's clinical presentation, you decide to contact medical control for guidance.

The physician advises you to catheterize the patient in an attempt to relieve any pressure caused by a full bladder and to transport for further evaluation and management of the blood pressure. While you explain the doctor's recommendation for treatment and transport, the patient's wife goes to get the catheterization kit. The patient informs you that he and his wife have discussed resuscitation measures in the event that they are required and that they wish to have everything attempted.

Reassessment	Recording Time: 12 Minutes
Skin	Flushed, warm, and diaphoretic about the face; cool, pale, and clammy elsewhere
Pulse	52 beats/min, regular
Blood pressure	208/120 mm Hg
Respirations	16 breaths/min, regular
Sao$_2$	98% on room air
ECG	Sinus bradycardia with no ectopy
Pupils	PERLA

4. Why did the doctor recommended catheterizing the patient's bladder prior to transport?

5. Why is it important that the patient's wishes for a full resuscitation be known?

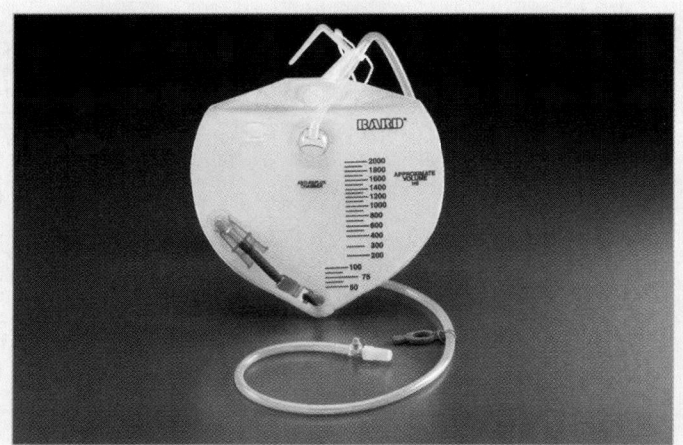

Figure 45-11 Urinary drainage bag.

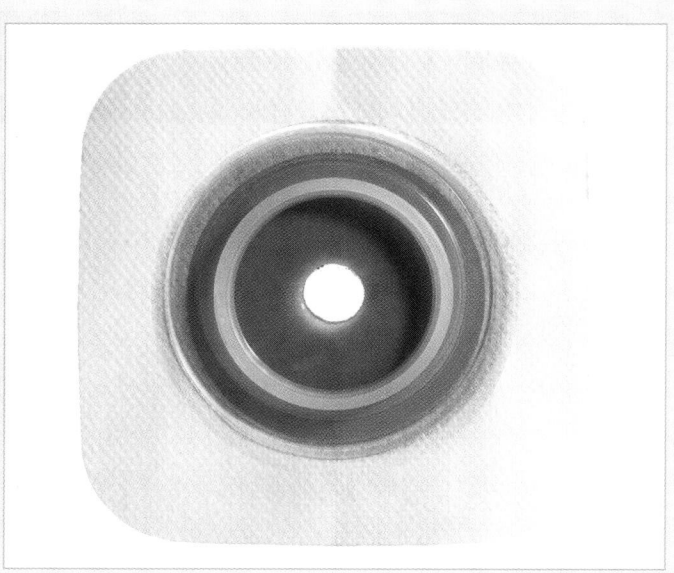

Figure 45-12 Ostomy skin wafer.

Courtesy of ConvaTec. ©/™ indicated a registered trademark of E.R. Squibb & Sons, LLC.

introduce bacteria. Unless the patient is immunocompromised, however, there is low risk that clean (rather than sterile) catheterization will cause an infection **Figure 45-11 ▲** .

Indwelling catheters have a greater likelihood of contributing to urinary tract infections. The bladder is normally closed to the outside by a sphincter at the bladder-urethra junction. Indwelling catheters keep the sphincter open and provide a continuous route of entry for bacteria. Due to the short urethra in the female, women are at greater risk for urinary tract infections than men. Given the ongoing risk of an infection with an indwelling catheter, urosepsis is one of the likely causes of septic shock in such patients.

The urge to urinate occurs when the bladder fills to about 150 mL of fluid. An extreme urge to urinate occurs when approximately 400 mL of fluid fills the bladder. In susceptible individuals (eg, those with a disruption in the spinal cord), a full bladder can lead to dangerously high blood pressure, which places the patient at risk for stroke.

Patients with small-bowel disease may need large portions of the small intestine removed (ileostomy). A stoma is constructed that connects the small intestine to the outside of the abdomen where the patient attaches a collection bag. The intestinal waste from an ileostomy is irritating to skin, as it contains some of the digestive juices. The bag must be emptied frequently.

A colostomy is a surgical opening in the large intestine that is brought to the surface of the abdomen to drain solid waste

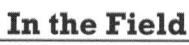

In the Field

Signs of potential failure of a gastrointestinal or genitourinary device in the home care setting include abdominal pain or distention, decreased or absent bowel sounds, bladder distention, dysuria, and changes in urinary output or color.

Figure 45-12 ▲ . The drainage varies from loose (if the colostomy is along the ascending colon) to soft (if the colostomy is along the transverse or descending colon). A temporary colostomy allows the bowel to rest and heal, and is intended to be reversed at a later date. In a permanent colostomy, stool is always diverted to the stoma.

Occasionally, the ureters will be brought to the surface to a stoma, and urine will then drain directly into an appliance. Such an ureterostomy differs from a suprapubic catheter in that the catheter is surgically placed into the bladder. In the latter case, the ureters remain intact and continue to drain the kidneys into the urinary bladder.

Signs and symptoms of a large-bowel obstruction include changes in stool (may be very watery), abdominal distention, and localized pain. Signs and symptoms of a small-bowel obstruction include diffuse pain, nausea, and vomiting (often containing fecal material). Bowel sounds may vary from hypoactive to high pitched and frequent.

A bladder overfilled with urine may appear as abdominal distention. If the bladder is distended, its upper margin can usually be palpated. In abdominal distention, no upper margin will be evident. Urine production depends on factors such as fluid intake, fluid losses other than urine, and the condition of the kidneys. Urine is normally clear yellow and sterile with a slight odor. A strong ammonia smell indicates a urinary tract infection.

Inserting a Nasogastric Tube

To insert a nasogastric tube in an adult, follow the steps presented in Chapter 11. Remember to explain what you are doing to the patient and be gentle.

Skill Drill 45-5: Catheterizing Adult Male Patient

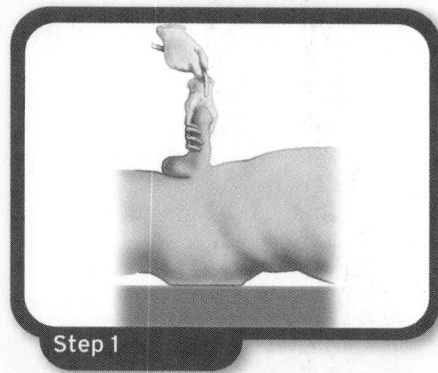

Step 1

Hold the penis at a 90° angle to the body and insert the catheter.

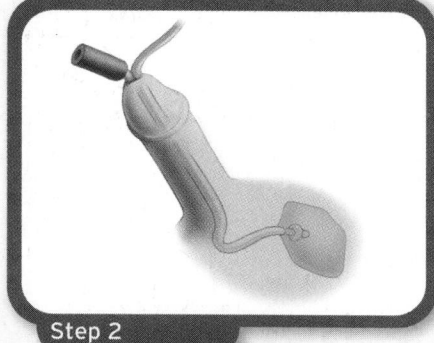

Step 2

Insert the catheter until the Y between the drainage port and the balloon port is at the tip of the penis. For a straight catheter, insert approximately 1″ more.

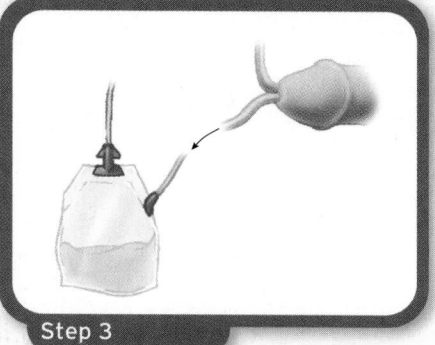

Step 3

Allow urine to drain.

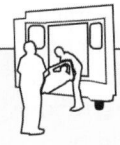

In the Field

When you are assessing bowel sounds, listen for 5 minutes in each abdominal quadrant. Have a quiet atmosphere and auscultate *before* you palpate the abdomen.

Inserting a Catheter

Patients who are not able to void (urinate) on their own may need to be catheterized. Catheters may remain in place (ie, indwelling catheters such as Foley catheters) or may be used intermittently (straight catheters). While the principles for catheterization remain the same for either gender, anatomy differences change the process.

To catheterize adult male patients, follow these steps **Skill Drill 45-5 ▲** :

1. Help position the patient supine with legs slightly spread apart. Maintain privacy as much as possible.
2. Wash your hands and apply a mask, goggles, and clean nonlatex gloves.
3. Open supplies including the urinary catheter and placement kit. Home care patients may reuse their catheters provided that they have been stored in a clean manner. Place necessary supplies onto a clean area within reach. If you are inserting an indwelling catheter, connect a syringe filled with saline to the balloon port. Also connect the indwelling catheter to the drainage system. There are

no connecting ports for either a balloon or a drainage bag on a straight catheter.

4. Wash the penis with soap and water (or have the patient do so if he is able), making sure that the foreskin has been retracted.
5. Coat the end of the catheter with a water-soluble gel. An anesthetic gel is preferred for patients with sensation in the penile area.
6. Hold the penis at a 90° angle to the body and insert the catheter **Step 1** .
7. When urine is evident in the tubing, insert the catheter until the Y between the drainage port and the balloon port is at the tip of the penis. For a straight catheter, insert approximately 1″ more **Step 2** .
8. Inflate the balloon and gently pull back on the catheter until you feel resistance, which indicates that the balloon is snug against the neck of the bladder. This step is unnecessary for a straight catheter.
9. Allow urine to drain. Note the amount and color **Step 3** .
10. To remove a catheter, remove the saline in the balloon port and pull back gently until the catheter is free of the tip of the penis. Never remove an indwelling catheter without using a syringe to remove the saline from the balloon, as it may damage the urinary sphincter. For a straight catheter, simply pull back gently to remove the catheter. Wash according to the home care instructions.
11. Remove your gloves and wash your hands, following BSI precautions.

Skill Drill 45-6: Catheterizing an Adult Female Patient

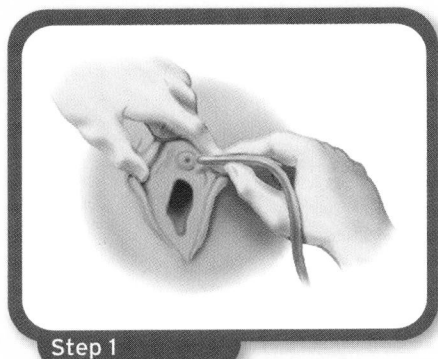

Step 1

Locate the urinary meatus anterior to the vagina and insert the catheter.

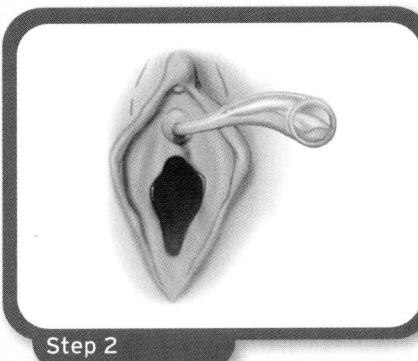

Step 2

When urine is evident in the tubing, insert the catheter another 1″ to 3″.

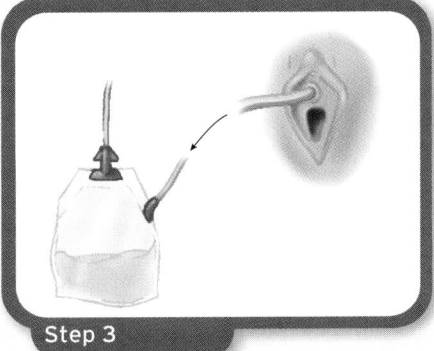

Step 3

Allow urine to drain.

12. If the catheter is to remain in place, secure it to the patient's leg according to the home care instructions.

13. Document the procedure and assessment on the PCR. To catheterize an adult female patient, follow these steps **Skill Drill 45-6 ▲** :

1. Help position the patient supine with legs spread apart or side lying with the top knee flexed. Maintain privacy as much as possible.

2. Wash your hands and apply clean nonlatex gloves.

3. Open supplies including the urinary catheter and placement kit. Home care patients may reuse their catheters provided that they have been stored in a clean manner. Place necessary supplies onto a clean area within reach. If you are inserting an indwelling catheter, connect a syringe filled with saline to the balloon port. Also connect the indwelling catheter to the drainage system. There are no connecting ports for either a balloon or a drainage bag on a straight catheter.

4. Wash the perineal area with soap and water (or have the patient do so if she is able). First cleanse the outer area of the perineum, and then spread the labia minora and thoroughly wash the mucosa surrounding the vagina and the urinary meatus. Dry with a clean towel.

5. Coat the end of the catheter with a water-soluble gel. An anesthetic gel is preferred for patients with sensation in the perineal area.

6. Locate the urinary meatus anterior to the vagina and insert the catheter **Step 1** .

7. When urine is evident in the tubing, insert the catheter another 1″ to 3″ **Step 2** .

8. Inflate the balloon and gently pull back on the catheter until you feel resistance, which indicates that the balloon is snug against the neck of the bladder. This step is unnecessary for a straight catheter.

9. Allow urine to drain. Note the amount and color **Step 3** .

10. To remove a catheter, remove the saline in the balloon port and pull back gently until the catheter is free of the tip of the meatus. Never remove an indwelling catheter without using a syringe to remove the saline from the balloon, as it may damage the urinary sphincter. For a straight catheter, simply pull back gently to remove the catheter. If the catheter is to be reused, it should be cleaned.

11. Remove your gloves and wash your hands.

12. If the catheter is to remain in place, secure it to the patient's leg or abdomen according to the patient's needs.

13. Document the procedure and assessment on the PCR.

Replacing an Ostomy Device

To replace an ostomy device, follow the steps in **Skill Drill 45-7 ▶** :

1. Help position the patient in a comfortable area in which to change the appliance and easily dispose of the contaminated articles.

2. Wash your hands and apply a mask, goggles, and clean nonlatex gloves.

3. Open supplies. Ostomy equipment includes a skin barrier called a wafer and one of several styles of drainage bags. Some bags can be opened along the bottom and emptied at regular intervals; others are sealed around a system similar to a urine drainage bag.

4. Empty/remove the current appliance and dispose of it appropriately **Step 1** .

5. Wash the area around the stoma with soap and water. Cleanse the stoma with water only, being careful not to rub or irritate the area **Step 2** .

6. Place a clean gauze pad over the stoma to prevent contamination of the clean skin with stool or urine (Step 3).

7. Cut the wafer to the correct size using the patient's measurement or tracing. Home care patients usually have the stoma already sized or have a tracing to cut a hole in the wafer large enough for the stoma but keeping exposed skin to a minimum (Step 4).

8. Attach the appliance to the wafer. Be sure the distal end is closed (Step 5).

9. Remove the gauze (Step 6).

10. Remove the paper backing from the wafer (Step 7).

11. Apply the appliance with the stoma centered in the wafer cutout (Step 8).

12. Remove your gloves and wash your hands.

13. Document the procedure and assessment on the PCR.

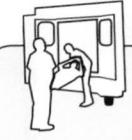

In the Field

Be careful not to cut the ostomy appliance when using trauma shears to cut away clothing. The drainage can contaminate wounds and damage intact skin.

Patients With Wounds and Acute Infections

Wounds associated with trauma or surgery result in a break in the skin. These wounds, which may be either intentional (as with surgery) or unintentional (as during trauma), then undergo healing—that is, regeneration of living tissue.

Factors that affect wound healing include nutritional status, activity level, medications (including use of nicotine, anti-inflammatory drugs, heparin, and chemotherapy), chronic illness or immobility, diabetes, and the presence (or absence) of infection.

Immunosuppressed patients—such as early transplant recipients or individuals with human immunodeficiency virus infection—are at greater risk of acquiring infections, including wound infections. Immunocompromised patients have alterations in their immunity that increase both the risk of infection and the ability to combat infection, especially respiratory infections. Fever is often the only sign of infection in the immunocompromised patient and always requires further investigation. Special care should be taken for protection of these patients.

Drainage from a wound (called exudate) consists of fluid and cells. Serous exudate is a clear, watery drainage. Purulent exudate is pus, which consists of white blood cells, liquefied dead tissue, and bacteria. The color of the exudate often provides a clue about the types of bacteria present. Sanguinous exudate is bloody; fresh blood is light red, while older blood is darker red.

Patients with vascular access devices are at increased risk for infections. Observe the device area for signs of infection, especially a hot to touch, reddened area that may indicate an abscess at the site. Practice good hand hygiene and site care when working with these devices.

Immobile patients with chronic illnesses are at high risk for skin breakdown, leaving them susceptible to infection. Perform a careful assessment of your patient's skin. Assess a surgical or treated wound by noting the following:

- **Appearance.** Healing appears as a pink to reddened area.
- **Size.** Measure the wound. Note any changes in size as described by the patient or caregiver.
- **Drainage.** Observe the color, consistency, odor, and number of gauze pads soaked in a timeframe to help measure the amount of drainage.
- **Swelling.** This can occur throughout the body (generalized) or in a specific area (localized). Generalized swelling or edema is a common sign in severely ill patients.
- **Pain.** Using a pain score, ask your patient to rate his or her level of pain; ask the patient or a family member for any observations of changes in level of pain. Many patients who are chronically ill may not be able to communicate their pain using a traditional 1 to 10 pain score, so be prepared to use a nonverbal scoring tool.
- **Drains or tubes.** Check the amount of drainage.
- **Temperature.** Warm to hot skin indicates a possible infection. Temperature regulation in many chronically ill or fragile patients is poor, however, so patients who have infections may not always feel warm to the touch or have a fever. Ask the patient or caregiver what is considered a normal temperature and what is different, if anything, today.

A wound with minor redness, slight warmth to the touch, and swelling may indicate a superficial infection. A painful reddened area that may have cracks or serous drainage, sometimes with red streaks extending from the area, may indicate that the patient has cellulitis. Patients with a fever and chills with an area that is hot to the touch, has purulent exudate, and is the source of pain may have a more serious infection. Cellulitis is usually treated with antibiotics, rest and elevation of the affected area, and warm compresses. Cellulitis may be more severe and require hospitalization in patients who have venous stasis, diabetes, or who are immunocompromised. If left untreated, wound infections in chronically ill patients may lead to sepsis—a serious systemic infection.

An important complication of wound healing is separation of the edges of the wound, called dehiscence. If the amount of drainage from a wound increases, especially 4 to 5 days after injury, dehiscence is likely.

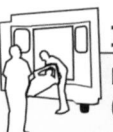

In the Field

Methicillin-resistant *Staphylococcus aureus* (MRSA) is a serious problem in the community, especially among chronically ill patients. MRSA can colonize the skin and body of an individual without causing sickness and, in this way, unknowingly be passed on to other individuals.

Skill Drill 45-7: Replacing an Ostomy Device

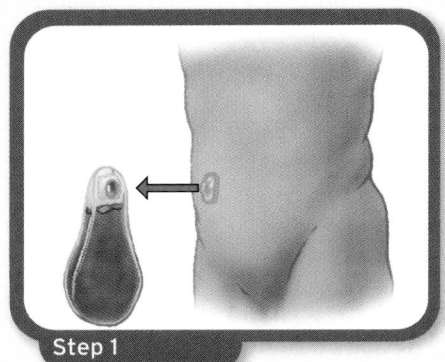

Step 1

Empty/remove the current appliance and dispose of it appropriately.

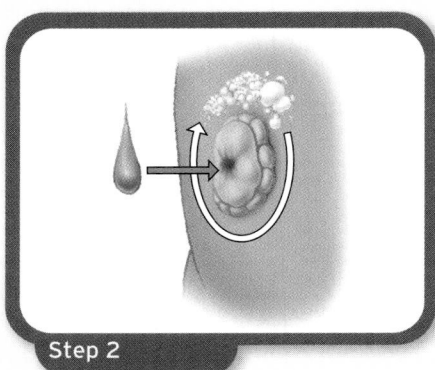

Step 2

Wash the area around the stoma with soap and water. Cleanse the stoma with water.

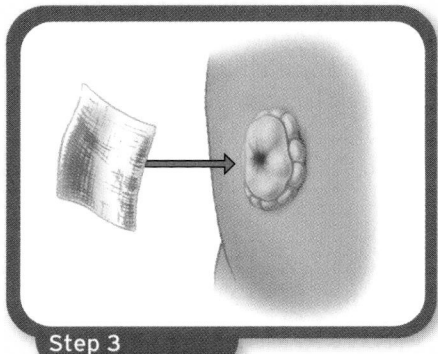

Step 3

Place a clean gauze pad over the stoma.

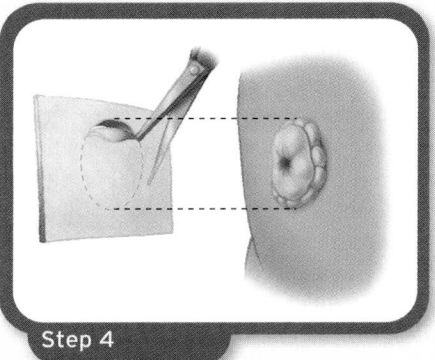

Step 4

Cut the wafer to the correct size using the patient's measurement or tracing.

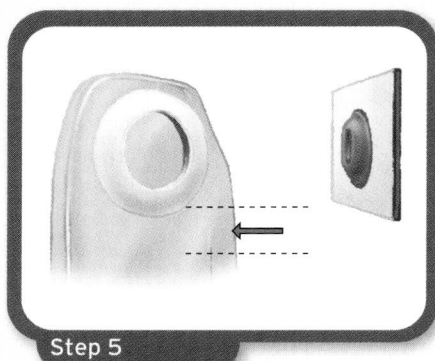

Step 5

Attach the appliance to the wafer.

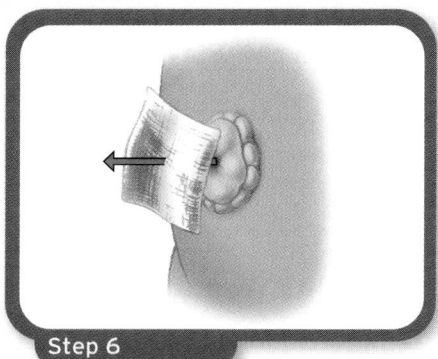

Step 6

Remove the gauze.

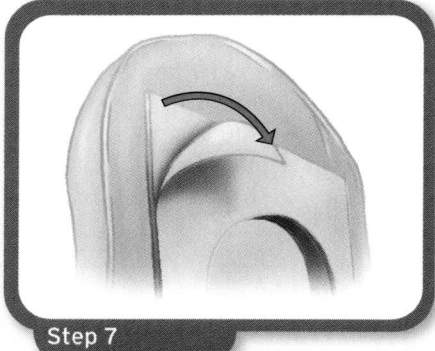

Step 7

Remove the paper backing from the wafer.

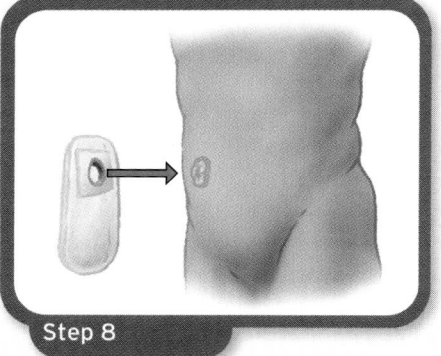

Step 8

Apply the appliance with the stoma centered in the wafer cutout.

Some wounds may be left open and unsutured to promote healing from within. In other cases, sutures or staples are used to hold the edges of a wound together; most are removed 7 to 10 days after repair. In contrast, stay sutures and retention sutures hold both skin and underlying fat or muscle together and may be left in place for 14 to 21 days.

Drains may also be sutured into place to allow liquids to escape and decrease tension on the sutures or staples. Drains are usually flat pieces of tubing that remain open on both ends. One end is placed deep within the wound; the other end lies on the skin, draining onto gauze dressing. Closed wound drainage systems rely on a tubing drain plus some type of negative pressure (suction). This kind of system prevents the entry of microorganisms into the drain and thus into the wound.

Wound Care

After exposing a wound for assessment, you should redress it to prevent further contamination. Encourage the patient to lie still while the wound is redressed. Apply a sterile dressing and secure it to the area prior to transport. This dressing should cover the surface of the wound and the surrounding area and should not be either too tight or too loose. You may need to apply a bulky dressing to a wound to help protect it during transfer and transport.

Always reassess the patient's pain level and tolerance to the dressing following the procedure. Patients with limited mobility may be uncomfortable during movement with a dressing in place. Providing reassurance, direction, and comfort to the patient and caregivers during these procedures will enhance their sense of control and comfort.

Maternal/Child Health Risks

Each year in the United States there are approximately 4 million births. More than a half million infants were born preterm in 2004, and infants were also more likely to be born low birth weight (< 2,500 g). In addition, the percentage of preterm births (infants born at less than 36 weeks of gestation) has increased slightly. Cesarean deliveries are also at an all-time high. Women may deliver at home, or may spend anywhere from a few hours to several days in a health care setting, typically a hospital birthing center. Each of these factors contributes to the increased need for home care for women and infants in the postpartum period.

Complications in the postpartum period include postpartum bleeding, depression, sepsis, pulmonary embolus, and infant septicemia. Postpartum bleeding or hemorrhage is the leading cause of maternal death. This occurs in as many as 10 out of 100 births. When you are obtaining the mother's history, asking her about postpartum bleeding in a previous pregnancy is important as a significant risk factor.

Pulmonary embolus is another complication that may occur in the postpartum period. The risk of pulmonary embolus is increased in both pregnancy and in the postpartum period. The incidence of thromboembolic disease in pregnancy has been reported to range from 1 case in 200 deliveries to 1 case in 1,400 deliveries and is caused by venous stasis, decreasing fibrinolytic activity, and increased procoagulant factors.

Depression that occurs during pregnancy or within a year after delivery is called perinatal depression, most commonly referred to as postpartum depression. During pregnancy the amount of estrogen and progesterone increases greatly. In the first 24 hours after childbirth, the amount of hormones rapidly drops back down to their normal prepregnancy levels. After pregnancy, similar hormonal changes may trigger symptoms of depression. The number of women affected with depression during this time is unknown, but some researchers suggest that depression is one of the most common complications during and after pregnancy. It is often not recognized or treated because normal changes during pregnancy such as fatigue, insomnia, strong emotional reactions, and changes in body weight may occur during pregnancy and after pregnancy. These same symptoms may also be signs of depression. The key to treatment is early recognition and referral.

Infants have immature physiology that can result in an inability to regulate temperature, adapt to respiratory problems, or respond to infection because of poorly functioning

You are the Provider Part 4

The patient's wife was able to catheterize her husband while he sat upright in his wheelchair. The catheter drained 800 mL of urine. An IV line was established in the right antecubital with an 18-gauge needle. During transport you note that the swelling in the patient's abdomen has almost resolved and it is now soft upon palpation. He states that his headache is almost relieved and that he no longer has blurred vision.

Upon arrival to the emergency department, the patient's symptoms have almost resolved. He is monitored in the emergency room and discharged after a short period of observation, with a diagnosis of autonomic hyperreflexia syndrome.

Reassessment	Recording Time: 18 Minutes
Skin	Pale, warm, and dry
Pulse	80 beats/min
Blood pressure	144/82 mm Hg
Respirations	16 breaths/min, unlabored
Sao₂	99% on room air
ECG	Sinus rhythm without ectopy

6. What is the pathophysiology of autonomic hyperreflexia syndrome?

7. What are signs and symptoms of autonomic hyperreflexia syndrome?

immune systems. All of these factors have an impact on sepsis, which is one of the most common causes of infant death.

In 2002, infant death from sepsis was 7 per 1,000 live births. Some pregnancy complications that can increase the risk of sepsis for a newborn include maternal bleeding, maternal fever, infection in the uterus, and premature rupture of membranes. Sepsis in newborns produces few symptoms and is difficult to determine. Frequently, these babies suddenly don't seem to be feeling well or "just don't look right" to those who care for them. Listen to the caregiver: any baby who has a change in mental status should be transported immediately for further evaluation and treatment.

Less than 1% of births occur unexpectedly at home. When an emergency home birth does occur, follow your usual paramedic practice and enjoy the experience. Once the baby has delivered, either before or on your arrival, a newborn examination should be conducted. Most newborns are healthy and need little treatment. Transport decisions should be based on local protocol and family requests. Discuss child safety restraint issues of newborns before you encounter an emergency delivery in the home. The five steps to follow in the approach to assessing a newborn are the same in any setting:

- Dry and warm the baby.
- Clear the airway.
- Assess breathing.
- Assess pulse rate.
- Assess color.

A depressed newborn does not respond to drying, warming, and clearing the airway. These babies require resuscitation.

Pediatric Apnea

Premature newborns or those with congenital heart, lung, or neurologic problems often require home care, including an apnea monitor. Healthy infants may experience periods of apnea, especially during sleep. If the apnea is prolonged, is frequent, or occurs with a drop in pulse rate or a change in skin color or muscle tone, it is not normal. Home monitoring of apnea may be indicated when an infant:

- Has unresolved apnea of prematurity at the time of hospital discharge.
- Has severe gastroesophageal reflux.
- Has a history of an apparent life-threatening event.
- Is the sibling of a baby who had sudden infant death syndrome.

Caregivers are taught to stimulate the infant if the low pulse rate or apnea alarm sounds; you may be called if stimulation doesn't work. Be prepared to provide positive-pressure ventila-

In the Field

False alarms are common with apnea monitors and may be caused by movement, loose lead wires, or improperly placed electrodes. When in doubt, follow your local EMS protocols and have the family contact the manufacturer of the device.

tion and remember that newborns—especially premature babies—have difficulty in controlling their body temperatures. Keep the infant warm, including covering the infant's head.

Hospice/Comfort Care

Patients in hospice care can experience pain and discomfort from tumor growth, treatment modalities (eg, radiation and chemotherapy), immobility, inflammation, or infection. Treatment of hospice patients is based on the type and severity of pain. Patients initially receive around-the-clock anti-inflammatory medications, often coupled with antianxiety or antiemetic agents. When this regimen no longer manages the pain, the patient may receive a mild opioid. A strong opioid may be added later, along with antianxiety and antiemetic medications.

Pain may also be managed by mechanical or electrical means. Transcutaneous electrical nerve stimulators relieve pain by competing for nerve transmission pathways with the painful stimulus. Less pain stimulation reaches the brain, so the patient feels less pain. In addition, simple comfort measures are important in providing pain reduction and comfort to the patient. Turning, positioning, and supporting body parts with blanket rolls or pillows can increase comfort. Maintaining a comfortable room temperature helps. Hands-on or energy-based therapies such as massage may be used.

Many health care providers are concerned that hospice patients may overdose on pain medications. This problem, however, is not as frequent as patients being undermedicated. If you suspect that a hospice patient has received too much medication, you should begin the assessment and treatment as for any other patient. Opioids affect the respiratory drive center, so pay close attention and care to breathing adequacy. Although naloxone can reverse the effects of opioids, the goal in these cases is to enable the patient to breathe sufficiently on his or her own. Complete reversal of the effects of the opioid will return the patient to intractable pain, initiation of the sympathetic response, and a sudden increase in blood pressure and pulse rate.

Progressive Dementia

Dementia is a progressive brain disorder with an insidious onset in which cognitive activities are lost first, followed by physical abilities. Causes of dementia may include Alzheimer's disease, Pick disease, Parkinson's disease, and stroke. Some nutritional disorders, such as Wernicke disease or Korsakoff psychosis, can also cause dementia.

Concerns regarding patients with dementia include injuries resulting from loss of judgment and insight, confusion when using medications, and becoming lost when leaving home or a familiar environment. Caregivers may also be at risk if the patient experiences paranoia. Early dementia can be managed in the home setting, but advanced dementia generally requires nursing home care.

Chronic Pain Management

Pain is a subjective term. *Nociception* is a term that more accurately describes the transmission of stimuli over specific nerve pathways. All nociceptors (ie, pain receptors) begin as free nerve endings and end in the dorsal (ascending) roots of the spinal cord. Some respond to mechanical damage, some to thermal damage, and some to chemical damage. The skin, joints, and musculature are well supplied with pain receptors, whereas the visceral organs have a limited number of pain receptors and the brain has no pain receptors. There are two major types of nociceptors: alpha (fast) fibers, which transmit a sharp, localized type of pain usually associated with an injury, and C (slow) fibers, which transmit a slow pain (often described as burning, throbbing, or achy) typically associated with long-term conditions.

Acute pain occurs immediately after an injury or surgery. Chronic pain occurs long after relief of the initiating cause is achieved; it may also be defined as pain lasting for 6 months or longer. Some research indicates that failure to treat acute pain adequately may lead to chronic pain.

The body perceives pain as a stressor. In response, it activates the sympathetic nervous system, leading to elevated blood pressure, tachycardia, and tachypnea. Energy stores are needed to maintain this sympathetic response, even though they could be better used for healing. Effective management of pain reduces energy consumption and allows for rest and healing.

Home Chemotherapy

Chemotherapy refers to the introduction of either single cytotoxic drugs or combinations of cytotoxic drugs into the body for the purpose of interrupting or eradicating malignant cellular growth. The many side effects of these treatments include alopecia (hair loss), anorexia, fatigue, leukopenia (decreased numbers of leukocytes), thrombocytopenia (decreased numbers of platelets), anemia, and increased risk of infections. During radiation therapy, painful blisters may develop at the treatment site.

Patients receiving chemotherapy routinely take multiple medications. Some of these drugs are given to battle the disease process, while others are intended to manage the symptoms of the side effects of chemotherapy. Analgesic medication patches and antiemetics are commonly prescribed. In addition, peripheral access devices may be surgically placed to aid in the delivery

of these medications. Use of these devices to deliver medication requires specialized training. Follow your local protocol or direction from medical control when using these devices.

Patients with cancer often have seriously depressed immune systems, owing to either the treatment regimen or the disease process. To safeguard patients from infection, wash your hands after contact and wear a mask. Reverse isolation, in which the patient wears a mask, is also suggested.

Transplant Recipients

Organ transplants are considered for the treatment of a failing organ or organs. The paramedic must remember that a patient who has recently undergone a transplant is at risk of infection and take steps to protect the patient—for example, by using reverse isolation, in which the patient wears a mask.

You should encourage transplant patients and caregivers to bring all medications and any other information to the hospital with them if transport is indicated.

Psychosocial Support

Adaptation and adjustment to a chronic illness do not occur all at once. Stages of adaptation and adjustment are varied and individual, and an unexpected event can trigger readjustment needs in a patient thought to have adjusted to his or her condition. When faced with such an illness, individuals are likely to proceed through a sense of loss or mourning that is similar to that experienced by survivors of a loved one's death Table 45-5 ▾ . The goal of adjustment is acceptance of the

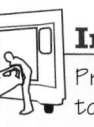

In the Field

Prehospital providers often find it most difficult to work with patients who are in the acceptance stage of the dying process because the patient appears to have given up. In chronic illness or during injury adjustment, this stage may be the easiest. Allow the patient to do as much as possible for himself or herself. Talk with the patient or caregiver so that you are aware of what the patient expects from your treatment.

Table 45-5	Stages of Adjustment to Chronic Illness	
Stages	**Behaviors**	**Paramedic Response**
Denial	Refusal to follow plan	Treat result of refusal; stay nonjudgmental/nonargumentative; educate/reinforce plan
Anger	Verbal or physical abuse	Anger is an acceptable emotion, abuse is not; set limits; retreat if the scene is unsafe; call for assistance; provide care when the scene becomes safe; document
Bargaining	Refusal to follow plan as part of bargain	Restate options; incorporate the bargain as possible
Withdrawal with depression	Profound sadness, reduction in interaction and eye contact, listlessness	Provide reassurance
Acceptance	Adaptive behaviors	Be supportive

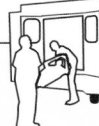

In the Field

A terminally ill patient has the following rights:
1. The right to know the truth
2. The right to confidentiality and privacy
3. The right to consent to treatment
4. The right to choose the place to die and the time of death
5. The right to determine the disposition of his or her body

Special Considerations

Paramedics must often assume the role of health educators. At the appropriate time during a call, encourage the caregiver to prepare a list including the following items:

- Telephone list of all family and friends who should be notified of a change in the patient's condition
- Current medications, ventilator settings, tracheostomy tube type and care, tube feeding type and amount, ostomy type and appliance

Community education includes the need for an emergency information form, such as the one developed by the American Academy of Pediatrics and the American College of Emergency Physicians.

condition and construction of a realistic life plan incorporating the new strengths and limitations.

Patients receiving home care are encouraged to make end-of-life decisions early in their care, if they haven't already. A durable power of attorney (DPOA; also called a health care proxy) allows a patient to appoint someone to make health care decisions in the event that he or she becomes incapacitated. The decisions covered by a DPOA include discontinuation of life support in the event of a terminal illness or injury, discontinuation and removal of life-sustaining equipment in the event of an irreversible coma, and termination of artificial nutrition and hydration. For more information, see Chapter 4.

A living will addresses the patient's wishes that life-sustaining measures be discontinued when there is no hope of recovery. A living will is not recognized in all states and provinces.

Do not resuscitate/do not attempt resuscitation (DNR/DNAR) and do not intubate forms are physician's orders to withhold life-sustaining treatment in the event of cardiac or respiratory arrest. These orders do *not* mean that no treatment should be given. That is, patients should receive pain medication, supplemental oxygen therapy, nutrition, and hydration as needed based on assessment. States and provinces may require that any such order be written on approved forms with witnesses present.

You are the Provider Summary

1. Does treating a patient with chronic health problems affect the way you deliver emergency care?

The emergency care given to a patient with a chronic illness is no different than the care given to a person who is acutely ill. What may change is the method of delivery. For example, medications may be administered through an indwelling catheter such a PICC line or oxygen therapy may be delivered via a tracheostomy tube.

2. What groups of patients are likely to benefit from home care?

Quite a few groups of patients benefit from home health care. As technology advances, the number of illnesses that can be treated at home is on the rise. For example, you might treat patient with spinal cord injuries, chronic neuromuscular disorders such as multiple sclerosis, respiratory illnesses such as cystic fibrosis, and patients with advanced heart failure. One important thing to remember is that there is no age limit to those receiving home health care, as diseases have no age barriers.

3. What type of equipment might you encounter with patients receiving home health care?

Just as the types of disease processes you will encounter are wide and varied, so is the type of equipment you might encounter. Common examples of equipment used in the home setting include tracheostomy tubes, ventilators, CPAP machines, urinary catheters, gastrostomy tubes, and indwelling IV catheters. A good rule of thumb to follow is: if you are unfamiliar with the equipment do not use it! Caregivers are excellent resources for you to use. Ask for help in understanding how a specific piece of equipment works. When you are in doubt how to use a piece of equipment, call medical control for guidance.

4. Why did the doctor recommended catheterizing the patient's bladder prior to transport?

Spinal cord injuries can make the body work in strange ways! In some spinal cord injury patients, the pressure of a full bladder can trigger a significant rise in blood pressure and decrease in blood pressure. If the pressure is not relieved, the hypertension can lead to further damage or death.

5. Why is it important that the patient's wishes for a full resuscitation be known?

Knowing a person's wishes regarding resuscitation is important because the person may have a completely different view of life with a chronic illness or injury. Your patient has had time to adjust to living as a quadriplegic and may view his life as meaningful and fulfilling in a new way. You must abide by your patient's wishes and not try to impose your impressions of how a person's life must be on the patient. Remember, what you may consider as a handicap may be considered a blessing to someone who is living with the condition.

6. What is the pathophysiology of autonomic hyperreflexia syndrome?

Autonomic hyperreflexia syndrome (also called autonomic dysreflexia) is seen in patients with a spinal cord injury above the T6 level. It results from a stimulus being introduced to areas of the body below the spinal cord. Common stimuli are the pressure caused by a distended bladder or rectum. The stimulus travels up the spinal cord until it becomes blocked, preventing it from reaching the brain. As a result, the sympathetic nerve receptors below the injury site cause a rise in blood pressure. This increase in pressure is then detected by the baroreceptors, which stimulate the parasympathetic nervous system in an attempt to lower the blood pressure. Since the signals cannot travel below the injury, the blood pressure remains elevated while the pulse rate decreases. If the blood pressure remains elevated it can become life-threatening.

7. What are signs and symptoms of autonomic hyperreflexia syndrome?

The signs and symptoms include paroxysmal hypertension (systolic pressure can reach as high as 300 mm Hg), pounding headache, blurred vision, sweating above the level of injury, increased nasal congestion, nausea, bradycardia, and a distended rectum or bladder.

Prep Kit

■ Ready for Review

- Breakthrough technologies, newer drugs, and research have combined to increase the average life expectancy. People who might have died of injuries or illnesses 50 years ago may now continue to lead satisfying and productive lives.
- Many of these patients require physical support and care of chronic illnesses—care that may take place in the home setting.
- In rehabilitation care, the focus is on restoration of a person with disabilities to his or her maximum potential along several fronts: physical, social, spiritual, psychological, and vocational areas.
- Chronically ill patients are cared for at home by a wide range of caregivers, who may include family members, unlicensed caregivers, licensed nonprofessional caregivers, licensed professionals, or a combination of these.
- Consumers of home health care are vulnerable, are frequently too sick to advocate for themselves, and may lack advocates. Paramedics have a unique opportunity to assist in securing additional resources, reporting to protective agencies, and offering guidance for in-home injury prevention.
- Many family members who care for chronically ill patients are medically sophisticated and are often the paramedic's best source of information and care guidelines.
- In the home care setting, you may encounter patients who are chronically ill or permanently injured, as well as those who have recently had a hospital stay, surgery, or a high-risk pregnancy. You may also encounter newborns with medical complications. Many of these patients experience similar physical problems regardless of the initial cause.
- Assessment of the chronic care patient follows the standard guidelines. Ask the caregivers how the patient's condition differs today.
- It is important to assess for airway patency in all patients, but especially in patients with artificial airways.
- Patients with respiratory compromise have the inability to adequately ventilate themselves. The home care treatment plan is designed to supplement the patient's loss of respiratory effort. Any stressor can tip the balance, increase the severity of signs and symptoms, and render the current respiratory support inadequate.
- Ventilators mechanically deliver air to the lungs. Home ventilators are smaller than most microwave ovens, use regular household electricity, and may include a battery backup.
- Patients who have chronic cardiovascular disease are often cared for in the home setting. Many patients have cardiac insufficiency or heart failure, an inability of the heart to keep up with the demands placed on it and failure of the heart to pump blood efficiently.
- Central venous catheters are used for many types of home care patients, including those receiving chemotherapy, long-term antibiotic therapy or pain management, high-concentration glucose solutions, and hemodialysis.
- A gastric tube may be placed when a patient cannot ingest fluids, food, or medications by mouth.
- Chronically ill patients and patients with neurologic damage may require a long-term indwelling urinary catheter or intermittent urinary catheterization.

- A wound with minor redness, slight warmth to the touch, and swelling may indicate a superficial infection. A painful reddened area with cracks, serous drainage, or red streaks extending from the area may indicate that the patient has cellulitis. Cellulitis may be more severe and require hospitalization in patients who have venous stasis, diabetes, or who are immunocompromised.
- Complications in the postpartum period that you may see in the field include postpartum bleeding, depression, sepsis, pulmonary embolus, and infant septicemia. You may also be called to assist with pediatric apnea monitors.
- Patients in hospice care can experience pain and discomfort from tumor growth, treatment modalities (eg, radiation and chemotherapy), immobility, inflammation, or infection. Treatment of hospice patients is based on the type and severity of pain.
- Patients receiving home care are encouraged to make end-of-life decisions early in their care. A durable power of attorney allows a patient to appoint someone to make health care decisions in the event that he or she becomes incapacitated.

■ Vital Vocabulary

chemotherapy The introduction of either single cytotoxic drugs or combinations of cytotoxic drugs into the body for the purpose of interrupting or eradicating malignant cellular growth.

chronic obstructive pulmonary disease (COPD) Illnesses that cause obstructive problems in the lower airways, including chronic bronchitis, emphysema, and sometimes asthma.

colostomy Establishment of an opening between the colon and the surface of the body for the purpose of providing drainage of the bowel.

dehiscence Separation of the edges of a wound.

dementia Chronic deterioration of mental functions.

Do Not Intubate Written documentation by a physician giving permission to medical personnel not to attempt intubation.

Do Not Resuscitate (DNR) Written documentation by a physician giving permission to medical personnel not to attempt resuscitation in the event of cardiac arrest.

ileostomy Surgical procedure to remove large portions of the small intestine.

laryngectomy A surgical procedure in which the larynx is removed.

negative-pressure ventilation Drawing of air into the lungs; airflow from a region of higher pressure (outside the body) to a region of lower pressure (the lungs); occurs during normal (unassisted breathing).

oxygen concentrators Large, electrical devices that concentrate the oxygen in ambient air and eliminate other gases

positive-pressure ventilation Forcing of air into the lungs.

purulent exudates Discharge that contains pus.

serous exudates Discharge that contains serum, a thin watery substance.

tidal volume Amount of air inhaled or exhaled during normal, quiet breathing; the volume of one breath.

tracheostomy Surgical opening into the trachea.

ureterostomy The formation of an opening to allow the passage of urine.

Assessment in Action

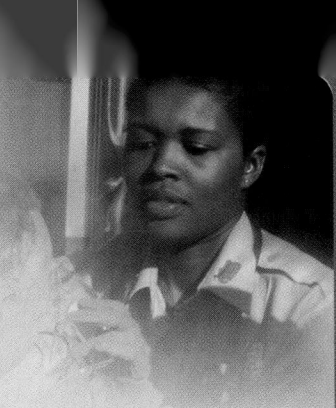

You are dispatched to the home of a 68-year-old man for an altered mental status. When you arrive on scene, you are greeted by his daughter, who tells you that the patient is an insulin-dependent diabetic whose blood sugar is 34. He is also a paraplegic from a traumatic accident 5 years before. His daughter tells you that the night before her father was experiencing upper body pain, which is typical, but it seemed to be worse yesterday. You administer IV therapy and provide dextrose. The patient becomes alert and oriented and refuses transport to the hospital. His only remaining complaint is his increased pain.

1. **Pain can be classified as _____ and _____.**
   A. Acute, surgical
   B. Chronic, traumatic
   C. Acute, chronic
   D. Subjective, stimuli

2. **Chronic pain is defined as:**
   A. pain lasting up to 3 months.
   B. pain lasting longer than 6 months.
   C. pain lasting only 2 months.
   D. pain lasting less than 3 months.

3. **The _____ nervous system is activated in the face of pain.**
   A. sympathetic
   B. parasympathetic
   C. cholinergic
   D. anticholinergic

4. **_____ is the more accurate term describing transmission of stimuli over specific nerve pathways.**
   A. Nociception
   B. Parasympathetic
   C. Sympathetic
   D. Receptor

5. **Management of pain _____, which allows for rest and healing.**
   A. increases energy consumption
   B. reduces energy consumption
   C. does nothing
   D. maintains the sympathetic response

6. **EMS providers must assume:**
   A. the patient is well cared for.
   B. the patient is being abused.
   C. the role of the legal guardian.
   D. the role of health educators.

7. **True or false? Conduct the initial assessment of the patient with chronic illness in the same way as for any other patient.**
   A. False
   B. True

Challenging Question

You are dispatched to the private residence of an 84-year-old man. When you arrive, the family greets you and tells you that the patient called 9-1-1 complaining of chest pain, but the patient has Alzheimer's disease. The family does not believe the patient has any complaints, and they do not want him transported to the hospital.

8. **What course of action should you take?**

■ Points to Ponder

You and your partner are dispatched to the home of a 72-year-old woman with a complaint of respiratory distress. When you arrive on scene, you are greeted by the patient's home health care provider. She tells you that the patient has terminal cancer. For the last 2 days, the patient has experienced an increase in shortness of breath. Her respiratory rate is 32 breaths/min; blood pressure, 100/60 mm Hg; pulse oximetry on room air, 91%; and pulse rate, 110 beats/min, sinus tachycardia on the monitor. The patient has breast cancer with metastasis to the lungs. Her family is in the process of placing the patient into hospice care, but the paperwork has not been completed yet.

Given the history of lung cancer and immunosuppression, what condition do you suspect? Should you transport the patient?

Issues: The Role of the Home Health Care Professional, Dealing With Family and Friends as Home Health Care Providers.

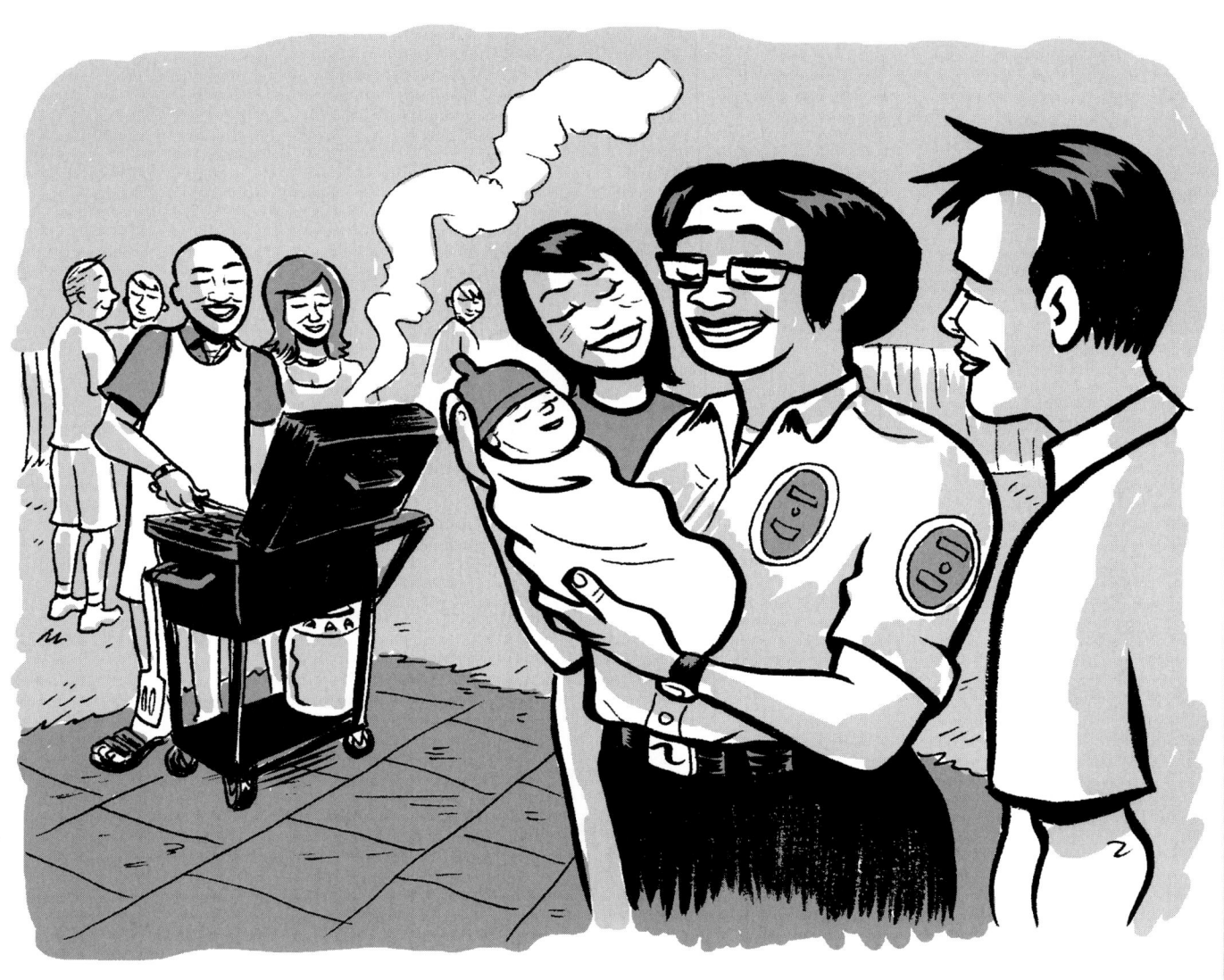

"It's not the ones you lose, but the ones you save by being there just when they needed you. We provide countless numbers of sons and daughters, husbands and wives, fathers and mothers with the precious gift of more time."

—Garry Briese

Operations

Section Editor: David L. Seabrook, MPA, EMT-P

46

Ambulance Operations

Objectives

Cognitive

8-1.1 Identify current local and state standards which influence ambulance design, equipment requirements and staffing of ambulances. (p 46.5)

8-1.2 Discuss the importance of completing an ambulance equipment/supply checklist. (p 46.6)

8-1.3 Discuss the factors to be considered when determining ambulance stationing within a community. (p 46.9)

8-1.4 Describe the advantages and disadvantages of air medical transport. (p 46.14)

8-1.5 Identify the conditions/situations in which air medical transport should be considered. (p 46.14)

Affective

8-1.6 Assess personal practices relative to ambulance operations which may affect the safety of the crew, the patient, and bystanders. (p 46.9, 46.10)

8-1.7 Serve as a role model for others relative to the operation of ambulances. (p 46.10)

8-1.8 Value the need to serve as the patient advocate to ensure appropriate patient transportation via ground or air. (p 46.14)

Psychomotor

8-1.9 Demonstrate how to place a patient in, and remove a patient from, an ambulance. (p 46.11)

Introduction

Driving an emergency vehicle is a tremendous responsibility. Not only do you have to be aware of the safety of your crew and passengers, but you are also responsible for the safe passage of other vehicles you encounter on the road. Activating the lights and sirens does not ensure that you will be heard or understood by other drivers. More importantly, the use of lights and sirens is usually only a request for the right of way.

History of Ground Ambulances

Over the years, much has changed in the way that patients are transported to emergency care facilities. During the French Revolutionary Wars (1790s), Dr. Dominique-Jean Larrey conceived the idea of a mobile transport system for casualties. The first vehicles used for this purpose were horse-drawn wagons called flying ambulances that were part of an ambulance corps. This ambulance corps consisted of a physician, a quartermaster, a noncommissioned officer, a drummer boy to carry bandages, and 24 infantrymen to protect them. Even with such a large entourage they were able to remove victims from the battlefield within 15 minutes   Figure 46-1 ▸ .

The first ambulances in the United States were commissioned in the 1860s. In 1864, Congress enacted "An Act to Establish a Uniform System of Ambulances in the Armies of the United States," which resulted in an organized system of patient transport for the military. Around that same time, civilian hospitals established their own ambulance services for the movement of patients. The first hospital credited with implementing this concept was New York City's Bellevue Hospital. It was not until 1899 that the first motorized vehicle was used. The Michael Reese Hospital in Chicago began operations featuring motorized travel, with vehicles that had a top speed of 16 mph. In 1937, the Hess and Eisenhardt Company built the first commercial ambulance.

Current standards for ambulances are determined by the US General Services Administration. Design and manufacturing specifications are outlined in the DOT KKK 1822 federal guidelines. These guidelines are reviewed and updated every 5 years based on recommendations from manufacturers and operators of the vehicles.

The original guidelines required that all ambulances be painted Omaha orange and white, allowing them to be easily recognized by other drivers. More recently, standards have been relaxed to allow for a variety of personalized paint schemes. The KKK Standards also established three major ambulance designs   Figure 46-2 ▾   and   Table 46-1 ▸ .

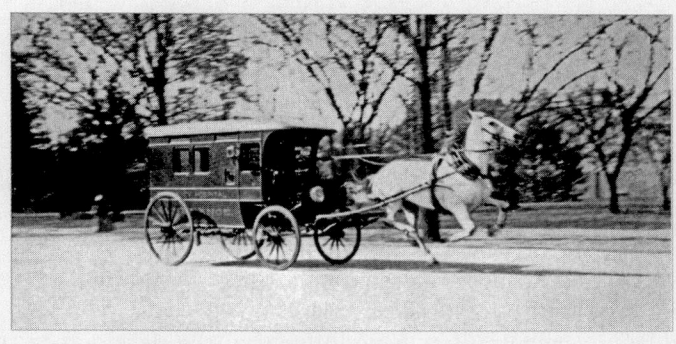

Figure 46-1 Horse-drawn carriage ambulance.

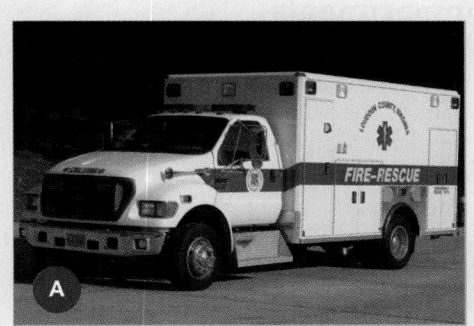
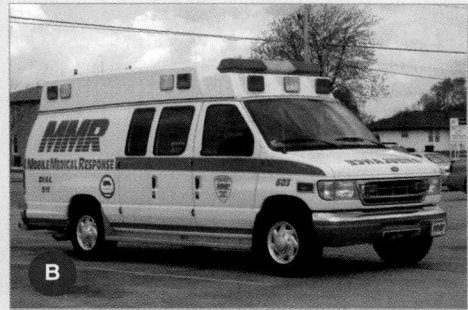
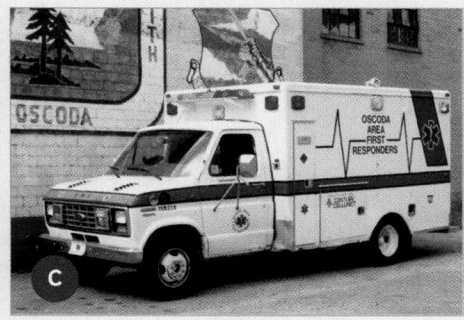

Figure 46-2 **A.** Type I (heavy duty). **B.** Type II. **C.** Type III.

You are the Provider Part 1

You and your partner have been dispatched to the scene of a multiple-vehicle collision on the interstate. Dispatch advises you that they have received several calls regarding the crash, with the potential for multiple victims. It is 3 PM and you realize that the school system in your area will be busy with traffic no matter which route you take.

1. What are some of the potential hazards you may encounter en route to the scene?
2. What dangers must be considered when approaching the scene with regard to parking and personnel protection?

Table 46-1	Basic Ambulance Designs
Type I	Conventional, truck-cab chassis with a modular ambulance body that can be transferred to a newer chassis as needed
Type II	Standard van, forward-control integral cab-body ambulance
Type III	Specialty van, forward-control integral cab-body ambulance

Improvements made to emergency vehicles over the years have not only made them safer for EMS personnel, but also more comfortable. Given the amount of time that personnel spend in their vehicles, even small improvements (eg, increased headroom in the patient compartment and safety nets on the squad bench) can make it easier to perform patient care activities with less fear of injury. Before padded cabinet corners were used, for example, many paramedics were injured when the vehicle was in motion.

Ambulance Equipment

The patient compartment of an ambulance can seem like a complicated place to someone who is not acquainted with the prehospital profession. Every inch of space is dedicated to storing or securing the equipment it takes to do the job well. Much like a jigsaw puzzle, everything must fit tightly together to prevent injury, yet be easily accessible.

Many organizations have influenced the development of the supplies and equipment carried on today's units. The Occupational Safety and Health Administration (OSHA) makes recommendations regarding infection control practices to include all areas of personnel protective equipment, sharps containers, and disinfecting equipment. The American College of Surgeons (ACS) developed the first standardized list of equipment to be carried on an ambulance in 1970 and continues to update these lists as technological advances are made in the field.

Checking the Ambulance

The paramedic must make sure that the ambulance carries the proper equipment. Getting ready to respond is just as important as providing patient care. The crew is also responsible for ensuring that the unit is capable of responding safely and efficiently to calls.

At the beginning of each shift, crew members must check the ambulance to ensure the proper equipment is available and in good working order. Each time supplies and equipment are used, they should be properly cleaned or replaced and returned to service for the next call. Medication expiration dates must be checked regularly to confirm that they have not

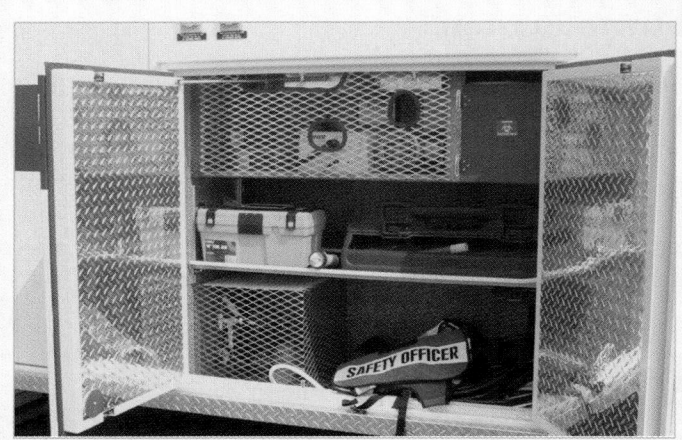

Figure 46-3 Equipment found in outside compartments.

Documentation and Communication

Because the mechanical aspects of emergency work such as driving and moving patients have an impact on your safety and the safety of others, your service should have specific procedures for daily inspections. Following these procedures protects you physically, and documenting your compliance is an important legal protection. Procedures should call for dating and either signing or initialing the check sheets. Store these sheets where they can be found later if needed.

expired. In addition, diagnostic equipment, such as defibrillators and pulse oximeters, must be tested or calibrated regularly.

Ambulance Compartments

All compartments in the ambulance should be checked regularly, both inside and out. Most ambulances carry stabilization and splinting equipment in the outside compartments for easy access when speed may be an important factor in patient care Figure 46-3 ▲ . Medications and temperature-sensitive equipment are generally stored in the patient compartment area. The following list gives some of the essential equipment that should be found on all emergency ambulances:

- Airway and ventilation equipment
- Basic wound care supplies
- Monitoring devices (eg, blood pressure cuffs, pulse oximeter, electrocardiogram monitor/defibrillator)
- Orthopaedic injury stabilizers
- Childbirth supplies
- Patient transfer equipment
- Medications

Understanding Your Ambulance

An ambulance needs to be able to do four things: start, steer, stop, and stay running Figure 46-4 ▶ . Any threat to one of

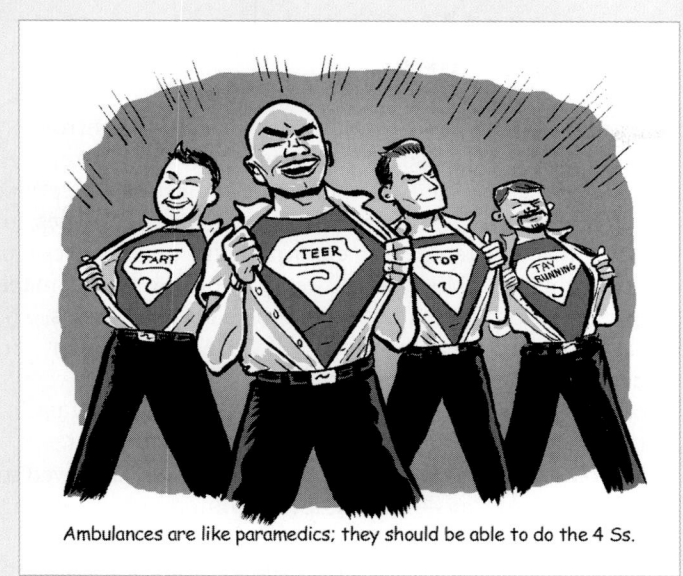

Ambulances are like paramedics; they should be able to do the 4 Ss.

Figure 46-4

the "four Ss" should prompt the operator to put the vehicle out of service immediately. Two other key functions that are especially important in extreme weather are adequate visibility (the wipers and lighting systems) and the internal environmental controls (heating and air conditioning).

Check It *Before* You Drive It

A standard daily checklist is essential to ensure the ambulance is in good operating order. The daily check should begin with a walk-around inspection to identify unreported body damage, major leaks, inoperative lighting, or damaged tires. A formal mechanical checklist should then guide you through a system-by-system inspection.

An operator should check the fuel levels first (many ambulances carry two fuel tanks). Next, the operator should check the motor oil prior to starting the engine. A gasoline-powered V8 motor typically contains 6 quarts; a diesel motor contains more than 12 quarts (all of which are critical to functioning). Make certain to consult your ambulance's owner's manual to learn the specifics of the engine. Check the oil not only to determine the level, but also for quality. Transmission fluid is often checked with the motor running and the gear selector in "park."

Lubricants of all kinds should feel slippery between the fingers, should appear clean, and should smell like fresh oil. Motor oil should be yellow or amber in a gasoline engine and may be gray or black in a diesel engine. It should never smell like fuel, which indicates that fuel is diluting the lubricant.

Transmission and steering fluids should be pink or yellow and should not smell like charcoal, which indicates that the fluids are burned. Brake fluid should be clear or yellow when fresh, but may be amber after a few years of service. Coolant may be either red or bright yellow-green. It is better to not uncap the brake fluid reservoir (because brake fluid absorbs moisture from the atmosphere) or the coolant reservoir, which

is pressurized (because hot coolant can expand rapidly and cause burns).

Look for leaks on the ground under the vehicle and inspect the inner surfaces of the tires to identify leakage of brake fluid or rear axle oil. The presence of water on the ground (eg, at the right front corner of the vehicle) is often a normal occurrence when the air conditioner has been operating.

Battery terminals should be clean, and the top surfaces of the batteries should be dry. The system voltage indicates battery condition at rest and alternator condition with the engine running. At rest, it should be between 12 and 12.5 volts; with the engine running, it should be between 13.5 and 14.5 volts. If the voltage rises to 15 volts or higher with the engine running, the alternator's voltage regulator has failed and should be replaced immediately. The ammeter measures electric current flow and indicates the condition of the battery and alternator simultaneously.

An odor like sewer gas may indicate that a battery has been boiling, perhaps because the system voltage is too high or the battery's resistance has dropped. An automotive battery is filled with concentrated sulfuric acid. When it boils, it produces sulfur dioxide (causing the odor) and pure hydrogen (odorless but highly explosive). The odor of sulfur dioxide should prompt you to take the vehicle out of service immediately, leave the hood closed, and avoid starting the engine.

Checking the brake and back-up lights requires the assistance of a second person unless the ambulance is backed up to a reflective surface like a window. Both are as essential to safe driving as the rest of the external lighting.

Check It *While* You Drive It

An ambulance has about a dozen different ways of warning you before something important fails.

Belt noise is a chirping or squealing sound, synchronous with engine speed (not road speed). It is usually related to a load on one of the appliances operated by a drive belt—the power steering pump, the water pump, the vacuum pump (in a diesel), or the alternator. Belt noise is always significant and will eventually keep an ambulance from operating. It does not necessarily warrant taking a unit out of service immediately.

Brake fade is a sensation that an ambulance has lost its power brakes. Its most common causes are overheating of brake surfaces, loss of vacuum, loss of brake fluid, wet or greasy brake drums, or a failed master cylinder. Even a single instance of brake fade warrants taking your vehicle out of service immediately.

Generally, you should not hear, smell, or feel a vehicle's brakes, with occasional exceptions. Cold brakes may squeak intermittently in wet weather. Some kinds of brake pads are equipped with "tell-tale tabs"—small aluminum projections that are designed to rub on the disk surfaces and squeak, warning an operator when the pads are nearing the end of their useful life. Otherwise, a consistent squeaking or grinding sound warrants immediate attention by a mechanic.

Brake pull is a sensation that, when you depress the brake pedal, someone is trying to jerk the steering wheel to the left or right. It can indicate brake fluid or grease on a brake pad, or it can result from a serious mechanical malfunction. Remove the vehicle from service immediately.

Drift is a finding that when you let go of the steering wheel, the vehicle consistently wanders left or right. Any vehicle may normally drift very slightly to the right, because most roads are built with a crown in the center (so water drains toward the gutters). A vehicle should not consistently drift to the left, however.

Steering pull is a persistent tug on the steering wheel that you can feel as the ambulance "drifts" to one side or the other. Its most common cause is uneven tire pressures (possibly a flat tire). Steering pull can also be caused by one or more misaligned wheels or another mechanical problem. It can cause loss of control in the event of a sudden stop. A vehicle's steering geometry is complex. To allow for its adjustment, the entire front suspension system is held together by clamps. Misalignment can occur when a vehicle hits a curb and dislodges one or more of these clamps. The result may be control problems as well as tire damage in short order.

A pulsating brake pedal—an up-and-down motion of the brake pedal during deceleration—is an abnormal condition, especially at low speeds. A pulsing brake pedal usually indicates warped brake rotors or drums, but can also suggest a bent wheel. This motion can be severe when the brakes are hot. This condition always warrants service.

Normally, little effort should be adequate to steer an ambulance. Excessive effort to steer is therefore a serious finding and can be caused by inadequate steering fluid or a failed power steering pump or drive belt.

Steering play is a sensation of looseness or sloppiness in a vehicle's steering. This finding is important when accompanied by clunking or banging noises during steering, and it should never be noticeable in a new vehicle. This problem is typically caused by wear, but it can also result from underinflated tires. This situation warrants immediate inspection of the ambulance.

Tire squeal is a singing sound that occurs when you turn the vehicle, especially at parking speeds. Squealing is normal on very smooth concrete, but not on asphalt. The most common cause is underinflated tires, but it can also result from misaligned wheels, especially in the presence of other signs. This situation warrants a mechanic's attention as soon as possible.

Wheel bounce is a vibration, synchronous with road speed, that you can feel in the steering wheel (suggesting a front wheel) or driver's seat (rear wheel). Wheel bounce is usually detectable at freeway speeds over 45 miles per hour. It suggests a defective shock absorber, a bubble in a tire, or an improperly balanced wheel.

Wheel wobble is a common finding at low speeds when a vehicle has a bent wheel. You normally detect wobble in the steering wheel if it involves a front wheel, or in the driver's seat if it is in the rear wheel. Potholes are the most common cause.

Ambulance Staffing and Development

Ambulance staffing has been a major source of controversy over the past decade. Escalating costs for medical care, fuel, and the financial burden of operating an ambulance service have prompted the development of alternative strategies for managing EMS systems. For example, the development of "high-performance EMS systems" represents an effort to maximize personnel productivity and minimize response times. The key factors that are analyzed in an effective, cost-efficient service are summarized below.

- **Response times.** High-performance systems typically use a fractile response time standard in which a significant fraction (usually 90%) of all responses must be achieved in an established time—for example, 8 minutes or less in an urban area. These standards are based on the recommendations of the Commission on the Accreditation of Ambulances (CAAS).
- **Productivity.** The EMS provider measures how many patient transports per hour each ambulance accomplishes (known as "unit-hour utilization").
- **Unit costs.** Determined by the cost to respond to each call as well as the actual number of hours the units were actively operating, these costs include the paramedics' salaries plus the operational cost of vehicles and equipment (gas, routine maintenance, and repairs).
- **Taxpayer subsidies.** The local government may make a financial commitment to help lower user fees. Some services also offer annual subscription fees in return for free services during the year.

Ambulance and EMS Systems

In the United States, most first-response emergency medical service is delivered by fire department personnel who are cross-trained in EMS. Some first responders are trained in BLS; others have ALS training. These responders may be paid or volunteer, and they typically respond from fire stations located throughout the community. Some fire services also operate the ambulance service.

In other communities, the ambulance service is provided by a private, for-profit enterprise. In some areas, a public agency (not part of the fire department) delivers ambulance service; this system is known as the third service delivery model. Another type of model involves a public–private partnership.

Staffing of ambulances may be variable between and within EMS systems. Some systems have two or even three paramedics on each ambulance. Others staff ambulances with EMT-Bs. Some systems employ a tiered response system that attempts to assign ALS ambulances only where they are needed.

System Status Management

System Status Management (SSM) is a concept that was developed by Jack Stout in 1983. The goals of SSM are to maximize efficiency and reduce response time. SSM uses historical data to determine ambulance service demands and then tries to take fluctuations in demand into consideration when organizing service. For example, an increased demand for service may be noted during certain hours of the day or in certain geographic locations. These demands are termed <u>peak loads</u>. In an urban area, the demand for ambulance service may be higher during the daytime but lighter during the night. SSM attempts <u>strategic deployment</u> of ambulance resources in order to minimize response times. The strategic deployment of an ambulance to a location, known as <u>posting</u>, can take advantage of developments in satellite vehicle location and GPS technologies.

Another component of SSM is peak demand staffing. Shift schedules are designed to provide a sufficient number of ambulances during peak load hours. For example, more ambulances might be staffed between noon and 6 PM than between midnight and 6 AM. One potentially negative aspect of SSM is the toll that it can take on personnel, who have less time to get out of the vehicle and relax in the ambulance station between calls.

Ambulance Stationing

The goals for establishing ambulance stations are to maximize efficiency and to minimize response times. In most urban and suburban areas, the distance factor may not be as important as the call volume. In a rural setting, both availability of first responders and distance may be equally important. Also, the district may have special facilities that create increased ambulance demand—long-term care facilities, for example. Other considerations in the design of ambulance stations include the need for maintenance of vehicles and equipment, storage, classrooms for training and meetings, and sleeping quarters for personnel who spend the night.

The Paramedic as an Emergency Health Care Professional

Paramedics working on an ambulance have a responsibility to conduct themselves as professionals. Even in times of severe stress or fatigue, the paramedic should act as an advocate for the patient. He or she should always seek to deliver high-quality care without regard to time of day,

Notes from Nancy
Even in times of severe stress or fatigue, you should act as an advocate for the patient.

the location of the call, or the appearance or conduct of the patient. Remember, you represent your service to the public, to your colleagues, and, most importantly, to patients and their families in their time of need.

Emergency Vehicle Operation

All the advances made in prehospital care mean nothing if you never arrive. Driving an emergency vehicle requires you to be aware of *all* dangers on the roadway, including some that are not factors when you drive your private vehicle. Knowing where to look for these dangers is your responsibility whenever you get behind the wheel of an ambulance.

Collision Prevention

According to the Department of Highway and Safety Administration's Fatality Analysis Reporting System (FARS), 300 fatal crashes involving ambulances occurred over the period 1991–2000 `Figure 46-5 ▼`. The most common causes for collisions were that the ambulance was not traveling in the proper lane or the operator was driving too fast.

A troubling fact is that nearly half of ambulance drivers involved in a collision had an earlier collision or moving violation in the 3 years prior to the incident. It is the responsibility of every ambulance service to ensure that personnel are not only safe drivers *before* they begin employment, but are given emergency vehicle operation courses *after* they are hired. Even

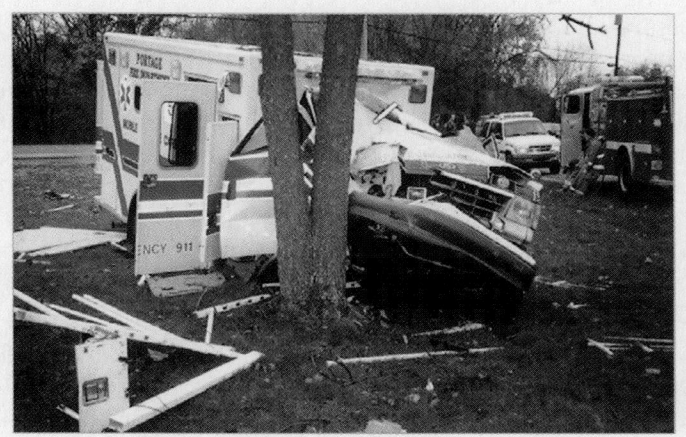

Figure 46-5 A wrecked ambulance.

You are the Provider Part 2

En route to the call you have received information from dispatch that the first responders are on the scene and report that you have a total of six vehicles involved with at least four pediatric patients with various degrees of injury.

3. How will knowing there are multiple patients, including children, affect your driving?
4. Where should the ambulance be positioned at the scene of a highway incident if you are the *first* to arrive?
5. Where should the ambulance be positioned at the scene of a highway incident if you are *not* the first to arrive?

46.10

if you are given specific exemptions to some traffic laws in an emergency, this privilege must be used sparingly.

Due Regard

Every state has laws regarding the use of lights and sirens when operating an emergency vehicle. The concept of due regard is an important part of those laws. Due regard means that you may use lights and sirens as a means to alert other drivers that you are in an emergency mode, but it does not exempt you from operating your vehicle with due regard for the safety of others.

Use of Escorts

It is typically *not* a good idea to follow another emergency vehicle, such as a police car, through traffic as an escort. Many drivers will see only the first set of lights and sirens and assume that the way is clear once that vehicle has passed. If you are following another emergency vehicle, leave enough space between the vehicles so that other drivers (and you) have enough time to react and safely stop should someone pull in front of you unexpectedly.

Another potential danger occurs when family members follow closely behind you on the way to the hospital. Both the ambulance and other drivers may have difficulty seeing the vehicles that are following. If you need to stop suddenly, there may be no time to react and the vehicle could collide with the ambulance. Instruct family members before you leave the scene that they cannot drive closely behind you.

Use of Lights and Sirens

Despite improvements in the sophistication of 9-1-1 answering systems and in the accuracy of telephone triage protocols, most EMS ambulances use their lights and sirens most of the time when responding to calls. In contrast, the decision to use lights and sirens when transporting patients to the hospital calls for judgment on the part of the paramedic. Only when transporting critical patients is the added hazard warranted. Even then, you must proceed with due regard for everyone's safety.

Driving to the Scene

When dispatched to an emergency, the paramedic must decide which route will be used to arrive at the scene safely. Avoid areas of heavy traffic if possible. School zones are especially dangerous at the beginning or ending of classes and should be avoided if possible. Be aware of construction zones in your area as well as railroad crossings. Know the best routes in your district before you head out.

The type of call can sometimes affect how you respond to it. When you hear that the call involves children or a severe trauma potential, you may want to drive with less caution, feeling that speed is more important than safety. Nothing will speed up a driver's adrenalin more than hearing that the call involves another public safety worker. As a professional, you must not let the nature of the call affect your judgment—always drive with caution.

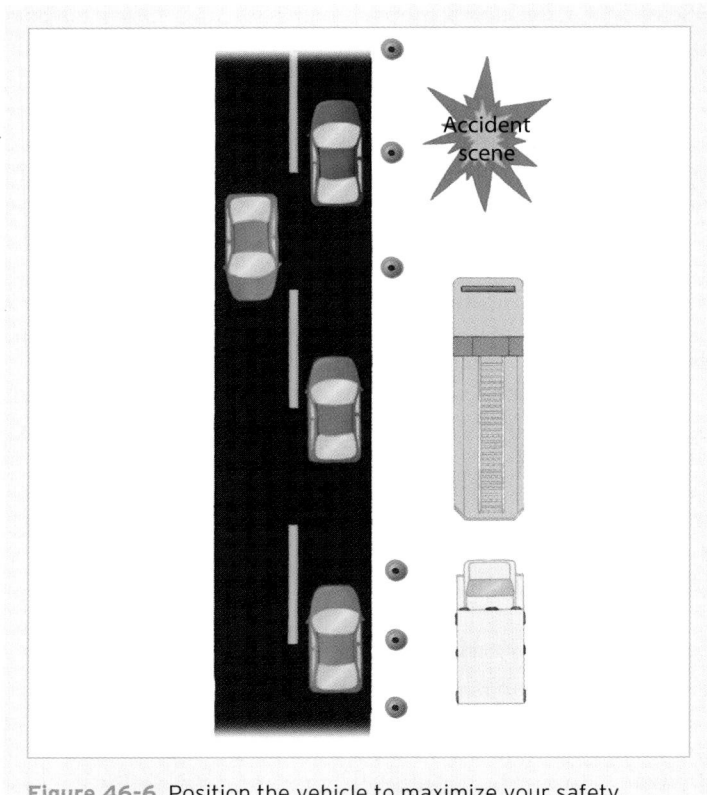

Figure 46-6 Position the vehicle to maximize your safety.

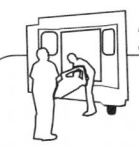

In the Field

Always brake in a straight line!

Parking at an Emergency Scene

Sometimes the general public complains about the way EMS inconveniences other drivers. It may be difficult to understand why people object to blocked roads when paramedics are working diligently to save people's lives. However, sometimes the ambulance *is* parked in such a way that it unnecessarily impedes traffic flow. If you need to park an ambulance in such a way to block a traffic lane for safety reasons, do it. At the same time, however, maintain concern for others who are not involved in the incident. For example, if you are parking in an apartment complex, be aware that other people may need to leave while you are inside and try not to block parked vehicles **Figure 46-6 ▲**.

When parking off the side of the road, you must be aware of the terrain **Figure 46-7 ▶**. In dry weather, the heat from underneath the vehicle could start a grass fire. In wet weather, the weight of the ambulance makes it susceptible to sinking into mud and getting stuck.

Parking on a roadway at night is especially dangerous. Some drivers may have their attention distracted by the scene,

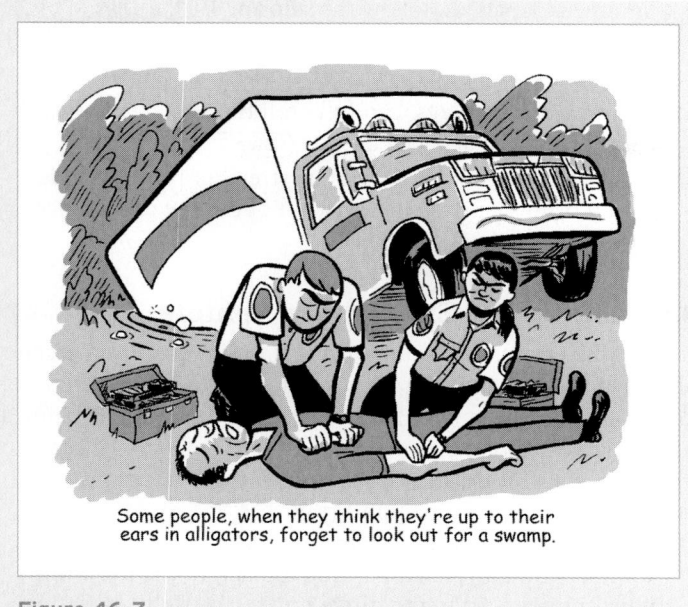

Some people, when they think they're up to their ears in alligators, forget to look out for a swamp.

Figure 46-7

Always secure the patient, either on a stretcher or in a seat, with shoulder and lap belts.

A person who is accompanying the patient should usually ride in the front passenger seat with seatbelt secured. There are reasonable exceptions to this rule, of course—for example, if the paramedic wants to keep the parent of a young child in the child's view or if the patient needs someone to translate what you say. When police presence is required, as when transporting a prisoner, the officer may need to ride in close proximity to the patient. In all cases, the riders should be secured into restraint devices, if possible. When transporting multiple patients in one ambulance, it is generally wise to load the most seriously injured last so that they will be unloaded first.

Depending on how the ambulance is equipped, follow the steps in **Skill Drill 46-1 ▼** to load a patient into an ambulance.

1. Tilt the head end of the main frame upward and place it into the patient compartment with the wheels on the floor. The two additional wheels that extend just below the head end are attached to the main frame and will enable this movement **Step 1**.

and they may drift toward and collide with a parked emergency vehicle. Sometimes it may be safer to use your emergency flashers instead of all the overhead flashers. Likewise, to avoid blinding oncoming traffic, it may be better to turn off the emergency vehicle's headlights when parked, especially if you are on a two-lane road.

Always wear visible protective clothing when you get out of the vehicle on roadways. Reflective vests are lightweight and have the added benefit of increasing visibility during the day as well as at night. Heavy protective clothing should also be considered when responding to collisions where extrication is being performed.

Loading and Unloading the Patient

When you are loading or unloading the ambulance, care must be taken to ensure that the patient is moved safely and quickly. Most patients will be loaded into the ambulance while on the stretcher. However, some can be allowed to enter the patient compartment with little assistance from the paramedic if it is safe to do so.

Skill Drill 46-1: Loading the Patient

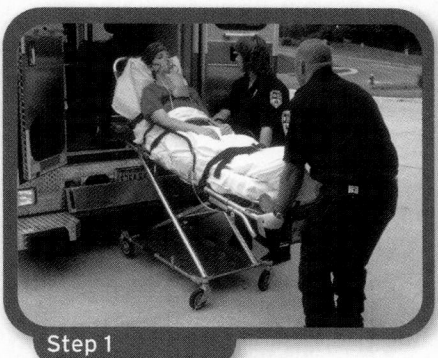

Step 1
Tilt the head of the cot upward, and place it into the patient compartment with the wheels on the floor.

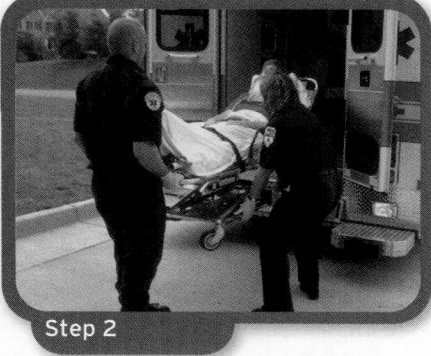

Step 2
The second paramedic on the side of the cot releases the undercarriage lock and lifts the undercarriage.

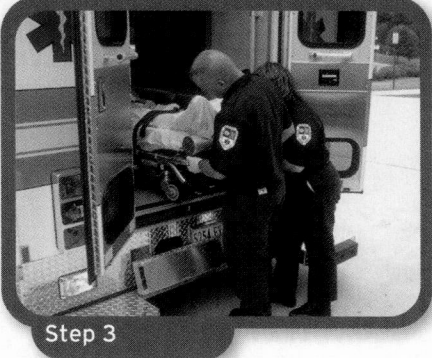

Step 3
Roll the cot into the back of the ambulance.

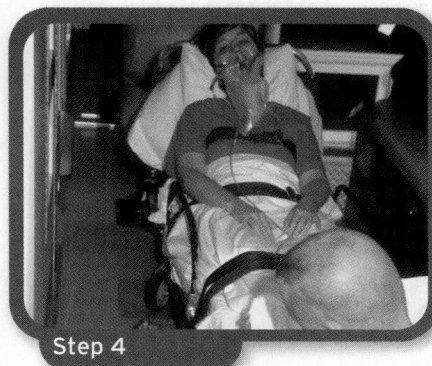

Step 4
Secure the cot to the brackets mounted in the ambulance.

2. With the patient's weight supported by the two head-end wheels and the paramedic at the foot end of the cot, move to the side of the main frame and release the undercarriage lock to lift the undercarriage up to its fully retracted position. The wheels of the undercarriage and the two head-end wheels of the main frame will now be on the same level (Step 2).

3. Roll the cot the rest of the way into the back of the ambulance, where it will rest on all six wheels (Step 3).

4. Secure the cot in the ambulance with the strong clamps that fasten around the undercarriage when the cot is pushed into them. The clamps are located in a rack on the floor or side of the patient compartment (Step 4).

Most ambulances have a system whereby one person can load the stretcher onto the ambulance. If this is the case, the ambulance is placed in the raised "load" position at the rear of the rig. Place the wheels on the head of the stretcher into the rig, and push forward while your partner lifts the wheels of the stretcher. Visually check to make sure all locks are engaged. Be sure to follow your district's protocols.

To unload a patient, follow the steps in (**Skill Drill 46-2** ◄):

1. Ensure that the patient is secured to the stretcher (Step 1).

2. Unlock the head and foot locks (Step 2).

3. Lifting with your legs, carefully roll the stretcher forward until the undercarriage engages (Step 3).

4. With your partner steadying the stretcher from the side, gently bring the stretcher forward out of the ambulance (Step 4).

Backing Up the Emergency Vehicle

Most EMS services have established a policy about emergency vehicle back up. Backing up a vehicle is the most common source of vehicle damage and may result in costly repairs. If possible, avoid situations in which the ambulance will have to be backed up. If it must be done, follow these rules:

- Use a spotter to guide you (**Figure 46-8** ▶).
- Agree with the spotter *before* you place the vehicle in reverse. You may be attempting to back to the left while your spotter is trying to direct you to the right.
- Keep your spotter in view at all times. If you lose sight of the spotter, stop until he or she is back in your line of sight.
  - Agree on hand signals with your spotter before moving. Some people have different ideas of which gesture means "Stop."
  - Keep your window cracked or rolled down when in motion. This may allow you to hear people warning you of unseen dangers.
  - Do a walk-around before getting behind the wheel and look up as well as down. Objects in the ground may not be visible once you start backing up.
  - Use audible warning devices whenever the ambulance is in motion.

Use of Safety Restraints

Standard operating procedures should mandate that everyone in the ambulance use seatbelts, not just the patient. Children should not be transported on the stretcher unless properly restrained. It is not advisable to use adult seatbelts for children. Many pediatric transport devices are available, and they

---

Skill Drill 46-2: Unloading a Patient

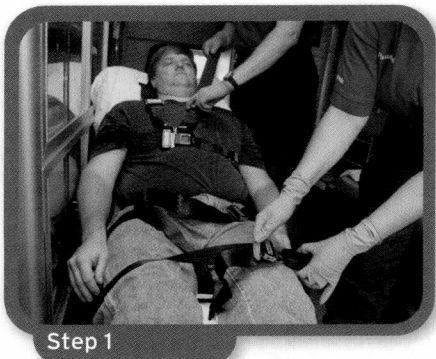

Step 1

Ensure that the patient is secured to the stretcher.

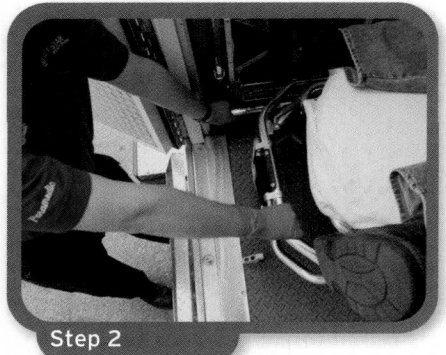

Step 2

Unlock the head and foot locks.

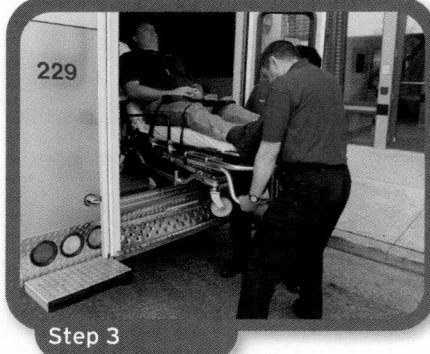

Step 3

Lifting with your legs, carefully roll the stretcher forward until the undercarriage engages.

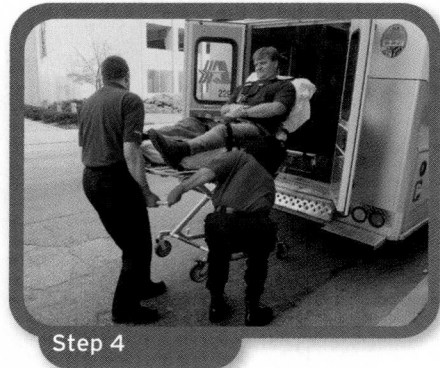

Step 4

With your partner steadying the stretcher from the side, gently bring the stretcher forward out of the ambulance.

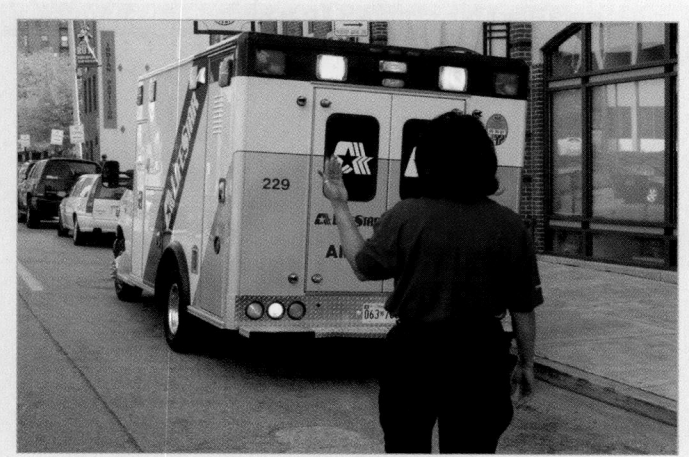

Figure 46-8 Always use a spotter when backing up the ambulance.

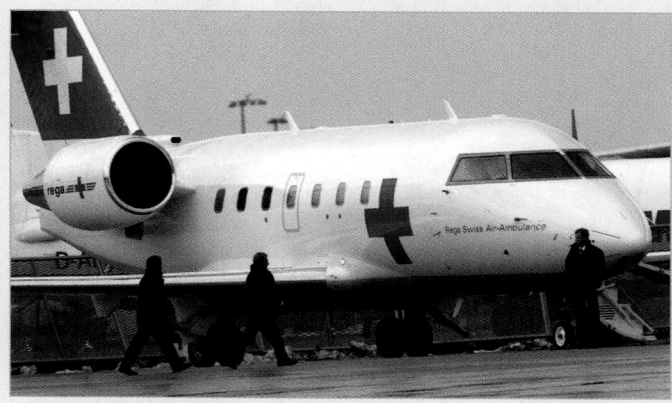

Figure 46-9 Fixed-winged aircraft.

should be used when appropriate. Of course, when you are driving the ambulance you should always use a seatbelt. Likewise, when you are providing treatment in the patient compartment you should use the restraints there.

Air Medical Transports

Air medical transport—especially the use of helicopters—has done much to speed up the transfer of patients from the trauma scene to definitive care. This mode of transport presents certain risks, however, and it is only appropriate in certain circumstances. Several factors must be considered before calling for an air ambulance: Does the patient's condition warrant the risk of using air medical transport? Will use of the air ambulance truly save the patient time in getting to definitive care once all other factors are considered?

Fixed-Wing Air Ambulances

The first fixed-winged airplane for military use was designed by Captain George H. R. Gosman and Lieutenant A. L. Rhodes at Fort Barrancas, Fla, in 1910. The plane flew 500 yards at a height of 100 feet before crashing. At the end of World War I, a Curtiss JN-4 Jenny biplane was converted to an air ambulance for the evacuation of wounded solders. So began the transition of ground transport to the use of air ambulances. Fixed-winged aircraft are used mainly for the transportation of patients over

long distances. EMS personnel are frequently called to transport these patients from the airfield to definitive care facilities Figure 46-9 ▲ .

The first use of a rotary-winged air ambulance occurred during the Burma Hump Airlift Operation in World War II. In 1943, the first "flight nurses," who were trained specifically to care for patients while in flight, graduated from Bowman Airfield in Kentucky. Civilian use of rotary-winged aircraft began in 1973, with St Anthony's Hospital in Denver sponsoring the Flight for Life program. Since then, these aircraft have become a standard of care for the transportation of clinically injured patients from the scene to a regional trauma center Figure 46-10 ▶ .

Advantages of Using Air Ambulances

Air ambulances have an advantage over ground transport in that they reduce transport time and may help the patient receive definitive treatment within the golden hour. The decision to use rotary-winged transport (helicopter) should be made as early in the call as possible. If, after patient assessment, it is determined that the helicopter is not needed, it can always be returned to service. Some districts have "automatic send helicopter" procedures written into their protocols.

You should weigh all the factors that involve time when deciding whether the helicopter is appropriate. The machine must be started, personnel and gear loaded, and sometimes great distances covered. Once the helicopter is at the scene, time must be allotted to land the aircraft and transfer the

You are the Provider Part 3

After a quick triage and assessment, you determine that air medical transportation is needed for the most critical patient. Dispatch advises you that a unit is en route and communication with you is being requested.

6. What information must you provide for the incoming helicopter?

7. How should EMS providers approach the helicopter that has landed?

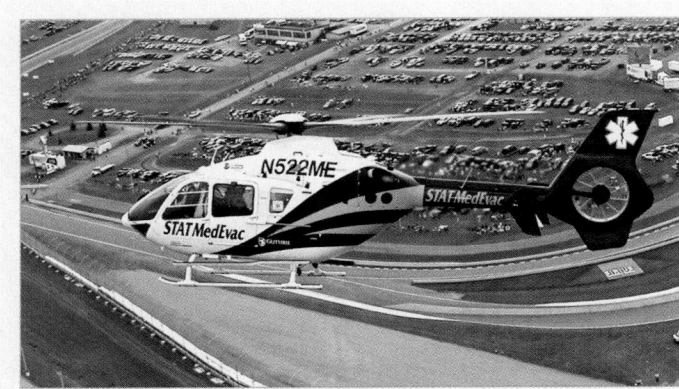

Figure 46-10 Rotary-wing air ambulance.

Table 46-3	**Disadvantages of Using an Air Ambulance**
	▪ Weather/environment
	▪ Altitude limitations
	▪ Airspeed limitations
	▪ Aircraft cabin size
	▪ Terrain
	▪ Cost
	▪ Patient's condition

Table 46-2	**Advantages of Using an Air Ambulance**
	▪ Specialized skills or equipment is needed
	▪ Rapid transport is possible
	▪ Can provide access to remote areas
	▪ Helicopter hospital helipads are available

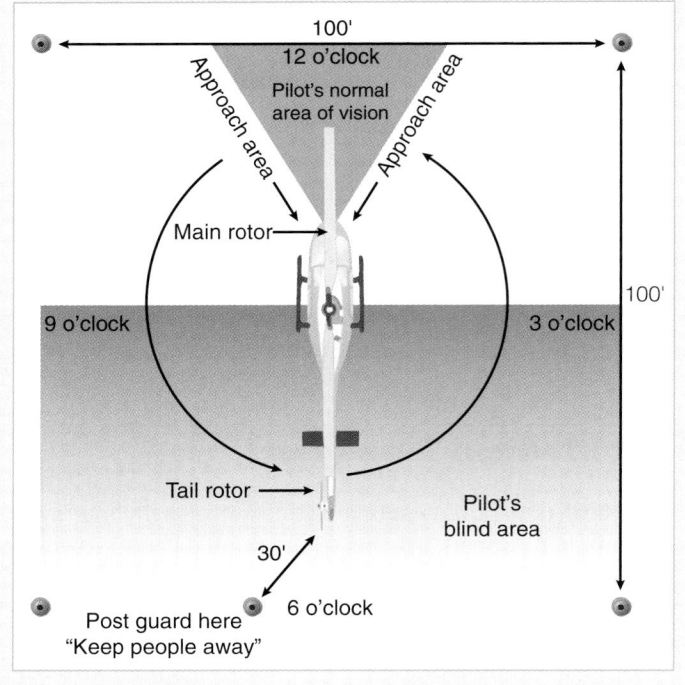

Figure 46-11 Landing zone with cones/warning devices in place.

patient to the air crew. Packaging the patient for air transport and loading the patient into the helicopter also require time. Especially in metropolitan areas, it can be difficult to justify use of the helicopter. Severe traffic congestion or prolonged extrication times may sometimes make the use of a helicopter appropriate in urban areas.

Use of an air ambulance may be warranted if the patient has a spinal injury and the terrain over which the patient must be carried is very rough. Even though the patient is stabilized, ground transport in a vehicle that is bouncing on the road could further injure the patient. The paramedic on scene is the best judge of the patient's transportation needs. **Table 46-2 ▲** summarizes the advantages of using an air ambulance.

Disadvantages of Using Air Ambulances

Patients in cardiac arrest or those who appear to be in pre-cardiac arrest should be transported by ground. Treating a patient in cardiac arrest in the helicopter is difficult due to space limitations.

In addition, air ambulances are usually restricted to flying under visual flight rules, so anything that interferes with visibility can make it too dangerous to fly. The terrain also may make it difficult to land the helicopter safely. Uneven ground and loose objects such as rocks or debris should be taken into account before attempting to land the aircraft. **Table 46-3 ▶** lists disadvantages of using the air ambulance.

Setting Up the Landing Zone

The landing zone should be large enough to accommodate a rotary-winged aircraft of any size; standard dimensions are

100′ × 100′. The landing zone must also be firm and level, with no loose objects or debris that might be pulled up into the rotors and engine, including clothing worn by emergency workers, such as caps and scarves, and IV poles. Remove the sheet from the stretcher before putting the backboard on it so that the sheet is not pulled up into the rotor blades when the patient-loaded backboard is removed. Be aware of wires overhead that might not be visible from the air, and remove all unnecessary vehicles and people from the landing site.

Mark the landing site with one visible light (preferably a strobe light) at each of the four corners **Figure 46-11 ▲**. Helicopters take off and land best into any existing wind, so it may be helpful to mark the side of prevailing winds with an extra strobe light. During a night landing, do not shine flashlights or spotlights up at the aircraft while it is descending; they may blind the pilot. Likewise, turn off headlights. Consider placing emergency vehicles under any overhead wires to signify the hazard.

Procedures for Landing

The most important function of the ground guide is to be aware of all hazards the pilot may not be able to see. Agree on communication channels before responding to an incident, and use standard "continue" and "abort" arm signals while at the scene (**Figure 46-12 ▶**). Wear eye protection against flying debris.

After the helicopter has landed, the paramedic should not approach the helicopter until signaled to do so by the pilot or a crewmember. If possible, all rotors should be stopped before you approach the aircraft. If the aircraft continues to operate in a "hot" mode (with rotor blades active), the tail rotor is the most dangerous part of the aircraft and should be avoided at all times. Always approach a helicopter from the front and keep the pilot in view at all times. Follow the air crew's instructions.

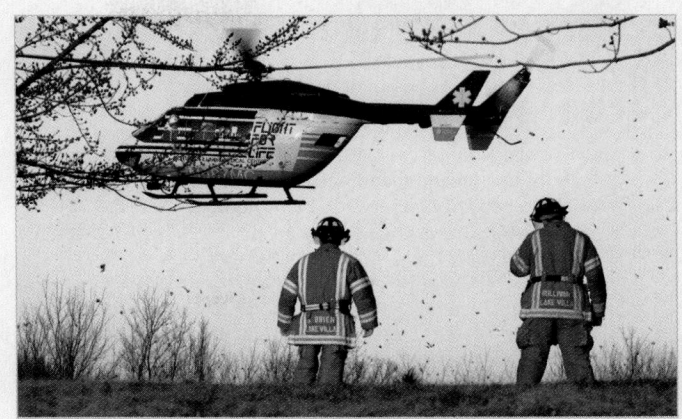

Figure 46-12 Personnel directing a helicopter for landing.

You are the Provider Summary

1. What are some of the potential hazards you may encounter en route to the scene?

Whenever an ambulance is en route to an emergency call, you must approach every intersection cautiously and with the thought that you could be meeting heavy traffic. In multiple-vehicle responses, always approach every intersection with caution and with the thought that you could be meeting another emergency vehicle at that intersection (police or fire).

2. What dangers must be considered upon approaching the scene with regard to parking and personnel protection?

Always approach the scene cautiously and with the thought that you could be meeting another emergency vehicle at the scene. If the scene has already been secured, park beyond the wreckage to prevent your ambulance from being exposed to the traffic. You may also receive arrival instructions if a first arriving EMS unit at the scene has already declared medical command. The arrival instructions may specify where the medical commander would like you to park your ambulance and to whom you should report. All EMS personnel should wear appropriate PPE such as gloves and possibly bunker gear, plus helmets when approaching the scene of a MVC.

3. How will knowing there are children involved affect your driving?

It should not affect your driving at all. Whenever the ambulance is on the road, day or night, turn on the headlights to increase visibility.

4. Where should the ambulance be positioned at the scene of a highway incident if you are the *first* to arrive?

If you are the first to arrive at the scene of a highway incident, take time to perform a scene size-up for potential hazards to you, your crew, and the patients. Consider establishing a danger zone, parking at least 100′ from the wreckage, upwind and uphill (if possible) to avoid fire or any escaping hazardous liquids or fumes, and deal with the traffic until the police arrive to relieve you of that task. If there is no fire or escaping liquids or fumes, park at least 50′ from the wreckage. Park in front of the wreckage if your ambulance is the first emergency vehicle on the scene so your warning lights can warn approaching motorists before flares can be set up.

5. Where should the ambulance be positioned at the scene of a highway incident if you are *not* the first to arrive?

If the scene has already been secured, park beyond the wreckage to prevent your ambulance from being exposed to the traf-

fic. You may also receive arrival instructions if the EMS unit first at the scene has already declared medical command. The arrival instructions may have specific instructions as to where the medical commander would like you to park your ambulance and to whom you should report.

6. What information must you provide for the incoming helicopter?

Once the decision has been made that a patient will be transported by helicopter, keep in mind any special considerations or limitations that will be necessary prior to loading the patient. The patient may need to be immobilized on a specific type of backboard that fits into the helicopter. Smaller helicopters only accept a specific size board. Larger helicopters may actually be able to take an entire stretcher. Some helicopter services have limitations on the length of the patient when supine, which could alter your method of immobilizing a fractured femur because a standard bipolar splint may extend the leg too long to fit in the helicopter. Methods of infection control and intubations will also be affected by air transport. Some flight crews may also need to intubate the patient prior to flight due to the limited area around the airway once the patient is on board the aircraft.

7. How should EMS providers approach the helicopter that has landed?

First, wait for the approval of the flight crew. Use extreme caution and follow the instructions that were discussed in your orientation with the flight crew prior to any actual calls involving patients. Some general rules to follow are listed below.

- Make sure all loose objects are secured, such as pillows and linens on your stretcher.
- Allow the flight crew to direct the loading of the patient.
- Approach in a crouched down position, as a sudden gust of wind can cause the main rotor of a helicopter to dip to a point as close as 4′ from the ground.
- If the helicopter is parked on a slight incline, approach it from the downhill side.
- Keep all traffic and vehicles 100′ or more away from the helicopter.
- Do not allow anyone to smoke within 200′ of the aircraft.

Prep Kit

◼ Ready for Review

- Federal Regulation DOT KKK 1822 sets the standards for ambulance design and manufacturing specifications.
- Three body style types are identified:
  - Type I: Conventional, truck-cab chassis with a modular ambulance body that can be transferred to a new chassis as needed
  - Type II: Standard van, forward-control integral cab-body ambulance
  - Type III: Specialty van, forward-control integral cab-body ambulance
- Check the ambulance at the beginning of every shift to ensure that all equipment is available and in good working order.
- Every ambulance needs to be able to do four things: start, steer, stop, and stay running.
- Preventive maintenance is just as important as operating skills. Looking for problems before the unit is in motion may prevent breakdowns while en route to calls.
- Any specific exemption from traffic laws does not negate the paramedic's responsibility to proceed with due regard to prevent ambulance collisions.
- Escorts should not be used due to the danger of motorists not seeing both the ambulance and the escort.
- Lights and sirens should be used when responding to emergencies but used sparingly when transporting a patient to the hospital.
- Avoid backing up the vehicle if possible. If it is necessary, use a spotter to assist in the procedure. Make sure everyone is clear on where the unit is to be placed and that hand signals used are agreed upon.
- All drivers and passengers should use safety restraints while a vehicle is in motion.
- Air transport should be considered whenever time is of the essence for the best patient outcome.

◼ Vital Vocabulary

belt noise A chirping or squealing sound, synchronous with engine speed.

brake fade A sensation that an ambulance has lost its power brakes.

brake pull A sensation that, when an operator depresses the brake pedal, the steering wheel is being pulled to the left or the right.

calibrated The diagnostic checking and synchronizing of digital or electronic equipment to assure that is in good working order and will measure accurately.

DOT KKK 1822 Federal standards that regulate the design and manufacturing guidelines of emergency ambulances.

drift A finding that when the operator lets go of the steering wheel, a vehicle consistently wanders left or right.

due regard Driving with awareness and responsibility for other drivers on the roadways when operating an ambulance in the emergency mode.

fractile response time A fraction (not average) of all emergency responses for the purpose of setting standards in response times.

landing zone Designated location for the landing of air ambulances.

peak loads A time of day or day of week in which the call volume is at its highest.

posting The placement of an ambulance at a specific geographic location in order to cover larger areas of territory and reduce response times.

specific exemptions Limited circumstances when an emergency vehicle operator can exceed the posted signage or speed limit.

steering play A sensation of looseness or sloppiness in a vehicle's steering.

steering pull A drift that is persistent enough so an operator can feel a tug on the steering wheel.

strategic deployment The staging of ambulances to strategic locations within a service area to allow for coverage of emergency calls.

Type I Ambulance Conventional, truck-cab chassis with a modular ambulance body that can be transferred to a new chassis as needed.

Type II Ambulance Standard van, forward-control integral cab-body ambulance.

Type III Ambulance Specialty van, forward-control integral cab-body ambulance.

wheel bounce A vibration, synchronous with road speed that can be felt in the steering wheel.

wheel wobble A common finding at low speeds when a vehicle has a bent wheel.

Assessment in Action

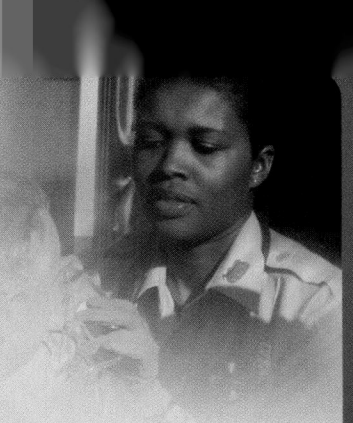

At the end of your shift you are dispatched to the scene of a vehicle that has crashed into a tree. When you arrive, you are approached by a fire fighter who tells you that the patient "is in there pretty good" and there will be a delay in accessing the patient due to extrication. You see that there is heavy damage to the driver's side of the vehicle. A post is crushed to the ground and the steering wheel and dashboard are crushing the patient in the vehicle. The patient appears unresponsive and copious amounts of blood are coming from his head. You notice a compound fracture of his left femur with extensive bleeding. You and your partner decide to request a Medevac due to the patient's condition and extended extrication time. After 15 minutes of extrication, you are able to free the patient from the vehicle. You secure the patient properly to a backboard and transfer him to the ambulance. While en route to the landing zone, you intubate him and start two large-bore IVs. When you arrive at the landing zone, the helicopter personnel are waiting for you.

1. **What was the advantage to using the Medevac for this patient?**
   A. Reduced transport time; it helped the patient receive definitive treatment within the golden hour.
   B. It was the end of your shift and you and your partner will be able to leave on time.
   C. You didn't have to deal with an unstable patient for the next 20 minutes while driving the patient to the hospital.
   D. The fire department and other personnel wanted to practice their helicopter landing skills.

2. **A landing zone should be large enough to accommodate a rotary-winged aircraft of any size; standard dimensions are:**
   A. 100´ × 50´.
   B. 150´ × 100´.
   C. 100´ × 100´.
   D. 75´ × 100´.

3. **While intubating this patient, you need to suction blood out of the airway. You were unable to find your suction unit. At the beginning of every shift you should:**
   A. check the ambulance to ensure the proper equipment is both available and in good working order.
   B. make sure that there is enough fuel and then go get coffee.
   C. document what the previous crew has to say about supplies and equipment.
   D. start your personal work that needs to get done before anything else.

4. **Which of the following safety measures should be used when approaching the helicopter to load the patient?**
   A. Approach the helicopter as soon as it lands.
   B. At least eight people should help load the aircraft.
   C. The aircraft should be approached from the front.
   D. The aircraft should be approached from the rear.

5. **While you were driving your vehicle to the call, your steering wheel was jerking to the left. What could this be?**
   A. Brake pull
   B. Brake fade
   C. Drift
   D. Steering pull

6. **The four things that every ambulance needs to be able to do are:**
   A. start, steer, stall, and stop.
   B. start, steer, stop, and stay running.
   C. steer, stop, start, and stage.
   D. start, stop, steer, and speed.

7. **Routine ambulance equipment checks are essential so that:**
   A. accurate patient billing and reimbursement can occur in a timely manner.
   B. essential equipment is available and in working order during patient care.
   C. state laws and regulations can be met and licensure can be maintained.
   D. disciplinary action will not be necessary if equipment failure occurs.

Challenging Question

You are the newly appointed director of your paramedic unit. Your first course of action is to begin replacing your fleet with new ambulances. You've never done this before and are not sure what needs to be done.

8. **What do you refer to that will provide you with the essential information you need to know?**

■ Points to Ponder

You are dispatched to a department store for a seizure. You are responding with lights and sirens. You make a right-hand turn onto a busy roadway. As you are approaching an intersection that has a blinking yellow-red light, you notice that you have the blinking yellow. There is a vehicle on your left at a corner that has the red blinking light as well as a stop sign. The driver of the vehicle begins to drive, then stops. You are aware of what he is doing and slow down. As he stops, you begin to accelerate through the intersection. At the last moment, the vehicle at the stop sign accelerates, trying to turn in front of you. You realize that a collision is unavoidable. You see another car approaching on the opposite side of the road so you cannot maneuver into the other lane.

You turn your wheels slightly to the right and strike the vehicle in the passenger's side corner panel. Why?

Issues: Assessing Personal Safety Practices While Operating Your Emergency Vehicle, Serving as a Role Model for Others in the Operations of Emergency Vehicles.

47 Medical Incident Command

Objectives

Cognitive

8-2.1   Explain the need for the incident management system (IMS)/incident command system (ICS) in managing emergency medical services incidents. (p 47.5)

8-2.2   Define the term multiple casualty incident (MCI). (p 47.4)

8-2.3   Define the term disaster management. (p 47.4)

8-2.4   Describe essential elements of scene size-up when arriving at a potential MCI. (p 47.9)

8-2.5   Describe the role of the paramedics and EMS systems in planning for MCIs and disasters. (p 47.5)

8-2.6   Define the following types of incidents and how they affect medical management:
- a. Open or uncontained incident
- b. Closed or contained incident (p 47.5)

8-2.7   Describe the functional components of the incident management system in terms of the following:
1. Command
2. Finance
3. Logistics
4. Operations
5. Planning (p 47.5–47.8)

8-2.8   Differentiate between singular and unified command and when each is most applicable. (p 47.5, 47.6)

8-2.9   Describe the role of command. (p 47.5)

8-2.10   Describe the need for transfer of command and procedures for transferring it. (p 47.6)

8-2.11   Differentiate between command procedures used at small, medium and large scale medical incidents. (p 47.5)

8-2.12   Explain the local/regional threshold for establishing command and implementation of the incident management system including threshold MCI declaration. (p 47.5)

8-2.13   List and describe the functions of the following groups and leaders in ICS as it pertains to EMS incidents:
- a. Safety
- b. Logistics
- c. Rehabilitation (rehab)
- d. Staging
- e. Treatment
- f. Triage
- g. Transportation
- h. Extrication/rescue
- i. Disposition of deceased (morgue)
- j. Communications (p 47.7–47.13)

8-2.14   Describe the methods and rationale for identifying specific functions and leaders for these functions in ICS. (p 47.5)

8-2.15   Describe the role of both command posts and emergency operations centers in MCI and disaster management. (p 47.5)

8-2.16   Describe the role of the physician at multiple casualty incidents. (p 47.11)

8-2.17   Define triage and describe the principles of triage. (p 47.13)

8-2.18   Describe the START (simple triage and rapid treatment) method of initial triage. (p 47.14)

8-2.19   Given a list of 20 patients with various multiple injuries, determine the appropriate triage priority with 90% accuracy. (p 47.13)

8-2.20   Given color coded tags and numerical priorities, assign the following terms to each:
- a. Immediate
- b. Delayed
- c. Hold
- d. Deceased (p 47.13)

8-2.21   Define primary and secondary triage. (p 47.13)

8-2.22   Describe when primary and secondary triage techniques should be implemented. (p 47.13)

8-2.23   Describe the need for and techniques used in tracking patients during multiple casualty incidents. (p 47.13–47.16)

8-2.24   Describe techniques used to allocate patients to hospitals and track them. (p 47.16)

8-2.25   Describe modifications of telecommunications procedures during multiple casualty incidents. (p 47.5, 47.6)

8-2.26   List and describe the essential equipment to provide logistical support to MCI operations to include:
- a. Airway, respiratory and hemorrhage control
- b. Burn management
- c. Patient packaging/ immobilization (p 47.7)

8-2.27   List the physical and psychological signs of critical incident stress. (p 47.11)

8-2.28   Describe the role of critical incident stress management sessions in MCIs. (p 47.16)

8-2.29   Describe the role of the following exercises in preparation for MCIs:
- a. Tabletop exercises
- b. Small and large MCI drills (p 47.5, 47.9)

Affective

8-2.30   Understand the rationale for initiating incident command even at a small MCI event. (p 47.5)

8-2.31   Explain the rationale for having efficient and effective communications as part of an incident command/ management system. (p 47.9, 47.10)

8-2.32   Explain why common problems of an MCI can have an adverse effect on an entire incident. (p 47.5, 47.6, 47.9, 47.16)

8-2.33   Explain the organizational benefits for having standard operating procedures (SOPs) for using the incident management system or incident command system. (p 47.5, 47.6)

Psychomotor

8-2.34 Demonstrate the use of local/regional triage tagging system used for primary and secondary triage. (p 47.12–47.14)

8-2.35 Given a simulated tabletop multiple casualty incident, with 5–10 patients:
  a. Establish unified or singular command
  b. Conduct a scene assessment
  c. Determine scene objectives
  d. Formulate an incident plan
  e. Request appropriate resources
  f. Determine need for ICS expansion and groups
  g. Coordinate communications and groups leaders
  h. Coordinate outside agencies (p 47.5–47.10)

8-2.36 Demonstrate effective initial scene assessment and update (progress) reports. (p 47.9)

8-2.37 Given a classroom simulation of a MCI with 5–10 patients, fulfill the role of triage group leader. (p 47.9)

8-2.38 Given a classroom simulation of a MCI with 5–10 patients, fulfill the role of treatment group leader. (p 47.9)

8-2.39 Given a classroom simulation of a MCI with 5–10 patients, fulfill the role of transportation group leader. (p 47.11)

Introduction

The most challenging situations you can be called to are disasters and mass-casualty incidents (MCIs). These incidents can be overwhelming because you will find a large number of patients and a lack of specialized equipment and/or adequate help. When you respond to an event with a large number of patients, you must use a systematic approach to manage the incident most efficiently. By learning to use the principles of the incident command system (ICS), you will be able to do the greatest good for the greatest number. As a paramedic, you will typically be assigned to work within the EMS/medical branch or group under an ICS, but you may be asked to function in other areas (which will be elaborated later in this chapter). To promote more efficient coordination of emergency incidents at the regional, state, and national levels, the National Incident Management System (NIMS) was developed. To reduce on-scene problems and to increase your efficiency, you should attend training and have a solid understanding of the basics of NIMS.

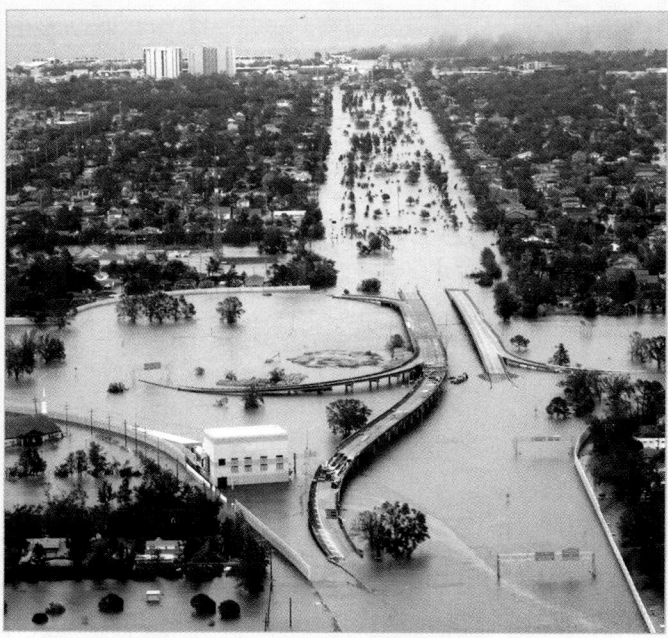

Figure 47-1 Disasters can overwhelm EMS resources and can damage critical infrastructure.

Disasters

Disasters overwhelm EMS and community resources because critical infrastructure has been damaged or destroyed Figure 47-1 ▶ . Critical infrastructure includes the electrical power grid, communication systems, fuel for vehicles, water, sewage removal, food, hospitals, and transportation systems. Disaster management requires planners to take a broad look at preparedness, planning, training, response, and after-action review.

Mass-Casualty Incidents

A mass-casualty incident (MCI) is an event in which the number of patients exceeds the resources available to the initial responders Figure 47-2 ▶ . Remember: a motor vehicle collision with several critical patients may be an MCI for a one-ambulance town. Although some EMS systems differentiate between MCIs and multiple-casualty incidents, in this chapter, either of these terms is considered an incident in which using the ICS will help paramedics work efficiently and effectively.

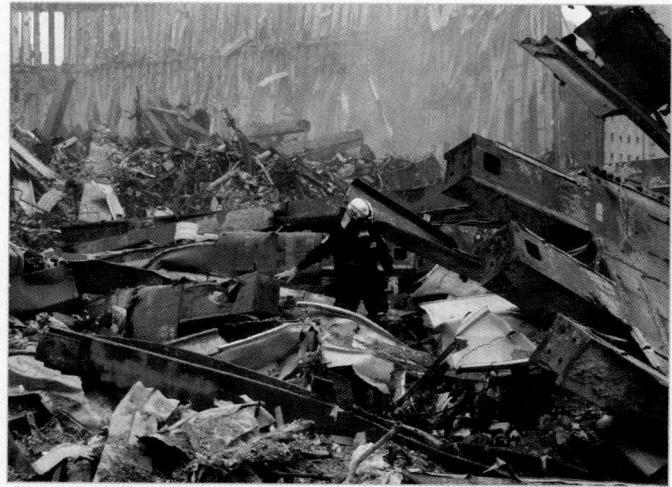

Figure 47-2 Mass-casualty incidents can be large, such as the attack on September 11, 2001, or can be much smaller in scope.

You are the Provider Part 1

You have been dispatched to the scene of a commercial plane down. You are the first responding rescue/EMS unit to arrive on the scene. There is no fire or other hazard noted initially. From inside the ambulance, you see approximately 30 to 40 victims walking or lying about the scene. As you arrive, 10 to 15 people approach your ambulance with cuts, bruises, and abrasions.

1. What is your plan of action?
2. Why is an incident command system (ICS) needed for handling major EMS incidents?
3. What is an "open" incident? What is a "closed" incident?

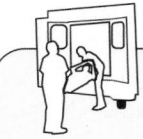

In the Field

Table-top MCI exercises are a helpful way for providers to learn their roles at an MCI.

Your response to MCIs will differ depending on the area of land covered by the incident and the location and how spread out your patients are. You should be able to recognize an MCI as an open (uncontained) incident or a closed (contained) incident. An open incident has a number of casualties not yet located when you answer the initial call. Rescuers may have to search for patients and then triage or treat them in multiple locations. There also may be an ongoing situation that produces more patients while you are at the scene, for example, school shootings, tornadoes, a hazardous materials release, or rising floodwaters.

A closed incident is a situation that is not expected to produce more patients than initially present. The patients can be triaged and treated as they are removed. Although a closed incident is often easier to handle, a closed incident may suddenly become an open incident.

Communities may establish different standards for what constitutes an MCI or for when to implement the ICS, but experience with previous MCIs is helpful in making the determination as well. Agencies and jurisdictions that regularly use the ICS will gain valuable experience and will be better prepared to respond to an MCI or a disaster. You can make significant contributions to the safety of your community by participating in disaster planning drills, table-top MCI exercises, and other ICS training opportunities.

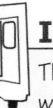

In the Field

The terminology used to describe an incident with multiple patients varies in different communities. Many communities use the term multiple-casualty incident to describe an emergency that involves more than one patient and the term mass-casualty incident to describe larger scale events, such as those with more than 20 patients. In this text, the term mass-casualty incident is used to describe any call that involves more than one patient or a situation that overwhelms your available resources.

▌The Incident Command System

It is important for you to be familiar with the terminology and concepts of the incident command system (ICS). As you know, communication is the building block of good patient care. Common terminology and the use of "clear text" communications (plain English as opposed to 10-codes) help responders from multiple agencies work efficiently together.

Using the ICS gives you a modular organizational structure that is built on the size and complexity of the incident. The goal of the ICS is to make the best use of your resources to manage the environment around the incident and to treat patients during an emergency. Make certain to follow your local standard operating procedures for establishing the ICS. The ICS is designed to control duplication of effort and freelancing, in which individual units or different organizations make independent and often inefficient decisions about the next appropriate action.

One of the organizing principles of the ICS is limiting the span of control of any one individual, keeping the supervisor/worker ratio at one supervisor for three to seven workers. A supervisor who finds that his or her effective span of control is exceeded, that is, has more than seven people reporting to him or her—needs to divide tasks and delegate supervision of some tasks to another person.

Organizational divisions may include sections, branches, divisions and groups, and resources ▶Figure 47-3 ▶. In some regions, emergency operations centers may exist. The centers are usually operated by city, state, or federal governments. These centers will usually only be activated in a large catastrophic event that may go on for days, that has hundreds of patients, and that taxes the whole system.

The individuals who will participate in the many tasks in an MCI or a disaster should use the ICS. You should find out from your service if one exists, who is in charge, how it is activated, and what your expected role will be.

ICS Roles and Responsibilities

There are many roles defined in the ICS. The general staff includes command, finance, logistics, operations, and planning. It is important for you to understand the specific duties of each and how they work in coordinating the response. Command functions include the public information officer (PIO), safety officer, and liaison officer.

Command

The incident commander (IC) is the person in charge of the overall incident. The IC will assess the incident, establish the strategic objectives and priorities, and develop a plan to manage the incident ▶Figure 47-4 ▶. The number of command duties (public information, safety, and liaison) the IC takes on often varies by the size of the incident. Small incidents often mean the IC will do it all. In an incident of medium size or complexity, the IC may delegate some functions but retain others. For example, at a motor vehicle collision with multiple patients, the IC may designate a safety officer or assign a PIO but maintain responsibility for the other command functions. In a complex situation, the IC may appoint team members to all of the command roles.

Large MCIs, such as a hazardous materials incident, require a multiagency or multijurisdiction response and need to use a unified command system. In this case, plans are drawn up in advance by all cooperating agencies that assume a shared

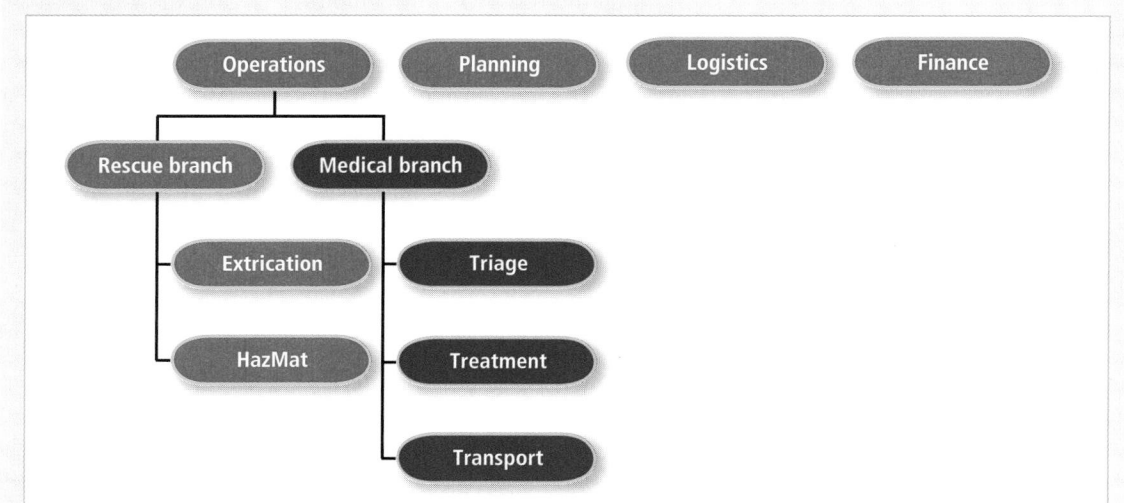

Figure 47-3 Incident command structure. Not all positions will be filled in every incident. However, the incident commander is ultimately responsible for all activity. Subordinates may be appointed to assist in managing the incident.

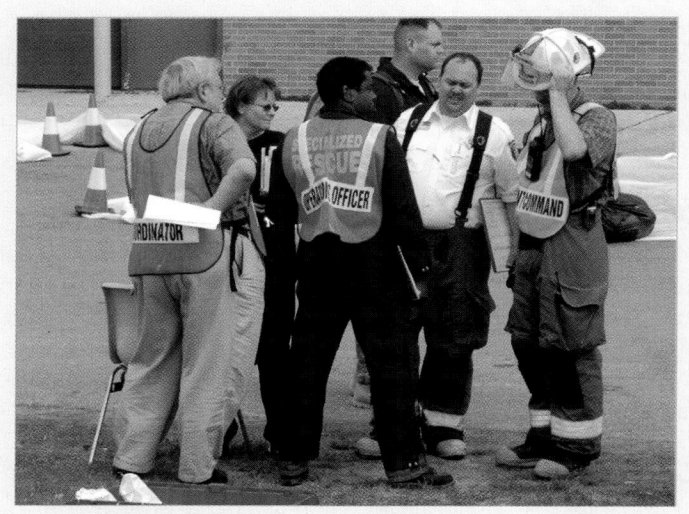

Figure 47-4 The person in command at an MCI oversees the incident and develops a plan for response.

sibility for incident management. Ideally, it is used for short duration, limited incidents that require the services of a single agency.

Your IC should be on or near the scene, where he or she can easily communicate with all emergency responders operating at the scene. It is important that you know who the IC is, where the command post is located, and how to communicate with your supervisor. If the incident is very large, you will be reporting to a supervisor working under the IC. (Remember the rule of span of control? The number of people who can be effectively supervised is between three and seven.) To make the IC easily identifiable, some type of garment can be worn, such as a brightly colored vest emblazoned with the word COMMAND. If the command post is set up in a vehicle, it should be well marked, and you should know its location. Make sure that your supervisor or the IC knows of any plans or operations before they are initiated.

This communication is particularly important if a transfer of command takes place. Because an MCI can be ever changing and ever increasing in scope, an IC may turn over command to someone with more experience in a critical area. This change, or transfer of command, must take place in an orderly manner and, if possible, face to face. In extreme situations, it could be done by phone, radio, or e-mail. Your agency should have standard operating procedures (SOPs) that govern the transfer of command. Make certain to follow those standard operating procedures. When an incident draws to a close, there should be a termination of command. Your agency should have demobilization procedures to implement as the situation de-escalates or comes to an end.

Finance

The finance section chief is responsible for documenting all expenditures at an incident for reimbursement. A financial person is not usually needed at smaller incidents, but larger incidents demand keeping track of personnel hours and expenditures for materials and supplies and reporting at meetings of the general staff. Responding agencies and organizations may be eligible for some types of reimbursement after the incident, and an efficient finance section chief will help your agency to succeed in the reimbursement process. Finance should be trained in the process of assessing expenditures with an eye to reimbursement long before an actual event.

responsibility for decision making and cooperation. The response plan should designate the lead and support agencies in several kinds of MCIs. (The hazardous materials team will take the lead in a chemical leak, for example. However, the medical team might take the lead in a multivehicle car crash.) Agencies bordering each other should practice often with each other to ensure that a unified command system will function well and that communication among the people involved is well established before a real incident occurs.

A single command system is one in which one person is in charge, even if multiple agencies respond. It is generally used with incidents in which one agency has the majority of respon-

Logistics

The logistics section or section chief has responsibility for communications equipment, facilities, food and water, fuel, lighting, and medical equipment and supplies for patients and emergency responders. Local standard operating procedures will list the medical equipment needed for the incident, depending on the type of incident. **Table 47-1 ▶** lists common MCI equipment and supplies. Logistics personnel are trained to find food, shelter, and health care for you and the other responders at the scene of an MCI **Figure 47-5 ▶**. In a large incident, it is often necessary for many people to handle logistics, even though only one person will report to the IC.

Operations

At a very large incident, the operations section is responsible for managing the tactical operations job usually handled by the IC on routine EMS calls. In a complex incident, however, the IC must coordinate with other agencies and the media, engage in strategic planning, and ensure that logistics are functioning effectively. In these cases, the IC should appoint an operations section chief. The operations section chief will supervise the people working at the scene of the incident, who will be assigned to branches, divisions, and groups. Operations personnel often have experience in management within EMS.

Planning

The planning section solves problems as they arise during the MCI. Planners obtain data about the problem, analyze the previous incident plan, and predict what or who is needed to make the new plan work. Planners need to work closely with the operations, finance, and, especially logistics sections. Planners can and should call on technical experts to help with the planning process. Planners will also set out a course for demobilizing the response when needed.

Command Staff

Three important positions that help the general staff (all staff described previously) and the IC are the safety officer, the

Table 47-1	MCI Equipment and Supplies*
Airway control	PPE (gloves, face shield, HEPA or N95 mask) Oral airways, nasal airways Suction units (manual units) Rigid tip Yankauer and flexible suction catheters LMA, Combitube, ET tubes* Laryngoscope and blades* Tube check, tube restraint, tape, syringes, stylet* End-tidal CO_2 device
Breathing	Pocket mask and one-way valve Bag-mask device(s) (adult and child), spare masks Oxygen delivery devices (nonrebreathing mask, cannula, extension tubing) Oxygen tank, regulator Occlusive dressings Large-bore IV catheter for thoracic decompression*
Circulation	Dressings, bandages, tape Sphygmomanometer, stethoscope Burn dressings, burn sheets, sterile water for irrigation One-handed tourniquets 1,000 mL bags of normal saline, IV start kits, catheters*
Disability	Rigid collars (one size fits all) Head beds, wide tape, backboard straps Flashlights, spare batteries
Exposure	Space blanket to cover patients Scissors
Logistic/Command	Sector vests (triage, treatment, transport, staging, command, rescue) Pads of paper, pencils, pens, markers Triage tags or kits used by your regional system Assessment cards

Note: The items denoted by * could be packaged in an ALS kit.

You are the Provider Part 2

As more units arrive on scene, you take on the role of triage officer. Patient 1 is bleeding from the nose.

Initial Assessment	Recording Time
Appearance	Pale, cool, dry skin
Level of consciousness	A (Alert to person, place, and day)
Airway	Open
Breathing	Adequate
Circulation	Pulse rapid, full, and regular

4. How should you triage this patient?
5. What is the difference between single and unified command?
6. What is "span of control"?

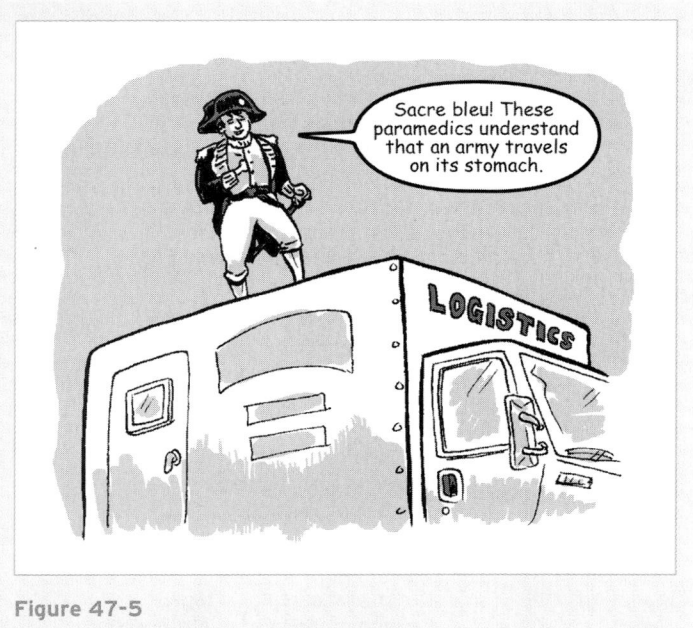

Figure 47-5

PIO, and the liaison officer. The safety officer monitors the scene for conditions or operations that may present a hazard to responders and patients. The safety officer may need to work with environmental health and hazardous materials specialists. The importance of the safety officer cannot be underestimated—he or she has the authority to stop an emergency operation whenever a rescuer is in danger. A safety officer should remove hazards to paramedics and patients before the hazards cause injury.

The public information officer (PIO) provides the public and media with clear and understandable information. A wise PIO positions his or her headquarters well away from the incident command post and, most important, away from the incident, to minimize distractions. Also, the PIO must keep the media safe and from becoming part of the incident. The designated PIO may work in cooperation with PIOs from other agencies in a joint information center (JIC). In some circumstances, the PIO/JIC may be responsible for disseminating a message designed to help a situation, prevent panic, and provide evacuation directions.

The liaison officer (LNO) relays information and concerns among command, the general staff, and other agencies. If an agency is not represented in the command structure, questions and input should be given through the LNO.

The NIMS

Although most incidents are handled at the local level, the president directed the Secretary of Homeland Security to implement the National Incident Management System (NIMS) in March 2004. Major incidents require the involvement and coordination of multiple jurisdictions, functional agencies, and

emergency response disciplines. NIMS provides a consistent nationwide template to enable federal, state, and local governments, as well as private-sector and nongovernmental organizations, to work together effectively and efficiently. NIMS is used to prepare for, prevent, respond to, and recover from domestic incidents, regardless of cause, size, or complexity, including acts of catastrophic terrorism.

Two important underlying principles of NIMS are flexibility and standardization. The organizational structure must be flexible enough to be rapidly adapted for use in any situation. NIMS provides standardization in terminology, resource classification, personnel training, certification, and more. Another important feature of NIMS is the concept of interoperability in which agencies of different types or from different jurisdictions can communicate with each other.

The ICS, which is the focus of this chapter, is one component of NIMS. The major NIMS components are:

- **Command and management.** The NIMS standardizes incident management for all hazards and across all levels of government. The NIMS standard incident command structures are based on three key constructs: ICS, multiagency coordination systems, and public information systems.
- **Preparedness.** NIMS establishes measures for all responders to incorporate into their systems in preparation to respond to all incidents at any time.
- **Resource management.** NIMS sets up mechanisms to describe, inventory, track, and dispatch resources before, during, and after an incident. NIMS also defines standard procedures to recover equipment used during the incident.
- **Communications and information management.** Effective communications and information management and sharing are critical aspects of domestic incident management. NIMS communications and information systems enable the essential functions needed to provide interoperability.
- **Supporting technologies.** NIMS promotes national standards and interoperability for supporting technologies to successfully implement NIMS and standard technologies for professions or incidents. It provides structure for the science and technology used in incident management.
- **Ongoing management and maintenance.** The US Department of Homeland Security will establish a multijurisdictional, multidisciplinary NIMS Integration Center. This center will provide strategic direction for and oversight of NIMS, supporting routine maintenance and continuous improvement of the system in the long-term.

EMS Response Within the ICS

Preparedness

Preparedness involves the decisions made and basic planning done before an incident occurs. Some parts of every country are prone to natural disasters, such as hurricanes, tornadoes, earthquakes, or wildfires. Therefore, preparedness in a given area would involve decisions and planning about the most likely natural disasters for the area, among other disasters.

Your EMS agency should have written disaster plans that you are regularly trained to carry out. A copy of the disaster plan should be kept in each EMS vehicle. EMS facilities should have disaster supplies for at least a 72-hour period of self-sufficiency. Your EMS service should have mutual aid agreements with surrounding organizations so that requests for help can be expedited in an emergency. All groups with mutual aid agreements should practice using the plans frequently. Organizations should share a list of resources with each other so they will know early on what they can access. Also, your local EMS organizations should develop an assistance program for the families of EMS responders. If EMS responders have concerns about their families during a disaster, their effectiveness on the job could be diminished.

Of course, you should have a personal disaster plan for your family. Families need to be prepared and know what to expect should you be required to be a disaster responder. You *are* up-to-date on immunizations for influenza, hepatitis A and B, and tetanus, aren't you?

Scene Size-up

You remember that sizing up a scene starts with dispatch. If dispatch information indicates a possible unsafe scene, you should stay away from the scene or get only close enough to make an assessment without putting yourself in harm's way. When you arrive first on the scene of an MCI, you will make an initial assessment and some preliminary decisions. The size-up will be driven by three basic questions that responders must ask themselves:

- *What do I have?*
- *What do I need to do?*
- *What resources do I need?*

These questions have a symbiotic relationship. The answer from one helps answer the others, and each represents a piece to the puzzle. Work as team when you answer these questions because missing just one safety issue early on can start a chain of problems.

What Do I Have?

Any call starts with scene safety, and you need to assess for hazards. Warn all other responders about hazardous materials, fuel spills, electrical hazards, or other safety concerns as soon as possible. Confirm the incident location. Establish whether the incident is open or closed. Estimate the number of casualties. Your immediate report to dispatch would be "Paramedic unit number one arriving on scene, multiple vehicles involved, full road blockage, no apparent hazards at this time, paramedic unit number one is assuming command."

What Do I Need to Do?

You should keep the following priorities in mind:

- Safety
- Incident stabilization
- Preservation of property and the environment

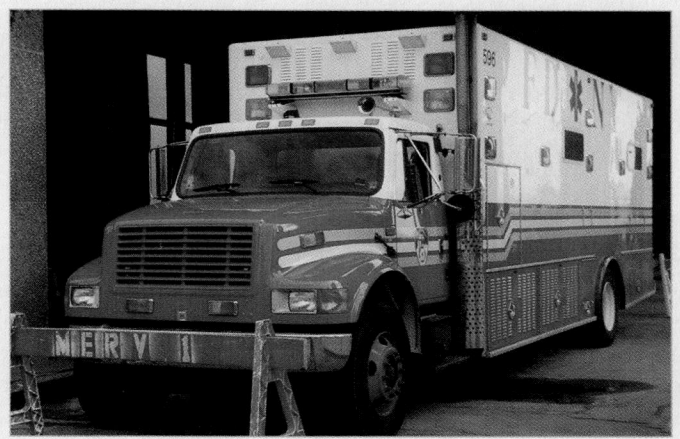

Figure 47-6 This mobile emergency room is staffed by EMTs, paramedics, and physicians who are able to provide advanced life support to multiple patients simultaneously on the scene of an MCI.

You need to consider these priorities in the order they are given. Safety is paramount. Safety includes your life, your partner's life, and other rescuers' lives. Then, consider the safety of the patient and any bystanders. This will be difficult for anyone dedicated to saving lives, but it is important to put yourself and your partner first—you have the skills, and bystanders usually don't; the situation can be far worse if you do not put yourself first. Often, if a responder is injured, other responders will focus on "their own," removing more available resources. You may have to initially work to isolate or stabilize the incident before providing care to injured persons, another difficult concept.

What Do I Need?

Decide what resources are needed. You may need more EMS responders, ambulances, or other forms of transportation. If extrication is required, a rescue unit and fire department response may be needed. If there are hazardous materials, get a hazardous materials team immediately. Many large EMS systems deploy specialized MCI units or mobile emergency room vehicles that are able to treat dozens of patients on the scene **Figure 47-6 ▲**.

Establishing Command

Once you have performed a good scene size-up and answered the three basic questions, command should be established,

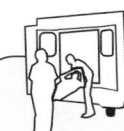

In the Field

Participating in a simulated table-top mass-casualty incident can help the paramedic better understand how command is established, the scene is assessed, how scene objectives are determined, how an incident plan is created, how resources are requested, when ICS needs to expand, how communication is coordinated, and how EMS works with other agencies during a large emergency.

notification to other responders should go out, and necessary resources should be requested. A command system ensures that resources are effectively and efficiently coordinated. Command must be established early, preferably by the first-arriving, most experienced public safety official. These officials may include police, fire, or EMS personnel and local government officials.

Communications

Communications is often the key problem at an MCI or a disaster. The infrastructure can be damaged, or communications capabilities can be overwhelmed. If possible, use face-to-face communications to limit radio traffic. Some organizations responding to a disaster might not know how to use a radio, and if you do use it, don't use codes or signals. Most communications problems should be worked out before a disaster happens by designating channels strictly for command during a disaster. Whatever form of communications equipment is used, it is imperative that it is reliable, durable, field-tested, and that there are backups in place if the primary communications system does not work. Some regions have mobile self-contained communications centers, whereas others use local radio groups such as HAM radio operators to assist with communications. Most important, your plan should include a "Plan B" in case of communications failure.

Medical Incident Command

What has traditionally been referred to as medical incident command is also known as the medical (or EMS) branch of the ICS   Figure 47-7 ▼ . At incidents that have a significant medical factor, the IC should appoint someone as the medical group or branch leader. This person will supervise the primary roles of the medical group—triage, treatment, and transport of the injured. The medical group leader should help ensure that EMS units responding to the scene are working within the ICS, each medical unit receives a clear assignment before beginning work at the scene, and personnel remain with their vehicle in the staging area until they are assigned their duties.   Figure 47-8 ▶ shows a diagram of an MCI with these areas.

Triage Unit

The triage officer is ultimately in charge of counting and prioritizing patients. During large incidents, a number of triage personnel may be needed. The primary duty of the triage unit is to ensure that every patient receives initial assessment of his or her condition. Paramedics doing triage will help move patients to the appropriate treatment sector. One of the most difficult parts of being a triage officer is that you must not begin treatment until all patients are triaged, or you will compromise your triage efforts.

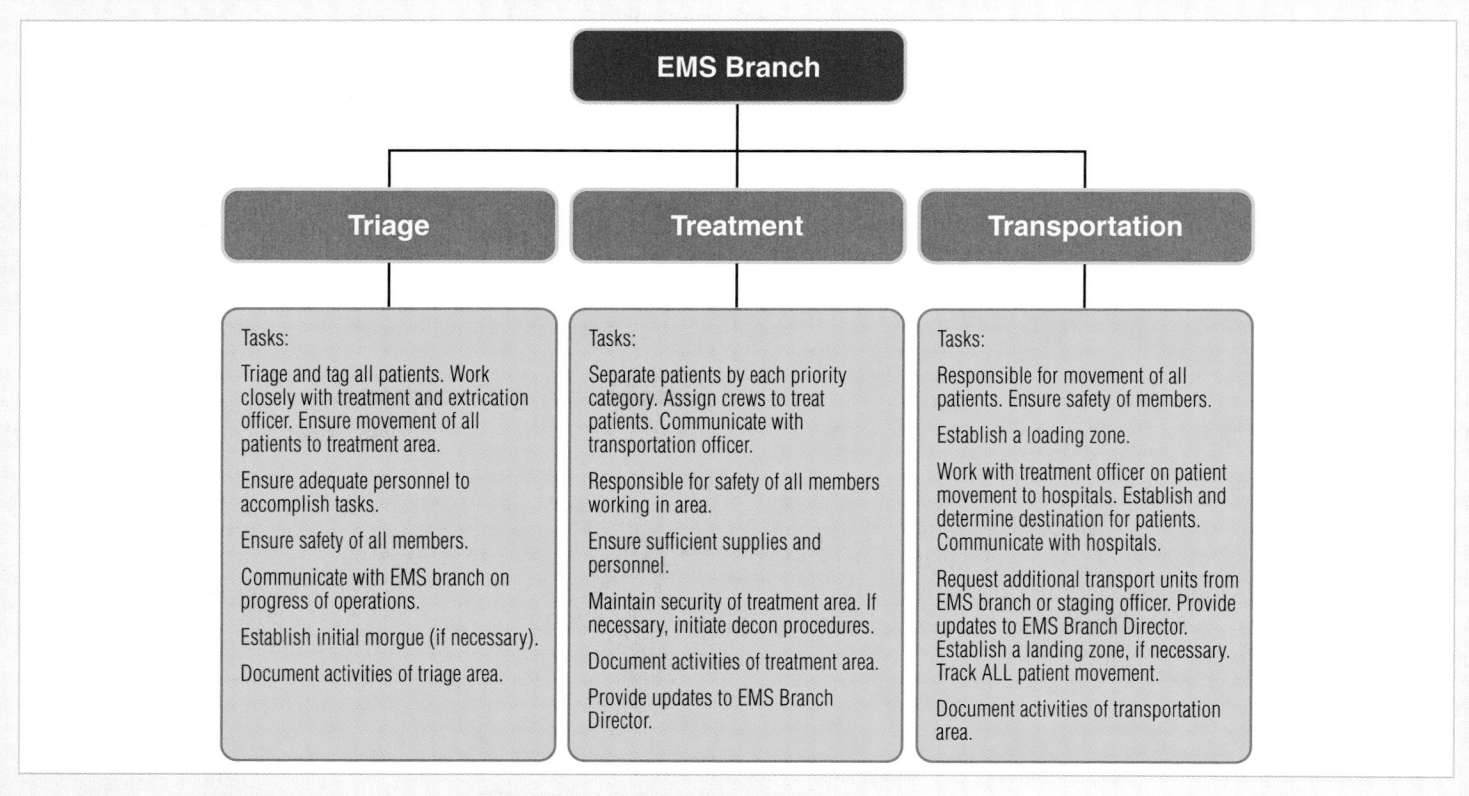

Figure 47-7 Components of the EMS branch within the incident management system.

Treatment Officer

The treatment officer will locate and set up the treatment area with a tier for each priority of patient. Treatment officers ensure that secondary triage of patients is performed and that adequate patient care is given as resources allow. Treatment officers also have a responsibility to assist with moving patients to the transportation area. As treatment officers supervise the responders, they must communicate with the medical group leaders to request sufficient quantities of supplies, including bandages, burn supplies, airway and respiratory supplies, and patient packaging equipment.

Transportation Officer

The transportation officer coordinates the transportation and distribution of patients to appropriate receiving hospitals. Transportation requires coordination with incident command to help ensure that enough personnel and ambulances are in staging or have been requested. A key role of the transportation officer is to communicate with the area hospitals to help determine where to transport the patients. Some regions may have planned for a designated hospital within a region to perform the coordination between hospitals on destination decisions. An MCI typically disrupts the everyday functioning of the region's trauma system, so good coordination is needed. The transportation officer documents and tracks the number of vehicles transporting, patients transported, and the facility destination of each vehicle and patient.

Staging Officer

A staging officer should be assigned when MCIs or scenes require response by numerous emergency vehicles or agencies. The vehicles cannot and should not drive into the scene of the MCI without direction from the staging officer. The staging area should be established away from the scene because the parked vehicles can be in the way. The staging officer locates an area to stage equipment and responders, tracks unit arrivals, and sends out vehicles as needed. This position plans for efficient access and exit from the disaster site and prevents traffic congestion among responding vehicles. The staging officer releases vehicles and supplies when ordered by command.

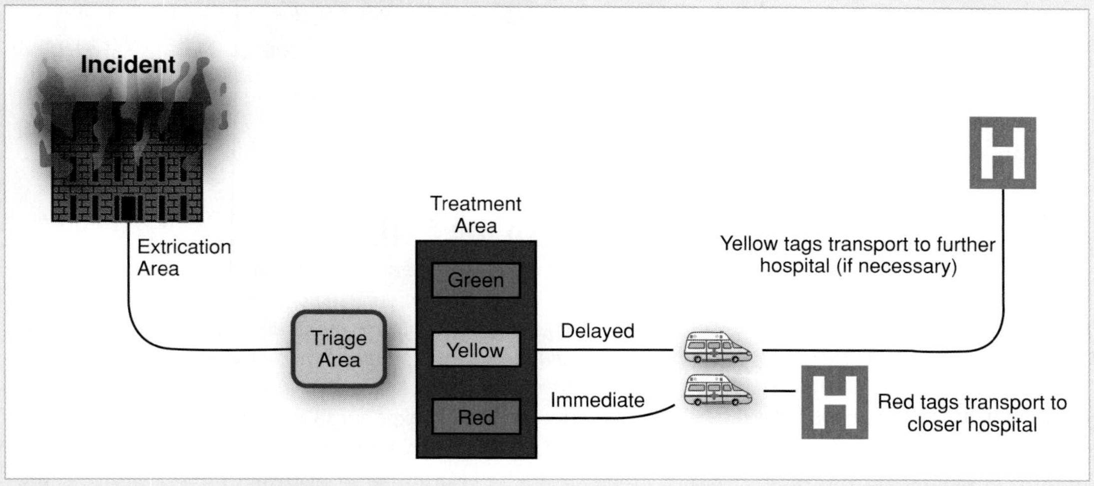

Physicians On Scene

In an MCI, some areas have plans in place for physicians on scene. Sometimes, even without a plan, the enormity of the situation may require that physicians be sent to the scene. Emergency physicians, especially, will have the ability to make difficult

Figure 47-8 Diagram of an MCI. The ICS established at the scene of a building fire may look similar to this diagram.

You are the Provider Part 3

A teenage boy is supine and unconscious. You find a nonsucking puncture wound in his chest.

Initial Assessment	Recording Time
Appearance	Pale, cool, moist skin
Level of consciousness	P (Responsive to painful stimuli)
Airway	Open
Breathing	Rapid, shallow, labored
Circulation	Radial pulse is rapid, weak, and regular

7. How should you triage this patient?

8. Why is there an essential need for common terminology in an ICS?

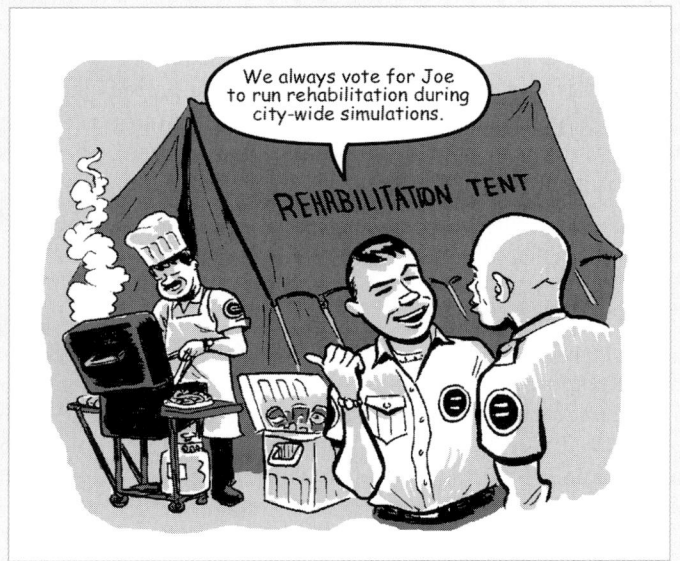

Figure 47-9

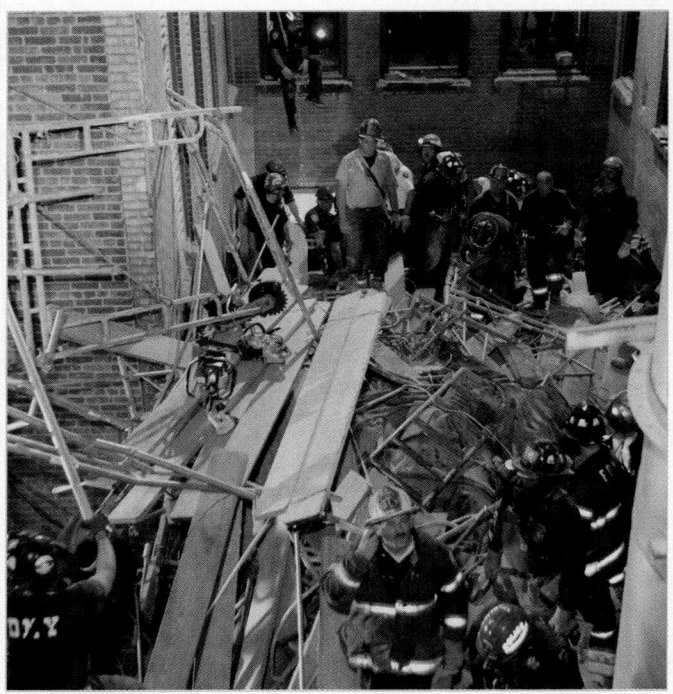

Figure 47-10 Some disasters will involve search and rescue or extrication.

triage decisions. They also provide secondary triage decisions in the treatment sector, deciding which priority patients are to be transported first. Physicians can provide on-scene medical direction for paramedics, and they can provide care in the treatment sector as appropriate.

Rehabilitation Officer

In disasters or situations that will last for extended periods, a rehabilitation section for the responders should be established. The rehabilitation officer should establish an area that provides protection for responders from the elements and the situation. The rehabilitation area should be located away from exhaust fumes and crowds (especially members of the media) and out of view of the scene itself. Rehabilitation is where a responder's needs for rest, fluids, food, and protection from the elements are met **Figure 47-9 ▲**. The rehabilitation officer must also monitor responders for signs of stress. These signs may include fatigue, altered thinking patterns, and complete collapse. You should remember that all EMS personnel should be responsible to be aware of signs of stress. Your service might consider having a defusing or debriefing team in this area. Responders should be encouraged to take advantage of these services but should never be forced to participate.

Extrication and Special Rescue

Some disasters require search and rescue or extrication of patients **Figure 47-10 ▶**. An extrication officer or rescue officer may need to be appointed. These officers determine the type of equipment and resources needed for the situation. In some incidents, victims may need to be extricated or rescued before they can be triaged and treated. Because extrication and rescue are medically complex, the officers will usually function under the EMS branch of the ICS. The extrication and rescue

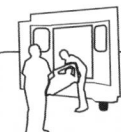 **In the Field**

MCIs and disasters take a physical and emotional toll on emergency responders. Make certain that you are medically evaluated if you have been injured, come into contact with any hazardous substance, or inhale any dust, fumes, or smoke. Often, the health effects of such exposures do not manifest for years and are difficult to link to a particular event. Also, be aware of signs of stress in yourself and in your coworkers. Take full advantage of the opportunity for stress debriefing after an incident.

officers identify the special equipment and personnel needed for the rescue. Extrication and rescue can be dangerous, so crew safety is of utmost importance.

Morgue Officer

In some disasters, there will be many dead patients. The morgue officer will work with area medical examiners, coroners, disaster mortuary assistance teams, and law enforcement agencies to coordinate removal of the bodies and even, possibly, body parts. The morgue officer should attempt to leave the dead victims in the location found, if possible, until a removal and storage plan can be determined. The location of victims may help in the identification of the dead victims in mass-fatality situations, or there may be crime scene considerations. If it is determined that a morgue area is needed, the morgue officer should ensure that the morgue is out of view of the living patients and other responders because the psychological impact could worsen the situation and that the morgue is secure from the public to prevent theft of any personal effects of the dead victims.

Triage

Triage simply means "to sort" your patients based on the severity of their injuries Figure 47-11 ▾ . The goal of doing the greatest good for the greatest number means that the triage assessment is brief and the patient condition categories are basic. Primary triage is the initial triage done in the field, whereas secondary triage is done as patients are brought to the treatment area. During primary triage, patients are briefly assessed and then identified in some way, such as by attaching a triage tag. The main information needed on the tag is a unique number and a triage category. Rapid and accurate

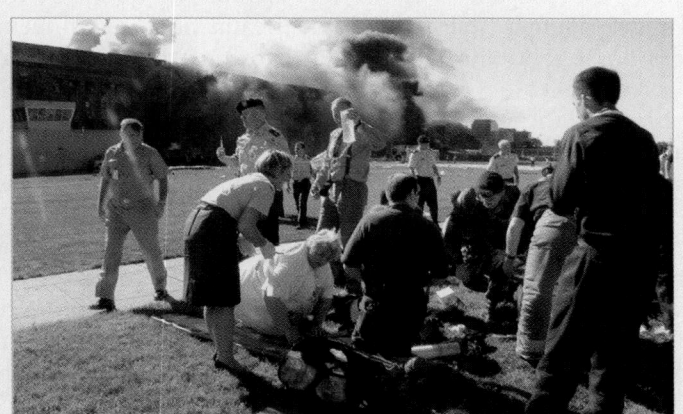

Figure 47-11 Triage is the process of sorting and prioritizing patients based on severity of conditions.

triage will help bring order to the chaos of the MCI scene. After the primary triage, the team leader should communicate the following information to the medical group leader.

- The total number of patients
- The number of patients in each of the triage categories
- Recommendations for extrication and movement of patients to the treatment area
- Resources needed to complete triage and begin movement of patients

Triage Categories

There are four common triage categories. They can be remembered using the mnemonic IDME, which stands for Immediate (red), Delayed (yellow), Minimal (green; hold), and Expectant (black; likely to die or dead) Table 47-2 ▾ . This is the order of priority for treatment and transport of the patients at an MCI.

Immediate (red-tag) patients are your first priority. They will need immediate care and transport. They usually have problems with the ABCs, head trauma, or signs and symptoms of shock.

Delayed (yellow-tag) patients are the second priority and will need treatment and transport, but it can be delayed. Patients usually have multiple injuries to bones or joints, including back injuries with or without spinal cord injury.

Minimal (green-tag) patients are the third priority. Patients may require no field or only "minimal" treatment. In some parts of the world, this is the hold category. These patients are the "walking wounded" at the scene. If they have any apparent injuries, they are usually soft-tissue injuries such as contusions, abrasions, and lacerations.

The last priority is the expectant (black-tag) patients who are dead or whose injuries are so severe that they have, at best, a minimal chance of survival. This category may include patients who are in cardiac arrest or who have an open head injury, for example. If you have limited resources, this category may also include patients in respiratory arrest. Patients in this

Table 47-2	Triage Priorities	
Triage Category	**Typical Injuries**

Red Tag: First Priority (immediate)
   Patients who need immediate care and transport.
   Treat these patients first, and transport as soon as possible.
	• Airway and breathing difficulties
	• Uncontrolled or severe bleeding
	• Severe medical problems
	• Signs of shock (hypoperfusion)
	• Severe burns
	• Open chest or abdominal injuries

Yellow Tag: Second Priority (delayed)
   Patients whose treatment and transport can
   be temporarily delayed.
	• Burns without airway problems
	• Major or multiple bone or joint injuries
	• Back injuries with or without spinal cord damage

Green Tag: Third Priority (walking wounded)
   Patients who require minimal or no treatment and
   transportation can be delayed until last.
	• Minor fractures
	• Minor soft-tissue injuries

Black Tag: Fourth Priority (expectant)
   Patients who are already dead or have little chance
   for survival. Treat salvageable patients before
   treating these patients.
	• Obvious death
	• Obviously nonsurvivable injury, such as major open brain trauma
	• Respiratory arrest (if limited resources)
	• Cardiac arrest

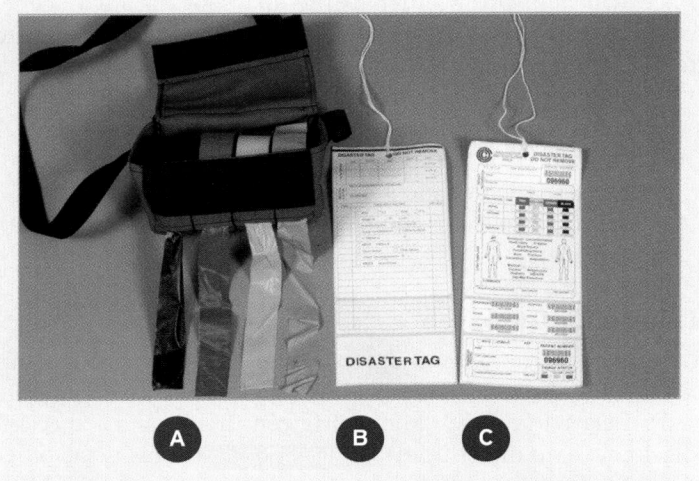

Figure 47-12 Triage tags (from left to right). **A.** Waterproof colored tape. **B.** Back of triage tag. **C.** Front of triage tag.

category receive treatment and transport only after patients in the other three categories have received care.

Triage Tags

Whatever triage system is used, it is vital that a patient has a tag or some type of label. Tagging patients early assists in tracking them and can help keep an accurate record of their condition. Triage tags should be weatherproof and easily read **Figure 47-12 ▲**. The patient tags or tape should be color-coded and should clearly show the category of the patients. The use of symbols and colors to indicate the triage categories is important in case some rescuers are color blind.

The tags will become part of the patient's medical record. Most have a tear-off receipt with a number correlating with the number on the tag. When torn off by the transportation officer, it will assist him or her in tracking a patient. If the patient is unconscious and cannot be identified at the scene, the tag will

be an identifier for tracking purposes. Some areas use digital photography of patients to assist in later identification. The photo is catalogued with the patient's tag number, and the patient's location is tracked with this. When family members are brought to crisis centers to help locate loved ones, the pictures may be of assistance. This technique has been used quite effectively in Europe and Israel with Polaroid and digital pictures. Another way of tracking and accounting for patients is to only issue 20 to 25 cards or tags at a time with a score card to mark how patients are triaged and their priority. When the medic returns for more tags, the scorecard will assist command to count the number of patients and assist command and the staff in developing a plan to respond and ensuring that appropriate resources are available or summoned. Whatever labeling system is used, it is imperative for the transportation officer to be able to identify which patient went by which unit and to which destination, as well as the priority of the patient's condition.

START Triage

START triage is one of the easiest methods of triage. START stands for Simple Triage And Rapid Treatment. The staff members at Hoag Memorial Hospital, Newport Beach, CA, are responsible for developing this method of triage. It is easily mastered with practice and will give you the ability to rapidly categorize patients at an MCI. START triage uses a limited assessment of the patient's ability to walk, respiratory status, hemodynamic status, and neurologic status.

The first step of the START triage system is performed on arrival at the scene by calling out to the disaster site, "If you can hear my voice and are able to walk . . ." and then directing patients to an easily identifiable landmark. The injured persons in this group are the "walking wounded" and are considered minimal priority, or third-priority patients.

The second step in the START process is directed toward nonwalking patients. You move to the first nonambulatory patient and assess the respiratory status. If the patient is not breathing, you should open the airway by using a simple man-

You are the Provider Part 4

A man has a 2′ long steel rod from the aircraft impaled in his thigh. There is minor bleeding from the wound; however, there is no apparent fracture.

Initial Assessment	Recording Time
Appearance	Pale, cool, dry skin
Level of consciousness	A (Alert to person, place, and day); feels pain
Airway	Open
Breathing	Rapid and deep
Circulation	Radial pulses are fast and regular

9. How should you triage this patient?
10. What is START?
11. What is the value of using triage tags?

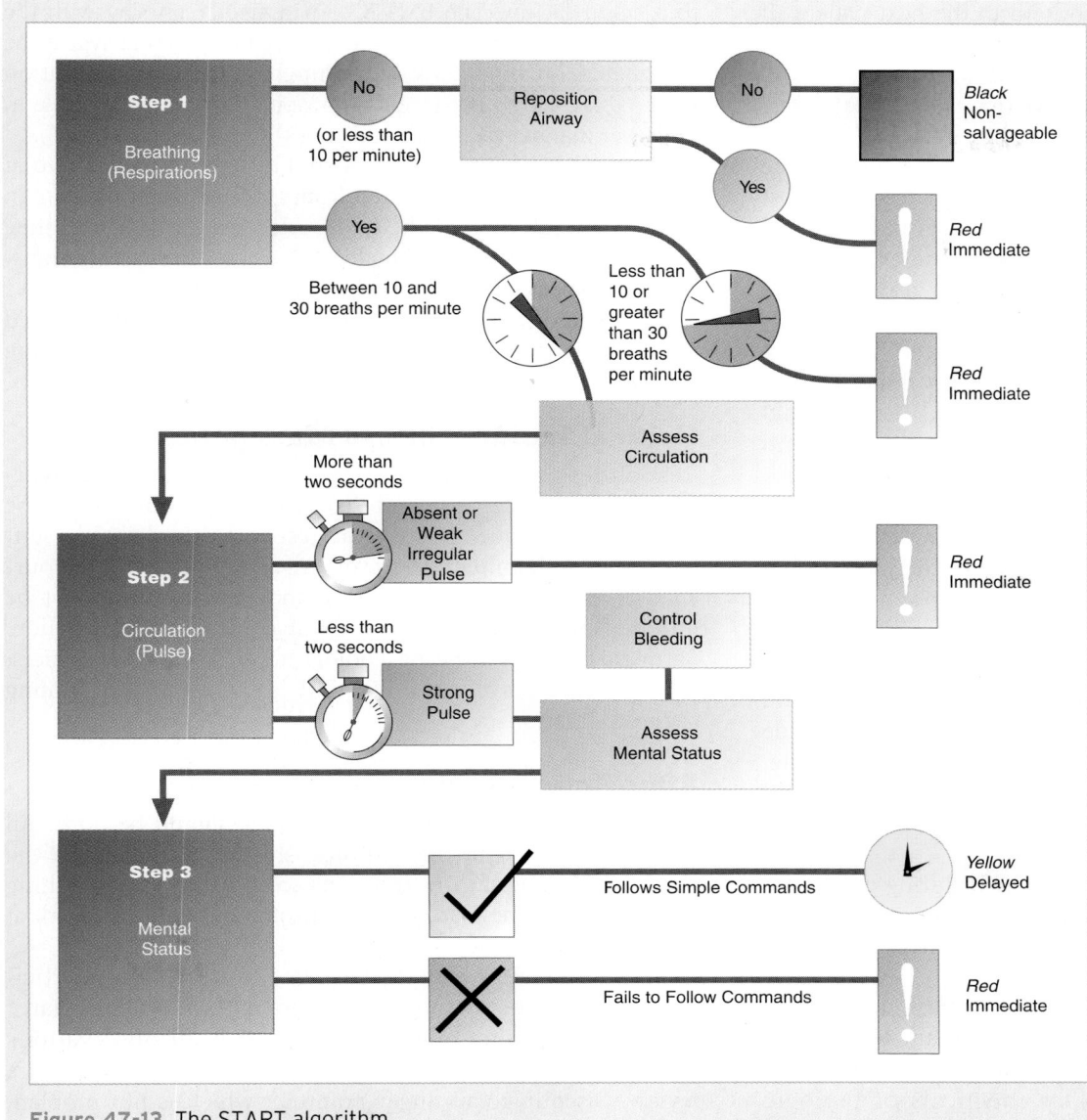

Figure 47-13 The START algorithm.

patient's ability to follow simple commands such as, "show me three fingers." This assessment establishes that the patient can understand and follow commands. A patient who is unconscious or cannot follow simple commands is an immediate priority patient. A patient who complies with a simple command should be triaged in the delayed category. The START system is shown in **Figure 47-13**.

JumpSTART Triage for Pediatric Patients

Lou Romig, MD, recognized that the START triage system does not take into account the physiologic and developmental differences of pediatric patients. She developed the JumpSTART triage system for pediatric patients. JumpSTART is intended for use in children younger than 8 years or who appear to weigh less than 100 pounds. As in START, the JumpSTART system begins by identifying the walking wounded. Infants or children not developed enough to walk or follow commands (including children with special needs) should be taken as soon as possible to the treatment sector for immediate secondary triage. This action assists in getting children who cannot take care of their own basic needs into a caregiver's hands. There are several differences within the respiratory status assessment compared with that in START. First, if you find that a pediatric patient is not breathing, immediately check the pulse. If there is no pulse, label the patient as expectant. If the patient is not breathing but has a pulse, open the airway with a manual maneuver. If the patient does not begin to breathe, give five rescue breaths and check respirations again. A child who does not begin to breathe should be labeled expectant. The primary reason for this difference is that the most common cause of cardiac arrest in children is respiratory arrest.

The next step of the JumpSTART process is to assess the approximate rate of respirations. A patient who is breathing less than 15 breaths/min or more than 45 breaths/min is tagged

ual maneuver. A patient who still does not begin to breathe is triaged as expectant (black). If the patient begins to breathe, tag him or her as immediate (red) and place in the recovery position and move on to the next patient.

If the patient is breathing, a quick estimation of the respiratory rate should be made. A patient who is breathing faster than 30 breaths per minute is triaged as an immediate priority (red). If the patient is breathing fewer than 30 breaths/min, move to the next step of the assessment.

The next step is to assess the hemodynamic status of the patient by checking for a radial pulse. An absent radial pulse implies the patient is hypotensive and should be triaged as an immediate priority. If the radial pulse is present, go to the next assessment.

The final assessment in START triage is to assess the patient's neurologic status, which simply means to assess the

as immediate priority, and you move on to the next patient. If the respirations are within the range of 15 to 45 breaths/min, the patient is assessed further.

The next assessment in JumpSTART triage is also the hemodynamic status of the patient. Just like in START, you are simply checking for a distal pulse. This does not need to be the brachial pulse; assess the pulse that you feel the most competent and comfortable checking. If there is an absence of a distal pulse, label the child as an immediate priority and move to the next patient. If the child has a distal pulse, move on to the next assessment.

The final assessment is for neurologic status. Because of the developmental differences in children, their responses will vary. For JumpSTART, a modified AVPU score is used. A child who is unresponsive or responds to pain by posturing or with incomprehensible sounds or is unable to localize pain is considered an immediate priority and tagged as such. A child who responds to pain by localizing it or withdrawing from it or is alert is considered a delayed priority patient. The JumpSTART system is shown in (Figure 47-14 ▶).

Triage Special Considerations

There are a few special situations in triage. Patients who are hysterical and disruptive to rescue efforts may need to be made an immediate priority and transported out of the disaster site, even if they are not seriously injured. Panic breeds panic, and this type of behavior could have a detrimental impact on other patients and on the rescuers.

A rescuer who becomes sick or injured during the rescue effort should be handled as an immediate priority and be transported off the site as soon as possible to avoid negative impact to the morale of remaining rescuers.

Hazardous materials and weapons of mass destruction incidents force the hazardous materials team to identify patients as contaminated or decontaminated before the regular triage process. Contamination by chemicals or biologic weapons in a treatment area, a hospital, or trauma center could obstruct all systems and organizations coping with the MCI. Bear in mind that some incidents may require multiple triage areas or teams because the victims are located far apart.

Transportation of Patients

All patients triaged as immediate (red) or delayed (yellow) should preferably be transported by ambulance. In extremely large situations, a bus may transport the walking wounded. If a bus is used for minimal priority patients, it is strongly suggested that they be transported to a hospital or clinic distant from the MCI or disaster site to avoid overwhelming the local area hospital resources. It is advisable when using a bus to plan for at least one EMT or paramedic to ride on the bus and to have an ambulance follow the bus. If a minimal patient's condition worsens, the patient could be moved to the ambulance and transported

to a closer facility. The EMT-B or paramedic can stay with the patients triaged as needing minimal care until their arrival at the designated hospital. Any worsening of a patient's condition must be relayed to the receiving hospital as soon as possible in whatever manner the incident dictates.

Immediate priority patients should be transported two at a time until all are transported from the site. Then patients in the delayed category can be transported two or three at a time until all are at a hospital. Finally, the slightly injured are transported. Expectant patients who are still alive would receive treatment and transport at this time. Dead victims are handled or transported according to the standing operating procedure for the area.

Critical Incident Stress Management

Responders at a disaster or an MCI may become overwhelmed. Critical incident stress management should be available and spoken about to all responders and should start within the rehabilitation sector. All responders are encouraged to participate, but stress management should not be imposed or forced. Forcing stress management can do more harm than good to the psychological well-being of rescuers. Some rescuers have the ability and resilience for self-healing in these situations.

After-Action Reviews

After any incident, an after-action review should be done. All agencies involved in the response should participate in the effort to improve future reactions to disasters. If something worked well in the plan, keep it. If something did not work at all, remove it or fix it.

No response is ever perfect, but it is up to all participants to keep perfecting their training, equipment, plans, and skills. Leaders in EMS suggest that all observations should be noted, in writing if possible, to allow future review. Discourage all finger pointing, which is not problem solving. All MCIs are different, and the way you react to each of them will be different, too.

▮ Conclusion

No paramedic ever wants the "Big One" to happen. These events can happen anywhere and at anytime. They can overwhelm EMS systems with huge demands on materials and people, and people can be affected physically and psychologically. By keeping the basic goal of "doing the most good for the most patients" in the forefront, developing plans, using the ICS, and applying a systematic approach to triage, even an MCI can be handled effectively. Practice plans often or on everyday smaller scale incidents, and they will become instinctive, which will help you use them in larger incidents.

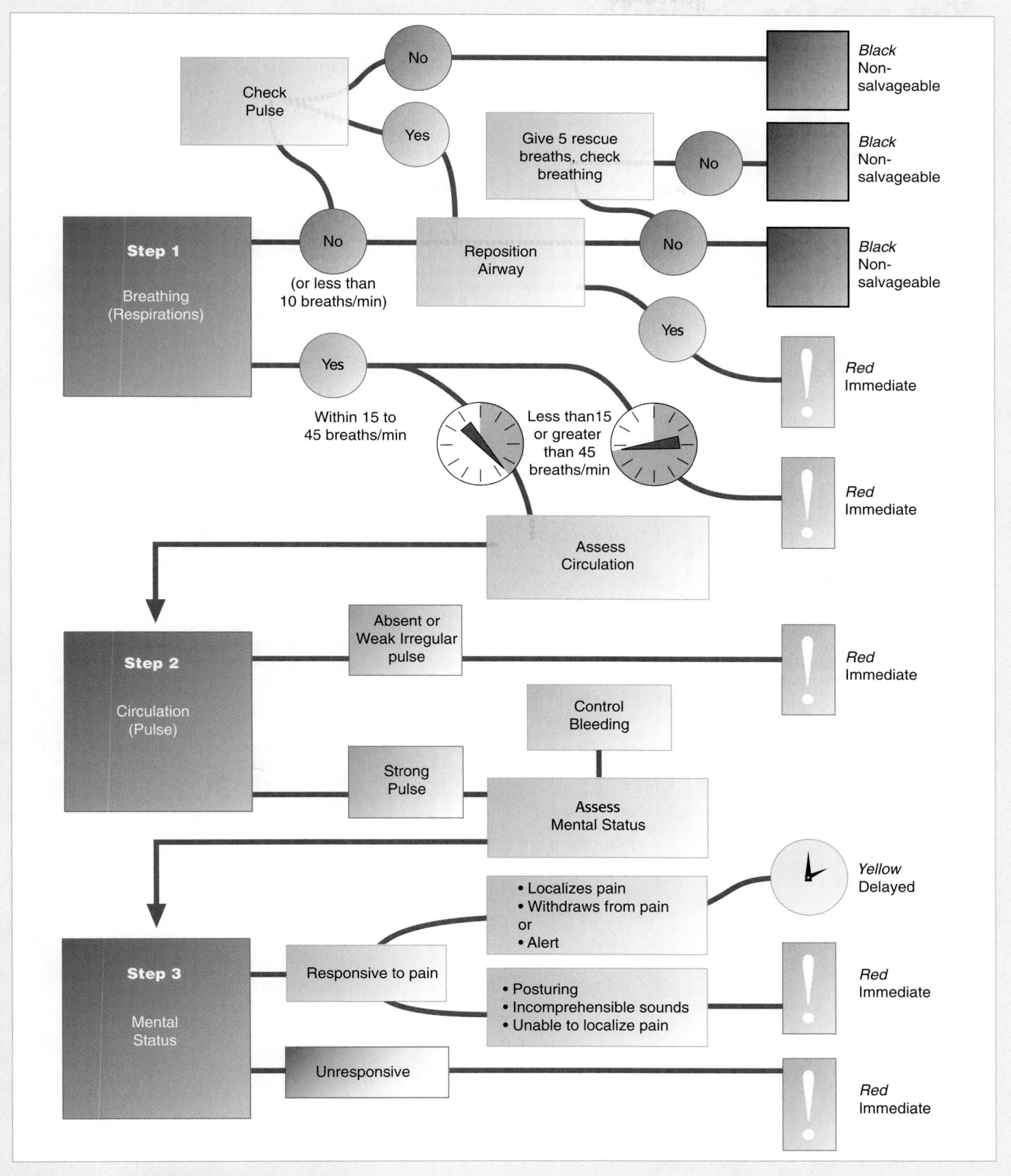

Figure 47-14 The JumpSTART algorithm.

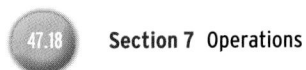

You are the Provider Summary

1. What is your plan of action?

Tag them green, and designate an area for them to be placed.

2. Why is an incident management system (IMS) needed for handling major EMS incidents?

Any incident that involves multiple units responding to an incident requires management of the resources and personnel for a timely and efficient operation. When multiple agencies, especially from different jurisdictions, are involved, it is even more urgent that a system be in place to manage the incident and coordinate the response. EMS providers are trained to manage a single patient with multiple priorities. This is practiced on a daily basis. When a situation arises in which multiple patients must be managed and multiple units are responding (not a daily practice), there must be an IMS that is simple and well understood by all providers. Each community needs to have an IMS that has been practiced and is understood by all of the providers in each of the agencies that may be asked to respond to any major incident.

3. What is an "open" incident? What is a "closed" incident?

An open incident has a number of casualties not yet located when you answer the initial call. Rescuers may have to search for patients and then triage or treat them in multiple locations. There may also be an ongoing situation that produces more patients while you are at the scene, for example, school shootings, tornadoes, a hazardous materials release, or rising floodwaters. A closed incident is a situation that is not expected to produce more patients than initially present. The patients can be triaged and treated as they are removed.

4. How should you triage this patient?

Yellow

5. What is the difference between single and unified command?

Single command usually only works well when there is one emergency service agency responsible for the entire operation and no need for other disciplines to be involved. A unified command structure is more common and a key component of an ICS. This means that all involved agencies contribute to the command process by determining the overall goals and objectives, joint planning for tactical activities, and maximizing the use of all assigned resources at the incident.

6. What is "span of control?"

Another key component of an ICS is the span of control. A manageable span of control is the number of subordinates that one supervisor can manage effectively. The desired range is from three to seven. It can be very easy to lose track of workers at an incident if they are not assigned to small units.

7. How should you triage this patient?

Red

8. Why is there an essential need for common terminology in an ICS?

Common terminology is needed because there may be units from many different jurisdictions. It is easier to use simple sector titles indicating the function they serve (that is, staging, command, operations, triage, treatment, transportation, extrication). An MCI is not the time to begin figuring out another agency's "code system." Plain English works best in these situations. It is much easier for responding units to report to the IC instead of trying to remember that the medic on unit 620 is the person commanding the EMS unit at the scene.

9. How should you triage this patient?

Yellow

10. What is START?

START is an acronym for Simple Triage And Rapid Treatment. This is a method of triaging developed in Newport Beach, CA, in the early 1980s. Under START, the first concept is to clear an area and tell all walking wounded to walk to that location. After clearing walking wounded patients from the scene, the next step is to triage each remaining patient, assessing their respiratory status, hemodynamic status, and mental status. Basically, patients who have adequate respiratory status and hemodynamic status and are alert are classified as "delayed." If they do not have an adequate respiratory status or hemodynamic status or are not alert, they are usually classified as "immediate." The START process permits a few rescuers to triage large numbers of patients very rapidly. If this is the system used in your region, check with your medical director for more specifics on how to use the system.

11. What is the value of triage tags?

Triage tags can be very useful tools. The hardest part is getting crews to start using them! Some EMS agencies have tag days in which all patients are tagged to give the crews practice using the tags. Typically, there are a few different types of triage tags commercially available for services to purchase. Some states have designed their own tags and issued supplies to all EMS agencies. One very useful aspect to triage tags is that they help to eliminate the need to reassess each patient over and over again. Once the patient is tagged, it is clear that an EMS provider has assessed the patient at least once.

Ready for Review

- Disaster management requires planners to take a broad look at preparedness, planning, training, response, and after-action review.
- A mass-casualty incident (MCI) is an event in which the number of patients exceeds the resources available to the initial responders.
- Using the incident command system (ICS) gives you a modular organizational structure that is built on the size and complexity of the incident.
- Major incidents require the involvement and coordination of multiple jurisdictions, functional agencies, and emergency response disciplines. The National Incident Management System (NIMS) is used to prepare for, prevent, respond to, and recover from domestic incidents, regardless of cause, size, or complexity, including acts of terrorism.
- Your EMS agency should have written disaster plans that you are regularly trained to carry out.
- What has traditionally been referred to as medical incident command is also known as the medical (or EMS) branch of the incident command system. At incidents that have a significant medical factor, the incident commander should appoint someone as the medical group or branch leader who will supervise triage, treatment, and transport of injured patients.
- The goal of triage is to do the greatest good for the greatest number. This means that the triage assessment is brief and patient condition categories are basic.

Vital Vocabulary

closed incident A contained incident in which patients are found in one focal location and the situation is not expected to produce more patients than initially present.

command In incident command, the position that oversees the incident, establishes the objectives and priorities, and from there develops a response plan.

critical infrastructure The external foundation in communities made up of structures and services critical in the day-to-day living activities of humans: energy sources, fuel, water, sewage removal, food, hospitals, and transportation systems.

demobilization The process of directing responders to return to their facilities when work at a disaster or mass-casualty incident has finished, at least for the particular responders.

disaster management A planned, coordinated response to a disaster that involves cooperation of multiple responders and agencies and enables effective triage and provision of care according to triage decisions.

disasters Widespread events that disrupt community resources and functions, in turn threatening public safety, lives, and property.

extrication officer In incident command, the person appointed to determine the type of equipment and resources needed for a situation involving extrication or special rescue; also called the rescue officer.

finance In incident command, the position in an incident responsible for accounting of all expenditures.

freelancing When individual units or different organizations make independent and often inefficient decisions about the next appropriate action.

incident commander (IC) The overall leader of the incident command system to whom commanders or leaders of incident command system divisions report.

incident command system (ICS) A system implemented to manage disasters and mass- and multiple-casualty incidents in which section chiefs, including finance, logistics, operations, and planning, report to the incident commander.

joint information center (JIC) An area designated by the incident commander, or a designee, in which public information officers from multiple agencies disseminate information about the incident.

JumpSTART triage A sorting system for pediatric patients less than 8 years old or weighing less than 100 pounds. There is a minor adaptation for infants since they cannot ambulate on their own.

liaison officer (LNO) In incident command, the person who relays information, concerns, and requests among responding agencies.

logistics In incident command, the position that helps procure and stockpile equipment and supplies during an incident.

mass-casualty incident (MCI) An emergency situation that can place great demand on the equipment or personnel of the EMS system or has the potential to overwhelm your available resources.

medical incident command A branch of operations in a unified command system, whose three designated sector positions are triage, treatment, and transport.

morgue officer In incident command, the person who works with area medical examiners, coroners, and law enforcement agencies to coordinate the disposition of dead victims.

National Incident Management System (NIMS) A Department of Homeland Security system designed to enable federal, state, and local governments and private-sector and nongovernmental organizations to effectively and efficiently prepare for, prevent, respond to, and recover from domestic incidents, regardless of cause, size, or complexity, including acts of catastrophic terrorism.

open incident An ongoing or uncontained incident in which rescuers will have to search for patients and then triage or treat them. The situation may produce more patients. Examples include school shootings, tornadoes, a hazardous materials release, and rising floodwaters.

operations In incident command, the position that carries out the orders of the commander to help resolve the incident.

planning In incident command, the position that ultimately produces a plan to resolve any incident.

primary triage A type of patient sorting used to rapidly categorize patients; the focus is on speed in locating all patients and determining an initial priority as their condition warrants.

public information officer (PIO) In incident command, the person who keeps the public informed and relates any information to the press.

rehabilitation officer In incident command, the person who establishes an area that provides protection for responders from the elements and the situation.

rescue officer In incident command, the person appointed to determine the type of equipment and resources needed for a situation involving extrication or special rescue; also called the extrication officer.

safety officer In incident command, the person who gives the "go ahead" to a plan or who may stop an operation when rescuer safety is an issue.

secondary triage A type of patient sorting used in the treatment sector that involves retriage of patients.

single command system A command system in which one person is in charge, generally used with small incidents that involve only one responding agency or one jurisdiction.

span of control In incident command, the subordinate positions under the commander's direction to which the workload is distributed; the supervisor/worker ratio.

staging officer In incident command, the person who locates an area to stage equipment and personnel and tracks unit arrival and deployment from the staging area.

START triage A patient sorting process that stands for simple triage and rapid treatment and uses a limited assessment of the patient's ability to walk, respiratory status, hemodynamic status, and neurologic status.

termination of command The end of the incident command structure when an incident draws to a close.

transfer of command In incident command, when an incident commander turns over command to someone with more experience in a critical area.

transportation officer In incident command, the person who coordinates transportation and distribution of patients to appropriate receiving hospitals.

treatment officer In incident command, the person responsible for locating, setting up, and supervising the treatment area.

triage To sort patients based on the severity of their conditions and prioritize them for care accordingly.

triage officer The person in charge of prioritizing patients, whose primary duty is to ensure that every patient receives initial triage.

unified command system A command system used in larger incidents in which there is a multiagency response or multiple jurisdictions are involved.

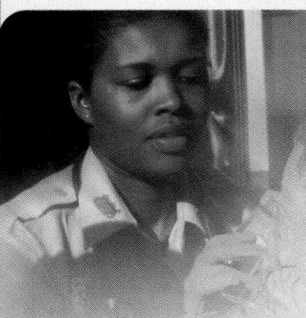

Assessment in Action

You are dispatched to a motor vehicle crash involving a commuter bus on the highway. You are the first unit on scene. When you exit your vehicle, you immediately begin your initial scene size-up. There are several walking wounded, and you are informed that the bus was full, was cut off by another vehicle, and swerved to the right. It traveled down an embankment, rolled over, and landed on its wheels. There are no other vehicles involved, but many people are exiting their vehicles to try to help.

1. **The first size-up radio report to your dispatcher is very important and should include all of the following, EXCEPT:**
   A. location of the triage sector.
   B. specific location of the incident.
   C. extent of the incident.
   D. approximate number of patients involved.

2. **As the first responder arriving at the scenario, you should ask yourself all of the following questions, EXCEPT:**
   A. What do I have?
   B. What do I need?
   C. What do I need to do it?
   D. When do shifts change?

3. **A mass-casualty incident is defined as:**
   A. the greatest challenge facing an EMS provider because the resources are severely limited initially.
   B. those things that are critical in the day-to-day living activities of humans, such as energy sources, fuel, water, sewage removal, food, hospitals, and transportation systems.
   C. an event in which the number of patients exceeds the number of patient care providers or the resources available to responders.
   D. the result of a natural or human-made disaster, subcategorized as open or closed.

4. **Regardless of the cause of this MCI, how would this scenario be subcategorized?**
   A. Closed incident
   B. Open incident
   C. Open-ended incident
   D. Human-made disaster

5. **As a result of the September 11, 2001, terrorist attacks, what system was created?**
   A. Federal Emergency of Management Agency
   B. Critical Incident Management System
   C. National Incident Management System
   D. Unified Command System

6. **What are the two types of incident management systems?**
   A. Single command and unified command systems
   B. Span of control and consolidated action systems
   C. Unified command and dual command systems
   D. Single command and multiple command systems

7. **What are the designated sector positions within medical incident command?**
   A. Triage
   B. Treatment
   C. Transportation
   D. All of the above

8. **What is span of control?**
   A. Individual units or different organizations making independent and often inefficient decisions about the next appropriate action
   B. Establishing the objectives and priorities by the person overseeing the incident
   C. The subordinate positions under a commander's direction to which the workload is distributed; the supervisor/worker ratio
   D. Assistance in procuring and stockpiling equipment

9. **The commander's support staff can be remembered by using the mnemonic:**
   A. C-LAP.
   B. C-ICS.
   C. C-ICE.
   D. C-FLOP.

10. **There are several positions that fall under the incident commander to assist him or her. They are:**
    A. safety officer.
    B. public information officer.
    C. liaison officer.
    D. all of the above.

You arrive to work your night shift. You learn the day crew has been at a structure fire all afternoon. Your supervisor tells you to go and relieve your coworkers. You arrive on scene and are asked to take over the triage sector. The off-going triage officer informs you that they have already triaged approximately 22 patients and that they are expecting another 15 to 20 victims. You've never done this before and are a little nervous. After taking in a few deep breathes, you begin your role.

11. **What is your role?**

■ Points to Ponder

You are dispatched to your local high school at 1:15 PM because of the smell of smoke. When you arrive, the local fire department is there assessing the situation. The cooking class left something burning on the stove and it caught fire. There are approximately 10 to 15 students who were in the classroom who are experiencing possible smoke inhalation symptoms.

What should you do first? Who should you contact?

Issues: Initiating Incident Command at Smaller Events, Knowing Your Department's Standard Operating Procedures for an MCI.

Objectives*

Cognitive

1. Define international and domestic terrorism. (p 48.3)
2. List the different terrorist agenda categories. (p 48.4)
3. Describe the threat levels (or colors) used by the Department of Homeland Security (DHS) to notify responders of the potential for a terrorist attack.
   a. SEVERE (RED)
   b. HIGH (ORANGE)
   c. ELEVATED (YELLOW)
   d. GUARDED (BLUE)
   e. LOW (GREEN) (p 48.6)
4. On the basis of DHS threat levels, discuss what actions the paramedic should take during the course of their work to heighten their ability to respond to and survive a terrorist attack. (p 48.7)
5. Recognize the hallmarks of a terrorist event. (p 48.6)
6. List potential terrorist targets and their vulnerability. (p 48.6)
7. Discuss these key principles to assuring responder safety at the scene of a terrorist event:
   a. Establishing scene safety
   b. Approaching the scene
   c. Protective measures
   d. Establishing a safety zone
   e. Ongoing reevaluation of scene safety
   f. Awareness of secondary devices (p 48.7, 48.8)
8. Discuss the following critical actions that the paramedic must perform to operate on the scene following a terrorist attack:
   a. Notification
   b. Establish command
   c. Patient management (p 48.7, 48.8)

9. Describe and list the four weapons of mass destruction (WMD). (p 48.4)
10. Describe historical events dealing with WMD. (p 48.4)
11. List nuclear/chemical/biological/explosive agents that may be used by a terrorist. (p 48.4, 48.5)
12. Describe the routes of exposure for chemical agents. (p 48.8)
13. Describe the routes of exposure for biological agents. (p 48.13)
14. Describe the routes of exposure for nuclear/radiological dispersal devices (RDD). (p 48.19)
15. Discuss the clinical manifestations of exposure to the various WMD agents. (p 48.8–48.20)
16. Describe the treatment to be rendered to a victim of a nuclear/chemical/biological/explosive attack. (p 48.8–48.20)

Affective

17. Discuss the "new age" terrorist's trend towards apocalyptic violence and indiscriminate death. (p 48.3, 48.4)
18. Explain the rationale behind not entering the WMD scene or being unable to treat contaminated patients, and the possible impact on the paramedic. (p 48.7, 48.8)

Psychomotor

19. Demonstrate the patient assessment skills to assist the patient involved in a nuclear/chemical/biological/explosive agent. (p 48.8–48.20)
20. Demonstrate the use of the nerve agent antidote (MARK 1) auto-injector kit. (p 48.11, 48.12)
21. Given a scenario of a terrorist event, establish scene safety and begin patient management. (p 48.7)

*All of these objectives are noncurriculum objectives.

Introduction

As a result of the increase in terrorist activity, it is possible that you may respond to a terrorist event during your career. International terrorists as well as domestic groups have increased their targeting of civilian populations with acts of terror. The question is not will terrorists strike again, but rather when and where they will strike. The paramedic must be mentally and physically prepared for the possibility of a terrorist event.

The use of weapons of mass destruction, or weapons of mass casualty, further complicates the management of the terrorist incident and places the paramedic in greater danger. Although it is difficult to anticipate and plan a response to many terrorist events, there are several key principles that apply to every response. This chapter describes how you can prepare to respond to these events by discussing types of terrorist events, personnel safety, and patient management. You will learn the signs, symptoms, and treatment of patients who have been exposed to nuclear, chemical, or biological agents or an explosive attack. At the end of this chapter, you will be able to answer the following key questions:

- What are your initial actions?
- Who should you notify, and what should you tell them?
- What type of additional resources might you require?
- How should you proceed to address the needs of the victims?
- How do you ensure your own and your partner's safety, as well as the safety of the victims?

- What is the clinical presentation of a patient exposed to a WMD?
- How are WMD patients to be assessed and treated?
- How do you avoid becoming contaminated or cross-contaminated with a WMD agent?

What Is Terrorism?

No one is quite sure who the first terrorist was, but terrorist forces have been at work since early civilizations. The US Department of Justice defines terrorism as a violent act dangerous to human life, in violation of the criminal laws of the United States or any segment to intimidate or coerce a government, the civilian population or any segment thereof, in furtherance of political or social objectives   Figure 48-1 ▶ . Today, terrorists pose a threat to nations and cultures everywhere. International terrorism has brought a new fear into the lives of many American citizens.

Modern-day terrorism is common in the Middle East, where terrorist groups have frequently attacked civilian populations. In Ireland terrorist groups have attacked the civilian population for decades under the guise of religious freedom. In Colombia, political terrorist groups target oil resources as a means to instill fear.

In the United States, domestic terrorists have struck multiple times within the last decade. The Centennial Park bombing during the 1996 Summer Olympics and the destruction of the

You are the Provider Part 1

You and your partner are dispatched to the Northside Regional Mall for a patient having a seizure. While en route dispatch informs you that they have received numerous 9-1-1 calls from within the mall. Callers are stating that a large number of people are vomiting and having seizures. Many appear to be unconscious.

Additional information received from dispatch states that mall security is reporting a high-pitched whistling sound, much like a gas leak. The HazMat team has been dispatched and has an established time of arrival (ETA) of 4 minutes. All units are given the order to not enter the mall until HazMat has evaluated the scene.

On arrival in the parking lot, you note that your supervisor is on the scene and has donned the "EMS Command" vest. Your supervisor, as well as numerous other responders from law enforcement, fire, and mall security, meets you at the front entrance. Your unit is assigned to report to the temporary field hospital that has been set up in a fast food restaurant across the street. As part of the START system, the "walking wounded" who have already exited the building were told to go to the fast food restaurant to be medically evaluated. There are a number of higher priority patients who are being evaluated or are yet to be evaluated pending authorization that the site is actually safe to enter, but they are clearly not your responsibility at this time.

Initial Assessment	Recording Time: 0 Minutes
Appearance	Female in her 30s who is pacing and appears to be crying
Level of consciousness	A (Alert to person, place, and day)
Airway	Open and clear
Breathing	Rapid and shallow
Circulation	Weak, slow radial pulse

1. What is your first priority at a call in this situation?
2. What does the dispatch information indicate as far as the need for additional resources?

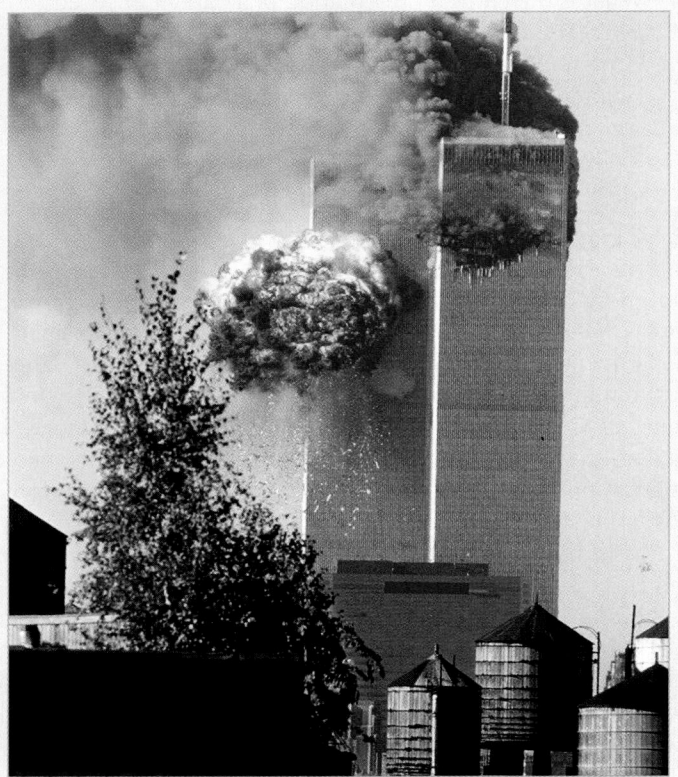

Figure 48-1 The September 11th attack on the World Trade Center accounted for the majority of the deaths caused by terrorists in 2001.

Alfred P. Murrah Federal Building in Oklahoma City in 1995 are examples. Terrorist organizations are generally categorized. Only a small percentage of groups, such as the following, actually turn towards terrorism as a means to achieve their goals:

1. **Violent religious groups/doomsday cults.** These include groups such as Aum Shinrikyo, who carried out chemical and biological attacks in Tokyo between 1994 and 1995. Some of these groups may participate in apocalyptic violence.

2. **Extremist political groups.** They may include violent separatist groups and those who seek political, religious, economic, and social freedom.

3. **Technology terrorists.** Those who attack a population's technological infrastructure as a means to draw attention to their cause, such as cyberterrorists.

4. **Single-issue groups.** These include anti-abortion groups, animal rights groups, anarchists, racists, or even ecoterrorists who threaten or use violence as a means to protect the environment.

Most terrorist attacks require the coordination of multiple terrorists or "actors" working together. Nineteen hijackers worked together to commit the worst act of terrorism in United States history on September 11, 2001. At least four terrorists worked together to commit the London Subway bombings on July 7, 2005. However, in a few instances there has been a single terrorist who struck with devastating results. Terrorists who acted alone carried out all of the Atlanta abortion clinic attacks, the 1996 Summer Olympics attack, and the Oklahoma City bombing.

Weapons of Mass Destruction

What Are Weapons of Mass Destruction?

A weapon of mass destruction (WMD), or weapon of mass casualty (WMC), is any agent designed to bring about mass death, casualties, and/or massive damage to property and infrastructure (bridges, tunnels, airports, and seaports). These instruments of death and destruction include biological, nuclear, chemical, and explosives/incendiary weapons. To date, the preferred WMD for terrorists has been explosive devices. Terrorist groups have favored tactics that use truck bombs or car or pedestrian suicide bombers. Many previous terrorist attempts to use either chemical or biological weapons to their full capacity have been unsuccessful. Nonetheless, as a paramedic you should understand the destructive potential of these weapons.

As discussed earlier, the motives and tactics of the new-age terrorist groups have begun to change. As with the doomsday cults, many terrorist groups participate in apocalyptic, indiscriminate killing. This doctrine of total carnage would make the use of WMDs highly desirable. WMDs are easy to obtain or create and are specifically geared toward killing large numbers of people. Had the proper techniques been used during the 1995 attack on the Tokyo subway, there may have been tens of thousands of casualties. With the fall of the former Soviet Union, the technology and expertise to produce WMDs may be available to terrorist groups with sufficient funding. Moreover, the technical recipes for making nuclear, biological, and chemical (NBC) weapons and explosive devices can be found readily on the Internet; in fact, they have even been published on terrorist group web sites.

There are five categories of terrorist incidents that first responder agencies may confront in the field. They are easily remembered with the mnemonic: BNICE as shown in **Table 48-1 ▼** .

Biological Terrorism/Warfare

Biological agents are organisms that cause disease or death. They are generally found in nature; for terrorist use, however, they are cultivated, synthesized, and mutated in a laboratory. The weaponization of biological agents is performed to artificially maximize the target population's exposure to the germ, thereby exposing the greatest number of people and achieving the desired result.

Table 48-1	The Categories of Terrorist Incidents
B	Biological
N	Nuclear
I	Incendiary
C	Chemical
E	Explosives

The primary types of biological agents that you may come into contact with during a biological event include:

- Viruses
- Bacteria
- Toxins

Nuclear/Radiological Terrorism

There have been only two publicly known incidents involving the use of a nuclear device. During World War II, Hiroshima and Nagasaki were devastated when they were targeted with nuclear bombs. It has been estimated that a death toll of 214,000 occurred due to the two bombs and their associated effects. The awesome destructive power demonstrated by the attack ended World War II and has served as a deterrent to nuclear war.

There are also nations that hold close ties with terrorist groups (known as state-sponsored terrorism) and have obtained some degree of nuclear capability. It is also possible for a terrorist to secure radioactive materials or waste to perpetrate an act of terror. Such materials are far easier for the determined terrorist to acquire and would require less expertise to use. The difficulties in developing a nuclear weapon are well documented. Radioactive materials, however, such as those in Radiological Dispersal Devices (RDDs), also known as "dirty bombs," can cause widespread panic and civil disturbances. More on these devices will be covered later in this chapter.

Chemical Terrorism/Warfare

Chemical agents are manmade substances that can have devastating effects on living organisms. They can be produced in liquid, powder, or vapor form depending on the desired route of exposure and dissemination technique. Developed during World War I, these agents have been implicated in thousands of deaths since being introduced on the battlefield, and since

then have been used to terrorize civilian populations. These agents consist of the following five categories:

- Vesicants or blister agents (ie, mustard gas and Lewisite)
- Respiratory or choking agents (ie, phosgene or chlorine)
- Nerve agents (ie, sarin, soman, tabun, or V agent)
- Metabolic or blood agents (ie, hydrogen cyanide, cyanogens chloride)
- Irritating agents (ie, mace, chloropicrin, tear gas, capsicum/pepper spray, and dibenzoxazepine)

Explosives/Incendiary Weapons

Explosives are the most likely method used by terrorists **Figure 48-2 ▸**. Incendiary weapons involve agents and chemicals used to start fires. Incendiary agents, such as acetone, can be combined with chemicals to produce explosives capable of massive destruction. Ranging from suicide bombings on public buses to trucks loaded with explosives set to go off in underground parking garages of government buildings, these explosions can be very

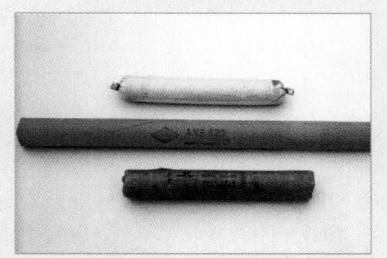

Figure 48-2 Every year, thousands of pounds of explosives are stolen.

destructive. According to the U.S. DOT, explosives are substances that fit into one of the following two categories:

- A substance or article, including a device designed to function by explosion
- A substance or article, including a device, which by chemical reaction within itself can function in a similar manner even if not designated to function by explosion, unless the substance or article is otherwise classified

You are the Provider Part 2

The HazMat team is on the scene and has entered the mall. The word is coming back through EMS Command that they believe a small canister of a nerve gas was released in the sporting goods store. The actual number of patients still inside the mall who are unconscious or may have had seizures is approximately eight patients. The HazMat team is attempting a rapid decontamination on these patients so they can be removed to the cold zone and lifesaving treatment begun. EMS Command has already been in contact with the poison control center and they have advised that all patients, even those who are alert like your patient, be evaluated for nerve agent symptoms (DUMBELS) and if necessary managed with a MARK 1 kit. You begin to evaluate your patient further and note she is still tearing and has vomited.

Vital Signs	Recording Time: 10 Minutes
Level of consciousness	Alert, with a Glasgow Coma Scale score of 15
Skin	Pale, warm and dry
Pulse	Weak radial at 52 beats/min
Respirations	12 breaths/min
Sao_2	97% with oxygen at 10 L/min via nonrebreathing mask

3. What precautions can you take to ensure your own safety?
4. What does your index of suspicion tell you about this scene?

Paramedic Response to Terrorism

Recognizing a Terrorist Event (Indicators)

Most acts of terror are <u>covert</u>, which means that the public safety community generally has no prior knowledge of the time, location, or nature of the attack. This element of surprise makes responding to an event more complex. You must constantly be aware of your surroundings and understand the possible risks for terrorism associated with certain locations, at certain times. It is therefore important that you know the current threat level issued by the federal government through the Department of Homeland Security (DHS).

The Homeland Security Advisory System alerts responders to the potential for an attack, although the specifics of the current threat will not be given. On the basis of the current threat level, the paramedic should take appropriate actions and precautions while continuing to perform daily duties and responding to calls. The system of colors is used to inform the public safety community of the climate of terrorism (derived from intelligence gathering and the amount of terrorist communication) and to heighten the awareness of the potential for a terrorist attack. The system is designed to save lives, including yours.

The DHS has not issued specific recommendations for EMS personnel to follow in response to the alert system. Follow your local protocols, policies, and procedures.

It is your responsibility to make sure you know the advisory level at the start of your workday. Daily newspapers, television news programs, and multiple web sites all give up-to-date information on the threat level. Many EMS organizations are starting to display the advisory system on boards where they can be seen once staff arrives for a shift.

Understanding and being aware of the current threat is only the beginning of responding safely to calls. Once you are on duty, you must be able to make appropriate decisions regarding the potential for a terrorist event. In determining the potential for a terrorist attack, on every call you should observe the following:

- **Type of location.** Is the location a monument, infrastructure, government building, or a specific type of location such as a temple? Is there a large gathering? Is there a special event taking place?
- **Type of call.** Is there a report of an explosion or suspicious device nearby? Does the call come into dispatch as someone having unexplained coughing and difficulty breathing? Are there reports of people fleeing the scene?
- **Number of patients.** Are there multiple patients with similar signs and symptoms? This is probably the single most important clue that a terrorist attack or an incident involving a WMD has occurred.

In the Field

One of the easiest ways to distinguish between a nonterrorist mass-casualty event and a terrorist event is that the intentional use of WMD affects multiple persons. These casualties will generally exhibit the same signs and symptoms. It is highly unlikely for more than one person to experience a seizure at any given time. It is not uncommon to find multiple patients complaining of difficulty breathing at the scene of a fire. However, the same report in the subway at rush hour, when no smell of smoke has been reported, is certainly cause for suspicion. In these situations, you must use good judgment and resist the urge to "rush in and help," especially when there are multiple victims from an unknown cause.

In the Field

The Department of Homeland Security Advisory System is posted daily to heighten awareness of the current terrorist threat Figure 48-3 .

SEVERE (red): Severe risk of terrorist attacks
HIGH (orange): High risk of terrorist attacks
ELEVATED (yellow): Significant risk of terrorist attacks
GUARDED (blue): General risk of terrorist attacks
LOW (green): Low risk of terrorist attacks

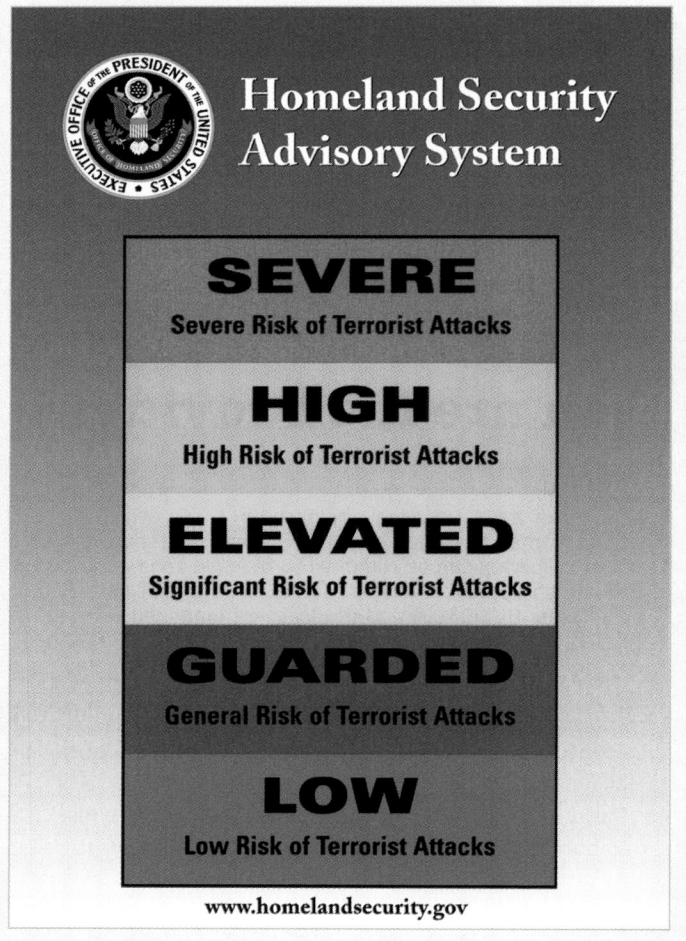

Figure 48-3 Homeland Security Advisory System.

- **Victims' statements.** This is probably the second best indication of a terrorist or WMD event. Are the patients fleeing the scene giving statements such as, "Everyone is passing out," "There was a loud explosion," or "There are a lot of people shaking on the ground." If so, something is occurring that you do not want to rush into, even if it is determined not to be a terrorist event.
- **Pre-incident indicators.** Is the terror alert level high (orange) or severe (red)? Has there been a recent increase in violent political activism? Are you aware of any credible threats made against the location, gathering, or occasion?

Response Actions

Once you suspect that a terrorist event has occurred or WMD have been used, there are certain actions to take to ensure that you will be safe and be in the proper position to help the community.

Scene Safety

Ensure that the scene is safe. If you have any doubt that it may not be safe, do not enter. When dealing with a WMD scene, it is safe to assume that you will not be able to enter where the event has occurred—nor do you want to. The best location for staging is upwind and uphill from the incident. Wait for assistance from those who are trained in assessing and managing WMD scenes Figure 48-4 ▾ . Also remember:

- Failure to park your vehicle at a safe location can place you and your partner in danger Figure 48-5 ▶ .
- If your vehicle is blocked in by other emergency vehicles or damaged by a secondary device (or event), you will be unable to provide patients with transportation, or escape yourself Figure 48-6 ▶ .

Responder Safety (Personnel Protection)

The best form of protection from a WMD agent is preventing yourself from coming into contact with the agent. The greatest threats facing a paramedic in a WMD attack are contamination and cross-contamination. Contamination with an agent occurs when you have direct contact with the WMD or are exposed to

it. Cross-contamination occurs when you come into contact with a contaminated person who has not yet been decontaminated.

Notification Procedures

When you suspect a terrorist or WMD event has taken place, notify the dispatcher, provided that communication is functioning properly. Vital information needs to be communicated effectively if you are to receive the appropriate assistance (see Chapter 16 for information on effective communication). Inform dispatch of the nature of the event, any additional resources that may be required, the estimated number of patients, and the upwind route of approach or optimal route of approach.

It is extremely important to establish a staging area, where other units will converge. Be mindful of access and exit routes when you direct units to respond to a location. It is unwise to have units respond to the front entrance of a hotel or apartment building that has had an explosion. Last, trained responders in the proper protective equipment are the only persons equipped to handle the WMD incident. These specialized units, traditionally hazardous materials (HazMat) teams, must be requested as early as possible due to the time required to

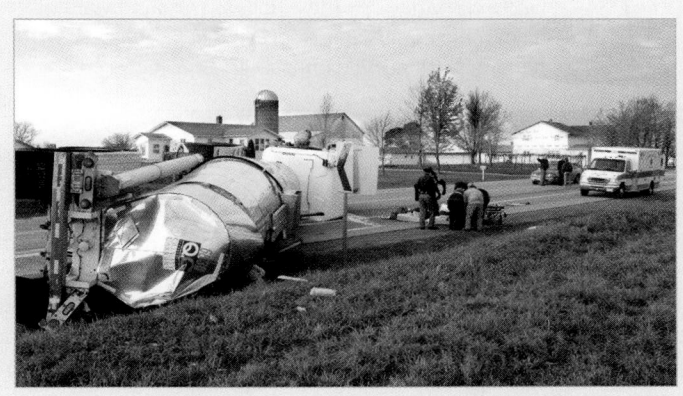

Figure 48-5 Park your vehicle at a safe location and distance.

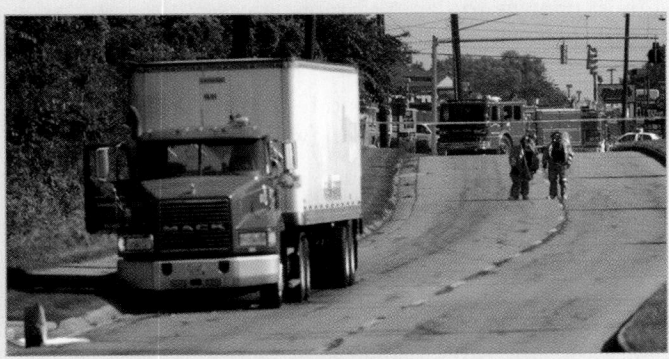

Figure 48-4 Improper staging of a mass-casualty scene could lead to injury or even death of EMS personnel. Wait for assistance from persons who are trained in assessing and managing such scenes.

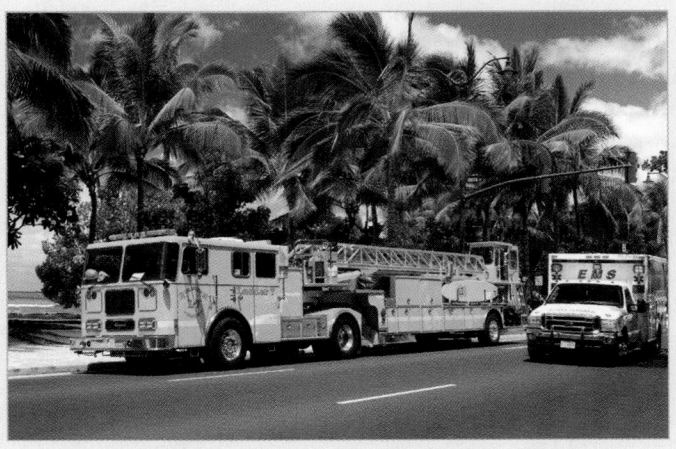

Figure 48-6 Make sure that your vehicle is not blocked in by other emergency vehicles.

assemble and dispatch the team and their equipment. Many jurisdictions share HazMat teams, and the team may have to travel a long distance to reach the location of the event. It is always better to be safe than sorry; call the team early and the outcome of the call will be more favorable. Keep in mind that there may be more than one type of device or agent present.

Establishing Command

The first arriving provider on the scene must begin to sort out the chaos and define his or her responsibilities under the Incident Command System (ICS). As the first person on scene, the paramedic may need to establish "EMS or Medical Command" until additional personnel arrive. Depending on the circumstances, you and other paramedics may function as medical branch officers, triage officers, treatment officers, transportation or logistic officers, or staff. If the ICS is already in place, then you should immediately seek out the medical staging officer to receive your assignment. The incident command system and its components are discussed in further detail in Chapter 47.

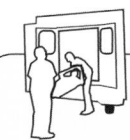

In the Field

Secondary devices may include various types of electronic equipment such as cell phones or pagers that are detonated when "answered."

Secondary Device or Event (Reassessing Scene Safety)

Terrorists have been known to plant additional explosives that are set to explode after the initial bomb. This type of secondary device is intended primarily to injure responders and to secure media coverage, because the media generally arrives on scene just after the initial response. Do not rely on others to secure your safety. It is every paramedic's responsibility to constantly assess and reassess the scene for safety. It is easy to overlook a suspicious package lying on the floor while you are treating casualties. Stay alert. Something as subtle as a change in the wind direction during a gas attack or an increase in the number of contaminated patients can place you in danger. Never become so involved with the tasks that you are performing that you do not look around and make sure that the scene remains safe.

In the Field

You are of no help to the public if you become a patient. More importantly, once you become a victim of the event, you place an additional burden on your fellow responders, who must treat you. Assess the scene and resist the urge to run in and help (do not develop tunnel vision). You may place your life and your partner in danger. Remember . . . do not become a victim.

Chemical Agents

Chemical agents are liquids or gases that are dispersed to kill or injure. Modern-day chemicals were first developed during the two World Wars. During the Cold War, many of these agents were perfected and stockpiled. While the United States has long renounced the use of chemical weapons, many nations still develop and stockpile them. These agents are deadly and pose a threat if acquired by terrorists.

Chemical weapons have several classifications. The properties or characteristics of an agent can be described as liquid, gas, or solid material. Persistency and volatility are terms used to describe how long the agent will stay on a surface before it evaporates. Persistent or nonvolatile agents can remain on a surface for long periods of time, usually longer than 24 hours. Nonpersistent or volatile agents evaporate relatively fast when left on a surface in the optimal temperature range. An agent that is described as highly persistent (such as VX, a nerve agent) can remain in the environment for weeks to months, whereas an agent that is highly volatile (such as sarin, also a nerve agent) will turn from liquid to gas (evaporate) within minutes to seconds.

Route of exposure is a term used to describe how the agent most effectively enters the body. Chemical agents can have either a vapor or contact hazard. Agents with a vapor hazard enter the body through the respiratory tract in the form of vapors. Agents with a contact hazard (or skin hazard) give off very little vapor or no vapors and enter the body through the skin.

Vesicants (Blister Agents)

The primary route of exposure of blister agents, or vesicants, is the skin (contact); however, if vesicants are left on the skin or clothing long enough, they produce vapors that can enter the respiratory tract. Vesicants cause burn-like blisters to form on the patient's skin as well as in the respiratory tract. The vesicant agents consist of sulfur mustard (H), Lewisite (L), and phosgene oxime (CX) (the symbols H, L, and CX are military designations for these chemicals). The vesicants usually cause the most damage to damp or moist areas of the body, such as the armpits, groin, and the respiratory tract. Signs of vesicant exposure on the skin include:

- Skin irritation, burning, and reddening
- Immediate intense skin pain (with L and CX)
- Formation of large blisters
- Gray discoloration of skin (a sign of permanent damage seen with L and CX)
- Swollen and closed or irritated eyes
- Permanent eye injury (including blindness)

If vapors were inhaled, the patient may experience the following:

- Hoarseness and stridor
- Severe cough
- Hemoptysis (coughing up of blood)
- Severe dyspnea

Sulfur mustard (agent H) is a brownish, yellowish oily substance that is generally considered very persistent. When released, mustard has the distinct smell of garlic or mustard and is quickly absorbed into the skin and/or mucous membranes. As the agent is absorbed into the skin, it begins an irreversible process of damage to the cells. Absorption through the skin or mucous membranes usually occurs within seconds, and damage to the underlying cells takes place within 1 to 2 minutes.

Mustard is considered a mutagen, which means that it mutates, damages, and changes the structures of cells. Eventually, cellular death will occur. On the surface, the patient will generally not produce any signs or symptoms until 4 to 6 hours after exposure (depending on concentration and amount of exposure) ▸ Figure 48-7 ▾ .

The patient will experience a progressive reddening of the affected area, which will gradually develop into large blisters. These blisters are very similar in shape and appearance to those

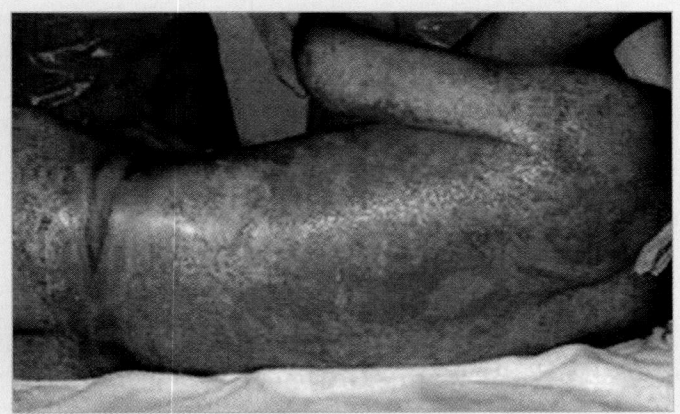

Figure 48-7 Skin damage resulting from exposure to sulfur mustard (agent H).

associated with thermal second-degree burns. The fluid within the blisters does not contain any of the agent; however, the skin covering the area is considered to be contaminated until decontamination by trained personnel has been performed.

Mustard also attacks vulnerable cells within the bone marrow and depletes the body's ability to reproduce white blood cells. As with burns, the primary complication associated with vesicant blisters is secondary infection. If the patient does survive the initial direct injury from the agent, the depletion of the white blood cells leaves the patient with a decreased resistance to infections. Although sulfur mustard is regarded as persistent, it does release enough vapors when dispersed to be inhaled. This creates upper and lower airway compromise. The result is damage and swelling of the airways. The airway compromise makes the patient's condition far more serious.

Lewisite (L) and phosgene oxime (CX) produce blister wounds very similar to mustard. They are highly volatile and have a rapid onset of symptoms, as opposed to the delayed onset seen with mustard. These agents produce immediate intense pain and discomfort when contact is made. The patient may have a grayish discoloration at the contaminated site. While tissue damage also occurs with exposure to these agents, they do not cause the secondary cellular injury that is associated with mustard.

Vesicant Agent Treatment

There are no antidotes for mustard or CX exposure. BAL (British Anti-Lewisite) is the antidote for agent L; however, it is not carried by civilian EMS. The paramedic must ensure that the patient has been decontaminated before ABCs are initiated. The patient may require prompt airway support if any agent has been inhaled, but this should not occur until after decontamination. Initiate transport and gain IV access as soon as possible. Generally, burn centers are best equipped to handle the wounds and subsequent infections produced by

You are the Provider Part 3

Your patient receives a rapid decontamination and she is now the first patient who is ready to be transported to the nearest facility. You are notified that the patient has been administered a nerve agent antidote or MARK 1 kit which involved auto-injectors of atropine and 2-PAM chloride. Your patient, who is a 30-year-old woman who was working in the mall when the incident took place, is still conscious, alert, and oriented. She is complaining of nausea and vomiting. She is experiencing excessive lacrimation and has already urinated twice while in the treatment area. She also has pinpoint pupils and denies any pertinent medical history.

Reassessment	Recording Time: 20 Minutes
Skin	Pale, warm, dry
Pulse	110 beats/min (after atropine), bounding, regular radial pulse
Blood pressure	150/92 mm Hg
Respirations	12 breaths/min
Sao$_2$	97% with supplemental oxygen at 12 L/min via nonrebreathing mask
ECG	Sinus tachycardia without ectopy

5. What could your patient's signs and symptoms represent?

6. What are your treatment options for this patient?

vesicants. Follow your local protocols when deciding what facility to transport the patient to.

Pulmonary Agents (Choking Agents)

The pulmonary agents are gases that cause immediate harm to persons exposed to them. The primary route of exposure for these agents is through the respiratory tract, which makes them an inhalation or vapor hazard. Once inside the lungs, they damage the lung tissue and fluid leaks into the lungs. Pulmonary edema develops in the patient, resulting in difficulty breathing due to the inability for air exchange. These agents produce respiratory-related symptoms such as dyspnea, tachypnea, and pulmonary edema. This class of chemical agents consists of chlorine (CL) and phosgene.

Chlorine (CL) was the first chemical agent ever used in warfare. It has a distinct odor of bleach and creates a green haze when released as a gas. Initially it produces upper airway irritation and a choking sensation. The patient may later experience:

- Shortness of breath
- Chest tightness
- Hoarseness and stridor due to upper airway constriction
- Gasping and coughing

With serious exposures, patients may experience pulmonary edema, complete airway constriction, and death. The fumes from a mixture of household bleach (CL) and ammonia create an acid gas that produces similar effects. Each year, such mixtures overcome hundreds of people when they try to mix household cleaners.

Phosgene should not be confused with phosgene oxime, a blistering agent, or vesicant. Not only has phosgene been produced for chemical warfare, but it is a product of combustion such as might be produced in a fire at a textile factory or house, or from metalwork or burning Freon (a liquid chemical used in refrigeration). Therefore, you may encounter a patient who was exposed to this gas during the course of a normal call or at a fire scene. Phosgene is a very potent agent that has a delayed onset of symptoms, usually hours. Unlike CL, when phosgene enters the body, it generally does not produce severe irritation, which would possibly cause the patient to leave the area or hold his or her breath. In fact, the odor produced by the chemical is similar to that of freshly mown grass or hay. The result is that much more of the gas is allowed to enter the body unnoticed. The initial symptoms of a mild exposure may include:

- Nausea
- Chest tightness
- Severe cough
- Dyspnea upon exertion

The patient with a severe exposure may present with dyspnea at rest and excessive pulmonary edema (the patient will actually expel large amounts of pulmonary edema from their lungs). The pulmonary edema that is seen with a severe exposure produces such large amounts of fluid from the lungs that the patient may actually become hypovolemic and subsequently hypotensive.

Pulmonary Agent Treatment

The best initial treatment for any pulmonary agent is to remove the patient from the contaminated atmosphere. This should be done by trained personnel in the proper PPE. Aggressive management of the ABCs should be initiated, paying particular attention to oxygenation, ventilation, and suctioning if required. Do not allow the patient to be active, as this will worsen the condition much faster. There are no antidotes to counteract the pulmonary agents. Performing the ABCs, gaining IV access, allowing the patient to rest in a position of comfort with the head elevated, and initiating rapid transport are the primary goals for care provided in the prehospital setting. Pharmacotherapy of this patient may include the standard treatment for bronchospasm, pulmonary edema, potential steroid use (per local medical direction) and positive-pressure ventilation with supplementary oxygen.

Nerve Agents

The nerve agents are among the most deadly chemicals developed. Designed to kill large numbers of people with small quantities, nerve agents can cause cardiac arrest within seconds to minutes of exposure. Nerve agents, discovered while in search of a superior pesticide, are a class of chemical called organophosphates, which are found in household bug sprays, agricultural pesticides, and some industrial chemicals, at far lower strengths than in nerve agents.

There are almost 900 different pesticides available for use in the United States. Approximately 37 of these belong to a class of insecticides known as organophosphates. The chemicals in this class kill insects by disrupting their brains and nervous systems. Unfortunately, these chemicals or nerve agents (at greater strengths) also can harm the brains and nervous systems of animals and humans. These chemicals block the essential enzyme in the nervous system called cholinesterase from working, causing the body's organs to become overstimulated and burn out.

G agents came from the early nerve agents, the G series, which were developed by German scientists (hence the G) in the period after WWI and into WWII. There are three G series agents, which are all designed with the same basic chemical structure with slight variations to produce different properties. The two variations of these agents are lethality and volatility. The following G agents are listed from high volatility to low volatility:

- **Sarin (GB).** Highly volatile colorless and odorless liquid. Turns from liquid to gas within seconds to minutes at room temperature. Highly lethal, with an LD_{50} of 1,700 mg/70 kg (about 1 drop, depending on the purity). The LD_{50} is the amount that will kill 50% of people who are exposed to this level. Sarin is primarily a vapor hazard, with the respiratory tract as the main route of entry. This agent is especially dangerous in enclosed environments such as office buildings, shopping malls, or subway cars. When this agent comes into contact with skin, it is quickly absorbed and evaporates. When sarin is on clothing, it has the effect of off-gassing, which means that the vapors are continuously released over a period of time (like perfume). This renders the patient as well as the patient's clothing contaminated.

- **Soman (GD).** Twice as persistent as sarin and five times as lethal. It has a fruity odor as a result of the type of alcohol used in the agent and generally has no color. This agent is both a contact and inhalation hazard that can enter the body through skin absorption and through the respiratory tract. A unique additive in GD causes it to bind to the cells that it attacks faster than any other agent. This irreversible binding is called aging, which makes it more difficult to treat patients who have been exposed.
- **Tabun (GA).** Approximately half as lethal as sarin and 36 times more persistent; under the proper conditions it will remain for several days. It also has a fruity smell and an appearance similar to sarin. The components used to manufacture GA are easy to acquire and the agent is easy to manufacture, which make it unique. GA is both a contact and inhalation hazard that can enter the body through skin absorption as well as through the respiratory tract.
- **V agent (VX).** Clear oily agent that has no odor and looks like baby oil. V agent was developed by the British after World War II and has similar chemical properties to the G series agents. The difference is that VX is over 100 times more lethal than sarin and is extremely persistent (**Figure 48-8**). In fact, VX is so persistent that given the proper conditions it will remain relatively unchanged for weeks to months. These properties make VX primarily a contact hazard, because it lets off very little vapor. It is easily absorbed into the skin, and the oily residue that remains on the skin's surface is extremely difficult to decontaminate.

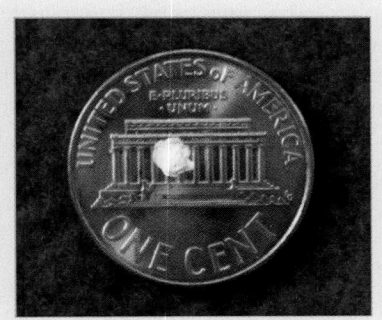

Figure 48-8 VX is the most toxic chemical ever produced. The dot on the penny demonstrates the amount needed to achieve the lethal dose.

Nerve agents all produce similar symptoms but have varying routes of entry. Nerve agents differ slightly in lethal concentration or dose and also differ in their volatility. Some agents are designed to become a gas quickly (nonpersistent or highly volatile), while others remain liquid for a period of time (persistent or nonvolatile). These agents have been used successfully in warfare and to date represent the only type of chemical agent that has been used successfully in a terrorist act. Once the agent has entered the body through skin contact or through the respiratory system, the patient will begin to exhibit a pattern of predictable symptoms. Like all chemical agents,

Table 48-2	Symptoms of Persons Exposed to Nerve Agents
Military Mnemonic: SLUDGEM	
S	Salivation
L	Lacrimation
U	Urination
D	Defecation
G	GI distress
E	Emesis
M	Miosis
Medical Mnemonic: DUMBELS	
D	Defecation
U	Urination
M	Miosis
B	Bradycardia, Bronchorrhea
E	Emesis
L	Lacrimation
S	Salivation

the severity of the symptoms will depend on the route of exposure and the amount of agent to which the patient was exposed. The resulting symptoms are described below using the military mnemonic SLUDGEM and the medical mnemonic DUMBELS. These two mnemonics are used to describe the symptoms of nerve agent exposure and are shown in **Table 48-2** . The medical mnemonic is more useful to you because it lists the more dangerous symptoms associated with exposure to nerve agents.

There are only a handful of medical conditions that are associated with the bilateral pinpoint constricted pupils (miosis) seen with nerve agent exposure. Conditions such as a suspected stroke, direct light to both eyes, and a drug overdose all can cause bilateral constricted pupils. You should therefore assess the patient for all of the SLUDGEM/DUMBELS signs and symptoms to determine whether the patient has been exposed to a nerve agent.

Miosis is the most common symptom of nerve agent exposure and can remain for days to weeks. This symptom, along with the others listed in Table 48-2, will help you recognize exposure to a nerve agent early. The seizures that are associated with nerve agent exposure are unlike those found in patients with a history of seizure. The patient will continue to seize until death or until treatment is given with a nerve agent antidote (MARK 1 or NAAK).

Nerve Agent Treatment (MARK 1/NAAK)

Fatalities from severe exposure occur as a result of respiratory complications, which lead to respiratory arrest. Once the patient has been decontaminated, the paramedic should be prepared to treat these patients aggressively, if they are to be saved. You can greatly increase the patient's chances of survival simply by providing airway and ventilatory support. As with all emergencies, managing the ABCs is the best and most important treatment that you can provide. Often patients exposed to these agents will begin seizing and will not stop. These patients will require administration of nerve agent antidote kits in addition to support of the ABCs.

Fortunately, there is an antidote for nerve agent exposure. MARK 1 kits, also known as Nerve Agent Antidote Kits (NAAK), contain two auto-injector medications: atropine and 2-PAM chloride (pralidoxime chloride). In some regions, the paramedic may carry MARK 1 kits on the unit and will be called upon to administer one or both of the antidotes. These medications are delivered using the same technique as the EpiPen auto-injector; however, multiple doses may need to be administered.

Atropine is used to block the nerve agent's overstimulation of the body. However, because the nerve agent may remain in the body for long periods of time, 2-PAM chloride is used to eliminate the agent from the body. The 2-PAM antidote is effective at relieving the respiratory muscle paralysis and twitching caused by the nerve agent. Many of the symptoms described in the DUMBELS mnemonic will be reversed with the use of atropine; however, many doses may need to be administered to see these results. If your service carries a nerve agent antidote, please refer to your medical director and local protocols for dose and usage information.

Table 48-3 has been provided for quick reference and comparison of the nerve agents.

In the Field

On March 20th, 1995, members of a Japanese cult released sarin (GB) in the Tokyo subway. The first arriving medical responders were met with chaos as hundreds and then thousands of people fled the subway system. Many were contaminated and showing signs and systems of nerve agent exposure. In the end more than 5,000 people sought medical care for exposure to sarin, and 12 people died. None of the EMS personnel wore protective clothing and most became cross-contaminated. Remember, you can avoid becoming exposed. Don't become a victim yourself!

Industrial Chemicals/Insecticides

As previously mentioned, the basic chemical ingredient in nerve agents is organophosphate. This is a common chemical that is used in lesser concentrations for insecticides. While industrial chemicals do not possess sufficient lethality to be effective WMDs, they are easy to acquire, inexpensive, and would have similar effects as the nerve agents. Crop-duster planes could be used to disseminate these chemicals. You should be cautious when responding to calls where insecticide equipment is stored and used, such as a farm or supply store that sells these products. The symptoms and medical management of patients poisoned by organophosphate insecticide are identical to those of the nerve agents.

Metabolic Agents (Cyanides)

Hydrogen cyanide (AC) and cyanogens chloride (CK) are both agents that affect the body's ability to use oxygen. Cyanide is a colorless gas that has an odor similar to almonds. The effects of the cyanides begin on the cellular level and are very rapidly seen at the organ system level. Beside the nerve agents, metabolic agents are the only chemical weapons known to kill within seconds to minutes. Unlike nerve agents, however, these deadly gases are commonly found in many industrial settings. Cyanides are produced in massive quantities throughout the United States every year for industrial uses such as gold and silver mining, photography, lethal injections, and plastics processing. They are often present in fires associated with textile or plastic factories. In fact, cyanide is naturally found in the pits of many fruits in very low doses. There is very little difference in the symptoms found between AC and CK. In low doses, these chemicals are associated with dizziness, light-headedness, headache, and vomiting. Higher doses will produce symptoms that include:

- Shortness of breath and gasping respirations
- Tachypnea
- Flushed skin color
- Tachycardia
- Altered mental status
- Seizures
- Coma
- Apnea
- Cardiac arrest

Table 48-3	Nerve Agents					
Name	Code Name	Odor	Special Features	Onset of Symptoms	Volatility	Route of Exposure
Tabun	GA	Fruity	Easy to manufacture	Immediate	Low	Both contact and vapor hazard
Sarin	GB	None (if pure) or strong	Will off-gas while on victim's clothing	Immediate	High	Primarily respiratory vapor hazard; extremely lethal if skin contact is made
Soman	GD	Fruity	Ages rapidly, making it difficult to treat	Immediate	Moderate	Contact with skin; minimal vapor hazard
V agent	VX	None	Most lethal chemical agent; difficult to decontaminate	Immediate	Very low	Contact with skin; no vapor hazard (unless aerosolized)

In the Field

Always make sure that your patients have been thoroughly decontaminated by trained personnel before you come into contact with them. Chemical agents are primarily a vapor hazard, and all of the patient's clothing must be removed to prevent off-gassing. Finally, never perform mouth-to-mouth or mouth-to-mask ventilation on a victim of a chemical agent. Many of the vapors may linger in the patient's airway and cross-contamination may occur.

The symptoms associated with the inhalation of a large amount of cyanide will all appear within several minutes. Death is likely unless the patient is treated promptly.

Cyanide Agent Treatment

Cyanide binds with the body's cells, preventing oxygen from being used. Several medications act as antidotes, but many services do not carry them. Once trained personnel wearing the proper PPE have removed the patient from the source of exposure, even if there is no liquid contamination, all of the patient's clothes must be removed to prevent off-gassing in the ambulance. Trained and protected personnel must decontaminate any patients who may have been exposed to liquid contamination before a paramedic can initiate treatment. Then you should support the patient's ABCs and gain IV access. Mild effects of cyanide exposure will generally resolve by simply removing the victim from the source of contamination and administering supplementary oxygen. Severe exposure, however, will require aggressive oxygenation and

perhaps ventilation with supplementary oxygen. Always use a bag-mask device or oxygen-powered ventilator device to ventilate a patient exposed to a metabolic agent. The agent can easily be passed on from the patient to the paramedic through mouth-to-mouth or mouth-to-mask ventilations. If no antidote is available, initiate transport immediately.

Table 48-4 ▾ summarizes the chemical agents. The odors of the particular chemicals are provided for informational purposes only. The sense of smell is a poor tool to use to determine whether there is a chemical agent present. Many persons are unable to smell the agents, and the odor could be derived from another source. This information is useful to you if you receive reports from victims claiming to smell bleach or garlic, for example. You should never enter a potentially hazardous area and "smell" to determine whether a chemical agent is present.

Biological Agents

Biological agents pose many difficult issues when used as a WMD. Biological agents can be almost completely undetectable. Also, most of the diseases caused by these agents will be similar to other minor illnesses commonly seen by paramedics.

Biological agents are grouped as viruses, bacteria, or neurotoxins and may be spread in various ways. Dissemination is the means by which a terrorist will spread the agent—for example, poisoning the water supply or aerosolizing the agent into the air or ventilation system of a building. A disease vector is an animal that spreads disease, once infected, to another animal. For example, the plague can be spread by infected rats,

Table 48-4	Chemical Agents					
Class	Military Designations	Odor	Lethality	Onset of Symptoms	Volatility	Primary Route of Exposure
Nerve agents	Tabun (GA) Sarin (GB) Soman (GD) VX	Fruity or none	Most lethal chemical agents can kill within minutes; effects are reversible with antidotes	Immediate	Moderate (GA, GD) Very high (GB) Low (VX)	Vapor hazard (GB) Both vapor and contact hazard (GA, GD) Contact hazard (VX)
Vesicants	Mustard (H) Lewisite (L) Phosgene oxime (CX)	Garlic (H) Geranium (L)	Causes large blisters to form on victims; may severely damage upper airway if vapors are inhaled; severe intense pain and grayish skin discoloration (L, CX)	Delayed (H) Immediate (L, CX)	Very low (H, L) Moderate (CX)	Primarily contact; with some vapor hazard
Pulmonary agents	Chlorine (CL) Phosgene (CG)	Bleach (CL) Cut grass (CG)	Causes irritation; choking (CL); severe pulmonary edema (CG)	Immediate (CL) Delayed (CG)	Very high	Vapor hazard
Cyanide agents	Hydrogen cyanide (AC) Cyanogens chloride (CK)	Almonds (AC) Irritating (CK)	Highly lethal chemical gases; can kill within minutes; effects are reversible with antidotes	Immediate	Very high	Vapor hazard

smallpox by infected persons, and West Nile virus by infected mosquitoes. How easily the disease is able to spread from one human to another human is called communicability. Some diseases, such as those caused by human immunodeficiency virus, are difficult to spread by routine contact. Therefore communicability is considered low. In other instances when communicability is high, such as with smallpox, the person is considered contagious. Typically, your BSI precautions are enough to prevent contamination from contagious biological organisms.

Incubation describes the period of time between the person becoming exposed to the agent and when symptoms begin. The incubation period is especially important for the paramedic to understand. Although your patient may not exhibit signs or symptoms, he or she may be contagious.

Paramedics need to be aware of when they should suspect the use of biological agents. If the agent is in the form of a powder, such as in the October 2001 incidents involving anthrax powder mailed in letters, the call must be handled by HazMat specialists. Patients who have come into direct contact with the agent need to be decontaminated before any EMS contact or treatment is initiated.

Viruses

Viruses are germs that require a living host to multiply and survive. A virus is a simple organism and cannot thrive outside of a host (living body). Once in the body, the virus will invade healthy cells and replicate itself to spread through the host. As the virus spreads, so does the disease that it carries. Viruses survive by moving from one host to another by using its transport system-vectors.

Viral agents that may be used during a biological terrorist release pose an extraordinary problem for health care providers, especially those in EMS. Although some viral agents do have vaccines, there is no treatment for a viral infection other than antivirals for some agents. Because of this characteristic, the following viruses have been used as terrorist agents.

Smallpox

Smallpox is a highly contagious disease. All forms of BSI precautions must be used to prevent cross-contamination to health care providers. Simply by wearing examination gloves, a HEPA-filtered respirator, and eye protection, you will greatly reduce your risk of contamination. The last natural case of smallpox in the world was seen in 1977. Before the rash and blisters show, the illness will start with a high fever and body aches and headaches. The patient's temperature is usually in the range of 101° to 104°F.

An easy, quick way to differentiate the smallpox rash from other skin disorders is to observe the size, shape, and location of the lesions. In smallpox, all the lesions are identical in their development. In other skin disorders, the lesions will be in various stages of healing and development. Smallpox blisters also begin on the face and extremities and eventually move toward the chest and abdomen. The disease is in its most contagious phase when the blisters begin to form (Figure 48-9 ▶).

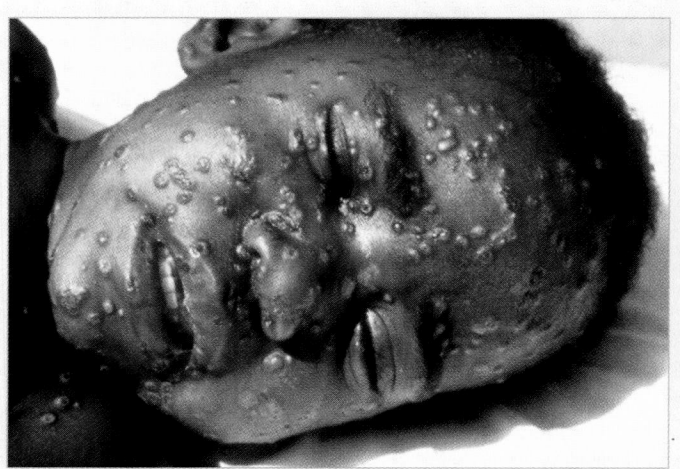

Figure 48-9 In smallpox, all the lesions are identical in their development. In other skin disorders, the lesions will be in various stages of healing and development.

Table 48-5	Characteristics of Smallpox
Dissemination	Aerosolized for warfare or terrorist uses
Communicability	High from infected individuals or items (such as blankets used by infected patients). Person-to-person transmission is possible.
Route of entry	Through inhalation of coughed droplets or direct skin contact with blisters
Signs and symptoms	Severe fever, malaise, body aches, headaches, small blisters on the skin, bleeding of the skin and mucous membranes. Incubation period is 10 to 12 days and the duration of the illness is approximately 4 weeks.
Medical management	BSI precautions. There is no specific treatment for smallpox victims. Patients should be provided with supportive care (ABCs).

Unprotected contact with these blisters will promote transmission of the disease. There is a vaccine to prevent smallpox; however, it has been linked to medical complications and in very rare cases death (Table 48-5 ▲). Vaccination against the disease is part of a national strategy to respond to a terrorist threat. Because the vaccine does have some risk, only first responders have been offered the vaccine. Should an outbreak occur, vaccine would be offered to people at risk.

Viral Hemorrhagic Fevers

Viral hemorrhagic fevers (VHF) consist of a group of diseases that include the Ebola, Rift Valley, and yellow fever viruses, among others. This group of viruses causes the blood in the body to seep out from the tissues and blood vessels

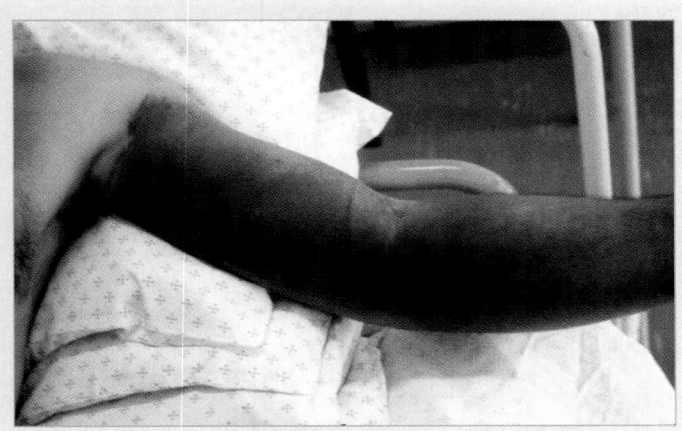

Figure 48-10 Viral hemorrhagic fevers cause the blood vessels and tissues to seep blood. The end result is ecchymosis, hemoptysis, and blood in the patient's stool. Notice the severe discoloration in this patient with Crimean Congo hemorrhagic fever, indicating internal bleeding.

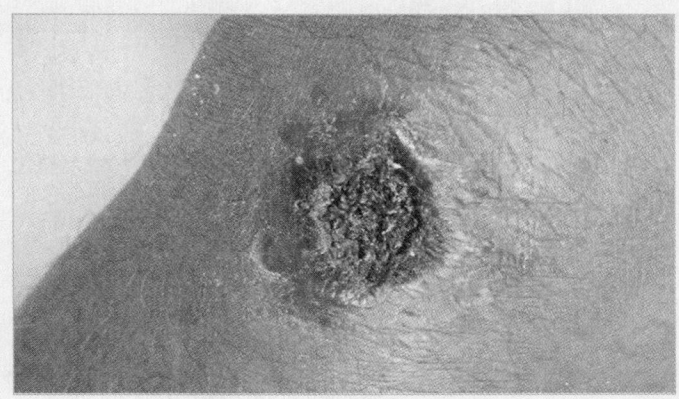

Figure 48-11 Cutaneous anthrax.

Table 48-6	Characteristics of Viral Hemorrhagic Fevers
Dissemination	Direct contact with an infected person's body fluids. It can also be aerosolized for use in an attack.
Communicability	Moderate from person to person or from contaminated items.
Route of entry	Direct contact with an infected person's body fluids.
Signs and symptoms	Sudden onset of fever, weakness, muscle pain, headache, and sore throat. All of these symptoms are followed by vomiting and as the virus runs it course, internal and external bleeding.
Medical management	BSI precautions. There is no specific treatment for viral hemorrhagic fever. Patients should be provided supportive care (ABCs) and treatment for shock and hypotension, if present.

Figure 48-10 ▲ . Initially, the patient will have flu-like symptoms, progressing to more serious symptoms such as internal and external hemorrhaging. Outbreaks are not uncommon in Africa and South America. Outbreaks in the United States, however, are extremely rare. All BSI precautions must be taken when treating these illnesses. Mortality rates can range from 5% to 90%, depending on the strain of virus, the patient's age and health condition, and the availability of a modern health care system Table 48-6 ▲ .

Bacteria

Unlike viruses, bacteria do not require a host to multiply and live. Bacteria are much more complex and larger than viruses and can grow up to 100 times larger than the largest virus.

Bacteria contain all the cellular structures of a normal cell and are completely self-sufficient. Most importantly, bacterial infections can be fought with antibiotics.

Most bacterial infections will generally begin with flu-like symptoms, which make it quite difficult to identify whether the cause is a biological attack or a natural epidemic. Biological agents have been developed and used for centuries during times of war.

Inhalation and Cutaneous Anthrax (Bacillus anthracis)

Anthrax is a deadly bacteria that lays dormant in a spore (protective shell). When exposed to the optimal temperature and moisture, the germ will be released from the spore. The routes of entry for anthrax are inhalation, cutaneous, or gastrointestinal (from consuming food that contain spores) Figure 48-11 ▲ . The inhalational form or pulmonary anthrax is the most deadly and often presents as a severe cold. Pulmonary anthrax infections are associated with a 90% death rate if untreated. Antibiotics can be used to treat anthrax successfully. There is also a vaccine to prevent anthrax infections Table 48-7 ▶ .

Plague—Bubonic/Pneumonic

Of all the infectious diseases known to humans, none has killed as many as the plague. The 14th century plague that ravaged Asia, the Middle East, and finally Europe (the Black Death) killed an estimated 33 to 42 million people. Later on, in the early 19th century, almost 20 million people in India and China perished due to plague. The plague's natural vectors are infected rodents and fleas. When a person is either bit by an infected flea or comes into contact with an infected rodent (or the waste of the rodent), the person can contract bubonic plague.

Bubonic plague infects the lymphatic system (a passive circulatory system in the body that bathes the tissues in lymph and works with the immune system). When this occurs, the patient's lymph nodes (area of the lymphatic system where infection-fighting cells are housed) become infected and grow. The glands of the nodes will grow large (up to the size of a tennis ball) and round, forming buboes Figure 48-12 ▶ . If left

Table 48-7	Characteristics of Anthrax
Dissemination	Aerosol
Communicability	Only in the cutaneous form (rare)
Route of entry	Through inhalation of spore or skin contact with spore or direct contact with skin wound (cutaneous)
Signs and symptoms	Flu-like symptoms, fever, respiratory distress with tachycardia, shock, pulmonary edema and respiratory failure after 3 to 5 days of flu-like symptoms
Medical management	Pulmonary/inhalation: BSI precautions, supplemental oxygen, ventilatory support for pulmonary edema or respiratory failure and transport. Cutaneous: BSI precautions, apply dry sterile dressing to prevent accidental contact with wound and fluids.

Table 48-8	Characteristics of Plague
Dissemination	Aerosol
Communicability	Bubonic: low, only from contact with fluid in buboe Pneumonic: high, from person to person
Route of entry	Ingestion, inhalation, or cutaneous
Signs and symptoms	Fever, headache, muscle pain and tenderness, pneumonia, shortness of breath, extreme lymph node pain and enlargement (bubonic)
Medical management	BSI, ABCs, provide supplemental oxygen, and transport

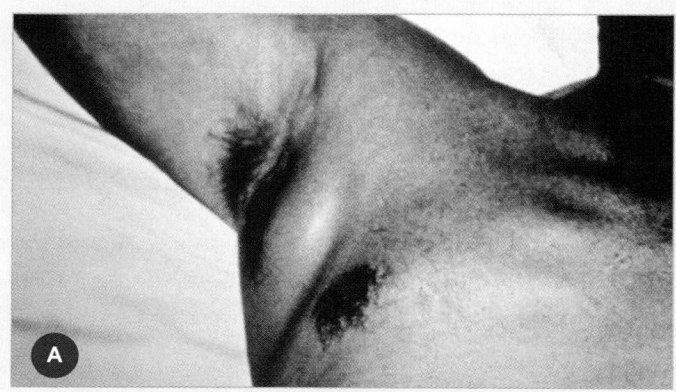

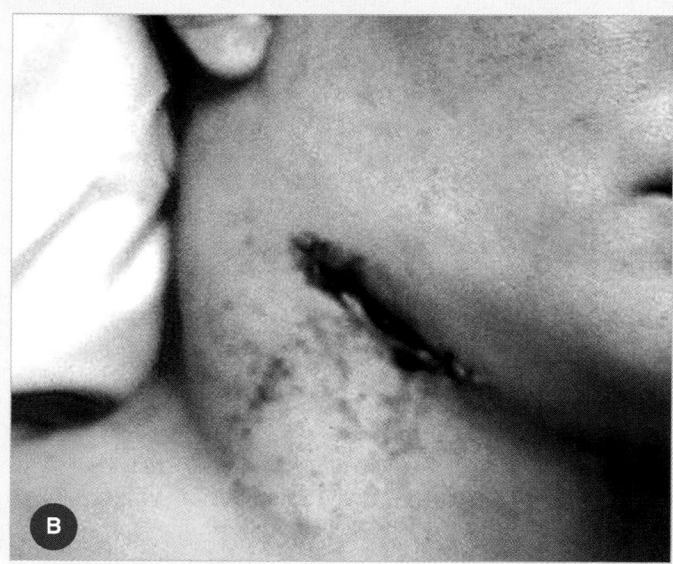

Figure 48-12 A. Plague buboe at lymph node under arm. **B.** Plague buboe at lymph node on neck.

untreated, the infection may spread through the body, leading to sepsis and possibly death. This form of plague is not contagious and is not likely to be seen in a bioterrorist incident.

Pneumonic plague is a lung infection, also known as plague pneumonia, that results from inhalation of plague bacteria. This form of the disease is contagious and has a much higher death rate than the bubonic form. This form of plague therefore would be easier to disseminate (aerosolized), has a higher mortality, and is contagious **Table 48-8 ▲** .

Neurotoxins

Neurotoxins are the most deadly substances known to humans. The strongest neurotoxin is 15,000 times more lethal than VX and 100,000 times more lethal than sarin. These toxins are produced from plants, marine animals, molds, and bacteria. The route of entry for these toxins is through ingestion, inhalation from aerosols, or injection. Unlike viruses and bacteria, neurotoxins are not contagious and have a faster onset of symptoms. Although these biological toxins have immense destructive potential, they have not been used successfully as a WMD.

Botulinum Toxin

The most potent neurotoxin is botulinum, which is produced by bacteria. When introduced into the body, this neurotoxin affects the nervous system's ability to function. Voluntary muscle control will diminish as the toxin spreads. Eventually the toxin will cause muscle paralysis that begins at the head and face and travels downward throughout the body. The patient's accessory muscles and diaphragm will become paralyzed, and the patient will go into respiratory arrest **Table 48-9 ▸** .

Ricin

While not as deadly as botulinum, ricin is still five times more lethal than VX. This toxin is derived from mash that is left from the castor bean **Figure 48-13 ▸** . When introduced into the body, ricin causes pulmonary edema and respiratory and circulatory failure leading to death **Table 48-10 ▸** .

The clinical picture depends on the route of exposure. The toxin is quite stable and extremely toxic by many routes of exposure, including inhalation. Perhaps 1 to 3 mg of ricin can kill an adult, and the ingestion of one seed can probably kill a child.

Table 48-9	Characteristics of Botulinum Toxin
Dissemination	Aerosol or food supply sabotage or injection
Communicability	None
Route of entry	Ingestion or gastrointestinal
Signs and symptoms	Dry mouth, intestinal obstruction, urinary retention, constipation, nausea and vomiting, abnormal pupil dilation, blurred vision, double vision, drooping eyelids, difficulty swallowing, difficulty speaking, and respiratory failure due to paralysis
Medical management	ABCs, provide supplemental oxygen and transport. Ventilatory support may be needed due to paralysis of the respiratory muscles. A vaccine is available.

Table 48-10	Characteristics of Ricin
Dissemination	Aerosol or contamination of a food or water supply by sabotage
Communicability	None
Route of entry	Inhalation, ingestion, injection
Signs and symptoms	Inhaled: Cough, difficulty breathing, chest tightness, nausea, muscle aches, pulmonary edema, and hypoxia Ingested: Nausea and vomiting, internal bleeding, and death Injection: No signs except swelling at the injection site and death
Medical management	ABCs. No treatment or vaccine exists.

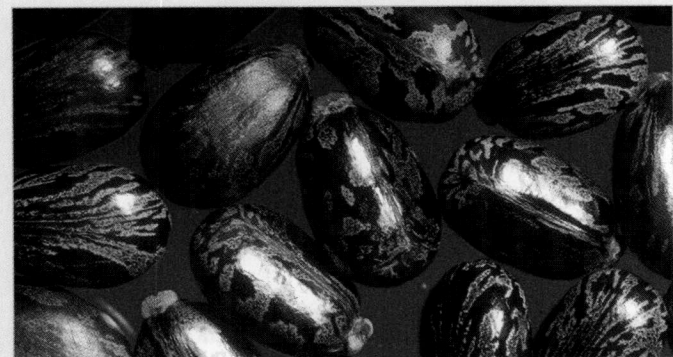

Figure 48-13 These seemingly harmless castor beans contain the key ingredient for ricin, one of the most potent toxins known to humans.

Although all parts of the castor bean are actually poisonous, it is the seeds that are the most toxic. Castor bean ingestion causes a rapid onset of nausea, vomiting, abdominal cramps, and severe diarrhea, followed by vascular collapse. Death usually occurs on the third day in the absence of appropriate medical intervention.

Ricin is least toxic by the oral route. This is probably a result of poor absorption in the gastrointestinal tract, some digestion in the gut, and, possibly, some expulsion of the agent as caused by the rapid onset of vomiting. Ingestion causes local hemorrhage and necrosis of the liver, spleen, kidney, and gastrointestinal tract. Signs and symptoms appear 4 to 8 hours after exposure.

Signs and symptoms of ricin ingestion are as follows:
- Fever
- Chills
- Headache
- Muscle aches
- Nausea
- Vomiting
- Diarrhea
- Severe abdominal cramping
- Dehydration
- Gastrointestinal bleeding
- Necrosis of liver, spleen, kidneys, and gastrointestinal tract

Inhalation of ricin causes nonspecific weakness, cough, fever, hypothermia, and hypotension. Symptoms occur about 4 to 8 hours after inhalation, depending on the inhaled dose. The onset of profuse sweating some hours later signifies the termination of the symptoms.

Signs and symptoms of ricin inhalation are as follows:
- Fever
- Chills
- Nausea
- Local irritation of eyes, nose, and throat
- Profuse sweating
- Headache
- Muscle aches
- Nonproductive cough
- Chest pain
- Dyspnea
- Pulmonary edema
- Severe lung inflammation
- Cyanosis
- Convulsions
- Respiratory failure

Treatment is supportive and includes both respiratory support and cardiovascular support as needed. Early intubation, ventilation, and positive end expiratory pressure, combined with treatment of pulmonary edema, are appropriate. Intravenous fluids and electrolyte replacement are useful for treating the dehydration caused by profound vomiting and diarrhea. **Table 48-11 ▶** summarizes the biological agents.

Other Paramedic Roles During a Biological Event
Syndromic Surveillance

Syndromic surveillance is the monitoring, usually by local or state health departments, of patients presenting to emergency departments and alternative care facilities, and the recording of EMS call volume and the use of over-the-counter medications. Patients with signs and symptoms that resemble influenza are particularly important. Local and state health departments monitor for an unusual influx of patients with these symptoms in hopes of catching an outbreak early. The EMS role in syndromic surveillance is a small one, yet valuable in the overall tracking of a biological terrorist event or infectious disease outbreak. Quality assurance and dispatch operations need to be aware of an unusual number of calls from patients with "unexplainable flu" coming from a particular region or community.

Points of Distribution

Points of distribution (PODs) (Strategic National Stockpile) are strategically placed facilities that have been pre-established for the mass distribution of antibiotics, antidotes, vaccinations, and other medications and supplies. These medications may be delivered in large containers known as "push packs" by the Centers for Disease Control and Prevention National Pharmaceutical Stockpile Figure 48-14 ▶ . These containers have a delivery time of 12 hours anywhere in the country and contain antibiotics, chemical antidotes, antitoxins, life-support medications, IV administration, airway maintenance supplies, and medical/surgical items. In some regions, local and state municipalities have started to stockpile their own supplies to reduce the time delay.

Paramedics may be called on to assist in the delivery of the medications to the public (depending on local emergency management planning). The paramedic's role may include triage, treatment of seriously ill patients, and patient transport to the hospital. Most plans for PODs include at least one ambulance on standby for the transport of seriously ill patients.

Table 48-11	Biological Agents			
Disease	**Transmission Person to Person**	**Incubation Period**	**Duration of Illness**	**Lethality (approximate case fatality rates)**
Inhalation anthrax	No	1 to 6 d	3 to 5 d (usually fatal if untreated)	High
Pneumonic plague	High	2 to 3 d	1 to 6 d (usually fatal)	High unless treated within 12 to 24 h
Smallpox	High	7 to 17 d (average 12 d)	4 wk	High to moderate
Viral hemorrhagic fevers	Moderate	4 to 21 d	Death between 7 to 16 d	High to moderate, depending on type of fever
Botulinum	No	1 to 5 d	Death in 24 to 72 h; lasts months if patient does not die	High without respiratory support
Ricin	No	18 to 24 h	Days; death within 10 to 12 d for ingestion	High

You are the Provider Part 4

Your patient has a patent airway. You immediately apply high-flow oxygen via a nonrebreathing mask. Lung sounds are raspy and moist sounding. Her oxygen saturation is at 97% on 15 L/min of oxygen. Since the patient report that you received from the HazMat team indicates that a nerve agent antidote kit was used on the patient, you will need to closely monitor her vital signs and watch to see if symptoms develop. Take along another MARK 1 kit and contact medical control once en route to the ED.

While en route your patient states that she does not feel right. She is becoming disoriented. She suddenly begins to have a seizure. You quickly place padding around the patient to keep her from injuring herself. She becomes incontinent.

Reassessment	**Recording Time: 30 Minutes**
Skin	Pale, warm, dry
Pulse	120 beats/min
Blood pressure	148/94 mm Hg
Respirations	12 breaths/min
Sao$_2$	96% with supplemental oxygen
ECG	Sinus tachycardia with an occasional PVC

7. What does the nerve agent antidote kit include?

8. Is this kit part of your local protocol in dealing with patients exposed to a nerve agent?

9. What is your next step in treatment?

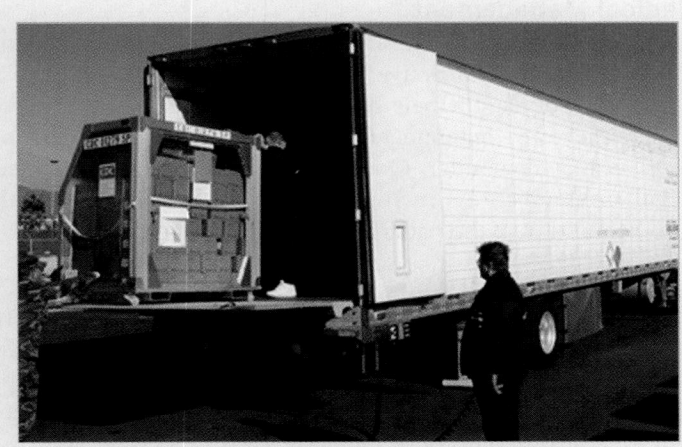

Figure 48-14 The Centers for Disease Control and Prevention Strategic National Stockpile can deliver one of many push packs to any location in the country within 12 hours of an emergency.

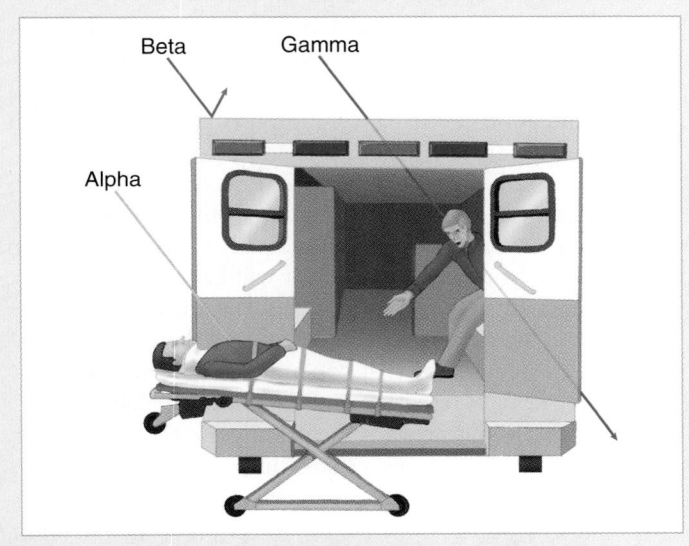

Figure 48-15 Alpha, beta, and gamma radiation.

Radiological/Nuclear Devices

What Is Radiation?

Ionizing radiation is energy that is emitted in the form of rays, or particles. This energy can be found in radioactive material, such as rocks and metals. Radioactive material is any material that emits radiation. This material is unstable, and attempts to stabilize itself by changing its structure is a natural process called decay. As the substance decays, it gives off radiation until it stabilizes. The process of radioactive decay can take from as little as minutes to billions of years; meanwhile, the substance remains radioactive.

The energy that is emitted from a strong radiological source is either alpha, beta, gamma (x-rays), or neutron radiation **Figure 48-15 ▲**. Alpha is the least harmful penetrating type of radiation and cannot travel fast or through most objects. In fact, a sheet of paper or the body's skin easily stops it. Beta radiation is slightly more penetrating than alpha and requires a layer of clothing to stop it. Gamma or x-rays are far faster and stronger than alpha and beta rays. These rays easily penetrate through the human body and require either several inches of lead or concrete to prevent penetration. Neutron energy is the fastest moving and most powerful form of radiation. Neutrons easily penetrate through lead and require several feet of concrete to stop them.

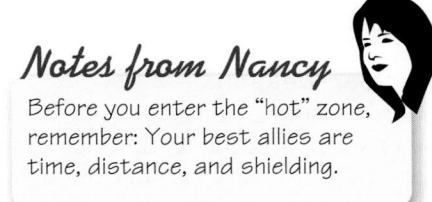

Notes from Nancy

Before you enter the "hot" zone, remember: Your best allies are time, distance, and shielding.

Sources of Radiological Material

There are thousands of radioactive materials found on the earth. These materials are generally used for purposes that benefit humankind, such as medicine, killing germs in food (irradiating), and construction work. Once radiological material has been used for its purpose, the material remaining is called radiological waste. Radiological waste remains radioactive but has no more usefulness. These materials can be found at:

- Hospitals
- Colleges and universities
- Chemical and industrial sites
- Power plants

Not all radioactive material is tightly guarded, and the waste is often not guarded. This makes use of radioactive material and substances appealing to terrorists.

Radiological Dispersal Devices

A radiological dispersal device (RDD) is any container that is designed to disperse radioactive material. This would generally require the use of a bomb, hence the nickname dirty bomb. A dirty bomb would carry the potential to injure victims with not only the radioactive material but also the explosive material used to deliver it. Just the thought of an RDD creates fear in a population, and so the ultimate goal of the terrorist—fear—is accomplished. In reality, however, the destructive capability of a dirty bomb is limited to the explosives that are attached to it. Therefore, if the explosive is sufficient to kill 10 persons without radioactive material, it will also kill 10 persons with the radioactive material added. There may be long-term injuries and illness associated with the use of an RDD, yet not much more than the bomb by itself would create. In short, the dirty bomb is an ineffective WMD.

Nuclear Energy

Nuclear energy is artificially made by altering (splitting) radioactive atoms. The result is an immense amount of energy that usually takes the form of heat. Nuclear material is used in medicine, weapons, naval vessels, and power plants. Nuclear material gives off all forms of radiation including neutrons (the most deadly

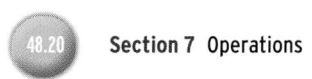

type). Like radioactive material, when nuclear material is no longer useful it becomes waste that is still radioactive.

Nuclear Weapons

The destructive energy of a nuclear explosion is unlike any other weapon in the world. That is why nuclear weapons are kept only in secure facilities throughout the world. There are nations that have ties to terrorists and that have actively attempted to build nuclear weapons. However, the ability of these nations to deliver a nuclear weapon, such as a missile or bomb, is as of yet, incomplete. There is also the deterrent of complete mutual annihilation. Therefore, the likelihood of a nuclear attack is extremely remote.

Unfortunately, due to the collapse of the former Soviet Union, the whereabouts of many small nuclear devices is unknown. These small suitcase-sized nuclear weapons are called Special Atomic Demolition Munitions (SADM). The SADM, or "suit-case nuke," was designed to destroy individual targets, such as important buildings, bridges, tunnels, or large ships. The estimate is that perhaps as many as 80 are missing as of 1998. No other information or updates on the whereabouts of these devices have been made public.

How Radiation Affects the Body

The effects of radiation exposure will vary depending on the amount of radiation that a person receives and the route of entry. Radiation can be introduced into the body by all routes of entry as well as through the body (irradiation). The patient can inhale radioactive dust from nuclear fallout or from a dirty bomb, or have radioactive liquid absorbed into the body through the skin. Once in the body, the radiation source will irradiate the person from within rather than from an external source (such as x-ray equipment). Some common signs of acute radiation sickness are nausea, vomiting, and diarrhea. Additional injuries will occur with a nuclear blast such as thermal and blast trauma, trauma from flying objects, and eye injuries.

Notes from Nancy

The farther away you get from a radioactive source the better, but moving even a small distance away reduces exposure a great deal.

Medical Management

Being exposed to a radiation source does not make a patient contaminated or radioactive. However, when patients have a radioactive source on their body (such as debris from a dirty bomb), they are contaminated and must be initially cared for by a HazMat responder. Once the patient is decontaminated and there is no threat to you, you may begin treatment with the ABCs and treat the patient for any burns or trauma.

Protective Measures

There are no suits or protective gear designed to completely shield from radiation. Those who work in high-risk areas do wear some protection (lead-lined suits); however this equipment is not available to the paramedic. The best ways to protect yourself from the effects of radiation are to use time and distance, and shield yourself in Level C protection from the source.

- **Time.** Radiation has a cumulative effect on the body. The less time that you are exposed to the source, the less the effects will be. If you realize that the patient is near a radiation source, leave the area immediately.
- **Distance.** Radiation is limited as to how far it can travel. Depending on the type of radiation, often moving only a few feet is enough to remove you from immediate danger. Alpha radiation cannot travel more than a few inches. You should take this into account when responding to a nuclear or radiological incident and make certain that responders are stationed far enough from the incident.
- **Shielding.** As discussed earlier, the path of all radiation can be stopped by a specific object. It will be impossible for you to recognize the type of radiation being emitted, or even from which direction it is coming. Therefore, you should always assume that you are dealing with the strongest form of radiation and use concrete shielding (such as buildings or walls) between yourself and the incident. The importance of shielding cannot be overemphasized. In one atomic test, a car was parked on the side of a house, opposite the direction of the oncoming blast. The house was completely destroyed, yet the car that was directly next to it sustained almost no damage.

You are the Provider Summary

1. What is your first priority at a call in this situation?

Since there are multiple patients and a potential hazard to the rescuers, the first priority is your personal safety and that of your crew. That is why it was smart to stage the units until more information was determined about the cause of the incident.

2. What does the dispatch information indicate as far as the need for additional resources?

The dispatch information paints a picture of multiple patients with medical complaints. While it is not uncommon to get multiple patients with traumatic complaints at a typical motor vehicle collision, we rarely get multiple patients with medical complaints unless there is something they all were exposed to causing the symptoms.

3. What precautions can you take to ensure your own safety?

Immediately make sure help is on the way with self-contained breathing apparatus (SCBA) and the appropriate level of Haz-Mat training. Each community has a plan and the best thing you can do at this point is don't just rush in, rather activate the plan.

4. What does your index of suspicion tell you about this scene?

The specifics are slowly being identified as the HazMat team identifies the product that the patients were exposed to. However, the slow pulse rate, vomiting, and tearing lead you in the direction of a nerve agent even before the actual substance is identified.

5. What could your patient's signs and symptoms represent?

As you have learned, patients who have been exposed to a nerve agent are likely to have the symptoms paramedics remember using the mnemonic DUMBELS. That stands for: Defecation, Urination, Miosis, Bradycardia/bronchorrhea, Emesis, Lacrimation, and Salivation.

6. What are your treatment options for this patient?

Always manage the ABCs and symptoms. In a case of suspected nerve gas exposure, contact medical direction or the poison control center for authorization to administer the MARK 1 kit, which usually consists of two auto-injectors: one with a high dose of atropine and the other with 2-PAM chloride (pralidoxime chloride). Then transport the patient with ongoing assessment and support of her ABCs.

7. What does the nerve agent antidote kit include?

The MARK 1 kit includes two auto-injectors, which contain a high dose of atropine and the other with 2-PAM chloride (pralidoxime chloride).

8. Is this kit part of your local protocol in dealing with patients exposed to a nerve agent?

If it is not, you should ask your medical director what the plan is for treating large numbers of patients who have been exposed to a nerve agent.

9. What are your next steps in treatment?

Ongoing assessment, manage the ABCs, and transport the patient. Depending on how fast she comes out of the seizure and how well she can ventilate, it may be necessary to consider intubation and the need to support or assist her ventilations with a bag-mask device and supplementary oxygen. Consult with medical control to consider the need to potentially medicate the patient for (1) nausea and vomiting, (2) developing fluid in the lungs, and (3) seizure activity if lengthy.

Prep Kit

■ Ready for Review

■ As a result of the increase in terrorist activity, it is possible that you could witness a terrorist event. You must be mentally and physically prepared for the possibility of a terrorist event.

■ The use of weapons of mass destruction or mass casualty further complicates the management of the terrorist incident. Be aware of your surroundings at all times. The best form of protection from a WMD agent is to avoid contact with the agent.

■ A WMD is any agent designed to bring about mass death, casualties, and/or massive damage to property and infrastructure (bridges, tunnels, airports, and seaports). These can be nuclear, chemical, biological, and explosive weapons.

■ Be aware of the current threat level issued by the federal government through the Department of Homeland Security (DHS). This threat level can be severe, high, elevated, guarded, or low. On the basis of the current threat level, take appropriate actions and precautions. Be aware of established policies that your organization may have regarding the current threat level.

■ Indicators that may give you clues as to whether the emergency is the result of an attack include the type of location, type of call, number of patients, patients' statements, and preincident indicators.

■ If you suspect that a terrorist or WMD event has occurred, ensure that the scene is safe. If you have any doubt that it may not be safe, do not enter. Wait for assistance.

■ Notification of the dispatcher is essential. Inform dispatch of the nature of the event, any additional resources that may be required, the estimated number of patients, and the upwind route of approach or optimal route of approach.

■ Establish a staging area, where other units will converge. Be mindful of access and exit routes.

■ Terrorists may set secondary devices to explode after the initial bomb, to injure responders and secure media coverage. Constantly assess and reassess the scene for safety.

■ Paramedics may be called upon to assist in the delivery of the medications to the public. The paramedic's role may include triage, treatment of seriously ill patients, and patient transport to the hospital.

■ Vital Vocabulary

alpha Type of energy that is emitted from a strong radiological source; it is the least harmful penetrating type of radiation and cannot travel fast or through most objects.

anthrax A deadly bacteria (Bacillus anthracis) that lays dormant in a spore (protective shell); the germ is released from the spore when exposed to the optimal temperature and moisture. The route of entry is inhalation, cutaneous, or gastrointestinal (from consuming food that contains spores).

bacteria Microorganisms that reproduce by binary fission. These single-cell creatures reproduce rapidly. Some can form spores (encysted variants) when environmental conditions are harsh.

beta Type of energy that is emitted from a strong radiological source; is slightly more penetrating than alpha, and requires a layer of clothing to stop it.

BNICE A mnemonic for the five types of terrorist incidents that first responder agencies may be confronted with in the field.

botulinum Produced by bacteria, this is a very potent neurotoxin. When introduced into the body, this neurotoxin affects the nervous system's ability to function and causes muscle paralysis.

buboes Enlarged lymph nodes (up to the size of tennis balls) that were characteristic of people infected with the bubonic plague.

bubonic plague An epidemic that spread throughout Europe in the Middle Ages, causing over 25 million deaths, also called the Black Death, transmitted by infected fleas and characterized by acute malaise, fever, and the formation of tender, enlarged, inflamed lymph nodes that appear as lesions, called buboes.

chlorine (CL) The first chemical agent ever used in warfare. It has a distinct odor of bleach, and creates a green haze when released as a gas. Initially it produces upper airway irritation and a choking sensation.

communicability Describes how easily a disease spreads from one human to another human.

contact hazard A hazardous agent that gives off very little or no vapors; the skin is the primary route for this type of chemical to enter the body; also called a skin hazard.

contagious A person infected with a disease that is highly communicable.

covert Act in which the public safety community generally has no prior knowledge of the time, location, or nature of the attack.

cross-contamination Occurs when a person is contaminated by an agent as a result of coming into contact with another contaminated person.

cyanide Agent that affects the body's ability to use oxygen. It is a colorless gas that has an odor similar to almonds. The effects begin on the cellular level and are very rapidly seen at the organ system level.

decay A natural process in which a material that is unstable attempts to stabilize itself by changing its structure.

dirty bomb Name given to a bomb that is used as a radiological dispersal device (RDD).

disease vector An animal that once infected, spreads a disease to another animal.

dissemination The means with which a terrorist will spread a disease, for example, by poisoning of the water supply, or aerosolizing the agent into the air or ventilation system of a building.

domestic terrorists Native citizens who carry out terrorist acts against their own country.

G agents Early nerve agents that were developed by German scientists in the period after WWI and into WWII. There are three such agents: sarin, soman, and tabun.

gamma (x-rays) Type of energy that is emitted from a strong radiological source that is far faster and stronger than alpha and beta rays. These rays easily penetrate through the human body and require either several inches of lead or concrete to prevent penetration.

incubation Describes the period of time from a person being exposed to a disease to the time when symptoms begin.

international terrorism Terrorism that is carried out by those not of the host's country; also known as cross-border terrorism.

ionizing radiation Energy that is emitted in the form of rays, or particles.

LD_{50} The amount of an agent or substance that will kill 50% of people who are exposed to this level.

Lewisite (L) A blistering agent that has a rapid onset of symptoms and produces immediate intense pain and discomfort on contact.

lymphatic system A passive circulatory system that transports a plasma-like liquid called lymph, a thin fluid that bathes the tissues of the body.

lymph nodes Area of the lymphatic system where infection-fighting cells are housed.

MARK 1 A nerve agent antidote kit containing two auto-injector medications, atropine and 2-PAM chloride (pralidoxime chloride); also known as a Nerve Agent Antidote Kit (NAAK).

miosis Bilateral pinpoint constricted pupils.

mutagen Substance that mutates, damages, and changes the structures of DNA in the body's cells.

NAAK A nerve agent antidote kit containing two auto-injector medications, atropine and 2-PAM chloride (pralidoxime chloride); also known as a MARK 1 kit.

nerve agents A class of chemicals called organophosphates; they function by blocking an essential enzyme in the nervous system, which causes the body's organs to become overstimulated and burn out.

neurotoxins Biological agents that are the most deadly substances known to humans; they include botulinum toxin and ricin.

neutron radiation Type of energy that is emitted from a strong radiological source; neutron energy is the fastest moving and most powerful form of radiation. Neutrons easily penetrate through lead, and require several feet of concrete to stop them.

off-gassing The emitting of an agent after exposure, for example from a person's clothes that have been exposed to the agent.

persistency Term used to describe how long a chemical agent will stay on a surface before it evaporates.

phosgene A pulmonary agent that is a product of combustion, such as might be produced in a fire at a textile factory or house, or from metalwork or burning Freon. Phosgene is a very potent agent that has a delayed onset of symptoms, usually hours.

phosgene oxime (CX) A blistering agent that has a rapid onset of symptoms and produces immediate intense pain and discomfort on contact.

pneumonic plague A lung infection, also known as plague pneumonia, that is the result of inhalation of plague bacteria.

points of distribution (PODs) Strategically placed facilities that have been pre-established for the mass distribution of antibiotics, antidotes, and vaccinations, along with other medications and supplies.

radioactive material Any material that emits radiation.

radiological dispersal device (RDD) Any container that is designed to disperse radioactive material.

ricin Neurotoxin derived from mash that is left from pressing oil from the castor bean; causes pulmonary edema and respiratory and circulatory failure, leading to death.

route of exposure Manner by which a toxic substance enters the body.

sarin (GB) A nerve agent that is one of the G agents; a highly volatile colorless and odorless liquid that turns from liquid to gas within seconds to minutes at room temperature.

secondary device Additional explosives used by terrorists, which are set to explode after the initial bomb.

smallpox A highly contagious disease; it is most contagious when blisters begin to form.

soman (GD) A nerve agent that is one of the G agents; twice as persistent as sarin and five times as lethal; it has a fruity odor as a result of the type of alcohol used in the agent, and is both a contact and inhalation hazard that can enter the body through skin absorption and through the respiratory tract.

Special Atomic Demolition Munitions (SADM) Small suitcase-sized nuclear weapons that were designed to destroy individual targets, such as important buildings, bridges, tunnels, or large ships.

state-sponsored terrorism Terrorism that is funded and/or supported by nations that hold close ties with terrorist groups.

sulfur mustard (H) A vesicant; it is a brownish-yellowish oily substance that is generally considered very persistent; has the distinct smell of garlic or mustard and, when released, it is quickly absorbed into the skin and/or mucous membranes and begins an irreversible process of damaging the cells.

syndromic surveillance The monitoring, usually by local or state health departments, of patients presenting to emergency departments and alternative care facilities, the recording of EMS call volume, and the use of over-the-counter medications.

tabun (GA) A nerve agent that is one of the G agents; is 36 times more persistent than sarin and approximately half as lethal; has a fruity smell and is unique because the components used to manufacture the agent are easy to acquire and the agent is easy to manufacture.

terrorism A violent act dangerous to human life, in violation of the criminal laws of the United States or any segment to intimidate or coerce a government, the civilian population or any segment thereof, in furtherance of political or social objectives.

V agent (VX) One of the G agents; it is a clear, oily agent that has no odor and looks like baby oil; over 100 times more lethal than sarin and is extremely persistent.

vapor hazard An agent that enters the body through the respiratory tract.

vesicants Blister agents; the primary route of entry for vesicants is through the skin.

viral hemorrhagic fevers (VHF) A group of diseases that include the Ebola, Rift Valley, and yellow fever viruses among others. This group of viruses causes the blood in the body to seep out from the tissues and blood vessels.

viruses Germs that require a living host to multiply and survive.

volatility Term used to describe how long a chemical agent will stay on a surface before it evaporates.

weapon of mass casualty (WMC) Any agent designed to bring about mass death, casualties, and/or massive damage to property and infrastructure (bridges, tunnels, airports, and seaports); also known as a weapon of mass destruction (WMD).

weapon of mass destruction (WMD) Any agent designed to bring about mass death, casualties, and/or massive damage to property and infrastructure (bridges, tunnels, airports, and seaports); also known as a weapon of mass casualty (WMC).

weaponization The creation of a weapon from a biological agent generally found in nature and that causes disease; the agent is cultivated, synthesized, and/or mutated to maximize the target population's exposure to the germ.

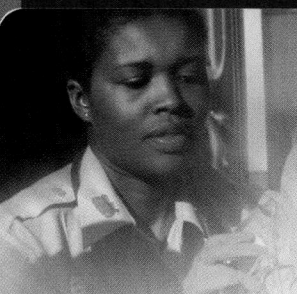

Assessment in Action

Events over the past decade have shown that terrorists, foreign and domestic, are willing to attack American interests at home and abroad. Terrorists now have access to a broad array of lethal materials worldwide and can strike a specific target at any given time. Terrorists are no longer limited to conventional weapons.

1. As a paramedic you must be familiar with the nonconventional agents that may be used in a WMD attack. All of the following are nonconventional weapons, EXCEPT:
   A. chemical.
   B. nuclear.
   C. biological.
   D. explosives.

2. A weapon of mass destruction is any agent that will bring about:
   A. mass casualty.
   B. mass death.
   C. massive damage to infrastructure.
   D. all of the above.

3. Terrorism carried out by individuals or groups who are not from the host country is known as:
   A. domestic terrorism.
   B. doomsday terrorism.
   C. international terrorism.
   D. Al Qaeda.

4. When you come on duty you are told during briefing that the Department of Homeland Security has posted the threat level to be yellow. What threat level does this color represent?
   A. Low
   B. Elevated
   C. High
   D. Severe

5. Chemical agents are manmade substances that can have devastating effects on living organisms. All of the following are agents that can be used for chemical warfare, EXCEPT:
   A. nerve agents.
   B. pulmonary agents.
   C. bacterial agents.
   D. blood agents.

6. Time, distance, and shielding are the three most important factors in staying safe when dealing with what type of WMD?
   A. Chemical weapon
   B. Radiological weapon
   C. Biological weapon
   D. Bacterial weapon

7. A chemical agent that is described as highly persistent can:
   A. evaporate relatively fast.
   B. remain in the environment for weeks to months.
   C. cause extensive blistering within minutes.
   D. all of the above.

Challenging Questions

You are responding to a train station where there was a reported small explosion. Dispatch reports there are now a number of patients complaining of difficulty breathing and nausea. As you walk into the station you observe that two patients are unconscious and seizing, while numerous others are pleading with you to help them.

8. What type of event do you suspect?

9. What concerns do you have for your safety?

■ Points to Ponder

You are responding to a WMD incident where a primary explosion has disseminated chemical agents at the State Bank. You are told by the Incident Commander (IC) to stage about two blocks from the incident location while they wait for the HazMat team to evaluate the situation. The staging area is near a park and the IC wants triage to be set up in the park. There are about 40 patients confirmed by the IC. A total of six ambulances within the city are responding.

What are your concerns with both the location of the triage area and the number of ambulances that are responding? What do you want to know about the chemical agent?

Issues: Scene Safety, Staging Location, Incident Commander, Need for Decontamination, Secondary Devices.

Objectives

Cognitive

8-3.1   Define the term rescue. (p 49.4)

8-3.2   Explain the medical and mechanical aspects of rescue situations. (p 49.4)

8-3.3   Explain the role of the paramedic in delivering care at the site of the injury, continuing through the rescue process and to definitive care. (p 49.4)

8-3.4   Describe the phases of a rescue operation. (p 49.6)

8-3.5   List and describe the types of personal protective equipment needed to safely operate in the rescue environment to include:
a. Head protection
b. Eye protection
c. Hand protection
d. Personal flotation devices
e. Thermal protection/layering systems
f. High visibility clothing
g. Specialized footwear (p 49.10)

8-3.6   Explain the differences in risk between moving water and flat water rescue. (p 49.21)

8-3.7   Explain the effects of immersion hypothermia on the ability to survive sudden immersion and self rescue. (p 49.21)

8-3.8   Explain the phenomenon of the cold protective response in cold water drowning situations. (p 49.21)

8-3.9   Identify the risks associated with low head dams and the rescue complexities they pose. (p 49.22)

8-3.10   Given a picture of moving water, identify and explain the following features and hazards associated with:
a. Hydraulics
b. Strainers
c. Dams/hydro-electric sites (p 49.22)

8-3.11   Explain why water entry or go techniques are methods of last resort. (p 49.23)

8-3.12   Explain the rescue techniques associated with reach-throw-row-go. (p 49.22)

8-3.13   Given a list of rescue scenarios, identify the patient survivability profile and which are rescue versus body recovery situations. (p 49.23)

8-3.14   Explain the self rescue position if unexpectedly immersed in moving water. (p 49.21)

8-3.15   Given a series of pictures identify which would be considered "confined spaces" and potentially oxygen deficient. (p 49.19)

8-3.16   Identify the hazards associated with confined spaces and risks posed to potential rescuers to include:
a. Oxygen deficiency
b. Chemical/toxic exposure/explosion
c. Engulfment
d. Machinery entrapment
e. Electricity (p 49.19)

8-3.17   Identify components necessary to ensure site safety prior to confined space rescue attempts. (p 49.20)

8-3.18   Identify the poisonous gases commonly found in confined spaces to include:
a. Hydrogen sulfide (H_2S)
b. Carbon dioxide (CO_2)
c. Carbon monoxide (CO)
d. Low/high oxygen concentrations (FiO_2)
e. Methane (CH_4)
f. Ammonia (NH_3)
g. Nitrogen dioxide (NO_2) (p 49.19, 49.20)

8-3.19   Explain the hazard of cave-in during trench rescue operations. (p 49.20)

8-3.20   Describe the effects of traffic flow on the highway rescue incident including limited access superhighways and regular access highways. (p 49.11)

8-3.21   List and describe the following techniques to reduce scene risk at highway incidents:
a. Apparatus placement
b. Headlights and emergency vehicle lighting
c. Cones, flares
d. Reflective and high visibility clothing (p 49.11, 49.12)

8-3.22   List and describe the hazards associated with the following auto/truck components:
a. Energy absorbing bumpers
b. Air bag/supplemental restraint systems
c. Catalytic converters and conventional fuel systems
d. Stored energy
e. Alternate fuel systems (p 49.12)

8-3.23   Given a diagram of a passenger auto, identify the following structures:
a. A, B, C, D posts
b. Fire wall
c. Unibody versus frame designs (p 49.12)

8-3.24   Describe methods for emergency stabilization using rope, cribbing, jacks, spare tire, and come-a-longs for vehicles found on their:
a. Wheels
b. Side
c. Roof
d. Inclines (p 49.12, 49.13)

8-3.25   Describe the electrical hazards commonly found at highway incidents (above and below ground). (p 49.9)

8-3.26   Explain the difference between tempered and safety glass, identify its locations on a vehicle and how to break it safely. (p 49.14, 49.15)

8-3.27   Explain typical door anatomy and methods to access through stuck doors. (p 49.14, 49.15)

8-3.28   Explain SRS or "air bag" systems and methods to neutralize them. (p 49.18)

8-3.29   Define the following terms:
a. Low angle
b. High angle
c. Belay
d. Rappel
e. Scrambling
f. Hasty rope slide (p 49.23, 49.24)

8-3.30 Describe the procedure for Stokes litter packaging for low angle evacuations. (p 49.27)

8-3.31 Explain the procedures for low angle litter evacuation to include:
a. Anchoring
b. Litter/rope attachment
c. Lowering and raising procedures (p 49.27)

8-3.32 Explain techniques to be used in non-technical litter carries over rough terrain. (p 49.24)

8-3.33 Explain non-technical high angle rescue procedures using aerial apparatus. (p 49.24)

8-3.34 Develop specific skill in emergency stabilization of vehicles and access procedures and an awareness of specific extrication strategies. (p 49.12)

8-3.35 Explain assessment procedures and modifications necessary when caring for entrapped patients. (p 49.15)

8-3.36 List the equipment necessary for an "off road" medical pack. (p 49.26)

8-3.37 Explain specific methods of improvisation for assessment, spinal immobilization and extremity splinting. (p 49.27)

8-3.38 Explain the indications, contraindications and methods of pain control for entrapped patients. (p 49.26)

8-3.39 Explain the need for and techniques of thermal control for entrapped patients. (p 49.26)

8-3.40 Explain the pathophysiology of "crush trauma" syndrome. (p 49.26)

8-3.41 Develop an understanding of the medical issues involved in providing care for a patient in a rescue environment. (p 49.26)

8-3.42 Develop proficiency in patient packaging and evacuation techniques that pertain to hazardous or rescue environments. (p 49.27)

8-3.43 Explain the different types of "Stokes" or basket stretchers and the advantages and disadvantages associated with each. (p 49.26)

Affective

None

Psychomotor

8-3.44 Using cribbing, ropes, lifting devices, spare tires, chains, and hand winches, demonstrate the following stabilization procedures:
a. Stabilization on all four wheels
b. Stabilization on its side
c. Stabilization on its roof
d. Stabilization on an incline/embankments (p 49.12)

8-3.45 Using basic hand tools demonstrate the following:
a. Access through a stuck door
b. Access through safety and tempered glass
c. Access through the trunk
d. Access through the floor
e. Roof removal
f. Dash displacement/roll-up
g. Steering wheel/column displacement
h. Access through the roof (p 49.13, 49.14, 49.16–49.18, 49.19)

8-3.46 Demonstrate methods of "Stokes" packaging for patients being:
a. Vertically lifted (high angle)
b. Horizontally lifted (low angle)
c. Carried over rough terrain (p 49.27)

8-3.47 Demonstrate methods of packaging for patients being vertically lifted without Stokes litter stretcher packaging. (p 49.27)

8-3.48 Demonstrate the following litter carrying techniques:
a. Stretcher lift straps
b. "Leap frogging"
c. Passing litters over and around obstructions (p 49.25, 49.26)

8-3.49 Demonstrate litter securing techniques for patients being evacuated by aerial apparatus. (p 49.25, 49.26)

8-3.50 Demonstrate in-water spinal immobilization techniques. (p 49.23, 49.24)

8-3.51 Demonstrate donning and properly adjusting a PFD. (p 49.10)

8-3.52 Demonstrate use of a throw bag. (p 49.22)

Introduction

"Rescue" means to deliver from danger or imprisonment. As EMS providers, we must remove from peril or confinement every patient we encounter. Prehospital providers can't simply push a button and magically transport patients to an emergency department—which means technically that every emergency scene is a rescue situation. Patients are found in every imaginable situation. Imagine you have a patient on the second floor of a three-story brick structure. This morbidly obese patient is lying on the floor of a half-bathroom in the back of the structure. Your assessment shows the patient is experiencing a myocardial infarction and acute exacerbation of chronic obstructive pulmonary disease (COPD). The treatment is easy, but the rescue is difficult. You must extricate this patient to your waiting squad with a monitor, two IVs, a nitro drip, and a continuous positive airway pressure machine attached **Figure 49-1 ▸**.

Rescue and removal of patients involves several steps. You must access the patient and then quickly assess him or her for medical/trauma complications to determine which treatments should be started. Treatment must begin at the site, but this is often difficult because of the circumstances surrounding the event. The patient must be released or removed from the entrapment, and medical care must continue throughout the incident. The most difficult process in any rescue is neither the rescue nor the treatment process, but rather the coordination and balance of both.

A technical rescue incident (TRI) is a complex rescue incident involving vehicles, water, trench collapse, confined spaces, or wilderness search and rescue that requires specially trained personnel and special equipment. This chapter

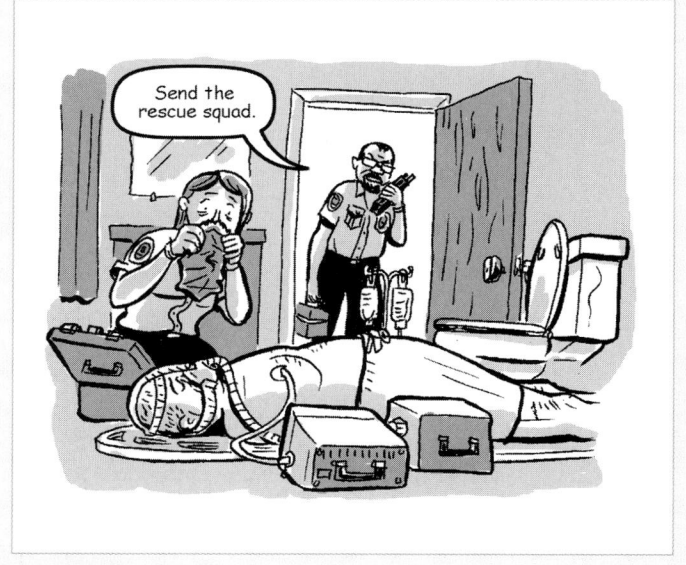

Figure 49-1

describes how to assist specially trained rescue personnel in carrying out the tasks, but it will not make you an expert in the skills that require specialized training.

Training in technical rescue areas is conducted at three levels:

- **Awareness.** This training level is an introduction to the topic, with an emphasis on recognizing the hazards, securing the scene, and calling for appropriate assistance. There is no actual use of rescue skills at the awareness level.
- **Operations.** Geared toward working in the "warm zone" of an incident (the area directly around the hazard area), this

You are the Provider Part 1

It's a blistering hot summer day in July. The meteorologist has warned people to stay indoors. The current temperature is 95°F with a heat index of 105°F. You and your partner make your way back to the station from the hospital after treating the third heat-related illness of the day. The two of you chuckle as a call is dispatched for the local police department regarding chickens in the road. Five minutes later your laughter is replaced by surprise as your unit is dispatched to the same location for a truck in a ditch.

Upon arrival, you and your partner are stunned as you navigate the unit through what appears to be at least 100 chickens wandering aimlessly across a two-lane paved road. Beyond the chickens, buried in a ditch, is a flatbed truck turned on its side. Wire mesh cages, feathers, and dead chickens are strewn about. The cab of the truck has landed on the driver's side with major intrusion into the driver's compartment and spidering of the windshield. Inside you find a middle-age man with active bleeding from a forehead laceration. He is screaming that he has severe abdominal pain and cannot move his legs, which are pinned beneath the dashboard. You let him know that help is there and advise him to keep as still as possible and not to move his neck. You decide to wait until fire department personnel advise you that the scene is safe prior to proceeding with patient care.

Initial Assessment	Recording Time: 0 Minutes
Appearance	Middle-aged man in obvious pain
Level of consciousness	A (Alert to person, place, and day)
Airway	Open
Breathing	Chest rise appears adequate
Circulation	Unable to assess

1. What are some examples of situations requiring special rescue teams?
2. Identify the ten steps of a special rescue sequence.

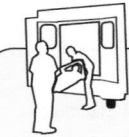

kind of training will allow you to directly assist those conducting the rescue operation.

- **Technician.** At this level, you are directly involved in the rescue operation itself. Training includes the use of specialized equipment, care of patients during the rescue, and management of the incident and of all personnel at the scene.

Most of the training and education EMS providers receive is aimed at the awareness level, enabling them to identify the hazards and secure the scene to prevent additional people from becoming patients. Your function as a paramedic in rescue operations depends on the type of services you provide and the level of expertise your com-

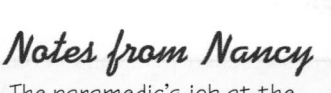

Notes from Nancy

The paramedic's job at the scene of an accident is to take care of the patients.

pany has attained. All providers must wear proper personal protective equipment (PPE) to allow them to access patients and safely administer treatment that will continue throughout the incident. Once the scene is safe, and the technical aspects of the patient rescue or extrication are understood, patient access and care can begin.

Types of Rescues

Most EMS departments respond to a variety of special rescue situations **Figure 49-2 ▶**, including vehicle, confined space, trench, water, and wilderness rescue. It's important for awareness-level responders to have an understanding of these types of rescues. Often, the first emergency unit to arrive at a rescue incident is an ambulance with EMS providers who may not be trained in special rescue techniques. The initial actions taken by paramedics may determine the safety of both patients and paramedics. They may also determine how efficiently the rescue is completed.

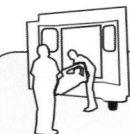

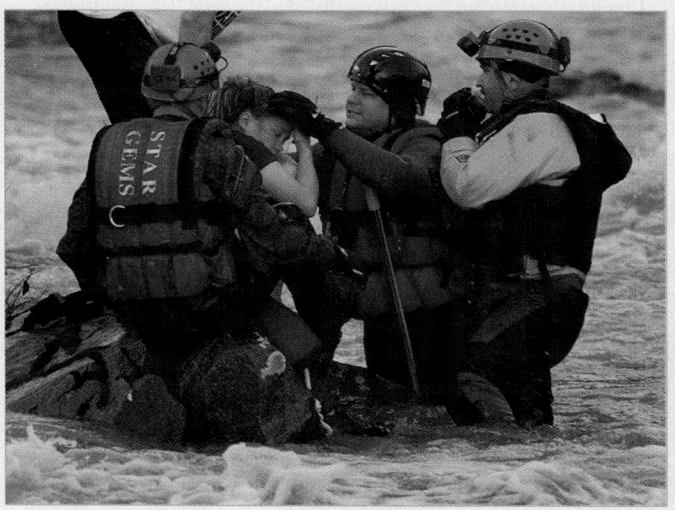

Figure 49-2 Most EMS departments respond to a variety of special rescue situations.

Guidelines for Operations

When assisting rescue team members, the following guidelines will prove useful:

- Be safe.
- Follow orders.
- Work as a team.
- Think.
- Follow the golden rule of public service.

Be Safe

Rescue situations have many hidden hazards, including oxygen-deficient atmospheres and strong water currents. Knowledge, education, and training are required to recognize the signs that indicate a hazardous rescue situation exists. Once the hazards are identified, determine what actions are necessary to ensure your own safety as well as the safety of your partner, the patients, and any bystanders. It requires experience and skill to determine that a rescue scene is not safe to enter, and that determination could save lives.

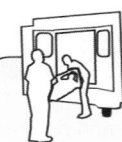

Follow Orders

The officers and the rescue teams you'll work with on special rescue incidents have received extensive specialized training. They've been chosen for those duties because they have experience and skills in a particular area of rescue. It's critical to follow the orders of personnel who understand exactly what needs to be done to ensure everyone's safety and to mitigate the dangers involved in the rescue situation. Follow their orders exactly as given. If you don't understand what's expected of you, *ask*. Have the orders clarified so you'll be able to complete your assigned task safely.

Work as a Team

Rescue efforts often require many people to complete a wide variety of tasks. Some personnel may be trained in specific tasks, such as rope rescue or swift water rescue. However, they can't do their jobs without the support and assistance of others. Rescue is a team effort, and you play an essential role on this team.

Think

As you're working on a rescue situation, you must constantly assess and reassess the scene. You may see something that the incident commander (IC) doesn't see. If you think your assigned task may be unsafe, bring it to the attention of the IC or safety officer. Don't try to reorganize the total rescue effort, as it's being directed by people who are highly trained and experienced, but don't ignore what's happening around you either. Observations that you should bring to the IC's attention include changing weather conditions that might affect the rescue scene operations, suspicious packages or items on the scene, and broken equipment.

Follow the Golden Rule of Public Service

When you're involved in carrying out a rescue effort, it's all too easy to concentrate on the technical aspects of the rescue and forget to focus on the scared person who needs your emotional

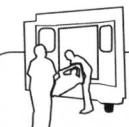

In the Field

F-A-I-L-U-R-E

The reasons for rescue failures can be referred to by the mnemonic "FAILURE":

F Failure to understand the environment, or underestimating it
A Additional medical problems not considered
I Inadequate rescue skills
L Lack of teamwork or experience
U Underestimating the logistics of the incident
R Rescue versus recovery mode not considered
E Equipment not mastered

support and encouragement. It's helpful to have a rescuer stay with the patient whenever possible, keeping the patient updated on which actions will be performed during the rescue process.

■ Steps of Special Rescue

The role of the paramedic in special rescue operations is often vague and can change as the rescue operation progresses. All EMS providers must have some formalized education or training in rescue techniques. This educational process is aimed at preparing responders to understand and identify potential hazards and to determine when it's safe or potentially unsafe to access and rescue patients. All prehospital providers will be involved with a rescue at some point in their careers, so they must be skilled in specialized patient packaging techniques to allow for a safe extrication and medical care.

You are the Provider Part 2

You are slightly relieved by the sound of the engine company sirens in the distance, but you know that you will require additional resources for extrication and transport. The closest rescue squad with extrication capabilities is 30 minutes away, and transport time to the trauma center is approximately 1 hour by ground. Your partner contacts dispatch and asks them to dispatch the rescue assignment for extrication assistance and a helicopter for transport.

After fire personnel stabilize the vehicle with cribbing and advise you that it is safe to gain access to the patient, you ask for assistance from one of the police officers to hold the patient's c-spine by leaning through the window on the driver's side of the cab. You are able to open the door on the passenger's side and carefully climb into the cab positioning yourself next to the patient. You introduce yourself to the patient, who tells you that he was driving down the road when he became "blinded by the sunlight" and ran off the road and landed in the ditch. The patient denies having any loss of consciousness, headache, dizziness, or visual disturbances. He has a medical history of panic attacks, for which he takes 40 mg of Prozac every day. He has no known drug allergies.

Vital Signs	Recording Time: 5 Minutes
Level of consciousness	Alert
Pulse	122 beats/min, strong and regular
Blood pressure	134/72 mm Hg
Respirations	22 breaths/min, nonlabored
Skin	Pink, warm, and slightly diaphoretic
Sao₂	95% on room air

3. Why is it important to maintain good communication with the patient during a special rescue incident?
4. What is the patient at risk of experiencing as a result of being pinned underneath the dashboard from the pelvis down?

Although special rescue situations may take many different forms, all rescuers should follow ten steps to perform these rescues in a safe, effective, and efficient manner:

1. Preparation
2. Response
3. Arrival and size-up
4. Stabilization
5. Access
6. Disentanglement
7. Removal
8. Transport
9. Security of the scene and preparation for the next call
10. Postincident analysis

Preparation

You can prepare for responses to emergency rescue incidents by training with fire departments and special rescue teams in your area. This educational process will prepare you to respond to a mutual aid call and teach you about the type of rescue equipment other departments have access to and the training levels of their personnel. Knowing the terminology used in the field will also make communicating with other rescuers easier and more effective.

Prior to any technical rescue call, your department must consider the following issues:

- Does the department have the personnel and equipment needed to handle a TRI from start to finish?
- What equipment and which personnel will the department send on a technical rescue call?
- Do members of the department know the potential hazard areas in their response area? Have they visited those areas with local representatives?

Response

A dispatch protocol should be established for a TRI. If your department has its own technical rescue team, it will usually respond with a rescue squad, an ambulance, fire engine company, and fire chief. Otherwise, it will respond with a medic unit, engine company, and chief. In many EMS departments, the rescue squad will come from an outside agency. Often, it is necessary to notify utility companies during a TRI and seek their assistance. Many technical rescues involve electricity, sewer pipes, or factors that may create the need for heavy equipment, to which utility companies have ready access.

Arrival and Size-up

Immediately upon arrival, the IC will assume command. A rapid and accurate scene size-up is needed to avoid placing rescuers in danger and to determine what additional resources may be needed. Providers must assess the extent of injuries and the number of patients; this information will then help to determine how many medic units and other resources are needed.

Do *not* rush into the incident scene until an assessment of the situation is complete. A paramedic approaching a trench collapse may cause further collapse. A paramedic entering a swiftly flowing river might be quickly knocked off his or her feet and carried downstream. A paramedic climbing into a well to evaluate an unconscious patient may be overcome by an oxygen-deficient atmosphere. EMS providers need to *stop and think about the dangers that may be present.* Don't make yourself part of the problem.

Stabilization

Once the resources are on the way and the scene is safe to enter, it's time to stabilize the incident. Look around you, identifying and evaluating the hazards at the scene, observing the geographical area, noting the routes of access and exit, observing weather and wind conditions, and considering evacuation problems and transport distances. Establish an outer perimeter to keep the public and media out of the staging area and maintain a smaller perimeter directly around the rescue. The rescue area is the area that surrounds the incident site (eg, collapsed structure, collapsed trench, hazardous spill area). The size of the rescue area is proportional to the hazards that exist.

As part of the stabilization effort, you should establish three controlled zones:

- **Hot zone.** For entry teams and rescue teams only. This zone immediately surrounds the dangers of the site (eg, hazardous materials releases) to protect personnel outside the zone.
- **Warm zone.** For properly trained and equipped personnel only. This zone is where personnel and equipment decontamination and hot zone support take place.
- **Cold zone.** For staging vehicles and equipment. This zone contains the command post. The public and the media should be kept clear of the cold zone at all times.

Police or fire line tape is often used to demarcate these controlled zones. Red tape is typically used for the hot zone, orange tape for the warm zone, and yellow tape for the cold zone. Of course, someone must ensure that the zones of the emergency scene are enforced. Scene control activities are sometimes assigned to law enforcement personnel.

During stabilization, atmospheric monitoring should be started to identify any immediately dangerous to life and health (IDLH) environments for rescuers and patients. After considering the type of incident, you may begin planning how to safely rescue patients. In a trench rescue, for example, you might set up ventilation fans for air flow, set up lights for visibility, and protect the trench from further collapse.

Access

With the scene stabilized, now you must gain access to the patient. How is he or she trapped? In a trench situation, the culprit may be a dirt pile. In a rope rescue, scaffolding may have fallen. In a confined space, a hazardous atmosphere may have caused the patient to collapse. To reach a patient who is buried or trapped beneath debris, it's sometimes necessary to dig a tunnel as a means of rescue and escape. Identify the actual reason for the rescue and work toward freeing the patient safely.

Communicate with patients at all times during the rescue to make sure they are not injured further by the rescue operation. Even if they're not injured, they need to be reassured that the team is working as quickly as possible to free them.

Emergency medical care should be initiated as soon as access to the patient is achieved. Technical rescue paramedics are crucial resources at TRIs; not only can these responders start IVs and treat medical conditions, but they also know how to deal with the special equipment being used and the procedures taking place around them. It's vitally important that the actions of EMS personnel be effectively coordinated into ongoing operations during rescue incidents. Their main functions are to treat patients and to stand by in case a rescue team member needs medical assistance. As soon as a rescue area is secured and stabilized, EMS personnel must be allowed access to the patients for medical assessment and stabilization. Some fire departments have trained paramedics to the technical rescue level so that they can enter hazardous areas and provide direct assistance to patients there. Throughout the course of the rescue operation, which may span many hours, EMS personnel must continually monitor and ensure the stability of all patients.

Gaining access to the patient depends on the type of incident. For example, in an incident involving a motor vehicle, its location and position, the damage to the vehicle, and the position of the patient are important considerations. The means of gaining access to the patient must also take into account the nature and severity of the patient's injuries. The chosen means of access may change during the course of the rescue as the nature or severity of the patient's injuries becomes apparent.

Disentanglement

Once precautions have been taken and the reason for entrapment has been identified, the patient needs to be freed as safely as possible. A team member should remain with the patient to direct the rescuers who are performing the disentanglement. In a trench incident, this would include digging either with a shovel or by hand to free the patient.

In a motor vehicle crash, the vehicle should be removed from around the patient rather than trying to remove the patient through the wreckage. Parts of the vehicle—for example, the steering wheel, seats, pedals, and dashboard—may trap the occupants. Disentanglement is the cutting of a vehicle (or machinery) away from trapped or injured patients, using extrication and rescue tools along with various extrication methods.

Removal

Once the patient has been disentangled, efforts shift to removing the patient **Figure 49-3**. In some instances, this may simply amount to having someone assist the patient up a ladder; in other situations, it may require removal with spinal immobilization due to possible injuries. A wide variety of

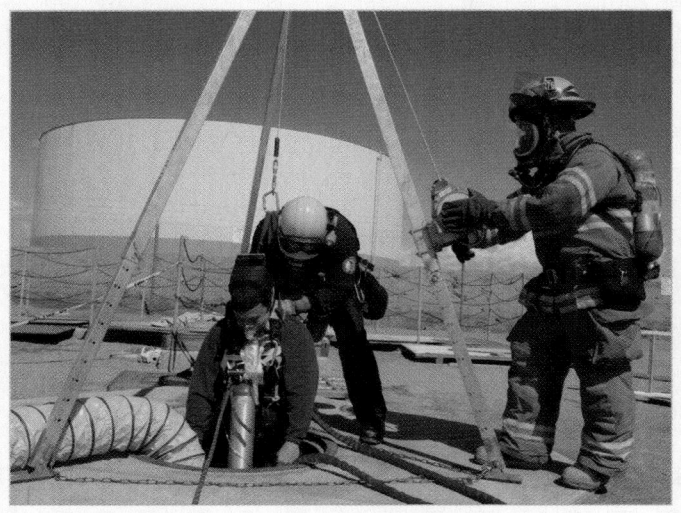

Figure 49-3 Patient removal.

equipment, including Stokes baskets, backboards, stretchers, and other immobilization devices, is used to remove injured patients from trenches, confined spaces, and elevated points.

Preparing the patient for removal involves maintaining continued control of all life-threatening problems, dressing all wounds, and immobilizing all suspected fractures and spinal injuries. The use of standard splints in confined areas is difficult and frequently impossible, but stabilization of the arms to the patient's trunk and of the legs to each other will often suffice until the patient is positioned on a long backboard, which may serve as the ultimate splint for the whole body. The short backboard is typically used for stabilization of a sitting patient.

Sometimes a patient must be removed quickly (rapid extrication; covered in Chapter 25) because his or her general condition is deteriorating and time does not permit meticulous splinting and dressing procedures. Quick removal may also occur if hazards are present, such as spilled gas or other materials that could endanger the patient or rescue personnel. The only time the patient should be moved prior to completion of initial care, assessment, stabilization, and treatment is when the patient's or emergency responder's life is in immediate danger.

Packaging is preparing the patient for movement as a unit. It is often accomplished by means of a long backboard or similar device. These boards are essential for moving patients with potential or actual spine injuries.

Rough-terrain rescues may require passing a multiple-person stretcher across rough terrain, fording streams, or climbing over rocks. These operations require at least one person to take each corner of the litter or backboard if possible. In extreme cases, a four-person team may have to hand a litter around or over obstacles to another team ("leapfrogging"). Rescues in rough terrain often require ingenuity to suspend or pad a stretcher so that the patient is provided with a reasonably comfortable ride. Padding may consist of inflated inner tubes, 4″ to 5″ foam padding, or loosely rolled blankets. This technique is superior to "slinging" the stretcher on straps, which may lead to excessive swaying and bouncing.

Transport

Once the patient has been removed from the hazard area, EMS will undertake transport to an appropriate medical facility. Depending on the severity of the patient's injuries and the distance to the medical facility, the type of transport will vary. For example, if a patient is critically injured or if the rescue is taking place some distance from the hospital, air transportation may be more appropriate than a ground ambulance.

In rough-terrain rescues, four-wheel drive, high-clearance vehicles may be required to transport patients on stretchers to an awaiting ambulance. Snowmobiles with attached sleds can be used to transport patients down snow-covered mountains. Helicopters are increasingly used for quick evacuation from remote areas, but they have their limitations in bad weather conditions.

▌General Rescue Scene Procedures

As a paramedic, you know that your own safety as well as the safety of your partner and the public is paramount. At a TRI, while you may be tempted to approach the patient or the accident area, it is critically important to slow down and properly evaluate the situation. Consider the potential general hazards and risks of utilities, confined spaces, and environmental conditions, as well as hazards that are IDLH. In confined-space rescue incidents, potential hazards may include deep or isolated spaces, multiple complicating hazards (eg, water or chemicals), failure of essential equipment or service, and environmental conditions (eg, snow or rain).

Approaching the Scene

Beginning with the initial dispatch of the rescue call, you should be compiling facts and impressions about the call. Scene size-up begins with the information gained from the person reporting the incident and then from the bystanders at the scene upon arrival.

The information gathered when an emergency call is received is important to the success of the rescue operation. Information collected should include the following:

- Location of the incident
- Nature of the incident (kinds and number of vehicles)
- Condition and position of patients
- Condition and position of vehicles
- Number of people trapped or injured and types of injuries
- Any specific or special hazard information
- Name of person calling and a number where the person can be reached

As you approach the scene of a TRI, however, you may not always know what kind of scene you are entering. Is it a construction scene? Do you see piles of dirt that would indicate a trench? What actions are the civilians taking? Are they attempt-ing to rescue trapped people, possibly placing themselves at considerable danger? Identify any life-threatening hazards, and take corrective measures to mitigate them. Determine whether the situation is a search, rescue, or recovery. If additional resources are needed, they should be ordered by the IC.

A scene size-up should include the initial and ongoing evaluation of the following issues:

- Scope and magnitude of the incident
- Risk and benefit analysis
- Number of known and potential patients
- Hazards
- Access to the scene
- Environmental factors
- Available and necessary resources
- Establishment of a control perimeter

Utility Hazards

In case of utility hazards, your goal is to control as many of the hazards as possible. Minimize all risks and ensure that all providers are using appropriate PPE. Are there any downed electrical wires near the scene Figure 49-4 ▾ ? Is equipment or machinery electrically charged so as to present a danger to the patient or the rescuers? The IC should ensure that the proper procedures are taken to shut off the utilities in the rescue area. Remember—utility hazards can be above or below ground, and the rescue situation will dictate which ones need to be addressed first.

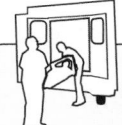

In the Field

Treat all downed wires as if they are charged (live) until you receive specific clearance from the electric company. Even if the lights are out along the street where the wires are down, never assume that the wires are dead. Be especially alert for downed wires after a storm that has blown down trees or tree limbs.

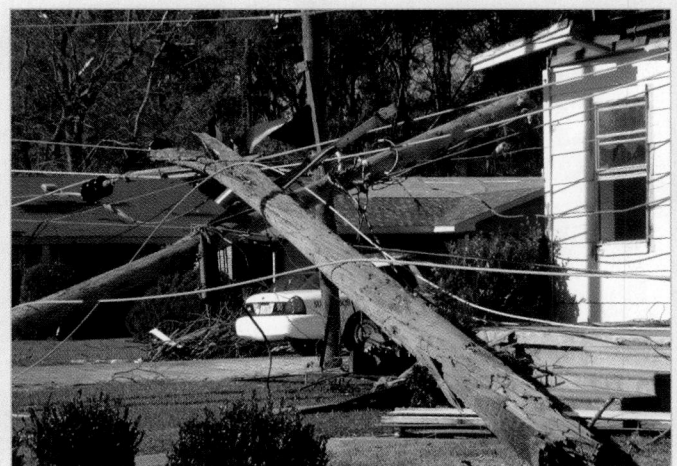

Figure 49-4 Downed electrical wires present a hazard.

Utility hazards require the assistance of trained personnel. For electrical hazards, such as downed lines, park at least one truck span away. Watch for falling utility poles; a damaged pole may bring other poles down with it. Don't touch any wires, power lines, or other electrical sources until they have been deenergized by a power company representative. It isn't just the wires that are hazardous; any metal that they touch is also energized. Metal fences or guardrails may become energized along their entire unbroken length. Be careful around running or standing water, as water is an excellent conductor of electricity.

Natural gas and liquefied petroleum gas are nontoxic but are classified as asphyxiates because they displace breathing air. In addition, both are explosive. If a call involves leaking gas, call the gas company immediately. If a patient has been overcome by leaking gas, wear positive-pressure self-contained breathing apparatus and remove the patient from the hazardous atmosphere before beginning treatment.

Scene Security

Has the area been secured to prevent people from entering? Coworkers, family members, and even other rescuers may unwittingly enter an unsafe scene and become patients themselves. The IC should coordinate with law enforcement to help secure the scene and control access. In addition, the fire department should implement a strict accountability system to control access to the rescue scene.

Protective Equipment

Most specialized teams carry items such as harnesses; smaller, lighter helmets; and jumpsuits that are easier to move in than turnout gear. For personnel who perform water rescues, the minimum PPE includes a personal flotation device (PFD), thermal protection, a helmet appropriate for water rescue, a cutting device, a whistle, and contamination protection (if necessary). Rescuers should use a properly sized PFD that is designed and certified for their specific mission. They must be familiar with the manufacturer's procedures for donning and removing (doffing) their PFD. All straps should be tightened with loose straps secured to prevent entanglement Figure 49-5 ◀ .

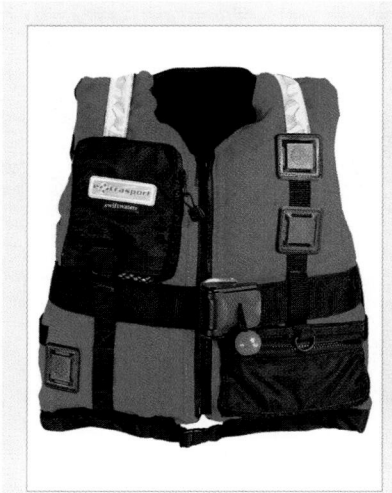

Figure 49-5 A PFD.

A handheld strobe light may help paramedics keep track of each other in a crowd or in rural or wilderness locations. When working along highways, they can hook these lights onto their belts or attach them to their upper arms to provide additional visibility to oncoming vehicles. Strobe lights are lightweight, quite durable, and readily visible at night at a distance of approximately 1 mile.

When considering the use of protective head gear, providers must use approved devices that meet certain standards and are appropriate for the rescue environment (eg, climbing helmets, fire fighter helmets). Footwear must be designed and certified for a specific rescue environment. The environment may require thermal protection (hot or cold), chemical protection, insole puncture barriers, and ankle support. Water rescue operations require specialized foot protection such as wetsuit-type booties. Providers must also consider the use of American National Standards Institute (ANSI)-approved safety glasses or goggles, puncture- or cut-resistant gloves, flame- or flash-protective clothing that is highly visible, and appropriate footwear to support ankles and provide traction. Other useful items that are easily carried by paramedics include binoculars, chalk or spray paint for marking searched areas, a compass for wilderness rescues, first aid kits, a whistle, a handheld global positioning system, and cyalume-type light sticks. The IC and the technical rescue team will help to determine what protective equipment you will need to wear while assisting.

Incident Management System

The first arriving officer immediately assumes command and starts using the incident management system (IMS). This step is critically important because many TRIs will eventually become very complex and require a large number of assisting units. Without the IMS in place, it will be difficult—if not impossible—to ensure the rescuers' safety.

Accountability

Accountability should be practiced at all emergencies, no matter how small. The accountability system is the single most important process to ensure rescuers' safety. It tracks the personnel on the scene, including their identities, assignments, and locations. This system ensures that only rescuers who have been given specific assignments are operating within the area where the rescue is taking place. By using an accountability system and working within the IMS, an IC can track the resources at the scene, task out assignments, and ensure that every person at the scene operates safely.

Patient Contact

At any rescue scene, you must try to communicate with the patient. Technical rescue situations often last for hours, with the patient being left alone for long periods of time. If at all possible, you should attempt to communicate via a radio, cell phone, or yelling. Reassure the patient that everything is being done to ensure his or her safety.

If you succeed in making contact, it's important to stay in communication with the patient. Ideally, someone should be assigned to talk to the patient, while others focus on making the rescue. Realize that the patient could be sick or injured and is probably frightened. If you are calm, your demeanor will in turn calm the patient:

- Make and keep eye contact with the patient.
- Tell the truth. Lying destroys trust and confidence. You may not always tell the patient everything, but if the patient asks a specific question, answer truthfully.
- Communicate at a level that the patient can understand.
- Be aware of your own body language.
- Always speak slowly, clearly, and distinctly.
- Use a patient's proper name. Use the patient's surname, preceded by the proper qualifier (ie, Mr. or Ms.).
- If a patient is hard of hearing, speak clearly and directly at the person, so that he or she can read your lips.
- Allow time for the patient to answer or respond to your questions.
- Try to make the patient comfortable and relaxed whenever possible.

Assisting Rescue Crews

If you will be assisting a technical rescue team, training with the team is probably the most important step you can take so that you can work together effectively during a TRI. Training allows you to get a feel for how the team members operate; likewise, they can get an idea of which duties they can trust you with. The more knowledge you have, the more you'll be able to do.

At any TRI, follow the IC's orders. Your ultimate goal is to protect the team and patients. No matter what type of rescue scene you enter, keep these three guidelines in mind:

- Approach the scene cautiously.
- Position apparatus properly.
- Assist specialized team members as needed.

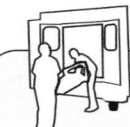

In the Field

Always assume that oncoming traffic can't see you, and act appropriately.

Vehicles

Determine where to locate your emergency vehicle, taking into account the safety of emergency workers, patients, and other motorists. Whenever possible, park emergency vehicles in a manner that will ensure safety and not disrupt traffic any more than necessary. Traffic flow is the largest single hazard associated with any operation that takes place on a highway. Provide a safe ambulance loading zone. On limited-access highways, keep vehicles and apparatus not directly involved in the rescue off the roadway. Have staging areas away from the scene. Don't hesitate to request that the road be closed if necessary.

Use large emergency vehicles to provide a barrier against motorists who fail to heed emergency warning lights. Many departments place apparatus at an angle to the crash. This position ensures that the apparatus is pushed to the side of a crash in the event that it is struck from behind. You can also place traffic cones or fusees to direct motorists away from the crash.

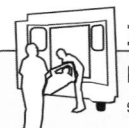

In the Field

Most newer cars and pickup trucks have driver-side and passenger-side airbags. Some newer vehicles have supplemental airbags in other places as well. Airbags that don't activate during a collision present a danger to rescuers until they're deactivated.

You are the Provider Part 3

A rapid trauma survey yields an actively bleeding 4″ laceration across the patient's forehead and diffuse abdominal tenderness. Assessment below the abdomen is not possible because the patient is pinned beneath the dashboard from the pelvis down. The patient is anxious about not being able to feel his legs. You do your best to reassure him that additional help is on its way and encourage him to focus on taking slow, deep breaths.

You place the patient on a nonrebreathing mask at 12 L/min of oxygen. Your partner applies a c-collar and manual c-spine continues to be held by the police officer. Bleeding from the forehead laceration is controlled with direct pressure and bandaging by one of the fire fighters. You are able to initiate a 16-gauge IV catheter in the right antecubital vein and begin a normal saline infusion at a keep-vein-open rate. Dispatch advises that the ETA for an additional unit is approximately 20 minutes and the ETA for the helicopter is approximately 10 minutes. Two of the fire fighters leave to establish a landing zone.

Reassessment	Recording Time: 13 Minutes
Skin	Pink, warm, and slightly diaphoretic
Pulse	130 breaths/min, strong and regular
Blood pressure	128/70 mm Hg
Respirations	22 breaths/min, regular
Sao$_2$	98% via nonrebreathing mask on 100% supplemental oxygen
ECG	Sinus tachycardia with no ectopy
Pupils	PERLA

5. What needs to be monitored on this patient?

You need to be visible at a crash scene. Use only essential warning lights, because too many lights tend to distract or confuse other drivers. Turn off headlights and consider the use of amber lighting at the scene. Your PPE should be bright to help ensure your visibility during daylight hours. Any PPE that is used at night needs to be equipped with reflective material to increase your visibility in the darkness. PPE must be worn at all motor vehicle crashes. Before exiting the ambulance at an emergency scene, be alert for any vehicles that might cause you injury. Don't assume that motorists will heed your warning lights, and let law enforcement personnel coordinate traffic control.

EMS providers must be aware of all potential hazards at rescue scenes—both obvious (eg, sharp metal and broken glass) and less obvious or hidden dangers. Downed power lines may fall from above, and underground electrical feeds may become exposed. Energy-absorbing bumpers can explode when subjected to heat and can spring out when loaded. Airbags or supplemental restraint systems (SRS) can deploy at any time after an accident and must be deactivated even if the power supply to the vehicle has been disconnected. Conventional fuel systems with highly flammable vapors may ignite if they come in contact with hot catalytic converters or heated engine components. New vehicles that use alternative fuel sources (eg, electric or propane-fueled vehicles) can also pose problems for rescuers. For example, providers must be aware of the electrical power, any storage cells, and high-pressure cylinders used in natural-gas–powered vehicles.

Vehicle-Related Terminology

To reduce confusion and mistakes at extrication scenes, it's important to use standardized terminology when referring to specific parts of vehicles. The front of a vehicle normally travels down the road first. The hood is located on the front of the vehicle. The rear of a vehicle is where the trunk is usually located.

The left side of a vehicle is on your left as you sit in the vehicle. In the United States and Canada, the driver's seat is on the left side of the vehicle. The right side of a vehicle is where the passenger's seat is located. Always refer to left and right as they relate to *the vehicle*—not as they refer to *your* left and right.

Vehicles contain A, B, C, and D posts, which are the vertical supports that hold up the roof and form the upright columns of the occupant cage. The A posts are located closest to the front of the vehicle; they form the sides of the windshield. In four-door vehicles, the B posts are located between the front and rear doors of a vehicle; in some vehicles, they don't reach all of the way to the roof. In four-door vehicles, the C posts are located behind the rear doors, if present. D posts can be found on larger vehicles such as sport utility vehicles and vans that have a passenger window on the side behind the rear doors. The D post is located behind the rear passenger windows.

The hood covers the engine compartment. The bulkhead divides the engine compartment from the passenger compartment. An insulating metal piece known as the firewall protects the passengers in the event of an engine fire. The passenger compartment includes the front and back seats. This part of a

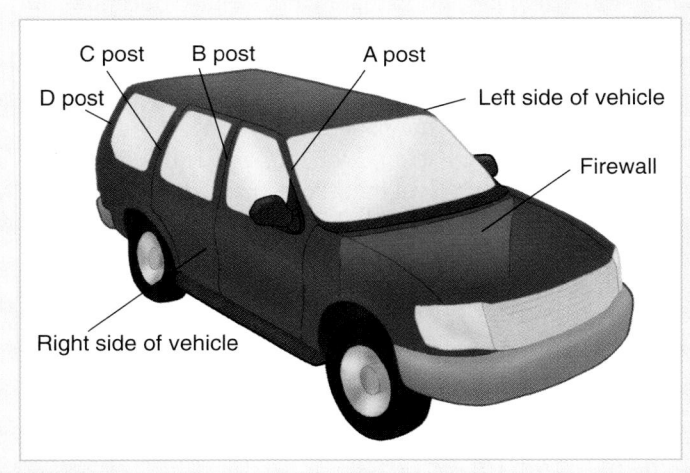

Figure 49-6 The anatomy of a vehicle.

vehicle is sometimes called the occupant cage or occupant compartment **Figure 49-6 ▲**.

There are two common types of vehicle frames: *platform frame* construction and *unibody* construction.

Platform frame construction uses beams to fabricate the load-bearing frame of a vehicle. The engine, transmission, and body components are then attached to this basic platform frame. This type of frame construction is found primarily in trucks and sport utility vehicles; it is rare in smaller passenger cars. Platform frame construction provides a structurally sound base for stabilizing the vehicle and an anchor point for attaching cables or extrication tools.

Unibody construction, which is used for most modern cars, combines the vehicle body and the frame into a single component. By folding multiple thicknesses of metal together, a column can be formed that is strong enough to serve as the frame for a lightweight vehicle. Unibody construction allows auto manufacturers to produce lighter weight vehicles. When extricating a person from such a vehicle, remember that unibody vehicles don't have the frame rails that are present with platform frame–constructed vehicles.

Vehicle Stabilization

Unstable objects pose a threat to both rescuers and victims of the crash. These objects—most often, the damaged vehicles—need to be stabilized before your approach.

Vehicles that end up on their wheels need to be stabilized with cribbing in the front and back of the wheels **Figure 49-7 ▶**. Cribbing is short lengths of robust timber (4″ × 4″) used to stabilize a vehicle. It prevents the vehicle from rolling backward or forward.

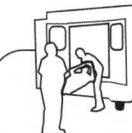

In the Field

Even vehicles that are positioned upright on all four wheels should be stabilized.

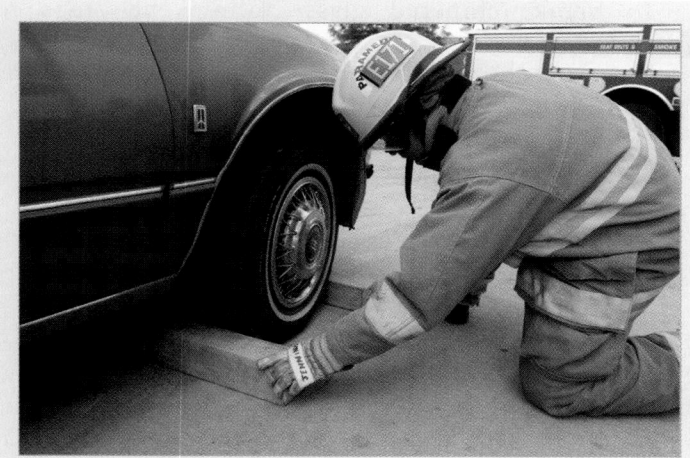

Figure 49-7 Cribbing.

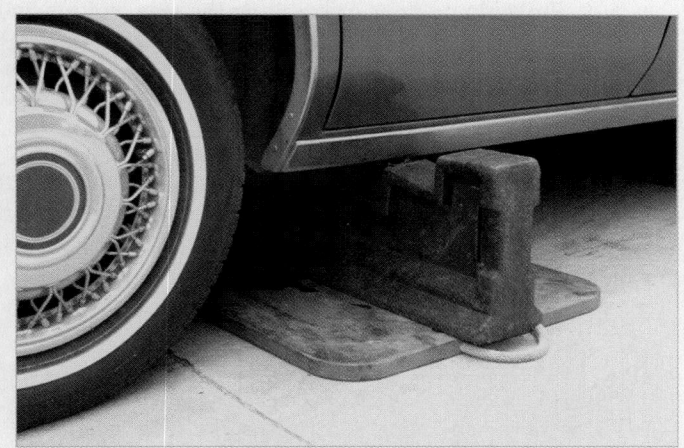

Figure 49-8 Step blocks can be used to stabilize a vehicle.

After the cribbing has been placed, a vehicle can still move because of the give and motion generated by the suspension system. This motion may occur as rescuers enter the vehicle and the patients are extricated from the vehicle, and it can cause further injuries to the patients of the crash. The suspension system of most vehicles can be stabilized with step blocks, which are stairstep-shaped blocks that are placed under the side of the vehicle. Place one step block toward the front of the vehicle and a second step block toward the rear of the vehicle Figure 49-8 ▲ . Once the step blocks are in place, the tires can be deflated by pulling out the valve stem with a pair of pliers or puncturing the tires. This creates a stable vehicle. If step blocks are not available or are not the right size, you can build a box crib by placing cribbing at right angles to the first layer of cribbing Figure 49-9 ▶ .

After a collision, some vehicles will come to rest on their roof or sides. These vehicles are very unstable, and the slightest weight on them can cause them to move. To stabilize these vehicles, use box cribs or step blocks on each end of the vehicle.

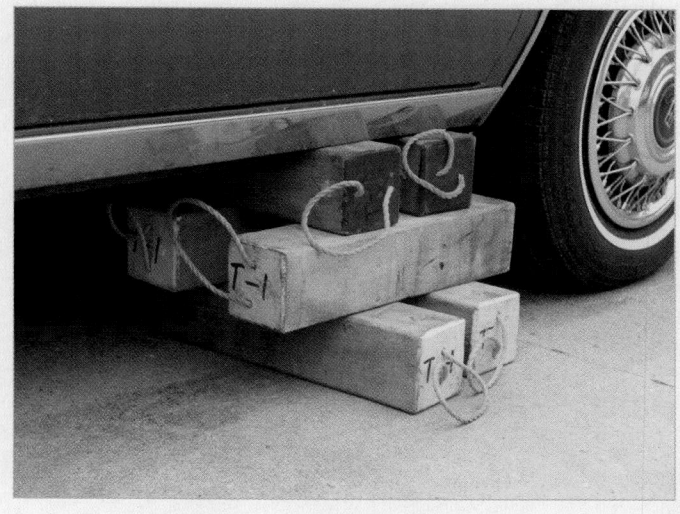

Figure 49-9 Box crib.

Wedges are used to snug loose cribbing under the load or when using lift airbags to fill the void between the crib and the object as it's raised. Wedges should be the same width as the cribbing, with the tapered end no less than 0.25″ thick. When the ends are less than 0.25″, the end will commonly fracture under a load.

Gain Access to the Patient
Open the Door
After stabilizing the vehicle, the simplest way to access a crash victim is to open a door. Try all of the doors first—even if they appear to be badly damaged. It's an embarrassing waste of time and energy to open a jammed door with heavy rescue equipment when another door can be opened easily and without any special equipment.

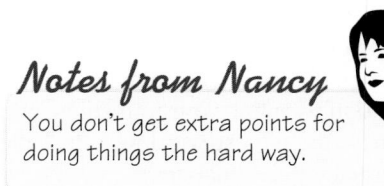

Notes from Nancy
You don't get extra points for doing things the hard way.

Attempt to unlock and open the least damaged door first. Make sure the locking mechanism is released. Try the outside and inside handles at the same time if possible.

If you have an open door but still need more room, have two rescuers lean against the door and push; most car doors will easily bend open, creating a much wider opening for patient removal.

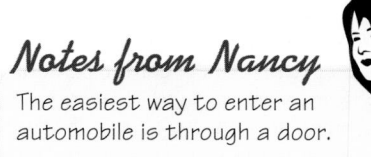

Notes from Nancy
The easiest way to enter an automobile is through a door.

Break Tempered Glass
If a patient's condition is serious enough to require immediate care and you can't enter the vehicle through a door, consider breaking a window. Don't try to break and enter through the

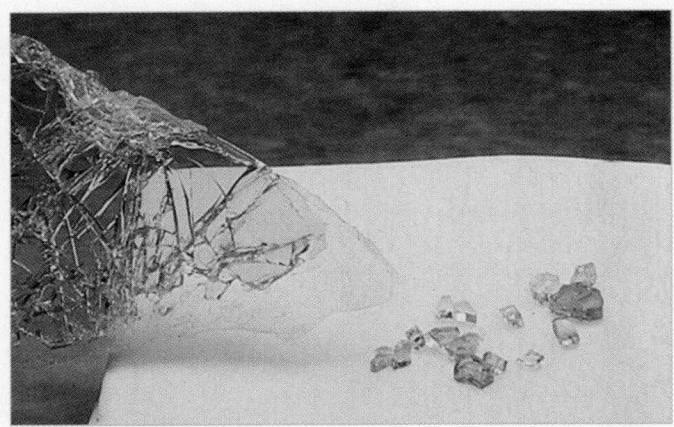

Figure 49-10 The two types of glass in vehicles: laminated glass (left) and tempered glass (right).

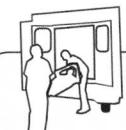

In the Field

Always warn trapped car passengers that you're going to break the glass!

windshield because it's made of laminated windshield glass, which is difficult to break. The side and rear windows are made of tempered glass, also known as safety glass, and will break easily into small pieces when hit with a sharp, pointed object such as a spring-loaded center punch or the point of an axe **Figure 49-10 ▲**. Because these windows do not pose as great a safety threat, they can be your primary access route.

If you must break a window to unlock a door or gain access, try to break one that's far away from the patient. If the patient's condition warrants your immediate entry, however, don't hesitate to break the closest window. Small pieces of tempered glass do not usually pose a danger to people trapped in cars.

Notes from Nancy

Don't use a sledgehammer to crack a walnut.

During this step of the rescue, all rescuers should be in proper PPE, including dust mask, safety glasses, or goggles. Attempt to lower windows as far as possible before breaking glass, and then select a spring-loaded center punch. If you're using something other than a spring-loaded center punch, always aim for a low corner. The window frame will help prevent the tool (such as an axe or screwdriver) from sailing into the vehicle and hitting the person inside. Personnel are given a verbal warning "Breaking glass," unless a stop/freeze call is made. After breaking the window, use your gloved hands to pull the remaining glass out of the window frame so it doesn't fall onto any passengers or injure any rescuers.

To break tempered glass, follow the steps in **Skill Drill 49-1 ▶**.

1. Ensure that the patient and rescuers are properly protected.
2. Place the center punch in the lower corner of the window and apply pressure until the spring is activated **Step 1**.
3. Press on the center punch to break the window **Step 2**.
4. Remove any loose glass around the window opening **Step 3**.
5. Follow this procedure until all glass has been removed **Step 4**.

Once you have removed the pieces of glass from the frame, try to unlock the door again. Release the locking mechanism, and then use both the inside and outside door handles at the same time. This action may force a jammed locking mechanism, even in a door that appears to be badly damaged.

Breaking the rear window will sometimes provide an opening large enough to enable a rescuer to reach a patient if there is no other rapid means for gaining access. Using the simple techniques of opening a door or breaking the rear window will enable you to gain access to most patients in vehicle crashes, even those in upside-down vehicles.

Force the Door

If you can't gain access to the vehicle by the methods already described, heavier extrication tools must be used to gain access to the patient. The most common technique is door displacement **Figure 49-11 ▼**. The opening and displacement of vehicle doors may be difficult and somewhat unpredictable, however.

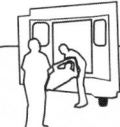

In the Field

To reduce the risk of tempered glass pieces falling on patients, cover the window with duct tape or shelf paper prior to breaking it. Most of the glass can be removed as a unit.

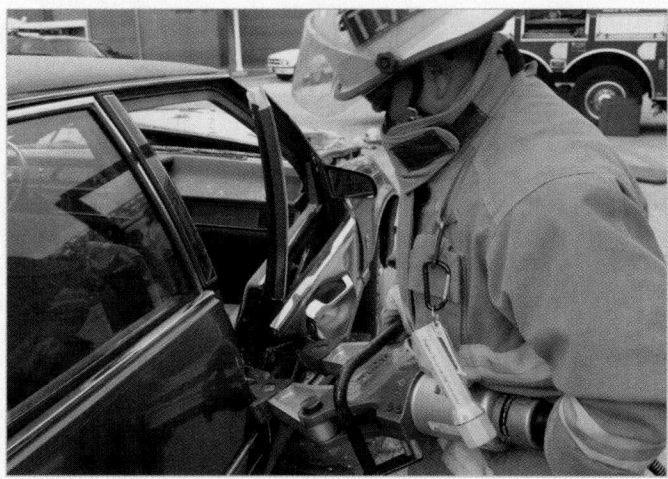

Figure 49-11 The most common technique for gaining access is door displacement.

Skill Drill 49-1: Breaking Tempered Glass

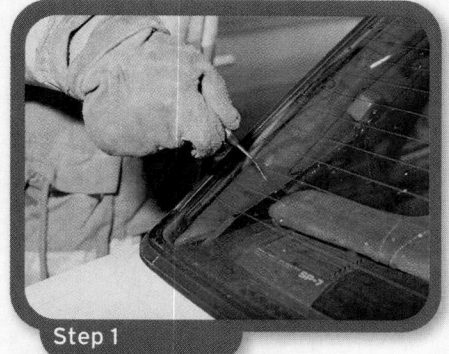

Step 1
Place the spring-loaded center punch at the lower corner of the window.

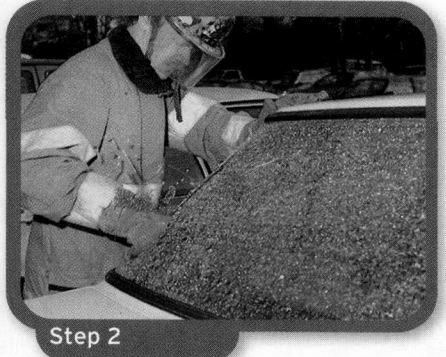

Step 2
Press on the center punch.

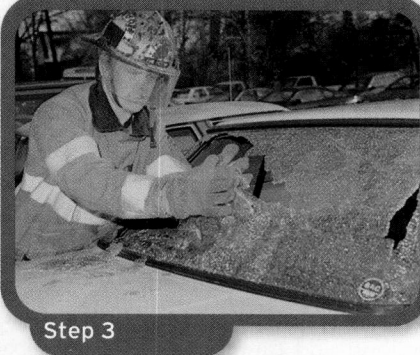

Step 3
Remove glass to the outside.

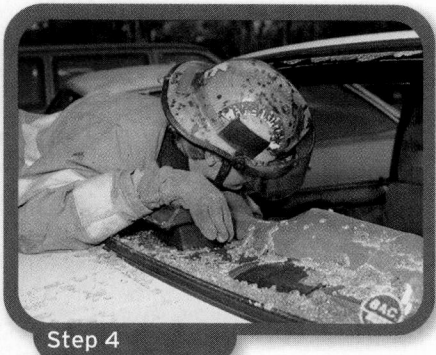

Step 4
Follow this procedure until all glass has been removed.

expose the hinges or door latch. Once the outer sheet metal has been exposed, close the tips of the spreader and remove them.

If the side bar is crushed onto the patient and the compartment is still intact, you should consider the "vertical crush" technique: Peel the door down and away from the patient with the jaws on the roof and the top of the door.

At this point, insert the closed tips onto the inner skin of the door and the door jamb just above the latch or hinges. Activate the spreader to extend the tips until the latch or hinge separates. When separating a door at the latch side, you can place 4″ × 4″ cribbing under the bottom of the door to hold it up and then start to separate the hinges of the door. When separating a door from the hinge side, place the spreader on the top of the bottom hinge. Use the hydraulic spreader to separate the door from the hinge. Once the hinges have separated, place 4″ × 4″ cribbing underneath the door to hold it in place while you work on the latch side of the door. Note that some hydraulic tools are capable of cutting door hinges.

Once the door has been removed, move it away from the vehicle, where it will not be a safety hazard to other rescuers.

Provide Initial Medical Care

As soon as you've secured access to the patient, a qualified emergency medical provider should begin to provide emergency medical care. Being trapped in a damaged vehicle is a frightening experience, so it's important that one caregiver remain with the patient and provide both emotional comfort and physical care. Patient care should occur simultaneously with extrication **Figure 49-12**. Although it may be necessary to delay some elements of these processes for a short period, it's important to work toward the goal of stabilizing the patient and removing him or her from the vehicle as quickly and safely as possible.

Notes from Nancy
A good extrication is a safe extrication.

Disentangle the Patient

The next step in the extrication sequence is disentangling the patient, a measure that seeks to remove those parts of the vehicle

When it's necessary to force a door to gain access to the patient, choose a door that will not endanger the safety of the patient. For example, don't try to force a door open if the patient is leaning against it.

Powered hydraulic tools are the most efficient and widely used tools for opening a jammed door that can be opened by releasing the door from the latch side or the hinge side of the door. The decision regarding which method to use will depend on the structure of the vehicle and the type of damage the door has sustained.

First, use a pry tool to bend the sheet metal away from the edge of the door where the spreader of the hydraulic tool is to be inserted. Next, place the spreader in a position so that it's not in the pathway that the door will take when the hinges or latch break. Don't stand in a position that might put you in danger. Activate the hydraulic tool to push apart the outer sheet metal skin of the vehicle to

Notes from Nancy
Try before you pry.

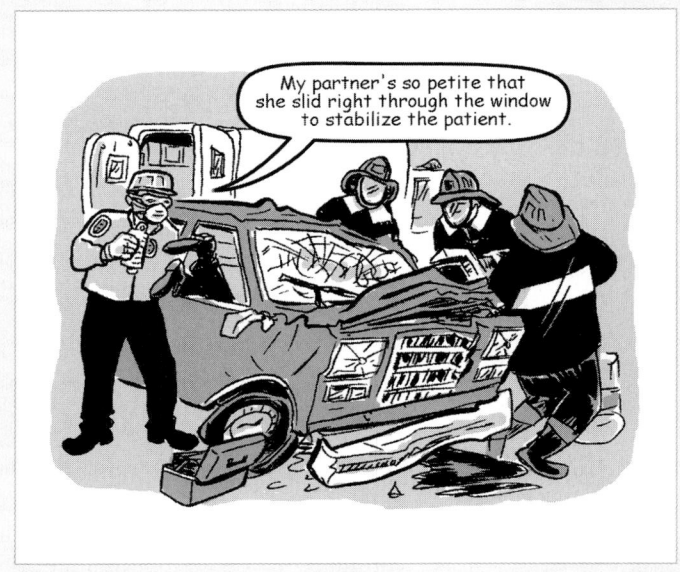

Figure 49-12

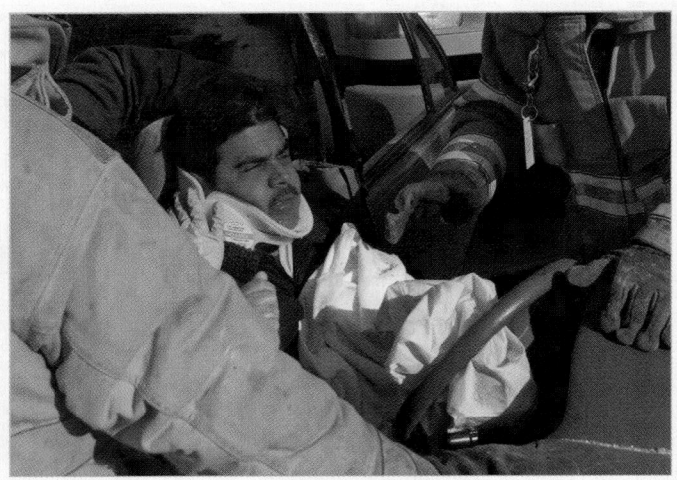

Figure 49-13 The driver may be trapped between the steering wheel and the back of the front seat.

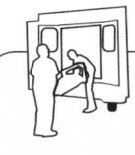

In the Field

If you're wearing a heavy coat for protection from the weather during a rescue operation, then the patient will also be cold if not covered with blankets.

that are trapping the patient. The goal here is to remove the sheet metal and plastic from around the patient—not to "cut the patient out of the vehicle."

Before attempting disentanglement, study the situation. What is trapping the patient in the vehicle? Perform only those disentanglement procedures that are necessary to remove the patient safely from the vehicle. The order in which these procedures are performed will be dictated by the specific conditions at the incident. Many times it will be necessary to perform one procedure before you can access the parts of the vehicle needed to perform another procedure.

As you work to disentangle the patient from the wrecked vehicle, protect the patient by covering him or her with a blanket or by using a backboard. Be sure that the patient understands what's being done—the sounds made by extrication procedures can be quite frightening for patients.

To learn all of the methods of disentangling a patient, you need to take an approved extrication course. The five procedures presented below are the ones that are most commonly performed.

Displace the Seat

In frontal and rear-end collisions, the vehicle may become compressed. As the front of the vehicle is pushed back, the space between the steering wheel and the seat becomes smaller. In some cases, the driver may be trapped between the steering

wheel and the back of the front seat   Figure 49-13 ▲ . Displacing the seat can relieve pressure on the driver and give rescuers more space for removal.

If it's necessary to displace a seat backward, start with the simplest steps. Many times you can gain some room by moving the seat backward on its track, especially with short drivers who have the seat forward. To move a seat back, first be sure that the patient is supported. With manually operated seats, you need to release the seat-adjusting lever and carefully slide the seat back as far as it will go. If the seat is electrically operated, check that the car has power, and engage the lever to electrically move the seat backward. With seats that have adjustable backs and adjustable heights, you can use these features to give the patient more room or lower the seat to help disentangle the patient.

If these methods are unsuccessful, perform a dash displacement. As a last resort, you can use a manual hydraulic spreader or a powered hydraulic tool to move the seat back. Place one tip of the hydraulic tool on the bottom of the seat. Avoid pushing on the seat channel that's attached to the floor of the vehicle. Place the other tip of the spreader at the bottom of the A-post door jamb. Support the patient carefully. Engage the seat adjustment lever on manually operated seats, and open the spreader in a careful and controlled fashion. The seat should move backward smoothly in a controlled manner.

In some cases, it may be helpful to remove the back of the seat. To do so, cut the upholstery away from the bottom of the seat back where it joins the main part of the seat. Use a reciprocating saw or a hydraulic cutter to cut the supports for the seat back. Be certain that the patient is supported and protected during this procedure.

Notes from Nancy

Remove the vehicle from the patient, not the patient from the vehicle.

Remove the Windshield

A second technique that's often part of disentanglement is the removal of glass. Removing the rear window, side glass, or windshield improves communication between rescue personnel inside the vehicle and personnel outside the vehicle. Sometimes all you need to do is to roll a window down. Open windows provide a good route for passing medical care supplies to the inside caregiver. When the roof of a vehicle must be removed, all of the glass must first be removed from the vehicle.

On most vehicles, the side windows and rear window are tempered glass that can be removed by striking the glass in a lower corner with a sharp object, such as a spring-loaded center punch. In contrast, windshields cannot be broken with a spring-loaded center punch. They consist of plastic laminated glass—a type of "sandwich," in which the two pieces of bread are thin sheets of specially constructed glass and the filling is a thin layer of a special flexible plastic. When laminated glass is struck by a sharp stone or by a spring-loaded center punch, a small mark is formed, but the structure of the glass remains intact. For this reason, the windshield must be removed in one large piece. The windshields of most passenger vehicles are glued in place with a strong, plastic-type adhesive.

Removing a windshield is an essential step before removing the roof of a vehicle. It will also provide added space when administering emergency medical care to an injured patient. The windshield of a damaged vehicle may be removed using either an axe or a saw.

To remove a windshield using an axe **Figure 49-14 ▶**, first be certain that the patient is protected from flying glass. One rescuer then begins to cut the top of the windshield at the center of the windshield, using short strokes of the axe. He or she continues cutting along the top of the windshield with the next cut down the side of the windshield close to the A post. Finally, the first rescuer cuts along the bottom of the windshield. At this point, the first rescuer stabilizes the half of the windshield that has been cut free. Next, a second rescuer starts

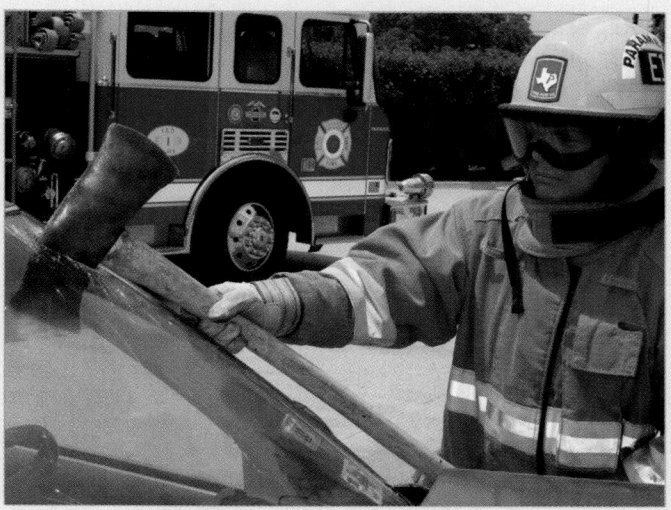

Figure 49-14 Removing the windshield with an axe.

at the top of the windshield where the initial cuts were made by the first rescuer. He or she cuts the second half of the windshield following the same sequence of cuts used by the first rescuer. The windshield is then lifted out of its frame and removed to a place where it will not present a safety hazard.

When using a saw, the windshield is removed by making the cuts in the same order as those made with an axe.

Displace the Dash

During a frontal collision, the vehicle's dash may be pushed down or backward. When a patient is trapped by the dash, you must remove it using a technique called the dash displacement or dash roll-up. The objective of the dash displacement is to lift the dash up and move it forward.

Dash displacement requires a cutting tool such as a hacksaw, reciprocating saw, air chisel, or hydraulic cutter. This cutting tool is used to make a cut on the A post. A mechanical

You are the Provider Part 4

About 10 minutes later the patient becomes extremely anxious and complains about excruciating abdominal pain. A reassessment of the abdomen shows marked distention and rigidity. The patient is becoming pale and increasingly diaphoretic. His radial pulses are weakening. He begs you to do something for the pain, although you have explained that you are not able to do so. Despite your best efforts to be reassuring, the patient's anxiety continues to escalate and he keeps repeating "I'm dying." You increase the flow of the IV and silently hope that additional help arrives soon. Off in the distance the whir of helicopter blades can be heard.

Reassessment	Recording Time: 23 Minutes
Skin	Pale, cool, and diaphoretic
Pulse	140 beats/min, carotid
Blood pressure	92/68 mm Hg
Respirations	20 breaths/min
Sao_2	97% on 100% supplemental oxygen
ECG	Sinus rhythm without ectopy

In the Field

Airbag Safety

- Steering wheels on most recently manufactured vehicles contain a driver's side airbag, which is a lifesaving safety feature for the occupants of the vehicle.
- If the airbag has deployed during the collision, it does not present a safety hazard for rescuers.
- If not deployed during the collision, an airbag presents a hazard for the passenger of the vehicle and for rescue personnel. It could potentially deploy if wires are cut or if it becomes activated during the rescue operation.
- If the airbag did not deploy, disconnect the battery and allow the airbag capacitor to discharge. The time required to discharge the capacitor varies from one model of airbag to another.
- Some newer-model vehicles have a switch mounted on or under the dash that allows drivers to disconnect or shut off the SRS.
- Don't place a hard object such as a backboard between the patient and an undeployed airbag.
- Don't attempt to cut a steering wheel if the airbag hasn't deployed.
- For your safety, never get in front of an undeployed airbag. You could suffer serious injury if it's unexpectedly activated.
- Some vehicles contain side-mounted airbags or curtains that provide lateral protection for passengers. Check vehicles for the presence of these devices.

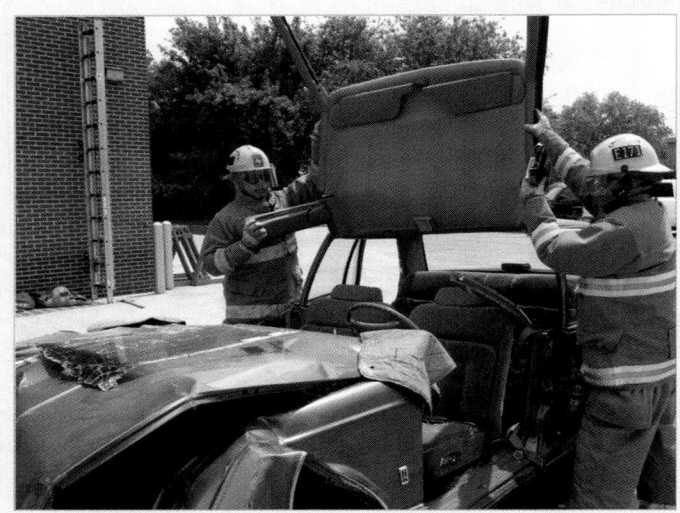

Figure 49-15 Removing the roof provides a large exit route for the patient.

Displace the Roof

Removing the roof of a vehicle allows equipment to be more easily passed in to the emergency medical provider. It also increases the amount of space available to perform medical care and increases the visibility and space for performing disentanglement. Both provider and patient will benefit from the fresh air supply, too. The increased space helps to reduce the feeling of panic caused by the confined space of the wrecked vehicle. Removing the roof also provides a large exit route for the patient **Figure 49-15 ▲** .

One method of displacing the roof is to cut the A posts and fold the roof back toward the rear of the vehicle. This method provides limited space and takes about the same time as removing the entire roof. Accordingly, in most cases, it's preferable to remove the entire roof.

Roof displacement can be accomplished with hand tools such as hacksaws, air chisels, or manual hydraulic cutters. Appropriate power tools include reciprocating saws and powered hydraulic cutters.

A key consideration in displacing the roof is to ensure the safety of rescuers and the patient inside the vehicle. In particular, as you cut the posts that support the roof, rescuers must support the roof to keep it from falling on the patient.

To displace the roof, first remove the glass to prevent it from falling on the patients. Cut the vehicle posts farthest away from the patient. Cut the posts at a level to ensure that the least amount of post will remain after roof removal. It's very important to cut the shoulder harness on seatbelts because they're attached to the roof in many cars and will be the only thing preventing roof removal. When cutting the wider rear posts, cut them at the narrowest point of the post. As each post is cut, a rescuer needs to support that post. Cut the post closest to the patient last. Working together, remove the roof and place it away from the vehicle, where it doesn't

high-lift jack or a hydraulic ram then pushes the dash forward, and cribbing maintains the opening made with these tools.

The first step of the dash displacement is to open both front doors. Tie them in the open position so they won't move as the dash is being displaced. Alternatively, you can remove the doors.

Next, place a backboard or other protective device between the patient and the bottom part of the A post, where the relief cut will be made. Cut the bottom of the A post where it meets the sill or floor of the vehicle. It's critical to make the cut perpendicular to the A post; failure to do so may cut the fuel or power line located in the rocker panels.

Place the base of a high-lift mechanical jack or a hydraulically powered ram at the base of the B post where the sill and the B post meet. Place the tip of the jack or ram at the bend in the A post, which is located toward the top of the A post. In a controlled manner, extend the jack or ram to push the dash up and off of the patient.

Once the dash has been removed, build a crib to hold the sill in the proper position and to prevent the dash from moving. You can then remove the jack or ram.

Performing dash displacement requires careful monitoring of the movement of the dash to be certain that it's moving away from the patient and that it isn't causing additional harm to the patient. Be sure that the patient is protected and have someone keep the patient updated on what is being done.

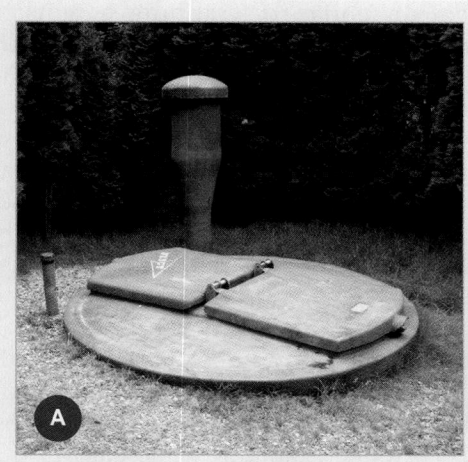
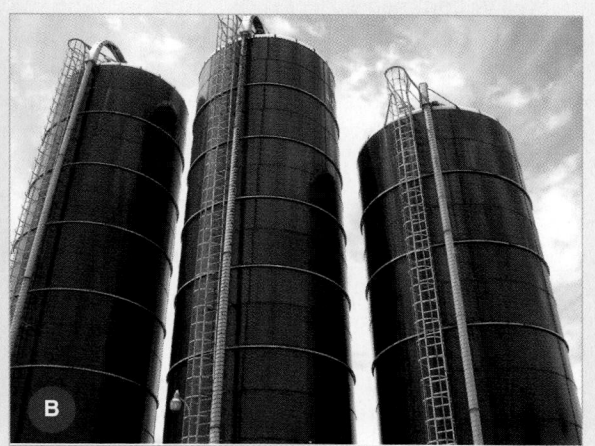

Figure 49-16 Confined spaces **A.** Below ground. **B.** Silo.

confined-space call is sometimes dispatched as a heart attack or medical illness call, because the caller assumes the person who entered a confined space and became unresponsive suffered a heart attack or medical illness.

Examples of Oxygen Deficiency/Poisonous Gases in Confined Spaces

Hydrogen sulfide (H_2S) is a colorless, toxic, flammable gas that is released when bacteria break down organic matter in the absence of oxygen. It can be found in swamps, standing water, sewers, volcanic gases, natural gas, and in some wells. Hydrogen sulfide is heavier than air and has a very pungent odor at first but deadens the sense of smell very quickly.

pose a safety hazard. Cover the sharp ends of the cut posts with a protective device.

Confined Spaces

A confined space is a location surrounded by a structure that isn't designed for continuous occupancy. Confined spaces have limited openings for entrance and exit. Confined spaces can occur in farm, commercial, and industrial settings. Structures such as grain silos, industrial pits, tanks, and below-ground structures are all considered confined spaces. Automobile trunks are also considered confined spaces. Cisterns, well casings, and septic tanks are also confined spaces that are found in many residential settings Figure 49-16 ▲ .

Confined spaces present a special hazard because they may have limited ventilation to provide for air circulation and exchange, which can make them an oxygen-deficient atmosphere, or they may contain poisonous gases. Entering a confined space without testing the atmosphere for safety and without the proper breathing apparatus can result in death. Additionally, there is a risk of fire and explosion in confined spaces because inadequate ventilation may trap flammable mixtures. Grain silos and trenches can suddenly become "quicksand" and lead to engulfment. Machinery may often have confined spaces containing augers or screws that can be hazardous to rescue workers. All rescue personnel must consider the potential for stored electrical energy in any machinery and should never attempt any rescue without being properly trained.

Don't be overwhelmed by the urgency to start treating patients; scene safety must always be considered first. A

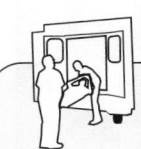
In the Field
Confined spaces such as manholes can be deceiving. They may look habitable but can contain minimal oxygen or deadly invisible toxins.

In the Field
More rescuers die in confined spaces than victims! Of all deaths in confined-space rescue incidents, 60% are rescuers. Do not enter a confined space without proper breathing apparatus and special training.

Carbon monoxide (CO) is a colorless, odorless, tasteless gas that can't be detected by your normal senses. Inhaling relatively small quantities of CO gas can result in severe poisoning because it binds to red blood cells about 200 to 250 times more readily than oxygen. Therefore, a small quantity of CO can "monopolize" the red blood cells and prevent them from transporting oxygen to all parts of the body. The signs and symptoms of CO poisoning include headache, nausea, disorientation, and unconsciousness.

Carbon dioxide (CO_2) is a colorless gas associated with asphyxiation risks. It is actually the end product of a metabolism process in which sugar and fats combine with oxygen. Carbon dioxide is used to make dry ice and is found in fire extinguishers. It produces a sour taste in the mouth and a stinging sensation in the nose and mouth.

Methane (CH_4)—the principal component of natural gas—isn't toxic but will cause burns if ignited. Flammable or explosive mixtures form at much lower concentrations than the concentrations at which asphyxiation risks arise. Methane is used as a fuel from natural gas fields but can also be generated from fermentation of organic matter (eg, manure, waste water, sludge, and municipal solid waste).

Ammonia (NH_3) is a toxic and corrosive chemical with a characteristic pungent odor. Because ammonia is lighter than air, it rises to the upper atmospheric level in confined spaces. It's typically found in rural areas and is used extensively for fertilizing agricultural crops.

Nitrogen dioxide (NO_2) is a reddish-brown gas that has a characteristic sharp, biting odor. It is most prominent in air pollution and is considered toxic by inhalation.

Safe Approach

As you approach a confined-space rescue scene, look for a bystander who might have witnessed the emergency. Information gathered prior to the technical rescue team's arrival will save valuable time during the actual rescue. Don't automatically assume that a person in a pit has simply suffered a heart attack; instead, assume that there's an IDLH atmosphere at any confined-space call. An IDLH atmosphere can immediately incapacitate anyone who enters the confined space without breathing protection. Toxic gases may be present, or oxygen levels may be insufficient to support life. Inevitably, it will take some time for qualified rescuers to arrive on the scene and prepare for a safe entry into the confined space. The victim of the original incident may have died before your arrival—don't put your life in danger for a dead patient.

Assisting Other Rescuers

You and your partner can prevent a confined-space incident from becoming worse by recognizing it, securing the scene, and ensuring that no one enters the space until additional rescue resources arrive. As highly trained personnel arrive, you may provide help by giving these rescuers a situation report.

The first responding rescuers must share whatever information is discovered at the rescue scene with the arriving crew. Anything that may be important to the response should be noted by the first arriving unit. Observed conditions should be compared to reported conditions, and a determination should be made as to the relative change over the time period. Whether an incident appears to be stable or has changed significantly since the first report will affect the operation strategy for the rescue. A size-up should be quickly completed immediately upon arrival, and this information should be relayed to the specialized rescue team members when they arrive at the scene. Other items of importance that should be included in a situation report are a description of any rescue attempts that have been made, exposures, hazards, extinguishment of fires, the facts and probabilities of the scene, the situation and resources of the fire company, the identity of any hazardous materials present, and a progress evaluation.

Confined-space rescues can be complex and can take a long time to complete. You may be asked to assist by bringing rescue equipment to the scene, maintaining a charged hose line, or providing crowd control. By understanding the hazards of confined spaces, you will be better prepared to assist a specialized team that's dealing with an emergency involving a confined space.

Trenches

Trench rescues may become necessary when earth is removed for placement of a utility line or for other construction and the

sides of the excavation collapse, trapping a worker **Figure 49-17 ▾**. Entrapments may also occur when children play around a pile of sand or earth that collapses. Unfortunately, many entrapments occur because the required safety precautions were not taken.

Whenever a collapse occurs, you need to understand that the collapsed product is unstable and prone to further collapse. Earth and sand are very heavy, and a person who's partly entrapped can't simply be pulled out. Instead, the patient must be carefully dug out after shoring has stabilized the sides of the excavation.

Vibration or additional weight on top of displaced earth will increase the probability of a secondary collapse. A secondary collapse occurs after the initial collapse; it can be caused by equipment vibration, personnel standing at the edge of the trench, or water eroding away the soil. Safe removal of trapped

> ### In the Field
>
> Most trench collapses occur in trenches less than 12′ deep and 6′ wide. Patients are suddenly covered with heavy soil, resulting in asphyxia. Specially trained rescuers should make safe access only after shoring is in place.

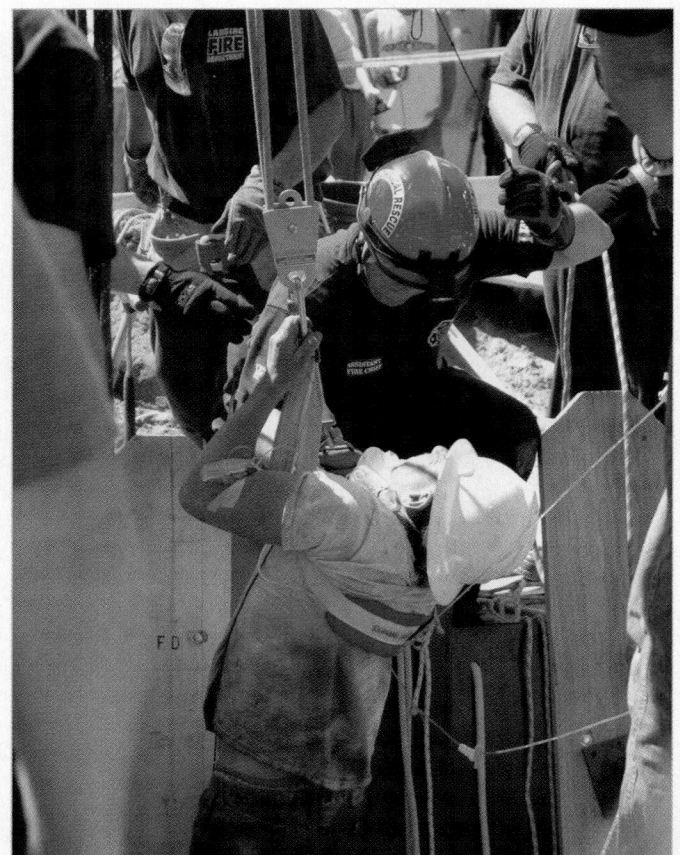

Figure 49-17 Trench rescue.

persons requires a special rescue team that is trained and equipped to erect shoring that will protect the rescuers and the entrapped person from secondary collapse.

Safety is of paramount importance when approaching a trench or excavation collapse. Walking close to the edge of a collapse can trigger a secondary collapse. Stay away from the edge of the site, and keep all workers and bystanders away. Vibration from equipment and machinery can cause secondary collapses, so shut off all heavy equipment. Vibrations caused by nearby traffic can also cause collapse, so it may be necessary to stop or divert traffic.

Soil that has been removed from the excavation and placed in a pile is called the spoil pile. This material is very unstable and may collapse if placed too close to the excavation. Avoid disturbing the spoil pile.

Make verbal contact with the trapped person if possible, but do *not* place yourself in danger while doing so. If you approach the trench, do so from the narrow end, where the soil will be more stable. However, it's best *not* to approach the trench unless absolutely necessary; EMS providers should stay out of a trench unless properly trained.

Provide reassurance by letting the trapped person know that a trained rescue team is on the way. By removing people from the edges of the excavation, shutting down machinery, and establishing contact with the patient, you start the rescue process.

You can also size up the scene, looking for evidence that would indicate where the trapped workers may be located. Hand tools and hard hats are one indicator of their presence. By questioning the workers, EMS providers may also determine where the patients were last seen.

Water

Almost all EMS departments may potentially be called to perform a water rescue—whether from a small stream, a large river, a lake, the ocean, a reservoir, or a swimming pool. A static source such as a lake may have no current and is considered flat water or slow moving. In contrast, a whitewater stream or flooded river may have a very swift current. During a flood, a dry wash in the desert can quickly become a raging monster.

Rescuers may suddenly find themselves immersed in moving water during a water rescue, so they should be aware of self-rescue techniques. A PFD is essential. In addition, if suddenly immersed in fast-moving water, rescuers should adopt the self-rescue position. The first step is to roll into a face-up arched position with the lower back higher than the feet to avoid subsurface objects. Keep the feet together and facing in the direction of travel (feet first) with arms to the side. Use the hands for changing direction to avoid objects and for diversion to a safe area. Keep the head down, with the chin tucked in. This posi-

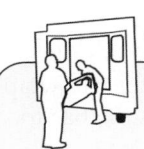

In the Field

Don't attempt a water rescue unless you are specially trained.

tion protects the rescuer's head, face, and lower back from striking objects and provides a means for controlling direction.

Cold Water Rescue

Water temperature varies widely by season and by geographical area. Even on warm days, water temperatures can be very low. Water causes heat loss 25 times greater than ambient air temperature. Indeed, any water temperature less than 98.6°F will cause hypothermia; patients who become hypothermic lose the ability to self-rescue. Maintaining body heat is critical because hypothermia becomes an immediate problem that progresses to unconsciousness and death. In extremely cold water (35°F), a submersion time of 15 to 20 minutes will cause the body to shut down and lead to death.

If you find yourself in cold water, make every effort to keep your face above water, protect your head, and assume the heat-escape-lessening position (HELP) **Figure 49-18 ▾** , which helps keep heat in the core of your body. Immersion victims should minimize movement and assume the HELP position. In a group, victims should huddle together to share body warmth.

In the Field

Humans can't maintain body heat in water that is less than 92°F. The colder the water, the faster the loss of heat. Compared with air, water causes a heat loss at a rate 25 times faster. Immersion for 15 to 20 minutes in 35°F water is likely to be fatal.

In water colder than 70°F (21°C), immersion victims may actually benefit from a phenomenon known as the cold protective response. Essentially, when a person is submerged in cold water, heat is conducted from the body to the water. The resulting hypothermia can protect vital organs from the lack of oxygen. In addition, exposure to cold water will occasionally activate certain primitive reflexes, which may preserve body functions for prolonged periods. In one case, a 2½-year-old girl

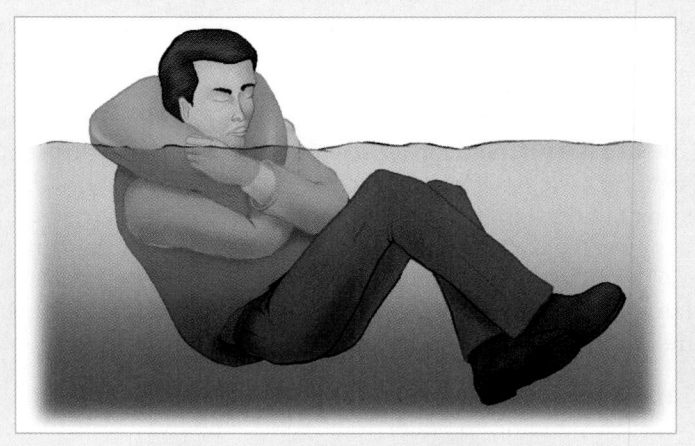

Figure 49-18 The heat-escape-lessening position (HELP).

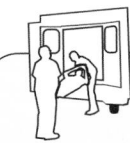

In the Field

The HELP position can decrease heat loss by 60% compared with treading water.

recovered after being submerged in cold water for at least 66 minutes. For this reason, you should continue to provide full resuscitative efforts for a victim of cold water submersion until the patient recovers or is pronounced dead by a physician (see Chapter 35 for a more detailed discussion of hypothermia).

Whenever a person dives or jumps into very cold water, the diving reflex (also known as the mammalian diving reflex)—the slowing of the heart rate caused by submersion in cold water—may cause immediate bradycardia. Although loss of consciousness may follow, the person may be able to survive for an extended time under water because of a lowering of the metabolic rate and decreased oxygen demand and consumption associated with hypothermia.

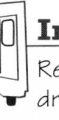

In the Field

Remember that hypothermic patients are dehydrated due to "cold diuresis," and should be removed from the water in a horizontal position to avoid orthostatic changes.

Other Water Rescue Situations

In North America, the most common swift water rescue scenario involves people who have attempted to drive vehicles through a pool of water created by a flooded stream. The vehicle stalls because of the depth of the water, leaving the vehicle occupants stranded in a rising stream with a swift current. If the water is high enough, the vehicle can be swept away. These incidents are especially dangerous for rescue personnel, because it is difficult to determine the depth of the water around the vehicle.

In surface water rescues, rescuers must consider hazards such as the dangerous hydraulics created by moving water as well as "strainers" (objects in the water such as trees, branches, debris, or wire mesh that can pose a serious pinning risk for rescuers). Dams and hydroelectric sites are also treacherous for even the most skilled rescuers. It's important to remember that the height of a dam does not indicate the degree of hazard to rescuers. Intakes at the base of a dam can act like strainers. Low-head dams are often associated with recirculating currents (sometimes referred to as a "boil") **Figure 49-19 ▸** . These currents can trap victims and unwary rescuers alike, forcing them underwater, away from the dam, and back to the surface again, where the cycle repeats itself. For this reason, low-head dams are often referred to as "drowning machines." Never underestimate the power or intensity of moving water.

Safe Approach

When responding to water rescue incidents, your safety and the safety of other rescuers are your primary concerns. Your

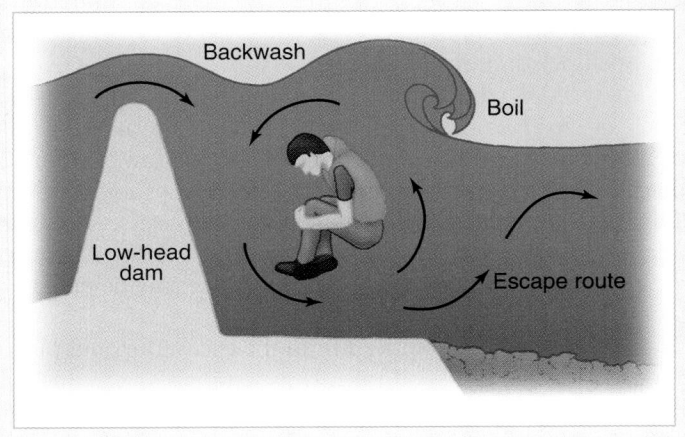

Figure 49-19 Recirculating current at a low-head dam.

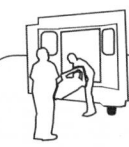

In the Field

The hydraulics of moving water change with variables such as depth, velocity, and obstruction to flow.

gear is not designed for water rescue activities. When working at a water rescue scene, you should use personal protective gear designed for water rescue. Whenever you are within 10′ of the water, you should wear an approved PFD. Shoes that provide solid traction are preferable to boots.

If you are part of the first arriving ambulance's crew, and the endangered people are in a vehicle or holding on to a tree or other solid object, try to communicate with them. Let them know that more help is on the way.

Don't exceed your level of training. If you can't swim, operating around or near water is not recommended. A person who is trained as a lifeguard for still water is not prepared to enter flowing water with a strong current, such as in a river, stream, or ocean. Make sure that bystanders don't try to rescue the patient and place themselves in a situation where they need to be rescued, too.

When you see a person struggling in the water, your first impulse may be to jump in to assist. However, that action may not result in a successful rescue and can endanger your life. The model most commonly used in water rescue is *reach-throw-row-go*:

- Attempt to *reach* out to the threatening person first, using any readily available object. If the person is close to shore, a branch, pole, oar, or paddle may be long enough.
- If you can't reach the person, *throw* something—for example, a life buoy or a throw bag (a small sack containing two ropes and a piece of foam). In an emergency situation, a rescuer opens the bag, pulls out enough rope to grasp firmly (some rescuers prefer to wrap the rope around their backs), and then throws the bag to the victim. The victim should be instructed to grab the

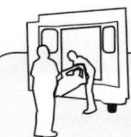

In the Field

Personal flotation devices (PFDs) that are not worn are not helpful!

rope and not the bag, because the bag may contain more rope that can uncoil.

- If you can't reach the person by throwing something that floats, you may be able to *row* out to the drowning person if a small boat or canoe is available. Do so only if you know how to operate or propel the craft properly. Protect yourself by wearing an approved PFD.
- As a last resort, *go* into the water to save the victim. Enter the water only if you are a capable swimmer trained in lifesaving techniques. Remove encumbering clothing before doing so, and take a flotation device with you if one is available.

Many departments in colder regions have developed specialized equipment to assist in ice rescues. Throwing a rope or flotation device may be helpful initially. Ladders can be used to distribute the weight of the rescuer on ice-covered water. Specially designed hose lines have been used with end-caps and an air line to create a flotation buoy. Special rescue suits are available to prevent hypothermia and provide flotation for the rescuer. If your department is involved in ice rescues, you should receive training in these specialized procedures.

Recovery Situations

On occasion, you may be called to the scene of a drowning and find that the patient is not floating or visible in the water. An organized rescue effort in these circumstances calls for personnel who are experienced with recovery techniques and equipment, including snorkels, masks, and scuba gear. As a last resort, when standard procedures for recovery are unsuccessful, you may have to use a grappling hook or large hook to drag the bottom for the victim. Although the hook could seriously wound the patient, it may be the only effective way to bring him or her to the surface for resuscitative efforts.

Spinal Incidents in Submersion Incidents

Submersion incidents may be complicated by spinal fractures and spinal cord injuries. You must assume that spinal injury exists with the following conditions:

- The submersion has resulted from a diving mishap or fall.
- The patient is unconscious, and no information is available to rule out the possibility of a mechanism causing neck injury.
- The patient is conscious but complains of weakness, paralysis, or numbness in the arms or legs.
- You suspect the possibility of spinal injury despite what witnesses say.

Most spinal injuries in diving incidents affect the cervical spine. When spinal injury is suspected, the neck must be protected from further injury. This means that you will have to sta-

bilize the suspected injury while the patient is still in the water. Follow the steps in ▶ Skill Drill 49-2 ▶ :

1. Turn the patient supine. Two rescuers are usually required to turn the patient safely, although in some cases one rescuer will suffice. Always rotate the entire upper half of the patient's body as a single unit. Twisting only the head, for example, may aggravate any injury to the cervical spine (Step 1).
2. Restore the airway and begin ventilation. Immediate ventilation is the primary treatment of all submersion patients as soon as the patient is face up in the water. Use a pocket mask if it is available. Have the other rescuer support the head and trunk as a unit while you open the airway and begin artificial ventilation (Step 2).
3. Float a buoyant backboard under the patient as you continue ventilation (Step 3).
4. Secure the trunk and head to the backboard to eliminate motion of the cervical spine. Do not remove the patient from the water until this is done (Step 4).
5. Remove the patient from the water, on the backboard (Step 5).
6. Cover the patient with a blanket. Give supplemental oxygen if the patient is breathing spontaneously. Begin CPR if there is no pulse. Effective cardiac compression or CPR is extremely difficult to perform when the patient is still in the water (Step 6).

Rope Rescue

Rope rescue skills are the most versatile and widely used technical rescue skills. Sometimes a rope rescue is performed to remove a person from a position of peril; at other times, rope rescues are needed to remove ill or injured persons—for example, from inside a tank.

Types of Rope Rescues

Rope rescue incidents are divided into low-angle and high-angle operations. <u>Low-angle operations</u> are situations where the slope of the ground over which the rescuers are working is less than 45°. In these cases, rescuers depend on the ground for their primary support, and the rope system serves as a secondary means of support. An example of a low-angle system is a rope stretched from the top of an embankment and used for support by rescuers who are carrying a patient up an incline.

Low-angle operations are used when the scene requires ropes to be used only as assistance to pull or haul up a patient or rescuer. They are usually necessary when adequate footing is not present, in areas such as a dirt or rock embankment. In

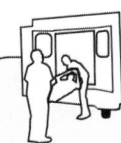

In the Field

There should be a minimum of six rescuers on the Stokes basket, and extra teams of six persons should be rotated when the patient needs to be carried a long distance.

Skill Drill 49-2: Stabilizing a Suspected Spinal Injury in the Water

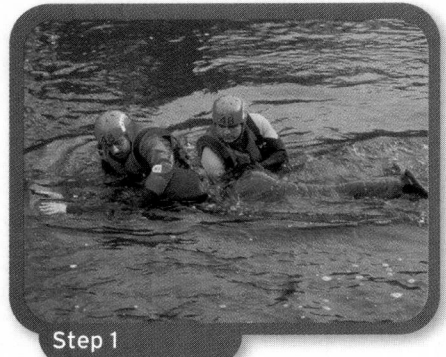

Step 1

Turn the patient to a supine position in the water by rotating the entire upper half of the body as a single unit.

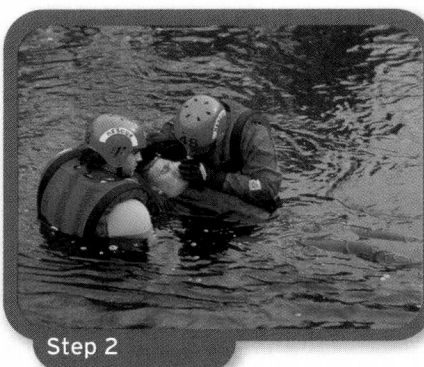

Step 2

As soon as the patient is turned, begin artificial ventilation using the mouth-to-mouth method or a pocket mask.

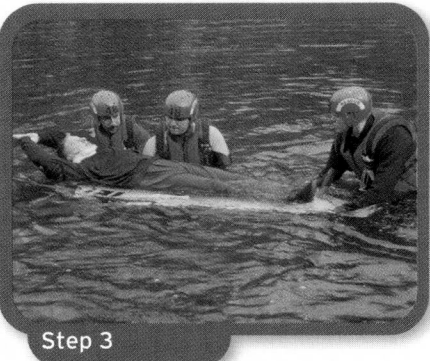

Step 3

Float a buoyant backboard under the patient.

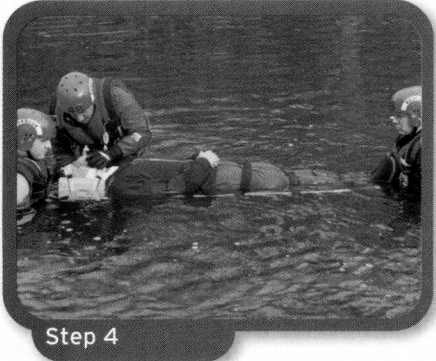

Step 4

Secure the patient to the backboard.

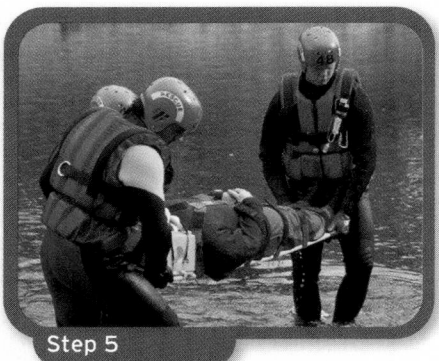

Step 5

Remove the patient from the water.

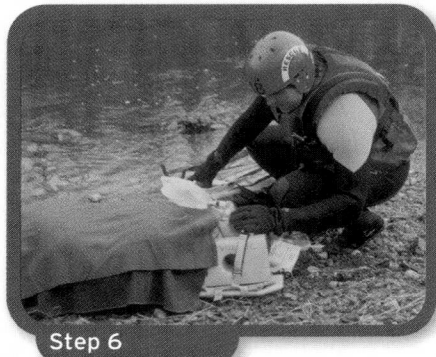

Step 6

Cover the patient with a blanket and apply oxygen if breathing. Begin CPR if breathing and a pulse are still absent.

such an incident, a rope will be tied to the rescuer's harness and the rescuer will climb the embankment by himself/herself, using the rope to keep from falling. Low-angle operations also include lifelines placed during ice or water rescues.

Ropes can also be used to assist in raising or lowering a Stokes basket. This technique frees the rescuers from having to carry all of the weight over rough terrain. Rescuers at the top of the embankment can help to pull up or lower the basket using a rope system.

When using any rope system to assist in rescue operations, a safety feature is to belay the rope. Belay in climbing is a technique of controlling the rope as it's fed out to the climbers. A critical part of the climbing system, it can be accomplished with a self-belay or a secondary lifeline. The use of belay systems has become a controversial issue in rescue, and their benefits are being researched. One potential complication is that belays depend on the angle of operations; as a consequence, the entire load may be transferred to the belay line. This could prove dangerous depending on the load and the length of rope.

Another aspect of climbing or rescue situations is the act of descending. In some descents, the angle is so severe that a technique known as rappelling is performed. To rappel is to descend on a fixed rope. Scrambling is a method used to ascend rocky faces and ridges and can be considered a cross between hill climbing (where an individual walks up a steep incline using both hands and feet) and rock climbing.

A hasty rope slide is a self-escape procedure when there is no other means of egress. This kind of semicontrolled fall without a descent device should not be attempted without proper training. The rope is wrapped around the back and under the arms or placed between the feet to provide resistance for slowing the rate of descent. Gloved hands are also effective for slowing the descent rate.

High-angle operations are situations where the slope of the ground is greater than 45°, and rescuers or patients are dependent on a life safety rope and not a fixed surface of support such as the ground. High-angle rescue techniques are used to raise or lower a person when other means of raising or lowering are not readily available. These rescues are extremely demanding and dangerous, and they should be attempted only by personnel who are thoroughly trained in proper procedure.

Safe Approach

If you respond to an incident that may require a rope rescue operation, consider both your safety and the safety of those around you. Rope rescues are among the most time-consuming calls that you will encounter. Extensive setup is necessary, and a considerable amount of equipment needs to be assembled prior to initiating any rescue. Protect your safety by remaining away from the area under the patient and away from any loose materials that might potentially fall. Work to control the scene so that bystanders move to an area where they will not be injured.

Wilderness Search and Rescue

Wilderness search and rescue (SAR) is an activity that is conducted by a limited number of departments. SAR missions consist of two parts: search (looking for a lost or overdue person) and rescue (removing a patient from a hostile environment).

Several types of situations may result in the initiation of SAR missions. Small children may wander off and be unable to find their way back to a known place. Older adults who are suffering from Alzheimer's disease may fail to remember where they're going and become lost. People who are hiking, hunting, or participating in other wilderness activities may become lost because they lack the proper training or equipment, because the weather changes unexpectedly, or if they become sick or injured.

Safe Approach

"Wilderness" can include many different environments, such as forests, mountains, deserts, natural parks, animal refuges, and rain forests. Depending on the terrain and environmental factors, the wilderness can be as little as a few minutes into the backcountry or a few feet off the roadway. Despite the short access time, the scene could require an extended evacuation and thus qualify as a wilderness incident. Examples of wilderness terrains include cliffs, steep slopes, rivers, streams, valleys, mountainsides, and beaches. Terrain hazards include cliffs, caves, wells, mines, avalanches, and rock slides.

When you participate in SAR missions, prepare for the weather conditions by bringing suitable clothing. Make sure that you don't exceed your physical limitations, and don't get in situations that are beyond your ability to handle in the wilderness. Call for a special wilderness rescue team, depending on the situation and your local protocols.

Using a Litter

Litters facilitate moving patients to a place of safety and can be used in a variety of situations. The manner in which a patient is packaged in a litter depends on his or her medical condition, the environment, and the manner in which the patient will be evacuated. Litters can be lifted by rope, carried by vehicles, or, most commonly, hand-carried by rescuers. In case of vertical evacuation, pack excess gear around the patient to prevent undue movement. While handling the patient, be sure to communicate and keep him or her apprised of the situation and your progress.

The standard litter carry involves a team of six to eight rescuers distributed around the litter, three or four to a side. Normally, the person at the front of the left side is in charge and directs the activities of the others. This method has the advantages of being fast, as little teamwork is required, and it usually gives the patient a comfortable ride. Its disadvantages include the fact that this carrying method is very tiring for the handlers, because it puts constant strain on certain muscles, and ground vision is difficult, especially at night; a handler can easily trip over a rock and drop the litter.

More than one team will be needed if the litter must be carried over a distance further than the team can cover in about 15 to 20 minutes. Team *leapfrogging* is a good method to use on long evacuations, ie, one team takes the litter for a given distance while the other team goes ahead to rest and preplan the next stretch. At the pass-off point, the first team advances to the next point for rest and planning.

When footing is highly unstable, an obstacle prevents the litter team from progressing, or falling becomes a possible hazard, the caterpillar or lap pass is a useful option. When the litter reaches the obstacle, the team pauses while every extra person lines up on the route ahead of the difficult terrain or obstacles. The rescuers form two lines facing each other about the width of the litter apart and alternate (in other words, they aren't all opposite

You are the Provider Part 5

The engine company has been on scene for 45 minutes and just finished widening access to the cab of the truck when the rescue company arrives. They are now ready to begin the process of removing the dashboard. Earplugs are provided for both you and the patient to protect your hearing from the hydraulic tools that will be used. A yellow blanket is placed over the two of you to prevent injury from debris. The helicopter crew is waiting, ready to assist in extrication and packaging.

Prior to the start of the dashboard removal you were able to increase the patient's blood pressure to 114/66 mm Hg. Your main concerns are keeping him calm and being prepared for the potential decline in his status once the dashboard is lifted off of his pelvis. It requires an additional 35 minutes to remove the dashboard. As feared, once the pressure of the dashboard is relieved from your patient's pelvis, he becomes pale and loses consciousness. One of the helicopter medics is able to palpate a weak carotid pulse. The patient is quickly but carefully moved over to the stretcher for resuscitative care by the flight crew. He is immediately intubated and has a second large-bore IV line placed.

Upon arrival to the trauma center, the patient is found to have a shattered pelvis, bilateral femur fractures, and a small subdural hematoma. He is evaluated in the emergency department and then taken promptly to the operating room for stabilization of his pelvis and lower extremities, and evacuation of the subdural hematoma.

each other). They usually sit down and try to make themselves as stable as possible. When everyone is set, rescuers pass the litter down between the two lines. As the litter passes a person, he or she gets up and carefully but quickly moves around the line in the direction of travel, and gets set to pass the litter again. Done correctly, this technique provides a very stable and secure passage.

Patient Care

Many medical and trauma conditions can and will be assessed during the rescue process. In confined-space rescues, especially with cave-ins and trench rescues, EMS providers need to consider the potential for crush injuries—in particular, the possibility of compartment syndrome. When human tissue goes without an adequate supply of oxygen-enriched blood, tissue (cells) continues to metabolize (produce energy) without oxygen (anaerobic metabolism), producing lactic acid as a by-product. When entrapped or compressed areas of the body are eventually reperfused, these metabolic by-products are released into the circulation. Treatment with high-flow oxygen therapy or positive-pressure ventilations, along with administration of sodium bicarbonate, can help to reverse the effects of respiratory and metabolic acidosis.

Pain Management

Patients involved in many rescue situations will be experiencing pain from injuries received during the incident. Pain control should take the form of nonpharmacologic methods such as splinting to minimize movement, gentle handling, or talking with patients to create a distraction during assessment and movement. EMS providers must also keep patients warm, as a shivering patient will aggravate pain with his or her every movement.

Pharmacologic treatment in the prehospital setting remains controversial, and providers should consult with their medical directors on issues related to pain management. All medications are contraindicated in patients with a known hypersensitivity to the drug. **Table 49-1 ▶** lists some of the medications that can be considered in the pain management of patients during rescue efforts. Because most analgesics have the potential to

induce nausea and vomiting, all medications must be administered slowly and use of antiemetics should be considered.

Medical Supplies

Table 49-2 ▶ lists the basic medical supplies that you should carry in an off-road medical pack.

Patient Packaging

A number of special patient packaging tools are available to help you extricate patients out of their situation and up, down, or out to your ambulance. The Stokes basket, for example, is a rigid framed structure that the patient is set into and then secured. It comes in two general types. The most common is the wire Stokes basket, which consists of a rigid metal (aluminum, steel, or titanium) frame and ribs with a chicken-wire mesh attached to the frame. The other style is the plastic or fiberglass Stokes basket, which consists of a steel or aluminum frame with a rigid plastic or fiberglass basket. Both types of Stokes baskets are available as one- or two-piece units that can be latched or joined together for easier packing into the rescue scene.

Table 49-1	Medications for Pain Management in Rescue Situations
Medication	**Characteristics**
Morphine sulfate	Narcotic analgesic and central nervous system depressant often used in the treatment of myocardial infarction, kidney stones, and pulmonary edema. It is contraindicated in patients who are volume-depleted or suffering from severe hypotension.
Meperidine (Demerol)	Narcotic analgesic and central nervous system depressant primarily used for the treatment of moderate to severe pain. It is relatively contraindicated in patients with undiagnosed abdominal pain and head injuries.
Nitrous oxide (Nitronox, Entonox)	This central nervous system depressant with analgesic properties is used for musculoskeletal pain, fractures, and burns. It should not be used in patients who can't follow verbal instructions, those with head injuries, COPD patients, and patients with thoracic injuries or possible pneumothorax. Use caution in environments less than 21°F, which could make administration difficult to impossible.
Fentanyl citrate (Sublimaze)	Unrelated to morphine but with similar analgesic effects, it is considered 50 to 100 times more potent than morphine; however, its duration of action is much shorter. It can be used for rapid-sequence intubation and severe pain, but is contraindicated with severe hemorrhage, shock, or known hypersensitivity.
Butorphanol tartrate (Stadol)	This synthetic analgesic, with effects equal to a large dose of morphine, is indicated for the treatment of moderate to severe pain, but is contraindicated in patients with undiagnosed abdominal pain and head injuries.
Nalbuphine (Nubain)	Synthetic analgesic with the same effects as morphine. Nubain has the hemodynamic effects of morphine and is used in patients with moderate to severe pain. Like morphine, Nubain is contraindicated in patients with undiagnosed abdominal pain and head injuries.
Ketorolac (Toradol)	Classified as a nonsteroidal anti-inflammatory drug (NSAID), ketorolac has analgesic, anti-inflammatory, and antipyretic effects. It is considered in controlling moderate to severe pain. Its only true contraindication is in patients with a known hypersensitivity to the drug and patients with reported allergies to aspirin or NSAIDs.

Table 49-2	Supplies for an Off-Road Medical Pack
• Vinyl or latex gloves • Face masks • Hand sanitizer • Mouth-to-mask resuscitation device • 1 triangular bandage (cravat) • Universal trauma dressings • 4″ × 4″ and 5″ × 9″ sterile dressings • Roller gauze bandage • Gauze-adhesive strips • Occlusive dressing for sealing chest wounds • Adhesive tape • Blankets • Cold packs • Alcohol pads • 1 12-mL or larger syringe for irrigation of wounds	• 2 glucose or energy gel packets • Heat packs • Abdominal dressing • Survival blanket • Scissors • Irrigation fluid or wound cleansing soap • Goggles • SAM splint • Steri-strips • Cervical collars • Blood pressure cuff • Rapid immobilization straps • Pocket flashlight • Batteries

The wire Stokes basket is more suitable for water rescue and helicopter hoist situations, as the wire mesh allows water or air to easily pass through it. Given that water weighs 8.37 pounds per gallon, this is a significant weight reduction. In the case of moving air (eg, a helicopter's rotor downwash) or moving water, such a basket allows the fluid to pass through it rather than spinning or dragging in response to the air or hydraulic forces being exerted on it.

Unfortunately, a wire Stokes basket catches every bit of debris and hooks on most any obstruction or obstacle. Thus for most other types of evacuations, a plastic or fiberglass Stokes basket is the superior choice as it more easily slides over the top of surfaces such as snow or debris, or down ladders.

Both types of Stokes baskets have a litter wheel device that can be attached to the bottom to facilitate movement over trails and low-level debris/screen. Also, both devices have minimal (or no) belts or straps to secure the patient into the basket. Instead, a number of patient packaging systems may be used, including those featuring 5- to 6-mm cord or 1″ tubular webbing. Each packaging system relies on the same basic principle: securing the patient's pelvis, which is the fulcrum of the body, into the Stokes basket. Separate securing techniques are then deployed to secure the patient's legs and/or chest, or to lash/lace the patient's entire body into the Stokes basket.

One difficulty that may arise is packaging the patient with a fractured pelvis, as these techniques will cause such a patient an incredible amount of pain. Indeed, any sort of patient packaging that involves first anchoring the pelvis will result in a significant amount of patient "discomfort."

One highly effective solution to this problem is to secure the patient in a full-body vacuum mattress. Once the patient is adequately splinted and secured in this device, then the mattress is placed and secured inside the Stokes basket. Now the main attachment/focal point is the entire vacuum splint and not the patient's broken pelvis.

Another difficulty frequently encountered is the need to transport a spine-immobilized patient in a Stokes basket. Some devices have a leg divider portion for the lower extremities that prohibits use of a backboard. Also, most backboards are too wide and their rectangular shape will not readily fit inside a Stokes basket.

There are two solutions to this problem. The first is to place the patient in a Kendrick Extrication Device (KED) rather than a backboard and then secure them into the Stokes basket. The second is to hold the cervical spine, surround the patient with enough rescuers to lift/levitate the patient up while maintaining spinal immobilization, slide the Stokes basket underneath the patient, and then lower the patient back down into the Stokes basket. The patient may then be secured, with the Stokes basket serving as the spinal immobilization device.

Once the patient has been safely extricated or evacuated, you can reverse the process and lower/secure the patient to a backboard in preparation for transportation. This consideration is especially important in a multiple-patient rescue scenario, as most rescue services possess only one or, at best, several Stokes baskets but have multiple backboards. Don't let the ambulance crew drive off with your Stokes basket unless you have a replacement for it. The loss of a specialized litter can put a rescue team out of service or necessitate having to improvise with alternative patient packaging.

When packaging a patient into a Stokes basket, you need to consider all of his or her needs. If you have placed the patient on supplemental oxygen, then the portable oxygen tank (preferably an aluminum one) must be secured in the litter as well. Likewise, the oxygen tubing to the mask or cannula must be secured, as it might potentially catch on a piece of debris or inadvertently become entangled in the raising or lowering system.

The same holds true for IVs. You don't want to rely on a gravity-fed system if possible: The IV tubing is just waiting for an opportunity to hang up on something at best, or to hang up on something and rip your hard-earned IV out of the patient at worst. If the patient requires an IV, use a pressure infuser and secure the IV and tubing along with the patient prior to extrication/transportation.

Stokes baskets are poor insulators. Thus, when packaging the patient into the Stokes basket, you must also protect him or her from the elements. Keep the patient (and any IV lines) warm.

If you will be transporting a patient through or out of an area where falling debris such as rocks, ice, or building material is a factor, you'll want to package your patient with head and eye protection. This may be as simple as placing a rock helmet and goggles or other protective glasses on the patient, or as comprehensive as using a litter shield to protect the patient's head and neck.

Some tight or confined spaces are so narrow that they can't accommodate the passage of a Stokes basket. Your patient, however, may require spinal immobilization. In such a case, the solution is a KED or KED/SKED combination.

A KED is an excellent spinal immobilization device that captures the three planes of the spinal column (ie, the head, shoulders, and pelvis). This narrow-profile device was originally designed by an EMT for extrication of Formula One race-car drivers. You apply the KED to the patient and then rig it for raising or lowering as you would an uninjured patient—namely, by using a seat harness and applying a chest harness around the patient and the KED.

Another option is to place the patient in a KED and then secure both into a SKED device. A SKED litter is the classic example of a flexible, wrap-around litter. It's essentially a drag sheet made from heavy-duty polyethylene plastic that wraps around (cocoons) the patient with prerigged securing and attachment points. It's a great tool for sliding patients through narrow passageways and over rough surfaces.

Adaptability and improvisation are an essential part of EMS patient care practices. In rescue and extrication situations, the patient's needs, your resources, and the techniques used can change as the rescue process develops. Should you find yourself at a rescue situation without all the necessary equipment, you may have to use your ingenuity to improvise the tools needed to get the patient to safety. If necessary, you can always rely on the technique of splinting one body part to another, by attaching upper extremities to the torso and lower legs to each other. This is a very effective means of splinting when no other devices are available.

You are the Provider Summary

1. What are some examples of situations requiring special rescue teams?

Special rescue teams are trained in specific areas such as cave rescue, dive rescue, confined space rescue, trench rescue, swift water rescue, rope rescue, and wilderness rescue. Being a member of a special rescue team requires personal dedication to maintaining personal fitness as well as to numerous hours of rigorous training.

2. Identify the ten steps of a special rescue sequence.

The ten steps of a special rescue sequence are as follows: (1) preparation, (2) response, (3) arrival and size-up, (4) stabilization, (5) access, (6) disentanglement, (7) removal, (8) transport, (9) security of the scene and preparation for the next call, and (10) postincident analysis.

3. Why is it important to maintain good communication with the patient during a special rescue incident?

Patients need to know that you are there and that everything possible is being done to remove them from the situation and provide the necessary care. In our case, communication is easily maintained because you are able to be in the vehicle with the patient. This is not possible in all special rescue incidents. Occasionally the patient or patients must remain alone for several hours while the scene is made safe and access can be made. This is a traumatic time for the patient. A reassuring voice can go a long way to helping keep the patient calm and maintain his or her level of confidence.

4. What is the patient at risk of experiencing as a result of being pinned underneath the dashboard from the pelvis down?

The patient is at risk for experiencing crush syndrome. While his inability to feel his legs may be the result of a spinal cord injury, lack of perfusion can also produce loss of sensation to the areas distal to the source of obstruction, which in this case is the dashboard.

5. What needs to be monitored on this patient?

In a word, SHOCK! Currently he is compensating for the injuries we suspect; at the very minimum you can suspect an abdominal bleed and fractured pelvis. There is no way of knowing how long his body can compensate for the blood loss. Also keep in mind that the dashboard is acting as a tourniquet. You need to anticipate that once the dashboard is removed from the pelvis and blood flow is restored to the lower extremities, the blood pressure might change significantly.

Prep Kit

Ready for Review

- "Rescue" means to deliver from danger or imprisonment.
- The most difficult process in any rescue is neither the rescue nor the treatment process, but rather the coordination and balance of both.
- A technical rescue incident (TRI) is a complex rescue incident involving vehicles, water, trench collapse, confined spaces, or wilderness search and rescue that requires specially trained personnel and special equipment.
- Technical rescue training occurs on three levels: awareness, operations, and technician. Most of the training and education EMS providers receive is aimed at the awareness level, enabling them to identify the hazards and secure the scene to prevent additional people from becoming patients.
- When assisting rescue team members, the following guidelines will prove useful:
  - Be safe.
  - Follow orders.
  - Work as a team.
  - Think.
  - Follow the golden rule of public service.
- Although special rescue situations may take many different forms, all rescuers should follow ten steps to perform these rescues in a safe, effective, and efficient manner:
  - Preparation
  - Response
  - Arrival and size-up
  - Stabilization
  - Access
  - Disentanglement
  - Removal
  - Transport
  - Security of the scene and preparation for the next call
  - Postincident analysis
- At a TRI, it is critically important to slow down and properly evaluate the situation. Consider the potential general hazards and risks of utilities, confined spaces, and environmental conditions, as well as hazards that are immediately dangerous to life and health (IDLH).
- The first arriving officer at a rescue scene should immediately assume command and starts using the incident management system (IMS). This step is critically important because many TRIs will eventually become very complex and require a large number of assisting units.
- Accountability should be practiced at all emergencies, no matter how small.
- Whenever possible, park emergency vehicles in a manner that will ensure safety and not disrupt traffic any more than necessary. Traffic flow is the largest single hazard associated with any operation that takes place on a highway.
- A confined space is a location surrounded by a structure that isn't designed for continuous occupancy. Confined spaces have limited openings for entrance and exit.
- Confined spaces present a special hazard because they may have limited ventilation to provide for air circulation and exchange, which can make them an oxygen-deficient atmosphere, or they may contain poisonous gases.
- Trench rescues may become necessary when earth is removed for placement of a utility line or for other construction and the sides of the excavation collapse, trapping a worker.
- Because almost all EMS providers have the potential to be called to a water rescue situation, you should know how to properly don a personal flotation device as well as how to use the self-rescue position.
- Rope rescue incidents are divided into low-angle and high-angle operations.
  - Low-angle operations are situations where the slope of the ground over which the rescuers are working is less than 45°. Low-angle operations are used when the scene requires ropes to be used only as assistance to pull or haul up a patient or rescuer.
  - High-angle operations are situations where the slope of the ground is greater than 45°, and rescuers or patients are dependent on a life safety rope and not a fixed surface of support such as the ground.
- Wilderness search and rescue (SAR) missions consist of two parts: search (looking for a lost or overdue person) and rescue (removing a patient from a hostile environment).
- Litters facilitate moving patients to a place of safety and can be used in a variety of situations. The manner in which a patient is packaged in a litter depends on his or her medical condition, the environment, and the manner in which the patient will be evacuated.
- Pain control in rescue situations should take the form of nonpharmacologic methods such as splinting to minimize movement, and gentle handling. Pharmacologic treatment in the prehospital setting remains controversial, and providers should consult with their medical directors on issues related to pain management.
- A number of special patient packaging tools are available to help extricate patients out of their situation and up, down, or out to the ambulance. The Stokes basket is an example of a packaging tool.

Vital Vocabulary

accountability system A method of accounting for all personnel at an emergency incident and ensuring that only personnel with specific assignments are permitted to work within the various zones.

awareness The first level of rescue training provided to all responders, with an emphasis on recognizing the hazards, securing the scene, and calling for appropriate assistance. There is no actual use of rescue skills.

belay Technique of controlling the rope as it is fed out to climbers.

cold protective response Phenomenon associated with cold water immersion in which reflexes in the body and a lowered metabolic rate help preserve basic body functions.

cold zone A safe area for those agencies involved in the operations; the incident commander (IC), command post, EMS providers, and other support functions necessary to control the incident should be located in the cold zone.

confined space A space with limited or restricted access that is not meant for continuous occupancy, such as a manhole, well, or tank.

cribbing Short lengths of wood that are used to stabilize vehicles.

entrapment A condition in which a patient is trapped by debris, soil, or other material and is unable to extricate himself or herself.

hasty rope slide Self-escape procedure when there is no other means of egress.

high-angle operations A rope rescue operation where the angle of the slope is greater than 45°; rescuers depend on life safety rope rather than a fixed support surface such as the ground.

hot zone The area immediately surrounding an incident site that is directly dangerous to life and health. All personnel working in the hot zone must wear complete and appropriate protective clothing and equipment. Entry requires approval by the IC or a designated sector officer. Complete backup, rescue, and decontamination teams must be in place at the perimeter before operations begin.

immediately dangerous to life and health (IDLH) An atmospheric concentration of any toxic, corrosive, or asphyxiant substance that poses an immediate threat to life or could cause irreversible or delayed adverse health effects. There are three general IDLH atmospheres: toxic, flammable, and oxygen-deficient.

laminated windshield glass Type of window glazing that incorporates a sheeting material that stops the glass from breaking into shards.

low-angle operations A rope rescue operation on a mildly sloping surface (less than 45°) or flat land where rescuers are dependent on the ground for their primary support, and the rope system is a secondary means of support.

operations The technical rescue training level geared toward working in the warm zone of an incident. Training at this level allows responders to directly assist those conducting the rescue operation and to use certain rescue skills and procedures.

personal flotation device (PFD) Also commonly known as a life vest, a PFD allows the body to float in water.

rappelling To descend on a fixed rope.

scrambling A method used to ascend rocky faces and ridges and can be considered a cross between hill climbing and rock climbing.

search and rescue (SAR) The process of locating and removing a patient from the wilderness.

secondary collapse A collapse that occurs following the primary collapse. This can occur in trench, excavation, and structural collapses.

self-rescue position Position used in fast-moving water rescue situations. The rescuer rolls into a face-up arched position with the lower back higher than the feet to avoid objects below the surface. The feet should be together and facing in the direction of travel (feet first), with arms at the sides.

shoring A method of supporting a trench wall or building components such as walls, floors, or ceilings using either hydraulic, pneumatic, or wood shoring systems. Shoring is used to prevent collapse.

spoil pile The pile of dirt that has been removed from an excavation. The pile may be unstable and prone to collapse.

step blocks Specialized cribbing assemblies made out of wood or plastic blocks in a step configuration.

technician The training level that provides a high level of competency in the various disciplines of technical or hazardous materials rescue for rescuers who will be directly involved in the rescue operation itself.

technical rescue incident (TRI) A complex rescue incident involving vehicles or machinery, water or ice, rope techniques, a trench or excavation collapse, confined spaces, a structural collapse, wilderness search and rescue, or hazardous materials, and which requires specially trained personnel and special equipment.

technical rescue team A group of rescuers specially trained in the various disciplines of technical rescue.

tempered glass A type of safety glass that is heat-treated so that it will break into small pieces.

warm zone The area located between the hot zone and the cold zone at an incident. Decontamination stations are located in the warm zone.

wedges Used to snug loose cribbing.

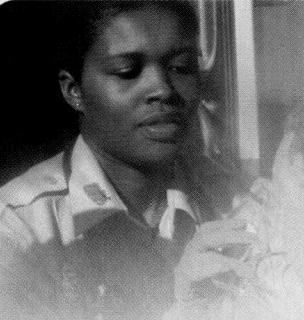

Assessment in Action

You are dispatched to the scene of a motor vehicle crash. Upon your arrival, you find a single-car motor vehicle crash involving one patient. You immediately notice parts of the vehicle that lie approximately 100′ away from the vehicle body. You safely and cautiously approach the vehicle, performing your mental scene size-up. The patient is heavily entrapped in the driver's seat of the vehicle. The truck company is preparing their jaws and other rescue equipment to extricate the patient from the vehicle. You notice the patient is gurgling and unconscious; you ask the incident commander approximately how long the extrication will take. They inform you that it will be at least 20 minutes due to the type of entrapment.

1. **At which three levels is training in technical rescue areas conducted?**
   A. Awareness, operations, training
   B. Awareness, technician, basic
   C. Awareness, operations, technician
   D. Awareness, basic level, advanced level

2. **Most of the training and education EMS providers receive is aimed at the _____ level.**
   A. basic
   B. operations
   C. technician
   D. awareness

3. **In a motor vehicle crash, what is the most important thing to remember?**
   A. The vehicle is to be removed from around the patient rather than trying to remove the patient through the wreckage.
   B. The patient is to be removed through the wreckage rather than trying to remove the vehicle from around the patient.
   C. You need to remove the patient immediately without any securing of the vehicle or scene size-up.
   D. Allow the family of the patient to climb into the car and be with the patient to calm him or her.

4. **The rescue operations commander informs you that the vehicle's A post has been crushed onto the patient's upper torso. You understand the A post to be:**
   A. between the front and rear doors of a vehicle.
   B. between the rear doors of the vehicle and the trunk.
   C. near the front bumper.
   D. closest to the front of the vehicle—it forms the sides of the windshield.

5. **You notice that the vehicle remains unstable and could pose a threat to the rescuers. What type of objects can be used to help support this vehicle?**
   A. Cribbing, wedges, or step blocks
   B. Cutting the battery cable
   C. Deflating the tires
   D. Removing the key from the ignition

6. **The next step after the extrication is completed is to:**
   A. perform patient care.
   B. disentangle the patient.
   C. displace the seat.
   D. remove the windshield.

Challenging Question

You are dispatched to the scene of a 25-year-old man who fell into a lake. The patient had been drinking alcohol heavily throughout the course of the day. The water is extremely cold, and the patient begins to panic.

7. **What should you do?**

Points to Ponder

Toward the end of your shift, you're dispatched to a residential area for a construction worker who fell into a pit. When you arrive on scene, you find a 30-year-old man lying in a prone position at the bottom of a dirt hole, which is about 10´ deep and 8´ wide. The fire department is shoring up the hole to allow you access to the patient.

You are told by his supervisors that the patient was climbing up a ladder while carrying a bucket; he slipped on the ladder and fell. His supervisor tells you that the patient initially was not responsive and stayed that way for approximately 2 minutes. The patient is verbally responsive now, and complains of back and head pain.

What PPE should you don?

Issues: Understanding What Your Needs Are at the Scene of a Technical Rescue Incident; Knowing What Information You Should Have at Initial Dispatch, En Route, and Arriving on Scene; Understanding the Importance of Scene Size-up.

50 Hazardous Materials Incidents

Objectives

Cognitive

8-4.1 Explain the role of the paramedic/EMS responder in terms of the following:
1. Incident size-up
2. Assessment of toxicologic risk
3. Appropriate decontamination methods
4. Treatment of semi-decontaminated patients
5. Transportation of semi-decontaminated patients (p 50.6, 50.13–50.16)

8-4.2 Size-up a hazardous materials (haz-mat) incident and determine the following:
1. Potential hazards to the rescuers, public and environment
2. Potential risk of primary contamination to patients
3. Potential risk of secondary contamination to rescuers (p 50.6)

8-4.3 Identify resources for substance identification, decontamination and treatment information including the following:
1. Poison control center
2. Medical control
3. Material safety data sheets (MSDS)
4. Reference textbooks
5. Computer databases (CAMEO)
6. CHEMTREC
7. Technical specialists
8. Agency for toxic substances and disease registry (p 50.6–50.8, 50.15)

8-4.4 Explain the following terms/concepts:
1. Primary contamination risk
2. Secondary contamination risk (p 50.11)

8-4.5 List and describe the following routes of exposure:
1. Topical
2. Respiratory
3. Gastrointestinal
4. Parenteral (p 50.11, 50.12)

8-4.6 Explain the following toxicologic principles:
1. Acute and delayed toxicity
2. Route of exposure
3. Local versus systemic effects
4. Dose response
5. Synergistic effects (p 50.11, 50.12)

8-4.7 Explain how the substance and route of contamination alters triage and decontamination methods. (p 50.13)

8-4.8 Explain the limitations of field decontamination procedures. (p 50.16)

8-4.9 Explain the use and limitations of personal protective equipment (PPE) in hazardous material situations. (p 50.10)

8-4.10 List and explain the common signs, symptoms, and treatment for the following substances:
1. Corrosives (acids/alkalis)
2. Pulmonary irritants (ammonia/chlorine)
3. Pesticides (carbamates/organophosphates)
4. Chemical asphyxiants (cyanide/carbon monoxide)
5. Hydrocarbon solvents (xylene, methlyene chloride) (p 50.15)

8-4.11 Explain the potential risk associated with invasive procedures performed on contaminated patients. (p 50.15)

8-4.12 Given a contaminated patient determine the level of decontamination necessary and:
1. Level of rescuer PPE
2. Decontamination methods
3. Treatment
4. Transportation and patient isolation techniques (p 50.13–50.16)

8-4.13 Identify local facilities and resources capable of treating patients exposed to hazardous materials. (p 50.15)

8-4.14 Determine the hazards present to the patient and paramedic given an incident involving hazardous materials. (p 50.16)

8-4.15 Define the following and explain their importance to the risk assessment process:
1. Boiling point
2. Flammable/explosive limits
3. Flash point
4. Ignition temperature
5. Specific gravity
6. Vapor density
7. Vapor pressure
8. Water solubility
9. Alpha radiation
10. Beta radiation
11. Gamma radiation (p 50.12, 50.13, 48.19)

8-4.16 Define the toxicologic terms and their use in the risk assessment process:
1. Threshold limit value (TLV)
2. Lethal concentration and doses (LD)
3. Parts per million/billion (ppm/ppb)
4. Immediately dangerous to life and health (IDLH)
5. Permissible exposure limit (PEL)
6. Short term exposure limit (TLV-STEL)
7. Ceiling level (TLV-C) (p 50.13)

8-4.17 Given a specific hazardous material be able to do the following:
1. Research the appropriate information about its physical and chemical characteristics and hazards
2. Suggest the appropriate medical response
3. Determine risk of secondary contamination (p 50.5, 50.10)

8-4.18 Determine the factors which determine where and when to treat a patient to include:
1. Substance toxicity
2. Patient condition
3. Availability of decontamination (p 50.12, 50.13)
8-4.19 Determine the appropriate level of PPE to include:
1. Types, application, use, and limitations
2. Use of chemical compatibility chart (p 50.10)
8-4.20 Explain decontamination procedures when functioning in the following modes:
1. Critical patient rapid two step decontamination process
2. Non-critical patient eight step decontamination process (p 50.13–50.15)
8-4.21 Explain specific decontamination procedures. (p 50.13–50.15)
8-4.22 Explain the four most common decontamination solutions used to include:
1. Water
2. Water and tincture of green soap
3. Isopropyl alcohol
4. Vegetable oil (p 50.13)
8-4.23 Identify the areas of the body difficult to decontaminate to include:
1. Scalp/hair
2. Ears/ear canals/nostrils
3. Axilla
4. Finger nails
5. Navel
6. Groin/buttocks/genitalia
7. Behind knees
8. Between toes, toe nails (p 50.14)
8-4.24 Explain the medical monitoring procedures of hazardous material team members to be used both pre and post entry, to include:
1. Vital signs
2. Body weight
3. General health
4. Neurologic status
5. ECG (p 50.16)

8-4.25 Explain the factors which influence the heat stress of hazardous material team personnel to include:
1. Hydration
2. Physical fitness
3. Ambient temperature
4. Activity
5. Level of PPE
6. Duration of activity (p 50.16)
8-4.26 Explain the documentation necessary for Haz-Mat medical monitoring and rehabilitation operations.
1. The substance
2. The toxicity and danger of secondary contamination
3. Appropriate PPE and suit breakthrough time
4. Appropriate level of decontamination
5. Appropriate antidote and medical treatment
6. Transportation method (p 50.16)
8-4.27 Given a simulated hazardous substance, use reference material to determine the appropriate actions. (p 50.6)
8-4.28 Integrate the principles and practices of hazardous materials response in an effective manner to prevent and limit contamination, morbidity, and mortality. (p 50.9)

Affective

None

Psychomotor

8-4.29 Demonstrate the donning and doffing of appropriate PPE. (p 50.14)
8-4.30 Set up and demonstrate an emergency two step decontamination process. (p 50.14)
8-4.31 Set up and demonstrate an eight step decontamination process. (p 50.14, 50.15)

Introduction

One of the inevitable consequences of living in an industrialized world is the proliferation of hazardous materials. The products of our civilization require the manufacture, transport, storage, use, and disposal of thousands of potentially toxic substances. Approximately 15,000 hazardous materials releases occur each year, with the great majority of these being highway transportation incidents. In 2005, the United States had more than 500 serious hazardous materials incidents, causing 31 fatalities and more than 700 injuries.

This chapter will take a broad look at some of the special considerations involved in responding to incidents that may involve hazardous materials. It is not intended to be a comprehensive coverage of hazardous materials. The general rule for EMS personnel responding to industrial, highway, and many other types of incidents is to maintain a high index of suspicion and to stay away from the hazardous materials incident.

Laws and Regulations

Training requirements and standards are put forth by the Occupational Safety and Health Administration (OSHA) in CFR 1910.120, *Hazardous Waste Operations and Emergency Response Standard* along with the 2002 edition of *NFPA 473: Standard for Competencies for EMS Personnel Responding to Hazardous Materials Incidents* published by the National Fire Protection Association (NFPA). All EMS personnel should receive training to the basic Awareness Level and those more involved (working on medical monitoring or decontamination of the team) will need to be trained to the Operations or Technician Level.

With Awareness Level training, you may be the first to discover a hazardous materials release. Topics covered in the course include recognizing potential hazards, initiating protective measures for yourself and your community, and requesting additional response resources.

The Operations Level (EMS/HM Level I Responder) of training will allow you to perform defensive actions against the hazardous material. You can perform patient care activities in the cold zone (the command and support center) at an incident for patients who no longer present a significant risk of secondary contamination.

The Technician Level (EMS/HM Level II Responder) of training will allow you to perform patient care activities in the warm zone at a hazardous materials incident, working with patients who may still present a significant risk of secondary contamination. At this level, you should be able to coordinate activities at a hazardous materials incident and provide medical support for hazardous materials teams.

Federal, state, and local rules govern the use, storage, and transportation of hazardous materials. These regulations are designed to improve the public's right to know and to help protect workers and emergency responders as they try to protect the public. Paramedics should become familiar with the laws of the states and localities in which they serve.

You are the Provider Part 1

You and a member of ABC Ambulance Service are responding to a chemical spill at a semiconductor manufacturing plant. Dispatch reports that there is one patient who has been removed from the structure by the HazMat entry team. When you arrive, you notice that the zones have been set up and the patient is just entering the cold zone from the decontamination corridor. The patient is conscious, well oriented, and answering all questions appropriately, although she is in pain. The HazMat officer reports that a forklift inside the building collided with some shelving, causing it to fall. The shelving stored several different chemicals.

You are handed a stack of MSDS that were provided by the manufacturing facility. Among the chemicals you notice a variety of acids (including 70% hydrofluoric, 10% sulfuric, and 20% acetic acid), 50% sodium hydroxide, a solvent, and methylene chloride.

The patient was the driver of the forklift. She is a 35-year-old woman who is conscious and experiencing minor pain. Fire department personnel on-scene currently are assisting ventilations with high-flow supplemental oxygen by nonrebreathing mask at 15 L/min.

Initial Assessment	Recording Time: 0 Minutes
Appearance	Entering the "cold zone" by fire personnel on-scene
Level of consciousness	A (Alert to person, place, and day)
Airway	Patent
Breathing	Rapid, shallow
Circulation	Slow, regular pulse; flushed skin

1. What is a hazardous material?
2. What is your role during a HazMat incident?
3. How would you manage this patient?

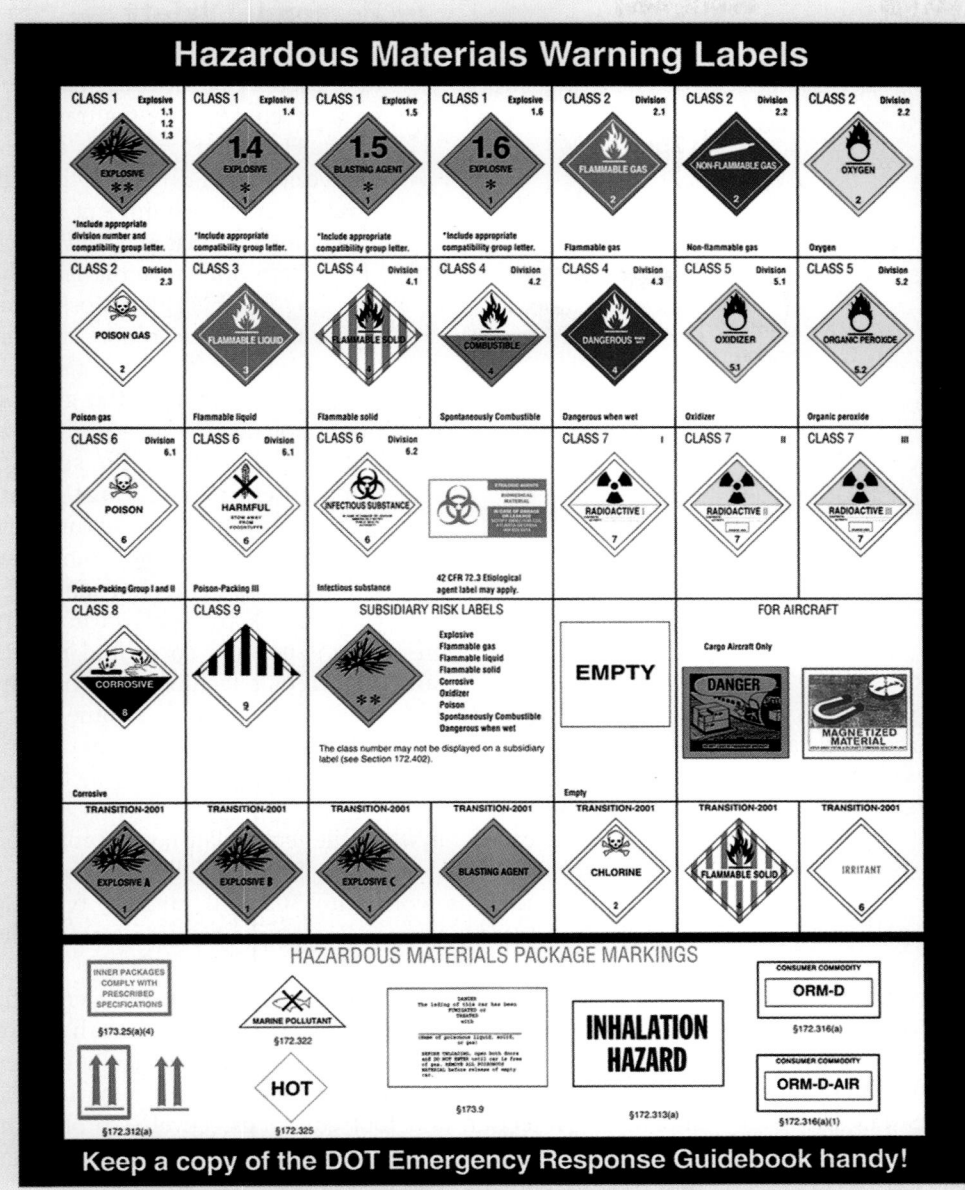

Figure 50-3 Hazardous materials warning labels.

treatment is provided. Both levels 1 and 2 are considered slightly hazardous but require use of self-contained breathing apparatus (SCBA) if you are going to come into contact with them. You would need training in using SCBA in a hazardous materials incident.

- **Level 3** includes materials that are extremely hazardous to health. Contact with these materials requires full protective gear so that none of your skin surface is exposed.
- **Level 4** includes materials that are so hazardous that minimal contact will cause death. For level 4 substances, you need specialized gear that is designed for protection against that particular hazard.

Table 50-1 ▼ further describes the four hazard classes.

Hazardous Materials Scene Management

To ensure efficiency and safety when responding to a potential hazardous materials incident, you should learn the concepts and principles of the National Incident Management System (NIMS) and the Incident Command System (ICS) discussed in Chapter 47. Hazardous materials incident management may seem laborious, slow, or cumbersome to you, but the potentially extreme hazards and the need to protect rescuers, other health care personnel, and the public from harm mandate a cautious approach.

Toxicity Level

Toxicity levels are measures of the health risk that a substance poses to someone who comes into contact with it. There are five toxicity levels: 0, 1, 2, 3, and 4. The higher the number, the greater the toxicity. Most ambulances are unlikely to have the specialized protective gear that would be required for dealing with any hazardous materials over Level 0.

- **Level 0** includes materials that would cause little, if any, health hazard if you came into contact with them. This is the only level that does not require special personal protection gear.
- **Level 1** includes materials that would cause irritation on contact but only mild residual injury, even without treatment.
- **Level 2** includes materials that could cause temporary damage or residual injury unless prompt medical

Table 50-1	Toxicity Levels of Hazardous Materials	
Level	**Health Hazard**	**Protection Needed**
0	Little or no hazard	None
1	Slightly hazardous	SCBA (level C suit, described below) only
2	Slightly hazardous	SCBA (level C suit) only
3	Extremely hazardous	Full protection, with no exposed skin (level A or B suit, described below)
4	Minimal exposure causes death	Special hazardous materials gear (level A suit)

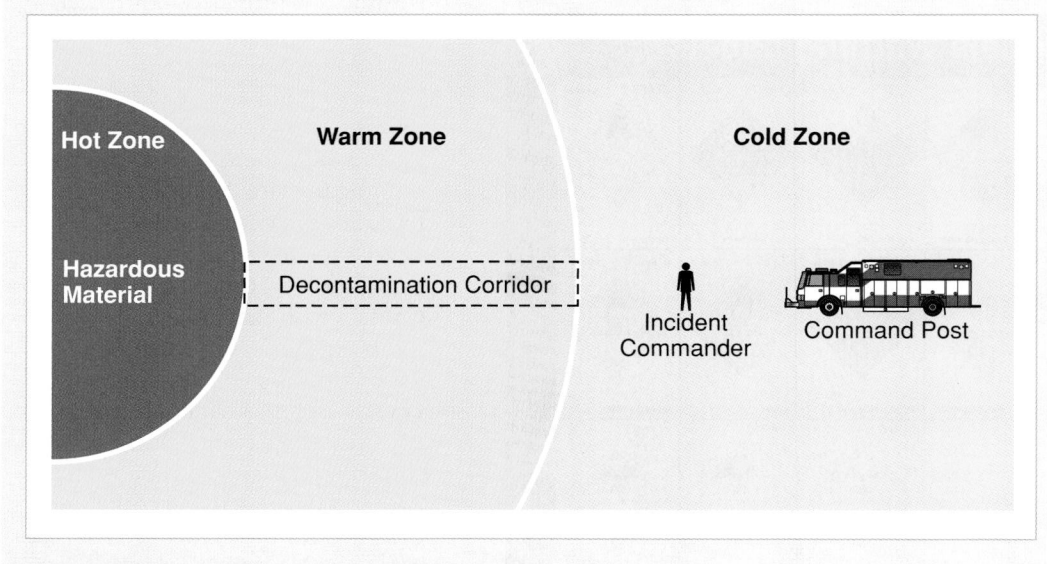

Figure 50-5 Hot, warm, and cold zones.

Establishing Safety Zones

If you discover that an ordinary ambulance call is really a hazardous materials incident, you must take the following steps:

- Notify your dispatcher and any other EMS, fire, or law enforcement responders that you can.
- Identify and tell the others what you observe about wind direction and terrain features.
- Approach and position yourself upwind and uphill from the scene.
- Keep in mind the rule of thumb (if you can't cover the scene with your thumb held at arm's length, you are too close to the hazardous material).
- Isolate the incident as much as possible to avoid the risk of further harm to other people—laypeople, EMS staff, fire fighters, and law enforcement. No one should risk life or health at a hazardous materials incident. The *Emergency Response Guidebook*, which you should carry in your vehicle, can help determine initial isolation distances.

As the hazardous materials incident progresses, hazardous materials specialists will establish several zones. Easy to remember, they're called the hot, warm, and cold zones. The hot zone is the contamination zone where only properly trained rescuers wearing appropriate personnel protective equipment (PPE) are allowed. The warm zone surrounds the hot zone. Typically the decontamination corridor is located in the warm zone. This zone should only be entered by trained hazardous materials specialists wearing appropriate PPE. Trained hazardous materials EMS workers may provide urgent life-saving care in the warm zone before patients are fully decontaminated. The cold zone provides a further buffer from the hazards present in the hot and warm zones. Paramedics normally perform triage and patient treatment in the cold zone **Figure 50-5 ▲** .

Personnel Safety

You should be familiar with the PPE used at hazardous materials scenes even if you are not trained to use it. Hazardous materials technicians call this PPE Level A through Level D, and the equipment is used depending on what and how much of the hazardous material is at the site **Figure 50-6 ▶** . Most paramedic ambulances do not carry this equipment.

Level A provides the greatest protection from exposure to hazardous substances. These suits look like an astronaut's suit because they are "fully encapsulating" **Figure 50-7 ▶** . Some hazardous materials technicians refer to Level A protection as fully encapsulating protection. These suits fully cover and protect the SCBA worn by hazardous materials technicians. The suits are rigorously tested by the manufacturers to determine resistance and permeability to many chemicals. Because they are so gas- and liquid-tight, you may be asked to monitor the technicians for heat stress.

Level B is called for when the technician needs protection from splashes and inhaled toxins. It is not fully encapsulating like Level A, and it is worn with SCBA. B suits are typically worn by the hazardous materials decontamination team in the warm zone.

Level C is designed to protect against a known agent. The equipment provides splash protection and is worn with an air-purifying respirator that must have filters specifically chosen to provide protection against the known agent. Offering eye and hand protection and foot coverings, Level C protection could be used during transport of patients with the potential of secondary contamination.

Level D is the level of PPE offered by fire fighters' turnout gear. It is typically not worn in hazardous materials incidents but may be used by some personnel in the cold zone.

The hazardous materials team should determine the appropriate PPE needed for a specific hazardous material. After identifying any hazardous material, the hazardous materials team will consult a permeability chart to determine breakthrough time for the fabrics the Level A suits are made of. The hazardous materials team will also determine which type of gloves and boots will be worn. The team might decide that a double or triple glove system is necessary for the incident.

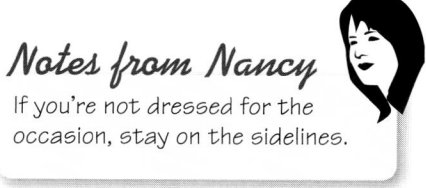

Notes from Nancy

If you're not dressed for the occasion, stay on the sidelines.

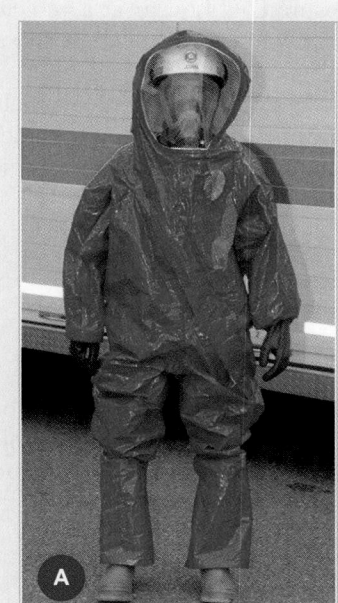 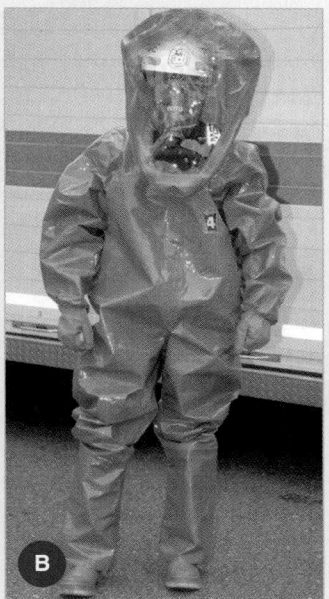 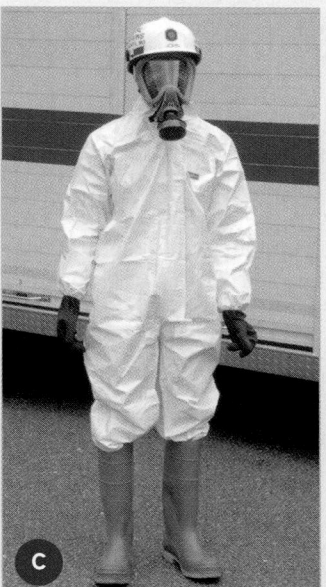 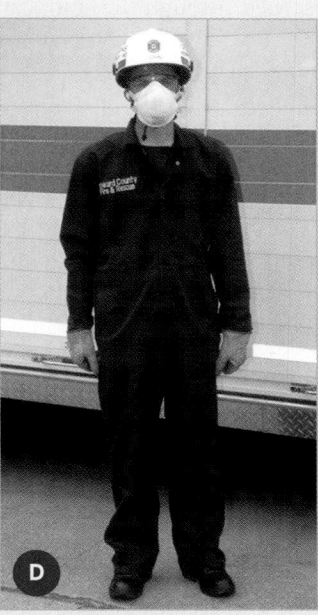

Figure 50-6 Four levels of protection. **A.** Level A protection. **B.** Level B protection. **C.** Level C protection. **D.** Level D protection.

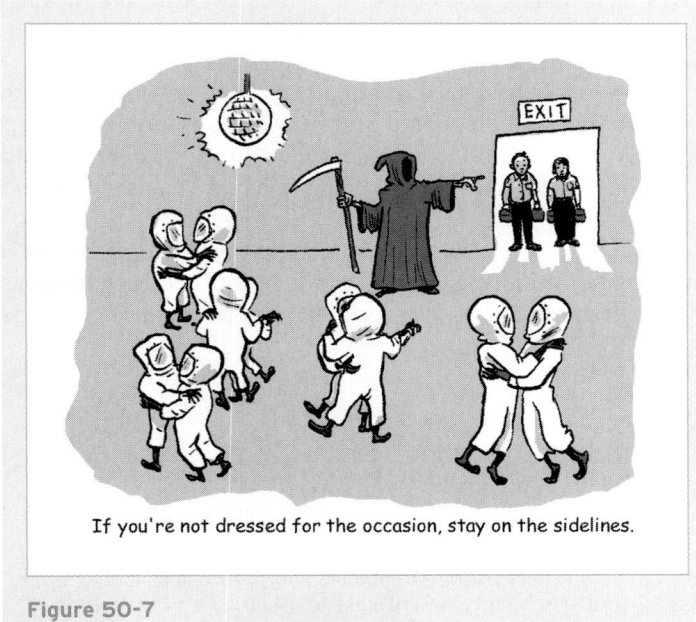

If you're not dressed for the occasion, stay on the sidelines.

Figure 50-7

Contamination and Toxicology

The dangers that hazardous materials present to the human body depend on the ability of the hazardous material to interfere with the body's processes. The bodily harm caused by a hazardous material is affected by the route of exposure, the dose and concentration, how long the toxin was in contact with the body, and whether it exhibits acute or delayed toxicity. If a patient has a chronic pre-existing condition, like a respiratory ailment, then a minor chlorine spill in an enclosed warehouse could prove to be more dangerous than would be expected.

Primary and Secondary Contamination

There are two basic types of contamination, primary and secondary. Primary contamination is the direct exposure of a patient to a hazardous material. Secondary contamination takes place when a hazardous material is transferred to a person from another person or from contaminated objects. Secondary contamination occurs when solids or liquids accumulate on a person, clothes, or an object, but doesn't normally occur with the diffusion of a toxic gas.

Routes of Exposure

The physical properties of hazardous materials and the physical surroundings at the hazardous materials spill can expose your patient in different ways. Air temperature, the concentration of the hazardous materials, and the amount of time that a patient is exposed will help you determine what your primary concern in treating your patient should be. If a material is not volatile and does not give off vapor but touches your patient's skin, it is called a dermal exposure. Many hazardous materials can be taken into other body systems through the skin. Skin conditions like abrasions may accelerate the absorption. Dermal exposure, also known as topical exposure, may result in only a local effect, such as reddening of the skin or the formation of blisters.

However, if the hazardous material is absorbed through the skin, a systemic effect may occur. Hazardous materials, when absorbed through the skin, can have a toxic effect on the neurologic, renal, or hepatic systems. These toxic effects may be seen immediately in the field, or may be delayed for hours or even years later with the appearance of a cancer. When the reaction shows up hours after your initial treatment, your careful medical records become invaluable to patients, who might not be able to speak for themselves. Your records should include a description of the scene, anything the hazardous materials team told you about what the toxin was, and how your patient looked initially.

Regardless of the route of exposure, the dose effect principle applies—the greater the length of time or the greater the concentration of the material, the greater the effect probably will be on the human body. For example, people who have a toxin briefly splashed on their skin will be exposed to a much lower dose of toxin than if they were lying in a puddle of that same toxin for 30 minutes. The cycle of poison action includes absorption into the body, delivery to target organs, and binding to the organs. The cycle continues with biotransformation and elimination of the toxin through the gastrointestinal, kidney, or respiratory systems. These concepts should be considered as decontamination decisions are made with the hazardous materials team.

In addition, paramedics should be aware that a synergistic effect may occur when two hazardous materials interact, producing a much greater impact than either substance alone. If your extrication patient is lying in a puddle of gasoline, his or her level of consciousness will be compounded if also exposed to carbon monoxide.

Respiratory exposure can be efficient, rapid, and lethal. Many hazardous gases, the gases formed when some liquids spill, or even dust-like powders can harm the respiratory membranes or be absorbed into the body by passing through the bronchial tree or alveoli directly into the bloodstream.

When hazardous materials are injected into the body or are absorbed through an open wound, this is known as par-enteral exposure. Parenteral exposure could occur at a vehicle collision if your patient has an open wound that is exposed to a toxin leaking from a container.

Gastrointestinal exposure occurs when your patient swallows a hazardous material like an organophosphate pesticide. You will need all your patient communication skills when assessing such a patient, because often the ingestion is deliberate.

Chemical and Toxicology Terminology

Learning some of the terms that describe the properties of hazardous materials and the toxicologic effects on people will help you as you work with others in handling a hazardous materials event.

Chemical Terms

When you are working at the scene of a hazardous materials event, you can often assess the scope of the problem by considering the physical properties of the toxin in relation to environmental factors. For example, if the liquid leaking from a tank has a high boiling point and the air temperature is low, then the paramedic will have less concern that the vapors of the liquid will be a respiratory hazard.

If vapors arise as a liquid turns to gas, it's important to know that as the air temperature becomes hotter, the vapor pressure of a hazardous material will also increase (as should your concern for more toxin being released to affect you and your patients).

Vapor density is another concept for figuring out where a gas or vapor might go. Vapor density compares the hazardous material gas to air (air has a vapor density of 1). If the toxic gas

You are the Provider Part 3

You monitor your patient's vital signs on the way to the hospital and note no further deterioration. You administer IV fluids at a KVO rate and monitor the ECG for further changes en route to the local trauma center.

On arrival at the trauma center, you and your partner provide a concise, complete report to the team, including the HazMat incident, your initial physical assessment, interventions, and the patient's response to your treatment. Patient care is assumed by the trauma team.

The patient is evaluated in the emergency department and found to have exposure to hydrofluoric acid and phenol.

Reassessment	Recording Time: 20 Minutes
Skin	Pink, warm, and dry
Pulse	100 beats/min, regular
Blood pressure	160/86 mm Hg
Respirations	30 breaths/min via nonrebreathing mask
Sao_2	100%
ECG	Sinus bradycardia with a first-degree heart block

7. What information about HazMat medical monitoring and rehabilitation operation must be documented?

is heavier than air, the toxin will sink into little valleys and ditches. But if the vapor rises and dissipates as it travels with the wind, then the vapor density is less than that of the air. This is why you are taught to approach a scene from upwind and uphill!

Of course, all bets are off if a fire is involved. If a hazardous material reaches a temperature at which its vapors can be ignited by a spark, then it has reached its flash point. If it gets warmer than the flash point, the vapors will burst into sustained burning; it has reached its ignition temperature. If the percentage concentration of the hazardous material as it mixes with air reaches its lower explosive limit (LEL), also known as lower flammable limit, then it can burn in the air (or explode). If the concentration of the hazardous material gets too high (or too "rich"), there will not be enough oxygen to support the combustion in air and the mixture has exceeded its upper explosive limit (UEL).

Hazardous materials teams can, in many cases, cool down the heat or dissipate the concentration of vapors by pouring on streams of cool water. However, before any water is applied, the hazardous materials team will make critical decisions about whether or not the material may be water reactive or water soluble. If they are going to use water, they will also determine the hazardous material's specific gravity—whether or not the hazardous material will sink or float in water.

Toxicology Terms

Chemistry experts and medical providers should communicate with each other using agreed-upon terms to describe the health hazards any incident might present. You will be a better reporter if you can master these terms for all the health care providers who will care for your patient in the hospital.

Safe and unsafe concentrations of various substances are often expressed in parts per billion (ppb) or parts per million (ppm). The threshold limit value (TLV) is the maximum concentration of a toxin that someone can be exposed to for a 40-hour work week. If you look up a chemical in a reference text and find that it has a very low ppb number for its TLV, this means it is more dangerous than if it had a high TLV. The threshold limit value short-term permissible limit (TLV-STEL) is the concentration that a person can be exposed to for a limited number of brief time periods (eg, four 15-minute exposures per day). The threshold limit value ceiling value (TLV-CL) is the concentration that a person should never be exposed to. A permissible exposure limit (PEL) is the maximum concentration of a chemical that a person may be exposed to under OSHA regulations. Sometimes you will hear the experts refer to the lethal dose or LD, which is the amount of the substance sure to cause death. You might hear the hazardous materials team refer to immediately dangerous to life and health (IDLH), which indicates that a respirator is mandatory. This means that the atmospheric concentration of any toxic, corrosive, or asphyxiant substance will pose an immediate threat to life, irreversible or delayed adverse effects, or serious interference for a team member's attempt to escape from the dangerous atmosphere.

Decontamination and Treatment

Treating hazardous materials patients can be a difficult and emotionally challenging experience. Remember, your safety comes first. *If you are first on the scene, you cannot immediately begin care.* Even when a patient is visible and in need of rescue, you must not rush in. Staying safe is a tough decision that requires discipline and emotional coolness. You must work as part of the team to prevent more casualties. Use the incident command system, which permits only properly trained and equipped hazardous materials personnel to enter the hot zone. Wait until your patients have been decontaminated. Then you can apply your knowledge and skills to actually treat the patient safely in a hands-on fashion.

Because hazardous materials can cause harmful effects, protecting the environment should be one of your considerations. If your patient's injuries are treated and not life-threatening, environmental issues should be a major consideration. You should take steps to prevent runoff during decontamination. If your patient is suffering, environmental considerations are still important but a lower priority than patient care.

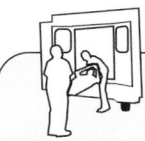

In the Field

Remember that no patient at a hazardous material incident is ever completely decontaminated. Always protect yourself first!

Decontamination

The team's approach to decontamination will depend on the type of hazardous material involved; the stability of the scene; and the number, condition, and location of patients. Decontamination is undertaken to reduce the dose of hazardous material in contact with the patient and decrease the risk of secondary contamination to others (including rescuers and hospital personnel). Protection of the environment during decontamination is important; plans should be made for containment of runoff.

There are four types of decontamination methods—dilution, absorption, neutralization, and disposal. Dilution uses copious amounts of water to flush the contaminant from the skin or eyes. This decreases the dose effect of the hazardous material on the patient. Sometimes a simple soap, such as tincture of green soap, is used in the decontamination process. Other decontamination agents are rarely used, however, isopropyl alcohol might be used to help with removal of isocyanates and vegetable oil is sometimes used if the contaminant is a water-reactive substance. Be cautious if you or any team member is using brushes; abrasion of a patient's skin increases the potential for hazardous material absorption.

Absorption is accomplished with large pads that the hazardous materials team carry to soak up liquid and remove it from the patient. Towels can also be used in the same way.

Neutralization involves the use of a chemical to change the hazardous material into less harmful substances. Neutralization is almost never used by hazardous materials teams because of the dangers of uncontrolled exothermic reactions. Disposal of as much clothing and equipment as possible to reduce the magnitude of the problem is another method of decontamination.

Emergency Decontamination in "Fast-Breaking" Situations

In some of the most difficult situations, you may be faced with the need to make an immediate decision about ambulatory patients who are approaching the ambulance, or who attempt to leave the scene to seek transportation despite being contaminated. In this case, you should provide patient assessment information to the incident commander, who is responsible for deciding whether to proceed with a rapid, emergency decontamination.

In such situations, you must still don appropriate PPE. Even if no respirator is available, the paramedic should take maximum barrier precautions. Put on turnouts or a splash-resistant (Tyvek) jumpsuit, eye protection, mask (such as a HEPA mask), and at least two layers of gloves. In addition, booties should be worn over footwear if possible. In general, nitrile gloves offer superior protection against many hazardous materials. Leather materials should be removed because these often absorb hazardous materials.

Once protected as much as possible, the paramedic should instruct patients to disrobe and remove as much of the hazardous materials from their bodies as they can. If you can, give the patients plastic bags in which they can place their personal belongings and clothing. If the hazardous material is a powder, then it should be brushed away first. If the hazardous material is water reactive, then no water should be used during decontamination. Most often, however, water is considered to be the universal decontamination solution. In any emergency decontamination method, you need to minimize the risk to yourself. This type of decontamination is also referred to as the two-step approach to decontamination. Unmanned hose streams can be set up by the fire department to douse patients with large amounts of water.

An example of such a set-up is the creation of an emergency decontamination corridor made by parking two fire engines parallel to each other and approximately 10 to 20 feet apart **Figure 50-8 ▶**. Nozzles can be attached to the side discharge ports of the engines and set to create a fine-particle fog-stream decontamination shower. Patients should disrobe on one end and enter the shower in single file. From a remote location, patients could be advised how to decontaminate and directed to pay special attention to the areas of the body that are difficult to rinse such as the axillae, between fingers and toes, around the groin, the scalp, and between the buttocks. Soap and soft brushes should be made available. At the other end of the shower corridor, towels, blankets, and temporary garments should be available. It is at the *end* of this corridor that you, the paramedic, would make initial contact with the

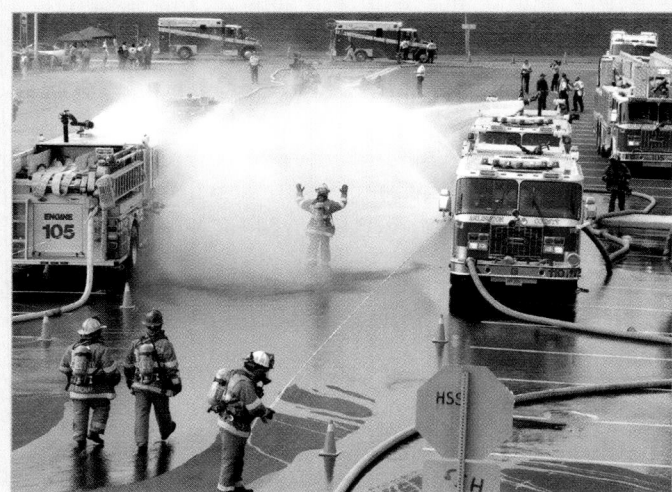

Figure 50-8 Emergency decontamination corridor.

patients and begin the triage process. Ideally, the runoff water from decontamination should be contained. At a minimum, the runoff should not be allowed to become a source of secondary contamination.

Technical Decontamination

You will hear the hazardous materials team refer to an "eight-step" process, which is only carried out by trained personnel.

1. Rescuers access the patients in the hot zone and remove as much of the contamination as possible as they move patients to the decontamination corridor.

2. Contaminated tools, equipment, and clothing should be left behind at the hot zone end of the decontamination corridor.

3. Patients and hazardous materials personnel are showered and washed using water, brushes, soap, or other appropriate decontamination agents to remove all surface contaminants. This is done with the assistance of other hazardous materials personnel who should wear not less than one step lower PPE than the entry team. This decontamination is done in a manner that will contain runoff. Often this is accomplished inside a small wading pool or other disposable basin. Any remaining clothing or jewelry is removed from the patients. At this point, the patients may be handed off to a separate decontamination team who should again wash the patients before they are handed off to medical personnel. Even at this point, the patients should not be considered fully decontaminated and paramedics should continue to wear PPE as they assess and treat the patients. Paramedics should stay alert for signs of an ongoing primary or potential secondary contamination problem.

4. Rescuers continue to decontaminate themselves. In this step, they remove their possibly contaminated SCBA.

5. Rescuers remove their contaminated protective clothing and equipment, placing these items into a bag or receptacle for later decontamination or disposal.

6. Depending on the potential of the situation, the rescuers may need to take off their clothing as well.

7. Personnel shower to further reduce the potential for contamination.

8. Entry team personnel undergo medical evaluation.

Treatment of Patients Exposed to Hazardous Materials

In general, the treatment of hazardous materials patients is straightforward. You can use many of the concepts learned in the chapters on burns and toxicology. There are some special considerations for hazardous materials patients, however. One of these is that invasive procedures should be minimized if possible. If you know from the hazardous materials team that your patient is contaminated, the process of endotracheal intubation may expose the patient to airway contamination. Placement of an IV may help contamination bypass the skin barrier. You will need to weigh the risks of invasive procedures against their benefits.

You should be familiar with references and how to access technical expertise when deciding how to treat patients from a hazardous materials incident. Some assistance may be obtained from the *Emergency Response Guidebook* and CHEMTREC. In addition, paramedics may consult with Poison Control Centers, the Agency for Toxic Substance Registry, and their local medical control. The hazardous materials team may have comprehensive reference textbooks that can guide the paramedic in treatment decisions and also be of assistance to emergency department physicians. Never forget that you are the eyes and ears of the physician in the field. Share the knowledge you've gained from the hazardous materials team for your patient's sake.

Corrosives: Acids and Bases

Corrosives are chemicals that include both acids and bases. Some examples are toilet bowl cleaner, lye, and hydrochloric acids. Acids have a low pH, while bases have a high pH. Agents with both high and low pH can cause severe burns. Signs and symptoms include skin irritation, reddening or other discoloration, and blistering. Exposure of fumes to mucous membranes can also cause burns, including severe life-threatening airway burns.

Decontamination of materials with a high pH will require considerably more time to flush from the skin. High pH materials have a soap-like resistance to being flushed from the skin as compared to low pH acids. Once the patient is decontaminated appropriately, treatment is symptomatic. Treat burns appropriately and consider transport to a burn center. Patients showing signs of pulmonary edema may need to be treated for this with furosemide, for example. However, paramedics should always consult medical control to determine the danger of a reaction between the drug and the contaminant.

Hydrocarbon Solvents

Many of these solvents give off potent vapors that can be inhaled and can also be absorbed through the skin. Respiratory exposure in particular can cause immediate pulmonary symptoms such as pulmonary edema. Prolonged dermal exposure can cause symptoms as well, including cardiac dysrhythmias and seizures.

Pulmonary Irritants

Many gases react with the moisture of mucous membranes to cause irritation ranging from minor to severe or choking. Examples of such gases are chlorine gas and ammonia. The first thing to do for your patients is to make sure they (and you as well) are away from the contamination and in fresh air. Removal of clothing may help dissipate trapped gases. Pulmonary edema should be treated according to protocols.

Pesticides

Exposure to organophosphate and carbamate pesticides can produce severe signs and symptoms. These hazardous materials interfere with the enzyme cholinesterase, which promotes uptake of the neurotransmitter acetylcholine. Runaway nerve stimulation produces a syndrome that is known by the mnemonic, SLUDGE (Salivation, Lacrimation, Urination, Gastrointestinal activity, and Emesis). Also look for excess pulmonary secretions. As always, paramedics should protect themselves from secondary contamination, including that from emesis when the exposure has been gastrointestinal. Treatment of organophosphate poisoning includes protection of the airway with possibly frequent suctioning, and the use of atropine to block the overstimulation of muscarinic receptors of the parasympathetic nervous system. The use of pralidoxime is recommended for organophosphate exposures but not for carbamates.

Chemical Asphyxiants

Any gas that displaces oxygen from the atmosphere is termed an asphyxiant. Colorless, odorless gases (eg, carbon monoxide and hydrogen sulfide) confined to an area may represent a deadly trap for would-be rescuers who rush in to help a collapsed victim. Substances known as chemical asphyxiants interfere with the utilization of oxygen at the cellular level; cyanide is a common example of such an agent. Hydrogen cyanide is used in many industrial processes. The release of cyanide in Bhopal, India, was a major hazardous materials incident that caused thousands of fatalities. Cyanide poisoning can also occur during exposure to the by-products of combustion at structure fires. Treatment of cyanide exposure begins with the use of amyl nitrite ampules that the patient should inhale for 15 seconds of every minute. This is followed by the IV administration of 300 mg of sodium nitrite, followed by 12.5 g of sodium thiosulfate. Another common exposure that results in a cellular respiratory failure is carbon monoxide. This gas ties up hemoglobin to the extent that oxygen in the blood becomes inaccessible to the cells. Treatment includes removal of the patient from the source and administration of 100% supplemental oxygen. Consider transport to a hospital with hyperbaric capability.

Transportation Considerations

The ideal transportation scenario at a hazardous materials incident would be to have a team of paramedics who were not involved with decontamination or cold zone patient treatment standing by to transport patients to the hospital emergency department. However, if the incident is a large one, the cold zone paramedics may well need to both treat and transport.

Paramedics should remember that patients received after field decontamination should not be assumed to be completely decontaminated. Accordingly, paramedics should take certain precautions to prepare themselves and their equipment for assuming care of the patient from the hazardous materials team and for getting the patient to the hospital. First, the paramedic should wear appropriate PPE. The hazardous materials team may be able to supply some of the PPE if the transporting paramedic does not have access to a splash-proof Tyvek jumpsuit, for example. The transporting paramedic should be given a complete report on what hazardous materials have been involved, what the patient's exposure has been, and what has been done to decontaminate and treat the patient. In no event should a transporting paramedic have to transport a patient if decontamination has not been sufficient for the driver to operate the ambulance. An example of insufficient decontamination would be when hazardous material on the patient continues to produce toxic gases.

Before receiving and transporting a patient exposed to hazardous material, the paramedic can do several things in preparation. One principle is to reduce the amount of supplies and equipment that the patient will come in contact with. You could remove the mattress from the stretcher because the patient will probably be carried on a backboard; removing the mattress will make later decontamination easier. In general, use as much disposal equipment as possible. Supplies and equipment inside the ambulance should be removed and set aside in a clean, safe place for later retrieval.

It is impractical and time-consuming to line the inside of the ambulance with plastic. Instead, plan to isolate the patient by wrapping him or her in a plastic barrier to reduce the potential for secondary contamination. A double-wrap procedure is preferable. In this procedure, the patient is first wrapped in a plastic blanket, preferably one that helps protect the patient from hypothermia. Then the patient is placed on a backboard and the backboard placed on the stretcher. Paramedics should know which hospitals in their area have facilities for receiving patients with possible hazardous materials contamination. The hospital should be given plenty of notice prior to the transport so that they can assemble the appropriately trained personnel and prepare equipment. Often hospitals will have a separate or dedicated treatment and decontamination room for these situations.

Medical Monitoring and Rehabilitation

You may be asked to assist with medical monitoring of the hazardous materials team. Rehabilitation (or "rehab") refers to the

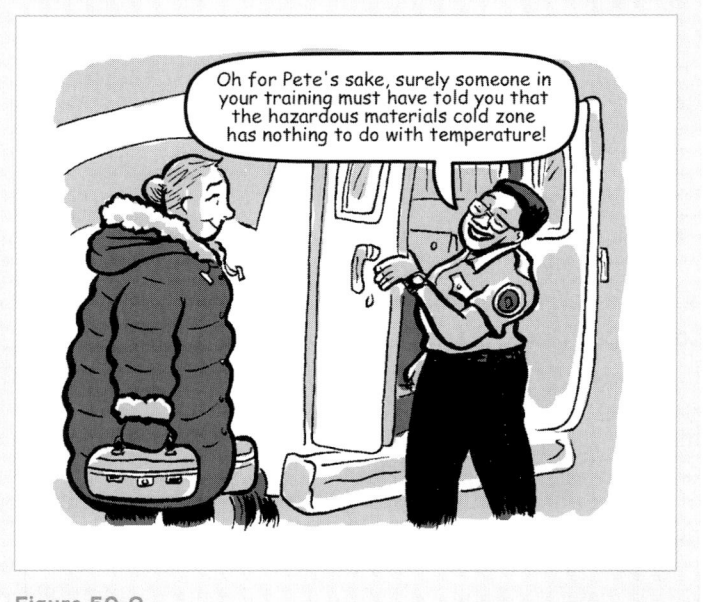

Figure 50-9

process through which hazardous materials entry teams are rested, rehydrated, and evaluated before being sent back into the hot zone. The PPE the team wears often causes heat stress, and of course the toxins the team is working with can cause serious health effects. Factors that influence hazardous materials team members' health include level of physical fitness, activity, level of PPE, and environment factors such as temperature.

Medical monitoring should include documentation of the incident factors including the hazardous materials involved, their toxic effects, what PPE was worn, its resistance to permeability with the hazardous materials, and what type of decontamination was used. You should have a plan for treatment, transport, and potential availability of antidotes in case a hazardous materials team member needs medical assistance.

You might be asked to assess hazardous materials team members before they suit up for entry into the hot zone and then again after they come out. Your assessment should include complete vital signs, as well as the ECG, temperature, and body weight. Team members should be encouraged to prehydrate with water or a sports drink. Working inside a Level A suit is like being inside a sauna, with no way to lose heat through evaporation, conduction, convection, or radiation. A useful fact that can help you with your assessment is that some hazardous materials teams keep a file of their members' baseline medical status. Be sure to ask for this information.

Before being allowed to re-enter the hot zone, the hazardous materials team should be evaluated by the paramedic in the rehab sector (located in the cold zone) for hydration status, vital signs, and any potential symptoms of exposure to the toxic agent the incident involves Figure 50-9 ▲ . Team members should take off their protective clothing and be given a chance to rest. Complete vital signs are again taken as well as other assessments, including neurologic assessment (eg, orientation to time, place, and events) as well as fine motor skills. Team members with elevated temperatures should be monitored closely for possible heat stroke. The loss of body weight is a direct correlation to the loss of fluids and the risk of dehydration and hypovolemia. Members should be encouraged to rehydrate by drinking water or other appropriate fluids. If there are abnormalities in vital signs or if the team member has signs or symptoms, they should not be allowed to return to work until their physical status returns to normal. An example of a hazardous materials team rehabilitation log that can assist paramedics in the hazardous materials rehab sector is shown in **Figure 50-10 ▸**.

HazMat Medical Monitoring Worksheet

Date:_____ Entry Person:_____

Incident #_____ Medical Monitor:_____

Important: HazMat team members shall not be allowed to don PPE if any of the following conditions are present: systolic BP < 100 or > 160, diastolic BP > 100, pulse rate > 120, oral temperature > 99.8°F, Respirations > 24. Medical monitors must read and be familiar with the "Medical Monitoring Guidelines" before beginning medical evaluations.

Pre-entry Evaluation
Before donning PPE, take and record baseline vital signs.

Time_____ BP_____ Pulse Rate_____ Resp._____ Oral Temp.____°F

Post-entry Evaluation
Immediately after doffing PPE, take vital signs and assess for hyperthermia.

Time_____ BP_____ Pulse Rate_____ Resp._____ Oral Temp.____°F

Re-entry Evaluation
Before redonning PPE, take vital signs and reassess for hyperthermia.
Entry person must remain in rehab for a minimum of 30 minutes between entries.

Time_____ BP_____ Pulse Rate_____ Resp._____ Oral Temp.____°F

HazMat Exposure Suspected?
Immediately contact HazMat Team Leader and see "HazMat Exposure Protocols."

Figure 50-10 Rehabilitation log.

You are the Provider Summary

1. What is a hazardous material?

The National Fire Protection Association (NFPA) 704 Hazardous Materials Classification defines a hazardous material (substance or waste) as: "Any substance that causes or may cause adverse effects on the health or safety of employees, the general public, or the environment; any biological agent and other disease-causing agent, or a waste or combination of wastes."

2. What is your role during a HazMat incident?

The role of EMS providers is to first keep themselves from being exposed or injured. Then a scene size-up is performed to assess for risks of primary or secondary contamination of the patient and the responders, determine the need for additional resources, and decide what safety parameters must be immediately established. Depending on the role your agency plays in local HazMat response plans and the level of training provided, you may also assess the level of decontamination, treatment, and transportation considerations.

3. How would you manage this patient?

Don the appropriate level PPE for the specific type of substance exposure. Then an initial assessment can be performed. If ambulatory, the patient should be instructed to remove all clothing and move to a predetermined decontamination center. Copious amounts of water are the decontamination solution of choice.

4. Evaluating the symptoms presented by this patient, what do you expect to be the primary offending chemical?

Phenol and hydrofluoric as well as sulfuric acids.

5. You have confirmed your diagnosis. Now how would you treat the patient? What supportive care would you use (include any drugs and dosages)?

- **Phenol.** Decontaminate initially with large volumes of water and then irrigate the burned area with mineral oil, olive oil, or isopropyl alcohol. Support respirations, control seizures, and manage ventricular ectopy with recognized means of treatment.
- **Bronchospasms secondary to toxic inhalation.** Immediately give 100% humidified oxygen. Issue an updraft of either metaproterenol (Alupent), albuterol (Proventil), or levalbuterol (Xopenex) by nebulizer. If wheezing continues, administer terbutaline (Brethine) 0.25 mL SQ.
- **Tachydysrhythmias.** Administer a 6-mg rapid IV push of adenosine (Adenocard) followed by a saline bolus.
- **Hydrofluoric acid.** Once the affected areas are decontaminated, the burned areas should be covered with calcium gluconate gel. If calcium gluconate is not available, Epsom salt (magnesium sulfate), magnesium-containing antacids such as Maalox or Mylanta, or Tums can be used as a topical agent.
  In the case of hydrofluoric acid burns, pain is an excellent indicator that the injury is continuing. If pain continues after calcium gluconate gel is applied, then calcium gluconate infiltration is needed. Calcium gluconate in a 5% solution is injected SQ in a volume of 0.5 mL every ¼″ into the burned area.
- **Cardiac symptoms of hypocalcemia.** Provide continuous monitoring of the ECG, watching for prolongation of the QT interval. Muscle contractions or cardiac arrest should be treated with an IV bolus of 5 mL 10% calcium chloride or 10 mL of 10% calcium gluconate. IV calcium should be considered for any patient with exposure to hydrofluoric acid in a concentration of greater than 10% over 5% or more of body surface area.

6. What resources can the EMS provider use to identify hazardous materials during the scene size-up?

There are several methods for identifying hazardous materials. Many EMS agencies are required to carry some form of reference to identify hazardous materials.

- *Emergency Response Guidebook:* Provides the names of substances, UN (United Nations) numbers, placard facsimiles, an emergency action guide, and evacuation and isolation information.
- NFPA 704 placard system: This is a fixed placard system used in many fixed facilities. The placards are colored and indicate specific hazards (red = fire hazard, blue = health hazard, and yellow = reactivity hazard).
- UN numbers and DOT placards: Placarding vehicles is required by law, but many owners do not comply.
- MSDS: Material Safety Data Sheets (MSDS) provide detailed information about a substance and are used when exposure occurs with that product. MSDS are used throughout the industry as a means of identifying chemicals and complying with employees' right to know. These must be readily available for employees to review.
- Packaging labels.
- Shipping papers: Carried by the shipper when transporting substances and contain the name of the product.
- Textbooks, handbooks.
- Dispatcher: When resources are not immediately available to the EMS provider, the dispatcher may be able to obtain information for you.
- Assistance from CHEMTREC (an information resource available through an 800 phone number with detailed information on the chemicals involved and their manufacturers).

7. What information about HazMat medical monitoring and rehabilitation operation must be documented?

The type of substance involved, its toxicity, and the danger of secondary contamination must be documented. Additional information to record includes appropriate PPE and suit break-through time, appropriate antidotes, medical treatment, and transportation method.

Prep Kit

■ Ready for Review

- Approximately 15,000 hazardous materials incidents occur each year.
- Handling hazardous materials emergencies requires specialized extra training and equipment.
- You should never enter a hazardous materials scene because specialized training and PPE are required.
- The three levels of hazardous materials training are: awareness, operations, and technician.
- Specific laws dictate that all paramedics should receive awareness level hazardous materials training.
- The great majority of hazardous materials emergencies are transportation incidents.
- When you are approaching transport incidents, especially those involving commercial vehicles, you should be alert for signs of hazardous materials.
- Signs of hazardous materials include vapor clouds, strange odors, spilled liquids, and multiple victims.
- Hazardous materials incident management follows NIMS and ICS principles.
- Hazardous material incidents have hot, warm, and cold zones.
- Without proper PPE, you should not enter the hot and warm zones.
- The four levels of hazardous materials PPE are level A, level B, level C, and level D.
- Sources of information about hazardous materials include placards, transport documents, and MSDS.
- Primary hazardous materials contamination comes from direct contact with the toxin.
- Secondary contamination is spread by people (patients, the hazardous materials team, or EMS providers), clothing, or objects.
- Effects from hazardous materials exposure may be local on the body or systemic.
- Routes of exposure include dermal, respiratory, parenteral, and gastrointestinal.
- Rescue and decontamination of victims is secondary to rescuer and public protection.
- Decontamination should be undertaken as a methodical eight-step process.
- In some situations, decontamination may have to be done rapidly in a two-step process.
- Treatment of hazardous materials victims is usually symptomatic and supportive of the ABCs.
- Invasive procedures should be minimized to avoid the risk of introducing contamination.
- Paramedics may be directed to support a hazardous materials operation with medical monitoring of the hazardous materials personnel.

■ Vital Vocabulary

absorption A type of decontamination that is done with large pads that the hazardous materials team carry to soak up liquid and remove it from the patient.

Agency for Toxic Substance Registry An information source for toxicologic effects of hazardous materials.

asphyxiant Any gas that displaces oxygen from the atmosphere; can be deadly if exposure occurs in a confined space.

Awareness Level The training level to which all EMS personnel should be trained; topics include recognizing potential hazards, initiating protective measures for yourself and your community, and requesting additional response resources.

bill of lading A document carried by drivers of commercial vehicles that should provide specific information about what is carried on the vehicle.

CAMEO Computer-Aided Management of Emergency Operations; a tool to help predict downwind concentrations of hazardous materials based on the input of environmental factors into a computer model.

carbon monoxide A chemical asphyxiant that results in a cellular respiratory failure; this gas ties up hemoglobin to the extent that oxygen in the blood becomes inaccessible to the cells.

chemical asphyxiants Substances that interfere with the utilization of oxygen at the cellular level.

CHEMTREC (Chemical Emergency Transportation Center) A resource available to emergency responders via telephone on a 24-hour basis.

cold zone The outermost zone of management at a hazardous materials scene; the area where paramedics typically first encounter the patient.

corrosives A class of chemicals with either high or low Ph levels. Exposure can cause severe soft-tissue damage.

cyanide A chemical asphyxiant used in many industrial processes; exposure can occur from by-products of combustion at structure fires.

decontamination The process of removing hazardous materials from the body or clothing of victims or rescuers. Includes the methods of dilution, absorption, disposal, and (in rare cases only) neutralization.

dermal exposure Skin exposure, also known as topical exposure. Some hazardous materials may be absorbed through the skin to produce a systemic effect.

dilution A type of decontamination method that uses copious amounts of water to flush the contaminant from the skin or eyes.

disposal A type of decontamination in which as much clothing and equipment as possible is disposed of to reduce the magnitude of the problem.

dose effect The principle that the longer a hazardous material is in contact with the body or the greater the concentration, the greater the effect will probably be.

Emergency Response Guidebook (ERG) A hazardous materials reference developed by the US Department of Transportation that provides valuable information about hazardous materials, isolation distances, etc; should be carried on every emergency response unit, and every paramedic should know how to use it.

flash point The temperature at which a vapor can be ignited by a spark.

gastrointestinal exposure Exposure to a hazardous material through intentional or unintentional swallowing of the substance.

hazardous material Any substance that is toxic, poisonous, radioactive, flammable, or explosive and causes injury or death with exposure.

hot zone The central area of a hazardous materials scene and the location of the greatest hazard.

ignition temperature The temperature at which a vapor will burst into sustained burning.

immediately dangerous to life and health (IDLH) A phrase that means the atmospheric concentration of any toxic, corrosive, or asphyxiant substance will pose an immediate threat to life, irreversible or delayed adverse effects, or serious interference for a team member attempting to escape from the dangerous atmosphere; a respirator is mandatory.

lethal dose (LD) Amount of a hazardous substance sure to cause death.

Level A The highest level of protective suit worn by hazardous materials personnel. Also referred to as fully encapsulating because the suit covers everything, including the breathing apparatus.

Level B PPE that is one step less protective than level A.

Level C A level of PPE that provides splash protection.

Level D The level of protection that fire fighter turnout gear provides.

local effect An effect of a hazardous material on the body that is limited to the area of contact.

lower explosive limit (LEL) The concentration of the hazardous material that can burn or explode in the air when it mixes with air.

Material Safety Data Sheets (MSDS) Information documents that are supposed to be kept on site at workplaces for every potentially hazardous chemical at the workplace.

medical monitoring The process of assessing the health status of hazardous materials team members before and after entry to a hazardous materials incident site.

neutralization A type of decontamination that uses one chemical to change the hazardous material into two less harmful substances; rarely used by hazardous materials teams.

Operations Level This training level, also called EMS/HM Level I Responder, allows providers to perform patient care activities in the cold zone (the command and support center) at an incident for patients who no longer present a significant risk of secondary contamination.

parenteral exposure Entry of a hazardous material into the bloodstream, either through force of injection or through an open wound.

permissible exposure limit (PEL) The maximum concentration of a chemical that a person may be exposed to under OSHA regulations.

ppb Parts per billion; an expression of concentration.

ppm Parts per million; an expression of concentration.

primary contamination An exposure that occurs with direct contact with the hazardous material.

respiratory exposure Exposure of the airways and lungs to a gas or vapor.

rule of thumb A reminder of the proper distance from a hazardous materials scene; the entire scene should be hidden by a thumb held at arm's length.

secondary contamination Exposure to a hazardous material by contact with a contaminated person or object.

SLUDGE An mnemonic that stands for salivation, lacrimation, urination, gastrointestinal activity, and emesis, which are the signs and symptoms that can be produced by exposure to organophosphate and carbamate pesticides or other nerve-stimulating agents.

specific gravity The measure that indicates whether or not a hazardous material will sink or float in water.

synergistic effect When two substances interact to produce an overall greater effect than either alone or combined.

systemic effect A physiologic effect on the entire body or one of the body's systems.

Technician Level This training level, also called EMS/HM Level II Responder, allows providers to perform patient care activities in the warm zone at a hazardous materials incident, working with patients who may still present a significant risk of secondary contamination.

threshold limit value (TLV) The concentration of a substance that is supposed to be safe for exposure no more than eight hours per day and forty hours per week.

threshold limit value ceiling level (TLV-CL) The concentration that a person should never be exposed to.

threshold limit value short-term exposure limit (TLV-STEL) The concentration of a substance that a worker can be exposed to for up to fifteen minutes but no more than four times per day with at least an hour between each exposure.

toxicity levels Measures of the risk that a hazardous material poses to the health of an individual who comes into contact with it.

upper explosive limit (UEL) The concentration of a hazardous material at which there is not enough oxygen to support the combustion in air.

vapor density A measure that compares the hazardous material gas to air; toxic gases that are heavier than air will sink, while vapors that are lighter than air will dissipate and travel with the wind.

vapor pressure The pressure exerted by a vapor when the liquid and vapor states of a material are in equilibrium; this measure changes as a material is heated.

warm zone The division of the HazMat scene that surrounds the hot zone and is inside the cold zone.

water reactive A property that indicates that a material will undergo a chemical reaction (for example, explosion) when mixed with water.

water soluble A property that indicates that a material can be dissolved in water.

waybill A cargo document kept by the conductor of a train.

www.Paramedic.EMSzone.com

Assessment in Action

You are dispatched to an overturned tractor trailer on a busy highway. When you arrive, you notice the truck is leaking something. You're not sure what it is. You immediately call for additional resources.

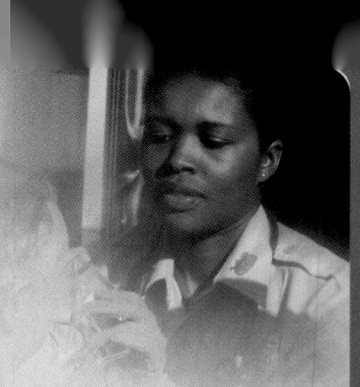

1. **On arrival, you see a placard with white and red stripes. This truck is most likely carrying:**
   A. oxidizers.
   B. flammable liquids.
   C. flammable solids.
   D. explosives.

2. **All EMS personnel should be trained to:**
   A. Technician Level.
   B. Operations Level.
   C. Hazard Level.
   D. Awareness Level.

3. **All of the following are responsibilities of hazardous material awareness-trained personnel, EXCEPT:**
   A. having knowledge of hazardous materials and risks involved in case of an accident.
   B. recognizing the need for additional resources.
   C. understanding the potential outcomes of a hazardous material incident.
   D. entering the hot zone and mitigating the incident.

4. **The standard rule of thumb for hazardous materials scene assessment is:**
   A. if the entire scene cannot be covered by your thumb held out at arm's length, then you are too close.
   B. approach should include stopping at a distance away.
   C. the identification of the hazardous material on scene.
   D. preparing the paramedic for the possible health risks.

5. **The guidebook that paramedics should have in their vehicle to help identify a hazardous material is the:**
   A. *Emergency Response Guidebook.*
   B. *Hazardous Material Textbook.*
   C. Material Safety Data Sheets.
   D. DOT truck placard chart.

6. **You should stay _____ from any hazardous material scene.**
   A. uphill and upwind
   B. downhill and downwind
   C. uphill and downwind
   D. upwind and downhill

7. **While on scene, to help get additional information regarding a specific chemical product, you may call:**
   A. CHEMTREC.
   B. FEMA.
   C. CDC.
   D. poison control.

8. **The measure of health risk that a substance poses to someone who comes into contact with it is called the:**
   A. health hazard.
   B. bill of lading.
   C. toxicity level.
   D. primary contamination.

9. **All concepts and principles of the _____ and the Incident Command System (ICS) should be applied to hazardous materials incidents.**
   A. National Incident Management Systems (NIMS)
   B. Federal Emergency Management Agency
   C. Secret Service
   D. Department of Transportation

10. **The type of personal protective equipment that provides the highest level of protection at a hazardous materials incident is known as:**
    A. Level A.
    B. Level B.
    C. Level C.
    D. Level D.

Challenging Questions

You are dispatched to a warehouse for three patients who are complaining of nausea, vomiting, diarrhea, and sweating. When you arrive on scene, you find the patients located outside on a bench. During your assessment, you note that the patients are also hypotensive and have constricted pupils. You begin to ask questions and you find out that this "warehouse" manufacturers pesticides.

11. **What should you immediately begin to suspect?**

12. **What treatment should you provide for these patients?**

■ Points to Ponder

You are dispatched to an explosion at an apartment complex. While you are en route, you see red balls of flames high in the air in the distance. When you arrive, several fire engines are already on scene. They are keeping you at a staging area until they figure out what happened and if any hazardous materials were involved.

What can you do while waiting for clearance? Once you can enter the scene, what precautions should you take?

Issues: Understanding What to Do at a Hazardous Materials Incident.

51 Crime Scene Awareness

Objectives

Cognitive

8-5.1 Explain how EMS providers are often mistaken for the police. (p 51.3)

8-5.2 Explain specific techniques for risk reduction when approaching the following types of routine EMS scenes:
 a. Highway encounters
 b. Violent street incidents
 c. Residences and "dark houses" (p 51.4, 51.7, 51.10)

8-5.3 Describe warning signs of potentially violent situations. (p 51.3)

8-5.4 Explain emergency evasive techniques for potentially violent situations, including:
 a. Threats of physical violence
 b. Firearms encounters
 c. Edged weapon encounters (p 51.7, 51.12)

8-5.5 Explain EMS considerations for the following types of violent or potentially violent situations:
 a. Gangs and gang violence
 b. Hostage/sniper situations
 c. Clandestine drug labs
 d. Domestic violence
 e. Emotionally disturbed people (p 37.12[e], 51.7–51.10)

8-5.6 Explain the following techniques:
 a. Field "contact and cover" procedures during assessment and care
 b. Evasive tactics
 c. Concealment techniques (p 51.11)

8-5.7 Describe police evidence considerations and techniques to assist in evidence preservation. (p 51.14)

Affective

None

Psychomotor

8-5.8 Demonstrate the following techniques:
 a. Field "contact and cover" procedures during assessment and care
 b. Evasive tactics
 c. Concealment techniques (p 51.11)

in preventing attacks with knives or other sharp objects. Again, the purpose of the distraction is to increase your chances of survival by giving you time to escape. The distraction does not have to be elaborate.

When something is coming at you, your initial instinct is to blink or flinch. Consider what happens when you are driving during a heavy rain and a passing vehicle throws water on your car's windshield. Even though you know the water is not going to hit you, you still blink or flinch when the water strikes the windshield. This is the reaction you want to provoke.

Throwing your patient care report pad at the person provides the same distraction as the water hitting the windshield. It interrupts the chain of events long enough to permit you to get out of the line of fire and run to safety.

Carry the clipboard in your left hand when you make an approach. Raise the pad to your left shoulder. If the patient takes aggressive action during your initial interview, be prepared to throw the pad directly at the aggressor's nose **Figure 51-21 ▶**. Use only a soft pad of paper for this technique. A hard object such as an aluminum report book or clipboard may cause needless injuries. The soft pad will not cause undue harm. If the person is reaching for a lighter instead of a weapon and you react by throwing the pad, you only have to apologize and explain. Explain that you have had calls during which the patient took aggressive action toward you, and you thought it was going to happen again.

After you throw the pad, do not wait for a reaction. As soon as it is out of your hand, turn toward your vehicle, get out of the possible line of fire, and run to safety.

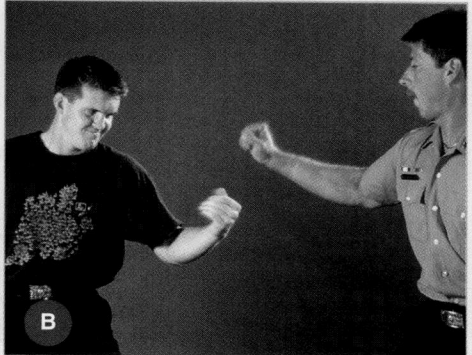

Figure 51-19 To break a hold, pull toward the thumb (**A**) and break the hold (**B**), turn, and run.

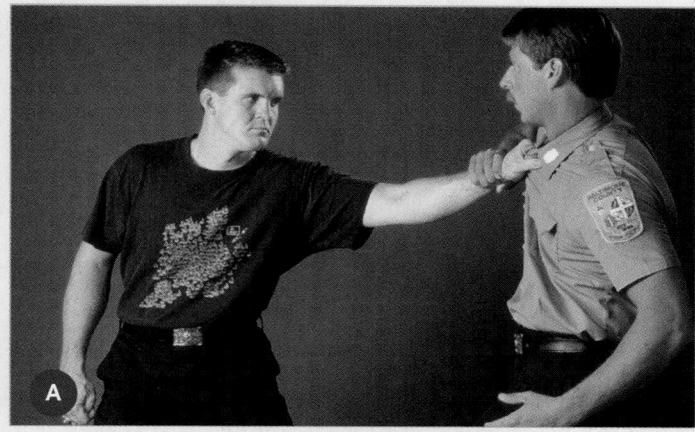

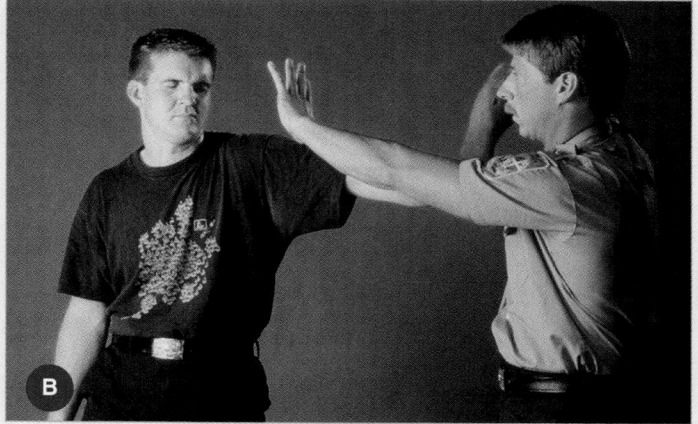

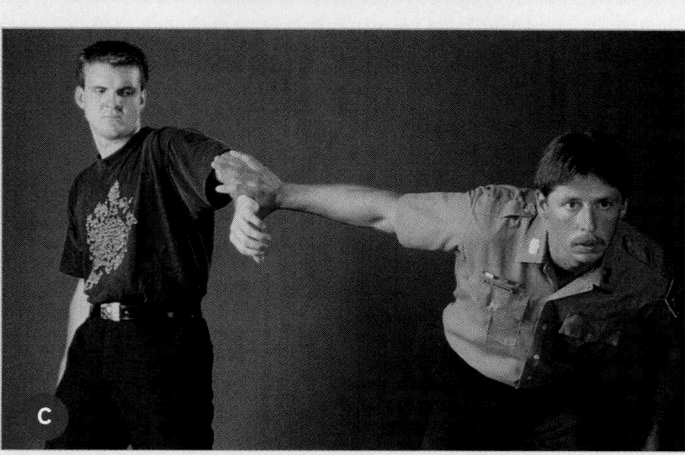

Figure 51-20 To break away from a person who has grabbed your shirt, do the following: **A.** Seize your attacker's hand and twist toward the thumb. **B.** Flash your free hand in the attacker's face, which will break the concentration long enough for you to escape. **C.** After you feel the grip relaxing on your shirt, twist your body away from your assailant and run to a safer area.

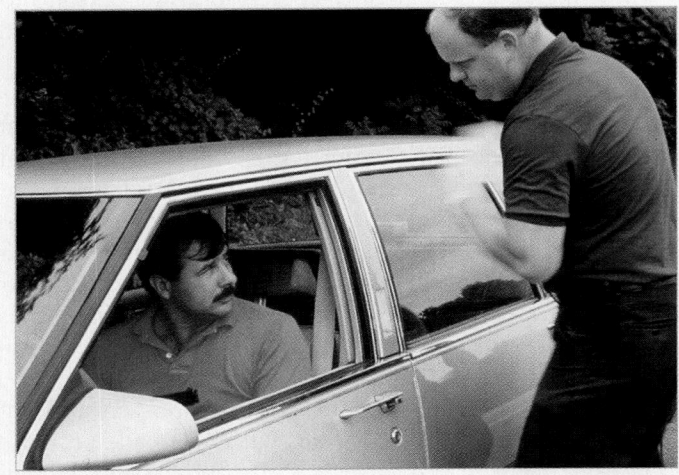

Figure 51-21 If aggressive action occurs, throw the pad directly at the nose of the aggressor.

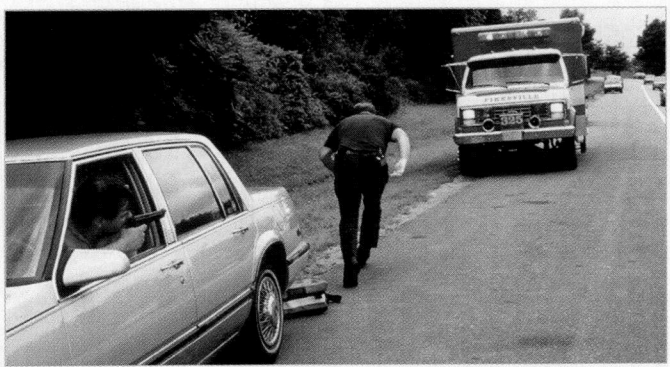

Figure 51-22 While the aggressor flinches and attempts to refocus, run toward the unit.

Put as much distance as possible between you and the aggressor. If possible, run to your vehicle Figure 51-22 . You can call for help or drive to a safer location. If you are cut off from the ambulance, evaluate the surrounding area for the best possible cover and concealment.

Use physical force as a defensive technique, not an aggressive motion. Properly executed defensive motions can be as effective as physical strikes and are easier to defend if you face civil liability charges.

The amount of defensive force needed to protect yourself varies with each incident. If you believe that your life is in imminent danger, any action that gets you out of the situation is a reasonable level of force.

Crime Scenes

As a paramedic, you will respond to assist the victims of violent crime. Clearly, your first responsibility, beyond that of personal safety, is to the patient. However, you also have a responsibility to the community at large. By assisting law enforcement personnel to maintain the integrity of the crime scene, you increase the probability that a suspect will be captured and convicted.

Preserving Evidence

Generally, there are two types of evidence: testimonial and real or physical. Testimonial evidence is the oral documentation by a witness of the facts. Real or physical evidence ties a suspect or a victim to a crime and includes body materials, objects, and impressions.

Follow law enforcement direction when you are asked to park in a specific area or to avoid a certain location. Officers may be attempting to safeguard tire imprints, bullet casings, or blood. Once you are at your patient's side, try to alter the scene as little as possible. Be mindful of bullet casings, weapons, blood spatter, and puddles. Whenever possible, walk around such evidence Figure 51-23 . Do not pick up expended cartridge casings to determine the caliber. Do not use telephones, flush toilets, or turn on water in a sink. In each case, valuable evidence can be lost. When you remove clothes to expose a wound, do not cut through bullet holes, knife cuts, or tears. Once the clothes are removed, do not shake them because valuables, including valuable trace evidence, may fall from the pockets to the floor.

You can be called to provide testimonial evidence in court regarding what you saw or heard at the scene of a crime. Because a criminal case might not go to trial for a year or more, it is imperative the incident be properly documented. Writing a complete report is the mark of a professional paramedic. Incomplete reports seldom keep anyone out of court.

You are the Provider Part 3

You retreat and stage a safe distance from the house. When law enforcement officers arrive, you brief them on the situation and wait until they have the scene secured. Once the law enforcement officers feel they have the scene secured, they have you enter the house and treat a badly beaten female patient. The officers tell you they have arrested a man with a handgun in his waistband, who had been beating the woman. You and your partner look at each other realizing the danger you would have placed yourself in had you elected to enter the house alone.

5. How can your approach to the scene be an important part of the scene size-up?
6. What would you or your partner have done if you elected to enter the house alone and found the gun in the patient's waist?

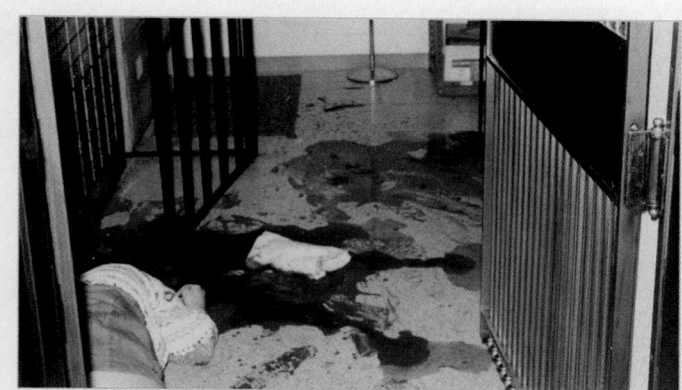

Figure 51-23 Do not disturb bullet casings, and avoid stepping in blood spatter and puddles.

Three elements require proper documentation: what you saw, what you heard, and the chain of custody. Documentation should include a description of the scene. How many patients? Was the victim supine or prone? Where was the weapon? Were any characteristics of the scene noteworthy? Do not draw conclusions or overstate facts. Any statements made by the patient during transfer to a medical facility should be documented.

Documentation and Communication

Remember to document as much as you can at the crime scene. Your documentation may become evidence in a court case. If you are called to testify, your documentation will help you remember the specifics of the call.

Documentation and Communication

Your report should answer the following questions.
- What did you see?
  - Overturned or damaged furniture
  - Weapons
  - Position of victim and other persons at the scene
- What did you hear?
  - Arguing or screams
  - Weapons being chambered or talk of the use of a weapon
  - Incriminating statements by persons on the scene
- What was done with evidence taken from the victim?
  - Clothing
  - Weapons (Law enforcement personnel should secure weapons whenever possible.)

As always, clearly note your actions on the scene.

You are the Provider Summary

1. Does the lack of violent incidents in your response district ensure your safety?

Absolutely not! Violence knows no geographic boundaries; it can happen anywhere and at any time. A statistically low rate of violence—although good—simply means that it's a matter of time before you are faced with such a call. It is crucial to remember that all calls you respond to pose a potential threat to your safety. It is your responsibility to carefully size up every scene—regardless of how docile it may appear—to ensure that you are not walking into a volatile situation.

2. What measures will you take to stay safe on this call?

First, you should request law enforcement response to the scene. You should exercise caution on every call; however, you should be especially cautious of calls in which the details are sketchy or unknown. A call for an "injured person" is very generic; it could range from a minor injury sustained during a family picnic to an intoxicated man with an assault rifle. You should also ask the dispatcher to attempt to gather more information about the call while you are en route; forewarned is forearmed. If this is not possible, err on the side of caution and stage in a safe place until law enforcement personnel arrive at the scene and ensure that it's safe.

3. What information can be obtained as you walk toward the house?

Screaming and profanity should immediately indicate that this is not a safe scene. Other signs of a violent situation include the sound of breaking glass, loud music, other unusual sounds, or an obvious struggle that you can see through a window. Keep your ears and eyes open at all times and never let your guard down.

4. What actions should you take in response to the hostilities heard from within the residence?

Unless you and your partner wish to become part of a situation that may result in your own deaths, it would be extremely wise to immediately withdraw from the scene and move to a place of safety. However, when doing so, you should back away from the residence. If you turn your back, and the person inside knows that you are there, you will never see an attack coming. Stage in a safe area and wait for law enforcement personnel to arrive.

5. How can your approach to the scene be an important part of the scene size-up?

Remember this: the life you save (or attempt to save) may take your own! Never hastily enter a scene without making a deliberate and concerted effort to look for safety hazards and taking appropriate action to buffer any hazards. This may include requesting law enforcement, fire personnel, the power company, or the animal warden. The scene size-up—with emphasis on remaining cognizant of threats to your safety—is not a one-time assessment; it is an ongoing process until the call has ended. Many scenes are safe initially, only to deteriorate with alarming speed and unpredictability.

6. What would you or your partner have done if you elected to enter the house alone and found the gun in the patient's waist?

The obvious must be pointed out: if you recognize that a scene is clearly unsafe (screaming and profane language should raise a red flag), then you will not be placed in such a situation. The answer to this question is "it depends." Can you egress before the person has a chance to draw the gun? Is there an escape route? If so, where is it in proximity to the person with the gun? Is there an object that you can use as cover if the person opens fire? Although you have no way of predicting how a person who is carrying a weapon is going to react or behave, you can safely assume that it will not be pleasant. If egression is not an option (ie, you are trapped in between the assailant and the door), try to remain calm and use your skills of diplomacy to assure the person that you are there to help.

Prep Kit

◼ Ready for Review

- No community, socioeconomic group, race, or religion is immune to violence. The use of sound survival skills will reduce the potential for you to fall victim to an act of violence while on an emergency call.
- Allow law enforcement personnel to secure the scene of violent incidents before you enter.
- Should violence erupt while you are on scene, retreat to a safe place and summon the police.

◼ Vital Vocabulary

clandestine drug laboratories Locations where illegal drugs such as methamphetamine, lysergic acid diethylamide (LSD), ecstasy, and phencyclidine hydrochloride (PCP) are manufactured.

concealment Protection from being seen.

contact and cover Technique that involves one paramedic making contact with the patient to provide care, while the second paramedic obtains patient information, gauges the level of tension, and warns his or her partner at the first sign of trouble.

cover Obstacles that are difficult or impossible for bullets to penetrate.

physical evidence The evidence that ties a suspect or victim to a crime. It may include body materials, objects, and impressions.

primary exit The main means of escape should violence erupt. This is usually the door you used to enter the building.

secondary exit Any other means of egress, including windows and rear doors.

SWAT-trained paramedics Specially trained medics who provide care for barricaded patients, patients being held hostage, and other special operations.

testimonial evidence The oral documentation by a witness of the facts of a criminal act.

tunnel vision Dangerous situation when a paramedic becomes so completely involved with patient care that he or she fails to see the possibility of physical harm to the patient or other care providers.

◼ Points to Ponder

You are dispatched to an assault on a corner in your local town. The local police department asks you to stage approximately two blocks away. After approximately 10 minutes, you are notified that the scene is safe. When you approach the patient, you see that he has two stab wounds to his chest. You and your partner provide spinal precautions and provide immediate lifesaving care to him. You transport him to the nearest trauma center.

What would you have done if you arrived at the scene before the police? If the perpetrator were on the scene, what would you do?

Issues: Potential Exposure to Scene Violence, How to Approach the Scene.

Assessment in Action

You and your partner are dispatched to the highway for an unconscious patient in a car. You are informed by your dispatch center that the scene appears to be safe. The person who called 9-1-1 was traveling in the opposite direction and noticed the vehicle pulled over on the shoulder of the highway.

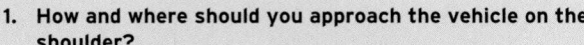

1. **How and where should you approach the vehicle on the shoulder?**
   - A. At a minimum of 15´ to the rear and a 20° angle
   - B. At a minimum of 15´ in front of the vehicle on a 1° angle
   - C. At a minimum of 15´ to the rear of the vehicle and on a 10° angle
   - D. At a minimum of a 10´ to the rear of the vehicle and on a 15° angle

2. **If you are the person riding in the passenger seat, how should you approach the vehicle?**
   - A. Proceed to the rear passenger side trunk area.
   - B. Proceed to the rear driver's side trunk area.
   - C. Proceed directly to the driver's side door.
   - D. Proceed directly to the passenger side door.

3. **Special attention should be taken when approaching:**
   - A. cars.
   - B. motorcycles.
   - C. SUVs.
   - D. vans.

4. **What should you do if the situation turns unsafe?**
   - A. Stay and deal with it.
   - B. Adapt and overcome.
   - C. Retreat from the scene.
   - D. Try to talk to the patient.

5. **Information that you need to give to your dispatcher if there is an unsafe condition includes all of the following, EXCEPT:**
   - A. the number of aggressors involved.
   - B. the patient's name and estimated transport time to the hospital.
   - C. the number and type of weapons involved, if any.
   - D. the make, color, body style and license number of the vehicle.

6. **True or false? Once on the scene, and there do not appear to be any threats to the EMS providers, you can move on to other things, such as treating the patient.**
   - A. True
   - B. False

7. **True or false? Only certain calls require a scene size-up for violence hazards.**
   - A. True
   - B. False

Challenging Question

You are dispatched to the scene of a pediatric pedestrian struck outside of an apartment complex. When you arrive on scene, you see an ambulance and a fire truck on scene already. You look for them and notice a crowd of approximately 100 angry individuals. You find a police officer and you ask her to lead you to where the patient is. When you arrive at the patient's side, you find the ambulance and fire crew. You immediately direct BLS to secure the patient, who appears to be stable, and transfer him to the ambulance.

8. **What dangers do large crowds pose to the EMS provider?**

A

Appendix A: Cardiac Life Support Fundamentals

Objectives

There are no DOT EMT-Paramedic objectives for this chapter, as current CPR training is a prerequisite and not a corequisite for all paramedic programs. This appendix is intended to address the following key areas:

1. Review the purpose of CPR. (p A.4)
2. Emphasize the importance of the links in the Chain of Survival to a successful code. (p A.3)
3. List the skill steps of one-rescuer and two-rescuer CPR for the adult, child, and infant patient. (p A.5)
4. Discuss the latest guidelines issued by the American Heart Association (December 2005) as they apply to the health care provider. (p A.4)
5. Review the management of a cardiac arrest based on analysis of the ECG as either a shockable (V-fib or V-tach) or a nonshockable (PEA or asystole) rhythm. (p A.13)
6. Review devices that may be useful adjuncts at a code to increase the probability of increasing the return of spontaneous circulation (ROSC). (p A.17)
7. Describe the typical roles of the code team leader and code team members at a resuscitation. (p A.19)
8. Discuss the value of scene choreography at a code. (p A.18)
9. Review a sample script for a typical prehospital cardiac arrest resuscitation. (p A.20)

Introduction

Paramedics and EMT-Bs are frequently dispatched to calls involving a cardiac arrest. An estimated 60% to 70% of all prehospital cardiac arrests occur in the home; the remainder occur in public places. Having a bystander who has initiated the proper care at the scene is definitely a plus—indeed, it often means the difference between life and death. Some paramedics might even find it difficult to remember successfully resuscitating a patient from cardiac arrest who did not either have citizen CPR or for whom the arrest was a witnessed event and an AED was immediately available.

This appendix explores planning for the resuscitation or "code," the roles of the code team leader and code team members, and ways that practice and planning can help increase your resuscitation success. The American Heart Association (AHA), in concert with the international resuscitation community, revises the guidelines for emergency cardiovascular care and CPR every 5 years. This appendix describes how your agency can incorporate the latest guidelines into your field codes.

Managing Cardiac Arrest

Survival for prehospital cardiac arrest averages 6.4% or less in most reports from the United States and Canada. According to the AHA, the "Chain of Survival" includes four essential links: early access, early CPR, early defibrillation, and early definitive care Figure A-1 ▶ . Those communities that have made survival of a prehospital cardiac arrest a benchmark for measurable improvements in their health care systems have worked hard on each of these links.

Improving the Response to Cardiac Arrest: The SMART Way

When you are undertaking a community-based program to improve survival of prehospital cardiac arrest, consider adopting the management acronym SMART to describe the program's objectives: Specific, Measurable, Attainable and Achievable, Realistic and Relevant, and Timely. Here are a few questions that progressive communities should ask:

- Is there a universal access number (ie, 9-1-1), and do all members of the public know how and when to use it?
- Are all the dispatchers/communicators trained in CPR telephone instruction?
- Is a community CPR training program readily available at all times of the day and days of the week at little to no cost for the citizens? If so, does the public know it is available? Have 10% to 20% of the population been trained? (Part of attaining this objective can be addressed by convincing the public to take the self-help approach to CPR training as provided by the 30-minute CPR Anytime program.)
- Is CPR a requirement to graduate high school?

You are the Provider Part 1

Jim, a 54-year-old man, is playing basketball in an adult league on a Saturday afternoon at the local elementary school. He leaves the game to get a drink and starts to feel dizzy as he returns to the court. He suddenly drops to his knees and then to the floor. Fortunately, one of his teammates, Tom, took a cardiopulmonary resuscitation (CPR) course about 2 months ago, so he takes charge of the situation. Tom orders a teammate, "Go call 9-1-1 and tell them we have a cardiac arrest." Next, he tells someone else, "Go search for an AED."

About 2 minutes pass as the nearest engine company, which was located only a few blocks away, arrives on the scene. Your paramedic rescue company is still responding from a few miles away.

Upon arrival of your medic unit, you are led into the court by a teammate. You hear over the radio that a supervisor is en route with a mechanical piston CPR device. As you approach the patient's side, you do a quick size-up of the scene for safety and potential hazards and then begin an initial assessment. Your general impression indicates a middle-aged, overweight male who is receiving good-quality CPR as judged by the counting you hear and the compressions. An EMT-B from the engine company is attaching the pads and cables to their AED. These cables can easily be switched to your monitor, but this can wait until after the first shock.

You note the following findings while getting an initial report.

Initial Assessment	Recording Time: 2 Minutes
Appearance	CPR is in progress, patient is not vomiting, and the belly is not distended
Level of consciousness	U (Unresponsive)
Airway	Open with a head tilt-chin lift
Breathing	Being ventilated with a bag-mask device with high-flow supplemental oxygen
Circulation	Receiving compressions at the two-rescuer rate/ratio

1. Arriving on the scene of an apparent cardiac arrest with bystanders who have initiated care, how should you evaluate the quality of the CPR?
2. Many elementary schools and public places have an AED available. How might that have helped in this situation?

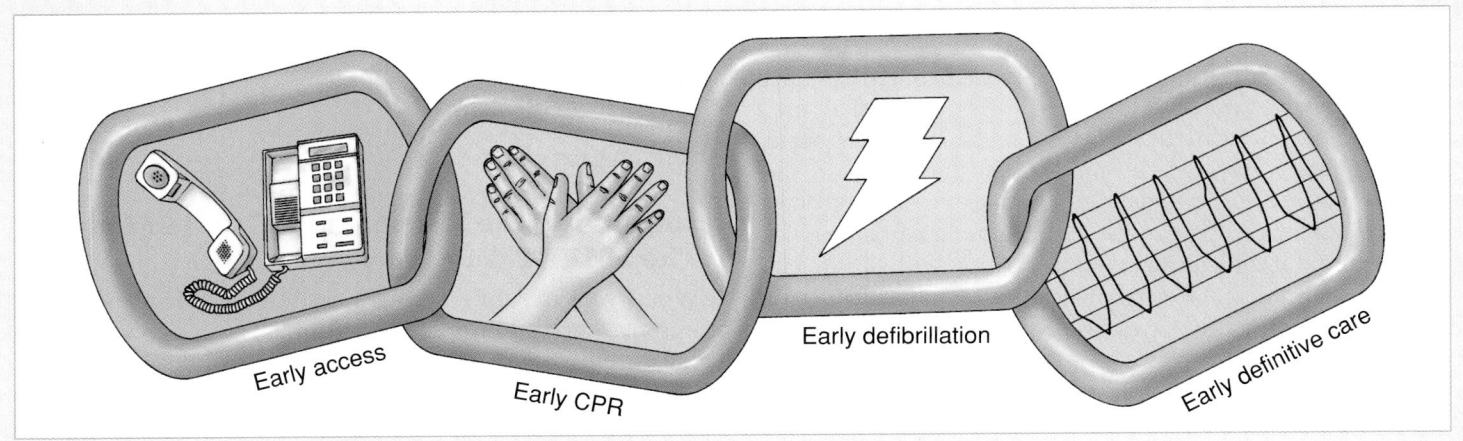

Figure A-1 The four links of the Chain of Survival.

- Are 100% of the responders to emergencies (police, fire, EMS) currently trained in CPR and the AED? Do all response vehicles have an AED?
- Are AEDs and qualified personnel who are trained in their use available in all locations of public assembly for more than 500 people or in high-risk locations?
- How long does it take for the first emergency responder to arrive on the scene? How long does it take for the paramedics to arrive?
- Is the EMS agency's medical director actively involved in reviewing all cardiac arrests and making quality improvements to the EMS system's response on a regular basis?
- Are the cardiac arrest events reported using the Recommended Guidelines for Uniform Reporting of Data from Out-of-Hospital Cardiac Arrest, "The Utstein Style" (approved by AHA and European Resuscitation Council in 1991), so your community's data can be compared to the data of other progressive communities?
- Do all hospitals you transport to participate in the National Registry of CardioPulmonary Resuscitation (NRCPR) data system? The NRCPR is the only national registry of in-hospital resuscitation events.

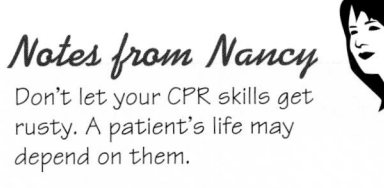

Notes from Nancy
Don't let your CPR skills get rusty. A patient's life may depend on them.

- How often does the code team practice its response and its teamwork in an effort to improve the success of future codes?

Guidelines 2005: A Reemphasis on Quality CPR

During the past 15 years the emphasis on quality CPR has seemed to slip as providers became more focused on intubation, drug administration, defibrillation, and other aspects of code management. Recent studies have shown that the quality

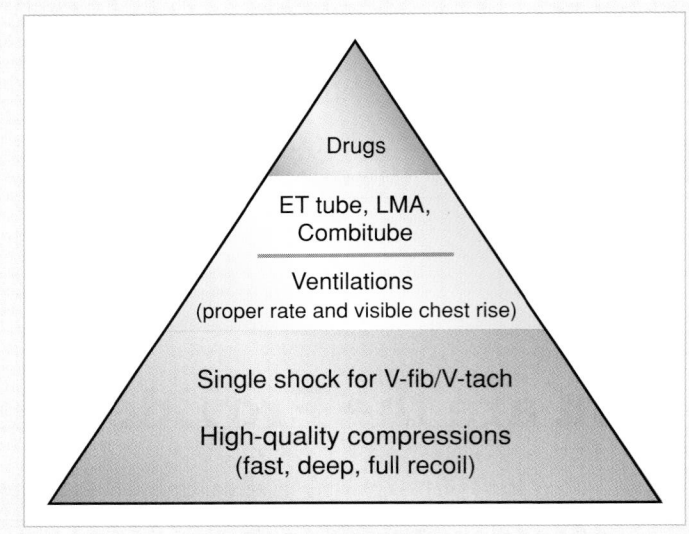

Figure A-2 The resuscitation pyramid. The success of a code relies on high-quality CPR.

of CPR is poor in both in-hospital and prehospital settings: The depth of compressions is inadequate, the rate of compressions is too slow, almost half the time no compressions are provided, the ventilations are too fast, and the chest is rarely allowed to fully recoil. Studies investigating the value of intubation and resuscitation drugs are inconclusive at best, but CPR is clearly important both before and after defibrillation. In addition, immediate CPR can double or triple the rate of survival from ventricular fibrillation (V-fib) sudden cardiac arrest.

The 2005 CPR guidelines reemphasize the importance of providing high-quality CPR (push hard and fast, and allow full chest recoil). In fact, the "resuscitation pyramid" is built on a strong base of high-quality CPR as illustrated in Figure A-2 ▲ . The recognition that a paramedic's best chance of succeeding at resuscitation hinges on continuous, uninterrupted high-quality CPR changes the focus of care. Mechanical piston CPR devices, such as the Thumper or the

AutoPulse device, have traditionally been used in the ambulance in some EMS systems during transport to the hospital. Today, given the renewed attention to high-quality CPR, the focus is on how to treat the patient using one of these devices as quickly as possible without any interruptions in manual CPR.

As you arrive on the scene of the code, you need to clearly understand that the success of the code relies on high-quality compressions and not on an IV, an ET tube, or any drug in your box. Work together with the BLS providers, assist them, compliment their efforts, and relieve them as they tire but do not interrupt or disrupt their efforts!

■ The Steps of CPR

The basic life support steps of CPR for the adult patient follow the algorithm shown in **Figure A-3 ▶**. They presume that an AED is not immediately available at the patient's side. Integration of the AED will be discussed later in this appendix. Health care providers (first responders, EMT-Bs, EMT-Intermediates, and paramedics) who work in the prehospital setting must be trained and prepared to provide either one-rescuer CPR or two-rescuer CPR as available personnel dictate.

In some instances, single-rescuer CPR may have been started before EMS personnel arrive. To help make CPR easier to learn, remember, and perform, the general public or "lay rescuers" are taught a universal compression–ventilation ratio of 30:2. They are not taught to take a pulse, to perform rescue breathing, or to perform two-rescuer CPR. Paramedics should be thrilled and thankful to arrive on the scene and find a bystander who is both properly trained and willing to provide CPR. Sadly, studies have shown that bystander CPR is performed in only one third or fewer of witnessed cardiac arrests and that when performed, even by health care providers, it is not done well. Bystanders who have been trained previously in CPR are often reluctant to begin this procedure for the following reasons:

- CPR steps may have been too complicated and included too many steps to remember. The 2005 guidelines made a significant effort to simplify the steps taught to the public.
- Training methods may have been inadequate, and skill retention typically declines very rapidly after a course. This issue is being studied to try to determine which methods of training will produce the greatest skill retention. A video-based watch-and-do method, as opposed to watch-then-do, has been incorporated into many course revisions.
- Some members of the public may be afraid of transmitted diseases and therefore may be reluctant to perform mouth-to-mouth resuscitation. Although the 2005 guidelines strongly emphasize that the risk of transmission of infection is very low, those who are still concerned are encouraged to use barrier devices. In addition, the technique of compression-only CPR is encouraged for those who are reluctant to do ventilations and for dispatcher-assisted CPR instruction.

Single-Rescuer CPR

Tom immediately began single-rescuer CPR when his teammate Jim dropped suddenly on the basketball court. The steps are shown in **Skill Drill A-1 ▶**.

1. Establish unresponsiveness. If there is no movement or response to shouting and shaking the adult patient, then the patient is considered "unresponsive."
   - If you are by yourself, phone 9-1-1 (or the emergency number) and make sure the AED is immediately available.
   - If there is a second rescuer, send him or her to call 9-1-1 (or the emergency number) and get the AED.
2. Open the airway **Step 1**. Use the head tilt–chin lift method unless trauma to the neck is suspected, in which case the jaw-thrust maneuver may be more appropriate.
3. Check for breathing **Step 2**. Look, listen, and feel for 5 seconds to a maximum of 10 seconds.
   - If there is no breathing, give two rescue breaths over 1 second each to achieve a visible chest rise. Do not over-ventilate the patient, as it can cause gastric distention and regurgitation.
   - If the patient is breathing or resumes effective breathing, place him or her in the recovery position and monitor closely.
4. Health care providers are taught to check for a carotid pulse in the adult for at least 5 seconds but to spend no more than 10 seconds trying to locate the pulse **Step 3**. Compressions are delivered in the center of the chest between the nipples with the heel of the hand and with the second hand on top of the first. Compressions on an adult should be provided at a rate of 100/min, pressing 1½″ to 2″ and ensuring full chest recoil after each compression.
   - If a pulse were present, the health care provider would provide one rescue breath every 5 to 6 seconds.
   - If no pulse were present, the health care provider would begin chest compressions **Step 4**. All compressors will eventually get tired. As help becomes available, be prepared to change compressors without interrupting compressions every 2 minutes.
5. Continue the cycles of 30 compressions (push hard and fast, and allow full chest recoil) and two breaths **Step 5** (1-second duration each to achieve visible chest rise) until the AED or defibrillator arrives.
6. Check the patient's rhythm **Step 6** once the AED arrives, with the least amount of interruption in chest compressions as possible.
   - If it is a shockable rhythm, administer a single shock, resume CPR immediately for five cycles (approximately 2 minutes), and then reanalyze the rhythm.
   - If it is not a shockable rhythm, resume CPR immediately for five cycles (approximately 2 minutes). Continue until ALS providers take over or the patient starts to move. The health care provider would determine whether the patient has a pulse at this point.

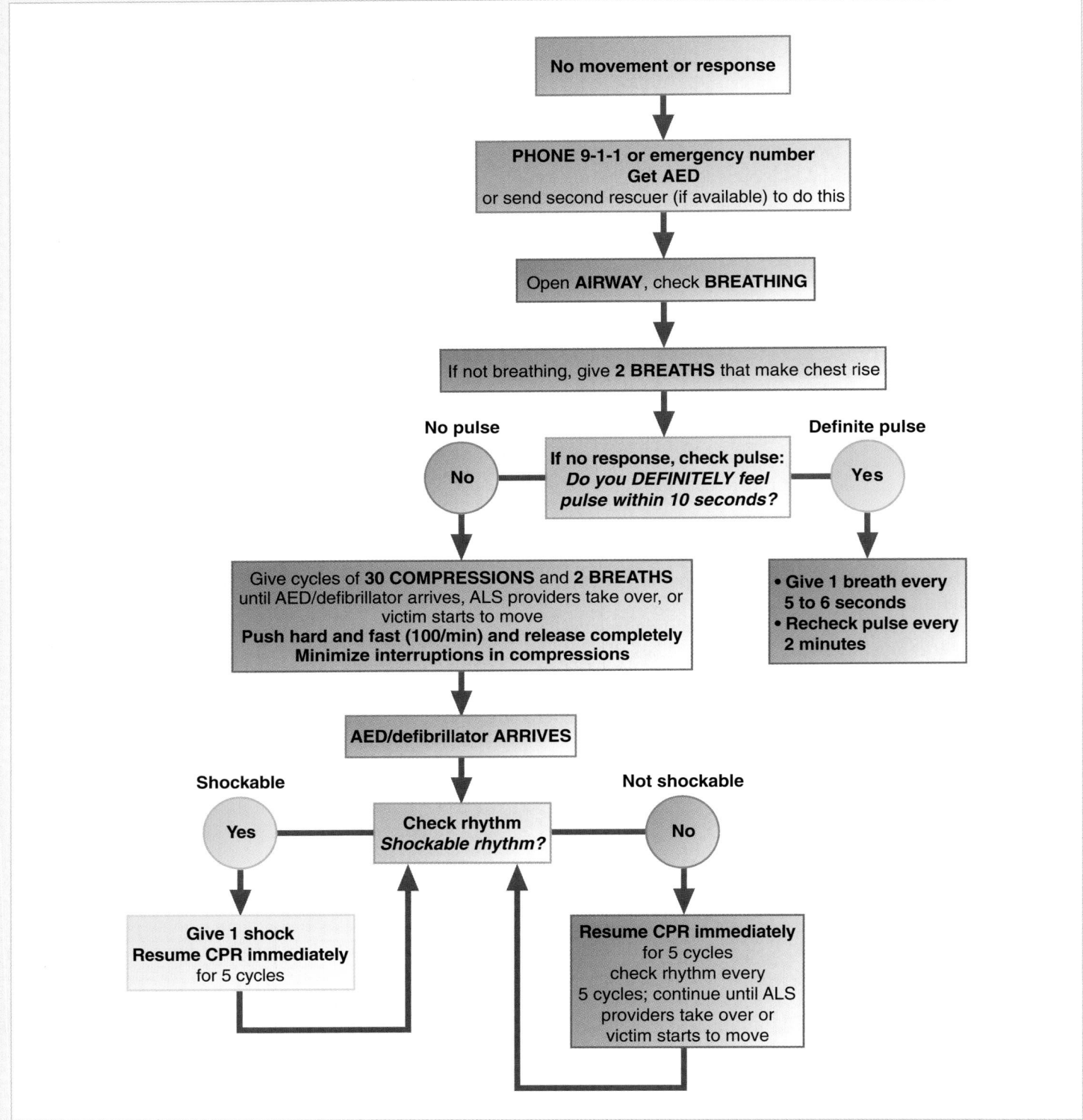

Figure A-3 The BLS adult health care provider algorithm.

Skill Drill A-1: Single-Rescuer Adult CPR

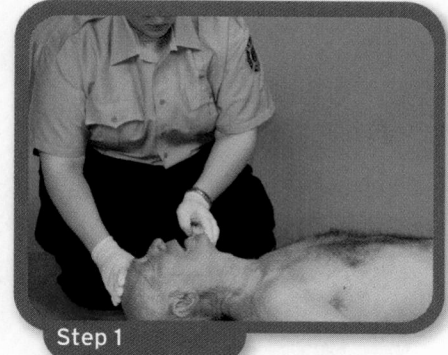

Step 1

Establish unresponsiveness. Open the airway.

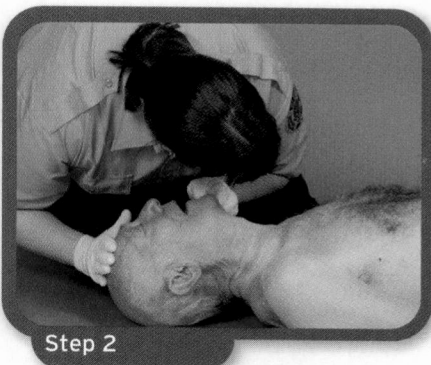

Step 2

Check for breathing (look, listen, and feel). If no breaths, administer two breaths, each 1 second, achieving visible chest rise.

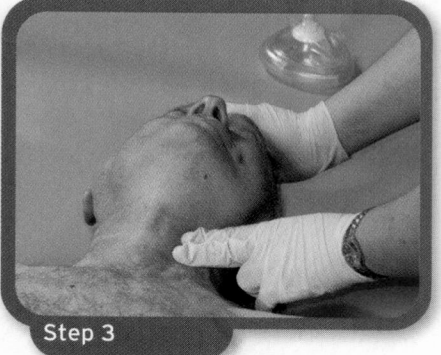

Step 3

Perform a carotid pulse check (maximum of 10 seconds).

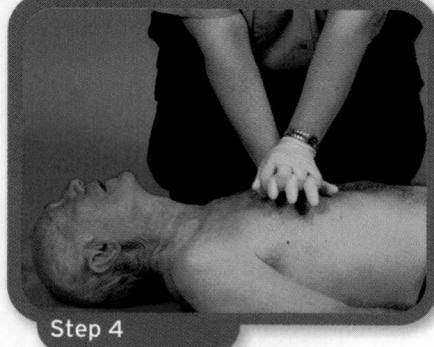

Step 4

Begin 30 compressions—center of the chest, push hard and fast (rate of 100/min), and allow full chest recoil.

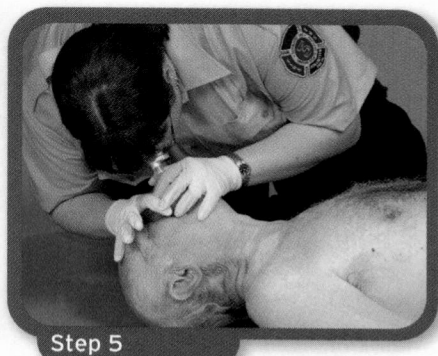

Step 5

Ventilate two times for 1 second each to achieve visible chest rise. Complete five cycles (approximately 2 minutes) and reassess the patient for a maximum of 10 seconds. If AED has arrived, attach it without interrupting compressions.

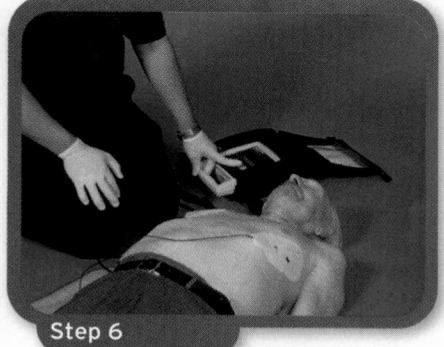

Step 6

Check the patient's rhythm.
If it is shockable, administer a single shock and then resume CPR immediately for five cycles. Reanalyze the rhythm.
If it is not shockable, resume CPR immediately for five cycles.

Two-Rescuer CPR

Two-rescuer adult CPR provides the same cycle of 30 compressions to every two breaths as in the single-rescuer technique. Because the work is split between the two rescuers, it is more efficient and there is less interruption in the chest compressions to provide the ventilations. If an advanced airway has been inserted, <u>asynchronous</u> compressions and ventilations are possible. That is, the compressor simply presses hard, fast, and with full chest recoil at the rate of 100/min while the ventilator provides one breath (over 1 second's time, while observing for visible chest rise) every 6 to 8 seconds.

When you are using the two-rescuer technique, rotate the compressor every 2 minutes. To do so, ask the bystander to continue to assist and kneel on the other side of the patient. Now you can have an "active compressor" and an "on-deck compressor" who is ready to take over after the five cycles or 2-minute interval. Studies of rescuer fatigue show that the compressor tires after 2 to 5 minutes and that the quality of compressions will suffer if the compressor is not replaced. The steps in two-rescuer CPR are outlined here and in **Skill Drill A-2 ▶**:

1. Establish unresponsiveness. Send a helper to phone 9-1-1 and get the AED.
2. Open the airway using the head tilt–chin lift maneuver **Step 1**.
3. Check for breathing (look, listen, and feel) **Step 2**. If there are no breaths, administer two breaths, each 1 second in duration and achieving visible chest rise.
4. The health care provider should perform a carotid pulse check for 5 seconds (maximum of 10 seconds) **Step 3**.
5. One rescuer begins 30 compressions—center of the chest, push hard and fast (rate of 100/min), and allow full chest

Skill Drill A-2: Two-Rescuer Adult CPR

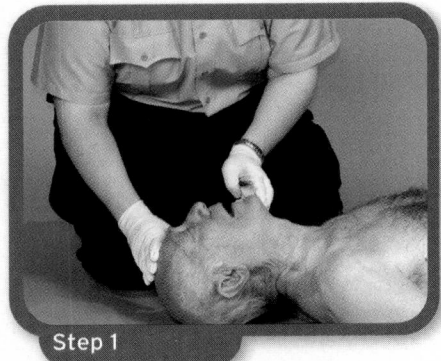

Step 1

Establish unresponsiveness. Open the airway.

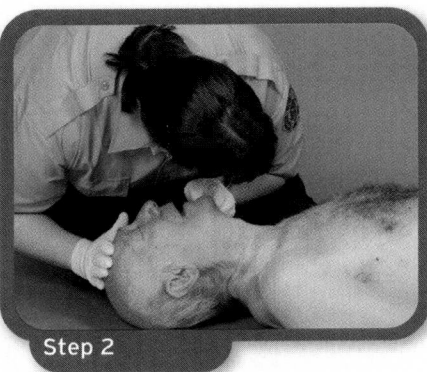

Step 2

Check for breathing. If there are no breaths, administer two breaths, each 1 second, achieving visible chest rise.

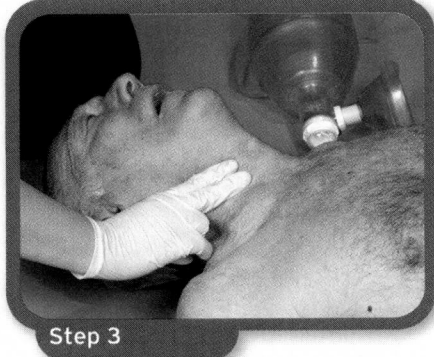

Step 3

Perform a carotid pulse check (maximum of 10 seconds).

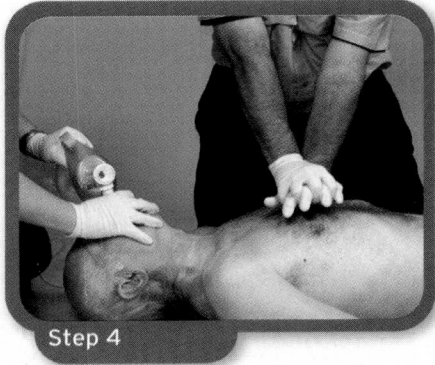

Step 4

One rescuer begins 30 compressions, counting out loud.

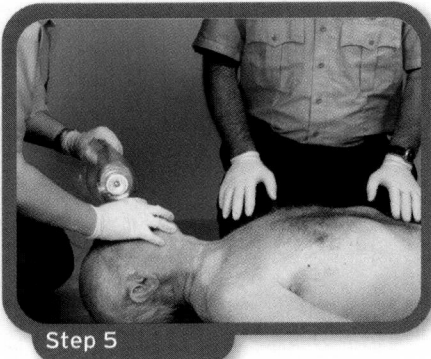

Step 5

Second rescuer ventilates two times and applies the AED pads while waiting. Complete five cycles and reassess the patient for a maximum of 10 seconds.

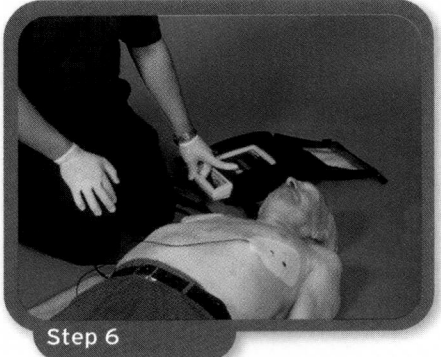

Step 6

Analyze the patient's ECG rhythm.
If it is shockable, administer a single shock at the device-specific dose. If it is nonshockable or immediately following the shock (unless the patient wakes up), begin five cycles of 30 compressions to two ventilations.
Repeat cycles of compressions/ventilations and AED shocks.

recoil (**Step 4**). Count out loud so the second rescuer is prepared to ventilate as you get to "28 and 29 and 30."

6. The second rescuer ventilates two times, each 1 second in duration and achieving visible chest rise (**Step 5**). The ventilator should use a bag-mask device with supplementary oxygen and an OPA. Position yourself approximately 18″ above the head of the supine patient to allow for the proper "E-C" or "OK" hand position and mask seal. During the waiting time, the second rescuer could apply the AED pads so it is ready to analyze at the 2-minute point.

7. Complete five cycles (approximately 2 minutes) and reassess the patient for a maximum of 10 seconds. If the AED has arrived and is attached, analyze the patient's ECG rhythm to determine whether it is shockable or nonshockable (**Step 6**).

8. If it is a shockable rhythm, administer a single shock at the device-specific dose (200 J is the default). Ensure that all parties are clear prior to administering the shock. ("I'm clear, you're clear, we're all clear.")

9. If it is a nonshockable rhythm or immediately following the shock (unless the patient wakes up), begin five cycles (approximately 2 minutes) of 30 compressions to two ventilations.

10. Repeat Steps 7, 8, and 9 until ALS arrives and takes over or the medical director orders otherwise. As additional help arrives, prepare for transport or contact medical control.

Note: Once an advanced airway has been inserted, the compressions and ventilations are no longer in cycles. Instead, they are asynchronous, with the compressor providing 100/min without pauses for breaths and the ventilator giving 8 to 10 breaths/min (every 6 to 8 seconds). The compressor will get tired so be prepared to switch compressors every 2 minutes with no more than 10-second pauses, if any.

▮ Modification in Technique for Children

Definitions

The age-old question raised to the pediatricians has been "For the purposes of resuscitation, what age defines a child?" Many pediatricians would simply say, "If the patient looks like a child, then he or she is a child; if the patient looks like an adult, then he or she is an adult." This vagueness is further complicated by the epidemic of childhood obesity in the United States. The 2005 guidelines use the following definitions of age groups for the purposes of resuscitation:

- **Newly born**—the infant at time of birth
- **Neonate**—the infant until discharge from the initial hospitalization

- **Infant**—younger than 1 year
- **Child**
  - health care providers: age 1 year to adolescence (signs of puberty or secondary sexual characteristic development)
  - lay rescuers: ages 1 to 8
- **Adult**—adolescent and older

This appendix concentrates on infant, child, and adult patients. The care of newly born and neonate patients is discussed in Chapter 40.

Child CPR

The technique of CPR has a few slight variations for children, as shown below in italics. **Skill Drill A-3 ▸** shows the steps of one-rescuer child CPR.

1. Establish unresponsiveness. If there is no movement or response to *tapping and asking loudly "Are you okay?"* the child is unresponsive.
   - Send someone to phone 9-1-1 (or the emergency number) and get the AED.
   - If you are a lone rescuer *for a sudden collapse,* phone 9-1-1 (or the emergency number) and get the AED.
   - If you are a lone rescuer and it was not a sudden collapse, proceed to the next step.

You are the Provider Part 2

During the first 2 minutes of CPR with Tom and the engine company EMT-Bs, a lot of teamwork has been going on. Tom is beginning to tire yet still wants to stay involved, so he becomes the "on-deck compressor." Another EMT-B has placed the AED next to Jim and relieved Tom; he becomes the compressor. Because Tom has been shown how to apply the AED electrodes, he is able to work around the compressor.

After approximately 2 minutes (five cycles) of CPR, a brief pause in care allows the team to analyze Jim's ECG. The AED begins to charge up, displaying a shockable rhythm such as ventricular fibrillation. In the meantime, Tom administers a few more compressions, and the ventilator removes the bag mask so oxygen does not flow near the patient. The EMT-B at the AED states, "I'm clear, you're clear, we're all clear," and proceeds to deliver a single shock. Jim's heavy body bounces on the hardwood floor but he does not awaken. The code team immediately begins the next five cycles of 30 compressions and two ventilations.

Vital Signs	Recording Time: 3 Minutes
Skin	Pale and clammy
Pulse	None palpable at carotid
Blood pressure	None
Respirations	Being ventilated with a bag-mask device

Previously, the duration of time from stopping compressions to analyzing to charging and providing the traditional three-shock series would have been almost 2 minutes of no chest compressions. No perfusion of the brain and vital organs occurs when there is no circulation from rescuers compressing the chest properly. Every pause in compressions, even when it lasts for as little as a few seconds, requires the next few compressions to reprime the pump. For this reason, a pause to analyze the rhythm should last no longer than 10 seconds without chest compressions.

When a patient has a shockable rhythm and does respond appropriately to a shock, it often takes a minute or so for return of spontaneous circulation (ROSC). Unless the patient actually wakes up, immediately after the shock the rescuers should begin CPR with chest compressions.

3. What should you do next as the paramedic on the scene?
4. What is the advantage to perfusion and chest compressions from inserting an advanced airway during two-rescuer CPR?

Skill Drill A-3: Single-Rescuer Child CPR

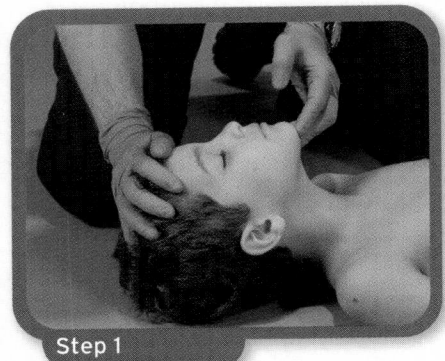

Step 1

Establish unresponsiveness. Open the airway.

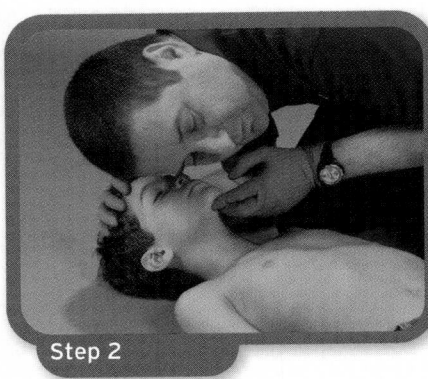

Step 2

Check for breathing (look, listen, and feel). If no breaths, administer two effective breaths.

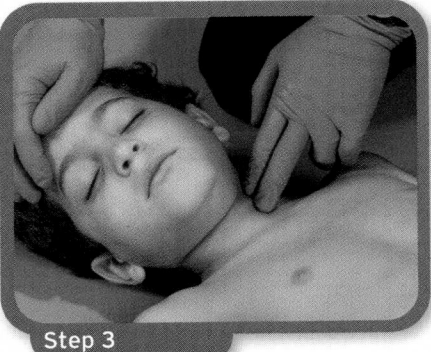

Step 3

Perform a carotid pulse check for 5 seconds (maximum of 10 seconds).

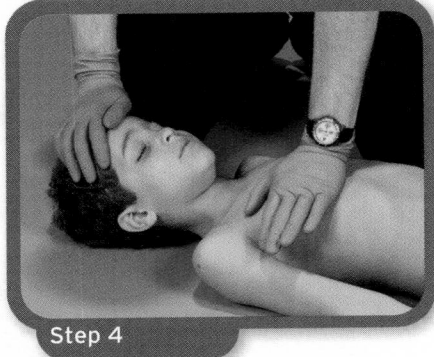

Step 4

Begin 30 compressions—center of the chest, push hard and fast (rate of 100/min), and allow full chest recoil—using either one or two hands depending on the child's size. Compress one third to one half the depth of the chest.

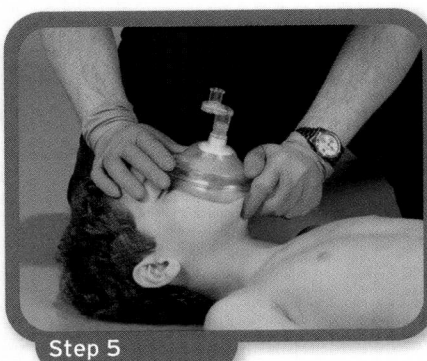

Step 5

Ventilate two times for 1 second each to achieve visible chest rise. Use a child-sized pocket mask with a one-way valve.

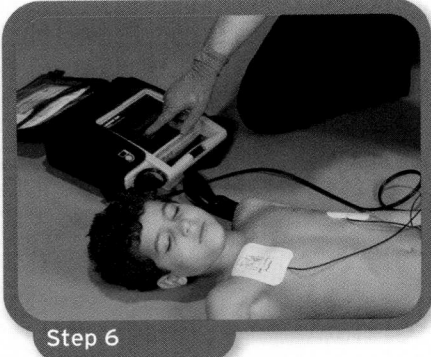

Step 6

Complete five cycles (approximately 2 minutes) and reassess the patient for a maximum of 10 seconds. If the AED has arrived, attach it, using child pads if the child is between 1 and 8 years old. Decrease the AED energy level. Analyze the rhythm.

If the rhythm is shockable, administer a single shock and then resume CPR immediately for five cycles. Reanalyze the rhythm.

If the rhythm is not shockable, resume CPR immediately for five cycles.

2. Open the airway (Step 1). Use the head tilt–chin lift method unless trauma to the neck is suspected, in which case the jaw-thrust maneuver may be more appropriate.

3. Check for breathing (Step 2). Look, listen, and feel for a maximum of 10 seconds.

- If there is no breathing, give two *effective* rescue breaths over 1 second each to achieve a visible chest rise. Do not over-ventilate the patient, as it can cause gastric distention and regurgitation. *Use a child-sized bag-mask* device with supplementary oxygen, implement an oropharyngeal airway, and position the second rescuer or ventilator approximately 18″ above the supine child's head. Use the "E-C" or "OK" method to ensure proper mask seal.

- If the patient is breathing or resumes effective breathing, place him or her in the recovery position and monitor closely.

4. At this point the lay rescuer begins compressions. Health care providers are taught to check for a carotid pulse in the child (as long as they do not exceed 10 seconds) (Step 3). Compressions are delivered in the center of the chest between the nipples with the heel of *either one hand or both hands as in the adult technique.* They should be provided at a rate of 100/min, pressing *one third to one half the depth of the chest* and ensuring full chest recoil after each compression (Step 4).

- If a pulse is present, the health care provider gives one rescue breath *every 3 to 5 seconds* (Step 5).

- If no pulse is present, the health care provider begins chest compressions. Be prepared to change compressors every 2 minutes.

5. *If not already done, phone 9-1-1 (or the emergency number) and get the AED.*

6. Continue the cycles of 30 compressions (push hard and fast, and allow full chest recoil) and two breaths (1-second duration each to achieve visible chest rise) until the AED or defibrillator arrives. *If there are two rescuers, health care providers are taught to give cycles of 15 compressions to two ventilations.*

7. Check the patient's rhythm once the AED arrives, with the least amount of interruption in chest compressions as possible (**Step 6**). *If the child is between 1 and 8 years old, use child pads if available. If the AED has a key or switch to deliver a child shock dose, activate it to decrease the energy level. If no child pads are available, use adult pads.*

- If there is a shockable rhythm, administer a single shock. Resume CPR immediately for five cycles (approximately 2 minutes), and then reanalyze the rhythm.
- If there is not a shockable rhythm, resume CPR immediately for five cycles (approximately 2 minutes). The public is trained to continue until ALS providers take over or the child starts to move. The health care provider would determine whether the patient has a pulse at this point.

Skill Drill A-4 ▶ shows the steps of two-rescuer child CPR, also summarized here.

1. Establish unresponsiveness, and send a helper to phone 9-1-1 and get the AED. If there is no helper, continue with the steps of CPR and then phone and look for an AED at the 2-minute point.

2. Open the airway using the head tilt–chin lift maneuver (**Step 1**).

3. Check for breathing (look, listen, and feel) (**Step 2**). If there are no breaths, administer two effective breaths, each lasting 1 second and achieving visible chest rise.

4. Perform a carotid pulse check (maximum of 10 seconds) (**Step 3**).

5. One rescuer begins 15 compressions—center of the chest, push hard and fast (rate of 100/min), and allow full chest recoil (**Step 4**). Count out loud so the second rescuer is prepared to ventilate as you get to "13 and 14 and 15."

6. The second rescuer ventilates two times, each lasting 1 second and achieving visible chest rise (**Step 5**). The ventilator should use a child-sized bag-mask device with supplementary oxygen and an OPA. Position yourself approximately 18″ above the head of the supine patient to allow for the proper "E-C" or "OK" hand position and mask seal. During the waiting time, the second rescuer could apply the AED pads so the AED is ready to analyze at the 2-minute point.

7. Complete five cycles (approximately 2 minutes) and reassess the patient for a maximum of 10 seconds. If the

AED has arrived and is attached, analyze the patient's ECG rhythm to determine whether it is shockable or nonshockable (**Step 6**). If the child is between 1 and 8 years old, use child pads if available. If the AED has a key or switch to deliver a child shock dose, activate it to decrease the energy level.

8. If there is a shockable rhythm, administer a single shock at the device-specific dose (200 J is the default). Ensure that all parties are clear prior to administering the shock. ("I'm clear, you're clear, we're all clear.")

9. If there is a nonshockable rhythm or immediately following the shock (unless the patient wakes up), begin five cycles (approximately 2 minutes) of 15 compressions to two ventilations.

10. Repeat Steps 7, 8, and 9 until ALS arrives and takes over or the medical director orders otherwise. As additional help arrives, prepare for transport or contact medical control.

Note: Once an advanced airway has been inserted, the compressions and ventilations are no longer in cycles. Instead, they are asynchronous with the compressor providing 100/min without pauses for breaths and the ventilator giving 8 to 10 breaths/min (every 6 to 8 seconds). Because the compressor will inevitably get tired, switch compressors every 2 minutes with no more than 10-second pauses, if any.

Infant CPR

The technique of CPR for an infant has a few slight variations (shown in italics below), as described in **Skill Drill A-5 ▶** .

1. Establish unresponsiveness. If there is no movement or response to *tapping and asking loudly "Are you okay?" you may consider flicking the infant's heels with your fingertips.* If there is no response, the infant is then considered unresponsive.

- Send someone to phone 9-1-1 (or the emergency number).
- If you are a lone rescuer, proceed to the next step.

2. Open the airway (**Step 1**). Use the head tilt–chin lift method (*do not hyperextend the neck*) unless trauma to the neck is suspected, in which case the jaw-thrust maneuver may be more appropriate.

3. Check for breathing (**Step 2**). Look, listen, and feel for a maximum of 10 seconds.

- If there is no breathing, give two *effective* rescue breaths with a barrier device or appropriate-size pocket mask over 1 second each to achieve a visible chest rise. Do not over-ventilate the patient, as it can cause gastric distention and regurgitation.

4. At this point, the lay rescuer begins compressions. Health care providers check for a *brachial or femoral pulse in the infant* as long as they do not spend more than 10 seconds trying to locate the pulse (**Step 3**). Compressions are delivered in the center of the chest just below the nipple line. *Use two fingers to compress.* Compressions on an infant should be provided at a rate of 100/min, pressing *one third*

Skill Drill A-4: Two-Rescuer Child CPR

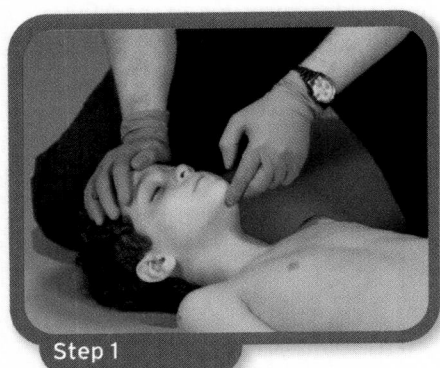

Step 1

Establish unresponsiveness. Open the airway.

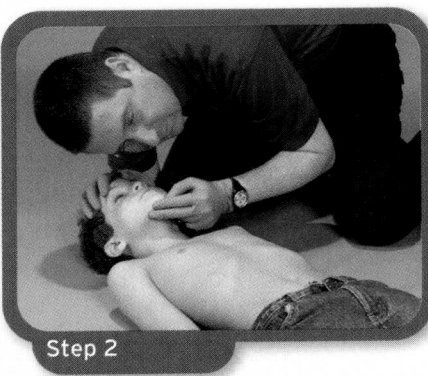

Step 2

Check for breathing (look, listen, and feel). If no breaths, administer two effective breaths.

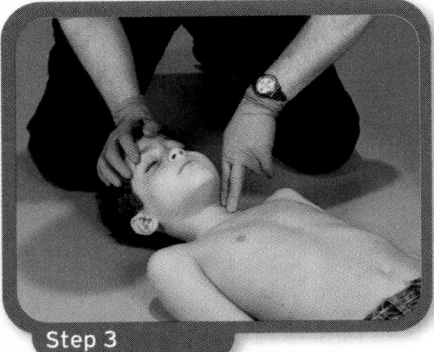

Step 3

Perform a carotid pulse check (maximum of 10 seconds).

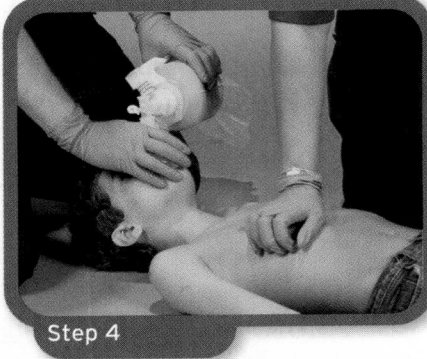

Step 4

One rescuer begins 15 compressions— center of the chest, push hard and fast (rate of 100/min) and allow full chest recoil.

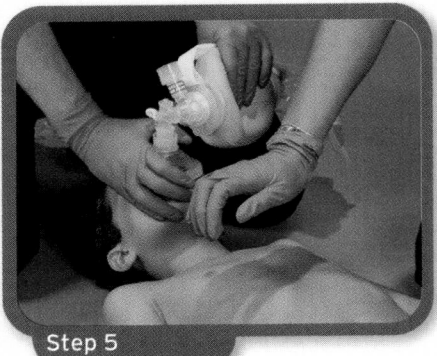

Step 5

The second rescuer ventilates two times for 1 second each to achieve visible chest rise. The ventilator should use a child-sized bag-mask device with supplementary oxygen and an oropharyngeal airway. Position yourself approximately 18″ above the head of the supine patient to allow for the proper hand position/mask seal.

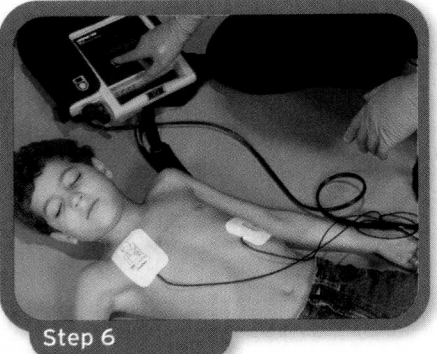

Step 6

Complete five cycles (approximately 2 minutes) and reassess the patient for a maximum of 10 seconds. If an AED has arrived and is attached, analyze the patient's ECG rhythm. Use child pads if the child is between 1 and 8 years old. Decrease the AED energy level.

If the rhythm is shockable, administer a single shock.

If the rhythm is not shockable or immediately following the shock, begin five cycles of 15 compressions to two ventilations.

to one half the depth of the chest and ensuring full chest recoil after each compression (Step 4).

- If a pulse is present, the health care provider provides one rescue breath *every 3 to 5 seconds.*
- If no pulse is present, the health care provider begins chest compressions. All compressors will inevitably get tired, so be prepared to change compressors without interrupting compressions every 2 minutes.

5. *If not already done, phone 9-1-1 (or the emergency number).*
6. Continue the cycles of 30 compressions (push hard and fast, and allow full chest recoil) and two breaths (1-second duration each to achieve visible chest rise) until the ALS unit arrives. If there are two rescuers, health care providers are taught to provide cycles of 15 compressions to

two ventilations. The compressions can be done using the two-hands encircling method (Figure A-4 ▶). Use of an AED is not recommended with an infant.

Defibrillation

Early in the steps of CPR, a rescuer or helper is sent to fetch the AED. Many communities have placed AEDs in public places such as health clubs, public pools, concert halls, sports venues, airports, schools, and government buildings.

The AED has been shown to be an effective lifesaving treatment for adults and children older than 1 year. The AEDs used on children from 1 to 8 years of age usually will have a pediatric-sized

2 minutes), move back to the shockable side of the algorithm. After each drug has been administered, allow it to circulate and then reanalyze the patient at the next 2-minute point.

Useful Adjuncts to Assist in the Return of Spontaneous Circulation

Several devices are available to provide feedback to rescuers on the quality of their compressions (rate, depth, and chest recoil). In addition, three devices hold considerable promise in improving the quality and consistency of the compressions as well as improving the blood flow during CPR: the impedance threshold device (ITD) and two mechanical compression adjuncts (AutoPulse, Thumper).

Impedance Threshold Device

The impedance threshold device (ITD) is marketed as the ResQPOD® in the United States. It has been shown to enhance the vacuum in the chest, which forms during the chest recoil phase of CPR. Imagine a bellows fanning a fireplace. As the bellows opens to its full size, it sucks in air. A similar process occurs when the chest wall re-expands—the vacuum that results pulls air into the lungs and blood back into the heart. An ITD selectively prevents that unnecessary air from rushing into the chest, maximizing the vacuum during the recoil phase of the compression. This results in enhanced return of blood that increases cardiac output, blood pressure, and perfusion to vital organs, and ultimately improves survival rates. Use of the ITD may therefore improve circulation during CPR and increase the return of spontaneous circulation in cardiac arrest patients. This device was given a strong recommendation (a Class IIa rating) by the AHA in its 2005 guidelines due to the strength of the available data on this point. As the patient's pulse returns, however, the ITD should be removed from the ventilation system because it is designed to be used in conjunction with compressions (Figure A-6 ▸).

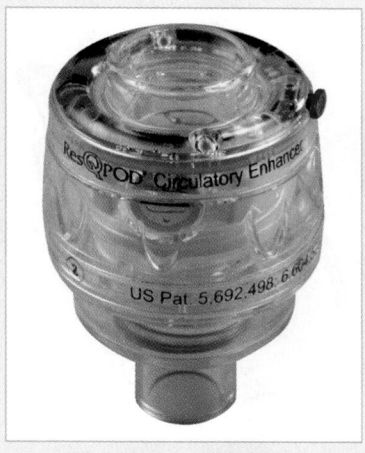

Figure A-6 The ResQPOD®, an impedance threshold device, improves perfusion during CPR.

Load-Distributing Band CPR Device

The AutoPulse device is designed to deliver consistent, uninterrupted chest compressions and therefore improve hemodynamics during cardiac arrest. This automated, portable device offers an easy-to-use, load-distributing LifeBand that squeezes the entire chest, thereby improving blood flow to the heart and brain during cardiac arrest (Figure A-7 ▸). Its use can also free up rescuers to focus on other lifesaving interventions and eliminate fatigue from the performance of CPR chest compressions.

The AutoPulse can be integrated into a code as follows:

1. Ensure that CPR is in progress and that effective, high-quality compressions are being provided.

You are the Provider Part 3

After providing CPR, two shocks with the AED, BLS airway management, an IV, a vasopressor, and then a third shock, the patient has a return of spontaneous circulation. He is being closely monitored and assisted with ventilation at 12 times/min because he is beginning to take some breaths on his own.

Reassessment	Recording Time: 10 Minutes
Level of consciousness	P (Responsive to painful stimuli)
Pulse	96 beats/min, regular
Blood pressure	110/70 mm Hg
Respirations	8 breaths/min, assisted to 12
Sao₂	96% being ventilated with supplemental oxygen
ECG	12-lead shows acute myocardial infarction

5. As this patient has experienced a return of spontaneous circulation prior to an advanced airway being placed, should one now be inserted?

6. If so, which device would be appropriate if experienced providers are present?

7. If you were using an impedance threshold device on the bag mask, should it be continued?

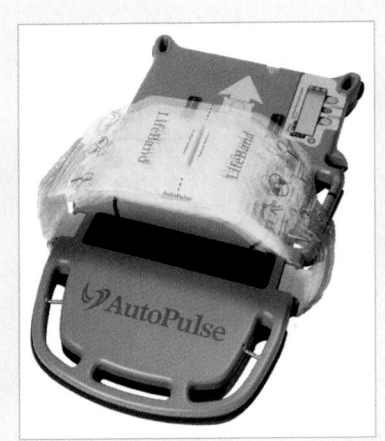

Figure A-7 The AutoPulse® non-invasive cardiac support pump.

2. Align the patient on the AutoPulse platform.

3. Close the LifeBand chest band over the patient's chest.

4. Press the start button (AutoPulse performs the compressions automatically).

5. Provide bag-mask ventilation at a rate of two ventilations for every 30 compressions. Each ventilation should be given over 1 second to provide visible chest rise.

6. If an advanced airway is in place (ETT, LMA, or Combitube), there are no longer cycles of compressions to ventilations. The compression rate is a continuous 100/min; the ventilation rate is 8 to 10/min.

7. After 2 minutes of CPR, reassess for pulse and/or shockable rhythm (maximum of 10 seconds).

Thumper CPR Device

The Thumper (**Figure A-8** ▾) is an adjunct to CPR that provides both continuous chest compressions (100/min) and ventilations. It can be used with a pocket mask or an advanced airway. Because this device is powered by oxygen and delivers oxygen when it ventilates, it does go through a large volume of oxygen. If you use the Thumper, plan to carry additional portable oxygen tanks equipped with high-pressure hose

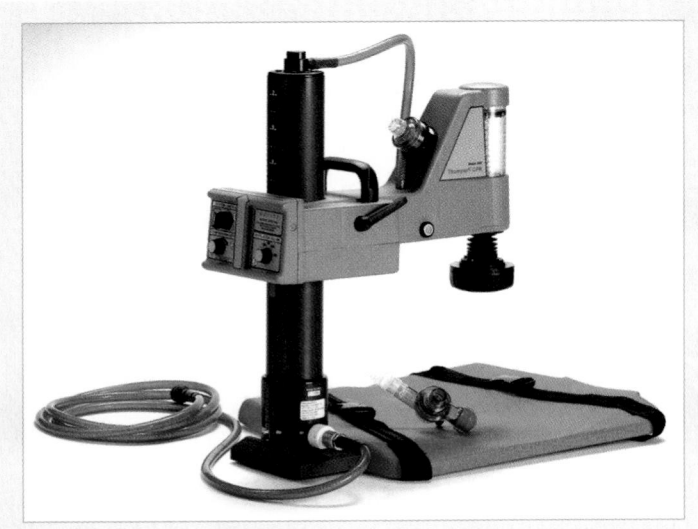

Figure A-8 The Thumper CPR system.

In the Field

Beware the Misplaced Tube!

The AHA's 2005 guidelines include recommendations on tube placement confirmation and continuous monitoring of the tube's position to avoid its dislodgment. To ensure that the tube is inserted in the correct location, after the tube is seen to pass through the vocal cords and the tube position is verified by chest expansion and auscultation during positive-pressure ventilation, the rescuer should obtain additional confirmation of placement using an end-tidal CO_2 or esophageal detection device. No single confirmation technique including clinical signs or the presence of water vapor in the tube, is completely reliable. Your initial techniques of verification should include the following measures:

- Direct visualization of the tube going through the vocal cords.
- Physical examination of the tube placement.
- Bilateral chest expansion.
- Five-point auscultation (two in each lung and epigastrium).
- Tube condensation.

Be sure to use one or more of the following techniques or devices upon initial placement and after any movement of the patient:

- Clinical assessment to confirm tube placement.
- Use of devices to confirm tube placement.
- Exhaled CO_2 devices.
- Esophageal detector devices.

adapters to facilitate rapid transfer of the gas. Use these high-pressure adapters in the ambulance and keep them available for use in the emergency department if the Thumper is used to transport the patient to the emergency department. The Thumper has been particularly useful in lengthy arrests (eg, hypothermic arrest), as it can produce excellent CPR compressions for a long time.

In the past, some services have reserved the use of the Thumper for transport to the hospital. Given that we now know how important high-quality compressions are to the success of the resuscitation, it makes much more sense for the code team to practice simulated codes to ensure they can apply the Thumper as early as possible without any interruptions in manual CPR.

Scene Choreography and Teamwork

During resuscitation, plenty of tasks need to be performed. This is where teamwork comes in. Teamwork divides the task while multiplying the chances for a successful resuscitation. There is a role for each health care provider who is committed to fulfilling his or her part. Experience tells us that teams who

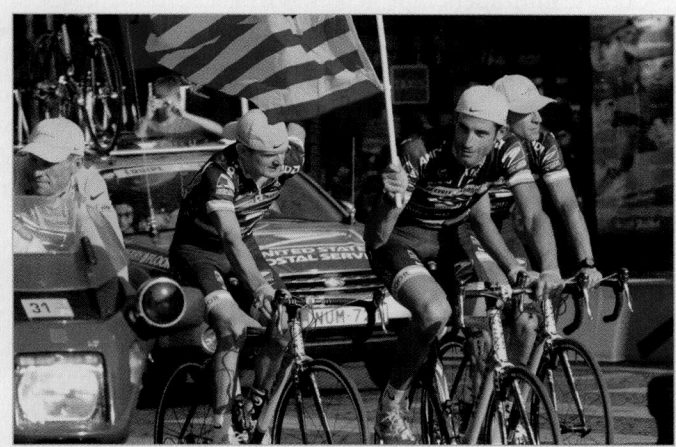

Figure A-9 Even though Lance Armstrong is the only household name on this team, cycling is a team sport.

practice together regularly are more successful in their resuscitation attempts.

Consider the following analogy from the world of sports. From 1999 to 2005, Lance Armstrong and his international team of cyclists set an unprecedented record by winning the Tour de France seven consecutive times Figure A-9 ▲. The Tour is a grueling 21-stage bike race traveling 3,607 km through the tallest mountains and smallest towns into Paris. Cycling is a *team sport*. Each member of the team has a specific role in maintaining the pace, blocking the wind, collecting water bottles and food bags, and helping the team succeed. All team members must be totally committed to the success of the team rather than to their own personal achievements.

The intense preparation and teamwork that characterize any type of high-level sports team hold a few pertinent lessons for code team members:

- Athletes do not only excel on their own. They need the support of their team and coach.
- The coach helps the team members understand the rules of the game and prepare for its challenges.
- The coach drills the athletes with routines or plays and provides constant feedback and plenty of practice opportunities to measure their progress.
- The team trains with the best equipment, eats nutritious meals, develops a positive mental attitude about winning, and gets plenty of rest after enduring rigorous demanding physical and mental exercise.
- When it is time to compete, team members are well prepared, on time, and ready to go. The coach can support

them from the sidelines and may offer signals and guidance or "plays" in some sports, but he or she can't compete for the team.

Code team members who are rested, fit, and well nourished, and who bring a positive attitude to their work, practice their skills, know the "plays," and work together as a team are on top of their game. They are ready to resuscitate patients. To be successful, your team needs to take the following steps:

- Know the plays expertly and automatically. This takes a lot of practice. When there are questions, use posters and pocket cards to explain and prepare.
- Listen to your "coaches." They have the best interests of the patients in mind—and your best interests, too.
- Have a "practice ethic." Pull out the manikins and run mock codes or simulations frequently. Collect data on the cumulative time of interruptions of compressions so that the team has feedback and can work to improve its performance.
- Remember that success equals practice, practice plus a positive mental attitude, well-designed plays (ie, algorithms), and excellent coaching.
- Recognize that the effectiveness of the team is not about you. It's about succeeding as a group. Patients are counting on you to get this right!

Code Team Member and Code Team Leader Roles

Whether you are a code team member or a code team leader, you should know both your own role and the roles of the other members of your code team during the resuscitation attempt. This will help you anticipate what steps are coming next and see how your role is an essential part of the resuscitation attempt. Whatever skills you are trained and appropriately authorized to perform, it is essential to the success of the resuscitation that you are prepared, have practiced regularly, have mastered the algorithms, and are committed to success.

Code Team Member Roles

A code team member may be called on to perform all of the following roles (and more):

- **Ventilator**—managing the airway. This team member's duties include suctioning the patient, applying cricoid pressure, ventilating the patient with a bag-mask device or ATV, inserting an advanced airway device (ie, LMA, ET

You are the Provider Part 4

Your patient experienced an acute myocardial infarction, which threw his heart into V-fib. Fortunately, his teammate responded quickly and initiated the links in the Chain of Survival. After a week in the hospital, the patient went home to his family with a supervised weight loss and exercise program.

tube, or Combitube), and maintaining manual in-line immobilization of the head and neck.

- **Active compressor**—providing high-quality chest compressions. The only responsibility of this team member is to compress for 2 minutes and be the on-deck compressor for 2 minutes.
- **On-deck compressor.** At the 2-minute point, this team member needs to be ready to relieve the compressor without any interruption in compressions. Other functions include assisting with application of mechanical CPR adjunct device (if available), checking on vital signs, and preparing the patient for transport.
- **Other support personnel**—responsible for analyzing the ECG and delivering shocks, gaining venous (IV or IO) access, providing documentation for the patient care report, and supporting family members.

Code Team Leader Roles

Every resuscitation team needs a leader to organize the efforts of the group in a manner similar to that of a conductor leading the individual musicians in an orchestra. Clearly the code team leader must know all of the specific skills and be able to perform each skill expertly—occasionally the code team leader will serve as the backup for a team member who may be having a tough time inserting a tube or gaining IV access. The code team leader is often responsible for making sure everything gets done at the right time in the right way, however.

The roles of the code team leader may include all of the following:

- Taking the patient's history and performing the physical exam.
- Interpreting the ECG.
- Keeping track of the time.
- Making a medication decision following the algorithm.
- Clearly delegating tasks to code team members.
- Completing documentation after the resuscitation attempt.
- Talking with medical control.
- Controlling the resuscitation scene.

 Controversies

To Terminate or Not to Terminate in the Field

Rescuers who begin BLS are taught to continue until one of the following events occurs:

- Effective spontaneous circulation and ventilation are restored.
- Care is transferred to a higher level of care provider, who in turn may determine whether the patient is not responsive to the resuscitative attempt.
- Reliable criteria indicating irreversible death are present.
- The rescuer is unable to continue because of exhaustion or the presence of dangerous environmental hazards or because continuation of the resuscitation effort places other lives in jeopardy.
- A valid DNR order is presented to the rescuers.

Code team leaders must also model excellent behavior and leadership skills for their team and all others who may be involved in the resuscitation. The code team leader should help train future team leaders, seek to improve the effectiveness of the entire team through continuous quality improvement, and practice after the resuscitation to help prepare for the next code.

The AHA's 2005 guidelines say the following about lengthy resuscitative efforts and transporting cardiac arrest patients:

- There are very few instances that require transporting a nontraumatic cardiac arrest patient who has failed a successfully executed prehospital ACLS resuscitation effort to an emergency department to continue the resuscitation attempt.
- In the absence of mitigating factors, prolonged resuscitative efforts are unlikely to be successful. If ROSC of any duration occurs, however, it may be appropriate to consider extending the resuscitative effort.
- Rare exceptions may include severe prehospital hypothermia (eg, submersion in icy water) and drug overdose. A successfully executed prehospital resuscitation includes an "adequate trial" of BLS and ALS.

Transporting a deceased patient who is refractory to proper BLS and ACLS is considered unethical. Protocols for pronouncement of death and appropriate transport of the body by non-EMS vehicles should be established.

■ A Plan for a Code

The following plan is merely an example and is not the "only way"; obviously, different communities have different resources that arrive at different times in different ways. The point is that you need a plan and you need to practice this plan diligently.

This example focuses on a prehospital EMS agency response to a cardiac arrest in a private home, assuming a five-person team that could arrive on different units (eg, EMT unit, paramedic unit, EMS field supervisor with a Thumper or other mechanical CPR-type device) at different times in the first few minutes. Roles for the adult scenario include Compressor 1, Compressor 2, Ventilator, Code Team Leader, and the EMS Field Supervisor:

- **Compressor 1.** Responsible for doing high-quality chest compressions (100/min, press hard and fast, and full chest recoil), stays in position and compresses for 2 minutes and then rests for 2 minutes (for the duration of the time the patient is pulseless), may assist with application of the Thumper (provided Compressor 2 is continuing uninterrupted compressions).
- **Compressor 2.** Responsible for doing high-quality chest compressions (100/min, press hard and fast, and full chest recoil), stays in position and compresses for 2 minutes and then rests for 2 minutes (for the duration of the time the patient is pulseless), may assist with application of the Thumper (provided Compressor 1 is continuing uninterrupted compressions).

- **Ventilator.** Responsible for providing ventilations (bag mask, oropharyngeal airway, oxygen) at a ratio of 30:2 ensuring visible chest rise with each ventilation (1 second in duration). May need to briefly suction the patient as necessary, and then as appropriate will switch over to the ATV. Will assist with the transition from BLS airway to advanced airway (not a high priority). Once an advanced airway is placed, ventilate 8 to 10 times/min to achieve visible chest rise over a 1-second duration for each ventilation.
- **Code team leader.** Responsible for initial ECG analysis and defibrillation with a single shock (200 J). Responsible for overall timing of the code and reassessment after 2 minutes of cycles of CPR with the interruption not to exceed 10 seconds. After the initial shock (or ascertaining "no shock" rhythm), proceed to establish IV or IO access (no medications down the tube), then begin a vasopressor every 3 to 5 minutes (1 mg epinephrine 1:10,000, with vasopressin as an acceptable substitute for the first or second—but not both—doses of epinephrine), help to transition the airway from BLS to an advanced airway (ET tube, Combitube, or LMA), and continue with single shocks every 2 minutes if patient is still in V-tach or V-fib.

Make the decision with input from the code team and medical control that the resuscitation should be terminated if there is no ROSC in the first 15 minutes. If there is ROSC, administer the appropriate antidysrrhythmic (eg, amiodarone, lidocaine), ensure appropriate ventilations, and assist the team in preparing for transport.

- **EMS field supervisor.** Bring in the Thumper and work with one of the compressors to transition the patient to mechanical CPR compressions with minimal interruption. Assist the medic with IV or IO, advanced airway placement, and preparation of medications, and contact medical control, per local protocols.

Vital Vocabulary

asynchronous In CPR, when two rescuers do ventilations and compressions individually and not timed or waiting for the other rescuer to pause.

code team leader The code team member who has the responsibility for managing the rescuers or team members during a cardiac arrest, as well as choreographing the effort of the group.

code team member A member of the resuscitation team trying to revive the patient.

You are the Provider Summary

1. Arriving on the scene of an apparent cardiac arrest with bystanders who have initiated care, how should you evaluate the quality of CPR?

Look at the depth of compressions, listen to hear if the compressor is counting to 30, and observe for full chest recoil.

2. Many elementary schools and public places have an AED available. How might that have helped in this situation?

The teammates could have quickly obtained the AED, and Tom could have used it within the first 4 minutes or the electrical phase of the arrest.

3. What should you do next as the paramedic on the scene?

Take over the role of the code team leader and focus on perfusion and choreographing the arrest.

4. What is the advantage to perfusion and chest compressions from inserting an advanced airway during two-rescuer CPR?

With an advanced airway inserted, the two rescuers can switch over to asynchronous CPR with compressions at 100/min and ventilations every 6 to 8 seconds.

5. As this patient experienced a return of spontaneous circulation prior to an advanced airway being placed, should one be inserted?

As time is available. As long as the patient will tolerate an ET tube and you have an experienced provider, it would be appropriate to insert one.

6. If so, which device would be appropriate if an experienced provider is present?

For the patient with ROSC and no gag reflex, the ET tube makes the most sense.

7. If you were using an impedance threshold device on the bag mask, should it be continued?

No. This device is designed for use with the patient in cardiac arrest during CPR. It should not be used after resuscitation.

Objectives

Cognitive

7-1.1   Explain how effective assessment is critical to clinical decision making. (p B.3)

7-1.2   Explain how the paramedic's attitude affects assessment and decision making. (p B.5)

7-1.3   Explain how uncooperative patients affect assessment and decision making. (p B.5)

7-1.4   Explain strategies to prevent labeling and tunnel vision. (p B.5)

7-1.5   Develop strategies to decrease environmental distractions. (p B.5)

7-1.6   Describe how manpower considerations and staffing configurations affect assessment and decision making. (p B.5)

7-1.7   Synthesize concepts of scene management and choreography to simulated emergency calls. (p B.10)

7-1.8   Explain the roles of the team leader and the patient care person. (p B.6)

7-1.9   List and explain the rationale for carrying the essential patient care items. (p B.7)

7-1.10   When given a simulated call, list the appropriate equipment to be taken to the patient. (p B.7)

7-1.11   Explain the general approach to the emergency patient. (p B.7)

7-1.12   Explain the general approach, patient assessment, differentials, and management priorities for patients with the following problems:
- a. Chest pain
- b. Medical and traumatic cardiac arrest
- c. Acute abdominal pain
- d. GI bleed
- e. Altered mental status
- f. Dyspnea
- g. Syncope
- h. Seizures
- i. Environmental or thermal problem
- j. Hazardous material or toxic exposure
- k. Trauma or multi trauma patients
- l. Allergic reactions
- m. Behavioral problems
- n. Obstetric or gynecological problems
- o. Pediatric patients (p B.8–B.11)

7-1.13   Describe how to effectively communicate patient information face to face, over the telephone, by radio, and in writing. (p B.19)

Affective

7-1.14   Appreciate the use of scenarios to develop high level clinical decision making skills. (p B.10)

7-1.15   Defend the importance of considering differentials in patient care. (p B.7)

7-1.16   Advocate and practice the process of complete patient assessment on all patients. (p B.3)

7-1.17   Value the importance of presenting the patient accurately and clearly. (p B.9)

Psychomotor

7-1.18   While serving as team leader, choreograph the EMS response team, perform a patient assessment, provide local/regionally appropriate treatment, present cases verbally and in writing given a moulaged and programmed simulated patient. (p B.6)

7-1.19   While serving as team leader, assess a programmed patient or mannequin, consider differentials, make decisions relative to interventions and transportation, provide the interventions, patient packaging and transportation, work as a team and practice various roles for the following common emergencies:
- a. Chest pain
- b. Cardiac arrest
  1. Traumatic arrest
  2. Medical arrest
- c. Acute abdominal pain
- d. GI bleed
- e. Altered mental status
- f. Dyspnea
- g. Syncope
- h. Seizure
- i. Thermal/environmental problem
- j. Hazardous materials/toxicology
- k. Trauma
  1. Isolated extremity fracture (tibia/fibula or radius/ulna)
  2. Femur fracture
  3. Shoulder dislocation
  4. Clavicular fracture or A-C separation
  5. Minor wound (no sutures required, sutures required, high risk wounds, with tendon and/or nerve injury)
  6. Spine injury (no neurologic deficit, with neurologic deficit)
  7. Multiple trauma—blunt
  8. Penetrating trauma
  9. Impaled object
  10. Elderly fall
  11. Athletic injury
  12. Head injury (concussion, subdural/epidural)
- l. Allergic reactions/bites/envenomation
  1. Local allergic reaction
  2. Systemic allergic reaction
  3. Envenomation
- m. Behavioral
  1. Mood disorders
  2. Schizophrenic and delusional disorders
  3. Suicidal
- n. Obstetrics/gynecology
  1. Vaginal bleeding
  2. Childbirth (normal and abnormal)
- o. Pediatric
  1. Respiratory distress
  2. Fever
  3. Seizures (p B.8–B.11)

Introduction

This appendix reviews the standardized approach to patient assessment, which is the format used and reinforced throughout each chapter of this text. Mastery of the standardized approach to patient assessment is a key clinical skill that helps characterize the best paramedics. Only after you have developed a strong foundation in patient assessment and broad clinical experience can you confidently make clinical judgments and adapt the standardized format to meet each patient's immediate needs.

This appendix also covers some of the finer points about assessment, dealing with people, and the importance of working as a team. Many of these strategies are presented throughout the text in the cases and will be used in the laboratory exercises in your paramedic training program.

Effective Assessment

The care that you provide is built on a strong base consisting of quality assessment of the patient. For this reason, much of your training program emphasizes assessment, and the scenarios or simulations you participate in during your classroom activities involve constant practice assessing patients. You simply cannot properly treat a patient without taking the time and effort to assess his or her situation. Likewise, you cannot obtain medical orders for patient treatment interventions or medication orders without first assessing the patient so you can report your findings.

Paramedics follow a uniform format to gather, evaluate, and synthesize the information. This consistency helps you, in consultation with medical control, make the right patient care management decisions and take the corresponding appropriate actions. Conversely, not doing an effective assessment can lead you down a bumpy road where the decision making can have disastrous results for the patient.

Accurate information is critical to your decision making. If an EMT-Basic or first responder is too embarrassed to admit he or she could not really hear the patient's blood pressure and makes up data, this "vital de jour" can lead to inappropriate decision making, poor patient care, or a lack of confidence in the provider's abilities. If you cannot feel, hear, or interpret essential information, such as vital signs, the best course is to immediately say you are having some difficulty obtaining the information and get some help. Perhaps the blood pressure is so low that it is not easy to hear or feel, or perhaps you are just having a bad day. It isn't always important that you make a mistake—it is what you do with your mistakes when they occur that is very important!

You are the Provider Part 1

After you check out the ambulance and grab a quick cup of coffee, it's 7:00 AM already. The pager tones go off, and the dispatcher alerts you to an incoming call. A head-on collision has just occurred in a suburban neighborhood not far from your station. The police, the fire department, a second ambulance, and a supervisor are all en route because they have received multiple calls on the crash that may involve a fire and entrapment.

The police arrive first and begin to control the flow of traffic. They report that the smoke was from an airbag, not a car fire. They notify the dispatcher to continue the response because there are two older patients, one in each vehicle, and it is not clear whether either is trapped. The fire department arrives next, and the incident command system is set up. The incident commander (IC) reports that there is no fire but a rescue company is needed to open the car doors. Both patients are conscious, elderly women. One patient may have her legs trapped; the other is very confused.

Your ambulance arrives next, and you size up the scene as you approach it. The mechanism of injury (MOI) is significant: There is a considerable amount of damage to the front ends of both vehicles, and the rear of the second vehicle has been pushed into a telephone pole. There are also some cracks in the windshield, which may explain the bleeding from the driver's head.

The IC fills you in on the details as you quickly don your personal protective gear—standard operating procedure at all collisions involving a rescue. The police officer said that one woman is acting as if she is highly intoxicated but he has not yet gotten a breathalyzer reading on her. The second ambulance and the supervisor are just arriving, so you are assigned to deal with the confused woman who, according to the police, "may have been the one to cause the crash."

Initial Assessment	Recording Time: 1 Minute
Appearance	A woman in her late 50s. She is bleeding from a head laceration, nervous, scared, and very confused.
Level of consciousness	V (Responsive to verbal stimuli); knows name, not sure of day or where she is
Airway	Open and clear
Breathing	Rapid but no obvious life threats at this time
Circulation	She has a weak radial pulse and no life-threatening bleeding.

1. What are some of the potential causes of a head-on collision in which the driver never hit the brakes?
2. What is the significance of the MOI in this collision for your patient?
3. If it is clear that your patient was not wearing a seatbelt, how could this fact change things?

In patient assessment, the history is critically important. Some experts believe that 80% of a medical diagnosis is based solely on the history and not on objective data, such as vital signs, laboratory test results, and ECGs. If you have gained a broad knowledge of diseases and medical conditions through your training, reading, and field experience, you will have many profiles with which you can compare the objective and subjective findings of the history. This "pattern recognition," helps you develop a "working differential diagnosis." With excellent history gathering and interviewing skills, you can focus the physical examination and assessment to arrive at the most accurate field diagnosis and assist emergency department (ED) staff in arriving at the admission diagnosis.

The Importance of the Physical Exam

The physical exam should be "vectored"—that is, focused on the body system that the chief complaint and history suggest is the source of the problem. **Table B-1 ▼** summarizes the types of physical exams that you have encountered in this text.

You will practice these physical exams as part of your training program numerous times until you master them. The exams will then be incorporated into classroom lab simulations of patient scenarios to help prepare you for their field application.

Observational studies show that paramedics who have clearly demonstrated in practical skills testing that they know the steps and sequences of the exams and know when they are supposed to use them nevertheless overlook the physical exams or apply them in only a cursory manner in the field. Ideally, your paramedic instructors and partners will model and instill excellent work habits and a practice ethic so that you will conduct the physical exams appropriately when your patient's condition warrants their use.

Developing an Action Plan

After you obtain subjective information from the patient through your interviewing skills (that is, OPQRST and SAMPLE) and then obtain objective findings by obtaining vital signs and other parameters (such as ECG, SpO_2, $ETCO_2$ blood glucose level, and other clinical findings), the next step is assessment and developing a treatment plan. The more extensive the knowledge base of clinical profiles (that is, typical clinical pictures) you have, the better your chances of making an accurate assessment. Pattern recognition and "gut instinct" based on lots of field experience have key roles in this decision process. Once the assessment has been completed, a treatment or action plan must be developed. Some of the treatment will have already begun if the initial assessment revealed life threats based on the patient's mental status or ABCs.

Your action plan for treatment of the patient must consider the priority and severity of the patient's condition, the environmental conditions, and the BLS and ALS treatment protocols used in your region. Many states have established a statewide BLS protocol but left the choice of ALS protocols to the regions of the state. Typically, the local or regional ALS protocols usually are built on the American Heart Association's adult and pediatric algorithms for acute coronary syndrome (ACS), stroke, dysrhythmias, or pulseless arrest. In addition, these protocols usually address the care of trauma patients following the standards and the appropriate field management requested by their trauma and burn centers. **Table B-2 ▼** shows an example of a statewide ALS protocol.

Some protocols are written in an assessment-based format in which the topics are typical assessment findings such as breathing difficulty, chest pain, and altered mental status. Most protocols—including the asthma, allergic reaction, head trauma, and suspected stroke protocols—involve a combination of assessment findings and presumptive clinical assessments (a "working field diagnosis"). You would need to arrive at the right clinical impression to know which protocol to use. In most protocols, a statement in the preface discusses the issue of clinical

Table B-1	Types of Physical Exams
Exam	**Description**
Rapid trauma exam/ assessment	Provided for a trauma patient with significant MOI
Rapid physical exam/ assessment	Provided for a medical patient who is not responsive
Detailed physical exam	Provided en route to the ED for a trauma patient with a significant MOI
Neurologic exam	Assesses the Cincinnati Stroke Scale, cranial nerves, and sensory and motor function in each extremity
Cardiopulmonary (heart/lungs) exam	Includes an assessment of the lung sounds, heart sounds, JVD (jugular venous distention), pedal edema, and ECG
Obstetric exam	Includes checking for crowning in a woman in labor
Other exams	For specific patient complaints

Table B-2	Florida ALS Protocol for Heat Stroke

Supportive Care

Trauma Supportive Care Protocol 2.1.4.

- Remove from warm environment and aggressively cool patient. Remove patient's clothing and wet patient directly with ice water. Also, turn A/C and fans on high and apply ice packs to head, neck, chest and groin.
- Monitor temperature. Cool patient to 102°F, then dry patient, remove ice packs, and turn off fans (avoid lowering temperature too much).

ALS Level 1

- Treat hypotension (systolic BP < 90 mm Hg) with IV fluids. Avoid using vasopressors and anticholinergic drugs (may potentiate heat stroke by inhibiting sweating). Administer fluid challenge of normal saline 500 mL IV.

ALS Level 2

None

judgment. Sometimes it takes this kind of clinical judgment to realize which specific protocol is the best to follow, especially when a patient has multiple presenting problems. Good judgment is developed over time and is based on supervised clinical experience plus common sense. Protocols have been described as "cookbooks for a thinking cook." Paramedics with good judgment know when and how to consult with medical direction to consider deviating from their cookbook.

Factors Affecting the Ability to Assess Patients and Make Decisions

Your attitude can significantly influence your assessment and decision-making abilities. We all have spent a good part of our lives developing attitudes, values, and biases—some helpful and some destructive. When you become a paramedic, you must leave your attitude and your ego at the door! Not everyone keeps their home the way you do, nor does every person look the same, act the same, or have the same values. Your patients' choices are not good or bad, just as yours are not good or bad. They just might be different from what you have become accustomed to. Steer clear of assigning "labels" to or stereotyping patients and their families. Referring to patients by derogatory names or slurs is disrespectful and distracting and often leads to a biased and incomplete assessment. Remember, patients call us to provide medical care—not to judge them or their families or their homes. Don't try to judge your patients, but rather treat their conditions as you would expect care to be provided to one of your loved ones.

Attempting to prejudge the situation or the patient leads to a form of myopia (tunnel vision), as if you have blinders on and miss everything in the periphery. This behavior can hamper your information gathering and cause you not to collect enough information for a thorough assessment. It is distracting and leads you to "lock on" to a field impression too early before you have analyzed all the facts. Such an inappropriate gut instinct can cause you to make poor judgments about a patient's medical condition based on past experiences. If you have collected insufficient information to recognize the patterns of injury or a medical condition, you may not be able to make an accurate assessment, or if you do, it will often take longer. Quality management of the patient depends on an accurate medical assessment, not whether you like the patient.

Uncooperative patients can be difficult to assess. When a patient is nasty, your first reaction may be to pack up and leave. Nevertheless, it is important to remember that this person may be "under the influence"—not necessarily of alcohol or drugs. Many patients who are acting out, belligerent, or restless may be reacting to a medical or traumatic situation such as hypoxia, hypovolemia, hypoglycemia, hypothermia, head injury, or concussion. Always rule out medical or traumatic causes for irritability and lack of cooperation before assuming the behavior is due to intoxication or a behavioral problem.

Sometimes patients have a very distracting injury, such as the fracture shown in Figure B-1 ▶ . Always follow the plan you have been taught: scene size-up, initial assessment (mental status, ABCs, priority decision), determination of the significance of the MOI, and then appropriate focused history and physical exam. Do not allow a distracting injury to divert your attention from the assessment plan. If necessary, temporarily cover the injury with a towel and continue your assessment! You will ultimately get to it at the proper point in the assessment. You do not want to treat the leg and lose the life because the patient was not breathing adequately.

The number of responders is a factor that definitely needs to be worked into the team's approach to patient assessment and management. Regardless of the various ways in which your local EMS system responds (one, two, or multiple tiers), once at the scene, the team can consist of two to four or more responders with varying levels of training. How the scene is managed, who the team leader is, and how assessment information is gathered (sequential versus simultaneous) needs to be practiced in advance. Patients dislike assessment by committee, in which two or more providers grill the patient at the same time. This practice can be confusing, often no one gets the entire story, and the patient may repeatedly be asked the same questions.

Sometimes the prehospital environment can prove a major distraction to your assessment. If you are prepared for the possibilities, you can consider strategies to deal with them proactively rather than reacting to them. Examples of environmental distracters include crowds, unruly bystanders, potentially violent or dangerous situations, high noise levels, and an excessive number of EMS providers at the scene. If the presence of too many people makes it difficult for you to do your job, politely ask them to wait elsewhere or release the extra responders from the scene. You might also move the patient into your "office" (the back of the ambulance). If an unruly crowd obstructs your assessment or rocks the ambulance, drive around the block!

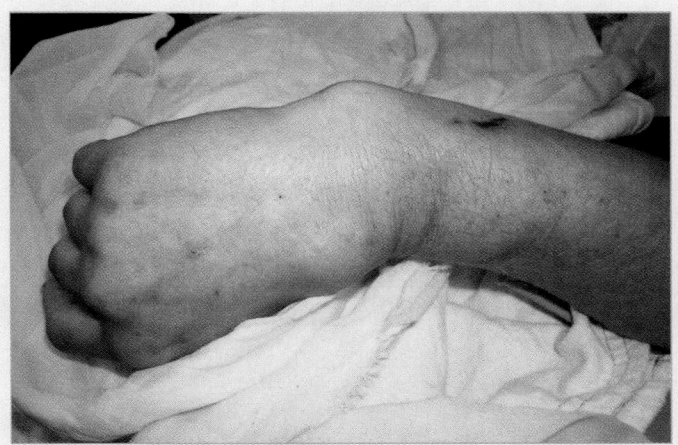

Figure B-1 This fracture is distracting but not an immediate life threat. Don't let it interfere with your initial assessment to locate the real life threats.

Finally, patient compliance issues may sometimes present obstacles to assessment and management. If the patient has difficulty confiding in you or any of the other rescuers, it can limit the information you have to make accurate decisions. Some patients simply will not tell you their medical history. Be careful not to spark this "problem" by displaying an attitude or body language that says you are disinterested or not really someone the patient can trust. Sensitivity to cultural and ethnic factors is also important and should be included in your training and classroom lab simulations.

Scene Choreography

The importance of a team leader choreographing the activities of the team at the scene of an emergency cannot be overstated. As described in Appendix A, the code team leader and code team members have specific roles that must be constantly practiced and carried out correctly to increase the success of prehospital resuscitations. Indeed, the role of the team leader is key to the coordinated effort of the entire team. Achieving this kind of coordination can be challenging when there are too few or too many responders at the scene. Clearly, the team gives its best response when a single leader manages and monitors the team's efforts with a clear understanding of the strategies, goals, and plans for the particular situation.

The team concept should be practiced not just for a cardiac arrest call. Instead, the team concept needs to be reinforced in the classroom lab setting with practice in numerous simulated responses. The team members and team leader will then be better prepared to respond quickly and effectively in the prehospital setting with real emergencies.

Practice is critically important, including practice in rotating roles and cross-training to assume various roles should the need arise. Some two-paramedic ambulance teams rotate responsibilities or roles by the call, with one partner being the driver/skills paramedic and the other the patient contact/assessment paramedic (team leader) who will ride in the patient compartment en route to the ED. If the call involves more team members, they are added to this basic response and one paramedic assumes the team leader role. If only two partners are on the scene, one establishes rapport and conducts the assessment of the patient, while the other handles the on-scene skills such as obtaining vital signs, applying oxygen, and inserting an IV. Because one paramedic will drive to the ED, he or she will most likely clean the stretcher and the back of the ambulance and prepare for the next call while the paramedic who rode with the patient to the ED gives the radio report, gives the face-to-face verbal report on arrival, and completes the patient care report (PCR).

Is this approach the perfect strategy for all EMS units? No, it is just one good way. Other strategies might work equally well. What is essential is that the roles have been practiced and worked out before arriving at the patient's side. If the team has a plan and the situation is complex, the responders have a basic starting point to adapt the response or actions to meet the challenges of the environment or situation.

Pull out the equipment, break into teams, and practice simulated responses with experienced educator/evaluators to document your actions for a post-simulation analysis. Discuss what went right and what did not, and figure out how improvements can be made to the equipment, the team members' performance, and their communication within the team, with patients and families, and with leadership. The next simulation—which could be the real thing—can flow smoothly and look as if it had been practiced a hundred times.

You are the Provider Part 2

From your initial patient assessment, it was clear that the patient is confused, yet the rest of the initial assessment seems unremarkable. Her chief complaint seems to be medical (altered mental status), so you proceed down the patient assessment algorithm and conduct a focused history and physical exam of a responsive medical patient—that is, you interview the patient and obtain a history before conducting the physical exam. Your partner obtains the baseline vital signs while you interview the patient.

Vital Signs	Recording Time: 4 Minutes
Skin	Pale, warm, and clammy
Pulse	118 beats/min; weak, regular rate
Blood pressure	110/70 mm Hg
Respirations	24 breaths/min and normal

4. What is the value of using mnemonics such as OPQRST and SAMPLE in your assessment?
5. If the patient had been "not responsive," which steps would your focused history and physical exam involve?

EMS Equipment

When Tom Wolfe wrote *The Right Stuff* in 1979, he was describing what it took to be one of the first seven astronauts selected by NASA for the space program. Similarly, a paramedic responding to emergency calls must carry the "right stuff"—that is, equipment that is packaged and at the patient's side when you need it. As paramedics, we always need to be prepared for the worst-case scenarios, which are threats to the patient's ABCs.

Not having equipment readily available compromises care. Consider a patient who has struck his head and has altered mental status. If he started vomiting and you did not have PPE (personal protective equipment) and a suction unit, the patient could easily aspirate.

Planning which EMS equipment to carry is a bit like traveling on a plane with only a carry-on bag that will fit in the overhead bin. You need to carry the essential items, downsize to facilitate rapid movement throughout the airport, and minimize the bulk and weight of the baggage. The essential equipment needs to be carried on every call to every patient's side. It includes the equipment to conduct the initial assessment and treat life threats you may find, as well as the cardiac monitor and defibrillator. **Table B-3 ▶** summarizes this set of equipment.

The specific equipment, bags, and boxes depend on your local protocols, standing order flexibility, the typical number of paramedic and EMT-B responders, and the difficulty in accessing the patient. Many EMS services continue to use the same plastic "fishing tackle" boxes that have long served as paramedic drug boxes.

General Approach to the Patient

Your general approach to the patient entails more than simply following the standardized assessment plan. You must have a calm demeanor, look the part, act the part, and have a kind manner. For some paramedics, these details come naturally; for others, they take practice. Practicing your approach is essential for ensuring that you can communicate effectively and provide the level of service patients expect to receive. Most patients are not in a position to rate your ability to conduct an accurate assessment, intubate, or insert an IV line (aside from how much it hurt or how big a mess you made), but they do gauge the quality of care in terms of the "people skills" provided and the level of compassion you showed.

Your approach to the patient should be planned in advance, in terms of which team member will do most of the talking and questioning and establish the rapport with the patient while the other team members focus on the necessary skills and equipment issues. Make sure you take in the right stuff and are ready to provide resuscitative care because confusion about equipment can unnecessarily add to the level of chaos. As the paramedic doing the assessment, you must carry on an active, concerned dialogue. Take notes—and listen to what the patient tells you!

Table B-3	Essential Equipment
Function	**Essential Items**
Airway control	PPE (gloves, face shield, and HEPA or N-95 mask) Oral airways, nasal airways Suction unit (electric or manual) Rigid tip Yankauer and flexible suction catheters LMA, Combitube, ET tubes Laryngoscope and blades Tube check, tube restraint, tape, syringes, stylet End-tidal carbon dioxide device
Breathing	Pocket mask and one-way valve Bag-mask ventilation device(s) (adult and child), spare masks Oxygen-delivery devices (nonrebreathing mask, cannula, extension tubing) Oxygen tank, regulator, transport ventilator Occlusive dressings Large-bore IV catheter for thoracic decompression Pulse oximeter
Circulation	Dressings, bandages, and tape Sphygmomanometer, stethoscope Assessment card and pen Impedance threshold device (ITD) and CPR prompt AED or manual defibrillator Drug box Glucometer Venous access supplies (IV and IO)
Disability and dysrhythmia	Rigid collars Flashlight ECG monitor
Exposure	Space blanket to cover the patient Scissors

Review of the Standardized Approach to Assessment

Throughout this book, we have emphasized using the same basic approach to the assessment of the patient. In summary, every scene gets a size-up to locate the hazards, recognize the MOI, and ensure you have the appropriate BSI and adequate help. The first assessment for every patient is the initial assessment, which is designed to find and deal with life threats. It includes the MS-ABC-priority elements: a check of the patient's mental status using AVPU; assessment and management of the airway, breathing, and circulation; and setting the priority as high or low for this specific patient. Next, the patient is classified as medical or trauma. Although there are some crossovers (such as a geriatric patient with a broken hip who had a syncopal episode), usually a patient will have one overwhelming problem type.

Trauma patients are further subclassified into one of two groups: those with a significant MOI and those without a significant MOI. A patient with a significant MOI will get a rapid trauma exam, with baseline vital signs and SAMPLE history being taken as you prepare the patient for transport. He or she will then get a detailed physical exam and ongoing assessment en route to the regional trauma center. For patients with a non-significant MOI, the exam focuses on the injured body part and then baseline vital signs, a SAMPLE history, and transport. These patients do not routinely receive a detailed physical exam, rather they receive an ongoing assessment en route to the ED.

Medical patients are likewise subclassified into two groups: those who are responsive and those who are not responsive. The focus in these cases is on the chief complaint, because your line of questioning will depend on how the patient presents. In all cases, you can use the OPQRST mnemonic to remember how to elaborate on the patient's chief complaint. The patient who does not respond appropriately (is not responsive) receives the same rapid exam that the trauma patient with significant MOI would receive, but it is termed the rapid physical exam in medical cases (rather than the rapid trauma exam, as in trauma cases). Next, baseline vital signs and a SAMPLE history are obtained; for a patient who is not responsive, this history may come from bystanders and family members. All medical patients receive an ongoing assessment en route to the ED.

A medical patient who is responsive will provide you with most of the information needed to arrive at a working field diagnosis if you ask the right questions. In a responsive patient, you should elaborate on the chief complaint, obtain baseline vital signs and a SAMPLE history, and conduct a physical exam that focuses on the body system involved in the chief complaint (such as a neurologic exam, a cardiopulmonary exam, or an obstetric exam). You can then conduct the ongoing assessment en route to the ED.

From a priority or sense of urgency perspective, some trauma patients have a significant MOI and some medical patients are not responsive; with these patients, you should take an urgent, rapid resuscitative approach. Conversely, with trauma patients without a significant MOI and medical patients who are responsive, you can take a slightly more contemplative and less rushed approach. Of course, we are still cognizant of the time with some responsive medical patients (such as for a possible MI or stroke)!

This approach to the patient assessment is the same for all levels of EMS providers. The only difference between assessment provided by emergency responders, EMT-Bs, EMT-Is, and paramedics is the addition of specific lab tests (such as blood glucose or ECG) and the clinical treatment prerogatives in your "toolbox."

Presenting the Patient

Your ability to present your patient to the next link in the chain of medical care can be a key element in ensuring continuity of care. Effective communication and transfer of the patient's assessment and management data are vital to prehospital caregivers and in-hospital providers who will ultimately be

You are the Provider Part 3

From your focused history and physical exam of the patient, you have learned that she is confused about the car crash and does not remember what happened. She is not sure if she passed out, although a bystander who heard the crash states that the patient was sleepy just after the accident.

The patient denies having any pain but thinks she is going to miss her morning meeting with her friends. By using the SAMPLE history, you find out that the patient has medication in her pocketbook, which is a clue that she has type 2 diabetes. The patient is not sure whether she had any breakfast this morning because she was running very late for her appointment.

You decide to obtain an ECG and a finger stick to check her blood glucose level. Your partner starts an IV. Her blood glucose level is very low, which is one of many possible explanations for her altered mental state.

After receiving 50 mL/25 mg of dextrose IV, the patient seems like a different person. She is alert and very apologetic about causing so much trouble. She says she must have forgotten to eat this morning because she was in a big rush to meet her friends. She asks you to contact her daughter who lives nearby and laughs as the police officer has her take a breathalyzer test, which is found to be negative. As you prepare to leave the scene, your patient inquires about the other woman whose car she hit. You are able to tell her that fortunately, after she was disentangled, the injuries were minor because she was wearing her seatbelt.

Vital Signs	Recording Time: 10 Minutes
Skin	Pale, warm, and clammy
Pulse	118 beats/min; weak, regular rate
Blood pressure	110/p mm Hg
Respirations	24 breaths/min; normal
Blood glucose	56 mg/dL

6. Why might you suspect that the patient has type 2 diabetes?

7. As long as she has a gag reflex, which medication options do you have?

responsible for the patient. Refining this skill is important so that the right amount of the right information is presented to the right person at the right time.

An Essential Skill

The number of calls involving other typical paramedic skills (such as IV insertion or drug administration) may be minimal compared with the number of times you must present the patient to another health care provider face-to-face, over the telephone, over the radio, or in writing on the PCR. Effective presentation and communications skills are essential for continuity of care and to establish trust and credibility with the medical control physician.

Good assessment and excellent presentation skills go hand in hand. After all, you can't report or treat anything that you haven't found! A good presentation suggests effective patient assessment; a poor presentation suggests poor assessment and care. The format that we use minimizes rambling and disjointed presentations that cover inconsequential information but omit vital information. Most health care providers are also programmed to mentally receive a patient presentation in a specific format. The format we recommend follows the SOAP mnemonic: Subjective information, Objective information, Assessment, and Plan for treatment.

A poor presentation can compromise the patient's care because the paramedic often relies on physician orders to administer specific medications and procedures. If the report was inaccurate or so disjointed that it was "not listened to" or understood by the physician, essential care may not be ordered when needed.

An effective patient presentation is concise, usually lasting about a minute. It should be free of medical jargon and follow the same basic information pattern (that is, the SOAP format). It should also include pertinent positives (such as dyspnea with clear lung sounds) and pertinent negatives (such as head injury with no loss of consciousness).

Components of an Effective Patient Presentation

The format for a radio report to medical control typically includes the following key components:

- Your unit identifier, level of training, and appropriate medical channel authorized for transmission
- Patient identification information, such as age, sex, and degree of distress
- The chief complaint or reason the ambulance was called
- The present illness or injury, which includes the MOI and an elaboration of the chief complaint using OPQRST
- The medical history obtained using the SAMPLE protocol
- Physical examination findings—pertinent positives and pertinent negatives
- Your assessment or working field diagnosis
- The treatment plan, including what has been done so far, what you will be doing, and any medical orders you are requesting
- Your estimated time of arrival (ETA) at the facility

Radio reports that do not involve medical control (BLS reports for notification) are usually briefer. Face-to-face reports are usually slightly more detailed, bringing the ED nurse or physician up-to-date on what has transpired during your care of the patient.

An example of a medical control radio report using this format follows:

Telemetry Dispatcher: *Go ahead, Medic 785. You are clear to transmit with MD 802 from Saint Peter's Hospital on Med Channel 2.*

Medic 785: *MD 802, this is Medic 785 on Med 2. How do you read?*

MD 802: *Medic 785, this is MD 802. You are loud and clear. Proceed with your transmission.*

Medic 785: *I am treating a 58-year-old male in moderate distress with a chief complaint of chest pain. He states it came on suddenly while shoveling snow. He describes the pain as "a crushing sensation under his breastbone" and states it radiates down his left arm. The pain is a 7 on 10, and he has had the pain for about 20 minutes. The patient states he has no relevant history and denies shortness of breath. He has an allergy to Novocain and takes 325 mg of aspirin daily and 10 mg of Lipitor (atorvastatin). He has a history of hypertension and high cholesterol with CAD (coronary artery disease) in his family. His last oral intake was lunch 3 hours ago and the 162 mg of chewable aspirin the dispatcher advised him to take before our arrival. The events leading up to the incident involved shoveling heavy snow.*

Physical exam reveals some crackles at the bases of both lungs, but no JVD or pedal edema. His vital signs are respirations of 20 and regular; pulse of 110, strong and regular; and a BP of 146/82 mm Hg. His pulse ox is 96 on a nonrebreathing mask. His ECG is sinus tach with no ectopy, but the 12-lead shows ST-segment elevation in V$_3$ and V$_4$ (a possible anterior wall MI). We are treating him as a rule-out MI and have administered morphine, oxygen, and nitro; aspirin was self-administered. We are currently transporting, and our plan is to continue monitoring him and go through the rest of the fibrinolytic checklist. We are requesting an order for 5 mg of metoprolol.

MD 802: *Medic 785, go ahead and administer 5 mg metoprolol and I will alert the cath lab staff right away.*

Medic 785: *Received. Be advised our ETA is 20 minutes.*

The keys to developing proficiency with a radio report or a face-to-face report are repetition and understanding the format. We suggest you use an assessment card that highlights the key areas of the radio report. Many pocket guides include this sample format for reference. Eventually, after much practice, you will no longer need the form or pocket guide to refer to because the communication format will be second nature. It is also helpful to practice giving radio reports for simulated patients into a cassette recorder. Soon you will notice that reports on real patients in the field come easily and flow off your tongue.

Simulations Using Common Complaints Found in the Prehospital Setting

Your paramedic program will offer scenario-based practice in the lab setting designed to help prepare you for the internship experience. These simulations take place after you have learned core paramedic skills (that is, ECG, IV, drug administration) and the treatment algorithms for complaints commonly encountered in the field. You will have the opportunity to work with the typical equipment and team members just as interactions would occur in the prehospital setting.

The goals of these simulations include practicing the teamwork, team leadership, and scene choreography discussed in this appendix. You will have many opportunities to work with the equipment and practice the assessment format and skills of paramedics. Likewise, you will have a chance to work on your leadership and decision-making abilities so you can provide interventions that are based on assessment and the treatment modalities in the regional treatment protocols and the ACLS algorithms. In addition, you will have ample opportunities to practice your verbal presentation skills and documentation using the PCR for review by your paramedic faculty.

Most simulations in the lab setting can be done on preprogrammed "patients" or manikins designed to allow you to use your core skills. Some paramedic programs use highly sophisti-

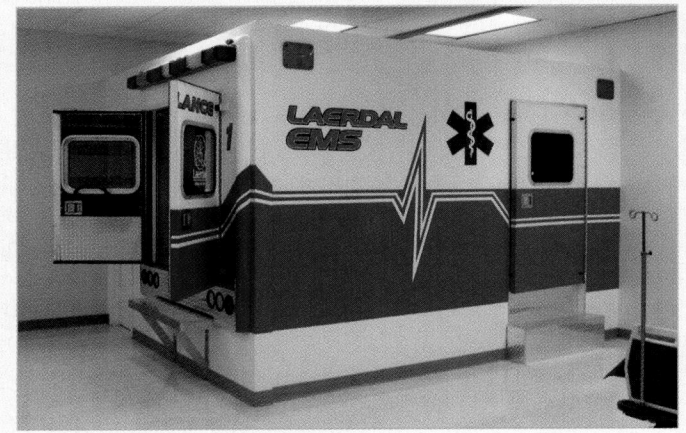

Figure B-2 This is an example of a simulations lab used in a number of paramedic training programs. The manikins and video can provide real-time feedback on changes in the "patient's" vital signs and reactions to your interventions.

cated training simulators and labs that provide realistic feedback to students on a real-time basis **Figure B-2 ▲**. Video has also been incorporated as a means of reviewing the simulations.

Ideally, simulations will include scenarios that allow you to practice each of the situations in **Table B-4 ▼**. It may be helpful to associate these scenarios with the treatment protocols and algorithms used in your EMS system.

Table B-4	Suggested Simulations				

Goals	Scenarios	Goals	Scenarios
Presenting Problem: Chest pain		**Presenting Problem: Cardiac arrest**	
Assess and manage	Stable with no dysrhythmias Stable bradycardia Unstable bradycardia (hypotension/ chest pain) Stable supraventricular tachycardia (SVT) Unstable SVT Stable ventricular tachycardia (VT) Unstable VT Ventricular ectopy Cardiogenic shock; hypotension	Assess and manage	Trauma arrest Medical arrest Ventricular fibrillation (VF)/VT PEA/asystole Termination of resuscitation No resuscitation indicated
		Identify/differentiate	Blunt trauma with tension pneumothorax Electrocution Drowning/submersion Hypothermia
Identify/differentiate	ACS Unstable angina Aortic aneurysm Pulmonary embolism Pneumothorax Esophageal rupture	**Abdominal pain**	
		Assess and manage	Acute abdominal pain Chronic abdominal pain
		Identify/differentiate	AMI Aortic aneurysm Renal colic Ruptured ectopic pregnancy Cholecystitis Appendicitis Hernia or intestinal obstruction

Table B-4 Suggested Simulations (continued)

Goals	Scenarios	Goals	Scenarios
Presenting Problem: GI bleeding		**Presenting Problem: Hazardous materials or toxicology**	
Identify/differentiate	Upper GI bleeding Lower GI bleeding	Assess and manage	Accidental toxic ingestion or inhalation Chemical burn or contact dermatitis Chemicals in the eyes Overdose or street drug use
Altered mental status		**Trauma**	
Identify/differentiate	Alcohol overdose Drug ingestion or overdose Idiopathic seizure disorder Hypoglycemia or hyperglycemia Stroke or TIA (transient ischemic attack) Head injury	Assess and manage	Isolated extremity fracture (tibia/fibula or radius/ulna) Femur fracture (hip, midshaft, supracondylar) Shoulder dislocation Clavicular fracture or AC separation Minor wounds Spinal injuries Multiple trauma, blunt Penetrating trauma Impaled object Fall of an older person Athletic injury Head injury
Dyspnea			
Identify/differentiate	Emphysema or chronic bronchitis Asthma or acute bronchospasm Acute pulmonary edema or left-sided heart failure ACS, AMI, or angina Foreign body airway obstruction Pneumonia Pulmonary embolism Spontaneous pneumothorax Hyperventilation syndrome/carpopedal spasm Smoke or toxic inhalation	Identify/differentiate	Minor wound, no sutures required Minor wound, sutures required High-risk wounds Wound with tendon and/or nerve injury Spine injury, with or without neurologic deficit Concussion Subdural or epidural hematoma
Syncope		**Allergic reactions, bites, envenomation**	
Identify/differentiate	Cardiac-related (such as bradycardia, heart block, reentry SVT, VT) Vascular or volume causes (such as medication-induced, hypovolemia, carotid sinus stimulation, orthostatic, vasovagal) Metabolic (hypoglycemic or hyperventilation) Neurogenic (TIA or seizure)	Assess and manage	Bee sting or other envenomation (such as from a pit viper) Spider or scorpion Human bite
		Identify/differentiate	Local allergic reaction and systemic allergic reaction
		Behavioral	
Seizure		Assess and manage	Mood disorders (depression, bipolar) Schizophrenic and delusional disorders Suicidal
Differentiate	Idiopathic Fever Neoplasms Infection Metabolic (such as hypoxia, hypoglycemia, thyrotoxicosis, hypocalcemia) Drug intoxication or withdrawal Head trauma Eclampsia Cerebral degenerative disease	**Obstetric/gynecologic**	
		Assess and manage	Vaginal bleeding Childbirth (normal and abnormal)
		Identify	Ectopic pregnancy
		Pediatric	
Environmental		Assess and manage	Respiratory distress, failure, and arrest Shock Cardiopulmonary failure and arrest Major trauma Fever Seizures
Assess and manage	Hypothermia Hyperthermia Superficial or deep frostbite Thermal burns Smoke inhalation Drowning/submersion	Identify/differentiate	Respiratory distress, failure, and arrest Upper airway obstruction and lower airway disease Cardiogenic vs noncardiogenic shock Major and minor trauma

You are the Provider Summary

1. What are some of the potential causes of a head-on collision in which the driver never hit the brakes?

Patients who suddenly lose consciousness, fall asleep at the wheel, commit suicide, or are highly intoxicated often veer off the road without hitting their brakes.

2. What is the significance of the MOI in this collision for your patient?

There was significant damage to the front of both vehicles, which means the patient's body may have absorbed significant energy in the form of blunt trauma. This possibility sets the tone of and priority for the assessment.

3. If it is clear that your patient was not wearing a seatbelt, how could this fact change things?

Without a seatbelt, the focus in a frontal collision is whether the patient took the up-and-over or down-and-under pathway in relationship to the dashboard and steering wheel. The up-and-over pathway is associated with head, neck, and chest injuries. The down-and-under pathway is associated with knee, leg, hip, and lower spine injuries.

4. What is the value of using mnemonics like the OPQRST and SAMPLE in your assessment?

The mnemonics help you remember key assessment questions during the focused history and physical exam. OPQRST is used to elaborate on the chief complaint. It stands for Onset; Provocation; Quality; Region, referral, or radiation; Severity; and Time. The SAMPLE history helps you obtain the patient's medical history. It stands for Signs/symptoms, Allergies, Medications, Pertinent past medical history (such as recent hospitalizations, diseases or conditions such as epilepsy, a heart condition, or diabetes), Last oral intake, and Events leading up to today's incident.

5. If the patient had been "not responsive," which steps would your focused history and physical exam have involved?

If your patient was not responsive, the focused history and physical exam would take a fast track that involves the rapid medical examination and the baseline vital signs. The SAMPLE history would be obtained from bystanders or family members because the patient was unable to talk. The rapid medical examination would be basically the same as the rapid trauma assessment which involves a quick hands-on examination of the head, neck, chest, abdomen, back, buttocks, and four extremities.

6. Why might you suspect that your patient has type 2 diabetes?

Because she has no obvious trauma and altered mental status, hypoglycemia is one of several differential diagnoses you might consider. The blood glucose test is a quick way to see exactly what her blood glucose level is. In this case, with a blood glucose level less than 70 mg/dL and her oral diabetic medications, you suspect type 2 diabetes. As a general rule, people with type 1 diabetes take insulin because their pancreas does not make insulin. People with type 2 diabetes usually regulate their blood glucose level with diet, exercise, and oral medications.

7. As long as she has a gag reflex, which medication options do you have?

When a person with diabetes has a gag reflex and altered mental status and the glucometer reads 56, you can administer glucose onto the gums with a tongue depressor or a small glass of juice with extra sugar added. If you have a good IV site that will not infiltrate, give 25 g D_{50} IV. Glucagon is another option.

Medication Formulary

Medication References

AHA Classification of Recommendations and Level of Evidence

A system of classifying recommendations based on strength of the supporting scientific evidence was used.

Class I This indicates that a treatment should be administered.

Class IIa This indicates that it is reasonable to administer treatment.

Class IIb This indicates that treatment may be considered.

Class III This indicates that treatment should NOT be administered. It is not helpful and may be harmful.

Class Indeterminate This indicates that either research is beginning on the treatment or that research is continuing on this treatment. There are no recommendations until further research is performed (eg, cannot recommend for or against).

Pregnancy Category Ratings for Drugs

Drugs have been categorized by the Food and Drug Administration (FDA) according to the level of risk to the fetus. These categories are listed for each herein under "Pregnancy Safety" and are interpreted as follows:

Category A Controlled studies in women fail to demonstrate a risk to the fetus in the first trimester, and there is no evidence of risk in later trimesters; the possibility of fetal harm appears to be remote.

Category B Either; (1) animal reproductive studies have not demonstrated a fetal risk but there are no controlled studies in women or, (2) animal reproductive studies have shown an adverse effect (other than decreased fertility) that was not confirmed in controlled studies on women in the first trimester and there is no evidence of risk in later trimesters.

Category C Either; (1) studies in animals have revealed adverse effects on the fetus and there are no controlled studies in women or, (2) studies in women and animals are not available. Drugs in this category should be given only if the potential benefit justifies the risk to the fetus.

Category D There is positive evidence of human fetal risk, but the benefits for pregnant women may be acceptable despite the risk, as in life-threatening diseases for which safer drugs cannot be used or are ineffective. An appropriate statement must appear in the "Warnings" section of the labeling of drugs in this category.

Category X Studies in animals and humans have demonstrated fetal abnormalities, there is evidence of fetal risk based on human experience, or both; the risk of using the drug in pregnant women clearly outweighs any possible benefit. The drug is contraindicated in women who are or may become pregnant. An appropriate statement must appear in the "Contraindications" section of the labeling of drugs in this category.

Federal "Controlled Substance Act of 1970" Schedule Summary

The Controlled Substances Act (CSA), Title II of the Comprehensive Drug Abuse Prevention and Control Act of 1970, is the legal foundation of the government's fight against abuse of drugs and other substances. This law is a consolidation of numerous laws regulating the manufacture and distribution of narcotics, stimulants, depressants, hallucinogens, anabolic steroids, and chemicals used in the illicit production of controlled substances. The Regulatory Agency is the DEA (Drug Enforcement Agency).

Schedule I The drug or other substance has a high potential for abuse. The drug or other substance has no currently accepted medical use in treatment in the United States. There is a lack of accepted safety for use of the drug or other substance under medical supervision. Some Schedule I substances are heroin, LSD, marijuana, and methaqualone.

Schedule II The drug or other substance has a high potential for abuse. The drug or other substance has a currently accepted medical use in treatment in the United States or a currently accepted medical use with severe restrictions. Abuse of the drug or other substance may lead to severe psychological or physical dependence. Schedule II substances include morphine, PCP, cocaine, methadone, and methamphetamine.

Schedule III The drug or other substance has a potential for abuse less than the drugs or other substances in Schedules I and II. The drug or other substance has a currently accepted medical use in treatment in the United States. Abuse of the drug or other substance may lead to moderate or low physical dependence or high psychological dependence. Anabolic steroids, codeine and hydrocodone with aspirin or Tylenol, and some barbiturates are Schedule III substances.

Schedule IV The drug or other substance has a low potential for abuse relative to the drugs or other substances in Schedule III. The drug or other substance has a currently accepted medical use in treatment in the United States. Abuse of the drug or other substance may lead to limited physical dependence or psychological dependence relative to the drugs or other substances in Schedule III. Included in Schedule IV are Darvon, Talwin, Equanil, Valium, and Xanax.

Schedule V The drug or other substance has a low potential for abuse relative to the drugs or other substances in Schedule IV. The drug or other substance has a currently accepted medical use in treatment in the United States. Abuse of the drug or other substance may lead to limited physical dependence or psychological dependence relative to the drugs or other substances in Schedule IV. Over-the-counter cough medicines with codeine are classified in Schedule V.

Weights and Measures

Commonly Used Prefixes		
Prefix Name	**Prefix Symbol**	**Prefix Value**
micro	μ	1/1,000,000 or 0.000001
milli	m	1/1,000 or 0.001
centi	c	1/100 or 0.01
kilo	k	1,000
mega	M	1 million or 1,000,000

Common Metric Conversions

Weight

1 kilogram (kg)	2.2 pounds (lb)
1 kilogram (kg)	1,000 grams (g or gm)
1 gram (g or gr)	1,000 milligrams (mg)
1 milligram (mg)	1,000 micrograms (μg or mcg)

Volume

1 liter (L)	1,000 milliliters or cubic centimeters (mL or cc)

Temperature

37° Celsius (°C)	98.6° Fahrenheit (°F)

Length

1 centimeter (cm)	10 millimeters (mm)
100 centimeters (cm)	1 meter (m)

Common Medical Abbreviations Related to Pharmacology

Common Medical Abbreviations Related to Pharmacology

ā	before		nitro	nitroglycerin
α	alpha		NKA	no known allergies
amp.	ampule		NKDA	no known diagnosed allergies
APAP	acetaminophen		NTG	nitroglycerin
ASA	aspirin		ø	null or none
β	beta		p̄	after
bid	Bis in die (twice a day)		pc	post cibos (after eating)
c̄	with		pedi	pediatric
caps	capsules		po	per os (by mouth)
cc	cubic centimeter		pr	per rectus (by rectum)
D/C	discontinue		prn	per re nata (when necessary)
dig	digitalis		q̄	quisque (every)
elix	elixir		qd	quisque die (every day)
ET	endotracheal		qh	quisque hora (every hour)
ETOH	ethyl alcohol		qid	quarter in die (four times a day)
g or gr	gram		qod	every other day
gtt	gutta (drop)		RL	Ringer's lactate
gtts	guttae (drops)		s̄	sine (without)
HHN	hand-held nebulizer		SC	subcutaneous
Hs	hora somni (at bedtime)		sol	solution
IC	intracardiac		SQ	subcutaneous
IM	intramuscular		stat	statim (now or immediately)
IO	intraosseous		SVN	small volume nebulizer
IV	intravenous		tid	ter in die (three times a day)
IVP	intravenous push		TKO	to keep open
IVPB	intravenous piggyback		u	unit
kg	kilogram		ut dict	ut dictum (as directed)
KO	keep open		®	registered trademark
KVO	keep vein open		♀	female
L or l	liter		♂	male
lb	pound		>	greater than
LR	lactated Ringer's		<	less than
MAX	maximum		≥	greater than or equal to
MDI	metered dose inhaler		≤	less than or equal to
μ	micro		≈	approximately
μgtt	microdrop		=	equal
μg or mcg	microgram		≠	not equal
mEq	milliequivalent		Δ	change(s)
mg	milligram		±	plus or minus
min	minute		°	degree(s)
mL	milliliter		™	trademark
MS or MSO4	morphine sulfate			

Drug Dosage Calculations

Terminology

Desired dose The quantity of a medication that is to be administered to a patient. This is usually expressed in milligrams, grams, or grains.

Concentration (of the medication on hand) The amount of a medication that is present in the ampule or vial. This is usually expressed in milligrams, grams, or grains.

Volume (of the medication on hand) The amount of a fluid that is present in the ampule or vial in which the medication is dissolved. This is usually expressed in milliliters or liters.

Formulas

$$\text{Concentration on hand} = \frac{\text{concentration on hand (mg)}}{\text{volume on hand (mL)}}$$

EXAMPLE

How many milligrams of medication "Q" are in each mL/cc. Medication "Q" is packaged 500 mg in 10 mL of saline.

$$\text{Concentration on hand} = \frac{\text{concentration on hand (500 mg)}}{\text{volume on hand (10 mL)}}$$

$$\text{Concentration on hand} = \frac{500 \text{ mg}}{10 \text{ mL}}$$

$$\text{Concentration on hand} = 50 \text{ mg/mL}$$

EXAMPLE

You are ordered to administer 70 mg of medication "Y" to a patient. The medication is prepared as follows, 100 mg in 5 mL of saline.

$$\text{Volume to be administered} = \frac{\text{volume on hand} \times \text{desired dose}}{\text{concentration on hand}}$$

$$\text{Volume to be administered} = \frac{\text{volume on hand (5 mL)} \times \text{desired dose (70 mg)}}{\text{concentration on hand (100 mg)}}$$

$$\text{Volume to be administered} = \frac{(5 \text{ mL}) \times (70 \text{ mg})}{(100 \text{ mg})}$$

Note: (mg) can be crossed out leaving the final units notation (mL).

$$\text{Volume to be administered} = \frac{350 \text{ mL}}{100}$$

$$\text{Volume to be administered} = 3.5 \text{ mL}$$

Intravenous Infusion Drip Rate Calculation

$$\text{Formula: Drops per minute (gtt/min)} = \frac{\text{total amount of fluid to be administered in mLL} \times \text{drop factor}^*}{\text{total time in minutes}}$$

*The drop factor for the IV tubing will be indicated on the package for the tubing. Standard values are as follows: 10, 15, and 20 gtt lines (macrodrip) and 50 or 60 gtt/mL lines (microdrip).

EXAMPLE

You are ordered to administer 1,000 mL of normal saline every 8 hours using a 10 gtt IV tubing set. Calculate the number of drops per minute.

Total volume: 1,000 mL

Drop factor: 10 gtt/mL

Total time: 8 hours × 60 = 480 minutes

$$\text{Drops per minute (gtt/min)} = \frac{\text{Total amount of fluid to be administered (1,000 mL)} \times \text{drop factor (10 gtt/mL)}}{\text{Total time in minutes (480)}}$$

$$\text{Drops per minute (gtt/min)} = \frac{(1,000 \text{ mL}) \times (10 \text{ gtt/mL})}{480 \text{ min}}$$

$$\text{Drops per minute (gtt/min)} = \frac{10,000}{480}$$

Drops per minute (gtt/min) = 20.83   Note: Round to the nearest drop

Drops per minute (gtt/min) = 21 gtt(s)/min

Medications
Reference for Medication Listings

Name of Medication (Other Common Names)

Class How the medication is categorized as compared to other medications. This is usually done by grouping those medications with similar characteristics, traits, or primary components.

Mechanism of action The manner of combination of parts, processes, etc., which form a common function.

Indications A circumstance that points to or shows the cause, pathology, treatment, or issue of an attack of disease; that which points out; that which serves as a guide or warning.

Contraindications Any condition, especially any condition of disease, which renders some particular line of treatment improper or undesirable.

Adverse reactions This is an abnormal or harmful effect to an organism caused by exposure to a chemical. It is indicated by some result such as death, a change in food or water consumption, altered body and organ weights, altered enzyme levels, or visible illness. An effect may be classed as adverse if it causes functional or anatomic damage, causes irreversible change in the homeostasis of the organism, or increases the susceptibility of the organism to other chemical or biologic stress. A nonadverse effect will usually be reversed when the organism is no longer being exposed to the chemical.

Drug interactions This refers to any potential effects that a medication may have when administered in conjunction or in the presence of another medication already in the patient's system, a medication delivery device, or fluid.

How supplied This is how the manufacturer packages the medication for distribution and sale. Typical methods of packaging are prefilled syringes, vials, or ampules.

Dosage and administration This is the typical or average volume of the medication that is to be administered to the patient and the route of introduction of the medication to the patient.

Duration of action Three values are given; (1) Onset: the estimated amount of time it will take for the medication to enter the body/system and begin to take effect, (2) Peak effect: the estimated amount of time it will take for the medication to have its greatest effect on the patient/system and (3) Duration: the estimated amount of time that the medication will have any effect on the patient/system.

Special considerations Additional pertinent information concerning a medication.

Activated Charcoal

Class Adsorbent.

Mechanism of action Adsorbs toxic substances from the gastrointestinal tract; onset of action is immediate.

Indications Most oral poisonings and medication overdoses; can be used after evacuation of poisons.

Contraindications Oral administration to comatose patient; after ingestion of corrosives, caustics, or petroleum distillates (ineffective and may induce vomiting); simultaneous administration with other oral drugs.

Adverse reactions May induce nausea and vomiting; may cause constipation; may cause black stools.

Drug interactions Bonds with and generally inactivates whatever it is mixed with, eg, syrup of ipecac.

How supplied 25 g (black powder)/125-mL bottle (200 mg/mL); 50 g (black powder)/250-mL bottle (200 mg/mL)

Dosage and administration *Note:* if not in premixed slurry, dilute with 1 part charcoal/4 parts water. *Adult:* 1–2 g/kg PO or via NGT. *Pediatric:* 1–2 g/kg PO or via NGT

Duration of action Depends on gastrointestinal function; will act until excreted.

Special considerations Often used in conjunction with magnesium citrate. Must be stored in a closed container. Does not adsorb cyanide, lithium, iron, lead, or arsenic.

Adenosine (Adenocard)

Class Endogenous nucleotide.

Mechanism of action Slows conduction time through the AV node; can interrupt re-entrant pathways; slows heart rate; acts directly on sinus pacemaker cells. Is drug of choice for re-entry SVT. Can be used diagnostically for stable, wide-complex tachycardias of unknown type after two doses of lidocaine.

Indications Conversion of PSVT to sinus rhythm. May convert re-entry SVT due to Wolff-Parkinson-White syndrome. Not effective in converting atrial fibrillation/flutter or V-tach.

Contraindications Second- or third-degree block or sick sinus syndrome, atrial flutter/atrial fibrillation, ventricular tachycardia, hypersensitivity to adenosine, poison-induced tachycardia.

Adverse reactions Facial flushing, shortness of breath, chest pain, headache, paresthesia, diaphoresis, palpitations, hypotension, nausea, metallic taste.

Drug interactions Methylxanthines (theophylline-like drugs) antagonize the effects of adenosine. Dipyridamole (Persantine) potentiates the effects of adenosine. Carbamazepine (Tegretol) may potentiate the AV node, blocking the effects of adenosine. May cause bronchoconstriction in asthmatic patients.

How supplied 3 mg/mL in 2-mL flip-top vials for IV injection

Dosage and administration *Adult:* 6 mg over 1–3 seconds, followed by a 20 mL saline flush and elevate extremity; if no response after 1–2 minutes, administer 12 mg over 1–3 seconds; maximum total dose, 30 mg; *Pediatric:* 0.1–0.2 mg/kg rapid IV; maximum single dose, 12 mg.

Duration of action Onset and peak effects in seconds; duration, 12 seconds.

Special considerations Short half-life limits side effects in most patients. Pregnancy safety: Category C.

Albuterol (Proventil, Ventolin)

Class Sympathomimetic, bronchodilator.

Mechanism of action Selective beta-2 agonist that stimulates adrenergic receptors of the sympathomimetic nervous system resulting in smooth muscle relaxation in the bronchial tree and peripheral vasculature.

Indications Treatment of bronchospasm in patients with reversible obstructive airway disease (COPD/asthma). Prevention of exercise-induced bronchospasm.

Contraindications Known prior hypersensitivity reactions to albuterol. Tachycardia arrhythmias, especially those caused by digitalis. Synergistic with other sympathomimetics.

Adverse reactions Often dose-related and include restlessness, tremors, dizziness, palpitations, tachycardia, nervousness, peripheral vasodilatation, nausea, vomiting, hyperglycemia, increased blood pressure, and paradoxical bronchospasm.

Drug interactions Tricyclic antidepressants may potentiate vasculature effects. Beta blockers are antagonistic. May potentiate hypokalemia caused by diuretics.

How supplied Solution for aerosolization: 0.5% (5 mg/mL). Metered dose inhaler: 90 µg/metered spray (17-g canister with 200 inhalations). Syrup: 2 mg/5 mL.

Dosage and administration *Adult:* Administer 2.5 mg. Dilute 0.5 mL of 0.5% solution for inhalation with 2.5 mL normal saline in nebulizer and administer over 10–15 minutes. MDI: 1–2 inhalations (90–180 µg). Five minutes between inhalations. *Pediatric:* Administer solution of 0.01–0.03 mL (0.05–0.15 mg/kg/dose diluted in 2 mL of 0.9% normal saline. May repeat every 20 minutes three times.

Duration of action Onset in 5–15 minutes with peak effect in 30 minutes to 2 hours and duration of 3–4 hours.

Special considerations Pregnancy safety: Category C. Antagonized by beta blockers (eg, Inderal, Lopressor). May precipitate angina pectoris and arrhythmias. Should only be administered by inhalation methodology in prehospital management.

Amiodarone (Cordarone, Pacerone)

Class Antiarrhythmic.

Mechanism of action Blocks sodium channels and myocardial potassium channels.

Indications V-fib/pulseless V-tach and unstable V-tach in patients refractory to other therapy.

Contraindications Known hypersensitivity, cardiogenic shock, sinus bradycardia, and second- or third-degree AV block (unless a functional pacemaker is available).

Adverse reactions Hypotension, bradycardia, prolongation of the P-R, QRS, and Q-T intervals.

Drug interactions Use with digoxin may cause digitalis toxicity. Antiarrhythmics may cause increased serum levels. Beta blockers and calcium channel blockers may potentiate bradycardia, sinus arrest, and AV heart blocks.

How supplied Ampules containing 150 mg/3 mL (50 mg/mL) and prefilled syringes containing 150 mg/3 mL (50 mg/mL).

Dosage and administration *Adult: V-fib/pulseless V-tach unresponsive to CPR, defibrillation, and vasopressors:* 300 mg IV/IO push (recommend dilution in 20–30 mL D$_5$W). Initial dose can be followed **one time** in 3–5 minutes at 150 mg IV/IO push. *Recurrent life-threatening ventricular arrhythmias:* Maximum cumulative dose is 2.2 g/24 hours, administered as follows: *Rapid infusion:* 150 mg IV/IO over 10 minutes (15 mg/min). May repeat rapid infusion (150 mg IV/IO) every 10 minutes as needed. *Slow infusion:* 360 mg IV/IO over 6 hours (1 mg/min). *Maintenance infusion:* 540 mg IV/IO over 18 hours (0.5 mg/min). **Pediatric:** *Refractory V-fib/pulseless V-tach:* 5 mg/kg IV/IO bolus. Can repeat the 5 mg/kg IV/IO bolus up to a total dose of 15 mg/kg per 24 hours. Maximum single dose is 300 mg. *Perfusing supraventricular and ventricular tachycardias:* Loading dose of 5 mg/kg IV/IO over 20–60 minutes (maximum single dose of 300 mg). Can repeat to maximum of 15 mg/kg per day.

Duration of action Onset: immediate with peak effect in 10–15 minutes. Duration of action: 30–45 minutes.

Special considerations Pregnancy safety: Category D. Monitor patient for hypotension. May worsen arrhythmias or precipitate new arrhythmias.

Amyl Nitrite, Sodium Nitrite, Sodium Thiosulfate (Cyanide Antidote Kit)

Class Antidote.

Mechanism of action Amyl nitrite: affinity for cyanide ions; reacts with hemoglobin to form methemoglobin (low toxicity); sodium nitrite: same as amyl nitrite; sodium thiosulfate: produces thiocyanate, which is then excreted.

Indications Cyanide or hydrocyanic acid poisoning.

Contraindications Not applicable.

Adverse reactions Excessive doses of amyl nitrite and sodium nitrite can produce severe, life-threatening methemoglobinemia. Use only recommended doses.

Drug interactions None.

How supplied Amyl nitrite: in capsules similar to ammonia capsules.

Dosage and administration *Adult:* Amyl nitrite: breathe 30 seconds out of every minute. Sodium thiosulfate and sodium nitrite: IV per antidote kit directions. *Pediatric:* Same as adult.

Duration of action Variable.

Special considerations Cyanide poisoning must be recognized quickly and treated quickly; if pulse persists, even in presence of apnea, prognosis is good with treatment. The antidote kit must be used in conjunction with administration of oxygen.

Aspirin

Class   Platelet inhibitor, anti-inflammatory agent.

Mechanism of action   Prostaglandin inhibition.

Indications   New onset chest pain suggestive of acute myocardial infarction. Signs and symptoms suggestive of recent cerebrovascular accident.

Contraindications   Hypersensitivity. Relatively contraindicated in patients with active ulcer disease or asthma.

Adverse reactions   Heartburn, GI bleeding, prolonged bleeding, nausea, and vomiting. Wheezing in allergic patients.

Drug interactions   Use with caution in patients allergic to NSAIDs.

How supplied   81-mg, 160-mg, or 325-mg tablets (chewable and standard).

Dosage and administration   160 mg to 325 mg PO (chewed if possible).

Duration of action   Onset: 30–45 minutes. Peak effect: variable. Duration: variable.

Special considerations   Pregnancy safety: Category D. Not recommended in pediatric population.

Atropine Sulfate

Class   Anticholinergic agent.

Mechanism of action   Parasympatholytic: inhibits action of acetylcholine at postganglionic parasympathetic neuroeffector sites. Increases heart rate in life-threatening bradyarrhythmias.

Indications   Hemodynamically unstable bradycardia, asystole, bradycardic (< 60 beats/min) pulseless electrical activity (PEA), organophosphate poisoning, bronchospastic pulmonary disorders.

Contraindications   Tachycardia, hypersensitivity, unstable cardiovascular status in acute hemorrhage and myocardial ischemia, narrow-angle glaucoma.

Adverse reactions   Headache; dizziness; palpitations; nausea and vomiting; tachycardia; arrhythmias; anticholinergic effects (blurred vision, dry mouth, urinary retention); paradoxical bradycardia when pushed slowly or at low doses; flushed, hot, dry skin.

Drug interactions   Potential adverse effects when administered with digoxin, cholinergics, physostigmine. Effects enhanced by antihistamines, procainamide, quinidine, antipsychotics, benzodiazepines, and antidepressants.

How supplied   Prefilled syringes: 1 mg in 10 mL (0.1 mg/mL). Nebulizer: 0.2% (1 mg in 0.5 mL) and 0.5% (2.5 mg in 0.5 mL).

Dosage and administration   *Adult: Asystole or bradycardic PEA:* 1 mg IV/IO push. May repeat every 3–5 minutes (if asystole or PEA persists) to a maximum of 3 doses (3 mg). Endotracheal administration: 2–3 mg diluted in 10 mL of water or normal saline. *Unstable bradycardia:* 0.5 mg IV/IO every 3–5 minutes as needed, not to exceed total dose of 3 mg. Use shorter dosing interval (3 minutes) and higher doses in severe clinical conditions. *Organophosphate poisoning:* Extremely large doses (2–4 mg or higher) may be needed. **Pediatric:** 0.02 mg/kg via IV/IO push; may double this dose for second IV/IO dose. *Minimum single dose:* 0.1 mg. *Maximum doses:* child single dose: 0.5 mg, child total dose: 1 mg, adolescent single dose: 1 mg, adolescent total dose: 2 mg. Endotracheal administration: 0.03 mg/kg (absorption may be unreliable).

Duration of action   Onset: immediate. Peak effect: rapid to 1–2 minutes. Duration: 2–6 hours.

Special considerations   Pregnancy safety: Category C. Moderate doses may cause pupillary dilation.

Benzocaine Spray (Hurricane)

Class   Topical anesthetic.

Mechanism of action   Stabilizes neuronal membrane.

Indications   Used as a lubricant and topical anesthetic to facilitate passage of diagnostic and treatment devices. Suppresses the pharyngeal and tracheal gag reflex.

Contraindications   Patients with a known hypersensitivity to benzocaine.

Adverse reactions   Methemoglobinemia has been reported following the use of benzocaine on extremely rare occasions.

Drug interactions   No significant interactions found or known.

How supplied   Multidose aerosol can, 20% benzocaine.

Dosage and administration   *Adult:* 0.5–1.0 second spray, repeat as needed. *Pediatric:* 0.25–0.5 second spray, repeat as needed.

Duration of action   Onset: Immediate. Peak effect: 30 seconds. Duration: 15 minutes.

Special considerations   Pregnancy safety: Category A. Topical use only, not for ocular use or injection.

Calcium Chloride

Class   Electrolyte.

Mechanism of action   Increases cardiac contractile state (positive inotropic effect). May enhance ventricular automaticity.

Indications   Hypocalcemia, hyperkalemia, magnesium sulfate overdose, calcium channel blocker overdose, adjunctive therapy in treatment of insect bites and stings.

Contraindications   Hypercalcemia, V-fib, digitalis toxicity.

Adverse reactions   Bradycardia, asystole, hypotension, peripheral vasodilation, metallic taste, local necrosis, coronary and cerebral artery spasm, nausea and vomiting.

Drug interactions   May worsen arrhythmias secondary to digitalis toxicity. May antagonize the effects of verapamil. Do not mix with or infuse immediately before or after sodium bicarbonate without intervening flush.

How supplied   Prefilled syringes containing a 10% solution in 10 mL (100 mg/mL).

Dosage and administration   *Adult:* 500 mg to 1,000 mg (5–10 mL of a 10% solution) IV/IO push for hyperkalemia and calcium channel blocker overdose. May be repeated as needed. *Pediatric:* 20 mg/kg (0.2 mL/kg) slow IV/IO push. Maximum 1 g dose; may repeat in 10 minutes.

Duration of action   Onset: 5–15 minutes. Peak effect: 3–5 minutes. Duration: 15–30 minutes, but may persist for 4 hours (dose dependent).

Special considerations   Pregnancy safety: Category C. Do not use routinely in cardiac arrest.

Dexamethasone Sodium Phosphate (Decadron, Hexadrol)

Class Corticosteroid.

Mechanism of action Suppresses acute and chronic inflammation; immunosuppressive effects.

Indications Anaphylaxis, asthma, spinal cord injury, croup, elevated intracranial pressure (prevention and treatment), as an adjunct to treatment of shock.

Contraindications Hypersensitivity to product.

Adverse reactions Hypertension, sodium and water retention, gastrointestinal bleeding, TB. None from single dose.

Drug interactions Calcium, metaraminol.

How supplied 100 mg/5-mL vials or 20 mg/1-mL vials.

Dosage and administration *Adult:* 10–100 mg IV (1 mg/kg slow IV bolus) (considerable variance through medical control). *Pediatric:* 0.25–1.0 mg/kg/dose IV, IO, IM.

Duration of action Onset: Hours. Peak effects: 8–12 hours. Duration: 24–72 hours.

Special considerations Pregnancy safety: unknown. Protect medication from heat. Toxicity and side effects with long-term use.

Dextrose

Class Carbohydrate, hypertonic solution.

Mechanism of action Rapidly increases serum glucose levels. Short-term osmotic diuresis.

Indications Hypoglycemia, altered level of consciousness, coma of unknown etiology, seizure of unknown etiology, status epilepticus.

Contraindications Intracranial hemorrhage.

Adverse reactions Extravasation leads to tissue necrosis. Warmth, pain, burning, thrombophlebitis, rhabdomyolysis, hyperglycemia.

Drug interactions Sodium bicarbonate, Coumadin.

How supplied 25 g/50-mL prefilled syringes (500 mg/mL)

Dosage and administration *Adult:* 12.5–25 g slow IV; may be repeated as necessary. *Pediatric:* 0.5–1 g/kg/dose slow IV; may be repeated as necessary.

Duration of action Onset: less than 1 minute. Peak effects: variable. Duration: variable.

Special considerations Administer thiamine prior to D_{50} in known alcoholic patients. Draw blood to determine glucose level before administering. Do not administer to patients with known CVA unless hypoglycemia documented.

Diazepam (Valium)

Class Benzodiazepine, sedative-hypnotic, anticonvulsant.

Mechanism of action Potentiates effects of inhibitory neurotransmitters. Raises seizure threshold. Induces amnesia and sedation.

Indications Acute anxiety states, acute alcohol withdrawal (delirium tremens), muscle relaxant, seizure activity, agitation. Analgesia for medical procedures (fracture reduction, cardioversion).

Contraindications Hypersensitivity, glaucoma, coma, shock, substance abuse, head injury.

Adverse reactions Respiratory depression, hypotension, drowsiness, ataxia, reflex tachycardia, nausea, confusion, thrombosis, and phlebitis.

Drug interactions Incompatible with most drugs, fluids.

How supplied 10 mg/5-mL prefilled syringes, ampules, vials, and Tubex.

Dosage and administration Seizure activity: *Adult:* 5–10 mg IV q 10–15 minutes prn (5 mg over 5 min)(maximum dose, 30 mg) Seizure activity: *Pediatric:* 0.2–0.5 mg slowly q 2–5 minutes up to 5 mg (maximum dose, 10 mg/kg). Rectal diazepam: 0.5 mg/kg via 2″ rectal catheter and flush with 2–3 mL air after administration. Sedation for cardioversion: 5–15 mg IV over 5–10 minutes prior to cardioversion.

Duration of action Onset: 1–5 minutes. Peak effect: Minutes. Duration: 20–50 minutes.

Special considerations Pregnancy safety: Category D. Short duration of anticonvulsant effect. Reduce dose 50% in elderly patient.

Digoxin (Lanoxin)

Class Inotropic agent.

Mechanism of action Rapid-acting cardiac glycoside with direct and indirect effects that increase force of myocardial contraction, increase refractory period of AV node, and increase total peripheral resistance.

Indications Congestive heart failure, re-entry SVT, especially atrial flutter and atrial fibrillation.

Contraindications Ventricular fibrillation, ventricular tachycardia, digitalis toxicity, hypersensitivity to digoxin.

Adverse reactions Headache, weakness, blurred yellow or green vision, confusion, seizures, arrhythmias, nausea, vomiting, and skin rash.

Drug interactions Amiodarone, verapamil, and quinidine may increase serum digoxin concentrations by 50%–70%. Concurrent use of digoxin and verapamil may lead to severe heart block. Diuretics may potentiate cardiac toxicity.

How supplied 2-mL ampules of 0.5 mg digoxin; also as tablets, capsules, and elixirs.

Dosage and administration *Adult:* Loading dose of 10 to 15 µg/kg. *Pediatric:* not recommended in the prehospital setting.

Duration of action Onset: IV: 5–30 minutes; Peak effect: 30–120 minutes. Duration: several days.

Special considerations Pregnancy safety: Category A. Patients receiving IV digoxin must be on a monitor. Patients with known renal failure are prone to digoxin toxicity. Hypokalemia, hypomagnesemia, and hypercalcemia potentiate digitalis toxicity. Use carefully in patients with Wolff-Parkinson-White Syndrome (ventricular arrhythmias).

Diltiazem Hydrochloride (Cardizem, Lyo-Ject)

Class Calcium channel blocker.

Mechanism of action Block influx of calcium ions into cardiac muscle; prevents spasm of coronary arteries. Arterial and venous vasodilator. Reduces preload and afterload. Reduces myocardial oxygen demand.

Indications Control of rapid ventricular rates due to atrial flutter, atrial fibrillation, and re-entry SVT; Angina pectoris.

Contraindications Hypotension, sick sinus syndrome, second- or third-degree AV block, cardiogenic shock, wide-complex tachycardias, poison/drug-induced tachycardia.

Adverse reactions Bradycardia, second- or third-degree AV blocks, chest pain, CHF, syncope. V-Fib, V-tach, nausea, vomiting, dizziness, dry mouth, dyspnea, headache.

Drug interactions Caution in patients using medications that affect cardiac contractility. In general, should not be used in patients on beta blockers.

How supplied 25 mg/5-mL vial; 50 mg/10-mL vial. Nonrefrigerated: Lyo-Ject syringe.

Dosage and administration *Adult:* Initial bolus: 0.25 mg/kg (average dose 15–20 mg) IV over 2 minutes. If inadequate response, may re-bolus in 15 minutes: 0.35 mg/kg (average dose 20–25 mg) IV over 2 minutes. Maintenance infusion of 5–15 mg/h. *Pediatric:* Not recommended.

Duration of action Onset: 2–5 minutes. Peak effect: variable. Duration: 1–3 hours.

Special considerations Pregnancy safety: Category C. Use with caution in patients with renal or hepatic dysfunction. PVCs may be noted at time of conversion of PSVT to sinus rhythm.

Diphenhydramine (Benadryl)

Class Antihistamine; anticholinergic.

Mechanism of action Blocks cellular histamine receptors; decreases vasodilation; decreases motion sickness. Reverses extrapyramidal reactions.

Indications Symptomatic relief of allergies, allergic reactions, anaphylaxis, acute dystonic reactions (phenothiazines). Blood administration reactions; used for motion sickness, hay fever.

Contraindications Asthma, glaucoma, pregnancy, hypertension, narrow angle glaucoma, infants, patients taking monoamine oxidase inhibitors (MAOIs).

Adverse reactions Sedation, hypotension, seizures, visual disturbances, vomiting, urinary retention, palpitations, arrhythmias, dry mouth and throat, and paradoxical CNS excitation in children.

Drug interactions Potentiates effects of alcohol and other anticholinergics, may inhibit corticosteroid activity; MAOIs prolong anticholinergic effects of diphenhydramine.

How supplied Tablets: 25, 50 mg; Capsules: 25, 50 mg; Prefilled syringes: 50- or 100-mg; vials (IV or IM); elixir, 12.5 mg/5 mL.

Dosage and administration *Adult:* 25–50 mg IM or IV or PO. *Pediatric:* 1–2 mg/kg IV, IO slowly or IM. If given PO: 5 mg/kg/24 hours.

Duration of action Onset: 15–30 minutes. Peak effect: 1 hour. Duration: 3–12 hours.

Special considerations Not used in infants or in pregnancy: Category B. If used in anaphylaxis, will be in conjunction with epinephrine, corticosteroids.

Dobutamine (Dobutrex)

Class Sympathomimetic, inotropic agent.

Mechanism of action Synthetic catecholamine. Increased myocardial contractility and stroke volume, increased cardiac output. Minimal chronotropic activity. Increases renal blood flow.

Indications Cardiogenic shock, CHF, left ventricular dysfunction. Often used in conjunction with other drugs.

Contraindications Tachyarrhythmias, IHSS, severe hypotension.

Adverse reactions May increase infarct size in patient with MI, headache, arrhythmias, hypertension, PVCs.

Drug interactions Incompatible with sodium bicarbonate and furosemide. Beta-blockers may blunt inotropic effects.

How supplied 250 mg/20-mL vials.

Dosage and administration *Adult:* IV infusion at 2–20 µg/kg/min titrated to desired effect. *Pediatric:* 2–20 µg/kg/min titrated to desired effect.

Duration of action Onset: 2 minutes. Peak effect: 10 minutes. Duration: 1–2 minutes after infusion discontinued.

Special considerations Pregnancy safety: not well established. Monitor blood pressure closely.

Dopamine (Intropin)

Class Sympathomimetic, inotropic agent.

Mechanism of action Immediate metabolic precursor to norepinephrine. Increases systemic vascular resistance, dilates renal and splanchnic vasculature. Increases myocardial contractility and stroke volume.

Indications Cardiogenic, septic or spinal shock, hypotension with low cardiac output states, distributive shock.

Contraindications Hypovolemic shock, pheochromocytoma, tachyarrhythmias, V-fib.

Adverse reactions Cardiac arrhythmias, hypertension, increased myocardial oxygen demand; extravasation may cause tissue necrosis.

Drug interactions Incompatible in alkaline solutions. MAOIs will enhance effects of dopamine. Bretylium may potentiate effect of dopamine. Beta blockers may antagonize effects of dopamine. When administered with phenytoin: may cause hypotension, bradycardia, and seizures.

How supplied 200 mg/5 mL–400 mg/5 mL prefilled syringes, ampules for IV infusion; 400 mg in 250-mL D_5W premixed solutions.

Dosage and administration *Adult:* 2–20 µg/kg/min titrated to patient response; *Pediatric:* 2–20 µg/kg/min titrated to patient response.

Duration of action Onset: 1–4 minutes. Peak effect: 5–10 minutes. Duration: Effects cease almost immediately after infusion is shut off.

Special considerations Pregnancy safety not established. Effects are dose-dependent. Dopaminergic response: 2–4 µg/kg/min: dilates vessels in kidneys; increased urine output. Beta-adrenergic response: 4–10 µg/kg/min: positive chronotropic and inotropic adrenergic response: 10–20 µg/kg/min: primarily alpha stimulant/vasoconstriction. Greater than 20 µg/kg/min: reversal of renal effects/override alpha effects. Always monitor drip rate. Avoid extravasation injury.

Epinephrine (Adrenalin)

Class   Sympathomimetic.

Mechanism of action   Direct-acting alpha- and beta-agonist. Alpha: vasoconstriction. Beta-1: positive inotropic, chronotropic, and dromotropic effects. Beta-2: bronchial smooth muscle relaxation and dilation of skeletal vasculature.

Indications   Cardiac arrest (V-fib/pulseless V-tach, asystole, PEA), symptomatic bradycardia as an alternative infusion to dopamine, severe hypotension secondary to bradycardia when atropine and transcutaneous pacing are unsuccessful, allergic reactions, anaphylaxis, asthma.

Contraindications   Hypertension, hypothermia, pulmonary edema, myocardial ischemia, hypovolemic shock.

Adverse reactions   Hypertension, tachycardia, arrhythmias, pulmonary edema, anxiety, restlessness, psychomotor agitation, nausea, headache, angina.

Drug interactions   Potentiates other sympathomimetics, deactivated by alkaline solutions (ie, sodium bicarbonate), monamine oxidase inhibitors (MAOIs) may potentiate effects, beta blockers may blunt effects.

How supplied   1:1,000 solution: ampules and vials containing 1 mg/mL. 1:10,000 solution: prefilled syringes containing 1 mg in 10 mL (0.1 mg/mL). Auto-injector (EpiPen): 0.5 mg/mL (1:2,000).

Dosage and administration   *Adult: Mild allergic reactions and asthma:* 0.3–0.5 mg (0.3–0.5 mL of 1:1,000) SC. *Anaphylaxis:* 0.1 mg (1 mL of 1:10,000) IV/IO over 5 minutes. *Cardiac arrest:* IV/IO dose: 1 mg (10 mL of 1:10,000 solution) every 3–5 minutes during resuscitation. Follow each dose with 20 mL flush and elevate arm for 10 to 20 seconds after dose. Higher dose: Higher doses (up to 0.2 mg/kg) may be used for specific indications (beta blocker or calcium channel blocker overdose). Continuous infusion: Add 1 mg (1 mL of 1:1,000 solution) to 500 mL normal saline or D_5W. Initial infusion rate of 1 µg/min titrated to effect (typical dose: 2–10 µg/min). Endotracheal (ET) dose: 2–2.5 mg diluted in 10 mL normal saline. *Profound bradycardia or hypotension:* 2–10 µg/min; titrate to patient response. **Pediatric:** *Mild allergic reactions and asthma:* 0.01 mg/kg (0.01 mL/kg) of 1:1,000 solution SC (maximum of 0.3 mL). *Cardiac arrest:* IV/IO dose: 0.01 mg/kg (0.1 mL/kg) of 1:10,000 solution every 3–5 minutes during arrest. All endotracheal (ET) doses: 0.1 mg/kg (0.1 mL/kg) of 1:1,000 solution. *Symptomatic bradycardia:* IV/IO dose: 0.01 mg/kg (0.1 mL/kg) of 1:10,000 solution. All endotracheal (ET) doses: 0.1 mg/kg (0.1 mL/kg) of 1:1,000 solution. *Continuous IV/IO infusion:* Begin with rapid infusion, then titrate to response. Typical initial infusion: 0.1–1 µg/min. Higher doses may be effective.

Duration of action   Onset: immediate. Peak effect: minutes. Duration: several minutes.

Special considerations   Pregnancy safety: Category C. May cause syncope in asthmatic children. May increase myocardial oxygen demand.

Epinephrine Racemic (Micronefrin, Vaponefrin)

Class   Sympathomimetic.

Mechanism of action   Stimulates beta-2 receptors in lungs: bronchodilatation with relaxation of bronchial smooth muscles. Reduces airway resistance. Useful in treating laryngeal edema; inhibits histamine release.

Indications   Bronchial asthma, prevention of bronchospasm. Croup, laryngotracheobronchitis, laryngeal edema.

Contraindications   Hypertension, underlying cardiovascular disease, epiglottitis.

Adverse reactions   Tachycardia, arrhythmias.

Drug interactions   MAOIs and bretylium may potentiate effects. Beta blockers may blunt effects.

How supplied   MDI: 0.16–0.25 mg/spray. Solution: 7.5, 15, 30 mL in 1%, 2.25% solutions

Dosage and administration   *Adult:* MDI: 2–3 inhalations, repeated every 5 minutes PRN. Solution: dilute 5 mL (1%) in 5.0 mL NS, administer over 15 minutes. *Pediatric:* Solution: dilute 0.25 mL (0.1%) in 2.5 mL NS (if less than 20 kg); dilute 0.5 mL in 2.5 mL NS (if 20–40 kg); dilute 0.75 mL in 2.5 mL NS (if greater than 40 kg). Administer by aerosolization.

Duration of action   Onset: within 5 minutes. Peak effect: 5–15 minutes. Duration: 1–3 hours.

Special considerations   May cause tachycardia and other arrhythmias. Monitor vital signs. Excessive use may cause bronchospasm.

Flumazenil (Romazicon)

Class   Benzodiazepine receptor antagonist.

Mechanism of action   Antagonizes the actions of benzodiazepines on the CNS.

Indications   Reversal of respiratory depression and sedative effects from pure benzodiazepine overdose.

Contraindications   Hypersensitivity, tricyclic antidepressant overdose, seizure-prone patients, coma of unknown etiology, benzodiazepine dependence.

Adverse reactions   Nausea, vomiting, agitation, injection site pain, visual disturbances, seizures, cutaneous vasodilation.

Drug interactions   Toxic effects of mixed-drug overdose (especially tricyclics).

How supplied   5 and 10 mL vials (0.1 mg/mL).

Dosage and administration   *Adult: First dose:* 0.2 mg IV/IO over 15 seconds. *Second dose:* 0.3 mg IV/IO over 30 seconds. If no response, give third dose. *Third dose:* 0.5 mg IV/IO over 30 seconds. If no response, repeat once every minute until adequate response or a total of 3 mg is given. **Pediatric:** Not recommended.

Duration of action   Onset: 1–2 minutes. Peak effect and duration: related to plasma concentration of benzodiazepines.

Special considerations   Pregnancy safety: Category C. Be prepared to manage seizures in patients who are physically dependent on benzodiazepines or who have ingested large doses of other drugs. Romazicon may precipitate withdrawal syndromes in patients dependent on benzodiazepines. Monitor patients for re-sedation and respiratory depression. Be prepared to assist ventilations.

Furosemide (Lasix)

Class Loop diuretic.

Mechanism of action Inhibits electrolyte reabsorption and promotes excretion of sodium, potassium, chloride.

Indications CHF, pulmonary edema, hypertensive crisis.

Contraindications Hypovolemia, anuria, hypotension (relative contraindication); hypersensitivity, hepatic coma.

Adverse reactions May exacerbate hypovolemia, hypokalemia, ECG changes, dry mouth, hypochloremia, hyponatremia, hyperglycemia (due to hemoconcentration).

Drug interactions Lithium toxicity may be potentiated by sodium depletion. Digitalis toxicity may be potentiated by potassium depletion.

How supplied 100 mg/5 mL, 20 mg/2 mL, 40 mg/4-mL vials.

Dosage and administration *Adult:* 0.5–1.0 mg/kg injected IV over 1 to 2 minutes. If no response, double the dose to 2 mg/kg over 1 to 2 minutes. *Pediatric:* 1 mg/kg/dose IV, IO.

Duration of action Onset: 5 minutes. Peak effects: 20–60 minutes. Duration: 4–6 hours.

Special considerations Pregnancy safety: Category C. Ototoxicity and deafness can occur with rapid administration. Should be protected from light.

Glucagon

Class Hyperglycemic agent, pancreatic hormone, insulin antagonist.

Mechanism of action Increases blood glucose level by stimulating glycogenolysis. Unknown mechanism of stabilizing cardiac rhythm in beta blocker overdose. Minimal positive inotropic and chronotropic response. Decreases gastrointestinal motility and secretions.

Indications Altered level of consciousness when hypoglycemia is suspected. May be used as inotropic agent in beta blocker overdose.

Contraindications Hyperglycemia, hypersensitivity.

Adverse reactions Nausea, vomiting, tachycardia, hypertension.

Drug interactions Incompatible in solution with most other substances. No significant drug interactions with other emergency medications.

How supplied 1-mg ampules (requires reconstitution with diluent provided)

Dosage and administration *Adult: Hypoglycemia:* 0.5–1 mg IM; may repeat in 7–10 minutes. *Calcium channel blocker or beta blocker overdose:* 3 mg initially, followed by infusion at 3 mg/hr as necessary. *Pediatric: Hypoglycemia:* 0.5–1 mg IM (for children < 20 kg). *Calcium channel blocker or beta blocker overdose:* not recommended.

Duration of action Onset: 1 minute. Peak effect: 30 minutes. Duration: variable (generally 9–17 minutes).

Special considerations Pregnancy safety: Category C. Ineffective if glycogen stores depleted. Should always be used in conjunction with 50% dextrose whenever possible. If patient does not respond to second dose glucagon, 50% dextrose must be administered.

Haloperidol (Haldol)

Class Tranquilizer, antipsychotic.

Mechanism of action Inhibits central nervous system (CNS) catecholamine receptors: strong antidopaminergic and weak anticholinergic. Acts on CNS to depress subcortical areas, mid-brain and ascending reticular activating system in the brain.

Indications Acute psychotic episodes.

Contraindications Agitation secondary to shock or hypoxia. Hypersensitivity.

Adverse reactions Extrapyramidal signs and symptoms, restlessness, spasms, Parkinson-like symptoms, drooling, dystonia, hypotension, orthostatic, hypotension, nausea, vomiting, blurred vision.

Drug interactions Enhanced CNS depression and hypotension in combination with alcohol. Antagonized amphetamines and epinephrine. Other CNS depressants may potentiate effects.

How supplied 5 mg/mL ampule.

Dosage and administration *Adult:* 2–5 mg IM every 30–60 minutes until sedation achieved. *Pediatric:* Not recommended.

Duration of action Onset: 10 minutes. Peak effect: 30–45 minutes. Duration: variable (generally 12–24 hours).

Special considerations Pregnancy safety: not established. Treat hypotension secondary to Haldol with fluids and norepinephrine, not epinephrine. Patient may also be taking Cogentin (benztropine mesylate) if on long-term therapy with Haldol.

Hydrocortisone Sodium Succinate (Solu-Cortef)

Class Corticosteroid

Mechanism of action Anti-inflammatory and immunosuppressive with salt-retaining actions.

Indications Shock due to acute adrenocortical insufficiency.

Contraindications None if given as single dose.

Adverse reactions Only for long-term use.

Drug interactions Incompatible with heparin and metaraminol.

How supplied 100-mg, 250-mg, or 500-mg vials.

Dosage and administration *Adult:* 4 mg/kg slow IV bolus. *Pediatric:* 0.16–1.0 mg/kg slow IV bolus.

Duration of action Onset: 1 hour. Peak effect: variable. Duration: 8–12 hours.

Special considerations May be used in status asthmaticus as a second-line drug.

Hydroxyzine (Atarax, Vistaril)

Class Antihistamine, antiemetic, antianxiety agent.

Mechanism of action Potentiates effects of analgesics; calming effect without impairing mental alertness.

Indications To potentiate the effects of analgesics; to control nausea and vomiting, anxiety reactions, and motion sickness; preoperative and postoperative sedation.

Contraindications Hypersensitivity.

Adverse reactions Dry mouth and drowsiness.

Drug interactions Potentiates the effects of CNS depressants such as narcotics, barbiturates, and alcohol.

How supplied 25 mg/mL or 50 mg/mL in 1-mL vials.

Dosage and administration *Adult:* 25–100 mg IM. *Pediatric:* 0.5–1.0 mg/kg/dose IM.

Duration of action Onset: IM: 15–30 minutes. Peak effect: 45 minutes to 1.5 hours. Duration: 4–6 hours.

Special considerations Should be given by IM injection only. Localized burning at injection site is common complaint.

Isoetharine (Bronchosol, Bronkometer)

Class Sympathomimetic.

Mechanism of action Beta-2 agonist; relaxes smooth muscle of bronchioles.

Indications Acute bronchial asthma, bronchospasm (especially in COPD patient).

Contraindications Use with caution in patients with diabetes, hyperthyroidism, cardiovascular and cerebrovascular disease.

Adverse reactions Dose-related tachycardia, palpitations, tremors, nervousness, nausea. Multiple doses can cause paradoxical bronchoconstriction.

Drug interactions Additive adverse effects if given with other beta-2 agonist drugs.

How supplied MDI; 2 mL unit dose of 1% solution.

Dosage and administration *Adult:* 1–2 inhalations with MDI. COPD: 2.5–5.0 mg (0.25 mL–0.5 mL) diluted in 3 mL normal saline (NS) and nebulized. *Pediatric:* 0.01 mL/kg; maximum dose: 0.5 mL diluted in 3 mL NS and nebulized.

Duration of action Onset: immediate. Peak effect: 5–15 minutes. Duration: 1–4 hours.

Special considerations None.

Ketorolac Tromethamine (Toradol IM)

Class Nonsteroidal anti-inflammatory (NSAID) analgesic.

Mechanism of action NSAID that also exhibits peripherally acting nonnarcotic analgesic activity by inhibiting prostaglandin synthesis.

Indications Short-term management of moderate to severe pain.

Contraindications Allergy to salicylates or other NSAIDs; patients with history of asthma; bleeding disorders, especially gastrointestinal (GI) related (peptic ulcer disease); renal failure.

Adverse reactions Anaphylaxis due to hypersensitivity, nausea, GI bleeding, sedation, hypotension or hypertension, rash, headache, edema.

Drug interactions May increase bleeding time in patients taking anticoagulants.

How supplied 15 or 30 mg in 1 mL or 60 mg in 2-mL vials.

Dosage and administration *Adult:* 30–60 mg IM. *Pediatric:* Not recommended.

Duration of action Onset: 10 minutes. Peak effect: 1–2 hours. Duration: 2–6 hours.

Special considerations Pregnancy safety: Category C. Use with caution in elderly patient. May be given IV in lower dosage (15–30 mg).

Labetolol (Normodyne, Trandate)

Class Selective alpha and nonselective beta-adrenergic blocker.

Mechanism of action Blood pressure reduced without reflex tachycardia; total peripheral resistance reduced without significant alteration in cardiac output.

Indications Moderate to severe hypertension.

Contraindications Bronchial asthma, CHF, cardiogenic shock, second- and third-degree heart block, bradycardia.

Adverse reactions Headache, dizziness, ventricular arrhythmias, hypotension, dyspnea, facial flushing, postural hypotension, diaphoresis, allergic reaction.

Drug interactions Trandate may block bronchodilator effects of beta-adrenergic agonists. NTG may augment hypotensive effects of Labetolol.

How supplied Trandate injection 5 mg/mL, 20 mL (100 mg) and 40 mL (200 mg) vials.

Dosage and administration *Adult:* 5–20 mg slow IV over 2 minutes (additional injections of 10–40 mg can be given at 10-minute intervals). Infusion: 2 mg/min titrated to acceptable supine blood pressure. *Pediatric:* safety not established.

Duration of action Onset: less than 5 minutes. Peak effect: variable. Duration: 3–6 hours.

Special considerations Pregnancy safety: Category C. Continuous monitoring of BP, pulse rate, and ECG. Observe for signs of CHF, bradycardia, bronchospasm. Should only be administered with patient in supine position.

Lidocaine Hydrochloride (Xylocaine)

Class Antiarrhythmic.

Mechanism of action Decreases automaticity by slowing the rate of phase 4 depolarization.

Indications Alternative to amiodarone in cardiac arrest from V-fib/pulseless V-tach, stable monomorphic V-tach, stable polymorphic V-tach with normal baseline QT interval.

Contraindications Hypersensitivity, second- and third-degree AV blocks in the absence of artificial pacemaker, Stokes-Adams syndrome, prophylactic use in AMI, wide-complex ventricular escape beats with bradycardia.

Adverse reactions Slurred speech, seizures (with high doses), altered mental status, confusion, lightheadedness, blurred vision, bradycardia.

Drug interactions Apnea induced with succinylcholine may be prolonged with high doses of lidocaine. Cardiac depression may occur in conjunction with IV phenytoin (Dilantin). Procainamide may exacerbate CNS effects. Metabolic clearance is decreased in patients with liver disease or in patients taking beta blockers.

How supplied 100 mg in 5-mL prefilled syringes and ampules (20 mg/mL), 1-g and 2-g additive syringes, 1-g and 2-g vials in 30 mL of solution.

Dosage and administration *Adult: Cardiac arrest from V-fib/pulseless V-tach:* Initial dose: 1–1.5 mg/kg IV/IO. Repeat dose: 0.5–0.75 mg/kg, repeated in 5–10 minutes to maximum dose of 3 mg/kg. Endotracheal (ET) dose: 2–4 mg/kg. *Stable V-tach, wide-complex tachycardia of uncertain type, significant ectopy:* Doses ranging from 0.5–0.75 mg/kg and up to 1–1.5 mg/kg may be used. Repeat 0.5–0.75 mg/kg every 5–10 minutes. Maximum total dose is 3 mg/kg. *Maintenance infusion:* 1–4 mg/min (30–50 µg/kg/min); can dilute in D_5W or normal saline. *Pediatric:* IV/IO dose: 1 mg/kg rapid IV/IO push. Maximum dose: 100 mg. *Continuous IV/IO infusion:* 20–50 µg/kg/min. Administer bolus dose (1 mg/kg) when infusion is initiated if bolus has not been given within previous 15 minutes. *Endotracheal (ET) dose:* 2–3 mg/kg.

Duration of action Onset: 1–3 minutes. Peak effect: 5–10 minutes. Duration: variable (15 minutes–2 hours).

Special considerations Pregnancy safety: Category B. Reduce maintenance infusions by 50% if patient is over 70 years of age, has liver or renal disease, or is in CHF or shock. A 75–100 mg bolus maintains blood levels for only 20 minutes (if not in shock). Exceedingly high doses of lidocaine can result in coma or death. Avoid lidocaine for reperfusion arrhythmias after fibrinolytic therapy. Cross-reactivity with other forms of local anesthetics.

Lorazepam (Ativan)

Class Benzodiazepine; sedative; anticonvulsant.

Mechanism of action Anxiolytic, anticonvulsant, and sedative effects; suppresses propagation of seizure activity produced by foci in cortex, thalamus, and limbic areas.

Indications Initial control of status epilepticus or severe recurrent seizures, severe anxiety, sedation.

Contraindications Acute narrow-angle glaucoma. Coma, shock, or suspected drug abuse.

Adverse reactions Respiratory depression, apnea, drowsiness, sedation, ataxia, psychomotor impairment, confusion, restlessness, delirium, hypotension, bradycardia.

Drug interactions May precipitate CNS depression if patient is already taking CNS depressant medications.

How supplied 2 and 4 mg/mL concentrations in 1 mL vials.

Dosage and administration *Note:* When given IV or IO, must dilute with equal volume of sterile water or sterile saline; When given IM, lorazepam is not to be diluted. *Adult:* 2–4 mg slow IV at 2 mg/min or IM; may repeat in 15–20 minutes to maximum dose of 8 mg. For sedation: 0.05 mg/kg up to 4 mg IM. *Pediatric:* 0.05–0.20 mg/kg slow IV, IO slowly over 2 minutes or IM; may repeat in 15–20 minutes to maximum dose of 0.2 mg/kg.

Duration of action Onset: 1–5 minutes. Peak effect: variable. Duration: 6–8 hours.

Special considerations Pregnancy safety: Category D. Monitor BP and respiratory rate during administration. Have advanced airway equipment readily available. Inadvertent arterial injection may result in vasospasm and gangrene. Lorazepam expires in 6 weeks if not refrigerated.

Magnesium Sulfate

Class Electrolyte.

Mechanism of action Reduces striated muscle contractions and blocks peripheral neuromuscular transmission by reducing acetylcholine release at the myoneural junction, manages seizures in toxemia of pregnancy, induces uterine relaxation, can cause bronchodilation after beta-agonists and anticholinergics have been used.

Indications Seizures of eclampsia (toxemia of pregnancy), torsade de pointes, hypomagnesemia, Class IIa agent for V-fib/pulseless V-tach that is refractory to lidocaine.

Contraindications Heart blocks, myocardial damage.

Adverse reactions CNS depression, facial flushing, diaphoresis, depressed reflexes, circulatory collapse, hypotension.

Drug interactions May enhance effects of other CNS depressants, serious changes in overall cardiac function may occur with cardiac glycosides.

How supplied 10%, 12.5%, 50% solution in 40, 80, 100, and 125 mg/mL.

Dosage and administration *Adult: Seizure activity associated with pregnancy:* 1–4 g IV/IO over 3 minutes; maximum dose of 30–40 g/day. *Cardiac arrest due to hypomagnesemia or torsade de pointes:* 1–2 g (2–4 mL of a 50% solution) diluted in 10 mL of D_5W IV/IO over 5–20 minutes. *Torsade de pointes with a pulse or AMI with hypomagnesemia:* Loading dose of 1–2 g mixed in 50–100 mL D_5W over 5–60 minutes IV. Follow with 0.5–1 g/hr IV (titrate to control torsade de pointes). *Pediatric:* IV/IO infusion: 25–50 mg/kg (maximum dose: 2 g) over 10–20 minutes; faster for torsade de pointes. *For asthma:* 25–50 mg/kg (maximum dose: 2 g) over 10–20 minutes.

Duration of action Onset: IV/IO: immediate, IM: 3–4 hours, Duration: 30 minutes (IV/IO), 3–4 hours (IM).

Special considerations Pregnancy safety: Category B. Recommended that the drug not be given in the 2 hours before delivery, if possible. IV calcium chloride or calcium gluconate should be available as a magnesium antagonist if needed. Use with caution in patients with renal failure.

Meperidine (Demerol)

Class Opioid analgesic.

Mechanism of action Synthetic opioid agonist that acts on opioid receptors to produce analgesia, euphoria, respiratory and physical depression; a schedule II drug with potential for physical dependency and abuse.

Indications Analgesia for moderate to severe pain.

Contraindications Hypersensitivity to narcotic agents, diarrhea caused by poisoning, patients taking MAOIs, during labor or delivery of a premature infant, undiagnosed abdominal pain or head injury.

Adverse reactions Respiratory depression, sedation, apnea, circulatory depression, arrhythmias, shock, euphoria, delirium, agitation, hallucinations, visual disturbances, coma, seizures, headache, facial flushing, increased ICP, nausea, vomiting.

Drug interactions Do not give concurrently with MAOIs (even with a dose in the last 14 days!). Exacerbates CNS depression when given with these medications.

How supplied 50/mL in 1-mL pre-filled syringes and Tubex.

Dosage and administration *Adult:* 50–100 mg IM, SC or 25–50 mg slowly IV. *Pediatric:* 1–2 mg/kg/dose IV, IO, IM, SC.

Duration of action Onset: IM: 10–45 minutes; IV: immediate. Peak effect: 30–60 minutes.

Special considerations Pregnancy safety: Category C. Use with caution in patients with asthma and COPD. May aggravate seizures in patients with known convulsive disorders. Naloxone should be readily available as antagonist.

Metaproterenol 5% (Alupent)

Class Sympathomimetic bronchodilator.

Mechanism of action Beta-2 agonist acts directly on bronchial smooth muscle causing relaxation of the bronchial tree and peripheral vasculature.

Indications Bronchial asthma, reversible bronchospasm secondary to bronchitis, COPD.

Contraindications Tachyarrhythmias, hypersensitivity, tachycardias due to digitalis toxicity.

Adverse reactions Tachyarrhythmias, anxiety, nausea, vomiting, restlessness, apprehension, palpitations, hypotension, coughing, facial flushing, diaphoresis.

Drug interactions Other sympathomimetics may exacerbate cardiovascular effects. MAOIs may potentiate hypotensive effects. Beta blockers may antagonize metaproterenol.

How supplied MDI: 0.65 mg/dose/spray (15-mL inhaler). Solution: 5% solution in bottles of 10 and 30 mL with calibrated dropper; Alupent inhalation solution unit-dose vial, 0.4% or 0.6%.

Dosage and administration *Adult:* MDI: 2–3 inhalations every 3–4 hours (2 minutes between inhalations). Inhalation solution 5%: via hand-held nebulizer 0.2–0.3 mL diluted in 2.5 mL saline. Inhalation solution unit-dose 0.4% or 0.6% vials: intermittent positive-pressure breathing device only: one vial/treatment. *Pediatric:* MDI: not recommended. Inhalation solution 5%: age 6–12 years: 0.1–0.2 mL diluted in 3 mL saline.

Duration of action Onset: 1 minute after inhalation. Peak effect: 45 minutes. Duration: 3–6 hours.

Special considerations Pregnancy safety: Category C. Monitor for hypotension or tachycardia. Use with caution in patients with diabetes mellitus and coronary artery disease.

Methylprednisolone (Solu-Medrol)

Class Anti-inflammatory glucocorticoid.

Mechanism of action Synthetic corticosteroid that suppresses acute and chronic inflammation; potentiates vascular smooth muscle relaxation by beta-adrenergic agonists.

Indications Acute spinal cord trauma, anaphylaxis, bronchodilator for unresponsive asthma.

Contraindications Premature infants, systemic fungal infections; use with caution in patients with gastrointestinal bleeding.

Adverse reactions Headache, hypertension, sodium and water retention. CHF, hypokalemia, alkalosis, peptic ulcer disease, nausea, vomiting.

Drug interactions Hypoglycemic responses to insulin and hypoglycemic agents may be blunted. Potassium-depleting agents may exacerbate hypokalemic effects.

How supplied 40-, 125-, 500- and 1,000-mg vials.

Dosage and administration *Adult:* Acute spinal cord injury: 30 mg/kg IV over 30 minutes followed by infusion: 5.4 mg/kg/h. Asthma, COPD: 1–2 mg/kg IV. *Pediatric:* Acute spinal cord trauma: 30 mg/kg IV over 30 minutes; infusion: 5.4 mg/kg/h. Asthma: 1–2 mg/kg/dose IV.

Duration of action Onset of action: 1–2 hours. Peak effects: variable. Duration of action: 8–24 hours.

Special considerations Pregnancy safety: not established. Not effective if spinal cord injury greater than 8 hours. Crosses the placenta and may cause fetal harm.

Midazolam (Versed)

Class Short-acting benzodiazepine CNS depressant.

Mechanism of action Anxiolytic and sedative properties similar to other benzodiazepines, memory impairment.

Indications Sedation, anxiolytic prior to endotracheal or nasotracheal intubation; administer for conscious sedation.

Contraindications Glaucoma, shock, coma, alcohol intoxication, overdose, depressed vital signs, concomitant use with other CNS depressants, barbiturates, alcohol, narcotics.

Adverse reactions Hiccough, cough, oversedation, nausea, vomiting, injection site pain, headache, blurred vision, hypotension, respiratory depression, and arrest.

Drug interactions Should not be used in patients who have taken a CNS depressant.

How supplied 2-, 5-, 10-mL vials (1 mg/mL); 1-, 2-, 5-, 10-mL vials (5 mg/mL).

Dosage and administration *Adult:* 2.0–2.5 mg slow IV over 2–3 minutes; may be repeated to total maximum: 0.1 mg/kg. *Pediatric:* Not recommended.

Duration of action Onset: 1–3 minutes, IV and dose dependent. Peak effect: variable. Duration: 2–6 hours, dose dependent.

Special considerations Pregnancy safety: Category D. Administer immediately prior to intubation procedure. Requires continuous monitoring of respiratory and cardiac function. Never administer as IV bolus.

Morphine Sulfate (Astramorph/PF and others)

Class   Opioid analgesic (schedule II narcotic).

Mechanism of action   Alleviates pain through CNS action, suppresses fear and anxiety centers in brain; depresses brain stem respiratory centers, increases peripheral venous capacitance and decreases venous return, decreases preload and afterload, which decreases myocardial oxygen demand.

Indications   Severe CHF, pulmonary edema, chest pain associated with acute MI, analgesia for moderate to severe acute and chronic pain (use with caution).

Contraindications   Head injury, exacerbated COPD, depressed respiratory drive, hypotension, undiagnosed abdominal pain, decreased level of consciousness, suspected hypovolemia, patients who have taken MAOIs within the past 14 days.

Adverse reactions   Respiratory depression, hypotension, decreased level of consciousness, nausea, vomiting, bradycardia, tachycardia, syncope, facial flushing, euphoria, bronchospasm, dry mouth.

Drug interactions   Potentiates sedative effects of phenothiazines. CNS depressant may potentiate effects of morphine. MAOIs may cause paradoxical excitation.

How supplied   10 mg in 1 mL of solution, ampules, and Tubex syringes.

Dosage and administration   *Adult:* Initial dose: 2–4 mg IV (over 1–5 minutes) every 5–30 minutes. *Repeat dose:* 2–8 mg at 5- to 15-minute intervals. ***Pediatric:*** 0.1–0.2 mg/kg per dose via IV, IO, IM, or SC; maximum dose of 5 mg.

Duration of action   Onset: immediate. Peak effect: 20 minutes. Duration: 2–7 hours.

Special considerations   Pregnancy safety: Category C. Morphine rapidly crosses the placenta. Safety in neonate not established. Use with caution in geriatric population and those with COPD, asthma. Vagotonic effect in patient with acute inferior MI (bradycardia, heart block). Naloxone should be readily available as an antidote.

Nalbuphine (Nubain)

Class   Opioid analgesic.

Mechanism of action   Activates opiate receptor in limbic system of CNS, analgesic similar to morphine on a milligram for milligram basis, agonist and antagonist properties; may be preferred for chest pain in setting of acute MI as it reduces the myocardial oxygen demand without reducing the blood pressure.

Indications   Chest pain associated with acute MI; moderate to severe acute pain; pulmonary edema, with or without associated chest pain (morphine remains first line).

Contraindications   Head injury or undiagnosed abdominal pain, diarrhea caused by poisoning, hypovolemia, hypotension.

Adverse reactions   Hypotension, bradycardia, facial flushing, respiratory depression, CNS depression, euphoria, paradoxical CNS stimulation, blurred vision.

Drug interactions   CNS depressants may potentiate effects.

How supplied   10 mg in 1-mL ampule (10 mg/mL), 20 mg in 1-mL ampule.

Dosage and administration   *Adult:* 2–5 mg slowly IV; may repeat 2-mg doses PRN to maximum dose of 10 mg. *Pediatric:* Not recommended.

Duration of action   Onset: 2–3 minutes. Peak effect: variable. Duration: 3–6 hours.

Special considerations   Pregnancy safety: Category B. Use with caution in patients with impaired respiratory function. May precipitate withdrawal syndromes in narcotic-dependent patients. Naloxone should be readily available.

Naloxone Hydrochloride (Narcan)

Class   Narcotic antagonist.

Mechanism of action   Competitive inhibition at narcotic receptor sites, reverse respiratory depression secondary to opiate drugs, completely inhibits the effect of morphine.

Indications   Opiate overdose, coma; complete or partial reversal of CNS and respiratory depression induced by opioids; decreased level of consciousness; coma of unknown origin; narcotic agonist for the following: morphine, heroin, hydromorphone (Dilaudid), methadone, meperidine (Demerol), paregoric, fentanyl (Sublimase), oxycodone (Percodan), codeine, propoxyphene (Darvon); narcotic agonist and antagonist for the following: Butorphanol (Stadol), pentazocine (Talwin), nalbuphine (Nubain).

Contraindications   Use with caution in narcotic-dependent patients; use with caution in neonates of narcotic-addicted mothers.

Adverse reactions   Withdrawal symptoms in the addicted patient, tachycardia, hypertension, arrhythmias, nausea, vomiting, diaphoresis.

Drug interactions   Incompatible with bisulfite and alkaline solutions.

How supplied   0.02 mg/mL (neonate); 0.4 mg/mL, 1 mg/mL; 2.0 mg/5-mL ampules; 2 mg/5-mL prefilled syringe.

Dosage and administration   *Adult:* 0.4–2.0 mg IV, IM, SC, or ET (diluted); minimum recommended dose, 2.0 mg; repeat at 5-minute intervals to a maximum dose of 10 mg (medical control may request higher amounts). Infusion: 2 mg in 500 mL of D_5W (4 µg/mL), infuse at 0.4 mg/h (100 mL/h). *Pediatric:* 0.1 mg/kg/dose IV, IM, SC, ET (diluted); maximum dose of 0.8 mg; if no response in 10 minutes, administer an additional 0.1 mg/kg/dose.

Duration of action   Onset: within 2 minutes. Peak effect: variable. Duration: 30–60 minutes.

Special considerations   Pregnancy safety: Category B. Seizures without causal relationship have been reported. May not reverse hypotension. Use caution when administering to narcotic addicts (potential violent behavior).

Nifedipine (Procardia)

Class   Calcium channel blocker.

Mechanism of action   Inhibits movement of calcium ions across cell membranes; calcium channel blocker, arterial and venous vasodilator; reduces preload and afterload; prevents coronary artery spasm and decreases total peripheral resistance; reduces myocardial oxygen demand; does not prolong AV nodal conduction.

Indications   Hypertensive crisis, angina pectoris, pulmonary edema (investigational).

Contraindications   Compensatory hypertension, hypotension, hypersensitivity.

Adverse reactions   Hypotension, CHF, headache, dizziness, lightheadedness, facial flushing, heat sensation, weakness, nausea, muscle cramps, mood changes, peripheral edema, myocardial infarction.

Drug interactions   Beta blockers may potentiate effects. Effects of theophylline may be increased. Antihypertensives may potentiate hypotensive effects.

How supplied   Soft gelatin capsules, 10–20 mg. Extended-release tablets, 30, 60, 90 mg.

Dosage and administration   *Adult:* 10 mg SL or buccal (puncture end of capsule with needle and squeeze; may administer SL or buccally or may have patient bite and swallow); may repeat in 30 minutes. *Pediatric:* Not recommended.

Duration of action   Onset: 15–30 minutes. Peak effect: 1–3 hours. Duration: 6–8 hours.

Special considerations   Pregnancy safety: Category C. Does not slow AV nodal activity. Have beta blocker available for control of reflex tachycardia. Use with caution in geriatric population; hypotension and angina pectoris may occur.

Nitroglycerin (Nitrostat, Tridil, and others)

Class   Vasodilator.

Mechanism of action   Smooth muscle relaxant acting on vascular, bronchial, uterine, and intestinal smooth muscle; dilation of arterioles and veins in the periphery; reduces preload and afterload; decreases the work load of the heart and, thereby, myocardial oxygen demand.

Indications   Acute angina pectoris, ischemic chest pain, hypertension, CHF, pulmonary edema.

Contraindications   Hypotension, hypovolemia; intracranial bleeding or head injury; previous administration of Viagra, Revatio, Levitra, Cialis, or similar agents within past 24 hours.

Adverse reactions   Headache, hypotension, syncope, reflex tachycardia, flushing, nausea, vomiting, diaphoresis, muscle twitching.

Drug interactions   Additive effects with other vasodilators; incompatible with other drugs IV.

How supplied   Tablets: 0.15 mg (1/400 grain); 0.3 mg (1/200 grain); 0.4 mg (1/150 grain); 0.6 mg (1/100 grain). NTG spray: 0.4 mg–0.8 mg under the tongue. NTG IV (Tridil).

Dosage and administration   *Adult:* Tablets: 0.3–0.4 mg SL; may repeat in 3–5 minutes to maximum of 3 doses. NTG spray: 0.4 mg under the tongue; 1–2 sprays. NTG IV infusion: begin at 10 to 20 µg/min; increase by 5–10 µg/min every 5 minutes until desired effect. *Pediatric:* Not recommended.

Duration of action   Onset: 1–3 minutes. Peak effect: 5–10 minutes. Duration: 20–30 minutes or if IV, 1–10 minutes after discontinuation of infusion.

Special considerations   Pregnancy safety: Category C. Hypotension more common in geriatric population. NTG decomposes if exposed to light or heat. Must be kept in airtight containers. Active ingredient may have a stinging effect when administered.

Nitropaste (Nitro-Bid Ointment)

Class   Vasodilator.

Mechanism of action   Same as NTG.

Indications   Angina pectoris and chest pain associated with acute MI.

Contraindications   Same as NTG.

Adverse reactions   Same as NTG.

Drug interactions   Same as NTG.

How supplied   2% solution of NTG in absorbent paste; 20-, 60-g tubes of paste with measuring applicators; transdermal units of varying doses.

Dosage and administration   *Adult:* Paste: Apply ½″ to ¾″ (1–2 cm), 15–30 mg, cover with wrap and secure with tape; maximum, 5″ (75 mg) per application. Transdermal: Apply unit to intact skin (usually chest wall) in varying doses. *Pediatric:* Not recommended.

Duration of action   Onset: 30 minutes. Peak effect: variable. Duration: 18–24 hours.

Special considerations   Pregnancy safety: Category C. Not of great value in prehospital arena. Avoid using fingers to spread paste. Store paste in cool place with tube tightly capped. Erratic absorption rates quite common.

Nitrous Oxide:Oxygen (50:50) (Nitronox)

Class   Gaseous analgesic and anesthetic.

Mechanism of action   Exact mechanism unknown; affects central nervous system phospholipids.

Indications   Moderate to severe pain, anxiety, apprehension.

Contraindications   Impaired level of consciousness, head injury, inability to comply with instructions; decompression sickness (nitrogen narcosis, air embolism, air transport); undiagnosed abdominal pain or marked distention, bowel obstruction; hypotension, shock, COPD (with history/suspicion of carbon dioxide retention); cyanosis; chest trauma with pneumothorax.

Adverse reactions   Dizziness, apnea, expansion of gas-filled pockets, cyanosis, nausea, vomiting, malignant hyperthermia, drowsiness, euphoria.

Drug interactions   None of significance.

How supplied   D and E cylinders (blue and green); of 50% nitrous oxide and 50% oxygen compressed gas.

Dosage and administration   *Adult:* (*Note:* Invert cylinder several times before use) Instruct the patient to inhale deeply through demand valve and mask or mouthpiece. *Pediatric:* Same as adult.

Duration of action   Onset: 2–5 minutes. Peak effect: variable. Duration: 2–5 minutes.

Special considerations   Pregnancy safety: Nitrous oxide increases the incidence of spontaneous abortion. Ventilate patient area during use. Nitrous oxide is a nonflammable and nonexplosive gas. Nitrous oxide is ineffective in 20% of the population.

Norepinephrine (Levophed, Levarterenol)

Class   Sympathomimetic.

Mechanism of action   Potent alpha-agonist resulting in intense vasoconstriction; positive chronotropic and increased inotropic effect (from 10% beta effects) with increased cardiac output.

Indications   Cardiogenic shock, significant hypotensive (< 70 mm Hg) states.

Contraindications   Hypotensive patients with hypovolemia, pregnancy (relative contraindication).

Adverse reactions   Headache, arrhythmias, tachycardia, reflex bradycardia; angina pectoris, hypertension; decreased blood flow to gastrointestinal tract, kidneys, skeletal muscle, and skin.

Drug interactions   Can be deactivated by alkaline solutions. Sympathomimetics and phosphodiesterase inhibitors may exacerbate arrhythmias. Bretylium may potentiate the effects of catecholamines.

How supplied   1-mg/mL, 4-mL ampules.

Dosage and administration   *Adult:* Dilute 8 mg in 500 mL of D_5W or 4 mg in 250 mL of D_5W (16 mg/mL); infuse by IV piggyback at 0.5–1.0 µg/min, titrated to improve blood pressure (up to 30 µg/min). *Pediatric:* 0.1–1.0 µg/min IV infusion, titrated to patient response.

Duration of action   Onset: 1–3 minutes. Peak effect: variable. Duration: 5–10 minutes and lasts only 1 minute after infusion discontinued.

Special considerations   Pregnancy safety: not established. May cause fetal anoxia when used in pregnancy. Must be infused through large stable vein to avoid tissue necrosis (antidote: local phentolamine injection). Often used with low-dose dopamine to spare renal and mesenteric blood flow.

Oral Glucose (Insta-Glucose)

Class   Hyperglycemic.

Mechanism of action   Provides quickly absorbed glucose to increase blood glucose levels.

Indications   Conscious patients with suspected hypoglycemia.

Contraindications   Decreased level of consciousness, nausea, vomiting.

Adverse reactions   Nausea, vomiting.

Drug interactions   None.

How supplied   Glucola: 300-mL bottles. Glucose pastes and gels in various forms.

Dosage and administration   *Adult:* Should be sipped slowly by patient until clinical improvement noted. *Pediatric:* Same as adult.

Duration of action   Onset: immediate. Peak effect: variable. Duration: variable.

Special considerations   As noted in indications section.

Oxygen

Class   Naturally occurring atmospheric gas.

Mechanism of action   Reverses hypoxemia.

Indications   Confirmed or expected hypoxemia, ischemic chest pain, respiratory insufficiency, prophylactically during air transport, confirmed or suspected carbon monoxide poisoning, all other causes of decreased tissue oxygenation, decreased level of consciousness.

Contraindications   Certain patients with COPD or emphysema who will not tolerate oxygen concentrations over 35%, hyperventilation.

Adverse reactions   Decreased level of consciousness and respiratory depression in patients with chronic carbon dioxide retention. Retrolental fibroplasia if give high concentrations to premature infants (maintain 30%-40% oxygen).

Drug interactions   None.

How supplied   Oxygen cylinders (usually green and white) of 100% compressed oxygen gas.

Dosage and administration   *Adult:* Cardiac arrest and carbon monoxide poisoning: 100%. Hypoxemia: 10–15 L/min via nonrebreathing mask. COPD: 1–6 L/min via nasal cannula or 28%–35% Venturi mask. Be prepared to provide ventilatory support if higher concentrations of oxygen needed. *Pediatric:* Same as for adult with exception of premature infant.

Duration of action   Onset: immediate. Peak effect: not applicable. Duration: Less than 2 minutes.

Special considerations   Be familiar with liter flow and each type of delivery device used. Supports possibility of combustion.

Oxytocin (Pitocin)

Class   Hormone.

Mechanism of action   Increases uterine contractions.

Indications   Postpartum hemorrhage after infant and placental delivery.

Contraindications   Presence of second fetus, unfavorable fetal position, hypersensitivity.

Adverse reactions   Hypotension, hypertension, tachycardia, arrhythmias, angina pectoris; anxiety, seizures, nausea, vomiting, uterine rupture; anaphylaxis.

Drug interactions   Other vasopressors may potentiate hypertension.

How supplied   10 USP units/1-mL ampule (10 U/mL) and prefilled syringe. 5 USP units/1-mL ampule (5 U/mL) and prefilled syringe.

Dosage and administration   IM administration: 3–10 units after delivery of placenta. IV administration: Mix 10–40 units in 1,000 mL of a nonhydrating diluent: Infused at 20–40 milliunits/min, titrated to severity of bleeding and uterine response.

Duration of action   Onset: IM: 3–5 minutes; IV: immediate. Peak effect: variable. Duration: IM; 30–60 minutes; IV: 20 minutes after infusion discontinued.

Special considerations   Pregnancy safety: not applicable. Monitor vital signs, including fetal heart rate and uterine tone closely.

Pancuronium (Pavulon)

Class Nondepolarizing neuromuscular blocker/paralytic.

Mechanism of action Binds to the receptor for acetylcholine at the neuromuscular junction.

Indications Induction or maintenance of paralysis after intubation to assist ventilations.

Contraindications Hypersensitivity, inability to control airway and support ventilations with oxygen and positive pressure, neuromuscular disease (myasthenia gravis), hepatic or renal failure.

Adverse reactions Apnea, weakness, salivation, premature ventricular contractions, tachycardia; transient hypotension, increased blood pressure; pain, burning at injection site.

Drug interactions Positive chronotropic drugs may potentiate tachycardia.

How supplied 4-mg/2-mL ampule.

Dosage and administration *Adult:* 0.1 mg/kg slow IV; repeat every 30–60 minutes PRN. *Pediatric:* 0.1 mg/kg slow IV, IO.

Duration of action Onset: 30 seconds. Peak effect: paralysis in 3–5 minutes. Duration: 45–60 minutes.

Special considerations Pregnancy safety: not established. If patient is conscious, explain the effect of the medication before administration and always sedate the patient before using pancuronium. Intubation and ventilatory support must be readily available. Monitor the patient carefully. Effects may be reversed with neostigmine (Prostigmin) 0.05 mg/kg and should be accompanied by atropine (0.5–1.2 mg IV). Pancuronium has no effect on consciousness or pain. Will not stop neuronal seizure activity. Pulse rate, cardiac output are increased. Decrease doses for patients with renal disease.

Phenobarbital (Luminal)

Class Barbiturate, anticonvulsant.

Mechanism of action Generally unknown but believed to reduce neuronal excitability by increasing the motor cortex threshold to electrical stimulation.

Indications Prevention and treatment of seizure activity; prophylaxis for febrile seizures; anxiety, apprehension; status epilepticus.

Contraindications Patients with porphyria, hypersensitivity, severe liver or respiratory diseases.

Adverse reactions Respiratory depression, hypotension, coma, bradycardia, nausea, vomiting; central nervous system (CNS) depression, ataxia, nystagmus, pupillary constriction; burning at injection site.

Drug interactions Effects potentiated by other CNS depressants, anticonvulsants, and MAOIs; incompatible with all other drugs; flush line before and after use.

How supplied Elixir: 20 mg/5 mL. Tablets: 8, 15, 30, 60, 90, 100 mg. Parenteral: 30, 60, 65 mg, 130 mg/mL ampule; dose may be diluted with 9 mL of D_5W (6.5, 13 mg/mL).

Dosage and administration *Adult:* 100–250 mg slow IV, or IM; may repeat as needed in 20–30 minutes. *Pediatric:* 10–20 mg/kg IV, IO (less than 1 mg/kg/min) or IM; repeat as needed in 20–30 minutes.

Duration of action Onset: 3–30 minutes. Peak effect: 30 minutes. Duration: 4–6 hours.

Special considerations Pregnancy safety: Category B. Potential for abuse. Carefully monitor vital signs. Use with caution in patients with pulmonary, cardiovascular, hepatic, or renal insufficiency. Use a large, stable vein for injection.

Phenytoin (Dilantin)

Class Anticonvulsant.

Mechanism of action Promotes sodium efflux from neurons, thereby stabilizing the neuron's threshold against excitability caused by excess stimulation; in similar fashion, decreases abnormal ventricular automaticity and decreases the refractory period in the myocardial conduction system.

Indications Prophylaxis and treatment of major motor seizures, digitalis-induced arrhythmias.

Contraindications Hypersensitivity, bradycardia, second- and third-degree heart block.

Adverse reactions Hypotension with too rapid IV push, heart block, arrhythmias, cardiovascular collapse, nausea, vomiting, ataxia, central nervous system depression, nystagmus, pain at injection site, respiratory depression.

Drug interactions Serum dilantin levels increased by: anticoagulants, tagamet, sulfonamides, salicylates. Metabolism increased by chronic alcohol use. Cardiac depressant effects increased by lidocaine, propranolol, and other beta blockers. Precipitation may occur when mixed with D_5W. Incompatible with many solutions and medications.

How supplied 50 mg/mL in 2- and 5-mL ampules, 2-mL prefilled syringes. May be diluted in normal saline (NS) (1–10 mg/mL); use in-line filter. *Note:* IV line should be flushed with 0.9% NS before and after drug administration.

Dosage and administration *Adult:* Seizures: 10–20 mg/kg slow IV, not to exceed 1 g or rate of 50 mg/min). Arrhythmias: 50–100 mg (diluted) slow IV every 5–15 min PRN; maximum, 1 g. *Pediatric:* Seizures: 10–20 mg/kg slow IV (1–3 mg/kg/min). Arrhythmias: 5 mg/kg slow IV; maximum, 1 g.

Duration of action Onset: 20–30 minutes for seizure disorder. Peak effect: 1–3 hours. Duration: 18–24 hours but as long as 15 days reported.

Special considerations Pregnancy safety: not established. Carefully monitor vital signs. Venous irritation may occur (use large stable vein).

Pralidoxime Chloride (2-PAM Chloride, Protopam)

Class Cholinesterase reactivator.

Mechanism of action Reactivation of cholinesterase to effectively act as an antidote to organophosphate pesticide poisoning. This action allows for destruction of accumulated acetylcholine at the neuromuscular junction.

Indications As an antidote in the treatment of poisoning by organophosphate pesticides and chemicals. In the prehospital arena, is used when atropine is or has become ineffective in management of organophosphate poisoning.

Contraindications Use with caution in patients with reduced renal function; patients with myasthenia gravis and organophosphate poisoning.

Adverse reactions Dizziness, blurred vision, diplopia, headache, drowsiness, nausea, tachycardia, hyperventilation, muscular weakness, excitement, and manic behavior.

Drug interactions No direct drug interactions; however, patients with organophosphate poisoning should not be given barbiturates, morphine, theophylline, aminophylline, succinylcholine, reserpine, and phenothiazines.

How supplied Emergency Single Dose Kit containing: One 20-mL vial of 1 g sterile protopam chloride. One 20-mL ampule of sterile diluent. Sterile, disposable 20-mL syringe. Needle and alcohol swab.

Dosage and administration *Note:* If Protopam is to be used, it should be administered almost simultaneously with atropine. *Adult:* Initial dose of 1–2 g as an IV infusion with 100 mL saline over 15–30 minutes. *Pediatric:* 20–40 mg/kg as IV infusion over 15–30 minutes. Doses may be repeated every 1 hour if muscle weakness persists. If IV administration is not feasible, IM or SC injection may be utilized.

Duration of action Onset: minutes. Peak effects: variable. Duration: variable.

Special considerations Pregnancy safety: unknown. Treatment will be most effective if given within a few hours after poisoning. Cardiac monitoring should be considered in all cases of severe organophosphate poisoning.

Procainamide (Pronestyl)

Class Antiarrhythmic.

Mechanism of action Suppresses phase 4 depolarization in normal ventricular muscle and Purkinje fibers, reducing ectopic pacemaker automaticity; suppresses intraventricular conduction.

Indications Stable monomorphic V-tach with normal QT interval, reentry SVT uncontrolled by vagal maneuvers and adenosine, stable wide-complex tachycardia of unknown origin, atrial fibrillation with rapid ventricular rate in patients with Wolff-Parkinson-White syndrome.

Contraindications Torsade de pointes, second- and third-degree AV block (without functional artificial pacemaker), digitalis toxicity, tricyclic antidepressant overdose.

Adverse reactions Widening of the PR, QRS, and QT intervals, AV heart block, hypotension, reflex tachycardia, bradycardia, nausea and vomiting.

Drug interactions May increase plasma levels of amiodarone and quinidine.

How supplied 1 g in 10-mL vials (100 mg/mL); 1 g in 2-mL vials (500 mg/mL) for infusion.

Dosage and administration *Adult: Recurrent V-fib/pulseless V-tach:* 20 mg/min IV infusion (maximum dose: 17 mg/kg). In urgent situations, up to 50 mg/min may be administered (maximum dose of 17 mg/kg). *Other indications:* 20 mg/min IV infusion until any **one** of the following occurs: arrhythmia suppression, hypotension, QRS widens by > 50% of its pre-treatment width, or total dose of 17 mg/kg has been given. *Maintenance infusion:* 1–4 mg/min (dilute in D5W or normal saline). *Pediatric:* Loading dose of 15 mg/kg IV/IO over 30–60 minutes.

Duration of action Onset: 10–30 minutes. Peak effect: variable. Duration: 3–6 hours.

Special considerations Pregnancy safety: Category C. Potent vasodilating and negative inotropic effects. Hypotension may occur with rapid infusion. Administer cautiously to patients with renal, hepatic, or cardiac insufficiency. Administer cautiously to patients with asthma or digitalis-induced arrhythmias.

Promethazine (Phenergan)

Class Antihistamine.

Mechanism of action H-1 receptor antagonist; blocks action of histamine; possesses sedative, anti-motion, antiemetic and anticholinergic activity; potentiates the effects of narcotics to induce analgesia.

Indications Nausea, vomiting, motion sickness; sedation for patients in labor; potentiation of analgesic effects of narcotics.

Contraindications Hypersensitivity, coma, CNS-depressed patients from alcohol, barbiturates, narcotics, Reye's syndrome.

Adverse reactions Sedation, dizziness, impairment of mental and physical ability, arrhythmias, nausea, vomiting, hyperexcitability; hallucinations, convulsions, and sudden death when used in children.

Drug interactions Additive with other CNS depressants. Increased extrapyramidal effects with MAOIs.

How supplied 25 and 50 mg/mL in 1-mL ampules and Tubex syringes.

Dosage and administration *Adult:* 12.5–25 mg IV, deep IM, PO, rectally. *Pediatric:* (greater than 2 years old) 0.25–0.5 mg/kg dose IM.

Duration of action Onset: IV: immediate. Peak effect: 30–60 minutes. Duration: 4–6 hours.

Special considerations Pregnancy safety: Category C. Use cautiously in patients with asthma, peptic ulcer disease and bone marrow suppression. Do not use in children with vomiting of unknown etiology. Avoid intra-arterial injection. IM injection is preferred route.

Vecuronium (Norcuron)

Class Paralytic agent.

Mechanism of action Nondepolarizing neuromuscular blocking agent, paralytic.

Indications To facilitate intubation, to terminate laryngospasm, to promote muscle relaxation, to facilitate electroconvulsive shock therapy.

Contraindications Acute narrow angle glaucoma, penetrating eye injuries, inability to control airway or support ventilations with oxygen and positive pressure, newborns, myasthenia gravis, hepatic or renal failure.

Adverse reactions Apnea, weakness, salivation, premature ventricular contractions, tachycardia, transient hypotension, increased blood pressure.

Drug interactions Use of inhalational anesthetics will enhance neuromuscular blockade.

How supplied 10 mg/10 mL vecuronium bromide vials with diluent. 20-mL vials (20 mg vecuronium) without diluent.

Dosage and administration *Adult:* 0.1 mg/kg IV push; maintenance dose within 25–40 minutes: 0.01–0.05 mg/kg IV push. *Pediatric:* 0.1 mg/kg IV, IO; maintenance dose within 20–35 minutes: 0.01–0.05 mg/kg IV push.

Duration of action Onset: 30 seconds. Peak effects: 2.5–3 minutes. Duration: 25–30 minutes.

Special considerations Pregnancy safety: Category C. If patient is conscious, explain the effect of the medication before administration and always sedate the patient before using vecuronium. Intubation and ventilatory support must be readily available. Monitor the patient carefully. Vecuronium has no effect on consciousness or pain. Will not stop neuronal seizure activity. Pulse rate, cardiac output are increased. Decrease doses for patients with renal disease.

Verapamil (Isoptin)

Class Antiarrhythmic.

Mechanism of action Calcium channel blocker, class IV antiarrhythmic, prolongs AV nodal refractory period, dilates coronary arteries and arterioles.

Indications PSVT, PAT, atrial fibrillation and atrial flutter with rapid ventricular response.

Contraindications Wolff-Parkinson-White syndrome, second-degree or third-degree AV block, sick sinus syndrome (unless patient has functioning pacemaker), hypotension, cardiogenic shock, severe CHF, pulmonary edema, patients receiving IV beta blockers, wide-complex tachycardias, children less than 12 months of age.

Adverse reactions Hypotension, AV block, bradycardia, asystole, dizziness, headache, nausea, vomiting, complete AV block, peripheral edema.

Drug interactions Increases serum concentration of digoxin. Beta-adrenergic blockers may have additive negative inotropic and chronotropic effects. Antihypertensives may potentiate hypotensive effects.

How supplied 5 mg/2 mL in 2-, 4-, 5-mL vials or 2-, 4-mL ampules.

Dosage and administration *Adult:* 2.5–5.0 mg IV bolus over 2 minutes (over 3 minutes in older patients). Repeat doses of 5–10 mg may be given every 15–30 minutes to a maximum of 20 mg. *Pediatric:* 0.1–0.2 mg/kg/dose IV, IO push over 2 minutes. Repeat dose in 30 minutes if not effective. (*Note:* not to be used in children less than 12 months of age.).

Duration of action Onset: 2–5 minutes. Peak effect: variable. Duration: 30–60 minutes.

Special considerations Pregnancy safety: Category C. Closely monitor patient's vital signs. Be prepared to resuscitate. AV block or asystole may occur as result of slowed AV conduction.

IV Solutions (Colloids and Crystalloids)

Colloids expand plasma volume by colloidal osmotic pressure. Colloids are most often used in hypovolemic shock states. Crystalloids are substances in solution that can diffuse through the intravascular compartment. Crystalloid solutions are used for electrolyte replacement, a route for medication, and short-term intravascular volume expansion.

Plasma Protein Fraction (Plasmanate)

Class   Natural colloid.

Mechanism of action   Plasmanate is a protein-containing colloid that remains in the intravascular compartment. It increases intravascular volume by attracting water from other fluid compartments by virtue of its colloid osmotic pressure.

Indications   Hypovolemic shock, especially burn shock; hypoproteinemia (low protein states)

Contraindications   There are no major contraindications to plasma protein fraction when used in the treatment of life-threatening hypovolemic states.

Adverse reactions   Chills, fever, urticaria (hives), nausea, and vomiting have all been reported with plasma protein fraction use.

Drug interactions   Solutions should not be mixed with or administered through the same administration sets as other intravenous fluids.

How supplied   Plasma protein fraction is supplied in 250- and 500-mL bottles of a 5% solution. An administration set is usually attached.

Dosage and administration   The plasma protein fraction infusion rate should be titrated according to the patient's hemodynamic response. In the management of shock secondary to burns, the physician's orders regarding the rate of administration must be closely followed. Standard formulas for IV fluid administration have been developed. The medical control physician will use these in judging the correct rate of intravenous administration.

Duration of action   24–36 hours.

Special considerations   Do not use if the solution is cloudy or if you see sedimentation.

Dextran

Class   Artificial colloid.

Mechanism of action   Dextran is a sugar-containing colloid used as an intravascular volume expander. It remains in the intravascular compartment for approximately 12 hours. It increases intravascular volume by attracting water from other fluid compartments by virtue of its colloid osmotic pressure.

Indications   Hypovolemic shock.

Contraindications   Dextran should not be administered to patients who have a known hypersensitivity to the drug. It should not be administered to patients suffering congestive heart failure, renal failure, or known bleeding disorders.

Adverse reactions   Rash, itching, dyspnea, chest tightness, and mild hypotension have all been reported with dextran use. The incidence of these side effects is, however, very low, and reactions are generally mild. Increased bleeding time has also been reported with dextran use due to its interference with platelet function.

Drug interactions   Dextran should not be administered to patients who are receiving anticoagulants as it significantly retards blood clotting.

How supplied   Dextran 40 and Dextran 70 are supplied in 250- and 500-mL bottles.

Dosage and administration   The dosage of dextran is titrated according to the patient's physiologic response.

Duration of action   8–12 hours.

Special considerations   In the management of burn shock, it is especially important to follow standard fluid resuscitation regimens to prevent possible circulatory overload.

Hetastarch (Hespan)

Class   Artificial colloid.

Mechanism of action   Hetastarch is a starch-containing colloid used as an intravascular volume expander. Following administration, the plasma volume is expanded slightly in excess of the volume of hetastarch administered. This effect has been observed for up to 24 to 36 hours. Hetastarch increases intravascular volume by virtue of its colloid osmotic pressure.

Indications   Hypovolemic shock, especially burn shock; septic shock.

Contraindications   There are no major contraindications to hetastarch when used in the management of life-threatening hypovolemic states.

Adverse reactions   Nausea, vomiting, mild febrile reactions, chills, itching, and urticaria (hives) have been reported with hetastarch administration. Severe anaphylactic reactions have been rarely reported.

Drug interactions   Hetastarch should not be administered to patients who are receiving anticoagulants.

How supplied   Sterile 6% hetastarch in 0.9% sodium chloride is supplied in 500-mL bottles.

Dosage and administration   The dosage of hetastarch is titrated according to the patient's physiologic response.

Duration of action   24–36 hours.

Special considerations   Pregnancy safety: Category C. Patients allergic to corn may be allergic to hetastarch.

Lactated Ringer's (Hartman's Solution)

Class   Isotonic crystalloid solution.

Mechanism of action   Lactated Ringer's replaces water and electrolytes.

Indications   Hypovolemic shock; keep open IV.

Contraindications   Lactated Ringer's should not be used in patients with congestive heart failure or renal failure.

Adverse reactions   Rare in therapeutic dosages.

Drug interactions   Few in the emergency setting.

How supplied   Lactated Ringer's is supplied in 250-, 500-, and 1,000-mL bags, IV infusion.

Dosage and administration   Hypovolemic shock; titrate according to patient's physiologic response.

Duration of action   Short-term therapy.

Special considerations   None.

5% Dextrose in Water (D₅W)

Class   Hypotonic dextrose-containing solution.

Mechanism of action D_5W provides nutrients in the form of dextrose as well as free water.

Indications   IV access for emergency drugs; for dilution of concentrated drugs for intravenous infusion.

Contraindications D_5W should not be used as a fluid replacement for hypovolemic states.

Adverse reactions   Rare in therapeutic dosages.

Drug interactions D_5W should not be used with phenytoin (Dilantin) or amrinone (Inocor).

How supplied D_5W is supplied in bags of 50, 100, 150, 250, 500, and 1,000 mL.

Dosage and administration D_5W is usually administered through a minidrip (60 drops/mL) set at a rate of "to keep open" (TKO).

Duration of action   Short-term therapy.

Special considerations   None.

10% Dextrose in Water (D₁₀W)

Class   Hypertonic dextrose-containing solution.

Mechanism of action $D_{10}W$ provides nutrients in the form of dextrose as well as free water.

Indications   Neonatal resuscitation, hypoglycemia.

Contraindications $D_{10}W$ should not be used as a fluid replacement for hypovolemic states.

Adverse reactions   Rare in therapeutic dosages.

Drug interactions   Should not be used with phenytoin (Dilantin) or amrinone (Inocor).

How supplied $D_{10}W$ is supplied in bags of 50, 100, 150, 250, 500, and 1,000 mL.

Dosage and administration   The administration rate of $D_{10}W$ will usually be dependent on the patient's condition.

Duration of action   Short-term therapy.

Special considerations   None.

0.9% Sodium Chloride (Normal Saline)

Class   Isotonic crystalloid solution.

Mechanism of action   Normal saline replaces water and electrolytes.

Indications   Heat-related problems (heat exhaustion, heat stroke), freshwater drowning, hypovolemia, diabetic ketoacidosis, keep open IV.

Contraindications   The use of 0.9% sodium chloride should not be considered in patients with congestive heart failure as circulatory overload can be easily induced.

Adverse reactions   Rare in therapeutic dosages.

Drug interactions   Few in the emergency setting.

How supplied   Normal saline is supplied in 250-, 500-, and 1,000-mL bags. Sterile normal saline for irrigation should not be confused with that designed for intravenous administration.

Dosage and administration   The specific situation being treated will dictate the rate in which normal saline will be administered. In severe heat stroke, diabetic ketoacidosis, and freshwater drowning, it is likely that you will be called on to administer the fluid quite rapidly. In other cases, it is advisable to administer the fluid at a moderate rate (for example, 100 mL/h).

Duration of action   Short-term therapy.

Special considerations   None.

0.45% Sodium Chloride (½ Normal Saline)

Class   Hypotonic crystalloid solution.

Mechanism of action   One-half normal saline replaces free water and electrolytes.

Indications   Patients with diminished renal or cardiovascular function for which rapid rehydration is not indicated.

Contraindications   Cases in which rapid rehydration is indicated.

Adverse reactions   Rare in therapeutic dosages.

Drug interactions   Few in the emergency setting.

How supplied   One-half normal saline is supplied in 250-, 500-, and 1,000-mL bags.

Dosage and administration   The specific situation and patient condition will dictate the rate at which one-half normal saline will be administered.

Duration of action   Short-term therapy.

Special considerations   None.

5% Dextrose in 0.45% Sodium Chloride ($D_5\frac{1}{2}NS$)

Class   Hypertonic dextrose-containing crystalloid solution.

Mechanism of action $D_5\frac{1}{2}NS$ replaces free water and electrolytes and provides nutrients in the form of dextrose.

Indications   Heat exhaustion, diabetic disorders; for use as a way to keep open solution in patients with impaired renal or cardiovascular function.

Contraindications $D_5\frac{1}{2}NS$ should not be used when rapid fluid resuscitation is indicated.

Adverse reactions   Rare in therapeutic dosages.

Drug interactions $D_5\frac{1}{2}NS$ should not be used with phenytoin (Dilantin) or amrinone (Inocor).

How supplied $D_5\frac{1}{2}NS$ is supplied in bags containing 250, 500, and 1,000 mL of the fluid.

Dosage and administration   The specific situation and patient condition will dictate the rate at which $D_5\frac{1}{2}NS$ should be administered.

Duration of action   Short-term therapy.

Special considerations   None.

5% Dextrose in 0.9% Sodium Chloride (D_5NS)

Class   Hypertonic dextrose-containing crystalloid solution.

Mechanism of action D_5NS replaces free water and electrolytes and provides nutrients in the form of dextrose.

Indications   Heat-related disorders, freshwater drowning, hypovolemia, peritonitis.

Contraindications D_5NS should not be administered to patients with impaired cardiac or renal function.

Adverse reactions   Rare in therapeutic dosages.

Drug interactions D_5NS should not be used with phenytoin (Dilantin) or amrinone (Inocor).

How supplied D_5NS is supplied in bags containing 250, 500, and 1,000 mL of the solution.

Dosage and administration   The specific situation and patient condition will dictate the rate at which D_5NS is given.

Duration of action   Short-term therapy.

Special considerations   None.

5% Dextrose in Lactated Ringer's (D_5LR)

Class   Hypertonic dextrose-containing crystalloid solution.

Mechanism of action D_5LR replaces water and electrolytes and provides nutrients in the form of dextrose.

Indications   Hypovolemic shock, hemorrhagic shock, certain cases of acidosis.

Contraindications D_5LR should not be administered to patients with decreased renal or cardiovascular function.

Adverse reactions   Rare in therapeutic dosages.

Drug interactions D_5LR should not be used with phenytoin (Dilantin) or amrinone (Inocor).

How supplied D_5LR is supplied in bags containing 250, 500, and 1,000 mL of the fluid.

Dosage and administration   In severe hypovolemic shock D_5LR should be infused through a large-bore catheter (14 or 16 gauge). This infusion should be administered "wide open" until a blood pressure of 100 mm Hg is achieved. When the blood pressure is attained, the infusions should be reduced to 100 mL/h. In other cases, the specific situation and patient condition will dictate the rate of administration.

Duration of action   Short-term therapy.

Special considerations   None.

Glossary

6 Ps of musculoskeletal assessment Pain, Paralysis, Parasthesias, Pulselessness, Pallor, and Pressure.

abandonment Abrupt termination of contact with the patient without giving the patient sufficient opportunity to find another suitable health care professional to take over his or her medical treatment.

abduction Movement away from the midline of the body.

aberrant conduction The abnormal conduction of the electrical impulse through the heart.

ABO system The antigen classification given to blood.

abortion Expulsion of the fetus, from any cause, before the 20th week of gestation.

abrasion An injury in which a portion of the body is denuded of epidermis by scraping or rubbing.

abruptio placenta A premature separation of the placenta from the wall of the uterus.

abscess A collection of pus in a sac, formed by necrotic tissues and an accumulation of white blood cells.

absence seizures The type of seizures characterized by a brief lapse of attention in which the patient may stare and not respond; formerly known as petit mal seizures.

absolute refractory period The early phase of cardiac repolarization, wherein the heart muscle cannot be stimulated to depolarize.

absorption The process by which a substance's molecules are moved from the site of entry or administration into the body and into systemic circulation.

absorption (hazardous materials) A type of decontamination that is done with large pads that the hazardous materials team carry to soak up liquid and remove it from the patient.

abuse Any form of maltreatment that results in harm or loss. Maltreatment may be physical, sexual, psychological, or financial/material.

acceleration The rate of change in velocity.

access port A sealed hub on an administration set designed for sterile access to the IV fluid.

accessory muscles Muscles not normally used during normal breathing; includes the sternocleidomastoid muscles of the neck.

accountability system A method of accounting for all personnel at an emergency incident and ensuring that only personnel with specific assignments are permitted to work within the various zones.

acetabulum The cup-shaped cavity in which the rounded head of the femur rotates.

acetylcholine (ACh) Chemical neurotransmitter of the parasympathetic nervous system.

acholic stools Light, clay-colored stools caused by liver failure.

acidosis A blood pH of less than 7.35. A pathologic condition resulting from the accumulation of acids in the body.

acquired immunity The immunity the body develops as part of exposure to an antigen.

acquired immunodeficiency syndrome (AIDS) The end-stage disease process caused by the human immunodeficiency virus (HIV). A person with this is extremely vulnerable to numerous bacterial, viral, and fungal infections that would not affect a person with an intact immune system.

acrocyanosis A decrease in the amount of oxygen delivered to the extremities. The hands and feet turn blue because of narrowing (constriction) of small arterioles (tiny arteries) toward the end of the arms and legs.

acromion Lateral extension of the scapula that forms the highest point of the shoulder.

activation Mediators of inflammation trigger the appearance of molecules known as selectins and integrins on the surfaces of endothelial cells and PMNs, respectively.

active hyperemia The dilation of arterioles after transient arteriolar constriction, which allows influx of blood under increased pressure.

active neglect The refusal or failure to fulfill a caregiving obligation; a conscious or intentional attempt to inflict physical or emotional stress. Examples include abandonment and denial of food or health-related services.

activities of daily living (ADLs) Normal everyday activities such as getting dressed, brushing teeth, taking out the garbage, etc.

acute coronary syndrome Term used to describe any group of clinical symptoms consistent with acute myocardial ischemia.

acute dystonic reaction A syndrome that may occur in patients taking typical antipsychotic agents. The patient develops muscle spasms of the neck, face, and back within a few days of starting treatment with the drug.

acute mountain sickness (AMS) An altitude illness characterized by headache plus at least one of the following: fatigue or weakness, gastrointestinal symptoms (nausea, vomiting or anorexia), dizziness or lightheadedness, or difficulty sleeping.

acute myocardial infarction (AMI) A condition present when a period of cardiac ischemia caused by sudden narrowing or complete occlusion of a coronary artery leads to death (necrosis) of myocardial tissue.

acute radiation syndrome The clinical course that usually begins within hours of exposure to a radiation source. Symptoms include nausea, vomiting, diarrhea, fatigue, fever, and headache. The long-term symptoms are dose-related and are hematopoietic and gastrointestinal.

acute renal failure (ARF) A sudden decrease in filtration through the glomeruli.

acute respiratory distress syndrome (ARDS) A respiratory syndrome characterized by respiratory insufficiency and hypoxemia.

adduction Movement toward the midline of the body.

adenoids Lymphatic tissues located on the posterior nasopharyngeal wall that filter bacteria.

adhesion The attachment of PMNs to endothelial cells, mediated by selectins and integrins.

adipose tissue A connective tissue containing large amounts of lipids. Also referred to as fat tissue.

administration set Tubing that connects to the IV bag access port and the catheter to deliver IV fluid.

adolescents Persons who are 12 to 18 years of age.

adrenal cortex The outer part of the adrenal glands that produces corticosteroids.

adrenal glands Endocrine glands located on top of the kidneys that release adrenaline when stimulated by the sympathetic nervous system.

adrenal medulla The inner portion of the adrenal glands that synthesizes, stores, and eventually releases epinephrine and norepinephrine.

adrenaline The hormone produced by the adrenal gland with alpha and beta sympathomimetic properties.

adrenergic Pertaining to nerves that release the neurotransmitter norepinephrine or noradrenaline (such as adrenergic nerves, adrenergic response). The term also pertains to the receptors acted on by norepinephrine, that is, the adrenergic receptors.

adrenocorticotropic hormone (ACTH) Hormone that targets the adrenal cortex to secrete cortisol (a glucocorticoid).

adult protective services (APS) Organizations that investigate cases involving abuse and neglect and provide case management services in some cases.

advance directive A written document that expresses the wants, needs, and desires of a patient in reference to future medical care; examples include living wills, do not resuscitate (DNR) orders, and organ donation.

adventitious A type of breath sound that occurs in addition to the normal breath sounds; examples are crackles and wheezes.

aerobic metabolism Metabolism that can proceed only in the presence of oxygen.

affect The outward expression of a person's mood.

afferent arteriole The structure in the kidney that supplies blood to the glomerulus.

afferent nerves The nerves that carry sensory impulses from all parts of the body to the brain.

affinity The force attraction between medications and receptors causing them to bind together.

afterdrop Continued fall in core temperature after a victim of hypothermia has been removed from a cold environment, due at least in part to the return of cold blood from the body surface to the body core.

afterload The pressure in the aorta against which the left ventricle must pump blood.

Agency for Toxic Substance Registry An information source for toxicologic effects of hazardous materials.

agitation Extreme restlessness and anxiety.

agnosia Inability to connect an object with its correct name.

agonal Pertaining to the period of dying.

agonal respirations Slow, shallow, irregular respirations or occasional gasping breaths; results from cerebral anoxia.

agonal rhythm A cardiac dysrhythmia seen just before the heart stops altogether; essentially asystole with occasional QRS complexes that are not associated with cardiac output.

agonist A substance that mimics the actions of a specific neurotransmitter or hormone by binding to the specific receptor of the naturally occurring substance.

agoraphobia Literally, "fear of the market-place"; fear of entering a public place from which escape may be impeded.

alarm reaction The body's first, "startle" response to a stressor.

alcoholism A state of physical and psychological addiction to ethanol.

aldosterone One of the two main hormones responsible for adjustments to the final composition of urine, aldosterone increases the rate of active resorption of sodium and chloride ions into the blood and decreases resorption of potassium.

alert and oriented (A x O) A determination made when assessing mental status by looking at whether the patient is oriented to four elements: person, place, time, and the event itself. Each element provides information about different aspects of the patient's memory.

alert response The first reaction in the alarm reaction, in which you immediately stop whatever you are doing and focus on the source of the stimulus.

alkalosis A pathologic condition resulting from the accumulation of bases in the body. A blood pH greater than 7.45.

allergen Any substance that causes a hypersensitivity reaction.

allergic reaction An abnormal immune response the body develops when reexposed to a substance or allergen.

allergy Hypersensitivity reaction to the presence of an agent (allergen) that is intrinsically harmless.

alpha Type of energy that is emitted from a strong radiological source; it is the least harmful penetrating type of radiation and cannot travel fast or through most objects.

alternative time sampling Time parameters that are set during a research project.

altitude illnesses Conditions caused by the effects from hypobaric (low atmospheric pressure) hypoxia on the CNS and pulmonary systems as result of unacclimatized people ascending to altitude; range from acute mountain sickness to high altitude cerebral edema (HACE) and high altitude pulmonary edema (HAPE).

alveolar ridges The ridges between the teeth, which are covered with thickened connective tissue and epithelium.

alveolar volume Volume of inhaled air that reaches the alveoli and participates in gas exchange; equal to tidal volume minus dead space volume and is approximately 350 mL in the average adult.

alveoli Sac-like units at the end of the bronchioles where gas exchange takes place (singular: alveolus).

Alzheimer's disease A progressive organic condition in which neurons die, causing dementia.

amenorrhea Absence of menstruation.

amnesia Loss of memory.

amniotic fluid A clear, slightly yellowish liquid that surrounds the unborn baby (fetus) during pregnancy; contained in the amniotic sac.

amniotic sac The fluid-filled, baglike membrane in which the fetus develops.

amphetamines A class of drugs that increase alertness and excitation (that is, stimulants); includes methamphetamine (crank or ice), methylenedioxyamphetamine (MDA, Adam), and methylenedioxymethamphetamine (MDMA, Eve, ecstasy).

ampules Small glass containers that are sealed and the contents sterilized.

amputation An injury in which part of the body is completely severed.

amyotrophic lateral sclerosis (ALS) Also known as Lou Gehrig's disease, this disease strikes the voluntary motor neurons, causing their death. It is characterized by fatigue and general weakness of muscle groups; eventually, the patient will not be able to walk, eat, or speak.

anaerobic metabolism The metabolism that takes place in the absence of oxygen; the principal product is lactic acid.

analgesia The absence of the sensation of pain.

analgesics A classification for medications that relieve pain, or induce analgesia.

anaphylactic shock A severe hypersensitivity reaction that involves bronchoconstriction and cardiovascular collapse.

anaphylaxis An extreme systemic form of an allergic reaction involving two or more body systems.

anatomic dead space Includes the trachea and larger bronchi. The air remaining in these areas is the result of residual gas in the upper airway at the end of inhalation.

androgens Male sex hormones that regulate body changes associated with sexual development (puberty), including growth spurts, deepening of the voice, growth of facial and pubic hair, and muscle growth and strength.

anemia A lower than normal hemoglobin or erythrocyte level.

anesthesia Lack of feeling within a body part.

anesthetic A type of medication intended to induce a loss of sensation to touch or pain.

aneurysm A swelling or enlargement of part of a blood vessel, resulting from weakening of the vessel wall.

anger A strong, negative emotion that may be a response to illness, and which could result in aggressive behavior on the part of the patient.

angina pectoris The sudden pain from myocardial ischemia, caused by diminished circulation to the cardiac muscle. The pain is usually substernal and often radiates to the arms, jaw, or abdomen and usually lasts 3 to 5 minutes and disappears with rest.

angioedema An allergic reaction that may cause profound swelling of the tongue and lips.

angiogenesis The growth of new blood vessels.

angiotensin converting enzyme (ACE) inhibitors Medications that suppress the conversion of angiotensin I to angiotensin II.

angiotensin II receptor antagonists Medications that are similar to ACE inhibitors but work by selectively blocking angiotensin II at their receptor sites.

angle of impact The angle at which an object hits another; this characterizes the force vectors involved and has a bearing on patterns of energy dissipation.

angle of Louis Prominence on the sternum that lies opposite the second intercostal space.

angulation The presence of an abnormal angle or bend in an extremity.

anion An ion that contains an overall negative charge.

anisocoria A condition in which the pupils are not of equal size.

anorexia nervosa An eating disorder in which a person diets by exerting extraordinary control over his or her eating, and loses weight to the point of jeopardizing his or her health and life.

anoxia An absence of oxygen.

antagonist A molecule that blocks the ability of a given chemical to bind to its receptor, preventing a biologic response.

antecubital The anterior aspect of the elbow.

antegrade amnesia Inability to remember from this point in time forward.

antepartum Before delivery.

anterior chamber The anterior area of the globe between the lens and the cornea that is filled with aqueous humor.

anterior cord syndrome A condition that occurs with flexion injuries or fractures resulting in the displacement of bony fragments into the anterior portion of the spinal cord; findings include paralysis below the level of the insult and loss of pain, temperature, and touch sensation.

anterior tibial artery The artery that travels through the anterior muscles of the leg and continues to the foot as the dorsalis pedis.

anterograde (posttraumatic) amnesia Loss of memory relating to events that occurred after the injury.

anthrax A deadly bacteria (*Bacillus anthracis*) that lays dormant in a spore (protective shell); the germ is released from the spore when exposed to the optimal temperature and moisture. The route of entry is inhalation, cutaneous, or gastrointestinal (from consuming food that contains spores).

antiarrhythmic medications The medications used to treat and prevent cardiac rhythm disorders.

antibiotic medications The medications that fight bacterial infection by killing the bacteria or by preventing multiplication of the bacteria to allow the body's immune system to overcome them.

antibodies Proteins secreted by certain immune cells that bind antigens to make them more visible to the immune system.

anticholinergic Of or pertaining to the blocking of acetylcholine receptors, resulting in inhibition of transmission of parasympathetic nerve impulses.

anticoagulant A substance that prevents blood from clotting.

anticoagulant drugs The medications used to prevent intravascular thrombosis by preventing blood coagulation in the vascular system.

anticonvulsant medications The medications used to treat seizures, which are believed to work by inhibiting the influx of sodium into cells.

antidiuretic hormone (ADH) One of the two main hormones responsible for adjustments to the final composition of urine, ADH causes ducts in the kidney to become more permeable to water.

antigen An agent that, when taken into the body, stimulates the formation of specific protective proteins called antibodies.

antihypertensives The medications used to control blood pressure.

antineoplastic medications The medications designed to combat cancer.

antiplatelet agents The medications that interfere with the collection of platelets.

antipsychotic drugs Medications used to control psychosis.

antiseptics Chemicals used to cleanse an area before performing an invasive procedure, such as starting an IV; not toxic to living tissues; examples include isopropyl alcohol and iodine.

anuria A complete stop in the production of urine.

anxiety disorder A mental disorder in which the dominant mood is fear and apprehension.

anxiolysis Relief of anxiety.

anxious avoidant attachment A bond between an infant and his or her parent or caregiver in which the infant is repeatedly rejected and develops an isolated lifestyle that does not depend upon the support and care of others.

aorta The largest artery in the body, originating from the left ventricle.

aortic valve The valve between the left ventricle and the aorta.

Apgar scoring system A scoring system for assessing the status of a newborn that assigns a number value to each of five areas of assessment.

aphasia The impairment of language that affects the production or understanding of speech and the ability to read or write.

aphonia Inability to speak.

apnea Respiratory pause greater than or equal to 20 seconds.

apneustic center Portion of the brain stem that influences the respiratory rate by increasing the number of inspirations per minute.

apoptosis Normal, genetically programmed cell death.

apparent life-threatening event (ALTE) An unexpected sudden episode of color change, tone change, or apnea that required mouth-to-mouth resuscitation or vigorous stimulation.

appendicular skeleton The part of the skeleton comprising the upper and lower extremities.

apraxia Inability to connect an object with its proper use.

aqueous humor The clear, watery fluid in the anterior chamber of the globe.

arachnoid The middle membrane of the three meninges that enclose the brain and spinal cord.

arrhythmias Disturbances in cardiac rhythm.

arterial air embolism Air bubbles in the arterial blood vessels.

arterial gas embolism (AGE) The resultant gaseous emboli from the forcing of gas into the pulmonary vasculature from barotrauma.

arteries The muscular, thick-walled blood vessels that carry blood away from the heart.

arteriole A small blood vessel that carries oxygenated blood, branching into yet smaller vessels called capillaries.

arteriosclerosis A pathologic condition in which the arterial walls become thickened and inelastic.

arthritis Joint inflammation that causes pain, swelling, stiffness, and decreased range of motion.

Arthus reaction A localized reaction involving vascular inflammation in response to an IgG-mediated allergic response.

articulations The locations where two or more bones meet; joints.

artifact An artificial product; in cardiology, is used to refer to noise or interference in an ECG tracing.

arytenoid cartilages Pyramid-like cartilaginous structures that form the posterior attachment of the vocal cords.

ascites Abnormal accumulation of fluid in the peritoneal cavity.

aseptic technique A method of cleansing used to prevent contamination of a site when performing an invasive procedure, such as starting an IV.

asphyxia Condition of severely deficient supply of oxygen to the body leading to end organ damage.

asphyxiant Any gas that displaces oxygen from the atmosphere; can be deadly if exposure occurs in a confined space.

aspiration Entry of fluids or solids into the trachea, bronchi, and lungs.

assault To create in another person a fear of immediate bodily harm or invasion of bodily security.

asthma A chronic inflammatory lower airway condition resulting in intermittent wheezing and excess mucus production.

asymmetric chest wall movement When one side of the chest moves less than the other; indicates decreased airflow into one lung.

asynchronous In CPR, when two rescuers do ventilations and compressions individually and not timed or waiting for the other rescuer to pause.

asystole The absence of ventricular contractions; a "straight-line ECG."

ataxia Inability to coordinate the muscles properly; often used to describe a staggering gait.

atelectasis Alveolar collapse that prevents use of that portion of the lung for ventilation and oxygenation.

atherosclerosis A disorder in which cholesterol and calcium build up inside the walls of the blood vessels, forming plaque, which eventually leads to partial or complete blockage of blood flow.

atlanto-occipital joint Joint formed at the articulation of the atlas of the vertebral column and the occipital bone of the skull.

atmosphere absolute (ATA) A measurement of ambient pressure; the weight of air at sea level.

atopic The medical term for having an allergic tendency.

atresia The process by which an oocyte dies.

atrial kick The addition to ventricular volume contributed by contraction of the atria.

atrioventricular (AV) node A specialized structure located in the AV junction that slows conduction through the AV junction.

atrioventricular (AV) valves The mitral and tricuspid valves.

atrophy Wasting away of a tissue.

atropine A parasympathetic blocker; opposes the action of acetylcholine on the heart and elsewhere, thereby allowing the body's natural sympathetic system to speed up the heart rate.

atropine-like effects Results of some antipsychotic medications that include side effects similar to atropine, resulting in dry mouth, blurred vision, urinary retention, and cardiac arrhythmias.

auditory ossicles The bones that function in hearing and are located deep within cavities of the temporal bone.

aura Sensations experienced before an attack occurs. Common in seizures and migraine headaches.

aural Pertaining to the ear.

auricle The large outside portion of the ear through which sound waves enter the ear; also called the pinna.

auscultation The method of listening to sounds within the body with a stethoscope.

autoantibodies Antibodies directed against the patient.

autocrine hormone A hormone that acts on the cell that has secreted it.

autoimmune disorders Disorders in which the body identifies its own antigen as a foreign body and activates the inflammatory system.

autoimmunity The production of antibodies or T cells that work against the tissues of a person's own body, producing autoimmune disease or a hypersensitivity reaction.

automatic transport ventilator (ATV) Portable mechanical ventilator attached to a control box that allows the variables of ventilation (eg, rate, tidal volume) to be set.

automaticity Spontaneous initiation of depolarizing electric impulses by pacemaker sites within the electric conduction system of the heart.

autonomic dysreflexia A potentially life-threatening late complication of spinal cord injury in which massive, uninhibited uncompensated cardiovascular response occurs due to stimulation of the sympathetic nervous system below the level of injury. Also known as autonomic hyperreflexia.

autonomic nervous system (ANS) A subdivision of the nervous system that controls primarily involuntary body functions. It comprises the sympathetic and parasympathetic nervous systems.

autoregulation An increase in mean arterial pressure to compensate for decreased cerebral perfusion pressure; compensatory response of the body to shunt blood to the brain; manifests clinically as hypertension.

autosomal dominant A pattern of inheritance that involves genes that are located on autosomes or the nonsex chromosomes. You only need to inherit a single copy of a particular form of a gene to show the trait.

autosomal recessive A pattern of inheritance that involves genes located on autosomes or the nonsex chromosomes. You must inherit two copies of a particular form of a gene to show the trait.

AV junction The atrioventricular junction; the portion of the electric conduction system of the heart located in the upper part of the interventricular septum that conducts the excitation impulse from the atria to the bundle of His.

avascular necrosis Tissue death resulting from the loss of blood supply.

avian (bird) flu A disease caused by a virus that occurs naturally in the bird population. Signs and symptoms include fever, sore throat, cough, and muscle aches.

AVPU A method of assessing mental status by determining whether a patient is Awake and alert, responsive to Verbal stimuli or Pain, or Unresponsive; used principally in the initial assessment.

avulsing A tearing away or forcible separation.

avulsion An injury that leaves a piece of skin or other tissue partially or completely torn away from the body.

avulsion fracture A fracture that occurs when a piece of bone is torn free at the site of attachment of a tendon or ligament.

Awareness Level The training level to which all EMS personnel should be trained; topics include recognizing potential hazards, initiating protective measures for yourself and your community, and requesting additional response resources.

axial skeleton The part of the skeleton comprising the skull, spinal column, and rib cage.

axilla The armpit.

axillary artery The artery that runs through the axilla, connecting the subclavian artery to the brachial artery.

axon Long, slender extension of a neuron (nerve cell) that conducts electrical impulses away from the neuronal soma.

azotemia Increased nitrogenous wastes in the blood.

Babinski reflex When the toe(s) moves upward in response to stimulation to the sole of the foot. Under normal circumstances, the toe(s) moves downward.

bacteria Small organisms that can grow and reproduce outside the human cell in the presence of the temperature and nutrients, and cause disease by invading and multiplying in the tissues of the host.

bacterial vaginosis An overgrowth of bacteria in the vagina, characterized by itching, burning, or pain, and possibly a "fishy" smelling discharge.

bag-mask device Manual ventilation device that consists of a bag, mask, reservoir, and oxygen inlet; capable of delivering up to 100% oxygen.

bandage Material used to secure a dressing in place.

barbiturates Any medications of a group of barbituric acid derivatives that act as central nervous system depressants and are used as sedatives or hypnotics.

barometric energy The energy that results from sudden changes in pressure as may occur in a diving accident or sudden decompression in an airplane.

barotrauma Injury resulting from pressure disequilibrium across body surfaces.

Bartholin glands The glands that secrete mucus for sexual lubrication.

basal ganglia Structures located deep within the cerebrum, diencephalon, and midbrain that have an important role in coordination of motor movements and posture.

basal metabolic rate (BMR) The heat energy produced at rest from normal body metabolic reactions, determined mostly by the liver and skeletal muscles.

base station Assembly of radio equipment consisting of at least a transmitter, receiver, and antenna connection at a fixed location.

basilar skull fractures Usually occur following diffuse impact to the head (such as falls, motor vehicle crashes); generally result from extension of a linear fracture to the base of the skull and can be difficult to diagnose with a radiograph (x-ray).

basophils White blood cells that work to produce chemical mediators during an immune response.

battery Unlawfully touching a person; this includes providing emergency care without consent.

Battle's sign Bruising over the mastoid bone behind the ear commonly seen following a basilar skull fracture; also called retroauricular ecchymosis.

Beck's triad The combination of a narrowed pulse pressure, muffled heart tones, and JVD associated with cardiac tamponade; usually resulting from penetrating chest trauma.

behavior The way people act or perform, for example how they react/respond to a situation.

behavioral emergencies An emergency in which the patient's presenting problem is some disorder of mood, thought, or behavior that interferes with their activities of daily living (ADLs).

belay Technique of controlling the rope as it is fed out to climbers.

Bell's palsy A temporary paralysis of the facial nerve (7th cranial nerve), which controls the muscles on each side of the face.

belt noise A chirping or squealing sound, synchronous with engine speed.

benzodiazepines Sedative-hypnotic drugs that provide muscle relaxation and mild sedation; includes drugs such as diazepam (Valium) and midazolam (Versed).

bereavement Sadness from loss; grieving.

beta Type of energy that is emitted from a strong radiological source; is slightly more penetrating than alpha, and requires a layer of clothing to stop it.

beta-2 agonists Pharmacologic agents that stimulate the beta-2 receptor sites found in smooth muscle; include common bronchodilators like albuterol and levalbuterol.

bigeminy An arrhythmia in which every other heartbeat is a premature contraction.

bill of lading A document carried by drivers of commercial vehicles that should provide specific information about what is carried on the vehicle.

bioavailability The amount of a medication that is still active once it reaches its target tissue.

biologic half-life The time it takes the body to eliminate half of the drug.

biomechanics The study of the physiology and mechanics of a living organism using the tools of mechanical engineering.

Biot respirations Characterized by an irregular rate, pattern, and volume of breathing with intermittent periods of apnea; results from increased intracranial pressure. Also called ataxic respirations.

biotelemetry Transmission of physiologic data, such as an ECG, from the patient to a distant point of reception (commonly referred to in EMS as "telemetry").

biotransformation A process by which a medication is chemically converted to a different compound or metabolite.

bipolar mood disorder A disorder in which a person alternates between mania and depression.

bivalent An ion that contains two charges.

blast front The leading edge of the shock wave.

blastocyst The term for an oocyte once it has been fertilized and multiplies into cells.

blind panic A fear reaction in which a person's judgment seems to disappear entirely; it is particularly dangerous because it may precipitate mass panic among others.

blinding The method of not giving the specifics of a project to the individuals participating in a research or study.

blood The fluid tissue that is pumped by the heart through the arteries, veins, and capillaries and consists of plasma and formed elements or cells, such as red blood cells, white blood cells, and platelets.

bloodborne pathogens Pathogenic microorganisms that are present in human blood and can cause disease in humans. These pathogens include, but are not limited to, hepatitis B virus (HBV) and human immunodeficiency virus (HIV).

blood pressure The pressure exerted by the pulsatile flow of blood against the arterial walls.

blood tubing A special type of macrodrip administration set designed to facilitate rapid fluid replacement by manual infusion of multiple IV bags or IV-blood replacement combinations.

bloody show A plug of mucus, sometimes mixed with blood, that is expelled from the dilating cervix and discharged from the vagina.

blow-by technique A method of delivering oxygen by holding a face mask or similar device near an infant's or a child's face; used when a nonrebreathing mask is not tolerated.

blowout fracture A fracture to the floor of the orbit usually caused by a blow to the eye.

blunt cardiac injury Contusion as the heart is compressed between the sternum and the spine.

blunt trauma Injury resulting from compression or deceleration forces, potentially crushing an organ or causing it to rupture.

BNICE A mnemonic for the five types of terrorist incidents that first responder agencies may be confronted with in the field.

body substance isolation (BSI) An infection control concept and practice that assumes that all body fluids are potentially infectious.

body In the context of the uterus, the portion below the fundus that begins to taper and narrow.

bolus A term used to describe "in one mass"; in medication administration, a single dose given by the IV or IO route; may be a small or large quantity of the drug.

bonding The formation of a close, personal relationship.

Bone Injection Gun (B.I.G.) A spring-loaded device that is used for inserting an IO needle into the proximal tibia in adult and pediatric patients.

bone marrow Specialized tissue found within bone.

borborygmi A bowel sound characterized by increased activity within the bowel.

borderline personality disorder A disorder characterized by disordered images of self, impulsive and unpredictable behavior, marked shifts in mood, and instability in relationships with others.

botulinum Produced by bacteria, this is a very potent neurotoxin. When introduced into the body, this neurotoxin affects the nervous system's ability to function and causes muscle paralysis.

botulism Poisoning from eating food containing botulinum toxin.

Bourdon-gauge flowmeter An oxygen flowmeter that is commonly used because it is not affected by gravity and can be placed in any position.

bowing fracture An incomplete fracture typically occurring in children in which the bone becomes bent as the result of a compressive force.

boxer's fracture A fracture of the head of the fifth metacarpal that usually results from striking an object with a clenched fist.

Boyle's law At a constant temperature, the volume of a gas is inversely proportional to its pressure (if you double the pressure on a gas, you halve its volume); written as PV = K, where P = pressure, V = volume, and K = a constant.

brachial artery The artery that runs through the arm and branches into the radial and ulnar arteries.

bradycardia A slow heart rate, less than 60 beats/min; a pulse rate of less than 100 beats/min in the newborn.

bradykinesia The slowing down of voluntary body movements. Found in Parkinson's disease.

brain Part of the central nervous system, located within the cranium and containing billions of neurons that serve a variety of vital functions.

brain stem The area of the brain between the spinal cord and cerebrum, surrounded by the cerebellum; controls functions that are necessary for life, such as respirations.

brake fade A sensation that an ambulance has lost its power brakes.

brake pull A sensation that, when an operator depresses the brake pedal, the steering wheel is being pulled to the left or the right.

breath-hold diving Also called free diving, this type of diving does not require any equipment, except sometimes a snorkel.

breech presentation A delivery in which the buttocks come out first.

brisance The shattering effect of a shock wave and its ability to cause disruption of tissues and structures.

bronchioles Subdivision of the smaller bronchi in the lungs; made of smooth muscle and dilate or constrict in response to various stimuli.

bronchiolitis A condition seen in children younger than 2 years, characterized by dyspnea and wheezing.

bronchoconstriction Narrowing of the bronchial tubes.

bronchodilation Widening of the bronchial tubes.

bronchospasm Severe constriction of the bronchial tree.

Brown-Sequard syndrome A condition associated with penetrating trauma with hemisection of the spinal cord and complete damage to all spinal tracts on the involved side.

bruit An abnormal "whoosh"-like sound of turbulent blood flow moving through a narrowed artery.

buboes Enlarged lymph nodes (up to the size of tennis balls) that were characteristic of people infected with the bubonic plague.

bubonic plague An epidemic that spread throughout Europe in the Middle Ages, causing over 25 million deaths, also called the Black Death, transmitted by infected fleas and characterized by acute malaise, fever, and the formation of tender, enlarged, inflamed lymph nodes that appear as lesions, called buboes.

buccal route A medication route in which medication is administered between the cheeks and gums.

buckle fracture A common incomplete fracture in children in which the cortex of the bone fractures from an excessive compression force.

buddy splinting Securing an injured digit to an adjacent uninjured one to allow the intact digit to act as a splint.

buffers Molecules that modulate changes in pH to keep it in the physiologic range.

bulimia nervosa An eating disorder characterized by consumption of large amounts of food, and for which the patient then sometimes compensates by using purging techniques.

bundle branch block A disturbance in electric conduction through the right or left bundle branch from the bundle of His.

bundle of His The portion of the electric conduction system in the interventricular septum that conducts the depolarizing impulse from the atrioventricular junction to the right and left bundle branches.

burn shock The shock or hypoperfusion caused by a burn injury and the tremendous loss of fluids.

burnout The exhaustion of physical or emotional strength.

BURP maneuver Acronym for Backward, Upward, Rightward Pressure.

bursa A fluid-filled sac located adjacent to joints that reduces the amount of friction between moving structures.

bursitis Inflammation of a bursa.

butterfly catheter   A rigid, hollow, venous cannulation device identified by its plastic "wings" that act as anchoring points for securing the catheter.

butyrophenones   Potent, effective sedatives; includes drugs such as haloperidol (Haldol) and droperidol (Inapsine).

caladium   A common houseplant that contains caladium oxalate crystals; ingestion leads to nausea, vomiting, and diarrhea.

calcaneous   The heel bone; the largest of the tarsal bones.

calcitonin   The hormone secreted by the thyroid gland that helps maintain normal calcium levels in the blood.

calcium channel blockers   The medications that suppress arrhythmias, provide more oxygen to the heart via coronary artery dilation, and reduce peripheral vascular resistance.

calibrated   The diagnostic checking and synchronizing of digital or electronic equipment to assure that is in good working order and will measure accurately.

calyces (singular: calyx)   Large urinary tubes that branch off the renal pelvis and connect with the renal pyramids to collect the urine draining from the collecting tubules.

CAMEO   Computer-Aided Management of Emergency Operations; a tool to help predict downwind concentrations of hazardous materials based on the input of environmental factors into a computer model.

cancellous bone   Trabecular or spongy bone.

cannulation   The insertion of a catheter, such as into a vein to allow for fluid flow.

capacitance vessels   The smallest venules.

cape cyanosis   Deep cyanosis of the face and neck and across the chest and back; associated with little or no blood flow; it is particularly ominous.

capillaries   Extremely narrow blood vessels composed of a single layer of cells through which oxygen and nutrients pass to the tissues. Capillaries form a network between arterioles and venules.

capillary refill time   A test done on the fingers or toes by briefly squeezing the toe or finger, then evaluating the time it takes for the pink color to return.

capnographer   Device that attaches in between the endotracheal tube and bag-mask device; contains colorimetric paper, which should turn yellow during exhalation, indicating proper tube placement.

capnometer   Device that attaches in the same way as a capnographer, but provides a light-emitting diode (LED) readout of the patient's exhaled carbon dioxide.

capsule   A cylindrical gelatin container enclosing a dose of medication.

carbon monoxide   A chemical asphyxiant that results in a cellular respiratory failure; this gas ties up hemoglobin to the extent that oxygen in the blood becomes inaccessible to the cells.

carboxyhemoglobin   Abnormal hemoglobin that is formed by the attachment of carbon monoxide to the hemoglobin molecule.

cardiac cycle   The period from one cardiac contraction to the next. Each cardiac cycle consists of ventricular contraction (systole) and relaxation (diastole).

cardiac glycosides   A classification of medications that naturally occur in plant substances and that block certain ionic pumps in the heart cells' membranes, which indirectly increases calcium concentrations; an example is digoxin.

cardiac output (CO)   Amount of blood pumped by the heart per minute, calculated by multiplying the stroke volume by the heart rate per minute.

cardiac tamponade   A condition in which the atria and right ventricle are collapsed by a collection of blood or other fluid within the pericardial sac, resulting in a diminished cardiac output.

cardiogenic shock   A condition caused by loss of 40% or more of the functioning myocardium; the heart is no longer able to circulate sufficient blood to maintain adequate oxygen delivery.

cardiopulmonary arrest   The sudden and often unexpected cessation of adequate cardiac output.

cardiovascular collapse   Failure of the heart and blood vessels; shock.

cardioversion   The use of a synchronized direct current (DC) electric shock to convert tachyarrhythmias (such as atrial flutter) to normal sinus rhythm.

carina   Point at which the trachea bifurcates (divides) into the left and right mainstem bronchi.

carpals   The eight small bones of the wrist.

carpopedal spasm   Contorted position of the hand in which the fingers flex in a clawlike attitude and the thumb curls toward the palm.

carrier   An individual who harbors an infectious agent and, although not personally ill, can transmit the infection to another person.

cartilage   Tough, elastic substance that covers opposable surfaces of moveable joints and forms part of the skeleton.

cartilaginous joints   Joints that are spanned completely by cartilage and allow for minimal motion.

castor bean   A seed that contains the poison ricin; causes a variety of toxic effects: burning of the mouth and throat; nausea, vomiting, diarrhea, and severe stomach pains; prostration; failing vision and kidney failure, which is the usual cause of death.

catatonic   Lacking expression or movement, or appearing rigid.

catatonic type   A type of schizophrenia in which the person displays odd motor activity, such as strange facial expression or rigidity.

catecholamines   Hormones produced by the adrenal medulla (epinephrine and norepinephrine) that assist the body in coping with physical and emotional stress by increasing the heart and respiratory rates and the blood pressure.

catheter shear   Occurs when a needle is reinserted into the catheter, and it slices through the catheter, creating a free-floating segment.

cation   An ion that contains an overall positive charge.

cauda equina   The location where the spinal cord separates, composed of nerve roots.

caustics   Chemicals that are acids or alkalis; cause direct chemical injury to the tissues they contact.

cavitation   Cavity formation; shock waves that push tissues in front of and lateral to the projectile and may not necessarily increase the wound size or cause permanent injury but can result in cavitation.

cell-mediated immunity   Immune process by which T-cell lymphocytes recognize antigens and then secrete cytokines (specifically lymphokines) that attract other cells or stimulate the production of cytotoxic cells that kill the infected cells.

cell signaling   The process by which cells communicate with one another.

cellular immunity   The immunity provided by special white blood cells called T cells that attack and destroy invaders.

cellular telephones   Low-power portable radios that communicate through an interconnected series of repeater stations called "cells."

Celsius scale   A scale for measuring temperature in which water freezes at 0° and boils at 100°.

central cord syndrome   A condition resulting from hyperextension injuries to the cervical area that cause damage with hemorrhage or edema to the central cervical segments; findings include greater loss of function in the upper extremities with variable sensory loss of pain and temperature.

central cyanosis   Bluish coloration of the skin due to the presence of deoxygenated hemoglobin in blood vessels near the skin surface.

central nervous system (CNS)   The system containing the brain and spinal cord.

central neurogenic hyperventilation   Deep, rapid respirations; similar to Kussmaul, but without an acetone breath odor; commonly seen following brain stem injury.

central shock   A term that describes shock secondary to central pump failure; it includes both cardiogenic shock and obstructive shock.

central venous catheter   A catheter inserted into the vena cava to permit intermittent or continuous monitoring of central venous pressure and to facilitate obtaining blood samples for chemical analysis.

central vision   The visualization of objects directly in front of you.

cerebellum   The region of the brain essential in coordinating muscle movements in the body; also called the athlete's brain.

cerebral concussion Occurs when the brain is jarred around in the skull; a mild diffuse brain injury that does not result in structural damage or permanent neurologic impairment.

cerebral contusion A focal brain injury in which brain tissue is bruised and damaged in a defined area.

cerebral cortex The largest portion of the cerebrum; regulates voluntary skeletal movement and one's level of awareness—a part of consciousness.

cerebral edema Cerebral water; causes or contributes to swelling of the brain.

cerebral palsy (CP) A developmental condition in which damage is done to the brain. It presents during infancy as delays in walking or crawling, and can take on a spastic form in which muscles are in a near constant state of contraction.

cerebral perfusion pressure (CPP) The pressure of blood flow through the brain; the difference between the mean arterial pressure (MAP) and intracranial pressure (ICP).

cerebrospinal fluid (CSF) Fluid produced in the ventricles of the brain that flows in the subarachnoid space and bathes the meninges.

cerebrospinal fluid shunts Tubes that drain fluid manufactured in the ventricles of the brain from the subarachnoid space to another part of the body outside of the brain, such as the peritoneum; lowers pressure in the brain.

cerebrospinal otorrhea Cerebrospinal fluid drainage from the ears.

cerebrospinal rhinorrhea Cerebrospinal fluid drainage from the nose.

cerebrovascular accident (CVA) An interruption of blood flow to the brain that results in the loss of brain function.

cerebrum The largest portion of the brain; responsible for higher functions, such as reasoning; divided into right and left hemispheres, or halves.

certified A title given when a person has shown that he or she has met requirements based on knowledge of certain facts.

cervical canal The interior of the cervix.

cervix The narrowest portion of the uterus that opens into the vagina.

chancre The primary hard lesion or ulcer of syphilis that occurs at the entry site of the infection.

chancroid A highly contagious sexually transmitted disease caused by the bacteria Haemophilus ducreyi, which causes painful sores (ulcers), usually of the genitals.

chemical asphyxiants Substances that interfere with the utilization of oxygen at the cellular level.

chemical energy The energy released as a result of a chemical reaction.

chemical mediators Chemicals that work to cause the immune or allergic response, for example, histamine.

chemical name A description of the drug's chemical composition and molecular structure.

chemoreceptors Monitor the levels of O_2, CO_2, and the pH of the CSF and then provide feedback to the respiratory centers to modify the rate and depth of breathing based on the body's needs at any given time.

chemotactic factors The factors that cause cells to migrate into an area.

chemotaxins Components of the activated complement system that attract leukocytes from the circulation to help fight infections.

chemotaxis The movement of additional white blood cells to an area of inflammation in response to the release of chemical mediators, such as neutrophils, injured tissue, and monocytes.

chemotherapy The introduction of either single cytotoxic drugs or combinations of cytotoxic drugs into the body for the purpose of interrupting or eradicating malignant cellular growth.

CHEMTREC (Chemical Emergency Transportation Center) A resource available to emergency responders via telephone on a 24-hour basis.

Cheyne-Stokes respirations Respirations that are fast and then become slow, with intervening periods of apnea; commonly seen following brain stem injury.

chickenpox A very contagious disease caused by varicella zoster virus, which is part of the herpes virus family, occurring most often in the winter and early spring.

chief complaint The problem for which the patient is seeking help.

child protective services (CPS) An agency that is the community legal organization responsible for protection, rehabilitation, and prevention of child maltreatment and neglect; it has the legal authority to temporarily remove from home children who are at risk for injury or neglect and to secure foster placement.

chlamydia A sexually transmitted disease caused by the bacterium Chlamydia trachomatis.

chlorine (CL) The first chemical agent ever used in warfare. It has a distinct odor of bleach, and creates a green haze when released as a gas. Initially it produces upper airway irritation and a choking sensation.

choanal atresia A narrowing or blockage of the nasal airway by membranous or bony tissue; a congenital condition, meaning it is present at birth.

cholestasis A common liver disease that occurs only during pregnancy, in which the flow of bile is altered resulting in acids being released into the bloodstream, causing profuse and painful itching.

cholinergic Fibers in the parasympathetic nervous system that release a chemical called acetylcholine.

chordae tendineae Fibrous strands shaped like umbrella stays that attach the free edges of the leaflets, or cusps, of the atrioventricular valves to the papillary muscles.

choroid plexus Specialized cells within the hollow areas in the ventricles of the brain that produce CSF.

chronic bronchitis Chronic inflammatory condition affecting the bronchi that is associated with excess mucous production that results from overgrowth of the mucous glands in the airways.

chronic hypertension A blood pressure that is equal to or greater than 140/90 mm Hg, which exists prior to pregnancy, occurs before the 20th week of pregnancy, or continues to persist postpartum.

chronic obstructive pulmonary disease (COPD) Illnesses that cause obstructive problems in the lower airways, including chronic bronchitis, emphysema, and sometimes asthma.

chronic renal failure (CRF) Progressive and irreversible inadequate kidney function due to permanent loss of nephrons.

chronotropic effect The rate of contraction of the heart.

chyme The partially digested food that exits the stomach, entering the duodenum.

cilia Hairlike microtubule projections on the surface of a cell that can move materials over the cell surface.

circumferential burns Burns on the neck or chest that may compress the airway or on an extremity that might act like a tourniquet.

circumflex coronary artery One of the two branches of the left main coronary artery.

circumstantial thinking Situation in which a patient includes many irrelevant details in his or her account of things.

civil suit An action instituted by a private individual or corporation against another private individual or corporation.

clandestine drug laboratories Locations where illegal drugs such as methamphetamine, lysergic acid diethylamide (LSD), ecstasy, and phencyclidine hydrochloride (PCP) are manufactured.

classic heat stroke Also called passive heat stroke, this is a serious heat illness that usually occurs during heat waves and is most likely to strike very old, very young, or bedridden people.

clavicle An S-shaped bone, also called the collarbone, that articulates medially with the sternum and laterally with the shoulder.

cleft lip An abnormal defect or fissure in the upper lip that failed to close during development. It is often associated with cleft palate.

cleft palate A fissure or hole in the palate (roof of the mouth) that forms a communicating pathway between the mouth and nasal cavities.

climacteric End phase of a woman's life menstrual cycle.

clitoris A small, cylindrical mass of erectile tissue and nerves located at the anterior junction of the labia minora, homologous to the glans penis of the male.

clonic activity Type of seizure movement involving the contraction and relaxation of muscle groups.

closed abdominal injury An injury in which there is soft-tissue damage inside the body, but the skin remains intact.

closed-ended question A question that is specific and focused, either demanding a yes or no answer, or an answer chosen from specific options.

closed fracture A fracture in which the skin is not broken.

closed incident A contained incident in which patients are found in one focal location and the situation is not expected to produce more patients than initially present.

closed wound An injury in which damage occurs beneath the skin or mucous membrane but the surface remains intact.

clotting factors Substances in the blood that are necessary for clotting; also called coagulation factors.

CNS stimulants Any medications or agents that increase brain activity.

coagulation Clotting.

coagulation system The system that forms blood clots in the body and facilitates repairs to the vascular tree.

cochlea The shell-shaped structure within the inner ear that contains the organ of Corti.

cochlear duct A canal within the cochlea that receives vibrations from the ossicles.

code team leader The code team member who has the responsibility for managing the rescuers or team members during a cardiac arrest, as well as choreographing the effort of the group.

code team member A member of the resuscitation team trying to revive the patient.

coin rubbing A cultural ritual intended to treat an illness by rubbing hot coins, often on the back, which produces rounded and oblong red, patchy, flat skin lesions.

cold diuresis Secretion of large amounts of urine in response to cold exposure and the consequent shunting of blood volume to the body core.

cold protective response Phenomenon associated with cold water immersion in which reflexes in the body and a lowered metabolic rate help preserve basic body functions.

cold zone A safe area for those agencies involved in the operations; the incident commander (IC), command post, EMS providers, and other support functions necessary to control the incident should be located in the cold zone.

collagen A protein that gives tensile strength to the connective tissues of the body.

collateral circulation The mesh of arteries and capillaries that furnishes blood to a segment of tissue whose original arterial supply has been obstructed.

colloid solutions Solutions that contain molecules (usually proteins) that are too large to pass out of the capillary membranes

and, therefore, remain in the vascular compartment.

colostomy Establishment of an opening between the colon and the surface of the body for the purpose of providing drainage of the bowel.

coma A state in which one does not respond to verbal or painful stimuli.

Combitube Multilumen airway device that consists of a single tube with two lumens, two balloons, and two ventilation ports; an alternative device if endotracheal intubation is not possible or has failed.

comedo A noninflammatory acne lesion.

command In incident command, the position that oversees the incident, establishes the objectives and priorities, and from there develops a response plan.

comminuted fracture A fracture in which the bone is broken into three or more pieces.

commotio cordis An event in which an often fatal cardiac dysrhythmia is produced by a sudden blow to the thoracic cavity.

communicability Describes how easily a disease spreads from one human to another human.

communicable disease A disease that can be transmitted from one person to another under certain conditions.

communicable period The period during which an infected person is capable of transmitting illness to someone else.

communication The transmission of information to another person—whether it be verbal or through body language.

compartment syndrome A condition that develops when edema and swelling result in increased pressure within soft tissues, causing circulation to be compromised, possibly resulting in tissue necrosis.

compensated shock The early stage of shock, in which the body can still compensate for blood loss.

complement system A group of plasma proteins whose function is to do one of three things: attract leukocytes to sites of inflammation, activate leukocytes, and directly destroy cells.

complete abortion Expulsion of all products of conception from the uterus.

complete fracture A fracture in which the bone is broken into two or more completely separate pieces.

complete spinal cord injury Total disruption of all tracts of the spinal cord, with all cord-mediated functions below the level of transection lost permanently.

complex febrile seizures An unusual form of seizures that occurs in association with a rapid increase in body temperature.

complex partial seizures Seizures characterized by alteration of consciousness with or without complex focal motor activity.

compound fracture An open fracture; a fracture beneath an open wound.

compulsion A repetitive action carried out to relieve the anxiety of obsessive thoughts.

computer-aided dispatch An automated computer system that processes the information received and assists the dispatcher with multiple functions and tasks.

concealment Protection from being seen.

concentration The total weight of a drug contained in a specific volume of liquid.

concentration gradient The natural tendency for substances to flow from an area of higher concentration to an area of lower concentration, within or outside the cell.

concept formation Pattern of understanding based on initially obtained information.

conduction Transfer of heat to a solid object or a liquid by direct contact.

conductive deafness A curable temporary condition, caused by an injury to the eardrum.

confabulation The invention of experiences to cover gaps in memory, seen in patients with certain organic brain syndromes.

confined space A space with limited or restricted access that is not meant for continuous occupancy, such as a manhole, well, or tank.

confrontation Interviewing technique in which the interviewer points out to the patient something of interest in his/her conversation or behavior.

confusion An impaired understanding of one's surroundings.

conjunctiva A thin, transparent membrane that covers the sclera and internal surfaces of the eyelids.

conjunctivitis An inflammation of the conjunctivae that usually is caused by bacteria, viruses, allergies, or foreign bodies; should be considered highly contagious; also called pink eye.

connective tissue Tissue that serves to bind various tissue types together.

consent Agreement by the patient to accept a medical intervention.

contact and cover Technique that involves one paramedic making contact with the patient to provide care, while the second paramedic obtains patient information, gauges the level of tension, and warns his or her partner at the first sign of trouble.

contact burn A burn produced by touching a hot object.

contact hazard A hazardous agent that gives off very little or no vapors; the skin is the primary route for this type of chemical to enter the body; also called a skin hazard.

contagious A person infected with a disease that is highly communicable.

contaminated The presence or the reasonably anticipated presence of blood or other potentially infectious materials on an item or surface.

contaminated stick The puncturing of an emergency care provider's skin with a needle or catheter that was used on a patient.

contraceptive device A device used to prevent pregnancy.

contractility The strength of heart muscle contractions.

contraindications In health care, conditions or factors that increase the risk involved in using a particular drug, carrying out a medical procedure, or engaging in a particular activity.

contusion A bruise; an injury that causes bleeding beneath the skin but does not break the skin.

convection Mechanism by which body heat is picked up and carried away by moving air currents.

convenience sampling A type of research in which subjects are manually assigned to a specific person or crew, rather than being randomly assigned; the least-preferred component of research.

conventional reasoning A type of reasoning in which a child looks for approval from peers and society.

conversion hysteria A reaction in which a person subconsciously transforms his or her anxiety into a bodily dysfunction; the person may be unable to see or hear or may become partially paralyzed.

cookbook medicine Treatment based on a protocol or algorithm without adequate knowledge of the patient being treated.

cor pulmonale Heart disease that develops secondary to a chronic lung disease, usually affecting primarily the right side of the heart.

core body temperature (CBT) The temperature in the part of the body comprising the heart, lungs, brain, and abdominal viscera.

cornea The transparent anterior portion of the eye that overlies the iris and pupil.

coronal suture The point where the parietal bones join with the frontal bone.

coronary arteries The blood vessels of the heart that supply blood to its walls.

coronary artery disease (CAD) A pathologic process caused by atherosclerosis that leads to progressive narrowing and eventual obstruction of the coronary arteries.

coronary sinus A large vessel in the posterior part of the coronary sulcus into which the coronary veins empty.

coronary sulcus The groove along the exterior surface of the heart that separates the atria from the ventricles.

corpus luteum The remains of a follicle after an oocyte has been released, and which secretes progesterone.

corrosives A class of chemicals with either high or low pH levels. Exposure can cause severe soft-tissue damage.

cortex Part of the internal anatomy of the kidney; the lighter-colored outer region closest to the capsule.

corticosteroids Hormones that regulate the body's metabolism, the balance of salt and water in the body, the immune system, and sexual function.

cortisol Hormone that stimulates most body cells to increase their energy production.

countercurrent multiplier The process in which the body produces either concentrated or diluted urine, depending on the body's needs.

coup-contrecoup injury Dual impacting of the brain into the skull; coup injury occurs at the point of impact; contrecoup injury occurs on the opposite side of impact, as the brain rebounds.

couplet Two premature ventricular contractions occurring sequentially.

cover Obstacles that are difficult or impossible for bullets to penetrate.

covert Act in which the public safety community generally has no prior knowledge of the time, location, or nature of the attack.

crackles Abnormal breath sounds that have a fine, crackling quality; previously called rales.

cranial vault The bones that encase and protect the brain, including the parietal, temporal, frontal, occipital, sphenoid, and ethmoid bones; also called the cranium or skull.

craniofacial disjunction A Le Fort III fracture; involves a fracture of all of the midfacial bones, thus separating the entire midface from the cranium.

crepitus A grating sensation made when two pieces of broken bone are rubbed together or subcutaneous emphysema is palpated.

cribbing Short lengths of wood that are used to stabilize vehicles.

cribriform plate A horizontal bone perforated with numerous foramina for the passage of the olfactory nerve filaments from the nasal cavity.

cricoid cartilage Forms the lowest portion of the larynx; also referred to as the cricoid ring; the first ring of the trachea and is the only upper airway structure that forms a complete ring.

cricoid pressure The application of posterior pressure to the cricoid cartilage; minimizes gastric distention and the risk of vomiting and aspiration during ventilation; also referred to as the Sellick maneuver.

cricothyroid membrane A thin, superficial membrane located between the thyroid and cricoid cartilages that is relatively avascular and contains few nerves; the site for emergency surgical and nonsurgical access to the airway.

criminal prosecution An action instituted by the government against a private individual for violation of criminal law.

crista galli A prominent bony ridge in the center of the anterior fossa and the point of attachment of the meninges.

critical incident An event that overwhelms the ability to cope with the experience, either at the scene or later.

critical incident stress debriefings (CISDs) A confidential peer group discussion in which specially trained teams work with emergency personnel who have been involved in traumatic calls or other painful incidents; CISDs usually occur within 24 to 72 hours of the incident.

critical infrastructure The external foundation in communities made up of structures and services critical in the day-to-day living activities of humans: energy sources, fuel, water, sewage removal, food, hospitals, and transportation systems.

critical minimum threshold Minimum cerebral perfusion pressure required to adequately perfuse the brain; 60 mm Hg in the adult.

cross-contamination Occurs when a person is contaminated by an agent as a result of coming into contact with another contaminated person.

cross-sectional research A type of research in which information is gathered from a group of individuals over a specific time frame.

cross-tolerance A form of drug tolerance in which patients who take a particular medication for an extended period can build up a tolerance to other medications in the same class.

croup A childhood viral disease characterized by edema of the upper airways with barking cough, difficult breathing, and stridor.

crown The part of the tooth that is external to the gum.

crowning The appearance of the infant's head at the vaginal opening during labor.

crush injury An injury in which the body or part of the body is crushed, preventing tissue function and, possibly, resulting in permanent tissue damage.

crush syndrome Significant metabolic derangement that can lead to renal failure and death. It develops when crushed extremities or other body parts remain trapped for prolonged periods.

crystalloid solutions Solutions of dissolved crystals (for example, salts or sugars) in water; contain compounds that quickly dissociate in solution.

cumulative effect An effect that occurs when several successive doses of a medication are administered or when absorption of a medication occurs faster than excretion or metabolism.

cupping The cultural practice of placing warm cups on the skin to pull out illness from the body. The red, flat, rounded skin lesions are often more intensely red at the borders.

current health status A composite picture of a number of factors in a patient's life, such as dietary habits, current medications, allergies, exercise, alcohol or tobacco use, recreational drug use, sleep patterns and disorders, and immunizations.

curved laryngoscope blade Also called the Macintosh blade; designed to fit into the vallecula, indirectly lifting the epiglottis and exposing the vocal cords.

Cushing's reflex The combination of a slowing pulse, rising blood pressure, and erratic respiratory patterns; a grave sign for patients with head trauma.

Cushing's syndrome A condition caused by an excess of cortisol production by the adrenal glands or by excessive use of cortisol or other similar steroid (glucocorticoid) hormones.

Cushing's triad Hypertension (with a widening pulse pressure), bradycardia, and irregular respirations; classic trio of findings associated with increased ICP.

cusps Points at the top of a tooth.

cutaneous Pertaining to the skin.

cyanide Agent that affects the body's ability to use oxygen. It is a colorless gas that has an odor similar to almonds. The effects begin on the cellular level and are very rapidly seen at the organ system level.

cyanosis A bluish-gray skin color that is caused by reduced levels of oxygen in the blood.

cystadenomas Fluid-filled cysts that form on the outer ovarian surface.

cystic fibrosis Chronic dysfunction of the endocrine system that affects multiple body systems, primarily the respiratory and digestive systems.

cytokines Products of cells that affect the function of other cells.

cytomegalovirus (CMV) A herpesvirus that can produce the symptoms of prolonged high fever, chills, headache, malaise, extreme fatigue, and an enlarged spleen.

D$_5$W An intravenous solution made up of 5% dextrose in water.

Dalton's law Each gas in mixture exerts the same partial pressure that it would exert if it were alone in the same volume, and the total pressure of a mixture of gases is the sum of the partial pressures of all the gases in the mixture.

damages Compensation for injury awarded by a court.

data interpretation The process of formulating a conclusion based on comparing the patient's condition with information from your training, education, and past experiences.

dead space The portion of the tidal volume that does not reach the alveoli and thus does not participate in gas exchange.

decay A natural process in which a material that is unstable attempts to stabilize itself by changing its structure.

deceleration A negative acceleration, that is, slowing down.

decerebrate (extensor) posturing Abnormal posture characterized by extension of the arms and legs; indicates pressure on the brain stem.

decision-making capacity The patient's ability to understand and process the information you give him or her about your proposed plan of care.

decompensated shock The late stage of shock, when blood pressure is falling.

decompression sickness (DCS) A broad range of signs and symptoms caused by nitrogen bubbles in blood and tissues coming out of solution on ascent.

decontamination The process of removing hazardous materials from the body or clothing of victims or rescuers. Includes the methods of dilution, absorption, disposal, and (in rare cases only) neutralization.

decorticate (flexor) posturing Abnormal posture characterized by flexion of the arms and extension of the legs; indicates pressure on the brain stem.

decussation Movement of nerves from one side of the brain to the opposite side of the body.

deep fascia A dense layer of fibrous tissue below the subcutaneous tissue; composed of tough bands of tissue that ensheath muscles and other internal structures.

deep frostbite A type of frostbite in which the affected part looks white, yellow-white, or mottled blue-white and is hard, cold, and without sensation.

deep vein thrombosis (DVT) The formation of a blood clot within the larger veins of an extremity, typically following a period of prolonged immobilization.

defamation Intentionally making a false statement, through written or verbal communication, which injures a person's good name or reputation.

defendant In a civil suit, the individual against whom a legal action is brought.

defense mechanisms Psychological ways to relieve stress; they are usually automatic or subconscious. Defense mechanisms include denial, regression, projection, and displacement.

defibrillation The use of an unsynchronized direct current (DC) electric shock to terminate ventricular fibrillation.

degloving A traumatic injury that results in the soft tissue of the hand being drawn downward like a glove being removed.

degranulate To release granules into the surrounding tissue.

dehydration Depletion of the body's systemic fluid volume.

delirium An acute confessional state characterized by global impairment of thinking, perception, judgment, and memory.

delirium tremens (DTs) A severe withdrawal syndrome seen in people with alcoholism who are deprived of ethyl alcohol; characterized by restlessness, fever, sweating, disorientation, agitation, and seizures; can be fatal if untreated.

delta wave The slurring of the upstroke of the first part of the QRS complex that occurs in Wolff-Parkinson-White syndrome.

delusion A fixed belief that is not shared by others of a person's culture or background and that can't be changed by reasonable argument; a false belief.

delusions of grandeur A state in which a person believes oneself to be someone of great importance.

delusions of persecution A state in which a person believes that others are plotting against him or her.

dementia The slow onset of progressive disorientation, shortened attention span, and loss of cognitive function.

demobilization The process of directing responders to return to their facilities when work at a disaster or mass-casualty incident has finished, at least for the particular responders.

dendrites Part of the neuron that receives impulses from the axon and contains vesicles for release of neurotransmitters.

denial An early response to a serious medical emergency, in which the severity of the emergency is diminished or minimized. Denial is the first coping mechanism for people who believe they are going to die.

dentin The principal mass of the tooth, which is made up of a material that is much more dense and stronger than bone.

depersonalization A type of dissociative disorder in which a person loses his or her sense of reality, and may experience events as being "dream-like."

depolarization The process of discharging resting cardiac muscle fibers by an electric impulse that causes them to contract.

depolarizing neuromuscular blocking agents Medications designed to keep muscles in a contracted state.

depressed skull fractures Result from high-energy direct trauma to a small surface area of the head with a blunt object (such as a baseball bat to the head); commonly result in bony fragments being driven into the brain, causing injury.

depression A persistent mood of sadness, despair, and discouragement; may be a symptom of many different mental and physical disorders, or it may be a disorder on its own.

depression fracture A fracture in which the broken region of the bone is pushed deeper into the body than the remaining intact bone.

derealization A symptom of a dissociative disorder in which objects seem to change size or shape; people may seem dead or behave like robots when viewed during a moment of acute stress.

dermal exposure Skin exposure, also known as topical exposure. Some hazardous materials may be absorbed through the skin to produce a systemic effect.

dermatomes Distinct areas of skin that correspond to specific spinal or cranial nerve levels where sensory nerves enter the CNS.

dermis The inner layer of skin, containing hair follicle roots, glands, blood vessels, and nerves.

dermoid cysts Ovarian cysts containing formational tissue, such as hair and teeth.

descriptive research A type of research in which an observation of an event is made, but without attempts to alter or change it.

designated infection control officer (DICO) An individual trained to ensure that proper postexposure medical treatment and counseling is provided to an exposed employee or volunteer.

desired dose The amount of a drug that the physician orders for a patient; the drug order.

desquamation The continuous shedding of the dead cells on the surface of the skin.

detailed physical exam The part of the assessment process in which a detailed area-by-area exam is performed on patients whose problems cannot be readily identified or when more specific information is needed about problems identified in the focused history and physical exam.

devascularization The loss of blood to a part of the body.

developmental disability Insufficient development of the brain, resulting in some level of dysfunction or impairment.

diabetes mellitus Disease characterized by the body's inability to sufficiently metabolize glucose. The condition occurs either because the pancreas doesn't produce enough insulin or the cells don't respond to the effects of the insulin that's produced.

diabetic ketoacidosis (DKA) A form of acidosis in uncontrolled diabetes in which certain acids accumulate when insulin is not available.

diaphragm Large skeletal muscle that plays a major role in breathing and separates the chest cavity from the abdominal cavity.

diaphragmatic hernia Passage of loops of bowel with or without other abdominal organs, through the diaphragm muscle; occurs as the bowel from the abdomen "herniates" upward through the diaphragm into the chest (thoracic) cavity.

diaphysis The shaft of a long bone.

diarrhea Liquid stool.

diastasis An increase in the distance between the two sides of a joint.

diastole The period of ventricular relaxation during which the ventricles passively fill with blood.

dieffenbachia A common houseplant that resembles "elephant ears"; ingestion leads to burns of the mouth and tongue and, possibly, paralysis of the vocal cords and nausea and vomiting; in severe cases, may be edema of the tongue and larynx, leading to airway compromise.

diencephalon The part of the brain between the brain stem and the cerebrum that includes the thalamus, the subthalamus, hypothalamus, and epithalamus.

diffuse axonal injury (DAI) Diffuse brain injury that is caused by stretching, shearing, or tearing of nerve fibers with subsequent axonal damage.

diffuse brain injury Any injury that affects the entire brain.

diffusion A process in which molecules move from an area of higher concentration to an area of lower concentration.

digital arteries The arteries that supply blood to the fingers and toes.

digital intubation Method of intubation that involves directly palpating the glottic structures and elevating the epiglottis with your middle finger while guiding the ET tube into the trachea by feel.

digitalis preparations The drugs used in the treatment of congestive heart failure and certain atrial arrhythmias.

diluent A solution (usually water or normal saline) used for diluting a medication.

dilution A type of decontamination method that uses copious amounts of water to flush the contaminant from the skin or eyes.

diplopia Double vision.

direct laryngoscopy Visualization of the airway with a laryngoscope.

dirty bomb Name given to a bomb that is used as a radiological dispersal device (RDD).

disaster management A planned, coordinated response to a disaster that involves cooperation of multiple responders and agencies and enables effective triage and provision of care according to triage decisions.

disasters Widespread events that disrupt community resources and functions, in turn threatening public safety, lives, and property.

disease vector An animal that once infected, spreads a disease to another animal.

disinfectants Chemicals used on nonliving objects to kill organisms; toxic to living tissues; examples include Virex, Cidex, and Microcide.

dislocation The displacement of a bone from its normal position within a joint.

disorganization A condition in which a person is characterized by uncontrolled and disconnected thought, is usually incoherent or rambling in speech, and may or may not be oriented to person and place.

disorganized symptoms Refers to erratic speech, emotional responses, and motor behavior.

disorganized type A type of schizophrenia in which the person usually displays the wrong emotion for a particular situation, often self-absorbed.

disorientation Confusion regarding a person's sense of who one is (person), where one is (place), and at what point in time one finds oneself (time).

dispatch To send to a specific destination or to send on a task.

displacement Redirection of an emotion from yourself to another person.

disposal A type of decontamination in which as much clothing and equipment as possible is disposed of to reduce the magnitude of the problem.

dissection In references to blood vessels, an aneurysm, or bulge, formed by the separation of the layers of an arterial wall.

disseminated intravascular coagulopathy (DIC) A life-threatening condition commonly found in severe trauma.

dissemination The means with which a terrorist will spread a disease, for example, by poisoning of the water supply, or aerosolizing the agent into the air or ventilation system of a building.

dissociation Feelings of being detached from yourself, as if you were dreaming.

distal convoluted tubule (DCT) Connects with the kidney's collecting tubules.

distractibility The patient's attention is easily diverted.

distraction injury An injury that results from a force that tries to increase the length of a body part or separate one body part from another.

distress A type of stress that a person finds overwhelming and debilitating.

distribution The movement and transportation of a medication throughout the bloodstream to tissues and cells of the body and, ultimately, to its target receptor.

distributive shock A condition that occurs when there is widespread dilation of the resistance vessels, the capacitance vessels, or both.

diuresis Secretion of large amounts of urine by the kidney.

diuretic medications The medications designed to promote elimination of excess salt and water by the kidneys.

diuretics Chemicals that increase urinary output.

Do Not Intubate forms Written documentation by a physician giving permission to medical personnel not to attempt intubation.

Do Not Resuscitate (DNR) forms Written documentation by a physician giving permission to medical personnel not to attempt resuscitation in the event of cardiac arrest.

Do Not Resuscitate (DNR) order A type of advance directive that describes which life-sustaining procedures should be performed in the event of a sudden deterioration in a patient's medical condition.

domestic terrorists Native citizens who carry out terrorist acts against their own country.

dopaminergic receptors The receptors believed to cause dilation of the renal, coronary, and cerebral arteries.

dorsal Referring to the back or posterior side of the body or an organ.

dorsiflex To bend the foot or hand backward.

dose effect The principle that the longer a hazardous material is in contact with the body or the greater the concentration, the greater the effect will probably be.

DOT KKK 1822 Federal standards that regulate the design and manufacturing guidelines of emergency ambulances.

Down syndrome A genetic chromosomal defect that can occur during fetal development and that results in mental retardation as well as certain physical characteristics, such as a round head with a flat occiput and slanted, wide-set eyes.

dressing Material used to directly cover a wound.

drift A finding that when the operator lets go of the steering wheel, a vehicle consistently wanders left or right.

drip chamber The area of the administration set where fluid accumulates so that the tubing remains filled with fluid.

dromotropic effect The effect on the velocity of conduction.

drowning The process of experiencing respiratory impairment from submersion or immersion in liquid.

drug Substance that has some therapeutic effect (such as reducing inflammation, fighting bacteria, or producing euphoria) when given in the appropriate circumstances and in the appropriate dose.

drug abuse Any use of drugs that causes physical, psychological, economic, legal, or social harm to the user or others affected by the user's behavior.

drug addiction A chronic disorder characterized by the compulsive use of a substance that results in physical, psychological, or social harm to the user who continues to use the substance despite the harm.

drug reconstitution Injecting sterile water or saline from one vial into another vial containing a powdered form of the drug.

ductus arteriosus A duct that is present before birth that connects the pulmonary artery to the aorta in order to move unoxygenated blood back to the placenta.

ductus venosus A duct that is present before birth that connects the placenta to the heart in order to move oxygenated blood to the fetus.

due process A right to a fair procedure for a legal action against a person or agency; has two components: Notice and Opportunity to be Heard.

due regard Driving with awareness and responsibility for other drivers on the roadways when operating an ambulance in the emergency mode.

duodenum The first part of the small intestine.

duplex Radio system using more than one frequency to permit simultaneous transmission and reception.

dura mater The outermost layer of the three meninges that enclose the brain and spinal cord; it is the toughest meningeal layer.

duration of action How long the medication concentration can be expected to remain above the minimum level needed to provide the intended action.

duty Legal obligation of public and certain other ambulance services to respond to a call for help in their jurisdiction.

dysconjugate gaze Paralysis of gaze or lack of coordination between the movements of the two eyes.

dysmenorrhea Painful menstruation.

dysphagia Difficulty in swallowing.

dysphonia Difficulty speaking.

dysplasia An alteration in the size, shape, and organization of cells.

dyspnea Any difficulty in respiratory rate, regularity, or effort.

dystonia Contractions of the body into a bizarre position.

early adults Persons who are 19 to 40 years of age.

ecchymosis Localized bruising or blood collection within or under the skin.

echolalia Meaningless echoing of the interviewer's words by the patient.

ecstasy A drug officially named methylenedioxymethamphetamine (MDMA) that is sometimes used to facilitate date rape; a methamphetamine derivative with hallucinogenic properties; street names include XTC, Adam, X, lover's speed, and clarity.

ectopic pregnancy A pregnancy in which the ovum implants somewhere other than the uterine endometrium.

edema A condition in which excess fluid accumulates in tissues, manifested by swelling.

efferent arteriole The structure in the kidney where blood drains from the glomerulus.

efferent nerves The nerves that carry messages from the brain to the muscles and all other organs of the body.

ejection fraction The portion of the blood ejected from the ventricle during systole.

elastin A protein that gives the skin its elasticity.

electrical alternans An ECG pattern in which the QRS vector changes with each heart beat. This pattern is pathognomonic for cardiac tamponade.

electrical conduction system In the heart, the specialized cardiac tissue that initiates and conducts electric impulses. The system includes the SA node, internodal atrial conduction pathways, atrioventricular junction, atrioventricular node, bundle of His, and the Purkinje network.

electrical energy The energy delivered in the form of high voltage.

electrolytes Charged atoms or compounds that result from the loss or gain of an electron. These are ions that the body uses to perform certain critical metabolic functions.

elixir A syrup with alcohol and flavoring added.

emancipated minor A person who is under the legal age in a given state but, because of other circumstances, is legally considered an adult.

embryo The fetus in the earliest stages after fertilization.

emergence phenomenon Nightmares associated with the use of ketamine.

emergency medical dispatch First aid instructions given by specially trained dispatchers to callers over the telephone while an ambulance is en route to the call.

emergency medical dispatcher (EMD) A person who receives information and relays that information in an organized manner during the emergency.

emergency medical services (EMS) A health care system designed to bring immediate on-scene care to those in need along with transport to a definitive medical care facility.

Emergency Response Guidebook (ERG) A hazardous materials reference developed by the US Department of Transportation that provides valuable information about hazardous materials, isolation distances, etc; should be carried on every emergency

response unit, and every paramedic should know how to use it.

emotional/mental impairment Illnesses that cause a person's emotions to become out of control.

emphysema Infiltration of any tissue by air or gas; a chronic obstructive pulmonary disease characterized by distention of the alveoli and destructive changes in the lung parenchyma.

EMTALA The Emergency Medical Treatment and Active Labor Act enacted in 1986 to combat the practice of patient dumping (hospitals refusing to admit seriously ill patients or women in labor who could not pay, forcing EMS providers to dump the patients at another hospital). EMTALA regulates hospitals that receive Medicare funding and severely fines hospitals or doctors who violate its provisions.

emulsion A preparation of one liquid (usually an oil) distributed in small globules in another liquid (usually water).

encoded A message is put into a code before it is transmitted.

endocardium The thin membrane lining the inside of the heart.

endocrine glands Glands that secrete or release chemicals that are used inside the body. Endocrine glands lack ducts and release hormones directly into the surrounding tissue and blood.

endocrine hormones Hormones that are carried to their target or cell group in the bloodstream.

endometriosis A condition in which endometrial tissue grows outside the uterus.

endometritis An inflammation of the endometrium that often is associated with a bacterial infection.

endometrium The inner mucous membrane of the uterus.

endoscopy The insertion of a flexible tube into the esophagus with the intent of visualizing and repairing damage or disease.

endosteum The inner lining of a hollow bone.

endothelial cells Specific types of epithelial cells that serve the function of lining the blood vessels.

endotoxin A toxin released by some bacteria when they die.

endotracheal (ET) tube Tube that is inserted into the trachea; equipped with a distal cuff, proximal inflation port, a 15/22-mm adapter, and cm markings on the side.

endotracheal intubation Passing an endotracheal (ET) tube through the glottic opening and sealing the tube with a cuff inflated against the tracheal wall.

end-tidal carbon dioxide The numeric percentage of carbon dioxide contained in the last few milliliters of the patient's exhaled air.

end-tidal carbon dioxide (ETCO$_2$) detectors Device that detects the presence of carbon dioxide in exhaled air.

enhanced 9-1-1 system An emergency call-in system in which additional information such as the phone number and location of the caller is recorded automatically through sophisticated telephone technology and the dispatcher need only confirm the information on the screen.

enteral route A route of medication administration that involves the medication passing through a portion of the gastrointestinal tract.

enterococcus A common, normal organism of the GI tract, urinary tract, and genitourinary tract, and which may become resistant to vancomycin.

entrapment A condition in which a patient is trapped by debris, soil, or other material and is unable to extricate himself or herself.

entry wound The point at which a penetrating object enters the body.

environmental emergencies Medical conditions caused or exacerbated by the weather, terrain, or unique atmospheric conditions such as high altitude or under water.

eosinophils Cells that make up approximately 1% to 3% of the leukocytes, which play a major role in allergic reactions and bronchoconstriction in an asthma attack.

epicardium The thin membrane lining the outside of the heart.

epidermis The outermost layer of the skin.

epidural hematoma An accumulation of blood between the skull and dura.

epigastric The right upper region of the abdomen directly inferior to the xyphoid process and superior to the umbilicus.

epiglottis Leaf-shaped cartilaginous structure that closes over the trachea during swallowing.

epiglottitis Inflammation of the epiglottis.

epinephrine Hormone produced by the adrenal medulla that plays a vital role in the function of the sympathetic nervous system.

epiphyseal plate The growth plate of a bone; a major site of bone development during childhood.

epiphyses The ends of a long bone.

episiotomy An incision in the perineal skin made to prevent tearing during childbirth.

epistaxis A nosebleed.

epithelialization The formation of fresh epithelial tissue to heal a wound.

epithelium Type of tissue that covers all external surfaces of the body.

Erb palsy Lack of movement at the shoulder due to nerve injury resulting from the stretching of the cervical nerve roots (C5 and C6 most commonly) during delivery of the baby's head during birth. The effect is usually transient, but can be permanent.

erythema Reddening of the skin.

erythrocytes Red blood cells.

escharotomy A surgical cut through the eschar or leathery covering of a burn injury to allow for swelling and minimize the potential for development of compartment syndrome in a circumferentially burned limb or the thorax.

esophageal detector device (EDD) Bulb or syringe that is attached to the proximal end of the ET tube; a device used to confirm proper ET tube placement.

estrogen One of the three major female hormones. At puberty, estrogen brings about the secondary sex characteristics.

ethical A behavior expected by an individual or group following a set of rules.

ethics A set of values in society that differentiates right from wrong.

etiology The cause of a disease process.

etomidate A nonnarcotic, nonbarbiturate hypnotic-sedative drug; also called Amidate.

eustress A type of stress that motivates an individual to achieve.

evaluation Collection of the methods, skills, and activities necessary to determine whether a service or program is needed, likely to be used, conducted as planned, and actually helps people.

evaporation The conversion of a liquid to a gas.

evisceration Displacement of an organ outside the body.

excretion The elimination of toxic or inactive metabolites from the body. This is primarily done by the kidneys, intestines, lungs, and assorted glands.

exertional heat stroke A serious type of heat stroke usually affecting young and fit people exercising in hot and humid conditions.

exertional hyponatremia A condition due to prolonged exertion in hot environments coupled with excessive hypotonic fluid intake that leads to nausea, vomiting, and, in severe cases, mental status changes and seizures.

exhalation Passive movement of air out of the lungs; also called expiration.

exit wound The point at which a penetrating object leaves the body, which may or may not be in a straight line from the entry wound.

exocrine glands Glands that excrete chemicals for elimination.

exocrine hormones Hormones that are secreted through ducts into an organ or onto epithelial surfaces.

exopthalmos Protrusion of the eyes from the normal position within the socket.

exotoxin A toxin that is secreted by living cells to aid in the death and digestion of other cells.

experimental research Describes a new product, skill, or idea that is undergoing research and will be trialed, with the effects evaluated.

expiration Passive movement of air out of the lungs; also called exhalation.

expiratory reserve volume The amount of air that you can exhale following a normal exhalation; average volume is about 1,200 mL.

expressed consent A type of informed consent that occurs when the patient does something, either through words or by taking some sort of action, that demonstrates permission to provide care.

expressive aphasia Damage to or loss of the ability to speak.

external auditory canal The area in which sound waves are received from the auricle (pinna) before they travel to the eardrum; also called the ear canal.

external ear One of three anatomic parts of the ear; it contains the pinna, the ear canal, and the external portion of the tympanic membrane.

external jugular (EJ) vein Large neck vein that is lateral to the carotid artery.

external os The junction where the uterus opens into the vagina.

external respiration The exchange of gases between the lungs and the blood cells in the pulmonary capillaries; also called pulmonary respiration.

extracellular fluid (ECF) The water outside the cells; accounts for 15% of body weight.

extract A concentrated preparation of a drug made by putting the drug into solution (in alcohol or water) and evaporating off the excess solvent to a prescribed standard.

extrication officer In incident command, the person appointed to determine the type of equipment and resources needed for a situation involving extrication or special rescue; also called the rescue officer.

extubation The process of removing the tube from an intubated patient.

eyelash reflex Contraction of the patient's lower eyelid when it is gently stroked; fairly reliable indicator of the presence or absence of an intact gag reflex.

EZ-IO A hand-held, battery-powered driver to which a special IO needle is attached; used for insertion of the IO needle into the proximal tibia of children and adults.

F.A.S.T.1 A sternal IO device used in adults; stands for First Access for Shock and Trauma.

facet joint The joint on which each vertebra articulates with adjacent vertebrae.

facial nerve The seventh cranial nerve; supplies motor activity to all muscles of facial expression, the sense of taste, and anterior two thirds of the tongue and cutaneous sensation to the external ear, tongue, and palate.

facilitation An interviewing technique in which the interviewer uses noncommittal words and gestures to encourage the patient to proceed.

Fahrenheit scale A scale for measuring temperature in which water freezes at 32° and boils at 212°.

fallopian tubes The vehicles of transportation of the ova from the ovaries to the uterus; also called oviducts.

false imprisonment The intentional and unjustified detention of a person against his or her will.

fascia The fiberlike connective tissue that covers arteries, veins, tendons, and ligaments.

fasciculations Characterized by brief, uncoordinated twitching of small muscle groups in the face, neck, trunk, and extremities; caused by the administration of depolarizing neuromuscular blocking agents (eg, succinylcholine).

fasciotomy   A surgical procedure that cuts away fascia to relieve pressure.

fatigue fractures   Fractures that result from multiple compressive loads.

fear   Also sometimes referred to as a phobia, this is an anxious feeling, usually about specific things or situations.

feculent   Smelling of feces.

Federal Communications Commission (FCC)   The federal agency that has jurisdiction over interstate and international telephone and telegraph services and satellite communications, all of which may involve EMS activity.

feedback inhibition   Negative feedback resulting in the decrease of an action in the body.

femoral artery   The main artery supplying the thigh and leg.

femoral shaft fractures   A break in the diaphysis of the femur.

femur   The proximal bone of the leg that extends from the pelvis to the knee.

fetus   The developing, unborn infant inside the uterus.

fibrin   A whitish, filamentous protein formed by the action of thrombin on fibrinogen. Fibrin is the protein that polymerizes (bonds) to form the fibrous component of a blood clot.

fibrinolysis cascade   The breakdown of fibrin in blood clots, and the prevention of the polymerization of fibrin into new clots.

fibrinolytic agents   The only medications available to dissolve blood clots after they have already formed; the drugs promote the digestion of fibrin.

fibrinolytic system   The mechanism by which fibrin undergoes dissolution owing to the action of enzymes; clots are destroyed.

fibrinolytic therapy   The therapy that uses medications that act to dissolve blood clots.

fibrous joints   The joints that contain dense fibrous tissue and allow for no motion.

fibula   The smaller of the two bones of the lower leg.

field diagnosis   A determination of what a paramedic thinks is the patient's current problem, usually based on the patient history and the chief complaint.

fight-or-flight syndrome   A physiologic response to a profound stressor that helps one deal with the situation at hand; features increased sympathetic tone and resulting in dilation of the pupils, increased heart rate, dilation of the bronchi, mobilization of glucose, shunting of blood away from the gastrointestinal tract and cerebrum, and increased blood flow to the skeletal muscles.

finance   In incident command, the position in an incident responsible for accounting of all expenditures.

first-degree heart block   A partial disruption of the conduction of the depolarizing impulse from the atria to the ventricles, causing prolongation of the P-R interval.

first stage of labor   The stage of labor that begins with the onset of regular labor pains,

crampy abdominal pains, during which the uterus contracts and the cervix effaces.

flail chest   An injury that involves two or more adjacent ribs fractured in two or more places, allowing the segment between the fractures to move independently of the rest of the thoracic cage.

flame burn   A thermal burn caused by flames touching the skin.

flash burn   An electrothermal injury caused by arcing of electric current.

flash chamber   The area of an IV catheter that fills with blood to help indicate when a vein is cannulated.

flash point   The temperature at which a vapor can be ignited by a spark.

flat   Used to describe behavior in which the patient doesn't seem to feel much of anything at all.

flat bones   Bones that are thin and broad, such as the scapula.

flexion injury   A type of injury that results from forward movement of the head, typically as the result of rapid deceleration, such as in a car crash, or with a direct blow to the occiput.

flight of ideas   Accelerated thinking in which the mind skips very rapidly from one thought to the next.

flow-restricted, oxygen-powered ventilation device (FROPVD)   Also referred to as a manually triggered ventilator or demand valve. Can be used to ventilate apneic or to administer supplemental oxygen to spontaneously breathing patients.

fluid extract   A concentrated form of a drug prepared by dissolving the crude drug in the fluid in which it is most readily soluble.

focal brain injury   A specific, grossly observable brain injury.

focused history and physical exam   The part of the assessment process in which the patient's major complaints or any problems that are immediately evident are further and more specifically evaluated.

focused physical exam   The exam done on a responsive medical patient, driven by the information gathered during the initial assessment and the history-taking phase.

follicle-stimulating hormone (FSH)   A hormone produced by the anterior pituitary gland which is important in the menstrual cycle.

fomite   An inanimate object contaminated with microorganisms that serves as a means of transmitting an illness.

fontanelles   The soft spots in the skull of a newborn and infant where the sutures of the skull have not yet grown together.

footling breech   A delivery in which one or both feet dangle through the vaginal opening.

foramen magnum   A large opening at the base of the skull through which the spinal cord exits the brain.

foramen ovale   An opening in the septum of the heart before birth, and which closes after birth.

foramina   Small natural openings, perforations, or orifices, such as in the bones of the cranial vault; plural of foramen.

Fowler's position   A sitting position with the head elevated to 90° (sitting straight upright).

foxglove   A plant that contains cardiac glycosides used in making digitalis; ingestion of leaves causes nausea, vomiting, diarrhea, abdominal cramps, hyperkalemia, and a variety of arrhythmias.

fractile response time   A fraction (not average) of all emergency responses for the purpose of setting standards in response times.

fraction of inspired oxygen (FiO$_2$)   The percentage of oxygen in inhaled air.

fracture   A break or rupture in the bone.

free-flow oxygen   Oxygen administered via oxygen tube and a cupped hand on patient's face.

freelancing   When individual units or different organizations make independent and often inefficient decisions about the next appropriate action.

free radicals   Molecules that are missing one electron in their outer shell.

frequency   In radio communications, the number of cycles per second of a signal, inversely related to the wavelength.

frontal lobe   The portion of the brain that is important in voluntary motor actions and personality traits.

frostbite   Localized damage to tissues resulting from prolonged exposure to extreme cold.

frostnip   Early frostbite, characterized by numbness and pallor without significant tissue damage.

fsw   Abbreviation for feet of seawater, an indirect measure of pressure under water.

full-thickness burn   A burn that extends through the epidermis and dermis into the subcutaneous tissues beneath; previously called a third-degree burn.

functional reserve capacity   The amount of air that can be forced from the lungs in a single exhalation.

fundus   The dome-shaped top of the uterus.

fungus (plural: fungi)   A small organism that can grow rapidly in the presence of nutrients and organic material, and can cause infection related to contact with decaying organic matter or from airborne spores in the environment such as molds.

G agents   Early nerve agents that were developed by German scientists in the period after WWI and into WWII. There are three such agents: sarin, soman, and tabun.

gag reflex   Automatic reaction when something touches an area deep in the oral cavity; helps protect the lower airway from aspiration.

gait   Walking pattern.

galea aponeurotica   Tough, tendinous layer of the scalp.

gamma (x-rays)   Type of energy that is emitted from a strong radiological source that is far faster and stronger than alpha and beta rays. These rays easily penetrate through the human body and require either several inches of lead or concrete to prevent penetration.

gamma-hydroxybutyric acid (GHB) A drug used to facilitate date rape; is colorless with a salty taste disguised when mixed with a drink; street names include Georgia home boy, grievous bodily harm, easy lay, G, scoop, liquid X, soap, and salty water.

ganglia Groupings of nerve cell bodies located in the peripheral nervous system.

gangrene An infection commonly caused by *C perfringens*. The result is tissue destruction and gas production that may lead to death.

Gardnerella **vaginitis** An infection caused by a bacterium that normally resides in the genital area in women but that can cause infection if the bacteria become too numerous; signs and symptoms include a vaginal odor that may be fishy, itching, irritation, and, possibly, a smooth, thin, sticky, white or gray discharge.

gastric distention Inflation of the patient's stomach with air.

gastric tubes Tubes that are commonly inserted in patients in the prehospital setting to decompress the stomach; can also be used to administer certain enteral medications.

gastroenteritis A term that comprises many types of infections and irritations of the gastrointestinal tract; symptoms include nausea and vomiting, fever, abdominal cramps, and diarrhea.

gastrointestinal exposure Exposure to a hazardous material through intentional or unintentional swallowing of the substance.

gauge The internal diameter of an IV catheter or needle.

general adaptation syndrome A three-stage description of the body's short-term and long-term reactions to stress.

general impression The overall initial impression that determines the priority for patient care; based on the patient's surroundings, the mechanism of injury, signs and symptoms, and the chief complaint.

generalized anxiety disorder (GAD) A disorder in which a person worries about everything for no particular reason, or their worrying is unproductive and they can't decide what to do about an upcoming situation.

generalized seizures The seizures characterized by manifestations that indicate involvement of both cerebral hemispheres.

generic drug A medication that is not patented.

generic name A general name for a drug that is not manufacturer-specific; usually the name given to the drug by the company that first manufactures it.

genital herpes An infection of the genitals, buttocks, or anal area caused by herpes simplex virus (HSV), which may cause sores of the genitals, mouth, or lips.

genital warts Warts caused by the human papillomavirus (HPV), a sexually transmitted disease; also called condylomata acuminata or venereal warts.

geriatrics The assessment and treatment of disease in someone 65 years or older.

gestation Period of time from conception to birth. For humans, the full period is normally 9 months.

gestational diabetes Diabetes that develops during pregnancy in women who did not have diabetes before pregnancy.

gestational hypertension High blood pressure that develops after the 20th week of pregnancy, in women with previously normal blood pressures, and resolves spontaneously in the postpartum period.

gestational period The time that it takes for the infant to develop in utero, normally 38 weeks.

glands Cells or organs that selectively remove, concentrate, or alter materials in the blood and then secrete them back into the body.

Glasgow Coma Scale (GCS) An evaluation tool used to determine level of consciousness, which evaluates and assigns point values (scores) for eye opening, verbal response, and motor response, which are then totaled; effective in helping predict patient outcomes.

glenoid fossa Socket in the scapula in which the head of the humerus rotates.

global aphasia Damage to or loss of both the ability to speak and the ability to understand speech.

globe The eyeball.

glomerular (Bowman's) capsule A double-layered cup with the inner layer infiltrating and surrounding the capillaries of the glomerulus.

glomerular filtration The first step in the formation of urine; calculated to determine renal function.

glomerular filtration rate (GFR) The rate at which blood is filtered through the glomerula.

glomerulus A tuft of capillaries located in the kidney that serve as the main filter for the blood in the kidney.

glossopharyngeal nerve Ninth cranial nerve; supplies motor fibers to the pharyngeal muscle, providing taste sensation to the posterior portion of the tongue, and carrying parasympathetic fibers to the parotid gland.

glottis The space in between the vocal cords that is the narrowest portion of the adult's airway; also called the glottic opening.

glucagon Hormone produced by the pancreas that is vital to the control of the body's metabolism and blood sugar level. Glucagon stimulates the breakdown of glycogen to glucose.

GnRF A chemical released by the hypothalamus that stimulates the release of follicle-stimulating hormone.

goals The end points toward which intervention efforts are directed. A statement of changes sought in an injury problem, stated in broad terms.

goblet cells Cells that produce a protective mucous lining.

gonads The reproductive glands; the main source of sex hormones.

gonorrhea A sexually transmitted disease which results in infection caused by the gonococcal bacteria, Neisseria gonorrhea. Signs and symptoms include pus-containing discharge from the urethra and painful urination in males, and signs and symptoms of an acute abdomen in females.

Good Samaritan law A statute providing limited immunity from liability to persons responding voluntarily and in good faith to the aid of an injured person outside the hospital.

gout A painful disorder characterized by the crystallization of uric acid within a joint.

granulocytes Cells that contain granules.

gravid The number of all pregnancies a woman has had, including those not necessarily carried to term.

gravidity A term used to refer to a uterus that contains a pregnancy, whatever the outcome.

gravity The acceleration of a body by the attraction of the earth's gravitational force, normally 32.2 ft/sec^2.

Greenfield filter A mesh filter placed in the inferior vena cava to catch blood clots in patients who are at high risk of pulmonary embolus.

greenstick fracture A type of fracture occurring most frequently in children in which there is incomplete breakage of the bone.

gross negligence Negligence that is willful, wanton, intentional, or reckless; a serious departure from the accepted standards.

ground substance Material between cells.

group B streptococcus (GBS) A bacteria that lives in the genitourinary and gastrointestinal tracts of normal healthy individuals, but which can cause life-threatening infections in newborn babies.

growth plates Structures located on either end of an infant's bone, which aid in lengthening bones as the child grows.

grunting A short, low-pitched sound at the end of exhalation, present in children with moderate to severe hypoxia; reflects poor gas exchange because of fluid in the lower airways and air sacs.

gtt A unit of measure that indicates drops.

guarding Contraction of the abdominal muscles in patients.

Guillain-Barré syndrome A disease of unknown etiology that causes paralysis that progresses from the feet to the head (ascending paralysis). If the paralysis reaches the diaphragm, the patient may require respiratory support.

gum bougie Also called the Eschmann stylet; a flexible device that is inserted in between the glottis under direct laryngoscopy. The ET tube is then threaded over the device, facilitating its entry into the trachea.

gut-associated lymphoid tissue (GALT) The lymphoid tissue that lies under the inner lining of the esophagus and intestines.

habituation The situation in which there is a physical tolerance and psychological dependence on a drug or drugs.

Haddon matrix A framework developed by William Haddon, Jr, MD as a method to generate ideas about injury prevention that address the host, agent, and environment and their impact in the pre-event, event, and post-event phases of the injury process.

hallucination A sense perception not founded on objective reality; a false perception.

hallucinogen An agent that produces false perceptions in any one of the five senses.

hantavirus Also known as hemorrhagic fever with renal syndrome, this is a type of virus found in wild rodents, which can also cause disease in humans, characterized by fever, headache, abdominal pain, loss of appetite, and vomiting.

hapten A substance that normally does not stimulate an immune response but can be combined with an antigen and at a later point initiate an antibody response.

hard palate The bony anterior part of the palate, which forms the roof of the mouth.

hasty rope slide Self-escape procedure when there is no other means of egress.

hazardous material Any substance that is toxic, poisonous, radioactive, flammable, or explosive and causes injury or death with exposure.

head bobbing A sign of increased work of breathing in which the head lifts and tilts back during inspiration, then moves forward during expiration.

head injury A traumatic insult to the head that may result in injury to soft tissue, bony structures, or the brain.

head tilt-chin lift maneuver Manual airway maneuver that involves tilting the head back while lifting up on the chin; used to open the airway of a semiconscious or unconscious nontrauma patient.

health care power of attorney A legal document that allows another person to make health care decisions for the patient, including withdrawal or withholding of care, when the patient is incapacitated.

health care professional A person who follows specific professional attributes that are outlined in this profession.

heart rate (HR) The number of heart contractions per minute.

heat cramps Acute and involuntary muscle pains, usually in the lower extremities, the abdomen, or both, that occur because of profuse sweating and subsequent sodium losses in sweat.

heat exhaustion A clinical syndrome characterized by volume depletion and heat stress that is thought to be a milder form of heat illness and on a continuum leading to heat stroke.

heat illness The increase in core body temperature due to inadequate thermolysis.

heat stroke The least common and most deadly heat illness, caused by a severe disturbance in thermoregulation, usually characterized by a core temperature of more than 104°F (40°C) and altered mental status.

heat syncope An orthostatic or near-syncopal episode that typically occurs in nonacclimated individuals who may be under heat stress.

Heimlich maneuver Abdominal thrusts performed to relieve a foreign body airway obstruction.

helminths Invertebrates with long, flexible, rounded, or flattened bodies, commonly called worms; a type of parasite.

helper T cells A type of T lymphocyte that is involved in both cell-mediated and antibody-mediated immune responses. It secretes cytokines that stimulate the B cells and other T cells.

hematemesis Vomit with blood. Can either be like coffee grounds in appearance, indicating partially digested blood, or bright red blood indicating current active bleeding.

hematochezia Blood with the stool that is separate. Caused by lower GI bleeds.

hematocrit The percentage of RBCs in total blood volume.

hematoma A localized collection of blood in the soft tissues as a result of injury or a broken blood vessel.

hematopoiesis The generation of blood cells.

hematopoietic system The system that includes all blood components and the organs involved in their development and production.

hematuria The presence of blood in the urine.

hemiparesis Weakness of one side of the body.

hemiplegia Paralysis of one side of the body.

hemochromatosis An inherited disease in which the body absorbs more iron than it needs and stores it in the liver, kidneys, and pancreas.

hemoglobin An iron-containing protein within red blood cells that has the ability to combine with oxygen.

hemolytic anemia A disease characterized by increased destruction of the red blood cells. It can occur from an Rh factor reaction, exposure to chemicals, or a disorder of the immune system.

hemolytic disorder A disorder relating to the breakdown of RBCs.

hemoperitoneum The presence of extravasated blood in the peritoneal cavity.

hemophilia A bleeding disorder that is primarily hereditary, in which clotting does not occur or occurs insufficiently.

hemopneumothorax A collection of blood and air in the pleural cavity.

hemoptysis Coughing up blood.

hemorrhage Profuse bleeding.

hemorrhagic One of the two main types of stroke; occurs as a result of bleeding inside the brain.

hemorrhagic cyst A blood-filled sac that forms when a blood vessel bursts in a cyst wall and the blood fills the sac.

hemostasis The body's natural blood-clotting mechanism.

hemothorax The collection of blood within the normally closed pleural space.

Henry's law The amount of gas dissolved in a liquid is directly proportional to the partial pressure of the gas above the liquid.

Hering-Breuer reflex The nervous system mechanism that terminates inhalation and prevents lung overexpansion.

hernia Protrusion of any organ through an opening into a body cavity where it does not belong.

herniation Process in which tissue is forced out of its normal position, such as when the brain is forced from the cranial vault, either through the foramen magnum or over the tentorium.

hertz (Hz) Unit of frequency equal to 1 cycle per second.

high-altitude cerebral edema (HACE) An altitude illness in which there is a change in mental status and/or ataxia in a person with AMS or the presence of mental status changes and ataxia in a person without AMS.

high-altitude pulmonary edema (HAPE) An altitude illness characterized by dyspnea at rest, cough, severe weakness, and drowsiness that may eventually lead to central cyanosis, audible rales or wheezing, tachypnea, and tachycardia.

high-angle operations A rope rescue operation where the angle of the slope is greater than 45°; rescuers depend on life safety rope rather than a fixed support surface such as the ground.

hilum Point of entry of all of the blood vessels and the bronchi into each lung.

hilus A cleft where the ureters, renal blood vessels, lymphatic vessels, and nerves enter and leave the kidney.

HIPAA The Health Insurance Portability and Accountability Act that was enacted in 1996, providing for criminal sanctions as well as for civil penalties for releasing a patient's protected health information (PHI) in a way not authorized by the patient.

histamine A chemical found in mast cells that, when released, causes vasodilation, capillary leaking, and bronchiole constriction.

history of the present illness Information about the chief complaint, obtained using the OPQRST mnemonic.

homeostasis A tendency to constancy or stability in the body's internal environment.

homeostatic mechanism The mechanism involving many parts of the body that maintain homeostasis.

hormones Proteins formed in specialized organs or glands and carried to another organ or group of cells in the same organism. Hormones regulate many body functions, including metabolism, growth, and temperature.

hospice An organization that provides end-of-life care to patients with terminal illnesses and their families.

host resistance One's ability to fight off infection.

hot zone The area immediately surrounding an incident site that is directly dangerous to life and health. All personnel working in the hot zone must wear complete and appropriate protective clothing and equipment. Entry requires approval by the IC or a designated sector officer. Complete backup, rescue, and decontamination teams must be in place at the perimeter before operations begin.

human chorionic gonadotropin hormone A hormone that sends signals to the corpus luteum that pregnancy has initiated.

human immunodeficiency virus (HIV) AIDS (acquired immunodeficiency syndrome) is caused by HIV, which kills or damages the cells in the body's immune system so that the body is unable to fight infections and certain cancers.

humerus The bone of the upper arm.

humoral immunity The use of antibodies dissolved in the plasma and lymph to destroy foreign substances.

hydrocarbons Compounds made up principally of hydrogen and carbon atom mostly obtained from the distillation of petroleum.

hydrocephalus The increased accumulation of cerebrospinal fluid within the ventricles of the brain.

hymen A membrane that protects the vaginal orifice before first intercourse.

hyoid bone A small, horseshoe-shaped bone to which the jaw, tongue, epiglottis, and thyroid cartilage attach.

hypercalcemia A condition in which calcium levels are elevated.

hypercarbia Increased carbon dioxide levels in the bloodstream.

hypercholesterolemia An elevated blood cholesterol level.

hyperemesis gravidarum A condition of persistent nausea and vomiting during pregnancy.

hyperesthesia Hyperacute pain to touch.

hyperextension Extension of a limb of other body part beyond its usual range of motion.

hyperglycemia Abnormally high blood glucose level.

hyperkalemia An increased level of potassium in the blood.

hypermagnesemia An increased serum magnesium level.

hypermenorrhea Menstrual blood flow that lasts several days longer than it should or flow that is abnormally excessive.

hypernatremia A blood serum sodium level greater than 148 mEq/L and a serum osmolarity greater than 295 mOsm/kg.

hyperosmolar hyperglycemic nonketotic coma (HHNC), also known as hyperosmolar nonketotic coma (HONK), is a metabolic derangement that occurs principally in patients with type 2 diabetes. The condition is characterized by hyperglycemia, hyperosmolarity, and an absence of significant ketosis.

hyperosmolar nonketotic coma (HONK), also known as hyperosmolar hyperglycemic nonketotic coma (HHNC), is a metabolic derangement that occurs principally in patients with type 2 diabetes. The condition is characterized by hyperglycemia, hyperosmolarity, and an absence of significant ketosis.

hyperperistalsis Increased movement within the bowel.

hyperphosphatemia An increased level of phosphate in the blood.

hyperplasia An increase in the actual number of cells in an organ or tissue, usually resulting in an increase in size of the organ or tissue.

hyperpyrexia A very high body temperature.

hypersensitivity Occurs when a patient reacts with exaggerated or inappropriate allergic symptoms after coming into contact with a substance the body perceives as harmful.

hypertension High blood pressure, usually a diastolic pressure greater than 90 mm Hg.

hyperthermia Unusually elevated body temperature.

hypertonic solution A solution that has a greater concentration of sodium than does the cell; the increased osmotic pressure can draw water out of the cell and cause it to collapse.

hypertrophic scar An abnormal scar with excess collagen that does not extend over the wound margins.

hypertrophy An increase in the size of the cells due to synthesis of more subcellular components, leading to an increase in tissue and organ size.

hyperventilation Occurs when CO_2 elimination exceeds CO_2 production.

hyphema Bleeding into the anterior chamber of the eye; results from direct ocular trauma.

hypnosis Altered consciousness often caused by hypnotic drugs, which are used to induce sleep.

hypocalcemia A low level of calcium in the blood.

hypocarbia Decreased CO_2 content in arterial blood.

hypoglossal nerve Twelfth cranial nerve; provides motor function to the muscles of the tongue and throat.

hypoglycemia A deficiency of glucose in the blood caused by too much insulin or too little glucose.

hypokalemia A low blood serum potassium level.

hypomagnesemia A decreased serum magnesium level.

hyponatremia A blood serum sodium level that is below 135 mEq/L and a serum osmolarity that is less than 280 mOsm/kg.

hypoperfusion A condition that occurs when the level of tissue perfusion decreases below that needed to maintain normal cellular functions.

hypoperistalsis Decreased bowel movement.

hypophosphatemia A decreased blood serum phosphate level.

hypothalamic-pituitary-adrenal (HPA) axis A major part of the neuroendocrine system that controls reactions to stress. It is the mechanism for a set of interactions among glands, hormones, and parts of the midbrain that mediate the general adaptation syndrome.

hypothalamus The most inferior portion of the diencephalon; responsible for control of many body functions, including heart rate, digestion, sexual development, temperature regulation, emotion, hunger, thirst, and regulation of the sleep cycle.

hypothermia Condition in which the core body temperature is significantly below normal.

hypotonia Low or poor muscle tone (floppy).

hypotonic solution A solution that has a lower concentration of sodium than does the cell; the increased osmotic pressure lets water flow into the cell, causing it to swell and possibly burst.

hypotonic solution A solution with an osmolarity lower than intracellular fluid.

hypoventilate To not move adequate volumes of gas; underventilate.

hypoventilation Occurs when CO_2 production exceeds the body's ability to eliminate it by ventilation.

hypovolemia An abnormal decrease in blood volume or, strictly speaking, an abnormal decrease in the volume of blood plasma.

hypovolemic shock A condition that occurs when the circulating blood volume is inadequate to deliver adequate oxygen and nutrients to the body.

hypoxemia A decrease in arterial oxygen levels.

hypoxia A lack of oxygen to the body's cells and tissues.

hypoxic drive Secondary control of breathing that stimulates breathing based on decreased PaO_2 levels.

hypoxic ischemic encephalopathy Damage to cells in the central nervous system (the brain and spinal cord) from inadequate oxygen.

iatrogenic response An adverse condition inadvertently induced in a patient by the treatment given.

icterus Jaundice; the yellow appearance of the skin and other tissues caused by an accumulation of bile pigments.

idiopathic Of no known cause.

idiosyncrasy An abnormal (and usually unexplained) reaction by a person to a medication, to which most other people do not react.

ignition temperature The temperature at which a vapor will burst into sustained burning.

ileostomy Surgical procedure to remove large portions of the small intestine.

ilium The broad, uppermost bone of the pelvis.

illicit In relation to drugs, illegal drugs such as marijuana, cocaine, and LSD.

illusion A misinterpretation of sensory stimuli.

immediately dangerous to life and health (IDLH) A phrase that means the atmospheric concentration of any toxic, corrosive, or asphyxiant substance will pose an immediate threat to life, irreversible or delayed adverse effects, or serious interference for a team member attempting to escape from the dangerous atmosphere; a respirator is mandatory.

immune response The body's defense reaction to any substance that is recognized as foreign.

immune system The body system that includes all of the structures and processes designed to mount a defense against foreign substances and disease-causing agents.

immunity The body's ability to protect itself from acquiring a disease.

immunity (legal) Legal protection from penalties that could normally be incurred under the law.

immunobiologic medications The medications that include serums, vaccines, and other immunizing agents.

immunodeficiency An abnormal condition in which some part of the body's immune system is inadequate, and consequently resistance to infectious disease is decreased.

immunogen An antigen that activates immune cells to generate an immune response against itself.

immunoglobulins Antibodies secreted by the B cells.

immunosuppressant medications The medications intended to inhibit the body's ability to attack the "foreign" organ or, in the case of autoimmune diseases, the medications that inhibit the body's attack on itself.

impacted fracture A broken bone in which the end of one bone becomes wedged into another bone, as could be the case in a fall from a significant height.

impaled object An object that has caused a puncture wound and remains embedded in the wound.

imperforate hymen A situation in which the hymen completely covers the vaginal orifice.

implementation plan A strategy for carrying out an intervention. Includes goals, objectives, activities, evaluation measures, resource assessment, and time line.

implied consent Assumption on behalf of a person unable to give consent that he or she would have done so.

implosion A bursting inward.

impulse control disorders A condition in which an individual lacks the ability to resist a temptation or can't stop acting on a drive.

inattention Used to describe patients with whom it is difficult to gain their attention or focus.

incidence The frequency with which a disease occurs.

incident command system (ICS) A system implemented to manage disasters and mass- and multiple-casualty incidents in which section chiefs, including finance, logistics, operations, and planning, report to the incident commander.

incident commander (IC) The overall leader of the incident command system to whom commanders or leaders of incident command system divisions report.

incision A wound usually made deliberately, as in surgery; a clean cut, as opposed to a laceration.

incomplete abortion Expulsion of the fetus which results in some products of conception remaining in the uterus.

incomplete fracture A fracture in which the bone does not fully break.

incomplete spinal cord injury Spinal cord injury in which there is some degree of cord-mediated function; initial dysfunction may be temporary and there may be potential for recovery.

incubation Describes the period of time from a person being exposed to a disease to the time when symptoms begin.

incubation period The time period between exposure to an organism and the first symptoms of illness, during which the organism multiplies within the body and starts to produce symptoms.

indications The reasons or conditions for which the medication is given.

indirect injury An injury that results from a force that is applied to one region of the body but leads to an injury in another area.

induced abortion Intentional expulsion of the fetus.

inevitable abortion A spontaneous abortion that cannot be prevented.

infants Persons who are from 1 month to 1 year of age.

infarction Death (necrosis) of a localized area of tissue caused by the cutting off of its blood supply.

infection The abnormal invasion of a host or host tissue by organisms such as bacteria, viruses, or parasites, with or without signs or symptoms of disease.

infectious hepatitis Another name for hepatitis A, an inflammation from a virus that causes mild fatigue, loss of appetite, fever, nausea, abdominal pain, and eventually, jaundice, dark-colored urine, and whitish stools.

inferential A research format that uses a hypothesis to prove one finding from another.

infiltration The escape of fluid into the surrounding tissue; the result of vein perforation during IV cannulation.

inflammatory response A reaction by tissues of the body to irritation or injury, characterized by pain, swelling, redness, and heat.

influenza The flu, a respiratory infection caused by a variety of viruses. It differs from the common cold in that the flu involves a fever, headache, and extreme exhaustion.

informed consent A patient's voluntary agreement to be treated after being told about the nature of the disease, the risks and benefits of the proposed treatment, alternative treatments, or the choice of no treatment at all.

ingestion Eating or drinking materials for absorption through the gastrointestinal tract.

inhalation Breathing into the lungs; a medication delivery route.

initial assessment The part of the assessment process that helps you identify immediately or potentially life-threatening conditions so that you can initiate lifesaving care.

injection When the skin is pierced, and foreign material is deposited into the skin.

injuries Any unintentional or intentional damage to the body resulting from acute exposure to thermal, mechanical, electrical, or chemical energy or from the absence of such essentials as heat or oxygen.

injury risk A potentially hazardous situation that puts people in a position in which they could be harmed.

injury surveillance The ongoing systematic collection, analysis, and interpretation of injury data essential to the planning, implementation, and evaluation of public health practice.

inner ear One of three anatomic parts of the ear; it consists of the cochlea and semicircular canals.

inotropic Affecting the contractility of muscle tissue, especially cardiac muscle.

inspection Looking at the patient, either in general or at a specific area (ie, a patient's overall appearance from the doorway, versus looking specifically at the chest wall for abnormalities/deformities).

inspiration The active process of moving air into the lungs; also called inhalation.

inspiratory reserve volume The amount of air that can be inhaled after a normal inhalation; the amount of air that can be inhaled in addition to the normal tidal volume.

institutional review board (IRB) A group or institution that follows a set of requirements for review that were devised by the US Public Health Service.

insulin Hormone produced by the pancreas that's vital to the control of the body's metabolism and blood sugar level. Insulin causes sugar, fatty acids, and amino acids to be taken up and metabolized by cells.

insulin resistance Condition in which the pancreas produces enough insulin but the body can't effectively utilize it.

integument The skin.

intension tremors Tremors that occur when trying to accomplish a task.

intentional injuries Injuries that are purposefully inflicted by a person on himself or herself or on another person. Examples include suicide or attempted suicide, homicide, rape, assault, domestic abuse, elder abuse, and child abuse.

intercostal nerves Nerves that innervate the external intercostal muscles, the muscles between the ribs.

intercostal retractions Skin sucking in between the ribs, seen when a patient creates increased negative intrathoracic pressure to breathe.

intercostal space The space between two ribs, named according to the number of the rib above it, that contains the intercostal muscles and neurovascular bundle.

interference A direct biochemical interaction between two drugs.

interferon Protein produced by cells in response to viral invasion. Interferon is released into the bloodstream or intercellular fluid to induce healthy cells to manufacture an enzyme that counters the infection.

interleukins Chemical substances that attract white blood cells to the sites of injury and bacterial invasion.

internal mucosa The inner layer of tissue in the fallopian tubes.

internal respiration The exchange of gases between the blood cells and the tissues; also called cellular respiration.

internal shunt Also called an arteriovenous (AV) fistula, this device is an artificial connection between a vein and an artery, usually in the forearm or upper arm.

international terrorism Terrorism that is carried out by those not of the host's country; also known as cross-border terrorism.

internodal pathways The three pathways of the electrical conduction system found in the atria that transmit the impulse from the SA node to the AV node.

interstitial fluid The water bathing the cells; accounts for about 10.5% of body weight; includes special fluid collections, such as cerebrospinal fluid and intraocular fluid.

interstitial nephritis A chronic inflammation of the interstitial cells surrounding the nephrons.

intertrochanteric fractures Fractures that occur in the region between the lesser and greater trochanters.

interventions Specific prevention measures or activities designed to meet a program objective. Categories include education/behavior change, enforcement/legislation, engineering/technology, and economic incentives.

interventricular septum A thick wall that separates the right and left ventricles.

intracellular fluid (ICF) The water contained inside the cells; normally accounts for 45% of body weight.

intracerebral hematoma Bleeding within the brain tissue (parenchyma) itself; also referred to as an intraparenchymal hematoma.

intracranial pressure (ICP) The pressure within the cranial vault; normally 0 to 15 mm Hg in adults.

intradermal the layer of the dermis, just beneath the epidermis; a medication delivery route.

intramuscular (IM) route A method of delivering a medication into the muscle of the body. This is accomplished by placing a needle into a muscle space and injecting the medication into the tissue.

intranasal Within the nose.

intraosseous Within the bone.

intraosseous (IO) infusion A technique of administering fluids, blood and blood products, and medications into the intraosseous space of a long bone, usually the proximal tibia.

intraosseous (IO) route A method of delivering a medication into the marrow cavity of a bone. This is accomplished by placing a

rigid needle into the marrow cavity and flushing a medication into the space.

intraosseous (IO) space The spongy cancellous bone of the epiphyses and the medullary cavity of the diaphysis, collectively.

intrapulmonary shunting Bypassing of oxygen-poor blood past nonfunctional alveoli.

intrarenal acute renal failure (IARF) A type of acute renal failure due to damage in the kidney itself, often caused by immune-mediated diseases, prerenal ARF, toxins, heavy metals, some medications, or some organic compounds.

intravascular fluid Plasma; the water within the blood vessels, which carries red blood cells, white blood cells, and vital nutrients; normally accounts for about 4.5% of body weight.

intravenous Within a vein.

intravenous (IV) therapy Cannulation of a vein with an IV catheter to access the patient's vascular system.

intussusception An event where one part of the intestine folds into another part of the intestines lead to a blockage.

iodine An essential element in the diet and an important component of thyroxine. Without the proper level of iodine intake, thyroxine can't be produced, and physical and mental growth are diminished.

ionic concentration The amount of charged particles found in a particular area.

ionizing radiation Energy that is emitted in the form of rays, or particles.

ions Charged atoms or compounds that result from the loss or gain of an electron.

iris The colored portion of the eye.

iron deficiency anemia The most common type of anemia in which iron stores are low or lacking and the serum iron concentration is low.

irregular bones Bones with unique shapes that allow them to perform a specific function and that do not fit into the other categories based on shape.

irreversible shock The final stage of shock, resulting in death.

ischemia Tissue anoxia from diminished blood flow to tissue, usually caused by narrowing or occlusion of the artery.

ischemic One of the two main types of stroke; occurs when blood flow to a particular part of the brain is cut off by a blockage (eg, a clot) inside a blood vessel.

ischium The lowermost dorsal bone of the pelvis.

islets of Langerhans A specialized group of cells in the pancreas where insulin and glucagon are produced.

isoelectric When referring to a wave, the wave is neither positive nor negative.

isoelectric line The baseline of the ECG.

isoimmunity Formation of antibodies or T cells that are directed against antigens or another person's cells.

isotonic crystalloids Intravenous solutions that do not cause a fluid shift into or out of

the cell; examples include normal saline and lactated Ringer's solutions.

isotonic solution A solution that has the same concentration of sodium as does the cell. In this case, water does not shift, and no change in cell shape occurs.

Jacksonian March The wave-like movement of a seizure from a point of focus to other areas of the brain.

jaundice The presence of excessive bile pigments in the bloodstream that give the skin, mucous membranes, and eyes a distinct yellow color; jaundice is often associated with liver disease.

jaw-thrust maneuver Manual airway maneuver that involves stabilizing the patient's head and thrusting the jaw forward; the preferred method of opening the airway of a semiconscious or unconscious trauma patient.

joint The point at which two or more bones articulate, or come together.

joint capsule A saclike envelope that encloses the cavity of a synovial joint.

joint information center (JIC) An area designated by the incident commander, or a designee, in which public information officers from multiple agencies disseminate information about the incident.

jugular vein distention (JVD) A prominence of the jugular veins due to increased volume or increased pressure within the central venous system or the thoracic cavity.

JumpSTART triage A sorting system for pediatric patients less than 8 years old or weighing less than 100 pounds. There is a minor adaptation for infants since they cannot ambulate on their own.

junctional rhythm An arrhythmia arising from ectopic foci in the area of the atrioventricular junction; often shows an absence of the P wave, a short P-R interval, or a P wave appearing after the QRS complex.

juxtaglomerular apparatus A structure formed at the site where the efferent arteriole and distal convoluted tubule meet.

Kehr's sign Left shoulder pain that may indicate a ruptured spleen.

keloid scar An abnormal scar commonly found in people with darkly pigmented skin. It extends over the wound margins.

ketamine A drug with sedative, analgesic, and hypnotic properties; created in the laboratory from phencyclidine (PCP).

ketamine hydrochloride A drug used to facilitate date rape but that is predominantly marketed in the United States as a veterinary anesthetic and is a phencyclidine hydrochloride derivative; street names include special K, vitamin K, cat Valium, and Fort Dodge.

kidneys Solid, bean-shaped organs located in the retroperitoneal space that filter blood and excrete body wastes in the form of urine.

kidney stones Solid crystalline masses formed in the kidney, resulting from an excess of insoluble salts or uric acid crystal-lizing in the urine; may become trapped any-where along the urinary tract.

kinetic energy   The energy associated with bodies in motion, expressed mathematically as half the mass times the square of the velocity.

kinetics   The study of the relationship among speed, mass, vector direction, and physical injury.

kinin system   A general term for a group of polypeptides that mediate inflammatory responses by stimulating visceral smooth muscle and relaxing vascular smooth muscle to produce vasodilation.

Klumpke paralysis   An injury of childbirth affecting the spinal nerves C7, C8, and T1 of the brachial plexus. It can be contrasted to Erb palsy, which affects C5 and C6.

Korotkoff sounds   Sounds related to blood pressure that are heard by stethoscope.

Kussmaul respirations   Deep, gasping respira-tions; common in diabetic coma (ketoacidosis).

kyphosis   Outward curve of the thoracic spine.

labia majora   Outer fleshy "lips" covered with pubic hair that protect the vagina.

labia minora   Inner fleshy "lips" devoid of pubic hair that protect the vagina.

labile   Used to describe a rapid shift in mood.

labor   The mechanism by which the baby and the placenta are expelled from the uterus.

laceration   A wound made by tearing or cut-ting tissues.

lacrimal apparatus   The structures in which tears are secreted and drained from the eye.

lactated Ringer's (LR) solution   A sterile isotonic crystalloid IV solution of specified amounts of calcium chloride, potassium chloride, sodium chloride, and sodium lac-tate in water.

lactic acid   A metabolic end product of the breakdown of glucose that accumulates when metabolism proceeds in the absence of oxygen.

lambdoid suture   The point where the occip-ital bones attach to the parietal bones.

lamina   Arise from the posterior pedicles and fuse to form the posterior spinous processes.

laminated windshield glass   Type of window glazing that incorporates a sheeting material that stops the glass from breaking into shards.

landing zone   Designated location for the landing of air ambulances.

landline   Communications system linked by wires, usually in reference to a conventional telephone system.

lantana   A perennial flowering shrub with clusters of red berries that can lead to serious and even fatal poisoning; Also known as red sage or wild sage; ingestion causes stomach upsets, muscle weakness, shock, and, some-times, death.

laryngeal mask airway (LMA)   Device that surrounds the opening of the larynx with an inflatable silicone cuff positioned in the hypopharynx; an alternative device to bag-mask ventilation.

laryngectomy   A surgical procedure in which the larynx is removed.

laryngoscope   Device that is used in con-junction with a laryngoscope blade in order to perform direct laryngoscopy.

laryngospasm   Severe constriction of the lar-ynx in response to allergy, noxious stimuli, or illness.

larynx   A complex structure formed by many independent cartilaginous structures that all work together; where the upper airway ends and the lower airway begins.

lassitude   Condition of listlessness and fatigue.

late adults   Persons who are 61 years old or older.

lateral compression   A force that is directed from the side toward the midline of the body.

law of conservation of energy   The principle that energy can be neither created nor destroyed, it can only change form.

LD$_{50}$ The amount of an agent or substance that will kill 50% of people who are exposed to this level.

Le Fort fractures   Maxillary fractures that are classified into three categories based on their anatomic location.

lead   Any one of the conductors, composed of two or more electrodes, in the ECG that shows the electrical conduction in the heart.

left atrium   The upper left chamber of the heart; receives blood from the pulmonary veins.

left ventricle   The thick-walled, muscular, lower left chamber of the heart; receives blood from the left atrium and pumps it out through the aorta into the systemic arteries.

lens   A transparent body within the globe that focuses light rays.

lethal dose (LD)   Amount of a hazardous substance sure to cause death.

leukemia   Cancer or malignancy of the blood-forming organs, particularly affecting the white blood cells that develop abnormally and/or excessively at the expense of normal blood cells.

leukocytes   The white blood cells responsi-ble for fighting off infection.

leukocytosis   Elevation of the white blood cell count often due to inflammation.

leukopenia   Reduction in the number of white blood cells.

leukotrienes   Arachidonic acid metabolites that function as chemical mediators of inflammation. Also known as slow-reacting substances of anaphylaxis (SRS-A).

Level A   The highest level of protective suit worn by hazardous materials personnel. Also referred to as fully encapsulating because the suit covers everything, including the breath-ing apparatus.

Level B   Personal protective equipment that is one step less protective than level A.

Level C   A level of personal protective equip-ment that provides splash protection.

Level D   The level of protection that fire fighter turnout gear provides.

Lewisite (L)   A blistering agent that has a rapid onset of symptoms and produces imme-diate intense pain and discomfort on contact.

liability   A finding in civil cases that the pre-ponderance of the evidence shows the defen-dant was responsible for the plaintiff's injuries.

liaison officer (LNO)   In incident command, the person who relays information, concerns, and requests among responding agencies.

libel   Making a false statement in written form that injures a person's good name.

lice   Tiny, wingless, parasitic insects that feed on the patient's blood. This infestation is easily spread through close personal contact. Several types exist: head, body, and pubic lice.

licensed   Similar to certified, a person who has shown a degree of competency in a spe-cific occupation and is granted ability to function through a governmental body.

licit   In relation to drugs, legalized drugs such as coffee, alcohol, and tobacco.

life expectancy   The average amount of years a person can be expected to live.

ligaments   Tough bands of tissue that con-nect bone to bone around a joint or support internal organs within the body.

ligand   Any molecule that binds a receptor leading to a reaction.

limb leads   The ECG leads attached to the limbs and that form the hexaxial system, dividing the heart along a coronal plane into the anterior and posterior segments.

limbic system   Structures within the cere-brum and diencephalon that influence emo-tions, motivation, mood, and sensations of pain and pleasure.

linear fracture   A fracture that runs parallel to the long axis of a bone.

linear skull fractures   Account for 80% of skull fractures; also referred to as nondis-placed skull fractures; commonly occur in the temporal-parietal region of the skull; not associated with deformities to the skull.

liniments   Liquid preparations of drugs for external use, usually to relieve some dis-comfort (such as pain, itching) or to protect the skin.

lithium   The cornerstone drug for the treat-ment of bipolar disorder.

living will   A type of advance directive, gen-erally requiring a precondition for withhold-ing resuscitation when the patient is incapacitated.

local anesthesia   A type of anesthesia that causes a loss of sensation to touch or pain at a specific isolated spot on the body where a procedure is to take place.

local effect (hazardous material)   An effect of a hazardous material on the body that is limited to the area of contact.

local effects   The effects that result from the direct application of a drug to a tissue, for example when lotions are applied to the skin to relieve itching.

local reaction When the body limits a response to a specific area after being exposed to a foreign substance.

logistics In incident command, the position that helps procure and stockpile equipment and supplies during an incident.

long bones Bones that are longer than they are wide.

loop diuretics Medications that inhibit the reabsorption of sodium and calcium ions and that can cause an excessive loss of potassium.

loop of Henle The U-shaped portion of the renal tubule that extends from the proximal to the distal convoluted tubule; concentrates the filtrate and converts it to urine.

loosening of associations A situation in which the logical connection between one idea and the next becomes obscure, at least to the listener.

lordosis Inward curve of the lumbar spine just above the buttocks. An exaggerated form of lordosis results in the condition known as swayback.

low-angle operations A rope rescue operation on a mildly sloping surface (less than 45°) or flat land where rescuers are dependent on the ground for their primary support, and the rope system is a secondary means of support.

lower explosive limit (LEL) The concentration of the hazardous material that can burn or explode in the air when it mixes with air.

lumen The inside diameter of an artery or other hollow structure.

Lund and Browder chart A detailed version of the rule of nines chart that takes into consideration the changes in body surface area brought on by growth.

lung compliance The ability of the alveoli to expand when air is drawn into the lungs, either during negative-pressure ventilation or positive-pressure ventilation.

luteinizing hormone (LH) Hormone that regulates the production of both eggs and sperm, as well as production of reproductive hormones.

Lyme disease A tick-borne disease which primarily affects the skin, heart, joints, and nervous system, and characterized by a round, red lesion or bull's-eye rash.

lymph A thin, watery fluid that bathes the tissues of the body.

lymphangitis Inflammation of a lymph channel.

lymphatic system A network of capillaries, vessels, ducts, nodes, and organs that helps to maintain the fluid environment of the body by producing lymph and transporting it through the body.

lymph nodes Area of the lymphatic system where infection-fighting cells are housed.

lymphoblasts Lymphocytes transformed because of stimulation by an antigen.

lymphocytes The white blood cells responsible for a large part of the body's immune protection.

lymphoid system The system primarily made up of the bone marrow, lymph nodes, and spleen that participates in formation of lymphocytes and immune responses.

lymphokines Cytokines released by lymphocytes, including many of the interleukins, gamma interferon, tumor necrosis factor beta, and chemokines.

lymphomas Malignant diseases that arise within the lymphoid system; includes non-Hodgkin and Hodgkin lymphomas.

macrodrip sets Administration sets named for the large orifice between the piercing spike and the drip chamber; allow for rapid fluid flow into the vascular system; allow 10 or 15 gtt/mL, depending on the manufacturer.

macrophages Cells that developed from the monocytes that provide the body's first line of defense in the inflammatory process.

Magill forceps A special type of forcep that is curved, thus allowing the paramedic to maneuver it in the airway.

malignant hyperthermia A condition that can result from common anesthesia medications (notably succinylcholine) and present with hyperthermia, muscular rigidity, altered mental status, and a hyperdynamic state.

malleolus The large, rounded bony protuberance on either side of the ankle joint.

mallet finger An avulsion fracture of the extensor tendon of the distal phalynx caused by jamming a finger into an object.

malocclusion Misalignment of the teeth.

malrotation A congenital anomaly of rotation of the midgut, the small bowel is found predominantly on the right side of the abdomen.

mandated reporter A category of professional required by some states to report suspicions of child maltreatment. Prehospital professionals may be included.

mandible The movable lower jaw bone.

mandibular nerve A sensory and motor nerve that supplies the muscles of chewing and skin of the lower lip, chin, temporal region, and part of the external ear.

mania A mental disorder characterized by abnormally exaggerated happiness, joy, or euphoria with hyperactivity, insomnia, and grandiose ideas.

manic-depressive illness A bipolar disorder in which mood fluctuates between depression and mania. The alterations in mood are usually episodic and recurrent.

manubrium The superior segment of the sternum; its lower border defines the angle of Louis.

march fractures *See* fatigue fractures.

margination Loss of fluid from the blood vessels into the tissue, causing the blood left in the vessels to have an increased viscosity, which in turn slows the flow of blood and produces stasis.

marijuana The dried leaves and flower buds of the *Cannabis sativa* plant that are smoked to achieve a high.

MARK 1 A nerve agent antidote kit containing two auto-injector medications, atropine and 2-PAM chloride (pralidoxime chloride); also known as a Nerve Agent Antidote Kit (NAAK).

mass-casualty incident (MCI) An emergency situation that can place great demand on the equipment or personnel of the EMS system or has the potential to overwhelm your available resources.

mast cells The cells that resemble basophils but do not circulate in the blood. Mast cells play a role in allergic reactions, immunity, and wound healing.

mastication The process of chewing with the teeth.

mastoid process A cone-shaped section of bone at the base of the temporal bone.

Material Safety Data Sheets (MSDS) Information documents that are supposed to be kept on site at workplaces for every potentially hazardous chemical at the workplace.

maxillary nerve A sensory nerve; supplies the skin on the posterior part of the side of the nose, lower eyelid, cheek, and upper lip.

mean The average number in a given research project.

mean arterial pressure (MAP) The average (or mean) pressure against the arterial wall during a cardiac cycle.

measles An infectious viral disease that occurs most often in late winter and spring. It begins with a fever followed by a cough, running nose, and pink eye. Then a rash spreads from the face and neck down the back and trunk.

mechanical energy The energy that results from motion (kinetic energy) or that is stored in an object (potential energy).

mechanism of action The way in which a medication produces the intended response.

mechanism of injury (MOI) The way in which traumatic injuries occur; the forces that act on the body to cause damage.

meconium A dark green material in the amniotic fluid that can indicate disease in the newborn; the meconium can be aspirated into the infant's lungs during delivery; the baby's first bowel movement.

median The midpoint number in a given research project.

mediastinitis Inflammation of the mediastinum, often a result of the gastric contents leaking into the thoracic cavity after esophageal perforation.

mediastinum Space within the chest that contains the heart, major blood vessels, vagus nerve, trachea, and esophagus; located between the two lungs.

medical ambiguity Uncertainty regarding the specific cause of the patient's condition.

medical asepsis A term applied to the practice of preventing contamination of the patient by using aseptic technique.

medical direction Direction given to an EMS service or provider by a physician.

medical incident command A branch of operations in a unified command system, whose three designated sector positions are triage, treatment, and transport.

medical monitoring The process of assessing the health status of hazardous materials team members before and after entry to a hazardous materials incident site.

Medical Practice Act   An act that usually defines the minimum qualifications of those who may perform various health services, defines the skills that each type of practitioner is legally permitted to use, and establishes a means of certification for different categories of health care professional.

medication   A licensed drug taken to cure or reduce symptoms of an illness or medical condition or as an aid in the diagnosis, treatment, or prevention of a disease or other abnormal condition.

medulla   Continuous inferiorly with the spinal cord; serves as a conduction pathway for ascending and descending nerve tracts; coordinates heart rate, blood vessel diameter, breathing, swallowing, vomiting, coughing, and sneezing. Also refers to part of the internal anatomy of the kidney; the middle layer.

medulla oblongata   The inferior portion of the midbrain, which serves as a conduction pathway for both ascending and descending nerve tracts.

medullary canal   The hollow center portion of a long bone.

melanin   The pigment that gives skin its color.

melena   Dark, tarry, very odorous stools caused by upper gastrointestinal bleeds.

membrane attack complex (MAC)   Molecules that insert themselves into the bacterial membrane, leading to weakened areas in the membrane.

menarche   The beginning phase of a woman's life cycle of menstruation.

meninges   A set of three tough membranes, the dura mater, arachnoid, and pia mater, that encloses the entire brain and spinal cord.

meningitis   An inflammation of the meningeal coverings of the brain and spinal cord; it is usually caused by a virus or bacterium.

meningococcal meningitis   An infection of the fluid of a person's spinal cord and the fluid that surrounds the brain. Sometimes referred to as spinal meningitis, it is caused by bacteria or virus. The viral type is less severe than the bacterial; the bacterial type can result in brain damage, hearing loss, learning disability, or death.

menopause   The ending phase of a woman's life cycle of menstruation.

menstrual cycle   The entire monthly cycle of menstruation from start to finish.

menstruation   Monthly flow of blood.

mental illness   A generic term for a variety of illnesses that result in emotional, cognitive, or behavioral dysfunction.

mental status examination (MSE)   A way of measuring the "mental vital signs" in a disturbed patient. The mnemonic COASTMAP can be used to conduct this exam, assessing consciousness, orientation, activity, speech, thought, memory, affect and mood, and perception.

mesentery   A membranous double fold of tissue in the abdomen that attaches various organs to the body wall.

metabolic   Pertaining to the breakdown of ingested foodstuffs into smaller and smaller molecules and atoms that are used as energy sources for cellular function.

metacarpals   The five bones that form the palm and back of the hand.

metaphysis   The region of the long bone between the epiphysis and diaphysis.

metaplasia   A reversible, cellular adaptation in which one adult cell type is replaced by another adult cell type.

metastasis   Change in location of a disease from one organ or part of the body to another. Often used to describe a cancer that has migrated to other parts of the body.

metatarsals   The five long bones extending from the tarsus to the phalanges of the foot.

metered-dose inhaler (MDI)   A pressurized canister that delivers a specific dose of a medication; commonly used for beta-agonist bronchodilators.

methamphetamine   A highly addictive drug in the amphetamine family.

metric system   A decimal system based on tens for the measurement of length, weight, and volume.

metrorrhagia   Irregular but frequent vaginal bleeding.

microdrip sets   Administration sets named for the small needlelike orifice between the piercing spike and the drip chamber; allow for carefully controlled fluid flow and are ideally suited for medication administration; allow for 60 gtt/mL.

micturition reflex   A spinal reflex that causes contraction of the bladder's smooth muscles, producing the urge to void as pressure is exerted on the internal urinary sphincter.

midbrain   The part of the brain that is responsible for helping to regulate level of consciousness.

middle adults   Persons who are 41 to 60 years of age.

middle ear   One of three anatomic parts of the ear; it consists of the inner portion of the tympanic membrane and the ossicles.

milk   In the context of pharmacology, an aqueous suspension of an insoluble drug.

milliequivalent (mEq)   Unit of measure for electrolytes.

minute volume   The amount of air that moves in and out of the respiratory tract per minute.

miosis   Bilateral pinpoint constricted pupils.

missed abortion   A situation in which a fetus has died during the first 20 weeks of gestation, but has remained in utero.

missile fragmentation   A primary mechanism of tissue disruption from certain rifles in which pieces of the projectile break apart, allowing the pieces to create their own separate paths through tissues.

mitochondria   The metabolic center or powerhouse of the cell. They are small and rod-shaped organelles.

mitral valve   The valve located between the left atrium and the left ventricle of the heart.

Mix-o-Vial   A single vial divided into two compartments by a rubber stopper; Solu-Medrol is stored this way.

mobile   In radio communications, a radio that is affixed to an EMS vehicle, but the vehicle can move around.

mobile intensive care units (MICUs)   An early title given to an ambulance-style unit.

mode   The most common number in any given research project.

molar pregnancy   Pregnancy in which there is a problem at the fertilization stage, with a malfunction of the egg or sperm that results in an abnormal placenta and a fetus with an abnormal chromosome count, or which results in an empty egg.

Mongolian spots   Blue-gray areas of discoloration of the skin caused by abnormal pigment, not by trauma or bruising.

monoamine oxidase inhibitors (MAOIs)   Psychiatric medication used primarily to treat atypical depression by increasing norepinephrine and serotonin levels in the central nervous system.

monocytes   Mononuclear phagocytic white blood cells derived from myeloid stem cells. They circulate in the bloodstream for about 24 hours and then move into tissues to mature into macrophages.

monomorphic   Having only one common shape.

mononucleosis   Infectious mononucleosis or mono (glandular fever), caused by the Epstein-Barr virus, is often called the kissing disease. It is also spread by coughing or sneezing.

monophonic   The sound of one note during wheezing, caused by the vibration of a single bronchus.

monovalent   An ion that contains one charge.

mons veneris   Also called the mons pubis, this is a rounded pad of fatty tissue that overlies the symphysis pubis and is anterior to the urethral and vaginal openings.

mood   A person's sustained and pervasive emotional state.

mood disorder   A group of disorders in which the disturbance of mood is accompanied by full or partial manic or depressive syndrome.

morality   Pertaining to conscience, conduct, and character.

morbidity   Number of nonfatally injured or disabled people. Usually expressed as a rate, meaning the number of nonfatal injuries in a certain population in a given time period divided by the size of the population.

morgue officer   In incident command, the person who works with area medical examiners, coroners, and law enforcement agencies to coordinate the disposition of dead victims.

moro reflex   An infant reflex in which, when an infant is caught off guard, the infant opens his or her arms wide, spreads the fingers, and seems to grab at things.

mortality   Deaths caused by injury and disease. Usually expressed as a rate, meaning the number of deaths in a certain population in a given time period divided by the size of the population.

mottling A condition of abnormal skin circulation, caused by vasoconstriction or inadequate circulation.

mucopolysaccharide gel One of the complex materials found, along with the collagen fibers and elastin fibers, in the dermis of the skin.

mucosal atomizer device (MAD) A device that attaches to the end of a syringe that is used to spray (atomize) certain medications via the intranasal route.

mucosal-associated lymphoid tissue (MALT) The lymphoid tissue associated with the skin and the respiratory, urinary, and reproductive traits as well as the tonsils.

multifocal Arising from or pertaining to many foci or locations.

multigravida A woman who has had two or more pregnancies, irrespective of the outcome.

multipara A woman who has had two or more deliveries.

multiple myeloma A disease in which an abnormal plasma cell infiltrates the bone marrow with a cancerous (neoplastic) cell, causing tumors to form inside the bones.

multiple-organ dysfunction syndrome (MODS) A progressive condition usually characterized by combined failure of several organs, such as the lungs, liver, and kidney, along with some clotting mechanisms, which occurs after severe illness or injury.

multiple sclerosis (MS) An autoimmune condition in which the body attacks the myelin of the brain and spinal cord, leading to gaps in the insulation normally provided by the myelin, causing scarring.

multiplex Method by which simultaneous transmission of voice and ECG signals can be achieved over a single radio frequency.

mumps A viral infection that primarily affects the parotid glands, which are one of the three pairs of salivary glands, causing swelling in front of the ears.

murmur An abnormal "whoosh"-like sound heard over the heart that indicates turbulent blood flow around a cardiac valve.

Murphy's eye An opening on the side of an endotracheal tube at its distal tip that enables ventilation to occur even if the tip becomes occluded by blood, mucus, or the tracheal wall.

Murphy's sign Pain when pressure is applied to the right upper quadrant of the abdomen in a specific manner; helps detect gallbladder problems.

muscarinic cholinergic antagonists Medications that block acetylcholine exclusively at the muscarinic receptors; an example is atropine.

muscle fatigue The condition that arises when a muscle depletes its supply of energy.

muscular dystrophy (MD) A nonneurologic condition of genetic origin in which defective DNA causes an error in the creation of muscle tissue, resulting in the degeneration of muscular tissue. This presents with progressive muscle weakness, delayed development

of muscle motor skills, ptosis, drooling, and poor muscle tone.

muscularis The middle layer of tissue in the fallopian tubes.

mutagen Substance that mutates, damages, and changes the structures of DNA in the body's cells.

mutism The absence of speech.

myasthenia gravis An abnormal condition characterized by the chronic fatigability and weakness of muscles, especially in the face and throat. It is the result of a defect in the conduction of nerve impulses at the nerve junction. This deficit is caused by a lack of acetylcholine.

myelin An insulating-type substance present in some neurons that allows the cell to consistently send its signal along the axon without "shorting out" or losing electricity to surrounding fluids and tissues.

myocardial contusion Blunt force injury to the heart that results in capillary damage, interstitial bleeding, and cellular damage in the area.

myocardial rupture An acute traumatic perforation of the ventricles, atria, intraventricular septum, intra-atrial septum, chordae, papillary muscles, or valves.

myocardium The cardiac muscle.

myoclonus Jerking motions of the body.

myoglobin A protein found in muscle that is released into the circulation after crush injury or other muscle damage and whose presence in the circulation may produce kidney damage.

myometrium The middle layer of tissue in the uterus.

myotomes Regions of the body innervated by the motor components of spinal nerves.

myxedema coma A rare condition that can occur in patients who have severe, untreated hypothyroidism.

NAAK A nerve agent antidote kit containing two auto-injector medications, atropine and 2-PAM chloride (pralidoxime chloride); also known as a MARK 1 kit.

narcotic The generic term for opiates and opioids, drugs that act as a CNS depressant and produce insensibility or stupor.

nasal cannula Delivers oxygen via two small prongs that fit into the patient's nostrils. With an oxygen flow rate of 1 to 6 L/min, the nasal cannula can deliver an oxygen concentration of 24% to 44%.

nasal cavity The chamber inside the nose that lies between the floor of the cranium and the roof of the mouth.

nasal flaring Intermittent outward movements of the nostrils with each inspiration; indicates an increase in the work needed to breathe.

nasal septum A rigid partition composed of bone and cartilage; divides the nasopharynx into two passages.

nasogastric (NG) tube Gastric tube is inserted into the stomach through the nose.

nasolacrimal duct The passage through which tears drain from the lacrimal sacs into the nasal cavity.

nasopharyngeal (nasal) airway A soft rubber tube about 6″ long that is inserted through the nose into the posterior pharynx behind the tongue, thereby allowing passage of air from the nose to the lower airway.

nasopharynx The nasal cavity; formed by the union of the facial bones.

nasotracheal intubation Insertion of an endotracheal tube into the trachea through the nose.

National Incident Management System (NIMS) A Department of Homeland Security system designed to enable federal, state, and local governments and private-sector and nongovernmental organizations to effectively and efficiently prepare for, prevent, respond to, and recover from domestic incidents, regardless of cause, size, or complexity, including acts of catastrophic terrorism.

native immunity A nonspecific cellular and humoral response that operates as the body's first line of defense against pathogens.

natural immunity The immunity the body develops as part of being exposed to an antigen and developing antibodies, for example, exposure to measles, having the measles, and developing immunity to the measles.

nature of illness (NOI) The general type of illness a patient is experiencing.

nebulizer A device for producing a fine spray or mist that is used to deliver inhaled medications.

necrosis The death of tissue, usually caused by a cessation of its blood supply.

needle cricothyrotomy Insertion of a 14- to 16-gauge over-the-needle IV catheter (angiocath) through the cricothyroid membrane and into the trachea.

needle decompression Also referred to as a needle thoracentesis, this procedure introduces a needle or angiocath into the pleural space in an attempt to relieve a tension pneumothorax.

needleless systems A device that does not use needles for: (1) collection of body fluids or withdrawal of body fluids after initial venous or arterial access is established; (2) administration of medication or fluids; or (3) any other procedure involving the potential for occupational exposure to bloodborne pathogens due to percutaneous injuries from contaminated sharps.

negative feedback The concept that once the desired effect of a process has been achieved, further action is inhibited until it is needed again; also called feedback inhibition.

negative-pressure ventilation Drawing of air into the lungs; airflow from a region of higher pressure (outside the body) to a region of lower pressure (the lungs); occurs during normal (unassisted) breathing.

negative symptoms Evidence of a disease or condition, noted by lack of normal circumstances, rather than the presence of new physical evidence or a physical change; with regard to schizophrenia, refers to a lack of normal behavior, and apathy, mutism, a flat affect, and a lack of interest in pleasure.

negative wave pulse The phase of an explosion in which pressure from the blast is less than atmospheric pressure.

neglect Refusal or failure on the part of the caregiver to provide life necessities, such as food, water, clothing, shelter, personal hygiene, medicine, comfort, and personal safety.

negligence Professional action or inaction on the part of the health care worker that does not meet the standard of ordinary care expected of similarly trained and prudent health care practitioners and that results in injury to the patient.

neologism An invented word that has meaning only to its inventor.

neonatal period The first month of life.

neonate Infant during the first month after birth.

neoplasms Tumors.

neoplastic cells Another term for cancerous cells.

neovascularization Development of vessels to aid in healing an injured soft tissue.

nephrons The structural and functional units of the kidney that form urine; composed of the glomerulus, the glomerular (Bowman's) capsule, the proximal convoluted tubule (PCT), loop of Henle, and the distal convoluted tubule (DCT).

nerve agents A class of chemicals called organophosphates; they function by blocking an essential enzyme in the nervous system, which causes the body's organs to become overstimulated and burn out.

neurogenic shock Circulatory failure caused by paralysis of the nerves that control the size of the blood vessels, leading to widespread dilation; seen in spinal cord injuries.

neuroleptic malignant syndrome (NMS) A condition caused by antipsychotic and even common antiemetic medications that presents with hyperthermia, muscular rigidity, altered mental status, and a hyperdynamic state.

neuromuscular blocking agents Medications that affect the parasympathetic nervous system by inducing paralysis.

neuronal soma The body of a neuron (nerve cell).

neurotoxins Biological agents that are the most deadly substances known to humans; they include botulinum toxin and ricin.

neurotransmission The process of chemical signaling between cells.

neurotransmitters Proteins that transmit signals between cells of the nervous system.

neurovascular bundle A closely placed grouping of an artery, vein, and nerve that lies beneath the inferior edge of a rib.

neurovascular compromise The loss of the nerve supply, blood supply, or both to a region of the body, typically distal to a site of injury; characterized by alterations in sensation, including numbness and tingling, or by a loss or decrease of motor function; vascular compromise is indicated by weak or absent pulses, poor skin color, and cool skin.

neutralization A type of decontamination that uses one chemical to change the hazardous material into two less harmful substances; rarely used by hazardous materials teams.

neutron radiation Type of energy that is emitted from a strong radiological source; neutron energy is the fastest moving and most powerful form of radiation. Neutrons easily penetrate through lead, and require several feet of concrete to stop them.

neutrophils Cells that make up approximately 55% to 70% of the leukocytes responsible in large part for the body's protection against infection. They are readily attracted by foreign antigens and destroy them by phagocytosis.

newborn Infant within the first few hours after birth.

Newton's first law of motion The principle that a body at rest will remain at rest unless acted on by an outside force.

Newton's second law of motion The principle that the force that an object can exert is the product of its mass times its acceleration.

nicotinic cholinergic antagonists Medications that block the acetylcholine only at nicotinic receptors.

nitrogen narcosis A state resembling alcohol intoxication produced by nitrogen gas dissolved in the blood at high ambient pressure; also called rapture of the deep.

noise In radio communications, interference in a radio signal.

nonbarbiturate hypnotics Medications designed to sedate without the side effects of a barbiturate.

nondepolarizing neuromuscular blocking agents Medications designed to cause temporary paralysis by binding in a competitive but nonstimulatory manner to part of the ACh receptor. Do not cause fasciculations.

nondisplaced fracture A break in which the bone remains aligned in its normal position.

nonelectrolytes Solutes that have no electrical charge; include glucose and urea; measured in milligrams (mg).

nonopioid analgesics Medications designed to relieve pain without the side effects of opioids.

nonrebreathing mask A combination mask and reservoir bag system. Oxygen fills a reservoir bag that is attached to the mask by a one-way valve. This permits the patient to inhale from the reservoir bag but not to exhale back into it. With a good mask-to-face seal and a flow rate of 15 L/min, it is capable of delivering up to 90% inspired oxygen.

nonspecific agents Medications that produce effects on different cells through a variety of mechanisms. Generally classified by the focus of action or specific therapeutic use.

nonsteroidal anti-inflammatory drugs (NSAIDs) Medications with analgesic and fever reducing properties.

norepinephrine A neurotransmitter and drug sometimes used in the treatment of shock; produces vasoconstriction through its alpha stimulator properties.

normal saline A solution of 0.9% sodium chloride; an isotonic crystalloid.

normal sinus rhythm The normal rhythm of the heart, wherein the excitation impulse arises in the SA node, travels through the internodal pathways to the atrioventricular junction, down the bundle of His, through the bundle branches, and into the Purkinje network without interference.

nosocomial infection An infection acquired from a health care setting.

nuchal rigidity A stiff or painful neck; commonly associated with meningitis.

nucleus A cellular organelle that contains the genetic information. The nucleus controls the function and structure of a cell.

nullipara A woman who has never delivered.

nursemaid's elbow The subluxation of the radial head that often results from pulling on an outstretched arm.

nystagmus The rhythmic shaking of the eyes.

obesity A term generally used when someone is 20% to 30% over their ideal weight.

objectives Specific, time-limited, and quantifiable statements that summarize an expected result of an intervention.

oblique fracture A fracture that travels diagonally from one side of the bone to the other.

obsession A persistent idea that a person cannot dismiss from his or her thoughts.

obstructive shock Shock that occurs when there is a block to blood flow in the heart or great vessels, causing an insufficient blood supply to the body's tissues.

obtunded A condition when the patient is dulled to pain and sensation.

occipital condyles Articular surfaces on the occipital bone where the skull articulates with the atlas on the vertebral column.

occipital lobe The portion of the brain that is responsible for the processing of visual information.

occiput The most posterior portion of the cranium.

occlusion Blockage, usually of a tubular structure such as a blood vessel or IV catheter.

ocular Pertaining to the eye.

oculomotor nerve Third cranial nerve; innervates the muscles that cause motion of the eyeballs and upper eyelid.

off-gassing The emitting of an agent after exposure, for example from a person's clothes that have been exposed to the agent.

official name The name listed in the United States Pharmacopeia (USP) once the generic name has been approved by the United States Adopted Name Council and the drug has been approved by the US Food and Drug Administration.

off-line medical control Medical direction given through a set of protocols, policies, and/or standards.

ointment A semisolid preparation for external application to the body, usually containing a medicinal substance.

olecranon The proximal bony projection of the ulna at the elbow; the part of the ulna that constitutes the "funny bone."

olfactory nerves Participates in the transmission of scent impulses.

oligohydramnios Decreased volume of amniotic fluid during a pregnancy; a risk factor associated with abnormalities of the urinary tract, postmaturity (birth after a prolonged pregnancy), and intrauterine growth retardation.

oliguria A decrease in urine output to the extent that total urine output drops below 500 mL/day.

ongoing assessment The part of the assessment process in which problems are reevaluated and responses to treatment are assessed.

online (direct) medical control Type of medical control in which the paramedic is in direct contact with a physician, usually via two-way radio or telephone.

onset of action The time needed for the concentration of the medication at the target tissue to reach the minimum effective level.

oocyte An egg produced from the female ovary.

open abdominal injury An injury in which there is a break in the surface of the skin or mucous membrane, exposing deeper tissue to potential contamination.

open book pelvic fracture A life-threatening fracture of the pelvis caused by a force that displaces one or both sides of the pelvis laterally and posteriorly.

open cricothyrotomy Also referred to as a surgical cricothyrotomy; an emergent procedure that involves incising the cricothyroid membrane with a scalpel and inserting an endotracheal or tracheostomy tube directly into the subglottic area of the trachea.

open-ended question A question that does not have a yes or no answer, and which does not give the patient specific options to choose from.

open fracture Any break in a bone in which the overlying skin has been damaged.

open incident An ongoing or uncontained incident in which rescuers will have to search for patients and then triage or treat them. The situation may produce more patients. Examples include school shootings, tornadoes, a hazardous materials release, and rising floodwaters.

open pneumothorax The result of a defect in the chest wall that allows air to enter the thoracic space.

open wound An injury in which there is a break in the surface of the skin or the mucous membrane, exposing deeper tissue to potential contamination.

operations The technical rescue training level geared toward working in the warm zone of an incident. Training at this level allows responders to directly assist those conducting the rescue operation and to use certain rescue skills and procedures.

Operations Level This training level, also called EMS/HM Level I Responder, allows providers to perform patient care activities in the cold zone (the command and support center) at an incident for patients who no longer present a significant risk of secondary contamination.

operations (incident command) The position that carries out the orders of the commander to help resolve the incident.

ophthalmic nerve A sensory nerve that supplies the skin of the forehead, the upper eyelid, and conjunctiva.

opiate Various alkaloids derived from the opium or poppy plant.

OPIM An acronym that stands for other potentially infectious materials. These include CSF, pericardial fluid, synovial fluid, pleural fluid, amniotic fluid, peritoneal fluid, and any fluid containing gross visible blood.

opioid A synthetic narcotic not derived from opium; potent analgesics with sedative properties, including drugs such as fentanyl (Sublimaze) and alfentanil (Alfenta).

opioid agonist-antagonists Medications designed to relieve pain without the side effects of opioids.

opioid agonists Chemicals that are similar to or derived from the opium plant.

opioid antagonists A classification of medications that reverses the effects of opioid drugs.

opsoninization Occurs when an antibody coats an antigen to facilitate its recognition by immune cells.

opthalmoscope An instrument used to look into a patient's eyes and view the retina and aqueous fluid; consists of a concave mirror and a battery-powered light that is usually contained in the handle.

optic nerve Either of the second cranial nerves that enter the eyeball posteriorly, through the optic foramen.

orbits Bony cavities in the frontal part of the skull that enclose and protect the eyes.

ordinary negligence Negligence that is a failure to act, or a simple mistake that causes harm to a patient.

organ of Corti A structure located in the cochlea that contains hairs that are stimulated by vibrations to form nerve impulses that travel to the brain and are perceived as sound.

organelles Internal cellular structures that carry out specific functions for the cell.

organic brain syndrome Temporary or permanent dysfunction of the brain, caused by a disturbance in the physical or physiologic functioning of brain tissue.

organophosphates A class of chemical found in many insecticides used in agriculture and in the home.

orientation A person's sense of who one is (person), where one is (place), and at what day of the week one finds oneself (day).

orogastric (OG) tube Gastric tube inserted into the stomach through the mouth.

oropharyngeal (oral) airway A hard plastic device that is curved in such a way that it fits over the back of the tongue with the tip in the posterior pharynx.

oropharynx Forms the posterior portion of the oral cavity, which is bordered superiorly by the hard and soft palates, laterally by the cheeks, and inferiorly by the tongue.

orotracheal intubation Insertion of an endotracheal tube into the trachea through the mouth.

orthopnea Severe dyspnea experienced when lying down and relieved by sitting or standing up.

orthostatic hypotension A drop in systolic blood pressure when moving from a sitting to a standing position.

orthostatic vital signs Assessing vital signs in two different patient positions to determine the degree of hypovolemia.

osmolarity The ability to influence the movement of water across a semipermeable membrane.

osmosis The movement of water across a semipermeable membrane (for example, the cell wall) from an area of lower to higher concentration of solute molecules.

ossicles The three small bones in the inner ear that transmit vibrations to the cochlear duct at the oval window.

ossification centers Areas where cartilage is transformed through calcification into a new area of bone.

osteoarthritis (OA) The degeneration of a joint surface caused by wear and tear that leads to pain and stiffness.

osteogenesis imperfecta A congenital bone disease that results in fragile bones.

osteomyelitis Inflammation of the bone due to infection; a potential complication of intraosseous infusion.

osteoporosis A condition characterized by decreased bone mass and density and increased susceptibility to fractures.

otoscope A tool used to examine the ears of a patient; consists of a head and a handle. The head contains an electric light source and a low-power magnifying lens.

outcome (impact) objectives State the intended effect of the program on participants or on the community in such terms as the participants' increased knowledge, changed behaviors or attitudes, or decreased injury rates.

oval window An oval opening between the middle ear and the vestibule.

ovaries Female gonads; ovaries release eggs and secrete the female hormones.

overhydration An increase in the body's systemic fluid volume.

overriding The overlap of a bone that occurs from the muscle spasm that follows a fracture, leading to a decrease in the length of the bone.

over-the-needle catheter A Teflon (plastic) catheter inserted over a hollow needle.

ovulation A process in which an ovum is released from a follicle.

ovum A mature oocyte.

oxygen concentrators Large, electrical devices that concentrate the oxygen in ambient air and eliminate other gases.

oxygen humidifier Small bottle of water through which the oxygen leaving the cylinder is moisturized before it reaches the patient.

oxygenation The process of delivering oxygen to the blood by diffusion from the alveoli following inhalation into the lungs.

oxyhemoglobin Hemoglobin that is occupied by oxygen.

P waves The first wave of the ECG complex, representing depolarization of the atria.

pacemaker The specialized tissue within the heart that initiates excitation impulses; an electronic device used to stimulate cardiac contraction when the electric conduction system of the heart is malfunctioning, especially in complete heart block. An electronic pacemaker consists of a battery-powered pulse generator and a wire that transmits the electric impulse to the ventricles.

palate Forms the roof of the mouth and separates the oropharynx and nasopharynx.

palatine bone An irregularly shaped bone found in the posterior part of the nasal cavity.

palatine tonsils One of three sets of lymphatic organs that comprise the tonsils; located in the back of the throat, on each side of the posterior opening of the oral cavity; help protect the body from bacteria introduced into the mouth and nose.

pallor Lack of color; paleness.

palmar grasp An infant reflex that occurs when something is placed in the infant's palm; the infant grasps the object.

palpation Physical touching for the purpose of obtaining information.

palpitations A sensation felt under the left breast of the heart "skipping a beat," usually caused by a premature ventricular contraction.

pancreas The digestive gland that secretes digestive enzymes into the duodenum through the pancreatic duct. The pancreas is considered both an endocrine gland and an exocrine gland.

pancuronium A nondepolarizing neuromuscular blocking agent; used to maintain paralysis following succinylcholine-facilitated intubation; also called Pavulon.

papillary muscles Protrusions of the myocardium into the ventricular cavities to which the chordae tendineae are attached.

para The number of pregnancies that resulted in the delivery of an infant or infants.

para-aminophenol derivatives Medications designed to reduce fevers and relieve pain.

paracrine hormones Hormones that diffuse through intracellular spaces to their target.

paralytics Also called neuromuscular blocking agents; paralyzes skeletal muscles; used in an emergency situation to facilitate intubation.

parameters Outlined measures that may be difficult to obtain in a research project.

paranasal sinuses The sinuses, or hollowed sections of bone in the front of the head, that are lined with mucous membrane and drain into the nasal cavity.

paranoid type A type of schizophrenia in which the person experiences delusions or hallucinations usually centered around a specific theme, where their cognitive functions remain intact.

paraplegia Paralysis of the lower part of the body.

parasite Any living organism in or on any other living creature; takes advantage of the host by feeding off cells and tissues.

parasthesias Tingling or sensory change.

parasympathetic nervous system A subdivision of the autonomic nervous system that is involved in control of involuntary, vegetative functions, mediated largely by the vagus nerve through the chemical acetylcholine.

parathyroid hormone (PTH) A hormone secreted by the parathyroids that acts as an antagonist to calcitonin. PTH is secreted when calcium blood levels are low.

parenchyma The substance of a gland or solid organ.

parenteral exposure Entry of a hazardous material into the bloodstream, either through force of injection or through an open wound.

parenteral routes Medication routes in which medications are administered via any route other than the alimentary canal (digestive tract), skin, or mucous membranes.

paresthesias Abnormal sensations such as burning, numbness, or tingling.

parietal lobe The portion of the brain that is the site for reception and evaluation of most sensory information, except smell, hearing, and vision.

parietal pain Pain caused by inflammation of the parietal peritoneum that is generally described as steady, aching, and aggravated by movement.

parietal pleura Thin membrane that lines the chest cavity.

parity The number of times a woman has delivered an infant or infants.

Parkinson's disease A neurologic condition in which the portion of the brain responsible for production of dopamine is damaged or overused, resulting in tremors.

Parkland formula A formula that recommends giving 4 mL of normal saline for each kilogram of body weight, multiplied by the percentage of body surface area burned; sometimes used to calculate fluid needs during lengthy transport times.

paroxysmal nocturnal dyspnea (PND) Severe shortness of breath occurring at night after several hours of recumbency, during which fluid pools in the lungs; the person is forced to sit up to breathe. PND is caused by left heart failure or decompensation of chronic obstructive pulmonary disease.

partial laryngectomy Surgical removal of a portion of the larynx.

partial pressure The amount of the total pressure contributed by various gases in solution.

partial rebreathing mask Similar to the nonrebreathing mask except that there is no one-way valve between the mask and the reservoir. Room air is not entrained with inspiration; however, residual expired air is mixed in the mask and rebreathed.

partial-thickness burn A burn that involves the epidermis and part of the dermis, characterized by pain and blistering; previously called a second-degree burn.

passive interventions Something that offers automatic protection from injury, often without requiring any conscious change of behavior by the individual; child-resistant bottles and air bags are some examples.

passive neglect An unintentional refusal or failure to fulfill a caregiving obligation, which results in physical or emotional distress. Examples include forgetting or isolating the person.

past medical history Information obtained during the patient history, such as the patient's general state of health, childhood and adult diseases, surgeries and hospitalizations, psychiatric and mental illnesses, or traumatic injuries, which may relate to the patient's current problem.

patch A connection between a telephone line and a radio communications system enabling a caller to get "on the air" by dialing into a special telephone.

patch (medication) A solid medication impregnated into a membrane or adhesive that is applied to the surface of the skin.

patella The kneecap.

patent Open.

pathologic fracture A fracture that occurs in an area of abnormally weakened bone.

pathophysiology The study of how normal physiologic processes are affected by disease.

pathway expansion The tissue displacement that occurs as a result of low-displacement shock waves that travel at the speed of sound in tissue.

patient autonomy The right to direct one's own care, and to decide how you want your end-of-life medical care provided.

patient history Information about the patient's chief complaint, present symptoms, and previous illnesses.

peak expiratory flow An approximation of the extent of bronchoconstriction; used to determine whether patients are improving with therapy (eg, inhaled bronchodilators).

peak loads A time of day or day of week in which the call volume is at its highest.

pectoral girdle The shoulder girdle.

Pediatric Assessment Triangle (PAT) An assessment tool that allows rapid formation of a general impression of the type and level of illness or injury in an infant or child without touching him or her; consists of assessing appearance, work of breathing, and circulation to the skin.

pedicles   Thick lateral bony struts that connect the vertebral body with spinous and transverse processes and make up the lateral and posterior portions of the spinal foramen; also, a narrow strip of tissue by which an avulsed piece of tissue remains connected to the body.

pelvic girdle   The large bone that arises in the area of the last nine vertebrae and sweeps around to form a complete ring.

pelvic inflammatory disease (PID)   An infection of the female upper organs of reproduction, specifically the uterus, ovaries, and fallopian tubes.

penetrating trauma   Injury caused by objects that pierce the surface of the body, such as knives and bullets, and damage internal tissues and organs.

Penrose drain   A type of surgical drain often used as a constricting band.

peptic ulcer disease (PUD)   Abrasion of the stomach or small intestine.

perception   The way a person processes the data supplied by the five senses.

percussion   Gently striking the surface of the body, typically overlying various body cavities to detect changes in the densities of the underlying structures.

percutaneous   Through the skin or mucous membrane.

percutaneous routes   The medication routes of any medication absorbed through the skin or a mucous membrane.

perfusion   The circulation of blood within an organ or tissue in adequate amounts to meet the cells' needs.

pericardial sac   The potential space between the layers of the pericardium.

pericardial tamponade   Impairment of diastolic filling of the right ventricle due to significant amounts of fluid in the pericardial sac surrounding the heart, leading to a decrease in the cardiac output.

pericardiocentesis   A procedure in which a needle or angiocath is introduced into the pericardial sac to relieve cardiac tamponade.

pericardium   The double-layered sac containing the heart and the origins of the superior vena cava, inferior vena cava, and pulmonary artery.

perimetrium   The outer protective layer of tissue in the uterus.

perineum   The area between the vaginal opening and the anus.

periorbital ecchymosis   Bruising under or around the orbits that is commonly seen following a basilar skull fracture; also called raccoon eyes.

periosteum   The fibrous tissue that covers bone.

peripheral nerves   All of the nerves of the body extending from the brain and spinal cord.

peripheral nervous system (PNS)   Consists of all nervous tissue outside of the brain and spinal cord and is subdivided into two divisions, the somatic and autonomic nervous systems. Consists of 31 pairs of spinal nerves and 12 pairs of cranial nerves, which may be sensory, motor, or connecting nerves.

peripheral neuropathy   A group of conditions in which the nerves leaving the spinal cord are damaged, resulting in distortion of signals to or from the brain. One type is diabetic, in which the peripheral nerves are damaged as blood glucose levels rise, causing loss of sensation, numbness, burning, pain, paresthesia, and muscle weakness.

peripheral shock   A term that describes shock secondary to peripheral circulatory abnormalities—includes both hypovolemic shock and distributive shock.

peripheral vein cannulation   Cannulating veins of the periphery, that is, those that can be seen and/or palpated. Examples of peripheral veins include those of the hand, arm, and lower extremity and the external jugular vein.

peripheral vision   Visualization of lateral objects while looking forward.

peristalsis   The rhythmic contractions of the intestines and esophagus that allow material to move.

peritoneum   A membrane in the abdomen encasing the liver, spleen, diaphragm, stomach, and transverse colon.

peritonitis   Inflammation of the peritoneum (the lining around the abdominal cavity) that results from either blood or hollow organ contents spilling into the abdominal cavity.

peritubular capillaries   A set of capillaries unique to the kidney that branch off from the efferent arteriole; the site of tubular resorption.

periumbilical   Pertaining to the area around the umbilicus (the navel).

permanent cavity   The path of crushed tissue produced by a missile traversing part of the body.

permissible exposure limit (PEL)   The maximum concentration of a chemical that a person may be exposed to under OSHA regulations.

perseveration   Repeating the same idea over and over again.

persistency   Term used to describe how long a chemical agent will stay on a surface before it evaporates.

persistent pulmonary hypertension   Delayed transition from fetal to neonatal circulation.

personal flotation device (PFD)   Also commonly known as a life vest, a PFD allows the body to float in water.

personality disorder   The term used to describe a condition a person has when he or she behaves or thinks in a way that is dysfunctional or causes distress to other people.

pertussis   An acute infectious disease characterized by a catarrhal stage, followed by a paroxysmal cough that ends in a whooping inspiration. Also called whooping cough.

petechiae   Tiny purple or red spots that appear on the skin due to bleeding within the skin or under mucous membranes.

petechial   Characterized by small purplish, nonblanching spots on the skin.

pH   The measure of acidity or alkalinity of a solution.

phagocyte   A kind of cell that engulfs and consumes foreign material such as microorganisms and debris.

phagocytosis   Process in which one cell eats or engulfs a foreign substance to destroy it.

phalanges   The bones of the fingers or toes.

pharmacodynamics   The branch of pharmacology that studies reactions between medications and living structures, including the processes of body responses to pharmacologic, biochemical, physiologic, and therapeutic effects.

pharmacokinetics   The study of the metabolism and action of medications with particular emphasis on the time required for absorption, duration of action, distribution in the body, and method of excretion.

pharmacology   The branch of medicine dealing with the actions of drugs in the body—therapeutic and toxic effects—and development and testing of new drugs and new uses of existing ones.

pharyngeotracheal lumen airway (PtL)   Multilumen airway device that consists of two tubes and two cuffs; an alternative device if endotracheal intubation is not possible or has failed.

pharynx   Throat.

phlebitis   Inflammation of the wall of a vein, sometimes caused by an IV line, manifested by tenderness, redness, and slight edema along part of the length of the vein.

phlebotomy   The withdrawal of blood from a vein.

phobia   An abnormal and persistent dread of a specific object or situation.

phosgene   A pulmonary agent that is a product of combustion, such as might be produced in a fire at a textile factory or house, or from metalwork or burning Freon. Phosgene is a very potent agent that has a delayed onset of symptoms, usually hours.

phosgene oxime (CX)   A blistering agent that has a rapid onset of symptoms and produces immediate intense pain and discomfort on contact.

phrenic nerves   Nerves that innervate the diaphragm.

physical dependence   A physiologic state of adaptation to a drug, usually characterized by tolerance to the drug's effects and a withdrawal syndrome if use of the drug is stopped, especially abruptly.

physical evidence   The evidence that ties a suspect or victim to a crime. It may include body materials, objects, and impressions.

physical examination   The process by which quantifiable, objective information is obtained from a patient about his or her overall state of health.

physiologic dead space   Additional dead space created by intrapulmonary obstructions or atelectasis.

physiologic fracture   A fracture that occurs when abnormal forces are applied to normal bone structures.

physis   The growth plate in long bones.

pia mater   The innermost of the three meninges that enclose the brain and spinal cord, it rests directly on the brain and spinal cord.

piercing spike   The hard, sharpened plastic spike on the end of the administration set designed to pierce the sterile membrane of the IV bag.

Pierre Robin sequence   A condition present at birth marked by a very small lower jaw (micrognathia). The tongue tends to fall back and downward (glossoptosis), and there is a cleft soft palate.

pill   A drug shaped into a ball or oval to be swallowed; often coated to disguise an unpleasant taste.

pinna   The large outside portion of the ear through which sound waves enter the ear; also called the auricle.

piriform fossa   Hollow pockets on the lateral sides of the glottic opening.

pituitary gland   Gland whose secretions control, or regulate, the secretions of other endocrine glands. Often called the "master gland."

placenta   The tissue attached to the uterine wall that nourishes the fetus through the umbilical cord.

placenta previa   A condition in which the placenta develops over and covers the cervix.

plaintiff   In a civil suit, the individual who brings a legal action against another individual.

planning   In incident command, the position that ultimately produces a plan to resolve any incident.

plantar   Referring to the sole of the foot.

plantar flexion   Bending of the foot toward the ground.

plaque   In cardiology, the white to yellow lesion found in atherosclerosis that is made up of lipids, cell debris, and smooth muscles cells; in older people, may also include calcium.

plasma   A component of blood, made of 92% water, 6% to 7% proteins, and electrolytes, clotting factors, and glucose; this makes up 55% of the total blood volume.

plasmin   A naturally occurring clot-dissolving enzyme, usually present in the body in its inactive form, plasminogen.

platelets   Small cells in the blood that are essential for clot formation.

pleura   Membrane lining the outer surface of the lungs (visceral pleura), the inner surface of the chest wall, and the thoracic surface of the diaphragm (parietal pleura).

pleural effusion   Excessive accumulation of fluid in the pleural space.

plexus   A cluster of nerve roots that permits peripheral nerve roots to rejoin and function as a group.

pneumonia   An inflammation of the lungs caused by bacteria, viruses, fungi, or other organisms.

pneumonic plague   A lung infection, also known as plague pneumonia, that is the result of inhalation of plague bacteria.

pneumonitis   Inflammation of the lung. Implies lung inflammation from an irritant such as a chemical, dust, or radiation, or from aspiration. When lung inflammation is caused by an infectious agent, it would typically be called pneumonia.

pneumotaxic center   Area of the brain stem that has an inhibitory influence on inspiration.

pneumothorax   The collection of air within the normally closed pleural space.

podocytes   Special cells in the inner membrane of the glomerulus that wrap around the capillaries in the glomerulus, forming filtration slits.

point of maximal impulse (PMI)   The palpable beat of the apex of the heart against the chest wall during ventricular contraction; normally palpated in the fifth left intercostal space in the midclavicular line.

point tenderness   The tenderness that is sharply localized at the site of the injury, found by gently palpating along the bone with the tip of one finger.

points of distribution (PODs)   Strategically placed facilities that have been pre-established for the mass distribution of antibiotics, antidotes, and vaccinations, along with other medications and supplies.

poison   A substance whose chemical action could damage structures or impair function when introduced into the body.

poliomyelitis   A viral infection that attacks the axons, especially motor axons, and destroys them, causing weakness, paralysis, and respiratory arrest. An effective vaccine has been developed and this disease is now rare.

polycythemia   An overabundance or production of RBCs, WBCs, and platelets, which makes the blood thick.

polyhydramnios   An excessive amount of amniotic fluid. May cause preterm labor.

polymenorrhea   Menstrual blood flow that occurs more often than a 24-day interval.

polymorphonuclear neutrophils (PMNs)   A type of white blood cell formed by bone marrow tissue that possesses a nucleus consisting of several parts or lobes connected by fine strands; a variety of leukocyte.

polypharmacy   Simultaneous use of many medications.

polyphonic   The sound of multiple notes during wheezing, caused by the vibrations of many bronchi.

polyuria   Frequent and plentiful urination.

pons   The portion of the brain stem that lies below the midbrain and contains nerve fibers that affect sleep and respiration.

popliteal artery   The artery in the area or space behind the knee joint.

portable   A hand-held radio that can be carried on a person and used for communications away from a vehicle.

portal vein   A large vessel created by the intersection of blood vessels from the GI system. The portal vein empties into the liver.

positive symptoms   Evidence of or physical change due to a disease or condition, which can be physically noted by the patient or health care provider; with regard to schizophrenia, refers to delusions and hallucinations.

positive wave pulse   The phase of the explosion in which there is a pressure front with a pressure higher than atmospheric pressure.

positive-pressure ventilation (PPV)   Method for assisting ventilation (bag-mask or intubated) with high-flow air or oxygen.

postconventional reasoning   A type of reasoning in which a child bases decisions upon his or her conscience.

posterior chamber   The posterior area of the globe between the lens and the iris.

posterior cord syndrome   A condition associated with extension injuries with isolated injury to the dorsal column; presents as decreased sensation to light touch, proprioception, and vibration while leaving most other motor and sensory functions intact.

posterior spinous process   Formed by the fusion of the posterior lamina, this is an attachment site for muscles and ligaments.

posterior tibial artery   The artery that travels through the calf muscles to the plantar aspect of the foot.

postictal   The period of time after a seizure during which the brain is reorganizing activity.

posting   The placement of an ambulance at a specific geographic location in order to cover larger areas of territory and reduce response times.

postpartum   After birth.

postpolio syndrome   A result of polio in which neurons break down and die, resulting in difficulty swallowing, weakness, fatigue, or breathing problems even after the patient has healed.

postrenal ARF   A type of acute renal failure caused by obstruction of urine flow from the kidneys, commonly caused by a blockage of the urethra by prostate enlargement, renal calculi, or strictures.

post-term   Any pregnancy that lasts more than 42 weeks.

posttraumatic stress disorder (PTSD)   A severe form of anxiety that stems from a traumatic experience. PTSD is characterized by the reliving of the stress and nightmares of the original situation.

postural hypotension   Symptomatic drop in blood pressure related to the patient's body position; detected by measuring pulse and blood pressure while the patient is lying supine, sitting up, and standing. An increase in pulse rate and a decrease in blood pressure in any one of these positions is considered a positive sign for this condition.

postural tremors Tremors that occur as the person holds a body part still.

posture The position of one's body.

potential energy The amount of energy stored in an object, the product of mass, gravity, and height, that is converted into kinetic energy and results in injury, such as from a fall.

potentiation In health care, the effect of increasing the potency or effectiveness of a drug or other treatment; may occur by administering two medications concurrently, and one increases the effect of the other.

powder A drug that has been ground into pulverized form.

ppb Parts per billion; an expression of concentration.

ppm Parts per million; an expression of concentration.

P-R interval The period between the beginning of the P wave (atrial depolarization) and the onset of the QRS complex (ventricular depolarization), signifying the time required for atrial depolarization and passage of the excitation impulse through the atrioventricular junction.

preconventional reasoning A type of reasoning in which a child acts almost purely to avoid punishment or to get what he or she wants.

precordial leads Another term used to describe the chest leads in an ECG.

preeclampsia A condition of late pregnancy that involves gradual onset of hypertension, headache, visual changes, and swelling of the hands and feet; also called pregnancy-induced hypertension or toxemia of pregnancy.

prefilled syringes Medication syringes that are prepackaged and prepared with a specific concentration.

preload The pressure under which the ventricle fills.

premature Underdeveloped; the condition of an infant born too soon. Refers to infants delivered before 37 weeks from the first day of the last menstrual period.

premenstrual syndrome (PMS) A cluster of all or some of the troubling symptoms that occur during a woman's menstrual phase that can include fluid retention, breast pain and tenderness, headache, severe cramping, and emotional changes, including agitation, irritability, depression, and anger.

prenatal The state of the pregnant woman before birth.

prepuce In the anatomy of the female genitalia, a layer of skin directly above the clitoris.

prerenal ARF A type of acute renal failure that is caused by hypoperfusion of the kidneys, resulting from hypovolemia (hemorrhage, dehydration), trauma, shock, sepsis, and heart failure (congestive heart failure,

myocardial infarction); often reversible if the underlying condition can be found and perfusion restored to the kidney.

presbycusis Progressive hearing loss, particularly in the high frequencies, along with lessened ability to discriminate between a particular sound and background noise.

preschoolers Persons who are 3 to 6 years of age.

pressure infuser device A sleeve that is placed around the IV bag and inflated to force fluid to flow from the IV bag and into the tubing.

pressure of speech Speech in which words seem to tumble out under immense emotional pressure.

pressure-compensated flowmeter An oxygen flowmeter that incorporates a float ball within a tapered calibrated tube. The float rises or falls according to the gas flow within the tube. Because this type of flowmeter is affected by gravity, it must remain in an upright position to obtain an accurate flow reading.

preterm Used to describe an infant delivered at less than 37 completed weeks.

prevalence The number of cases of a disease in a specific population over time.

primary adrenal insufficiency Also known as Addison's disease. A rare condition in which the adrenal glands produce an insufficient amount of adrenal hormones.

primary apnea Apnea caused by oxygen deprivation; usually corrected with stimulation, such as drying or slapping the newborn's feet. Primary apnea is typically preceded by an initial period of rapid breathing.

primary brain injury An injury to the brain and its associated structures that is a direct result of impact to the head.

primary contamination An exposure that occurs with direct contact with the hazardous material.

primary exit The main means of escape should violence erupt. This is usually the door you used to enter the building.

primary injury prevention Keeping an injury from occurring.

primary respiratory drive Normal stimulus to breathe; based on fluctuations in $PaCO_2$ and pH of the CSF.

primary response The first encounter with the foreign substance to begin the immune response.

primary spinal cord injury Injury to the spinal cord that is a direct result of trauma, for example transection of the spinal cord from penetrating trauma or displacement of ligaments and bone fragments, resulting in compression of the spinal cord.

primary triage A type of patient sorting used to rapidly categorize patients; the focus is on speed in locating all patients and determining an initial priority as their condition warrants.

primigravida First pregnancy.

primipara A woman who has had one delivery only.

primitive reflexes Reflex reactions such as Babinski, grasping, and sucking signs normally found in very young patients.

process objectives State how a program will be implemented, describing the service to be provided, the nature of the service, and to whom it will be directed.

prodrome The early signs and symptoms that occur before a disease or condition fully appears, eg, dizziness before fainting.

profession A specialized set of knowledge, skills, and/or expertise.

professional A person who follows expected standards and performance parameters in a specific profession.

progesterone One of the three major female hormones.

projection Blaming unacceptable feelings, motives, or desires on others.

prolapsed cord When the umbilical cord presents itself outside of the uterus while the fetus is still inside; an obstetric emergency during pregnancy or labor that acutely endangers the life of the baby; can happen when the water breaks and with the gush of water the cord comes along.

pronation The act of turning the palm of the hand backward or downward, performed by internal rotation of the forearm.

proprioception The ability to perceive the position and movement of one's body or limbs.

prospective research Specific reason a task or research will be performed before it is started.

prostaglandins A group of lipids that act as chemical messengers.

protocol A treatment plan developed for a specific illness or injury.

protozoans Single-celled, usually microscopic, eukaryotic organisms such as amoebas, ciliates, flagellates, and sporozoans; a type of parasite.

protuberant A convex or distended shape of the abdomen. This can be caused by edema.

proximal convoluted tubule (PCT) One of two complex sections of the nephron, the PCT includes an enlargement at the end called the glomerular capsule.

proximate cause The specific reason that an injury occurred; one of the items that must be proven in order for a paramedic to be held liable for negligence.

pruritus Unspecified itching.

pseudocyesis A false pregnancy that develops all the typical signs and symptoms of true pregnancy, but in which no actual pregnancy exists.

pseudomembrane A false membrane formed by a dead tissue layer. Seen in the posterior pharynx of patients with diphtheria.

psychiatric emergency An emergency in which abnormal behavior threatens an individual's health and safety or the health and safety of another person, for example when a person becomes suicidal, homicidal, or has a psychotic episode.

psychological dependence The emotional state of craving a drug to maintain a feeling of well-being.

psychosis A mental disorder characterized by loss of contact with reality.

psychotropic drugs Drugs that affect mood, thought, or behavior.

ptosis Drooping of an eyelid.

pubic symphysis The midline articulation of the pubic bones.

pubis One of two bones that form the anterior portion of the pelvic ring.

public information officer (PIO) In incident command, the person who keeps the public informed and relates any information to the press.

pudendum The female external genitalia.

pulmonary artery One of two arteries that carry deoxygenated blood from the right ventricle to the lungs.

pulmonary blast injuries Pulmonary trauma resulting from short-range exposure to the detonation of high explosives.

pulmonary circulation The flow of blood from the right ventricle through the pulmonary arteries and all of their branches and capillaries in the lungs and back to the left atrium through the venules and pulmonary veins; also called the lesser circulation.

pulmonary contusion Injury to the lung parenchyma that results in capillary hemorrhage into the tissue.

pulmonary edema Congestion of the pulmonary air spaces with exudate and foam, often secondary to left heart failure.

pulmonary embolism Obstruction of a pulmonary artery or arteries by solid, liquid, or gaseous material swept through the right side of the heart into the lungs.

pulmonary hypertension Elevated blood pressure in the pulmonary arteries from constriction; causes problems with the blood flow in the lungs, and makes the heart work harder.

pulmonary overpressurization syndrome Also called "POPS" or "burst lung," this diving emergency can occur during ascent and can cause pneumothorax, mediastinal and subcutaneous emphysema, alveolar hemorrhage, and the lethal arterial gas embolism (AGE).

pulmonary route A medication route in which medication is administered directly to the pulmonary system through inhalation or injection.

pulmonary veins The vessels that carry oxygenated blood from the lungs to the left atrium.

pulmonic valve The valve between the right ventricle and the pulmonary artery.

pulp Specialized connective tissue within the pulp cavity of a tooth.

pulse oximeter Device that measures oxygen saturation.

pulse oximetry An assessment tool that measures oxygen saturation of hemoglobin in the capillary beds.

pulse pressure The difference between the systolic and diastolic pressures.

pulsus paradoxus A drop in the systolic BP of 10 mm Hg or more; commonly seen in patients with pericardial tamponade or severe asthma.

pulvule A solid medication form that resembles a capsule but it is not made of gelatin and does not separate.

puncture wound A stab injury from a pointed object, such as a nail or a knife.

pupil The circular opening in the center of the eye through which light passes to the lens.

Purkinje fibers A system of fibers in the ventricles that conducts the excitation impulse from the bundle branches to the myocardium.

purpuric Pertaining to bruising of the skin.

purulent Full of pus; having the character of pus.

purulent exudates Discharge that contains pus.

push-to-talk Commonly abbreviated as PTT, a method for communicating on a half-duplex communications system by pushing a button on the communication device to send and releasing the button to receive.

pyelonephritis Inflammation of the kidney linings.

pylorus A circumferential muscle at the end of the stomach that acts as a valve between the stomach and duodenum.

pyriform fossae Two pockets of tissue on the lateral borders of the larynx.

pyrogenic reaction A reaction characterized by an abrupt temperature elevation (as high as 106°F [41°C]) with severe chills, backache, headache, weakness, nausea, and vomiting; a potential complication of IV or IO therapy.

pyrogens Chemicals or proteins that travel to the brain and affect the hypothalamus, and stimulate a rise in the body's core temperature.

QRS complex Deflections of the ECG produced by ventricular depolarization.

quadriplegia Paralysis of all four extremities and the trunk.

qualified immunity Protection in which the paramedic is only held liable when the plaintiff can show that the paramedic violated clearly established law of which he or she should have known.

qualitative A type of descriptive statistic in research that does not use numerical information.

quantitative A type of measurement in research that uses a mean, median, and mode.

rabies A fatal infection of the central nervous system caused by a bite from an animal that has been infected with the rabies virus.

raccoon eyes Bruising under or around the orbits that is commonly seen following a basilar skull fracture; also called periorbital ecchymosis.

radial artery The artery pertaining to the wrist.

radiation Emission of heat from an object into surrounding, colder air.

radioactive material Any material that emits radiation.

radiological dispersal device (RDD) Any container that is designed to disperse radioactive material.

radiopaque Feature of an IV catheter (or any other object) that allows it to appear on an x-ray.

radius The bone on the thumb side of the forearm.

rales Old terminology for abnormal breath sounds that have a fine, crackling quality; now called crackles.

randomly A way of choosing subjects for a research project without specific reasons.

range of motion (ROM) The arc of movement of an extremity at a joint in a particular direction.

rape Sexual intercourse inflicted forcibly on another person, against that person's will.

rapid trauma assessment A unique and specialized assessment performed between the initial assessment and the focused physical exam of a trauma patient, usually on patients with a significant mechanism of injury, assessing specific parts of the entire body.

rapid-sequence intubation (RSI) A specific set of procedures, combined in rapid succession, to induce sedation and paralysis and intubate a patient quickly.

rappelling To descend on a fixed rope.

reactive airway disease A term used to describe any condition that causes hyperreactive bronchioles and bronchospasm.

recall The ability to retrieve a specific piece of stored information on demand.

recanalization The opening up of new channels through a blocked artery.

receptive aphasia Damage to or loss of the ability to understand speech.

receptors Specialized areas in tissues that initiate certain actions after specific stimulation.

reciprocity The process of granting licensing or certification to a provider from another state or agency.

recognition The ability to identify information that one has encountered before.

recovery position Left-lateral recumbent position; used in all semiconscious and unconscious nontrauma patients, who are able to maintain their own airway spontaneously and are breathing adequately.

recruitment The process of signaling additional muscle fibers to contract to create a more forceful contraction.

referred pain Pain that originates in one area of the body but is interpreted as coming from a different area of the body.

reflexes Involuntary motor responses to specific sensory stimuli, such as a tap on the knee or stroking the eyelash.

refractory period A short period immediately after depolarization in which the myocytes are not yet repolarized and are unable to fire or conduct an impulse.

regional anesthesia A type of anesthesia that focuses on a particular portion of the body, such as the legs or the arms.

registration Giving information that will be stored in some form of record book or the ability to add new items to the cerebral data bank.

regression A return to more childish behavior while under stress.

rehabilitation officer In incident command, the person who establishes an area that provides protection for responders from the elements and the situation.

relative refractory period That period in the cell-firing cycle at which it is possible but difficult to restimulate the cell to fire another impulse.

renal columns Inward extensions of cortical tissue that surround the renal pyramids.

renal dialysis A technique for "filtering" the blood of its toxic wastes, removing excess fluids, and restoring the normal balance of electrolytes.

renal fascia Dense, fibrous connective tissue that anchors the kidney to the abdominal wall.

renal pelvis Part of the internal anatomy of the kidney; a flat, funnel-shaped tube filling the sinus at the level of the hilus.

renal pyramids Parallel cone-shaped bundles of urine-collecting tubules that are located in the medulla of the kidneys.

renin A hormone produced by cells in the juxtaglomerular apparatus when the blood pressure is low.

renin-angiotensin-aldosterone system (RAAS) A complex feedback mechanism responsible for the kidney's regulation of sodium in the body.

repeater Miniature transmitter that picks up a radio signal and rebroadcasts it, extending the range of a radio communications system.

reperfusion The resumption of blood flow through an artery.

rescue officer In incident command, the person appointed to determine the type of equipment and resources needed for a situation involving extrication or special rescue; also called the extrication officer.

reservoir In the context of communicable disease, a place where organisms may live and multiply.

residual volume The air that remains in the lungs after maximal expiration.

resistance vessels The smallest arterioles.

respiration The exchange of gases between a living organism and its environment.

respiratory arrest The absence of respirations with detectable cardiac activity.

respiratory distress A clinical state characterized by increased respiratory rate, effort, and work of breathing.

respiratory exposure Exposure of the airways and lungs to a gas or vapor.

respiratory failure A clinical state of inadequate oxygenation, ventilation, or both.

respiratory syncytial virus (RSV) A labile paramyxovirus that produces its characteristic fusion of human cells in a tissue culture known as the syncytial effect. Two subtypes, A and B, have been identified. RSV can affect both the upper and lower respiratory tracts but is more prevalent with the lower, causing pneumonias and bronchiolitis.

restlessness A situation in which the patient can't sit still.

rest tremors Tremors that occur when the body part is not in motion.

retardation of thought The patient seems to take a very long time to get from one thought to the next.

retention The ability to store items in an accessible place in the mind.

reticular activating system (RAS) Located in the upper brain stem; responsible for maintenance of consciousness, specifically one's level of arousal.

reticuloendothelial system The system in the body that is primarily used to defend against infection.

retina A delicate 10-layered structure of nervous tissue located in the rear of the interior of the globe that receives light and generates nerve signals that are transmitted to the brain through the optic nerve.

retinal detachment Separation of the inner layers of the retina from the underlying choroid, the vascular membrane that nourishes the retina.

retinopathy of prematurity A disease of the eye that affects prematurely born babies, thought to be caused by disorganized growth of retinal blood vessels resulting in scarring and retinal detachment; can lead to blindness in serious cases.

retractions Physical drawing in of the chest wall between the ribs that occurs with increased work of breathing.

retrograde amnesia Loss of memory relating to events that occurred before the injury.

retroperitoneal space The area in the abdomen containing the aorta, vena cava, pancreas, kidneys, ureters, and portions of the duodenum and large intestine.

retrospective research Research performed from current available information.

retrosternal Situated or occurring behind the sternum.

review of systems A systematic survey of the patient's symptoms according to the major organ systems.

Rh factor A protein found on the red blood cells of most people; when a woman without this protein is impregnated by a man with this protein, the woman's body can create antibodies against the protein and attack future pregnancies.

rhabdomyolysis The destruction of muscle tissue leading to a release of potassium and myoglobin.

rheumatoid arthritis (RA) An inflammatory disorder that affects the entire body and leads to degeneration and deformation of joints.

rhonchi Rattling respiratory sounds that may resemble snoring; also called crackles.

rhonchus A coarse, low-pitched breath sound heard in patients who have chronic mucus in the airways (plural: rhonchi).

ribonucleic acid (RNA) Nucleic acid associated with controlling cellular activities.

ricin Neurotoxin derived from mash that is left from pressing oil from the castor bean; causes pulmonary edema and respiratory and circulatory failure, leading to death.

right atrium The upper right chamber of the heart; receives blood from the venae cavae and supplies blood to the right ventricle.

right ventricle The lower right chamber of the heart; receives blood from the right atrium and pumps blood out through the pulmonic valve into the pulmonary artery.

risk factors Characteristics of people, behaviors, or environments that increase the chances of disease or injury. Some examples are alcohol use, poverty, or gender.

Rohypnol A benzodiazepine used to facilitate date rape and that can create memory loss; street names include roofies, roof, roachies, rocha, and Mexican Valium.

rooting reflex An infant reflex that occurs when something touches an infant's cheek, and the infant instinctively turns his head toward the touch.

rotation-flexion injury A type of injury typically resulting from high acceleration forces; can result in a stable unilateral facet dislocation in the cervical spine.

round bones The small bones that are found adjacent to joints that assist with motion.

route of exposure Manner by which a toxic substance enters the body.

R-R interval The period between the onset of one QRS complex and the onset of the next QRS complex.

rubella A viral disease similar to measles, best known by the distinctive red rash on the skin. It is not nearly as infectious or severe as measles.

rubor Redness; one of the classic signs of inflammation.

rubs Lung sound produced by a partial loss of intrapleural integrity, when an abnormal collection of fluid has accumulated between a portion of the visceral and parietal pleura, resulting in "pleuritic" pain and a perceived rub on auscultation.

rule of nines A system that assigns percentages to sections of the body, allowing calculation of the amount of skin surface involved in the burn area.

rule of palm A system that estimates total body surface area burned by comparing the affected area with the size of the patient's palm, which is roughly equal to 1% of the patient's total body surface area.

rule of thumb A reminder of the proper distance from a hazardous materials scene; the entire scene should be hidden by a thumb held at arm's length.

ruptured ovarian cyst A fluid-filled sac within the ovary that bursts from internal pressure.

ST segment The interval between the end of the QRS complex and the beginning of the T wave; often elevated or depressed with respect to the isoelectric line when there is significant myocardial ischemia.

sacroiliac joints The points of attachment of the ilium to the sacrum.

safe residual pressure A term that implies that it is unsafe to continue using an oxygen cylinder with a pressure of less than 200 psi.

safety officer In incident command, the person who gives the "go ahead" to a plan or who may stop an operation when rescuer safety is an issue.

sagittal suture The point of the skull where the parietal bones join.

salicylates Aspirinlike drugs.

saline locks Special types of IV devices that eliminate the need to hang a bag of IV fluid; also called a buff cap or INT (intermittent); commonly used for patients who do not require fluid boluses but may require medication therapy.

sampling errors Expected errors that occur in the sampling phase of research.

sarin (GB) A nerve agent that is one of the G agents; a highly volatile colorless and odorless liquid that turns from liquid to gas within seconds to minutes at room temperature.

saturation diving A type of diving in which the diver remains at depth for prolonged periods.

scabies An infestation of the skin with the mite Sarcoptes scabei. It spreads rapidly when there is skin-to-skin contact.

scald burn A burn produced by hot liquids.

scaphoid A concave shape of the abdomen. This can be caused by evisceration.

scaphoid (bone) The wrist bone that is found just beyond that most distal portion of the radius.

scapula A large, flat, triangular bone along the posterior thorax that articulates with the clavicle and humerus.

scar revision A surgical procedure to improve the appearance of a scar, reestablish function, or correct disfigurement from soft-tissue damage, surgical incision, or lesion.

scene size-up A quick assessment of the scene and its surroundings made to provide information about scene safety and the mechanism of injury or nature of illness, before you enter and begin patient care.

school age A person who is 6 to 12 years of age.

sclera The white part of the eye.

scoliosis Sideways curvature of the spine.

scope of practice What a state permits a paramedic practicing under its license or certification to do.

scrambling A method used to ascend rocky faces and ridges and can be considered a cross between hill climbing and rock climbing.

search and rescue (SAR) The process of locating and removing a patient from the wilderness.

sebaceous gland A gland located in the dermis that secretes sebum.

sebum An oily substance secreted by sebaceous glands.

second stage of labor The stage of labor in which the baby's head enters the birth canal, during which contractions become more intense and more frequent.

secondary apnea When asphyxia continues after primary apnea, infant responds with a period of gasping respirations, falling pulse rate and falling blood pressure.

secondary brain injury The "after effects" of the primary injury; includes abnormal processes such as cerebral edema, increased intracranial pressure, cerebral ischemia and hypoxia, and infection; onset is often delayed following the primary brain injury.

secondary collapse A collapse that occurs following the primary collapse. This can occur in trench, excavation, and structural collapses.

secondary contamination Exposure to a hazardous material by contact with a contaminated person or object.

secondary device Additional explosives used by terrorists, which are set to explode after the initial bomb.

secondary exit Any other means of egress, including windows and rear doors.

secondary injury prevention Reducing the effects of an injury that has already happened.

secondary response The body's reaction when it is exposed to an antigen for which it already has antibodies, in which it responds by killing the invading substance.

secondary spinal cord injury Injury to the spinal cord, thought to be the result of multiple factors that result in a progression of inflammatory responses from primary spinal cord injury.

secondary triage A type of patient sorting used in the treatment sector that involves retriage of patients.

secretory phase The second phase of the menstrual cycle.

secure attachment A bond between an infant and his or her parent or caregiver, in which the infant understands that his parents or caregivers will be responsive to his needs and take care of him when he needs help.

sedation Reduction of a patient's anxiety, induction of amnesia, and suppression of the gag reflex.

sedative-hypnotic A drug used to reduce anxiety, calm agitated patients, and help produce drowsiness and sleep (CNS depressants).

segmental fracture A bone that is broken in more than one place.

seizure A paroxysmal alteration in neurologic function, ie, behavioral and/or autonomic function.

selective serotonin reuptake inhibitors (SSRIs) A class of antidepressants that inhibit the reuptake of serotonin.

self-contained underwater breathing apparatus The expansion of the acronym (SCUBA) for specialized underwater breathing equipment.

self-rescue position Position used in fast-moving water rescue situations. The rescuer rolls into a face-up arched position with the lower back higher than the feet to avoid objects below the surface. The feet should be together and facing in the direction of travel (feet first), with arms at the sides.

self-sealing blood tubes Glass tubes with self-sealing rubber caps; used to obtain blood samples for laboratory analysis.

Sellick maneuver The application of posterior pressure to the cricoid cartilage to minimize the risk of regurgitation during positive-pressure ventilation; also referred to as cricoid pressure.

semilunar valves The two valves, the aortic and pulmonic, that divide the heart from the aorta and pulmonary arteries.

sensitivity The ability to recognize a foreign substance the next time it is encountered.

sensitization Developing sensitivity to a substance that initially caused no allergic reaction.

sensorineural deafness A permanent lack of hearing caused by a lesion or damage of the inner ear.

sepsis A pathologic state, usually in a febrile patient, resulting from the presence of invading microorganisms or their toxic products in the bloodstream.

septic abortion A life-threatening emergency in which the uterus becomes infected following any type of abortion.

septic shock Shock that occurs as a result of widespread infection, usually bacterial. Untreated, the result is multiple organ dysfunction syndrome (MODS) and often death.

seropositive Having a positive blood test for an infectious agent, such as HIV or hepatitis B or C virus.

serosa The outermost layer of tissue in the fallopian tubes.

serotonin A vasoactive amine that increases vascular permeability to cause vasodilation.

serotonin syndrome An idiosyncratic complication that occurs with antidepressant therapy in which patients have lower extremity muscle rigidity, confusion or disorientation, and/or agitation.

serous exudates Discharge that contains serum, a thin watery substance.

serum hepatitis The hepatitis type B virus (HBV), which is transmitted through sexual contact, blood transfusion, or puncture of the skin with contaminated needles, and whose signs and symptoms include loss of appetite, nausea, vomiting, general fatigue and malaise, low-grade fever, vague abdominal discomfort, and sometimes aching in the joints. Eventually, jaundice will occur.

serum sickness   A condition in which antigen antibody complexes formed in the bloodstream deposit in sites around the body, most notably in the kidney, with resultant inflammatory reactions.

severe acute respiratory syndrome (SARS)   Potentially life-threatening viral infection that usually starts with flu-like symptoms.

sexual assault   An attack against a person that is sexual in nature, the most common of which is rape.

sexually transmitted diseases (STDs)   A group of diseases usually acquired by sexual contact, and which include gonorrhea, syphilis, chlamydia, scabies, pubic lice, herpes, hepatitis, and HIV infection.

shaken baby syndrome   A syndrome seen in abused infants and children; the patient has been subjected to violent, whiplash-type shaking injuries inflicted by the abusing individual that may cause coma, seizures, and increased intracranial pressure due to tearing of the cerebral veins with consequent bleeding into the brain.

shallow water blackout   A diving emergency that occurs when a person hyperventilates just before submerging underwater and loses consciousness before resurfacing due to hypoxemia and cerebral vasoconstriction.

sharps   Any contaminated item that can cause injury; includes IV needles and catheters, broken ampules or vials, or anything else that can penetrate or lacerate the skin.

shearing   An applied force or pressure exerted against the surface and layers of the skin as tissues slide in opposite but parallel planes.

Shiley   A type of tracheostomy tube.

shock   An abnormal state associated with inadequate oxygen and nutrient delivery to the metabolic apparatus of the cell.

shoring   A method of supporting a trench wall or building components such as walls, floors, or ceilings using either hydraulic, pneumatic, or wood shoring systems. Shoring is used to prevent collapse.

short bones   The bones that are nearly as wide as they are long.

shunt   Situation in which a portion of the output of the right side of the heart reaches the left side of the heart without being oxygenated in the lungs; may be caused by atelectasis, pulmonary edema, or a variety of other conditions. In hemodialysis, an anastomosis between a peripheral artery and vein.

sickle cell disease   A disease that causes red blood cells to be misshapen, resulting in poor oxygen-carrying capability and potentially resulting in lodging of the red blood cells in blood vessels or the spleen.

side effects   Reactions that can manifest as signs or symptoms that are not desired but are expected based on how the medication works.

signs   Indications of illness or injury that the examiner can see, hear, feel, smell, and so on.

silver fork deformity   The dorsal deformity of the forearm that results from a Colles fracture.

simple face mask   A full mask enclosure with open side ports. Room air is drawn in through the side ports on inhalation, diluting the concentration of inspired oxygen. Exhaled air is vented through holes on each side of the mask. The simple face mask will deliver between 40% and 60% oxygen at 10 L/min.

simple febrile seizures   A brief, self-limited, generalized seizure in a previously healthy child between the ages of 6 months and 6 years that is associated with the onset of or sudden increase in fever.

simple partial seizures   Focal seizures that involve a motor or sensory abnormality in a patient who remains conscious.

simple phobia   A fear that is focused on one class of objects (eg, mice, spiders, dogs) or situations (eg, high places, darkness, flying).

simplex   Method of radio communication using a single frequency that enables transmission or reception of voice or an ECG signal but is incapable of simultaneous transmission and reception.

single command system   A command system in which one person is in charge, generally used with small incidents that involve only one responding agency or one jurisdiction.

sinoatrial (SA) node   The dominant pacemaker of the heart, located at the junction of the superior vena cava and the right atrium.

sinus arrhythmia   A slight irregularity of the heart rate caused by changes in parasympathetic tone during breathing.

sinus bradycardia   A sinus rhythm with a heart rate less than 60 beats/min.

sinus tachycardia   A sinus rhythm with a heart rate greater than 100 beats/min.

sinuses   Cavities formed by the cranial bones that trap contaminants from entering the respiratory tract and act as tributaries for fluid to and from the eustachian tubes and tear ducts.

skeletal muscle   Muscle that is attached to bones and usually crosses at least one joint; striated or voluntary muscle.

skeletal muscle relaxants   Medications that provide relief of skeletal muscle spasms.

skull   The structure at the top of the axial skeleton that houses the brain and consists of 28 bones that comprise the auditory ossicles, the cranium, and the face.

slander   Verbally making a false statement that injures a person's good name.

slow-reacting substances of anaphylaxis (SRS-A)   Biologically active compounds derived from arachidonic acid called leukotrienes.

SLUDGE   An mnemonic that stands for salivation, lacrimation, urination, gastrointestinal activity, and emesis, which are the signs and symptoms that can be produced by exposure to organophosphate and carbamate pesticides or other nerve-stimulating agents.

small for gestational age   An infant whose size and weight are considerably less than the average for babies of the same age.

smallpox   A highly contagious disease; it is most contagious when blisters begin to form.

smooth muscle   Nonstriated involuntary muscle found in vessel walls, glands, and the gastrointestinal tract.

sniffing position   An upright position in which the patient's head and chin are thrust slightly forward to keep the airway open; appears to be sniffing.

snoring   Noise made on inhalation when the upper airway is partially obstructed by the tongue.

snuffbox   The region at the base of the thumb where the scaphoid may be palpated.

sodium channel blockers   Antiarrhythmic medications that slow conduction through the heart.

sodium-potassium (Na+-K+) pump   The mechanism by which the cell brings in two potassium (K+) ions and releases three sodium (Na+) ions.

solute   The dissolved particles contained in the solvent.

solution   A liquid containing one or more chemical substances entirely dissolved, usually in water.

solvent   The fluid that does the dissolving, or the solution that contains the dissolved components.

soman (GD)   A nerve agent that is one of the G agents; twice as persistent as sarin and five times as lethal; it has a fruity odor as a result of the type of alcohol used in the agent, and is both a contact and inhalation hazard that can enter the body through skin absorption and through the respiratory tract.

somatic motor neurons   The nerve fibers that transmit impulses to a muscle.

somatoform disorder   A condition in which a person is overly concerned with physical health and appearance to the point that it dominates his or her life; an example is hypochondria.

source individual   Any individual, living or dead, whose blood or other potentially infectious materials may be a source of occupational exposure to the member/volunteer. Examples include, but are not limited to, hospital and clinic patients; clients in institutions for the developmentally disabled; trauma victims; clients of drug and alcohol treatment facilities; residents of hospices and nursing homes; human remains; and individuals who donate or sell blood or blood components.

spacer A device that collects medication as it is released from the canister of a metered-dose inhaler, allowing more to be delivered to the lungs and less to be lost to the environment.

spalling Delaminating or breaking off into chips and pieces.

span of control In incident command, the subordinate positions under the commander's direction to which the workload is distributed; the supervisor/worker ratio.

Special Atomic Demolition Munitions (SADM) Small suitcase-sized nuclear weapons that were designed to destroy individual targets, such as important buildings, bridges, tunnels, or large ships.

specific agents Medications that bring about an identifiable mechanism with unique receptors for the agent.

specific exemptions Limited circumstances when an emergency vehicle operator can exceed the posted signage or speed limit.

specific gravity The measure that indicates whether or not a material will sink or float in water.

spina bifida The most common permanently disabling birth defect in which, during the first month of pregnancy, the spinal column of the fetus does not close properly or completely and vertebrae do not develop, leaving a portion of the spinal cord exposed.

spinal cord The part of the central nervous system that extends downward from the brain through the foramen magnum and is protected by the spine.

spinal shock The temporary local neurologic condition that occurs immediately after spinal trauma; swelling and edema of the spinal cord begin immediately after injury, with severe pain and potential paralysis.

spiral fracture A break in a bone that appears like a spring on a radiograph.

spirits A preparation of a volatile substance dissolved in alcohol.

spoil pile The pile of dirt that has been removed from an excavation. The pile may be unstable and prone to collapse.

spondylosis Immobility and consolidation of a vertebral joint.

spontaneous abortion Expulsion of the fetus that occurs naturally; also called miscarriage.

sprains Injuries, including a stretch or a tear, to the ligaments of a joint that commonly lead to pain and swelling.

stable angina Angina pectoris characterized by periodic pain with a predictable pattern.

staging officer In incident command, the person who locates an area to stage equipment and personnel and tracks unit arrival and deployment from the staging area.

standard deviation In research this outlines how much change from the mean is expected.

standard of care What a reasonable paramedic with training would do in the same or a similar situation.

standard precautions The new term used to describe the infection control practices that will reduce the opportunity for exposure of providers in the daily care of patients.

standing order A form of off-line or indirect medical control; a written document signed by the EMS system's medical director that outlines specific directions, permissions, and sometimes prohibitions regarding patient care that is rendered prior to contacting medical control.

Staphylococcus aureus A strain of bacteria that became resistant to the drug methicillin, creating a new strain called methicillin-resistant *Staphylococcus aureus;* symptoms include infection and possibly localized skin abscesses and cellulites, empyemas, and endocarditis.

START triage A patient sorting process that stands for simple triage and rapid treatment and uses a limited assessment of the patient's ability to walk, respiratory status, hemodynamic status, and neurologic status.

state-sponsored terrorism Terrorism that is funded and/or supported by nations that hold close ties with terrorist groups.

status asthmaticus A severe, prolonged asthma attack that cannot be broken with epinephrine.

status epilepticus A state of continuous seizures or multiple seizures without a return to consciousness for 20 minutes.

steam burn A burn that has been caused by direct exposure to hot steam exhaust, as from a broken pipe.

steatorrhea Foamy, fatty stools caused by liver failure or gallbladder problems.

steering play A sensation of looseness or sloppiness in a vehicle's steering.

steering pull A drift that is persistent enough so an operator can feel a tug on the steering wheel.

stem cells Cells that can develop into other types of cells in the body.

stenosis Narrowing.

step blocks Specialized cribbing assemblies made out of wood or plastic blocks in a step configuration.

stereotyped activity Repetitive movements that don't appear to serve any purpose.

sterile The destruction of all living organisms; achieved by using heat, gas, or chemicals.

sternum Also known as the breastbone, this bony structure along the midline of the thorax provides a point of anterior attachment for the thoracic cage.

stimulants An agent that increases the level of body activity.

stoma A small opening, especially an artificially created opening, such as that made by tracheostomy.

straddle fracture A fracture of the pelvis that results from landing on the perineal region.

straight laryngoscope blade Also called the Miller blade; designed to lift the epiglottis and expose the vocal cords.

strain Stretching or tearing of a muscle by excessive stretching or overuse.

strategic deployment The staging of ambulances to strategic locations within a service area to allow for coverage of emergency calls.

stratum basalis A permanent mucous membrane that makes up part of the outer endometrium.

stratum functionalis An inner mucous membrane that makes up part of the endometrium, and which is renewed following menstruation.

stress A nonspecific response of the body to any demand made upon it.

stress fracture A fracture that results from exaggerated stress on the bone caused by unusually rapid muscle development.

stressor Any agent or situation that causes stress.

striae Stretch marks on the abdomen caused by size changes.

striated muscle Skeletal muscle that is under voluntary control.

stridor A harsh, high-pitched, crowing inspiratory sound, such as the sound often heard in acute laryngeal obstruction.

stroke volume (SV) The volume of blood pumped forward with each ventricular contraction.

stylet A semirigid wire that is inserted into the ET tube to mold and maintain the shape of the tube.

subarachnoid hemorrhage Bleeding into the subarachnoid space, where the cerebrospinal fluid (CSF) circulates.

subarachnoid space The space located between the pia mater and the arachnoid mater.

subclavian artery The artery that travels from the aorta to each upper extremity.

subconjunctival hematoma The collection of blood within the sclera of the eye, presenting as a bright red patch of blood over the sclera but not involving the cornea.

subcutaneous Beneath the skin.

subcutaneous emphysema A physical finding of air within the subcutaneous tissue.

subcutaneous (SC or SQ) route A medication route in which injections are given beneath the skin into the fat or connective tissue immediately underlying it.

subdural hematoma An accumulation of blood beneath the dura but outside the brain.

subglottic space The narrowest part of the pediatric airway.

sublingual (SL) A medication route in which medication is administered under the tongue.

subluxation A partial or incomplete dislocation.

substance abuse   Use of a substance that disrupts activities of daily living.

substance dependence   Use of a substance that results in addiction and physiologic dependence on the substance.

substance intoxication   Use of a substance that results in impaired thinking and motor function.

substance use   Use of moderate amounts of a substance without seriously affecting activities of daily living.

subthalamus   The part of the diencephalon that is involved in controlling motor functions.

succinylcholine chloride   A depolarizing neuromuscular blocker frequently used as the initial paralytic during rapid-sequence intubation; causes muscle fasciculations; also referred to as Anectine.

sucking reflex   An infant reflex in which the infant starts sucking when his or her lips are stroked.

sudden infant death syndrome (SIDS)   The abrupt and unexplained death of an apparently healthy child younger than 1 year.

suicide   Any willful act designed to bring an end to one's own life.

sulfur mustard (H)   A vesicant; it is a brownish-yellowish oily substance that is generally considered very persistent; has the distinct smell of garlic or mustard and, when released, it is quickly absorbed into the skin and/or mucous membranes and begins an irreversible process of damaging the cells.

summation effect   The process whereby multiple medications can produce a response that the individual medications alone do not produce.

superficial burn   A burn involving only the epidermis, producing very red, painful skin; previously called a first-degree burn.

superficial frostbite   A type of frostbite characterized by altered sensation (numbness, tingling, or burning) and white, waxy skin that is firm to palpation, but the underlying tissues remain soft.

supination   To turn the forearm laterally so that the palm faces forward (if standing) or upward (if lying supine).

supine hypotensive syndrome   Low blood pressure resulting from compression of the inferior vena cava by the weight of the pregnant uterus when the mother is supine.

suppository   A drug mixed in a firm base that melts at body temperature and is shaped to fit the rectum, urethra, or vagina.

supracondylar fractures   Fractures of the distal humerus that occur just proximal to the elbow.

supraglottic   Located above the glottic opening, as in the upper airway structures.

suprapubic   The region of the abdomen superior to the pubic bone and inferior to the umbilicus.

suprasternal notch   The indentation formed by the superior border of the manubrium and the clavicles, often used as a landmark for procedures such as subclavian vein access.

supraventricular tachycardia (SVT)   An abnormal heart rhythm with a rapid, narrow QRS complex.

surface-tended diving   A type of diving in which air is piped to the diver through a tube from the surface.

surfactant   A liquid protein substance that coats the alveoli in the lungs, decreases alveolar surface tension, and keeps the alveoli expanded; a low level in a premature baby contributes to respiratory distress syndrome.

surrogate decision maker   A person designated by a patient to make health care decisions for them when they are unable to make decisions for themselves.

suspension   A preparation of a finely divided drug intended to be (or already) incorporated in a suitable liquid.

SWAT-trained paramedics   Specially trained medics who provide care for barricaded patients, patients being held hostage, and other special operations.

sympathetic blocking agent   An antihypertensive medication that decreases cardiac output and rennin secretions.

sympathetic eye movement   The movement of both eyes in unison.

sympathetic nervous system   Subdivision of the autonomic nervous system that governs the body's fight-or-flight reactions by inducing smooth muscle contraction or relaxation of the blood vessels and bronchioles.

sympathomimetics   The medications administered to stimulate the sympathetic nervous system.

symptoms   The pain, discomfort, or other abnormality that the patient feels.

synapses   Gaps between nerve cells across which nervous stimuli are transmitted.

synchronized cardioversion   The timed delivery of energy into the myocardium to correct rapid, regular cardiac rhythms in patients who are in unstable condition.

syncopal episodes   Fainting; brief losses of consciousness caused by transiently inadequate blood flow to the brain.

syncope   Fainting; brief loss of consciousness caused by transiently inadequate blood flow to the brain.

syndromic surveillance   The monitoring, usually by local or state health departments, of patients presenting to emergency departments and alternative care facilities, the recording of EMS call volume, and the use of over-the-counter medications.

synergism   An interaction of two or more medications that results in an effect that is greater than the sum of their effects if taken independently.

synovial joints   Joints that permit movement of the component bones.

synovial membrane   The lining of a joint that secretes synovial fluid into the joint space.

syphilis   A sexually transmitted disease caused by the spiral-shaped bacteria *Treponema pallidum* and whose signs and symptoms include an ulcerative lesion or chancre of the skin or mucous membrane at the site of infection, commonly in the genital region.

syrup   A drug suspended in sugar and water to improve its taste.

systematic sampling   A computer-generated list of subjects or groups for research.

systemic anesthesia   A type of anesthesia often done through the inhalation of volatile vaporized liquids and predominantly reserved for operating room use; also called general anesthesia.

systemic circulation   The flow of blood from the left ventricle through the aorta, to all of its branches and capillaries in the tissues, and back to the right atrium through the venules, veins, and venae cavae; also called the greater circulation.

systemic complications   Reactions that affect systems of the body.

systemic effect   A physiologic effect on the entire body or one of the body's systems.

systemic effects   The effects that occur after the drug is absorbed by any route and distributed by the bloodstream; almost invariably involve more than one organ.

systemic reaction   A reaction that occurs throughout the body, possibly affecting multiple body systems.

systole   The period during which the ventricles contract.

T killer cells   Cells released during a type IV allergic reaction that kill antigen-bearing target cells.

T wave   The upright, flat, or inverted wave following the QRS complex of the ECG, representing ventricular repolarization.

tablet   A powdered drug that has been molded or compressed into a small disk.

tabun (GA)   A nerve agent that is one of the G agents; is 36 times more persistent than sarin and approximately half as lethal; has a fruity smell and is unique because the components used to manufacture the agent are easy to acquire and the agent is easy to manufacture.

tachycardia   A rapid heart rate, more than 100 beats/min.

tachyphylaxis   A condition in which the patient rapidly becomes tolerant to a medication.

tactile fremitus   Vibrations in the chest as the patient breathes.

talus   The bone of the foot that articulates with the tibia.

tangential thinking   Leaving the current topic midconversation to talk about something else, inhibiting interpersonal communication.

target tissues   Tissues to which hormones are directed to act on.

tarsals   The ankle bones.

technical rescue incident (TRI) A complex rescue incident involving vehicles or machinery, water or ice, rope techniques, a trench or excavation collapse, confined spaces, a structural collapse, wilderness search and rescue, or hazardous materials, and which requires specially trained personnel and special equipment.

technical rescue team A group of rescuers specially trained in the various disciplines of technical rescue.

technician The training level that provides a high level of competency in the various disciplines of technical or hazardous materials rescue for rescuers who will be directly involved in the rescue operation itself.

tempered glass A type of safety glass that is heat-treated so that it will break into small pieces.

temporal lobe The portion of the brain that has an important role in hearing and memory.

temporomandibular joint (TMJ) The joint between the temporal bone and the posterior condyle that allows for movements of the mandible.

ten-code A radio code system using the number 10 plus another number.

tendinitis Inflammation of a tendon that most commonly results from overuse.

tendons The fibrous portions of muscle that attach to bone.

tension lines The pattern of tautness of the skin, which is arranged over body structures and affects how well wounds heal.

tension pneumothorax A life-threatening collection of air within the pleural space; the volume and pressure have both collapsed the involved lung and caused a shift of the mediastinal structures to the opposite side.

tenting A condition in which the skin slowly retracts after being pinched and pulled away slightly from the body; a sign of dehydration.

tentorium A structure that separates the cerebral hemispheres from the cerebellum and brain stem.

term Used to describe an infant delivered at 38 to 42 weeks of gestation.

terminal drop hypothesis The theory that a person's mental function declines in the last 5 years of life.

terminal illness A sickness that the patient cannot be cured of; death is imminent.

termination of action The amount of time after the medication's concentration falls below the minimum effective level until it is eliminated from the body.

termination of command The end of the incident command structure when an incident draws to a close.

terrorism A violent act dangerous to human life, in violation of the criminal laws of the United States or any segment to intimidate or coerce a government, the civilian population or any segment thereof, in furtherance of political or social objectives.

testes Male gonads located in the scrotum that produce hormones called androgens.

testimonial evidence The oral documentation by a witness of the facts of a criminal act.

testosterone The most important androgen in men.

tetanus A disease caused by spores that enter the body through a puncture wound contaminated with animal feces, street dust, or soil, or which can enter through contaminated street drugs, and whose signs and symptoms include pain at the wound site and painful muscle contractions in the neck and trunk muscles.

thalamus The part of the diencephalon that processes most sensory input and influences mood and general body movements, especially those associated with fear or rage.

thalassemia A type of anemia in which not enough hemoglobin is produced, or the hemoglobin is defective.

theophylline A naturally occurring alkaloid found in a variety of plants (such as tea leaves).

therapeutic The desired or intended action of a medication.

therapeutic index The ratio of a drug's lethal dose for 50% (LD50) of the population to its effective dose for 50% (ED50) of the population; a medication's margin of safety.

therapy regulator Attaches to the stem of the oxygen cylinder, and reduces the high pressure of gas to a safe range (about 50 psi).

thermal burn An injury caused by radiation or direct contact with a heat source on the skin.

thermogenesis The production of heat in the body.

thermolysis The liberation of heat from the body.

thermoregulation The process by which the body maintains temperature through a combination of heat gain by metabolic processes and muscular movement and heat loss through respiration, evaporation, conduction, convection, and perspiration.

thiazides A type of diuretic medication that specifically controls the sodium and water quantities excreted by the kidneys.

third spacing The shifting of fluid into the tissues, creating edema.

third stage of labor The stage of labor in which the placenta is expelled.

Thompson test Squeezing of the calf muscle to evaluate for plantar flexion of the foot to determine whether the Achilles tendon is intact.

thoracic inlet The superior aspect of the thoracic cavity, this ring-like opening is created by the first vertebral vertebra, the first rib, the clavicles, and the manubrium.

thorax The part of the body between the neck and the diaphragm, encased by the ribs.

thought broadcasting The belief that others can hear one's thoughts.

thought control The belief that outside forces are controlling one's thoughts.

thought insertion The belief that thoughts are being thrust into one's mind by another person.

thought withdrawal The belief that thoughts are being removed from one's mind.

threatened abortion Expulsion of the fetus that is attempting to take place but has not occurred yet; usually occurs in the first trimester.

threshold limit value (TLV) The concentration of a substance that is supposed to be safe for exposure no more than 8 hours per day and 40 hours per week.

threshold limit value ceiling level (TLV-CL) The concentration that a person should never be exposed to.

threshold limit value short-term exposure limit (TLV-STEL) The concentration of a substance that a worker can be exposed to for up to 15 minutes but no more than four times per day with at least an hour between each exposure.

thrombin An enzyme that causes the conversion of fibrinogen to fibrin, which binds to the platelet plugs, forming the final mature blood clot.

thrombocytes Platelets.

thrombocytopenia Reduction in the number of platelets.

thromboembolic disease The condition in which a patient has a DVT or pulmonary embolism.

thrombophlebitis Inflammation of a vein.

through-the-needle catheters Plastic catheters inserted through a hollow needle; referred to as Intracaths.

thyroid Large gland located at the base of the neck that produces and excretes hormones that influence growth, development, and metabolism.

thyroid cartilage The main supporting cartilage of the larynx; a shield-shaped structure formed by two plates that join in a "V" shape anteriorly to form the laryngeal prominence known as the Adam's apple.

thyroid-stimulating hormone (TSH) Hormone that controls the release of thyroid hormone from the thyroid gland.

thyroid storm A rare, life-threatening condition that may occur in patients with thyrotoxicosis. The condition is usually triggered by a stressful event or increased volume of thyroid hormones in the circulation.

thyrotoxicosis A toxic condition caused by excessive levels of circulating thyroid hormone.

thyroxine The body's major metabolic hormone. Thyroxine stimulates energy production in cells, which increases the rate at which the cells consume oxygen and use carbohydrates, fats, and proteins.

tibia The shin bone.

tidal volume A measure of the depth of breathing; the volume of air that is inhaled or exhaled during a single respiratory cycle.

tincture A dilute alcoholic extract of a drug.

toddlers Persons who are 1 to 3 years of age.

tokolytics Drugs used to delay preterm labor.

tolerance Physiologic adaptation to the effects of a drug such that increasingly larger doses of the drug are required to achieve the same effect.

tongue-jaw lift maneuver A manual maneuver that involves grasping the tongue and jaw and lifting; commonly used to suction the airway and to place certain airway devices.

tonic activity Type of seizure movement involving the constant contraction and trembling of muscle groups.

tonic-clonic seizures Seizures that feature rhythmic back-and-forth motion of an extremity and body stiffness.

tonicity The osmotic pressure of a solution, based on the relationship between sodium and water inside and outside the cell, that takes advantage of their chemical and osmotic properties to move water to areas of higher sodium concentration.

tonsils Lymphatic tissues that are located in the posterior pharynx; they help to trap bacteria.

tonsil-tip catheter A hard or rigid suction catheter; also called a Yankauer catheter.

tort A wrongful act that gives rise to a civil suit.

torus fracture *See* buckle fracture.

total body surface area (TBSA) Used in the calculation of a burn injury to determine the percentage of the surface of the patient's body that has been injured. This is commonly estimated by using the rule of palm or the rule of nines.

total body water (TBW) Total amount of water in the human body; accounts for approximately 60% of the weight of an average man; divided into various compartments.

total laryngectomy Surgical removal of the entire larynx.

total lung capacity The total volume of air that the lungs can hold; approximately 6 L in the average adult male.

toxic shock syndrome (TSS) A form of septic shock caused by *Streptococcus pyogenes* (group A strep) or *Staphylococcus aureus;* initial symptoms include syncope, myalgia, diarrhea, vomiting, headache, fever, and sore throat.

toxicity levels Measures of the risk that a hazardous material poses to the health of an individual who comes into contact with it.

toxicologic emergencies Medical emergencies caused by toxic agents such as poison.

toxidrome The syndrome-like symptoms of a poisonous agent.

toxoid A modified bacterial toxin that has been made nontoxic but retains the ability to stimulate the formation of antibodies.

trachea The conduit for all entry into the lungs; a tubular structure that is approximately 10 to 12 cm in length and is composed of a series of C-shaped cartilaginous rings; also called the windpipe.

tracheal transection Traumatic separation of the trachea from the larynx.

tracheobronchial suctioning Passing a suction catheter into the endotracheal tube to remove pulmonary secretions.

tracheostomy Surgical opening into the trachea.

tracheostomy tube Plastic tube placed within the tracheostomy site (stoma).

track marks The visible scars from repeated cannulation of a vein; commonly associated with illicit drug use.

trade name The brand name registered to a specific manufacturer or owner; also called proprietary name.

transceiver A radio transmitter and receiver housed in a single unit; a two-way radio.

transdermal Across the skin; a medication delivery route.

transdermal route A medication route generally performed by placing medication directly onto the patient's skin.

transfer of command In incident command, when an incident commander turns over command to someone with more experience in a critical area.

transient ischemic attack (TIA) A disorder of the brain in which brain cells temporarily stop working because of insufficient oxygen, causing stroke-like symptoms that resolve completely within 24 hours of onset.

transillumination intubation Method of intubation that uses a lighted stylet to guide the endotracheal tube into the trachea.

translaryngeal catheter ventilation Used in conjunction with needle cricothyrotomy to ventilate a patient; requires a high-pressure jet ventilator.

transmigration (diapedesis) The PMNs permeate through the vessel wall, moving into the interstitial space.

transportation officer In incident command, the person who coordinates transportation and distribution of patients to appropriate receiving hospitals.

transverse fracture A fracture that runs in a straight line from one edge of the bone to the other and that is perpendicular to each edge.

transverse presentation A delivery in which the fetus lies crosswise in the uterus; one hand may protrude through the vagina.

transverse spinous process The junction of each pedicle and lamina on each side of a vertebra; these project laterally and posteriorly and form points of attachment for muscles and ligaments.

trauma Acute physiologic and structural change that occurs in a victim as a result of the rapid dissipation of energy delivered by an external force.

trauma systems The collaboration of prehospital and in-hospital medicine that focuses on optimizing the use of resources and assets of each with a primary goal of reducing the mortality and morbidity of trauma patients.

traumatic asphyxia A pattern of injuries seen after a severe force is applied to the thorax, forcing blood from the great vessels and back into the head and neck.

traumatic brain injury (TBI) A traumatic insult to the brain capable of producing physical, intellectual, emotional, social, and vocational changes.

treatment officer In incident command, the person responsible for locating, setting up, and supervising the treatment area.

trench foot A process similar to frostbite but caused by prolonged exposure to cool, wet conditions.

triage To sort patients based on the severity of their conditions and prioritize them for care accordingly.

triage officer The person in charge of prioritizing patients, whose primary duty is to ensure that every patient receives initial triage.

trichomoniasis A parasitic infection.

tricuspid valve The valve between the right atrium and right ventricle of the heart.

tricyclic antidepressants (TCAs) A group of drugs used to treat severe depression and manage pain; minimal dosing errors can cause toxic results.

trigeminal nerve Fifth cranial nerve; supplies sensation to the scalp, forehead, face, and lower jaw and innervates the muscles of mastication, the throat, and the inner ear.

trigeminy A premature complex in every third heartbeat.

tripoding An abnormal position to keep the airway open; involves leaning forward onto two arms stretched forward.

trismus Clenched teeth caused by spasms of the jaw muscles; occurs during seizures and head injuries.

trunking Sharing of radio frequencies by multiple agencies or systems.

trust and mistrust A phrase that refers to a stage of development from birth to approximately 18 months of age, during which infants gain trust of their parents or caregivers if their world is planned, organized, and routine.

tuberculin skin test A test to determine if a person has ever been infected with tuberculosis.

tuberculosis (TB) A chronic bacterial disease caused by *Mycobacterium tuberculosis* that usually affects the lungs but can also affect other organs such as the brain or kidneys; may be characterized by a persistent cough, night sweats, headache, weight loss, hemoptysis, or chest pain.

tubo-ovarian abscess   An infectious mass growing within the ovaries and fallopian tubes.

tubules   Sections of the kidney where the filtration of wastes, electrolytes, and water is controlled.

tunica adventitia   The outer layer of tissue of a blood vessel wall, composed of elastic and fibrous connective tissue.

tunica intima   The smooth, thin, inner lining of a blood vessel.

tunica media   The middle and thickest layer of tissue of a blood vessel wall, composed of elastic tissue and smooth muscle cells that allow the vessel to expand or contract in response to changes in blood pressure and tissue demand.

tunnel vision   Dangerous situation when a paramedic becomes so completely involved with patient care that he or she fails to see the possibility of physical harm to the patient or other care providers.

turbinates   Three bony shelves that protrude from the lateral walls of the nasal cavity and extend into the nasal passageway, parallel to the nasal floor; serve to increase the surface area of the nasal mucosa, thereby improving the processes of warming, filtering, and humidification of inhaled air.

turgor   Loss of elasticity in the skin.

twisting injuries   Injuries that commonly occur during athletic activities in which an extremity rotates around a planted foot or hand.

tympanic membrane   The eardrum; a thin, semitransparent membrane in the middle ear that transmits sound vibrations to the internal ear by means of the auditory ossicles.

type 1 diabetes   The type of diabetic disease that usually starts in childhood and requires daily injections of supplemental synthetic insulin to control blood glucose. Sometimes called juvenile or juvenile-onset diabetes.

type 2 diabetes   The type of diabetic disease that usually starts in later life and often can be controlled through diet and oral medications. Sometimes called adult-onset diabetes.

Type I Ambulance   Conventional, truck-cab chassis with a modular ambulance body that can be transferred to a new chassis as needed.

Type II Ambulance   Standard van, forward-control integral cab-body ambulance.

Type III Ambulance   Specialty van, forward-control integral cab-body ambulance.

U wave   A small flat wave sometimes seen after the T wave and before the next P wave.

ulna   The larger bone of the forearm, on the side opposite the thumb.

ulnar artery   The artery of the forearm that travels along its medial aspect.

ultrahigh frequency (UHF) band   The portion of the radio frequency spectrum between 300 and 3,000 mHz.

umbilical   The region of the abdomen surrounding the umbilicus.

umbilical cord   The conduit connecting mother to infant via the placenta; contains two arteries and one vein.

umbilical vein   Blood vessel in umbilical cord used to administer emergency medications.

unblinded study   A type of study in which the subjects are advised of all aspects of the study.

undifferentiated type   Schizophrenia that does not fit neatly into another category.

unified command system   A command system used in larger incidents in which there is a multiagency response or multiple jurisdictions are involved.

unifocal   Arising from a single site.

unintentional injuries   Injuries that occur without intent to harm (commonly called accidents). Some examples are motor vehicle crashes, poisonings, drownings, falls, and most burns.

universal precautions   Protective measures that have traditionally been developed by the Centers for Disease Control and Prevention (CDC) for use in dealing with objects, blood, body fluids, or other potential exposure risks of communicable disease.

unstable angina   Angina pectoris characterized by a changing, unpredictable pattern of pain, which may signal an impending acute myocardial infarction.

upper airway   Consists of all anatomic airway structures above the level of the vocal cords.

upper explosive limit (UEL)   The concentration of a hazardous material at which there is not enough oxygen to support the combustion in air.

uremia   Severe kidney failure resulting in the buildup of waste products within the blood. Eventually brain functions will be impaired.

uremic frost   A powdery buildup of uric acid, especially around the face.

ureters   A pair of thick-walled, hollow tubes that transport urine from the kidneys to the bladder.

urethra   A hollow, tubular structure that drains urine from the bladder, passing it outside of the body.

uricosuric medications   The medications designed to lower the uric acid level in the blood by increasing the excretion by the kidneys into the urine.

urinary bladder   A hollow, muscular sac in the midline of the lower abdominal area that stores urine until it is released from the body.

urinary tract infections (UTIs)   Infections, usually of the lower urinary tract (urethra and bladder), which occur when normal flora bacteria enter the urethra and grow.

urine   Liquid waste products filtered out of the body by the urinary system.

urticaria   Multiple small, raised areas on the skin that may be one of the warning signs of impending anaphylaxis. Also known as hives.

uterine cavity   The interior of the body of the uterus.

uterine inversion   A potentially fatal complication of childbirth in which the placenta fails to detach properly and results in the uterus turning inside-out.

uterus   A muscular inverted pear-shaped organ, that lies situated between the urinary bladder and the rectum.

uvula   A soft-tissue structure that resembles a punching bag; located in the posterior aspect of the oral cavity, at the base of the tongue.

V agent (VX)   One of the G agents; it is a clear, oily agent that has no odor and looks like baby oil; it is over 100 times more lethal than sarin and is extremely persistent.

vaccine   A suspension of whole (live or inactivated) or fractionated bacteria or viruses that have been made nonpathogenic; given to induce an immune response and prevent disease.

Vacutainer   A cylindrical device that attaches to an 18- or 20-gauge sampling needle; accommodates self-sealing blood tubes when obtaining blood samples.

vagina   The lower portion of the birth canal, which also serves as a passage for menstrual bleeding.

vaginal yeast infection   An infection caused by the fungus Candida albicans, in which fungi overpopulate the vagina.

vagus nerve   The 10th cranial nerve, the chief mediator of the parasympathetic nervous system.

vallecula   An anatomic space, or "pocket," located between the base of the tongue and the epiglottis; an important anatomic landmark for endotracheal intubation.

Valsalva maneuver Forced exhalation against a closed glottis, the effect of which is to stimulate the vagus nerve and, thereby, slow the heart rate.

vapor A gaseous medication form primarily used in operating room anesthesia.

vapor density A measure that compares the hazardous material gas to air; toxic gases that are heavier than air will sink, while vapors that are lighter than air will dissipate and travel with the wind.

vapor hazard An agent that enters the body through the respiratory tract.

vapor pressure The pressure exerted by a vapor when the liquid and vapor states of a material are in equilibrium; this measure changes as a material is heated.

vasa recta A series of peritubular capillaries that surround the loop of Henle, into which water moves after passing through the descending and ascending limbs of the loop of Henle.

vasculitis An inflammation of the blood vessels.

vasoactive amines Substances such as histamine and serotonin that increase vascular permeability.

vasoconstriction Narrowing of a blood vessel, such as with hypoperfusion or cold extremities.

vasodilatation Widening of a blood vessel.

vasodilator medications The medications that work on the smooth muscles of the arterioles and/or the veins.

vecuronium A nondepolarizing neuromuscular blocking agent; used to maintain paralysis following succinylcholine-facilitated intubation; also called Norcuron.

veins The blood vessels that carry blood to the heart.

velocity The speed of an object in a given direction.

venae cavae The largest veins of the body; they return blood to the right atrium.

venous thrombosis The development of a stationary blood clot in the venous circulation.

ventilation The process of eliminating carbon dioxide from the blood by diffusion into the alveoli and exhalation from the lungs.

ventilation-perfusion mismatch A pathologic state in which the oxygen entering the lungs is not mixing properly with the blood circulating through the lungs.

ventricles Specialized hollow areas in the brain.

Venturi mask A mask that has a number of interchangeable adapters that draws room air into the mask along with the oxygen flow; allows for the administration of highly specific oxygen concentrations.

venules Very small veins.

vertebral body Anterior weight-bearing structure in the spine made of cancellous bone and surrounded by a layer of hard, compact bone that provides support and stability.

vertical compression A type of injury typically resulting from a direct blow to the crown of the skull or rapid deceleration from a fall through the feet, legs, and pelvis, possibly causing a burst fracture or disk herniation.

vertical shear The type of pelvic fracture that occurs when a massive force displaces the pelvis superiorly.

very high frequency (VHF) band The portion of the radio frequency spectrum between 30 and 150 mHz.

vesicants Blister agents; the primary route of entry for vesicants is through the skin.

vesicle A tiny fluid-filled sac; a small blister.

vestibule A cleft between the labia minora, where the urethral opening (orifice), the vaginal opening (orifice), and the hymen are located.

vials Small glass or plastic bottles that contain medication; may contain single or multiple doses.

viral hemorrhagic fevers (VHF) A group of diseases that include the Ebola, Rift Valley, and yellow fever viruses among others. This group of viruses causes the blood in the body to seep out from the tissues and blood vessels.

viral hepatitis An inflammation of the liver produced by one of five distinct forms a virus—A, B, C, D, and E. The five types differ in transmission but present with the same signs and symptoms.

virulence A measure of the disease-causing ability of a microorganism. Also refers to the ability of an organism to survive outside the living host.

virus A small organism that can only multiply inside a host, such as a human, and cause disease.

visceral pain Crampy, aching pain deep within the body, the source of which is usually hard to pinpoint; common with urologic problems.

visceral pleura Thin membrane that lines the lungs.

visual acuity (VA) The ability or inability to see, and how well one can see.

visual cortex The area in the brain where signals from the optic nerve are converted into visual images.

vitreous humor A jellylike substance found in the posterior compartment of the eye between the lens and the retina.

vocal cords White bands of tough tissue that are the lateral borders of the glottis.

volar Pertaining to the palm or sole; referring to the flexor surfaces of the forearm, wrist, or hand.

volatility Term used to describe how long a chemical agent will stay on a surface before it evaporates.

Volkmann contracture Deformity of the hand, fingers, and wrist resulting from damage to forearm muscles; develops from muscle ischemia and is associated with compartment syndrome.

voluntary muscle Muscle that can be controlled by a person.

Volutrol A special type of microdrip set that features a 100- or 200-mL calibrated drip chamber; used for fluid regulation in patients prone to circulatory overload, such as pediatric and elderly patients; also called a Buretrol.

Waddell triad A pattern of automobile-pedestrian injuries in children and people of short stature in which (1) the bumper hits pelvis and femur, (2) the chest and abdomen hit the grille or low hood, and (3) the head strikes the ground.

warm zone The area located between the hot zone and the cold zone at an incident. Decontamination stations are located in the warm zone.

water reactive A property that indicates that a material will undergo a chemical reaction (for example, explosion) when mixed with water.

water soluble A property that indicates that a material can be dissolved in water.

wavelength The distance in a propagating wave from one point to the corresponding point on the next wave.

waybill A cargo document kept by the conductor of a train.

weapon of mass casualty (WMC) Any agent designed to bring about mass death, casualties, and/or massive damage to property and infrastructure (bridges, tunnels, airports, and seaports); also known as a weapon of mass destruction (WMD).

weapon of mass destruction (WMD) Any agent designed to bring about mass death, casualties, and/or massive damage to property and infrastructure (bridges, tunnels, airports, and seaports); also known as a weapon of mass casualty (WMC).

weaponization The creation of a weapon from a biological agent generally found in nature and that causes disease; the agent is cultivated, synthesized, and/or mutated to maximize the target population's exposure to the germ.

wedges   Used to snug loose cribbing.

West Nile virus (WNV)   A type of virus that is transmitted by mosquitos, and which usually only causes mild disease in humans, but can cause encephalitis, meningitis, or death. Symptoms, if exhibited, include fever, headache, body rash, and swollen lymph glands.

wheel bounce   A vibration, synchronous with road speed that can be felt in the steering wheel.

wheel wobble   A common finding at low speeds when a vehicle has a bent wheel.

wheezing   The production of whistling sounds during expiration such as occurs in asthma and bronchiolitis.

whiplash   An injury to the cervical vertebrae or their supporting ligaments and muscles, usually resulting from sudden acceleration or deceleration.

whistle-tip catheters   Soft plastic, nonrigid catheters; also called French catheters.

windchill factor   The factor that takes into account the temperature and wind velocity in calculating the effect of a given ambient temperature on living organisms.

withdrawal syndrome   A predictable set of signs and symptoms, usually involving altered central nervous system activity, that occurs after the abrupt cessation of a drug or after rapidly decreasing the usual dosage of a drug.

Wolff-Parkinson-White (WPW) syndrome   A syndrome characterized by short P-R intervals, delta waves, nonspecific ST-T wave changes, and paroxysmal episodes of tachycardia caused by the presence of an accessory pathway.

xanthines   A classification of medications that affect the respiratory smooth muscle and that relax bronchiole smooth muscles, stimulate cardiac muscle, and stimulate the central nervous system.

xyphoid process   An inferior segment of the sternum often used as a landmark for CPR.

years of potential life lost   A way of measuring and comparing the overall impact of deaths resulting from different causes. It is calculated based on a fixed age minus the age at death. Usually the fixed age is 65 or 70 or the life expectancy of the group in question.

zone of coagulation   The reddened area surrounding the leathery and sometimes charred tissue that has sustained a full-thickness burn.

zone of hyperemia   In a thermal burn, the area that is least affected by the burn injury.

zone of stasis   The peripheral area surrounding the zone of coagulation that has decreased blood flow and inflammation. This area can undergo necrosis within 24 to 48 hours after the injury, particularly if perfusion is compromised due to burn shock.

zygomatic arch   The bone that extends along the front of the skull below the orbit.

Index

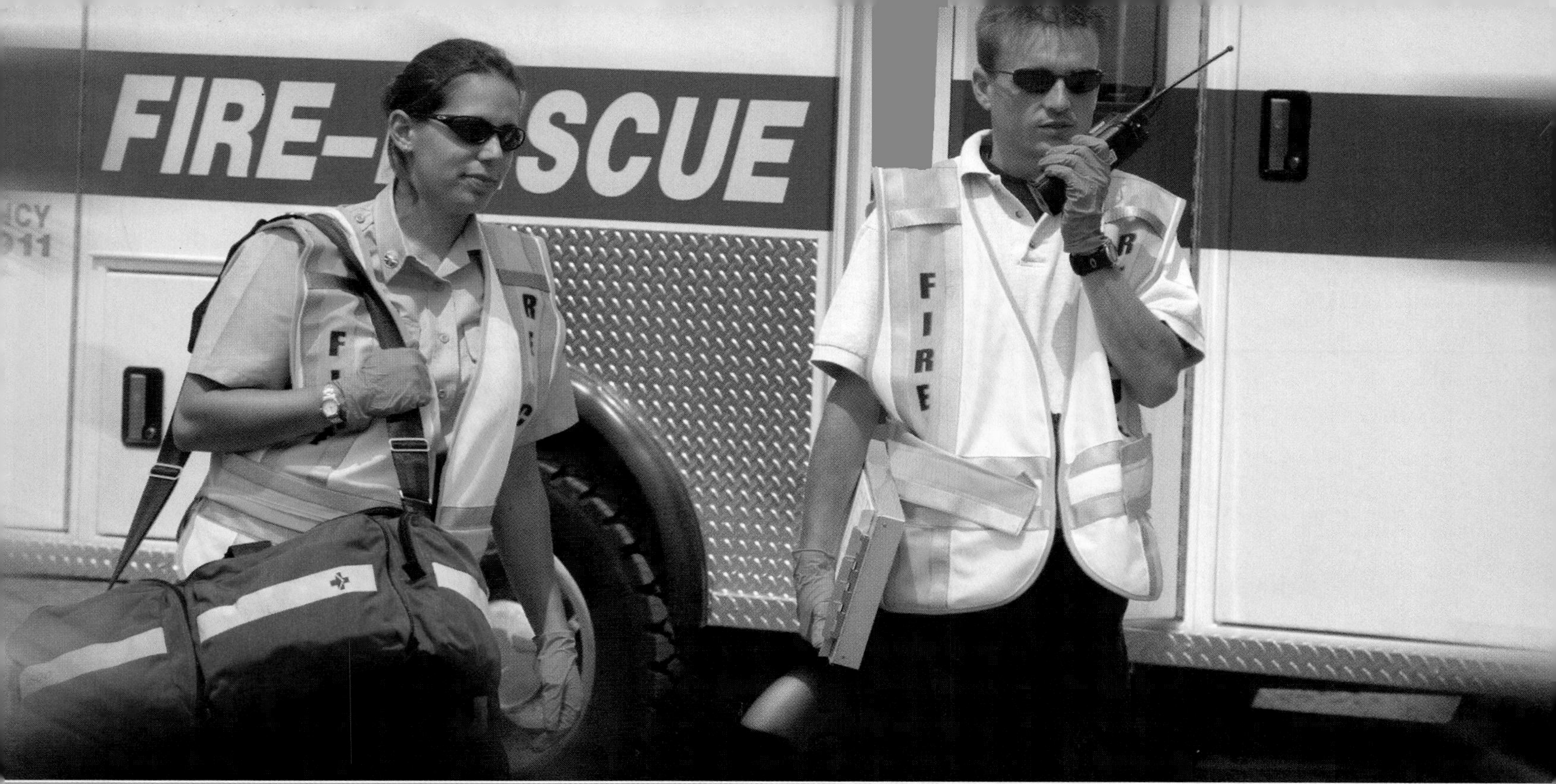

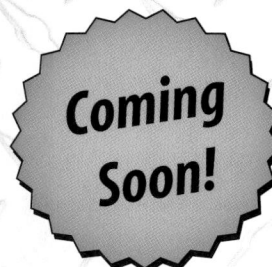
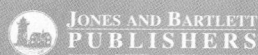

Paramedic Resources from

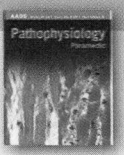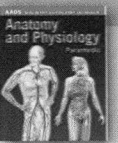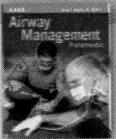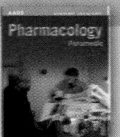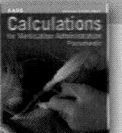

AAOS Paramedic Series

Written for paramedics by paramedics, this series uses a case-based approach to help future paramedics develop analytical skills, while learning the content of airway management, anatomy and physiology, and pathophysiology.

Paramedic: Pathophysiology
American Academy of Orthopaedic Surgeons, Bob Elling, MPA, REMT-P, Kirsten M. Elling, BS, REMT-P, Mikel A. Rothenberg, MD
ISBN-13: 978-0-7637-3765-8 • ISBN-10: 0-7637-3765-8 • $52.95* • Paperback
320 pages © 2006

Paramedic: Anatomy and Physiology
American Academy of Orthopaedic Surgeons, Bob Elling, MPA, REMT-P, Kirsten M. Elling, BS, REMT-P, Mikel A. Rothenberg, MD
ISBN-13: 978-0-7637-3792-4 • ISBN-10: 0-7637-3792-5 • $52.95* • Paperback
320 Pages © 2004

Paramedic: Airway Management
American Academy of Orthopaedic Surgeons, Gregg Margolis, MS, NREMT-P
ISBN-13: 978-0-7637-1327-0 • ISBN-10: 0-7637-1327-9 • $52.95* • Paperback
332 Pages © 2004

Coming Soon

Paramedic: Pharmacology
American Academy of Orthopaedic Surgeons, Bob Elling, MPA, REMT-P, Kirsten M. Elling, BS, REMT-P
ISBN-13: 978-0-7637-5119-7
ISBN-10: 0-7637-5119-7
$52.95* · Paperback · 150 Pages
© 2008

Paramedic: Calculations for Medication Administration
American Academy of Orthopaedic Surgeons, Mithriel Salmon, B.S.M.T. (ASCP), LP, NREMT-P
ISBN-13: 978-0-7637-4683-4
SBN-10: 0-7637-4683-5
$47.95* · Paperback · 200 Pages
© 2008

12-Lead Series

Become a fully advanced interpreter of ECGs with this series! Using hundreds of four-color graphics and full-size rhythm strips, these texts help students with little or no knowledge of electrocardiology become adept at reading and interpreting ECGs.

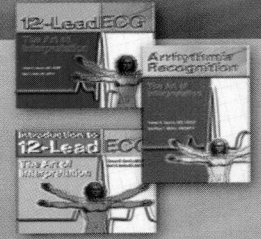

12-Lead ECG: The Art of Interpretation
Tomas B. Garcia, MD, Neil Holtz, BS, EMT-P
ISBN-13: 978-0-7637-1284-6
ISBN-10: 0-7637-1284-1
$49.95* • Paperback • 536 Pages
© 2001

Introduction to 12-Lead ECG: The Art of Interpretation
Tomas B. Garcia, MD, Neil Holtz, BS, EMT-P
ISBN-13: 978-0-7637-1961-6
ISBN-10: 0-7637-1961-7
$39.95* • Paperback • 236 Pages
© 2003

Arrhythmia Recognition: The Art of Interpretation
Tomas B. Garcia, MD, Geoffrey T. Miller, NREMT-P
ISBN-13: 978-0-7637-2246-3
ISBN-10: 0-7637-2246-4
$64.95* • Paperback • 633 Pages
© 2004

Image © Steve L. Smith

Jones and Bartlett Publishers

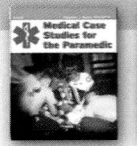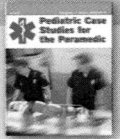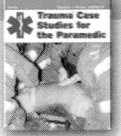

Case Studies for the Paramedic Series

Performing a systematic patient assessment and determining appropriate treatment is the most vital and complicated part of a paramedic's job. To help teach and refresh assessment and treatment decision-making principles, each book in this series provides 20 detailed scenarios to realistically test and refine paramedic assessment skills without actually being in the field.

Medical Case Studies for the Paramedic
American Academy of Orthopaedic Surgeons, Stephen J. Rahm, NREMT-P
ISBN-13: 978-0-7637-2581-5 • ISBN-10: 0-7637-2581-1 • $37.95* • Paperback • 196 Pages • © 2004

Pediatric Case Studies for the Paramedic
American Academy of Orthopaedic Surgeons, Stephen J. Rahm, NREMT-P
ISBN-13: 978-0-7637-2582-X • ISBN-10: 0-7637-2582-X • $37.95* • Paperback • 200 Pages • © 2006

Trauma Case Studies for the Paramedic
American Academy of Orthopaedic Surgeons, Stephen J. Rahm. NREMT-P
ISBN-13: 978-0-7637-2583-9 • ISBN-10: 0-7637-2583-8 • $37.95* • Paperback • 200 Pages • © 2005

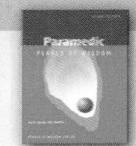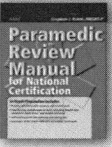

Paramedic Review Manuals

Help students prepare for state and national exams with these review manuals. The *Paramedic Review Manual* includes the same types of skill-based and multiple choice questions they are likely to encounter on national exams, while *Pearls of Wisdom* is written in a rapid-fire question and answer format perfect for reviewing for any exam or simply brushing up on paramedic knowledge.

Paramedic Pearls of Wisdom, Second Edition
Guy Haskell, PhD, NREMT-P
ISBN-13: 978-0-7637-3870-9 • ISBN-10: 0-7637-3870-0 • $34.95* • Paperback • 520 Pages • © 2006

Paramedic Review Manual for National Certification
American Academy of Orthopaedic Surgeons, Stephen J. Rahm, NREMT-P
ISBN-13: 978-0-7637-4407-6 • ISBN-10: 0-7637-4407-7 • $29.95* • Paperback • 156 Pages • © 2004

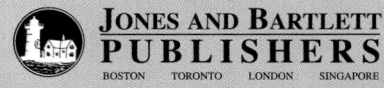

JONES AND BARTLETT
PUBLISHERS
BOSTON   TORONTO   LONDON   SINGAPORE

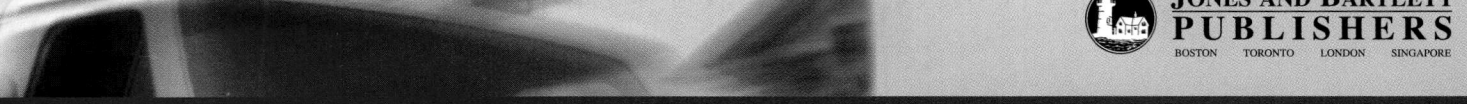

from first aid and CPR to paramedic, please visit www.EMSzone.com today!